16th Edition

HARRISON'S
PRINCIPLES OF
Internal
Medicine

EDITORS OF PREVIOUS EDITIONS

T. R. HARRISON
Editor-in-Chief, Editions 1, 2, 3, 4, 5

W. R. RESNICK
Editor, Editions 1, 2, 3, 4, 5

M. M. WINTROBE
Editor, Editions 1, 2, 3, 4, 5
Editor-in-Chief, Editions 6, 7

G. W. THORN
Editor, Editions 1, 2, 3, 4, 5, 6, 7
Editor-in-Chief, Edition 8

R. D. ADAMS
Editor, Editions 2, 3, 4, 5, 6, 7, 8, 9, 10

P. B. BEESON
Editor, Editions 1, 2

I. L. BENNETT, JR.
Editor, Editions 3, 4, 5, 6

E. BRAUNWALD
Editor, Editions 6, 7, 8, 9, 10, 12, 13, 14
Editor-in-Chief, Edition 11, 15

K. J. ISSELBACHER
Editor, Editions 6, 7, 8, 10, 11, 12, 14
Editor-in-Chief, Editions 9, 13

R. G. PETERSDORF
Editor, Editions 6, 7, 8, 9, 11, 12, 13
Editor-in-Chief, Edition 10

J. D. WILSON
Editor, Editions 9, 10, 11, 13, 14
Editor-in-Chief, Edition 12

J. B. MARTIN
Editor, Editions 10, 11, 12, 13, 14

A. S. FAUCI
Editor, Editions 11, 12, 13, 15
Editor-in-Chief, Edition 14

R. ROOT
Editor, Edition 12

D. L. KASPER
Editor, Editions 13, 14, 15

S. L. HAUSER
Editor, Edition 14, 15

D. L. LONGO
Editor, Edition 14, 15

J. L. JAMESON
Editor, Edition 15

16th Edition

HARRISON'S
PRINCIPLES OF
Internal
Medicine

Editors

DENNIS L. KASPER, MD

William Ellery Channing Professor of Medicine,
Professor of Microbiology and Molecular Genetics,
Harvard Medical School; Director, Channing
Laboratory, Department of Medicine, Brigham and
Women's Hospital, Boston

ANTHONY S. FAUCI, MD

Chief, Laboratory of Immunoregulation; Director,
National Institute of Allergy and Infectious Diseases,
National Institutes of Health, Bethesda

DAN L. LONGO, MD

Scientific Director, National Institute on Aging,
National Institutes of Health,
Bethesda and Baltimore

EUGENE BRAUNWALD, MD

Distinguished Hersey Professor of Medicine,
Harvard Medical School; Chairman, TIMI Study Group,
Brigham and Women's Hospital, Boston

STEPHEN L. HAUSER, MD

Robert A. Fishman Distinguished Professor and Chairman,
Department of Neurology,
University of California San Francisco, San Francisco

J. LARRY JAMESON, MD, PhD

Irving S. Cutter Professor and Chairman,
Department of Medicine,
Northwestern University Feinberg School of Medicine;
Physician-in-Chief, Northwestern
Memorial Hospital, Chicago

Volume I

McGraw-Hill
MEDICAL PUBLISHING DIVISION

New York   Chicago   San Francisco   Lisbon   London   Madrid
Mexico City   Milan   New Delhi   San Juan   Seoul   Singapore   Sydney   Toronto

Harrison's
PRINCIPLES OF INTERNAL MEDICINE
Sixteenth Edition

34567890 DOWDOW 098765

ISBN 0-07-140235-7 (Combo)

ISBN 0-07-139140-1 (Set)
ISBN 0-07-139141-X (Vol. I)
ISBN 0-07-139142-8 (Vol. II)

FOREIGN LANGUAGE EDITIONS

Arabic (13e): McGraw-Hill Libri Italia srl (est. 1996)
Chinese Long Form (15e): McGraw-Hill International Enterprises, Inc., Taiwan
Chinese Short Form (15e): McGraw-Hill Education (Asia), Singapore
Croatian (13e): Placebo, Split, Croatia
French (15e): Medecine-Sciences Flammarion, Paris, France
German (15e): ABW Wissenschaftsverlagsgesellschaft mbH, Berlin, Germany
Greek (15e): Parissianos, S.A., Athens, Greece
Italian (15e): The McGraw-Hill Companies, Srl, Milan, Italy
Japanese (15e): MEDSI-Medical Sciences International Ltd, Tokyo, Japan

Korean (15e): McGraw-Hill Korea, Inc., Seoul, Korea
Polish (14e): Czelej Publishing Company, Lubin, Poland (est. 2000)
Portuguese (15e): McGraw-Hill Interamericana do Brazil, Rio de Janeiro, Brazil
Romanian (14e): Teora Publishers, Bucharest, Romania (est. 2000)
Serbian (15e): Publishing House Romanov, Bosnia & Herzegovina, Republic of Serbska
Spanish (15e): McGraw-Hill Interamericana de Espana S.A., Madrid, Spain
Turkish (15e): Nobel Tip Kitabevleri, Ltd., Istanbul, Turkey
Vietnamese (15e): McGraw-Hill Education (Asia), Singapore

This book was set in Times Roman by Progressive Information Technologies. The editors were Martin Wonsiewicz and Mariapaz Ramos Englis. The production director was Robert Laffler. The index was prepared by Barbara Littlewood. The text designer was Marsha Cohen/Parallelogram Graphics. Art director: Libby Pisacreta; cover design by Janice Bielawa. Medical illustrator: Jay McElroy, MAMS.

R. R. Donnelley and Sons, Inc., was the printer and binder.

Cover illustrations courtesy of Raymond J. Gibbons, MD; George V. Kelvin; Robert S. Hillman, MD; and Marilu Gorno-Tempini, MD.

Library of Congress Cataloging-in-Publication Data

Harrison's principles of internal medicine—16th ed./editors, Dennis L. Kasper . . . [et al.].   p. cm.
    Includes bibliographical references and index.
    ISBN 0-07-139140-1 (set)—ISBN 0-07-139141-X (v. 1)—ISBN 0-07-139142-8 (v. 2)—ISBN 0-07-140235-7 (combo)
    1. Internal medicine. I. Title: Principles of internal medicine. II. Kasper, Dennis L. III. Harrison, Tinsley Randolph, 1900– Principles of internal medicine.
    [DNLM: 1. Internal Medicine. WB 115 H322 2005]
    RC46.H333 2005
    616—dc21

2004044931

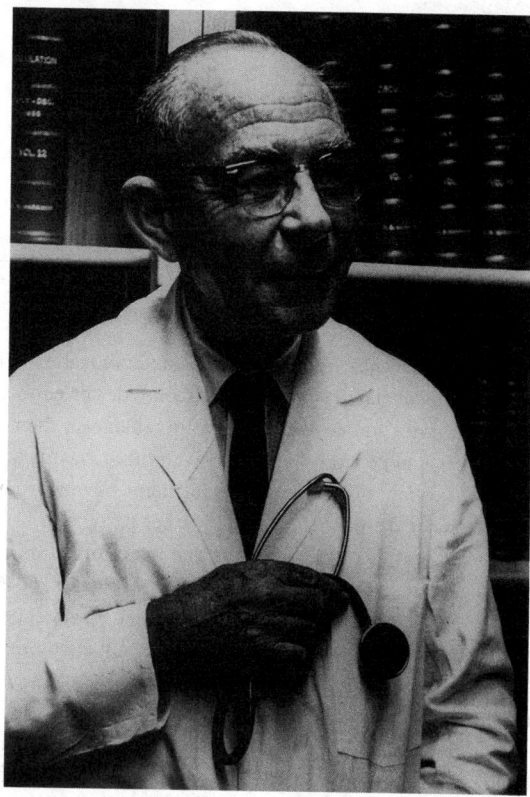

Tinsley R. Harrison

The 16th Edition of Harrison's Principles of Internal Medicine is dedicated to Tinsley R. Harrison, the founding editor and Editor-in-Chief for the first five editions.

From time to time a personality scintillates across the medical firmament who dazzles all beholders. Tinsley Harrison was such a person. A delightful, vivacious, passionate physician, he stimulated everyone with whom he came into contact, and he placed an indelible stamp on the medical events of his day.

Tinsley Randolph Harrison was born in Talladega, Alabama, on March 18, 1900. His father, Groce Harrison, was a sixth-generation physician, a student of William Osler who inculcated Osler's values into his son from an early age. Tinsley earned his undergraduate degree from the University of Michigan and his M.D. from Johns Hopkins School of Medicine. After a medical residency at the Peter Bent Brigham Hospital in Boston, where he developed his life-long interest in cardiovascular science and medicine, and additional training at Hopkins, Dr. Harrison served as chief medical resident and then joined the faculty of Vanderbilt University School of Medicine. His Chief of Medicine there, Canby Robinson, described him as "a human dynamo with unbounded energy." After a brief period of private practice, which Harrison later described as "perhaps the greatest educational experience of my entire life," he served successively as chair of medicine at Bowman-Gray School of Medicine, Winston-Salem, North Carolina; the Southwestern Medical School in Dallas, Texas; and the University of Alabama, Birmingham. He played a key role in organizing the Bowman-Gray and Southwestern medical schools. He also served as Dean of Southwestern and the University of Alabama and as Chief of Cardiology at the latter. Dr. Harrison died in Birmingham, on August 4, 1978.

For decades he was an active experimentalist, and his important contributions to the understanding of the pathophysiology of heart failure were all the more remarkable because they were obtained before the availability of measurements of intracardiac pressures, cardiac output, and regional blood flow. Harrison's research involved both basic studies in cardiovascular physiology as well as clinical research and were summarized in a classic text *Failure of the Circulation*. He was

a founding member of the Council of the National Heart Institute and served as president of the American Society for Clinical Investigation and of the American Heart Association. Tinsley Harrison received the Gold Heart Award from the latter, the Kober Medal of the Association of American Physicians, and the Distinguished Teacher Award of the American College of Physicians. Few people of his generation surpassed him as a bedside teacher.

In 1945, stimulated by the publisher Blakiston, Harrison conceived of a new type of textbook of internal medicine, in which both of his interests—clinical medicine and the pathophysiologic mechanisms of disease—would be as closely interwoven as they were in his mind. He immediately recruited an editorial team; Harrison authored or co-authored almost the entire cardiovascular section. By 1950, the first edition of *Principles of Internal Medicine* was published.

Although Harrison was a distinguished investigator, teacher, academic leader, and editor, he was first and foremost a masterful physician who excelled in the care of the sick. The individual patient was always in the center of the stage. To put the disease first, to refer to the patient as "a case," would arouse Harrison's wrath. The words that he penned for the first edition of this book reflect the importance he attached to his role as a physician.

No greater opportunity or obligation can fall the lot of a human being than to be a physician. In the care of the suffering he needs technical skill, scientific knowledge, and human understanding. He who uses these with courage, humility, and wisdom will provide a unique service for his fellow man and will build an enduring edifice of character within himself. The physician should ask of his destiny no more than this, and he should be content with no less.

These words express the philosophy of the original editors and of all those who have followed.

It is to the memory of this great physician, teacher, investigator, and editor, whose life and works have so inspired us, that this sixteenth edition of *Harrison's Principles of Internal Medicine* is dedicated.

THE EDITORS

CONTENTS

Part Six
INFECTIOUS DISEASES

Part Ten

CRITICAL CARE MEDICINE

Part Eleven

DISORDERS OF THE KIDNEY AND URINARY TRACT

Part Twelve

DISORDERS OF THE GASTROINTESTINAL SYSTEM

Part Fifteen
NEUROLOGIC DISORDERS

Part Sixteen
POISONING, DRUG OVERDOSE, AND ENVENOMATION

CONTRIBUTORS

Numbers in brackets refer to chapters written or co-written by the contributor.

ELIAS ABRUTYN, MD
Professor of Medicine and Public Health, Associate Provost and Associate Dean for Faculty Affairs; Interim Chief, Infectious Diseases, Drexel University College of Medicine, Philadelphia [124,125]

JOHN C. ACHERMANN, MRCP, MRCPCH, MD
Wellcome Trust Clinician Scientist, Department of Medicine and Institute of Child Health, University College London, London, UK [328]

JOHN W. ADAMSON, MD
Executive Vice President for Research, Director, Blood Research Institute, Blood Center of Southeastern Wisconsin, Milwaukee [52, 90]

DAVID A. AHLQUIST, MD
Professor of Medicine, Mayo Clinic College of Medicine; Consultant in Gastroenterology, Division of Gastroenterology and Hepatology, Mayo Clinic, Rochester [35]

LEENA ALA-KOKKO, MD, PhD
Professor of Medicine, Center for Gene Therapy, Tulane University Health Sciences Center, New Orleans [342]

KENNETH C. ANDERSON, MD
Chief, Division of Hematologic Neoplasia; Director, Jerome Lipper Multiple Myeloma Center, Dana-Farber Cancer Institute; Kraft Family Professor of Medicine, Harvard Medical School, Boston [98, 99]

ELLIOTT M. ANTMAN, MD
Professor of Medicine, Harvard Medical School; Director, Samuel A. Levine Cardiac Unit, Brigham and Women's Hospital, Boston [228]

FREDERICK R. APPELBAUM, MD
Member and Director, Clinical Research Division, Fred Hutchinson Cancer Research Center; Professor and Head, Division of Medical Oncology, University of Washington School of Medicine, Seattle [100]

GORDON L. ARCHER, MD
Professor of Medicine and Microbiology/Immunology; Chair, Division of Infectious Diseases, Department of Medicine, Virginia Commonwealth University Medical Center, Richmond [118]

JAMES O. ARMITAGE, MD
Joe Shapiro Professor of Medicine, University of Nebraska, Omaha [97]

ARTHUR K. ASBURY, MD
Van Meter Professor of Neurology Emeritus, University of Pennsylvania School of Medicine, Philadelphia [22, 363, 365]

JOHN R. ASPLIN, MD
Assistant Professor of Medicine, Section of Nephrology, University of Chicago Pritzker School of Medicine, Chicago [265, 268]

JOHN C. ATHERTON, MD
Professor of Gastroenterology, Wolfson Digestive Diseases Centre and Institute of Infections, Immunity and Inflammation, University of Nottingham, Nottingham, England [135]

PAUL S. AUERBACH, MD, MS
Clinical Professor of Surgery, Department of Surgery, Division of Emergency Medicine, Stanford University School of Medicine, Los Altos [378]

K. FRANK AUSTEN, MD
AstraZeneca Professor of Respiratory and Inflammatory Diseases, Harvard Medical School; Director, Inflammation and Allergic Diseases Research Section, Division of Rheumatology, Immunology, and Allergy, Department of Medicine, Brigham and Women's Hospital, Boston [298]

BERNARD M. BABIOR, MD, PhD
Professor and Head, Division of Biochemistry, Department of Molecular and Experimental Medicine, The Scripps Research Institute, La Jolla [92]

LINDSEY R. BADEN, MD
Assistant Professor of Medicine, Harvard Medical School; Division of Infectious Diseases, Brigham and Women's Hospital, Boston [162]

KAMAL F. BADR, MD
Professor and Chair, Department of Internal Medicine, American University of Beirut (Lebanon); Attending Physician, American University of Beirut Medical Center, Beirut, Lebanon [267]

DONALD S. BAIM, MD
Professor of Medicine, Harvard Medical School; Director, Center for Integration of Medicine and Innovative Technology, Brigham and Women's Hospital, Boston [212, 229]

ROBERT L. BARBIERI, MD
Kate Macy Ladd Professor of Obstetrics, Gynecology, and Reproductive Biology, Harvard Medical School; Chairman, Obstetrics and Gynecology, Brigham and Women's Hospital, Boston [6]

TAMAR F. BARLAM, MD
Associate Professor of Medicine, Boston University School of Medicine, Boston [106, 131]

KENNETH J. BART, MD
Director, Graduate School of Public Health, Professor of Epidemiology and Biostatistics, San Diego State University, San Diego [107]

SHARI S. BASSUK, ScD
Epidemiologist, Division of Preventive Medicine, Brigham and Women's Hospital, Boston [327]

M. FLINT BEAL, MD
Anne Parrish Titzel Professor and Chair, Department of Neurology and Neuroscience, Weill Medical College of Cornell University; Neurologist-in-Chief, New York Presbyterian Hospital, New York [345, 355]

NICHOLAS J. BEECHING, FRCP, FRACP, DCH, DTM&H
Senior Lecturer in Infectious Diseases, Liverpool School of Tropical Medicine; Clinical Lead, Tropical and Infectious Disease Unit, Royal Liverpool University Hospital, Liverpool, United Kingdom [141]

ROBERT S. BENJAMIN, MD
Professor of Medicine, Chairman, Department of Sarcoma Medical Oncology, The University of Texas MD Anderson, Houston [84]

JOHN E. BENNETT, MD
Head, Clinical Mycology Section, Laboratory of Clinical Investigation, National Institute of Allergy and Infectious Diseases, National Institutes of Health, Potomac [182–190]

EDWARD J. BENZ, JR., MD
Richard and Susan Smith Professor of Medicine, Professor of Pediatrics, Professor of Pathology, Harvard Medical School; President and CEO, Dana-Farber Cancer Institute; Director, Dana-Farber/Harvard Cancer Center, Boston [91]

SHALENDAR BHASIN, MD
Professor of Medicine, University of California Los Angeles School of Medicine; Chief, Division of Endocrinology, Charles R. Drew University, Los Angeles [325]

DAVID R. BICKERS, MD
Carl Truman Nelson Professor and Chair, Department of Dermatology, College of Physicians and Surgeons, Columbia University Medical Center, New York [51]

HENRY J. BINDER, MD
Professor of Medicine, Professor of Cellular and Molecular Physiology, Yale University, New Haven [275]

THOMAS D. BIRD, MD
Professor of Neurology and Medicine, University of Washington; Veterans Affairs Puget Sound Medical Center, Seattle [350, 364]

NEIL R. BLACKLOW, MD
Chairman Emeritus, Department of Medicine, Professor of Medicine, University of Massachusetts Medical School, Worcester; Visiting Professor of Medicine, Harvard Medical School, Boston [168]

MARTIN J. BLASER, MD
Chairman, Department of Medicine, Frederick H. King Professor of Internal Medicine; Professor of Microbiology, New York University School of Medicine, New York [135, 139]

CLARA D. BLOOMFIELD, MD
William G. Pace III Professor of Cancer Research, Cancer Scholar and Senior Advisor, The Ohio State University Comprehensive Cancer and The Arthur G. James Cancer Hospital and Richard J. Solove Research Institute, Columbus [96]

RICHARD S. BLUMBERG, MD
Chief, Division of Gastroenterology, Hepatology, and Endoscopy, Brigham and Women's Hospital, Boston [276]

DAVID M. BODINE, PhD
Chief, Hematopoiesis Section, Genetics and Molecular Biology Branch, National Human Genome Research Institute, Bethesda [59]

JEAN L. BOLOGNIA, MD
Professor of Dermatology, Yale University School of Medicine, New Haven [48]

GEORGE J. BOSL, MD
Chairman, Department of Medicine, Memorial Sloan-Kettering Cancer Center; Professor of Medicine, Weill Medical College of Cornell University, New York [82]

RICHARD C. BOUCHER JR., MD
William Rand Kenan Professor of Medicine, University of North Carolina at Chapel Hill; Director, University of North Carolina Cystic Fibrosis Center, Chapel Hill [241]

KAREN D. BRADSHAW, MD
Professor of Obstetrics/Gynecology and Surgery, Helen J. and Robert S. Strauss and Diana K. and Richard C. Strauss Distinguished Professor in Women's Health, The University of Texas Southwestern Medical Center, Dallas [326]

HUGH R. BRADY, MD, PhD, FRCPI
Professor and Head, Department of Medicine and Therapeutics, University College Dublin, Dublin, Ireland [260, 264]

KENNETH D. BRANDT, MD
Professor of Medicine and Professor of Orthopaedic Surgery, Indiana University School of Medicine; Director, Indiana University Multipurpose Arthritis and Musculoskeletal Diseases Center, Indianapolis [312]

EUGENE BRAUNWALD, MD, MA(Hon), MD(Hon), ScD(Hon)
Distinguished Hersey Professor of Medicine, Harvard Medical School; Chairman, TIMI Study Group, Brigham and Women's Hospital, Boston [29, 31, 32, 208, 209, 215, 216, 219, 221, 222, 226–228]

IRWIN M. BRAVERMAN, MD
Professor of Dermatology, Yale University School of Medicine, New Haven [48]

OTIS W. BRAWLEY, MD
Professor of Hematology, Oncology, and Epidemiology, Emory University Medical School; Associate Director, Population Sciences and Cancer Control Program, Winship Cancer Institute, Atlanta [67]

JOEL G. BREMAN, MD, DTPH
Senior Scientific Advisor, Fogarty International Center, National Institutes of Health, Bethesda [195]

BARRY M. BRENNER, MD, DSc(Hon), DMSc(Hon)
Samuel A. Levine Professor of Medicine, Harvard Medical School; Director Emeritus, Renal Division, Brigham and Women's Hospital, Boston [40, 41, 259–262, 264, 266, 267, 270]

ROBERT M. BRENNER, MD
Associate Medical Director, Clinical Research, Amgen In., Thousand Oaks, California [259]

GEORGE J. BREWER, MD
Morton S. and Henrietta K. Sellner Active Emeritus Professor of Human Genetics, Active Emeritus Professor of Internal Medicine, University of Michigan Medical School, Ann Arbor [339]

F. RICHARD BRINGHURST, MD
Associate Professor of Medicine, Harvard Medical School, Boston [331]

CLAIRE V. BROOME, MD
Senior Advisor, Centers for Disease Control and Prevention, Atlanta [123]

ROBERT H. BROWN, JR., MD, DPHil
Associate Neurologist, Massachusetts General Hospital; Professor of Neurology, Harvard Medical School, Boston [353, 368]

GREGORY BULKLEY, MD
Mark M. Ravitch Professor of Surgery, The Johns Hopkins University School of Medicine, Baltimore [279]

H. FRANKLIN BUNN, MD
Professor of Medicine, Harvard Medical School, Boston [92, 93]

DAVID M. BURNS, MD
Professor of Family and Preventive Medicine, Professor of Medicine, University of California San Diego, San Diego [375]

MICHAEL J. BURNS, MD
Assistant Professor of Medicine, Harvard Medical School, Boston [377]

JOAN R. BUTTERTON, MD, DTM&H
Assistant Professor of Medicine, Harvard Medical School; Assistant in Medicine, Infectious Disease Division, Massachusetts General Hospital, Boston [113]

JOHN C. BYRD, MD
D. Warren Brown Professor of Leukemia Research, Associate Professor of Medicine and Medical Chemistry, The Ohio State University; Director of Hematologic Malignancies, Division of Hematology and Oncology, James Cancer Hospital and Solove Research Institute, Columbus [96]

STEPHEN B. CALDERWOOD, MD
Chief, Division of Infectious Diseases, Massachusetts General Hospital; Professor of Medicine (Microbiology and Molecular Genetics), Harvard Medical School, Boston [113]

MICHAEL V. CALLAHAN, MD, MSPH, DTM&H
Program Leader, Biological Threat Defense, Center for Integration of Medicine and Innovative Technologies, Massachusetts General Hospital, Boston [18]

MICHAEL CAMILLERI, MD
Atherton and Winifred W. Bean Professor, Professor of Medicine and Physiology, Mayo Clinic College of Medicine; Consultant in Gastroenterology, Mayo Clinic, Rochester [35]

G. DOUGLAS CAMPBELL, MD
Professor of Medicine, Director, Division of Pulmonary, Critical Care, and Sleep Medicine, University of Mississippi School of Medicine, Jackson [239]

GRANT L. CAMPBELL, MD, PhD
Chief, Epidemiology Activity, Arbovirus Diseases Branch, Division of Vector-Borne Infectious Diseases, National Center for Infectious Diseases, Centers for Disease Control and Prevention, Fort Collins [143]

CHRISTOPHER P. CANNON, MD
Associate Professor of Medicine, Harvard Medical School; Senior Investigator, TIMI Study Group, Cardiovascular Division, Brigham and Women's Hospital, Boston [227]

MARK D. CARLSON, MD
Professor of Medicine, Associate Vice President for Government Relations, Case Western Reserve University; Associate Dean, Case School of Medicine, Cleveland [20]

CHARLES B. CARPENTER, MD
Professor of Medicine, Harvard Medical School; Senior Physician, Brigham and Women's Hospital, Boston [263]

BRUCE R. CARR, MD
Professor and Director, Division of Reproductive Endocrinology and Infertility; Holder, Paul C. MacDonald Distinguished Chair in Obstetrics and Gynecology, The University of Texas Southwestern Medical Center, Dallas [326]

AGUSTIN CASTELLANOS, MD
Professor of Medicine; Director, Clinical Electrophysiology, University of Miami School of Medicine, Miami [256]

PHILIP F. CHANCE, MD
Professor of Pediatrics and Neurology, University of Washington School of Medicine; Chief, Division of Genetics and Development, Children's Hospital and Regional Medical Center, Seattle [364]

FENG-YEE CHANG, MD
Professor, Department of Medicine, National Defense Medical Center; Chief, Division of Infectious Diseases and Tropical Medicine, Department of Internal Medicine, Tri-Service General Hospital, Taipei, Taiwan [132]

YUAN-TSONG CHEN, MD, PhD
Professor and Chief, Division of Medical Genetics, Duke University Medical Center; Director, Institute of Biomedical Sciences, Durham [341]

JOHN S. CHILD, MD
Streisand Professor of Medicine/Cardiology; Co-Chief, Division of Cardiology, David Geffen School of Medicine at UCLA; Director, Ahmanson/UCLA Adult Congenital Heart Disease Center, UCLA Medical Center, Los Angeles [218]

KATARINA G. CHILLER, MD
Assistant Professor, Department of Dermatology, Emory University, Atlanta [73]

OLIVIER M. CHOSIDOW, MD, PhD
Department of Internal Medicine, Hôpital Pitié-Salpêtrière, Paris, France [50]

RAYMOND T. CHUNG, MD
Assistant Professor of Medicine, Harvard Medical School; Director, Hepatology Source, Medical Director, Lung Transplant Program, Associate Physician, Massachusetts General Hospital, Boston [289]

FREDRIC L. COE, MD
Professor of Medicine and Physiology, University of Chicago Pritzker School of Medicine, Chicago [265, 268]

ALAN S. COHEN, MD
Distinguished Professor of Medicine in Rheumatology, Emeritus, Boston University School of Medicine, Boston [310]

JEFFREY I. COHEN, MD
Head, Medical Virology Section, Laboratory of Infectious Diseases, National Institute of Allergy and Infectious Diseases, National Institutes of Health, Bethesda [165, 175]

FRANCIS S. COLLINS, MD, PhD
Director, National Human Genome Research Institute, National Institutes of Health, Bethesda [68]

WILSON S. COLUCCI, MD, FACC, FAHA
Thomas J. Ryan Professor of Medicine, Boston University School of Medicine; Chief, Cardiovascular Medicine, Boston University Medical Center, Boston [223]

JOEL D. COOPER, MD
Evarts A. Graham Professor of Surgery, Department of Surgery, Division of Cardiothoracic Surgery, Washington University School of Medicine, St. Louis [248]

MAX D. COOPER, MD
Professor of Medicine, Pediatrics, and Microbiology; Howard Hughes Medical Institute Investigator, University of Alabama at Birmingham, Birmingham [297]

MICHAEL J. CORBEL, PhD, DSc(Med), FIBiol, FRCPath
Head, Division of Bacteriology, National Institute for Biological Standards and Control, Potters Bar, United Kingdom [141]

LAWRENCE COREY, MD
Professor, Medicine and Laboratory Medicine; Head, Virology Division, University of Washington; Head, Program in Infectious Diseases, Fred Hutchinson Cancer Research Center, Seattle [163, 179]

FELICIA COSMAN, MD
Associate Professor of Clinical Medicine, Columbia University College of Physicians and Surgeons; Medical Director, Clinical Research Center, Helen Hayes Hospital, West Haverstraw, New York [333]

MARK A. CREAGER, MD
Professor of Medicine, Harvard Medical School; Physician, Brigham and Women's Hospital, Boston [231, 232]

PHILIP E. CRYER, MD
Irene E. and Michael M. Karl Professor of Endocrinology and Metabolism in Medicine, Washington University School of Medicine, St. Louis [324]

RONALD G. CRYSTAL, MD
Professor and Chair, Department of Genetic Medicine, Weill Medical College of Cornell University; Chief, Division of Pulmonary and Critical Care Medicine, New York Presbyterian Hospital-Weill Cornell Medical Center, New York [309]

JOHN J. CUSH, MD
Medical Director, Arthritis Center, Presbyterian Hospital of Dallas, Dallas [311]

CHARLES A. CZEISLER, MD, PhD
Professor of Medicine, Harvard Medical School; Chief, Division of Sleep Medicine; Director, Sleep Disorders and Circadian Medicine, Brigham and Women's Hospital, Boston [24]

MARINOS C. DALAKAS, MD
Professor of Neurology; Chief, Neuromuscular Diseases Section, National Institute of Neurological Disorders and Stroke, National Institutes of Health, Bethesda [369]

JOSEP DALMAU, MD, PhD
Associate Professor of Neurology, Department of Neurology, University of Pennsylvania, Philadelphia [87]

DANIEL F. DANZL, MD
Professor and Chair, Department of Emergency Medicine, University of Louisville School of Medicine, Louisville [19]

ROBERT B. DAROFF, MD
Professor of Neurology and Associate Dean, Case Western Reserve University School of Medicine, Cleveland [20]

CHARLES E. DAVIS, MD
Professor of Pathology and Medicine Emeritus, University of California San Diego School of Medicine; Director Emeritus, Microbiology Laboratory, University of California San Diego Medical Center, San Diego [192]

STEVEN R. DEITCHER, MD
Head, Section of Hematology and Coagulation Medicine, Department of Hematology-Medical Oncology, The Cleveland Clinic Foundation, Cleveland [103]

JOHN DEL VALLE, MD
Professor and Senior Associate Chair of Medicine, Graduate Medical Education, Department of Internal Medicine, University of Michigan Health System, Ann Arbor [274]

MAHLON R. DELONG, MD
Timmie Professor of Neurology; Director of Neuroscience, Emory University School of Medicine, Atlanta [351]

MARIE B. DEMAY, MD
Associate Professor of Medicine, Harvard Medical School, Boston [331]

BRADLEY M. DENKER, MD
Assistant Professor of Medicine, Harvard Medical School; Associate Physician, Brigham and Women's Hospital, Boston [40]

DAVID T. DENNIS, MD, MPH
Faculty Affiliate, Department of Microbiology, Colorado State University; Medical Epidemiologist, Division of Vector-Borne Infectious Diseases, Centers for Disease Control and Prevention, Fort Collins [143, 156]

ROBERT J. DESNICK, MD, PhD
Professor and Chair, Department of Human Genetics, Mount Sinai School of Medicine of New York University, New York [337]

BETTY DIAMOND, MD
Chief, Division of Rheumatology, Department of Microbiology and Immunology, Albert Einstein College of Medicine, New York [299]

JULES L. DIENSTAG, MD
Professor of Medicine, Harvard Medical School; Physician, Massachusetts General Hospital, Boston [78, 285–287, 291]

WILLIAM P. DILLON, MD
Professor of Radiology, Section Chief, Neuroradiology, Vice-Chair for Research Radiology, University of California San Francisco, San Francisco [347]

CHARLES A. DINARELLO, MD
Professor of Medicine, University of Colorado Health Sciences Center, Denver [16]

ROBERT G. DLUHY, MD
Professor of Medicine, Harvard Medical School, Brigham and Women's Hospital, Boston [321]

RAPHAEL DOLIN, MD
Maxwell Finland Professor of Medicine (Microbiology and Molecular Genetics); Dean for Academic and Clinical Programs, Harvard Medical School, Boston [162, 170, 171]

DAVID M. DOSA, MD, MPH
Assistant Professor of Medicine, Brown Medical School; Division of Geriatrics, Rhode Island Hospital, Providence [8]

DANIEL B. DRACHMAN, MD
Professor of Neurology and Neuroscience; WW Smith Charitable Foundation Professor of Neuroimmunology; Director, Neuromuscular Unit, The Johns Hopkins University School of Medicine, Baltimore [366]

JEFFREY M. DRAZEN, MD
Professor of Medicine, Harvard Medical School, Boston [233–235, 252]

THOMAS D. DuBOSE, JR., MD
Professor and Chair, Department of Internal Medicine, Professor, Department of Physiology and Pharmacology, Wake Forest University School of Medicine, Winston-Salem [42]

J. STEPHEN DUMLER, MD
Professor, Division of Medical Microbiology, Department of Pathology and the Program in Cellular and Molecular Medicine, The Johns Hopkins University School of Medicine; Department of Molecular Microbiology and Immunology, The Johns Hopkins University Bloomberg School of Public Health, Baltimore [158]

ANDREA E. DUNAIF, MD
Charles F. Kettering Professor of Medicine, Northwestern University Feinberg School of Medicine; Chief, Division of Endocrinology, Metabolism and Molecular Medicine, Northwestern University, Chicago [5]

SAMUEL C. DURSO, MD
Associate Professor of Medicine, Division of Geriatric Medicine and Gerontology, The Johns Hopkins University School of Medicine; Deputy Director of Education, Co-Director Fellowship Training Program, Director of Ambulatory Clinical Services, Baltimore [28]

JANICE P. DUTCHER, MD
Professor of Medicine, New York Medical College; Associate Director, Clinical Affairs, Our Lady of Mercy Cancer Center, Bronx [88]

JOHANNA T. DWYER, DSc
Professor of Medicine and Community Health, Tufts University School of Medicine and Friedman School of Nutrition; Director, Frances Stern Nutrition Center; Tufts-New England Medical Center Senior Scientist; Nutritional Epidemiology Program, Jean Mayer USDA Human Nutrition Center on Aging at Tufts, Boston [60]

VICTOR J. DZAU, MD
Hershey Professor of Medicine, Harvard Medical School; Chairman, Department of Medicine and Director of Research, Brigham and Women's Hospital, Boston [231, 232]

JEFFERY S. DZIECZKOWSKI, MD
Physician, New Britain General Hospital, New Britain [99]

J. DONALD EASTON, MD
Professor and Chair, Department of Clinical Neurosciences, Brown Medical School and Rhode Island Hospital, Providence [349]

DAVID A. EHRMANN, MD
Associate Professor, Section of Endocrinology, Department of Medicine, University of Chicago Pritzker School of Medicine, Chicago [44]

EZEKIEL J. EMANUEL, MD, PhD
Chief, Department of Clinical Bioethics, Warren G. Magnuson Clinical Center, National Institutes of Health, Bethesda [9]

LINDA L. EMANUEL, MD
Buehler Professor of Geriatric Medicine, Director, Buehler Center on Aging, Northwestern University School of Medicine, Chicago [9]

JOHN W. ENGSTROM, MD
Professor of Neurology; Vice Chairman, Residency Program Director, University of California San Francisco, San Francisco [15, 354]

ANTHONY S. FAUCI, MD
Chief, Laboratory of Immunoregulation; Director, National Institute of Allergy and Infectious Diseases, National Institutes of Health, Bethesda [172, 173, 205, 295, 306]

MURRAY J. FAVUS, MD
Professor of Medicine, University of Chicago Pritzker School of Medicine, Division of Biological Sciences, Chicago [268, 334]

ROBERT G. FENTON, MD, PhD
Associate Professor of Medicine, University of Maryland Greenebaum Cancer Center, Baltimore [69]

HOWARD L. FIELDS, MD, PhD
Professor of Neurology and Physiology, University of California San Francisco, San Francisco [11]

GREGORY A. FILICE, MD
Chief, Infectious Disease Section, Veterans Affairs Medical Center; Associate Professor, Department of Medicine, University of Minnesota, Minneapolis [146]

ROBERT W. FINBERG, MD
Professor and Chair, Department of Medicine, University of Massachusetts Medical School, Worcester [72, 117]

JOYCE D. FINGEROTH, MD
Assistant Professor of Medicine, Harvard Medical School; Division of Infectious Diseases, Beth Israel Deaconess Medical Center, Boston [117]

NAOMI D.L. FISHER, MD
Assistant Professor, Harvard Medical School; Director, Hypertension Service, Brigham and Women's Hospital, Boston [230]

JEFFREY S. FLIER, MD
Chief Academic Officer, Beth Israel Deaconess Medical Center; George C. Reisman Professor of Medicine, Harvard Medical School, Boston [64]

SONIA FRIEDMAN, MD
Instructor of Medicine, Harvard Medical School; Associate Physician, Brigham and Women's Hospital, Boston [276]

WILLIAM F. FRIEDMAN, MD
JH Nicholson Professor of Pediatrics (Cardiology); Senior Associate Dean for Academic Affairs, David Geffen School of Medicine at UCLA, Los Angeles [218]

ROBERT F. GAGEL, MD
Professor of Medicine and Head, Division of Internal Medicine, University of Texas MD Anderson Cancer Center, Houston [330]

JOHN I. GALLIN, MD
Director, NIH Warren Grant G. Magnuson Clinical Center; NIH Associate Director for Clinical Research; Chief Laboratory of Host Defenses, National Institute of Allergy and Infectious Diseases, National Institutes of Health, Bethesda [55]

SUSAN L. GEARHART, MD
Assistant Professor of Surgery, The Johns Hopkins University School of Medicine, Baltimore [279]

ROBERT H. GELBER, MD
Leonard Wood Memorial Scientific Director, American Leprosy Foundation; Clinical Professor of Medicine and Dermatology, University of California San Francisco, San Francisco [151]

JEFFREY A. GELFAND, MD
Visiting Professor of Medicine, Harvard Medical School; Professor of Medicine, Tufts University School of Medicine; Physician, Infectious Diseases Unit, Department of Medicine, Massachusetts General Hospital, Boston [16, 18]

DALE N. GERDING, MD
Chief, Medical Service, VA Chicago Health Care System—Lakeside Division; Professor and Associate Chairman, Department of Medicine, The Feinberg School of Medicine, Northwestern University, Chicago [114]

ANNE A. GERSHON, MD
Professor of Pediatrics; Director, Division of Pediatric Infectious Diseases, Columbia University Medical Center, New York [176–178]

MARC GHANY, MD
Medical Staff Fellow, Liver Diseases Section, Digestive Diseases Branch, National Institute of Diabetes and Digestive and Kidney Diseases, National Institutes of Health, Bethesda [282]

RAYMOND J. GIBBONS, MD
Arthur M. and Gladys D. Gray Professor of Medicine, Mayo Clinic College of Medicine, Rochester [211]

BRUCE C. GILLILAND, MD
Professor of Medicine and Laboratory Medicine, University of Washington School of Medicine, Seattle [303, 308, 315, 316]

ROGER I. GLASS, MD, PhD
Viral Gastroenteritis Section, Centers for Disease Control and Prevention, Atlanta [174]

ELI GLATSTEIN, MD
Morton M. Kligerman Professor and Vice Chairman, Clinical Director, Department of Radiation Oncology, University of Pennsylvania Medical Center, Philadelphia [71, 207]

ROBERT M. GLICKMAN, MD
Professor of Medicine and Dean, New York University School of Medicine; CEO New York University Hospitals Center, New York [39]

JAMES F. GLOCKNER, MD
Assistant Professor of Radiology, Mayo Clinic College of Medicine; Consultant, Department of Radiology, Mayo Clinic, Rochester [211]

ARY L. GOLDBERGER, MD
Associate Professor of Medicine, Harvard Medical School; Director, Margret and H.A. Rey Institute for Nonlinear Dynamics in Medicine, Beth Israel Deaconess Medical Center, Boston [210]

SAMUEL Z. GOLDHABER, MD
Associate Professor of Medicine, Harvard Medical School; Director, Venous Thromboembolism Research Group, Director, Anticoagulation Service and Staff Cardiologist, Brigham and Women's Hospital, Boston [244]

RALPH GONZALES, MD, MSPH
Associate Professor of Medicine, Epidemiology and Biostatistics, University of California San Francisco, San Francisco [27]

DOUGLAS S. GOODIN, MD
Professor of Neurology, University of California San Francisco, San Francisco [359]

RAJ K. GOYAL, MD
Mallinckrodt Professor of Medicine, Harvard Medical School, Boston [33, 273]

GREGORY A. GRABOWSKI, MD
Director, Division and Program in Human Genetics, Cincinnati Children's Hospital Research Foundation; Professor, Department of Pediatrics, and Molecular Genetics and Biochemistry, University of Cincinnati College of Medicine, Cincinnati [340]

JACOB GREEN, MD
Associate Professor of Medicine, Department of Nephrology, Technion Faculty of Medicine, Haifa, Israel [261]

NORTON J. GREENBERGER, MD
Professor of Medicine, Harvard Medical School; Senior Physician, Brigham and Women's Hospital, Boston [292–294]

DAVID E. GRIFFITH, MD
Director of Tuberculosis Services and Professor of Medicine, University of Texas Health Center, Tyler [149]

WILLIAM GROSSMAN, MD
Myer Friedman Distinguished Professor of Medicine, University of California San Francisco; Chief of Cardiology, University of California San Francisco Medical Center, San Francisco [212]

RASIM GUCALP, MD
Associate Professor of Medicine, Department of Oncology, Montefiore Medical Center, Albert Einstein College of Medicine, New York [88]

BEVRA HANNAHS HAHN, MD
Professor of Medicine, David Geffen School of Medicine at the University of California Los Angeles, Los Angeles [300]

STEPHEN M. HAHN, MD
Associate Professor, Department of Radiation Oncology, Division of Hematology Oncology, University of Pennsylvania, Philadelphia [71]

JANET E. HALL, MD
Associate Professor of Medicine, Harvard Medical School; Assistant Physician, Massachusetts General Hospital, Boston [45]

JESSE B. HALL, MD
Section Chief, Pulmonary and Critical Care Medicine; Professor of Medicine, Anesthesia and Critical Care, University of Chicago, Chicago [249]

SCOTT A. HALPERIN, MD
Professor of Pediatrics; Associate Professor of Microbiology and Immunology, Dalhousie University, Halifax, Nova Scotia, Canada [133]

CHARLES H. HALSTED, MD
Professor of Internal Medicine and Nutrition, University of California-Davis School of Medicine, Davis [62]

ROBERT I. HANDIN, MD
Professor of Medicine, Harvard Medical School, Boston [53, 101, 102]

CATHLEEN A. HANLON, VMD, PhD
Veterinary Medical Officer, Rabies Section, Centers for Disease Control and Prevention, Atlanta [179]

GAVIN HART, MD, MPH
Director, STD Services, Royal Adelaide Hospital; Clinical Associate Professor, School of Medicine, Flinders University, Adelaide, South Australia, Australia [145]

WILLIAM L. HASLER, MD
Associate Professor of Internal Medicine, Division of Gastroenterology, University of Michigan Medical Center, Ann Arbor [34, 271]

TERRY J. HASSOLD, PhD
Professor of Genetics, Case Western Reserve University School of Medicine, Cleveland [57]

STEPHEN L. HAUSER, MD
Robert A. Fishman Distinguished Professor and Chairman, Department of Neurology, University of California San Francisco, San Francisco [345, 346, 355, 356, 365]

EDWARD B. HAYES, MD
Medical Epidemiologist, Division of Vector-Borne Infectious Diseases, Centers for Disease Control and Prevention, Fort Collins [156]

BARTON F. HAYNES, MD
Frederic M. Hanes Professor of Medicine, Professor of Immunology, Duke University School of Medicine, Durham [295]

J. CLAUDE HEMPHILL III, MD
Assistant Professor of Neurology, University of California San Francisco; Director, Neurovascular and Neurocritical Care Program, San Francisco General Hospital, San Francisco [258]

PATRICK H. HENRY, MD
Principal Investigator, St. Louis-Cape Girardeau Community Clinical Oncology Program, St. Louis [54]

BARBARA L. HERWALDT, MD, MPH
Medical Epidemiologist, Division of Parasitic Diseases, Centers for Disease Control and Prevention, Atlanta [196]

MARTIN S. HIRSCH, MD
Professor of Medicine, Harvard Medical School; Professor of Immunology and Infectious Diseases, Harvard School of Public Health; Director of Clinical AIDS Research, Massachusetts General Hospital, Boston [166]

HELEN HASKELL HOBBS, MD
Investigator, Howard Hughes Medical Institute; Professor of Internal Medicine and Molecular Genetics, University of Texas Southwestern Medical Center, Dallas [335]

JUDITH S. HOCHMAN, MD, FACC
Harold Snyder Family Professor of Cardiology; Clinical Chief, Division of Cardiology; Director, Cardiovascular Clinical Research, New York University School of Medicine, New York [255]

STEVEN M. HOLLAND, MD
Senior Investigator and Head, Immunopathogenesis Unit, Clinical Pathophysiology Section, Laboratory of Host Defenses, National Institute of Allergy and Infectious Diseases, National Institute of Health, Bethesda [55]

KING K. HOLMES, MD, PhD
Professor of Medicine; Director, Center for AIDS and Sexually Transmitted Diseases, University of Washington, Seattle [115]

RANDALL K. HOLMES, MD, PhD
Professor and Chair, Department of Microbiology, University of Colorado Health Sciences Center, Denver [122]

JAY H. HOOFNAGLE, MD
Director, Liver Disease Research Branch, Division of Digestive Diseases and Nutrition, National Institute of Diabetes and Digestive and Kidney Diseases, National Institutes of Health, Bethesda [282]

ROBERT J. HOPKIN, MD
Assistant Professor of Clinical Pediatrics, The University of Cincinnati College of Medicine; Division and Program in Human Genetics, Cincinnati Children's Hospital Research Foundation, Cincinnati [340]

JONATHAN C. HORTON, MD, PhD
William F. Hoyt Professor of Neuro-Ophthalmology, Departments of Ophthalmology, Neurology, and Physiology, University of California San Francisco, San Francisco [25]

LYN HOWARD, MB, FRCP
Emeritus Professor of Medicine, Associate Professor of Pediatrics, Albany Medical College, Albany [63]

HOWARD HU, MD, MPH, ScD
Professor of Occupational and Environmental Medicine, Department of Environmental Health, Harvard School of Public Health; Associate Physician Channing Laboratory, Department of Medicine, Brigham and Women's Hospital; Associate Professor of Medicine, Harvard Medical School, Boston [376]

GARY W. HUNNINGHAKE, MD
Sterba Professor of Medicine, Director, Division of Pulmonary Critical Care and Occupational Medicine; Director, Graduate Program in Translational Biomedical Research, University of Iowa College of Medicine, Iowa City [237]

SHARON A. HUNT, MD
Professor, Division of Cardiovascular Medicine, Stanford University, Stanford [217]

CHARLES G. HURST, MD
Chief, Chemical Casualty Care Division, US Army Medical Research Institute of Chemical Defense, Maryland [206]

DAVID H. INGBAR, MD
Professor, Medicine Physiology and Pediatrics; Director, Pulmonary Allergy and Critical Care Division, University of Minnesota, Minneapolis [255]

EDWARD P. INGENITO, MD, PhD
Associate Physician, Brigham and Women's Hospital; Adjunct Assistant Professor, Harvard Medical School, Boston [250, 252]

ROLAND H. INGRAM, JR., MD
Martha West Looney Professor Emeritus, Emory University School of Medicine, Atlanta [29]

MARK A. ISRAEL, MD
Professor of Pediatrics and Genetics, Dartmouth Medical School; Director, Norris Cotton Cancer Center, Dartmouth–Hitchcock Medical Center, Lebanon [358]

KURT J. ISSELBACHER, MD
Distinguished Mallinckrodt Professor of Medicine, Harvard Medical School; Physician and Director, Massachusetts General Hospital Cancer Center, Boston [78, 285–287]

RICHARD F. JACOBS, MD
Horace C. Cabe Professor of Pediatrics, University of Arkansas for Medical Sciences College of Medicine; Chief, Pediatric Infectious Diseases, Arkansas Children's Hospital, Little Rock [142]

J. LARRY JAMESON, MD, PhD
Irving S. Cutter Professor and Chair, Department of Medicine, Northwestern University Feinberg School of Medicine; Physician-in-Chief, Northwestern Memorial Hospital, Chicago [56, 58, 59, 86, 317, 318, 320, 325, 328]

JAMES L. JANUZZI, JR., MD
Assistant Professor of Medicine, Harvard Medical School; Assistant Physician, Division of Cardiology and Department of Medicine, Massachusetts General Hospital, Boston [Appendices]

ROBERT T. JENSEN, MD
Chief, Digestive Diseases Branch, National Institute of Diabetes and Digestive and Kidney Diseases, National Institutes of Health, Bethesda [329]

BRUCE E. JOHNSON, MD
Associate Professor of Medicine, Brigham and Women's Hospital and Harvard Medical School; Program Director, Lowe Center for Thoracic Oncology, Dana-Farber Cancer Institute, Boston [86]

STUART JOHNSON, MD
Attending Physician, Hines VA Hospital; Associate Professor, Department of Medicine, Stritch School of Medicine, Loyola University, Maywood, IL [114]

S. CLAIBORNE JOHNSTON, MD, PhD
Associate Professor of Neurology and Epidemiology; Director, Stroke Service, University of California San Francisco, San Francisco [349]

MARK E. JOSEPHSON, MD
Professor of Medicine, Harvard Medical School; Chief, Cardiovascular Division, Beth Israel Deaconess Medical Center; Director, Harvard-Thorndike Electrophysiology Institute and Arrhythmia Service, Boston [213, 214]

JORGE L. JUNCOS, MD
Associate Professor of Neurology, Emory University School of Medicine; Director of Neurology, Wesley Woods Hospital, Atlanta [351]

EDWARD L. KAPLAN, MD
Professor of Pediatrics, University of Minnesota Medical School, Minneapolis [302]

MARSHALL M. KAPLAN, MD
Professor of Medicine, Tufts University School of Medicine, Boston [38, 283]

ADOLF W. KARCHMER, MD
Professor of Medicine, Harvard Medical School; Chief, Division of Infectious Diseases, Beth Israel Deaconess Medical Center, Boston [109]

DENNIS L. KASPER, MD, MA(Hon)
William Ellery Channing Professor of Medicine, Professor of Microbiology and Molecular Genetics, Harvard Medical School; Director, Channing Laboratory, Department of Medicine, Brigham and Women's Hospital, Boston [104, 106, 112, 126, 131, 148]

LLOYD H. KASPER, MD
Professor of Medicine (Neurology) and Microbiology/Immunology; Director, Multiple Sclerosis Center, Dartmouth Medical School, Lebanon [198]

DANIEL L. KASTNER, MD, PhD
Chief, Genetics and Genomics Branch, National Institute of Arthritis and Musculoskeletal and Skin Diseases, National Institutes of Health, Bethesda [278]

ELAINE T. KAYE, MD
Clinical Instructor in Dermatology, Harvard Medical School; Assistant in Medicine, Department of Medicine, Children's Hospital Medical Center, Boston [17]

KENNETH M. KAYE, MD
Assistant Professor of Medicine, Harvard Medical School; Associate Physician, Division of Infectious Diseases, Brigham and Women's Hospital, Boston [17]

GERALD T. KEUSCH, MD
Assistant Provost and Associate Dean for Global Health; Professor of Medicine and International Health, Boston University Medical Campus and School of Public Health, Boston [107, 138, 140]

JAY S. KEYSTONE, MD, MSC(CTM), FRCPC
Professor of Medicine, University of Toronto; Tropical Disease Unit, Division of Infectious Disease, Toronto General Hospital, University Health Network, Toronto, Ontario, Canada [108]

ELLIOTT KIEFF, MD, PhD
Harriet Ryan Albee Professor of Medicine and Microbiology and Molecular Genetics, Harvard Medical School; Senior Physician, Brigham and Women's Hospital, Boston [161]

TALMADGE E. KING, JR., MD
The Constance B. Wofsy Distinguished Professor and Vice Chairman, Department of Medicine, University of California San Francisco; Chief, Medical Services, San Francisco General Hospital, San Francisco [243]

LOUIS V. KIRCHHOFF, MD, MPH
Professor, Departments of Internal Medicine and Epidemiology, University of Iowa; Staff Physician, Department of Veterans Affairs Medical Center, Iowa City [197]

JOEL N. KLINE, MD, MS
Professor, Director, University of Iowa Adult Asthma Center, University of Iowa College of Medicine, Iowa City [237]

HOWARD K. KOH, MD, PhD
Professor and Associate Dean, Harvard School of Public Health, Boston [73]

DENNIS J. KOPECKO, PhD
Chief, Laboratory of Enteric and Sexually Transmitted Diseases, Center for Biologics Evaluation and Research, National Institutes of Health, Bethesda [138]

PETER KOPP, MD
Associate Professor, Division of Endocrinology, Metabolism, and Molecular Medicine, Northwestern University Feinberg School of Medicine, Chicago [56]

WALTER J. KOROSHETZ, MD
Vice Chair, Neurology Service, Massachusetts General Hospital, Associate Professor of Neurology, Harvard Medical School, Boston [361]

PHYLLIS E. KOZARSKY, MD
Professor of Medicine/Infectious Diseases, Emory University School of Medicine; Chief, Traveler's Health, Division of Global Migration and Quarantine, Centers for Disease Control and Prevention, Atlanta [108]

BARNETT S. KRAMER, MD, MPH
Associate Director for Disease Prevention, National Institutes of Health; Clinical Professor of Medicine, Uniformed Services University of the Health Sciences, Bethesda [67]

STEPHEN M. KRANE, MD
Persis, Cyrus, and Marlow B. Harrison Professor of Medicine, Harvard Medical School; Physician and Chief, Arthritis Unit, Massachusetts General Hospital, Boston [331]

ALEXANDER KRATZ, MD, PhD, MPH
Assistant Professor of Pathology, Harvard Medical School; Director, Clinical Hematology Laboratory, Massachusetts General Hospital [Appendices]

JOHN P. KRESS, MD
Assistant Professor of Medicine, University of Chicago Pritzker School of Medicine, Chicago [249]

HENRY M. KRONENBERG, MD
Professor of Medicine, Harvard Medical School; Chief, Endocrine Unit, Massachusetts General Hospital, Boston [331]

LOREN LAINE, MD
Professor of Medicine, Gastrointestinal Division, Department of Medicine, Keck School of Medicine, University of Southern California School of Medicine, Los Angeles [37]

ANIL K. LALWANI, MD
Mendik Foundation Professor and Chair, Department of Otolaryngology; Professor of Physiology and Neuroscience, New York University School of Medicine, New York [26]

LEWIS LANDSBERG, MD
Professor of Medicine, Dean and Vice President for Medical Affairs, Northwestern University Feinberg School of Medicine, Chicago [322]

H. CLIFFORD LANE, MD
Head, Clinical and Molecular Retrovirology Section, Laboratory of Immunoregulation; Clinical Director, National Institute of Allergy and Infectious Diseases, National Institutes of Health, Bethesda [173, 205]

CAROL A. LANGFORD, MD
Senior Investigator, Immunologic Diseases Section, NIAID, NIH, Bethesda [306]

THOMAS J. LAWLEY, MD
Dean, Emory University School of Medicine, Atlanta [46, 47, 49]

THOMAS H. LEE, MD
Associate Professor of Medicine, Harvard Medical School; Chief Executive Officer, Partners Community Health Care, Inc; Network President, Partners Health Care, Boston [12]

OFER LEHAVI, MD
Attending Physician, Department of Obstetrics and Gynecology, Tel-Aviv Medical Center, Israel [207]

CAMMIE F. LESSER, MD, PhD
Assistant Professor in Medicine, Harvard Medical School, Cambridge [137]

BRUCE D. LEVY, MD, FACP
Assistant Professor of Medicine, Harvard Medical School; Pulmonary and Critical Care Medicine, Brigham and Women's Hospital, Boston [251]

KENT B. LEWANDROWSKI, MD
Associate Chief of Pathology, Director, Core Laboratory, Massachusetts General Hospital; Associate Professor, Harvard Medical School, Boston [Appendices]

PETER LIBBY, MD
Mallinckrodt Professor of Medicine, Harvard Medical School; Chief, Cardiovascular Medicine, Brigham and Women's Hospital, Boston [224, 225]

RICHARD W. LIGHT, MD
Professor of Medicine, Vanderbilt University, Nashville [245]

CRAIG LILLY, MD
Associate Professor of Medicine, Harvard Medical School; Division of Pulmonary and Critical Care, Department of Medicine, Brigham and Women's Hospital, Boston [250]

CHRISTOPHER H. LINDEN, MD
Professor, Department of Emergency Medicine, Division of Medical Toxicology, University of Massachusetts Medical School, Worcester [377]

ROBERT LINDSAY, MD, PhD
Professor of Clinical Medicine, Columbia University College of Physicians and Surgeons; Chief, Internal Medicine, Helen Hayes Hospital, West Haverstraw, New York [333]

MARC E. LIPPMAN, MD
John G. Searle Professor and Chair, Department of Internal Medicine, University of Michigan Health System, Ann Arbor [76]

PETER E. LIPSKY, MD
Scientific Director, National Institute of Arthritis and Musculoskeletal and Skin Diseases, National Institutes of Health, Bethesda [299, 301, 311]

DAN L. LONGO, MD
Scientific Director, National Institute on Aging, National Institutes of Health, Bethesda and Baltimore [52, 54, 66, 69, 70, 89, 97, 98, 172]

NICOLA LONGO, MD, PhD
Professor of Pediatrics and Director, Metabolic Service, Division of Medical Genetics, Department of Pediatrics, University of Utah, Salt Lake City [343, 344]

DONALD E. LOW, MD
Chief, Department of Medicine, Toronto Medical Laboratories and Mount Sinai Hospital; Professor of Medicine and Microbiology, University of Toronto, Toronto, Ontario, Canada [239]

PHILLIP A. LOW, MD
Professor of Neurology, Mayo Medical School; Chairman, Division of Clinical Neurophysiology; Consultant in Neurology, Mayo Clinic, Rochester [354]

DANIEL H. LOWENSTEIN, MD
Professor of Neurology, Vice Chairman, Department of Neurology; Director, Physician-Scientist Education and Training Program; Director UCSF Epilepsy Center, University of California San Francisco, San Francisco [346, 348]

FRANKLIN D. LOWY, MD
Professor of Medicine and Physiology, Columbia University, New York [120]

SHEILA A. LUKEHART, PhD
Research Professor, University of Washington, Seattle [153,154]

LAWRENCE C. MADOFF, MD
Assistant Professor of Medicine, Harvard Medical School; Associate Physician, Brigham and Women's Hospital, Boston [104, 126, 314]

JAMES H. MAGUIRE, MD
Chief, Parasitic Diseases Branch, Centers for Disease Control and Prevention, Atlanta [111, 314, 379]

ADEL A. F. MAHMOUD, MD, PhD
President, Merck Vaccines, Merck & Co., Inc.; Adjunct Professor of Medicine, Case Western Reserve University, Whitehouse Station [203]

RONALD V. MAIER, MD
Professor and Vice Chair, Surgery, University of Washington; Surgeon-in-Chief, Harborview Medical Center, Seattle [253]

MARK E. MAILLIARD, MD
Associate Professor, Department of Internal Medicine, University of Nebraska College of Medicine; Chief, Section of Gastroenterology, Omaha Veterans Affairs Medical Center, Omaha [288]

JOANN E. MANSON, MD, DRPH
Professor of Medicine and the Elizabeth F. Brigham Professor of Women's Health, Harvard Medical School; Chief, Division of Preventive Medicine, Brigham and Women's Hospital, Boston [327]

ELEFTHERIA MARATOS-FLIER, MD
Associate Professor of Medicine, Harvard Medical School; Chief, Obesity Section, Joslin Diabetes Center, Boston [64]

DANIEL B. MARK, MD, MPH
Professor of Medicine, Duke University Medical Center; Director, Outcomes Research, Duke Clinical Research Institute, Durham [2]

THOMAS J. MARRIE, MD, FRCPC
Professor, Department of Medicine, Dean Faculty of Medicine and Dentistry, University of Alberta, Edmonton, Alberta, Canada [158, 239]

GARY J. MARTIN, MD
Raymond J. Lagenback, MD, Professor of Medicine, Vice Chairman, Department of Medicine, Northwestern University Feinberg School of Medicine, Chicago [4]

JOSEPH B. MARTIN, MD, PhD, MA(Hon)
Dean of the Faculty of Medicine; Caroline Shields Walker Professor of Neurobiology and Clinical Neuroscience, Harvard Medical School, Boston [11, 346]

ROBERT J. MAYER, MD
Vice Chair for Academic Affairs; Director, Center for Gastrointestinal Oncology, Dana-Farber Cancer Institute; Professor of Medicine, Harvard Medical School, Boston [77, 79]

CALVIN O. McCALL, MD
Assistant Professor of Dermatology, Department of Dermatology, Emory University School of Medicine, Atlanta [47]

WILLIAM M. McCORMACK, MD
Professor of Medicine; Chief, Infectious Diseases Division, State University of New York Downstate Medical Center, New York [159]

E. REGIS McFADDEN, JR., MD
Argyl J. Beams Professor of Medicine, MetroHealth Medical Center, Cleveland [236]

RONALD D.G. McKAY, PhD
Chief, Laboratory of Molecular Biology, National Institute of Neurologic Disorders and Stroke, NIH, Bethesda [59]

KEVIN T. McVARY, MD
Associate Professor of Urology, Northwestern University Feinberg School of Medicine, Chicago [43]

NANCY K. MELLO, PhD
Professor of Psychology, Harvard Medical School, Boston [374]

SHLOMO MELMED, MD
Professor and Associate Dean, David Geffen School of Medicine at University of California Los Angeles; Senior Vice President and Chief Academic Officer at Cedars-Sinai Medical Center, Los Angeles [318]

JERRY R. MENDELL, MD
Helen C. Kurtz Professor and Chairman of Neurology, Ohio State University, Columbus [367, 368]

JACK H. MENDELSON, MD
Professor of Psychiatry (Neuroscience), Harvard Medical School, Belmont [374]

M. -MARSEL MESULAM, MD
Ruth and Evelyn Dunbar Professor of Neurology and Psychiatry; Director, Center for Behavioral and Cognitive Neurology; Director, Alzheimer's Program, Northwestern University Feinberg School of Medicine, Chicago [23]

SUSAN MIESFELDT, MD
Maine Center for Cancer Medicine and Blood Disorders, Scarborough [58]

EDGAR L. MILFORD MD
Associate Professor of Medicine, Harvard Medical School; Brigham and Women's Hospital, Boston [263]

BRUCE L. MILLER, MD
AW and Mary Margaret Clausen Distinguished Chair, Professor of Neurology, University of California San Francisco, San Francisco [350, 362]

MARK MILLER, MD
Associate Director for Research; Director, Division of International Epidemiology and Population Studies, Fogarty International Center, National Institutes of Health, Bethesda [107]

SAMUEL I. MILLER, MD
Professor of Medicine, Microbiology, and Genome Sciences, University of Washington, Seattle [137]

JOHN D. MINNA, MD
Professor of Internal Medicine and Pharmacology; Director, Hamon Center for Therapeutic Oncology Research, University of Texas Southwestern Medical Center, Dallas [75]

THOMAS A. MOORE, MD, FACP
Clinical Associate Professor of Medicine, University of Kansas School of Medicine, Wichita [193]

PAT J. MORIN, PhD
Investigator, National Institute on Aging, National Institutes of Health; Assistant Professor, Department of Pathology, The Johns Hopkins School of Medicine, Baltimore [68]

ROBERT J. MOTZER, MD
Attending Physician, Memorial Sloan-Kettering Cancer Center; Professor of Medicine, Weill Medical College of Cornell University, New York [80, 82]

HARALAMPOS M. MOUTSOPOULOS, MD
Professor and Director, Department of Pathophysiology, National University School of Medicine; President of the National Organization for Medicines, Athens, Greece [304, 307]

ROBERT S. MUNFORD, MD
Jan and Henri Bromberg Professor of Internal Medicine, University of Texas Southwestern Medical Center, Dallas [127, 254]

TIMOTHY F. MURPHY, MD
Distinguished Professor of Medicine; Chief, Division of Infectious Diseases, State University of New York at Buffalo, Buffalo [130]

DANIEL M. MUSHER, MD
Chief, Infectious Diseases Section, Veterans Affairs Medical Center; Professor of Medicine, Professor of Molecular Virology and Immunology, Baylor College of Medicine, Houston [119, 129]

ROBERT J. MYERBURG, MD
Lemberg Professor of Medicine and Physiology, Director, Division of Cardiology, University of Miami School of Medicine; American Heart Association Chair in Cardiovascular Research, Miami [256]

GERALD T. NEPOM, MD, PhD
Director, Benaroya Research Institute at Virginia Mason; Professor (Affiliate), Department of Immunology, University of Washington School of Medicine, Seattle [296]

JONATHAN NEWMARK, MD
Chief, Operations, Chemical Casualty Care, US Army Medical Research Institute of Chemical Defense, Maryland [206]

RICHARD A. NISHIMURA, MD
Judd and Mary Morris Leighton Professor of Cardiovascular Diseases, Mayo Clinic College of Medicine, Rochester [211]

ROBERT L. NORRIS, MD
Associate Professor of Surgery, Department of Surgery, Division of Emergency Medicine, Stanford University School of Medicine, Stanford [378]

THOMAS B. NUTMAN, MD
Head, Helminth Immunology Section, and Head, Clinical Parasitology Unit, Laboratory of Parasitic Diseases, National Institute of Allergy and Infectious Diseases, National Institutes of Health, Bethesda [201, 202]

RICHARD J. O'BRIEN, MD
Head of Scientific Evaluation, Foundation for Innovative New Diagnostics, Geneva, Switzerland [150]

CHRISTOPHER A. OHL, MD
Associate Professor of Medicine, Section of Infectious Diseases, Wake Forest University School of Medicine; Director, Center for Antimicrobial Utilization, Stewardship, and Epidemiology, Baptist Medical Center, Winston-Salem [136]

RICHARD K. OLNEY, MD
Professor of Neurology, University of California San Francisco, San Francisco [21]

YVONNE M. O'MEARA, MD, FRCPI
Senior Lecturer in Medicine, University College Dublin; Consultant Nephrologist, Mater Misericordiae Hospital, Dublin, Ireland [264]

ROBERT A. O'ROURKE, MD
Charles Conrad Brown Distinguished Professor of Cardiovascular Science, University of Texas Health Science Center at San Antonio, San Antonio [209]

CHUNG OWYANG, MD
Professor of Internal Medicine, H. Marvin Pollard Collegiate Professor and Chief, Division of Gastroenterology, Department of Internal Medicine, University of Michigan Medical Center, Ann Arbor [271, 277]

UMESH D. PARASHAR, MBBS, MPH
Medical Epidemiologist, Respiratory and Enteric Viruses Branch, Centers for Disease Control and Prevention, Atlanta [174]

JEFFREY PARSONNET, MD
Associate Professor of Medicine and of Microbiology, Dartmouth Medical School; Staff Physician, Infectious Diseases Section, Dartmouth-Hitchcock Medical Center, Lebanon [111]

SHREYASKUMAR R. PATEL, MD
Associate Professor of Medicine, Deputy Chairman, Department of Sarcoma Medical Oncology, University of Texas, MD Anderson Cancer Center, Houston [84]

G. ALEXANDER PATTERSON, MD
Joseph C. Bancroft Professor of Surgery, Department of Surgery, Division of Cardiothoracic Surgery, Washington University School of Medicine, St. Louis [248]

GUSTAV PAUMGARTNER, MD
Professor of Medicine, Ludwig Maximiliam University of Munich, Durchwal, Germany [292]

MICHAEL C. PERRY, MD, FACP
Professor of Internal Medicine, Director, Division of Hematology/ Oncology, Nellie B. Smith Chair of Oncology, University of Missouri/ Ellis Fischer Cancer Center, Columbia [89]

CLARENCE J. PETERS, MD
John Sealy Distinguished University Chair in Tropical and Emerging Virology, Director for Biodefense, Center for Biodefense and Emerging Infectious Diseases, University of Texas Medical Branch in Galveston, Galveston [180, 181]

ELIOT A. PHILLIPSON, MD
Sir John and Lady Eaton Professor and Chair, Department of Medicine, University of Toronto, Toronto, Ontario, Canada [246, 247]

GERALD B. PIER, PhD
Professor of Medicine (Microbiology and Molecular Genetics), Harvard School of Medicine, Boston [105]

DANIEL K. PODOLSKY, MD
Mallinckrodt Professor of Medicine, Harvard Medical School; Chief, Gastroenterology, Massachusetts General Hospital, Boston [289, 290]

RONALD E. POLK, Pharm. D.
Professor of Pharmacy and Medicine, Chair, Department of Pharmacy, School of Pharmacy, Virginia Commonwealth University, Richmond [118]

MATTHEW POLLACK, MD
Professor of Medicine, Uniformed Services University; F. Edward Hébert School of Medicine; Attending Staff Physician, Internal Medicine and Infectious Diseases, National Naval Medical Center, Bethesda [136]

RICHARD J. POLLACK, PhD
Instructor of Tropical Public Health, Department of Immunology and Infectious Diseases, Harvard School of Public Health, Boston [379]

JOHN T. POTTS, JR., MD
Jackson Distinguished Professor of Clinical Medicine, Harvard Medical School, Boston [332]

LAWRIE W. POWELL, MD, PhD
Professor of Medicine, The University of Queensland and The Royal Brisbane and Women's Hospital, Brisbane, Queensland, Australia [336]

ALVIN C. POWERS, MD
Ruth K. Scoville Professor of Medicine, Division of Diabetes, Endocrinology, and Metabolism, Vanderbilt University Medical Center; Chief, Diabetes and Endocrinology Section, VA Tennessee Valley Healthcare System, Nashville [323]

DANIEL S. PRATT, MD
Assistant Professor of Medicine, Tufts University School of Medicine; Medical Director of Liver Transplantation, New England Medical Center, Boston [38, 283]

DANIEL T. PRICE, MD
Assistant Professor of Medicine, Boston University School of Medicine; Staff Physician, Boston Veterans Affairs Medical Center, West Roxbury [223]

DARWIN J. PROCKOP, MD, PhD
Director of Center for Gene Therapy and Professor of Biochemistry, Tulane Health Sciences Center, New Orleans [342]

STANLEY B. PRUSINER, MD
Director, Institute for Neurodegenerative Diseases; Professor, Departments of Neurology, Biochemistry and Biophysics, University of California San Francisco, San Francisco [362]

DANIEL J. RADER, MD
Associate Professor, Department of Medicine, University of Pennsylvania School of Medicine, Philadelphia [335]

SANJAY RAM, MD
Assistant Professor of Medicine, Section of Infectious Diseases, Boston University School of Medicine and Boston Medical Center, Boston [128]

DIDIER RAOULT, MD
Professor of Medicine, Unité des Rickettsies, School of Medicine, University of Aux-Marseille, Marseille, France [158]

NEIL H. RASKIN, MD
Professor of Neurology, University of California San Francisco, San Francisco [14]

MARIO C. RAVIGLIONE, MD
Director, Stop TB Department, World Health Organization, Geneva, Switzerland [150]

SHARON L. REED, MD
Professor of Pathology and Medicine, Director, Microbiology and Virology Laboratories, University of California Medical Center, San Diego [194]

ANTONIO J. REGINATO, MD
Professor of Medicine; Head, Division of Rheumatology, Cooper University Medical Center, Robert Wood Johnson Medical School at Camden, Camden [313]

RICHARD C. REICHMAN, MD
Professor of Medicine, Microbiology and Immunology; Head, Infectious Diseases Unit, Senior Associate Dean for Clinical Research, University of Rochester School of Medicine and Dentistry, Rochester [169]

CAROL M. REIFE, MD
Assistant Professor of Medicine, Jefferson Medical College of Thomas Jefferson University, Philadelphia [36]

JOHN J. REILLY, MD
Associate Professor of Medicine, Harvard Medical School; Clinical Director, Pulmonary and Critical Care Medicine, Brigham and Women's Hospital, Boston [242]

JOHN T. REPKE, MD, FACOG
Professor and Chair, Department of Obstetrics and Gynecology, Pennsylvania State University College of Medicine; Obstetrician-Gynecologist In-Chief, The Milton S. Hershey Medical Center, Hershey [6]

NEIL M. RESNICK, MD
Professor of Medicine, University of Pittsburgh School of Medicine; Chief, Division of Geriatric Medicine, University of Pittsburgh Institute on Aging, Pittsburgh [8]

VICTOR I. REUS, MD
Professor of Psychiatry, University of California San Francisco; Medical Director, Langley Porter Hospital, San Francisco [371]

C. FORDHAM VON REYN, MD
Professor of Medicine, Chief, Infectious Diseases and International Health, Dartmouth Medical School, Lebanon [152]

PETER A. RICE, MD
Professor of Medicine and Chief, Section of Infectious Diseases, Boston University Medical Center, Boston [128]

STUART RICH, MD
Professor of Medicine, Rush University Medical, Chicago [220]

GARY S. RICHARDSON, MD
Assistant Professor of Psychiatry, Case Western Reserve University, Cleveland; Senior Research Scientist, Sleep Disorders and Research Center, Henry Ford Hospital, Detroit [24]

GARY L. ROBERTSON, MD
Professor of Medicine and Neurology, Northwestern University Feinberg School of Medicine, Chicago [319]

DAN M. RODEN, MD
Professor of Medicine and Pharmacology; Chief, Division of Clinical Pharmacology, Vanderbilt University School of Medicine, Nashville [3]

JAMES A. ROMANO, JR., PhD
Commander, US Army Medical Research Institute of Chemical Defense, Maryland [206]

KAREN L. ROOS, MD
John and Nancy Nelson Professor of Neurology, Indiana University School of Medicine, Indianapolis [360]

ALLAN H. ROPPER, MD
Professor and Chairman of Neurology, Tufts University School of Medicine; Chief, Department of Neurology, St. Elizabeth's Medical Center, Boston [257, 356, 357]

ROGER N. ROSENBERG, MD
Zale Distinguished Chair and Professor of Neurology, University of Texas Southwestern Medical Center at Dallas; Attending Neurologist, Parkland Memorial Hospital and Zale-Lipsky University Hospital, Dallas [352]

MYRNA R. ROSENFELD, MD, PhD
Associate Professor of Neurology, Department of Neurology, University of Pennsylvania, Philadelphia [87]

WENDELL ROSSE, MD
Florence Reynaud McAlister Professor of Medicine and Medical Research, Department of Medicine, Duke University Medical School, Durham [93]

MICHAEL A. RUBIN, MD, PhD
Assistant Professor, Internal Medicine, Division of Infectious Diseases, Division of Clinical Epidemiology, Salt Lake City [27]

ROBERT M. RUSSELL, MD
Professor, Friedman School of Nutrition Science and Policy; Director and Scientist, Jean Mayer USDA Human Nutrition Center on Aging at Tufts, Boston [61]

THOMAS A. RUSSO, MD, CM
Assistant Professor of Medicine, Division of Infectious Diseases, Department of Medicine, State University of New York at Buffalo; Veterans Affairs Medical Center, Buffalo [134, 147]

STEPHEN M. SAGAR, MD
Professor of Neurology, Case Western Reserve School of Medicine; Director of Neuro-Oncology, Ireland Cancer Center, University Hospitals of Cleveland, Cleveland [358]

MERLE A. SANDE, MD
Professor of Medicine, University of Utah School of Medicine; President, Academic Alliance for AIDS Care and Prevention in Africa Foundation, Salt Lake City [27]

EDWARD A. SAUSVILLE, MD, PhD
Associate Director for Clinical Research, Greenebaum Cancer Center, University of Maryland, Baltimore [70]

MOHAMED H. SAYEGH, MD
Associate Professor of Medicine, Harvard Medical School; Director, Transplantation Research Center, Brigham and Women's Hospital and Children's Hospital, Boston [263]

HOWARD I. SCHER, MD
D. Wayne Calloway Chair in Urologic Oncology, Attending Physician and Chief, Genitourinary Oncology Service, Department of Medicine, Memorial Sloan-Kettering Cancer Center; Professor of Medicine, Weill Medical College of Cornell University, New York [80, 81]

HARRY W. SCHROEDER, JR., MD, PhD
Professor of Medicine and Microbiology, University of Alabama at Birmingham, Birmingham [297]

ANNE SCHUCHAT, MD
Chief, Respiratory Diseases Branch, National Center for Infectious Diseases, Centers for Disease Control and Prevention, Atlanta [123]

MARC A. SCHUCKIT, MD
Professor of Psychiatry, University of California, San Diego; Director, Alcohol Research Center; Director, Alcohol and Drug Treatment Program, Veterans Affairs San Diego Healthcare System, San Diego [372, 373]

STUART SCHWARTZ, PhD
Professor of Genetics and Oncology, Center for Human Genetics Laboratory, Cleveland [57]

DAVID S. SEGAL, PhD
Professor of Psychiatry, University of California San Diego, La Jolla [373]

JULIAN L. SEIFTER, MD
Associate Professor of Medicine, Harvard Medical School; Physician, Brigham and Women's Hospital, Boston [270]

ANDREW P. SELWYN, MD
Professor of Medicine, Harvard Medical School; Physician, Brigham and Women's Hospital, Boston [226]

STEVEN D. SHAPIRO, MD
Parker B. Francis Professor of Medicine, Harvard Medical School and Brigham and Women's Hospital, Boston [242, 250, 251]

STEVEN I. SHERMAN, MD
Associate Professor, University of Texas M.D. Anderson Cancer Center; Adjunct Associate Professor, Baylor College of Medicine, Houston [330]

WILLIAM SILEN, MD
Johnson and Johnson Distinguished Professor of Surgery, Emeritus, Harvard Medical School, Boston [13, 280, 281]

EDWIN K. SILVERMAN, MD, PhD
Assistant Professor of Medicine, Harvard Medical School; Brigham and Women's Hospital, Boston [242]

GARY G. SINGER, MD
Assistant Professor of Medicine, Washington University School of Medicine; Associate Director, Transplant Nephrology, Barnes Jewish Hospital, St. Louis [41]

AJAY K. SINGH, MD
Associate Professor of Medicine, Harvard Medical School; Director of Clinical Nephrology, Brigham and Women's Hospital, Boston [262]

JEAN DOW SIPE, PhD
Professor Emeritus, Boston University School of Medicine; Scientific Review Administrator, National Institutes of Health, Bethesda [310]

KARL SKORECKI, MD
Annie Chutick Professor of Medicine, Bruce Rappaport Faculty of Medicine, Technion-Israel Institute of Technology; Director, Department of Nephrology and Molecular Medicine, Rambam Medical Center, Haifa, Israel [261]

GERALD W. SMETANA, MD
Associate Professor of Medicine, Harvard Medical School; Division of General Medicine and Primary Care, Beth Israel Deaconess Medical Center, Boston [7]

PATRICK M. SLUSS, PhD
Director, Immunodiagnostics Laboratory, Department of Pathology, Massachusetts General Hospital; Assistant Professor, Harvard Medical School, Boston [Appendices]

WADE S. SMITH, MD
Associates Professor of Neurology; Director, Neurointensive Care Service, University of California San Francisco, San Francisco [349]

MICHAEL C. SNELLER, MD
Chief of Immunologic Diseases Section, NIAID, NIH, Bethesda [306]

JAMES B. SNOW, JR., MD
Professor Emeritus, Department of Otorhinolaryngology, University of Pennsylvania; former Director, National Institute on Deafness and Other Communication Disorders, National Institutes of Health, Bethesda [26]

ARTHUR J. SOBER, MD
Professor of Dermatology, Harvard Medical School; Associate Chief of Dermatology, Massachusetts General Hospital, Boston [73]

MICHAEL F. SORRELL, MD
Robert L. Grissom Professor of Medicine; Chief, Section of Gastroenterology and Hepatology, and Medical Director, Liver Transplantation, University of Nebraska Medical Center, Omaha [288]

PETER SPEELMAN, MD, PhD
Professor of Internal Medicine, Division of Infectious Diseases, Tropical Medicine and AIDS, Department of Internal Medicine, Academic Medical Center, University of Amsterdam, Amsterdam, The Netherlands [155]

FRANK E. SPEIZER, MD
Edward H. Kass Professor of Medicine, Harvard Medical School; Co-Director, Channing Laboratory, Brigham and Women's Hospital; Professor of Environmental Science, Harvard School of Public Health, Boston [238]

ANDREW SPIELMAN, ScD
Professor of Tropical Public Health, Harvard School of Public Health, Boston [379]

JERRY L. SPIVAK, MD
Professor of Medicine and Oncology, Johns Hopkins University School of Medicine, Baltimore [95]

WALTER E. STAMM, MD
Professor of Medicine and Head, Division of Allergy and Infectious Diseases, University of Washington School of Medicine, Seattle [160, 269]

ALLEN C. STEERE, MD
Professor of Medicine, Harvard Medical School; Director of Rheumatology, Massachusetts General Hospital, Boston [157]

DAVID S. STEPHENS, MD
Director, Division of Infectious Diseases, Emory University Hospital; Stephen W. Schwarzmann Professor and Executive Vice Chair, Department of Medicine, Emory University School of Medicine, Atlanta [127]

ROBERT S. STERN, MD
Carl J. Herzog Professor of Dermatology, Harvard Medical, Boston [50]

DENNIS L. STEVENS, MD, PhD
Professor of Medicine, University of Washington School of Medicine, Seattle; Chief, Infectious Diseases, VA Medical Center, Boise [110]

RICHARD M. STONE, MD
Clinical Director, Adult Leukemia Program, Dana-Farber Cancer Institute/Brigham and Women's Hospital; Associate Professor of Medicine, Harvard Medical School, Boston [85]

STEPHEN E. STRAUS, MD
Senior Investigator, Laboratory of Clinical Investigation, National Institute of Allergy and Infectious Diseases; Director, National Center for Complementary and Alternative Medicine, National Institutes of Health, Bethesda [10, 370]

MORTON N. SWARTZ, MD
Professor, Department of Medicine, Harvard Medical School; Chief Emeritus, Infectious Disease, Chief, James Jackson Firm Medical Services, Massachusetts General Hospital, Boston [361]

A. JAMIL TAJIK, MD
Thomas J. Watson, Jr., Professor; Professor of Medicine and Pediatrics, Mayo Clinic College of Medicine Chair (Emeritus); Division of Cardiovascular Diseases and Internal Medicine; Consultant, Section of Pediatric Cardiology, Mayo Clinic, Minnesota [211]

JOEL D. TAUROG, MD
Professor of Internal Medicine, and William M. and Gatha Burnett Professor for Arthritis Research, University of Texas Southwestern Medical Center, Dallas [296, 305]

SCOTT J. THALER, MD
Chief Medical Officer, AERAS Global TB Vaccine Foundation, Bethesda [314]

ZELIG A. TOCHNER, MD
Associate Professor, Department of Radiation Oncology, University of Pennsylvania Medical Center, Philadelphia [207]

LUCY STUART TOMPKINS, MD
Professor of Medicine (Infectious Diseases and Geographic Medicine), Professor of Microbiology, Immunology and Pathology, Stanford University School of Medicine, Stanford [144]

MARK TOPAZIAN, MD
Associate Professor of Medicine, Yale University School of Medicine; Assistant Director, Gastrointestinal Procedure Center, Yale New Haven Hospital, New Haven [272]

PHILLIP P. TOSKES, MD
Professor of Medicine and Director, Division of Gastroenterology, Hepatology and Nutrition; Associate Chairman for Clinical Affairs, Department of Medicine, University of Florida, Gainesville [293, 294]

JEFFREY M. TRENT, PhD
President and Scientific Director; Senior Investigator, Molecular Diagnostics and Target Validation Division, T-Gen, Phoenix [68]

ELBERT P. TRULOCK, MD
Rosemary and I. Jerome Flance Professor of Pulmonary Medicine, Washington University School of Medicine; Medical Director, Lung Transplantation Program, Barnes-Jewish Hospital, St. Louis [248]

KENNETH L. TYLER, MD
Reuler-Lewin Family Professor of Neurology; Professor of Medicine, Microbiology and Immunology, University of Colorado Health Sciences Center; Chief, Neurology Service, Denver VA Medical Center, Denver [360]

BERT VOGELSTEIN, MD
Professor of Oncology and Pathology, Howard Hughes Investigator, The Sidney Kimmel Comprehensive Cancer Center, The Johns Hopkins University School of Medicine, Baltimore [68]

EVERETT E. VOKES, MD
Director, Section of Hematology/Oncology; John E. Ultmann Professor of Medicine and Radiation Oncology, University of Chicago, Chicago [74]

TAMARA J. VOKES, MD
Assistant Professor of Clinical Medicine, University of Chicago Pritzker School of Medicine, Chicago [334]

MATTHEW K. WALDOR, MD, PhD
Associate Professor of Medicine and Microbiology, Tufts University School of Medicine, Boston [140]

DAVID H. WALKER, MD
Professor and Chairman, Department of Pathology; Director, WHO Collaborating Center for Tropical Diseases, University of Texas Medical Branch, Galveston [158, 239]

RICHARD J. WALLACE, JR., MD
Chairman, Department of Microbiology, John Chapman Professorship in Microbiology, Professor of Medicine, University of Texas Health Center, Tyler [149]

B. TIMOTHY WALSH, MD
Ruane Professor of Psychiatry, College of Physicians and Surgeons, Columbia University; Director, Eating Disorders Research Unit, New York State Psychiatric Institute, New York [65]

PETER D. WALZER, MD
Associate Chief of Staff for Research, Cincinnati VA Medical Center; Professor of Medicine, University of Cincinnati, Cincinnati [191]

FREDERICK C.S. WANG, MD
Associate Professor of Medicine, Harvard Medical School; Medical Director, Clinical Virology Laboratory, Brigham and Women's Hospital, Boston [161,167]

CARL V. WASHINGTON, JR., MD
Assistant Professor of Dermatology, Emory University School of Medicine; Director, Mohs Surgery Unit, The Emory Clinic, Atlanta [73]

ANTHONY P. WEETMAN, MD, DSc
Professor of Medicine and Dean, University of Sheffield Medical School; Consultant Physician, Northern General Hospital, Sheffield, UK [320]

STEVEN E. WEINBERGER, MD
Professor of Medicine, Harvard Medical School; Senior Vice President, Medical Knowledge and Education Division, American College of Physicians, Philadelphia [30, 233–235, 240]

ROBERT A. WEINSTEIN, MD
Professor of Medicine, Rush Medical College; Chair, Infectious Diseases, Cook County Hospital; Chief Operating Officer, The CORE Center, Chicago [116]

PETER F. WELLER, MD, FACP
Professor of Medicine, Harvard Medical School; Co-Chief, Infectious Diseases Division; Chief, Allergy and Inflammation Division; Senior Vice Chair of Research, Department of Medicine, Beth Israel Deaconess Medical Center, Boston [199–202, 204]

MICHAEL R. WESSELS, MD
Professor of Pediatrics and Medicine (Microbiology and Molecular Genetics), Harvard Medical School; Chief, Division of Infectious Diseases, Children's Hospital, Boston [121]

LEE M. WETZLER, MD
Associate Professor of Medicine and Microbiology, Boston University School of Medicine, Boston [127]

MEIR WETZLER, MD
Associate Professor of Medicine, Roswell Park Cancer Institute, Buffalo [96]

A. CLINTON WHITE, JR., MD
Professor, Infectious Diseases Section, Department of Medicine, Baylor College of Medicine, Houston [204]

NICHOLAS J. WHITE, MD, DSc
Professor of Tropical Medicine, Mahidol University, Bangkok, Thailand; and Oxford University, Oxford, UK [195]

RICHARD J. WHITLEY, MD
Loeb Eminent Scholar in Pediatrics; Professor of Pediatrics, Microbiology, Medicine, and Neurosurgery, University of Alabama at Birmingham, Birmingham [164]

GORDON H. WILLIAMS, MD
Professor of Medicine, Harvard Medical School; Chief, Cardiovascular Endocrinology Section, Brigham and Women's Hospital, Boston [230, 321]

JOHN W. WINKELMAN, MD, PhD
Assistant Professor of Psychiatry, Harvard Medical School; Medical Director, Sleep Health Center, Brigham and Women's Hospital, Boston [24]

BRUCE U. WINTROUB, MD
Professor and Chair of Dermatology, Associate Dean, School of Medicine, University of California San Francisco, San Francisco [50]

ALLAN W. WOLKOFF, MD
Professor of Medicine and Anatomy and Structural Biology, Albert Einstein College of Medicine, New York [284]

ROBERT L. WORTMANN, MD
Professor and Chair, Department of Internal Medicine, University of Oklahoma College of Medicine, Tulsa [338]

JOSHUA WYNNE, MD, MBA, MPH
Professor of Medicine, Wayne State University; Attending Physician, Detroit Medical Center, Detroit [221]

KIM B. YANCEY, MD
Professor and Chair, Department of Dermatology, Medical College of Wisconsin, Milwaukee [46, 49]

JAMES B. YOUNG, MD
Professor of Medicine, Executive Associate Dean for Faculty Affairs, Northwestern University Feinberg School of Medicine, Chicago [322]

NEAL S. YOUNG, MD
Chief, Hematology Branch, National Heart, Lung and Blood Institute, National Institutes of Health, Bethesda [94]

ROBERT C. YOUNG, MD
President, Fox Chase Cancer Center, Philadelphia [83]

ALAN S.L. YU, MD, BChir
Assistant Professor of Medicine, University of Southern California Keck School of Medicine, Los Angeles [266]

VICTOR L. YU, MD
Professor of Medicine, University of Pittsburgh; Chief, Infectious Disease Section, VA Medical Center, Pittsburgh [132]

DORI F. ZALEZNIK, MD
Associate Clinical Professor of Medicine, Harvard Medical School; Senior Physician, Beth Israel Deaconess Medical Center, Boston [112]

PETER J. ZIMETBAUM, MD
Assistant Professor of Medicine, Harvard Medical School; Beth Israel Deaconess Medical Center, Boston [213, 214]

The first edition of *Harrison's Principles of Internal Medicine* was published more than half a century ago. Over the decades, this textbook has evolved to reflect the continuing advances in the field of internal medicine and to meet the growing information base required of medical students and clinical practitioners. The users of this sixteenth edition of *Harrison's* will not even have to open the volume to see that it marks a transition point in the book's history. The new cover is only the most obvious indication of a new direction for *Harrison's*.

In shaping and revising this new version, the Editors have committed themselves to making the textbook as useful as possible to students and practitioners coping with the demands of modern medicine. The growth of evidence-based medicine, the prominence of managed care, and the explosion of information in fundamental areas such as the genetics of disease are only three of the many factors that make these demands different from those faced by physicians only a decade ago. Just as the cover retains key elements of the classic book, the content of the sixteenth edition retains the essential facts that remain clinically useful and important. However, through modifications in both its format and its content, the new *Harrison's* addresses the changing needs of its readers.

The sixteenth edition of *Harrison's* has a full-color format that facilitates quick reference and allows the inclusion of hundreds more high-quality illustrations than in previous editions. We expect that the reader's convenience will be well served by the placement of color illustrations within the chapters rather than in the separate color atlas used in earlier editions. While providing the basic-science information that is critical to an understanding of biology and pathophysiology, this edition focuses more directly and extensively than ever on crucial aspects of clinical practice. Areas of emphasis include the approach to the patient, differential diagnosis, state-of-the-art treatment options, and disease prevention. Key topics, such as the immune system and HIV infection/AIDS, are covered in chapters amounting to "mini-textbooks." New sections offer information on the formidable challenges posed by critical care medicine and by the threat of bioterrorism. New chapters provide coverage of highly relevant clinical topics such as disease screening, perimenopausal management and hormone replacement therapy, and end-of-life care. Virtually every chapter in this edition has been substantially rewritten, and 46 chapters either are entirely new or have new authors.

These are only highlights of the changes that the Editors hope will make the new *Harrison's* a helpful tool—not only for the student who needs an expert source of basic knowledge in internal medicine, but also for the pressured practitioner who needs a clear, concise, and balanced distillation of the best information on which to base daily clinical decisions.

Part One, "Introduction to Clinical Medicine," contains a new chapter that provides practical information about the screening approaches that every internist should consider for routine health maintenance. This chapter discusses the principles and guidelines used in screening for common conditions such as cancer, hypertension, lipid disorders, and osteoporosis. Another new chapter offers a pragmatic approach to the medical evaluation of patients who are about to undergo surgical procedures. In light of the growth of the hospice movement and the increased awareness of the sensitive issues—physical, mental, social, and existential—that surround end-of-life care, a new chapter on this complex topic provides insights, information, and guidance to practitioners dealing with dying patients and their families. The chapter on women's health has been entirely revised and offers a broad overview of the approach to disorders that affect women disproportionately.

Part Two, "Cardinal Manifestations and Presentation of Diseases,"

serves as a comprehensive introduction to clinical medicine as well as a practical guide to the care of patients with these manifestations. Each section focuses on a particular group of disorders, examining the concepts of pathophysiology and differential diagnosis that must be considered in caring for patients with these common clinical presentations. Major symptoms are reviewed and correlated with specific disease states, and clinical approaches to patients presenting with these symptoms are summarized. Every chapter has been updated, and three chapters have new authors. The chapter on sexual dysfunction now addresses disorders in both men and women.

Given the rapid advances in human genetics over the past several years, Part Three, "Genetics and Disease," has once again been completely updated. The material included in this edition is strongly geared toward clinical practice, in which genetic information increasingly comes into play. The new chapter on stem cell and gene transfer in clinical medicine addresses a timely and controversial topic, defining different types of stem cells and discussing their potential clinical applications.

Part Four, "Nutrition," covers nutritional considerations related to clinical medicine. Areas of focus include nutritional and dietary assessment, nutritional requirements, protein-energy malnutrition, eating disorders, obesity, and enteral and parenteral nutrition therapy.

The core of *Harrison's* continues to encompass the disorders of the organ systems and is contained in Parts Five through Sixteen. These sections include succinct accounts of the pathophysiology of diseases involving the major organ systems as well as infectious diseases, with an emphasis on clinical manifestations, diagnostic procedures, differential diagnosis, and treatment strategies and guidelines.

Part Five, "Oncology and Hematology," includes four chapters by new authors. An increasing proportion of patients who develop cancer are being cured. It is important to detect late consequences as early as possible in their natural history to optimize outcome. The chapter on the late consequences of cancer and its treatment helps physicians following such patients to know what to look for in addition to a recurrence of the cancer. Advances in the management of many cancers are highlighted—for example, the dramatic impact of imatinib mesylate (Gleevec) on chronic myeloid leukemia and gastrointestinal stromal cell tumors and the role of rituximab in the management of lymphoma and autoimmune diseases. The chapter delineating the principles of radiation therapy has been entirely rewritten by Eli Glatstein and is a companion piece to this author's chapter on radiation bioterrorism in Part Seven (see below). The hematology section features the World Health Organization's new classification of lymphoid and myeloid neoplasms. One of the most rapidly expanding areas of medicine is the development of novel agents to interfere with blood coagulation. With a new author who is an expert in this field, the chapter on anticoagulant, fibrinolytic, and antiplatelet therapy reviews all these new products and their indications.

Part Six, "Infectious Diseases," summarizes the latest information on pathology, genetics, and epidemiology while focusing sharply on the needs of clinicians who must accurately diagnose and treat infections under time pressure and cost constraints. In particular, the inclusion of dozens more illustrations in full color provides easily accessible information to assist clinicians with these challenges. Specific recommendations are provided for therapeutic regimens, including the drug of choice, dose, duration, and alternatives. Current trends in antimicrobial resistance are presented and considered in light of their impact on therapeutic choices. A new chapter offers key information on the management of the complex clinical issues raised by *Clostridium difficile*–associated disease, including pseudomembranous colitis. New authors cover the latest advances in the management of diseases caused by staphylococci and nontuberculous mycobacteria, viral gastroenteritis, and brucellosis. The superb chapter by Raphael Dolin on common viral respiratory infections has been expanded to include thorough coverage of severe acute respiratory syndrome (SARS). Now placed in a separate section with the overview of the human retroviruses, the chapter on HIV infection and AIDS by Anthony S. Fauci and H. Clifford Lane has been completely revised and updated, with an emphasis on therapeutic strategies. This chapter is widely considered to be a classic in the field; its clinically pragmatic focus in combination with its comprehensive and analytical approach to the pathogenesis of HIV disease has allowed its use as the sole complete reference on HIV/AIDS in medical schools.

In recent years, physicians have found themselves on the front line of response to bioterrorist attacks around the world. Since the attacks on the United States on September 11, 2001, and the subsequent anthrax attacks, the nation has been preparing for the further attacks that will inevitably come. Part Seven, "Bioterrorism and Clinical Medicine," consists of entirely new material written by authorities in three areas of bioterrorism: microbial, chemical, and radiation. Edited by *Harrison's* editor Anthony S. Fauci, these chapters are written succinctly and include easily readable charts, tables, and algorithms; their goal is to confer an understanding of the pathogenesis, diagnosis, treatment, and prognosis of the diseases in question.

Part Eight, "Disorders of the Cardiovascular System," is once again edited by the preeminent expert in the field, Eugene Braunwald. A new chapter covers the clinically important topics of unstable angina and non-ST-segment elevation myocardial infarction; three other chapters have new authors; and every chapter has been revised to reflect the latest trends and strategies for management. These include primary percutaneous coronary intervention for ST-segment elevation myocardial infarction as well as new drugs and devices for the treatment of heart failure.

Enormous strides have been made in the use of lung transplantation for selected patients with end-stage, irreversible, pulmonary parenchymal and vascular disease. Part Nine, "Disorders of the Respiratory System," includes a chapter by a new author that focuses on the selection of patients for this intervention. New authors have also taken on the broad topic of pneumonia and lung abscess, providing focus and a clinical perspective to help the reader grasp the central issues involved in the diagnosis and management of both community-acquired and nosocomial disease.

With advances in health care delivery and pressures aimed at cost containment, critical care units account for a growing percentage of hospital beds. Part Ten, "Critical Care Medicine," is a new section of *Harrison's* that is devoted to the provision of optimal care in this medical setting of growing importance. Incorporating both new chapters and refocused chapters on topics covered in previous editions, this part deals with three main areas: respiratory critical care, shock and cardiac arrest, and neurologic critical care. The approach to the patient and the central tenets underlying critical care are at the heart of this part of the sixteenth edition.

Part Eleven, "Disorders of the Kidney and Urinary Tract," includes contributions from several new authors and, as in previous editions, provides a thorough overview of the urinary-tract disorders encountered in internal medicine.

Part Twelve, "Disorders of the Gastrointestinal System," includes a new chapter on familial Mediterranean fever. The chapter on the approach to the patient with gastrointestinal disease has been completely reworked by a new author, as has the chapter on diverticular and vascular disease of the bowel. The chapters on the various categories of viral hepatitis have been extensively revised and updated to reflect breakthrough advances in treatment.

The first chapter in Part Thirteen, "Disorders of the Immune System, Connective Tissue, and Joints," provides an introduction to the immune system that has become a classic in its field and is often used as the textbook of immunology in postgraduate and medical school courses. This chapter combines an in-depth description and analysis of the principles of basic immunology with an easy flow into the application of these principles to clinical disease states. Its description of the relationship of innate to adaptive immunity is a model for understanding the intricacies of the human immune system. Once again, the authors have extensively revised this chapter to bring it up to date with regard to recent rapid advances in both basic and clinical immunology. In the section on disorders of immune-mediated injury, the spondyloarthropathies have been grouped together in one chapter that clearly and comprehensively discusses the similarities and dissimilarities among the various diseases in this category. The breakthrough advances in immunomodulatory therapy that have been realized in rheumatology over the past few years are captured in the spondyloarthropathy chapters and in the extensively revised chapters on rheumatoid arthritis and systemic lupus erythematosus. A new chapter covers fibromyalgia, arthritis associated with systemic disease, and other arthritides.

Part Fourteen, "Endocrinology and Metabolism," includes six chapters with new authors as well as a timely new chapter on the perimenopause transition and hormone replacement therapy. The writing of the latter chapter coincided with publication of results from the Women's Health Initiative that unexpectedly showed an increased risk of cardiovascular disease among women who received estrogen treatment. The author reviews the literature in this area and provides practical algorithms for the management of patients during this transition. The new authors of the chapter on disorders of sexual differentiation highlight novel insights derived from elucidation of the genetic basis of sex determination. The outstanding new review of bone and mineral metabolism lays a superb foundation for an understanding of the pathophysiology and treatment of various metabolic bone diseases. The newly authored version of the chapter on disorders of lipoprotein metabolism offers a much sharper focus on the classification, diagnosis, and treatment of disorders of cholesterol and triglyceride metabolism, emphasizing the use of statins for the reduction of cardiovascular risk. The new chapter on Wilson disease reports on the substantially modified treatment recommendations for this entity.

Part Fifteen, "Neurologic Disorders," has been extensively updated. A comprehensive new chapter on Alzheimer's disease and related dementias summarizes the recent explosion of knowledge on this topic, highlighting the new understanding of the genetics of these dementias and the molecules that trigger them as well as providing a clinical guide to diagnosis, differential diagnosis, and the latest treatments. The new chapter on Parkinson's disease reviews the recent genetic findings and provides an authoritative approach to therapy, including surgical options. The chapter on cerebrovascular diseases has been extensively rewritten, offering an evidence-based approach to the treatment and prevention of stroke, the third leading killer in the Western world. The updated chapter on multiple sclerosis presents the most recent advances in therapy and a practical approach to management of different stages of the disease. Finally, the recognition of bovine spongiform encephalopathy in many regions of the world has focused the global health care community on the biology and clinical manifestations of prion diseases; the sixteenth edition of *Harrison's* includes a comprehensive review of this subject by Nobel Laureate Stanley Prusiner.

Part Sixteen, "Poisoning, Drug Overdose, and Envenomation," has been thoroughly revised and streamlined to focus on the topics most relevant to internal medicine.

In view of the requirements for continuing education for licensure and relicensure as well as the emphasis on certification and recertification, a revision of the PreTest Self-Assessment and Review will again be published with this edition. This volume is in the capable hands of a new author, Dr. Charles Wiener from Johns Hopkins. It consists of several hundred questions based on the sixteenth edition of *Harrison's*, along with answers and explanations for the answers. The *Companion Handbook*, which was pioneered as a supplement to the eleventh edition of *Harrison's*, has been reworked as a concise quick-reference clinical manual; the *Manual of Medicine* will appear shortly after the publication of this edition, along with a PDA version, *Harrison's OnHand*. In 1998, *Harrison's* went online to provide a "living" textbook of internal medicine. In addition to permitting full search capabilities of the text, *Harrison's Online* offers frequent updates, reports of clinical trials, practice guidelines, online lectures, and concise reviews of timely topics as well as additional and updated references (with links to MEDLINE abstracts) and illustrations.

We wish to express our appreciation to our many associates and colleagues, who, as experts in their fields, have offered us constructive criticism and helpful suggestions. We acknowledge especially the contributions of the following individuals: Joseph Alpert, Michael Bray, Mark D. Carlson, Daniel H. Lowenstein, Lawrence C. Madoff, Thomas R. Martin, Chung Owyang, Alice Pau, and Mary Wright.

We thank in particular Kenneth and Elaine Kaye and Lindsey Baden, who gathered many high-quality illustrations of infectious disease manifestations. We also express our gratitude to Eileen J. Scott, who has applied her editorial expertise to the past six editions of *Harrison's*, and Marsha Cohen, who has been the text and cover designer for the past five editions.

This book could not have been edited without the dedicated help of our co-workers in the editorial offices of the individual editors. We are especially indebted to Patricia L. Duffey, Gregory K. Folkers, Sarah Matero, Julie B. McCoy, Jaylyn Olivo, Elizabeth Robbins, Leslie Runnels, Kathryn Saxon, Marie Scurti, and Sue Anne Tae.

Finally, we continue to be highly indebted to three outstanding members of the McGraw-Hill organization: Mariapaz Ramos Englis, Senior Managing Editor; Robert Laffler, Production Director; and Martin J. Wonsiewicz, Publisher. They are an effective team who have given the Editors constant encouragement and sage advice. They have been instrumental in guiding the many changes instituted with this edition of *Harrison's* and in bringing this volume to fruition in a timely manner.

THE EDITORS

1 THE PRACTICE OF MEDICINE
The Editors

WHAT IS EXPECTED OF THE PHYSICIAN The accelerating pace of change in medicine stems from an explosion of scientific information and the need to blend this information into the art and practice of medicine.

The role of *science in medicine* is clear. Science-based technology and deductive reasoning form the foundation for the solution to many clinical problems. Spectacular advances in genetics, biochemistry, and imaging techniques allow access to the innermost parts of the cell and the most remote recesses of the body. Revelations about the nature of genes and single cells have opened the portal for formulating a new molecular basis for the physiology of systems. These physiologic insights will undoubtedly result in a better understanding of complex disease processes and new approaches to disease treatment and prevention. Highly advanced therapeutic maneuvers are increasingly a major part of medical practice. Yet skill in the most sophisticated application of laboratory technology and in the use of the latest therapeutic modality alone does not make a good physician.

The editors of the first edition of this book articulated well the responsibility of the physician in interacting with the patient:

> *No greater opportunity, responsibility, or obligation can fall to the lot of a human being than to become a physician. In the care of the suffering, [the physician] needs technical skill, scientific knowledge, and human understanding. . . . Tact, sympathy, and understanding are expected of the physician, for the patient is no mere collection of symptoms, signs, disordered functions, damaged organs, and disturbed emotions. [The patient] is human, fearful, and hopeful, seeking relief, help, and reassurance.*

When a patient poses challenging clinical problems, an effective physician must be able to identify the crucial elements in a complex history and physical examination and to extract the key laboratory results from the crowded computer printouts of data in order to determine whether to "treat" or to "watch." Deciding whether a clinical clue is worth pursuing or should be dismissed as a "red herring" and weighing whether a proposed treatment entails a greater risk than the disease itself are essential judgments that the skilled clinician must make many times each day. This combination of medical knowledge, intuition, experience, and judgment defines the *art of medicine*, which is as necessary to the practice of medicine as is a sound scientific base.

THE PATIENT-PHYSICIAN RELATIONSHIP: A HUMANE APPROACH IN THE FACE OF CHANGE In this era of "techno-medicine," physicians need to approach patients not as "cases" or "diseases" but as individuals whose problems all too often transcend their physical complaints. Most patients are anxious and fearful. Physicians should instill confidence and should be reassuring (as depicted humorously in Fig. 1-1) but should never be arrogant. A professional attitude, coupled with warmth and openness, can do much to alleviate anxiety and to encourage patients to share all aspects of their medical history. Whatever the patient's attitude, the physician needs to consider the setting in which an illness occurs—in terms not only of the patients themselves but also of their familial, social, and cultural backgrounds. The ideal patient-physician relationship is based on thorough knowledge of the patient, on mutual trust, and on the ability to communicate.

Technological Complexity and Managed Care The one-to-one patient-physician relationship, which has traditionally characterized the practice of medicine, is increasingly in jeopardy because of the growing complexity of medicine and the changes in health care delivery systems. Often the management of an individual patient is a team effort involving a number of physicians and other professional personnel. Increasingly, hospitalists assume the responsibility for patient management in the inpatient setting. The patient can benefit greatly from effective collaboration among health care professionals, but *it is the duty of the patient's principal physician to provide guidance through an illness*. To carry out this difficult task, this physician must be familiar with the techniques, skills, and objectives of specialist physicians and of colleagues in the fields allied to medicine. In giving the patient an opportunity to benefit from scientific advances, the primary physician must retain responsibility for the major decisions concerning diagnosis and treatment.

The practice of medicine in a managed-care setting puts additional stress on the patient-physician relationship. Whatever the potential advantages of organized medical groups such as health maintenance organizations (HMOs), there are also drawbacks, including the loss of the clear identification of the physician who is primarily and continuously responsible for the patient. Even under these circumstances, it is essential for each patient to have a physician who has an overview of the problems and who is familiar with the patient's reaction to the illness, the drugs the patient is given, and the challenges the patient faces. Moreover, in managed-care settings, many physicians must treat patients within a restricted time frame, with limited access to specialists, and under organizational guidelines that may compromise their ability to exercise their individual clinical judgment. As difficult as these restrictions may be, it is the ultimate responsibility of the physician, in close consultation with the patient, to determine what is best for the patient. This responsibility cannot be relinquished in the name of compliance with organizational guidelines.

The Modern Hospital Environment The physician must be aware that the hospital is an intimidating environment for most individuals. Hospitalized patients find themselves surrounded by air jets, buttons, and lights; invaded by tubes and wires; and beset by the numerous members of the health care team—nurses, nurses' aides, physicians' assistants, social workers, technologists, physical therapists, medical students, house officers, attending and consulting physicians, and many others. They may be transported to special laboratories and imaging facilities replete with blinking lights, strange sounds, and unfamiliar personnel; they may be obliged to share a room with other patients who have their own health problems. It is little wonder that

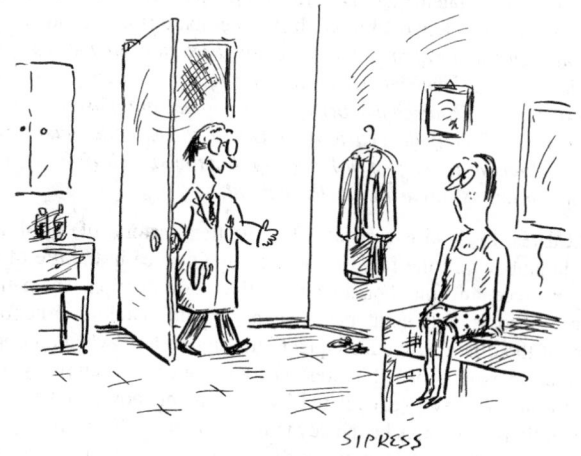

SIPRESS

"Let the healing begin!"

FIGURE 1-1 Although physicians must be confident and reassuring, it may be possible to go too far. (*The New Yorker Collection 2000, David Sipress, from cartoonbank.com. All Rights Reserved.*)

patients may lose their sense of reality. A strong personal relationship with the physician helps to sustain the patient in such a stressful situation.

Societal Trends   Many trends in contemporary society tend to make medical care impersonal. These trends, some of which have been mentioned already, include (1) vigorous efforts to reduce the escalating costs of health care; (2) the growing number of managed-care programs, which are intended to reduce costs but in which the patient may have little choice in selecting a physician or in seeing that physician consistently; (3) increasing reliance on technological advances and computerization for many aspects of diagnosis and treatment; (4) increased geographic mobility of both patients and physicians; (5) the need for numerous physicians to be involved in the care of most patients who are seriously ill; and (6) an increasing tendency on the part of patients to express their frustrations with the health care system through malpractice suits.

Given these changes in the medical care system, it is a major challenge for physicians to maintain the *humane* aspects of medical care. The American Board of Internal Medicine, working together with the American College of Physicians–American Society of Internal Medicine and the European Federation of Internal Medicine, has published a *Charter on Medical Professionalism* that underscores three main principles in physicians' contract with society: (1) the primacy of patient welfare, (2) patient autonomy, and (3) social justice. The humanistic qualities of a physician must encompass integrity, respect, and compassion. Availability, the expression of sincere concern, the willingness to take the time to explain all aspects of the illness, and a nonjudgmental attitude when dealing with patients whose cultures, lifestyles, attitudes, and values differ from those of the physician are just a few of the characteristics of the humane physician. Every physician will, at times, be challenged by patients who evoke strongly negative or positive emotional responses. Physicians should be alert to their own reactions to such patients and situations and should consciously monitor and control their behavior so that the patient's best interest remains the principal motivation for their actions at all times.

An important aspect of patient care involves an appreciation of the "quality of life," a subjective assessment of what each patient values most. Such an assessment requires detailed, sometimes intimate knowledge of the patient, which can usually be obtained only through deliberate, unhurried, and often repeated conversations. It is in these situations that the time constraints of a managed-care setting may prove particularly problematic. Time pressures will always threaten these interactions but do not diminish the importance of understanding patients' priorities from their point of view.

The famous statement of Dr. Francis Peabody is even more relevant today than when delivered more than three-quarters of a century ago:

> *The significance of the intimate personal relationship between physician and patient cannot be too strongly emphasized, for in an extraordinarily large number of cases both the diagnosis and treatment are directly dependent on it. One of the essential qualities of the clinician is interest in humanity,* **for the secret of the care of the patient is in caring for the patient**.

CLINICAL SKILLS ■ History-Taking   The written history of an illness should embody all the facts of medical significance in the life of the patient. Recent events should be given the most attention. The patient should, at some early point, have the opportunity to tell his or her own story of the illness without frequent interruption and, when appropriate, receive expressions of interest, encouragement, and empathy from the physician. Any event related by the patient, however trivial or apparently remote, may be the key to the solution of the medical problem. In general, only patients who feel comfortable will provide the physician with complete information.

An informative history is more than an orderly listing of symptoms; something is always gained by listening to patients and noting the way in which they describe their symptoms. Inflections of voice, facial expression, gestures, and attitude may reveal important clues to the meaning of the symptoms to the patient. Because patients vary in their medical sophistication and ability to recall facts, the reported medical history should be corroborated whenever possible. The family and social history can also provide important insights into the types of diseases that should be considered. In listening to the history, the physician discovers not only something about the disease but also something about the patient. The process of history-taking provides an opportunity to observe the patient's behavior and to watch for features to be pursued more thoroughly during the physical examination.

The very act of eliciting the history provides the physician with the opportunity to establish or enhance the unique bond that is the basis for the ideal patient-physician relationship. It is helpful to develop an appreciation of the patient's perception of the illness, the patient's expectations of the physician and the medical care system, and the financial and social implications of the illness to the patient. The confidentiality of the patient-physician relationship should be emphasized, and the patient should be given the opportunity to identify any aspects of the history that should not be disclosed to others.

Physical Examination   Physical signs are objective indications of disease whose significance is enhanced when they confirm a functional or structural change already suggested by the patient's history. At times, however, the physical signs may be the only evidence of disease.

The physical examination should be performed methodically and thoroughly, with consideration for the patient's comfort and modesty. Although attention is often directed by the history to the diseased organ or part of the body, the examination of a new patient must extend from head to toe in an objective search for abnormalities. Unless the physical examination is systematic, important segments may be omitted. The results of the examination, like the details of the history, should be recorded at the time they are elicited, not hours later when they are subject to the distortions of memory. Skill in physical diagnosis is acquired with experience, but it is not merely technique that determines success in eliciting signs. The detection of a few scattered petechiae, a faint diastolic murmur, or a small mass in the abdomen is not a question of keener eyes and ears or more sensitive fingers but of a mind alert to these findings. Since physical findings are subject to changes, the physical examination should be repeated as frequently as the clinical situation warrants.

Laboratory Tests and Imaging Studies   The availability of a wide array of laboratory tests has increased our reliance on these studies for the solution of clinical problems. The accumulation of laboratory data does not relieve the physician from the responsibility of careful observation, examination, and study of the patient. It is also essential to bear in mind the limitations of such tests. By virtue of their impersonal quality, complexity, and apparent precision, they often gain an aura of authority regardless of the fallibility of the tests themselves, the instruments used in the tests, and the individuals performing or interpreting them. Physicians must weigh the expense involved in the laboratory procedures they order relative to the value of the information they are likely to provide.

Single laboratory tests are rarely ordered. Rather, physicians generally request "batteries" of multiple tests, which are often useful. For example, abnormalities of hepatic function may provide the clue to such nonspecific symptoms as generalized weakness and increased fatigability, suggesting the diagnosis of chronic liver disease. Sometimes a single abnormality, such as an elevated serum calcium level, points to particular diseases, such as hyperparathyroidism or underlying malignancy.

The thoughtful use of screening tests should not be confused with indiscriminate laboratory testing. The use of screening tests is based on the fact that a group of laboratory determinations can be carried out conveniently on a single specimen at relatively low cost. Screening tests are most useful when they are directed toward common diseases or disorders and when their results indicate other useful tests or interventions that may be costly to perform. Biochemical measurements, together with simple laboratory examinations such as blood count, urinalysis, and sedimentation rate, often provide the major clue to the presence of a pathologic process. At the same time, the physician must learn to evaluate occasional abnormalities among the screening tests that may not necessarily connote significant disease. An in-depth workup following a report of an isolated laboratory abnormality in a person who is otherwise well is almost invariably wasteful and unproductive. Among the more than 40 tests that are routinely performed, one or two are often slightly abnormal. If there is no suspicion of an underlying illness, these tests are ordinarily repeated to ensure that the abnormality does not represent a laboratory error. If an abnormality is confirmed, it is important to consider its potential significance in the context of the patient's condition and other test results.

The technical capability of imaging studies is one of the most rapidly advancing areas of medicine. These tests provide remarkably detailed anatomical information that can be a pivotal factor in medical decision-making. Ultrasonography, a variety of isotopic scans, computed tomography, magnetic resonance imaging, and positron emission tomography have benefited patients by opening new diagnostic vistas and by largely supplanting older, more invasive approaches. In our effort to make diagnoses quickly, it is tempting to order a battery of imaging studies. All physicians have had cases in which imaging studies turned up findings leading to an unexpected diagnosis. Nonetheless, patients must endure each of these tests, and the added cost of unnecessary testing is substantial. A skilled physician must learn to use these powerful diagnostic tools judiciously, always asking whether the results will alter management and benefit the patient.

PRINCIPLES OF PATIENT CARE ■ Evidence-Based Medicine

Sackett has defined evidence-based medicine as "the conscientious, explicit and judicious use of current best evidence in making decisions about the care of individual patients." Rigorously obtained evidence is contrasted with anecdotal experience, which is often biased. Even the most experienced physicians can be influenced by recent experiences with selected patients, unless they are attuned to the importance of using larger, more objective studies for making decisions. The prospectively designed, double-blind, randomized clinical trial represents the "gold standard" for providing evidence regarding therapeutic decisions. →*For a more complete discussion of evidence-based medicine, see Chap. 2.*

Practice Guidelines

The intelligent and cost-effective practice of medicine consists of making diagnostic and therapeutic choices that are most appropriate to a particular patient and clinical situation. Professional organizations and government agencies are developing formal clinical-practice guidelines in an effort to aid physicians and other caregivers in this endeavor. As the evidence base of medicine increases, guidelines can provide a useful framework for managing patients with particular diagnoses or symptoms. They can protect patients—particularly those with inadequate health care benefits—from receiving substandard care. Guidelines can also protect conscientious caregivers from inappropriate charges of malpractice and society from the excessive costs associated with the overuse of medical resources. On the other hand, clinical guidelines tend to oversimplify the complexities of medicine. Groups with differing perspectives may develop divergent recommendations regarding issues as basic as the need for periodic sigmoidoscopy in middle-aged persons. Furthermore, guidelines do not—and cannot be expected to—take into account the uniqueness of each individual and of his or her illness. The challenge for the physician is to integrate into clinical practice the useful recommendations offered by the experts who prepare clinical practice guidelines without accepting them blindly or being inappropriately constrained by them.

Medical Decision-Making

Medical decision-making occurs throughout the diagnostic and treatment process. It involves the ordering of additional tests, requests for consults, and decisions regarding prognosis and treatment. This process requires an in-depth understanding of the pathophysiology and natural history of disease. It is for this reason that these topics are strongly emphasized in this textbook. As described above, medical decision-making should be evidence-based so that patients derive the full benefit of the scientific knowledge available to physicians. Formulating a differential diagnosis requires not only a broad knowledge base but also the ability to assess the relative probabilities of various diseases and to understand the significance of missing diagnoses that may be less likely. Arriving at a diagnosis requires the application of the scientific method. Hypotheses are formed, data are collected, and objective conclusions are reached concerning whether to accept or reject a particular diagnosis. Analysis of the differential diagnosis is an iterative process. As new information or test results are acquired, the group of disease processes being considered can be contracted or expanded appropriately.

Despite the importance of evidence-based medicine, much of medical decision-making relies on judgment—a process that is difficult to quantify or even to assess qualitatively. Especially when a relevant evidence base is unavailable, physicians must use their knowledge and experience as a basis for weighing known factors along with the inevitable uncertainties and then making a sound judgment. Several quantitative tools may be invaluable in synthesizing the available information, including diagnostic tests, Bayes' theorem, and multivariate statistical models. *Diagnostic tests* serve to reduce uncertainty about a diagnosis or prognosis in a particular individual and to help the physician decide how best to manage that individual's condition. Not only laboratory tests and procedures but also the history and the physical examination can be considered part of the battery of diagnostic tests. The accuracy of a given test is ascertained by determining its sensitivity (true positive rate) and specificity (true negative rate) as well as the predictive value of a positive and negative result. *Bayes' theorem* uses information on a test's sensitivity and specificity, in conjunction with the pretest probability of a diagnosis, to determine mathematically the posttest probability of the diagnosis. More complex clinical problems can be approached with *multivariate statistical models*, which generate highly accurate information even when multiple factors are acting individually or together to affect disease risk, progression, or response to treatment. Studies comparing the performance of statistical models with that of expert clinicians have documented equivalent accuracy, although the models tend to be more consistent. Thus multivariate statistical models may be particularly helpful to less experienced clinicians.

Information technology is playing an ever-increasing role in medicine. Laboratory data are accessed almost universally through computers. Many medical centers now have electronic medical records, computerized order entry, and bar-coded tracking of medications. Some of these systems are interactive and provide reminders or warn of potential medical errors. Nonetheless, at this point, clinical decisions are still best made by the physician. Many decisions are not easily compacted into practice guidelines or computerized approaches. Clinical knowledge and an understanding of the patient's needs, supplemented by quantitative tools, still seem to represent the best approach to practicing medicine.

Assessing the Outcome of Treatment

Clinicians generally use *objective* and readily measurable parameters to judge the outcome of a therapeutic intervention. For example, findings on physical or laboratory examination—such as the level of blood pressure, the patency of a coronary artery on an angiogram, or the size of a mass on a radiologic examination—can provide information of critical importance. However, patients usually seek medical attention for *subjective* reasons; they wish to obtain relief from pain, to preserve or regain function, and to enjoy life. The components of a patient's health status or quality of life can include bodily comfort, capacity for physical activity, personal and professional function, sexual function, cognitive function, and overall perception of health. Each of these important areas can be assessed by means of structured interviews or specially designed questionnaires. Such assessments also provide useful parameters by which the physician can judge the patient's subjective view of his or her disability and the response to treatment, particularly in chronic illness.

The practice of medicine requires consideration and integration of both objective and subjective outcomes.

Care of the Elderly   Over the next several decades, the practice of medicine will be greatly influenced by the health care needs of the growing elderly population. In the United States the population over age 65 will almost triple over the next 30 years. The physician must understand and appreciate the decline in physiologic reserve associated with aging; the different responses of the elderly to common diseases; and disorders that occur commonly with aging, such as depression, dementia, frailty, urinary incontinence, and fractures. →*For a more complete discussion of medical care for the elderly, see Chap. 8.*

Diseases in Women versus Men   In the past, many epidemiologic studies and clinical trials focused on men. More recently, studies have included representative numbers of women, and some, like the Women's Health Initiative, have specifically addressed women's health issues. Significant sex differences exist in diseases that afflict both men and women. Ongoing study should enhance our understanding of the mechanisms of sex differences in the course and outcome of certain diseases. →*For a more complete discussion of women's health, see Chap. 5.*

Medical Errors   A report from the Institute of Medicine concluded that "to err is human" but called for an ambitious agenda to reduce medical-error rates and improve patient safety by designing and implementing fundamental changes in health care systems. Adverse drug reactions occur in at least 5% of hospitalized patients, and the incidence increases with use of a large number of drugs. No matter what the clinical situation, it is the responsibility of the physician to use powerful therapeutic measures wisely, with due regard for their beneficial action, potential dangers, and cost. It is also the responsibility of hospitals and health care organizations to develop systems to reduce risk and ensure patient safety. Medication errors can be reduced through the use of ordering systems that eliminate misreading of handwriting and through vigilance regarding dilution errors. Implementation of infection-control systems, enforcement of hand-washing protocols, and careful oversight of antibiotic use can minimize complications of nosocomial infections. The harm that a physician can do is not limited to the imprudent use of medication or procedures. Equally important are ill-considered or unjustified remarks. Many a patient has developed a cardiac neurosis because the physician ventured a grave prognosis on the basis of a misinterpreted finding of a heart murmur.

Informed Consent and Respect for the Patient's Autonomy   The fundamental principles of medical ethics are to act in the patient's best interest and to respect the patient's autonomy. Most patients possess only limited medical knowledge and must rely on their physicians for advice. Confusion or even disagreement about approaches to disease management may arise (see also "Medicine on the Internet," below), and—in the end—the patient's informed choices must prevail. Physicians must respect their patients' autonomy, fully discussing the alternatives for care and the risks, benefits, and likely consequences of each alternative.

When patients require diagnostic and therapeutic procedures that are painful and that pose some risk, they are generally required to sign a consent form. In such cases, it is particularly important for the patient to understand clearly the risks entailed in these procedures; this is the definition of *informed consent*. It is incumbent on the physician to explain the procedures in a clear and understandable manner and to ascertain that the patient comprehends both the nature of the procedure and the attendant risks. The dread of the unknown that is inherent in hospitalization can be mitigated by such explanations.

Incurable Disorders and Death   No problem is more distressing than that presented by the patient with an incurable disease, particularly when premature death is inevitable. What should the patient and family be told? What measures should be taken to maintain life? What can be done to maintain the quality of life? How is death to be defined?

Although some would argue otherwise, there is no ironclad rule that the patient must immediately be told "everything," even if the patient is an adult with substantial family responsibilities. How much is told should depend on the individual's ability to deal with the possibility of imminent death; often this capacity grows with time, and, whenever possible, gradual rather than abrupt disclosure is the best strategy. A wise and insightful physician is often guided by an understanding of what a patient wants to know and when he or she wants to know it. The patient's religious beliefs may also be taken into consideration. The patient must be given an opportunity to talk with the physician and ask questions. Patients may find it easier to share their feelings about death with their physician, who is likely to be more objective and less emotional, than with family members. As William Osler wrote: "One thing is certain; it is not for you to don the black cap and, assuming the judicial function, take hope away from any patient." Even when the patient directly inquires, "Am I dying?" the physician must attempt to determine whether this is a request for information or a demand for reassurance. Only open communication between the patient and the physician can resolve this question and guide the physician in what to say and how to say it.

The physician should provide or arrange for emotional, physical, and spiritual support and must be compassionate, unhurried, and open. There is much to be gained by the laying on of hands. Pain should be adequately controlled, human dignity maintained, and isolation from the family avoided. These aspects of care tend to be overlooked in hospitals, where the intrusion of life-sustaining apparatus can so easily detract from attention to the whole person and encourage concentration instead on the life-threatening disease, against which the battle will ultimately be lost in any case. In the face of terminal illness, the goal of medicine must shift from *cure* to *care*, in the broadest sense of the term. In offering care to the dying patient, the physician must be prepared to provide information to family members and to deal with their guilt and grief. It is important for the doctor to assure the family that everything possible has been done. →*For a more complete discussion of end-of-life care, see Chap. 9.*

THE EXPANDING ROLE OF THE PHYSICIAN ■ **Genetics and Medicine**   The genomic era is leading to a revolution in the practice of medicine. The sequencing of the entire human genome has set researchers on the path to elucidating the genetic components of common chronic diseases—hypertension, diabetes, atherosclerosis, many cancers, autoimmune disorders, dementias, and behavioral disorders. Forthcoming information should make it possible to determine individual susceptibility to these conditions early in life and to implement individualized prevention programs. Subclassification of many diseases on a genetic basis may allow the selection of appropriate therapy for each patient. As the response to drugs becomes more predictable, pharmacotherapy should become more rational.

Patients will be best served if physicians play an active role in applying this powerful, sensitive new information rather than being passive bystanders who are intimidated by the new technology. This is a rapidly evolving field, and physicians and other health care professionals must continue to educate themselves so that they can apply this new knowledge to the benefit of their patients' health and well-being. Genetic testing requires wise counsel based on an understanding of the value and limitations of the tests as well as the implications of their results for specific individuals. →*For a more complete discussion of the use of genetic testing, see Chap. 58.*

Medicine on the Internet   The explosion in use of the Internet through personal computers is having an important influence on health care. The Internet makes a wide range of information available to physicians and patients almost instantaneously at any time of the day or night and from anywhere in the world. This medium holds enormous potential for delivering up-to-date information, practice guidelines, state-of-the-art conferences, journal contents, textbooks (including this text), and direct communications with other physicians and specialists, thereby expanding the depth and breadth of information available to the physician about the diagnosis and care of patients. Most medical journals are now accessible online, providing rapid and comprehensive sources of information.

Patients, too, are turning to the Internet in increasing numbers to derive information about their illnesses and therapies and to join Internet-based support groups. Physicians are increasingly challenged by dealing with patients who arrive with sophisticated information about their illness. It is difficult, however, for patients to put this sometimes-alarming information into context, and the physician plays an invaluable role by encouraging patient education but helping the patient to assimilate new information and apply it to a particular circumstance.

A critically important caveat is that virtually anything can be published on the Internet, with easy circumvention of the peer-review process that is an essential feature of quality publications. Physicians or patients who search the Internet for medical information must be aware of this danger. Notwithstanding this limitation, appropriate use of the Internet is revolutionizing information access for physicians and patients and is a positive force in the practice of medicine.

Delivering Cost-Effective Medical Care   As the cost of medical care has risen, it has become necessary to establish priorities in the expenditure of resources. In some instances, preventive measures offer the greatest return for the expenditure; outstanding examples include vaccination, improved sanitation, reduction in accidents and occupational hazards, and biochemical- and DNA-based screening of newborns. As one more specific example, the detection of phenylketonuria by newborn screening may result in a net saving of many thousands of dollars.

As resources become increasingly constrained, society must weigh the benefits of performing costly procedures that provide only a limited increase in life expectancy against the pressing need for more primary care for those persons who do not have adequate access to medical services. For the individual patient, it is important to reduce costly hospital admissions as much as possible if total health care is to be affordable. This policy, of course, depends on close cooperation among patients, their physicians, employers, payers, and government. It is equally important for physicians to know the cost of the diagnostic procedures they order and the drugs and other therapies they prescribe and to monitor both costs and effectiveness. The medical profession should provide leadership and guidance to the public in matters of cost control, and physicians must take this responsibility seriously without being or seeming to be self-serving. However, the economic aspects of health care delivery must not interfere with the welfare of patients. The patient must be able to rely on the individual physician as his or her principal advocate in matters of health care.

Accountability   As the public has become more educated and more sophisticated regarding health-related issues, expectations of the health care system in general and of physicians in particular have risen. Physicians are expected to maintain mastery of rapidly advancing fields (the *science* of medicine) while considering their patients' unique needs (the *art* of medicine). Thus, physicians are held accountable not only for the technical aspects of the care that they provide but also for their patients' satisfaction with the delivery and costs of care.

In the United States, there are increasing demands for physicians to account for the way in which they practice medicine by meeting certain standards prescribed by federal and state governments. The hospitalization of patients whose health care costs are reimbursed by the government and other third parties is subjected to utilization review. Thus the physician must defend the cause for and duration of a patient's hospitalization if it falls outside certain "average" standards. Authorization for reimbursement is increasingly based on documentation of the nature and complexity of an illness, as reflected by recorded elements of the history and physical examination. The purpose of these regulations is both to improve standards of health care and to contain spiraling health care costs. This type of review is being extended to all phases of medical practice and is profoundly altering the practice of medicine. Physicians are also expected to give evidence of their continuing competence through mandatory continuing education, patient-record audits, recertification by examination, or relicensing.

Continued Learning   The conscientious physician must be a perpetual student because the body of medical knowledge is constantly expanding and being refined. The profession of medicine should be inherently linked to a career-long thirst for new information that can be used for the good of the patient. It is the responsibility of a physician to pursue new knowledge continually by reading, attending conferences and courses, and consulting colleagues and the Internet. This is often a difficult task for a busy practitioner; however, such a commitment to continued learning is an integral part of being a physician and must be given the highest priority.

Research and Teaching   The title *doctor* is derived from the Latin *docere*, "to teach," and physicians should share information and medical knowledge with colleagues, with students of medicine and related professions, and with their patients (Fig. 1-2). The practice of medicine is dependent on the sum total of medical knowledge, which in turn is based on an unending chain of scientific discovery, clinical observation, analysis, and interpretation. Advances in medicine depend on the acquisition of new information, i.e., on research, which often involves patients; improved medical care requires the transmission of this information. As part of broader societal responsibilities, the physician should encourage patients to participate in ethical and properly approved clinical investigations if they do not impose undue hazard, discomfort, or inconvenience. On the other hand, physicians engaged in clinical research must be alert to potential conflicts of interest between their research goals and their obligations to individual patients; the best interests of the patient must always take priority. To quote William Osler:

To wrest from nature the secrets which have perplexed philosophers in all ages, to track to their sources the causes of disease, to correlate the vast stores of knowledge, that they may be quickly

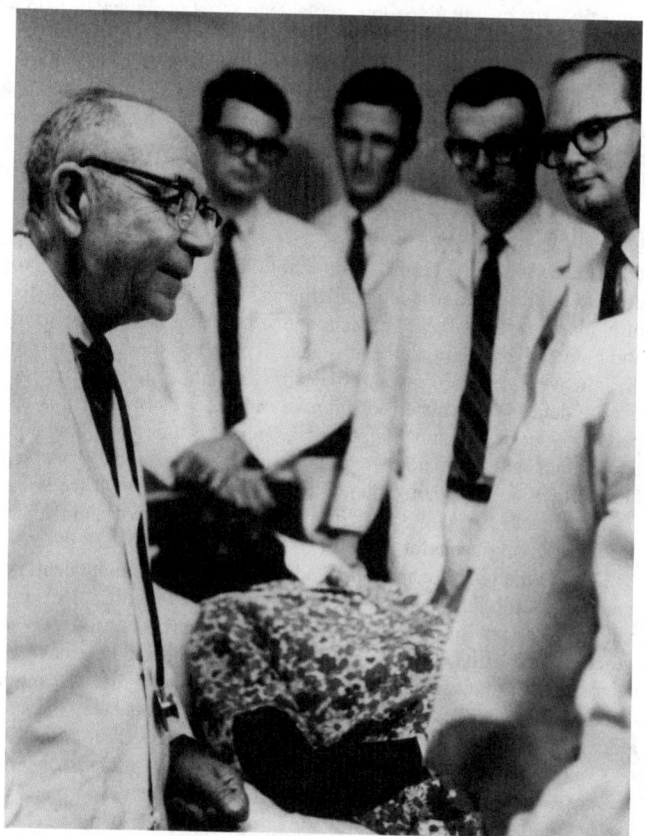

FIGURE 1-2   Dr. Tinsley R. Harrison instructing students at a patient's bedside. Dr. Harrison was the editor-in-chief of the first five editions of this textbook. (*Photo reprinted with permission from the UAB Archives, University of Alabama at Birmingham.*)

available for the prevention and cure of disease—these are our ambitions.

FURTHER READING

COLLINS FS: Shattuck Lecture: Medical and societal consequences of the Human Genome Project. N Engl J Med 341:28, 1999

COUNCIL ON GRADUATE MEDICAL EDUCATION: *Thirteenth Report: Physi-cian Education for a Changing Health Care Environment.* US Department of Health and Human Services, March 1999

LUDMERER KM: *Time to Heal: American Medical Education from the Turn of the Century to the Era of Managed Care.* New York, Oxford, 1999

PROJECT OF THE ABIM FOUNDATION, ACP-ASIM FOUNDATION, AND EUROPEAN FEDERATION OF INTERNAL MEDICINE: Medical professionalism in the new millennium: A physician charter. Ann Intern Med 136:243, 2002

SACKETT DL et al: *Evidence Based Medicine: How to Practise and Teach EBM.* London, Churchill Livingstone, 1997

2 DECISION-MAKING IN CLINICAL MEDICINE
Daniel B. Mark

To the medical student who requires 2 h to collect a patient's history and perform a physical examination, and several additional hours to organize them into a coherent presentation, the experienced clinician's ability to reach a diagnosis and decide on a management plan in a fraction of the time seems extraordinary. While medical knowledge and experience play a significant role in the senior clinician's ability to arrive at a differential diagnosis and plan quickly, much of the process involves skill in clinical decision-making. The first goal of this chapter is to provide an introduction to the study of clinical reasoning.

Equally bewildering to the student are the proper use of diagnostic tests and the integration of the results into the clinical assessment. The novice medical practitioner typically uses a "shotgun" approach to testing, hoping to a hit a target without knowing exactly what that target is. The expert, on the other hand, usually has a specific target in mind and efficiently adjusts the testing strategy to it. The second goal of this chapter is to review briefly some of the crucial basic statistical concepts that govern the proper interpretation and use of diagnostic tests; quantitative tools available to assist in clinical decision-making will also be discussed.

Evidence-based medicine is the term used to describe the integration of the best available research evidence with clinical judgment and experience in the care of patients. The third goal of this chapter is to provide a brief overview of some of the tools of evidence-based medicine.

CLINICAL DECISION-MAKING

CLINICAL REASONING The most important clinical actions are not procedures or prescriptions but the judgments from which all other aspects of clinical medicine flow. In the modern era of large randomized trials and evidence-based medicine, it is easy to overlook the importance of this elusive mental activity and focus instead on the algorithmic practice guidelines constructed to improve care. One reason for this apparent neglect is that much more research has been done on how doctors *should* make decisions (e.g., using a Bayesian model discussed below) than on how they actually *do*. Thus, much of what we know about clinical reasoning comes from empirical studies of nonmedical problem-solving behavior.

Despite the great technological advances of the twentieth century, uncertainty still plays a pivotal role in all aspects of medical decision-making. We may know that a patient does not have long to live, but we cannot be certain how long. We may prescribe a potent new receptor blocker to reverse the course of a patient's illness, but we cannot be certain that the therapy will achieve the desired result and that result alone. Uncertainty in medical outcomes creates the need for probabilities and other mathematical/statistical tools to help guide decision-making. (These tools are reviewed later in the chapter.)

Uncertainty is compounded by the information overload that characterizes modern medicine. Today's experienced clinician needs close to 2 million pieces of information to practice medicine. Doctors subscribe to an average of 7 journals, representing over 2500 new articles each year. Computers offer the obvious solution both for management of information and for better quantitation and management of the daily uncertainties of medical care. While the technology to computerize medical practice is available, many practical problems remain to be solved before patient information can be standardized and integrated with medical evidence on a single electronic platform.

The following three examples introduce the subject of clinical reasoning:

- A 46-year-old man presents to his internist with a chief complaint of hemoptysis. The physician knows that the differential diagnosis of hemoptysis includes over 100 different conditions, including cancer and tuberculosis (Chap. 30). The examination begins with some general background questions, and the patient is asked to describe his symptoms and their chronology. By the time the examination is completed, and even before any tests are run, the physician has formulated a working diagnostic hypothesis and planned a series of steps to test it. In an otherwise healthy and nonsmoking patient recovering from a viral bronchitis, the doctor's hypothesis would be that the acute bronchitis is responsible for the small amount of blood-streaked sputum the patient observed. In this case, a chest x-ray may provide sufficient reassurance that a more serious disorder is not present.

- A second 46-year-old patient with the same chief complaint who has a 100-pack-year smoking history, a productive morning cough, and episodes of blood-streaked sputum may generate the principal diagnostic hypothesis of carcinoma of the lung. Consequently, along with the chest x-ray, the physician obtains a sputum cytology examination and refers this patient for fiberoptic bronchoscopy.

- A third 46-year-old patient with hemoptysis who is from a developing country is evaluated with an echocardiogram as well, because the physician thinks she hears a soft diastolic rumble at the apex on cardiac auscultation, suggesting rheumatic mitral stenosis.

These three simple vignettes illustrate two aspects of expert clinical reasoning: (1) the use of cognitive shortcuts as a way to organize the complex unstructured material that is collected in the clinical evaluation, and (2) the use of diagnostic hypotheses to consolidate the information and indicate appropriate management steps.

THE USE OF COGNITIVE SHORTCUTS Cognitive shortcuts or rules of thumb, sometimes referred to as *heuristics*, can help solve complex problems, of the sort encountered daily in clinical medicine, with great efficiency. Clinicians rely on three basic types of heuristics. When assessing a patient, clinicians often weigh the probability that this patient's clinical features match those of the class of patients with the leading diagnostic hypotheses being considered. In other words, the clinician is searching for the diagnosis for which the patient appears to be a representative example; this cognitive shortcut is called the *representativeness heuristic.*

It may take only a few characteristics from the history for an expert clinician using the representativeness heuristic to arrive at a sound diagnostic hypothesis. For example, an elderly patient with new-onset fever, cough productive of copious sputum, unilateral pleuritic chest pain, and dyspnea is readily identified as fitting the pattern for acute pneumonia, probably of bacterial origin. Evidence of focal pulmonary consolidation on the physical examination will increase the clinician's confidence in the diagnosis because it fits the expected pattern of acute bacterial pneumonia. Knowing this allows the experienced clinician to conduct an efficient, directed, and therapeutically productive patient evaluation although there may be little else in the history or physical examination of direct relevance. The inexperienced medical student or resident, who has not yet learned the patterns most prevalent in clinical medicine, must work much harder to achieve the same result and is often at risk of missing the important clinical problem in a sea of compulsively collected but unhelpful data.

However, physicians using the representativeness heuristic can reach erroneous conclusions if they fail to consider the underlying prevalence of two competing diagnoses (i.e., the prior, or pretest, probabilities). Consider a patient with pleuritic chest pain, dyspnea, and a low-grade fever. A clinician might consider acute pneumonia and acute pulmonary embolism to be the two leading diagnostic alternatives. Using the representativeness heuristic, the clinician might judge both diagnostic candidates to be equally likely, although to do so would be wrong if pneumonia was much more prevalent in the underlying population. Mistakes may also result from a failure to consider that a pattern based on a small number of prior observations will likely be less reliable than one based on larger samples.

A second commonly used cognitive shortcut, the *availability heuristic*, involves judgments made on the basis of how easily prior similar cases or outcomes can be brought to mind. For example, the experienced clinician may recall 20 elderly patients seen over the past few years who presented with painless dyspnea of acute onset and were found to have acute myocardial infarction. The novice clinician may spend valuable time seeking a pulmonary cause for the symptoms before considering and discovering the cardiac diagnosis. In this situation, the patient's clinical pattern does not fit the expected pattern of acute myocardial infarction, but experience with this atypical presentation, and the ability to recall it, can help direct the physician to the diagnosis.

Errors with the availability heuristic can come from several sources of recall bias. For example, rare catastrophes are likely to be remembered with a clarity and force out of proportion to their value, and recent experience is, of course, easier to recall and therefore more influential on clinical judgments.

The third commonly used cognitive shortcut, the *anchoring heuristic*, involves estimating a probability by starting from a familiar point (the anchor) and adjusting to the new case from there. Anchoring can be a powerful tool for diagnosis but is often used incorrectly. For example, a clinician may judge the probability of coronary artery disease (CAD) to be very high after a positive exercise thallium test, because the prediction has been anchored to the test result ("positive test = high probability of CAD"). Yet, as discussed below, this prediction would be inaccurate if the clinical (pretest) picture of the patient being tested indicates a low probability of disease (e.g., a 30-year-old woman with no risk factors). As illustrated in this example, anchors are not necessarily the same as the pretest probability (see "Measures of Disease Probability and Bayes' Theorem," below).

DIAGNOSTIC HYPOTHESIS GENERATION Cognitive scientists studying the thought processes of expert clinicians have observed that clinicians group data into packets, or "chunks," which are stored in their memories and manipulated to generate diagnostic hypotheses. Because short-term memory can typically hold only 7 to 10 items at a time, the number of packets that can be actively integrated into hypothesis-generating activities is similarly limited. The cognitive shortcuts discussed above play a key role in the generation of diagnostic hypotheses, many of which are discarded as rapidly as they are formed.

A diagnostic hypothesis sets a context for diagnostic steps to follow and provides testable predictions. For example, if the enlarged and quite tender liver felt on physical examination is due to acute hepatitis (the hypothesis), certain specific liver function tests should be marked-

edly elevated (the prediction). If the tests come back normal, the hypothesis may need to be discarded or substantially modified.

One of the factors that makes teaching diagnostic reasoning so difficult is that expert clinicians do not follow a fixed pattern in patient examinations. From the outset, they are generating, refining, and discarding diagnostic hypotheses. The questions they ask in the history are driven by the hypotheses they are working with at the moment. Even the physical examination is driven by specific questions rather than a preordained checklist. While the student is palpating the abdomen of the alcoholic patient, waiting for a finding to strike him, the expert clinician is on a focused search mission. Is the spleen enlarged? How big is the liver? Is it tender? Are there any palpable masses or nodules? Each question focuses the attention of the examiner to the exclusion of all other inputs until answered, allowing the examiner to move on to the next specific question.

Negative findings are often as important as positive ones in establishing and refining diagnostic hypotheses. Chest discomfort that is not provoked or worsened by exertion in an active patient reduces the likelihood that chronic ischemic heart disease is the underlying cause. The absence of a resting tachycardia and thyroid gland enlargement reduces the likelihood of hyperthyroidism in a patient with paroxysmal atrial fibrillation.

The acuity of a patient's illness can play an important role in overriding considerations of prevalence and other issues described above. For example, clinicians are taught to consider aortic dissection routinely as a possible cause of acute severe chest discomfort along with myocardial infarction, even though the typical history of dissection is different from myocardial infarction and dissection is far less prevalent (Chap. 231). This recommendation is based on the recognition that a relatively rare but catastrophic diagnosis like aortic dissection is very difficult to make unless it is explicitly considered. If the clinician fails to elicit any of the characteristic features of dissection by history and finds equivalent blood pressures in both arms and no pulse deficits, he or she may feel comfortable in discarding the aortic dissection hypothesis. If, however, the chest x-ray shows a widened mediastinum, the hypothesis may be reinstated and a diagnostic test ordered [e.g., thoracic computed tomography (CT) scan, transesophageal echocardiogram] to evaluate it more fully. In nonacute situations, the prevalence of potential alternative diagnoses should play a much more prominent role in diagnostic hypothesis generation.

Generation of Diagnostic Hypotheses Because the generation and evaluation of appropriate diagnostic hypotheses is a skill that not all clinicians possess to an equal degree, errors in this process can occur; in the patient with serious acute illness these may lead to tragic consequences. Consider the following hypothetical example. A 45-year-old male patient with a 3-week history of a "flulike" upper respiratory infection (URI) presented to his physician with symptoms of dyspnea and a productive cough. Based on the presenting complaint, the clinician pulled out a "URI Assessment Form" to improve quality and efficiency of care. The physician quickly completed the examination components outlined on this structured form, noting in particular the absence of fever and a clear chest examination. He then prescribed an antibiotic for presumed bronchitis, showed the patient how to breathe into a paper bag to relieve his "hyperventilation," and sent him home with the reassurance that his illness was not serious. After a sleepless night with significant dyspnea unrelieved by rebreathing into a bag, the patient developed nausea and vomiting and collapsed. He was brought into the Emergency Department in cardiac arrest and could not be resuscitated. Autopsy showed a posterior wall myocardial infarction and a fresh thrombus in an atherosclerotic right coronary artery. What went wrong? The clinician decided, even before starting the history, that the patient's complaints were not serious. He therefore felt confident that he could perform an abbreviated and focused examination using the URI assessment protocol rather than considering the full range of possibilities and performing appropriate tests to confirm or refute his initial hypotheses. In particular, by concentrating on the "URI," the clinician failed to elicit the full dyspnea history, which would have suggested a far more serious disorder, and neglected to search for other symptoms that could have directed him to the correct diagnosis.

This example illustrates how patients can diverge from textbook symptoms and the potential consequences of being unable to adapt the diagnostic process to real-world challenges. The expert, while recognizing that common things occur commonly, approaches each evaluation on high alert for clues that the initial diagnosis may be wrong. Patients often provide information that "does not fit" with any of the leading diagnostic hypotheses being considered. Distinguishing real clues from false trails can only be achieved by practice and experience. A less experienced clinician who tries to be too efficient (as in the above example) can make serious judgment errors. Furthermore, the value of conducting a rapid systematic clinical survey of symptoms and organ systems to avoid missing important but inapparent clues cannot be overstated.

MAJOR INFLUENCES ON CLINICAL DECISION-MAKING More than a decade of research on variations in clinician practice patterns has shed much light on forces that shape clinical decisions. The use of heuristic "shortcuts," as detailed above, provides a partial explanation, but several other key factors play an important role in shaping diagnostic hypotheses and management decisions. These factors can be grouped conceptually into three overlapping categories: (1) factors related to physician personal characteristics and practice style, (2) factors related to the practice setting, and (3) economic incentive factors.

Practice Style Factors One of the key roles of the physician in medical care is to serve as the patient's agent to ensure that necessary care is provided at a high level of quality. Factors that influence this role include the physician's knowledge, training, and experience. It is obvious that physicians cannot practice evidence-based medicine (EBM; described later in the chapter) if they are unfamiliar with the evidence. As would be expected, specialists generally know the evidence in their field better than do generalists. Surgeons may be more enthusiastic about recommending surgery than medical doctors because their belief in the beneficial effects of surgery is stronger. For the same reason, invasive cardiologists are much more likely to refer chest pain patients for diagnostic catheterization than are noninvasive cardiologists or generalists. The physician beliefs that drive these different practice styles are based on personal experience, recollection, and interpretation of the available medical evidence. For example, heart failure specialists are much more likely than generalists to achieve target angiotensin-converting enzyme (ACE) inhibitor therapy in their heart failure patients because they are more familiar with what the targets are (as defined by large clinical trials), have more familiarity with the specific drugs (including dosages and side effects), and are less likely to overreact to foreseeable problems in therapy such as a rise in creatinine levels or symptomatic hypotension. Other intriguing research has shown a wide distribution of acceptance times of antibiotic therapy for peptic ulcer disease following widespread dissemination of the "evidence" in the medical literature. Some gastroenterologists accepted this new therapy before the evidence was clear (reflecting, perhaps, an aggressive practice style), and some gastroenterologists lagged behind (a conservative practice style, associated in this case with older physicians). As a group, internists lagged several years behind gastroenterologists.

The opinion of influential leaders can also have an important effect on practice patterns. Such influence can occur at both the national level (e.g., expert physicians teaching at national meetings) and the local level (e.g., local educational programs, "curbside consultants"). Opinion leaders do not have to be physicians. When conducting rounds with clinical pharmacists, physicians are less likely to make medication errors and more likely to use target levels of evidence-based therapies.

The patient's welfare is not the only concern that drives clinical decisions. The physician's perception about the risk of a malpractice suit resulting from either an erroneous decision or a bad outcome creates a style of practice referred to as *defensive medicine*. This practice involves using tests and therapies with very small marginal returns to preclude future criticism in the event of an adverse outcome. For example, a 40-year-old woman who presents with a long-standing history of intermittent headache and a new severe headache along with a normal neurologic examination has a very low likelihood of structural intracranial pathology. Performance of a head CT or magnetic resonance imaging (MRI) scan in this situation would constitute defensive medicine. On the other hand, the results of the test could provide reassurance to an anxious patient.

Practice Setting Factors Factors in this category relate to the physical resources available to the physician's practice and the practice environment. *Physician-induced demand* is a term that refers to the repeated observation that physicians have a remarkable ability to accommodate to and employ the medical facilities available to them. A classic early study in this area showed that physicians in Boston had an almost 50% higher hospital admission rate than did physicians in New Haven, despite there being no obvious differences in the health of the cities' inhabitants. The physicians in New Haven were not aware of using fewer hospital beds for their patients, nor were the Boston physicians aware of using less stringent criteria to admit patients. In both cities, physicians unconsciously adopted their practice styles to the available level of hospital beds.

Other environmental factors that can influence decision-making include the local availability of specialists for consultations and procedures, "high tech" facilities such as angiography suites, a heart surgery program, and MRI machines.

Economic Incentives Economic incentives are closely related to the other two categories of practice-modifying factors. Financial issues can exert both stimulatory and inhibitory influences on clinical practice. In general, physicians are paid on a fee-for-service, capitation, or salary basis. In fee-for-service, the more the physician does, the more the physician gets paid. The incentive in this case is to do more. When fees are reduced (discounted fee-for-service), doctors tend to increase the number of services billed for. Capitation, in contrast, provides a fixed payment per patient per year, encouraging physicians to take on more patients but to provide each patient with fewer services. Expensive services are more likely to be affected by this type of incentive than inexpensive preventive services. Salary compensation plans pay physicians the same regardless of the amount of clinical work performed. The incentive here is to see fewer patients.

In summary, expert clinical decision-making can be appreciated as a complex interplay between cognitive devices used to simplify large amounts of complex information interacting with physician biases reflecting education, training, and experience, all of which are shaped by powerful, sometimes perverse, external forces. In the next section, a set of statistical tools and concepts that can assist in making clinical decisions under uncertainty are reviewed.

QUANTITATIVE METHODS TO AID CLINICAL DECISION-MAKING

The process of medical decision-making can be divided into two parts: (1) defining the available courses of action and estimating the likely outcomes with each, and (2) assessing the desirability of the outcomes. The former task involves integrating key information about the patient along with relevant evidence from the medical literature to create the structure of a decision problem. The remainder of this chapter will review some quantitative tools available to assist the clinician in these activities. These tools can be divided into those that assist the clinician in making better outcome predictions, which are then used to make decisions, and those that support the decision process directly. While these tools are not yet used routinely in daily clinical practice, the computerization of medicine is creating the required platform for their future widespread dissemination.

QUANTITATIVE MEDICAL PREDICTIONS ■ Diagnostic Testing The purpose of performing a test on a patient is to reduce uncertainty about the patient's diagnosis or prognosis and to aid the clinician in making management decisions. Although diagnostic tests are commonly thought of as laboratory tests (e.g., measurement of serum amylase level) or procedures (e.g., colonoscopy or bronchoscopy), any technology that changes our understanding of the patient's problem qualifies as a diagnostic test. Thus, even the history and physical examination can be considered a form of diagnostic test. In clinical medicine, it is common to reduce the results of a test to a dichotomous outcome, such as positive or negative, normal or abnormal. In many cases, this simplification results in the waste of useful information. However, such simplification makes it easier to demonstrate some of the quantitative ways in which test data can be used.

To characterize the accuracy of diagnostic tests, four terms are routinely used (Table 2-1). The *true-positive rate*, i.e., the sensitivity, provides a measure of how well the test correctly identifies patients with disease. The *false-negative rate* is calculated as (1 − sensitivity). The *true-negative rate*, i.e., the specificity, reflects how well the test correctly identifies patients without disease. The *false-positive rate* is (1 − specificity). A perfect test would have a sensitivity of 100% and a specificity of 100% and would completely separate patients with disease from those without it.

Calculating sensitivity and specificity require selection of a cut-point value for the test, called the *positivity criterion*, to define the threshold value at or above which the test is considered "positive." As the cutpoint is moved to improve sensitivity, specificity typically falls and vice versa. This dynamic tradeoff between more accurate identification of subjects with disease versus those without disease is often displayed graphically as a receiver operating characteristic (ROC) curve (Fig. 2-1). An ROC curve plots sensitivity (*y*-axis) versus 1 − specificity (*x*-axis). Each point on the curve represents a potential cutpoint with an associated sensitivity and specificity value. The area under the ROC curve is often used as a quantitative measure of the information content of a test. Values range from 0.5 (no diagnostic information at all, test is equivalent to flipping a coin) to 1.0 (perfect test).

In the testing literature, ROC areas are often used to compare alternative tests that can be used for a particular diagnostic problem. The test with the highest area (i.e., closest to 1.0) is presumed to be the most accurate. However, ROC curves are not a panacea for evaluation of diagnostic test utility. Like Bayes' theorem (discussed below), they are typically focused on only one possible test parameter (e.g., ST-segment response in a treadmill exercise test) to the exclusion of other potentially relevant data. In addition, ROC area comparisons do not simulate the way test information is actually used in clinical practice. Finally, biases in the underlying population used to generate the ROC curves (e.g., related to an unrepresentative test sample) can bias the ROC area and the validity of a comparison among tests.

Measures of Disease Probability and Bayes' Theorem Unfortunately, there are no perfect tests; after every test is completed the true disease state of the patient remains uncertain. Quantitating this residual uncertainty

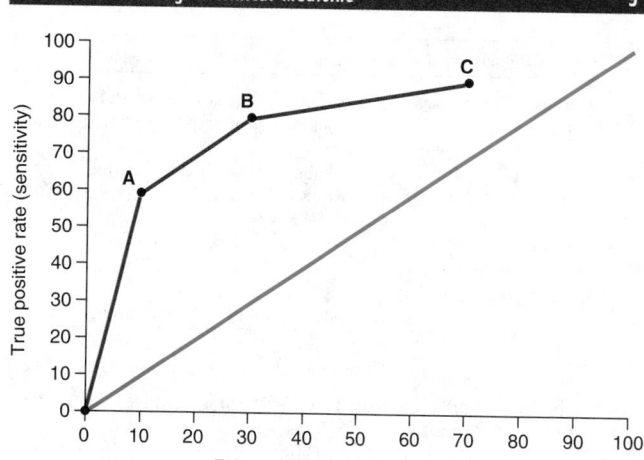

FIGURE 2-1 The receiver operating characteristic (ROC) curves for a hypothetical diagnostic test. The ROC curve illustrates the trade off that occurs between improved test sensitivity (accurate detection of patients with disease) and improved test specificity (accurate detection of patients without disease), as the test value defining when the test turns from "negative" to "positive" is varied. The 45° line indicates a test with no information (sensitivity = specificity at every test value). Point A indicates a test positivity criterion that has good specificity (90%) but poor sensitivity (60%). Point C indicates a test positivity criterion with the reverse problem: good sensitivity (90%) but poor specificity (30%). Point B may therefore represent the best compromise for clinical use.

can be done with Bayes' theorem. This theorem provides a simple mathematical way to calculate the posttest probability of disease from three parameters: the pretest probability of disease, the test sensitivity, and the test specificity (Table 2-2). The pretest probability is a quantitative expression of the confidence in a diagnosis before the test is performed. In the absence of more relevant information it is usually estimated from the prevalence of the disease in the underlying population. For some common conditions, such as CAD, nomograms and statistical models have been created to generate better estimates of pretest probability from elements of the history and physical examination. The posttest probability, then, is a revised statement of the confidence in the diagnosis, taking into account what was known both before and after the test.

To understand conceptually how Bayes' theorem creates this revised confidence statement, it is useful to examine a nomogram version of Bayes' theorem that uses the same three parameters to predict the posttest probability of disease (Fig. 2-2). In this nomogram, the accuracy of the diagnostic test in question is summarized by the likelihood ratio for a positive test, which is the ratio of the true-positive rate to the false-positive rate [or sensitivity/(1 − specificity)]. For example, a test with a sensitivity of 0.90 and a specificity of 0.90 has a likelihood ratio of 0.90/(1 − 0.90), or 9. Thus, for this hypothetical test, a "positive" result is 9 times more likely in a patient with the disease than in a patient without it. The more accurate the test, the higher the likelihood ratio. However, if sensitivity is excellent but specificity is less so, the likelihood ratio will be substantially reduced (e.g., with a 90% sensitivity but a 60% specificity, the likelihood ratio is 2.25). Most tests in medicine have likelihood ratios for a positive result between 1.5 and 20.

Applications to Diagnostic Testing in CAD Consider two tests commonly used in the diagnosis of CAD, an exercise treadmill and an exercise thallium-201 single photon emission CT (SPECT) test (Chap. 226). Meta-analysis has shown the treadmill to have an average sensitivity of 66% and an average specificity of 84%, yielding a likelihood ratio of 4.1 [0.66/(1 − 0.84)]. If we use this test on a patient with a pretest probability of CAD of 10%, the posttest probability of disease following a positive result rises only to about 30%. If a patient with a pretest probability of CAD of 80% has a positive test result, the posttest probability of disease is about 95%.

TABLE 2-1 *Measures of Diagnostic Test Accuracy*

Test Result	Disease Status	
	Present	*Absent*
Positive	True-positive (*TP*)	False-positive (*FP*)
Negative	False-negative (*FN*)	True-negative (*TN*)

IDENTIFICATION OF PATIENTS WITH DISEASE

True-positive rate (sensitivity) = $TP/(TP + FN)$
False-negative rate = $FN/(TP + FN)$
True-positive rate = 1 − false-negative rate

IDENTIFICATION OF PATIENTS WITHOUT DISEASE

True-negative rate (specificity) = $TN/(TN + FP)$
False-positive rate = $FP/(TN + FP)$
True-negative rate = 1 − false-positive rate

TABLE 2-2   *Measures of Disease Probability*

Pretest probability of disease = probability of disease before test is done. May use population prevalence of disease or more patient-specific data to generate this probability estimate.

Posttest probability of disease = probability of disease accounting for both pretest probability and test results. Also called predictive value of the test.

Bayes' theorem

  Computational version:

    Posttest probability =

$$\frac{\text{Pretest probability} \times \text{test sensitivity}}{\begin{array}{c}\text{Pretest probability} \times \text{test sensitivity} + \\ (1 - \text{disease prevalence}) \times \text{test false-positive rate}\end{array}}$$

  Example [with a pretest probability of 0.50 and a "positive" diagnostic test result (test sensitivity = 0.90, test specificity = 0.90)]:

$$\text{Posttest probability} = \frac{(0.50)(0.90)}{(0.50)(0.90) + (0.50)(0.10)}$$
$$= 0.90$$

The exercise thallium SPECT test is a more accurate test for the diagnosis of CAD. For our purposes, assume that it has both a sensitivity and specificity of 90%, yielding a likelihood ratio of 9.0 [0.90/(1 − 0.90)]. If we again test our low pretest probability patient and he has a positive test, using Fig. 2-2 we can demonstrate that the posttest probability of CAD rises from 10 to 50%. However, from a decision-making point of view, the more accurate test has not been able to improve diagnostic confidence enough to change management. In fact, the test has moved us from being fairly certain that the patient did not have CAD to being completely undecided (a 50:50 chance of disease). In a patient with a pretest probability of 80%, using the more accurate thallium SPECT test raises the posttest probability to 97% (compared with 95% for the exercise treadmill). Again, the more accurate test does not provide enough improvement in posttest confidence to alter management, and neither test has improved much upon what was known from clinical data alone.

If the pretest probability is low (e.g., 20%), even a positive result on a very accurate test will not move the posttest probability to a range high enough to rule in disease (e.g., 80%). Conversely, with a high pretest probability, a negative test will not adequately rule out disease. Thus, the largest gain in diagnostic confidence from a test occurs when the clinician is most uncertain before performing it (e.g., pretest probability between 30 and 70%). For example, if a patient has a pretest probability for CAD of 50%, a positive exercise treadmill test will move the posttest probability to 80% and a positive exercise thallium SPECT test will move it to 90% (Fig. 2-2).

Bayes' theorem, as presented above, employs a number of important simplifications that should be considered. First, few tests have only two useful outcomes, positive or negative, and many tests provide numerous pieces of data about the patient. Even if these can be integrated into a summary result, multiple levels of useful information may be present (e.g., strongly positive, positive, indeterminate, negative, strongly negative). While Bayes' theorem can be adapted to this more detailed test result format, it is computationally complex to do so. Second, Bayes' theorem assumes that the information from the test is completely unique and nonoverlapping with information used to estimate the pretest probability. This independence assumption, however, is often wrong. In many cases, test results are correlated with patient characteristics. For example, the findings of cardiomegaly and pulmonary edema on chest x-ray are correlated with the historic features of heart failure and with the physical findings of a displaced left ventricular apical impulse, an S_3 gallop, and rales. The unique predictive information contributed by the test in this case (the chest x-ray) is only a fraction of its total information because much had already been learned about the probability of heart failure before the test was done.

Finally, it has long been thought that sensitivity and specificity are

prevalence-independent parameters of test accuracy, and many texts still make this assertion. This statistically useful assumption, however, is clinically wrong. For example, a treadmill exercise test has a sensitivity in a population of patients with one-vessel CAD of around 30%, whereas the sensitivity in severe three-vessel CAD approaches 80%. Thus, the best estimate of sensitivity to use in a particular decision will often vary depending on the distribution of disease stages present in the tested population. A hospitalized population typically has a higher prevalence of disease and in particular a higher prevalence of more advanced disease stages than an outpatient population. As a consequence, test sensitivity will tend to be higher in hospitalized patients, whereas test specificity will be higher in outpatients.

Statistical Prediction Models   Bayes' theorem, as presented above, deals with a clinical prediction problem that is unrealistically simple relative to most problems a clinician faces. Prediction models, based on multivariable statistical models, can handle much more complex problems and substantially enhance predictive accuracy for specific situations. Their particular advantage is the ability to take into account many overlapping pieces of information and assign a relative weight to each based on its unique contribution to the prediction in question. For example, a logistic regression model to predict the probability of CAD takes into account all of the relevant independent factors from the clinical examination and diagnostic testing instead of the small handful of data that clinicians can manage in their heads or with Bayes' theorem. However, despite this strength, the models are too complex computationally to use without a calculator or computer (although this limit may be overcome when medicine is practiced from a fully computerized platform). To date, only a handful of prediction models have been developed and properly validated. The importance of independent validation in a population separate from the one used to develop the model cannot be overstated. Unfortunately, most published models have not been properly validated, making their utility in clinical practice uncertain at best.

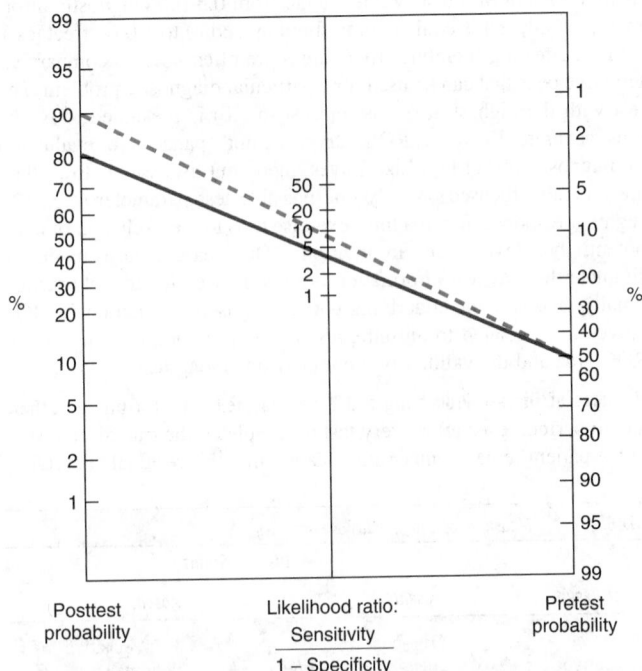

FIGURE 2-2   Nomogram version of Bayes' Theorem used to predict the posttest probability of disease (left-hand scale) using the pretest probability of disease (right-hand scale) and the likelihood ratio for a positive test (middle scale). The likelihood ratio is calculated as the sensitivity/(1 − specificity). To use, place a straightedge connecting the pretest probability and the likelihood ratio, and read off the posttest probability. This figure illustrates the value of a positive exercise treadmill test (likelihood ratio 4) and a positive exercise thallium SPECT study (likelihood ratio 9) in the patient with a pretest probability of coronary artery disease of 50%. Treadmill results shown in solid line; thallium results in dashed line. *(Adapted from Fagan TJ: N Engl J Med 293:257, 1975. Copyright 1975, Massachusetts Medical Society. All rights reserved.)*

When statistical models have been compared directly with expert clinicians, they have been found to be more consistent, as would be expected, but not significantly more accurate. Their biggest promise, then, would seem to be to make less-experienced clinicians more accurate predictors of outcome.

DECISION SUPPORT TOOLS

DECISION SUPPORT SYSTEMS Over the past 30 years, many attempts have been made to develop computer systems to help clinicians make decisions and manage patients. Conceptually, computers offer a very attractive way to handle the vast information load that today's physicians face. The computer can help by making accurate predictions of outcome, simulating the whole decision process, or providing algorithmic guidance. Computer-based predictions using Bayesian or statistical regression models inform a clinical decision but do not actually reach a "conclusion" or "recommendation." Artificial intelligence systems attempt to simulate or replace human reasoning with a computer-based analogue. To date, such approaches have achieved only limited success. Reminder or protocol-directed systems do not make predictions but use existing algorithms, such as practice guidelines, to guide clinical practice. In general, however, decision support systems have shown little impact on practice. Reminder systems, although not yet in widespread use, have shown the most promise, particularly in correcting drug dosing and in promoting guideline adherence. The full potential of these approaches will only be achieved when computers are fully integrated into medical practice.

DECISION ANALYSIS Compared with the methods discussed above, decision analysis represents a completely different approach to decision support. Its principal application is in decision problems that are complex and involve a substantial risk, a high degree of uncertainty in some key area, or an idiosyncratic feature that does not "fit" the available evidence. Three general steps are involved. First, the decision problem must be clearly defined. Second, the elements of the decision must be made explicit. This involves specifying the alternatives being considered, their relevant outcomes, the probabilities attached to each outcome, and the relative desirability (called "utility") of each outcome. Cost can also be assigned to each branch of the decision tree, allowing calculation of cost effectiveness. Finally, the decision tree must be "analyzed" to find the strategy with the best expected outcome.

An example of a decision tree used to evaluate strategies for management of the risk of infective endocarditis after catheter-associated *Staphylococcus aureus* bacteremia is shown in Fig. 2-3. Approximately 35,000 cases of *S. aureus* bacteremia occur each year in the United States. The development of complicating endocarditis, which occurs in about 6% of cases, is associated with high morbidity (31% mortality, 21% stroke rate) and medical costs. The three choices for management of the bacteremia are (1) transesophageal echocardiography (TEE), (2) a 4-week course of intravenous antibiotics (long-course), or (3) a 2-week course of intravenous antibiotics (short-course). In the TEE strategy, a 4-week course of antibiotics is given if endocarditis is evident and a 2-week course is given if it is not. With each strategy, there is a risk that the patient will develop endocarditis with or without major complications. In this analysis, the longest quality-adjusted survival (5.47 quality-adjusted life-years) was associated with the 4-week antibiotic course strategy, which also had the highest costs ($14,136 per patient), whereas the lowest costs ($9830 per patient) and worst outcomes (5.42 quality-adjusted life-years) were associated with the 2-week antibiotic course strategy. From a clinical

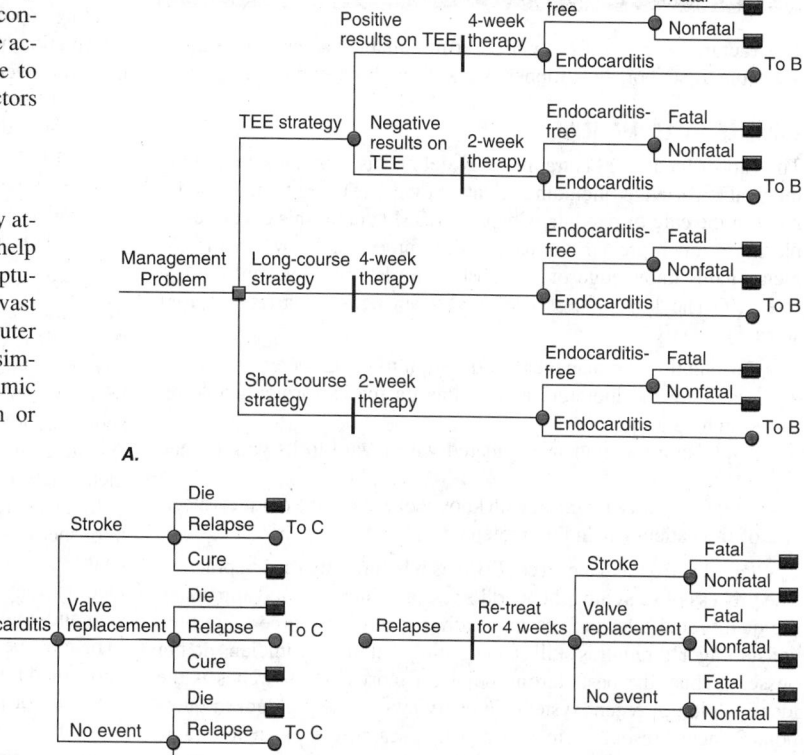

FIGURE 2-3 Decision model used to evaluate strategies for management of the risk of infective endocarditis after catheter-associated *Staphylococcus aureus* bacteremia. The square node indicates a decision between possible management strategies. Round nodes represent chance events, and rectangular (or terminal) nodes indicate the outcomes of interest. All nonterminal chance nodes in the main tree (structure A) enter substructure B. All nonterminal chance nodes in substructure B enter substructure C. TEE, transesophageal echocardiography. (*From Rosen AB et al: Ann Intern Med 130:810, 1999, with permission.*)

point of view (ignoring costs), the 4-week antibiotic course was best. From a cost-effectiveness point of view, the TEE strategy (5.46 quality-adjusted life-years and $10,051 per patient costs) provided the best balance of added benefits and costs. Thus, decision analysis can be extremely helpful in clarifying tradeoffs in outcomes and costs in difficult management areas where it is highly unlikely that an adequate randomized trial will ever be done, such as the above.

Filling in the Decision Tree The data needed to fill in a decision tree (Fig. 2-3) are typically cobbled together from a variety of sources, including the literature (randomized trials, meta-analyses, observational studies) and expert opinion. Once the decision tree is finished, the decision is "analyzed" by calculating the average value of each limb of the tree. The decision arm with the highest net value (or expected utility) is the preferred choice. The value of this exercise, however, is not so much in developing a prescription for action as it is in exploring the key elements and pressure points of a complex or difficult decision. The process of building the decision tree forces the analyst to be explicit about the choices being considered and all their relevant outcomes. Areas of high uncertainty are readily identified. Sensitivity analyses are an integral part of decision analysis and involve systematically varying the value of each key parameter in the model alone (one-way sensitivity analysis), in pairs (two-way), or in higher combinations (multivariable) to assess the impact on choice of preferred management strategy. In the above example, varying the incidence of endocarditis resulting from *S. aureus* bacteremia from 3% to >50% had no impact on the choice of TEE as the preferred strategy.

User-friendly personal computer–based software packages now make the creation and analysis of decision trees much more straightforward than in the past. However, the process is still far too cumbersome and time-consuming to be used on a routine basis. When medicine is practiced from a fully computerized platform, a library of prestructured decision trees with user-modifiable values can be made available to support practitioners working with individual patients.

EVIDENCE-BASED MEDICINE

The "art of medicine" is traditionally defined as a practice combining medical knowledge (including scientific evidence), intuition, and judgment in the care of patients (Chap. 1). EBM updates this construct by placing a much greater emphasis on the processes by which the clinician gains knowledge of the most up-to-date and relevant clinical research. The key processes of EBM can be summarized in four steps:

1. Formulating the management question to be answered
2. Searching the literature and on-line databases for applicable research data
3. Appraising the evidence gathered with regard to its validity and relevance
4. Integrating this appraisal with knowledge about the unique aspects of the patient (including preferences).

Steps 2 and 3 are the heart of EBM as it is currently used in practice. The process of searching the world's research literature and appraising the quality and relevance of studies thus identified can be quite time consuming and requires skills and training that many clinicians do not possess. Thus, the best starting point for most EBM searches is the identification of recent systematic overviews of the problem in question. Selected resources to assist in this search are listed in (Table 2-3).

Generally, the EBM tools listed in Table 2-3 provide access to research information in one of two forms. The first, primary research reports, is the original peer-reviewed research work that is published in medical journals. Initial access to this information in an EBM search may be gained through MEDLINE, which provides access to a huge amount of data in abstract form. The difficulty with MEDLINE is locating reports that are on point in a sea of irrelevant or unhelpful information and being reasonably certain that important reports have not been overlooked. The second form, systematic reviews, comprehensively summarizes the available evidence on a particular topic up to a certain date and provides the interpretation of the reviewer. Explicit criteria are used to find all the relevant scientific research and grade its quality. The prototype for this kind of resource is the Cochrane Database of Systematic Reviews. One of the key components of a systematic review is a meta-analysis.

Meta-analysis This is research done on research data for the purpose of combining and summarizing the available evidence quantitatively. Although it can be used to combine nonrandomized studies, meta-analysis is most valuable when used to summarize all the randomized trials on a particular therapeutic problem. Ideally, unpublished trials should be identified and included to avoid publication bias (i.e., only "positive" trials tend to get published). Furthermore, some of the best meta-analyses obtain and analyze the raw patient-level data from the individual trials rather than working only with what is available in the published reports of each trial. Importantly, not all published meta-analyses are reliable sources of evidence on a particular problem. Their methodology must be carefully scrutinized to ensure proper study design and analysis. The results of a well done meta-analysis are likely to be most persuasive if it includes at least several large-scale, properly performed randomized trials. In many cases, where the available trials are small or poorly done, the best that may be concluded is that substantial additional trials are required to reach a reliable conclusion about a particular therapy.

Meta-analyses typically focus on summary measures of relative treatment benefit, such as odds ratios or relative risks. Clinicians should also examine what absolute risk reduction (ARR) can be expected from the therapy. A useful summary metric of absolute treatment benefit is the number needed to treat (NNT) to prevent one adverse outcome event (e.g., death, stroke). NNT is simply $1/ARR$. For example, if a hypothetical therapy reduced mortality over a 5-year follow-up by 33% (the relative treatment benefit) from 12% (control arm) to 8% (treatment arm), the absolute risk reduction would be $12\% - 8\% = 4\%$ and the $NNT = \frac{1}{4}$ or 25. Thus, we would need to treat 25 patients for 5 years to prevent 1 death. If we applied our hypothetical treatment to a lower risk population, say with a 6% 5-year mortality, the 33% relative treatment benefit would reduce absolute mortality by 2% (from 6% to 4%) and the NNT for the same therapy in this different group of patients would be 50.

CONCLUSIONS

In this era of evidence-based medicine, it is tempting to think that all the difficult decisions practitioners face have been or soon will be solved and digested into practice guidelines and computerized reminders. However, EBM provides practitioners with an ideal rather than a finished set of tools with which to manage patients. The significant contribution of EBM has been to promote the development of more powerful and user-friendly EBM tools that can be accessed by the busy practitioners. This is an enormously important contribution that is slowly changing the way medi-

---

TABLE 2-3 *Selected Tools for Finding the Evidence in Evidence-Based Medicine*

Name	Description	Web Address	Availability
Evidence-Based Medicine Reviews	Comprehensive electronic database that combines and integrates: 1. The Cochrane Database of Systematic Reviews 2. ACP Journal Club 3. The Database of Abstracts of Reviews of Effectiveness	www.ovid.com	Subscription required; available through medical center libraries and other institutions
Cochrane Library	Collection of EBM databases including The Cochrane Database of Systematic Reviews—full text articles reviewing specific health care topics	www.cochrane.org	Subscription required; abstracts of systematic reviews available free online; some countries have funding to provide free access to all residents
ACP Journal Club	Collection of summaries of original studies and systematic reviews; published bimonthly; all data since 1991 available on Web site, updated yearly	www.acpic.org	Subscription required
Clinical Evidence	Monthly updated directory of concise overviews of common clinical interventions	www.clinicalevidence.com	Subscription required; free access for UK and for developing countries
MEDLINE	National Library of Medicine database with citations back to 1966	www.nlm.nih.gov	Free via Internet

Note: ACP, American College of Physicians; EBM, evidence-based medicine.

cine is practiced. One of the repeated admonitions of EBM pioneers has been to replace reliance on the local "gray-haired expert" (who may be often wrong but rarely in doubt) with a systematic search for and evaluation of the evidence. But EBM has not eliminated the need for subjective judgments; each systematic review presents the interpretation of an "expert," whose biases remain largely invisible to the consumer of the review. In addition, meta-analyses cannot generate evidence where there are no adequate randomized trials, and most of what clinicians face will never be thoroughly tested in a randomized trial. For the foreseeable future, excellent clinical reasoning skills and experience supplemented by well-designed quantitative tools and a keen appreciation for individual patient preferences will continue to be of paramount importance in the professional life of medical practitioners.

FURTHER READING

BALK EM et al: Correlation of quality measures with estimates of treatment effect in meta-analyses of randomized controlled trials. JAMA 287:2973, 2002

NAYLOR CD: Gray zones of clinical practice: Some limits to evidence-based medicine. Lancet 345:840, 1995

POYNARD T et al: Truth survival in clinical research: An evidence-based requiem? Ann Intern Med 136:888; 2002

SACKETT DL et al: *Evidence-Based Medicine: How to Practice and Teach EBM.* 2d ed. London, Churchill Livingstone, 2000

SCHULMAN KA et al: The effect of race and sex on physicians' recommendations for cardiac catheterization. N Engl J Med 340:618, 1999

3 PRINCIPLES OF CLINICAL PHARMACOLOGY
Dan M. Roden

Drugs are the cornerstone of modern therapeutics. Nevertheless, it is well recognized among physicians and among the lay community that the outcome of drug therapy varies widely among individuals. While this variability has been perceived as an unpredictable, and therefore inevitable, accompaniment of drug therapy, this is not the case. The goal of this chapter is to describe the principles of clinical pharmacology that can be used for the safe and optimal use of available and new drugs.

Drugs interact with specific target molecules to produce their beneficial and adverse effects. The chain of events between administration of a drug and production of these effects in the body can be divided into two important components, both of which contribute to variability in drug actions. The first component comprises the processes that determine drug delivery to, and removal from, molecular targets. The resultant description of the relationship between drug concentration and time is termed *pharmacokinetics*. The second component of variability in drug action comprises the processes that determine variability in drug actions despite equivalent drug delivery to effector drug sites. This description of the relationship between drug concentration and effect is termed *pharmacodynamics*. As discussed further below, pharmacodynamic variability can arise as a result of variability in function of the target molecule itself or of variability in the broad biologic context in which the drug-target interaction occurs to achieve drug effects.

Two important goals of the discipline of clinical pharmacology are (1) to provide a description of conditions under which drug actions vary among human subjects; and (2) to determine mechanisms underlying this variability, with the goal of improving therapy with available drugs as well as pointing to new drug mechanisms that may be effective in the treatment of human disease. The first steps in the discipline were empirical descriptions of the influence of disease X on drug action Y or of individuals or families with unusual sensitivities to adverse drug effects. These important descriptive findings are now being replaced by an understanding of the molecular mechanisms underlying variability in drug actions. Thus, the effects of disease, drug coadministration, or familial factors in modulating drug action can now be reinterpreted as variability in expression or function of specific genes whose products determine pharmacokinetics and pharmacodynamics. Nevertheless, it is the personal interaction of the patient with the physician or other health care provider that first identifies unusual variability in drug actions; maintained alertness to unusual drug responses continues to be a key component of improving drug safety.

Unusual drug responses, segregating in families, have been recognized for decades and initially defined the field of *pharmacogenetics*. Now, with an increasing appreciation of common polymorphisms across the human genome, comes the opportunity to reinterpret descriptive mechanisms of variability in drug action as a consequence of specific DNA polymorphisms, or sets of DNA polymorphisms, among individuals. This approach defines the nascent field of *pharmacogenomics*, which may hold the opportunity of allowing practitioners to integrate a molecular understanding of the basis of disease with an individual's genomic makeup to prescribe personalized, highly effective, and safe therapies.

INDICATIONS FOR DRUG THERAPY It is self-evident that the benefits of drug therapy should outweigh the risks. Benefits fall into two broad categories: those designed to alleviate a symptom, and those designed to prolong useful life. An increasing emphasis on the principles of evidence-based medicine and techniques such as large clinical trials and meta-analyses have defined benefits of drug therapy in specific patient subgroups. Establishing the balance between risk and benefit is not always simple: for example, therapies that provide symptomatic benefits but shorten life may be entertained in patients with serious and highly symptomatic diseases such as heart failure or cancer. These decisions illustrate the continuing highly personal nature of the relationship between the prescriber and the patient.

Some adverse effects are so common, and so readily associated with drug therapy, that they are identified very early during clinical use of a drug. On the other hand, serious adverse effects may be sufficiently uncommon that they escape detection for many years after a drug begins to be widely used. The issue of how to identify rare but serious adverse effects (that can profoundly affect the benefit-risk perception in an individual patient) has not been satisfactorily resolved. Potential approaches range from an increased understanding of the molecular and genetic basis of variability in drug actions to expanded postmarketing surveillance mechanisms. None of these have been completely effective, so practitioners must be continuously vigilant to the possibility that unusual symptoms may be related to specific drugs, or combinations of drugs, that their patients receive.

Beneficial and adverse reactions to drug therapy can be described by a series of dose-response relations (Fig. 3-1). Well-tolerated drugs demonstrate a wide margin, termed the *therapeutic ratio*, *therapeutic index*, or *therapeutic window*, between the doses required to produce a therapeutic effect and those producing toxicity. In cases where there is a similar relationship between plasma drug concentration and effects, monitoring plasma concentrations can be a highly effective aid in managing drug therapy, by enabling concentrations to be maintained above the minimum required to produce an effect and below the concentration range likely to produce toxicity. Such monitoring has been most widely used to guide therapy with specific agents, such as certain antiarrhythmics, anticonvulsants, and antibiotics. Many of the principles in clinical pharmacology and examples outlined below—that can

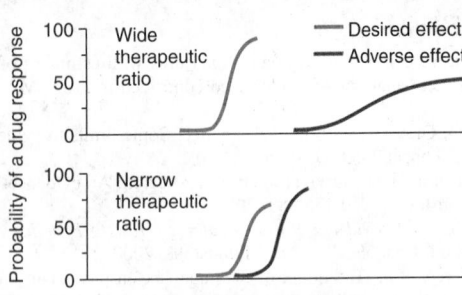

FIGURE 3-1 The concept of a therapeutic ratio. Each panel illustrates the relationship between increasing dose and cumulative probability of a desired or adverse drug effect. *Top.* A drug with a wide therapeutic ratio, i.e., a wide separation of the two curves. *Bottom* A drug with a narrow therapeutic ratio; here, the likelihood of adverse effects at therapeutic doses is increased because the curves are not well separated. Further, a steep dose-response curve for adverse effects is especially undesirable, as it implies that even small dosage increments may sharply increase the likelihood of toxicity. When there is a definable relationship between drug concentration (usually measured in plasma) and desirable and adverse effect curves, concentration may be substituted on the abscissa. Note that not all patients necessarily demonstrate a therapeutic response (or adverse effect) at any dose, and that some effects (notably some adverse effects) may occur in a dose-independent fashion.

be applied broadly to therapeutics—have been developed in these arenas.

PRINCIPLES OF PHARMACOKINETICS

The processes of absorption, distribution, metabolism, and elimination—collectively termed *drug disposition*—determine the concentration of drug delivered to target effector molecules. Mathematical analysis of these processes can define specific, and clinically useful, parameters that describe drug disposition. This approach allows prediction of how factors such as disease, concomitant drug therapy, or genetic variants affect these parameters, and how dosages therefore should be adjusted. In this way, the chances of undertreatment due to low drug concentrations or adverse effects due to high drug concentrations can be minimized.

BIOAVAILABILITY When a drug is administered intravenously, each drug molecule is by definition available to the systemic circulation. However, drugs are often administered by other routes, such as orally, subcutaneously, intramuscularly, rectally, sublingually, or directly into desired sites of action. With these other routes, the amount of drug actually entering the systemic circulation may be less than with the intravenous route. The fraction of drug available to the systemic circulation by other routes is termed *bioavailability*. Bioavailability may be <100% for two reasons: (1) absorption is reduced, or (2) the drug undergoes metabolism or elimination prior to entering the systemic circulation. Bioavailability (*F*) is defined as the area under the time-concentration curve (*AUC*) after a drug dose, divided by *AUC* after the same dose intravenously (Fig. 3-2*A*).

Absorption Drug administration by nonintravenous routes often involves an absorption process characterized by the plasma level increasing to a maximum value at some time after administration and then declining as the rate of drug elimination exceeds the rate of absorption (Fig. 3-2*A*). Thus, the peak concentration is lower and occurs later than after the same dose given by rapid intravenous injection. The extent of absorption may be reduced because a drug is incompletely released from its dosage form, undergoes destruction at its site of administration, or has physicochemical properties such as insolubility that prevent complete absorption from its site of administration.

The rate of absorption can be an important consideration for determining a dosage regimen, especially for drugs with a narrow therapeutic ratio. If absorption is too rapid, then the resulting high concentration may cause adverse effects not observed with a more slowly absorbed formulation. At the other extreme, slow absorption is

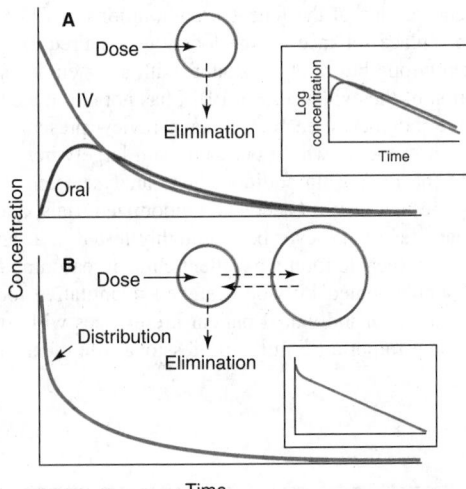

FIGURE 3-2 Idealized time-plasma concentration curves after a single dose of drug. *A.* The time course of drug concentration after an instantaneous intravenous (IV) bolus or an oral dose in the one-compartment model shown. The area under the time-concentration curve is clearly less with the oral drug than the IV, indicating incomplete bioavailability. Note that despite this incomplete bioavailability, concentration after the oral dose can be higher than after the IV dose at some time points. The inset shows that the decline of concentrations over time is linear on a log-linear plot, characteristic of first-order elimination, and that oral and IV drug have the same elimination (parallel) time course. *B.* The decline of central compartment concentration when drug is both distributed to and from a peripheral compartment and eliminated from the central compartment. The rapid initial decline of concentration reflects not drug elimination but distribution.

deliberately designed into "slow-release" or "sustained-release" drug formulations in order to minimize variation in plasma concentrations during the interval between doses, because the drug's rate of elimination is offset by an equivalent rate of absorption controlled by formulation factors (Fig. 3-3).

Presystemic Metabolism or Elimination When a drug is administered orally, it must transverse the intestinal epithelium, the portal venous system, and the liver prior to entering the systemic circulation (Fig. 3-4). At each of these sites, drug availability may be reduced; this mechanism of reduction of systemic availability is termed *presystemic elimination*, or *first-pass elimination*, and its efficiency assessed as extraction ratio. Uptake into the enterocyte is a combination of passive and active processes, the latter mediated by specific drug uptake transport molecules. Once a drug enters the enterocyte, it may undergo metabolism, be transported into the portal vein, or undergo excretion back into the intestinal lumen. Both excretion into the intestinal lumen and metabolism decrease systemic bioavailability. Once a drug passes this enterocyte barrier, it may also undergo uptake (again often by specific uptake transporters such as the organic cation transporter or organic anion transporter) into the hepatocyte, where bioavailability can be further limited by metabolism or excretion into the bile.

The drug transport molecule that has been most widely studied is

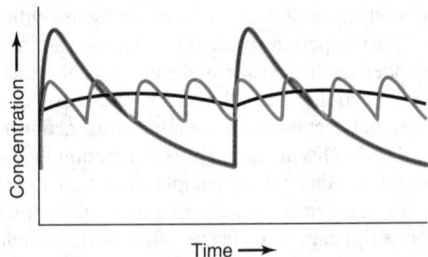

FIGURE 3-3 Concentration excursions between doses at steady state as a function of dosing frequency. With less frequent dosing (blue), excursions are larger; this is acceptable with a wide therapeutic ratio drug (Fig. 3-1). For narrower therapeutic ratio drugs, more frequent dosing (red) may be necessary to avoid toxicity and maintain efficacy. Another approach is use of a sustained-release formulation (black) that in theory results in very small excursions even with infrequent dosing.

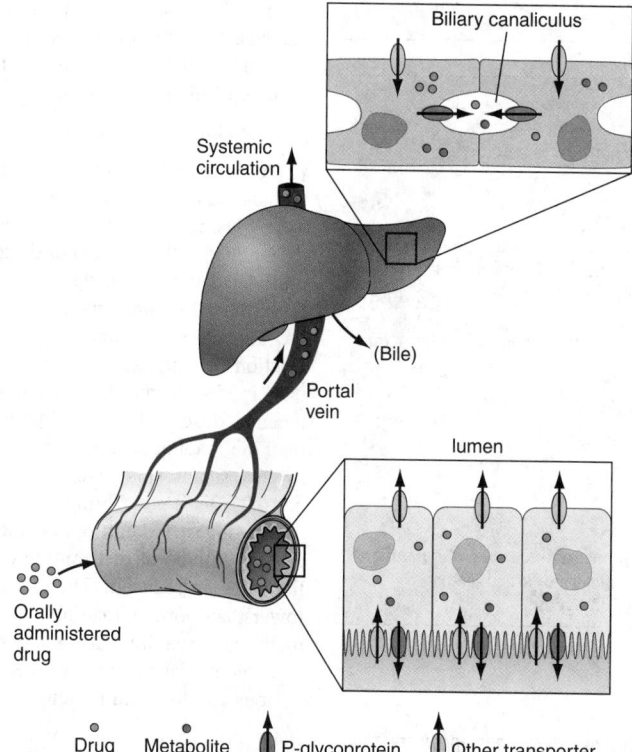

FIGURE 3-4 Mechanism of presystemic clearance. After drug enters the enterocyte, it can undergo metabolism, excretion into the intestinal lumen, or transport into the portal vein. Similarly, the hepatocyte may accomplish metabolism and biliary excretion prior to the entry of drug and metabolites to the systemic circulation. *[Adapted by permission from DM Roden, in DP Zipes, J Jalife (eds): Cardiac Electrophysiology: From Cell to Bedside, 4th ed. Philadelphia, Saunders, 2003. Copyright 2003 with permission from Elsevier.]*

P-glycoprotein, the product of the normal expression of the *MDR1* gene. P-glycoprotein is expressed on the apical aspect of the enterocyte and on the canalicular aspect of the hepatocyte (Fig. 3-4); in both locations, it serves as an efflux pump, thus limiting availability of drug to the systemic circulation.

Most drug metabolism takes place in the liver, although the enzymes accomplishing drug metabolism may be expressed, and hence drug metabolism may take place, in multiple other sites, including kidney, intestinal epithelium, lung, and plasma. Drug metabolism is generally conceptualized as "phase I," which generally results in more polar metabolites that are more readily excreted, and "phase II," during which specific endogenous compounds are conjugated to the drugs or their metabolites, again to enhance polarity and thus excretion. The major process during phase I is drug oxidation, generally accomplished by members of the cytochrome P450 (CYP) monooxygenase superfamily. CYPs that are especially important for drug metabolism (Table 3-1) include CYP3A4, CYP3A5, CYP2D6, CYP2C9, CYP2C19, CYP1A2, and CYP2E1, and each drug may be a substrate for one or more of these enzymes. The enzymes that accomplish phase II reactions include glucuronyl-, acetyl-, sulfo- and methyltransferases. Drug metabolites may exert important pharmacologic activity, as discussed further below.

Clinical Implications of Altered Bioavailability Some drugs undergo near-complete presystemic metabolism and thus cannot be administered orally. Lidocaine is an example; the drug is well absorbed but undergoes near-complete extraction in the liver, so only lidocaine metabolites (which may be toxic) appear in the systemic circulation following administration of the parent drug. Similarly, nitroglycerin cannot be used orally because it is completely extracted prior to reaching the systemic circulation. The drug is therefore used by the sublingual or transdermal routes, which bypass presystemic metabolism.

Other drugs undergo very extensive presystemic metabolism but can still be administered by the oral route, using much higher doses

than those required intravenously. Thus, a typical intravenous dose of verapamil would be 1 to 5 mg, compared to the usual single oral dose of 40 to 120 mg. Even small variations in the presystemic elimination of very highly extracted drugs such as propranolol or verapamil can cause large interindividual variations in systemic availability and effect. Oral amiodarone is 35 to 50% bioavailable because of poor solubility. Therefore, prolonged administration of usual oral doses by the intravenous route would be inappropriate. Administration of low-dose aspirin can result in exposure of cyclooxygenase in platelets in the portal vein to the drug, but systemic sparing because of first-pass deacylation in the liver. This is an example of presystemic metabolism being exploited to therapeutic advantage.

FIRST-ORDER DISTRIBUTION AND ELIMINATION Most pharmacokinetic processes are first order; i.e., the rate of the process depends on the amount of drug present. In the simplest pharmacokinetic model (Fig. 3-2A), a drug bolus is administered instantaneously to a central compartment, from which drug elimination occurs as a first-order process. The first-order (concentration-dependent) nature of drug elimination leads directly to the relationship describing drug concentration (C) at any time (t) following the bolus:

$$C = (\text{dose}/V_c) \cdot e^{(-0.69t/t_{1/2})}$$

where V_c is the volume of the compartment into which drug is delivered and $t_{1/2}$ is elimination half-life. As a consequence of this relationship, a plot of the logarithm of concentration vs time is a straight line (Fig. 3-2A, inset). *Half-life* is the time required for 50% of a first-order process to be complete. Thus, 50% of drug elimination is accomplished after one drug elimination half-life; 75% after two; 87.5% after three, etc. In practice, first-order processes such as elimination are near-complete after four to five half-lives.

In some cases, drug is removed from the central compartment not only by elimination but also by distribution into peripheral compartments. In this case, the plot of plasma concentration vs time after a bolus demonstrates two (or more) exponential components (Fig. 3-2B). In general, the initial rapid drop in drug concentration represents not elimination but drug distribution into and out of peripheral tissues (also first-order processes), while the slower component represents drug elimination; the initial precipitous decline is usually evident with administration by intravenous but not other routes. Drug concentrations at peripheral sites are determined by a balance between drug distribution to and redistribution from peripheral sites, as well as by elimination. Once the distribution process is near-complete (four to five distribution half-lives), plasma and tissue concentrations decline in parallel.

Clinical Implications of Half-Life Measurements The elimination half-life not only determines the time required for drug concentrations to fall to near-immeasurable levels after a single bolus, but it is the key determinant of the time required for steady-state plasma concentrations to be achieved after any change in drug dosing (Fig. 3-5). This applies to the initiation of chronic drug therapy (whether by multiple oral doses or by continuous intravenous infusion), a change in chronic drug dose or dosing interval, or discontinuation of drug. When drug effect parallels drug concentrations, the time required for a change in drug dosing to achieve a new level of effect is therefore determined by the elimination half-life.

During chronic drug administration, a point is reached at which the amount of drug administered per unit time equals drug eliminated per unit time, defining the *steady state*. With a continuous intravenous infusion, plasma concentrations at steady state are stable, while with chronic oral drug administration, plasma concentrations vary during the dosing interval but the time-concentration profile between dosing intervals is stable (Fig. 3-5).

DRUG DISTRIBUTION Distribution from central to peripheral sites, or from extracellular to intracellular sites, can be accomplished by passive mechanisms such as diffusion or by specific drug transport mech-

TABLE 3-1 Molecular Pathways Mediating Drug Disposition[a]

Molecule	Substrates[c]	Inhibitors[c]
CYP3A	Calcium channel blockers; antiarrhythmics (lidocaine, quinidine, mexiletine); HMG-CoA reductase inhibitors ("statins"; see text); cyclosporine, tacrolimus; indinavir, saquinavir, ritonavir	Amiodarone; ketoconazole; itraconazole; erythromycin, clarithromycin; ritonavir
CYP2D6[b]	Timolol, metoprolol, carvedilol; phenformin; codeine; propafenone, flecainide; tricyclic antidepressants; fluoxetine, paroxetine	Quinidine (even at ultralow doses); tricyclic antidepressants; fluoxetine, paroxetine
CYP2C9[b]	Warfarin; phenytoin; glipizide; losartan	Amiodarone; fluconazole; phenytoin
CYP2C19[b]	Omeprazole; mephenytoin	
Thiopurine S-methyltransferase[b]	6-Mercaptopurine, azathioprine	
N-acetyl transferase[b]	Isoniazid; procainamide; hydralazine; some sulfonamides	
UGT1A1[b]	Irinotecan	
Pseudocholinesterase[b]	Succinylcholine	
P-glycoprotein	Digoxin; HIV protease inhibitors; many CYP3A substrates	Quinidine; amiodarone; verapamil; cyclosporine; itraconazole; erythromycin

[a] A listing of CYP substrates, inhibitors, and inducers is maintained at *http://medicine.iupui.edu/flockhart/clinlist.html*.

[b] Clinically important genetics variants described.

[c] Inhibitors affect the molecular pathway and thus may affect substrate.

anisms that are only now being defined at the molecular level. Models such as those shown in Fig. 3-2 allow derivation of a volume term for each compartment. These volumes rarely have any correspondence to actual physiologic volumes, such as plasma volume or total-body water volume. For many drugs the central volume may be viewed conveniently as a site in rapid equilibrium with plasma. Central volumes and volume of distribution at steady state can be used to estimate tissue drug uptake and, in some cases, to adjust drug dosage in disease. In a typical 70-kg human, plasma volume is ~3 L, blood volume is ~5.5 L, and extracellular water outside the vasculature is ~42 L. The volume of distribution of drugs extensively bound to plasma proteins but not to tissue components approaches plasma volume; warfarin is an example. However, for most drugs, the volume of distribution is far greater than any physiologic space. For example, the volume of distribution of digoxin and tricyclic antidepressants is hundreds of liters, obviously exceeding total-body volume. This indicates that these drugs are largely distributed outside the vascular system, and the proportion of the drug present in the plasma compartment is low. As a consequence, such drugs are not readily removed by dialysis, an important consideration in overdose.

Clinical Implications of Drug Distribution Digoxin accesses its cardiac site of action slowly, over a distribution phase of several hours. Thus after an intravenous dose, plasma levels fall but those at the site of action increase over hours. Only when distribution is near-complete does the concentration of digoxin in plasma reflect pharmacologic effect. For this reason, there should be a 6- to 8-h wait after administration before plasma levels of digoxin are measured as a guide to therapy.

Animal models have suggested, and clinical studies are confirming, that limited drug penetration into the brain, the "blood-brain barrier," often represents a robust P-glycoprotein-mediated efflux process from capillary endothelial cells in the cerebral circulation. Thus drug distribution into the brain may be modulated by changes in P-glycoprotein function.

LOADING DOSES For some drugs, the indication may be so urgent that the time required to achieve steady-state concentrations may be too long. Under these conditions, administration of "loading" dosages may result in more rapid elevations of drug concentration to achieve therapeutic effects earlier than with chronic maintenance therapy (Fig. 3-5). Nevertheless, the time required for true steady state to be achieved is still determined only by elimination half-life. This strategy is only appropriate for drugs exhibiting a defined relationship between drug

dose and effect. A loading dose can be estimated from the desired plasma level (*C*) and the apparent volume of distribution (*V*):

$$\text{Loading dose} = C \times V$$

Alternatively, the loading amount required to achieve steady-state plasma levels can also be determined if the fraction of drug eliminated during the dosing interval and the maintenance dose are known. For example, if the fraction of digoxin eliminated daily is 35% and the planned maintenance dose is 0.25 mg daily, then the loading dose required to achieve steady-state levels would be $(0.25/0.35) \approx 0.75$ mg.

In congestive heart failure, the central volume of distribution of lidocaine is reduced. Therefore, lower-than-normal loading regimens are required to achieve equivalent plasma drug concentrations and to avoid toxicity.

RATE OF INTRAVENOUS ADMINISTRATION Although the simulations in Fig. 3-2 use a single intravenous bolus, this is very rarely appropriate in practice because side effects related to transiently very high concentrations can result. Rather, drugs are more usually administered orally or as a slower intravenous infusion. Thus, administration of a full loading dose of lidocaine (3 to 4 mg/kg) as a single bolus often results transiently in very high concentrations, with a risk of adverse effects such as seizures. Since the distribution half-life of the drug is 8 min, a more appropriate loading regimen is the same dose, administered as two to four divided boluses every 8 min, or a rapid infusion (e.g., 10 mg/min for 20 min).

Some drugs are so predictably lethal when infused too rapidly that special precautions should be taken to prevent accidental boluses. For example, solutions of potassium for intravenous administration >20

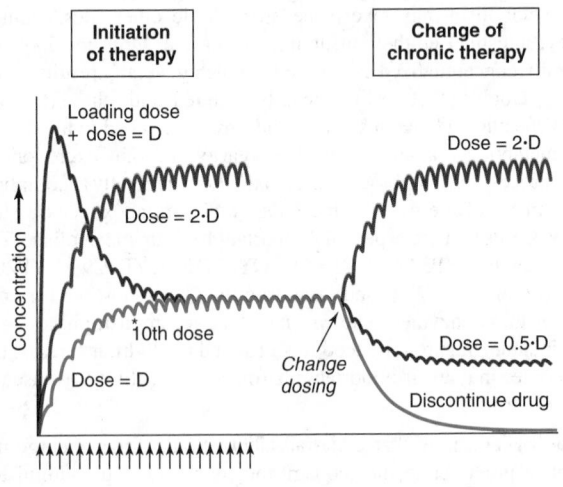

FIGURE 3-5 Drug accumulation to steady state. In this simulation, drug was administered (arrows) at intervals = 50% of the elimination half-life. Steady state is achieved during initiation of therapy after ~5 elimination half-lives, or 10 doses. A loading dose did not alter the eventual steady state achieved. A doubling of the dose resulted in a doubling of the steady state but the same time course of accumulation. Once steady state is achieved, a change in dose (increase, decrease, or drug discontinuation) results in a new steady state in ~5 elimination half-lives. [*Adapted by permission from DM Roden, in DP Zipes, J Jalife (eds): Cardiac Electrophysiology: From Cell to Bedside, 4th ed. Philadelphia, Saunders, 2003. Copyright 2003 with permission from Elsevier.*]

meq/L should be avoided in all but the most exceptional and carefully monitored circumstances. This minimizes the possibility of cardiac arrest, which can occur as a result of accidental increases in infusion rates of more concentrated solutions.

Procainamide, which is almost totally absorbed after oral administration, can be given orally as a single 1000-mg loading dose with little risk of hypotension. However, administration by the intravenous route is more safely accomplished by giving the dose in fractions of about 100 mg at 5-min intervals or, more conveniently, as a 20-mg/min infusion over 50 min to avoid hypotension during the distribution phase.

As these examples illustrate, excessively rapid administration of many drugs can lead to catastrophic consequences that result from high concentrations in the blood during the distribution phase. In contrast, for some centrally active drugs, the higher concentration of drug during the distribution phase after intravenous administration is used to advantage. The use of midazolam for intravenous sedation, for example, depends upon its rapid uptake by the brain during the distribution phase to produce sedation quickly, with subsequent egress from the brain during the redistribution of the drug as equilibrium is achieved.

Similarly, adenosine must be administered as a rapid bolus in the treatment of reentrant supraventricular tachycardias (Chap. 214), to prevent elimination by very rapid ($t_{\frac{1}{2}}$ of seconds) uptake into erythrocytes and endothelial cells before the drug can reach its clinical site of action, the atrioventricular node.

PLASMA PROTEIN BINDING Many drugs circulate in the plasma partly bound to plasma proteins. Since only unbound (free) drug can distribute to sites of pharmacologic action, drug response is related to the free rather than the total circulating plasma drug concentration. In most cases, the degree of binding is fairly constant across the therapeutic concentration range; in this case, when plasma drug concentration is used to adjust doses, total levels in plasma can be used without resulting in significant error.

Clinical Implications of Altered Protein Binding For drugs that are normally highly bound to plasma proteins (>90%), small changes in the extent of binding (e.g., due to disease) produce a large change in the amount of unbound drug, and hence drug effect. The acute-phase reactant α_1-acid glycoprotein binds to basic drugs, such as lidocaine or quinidine, and is increased in a range of common conditions, including myocardial infarction, surgery, neoplastic disease, rheumatoid arthritis, and burns. This increased binding can lead to reduced pharmacologic effects at therapeutic concentrations of total drug. Conversely, conditions such as hypoalbuminemia, liver disease, and renal disease can decrease the extent of drug binding, particularly of acidic and neutral drugs, such as phenytoin. Here, plasma concentration of free drug is increased, so drug efficacy and toxicity are enhanced if total (free + bound) drug is used to monitor therapy.

CLEARANCE When drug is eliminated from the body, the amount of drug in the body declines over time. An important concept in quantifying this reduction is to consider that drug concentration at the beginning and end of a time period are unchanged, and that a specific volume of the body has been "cleared" of the drug during that time period. This defines clearance as volume/time. Clearance is a measure of the efficiency of drug removal that encompasses both drug metabolism as well as drug excretion.

Clinical Implications of Altered Clearance ■ *ADJUSTING DRUG DOSAGES* While elimination half-life determines the time required to achieve steady-state plasma concentrations (C_{ss}), the *magnitude* of that steady state is determined by clearance (Cl) and dose alone. For a drug administered as an intravenous infusion, this relationship is

$$C_{ss} = \text{dosing rate}/Cl \quad \text{or} \quad \text{dosing rate} = Cl \times C_{ss}$$

When drug is administered orally, the average plasma concentration within a dosing interval ($C_{avg,ss}$) replaces C_{ss}, and bioavailability (F) must be included:

$$F \times \text{dosing rate} = Cl \times C_{avg,ss}$$

Genetic variants, drug interactions, or diseases that reduce the activity of drug-metabolizing enzymes or excretory mechanisms may lead to decreased clearance and hence a requirement for downward dose adjustment to avoid toxicity. Genetic variants may reduce expression of CYPs (or other drug-metabolizing enzymes) or may result in normal expression of enzymes that have reduced function; in either case, dose requirements may need to be reduced. Conversely, some drug interactions and genetic variants increase CYP expression, and hence increased drug dosage may be necessary to maintain a therapeutic effect.

Clearance varies among drugs but is constant for most drugs over the therapeutic range of concentrations. In some cases, elimination becomes saturated at high doses, and the process then occurs at a fixed amount per unit time (zero order). With such nonlinear elimination kinetics, an increase in drug dosage is followed by a disproportionate rise in drug concentration, which can carry a risk of toxicity. Drugs that undergo zero-order elimination at therapeutic dosages include phenytoin, theophylline, and ethanol. Monitoring plasma concentrations of these agents is an indispensable guide to adjusting dose.

THE CONCEPT OF HIGH-RISK PHARMACOKINETICS Many drugs undergo elimination by multiple drug-metabolizing or excretory pathways. In this case, absence of one pathway (due to a genetic variant or drug interaction) may not have a large impact on drug concentrations or drug actions. However, other drugs utilize a single pathway exclusively for drug elimination. Under this scenario, any condition that inhibits that pathway (be it disease-related, genetic, or due to a drug interaction) can lead to dramatic changes in drug concentrations and hence effect. Examples of this phenomenon are discussed further below and include digoxin toxicity when P-glycoprotein, the major route of digoxin elimination, is inhibited and potentially fatal bone marrow aplasia due to azathioprine or 6-mercaptopurine in patients with genetically determined absence of function of thiopurine *S*-methyltransferase (TPMT). A dual-pathway example is the antiarrhythmic flecainide, which is eliminated by both renal excretion and CYP2D6-mediated metabolism. Rare patients with both renal dysfunction and absent CYP2D6 activity (on a genetic basis or because of drug interactions) may develop severe adverse reactions related to high plasma concentrations.

ACTIVE DRUG METABOLITES A major role of drug metabolism is generation of more polar compounds that then readily undergo renal or biliary excretion. From an evolutionary point of view, drug metabolism probably developed as a defense against noxious xenobiotics (foreign substances, e.g., from plants) to which our ancestors inadvertently exposed themselves. The organization of the drug uptake and efflux pumps, and the location of drug metabolism in the intestine and liver prior to drug entry to the systemic circulation (Fig. 3-4), support this idea of a primitive protective function.

However, drug metabolites are not necessarily pharmacologically inactive. Metabolites may produce effects similar to, overlapping with, or distinct from those of the parent drug. For example, *N*-acetylprocainamide (NAPA) is a major metabolite of the antiarrhythmic procainamide. While it exerts antiarrhythmic effects, its electrophysiologic properties differ from those of the parent drug. Indeed, NAPA accumulation is the usual explanation for marked QT prolongation and torsades de pointes ventricular tachycardia (Chap. 214) during therapy with procainamide. Thus, the common laboratory practice of adding procainamide to NAPA concentrations to estimate a total therapeutic effect is inappropriate.

Some drugs are administered in an inactive form and require metabolism to generate active metabolites that mediate the drug effects. Examples include many angiotensin-converting enzyme (ACE) inhibitors and the analgesic codeine (whose active metabolite morphine probably underlies the opioid effect during codeine administration). Codeine and procainamide metabolism are also variable on a genetic basis, further contributing to variability in drug effects. Drug metabolism has also been implicated in bioactivation of procarcinogens and in generation of reactive metabolites that mediate certain adverse drug effects (e.g., acetaminophen hepatotoxicity, discussed below).

PRINCIPLES OF PHARMACODYNAMICS

Once a drug accesses a molecular site of action, it alters the function of that molecular target, with the ultimate result of a drug effect that the patient or physician can perceive. For drugs used in the urgent treatment of acute symptoms, little or no delay is anticipated (or desired) between the drug-target interaction and the development of a clinical effect. Examples include vascular thrombosis, shock, malignant hypertension, status epilepticus, or arrhythmias. For many conditions, however, the indication for therapy is less urgent, and in fact a delay between the interaction of a drug with its pharmacologic target(s) and a clinical effect is common. Pharmacokinetic mechanisms that can contribute to such a delay include uptake into peripheral compartments or generation and accumulation of active metabolites. A common pharmacodynamic mechanism is that the clinical effect develops as a downstream consequence of the initial molecular effect the drug produces. Thus, administration of a proton-pump inhibitor or an H_2-receptor blocker produces an immediate increase in gastric pH but ulcer healing that is delayed. Cancer chemotherapy inevitably produces delayed therapeutic effects, often long after drug is undetectable in plasma and tissue. Translation of a molecular drug action to a clinical effect can thus be highly complex and dependent on the details of the pathologic state being treated. These complexities have made pharmacodynamics and its variability less amenable than pharmacokinetics to rigorous mathematical analysis. Nevertheless, some clinically important principles can be elucidated.

A therapeutic drug effect assumes the presence of underlying pathophysiology. Thus, a drug may produce no action, or a different spectrum of actions, in unaffected individuals compared to patients. Further, concomitant disease can complicate interpretation of response to drug therapy, especially adverse effects. For example, increasing dyspnea in a patient with chronic lung disease receiving amiodarone therapy could be due to drug, underlying disease, or an intercurrent cardiopulmonary problem. Thus the presence of chronic lung disease, and interpretation of the symptom of increasing dyspnea, is one factor that should be considered in selection of antiarrhythmic therapies. Similarly, high doses of anticonvulsants such as phenytoin may cause neurologic symptoms, which may be confused with the underlying neurologic disease.

The concept that a drug interacts with a specific molecular receptor does not imply that the drug effect will be constant over time, even if stable drug and metabolite concentrations are maintained. The drug-receptor interaction occurs in a complex biologic milieu that itself can vary to modulate the drug effect. For example, ion channel blockade by drugs, an important anticonvulsant and antiarrhythmic effect, is often modulated by membrane potential, itself a function of factors such as extracellular potassium or ischemia. Thus, the effects of these drugs may vary depending on the external milieu. Receptors may be up- or downregulated by disease or by the drug itself. For example, β-adrenergic blockers upregulate β-receptor density during chronic therapy. While this effect does not usually result in resistance to the therapeutic effect of the drugs, it may produce severe β agonist–mediated effects (such as hypertension or tachycardia) if the blocking drug is abruptly withdrawn.

PRINCIPLES OF DOSE SELECTION

The desired goal of therapy with any drug is to maximize the likelihood of a beneficial effect while minimizing the risk of adverse effects. Previous experience with the drug, in controlled clinical trials or in postmarketing use, defines the relationships between dose (or plasma concentration) and these dual effects and provides a starting point for initiation of drug therapy.

Figure 3-1 illustrates the relationships among dose, plasma concentrations, efficacy, and adverse effects and carries with it several important implications:

1. *The target drug effect should be defined when drug treatment is started.* With some drugs, the desired effect may be difficult to measure objectively, and the onset of efficacy can be delayed for weeks or months; drugs used in the treatment of cancer and psychiatric disease are examples. Sometimes, a drug is used to treat a symptom, such as pain or palpitations, and here it is the patient who will report whether the selected dose is effective. In yet other settings, such as anticoagulation or hypertension, the desired response is readily measurable.

2. *The nature of anticipated toxicity often dictates the starting dose.* If side effects are minor, it may be acceptable to start at a dose highly likely to achieve efficacy and downtitrate if side effects occur. However, this approach is rarely if ever justified if the anticipated toxicity is serious or life-threatening; in this circumstance, it is more appropriate to initiate therapy with the lowest dose that may produce a desired effect.

3. *The above considerations do not apply if these relationships between dose and effects cannot be defined.* This is especially relevant to some adverse drug effects (discussed in further detail below) whose development is not readily related to drug dose.

4. *If a drug dose does not achieve its desired effect, a dosage increase is justified only if toxicity is absent and the likelihood of serious toxicity is small.* For example, a small percentage of patients with strong seizure foci require plasma levels of phenytoin >20 $\mu g/mL$ to control seizures. Dosages to achieve this effect may be appropriate, if tolerated. Conversely, clinical experience with flecainide suggests that levels >1000 ng/mL, or dosages >400 mg/d, may be associated with an increased risk of sudden death; thus dosage increases beyond these limits are ordinarily not appropriate, even if the higher dosage appears tolerated.

Other mechanisms that can lead to failure of drug effect should also be considered; drug interactions and noncompliance are common examples. This is one situation in which measurement of plasma drug concentrations, if available, can be especially useful. Noncompliance is an especially frequent problem in the long-term treatment of diseases such as hypertension and epilepsy, occurring in $\geq25\%$ of patients in therapeutic environments in which no special effort is made to involve patients in the responsibility for their own health. Multidrug regimens with multiple doses per day are especially prone to noncompliance.

Monitoring response to therapy, by physiologic measures or by plasma concentration measurements, requires an understanding of the relationships between plasma concentration and anticipated effects. For example, measurement of QT interval is used during treatment with sotalol or dofetilide to avoid marked QT prolongation that can herald serious arrhythmias. In this setting, evaluating the electrocardiogram at the time of anticipated peak plasma concentration and effect (e.g., 1 to 2 h postdose at steady state) is most appropriate. Maintained high aminoglycoside levels carry a risk of nephrotoxicity, so dosages should be adjusted on the basis of plasma concentrations measured at trough (predose). On the other hand, ensuring aminoglycoside efficacy is accomplished by adjusting dosage so that peak drug concentrations are above a minimal antibacterial concentration. For dose adjustment of other drugs (e.g., anticonvulsants, antiarrhythmics), concentration should be measured at its lowest during the dosing interval, just prior to a dose at steady state (Fig. 3-5), to ensure a maintained therapeutic effect.

CONCENTRATION OF DRUGS IN PLASMA AS A GUIDE TO THERAPY Factors such as interactions with other drugs, disease-induced alterations in elimination and distribution, and genetic variation in drug disposition combine to yield a wide range of plasma levels in patients given the same dose. Hence, if a predictable relationship can be established between plasma drug concentration and beneficial or adverse drug effect, measurement of plasma levels can provide a valuable tool to guide selection of an optimal dose. This is particularly true when there is a narrow range between the plasma levels yielding therapeutic and adverse effects, as with digoxin, theophylline, some antiarrhythmics, aminoglycosides, cyclosporine, and anticonvulsants. The common situation of first-order elimination implies that average, maximum, and minimum steady-state concentrations are related linearly to the dosing rate. Accordingly, the maintenance dose may be adjusted on the basis of the ratio between the desired and measured concentrations *at steady state*; for example if a doubling of the steady-state plasma concentration is desired, the dose should be doubled.

For drugs that have zero-order kinetics (e.g., phenytoin and theophylline), plasma concentrations change disproportionately more than the alteration in the dosing rate. In this situation, changes in dose should be small to minimize the degree of unpredictability, and plasma concentration monitoring should be used to ensure that dose modification achieves the desired level.

DETERMINATION OF MAINTENANCE DOSE An increase in dosage is usually best achieved by changing the drug dose but not the dosing interval, e.g., by giving 200 mg every 8 h instead of 100 mg every 8 h. However, this approach is acceptable only if the resulting maximum concentration is not toxic and the trough value does not fall below the minimum effective concentration for an undesirable period of time. Alternatively, the steady state may be changed by altering the frequency of intermittent dosing but not the size of each dose. In this case, the magnitude of the fluctuations around the average steady-state level will change—the shorter the dosing interval, the smaller the difference between peak and trough levels (Fig. 3-3).

Fluctuation within a dosing interval is determined by the relationship between the dosing interval and the drug's half-life. If the dosing interval is equal to the drug's half-life, fluctuation is about twofold, which is usually acceptable. With drugs that have a low therapeutic ratio, dosage changes should be conservative (<50% dose change) and not more frequent than every three to four half-lives. Other drugs, such as many antihypertensives, have little dose-related toxicity so the therapeutic ratio is large. Even if drug is eliminated rapidly, it can be given infrequently. Thus, 75 mg of captopril will result in reduced blood pressure for up to 12 h, even though captopril elimination half-life is about 2 h; this is because the dose raises the concentration of drug in plasma many times higher than the threshold for its pharmacologic effect.

EFFECTS OF DISEASE ON DRUG CONCENTRATION AND RESPONSE

RENAL DISEASE Renal excretion of parent drug and metabolites is generally accomplished by glomerular filtration and by specific drug transporters, only now being identified. If a drug or its metabolites are primarily excreted through the kidneys and increased drug levels are associated with adverse effects, drug dosages must be reduced in patients with renal dysfunction to avoid toxicity. The antiarrhythmics dofetilide and sotalol undergo predominant renal excretion and carry a risk of QT prolongation and arrhythmias if doses are not reduced in renal disease. Thus, in end-stage renal disease, sotalol can be given as 40 mg after dialysis (every second day), compared to the usual daily dose, 80 to 120 mg every 12 h. The narcotic analgesic meperidine undergoes extensive hepatic metabolism, so that renal failure has little effect on its plasma concentration. However, its metabolite, normeperidine, does undergo renal excretion, accumulates in renal failure, and probably accounts for the signs of central nervous system excitation, such as irritability, twitching, and seizures, that appear when multiple doses of meperidine are administered to patients with renal disease. Protein binding of some drugs (e.g., phenytoin) may be altered in uremia, so measuring free drug concentration may be desirable.

In non-end-stage renal disease, changes in renal drug clearance are generally proportional to those in creatinine clearance, which may be measured directly or estimated from the serum creatinine (Chap. 259). This estimate, coupled with the knowledge of how much drug is normally excreted renally vs nonrenally, allows an estimate of the dose adjustment required. In practice, most decisions involving dosing adjustment in patients with renal failure use published recommended adjustments in dosage or dosing interval based on the severity of renal

dysfunction indicated by creatinine clearance. Any such modification of dose is a first approximation and should be followed by plasma concentration data (if available) and clinical observation to further optimize therapy for the individual patient.

LIVER DISEASE In contrast to the predictable decline in renal clearance of drugs in renal insufficiency, the effects of hepatitis or cirrhosis on drug disposition range from impaired to increased drug clearance, in an unpredictable fashion. Standard tests of liver function are not useful in adjusting doses. First-pass metabolism may decrease, and thus oral bioavailability increase, as a consequence of disrupted hepatocyte function, altered liver architecture, and portacaval shunts. The oral availability for high-first-pass drugs such as morphine, meperidine, midazolam, and nifedipine is almost doubled in patients with cirrhosis, compared to those with normal liver function. Therefore, the size of the oral dose of such drugs should be reduced in this setting.

HEART FAILURE AND SHOCK Under conditions of decreased tissue perfusion, the cardiac output is redistributed to preserve blood flow to the heart and brain at the expense of other tissues (Chap. 216). As a result, drugs may be distributed into a smaller volume of distribution, higher drug concentrations will be present in the plasma, and the tissues that are best perfused (the brain and heart) will be exposed to these higher concentrations. If either the brain or heart is sensitive to the drug, an alteration in response will occur. As well, decreased perfusion of the kidney and liver may impair drug clearance. Thus, in severe congestive heart failure, in hemorrhagic shock, and in cardiogenic shock, response to usual drug doses may be excessive, and dosage reduction may be necessary. For example, the clearance of lidocaine is reduced by about 50% in heart failure, and therapeutic plasma levels are achieved at infusion rates only about half those usually required. The volume of distribution of lidocaine is also reduced, so loading regimens should be reduced.

DRUG USE IN THE ELDERLY Aging results in changes in organ function, especially of the organs involved in drug disposition. Therefore, pharmacokinetics are often different in elderly individuals than in younger adults. In the elderly, multiple pathologies and medications used to treat them result in more drug interactions and adverse effects.

Even in the absence of kidney disease, renal clearance may be reduced by 35 to 50% in elderly patients. Dosage adjustments are therefore necessary for drugs that are eliminated mainly by the kidneys. Because muscle mass and therefore creatinine production are reduced in older individuals, a normal serum creatinine concentration can be present even though creatinine clearance is impaired; dosages should be adjusted on the basis of creatinine clearance, as discussed above. Aging also results in a decrease in the size of and blood flow to the liver and possibly in the activity of hepatic drug-metabolizing enzymes; accordingly, the hepatic clearance of some drugs is impaired in the elderly. As with liver disease, these changes are not readily predicted.

Elderly patients may display altered drug sensitivity. Examples include increased analgesic effects of opioids, increased sedation from benzodiazepines and other CNS depressants, and increased risk of bleeding while receiving anticoagulant therapy, even when clotting parameters are well controlled. Exaggerated responses to cardiovascular drugs are also common because of the impaired responsiveness of normal homeostatic mechanisms. Conversely, the elderly display decreased sensitivity to β-adrenergic receptor blockers.

Adverse drug reactions are especially common in the elderly, because of altered pharmacokinetics and pharmacodynamics, the frequent use of multidrug regimens, and concomitant disease. For example, use of long half-life benzodiazepines is linked to the occurrence of hip fractures in elderly patients, perhaps reflecting both a risk of falls from these drugs (due to increased sedation) and the increased incidence of osteoporosis in elderly patients. In population surveys of the noninstitutionalized elderly, as many as 10% had at least one adverse drug reaction in the previous year.

Accordingly, optimization of drug therapy in the elderly, particularly in frail patients, is often difficult, as these multiple factors accentuate interindividual variability in drug response. Initial doses should be less than the usual adult dosage and should be increased slowly. The number of medications, and doses per day, should be kept as low as possible.

GENETIC DETERMINANTS OF THE RESPONSE TO DRUGS

PRINCIPLES OF GENETIC VARIATION AND HUMAN TRAITS (See also Chap. 58) Variants in the human genome resulting in variation in level of expression or function of molecules important for pharmacokinetics and pharmacodynamics are increasingly recognized. These may be mutations (very rare variants, often associated with disease) or polymorphisms, variants that are much more common in a population. Variants may occur at a single nucleotide or involve insertion or deletion of one or more nucleotides. They may be in the exons (coding regions) or introns. Exonic polymorphisms may or may not alter the encoded protein, and variant proteins may or may not display altered function. Similarly, polymorphisms in intronic regions (including those that regulate gene expression) may or may not alter protein level.

As variation in the human genome is increasingly well documented, associations are being described between polymorphisms and various traits (including response to drug therapy). Some of these rely on well-developed chains of evidence, including in vitro studies demonstrating variant protein function, familial aggregation of variant allele with the trait, and association studies in large populations. In other cases, the associations are less compelling. Identifying "real" associations is one challenge that must be overcome before genomics, and in particular the concept of genotyping to identify optimal drugs (or dosages) in individual patients prior to prescribing, can be considered for widespread clinical practice. Nevertheless, the appeal of this approach is considerable.

Rates of drug efficacy and adverse effects often vary among ethnic groups. Many explanations for such differences are plausible; genomic approaches have now established that functionally important variants determining differences in drug response often display differing distributions among ethnic groups. This finding may have importance for drug use among ethnic groups, as well as in drug development.

GENETICALLY DETERMINED DRUG DISPOSITION AND VARIABLE EFFECTS The concept that genetically determined variations in drug metabolism might be associated with variant drug levels, and hence effect, was advanced at the end of the nineteenth century, and the first examples of familial clustering of unusual drug responses due to this mechanism were noted in the mid-twentieth century. Clinically important genetic variants have been described in multiple molecular pathways of drug disposition (Table 3-1). These variants are identified either by directly establishing DNA sequence (genotyping) or by phenotyping: exposing a large group of otherwise healthy subjects to a specific probe substrate for the metabolizing enzyme under study and observing the distribution of activity (Fig. 3-6). A distinct multimodal distribution argues for a predominant effect of variants in a single gene in the metabolism of that substrate. Individuals with two alleles (variants) encoding for nonfunctional protein make up one group, often termed *poor metabolizers* (PM phenotype); many variants can produce such a loss of function, complicating the use of genotyping in clinical practice. Individuals with one functional allele make up a second (*intermediate metabolizers*), and those with two functional alleles a third (*extensive metabolizers*, EMs). On the other hand, a unimodal distribution of activity argues against the presence of important single loss-of-function alleles in the population under study.

Transferase Variants Of the variants in genes encoding drug-metabolizing enzymes that have been described to date, one, in the *TPMT* gene, has been adopted as routine clinical practice in some specialized centers. TPMT bioinactivates the antileukemic drug 6-mercaptopurine. Further, 6-mercaptopurine is itself an active metabolite of the immunosuppressive azathioprine. Homozygotes for alleles encoding the inactive TPMT (1 in 300 individuals) predictably exhibit severe and potentially fatal pancytopenia on standard doses of azathioprine or 6-mercaptopurine. On the other hand, homozygotes for fully functional alleles may display less anti-inflammatory or antileukemic effect with the drugs. These data illustrate the potential power of a genomic approach to optimize therapy, especially in the setting of high-risk pharmacokinetics.

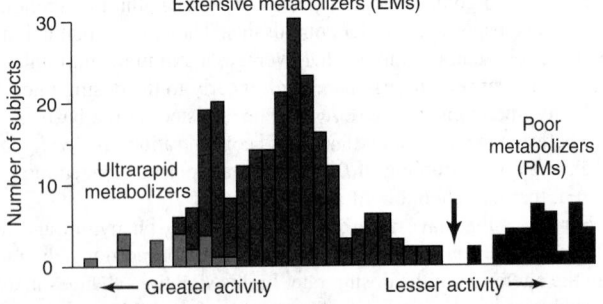

FIGURE 3-6   CYP2D6 metabolic activity was assessed in 290 subjects by administration of a test dose of a probe substrate and measurement of urinary formation of the CYP2D6-generated metabolite. The heavy arrow indicates a clear antimode, separating poor metabolizer subjects (black), with two loss-of-function CYP2D6 alleles. Individuals with one or two functional alleles are grouped together as extensive metabolizers (blue). Also shown are ultrarapid metabolizers, with 2 to 11 functional copies of the gene (red) and 12 functional copies (green), displaying the greatest enzyme activity. *(Adapted by permission from M-L Dahl et al: J Pharmacol Exp Ther 274:516, 1995.)*

N-acetylation is catalyzed by hepatic *N*-acetyl transferase (NAT), which actually represents the activity of two genes, *NAT-1* and *NAT-2*. Both enzymes transfer an acetyl group from acetyl coenzyme A to the drug; NAT-1 activity is generally constant, while polymorphisms in *NAT-2* result in individual differences in the rate at which drugs are acetylated and thus define "rapid acetylators" and "slow acetylators." Slow acetylators make up ~50% of European- and African-derived populations but are less common among Asians.

Slow acetylators have an increased incidence of the drug-induced lupus syndrome during procainamide and hydralazine therapy and of hepatitis with isoniazid. Induction of CYPs (e.g., by rifampin) also increases the risk of isoniazid-related hepatitis, likely reflecting generation of reactive metabolites of acetylhydrazine, itself an isoniazid metabolite.

Polymorphisms that reduce transcription of uridine diphosphate glucuronosyltransferase (*UGT1A1*) cause benign hyperbilirubinemia (Gilbert's disease; Chap. 284). These have also been associated with diarrhea and increased bone marrow depression with the antineoplastic irinotecan, whose active metabolite is normally detoxified by this pathway.

CYP Variants   CYP3A4 is the most abundant hepatic and intestinal CYP and is also the enzyme responsible for metabolism of the greatest number of drugs in therapeutic use. CYP3A4 activity is highly variable (up to an order of magnitude) among individuals, but the distribution is unimodal, suggesting that the variability does not arise from variants in the *CYP3A4* gene. The mechanisms underlying this variability are not yet well understood. A closely related gene, encoding CYP3A5 (which shares substrates with CYP3A4), does display loss-of-function variants, especially in African-derived populations. CYP3A refers to both enzymes.

CYP2D6 accounts for very little total hepatic CYP by weight but is second to CYP3A4 in the number of commonly used drugs that it metabolizes. CYP2D6 is polymorphically distributed, with about 7% of European- and African-derived populations (but very few Asians) displaying the PM phenotype (Fig. 3-6). Over 70 loss-of-function variants in the CYP2D6 gene have been described; the PM phenotype arises in individuals with two such alleles. In addition, individuals with multiple functional copies of the CYP2D6 gene (ultrarapid metabolizers) have been identified, particularly among northern Africans. CYP2D6 represents the main metabolic pathway for a number of drugs

(Table 3-1). Codeine is biotransformed by CYP2D6 to the potent active metabolite morphine, so its effects are blunted in PMs and exaggerated in ultrarapid metabolizers. With beta blockers metabolized by CYP2D6 (including ophthalmic timolol and the antiarrhythmic propafenone), PM subjects display greater signs of beta blockade (including bradycardia and bronchospasm) than EMs. Further, in EM subjects, propafenone elimination becomes nonlinear at higher doses so, for example, a tripling of the dose may lead to a tenfold increase in drug concentration. The oral hypoglycemic agent phenformin was withdrawn because it occasionally caused profound lactic acidosis; this likely arose as a result of high concentrations in CYP2D6 PMs. Ultrarapid metabolizers may require very high dosages of tricyclic antidepressants to achieve a therapeutic effect, and with codeine may display transient euphoria and nausea due to very rapid generation of morphine.

The PM phenotype for CYP2C19 is common (20%) among Asians, and rarer (3 to 5%) in European-derived populations. The impact of polymorphic CYP2C19-mediated metabolism has been demonstrated with the proton pump inhibitor omeprazole, where ulcer cure rates with "standard" dosages were markedly lower in EM patients (29%) than in PMs (100%). Thus, understanding the importance of this polymorphism would have been important in developing the drug, and knowing a patient's CYP2C19 genotype should improve therapy.

There are common allelic variants of *CYP2C9* that encode proteins with loss of catalytic function. These variant alleles are associated with a requirement for lower maintenance dose of warfarin. In rarer (<2%) individuals homozygous for these variant alleles, maintenance warfarin dosages may be difficult to establish, and the risk of bleeding complications appears increased. Similarly, patients with loss-of-function CYP2C9 alleles display increased rates of neurologic complications with phenytoin and of hypoglycemia with glipizide.

VARIABILITY IN THE MOLECULAR TARGETS WITH WHICH DRUGS INTERACT
As molecular approaches identify specific gene products as targets of drug action, polymorphisms that alter the expression or function of these drug targets—and thus modulate their actions in patients—are also being recognized. For example, genome-wide searches in families with premature Alzheimer's disease have associated variants in the *APOE* locus with the disease (Chap. 350). The *E4* allele of the gene has been associated with a worse prognosis, a finding that has been attributed to reduced expression of choline acetyltransferase. Further, this polymorphism is also linked to response to the acetylcholinesterase inhibitor tacrine; a beneficial response appears to be more common in patients with the prognostically more benign *APOE2* or *APOE3* alleles (in which the target molecule is expressed more abundantly).

Multiple polymorphisms identified in the β_2-adrenergic receptor appear to be linked to specific phenotypes in asthma and congestive heart failure, diseases in which β_2-receptor function might be expected to determine prognosis. Polymorphisms in the β_2-receptor gene have also been associated with response to inhaled β_2-receptor agonists, while those in the β_1-adrenergic receptor gene have been associated with variability in heart rate slowing and blood pressure lowering. Similarly, response to the 5-lipoxygenase inhibitor zileuton in asthma has been linked to polymorphisms that determine the expression level of the 5-lipoxygenase gene. Herceptin, which potentiates anthracycline-related cardiotoxicity, is ineffective in breast cancers that do not express the herceptin receptor; thus, "genotyping" the tumor is a mechanism to avoid potentially toxic therapy in patients who would derive no benefit.

Drugs may also interact with genetic pathways of disease, to elicit or exacerbate symptoms of the underlying conditions. In the porphyrias, CYP inducers are thought to increase the activity of enzymes proximal to the deficient enzyme, exacerbating or triggering attacks (Chap. 337). Deficiency of glucose-6-phosphate dehydrogenase (G6PD), most often in individuals of African or Mediterranean descent, increases risk of hemolytic anemia in response to primaquine and a number of other drugs that do not cause hemolysis in patients with adequate quantities of this enzyme (Chap. 93). Patients with mutations in the ryanodine

receptor that controls intracellular calcium in skeletal muscle and other tissues may be asymptomatic until exposed to certain general anesthetics, which trigger the syndrome of malignant hyperthermia. Certain antiarrhythmics and other drugs can produce marked QT prolongation and torsades de pointes (Chap. 214), and in some patients this adverse effect represents unmasking of previously subclinical congenital long QT syndrome.

POLYMORPHISMS THAT MODULATE THE BIOLOGIC CONTEXT WITHIN WHICH THE DRUG-TARGET INTERACTIONS OCCUR The interaction of a drug with its molecular target is translated into a clinical action in a complex biologic milieu that is itself often perturbed by disease. Thus, polymorphisms that determine variability in this biology may profoundly influence drug response, although the genes involved are not themselves directly targets of drug action. The common insertion/deletion (I/D) polymorphism in the ACE gene determines prognosis in many types of heart disease, including heart failure. In patients with heart failure treated with β-adrenergic blockers, the best response to therapy has been associated with the DD genotype, the group with the worst prognosis. The mechanism underlying this outcome is uncertain, but a direct effect of beta blockers on ACE seems unlikely; rather the I/D genotype likely affects the biology of heart failure to allow an improved response to beta blockers. Similarly, polymorphisms in genes important for lipid homeostasis (such as the ABCA1 transporter and the cholesterol ester transport protein) modulate response to HMG-CoA reductase inhibitors. In one large study, the combination of diuretic use combined with a variant in the adducin gene (encoding a cytoskeletal protein important for renal tubular sodium absorption) decreased stroke or myocardial infarction risk, while neither factor alone has an effect. Common polymorphisms in ion channel genes that are not themselves the target of QT-prolonging drugs may nevertheless influence the extent to which those drugs affect the electrocardiogram and produce arrhythmias.

PROSPECTS FOR INCORPORATING GENETIC INFORMATION INTO CLINICAL PRACTICE
These and many other examples of associations between specific genotypes and drug responses raise the tantalizing prospect that patients will undergo routine genotyping for loci known to modulate drug levels or response prior to receiving a prescription. The twin goals are to identify patients likely to exhibit adverse effects and those most likely to respond well. Obstacles that must be overcome before this vision becomes a reality include replication of even the most compelling associations, demonstrations of cost-effectiveness, development of readily useable genotyping technologies, and ethical issues involved in genotyping. While these barriers seem daunting, the field is very young and evolving rapidly. Indeed, one major result of understanding of the role of genetics in drug action has been improved screening of drugs during the development process to reduce the likelihood of highly variable metabolism or unanticipated toxicity (such as torsades de pointes).

INTERACTIONS BETWEEN DRUGS

Drug interactions can complicate therapy by adversely increasing or decreasing the action of a drug; interactions may be based on changes in drug disposition or in drug response in the absence of changes in drug levels. *Interactions must be considered in the differential diagnosis of any unusual response occurring during drug therapy.* Prescribers should recognize that patients often come to them with a legacy of drugs acquired during previous medical experiences, often with multiple physicians who may not be aware of all the patient's medications. A meticulous drug history should include examination of the patient's medications and, if necessary, calls to the pharmacist to identify prescriptions. It should also address the use of agents not often volunteered during questioning, such as over-the-counter (OTC) drugs, health food supplements, and topical agents such as eye drops. Lists of interactions are available from a number of electronic sources. The practicing physician cannot be expected to memorize these. How-

Drug	Mechanism	Examples
Antacids; bile acid sequestrants	Reduced absorption	Antacids/tetracyclines; cholestryamine/digoxin
Proton pump inhibitors; H_2-receptor blockers	Altered gastric pH	Ketoconazole absorption decreased
Rifampin; carbamazepine; barbiturates; phenytoin; St. John's wort; glutethimide	Induction of hepatic metabolism	Decreased concentration and effects of: warfarin; quinidine; cyclosporine; losartan
Tricyclic antidepressants; fluoxetine; quinidine	Inhibitors of CYP2D6	Increased beta blockade; decreased codeine effect
Cimetidine	Inhibitor of multiple CYPs	Increased concentration and effects of: warfarin; theophylline; phenytoin
Ketoconazole, itraconazole; erythromycin, clarithromycin; calcium channel blockers; ritonavir	Inhibitor of CYP3A	Increased concentration and toxicity of: some HMG-CoA reductase inhibitors; cyclosporine; cisapride, terfenadine (now withdrawn) Increased concentration and effects of: indinavir (with ritonavir); Decreased clearance and dose requirement for: cyclosporine (with calcium channel blockers)
Allopurinol	Xanthine oxidase inhibitor	Azathioprine and 6-mercaptopurine toxicity
Amiodarone	Inhibitor of many CYPs and of P-glycoprotein	Decreased clearance (risk of toxicity) for: warfarin; digoxin; quinidine
Gemfibrozil (and other fibrates)	CYP3A inhibition	Rhabdomyolysis when co-prescribed with some HMG-CoA reductase inhibitors
Quinidine; amiodarone; verapamil; cyclosporine; itraconazole; erythromycin	P-glycoprotein inhibition	Risk of digoxin toxicity
Phenylbutazone, probenecid; salicylates	Inhibition of renal tubular transport	Salicylates → increased risk of methotrexate toxicity

ever, certain drugs consistently run the risk of generating interactions, through mechanisms that are well understood; examples (not an exhaustive listing) are presented below and in Table 3-2. When such drugs are started or stopped, prescribers must be especially alert to the possibility of interactions.

PHARMACOKINETIC INTERACTIONS CAUSING DIMINISHED DRUG DELIVERY TO TARGET SITES ■ Impaired Gastrointestinal Absorption Aluminum ions, present in antacids, can form insoluble chelates with the tetracyclines, preventing their absorption. Kaolin-pectin suspensions bind digoxin, and when the substances are administered together, digoxin absorption is reduced by about one-half. Resins that sequester bile acids in the gut can bind other drugs, such as digoxin. Ketoconazole is a weak base that dissolves well only at acidic pH. Histamine H_2 receptor antagonists and proton pump inhibitors reduce gastric acidity and thus impair the dissolution and absorption of ketoconazole.

Induction of CYP or Transporter Activity Expression of some genes responsible for drug elimination, notably *CYP3A* and *MDR1*, can be markedly increased by "inducing" drugs, such as rifampin, carbamazepine, phenytoin, St. John's wort, and glutethimide and by smoking, exposure to chlorinated insecticides such as DDT (CYP1A2), and chronic alcohol ingestion. One mechanism for this coordinate induction of multiple pathways is increased expression of common transcription factors (e.g., hepatocyte nuclear factor 4α). Administration of inducing agents lowers plasma levels over 2 to 3 weeks as gene expression is increased. This alters the effects of many drugs, including warfarin, quinidine, mexiletine, verapamil, ketoconazole, itraconazole, cyclosporine, dexamethasone, methylprednisolone, prednisolone (the active metabolite of prednisone), oral contraceptive steroids, methadone, and metronidazole. These interactions all have obvious clinical significance. Further, if a drug dose is stabilized in the presence of an inducer which is subsequently stopped, major toxicity can occur as clearance returns to preinduction levels and drug concentrations rise. This is a particular problem with narrow-therapeutic-ratio drugs such as warfarin and some antiarrhythmics. Individuals vary in the extent to which drug metabolism can be induced, likely through genetic mechanisms.

Inhibition of Cellular Uptake or Binding Tricyclic antidepressants, doxepin, and chlorpromazine are potent inhibitors of norepinephrine uptake into adrenergic neurons and prevent the uptake of the guanidinium antihypertensive agents (such as guanethidine and guanadrel), thereby abolishing their antihypertensive effects. Similarly, the antihypertensive effect of clonidine is partially antagonized by tricyclic antidepressants.

PHARMACOKINETIC INTERACTIONS CAUSING INCREASED DRUG DELIVERY TO TARGET SITES ■ Inhibition of Drug Metabolism Inhibition of drug metabolism can lead to reduced clearance, prolonged half-life, accumulation of drug during maintenance therapy, and thus adverse effects. In contrast to induction, new protein synthesis is not involved, and the effect develops as drug and any inhibitor metabolites accumulate (a function of their elimination half-lives). Since shared substrates of a single enzyme can compete for access to the active site of the protein, many CYP substrates can also be considered inhibitors. However, some drugs are especially potent as inhibitors (and occasionally may not even be substrates); it is in the use of agents of the latter type that clinicians must be most alert to the potential for interactions.

Cimetidine (but not other H_2-receptor blockers) is a potent inhibitor of the oxidative metabolism of many drugs, including warfarin, quinidine, nifedipine, lidocaine, theophylline, and phenytoin. Severe adverse reactions can develop as a consequence.

The antifungal agents ketoconazole and itraconazole are potent inhibitors of enzymes in the CYP3A family. When fluconazole levels are elevated as a result of higher doses and/or renal insufficiency, this drug can also inhibit CYP3A. The macrolide antibiotics erythromycin and clarithromycin inhibit CYP3A4 to a clinically significant extent, but azithromycin does not. Some of the calcium channel blockers, including diltiazem, nicardipine, and verapamil can also inhibit CYP3A, as can some of the enzyme's substrates, such as cyclosporine. Examples of CYP3A substrates also include quinidine, lovastatin, simvastatin, atorvastatin, nifedipine, lidocaine, erythromycin, methylprednisolone, carbamazepine, midazolam, and triazolam.

Phenytoin, an inducer of many systems including CYP3A, inhibits CYP2C9. CYP2C9 metabolism of losartan to its active metabolite is inhibited by phenytoin, with potential loss of antihypertensive effect.

Accumulation of the prokinetic drug cisapride and the antihistamine terfenadine due to CYP3A inhibition led to QT prolongation and torsades de pointes. Measures to prevent co-prescription of these agents with CYP3A inhibitors were unsuccessful, and alternative safer agents were developed, so these drugs were eventually withdrawn.

Cyclosporine can cause serious toxicity when its metabolism via CYP3A4 is inhibited by erythromycin, ketoconazole, diltiazem, nicardipine, or verapamil. The risk of myopathy with some HMG-CoA reductase inhibitors (lovastatin, simvastatin, atorvastatin) is thought to be increased by CYP3A4 inhibition. One agent in this class, cerivastatin, was withdrawn because of an especially high incidence of this adverse effect, although cellular studies suggest inhibition of other pathways may have also contributed in this case. The antiviral ritonavir is a very potent CYP3A4 inhibitor that is often added to anti-HIV regimens not because of its antiviral effects but because it decreases clearance, and hence increases efficacy, of other anti-HIV agents. Grapefruit (but not orange) juice inhibits CYP3A, especially at high doses; patients receiving drugs where even modest CYP3A inhibition may increase the risk of adverse effects (e.g., cyclosporine, some HMG-CoA reductase inhibitors) should therefore avoid grapefruit juice.

CYP2D6 is markedly inhibited by quinidine and is also blocked by a number of neuroleptic drugs, such as chlorpromazine and haloperidol, and by fluoxetine. The analgesic effect of codeine depends on its metabolism to morphine via CYP2D6. Thus, quinidine reduces the analgesic efficacy of codeine in EMs. Since desipramine is cleared largely by metabolism via CYP2D6 in EMs, its levels are increased substantially by concurrent administration of quinidine, fluoxetine, or the neuroleptic drugs that inhibit CYP2D6. Clinical consequences of fluoxetine's interaction with CYP2D6 substrates may not be apparent for weeks after the drug is started, because of its very long half-life and slow generation of a CYP2D6-inhibiting metabolite.

6-Mercaptopurine, the active metabolite of azathioprine, is metabolized not only by TPMT but also by xanthine oxidase. When allopurinol, a potent inhibitor of xanthine oxidase, is administered with standard doses of azathioprine or 6-mercaptopurine, life-threatening toxicity (bone marrow suppression) can result.

Inhibition of Drug Transport The best studied example is P-glycoprotein (Fig. 3-4). Quinidine inhibits P-glycoprotein function in vitro, and it now appears that the long-recognized doubling of plasma digoxin when quinidine is coadministered reflects this action in vivo, particularly since the effects of quinidine (increased digoxin bioavailability and reduced renal and hepatic secretion) occur at the sites of P-glycoprotein expression. Many other drugs also elevate digoxin concentrations (e.g., amiodarone, verapamil, cyclosporine, itraconazole, and erythromcyin), and a similar mechanism seems likely. Reduced CNS penetration of multiple HIV protease inhibitors (with the attendant risk of facilitating viral replication in a sanctuary site) appears attributable to P-glycoprotein-mediated exclusion of the drug from the CNS; thus inhibition of P-glycoprotein has been proposed as a therapeutic approach to enhance drug entry to the CNS.

A number of drugs are secreted by the renal tubular transport systems for organic anions. Inhibition of these systems can cause excessive drug accumulation. Salicylate, for example, reduces the renal clearance of methotrexate, an interaction that may lead to methotrexate toxicity. Renal tubular secretion contributes substantially to the elimination of penicillin, which can be inhibited (to increase its therapeutic effect) by probenecid.

Inhibition of the tubular cation transport system by cimetidine decreases the renal clearance of dofetilide and of procainamide and its active metabolite NAPA.

DRUG INTERACTIONS NOT MEDIATED BY CHANGES IN DRUG DISPOSITION Drugs may act on separate components of a common process to generate effects greater than either has alone. For example, although small doses of aspirin (<1 g daily) do not alter the prothrombin time appreciably in patients who are receiving warfarin therapy, aspirin nevertheless increases the risk of bleeding in these patients because it inhibits platelet aggregation. Thus the combination of impaired functions of platelets and of the clotting system, while useful in some patients, also increases the potential for hemorrhagic complications. Similarly, the use of other anticlotting agents (heparin, glycoprotein IIb/IIIa inhibitors, clopidogrel) with aspirin improves outcomes in acute coronary syndromes, while exacerbating this bleeding tendency.

Nonsteroidal anti-inflammatory drugs (NSAIDs) cause gastric ulcers, and, in patients treated with warfarin, the risk of bleeding from a peptic ulcer is increased almost threefold by concomitant use of a NSAID.

Indomethacin, piroxicam, and probably other NSAIDs antagonize the antihypertensive effects of β-adrenergic receptor blockers, diuretics, ACE inhibitors, and other drugs. The resulting elevation in blood pressure ranges from trivial to severe. This effect is not seen with aspirin and sulindac but has been found with cyclooxygenase-2 inhibitors (celecoxib, rofecoxib).

Torsades de pointes during administration of QT-prolonging antiarrhythmics (quinidine, sotalol, dofetilide) occur much more frequently in those patients receiving diuretics, probably reflecting hypokalemia. In vitro, hypokalemia not only prolongs the QT interval in the absence of drug but also potentiates drug block of ion channels that results in QT prolongation. Also, some diuretics have direct electrophysiologic actions that prolong QT.

The administration of supplemental potassium leads to more frequent and more severe hyperkalemia when potassium elimination is reduced by concurrent treatment with ACE inhibitors, spironolactone, amiloride, or triamterene.

The pharmacologic effects of sildenafil result from inhibition of the phosphodiesterase type 5 isoform that inactivates cyclic GMP in the vasculature. Nitroglycerin and related nitrates used to treat angina produce vasodilation by elevating cyclic GMP. Thus, coadministration of these nitrates with sildenafil can cause profound hypotension, which can be catastrophic in patients with coronary disease.

Sometimes, combining drugs can increase overall efficacy and/or reduce drug-specific toxicity. Such therapeutically useful interactions are described in chapters dealing with specific disease entities, elsewhere in this text.

ADVERSE REACTIONS TO DRUGS

The beneficial effects of drugs are coupled with the inescapable risk of untoward effects. The morbidity and mortality from these untoward effects often present diagnostic problems because they can involve every organ and system of the body and are frequently mistaken for signs of underlying disease. Major advances in the investigation, development, and regulation of drugs ensure in most instances that drugs are uniform, effective, and relatively safe and that their recognized hazards are publicized. However, prior to regulatory approval and marketing, new drugs are tested in relatively few patients who tend to be less sick and to have fewer concomitant diseases than those patients who subsequently receive the drug therapeutically. Because of the relatively small number of patients studied in clinical trials, and the selected nature of these patients, rare adverse effects may not be detected prior to a drug's approval, and physicians therefore need to be cautious in the prescription of new drugs and alert for the appearance of previously unrecognized adverse events. Often, these adverse reactions are rare, such as hematologic abnormalities, arrhythmias, hepatitis, or renal dysfunction. In these cases, often (but inappropriately) labeled "idiosyncratic," elucidating underlying mechanisms can assist development of safer compounds or allow a patient subset at especially high risk to be excluded from drug exposure. National adverse reaction reporting systems, such as those operated by the U.S. Food and Drug Administration (suspected adverse reactions can be reported online at *http://www.fda.gov/medwatch/report/hcp.htm*) and the Committee on Safety of Medicines in Great Britain, can prove useful. The publication or reporting of a newly recognized adverse reaction can in a short time stimulate many similar such reports of reactions that previously had gone unrecognized.

Occasionally, "adverse" effects may be exploited to develop an entirely new indication for a drug. Unwanted hair growth during minoxidil treatment of severely hypertensive patients led to development of the drug for hair growth. Sildenafil was initially developed as an antianginal, but its effects to alleviate erectile dysfunction not only led to a new drug indication but also to increased understanding of the role of type 5 phosphodiesterase in erectile tissue. These examples further reinforce the concept that prescribers must remain vigilant to the possibility that unusual symptoms may reflect unappreciated drug effects.

The large number and variety of drugs and herbal remedies available OTC as well as by prescription make it impossible for patient or physician to obtain or retain the knowledge necessary to use all drugs well. It is understandable, therefore, that many OTC drugs are used unwisely by the public and that restricted drugs may be prescribed incorrectly by physicians.

Some 25 to 50% of patients make errors in self-administration of prescribed medicines, and these errors can be responsible for adverse drug effects. Elderly patients are the group most likely to commit such errors, perhaps in part because they consume more medicines. One-third or more of patients also may not take their prescribed medications. Similarly, patients commit errors in taking OTC drugs by not reading or following the directions on the containers. Physicians must recognize that providing directions with prescriptions does not always guarantee compliance.

In hospital, drugs are administered in a controlled setting, and patient compliance is, in general, ensured. Errors may occur nevertheless—the wrong drug or dose may be given or the drug may be given to the wrong patient—and improved drug distribution and administration systems are addressing this problem. On the other hand, there are no easy means for controlling how ambulatory patients take prescription or OTC drugs.

EPIDEMIOLOGY   Patients receive, on average, 10 different drugs during each hospitalization. The sicker the patient, the more drugs are given, and there is a corresponding increase in the likelihood of adverse drug reactions. When <6 different drugs are given to hospitalized patients the probability of an adverse reaction is ~5%, but if >15 drugs are given, the probability is >40%. Retrospective analyses of ambulatory patients have revealed adverse drug effects in 20%. Serious adverse reactions are also well recognized with "herbal" remedies and OTC compounds: examples include kava-associated hepatotoxicity, L-tryptophan-associated eosinophilia-myalgia, and phenylpropanolamine-associated stroke, each of which has caused fatalities.

A 2000 Institute of Medicine report indicated that 7000 Americans die annually because of medication errors, that 2 to 3% of hospital admissions are for illnesses attributed to drugs, that the in-hospital cost was >$2 billion, and that this represents a tiny fraction of the overall problem of medication errors and its costs. A small group of widely used drugs accounts for a disproportionate number of reactions. Aspirin and other NSAIDs, analgesics, digoxin, anticoagulants, diuretics, antimicrobials, glucocorticoids, antineoplastics, and hypoglycemic agents account for 90% of reactions, although the drugs involved differ between ambulatory and hospitalized patients.

ETIOLOGY   Most adverse drug reactions are preventable, and recent studies using a systems analysis approach suggest that the most common system failure associated with an adverse drug reaction is the failure to disseminate knowledge about drugs to individuals who prescribe and administer them. Most adverse reactions may be classified in two groups. The most frequent ones result from exaggeration of an intended pharmacologic action of the drug, and the underlying mechanisms have been discussed above. Other adverse reactions ensue from toxic effects unrelated to the intended pharmacologic actions. The latter effects are often unpredictable and frequently severe, and result from recognized as well as undiscovered mechanisms.

TOXICITY UNRELATED TO A DRUG'S PRIMARY PHARMACOLOGIC ACTIVITY ■ Cytotoxic Reactions   Drug or more commonly reactive metabolites generated by CYPs can covalently bind to tissue macromolecules (such as proteins or DNA) to cause tissue toxicity. Because of the reactive nature of these metabolites covalent binding often occurs close to the site of production; this is typically the liver, although CYPs are found in other tissues as well.

The most common cause of drug-induced hepatotoxicity is acetaminophen overdosage. Normally, reactive metabolites are detoxified by combining with hepatic glutathione. When glutathione becomes exhausted, the metabolites bind instead to hepatic protein, with resultant hepatocyte damage. The hepatic necrosis produced by the ingestion of acetaminophen can be prevented, or at least attenuated, by the administration of substances such as N-acetylcysteine that reduce the binding of electrophilic metabolites to hepatic proteins. The risk of hepatic necrosis is increased in patients receiving drugs such as phenobarbital or phenytoin that increase the rate of drug metabolism or ethanol that exhaust glutathione stores. Such toxicity has even occurred with therapeutic dosages, so patients at risk through these mechanisms should be warned.

Immunologic Mechanisms   Most pharmacologic agents are small molecules with low molecular weights (<2000) and thus are poor immunogens. Generation of an immune response to a drug therefore usually requires in vivo activation and covalent linkage to protein, carbohydrate, or nucleic acid.

Drug stimulation of antibody production may mediate tissue injury by several mechanisms. The antibody may attack the drug when the drug is covalently attached to a cell, and thereby destroy the cell. This occurs in penicillin-induced hemolytic anemia. Antibody-drug-antigen complexes may be passively adsorbed by a bystander cell, which is then destroyed by activation of complement; this occurs in quinine- and quinidine-induced thrombocytopenia. Heparin-induced thrombocytopenia arises when antibodies against complexes of platelet factor 4 peptide and heparin generate immune complexes that activate platelets; thus the thrombocytopenia is accompanied by "paradoxical" thrombosis and is treated with thrombin inhibitors. Drugs or their reactive metabolites may alter a host tissue, rendering it antigenic and eliciting autoantibodies. For example, hydralazine and procainamide (or their reactive metabolites) can chemically alter nuclear material, stimulating the formation of antinuclear antibodies and occasionally causing lupus erythematosus. Autoantibodies can be elicited by drugs that neither interact with the host antigen nor have any chemical similarity to the host tissue; for example, the antihypertensive α-methyldopa frequently stimulates the formation of antibodies to host erythrocytes, yet the drug neither attaches to the erythrocyte nor shares any chemical similarities with the antigenic determinants on the erythrocyte. Drug-induced pure red cell aplasia (Chap. 94) is due to an immune-based drug reaction. Red cell formation in bone marrow cultures can be inhibited by phenytoin and purified IgG obtained from a patient with pure red cell aplasia associated with phenytoin.

Serum sickness (Chap. 298) results from the deposition of circulating drug-antibody complexes on endothelial surfaces. Complement activation occurs, chemotactic factors are generated locally, and an inflammatory response develops at the site of complex entrapment. Arthralgias, urticaria, lymphadenopathy, glomerulonephritis, or cerebritis may result. Foreign proteins (vaccines, streptokinase, therapeutic antibodies) and antibiotics are common causes. Many drugs, particularly antimicrobial agents, ACE inhibitors, and aspirin, can elicit anaphylaxis, with production of IgE, which binds to mast cell membranes. Contact with a drug antigen initiates a series of biochemical events in the mast cell and results in the release of mediators that can produce the characteristic urticaria, wheezing, flushing, rhinorrhea, and (occasionally) hypotension.

Drugs may also elicit cell-mediated immune responses. Topically administered substances may interact with sulfhydryl or amino groups in the skin and react with sensitized lymphocytes to produce the rash characteristic of contact dermatitis. Other types of rashes may also result from the interaction of serum factors, drugs, and sensitized lymphocytes.

DIAGNOSIS AND TREATMENT OF ADVERSE DRUG REACTIONS   The manifestations of drug-induced diseases frequently resemble those of other diseases, and a given set of manifestations may be produced by different and dissimilar drugs. Recognition of the role of a drug or drugs in an illness depends on appreciation of the possible adverse reactions to drugs in any disease, on identification of the temporal relationship between drug administration and development of the illness, and on familiarity with the common manifestations of the drugs. Many associations between particular drugs and specific reactions have been described, but there is always a "first time" for a novel association, and any drug should be suspected of causing an adverse effect if the clinical setting is appropriate.

Illness related to a drug's intended pharmacologic action is often more easily recognized than illness attributable to immune or other mechanisms. For example, side effects such as cardiac arrhythmias in patients receiving digitalis, hypoglycemia in patients given insulin, and bleeding in patients receiving anticoagulants are more readily related to a specific drug than are symptoms such as fever or rash, which may be caused by many drugs or by other factors.

Electronic sources of adverse drug reactions can be useful (e.g., *http://www.hc-sc.gc.ca/hpb-dgps/therapeut/htmleng/cadrnwsletter.html*). However, exhaustive compilations often provide little sense of perspective in terms of frequency and seriousness, which can vary considerably among patients.

Eliciting a drug history from patients is important for diagnosis. Attention must be directed to OTC drugs and herbal preparations as well as to prescription drugs. Each type can be responsible for adverse drug effects, and adverse interactions may occur between OTC drugs and prescribed drugs. Loss of efficacy of oral contraceptives or cyclosporine by concurrent use of St. John's wort are examples. In addition, it is common for patients to be cared for by several physicians, and duplicative, additive, counteractive, or synergistic drug combinations may therefore be administered if the physicians are not aware of the patients' drug histories. Every physician should determine what drugs a patient has been taking, at least during the preceding 30 days, before prescribing any medications. A frequently overlooked source of additional drug exposure is topical therapy; for example, a patient complaining of bronchospasm may not mention that an ophthalmic beta blocker is being used unless specifically asked. A history of previous adverse drug effects in patients is common. Since these patients have shown a predisposition to drug-induced illnesses, such a history should dictate added caution in prescribing drugs.

Laboratory studies may include demonstration of serum antibody in some persons with drug allergies involving cellular blood elements, as in agranulocytosis, hemolytic anemia, and thrombocytopenia. For example, both quinine and quinidine can produce platelet agglutination in vitro in the presence of complement and the serum from a patient who has developed thrombocytopenia following use of this drug. Biochemical abnormalities such as G6PD deficiency, serum pseudocholinesterase level, or genotyping may also be useful in diagnosis, often after an adverse effect has occurred in the patient or a family member.

Once an adverse reaction is suspected, discontinuation of the suspected drug followed by disappearance of the reaction is presumptive evidence of a drug-induced illness. Confirming evidence may be sought by cautiously reintroducing the drug and seeing if the reaction reappears. However, that should be done only if confirmation would be useful in the future management of the patient and if the attempt would not entail undue risk. With concentration-dependent adverse reactions, lowering the dosage may cause the reaction to disappear, and raising it may cause the reaction to reappear. When the reaction is thought to be allergic, however, readministration of the drug may be hazardous, since anaphylaxis may develop. Readministration is unwise under these conditions unless no alternative drugs are available and treatment is necessary.

If the patient is receiving many drugs when an adverse reaction is suspected, the drugs likeliest to be responsible can usually be identified. All drugs may be discontinued at once or, if this is not practical, they should be discontinued one at a time, starting with the one that is most suspect, and the patient observed for signs of improvement.

The time needed for a concentration-dependent adverse effect to disappear depends on the time required for the concentration to fall below the range associated with the adverse effect; that, in turn, depends on the initial blood level and on the rate of elimination or metabolism of the drug. Adverse effects of drugs with long half-lives take a considerable time to disappear.

SUMMARY

Modern clinical pharmacology aims to replace empiricism in the use of drugs with therapy based on in-depth understanding of factor(s) that determine an individual's response to drug treatment. Molecular pharmacology, pharmacokinetics, genetics, clinical trials, and the educated prescriber all contribute to this process. No drug response should ever be termed "idiosyncratic"; all responses have a mechanism whose understanding will help guide further therapy with that drug or successors. This rapidly expanding understanding of variability in drug actions makes the process of prescribing drugs increasingly daunting for the practitioner. However, fundamental principles should guide this process:

- The benefits of drug therapy, however defined, should always outweigh the risk.
- The smallest dosage necessary to produce the desired effect should be used.
- The number of medications and doses per day should be minimized.
- Although the literature is rapidly expanding, accessing it is becoming easier; tools such as computers and hand-held devices to search databases of literature and unbiased opinion will become increasingly commonplace.
- Genetics play a role in determining variability in drug response and may become a part of clinical practice
- Prescribers should be particularly wary when adding or stopping specific drugs that are especially liable to provoke interactions and adverse reactions.
- Prescribers should use only a limited number of drugs, with which they are thoroughly familiar.

ACKNOWLEDGMENT

The author acknowledges John A. Oates, Grant Wilkinson, and Alastair Wood who wrote chapters on this material for previous editions; some of their text have been retained.

FURTHER READING

EVANS WE, JOHNSON JA: Pharmacogenomics: The inherited basis for interindividual differences in drug response. Annu Rev Genom Hum Genet 2: 9, 2001

HIGASHI MK et al: Association between CYP2C9 genetic variants and anticoagulation-related outcomes during warfarin therapy. JAMA 287:1690, 2002

MCLEOD HL, EVANS WE: Pharmacogenomics: Unlocking the human genome for better drug therapy. Annu Rev Pharmacol Toxicol 41:101, 2001

PSATY BM et al: Diuretic therapy, the alpha-adducin gene variant, and the risk of myocardial infarction or stroke in persons with treated hypertension. JAMA 287:1680, 2002

WILKINSON GR: Pharmacokinetics: The dynamics of drug absorption, distribution, and elimination, in JG Hardman, LE Limbird (eds). *Goodman and Gilman's The Pharmacological Basis of Therapeutics*, 9th ed, New York, McGraw-Hill, 2001, pp 3–30

WOOD AJ et al: Making medicines safer: The need for an independent drug safety board. N Engl J Med 339:1851, 1998

A primary goal of health care is to prevent disease or to detect it early enough that interventions will be more effective. Strategies for disease screening and prevention are driven by evidence that testing and interventions are practical and effective. Most screening tests are currently based on readily available and inexpensive biochemical (e.g., cholesterol), physiologic (e.g., blood pressure), radiologic (e.g., mammogram), or tissue specimens (e.g., Pap smear). In the future, it is anticipated that genetic testing will play an increasingly important role for predicting disease risk (Chap. 58). However, such tests are not widely used except for individuals at risk for high-penetrance genes based on family or ethnic history (e.g., *BRCA1*, *BRCA2*). The identification of low-penetrance but high-frequency genes that cause common disorders such as diabetes or hypertension offers the possibility of new genetic tests. However, any new screening test, whether based on genetic or other methods, must be subjected to rigorous evaluation of its sensitivity, specificity, impact on disease, and cost-effectiveness. Physicians and patients are continuously introduced to new screening tests, often in advance of complete evaluation. For example, the use of whole-body computed tomography imaging has been advocated as a means to screen for a variety of disorders. Though appealing in concept, there is currently no evidence to justify this approach, which is associated with high cost and a substantial risk of false-positive results.

This chapter will review the basic principles of screening and strategies for measuring the impact of screening and prevention and will provide a summary of recommendations for screening and prevention in the primary care setting. Recommendations for specific disorders, such as cardiovascular disease, diabetes, or cancer, are provided in the chapters dedicated to these topics.

BASIC PRINCIPLES OF SCREENING In general, screening is most effective when applied to relatively common disorders that carry a large disease burden (Table 4-1). The five leading causes of mortality in the United States are heart diseases, malignant neoplasms, accidents, cerebrovascular diseases, and chronic obstructive pulmonary disease. Thus, many prevention strategies are targeted at these conditions.

A primary goal of screening is the early detection of a risk factor or disease at a stage when it can be corrected or cured. For example, most cancers have a better prognosis when identified as premalignant lesions or when they are still resectable. Similarly, early identification of hypertension or hyperlipidemia allows therapeutic interventions that reduce the risk of cardiovascular or cerebrovascular events. However, early detection does not necessarily influence survival. For example, in some studies of lung cancer screening, tumors are identified at an earlier stage, but overall mortality does not differ between screened and unscreened populations. The apparent improvement in 5-year survival rates can be attributed to the detection of smaller tumors rather than a real change in clinical course after diagnosis. Similarly, the detection of prostate cancer may not lead to a mortality difference because the disease is often indolent and competing morbidities, such as coronary artery disease, may ultimately cause mortality (Chap. 67).

Disorders with a long latency period increase the potential gains associated with detection. For example, cancer of the cervix has a long latency between dysplasia and invasive carcinoma, providing an opportunity for detection by routine screening. Similarly, an adenoma-tous polyp progresses to invasive colon cancer over 4 to 12 years, allowing an opportunity to detect early lesions by fecal occult blood testing or endoscopy. On the other hand, breast cancer screening in premenopausal women is more challenging because of the relatively short interval between development of a localized breast cancer and metastasis to regional nodes (estimated to be ~12 months).

METHODS OF MEASURING HEALTH BENEFITS It is not practical to perform all possible screening procedures. For example, screening for laryngeal cancer in smokers is not currently recommended. It is necessary to examine the strength of evidence in favor of screening measures relative to the cost and risk of false-positive tests. For example, should ultrasound be used to screen for ovarian cancer in average-risk women? It is currently estimated that the unnecessary laparotomies triggered by finding benign ovarian masses would actually cause more harm than the benefit derived from detecting the occasional curable ovarian cancer.

A variety of end points are used to assess the potential gain from screening and prevention interventions:

1. *The number of subjects screened to alter the outcome in one individual.* It is estimated, for example, that 731 women aged 65 to 69 would need to be screened by dual-energy x-ray absorptiometry (DEXA) and then treated appropriately to prevent one hip fracture from osteoporosis.

2. *The absolute and relative impact of screening on disease outcome.* A meta-analysis of Swedish mammography trials (ages 40 to 70) found that ~1.2 fewer women per thousand would die from breast cancer if they were screened over a 12-year period. By comparison, ~3 lives per 1000 might be saved from colon cancer in a population (ages 50 to 75) screened with annual fecal occult blood testing (FOBT) over a 13-year period. Based on this analysis, colon cancer screening may actually save more women's lives than mammography. The impact of FOBT (8.8/1000 versus 5.9/1000) might be stated as either 3 lives per 1000, or as a 30% reduction in colon cancer death; thus, it is important to consider both the relative and absolute impact on numbers of lives saved.

3. *The cost per year of life saved.* This is used to assess the effectiveness of many screening and prevention strategies. Typically, strategies that cost <\$30,000 to \$50,000 per year of life saved are considered "cost effective" (Chap. 2). For example, using alendronate to treat 65-year-old women with osteoporosis approaches this threshold of approximately \$30,000 per year of life saved.

4. *Increase in average life expectancy for a population.*

Predicted increases in life expectancy for various screening procedures are listed in Table 4-2. It should be noted, however, that the life expectancy increase is an average that applies to a population and not to an individual. In reality, the vast majority of the screened population does not derive any benefit and possibly incurs a slight risk

TABLE 4-1 *Lifetime Cumulative Risk*

Breast cancer for women	10%
Colon cancer	6%
Cancer of the cervix for women[a]	2%
Domestic violence for women	Up to 15%
Hip fracture for Caucasian women	16%

[a] Assuming an unscreened population.

TABLE 4-2 *Estimated Average Increase in Life Expectancy for a Population*

Screening Procedure	Average Increase
Mammography:	
Women, 40–50 years	0–5 days
Women, 50–70 years	1 month
Pap smears, age 18–65	2–3 months
Screening treadmill for a 50-year-old (asymptomatic) man	8 days
PSA and digital rectal exam for a man >50 years	Up to 2 weeks
Getting a 35-year-old smoker to quit	3–5 years
Beginning regular exercise for a 40-year-old man (30 min 3 times a week)	9 months to 2 years

Note: PSA, prostate-specific antigen.

from false-positive results. A small subset of patients, however, will benefit greatly from being screened. For example, Pap smears do not benefit the 98% of women who never develop cancer of the cervix. However, for the 2% who would develop localized cervical cancer, Pap smears may add as much as 25 years to their lives. Some studies suggest that a 1-month gain of life expectancy is a reasonable goal for a population-based preventive strategy.

The U.S. Preventive Services Task Force provides recommendations for evidence-based screening (Table 4-3). In addition to these population-based guidelines, it is reasonable to consider family and social history to identify individuals with special risk (*www.ahrq.gov/clinic/uspstfix.htm*). For example, when there is a significant family history of breast, colon, or prostate cancer, it is prudent to initiate screening about 10 years before the age when the youngest family member developed cancer. Screening should also be considered for many other com-

TABLE 4-3 *Clinical Preventive Services for Normal-Risk Adults Recommended by the U.S. Preventive Services Task Force*

Test or Disorder	Population,[a] Years	Frequency	Chapter Reference
Blood pressure, height and weight	>18	Periodically	64
Cholesterol	Men > 35	Every 5 years	225
	Women > 45	Every 5 years	
Diabetes	>45 or earlier, if there are additional risk factors	Every 3 years	323
Pap smear	Within 3 years of onset of sexual activity or 21–65	Every 1–3 years	67
Chlamydia	Women 18–25	Every 1–2 years	160
Mammography[a]	Women > 40	Every 1–2 years	67, 76
Colorectal cancer[a]	>50		67, 77
fecal occult blood and/or		Every year	
sigmoidoscopy or		Every 5 years	
colonoscopy		Every 10 years	
Osteoporosis	Women > 65; >60 at risk	Periodically	333
Alcohol use	>18	Periodically	372
Vision, hearing	>65	Periodically	25, 26
Adult immunization			107, 108
Tetanus-diptheria (Td)	>18	Every 10 years	
Varicella (VZV)	Susceptibles only, >18	Two doses	
Measles, mumps, rubella (MMR)	Women, childbearing age	One dose	
Pneumococcal	>65	One dose	
Influenza	>50	Yearly	

[a] Screening is performed earlier and more frequently when there is a strong family history. Randomized, controlled trials have documented that fecal occult blood testing (FOBT) confers a 15 to 30% reduction in colon cancer mortality. Although randomized trials have not been performed for sigmoidoscopy or colonoscopy, well-designed case-control studies suggest similar or greater efficacy relative to FOBT.
Note: Prostate-specific antigen (PSA) testing is capable of enhancing the detection of early-stage prostate cancer, but evidence is inconclusive that it improves health outcomes. PSA testing is recommended by several professional organizations and is widely used in clinical practice, but it is not currently recommended by the U.S. Preventive Services Task Force (Chap. 81).
Source: Adapted from the U.S. Preventive Services Task Force, 1996. *Guide to Clinical Prevention Services*, 3d ed (*www.ahrq.gov/clinic/uspstfix.htm*)

mon disorders pending the development of further evidence. Three examples are screening for diabetes (using fasting blood glucose), domestic violence, and features of depression.

Cost-Effectiveness Screening techniques must be cost effective, if they are to be applied to large populations. Costs include not only the expense of testing but also time away from work and potential risks. When the risk-to-benefit ratio is less favorable, it is useful to provide information to patients and factor their perspectives into the decision-making process. For example, many expert groups, including the U.S. Preventive Services Task Force, recommend an individualized discussion about prostate cancer screening, as the decision-making process is complex and relies heavily on personal issues. Although the early detection of prostate cancer may intuitively seem desirable, risks include false-positive results that can lead to anxiety and unnecessary surgery. Potential complications from surgery and radiation treatment include erectile dysfunction, urinary incontinence, and bowel dysfunction. Some men may decline screening, while others may be more willing to accept the risks of an early detection strategy. Another example of shared decision-making is the choice of colon cancer screening techniques (Chap. 67). In controlled studies, the use of annual FOBT reduces colon cancer deaths by 15 to 30%. Flexible sigmoidoscopy reduces colon cancer deaths by ~60%. Colonoscopy offers the same, or greater, benefit than flexible sigmoidoscopy, but its use incurs additional costs and risks. These screening procedures have not been directly compared in the same population, but the estimated cost to society is similar—$10,000 to $25,000 per year of life saved. Thus, while one patient may prefer the ease of preparation, less time disruption, and the lower risk of flexible sigmoidoscopy, others may prefer the sedation and thoroughness of colonscopy.

When considering the impact of screening tests, it is important to recognize that tobacco and alcohol use, diet, and exercise represent the vast majority of factors that influence preventable deaths. Perhaps the single greatest preventive health care measure is to help patients quit smoking (Chap. 375).

COMMONLY ENCOUNTERED ISSUES Despite compelling evidence that prevention strategies can have major health care benefits, implementation of these services is challenging because of competing demands on physician and patient time and because of gaps in health care reimbursement. Moreover, efforts to reduce disease risk frequently involve behavior changes (e.g., weight loss, exercise, seatbelts) or managing addictive conditions (e.g., tobacco and alcohol use) that are often recalcitrant to intervention. Public education and economic incentives are often useful, in addition to counseling by health care providers (Table 4-4).

A number of techniques can assist the physician with the growing number of recommended screening tests. An appropriately configured electronic medical record can provide reminder systems that make it easier for physicians to track and meet guidelines. Some systems pro-

TABLE 4-4 *Counseling to Prevent Disease*

Topic	Chapter Reference
Tobacco cessation	375
Drug and alcohol use	372, 373
Nutrition to maintain caloric balance and vitamin intake	60
Calcium intake in women > 18 years	333
Folic acid: Women of childbearing age	61
Oral health	28
Aspirin use to prevent cardiovascular disease in selected men >40 years and women >50 years	225
Chemoprevention of breast cancer in women at high risk	76
STDs and HIV prevention	115, 173
Physical activity	
Sun exposure	51
Injury prevention (loaded handgun, seat belts, bicycle helmet)	
Issues in the elderly	8
Polypharmacy	
Fall prevention	
Hot water heater <120°	
Vision, hearing, dental evaluations	
Immunizations (pneumococcal, influenza)	

Note: STDs, sexually transmitted diseases.

vide patients with secure access to their medical records, providing an additional means to ensure compliance with routine screening. Systems that provide nurses and other staff with standing orders are effective for smoking prevention and immunizations. The Agency for Healthcare Research and Quality and the Centers for Disease Control and Prevention have developed flow sheets as part of their "Put Prevention into Practice" program (*http://www.ahcpr.gov/clinic/ppipix.htm*).

A routine health care examination should be performed every 1 to 3 years before age 50 and every year thereafter. History should include medication use (prescription and nonprescription), allergies, dietary history, use of alcohol and tobacco, sexual practices, and a thorough family history, if not obtained previously. Routine measurements should include assessments of height, weight (body mass index, BMI), and blood pressure, in addition to the relevant physical examination. The increasing incidence of skin cancer underscores the importance of screening for suspicious skin lesions. Hearing and vision should be tested after age 65, or earlier if the patient describes difficulties. Other gender- and age-specific examinations are listed in Table 4-3. Counseling and instruction about self-examination (e.g., skin, breast) can be provided during the routine examination.

Many patients see a physician for ongoing care of chronic illnesses, and this visit provides an opportunity to include a "measure of prevention" for other health problems. For example, the patient seen for management of hypertension or diabetes can have breast cancer screening incorporated into one visit and a discussion about colon cancer screening at the next visit. Other patients may respond more favorably to a clearly defined visit that addresses all relevant screening and prevention interventions. In some patients, because of age or co-morbidities, it may be appropriate to abandon certain screening and prevention activities, although there are fewer data about when to "sunset" these services. The risk of certain cancers, like cancer of the cervix, ultimately declines, and it is reasonable to cease Pap smears after about age 65, if previous recent Pap smears have been negative. For breast, colon, and prostate cancer, it is reasonable to reevaluate the need for screening after about age 75. For some older patients with advanced diseases such as severe chronic obstructive pulmonary disease or congestive heart failure or who are immobile, the benefit of some screening procedures is low, and other priorities emerge when life expectancy is <10 years. This shift in focus needs to be done tactfully and allows greater focus on the conditions likely to impact quality and length of life.

FURTHER READING

BLUMENTHAL RS et al: Detecting occult coronary artery disease in a high-risk asymptomatic population. Circulation 107:702, 2003

CLINICAL PREVENTIVE SERVICES FOR NORMAL-RISK ADULTS RECOMMENDED BY THE U.S. PREVENTIVE SERVICES TASK FORCE. Put Prevention into Practice, January 2003. Agency for Healthcare Research and Quality, Rockville, MD. *www.ahrq.gov/ppip/adulttm.htm*

RANSOHOFF DF, SANDLER RS: Clinical practice: Screening for colorectal cancer. N Engl J Med 346:40, 2002

U.S. PREVENTIVE SERVICES TASK FORCE: *Guide to Clinical Preventive Services*, 3d ed. Baltimore, Williams & Wilkins, 1996

WRIGHT JC, WEINSTEIN MC: Gains in life expectancy from medical interventions—standardizing data on outcomes. N Engl J Med 339:380, 1998

5 WOMEN'S HEALTH
Andrea Dunaif

The study of biologic differences between sexes has emerged as a distinct scientific discipline in the United States. A report from the Institute of Medicine (IOM) found that sex has a broad impact on biologic and disease processes and succinctly concluded—sex matters. The National Institutes of Health established the Office of Research on Women's Health in 1990 to develop an agenda for future research in the field. In parallel, women's health is developing as a new clinical discipline with a focus on disorders that are disproportionately represented in women. The integration of women's health into internal medicine and other specialties has been accompanied by novel approaches to health care delivery, including greater attention to patient education and involvement in disease prevention and medical decision-making.

The IOM report recommended the terms *sex difference* to describe biologic processes that differ between males and females and *gender difference* for features related to social influences. This chapter highlights representative examples of sex differences in selected medical areas. Disorders discussed in this section are reviewed in detail in other chapters.

DISEASE RISK: REALITY AND PERCEPTION   The leading causes of death are the same in women and men: (1) heart disease, (2) cancer, and (3) cerebrovascular disease (Table 5-1; Fig. 5-1). The leading cause of cancer death, lung cancer, is the same in both sexes. Breast cancer is the second leading cause of cancer death in women but with rates that are 35% lower than those for lung cancer. Men are substantially more likely to die from suicide, homicide, and accidents than women.

Women's risk for many diseases increases at menopause, which occurs at a median age of 51.4 years. In the industrialized world, women spend one-third of their lives in the postmenopausal period. Estrogen levels fall abruptly at menopause, inducing a variety of physiologic and metabolic responses. Rates of cardiovascular disease increase and bone density begins to decrease after menopause. Nevertheless, in the United States women live on average 5.7 years longer than men, with a life expectancy of 79.5 years compared to 73.8 years in men. Elderly women outnumber elderly men, so that age-related conditions, such as hypertension, have a female preponderance.

Women's perception of disease risk is often inaccurate; <10% know that cardiovascular disease is the leading cause of death in women. The condition that they fear most is breast cancer, despite the fact that death rates from breast cancer have been falling since the 1990s. In any given decade of life, a woman's risk for breast cancer never exceeds 1 in 34. Although a woman's lifetime risk of developing breast cancer if she lives past 85 years is about 1 in 9, it is much more likely that she will die from cardiovascular disease than from breast cancer. In other words, many elderly women have breast cancer but die from other causes. Similarly, only 26% of women are aware that lung cancer is the leading cause of cancer death in women. These misconceptions are unfortunate as they perpetuate inadequate attention to modifiable risk factors, such as dyslipidemia, hypertension, and cigarette smoking. Physicians are also less likely to recognize women's risk for cardiovascular disease. When presented with actors portraying patients with chest pain, physicians' estimates for probability of coronary heart disease (CHD) were significantly lower for women than for men and were lower for black women than for white women. These perceptions on the part of both the patient and her physician lead to important differences in cardiac care that are discussed below.

SEX DIFFERENCES IN HEALTH AND DISEASE ■ Alzheimer's Disease (See also Chap. 350)   Alzheimer's disease (AD) affects approximately twice as many women as men. Because the risk for AD increases with age, part of this sex difference is accounted for by the fact that women live longer than men. However, additional factors likely contribute to the increased risk for AD in women. There are sex differences in brain size, structure, and functional organization. There is emerging evidence for sex-specific differences in gene expression, not only for genes on the X and Y chromosomes but also for some autosomal genes. Estrogens have pleiotropic genomic and nongenomic effects on the central nervous system, including neurotrophic actions in key areas involved in cognition and memory. Women with AD have lower endogenous estrogen levels compared to women without AD. These observations have led to the hypothesis that estrogen is neuroprotective.

Some studies have suggested that estrogen administration improves cognitive function in nondemented postmenopausal women as well as in women with AD, and several observational studies have suggested that postmenopausal hormone therapy (PHT) may decrease the risk of AD. However, recent placebo-controlled trials have found no improvement in disease progression or cognitive function after up to 15 months of PHT in women with AD. The findings in these observational studies may be confounded by the fact that PHT users are better educated and have higher socioeconomic status, both of which are associated with a decreased risk of AD. An ancillary study of the Women's Health Initiative (WHI) randomized clinical trial, the WHI Memory Study, is prospectively evaluating the impact of PHT on cognitive function and the development of AD in women 65 to 79 years of age at the time of enrollment. The results of this study should be available in 2007.

Coronary Heart Disease
(See also Chap. 226)   There are major sex differences in CHD, the leading cause of death in men and women in the United States. CHD death rates have been falling in men over the past 30 years but they have been increasing in women.

CHD presents differently in women, who are usually 10 to 15 years older than their male counterparts and are more likely to have comorbidities, such as hypertension, congestive heart failure, and diabetes. In the Framingham study, angina was the most frequent initial symptom of CHD in women, whereas myocardial infarction was the most frequent initial presentation in men. Women more often have atypical symptoms, such as nausea, vomiting, indigestion, and upper back pain.

Women with myocardial infarction are more likely to present with cardiac arrest or cardiogenic shock, whereas men are more likely to present with ventricular tachycardia. Further, younger women with myocardial infarction are more likely to die than men of similar age, with women under <50 experiencing twice the mortality rate of men, even after adjustment for differences in disease severity and management. Indeed, the younger the woman, the greater the risk of death from myocardial infarction compared to men (Fig. 5-2).

Physicians are less likely to suspect heart disease in women with chest pain and are less likely to perform diagnostic and therapeutic cardiac procedures in women. In addition, there are sex differences in the accuracy of certain diagnostic procedures. The exercise electrocardiogram has substantial false-positive as well as false-negative rates in women compared to men. Women are less likely to receive therapies such as angioplasty, thrombolytic therapy, coronary artery bypass grafts, beta-blockers, or aspirin. There are also sex differences in outcomes when women with CHD do receive therapeutic interventions. Women undergoing coronary artery bypass graft surgery have more advanced disease, a higher periop-

erative mortality rate, less relief of angina, and less graft patency; however, 5- and 10-year survival rates are similar. Women undergoing percutaneous transluminal coronary angioplasty have lower rates of initial angiographic and clinical success than men, but they also have a lower rate of restenosis and a better long-term outcome. Women may benefit less and have more frequent serious bleeding complications from thrombolytic therapy than do men. Factors such as older age, more comorbid conditions, and more severe CHD in women at the time of events or procedures appear to account in part for the observed sex differences.

Elevated cholesterol levels, hypertension, smoking, obesity, low high-density lipoprotein (HDL) cholesterol levels, diabetes, and lack of physical activity are important risk factors for CHD in both men and women. Total triglyceride levels are an independent risk factor for CHD in women but not in men. Low HDL-cholesterol and diabetes are more important risk factors for CHD in women than in men. Smoking is an important risk factor for CHD in women—it accelerates atherosclerosis, exerts direct negative effects on cardiac function, and is associated with an earlier age of menopause. Cholesterol-lowering drugs are equally effective in men and women for primary and sec-

TABLE 5-1   *Deaths and Percent of Total Deaths for the Ten Leading Causes of Death by Sex in the United States, 2000*

Cause of Death	Women			Men		
	Rank	Deaths	Percent of Total Deaths	Rank	Deaths	Percent of Total Deaths
Diseases of heart	1	365,953	29.9	1	344,807	29.3
Malignant neoplasms	2	267,009	21.8	2	286,082	24.3
Cerebrovascular diseases	3	102,892	8.4	3	64,769	5.5
Chronic lower respiratory diseases	4	62,005	5.1	5	60,004	5.1
Diabetes mellitus	5	37,699	3.1	6	31,602	2.7
Influenza and pneumonia	6	36,655	3.0	7	28,658	2.4
Alzheimer's disease	7	35,120	2.9	—	14,438	1.2
Accidents	8	34,083	2.8	4	63,817	5.4
Nephritis, nephrotic syndrome, and nephrosis	9	19,440	1.6	9	17,811	1.5
Septicemia	10	17,687	1.4	—	13,537	1.1
Intentional self-harm	—	5732	0.5	8	23,618	2.0
Chronic liver disease and cirrhosis	—	9338	0.8	10	17,214	1.5

Source: Data from National Vital Statistics Report, Vol. 50, No. 16, September 16, 2002, *www.cdc.gov/nchs/data/nvsr/nvsr50/nvsr50_16.pdf*

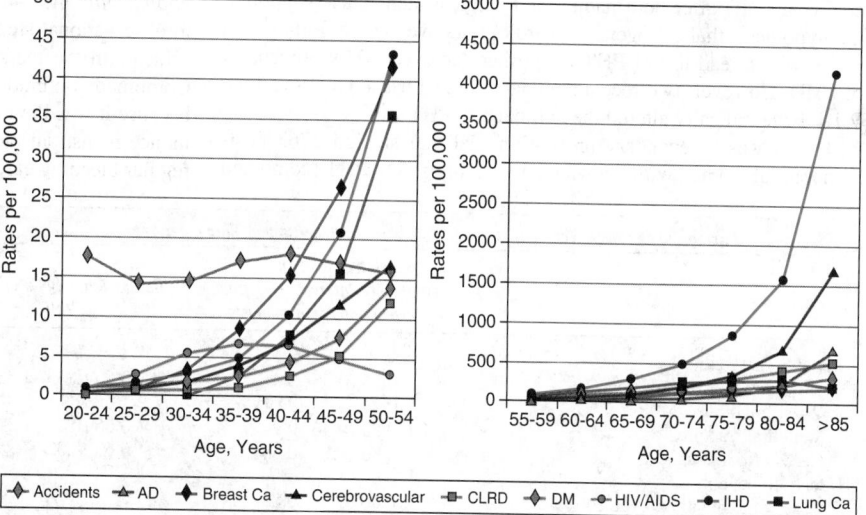

—◆— Accidents —▲— AD —◆— Breast Ca —▲— Cerebrovascular —■— CLRD —◆— DM —●— HIV/AIDS —●— IHD —■— Lung Ca

FIGURE 5-1   Death rates per 100,000 population for 1999 by 5-year age groups in U.S. women; note that the scale of the y-axis is increased by tenfold in the graph on the right compared to that on the left. Accidents and HIV/AIDS are the leading causes of death in young women 20 to 34 years of age. Accidents, breast cancer, and ischemic heart disease (IHD) are the leading causes of death in women 35 to 44 years of age. Breast cancer is the leading cause of death in women 45 to 49 years of age, and IHD becomes the leading cause of death in women beginning at 50 years of age. In older women, IHD remains the leading cause of death, cerebrovascular disease becomes the second leading cause of death, and lung cancer is the leading cause of cancer-related deaths. AD, Alzheimer's disease; Ca, cancer; CLRD, chronic lower respiratory disease; DM, diabetes mellitus; IHD, ischemic heart disease. (*Data adapted from www.cdc.gov/nchs/data/sttab/vs00199_tabl21or.pdf.*) (Writing Group for the Women's Health Initiative Investigation, JAMA 288:321, 2002. Copyright © 2002, American Medical Association.)

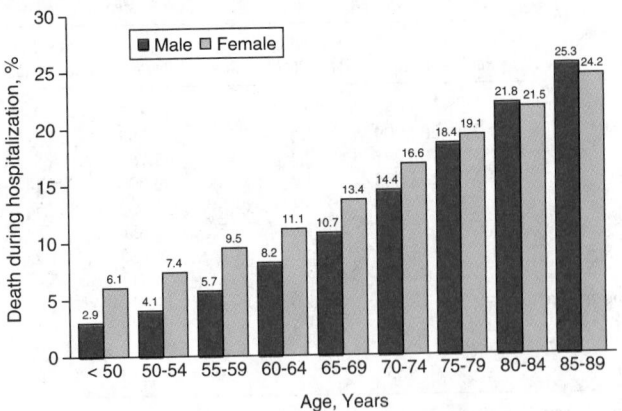

FIGURE 5-2   Rates of death during hospitalization for myocardial infarction among women and men according to age. The overall mortality rate during hospitalization was 16.7% among women and 11.5% among men but was twice the rate in women <50 years compared to men in the same age range. The interaction between sex and age was significant (*p* < .001). (*From V Vaccarino et al: N Engl J Med 341:217, 1999; with permission.*)

ondary prevention of CHD. However, because of perceptions that women are at lower risk for CHD, they receive fewer interventions for modifiable risk factors than do men. Secondary prevention in women with known CHD is also suboptimal. At baseline, only about 30% of women enrolled in the Heart and Estrogen/progestin Replacement Study (HERS), a secondary prevention trial in women with established CHD, were taking beta blockers, and only 45% received lipid-lowering medications.

Effect of Hormone Replacement Therapy on Cardiovascular Disease (See also Chap. 327)   Until recently, it was widely believed that the sex-specific effects of gonadal steroids on the cardiovascular system and lipid metabolism accounted for the different rates of CHD in women compared to men. Estrogen increases HDL and lowers low-density lipoprotein (LDL), whereas androgens have the opposite effect. Estrogen has direct vasodilatory effects on the vascular endothelium, enhances insulin sensitivity, and has antioxidant properties. The striking increase in CHD after both natural and surgical menopause supported the hypothesis that estrogens are cardioprotective. These findings led to the widespread use of PHT for primary and secondary prevention of CHD. However, two recent landmark clinical trials, HERS and the WHI, have radically altered the approach to PHT.

HERS was a secondary prevention trial that studied 2763 postmenopausal women with known CHD randomized to PHT (combined continuous conjugated equine estrogen, 0.625 mg qd, and medroxy-progesterone acetate, 2.5 mg qd) or to placebo for an average of 4.1 years. Unexpectedly, there was a 50% increase in CHD events in the first year of the trial in the PHT group. The lack of a beneficial effect on CHD events occurred in the face of a significant increase in HDL-cholesterol and fall in LDL-cholesterol levels in the PHT group. The HERS II data show no difference in CHD events after an additional 2.7 years of follow-up.

The WHI trial randomized 16,608 women 50 to 79 years of age: 8506 to estrogen plus progestin and 8102 to placebo. It was halted in May 2002 after an average follow-up of 5.2 years because women receiving PHT had an increased risk of invasive breast cancer, and an overall assessment of outcomes showed more risk than benefit. Compared to women in the placebo group, women in the PHT group had a 26% higher rate of breast cancer, a 29% higher rate of CHD, a 41% higher rate of stroke, and a greater than twofold increase in pulmonary embolism (Table 5-2). There was no difference in the rate of endometrial cancer in the PHT group compared to the placebo group. There was a 33% reduction in the rate of hip fractures and a 37% reduction in the rate of colon cancer in the PHT group. Despite these beneficial effects, the global index of outcomes showed that the PHT group had a 15% higher rate of adverse events compared to the placebo group. Nevertheless, the absolute risk of PHT is relatively small. In 10,000 women receiving PHT compared to those receiving placebo, one would predict that over 1 year there might be eight more invasive breast cancers, seven more CHD events, eight more strokes, eight more pulmonary embolic events, but six fewer colon cancers and five fewer hip fractures. An estrogen-only arm of this study is ongoing.

Why did the results of these randomized clinical trials differ so markedly from those of observational studies of PHT? Women placed on PHT tend to have higher socioeconomic status, more education, lower body weight and blood pressure, and more favorable lipid profiles than nonusers—all factors that independently decrease the risk of CHD. This phenomenon has been called the *healthy user effect*. Physicians may also choose to prescribe PHT to women they deem to be healthier. Women at risk for certain conditions, such as breast cancer, may not be placed on PHT, which could decrease the number of PHT-associated cases of breast cancer in observational studies. In addition, individuals who continue to take medication, including placebo, have decreased overall mortality. This phenomenon is known as *compliance bias* and could contribute to the better outcomes for PHT users in observational studies. It is also possible that the type of PHT was a factor in the paradoxical results of the randomized clinical trials. Combined continuous estrogen plus progestin was used in both trials, because it was the most widely prescribed preparation and it does not induce menstrual bleeding (although many women do experience irregular bleeding early in therapy), permitting blinding of the trial. The progestin used was medroxyprogesterone acetate, which has been shown to have a number of adverse metabolic effects, such as antagonizing the beneficial effects of estrogen on lipids and insulin sensitivity. Progestins may also abolish the beneficial direct vascular actions of estrogen and increase the risk for breast cancer. The estrogen-alone component of the WHI will determine whether the progestin accounted for the increased risk of PHT. The oral route of administration results in first-pass hepatic metabolism that induces the production of several clotting factors. It remains possible that more physiologic PHT, such as transdermal estradiol, may not have the adverse effects of other forms of PHT. This hypothesis needs to be tested in randomized clinical trials.

TABLE 5-2 Hormone Replacement Therapy Use in 10,000 Women: Benefits and Harms per Year		
	Relative Risk [95% Confidence Interval (CI)] from Review and Meta-analysis	Hazard Ratio (95% CI) from WHI
Benefits (prevention)		
Hip fractures	0.76 (0.56–1.01)	0.66 (0.33–1.33)
Wrist fractures	0.44 (0.23–0.84)	NA
Vertebral fractures	0.60 (0.36–0.99)	0.66 (0.32–1.34)
Cases of colon cancer	0.80 (0.74–0.86)	0.63 (0.32–1.24)
Uncertain benefits		
Cases of dementia prevented	0.66 (0.53–0.82)	NA
Harms (caused)		
Coronary heart disease	0.91 (0.67–1.33)	1.29 (1.02–1.63)
Strokes	1.12 (1.01–1.23)	1.41 (0.86–2.31)
Thromboembolic events	2.14 (1.64–2.81)	2.11 (1.26–3.55)
Thromboembolic events during first year	3.49 (2.33–5.59)	NA
Breast cancer cases (<5 years' use)	1.0 to 1.14	NA
Breast cancer cases (5 years' use)	1.23 to 1.35	1.26 (1.00–1.59)
Cholecystitis cases (<5 years' use)	1.8 (1.6–2.0)	NA
Cholecystitis cases (5 years' use)	2.5 (2.0–2.9)	NA

Note: WHI, Women's Health Initiative; NA, not applicable.   *Source*: From Nelson, with permission.

Diabetes Mellitus (See also Chap. 323) Women are more sensitive to insulin than men. Despite this, the prevalence of type 2 diabetes mellitus (DM) is higher in women, in part related to the higher prevalence of obesity among women. Polycystic ovary syndrome and gestational diabetes mellitus—common conditions in premenopausal women—are associated with a significantly increased risk for type 2 DM. Premenopausal women with DM lose the cardioprotective effect of female sex and have identical rates of CHD to those in males. This finding is partially explained by the coexistence of several CHD risk factors: obesity, hypertension, and dyslipidemia. Premenopausal women with DM also have impaired endothelial function and reduced coronary vasodilatory responses, which may predispose to cardiovascular complications.

Hypertension (See also Chap. 230) After age 60 years, hypertension is more common in U.S. women than in men, largely because of the high prevalence of hypertension in older age groups and the longer survival of women. Isolated systolic hypertension is present in 30% of women >60 years. Sex hormones affect blood pressure. Both normotensive and hypertensive women have higher blood pressure levels during the follicular than during the luteal phase. In the Nurses Health Study, the relative risk of hypertension was 1.8 in current users of oral contraceptives, but this risk is lower with the newer low-dose contraceptive preparations. PHT is not associated with hypertension. Among secondary causes of hypertension, there is a female preponderance of renal artery fibromuscular dysplasia.

The benefits of treatment for hypertension have been dramatic in both women and men. In a meta-analysis of the effects of hypertension treatment, the Individual Data Analysis of Antihypertensive Intervention Trial found a reduction of risk for stroke and for major cardiovascular events in women. The effectiveness of various antihypertensive drugs appears to be comparable in women and men; however, women may experience more side effects. For example, women are more likely to develop cough with angiotensin-converting enzyme inhibitors.

Autoimmune Disorders (See also Chap. 299) Most autoimmune disorders occur more commonly in women than in men; these include autoimmune thyroid and liver diseases, lupus, rheumatoid arthritis, scleroderma, multiple sclerosis, and idiopathic thrombocytopenic purpura. However, there is no sex difference in the incidence of type 1 DM, and ankylosing spondylitis occurs more commonly in men. There are relatively few differences in bacterial disease infection rates in men and women. In general, sex differences in viral diseases can be accounted for by differences in behaviors, such as exposures or rates of immunization. There are, however, sex differences in HIV infection (see below). Sex differences in both immune responses and adverse reactions to vaccines have been reported. For example, there is a female preponderance of postvaccination arthritis.

The mechanisms for these sex differences remain obscure. Adaptive immune responses are more robust in women than in men, which may be explained by the stimulatory actions of estrogens and the inhibitory actions of androgens on the cellular mediators of immunity. Consistent with an important role for gonadal hormones, there is variation in immune responses during the menstrual cycle, and the activity of certain autoimmune disorders is altered by castration or pregnancy (e.g., rheumatoid arthritis and multiple sclerosis may remit during pregnancy). Nevertheless, the majority of studies show that exogenous estrogens and progestins in the form of PHT or oral contraceptives do not alter autoimmune disease incidence or activity. Exposure to fetal antigens, including circulating fetal cells that persist in certain tissues, has been speculated to increase the risk of autoimmune responses. There is clearly an important genetic component to autoimmunity, as indicated by the familial clustering and HLA association of many such disorders. However, HLA types are not sexually dimorphic.

HIV Infection (See also Chap. 173) AIDS is an important cause of death in younger women (Fig. 5-1). Heterosexual contact with an at-risk partner is the fastest-growing transmission category, and women are twice as likely as men to be infected by a partner. Women are also more likely to be infected by multiple variants of the virus than men. Women with HIV have more rapid decreases in their CD4 cell counts than men. Compared with men, HIV-infected women more frequently develop candidiasis, but Kaposi's sarcoma is less common than in men.

Other sexually transmitted diseases, such as chlamydial infection and gonorrhea, are important causes of infertility in women, and papilloma virus infection predisposes to cervical cancer.

Osteoporosis (See also Chap. 333) Osteoporosis is much more prevalent in postmenopausal women than in age-matched men, and osteoporotic hip fractures are a major cause of morbidity in elderly women. Men accumulate more bone mass, and lose bone more slowly, than women. Sex differences in bone mass are found as early as infancy. Calcium intake, vitamin D, and estrogen all play important roles in bone formation and bone loss. Particularly during adolescence, calcium intake is an important determinant of peak bone mass. Vitamin D deficiency is surprisingly common in elderly women, occurring in >40% of women living in northern latitudes. Receptors for estrogens and androgens have been identified in bone. Estrogen deficiency is associated with increased osteoclast activity and a decreased number of bone-forming units, leading to net bone loss. The aromatase enzyme, which converts androgens to estrogens, is also present in bone. Recent studies show that estrogen is an important determinant of bone mass in men (derived from the aromatization of androgens) as well as in women.

Pharmacology On average, women have lower body weights, smaller organs, higher percent body fat, and lower total body water than men. There are also important sex differences in drug action and metabolism that are not accounted for by these differences in body size and composition. Gonadal steroids alter the binding and metabolism of a number of drugs. Further, menstrual cycle phase and pregnancy can alter drug action. Women require lower doses of neuroleptics to control schizophrenia. Women awaken from anesthesia faster than men given the same doses of anesthetics. Women also take more medications than men, including over-the-counter formulations and supplements. The greater use of medications combined with these biologic differences may account for the reported higher frequency of adverse drug reactions in women than in men.

Psychological Disorders (See also Chap. 371) Depression, anxiety, and affective and eating disorders (bulimia and anorexia nervosa) are more common in women than in men. Epidemiologic studies from both developed and developing nations consistently find major depression to be twice as common in women as in men, with the sex difference becoming evident in early adolescence. Depression occurs in 10% of women during pregnancy and in 10 to 15% of women during the postpartum period. There is a high likelihood of recurrence of postpartum depression with subsequent pregnancies. The incidence of major depression diminishes after age 45 years and does not increase with the onset of menopause. Depression in women appears to have a worse prognosis than in men; episodes last longer and there is a lower rate of spontaneous remission. Schizophrenia and bipolar disorders occur at equal rates in men and women, although there may be sex differences in symptoms.

Both biologic and social factors account for the greater prevalence depressive disorders in women. Men have higher levels of the neurotransmitter serotonin. Gonadal steroids also affect mood, and fluctuations during the menstrual cycle have been linked to symptoms of premenstrual syndrome.

Substance Abuse and Tobacco (See also Chaps. 372 and 375) Substance abuse is more common in men than women. However, one-third of Americans who suffer from alcoholism are women. Women alcoholics are less likely to be diagnosed than men. A greater proportion of men than women seek help for alcohol and drug abuse. Men are more likely to go to an alcohol or drug treatment facility, while women tend to approach a primary care physician or mental health professional for help under the guise of a psychosocial problem. Late-life alcoholism is more common in women than men. On average, alcoholic women drink less than alcoholic men but exhibit the same degree of impairment. Blood alcohol levels are higher in women than in men after drinking equivalent amounts of alcohol, adjusted for body weight. This greater bioavailability of alcohol in women is due both to the smaller volume of distribution and the slower gastric metabolism of alcohol secondary to lower activity of gastric alcohol dehydrogenase than in men. In addition, alcoholic women are more likely to abuse tranquilizers, sedatives, and amphetamines. Women alcoholics have a higher mortality rate than do nonalcoholic women and alcoholic men. Women also appear to develop alcoholic liver disease and other alcohol-related diseases with shorter drinking histories and lower levels of alcohol consumption. Alcohol abuse also poses special risks to a woman, adversely affecting fertility and the health of the baby (fetal alcohol syndrome). Even moderate alcohol use increases the risk of breast cancer, hypertension, and stroke in women.

More men than women smoke tobacco, but the prevalence of smoking is declining faster in men than women. Smoking markedly increases the risk of cardiovascular disease in premenopausal women and is also associated with a decrease in the age of menopause. Women who smoke are more likely to develop chronic obstructive pulmonary disease and lung cancer than men and at lower levels of tobacco exposure.

Violence Against Women (See also Chap. 371)   Domestic violence is the most common cause of physical injury in women, exceeding the combined incidence of all other types of injury (such as from rape, mugging, and auto accidents). Sexual assault is one of the most common crimes against women. One in five adult women in the United States reports having experienced sexual assault during her lifetime. Adult women are much more likely to be raped by a spouse, ex-spouse, or acquaintance than by a stranger. Domestic violence may be an unrecognized feature of certain clinical presentations such as chronic abdominal pain, headaches, substance abuse, and eating disorders, in addition to more obvious manifestations such as trauma.

SUMMARY   Women's health has become a mature discipline over the past decade. The importance of sex differences in biologic processes is now recognized. It is clear that understanding the mechanisms of these differences will have an impact not only on women's but also on men's health. For example, estrogen is now recognized as an important regulator of bone density in men as well as in women. Elucidating the biology of sex hormone action has resulted in the design of drugs with tissue-specific hormone agonist and antagonist effects. These discoveries will make it feasible to selectively modulate the actions of sex hormones in both women and men to prevent and treat disease.

ACKNOWLEDGMENT
The author wishes to acknowledge the contributions of Dr. Anthony Komaroff and Dr. Celeste Robb-Nicholson to this chapter in previous editions of the text.

FURTHER READING

HASELTINE FP, JACOBSON BG (eds): Women's health research: An introduction, in *Women's Health Research: A Medical and Policy Primer.* Washington, DC, American Psychiatric Press, 1997, pp 1–26

HULLEY SH et al: Randomized trial of estrogen plus progestin for secondary prevention of coronary heart disease in postmenopausal women. JAMA 280:605, 1998

NELSON HD et al: Postmenopausal hormone replacement therapy (scientific review). JAMA 288:872, 2002

WIZEMANN TM, PARDUE M-L (eds): *Exploring the Biological Contributions to Human Health: Does Sex Matter?* Washington, DC, National Academy of Sciences, 2001

WRITING GROUP FOR THE WOMEN'S HEALTH INITIATIVE INVESTIGATORS: Risk and benefits of estrogen plus progestin in healthy postmenopausal women: Principal results from the women's health initiative randomized controlled trial. JAMA 288:321, 2002

6 MEDICAL DISORDERS DURING PREGNANCY
Robert L. Barbieri, John T. Repke

Approximately 4 million births occur in the United States each year. A significant proportion of these are complicated by one or more medical disorders. Two decades ago, many medical disorders were contraindications to pregnancy. Advances in obstetrics, neonatology, obstetric anesthesiology, and medicine have increased the expectation that pregnancy will result in an excellent outcome for both mother and fetus despite most of these conditions. Successful pregnancy requires important physiologic adaptations, such as a marked increase in cardiac output. Medical problems that interfere with the physiologic adaptations of pregnancy increase the risk for poor pregnancy outcome; conversely, in some instances pregnancy may adversely impact an underlying medical disorder.

HYPERTENSION (See also Chap. 230)   In pregnancy, cardiac output increases by 40%, most of which is due to an increase in stroke volume. Heart rate increases by approximately 10 beats per minute during the third trimester. In the second trimester of pregnancy, systemic vascular resistance decreases and this is associated with a fall in blood pressure. During pregnancy, a blood pressure of 140/90 mmHg is considered to be abnormally elevated and is associated with a marked increase in perinatal morbidity and mortality. In all pregnant women, the measurement of blood pressure should be performed in the sitting position, because for many the lateral recumbent position is associated with a blood pressure lower than that recorded in the sitting position. The diagnosis of hypertension requires the measurement of two elevated blood pressures, at least 6 h apart. Hypertension during pregnancy is usually caused by preeclampsia, chronic hypertension, gestational hypertension, or renal disease.

Preeclampsia   Approximately 5 to 7% of all pregnant women develop *preeclampsia*, the new onset of hypertension (blood pressure > 140/90 mmHg), proteinuria (>300 mg/24 h), and pathologic edema during gestation. Although the precise placental factors that cause preeclampsia are unknown, the end result is vasospasm and endothelial injury in multiple organs. Excessive placental secretion of an fms-like tyrosine kinase 1 may contribute to the endothelial dysfunction, hypertension, and proteinuria observed in preeclampsia. Glomerular endothelial cells demonstrate swelling and encroach on the vascular lumen. Preeclampsia is associated with abnormalities of cerebral circulatory autoregulation, which increase the risk of stroke at near-normal blood pressures. Risk factors for the development of preeclampsia include nulliparity, diabetes mellitus, a history of renal disease or chronic hypertension, a prior history of preeclampsia, extremes of maternal age (>35 years or <15 years), obesity, factor V Leiden mutation, angiotensinogen gene T235, antiphospholipid antibody syndrome, and multiple gestation.

There are no well-established strategies for the prevention of preeclampsia. Clinical trials have demonstrated that low-dose aspirin treatment does *not* prevent preeclampsia in either low- or high-risk women. Two meta-analyses reported that dietary calcium supplementation appeared to be effective in reducing the risk of developing preeclampsia. Subsequently, however, a large randomized clinical trial in low-risk women did not demonstrate a protective effect of calcium supplementation. Therefore, calcium supplementation *may* be considered in women at high risk for preeclampsia (see above). The observation that dietary intervention may reduce the risk of hypertension in men and nonpregnant women raises the possibility that dietary manipulations will be discovered that reduce the risk of preeclampsia.

Severe preeclampsia is the presence of new-onset hypertension and proteinuria accompanied by central nervous system dysfunction (headaches, blurred vision, seizures, coma), marked elevations of blood pressure (>160/110 mmHg), severe proteinuria (>5 g/24 h), oliguria or renal failure, pulmonary edema, hepatocellular injury (ALT > 2 × the upper limits of normal), thrombocytopenia (platelet count < 100,000/μL), or disseminated intravascular coagulation. Women with *mild preeclampsia* are those with the diagnosis of new-onset hypertension, proteinuria, and edema without evidence of severe preeclampsia. The HELLP (*h*emolysis, *e*levated *l*iver enzymes, *l*ow *p*latelets) syndrome is a special subgroup of severe preeclampsia and is a major cause of morbidity and mortality in this disease. The presence of platelet dysfunction and coagulation disorders further increases the risk of stroke.

℞ TREATMENT

Preeclampsia resolves within a few weeks after delivery. For pregnant women with preeclampsia prior to 37 weeks' gestation, delivery reduces the mother's morbidity but exposes the fetus to the risk of premature delivery. The management of preeclampsia is challenging because it requires the clinician to balance the health of both mother and fetus simultaneously and to make management decisions that afford both the best opportunities for infant survival. In general, prior to term, women with *mild* preeclampsia can be managed conservatively with bed rest, close monitoring of blood pressure and renal function, and careful fetal surveillance. For women with *severe* preeclampsia, delivery is recommended after 32 weeks' gestation. This reduces maternal morbidity and slightly increases the risks associated with prematurity for the newborn. Prior to 32 weeks' gestation, the risks of prematurity for the fetus are great, and some authorities recommend conservative management to allow for continued fetal maturation. Expectant management of severe preeclampsia remote from term affords some benefits for the fetus with significant risks for the mother. Such management should be restricted to tertiary care centers where maternal-fetal medicine, neonatal medicine, and critical care medicine expertise are available.

The definitive treatment of preeclampsia is delivery of the fetus and placenta. For women with severe preeclampsia, aggressive management of blood pressures > 160/110 mmHg reduces the risk of cerebrovascular accidents.

Intravenous labetalol or hydralazine are the drugs most commonly used to manage preeclampsia. Alternative agents such as calcium channel blockers may be used. Elevated arterial pressure should be reduced slowly to avoid hypotension and a decrease in blood flow to the fetus. *Angiotensin-converting enzyme (ACE) inhibitors as well as angiotensin-receptor blockers should be avoided in the second and third trimesters of pregnancy because of their adverse effects on fetal development.* Pregnant women treated with ACE inhibitors often develop oligohydramnios, which may be caused by decreased fetal renal function.

Magnesium sulfate is the treatment of choice for the prevention and treatment of eclamptic seizures. Two large randomized clinical trials have demonstrated the superiority of magnesium sulfate over phenytoin and diazepam, and a recent large randomized clinical trial has demonstrated the efficacy of magnesium sulphate in reducing the risk of seizure and possible reducing the risk of maternal death. Magnesium may prevent seizures by interacting with *N*-methyl-D-aspartate (NMDA) receptors in the central nervous system. Given the difficulty of predicting eclamptic seizures on the basis of disease severity, it is recommended that once the decision to proceed with delivery is made, all patients carrying a diagnosis of preeclampsia be treated with magnesium sulfate (see Guideline).

REGIMENS FOR THE ADMINISTRATION OF MAGNESIUM SULFATE FOR SEIZURE PROPHYLAXIS IN WOMEN IN LABOR WITH PREECLAMPSIA

Intramuscular	Intravenous
10 g (5 g IM deep in each buttock)[a]	6-g bolus over 15 min
5 g IM deep q4h, alternating sides	1–3 g/h by continuous infusion pump
	May be mixed in 100 mL crystalloid; if given by intravenous push, make up as 20% solution; push at maximum rate of 1g/min
	40-g MgSO$_4$·7H$_2$O in 1000 mL Ringers lactate; run at 25–75 mL/h (1–3 g/h)[a]

[a] Made up as 50% solution

Chronic Essential Hypertension Pregnancy complicated by chronic essential hypertension is associated with intrauterine growth restriction and increased perinatal mortality. Pregnant women with chronic hypertension are at increased risk for superimposed preeclampsia and abruptio placenta. Women with chronic hypertension should have a thorough prepregnancy evaluation, both to identify remediable causes of hypertension and to ensure that the prescribed antihypertensive agents are not associated with an adverse outcome of pregnancy (e.g., ACE inhibitors, angiotensin-receptor blockers). α-Methyldopa and labetalol are the most commonly used medications for the treatment of chronic hypertension in pregnancy. Baseline evaluation of renal function is necessary to help differentiate the effects of chronic hypertension versus superimposed preeclampsia should the hypertension worsen during pregnancy. There are no convincing data that demonstrate that treatment of mild chronic hypertension improves perinatal outcome.

Gestational Hypertension This is the development of elevated blood pressure during pregnancy or in the first 24 h post partum in the absence of preexisting chronic hypertension and other signs of preeclampsia. Uncomplicated gestational hypertension that does not progress to preeclampsia has not been associated with adverse pregnancy outcome or adverse long-term prognosis.

RENAL DISEASE (See also Chaps. 259 and 267) Normal pregnancy is characterized by an increase in glomerular filtration rate and creatinine clearance. This occurs secondary to a rise in renal plasma flow and increased glomerular filtration pressures. Patients with underlying renal disease and hypertension may expect a worsening of hypertension during pregnancy. If superimposed preeclampsia develops, the additional endothelial injury results in a capillary leak syndrome that may make the management of these patients challenging. In general, patients with underlying renal disease and hypertension benefit from more aggressive management of blood pressure than do those with gestational hypertension. Preconception counseling is also essential for these patients so that accurate risk assessment can occur prior to the establishment of pregnancy and important medication changes and adjustments can be made. In general, a prepregnancy serum creatinine level <133 μmol/L (<1.5 mg/dL) is associated with a favorable prognosis. When renal disease worsens during pregnancy, close collaboration between the nephrologist and the maternal-fetal medicine specialist is essential so that decisions regarding delivery can be weighed in the context of sequelae of prematurity for the neonate versus long-term sequelae for the mother with respect to future renal function.

Post-Renal Transplant Successful pregnancy after renal transplantation has been reported increasingly. Predictors for success include a normally functioning transplanted kidney, absence of rejection for at least 2 years prior to the pregnancy, absence of hypertension, and preferably minimal doses of immunosuppressant medications. Pregnancies in women using cyclosporine are more likely to be complicated by renal insufficiency and/or the development of hypertension. Such patients require very careful maternal and fetal surveillance. Nearly half of these pregnancies deliver preterm, and 20% of neonates are small for their gestational age. Rejection occurs in ~10% of pregnancies, and ~15% of patients will have deterioration in their renal function that persists after delivery. While pregnancy is generally well tolerated in renal transplant recipients, controversy remains as to whether or not deterioration of graft function is accelerated by pregnancy. More aggressive management of blood pressure has been suggested in this group of patients in an effort to protect the grafted kidney.

Systemic Lupus Erythematosus (SLE)

Another subset of patients with chronic renal disease and hypertension are those patients whose pregnancies are complicated by SLE (Chap. 300). In the past, SLE was considered to be a contraindication to pregnancy. With improved understanding of the effects of SLE on pregnancy, and vice versa, and with improved pharmacologic methods for managing SLE, successful pregnancy outcome is likely. Good prognostic factors for establishment of pregnancy in the presence of SLE are as follows:

1. Disease quiescence > 6 months
2. Normal blood pressure (with or without medication)
3. Normal renal function [creatinine < 133 μmol/L (< 1.5 mg/dL)]
4. Absence of antiphospholipid antibodies
5. Minimal or no need for immunosuppressive drugs
6. Absence of prior adverse reproductive outcome

Previously a point of controversy, there is now increasing consensus that pregnancy and the postpartum period are times of increased lupus activity. In severe flares early in gestation, pregnancy termination is often recommended. If pregnancy termination is not an option, then medical therapy to manage the lupus flare should not be influenced by the pregnancy, provided informed consent for treatment is obtained from the patient. Pulsed glucocorticoid therapy, azathioprine, hydroxychloroquine, and cyclophosphamide have all been used successfully in pregnancy.

CARDIAC DISEASE ■ Valvular Heart Disease

(See also Chap. 219) This is the most common cardiac problem complicating pregnancy.

MITRAL STENOSIS This is the valvular disease most likely to cause death during pregnancy. The pregnancy-induced increase in blood volume, cardiac output, and tachycardia can cause pulmonary edema in women with mitral stenosis. Pregnancy associated with long-standing mitral stenosis may result in pulmonary hypertension. Sudden death has been reported when hypovolemia has been allowed to occur in this condition. Careful control of heart rate, especially during labor and delivery, minimizes the impact of tachycardia and reduced ventricular filling times on cardiac function. Pregnant women with mitral stenosis are at increased risk for the development of atrial fibrillation and other tachyarrythmias. Medical management of severe mitral stenosis and atrial fibrillation with digoxin and beta blockers is recommended. Balloon valvulotomy can be carried out during pregnancy.

MITRAL REGURGITATION AND AORTIC REGURGITATION These are both generally well tolerated during pregnancy. The pregnancy-induced decrease in systemic vascular resistance reduces the risk of cardiac failure with these conditions. As a rule, mitral valve prolapse does not present problems for the pregnant patient, and aortic stenosis, unless very severe, is well tolerated. In the most severe cases of aortic stenosis, limitation of activity or balloon valvuloplasty may be indicated.

For women with artificial valves contemplating pregnancy, it is important that warfarin be stopped and heparin initiated prior to conception. Warfarin therapy during the first trimester of pregnancy has been associated with fetal chondrodysplasia punctata. In the second and third trimester of pregnancy, warfarin may cause fetal optic atrophy and mental retardation. For women with prosthetic heart valves, prophylaxis against thrombosis with low-molecular-weight heparin (LMWH) is not recommended due to reports of valvular thrombosis

despite adequate anticoagulation. Prophylaxis with unfractionated heparin is recommended for this group of women.

Congenital Heart Disease

(See also Chap. 218) The presence of a congenital cardiac lesion in the mother increases the risk of congenital cardiac disease in the newborn. Prenatal screening of the fetus for congenital cardiac disease with ultrasound is recommended. Atrial or ventricular septal defect is usually well tolerated during pregnancy in the absence of pulmonary hypertension, provided that the woman's prepregnancy cardiac status is favorable. Use of air filters on intravenous sets during labor and delivery in patients with intracardiac shunts is generally recommended.

Other Cardiac Disorders

Supraventricular tachycardia (Chap. 214) is a common cardiac complication of pregnancy. Treatment is the same as in the nonpregnant patient, and fetal tolerance of medications such as adenosine and calcium channel blockers is acceptable. When necessary, electrocardioversion may be performed and is generally well tolerated by mother and fetus.

Peripartum cardiomyopathy (Chap. 221) is a rare disorder of pregnancy associated with myocarditis, and its etiology remains unknown. Treatment is directed toward symptomatic relief and improvement of cardiac function. Many patients recover completely; others are left with a progressive dilated cardiomyopathy. Recurrence in a subsequent pregnancy has been reported, and women should be counseled to avoid pregnancy after a diagnosis of peripartum cardiomyopathy.

Specific High-Risk Cardiac Lesions ■ *MARFAN SYNDROME*

(See also Chap. 342) This is an autosomal dominant disease, associated with a high risk of maternal morbidity. Approximately 15% of pregnant women with Marfan syndrome develop a major cardiovascular manifestation during pregnancy, with almost all women surviving. An aortic root diameter <40 mm is considered to be associated with a favorable outcome of pregnancy. Prophylactic therapy with beta blockers has been advocated, although large-scale clinical trials in pregnancy have not been performed.

PULMONARY HYPERTENSION (See also Chap. 220) Maternal mortality in the setting of severe pulmonary hypertension is high, and primary pulmonary hypertension is a contraindication to pregnancy. Termination of pregnancy may be advisable in these circumstances to preserve the life of the mother. In the Eisenmenger syndrome, i.e., the combination of pulmonary hypertension with right-to-left shunting due to congenital abnormalities (Chap. 218), maternal and fetal death occur frequently. Systemic hypotension may occur after blood loss, prolonged Valsalva maneuver, or regional anesthesia; sudden death secondary to hypotension is a dreaded complication. Management of these patients is challenging, and invasive hemodynamic monitoring during labor and delivery is generally recommended.

In patients with pulmonary hypertension, vaginal delivery is less stressful hemodynamically than Cesarean section, which should be reserved for accepted obstetric indications.

DEEP VENOUS THROMBOSIS AND PULMONARY EMBOLISM

(See also Chaps. 232 and 244) A hypercoagulable state is characteristic of pregnancy, and deep venous thrombosis (DVT) is a common complication. Indeed, pulmonary embolism is the most common cause of maternal death in the United States. In pregnant women, DVT occurs much more commonly in the left leg than in the right leg, due to the compression of the left iliac vein by the right iliac artery and the uterus. Activated protein C resistance caused by the factor V Leiden mutation increases the risk for DVT and pulmonary embolism during pregnancy. Approximately 25% of women with DVT during pregnancy carry the factor V Leiden allele. The presence of the factor V Leiden mutation also increases the risk for severe preeclampsia. If the fetus carries a factor V Leiden mutation, the risk of extensive placental infarction is very high. Additional genetic mutations associated with DVT during pregnancy include the prothrombin G20210A mutation (heterozygotes and homozygotes) and the methylenetetrahydrofolate reductase C677T mutation (homozygotes).

TREATMENT

Aggressive diagnosis and management of DVT and suspected pulmonary embolism optimize the outcome for mother and fetus. In general, all diagnostic and therapeutic modalities afforded the nonpregnant patient should be utilized in pregnancy. Anticoagulant therapy with LMWH or unfractionated heparin is indicated in pregnant women with DVT. LMWH may be associated with an increased risk of epidural hematoma in women receiving an epidural anesthetic in labor. One approach to this problem is to switch from LMWH heparin to unfractionated heparin about 2 weeks before the anticipated delivery date. Warfarin therapy is contraindicated in the first trimester due to its association with fetal chondrodysplasia punctata. In the second and third trimesters, warfarin may cause fetal optic atrophy and mental retardation. When DVT occurs in the postpartum period, LMWH therapy for 7 to 10 days may be followed by warfarin therapy for 3 to 6 months. Warfarin is not contraindicated in breast-feeding women.

ENDOCRINE DISORDERS ■ Diabetes Mellitus (See also Chap. 323) In pregnancy, the fetoplacental unit induces major metabolic changes, the purpose of which is to shunt glucose and amino acids to the fetus while the mother uses ketones and triglycerides to fuel her metabolic needs. These metabolic changes are accompanied by maternal insulin resistance, caused in part by placental production of steroids, a growth hormone variant, and placental lactogen. Although pregnancy has been referred to as a state of accelerated starvation, it is better characterized as accelerated ketosis. In pregnancy, after an overnight fast, plasma glucose is lower by 0.8 to 1.1 mmol/L (15 to 20 mg/dL) than in the nonpregnant state. This is due to the use of glucose by the fetus. In early pregnancy, fasting may result in circulating glucose concentrations in the range of 2.2 mmol/L (40 mg/dL) and may be associated with symptoms of hypoglycemia. In contrast to the decrease in maternal glucose concentration, plasma hydroxybutyrate and acetoacetate levels rise to two to four times normal after a fast.

TREATMENT

Pregnancy complicated by diabetes mellitus is associated with higher maternal and perinatal morbidity and mortality rates. Preconception counseling and treatment are important for the diabetic patient contemplating pregnancy. Optimizing preconception glucose control and attention to other dietary needs such as appropriate levels of folate can significantly reduce the risk of congenital fetal malformations. Folate supplementation reduces the incidence of fetal neural tube defects, which occur with greater frequency in fetuses of diabetic mothers. In addition, optimizing glucose control during key periods of organogenesis reduces other congenital anomalies including sacral agenesis, caudal dysplasia, renal agenesis, and ventricular septal defect.

Once pregnancy is established, glucose control should be managed more aggressively than in the nonpregnant state. In addition to dietary changes, this requires more frequent blood glucose monitoring and often involves additional injections of insulin or conversion to an insulin pump. Fasting blood glucose levels should be maintained at <5.8 mmol/L (<105 mg/dL) with no values exceeding 7.8 mmol/L (140 mg/dL). Commencing in the third trimester, regular surveillance of maternal glucose control as well as assessment of fetal growth (obstetric sonography) and fetoplacental oxygenation (fetal heart rate monitoring or biophysical profile) optimize pregnancy outcome. Pregnant diabetic patients without vascular disease are at greater risk for delivering a macrosomic fetus, and attention to fetal growth via clinical and ultrasound examinations is important. Fetal macrosomia is associated with an increased risk of maternal and fetal birth trauma. Pregnant women with diabetes have an increased risk of developing preeclampsia, and those with vascular disease are at greater risk for developing intrauterine growth restriction, which is associated with an increased risk of fetal and neonatal death. Excellent pregnancy outcomes in patients with diabetic nephropathy and proliferative retinopathy have been reported with aggressive glucose control and intensive maternal and fetal surveillance.

Glycemic control may become more difficult to achieve as pregnancy progresses. Because of delayed pulmonary maturation of the fetuses of diabetic mothers, early delivery should be avoided unless there is biochemical evidence of fetal lung maturity. In general, efforts to control glucose and maintain the pregnancy until the estimated date of delivery result in the best overall outcome for both mother and newborn.

Gestational Diabetes All pregnant women should be screened for gestational diabetes unless they are in a low-risk group. Women at low risk for gestational diabetes are those <25 years of age; those with a body mass index <25 kg/m^2, no maternal history of macrosomia or gestational diabetes, and no diabetes in a first-degree relative; and those not members of a high-risk ethnic group (African American, Hispanic, Native American). A typical two-step strategy for establishing the diagnosis of gestational diabetes involves administration of a 50-g oral glucose challenge with a single serum glucose measurement at 60 min. If the plasma glucose is < 7.8 mmol/L (<140 mg/dL), the test is considered normal. Serum glucose > 7.8 mmol/L (>140 mg/dL) warrants administration of a 100-g oral glucose challenge with serum glucose measurements obtained in the fasting state, and at 1, 2, and 3 h. Normal values are plasma glucose concentrations <5.8 mmol/L (<105 mg/dL), 10.5 mmol/L (190 mg/dL), 9.1 mmol/L (165 mg/dL), and 8.0 mmol/L (145 mg/dL), respectively.

Pregnant women with gestational diabetes are at increased risk of preeclampsia, delivering infants who are large for their gestational age, and birth lacerations. Their fetuses are at risk of hypoglycemia and birth trauma (brachial plexus) injury.

TREATMENT

Gestational diabetes is first treated with dietary measures. Inability to maintain fasting glucose concentrations <5.8 mmol/L (<105 mg/dL) or 2-h postprandial glucose concentrations <6.7 mmol/L (<120 mg/dL) should prompt initiation of insulin therapy. Patients with a diagnosis of gestational diabetes will benefit from postpartum follow-up as they are at increased risk for developing type 2 diabetes.

Thyroid Disease (See also Chap. 320) In pregnancy, the estrogen-induced increase in thyroxine-binding globulin causes an increase in circulating levels of total T_3 and total T_4. The normal range of circulating levels of free T_4, free T_3, and thyroid stimulating hormone (TSH) remain unaltered by pregnancy.

The thyroid gland normally enlarges during pregnancy. Maternal hyperthyroidism occurs at a rate of approximately 2 per 1000 pregnancies and is generally well tolerated by pregnant women. Clinical signs and symptoms should alert the physician to the occurrence of this disease. Many of the physiologic adaptations to pregnancy may mimic subtle signs of hyperthyroidism. Although pregnant women are able to tolerate mild hyperthyroidism without adverse sequelae, more severe hyperthyroidism can cause spontaneous abortion or premature labor, and thyroid storm is associated with a significant risk of maternal mortality.

TREATMENT

Hyperthyroidism in pregnancy should be aggressively evaluated and treated. The treatment of choice is propylthiouracil. Because it crosses the placenta, the minimum effective dose should be used to maintain free T_4 in the upper normal range. Methimazole crosses the placenta to a greater degree than propylthiouracil and has been associated with fetal aplasia cutis. Radioiodine should not be used during pregnancy, either for scanning or treatment, because of effects on the fetal thyroid. In emergent circumstances, additional treatment with beta blockers and a saturated solution of potassium iodide may be necessary. Hyperthyroidism is most difficult to control in the first trimester of pregnancy and easiest to control in the third trimester.

The goal of therapy for *hypothyroidism* is to maintain the serum

TSH in the normal range, and thyroxine is the drug of choice. Children born to women with an elevated serum TSH (and a normal total thyroxine) during pregnancy have impaired performance on neuropsychologic tests. During pregnancy, the dose of thyroxine required to keep the TSH in the normal range rises. In one study, the mean replacement dose of thyroxine required to maintain the TSH in the normal range was 0.1 mg daily before pregnancy, and it increased to 0.15 mg daily during pregnancy.

HEMATOLOGIC DISORDERS　Pregnancy has been described as a state of physiologic anemia. Part of the reduction in hemoglobin concentration is dilutional, but iron and folate deficiencies are the major causes of correctable anemia during pregnancy. Folic acid food supplementation implemented in 1998 has reduced the risk of fetal neural tube defects.

In populations at high risk for hemoglobinopathies (Chap. 91), hemoglobin electrophoresis should be performed as part of the prenatal screen. Hemoglobinopathies can be associated with increased maternal and fetal morbidity and mortality. Management is tailored to the specific hemoglobinopathy and is generally the same for both pregnant and nonpregnant women. Prenatal diagnosis of hemoglobinopathies in the fetus is readily available and should be discussed with prospective parents either prior to or early in pregnancy.

Thrombocytopenia occurs commonly during pregnancy. The majority of cases are benign gestational thrombocytopenias, but the differential diagnosis should include immune thrombocytopenia (Chap. 101) and preeclampsia. Maternal thrombocytopenia may also be caused by catastrophic obstetric events such as retention of a dead fetus, sepsis, abruptio placenta, and amniotic fluid embolism.

NEUROLOGIC DISORDERS　Headache appearing during pregnancy is usually due to migraine (Chap. 14), a condition that may worsen, improve, or be unaffected by pregnancy. A new or worsening headache, particularly if associated with visual blurring, may signal eclampsia (above) or pseudotumor cerebri (benign intracranial hypertension; Chap. 25); diplopia due to a sixth nerve palsy suggests pseudotumor cerebri. The risk of seizures in patients with epilepsy increases in the postpartum period but not consistently during pregnancy; management is discussed in Chap. 348. The risk of stroke is generally thought to increase during pregnancy because of a hypercoagulable state; however, studies suggest that the period of risk occurs primarily in the postpartum period and that both ischemic and hemorrhagic strokes may occur at this time. Guidelines for use of heparin therapy are summarized above (see "Deep Venous Thrombosis and Pulmonary Embolism"); warfarin is teratogenic and should be avoided. The onset of a new movement disorder during pregnancy suggests chorea gravidarum, a variant of Sydenham's chorea associated with rheumatic fever and streptococcal infection (Chap. 121); the chorea may recur with subsequent pregnancies. Patients with preexisting multiple sclerosis (Chap. 359) experience a gradual decrease in the risk of relapses as pregnancy progresses and, conversely, an increase in attack risk during the postpartum period. Beta interferons should *not* be administered to pregnant MS patients, but moderate or severe relapses can be safely treated with pulse glucocorticoid therapy. Finally, certain tumors, particularly pituitary adenoma and meningioma (Chap. 358), may manifest during pregnancy because of accelerated growth, possibly driven by hormonal factors.

Peripheral nerve disorders associated with pregnancy include Bell's palsy (idiopathic facial paralysis, Chap. 363), which is approximately threefold more likely to occur during the third trimester and immediate postpartum period than in the general population. Therapy with glucocorticoids should follow the guidelines established for nonpregnant patients; however, acyclovir should probably be avoided, particularly during the first two trimesters. Entrapment neuropathies (Chap. 363) are common in the later stages of pregnancy, presumably as a result of fluid retention. Carpal tunnel syndrome (median nerve) presents as pain and paresthesia in the hand, often worse at night, and later with weakness in the thenar muscles. Treatment is generally conservative;

wrist splints may be helpful, and glucocorticoid injections or surgical section of the carpal tunnel can usually be postponed. Meralgia paresthetica (lateral femoral cutaneous nerve) consists of pain and numbness in the lateral aspect of the thigh without weakness. Patients are usually reassured to learn that these symptoms are benign and can be expected to remit spontaneously after the pregnancy has been completed.

Judicious use of neuroimaging procedures is reasonable during pregnancy. Some centers require that formal consent be obtained from pregnant patients before magnetic resonance imaging (MRI) scans are administered. Experimental data indicate that high-field-strength MRI may be teratogenic to rodents; however, studies in pregnant MRI technicians have failed to show any risk to the fetus, even with chronic exposure. The paramagnetic MRI contrast agent gadolinium is usually not administered, particularly during the first trimester, because it crosses the blood-brain barrier. Computed tomography scanning of the brain is also considered safe, particularly as the procedure is fast, little radioactive scatter is produced, and pelvic contents are easily shielded; iodinated contrast media should be avoided whenever possible.

GASTROINTESTINAL AND LIVER DISEASE　Up to 90% of pregnant women experience nausea and vomiting during the first trimester of pregnancy. Occasionally, hyperemesis gravidarum requires hospitalization to prevent dehydration, and sometimes parenteral nutrition is required.

Crohn's disease may be associated with exacerbations in the second and third trimesters. Ulcerative colitis is associated with disease exacerbations in the first trimester and during the early postpartum period. Medical management of these diseases during pregnancy is identical to the management in the nonpregnant state (Chap. 276).

Exacerbation of gall bladder disease is commonly observed during pregnancy. In part this may be due to pregnancy-induced alteration in the metabolism of bile and fatty acids. Intrahepatic cholestasis of pregnancy is generally a third-trimester event. Profound pruritus may accompany this condition, and it may be associated with increased fetal mortality. It has been suggested that placental bile salt deposition may contribute to progressive uteroplacental insufficiency. Therefore, regular fetal surveillance should be undertaken once the diagnosis of intrahepatic cholestasis is made. Favorable results with ursodiol have been reported.

Acute fatty liver is a rare complication of pregnancy. Frequently confused with the HELLP syndrome (see "Preeclampsia," above) and severe preeclampsia, the diagnosis of acute fatty liver of pregnancy may be facilitated by imaging studies and laboratory evaluation. Acute fatty liver of pregnancy is generally characterized by markedly increased levels of bilirubin and ammonia and by hypoglycemia. Management of acute fatty liver of pregnancy is supportive; recurrence in subsequent pregnancies has been reported.

All pregnant women should be screened for hepatitis B. This information is important for pediatricians after delivery of the infant. All infants receive hepatitis B vaccine. Infants born to mothers who are carriers of hepatitis B surface antigen should also receive hepatitis B immune globulin as soon after birth as possible and preferably within the first 72 h.

INFECTIONS ■ Bacterial Infections　Other than bacterial vaginosis, the most common bacterial infections during pregnancy involve the urinary tract (Chap. 269). Many pregnant women have asymptomatic bacteriuria, most likely due to stasis caused by progestational effects on ureteral and bladder smooth muscle and to compression effects of the enlarging uterus. In itself, this condition is not associated with an adverse outcome of pregnancy. However, if asymptomatic bacteriuria is left untreated, symptomatic pyelonephritis may occur. Indeed, ~75% of cases of pregnancy-associated pyelonephritis are the result of untreated asymptomatic bacteriuria. All pregnant women should be screened with a urine culture for asymptomatic bacteriuria at the first prenatal visit. Subsequent screening with nitrite/leukocyte esterase strips is indicated for high-risk women, such as those with sickle cell trait or a history of urinary tract infections. All women with positive screens should be treated.

Because of the association between bacterial vaginosis and preterm delivery, screening for bacterial vaginosis has been used in an effort to reduce risk. However, standard treatment for bacterial vaginosis does not reduce the risk of preterm delivery.

Abdominal pain and fever during pregnancy create a clinical dilemma. The diagnosis of greatest concern is intrauterine amniotic infection. While amniotic infection most commonly follows rupture of the membranes, this is not always the case. In general, antibiotic therapy is not recommended as a temporizing measure in these circumstances. If intrauterine infection is suspected, induced delivery with concomitant antibiotic therapy is generally indicated. Intrauterine amniotic infection is most often caused by pathogens such as *Escherichia coli* and group B streptococcus. In high-risk patients at term or in preterm patients, routine intrapartum prophylaxis of group B streptococcal (GBS) disease is recommended. Penicillin G and ampicillin are the drugs of choice. In penicillin-allergic patients, clindamycin is recommended. Recently, it has been reported that universal screening of pregnant women for GBS disease may be superior to treatment based on presence of risk factors alone.

Postpartum infection is a significant cause of maternal morbidity and mortality. While rare after vaginal delivery, postpartum endomyometritis develops in 5% of patients having elective repeat cesarean section and in 25% of patients after emergency cesarean section following prolonged labor. Prophylactic antibiotics should be given to all patients undergoing cesarean section. As most cases of postpartum endomyometritis are polymicrobial, broad-spectrum antibiotic coverage with a penicillin, aminoglycoside, and metronidazole is recommended (Chap. 148). Most cases resolve within 72 h. Women who do not respond to antibiotic treatment for postpartum endomyometritis should be evaluated for septic pelvic thrombophlebitis. Imaging studies may be helpful in establishing the diagnosis, which is primarily a clinical diagnosis of exclusion. Patients with septic pelvic thrombophlebitis generally have tachycardia out of proportion to their fever and respond rapidly to intravenous administration of heparin.

All patients are screened prenatally for gonorrhea and chlamydial infections, and the detection of either should result in prompt treatment. Ceftriaxone and azithromycin are the agents of choice (Chaps. 128 and 160).

Viral Infections ■ *CYTOMEGALOVIRUS INFECTION* Viral infection in pregnancy presents a significant challenge. The most common cause of congenital viral infection in the United States is cytomegalovirus (CMV) (Chap. 166). As many as 50 to 90% of women of childbearing age have antibodies to CMV, but only rarely does CMV reactivation result in neonatal infection. More commonly, primary CMV infection during pregnancy creates a risk of congenital CMV. No currently accepted treatment of CMV during pregnancy has been demonstrated to protect the fetus effectively. Moreover, it is impossible to predict which fetus will sustain life-threatening CMV infection. Severe CMV disease in the newborn is characterized most often by petechiae, hepatosplenomegaly, and jaundice. Chorioretinitis, microcephaly, intracranial calcifications, hepatitis, hemolytic anemia, and purpura may also develop. Central nervous system involvement, resulting in the development of psychomotor, ocular, auditory, and dental abnormalities over time, has been described.

RUBELLA (See also Chap. 177)   Rubella virus is a known teratogen; first-trimester rubella carries a high risk of fetal anomalies, though the risk decreases significantly later in pregnancy. Congenital rubella may be diagnosed by percutaneous umbilical blood sampling with the detection of IgM antibodies in fetal blood. All pregnant women should be screened for their immune status to rubella. Indeed, all women of childbearing age, regardless of pregnancy status, should have their immune status for rubella verified and be immunized if necessary. The incidence of congenital rubella in the United States is extremely low.

HERPESVIRUS (See also Chap. 163)   The acquisition of genital herpes during pregnancy is associated with spontaneous abortion, prematurity, and congenital and neonatal herpes. A recent cohort study of pregnant women without evidence of previous herpes infection demonstrated that ~2% of the women acquired a new herpes infection during the pregnancy. Approximately 60% of the newly infected women had no clinical symptoms. Infection occurred equally in all three trimesters. If herpes seroconversion occurred early in pregnancy, the risk of transmission to the newborn was very low. In women who acquired genital herpes shortly before delivery, the risk of transmission was high. The risk of active genital herpes lesions at term can be reduced by prescribing acyclovir for the last 4 weeks of pregnancy to women who have had their first episode of genital herpes during the pregnancy. However, whether or not this strategy results in less viral shedding or enhanced fetal protection at delivery remains to be determined.

Herpesvirus infection in the newborn can be devastating. Disseminated neonatal herpes carries with it high mortality and morbidity rates from central nervous system involvement. It is recommended that pregnant women with active genital herpes lesions at the time of presentation in labor be delivered by cesarean section.

PARVOVIRUS (See also Chap. 168)   Parvovirus infection (human parvovirus B19) may occur during pregnancy. It rarely causes sequelae, but susceptible women infected during pregnancy may be at risk for fetal hydrops secondary to erythroid aplasia and profound anemia.

TOXOPLASMOSIS (See also Chap. 198)   In the United States, approximately 70% of women of childbearing age are susceptible to *Toxoplasma*. Most primary infections of toxoplasmosis in the United States come from eating undercooked meat. The diagnosis of congenital toxoplasmosis is possible through sampling of fetal umbilical blood. If there is no evidence of placental/fetal infection, single-drug treatment with spiramycin is recommended. Triple-drug therapy with spiramycin, pyrimethamine, and sulfa is recommended if there is evidence of fetal infection and the woman does not wish to terminate the pregnancy or cannot terminate it because of advanced gestational age. Prenatal treatment has been shown to reduce the number of infants with severe infection.

HUMAN IMMUNODEFICIENCY VIRUS (HIV) (See also Chap. 173)   The predominant cause of HIV infection in children is transmission of the virus from the mother to the newborn during the perinatal period. Exposures, which increase the risk of mother-to-child transmission, include vaginal delivery, preterm delivery, trauma to the fetal skin, and maternal bleeding. Additionally, recent infection with high maternal viral load, low maternal CD4+T cell count, prolonged labor, prolonged length of membrane rupture, and the presence of other genital tract infections, such as syphilis or herpes, increase the risk of transmission. Breast feeding may also transmit HIV to the newborn and is therefore contraindicated in most developed countries for HIV-infected mothers. There is no clear evidence to suggest that the course of HIV disease is altered by pregnancy. There is also no clear evidence to suggest that uncomplicated HIV disease adversely impacts pregnancy other than by its inherent infection risk.

℞ TREATMENT

The majority of cases of mother-to-child (vertical) transmission of HIV-1 occur during the intrapartum period. Mechanisms of vertical transmission include infection after rupture of the membranes and direct contact of the fetus with infected secretions or blood from the maternal genital tract. In women with HIV infection who are not receiving antiretroviral therapy, the rate of vertical transmission is approximately 25%. Cesarean section and treatment with zidovudine, administered both before and during delivery, decrease the rate of vertical transmission. In a meta-analysis, zidovudine treatment of both the mother during the prenatal and intrapartum periods and the neonate at birth reduced the risk of vertical transmission to 7.3%. The combination of elective cesarean section plus zidovudine treatment reduced the risk of vertical transmission to 2%. The role of multiple drug therapy during pregnancy has not yet been established, pending safety data for the neonate.

SUMMARY Maternal mortality has decreased steadily during the past 60 years. The maternal death rate has decreased from nearly 600/100,000 live births in 1935 to 8.5/100,000 live births in 1996. The most common causes of maternal death in the United States today are, in decreasing order of frequency, thromboembolic disease, hypertension, ectopic pregnancy, and hemorrhage. With improved diagnostic and therapeutic modalities as well as with advances in the treatment of infertility, more patients with medical complications will be seeking, and be in need of, complex obstetric care. Improving outcome of pregnancy in these women will be best obtained by assembling a team of internists and specialists in maternal-fetal medicine (high-risk obstetrics) to counsel these patients about the risks of pregnancy and to plan their treatment prior to conception. The importance of preconception counseling cannot be overstated. It is the responsibility of all physicians caring for women in the reproductive age group to assess their patient's reproductive plans as part of their overall health evaluation.

FURTHER READING

HADDOW JE et al: Maternal thyroid deficiency during pregnancy and subsequent neuropsychological development of the child. N Engl J Med 41:549, 1999

HIRSCH DR et al: Pulmonary embolism and deep venous thrombosis during pregnancy or oral contraceptive use: Prevalence of factor V Leiden. Am Heart J 131:1145, 1996

INTERNATIONAL PERINATAL HIV GROUP: The mode of delivery and the risk of vertical transmission of human immunodeficiency virus type 1—a meta-analysis of 15 prospective cohort studies. N Engl J Med 340:977, 1999

MAYNARD SE: Excess placental soluble fms-like tyrosine kinase 1 (sFlt1) may contribute to endothelial dysfunction, hypertension, and proteinuria in preeclampsia. J Clin Invest 111:649, 2003

RIDKER PM et al: Factor V Leiden mutation as a risk factor for recurrent pregnancy loss. Ann Intern Med 128:1000, 1998

SCHRAG SJ et al: A population-based comparison of strategies to prevent early-onset group B streptococcal disease in neonates. N Engl J Med 347:233, 2002

SCOTT LL et al: Acyclovir suppression to prevent cesarean delivery after first episode genital herpes. Obstet Gynecol 87:69, 1996

SIBAI BM: Chronic hypertension in pregnancy. Obstet Gynecol 100:369, 2002

THE MAGPIE TRIAL COLLABORATIVE GROUP: Do women with pre-eclampsia, and their babies, benefit from magnesium sulfate? The Magpie Trial: A randomised placebo-controlled trial. Lancet 359:1877, 2002

7 MEDICAL EVALUATION OF THE SURGICAL PATIENT
Gerald W. Smetana

Most individuals will require surgery at some point in their lifetimes. In the United States, surgeons performed 18 million inpatient operations in 2000; ambulatory surgery accounted for a substantial number of additional procedures. Preoperative medical consultation is, therefore, a common activity for practicing internists. However, many internists may be uncomfortable in this role as the process of preoperative risk stratification is not intuitive and relies heavily on a highly specialized literature that is not common knowledge among practicing clinicians.

The role of the medical consultant is to determine the presence of known or unrecognized comorbid disease or other factors that may increase risk of morbidity or mortality from baseline and to recommend strategies to reduce the risk and optimize the patient's condition before operation. This knowledge informs the discussion of risks and benefits for the patient and surgeon. Such consultations may range from the routine evaluation of a healthy patient before minor surgery to confirmation of high risk in a moribund patient undergoing emergency surgery for a life-threatening illness. Overall morbidity and mortality from surgery is low. Studies have demonstrated surgical mortality rates of 1% across all procedures for unselected patients. Mortality for the subset of patients undergoing ambulatory surgery is substantially lower. Surgeons select patients for ambulatory surgery when the combination of a lower risk procedure and few patient-related comorbidities suggests a low risk of adverse outcomes. Mortality in this group of patients is approximately 0.01%.

The most important contributions to postoperative morbidity and mortality are cardiac and pulmonary complications; each occurs in approximately 5% of all patients undergoing an operation. This chapter will review preoperative risk assessment and risk-reduction strategies for healthy patients and for the major categories of adverse outcomes and medical comorbidities—cardiac complications, pulmonary complications, and diabetes mellitus. Two other important perioperative considerations, venous thromboembolism prophylaxis (Chaps. 232 and 244) and endocarditis prophylaxis (Chap. 109), are discussed elsewhere in this text.

ANESTHETIC PHYSIOLOGY Modern anesthesia is extremely safe. Mortality among healthy patients undergoing surgery is low; estimates range from 0.01 to 0.03%. Patient- and procedure-related factors are more important contributors to perioperative morbidity than is anesthesia itself. Inhalational anesthetic agents have predictable physiologic effects. All inhalational anesthetic agents are myocardial depressants. While not clinically significant in healthy patients, this effect leads to a dependence on cardiac preload that may cause an accentuated response to the induction of anesthesia in patients who are volume-depleted due to illness or overdiuresis or who have left ventricular dysfunction. Anesthesia leads to a decrease in lung volumes. Both vital capacity and functional residual capacity decrease by one-third in abdominal surgery. This results from diaphragmatic dysfunction, decreased mucociliary clearance, loss of sighing breaths, and depression of the ventilatory response to hypoxemia and hypercarbia. This decrease in lung volumes may lead to atelectasis and is a principal factor leading to the development of postoperative pulmonary complications.

Controversy has long existed regarding the relative safety of general versus spinal or epidural anesthesia in patients at risk for postoperative cardiac or pulmonary complications. In a recent large meta-analysis of randomized controlled trials of anesthetic technique, patients who were randomized to spinal or epidural anesthesia as a component of their anesthesia had significantly lower rates of venous thromboembolism, pneumonia, respiratory depression, myocardial infarction, or death than patients receiving general anesthesia exclusively; relative risk reductions ranged from 30 to 55%. Clinicians should recommend spinal or epidural anesthesia, when possible, for patients at high risk for postoperative medical complications.

EVALUATION OF THE HEALTHY PATIENT Given the very low risk of complications among healthy patients undergoing surgery, additional clinical evaluation only rarely identifies patients at higher than average risk. Furthermore, due to the low prior probability of adverse events, most abnormal results from potential preoperative tests are false-positive tests. These results often contribute little to the estimation of risk, may increase patient and physician anxiety, lead to additional invasive tests that carry risk, and may increase medicolegal liability due to the possibility of abnormal test results that are ignored. A careful screening history and physical examination are the most important parts of the preoperative assessment of patients who report that they are healthy.

The history should focus on symptoms that suggest the possibility of occult cardiac or pulmonary disease. Many institutions have developed simple preoperative screening questionnaires for this purpose;

several of these instruments have been validated and shown to correctly identify most patients at higher than average risk. For example, in one study of a screening questionnaire, clinical evaluation by an anesthesiologist determined that only 2% of patients had negative responses to the questionnaire yet would have benefited from a more detailed clinical evaluation. Table 7-1 lists the questions on this validated questionnaire.

It is particularly important to query the patient about exercise capacity and to determine the reason for exercise intolerance, if present. For example, one report confirmed that a patient's self-report of the inability to walk at least four blocks on level ground or to climb at least two flights of stairs predicts a twofold increase in cardiac and all serious postoperative complications. One should inquire specifically about chest pain or shortness of breath with activity and about chronic cough. The history should also include a review of medications (both prescription and over the counter), any previous operations or important medical problems, alcohol use, the possibility of pregnancy in reproductive-age women, previous adverse responses to anesthesia or surgery, and a family history of anesthetic reactions (that might suggest malignant hyperthermia).

Age appears to be a minor risk factor for both pulmonary and cardiac complications. Most of the risk attributed to age can be explained by medical comorbidities that are more common with advancing age. In the few studies that have looked at this question, younger and older patients with a similar burden of medical comorbidities appear to have a similar risk of postoperative complications. While counterintuitive, obesity does *not* appear to be a risk factor for cardiac or pulmonary complications or perioperative mortality.

Clinicians should not routinely obtain laboratory testing before surgery. Rather, tests should be requested selectively based on patient- or procedure-related factors that predict a higher likelihood of an abnormal result that may potentially influence perioperative management. Many studies have shown the very limited value of preoperative testing (laboratory testing, urinalysis, electrocardiogram, and chest radiograph) of healthy patients. In most reports, <1% of all routine preoperative tests are abnormal and could potentially influence management; most of these can be predicted by clinical evaluation. Among patients undergoing low-risk surgery, such as cataract surgery, there is no difference in morbidity or mortality between patients who undergo routine preoperative testing and those who do not undergo such testing. When clinicians do choose to obtain preoperative tests, tests obtained within the previous 4 months may be safely used as preoperative tests, assuming there has been no change in the patient's clinical condition. Table 7-2 lists recommendations for specific tests in healthy patients based on the incidence of abnormalities that influence management and the predictive value of an abnormal test. The positive and negative likelihood ratios refer to the change in the odds of an adverse postoperative event if the test result is abnormal or normal, respectively.

CARDIAC RISK ASSESSMENT

Cardiac complications are the most important source of perioperative morbidity and may occur even in patients previously unknown to have heart disease. Therefore, an assessment of cardiac risk must be part of every preoperative medical evaluation. In general, low-risk patients may proceed without further evaluation; high-risk patients will require treatment to reduce the risk of complications regardless of the results of preoperative cardiac testing; and intermediate-risk patients will benefit most from additional testing to stratify risk before surgery.

CARDIAC RISK INDICES In most cases, one can confidently estimate risk through a careful history and physical examination and application of a cardiac risk index. The science of cardiac risk stratification began with the landmark study of Goldman and colleagues in 1977 that identified risk factors among the history, physical examination, electrocardiogram, general medical status, and type of surgical procedure. More recently, the revised cardiac risk index of Lee and colleagues has been shown to outperform the original index and other available risk-stratification tools and is now the preferred tool for initial risk stratification before noncardiac surgery (Table 7-3). This index resulted from a multivariate analysis of patients undergoing elective noncardiac surgery and includes six independent factors that predict risk of postoperative cardiac complications. As all of these factors were associated with a similar odds ratio for complications (range, 1.9 to 3.2), each factor is assigned one point in the revised cardiac risk index. Predictive factors include high-risk surgery (intraperitoneal, intrathoracic, or suprainguinal vascular procedures), ischemic heart disease, a history of congestive heart failure, a history of symptomatic cerebrovascular disease, insulin therapy for diabetes mellitus, or a preoperative serum creatinine >177 μmol/L (>2.0 mg/dL). Risk classes result from the total number of points (of six possible points). Risk increases substantially when two points exist; the greatest risk is for patients with three or more points.

Several factors that increase the likelihood of coronary artery disease (CAD) nonetheless do not increase the risk of postoperative cardiac complications. Factors that do *not* appear to increase risk include obesity, stable hypertension with a diastolic blood pressure of <110 mmHg, elevated cholesterol, bundle branch block, and cigarette smoking.

After application of the revised cardiac risk index (Table 7-3) to

---

TABLE 7-1 Suggested Preoperative Screening Questionnaire[a]

1. Have you ever had a heart attack?
2. Have you ever had heart trouble?
3. Have you ever had heart failure?
4. Have you ever had fluid in your lungs?

5. Do you have a heart murmur?
6. Did you have rheumatic fever as a child?

7. Do you ever have chest pain, angina, or chest tightness?
8. Have you ever been treated for an irregular heartbeat?
9. Do you have high blood pressure?

10. Do you ever have difficulty with your breathing?
11. Do you have asthma, bronchitis, or emphysema?
12. Do you cough frequently?
13. Does climbing one flight of stairs make you short of breath?
14. Does walking one city block make you short of breath?
15. Do you now or have you recently smoked cigarettes? If yes, how many packs per day? For how many years?
16. Do you have liver disease, or a history of jaundice or hepatitis?
17. Do you drink more than three drinks of alcohol per day? If yes, how many per week?
18. Do you have indigestion, heartburn, or a hiatus hernia?

19. Do you have a history of thyroid problems?
20. Do you have diabetes?
21. Do you have a kidney problem?
22. Do you have numbness or weakness of your arms or legs?
23. Do you have epilepsy, blackouts, or seizures?
24. Have you had problems with blood clots, or excessive bleeding?
25. Do you have any other important medical problems? Please list.
26. Have you ever had an anesthetic? If yes, when was your last one?
27. Have you or any member of your family had a reaction to an anesthetic?
28. Do you have arthritis or pain in your neck or jaw?
29. Do you have dentures, capped or loose teeth?
30. Do you think you may be pregnant?
31. Have you taken prednisone, steroid medications, or cortisone-like drugs in the past year?
32. Please list any food or medications allergies that you have.
33. Please list any medications you are currently taking.
34. Please list any operations you have had in the past.
35. If this is the day of your surgery, when did you last eat or drink?
36. Age: Weight: Height:

[a] Patients who answer yes to any of questions #1–8, 10–14, 16, 19–25, or 30 should receive a complete history and physical examination as part of the preoperative evaluation.
Source: From NH Badner et al: Can J Anaesth 45:87, 1998, with permission.

TABLE 7-2 *Recommendations for Preoperative Laboratory Testing for Healthy Patients*

Test	Incidence of Abnormalities That Influence Management, %	Likelihood Ratio [+]	Likelihood Ratio [−]	Indications
Hemoglobin	0.1	3.3	0.9	Anticipated major blood loss or symptoms of anemia
White blood cell count	0.0	0	1	Symptoms suggest infection, myeloproliferative disorder, or myelotoxic medications
Platelet count	0.0	0	1	History of bleeding diathesis, myeloproliferative disorder, or myelotoxic medications
Prothrombin time (PT)	0.0	0	1.01	History of bleeding diathesis, chronic liver disease, malnutrition, recent or long-term antibiotic use
Partial thromboplastin time (PTT)	0.1	1.7	0.86	History of bleeding diathesis
Electrolytes	1.8	4.3	0.8	Known renal insufficiency, congestive heart failure, medications that affect electrolytes
Renal function	2.6	3.3	0.81	Age > 50 years, hypertension, cardiac disease, major surgery, medications that may affect renal function
Glucose	0.5	1.6	0.85	Obesity or known diabetes
Liver function tests	0.1			No indication; consider albumin measurement for major surgery or chronic illness
Urinalysis	1.4	1.7	0.97	No indication
Electrocardiogram	2.6	1.6	0.96	Men > 40 years, women > 50 years, known CAD, diabetes, or hypertension
Chest radiograph	3.0	2.5	0.72	Age > 50 years, known cardiac or pulmonary disease, symptoms or exam suggest cardiac or pulmonary disease

Note: CAD, coronary artery disease.
Source: Reprinted from Smetana and Macpherson, with permission from Elsevier Science.

stratify risk, clinicians should apply one of the established cardiac risk guidelines to determine the optimal strategy for additional testing and risk reduction strategies. Both the American College of Physicians (ACP) and the American Heart Association/American College of Cardiology (AHA/ACC) have published guidelines that suggest criteria for additional cardiac testing for selected patients before surgery and treatment strategies to reduce risk in high-risk patients. The ACP guideline is more clinically based and easier to use but does not incorporate the revised cardiac risk index, which was published after its

TABLE 7-3 *The Revised Cardiac Risk Index*

Factor	Adjusted Odds Ratio (OR) for Cardiac Complications in Derivation Cohort
1. High-risk surgery	2.8
2. Ischemic heart disease	2.4
3. History of congestive heart failure	1.9
4. History of cerebrovascular disease	3.2
5. Insulin therapy for diabetes mellitus	3.0
6. Preoperative serum creatinine > 2.0 mg/dL	3.0

Class	Number of Factors	Cardiac Complication Rates, % Derivation Cohort	Cardiac Complication Rates, % Validation Cohort
I	0	0.5	0.4
II	1	1.3	0.9
III	2	3.6	6.6
IV	3–6	9.1	11.0

Source: Adapted from Lee et al, with permission.

release (Fig. 7-1). One can use elements of the ACP guideline along with more recent data to suggest that the first step would be to apply the revised cardiac risk index. Low-risk patients (class I) undergoing nonvascular surgery may proceed without additional evaluation. Additional noninvasive cardiac testing is appropriate for intermediate-risk patients (class II) undergoing vascular surgery. All high-risk patients (classes III and IV) should receive treatment to reduce risk (discussed below).

The AHA/ACC guideline is more complicated and relies on three separate factors: (1) clinical predictors (such as those in the revised cardiac risk index; Table 7-3), (2) functional capacity, and (3) procedure-specific risks. Examples of major clinical predictors include unstable coronary syndromes, recent myocardial infarction with evidence of ischemic risk, and decompensated congestive heart failure. Functional capacity is considered poor if patients are unable to perform activities requiring expenditure of at least four metabolic equivalents (METs). Examples in daily life include climbing one flight of stairs, doing light housework, or walking at least two blocks on level ground. Procedure-specific risks go beyond the high-risk categories defined in the revised cardiac risk index to identify low- and intermediate-risk procedures. This guideline recommends noninvasive cardiac testing for any patient with at least two of the following: (1) intermediate clinical predictors, (2) poor functional capacity, and (3) high-risk surgery.

EVALUATION BEFORE VASCULAR SURGERY Cardiac risk indices are unable to identify a subset of patients at low risk for cardiac complications after vascular surgery. This is due to the observation that the risk factors for peripheral vascular disease and CAD are the same. Therefore, patients undergoing arterial surgery are much more likely to have CAD than are patients undergoing general surgical procedures such as cholecystectomy, for example. As the prior probability of CAD is higher among such patients (92% in one angiographic study), even patients with low scores on cardiac risk indices have substantial risk for postoperative cardiac complications. Additional testing is necessary to estimate risk in these patients. Pharmacologic stress tests have been used widely to estimate cardiac risk before vascular surgery. Dipyridamole-thallium testing and dobutamine stress echocardiography have been studied most extensively. The test characteristics of the two tests are similar. Each has a negative predictive value of 95 to 100% but a positive predictive value for postoperative cardiac complications of only 10 to 20% for patients undergoing major vascular operations. As the predictive performances of these two tests are similar, clinicians may consider them to be interchangeable, and the selection of one test over the other depends on local availability and expertise.

Given the low predictive value when used in unselected patients before vascular surgery, clinicians may incorporate clinical factors to identify an intermediate probability group that will benefit most from noninvasive testing. Several strategies exist; the most widely used are the "Eagle" criteria that include Q waves on the electrocardiogram, age > 70 years, angina, ventricular ectopy requiring treatment, and diabetes requiring treatment. Patients who have none of these factors have a low risk of adverse events and can proceed without further evaluation. Those with three to five factors are at high risk and need no risk refinement by further study. Those with one to two factors benefit the most from noninvasive testing.

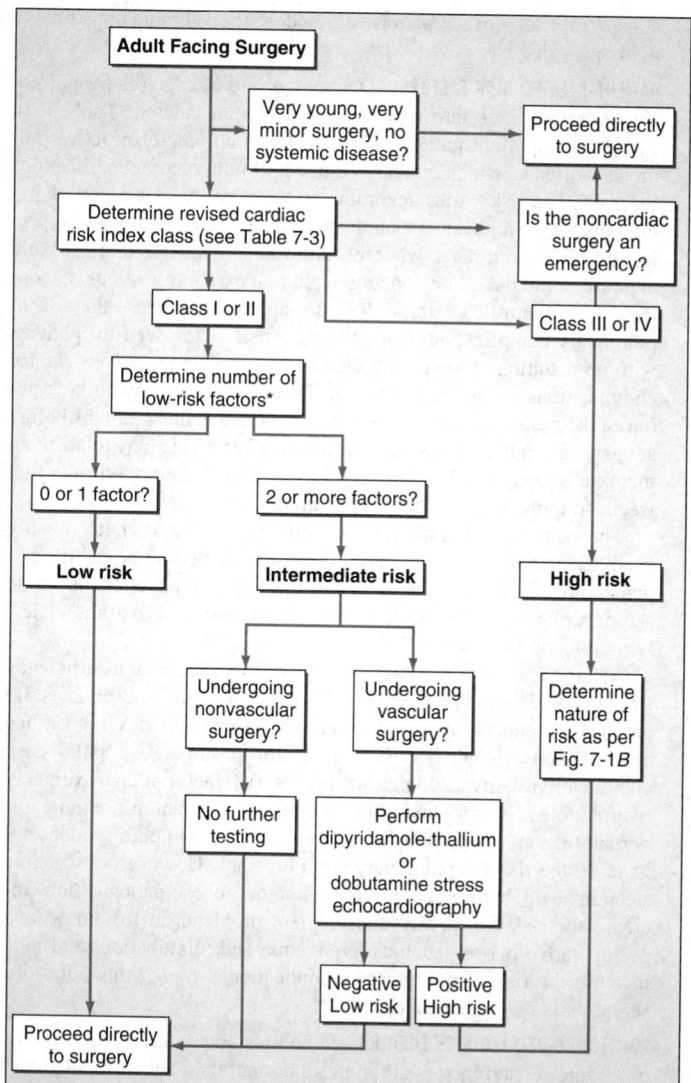

A.

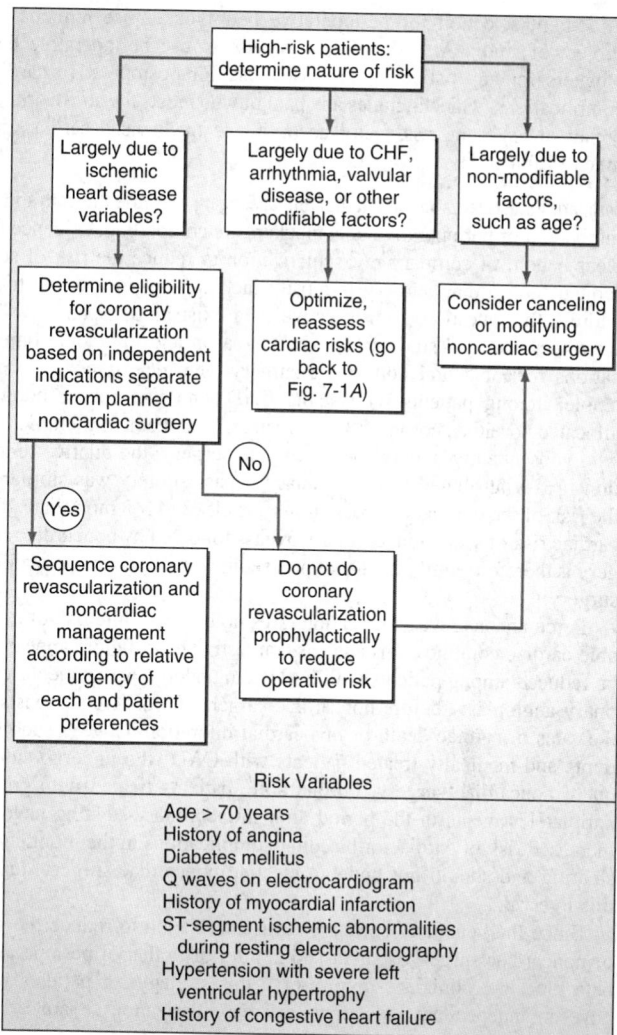

B.

FIGURE 7-1 American College of Physicians' guidelines for cardiac evaluation before noncardiac surgery. *A.* Guidelines for all adults facing surgery. *B.* Guidelines for high-risk patients. *Clinicians may use the revised cardiac risk index (Table 7-3) in place of the modified cardiac risk index for this guideline, which has been shown since the 1997 publication of the ACP guideline to be a superior tool for risk stratification. In addition, broader use of perioperative beta blockers is supported by recent studies, as described in the text. ACP, American College of Physicians; CHF, congestive heart failure; DSE, dobutamine stress echocardiography; DTI, dipyridamole-thallium imaging. (*Reprinted with permission from American College of Physicians: Ann Intern Med 127: 309, 1997.*)

STRATEGIES TO REDUCE CARDIAC RISK After identifying patients whose risk of postoperative cardiac complications is above average, one must identify interventions and strategies to reduce risk, assuming that the risk is not so high that one would consider cancelation of surgery. As a recent myocardial infarction increases the risk of adverse events, one should delay elective surgery until at least 6 months after myocardial infarction. If an operation is necessary during this interval, a functional test such as an exercise test may stratify risk and identify a subset of patients with good exercise capacity and no inducible ischemia who may consider proceeding to surgery. Active congestive heart failure increases risk, and appropriate treatment of pulmonary congestion, including diuretic therapy, will reduce this risk. One should not diurese to the point of orthostatic hypotension as this may increase the risk of hypotension with anesthetic induction.

The risk attributed to aortic stenosis is controversial. While this was an important factor in the original Goldman cardiac risk index, recent retrospective uncontrolled studies suggest that even patients with critical aortic stenosis may undergo noncardiac surgery with an acceptable degree of risk. One should evaluate the severity of aortic stenosis in all patients suspected of having symptoms caused by their valvular disease. The indication for surgical treatment of aortic ste-

nosis is the same as for patients who are not contemplating noncardiac surgery.

When risk is due to a high-risk operation, and few opportunities exist to otherwise reduce risk, clinicians may consider the possibility of an alternate lower risk procedure, if such a procedure exists.

Perioperative Beta Blockers The most important recent observation in the field of perioperative cardiac risk is that perioperative beta blockers markedly reduce the risk of cardiac complications in selected patients. Four separate large-scale randomized trials have now addressed the benefit of this intervention. In two of the trials, all patients had either known CAD or at least two of the following risk factors: age ≥ 65 years, hypertension, current cigarettes use, total cholesterol ≥ 6.2 mmol/L (≥240 mg/dL), and diabetes mellitus. Many patients in clinical practice would meet these broad inclusion criteria. The other trials evaluated patients undergoing vascular surgery with at least one additional risk factor or preoperative ischemia demonstrated by Holter monitoring. The results of these trials show reductions in the rate of postoperative myocardial infarction and cardiac death from 55 to 93%. The number of such patients needed to treat to prevent one event range from 2.5 to 8.3, indicating a strong effect on reducing risk.

Patient selection for perioperative beta-blocker use remains the subject of study. At this point, it is wise to use perioperative beta blockers for any patient at increased risk for postoperative cardiac complications, which includes any patient who meets the above criteria or has at least one risk factor according to the revised cardiac risk index (Table 7-3).

Coronary Revascularization Before Noncardiac Surgery   While the data showing benefit of perioperative beta blockers are compelling, evidence for clear benefit of coronary revascularization to reduce the risk of subsequent noncardiac surgery is mostly lacking. No prospective trials address this question. Retrospective data exist among patients who were recruited and studied for another reason and in whom complications for incidental noncardiac surgery were determined. For example, among patients with stable CAD who had been randomly allocated to either coronary bypass surgery or medical therapy, and who subsequently underwent noncardiac surgery, the relative reduction in risk attributed to the coronary bypass surgery was similar to the risk of the coronary bypass surgery itself (2 to 3% mortality). The cardiac risk of sequential coronary bypass followed by noncardiac surgery is therefore similar to that of proceeding directly to the noncardiac surgery.

Percutaneous revascularization fares no better. While risk of treatable cardiac complications such as congestive heart failure appears to be reduced among patients with CAD who undergo percutaneous coronary angioplasty before noncardiac surgery, no difference exists in the rates of cardiac death or myocardial infarction between such patients and medically treated patients with CAD who undergo subsequent noncardiac surgery. Furthermore, patients treated with potent antiplatelet agents in the period after intracoronary stenting have an increased risk of cardiac or bleeding complications in the month after stenting and should not undergo elective noncardiac surgery during this interval.

Since the benefit of coronary revascularization to reduce the risk of noncardiac surgery is small and is inferior to that of perioperative beta blockers, clinicians may reserve this strategy for patients who have an independent indication for revascularization separate from their need for noncardiac surgery.

PREOPERATIVE PULMONARY EVALUATION

While estimation of cardiac risk is rightfully a major focus of the preoperative evaluation, clinicians may be surprised to learn that postoperative pulmonary complications are as prevalent as cardiac complications and contribute equally to morbidity, mortality, and length of hospital stay. Therefore, estimation of the risk of pulmonary complications is a necessary part of the preoperative evaluation. Important postoperative pulmonary complications include pneumonia, respiratory failure with prolonged mechanical ventilation, atelectasis, bronchospasm, and exacerbation of underlying chronic obstructive pulmonary disease.

PATIENT-RELATED RISK FACTORS   One may group risk factors for pulmonary complications into patient- and procedure-related (Table 7-4). The most important patient-related factor is chronic obstructive pulmonary disease, which increases the risk of pulmonary complications fourfold. The risk varies according to the severity of the underlying lung disease. On physical examination, decreased breath sounds, prolonged expiration, rales, wheezes, and rhonchi each predict a sixfold increase in the risk of postoperative pulmonary complications. In contrast, well-controlled asthma does not appear to increase the risk of pulmonary complications. Smoking is a risk factor even for patients with no resulting chronic lung disease; the reported relative risks for complications range from 1.5 to 4. However, patients who have reduced their cigarette use or stopped completely in the 2 months before surgery have a higher risk than current smokers. This may relate to an increase in cough and sputum production that is common in the first weeks to months after cigarette cessation.

The risk of viral respiratory infections is unknown but probably small. Bacterial lower respiratory infections, including bronchitis and pneumonia, do increase the risk of pulmonary complications. In these settings, clinicians should delay elective surgery and treat the underlying infection.

Metabolic factors shown to increase risk include renal insufficiency [BUN > 10.7 mmol/L (>30 mg/dL)] and albumin < 30 g/L (<3.0 g/dL). Poor functional capacity, known to increase risk for cardiac complications, is also a risk factor for postoperative pulmonary complications. Advanced age is a modest risk factor of approximately twofold; other patient- and procedure-related risk factors are more important than age. Surprisingly, obesity, even morbid obesity, does not increase the risk for pulmonary complications. However, obstructive sleep apnea, which is more common among obese patients, does increase the risk for airway management problems in the immediate postoperative period (such as hypoxemia and reintubation) and may increase the risk of pulmonary complications, though this latter observation is not well established.

PROCEDURE-RELATED RISK FACTORS   In contrast to cardiac complications, procedure-related factors are more important than patient-related factors in predicting the risk of pulmonary complications. The most important factor is the surgical site. Risk increases as the incision approaches the diaphragm. The highest risk is for upper abdominal, thoracic, and abdominal aortic aneurysm surgery. Depending on the series, studies have shown complication of rates of 20 to 40% for these procedures. There is lower risk for lower abdominal surgery and peripheral vascular surgery. Laparoscopic abdominal surgeries carry a much lower risk of pulmonary complications (1%). Pulmonary complications are rare for surgeries outside of the chest and abdomen. Other procedure-related factors include prolonged surgical duration (>3 h), general anesthesia, emergency surgery, and the use of long-acting neuromuscular blockers such as pancuronium during anesthesia.

PREOPERATIVE PULMONARY FUNCTION TESTING (See also Chap. 234)   The role of preoperative pulmonary function testing is debated. While such testing is necessary before planned lung resection (this is not the subject of this chapter), its value before other high-risk surgeries is less clear. The most commonly performed tests in this setting are simple spirometry including forced expiratory capacity in 1 s (FEV_1) and forced vital capacity (FVC). Advocates of testing suggest that clinical decision-making and patient selection for surgery may be influenced by such test results. However, most reports demonstrate that clinical factors (as described above in patient- and procedure-related risk factor sections) are as or more helpful in the estimation of risk than spirometry. Preoperative spirometry could be potentially useful were it to identify either high-risk patients who would escape clinical detection or those patients whose risk of proceeding to surgery would be prohibitive. Neither of these criteria is met.

Several reports have shown that clinical factors correctly identify

---

TABLE 7-4   *Risk Factors for Postoperative Pulmonary Complications*

Patient-Related Risk Factors	Procedure-Related Risk Factors
Chronic obstructive pulmonary disease	Surgical site:
	Thoracic surgery
Cigarette use < 8 weeks before surgery	Abdominal aortic aneurysm surgery
ASA class > 2	Upper abdominal surgery
Goldman class 2–4[a]	Neurosurgery
Age > 60	Peripheral vascular surgery
Dependent functional status	General anesthesia
Albumin < 3.0 g/dL	Pancuronium use
Blood urea nitrogen > 30 mg/dL	Emergency surgery
Abnormal chest radiograph	Surgery lasting > 3 hours

[a] Goldman cardiac risk index. Of four classes possible; class 4 represents the highest risk.
Note: ASA, American Society of Anesthesiologists.
Source: Reprinted from GW Smetana: Clin Geriatr Med 19:35, 2003, with permission from Elsevier Science.

patients at high risk for postoperative pulmonary complications and that there is no substantial incremental value of preoperative spirometry as a risk-stratification tool. While abnormal spirometry, in some studies, does predict risk, these patients would have been identified based on clinical criteria alone. As to prohibitive risk, it is now clear that even patients with spirometric values previously thought to represent an absolute contraindication to surgery (e.g., $FEV_1 < 1$ L or 50% predicted) can proceed to surgery with an acceptable degree of risk if the indication for surgery is compelling and if every effort is made to reduce postoperative pulmonary complications (see below). Evidence for the benefit of preoperative arterial blood gas analysis is even weaker and is based on small case series. No reports have shown that such studies are superior to clinical evaluation before high-risk nonpulmonary surgery. There is, therefore, no role for routine preoperative arterial blood gas analysis in high-risk patients.

STRATEGIES TO REDUCE POSTOPERATIVE PULMONARY COMPLICATIONS Most risk-reduction strategies follow logically from the above risk factors. One should recommend cigarette cessation for at least 8 weeks before elective surgery. Cessation for briefer periods may increase risk. Clinicians should treat patients with chronic obstructive pulmonary disease or asthma in the usual fashion so as to maximally reduce airflow obstruction. The treatment strategies are identical to those used in patients who are not preparing for surgery. Patients with asthma should be free of wheezes and have a peak flow of at least 80% of the predicted value or of personal best. Antibiotics should be reserved for patients with bacterial lower respiratory tract infection, as their indiscriminate use does not reduce risk. Intraoperative strategies include epidural or spinal anesthesia when feasible, the avoidance of pancuronium as a neuromuscular blocker in high-risk patients, and the use of shorter duration or laparoscopic procedures.

Postoperative strategies include lung expansion maneuvers and pain control. Lung expansion maneuvers reduce risk by minimizing the expected fall in lung volumes (particularly for thoracic and upper abdominal surgery) that contribute importantly to the risk of complications. These strategies include deep breathing exercises (a component of chest physical therapy) and incentive spirometry and effort-independent strategies such as continuous positive airway pressure (CPAP) (Chap. 252). Deep breathing exercises and incentive spirometry are equally effective; each reduces risk by one half. CPAP should be reserved for patients who cannot cooperate with the other maneuvers as it is more costly and carries some risk of barotrauma.

Pain control strategies decrease splinting and improve the ability to take deep breaths; they reduce pulmonary complications by these mechanisms. Epidural analgesia with local anesthetics reduces complication rates in patients undergoing abdominal, thoracic, and aortic surgery. Intercostal nerve blocks may also be beneficial, but the effect did not reach statistical significance in a large well-designed meta-analysis.

DIABETES MELLITUS (See also Chap. 323)

The most important perioperative risk attributable to diabetes mellitus is that of cardiac complications. This is due to the higher prevalence of CAD, both known and clinically inapparent, among patients with diabetes than among the general population. Therefore, the principal goal of the preparation of patients with diabetes before surgery is a careful assessment of cardiac risk, as described above. Diabetes also increases the risk of surgical wound infections. For the subset of patients with diabetic neuropathy, there is additional risk for aspiration of gastric contents during anesthesia if gastroparesis is present, and for blood pressure lability during surgery if autonomic neuropathy exists.

Strategies to control blood sugar in the perioperative period must balance the risk of hyperglycemia due to the stress of surgery and anesthesia and the need for patients to fast before surgery that may increase the risk of hypoglycemia. One achieves this balance through frequent monitoring and the use of short-acting insulin as needed to achieve blood sugar goals. Optimal perioperative blood sugars are between 120 and 200 mg/dL. Patients who are diet-controlled may proceed to surgery without additional treatment of blood sugar other than careful perioperative monitoring of blood sugar by fingerstick. Those who receive oral hypoglycemic agents should hold their medication on the morning of surgery (with the exception of metformin, which should be stopped the day before to minimize the risk of lactic acidosis). One treats these patients as needed with short-acting insulin on a sliding scale based on frequent monitoring. Intravenous fluids for oral agent– and insulin-treated patients should include glucose to decrease the risk for lipolysis and ketone production.

Controversy exists as to whether patients with insulin-requiring diabetes should be treated with a continuous insulin infusion in the perioperative period versus the conventional use of one-half of the patient's usual morning long-acting insulin dose on the morning of surgery followed by a sliding scale of regular insulin based on frequent monitoring. Patients undergoing coronary bypass grafting have a lower incidence of sternal wound infections when managed with continuous infusion insulin to achieve tight perioperative blood sugar control. Among seriously ill patients who require prolonged mechanical ventilation after surgery, intensive continuous infusion insulin to achieve near-normal blood sugars reduces overall mortality when compared to a less intensive continuous infusion insulin strategy. Until further data are available, it is reasonable to recommend continuous infusion insulin in the perioperative period for patients undergoing prolonged major surgery, cardiac surgery, or emergent surgery with metabolic abnormalities or who will require prolonged mechanical ventilation after surgery.

FURTHER READING

AUERBACH AD, GOLDMAN L: Beta-blockers and reduction of cardiac events in noncardiac surgery: Scientific review. JAMA 1987:1435, 2002

EAGLE KA et al: ACC/AHA guideline update for perioperative cardiovascular evaluation for noncardiac surgery. Executive summary: A report of the American College of Cardiology/American Heart Association Task Force on Practice Guidelines (Committee to Update the 1996 Guidelines on Perioperative Cardiovascular Evaluation for Noncardiac Surgery). Circulation 105:1257, 2002

LEE TH et al: Derivation and prospective validation of a simple index for prediction of cardiac risk of major noncardiac surgery. Circulation 100: 1043, 1999

PALDA VA, DETSKY AS: Perioperative assessment and management of risk from coronary artery disease. Ann Intern Med 127:313, 1997

SMETANA GW: Preoperative pulmonary evaluation. N Engl J Med 340:937, 1999

———, MACPHERSON DS: The case against routine preoperative laboratory testing. Med Clin North Am 87:7, 2003

8 GERIATRIC MEDICINE
Neil M. Resnick, David Dosa

Of all the people who have ever lived to age 65, more than half are now alive. This statistic has important demographic and economic implications, and its impact on medical care is also substantial.

BIOLOGY OF AGING

Numerous molecular concomitants of aging have been described. For instance, there is an increase in chromosome structural abnormalities, DNA cross-linking, and frequency of single-strand breaks; a decline in DNA methylation; and loss of DNA telomeric sequences. The primary structure of proteins is unaltered, but there is an increase in posttranslational changes, deamidation, oxidation, cross-linking, and nonenzymatic glycation. Mitochondrial structure deteriorates, albeit not universally.

However, the biologic changes are clearer than the mechanisms that mediate them. In fact, although the senescent phenotype appears to be ubiquitous, biologists disagree about whether senescence even exists beyond zoos and civilized societies and whether it occurs at all in many species. There is little evolutionary rationale for a process that happens after reproduction is complete, particularly one associated with such a long and complex course. In nature, senescence is most notable for its absence; nearly all animals die of predation, disease, or environmental hazards rather than aging. The argument that different species have different maximum life spans can be explained without invoking a specific aging process: while growth and development are based on a genetic template, aging may reflect merely the accumulation of random damage rather than a specific mechanism.

If aging exists as a distinct process, there is consensus that the mechanisms are likely multifactorial, environmentally influenced, and species-specific, if not organ- and cell-specific, making the paucity of available human data particularly problematic. As a result, there are nearly as many theories of aging as investigators. Most theories overlap or are not mutually exclusive, and none is completely compatible with the dearth of data. As a group, the theories can be divided into two broad categories, based on whether they attribute aging to a genetic program or to progressive and random damage to homeostatic systems.

GENETIC THEORIES OF AGING   Enthusiasm for genetic theories of aging is fueled by several observations, including the dramatic species-specific differences in maximal life span, the strong correlation with survival among monozygotic compared to dizygotic twins, and the fact that single mutations can prolong life span by >50% in some nematodes, flies, and mice. However, all genetic theories must account for the fact that evolutionary selection pressure is minimal following completion of reproduction. Three genetic theories have recently been advanced, but few relevant data have yet been accrued. The first theory suggests that, since animals usually succumb to natural forces long before reaching their maximal life span, aging might reflect mutations that impair long-term survival. These mutations would accumulate in the genome because there is no selection pressure to delete them. A second theory, "pleiotropic antagonism," proposes that aging may be caused by the late and deleterious effects of genes that are conserved because of the survival advantages they confer prior to reproduction. The third theory applies to ecological niches where extrinsic hazards are relatively low. In such an environment, evolution might select for mutations that retard the aging process since these might allow an animal to produce and protect many more litters. In support of this theory, the rate of aging in an isolated clan of Virginia opossums was calculated to be roughly half of that seen in their less fortunate cousins.

The Random Damage Theories   These are based on the possibility that the balance between ongoing damage and repair is disrupted. The theories differ in the emphasis placed on increased damage (e.g., by free radicals, oxidation, or glycation) versus deficient repair, as well as in the mechanisms that might mediate each. However, all share the observation that cell and organ repair capacity declines with age. Some 40 years ago, Hayflick and Moorehead observed that the number of replications among cultured cells is finite. Subsequent research revealed that this replicative senescence was due to arrest of the cell cycle at the G_1/S phase, the point at which DNA synthesis begins. Recently, cell replication has also been linked to the length of telomeric DNA. Present at the termini of chromosomes, telomeric DNA prevents chromosomal instability, fragmentation, and rearrangement; anchors chromosomes to nuclear matrix; and provides a buffer between coding regions of DNA and the ends of the chromosomes. In addition, telomeric DNA is necessary for cell division. With each cell division, however, roughly 50 of the total 2000 base pairs of the telomere are lost. Telomeric shortening might thus result in loss of gene accessibility, which is necessary to repair ongoing cell damage caused by metabolism. Together with cytoplasmic factors mediating arrest of DNA synthesis, telomeric shortening could also limit the cell's ability to divide and thereby replace cells lost to apoptosis.

Many mechanisms previously postulated to mediate aging have not been borne out, including the somatic mutation theory (in which aging would result from cumulative spontaneous mutations), the error catastrophe theory (in which aging would result from errors in the synthesis of proteins critical to the synthesis of genetic material or protein-synthesizing machinery), and the intrinsic mutagenesis theory (in which aging is the result of ongoing intrinsic DNA rearrangements).

To date, the only intervention known to delay aging is caloric restriction. The salutary effect of restricting caloric intake by 30 to 40% has been documented in multiple species, from single-cell organisms to rodents. In rodents, it not only increases average life expectancy and maximum life span but also delays the onset of some typical age-associated diseases as well as deterioration of physiologic systems (e.g., immune responsiveness, glucose metabolism, muscle atrophy). Moreover, its impact is evident in both mitotic and postmitotic cells, in gene expression, and in protein turnover and cross-linking. Although the mechanism is still not determined, it is specific to caloric restriction rather than to reduction of any dietary component (e.g., fat intake) or supplements with vitamins or antioxidants. Unfortunately, adequate data from primates are still limited, and the effect of caloric restriction in humans is still unknown.

PRINCIPLES OF GERIATRIC MEDICINE

Despite the biologic controversy, from a physiologic standpoint human aging is characterized by progressive constriction of the homeostatic reserve of every organ system. This decline, often referred to as *homeostenosis*, is evident by the third decade and is gradual and progressive, although the rate and extent of decline vary. The decline of each organ system (Table 8-1) appears to occur independently of changes in other organ systems and is influenced by diet, environment, and personal habits as well as by genetic factors.

Several important principles follow from these facts: (1) Individuals become more dissimilar as they age, belying any stereotype of aging; (2) an *abrupt* decline in any system or function is always due to disease and not to "normal aging"; (3) "normal aging" can be attenuated by modification of risk factors (e.g., increased blood pressure, smoking, sedentary lifestyle); and (4) "healthy old age" is not an oxymoron. In fact, *in the absence of disease, the decline in homeostatic reserve causes no symptoms and imposes few restrictions on activities of daily living regardless of age*.

Appreciation of these facts may make it easier to understand the striking increases that have occurred in life expectancy. Average life expectancy is now 18 years at age 65, 11 years at age 75, 6 years at age 85, 4 years at age 90, and 2 years at age 100. Moreover, the bulk of these years is characterized by a lack of significant impairment (Table 8-2). Even beyond age 85, only 30% of people are impaired in any activity required for daily living and only 20% reside in a nursing home. Yet, as individuals age they are more likely to suffer from disease, disability, and the side effects of drugs, all of which, when combined with the decrease in physiologic reserve, make the older person more vulnerable to environmental, pathologic, and pharmacologic challenges.

The following concepts underlie the remainder of the chapter:

1. Disease presentation is often atypical in the elderly, especially in those >75 to 80 years old. Homeostatic strain caused by onset of a new disease often leads to symptoms associated with a different organ system, particularly one compromised by preexisting disease. For example, fewer than one-fourth of older patients with hyperthyroidism present with goiter, tremor, and exophthalmos; more likely are atrial fibrillation, confusion, depression, syncope, and weakness. Significantly, because the "weakest link" is so often the brain, the lower urinary tract, or the cardiovascular or musculoskeletal system, a limited number of presenting symptoms predominate—acute confusion, depression, incontinence, falling, and syncope—no matter

TABLE 8-1 *Selected Age-Related Changes and Their Consequences*

Organ/System	Age-Related Physiologic Change[a]	Consequences of Age-Related Physiologic Change	Consequences of Disease, not Age
General	↑Body fat ↓Total body water	↑Volume of distribution for fat-soluble drugs ↓Volume of distribution for water-soluble drugs	Obesity Anorexia
Eyes/ears	Presbyopia Lens opacification ↓High-frequency acuity	↓Accommodation ↑Susceptibility to glare Need for increased illumination Difficulty discriminating words if background noise is present	Blindness Deafness
Endocrine	Impaired glucose homeostasis ↓Thyroxine clearance (and production) ↑ADH, ↓renin, and ↓aldosterone ↓Testosterone ↓Vitamin D absorption and activation	↑Glucose level in response to acute illness ↓T_4 dose required in hypothyroidism Osteopenia	Diabetes mellitus Thyroid dysfunction ↓Na^+, ↑K^+ Impotence Osteomalacia, fracture
Respiratory	Decreased cough reflex ↓Lung elasticity and ↑chest wall stiffness Decreased DL_{CO}	Microaspiration Ventilation/perfusion mismatch and ↓P_{O_2} Decreased resting P_{O_2}	Aspiration pneumonia Dyspnea, hypoxia Dyspnea
Cardiovascular	↓Arterial compliance and ↑ systolic BP →LVH ↓β-adrenergic responsiveness ↓Baroreceptor sensitivity and ↓SA node automaticity	Hypotensive response to ↑HR, volume depletion, or loss of atrial contraction ↓Cardiac output and HR response to stress Impaired blood pressure response to standing, volume depletion	Syncope Heart failure Heart block
Gastrointestinal	↓Hepatic function ↓Gastric acidity ↓Colonic motility ↓Anorectal function	Delayed metabolism of some drugs ↓Ca^{2+} absorption on empty stomach Constipation	Cirrhosis Osteoporosis, B_{12} deficiency Fecal impaction Fecal incontinence
Hematologic/immune system	↓Bone marrow reserve(?) ↓T cell function ↑Autoantibodies	False-negative PPD response False-positive rheumatoid factor, antinuclear antibody	Anemia Autoimmune disease
Renal	↓GFR ↓Urine concentration/dilution (see also "Endocrine")	Impaired excretion of some drugs Delayed response to salt or fluid restriction/ overload; nocturia	↑Serum creatinine ↓↑Na^+
Genitourinary	Vaginal/urethral mucosal atrophy Prostate enlargement	Dyspareunia, bacteriuria ↑Residual urine volume	Symptomatic UTI Urinary incontinence; urinary retention
Musculoskeletal	↓Lean body mass, muscle ↓Bone density	 Osteopenia	Functional impairment Hip fracture
Nervous system	Brain atrophy ↓Brain catechol synthesis ↓Brain dopaminergic synthesis ↓Righting reflexes ↓Stage 4 sleep Impaired thermal regulation	Benign senescent forgetfulness Stiffer gait ↑Body sway Early wakening, insomnia Lower resting temperature	Dementia, delirium Depression Parkinson's disease Falls Sleep apnea Hypothermia, hyperthermia

[a] Changes generally observed in healthy elderly subjects free of symptoms and detectable disease in the organ system studied. The changes are usually important only when the system is stressed or other factors are added (e.g., drugs, disease, or environmental challenge); they rarely result in symptoms otherwise.

Abbreviations: T_4, thyroxine; BP, blood pressure; HR, heart rate; ADH, antidiuretic hormone; GFR, glomerular filtration rate; LVH, left ventricular hypertrophy; PPD, purified protein derivative; UTI, urinary tract infection.

what the underlying disease. Thus for the most common geriatric syndromes, regardless of the presenting symptom, the differential diagnosis is often largely similar. The corollary is equally important: The organ system usually associated with a particular symptom is less likely to be the source of that symptom in older individuals than in younger ones. Compared with middle-aged individuals, for example, acute confusion in older patients is less often due to a new brain lesion, depression to a psychiatric disorder, incontinence to bladder dysfunction, falling to a neuropathy, or syncope to heart disease.

2. Because of decreased physiologic reserve, older patients often develop symptoms at an earlier stage of their disease (Fig. 8-1). For example, heart failure may be precipitated by mild hyperthyroidism, cognitive dysfunction by mild hyperparathyroidism, urinary retention by mild prostatic enlargement, and nonketotic hyperosmolar coma by

TABLE 8-2 *Life Expectancy and Number of Remaining Years Free of Dependency in Activities of Daily Living*

Age	Life Expectancy[a], av		Disability-Free Years Remaining	
	Men	Women	Men	Women
65–69	13	20	9	11
70–74	12	16	8	8
75–79	10	13	7	7
80–84	7	10	5	5
≥85	7	8	3	3

[a] For independent noninstitutionalized elderly men and women in Massachusetts. Longevity and disability-free longevity are surprisingly long and must be incorporated into treatment decisions. All figures rounded to nearest year. See text for more recent data on longevity alone.

Source: S Katz et al: N Engl J Med 309:1218, 1983.

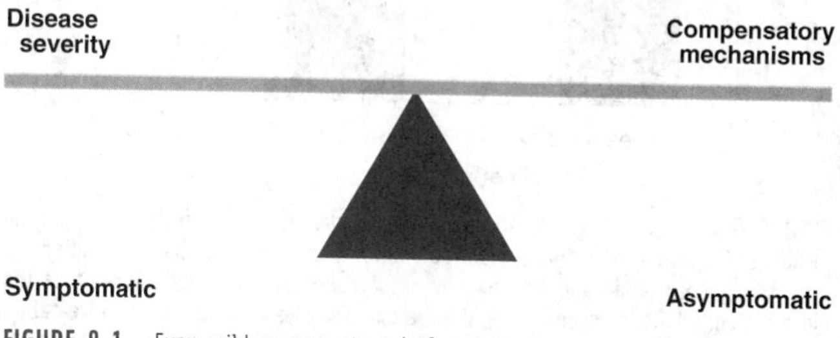

FIGURE 8-1 Even mild organ system dysfunction may cause symptoms if compensatory mechanisms are impaired. (*From NM Resnick: JAMA 276:1832, 1996.*)

mild glucose intolerance. Paradoxically, therefore, treatment of the underlying disease may be easier because it is frequently less advanced at the time of presentation. A corollary is that drug side effects can occur with drugs and drug doses unlikely to produce side effects in younger people. For instance, a sedating antihistamine (e.g., diphenhydramine) may cause confusion, loop diuretics may precipitate urinary incontinence, digoxin may induce depression even with normal serum levels, and over-the-counter sympathomimetics may precipitate urinary retention in men with mild prostatic obstruction.

Unfortunately, the predisposition to develop symptoms at an earlier stage of disease is often offset by two factors. First, symptoms may present later if there is functional limitation in another system. Coronary artery disease or aortic stenosis may not cause symptoms as early in patients whose mobility is compromised by arthritis. Second, a change in illness behavior occurs with age. Raised at a time when symptoms and debility were accepted as normal consequences of aging, the elderly are less likely to seek attention until symptoms become disabling. Thus, any symptom, particularly those associated with a change in functional status, must be taken seriously and evaluated promptly.

3. Since many homeostatic mechanisms may be compromised concurrently, there are usually multiple abnormalities amenable to treatment, and small improvements in each may yield dramatic benefits overall. For instance, cognitive impairment in patients with Alzheimer's disease may respond much better to interventions that alleviate comorbidity than to prescription of a cholinesterase inhibitor (Fig. 8-2). Similar approaches apply to most other geriatric syndromes, including falls, incontinence, depression, delirium, syncope, and fracture. In each case, substantial functional improvement can result from treating the contributing factors even if—as in Alzheimer's disease—the disease itself is largely untreatable.

4. Many findings that are abnormal in younger patients are relatively common in older people—e.g., bacteriuria, premature ventricular contractions, low bone mineral density, impaired glucose tolerance, and uninhibited bladder contractions. However, they may not be responsible for a particular symptom but only be incidental findings that result in missed diagnoses and misdirected therapy. For instance, the finding of bacteriuria should not end the search for a source of fever in an acutely ill older patient, nor should an elevated random blood sugar—especially in an acutely ill patient—be incriminated as the cause of neuropathy. On the other hand, certain other abnormalities must not be dismissed as due to old age—e.g., there is no anemia, impotence, depression, or confusion of old age.

5. Because symptoms in older people are often due to multiple causes, the diagnostic "law of parsimony" often does not apply. For instance, fever, anemia, retinal embolus, and a heart murmur prompt almost a reflex diagnosis of infective endocarditis in a younger patient but may reflect aspirin-induced blood loss, a cholesterol embolus, insignificant aortic sclerosis, and a viral illness in an older patient. Moreover, even when the diagnosis is correct, treatment of a single disease in an older patient is unlikely to result in cure. For instance, in a younger patient, incontinence due to involuntary bladder contractions is treated effectively with a bladder relaxant medication. However, in an older patient with the same condition but who also has fecal impaction, takes medications that cloud the sensorium, and suffers from arthritis-associated impairments of mobility and manual dexterity, treatment of the bladder spasms alone is unlikely to restore continence. On the other hand, disimpaction, discontinuation of the offending medications, and treatment of the arthritis are likely to restore continence without the need for a bladder relaxant. Failure to recognize these principles often leads to prescribing "ineffective" therapy and to unjustified therapeutic nihilism toward older patients.

6. Because the older patient is more likely to suffer the adverse consequences of disease, treatment—and even prevention—may be equally or even more effective. For instance, the survival benefits of exercise, as well as thrombolysis and beta-blocker therapy after a myocardial infarction, are as impressive in older patients as in younger ones; and treatment of hypertension and transient ischemic attacks, as well as immunization against influenza and pneumococcal pneumonia, are more effective in older patients. A proactive approach is even more effective in acute care, in which it decreases the risk of delirium by 30 to 60%. In the outpatient setting, such an approach can delay functional decline and institutionalization. In addition, prevention in older patients must often be seen in a broader context. For instance, although interventions to increase bone density may be limited in older patients, fracture may still be prevented by efforts to improve balance, strengthen legs, reduce peripheral edema, treat other contributing medical conditions, replete nutritional deficits, eliminate environmental hazards, and remove adverse medications—not so much those that affect bone metabolism, but rather those that induce orthostasis, confusion, and extrapyramidal stiffness.

In summary, optimal treatment of the older patient generally requires treating much more than the organ system usually associated with the disease or symptom, and often permits ignoring that system entirely.

EVALUATION   Evaluation of the older patient can be time-consuming, even when it is tailored to the problem. Yet, such initial investment can reduce subsequent morbidity and resource utilization and enhance patient and physician satisfaction. Additionally, the assessment can often be accomplished over several visits. Moreover, much can be gleaned from questionnaires filled out by the patient or caregiver in advance as well as from observation. For instance, greeting the patient in the waiting room allows the physician to note affective and cognitive response, the strength of the handshake, the ease of rising from a chair without using the arms, the length and steadiness of the stride, and the ability to follow directions to the examining room and to sit down safely in the examining room chair. Observing the patient dress or undress can also enhance detection of impaired cognition, fine motor skills, balance, and judgment. Such observations often provide more information than standard examinations and can shorten the clinical evaluation.

HISTORY-TAKING IN ELDERLY PATIENTS   Most older patients are able to provide a reliable medical history; however, a multitude of complaints may make obtaining a history more difficult. If the patient is unable to comprehend or communicate, data should be sought from family, friends, and caregivers. The history should also include drug and alcohol ingestion, dietary patterns, falling, incontinence, sexual dysfunction, depression, and anxiety.

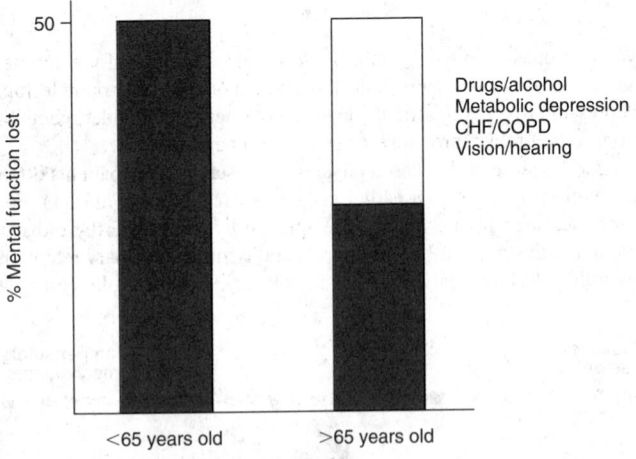

FIGURE 8-2   Although young and old patients may appear to suffer equally from Alzheimer's disease, its extent in older patients is often magnified by comorbidity and drug use. Identification and treatment of these contributing factors will improve the older patient's function even though the Alzheimer's disease is inadequately treatable. CHF, congestive heart failure; COPD, chronic obstructive pulmonary disease. (*From NM Resnick, ER Marcantonio: Lancet 350:1175, 1997.*)

Advance Directives All older patients should be asked whether they have drafted advance health care directives, and, if they have, a copy should be placed in the record. Such directives may consist of a health care proxy or durable power of attorney for health care, in which patients designate a surrogate decision-maker who makes health care decisions if the patient cannot, and/or a living will or medical directive, in which patients specify their desires for treatment in specific situations if they cannot communicate at the critical time.

Whether or not the patient has formally drafted these directives, it is useful to indicate in the record who should make health care decisions if the patient is no longer able to do so. Patients should then be encouraged to discuss their thoughts with the physician as well as the designated proxy. It is not feasible to cover all possible future complications in such discussions. Ascertaining patients' perspectives on specific interventions, such as resuscitation or intubation, is also difficult because preferences will likely differ depending on prognosis. For instance, a patient may not be interested in feeding tube placement following a massive stroke with little chance of recovery but would prefer the same intervention if it is short-term and helps ensure more rapid and complete recovery from an intercurrent illness such as pneumonia. More useful is a discussion that uses open-ended questions and empathic comments to elicit the patient's values and goals. Moreover, for any given condition, preferences may differ depending on baseline clinical status. For robust elderly individuals, recovery is a realistic goal, albeit the odds of complications are higher than for younger individuals. For the frail elderly patient with comorbidity that impairs functional status, reduction or alleviation of symptoms may be the goal. For patients with advanced dementia or terminal illness, maximizing comfort may be the most appropriate strategy. In each situation, however, early elicitation of a patient's preferences and values—when the patient can still state them—can often help both physicians and families in subsequent difficult decisions by giving surrogate decision-makers the sense that they are doing as the patient would have wanted.

PHYSICAL EXAMINATION Certain features of the examination should receive special attention, depending in part on clues from the history. Weight and postural blood pressure should be measured at most visits. Vision and hearing should be checked; if hearing is impaired, excess cerumen should be removed from the external auditory canals prior to audiologic referral. Denture fit should be assessed, and the oral cavity should be inspected with the dentures removed. Although thyroid disease becomes more common with age, the sensitivity and specificity of related findings are substantially lower than in younger individuals; consequently, the physical examination can rarely corroborate or exclude thyroid dysfunction in older patients. The breasts should not be overlooked, since older women are more likely to have breast cancer and less likely to do breast self-examination. The systolic murmur of aortic sclerosis is common and may be difficult to differentiate from aortic stenosis, especially since the presence of a fourth heart sound in an elderly person does not imply significant cardiac disease, and the carotid upstroke normally increases owing to age-related arterial stiffening.

In inactive patients and those with fecal or urinary incontinence, one should check for fecal impaction. In patients with urinary incontinence—especially men—a distended bladder must be looked for, since it may be the only finding in urinary retention; perineal sensation and the bulbocavernosus reflex should also be tested. Patients who fall should be observed standing up from a chair, bending down, reaching up, walking 3 m (10 ft), turning, returning, and sitting again; abnormalities of gait and balance should be evaluated with the patient's eyes open and closed and in response to a sternal push. It should be appreciated that "frontal release signs" (e.g., "snout," "glabellar," or palmomental reflexes) and absent ankle jerks and vibratory sense in the feet may be normal in the elderly.

MENTAL STATUS EXAMINATION In addition to evaluating mood and affect, some form of cognitive testing is essential in all elderly patients, even if it involves only checking different components of the history for consistency. People with mild degrees of dementia usually retain their

social graces and may mask intellectual impairment by a cheerful and cooperative manner. Thus, the examiner should always probe for content. For patients who follow the news, one can ask what stories they are particularly interested in and why; the same applies to reading, social events—even the soap operas on television.

If there is any suspicion of a cognitive deficit after this kind of conversational probing, further questioning is indicated. An examination that tests only orientation as to person, place, and time is insufficient to detect mild or moderate intellectual impairment. As a quick screen, simply assessing orientation and asking the patient to draw a clock with the hands at a set time (e.g., 10 min before 2:00) can be very informative regarding cognitive status, visuospatial deficits, ability to comprehend and execute instructions in logical sequence, and presence or absence of perseveration. For slightly more detailed examinations, many practical mental status tests are available. The most widely used is the Mini-Mental Status Examination of Folstein (Chap. 257), which provides a numerical score that can be obtained in 5 to 10 min. Regardless of the test employed, the total score is less useful diagnostically than is knowledge of the specific domain of the deficit. As a general rule, disproportionate difficulty with immediate recall (e.g., of a list of three items) suggests depression, while predominant difficulty with recalling the items 5 min later suggests dementia. For patients with deficits of attention—recognized by inability to spell simple words backwards, repeat five digits, or recite the months of the year backwards—delirium is probably present, and the accuracy of the remainder of the test is dubious. However, the test can be interpreted accurately only in the context of a comprehensive evaluation.

EVALUATION OF FUNCTIONAL CAPACITY Medical problem lists, a standard tool for assessing and following younger patients, often prove inadequate for older patients. Heart failure, stroke, and prostate cancer can describe a bedbound institutionalized person as well as a Supreme Court justice. Thus, it is essential to ascertain the patient's degree of functional incapacity owing to both medical and psychosocial problems. The functional assessment includes determination of the patient's ability to perform basic activities of daily life (ADL), which are those needed for personal self-care, as well as the ability to perform more complex tasks required for independent living, the instrumental activities of daily living (IADL). ADLs include bathing, dressing, toileting, feeding, getting in and out of chairs and bed, and walking. IADLs include shopping, cooking, money management, housework, using a telephone, and traveling outside the home. For frail patients, an assessment in the home by a trained observer may be required, but for most patients a questionnaire dealing with these activities can be completed by the family or patient. In either case, the physician must determine the cause of any impairment and whether it can be treated. Assessment should conclude with determination of the socioeconomic circumstances and social support systems.

MANAGEMENT OF COMMON GERIATRIC CONDITIONS

Diseases more common in the elderly are covered elsewhere in the text. The medical problems discussed below do not usually present as clear-cut organ-specific diagnoses and are most common in the frail elderly, especially those over 80 years of age.

INTELLECTUAL IMPAIRMENT The predominant causes of impaired mentation in older patients are delirium, dementia, and depression. Each condition is covered elsewhere in the text in detail (Chaps. 257 and 350), but their management in the elderly is discussed here.

Differentiating the causes of impaired mentation is important, but in older patients they frequently coexist. Thus, the most important first step is to search for and correct all factors that may contribute to cognitive impairment, even in patients with dementia (Fig. 8-2). Evidence of dangerous behavior should also be sought (e.g., leaving the stove on, wandering, and getting lost), and plans should be devised to deal with it. Although there is no definitive treatment for Alzheimer's disease, it is important to detect. Such knowledge allows the physician to discontinue all unnecessary medications, identify and treat new intercurrent illness, and search for alternative ways to obtain the interval history and to ensure that the patient's medications are taken correctly. In addition, the physician should help the family and patient predict and deal with the disease; indeed, the family often needs the physician's support more than the patient does.

Rx TREATMENT

Community services should be suggested as needed, including a visiting nurse, a home health aide to assist with personal hygiene, a homemaker to assist with housework, meal delivery, transportation services, day health centers, and respite care to ease the burden on family members. Support groups such as the Alzheimer's Association are often of value to the family and help them to anticipate problems. Signs of patient abuse by an overstressed caregiver should be watched for. Legal counsel should be recommended to help the patient and family devise plans for ongoing management and ultimate disposition of assets. Assessment of driving safety may be warranted and can often be completed at a driving school or rehabilitation center. Advance directives should be sought as soon as possible while the patient can still participate.

Cholinesterase inhibitors (e.g., donepezil, galantamine, and rivastigmine) can slow clinical progression and ameliorate behavior. However, they are expensive, their efficacy is modest, their utility for more than a year is largely unstudied, and their side effects (nausea, diarrhea, insomnia, dizziness, and confusion) are common, particularly at the higher dosages often needed. Thus, goals should be agreed upon prior to therapy. If they are not met within 3 to 6 months at maximum dosage, consideration may be given to discontinuing therapy. Patients should be monitored for decline when cholinesterase inhibitors are stopped, since this may point to a previously unrecognized therapeutic benefit.

Finally, abrupt worsening of mentation or the onset of disruptive behavior should always prompt a search for new illness or medication. Exacerbation of cognitive dysfunction may occur with mild infections (e.g., subungual toe abscess, vaginitis, or pressure ulcer); with "therapeutic" levels of many drugs; with use of nonprescribed drugs or alcohol; with modest abnormalities of serum sodium, calcium, glucose, or thyroxine; with mild hypoxia; with borderline nutritional deficiencies; with subdural hematoma or "minor" stroke; and with the development of fecal impaction, urinary retention, pain, or change in environment, particularly in frail older patients. However, if a cause is not found and behavior does not respond to environmental manipulation (e.g., ignoring the behavior, distracting the patient, addressing situational "triggers," and providing a calm environment), low doses of an antipsychotic medication may be helpful (e.g., haloperidol, 0.25 to 2 mg/d orally; see below). Of note, feeding tubes inserted into patients with advanced dementia do not prolong life, prevent aspiration, or promote healing of pressure ulcers.

DEPRESSION   Depression of significant degree occurs in 5 to 10% of community-dwelling elderly but is often overlooked. At highest risk are individuals with recent medical illness (e.g., stroke or fracture), bereavement, lack of social supports, recent nursing home admission, or psychiatric history (including alcohol abuse). The diagnosis requires the presence of a depressed mood for at least two consecutive weeks plus at least four of the following eight symptoms: sleep disturbance, lack of interest, feelings of guilt, decreased energy, decreased concentration, decreased appetite, psychomotor agitation/retardation, and suicidal ideation. Also helpful diagnostically are a personal or family history of depression, anhedonia (loss of pleasure), and past response to an antidepressant. It is essential to bear in mind that depression in older patients is often caused or contributed to by drugs or a systemic illness. It is also important to recognize that the risk of suicide is highest in older adults. Although "subsyndromal" depression (fewer than four of the above symptoms) also causes substantial morbidity and health resource utilization, it appears to be less responsive than major depression to therapy.

Rx TREATMENT

For the hospitalized patient in whom acute depression delays recovery or rehabilitation—when correction of medical and pharmacologic contributing factors is ineffective and there is no prior history of mania or major depression—methylphenidate, 5 to 10 mg at 8 A.M. and noon (to avoid insomnia) is often very effective, with benefits discernible within a few days. For patients with major depression, there is no ideal antidepressant drug. All are about equally effective, but the side effects differ (see below and Chap. 371). Consequently, one should become familiar with more than one agent with proven efficacy in older adults (e.g., sertraline, citalopram, bupropion, venlafaxine, mirtazapine, and nortriptyline). Because of its potent anticholinergic and orthostatic side effects, amitriptyline should be avoided whenever possible in older patients. Initial low dosages should be increased slowly to avoid serious side effects; low doses of each medication (e.g., nortriptyline, 10 to 50 mg daily; desipramine, 25 to 75 mg daily; or sertraline 50 to 150 mg daily) are often effective in the elderly, especially when combined with psychotherapy. All of the selective serotonin reuptake inhibitors (SSRIs) and venlafaxine may cause hyponatremia due to the syndrome of inappropriate diuretic hormone (SIADH), and all, like the tricyclic antidepressants, may cause falls. Adverse drug reactions should not be assumed to be due to the aging process.

Treatment should be continued for up to a year after remission of the first episode of depression because relapse rates are higher in the elderly. Consideration for indefinite antidepressant therapy should be given to patients with two or more relapses. For those with psychotic depression, refractory depression, or depression where a definitive, rapid response is required (e.g., extreme frailty, actively suicidal), electroconvulsive therapy is usually well tolerated and highly effective in elderly patients.

URINARY INCONTINENCE ■ Transient Incontinence (Table 8-3)   Because urinary continence requires adequate mobility, mentation, motivation, and manual dexterity—in addition to integrated control of the lower urinary tract—problems outside the bladder can result in incontinence.

1. *Delirium.* A clouded sensorium impedes recognition of both the need to void and the location of the nearest toilet; once delirium clears, incontinence resolves.
2. *Infection.* Symptomatic urinary tract infection commonly causes or contributes to incontinence; asymptomatic infection does not.
3. *Atrophic urethritis/vaginitis.* Atrophic urethritis/vaginitis, characterized by the presence of vaginal telangiectasia, petechiae, erythema, or friability, commonly contributes to incontinence in women and responds to a several-month course of low-dose estrogen or vaginal estrogen creams.

TABLE 8-3   Classification of Incontinence

TRANSIENT
Delirium/confusional state
Infection—urinary (symptomatic)
Atrophic urethritis/vaginitis
Pharmaceuticals
Psychological, especially depression
Excessive urine output (e.g., CHF, hyperglycemia)
Restricted mobility
Stool impaction

ESTABLISHED
Detrusor overactivity
Detrusor underactivity
Urethral obstruction
Urethral incompetence

Note: CHF, congestive heart failure.
Source: Adapted from NM Resnick: Medical Grand Rounds 3:281, 1984.

4. *Pharmaceutical.* The drugs most commonly causing transient incontinence are listed in Table 8-4.

5. *Psychological.* Depression and psychosis are uncommon but treatable causes.

6. *Excess urine output.* Excess urine output may overwhelm the ability to reach a toilet in time. Causes include diuretics, alcohol, excess fluid intake, and metabolic abnormalities (e.g., hyperglycemia, hypercalcemia, diabetes insipidus); nocturnal incontinence may also result from mobilization of peripheral edema.

7. *Restricted mobility.* If mobility cannot be improved, access to a urinal or commode may restore continence. (See "Immobility," below.)

8. *Stool impaction.* This is a common cause of urinary incontinence, especially in hospitalized or immobile patients. Although the mechanism is unknown, a clue to its presence is the coexistence of both urinary and fecal incontinence. Disimpaction restores continence.

Established Incontinence (Table 8-3) The causes of established incontinence include irreversible functional deficits, such as *end-stage* Alzheimer's disease, and intrinsic lower urinary tract dysfunction. Lower

urinary tract dysfunction should be sought after transient causes have been excluded.

DETRUSOR OVERACTIVITY This disorder (involuntary bladder contraction) accounts for two-thirds of geriatric incontinence in both sexes, regardless of whether patients are demented. Detrusor overactivity can be diagnosed presumptively in a woman when leakage occurs in the absence of stress maneuvers or urinary retention and is preceded by the abrupt onset of an intense urge to urinate that cannot be forestalled. In men, the symptoms are similar, but since detrusor overactivity often coexists with urethral obstruction, urodynamic testing should be done if prescription of a bladder relaxant is planned. Because detrusor overactivity may also be due to bladder stones or tumor, the abrupt onset of otherwise unexplained urge incontinence—especially if accompanied by perineal/suprapubic discomfort or sterile hematuria—should prompt cystoscopy and cytologic examination.

℞ TREATMENT

The cornerstone of treatment is behavioral therapy with or without biofeedback. Patients without dementia are instructed to void every 1 to 2 h (while awake only) and to suppress urgency in between; once daytime continence is restored, the interval between voiding can be progressively increased. Demented patients are "prompted" to void at similar intervals. When drugs are necessary, they should be added to these regimens and monitored to avoid inducing urinary retention. Effective drugs include oxybutynin (2.5 to 5 mg three or four times daily, or sustained release, 5 to 20 mg once daily) and tolterodine (1 to 2 mg twice daily or 2 to 4 mg once daily). If prescribed for older patients, desmopressin should be used cautiously—especially in the setting of renal insufficiency or heart failure—and it probably should not be given to patients with hyponatremia or urine output >2500 mL/d. Alternative treatments, such as neuromodulation, botulinum toxin injections, and stem cell therapy, are under investigation.

Indwelling catheterization is rarely indicated for detrusor overactivity. If all measures fail, an external collection device or protective pad or undergarment may be required.

STRESS INCONTINENCE This disorder, the second most common cause of established incontinence in older women (it is rare in men), is characterized by symptoms and evidence of *instantaneous* leakage of urine in response to stress. Leakage is worse or occurs only during the day unless another abnormality (e.g., detrusor overactivity) is also present. On examination, with the bladder full and the perineum relaxed, instantaneous leakage upon coughing strongly suggests stress incontinence, especially if it reproduces symptoms and if urinary retention has been excluded by a postvoiding residual determination; a several-second delay suggests that leakage is instead caused by an involuntary bladder contraction induced by coughing.

℞ TREATMENT

Surgery is the most effective treatment. For women who can comply indefinitely, pelvic muscle exercises are an option for mild to moderate stress incontinence, but they often require specialized training using vaginal cones or biofeedback. Occasionally, a pessary or even a tampon (for women with vaginal stenosis) provides some relief.

URETHRAL OBSTRUCTION Rarely present in women, urethral obstruction (due to prostatic enlargement, urethral stricture, bladder neck contracture, or prostate cancer) is the second most common cause of established incontinence in older men. It can present as dribbling incontinence after voiding, urge incontinence due to detrusor overactivity (which coexists in two-thirds of cases), or overflow incontinence due to urinary retention. Renal ultrasound is recommended to exclude hydronephrosis in men whose postvoiding residual volume exceeds 100 to 200 mL; in older men for whom surgery is planned, urodynamic confirmation of obstruction is strongly advised.

TABLE 8-4	*Commonly Used Medications That May Affect Continence*	
Type of Medication	Examples	Potential Effects on Continence
Sedatives/hypnotics	Long-acting benzodiazepines (e.g., diazepam, flurazepam)	Sedation, delirium, immobility
Alcohol		Polyuria, frequency, urgency, sedation, delirium, immobility
Anticholinergics	Dicyclomine, disopyramide, sedating antihistamines	Urinary retention, overflow incontinence, delirium, impaction
Antipsychotics	Thioridazine, haloperidol	Anticholinergic actions, sedation, rigidity, immobility
Tricyclic antidepressants	Amitriptyline, desipramine	Anticholinergic actions, sedation
Antiparkinsonians	Trihexyphenidyl, benztropine mesylate (not L-dopa/selegiline)	Anticholinergic actions, sedation
Narcotic analgesics	Opiates	Urinary retention, fecal impaction, sedation, delirium
α-Adrenergic antagonists	Prazosin, terazosin, doxazosin	Urethral relaxation may precipitate stress incontinence in women
α-Adrenergic agonists	Nasal decongestants	Urinary retention in men
Calcium channel blockers	All dihydropyridines[a]	Urinary retention; nocturnal diuresis due to fluid retention
Potent diuretics	Furosemide, bumetanide	Polyuria, frequency, urgency
Angiotensin-converting enzyme inhibitors	Captopril, enalapril, lisinopril	Drug-induced cough can precipitate stress incontinence in women and in some men with prior prostatectomy
Thiazolidinediones	Rosiglitazone	Nocturnal diuresis due to fluid retention
Cyclooxygenase 2 selective NSAIDs	Rofecoxib, celecoxib	Nocturnal diuresis due to fluid retention
Vincristine		Urinary retention

[a] Examples include nifedipine, nicardipine, israpidine, felodipine, nimodipine.
Source: Adapted from NM Resnick, in *Current Medical Diagnosis and Treatment*, LT Tierney et al (eds), Norwalk, Appleton & Lange, 1993.

Risk Factor	Interventions Medical	Rehabilitative or Environmental
Reduced visual acuity, dark adaptation, and perception	Refraction; cataract extraction	Home safety assessment
Reduced hearing	Removal of cerumen; audiologic evaluation	Hearing aid if appropriate (with training); reduction in background noise
Vestibular dysfunction	Avoidance of drugs affecting the vestibular system; neurologic or ear, nose, and throat evaluation, if indicated	Habituation exercises
Proprioceptive dysfunction, cervical degenerative disorders, and peripheral neuropathy	Screening for vitamin B_{12} deficiency and cervical spondylosis	Balance exercises; appropriate walking aid; correctly sized footwear with firm soles; home safety assessment
Dementia	Detection of reversible causes; avoidance of sedative or centrally acting drugs	Supervised exercise and ambulation; home safety assessment
Musculoskeletal disorders	Appropriate diagnostic evaluation	Balance-and-gait training; muscle-strengthening exercises; appropriate walking aid; home safety assessment
Foot disorders (calluses, bunions, deformities, edema)	Shaving of calluses; bunionectomy; treatment of edema	Trimming of nails; appropriate footwear
Postural hypotension	Assessment of medications; rehydration; possible alteration in situational factors (e.g., meals, change of position)	Dorsiflexion exercises; pressure-graded stockings; elevation of head of bed; use of tilt table if condition is severe
Use of medications (sedatives: benzodiazepines, phenothiazines, antidepressants; antihypertensives; others: antiarrhythmics, anticonvulsants, diuretics, alcohol)	Steps to be taken: 1. Attempted reduction in the total number of medications taken 2. Assessment of risks and benefits of each medication 3. Selection of medication, if needed, that is least centrally acting, least associated with postural hypotension, and has shortest action 4. Prescription of lowest effective dose 5. Frequent reassessment of risks and benefits	

Source: After ME Tinetti and M Speechley, N Engl J Med 320:1055, 1989.

℞ TREATMENT

Surgical decompression is the most effective treatment for obstruction, especially if there is urinary retention. For a nonoperative candidate, intermittent or indwelling catheterization is used; a condom catheter is contraindicated when urinary retention is present. For a man with prostatic obstruction who is not in retention, treatment with an α-adrenergic antagonist (e.g., terazosin, 5 to 10 mg daily, or tamsulosin, 0.4 to 0.8 mg daily) may lessen symptoms in a few weeks. The 5α-reductase inhibitor finasteride may ameliorate symptoms in a third or more of patients, but its impact is less and not apparent for many months. Combined treatment with finasteride and either terazosin or tamsulosin has proved no better than treatment with an alpha blocker alone in most men.

DETRUSOR UNDERACTIVITY Whether idiopathic or due to sacral lower motor nerve dysfunction, this is the least common cause of incontinence (<10% of cases). When it causes incontinence, detrusor underactivity is associated with urinary frequency, nocturia, and frequent leakage of small amounts. The elevated postvoiding residual volume (generally >450 mL) distinguishes it from detrusor overactivity and stress incontinence, but only urodynamic testing (rather than cystoscopy or intravenous urography) differentiates it from urethral obstruction in

men; such testing is not usually required in women, in whom obstruction is rare.

℞ TREATMENT

For the patient with a poorly contractile bladder, augmented voiding techniques (e.g., double voiding or applying suprapubic pressure) are often effective; pharmacologic agents (e.g., bethanechol) are rarely effective. If further emptying is needed or for the patient with an acontractile bladder, intermittent or indwelling catheterization is the only option. Antibiotics should be used for symptomatic upper tract infection, or as prophylaxis for recurrent symptomatic infections only in a patient using intermittent catheterization; they should not be used as prophylaxis with an indwelling catheter.

FALLS Falls are a major problem for elderly people, especially women. Some 30% of community-dwelling elderly individuals fall each year, and the proportion increases with age. Nonetheless, falling must *not* be viewed as accidental, inevitable, or untreatable.

Causes of Falls Balance and ambulation require a complex interplay of cognitive, sensory, neuromuscular, and cardiovascular function and the ability to adapt rapidly to an environmental challenge. With age, balance becomes impaired and sway increases. The resulting vulnerability predisposes the older person to fall when challenged by an additional insult to *any* of these systems. Thus, a seemingly minor fall may be due to a serious problem, such as pneumonia or a myocardial infarction.

Much more commonly, however, falls are due to the complex interaction between a variably impaired patient and an environmental challenge. While a warped floorboard may pose little problem for a vigorous, unmedicated, alert person, it may be sufficient to precipitate a fall and hip fracture in the patient with impaired vision, strength, balance, or cognition. Thus, falls in older people are rarely due to a single cause, and effective prevention entails a comprehensive assessment of the patient's intrinsic deficits (usually diseases and medications), the routine activities, and the environmental obstacles.

Intrinsic deficits are those that impair sensory input, judgment, blood pressure regulation, reaction time, and balance and gait (Table 8-5). Medications and alcohol use are among the most common, significant, and reversible causes of falling. Other treatable contributors include postprandial hypotension (which peaks 30 to 60 min after a meal), insomnia, urinary urgency, foot problems, and peripheral edema [which can burden impaired leg strength and gait with an additional 2 to 5 kg (5 to 10 lb)].

Environmental obstacles are listed in Table 8-6. Since most falls occur in or around the home, a visit by a visiting nurse, physical therapist, or physician often reaps substantial dividends.

Complications of Falls and Treatment One out of four people who fall suffers serious injury. About 5% of falls result in fractures, and an equal proportion cause serious soft tissue damage. Falls are the sixth leading cause of death for older people and a contributing factor in

TABLE 8-6 *Environmental Factors Affecting the Risk of Falling*

Environmental Area or Factor	Objective and Recommendations
All areas	
Lighting	Adequacy of illumination (older people need twice as much as younger people); absence of glare and shadows; accessible switches at room entrances; night light in bedroom, hall, bathroom
Floors	Nonskid backing for throw rugs; carpet edges tacked down; carpets with shallow pile; nonskid wax on floors; cords out of walking path; small objects (e.g., clothes, shoes) off floor
Stairs	Lighting sufficient, with switches at top and bottom of stairs; securely fastened bilateral handrails that stand out from wall; top and bottom steps marked with bright, contrasting tape; stair rises of no more than 6 in; steps in good repair; no objects stored on steps
Kitchen	Items stored so that reaching up and bending over are not necessary; secure step stool available if climbing is necessary; firm, nonmovable table
Bathroom	Grab bars for tub, shower, and toilet; nonskid decals or rubber mat in tub or shower; shower chair with handheld shower; nonskid rugs; raised toilet seat; door locks removed to ensure access in an emergency
Yard and entrances	Repair of cracks in pavement, holes in lawn; removal of rocks, tools, and other tripping hazards; well-lit walkways, free of ice and wet leaves; stairs and steps as above
Institutions	All the above; bed at proper height (not too high or low); spills on floor cleaned up promptly; appropriate use of walking aids and wheelchairs
Footwear	Shoes with firm, nonskid, nonfriction soles; low heels (unless person is accustomed to high heels); avoidance of walking in stocking feet or loose slippers

Source: After ME Tinetti and M Speechley, N Engl J Med 320:1055, 1989.

40% of admissions to nursing homes. Resultant hip problems and fear of falls are major causes of loss of independence.

Subdural hematoma is a treatable but easily overlooked complication of falls that must be considered in any elderly patient presenting with new neurologic signs, including confusion alone, even in the absence of a headache. Dehydration, electrolyte imbalance, pressure sores, rhabdomyolysis, and hypothermia may also occur and endanger the patient's life following a fall.

The risk of falling is related to the number of contributory conditions. Because the relationship is multiplicative rather than additive, however, even minor improvement in a number of these factors will reduce the risk substantially. In addition, gait training by a physical therapist often alleviates fear of falling. For those willing to wear them, hip pads have proved effective in two European trials, but the efficacy and acceptability of pads available in the United States are not yet established. Ensuring the availability of phones at floor level, a portable phone, or a lightweight radio call system is also important, as is detection and treatment of osteoporosis.

IMMOBILITY The main causes of immobility are weakness, stiffness, pain, imbalance, and psychological problems. Weakness may result from disuse of muscles, malnutrition, electrolyte disturbances, anemia, neurologic disorders, or myopathies. The most common cause of stiffness in the elderly is osteoarthritis; however, Parkinson's disease, rheumatoid arthritis, gout, pseudogout, and antipsychotic drugs such as haloperidol may also contribute. Pain, whether from bone (e.g., osteoporosis, osteomalacia, Paget's disease, metastatic bone cancer, trauma), joints (e.g., osteoarthritis, rheumatoid arthritis, gout), bursa, muscle (e.g., polymyalgia rheumatica, intermittent claudication, or "pseudoclaudication"), or foot problems may immobilize the patient.

Imbalance and fear of falling are major causes of immobilization. Imbalance may result from general debility, neurologic causes (e.g.,

stroke; loss of postural reflexes; peripheral neuropathy due to diabetes mellitus, alcohol, or malnutrition; and vestibulocerebellar abnormalities), orthostatic or postprandial hypotension, or drugs (e.g., diuretics, antihypertensives, neuroleptics, and antidepressants) or may occur following prolonged bed rest. Psychological conditions such as severe anxiety or depression may also contribute to immobilization.

Consequences In addition to thrombophlebitis and pulmonary embolus, there are multiple hazards of bed rest in the elderly. Deconditioning of the cardiovascular system occurs within days and involves fluid shifts, fluid loss, decreased cardiac output, decreased peak oxygen uptake, and increased resting heart rate. Striking changes also occur in skeletal muscle. At the cellular level, intracellular ATP and glycogen concentrations decrease, rates of protein degradation increase, and contractile velocity and strength decline, while at the whole-muscle level, atrophy, weakness, and shortening are seen. Pressure sores are another serious complication; mechanical pressure, moisture, friction, and shearing forces all predispose to their development. As a result, within days of being confined to bed, the risk of postural hypotension, falls, and skin breakdown rises. Moreover, these changes usually take weeks to months to reverse.

℞ TREATMENT

The most important step is preventive—to avoid bedrest whenever possible. When it cannot be avoided, several measures can be employed to minimize its consequences. Patients should be positioned as close to the upright position as possible several times daily. Range-of-motion exercises should begin immediately, and the skin over pressure points should be inspected frequently. Isometric and isotonic exercises should be performed while the patient is in bed, and whenever possible patients should assist their own positioning, transferring, and self-care. As mobility becomes feasible, graduated ambulation should begin. For individuals confined to a wheelchair, ring-shaped devices ("donuts") should not be used to prevent pressure ulcers since they cause venous congestion and edema and actually increase the risk.

If a pressure ulcer develops, therapy depends on its stage. Stage 1 ulcers are characterized by nonblanchable erythema of intact skin; stage 2 lesions involve an ulcer of the epidermis, dermis, or both; stage 3 ulcers extend to the subcutaneous tissue; and stage 4 lesions involve muscle, bone, and/or the supporting tissues. For stage 1 lesions, eliminating excess pressure and ensuring adequate nutrition and hygiene are sufficient. For the remaining types, the caregiver must also ensure that the wound stays clean and moist; thus, if saline dressings are used they should be changed when they are damp rather than dry. Synthetic dressings are more expensive than saline but are more effective because they require fewer changes (with less disruption of reepithelialization) and protect against contamination. Because bacterial colonization of pressure ulcers is universal, swab cultures should not be performed and topical treatment should be considered only for patients whose ulcers have not healed after 2 weeks of therapy. By contrast, associated cellulitis, osteomyelitis, or sepsis requires systemic therapy after cultures of blood and the wound border (by needle aspiration or biopsy) have been obtained. Surgical or enzymatic debridement is required for stage 3 and 4 lesions. In addition to a daily multivitamin, prescribing vitamin C (500 mg twice daily) is also useful. For debilitated patients, special mattresses are beneficial, including those that reduce pressure (e.g., static air mattress or foam) and those that relieve it (e.g., dynamic units that sequentially inflate and deflate).

In addition to treating all identified factors that contribute to immobility, consultation with a physical therapist should be sought. Installing handrails, lowering the bed, and providing chairs of proper height with arms and rubber skid guards may allow the patient to be safely mobile in the home. A properly fitted cane or walker may be helpful.

IATROGENIC DRUG REACTIONS   For several reasons, older patients are two or three times more likely to have adverse drug reactions (Chap. 3). Drug clearance is often markedly reduced. This is due to a decrease in renal plasma flow and glomerular filtration rate and a reduced hepatic clearance. The last is due to a decrease in activity of the drug-metabolizing microsomal enzymes and an overall decline in blood flow to the liver with aging. The volume of distribution of drugs is also affected, since the elderly have a decrease in total-body water and a relative increase in body fat. Thus, water-soluble drugs become more concentrated, and fat-soluble drugs have longer half-lives. In addition, serum albumin levels decline, particularly in sick patients, so that there is a decrease in protein binding of some drugs (e.g., warfarin, phenytoin), leaving more free (active) drug available. Thus, a lower/total serum drug level, as assessed by routine assays, may be an appropriate level in older patients.

In addition to impaired drug clearance, which alters pharmacokinetics, older patients have altered responses to similar serum drug levels, a phenomenon known as *altered pharmacodynamics*. They are more sensitive to some drugs (e.g., opiates, anticoagulants) and less sensitive to others (e.g., β-adrenergic agents). Finally, the older patient with multiple chronic conditions is likely to be taking several drugs, including nonprescribed agents. Thus, adverse drug reactions and dosage errors are more likely to occur, especially if the patient has visual, hearing, or memory deficits. Nonetheless, because undertreatment of older patients is as problematic as overtreatment, these caveats should not deter prescription of appropriate therapy.

Precautions to Avoid Drug Toxicity   ■   *DRUG SELECTION AND ADMINISTRATION* Before initiating treatment, the physician should first ensure that the symptom requiring treatment is not itself due to another drug. For example, antipsychotic agents can cause symptoms that mimic depression (flat affect, restlessness, and pacing); such symptoms should prompt lowering of the dose rather than initiation of an antidepressant. In addition, drug therapy should be employed only after nonpharmacologic means have been considered or tried and only when the benefit clearly outweighs the risk.

Once pharmacotherapy has been decided upon, it should begin at less than the usual adult dosage and the dose should be increased slowly. However, given the marked variability in pharmacokinetics and pharmacodynamics in the elderly, dose escalation should continue until either a successful endpoint is reached or an intolerable side effect is encountered. The final dosage schedule should be kept as simple as possible, and the number of pills should be kept as low as possible. Serum drug levels are often useful in older patients, especially for monitoring drugs with narrow therapeutic indices such as phenytoin, theophylline, quinidine, aminoglycosides, lithium, and psychotropic agents such as nortriptyline. However, toxicity can occur even with "normal" therapeutic levels of some drugs (e.g., digoxin, phenytoin). Potential drug interactions should be searched for at every visit.

Over-the-Counter Agents   Nearly three-quarters of the elderly regularly use nonprescribed drugs, many of which cause significant symptoms and/or interact with other medications. Frequent offenders include nonprescribed agents for insomnia (most of which are anticholinergics), and nonsteroidal anti-inflammatory drugs (NSAIDs), which can hamper control of hypertension in addition to causing renal dysfunction and gastrointestinal bleeding. Gingko biloba, increasingly used as a "memory booster," may interfere with previously stable anticoagulation regimens. Because older patients often consider such agents "nostrums" rather than drugs, the physician must ask about them directly.

Sedative-Hypnotics   If nonpharmacologic treatment of insomnia is unsuccessful, low-dose and short-term or intermittent use of an intermediate-acting agent whose metabolism is not affected by age (e.g., oxazepam, 10 to 30 mg/d) may be useful. Because of the increased risk of confusion and other adverse effects, benzodiazepines with either short (e.g., triazolam) or long duration of action (e.g., flurazepam

and diazepam) should be avoided. Barbiturates should be avoided for the same reasons. A tricyclic antidepressant should not be prescribed for insomnia unless the patient is depressed.

Antibiotics   Serum creatinine is not a good index of renal function in old people; however, when it is elevated, special care must be taken with the administration of drugs normally excreted by the kidneys. Concentrations of relevant antibiotics should be measured directly.

Cardiac Drugs   In older patients, digitalis, procainamide, and quinidine have prolonged half-lives and narrow therapeutic windows; toxicity is common at the usual dosages. For example, digoxin toxicity—especially anorexia, confusion, or depression—can occur even with therapeutic digoxin levels.

H₂ Receptor Antagonists   Most of these agents interfere with hepatic metabolism of other drugs, and all can produce confusion in the elderly. Because they are renally excreted, lower doses should be used to minimize the risk of toxicity in older individuals.

Antipsychotics and Tricyclic Antidepressants   These drugs can produce anticholinergic side effects in old people (e.g., confusion, urinary retention, constipation, dry mouth). These can be minimized by switching to a nonanticholinergic agent (e.g., sertraline or citalopram) or one with less anticholinergic effect (e.g., olanzapine, nortriptyline). In general, the least potent agents for psychosis (e.g., chlorpromazine) have the most sedating and anticholinergic effects and are the most likely to induce postural hypotension. By contrast, the most potent antipsychotic agents (e.g., haloperidol) have the least sedating, anticholinergic, and hypotensive side effects but cause extrapyramidal side effects, including dystonia, akathisia, rigidity, and tardive dyskinesia. The newer potent antipsychotics (e.g., risperidone, olanzapine, quetiapine, and clozapine) are relative exceptions to this rule. More specific for serotonin than dopamine D_2 receptors, these medications may be safer for older demented patients, especially those with hallucinations associated with Lewy body dementia or in those receiving therapy for Parkinson's disease. Unfortunately, even these newer drugs lose their specificity at the higher doses that are commonly required in clinical practice. Thus all of these agents are potentially toxic. Moreover, since both depression and agitation often remit spontaneously, cautious discontinuation of these drugs should be considered periodically.

Glaucoma Medications   Both topical beta blockers and carbonic anhydrase inhibitors can cause systemic side effects. The latter can cause malaise and anorexia independent of the induced metabolic acidosis.

Anticoagulants   Elderly patients benefit from anticoagulation as much as do younger individuals but are more vulnerable to serious bleeding and drug interactions. Hence, more careful monitoring and aiming for the lower boundary of the therapeutic window are advisable.

Analgesics   Both propoxyphene and meperidine are associated with a disproportionate risk of delirium, and propoxyphene also increases the risk of hip fracture. Of the NSAIDs, indomethacin is most likely to induce confusion, fluid retention, and gastrointestinal bleeding. Each of these agents should be avoided in the elderly. Cyclooxygenase 2 (COX-2) inhibitors are safer than nonselective NSAIDs for older adults. However, they are more expensive and can cause fluid retention with consequent worsening of hypertension and nocturnal incontinence.

Avoidance of Overtreatment   Drugs are frequently not indicated in some common clinical situations. For instance, antibiotics need not be given for asymptomatic bacteriuria unless obstructive uropathy, other anatomic abnormalities, or stones are also present. Ankle edema is often due to venous insufficiency, drugs such as NSAIDs or some calcium antagonists, or even inactivity or malnutrition in chairbound patients. Diuretics are usually not indicated unless edema is associated with heart failure. Fitted, pressure gradient stockings are often helpful. For claudication, regular exercise should be prescribed before cilostazol. Finally, since older patients generally tolerate aspirin and other NSAIDs less well than do younger patients, localized pain should be treated when possible with local measures such as injection, physical therapy, heat, ultrasound, or transcutaneous electrical stimulation (Chap. 11).

PREVENTION

Much can be done to prevent the progression and even the onset of disease in older persons. Even when the relative benefit of an intervention is less than in younger adults, its absolute impact is often greater in the elderly because their baseline risk is higher. However, while reductions of mortality and morbidity are valuable goals for older adults, prevention must also encompass preservation of function and quality of life. Moreover, because preventive interventions are often associated with discomfort, risk, and expense, it is important to ensure that the patient believes the benefit is worth the effort.

Certain recommendations are straightforward. Dietary inadequacies should be corrected. Daily calcium intake should approximate 1500 mg, and most elderly people should take 400 to 800 IU of vitamin D daily (contained in one to two multivitamin tablets). Tobacco and alcohol use should be minimized, since the benefits of discontinuing these accrue even to individuals over age 65. Because of the prevalence, functional impact, and ease of treatment, glaucoma should be screened for, and visual and auditory impairment should be corrected. Dentures should be assessed for their fit, and oral lesions beneath them should be detected. Because thyroid dysfunction is more prevalent in the elderly, difficult to detect clinically, and treatable, serum levels of thyroid-stimulating hormone should be measured at least once in asymptomatic older people and probably every 3 to 5 years thereafter. All older women should be screened for osteoporosis. The importance of reviewing all of a patient's medications and discontinuing them whenever feasible cannot be overemphasized.

Exercise should be encouraged not only because of its beneficial effects of blood pressure, cardiovascular conditioning, glucose homeostasis, bone density, insomnia, functional status, and even longevity, but also because it may improve mood and social interaction, reduce constipation, and prevent falls. Resistance training should be encouraged as much as a walking program. Sophisticated screening tests are generally not required. Spinal flexion exercises should be avoided in patients with osteopenia.

Immunizations for influenza, pneumococcal pneumonia, and tetanus should be current. Purified protein derivative (PPD) testing should be done on residents of chronic care facilities and on others at high risk of tuberculosis; those who have recently converted probably should be treated. Since responsiveness wanes with age, the test, if negative, should be repeated in a week.

Hypertension, whether isolated systolic hypertension or combined systolic and diastolic hypertension, should be treated as outlined in Chap. 230.

Serum cholesterol should be measured in patients with established coronary heart disease. Older adults with cardiovascular risk factors experience a similar benefit from statin therapy as younger adults (Chap. 225). Low-dose aspirin is likely useful for primary prevention among those at highest risk for coronary and cerebrovascular disease, but the relative risks and benefits must be considered on an individual basis.

Cancer screening is warranted. A Papanicolaou test should be done in women who have not had one before, since the incidence of cervical carcinoma and associated death increases with age; it should be repeated triennially in all older women unless two previous tests have been normal. Screening for colon cancer is warranted until a minimum age of 80 to 85, at least in community-dwelling elderly, although the optimal method is unclear. Because older women with breast cancer are more likely to die of *of* it than *with* it, screening mammography is indicated every 1 to 2 years, at least until age 75, and thereafter if a positive finding would result in therapeutic intervention.

Perhaps the most valuable preventive measure in the elderly is to take a careful history, focusing not only on the "chief complaint" but also on common and often hidden conditions such as falls, confusion, depression, alcohol abuse, sexual dysfunction, and incontinence. In addition, one should always anticipate the complications for which the specific patient is at risk and take steps to avert them. For instance, a patient with cognitive impairment who smokes is at risk not only for lung cancer but also for starting a fire, and a patient who requires narcotics is at risk for fecal impaction, delirium, urinary retention, and confusion. Community-dwelling patients who are at highest risk of rapid deterioration and institutionalization and who should be monitored more closely include those over age 80, those who live alone, those who are bereaved or depressed, and those who are intellectually impaired.

FURTHER READING

BLAZER DG: Depression in late life: Review and commentary. J Gerontol A Biol Sci Med Sci 58A:249, 2003

BURGIO KL et al: Behavioral training with and without biofeedback in the treatment of urge incontinence in older women. A randomized controlled trial. JAMA 288:2293, 2002

CUMMINGS JL, COLE G: Alzheimer's disease. JAMA 287:2335, 2002

DUBINSKI RM et al: Practice parameter: Risk of driving and Alzheimer's disease (an evidence-based review): Report of the Quality Standards Subcommittee of the American Academy of Neurology. Neurology 54:2205, 2000

GILLICK MR: Choosing appropriate medical care for the elderly. J Am Med Dir Assoc 2:305, 2001

KANNUS P et al: Prevention of hip fracture in elderly people with the use of a hip protector. N Engl J Med 343:1506, 2000

KIRKLAND JL: The biology of senescence: Potential for prevention of disease. Clin Geriatr Med 18:383, 2002

MARCANTONIO ER et al: Reducing delirium after hip fracture. A randomized trial. J Am Geriatr Soc 49:516, 2001

SCIENTIFIC COMMITTEE OF THE FIRST INTERNATIONAL CONSULTATION ON INCONTINENCY: Assessment and treatment of urinary incontinence. Lancet 355:2153, 2000

SHEPHERD J et al: Pravastatin in elderly individuals at risk of vascular disease (PROSPER): A randomised controlled trial. Lancet 360:1623, 2002

TINETTI MP: Preventing falls in elderly persons. N Engl J Med 348:42, 2003

TRINH N-H et al: Efficacy of cholinesterase inhibitors in the treatment of neuropsychiatric symptoms and functional impairment in Alzheimer disease: A meta-analysis. JAMA 289:210, 2003

US PREVENTIVE SERVICES TASK FORCE: Screening for osteoporosis in postmenopausal women: Recommendations and rationale. Ann Intern Med 137:526, 2002

WALTER LC, COVINSKY KE: Cancer screening in elderly patients. A framework for individualized decision making. JAMA 285:2750, 2001

9 PALLIATIVE AND END-OF-LIFE CARE
Ezekiel J. Emanuel, Linda L. Emanuel

EPIDEMIOLOGY

In 2000, 2,403,351 people died in the United States (Table 9-1). Over 70% of all deaths occur in people >65 years of age. The epidemiology of mortality is similar in most developed countries; cardiovascular diseases and cancer are the predominant killers, a marked change since 1900, when heart disease caused ~8% of all deaths and cancer accounted for <4% of all deaths. In 2000, AIDS accounted for <1% of all deaths, although among those aged 35 to 44, it remains a leading cause of death.

While precise statistics are not available, it is estimated that in developed countries ~70% of all deaths are preceded by a disease or condition such that it is reasonable to plan for dying in the foreseeable future. Cancer has served as the paradigm for terminal care, but it is not the only type of illness with a recognizable and predictable terminal phase. Since congestive heart failure, chronic obstructive pul-

TABLE 9-1 Ten Leading Causes of Death in the United States and Britain

	United States			Britain	
Cause of Death	Number of Deaths	Percent or Total	Number of Deaths Among People ≥65 Years of Age	Number of Deaths	Percent of Total
All deaths	2,403,351	100	1,799,825	535,664	100
Heart disease	710,760	29.6	593,707	108,418	20.2
Cancer	553,091	23.0	392,366	132,793	24.8
Stroke	167,661	7.0	148,045	52,516	9.8
Chronic obstructive pulmonary disease	122,009	5.1	106,375	23,538	4.4
Accidents	97,900	4.1	31,051	10,733	2.0
Diabetes	69,301	2.9	52,414	5,773	1.1
Pneumonia/influenza	65,313	2.7	58,557	56,329	10.5
Alzheimer's disease	49,558	2.1	48,993	14,082	2.6
Nephritis, nephritic syndrome, nephrosis	37,251	1.5	31,225	7,270	1.4
Septicemia	31,224	1.4	24,786	3,410	0.6

Source: National Center for Health Statistics (2000) *www.cdc.gov/nchs*; National Statistics (Great Britain) www.statistics.gov.uk.

monary disease (COPD), chronic liver failure, and many other conditions have recognizable terminal phases, a systematic approach to end-of-life care should be part of all medical specialties. Many patients with advanced illness can also benefit from palliative care long before the terminal phases of their illnesses.

Over the past few decades in the United States, a significant change in the site of death has occurred that coincides with patient and family preferences. Nearly 60% of Americans died as inpatients in hospitals in 1980. By 2000, the trend was reversing, with ~40% of Americans dying as hospital inpatients (Fig. 9-1). This shift has been most dramatic for people dying from cancer and COPD and for younger and very old individuals. In the past decade, it is associated with the increased use of hospice care; in 2000, ~20% of all decedents in the United States received such care. Cancer patients currently constitute >70% of hospice users, with 33 to 50% of all terminal cancer patients receiving hospice care. About 90% of patients receiving hospice care die out of the hospital. Consequently, providing optimal palliative and end-of-life care requires ensuring appropriate services in a variety of settings, including noninstitutional settings.

HOSPICE AND THE PALLIATIVE CARE FRAMEWORK

Central to this type of care is an interdisciplinary team approach that typically encompasses pain and symptom management, spiritual and psychological care for the patient, and support for family caregivers.

Terminally ill patients have a wide variety of advanced diseases, often with multiple symptoms demanding relief, and require noninvasive therapeutic regimens to be delivered in a commodious care setting. Fundamental to ensuring quality palliative and end-of-life care

is a focus on four broad domains: (1) physical symptoms; (2) mental or psychological symptoms; (3) social needs that include interpersonal relationships, caregiving, and economic concerns; and (4) existential or spiritual needs.

A whole-person assessment screens for and evaluates needs in each of these four domains. Goals for care are established in discussion with the patient and/or family based on the assessment in each of these domains. Interventions are aimed at improving or managing symptoms and needs. While physicians are responsible for certain especially technical interventions, and for coordinating the interventions, they cannot be responsible for providing all of them. Since failing to address any one of the domains is likely to preclude a good death, a well coordinated, effectively communicating interdisciplinary team takes on special importance in end-of-life care.

ASSESSMENT AND CARE PLANNING ■ **Whole-Person Assessment** Standardized methods for conducting a whole-person assessment focus on evaluating the patient's condition in all four domains affected by illness: physical, mental, social, and spiritual. The assessment of physical and mental symptoms should follow a modified version of the traditional medical history and physical examination that emphasizes symptoms. Questions should aim at elucidating symptoms but also discerning sources of suffering and how much these symptoms interfere with the patient's life. Standardized assessment questions are available from scales such as the Memorial Symptom Assessment Scale. Using such scales ensures that the assessment is comprehensive and does not just focus on pain and a few other physical symptoms. Invasive tests are best avoided in end-of-life care, and even minimally invasive tests should be carefully evaluated for their benefit-to-burden ratio for the patient. Aspects of the physical examination that are uncomfortable and unlikely to yield useful information can also be omitted.

Regarding social needs, health care providers should assess the status of important relationships, financial burdens, care-giving needs, and access to medical care. Relevant questions will include: *How often is there someone to feel close to? How much help do you need with things like getting meals or getting around? How much trouble do you have getting the medical care you need?* In the area of existential needs, providers should assess distress and the patient's sense of being emotionally and existentially settled and of finding purpose or meaning. Helpful assessment questions can include: *How much are you able to find meaning since your illness began?* In addition, it can be helpful to ask about how well the patient perceives his or her care to be: *How much do you feel your doctors and nurses respect you? How clear is the information from us about what to expect regarding your illness? How much do you feel that the medical care you are getting fits with your goals?* If concern is detected in any of these areas, deeper evaluative questions are warranted.

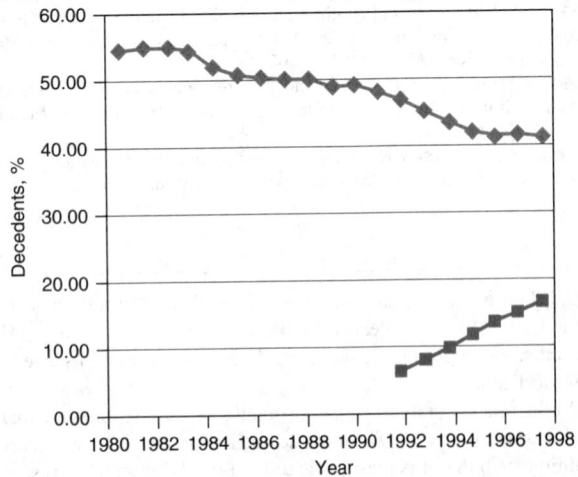

FIGURE 9-1 Graph showing trends in the site of death in the past two decades. ◆, percentage of hospital inpatient deaths; ■, percentage of decedents enrolled in a hospice.

Communication Foremost is to ensure empathetic and effective communication. When an illness is life-threatening, there are many emotionally charged and potentially conflict-creating moments, collectively called "bad news" situations, in which good communication skills are essential. These moments include communicating to the patient and/or family about a terminal diagnosis, the patient's prognosis, any treatment failures, deemphasizing efforts to cure and prolong life while focusing more on symptom management and palliation, advance care planning, and the patient's actual death.

Just as surgeons plan and prepare for major operations or investigators rehearse a presentation of research results, physicians and health care providers caring for patients with advanced illness must develop a practiced approach to sharing important information and planning interventions. In addition, families identify as important not only how well the physician was prepared to deliver bad news but also the setting in which it was delivered. For instance, 27% of families making critical decisions for patients in the intensive care unit (ICU) desired better and more private physical space to communicate with physicians, and 48% found having clergy present reassuring.

An organized and effective procedure for communicating bad news with seven steps goes by the acronym P-SPIKES: (1) *p*repare for the discussion, (2) *s*et up a suitable environment, (3) begin the discussion

by finding out what the *p*atient and/or family understand, (4) determine how they will comprehend new *i*nformation best and how much they want to know, (5) provide needed new *k*nowledge accordingly, (6) allow for *e*motional responses; and (7) *s*hare plans for the next steps in care. Table 9-2 provides a summary of these steps along with suggested phrases and underlying rationales for each.

Continuous Goal Assessment Major barriers to ensuring quality palliative and end-of-life care include difficulty in providing an accurate prognosis and emotional resistance of patients and their families to accepting the implications of a poor prognosis. A practical solution to these barriers is to integrate palliative care with curative care regardless of prognosis. With this approach, palliative care no longer conveys the message of failure, having no more treatments, or "giving up hope." Fundamental to integrating palliative care with curative therapy is to include continuous goal assessment as part of the routine patient reassessment that occurs at most patient-physician encounters.

Goals for care are numerous, ranging from cure of a specific dis-

TABLE 9-2 Elements of Communicating Bad News—the P-SPIKES Approach

Acronym	Steps	Aim of the Interaction	Preparations, Questions, or Phrases
P	Preparation	Mentally prepare for the interaction with the patient and/or family.	Review what information needs to be communicated. Plan how you will provide emotional support. Rehearse key steps and phrases in the interaction.
S	Setting of the interaction	Ensure the appropriate setting for a serious and emotionally charged discussion.	Ensure patient, family, and appropriate social supports are present. Devote sufficient time—do not squeeze in a discussion. Ensure privacy and prevent interruptions by people or beeper. Bring a box of tissues.
P	Patient's perception and preparation	Begin the discussion by establishing the baseline and whether the patient and family can grasp the information. Ease tension by having the patient and family contribute.	Start with open-ended questions to encourage participation. Possible phrases to use: *What do you understand about your illness? When you first had symptom X, what did you think it might be? What did Dr. X tell you when he sent you here? What do you think is going to happen?*
I	Invitation and information needs	Discover what information needs the patient and/or family have and what limits they want regarding the bad information.	Possible phrases to use: *If this condition turns out to be something serious, do you want to know? Would you like me to tell you the full details of your condition? If not, then who would you like me to talk to?*
K	Knowledge of the condition	Provide the bad news or other information to the patient and/or family sensitively.	Do not just dump the information on the patient and family. Interrupt and check that the patient and family are understanding. Possible phrases to use: *I feel badly to have to tell you this, but . . . Unfortunately, the tests showed . . . I'm afraid the news is not good . . .*
E	Empathy and exploration	Identify the cause of the emotions—e.g., poor prognosis. Empathize with the patient and/or family's feeling. Explore by asking open-ended questions.	Strong feelings in reaction to bad news are normal. Acknowledge what the patient and family are feeling. Remind them such feelings are normal, even if frightening. Give them time to respond. Remind patient and family you won't abandon them. Possible phrases to use: *I imagine this is very hard for you. You look very upset. Tell me how you are feeling. I wish the news were different. I'll do whatever I can to help you.*
S	Summary and strategic planning	Delineate for the patient and the family the next steps, including additional tests or interventions.	It is the unknown and uncertain that increase anxiety. Recommend a schedule with goals and landmarks. Provide your rationale for the patient and/or family to accept (or reject). If the patient and/or family are not ready to discuss the next steps, schedule a follow-up visit.

Source: Adapted from Buckman.

ease, to relief of a symptom, to delaying the course of an incurable disease, to adapting to progressive disability without disrupting the family, to finding peace of mind or personal meaning, to dying in a manner that leaves loved ones with a positive "departure memory." Discernment of goals for care can be approached through a seven-step protocol: (1) ensure that information is as complete as reasonably possible and understood by all relevant parties (see above); (2) explore what the patient and/or family are hoping for while identifying relevant and realistic goals; (3) share all the options with the patient and family; (4) respond with empathy as they adjust to declining expectations; (5) make a plan, emphasizing what can be done toward the realistic goals; (6) follow through with the plan; and (7) review and revise this plan periodically, considering at every encounter whether the goals of care should be reviewed with the patient and/or family. If a patient or family member has difficulty letting go of an unrealistic goal, suggest that, while hoping for the best, it is still prudent to have a plan for other outcomes as well.

Advance Care Planning ■ *PRACTICES* Advance care planning is a process of planning for future medical care in case the patient becomes incapable of making medical decisions. Ideally, such planning would occur before a health care crisis or the terminal phase of an illness. Unfortunately, diverse barriers prevent this. While 80% of Americans endorse advance care planning and completing living wills, only 20% have actually done so. Most patients expect physicians to initiate advance care planning and will wait for physicians to broach the subject. Patients also wish to discuss advance care planning with their family.

Yet patients with unrealistic expectations are significantly more likely to prefer aggressive treatments. Fewer than one-third of health care providers have completed advance care planning for themselves. Hence, a good first step is for health care providers to complete advance care planning for themselves. This makes providers aware of the critical choices in the process and the issues that are especially charged and allows them to tell their patients truthfully that they have done this themselves.

Steps in effective advance care planning center on (1) introducing the topic, (2) structuring a discussion, (3) reviewing plans that have been discussed by the patient and family, (4) documenting the plans, (5) updating them periodically, and (6) implementing the advance care directive (Table 9-3). The main barriers to advance care planning are problems in raising the topic and structuring a succinct discussion. Raising the topic can be done efficiently as a routine matter that is recommended for all patients, analogous to purchasing insurance or estate planning. It can be reassuring and effective if the physician has completed his or her own advance care directive.

Structuring a focused discussion is the central skill. Identify the health care proxy and recommend his or her involvement in the advance care planning process. Select a worksheet, preferably one that has been evaluated and demonstrated to produce reliable and valid expressions of patient preferences, and orient the patient and proxy to it. Such worksheets exist both for general and disease-specific situations. Discuss with the patient and proxy one scenario as an example to demonstrate how to think about the issues. It is often helpful to begin with a scenario in which the patient is likely to have settled preferences, such as being in a persistent vegetative state. Once the

TABLE 9-3 *Steps in Advance Care Planning*

Step	Goals to be Achieved and Measures to Cover	Useful Phrases or Points to Make
Introducing advance care planning	Ask the patient what he or she knows about advance care planning and if he or she has already completed an advanced care directive. Indicate that you as a physician have completed advance care planning. Indicate that you try to perform advance care planning with all patients regardless of prognosis. Explain the goals of the process as empowering the patient and ensuring you and the proxy understand the patient's preferences. Provide the patient relevant literature including the advance care directive that you prefer to use. Recommend the patient identify a proxy decision-maker who should attend the next meeting.	*I'd like to talk with you about something I try to discuss with all my patients. It's called advance care planning. In fact, I feel that this is such an important topic that I have done this myself. Are you familiar with advance care planning or living wills?* *Have you thought about the type of care you would want if you ever became too sick to speak for yourself? That is the purpose of advance care planning.* *There is no change in health that we have not discussed. I am bringing this up now because it is sensible for everyone, no matter how well or ill, old or young.* Have many copies of advance care directives available, including in the waiting room, for patients and families.
Structured discussion of scenarios and patient	Affirm that the goal of the process is to follow the patient's wishes if the patient looses decision-making capacity. Elicit the patient's overall goals related to health care. Elicit the patient's preferences for specific interventions in a few salient and common scenarios. Help the patient define the threshold for withdrawing and withholding interventions. Define the patient's preference for the role of the proxy.	Use a structure worksheet with typical scenarios. Begin the discussion with persistent vegetative state and consider other scenarios, such as recovery from and acute event with serious disability, asking the patient about his or her preferences regarding specific interventions, such as ventilators, nasogastric feedings, and CPR proceeding to less-invasive interventions, such as blood transfusions and antibiotics.
Review the patient's preferences	After the patient has made choices of interventions, review them to ensure they are consistent and the proxy is aware of them.	
Document the patient's preferences	Formally complete the advance care directive and have witness sign it. Provide a copy for the patient and the proxy. Insert a copy into the patient's medical record.	
Update the directive	Periodically, and with major changes in health status, review with the patient the existing choice made and make any modifications.	
Apply the directive	The directive goes into effect only when the patient becomes unable to make medical decisions for him- or herself. Re-read the directive to be sure about its content. Discuss your proposed actions based on the directive with the proxy.	

Note: CPR, cardiopulmonary resuscitation.

patient's preferences for interventions in this scenario are determined, suggest that the patient and proxy discuss and complete the worksheet for the others. If appropriate, suggest they involve family members in the discussion. On a return visit, go over the patient's preferences, checking and resolving any inconsistencies. After having the patient and proxy sign the document, place it in the medical chart and be sure that copies are provided to relevant family members and care sites. Since patients' preferences can change, these documents need to be reviewed periodically or after an illness episode or personal experience.

TYPES OF DOCUMENTS Advance care planning documents are of two broad types. The first includes living wills or instructional directives; these are advisory documents that describe the types of decisions that should direct care. Some are more specific, delineating different scenarios and interventions for the patient to choose from. Among these, some are for general use and others are designed for use by patients with a specific type of disease, such as cancer or HIV. Less specific directives can be general statements of not wanting life-sustaining interventions or forms that describe the values that should guide specific terminal care decisions. Health care proxy designation directives appoint an individual to make decisions. The choice is not either-or; a combined directive that both directs care and designates a proxy is often utilized, and the directive should clearly indicate whether the specified patient preferences or the proxy's choice should take precedence if they conflict.

A potentially misleading distinction relates to statutory as opposed to advisory documents. Statutory documents are drafted to fulfill relevant state laws. They tend to be written with the goal of protecting the clinician from legal action if they follow the patient's stated wishes. Advisory documents are drafted to reflect the patient's wishes. Both are legal, the first under state law, and the latter under common or constitutional law.

LEGAL ASPECTS As of 2003, 47 states and the District of Columbia had enacted living will legislation. Many states have their own statutory forms. Massachusetts, Michigan, and New York do not have living will laws. However, like all other states except Alaska, these states have enacted durable power of attorney for health care laws that permit patients to designate a proxy decision maker with authority to terminate life-sustaining treatments. Only in Alaska does the law prohibit proxies from terminating life-sustaining treatments.

The U.S. Supreme Court has ruled that patients have a constitutional right to decide about refusing and terminating medical interventions, including life-sustaining interventions, and that mentally incompetent patients can exercise this right by providing "clear and convincing evidence" of their preferences. Since advance care directives permit patients to provide such evidence, commentators agree that they are constitutionally protected. Most commentators believe that a state is required to honor any clear advance care directive. Many states explicitly honor out-of-state directives. If a patient is not using a statutory form, then a statutory form should be attached to the advance care directive being used.

INTERVENTIONS

PHYSICAL SYMPTOMS AND THEIR MANAGEMENT Great emphasis has been placed on addressing dying patients' pain. Some institutions have made it a fifth vital sign. While good end-of-life care requires good pain management, it also requires more. The frequency of symptoms varies by disease and other factors. The most common physical and psychological symptoms among all terminally ill patients include pain, fatigue, insomnia, anorexia, dyspnea, depression, anxiety, and nausea and vomiting. In the last days of life, terminal delirium is also common. Assessments of patients with advanced cancer have shown that patients experienced an average of 11.5 different physical and psychological symptoms (Table 9-4).

Evaluations to determine the etiology of these symptoms should be limited to the history and physical examination. Only in rare cases will radiologic or other diagnostic examinations provide sufficient ben-

TABLE 9-4 *Common Physical and Psychological Symptoms of Terminally Ill Patients*

Physical Symptoms	Psychological Symptoms
Pain	Anxiety
Fatigue and weakness	Depression
Dyspnea	Hopelessness
Insomnia	Meaninglessness
Dry mouth	Irritability
Anorexia	Impaired concentration
Nausea and vomiting	Confusion
Constipation	Delirium
Cough	
Swelling of arms or legs	
Itching	
Diarrhea	
Dysphagia	
Dizziness	
Loss of libido	
Fecal and urinary incontinence	
Numbness/tingling in hands/feet	

efit in directing optimal palliative care to warrant the risks, discomfort, and inconvenience to the seriously ill patient. Only a few of the common symptoms presenting difficult management issues will be addressed in this chapter. →*Management of other symptoms, such as nausea and vomiting, insomnia, and diarrhea can be found in Chaps. 34 and 66, Chap. 24, and Chap. 35, respectively.*

Pain ■ *FREQUENCY* The frequency of pain among terminally ill patients varies widely. The proportion of advanced cancer patients experiencing substantial pain is reported to range from 36 to 90%. In the SUPPORT study of hospitalized patients with diverse conditions and an estimated survival of ≤6 months, 22% reported moderate to severe pain, and caregivers of these patients reported that 50% had similar levels of pain during the last few days of life.

ETIOLOGY Nociceptive pain is the result of direct mechanical or chemical stimulation of nociceptors and normal neural signaling to the brain. It tends to be localized, aching, throbbing, and cramping. The classic example is bone metastases. *Visceral pain* is caused by nociceptors in gastrointestinal, respiratory, and other organ systems. It is a deep or colicky type of pain classically associated with pancreatitis, myocardial infarction, or tumor invasion of viscera. *Neuropathic pain* arises from disordered, ectopic nerve signals. It is burning or shocklike pain. Classic cases are post-stroke pain and tumor invasion of the brachial plexus. Well-recognized pain syndromes are associated with peripheral neuropathy after chemotherapy or surgery.

ASSESSMENT Pain is a subjective experience. Depending upon the patient's circumstances, perspective, and physiologic condition, the same insult can produce different levels of reported pain and need for pain relief. Systematic assessment includes eliciting the following: (1) periodicity—continuous, with or without exacerbations, or incident; (2) location; (3) intensity; (4) modifying factors; (5) effects of treatments; (6) functional impact; and (7) impact on patient. Several validated pain assessment measures may be used, such as the Visual Analogue Scale, the Brief Pain Inventory, and the pain component of the Memorial Symptom Assessment Scale. Frequent reassessments are essential to assess the effects of interventions.

INTERVENTIONS Interventions for pain must be tailored to each individual with the goal of preempting chronic pain and relieving breakthrough pain. At the end of life, there is no reason to doubt the patient's report of pain. Pain medications are the cornerstone of management. If these are failing and nonpharmacologic interventions—including radiotherapy, anesthetic or neurosurgical procedures, such as peripheral nerve blocks or epidural morphine—are required, a pain consultation is appropriate.

Pharmacologic interventions follow the World Health Organization three-step approach involving nonopioid analgesics, mild opioids, and strong opioids, with or without adjuvants (Chap. 11). Nonopioid analgesics, especially nonsteroidal anti-inflammatory drugs, are the initial treatments for mild pain. They work primarily by inhibiting peripheral prostaglandins, reducing inflammation, but may also have central nervous system (CNS) effects. They have a ceiling effect. Ibuprofen, up to 1600 mg/d, has a minimal risk of bleeding and renal impairment and is a good initial choice.

If nonopioid analgesics are insufficient, then opioids should be introduced. They work by interacting with mu opioid receptors in the CNS to activate pain-inhibitory neurons; most are receptor antagonists. The mixed agonist/antagonist opioids useful for post-acute pain should not be used for the chronic pain in end-of-life care. Weak opioids, such as codeine, should be used initially. However, if the weak opioids are escalated and also fail to relieve pain sufficiently, then strong opioids, such as morphine 5 to 10 mg every 4 h, should be used. Nonopioid analgesics should be combined with opioids because they potentiate the effect of opioids.

For continuous pain, the opioids should be administered on a regular, around-the-clock basis consistent with their duration of analgesia. They should not be provided only when the patient experiences pain; the goal is to prevent patients from experiencing pain. Patients should also be provided rescue medication, such as liquid morphine, for breakthrough pain and should be instructed to take one-half of the standing opioid dose. Patients should be informed that using the rescue medication does not obviate their taking the next standard dose of pain medication. If after 24 h the patient's pain remains uncontrolled and recurs before the next dose, requiring the patient to utilize the rescue medication, increase the daily opioid dose by the total dose of rescue medications used by the patient, or by 50% for moderate pain and 100% for severe pain of the standing opioid daily dose.

It is inappropriate to start with extended-release preparations. Once pain relief is obtained, then switch to extended-release preparations. Even with a stable extended-release preparation regimen, the patient may have incident pain, such as pain during dressing changes. Short-acting preparations should be used to cover such predictable episodes.

Because of differences in opioid receptors, cross-tolerance among opioids is incomplete and patients may experience different side effects with different opioids. Therefore, if a patient is not experiencing pain relief or is experiencing too many side effects, change to another opioid preparation. When switching, begin with ≥50% of the published equianalgesic dose of the new opioid. (Starting at 25% of the equianalgesic dose is inadequate for terminally ill patients.) Opioids have no ceiling effect; therefore, there is no maximum dose no matter how many milligrams the patient is receiving. The appropriate dose is the dose needed to achieve pain relief. Addiction or excessive respiratory depression is extremely unlikely in the terminally ill; fear of these side effects should neither prevent escalating opioid medications when the patient is experiencing insufficient pain relief nor justify using opioid antagonists, such as naloxone.

Opioid side effects should be anticipated and treated preemptively. Nearly all patients experience constipation that can be quite debilitating (see below). Failure to prevent constipation often results in noncompliance with narcotic therapy. About a third of patients experience nausea and vomiting, but tolerance develops, usually within a week. Therefore, when beginning opioids, an antiemetic, such as metoclopramide or a serotonin antagonist, should be prescribed prophylactically and stopped after 1 week. Drowsiness, a common side effect of opioids, also abates within a week. During this period, drowsiness can be treated with psychostimulants, such as dextroamphetamine or methylphenidate. Anecdotal reports suggest that donepezil may also be helpful for opiate-induced drowsiness. Metabolites of morphine and most opioids are cleared renally; doses may need to be adjusted for renal failure.

Patients and families may withhold the prescribed opioids for fear of addiction or dependence. Physicians and health care providers must reassure patients and families that the patient will not become addicted or dependent upon the opioids if used as prescribed for pain relief; this fear should not prevent the patient from taking the medications around the clock.

Seriously ill patients with chronic pain relief rarely if ever become addicted. Suspicion of addiction should not be a reason to withhold pain medications from terminally ill patients. However, diversion of drugs for use by other family members or illicit sale may occur. If this occurs, it should be managed in a way that does not inflict unnecessary pain on the dying patient. Contract writing with the patient and family can help. If that fails, transfer to a safe facility may be necessary.

Tolerance is the need for increasing medication dosage for the same pain relief without a change in disease. In the case of patients with advanced disease, the need for increasing opioid dosage for pain relief is usually caused by disease progression rather than tolerance. Physical dependence is indicated by symptoms from the abrupt withdrawal of opioids and should not be confused with addiction.

Adjuvant analgesic medications are nonopioids that potentiate the analgesic effects of opioids. In the management of neuropathic pain, tricyclic antidepressants, such as desipramine, which has fewer side effects than other tricyclic antidepressants, can begin to work in a few days at doses of 10 to 25 mg before bedtime. Similarly, anticonvulsants, especially gabapentin (begun at 100 mg tid and titrated up by 100 mg tid until relief, with usual doses between 300 mg and 1200 mg tid) or carbamazepine, have shown effectiveness in relief of neuropathic pain. Glucocorticoids, preferably dexamethasone provided once a day, can be useful in reducing inflammation that causes pain while elevating mood, energy, and appetite. Other drugs, including clonidine and baclofen, can be effective in pain relief. These drugs are adjuvants and should all be used in conjunction with—not instead of—opioids. Methadone, carefully dosed, has activity at the N-methyl D-aspartamate (NMDA) receptor and is useful for complex pain syndromes and neuropathic pain.

Radiation therapy can treat bone pain from single metastatic lesions. Bone pain from multiple metastases can be amenable to radiopharmaceuticals, such as strontium 89 and samarium 153. Pamidronate (90 mg every 4 weeks) and calcitonin (200 IU intranasally once or twice a day) can also provide relief from bone pain.

Constipation ■ *FREQUENCY*   Constipation is reported in up to 90% of terminally ill patients.

ETIOLOGY   While hypercalcemia and other factors can cause constipation, it is a predictable consequence of the use of opioids for the relief of pain and dyspnea and of tricyclic antidepressants, from their anticholinergic effects, as well as of the inactivity and poor diet that are common among seriously ill patients. If untreated, constipation can cause substantial pain, vomiting, impaction, and mental confusion. Whenever opioids, tricyclic antidepressants, and other medications known to cause constipation are used, preemptive cathartic treatment should be instituted.

ASSESSMENT   Establish the patient's previous bowel habits, including the frequency, consistency, and volume. Abdominal and rectal examinations should be performed to exclude impaction or acute abdomen. Radiographic assessments beyond a simple flat plate of the abdomen are rarely necessary except when obstruction cannot be definitively excluded.

INTERVENTION   While physical activity, adequate hydration, and dietary treatments with fiber and roughage can be helpful, each is limited in its effectiveness for most seriously ill patients, and roughage may exacerbate problems if impaired motility is the etiology. Fiber is contraindicated in the presence of opioid use. Stimulant and osmotic laxatives, stool softeners, fluids, and enemas are the mainstay of therapy (Table 9-5). When preventing constipation from opioids and other medications, a combination of a laxative and stool softener should be utilized. If after several days of treatment a bowel movement has not occurred, a rectal examination to remove impacted stool and to place a suppository is necessary. For patients with impending bowel obstruction or gastric stasis, octreotide to reduce secretions can be helpful.

Dyspnea ■ FREQUENCY Dyspnea is a subjective experience of being short of breath. Nearly 75% of dying patients experience dyspnea. Dyspnea is among the most distressing of physical symptoms, even more distressing than pain.

ASSESSMENT As with pain, dyspnea is a subjective experience that may not correlate with objective measures of P_{O_2}, P_{CO_2}, or respiratory rate. Consequently, measurements, much less repeated measurements, of oxygen saturation through pulse oximetry or blood gases are rarely helpful. Reversible or treatable causes of dyspnea include infection, pleural effusions, pulmonary emboli, or lung tumor encroachment on the airway. However, the risk-benefit ratio of the diagnostic and therapeutic interventions for patients with little time left to live must be carefully considered before undertaking diagnostic steps. Frequently, secondary etiologies cannot be identified, and dyspnea is the consequence of progression of the underlying disease that cannot be treated. The anxiety caused by dyspnea and the choking sensation can significantly exacerbate the underlying dyspnea in a negative reinforcing cycle.

INTERVENTIONS When reversible or treatable etiologies are diagnosed, they should be treated as long as the side effects of treatment, such as repeated drainage of effusions or anticoagulants, are less bothersome than the dyspnea itself. Usually, treatment will be symptomatic (Table 9-6). Low-dose opioids reduce the sensitivity of the central respiratory center and the sensation of dyspnea. If patients are not receiving opioids, weak opioids can be initiated; if patients are already receiving opioids, then morphine should be used. Benzodiazepines are helpful if anxiety is present. If the patient has a history of COPD, bronchodilators may also be helpful, as may glucocorticoids. Secretions can be dried with scopolamine. Oxygen can be used, although it may only be an expensive placebo. Medical staff should sit the patient upright, remove smoke or other irritants such as perfume, ensure a supply of fresh air with sufficient humidity, and minimize other factors that can increase anxiety.

Fatigue ■ FREQUENCY Fatigue and weakness are the most common symptoms of terminally ill patients. More than 90% of the terminally ill experience fatigue and/or weakness. Fatigue is frequently cited as among the most distressing of symptoms.

ETIOLOGY The multiple causes of fatigue in the terminally ill can be categorized as resulting from the underlying disease; from disease-induced factors, such as tumor necrosis factor and other cytokines; and from secondary factors such as cachexia, dehydration, anemia, infection, hypothyroidism, and drug side effects. Apart from low caloric intake, loss of muscle mass and changes in muscle enzymes may play an important role in fatigue of terminal illness. The importance of changes in the CNS, especially the reticular activating system, have been hypothesized based on reports of fatigue in patients receiving cranial radiation, experiencing depression, or with chronic pain in the absence of cachexia or other physiologic changes. Finally, depression and other causes of psychological distress can contribute to fatigue.

ASSESSMENT Fatigue is subjective; objective changes, even in body weight, may be absent. Consequently, assessment must rely on patient self-reporting. Scales used to measure fatigue, such as the Edmonton Functional Assessment Tool, the Fatigue Self-Report scales, or the Rhoten Fatigue scale, are usually appropriate for research rather than clinical purposes. In clinical practice, a simple performance assessment such as the Karnofsky Performance Status or the Eastern Cooperative Oncology Group's question "How much of the day does the patient spend in bed?" may be the best measure. In this 0 to 4 performance status assessment, a 0 = normal activity, 1 = symptomatic without being bedridden, 2 = requiring some, but <50%, bed time, 3 = bedbound more than half the day, and 4 = bedbound all the time. Such a scale allows for assessment over time and by third parties.

INTERVENTION At the end of life, fatigue will not be "cured." The goal is the ameliorate it and adjust expectations. Behavioral interventions should be utilized to avoid blaming the patient for inactivity, and to educate both the family and patient that the underlying disease causes physiologic changes producing low energy levels. Understanding that the problem is physiologic not psychological can help to alter expectations regarding the patient's level of physical activity. Practically, this may mean reducing routine activities, such as housework and cooking, or social events outside the house, and making it acceptable to receive guests lying on a couch. At the same time, institution of exercise regimens that are possible can raise endorphins, reduce muscle wasting, and reduce the risk of depression. In addition, ensuring good hydration without worsening edema may help reduce fatigue. Discontinuing medications that worsen fatigue, such as cardiac medications or even opioids, if pain is well controlled, may help.

TABLE 9-5 Medications for the Management of Constipation

Intervention	Dose	Comment
Stimulant laxatives		These agents directly stimulate peristalsis and may
Prune juice	120–240 mL/d	reduce colonic absorption of water.
Senna (Senokot)	2–4 tablets PO per day	Work in 6 to 12 h.
Bisacodyl	5–15 mg/d PO, PR	
Osmotic laxatives		These agents are not absorbed. They attract and
Lactulose	15–30 mL PO q4–8h	retain water in the gastrointestinal tract.
Magnesium hydroxide	15–30 mL/d PO	Lactulose may cause flatulence and bloating.
(Milk of Magnesia)		Lactulose works in 1 day;
Magnesium citrate	125–250 mL/d PO	Magnesium products in 6 h.
Stool softeners		These agents work by increasing water secretion
Sodium docusate (Colace)	300–600 mg/d PO	and as detergents increasing water penetration in
Calcium docusate	300–600 mg/d PO	to the stool.
		Work in 1 to 3 days.

TABLE 9-6 Medications for the Management of Dyspnea

Intervention	Dose	Comments
Weak opioids		For patients with mild dyspnea
Codeine (or codeine with 325 mg acetaminophen)	30 mg PO q4h	For opioid-naïve patient
Hydrocodone	5 mg PO q4h	
Strong opioids		For opioid-naïve patients with
Morphine	5–10 mg PO q4h	moderate to severe dyspnea
	30–50% of baseline opioid dose q4h	For patients already taking opioids for pain or other symptoms
Oxycodone	5–10 mg PO q4h	
Hydromorphone	1–2 mg PO q4h	
Anxiolytics		Give a dose every hour until the
Lorazepam	0.5–2.0 mg PO/SL/IV qh then q4–6h	patient is relaxed, then provide a dose for maintenance
Diazepam	5–10 mg PO or IV qh then q6–18h	
Clonazepam	0.25–2.0 mg PO q12h	
Midazolam	0.5 mg IV q15min	

Only a few pharmacologic interventions target fatigue and weakness. Glucocorticoids can increase energy and enhance mood. Dexamethasone is preferred for its once-a-day dosing and minimal mineralocorticoid activity. However, use for >1 month tends to diminish the positive effects. Psychostimulants, such as dextroamphetamine (5 to 10 mg orally) and methylphenidate (2.5 to 5 mg orally), can also enhance energy levels. Dosages should be given in the morning and at noon, otherwise they can cause counterproductive insomnia. Modafinil, developed for narcolepsy, has shown some promise in the treatment of fatigue. Its precise role in the fatigue at the end of life is yet to be determined.

MENTAL SYMPTOMS AND THEIR MANAGEMENT ■ Depression ■ *FREQUENCY*
Depression at the end of life presents an apparently paradoxical situation. Many people believe that depression is normal among seriously ill patients because they are dying. People frequently say "wouldn't you be depressed?" Depression is not a necessary part of terminal illness and constitutes needless suffering. While sadness, anxiety, anger, and irritability are normal responses to a serious condition, they are typically of modest intensity and transient. Persistent sadness and anxiety are abnormal and suggestive of major depression. While as many as 75% of terminally ill patients experience depressive symptoms, <25% of terminally ill patients have major depression.

ETIOLOGY Previous history of depression, family history of depression or manic-depression, and prior suicide attempts are associated with increased risk for depression among terminally ill patients. Other symptoms, such as pain and fatigue, are associated with higher rates of depression; uncontrolled pain can exacerbate depression, and depression can cause patients to be more distressed by pain. Many medications used in the terminal stages, including glucocorticoids, and some anticancer agents, such as tamoxifen, interleukin 2, interferon α, and vincristine, are also associated with depression. Some terminal conditions, such as pancreatic cancer and certain strokes, have been reported to be associated with higher rates of depression, although this is controversial. Finally, depression may be attributable to grief over the loss of a role or function, social isolation, or loneliness.

ASSESSMENT Diagnosing depression among patients at the end of life is complicated because many of the vegetative symptoms contained in the DSM IV criteria—insomnia, anorexia and weight loss, fatigue, decreased libido, and difficulty concentrating—are associated with the dying process itself. The assessment of depression in seriously ill patients must focus on the dysphoric mood, helplessness, hopelessness, and lack of interest and enjoyment. The single questions "how often do you feel downhearted and blue?" (more than a good bit of the time or similar responses) or "do you feel depressed most of the time?" are appropriate for screening.

Certain conditions may be confused with depression. Endocrinopathies, such as hypothyroidism or Cushing's syndrome, electrolyte abnormalities such as hypercalcemia, and akathisia, especially from dopamine blocking antiemetics such as metoclopramide and prochlorperazine, can mimic depression and should be excluded.

INTERVENTIONS Physicians must treat any physical symptom, such as pain, that may be causing or exacerbating depression. Nonpharmacologic interventions, including group or individual psychological counseling, and behavioral therapies, such as relaxation or imagery, can be helpful, especially in combination with drug therapy.

Pharmacologic interventions remain the core of therapy. The same medications are used to treat depression in terminally ill as in non-terminally ill patients. Psychostimulants may be preferred for patients with a poor prognosis or for those with fatigue or opioid-induced somnolence. Psychostimulants are comparatively fast acting, working within a few days. Dextroamphetamine or methylphenidate should be started at 2.5 to 5.0 mg in the morning and at noon, the same starting dosages used for treating fatigue. The dose can be escalated up to 15 mg twice a day; higher doses are only rarely necessary. Pemoline

is a nonamphetamine psychostimulant with minimal abuse potential. It is also effective as an antidepressant beginning at 18.75 mg in the morning and at noon. Because it can be absorbed through the buccal mucosa, it is preferred for patients with intestinal obstruction or dysphagia. If used for prolonged periods, liver function must be monitored. The psychostimulants can also be combined with more traditional antidepressants, while waiting for the latter to become effective, and then tapered after a few weeks if necessary. Psychostimulants have side effects, particularly initial anxiety, insomnia, and rarely paranoia, which may necessitate lowering the dose or discontinuing treatment. A newer, promising agent is mirtazepine starting at 7.5 mg before bed. It is sedating and has antiemetic and anxiolytic properties with few drug interactions. Its side effect of weight gain may also be beneficial for seriously ill patients, and it is available in orally disintegrating tablets.

For patients with a prognosis of several months or longer, selective serotonin reuptake inhibitors, including fluoxetine, sertraline, and citalopram, and serotonin-noradrenaline reuptake inhibitors, such as venlafaxine, are the preferred treatment because of their efficacy and comparatively few side effects. Because low doses of these medications may be effective for seriously ill patients, use half the usual starting dose for healthy adults. The starting dose for fluoxetine is 10 mg once a day. In most cases, once-a-day dosing is possible.

Atypical antidepressants are recommended only in selected circumstances, usually with the assistance of a specialty consultation. Trazadone can be an effective antidepressant but is sedating and can cause orthostatic hypotension and priapism. Therefore, it should be used only when a sedating effect is desired. In addition to its antidepressant effects, bupropion is energizing, making it useful for depressed patients suffering from fatigue. However, it can cause seizures, preventing its use for patients with a risk of CNS neoplasms or terminal delirium. Finally, alprazolam, a benzodiazepine, starting at 0.25 to 1.0 mg three times a day, can be effective in seriously ill patients suffering from a combination of anxiety and depression. While it is potent and works quickly, it has many drug interactions and may cause delirium, especially among very ill patients, because of its strong binding to the benzodiazepine-GABA receptor complex.

Unless used as adjuvants for the treatment of pain, tricyclic antidepressants are not recommended. Similarly the monoamine oxidase inhibitors are not recommended because of their side effects and dangerous drug interactions.

Delirium ■ *FREQUENCY* In the weeks or months before death, delirium is uncommon, although it may be significantly underdiagnosed. However, delirium becomes relatively common in the hours and days immediately before death. As many as 85% of patients in the active stages of dying from cancer may experience terminal delirium.

ETIOLOGY Delirium is a global cerebral dysfunction characterized by alterations in cognition and consciousness. It is frequently preceded by anxiety, changes in sleep patterns (especially reversal of day and night), and decreased attention. In contrast to dementia, delirium has an acute onset and is reversible, although reversibility may be more theoretical than real for patients near death. It is possible to have delirium in a patient with dementia.

Causes of delirium include metabolic encephalopathy arising from liver failure, hypoxemia, or sepsis; electrolyte imbalances such as hypercalcemia; nutritional deficiencies such as vitamin B_{12} deficiency; paraneoplastic syndromes; and primary brain tumors or brain metastases. Commonly, among dying patients, delirium can be caused by side effects of treatments, including radiation for brain metastases, and medications, including opioids, glucocorticoids, anticholinergic drugs, antihistamines, antiemetics, and many chemotherapeutic agents. In many terminally ill patients, the etiology will be multifactorial; e.g., dehydration may exacerbate opioid-induced delirium.

ASSESSMENT Delirium should be recognized in any terminally ill patient with new onset of disorientation, impaired cognition, somnolence, fluctuating levels of consciousness, or delusions, with or without agitation. Delirium must be distinguished from acute anxiety and depression, as well as dementia. In some cases, use of formal assessment tools such as the Mini-Mental Status Examination (which does not distinguish delirium from dementia) or the Delirium Rating Scale (which does distinguish delirium from dementia) may be helpful in distinguishing delirium from other processes. The patient's list of medications must be carefully evaluated. Nonetheless, a reversible etiologic factor for delirium is found in fewer than half of terminally ill patients. Because most terminally ill patients experiencing delirium will be very close to death and may be at home, extensive diagnostic evaluations, such as lumbar punctures or neuroradiologic examinations, are usually inappropriate.

INTERVENTIONS One of the most important objectives of terminal care is to provide terminally ill patients the lucidity to say goodbye to the people they love. Delirium, especially with agitation during the final days, is distressing to family and caregivers. A strong determinant of bereavement difficulties is witnessing a difficult death. Thus, terminal delirium should be treated aggressively.

At the first sign of delirium, such as day-night reversal with slight changes in mentation, let the family know that it is time to be sure that everything they want to have said has been said. The family should be informed that delirium is common just before death.

If medications such as opioids are suspected of being a cause of the delirium, then unnecessary agents should be discontinued. Other reversible causes such as constipation, urinary retention, and metabolic abnormalities should be treated. Supportive measures aimed at providing a familiar environment should be instituted, including restricting visits only to individuals with whom the patient is familiar and eliminating new experiences; orienting the patient, if possible, by providing a clock and calendar; and gently correcting the patient's hallucinations or cognitive mistakes.

Pharmacologic management focuses on the use of neuroleptics and, in the extreme, anesthetics (Table 9-7). Haloperidol remains first-line therapy. Usually, patients can be controlled with a low dose (1 to 3 mg/d), although some may require as much as 20 mg/d. It can be administered orally, subcutaneously, or intravenously. Intramuscular injections should not be used, except when it is the only way to get a patient under control. Chlorpromazine (10 to 25 mg every 4 to 6 h) can be useful if sedation is desired. Dystonic reactions resulting from dopamine blockade are a side effect of neuroleptics, although they are reported to be rare when used to treat terminal delirium. The new atypical neuroleptics—risperidone and olanzapine—have also been used successfully and are especially helpful for patients with longer anticipated life spans since they are less likely to cause dysphoria and have a lower risk of dystonic reactions. If patients develop dystonic reactions, benztropine should be administered. Neuroleptics may be combined with lorazepam to reduce agitation when the delirium is the result of alcohol or sedative withdrawal.

If no response to first-line therapy is seen, a specialty consultation should be obtained with a change to a different medication. If patients fail to improve after a second neuroleptic, then sedation with an anesthetic such as propofol or continuous-infusion midazolam may be

necessary. By some estimates, at the very end of life as many as 25% of patients experiencing delirium, especially restless delirium with myoclonus or convulsions, may require sedation.

Physical restraints should be used with great reluctance only when the patient's violence is threatening to self or others. If used, their appropriateness should be reevaluated frequently.

SOCIAL NEEDS AND THEIR MANAGEMENT ■ Financial Burdens ■ *FREQUENCY* Dying can impose substantial economic strains on patients and families, causing distress. In the United States, with one of the least comprehensive health insurance systems among the developed countries, about 20% of terminally ill patients and their families spend >10% of family income on health care costs over and above health insurance premiums. Between 10 and 30% of families sell assets, use savings, or take out a mortgage to pay for the patient's health care costs. Nearly 40% of terminally ill patients in the United States report that the cost of their illness is a moderate or great economic hardship for their family.

The patient is likely to reduce and stop working. In 20% of cases, a family member of the terminally ill patient stops working to provide care. The major underlying causes of economic burden are related to poor physical functioning and care needs, such as the need for housekeeping, nursing, and personal care. More debilitated patients and poor patients experience greater economic burdens.

INTERVENTION The economic burden should not be ignored as a private matter. It has been associated with a number of adverse health outcomes, including preferring comfort care over life-prolonging care as well as consideration of euthanasia or physician-assisted suicide. Economic burdens tend to increase the psychological distress of families and caregivers of terminally ill patients. Assistance from a social worker, early on if possible, to ensure access to all available benefits may be helpful. Many people and health care providers are unaware of options for long-term care insurance, respite care, the Family Medical Leave Act, and other sources of assistance.

Relationships ■ *FREQUENCY* Settling personal issues and closing the narrative of lived relationships are universal needs. When asked if sudden death or death after an illness is preferable, respondents often initially select the former but soon change to the latter as they reflect on the importance of saying goodbye. Bereaved family members who have not had the chance to say goodbye often have a more difficult grief process.

INTERVENTION Care of seriously ill patients requires efforts to facilitate the types of encounters and time spent with family and friends that are necessary to meet these needs. Family and close friends may need to be accommodated with unrestricted visiting hours, which perhaps may include sleeping near the patient even in otherwise regimented institutional settings. Physicians and health care providers may facilitate and resolve strained interactions between the patient and other family members. Assistance for patients and family members who are unsure about how to create or help preserve memories, whether by providing raw materials such as a scrap book or memory box or by offering them suggestions and informational resources, can be deeply appreciated. Taking photographs and creating videos can be especially helpful to terminally ill patients who have younger children or grandchildren.

Family Caregivers ■ *FREQUENCY* Caring for seriously ill patients places a heavy burden on families. Families are frequently required to provide transportation and homemaking as well as other services. Typically, paid professionals such as home health nurses and hospice workers supplement family care; only about a quarter of all care giving is exclusively paid professional assistance. The trend toward more out-of-hospital deaths will increase reliance on families for end-of-life care.

Three-quarters of the caregivers of terminally ill patients are women—wives, daughters, and even sisters. Since many are widowed, women themselves tend to be able to rely less on family for care-

TABLE 9-7 Medications for the Management of Delirium	
Interventions	**Dose**
Neuroleptics	
Haloperidol	0.5–5 mg q2–12h, PO/IV/SC/IM
Thioridazine	10–75 mg q4–8h, PO
Chlorpromazine	12.5–50 mg q4–12h, PO/IV/IM
Molindone	10–50 mg q8–12h, PO
Atypical neuroleptics	
Olanzapine	2.5–5 mg qd, PO
Risperidone	1–3 mg q12h, PO
Anxiolytics	
Lorazepam	0.5–2 mg q1–4h, PO/IV/IM
Midazolam	1–5 mg/h continuous infusion, IV/SC
Anesthetics	
Propofol	0.3–2.0 mg/h continuous infusion, IV

giving assistance and may need more paid assistance. About 20% of terminally ill patients report substantial unmet needs for nursing and personal care.

INTERVENTION It is imperative to inquire about unmet needs and to try to ensure those needs are met either through the family or paid professional services when possible. Community assistance through houses of worship or other community groups can often be mobilized by one or two phone calls from the medical team to someone the patient or family identifies.

EXISTENTIAL NEEDS AND THEIR MANAGEMENT ■ FREQUENCY Religion and spirituality are often important to dying patients. Nearly 70% of patients report becoming more religious or spiritual when they became terminally ill, and many find comfort in various religious or spiritual practices such as prayer. However, ~20% of terminally ill patients become less religious, frequently feeling somehow cheated or betrayed by becoming terminally ill. For other patients, the need is for existential meaning and purpose that is distinct from and maybe even antithetical to religion or spirituality.

ASSESSMENT Health care providers are often hesitant about involving themselves in the religious, spiritual, and existential experiences of their patients, because it may seem private, related to alternative lifestyles, or "soft." But physicians and other members of the interdisciplinary team should be able to at least detect spiritual and existential needs. Screening questions have been developed for a physician's spiritual history taking. Spiritual distress can amplify other types of suffering and even masquerade as intractable physical pain, anxiety, or depression, for instance. The screening questions in the whole-person assessment are usually sufficient. Deeper evaluation and intervention are rarely appropriate for the physician unless no other member of an interdisciplinary team is available or suitable. Pastoral care providers may be helpful, whether from the medical institution or the patient's community.

INTERVENTION Precisely how religious practices, spirituality, and existential explorations can be facilitated and improve end-of-life care is not well established. In one study, only 36% of respondents indicated that a clergy member would be comforting. Nevertheless, this increase in religious and spiritual interest among a substantial fraction of dying patients suggests inquiring of individual patients how this need can be addressed.

MANAGING THE LAST STAGES

WITHDRAWING AND WITHHOLDING LIFE-SUSTAINING TREATMENT ■ LEGAL
ASPECTS For centuries, it has been deemed ethical to withhold or withdraw life-sustaining interventions. The current legal consensus is that patients have a constitutional and common law right to refuse medical interventions (Table 9-8). Courts have held that incompetent patients have a right to refuse medical interventions. For patients who are incompetent and terminally ill and who have not completed an advance care directive, next of kin can exercise this right, although this may be restricted in some states depending how clear and convincing the evidence is of the patient's preferences. Courts are limiting families' ability to terminate life-sustaining treatments from patients who are conscious, incompetent, but not terminally ill. In theory, patients' right to refuse medical therapy can be limited by four countervailing interests: (1) preservation of life, (2) prevention of suicide, (3) protection of third parties such as children, and (4) preserving the integrity of the medical profession. In practice, these interests almost never override the right of competent patients and incompetent patients who have left explicit and advance care directives.

Regarding incompetent patients who either appointed a proxy without specific indications of their wishes or who never completed an advance care directive, three criteria have been suggested to guide the decision to terminate medical interventions. Some commentators suggest that ordinary care should be administered but extraordinary care

could be terminated. Because the ordinary/extraordinary distinction is too vague, courts and commentators widely agree that it should not be used to justify decisions about stopping treatment. Many courts have advocated use of the substituted-judgment criterion, which holds that the proxy decision-makers should try to imagine what the incompetent patient would do if he or she were competent. However, most proxies, even close family members, cannot accurately predict what the patient would have wanted. Therefore, substituted judgment becomes more of a guessing game than a way of fulfilling the patient's wishes. Finally, the best-interests criterion holds that proxies should evaluate treatments by balancing their benefits and risks and select those treatments in which the benefits maximally outweigh the burdens of treatment. Yet, as many family conflicts reveal, different individuals can have very different views of what is in the patient's best interests. Indeed, this criterion has been criticized because no objective way exists of determining the balance between benefits and burdens; it depends on a patient's personal values. As a matter of practice, physicians rely on family members to make decisions that they feel are best and object only if these decisions seem to demand treatments that the physicians consider not beneficial.

PRACTICES Withholding and withdrawing acutely life-sustaining medical interventions from terminally ill patients are now standard practice. More than 90% of American patients die without cardiopulmonary resuscitation (CPR), and just as many forgo other potentially life-sustaining interventions. For instance, during 1987 to 1988 in ICUs, CPR was performed 49% of the time, but only 10% of the time in 1992 to 1993. On average, 3.8 interventions, such as vasopressors and transfusions, were stopped from each dying ICU patient.

Mechanical ventilation may be the most challenging intervention to withdraw. The two approaches are *terminal extubation*, which is the removal of the endotracheal tube, and *terminal wean*, which is the gradual reduction of the FI_{O_2} or ventilator rate. One-third of ICU physicians prefer to use the terminal wean technique, while 13% extubate; the majority of physicians utilize both techniques. Some recommend the terminal wean because patients do not develop upper airway obstruction and the distress caused by secretions or stridor; however, terminal weaning can prolong the dying process. To ensure comfort for conscious or semiconscious patients before withdrawal of the ventilator, neuromuscular blocking agents should be terminated and sedatives and analgesics administered. Removing the neuromuscular blocking agents permits patients to show discomfort, facilitating the titration of sedatives and analgesics; it also permits interactions between patients and their families. A common practice is to inject a bolus of midazolam (2 to 4 mg) before withdrawal followed by 5 to 10 mg of morphine and continuous infusion of morphine (50% of the bolus dose per hour) during weaning. Additional boluses of morphine or increases in the infusion rate should be administered for any distress. Higher doses will be needed for patients already receiving anxiolytics and opioids. Families need to be warned that up to 10% of patients unexpectedly survive for 1 day or more after mechanical ventilation is stopped.

FUTILE CARE Beginning in late 1980s, some commentators argued that physicians could terminate futile treatments demanded by families of terminally ill patients. No objective definition or standard of futility exists. Physiologic futility means that an intervention will have no physiologic effect. Some have defined qualitative futile treatments as those that "fail to end a patient's total dependence on intensive medical care." Quantitative futility occurs "when physicians conclude (either through personal experience, experiences shared with colleagues, or consideration of reported empiric data) that in the last 100 cases, a medical treatment has been useless." The term conceals subjective value judgments about when a treatment is "not beneficial." Deciding whether a treatment that obtains an additional 6 weeks of life or a 1% survival advantage confers benefit depends upon patients' preferences and goals. Furthermore, physicians' predictions of when treatments were futile deviated markedly from the quantitative definition. When residents thought CPR was quantitatively futile, more than one in five

TABLE 9-8 *Major Legal Cases Regarding the Withholding or Withdrawing of Medical Interventions*

Case and Citation	Year	State	Facts	Decision
In re Quinlan 70 N.J. 10	1976	NJ	21-year-old woman in a persistent vegetative state dependent on a respirator, artificial nutrition, and hydration.	The right to privacy includes a right to refuse medical care and extends to incompetent patients. Patient's guardian can withdraw her respirator. No need for judicial review in most cases.
Superintendent of Belchertown v Saikewicz 373 Mass 728	1977	MA	67-year-old retarded man with a mental age of 2 years 8 months who had always lived in a state institution develops acute myelomonocytic leukemia. Does he have to receive chemotherapy?	All persons including incompetent persons have the right to refuse medical treatment. Using substituted judgment, the court determined that the patient would not want chemotherapy.
In re Eichner (Brother Fox) 52 NY 2d 262	1981	NY	83-year-old priest was in a persistent vegetative state after a cardiac arrest. Prior to the event, he had publicly stated that he would not want to be respirator-dependent if he were vegetative.	Patients have the right to determine the course of their own medical care. Patient's wishes were known, even if not expressed in writing. Respirator should be withdrawn.
In re Conroy 98 N.J. 321	1985	NJ	84-year-old bedridden, totally impaired woman with organic brain syndrome fed by a nasogastric tube. Her nephew requests removal of the tube.	Nasogastric tube feedings are medical interventions that can be withdrawn.
Brophy v New England Sinai Hospital 398 Mass 417	1986	MA	49-year-old man in persistent vegetative state after a ruptured aneurysm; maintained by gastric tube feedings. He had no written living will, but he had explicitly stated that he would never want to live on life support systems.	Common law and the constitutional right of privacy given a person the right to refuse medical treatment. The patient's wishes are clearly known from explicit conversations. The gastric tube can be withdrawn.
Bouvia v Superior Court 225 Cal Rptr 297	1986	CA	29-year-old mentally competent woman with cerebral palsy that left her almost completely immobile and totally unable to care for herself. She requests a nasogastric tube to supplement her inadequate oral intake be withdrawn.	The patient has the "right to refuse any medical treatment even that which may save or prolong her life."
In re Jobes 108 N.J. 394	1987	NJ	32-year-old woman in a permanent vegetative state, receiving J-tube feedings. Her husband and parents request withdrawal of the feedings. She left no clear written or verbal indication of her wishes.	Incompetent patients have the right to refuse medical care even if they have left no clear indication of their wishes. Using substituted judgment the family can exercise her right to withdraw the J-tube feedings.
Cruzan v Director of Missouri Department of Health 110 S. Ct. 2841	1990	U.S.	33-year-old woman in a persistent vegetative state maintained by gastric tube nutrition and hydration. Her parents requested that these tube feedings be terminated.	By 8 to 1, the Supreme Court ruled that patients have a constitutional right to refuse medical care and that this applies to artificial nutrition and hydration. If there was no clear and convincing written or verbal statement of the patient's wishes, states could regulate how families exercise the right.
In re Helga Wanglie Fourth judicial district PX-91-283. Minnesota (Hennepin County)	1991	MN	85-year-old woman in a persistent vegetative state. After months, physicians suggested withdrawal of life-sustaining treatment because the patient was receiving no benefit. The family refused withdrawal.	The husband should represent the patient's interests, and his refusal to discontinue the respirator is binding.
Wendland v. Wendland 110 Cal Rptr 2d. 412	2001	CA	42-year-old conscious man with severe cognitive impairments, hemiparesis, and limited communication who was not terminally ill required feeding tube. The feeding tube fell out and needed to be replaced. After authorizing replacement of the feeling tube 3 times, wife refused replacement.	Patients have a right to refuse all medical treatments including life-sustaining treatments. This right can be exercised for mentally incompetent patients through advance care directives. For patients who are terminally ill, in persistent vegetative state, or comatose who have not completed an advance care directive, proxies who have not been formally appointed can terminate interventions. However, for mentally incompetent but conscious patients "clear and convincing" evidence is needed of the patient's wishes before life-sustaining treatment can be stopped.

patients had a >10% chance of survival to hospital discharge. Quantitative futility rarely applies in ICU settings. Most commentators reject using futility as a criterion of withdrawing care.

EUTHANASIA AND PHYSICIAN-ASSISTED SUICIDE Euthanasia and physician-assisted suicide are defined in Table 9-9. Terminating life-sustaining care and providing opioid medications to manage symptoms have long been considered ethical by the medical profession and legal by courts and should not be confused with euthanasia or physician-assisted suicide.

LEGAL ASPECTS Euthanasia is legal in the Netherlands and Belgium. Euthanasia was legalized in the Northern Territory of Australia but then repealed. Euthanasia is not legal in any state in the United States. Physician-assisted suicide is legal in Oregon but only if multiple criteria are met and then only after a process that includes a 15-day waiting period. In Switzerland, a layperson can legally assist suicide.

In all other countries and all other states in the United States, physician-assisted suicide and euthanasia are illegal explicitly or by common law.

PRACTICES Fewer than 10 to 20% of terminally ill patients actually consider euthanasia and/or physician-assisted suicide for themselves. In the Netherlands and Oregon, >70% of patients utilizing these interventions are dying of cancer; <5% of deaths by euthanasia or physician-assisted suicide involve patients with AIDS or amyotrophic lateral sclerosis. In the Netherlands, if all legal and illegal acts are grouped, euthanasia and physician-assisted suicide account for <3.5% of all deaths. In Oregon, ~0.1% of patients die by physician-assisted suicide, although many commentators suspect this is an undercount of actual cases.

Pain is not a primary motivator for patients' requests for or interest in euthanasia and/or physician-assisted suicide. Among the first patients to receive physician-assisted suicide in Oregon, only 1 patient

TABLE 9-9   *Definitions of Assisted Suicide and Euthanasia*

Term	Definition	Legal Status
Voluntary active euthanasia	Intentionally administering medications or other interventions to cause the patient's death with the patient's informed consent	Netherlands Belgium
Involuntary active euthanasia	Intentionally administering medications or other interventions to cause the patient's death when the patient was competent to consent but did not–e.g., the patient may not have been asked	Nowhere
Nonvoluntary active euthanasia	Intentionally administering medications or other interventions to cause the patient's death when the patient was incompetent and was mentally incapable of consenting—e.g., the patient might have been in a coma	Nowhere
Passive euthanasia	Withholding or withdrawing life-sustaining medical treatments from a patient to let him or her die (terminating life-sustaining treatments)	Everywhere
Indirect euthanasia	Administering opioids or other medications to relieve pain, dyspnea, or other symptoms with the incidental consequence of causing sufficient respiratory depression to result in the patient's death	Everywhere
Physician-assisted suicide	A physician provides medications or other interventions to a patient with the understanding that the patient can use them to commit suicide	Oregon Netherlands Belgium Switzerland

of 15 had inadequate pain control compared to 15 of 43 patients in a control group experiencing inadequate pain relief. Depression, hopelessness, and, more vaguely, worries about loss of dignity or autonomy appear to be the primary factors motivating a desire for euthanasia or physician-assisted suicide.

Euthanasia and physician-assisted suicide are no guarantee of a painless, quick death. Data from the Netherlands indicate that in as many as 20% of cases technical and other problems arose, including patients waking from coma, not becoming comatose, regurgitating medications, and a prolonged time to death. Problems were significantly more common in physician-assisted suicide, sometimes requiring the physician to intervene and provide euthanasia.

After receiving a request for euthanasia and/or physician-assisted suicide, health care providers should carefully clarify the request with empathic, open-ended questions to help elucidate the underlying cause for the request such as: "What makes you want to consider this option?" Endorsing either moral opposition or moral support for the act tends to be counterproductive, either lending an impression of being judgmental or of endorsing the idea that the patient's life is worthless. Health care providers must reassure the patient of continued care and commitment. The patient should be educated about alternative, less controversial options, such as symptom management and withdrawing any unwanted treatments; the reality of euthanasia and/or physician-assisted suicide, since the patient is likely to have misconceptions about its effectiveness; and also the legal implications of the choice. Depression, hopelessness, and other symptoms of psychological distress as well as physical suffering and economic burdens are likely factors motivating the request, and such factors should be assessed and treated aggressively. After these interventions and clarification of options, most patients proceed with a less controversial approach of declining life-sustaining interventions, possibly including refusal of nutrition and hydration.

CARE DURING THE LAST HOURS   Most laypersons have limited experiences with the actual dying process and death. They frequently do not know what to expect of the final hours, and afterwards. Therefore, the family and other caregivers must be prepared, especially if the plan is for the patient to die at home.

Patients in the last days of life experience extreme weakness and fatigue and become bedbound; this can lead to bedsores. They stop eating and drinking with drying of mucosal membranes and dysphagia. Careful attention to oral swabbing, lubricants for lips, and use of artificial tears can provide a form of care to substitute for attempts at feeding the patient. With loss of the gag reflex and dysphagia, patients may also experience accumulation of oral secretions, producing noises during respiration sometimes called "the death rattle." Scopolamine can reduce the secretions. Patients also experience changes in respiration with periods of apnea or Cheyne-Stokes breathing. Decreased intravascular volume and cardiac output causes tachycardia, hypotension, peripheral coolness, and livedo reticularis (skin mottling). Patients can also have urinary and, less frequently, fecal incontinence. Changes in consciousness and neurologic function generally lead to two different paths to death (Fig. 9-2).

Each of these terminal changes can cause patients and families distress, requiring reassurance and targeted interventions (Table 9-10). Informing families that these changes might occur, and even providing them an information sheet, can help to preempt problems and minimize distress. Understanding that patients stop eating because they are dying, not dying because they have stopped eating, can reduce family and caregiver anxiety. Similarly, informing the family and caregivers that the "death rattle" may occur and that it is not indicative of suffocation or choking can reduce their preoccupation with the breathing sounds.

Families and caregivers can also feel guilty about stopping treatments, fearing that they are "killing" the patient. This may lead to demands for interventions that may be ineffective. In such cases, the

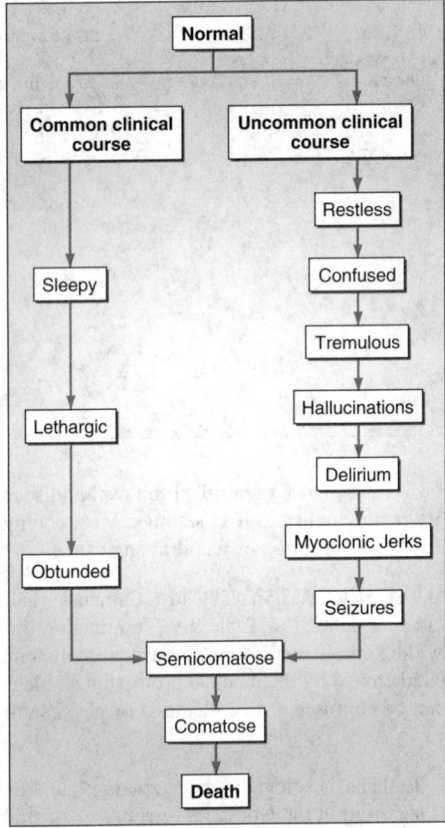

FIGURE 9-2   Common and uncommon clinical courses in the last days of terminally ill patients. (*Adapted from FD Ferris et al: Module 4: Palliative care, in Comprehensive Guide for the Care of Persons with HIV Disease. Toronto: Mt. Sinai Hospital and Casey Hospice, 1995, at www.cpsonline.info/content/resources/hivmodule4.html*)

TABLE 9-10 Managing Changes in the Patient's Condition during the Final Days and Hours

Changes in the Patient's Condition	Potential Complication	Family's Possible Reaction and Concern	Advice and Intervention
Profound fatigue	Bedbound with development of pressure ulcers that are prone to infection, malodor, and pain, and joint pain	Patient is lazy and giving up.	Reassure family and caregivers that terminal fatigue will not respond to interventions and should not be resisted. Use an air mattress if necessary.
Anorexia	None	Patient is giving up; patient will suffer from hunger and will starve to death.	Reassure family and caregivers that the patient is not eating because he or she is dying; not eating at the end of life does not cause suffering or death. Forced feeding, whether oral, parenteral, or enteral, does not reduce symptoms or prolong life.
Dehydration	Dry mucosal membranes (see below)	Patient will suffer from thirst and die of dehydration.	Reassure family and caregivers that terminal dehydration does not cause suffering because patients lose consciousness before any symptom distress. Intravenous hydration can worsen symptoms of dyspnea by pulmonary edema and peripheral edema as well as prolong dying process.
Dysphagia	Inability to swallow oral medications needed for palliative care		Do not force oral intake. Discontinue unnecessary medications that may have been continued including antibiotics, diuretics, anti-depressants, and laxatives. If swallowing pills is difficult, convert essential medications (analgesics, antiemetics, anxiolytics, and psychotropics) to oral solutions, buccal, sublingual, or rectal administration.
"Death rattle"—noisy breathing		Patient is choking and suffocating.	Reassure the family and caregivers that this is caused by secretions in the oropharynx and the patient is not choking. Reduce secretions with scopolamine (0.2–0.4 mg SC q4h or 1–3 patches q3d) Reposition patient to permit drainage of secretions. Do not suction. Suction can cause patient and family discomfort, and is usually ineffective.
Apnea, Cheyne-Stokes respirations, dyspnea		Patient is suffocating.	Reassure family and caregivers that unconscious patients do not experience suffocation or air hunger. Apneic episodes are frequently a premorbid change. Opioids or anxiolytics may be used for dyspnea. Oxygen is unlikely to relieve dyspneic symptoms and may prolong the dying process.
Urinary or fecal incontinence	Skin breakdown if days until death Potential transmission of infectious agents to caregivers	Patient is dirty, malodorous, and physically repellent.	Remind family and caregivers to use universal precautions. Frequent changes of bedclothes and bedding. Use diapers, urinary catheter, or rectal tube if diarrhea or high urine flow occur.
Agitation or delirium	Day/night reversal Hurt self or caregivers	Patient is in horrible pain and going to have a horrible death.	Reassure family and caregivers that agitation and delirium do not necessarily connote physical pain. Depending upon the prognosis and goals of treatment, consider evaluating for causes of delirium and modify medications. Manage symptoms with haloperidol, chlorpromazine, diazepam, or midazolam.
Dry mucosal membranes	Cracked lips, mouth sores, and candidiasis can also cause pain. Malodor	Patient may be malodorous, physically repellent.	Use baking soda mouthwash or saliva preparation q15–30min. Use topical nystatin for candidiasis. Coat lips and nasal mucosa with petroleum jelly q60–90min. Use ophthalmic lubricants q4h or artificial tears q30min.

physician should remind the family and caregivers about the inevitability of events, the palliative goals, and that interventions may prolong the dying process and cause discomfort. Physicians should also emphasize that withholding treatments is both legal and ethical, and that they are not the cause of the patient's death. This reassurance may need to be provided multiple times.

Hearing and touch are said to be the last senses to stop functioning. Therefore, families and caregivers should be permitted to communicate with the dying patient. Encouraging them to talk directly to the patient, even if he or she is unconscious, and hold the patient's hand or demonstrate affection in other ways can be an effective way to channel their urge "to do something" for the patient.

When the plan is for the patient to die at home, the physician must inform the family and caregivers how to determine that the patient has died. The cardinal signs are cessation of cardiac function and respiration; the pupils become fixed; the body becomes cool, ashen white, and waxy; muscles relax; and incontinence may occur. Remind the family and caregivers that the eyes may remain open even when the patient has died because the retroorbital fat pad may be depleted permitting the orbit to fall posteriorly, which makes it difficult for the eyelids to cover the eyeball.

The physician should establish a plan of who the family or caregivers will contact when the patient is dying and has died. Without a plan, they may panic and call 911, unleashing a cascade of unwanted events from arrival of emergency personal and resuscitation to hospital admission. The family and caregivers should be instructed to contact the hospice (if one is involved), the covering physician, or the on-call member of the palliative care team. They should also be told that the coroner need not be called, unless the state requires it for all deaths. Unless foul play is suspected, the health care team need not contact the coroner either.

Just after the patient dies, even the best-prepared family may experience shock and loss and be emotionally distraught. They need time to assimilate the event and be comforted. Health care providers should write a bereavement card or letter to the family. The purpose is to communicate about the patient, perhaps emphasizing the patient's virtues, the honor it was to care for the patient, and express concern for the family's hardship. Many physicians attend the funerals of their patients. While this is beyond any medical obligation, the presence of the physician can be a source of support to the grieving family, and the funeral provides an opportunity for closure for the physician.

Death is a strong predictor of poor health, and even mortality, for the surviving spouse. It may be important to alert the spouse's physician about the death to be aware of symptoms that might require professional attention.

PALLIATIVE CARE SERVICES: HOW AND WHERE

Determining the best approach to providing palliative care to patients will depend upon patient preferences, the availability of caregivers and specialized services in close proximity, institutional resources, and reimbursement. A hospice is a leading, but not the only, model of palliative care services. In the United States, Medicare pays for hospice services under Part A, the hospital insurance part of reimbursement. Two physicians must certify that the patient has a prognosis of ≤6 months, if the disease runs its usual course. Prognoses are probabilistic by their nature; patients are not required to die within 6 months but rather to have a condition from which half the individuals with it would be dead within 6 months. Patients sign a hospice enrollment form that states their intent to forgo curative services related to their terminal illness, but they can still receive medical services for other comorbid conditions. Patients can also un-enroll and re-enroll later; the hospice Medicare benefit can be revoked later to secure traditional Medicare benefits. Payments to the hospice are per diem, not fee-for-service. Payments are intended to cover physician services for the medical direction of the care team; regular home care visits by registered nurses and licensed practical nurses; home health aid and homemaker services; dietary counseling; chaplain services; social work services; bereavement counseling; and medical equipment, supplies, and medications. Additional clinical care, including services of the primary physician, is covered by Medicare Part B even while the hospice Medicare benefit is in place.

By 1996, the mean length of enrollment in a hospice was 65 days, with the median being <24 days. Since then, it appears the length of enrollment is declining. Such short stays create barriers to establishing high-quality palliative services in patients' homes and also place financial strains on hospice providers since the initial assessments and institution of care plans are resource intensive. Physicians should initiate early referrals to the hospice to allow more time for patients to receive palliative care.

Hospice care has been the main way of securing palliative services for terminally ill patients. However, efforts are now being made to ensure continuity of palliative care across settings and through time. Palliative care services are becoming available as consultative services in hospitals, in day care and other outpatient settings, and in nursing homes. In the United States, while the vast majority of hospice care is provided in residential homes, just over 10% now occurs in nursing homes. Palliative care consultations for non-hospice patients can be billed as for other consultations under Medicare Part B, the physician reimbursement part. Many believe palliative care should be offered to patients regardless of their prognosis. A patient and his or her family should not have to make a "curative vs. palliative care" decision because it is rarely psychologically possible to make such a decisive switch to embracing mortality.

FUTURE DIRECTIONS

OUTCOME MEASURES Care near the end of life cannot be measured by most of the available validated outcome measures since palliative care does not consider death a bad outcome. Similarly, the family and patients receiving end-of-life care may not desire the elements elicited in current quality-of-life measurements. Symptom control, enhanced family relationships, and quality of bereavement are difficult to measure and are rarely the primary focus of carefully developed or widely used outcome measures. Nevertheless, outcomes are as important in end-of-life care as in any other field of medical care. Specific end-of-life care instruments are being developed both for assessment, such as The Brief Hospice Inventory and NEST (*n*eeds near the *e*nd of life *s*creening *t*ool), and for outcome measures, such as the Palliative Care Outcomes Scale. The field of end-of-life care is ready to enter an era of evidence-based practice and continuous improvement through clinical trials.

FURTHER READING

AMERICAN SOCIETY OF CLINICAL ONCOLOGY: *Optimizing Cancer Care— The Importance of Symptom Management*, vols 1 and 2. Alexandria, Virginia, ASCO, 2001

BUCKMAN R: *How to Break Bad News: A Guide for Health Care Professionals*. Baltimore, Johns Hopkins University Press, 1992

LEVY MH: Pharmacologic treatment of cancer pain. N Engl J Med 335:1124, 1996

NCCN: The National Comprehensive Cancer Network (NCCN) palliative care guidelines. 2002: *www.nccn.org*

THE PALLIATIVE CARE GUIDELINES GROUP OF THE AMERICAN HOSPICE FOUNDATION: *Integrating Palliative Care into Disease Management Guidelines*. American Hospice Foundation, Washington, DC, 2003

www.epec.net
www.eperc.mcw.edu
www.partnershipforcaring.org

---

10   COMPLEMENTARY AND ALTERNATIVE MEDICINE
Stephen E. Straus

BACKGROUND Medicine, not long ago the domain of solitary generalists and their nurse assistants, now engages scores of specialists and allied professionals—radiation physicists, cytologists, nurse practitioners, psychiatric social workers, dental hygienists, and many more—who wield tools of unprecedented ability to extend life and sustain its quality. This evolution of the health care system has been achieved, in part, by a formidable enterprise of critical observation and formal investigation that disproves some once-accepted practices and stimulates emergence of new approaches that compete for acceptance. One need only peruse the serial editions of this textbook to comprehend the scope of these changes.

Other factors have also affected evolutionary changes in medicine. Immigration and related demographic changes yield increasingly diverse populations who value their own traditions. People's expectations of health and the nature of the health care system itself have been altered by unprecedented access to sources of information, goods, and services; the disposable income to afford them, and a patchwork quilt of regulations and laws that constrain medical practice on the one hand and facilitate increased choice in health care on the other. The emergence of complementary and alternative medicine is one manifestation of these changes in health care.

DEFINITIONS In every generation, medical practices exist that are not accepted by the mainstream: they are viewed with suspicion and dismissed as implausible or irrational. For a time, approaches that evoked some appeal, but which had not been thoroughly tested, were deemed *unconventional*. Over the past decade or so, they have been called complementary or alternative medicine (CAM), to reflect their use as adjuncts to, or as substitutes for, more generally accepted practices, respectively. CAM does not encompass practices that have yet to be translated fully from the laboratory into the clinic, nor practices that were well studied and disproved, but which manage to persist in some fashion nonetheless. Rather, CAM entails approaches with surprising pervasiveness, many of which can claim at least some evidentiary support. Until recently, CAM could also be defined as practices that are not widely taught in medical schools or reimbursed. However, medical students increasingly seek and receive some instruction about CAM, while third-party payers have identified in CAM a marketing tool to attract new, well-heeled clients. In the past few years, another term has been coined—*integrative medicine*—to suggest encouragingly that some CAM approaches, and the practitioners who deliver them, will be shown worthy of being added to the health care repertoire.

SCOPE   The myriad practices and products that encompass CAM (Table 10-1) can be organized into five somewhat overlapping domains. Special diets, high doses of vitamins and minerals, and extracts of animal or botanical products are grouped together as *biologically based* CAM approaches. Massage, osteopathic and chiropractic manipulation, and cranial-sacral therapies are grouped as *manipulative and body-based* CAM approaches. Diverse forms of meditation, various uses of biofeedback, and hypnosis are considered *mind-body* approaches. All three of these CAM domains have well-accepted analogues in conventional medicine—low-fat, low-cholesterol diets; physical therapy; psychotherapy; to name but a few.

The fourth domain is known as *energy medicine*, to reflect its exploitation of veritable or putative energy fields. Today, magnets are

increasingly popular health products. Over 2000 years ago, however, while Greek physicians believed that health requires a balance of vital humors, Asian practitioners postulated the flow and balance of vital energies and described tools to restore them. Acupuncture aims to correct energies that flow through special meridians, or channels. Reiki, a Japanese approach, and healing touch, a modern variant, purport to diagnose and correct one's energy by passing the hands of an adept therapist over the patient.

The fifth domain, termed *alternative systems of medicine*, combines elements of the four other domains and aims to provide primary approaches to all health needs, rather than just adjunctive solutions to them. Western variants include practices developed by Native Americans, homeopathy, and naturopathic medicine. Eastern variants such as Ayurvedic medicine of India, traditional Chinese medicine, and Tibetan medicine are rich in their use of meditative exercises and herbal products.

PATTERNS OF USE   Despite its enormous success, contemporary western biomedicine has features that can discourage patients: many diseases, especially chronic ones, are not cured or even adequately ameliorated; existing treatments can impose serious adverse reactions; and the care is fragmented and impersonal. CAM, despite its lack of proof, appeals to many because its practitioners are optimistic. They spend a lot of time talking with and touching their patients. CAM empowers patients to make their own health choices, its natural products are believed to be inherently healthier and safer than synthetic ones, and care is pro-

TABLE 10-1 *Some Complementary and Alternative Medical Practices*	
Type	**Description**
Acupuncture	A Chinese medical practice that involves the insertion of hair-thin needles into nonanatomic energy channels, called meridians
Alexander technique	A movement therapy that emphasizes efficient use of muscles to relieve pain, decrease skeletal strain, and improve posture
Anthroposophic medicine	A spiritually based system of medicine that incorporates herbs, homeopathy, diet, and a movement therapy called eurythmy
Aromatherapy	The use of essential plant oils (distilled concentrates) in massage, baths, or inhalation
Ayurvedic medicine	The major East Indian traditional medicine system, utilizing pulse and tongue diagnosis; treatment includes diet, exercise, herbs, oil massages, and elimination regimens (utilizing emetics, diarrheals, etc.)
Bach flower remedies	Dilute flower infusions used to treat emotional conditions
Biofeedback	The use of machinery that translates physiologic processes into audio or visual signals
Chiropractic	Adjustments of spinal vertebrae in an effort to affect neuromuscular function
Cranial-sacral therapy	Gentle manipulation of the cranium and spine
Curanderismo	A spiritual healing tradition common in Mexican-American communities that utilizes ritual cleansing, herbs and incantations
Dance therapy	Therapeutic method that uses movement to facilitate emotional expression and release
Feldenkrais bodywork	Highly structured movement sequences that emphasize proper head positioning
Guided imagery	The use of imagination to invoke specific images that are hoped to affect physiologic function
Hydropathy	Treatment utilizing water at various temperatures, sometimes aerated or under pressure, sometimes with added salts or other substances
Hypnosis	The induction of an altered of mind within which a subject becomes receptive to specific suggestions
Massage	The use of specific gliding and kneading strokes and friction to achieve muscle relaxation
Meditation	A process by which one tries to achieve awareness without thought
Music therapy	Singing, playing instruments, or listening to music
Naturopathy	A mixture of modalities that may include herbs, homeopathy, acupuncture, hydropathy, diet, and exercise
Native American medicine	Diverse systems, many of which incorporate prayer, chant, music, healing ceremonies, counseling, herbs, laying on of hands, and smudging (ritual cleansing with smoke from sacred plants)
Osteopathy	A medical field incorporating manipulative techniques for correcting abnormalities of the musculoskeletal system
Reflexology/zone therapy	Manual stimulation of points on the hands or feet, believed to affect distant organs
Rolfing/structural integration	A manual therapy that attempts to realign the body by deep tissue manipulation of fasciae
Shiatsu/acupressure	Finger pressure at points along nonanatomic meridians
Siddha medicine	An East Indian medical system (prevalent among Tamil-speaking people) utilizing breathing techniques, incantations, herbs, and muppu (a tri-salt preparation)
T'ai chi ch'aun	Chinese dancelike exercises described as a "moving meditation"
Therapeutic touch	Secular version of the laying on hands, described as a "healing meditation" (a tri-salt preparation)
Tibetan medicine	A medical system that utilizes diagnosis by pulse and urine examination; therapies include herbs, diet, and massage
Traditional Chinese medicine	A medical system that utilizes examination of the tongue and pulses for diagnosis and acupuncture, herbal mixtures, massage, exercise, and diet
Trager bodywork	Light massage combined with gentle passive movements to help patients maximize freedom of movement
Unani medicine	An East Indian medial system, derived from Persian medicine, practiced primarily in the Muslim community
Yoga	An Indian practice that includes postures (asanas), breathing exercises (pranayama), and cleansing practices (kriyas)

vided in a "holistic" fashion, meaning that the broader medical, social, and emotional contexts of illness are considered in designing the treatment plan.

The very first large survey by Eisenberg in 1993 surprised the medical community by showing that >30% of Americans use CAM approaches. Countless studies since then have extended these conclusions by surveying specific demographic groups and patient populations. The Centers for Disease Control and Prevention (CDC) study of nearly 31,000 American adults revealed that in 1999 29% had used one or more modalities, with spiritual approaches, herbal medicine, chiropractic, and massage being the most prevalent. Over 1% underwent acupuncture treatment that year. Surveys among patients with cancer showed that 30 to 86% used CAM, with highest rates in those with more advanced disease and undergoing aggressive treatments. Similarly, among AIDS patients, 36 to 91% are reported to use CAM. In devastating chronic illnesses like these, CAM is called upon to provide hope of cures when conventional medicine cannot, to extend life, to ameliorate treatment side effects, and to provide emotional and physical comfort. While somewhat subject to vagaries of definition as to what counts as a CAM treatment, surveys have shown that Americans are willing to pay for these services out of pocket, with an estimated $7 billion each year on vitamins and mineral supplements, $4 billion on herbals and other natural products, and nearly $4 billion more on sports supplements. Eisenberg reported that total CAM expenditures in 1997 approached $30 billion, with more visits to practitioners for CAM services than to physicians in general.

FIELDS OF PRACTICE ■ Osteopathic Medicine   Founded in 1892 in the American heartland by the physician Andrew Taylor Still, osteopathic medicine was based originally on the belief that manipulation of soft tissue and bone can correct a wide range of diseases of the musculoskeletal and other organ systems. Over the ensuing century, osteopathy evolved progressively towards conventional (allopathic) medicine. Today, the training, practice, credentialing, licensure, and reimbursement of osteopathic physicians is virtually indistinguishable from those of allopathic physicians, with 4 years of osteopathic medical school followed by specialty and subspecialty training and certification by organizations such as the American Board of Internal Medicine. Some osteopathic physicians continue to practice spinal manipulation, primarily as a tool to address specific musculoskeletal complaints.

Chiropractic Medicine   In 1895, Daniel David Palmer founded in Missouri the first school of chiropractic medicine to teach manipulation of the spine. Palmer believed that subluxations, or partial dislocations of vertebrae, cause disease by impinging on key nerve roots. Today, chiropractors undertake 5 years of training in basic and relevant clinical sciences. Increasingly, they complete additional postgraduate training in radiology and outpatient therapeutics, primarily of musculoskeletal conditions, although within the discipline there are factions that continue to perform manipulation for many other pathologic entities. Chiropractors also advise on nutrition, exercise, and other health maintenance approaches. Over 70,000 doctors of chiropractic medicine are licensed to practice in all states and the District of Columbia.

Acupuncture   A venerable component of traditional Chinese medicine, acupuncture has emerged in recent decades as a free-standing clinical discipline. Over 3000 American physicians have acquired targeted postgraduate training that permits them to practice acupuncture in over 40 states and the District of Columbia. Over 4000 non-MDs have taken far more extended training, leading to licensure to practice independently or under the supervision of a physician.

Massage Therapy   Drawing upon millennia of empirical knowledge, some 80 American schools instruct students in an array of the soft tissue manipulative approaches that constitute massage. Thirty-one states and the District of Columbia license trainees to perform therapeutic massage.

Naturopathic Medicine   Eleven states license practitioners of naturopathy, a discipline that emerged in central Europe in the late eighteenth century. That conventional treatments of the day were usually ineffective, if not overtly harmful, stimulated the search for safer and more "natural" approaches—naturopathy is one of them. The concept underlying this discipline is that the body possesses powerful mechanisms for self-healing that a properly instructed practitioner could harness. About 1400 naturopathic physicians have completed 4 years of education in basic and clinical sciences and are licensed to manage a predominantly outpatient population. Conventional and unconventional diagnostic tests and medications are prescribed with an emphasis on relatively low doses of drugs, herbal medicines, special diets, and exercises.

Homeopathic Medicine   The late eighteenth century also witnessed the emergence of homeopathy, another discipline that reacted to toxicity of the allopathic approaches of the day. It was developed by Samuel Hahnemann, a German physician, who postulated that substances that cause particular side effects in a well person may be used to treat or prevent such symptoms in an ill person if administered in miniscule amounts—what is known as "the doctrine of similars." For example, contact with poison ivy (*Rhus toxicodendron*) causes an itchy, blistering rash. Highly diluted extracts of poison ivy are recommended to treat chickenpox. The nascent field of homeopathy used blinded tests on volunteers, presaging to some extent the use of placebo-controlled trials, to prove which materials were the most able to induce or relieve symptoms. By the mid-nineteenth century homeopathy had gained considerable presence in the American medical establishment and may, in fact, have facilitated the development of immunization and allergen desensitization, both of which utilize very small quantities of materials to elicit measurable biologic outcomes. Today, however, homeopathy is accepted less fully in the United States than in some other countries: it is the largest of all CAM practices in the United Kingdom, Germany, and France and is widely used in India. Only three states license the practice of homeopathy. The relative decline of homeopathy relates, at least in part, to the field's inability to articulate a rational mechanism as to why products that are diluted more than 10^{60}-fold, vastly greater than Avogadro's number, could incite biologic effects. Nonetheless, homeopathic remedies are readily available and commonly recommended by naturopathic physicians and other licensed and unlicensed practitioners.

Other Disciplines   There are numerous other CAM practices, among which some involve formal training, such as that leading to a Doctorate of Oriental Medicine, or extended apprenticeships, as in learning herbal medicine. Unfortunately, most of the other fields have no agreed upon practice standards, credentialing processes, requirements for continuing education, or accountability.

REGULATION   As indicated above, some CAM disciplines are carefully regulated. CAM products, however, are not strongly regulated. Herbal medicines, and dietary supplements more generally, occupy a unique regulatory status that affords the public remarkable freedom of choice but also many undesired challenges, summarized below. Elements of virtually all traditional healing approaches, herbal medicines were presumed safe long before the implementation of stringent drug regulations by the U.S. Food and Drug Administration (FDA). In 1994, the United States Congress passed the Dietary Supplements Health and Education Act (DSHEA) that permits sale of dietary supplements "over-the-counter," as it were, but without the requirement imposed on manufacturers of prescription or classic over-the-counter drugs to prove their products to be safe and effective before marketing. Supplements can be removed by the FDA from the market only if they are proven to be hazardous. Dietary supplements, however, cannot legally claim to prevent or treat any disease. They can, however, claim to maintain "normal structure and function" of body systems. For example, a product cannot claim to treat arthritis, but it can claim to maintain "normal joint health."

Homeopathic products predate FDA drug regulations and are sold with no requirement that they be proven effective. It would be reasonable to assume, however, given the extent to which homeopathic products are diluted, that most of them are safe.

SAFETY Despite their lack of apparent toxicities, homeopathic products, like all other CAM products and practices, do convey one type of risk, namely, that people will pursue them in lieu of more conventional modalities that are proven to be beneficial. Members of the public have considerable freedom to determine what is in their own best interest, even if those decisions deny them effective treatment, although the courts have found the rights of parents to withhold treatment of their children to be limited in instances of life-threatening illnesses. Investigators, however, have a broad ethical obligation to not withhold proven treatments for serious illnesses for the sake of testing unproven ones.

Additional risks are imposed by the use of other CAM approaches: injuries inflicted by a practice, inherent toxicities of the modality, and interference by the modality with more conventional treatments.

Injury Physical and manipulative interventions can harm patients. In past decades, reused acupuncture needles transmitted hepatitis B virus infection; today, the standard of care requires disposable needles. Aggressive massage can cause soft tissue injuries. Spinal manipulation of patients with unrecognized vertebral lesions has been associated with cord injuries, and cervical manipulation has been associated with stroke. These appear to be rare events.

Inherent Toxicity While the public may believe that "natural" equates with "safe," it is abundantly clear that natural products can be toxic. Misidentification of medicinal mushrooms has led to liver failure. Contamination of tryptophan supplements caused the eosinophilia-myalgia syndrome. Herbal products containing particular species of *Aristolochia* were associated with genitourinary malignancies. In 2001, extracts of kava, long used by Pacific Islanders for its mild anxiolytic and sedative properties, were associated with fulminant liver failure. A number of products, including the popular *Ginkgo biloba*, are known to prolong bleeding times and have been associated with postoperative hemorrhage. Among the most controversial is *Ephedra sinica*, or ma huang, a product used in traditional Chinese medicine for short-term treatment of asthma and bronchial congestion. The scientific basis for these indications was revealed when ephedra was shown to contain the ephedrine alkaloids, especially ephedrine and pseudoephedrine. With the promulgation of the DSHEA regulations, supplements containing ephedra and herbs rich in caffeine flooded the U.S. marketplace, claiming to promote weight loss and to enhance athletic performance. Reports of severe and fatal adverse events in young and, in some cases, well-known Americans led to calls for removal of ephedra-containing supplements.

Herbal-Drug Interactions The constituents of natural products may not only be toxic but may also interfere with the metabolism of life-saving drugs. This effect was illustrated most profoundly with the demonstration in 2000 that consumption of St.-John's-wort interferes with the bioavilability of the HIV protease inhibitor indinavir. Later studies showed its similar interference with metabolism of topoisomerase inhibitors such as irinotecan, with cyclosporine, and with many other drugs. The breadth of interference stems from the ability of hyperforin in St.-John's-wort to upregulate expression of the pregnane X receptor, a promiscuous nuclear regulatory factor that promotes the expression of many hepatic oxidative, conjugative, and efflux enzymes engaged in drug and food metabolism.

ACQUIRING EVIDENCE CAM evolved through an entirely different epistemologic framework than contemporary biomedicine. Empirical observations of individual patients constitute the primary evidentiary base on which CAM practices are guided and taught. Nonetheless, over the past few decades, thousands of studies have been performed of various CAM approaches, including hundreds of trials involving herbals, acupuncture, or homeopathy. To date, however, no single approach has been proven effective in a convincing way. (If they had, the practice would no longer be considered CAM!) Several factors contribute to this lack of convincing evidence. The vast majority of

CAM studies have been seriously flawed by lack of appropriate controls, bias on the part of the investigators, small sample sizes, reliance on highly subjective and nonvalidated measures of benefit, and by inappropriate statistical tests.

There are in addition, a series of methodologic issues that challenge even the better-designed CAM studies. No uniform practice guidelines exist, and the herbal products marketed in the United States are highly variable in quality and composition. Some CAM practices are not amenable to blinding. For example, both the patient and the practitioner would know if spinal manipulation had been performed. These problems are not unique to CAM, however, as they also complicate attempts to study conventional practices such as psychotherapy or surgery. Efforts are now being made to randomize patients to other equally demanding control interventions, and acupuncture at traditional needling points is being compared to needling at what are arguably irrelevant points.

Even with ongoing improvements in study design and conduct, issues of belief stand in the way of comprehending and accepting the results of some CAM studies. Many physicians are reluctant to believe positive outcomes of exotic approaches that have not emerged through the classic experimental paradigm by which drugs and biological agents are now developed, namely, the orderly progression from preclinical testing through three phases of clinical trials. More importantly, it is difficult to accept results that are counterintuitive or whose mechanism cannot be rationally explained. A powerful example of this dilemma involves studies of homeopathy. Some clinical trials of homeopathy for asthma, infantile diarrhea, and other common conditions reported positive results. Two systematic reviews of homeopathy trials gleaned an overall favorable impression of the clinical trials data, concluding that the treatments were more beneficial than placebo. Even the best trials and these reviews have been criticized on methodologic grounds. It remains unclear what evidence could compel a tidal change in belief about the benefits of homeopathy when there remain no cogent explanations for how substances diluted to the point at which only solute remains could exert physiologic effects.

By contrast, while methodologic problems continue to plague acupuncture trials, belief has been growing even in academic centers that acupuncture may be effective. The emerging acceptance of acupuncture may result, in part, from its widespread availability and use in the United States today: the CDC estimated that >1% of adult Americans received acupuncture treatments in 1999. Acupuncturists are now practicing within major medical centers, providing an ancillary approach to pain management. Yet, its acceptance may stem from more than just its communal appeal. Since the mid-1970s, studies have revealed palatable explanations for how needling may moderate pain and, not just by rephrasing the traditional explanation that acupuncture restores the flow of vital energies along meridians, for which there remain no known anatomic correlates. Rather, biochemical and imaging studies have shown that needling triggers the release of endogenous opioids that bind to specific receptors in the very brain regions that mediate the beneficial effects of narcotic analgesics.

EXISTING EVIDENCE Numerous CAM approaches lack coherent explanations and any credible body of data regarding their safety and effectiveness. And, while it is difficult to conclude decisively that an approach lacks any merit, it is quite feasible to discern that its effect size, or degree of benefit, is too small to be worth pursuing further. Over the past century, many approaches failed—one need only think back to the exotic electrical devices, procedures, and tonics that fell out of fashion. Two questions are often asked: (1) Whether any of the more contemporary CAM modalities deserve to be rejected? (2) Whether data showing it to be ineffective would change anyone's mind about using it? The case of laetrile is instructive in this regard. This extract of apricot seeds was touted in the 1970s as a cure for solid tumors. Thousands crossed the Mexican border to be treated. The lack of any positive preclinical data discouraged oncologists from agreeing to study laetrile, until public pressure required that an answer be obtained. Two studies in the 1980s showed no benefit of laetrile treatment. Today, some continue to seek the product, but the numbers are vastly smaller than before meaningful data were obtained. A similar fate befell a cocktail of drugs used for cancer patients through the 1970s and 1980s by Dr. Luigi DiBella in Italy, once large studies revealed it to have no detectable impact on the course of a variety of advanced cancers.

In contrast, modalities that have been well tested and found ineffective are still in fairly common practice. For example, the renowned biochemist and peace activist Linus Pauling proclaimed vitamin C to be the answer to the common cold. Numerous, high-quality studies failed to demonstrate clinically important effects of vitamin C in preventing or treating viral colds. The early studies were criticized for using too little of the vitamin, yet doses that well exceeded its bioavailability also proved negative. Nonetheless, ingestion of extra vitamin C remains a common habit in individuals who perceive the onset of cold symptoms. For most people, this practice is wasteful but not harmful; however, people with iron overload (either hemochromatosis or chronic transfusion requirement) can be damaged by vitamin C, which generates free radicals in the setting of iron excess.

Despite the failure of some CAM approaches, early studies have yielded positive or at least encouraging data for a number of them. Good sources of information include the Natural Medicines Comprehensive Database (www.NaturalDatabase.com) and National Institutes of Health (NIH) websites such as http://ods.od.nih.gov; http://nccam.nih.gov/health/ and http://www3.cancer.gov/occam/information.html.

Vitamins/Minerals

- *Vitamin A:* Massive studies in a number of developing nations proved that vitamin A deficiency is prevalent and associated with increased risks of mortality in young children. Prospective trials showed that 100,000 to 200,000 IU of vitamin A twice a year can reduce the overall death rate significantly.
- *Folic Acid:* Rates of neural tube defects are significantly diminished if the diet is supplemented with folic acid during pregnancy.
- *Folic acid, vitamin B_6, and vitamin B_{12}:* Randomized, double-blind, controlled trials suggest that this vitamin combination lowers serum homocysteine levels and the risk of myocardial infarction.
- *Vitamins C and E, β-carotene, and zinc:* A large, randomized controlled trial showed that these supplements combined reduce the progression of age-related macular degeneration.

Even vitamins and minerals, which are presumed safe in moderate doses, can have unexpected adverse effects. Two large controlled trials of β-carotene for prevention of cancer or retinal diseases found increased rates of lung cancer in those randomized to the supplement. Ongoing are large prospective trials seeking benefits from ingestion of supplements on rates of prostate cancer (vitamin E and selenium) and Alzheimer's disease (vitamin E).

Herbals and Other Natural Products

- *Glucosamine and/or chondroitin sulfate:* Systematic surveys of controlled trials concluded that these products of animal joints are superior to placebo in improving performance and slowing the narrowing of the joint space in patients with osteoarthritis of the knee.
- *Ginkgo biloba:* Americans consumed nearly $250 million of this herbal product in 2000. The literature shows no evidence that it improves cognition, but it may decrease the risk of dementia.
- *Saw palmetto (Serenoa repens)* and *African plum (Pygeum africanum):* Each of these botanicals is likely effective for the symptomatic treatment of benign prostatic hyperplasia. Sales of saw palmetto are growing, with an estimated $131 million of the product consumed by Americans in 2000.
- *St.-John's-wort (Hypericum perforatum):* Among the most popular herbal product worldwide, numerous small studies and systematic reviews suggested it to benefit patients with a wide range of depressive syndromes. High-quality, randomized, placebo-controlled trials, found St.-John's-wort to not be superior to placebo for treatment of major depression of moderate severity, a spectrum of illness that clearly warrants professional evaluation and treatment.
- *Echinacea species: Echinacea* roots are widely used to treat or prevent respiratory infections, with over $200 million in sales in 2000. Although in vitro studies have shown that *Echinacea* constituents stimulate humoral and cellular immune responses, systematic reviews of the clinical trials have not concluded that they are beneficial.

Other Modalities

- *Acupuncture:* A frequently cited NIH-led consensus development conference in 1997 concluded that evidence exists that acupuncture relieves nausea from chemotherapy and pain following extraction of molars. Some subsequent studies have confirmed these earlier impressions regarding acute nausea and vomiting, but the data regarding pain management have been mixed, with little evidence that it benefits neuropathic pain.
- *Mind-body medicine:* Clinical trials support the use of biofeedback for incontinence, headache, and stroke rehabilitation. Hypnosis may be beneficial in relieving pain due to minor surgical interventions, chemotherapy-associated nausea, and irritable bowel syndrome.
- *Spinal manipulation:* Systematic reviews of fairly well designed trials concluded that chiropractic or osteopathic manipulation provides significant improvement for patients with uncomplicated acute back pain. No proof exists that they are superior to, or more cost-effective than, other conventional approaches, nor do they alter the long-term outcome.

SUMMARY   An array of unproven modalities will always be used by the patients under our care. Physicians must approach each encounter as an opportunity to better understand patients, their beliefs, and their expectations and as an opportunity to help guide their choices in a constructive way. Many of these choices are entirely innocuous and can be accommodated in the context of the larger diagnostic and therapeutic intervention. Some should be actively discouraged. Along the way, scientific evidence will drive many CAM approaches out of favor. Some modalities will garner sufficient support to become part of mainstream care: the next generation of physicians will never know they were once controversial.

FURTHER READING

DE SMET PA: Herbal remedies. N Engl J Med 347:2046, 2002

EISENBERG DM et al: Trends in alternative medicine use in the United States, 1990–1997: Results of a follow-up national survey. JAMA 280:1569, 1998

ENGEL L, STRAUS SE: Development of therapeutics: Opportunities within complementary and alternative medicine. Nat Rev Drug Discov 1:229, 2002

KAPTCHUK TJ: Acupuncture: Theory, efficacy and practice. Ann Intern Med 136:374, 2002

KINSEL JF, STRAUS SE: Complementary and alternative therapeutics: rigorous research is needed to support claims. Annu Rev Pharmacol Toxicol 43:463, 2003

RICHARDSON MA, STRAUS SE: Complementary and alternative medicine: Opportunities and challenges for cancer management and research. Semin Oncol 29:531, 2002

11 | PAIN: PATHOPHYSIOLOGY AND MANAGEMENT
Howard L. Fields, Joseph B. Martin

The task of medicine is to preserve and restore health and to relieve suffering. Understanding pain is essential to both these goals. Because pain is universally understood as a signal of disease, it is the most common symptom that brings a patient to a physician's attention. The function of the pain sensory system is to protect the body and maintain homeostasis. It does this by detecting, localizing, and identifying tissue-damaging processes. Since different diseases produce characteristic patterns of tissue damage, the quality, time course, and location of a patient's pain complaint and the location of tenderness provide important diagnostic clues and are used to evaluate the response to treatment. Once this information is obtained, it is the obligation of the physician to provide rapid and effective pain relief.

THE PAIN SENSORY SYSTEM

Pain is an unpleasant sensation localized to a part of the body. It is often described in terms of a penetrating or tissue-destructive process (e.g., stabbing, burning, twisting, tearing, squeezing) and/or of a bodily or emotional reaction (e.g., terrifying, nauseating, sickening). Furthermore, any pain of moderate or higher intensity is accompanied by anxiety and the urge to escape or terminate the feeling. These properties illustrate the duality of pain: it is both sensation and emotion. When acute, pain is characteristically associated with behavioral arousal and a stress response consisting of increased blood pressure, heart rate, pupil diameter, and plasma cortisol levels. In addition, local muscle contraction (e.g., limb flexion, abdominal wall rigidity) is often present.

PERIPHERAL MECHANISMS ■ The Primary Afferent Nociceptor A peripheral nerve consists of the axons of three different types of neurons: primary sensory afferents, motor neurons, and sympathetic postganglionic neurons (Fig. 11-1). The cell bodies of primary afferents are located in the dorsal root ganglia in the vertebral foramina. The primary afferent axon bifurcates to send one process into the spinal cord and the other to innervate tissues. Primary afferents are classified by their diameter, degree of myelination, and conduction velocity. The largest-diameter fibers, A-beta (Aβ), respond maximally to light touch and/or moving stimuli; they are present primarily in nerves that innervate the skin. In normal individuals, the activity of these fibers does not produce pain. There are two other classes of primary afferents: the small-diameter myelinated A-delta (Aδ) and the unmyelinated (C fiber) axons (Fig. 11-1). These fibers are present in nerves to the skin and to deep somatic and visceral structures. Some tissues, such as the cornea, are innervated only by Aδ and C afferents. Most Aδ and C afferents respond maximally only to intense (painful) stimuli and produce the subjective experience of pain when they are electrically stimulated; this defines them as *primary afferent nociceptors* (*pain receptors*). The ability to detect painful stimuli is completely abolished when Aδ and C axons are blocked.

Individual primary afferent nociceptors can respond to several different types of noxious stimuli. For example, most nociceptors respond to heating, intense mechanical stimuli such as a pinch, and application of irritating chemicals.

Sensitization When intense, repeated, or prolonged stimuli are applied to damaged or inflamed tissues the threshold for activating primary afferent nociceptors is lowered and the frequency of firing is higher for all stimulus intensities. Inflammatory mediators such as bradykinin, some prostaglandins, and leukotrienes contribute to this process, which is called *sensitization*. In sensitized tissues normally innocuous stimuli can produce pain. Sensitization is a clinically important process that contributes to tenderness, soreness, and hyperalgesia. A striking example of sensitization is sunburned skin, in which severe pain can be produced by a gentle slap on the back or a warm shower.

Sensitization is of particular importance for pain and tenderness in deep tissues. Viscera are normally relatively insensitive to noxious mechanical and thermal stimuli, although hollow viscera do generate significant discomfort when distended. In contrast, when affected by a disease process with an inflammatory component, deep structures such as joints or hollow viscera characteristically become exquisitely sensitive to mechanical stimulation.

A large proportion of Aδ and C afferents innervating viscera are completely insensitive in normal noninjured, noninflamed tissue. That is, they cannot be activated by known mechanical or thermal stimuli and are not spontaneously active. However, in the presence of inflammatory mediators, these afferents become sensitive to mechanical stimuli. Such afferents have been termed *silent nociceptors*, and their characteristic properties may explain how under pathologic conditions the relatively insensitive deep structures can become the source of severe and debilitating pain and tenderness. Low pH, prostaglandins, leukotrienes, and other inflammatory mediators such as bradykinin play a significant role in sensitization.

Nociceptor-Induced Inflammation One important concept to emerge in recent years is that afferent nociceptors also have a neuroeffector func-

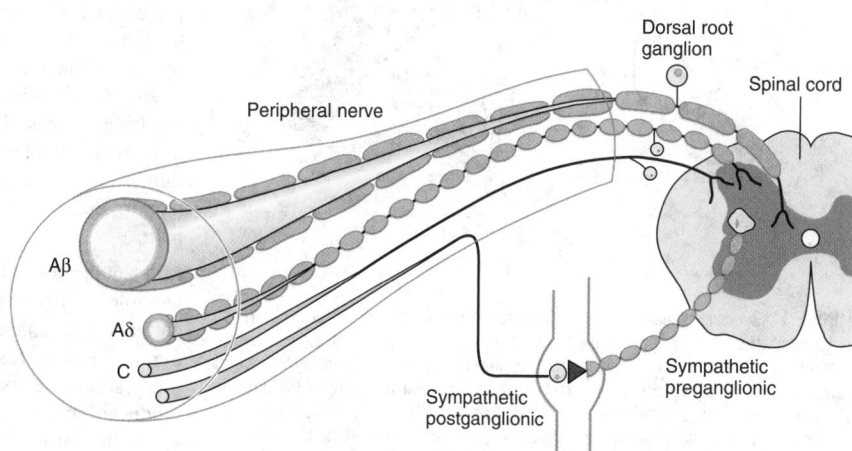

FIGURE 11-1 Components of a typical cutaneous nerve. There are two distinct functional categories of axons: primary afferents with cell bodies in the dorsal root ganglion, and sympathetic postganglionic fibers with cell bodies in the sympathetic ganglion. Primary afferents include those with large-diameter myelinated (Aβ), small-diameter myelinated (Aδ), and unmyelinated (C) axons. All sympathetic postganglionic fibers are unmyelinated.

tion. Most nociceptors contain polypeptide mediators that are released from their peripheral terminals when they are activated (Fig. 11-2). An example is substance P, an 11-amino-acid peptide. Substance P is released from primary afferent nociceptors and has multiple biologic activities. It is a potent vasodilator, degranulates mast cells, is a chemoattractant for leukocytes, and increases the production and release of inflammatory mediators. Interestingly, depletion of substance P from joints reduces the severity of experimental arthritis. Primary afferent nociceptors are not simply passive messengers of threats to tissue injury but also play an active role in tissue protection through these neuroeffector functions.

CENTRAL MECHANISMS ■ **The Spinal Cord and Referred Pain**   The axons of primary afferent nociceptors enter the spinal cord via the dorsal root. They terminate in the dorsal horn of the spinal gray matter (Fig. 11-3). The terminals of primary afferent axons contact spinal neurons that transmit the pain signal to brain sites involved in pain perception. The axon of each primary afferent contacts many spinal neurons, and each spinal neuron receives convergent inputs from many primary afferents.

The convergence of sensory inputs to a single spinal pain-transmission neuron is of great importance because it underlies the phenomenon of referred pain. All spinal neurons that receive input from

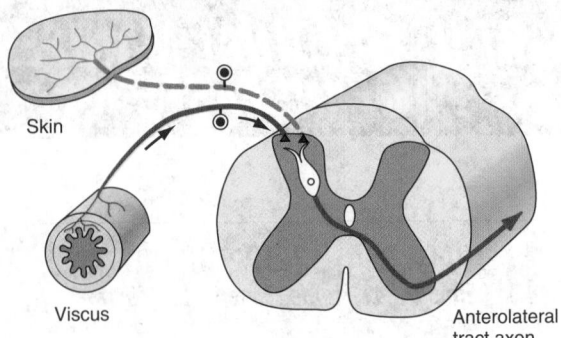

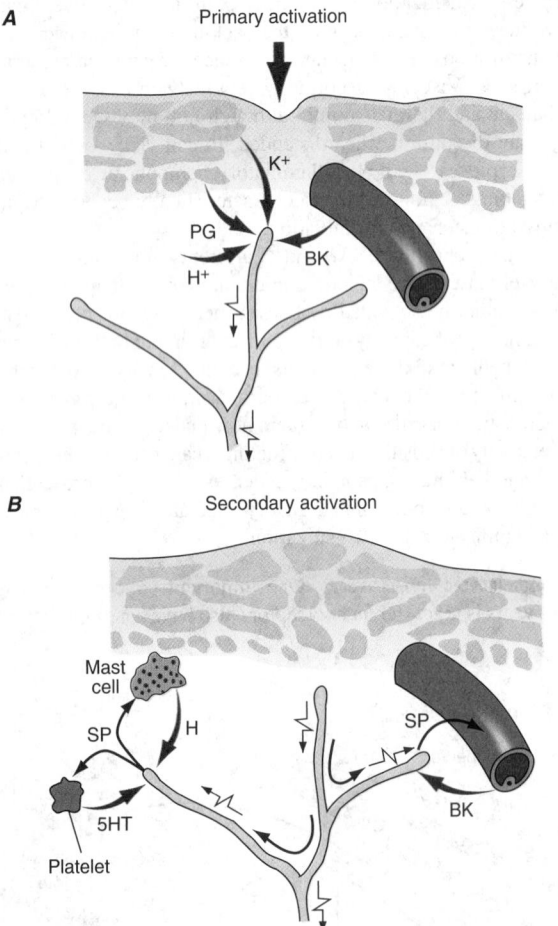

A   Primary activation

B   Secondary activation

Mast cell

SP   H   SP

5HT   BK

Platelet

FIGURE 11-2   Events leading to activation, sensitization, and spread of sensitization of primary afferent nociceptor terminals. *A.* Direct activation by intense pressure and consequent cell damage. Cell damage induces lower pH (H^+) and leads to release of potassium (K^+) and to synthesis of prostaglandins (PG) and bradykinin (BK). Prostaglandins increase the sensitivity of the terminal to bradykinin and other pain-producing substances. *B.* Secondary activation. Impulses generated in the stimulated terminal propagate not only to the spinal cord but also into other terminal branches where they induce the release of peptides, including substance P (SP). Substance P causes vasodilation and neurogenic edema with further accumulation of bradykinin. Substance P also causes the release of histamine (H) from mast cells and serotonin (5HT) from platelets.

FIGURE 11-3   The convergence-projection hypothesis of referred pain. According to this hypothesis, visceral afferent nociceptors converge on the same pain-projection neurons as the afferents from the somatic structures in which the pain is perceived. The brain has no way of knowing the actual source of input and mistakenly "projects" the sensation to the somatic structure.

the viscera and deep musculoskeletal structures also receive input from the skin. The convergence patterns are determined by the spinal segment of the dorsal root ganglion that supplies the afferent innervation of a structure. For example, the afferents that supply the central diaphragm are derived from the third and fourth cervical dorsal root ganglia. Primary afferents with cell bodies in these same ganglia supply the skin of the shoulder and lower neck. Thus sensory inputs from both the shoulder skin and the central diaphragm converge on pain-transmission neurons in the third and fourth cervical spinal segments. *Because of this convergence and the fact that the spinal neurons are most often activated by inputs from the skin, activity evoked in spinal neurons by input from deep structures is mislocalized by the patient to a place that is roughly coextensive with the region of skin innervated by the same spinal segment.* Thus inflammation near the central diaphragm is usually reported as discomfort near the shoulder. This spatial displacement of pain sensation from the site of the injury that produces it is known as *referred pain.*

Ascending Pathways for Pain   A majority of spinal neurons contacted by primary afferent nociceptors send their axons to the contralateral thalamus. These axons form the contralateral spinothalamic tract, which lies in the anterolateral white matter of the spinal cord, the lateral edge of the medulla, and the lateral pons and midbrain. The spinothalamic pathway is crucial for pain sensation in humans. Interruption of this pathway produces permanent deficits in pain and temperature discrimination.

Spinothalamic tract axons ascend to several regions of the thalamus. There is tremendous divergence of the pain signal from these thalamic sites to broad areas of the cerebral cortex that subserve different aspects of the pain experience (Fig. 11-4). One of the thalamic projections is to the somatosensory cortex. This projection mediates the purely sensory aspects of pain, i.e., its location, intensity, and quality. Other thalamic neurons project to cortical regions that are linked to emotional responses, such as the cingulate gyrus and other areas of the frontal lobes. These pathways to the frontal cortex subserve the affective or unpleasant emotional dimension of pain. This affective dimension of pain produces suffering and exerts potent control of behavior. Because of this dimension, fear is a constant companion of pain.

PAIN MODULATION   The pain produced by similar injuries is remarkably variable in different situations and in different individuals. For example, athletes have been known to sustain serious fractures with only minor pain, and Beecher's classic World War II survey revealed that many soldiers in battle were unbothered by injuries that would have produced agonizing pain in civilian patients. Furthermore, even the suggestion of relief can have a significant analgesic effect (placebo). On the other hand, many patients find even minor injuries (such as venipuncture) frightening and unbearable, and the expectation of pain has been demonstrated to induce pain without a noxious stimulus.

The powerful effect of expectation and other psychological varia-

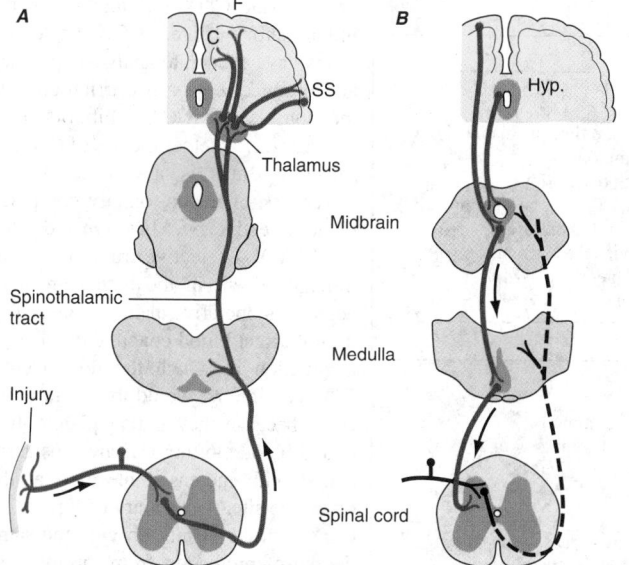

FIGURE 11-4 *A.* Transmission system for nociceptive messages. Noxious stimuli activate the sensitive peripheral ending of the primary afferent nociceptor by the process of transduction. The message is then transmitted over the peripheral nerve to the spinal cord, where it synapses with cells of origin of the major ascending pain pathway, the spinothalamic tract. The message is relayed in the thalamus to the anterior cingulate (C), frontal insular (F), and somatosensory cortex (SS). *B.* Pain-modulation network. Inputs from frontal cortex and hypothalamus (Hyp.) activate cells in the midbrain that control spinal pain-transmission cells via cells in the medulla.

bles on the perceived intensity of pain implies the existence of brain circuits that can modulate the activity of the pain-transmission pathways. One of these circuits has links in the hypothalamus, midbrain, and medulla, and it selectively controls spinal pain-transmission neurons through a descending pathway (Fig. 11-4).

Human brain imaging studies have implicated this pain-modulating circuit in the pain-relieving effect of attention, suggestion, and opioid analgesic medications. Furthermore, each of the component structures of the pathway contains opioid receptors and is sensitive to the direct application of opioid drugs. In animals, lesions of the system reduce the analgesic effect of systemically administered opioids such as morphine. Along with the opioid receptor, the component nuclei of this pain-modulating circuit contain endogenous opioid peptides such as the enkephalins and β-endorphin.

The most reliable way to activate this endogenous opioid-mediated modulating system is by prolonged pain and/or fear. There is evidence that pain-relieving endogenous opioids are released following surgical procedures and in patients given a placebo for pain relief.

Pain-modulating circuits can enhance as well as suppress pain. Both pain-inhibiting and pain-facilitating neurons in the medulla project to and control spinal pain-transmission neurons. Since pain-transmission neurons can be activated by modulatory neurons, it is theoretically possible to generate a pain signal with no peripheral noxious stimulus. In fact, functional imaging studies have demonstrated increased activity in this circuit during migraine headache. A central circuit that facilitates pain could account for the finding that pain can be induced by suggestion and could provide a framework for understanding how psychological factors can contribute to chronic pain.

NEUROPATHIC PAIN Lesions of the peripheral or central nervous pathways for pain typically result in a loss or impairment of pain sensation. Paradoxically, damage or dysfunction of these pathways can produce pain. For example, damage to peripheral nerves, as occurs in diabetic neuropathy, or to primary afferents, as in herpes zoster, can result in pain that is referred to the body region innervated by the damaged nerves. Though rare, pain may also be produced by damage to the central nervous system, particularly the spinothalamic pathway or thalamus. Such neuropathic pains are often severe and are notoriously intractable to standard treatments for pain.

Neuropathic pains typically have an unusual burning, tingling, or electric shock–like quality and may be triggered by very light touch. These features are rare in other types of pain. On examination, a sensory deficit is characteristically present in the area of the patient's pain. Hyperpathia is also characteristic of neuropathic pain; patients often complain that the very lightest moving stimuli evoke exquisite pain (allodynia). In this regard it is of clinical interest that a topical preparation of 5% lidocaine in patch form is effective for patients with postherpetic neuralgia who have prominent allodynia.

A variety of mechanisms contribute to neuropathic pain. As with sensitized primary afferent nociceptors, damaged primary afferents, including nociceptors, become highly sensitive to mechanical stimulation and begin to generate impulses in the absence of stimulation. There is evidence that this increased sensitivity and spontaneous activity is due to an increased concentration of sodium channels. Damaged primary afferents may also develop sensitivity to norepinephrine. Interestingly, spinal cord pain-transmission neurons cut off from their normal input may also become spontaneously active. Thus both central and peripheral nervous system hyperactivity contribute to neuropathic pain.

Sympathetically Maintained Pain Patients with peripheral nerve injury can develop a severe burning pain (causalgia) in the region innervated by the nerve. The pain typically begins after a delay of hours to days or even weeks. The pain is accompanied by swelling of the extremity, periarticular osteoporosis, and arthritic changes in the distal joints. The pain is dramatically and immediately relieved by blocking the sympathetic innervation of the affected extremity. Damaged primary afferent nociceptors acquire adrenergic sensitivity and can be activated by stimulation of the sympathetic outflow. A similar syndrome called *reflex sympathetic dystrophy* can be produced without obvious nerve damage by a variety of injuries, including fractures of bone, soft tissue trauma, myocardial infarction, and stroke (Chap. 354). Although the pathophysiology of this condition is poorly understood, the pain and the signs of inflammation are rapidly relieved by blocking the sympathetic nervous system. This implies that sympathetic activity can activate undamaged nociceptors when inflammation is present. Signs of sympathetic hyperactivity should be sought in patients with posttraumatic pain and inflammation and no other obvious explanation.

℞ TREATMENT

ACUTE PAIN The ideal treatment for any pain is to remove the cause; thus diagnosis should always precede treatment planning. Sometimes treating the underlying condition does not immediately relieve pain. Furthermore, some conditions are so painful that rapid and effective analgesia is essential (e.g., the postoperative state, burns, trauma, cancer, sickle cell crisis). Analgesic medications are a first line of treatment in these cases, and all practitioners should be familiar with their use.

Aspirin, Acetaminophen, and Nonsteroidal Anti-Inflammatory Agents (NSAIDS) These drugs are considered together because they are used for similar problems and may have a similar mechanism of action (Table 11-1). All these compounds inhibit cyclooxygenase (COX), and, except for acetaminophen, all have anti-inflammatory actions, especially at higher dosages. They are particularly effective for mild to moderate headache and for pain of musculoskeletal origin.

Since they are effective for these common types of pain and are available without prescription, COX inhibitors are by far the most commonly used analgesics. They are absorbed well from the gastrointestinal tract and, with occasional use, side effects are minimal. With chronic use, gastric irritation is a common side effect of aspirin and NSAIDs and is the problem that most frequently limits the dose that can be given. Gastric irritation is most severe with aspirin, which may cause erosion of the gastric mucosa, and because aspirin irreversibly acetylates platelets and thereby interferes with coagulation of the blood, gastrointestinal bleeding is a risk. The NSAIDs are less prob-

TABLE 11-1 *Drugs for Relief of Pain*

Generic Name	Dose, mg	Interval	Comments
NONNARCOTIC ANALGESICS: USUAL DOSES AND INTERVALS			
Acetylsalicylic acid	650 PO	q 4 h	Enteric-coated preparations available
Acetaminophen	650 PO	q 4 h	Side effects uncommon
Ibuprofen	400 PO	q 4–6 h	Available without prescription
Naproxen	250–500 PO	q 12 h	Delayed effects may be due to long half-life
Fenoprofen	200 PO	q 4–6 h	Contraindicated in renal disease
Indomethacin	25–50 PO	q 8 h	Gastrointestinal side effects common
Ketorolac	15–60 IM	q 4–6 h	Available for parenteral use (IM)
Celecoxib	100–200 PO	q 12–24 h	Useful for arthritis

Generic Name	Parenteral Dose, mg	PO Dose, mg	Comments
NARCOTIC ANALGESICS: USUAL DOSES AND INTERVALS			
Codeine	30–60 q 4 h	30–60 q 4 h	Nausea common
Oxycodone	—	5–10 q 4–6 h	Usually available with acetaminophen or aspirin
Morphine	10 q 4 h	60 q 4 h	
Morphine sustained release	—	30–200 bid to tid	Oral slow-release preparation
Hydromorphone	1–2 q 4 h	2–4 q 4 h	Shorter acting than morphine sulfate
Levorphanol	2 q 6–8 h	4 q 6–8 h	Longer acting than morphine sulfate; absorbed well PO
Methadone	10 q 6–8 h	20 q 6–8 h	Delayed sedation due to long half-life
Meperidine	75–100 q 3–4 h	300 q 4 h	Poorly absorbed PO; normeperidine a toxic metabolite
Butorphanol	—	1–2 q 4 h	Intranasal spray
Fentanyl	25–100 μg/h	—	72 h Transdermal patch
Tramadol	—	50–100 q 4–6 h	Mixed opioid/adrenergic action

Generic Name	Uptake Blockade 5-HT	Uptake Blockade NE	Sedative Potency	Anticholinergic Potency	Orthostatic Hypotension	Cardiac Arrhythmia	Ave. Dose, mg/d	Range, mg/d
ANTIDEPRESSANTS[a]								
Doxepin	++	+	High	Moderate	Moderate	Less	200	75–400
Amitriptyline	++++	++	High	Highest	Moderate	Yes	150	25–300
Imipramine	++++	++	Moderate	Moderate	High	Yes	200	75–400
Nortriptyline	+++	++	Moderate	Moderate	Low	Yes	100	40–150
Desipramine	+++	++++	Low	Low	Low	Yes	150	50–300
Venlafaxine	+++	++	Low	None	None	No	150	75–400

Generic Name	PO Dose, mg	Interval	Generic Name	PO Dose, mg	Interval
ANTICONVULSANTS AND ANTIARRHYTHMICS[a]					
Phenytoin	300	daily/qhs	Clonazepam	1	q 6 h
Carbamazepine	200–300	q 6 h	Mexiletine	150–300	q 6–12 h
Oxcarbazine	300	bid	Gabapentin[b]	600–1200	q 8 h

[a] Antidepressants, anticonvulsants, and antiarrhythmics have not been approved by the U.S. Food and Drug Administration (FDA) for the treatment of pain.

[b] Gabapentin in doses up to 1800 mg/d is FDA approved for postherpetic neuralgia.

Note: 5-HT, serotonin; NE, norepinephrine.

lematic, but their risk in this regard is still significant. In addition to their well known gastrointestinal toxicity, nephrotoxicity is a significant problem for patients using NSAIDs on a chronic basis, and patients at risk for renal insufficiency should be monitored closely. NSAIDs also cause an increase in blood pressure in a significant number of individuals. Long-term treatment with NSAIDs requires regular blood pressure monitoring and treatment if necessary. Although toxic to the liver when taken in a high dose, acetaminophen rarely produces gastric irritation and does not interfere with platelet function.

The introduction of a parenteral form of NSAID, ketorolac, extends the usefulness of this class of compounds in the management of acute severe pain. Ketorolac is sufficiently potent and rapid in onset to supplant opioids for many patients with acute severe headache and musculoskeletal pain.

There are two major classes of COX: COX-1 is constitutively ex-pressed, and COX-2 is induced in the inflammatory state. COX-2-selective drugs have moderate analgesic potency and produce less gastric irritation than the nonselective COX inhibitors. It is not yet clear whether the use of COX-2-selective drugs is associated with a lower risk of nephrotoxicity compared to nonselective NSAIDs. On the other hand, COX-2-selective drugs offer a significant benefit in the management of acute postoperative pain because they do not affect blood coagulation. This is a situation in which the nonselective COX inhibitors would be contraindicated because they impair platelet-mediated blood clotting and are thus associated with increased bleeding at the operative site. A corollary of this is that COX-2 drugs do not provide the same degree of protection from thromboembolic cardiovascular adverse events such as myocardial infarction. In fact, in patients treated for arthritis, those treated with naproxen had significantly fewer adverse thromboembolic events than those treated with rofecoxib, a selective COX-2 inhibitor.

Opioid Analgesics Opioids are the most potent pain-relieving drugs currently available. Furthermore, of all analgesics, they have the broadest range of efficacy, providing the most reliable and effective method for rapid pain relief. Although side effects are common, they are usually not serious except for respiratory depression and can be reversed rapidly with the narcotic antagonist naloxone. The physician should not hesitate to use opioid analgesics in patients with acute severe pain. Table 11-1 lists the most commonly used opioid analgesics.

Opioids produce analgesia by actions in the central nervous system. They activate pain-inhibitory neurons and directly inhibit pain-transmission neurons. Most of the commercially available opioid analgesics act at the same opioid receptor (mu receptor), differing mainly in potency, speed of onset, duration of action, and optimal route of administration. Although the dose-related side effects (sedation, respiratory depression, pruritus, constipation) are similar among the different opioids, some side effects are due to accumulation of nonopioid metabolites that are unique to individual drugs. One striking example of this is normeperidine, a metabolite of meperidine. Normeperidine produces hyperexcitability and seizures that are not reversible with naloxone. Normeperidine accumulation is increased in patients with renal failure.

The most rapid relief with opioids is obtained by intravenous administration; relief with oral administration is significantly slower. Common acute side effects include nausea, vomiting, and sedation. The most serious side effect is respiratory depression. Patients with any form of respiratory compromise must be kept under close observation following opioid administration; an oxygen saturation monitor may be useful. The opioid antagonist, naloxone, should be readily available. Opioid effects are dose-related, and there is great variability among patients in the doses that relieve pain and produce side effects. Because of this, initiation of therapy requires titration to optimal dose and interval. The most important principle is to provide adequate pain relief. This requires determining whether the drug has adequately relieved the pain and the duration of the relief. *The most common error made by physicians in managing severe pain with opioids is to prescribe an inadequate dose. Since many patients are reluctant to complain, this practice leads to needless suffering.* In the absence of sedation at the expected time of peak effect, a physician should not hesitate to repeat the initial dose to achieve satisfactory pain relief.

An innovative approach to the problem of achieving adequate pain relief is the use of patient-controlled analgesia (PCA). PCA requires a device that delivers a baseline continuous dose of an opioid drug, and preprogrammed additional doses whenever the patient pushes a button. The device can be programmed to limit the total hourly dose so that overdosing is impossible. The patient can then titrate the dose to the optimal level. This approach is used most extensively for the management of postoperative pain, but there is no reason why it should not be used for any hospitalized patient with persistent severe pain. PCA is also used for short-term home care of patients with intractable pain, such as is caused by metastatic cancer.

Many physicians, nurses, and patients have a certain trepidation about using opioids that is based on an exaggerated fear of addiction. In fact, there is a vanishingly small chance of patients becoming addicted to narcotics as a result of their appropriate medical use.

The availability of new routes of administration has extended the usefulness of opioid analgesics. Most important is the availability of spinal administration. Opioids can be infused through a spinal catheter placed either intrathecally or epidurally. By applying opioids directly to the spinal cord, regional analgesia can be obtained using a relatively low total dose. In this way, such side effects as sedation, nausea, and respiratory depression can be minimized. This approach has been used extensively in obstetric procedures and for lower-body postoperative pain. Opioids can also be given intranasally (butorphanol), rectally, and transdermally (fentanyl), thus avoiding the discomfort of frequent injections in patients who cannot be given oral medication. The fentanyl transdermal patch has the advantage of providing fairly steady plasma levels, which maximizes patient comfort.

OPIOID AND CYCLOOXYGENASE INHIBITOR COMBINATIONS   When used in combination, opioids and COX inhibitors have additive effects. Because a lower dose of each can be used to achieve the same degree of pain relief and their side effects are nonadditive, such combinations can be used to lower the severity of dose-related side effects. Fixed-ratio combinations of an opioid with acetaminophen carry a special risk. Dose escalation as a result of increased severity of pain or decreased opioid effect as a result of tolerance may lead to levels of acetaminophen that are toxic to the liver.

CHRONIC PAIN

Managing patients with chronic pain is intellectually and emotionally challenging. The patient's problem is often difficult to diagnose; such patients are demanding of the physician's time and often appear emotionally distraught. The traditional medical approach of seeking an obscure organic pathology is usually unhelpful. On the other hand, psychological evaluation and behaviorally based treatment paradigms are frequently helpful, particularly in the setting of a multidisciplinary pain-management center.

There are several factors that can cause, perpetuate, or exacerbate chronic pain. First, of course, the patient may simply have a disease that is characteristically painful for which there is presently no cure. Arthritis, cancer, migraine headaches, fibromyalgia, and diabetic neuropathy are examples of this. Second, there may be secondary perpetuating factors that are initiated by disease and persist after that disease has resolved. Examples include damaged sensory nerves, sympathetic efferent activity, and painful reflex muscle contraction. Finally, a variety of psychological conditions can exacerbate or even cause pain.

There are certain areas to which special attention should be paid in the medical history. Because depression is the most common emotional disturbance in patients with chronic pain, patients should be questioned about their mood, appetite, sleep patterns, and daily activity. A simple standardized questionnaire, such as the Beck Depression Inventory, can be a useful screening device. It is important to remember that major depression is a common, treatable, and potentially fatal illness.

Other clues that a significant emotional disturbance is contributing to a patient's chronic pain complaint include: pain that occurs in multiple unrelated sites; a pattern of recurrent, but separate, pain problems beginning in childhood or adolescence; pain beginning at a time of emotional trauma, such as the loss of a parent or spouse; a history of physical or sexual abuse; and past or present substance abuse.

On examination, special attention should be paid to whether the patient guards the painful area and whether certain movements or postures are avoided because of pain. Discovering a mechanical component to the pain can be useful both diagnostically and therapeutically. Painful areas should be examined for deep tenderness, noting whether this is localized to muscle, ligamentous structures, or joints. Chronic myofascial pain is very common, and in these patients deep palpation may reveal highly localized trigger points that are firm bands or knots in muscle. Relief of the pain following injection of local anesthetic into these trigger points supports the diagnosis. A neuropathic component to the pain is indicated by evidence of nerve damage, such as sensory impairment, exquisitely sensitive skin, weakness and muscle atrophy, or loss of deep tendon reflexes. Evidence suggesting sympathetic nervous system involvement includes the presence of diffuse swelling, changes in skin color and temperature, and hypersensitive skin and joint tenderness compared with the normal side. Relief of the pain with a sympathetic block is diagnostic.

A guiding principle in evaluating patients with chronic pain is to assess both emotional and organic factors before initiating therapy. Addressing these issues together, rather than waiting to address emotional issues after organic causes of pain have been ruled out, improves compliance in part because it assures patients that a psychological evaluation does not mean that the physician is questioning the validity of their complaint. Even when an organic cause for a patient's pain can be found, it is still wise to look for other factors. For example, a cancer patient with painful bony metastases may have additional pain due to nerve damage and may also be depressed. Optimal therapy requires that each of these factors be looked for and treated.

℞ TREATMENT

Once the evaluation process has been completed and the likely causative and exacerbating factors identified, an explicit treatment plan should be developed. An important part of this process is to identify specific and realistic functional goals for therapy, such as getting a good night's sleep, being able to go shopping, or returning to work. A multidisciplinary approach that utilizes medications, counseling, physical therapy, nerve blocks, and even surgery may be required to improve the patient's quality of life. There are also some newer, relatively invasive procedures that can be helpful for some patients with intractable pain. These procedures include implanting intraspinal cannulae to deliver morphine or intraspinal electrodes for spinal stimulation. There are no set criteria for predicting which patients will respond to these procedures. They are generally reserved for patients who have not responded to conventional pharmacologic approaches. Referral to a multidisciplinary pain clinic for a full evaluation should precede any of these procedures. Such referrals are clearly not necessary for all chronic pain patients. For some, pharmacologic management alone can often provide adequate relief.

ANTIDEPRESSANT MEDICATIONS   The tricyclic antidepressants (TCAs; Table 11-1) are extremely useful for the management of patients with chronic pain. Although developed for the treatment of depression, the tricyclics have a spectrum of dose-related biologic activities that include the production of analgesia in a variety of clinical conditions. Although the mechanism is unknown, the analgesic effect of TCAs has a more rapid onset and occurs at a lower dose than is typically required for the treatment of depression. Furthermore, patients with chronic pain who are not depressed obtain pain relief with antidepressants. There is evidence that tricyclic drugs potentiate opioid analgesia, so they are useful adjuncts for the treatment of severe persistent pain such as occurs with malignant tumors. Table 11-2 lists some of the painful conditions that respond to tricyclics. TCAs are of particular value in the management of neuropathic pain such as occurs in diabetic neuropathy and postherpetic neuralgia, for which there are few other therapeutic options.

The TCAs that have been shown to relieve pain have significant side effects (Table 11-1; Chap. 371). Some of these side effects, such as orthostatic hypotension, cardiac conduction delay, memory impairment, constipation, and urinary retention, are particularly problematic in elderly patients, and several are additive to the side effects of opioid analgesics. The serotonin-selective reuptake inhibitors such as fluoxetine (Prozac) have fewer and less serious side effects than TCAs, but they are much less effective for relieving pain. It is of interest that venlafaxine (Effexor), a nontricyclic antidepressant that blocks both serotonin and norepinephrine reuptake, appears to retain most of the pain-relieving effect of TCAs with a side-effect profile more like that of the serotonin-selective reuptake inhibitors. The drug may be particularly useful in patients who cannot tolerate the side effects of tricyclics.

ANTICONVULSANTS AND ANTIARRHYTHMICS (Table 11-1) These drugs are useful primarily for patients with neuropathic pain. Phenytoin (Dilantin) and carbamazepine (Tegretol) were first shown to relieve the pain of trigeminal neuralgia. This pain has a characteristic brief, shooting, electric shock–like quality. In fact, anticonvulsants seem to be helpful largely for pains that have such a lancinating quality. A new-generation anticonvulsant, gabapentin (Neurontin), is effective for a broad range of neuropathic pains.

Antiarrhythmic drugs such as low-dose lidocaine and mexiletine (Mexitil) can also be effective for neuropathic pain. These drugs block the spontaneous activity of damaged primary afferent nociceptors.

CHRONIC OPIOID MEDICATION The long-term use of opioids is accepted for patients with pain due to malignant disease. Although opioid use for chronic pain of nonmalignant origin is controversial, it is clear that for many such patients opioid analgesics are the best available option. This is understandable since opioids are the most potent and have the broadest range of efficacy of any analgesic medications. Although addiction is rare in patients who first use opioids for pain relief, some degree of tolerance and physical dependence are likely with long-term use. Therefore, before embarking on opioid therapy, other options should be explored, and the limitations and risks of opioids should be explained to the patient. It is also important to point out that some opioid analgesic medications have mixed agonist-antagonist properties (e.g., pentazocine and butorphanol). From a practical standpoint, this means that they may worsen pain by inducing an abstinence syndrome in patients who are physically dependent on other opioid analgesics.

With long-term outpatient use of orally administered opioids, it is desirable to use long-acting compounds such as levorphanol, methadone, or sustained-release morphine (Table 11-1). Transdermal fentanyl is another excellent option. The pharmacokinetic profile of these drug preparations enables prolonged pain relief, minimizes side effects such as sedation that are associated with high peak plasma levels, and reduces the likelihood of rebound pain associated with a rapid fall in plasma opioid concentration. Constipation is a virtually universal side effect of opioid use and should be treated expectantly.

It is worth emphasizing that many patients, especially those with chronic pain, seek medical attention primarily because they are suffering and because only physicians can provide the medications required for their relief. A primary responsibility of all physicians is to minimize the physical and emotional discomfort of their patients. Familiarity with pain mechanisms and analgesic medications is an important step toward accomplishing this aim.

FURTHER READING

CRAIG AD: How do you feel? Interoception: The sense of the physiological condition of the body. Nat Rev Neurosci:655, 2002

PETROVIC P et al: Placebo and opioid analgesia—imaging a shared neuronal network. Science:1737, 2002

TABLE 11-2 *Painful Conditions that Respond to Tricyclic Antidepressants*

Postherpetic neuralgia[a]	Rheumatoid arthritis[a,b]
Diabetic neuropathy[a]	Chronic low back pain[b]
Tension headache[a]	Cancer
Migraine headache[a]	Central post-stroke pain

[a] Controlled trials demonstrate analgesia.
[b] Controlled studies indicate benefit but not analgesia.

12 CHEST DISCOMFORT AND PALPITATIONS
Thomas H. Lee

CHEST DISCOMFORT

Chest discomfort is one of the most common challenges for clinicians in the office or emergency department. The differential diagnosis includes conditions affecting organs throughout the thorax and abdomen, with prognostic implications that vary from benign to life-threatening (Table 12-1). Failure to recognize potentially serious conditions such as acute ischemic heart disease, aortic dissection, tension pneumothorax, or pulmonary embolism can lead to serious complications, including death. Conversely, overly conservative management of low-risk patients leads to unnecessary hospital admissions, tests, procedures, and anxiety.

CAUSES OF CHEST DISCOMFORT

MYOCARDIAL ISCHEMIA AND INJURY (See also Chap. 226) Myocardial ischemia occurs when the oxygen supply to the heart is not sufficient

TABLE 12-1 *Differential Diagnoses of Patients Admitted to Hospital with Acute Chest Pain Ruled Not Myocardial Infarction*

Diagnosis	Percent
Gastroesophageal disease[a]	42
Gastroesophageal reflux	
Esophageal motility disorders	
Peptic ulcer	
Gallstones	
Ischemic heart disease	31
Chest wall syndromes	28
Pericarditis	4
Pleuritis/pneumonia	2
Pulmonary embolism	2
Lung cancer	1.5
Aortic aneurysm	1
Aortic stenosis	1
Herpes zoster	1

[a] In order of frequency.
Source: Fruergaard P et al: Eur Heart J 17:1028, 1996.

to meet metabolic needs. This mismatch can result from a decrease in oxygen supply, a rise in demand, or both. The most common underlying cause of myocardial ischemia is obstruction of coronary arteries by atherosclerosis; in the presence of such obstruction, transient ischemic episodes are usually precipitated by an increase in oxygen demand as a result of physical exertion. However, ischemia can also result from psychological stress, fever, or large meals or from compromised oxygen delivery due to anemia, hypoxia, or hypotension. Ventricular hypertrophy due to valvular heart disease, hypertrophic cardiomyopathy, or hypertension can predispose the myocardium to ischemia because of impaired penetration of blood flow from epicardial coronary arteries to the endocardium.

Angina Pectoris   The chest discomfort of myocardial ischemia is a visceral discomfort that is usually described as a heaviness, pressure, or squeezing (Table 12-2). Other common adjectives for anginal pain are burning and aching. Some patients deny any "pain" but may admit to dyspnea or a vague sense of anxiety. The word "sharp" is sometimes used by patients to describe intensity rather than quality.

The location of angina pectoris is usually retrosternal; most patients do not localize the pain to any small area. The discomfort may radiate to the neck, jaw, teeth, arms, or shoulders, reflecting the common origin in the posterior horn of the spinal cord of sensory neurons supplying the heart and these areas. Some patients present with aching in sites of radiated pain as their only symptoms of ischemia. Occasional patients report epigastric distress with ischemic episodes. Less common is radiation to below the umbilicus or to the back.

Stable angina pectoris usually develops gradually with exertion, emotional excitement, or after heavy meals. Rest or treatment with sublingual nitroglycerin typically leads to relief within several minutes. In contrast, pain that is fleeting (lasting only a few seconds) is rarely ischemic in origin. Similarly, pain that lasts for several hours is unlikely to represent angina, particularly if the patient's electrocardiogram does not show evidence of ischemia.

Anginal episodes can be precipitated by any physiologic or psychological stress that induces tachycardia. Most myocardial perfusion occurs during diastole, when there is minimal pressure opposing coronary artery flow from within the left ventricle. Since tachycardia decreases the percentage of the time in which the heart is in diastole, it decreases myocardial perfusion.

TABLE 12-2   *Typical Clinical Features of Major Causes of Acute Chest Discomfort*

Condition	Duration	Quality	Location	Associated Features
Angina	More than 2 and less than 10 min	Pressure, tightness, squeezing, heaviness, burning	Retrosternal, often with radiation to or isolated discomfort in neck, jaw, shoulders, or arms—frequently on left	Precipitated by exertion, exposure to cold, psychologic stress S4 gallop or mitral regurgitation murmur during pain
Unstable angina	10–20 min	Similar to angina but often more severe	Similar to angina	Similar to angina, but occurs with low levels of exertion or even at rest
Acute myocardial infarction	Variable; often more than 30 min	Similar to angina but often more severe	Similar to angina	Unrelieved by nitroglycerin May be associated with evidence of heart failure or arrhythmia
Aortic stenosis	Recurrent episodes as described for angina	As described for angina	As described for angina	Late-peaking systolic murmur radiating to carotid arteries
Pericarditis	Hours to days; may be episodic	Sharp	Retrosternal or toward cardiac apex; may radiate to left shoulder	May be relieved by sitting up and leaning forward Pericardial friction rub
Aortic dissection	Abrupt onset of unrelenting pain	Tearing or ripping sensation; knifelike	Anterior chest, often radiating to back, between shoulder blades	Associated with hypertension and/or underlying connective tissue disorder, e.g., Marfan syndrome Murmur of aortic insufficiency, pericardial rub, pericardial tamponade, or loss of peripheral pulses
Pulmonary embolism	Abrupt onset; several minutes to a few hours	Pleuritic	Often lateral, on the side of the embolism	Dyspnea, tachypnea, tachycardia, and hypotension
Pulmonary hypertension	Variable	Pressure	Substernal	Dyspnea, signs of increased venous pressure including edema and jugular venous distention
Pneumonia or pleuritis	Variable	Pleuritic	Unilateral, often localized	Dyspnea, cough, fever, rales, occasional rub
Spontaneous pneumothorax	Sudden onset; several hours	Pleuritic	Lateral to side of pneumothorax	Dyspnea, decreased breath sounds on side of pneumothorax
Esophageal reflux	10–60 min	Burning	Substernal, epigastric	Worsened by postprandial recumbency Relieved by antacids
Esophageal spasm	2–30 min	Pressure, tightness, burning	Retrosternal	Can closely mimic angina
Peptic ulcer	Prolonged	Burning	Epigastric, substernal	Relieved with food or antacids
Gallbladder disease	Prolonged	Burning, pressure	Epigastric, right upper quadrant, substernal	May follow meal
Musculoskeletal disease	Variable	Aching	Variable	Aggravated by movement May be reproduced by localized pressure on examination
Herpes zoster	Variable	Sharp or burning	Dermatomal distribution	Vesicular rash in area of discomfort
Emotional and psychiatric conditions	Variable; may be fleeting	Variable	Variable; may be retrosternal	Situational factors may precipitate symptoms Anxiety or depression often detectable with careful history

Unstable Angina and Myocardial Infarction (See also Chaps. 227 and 228) Patients with these acute ischemic syndromes usually complain of symptoms similar in quality to angina pectoris, but more prolonged and severe. The onset of these syndromes may occur with the patient at rest, or awakened from sleep, and sublingual nitroglycerin may lead to transient or no relief. Accompanying symptoms may include diaphoresis, dyspnea, nausea, and light-headedness.

The physical examination may be completely normal in patients with chest discomfort due to ischemic heart disease. Careful auscultation during ischemic episodes may reveal a third or fourth heart sound, reflecting myocardial systolic or diastolic dysfunction. A transient murmur of mitral regurgitation suggests ischemic papillary muscle dysfunction. Severe episodes of ischemia can lead to pulmonary congestion and even pulmonary edema.

Other Cardiac Causes Myocardial ischemia caused by hypertrophic cardiomyopathy, aortic stenosis, or other conditions leads to angina pectoris similar to that caused by coronary atherosclerosis. In such cases, a systolic murmur or other findings usually suggest the abnormalities other than coronary atherosclerosis that may be contributing to the patient's symptoms. Some patients with chest pain and normal coronary angiograms have functional abnormalities of the coronary circulation, ranging from coronary spasm visible on coronary angiography to abnormal vasodilator responses and heightened vasoconstrictor responses. The term "Syndrome X" is used to describe patients with angina-like chest pain and ischemic-appearing ST segment depression during stress despite normal coronary arteriograms. Some data indicate that many such patients have limited changes in coronary flow in response to pacing stress or coronary vasodilators. Despite the possibility that chest pain may be due to myocardial ischemia in such patients, their prognosis is excellent.

PERICARDITIS (See also Chap. 222) The pain in pericarditis is believed to be due to inflammation of the adjacent parietal pleura, since most of the pericardium is believed to be insensitive to pain. Thus, infectious pericarditis, which usually involves adjoining pleura surfaces, tends to be associated with pain, while conditions that cause only local inflammation (e.g., myocardial infarction or uremia) and cardiac tamponade tend to result in mild or no chest pain.

The adjacent parietal pleura receives its sensory supply from several sources, so the pain of pericarditis can be experienced in areas ranging from the shoulder and neck to the abdomen and back. Most typically, the pain is retrosternal and is aggravated by coughing, deep breaths, or changes in position—all of which lead to movements of pleural surfaces. The pain is often worse in the supine position and relieved by sitting upright and leaning forward. Less common is a steady aching discomfort that mimics acute myocardial infarction.

DISEASES OF THE AORTA (See also Chap. 231) *Aortic dissection* is a potentially catastrophic condition that is due to spread within the wall of the aorta of a subintimal hematoma. The hematoma may begin with a tear in the intima of the aorta or with rupture of the vasa vasorum within the aortic media. This syndrome can occur with trauma to the aorta, including motor vehicle accidents or medical procedures in which catheters or intraaortic balloon pumps damage the intima of the aorta. Nontraumatic aortic dissections are rare in the absence of hypertension and/or conditions associated with deterioration of the elastic or muscular components of the media within the aorta's wall. Cystic medial degeneration is a feature of several inherited connective tissue diseases, including Marfan and Ehlers-Danlos syndromes. About half of all aortic dissections in women under 40 years of age occur during pregnancy.

Almost all patients with acute dissections present with severe chest pain, although some patients with chronic dissections are identified without associated symptoms. Unlike the pain of ischemic heart disease, symptoms of aortic dissection tend to reach peak severity immediately, often causing the patient to collapse from its intensity. The adjectives used to describe the pain reflect the process occurring within the wall of the aorta—"ripping" and "tearing"—and the location usually correlates with the site and extent of the dissection. Thus, dissections that begin in the ascending aorta and extend to the descending aorta tend to cause pain in the front of the chest that extends into the back, between the shoulder blades.

Physical findings may also reflect extension of the aortic dissection that compromises flow into arteries branching off the aorta. Thus, loss of a pulse in one or both arms, cerebrovascular accident, or paraplegia can all be catastrophic consequences of aortic dissection. Hematomas that extend proximally and undermine the coronary arteries or aortic valve apparatus may lead to acute myocardial infarction or acute aortic insufficiency. Rupture of the hematoma into the pericardial space leads to pericardial tamponade.

Another abnormality of the aorta that can cause chest pain is a *thoracic aortic aneurysm*. Aortic aneurysms are frequently asymptomatic but can cause chest pain and other symptoms by compressing adjacent structures. This pain tends to be steady, deep, and sometimes severe.

PULMONARY EMBOLISM (See also Chap. 244) Chest pain due to pulmonary embolism is believed to be due to distention of the pulmonary artery or infarction of a segment of the lung adjacent to the pleura. Massive pulmonary emboli may lead to substernal pain that is suggestive of acute myocardial infarction. More commonly, smaller emboli lead to focal pulmonary infarctions that cause pain that is lateral and pleuritic. Associated symptoms include dyspnea and, occasionally, hemoptysis. Tachycardia is usually present. Although not always present, certain characteristic ECG changes can support the diagnosis.

PNEUMOTHORAX (See also Chap. 245) Sudden onset of pleuritic chest pain and respiratory distress should lead to consideration of spontaneous pneumothorax, as well as pulmonary embolism. Such events may occur without a precipitating event in people without lung disease, or as a consequence of underlying lung disorders.

PNEUMONIA OR PLEURITIS (See also Chaps. 239 and 245) Lung diseases that damage and cause inflammation of the pleura of the lung usually cause a sharp, knifelike pain that is aggravated by inspiration or coughing.

GASTROINTESTINAL CONDITIONS (See also Chap. 273) Esophageal pain from acid reflux from the stomach, spasm, obstruction, or injury can be difficult to discern from myocardial syndromes. Acid reflux typically causes a deep burning discomfort that may be exacerbated by alcohol, aspirin, or some foods; this discomfort is often relieved by antacid or other acid-reducing therapies. Acid reflux tends to be exacerbated by lying down and may be worse in early morning when the stomach is empty of food that might otherwise absorb gastric acid.

Esophageal spasm may occur in the presence or absence of acid reflux, and leads to a squeezing pain indistinguishable from angina. Prompt relief of esophageal spasm is often provided by antianginal therapies such as sublingual nifedipine, further promoting confusion between these syndromes. Chest pain can also result from injury to the esophagus, such as a Mallory-Weiss tear caused by severe vomiting.

Chest pain can result from diseases of the gastrointestinal tract below the diaphragm, including *peptic ulcer disease*, *biliary disease*, and *pancreatitis*. These conditions usually cause abdominal pain as well as chest discomfort; symptoms are not likely to be associated with exertion. The pain of ulcer disease typically occurs 60 to 90 min after meals, when postprandial acid production is no longer neutralized by food in the stomach. Cholecystitis usually causes a pain that is described as aching, occurring an hour or more after meals.

NEUROMUSCULOSKELETAL CONDITIONS *Cervical disk disease* can cause chest pain by compression of nerve roots. Pain in a dermatomal distribution can also be caused by *intercostal muscle cramps* or by *herpes zoster*. Chest pain symptoms due to herpes zoster may occur before skin lesions are apparent.

Costochondral and *chondrosternal syndromes* are the most common causes of anterior chest musculoskeletal pain. Only occasionally are physical signs of costochondritis such as swelling, redness, and warmth (Tietze's syndrome) present. The pain of such syndromes is usually fleeting and sharp, but some patients experience a dull ache that lasts for hours. Direct pressure on the chondrosternal and costochondral junctions may reproduce the pain from these and other musculoskeletal syndromes. Arthritis of the shoulder and spine and bursitis may also cause chest pain. Some patients who have these conditions and myocardial ischemia blur and confuse symptoms of these syndromes.

EMOTIONAL AND PSYCHIATRIC CONDITIONS As many as 10% of patients who present to emergency departments with acute chest pain have panic disorder or other emotional conditions. The symptoms in these populations are highly variable, but frequently the discomfort is described as visceral tightness or aching that lasts more than 30 min. Some patients offer other atypical descriptions, such as pain that is fleeting, sharp, and/or localized to a small region. The electrocardiogram in patients with emotional conditions may be difficult to interpret if hyperventilation causes ST-T-wave abnormalities. A careful history may elicit clues of depression, prior panic attacks, somatization, agoraphobia, or other phobias.

APPROACH TO THE PATIENT

The evaluation of the patient with chest discomfort must accommodate two goals—determining the diagnosis and assessing the safety of the immediate management plan. The latter issue is often dominant when the patient has acute chest discomfort, such as patients seen in the emergency department. In such settings, the clinician must focus first on identifying patients who require aggressive interventions to diagnose or manage potentially life-threatening conditions, including acute ischemic heart disease, acute aortic dissection, pulmonary embolism, and tension pneumothorax. If such conditions are unlikely, the clinician must address questions such as the safety of discharge to home, admission to a non-coronary care unit facility, or immediate exercise testing. Table 12-3 displays a sequence of questions that can be used in the evaluation of the patient with chest discomfort, with the diagnostic entities that are most important for consideration at each stage of the evaluation.

ACUTE CHEST DISCOMFORT In patients with acute chest discomfort, the clinician must first assess the patient's respiratory and hemodynamic status. If either is compromised, initial management should focus on stabilizing the patient before the diagnostic evaluation is pursued. If, however, the patient does not require emergent interventions, then a focused history, physical examination,

and laboratory evaluation should be performed to assess the patient's risk of life-threatening conditions.

The *history* should include questions about the quality and location of the chest discomfort (Table 12-2). The patient should also be asked about the nature of onset of the pain and its duration. Myocardial ischemia is usually associated with a gradual intensification of symptoms over a period of minutes. Pain that is fleeting or that lasts hours without being associated with electrocardiographic changes is not likely to be ischemic in origin. Although the presence of risk factors for coronary artery disease may heighten concern for this diagnosis, the absence of such risk factors does not lower the risk for myocardial ischemia enough to be used to justify a decision to discharge a patient.

Wide radiation of chest pain increases probability that pain is due to myocardial infarction. Radiation of chest pain to the left arm is common with acute ischemic heart disease, but radiation to the right arm is also consistent with this diagnosis. Right shoulder pain is common with acute cholecystitis, but this syndrome is usually accompanied by pain that is located in the abdomen rather than chest. Chest pain that radiates between the scapulae raises the question of aortic dissection.

The *physical examination* should include evaluation of blood pressure in both arms and of pulses in both legs. Poor perfusion of a limb may be due to an aortic dissection that has compromised flow to an artery branching from the aorta. Chest auscultation may reveal diminished breath sounds; a pleural rub; or evidence of pneumothorax, pulmonary embolism, pneumonia, or pleurisy. Tension pneumothorax may lead to a shift in the trachea from the midline, away from the side of the pneumothorax. The cardiac examination should seek pericardial rubs, systolic and diastolic murmurs, and third or fourth heart sounds. Pressure on the chest wall may reproduce symptoms in patients with musculoskeletal causes of chest pain; it is important that the clinician ask the patient if the chest pain syndrome is being completely reproduced before drawing too much reassurance that more serious underlying conditions are not present.

An *electrocardiogram* is an essential test for adults with chest discomfort that is not due to an obvious traumatic cause. In such patients, the presence of electrocardiographic changes consistent with ischemia or infarction (Chap. 210) is associated with high risks of acute myocardial infarction or unstable angina (Table 12-4); such patients should be admitted to a unit with electrocardiographic monitoring and the capacity to respond to a cardiac arrest. The absence of such changes does not exclude acute ischemic heart

TABLE 12-3   Considerations in the Assessment of the Patient with Chest Pain

1. Could the chest discomfort be due to an acute, potentially life-threatening condition that warrants immediate hospitalization and aggressive evaluation?

Acute ischemic heart disease	Pulmonary embolism
Aortic dissection	Spontaneous pneumothorax

2. If not, could the discomfort be due to a chronic condition likely to lead to serious complications?

    Stable angina
    Aortic stenosis
    Pulmonary hypertension

3. If not, could the discomfort be due to an acute condition that warrants specific treatment?

    Pericarditis
    Pneumonia/pleuritis
    Herpes zoster

4. If not, could the discomfort be due to another treatable chronic condition?

Esophageal reflux	Cervical disk disease
Esophageal spasm	Arthritis of the shoulder or spine
Peptic ulcer disease	Costochondritis
Gallbladder disease	Other musculoskeletal disorders
Other gastrointestinal conditions	Anxiety state

TABLE 12-4   Prevalence of Myocardial Infarction and Unstable Angina Among Subsets of Patients with Acute Chest Pain in the Emergency Department

	Prevalence	
Finding	Myocardial Infarction, %	Unstable Angina, %
ST elevation (≥1 mm) or Q waves on ECG not known to be old	79	12
Ischemia or strain on ECG not known to be old (ST depression ≥1 mm or ischemic T waves)	20	41
None of the preceding ECG changes but a prior history of angina or myocardial infarction (history of heart attack or nitroglycerin use)	4	51
None of the preceding ECG changes and no prior history of angina or myocardial infarction (history of heart attack or nitroglycerin use)	2	14

Note: ECG, electrocardiogram.
Source: Unpublished data from Brigham and Women's Hospital Chest Pain Study, 1997–1999.

disease, but the risk of life-threatening complications is low for patients with normal electrocardiograms or only nonspecific ST-T-wave changes. If these patients are not considered appropriate for immediate discharge, they are often candidates for early or immediate exercise testing.

Markers of myocardial injury are often obtained in the emergency department evaluation of acute chest discomfort. The most commonly used markers are creatine kinase (CK), CK-MB, and the cardiac troponins (I and T). Rapid bedside assays of the cardiac troponins have been developed and shown to be sufficiently accurate to predict prognosis and guide management. Some data support the use of other markers, such as serum myoglobin, C-reactive protein (CRP), and B-type natriuretic peptide (BNP); their roles are the subject of ongoing research. Single values of any of these markers do not have high sensitivity for acute myocardial infarction or for prediction of complications. Hence, decisions to discharge patients home should not be made on the basis of single negative values of these tests.

Provocative tests for coronary artery disease are not appropriate for patients with ongoing chest pain. In such patients, rest myocardial perfusion scans can be considered; a normal scan reduces the likelihood of coronary artery disease, and can help avoid admission of low-risk patients to the hospital. Clinicians frequently employ therapeutic trials with sublingual nitroglycerin or antacids or, in the stable patient seen in the office setting, a proton pump inhibitor. A common error is to assume that a response to any of these interventions clarifies the diagnosis. While such information is often helpful, the patient's response may be due to the placebo effect. Hence, myocardial ischemia should never be considered excluded solely because of a response to antacid therapy. Similarly, failure of nitroglycerin to relieve pain does not exclude the diagnosis of coronary disease.

If the patient's history or examination is consistent with aortic dissection, imaging studies to evaluate the aorta must be pursued promptly because of the high risk of catastrophic complications with this condition. A chest x-ray is not sufficient to exclude this diagnosis. Appropriate tests include a chest computed tomography scan with contrast or a magnetic resonance imaging scan in patients who are hemodynamically stable, or a transesophageal echocardiogram in patients who are less stable. Aortic angiography is no longer a first test at most institutions.

Acute pulmonary embolism should be considered in patients with respiratory symptoms, pleuritic chest pain, hemoptysis, or a history of venous thromboembolism or coagulation abnormalities. Initial tests usually include a lung scan and/or pulmonary arteriography.

If patients with acute chest discomfort show no evidence of life-threatening conditions, the clinician should then focus on serious chronic conditions with the potential to cause major complications, the most common of which is stable angina. Early use of exercise electrocardiography, stress echocardiography, or stress perfusion imaging for such patients, whether in the office or the emergency department, is now an accepted management strategy for low-risk patients. Exercise testing is not appropriate, however, for patients who (1) report pain that is believed to be ischemic occurring at rest or (2) have electrocardiographic changes not known to be old that are consistent with ischemia.

Patients with sustained chest discomfort who do not have evidence for life-threatening conditions should be evaluated for evidence of conditions likely to benefit from acute treatment (Table 12-3). Pericarditis may be suggested by the history, physical examination, and electrocardiogram (Table 12-2). Clinicians should carefully assess blood pressure patterns and consider echocardiography in such patients to detect evidence of impending pericardial tamponade. Chest x-rays can be used to evaluate the possibility of pulmonary disease.

GUIDELINES AND CRITICAL PATHWAYS FOR ACUTE CHEST PAIN

Guidelines for the initial evaluation for patients with acute chest pain have been developed by the American College of Cardiology, American Heart Association, and other organizations. These guidelines recommend performance of an electrocardiogram for virtually all patients with chest pain who do not have an obvious noncardiac cause of their pain, and performance of a chest x-ray for patients with signs or symptoms consistent with congestive heart failure, valvular heart disease, pericarditial disease, or aortic dissection or aneurysm.

Other organizations, including the Agency for Health Care Policy and Research (AHCPR) and the National Heart Attack Alert Program, have also issued guidelines for management of patients with a high probability of acute ischemic heart disease. In these and other guidelines, patients with possible or probable acute myocardial infarction as suggested by the description of their pain or ECG findings are expected to be admitted to the hospital. The AHCPR guidelines for unstable angina note that not all patients with that syndrome require admission but recommend that patients with unstable angina be monitored electrocardiographically during their evaluation; that those with ongoing rest pain should be placed at bed rest during the initial phase of stabilization.

The American Heart Association has published guidelines for the use of exercise testing in the emergency department. These recommendations include having two sets of cardiac enzymes or troponins at 4-h intervals that are normal; an ECG at presentation and preexercise ECG that shows no significant change; absence of rest ECG abnormalities that preclude accurate interpretation of an exercise ECG; and absence of ischemic chest pain at the time of exercise testing or during the observation period after admission to the emergency department.

Many medical centers have adopted critical pathways and other forms of guidelines to increase efficiency and to expedite the treatment of patients with high-risk acute ischemic heart disease syndromes. These guidelines emphasize the following strategies:

- Rapid identification and treatment of patients for whom emergent reperfusion therapy, either via percutaneous coronary interventions or thrombolytic agents, is likely to lead to improved outcomes.
- Triage to non-coronary care unit monitored facilities such as intermediate care units or chest pain units of patients with a low risk for complications, such as patients without new ischemic changes on their electrocardiograms and without ongoing chest pain. Such patients can usually be safely observed in non-coronary care unit settings, undergo early exercise testing, or be discharged home. Risk stratification can be assisted through use of prospectively validated multivariate algorithms that have been published for acute ischemic heart disease and its complications.
- Shortening lengths of stay in the coronary care unit and hospital. Recommendations regarding the minimum length of stay in a monitored bed for a patient who has no further symptoms have decreased in recent years to 12 h or less if exercise testing or other risk stratification technologies are available.

NONACUTE CHEST DISCOMFORT

The management of patients who do not require admission to the hospital or who no longer require inpatient observation should seek to identify the cause of the symptoms and the likelihood of major complications. Cost-effectiveness analyses support use of noninvasive testing for coronary disease, such as exercise electrocardiography and stress echocardiography. These tests serve both to diagnose coronary disease and to identify patients with high-risk forms of coronary disease who may benefit from revascularization. Gastrointestinal causes of chest pain can be evaluated via endoscopy or radiology studies, or with trials of medical therapy. Emotional and psychiatric conditions warrant appropriate evaluation and treatment; randomized trial data indicate that cognitive therapy and group interventions lead to decreases in symptoms for such patients.

PALPITATIONS

Palpitations are characterized by an awareness of the beating of the heart. Patients commonly describe "pounding" or "fluttering" heart beats or report a sensation that the heart is stopping or skipping beats. These symptoms may be caused by a change in the heart's rhythm or rate or by an increase in the force of its contractions. In many cases, this awareness reflects lack of competing sensory stimuli, such as when a person is lying in bed, unable to sleep.

Palpitations are often manifestations of psychiatric conditions, the most common of which are depression and panic disorder. For example, in one study of outpatients referred for ambulatory electrocardiographic monitoring to evaluate palpitations, 19% were found to have a psychiatric disorder. Patients with psychiatric disorders were more likely than other patients to report that their palpitations lasted longer than 15 min or were accompanied by ancillary symptoms. In this study, physicians usually recognized the emotional basis of the patients' symptoms but frequently did not refer the patient for specific therapy.

Palpitations can also be caused by virtually any cardiac arrhythmia as well as by other cardiac and noncardiac conditions. A markedly enlarged left ventricle can cause awareness of the heart beat by contact with the chest wall. Any condition associated with increased catecholamine levels can lead to palpitations both by increasing the forcefulness of cardiac contractions and by increasing the rate of premature beats.

Palpitations can be intermittent or sustained and regular or irregular. Patients with this complaint should be asked to describe their palpitations' onset, duration, associated symptoms, and the circumstances in which they occur. Abrupt onset and termination after several minutes may reflect a sustained ventricular or supraventricular tachyarrhythmia. Gradual onset and termination of a pounding heart beat is more consistent with sinus tachycardia. Patients should try to replicate the rhythm of their palpitations by tapping on a table. This maneuver can help the physician determine the nature of any cardiac arrhythmia. Patients should also be taught to take their pulse so that they can more accurately report their approximate heart rate and whether the rhythm was regular.

DIFFERENTIAL DIAGNOSIS

Patients who report "skipped" beats or a "flopping" sensation often have atrial or ventricular extrasystoles (Chap. 214). These premature beats are followed by a compensatory pause, and the first heart beat after the pause may be unusually strong due to increased left ventricular volume and enhanced contractility (a phenomenon called *postextrasystolic potentiation*). Sustained bursts of rapid heart beats may be due to ventricular or supraventricular tachyarrhythmias. A sustained irregular rhythm suggests atrial fibrillation.

Conditions that cause marked left ventricular enlargement such as aortic regurgitation can cause an awareness of the heart beat that is sometimes positional. Presumably because of associated arrhythmias, hypertrophic cardiomyopathy, mitral valve prolapse, and other cardiac structural abnormalities are also associated with palpitations.

Palpitations can also be a prominent symptom in noncardiac conditions, including thyrotoxicosis, hypoglycemia, pheochromocytoma, and fever. The physiologic basis of palpitations with these conditions is either arrhythmia or increased catecholamine levels leading to greater myocardial contractility. Drugs that can precipitate arrhythmias and palpitations include tobacco, coffee, tea, alcohol, epinephrine, ephedrine, aminophylline, and atropine.

APPROACH TO THE PATIENT

The first goal in the evaluation of patients with palpitations is to exclude the possibility of life-threatening arrhythmias. The risk for such arrhythmias is highest in patients with coronary artery disease, congestive heart failure, or other structural cardiac abnormalities. The history, physical examination, and electrocardiogram should therefore be focused on stratifying patients according to the risk of such conditions. Palpitations are also more likely to reflect serious arrhythmias if they are associated with symptoms that suggest hemodynamic compromise, such as syncope, light-headedness, dizziness, or shortness of breath.

The most common first test after the initial evaluation of palpitations is continuous electrocardiographic (Holter) monitoring. This test is especially useful if patients have unexplained palpitations that recur frequently. For patients with more sporadic palpitations, a variety of new technologies have become available to allow capture of ECG tracings at the time of their symptoms. These technologies include loop recorders, that can freeze the last several minutes of data when the patient presses a button, and telephonic monitors, which can be used to "call in" tracings when symptoms occur. For patients who require very long-term monitoring, implantable loop recorders are available. If episodes are associated with physical stress, exercise electrocardiography can be used in an attempt to elicit an arrhythmia.

Most patients with palpitations do not have evidence of major arrhythmias or abnormal physiologic conditions associated with increased catecholamine levels. Patients with emotional or psychological causes of palpitations should be evaluated for possible cognitive and pharmaceutical therapy. Drugs and medications that may precipitate palpitations should be eliminated or reduced. A trial of beta blockers is often successful in reducing premature beats and symptoms. Regardless of the cause and treatment, the clinician should remain aware that palpitations are extremely bothersome symptoms for patients. Reassurance that a comprehensive evaluation has been performed and that the palpitations do not adversely affect the patient's prognosis is a critical part of the patient's care.

FURTHER READING

BARSKY AJ et al: Somatized psychiatric disorder presenting as palpitations. Arch Intern Med 156:1102, 1996

BRAUNWALD E et al: ACC/AHA guideline update for the management of patients with unstable angina and non-ST-segment elevation myocardial infarction, 2002: Summary article. J Am Coll Cardiol 40:1366, 2002

CANNON CP et al: National Heart Attack Alert Program (NHAAP) Coordinating Committee Critical Pathways Writing Group. Critical pathways for management of patients with acute coronary syndromes: An assessment by the National Heart Attack Alert Program. Am Heart J 143:777, 2002

GIBSON PB, et al: Low event rate for stress-only perfusion imaging in patients evaluated for chest pain. J Am Coll Cardiol 39:999, 2002

HAMM CW: Cardiac biomarkers for rapid evaluation of chest pain. Circulation 104:1454, 2001

MARTINEZ E, et al: The observation unit: A new interface between inpatient and outpatient care. Am J Med 110:274:2001

NG SM, et al: Ninety-minute accelerated critical pathway for chest pain evaluation. Am J Cardiol 88:611:2001

POPE JH, et al: Missed diagnoses of acute cardiac ischemia in the emergency department. N Engl J Med 342:1163, 2000

STEIN RA, et al: Safety and utility of exercise testing in emergency room chest pain centers: An advisory from the Committee on Exercise, Rehabilitation, and Prevention Council on Clinical Cardiology, American Heart Association. Circulation 102:1463, 2000

VAN PESKI-OOSTERBAAN AS et al: Cognitive-behavioral therapy for noncardiac chest pain: A randomized trial. Am J Med 106:424, 1999

WEBER BE, KAPOOR WN: Evaluation and outcomes of patients with palpitations. Am J Med 100:138, 1996

13 ABDOMINAL PAIN
William Silen

The correct interpretation of acute abdominal pain is challenging. Since proper therapy may require urgent action, the unhurried approach suitable for the study of other conditions is sometimes denied. Few other clinical situations demand greater judgment, because the most catastrophic of events may be forecast by the subtlest of symptoms and signs. A meticulously executed, detailed history and physical examination are of great importance. The etiologic classification in Table 13-1, although not complete, forms a useful basis for the evaluation of patients with abdominal pain.

The diagnosis of "acute or surgical abdomen" is not an acceptable one because of its often misleading and erroneous connotation. The most obvious of "acute abdomens" may not require operative intervention, and the mildest of abdominal pains may herald an urgently correctable lesion. Any patient with abdominal pain of recent onset requires early and thorough evaluation and accurate diagnosis.

SOME MECHANISMS OF PAIN ORIGINATING IN THE ABDOMEN ■ Inflammation of the Parietal Peritoneum The pain of parietal peritoneal inflammation is steady and aching in character and is located directly over the inflamed area, its exact reference being possible because it is transmitted by somatic nerves supplying the parietal peritoneum. The intensity of the pain is dependent on the type and amount of material to which the peritoneal surfaces are exposed in a given time period. For example, the sudden release into the peritoneal cavity of a small quantity of *sterile* acid gastric juice causes much more pain than the same amount

TABLE 13-1 *Some Important Causes of Abdominal Pain*

PAIN ORIGINATING IN THE ABDOMEN

1. Parietal peritoneal inflammation
   a. Bacterial contamination, e.g., perforated appendix, pelvic inflammatory disease
   b. Chemical irritation, e.g., perforated ulcer, pancreatitis, mittelschmerz
2. Mechanical obstruction of hollow viscera
   a. Obstruction of the small or large intestine
   b. Obstruction of the biliary tree
   c. Obstruction of the ureter
3. Vascular disturbances
   a. Embolism or thrombosis
   b. Vascular rupture
   c. Pressure or torsional occlusion
   d. Sickle cell anemia
4. Abdominal wall
   a. Distortion or traction of mesentery
   b. Trauma or infection of muscles
5. Distention of visceral surfaces, e.g., hepatic or renal capsules

PAIN REFERRED FROM EXTRAABDOMINAL SOURCE

1. Thorax, e.g., pneumonia, referred pain from coronary occlusion
2. Spine, e.g., radiculitis from arthritis, herpes zoster
3. Genitalia, e.g., torsion of the testicle

METABOLIC CAUSES

1. Exogenous
   a. Black widow spider bite
   b. Lead poisoning and others
2. Endogenous
   a. Uremia
   b. Diabetic ketoacidosis
   c. Porphyria
   d. Allergic factors (C'1 esterase inhibitor deficiency)

NEUROGENIC CAUSES

1. Organic
   a. Tabes dorsalis
   b. Herpes zoster
   c. Causalgia and others
2. Functional

of grossly contaminated neutral feces. Enzymatically active pancreatic juice incites more pain and inflammation than does the same amount of sterile bile containing no potent enzymes. Blood and urine are often so bland as to go undetected if their contact with the peritoneum has not been sudden and massive. In the case of bacterial contamination, such as in pelvic inflammatory disease, the pain is frequently of low intensity early in the illness until bacterial multiplication has caused the elaboration of irritating substances.

The rate at which the irritating material is applied to the peritoneum is important. Perforated peptic ulcer may be associated with entirely different clinical pictures dependent only on the rapidity with which the gastric juice enters the peritoneal cavity.

The pain of peritoneal inflammation is invariably accentuated by pressure or changes in tension of the peritoneum, whether produced by palpation or by movement, as in coughing or sneezing. The patient with peritonitis lies quietly in bed, preferring to avoid motion, in contrast to the patient with colic, who may writhe incessantly.

Another characteristic feature of peritoneal irritation is tonic reflex spasm of the abdominal musculature, localized to the involved body segment. The intensity of the tonic muscle spasm accompanying peritoneal inflammation is dependent on the location of the inflammatory process, the rate at which it develops, and the integrity of the nervous system. Spasm over a perforated retrocecal appendix or perforated ulcer into the lesser peritoneal sac may be minimal or absent because of the protective effect of overlying viscera. A slowly developing process often greatly attenuates the degree of muscle spasm. Catastrophic abdominal emergencies such as a perforated ulcer may be associated with minimal or no detectable pain or muscle spasm in obtunded, seriously ill, debilitated elderly patients or in psychotic patients.

Obstruction of Hollow Viscera The pain of obstruction of hollow abdominal viscera is classically described as intermittent, or colicky. Yet the lack of a truly cramping character should not be misleading, because distention of a hollow viscus may produce steady pain with only very occasional exacerbations. It is not nearly as well localized as the pain of parietal peritoneal inflammation.

The colicky pain of obstruction of the small intestine is usually periumbilical or supraumbilical and is poorly localized. As the intestine becomes progressively dilated with loss of muscular tone, the colicky nature of the pain may diminish. With superimposed strangulating obstruction, pain may spread to the lower lumbar region if there is traction on the root of the mesentery. The colicky pain of colonic obstruction is of lesser intensity than that of the small intestine and is often located in the infraumbilical area. Lumbar radiation of pain is common in colonic obstruction.

Sudden distention of the biliary tree produces a steady rather than colicky type of pain; hence the term *biliary colic* is misleading. Acute distention of the gallbladder usually causes pain in the right upper quadrant with radiation to the right posterior region of the thorax or to the tip of the right scapula, and distention of the common bile duct is often associated with pain in the epigastrium radiating to the upper part of the lumbar region. Considerable variation is common, however, so that differentiation between these may be impossible. The typical subscapular pain or lumbar radiation is frequently absent. Gradual dilatation of the biliary tree, as in carcinoma of the head of the pancreas, may cause no pain or only a mild aching sensation in the epigastrium or right upper quadrant. The pain of distention of the pancreatic ducts is similar to that described for distention of the common bile duct but, in addition, is very frequently accentuated by recumbency and relieved by the upright position.

Obstruction of the urinary bladder results in dull suprapubic pain, usually low in intensity. Restlessness without specific complaint of pain may be the only sign of a distended bladder in an obtunded patient. In contrast, acute obstruction of the intravesicular portion of the ureter is characterized by severe suprapubic and flank pain that radiates to the penis, scrotum, or inner aspect of the upper thigh. Obstruction of the ureteropelvic junction is felt as pain in the costovertebral angle, whereas obstruction of the remainder of the ureter is associated with flank pain that often extends into the same side of the abdomen.

Vascular Disturbances A frequent misconception, despite abundant experience to the contrary, is that pain associated with intraabdominal vascular disturbances is sudden and catastrophic in nature. The pain of embolism or thrombosis of the superior mesenteric artery or that of impending rupture of an abdominal aortic aneurysm certainly may be severe and diffuse. Yet, just as frequently, the patient with occlusion of the superior mesenteric artery has only mild continuous diffuse pain for 2 or 3 days before vascular collapse or findings of peritoneal inflammation appear. The early, seemingly insignificant discomfort is caused by hyperperistalsis rather than peritoneal inflammation. Indeed, absence of tenderness and rigidity in the presence of continuous, diffuse pain in a patient likely to have vascular disease is quite characteristic of occlusion of the superior mesenteric artery. Abdominal pain with radiation to the sacral region, flank, or genitalia should always signal the possible presence of a rupturing abdominal aortic aneurysm. This pain may persist over a period of several days before rupture and collapse occur.

Abdominal Wall Pain arising from the abdominal wall is usually constant and aching. Movement, prolonged standing, and pressure accentuate the discomfort and muscle spasm. In the case of hematoma of the rectus sheath, now most frequently encountered in association with anticoagulant therapy, a mass may be present in the lower quadrants of the abdomen. Simultaneous involvement of muscles in other parts of the body usually serves to differentiate myositis of the abdominal wall from an intraabdominal process that might cause pain in the same region.

REFERRED PAIN IN ABDOMINAL DISEASES Pain referred to the abdomen from the thorax, spine, or genitalia may prove a vexing diagnostic problem, because diseases of the upper part of the abdominal cavity such as acute cholecystitis or perforated ulcer are frequently associated with intrathoracic complications. A most important, yet often forgotten, dictum is that the possibility of intrathoracic disease must be considered in every patient with abdominal pain, especially if the pain is in the upper part of the abdomen. Systematic questioning and examination directed toward detecting myocardial or pulmonary infarction, pneumonia, pericarditis, or esophageal disease (the intrathoracic diseases that most often masquerade as abdominal emergencies) will often provide sufficient clues to establish the proper diagnosis. Diaphragmatic pleuritis resulting from pneumonia or pulmonary infarction may cause pain in the right upper quadrant and pain in the supraclavicular area, the latter radiation to be distinguished from the referred subscapular pain caused by acute distention of the extrahepatic biliary tree. The ultimate decision as to the origin of abdominal pain may require deliberate and planned observation over a period of several hours, during which repeated questioning and examination will provide the diagnosis or suggest the appropriate studies.

Referred pain of thoracic origin is often accompanied by splinting of the involved hemithorax with respiratory lag and decrease in excursion more marked than that seen in the presence of intraabdominal disease. In addition, apparent abdominal muscle spasm caused by referred pain will diminish during the inspiratory phase of respiration, whereas it is persistent throughout both respiratory phases if it is of abdominal origin. Palpation over the area of referred pain in the abdomen also does not usually accentuate the pain and in many instances actually seems to relieve it. Thoracic and abdominal disease frequently coexist and may be difficult or impossible to differentiate. For example, the patient with known biliary tract disease often has epigastric pain during myocardial infarction, or biliary colic may be referred to the precordium or left shoulder in a patient who has suffered previously from angina pectoris. →*For an explanation of the radiation of pain to a previously diseased area, see Chap. 11.*

Referred pain from the spine, which usually involves compression or irritation of nerve roots, is characteristically intensified by certain motions such as cough, sneeze, or strain and is associated with hyperesthesia over the involved dermatomes. Pain referred to the abdo-

men from the testicles or seminal vesicles is generally accentuated by the slightest pressure on either of these organs. The abdominal discomfort is of dull aching character and is poorly localized.

METABOLIC ABDOMINAL CRISES Pain of metabolic origin may simulate almost any other type of intraabdominal disease. Several mechanisms may be at work. In certain instances, such as hyperlipidemia, the metabolic disease itself may be accompanied by an intraabdominal process such as pancreatitis, which can lead to unnecessary laparotomy unless recognized. $C'1$ esterase deficiency associated with angioneurotic edema is often associated with episodes of severe abdominal pain. Whenever the cause of abdominal pain is obscure, a metabolic origin always must be considered. Abdominal pain is also the hallmark of familial Mediterranean fever (Chap. 278).

The problem of differential diagnosis is often not readily resolved. The pain of porphyria and of lead colic is usually difficult to distinguish from that of intestinal obstruction, because severe hyperperistalsis is a prominent feature of both. The pain of uremia or diabetes is nonspecific, and the pain and tenderness frequently shift in location and intensity. Diabetic acidosis may be precipitated by acute appendicitis or intestinal obstruction, so if prompt resolution of the abdominal pain does not result from correction of the metabolic abnormalities, an underlying organic problem should be suspected. Black widow spider bites produce intense pain and rigidity of the abdominal muscles and back, an area infrequently involved in intraabdominal disease.

NEUROGENIC CAUSES Causalgic pain may occur in diseases that injure sensory nerves. It has a burning character and is usually limited to the distribution of a given peripheral nerve. Normal stimuli such as touch or change in temperature may be transformed into this type of pain, which is frequently present in a patient at rest. The demonstration of irregularly spaced cutaneous pain spots may be the only indication of an old nerve lesion underlying causalgic pain. Even though the pain may be precipitated by gentle palpation, rigidity of the abdominal muscles is absent, and the respirations are not disturbed. Distention of the abdomen is uncommon, and the pain has no relationship to the intake of food.

Pain arising from spinal nerves or roots comes and goes suddenly and is of a lancinating type (Chap. 15). It may be caused by herpes zoster, impingement by arthritis, tumors, herniated nucleus pulposus, diabetes, or syphilis. It is not associated with food intake, abdominal distention, or changes in respiration. Severe muscle spasm, as in the gastric crises of tabes dorsalis, is common but is either relieved or is not accentuated by abdominal palpation. The pain is made worse by movement of the spine and is usually confined to a few dermatomes. Hyperesthesia is very common.

Pain due to functional causes conforms to none of the aforementioned patterns. Mechanism is hard to define. Irritable bowel syndrome (IBS) is a functional gastrointestinal disorder characterized by abdominal pain and altered bowel habits. The diagnosis is made on the basis of clinical criteria (Chap. 277) and after exclusion of demonstrable structural abnormalities. The episodes of abdominal pain are often brought on by stress, and the pain varies considerably in type and location. Nausea and vomiting are rare. Localized tenderness and muscle spasm are inconsistent or absent. The causes of IBS or related functional disorders are not known.

APPROACH TO THE PATIENT

Few abdominal conditions require such urgent operative intervention that an orderly approach need be abandoned, no matter how ill the patient. Only those patients with exsanguinating intraabdominal hemorrhage (e.g., ruptured aneurysm) must be rushed to the operating room immediately, but in such instances, only a few minutes are required to assess the critical nature of the problem. Under these circumstances, all obstacles must be swept aside, adequate venous access for fluid replacement obtained, and the operation begun. Many patients of this type have died in the radiology department or the emergency room while awaiting such unnecessary examinations as electrocardiograms or abdominal films. *There are no contraindications to operation when massive intraabdominal hemorrhage is present.* This situation fortunately is relatively rare. These comments do not pertain to gastrointestinal hemorrhage, which can often be managed by other means (Chap. 37).

Nothing will supplant an orderly, painstakingly *detailed history*, which is far more valuable than any laboratory or radiographic examination. This kind of history is laborious and time-consuming, making it not especially popular, even though a reasonably accurate diagnosis can be made on the basis of the history alone in the majority of cases. Computer-aided diagnosis of abdominal pain provides no advantage over clinical assessment alone. In cases of *acute* abdominal pain, a diagnosis is readily established in most instances, whereas success is not so frequent in patients with *chronic* pain. IBS is one of the most common causes of abdominal pain and must always be kept in mind (Chap. 277). The *chronological sequence of events* in the patient's history is often more important than emphasis on the location of pain. If the examiner is sufficiently open-minded and unhurried, asks the proper questions, and listens, the patient will usually provide the diagnosis. Careful attention should be paid to the extraabdominal regions that may be responsible for abdominal pain. An accurate menstrual history in a female patient is essential. Narcotics or analgesics should *not* be withheld until a definitive diagnosis or a definitive plan has been formulated; obfuscation of the diagnosis by adequate analgesia is unlikely.

In the examination, simple critical inspection of the patient, e.g., of facies, position in bed, and respiratory activity, may provide valuable clues. The amount of information to be gleaned is directly proportional to the *gentleness* and thoroughness of the examiner. Once a patient with peritoneal inflammation has been examined brusquely, accurate assessment by the next examiner becomes almost impossible. Eliciting rebound tenderness by sudden release of a deeply palpating hand in a patient with suspected peritonitis is cruel and unnecessary. The same information can be obtained by gentle percussion of the abdomen (rebound tenderness on a miniature scale), a maneuver that can be far more precise and localizing. Asking the patient to cough will elicit true rebound tenderness without the need for placing a hand on the abdomen. Furthermore, the forceful demonstration of rebound tenderness will startle and induce protective spasm in a nervous or worried patient in whom true rebound tenderness is not present. A palpable gallbladder will be missed if palpation is so brusque that voluntary muscle spasm becomes superimposed on involuntary muscular rigidity.

As in history taking, there is no substitute for sufficient time spent in the examination. Abdominal signs may be minimal but nevertheless, if accompanied by consistent symptoms, may be exceptionally meaningful. Abdominal signs may be virtually or totally absent in cases of pelvic peritonitis, so careful *pelvic and rectal examinations are mandatory in every patient with abdominal pain.* Tenderness on pelvic or rectal examination in the absence of other abdominal signs can be caused by operative indications such as perforated appendicitis, diverticulitis, twisted ovarian cyst, and many others.

Much attention has been paid to the presence or absence of peristaltic sounds, their quality, and their frequency. Auscultation of the abdomen is one of the least revealing aspects of the physical examination of a patient with abdominal pain. Catastrophes such as strangulating small intestinal obstruction or perforated appendicitis may occur in the presence of normal peristaltic sounds. Conversely, when the proximal part of the intestine above an obstruction becomes markedly distended and edematous, peristaltic sounds may lose the characteristics of borborygmi and become

weak or absent, even when peritonitis is not present. It is usually the severe chemical peritonitis of sudden onset that is associated with the truly silent abdomen. Assessment of the patient's state of hydration is important.

Laboratory examinations may be of great value in assessment of the patient with abdominal pain, yet with few exceptions they rarely establish a diagnosis. Leukocytosis should never be the single deciding factor as to whether or not operation is indicated. A white blood cell count >20,000/μL may be observed with perforation of a viscus, but pancreatitis, acute cholecystitis, pelvic inflammatory disease, and intestinal infarction may be associated with marked leukocytosis. A normal white blood cell count is not rare in cases of perforation of abdominal viscera. The diagnosis of anemia may be more helpful than the white blood cell count, especially when combined with the history.

The urinalysis may reveal the state of hydration or rule out severe renal disease, diabetes, or urinary infection. Blood urea nitrogen, glucose, and serum bilirubin levels may be helpful. Serum amylase levels may be increased by many diseases other than pancreatitis, e.g., perforated ulcer, strangulating intestinal obstruction, and acute cholecystitis; thus, elevations of serum amylase do not rule out the need for an operation. The determination of the serum lipase may have greater accuracy than that of the serum amylase.

Plain and upright or lateral decubitus radiographs of the abdomen may be of value in cases of intestinal obstruction, perforated ulcer, and a variety of other conditions. They are usually unnecessary in patients with acute appendicitis or strangulated external hernias. In rare instances, barium or water-soluble contrast study of the upper part of the gastrointestinal tract may demonstrate partial intestinal obstruction that may elude diagnosis by other means. If there is any question of obstruction of the colon, oral administration of barium sulfate should be avoided. On the other hand, in cases of suspected colonic obstruction (without perforation), contrast enema may be diagnostic.

In the absence of trauma, peritoneal lavage has been replaced as a diagnostic tool by ultrasound, computed tomography (CT), and laparoscopy. Ultrasonography has proved to be useful in detecting an enlarged gallbladder or pancreas, the presence of gallstones, an enlarged ovary, or a tubal pregnancy. Laparoscopy is especially helpful in diagnosing pelvic conditions, such as ovarian cysts, tubal pregnancies, salpingitis, and acute appendicitis. Radioisotopic scans (HIDA) may help differentiate acute cholecystitis from acute pancreatitis. A CT scan may demonstrate an enlarged pancreas, ruptured spleen, or thickened colonic or appendiceal wall and streaking of the mesocolon or mesoappendix characteristic of diverticulitis or appendicitis.

Sometimes, even under the best circumstances with all available aids and with the greatest of clinical skill, a definitive diagnosis cannot be established at the time of the initial examination. Nevertheless, despite lack of a clear anatomic diagnosis, it may be abundantly clear to an experienced and thoughtful physician and surgeon that on clinical grounds alone operation is indicated. Should that decision be questionable, watchful waiting with repeated questioning and examination will often elucidate the true nature of the illness and indicate the proper course of action.

FURTHER READING

CERVERO F, LAIRD JM: Visceral pain. Lancet 353:2145, 1999

JONES PF: Suspected acute appendicitis: Trends in management over 30 years. Br J Surg 88:1570, 2001

MARCO CA et al: Abdominal pain in geriatric emergency patients: Variables associated with adverse outcome. Acad Emerg Med 5:1163, 1998

TAIT IS et al: Do patients with abdominal pain wait unduly long for analgesia? J R Coll Surg Edinb 44:181, 1999

TAOUREL P et al: Acute abdomen of unknown origin: Impact of CT on diagnosis and management. Gastrointest Radiol 17:287, 1992

14 | HEADACHE
Neil H. Raskin

Few of us are spared the experience of head pain. As many as 90% of individuals have at least one headache per year. Severe, disabling headache is reported to occur at least annually by 40% of individuals worldwide. A useful classification of the many causes of headache is shown in Table 14-1. Headache is usually a benign symptom, but occasionally it is the manifestation of a serious illness such as brain tumor, subarachnoid hemorrhage, meningitis, or giant cell arteritis. In emergency settings, approximately 5% of patients with headache are found to have a serious underlying neurologic disorder. Therefore, it is imperative that the serious causes of headache be diagnosed rapidly and accurately.

PAIN-SENSITIVE STRUCTURES OF THE HEAD

Pain usually occurs when peripheral nociceptors are stimulated in response to tissue injury, visceral distension, or other factors (Chap. 11). In such situations, pain perception is a normal physiologic response mediated by a healthy nervous system. Pain can also result when pain-sensitive pathways of the peripheral or central nervous system are damaged or activated inappropriately. Headache may originate from either or both mechanisms. Relatively few cranial structures are pain-sensitive: the scalp, middle meningeal artery, dural sinuses, falx cerebri, and the proximal segments of the large pial arteries. The ventricular ependyma, choroid plexus, pial veins, and much of the brain parenchyma are pain-insensitive. Electrical stimulation of the midbrain

in the region of the dorsal raphe has resulted in migraine-like headaches. Thus, whereas most of the brain is insensitive to electrode probing, a site in the midbrain represents a possible source of headache generation. Sensory stimuli from the head are conveyed to the central nervous system via the trigeminal nerves for structures above the tentorium in the anterior and middle fossae of the skull, and via the first three cervical nerves for those in the posterior fossa and the inferior surface of the tentorium.

Headache can occur as the result of (1) distention, traction, or dilation of intracranial or extracranial arteries; (2) traction or displacement of large intracranial veins or their dural envelope; (3) compression, traction, or inflammation of cranial and spinal nerves; (4) spasm, inflammation, or trauma to cranial and cervical muscles; (5) meningeal irritation and raised intracranial pressure; or (6) other possible mechanisms such as activation of brainstem structures.

GENERAL CLINICAL CONSIDERATIONS

The quality, location, duration, and time course of the headache and the conditions that produce, exacerbate, or relieve it should be carefully reviewed. Ascertaining the *quality* of cephalic pain is occasionally helpful for diagnosis. Most tension-type headaches are described as tight "bandlike" pain or as dull, deeply located, and aching pain. Jabbing, brief, sharp cephalic pain, often occurring multifocally (ice pick–like pain), is usually benign. A throbbing quality and tight muscles about the head, neck, and shoulder girdle are common nonspecific accompaniments of migraine headaches.

Pain *intensity* rarely has diagnostic value, although from the patient's perspective, it is the single aspect of pain that is most important.

TABLE 14-1 *International Headache Society Classification of Headache*

1. **Migraine**
   Migraine without aura
   Migraine with aura
   Ophthalmoplegic migraine
   Retinal migraine
   Childhood periodic syndromes that may be precursors to or associated with migraine
   Migrainous disorder not fulfilling above criteria
2. **Tension-type headache**
   Episodic tension-type headache
   Chronic tension-type headache
3. **Cluster headache and chronic paroxysmal hemicrania**
   Cluster headache
   Chronic paroxysmal hemicrania
4. **Miscellaneous headaches not associated with structural lesion**
   Idiopathic stabbing headache
   External compression headache
   Cold stimulus headache
   Benign cough headache
   Benign exertional headache
   Headache associated with sexual activity
5. **Headache associated with head trauma**
   Acute posttraumatic headache
   Chronic posttraumatic headache
6. **Headache associated with vascular disorders**
   Acute ischemic cerebrovascular disorder
   Intracranial hematoma
   Subarachnoid hemorrhage
   Unruptured vascular malformation
   Arteritis
   Carotid or vertebral artery pain
   Venous thrombosis
   Arterial hypertension
   Other vascular disorder
7. **Headache associated with nonvascular intracranial disorder**
   High CSF pressure
   Low CSF pressure
   Intracranial infection

7. **Headache associated with nonvascular intracranial disorder (cont.)**
   Sarcoidosis and other noninfectious inflammatory diseases
   Related to intrathecal injections
   Intracranial neoplasm
   Associated with other intracranial disorder
8. **Headache associated with substances or their withdrawal**
   Headache induced by acute substance use or exposure
   Headache induced by chronic substance use or exposure
   Headache from substance withdrawal (acute use)
   Headache from substance withdrawal (chronic use)
9. **Headache associated with noncephalic infection**
   Viral infection
   Bacterial infection
   Other infection
10. **Headache associated with metabolic disorder**
    Hypoxia
    Hypercapnia
    Mixed hypoxia and hypercapnia
    Hypoglycemia
    Dialysis
    Other metabolic abnormality
11. **Headache or facial pain associated with disorder of facial or cranial structures**
    Cranial bone
    Eyes
    Ears
    Nose and sinuses
    Teeth, jaws, and related structures
    Temporomandibular joint disease
12. **Cranial neuralgias, nerve trunk pain, and deafferentation pain**
    Persistent (in contrast to ticlike) pain of cranial nerve origin
    Trigeminal neuralgia
    Glossopharyngeal neuralgia
    Nervus intermedius neuralgia
    Superior laryngeal neuralgia
    Occipital neuralgia
    Central causes of head and facial pain other than tic douloureux
13. **Headache not classifiable**

Note: CSF, cerebrospinal fluid.
Source: After J Olesen: Cephalalgia 8(Suppl 7):1, 1988.

Although meningitis, subarachnoid hemorrhage, and cluster headache produce intense cranial pain, most patients entering emergency departments with the most severe headache of their lives usually have migraine. Contrary to common belief, the headache produced by a brain tumor is not usually distinctive or severe.

Data regarding *location* of headache may be informative. If the source is an extracranial structure, as in giant cell arteritis, the correspondence with the site of pain is fairly precise. Inflammation of an extracranial artery causes pain and exquisite tenderness localized to the site of the vessel. Lesions of paranasal sinuses, teeth, eyes, and upper cervical vertebrae induce less sharply localized pain, but pain that is still referred in a regional distribution. Intracranial lesions in the posterior fossa cause pain that is usually occipitonuchal, and supratentorial lesions most often induce frontotemporal pain.

Duration and *time-intensity* curves of headaches are diagnostically useful. A ruptured aneurysm results in head pain that peaks in an instant, thunderclap-like; much less often, unruptured aneurysms may signal their presence in the same way. Cluster headache attacks reach their peak over 3 to 5 min, remain at maximal levels for about 45 min, and then taper off. Migraine attacks build up over hours, are maintained for several hours to days, and are characteristically relieved by sleep. Sleep disruption and early morning headaches that improve during the day are characteristics of headaches produced by brain tumors or other disorders that produce increased intracranial pressure.

Facial pain must be distinguished from headache. Trigeminal and, less commonly, glossopharyngeal neuralgia are frequent causes of facial pain (Chap. 355). *Neuralgias* are painful disorders characterized by paroxysmal, fleeting, often electric shock–like episodes that are frequently caused by demyelinating lesions of nerves (the trigeminal or glossopharyngeal nerves in cranial neuralgias). Certain maneuvers characteristically trigger paroxysms of pain. However, the most common cause of facial pain by far is dental; provocation by hot, cold, or sweet foods is typical. The application of a cold stimulus will repeatedly induce dental pain, whereas in neuralgic disorders, a refractory period usually occurs after the initial response so that pain cannot be repeatedly induced.

The effect of eating on facial pain may provide insight into its cause. Is it the chewing, swallowing, or taste of the food that elicits pain? Chewing suggests trigeminal neuralgia, temporomandibular joint dysfunction, or giant cell arteritis ("jaw claudication"), whereas swallowing *and* taste provocation suggest glossopharyngeal neuralgia. Pain with swallowing is common in patients with carotidynia (see below) because the inflamed, tender carotid artery abuts the esophagus during deglutition.

Many patients with facial pain do not experience stereotypic neuralgias; the term *atypical facial pain* has been used in this setting. Vague, poorly localized, continuous facial pain is characteristic of nasopharyngeal carcinoma; a burning pain often develops as deafferentation occurs and evidence of cranial neuropathy appears. Burning facial pain may also occur with tumors of the fifth cranial nerve (meningioma or schwannoma) or with lesions of the pons that interrupt the dorsal root entry zone of the nerve (multiple sclerosis). In patients with facial pain, the finding of objective sensory loss is an important clue to a serious underlying disorder. Occasionally, the cause of a pain problem cannot be resolved promptly, necessitating periodic follow-up until further signs appear.

CLINICAL EVALUATION OF ACUTE, NEW-ONSET HEADACHE

Patients who present with their first severe headache raise entirely different diagnostic possibilities than those with recurrent headaches over many years. In new-onset and severe headaches, the probability of finding a potentially serious cause is considerably greater than in recurrent headache. When a patient complains of an acute, new-onset headache, a number of causes should be considered including meningitis, subarachnoid hemorrhage, epidural or subdural hematoma, glaucoma, and purulent sinusitis. Clinical features of acute, new-onset

TABLE 14-2 *Headache Symptoms That Suggest a Serious Underlying Disorder*

"Worst" headache ever
First severe headache
Subacute worsening over days or weeks
Abnormal neurologic examination
Fever or unexplained systemic signs
Vomiting precedes headache
Induced by bending, lifting, cough
Disturbs sleep or presents immediately upon awakening
Known systemic illness
Onset after age 55

headache caused by serious underlying conditions are summarized in Table 14-2.

A complete neurologic examination is an essential first step in the evaluation. In most cases, an abnormal examination should be followed by a computed tomography (CT) or a magnetic resonance imaging (MRI) study. As a screening procedure for intracranial pathology in this setting, CT and MRI methods appear to be equally sensitive. A general evaluation of acute headache might include the investigation of cardiovascular and renal status by blood pressure monitoring and urine examination; eyes by fundoscopy, intraocular pressure measurement, and refraction; cranial arteries by palpation; and cervical spine by the effect of passive movement of the head and imaging.

The psychological state of the patient should also be evaluated since a relationship exists between head pain and depression. Many patients in chronic daily pain cycles become depressed; moreover, there is a greater-than-chance coincidence of migraine with both bipolar (manic-depressive) and unipolar major depressive disorders. Drugs with antidepressant actions are also effective in the prophylactic treatment of both tension-type headache and migraine.

Underlying recurrent headache disorders may be activated by pain that follows otologic or endodontic surgical procedures. Thus, pain about the head as the result of diseased tissue or trauma may reawaken an otherwise quiescent migrainous syndrome. Treatment of the headache is largely ineffective until the cause of the primary problem is addressed.

Serious underlying conditions that are associated with headache are described below and in Table 14-3.

MENINGITIS In general, acute, severe headache with stiff neck and fever suggests meningitis. Lumbar puncture is mandatory. Often there is striking accentuation of pain with eye movement. Meningitis is par-

TABLE 14-3 *Symptoms of Serious Underlying Causes of Headache*

Cause	Symptoms
Meningitis	Nuchal rigidity, headache, photophobia, and prostration; may not be febrile. Lumbar puncture is diagnostic.
Intracranial hemorrhage	Nuchal rigidity and headache; may not have clouded consciousness or seizures. Hemorrhage may not be seen on CT scan. Lumbar puncture shows "bloody tap" that does not clear by the last tube. A fresh hemorrhage may not be xanthochromic.
Brain tumor	May present with prostrating pounding headaches that are associated with nausea and vomiting. Should be suspected in progressively severe new "migraine" that is invariably unilateral.
Temporal arteritis	May present with a unilateral pounding headache. Onset generally in older patients (>50 years) and frequently associated with visual changes. The erythrocyte sedimentation rate is the best screening test and is usually markedly elevated (i.e., >50). Definitive diagnosis can be made by arterial biopsy.
Glaucoma	Usually consists of severe eye pain. May have nausea and vomiting. The eye is usually painful and red. The pupil may be partially dilated.

Note: CT, computed tomography.

ticularly easy to mistake for migraine in that the cardinal symptoms of pounding headache, photophobia, nausea, and vomiting are present. →*A detailed discussion of meningitis can be found in Chaps. 360 and 361.*

INTRACRANIAL HEMORRHAGE In general, acute, severe headache with stiff neck but without fever suggests subarachnoid hemorrhage. A ruptured aneurysm, arteriovenous malformation, or intraparenchymal hemorrhage may also present with headache alone. Rarely, if the hemorrhage is small or below the foramen magnum, the head CT scan can be normal. Therefore, a lumbar puncture may be required to make the definitive diagnosis of a subarachnoid hemorrhage. →*A detailed discussion of intracranial hemorrhage can be found in Chap. 349.*

BRAIN TUMOR Approximately 30% of patients with brain tumors consider headache to be their chief complaint. The head pain is usually nondescript—an intermittent deep, dull aching of moderate intensity, which may worsen with exertion or change in position and may be associated with nausea and vomiting. This pattern of symptoms results from migraine far more often than from brain tumor. Headache of brain tumor disturbs sleep in about 10% of patients. Vomiting that precedes the appearance of headache by weeks is highly characteristic of posterior fossa brain tumors. A history of amenorrhea or galactorrhea should lead one to question whether a prolactin-secreting pituitary adenoma (or the polycystic ovary syndrome) is the source of headache. Headache arising de novo in a patient with known malignancy suggests either cerebral metastases and/or carcinomatous meningitis. Head pain appearing abruptly after bending, lifting, or coughing can be due to a posterior fossa mass (or a Chiari malformation). →*A detailed discussion of brain tumors can be found in Chap. 358.*

TEMPORAL ARTERITIS (See also Chaps. 25 and 306) Temporal (giant cell) arteritis is an inflammatory disorder of arteries that frequently involves the extracranial carotid circulation. This is a common disorder of the elderly; its annual incidence is 77:100,000 in individuals aged 50 and older. The average age of onset is 70 years, and women account for 65% of cases. About half of patients with untreated temporal arteritis develop blindness due to involvement of the ophthalmic artery and its branches; indeed, the ischemic optic neuropathy induced by giant cell arteritis is the major cause of rapidly developing bilateral blindness in patients >60 years. Because treatment with glucocorticoids is effective in preventing this complication, prompt recognition of this disorder is important.

Typical presenting symptoms include headache, polymyalgia rheumatica (Chap. 306), jaw claudication, fever, and weight loss. Headache is the dominant symptom and often appears in association with malaise and muscle aches. Head pain may be unilateral or bilateral and is located temporally in 50% of patients but may involve any and all aspects of the cranium. Pain usually appears gradually over a few hours before peak intensity is reached; occasionally, it is explosive in onset. The quality of pain is only seldom throbbing; it is almost invariably described as dull and boring with superimposed episodic ice pick–like lancinating pains similar to the sharp pains that appear in migraine. Most patients can recognize that the origin of their head pain is superficial, external to the skull, rather than originating deep within the cranium (the pain site for migraineurs). Scalp tenderness is present, often to a marked degree; brushing the hair or resting the head on a pillow may be impossible because of pain. Headache is usually worse at night and is often aggravated by exposure to cold. Reddened, tender nodules or red streaking of the skin overlying the temporal arteries may be found in patients with headache, as is tenderness of the temporal or, less commonly, the occipital arteries.

The erythrocyte sedimentation rate (ESR) is often, though not always, elevated; a normal ESR does not exclude giant cell arteritis. A temporal artery biopsy and treatment with prednisone at 80 mg daily for the first 4 to 6 weeks should be initiated when clinical suspicion is high. The prevalence of migraine among the elderly is substantial, considerably higher than that of giant cell arteritis. Migraineurs often report amelioration of their headaches with prednisone, so that one must be cautious about interpreting the therapeutic response.

GLAUCOMA Glaucoma may present with a prostrating headache associated with nausea and vomiting. The history will usually reveal that the headache started with severe eye pain. On physical examination, the eye is often red with a fixed, moderately dilated pupil. →*A discussion of glaucoma can be found in Chap. 25.*

OTHER CAUSES OF HEADACHE ■ **Systemic Illness** There is hardly any illness that is never manifested by headache; however, some illnesses are frequently associated with headache. These include infectious mononucleosis, systemic lupus erythematosus, chronic pulmonary failure with hypercapnia (early morning headaches), Hashimoto's thyroiditis, inflammatory bowel disease, many of the illnesses associated with HIV, and the acute blood pressure elevations that occur in pheochromocytoma and in malignant hypertension. The last two examples are the exceptions to the generalization that hypertension per se is a very uncommon cause of headache; diastolic pressures of at least 120 mmHg are requisite for hypertension to cause headache. Persistent headache and fever are often the manifestations of an acute systemic viral infection; if the neck is supple in such a patient, lumbar puncture may be deferred. Some drugs and drug-withdrawal states, e.g., oral contraceptives, ovulation-promoting medications, and glucocorticoid withdrawal, are also associated with headache in some individuals.

Idiopathic Intracranial Hypertension (Pseudotumor Cerebri) Headache, clinically resembling that of brain tumor, is a common presenting symptom of pseudotumor cerebri, a disorder of raised intracranial pressure probably resulting from impaired cerebrospinal fluid (CSF) absorption by the arachnoid villi. Morning headaches that are worsened by coughing and straining are typical. The pain is sometimes retroocular and worsened by eye movements. Transient visual obscurations and papilledema with enlarged blind spots and loss of peripheral visual fields are additional manifestations. Most patients are young, female, and obese. They often have a history of exposure to provoking agents such as vitamin A and glucocorticoids. →*Treatment of idiopathic intracranial hypertension is discussed in Chap. 25.*

Cough A male-dominated (4:1) syndrome, cough headache is characterized by transient, severe head pain upon coughing, bending, lifting, sneezing, or stooping. Head pain persists for seconds to a few minutes. Many patients date the origins of the syndrome to a lower respiratory infection accompanied by severe coughing or to strenuous weight-lifting programs. Headache is usually diffuse but is lateralized in about one-third of patients. The incidence of serious intracranial structural anomalies causing this condition is about 25%; the Chiari malformation (Chap. 356) is a common cause. Thus, MRI is indicated for most patients with cough headache. The benign disorder may persist for a few years; it responds dramatically to indomethacin at doses ranging from 50 to 200 mg daily. Approximately half of patients will also show a response to therapeutic lumbar puncture with removal of 40 mL of CSF.

Many patients with migraine note that attacks of headache may be provoked by *sustained* physical exertion, such as during the third mile of a 5-mile run. Such headaches build up over hours, in contrast to cough headache. The term *effort migraine* has been used for this syndrome to avoid the ambiguous term *exertional headache.*

Lumbar Puncture Headache following lumbar puncture usually begins within 48 h but may be delayed for up to 12 days. Its incidence is between 10 and 30%. Head pain is dramatically positional; it begins when the patient sits or stands upright; there is relief upon reclining or with abdominal compression. The longer the patient is upright, the longer the latency before head pain subsides. It is worsened by head shaking and jugular vein compression. The pain is usually a dull ache but may be throbbing; its location is occipitofrontal. Nausea and stiff neck often accompany headache, and occasional patients report blurred vision, photophobia, tinnitus, and vertigo. The symptoms resolve over a few days but may on occasion persist for weeks to months.

Loss of CSF volume decreases the brain's supportive cushion, so

TABLE 14-4 *Drugs Effective in the Treatment of Tension-Type Headache*

Drug	Trade Name	Dosage
NONSTEROIDAL ANTI-INFLAMMATORY AGENTS		
Acetaminophen	Tylenol, generic	650 mg PO q4–6h
Aspirin	Generic	650 mg PO q4–6h
Diclofenac	Cataflam, generic	50–100 mg q4–6h (max 200 mg/d)
Ibuprofen	Advil, Motrin, Nuprin, generic	400 mg PO q3–4h
Naproxen sodium	Aleve, Anaprox, generic	220–550 mg bid
COMBINATION ANALGESICS		
Acetaminophen, 325 mg, *plus* butalbital, 50 mg	Phrenilin, generic	1–2 tablets; max 6 per day
Acetaminophen, 650 mg, *plus* butalbital, 50 mg	Phrenilin Forte	1 tablet; max 6 per day
Acetaminophen, 325 mg, *plus* butalbital, 50 mg, *plus* caffeine, 40 mg	Fioricet; Esgic, generic	1–2 tablets; max 6 per day
Acetaminophen, 500 mg, *plus* butalbital, 50 mg, *plus* caffeine, 40 mg	Esgicplus	1–2 tablets; max 6 per day
Aspirin, 325 mg, *plus* butalbital, 50 mg, *plus* caffeine, 40 mg	Fiorinal	1–2 tablets; max 6 per day
Aspirin, 650 mg, *plus* butalbital, 50 mg	Axotal	1 tablet q4h; max 6 per day
PROPHYLACTIC MEDICATIONS		
Amitriptyline	Elavil, generic	10–50 mg at bedtime
Doxepin	Sinequan, generic	10–75 mg at bedtime
Nortriptyline	Pamelor, generic	25–75 mg at bedtime

that when a patient is upright there is probably dilation and tension placed on the brain's anchoring structures, the pain-sensitive dural sinuses, resulting in pain. Intracranial hypotension often occurs, but severe lumbar puncture headache may be present even in patients who have normal CSF pressure.

Treatment with intravenous caffeine sodium benzoate given over a few minutes as a 500-mg dose will promptly terminate headache in 75% of patients; a second dose given in 1 h brings the total success rate to 85%. An epidural blood patch accomplished by injection of 15 mL of autologous whole blood rarely fails for those who do not respond to caffeine. The mechanism for these treatment effects is not straightforward. The blood patch has an *immediate* effect, making it unlikely that sealing off a dural hole with blood clot is its mechanism of action.

Postconcussion Following seemingly trivial head injuries and particularly after rear-end motor vehicle collisions, many patients report varying combinations of headache, dizziness, vertigo, and impaired memory. Anxiety, irritability, and difficulty with concentration are other hallmarks of this syndrome. Symptoms may remit after several weeks or persist for months and even years after the injury. Postconcussion headaches may occur whether or not a person was rendered unconscious by head trauma. Typically, the neurologic examination is normal with the exception of the behavioral abnormalities, and CT or MRI studies are unrevealing. Chronic subdural hematoma may on occasion mimic this disorder. Although the cause of postconcussive headache disorder is not known, it should not in general be viewed as a primary psychological disturbance. It often persists long after the settlement of pending lawsuits. The treatment is symptomatic support. Repeated encouragement that the syndrome eventually remits is important.

Coital Headache This is another male-dominated (4:1) syndrome. Attacks occur periorgasmically, are very abrupt in onset, and subside in a few minutes if coitus is interrupted. These are nearly always benign events and usually occur sporadically; if they persist for hours or are accompanied by vomiting, subarachnoid hemorrhage must be excluded (Chap. 349).

PRINCIPAL CLINICAL VARIETIES OF RECURRENT HEADACHE

There is usually little difficulty in diagnosing the serious types of headaches listed above because of the clues provided by the associated symptoms and signs. It is when headache is chronic, recurrent, and unattended by other important signs of disease that the physician faces a challenging and unique medical problem. The following sections describe a variety of headache types, ranging from the most common (e.g., migraine) to rare causes of recurrent headache.

TENSION-TYPE HEADACHE The term *tension-type headache* is still commonly used to describe a chronic head pain syndrome characterized by bilateral tight, bandlike discomfort. Patients may report that the head feels as if it is in a vise or that the posterior neck muscles are tight. The pain typically builds slowly, fluctuates in severity, and may persist more or less continuously for many days. Exertion does not usually worsen the headache. The headache may be episodic or chronic (i.e., present >15 days per month). Tension-type headache is common in all age groups, and females tend to predominate. In some patients, anxiety or depression coexist with tension headache.

The pathophysiologic basis of tension-type headache remains unknown. Many investigators believe that periodic tension headache is biologically indistinguishable from migraine, whereas others believe that tension-type headache and migraine are two distinct clinical entities. Abnormalities of cervical and temporal muscle contraction are likely to exist, but the exact nature of the dysfunction has not yet been elucidated.

Relaxation almost always relieves tension-type headaches. Patients should be encouraged to find a means of relaxation, which, for a given individual, could include bed rest, massage, and/or formal biofeedback training. Pharmacologic treatment consists of either simple analgesics and/or muscle relaxants. Ibuprofen and naproxen sodium are useful treatments for most individuals. When simple over-the-counter analgesics such as acetaminophen, aspirin, ibuprofen, and/or other nonsteroidal anti-inflammatory drugs (NSAIDs) alone fail, the addition of butalbital and caffeine (in a combination compound such as Fiorinal, Fioricet) to these analgesics may be effective. A list of commonly used analgesics for tension-type headaches is presented in Table 14-4. For chronic tension-type headache, prophylactic therapy is recommended. Low doses of amitriptyline (10 to 50 mg at bedtime) can provide effective prophylaxis.

MIGRAINE Migraine, the most common cause of headache, afflicts approximately 15% of women and 6% of men. A useful definition of migraine is a benign and recurring syndrome of headache, nausea, vomiting, and/or other symptoms of neurologic dysfunction in varying admixtures (Table 14-5). Migraine can often be recognized by its activators (red wine, menses, hunger, lack of sleep, glare, estrogen, worry, perfumes, let-down periods) and its deactivators (sleep, pregnancy, exhilaration, triptans). A classification of the many subtypes of migraine, as defined by the International Headache Society, is shown in Table 14-1.

Severe headache attacks, regardless of cause, are more likely to be described as throbbing and associated with vomiting and scalp tenderness. Milder headaches tend to be nondescript—tight, bandlike discomfort often involving the entire head—the profile of tension-type headache.

Pathogenesis ■ *GENETIC BASIS OF MIGRAINE* Migraine has a definite genetic predisposition. Specific mutations leading to *rare* causes of vascular headache have been identified (Table 14-6). For example, the MELAS syndrome consists of a *m*itochondrial *e*ncephalomyopathy, *l*actic *a*cidosis, and *s*troke-like episodes and is caused by an A → G point mutation in the mitochondrial gene encoding for tRNA$^{Leu(UUR)}$ at nucleotide position 3243. Episodic migraine-like headaches are another

TABLE 14-5 *Symptoms Accompanying Severe Migraine Attacks in 500 Patients*

Symptom	Patients Affected, %
Nausea	87
Photophobia	82
Lightheadedness	72
Scalp tenderness	65
Vomiting	56
Visual disturbances	36
Photopsia	26
Fortification spectra	10
Paresthesias	33
Vertigo	33
Alteration of consciousness	18
Syncope	10
Seizure	4
Confusional state	4
Diarrhea	16

Source: From NH Raskin, *Headache*, 2d ed. New York, Churchill Livingston, 1998; with permission.

common clinical feature of this syndrome, especially early in the course of the disease. The genetic pattern of mitochondrial disorders is unique, since only mothers transmit mitochondrial DNA. Thus, all children of mothers with MELAS syndrome are affected with the disorder.

Familial hemiplegic migraine (FHM) is characterized by episodes of recurrent hemiparesis or hemiplegia during the aura phase of a migraine headache. Other associated symptoms may include hemianesthesia or paresthesias; hemianopic visual field disturbances; dysphasia; and variable degrees of drowsiness, confusion, and/or coma. In severe attacks, these symptoms can be quite prolonged and persist for days or weeks, but characteristically they last for only 30 to 60 min and are followed by a unilateral throbbing headache.

Approximately 50% of cases of FHM appear to be caused by mutations within the CACNL1A4 gene on chromosome 19, which encodes a P/Q type calcium channel subunit expressed only in the central nervous system. The gene is very large (>300 kb in length) and consists of 47 exons. Four distinct point mutations have been identified within the gene (in five different families) that cosegregate with the clinical diagnosis of FHM. Analysis of haplotypes in the two families with the same mutation suggest that each mutation arose independently rather than representing a founder effect. CACNL1A4 is likely to play a role in calcium-induced neurotransmitter release and/or contraction of smooth muscle. Different mutations within this gene are the cause of two other neurogenetic disorders, spinocerebellar ataxia type 6 and episodic ataxia type 2 (Chap. 352).

In a genetic association study, a *Nco*I polymorphism in the gene encoding the D_2 dopamine receptor (DRD2) was overrepresented in a population of patients with migraine with aura compared to a control group of nonmigraineurs, suggesting that susceptibility to migraine with aura is modified by certain DRD2 alleles. In a Sardinian population, an association between different DRD2 alleles and migraine has also been demonstrated. These initial studies suggest that variations in dopamine receptor regulation and/or function may alter susceptibility to migraine since molecular variations within the DRD2 gene have been associated with variations in dopaminergic function. However, since not all individuals with the implicated DRD2 genotypes suffer from migraine with aura, additional genes or factors must also be involved. Migraine is likely to be a complex disorder with polygenic inheritance and a strong environmental component.

THE VASCULAR THEORY OF MIGRAINE It was widely held for many years that the headache phase of migrainous attacks was caused by extracranial vasodilatation and that the neurologic symptoms were produced by intracranial vasoconstriction (i.e., the "vascular" hypothesis of migraine). Regional cerebral blood flow studies have shown that in patients with classic migraine there is, during attacks, a modest cortical hypoperfusion that begins in the visual cortex and spreads forward at a rate of 2 to 3 mm/min. The decrease in blood flow averages 25 to 30% (insufficient to explain symptoms on the basis of ischemia) and progresses anteriorly in a wavelike fashion independent of the topography of cerebral arteries. The wave of hypoperfusion persists for 4 to 6 h, appears to follow the convolutions of the cortex, and does not cross the central or lateral sulcus, progressing to the frontal lobe via the insula. Perfusion of subcortical structures is normal. Contralateral neurologic symptoms appear during temporoparietal hypoperfusion; at times, hypoperfusion persists in these regions after symptoms cease. More often, frontal spread continues as the headache phase begins. A few patients with classic migraine show no flow abnormalities; an occasional patient has developed focal ischemia sufficient to cause symptoms. However, focal ischemia does not appear to be *necessary* for focal symptoms to occur.

The ability of these changes to induce the symptoms of migraine has been questioned. Specifically, the decrease in blood flow that is observed does not appear to be significant enough to cause focal neurologic symptoms. Second, the increase in blood flow per se is not painful, and vasodilatation alone cannot account for the local edema and focal tenderness often observed in migraineurs. Moreover, in migraine without aura, no flow abnormalities are usually seen. Thus, it is unlikely that simple vasoconstriction and vasodilatation are the fundamental pathophysiologic abnormalities in migraine. However, it is clear that cerebral blood flow is altered during certain migraine attacks, and these changes may explain some, but clearly not all, of the clinical syndrome of migraine.

THE NEURONAL THEORY OF MIGRAINE Fortification spectrum is a migraine aura characterized by a slowly enlarging visual scotoma with luminous edges (see below). It is believed to result from *spreading depression*, a slowly moving (2 to 3 mm/min), potassium-liberating depression of cortical activity, preceded by a wavefront of increased metabolic activity. Spreading depression can be produced by a variety of experimental stimuli, including hypoxia, mechanical trauma, and the topical application of potassium. These observations suggest that neuronal abnormalities could be the cause of a migraine attack.

Physiologically, electrical stimulation near dorsal raphe neurons in the upper brainstem can result in migraine-like headaches. Blood flow in the pons and midbrain increases focally during migraine headache episodes; this alteration probably results from increased activity of cells in the dorsal raphe and locus coeruleus. There are projections from the dorsal raphe that terminate on cerebral arteries and alter cerebral blood flow. There are also major projections from the dorsal raphe to important visual centers, including the lateral geniculate body, superior colliculus, retina, and visual cortex. These various serotonergic projections may represent the neural substrate for the circulatory and visual characteristics of migraine. The dorsal raphe cells stop firing during deep sleep, and sleep is known to ameliorate migraine; the antimigraine prophylactic drugs also inhibit activity of the dorsal raphe cells through a direct or indirect agonist effect.

Positron emission tomography (PET) scan studies have demon-

TABLE 14-6 *Migraine Genetics*

Gene (Locus)	Function of Gene	Clinical Syndrome	Comment
tRNA^{Leu(UUR)} (mitochondrial)	Unknown	MELAS syndrome	Extremely rare syndrome
CACNL1A4 (19p13)	P/Q calcium channel regulating neurotransmitter release	Familial hemiplegic migraine (FHM)	Mutations account for approximately 50% of FHM cases
DRD2 (11q23)	G protein–coupled D_2 receptor for dopamine	Migraine	Positive association reported in two independent laboratories

Note: MELAS, mitochondrial encephalomyopathy, lactic acidosis, and stroke-like episodes.

strated that midbrain structures near the dorsal raphe are activated during a migraine attack. In one study of acute migraine, an injection of sumatriptan relieved the headache but did not alter the brainstem changes noted on the PET scan. These data suggest that a "brainstem generator" may be the cause of migraine and that certain antimigraine medications may not interfere with the underlying pathologic process in migraine.

THE TRIGEMINOVASCULAR SYSTEM IN MIGRAINE Activation of cells in the trigeminal nucleus caudalis in the medulla (a pain-processing center for the head and face region) results in the release of vasoactive neuropeptides, including substance P and calcitonin gene–related peptide, at vascular terminations of the trigeminal nerve. These peptide neurotransmitters have been proposed to induce a sterile inflammation that activates trigeminal nociceptive afferents originating on the vessel wall, further contributing to the production of pain. This provides a potential mechanism for the soft tissue swelling and tenderness of blood vessels that accompany migraine attacks. However, numerous pharmacologic agents that are effective in preventing or reducing inflammation in this animal model (e.g., selective 5-HT$_{1D}$ agonists, NK-1 antagonists, endothelin antagonists) have failed to demonstrate any clinical efficacy in migraine trials.

5-HYDROXYTRYPTAMINE IN MIGRAINE Pharmacologic and other data point to the involvement of the neurotransmitter 5-hydroxytryptamine (5-HT; also known as serotonin) in migraine. Approximately 40 years ago, methysergide was found to antagonize certain peripheral actions of 5-HT and was introduced as the first drug capable of preventing migraine attacks. Subsequently, it was found that platelet levels of 5-HT fall consistently at the onset of headache and that drugs that cause 5-HT to be released may trigger migrainous episodes. Such changes in circulating 5-HT levels proved to be pharmacologically trivial, however, and interest in the humoral role of 5-HT in migraine declined.

More recently, interest in the role of 5-HT in migraine has been renewed due to the introduction of the triptan class of antimigraine drugs. The triptans are designed to stimulate selectively a particular subpopulation of 5-HT receptors. At least 14 specific 5-HT receptors exist in humans. The triptans (e.g., naratriptan, rizatriptan, sumatriptan, and zolmitriptan) are potent agonists of 5-HT$_{1B}$, 5-HT$_{1D}$, and 5-HT$_{1F}$ receptors and are less potent at 5-HT$_{1A}$ and 5-HT$_{1E}$ receptors. A growing body of data indicates that the antimigraine efficacy of the triptans relates to their ability to stimulate 5-HT$_{1B}$ receptors, which are located on both blood vessels and nerve terminals. Selective 5-HT$_{1D}$ receptor agonists have, thus far, failed to demonstrate clinical efficacy in migraine. Triptans that are weak 5-HT$_{1F}$ agonists are also effective in migraine; however, only 5-HT$_{1B}$ efficacy is currently thought to be essential for antimigraine efficacy.

DOPAMINE IN MIGRAINE A growing body of biologic, pharmacologic, and genetic data supports a role for dopamine in the pathophysiology of certain subtypes of migraine. Most migraine symptoms can be induced by dopaminergic stimulation. Moreover, there is dopamine receptor hypersensitivity in migraineurs, as demonstrated by the induction of yawning, nausea, vomiting, hypotension, and other symptoms of a migraine attack by dopaminergic agonists at doses that do not affect nonmigraineurs. Conversely, dopamine receptor antagonists are effective therapeutic agents in migraine, especially when given parenterally or concurrently with other antimigraine agents. As noted above, genetic data also suggest that molecular variations within dopamine receptor genes play a modifying role in the pathophysiology of migraine with aura. Therefore, modulation of dopaminergic neurotransmission should be considered in the therapeutic management of migraine.

THE SYMPATHETIC NERVOUS SYSTEM IN MIGRAINE Alterations occur within the sympathetic nervous system (SNS) of migraineurs before, during, and between migraine attacks. Factors that activate the SNS are all triggers for migraine. Specific examples include environmental changes (e.g., stress, sleep patterns, hormonal shifts, hypoglycemia) and agents that cause release and a secondary depletion of peripheral catecholamines (e.g., tyramine, phenylethylamine, fenfluramine, m-chlorophenylpiperazine, and reserpine). By contrast, effective therapeutic approaches to migraine share an ability to mimic and/or enhance the effects of norepinephrine in the peripheral SNS. For example, norepinephrine itself, sympathomimetics (e.g., isometheptene), monoamine oxidase inhibitors (MAOIs), and reuptake blockers alleviate migraine. Dopamine antagonists, prostaglandin synthesis inhibitors, and adenosine antagonists are pharmacologic agents effective in the acute treatment of migraine. These drugs block the negative feedback inhibition or norepinephrine release induced by endogenous dopamine, prostaglandins, and adenosine. Therefore, migraine susceptibility may relate to genetically based variations in the ability to maintain adequate concentrations of certain neurotransmitters within postganglionic sympathetic nerve terminals. This hypothesis has been called the *empty neuron theory* of migraine.

Clinical Features ■ *MIGRAINE WITHOUT AURA (COMMON MIGRAINE)* In this syndrome no focal neurologic disturbance precedes the recurrent headaches. Migraine without aura is by far the more frequent type of vascular headache. The International Headache Society criteria for migraine include moderate to severe head pain, pulsating quality, unilateral location, aggravation by walking stairs or similar routine activity, attendant nausea and/or vomiting, photophobia and phonophobia, and multiple attacks, each lasting 4 to 72 h.

MIGRAINE WITH AURA (CLASSIC MIGRAINE) In this syndrome headache is associated with characteristic premonitory sensory, motor, or visual symptoms. Focal neurologic disturbances are more common during headache attacks than as prodromal symptoms. Focal neurologic disturbances without headache or vomiting have come to be known as *migraine equivalents* or *migraine accompaniments* and appear to occur more commonly in patients between the ages of 40 and 70 years. The term *complicated migraine* has generally been used to describe migraine with dramatic transient focal neurologic features or a migraine attack that leaves a persisting residual neurologic deficit.

The most common premonitory symptoms reported by migraineurs are visual, arising from dysfunction of occipital lobe neurons. Scotomas and/or hallucinations occur in about one-third of migraineurs and usually appear in the central portions of the visual fields. A highly characteristic syndrome occurs in about 10% of patients; it usually begins as a small paracentral scotoma, which slowly expands into a "C" shape. Luminous angles appear at the enlarging outer edge, becoming colored as the scintillating scotoma expands and moves toward the periphery of the involved half of the visual field, eventually disappearing over the horizon of peripheral vision. The entire process lasts 20 to 25 min. This phenomenon is pathognomonic for migraine and has never been described in association with a cerebral structural anomaly. It is commonly referred to as a *fortification spectrum* because the serrated edges of the hallucinated "C" seemed to resemble a fortified town with bastions around it; spectrum is used in the sense of an apparition or specter.

BASILAR MIGRAINE Symptoms referable to a disturbance in brainstem function, such as vertigo, dysarthria, or diplopia, occur as the only neurologic symptoms of the attack in about 25% of patients. A dramatic form of basilar migraine (Bickerstaff's migraine) occurs primarily in adolescent females. Episodes begin with total blindness accompanied or followed by admixtures of vertigo, ataxia, dysarthria, tinnitus, and distal and perioral paresthesias. In about one-quarter of patients, a confusional state supervenes. The neurologic symptoms usually persist for 20 to 30 min and are generally followed by a throbbing occipital headache. This basilar migraine syndrome is now known also to occur in children and in adults over age 50. An altered sensorium may persist for as long as 5 days and may take the form of confusional states superficially resembling psychotic reactions. Full recovery after the episode is the rule.

CAROTIDYNIA The carotidynia syndrome, sometimes called *lower-half headache* or *facial migraine*, is most common among older patients, with the incidence peaking in the fourth through sixth decades. Pain is usually located at the jaw or neck, although sometimes periorbital or maxillary pain occurs; it may be continuous, deep, dull, and aching, and it becomes pounding or throbbing episodically. There are often superimposed sharp, ice pick–like jabs. Attacks occur one to several times per week, each lasting several minutes to hours. Tenderness and prominent pulsations of the cervical carotid artery and soft tissue swelling overlying the carotid are usually present ipsilateral to the pain; many patients also report throbbing ipsilateral headache concurrent with carotidynia attacks as well as between attacks. Dental trauma is a common precipitant of this syndrome. Carotid artery involvement also appears to be common in the more traditional forms of migraine; over 50% of patients with frequent migraine attacks are found to have carotid tenderness at several points on the side most often involved during hemicranial migraine attacks.

℞ TREATMENT

Nonpharmacologic Approaches for All Migraineurs Migraine can often be managed to some degree by a variety of nonpharmacologic approaches (Table 14-7). The measures that apply to a given individual should be used routinely since they provide a simple, cost-effective approach to migraine management. Patients with migraine do not encounter more stress than headache-free individuals; overresponsiveness to stress appears to be the issue. Since the stresses of everyday living cannot be eliminated, lessening one's response to stress by various techniques is helpful for many patients. These include yoga, transcendental meditation, hypnosis, and conditioning techniques such as biofeedback. For most patients, this approach is, at best, an adjunct to pharmacotherapy. Avoidance of migraine trigger factors may also provide significant prophylactic benefits. Unfortunately, these measures are unlikely to prevent all migraine attacks. When these measures fail to prevent an attack, pharmacologic approaches are then needed to abort an attack.

Pharmacologic Treatment of Acute Migraine The mainstay of pharmacologic therapy is the judicious use of one or more of the many drugs that are effective in migraine. The selection of the optimal regimen for a given patient depends on a number of factors, the most important of which is the severity of the attack (Table 14-8). Mild migraine attacks can usually be managed by oral agents; the average efficacy rate is 50 to 70%. Severe migraine attacks may require parenteral therapy. Most drugs effective in the treatment of migraine are members of one of three major pharmacologic classes: anti-inflammatory agents, 5-HT$_1$ agonists, and dopamine antagonists.

Table 14-9 lists specific drugs effective in migraine. In general, an adequate dose of whichever agent is chosen should be used as soon as possible after the onset of an attack. If additional medication is required within 60 min because symptoms return or have not abated, the initial dose should be increased for subsequent attacks. Migraine therapy must be individualized for each patient; a standard approach for all patients is not possible. A therapeutic regimen may need to be

TABLE 14-8 *A Staged Approach to Migraine Pharmacotherapy*

Stage	Diagnosis	Therapies
Mild migraine	Occasional throbbing headaches	NSAIDs
		Combination analgesics
	No major impairment of functioning	Oral 5-HT$_1$ agonists
Moderate migraine	Moderate or severe headaches	Oral, nasal, or SC 5-HT$_1$ agonists
	Nausea common	Oral dopamine antagonists
	Some impairment of functioning	
Severe migraine	Severe headaches >3 times per month	SC, IM, or IV 5-HT$_1$ agonists
	Significant functional impairment	IM or IV dopamine antagonists
	Marked nausea and/or vomiting	Prophylactic medications

Note: NSAIDs, nonsteroidal anti-inflammatory drugs; 5-HT, 5-hydroxytryptamine.

constantly refined and personalized until one is identified that provides the patient with rapid, complete, and consistent relief with minimal side effects.

NONSTEROIDAL ANTI-INFLAMMATORY AGENTS Both the severity and duration of a migraine attack can be reduced significantly by anti-inflammatory agents. Indeed, many undiagnosed migraineurs are self-treated with nonprescription anti-inflammatory agents (Table 14-4). A general consensus is that NSAIDs are most effective when taken early in the migraine attack. However, the effectiveness of anti-inflammatory agents in migraine is usually less than optimal in moderate or severe migraine attacks. The combination of acetaminophen, aspirin, and caffeine (Excedrin Migraine) has been approved for use by the U.S. Food and Drug Administration (FDA) for the treatment of mild to moderate migraine. The combination of aspirin and metoclopramide has been shown to be equivalent to a single dose of sumatriptan. Major side effects of NSAIDs include dyspepsia and gastrointestinal irritation.

5-HT$_1$ AGONISTS ■ *Oral* Stimulation of 5-HT$_1$ receptors can stop an acute migraine attack. Ergotamine and dihydroergotamine are nonselective receptor agonists, while the series of drugs known as triptans are selective 5-HT$_1$ receptor agonists. A variety of triptans (e.g., naratriptan, rizatriptan, sumatriptan, zolmitriptan, almotriptan, frovatriptan) are now available for the treatment of migraine (Table 14-9).

Each of the triptan class of drugs has similar pharmacologic properties but varies slightly in terms of clinical efficacy. Rizatriptan and almotriptan are the fastest acting and most efficacious of the triptans currently available in the United States. Sumatriptan and zolmitriptan have similar rates of efficacy as well as time to onset, whereas naratriptan and frovatriptan are the slowest acting and the least efficacious. Clinical efficacy appears to be related more to the t_{max} (time to peak plasma level) than to the potency, half-life, or bioavailability (Table 14-10). This observation is in keeping with a significant body of data indicating that faster-acting analgesics are more efficacious than slower-acting agents.

Unfortunately, monotherapy with a selective oral 5-HT$_1$ agonist does not result in rapid, consistent, and complete relief of migraine in all patients. Triptans are not effective in migraine with aura unless given after the aura is completed and the headache initiated. Side effects, although often mild and transient, occur in up to 89% of patients. Moreover, 5-HT$_1$ agonists are contraindicated in individuals with a history of cardiovascular disease. Recurrence of headache is a major limitation of triptan use, and occurs at least occasionally in 40 to 78% of patients.

Ergotamine preparations offer a nonselective means of stimulating 5-HT$_1$ receptors. A nonnauseating dose of ergotamine should be sought since a dose that provokes nausea is too high and may intensify head pain. Except for a sublingual formulation of ergotamine (Ergo-

TABLE 14-7 *Nonpharmacologic Approaches to Migraine*

Identify and then avoid trigger factors such as:
  Alcohol (e.g., red wine)
  Foods (e.g., chocolate, certain cheeses, monosodium glutamate, nitrate-containing foods)
  Hunger (avoid missing meals)
  Irregular sleep patterns (both lack of sleep and excessive sleep)
  Organic odors
  Sustained exertion
  Acute changes in stress levels
  Miscellaneous (glare, flashing lights)
Attempt to manage environmental shifts such as:
  Time zone shifts
  High altitude
  Barometric pressure changes
  Weather changes
Assess menstrual cycle relationship

TABLE 14-9 *Treatment of Acute Migraine*

Drug	Trade Name	Dosage
NSAIDS		
Acetaminophen, aspirin, caffeine	Excedrin Migraine	Two tablets or caplets q6h (max 8 per day)
5-HT₁ AGONISTS		
Oral		
Ergotamine	Ergomar	One 2 mg sublingual tablet at onset and q1/2h (max 3 per day, 5 per week)
Ergotamine 1 mg, caffeine 100 mg	Ercaf, Wigraine	One or two tablets at onset, then one tablet q1/2h (max 6 per day, 10 per week)
Naratriptan	Amerge	2.5 mg tablet at onset; may repeat once after 4 h
Rizatriptan	Maxalt, Maxalt-MLT	5 to 10 mg tablet at onset; may repeat after 2 h (max 30 mg/d)
Sumatriptan	Imitrex	50 to 100 mg tablet at onset; may repeat after 2 h (max 200 mg/d)
Zolmitriptan	Zomig, Zomig Rapimelt	2.5 mg tablet at onset; may repeat after 2 h (max 10 mg/d)
Nasal		
Dihydroergotamine	Migranal Nasal Spray	Prior to nasal spray, the pump must be primed 4 times; one spray (0.5 mg) is administered followed, in 15 min, by a second spray
Sumatriptan	Imitrex Nasal Spray	5 to 20 mg intranasal spray as 4 sprays of 5 mg or a single 20 mg spray (may repeat once after 2 h, not to exceed a dose of 40 mg/d)
Parenteral		
Dihydroergotamine	DHE-45	1 mg IV, IM, or SC at onset and q1h (max 3 mg/d, 6 mg per week)
Sumatriptan	Imitrex Injection	6 mg SC at onset (may repeat once after 1 h for max of two doses in 24 h)
DOPAMINE ANTAGONISTS		
Oral		
Metoclopramide	Reglan,[a] generic[a]	5–10 mg/d
Prochlorperazine	Compazine,[a] generic[a]	1–25 mg/d
Parenteral		
Chlorpromazine	Generic[a]	0.1 mg/kg IV at 2 mg/min; max 35 mg/d
Metoclopramide	Reglan,[a] generic	10 mg IV
Prochlorperazine	Compazine,[a] generic[a]	10 mg IV
OTHER		
Oral		
Acetaminophen, 325 mg, *plus* dichloralphenazone, 100 mg, *plus* isometheptene, 65 mg	Midrin, Duradrin, generic	Two capsules at onset followed by 1 capsule q1h (max 5 capsules)
Nasal		
Butorphanol	Stadol[a]	1 mg (1 spray in 1 nostril), may repeat if necessary in 1–2 h
Parenteral		
Narcotics	Generic[a]	Multiple preparations and dosages; see Table 11-1.

[a] Not specifically indicated by the U.S. Food and Drug Administration for migraine.
Note: NSAIDs, nonsteroidal anti-inflammatory drugs; 5-HT, 5-hydroxytryptamine.

mar), oral formulations of ergotamine also contain 100 mg caffeine (theoretically to enhance ergotamine absorption and possibly to add additional vasoconstrictor activity). The average oral ergotamine dose for a migraine attack is 2 mg. Since the clinical studies demonstrating the efficacy of ergotamine in migraine predated the clinical trial methodologies used with the triptans, it is difficult to assess the clinical efficacy of ergotamine versus the triptans. In general, ergotamine appears to have a much higher incidence of nausea than triptans, but less headache recurrence.

Nasal The fastest acting nonparenteral antimigraine therapies that can be self-administered include nasal formulations of dihydroergotamine (Migranal) or sumatriptan (Imitrex Nasal). The nasal sprays result in substantial blood levels within 30 to 60 min. However, the nasal formulations suffer from inconsistent dosing, poor taste, and variable efficacy. Although in theory the nasal sprays might provide faster and more effective relief of a migraine attack than oral formulations, their reported efficacy is only approximately 50 to 60%.

Parenteral Parenteral administration of drugs such as dihydroergotamine (DHE-45 Injectable) and sumatriptan (Imitrex SC) is approved by the FDA for the rapid relief of a migraine attack. Peak plasma levels of dihydroergotamine are achieved 3 min after intravenous dosing, 30 min after intramuscular dosing, and 45 min after subcutaneous dosing. If an attack has not already peaked, subcutaneous or intramuscular administration of 1 mg dihydroergotamine suffices for about 80 to 90% of patients. Sumatriptan, 6 mg subcutaneously, is effective in approximately 70 to 80% of patients.

DOPAMINE ANTAGONISTS ◼ *Oral* Oral dopamine antagonists should be considered as adjunctive therapy in migraine. Drug absorption is impaired during migrainous attacks because of reduced gastrointestinal motility. Delayed absorption occurs in the absence of nausea and is related to the severity of the attack and not its duration. Therefore, when oral NSAIDs and/or triptan agents fail, the addition of a dopamine antagonist such as metoclopramide, 10 mg, should be considered to enhance gastric absorption. In addition, dopamine antagonists decrease nausea/vomiting and restore normal gastric motility.

Parenteral Parenteral dopamine antagonists (e.g., chlorpromazine, prochlorperazine, metoclopramide) can also provide significant acute relief of migraine; they can be used in combination with parenteral 5-HT₁ agonists. A common intravenous protocol used for the treatment of severe migraine is the administration over 2 min of a mixture of 5 mg of prochlorperazine and 0.5 mg of dihydroergotamine.

OTHER MEDICATIONS FOR ACUTE MIGRAINE ◼ *Oral* The combination of acetaminophen, dichloralphenazone, and isometheptene (i.e., Midrin, Duradrin, generic), one to two capsules, has been classified by the FDA as "possibly" effective in the treatment of migraine. Since the clinical studies demonstrating the efficacy of this combination analgesic in migraine predated the clinical trial methodologies used with

TABLE 14-10 *Comparative Pharmacology of Oral Triptans[a]*

Drug and Dose, mg	t_{max}, h	$t_{1/2}$, h	Oral Bioavailability, %	Clinical Efficacy at 2 h, %
Rizatriptan, 10	1–2	2–3	45	71
Zolmitriptan, 2.5	2	2.5–3	44	65
Sumatriptan, 50	2–3	2	14	61
Naratriptan, 2.5	2–4	5–6	68	45
Frovatriptan, 2.5	2–3	26	25	43
Almotriptan, 12.5	2–3	3	70	58

[a] Data adapted from package inserts approved by the U.S. Food and Drug Administration.

the triptans, it is difficult to assess the clinical efficacy of this sympathomimetic compound in comparison to other agents.

Nasal   A nasal preparation of butorphanol is available for the treatment of acute pain. As with all narcotics, the use of nasal butorphanol should be limited to a select group of migraineurs, as described below.

Parenteral   Narcotics are effective in the acute treatment of migraine. For example, intravenous meperidine (Demerol), 50 to 100 mg, is given frequently in the emergency room. This regimen "works" in the sense that the pain of migraine is eliminated. However, this regimen is clearly suboptimal in patients with recurrent headache for two major reasons. First, narcotics do not treat the underlying headache mechanism; rather, they act at the thalamic level to alter pain sensation. Second, the recurrent use of narcotics can lead to significant problems. In patients taking oral narcotics such as oxycodone (Percodan) or hydrocodone (Vicodin), narcotic addiction can greatly confuse the treatment of migraine. The headache that results from narcotic craving and/or withdrawal can be difficult to distinguish from chronic migraine. Therefore, it is recommended that narcotic use in migraine be limited to patients with severe, but infrequent, headaches that are unresponsive to other pharmacologic approaches.

Prophylactic Treatment of Migraine   A substantial number of drugs are now available that have the capacity to stabilize migraine (Table 14-11). The decision of whether to use this approach depends on the frequency of attacks and on how well acute treatment is working. The occurrence of at least three attacks per month could be an indication for this approach. Drugs must be taken daily, and there is usually a lag of at least 2 to 6 weeks before an effect is seen. The drugs that have been approved by the FDA for the prophylactic treatment of migraine include propranolol, timolol, sodium valproate, and methysergide. In addition, a number of other drugs appear to display prophylactic efficacy. This group of drugs includes amitriptyline, nortriptyline, verapamil, phenelzine, gabapentin, and cyproheptadine. Phenelzine and methysergide are usually reserved for recalcitrant cases because of their serious potential side effects. Phenelzine is an MAOI; therefore, tyramine-containing foods, decongestants, and meperidine are contraindicated. Methysergide may cause retroperitoneal or cardiac valvular fibrosis when it is used for >8 months, thus monitoring is required for patients using this drug; the risk of the fibrotic complication is about 1:1500 and is likely to reverse after the drug is stopped.

The probability of success with any one of the antimigraine drugs is 50 to 75%; thus, if one drug is assessed each month, there is a good chance that effective stabilization will be achieved within a few months. Many patients are managed adequately with low-dose amitriptyline, propranolol, or valproate. If these agents fail or lead to un-

acceptable side effects, then methysergide or phenelzine can be used. Once effective stabilization is achieved, the drug is continued for 5 to 6 months and then slowly tapered to assess the continued need. Many patients are able to discontinue medication and experience fewer and milder attacks for long periods, suggesting that these drugs may alter the natural history of migraine.

CLUSTER HEADACHE   A variety of names have been used for this condition, including *Raeder's syndrome*, *histamine cephalalgia*, and *sphenopalatine neuralgia*. *Cluster headache* is a distinctive and treatable vascular headache syndrome. The episodic type is most common and is characterized by one to three short-lived attacks of periorbital pain per day over a 4- to 8-week period, followed by a pain-free interval that averages 1 year. The chronic form, which may begin de novo or several years after an episodic pattern has become established, is characterized by the absence of sustained periods of remission. Each type may transform into the other. Men are affected seven to eight times more often than women; hereditary factors are usually absent. Although the onset is generally between ages 20 and 50, it may occur as early as the first decade of life. Propranolol and amitriptyline are largely ineffective. Lithium is beneficial for cluster headache and ineffective in migraine. The cluster syndrome is thus clinically, genetically, and therapeutically different from migraine. Nevertheless, mixed features of the two disorders are occasionally present, suggesting some common elements to their pathogenesis.

Clinical Features   Periorbital or, less commonly, temporal pain begins without warning and reaches a crescendo within 5 min. It is often excruciating in intensity and is deep, nonfluctuating, and explosive in quality; only rarely is it pulsatile. Pain is strictly unilateral and usually affects the same side in subsequent months. Attacks last from 30 min to 2 h; there are often associated symptoms of homolateral lacrimation, reddening of the eye, nasal stuffiness, lid ptosis, and nausea. Alcohol provokes attacks in about 70% of patients but ceases to be provocative when the bout remits; this on-off vulnerability to alcohol is pathognomonic of cluster headache. Only rarely do foods or emotional factors precipitate pain, in contrast to migraine.

There is a striking periodicity of attacks in at least 85% of patients. At least one of the daily attacks of pain recurs at about the same hour each day for the duration of a cluster bout. Onset is nocturnal in about 50% of the cases, and then the pain usually awakens the patient within 2 h of falling asleep.

Pathogenesis   No consistent cerebral blood flow changes accompany attacks of pain. Perhaps the strongest evidence for a central mechanism is the periodicity of attacks; the existence of a central mechanism is also suggested by the observation that autonomic symptoms that accompany the pain are bilateral and are more severe on the painful side. The hypothalamus is probably the site of activation in this disorder. The posterior hypothalamus contains cells that regulate autonomic functions, and the anterior hypothalamus contains cells (in the suprachiasmatic nuclei) that constitute the principal circadian pacemaker in mammals. Activation of both is necessary to explain the symptoms of cluster headache. The pacemaker is modulated via serotonergic dorsal raphe projections. It can be concluded tentatively that both migraine and cluster headache result from abnormal serotonergic neurotransmission, albeit at different loci.

Rx TREATMENT

The most satisfactory treatment is the administration of drugs to prevent cluster attacks until the bout is over. Effective prophylactic drugs are prednisone, lithium, methysergide, ergotamine, sodium valproate, and verapamil. Lithium (600 to 900 mg daily) appears to be particularly useful for the chronic form of the disorder. A 10-day course of prednisone, beginning at 60 mg daily for 7 days followed by a rapid taper, may interrupt the pain bout for many patients. When ergotamine is used, it is most effective when given 1 to 2 h before an expected

TABLE 14-11   *Drugs Effective in the Prophylactic Treatment of Migraine*

Drug	Trade Name	Dosage
β-Adrenergic agents		
Propranolol	Inderal	80–320 mg qd
	Inderal LA	
Timolol	Blocadren	20–60 mg qd
Anticonvulsants		
Sodium valproate	Depakote	250 mg bid (max 1000 mg/d)
Tricyclic antidepressants		
Amitriptyline	Elavil,[a] generic	10–50 mg qhs
Nortriptyline	Pamelor,[a] generic	25–75 mg qhs
Monoamine oxidase inhibitors		
Phenelzine	Nardil[a]	15 mg tid
Serotonergic drugs		
Methysergide	Sansert	4–8 mg qd
Cyproheptadine	Periactin[a]	4–16 mg qd
Other		
Verapamil	Calan[a]	80–480 mg qd
	Isoptin[a]	

[a] Not specifically indicated for migraine by the U.S. Food and Drug Administration.

attack. Patients who use ergotamine daily must be educated regarding the early symptoms of ergotism, which may include vomiting, numbness, tingling, pain, and cyanosis of the limbs; a weekly limit of 14 mg should be adhered to.

For the attacks themselves, oxygen inhalation (9 L/min via a loose mask) is the most effective modality; 15 min of inhalation of 100%

oxygen is often necessary. Sumatriptan, 6 mg subcutaneously, will usually shorten an attack to 10 to 15 min.

FURTHER READING

FERRARI MD et al: Oral triptans in acute migraine treatment: A meta-analysis of 53 trials. Lancet 358:1668, 2001

GOADSBY PJ: Serotonin 5-HT 1B/1D receptor agonists in migraine. CNS Drugs 10:271, 1998

LODER E: Safety of sumatriptan in pregnancy. CNS Drugs 17:1, 2003

---

15 BACK AND NECK PAIN
John W. Engstrom

The importance of back and neck pain in our society is underscored by the following: (1) the cost of back pain in the United States is between $20 and $50 billion annually, (2) back symptoms are the most common cause of disability in patients under 45 years of age, (3) low back pain is the second most common reason for visiting a physician in the United States, and (4) approximately 1% of the U.S. population is chronically disabled because of back pain.

ANATOMY OF THE SPINE

The anterior portion of the spine consists of cylindrical vertebral bodies separated by intervertebral disks and held together by the anterior and posterior longitudinal ligaments. The intervertebral disks are composed of a central gelatinous nucleus pulposus surrounded by a tough cartilagenous ring, the annulus fibrosis; disks are responsible for 25% of spinal column length (Figs. 15-1 and 15-2). The disks are largest in the cervical and lumbar regions where movements of the spine are greatest. The disks are elastic in youth and allow the bony vertebrae to move easily upon each other. Elasticity is lost with age. The function of the anterior spine is to absorb the shock of body movements such as walking and running.

The posterior portion of the spine consists of the vertebral arches and seven processes. Each arch consists of paired cylindrical pedicles anteriorly and paired laminae posteriorly. The vertebral arch gives rise to two transverse processes laterally, one spinous process posteriorly, plus two superior and two inferior articular facets. The functions of the posterior spine are to protect the spinal cord and nerves within the spinal canal and to stabilize the spine by providing sites for the attachment of muscles and ligaments. The contraction of muscles attached to the spinous and transverse processes produces a system of pulleys and levers that results in flexion, extension, and lateral bending movements of the spine.

Nerve root injury (*radiculopathy*) is a common cause of neck, arm, low back, and leg pain. The nerve roots exit at a level above their respective vertebral bodies in the cervical region (the C7 nerve root exits at the C6-C7 level) and below their respective vertebral bodies in the thoracic and lumbar regions (the T1 nerve root exits at the T1-T2 level). The cervical nerve roots follow a relatively short intraspinal course before exiting. By contrast, because the spinal cord ends at the vertebral L1 or L2 level, the lumbar nerve roots follow a long intraspinal course and can be injured anywhere from the upper lumbar spine to their exit at the intervertebral foramen. For example, it is common for disk herniation at the L4-L5 level to produce compression of the S1 nerve root (Fig. 15-3).

Pain-sensitive structures in the spine include the periosteum of the vertebrae, dura, facet joints, annulus fibrosus of the intervertebral disk, epidural veins, and the posterior longitudinal ligament. The nucleus pulposus of the intervertebral disk is not pain-sensitive under normal circumstances. Pain sensation is conveyed by the sinuvertebral nerve that arises from the spinal nerve at each spine segment and reenters the spinal canal through the intervertebral foramen at the same level. Disease of these diverse pain-sensitive spine structures may explain many cases of back pain without nerve root compression. The lumbar and cervical spine possess the greatest potential for movement and injury.

APPROACH TO THE PATIENT

Types of Back Pain   Understanding the type of pain experienced by the patient is the essential first step. Attention is also focused on identification of risk factors for serious underlying diseases.

Local pain is caused by stretching of pain-sensitive structures that compress or irritate sensory nerve endings. The site of the pain is near the affected part of the back.

Pain referred to the back may arise from abdominal or pelvic viscera. The pain is usually described as primarily abdominal or pelvic but is accompanied by back pain and usually unaffected by posture. The patient may occasionally complain of back pain only.

Pain of spine origin may be located in the back or referred to the buttocks or legs. Diseases affecting the upper lumbar spine tend to refer pain to the lumbar region, groin, or anterior thighs. Diseases affecting the lower lumbar spine tend to produce pain referred to the buttocks, posterior thighs, or rarely the calves or feet. Provocative injections into the pain-sensitive structures of the spine may produce leg pain that does not follow a dermatomal distribution. This "sclerotomal" pain may explain instances in which back and leg pain is unaccompanied by evidence of nerve root compression.

Radicular back pain is typically sharp and radiates from the spine to the leg within the territory of a nerve root (see "Lumbar Disk Disease," below). Coughing, sneezing, or voluntary contraction of abdominal muscles (lifting heavy objects or

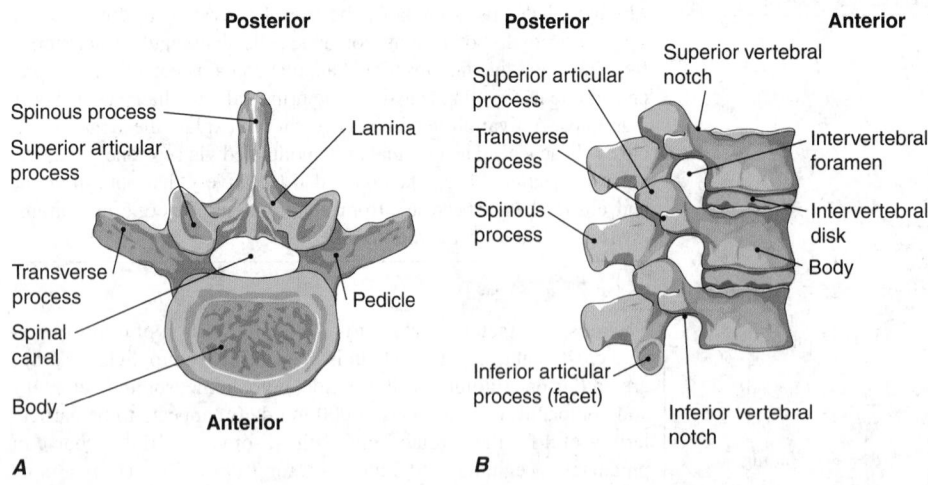

FIGURE 15-1 Vertebral anatomy. (*From A Gauthier Cornuelle, DH Gronefeld: Radiographic Anatomy Positioning. New York, McGraw-Hill, 1998, with permission.*)

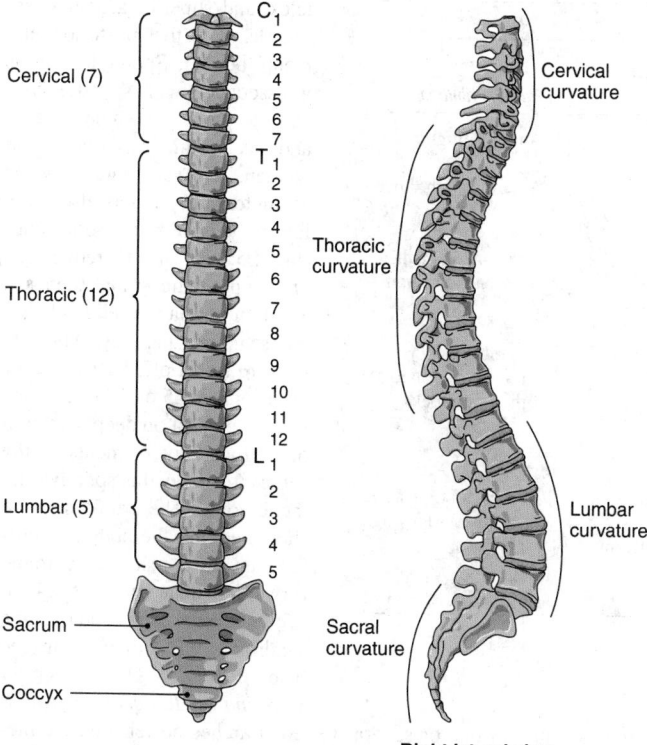

Cervical (7)

C1
2
3
4
5
6
7

Cervical curvature

T1
2
3
4
5
6
7
8
9
10
11
12

Thoracic (12)

Thoracic curvature

L1
2
3
4
5

Lumbar (5)

Lumbar curvature

Sacrum

Sacral curvature

Coccyx

Right lateral view

FIGURE 15-2 Spinal column. (*From A Gauthier Cornuelle, DH Gronefeld: Radiographic Anatomy Positioning. New York, McGraw-Hill, 1998, with permission.*)

tures). Knowledge of the circumstances associated with the onset of back pain is important when weighing possible serious underlying causes for the pain. Some patients involved in accidents or work-related injuries may exaggerate their pain for the purpose of compensation or for psychological reasons.

Examination of the Back A physical examination that includes the abdomen and rectum is advisable. Back pain referred from visceral organs may be reproduced during palpation of the abdomen [pancreatitis, abdominal aortic aneurysm (AAA)] or percussion over the costovertebral angles (pyelonephritis, adrenal disease).

The normal spine has a thoracic kyphosis, lumbar lordosis, and cervical lordosis. Exaggeration of these normal alignments may result in hyperkyphosis (lameback) of the thoracic spine or hyperlordosis (swayback) of the lumbar spine. Spasm of lumbar paraspinal muscles results in flattening of the usual lumbar lordosis. Inspection may reveal lateral curvature of the spine (scoliosis) or an asymmetry in the paraspinal muscles, suggesting muscle spasm. Taut paraspinal muscles limit motion of the lumbar spine. Back pain of bony spine origin is often reproduced by palpation or percussion over the spinous process of the affected vertebrae.

Forward bending is frequently limited by paraspinal muscle spasm. Flexion of the hips is normal in patients with lumbar spine disease, but flexion of the lumbar spine is limited and sometimes painful. Lateral bending to the side opposite the injured spinal element may stretch the damaged tissues, worsen pain, and limit motion. Hyperextension of the spine (with the patient prone or standing) is limited when nerve root compression or bony spine disease is present.

Pain from hip disease may resemble the pain of lumbar spine disease. Hip pain can be reproduced by internal and external rotation at the hip with the knee and hip in flexion (Patrick sign) and by tapping the heel with the examiner's palm while the leg is extended.

With the patient lying flat, passive flexion of the extended leg at the hip stretches the L5 and S1 nerve roots and the sciatic nerve. Passive dorsiflexion of the foot during the maneuver adds to the stretch. While flexion to at least 80° is normally possible without causing pain, tight hamstrings may be a source of pain in some patients. The *straight leg–raising (SLR)* test is positive if the maneuver reproduces the patient's usual back or limb pain. Eliciting the SLR sign in the sitting position may help determine if the finding is reproducible. The patient may describe pain in the low back, buttocks, posterior thigh, or lower leg, but the key feature is reproduction of the patient's usual pain. The *crossed SLR sign* is positive when flexion of one leg reproduces the pain in the opposite leg or buttocks. The crossed SLR sign is less sensitive but more specific for disk herniation than the SLR sign. The nerve or nerve root lesion is always on the side of the pain. The *reverse SLR sign* is elicited by standing the patient next to the examination table and passively extending each leg. This maneuver, which stretches the L2-L4 nerve roots and the femoral nerve, is considered positive if the patient's usual back or limb pain is reproduced.

The neurologic examination includes a search for weakness, muscle atrophy, focal reflex changes, diminished sensation in the legs, and signs of spinal cord injury. The examiner should be alert to the possibility of breakaway weakness, defined as fluctuating levels of strength in one or more muscle groups on examination. The weakness may be due to pain or a combination of pain and underlying true weakness. Breakaway weakness without pain is due to lack of effort. In uncertain cases, electromyography (EMG) can determine whether or not true weakness is present. Findings with specific nerve root lesions are shown in Table 15-1 and are discussed below.

straining at stool) may elicit the radiating pain. The pain may increase in postures that stretch the nerves and nerve roots. Sitting stretches the sciatic nerve (L5 and S1 roots) because the nerve passes posterior to the hip. The femoral nerve (L2, L3, and L4 roots) passes anterior to the hip and is not stretched by sitting. The description of the pain alone often fails to distinguish clearly between sclerotomal pain and radiculopathy.

Pain associated with muscle spasm, although of obscure origin, is commonly associated with many spine disorders. The spasms are accompanied by abnormal posture, taut paraspinal muscles, and dull pain.

Back pain at rest or unassociated with specific postures should raise the index of suspicion for an underlying serious cause (e.g., spine tumor, fracture, infection, or referred pain from visceral struc-

Laboratory, Imaging, and EMG Studies Routine laboratory studies such as a complete blood count, erythrocyte sedimentation rate, chem-

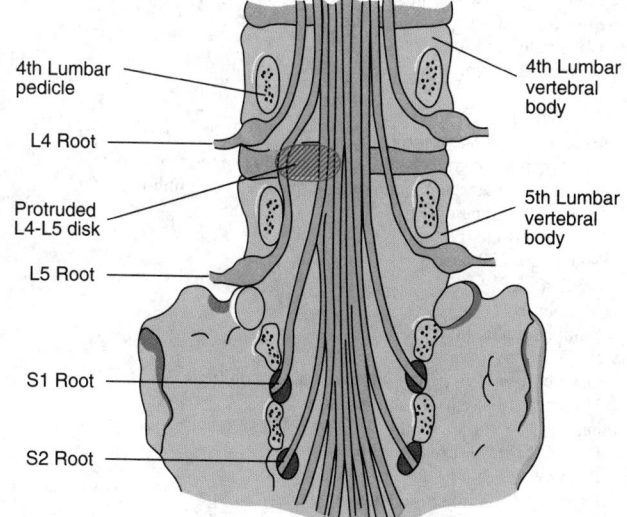

4th Lumbar pedicle

4th Lumbar vertebral body

L4 Root

Protruded L4-L5 disk

5th Lumbar vertebral body

L5 Root

S1 Root

S2 Root

FIGURE 15-3 Compression of L5 and S1 roots by herniated disk. (*From RD Adams et al: Principles of Neurology, 7th ed. New York, McGraw-Hill, 1997, with permission.*)

TABLE 15-1 *Lumbosacral Radiculopathy—Neurologic Features*

Lumbosacral Nerve Roots	Examination Findings				Pain Distribution
	Reflex	Sensory	Motor		Pain Distribution
L2[a]	—	Upper anterior thigh	Psoas (hip flexion)		Anterior thigh
L3[a]	—	Lower anterior thigh Anterior knee	Psoas (hip flexion) Quadriceps (knee extension) Thigh adduction		Anterior thigh, knee
L4[a]	Quadriceps (knee)	Medial calf	Quadriceps (knee extension)[b] Thigh adduction Tibialis anterior (foot dorsiflexion)		Knee, medial calf Anterolateral thigh
L5[c]	—	Dorsal surface—foot Lateral calf	Peroneii (foot eversion)[b] Tibialis anterior (foot dorsiflexion) Gluteus medius (hip abduction) Toe dorsiflexors		Lateral calf, dorsal foot, posterolateral thigh, buttocks
S1[c]	Gastrocnemius/soleus (ankle)	Plantar surface—foot Lateral aspect—foot	Gastrocnemius/soleus (foot plantar flexion)[b] Abductor hallucis (toe flexors)[b] Gluteus maximus (hip extension)		Bottom foot, posterior calf, posterior thigh, buttocks

[a] Reverse straight leg–raising sign present—see "Examination of the Back."
[b] These muscles receive the majority of innervation from this root.
[c] Straight leg–raising sign present—see "Examination of the Back."

istry panel, and urinalysis are rarely needed for the initial evaluation of nonspecific ALBP (3 months). If risk factors for a serious underlying disease are present, then laboratory studies (guided by the history and examination) are indicated.

Plain films of the lumbar or cervical spine are helpful when risk factors for vertebral fracture (trauma, chronic steroid use) are present. In the absence of risk factors, routine x-rays of the lumbar spine in nonspecific ALBP are expensive and rarely helpful. Magnetic resonance imaging (MRI) and computed tomography (CT)–myelography are the radiologic tests of choice for evaluation of most serious diseases involving the spine. MRI is superior for the definition of soft tissue structures, whereas CT-myelography provides optimal imaging of bony lesions and is tolerated by claustrophobic patients. With rare exceptions, conventional myelography and bone scan are inferior to MRI and CT-myelography.

EMG can be used to assess the functional integrity of the peripheral nervous system (Chap. 363). Sensory nerve conduction studies are normal when focal sensory loss is due to nerve root damage because the nerve roots are proximal to the nerve cell bodies in the dorsal root ganglia. The diagnostic yield of needle EMG is higher than that of nerve conduction studies for radiculopathy. Denervation changes in a myotomal (segmental) distribution are detected by sampling multiple muscles supplied by different nerve roots and nerves; the pattern of muscle involvement indicates the nerve root(s) responsible for the injury. Needle EMG provides objective information about motor nerve fiber injury when the clinical evaluation of weakness is limited by pain or poor effort. EMG and nerve conduction studies will be normal when only limb pain or sensory nerve root injury or irritation is present. Mixed nerve somatosensory evoked potentials and F-wave studies are of uncertain value in the evaluation of radiculopathy.

CAUSES OF BACK PAIN (Table 15-2)

CONGENITAL ANOMALIES OF THE LUMBAR SPINE *Spondylolysis* is a bony defect in the pars interarticularis (a segment near the junction of the pedicle with the lamina) of the vertebra; the etiology may be a stress fracture in a congenitally abnormal segment. The defect (usually bilateral) is best visualized on oblique projections in plain x-rays or by CT scan and occurs in the setting of a single injury, repeated minor injuries, or growth.

Spondylolisthesis is the anterior slippage of the vertebral body, ped-

icles, and superior articular facets, leaving the posterior elements behind. Spondylolisthesis is associated with spondylolysis and degenerative spine disease and occurs more frequently in women. The slippage may be asymptomatic but may also cause low back pain, nerve root injury (the L5 root most frequently), or symptomatic spinal stenosis. Tenderness may be elicited near the segment that has "slipped" forward (most often L4 on L5 or occasionally L5 on S1). A "step" may be present on deep palpation of the posterior elements of the segment above the spondylolisthetic joint. The trunk may be shortened and the abdomen protuberant as a result of extreme forward displacement of L4 on L5; in severe cases cauda equina syndrome (CES) may occur (see below).

Spina bifida occulta is a failure of closure of one or several vertebral arches posteriorly; the meninges and spinal cord are normal. A dimple or small lipoma may overlie the defect. Most cases are asymptomatic and discovered incidentally during evaluation for back pain.

Tethered cord syndrome usually presents as a progressive cauda

TABLE 15-2 *Causes of Low Back and Neck Pain*

Congenital/developmental
  Spondylolysis and spondylolisthesis[a]
  Kyphoscoliosis[a]
  Spina bifida occulta[a]
  Tethered spinal cord[a]
Minor trauma
  Strain or sprain
  Whiplash injury[b]
Fractures
  Traumatic—falls, motor vehicle accidents
  Atraumatic—osteoporosis, neoplastic infiltration, exogenous steroids
Intervertebral disk herniation
Degenerative
  Disk-osteophyte complex
  Internal disk disruption
  Spinal stenosis with neurogenic claudication[a]
  Uncovertebral joint disease[b]
  Atlantoaxial joint disease (e.g., rheumatoid arthritis)[a]
Arthritis
  Spondylosis
  Facet or sacroiliac arthropathy
  Autoimmune (e.g., ankylosing spondylitis, Reiter's syndrome)
Neoplasms—metastatic, hematologic, primary bone tumors
Infection/inflammation
  Vertebral osteomyelitis
  Spinal epidural abscess
  Septic disk
  Meningitis
  Lumbar arachnoiditis[a]
Metabolic
  Osteoporosis—hyperparathyroidism, immobility
  Osteosclerosis (e.g., Paget's disease)
Other
  Referred pain from visceral disease
  Postural
  Psychiatric, malingering, chronic pain syndromes
  Vertebral artery dissection[a]

[a] Low back pain only.
[b] Neck pain only.

equina disorder (see below), although myelopathy may also be the initial manifestation. The patient is often a young adult who complains of perineal or perianal pain, sometimes following minor trauma. Neuroimaging studies reveal a low-lying conus (below L1-L2) and a short and thickened filum terminale.

TRAUMA A patient complaining of back pain and inability to move the legs may have a spinal fracture or dislocation and, with fractures above L1, spinal cord compression. Care must be taken to avoid further damage to the spinal cord or nerve roots by immobilizing the back pending results of x-rays.

Sprains and Strains The terms *low back sprain*, *strain*, or *mechanically induced muscle spasm* refer to minor, self-limited injuries associated with lifting a heavy object, a fall, or a sudden deceleration such as in an automobile accident. These terms are used loosely and do not clearly describe a specific anatomic lesion. The pain is usually confined to the lower back, and there is no radiation to the buttocks or legs. Patients with paraspinal muscle spasm often assume unusual postures.

Traumatic Vertebral Fractures Most traumatic fractures of the lumbar vertebral bodies result from injuries producing anterior wedging or compression. With severe trauma, the patient may sustain a fracture-dislocation or a "burst" fracture involving the vertebral body and posterior elements. Traumatic vertebral fractures are caused by falls from a height (a pars interarticularis fracture of the L5 vertebra is common), sudden deceleration in an automobile accident, or direct injury. Neurologic impairment is common, and early surgical treatment is indicated.

LUMBAR DISK DISEASE This is a common cause of chronic or recurrent low back and leg pain (Fig. 15-4). Disk disease is most likely to occur at the L4-L5 and L5-S1 levels, but upper lumbar levels are involved occasionally. The cause is often unknown; the risk is increased in overweight individuals. Disk herniation is unusual prior to age 20 and is rare in the fibrotic disks of the elderly. Degeneration of the nucleus pulposus and the annulus fibrosus increases with age and may be asymptomatic or painful. The pain may be located in the low back only or referred to the leg, buttock, or hip. A sneeze, cough, or trivial movement may cause the nucleus pulposus to prolapse, pushing the frayed and weakened annulus posteriorly. With severe disk disease, the nucleus may protrude through the annulus (herniation) or become extruded to lie as a free fragment in the spinal canal.

The mechanism by which intervertebral disk injury causes back

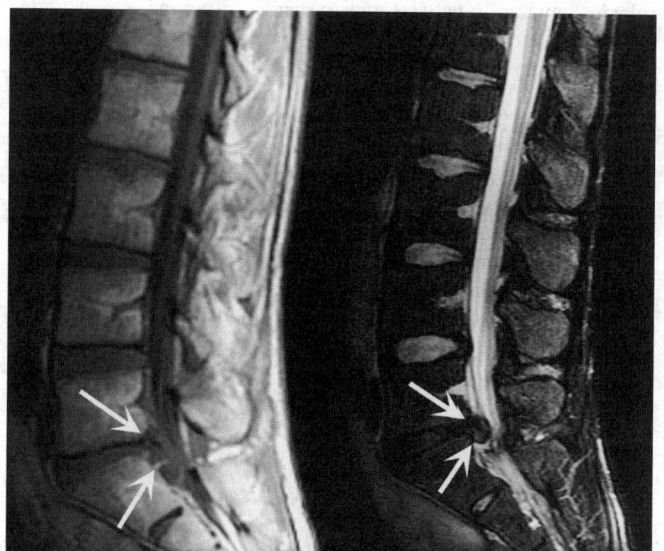

FIGURE 15-4 MRI of lumbar herniated disk; left S1 radiculopathy. Sagittal T1-weighted image on the left with arrows outlining disk margins. Sagittal T2 image on the right reveals a protruding disk at the L5-S1 level (*arrows*), which displaces the central thecal sac.

pain is controversial. The inner annulus fibrosus and nucleus pulposus are normally devoid of innervation. Inflammation and production of proinflammatory cytokines within the protruding or ruptured disk may trigger or perpetuate back pain. Ingrowth of nociceptive (pain) nerve fibers into inner portions of a diseased disk may be responsible for chronic "diskogenic" pain. Nerve root injury (radiculopathy) from disk herniation may be due to compression, inflammation, or both; pathologically, demyelination and axonal loss are usually present.

Symptoms of a ruptured disk include back pain, abnormal posture, limitation of spine motion (particularly flexion), or radicular pain. A dermatomal pattern of sensory loss or a reduced or absent deep tendon reflex is more suggestive of a specific root lesion than the pattern of pain. Motor findings (focal weakness, muscle atrophy, or fasciculations) occur less frequently than sensory or reflex changes. Symptoms and signs are usually unilateral, but bilateral involvement does occur with large central disk herniations that compress several nerve roots at the same level. Clinical manifestations of specific nerve root lesions are summarized in Table 15-1. There is evidence to suggest that lumbar disk herniation with a nonprogressive nerve root deficit can be managed nonsurgically. The size of the disk protrusion may naturally decrease over time.

The differential diagnosis includes a variety of serious and treatable conditions, including epidural abscess, hematoma, or tumor. Fever, constant pain uninfluenced by position, sphincter abnormalities, or signs of spinal cord disease suggest an etiology other than lumbar disk disease. Bilateral absence of ankle reflexes can be a normal finding in old age or a sign of bilateral S1 radiculopathy. An absent deep tendon reflex or focal sensory loss may reflect injury to a nerve root, but other sites of injury along the nerve must also be considered. For example, an absent knee reflex may be due to a femoral neuropathy rather than an L4 nerve root injury. A loss of sensation over the foot and distal lateral calf may result from a peroneal or lateral sciatic neuropathy rather than an L5 nerve root injury. Focal muscle atrophy may reflect a nerve root or peripheral nerve injury, an anterior horn cell disease, or disuse.

An MRI scan or CT-myelogram is necessary to establish the location and type of pathology. Simple MRI yields exquisite views of intraspinal and adjacent soft tissue anatomy. Bony lesions of the lateral recess or intervertebral foramen may be seen with optimal clarity on CT-myelographic studies. The correlation of neuroradiologic findings to symptoms, particularly pain, is not simple. Contrast-enhancing tears in the annulus fibrosus or disk protrusions are widely accepted as common sources of back pain; however, one study found that over half of asymptomatic adults have similar findings. Asymptomatic disk protrusions are also common, and these abnormalities may enhance with contrast. Furthermore, in patients with known disk herniation treated either medically or surgically, persistence of the herniation 10 years later had no relationship to the clinical outcome. MRI findings of disk protrusion, tears in the annulus fibrosus, or contrast enhancement are common incidental findings that by themselves should not dictate management decisions for patients with back pain.

There are four indications for intervertebral disk surgery: (1) progressive motor weakness from nerve root injury demonstrated on clinical examination or EMG, (2) bowel or bladder disturbance or other signs of spinal cord compression, (3) incapacitating nerve root pain despite conservative treatment for at least 4 weeks, and (4) recurrent incapacitating pain despite conservative treatment. The latter two criteria are more subjective and less well established than the others. Surgical treatment should also be considered if the pain and/or neurologic findings do not substantially improve over 4 to 12 weeks.

The usual surgical procedure is a partial hemilaminectomy with excision of the prolapsed disk. Fusion of the involved lumbar segments is considered only if significant spinal instability is present (i.e., degenerative spondylolisthesis or isthmic spondylolysis).

CES is an injury of multiple lumbosacral nerve roots within the spinal canal. Low back pain, weakness and areflexia in the lower extremities, saddle anesthesia, and loss of bladder function may occur. The problem must be distinguished from disorders of the lower spinal cord (conus medullaris syndrome), acute transverse myelitis (Chap. 356), and Guillain-Barré syndrome (Chap. 365). Combined involvement of the conus medullaris and cauda equina can occur. CES is commonly due to a ruptured lumbosacral intervertebral disk, lumbosacral spine fracture, hematoma within the spinal canal (e.g., following lumbar puncture in patients with coagulopathy), compressive tumors, or other mass lesions. Treatment options include surgical decompression, sometimes urgently in an attempt to restore or preserve motor or sphincter function, or palliative radiotherapy or chemotherapy for metastatic tumors.

DEGENERATIVE CONDITIONS   *Lumbar spinal stenosis* describes a narrowed lumbar spinal canal. When severe, neurogenic claudication, consisting of back and buttock or leg pain induced by walking or standing and relieved by sitting, can occur. Symptoms in the legs are usually bilateral. Unlike vascular claudication, symptoms are often provoked by standing without walking. Unlike lumbar disk disease, symptoms are usually relieved by sitting. Focal weakness, sensory loss, or reflex changes may occur when spinal stenosis is associated with radiculopathy. Severe neurologic deficits, including paralysis and urinary incontinence, occur rarely. Spinal stenosis can be acquired (75%), congenital, or due to a combination of the two causes. Congenital forms (achondroplasia, idiopathic) are characterized by short, thick pedicles that produce both spinal canal and lateral recess stenosis. Acquired factors that may contribute to spinal stenosis include degenerative diseases (spondylosis, spondylolisthesis, scoliosis), trauma, spine surgery (postlaminectomy, fusion), metabolic or endocrine disorders (epidural lipomatosis, osteoporosis, acromegaly, renal osteodystrophy, hypoparathyroidism), and Paget's disease. MRI or CT-myelography provide the best definition of the abnormal anatomy (Fig. 15-5).

Conservative treatment of symptomatic spinal stenosis includes nonsteroidal anti-inflammatory drugs (NSAIDs), exercise programs, and symptomatic treatment of acute pain exacerbations. Surgical therapy is considered when medical therapy does not relieve pain sufficiently to allow for activities of daily living or when significant focal neurologic signs are present. Between 65 and 80% of properly selected patients treated surgically experience 75% relief of back and leg pain. Up to 25% develop recurrent stenosis at the same spinal level or an adjacent level 5 years after the initial surgery; recurrent symptoms usually respond to a second surgical decompression.

Facet joint hypertrophy can produce unilateral radicular symptoms or signs due to bony compression, that are indistinguishable from disk-related radiculopathy. Patients may exhibit stretch signs, focal motor

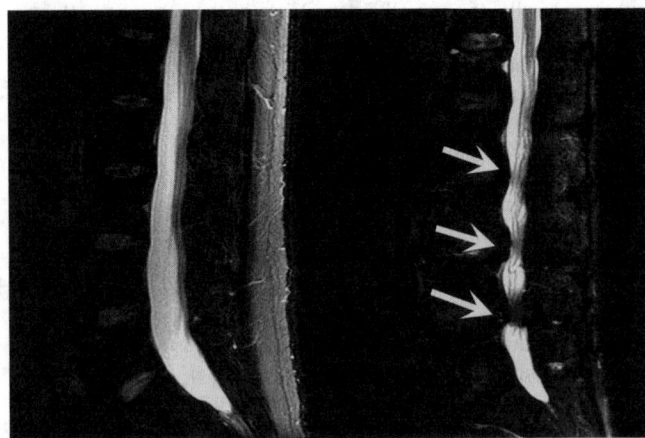

FIGURE 15-5   Spinal stenosis. Sagittal T2 fast spin echo magnetic resonance imaging of a normal (*left*) and stenotic (*right*) lumbar spine, revealing multifocal narrowing (*arrows*) of the cerebrospinal fluid spaces surrounding the nerve roots within the thecal sac.

weakness, hyporeflexia, or dermatomal sensory loss. Hypertrophic superior or inferior facets can often be visualized radiologically. Foraminotomy results in long-term relief of leg and back pain in 80 to 90% of patients.

ARTHRITIS   *Spondylosis*, or osteoarthritic spine disease, typically occurs in later life and primarily involves the cervical and lumbosacral spine. Patients often complain of back pain that is increased by motion and associated with stiffness or limitation of motion. The relationship between clinical symptoms and radiologic findings is usually not straightforward. Pain may be prominent when x-ray findings are minimal; alternatively, large osteophytes can be seen in asymptomatic patients in middle and later life. Hypertrophied facets and osteophytes may compress nerve roots in the lateral recess or intervertebral foramen. Osteophytes arising from the vertebral body may cause or contribute to central spinal canal stenosis. Loss of intervertebral disk height reduces the vertical dimensions of the intervertebral foramen; the descending pedicle may compress the nerve root exiting at that level. Rarely, osteoarthritic changes in the lumbar spine compress the cauda equina.

Ankylosing Spondylitis   (See also Chap. 305)   This distinctive arthritic spine disease typically presents with the insidious onset of low back and buttock pain. Patients are often males below age 40. Associated features include morning back stiffness, nocturnal pain, pain unrelieved by rest, an elevated sedimentation rate, and the histocompatibility antigen HLA-B27. Onset at a young age and back pain improving with exercise is characteristic. Loss of the normal lumbar lordosis and exaggeration of thoracic kyphosis are seen as the disease progresses. Inflammation and erosion of the outer fibers of the annulus fibrosus at the point of contact with the vertebral body are followed by ossification and bony growth that bridges adjacent vertebral bodies and reduces spine mobility in all planes. Radiologic hallmarks are periarticular destructive changes, sclerosis of the sacroiliac joints, and bridging of vertebral bodies to produce the fused "bamboo spine." Similar restricted movements may accompany Reiter's syndrome, psoriatic arthritis, and chronic inflammatory bowel disease. Stress fractures through the spontaneously ankylosed posterior bony elements of the rigid, osteoporotic spine may produce focal pain, spinal cord compression, or CES. Atlantoaxial subluxation with spinal cord compression occasionally occurs. Ankylosis of the ribs to the spine and a decrease in the height of the thoracic spine may compromise respiratory function.

NEOPLASMS   (See also Chap. 358)   Back pain is the most common neurologic symptom in patients with systemic cancer and is usually due to vertebral metastases. Metastatic carcinoma (breast, lung, prostate, thyroid, kidney, gastrointestinal tract), multiple myeloma, and non-Hodgkin's and Hodgkin's lymphomas frequently involve the spine. Back pain may be the presenting symptom. The pain tends to be constant, dull, unrelieved by rest, and worse at night. In contrast, mechanical low back pain usually improves with rest. Plain x-rays usually, but not always, show destructive lesions in one or several vertebral bodies without disk space involvement. MRI or CT-myelography are the studies of choice when spinal metastasis is suspected. MRI is usually preferred, but the procedure of choice is the study most rapidly available because the patient's condition may worsen quickly.

INFECTIONS/INFLAMMATION   *Vertebral osteomyelitis* is usually caused by staphylococci, but other bacteria or the tubercle bacillus (Pott's disease) may be responsible. A primary source of infection, most often the urinary tract, skin, or lungs, can be identified in 40% of patients. Intravenous drug use is a well-recognized risk factor. Back pain exacerbated by motion and unrelieved by rest, spine tenderness over the involved spine segment, and an elevated erythrocyte sedimentation rate are the most common findings. Fever or an elevated white blood cell count are found in a minority of patients. Plain radiographs may show a narrowed disk space with erosion of adjacent vertebrae; however, these diagnostic changes may take weeks or months to appear. MRI and CT are sensitive and specific for osteomyelitis; CT may be more readily available in emergency settings and better tolerated by some patients with severe back pain.

Spinal epidural abscess (Chap. 356) presents with back pain (aggravated by movement or palpation) and fever. Signs of nerve root injury or spinal cord compression may be present. The abscess may track over multiple spinal levels and is best delineated by spine MRI.

Lumbar adhesive arachnoiditis with radiculopathy is due to fibrosis following inflammation within the subarachnoid space. The fibrosis results in nerve root adhesions, producing back and leg pain associated with motor, sensory, or reflex changes. Myelography-induced arachnoiditis has become rare with the abandonment of oil-based contrast. Other causes of arachnoiditis include multiple lumbar operations, chronic spinal infections, spinal cord injury, intrathecal hemorrhage, intrathecal injection of glucocorticoids or anesthetics, and foreign bodies. The MRI may show nerve roots that clump together centrally and adhere to the dura peripherally, or loculations of cerebrospinal fluid within the thecal sac. Treatment is often unsatisfactory. Microsurgical lysis of adhesions, dorsal rhizotomy, and dorsal root ganglionectomy have resulted in poor outcomes. Dorsal column stimulation for pain relief has produced varying results. Epidural injections of glucocorticoids have been of limited value.

METABOLIC CAUSES ■ Osteoporosis and Osteosclerosis

Immobilization or underlying systemic disorders such as osteomalacia, hyperparathyroidism, hyperthyroidism, multiple myeloma, metastatic carcinoma, or glucocorticoid use may accelerate osteoporosis and weaken the vertebral body. The most common causes of atraumatic vertebral body fractures are postmenopausal (type 1) or senile (type 2) osteoporosis (Chap. 333). Compression fractures occur in up to half of patients with severe osteoporosis, and those who sustain a fracture have a 4.5-fold increased risk for recurrence. The sole manifestation of a compression fracture may be localized aching (often after a trivial injury) that is exacerbated by movement. Other patients experience radicular pain only. Focal tenderness to palpation is common. The clinical context, neurologic signs, and x-ray appearance of the spine establish the diagnosis. When compression fractures are found, treatable risk factors should be sought. Antiresorptive drugs including bisphosphonates (e.g., alendronate), transdermal estrogen, and tamoxifen have been shown to reduce the risk of osteoporotic fractures. Compression fractures above the midthoracic region suggest malignancy; if tumor is suspected, a bone biopsy or diagnostic search for a primary tumor is indicated.

Interventions [percutaneous vertebroplasty (PVP), kyphoplasty] exist for osteoporotic compression fractures associated with debilitating pain. Candidates for PVP should have midline pain, focal tenderness over the spinous process of the affected vertebral body, <80% loss of vertebral body height, and onset of symptoms within the prior 4 months. The technique consists of injection of polymethylmethacrylate, under fluoroscopic guidance, into the affected vertebral body. Rare major complications include extravasation of cement into the epidural space (resulting in myelopathy) or fatal pulmonary embolism from migration of cement into paraspinal veins. Approximately three-quarters of patients who meet selection criteria have reported enhanced quality of life. Relief of pain following PVP has also been reported in patients with vertebral metastases, myeloma, or hemangiomas.

Osteosclerosis (abnormally increased bone density) is readily identifiable on routine x-ray studies (e.g., Paget's disease) and may or may not produce back pain. Spinal cord or nerve root compression may result from bony encroachment on the spinal canal or intervertebral foramina. Single dual-beam photon absorptiometry or quantitative CT can be used to detect small changes in bone mineral density. →*For further discussion of these bone disorders, see Chaps. 332–334.*

REFERRED PAIN FROM VISCERAL DISEASE

Diseases of the thorax, abdomen, or pelvis may refer pain to the posterior portion of the spinal segment that innervates the diseased organ. Occasionally, back pain may be the first and only sign. Upper abdominal diseases generally refer pain to the lower thoracic or upper lumbar region (eighth thoracic to the first and second lumbar vertebrae), lower abdominal diseases to the lumbar region (second to fourth lumbar vertebrae), and pelvic diseases to the sacral region. Local signs (pain with spine palpation, paraspinal muscle spasm) are absent, and minimal or no pain accompanies normal spine movements.

Low Thoracic or Lumbar Pain with Abdominal Disease Peptic ulcers or tumors of the posterior wall of the stomach or duodenum typically produce epigastric pain (Chaps. 77 and 274), but midline back or paraspinal pain may occur if retroperitoneal extension is present. Back pain due to peptic ulcer may be precipitated by ingestion of an orange, alcohol, or coffee and relieved by food or antacids. Fatty foods are more likely to induce back pain associated with biliary disease. Diseases of the pancreas produce back pain to the right of the spine (head of the pancreas involved) or to the left (body or tail involved). Pathology in retroperitoneal structures (hemorrhage, tumors, pyelonephritis) produces paraspinal pain that radiates to the lower abdomen, groin, or anterior thighs. A mass in the iliopsoas region often produces unilateral lumbar pain with radiation toward the groin, labia, or testicles. The sudden appearance of lumbar pain in a patient receiving anticoagulants suggests retroperitoneal hemorrhage.

Isolated low back pain occurs in 15 to 20% of patients with a contained rupture of an abdominal aortic aneurysm (AAA). The classic clinical triad of abdominal pain, shock, and back pain in an elderly man occurs in <20% of patients. Two of these three features are present in two-thirds of patients, and hypotension is present in half. The typical patient is an elderly male smoker with back pain. The diagnosis is initially missed in at least one-third of patients because the symptoms and signs can be nonspecific. Common misdiagnoses include nonspecific back pain, diverticulitis, renal colic, sepsis, and myocardial infarction. A careful abdominal examination revealing a pulsatile mass (present in 50 to 75% of patients) is an important physical finding. Patients with suspected AAA should be evaluated with ultrasound, CT, or MRI (Chap. 231).

Inflammatory bowel disorders (colitis, diverticulitis) or cancers of the colon may produce lower abdominal pain, midlumbar back pain, or both. The pain may have a beltlike distribution around the body. A lesion in the transverse or proximal descending colon may refer pain to the middle or left back at the L2-L3 level. Lesions of the sigmoid colon may refer pain to the upper sacral or midline suprapubic regions or left lower quadrant of the abdomen.

Sacral Pain with Gynecologic and Urologic Disease Pelvic organs rarely cause low back pain, except for gynecologic disorders involving the uterosacral ligaments. The pain is referred to the sacral region. Endometriosis or cancers of the uterus may invade the uterosacral ligaments; malposition of the uterus may cause uterosacral ligament traction. Pain associated with endometriosis is typically premenstrual and often continues until it merges with menstrual pain. Malposition of the uterus (retroversion, descensus, and prolapse) may produce sacral pain after prolonged standing.

Menstrual pain may be felt in the sacral region. The poorly localized, cramping pain can radiate down the legs. Pain due to neoplastic infiltration of nerves is typically continuous, progressive in severity, and unrelieved by rest at night. Less commonly, radiation therapy of pelvic tumors may produce sacral pain from late radiation necrosis of tissue or nerves. Low back pain that radiates into one or both thighs is common in the last weeks of pregnancy.

Urologic sources of lumbosacral back pain include chronic prostatitis, prostate cancer with spinal metastasis, and diseases of the kidney and ureter. Lesions of the bladder and testes do not usually produce back pain. The diagnosis of metastatic prostate carcinoma is established by rectal examination, spine imaging studies (MRI or CT), and measurement of prostate-specific antigen (Chap. 81). Infectious, inflammatory, or neoplastic renal diseases may produce ipsilateral lumbosacral pain, as can renal artery or vein thrombosis. Paraspinal lumbar pain may be a symptom of ureteral obstruction due to nephrolithiasis.

OTHER CAUSES OF BACK PAIN ■ **Postural Back Pain** There is a group of patients with nonspecific CLBP in whom no anatomic or pathologic lesion can be found despite exhaustive investigation. These individuals complain of vague, diffuse back pain with prolonged sitting or standing that is relieved by rest. The physical examination is unrevealing except for "poor posture." Imaging studies and laboratory evaluations are normal. Exercises to strengthen the paraspinal and abdominal muscles are sometimes therapeutic.

Psychiatric Disease CLBP may be encountered in patients who seek financial compensation, in malingerers, or in those with concurrent substance abuse, chronic anxiety states, or depression. Many patients with CLBP have a history of psychiatric illness (depression, anxiety, substance abuse) or childhood trauma (physical or sexual abuse) that antedates the onset of back pain. Preoperative psychological assessment has been used to exclude patients with marked psychological impairments; these patients are likely to have a poor surgical outcome.

Unidentified The cause of low back pain occasionally remains unclear. Some patients have had multiple operations for disk disease but have persistent pain and disability. The original indications for surgery may have been questionable, with back pain only, no definite neurologic signs, or a minor disk bulge noted on CT or MRI. Scoring systems based upon neurologic signs, psychological factors, physiologic studies, and imaging studies have been devised to minimize the likelihood of unsuccessful surgical explorations.

℞ TREATMENT

Acute Low Back Pain A practical approach to the management of low back pain is to consider acute and chronic presentations separately. ALBP is defined as pain of <3 months duration. Full recovery can be expected in 85% of adults with ALBP unaccompanied by leg pain. Most have purely "mechanical" symptoms—i.e., pain that is aggravated by motion and relieved by rest.

Observational studies have been used to justify a minimalist approach to this problem. These studies share a number of limitations: (1) a true placebo control group is often lacking; (2) patients who consult different provider groups (generalists, orthopedists, neurologists) are assumed to have similar etiologies for their back pain; (3) no information is provided about the details of treatment; and (4) no attempt to tabulate serious causes of ALBP is made.

The algorithms for the treatment of back pain (Fig. 15-6) draw from published guidelines. However, since CPGs are based on incomplete evidence, guidelines should not substitute for clinical judgment.

The initial assessment excludes serious causes of spine pathology that require urgent intervention, including infection, cancer, and trauma. Risks factors for a possible serious underlying cause of back pain include: age >50 years, prior diagnosis of cancer or other serious medical illness, bed rest without relief, duration of pain >1 month, urinary incontinence or recent nocturia, focal leg weakness or numbness, pain radiating into the leg(s) from the back, intravenous drug use, chronic infection (pulmonary or urinary), pain increasing with standing and relieved by sitting, history of spine trauma, and glucocorticoid use. Worrisome signs include unexplained fever, unexplained weight loss, positive SLR sign or reverse SLR sign, crossed SLR sign, percussion tenderness over the spine or costovertebral angle, an abdominal mass (pulsatile or nonpulsatile), a rectal mass, focal sensory loss (saddle anesthesia or focal limb sensory loss), leg weakness, spasticity, or reflex asymmetry. Laboratory studies are unnecessary unless a serious underlying cause is suspected. Plain spine films are rarely indicated in the first month of symptoms unless a spine fracture is suspected.

Clinical trials have shown no benefit of prolonged (>2 days) bed rest for uncomplicated ALBP. There is evidence that bed rest is also ineffective for patients with sciatica or for acute back pain with findings of nerve root injury. Theoretical advantages of early ambulation

for ALBP include maintenance of cardiovascular conditioning, improved disk and cartilage nutrition, improved bone and muscle strength, and increased endorphin levels. A trial examining the effects of a program of early vigorous exercise was negative, but the benefits of less vigorous exercise or other exercise programs are unknown. The early resumption of normal physical activity (without heavy manual labor) is likely to be beneficial. Traction for ALBP is not effective, as shown in well-designed clinical trials that include a "sham" traction control group. Despite this knowledge, in one survey physicians identified strict bed rest for 3 days, trigger point injections (see below), and physical therapy (PT) as beneficial for ALBP. In many instances, the behavior of treating physicians does not reflect the current medical literature.

Proof is lacking to support the treatment of acute back and neck pain with acupuncture, transcutaneous electrical nerve stimulation, massage, ultrasound, diathermy, or electrical stimulation. Cervical collars can be modestly helpful by limiting spontaneous and reflex neck movements that exacerbate pain. Evidence regarding the efficacy of ice or heat is lacking, but these interventions are optional given the lack of negative evidence, low cost, and low risk. Biofeedback has not been studied rigorously. Facet joint, trigger point, and ligament injections are not recommended.

A role for modification of posture has not been validated by rigorous clinical studies. As a practical matter, temporary suspension of activity known to increase mechanical stress on the spine (heavy lifting, prolonged sitting, bending or twisting, straining at stool) may be helpful.

Education is an important part of treatment. Satisfaction and the likelihood of follow-up increase when patients are educated about prognosis, treatment methods, activity modifications, and strategies to prevent future exacerbations. In one study, patients who felt they did not receive an adequate explanation for their symptoms wanted further diagnostic tests. Evidence for the efficacy of structured education programs ("back school") is inconclusive; in one study, patients attending back school had a shorter duration of sick leave during the initial episode but not during subsequent episodes. Randomized studies of back school for primary prevention of low back injury and pain have failed to demonstrate any benefit.

NSAIDs and acetaminophen are effective over-the-counter agents for ALBP. Muscle relaxants (cyclobenzaprine, methocarbamol) provide short-term (4 to 7 days) benefit, but drowsiness limits daytime use. Opioid analgesics are no more effective than NSAIDs or acetaminophen for initial treatment of ALBP, nor do they increase the likelihood of return to work. Short-term use of opioids in patients unresponsive to or intolerant of acetaminophen or NSAIDs may be helpful. There is no evidence to support the use of oral glucocorticoids or tricyclic antidepressants for ALBP.

Epidural glucocorticoids may occasionally produce short-term pain relief in ALBP and radiculopathy, but proof is lacking for pain relief beyond 1 month. Epidural anesthetics, glucocorticoids, or opioids are not indicated in the initial treatment of ALBP without radiculopathy. Diagnostic nerve root blocks have been advocated to determine if pain originates from a specific nerve root. However, improvement may result even when the nerve root is not responsible for the pain syndrome; this may occur with placebo effects, painful lesions located distally along the peripheral nerve, or anesthesia of the sinuvertebral nerve. Therapeutic nerve root blocks with injection of glucocorticoids and a local anesthetic is an option after conservative measures fail, particularly when temporary relief of pain is necessary.

A short course of spinal manipulation or PT for symptomatic relief of uncomplicated ALBP is an option. A prospective, randomized study comparing PT, chiropractic manipulation, and education interventions for patients with ALBP found modest trends toward benefit with both PT and chiropractic manipulation at 1 year. Costs per year were equivalent in the PT/chiropractic group and ~$280 less for the group treated with the education booklet alone. The value of such treatment beyond 1 year is unknown. Similarly, the specific PT or chiropractic protocols that may provide benefit have not been fully defined.

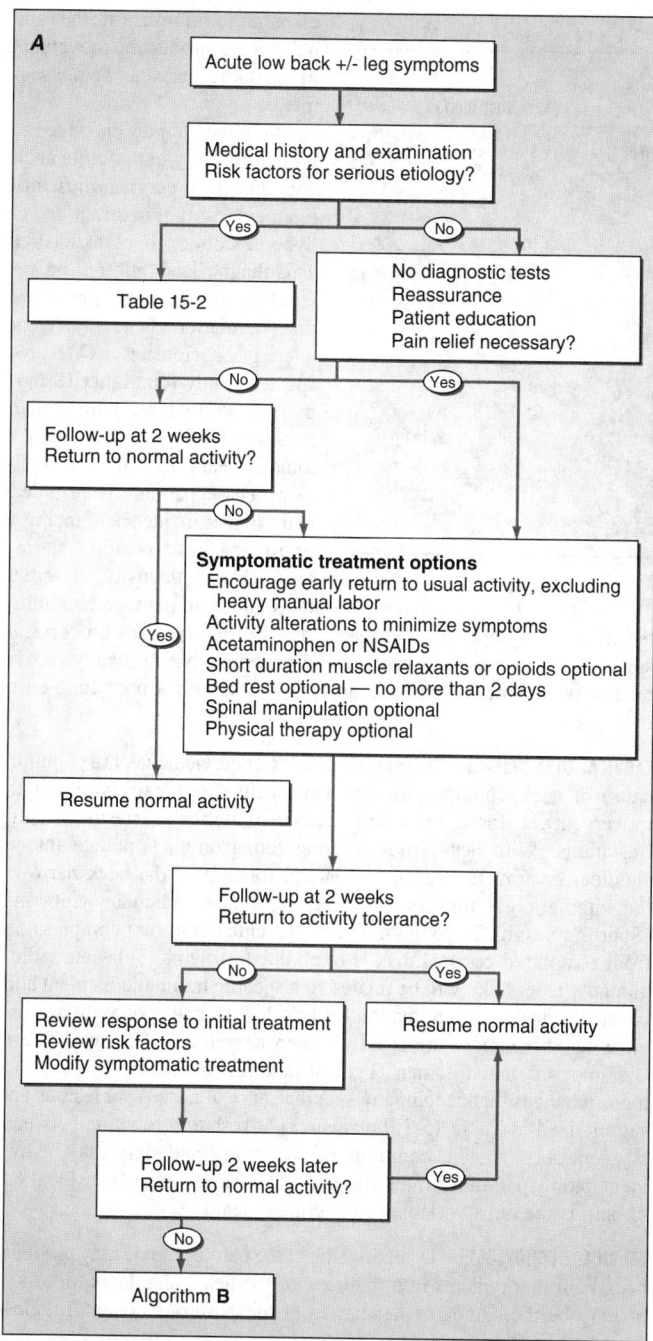

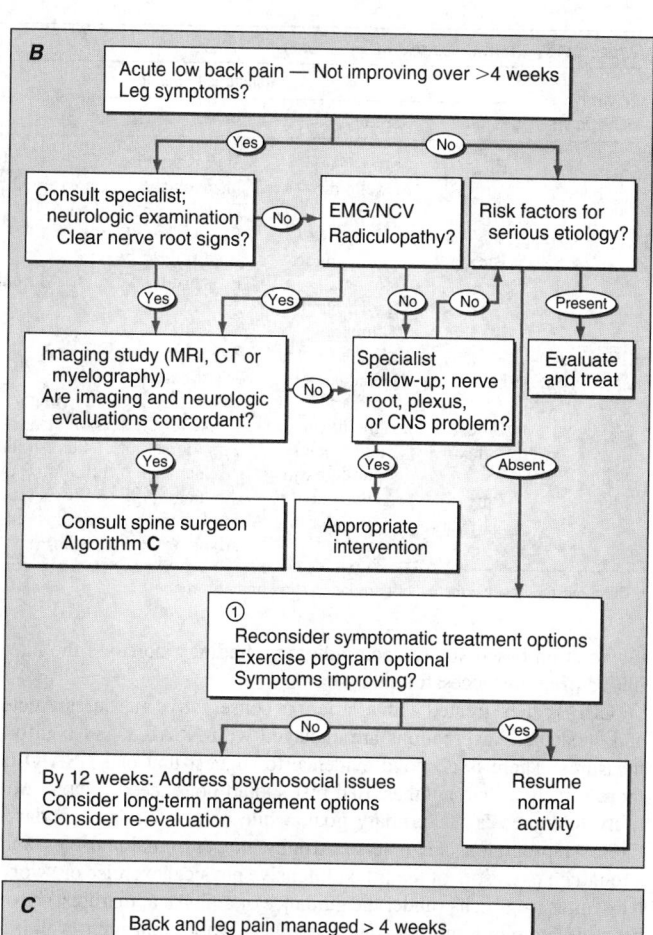

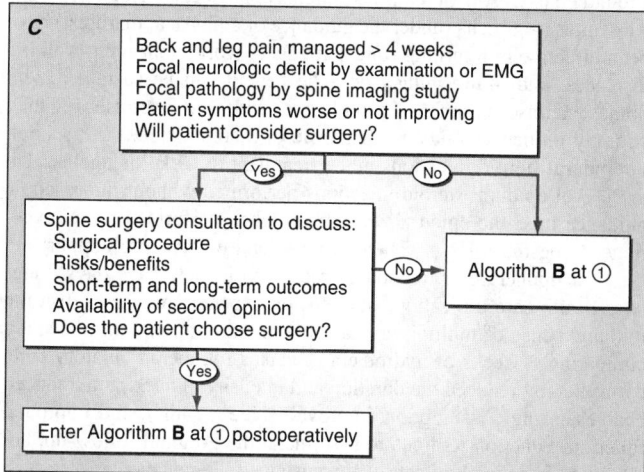

FIGURE 15-6 Algorithms for management of acute low back pain, age ≥ 18 years. *A.* Symptoms <3 months, first 4 weeks. *B.* Management weeks 4–12. ①, entry point from Algorithm *C* postoperatively or if patient declines surgery. *C.* Surgical options. (NSAIDs, nonsteroidal anti-inflammatory drugs; CBC, complete blood count; ESR, eryth- rocyte sedimentation rate; UA, urinalysis; EMG, electromyography; NCV, nerve conduc- tion velocity studies; MRI, magnetic resonance imaging; CT, computed tomography; CNS, central nervous system.)

Chronic Low Back Pain CLBP, defined as pain lasting >12 weeks, ac- counts for 50% of total back pain costs. Overweight individuals appear to be at particular risk. Other risk factors include: female gender, older age, prior history of back pain, restricted spinal mobility, pain radiating into a leg, high levels of psychological distress, poor self-rated health, minimal physical activity, smoking, job dissatisfaction, and wide- spread pain. Combinations of these premorbid factors have been used to predict which individuals with ALBP are likely to develop CLBP. The initial approach to these patients is similar to that for ALBP, and the differential diagnosis is similar. Treatment of this heterogeneous group of patients is directed toward the underlying cause when known; the ultimate goal is to restore function to the greatest extent possible.

Many conditions that produce CLBP can be identified by a com- bination of neuroimaging and electrophysiologic studies. Spine MRI or CT-myelography are the techniques of choice but are generally not indicated within the first month after initial evaluation in the absence of risk factors for a serious underlying cause. Imaging studies should be performed only in circumstances where the results are likely to influence surgical or medical treatment.

Diskography provides no additional anatomic information beyond what is available by MRI. Reproduction of the patient's typical pain with the injection is often used as evidence that a specific disk is the pain generator, but it is not known whether this information has any value in selecting candidates for surgery. There is no proven role for thermography in the assessment of radiculopathy.

The diagnosis of nerve root injury is most secure when the history, examination, results of imaging studies, and the EMG are concordant. The correlation between CT and EMG for localization of nerve root injury is between 65 and 73%. Up to one-third of asymptomatic adults have a disk protrusion detected by CT or MRI scans. Thus, surgical

TABLE 15-3 Cervical Radiculopathy—Neurologic Features

Cervical Nerve Roots	Examination Findings			Pain Distribution
	Reflex	Sensory	Motor	
C5	Biceps	Over lateral deltoid	Supraspinatus[a] (initial arm abduction) Infraspinatus[a] (arm external rotation) Deltoid[a] (arm abduction) Biceps (arm flexion)	Lateral arm, medial scapula
C6	Biceps	Thumb, index fingers Radial hand/ forearm	Biceps (arm flexion) Pronator teres (internal forearm rotation)	Lateral forearm, thumb, index finger
C7	Triceps	Middle fingers Dorsum forearm	Triceps[a] (arm extension) Wrist extensors[a] Extensor digitorum[a] (finger extension)	Posterior arm, dorsal forearm, lateral hand
C8	Finger flexors	Little finger Medial hand and forearm	Abductor pollicis brevis (abduction D1) First dorsal interosseous (abduction D2) Abductor digiti minimi (abduction D5)	4th and 5th fingers, medial forearm
T1	Finger flexors	Axilla and medial arm	Abductor pollicis brevis (abduction D1) First dorsal interosseous (abduction D2) Abductor digiti minimi (abduction D5)	Medial arm, axilla

[a] These muscles receive the majority of innervation from this root.

intervention based solely upon radiologic findings increases the likelihood of an unsuccessful outcome.

CLBP can be treated with a variety of conservative measures. Acute and subacute exacerbations are managed with NSAIDs and comfort measures. There is no good evidence to suggest that one NSAID is more effective than another. Bed rest should not exceed 2 days. Activity tolerance is the primary goal, while pain relief is secondary. Exercise programs can reverse atrophy in paraspinal muscles and strengthen extensors of the trunk. Intensive physical exercise or "work hardening" regimens (under the guidance of a physical therapist) have been effective in returning some patients to work, improving walking distances, and diminishing pain. The benefit can be sustained with home exercise regimens; compliance with the exercise regimen strongly influences outcome. The role of manipulation, back school, or epidural steroid injections in the treatment of CLBP is unclear. Up to 30% of epidural steroid injections performed without fluoroscopic guidance miss the epidural space even when performed by an experienced anesthesiologist. There is no strong evidence to support the use of acupuncture or traction. A reduction in sick leave days, long-term health care utilization, and pension expenditures may offset the initial expense of multidisciplinary treatment programs. In one study comparing 3 weeks of hydrotherapy versus routine ambulatory care, hydrotherapy reduced the duration and intensity of back pain, reduced analgesic drug consumption, improved spine mobility, and improved function. Function returned to baseline at the 9-month follow-up, but all other beneficial effects were sustained. Percutaneous electrical nerve stimulation (PENS) has been shown to provide significant short-term relief of CLBP, but additional studies regarding its long-term efficacy and cost are needed.

PAIN IN THE NECK AND SHOULDER (Table 15-2)

Neck pain, which usually arises from diseases of the cervical spine and soft tissues of the neck, is common (4.6% of adults in one study). Neck pain arising from the cervical spine is typically precipitated by movements and may be accompanied by focal tenderness and limitation of motion. Pain arising from the brachial plexus, shoulder, or peripheral nerves can be confused with cervical spine disease, but the history and examination usually identify a more distal origin for the pain. Cervical spine trauma, disk disease, or spondylosis may be asymptomatic or painful and can produce a myelopathy, radiculopathy, or both. The nerve roots most commonly affected are C7 and C6.

TRAUMA TO THE CERVICAL SPINE Trauma to the cervical spine (fractures, subluxation) places the spinal cord at risk for compression. Motor vehicle accidents, violent crimes, or falls account for 87% of spinal cord injuries (Chap. 356). Immediate immobilization of the neck is essential to minimize further spinal cord injury from movement of unstable cervical spine segments.

Whiplash injury is due to trauma (usually automobile accidents) causing cervical musculoligamental sprain or strain due to hyperflexion or hyperextension. This diagnosis should not be applied to patients with fractures, disk herniation, head injury, or altered consciousness. One prospective study found that 18% of patients with whiplash injury had persistent injury-related symptoms 2 years after the car accident. These patients were older, had a higher incidence of inclined or rotated head position at impact, greater intensity of initial neck and head pain, greater number of initial symptoms, and more osteoarthritic changes on cervical spine x-rays at baseline compared to patients who ultimately recovered. Severe initial symptoms are associated with a poor long-term outcome.

CERVICAL DISK DISEASE Herniation of a lower cervical disk is a common cause of neck, shoulder, arm, or hand pain. Neck pain (worse with movement), stiffness, and a limited range of motion are the usual manifestations. With nerve root compression, pain may radiate into a shoulder or arm. Extension and lateral rotation of the neck narrows the intervertebral foramen and may reproduce radicular symptoms (Spurling's sign). In young individuals, acute nerve root compression from a ruptured cervical disk is often due to trauma. Subacute radiculopathy is less likely to be related to a specific traumatic incident and is usually due to a combination of disk disease and spondylosis. Cervical disk herniations are usually posterolateral near the lateral recess and intervertebral foramen. Typical patterns of reflex, sensory, and motor changes that accompany specific cervical nerve root lesions are summarized in Table 15-3; however, (1) overlap in function between adjacent nerve roots is common, (2) symptoms and signs may be evident in only part of the injured nerve root territory, and (3) the location of pain is the most variable of the clinical features.

CERVICAL SPONDYLOSIS Osteoarthritis of the cervical spine may produce neck pain that radiates into the back of the head, shoulders, or arms, or may be the source of headaches in the posterior occipital region (supplied by the C2-C4 nerve roots). Osteophyte formation in the lateral recess or hypertrophic facet joints may produce a monoradiculopathy (Fig. 15-7). Narrowing of the spinal canal by osteophytes, ossification of the posterior longitudinal ligament, or a large central disk may compress the cervical spinal cord. Combinations of radiculopathy and myelopathy also occur. An electrical sensation elicited by neck flexion and radiating down the spine from the neck (Lhermitte's symptom) usually indicates involvement of the cervical or upper thoracic (T1-T2) spine. When little or no neck pain accompanies the cord compression, the diagnosis may be confused with amyotrophic lateral sclerosis (Chap. 353), multiple sclerosis (Chap. 359), spinal cord tumors, or syringomyelia (Chap. 356). The possibility of treatable cervical spondylosis must be considered even when the patient presents with leg complaints only. In other cases, an unrelated lumbar radiculopathy or polyneuropathy may mask signs of an associated cervical myelopathy. MRI or CT-myelography can define the anatomic abnormalities, and EMG and nerve conduction studies can localize and assess the severity of the nerve root injury.

OTHER CAUSES OF NECK PAIN *Rheumatoid arthritis* (RA) (Chap. 301) of the cervical apophyseal joints produces neck pain, stiffness, and limitation of motion. In typical cases with symmetric inflammatory polyarthritis, the diagnosis of RA is straightforward. In advanced RA, synovitis of the atlantoaxial joint (C1-C2; Fig. 15-2) may damage the transverse ligament of the atlas, producing forward displacement of the atlas on the axis (atlantoaxial subluxation). Radiologic evidence of atlantoaxial subluxation occurs in 30% of patients with RA. Not surprisingly, the degree of subluxation correlates with the severity of erosive disease. When subluxation is present, careful neurologic assessment is important to identify early signs of myelopathy. Occasional patients develop high spinal cord compression leading to quadriparesis, respiratory insufficiency, and death. Low back pain is common in RA; however, the frequency of facet disease, fracture, and spondylolisthesis is no greater than in controls with mechanical low back pain.

Ankylosing spondylitis can cause neck pain and on occasion atlantoaxial subluxation; when spinal cord compression is present or threatened, surgical intervention is indicated. *Herpes zoster* produces acute posterior occipital or neck pain prior to the outbreak of vesicles. *Neoplasms* metastatic to the cervical spine, *infections* (osteomyelitis and epidural abscess), and *metabolic bone diseases* may also be the cause of neck pain. Neck pain may also be referred from the heart with coronary artery ischemia (cervical angina syndrome).

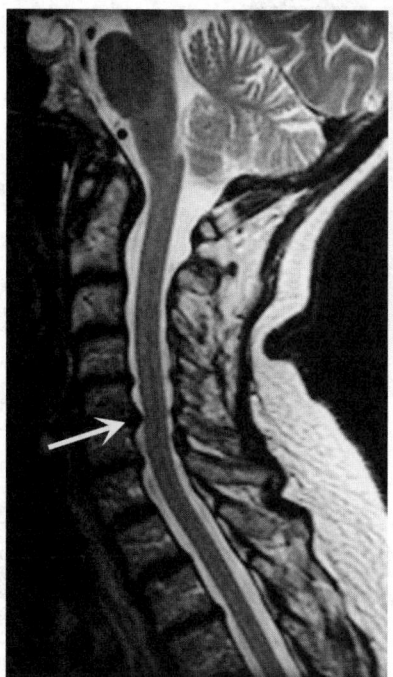

A

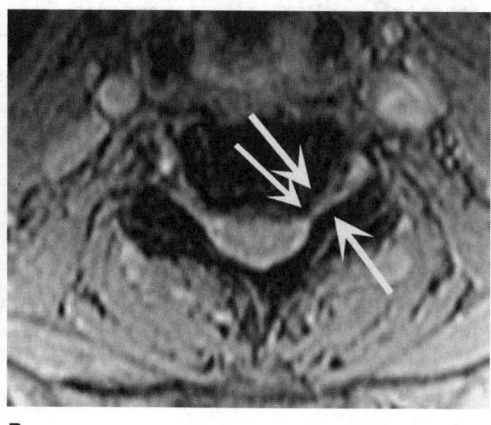

B

FIGURE 15-7 Cervical spondylosis; left C6 radiculopathy. *A.* Sagittal T2 fast spin echo magnetic resonance imaging reveals a hypointense osteophyte that protrudes from the C5-C6 level into the thecal sac, displacing the spinal cord posteriorly (*white arrow*). *B.* Axial 2-mm section from a 3-D volume gradient echo sequence of the cervical spine. The high signal of the right C5-C6 intervertebral foramen contrasts with the narrow high signal of the left C5-C6 intervertebral foramen produced by osteophytic spurring (*arrows*).

THORACIC OUTLET The thoracic outlet contains the first rib, the subclavian artery and vein, the brachial plexus, the clavicle, and the lung apex. Injury to these structures may result in postural or movement-induced pain around the shoulder and supraclavicular region. *True neurogenic thoracic outlet syndrome* (TOS) results from compression of the lower trunk of the brachial plexus or ventral rami of the C8 or T1 nerve roots by an anomalous band of tissue connecting an elongate transverse process at C7 with the first rib. Signs include weakness of intrinsic muscles of the hand and diminished sensation on the palmar aspect of the fourth and fifth digits. EMG and nerve conduction studies confirm the diagnosis. Treatment consists of surgical division of the anomalous band. The weakness and wasting of intrinsic hand muscles typically does not improve, but surgery halts the insidious progression of weakness. *Arterial TOS* results from compression of the subclavian artery by a cervical rib; the compression results in poststenotic dilatation of the artery and thrombus formation. Blood pressure is reduced in the affected limb, and signs of emboli may be present in the hand; neurologic signs are absent. Ultrasound can confirm the diagnosis noninvasively. Treatment is with thrombolysis or anticoagulation (with or without embolectomy) and surgical excision of the cervical rib compressing the subclavian artery or vein. *Disputed TOS* includes a large number of patients with chronic arm and shoulder pain of unclear cause. The lack of sensitive and specific findings on physical examination or laboratory markers for this condition frequently results in diagnostic uncertainty. The role of surgery in disputed TOS is controversial. Multidisciplinary pain management is a conservative approach, although treatment is often unsuccessful.

BRACHIAL PLEXUS AND NERVES Pain from injury to the brachial plexus or peripheral nerves of the arm can occasionally mimic pain of cervical spine origin. Neoplastic infiltration of the lower trunk of the brachial plexus may produce shoulder pain radiating down the arm, numbness of the fourth and fifth fingers, and weakness of intrinsic hand muscles innervated by the ulnar and median nerves. Postradiation fibrosis (breast carcinoma is the most common setting) may produce similar findings, although pain is less often present. A Pancoast tumor of the lung (Chap. 75) is another cause and should be considered, especially when a Horner's syndrome is present. *Suprascapular neuropathy* may produce severe shoulder pain, weakness, and wasting of the supraspinatous and infraspinatous muscles. *Acute brachial neuritis* is often confused with radiculopathy. It consists of the acute onset of severe shoulder or scapular pain followed over days to weeks by weakness of the proximal arm and shoulder girdle muscles innervated by the upper brachial plexus. The onset is often preceeded by an infection or immunization. Complete recovery occurs in 75% of patients after 2 years and in 89% after 3 years. Occasional cases of carpal tunnel syndrome produce pain and paresthesias extending into the forearm, arm, and shoulder resembling a C5 or C6 root lesion. Lesions of the radial or ulnar nerve can mimic a radiculopathy at C7 or C8, respectively. EMG and nerve conduction studies can accurately localize lesions to the nerve roots, brachial plexus, or peripheral nerves. →*For further discussion of peripheral nerve disorders, see Chap. 363.*

SHOULDER Pain from the shoulder can be difficult to distinguish from neck pain. If symptoms and signs of radiculopathy are absent, then the differential diagnosis includes mechanical shoulder pain (tendonitis, bursitis, rotator cuff tear, dislocation, adhesive capsulitis, and cuff impingement under the acromion) and referred pain (subdiaphragmatic irritation, angina, Pancoast tumor). Mechanical pain is often worse at night, associated with local shoulder tenderness and aggravated by abduction, internal rotation, or extension of the arm. Pain from shoulder disease may on occasion radiate into the arm or hand, but sensory, motor, and reflex changes are absent.

℞ TREATMENT

There are few well-designed clinical trials that address optimal treatment of neck pain. Symptomatic treatment can include the use of analgesic medications and/or a soft cervical collar. Current indications for cervical disk surgery are similar to those for lumbar disk surgery; because of the risk of spinal cord injury with cervical spine disease, an aggressive approach is generally indicated whenever spinal cord injury is threatened. Surgical management of cervical herniated disks usually consists of an anterior approach with diskectomy followed by anterior interbody fusion. A simple posterior partial laminectomy with diskectomy is an acceptable alternative approach. The risk of subsequent radiculopathy or myelopathy at cervical segments adjacent to the fusion is ~3% per year and 26% per decade. Although this risk is

103

sometimes portrayed as a late complication of surgery, it may also reflect the natural history of degenerative cervical spine disease. Non-progressive cervical radiculopathy (associated with a focal neurologic deficit) due to a herniated cervical disk may be treated conservatively with a high rate of success. Cervical spondylosis with bony, compressive cervical radiculopathy is generally treated with surgical decompression to forstall the progression of neurologic signs. Cervical spondylotic myelopathy is typically managed with either anterior decompression and fusion or laminectomy. Outcomes in both surgical groups vary, but late functional deterioration occurs in 20 to 30% of patients; a prospective, controlled study comparing different surgical interventions is needed.

FURTHER READING

ATLAS SJ, NARDIN RA: Evaluation and treatment of low back pain: An evidence-based approach to clinical care. Muscle and Nerve 27:265, 2003

CASSIDY JD et al: Effect of eliminating compensation for pain and suffering on the outcome of insurance claims for whiplash injury. N Engl J Med 342: 1179, 2000

HASSETT G et al: Risk factors for progression of lumbar spine disc degeneration. Arthritis Rheum 48:3112, 2003

Section 2   Alterations in Body Temperature

16 | FEVER AND HYPERTHERMIA
Charles A. Dinarello, Jeffrey A. Gelfand

Body temperature is controlled by the hypothalamus. Neurons in both the preoptic anterior hypothalamus and the posterior hypothalamus receive two kinds of signals: one from peripheral nerves that reflect warmth/cold receptors and the other from the temperature of the blood bathing the region. These two types of signals are integrated by the thermoregulatory center of the hypothalamus to maintain normal temperature. In a neutral environment, the metabolic rate of humans consistently produces more heat than is necessary to maintain the core body temperature at 37°C.

A normal body temperature is ordinarily maintained, despite environmental variations, because the hypothalamic thermoregulatory center balances the excess heat production derived from metabolic activity in muscle and the liver with heat dissipation from the skin and lungs. According to studies of healthy individuals 18 to 40 years of age, the mean oral temperature is 36.8° ± 0.4°C (98.2° ± 0.7°F), with low levels at 6 A.M. and higher levels at 4 to 6 P.M. The maximum normal oral temperature is 37.2°C (98.9°F) at 6 A.M. and 37.7°C (99.9°F) at 4 P.M.; these values define the 99th percentile for healthy individuals. In light of these studies, *an A.M. temperature of >37.2°C (>98.9°F) or a P.M. temperature of >37.7°C (>99.9°F) would define a fever.* The normal daily temperature variation is typically 0.5°C (0.9°F). However, in some individuals recovering from a febrile illness, this daily variation can be as great as 1.0°C. During a febrile illness, diurnal variations are usually maintained but at higher levels. Daily temperature swings do not occur in patients with hyperthermia (see below). Rectal temperatures are generally 0.4°C (0.7°F) higher than oral readings. The lower oral readings are probably attributable to mouth breathing, which is a particularly important factor in patients with respiratory infections and rapid breathing. Lower esophageal temperatures closely reflect core temperature. Tympanic membrane (TM) thermometers measure radiant heat energy from the tympanic membrane and nearby ear canal and display that absolute value (unadjusted mode) or a value automatically calculated from the absolute reading on the basis of nomograms relating the radiant temperature measured to actual core temperatures obtained in clinical studies (adjusted mode). These measurements, although convenient, may be more variable than directly determined oral or rectal values. Studies in adults show that readings are lower with unadjusted-mode than with adjusted-mode TM thermometers and that unadjusted-mode TM values are 0.8°C (1.6°F) lower than rectal temperatures.

In women who menstruate, the A.M. temperature is generally lower in the 2 weeks before ovulation; it then rises by about 0.6°C (1°F) with ovulation and remains at that level until menses occur. Seasonal variation in body temperature has been described but may reflect a metabolic change and is not common. Body temperature is elevated in the postprandial state. Pregnancy and endocrinologic dysfunction also affect body temperature. The daily temperature variation appears to be fixed in early childhood; in contrast, elderly individuals can exhibit a reduced ability to develop fever, with only a modest fever even in severe infections.

FEVER VERSUS HYPERTHERMIA

FEVER   Fever is an elevation of body temperature that exceeds the normal daily variation and occurs *in conjunction with an increase in the hypothalamic set point*—for example, from 37°C to 39°C. This shift of the set point from "normothermic" to febrile levels very much resembles the resetting of the home thermostat to a higher level in order to raise the ambient temperature in a room. Once the hypothalamic set point is raised, neurons in the vasomotor center are activated and vasoconstriction commences. The individual first notices vasoconstriction in the hands and feet. Shunting of blood away from the periphery to the internal organs essentially decreases heat loss from the skin, and the person feels cold. For most fevers, body temperature increases by 1° to 2°C. Shivering, which increases heat production from the muscles, may begin at this time; however, shivering is not required if heat conservation mechanisms raise blood temperature sufficiently. Heat production from the liver also increases. In humans, behavior (e.g., putting on more clothing or bedding) helps raise body temperature.

The processes of heat conservation (vasoconstriction) and heat production (shivering and increased metabolic activity) continue until the temperature of the blood bathing the hypothalamic neurons matches the new thermostat setting. Once that point is reached, the hypothalamus maintains the temperature at the febrile level by the same mechanisms of heat balance that are operative in the afebrile state. When the hypothalamic set point is again reset downward (due to either a reduction in the concentration of pyrogens or the use of antipyretics), the processes of heat loss through vasodilation and sweating are initiated. Loss of heat by sweating and vasodilation continues until the blood temperature at the hypothalamic level matches the lower setting.

A fever of >41.5°C (>106.7°F) is called *hyperpyrexia*. This extraordinarily high fever can develop in patients with severe infections but most commonly occurs in patients with central nervous system (CNS) hemorrhages. In the preantibiotic era, fever due to a variety of infectious diseases rarely exceeded 106°F, and there has been speculation that this natural "thermal ceiling" is mediated by neuropeptides functioning as central antipyretics.

In some rare cases, the hypothalamic set point is elevated as a result of local trauma, hemorrhage, tumor, or intrinsic hypothalamic malfunction. The term *hypothalamic fever* is sometimes used to describe elevated temperature caused by abnormal hypothalamic function. However, most patients with hypothalamic damage have *sub*normal, not *supra*normal, body temperatures.

HYPERTHERMIA Hyperthermia is characterized by *an unchanged (normothermic) setting of the thermoregulatory center* in conjunction with an uncontrolled increase in body temperature that exceeds the body's ability to lose heat. Exogenous heat exposure and endogenous heat production are two mechanisms by which hyperthermia can result in dangerously high internal temperatures. Excessive heat production can easily cause hyperthermia despite physiologic and behavioral control of body temperature. For example, work or exercise in hot environments can produce heat faster than peripheral mechanisms can lose it.

Although most patients with elevated body temperature have fever, there are a few circumstances in which elevated temperature represents not fever but hyperthermia (Table 16-1). *Heat stroke*, caused by thermoregulatory failure in association with a warm environment, may be categorized as exertional or nonexertional. *Exertional heat stroke* typically occurs in younger individuals exercising at ambient temperatures and/or humidities that are higher than normal. In a dry environment and at maximal efficiency, sweating can dissipate ~600 kcal/h, requiring the production of >1 L of sweat. Even in normal individuals, dehydration or the use of common medications (e.g., over-the-counter antihistamines with anticholinergic side effects) may help to precipitate exertional heat stroke. *Nonexertional* or *classic heat stroke* typically occurs in either very young or elderly individuals, particularly during heat waves. According to the Centers for Disease Control and Prevention (CDC), there were 7000 deaths attributed to heat injury in the United States from 1979 to 1997. The elderly, the bedridden, persons taking anticholinergic or antiparkinsonian drugs or diuretics, and individuals confined to poorly ventilated and non-air-conditioned environments are most susceptible.

Drug-induced hyperthermia has become increasingly common as a result of the increased use of prescription psychotropic drugs and illicit drugs. Drug-induced hyperthermia may be caused by monoamine oxidase inhibitors (MAOIs), tricyclic antidepressants, and amphetamines and by the illicit use of phencyclidine (PCP), lysergic acid diethylamide (LSD), methylenedioxymethamphetamine (MDMA, "ecstasy"), or cocaine.

Malignant hyperthermia occurs in individuals with an inherited abnormality of skeletal-muscle sarcoplasmic reticulum that causes a rapid increase in intracellular calcium levels in response to halothane

---

TABLE 16-1 Causes of Hyperthermia Syndromes

HEAT STROKE

Exertional: Exercise in higher-than-normal heat and/or humidity
Nonexertional: Anticholinergics, including antihistamines; antiparkinsonian drugs; diuretics; phenothiazines

DRUG-INDUCED HYPERTHERMIA

Amphetamines, cocaine, phencyclidine (PCP), methylenedioxymethamphetamine (MDMA; "ecstasy"), lysergic acid diethylamide (LSD), salicylates, lithium, anticholinergics, sympathomimetics

NEUROLEPTIC MALIGNANT SYNDROME

Phenothiazines; butyrophenones, including haloperidol and bromperidol; fluoxetine; loxapine; tricyclic dibenzodiazepines; metoclopramide; domperidone; thiothixene; molindone; withdrawal of dopaminergic agents

SEROTONIN SYNDROME

Selective serotonin reuptake inhibitors (SSRIs), monoamine oxidase inhibitors (MAOIs), tricyclic antidepressants

MALIGNANT HYPERTHERMIA

Inhalational anesthetics, succinylcholine

ENDOCRINOPATHY

Thyrotoxicosis, pheochromocytoma

CENTRAL NERVOUS SYSTEM DAMAGE

Cerebral hemorrhage, status epilepticus, hypothalamic injury

Source: After FJ Curley, RS Irwin, JM Rippe et al (eds): *Intensive Care Medicine*, 3d ed. Boston, Little, Brown, 1996.

---

and other inhalational anesthetics or to succinylcholine. Elevated temperature, increased muscle metabolism, muscle rigidity, rhabdomyolysis, acidosis, and cardiovascular instability develop rapidly. This condition is often fatal. The *neuroleptic malignant syndrome* (NMS) occurs in the setting of neuroleptic agent use (antipsychotic phenothiazines, haloperidol, prochlorperazine, metoclopramide) or the withdrawal of dopaminergic drugs and is characterized by "lead-pipe" muscle rigidity, extrapyramidal side effects, autonomic dysregulation, and hyperthermia. This disorder appears to be caused by the inhibition of central dopamine receptors in the hypothalamus, which results in increased heat generation and decreased heat dissipation. The *serotonin syndrome*, seen with selective serotonin uptake inhibitors (SSRIs), MAOIs, and other serotonergic medications, has many overlapping features, including hyperthermia, but may be distinguished by the presence of diarrhea, tremor, and myoclonus rather than the lead-pipe rigidity of NMS. Thyrotoxicosis and pheochromocytoma can also cause increased thermogenesis.

It is important to distinguish between fever and hyperthermia since hyperthermia can be rapidly fatal and characteristically does not respond to antipyretics. However, there is no rapid way to make this distinction. Hyperthermia is often diagnosed on the basis of the events immediately preceding the elevation of core temperature—e.g., heat exposure or treatment with drugs that interfere with thermoregulation. However, in addition to the clinical history of the patient, the physical aspects of some forms of hyperthermia may alert the clinician. For example, in patients with heat stroke syndromes and in those taking drugs that block sweating, the skin is hot but dry. Moreover, antipyretics do not reduce the elevated temperature in hyperthermia, whereas in fever—and even in hyperpyrexia—adequate doses of either aspirin or acetaminophen usually result in some decrease in body temperature.

PATHOGENESIS OF FEVER

PYROGENS The term *pyrogen* is used to describe any substance that causes fever. *Exogenous* pyrogens are derived from outside the patient; most are microbial products, microbial toxins, or whole microorganisms. The classic example of an exogenous pyrogen is the lipopolysaccharide endotoxin produced by all gram-negative bacteria. Endotoxins are potent not only as pyrogens but also as inducers of various pathologic changes in gram-negative infections. Another group of potent bacterial pyrogens is produced by gram-positive organisms and includes the enterotoxins of *Staphylococcus aureus* and the group A and B streptococcal toxins, also called *superantigens*. One staphylococcal toxin of clinical importance is the toxic shock syndrome toxin associated with isolates of *S. aureus* from patients with toxic shock syndrome. Like the endotoxins of gram-negative bacteria, the toxins produced by staphylococci and streptococci cause fever in experimental animals when injected intravenously at concentrations of <1 μg/kg of body weight. Endotoxin is a highly pyrogenic molecule in humans: a dose of 2 to 3 ng/kg produces fever and generalized symptoms of malaise in volunteers.

PYROGENIC CYTOKINES Cytokines are small proteins (molecular mass, 10,000 to 20,000 Da) that regulate immune, inflammatory, and hematopoietic processes. For example, stimulation of lymphocyte proliferation during an immune response to vaccination is the result of the cytokines interleukin (IL) 2, IL-4, and IL-6. Another cytokine, granulocyte colony-stimulating factor, stimulates granulocytopoiesis in the bone marrow. Some cytokines cause fever and hence are called *pyrogenic cytokines*. From a historic point of view, the field of cytokine biology began in the 1940s with laboratory investigations into fever induction by products of activated leukocytes. These fever-producing molecules were called *endogenous pyrogens*.

The known pyrogenic cytokines include IL-1, IL-6, tumor necrosis factor (TNF), ciliary neurotropic factor (CNTF), and interferon (IFN) α. Others probably exist, although IL-18—a member of the IL-1 family—does not appear to be a pyrogenic cytokine. Each cytokine is encoded by a separate gene, and each pyrogenic cytokine has been shown to cause fever in laboratory animals and in humans. When injected into humans, IL-1, IL-6, and TNF produce fever at low doses (10 to 100 ng/kg).

The synthesis and release of endogenous pyrogenic cytokines are induced by a wide spectrum of exogenous pyrogens, most of which have recognizable bacterial or fungal sources. Viruses also induce pyrogenic cytokines by infecting cells. However, in the absence of microbial infection, inflammation, trauma, tissue necrosis, or antigen-antibody complexes can induce the production of IL-1, TNF, and/or IL-6, which—individually or in combination—trigger the hypothalamus to raise the set point to febrile levels. The cellular sources of pyrogenic cytokines are primarily monocytes, neutrophils, and lymphocytes, although many other types of cells can synthesize these molecules when stimulated.

ELEVATION OF THE HYPOTHALAMIC SET POINT BY CYTOKINES   During fever, levels of prostaglandin E_2 (PGE_2) are elevated in hypothalamic tissue and the third cerebral ventricle. The concentrations of PGE_2 are highest near the circumventricular vascular organs (organum vasculosum of lamina terminalis)—networks of enlarged capillaries surrounding the hypothalamic regulatory centers. Destruction of these organs reduces the ability of pyrogens to produce fever. Most studies in animals have failed to show, however, that pyrogenic cytokines pass from the circulation into the brain itself. Thus, it appears that both exogenous and endogenous pyrogens interact with the endothelium of these capillaries and that this interaction is the first step in initiating fever—i.e., in raising the set point to febrile levels.

The key events in the production of fever are illustrated in Fig. 16-1. As has been mentioned, several cell types can produce pyrogenic cytokines. Pyrogenic cytokines such as IL-1, IL-6, and TNF are released from the cells and enter the systemic circulation. Although the systemic effects of these circulating cytokines lead to fever by inducing the synthesis of PGE_2, they also induce PGE_2 in peripheral tissues. The increase in PGE_2 in the periphery accounts for the nonspecific myalgias and arthralgias that often accompany fever. However, it is the induction of PGE_2 in the brain that starts the process of raising the hypothalamic set point for core temperature.

There are four receptors for PGE_2, and each signals the cell in different ways. Of the four receptors, the third (EP-3) is essential for fever: when the gene for this receptor is deleted in mice, no fever follows the injection of IL-1 or endotoxin. Deletion of the other PGE_2 receptor genes leaves the fever mechanism intact. Although PGE_2 is essential for fever, it is not a neurotransmitter. Rather, the release of PGE_2 from the brain side of the hypothalamic endothelium triggers the PGE_2 receptor on glial cells, and this stimulation results in the rapid release of cyclic adenosine 5'-monophosphate (cyclic AMP), which is a neurotransmitter. As shown in Fig. 16-1, the release of cyclic AMP from the glial cells activates neuronal endings from the thermoregulatory center that extend into the area. The elevation of cyclic AMP is thought to account for changes in the hypothalamic set point either directly or indirectly by inducing the release of neurotransmitters. Distinct receptors for microbial products (such as endotoxins) from gram-negative bacteria and for teichoic acids from gram-positive bacteria are located on the hypothalamic endothelium. These receptors are called *Toll-like receptors* and are similar in many ways to IL-1 receptors. The direct activation of Toll-like receptors also results in PGE_2 production and fever.

PRODUCTION OF CYTOKINES IN THE CNS   Several viral diseases produce active infection in the brain. Glial and possibly neuronal cells synthesize IL-1, TNF, and IL-6. CNTF is also synthesized by neural as well as neuronal cells. What role in the production of fever is played by these cytokines produced in the brain itself? In experimental animals, the concentrations of cytokine required to cause fever are several orders of magnitude lower with direct injection into the brain than with intravenous injection. Therefore, CNS production of these cytokines apparently can raise the hypothalamic set point, bypassing the circumventricular organs involved in fever caused by circulating cytokines. CNS cytokines may account for the hyperpyrexia of CNS hemorrhage, trauma, or infection.

APPROACH TO THE PATIENT

History   It is in the diagnosis of a febrile illness that the science and art of medicine come together (see also Chaps. 1, 18, and 106). In no other clinical situation is a meticulous history more important. Painstaking attention must be paid to the chronology of symptoms in relation to the use of prescription drugs (including drugs, supplements, or herbs taken without a physician's supervision) or treatments such as surgical or dental procedures. The exact nature of any prosthetic materials and/or implanted devices should be ascertained. A careful occupational history should include exposures to animals; toxic fumes; potential infectious agents; possible antigens; or other febrile or infected individuals in the home, workplace, or school. A history of the geographic areas in which the patient has lived and a travel history should include locations during military service. Information on unusual hobbies, dietary proclivities (such as raw or poorly cooked meat, raw fish, and unpasteurized milk or cheeses), and household pets should be elicited, as should that on sexual orientation and practices, including precautions taken or omitted. Attention should be directed to the use of tobacco, marijuana, intravenous drugs, or alcohol; trauma; animal bites; tick or other insect bites; and prior transfusions, immunizations, drug allergies, or hypersensitivities. A careful family history should include information on family members with tuberculosis, other febrile or infectious diseases, arthritis or collagen vascular disease, or unusual familial symptomatology such as deafness, urticaria, fevers and polyserositis, bone pain, or anemia. Ethnic origin may be critical. For example, blacks are more likely than persons in other groups to have hemoglobinopathies. Turks, Arabs, Armenians, and Sephardic Jews are especially likely to have familial Mediterranean fever (Chap. 278).

Physical Examination   A meticulous physical examination should be repeated on a regular basis. All the vital signs are relevant. The temperature may be taken orally or rectally, but the site used should be consistent. Axillary temperatures are notoriously unreliable. Special attention should be paid to the skin, lymph nodes, eyes, nail beds, cardiovascular system, chest, abdomen, musculoskeletal system, and nervous system. Rectal examination is imperative. The penis, prostate, scrotum, and testes should be examined carefully and the foreskin, if present, retracted. Pelvic examination must be part of every complete physical examination of a woman, with a

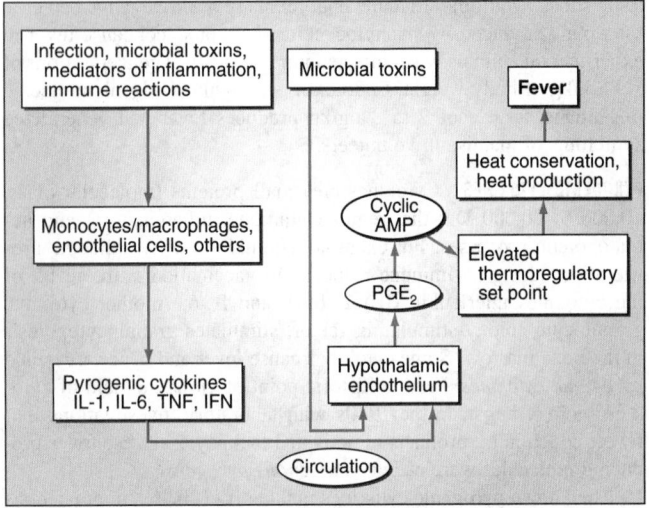

FIGURE 16-1   *Chronology of events required for the induction of fever. Abbreviations: AMP, adenosine 5'-monophosphate; IFN, interferon; IL, interleukin; PGE_2, prostaglandin E_2; TNF, tumor necrosis factor.*

search for such causes of fever as pelvic inflammatory disease and tubo-ovarian abscess.

Laboratory Tests Few signs and symptoms in medicine have as many diagnostic possibilities as fever. If the history, epidemiologic situation, or physical examination suggests more than a simple viral illness or streptococcal pharyngitis, then laboratory testing is indicated. The tempo and complexity of the workup will depend on the pace of the illness, diagnostic considerations, and the immune status of the host. If findings are focal or if the history, epidemiologic setting, or physical examination suggests certain diagnoses, the laboratory examination can be focused. If fever is undifferentiated, the diagnostic nets must be cast farther, and certain guidelines are indicated, as follows.

CLINICAL PATHOLOGY The workup should include a complete blood count; a differential count should be performed manually or with an instrument sensitive to the identification of eosinophils, juvenile or band forms, toxic granulations, and Döhle bodies, the last three of which are suggestive of bacterial infection. Neutropenia may be present with some viral infections, particularly parvovirus B19 infection; drug reactions; systemic lupus erythematosus; typhoid; brucellosis; and infiltrative diseases of the bone marrow, including lymphoma, leukemia, tuberculosis, and histoplasmosis. Lymphocytosis may occur with typhoid, brucellosis, tuberculosis, and viral disease. Atypical lymphocytes are documented in many viral diseases, including infection with Epstein-Barr virus, cytomegalovirus, or HIV; dengue; rubella; varicella; measles; and viral hepatitis. This abnormality also occurs in serum sickness and toxoplasmosis. Monocytosis is a feature of typhoid, tuberculosis, brucellosis, and lymphoma. Eosinophilia may be associated with hypersensitivity drug reactions, Hodgkin's disease, adrenal insufficiency, and certain metazoan infections. If the febrile illness appears to be severe or is prolonged, the smear should be examined carefully for malarial or babesial pathogens (where appropriate) as well as for classic morphologic features, and the erythrocyte sedimentation rate should be determined. Urinalysis, with examination of urinary sediment, is indicated. It is axiomatic that any abnormal fluid accumulation (pleural, peritoneal, joint), even if previously sampled, merits reexamination in the presence of undiagnosed fever. Joint fluids should be examined for bacteria as well as crystals. Bone marrow biopsy (not simple aspiration) for histopathologic studies (as well as culture) is indicated when marrow infiltration by pathogens or tumor cells is possible. Stool should be inspected for occult blood; an inspection for fecal leukocytes, ova, or parasites also may be indicated.

CHEMISTRY Electrolyte, glucose, blood urea nitrogen, and creatinine levels should be measured. Liver function tests are usually indicated if efforts to identify the cause of fever do not point to the involvement of another organ. Additional assessments (e.g., measurement of creatinine phosphokinase or amylase) can be added as the workup progresses.

MICROBIOLOGY Smears and cultures of specimens from the throat, urethra, anus, cervix, and vagina should be assessed when there are no localizing findings or when findings suggest the involvement of the pelvis or the gastrointestinal tract. If respiratory tract infection is suspected, sputum evaluation (Gram's staining, staining for acid-fast bacilli, culture) is indicated. Cultures of blood, abnormal fluid collections, and urine are indicated when fever is thought to reflect more than uncomplicated viral illness. Cerebrospinal fluid should be examined and cultured if meningismus, severe headache, or a change in mental status is noted.

RADIOLOGY A chest x-ray is usually part of the evaluation for any significant febrile illness.

Outcome of Diagnostic Efforts In most cases of fever, either the patient recovers spontaneously or the history, physical examination, and initial screening laboratory studies lead to a diagnosis. When

fever continues for 2 to 3 weeks, during which time repeat physical examinations and laboratory tests are unrevealing, the patient is provisionally diagnosed as having fever of unknown origin (Chap. 18).

℞ TREATMENT

The Decision to Treat Fever Most fevers are associated with self-limited infections, most commonly of viral origin. In these cases, the general cause of the fever is easily identified. The routine use of antipyretics given automatically as "standing," "routine," or "prn" orders to treat low-grade fevers in adult patients on hospital wards is entirely unacceptable. This practice masks not only fever but also other important clinical indicators of a patient's course. For example, the daily highs and lows of normal temperature are exaggerated in most fevers, but the usual times of peak and trough temperatures may be reversed in typhoid fever and disseminated tuberculosis. Temperature-pulse dissociation (relative bradycardia) occurs in typhoid fever, brucellosis, leptospirosis, some drug-induced fevers, and factitious fever. In newborns, the elderly, patients with chronic renal failure, and patients taking glucocorticoids, fever may not be present despite infection, or core temperature may be hypothermic. Hypothermia is observed in patients with septic shock.

Some febrile diseases have characteristic patterns. With *relapsing* fevers, febrile episodes are separated by intervals of normal temperature; when paroxysms occur on the first and third days, the fever is called *tertian*. *Plasmodium vivax* causes tertian fevers. *Quartan* fevers are associated with paroxysms on the first and fourth days and are seen with *P. malariae*. Other relapsing fevers are related to *Borrelia* infections and rat-bite fever, which are both associated with days of fever followed by a several-day afebrile period and then a relapse of days of fever. Pel-Ebstein fever, with fevers lasting 3 to 10 days followed by afebrile periods of 3 to 10 days, is classic for Hodgkin's disease and other lymphomas. Another characteristic fever is that of cyclic neutropenia, in which fevers occur every 21 days and accompany the neutropenia. There is no periodicity of fever in patients with familial Mediterranean fever (Chap. 278).

Mechanisms of Antipyretic Agents The synthesis of PGE_2 depends on the constitutively expressed enzyme cyclooxygenase. The substrate for cyclooxygenase is arachidonic acid released from the cell membrane, and this release is the rate-limiting step in the synthesis of PGE_2. Inhibitors of cyclooxygenase are potent antipyretics. The antipyretic potency of various drugs is directly correlated with the inhibition of brain cyclooxygenase. Acetaminophen is a poor cyclooxygenase inhibitor in peripheral tissue and is without noteworthy anti-inflammatory activity; in the brain, however, acetaminophen is oxidized by the p450 cytochrome system, and the oxidized form inhibits cyclooxygenase activity. Moreover, in the brain, the inhibition of another enzyme, COX-3, by acetaminophen may account for the antipyretic effect of this agent. However, COX-3 is not found outside the CNS.

Oral aspirin and acetaminophen are equally effective in reducing fever in humans. Nonsteroidal anti-inflammatory agents (NSAIDs) such as indomethacin and ibuprofen are also excellent antipyretics. Chronic high-dose therapy with antipyretics such as aspirin or the NSAIDs used in arthritis does not reduce normal core body temperature. Thus, PGE_2 appears to play no role in normal thermoregulation.

As effective antipyretics, glucocorticoids act at two levels. First, similar to the cyclooxygenase inhibitors, glucocorticoids reduce PGE_2 synthesis by inhibiting the activity of phospholipase A_2, which is needed to release arachidonic acid from the cell membrane. Second, glucocorticoids block the transcription of the mRNA for the pyrogenic cytokines.

Indications and Regimens for the Treatment of Fever The objectives in treating fever are first to reduce the elevated hypothalamic set point and second to facilitate heat loss. There is no evidence that fever itself facilitates the recovery from infection or acts as an adjuvant to the immune system. In fact, peripheral PGE_2 production is a potent immunosuppressant. Hence, treating fever and its symptoms does no harm and does not slow the resolution of common viral and bacterial infections. Reducing fever with antipyretics also reduces systemic symptoms of headache, myalgias, and arthralgias.

Oral aspirin and NSAIDs effectively reduce fever but can adversely affect platelets and the gastrointestinal tract. Therefore, acetaminophen is preferred to all of these agents as an antipyretic. In children, acetaminophen must be used because aspirin increases the risk of Reye's syndrome. If the patient cannot take oral antipyretics, parenteral preparations of NSAIDs and rectal suppository preparations of various antipyretics can be used.

Treatment of fever in some groups of patients is recommended. Fever increases the demand for oxygen (i.e., for every increase of 1°C over 37°C, there is a 13% increase in oxygen consumption) and can aggravate preexisting cardiac, cerebrovascular, or pulmonary insufficiency. Elevated temperature can induce mental changes in patients with organic brain disease. Children with a history of febrile or nonfebrile seizure should be aggressively treated to reduce fever, although it is unclear what triggers the febrile seizure and there is no correlation between absolute temperature elevation and onset of a febrile seizure in susceptible children.

In hyperpyrexia, the use of cooling blankets facilitates the reduction of temperature; however, cooling blankets should not be used without oral antipyretics. In hyperpyretic patients with CNS disease or trauma, reducing core temperature mitigates the ill effects of high temperature on the brain.

Treating Hyperthermia A high core temperature in a patient with an appropriate history (e.g., environmental heat exposure or treatment with anticholinergic or neuroleptic drugs, tricyclic antidepressants, succinylcholine, or halothane) along with appropriate clinical findings (dry skin, hallucinations, delirium, pupil dilation, muscle rigidity, and/or elevated levels of creatine phosphokinase) suggests hyperthermia.

The attempt to lower the already normal hypothalamic set point is of little use. Physical cooling with sponging, fans, cooling blankets, and even ice baths should be initiated immediately in conjunction with the administration of intravenous fluids and appropriate pharmacologic agents (see below). If insufficient cooling is achieved by external means, internal cooling can be achieved by gastric or peritoneal lavage with iced saline. In extreme circumstances, hemodialysis or even cardiopulmonary bypass with cooling of blood may be performed.

Malignant hyperthermia should be treated immediately with cessation of anesthesia and intravenous administration of dantrolene sodium. The recommended dose of dantrolene is 1 to 2.5 mg/kg of body weight given intravenously every 6 h for at least 24 to 48 h—until oral dantrolene can be administered, if needed. Procainamide should also be administered to patients with malignant hyperthermia because of the likelihood of ventricular fibrillation in this syndrome. Dantrolene at similar doses is indicated in NMS and in drug-induced hyperthermia and may even be useful in the hyperthermia of the serotonin syndrome and thyrotoxicosis. NMS may also be treated with bromocriptine, levodopa, amantadine, or nifedipine or by induction of muscle paralysis with curare and pancuronium. Tricyclic antidepressant overdose may be treated with physostigmine.

FURTHER READING

BOUCHAMA A, KNOCHEL JP: Heat stroke. N Engl J Med 346:1978, 2002
CHANDRASEKHARAN NV et al: COX-3, a cyclooxygenase-1 variant inhibited by acetaminophen and other analgesic/antipyretic drugs: Cloning, structure, and expression. Proc Natl Acad Sci USA 99:13926, 2002
DINARELLO CA: Proinflammatory cytokines. Chest 118:503, 2000
NETEA MG et al: Circulating cytokines as mediators of fever. Clin Infect Dis 31:178, 2000
USHIKUBI F et al: Impaired febrile response in mice lacking the prostaglandin E receptor subtype EP3. Nature 395:281, 1998
YANG RB et al: Toll-like receptor-2 mediates lipopolysaccharide-induced cellular signaling. Nature 395:284, 1998

17 FEVER AND RASH
Elaine T. Kaye, Kenneth M. Kaye

The acutely ill patient with fever and rash often presents a diagnostic challenge for physicians. The distinctive appearance of an eruption in concert with a clinical syndrome may facilitate a prompt diagnosis and the institution of life-saving therapy or critical infection-control interventions.

APPROACH TO THE PATIENT

A thorough history of patients with fever and rash includes the following relevant information: immune status, medications taken within the previous month, specific travel history, immunization status, exposure to domestic pets and other animals, history of animal or arthropod bites, existence of cardiac abnormalities, presence of prosthetic material, recent exposure to ill individuals, and exposure to sexually transmitted diseases. The history should also include the site of onset of the rash and its direction and rate of spread.

A thorough physical examination entails close attention to the rash, with an assessment and precise definition of its salient features. First, it is critical to determine the *type* of lesions that make up the eruption. *Macules* are flat lesions defined by an area of changed color (i.e., a blanchable erythema). *Papules* are raised, solid lesions <5 mm in diameter; *plaques* are lesions >5 mm in diameter with a flat, plateau-like surface; and *nodules* are lesions >5 mm in diameter with a more rounded configuration. *Wheals* (urticaria, hives) are papules or plaques that are pale pink and may appear annular (ringlike) as they enlarge; classic (nonvasculitic) wheals are transient, lasting only 24 to 48 h in any defined area.

Vesicles (<5 mm) and *bullae* (>5 mm) are circumscribed, elevated lesions containing fluid. *Pustules* are raised lesions containing purulent exudate; vesicular processes such as varicella or herpes simplex may evolve to pustules. *Nonpalpable purpura* is a flat lesion that is due to bleeding into the skin; if <3 mm in diameter, the purpuric lesions are termed *petechiae*; if >3 mm, they are termed *ecchymoses*. *Palpable purpura* is a raised lesion that is due to inflammation of the vessel wall (vasculitis) with subsequent hemorrhage. An *ulcer* is a defect in the skin extending at least into the upper layer of the dermis, and an *eschar* (tâche noire) is a necrotic lesion covered with a black crust.

Other pertinent features of rashes include their *configuration* (i.e., annular or target), the *arrangement* of their lesions, and their *distribution* (i.e., central or peripheral). →*For further discussion, see Chaps. 46 and 48.*

CLASSIFICATION OF RASH

This chapter reviews rashes that reflect systemic disease, but it does not include localized skin eruptions (i.e., cellulitis, impetigo) that may also be associated with fever (Chap. 110). Rashes are classified herein on the basis of the morphology and distribution of lesions. For practical purposes, this classification system is based on the most typical disease presentations. However, morphology may vary as rashes evolve, and the presentation of diseases with rashes is subject to many variations (Chap. 48). For instance, the classic petechial rash of Rocky Mountain spotted fever (RMSF; Chap. 158) may initially consist of blanchable erythematous macules distributed peripherally; at times, the rash associated with RMSF may not be predominantly acral, or a rash may not develop at all.

Diseases with fever and rash may be classified by type of eruption: centrally distributed maculopapular, peripheral, confluent desquamative erythematous, vesiculobullous, urticarial, nodular, purpuric, ulcerated, or eschars (Table 17-1). For a more detailed discussion of each disease associated with a rash, the reader is referred to the chapter dealing with that specific disease. (Reference chapters are cited in the text and listed in Table 17-1.)

CENTRALLY DISTRIBUTED MACULOPAPULAR ERUPTIONS Centrally distributed rashes, in which lesions are primarily truncal, are the most common type of eruption. The rash of *measles* (rubeola) starts at the hairline 2 to 3 days into the illness and moves down the body, sparing the palms and soles (Chap. 176). It begins as discrete erythematous lesions, which become confluent as the rash spreads. Koplik's spots (1- to 2-mm white or bluish lesions with an erythematous halo on the buccal mucosa) are pathognomonic for measles and are generally seen during the first 2 days of symptoms. They should not be confused with Fordyce's spots (ectopic sebaceous glands), which have no erythematous halos and are found in the mouth of healthy individuals. Koplik's spots may briefly overlap with the measles exanthem.

German measles (rubella) also spreads from the hairline downward; unlike that of measles, however, the rash of rubella tends to clear from originally affected areas as it migrates and may be pruritic (Chap. 177). Forchheimer spots (palatal petechiae) may develop but are nonspecific since they also develop in mononucleosis (Chap. 165) and scarlet fever (Chap. 121). Postauricular and suboccipital adenopathy and arthritis are common among adults with German measles. Exposure of pregnant women to ill individuals should be avoided, as rubella causes severe congenital abnormalities. Numerous strains of enteroviruses (Chap. 175), primarily echoviruses and coxsackieviruses, cause nonspecific syndromes of fever and eruptions that may mimic rubella or measles. Patients with infectious mononucleosis caused by Epstein-Barr virus (Chap. 165) or with primary infection caused by HIV (Chap. 173) may exhibit pharyngitis, lymphadenopathy, and a nonspecific maculopapular exanthem.

The rash of *erythema infectiosum* (fifth disease), which is caused by human parvovirus B19, primarily affects children 3 to 12 years old; it develops after fever has resolved as a bright blanchable erythema on the cheeks ("slapped cheeks") with perioral pallor (Chap. 168). A more diffuse rash (often pruritic) appears the next day on the trunk and extremities and then rapidly develops into a lacy reticular eruption that may wax and wane (especially with temperature change) over 3 weeks. Adults with fifth disease often have arthritis, and fetal hydrops can develop in association with this condition in pregnant women.

Exanthem subitum (roseola) is caused by human herpesvirus 6 and is most common among children <3 years of age (Chap. 166). As in erythema infectiosum, the rash usually appears after fever has subsided. It consists of 2- to 3-mm rose-pink macules and papules that rarely coalesce, occur initially on the trunk and sometimes on the extremities (sparing the face), and fade within 2 days.

Although drug reactions have many manifestations, including urticaria, exanthematous *drug-induced eruptions* (Chap. 50) are most common and are often difficult to distinguish from viral exanthems. Eruptions elicited by drugs are usually more intensely erythematous and pruritic than viral exanthems, but this distinction is not reliable. A history of new medications and an absence of prostration may help to distinguish a drug-related rash from an eruption of another etiology. Rashes may persist for up to 2 weeks after administration of the offending agent is discontinued. Certain populations are more prone than others to drug rashes. Of HIV-infected patients, 50 to 60% develop a rash in response to sulfa drugs; 50 to 100% of patients with mononucleosis due to Epstein-Barr virus develop a rash when given ampicillin.

Rickettsial illnesses (Chap. 158) should be considered in the evaluation of individuals with centrally distributed maculopapular eruptions. The usual setting for *epidemic typhus* is a site of war or natural disaster in which people are exposed to body lice. A diagnosis of recrudescent typhus should be considered in European immigrants to the United States. However, an indigenous form of typhus, presumably transmitted by flying squirrels, has been reported in the southeastern United States. *Endemic typhus* or *leptospirosis* (the latter caused by a spirochete; Chap. 155) may be seen in urban environments where rodents proliferate. Outside the United States, other rickettsial diseases cause a spotted-fever syndrome and should be considered in residents of or travelers to endemic areas. Similarly, *typhoid fever*, a nonrickettsial disease caused by *Salmonella typhi* (Chap. 137), is usually acquired during travel outside the United States. Dengue fever, caused by a mosquito-transmitted flavivirus, occurs in tropical and subtropical regions of the world (Chap. 180).

Some centrally distributed maculopapular eruptions have distinctive features. Erythema chronicum migrans (ECM), the rash of Lyme disease (Chap. 157), typically manifests as singular or multiple annular plaques. Untreated ECM lesions usually fade within a month but may persist for more than a year. *Erythema marginatum*, the rash of acute rheumatic fever (Chap. 302), has a distinctive pattern of enlarging and shifting transient annular lesions.

Collagen vascular diseases may cause fever and rash. Patients with *systemic lupus erythematosus* (Chap. 300) typically develop a sharply defined, erythematous eruption in a butterfly distribution on the cheeks (malar rash) as well as many other skin manifestations. *Still's disease* (Chap. 316) manifests as an evanescent salmon-colored rash on the trunk and proximal extremities that coincides with fever spikes.

PERIPHERAL ERUPTIONS These rashes are alike in that they are most prominent peripherally or begin in peripheral (acral) areas before spreading centripetally. Early diagnosis and therapy are critical in RMSF (Chap. 158) because of its grave prognosis if untreated. Lesions evolve from macular to petechial, start on the wrists and ankles, spread centripetally, and appear on the palms and soles only later in the disease. The rash of *secondary syphilis* (Chap. 153), which may be generalized but is prominent on the palms and soles, should be considered in the differential diagnosis of pityriasis rosea, especially in sexually active patients. *Atypical measles* (Chap. 176) is seen in individuals contracting measles who received the killed measles vaccine between 1963 and 1967 in the United States and who were not subsequently protected with the live vaccine. *Hand-foot-and-mouth disease* (Chap. 175), most commonly caused by coxsackievirus A16, is distinguished by tender vesicles distributed peripherally and in the mouth; outbreaks commonly occur within families. The classic target lesions of *erythema multiforme* appear symmetrically on the elbows, knees, palms, and soles. In relatively severe cases, these lesions may spread diffusely and involve mucosal surfaces (Stevens-Johnson syndrome). Lesions may develop on the hands and feet in *endocarditis* (Chap. 109).

CONFLUENT DESQUAMATIVE ERYTHEMAS These eruptions consist of diffuse erythema frequently followed by desquamation. The eruptions caused by group A *Streptococcus* or *Staphylococcus aureus* are toxin mediated. Certain disease features may provide diagnostic clues. *Scarlet fever* (Chap. 121) usually follows pharyngitis; patients have a facial flush, a "strawberry" tongue, and accentuated petechiae in body folds (Pastia's lines). *Kawasaki disease* (Chaps. 48 and 306) presents in the pediatric population as fissuring of the lips, a strawberry tongue, conjunctivitis, adenopathy, and sometimes cardiac abnormalities. *Streptococcal toxic shock syndrome* (Chap. 121) manifests with hypotension, multiorgan failure, and often a severe group A streptococcal infection (e.g., necrotizing fasciitis). *Staphylococcal toxic shock syndrome* (Chap. 120) also presents with hypotension and multiorgan failure, but usually only *S. aureus* colonization—not a severe *S. aureus* infection—is documented. *Staphylococcal scalded-skin syndrome* (Chap. 120) is seen primarily in children and in immunocompromised adults. Generalized erythema is often evident during the prodrome of fever and malaise; profound tenderness of the skin is distinctive. In the exfoliative stage, the skin can be induced to form bullae with light lateral pressure (Nikolsky's sign). In a mild form, a scarlatiniform eruption mimics scarlet fever, but the patient does not exhibit a straw-

TABLE 17-1 *Diseases Associated with Fever and Rash*

Disease	Etiology	Description	Group Affected/ Epidemiologic Factors	Clinical Syndrome	Chapter
CENTRALLY DISTRIBUTED MACULOPAPULAR ERUPTIONS					
Measles (rubeola, first disease)	Paramyxovirus	Discrete lesions that become confluent as rash spreads from hairline downward, sparing palms and soles; lasts ≥3 days; Koplik's spots	Nonimmune individuals	Cough, conjunctivitis, coryza, severe prostration	176
German measles (rubella, third disease)	Togavirus	Spreads from hairline downward, clearing as it spreads; Forchheimer spots	Nonimmune individuals	Adenopathy, arthritis	177
Erythema infectiosum (fifth disease)	Human parvovirus B19	Bright-red "slapped-cheek" appearance followed by lacy reticular rash that waxes and wanes over 3 weeks	Most common in children aged 3–12 years; occurs in winter and spring	Mild fever; arthritis in adults; rash follows resolution of fever	168
Exanthem subitum (roseola, sixth disease)	Human herpesvirus 6	Diffuse maculopapular eruption (sparing face); resolves within 2 days	Usually affects children <3 years old	Rash following resolution of fever; similar to Boston exanthem (echovirus 16)	166
Primary HIV infection	HIV	Nonspecific diffuse macules and papules; may be urticarial; oral or genital ulcers in some cases	Individuals recently infected with HIV	Pharyngitis, adenopathy, arthralgias	173
Infectious mononucleosis	Epstein-Barr virus	Diffuse maculopapular eruption (10–15% of cases; 90% if ampicillin is given); urticaria in some cases; periorbital edema (50%); palatal petechiae (25%)	Adolescents, young adults	Hepatosplenomegaly, pharyngitis, cervical lymphadenopathy, atypical lymphocytosis, heterophile antibody	165
Other viral exanthems	Echoviruses 2, 4, 9, 11, 16, 19, and 25; coxsackieviruses A9, B1, and B5; etc.	Skin findings mimicking rubella or measles	Affect children more commonly than adults	Nonspecific viral syndromes	175
Exanthematous drug-induced eruption	Drugs (antibiotics, anticonvulsants, diuretics, etc.)	Intensely pruritic, bright-red macules and papules, symmetric on trunk and extremities; may become confluent	Occurs 2–3 d after exposure in previously sensitized individuals; otherwise, after 2–3 weeks (but can occur anytime, even shortly after drug is discontinued)	Variable findings: fever and eosinophilia	50
Epidemic typhus	*Rickettsia prowazekii*	Maculopapular eruption appearing in axillae, spreading to trunk and later to extremities; usually spares face, palms, soles; evolves from blanchable macules to confluent eruption with petechiae; rash evanescent in recrudescent typhus (Brill-Zinsser disease)	Exposure to body lice; occurrence of recrudescent typhus as relapse after 30–50 years	Headache, myalgias; 10–40% mortality if untreated; milder clinical presentation in recrudescent form	158
Endemic (murine) typhus	*Rickettsia typhi*	Maculopapular eruption, usually sparing palms, soles	Exposure to rat or cat fleas	Headache, myalgias	158
Scrub typhus	*Orientia tsutsugamushi*	Diffuse macular rash starting on trunk; eschar at site of mite bite	Endemic in South Pacific, Australia, Asia; transmitted by mites	Headache, myalgias, regional adenopathy; mortality up to 30% if untreated	158
Rickettsial spotted fevers	*Rickettsia conorii* (boutonneuse fever), *Rickettsia australis* (North Queensland tick typhus), *Rickettsia sibirica* (Siberian tick typhus), and others	Eschar common at bite site; maculopapular (rarely, vesicular and petechial) eruption on proximal extremities, spreading to trunk and face	Exposure to ticks; *R. conorii* in Mediterranean region, India, Africa; *R. australis* in Australia; *R. sibirica* in Siberia, Mongolia	Headache, myalgias, regional adenopathy	158
Human monocytotropic ehrlichiosis[a]	*Ehrlichia chaffeensis*	Maculopapular eruption (40% of cases), involves trunk and extremities; may be petechial	Tick-borne; most common in U.S. Southeast, southern Midwest, and mid-Atlantic regions	Headache, myalgias, leukopenia	158
Leptospirosis	*Leptospira interrogans*	Maculopapular eruption; conjunctivitis; scleral hemorrhage in some cases	Exposure to water contaminated with animal urine	Myalgias; aseptic meningitis; *fulminant form*: icterohemorrhagic fever (Weil's disease)	155

(continued)

TABLE 17-1—(Continued)

Disease	Etiology	Description	Group Affected/ Epidemiologic Factors	Clinical Syndrome	Chapter
Lyme disease	*Borrelia burgdorferi*	Papule expanding to erythematous annular lesion with central clearing (erythema chronicum migrans or ECM; average diameter, 15 cm), sometimes with concentric rings, sometimes with indurated or vesicular center; multiple secondary ECM lesions in some cases	Bite of tick vector	Headache, myalgias, chills, photophobia occurring acutely; CNS disease, myocardial disease, arthritis weeks to months later in some cases	157
Typhoid fever	*Salmonella typhi*	Transient, blanchable erythematous macules and papules, 2–4 mm, usually on trunk (rose spots)	Ingestion of contaminated food or water (rare in U.S.)	Variable abdominal pain and diarrhea; headache, myalgias, hepatosplenomegaly	137
Dengue fever[b]	Dengue virus (4 serotypes; flaviviruses)	Rash in 50% of cases; initially diffuse flushing; midway through illness, onset of maculopapular rash, which begins on trunk and spreads centrifugally to extremities and face; pruritus, hyperesthesia in some cases; after defervescence, petechiae on extremities in some cases	Occurs in tropics and subtropics; transmitted by mosquito	Headache, musculoskeletal pain ("breakbone fever"); leukopenia; occasionally biphasic ("saddleback") fever	180
Rat-bite fever (sodoku)	*Spirillum minus*	Eschar at bite site; then blotchy violaceous or red-brown rash involving trunk and extremities	Rat bite; primarily found in Asia; rare in U.S.	Regional adenopathy, recurrent fevers if untreated	. . .
Relapsing fever	*Borrelia* species	Central rash at end of febrile episode; petechiae in some cases	Exposure to ticks or body lice	Recurrent fever, headache, myalgias, hepatosplenomegaly	156
Erythema marginatum (rheumatic fever)	Group A *Streptococcus*	Erythematous annular papules and plaques occurring as polycyclic lesions in waves over trunk, proximal extremities; evolving and resolving within hours	Patients with rheumatic fever	Pharyngitis preceding polyarthritis, carditis, subcutaneous nodules, chorea	302
Systemic lupus erythematosus	Autoimmune disease	Macular and papular erythema, often in sun-exposed areas; discoid lupus lesions (local atrophy, scale, pigmentary changes); periungual telangiectasis; malar rash; vasculitis sometimes causing urticaria, palpable purpura; oral erosions in some cases	Most common in young to middle-aged women; flares precipitated by sun exposure	Arthritis; cardiac, pulmonary, renal, hematologic, and vasculitic disease	300
Still's disease	Autoimmune disease	Transient 2- to 5-mm erythematous papules appearing at height of fever on trunk, proximal extremities; lesions evanescent	Children and young adults	High spiking fever, polyarthritis, splenomegaly; erythrocyte sedimentation rate, >100 mm/h	316
Arcanobacterial pharyngitis	*Arcanobacterium (Corynebacterium) haemolyticum*	Diffuse, erythematous, maculopapular eruption involving trunk and proximal extremities; may desquamate	Children and young adults	Exudative pharyngitis, lymphadenopathy	122
PERIPHERAL ERUPTIONS					
Chronic meningococcemia, disseminated gonococcal infection[c]	—	—	—	—	127, 128
Rocky Mountain spotted fever	*Rickettsia rickettsii*	Rash beginning on wrists and ankles and spreading centripetally; appears on palms and soles later in disease; lesion evolution from blanchable macules to petechiae	Tick vector; widespread but more common in southeastern and southwest-central U.S.	Headache, myalgias, abdominal pain; mortality up to 40% if untreated	158
Secondary syphilis	*Treponema pallidum*	Coincident primary chancre in 10% of cases; copper-colored, scaly papular eruption, diffuse but prominent on palms and soles; rash never vesicular in adults; condyloma latum, mucous patches, and alopecia in some cases	Sexually transmitted	Fever, constitutional symptoms	153

(continued)

TABLE 17-1 *Diseases Associated with Fever and Rash*—(continued)

Disease	Etiology	Description	Group Affected/ Epidemiologic Factors	Clinical Syndrome	Chapter
Atypical measles	Paramyxovirus	Maculopapular eruption beginning on distal extremities and spreading centripetally; may evolve into vesicles or petechiae; edema of extremities; Koplik's spots absent	Individuals contracting measles who received killed measles vaccine in 1963–1967 in U.S. without subsequent live vaccine	Headache, nodular pneumonia	176
Hand-foot-and-mouth disease	Coxsackievirus A16 most common cause	Tender vesicles, erosions in mouth; 0.25-cm papules on hands and feet with rim of erythema evolving into tender vesicles	Summer and fall; primarily children <10 years old; multiple family members	Transient fever	175
Erythema multiforme	Drugs, infection, idiopathic causes	Target lesions (central erythema surrounded by area of clearing and another rim of erythema) up to 2 cm; symmetric on knees, elbows, palms, soles; may become diffuse; may involve mucosal surfaces (Stevens-Johnson syndrome if 2 or more mucosal sites involved)	Drug intake (i.e., sulfa, phenytoin, penicillin); herpes simplex virus or *Mycoplasma pneumoniae* infection	Varies with predisposing factor	—[d]
Rat-bite fever (Haverhill fever)	*Streptobacillus moniliformis*	Maculopapular eruption over palms, soles, and extremities, tends to be more severe at joints; eruption sometimes becoming generalized; may be purpuric; may desquamate	Rat bite, ingestion of contaminated food	Myalgias; arthritis (50%); fever recurrence in some cases	. . .
Bacterial endocarditis	*Streptococcus, Staphylococcus,* etc.	*Subacute course:* Osler's nodes (tender pink nodules on finger or toe pads); petechiae on skin and mucosa; splinter hemorrhages. *Acute course (S. aureus):* Janeway lesions (painless erythematous or hemorrhagic macules, usually on palms and soles)	Abnormal heart valve, intravenous drug use	New heart murmur	109

CONFLUENT DESQUAMATIVE ERYTHEMAS

Disease	Etiology	Description	Group Affected/ Epidemiologic Factors	Clinical Syndrome	Chapter
Scarlet fever (second disease)	Group A *Streptococcus* (pyrogenic exotoxins A, B, C)	Diffuse blanchable erythema beginning on face and spreading to trunk and extremities; circumoral pallor; "sandpaper" texture to skin; accentuation of linear erythema in skin folds (Pastia's lines); enanthem of white evolving into red "strawberry" tongue; desquamation in second week	Most common in children aged 2–10 years; usually follows group A streptococcal pharyngitis	Fever, pharyngitis, headache	121
Kawasaki disease	Idiopathic causes	Rash similar to scarlet fever (scarlatiniform) or erythema multiforme; fissuring of lips, strawberry tongue; conjunctivitis; edema of hands, feet; desquamation later in disease	Children <8 years	Cervical adenopathy, pharyngitis, coronary artery vasculitis	48, 306
Streptococcal toxic shock syndrome	Group A *Streptococcus* (associated with pyrogenic exotoxin A and/or B or certain M types)	When present, rash often scarlatiniform	May occur in setting of severe group A streptococcal infections, such as necrotizing fasciitis, bacteremia, pneumonia	Multiorgan failure, hypotension; 30% mortality rate	121
Staphylococcal toxic shock syndrome	*S. aureus* (toxic shock syndrome toxin 1, enterotoxin B or C)	Diffuse erythema involving palms; pronounced erythema of mucosal surfaces, conjunctivitis; desquamation 7–10 days into illness	Colonization with toxin-producing *S. aureus*	Fever >39°C (102°F), hypotension, multiorgan dysfunction	120
Staphylococcal scalded-skin syndrome	*S. aureus,* phage group II	Diffuse tender erythema, often with bullae and desquamation; Nikolsky's sign	Colonization with toxin-producing *S. aureus;* occurs in children <10 years old (termed "Ritter's disease" in neonates) or adults with renal dysfunction	Irritability; nasal or conjunctival secretions	120

(continued)

TABLE 17-1—(Continued)

Disease	Etiology	Description	Group Affected/ Epidemiologic Factors	Clinical Syndrome	Chapter
Exfoliative erythroderma syndrome	Underlying psoriasis, eczema, drug eruption, mycosis fungoides	Diffuse erythema (often scaling) interspersed with lesions of underlying condition	Usually occurs in adults over age 50; more common in men	Fever, chills (i.e., difficulty with thermoregulation); lymphadenopathy	47, 50
Toxic epidermal necrolysis	Drugs, other causes (infection, neoplasm, graft-vs.-host disease)	Diffuse erythema or target-like lesions progressing to bullae, with sloughing and necrosis of entire epidermis; Nikolsky's sign	Uncommon in children; more common in patients with HIV infection or graft-vs.-host disease	Dehydration, sepsis sometimes resulting from lack of normal skin integrity; 25% mortality	50

VESICULOBULLOUS ERUPTIONS

Disease	Etiology	Description	Group Affected/ Epidemiologic Factors	Clinical Syndrome	Chapter
Hand-foot-and-mouth syndrome[e]; staphylococcal scalded-skin syndrome, toxic epidermal necrolysis[f]	—	—	—	—	—[d]
Varicella (chickenpox)	Varicella-zoster virus	Macules (2–3 mm) evolving into papules, then vesicles (sometimes umbilicated), on an erythematous base ("dewdrops on a rose petal"); pustules then forming and crusting; lesions appearing in crops; may involve scalp, mouth; intensely pruritic	Usually affects children; 10% of adults susceptible; most common in late winter and spring	Malaise; mild disease in healthy children; more severe disease with complications in adults and immunocompromised children	164
Variola (smallpox)	Variola major virus	Red macules on tongue, palate evolving to papules and vesicles; skin macules evolving to papules, then vesicles, then pustules over 1 week, with subsequent lesion crusting; lesions initially appearing on face and spreading centrifugally from trunk to extremities; differs from varicella in that (1) skin lesions in any given area are at same stage of development and (2) there is a prominent distribution of lesions on face and extremities (including palms, soles) as opposed to prominent rash on trunk	Nonimmune individuals exposed to smallpox	Prodrome of fever, headache, backache, myalgias; vomiting in 50% of cases	205
Disseminated herpesvirus infection	Varicella-zoster virus or herpes simplex virus (HSV)	Individual lesions similar for varicella-zoster and HSV; *zoster cutaneous dissemination*: >25 lesions extending outside involved dermatome; *HSV*: extensive, progressive mucocutaneous lesions in some cases; HSV lesions sometimes disseminate in eczematous skin (eczema herpeticum); HSV visceral dissemination may occur with only limited skin lesions	Immunosuppressed individuals, eczema	Visceral organ involvement (especially liver) in some cases	163, 164, 360
Rickettsialpox	*Rickettsia akari*	Eschar found at site of mite bite; generalized rash involving face, trunk, extremities; may involve palms and soles; <100 papules and plaques (2–10 mm); tops of lesions develop vesicles that may evolve into pustules	Seen in urban settings; transmitted by mouse mites	Headache, myalgias, regional adenopathy; mild disease	158
Disseminated *Vibrio vulnificus* infection	*V. vulnificus*	Erythematous lesions evolving into hemorrhagic bullae and then into necrotic ulcers	Patients with cirrhosis, diabetes, renal failure; exposure by ingestion of contaminated saltwater seafood	Hypotension; 50% mortality	140
Ecthyma gangrenosum	*Pseudomonas aeruginosa*, other gram-negative rods, fungi	Indurated plaque evolving into hemorrhagic bulla or pustule that sloughs, resulting in eschar formation; erythematous halo; most common in axillary, groin, perianal regions	Usually affects neutropenic patients; occurs in up to 28% of individuals with *Pseudomonas* bacteremia	Clinical signs of sepsis	136

(continued)

TABLE 17-1 *Diseases Associated with Fever and Rash*—(continued)

Disease	Etiology	Description	Group Affected/ Epidemiologic Factors	Clinical Syndrome	Chapter
URTICARIAL ERUPTIONS					
Urticarial vasculitis	Serum sickness, often due to infection (including hepatitis B viral, enteroviral, parasitic), drugs (including penicillins, sulfonamides, salicylates, barbiturates); connective tissue disease; idiopathic causes	Erythematous, circumscribed areas of edema; occasionally indurated; pruritic or burning; lesions sometimes purpuric; individual lesions lasting up to 5 days	In serum sickness, occurs 8–14 days after antigen exposure in nonsensitized individuals; may occur within 36 h in sensitized individuals	Malaise, lymphadenopathy, myalgias, arthralgias	306[d]
NODULAR ERUPTIONS					
Disseminated infection	Fungi (e.g., candidiasis, histoplasmosis, cryptococcosis, sporotrichosis, coccidioi-domycosis); mycobacteria	Subcutaneous nodules (up to 3 cm); fluctuance, draining common with mycobacteria; necrotic nodules (extremities, periorbital or nasal regions) common with *Aspergillus, Mucor*	Immunocompromised hosts (i.e., bone marrow transplant recipients, patients undergoing chemotherapy, HIV-infected patients, alcoholics)	Features vary with organism	—[d]
Erythema nodosum (septal panniculitis)	Infections (e.g., streptococcal, fungal, mycobacterial, yersinial); drugs (e.g., sulfas, penicillins, oral contraceptives); sarcoidosis; idiopathic causes	Large, violaceous, nonulcerative, subcutaneous nodules; exquisitely tender; usually on lower legs but also on upper extremities	More common in females 15–30 years old	Arthralgias (50%); features vary with associated condition	—[d]
Sweet's syndrome (acute febrile neutrophilic dermatosis)	Yersinial infection; lymphoproliferative disorders; idiopathic causes	Tender red or blue edematous nodules giving impression of vesiculation; usually on face, neck, upper extremities; when on lower extremities, may mimic erythema nodosum	More common in women and in persons 30–60 years old; 20% of cases associated with malignancy (men and women equally affected in this group)	Headache, arthralgias, leukocytosis	48
Bacillary angiomatosis	*Bartonella henselae* or *Bartonella quintana*	Many forms, including erythematous, smooth vascular nodules; friable, exophytic lesions; erythematous plaques (may be dry, scaly); subcutaneous nodules (may be erythematous)	Usually in HIV infection	Peliosis of liver and spleen in some cases; lesions may involve multiple organs; bacteremia	144
PURPURIC ERUPTIONS					
Rocky Mountain spotted fever, rat-bite fever, endocarditis[e]; epidemic typhus[g]; dengue fever	—	—	—	—	—[d]
Acute meningococcemia	*Neisseria meningitidis*	Petechiae rapidly becoming numerous, sometimes enlarging and becoming vesicular; trunk, extremities most commonly involved; may appear on face, hands, feet; may include purpura fulminans reflecting disseminated intravascular coagulation (see below)	Most common in children, individuals with asplenia or terminal complement component deficiency (C5-C8)	Hypotension, meningitis (sometimes preceded by upper respiratory infection)	127

(continued)

TABLE 17-1—(Continued)

Disease	Etiology	Description	Group Affected/ Epidemiologic Factors	Clinical Syndrome	Chapter
Purpura fulminans	Severe disseminated intravascular coagulation	Large ecchymoses with sharply irregular shapes evolving into hemorrhagic bullae and then into black necrotic lesions	Individuals with sepsis (e.g., involving *N. meningitidis*), malignancy, or massive trauma; asplenic patients at high risk for sepsis	Hypotension	127, 254
Chronic meningococcemia	*N. meningitidis*	Variety of recurrent eruptions, including pink maculopapular; nodular (usually on lower extremities); petechial (sometimes developing vesicular centers); purpuric areas with pale blue-gray centers	Individuals with complement deficiencies	Fevers, sometimes intermittent; arthritis, myalgias, headache	127
Disseminated gonococcal infection	*Neisseria gonorrhoeae*	Papules (1–5 mm) evolving over 1–2 days into hemorrhagic pustules with gray necrotic centers; hemorrhagic bullae occurring rarely; lesions (usually fewer than 40) distributed peripherally near joints (more commonly on upper extremities)	Sexually active individuals (more often females), some with complement deficiency	Low-grade fever, tenosynovitis, arthritis	128
Enteroviral petechial rash	Usually echovirus 9 or coxsackievirus A9	Disseminated petechial lesions (may also be maculopapular, vesicular, or urticarial)	Often occurs in outbreaks	Pharyngitis, headache; aseptic meningitis with echovirus 9	175
Viral hemorrhagic fever	Arboviruses and arenaviruses	Petechial rash	Residence in or travel to endemic areas or other virus exposure	Triad of fever, shock, hemorrhage from mucosa or gastrointestinal tract	180, 181
Thrombotic thrombocytopenic purpura/hemolytic-uremic syndrome	Idiopathic, *Escherichia coli* O157:H7 (Shiga toxin), drugs	Petechiae	Individuals with *E. coli* O157:H7 gastroenteritis (especially children), cancer chemotherapy, HIV infection, autoimmune diseases; pregnant/ postpartum women	Fever (not always present), hemolytic anemia, thrombocytopenia, renal dysfunction, neurologic dysfunction; coagulation studies normal	48, 93, 101, 134, 138
Cutaneous small-vessel vasculitis (leukocytoclastic vasculitis)	Infections (including group A *Streptococcus*, viral hepatitis), drugs, chemicals, food allergens, idiopathic causes	Palpable purpuric lesions appearing in crops on legs or other dependent areas; may become vesicular or ulcerative; usually resolve over 3–4 weeks	Occurs in a wide spectrum of diseases, including connective tissue disease, cryoglobulinemia, malignancy, Henoch-Schönlein purpura (HSP); more common in children	Fever, malaise, arthralgias, myalgias; systemic vasculitis in some cases; renal, joint, and gastrointestinal involvement commonly seen in HSP	48

ERUPTIONS WITH ULCERS AND/OR ESCHARS

Disease	Etiology	Description	Group Affected/ Epidemiologic Factors	Clinical Syndrome	Chapter
Scrub typhus, rickettsial spotted fevers, rat-bite fever[g]; rickettsialpox, ecthyma gangrenosum[h]	—	—	—	—	—[d]
Tularemia	*Francisella tularensis*	Ulceroglandular form: erythematous, tender papule evolves into necrotic, tender ulcer with raised borders; in 35% of cases, eruptions (maculopapular, vesiculopapular, acneiform, urticarial, erythema nodosum, or erythema multiforme) may occur	Exposure to ticks, biting flies, infected animals	Fever, headache, lymphadenopathy	142
Anthrax	*Bacillus anthracis*	Pruritic papule enlarging and evolving into a 1- by 3-cm painless ulcer surrounded by vesicles and then developing a central eschar with edema; residual scar	Exposure to infected animals or animal products or other exposure to anthrax spores	Lymphadenopathy, headache	205

[a] In human granulocytotropic ehrlichiosis, or anaplasmosis (caused by *Anaplasma phagocytophila*; most common in the upper midwestern and northeastern regions of the United States), rash is rare.

[b] See "Viral hemorrhagic fever" under "Purpuric eruptions" for dengue hemorrhagic fever/dengue shock syndrome.

[c] See "Purpuric eruptions."

[d] See etiology-specific chapters.

[e] See "Peripheral eruptions."

[f] See "Confluent desquamative erythemas."

[g] See "Centrally distributed maculopapular eruptions."

[h] See "Vesiculobullous eruptions."

berry tongue or circumoral pallor. In contrast to the staphylococcal scalded-skin syndrome, in which the cleavage plane is superficial in the epidermis, *toxic epidermal necrolysis* (Chap. 50) involves sloughing of the entire epidermis, resulting in severe disease. *Exfoliative erythroderma syndrome* (Chaps. 47 and 50) is a serious reaction associated with systemic toxicity that is often due to eczema, psoriasis, mycosis fungoides, or a severe drug reaction.

VESICULOBULLOUS ERUPTIONS *Varicella* (Chap. 164) is highly contagious, often occurring in winter or spring. At a given time within a given region of the body, varicella lesions are in different stages of development. In immunocompromised hosts, varicella vesicles may lack the characteristic erythematous base or may appear hemorrhagic. Lesions of *variola* (smallpox; Chap. 205) appear similar to those of varicella but are all at the same stage of development in a given region of the body. Variola lesions are most prominent on the face and extremities, while varicella lesions are most prominent on the trunk. *Rickettsialpox* (Chap. 158) is often documented in urban settings and is characterized by vesicles. It can be distinguished from varicella by an eschar at the site of the mouse-mite bite and the papule/plaque base of each vesicle. Disseminated *Vibrio vulnificus* infection (Chap. 140) or *ecthyma gangrenosum* due to *Pseudomonas aeruginosa* (Chap. 136) should be considered in immunosuppressed individuals with sepsis and hemorrhagic bullae.

URTICARIAL ERUPTIONS Individuals with classic urticaria ("hives") usually have a hypersensitivity reaction without associated fever. In the presence of fever, urticarial eruptions are usually due to *urticarial vasculitis* (Chap. 306). Unlike individual lesions of classic urticaria, which last up to 48 h, these lesions may last up to 5 days. Etiologies include serum sickness (often induced by drugs such as penicillins, sulfas, salicylates, or barbiturates), connective-tissue disease (e.g., systemic lupus erythematosus or Sjögren's syndrome), and infection (e.g., with hepatitis B virus, enteroviruses, or parasites). Malignancy may be associated with fever and chronic urticaria (Chap. 48).

NODULAR ERUPTIONS In immunocompromised hosts, nodular lesions often represent disseminated infection. Patients with disseminated *candidiasis* (often due to *Candida tropicalis*) may have a triad of fever, myalgias, and eruptive nodules (Chap. 187). Disseminated *cryptococcosis* lesions (Chap. 186) may resemble molluscum contagiosum. Necrosis of nodules should raise the suspicion of *aspergillosis* (Chap. 188) or *mucormycosis* (Chap. 189). *Erythema nodosum* presents with exquisitely tender nodules on the lower extremities. *Sweet's syndrome* (Chap. 48) should be considered in individuals with multiple nodules and plaques, often so edematous that they give the appearance of vesicles or bullae. Sweet's syndrome may affect either healthy individuals or persons with lymphoproliferative disease.

PURPURIC ERUPTIONS *Acute meningococcemia* (Chap. 127) classically presents in children as a petechial eruption, but initial lesions may appear as blanchable macules or urticaria. RMSF should be considered in the differential diagnosis of acute meningococcemia. *Echovirus 9 infection* (Chap. 175) may mimic acute meningococcemia; patients should be treated as if they have bacterial sepsis since prompt differentiation of these conditions may be impossible. Large ecchymotic areas of *purpura fulminans* (Chaps. 127 and 254) reflect severe underlying disseminated intravascular coagulation, which may be due to infectious or noninfectious causes. The lesions of *chronic meningococcemia* (Chap. 127) may have a variety of morphologies, including petechial. Purpuric nodules may develop on the legs and resemble erythema nodosum but lack its exquisite tenderness. Lesions of *disseminated gonococcemia* (Chap. 128) are distinctive, sparse, countable hemorrhagic pustules, usually located near joints. The lesions of chronic meningococcemia and those of gonococcemia may be indistinguishable in terms of appearance and distribution. *Viral hemorrhagic fever* (Chaps. 180 and 181) should be considered in patients with an appropriate travel history and a petechial rash. *Thrombotic thrombocytopenic purpura* (Chaps. 48, 93, and 101) and *hemolytic-uremic syndrome* (Chaps. 101, 134, and 138) are closely related and are noninfectious causes of fever and petechiae. *Cutaneous small-vessel vasculitis* (*leukocytoclastic vasculitis*) typically manifests as palpable purpura and has a wide variety of causes (Chap. 48).

ERUPTIONS WITH ULCERS OR ESCHARS The presence of an ulcer or eschar in the setting of a more widespread eruption can provide an important diagnostic clue. For example, the presence of an eschar may suggest the diagnosis of scrub typhus or rickettsialpox (Chap. 158) in the appropriate setting. In other illnesses (e.g., anthrax; Chap. 205), an ulcer or eschar may be the only skin manifestation.

FURTHER READING

CHERRY JD: Contemporary infectious exanthems. Clin Infect Dis 16:199, 1993
———: Cutaneous manifestations of systemic infections, in *Textbook of Pediatric Infectious Diseases*, vol. 1, 3d ed, RD Feigin and JD Cherry (eds). Philadelphia, Saunders, 1992, pp 755–782
EICHENFIELD LF et al (eds): *Textbook of Neonatal Dermatology*, Philadelphia, Saunders, 2001
FREEDBERG IM et al (eds): *Fitzpatrick's Dermatology in General Medicine*, 6th ed. New York, McGraw-Hill, 2003
LEVIN S, GOODMAN LJ: An approach to acute fever and rash (AFR) in the adult. Curr Clin Top Infect Dis 15:19, 1995
SCHLOSSBERG D: Fever and rash. Infect Dis Clin North Am 10:101, 1996
WEBER DJ et al: The acutely ill patient with fever and rash, in *Principles and Practice of Infectious Diseases*, vol 1, 5th ed, GL Mandell et al (eds). Philadelphia, Churchill Livingstone, 2000, pp 633–50

18 FEVER OF UNKNOWN ORIGIN
Jeffrey A. Gelfand, Michael V. Callahan

DEFINITION AND CLASSIFICATION *Fever of unknown origin* (FUO) was defined by Petersdorf and Beeson in 1961 as (1) temperatures of >38.3°C (>101°F) on several occasions; (2) a duration of fever of >3 weeks; and (3) failure to reach a diagnosis despite 1 week of inpatient investigation. While this classification has stood for more than 30 years, Durack and Street have proposed a new system for classification of FUO: (1) classic FUO; (2) nosocomial FUO; (3) neutropenic FUO; and (4) FUO associated with HIV infection (Table 18-1).

Classic FUO corresponds closely to the earlier definition of FUO, differing only with regard to the prior requirement for 1 week's study in the hospital. The new definition is broader, stipulating three outpatient visits or 3 days in the hospital without elucidation of a cause or 1 week of "intelligent and invasive" ambulatory investigation. In

nosocomial FUO, a temperature of ≥38.3°C (≥101°F) develops on several occasions in a hospitalized patient who is receiving acute care and in whom infection was not manifest or incubating on admission. Three days of investigation, including at least 2 days' incubation of cultures, is the minimum requirement for this diagnosis. *Neutropenic FUO* is defined as a temperature of ≥38.3°C (≥101°F) on several occasions in a patient whose neutrophil count is <500/μL or is expected to fall to that level in 1 to 2 days. The diagnosis of neutropenic FUO is invoked if a specific cause is not identified after 3 days of investigation, including at least 2 days' incubation of cultures. *HIV-associated FUO* is defined by a temperature of ≥38.3°C (≥101°F) on several occasions over a period of >4 weeks for outpatients or >3 days for hospitalized patients with HIV infection. This diagnosis is invoked if appropriate investigation over 3 days, including 2 days' incubation of cultures, reveals no source.

Adoption of these categories of FUO on a wide scale in the literature would allow a more rational compilation of data regarding these

TABLE 18-1 Categories of FUO[a]

| Feature | Category of FUO | | | |
	Nosocomial	Neutropenic	HIV-Associated	Classic
Patient's situation	Hospitalized, acute care, no infection when admitted	Neutrophil count either <500/μL or expected to reach that level in 1–2 days	Confirmed HIV-positive	All others with fevers for ≥3 weeks
Duration of illness while under investigation	3 days[b]	3 days[b]	3 days[b] (or 4 weeks as outpatient)	3 days[b] or three outpatient visits
Examples of cause	Septic thrombophlebitis, sinusitis, *Clostridium difficile* colitis, drug fever	Perianal infection, aspergillosis, candidemia	MAI[c] infection, tuberculosis, non-Hodgkin's lymphoma, drug fever	Infections, malignancy, inflammatory diseases, drug fever

[a] All require temperatures of ≥38.3°C (≥101°F) on several occasions.
[b] Includes at least 2 days' incubation of microbiology cultures.
[c] *M. avium/M. intracellulare.*

Source: Modified from DT Durack, AC Street, in JS Remington, MN Swartz (eds): *Current Clinical Topics in Infectious Diseases.* Cambridge, MA, Blackwell, 1991.

disparate groups. In the remainder of this chapter, the discussion will focus on classic FUO unless otherwise specified.

CAUSES OF CLASSIC FUO Table 18-2 summarizes the findings of several large studies of FUO carried out since the advent of the antibiotic era, including a prospective study of 167 adult patients with FUO encompassing all 8 university hospitals in the Netherlands and using a standardized protocol in which the first author reviewed every patient. Coincident with the widespread use of antibiotics, increasingly useful diagnostic technologies—both noninvasive and invasive—have been developed. Newer studies reflect not only changing patterns of disease but also the impact of diagnostic techniques that make it possible to eliminate many patients with specific illness from the FUO category. The ubiquitous use of potent broad-spectrum antibiotics may have decreased the number of infections causing FUO. The wide availability of ultrasonography, computed tomography (CT), magnetic resonance imaging (MRI), radionuclide scanning, and positron emission tomography (PET) scanning has enhanced the detection of occult neoplasms and lymphomas in patients previously thought to have FUO. Likewise, the widespread availability of highly specific and sensitive immunologic testing has reduced the number of undetected cases of systemic lupus erythematosus and other autoimmune diseases.

Infections, especially extrapulmonary tuberculosis, remain the leading diagnosable cause of FUO. Prolonged mononucleosis syndromes caused by Epstein-Barr virus, cytomegalovirus (CMV), or HIV are conditions whose consideration as a cause of FUO is sometimes confounded by delayed antibody responses. Intraabdominal abscesses (sometimes poorly localized) and renal, retroperitoneal, and paraspinal abscesses continue to be difficult to diagnose. Renal malacoplakia, with submucosal plaques or nodules involving the urinary tract, may cause FUO and is often fatal if untreated. It is associated with coliform infection, is seen most often in patients with defects of intracellular bacterial killing, and is treated with fluoroquinolones or trimethoprim-sulfamethoxazole. Occasionally, other organs may be involved. Osteomyelitis, especially where prosthetic devices have been implanted, and infective endocarditis must be considered. Although true culture-negative infective endocarditis is rare, one may be misled by slow-growing organisms of the HACEK group (*Haemophilus aphrophilus*, *Actinobacillus actinomycetemcomitans*, *Cardiobacterium hominis*, Ei-

kenella corrodens, and Kingella kingae; Chap. 131), *Bartonella* spp. (previously *Rochalimaea*), *Legionella* spp., *Coxiella burnetii*, *Chlamydia psittaci*, and fungi. Prostatitis, dental abscesses, sinusitis, and cholangitis continue to be sources of occult fever.

Fungal disease, most notably histoplasmosis involving the reticuloendothelial system, may cause FUO. FUO with headache should prompt examination of spinal fluid for *Cryptococcus neoformans*. Malaria (which may result from transfusion, the failure to take a prescribed prophylactic agent, or infection with a drug-resistant strain) continues to be a cause, particularly of asynchronous FUO. A related protozoan species, *Babesia*, may cause FUO and is increasing in geographic distribution and in incidence, especially among the elderly and immunosuppressed.

In most earlier series, neoplasms were the next most common cause of FUO after infections (Table 18-2). In the two most recent series, a decrease in the percentage of FUO cases due to malignancy was attributed to improvement in diagnostic technologies—in particular, high-resolution tomography and tumor antigen assays. This observation does not diminish the importance of considering neoplasia in the initial diagnostic evaluation of a patient with fever. A number of patients in these series had temporal arteritis, adult Still's disease, drug-related fever, and factitious fever. In recent series, ~25 to 30% of cases of FUO have remained undiagnosed. The general term *noninfectious inflammatory diseases* applies to systemic rheumatologic or vasculitic diseases such as polymyalgia rheumatica, lupus, and adult Still's disease as well as to granulomatous diseases such as sarcoidosis and Crohn's and granulomatous hepatitis. Table 18-3 shows the 10 leading causes of FUO identified in an investigation at several U.S. community hospitals; the method of classification—i.e., "lumping or splitting" of specific entities—can skew rank.

In the elderly, multisystem disease is the most frequent cause of FUO, giant cell arteritis being the leading etiologic entity in this category. Tuberculosis is the most common infection causing FUO in the elderly, and colon cancer is an important cause of FUO with malignancy in this age group.

Many diseases have been grouped in the various studies as "miscellaneous." On this list are drug fever, pulmonary embolism, factitious fever, the hereditary periodic fever syndromes (familial

TABLE 18-2 Classic FUO in Adults

Authors (Year of Publication)	Years of Study	No. of Cases	Infections (%)	Neoplasms (%)	Noninfectious Inflammatory Diseases (%)	Miscellaneous Causes (%)	Undiagnosed Causes (%)
Petersdorf and Beeson (1961)	1952–1957	100	36	19	19[a]	19[a]	7
Larson and Featherstone (1982)	1970–1980	105	32	20	16[a]	11[a]	7
Knockaert and Vanneste (1992)	1980–1989	199	22.5	7	23[a]	21.5[a]	25.5
DeKleijn et al. (1997, Part I)	1992–1994	167	26	12.5	24	8	30

[a] Authors' raw data retabulated to conform to altered diagnostic categories.

Source: Modified from DeKleijn et al., 1997 (Part I).

TABLE 18-3 *Ten Leading Causes of Classic FUO among Adults at Community Hospitals in the United States*

Cause	% of Total
Lymphoma	16
Collagen vascular disease	16
Abscess	13
Undiagnosed cause	9
Solid tumor	8
Thrombosis or hematoma	7
Granulomatous disease, nonmycobacterial	5
Endocarditis	5
Mycobacterial disease	5
Viral disease	5
Remaining causes	11
	100

Source: Adapted from Kazanjian, 1992.

Mediterranean fever, hyper-IgD syndrome, tumor necrosis factor receptor–associated periodic syndrome), familial cold urticaria, the Muckle-Wells syndrome, and Fabry's disease.

A drug-related etiology must be considered in any case of prolonged fever. Any febrile pattern may be elicited by a drug, and both relative bradycardia and hypotension are uncommon. Eosinophilia and/or rash is found in only one-fifth of patients with drug fever, which usually begins 1 to 3 weeks after the start of therapy and remits 2 to 3 days after therapy is stopped. Virtually all classes of drugs cause fever, but antimicrobial agents (especially β-lactam antibiotics), cardiovascular drugs (e.g., quinidine), antineoplastic drugs, and drugs acting on the central nervous system (e.g., phenytoin) are particularly common causes.

It is axiomatic that, as the duration of fever increases, the likelihood of an infectious cause decreases, even for the more indolent infectious etiologies (e.g., brucellosis, paracoccidioidomycosis, *Plasmodium malariae*) (Table 18-4). In a series of 347 patients referred to the National Institutes of Health from 1961 to 1977, only 6% had an infection. A significant proportion (9%) had factitious fevers—i.e., fevers due either to false elevations of temperature or to self-induced disease. A substantial number of these factitious cases were in young women in the health professions. It is worth noting that 8% of the patients with prolonged fevers (some of whom had completely normal liver function studies) had granulomatous hepatitis, and 6% had adult Still's disease. After prolonged investigation, 19% of cases still had no specific diagnosis. A total of 27% of patients had no actual fever during inpatient observation or had an exaggerated circadian temperature rhythm without chills, elevated pulse, or other abnormalities.

The conditions that may be considered in a differential diagnosis of classic FUO in adults are listed in Table 18-5. This list applies strictly to the United States; the frequency of global travel underscores the need for a detailed travel history, and the continuing emergence of new infectious diseases makes this listing potentially incomplete. Increased international and domestic terrorist activity involving the intentional release of infectious agents, many of which cause illnesses presenting with prolonged fever, further underscores the need for obtaining an insightful environmental, occupational, and professional history, with early notification of public health authorities in cases of suspicious etiology (Chap. 205).

SPECIALIZED DIAGNOSTIC STUDIES ■ Classic FUO A stepwise flow chart depicting the diagnostic workup and therapeutic management of FUO is provided in Fig. 18-1. In this flow chart, reference is made to "potentially diagnostic clues," as outlined by DeKleijn and colleagues; these clues may be key findings in the history (e.g., travel), localizing signs, or key symptoms. Certain specific diagnostic maneuvers become critical in dealing with prolonged fevers. If factitious fever is suspected, electronic thermometers should be used, temperature-taking should be supervised, and simultaneous urine and body temperatures

should be measured. Thick blood smears should be examined for *Plasmodium*; thin blood smears, prepared with proper technique and quality stains and subjected to expert microscopy, should be used to speciate *Plasmodium* and to identify *Babesia*, *Trypanosoma*, *Leishmania*, *Rickettsia*, and *Borrelia*. Any tissue removed during prior relevant surgery should be reexamined; slides should be requested, and, if need be, paraffin blocks of fixed pathologic material should be reexamined and additional special studies performed. Relevant x-rays should be reexamined; reviewing of prior radiologic reports may be insufficient. Serum should be set aside in the laboratory as soon as possible and retained for future examination for rising antibody titers. *Febrile agglutinins* is a vague term that in most laboratories refers to serologic studies for salmonellosis, brucellosis, and rickettsial diseases. These studies are seldom useful, having low sensitivity and variable specificity. Multiple blood samples (no fewer than three and rarely more than six, including samples for anaerobic culture) should be cultured in the laboratory for at least 2 weeks to ensure that any HACEK group organisms that may be present have ample time to grow (Chap. 131). Lysis-centrifugation blood culture techniques should be employed in cases where prior antimicrobial therapy or fungal or atypical mycobacterial infection is suspected. Blood culture media should be supplemented with L-cysteine or pyridoxal to assist in the isolation of nutritionally variant streptococci. It should be noted that sequential cultures positive for multiple organisms may reflect self-injection of contaminated substances. Urine cultures, including cultures for mycobacteria, fungi, and CMV, are indicated. In the setting of recurrent fevers with lymphocytic meningitis (Mollaret's meningitis), cerebrospinal fluid can be tested for herpesvirus, with use of polymerase chain reaction (PCR) to amplify and detect viral nucleic acid (Chap. 163).

In any FUO workup, the erythrocyte sedimentation rate (ESR) should be determined. Striking elevation of the ESR and anemia of chronic disease are frequently seen in association with giant cell arteritis or polymyalgia rheumatica, common causes of FUO in patients >50 years of age. Still's disease is also suggested by elevations of ESR, leukocytosis, and anemia and is often accompanied by arthralgias, polyserositis (pleuritis, pericarditis), lymphadenopathy, splenomegaly, and rash. C-reactive protein may be a useful cross-reference for the ESR and is a more sensitive and specific indicator of an "acute-phase" inflammatory metabolic response. Antinuclear antibody, antineutrophil cytoplasmic antibody, rheumatoid factor, and serum cryoglobulins should be measured to rule out other collagen vascular diseases and vasculitis. Elevated levels of angiotensin-converting enzyme in serum may point to sarcoidosis. With rare exceptions, the intermediate-strength purified protein derivative (PPD) skin test should be used to screen for tuberculosis in patients with classic FUO. Concurrent control tests, such as the mumps skin test antigen (Aventis-Pasteur, Swiftwater, PA), should be employed. It should be kept in mind that both the PPD skin test and control tests may yield negative results in miliary tuberculosis, sarcoidosis, Hodgkin's disease, malnutrition, or AIDS. Noninvasive procedures should include an upper

TABLE 18-4 *Causes of FUO Lasting >6 Months*

Cause	Cases, %
None identified	19
Miscellaneous causes	13
Factitious causes	9
Granulomatous hepatitis	8
Neoplasm	7
Still's disease	6
Infection	6
Collagen vascular disease	4
Familial Mediterranean fever	3
No fever[a]	27

[a] No actual fever observed during 2 to 3 weeks of inpatient observation. Includes patients with exaggerated circadian rhythm.

Source: From a study of 347 patients referred to the National Institutes of Health from 1961 to 1977 with a presumptive diagnosis of FUO of >6 months' duration (Aduan et al.)

TABLE 18-5 *Causes of FUO in Adults in the United States*

INFECTIONS

Localized pyogenic infections
- Appendicitis
- Cat-scratch disease
- Cholangitis
- Cholecystitis
- Dental abscess
- Diverticulitis/abscess
- Lesser sac abscess
- Liver abscess
- Mesenteric lymphadenitis
- Osteomyelitis
- Pancreatic abscess
- Pelvic inflammatory disease
- Perinephric/intrarenal abscess
- Prostatic abscess
- Renal malacoplakia
- Sinusitis
- Subphrenic abscess
- Suppurative thrombophlebitis
- Tuboovarian abscess

Intravascular infections
- Bacterial aortitis
- Bacterial endocarditis
- Vascular catheter infection

Systemic bacterial infections
- Bartonellosis
- Brucellosis
- *Campylobacter* infection
- Cat-scratch disease/bacillary angiomatosis (*B. henselae*)
- Gonococcemia
- Legionnaires' disease
- Leptospirosis
- Listeriosis
- Lyme disease
- Melioidosis
- Meningococcemia
- Rat-bite fever
- Relapsing fever
- Salmonellosis
- Syphilis
- Tularemia
- Typhoid fever
- Vibriosis
- *Yersinia* infection

Mycobacterial infections
- *M. avium/M. intracellulare* infections
- Other atypical mycobacterial infections
- Tuberculosis

Fungal infections
- Aspergillosis
- Blastomycosis
- Candidiasis
- Coccidioidomycosis
- Cryptococcosis
- Histoplasmosis
- Mucormycosis
- Paracoccidioidomycosis
- Sporotrichosis

Other bacterial infections
- Actinomycosis
- Bacillary angiomatosis
- Nocardiosis
- Whipple's disease

Rickettsial infections
- Anaplasmosis
- Ehrlichiosis
- Murine typhus
- Q fever
- Rickettsialpox
- Rocky Mountain spotted fever

Mycoplasmal infections

Chlamydial infections
- Lymphogranuloma venereum
- Psittacosis
- TWAR (*C. pneumoniae*) infection

Viral infections
- Colorado tick fever
- Coxsackievirus group B infection
- Cytomegalovirus infection
- Dengue
- Epstein-Barr virus infection
- Hepatitis A, B, C, D, and E
- Human herpesvirus 6 infection
- Human immunodeficiency virus infection
- Lymphocytic choriomeningitis
- Parvovirus B19 infection

Parasitic infections
- Amebiasis
- Babesiosis
- Chagas' disease
- Leishmaniasis
- Malaria
- *Pneumocystis* infection
- Strongyloidiasis
- Toxocariasis
- Toxoplasmosis
- Trichinosis

Presumed infections, agent undetermined
- Kawasaki's disease (mucocutaneous lymph node syndrome)
- Kikuchi's necrotizing lymphadenitis

NEOPLASMS

Malignant
- Colon cancer
- Gall bladder carcinoma
- Hepatoma
- Hodgkin's lymphoma
- Immunoblastic T-cell lymphoma
- Leukemia
- Lymphomatoid granulomatosis
- Malignant histiocytosis
- Non-Hodgkin's lymphoma
- Pancreatic cancer
- Renal cell carcinoma
- Sarcoma

Benign
- Atrial myxoma
- Castleman's disease
- Renal angiomyolipoma

HABITUAL HYPERTHERMIA

(Exaggerated circadian rhythm)

COLLAGEN VASCULAR/HYPERSENSITIVITY DISEASES

- Adult Still's disease
- Behçet's disease
- Erythema multiforme
- Erythema nodosum
- Giant cell arteritis/polymyalgia rheumatica
- Hypersensitivity pneumonitis
- Hypersensitivity vasculitis
- Mixed connective-tissue disease
- Polyarteritis nodosa
- Relapsing polychondritis
- Rheumatic fever
- Rheumatoid arthritis
- Schnitzler's syndrome
- Systemic lupus erythematosus
- Takayasu's aortitis
- Weber-Christian disease
- Wegener's granulomatosis

GRANULOMATOUS DISEASES

- Crohn's disease
- Granulomatous hepatitis
- Midline granuloma
- Sarcoidosis

MISCELLANEOUS CONDITIONS

- Aortic dissection
- Drug fever
- Gout
- Hematomas
- Hemoglobinopathies
- Laennec's cirrhosis
- PFPA syndrome: periodic fever, adenitis, pharyngitis, aphthae
- Postmyocardial infarction syndrome
- Recurrent pulmonary emboli
- Subacute thyroiditis (de Quervain's)
- Tissue infarction/necrosis

INHERITED AND METABOLIC DISEASES

- Adrenal insufficiency
- Cyclic neutropenia
- Deafness, urticaria, and amyloidosis
- Fabry's disease
- Familial cold urticaria
- Familial Mediterranean fever
- Hyperimmunoglobulinemia D and periodic fever
- Muckle-Wells syndrome
- Tumor necrosis factor receptor–associated periodic syndrome
- Type V hypertriglyceridemia

THERMOREGULATORY DISORDERS

Central
- Brain tumor
- Cerebrovascular accident
- Encephalitis
- Hypothalamic dysfunction

Peripheral
- Hyperthyroidism
- Pheochromocytoma

FACTITIOUS FEVERS

"AFEBRILE" FUO (<38.3°C)

Source: Modified from RK Root, RG Petersdorf, in JD Wilson et al (eds): *Harrison's Principles of Internal Medicine*, 12th ed. New York, McGraw-Hill, 1991.

gastrointestinal contrast study with small-bowel follow-through and colonoscopy to examine the terminal ileum and cecum. Chest x-rays should be repeated if new symptoms arise. Sputum should be induced with an ultrasonic nebulizer for cultures and cytology. If there are pulmonary signs or symptoms, bronchoscopy with bronchoalveolar lavage for cultures and cytology should be considered. High-resolution spiral CT of the chest and abdomen should be performed with both intravenous and oral contrast. If a spinal or paraspinal lesion is sus-

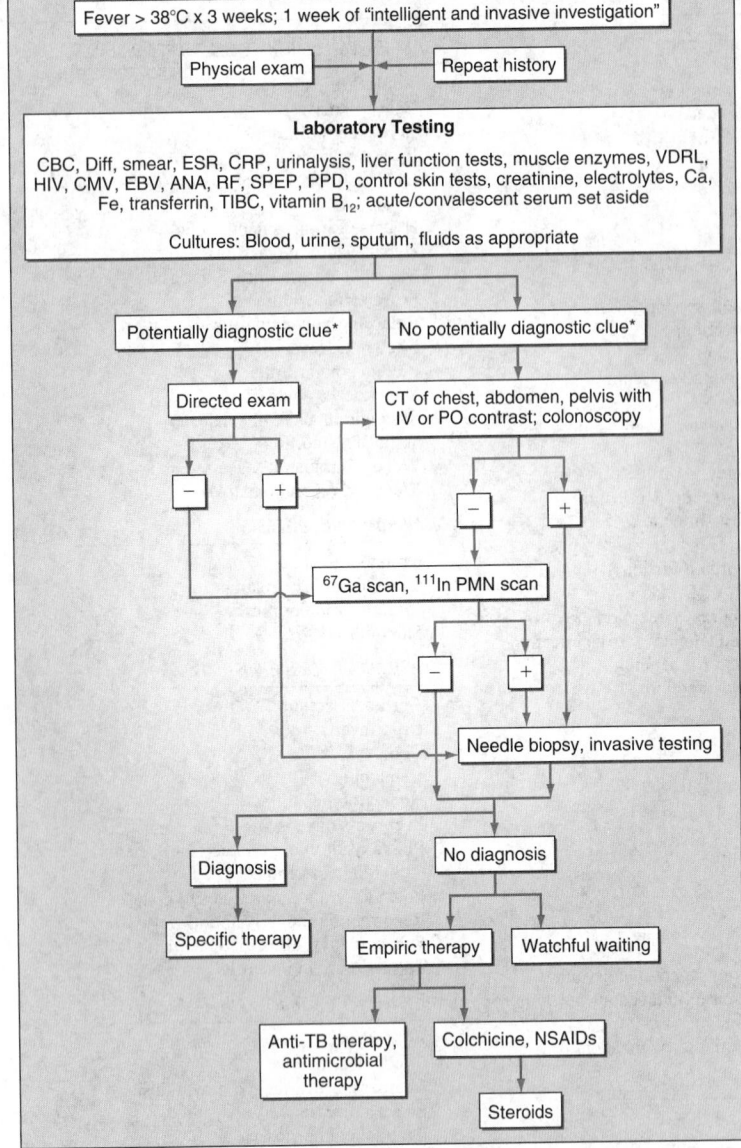

FIGURE 18-1 Approach to the patient with classic FUO. *"Potentially diagnostic clues," as outlined by DeKleijn and colleagues (1997, Part II), may be key findings in the history, localizing signs, or key symptoms. Abbreviations: ANA, antinuclear antibody; CBC, complete blood count; CMV, cytomegalovirus; CRP, C-reactive protein; CT, computed tomography; Diff, differential; EBV, Epstein-Barr virus; ESR, erythrocyte sedimentation rate; NSAIDs, nonsteroidal anti-inflammatory drugs; PMN, polymorphonuclear leukocyte; PPD, purified protein derivative; RF, rheumatoid factor; SPEP, serum protein electrophoresis; TB, tuberculosis; TIBC, total iron-binding capacity; VDRL, Venereal Disease Research Laboratory test.

Within the figure:

Fever > 38°C x 3 weeks; 1 week of "intelligent and invasive investigation"

Physical exam — Repeat history

Laboratory Testing
CBC, Diff, smear, ESR, CRP, urinalysis, liver function tests, muscle enzymes, VDRL, HIV, CMV, EBV, ANA, RF, SPEP, PPD, control skin tests, creatinine, electrolytes, Ca, Fe, transferrin, TIBC, vitamin B_{12}; acute/convalescent serum set aside

Cultures: Blood, urine, sputum, fluids as appropriate

Potentially diagnostic clue* / No potentially diagnostic clue*

Directed exam / CT of chest, abdomen, pelvis with IV or PO contrast; colonoscopy

^{67}Ga scan, ^{111}In PMN scan

Needle biopsy, invasive testing

Diagnosis / No diagnosis

Specific therapy / Empiric therapy / Watchful waiting

Anti-TB therapy, antimicrobial therapy / Colchicine, NSAIDs

Steroids

---

pected, however, MRI is preferred. MRI may be superior to CT in demonstrating intraabdominal abscesses and aortic dissection, but the relative utility of MRI and CT in the diagnosis of FUO is unknown. At present, abdominal CT with contrast should be used unless MRI is specifically indicated. Arteriography may be useful for patients in whom systemic necrotizing vasculitis is suspected. Saccular aneurysms may be seen, most commonly in renal or hepatic vessels, and may permit diagnosis of arteritis when biopsy is difficult. Ultrasonography of the abdomen is useful for investigation of the hepatobiliary tract, kidneys, spleen, and pelvis. Echocardiography may be helpful in an evaluation for bacterial endocarditis, pericarditis, nonbacterial thrombotic endocarditis, and atrial myxomas. Transesophageal echocardiography is especially sensitive for these lesions.

Radionuclide scanning procedures using technetium (Tc) 99m sulfur colloid, gallium (Ga) 67 citrate, or indium (In) 111–labeled leukocytes may be useful in identifying and/or localizing inflammatory processes. In one study, Ga scintigraphy yielded useful diagnostic information in almost one-third of cases, and it was suggested that this procedure might actually be used before other imaging techniques if no specific organ is suspected of being abnormal. It is likely that PET scanning, which provides quicker results (hours vs days), will prove even more sensitive and specific than ^{67}Ga scanning in FUO. ^{99m}Tc bone scan should be undertaken to look for osteomyelitis or bony metastases; ^{67}Ga scan may be used to identify sarcoidosis (Chap. 309) or *Pneumocystis* (Chap. 191) in the lungs or Crohn's disease (Chap. 276) in the abdomen. ^{111}In-labeled white blood cell (WBC) scan may be used to locate abscesses. With these scans, false-positive and false-negative findings are common.

Biopsy of the liver and bone marrow should be considered in the workup of FUO if the studies mentioned above are unrevealing and if fever is prolonged. Granulomatous hepatitis has been diagnosed by liver biopsy, even when liver enzymes are normal and no other diagnostic clues point to liver disease. All biopsy specimens should be cultured for bacteria, mycobacteria, and fungi. Likewise, in the absence of clues pointing to the bone marrow, bone marrow biopsy (not simple aspiration) for histology and culture has yielded diagnoses late in the workup. When possible, a section of the tissue block should be retained for further sections or stains. PCR technology makes it potentially possible to identify and speciate mycobacterial DNA in paraffin-embedded, fixed tissues at some research centers. Thus, in some cases, a retrospective diagnosis can be made on the basis of studies of long-fixed pathologic tissues. In a patient over age 50 (or occasionally in a younger patient) with the appropriate symptoms and laboratory findings, "blind biopsy" of one or both temporal arteries may yield a diagnosis of arteritis. Tenderness or decreased pulsation, if noted, should guide the selection of a site for biopsy. Lymph node biopsy may be helpful if nodes are enlarged, but inguinal nodes are often palpable and are seldom diagnostically useful.

Exploratory laparotomy has been performed when all other diagnostic procedures fail but has largely been replaced by imaging and guided-biopsy techniques. Laparoscopic biopsy may provide more adequate guided sampling of lymph nodes or liver.

Nosocomial FUO (See also Chap. 116) The primary considerations in diagnosing nosocomial FUO are the underlying susceptibility of the patient coupled with the potential complications of hospitalization. The original surgical or procedural field is the place to begin a directed physical and laboratory examination for abscesses, hematomas, or infected foreign bodies. More than 50% of patients with nosocomial FUO are infected, and intravascular lines, septic phlebitis, and prostheses are all suspect. In this setting, the approach is to focus on sites where occult infections may be sequestered, such as the sinuses of intubated patients or a prostatic abscess in a man with a urinary catheter. *Clostridium difficile* colitis may be associated with fever and leukocytosis before the onset of diarrhea. In ~25% of patients with nosocomial FUO, the fever has a noninfectious cause. Among these causes are acalculous cholecystitis, deep-vein thrombophlebitis, and pulmonary embolism. Drug fever, transfusion reactions, alcohol/drug withdrawal, adrenal insufficiency, thyroiditis, pancreatitis, gout, and pseudogout are among the many possible causes to consider. As in classic FUO, repeated meticulous physical examinations, coupled with focused diagnostic techniques, are imperative. Multiple blood, wound, and fluid cultures are mandatory. The pace of diagnostic tests is accelerated, and the threshold for procedures—CT scans, ultrasonography, ^{111}In-WBC scans, noninvasive venous studies—is low. Even so, 20% of cases of nosocomial FUO may go undiagnosed.

Like diagnostic measures, therapeutic maneuvers must be swift and decisive, as many patients are already critically ill. Intravenous lines must be changed (and cultured), drugs stopped for 72 h, and empirical therapy started if bacteremia is a threat. In many hospital settings, empirical antibiotic coverage for nosocomial FUO now includes vancomycin for coverage of methicillin-resistant *Staphylococcus aureus* as well as broad-spectrum gram-negative coverage with piperacillin/tazobactam, ticarcillin/clavulanate, imipenem, or meropenem. Practice guidelines covering many of these issues have been published jointly by the Infectious Diseases Society of America (IDSA) and the Society for Critical Care Medicine and can be accessed on the IDSA website (www.journals.uchicago.edu/IDSA/guidelines).

Neutropenic FUO (See also Chap. 72)   Neutropenic patients are susceptible to focal bacterial and fungal infections, to bacteremic infections, to infections involving catheters (including septic thrombophlebitis), and to perianal infections. *Candida* and *Aspergillus* infections are common. Infections due to herpes simplex virus or CMV are sometimes causes of FUO in this group. While the duration of illness may be short in these patients, the consequences of untreated infection may be catastrophic; 50 to 60% of febrile neutropenic patients are infected, and 20% are bacteremic. The IDSA has published extensive practice guidelines covering these critically ill neutropenic patients; these guidelines appear on the website cited in the previous section. In these patients, severe mucositis, quinolone prophylaxis, colonization with methicillin-resistant *S. aureus*, obvious catheter-related infection, or hypotension dictates the use of vancomycin plus ceftazidime, cefepime, or a carbapenem with or without an aminoglycoside to provide empirical coverage for bacterial sepsis.

HIV-Associated FUO   HIV infection alone may be a cause of fever. Infection due to *Mycobacterium avium* or *Mycobacterium intracellulare*, tuberculosis, toxoplasmosis, CMV infection, *Pneumocystis* infection, salmonellosis, cryptococcosis, histoplasmosis, non-Hodgkin's lymphoma, and (of particular importance) drug fever are all possible causes of FUO. Mycobacterial infection can be diagnosed by blood cultures and by liver, bone marrow, and lymph node biopsies. Chest CT should be performed to identify enlarged mediastinal nodes. Serologic studies may reveal cryptococcal antigen, and ^{67}Ga scan may help identify *Pneumocystis* pulmonary infection. More than 80% of HIV patients with FUO are infected, but drug fever and lymphoma remain important considerations. →*Treatment of HIV-associated FUO depends on many factors and is discussed in Chap. 173.*

℞ TREATMENT

The focus here is on classic FUO. Other modifiers of FUO—neutropenia, HIV infection, a nosocomial setting—all vastly modify the risk equation and dictate therapy based on the probability of various causes of fever and on the calculated risks and benefits of a guided empirical approach. The age and physical state of the patient are factors as well: the frail elderly patient may merit a trial of empirical therapy earlier than the robust young adult.

The emphasis in patients with classic FUO is on continued observation and examination, with the avoidance of "shotgun" empirical therapy. Antibiotic therapy (even that for tuberculosis) may irrevocably alter the ability to culture fastidious bacteria or mycobacteria and delineate ultimate cause. However, vital-sign instability or neutropenia is an indication for empirical therapy with a fluoroquinolone plus piperacillin or the regimen mentioned above, for example. Cirrhosis, asplenia, intercurrent immunosuppressive drug use, or recent exotic travel may all tip the balance toward earlier empirical anti-infective therapy. If the PPD skin test is positive or if granulomatous hepatitis or other granulomatous disease is present with anergy (and sarcoid seems unlikely), then a therapeutic trial with isoniazid and rifampin (and possibly a third drug) should be undertaken, with treatment usually continued for up to 6 weeks. A failure of the fever to respond over this period suggests an alternative diagnosis.

The response of rheumatic fever and Still's disease to aspirin and nonsteroidal anti-inflammatory agents (NSAIDs) may be dramatic. The effects of glucocorticoids on temporal arteritis, polymyalgia rheumatica, and granulomatous hepatitis are equally dramatic. Colchicine is highly effective in preventing attacks of familial Mediterranean fever but is of little use once an attack is well under way. The ability of glucocorticoids and NSAIDs to mask fever while permitting the spread of infection dictates that their use be avoided unless infection has been largely ruled out and unless inflammatory disease is both probable and debilitating or threatening.

When no underlying source of FUO is identified after prolonged observation (>6 months), the prognosis is generally good, however vexing the fever may be to the patient. Under such circumstances, debilitating symptoms are treated with NSAIDs, and glucocorticoids are the last resort. The initiation of empirical therapy does not mark the end of the diagnostic workup; rather, it commits the physician to continued thoughtful reexamination and evaluation. Patience, compassion, equanimity, and intellectual flexibility are indispensable attributes for the clinician in dealing successfully with FUO.

ACKNOWLEDGMENT
Sheldon M. Wolff, MD, now deceased, was an author of a previous version of this chapter. It is to his memory that the chapter is dedicated.

FURTHER READING

ADUAN R et al: Prolonged fever of unknown origin. Clin Res 26:558A, 1978

DEKLEIJN EMHA et al: Fever of unknown origin (FUO): I. A prospective multicenter study of 167 patients with FUO, using fixed epidemiologic entry criteria. Medicine 76:392, 1997

——— et al: Fever of unknown origin (FUO): II. Diagnostic procedures in a prospective multicenter study of 167 patients. Medicine 76:401, 1997

HIRSCHMANN JV: Fever of unknown origin in adults. Clin Infect Dis 24:291, 1997

HOEN B et al: The Duke criteria for diagnosing infective endocarditis are specific: Analysis of 100 patients with acute fever or fever of unknown origin. Clin Infect Dis 23:298, 1996

HUGHES WT et al: 2002 guidelines for the use of antimicrobial agents in neutropenic patients with cancer. Clin Infect Dis 34:730, 2002

KAZANJIAN PH: Fever of unknown origin: Review of 86 patients treated in community hospitals. Clin Infect Dis 15:968, 1992

KNOCKAERT DC et al: Long-term follow-up of patients with undiagnosed fever of unknown origin. Arch Intern Med 156:618, 1996

O'GRADY NP et al: Practice guidelines for evaluating new fever in critically ill adult patients. Clin Infect Dis 26:1042, 1998

PETERSDORF RC, BEESON PB: Fever of unexplained origin. Medicine 40:1, 1961

19 HYPOTHERMIA AND FROSTBITE
Daniel F. Danzl

HYPOTHERMIA

Accidental hypothermia occurs when there is an unintentional drop in the body's core temperature below 35°C (95°F). At this temperature, many of the compensatory physiologic mechanisms to conserve heat begin to fail. *Primary accidental hypothermia* is a result of the direct exposure of a previously healthy individual to the cold. The mortality rate is much higher for those patients who develop *secondary hypothermia* as a complication of a serious systemic disorder.

CAUSES

Primary accidental hypothermia is geographically and seasonally pervasive. Although most cases occur in the winter months and in colder climates, it is surprisingly common in warmer regions as well. Multiple variables make individuals at the extremes of age, the elderly and neonates, particularly vulnerable to hypothermia (Table 19-1). The

TABLE 19-1   Risk Factors for Hypothermia

Age extremes	Endocrine-related
Elderly	Hypoglycemia
Neonates	Hypothyroidism
Outdoor exposure	Adrenal insufficiency
Occupational	Hypopituitarism
Sports-related	Neurologic-related
Inadequate clothing	Stroke
Drugs and intoxicants	Hypothalamic disorders
Ethanol	Parkinson's disease
Phenothiazines	Spinal cord injury
Barbiturates	Multisystem
Anesthetics	Malnutrition
Neuromuscular blockers	Sepsis
Others	Shock
	Hepatic or renal failure
	Burns and exfoliative dermatologic
	disorders
	Immobility or debilitation

elderly have diminished thermal perception and are more susceptible to immobility, malnutrition, and systemic illnesses that interfere with heat generation or conservation. Dementia, psychiatric illness, and socioeconomic factors often compound these problems by impeding adequate measures to prevent hypothermia. Neonates have high rates of heat loss because of their increased surface-to-mass ratio and their lack of effective shivering and adaptive behavioral responses. In addition, malnutrition can contribute to heat loss because of diminished subcutaneous fat and because of its association with depleted energy stores used for thermogenesis.

Individuals whose occupations or hobbies entail extensive exposure to cold weather are clearly at increased risk for hypothermia. Military history is replete with hypothermic tragedies. Hunters, sailors, skiers, and climbers also are at great risk of exposure, whether it involves injury, changes in weather, or lack of preparedness.

Ethanol causes vasodilatation (which increases heat loss), reduces thermogenesis and gluconeogenesis, and may impair judgment or lead to obtundation. Phenothiazines, barbiturates, benzodiazepines, cyclic antidepressants, and many other medications reduce centrally mediated vasoconstriction. Up to one-quarter of patients admitted to an intensive care unit because of drug overdose are hypothermic. Anesthetics can block the shivering responses; their effects may be compounded when patients are not covered adequately in the operating or recovery rooms.

Several types of endocrine dysfunction can lead to hypothermia. Hypothyroidism—particularly when extreme, as in myxedema coma—reduces the metabolic rate and impairs thermogenesis and behavioral responses. Adrenal insufficiency and hypopituitarism can also increase susceptibility to hypothermia. Hypoglycemia, most commonly caused by insulin or oral hypoglycemic drugs, is associated with hypothermia, in part the result of neuroglycopenic effects on hypothalamic function. Increased osmolality and metabolic derangements associated with uremia, diabetic ketoacidosis, and lactic acidosis can lead to altered hypothalamic thermoregulation.

Neurologic injury from trauma, cerebrovascular accident, subarachnoid hemorrhage, or hypothalamic lesions increases susceptibility to hypothermia. Agenesis of the corpus callosum, or Shapiro syndrome, is one cause of episodic hypothermia, characterized by profuse perspiration followed by a rapid fall in temperature. Acute spinal cord injury disrupts the autonomic pathways that lead to shivering and prevents cold-induced reflex vasoconstrictive responses.

Hypothermia associated with sepsis is a poor prognostic sign. Hepatic failure causes decreased glycogen stores and gluconeogenesis, as well as a diminished shivering response. In acute myocardial infarction associated with low cardiac output, hypothermia may be reversed after adequate resuscitation. With extensive burns, psoriasis, erythrodermas,

and other skin diseases, increased peripheral blood flow leads to excessive heat loss.

THERMOREGULATION

Heat loss occurs through five mechanisms: radiation (55 to 65% of heat loss), conduction (10 to 15% of heat loss, but much greater in cold water), convection (increased in the wind), respiration, and evaporation (which are affected by the ambient temperature and the relative humidity).

The preoptic anterior hypothalamus normally orchestrates thermoregulation (Chap. 16). The immediate defense of thermoneutrality is via the autonomic nervous system, whereas delayed control is mediated by the endocrine system. Autonomic nervous system responses include the release of norepinephrine, increased muscle tone, and shivering, leading to thermogenesis and an increase in the basal metabolic rate. Cutaneous cold thermoreception causes direct reflex vasoconstriction to conserve heat. Prolonged exposure to cold also stimulates the thyroid axis, leading to an increased metabolic rate.

CLINICAL PRESENTATION

In most cases of hypothermia, the history of exposure to environmental factors, such as prolonged exposure to the outdoors without adequate clothing, makes the diagnosis straightforward. In urban settings, however, the presentation is often more subtle and other disease processes, toxin exposures, or psychiatric diagnoses should be considered.

After initial stimulation by hypothermia, there is progressive depression of all organ systems. The timing of the appearance of these clinical manifestations varies widely (Table 19-2). Without knowing the core temperature, it can be difficult to interpret other vital signs. For example, a tachycardia disproportionate to the core temperature suggests secondary hypothermia resulting from hypoglycemia, hypovolemia, or a toxin overdose. Because carbon dioxide production declines progressively, the respiratory rate should be low; persistent hyperventilation suggests a central nervous system (CNS) lesion or one of the organic acidoses. A markedly depressed level of consciousness in a patient with mild hypothermia should raise suspicion of an overdose or CNS dysfunction due to infection or trauma.

Physical examination findings can also be altered by hypothermia. For instance, the assumption that areflexia is solely attributable to hypothermia can obscure and delay the diagnosis of a spinal cord lesion. Patients with hypothermia may be confused or combative; these symptoms abate more rapidly with rewarming than with the use of restraints. A classic example of maladaptive behavior in patients with hypothermia is paradoxical undressing, which involves the inappropriate removal of clothing in response to a cold stress. The cold-induced ileus and abdominal rectus spasm can mimic, or mask, the presentation of an acute abdomen (Chap. 13).

When a patient in hypothermic cardiac arrest is first discovered, cardiopulmonary resuscitation is indicated, unless (1) a do-not-resuscitate status is verified, (2) obviously lethal injuries are identified, or (3) the depression of a frozen chest wall is not possible. As the resuscitation proceeds, the prognosis is grave if there is evidence of widespread cell lysis, as reflected by potassium levels exceeding 10 meq/L. Other findings that may preclude continuing resuscitation include a core temperature $<12°C$, a pH <6.5, or evidence of intravascular thrombosis with a fibrinogen value <50 mg/dL. The decision to terminate resuscitation before rewarming the patient past 33°C is extremely difficult. There are no validated prognostic indicators for recovery from hypothermia. A history of asphyxia with secondary cooling is the most important negative predictor of survival.

DIAGNOSIS AND STABILIZATION

Hypothermia is confirmed by measuring the core temperature, preferably at two sites. Rectal probes should be placed to a depth of 15 cm and not adjacent to cold feces. A simultaneous esophageal probe should be placed 24 cm below the larynx; it may read falsely high during heated inhalation therapy. Relying solely on infrared tympanic thermography is not advisable.

TABLE 19-2 *Physiologic Changes Associated with Hypothermia*

Severity	Body Temperature	Central Nervous System	Cardiovascular	Respiratory	Renal and Endocrine	Neuromuscular
Mild	35°C (95°F)–32.2°C (90°F)	Linear depression of cerebral metabolism; amnesia; apathy; dysarthria; impaired judgment; maladaptive behavior	Tachycardia, then progressive bradycardia; cardiac-cycle prolongation; vasoconstriction; increase in cardiac output and blood pressure	Tachypnea, then progressive decrease in respiratory minute volume; declining oxygen consumption; bronchorrhea; bronchospasm	Diuresis; increase in catecholamines, adrenal steroids, triiodothyronine and thyroxine; increase in metabolism with shivering	Increased preshivering muscle tone, then fatiguing, shivering-induced thermogenesis; ataxia
Moderate	<32.2°C (90°F)–28°C (82.4°F)	EEG abnormalities; progressive depression of level of consciousness; pupillary dilatation; paradoxical undressing; hallucinations	Progressive decrease in pulse and cardiac output; increased atrial and ventricular arrhythmias; nonspecific and suggestive (J-wave) ECG changes; prolonged systole	Hypoventilation; 50% decrease in carbon dioxide production per 8°C drop in temperature; absence of protective airway reflexes; 50% decrease in oxygen consumption	50% increase in renal blood flow; renal autoregulation intact; impaired insulin action	Hyporeflexia; diminishing shivering-induced thermogenesis; rigidity
Severe	<28°C (82.4°F)	Loss of cerebrovascular autoregulation; decline in cerebral blood flow; coma; loss of ocular reflexes; progressive decrease in EEG	Progressive decreases in blood pressure, heart rate, and cardiac output; reentrant dysrhythmias; decreased ventricular arrhythmia threshold; asystole	Pulmonic congestion and edema; 75% decrease in oxygen consumption; apnea	Decrease in renal blood flow parallels decrease in cardiac output; extreme oliguria; poikilothermia; 80% decrease in basal metabolism	No motion; decreased nerve-conduction velocity; peripheral areflexia

Source: From DF Danzl, RS Pozos: N Engl J Med 331:1756, 1994. Copyright 1994, Massachusetts Medical Society. All rights reserved.

After a diagnosis of hypothermia is established, cardiac monitoring should be instituted, along with attempts to limit further heat loss. If the patient is in ventricular fibrillation, one sequence of 3 defibrillation attempts (2 J/kg) should be administered. Supplemental oxygenation is always warranted, since tissue oxygenation is adversely affected by the leftward shift of the oxyhemoglobin dissociation curve. Pulse oximetry may be unreliable in patients with vasoconstriction. If protective airway reflexes are absent, gentle endotracheal intubation should be performed. Adequate pre-oxygenation will prevent ventricular arrhythmias. Although cardiac pacing for hypothermic bradydysrhythmias is rarely indicated, the transthoracic technique appears preferable to the transvenous.

Insertion of a gastric tube prevents dilatation secondary to decreased bowel motility. Indwelling bladder catheters facilitate monitoring of cold-induced diuresis. Dehydration is commonly encountered with chronic hypothermia, and most patients benefit from a bolus of crystalloid. Normal saline is preferable to lactated Ringer's solution, as the liver in hypothermic patients inefficiently metabolizes lactate. The placement of a pulmonary artery catheter, although of potential value, risks perforation of the less compliant pulmonary artery. Insertion of a central venous catheter into the cold right atrium should be avoided, since this can precipitate arrhythmias.

Arterial blood gases should not be corrected for temperature (Chap. 42). An uncorrected pH of 7.42 and a P_{CO_2} of 40 mmHg reflects appropriate alveolar ventilation and acid-base balance at any core temperature. Acid-base imbalances should be corrected gradually, since the bicarbonate buffering system is inefficient. A common error is overzealous hyperventilation in the setting of depressed CO_2 production. When the P_{CO_2} decreases 10 mmHg at 28°C, it doubles the pH increase of 0.08 that occurs at 37°C.

The severity of anemia may be underestimated because the hematocrit increases 2% for each 1°C drop in temperature. White blood cell sequestration and bone marrow suppression are common, potentially masking an infection. Although hypokalemia is more common in chronic hypothermia, hyperkalemia also occurs; the expected electrocardiographic changes can be obscured by hypothermia. Patients with renal insufficiency, metabolic acidoses, or rhabdomyolysis are at greatest risk for electrolyte disturbances.

Coagulopathies are common because cold inhibits the enzymatic reactions required for activation of the intrinsic cascade. In addition, the production of thromboxane B_2 by platelets is temperature-dependent, and platelet function is impaired. The administration of platelets and fresh frozen plasma is, therefore, not effective. The prothrombin or partial thromboplastin times reported by the laboratory appear deceptively normal and contrast with the observed in vivo coagulopathy. This contradiction appears because all coagulation tests are routinely performed at 37°C, and the enzymes are thus rewarmed.

REWARMING STRATEGIES

The key initial decision is whether to rewarm the patient passively or actively. *Passive external rewarming* simply involves covering and insulating the patient in a warm environment. With the head also covered, the rate of rewarming is usually 0.5° to 2.0°C per hour. This technique is ideal for previously healthy patients who develop acute, mild primary accidental hypothermia. The patient must have sufficient glycogen to support endogenous thermogenesis.

There are reservations about the application of heat directly to the extremities of patients with chronic severe hypothermia. Extinguishing peripheral vasoconstriction in the dehydrated patient may precipitate core temperature "afterdrop"—the continual decline in the core temperature after removal of the patient from the cold. Truncal heat application may minimize the risk of afterdrop.

Active rewarming is necessary under the following circumstances: core temperature <32°C (poikilothermia), cardiovascular instability, age extremes, CNS dysfunction, endocrine insufficiency, or any suspicion of secondary hypothermia. *Active external rewarming* is best accomplished with forced-air heating blankets. Other options include radiant heat sources and hot packs. Monitoring a patient with hypothermia in a heated tub is extremely difficult. Electric blankets should be avoided because vasoconstricted skin is easily burned.

There are numerous widely available *active core rewarming* options. Airway rewarming with heated humidified oxygen (40° to 45°C) is a convenient option via mask or endotracheal tube. Although airway rewarming provides less heat than some other forms of active core rewarming, it eliminates respiratory heat loss and adds 1° to 2°C to the overall rewarming rate. Crystalloids should be heated to 40° to 42°C. The quantity of heat provided is significant only during massive volume resuscitation. The most efficient method for heating and delivering fluid or blood is with a countercurrent in-line heat exchanger. Heated irrigation of the gastrointestinal tract or bladder transfers minimal heat because of the limited available surface area. These methods should be reserved for patients in cardiac arrest and then used in combination with all available active rewarming techniques. Closed thoracic lavage is far more efficient in severely hypothermic patients with cardiac arrest. The hemithoraces are irrigated through two large-bore thoracostomy tubes that are inserted into the left or both of the hemithoraces. Thoracostomy tubes should not be placed in the left chest of a spontaneously perfusing patient for purposes of rewarming. Peritoneal lavage with the dialysate at 40° to 45°C efficiently transfers heat when delivered through two catheters with outflow suction. Like peritoneal dialysis, standard hemodialysis is especially useful for patients with electrolyte abnormalities, rhabdomyolysis, or toxin ingestions. The efficacy of arteriovenous anastomoses rewarming, which provides exogenous heat by immersion of the hands, forearms, feet, and calves in 44° to 45°C water, is unclear.

There are four extracorporeal blood rewarming options, which should be considered in severely hypothermic patients, especially those with *primary accidental hypothermia* (Table 19-3). Cardiopulmonary bypass should be considered in nonperfusing patients without documented contraindications to resuscitation. Circulatory support may also be the only effective option in patients with completely frozen extremities, or those with significant tissue destruction coupled with rhabdomyolysis. There is no evidence that extremely rapid rewarming improves survival in perfusing patients. The best strategy is usually a combination of passive, truncal active, and active core rewarming techniques.

DRUG THERAPY

When a patient is hypothermic, target organs and the cardiovascular system respond minimally to most medications. Moreover, cumulative doses can cause toxicity during rewarming because of increased binding of drugs to proteins, and impaired metabolism and excretion. As an example, the administration of repeated doses of digoxin or insulin would be ineffective while the patient is hypothermic, and the residual drugs are potentially toxic during rewarming.

Achieving a mean arterial pressure of at least 60 mmHg should be an early objective. If the hypotension does not respond to crystalloid/colloid infusion and rewarming, low-dose dopamine (2 to 5 μg/kg per min) support should be considered. Perfusion of the vasoconstricted cardiovascular system may also be improved with low-dose IV nitroglycerin.

Atrial arrhythmias should initially be monitored without intervention, as the ventricular response will be slow, and most will convert spontaneously during rewarming. The role of prophylaxis and treatment of ventricular arrhythmias is problematic. Preexisting ventricular ectopy may be suppressed by hypothermia, and reappear during rewarming. None of the class I agents has proved to be safe and efficacious. When available, bretylium tosylate was the class III ventricular antiarrhythmic of choice. Although class III agents such as bretylium possess direct antifibrillatory action, there is no evidence that amiodarone is safe.

Initiating empirical therapy for adrenal insufficiency is usually not

TABLE 19-3 *Options for Extracorporeal Rewarming*

Extracorporeal Rewarming (ECR) Technique	Considerations
Venovenous (VV)	Circuit—CV catheter to CV or peripheral catheter No oxygenator/circulatory support Flow rates 150–400 mL/min ROR 2°–3°C/h
Hemodialysis (HD)	Circuit—single-or dual-vessel cannulation Stabilizes electrolyte or toxicologic abnormalities Exchange cycle volumes 200–500 mL/min ROR 2°–3°C/h
Continuous arteriovenous rewarming (CAVR)	Circuit—percutaneous 8.5 Fr femoral catheters Requires BP 60 mmHg systolic No perfusionist/pump/anticoagulation Flow rates 225–375 mL/min ROR 3°–4°C/h
Cardiopulmonary bypass (CPB)	Circuit—full circulatory support with pump and oxygenator Perfusate-temperature gradient (5°–10°C) Flow rates 2–7 L/min (ave. 3–4) ROR up to 9.5°C/h

Note: BP, blood pressure; CV, central venous; ROR, rate of rewarming.

warranted unless there is a history suggesting steroid dependence, hypoadrenalism, or a failure to rewarm with standard therapy. However, the administration of parenteral levothyroxine to euthyroid patients with hypothermia is potentially hazardous. Because laboratory results can be delayed and confounded by the presence of the sick euthyroid syndrome (Chap. 320), historic clues or physical findings suggestive of hypothyroidism should be sought. When myxedema is the cause of hypothermia, the relaxation phase of the Achilles reflex is prolonged more than the contraction phase.

Hypothermia obscures most of the symptoms and signs of infection, notably fever and leukocytosis. Shaking rigors from infection may be mistaken for shivering. Except in mild cases, extensive cultures and repeated physical examinations are essential. Unless an infectious source is identified, empirical antibiotic prophylaxis is most warranted in the elderly, neonates, and immunocompromised patients.

Preventive measures should be discussed with high-risk individuals, such as the elderly or people whose work frequently exposes them to extreme cold. The importance of layered clothing and headgear, adequate shelter, increased caloric intake, and the avoidance of ethanol should be emphasized, along with access to rescue services.

FROSTBITE

Peripheral cold injuries include both freezing and nonfreezing injuries to tissue. Tissue freezes quickly when in contact with thermal conductors such as metal or volatile solutions. Other predisposing factors include constrictive clothing or boots, immobility, or vasoconstrictive medications. Frostbite occurs when the tissue temperature drops below 0°C. Ice crystal formation subsequently distorts and destroys the cellular architecture. Once the vascular endothelium is damaged, stasis progresses rapidly to microvascular thrombosis. After the tissue thaws, there is progressive dermal ischemia. The microvasculature begins to collapse, arteriovenous shunting increases tissue pressures, and edema forms. Finally, thrombosis, ischemia, and superficial necrosis appear. The development of mummification and demarcation may take weeks to months.

CLINICAL PRESENTATION

The initial presentation of frostbite can be deceptively benign. The symptoms always include a sensory deficiency affecting light touch, pain, and temperature perception. The acral areas and distal extremities are the most common insensate areas. Some patients complain of a clumsy or "chunk of wood" sensation in the extremity.

Deep frostbitten tissue can appear waxy, mottled, yellow, or violaceous-white. Favorable presenting signs include some warmth or sensation with normal color. The injury is often superficial if the subcutaneous tissue is pliable or if the dermis can be rolled over boney prominences.

Clinically, it is most practical to classify frostbite as superficial or deep. Superficial does not entail tissue loss. Classically, frostbite is retrospectively graded like a burn once the resultant pathology is demarcated over time. First-degree frostbite causes only anesthesia and erythema. The appearance of superficial vesiculation surrounded by edema and erythema is considered second degree (Fig. 19-1). Hemorrhagic vesicles reflect a serious injury to the microvasculature, and indicate third-degree frostbite. Fourth-degree injuries damage subcuticular, muscular, and osseous tissues.

The two most common nonfreezing peripheral cold injuries are *chilblain (pernio)* and *immersion (trench) foot.* Chilblain results from neuronal and endothelial damage induced by repetitive exposure to dry cold. Young females, particularly those with a history of Raynaud's phenomenon, are at greatest risk. Persistent vasospasticity and

TABLE 19-4 *Treatment for Frostbite*

Before Thawing	During Thawing	After Thawing
Remove from environment	Consider parenteral analgesia and ketorolac	Gently dry and protect part; elevate; pledgets between toes, if macerated
Prevent partial thawing and refreezing	Administer ibuprofen, 400 mg PO	If clear vesicles are intact, aspirate or the fluid will reabsorb in days; if broken, debride and dress with antibiotic or sterile aloe vera ointment
Stabilize core temperature and treat hypothermia	Immerse part in 37°–40°C (thermometer-monitored) circulating water containing an antiseptic soap until distal flush (10–45 min)	Leave hemorrhagic vesicles intact to prevent dessication and infection
Protect frozen part—no friction or massage	Encourage patient to gently move part	Continue ibuprofen 400 mg PO (12 mg/kg per day) q8–12h
Address medical or surgical conditions	If pain is refractory, reduce water temperature to 33°–37°C and administer parenteral narcotics	Consider tetanus and streptococcal prophylaxis; elevate part
		Hydrotherapy at 37°C

vasculitis can cause erythema, mild edema, and pruritus. Eventually plaques, blue nodules, and ulcerations develop. These lesions typically involve the dorsa of the hands and feet. In contrast, immersion (trench) foot results from repetitive exposure to wet cold above the freezing point. The feet initially appear cyanotic, cold, and edematous. The subsequent development of bullae is often indistinguishable from frostbite. This vesiculation rapidly progresses to ulceration and liquefaction gangrene. Patients with milder cases complain of hyperhidrosis, cold sensitivity, and painful ambulation for many years.

℞ TREATMENT

Frozen tissue should be rapidly and completely thawed by immersion in circulating water at 37° to 40°C. Rapid rewarming often produces an initial hyperemia. The early formation of clear distal large blebs is more favorable than smaller proximal dark hemorrhagic blebs. A common error is the premature termination of thawing, since the reestablishment of perfusion is intensely painful. Parenteral narcotics will be necessary with deep frostbite. If cyanosis persists after rewarming, the tissue compartment pressures should be monitored carefully.

Numerous experimental antithrombotic and vasodilatory treatment regimens have been evaluated. There is no conclusive evidence that dextran, heparin, steroids, calcium channel blockers, or hyperbaric oxygen salvage tissue. A treatment protocol for frostbite is summarized in Table 19-4.

Unless infection develops, any decision regarding debridement or amputation should be deferred until there is clear evidence of demarcation, mummification, and sloughing. The most common symptomatic sequelae reflect neuronal injury and the persistently abnormal sympathetic tone, including paresthesias, thermal misperception, and hyperhidrosis. Delayed findings include nail deformities, cutaneous carcinomas, and epiphyseal damage in children.

FURTHER READING

CAUCHY E et al: Retrospective study of 70 cases of severe frostbite lesions: A proposed new classification scheme. Wilderness Environ Med 12:248, 2001

DANZL DF: Hypothermia. Semin Respir Crit Care Med 23:57, 2002

GIESBRECHT GG: Cold stress, near drowning and accidental hypothermia: A review. Aviat Space Environ Med 71:733, 2000

VASSAL T et al: Severe accidental hypothermia treated in an ICU: Prognosis and outcome. Chest 120:1998, 2001

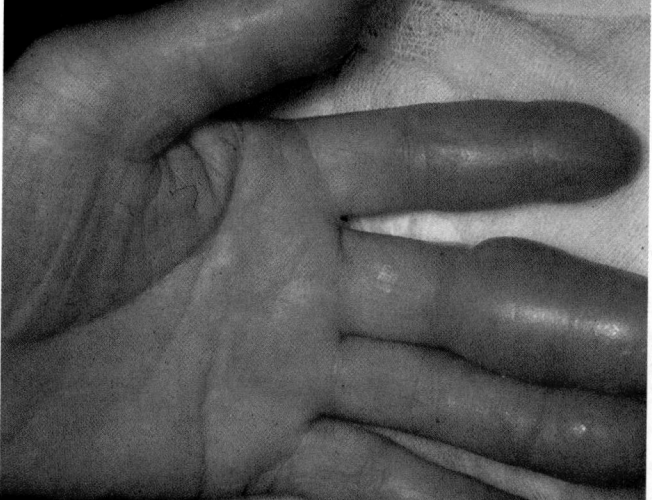
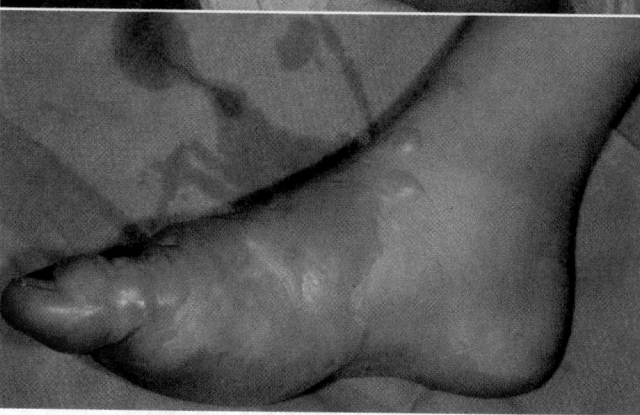

FIGURE 19-1 Frostbite with vesiculation, surrounded by edema and erythema.

20 | SYNCOPE, FAINTNESS, DIZZINESS, AND VERTIGO
Robert B. Daroff, Mark D. Carlson

SYNCOPE

Syncope is defined as transient loss of consciousness due to reduced cerebral blood flow. Syncope is associated with postural collapse and spontaneous recovery. It may occur suddenly, without warning, or may be preceded by symptoms of faintness ("presyncope"). These include lightheadedness, "dizziness" without true vertigo, a feeling of warmth, diaphoresis, nausea, and visual blurring occasionally proceeding to blindness. Presyncopal symptoms vary in duration and may increase in severity until loss of consciousness occurs or may resolve prior to loss of consciousness if the cerebral ischemia is corrected. The differentiation of syncope from seizure is an important, sometimes difficult, diagnostic problem.

Syncope may be benign when it occurs as a result of normal cardiovascular reflex effects on heart rate and vascular tone, or serious when due to a life-threatening arrhythmia. Syncope may occur as a single event or may be recurrent. Recurrent, unexplained syncope, particularly in an individual with structural heart disease, is associated with a high risk of death (40% mortality within 2 years).

PATHOPHYSIOLOGY Syncope results from a sudden impairment of brain metabolism, usually brought about by hypotension with reduction of cerebral blood flow. Several mechanisms subserve circulatory adjustments to the upright posture. Approximately three-fourths of the systemic blood volume is contained in the venous bed, and any interference in venous return may lead to a reduction in cardiac output. Cerebral blood flow may still be maintained as long as systemic arterial vasoconstriction occurs, but when this adjustment fails, serious hypotension, with resultant cerebral underperfusion to less than half of normal, results in syncope. Normally, the pooling of blood in the lower parts of the body is prevented by (1) pressor reflexes that induce constriction of peripheral arterioles and venules, (2) reflex acceleration of the heart by means of aortic and carotid reflexes, and (3) improvement of venous return to the heart by activity of the muscles of the limbs. Tilting a normal person upright on a tilt table causes some blood to accumulate in the lower limbs and diminishes cardiac output slightly; this may be followed by a slight transitory fall in systolic blood pressure. In a patient with defective vasomotor reflexes, however, tilt table testing may produce an abrupt and sustained fall in blood pressure, precipitating a faint.

CAUSES OF SYNCOPE Transiently decreased cerebral blood flow is usually due to one of three general mechanisms: disorders of vascular tone or blood volume, cardiovascular disorders including cardiac arrhythmias, or cerebrovascular disease (Table 20-1). Not infrequently, however, the cause of syncope is multifactorial.

Disorders of Vascular Tone or Blood Volume Disorders of autonomic control of the heart and circulation share common pathophysiologic mechanisms: a cardioinhibitory component (e.g., bradycardia due to increased vagal activity), a vasodepressor component (e.g., inappropriate vasodilatation due to sympathetic withdrawal), or both.

NEUROCARDIOGENIC (VASOVAGAL AND VASODEPRESSOR) SYNCOPE The term *neurocardiogenic* is generally used to encompass both vasovagal and vasodepressor syncope. Strictly speaking, vasovagal syncope is associated with both sympathetic withdrawal (vasodilatation) and increased parasympathetic activity (bradycardia), whereas vasodepressor syncope is associated with sympathetic withdrawal alone.

These forms of syncope are the common faint that may be experienced by normal persons and account for approximately half of all episodes of syncope. Neurocardiogenic syncope is frequently recurrent and commonly precipitated by a hot or crowded environment, alcohol,

extreme fatigue, severe pain, hunger, prolonged standing, and emotional or stressful situations. Episodes are often preceded by a presyncopal prodrome lasting seconds to minutes, and rarely occur in the supine position. The individual is usually sitting or standing and experiences weakness, nausea, diaphoresis, lightheadedness, blurred vision, and often a forceful heart beat with tachycardia followed by cardiac slowing and decreasing blood pressure prior to loss of consciousness. The individual appears pale or ashen; in dark-skinned individuals, the pallor may only be notable in the conjunctivae and lips. Patients with a gradual onset of presyncopal symptoms have time to

---

TABLE 20-1   *Causes of Syncope*

I. Disorders of vascular tone or blood volume
  A. Vasovagal (vasodepressor, neurocardiogenic)
  B. Postural (orthostatic) hypotension
    1. Drug induced (especially antihypertensive or vasodilator drugs)
    2. Peripheral neuropathy (diabetic, alcoholic, nutritional, amyloid)
    3. Idiopathic postural hypotension
    4. Multisystem atrophies
    5. Physical deconditioning
    6. Sympathectomy
    7. Acute dysautonomia (Guillain-Barré syndrome variant)
    8. Decreased blood volume (adrenal insufficiency, acute blood loss, etc.)
  C. Carotid sinus hypersensitivity
  D. Situational
    1. Cough
    2. Micturition
    3. Defecation
    4. Valsalva
    5. Deglutition
  E. Glossopharyngeal neuralgia
II. Cardiovascular disorders
  A. Cardiac arrhythmias (Chaps. 213 and 214)
    1. Bradyarrhythmias
      a. Sinus bradycardia, sinoatrial block, sinus arrest, sick-sinus syndrome
        Atrioventricular block
    2. Tachyarrhythmias
      a. Supraventricular tachycardia with structural cardiac disease
      b. Atrial fibrillation associated with the Wolff-Parkinson-White syndrome
      c. Atrial flutter with 1:1 atrioventricular conduction
      d. Ventricular tachycardia
  B. Other cardiopulmonary etiologies
    1. Pulmonary embolism
    2. Pulmonary hypertension
    3. Atrial myxoma
    4. Myocardial disease (massive myocardial infarction)
    5. Left ventricular myocardial restriction or constriction
    6. Pericardial constriction or tamponade
    7. Aortic outflow tract obstruction
    8. Aortic valvular stenosis
    9. Hypertrophic obstructive cardiomyopathy
III. Cerebrovascular disease (Chap. 349)
  A. Vertebrobasilar insufficiency
  B. Basilar artery migraine
IV. Other disorders that may resemble syncope
  A. Metabolic
    1. Hypoxia
    2. Anemia
    3. Diminished carbon dioxide due to hyperventilation
    4. Hypoglycemia
  B. Psychogenic
    1. Anxiety attacks
    2. Hysterical fainting
  C. Seizures

protect themselves against injury; in others, syncope occurs suddenly, without warning.

The depth and duration of unconsciousness vary. Sometimes the patient remains partly aware of the surroundings, or there may be complete unresponsiveness. The unconscious patient usually lies motionless with skeletal muscles relaxed, but a few clonic jerks of the limbs and face may occur. Sphincter control is usually maintained, in contrast to a seizure. The pulse may be feeble or apparently absent, the blood pressure low or undetectable, and breathing may be almost imperceptible. The duration of unconsciousness is rarely longer than a few minutes if the conditions that provoke the episode are reversed. Once the patient is placed in a horizontal position, the strength of the pulse improves, color begins to return to the face, breathing becomes quicker and deeper, and consciousness is restored. Some patients may experience a sense of residual weakness after regaining consciousness, and rising too soon may precipitate another faint. Unconsciousness may be prolonged if an individual remains upright, thus it is essential that individuals with vasovagal syncope assume a recumbant position as soon as possible. Although commonly benign, neurocardiogenic syncope can be associated with prolonged asystole and hypotension, resulting in injury.

The syncope often occurs in this setting of increased peripheral sympathetic activity and venous pooling. Under these conditions, vigorous myocardial contraction of a relatively empty left ventricle activates myocardial mechanoreceptors and vagal afferent nerve fibers that inhibit sympathetic activity and increase parasympathetic activity. The resultant vasodilatation and bradycardia induce hypotension and syncope. Although the reflex involving myocardial mechanoreceptors is the mechanism usually accepted as responsible for neurocardiogenic syncope, other reflexes may also be operative. Patients with transplanted (denervated) hearts have experienced cardiovascular responses identical to those present during neurocardiogenic syncope. This should not be possible if the response depends solely on the reflex mechanisms described above, unless the transplanted heart has become reinnervated. Moreover, neurocardiogenic syncope often occurs in response to stimuli (fear, emotional stress, or pain) that may not be associated with venous pooling in the lower extremities, which suggests a cortical component to the reflex. Thus, a variety of afferent and efferent responses may cause neurocardiogenic syncope.

As distinct from the peripheral mechanisms, the central nervous system (CNS) mechanisms responsible for neurocardiogenic syncope are uncertain, but a sudden surge in central serotonin levels may contribute to the sympathetic withdrawal. Endogenous opiates (endorphins) and adenosine are also putative participants in the pathogenesis.

POSTURAL (ORTHOSTATIC) HYPOTENSION This occurs in patients who have a chronic defect in, or variable instability of, vasomotor reflexes. Systemic arterial blood pressure falls on assumption of upright posture due to loss of vasoconstriction reflexes in resistance and capacitance vessels of the lower extremities. Although the syncopal attack differs little from vasodepressor syncope, the effect of posture is critical. Sudden rising from a recumbent position or standing quietly are precipitating circumstances. *Orthostatic hypotension may be the cause of syncope in up to 30% of the elderly; polypharmacy with antihypertensive or antidepressant drugs is often a contributor in these patients.*

Postural syncope may occur in otherwise normal persons with defective postural reflexes. Patients with *idiopathic postural hypotension* may be identified by a characteristic response to upright tilt on a table. Initially, the blood pressure diminishes slightly before stabilizing at a lower level. Shortly thereafter, the compensatory reflexes fail and the arterial pressure falls precipitously. The condition is often familial.

Orthostatic hypotension, often accompanied by disturbances in sweating, impotence, and sphincter difficulties, is also a primary feature of autonomic nervous system disorders (Chap. 354). The most common causes of neurogenic orthostatic hypotension are chronic diseases of the peripheral nervous system that involve postganglionic unmyelinated fibers (e.g., diabetic, nutritional, and amyloid polyneuropathy). Much less common are the multiple system atrophies; these

are CNS disorders in which orthostatic hypotension is associated with (1) parkinsonism (Shy-Drager syndrome), (2) progressive cerebellar degeneration, or (3) a more variable parkinsonian and cerebellar syndrome (striatonigral degeneration) (Chap. 351). A rare, acute postganglionic dysautonomia may represent a variant of Guillain-Barré syndrome (Chap. 365).

There are several additional causes of postural syncope: (1) After physical deconditioning (such as after prolonged illness with recumbency, especially in elderly individuals with reduced muscle tone) or after prolonged weightlessness, as in space flight; (2) after sympathectomy that has abolished vasopressor reflexes; and (3) in patients receiving antihypertensive or vasodilator drugs and those who are hypovolemic because of diuretics, excessive sweating, diarrhea, vomiting, hemorrhage, or adrenal insufficiency.

CAROTID SINUS HYPERSENSITIVITY Syncope due to carotid sinus hypersensitivity is precipitated by pressure on the carotid sinus baroreceptors, which are located just cephalad to the bifurcation of the common carotid artery. This typically occurs in the setting of shaving, a tight collar, or turning the head to one side. Carotid sinus hypersensitivity occurs predominantly in men $\geq$50 years old. Activation of carotid sinus baroreceptors gives rise to impulses carried via the nerve of Hering, a branch of the glossopharyngeal nerve, to the medulla oblongata. These afferent impulses activate efferent sympathetic nerve fibers to the heart and blood vessels, cardiac vagal efferent nerve fibers, or both. In patients with carotid sinus hypersensitivity, these responses may cause sinus arrest or atrioventricular (AV) block (a cardioinhibitory response), vasodilatation (a vasodepressor response), or both (a mixed response). The mechanisms responsible for the syndrome are not clear, and validated diagnostic criteria do not exist; some authorities have questioned its very existence.

SITUATIONAL SYNCOPE A variety of activities, including cough, deglutition, micturition, and defecation, are associated with syncope in susceptible individuals. These syndromes are caused, at least in part, by abnormal autonomic control and may involve a cardioinhibitory response, a vasodepressor response, or both. Cough, micturition, and defecation are associated with maneuvers (such as Valsalva, straining, and coughing) that may contribute to hypotension and syncope by decreasing venous return. Increased intracranial pressure secondary to the increased intrathoracic pressure may also contribute by decreasing cerebral blood flow.

Cough syncope typically occurs in men with chronic bronchitis or chronic obstructive lung disease during or after prolonged coughing fits. Micturition syncope occurs predominantly in middle-aged and older men, particularly those with prostatic hypertrophy and obstruction of the bladder neck; loss of consciousness usually occurs at night during or immediately after voiding. Deglutition syncope and defecation syncope occur in men and women. Deglutition syncope may be associated with esophageal disorders, particularly esophageal spasm. In some individuals, particular foods and carbonated or cold beverages initiate episodes by activating esophageal sensory receptors that trigger reflex sinus bradycardia or AV block. Defecation syncope is probably secondary to a Valsalva maneuver in older individuals with constipation.

GLOSSOPHARYNGEAL NEURALGIA Syncope due to glossopharyngeal neuralgia (Chap. 355) is preceded by pain in the oropharynx, tonsillar fossa, or tongue. Loss of consciousness is usually associated with asystole rather than vasodilatation. The mechanism is thought to involve activation of afferent impulses in the glossopharyngeal nerve that terminate in the nucleus solitarius of the medulla and, via collaterals, activate the dorsal motor nucleus of the vagus nerve.

CARDIOVASCULAR DISORDERS Cardiac syncope results from a sudden reduction in cardiac output, caused most commonly by a cardiac arrhythmia. In normal individuals, heart rates between 30 and 180 beats/min do not reduce cerebral blood flow, especially if the person is in the supine position. As the heart rate decreases, ventricular filling time and stroke volume increase to maintain normal cardiac output. At rates <30 beats/min, stroke volume can no longer increase to compensate adequately for the decreased heart rate. At rates greater than ~180 beats/min, ventricular filling time is inadequate to maintain adequate stroke volume. In either case, cerebral hypoperfusion and syncope may occur. Upright posture; cerebrovascular disease; anemia; loss of atrioventricular synchrony; and coronary, myocardial, or valvular disease all reduce the tolerance to alterations in rate.

Bradyarrhythmias (Chap. 213) may occur as a result of an abnormality of impulse generation (e.g., sinoatrial arrest) or impulse conduction (e.g., AV block). Either may cause syncope if the escape pacemaker rate is insufficient to maintain cardiac output. Syncope due to bradyarrhythmias may occur abruptly, without presyncopal symptoms, and recur several times daily. Patients with *sick sinus syndrome* may have sinus pauses (>3 s), and those with syncope due to high-degree AV block (*Stokes-Adams-Morgagni syndrome*) may have evidence of conduction system disease (e.g., prolonged PR interval, bundle branch block). However, the arrhythmia is often transitory, and the surface electrocardiogram or continuous electrocardiographic monitor (Holter monitor) taken later may not reveal the abnormality. The *bradycardia-tachycardia syndrome* is a common form of sinus node dysfunction in which syncope generally occurs as a result of marked sinus pauses, some following termination of paroxysms of atrial tachyarrhythmias. Drugs are a common cause for bradyarrhythmias, particularly in patients with underlying structural heart disease. Digoxin, β-adrenergic receptor antagonists, calcium channel blockers, and many antiarrhythmic drugs may suppress sinoatrial node impulse generation or slow AV nodal conduction.

Syncope due to a *tachyarrhythmia* (Chap. 214) is usually preceded by palpitation or lightheadedness but may occur abruptly with no warning symptoms. *Supraventricular tachyarrhythmias* are unlikely to cause syncope in individuals with structurally normal hearts but may if they occur in patients with (1) heart disease that also compromises cardiac output, (2) cerebrovascular disease, (3) a disorder of vascular tone or blood volume, or (4) a rapid ventricular rate. These tachycardias result most commonly from paroxysmal atrial flutter, atrial fibrillation, or reentry involving the AV node or accessory pathways that bypass part or all of the AV conduction system. Patients with the *Wolff-Parkinson-White syndrome* may experience syncope when a very rapid ventricular rate occurs due to reentry across an accessory AV connection.

In patients with structural heart disease, ventricular tachycardia is a common cause of syncope, particularly in patients with a prior myocardial infarction. Patients with aortic valvular stenosis and hypertrophic obstructive cardiomyopathy are also at risk for ventricular tachycardia. Individuals with abnormalities of ventricular repolarization (prolongation of the QT interval) are at risk to develop polymorphic ventricular tachycardia (*torsades de pointes*). Those with the inherited form of this syndrome often have a family history of sudden death in young individuals. Genetic markers can identify some patients with familial long-QT syndrome, but the clinical utility of these markers remains unproven. Drugs (i.e., certain antiarrhythmics and erythromycin) and electrolyte disorders (i.e., hypokalemia, hypocalcemia, hypomagnesemia) can prolong the QT interval and predispose to torsades de pointes. Antiarrhythmic medications may precipitate ventricular tachycardia, particularly in patients with structural heart disease.

In addition to arrhythmias, syncope may also occur with a variety of structural cardiovascular disorders. Episodes are usually precipitated when the cardiac output cannot increase to compensate adequately for peripheral vasodilatation. Peripheral vasodilatation may be appropriate, such as following exercise, or may occur due to inappropriate activation of left ventricular mechanoreceptor reflexes, as occurs in aortic outflow tract obstruction (aortic valvular stenosis or hypertrophic obstructive cardiomyopathy). Obstruction to forward flow is the most common reason that cardiac output cannot increase. Pericar-

dial tamponade is a rare cause of syncope. Syncope occurs in up to 10% of patients with massive pulmonary embolism and may occur with exertion in patients with severe primary pulmonary hypertension. The cause is an inability of the right ventricle to provide appropriate cardiac output in the presence of obstruction or increased pulmonary vascular resistance. Loss of consciousness is usually accompanied by other symptoms such as chest pain and dyspnea. Atrial myxoma, a prosthetic valve thrombus, and, rarely, mitral stenosis may impair left ventricular filling, decrease cardiac output, and cause syncope.

Cerebrovascular Disease Cerebrovascular disease alone rarely causes syncope but may lower the threshold for syncope in patients with other causes. The vertebrobasilar arteries, which supply brainstem structures responsible for maintaining consciousness, are usually involved when cerebrovascular disease causes or contributes to syncope. An exception is the rare patient with tight bilateral carotid stenosis and recurrent syncope, often precipitated by standing or walking. Most patients who experience lightheadedness or syncope due to cerebrovascular disease also have symptoms of focal neurologic ischemia, such as arm or leg weakness, diplopia, ataxia, dysarthria, or sensory disturbances. Basilar artery migraine is a rare disorder that causes syncope in adolescents.

DIFFERENTIAL DIAGNOSIS ■ **Anxiety Attacks and the Hyperventilation Syndrome** Anxiety, such as occurs in panic attacks, is frequently interpreted as a feeling of faintness or dizziness resembling presyncope. The symptoms are not accompanied by facial pallor and are not relieved by recumbency. The diagnosis is made on the basis of the associated symptoms such as a feeling of impending doom, air hunger, palpitations, and tingling of the fingers and perioral region. Attacks can often be reproduced by hyperventilation, resulting in hypocapnia, alkalosis, increased cerebrovascular resistance, and decreased cerebral blood flow. The release of epinephrine also contributes to the symptoms.

Seizures A seizure may be heralded by an aura, which is caused by a focal seizure discharge and hence has localizing significance (Chap. 348). The aura is usually followed by a rapid return to normal or by a loss of consciousness. Injury from falling is frequent in a seizure and rare in syncope, since only in generalized seizures are protective reflexes abolished instantaneously. Sustained tonic-clonic movements are characteristic of convulsive seizures but brief clonic, or tonic-clonic, seizure-like activity can accompany fainting episodes. The period of unconsciousness tends to be longer in seizures than in syncope. Urinary incontinence is frequent in seizures and rare in syncope. The return of consciousness is prompt in syncope, slow after a seizure. Mental confusion, headache, and drowsiness are common sequelae of seizures, whereas physical weakness with a clear sensorium characterizes the postsyncopal state. Repeated spells of unconsciousness in a young person at a rate of several per day or month are more suggestive of epilepsy than syncope. See Table 348-7 for a comparison of seizures and syncope.

Hypoglycemia Severe hypoglycemia is usually due to a serious disease such as a tumor of the islets of Langerhans; advanced adrenal, pituitary, or hepatic disease; or to excessive administration of insulin.

Acute Hemorrhage Hemorrhage, usually within the gastrointestinal tract, is an occasional cause of syncope. In the absence of pain and hematemesis, the cause of the weakness, faintness, or even unconsciousness may remain obscure until the passage of a black stool.

Hysterical Fainting The attack is usually unattended by an outward display of anxiety. Lack of change in pulse and blood pressure or color of the skin and mucous membranes distinguish it from the vasodepressor faint.

APPROACH TO THE PATIENT

The diagnosis of syncope is often challenging. The cause may only be apparent at the time of the event, leaving few, if any, clues when the patient is seen later by the physician. The physician should think first of those causes that constitute a therapeutic emergency. Among them are massive internal hemorrhage or myocardial infarction, which may be painless, and cardiac arrhythmias. In elderly persons, a sudden faint, without obvious cause, should arouse the suspicion of complete heart block or a tachyarrhythmia, even though all findings are negative when the patient is seen.

Figure 20-1 depicts an algorithmic approach to syncope. A careful history is the most important diagnostic tool, both to suggest the correct cause and to exclude important potential causes (Table 20-1). The nature of the events and their time course immediately prior to, during, and after an episode of syncope often provide valuable etiologic clues. Loss of consciousness in particular situations, such as during venipuncture, micturition, or with volume depletion, suggests an abnormality of vascular tone. The position of the patient at the time of the syncopal episode is important; syncope in the supine position is unlikely to be vasovagal and suggests an arrhythmia or a seizure. Syncope due to carotid sinus syndrome may occur when the individual is wearing a shirt with a tight collar, turning the head (turning to look while driving in reverse), or manipulating the neck (as in shaving). The patient's medications must be noted, including nonprescription drugs or health store supplements, with particular attention to recent changes.

The physical examination should include evaluation of heart rate and blood pressure in the supine, sitting, and standing positions. In patients with unexplained recurrent syncope, an attempt to reproduce an attack may assist in diagnosis. Anxiety attacks induced by hyperventilation can be reproduced readily by having the patient breathe rapidly and deeply for 2 to 3 min. Cough syncope may be reproduced by inducing the Valsalva maneuver. Carotid sinus massage should generally be avoided, even in patients with suspected carotid sinus hypersensitivity; it is a risky procedure that can cause a transient ischemic attack (TIA) or stroke in individuals with carotid atheromas.

Diagnostic Tests The choice of diagnostic tests should be guided by the history and the physical examination. Measurements of serum electrolytes, glucose, and the hematocrit are usually indicated. Cardiac enzymes should be evaluated if myocardial ischemia is suspected. Blood and urine toxicology screens may reveal the presence of alcohol or other drugs. In patients with possible adrenocortical insufficiency, plasma aldosterone and mineralocorticoid levels should be obtained.

Although the surface electrocardiogram is unlikely to provide a definitive diagnosis, it may provide clues to the cause of syncope *and should be performed in almost all patients*. The presence of conduction abnormalities (PR prolongation and bundle branch block) suggests a bradyarrhythmia, whereas pathologic Q waves or prolongation of the QT interval suggests a ventricular tachyarrhythmia. Inpatients should undergo continuous electrocardiographic monitoring; outpatients should wear a Holter monitor for 24 to 48 h. Whenever possible, symptoms should be correlated with the occurrence of arrhythmias. Continuous electrocardiographic monitoring may establish the cause of syncope in as many as 15% of patients. Cardiac event monitors may be useful in patients with infrequent symptoms, particularly in patients with presyncope. The presence of a late potential on a signal-averaged electrocardiogram is associated with increased risk for ventricular tacharrhythmias in patients with a prior myocardial infarction. Low-voltage (visually inapparent) T wave alternans is also associated with development of sustained ventricular arrhythmias.

Invasive cardiac electrophysiologic testing provides diagnostic and prognostic information regarding sinus node function, AV conduction, and supraventricular and ventricular arrhythmias (Chaps. 213 and 214). Prolongation of the sinus node recovery time (>1500 ms) is a specific finding (85 to 100%) for diagnosis of sinus node dysfunction but has a low sensitivity; continuous electrocardiographic monitoring is usually more effective for diagnosing this abnormality. Prolongation of the HV interval and conduction block below the His bundle indicate that His-Purkinje disease may be responsible for syncope. Programmed stimulation for ventricular arrhythmias is most useful in patients who have experienced a myocardial infarction; the sensitivity and specificity of this technique is lower in patients with normal hearts or those with heart disease other than coronary artery disease.

Upright tilt table testing is indicated for recurrent syncope, a single syncopal episode that caused injury, or a single syncopal event in a "high-risk" setting (pilot, commercial vehicle driver, etc.), whether or not there is a history of preexisting heart disease or prior vasovagal episodes. In susceptible patients, upright tilt at an angle between 60 and 80° for 30 to 60 min induces a vasovagal episode. The protocol can be shortened if upright tilt is combined with administration of drugs that cause venous pooling or increase adrenergic stimulation (isoproterenol, nitroglycerin, edrophonium, or adenosine). The sensitivity and specificity of tilt table testing is difficult to ascertain because of the lack of validated criteria. Moreover, the reflexes responsible for vasovagal syncope can be elicited in most, if not all, individuals given the appropriate stimulus. The reported accuracy of the test ranges from 30 to 80%, depending on the population studied and the techniques used. Whereas the reproducibility of a negative test is 85 to 100%, the reproducibility of a positive tilt table test is only between 62 and 88%.

A variety of other tests may be useful to determine the presence of structural heart disease that may cause syncope. The echocardiogram with Doppler examination detects valvular, myocardial, and pericardial abnormalities. The echocardiogram is the "gold standard" for the diagnosis of hypertrophic cardiomyopathy and atrial myxoma. Cardiac cine magnetic resonance (MR) imaging provides an alternative noninvasive modality that may be useful for patients in whom diagnostic-quality echocardiographic images cannot be obtained. This test is also indicated for patients suspected of having arrhythmogenic right ventricular dysplasia or right ventricular outflow tract ventricular tachycardia. Both are associated

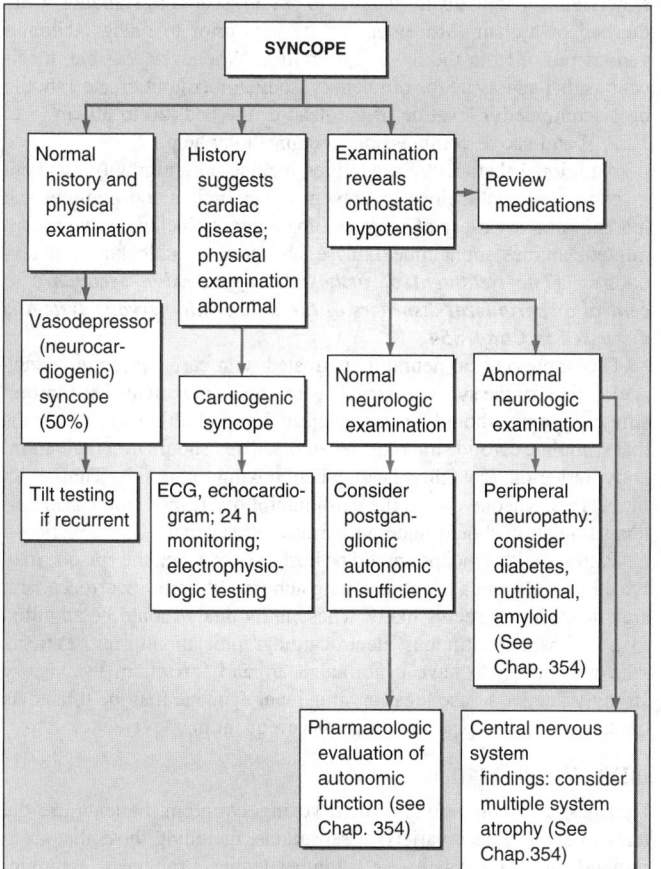

FIGURE 20-1 Approach to the patient with syncope.

with right ventricular structural abnormalities that are better visualized on MR imaging than by echocardiogram. Exercise testing may detect ischemia or exercise-induced arrhythmias. In some patients, cardiac catheterization may be necessary to diagnose the presence or severity of coronary artery disease or valvular abnormalities. Ultrafast computed tomographic scan, ventilation-perfusion scan, or pulmonary angiography is indicated in patients in whom syncope may be due to pulmonary embolus.

In possible cases of cerebrovascular syncope neuroimaging tests may be indicated, including Doppler ultrasound studies of the carotid and vertebrobasilar systems, MR imaging, MR angiography, and x-ray angiography of the cerebral vasculature (Chap. 349). Electroencephalography is indicated if seizures are suspected.

Rx TREATMENT

The treatment of syncope is directed toward the underlying cause. This discussion will focus on disorders of autonomic control. →*Arrhythmias are discussed in Chaps. 213 and 214, valvular heart diseases in Chap. 219, and cerebrovascular disorders in Chap. 349.*

Certain precautions should be taken regardless of the cause of syncope. At the first sign of symptoms, patients should make every effort to avoid injury should they lose consciousness. Patients with frequent episodes, or those who have experienced syncope without warning symptoms, should avoid situations in which sudden loss of consciousness might result in injury (e.g., climbing ladders, swimming alone, operating heavy machinery, driving). Patients should lower their head to the extent possible and preferably should lie down. Lowering the head by bending at the waist should be avoided because it may further compromise venous return to the heart. When appropriate, family members or other close contacts should be educated as to the problem. This will ensure appropriate therapy and may prevent delivery of inappropriate therapy (chest compressions associated with cardiopulmonary resuscitation) that may inflict trauma.

Patients who have lost consciousness should be placed in a position that maximizes cerebral blood flow, offers protection from trauma, and secures the airway. Whenever possible, the patient should be placed supine with the head turned to the side to prevent aspiration and the tongue from blocking the airway. Assessment of the pulse and direct cardiac auscultation may assist in determining if the episode is associated with a bradyarrhythmia or tachyarrhythmia. Clothing that fits tightly around the neck or waist should be loosened. Peripheral stimulation, such as by sprinkling cold water on the face, may be helpful. Patients should not be given anything by mouth or be permitted to rise until the sense of physical weakness has passed.

Patients with vasovagal syncope should be instructed to avoid situations or stimuli that have caused them to lose consciousness and to assume a recumbent position when premonitory symptoms occur. These behavioral modifications alone may be sufficient for patients with infrequent and relatively benign episodes of vasovagal syncope, particularly when loss of consciousness occurs in response to a specific stimulus. Tilt training (standing and leaning against a wall for progressively longer periods each day) has been used with limited success, particularly for those patients who have profound orthostatic intolerance. Episodes associated with intravascular volume depletion may be prevented by salt and fluid loading prior to provocative events.

Prescription drug therapy may be necessary when vasovagal syncope is resistant to these measures, when episodes occur frequently, or when syncope is associated with a significant risk for injury. β-Adrenergic receptor antagonists (metoprolol, 25 to 50 mg bid; atenolol, 25 to 50 mg qd; or nadolol, 10 to 20 mg bid; all starting doses), the most widely used agents, mitigate the increase in myocardial contractility that stimulates left ventricular mechanoreceptors and also block central serotonin receptors. Serotonin reuptake inhibitors (paroxetine, 20 to 40 mg qd; or sertraline, 25 to 50 mg qd), appear to be effective for some patients. Bupropion SR (150 mg qd), another antidepressant, has also been used with success. β-Adrenergic receptor antagonists and serotonin reuptake inhibitors are well tolerated and are often used as first-line agents for younger patients. Hydrofludrocortisone (0.1 to 0.2 mg qd), a mineralocorticoid, promotes sodium retention, volume expansion, and peripheral vasoconstriction by increasing β-receptor sensitivity to endogenous catecholamines. Hydrofludrocortisone is useful for patients with intravascular volume depletion and those who also have postural hypotension. Proamatine (2.5 to 10 mg bid or tid), an α-agonist, has been used as a first-line agent for some patients. In a recent randomized controlled trial, proamatine was more effective than placebo in preventing syncope during an upright tilt-test. However, in some patients, proamatine and hydrofludrocortisone may increase resting supine systemic blood pressure, a property that may be problematic for those with hypertension.

Disopyramide (150 mg bid), a vagolytic antiarrhythmic drug with negative inotropic properties, and another vagolytic, transdermal scopolamine, have been used to treat vasovagal syncope, as have theophylline and ephedrine. Side effects associated with these drugs have limited their use for this indication. Disopyramide is a type 1A antiarrhythmic drug and should be used with great caution, if at all, in patients who are at risk for ventricular arrhythmias. Although several clinical trials have suggested that pharmacologic therapy for vasovagal syncope is effective, long-term prospective randomized controlled trials have yet to be completed.

Permanent dual-chamber cardiac pacing is effective for patients with frequent episodes of vasovagal syncope and is indicated for those with prolonged asystole associated with vasovagal episodes. Patients in whom vasodilatation contributes to loss of consciousness may also experience symptomatic benefit from permanent pacing. Pacemakers that can be programmed to transiently pace at a high rate (90 to 100 beats/min) after a profound drop in the patient's intrinsic heart rate are most effective.

Patients with orthostatic hypotension should be instructed to rise slowly and systematically (supine to seated, seated to standing) from the bed or a chair. Movement of the legs prior to rising facilitates venous return from the lower extremities. Whenever possible, medications that aggravate the problem (vasodilators, diuretics, etc.) should be discontinued. Elevation of the head of the bed [20 to 30 cm (8 to 12 in.)] and use of compression stockings may help.

Additional therapeutic modalities include an antigravity or g suit or compression stockings to prevent lower limb blood pooling; salt loading; and a variety of pharmacologic agents including sympathomimetic amines, monamine oxidase inhibitors, beta blockers, and levodopa. →*The treatment of orthostatic hypotension secondary to central or peripheral disorders of the autonomic nervous system is discussed in Chap. 354.*

Glossopharyngeal neuralgia is treated with carbamazepine, which is effective for the syncope as well as for the pain. Patients with carotid sinus syndrome should be instructed to avoid clothing and situations that stimulate carotid sinus baroreceptors. They should turn their entire body, rather than just their head, when looking to the side. Those with intractable syncope due to the cardioinhibitory response to carotid sinus stimulation should undergo permanent pacemaker implantation.

Patients with syncope should be hospitalized when the episode may have resulted from a life-threatening abnormality or if recurrence with significant injury seems likely. These individuals should be admitted to a bed with continuous electrocardiographic monitoring. Patients who are known to have a normal heart and for whom the history strongly suggests vasovagal or situational syncope may be treated as outpatients if the episodes are neither frequent nor severe.

DIZZINESS AND VERTIGO

Dizziness is a common and often vexing symptom. Patients use the term to encompass a variety of sensations, including those that seem semantically appropriate (e.g., lightheadedness, faintness, spinning, giddiness) and those that are misleadingly inappropriate, such as mental confusion, blurred vision, headache, or tingling. Moreover, some individuals with gait disorders caused by peripheral neuropathy, myelopathy, spasticity, parkinsonism, or cerebellar ataxia complain of "dizziness" despite the absence of vertigo or other abnormal cephalic sensations. In this context, the term *dizziness* is being used to describe disturbed ambulation. There may be mild associated lightheadedness, particularly with impaired sensation from the feet or poor vision; this is known as *multiple-sensory-defect dizziness* and occurs in elderly individuals who complain of dizziness only when walking. Decreased position sense (secondary to neuropathy or myelopathy) and poor vision (from cataracts or retinal degeneration) create an overreliance on the aging vestibular apparatus. A less precise but sometimes comforting designation to patients is *benign dysequilibrium of aging*. Thus, a careful history is necessary to determine exactly what a patient who states, "Doctor, I'm dizzy," is experiencing. After eliminating the misleading symptoms or gait disturbance, "dizziness" usually means either *faintness* (presyncope) or *vertigo* (an illusory or hallucinatory sense of movement of the body or environment, most often a feeling of spinning). Operationally, after obtaining the history, dizziness may be classified into three categories: (1) faintness, (2) vertigo, and (3) miscellaneous head sensations.

FAINTNESS Prior to an actual faint (syncope), there are often prodromal presyncopal symptoms (faintness) reflecting ischemia to a degree insufficient to impair consciousness (see above).

VERTIGO Vertigo is usually due to a disturbance in the vestibular system. The end organs of this system, situated in the bony labyrinths of the inner ears, consist of the three semicircular canals and the otolithic apparatus (utricle and saccule) on each side. The canals transduce angular acceleration, while the otoliths transduce linear acceleration and the static gravitational forces that provide a sense of head position in space. The neural output of the end organs is conveyed to the vestibular nuclei in the brainstem via the eighth cranial nerves. The principal projections from the vestibular nuclei are to the nuclei of cranial nerves III, IV, and VI; spinal cord; cerebral cortex; and cerebellum. The vestibuloocular reflex (VOR) serves to maintain visual stability during head movement and depends on direct projections from the vestibular nuclei to the sixth cranial nerve (abducens) nuclei in the pons and, via the medial longitudinal fasciculus, to the third (oculomotor) and fourth (trochlear) cranial nerve nuclei in the midbrain. These connections account for the nystagmus (to-and-fro oscillation of the eyes) that is an almost invariable accompaniment of vestibular dysfunction. The vestibular nerves and nuclei project to areas of the cerebellum (primarily the flocculus and nodulus) that modulate the VOR. The vestibulospinal pathways assist in the maintenance of postural stability. Projections to the cerebral cortex, via the thalamus, provide conscious awareness of head position and movement.

The vestibular system is one of three sensory systems subserving spatial orientation and posture; the other two are the visual system (retina to occipital cortex) and the somatosensory system that conveys peripheral information from skin, joint, and muscle receptors. The three stabilizing systems overlap sufficiently to compensate (partially or completely) for each other's deficiencies. Vertigo may represent either physiologic stimulation or pathologic dysfunction in any of the three systems.

Physiologic Vertigo This occurs in normal individuals when (1) the brain is confronted with a mismatch among the three stabilizing sensory systems; (2) the vestibular system is subjected to unfamiliar head movements to which it is unadapted, such as in seasickness; (3) unusual head/neck positions, such as the extreme extension when painting a ceiling; or (4) following a spin. Intersensory mismatch explains carsickness, height vertigo, and the visual vertigo most commonly experienced during motion picture chase scenes; in the latter, the visual sensation of environmental movement is unaccompanied by concomitant vestibular and somatosensory movement cues. *Space sickness*, a frequent transient effect of active head movement in the weightless zero-gravity environment, is another example of physiologic vertigo.

Pathologic Vertigo This results from lesions of the visual, somatosensory, or vestibular systems. Visual vertigo is caused by new or incorrect spectacles or by the sudden onset of an extraocular muscle paresis with diplopia; in either instance, CNS compensation rapidly counteracts the vertigo. Somatosensory vertigo, rare in isolation, is usually due to a peripheral neuropathy or myelopathy that reduces the sensory input necessary for central compensation when there is dysfunction of the vestibular or visual systems.

The most common cause of pathologic vertigo is vestibular dysfunction involving either its end organ (labyrinth), nerve, or central connections. The vertigo is frequently accompanied by nausea, jerk nystagmus, postural unsteadiness, and gait ataxia. Since vertigo increases with rapid head movements, patients tend to hold their heads still.

LABYRINTHINE DYSFUNCTION This causes severe rotational or linear vertigo. When rotational, the hallucination of movement, whether of environment or self, is directed away from the side of the lesion. The fast phases of nystagmus beat away from the lesion side, and the tendency to fall is toward the side of the lesion, particularly in darkness or with the eyes closed.

Under normal circumstances, when the head is straight and immobile, the vestibular end organs generate a tonic resting firing frequency that is equal from the two sides. With any rotational acceleration, the anatomic positions of the semicircular canals on each side necessitate an increased firing rate from one and a commensurate decrease from the other. This change in neural activity is ultimately projected to the cerebral cortex, where it is summed with inputs from the visual and somatosensory systems to produce the appropriate conscious sense of rotational movement. After cessation of movement, the firing frequencies of the two end organs reverse; the side with the initially increased rate decreases, and the other side increases. A sense of rotation in the opposite direction is experienced; since there is no actual head movement, this hallucinatory sensation is *physiologic postrotational vertigo*.

Any disease state that changes the firing frequency of an end organ, producing unequal neural input to the brainstem and ultimately the cerebral cortex, causes vertigo. The symptom can be conceptualized as the cortex inappropriately interpreting the abnormal neural input as indicating actual head rotation. Transient abnormalities produce short-lived symptoms. With a fixed unilateral deficit, central compensatory mechanisms ultimately diminish the vertigo. Since compensation depends on the plasticity of connections between the vestibular nuclei and the cerebellum, patients with brainstem or cerebellar disease have diminished adaptive capacity, and symptoms may persist indefinitely. Compensation is always inadequate for severe fixed bilateral lesions despite normal cerebellar connections: these patients are permanently symptomatic.

Acute unilateral labyrinthine dysfunction is caused by infection, trauma, and ischemia. Often, no specific etiology is uncovered, and the nonspecific terms *acute labyrinthitis*, *acute peripheral vestibulopathy*, or *vestibular neuritis* are used to describe the event. The vertiginous attacks are brief and leave the patient with mild vertigo for several days. Infection with herpes simplex virus type 1 has been implicated. It is impossible to predict whether a patient recovering from the first bout of vertigo will have recurrent episodes.

Labyrinthine ischemia, presumably due to occlusion of the labyrinthine branch of the internal auditory artery, may be the sole manifestation of vertebrobasilar insufficiency (Chap. 349); patients with this syndrome present with the abrupt onset of severe vertigo, nausea, and vomiting, but without tinnitus or hearing loss.

Acute bilateral labyrinthine dysfunction is usually the result of toxins such as drugs or alcohol. The most common offending drugs are the aminoglycoside antibiotics that damage the hair cells of the vestibular end organs and may cause a permanent disorder of equilibrium.

Recurrent unilateral labyrinthine dysfunction, in association with signs and symptoms of cochlear disease (progressive hearing loss and tinnitus), is usually due to Ménière's disease (Chap. 26). When auditory manifestations are absent, the term *vestibular neuronitis* denotes recurrent monosymptomatic vertigo. TIAs of the posterior cerebral circulation (vertebrobasilar insufficiency) only infrequently cause recurrent vertigo without concomitant motor, sensory, visual, cranial nerve, or cerebellar signs (Chap. 349).

Positional vertigo is precipitated by a recumbent head position, either to the right or to the left. Benign paroxysmal positional (or positioning) vertigo (BPPV) of the posterior semicircular canal is particularly common. Although the condition may be due to head trauma, usually no precipitating factors are identified. It generally abates spontaneously after weeks or months. The vertigo and accompanying nystagmus have a distinct pattern of latency, fatigability, and habituation that differs from the less common central positional vertigo (Table 20-2) due to lesions in and around the fourth ventricle. Moreover, the pattern of nystagmus in posterior canal BPPV is distinctive. When supine, with the head turned to the side of the offending ear (bad ear down), the lower eye displays a large-amplitude torsional nystagmus, and the upper eye has a lesser degree of torsion combined with upbeating nystagmus. If the eyes are directed to the upper ear, the vertical nystagmus in the upper eye increases in amplitude. Mild dysequilibrium when upright may also be present.

A *perilymphatic fistula* should be suspected when episodic vertigo is precipitated by Valsalva or exertion, particularly upon a background of a stepwise progressive sensory-neural hearing loss. The condition is usually caused by head trauma or barotrauma or occurs after middle ear surgery.

VERTIGO OF VESTIBULAR NERVE ORIGIN   This occurs with diseases that involve the nerve in the petrous bone or the cerebellopontine angle. Although less severe and less frequently paroxysmal, it has many of the characteristics of labyrinthine vertigo. The adjacent auditory division of the eighth cranial nerve is usually affected, which explains the frequent association of vertigo with unilateral tinnitus and hearing loss. The most common cause of eighth cranial nerve dysfunction is a tumor, usually a schwannoma (*acoustic neuroma*) or a meningioma. These tumors grow slowly and produce such a gradual reduction of labyrinthine output that central compensatory mechanisms can prevent or minimize the vertigo; auditory symptoms of hearing loss and tinnitus are the most common manifestations.

CENTRAL VERTIGO   Lesions of the brainstem or cerebellum can cause acute vertigo, but associated signs and symptoms usually permit distinction from a labyrinthine etiology (Table 20-3). Occasionally, an acute lesion of the vestibulocerebellum may present with monosymptomatic vertigo indistinguishable from a labyrinthopathy.

Vertigo may be a manifestation of a migraine aura (Chap. 14), but some patients with migraine have episodes of vertigo unassociated with their headaches. Antimigrainous treatment should be considered in such patients with otherwise enigmatic vertiginous episodes.

Vestibular epilepsy, vertigo secondary to temporal lobe epileptic activity, is rare and almost always intermixed with other epileptic manifestations.

TABLE 20-2   *Benign Paroxysmal Positional Vertigo and Central Positional Vertigo*

Features	BPPV	Central
Latency[a]	3–40 s	None: immediate vertigo and nystagmus
Fatigability[b]	Yes	No
Habituation[c]	Yes	No
Intensity of vertigo	Severe	Mild
Reproducibility[d]	Variable	Good

[a] Time between attaining head position and onset of symptoms.
[b] Disappearance of symptoms with maintenance of offending position.
[c] Lessening of symptoms with repeated trials.
[d] Likelihood of symptom production during any examination session.

TABLE 20-3   *Differentiation of Peripheral and Central Vertigo*

Sign or Symptom	Peripheral (Labyrinth)	Central (Brainstem or Cerebellum)
Direction of associated nystagmus	Unidirectional; fast phase opposite lesion[a]	Bidirectional or unidirectional
Purely horizontal nystagmus without torsional component	Uncommon	Common
Vertical or purely torsional nystagmus	Never present	May be present
Visual fixation	Inhibits nystagmus and vertigo	No inhibition
Severity of vertigo	Marked	Often mild
Direction of spin	Toward fast phase	Variable
Direction of fall	Toward slow phase	Variable
Duration of symptoms	Finite (minutes, days, weeks) but recurrent	May be chronic
Tinnitus and/or deafness	Often present	Usually absent
Associated central abnormalities	None	Extremely common
Common causes	Infection (labyrinthitis), Ménière's, neuronitis, ischemia, trauma, toxin	Vascular, demyelinating, neoplasm

[a] In Ménière's disease, the direction of the fast phase is variable.

PSYCHOGENIC VERTIGO   This is usually a concomitant of panic attacks (Chap. 371) or agoraphobia (fear of large open spaces, crowds, or leaving the safety of home) and should be suspected in patients so "incapacitated" by their symptoms that they adopt a prolonged housebound status. Most patients with organic vertigo attempt to function despite their discomfort. Organic vertigo is accompanied by nystagmus; a psychogenic etiology is almost certain when nystagmus is absent during a vertiginous episode.

Miscellaneous Head Sensations   This designation is used, primarily for purposes of initial classification, to describe dizziness that is neither faintness nor vertigo. Cephalic ischemia or vestibular dysfunction may be of such low intensity that the usual symptomatology is not clearly identified. For example, a small decrease in blood pressure or a slight vestibular imbalance may cause sensations different from distinct faintness or vertigo but that may be identified properly during provocative testing techniques (see below). Other causes of dizziness in this category are hyperventilation syndrome, hypoglycemia, and the somatic symptoms of a clinical depression; these patients should all have normal neurologic examinations and vestibular function tests. Depressed patients often insist that the depression is "secondary" to the dizziness.

APPROACH TO THE PATIENT

The most important diagnostic tool is a detailed history focused on the meaning of "dizziness" to the patient. Is it faintness (presyncope)? Is there a sensation of spinning? If either of these is affirmed and the neurologic examination is normal, appropriate investigations for the multiple causes of cephalic ischemia or vestibular dysfunction are undertaken.

When the meaning of "dizziness" is uncertain, provocative tests may be helpful. These office procedures simulate either cephalic ischemia or vestibular dysfunction. Cephalic ischemia is obvious if the dizziness is duplicated during maneuvers that produce orthostatic hypotension. Further provocation involves the Valsalva maneuver, which decreases cerebral blood flow and should reproduce ischemic symptoms.

Hyperventilation is the cause of dizziness in many anxious individuals; tingling of the hands and face may be absent. Forced hyperventilation for 1 min is indicated for patients with enigmatic dizziness and normal neurologic examinations.

The simplest provocative test for vestibular dysfunction is rapid rotation and abrupt cessation of movement in a swivel chair. This always induces vertigo that the patients can compare with their symptomatic dizziness. The intense induced vertigo may be unlike the spontaneous symptoms, but shortly thereafter, when the vertigo has all but subsided, a lightheadedness supervenes that may be identified as "my dizziness." When this occurs, the dizzy patient, originally classified as suffering from "miscellaneous head sensations," is now properly diagnosed as having mild vertigo secondary to a vestibulopathy.

Patients with symptoms of positional vertigo should be appropriately tested (Table 20-2). A final provocative and diagnostic vestibular test, requiring the use of Frenzel eyeglasses (self-illuminated goggles with convex lenses that blur out the patient's vision, but allow the examiner to see the eyes greatly magnified), is vigorous head shaking in the horizontal plane for about 10 s. If nystagmus develops after the shaking stops, even in the absence of vertigo, vestibular dysfunction is demonstrated. The maneuver can then be repeated in the vertical plane. If the provocative tests establish the dizziness as a vestibular symptom, an evaluation of vestibular vertigo is undertaken.

Evaluation of Patients with Pathologic Vestibular Vertigo The evaluation depends on whether a central etiology is suspected (Table 20-3). If so, MR imaging of the head is mandatory. Such an examination is rarely helpful in cases of recurrent monosymptomatic vertigo with a normal neurologic examination. Typical BPPV requires no investigation after the diagnosis is made (Table 20-2).

Vestibular function tests serve to (1) demonstrate an abnormality when the distinction between organic and psychogenic is uncertain, (2) establish the side of the abnormality, and (3) distinguish between peripheral and central etiologies. The standard test is electronystagmography (calorics), where warm and cold water (or air) are applied, in a prescribed fashion, to the tympanic membranes, and the slow-phase velocities of the resultant nystagmus from the two are compared. A velocity decrease from one side indicates hypofunction ("canal paresis"). An inability to induce nystagmus with ice water denotes a "dead labyrinth." Some institutions have the capability of quantitatively determining various aspects of the VOR using computer-driven rotational chairs and precise oculographic recording of the eye movements.

CNS disease can produce dizzy sensations of all types. Consequently, a neurologic examination is always required even if the history or provocative tests suggest a cardiac, peripheral vestibular, or psychogenic etiology. Any abnormality on the neurologic examination should prompt appropriate neurodiagnostic studies.

℞ TREATMENT

Treatment of acute vertigo consists of bed rest (1 to 2 days maximum) and vestibular suppressant drugs such as antihistaminics (meclizine, dimenhydrinate, promethazine), tranquilizers with GABA-ergic effects (diazepam, clonazepam), phenothiazines (prochlorperazine), or glucocorticoids (Table 20-4). If the vertigo persists beyond a few days, most authorities advise ambulation in an attempt to induce central compensatory mechanisms, despite the short-term discomfort to the patient. Chronic vertigo of labyrinthine origin may be treated with a systematized vestibular rehabilitation program to facilitate central compensation.

BPPV is often self-limited but, when persistent, may respond dramatically to specific repositioning exercise programs designed to empty particulate debris from the posterior semicircular canal. One of

TABLE 20-4 *Treatment of Vertigo*

Agent[a]	Dose[b]
Antihistamines	
Meclizine	25–50 mg 3 times/day
Dimenhydrinate	50 mg 1–2 times/day
Promethazine[c]	25–50-mg suppository or IM
Benzodiazepines	
Diazepam	2.5 mg 1–3 times/day
Clonazepam	0.25 mg 1–3 times/day
Phenothiazines	
Prochlorperazine[c]	5 mg IM or 25-mg suppository
Anticholinergic[d]	
Scopolamine transdermal	Patch
Sympathomimetics[d]	
Ephedrine	25 mg/d
Combination preparations[d]	
Ephedrine and promethazine	25 mg/d of each
Exercise therapy	
Repositioning maneuvers[e]	
Vestibular rehabilitation[f]	
Other	
Diuretics or low-salt (1 g/d) diet[g]	
Antimigrainous drugs[h]	
Inner ear surgery[i]	
Glucocorticoids[c]	

[a] All listed drugs are U.S. Food and Drug Administration approved, but most are not approved for the treatment of vertigo.
[b] Usual oral (unless otherwise stated) starting dose in adults; maintenance dose can be reached by a gradual increase.
[c] For acute vertigo only.
[d] For motion sickness only.
[e] For benign paroxysmal positional vertigo.
[f] For vertigo other than Ménière's and positional.
[g] For Ménière's disease.
[h] For migraine-associated vertigo (see Chap. 14 for a listing of prophylactic antimigrainous drugs).
[i] For perilymphatic fistula and refractory cases of Ménière's disease.

these exercises, the Epley procedure, is graphically demonstrated, in four languages, on a website for use in both physician's offices and self-treatment (*www.charite.de/ch/neuro/vertigo.html*).

Prophylactic measures to prevent recurrent vertigo are variably effective. Antihistamines are commonly utilized but are of limited value. Ménière's disease may respond to a diuretic or, more effectively, to a very low salt diet (1 g/d). Recurrent episodes of migraine-associated vertigo should be treated with antimigrainous therapy (Chap. 14). There are a variety of inner ear surgical procedures for refractory Ménière's disease, but these are only rarely necessary.

Helpful websites for both physicians and vertigo patients are: *www.iVertigo.net* and *www.tchain.com.*

FURTHER READING

KAPOOR WN: Current evaluation in management of syncope. Circulation 106: 1606, 2002

KAUFMAN H et al: Midodrine in neurally mediated syncope: A double-blind, randomized, crossover study. Ann Neurol 52:342, 2002

KAUFMAN NH, BHATTACHARYA K: Diagnosis and treatment of neurally mediated syncope. The Neurologist 8:175, 2002

MAISEL W, STEBENSON W: Syncope—getting to the heart of the matter. N Engl J Med 347:931, 2002

SOTERIADES E et al: Incidence and prognosis of syncope. N Engl J Med 347: 878, 2002

Normal motor function requires integrated muscle activity with appropriate modulation by neuronal activity in the cerebral cortex, basal ganglia, cerebellum, and spinal cord. Symptoms and signs of motor system dysfunction may include weakness, fatigue, myalgias, spasms, cramps, dyskinetic movement, ataxia, imbalance, or disorders in the initiation or planning of movement.

WEAKNESS

Weakness is a reduction in normal power of one or more muscles. Limitation in rising from a seated position or combing hair suggests proximal weakness, whereas slapping of the feet while walking or limitation in opening jars suggests distal weakness. Increased fatigability or limitation in function due to pain is often confused with weakness by patients. *Increased fatigability* is the inability to sustain the performance of an activity that should be normal for a person of the same age, gender, and size.

Paralysis and the suffix "-plegia" indicate weakness that is so severe that it is complete or nearly complete. "Paresis" refers to weakness that is mild or moderate. The prefix "hemi-" refers to one half of the body, "para-" to both legs, and "quadri-" to all four limbs.

Tone is the resistance of a muscle to passive stretch. Central nervous system (CNS) abnormalities that cause weakness generally produce *spasticity*, an increase in tone due to upper motor neuron disease. Spasticity is velocity-dependent, has a sudden release after reaching a maximum (the "clasp-knife" phenomenon), and predominantly affects antigravity muscles (i.e., upper limb flexors and lower limb extensors). Spasticity is distinct from rigidity and paratonia, two other types of increased tone. *Rigidity* is increased tone that is present throughout the range of motion (a "lead pipe" or "plastic" stiffness) and affects flexors and extensors equally. In some patients, rigidity has a cogwheel quality that is enhanced by voluntary movement of the contralateral limb (reinforcement). Rigidity occurs with certain extrapyramidal disorders such as Parkinson's disease. *Paratonia*, also referred to as *gegenhalten*, is increased tone that varies irregularly in a manner that may seem related to the degree of relaxation, is present throughout the range of motion, and affects flexors and extensors equally. Paratonia usually results from disease of the frontal lobes. Weakness with decreased tone (flaccidity) or normal tone occurs with disorders of the *motor unit*, that is, a single lower motor neuron and all of the muscle fibers it innervates.

Three basic patterns of weakness can usually be recognized based on the signs summarized in Table 21-1. One results from upper motor neuron pathology, and the other two from disorders of the motor unit (lower motor neuron and myopathic weakness). Fasciculations and early atrophy help to distinguish lower motor neuron (neurogenic) weakness from myopathic weakness. A *fasciculation* is a visible or palpable twitch within a single muscle due to the spontaneous discharge of one motor unit. Lower motor neuron weakness also produces more prominent hypotonia and greater depression of tendon reflexes than does myopathic weakness.

PATHOGENESIS ■ Upper Motor Neuron Weakness

This pattern of weakness results from disorders that affect the upper motor neurons or their axons in the cerebral cortex, subcortical white matter, internal capsule, brainstem, or spinal cord (Fig. 21-1). Upper motor neuron lesions produce weakness through decreased activation of the lower motor neurons. In general, distal muscle groups are affected more severely than proximal ones, and axial movements are spared unless the lesion is severe and bilateral. With corticobulbar involvement, weakness is usually observed only in the lower face and tongue; extraocular, upper facial, pharyngeal, and jaw muscles are almost always spared. With bilateral corticobulbar lesions, *pseudobulbar palsy* often develops, in which dysarthria, dysphagia, dysphonia, and emotional lability accompany bilateral facial weakness. Spasticity accompanies upper motor

neuron weakness but may not be present in the acute phase. Upper motor neuron lesions also affect the ability to perform rapid repetitive movements. Such movements are slow and coarse, but normal rhythmicity is maintained. Finger-nose-finger and heel-knee-shin are performed slowly but adequately.

Lower Motor Neuron Weakness This pattern results from disorders of cell bodies of lower motor neurons in the brainstem motor nuclei and the anterior horn of the spinal cord, or from dysfunction of the axons of these neurons as they pass to skeletal muscle (Fig. 21-2). Weakness is due to a decrease in the number of motor units that can be activated, through a loss of the α motor neurons or disruption of their connections to muscle. With a decreased number of motor units, fewer muscle fibers are activated with full effort and maximum power is reduced. Loss of γ motor neurons does not cause weakness but decreases tension on the muscle spindles, which decreases muscular tone and contributes to less active tendon reflexes on examination. An absent tendon stretch reflex suggests involvement of the spindle afferent fibers.

When a motor unit becomes diseased, especially in anterior horn cell diseases, it may spontaneously discharge, producing a *fasciculation*. These isolated small twitches may be seen or felt clinically or recorded by electromyography (EMG). When α motor neurons or their axons degenerate, the denervated muscle fibers spontaneously discharge in a manner that cannot be seen or felt but can be recorded with EMG. These small single muscle fiber discharges are called *fibrillation potentials*. If lower motor neuron weakness is present, recruitment of motor units is delayed or reduced, with fewer than normal activated at a given discharge frequency. This contrasts with upper motor neuron weakness, in which a normal number of motor units are activated at a given frequency but in which the maximum discharge frequency is decreased.

Myopathic Weakness This pattern of weakness is produced by disorders within the motor unit that affect the muscle fibers or the neuromuscular junctions.

Two types of muscle fibers exist. Type I muscle fibers are rich in mitochondria and oxidative enzymes, produce relatively low force, but have low energy demands that can be supplied by ongoing aerobic metabolism. They produce sustained postural and nonforceful movements. Type II muscle fibers are rich in glycolytic enzymes, can produce relatively high force, but have high energy demands that cannot be supplied for long by ongoing aerobic metabolism. Thus, these units can be activated maximally for only brief periods of time to produce high-force movements.

For graded voluntary movements, type I muscle fibers are activated earlier in recruitment. For each muscle fiber, if the nerve terminal releases a normal number of acetylcholine molecules presynaptically and a sufficient number of postsynaptic acetylcholine receptors are opened, the end plate reaches threshold and thereby generates an action potential that spreads across the muscle fiber membrane and into the transverse tubular system. This electrical excitation activates intracel-

TABLE 21-1 *Signs That Distinguish Patterns of Weakness*			
Sign	Upper Motor Neuron	Lower Motor Neuron	Myopathic
Atrophy	None	Severe	Mild
Fasciculations	None	Common	None
Tone	Spastic	Decreased	Normal/decreased
Distribution of weakness	Pyramidal/regional	Distal/segmental	Proximal
Tendon reflexes	Hyperactive	Hypoactive/absent	Normal/hypoactive
Babinski's sign	Present	Absent	Absent

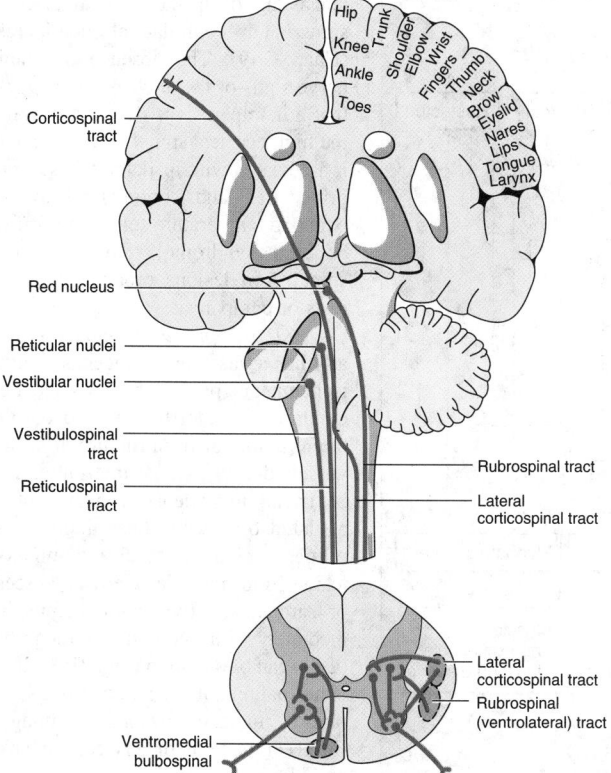

FIGURE 21-1 The corticospinal and bulbospinal upper motor neuron pathways. Upper motor neurons have their cell bodies in layer V of the primary motor cortex (the precentral gyrus, or Brodmann's area 4) and in the premotor and supplemental motor cortex (area 6). The upper motor neurons in the primary motor cortex are somatotopically organized as illustrated on the right side of the figure.

Axons of the upper motor neurons descend through the subcortical white matter and the posterior limb of the internal capsule. Axons of the *pyramidal* or *corticospinal system* descend through the brainstem in the cerebral peduncle of the midbrain, the basis pontis, and the medullary pyramids. At the cervicomedullary junction, most pyramidal axons decussate into the contralateral corticospinal tract of the lateral spinal cord, but 10 to 30% remain ipsilateral in the anterior spinal cord. Pyramidal neurons make direct monosynaptic connections with lower motor neurons. They innervate most densely the lower motor neurons of hand muscles and are involved in the execution of learned, fine movements. Corticobulbar neurons are similar to corticospinal neurons but innervate brainstem motor nuclei.

Bulbospinal upper motor neurons influence strength and tone but are not part of the pyramidal system. The descending *ventromedial bulbospinal pathways* originate in the tectum of the midbrain (tectospinal pathway), the vestibular nuclei (vestibulospinal pathway), and the reticular formation (reticulospinal pathway). These pathways influence axial and proximal muscles and are involved in the maintenance of posture and integrated movements of the limbs and trunk. The descending *ventrolateral bulbospinal pathways*, which originate predominantly in the red nucleus (rubrospinal pathway), facilitate distal limb muscles. The bulbospinal system is sometimes referred to as the *extrapyramidal upper motor neuron system*. In all figures, nerve cell bodies and axon terminals are shown, respectively, as closed circles and forks.

lular events that produce an energy-dependent contraction of the muscle fiber (excitation-contraction coupling).

Myopathic weakness is produced by a decrease in the number or contractile force of muscle fibers activated within the motor unit. With muscular dystrophies, inflammatory myopathies, or myopathies with muscle fiber necrosis, decreased numbers of muscle fibers survive within many motor units. As demonstrated with EMG, the size of each motor unit action potential is decreased so that motor units must be recruited more rapidly than normal to produce the power necessary for a certain movement. Neuromuscular junction diseases such as myasthenia gravis produce weakness in a similar manner, although the loss of muscle fibers within the motor unit is functional rather than actual. Furthermore, the number of muscle fibers activated can vary over time, depending on the state of rest of the neuromuscular junctions. Thus, fatigable weakness is suggestive of myasthenia gravis or another neuromuscular junction disease. Some myopathies produce weakness

through loss of contractile force of muscle fibers or through relatively selective involvement of the type II muscle fibers. These may not affect the size of individual motor unit action potentials observed with EMG and are detected by a discrepancy between the electrical activity and force of a muscle.

Integrated Movements Most purposeful movements require the integrated coordination of many muscle groups. Consider a simple movement, such as grasping a ball. The primary movement is a flexion of the thumb and fingers of one hand, with opposition of the thumb and little finger. This requires the contraction of several muscles, including flexor digitorum superficialis, flexor digitorum profundus, flexor pollicis longus, flexor pollicis brevis, opponens pollicis, and opponens digiti minimi. The prime movers for this action are called *agonists*. In order for the grasping to be smooth and forceful, the thumb and finger extensors need to relax at the same rate as the flexors contract. The muscles that act in a directly opposing manner to the agonists are *antagonists*. A secondary action of the thumb and finger flexors is to flex the wrist; because wrist flexion tends to weaken finger flexion if both occur, activation of wrist extensors assists the grasping movement. Muscles that produce such complementary movements are *synergists*. Finally, the arm needs to be held in a stable position as the grasp occurs, so that the ball is not knocked away before it is secured. Muscles that stabilize the arm position are *fixators*.

The coordination of activity by agonists, antagonists, synergists, and fixators is regulated by a three-level hierarchy of motor control. The lowest level of control is mediated through segmental reflexes in the spinal cord. These reflexes facilitate agonists and reciprocally inhibit the antagonists. Spinal segments also control rhythmic patterns of movement that involve more than a single pair of agonists and antagonists. For example, the lumbosacral spinal cord contains the basic programming for cyclical stepping movements that involve the synergistic activation of different muscle groups over time. The intermediate level of control is mediated through the descending bulbo-

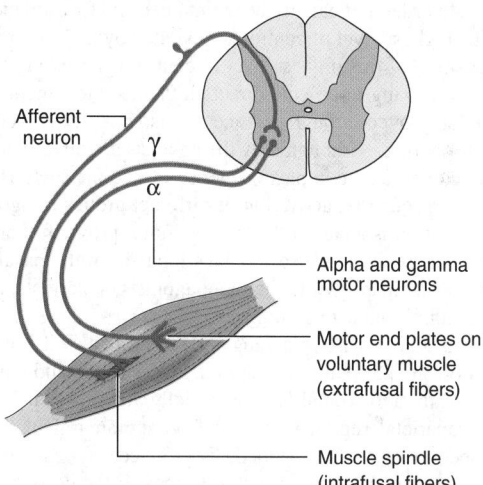

FIGURE 21-2 Lower motor neurons are divided into α and γ types. The larger α motor neurons are more numerous and innervate the extrafusal muscle fibers of the motor unit. Loss of α motor neurons or disruption of their axons produces lower motor neuron weakness. The smaller, less numerous γ motor neurons innervate the intrafusal muscle fibers of the muscle spindle and contribute to normal tone and stretch reflexes. The α motor neuron receives direct excitatory input from corticomotoneurons and primary muscle spindle afferents. The α and γ motor neurons also receive excitatory input from other descending upper motor neuron pathways, segmental sensory inputs, and interneurons. The α motor neurons receive direct inhibition from Renshaw cell interneurons, and other interneurons indirectly inhibit the α and γ motor neurons.

A tendon reflex requires the function of all illustrated structures. A tap on a tendon stretches muscle spindles (which are tonically activated by γ motor neurons) and activates the primary spindle afferent neurons. These stimulate the α motor neurons in the spinal cord, producing a brief muscle contraction, which is the familiar tendon reflex.

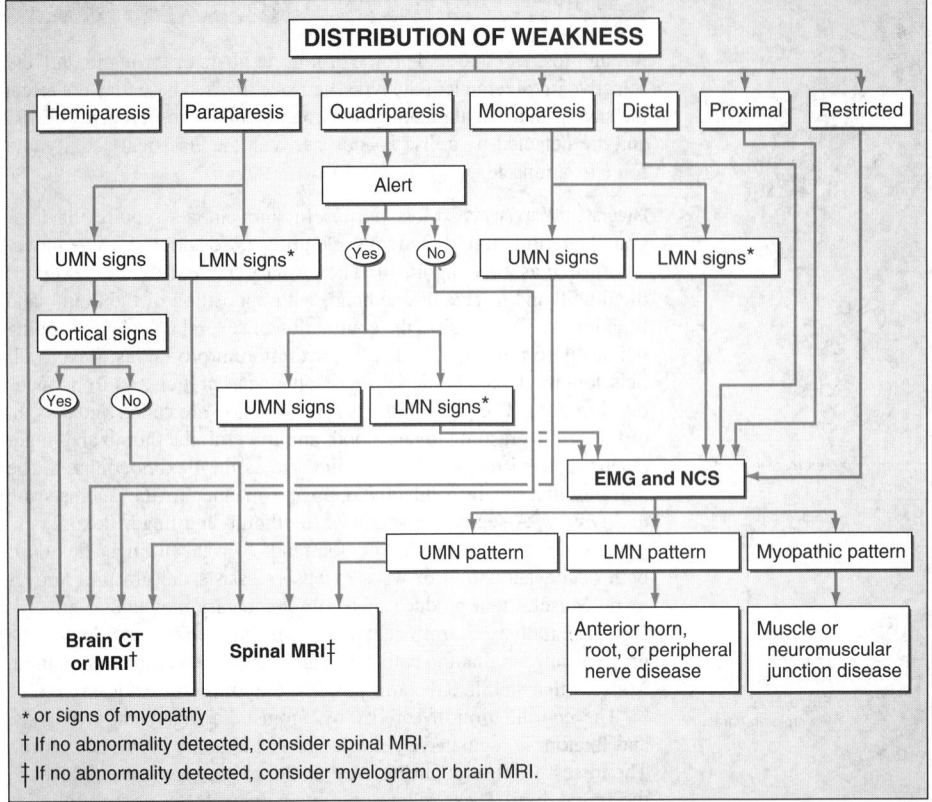

FIGURE 21-3 An algorithm for the initial workup of a patient with weakness. CT, computed tomography; EMG, electromyography; LMN, lower motor neuron; MRI, magnetic resonance imaging; NCS, nerve conduction studies; UMN, upper motor neuron.

Within the figure:

DISTRIBUTION OF WEAKNESS

Hemiparesis | Paraparesis | Quadriparesis | Monoparesis | Distal | Proximal | Restricted

Alert — Yes / No

UMN signs | LMN signs* | UMN signs | LMN signs*

Cortical signs — Yes / No

UMN signs | LMN signs*

EMG and NCS

UMN pattern | LMN pattern | Myopathic pattern

Brain CT or MRI† | Spinal MRI‡

Anterior horn, root, or peripheral nerve disease | Muscle or neuromuscular junction disease

* or signs of myopathy
† If no abnormality detected, consider spinal MRI.
‡ If no abnormality detected, consider myelogram or brain MRI.

---

spinal pathways, which integrate visual, proprioceptive, and vestibular feedback into the execution of an action. For example, the locomotor center in the midbrain is required to modify the cyclical stepping movements in order that balance be maintained and forward movement occurs. The highest level of control is mediated by the cerebral cortex. Superimposition of this highest level of control is necessary for activities such as walking to be goal-directed. Precise movements that are learned and improved through practice are also initiated and controlled by the motor cortex. Although only the agonists are directly activated, during the course of a complex sequence of actions such as playing the piano, the sequential activation of different groups of agonists for each note or chord is a part of the learned motor program. Further, the execution of these actions also involves input from the basal ganglia and cerebellar hemispheres to facilitate agonists, synergists, and fixators and to inhibit undesired antagonists.

Apraxia is a disorder of planning and initiating a skilled or learned movement (Chap. 23). Unilateral apraxia of the right hand may be due to a lesion of the left frontal lobe (especially anterior or inferior), the left temporoparietal region (especially the supramarginal gyrus), or their connections. Left body apraxia is produced by lesions of these regions in the right hemisphere or by lesions in the corpus callosum that disconnect the right temporoparietal or frontal regions from those on the left. Bilateral apraxia is often due to bilateral frontal lobe lesions or diffuse bilateral hemispheric disease.

Hemiparesis Hemiparesis results from an upper motor neuron lesion above the midcervical spinal cord; most lesions that produce hemiparesis are located above the foramen magnum. The presence of language disorders, cortical sensory disturbances, cognitive abnormalities, disorders of visual-spatial integration, apraxia, or seizures indicates a cortical lesion. Homonymous visual field defects reflect either a cortical or a subcortical hemispheric lesion. A "pure motor" hemiparesis of the face, arm, and/or leg is due to a small, discrete lesion in the posterior limb of the internal capsule, cerebral peduncle, or upper pons. Some brainstem lesions produce "crossed paralyses,"

consisting of ipsilateral cranial nerve signs and contralateral hemiparesis (Chap. 349). The absence of cranial nerve signs or facial weakness suggests that a hemiparesis is due to a lesion in the high cervical spinal cord, especially if associated with ipsilateral loss of proprioception and contralateral loss of pain and temperature sense (the Brown-Séquard syndrome). However, most spinal cord lesions produce quadriparesis or paraparesis.

Acute or episodic hemiparesis usually has a vascular pathogenesis, either ischemia or a primary hemorrhage. Less commonly, hemorrhage may occur into brain tumors or from rupture of normal vessels due to trauma; the trauma may be trivial in patients who are anticoagulated or elderly. Less likely possibilities include a focal inflammatory lesion from multiple sclerosis, abscess, or sarcoidosis. Evaluation begins immediately with a computed tomography (CT) scan of the brain (Fig. 21-3). If CT is normal and an ischemic stroke is unlikely, magnetic resonance imaging (MRI) of the brain or cervical spine may be indicated.

Subacute hemiparesis that evolves over days or weeks has an extensive differential diagnosis. A common cause is subdural hematoma; this readily treatable condition must always be considered, especially in elderly or anticoagulated patients, even in the absence of a history of trauma. Infectious possibilities include cerebral bacterial abscess, fungal granuloma or meningitis, and parasitic infection. Weakness from primary and metastatic neoplasms may evolve over days to weeks. AIDS may present with subacute hemiparesis due to toxoplasmosis or primary CNS lymphoma. Noninfectious inflammatory processes, such as multiple sclerosis or, less commonly, sarcoidosis, are further considerations. If the brain MRI is normal and if cortical and hemispheric signs are not present, MRI of the cervical spine may be required.

Chronic hemiparesis that evolves over months is usually due to a neoplasm, an unruptured arteriovenous malformation, a chronic subdural hematoma, or a degenerative disease. The initial diagnostic test is often an MRI of the brain, especially if the clinical findings suggest brainstem pathology. If MRI of the brain is normal, the possibility of a foramen magnum or high cervical spinal cord lesion should be considered.

Paraparesis An intraspinal lesion at or below the upper thoracic spinal cord level is most commonly responsible. A sensory level over the trunk identifies the approximate level of the cord lesion. Paraparesis can also result from lesions at other locations that disturb upper motor neurons (especially parasagittal lesions and hydrocephalus) and lower motor neurons (anterior horn cell disorders, cauda equina syndromes, and occasionally peripheral neuropathies).

Acute or episodic paraparesis due to spinal cord disease may be difficult to distinguish from disorders affecting lower motor neurons or cerebral hemispheres. Recurrent episodes of paraparesis are often due to multiple sclerosis or to vascular malformations of the spinal cord. With acute spinal cord disease, the upper motor neuron deficit is usually associated with incontinence and a sensory disturbance of the lower limbs that extends rostrally to a level on the trunk; tone is typically flaccid, and tendon reflexes absent. In such cases, the diagnostic approach begins with an imaging study of the spinal cord (Fig. 21-3). Compressive lesions (particularly epidural tumor, abscess, or hematoma), spinal cord infarction (proprioception is usually spared), an arteriovenous fistula or other vascular anomaly, and transverse myelitis, among other causes, may be responsible (Chap. 356). Diseases of the cerebral hemispheres that produce acute paraparesis include anterior cerebral artery ischemia (shoulder shrug also affected), superior sagittal sinus or cortical venous thrombosis, and acute hydrocephalus. If upper motor neuron signs are associated with drowsiness, confusion, seizures, or other hemispheric signs but not a sensory level over the trunk, the diagnostic approach starts with an MRI of the brain. Paraparesis is part of the cauda equina syndrome, which may result from trauma to the low back, a midline disk herniation, or intraspinal tumor; although sphincters are affected, hip flexion is often spared, as is sensation over the anterolateral thighs. Rarely, paraparesis is caused by a rapidly evolving peripheral neuropathy such as Guillain-Barré syndrome (Chap. 365) or by a myopathy (Chap. 368). In such cases, electrophysiologic studies are diagnostically helpful and refocus the subsequent evaluation.

Subacute or chronic paraparesis with spasticity is caused by upper motor neuron disease. When there is associated lower limb sensory loss and sphincter involvement, a chronic spinal cord disorder is likely; these are discussed in Chap. 356. The clinical approach begins with an MRI of the spinal cord. If the imaging study is normal and spasticity is present, MRI of the brain may be indicated. If hemispheric signs are present, parasagittal meningioma or chronic hydrocephalus is likely and MRI of the brain is the initial test. In the rare situation when chronic paraparesis is due to lower motor neuron or myopathic etiology, the localization is usually suspected on clinical grounds by the absence of spasticity and confirmed by EMG and nerve conduction tests.

Quadriparesis or Generalized Weakness Generalized weakness may be due to disorders of the CNS or of the motor unit. Although the terms *quadriparesis* and *generalized weakness* are often used interchangeably, quadriparesis is more often chosen when an upper motor neuron cause is suspected and generalized weakness when a disease of the motor unit is likely. Weakness from CNS disorders is usually associated with changes in consciousness or cognition, with increased muscle tone and muscle stretch reflexes, and with alterations of sensation. Most neuromuscular causes of generalized weakness are associated with normal mental function, diminished muscle tone, and hypoactive muscle stretch reflexes. Exceptions are some causes of acute quadriparesis due to upper motor neuron disorders in which transient hypotonia is present. The major causes of intermittent weakness are listed in Table 21-2. A patient with generalized fatigability without objective weakness may have the chronic fatigue syndrome (Chap. 370).

ACUTE QUADRIPARESIS Acute quadriparesis with onset over minutes may result from disorders of upper motor neurons (e.g., anoxia, hypotension, brainstem or cervical cord ischemia, trauma, and systemic metabolic abnormalities) or muscle (electrolyte disturbances, certain inborn errors of muscle energy metabolism, toxins, or periodic paralyses). Onset over hours to weeks may, in addition to the above, be due to lower motor neuron disorders. Guillain-Barré syndrome (Chap. 365)

---

is the most common lower motor neuron weakness that progresses over days to 4 weeks; the finding of an elevated protein level in the cerebrospinal fluid is helpful but may be absent early in the course. If stupor or coma is present, the evaluation begins with a CT scan of the brain. If upper motor neuron signs are present but the patient is alert, the initial test is usually an MRI of the cervical cord. If weakness is lower motor neuron, myopathic, or uncertain in origin, the clinical approach begins with blood studies for muscle enzymes and electrolytes and an EMG and nerve conduction study.

SUBACUTE OR CHRONIC QUADRIPARESIS When quadriparesis due to upper motor neuron disease develops over weeks, months, or years, the distinction among disorders of the cerebral hemispheres, brainstem, and cervical spinal cord is usually possible by clinical criteria alone. The diagnostic approach begins with an MRI of the clinically suspected site of pathology. Lower motor neuron disease usually presents with weakness that is most profound distally, whereas myopathic weakness is typically proximal; the evaluation then begins with EMG and nerve conduction studies.

Monoparesis This is usually due to lower motor neuron disease, with or without associated sensory involvement. Upper motor neuron weakness occasionally presents with a monoparesis of distal and nonantigravity muscles. Myopathic weakness is rarely limited to one limb.

ACUTE MONOPARESIS Distinguishing between upper and lower motor neuron disorders may be difficult clinically because tone and reflexes are frequently decreased in both at presentation. If the weakness is predominantly in distal and nonantigravity muscles and not associated with sensory impairment or pain, focal cortical ischemia is likely (Chap. 349); in this setting, diagnostic possibilities are similar to those for acute hemiparesis. Sensory loss and pain usually accompany acute lower motor neuron weakness. The distribution of weakness is commonly localized to a single nerve root or peripheral nerve within one limb but occasionally reflects involvement of the brachial or lumbosacral plexus. If lower motor neuron weakness is suspected, or if the pattern of weakness is uncertain, the clinical approach begins with an EMG and nerve conduction study.

SUBACUTE OR CHRONIC MONOPARESIS Weakness with atrophy of one limb that develops over weeks or months is almost always lower motor neuron in origin. If the weakness is associated with numbness, a peripheral nerve or spinal root origin is likely; uncommonly, the brachial or lumbosacral plexus is affected. If numbness is absent, anterior horn cell disease is likely. In either case, an electrodiagnostic study is indicated. If upper rather than lower motor neuron signs are present, a tumor, vascular malformation, or other cortical lesion affecting the precentral gyrus may be responsible. Alternatively, if the leg is affected, a small thoracic cord lesion, often a tumor or multiple sclerosis, may be present. In these situations, the approach begins with an imaging study of the suspicious area.

Distal Weakness Involvement of two or four limbs distally suggests lower motor neuron or peripheral nerve disease. Acute distal lower limb weakness occurs occasionally from an acute toxic polyneuropathy or cauda equina syndrome. Distal symmetric weakness usually develops over weeks, months, or years and is due to metabolic, toxic, hereditary, degenerative, or inflammatory diseases of peripheral nerves (Chap. 363). With peripheral nerve disease, weakness is usually less severe than numbness. Anterior horn cell disease may begin distally but is typically asymmetric and is not associated with numbness (Chap. 353). Rarely, myopathies also present with distal weakness (Chap. 368). The first step in evaluation is an electrophysiologic study (Fig. 21-3).

Proximal Weakness Proximal weakness of two or four limbs suggests a disorder of muscle or, less commonly, neuromuscular junction or anterior horn cell. Myopathy often produces symmetric weakness of the pelvic or shoulder girdle muscles (Chap. 368). Diseases of the

---

TABLE 21-2 Causes of Episodic Generalized Weakness
1. Electrolyte disturbances, e.g., hypokalemia, hyperkalemia, hypercalcemia, hypernatremia, hyponatremia, hypophosphatemia, hypermagnesemia
2. Muscle disorders
a. Channelopathies (periodic paralyses)
b. Metabolic defects of muscle (impaired carbohydrate or fatty acid utilization; abnormal mitochondrial function)
3. Neuromuscular junction disorders
a. Myasthenia gravis
b. Lambert-Eaton myasthenic syndrome
4. Central nervous system disorders
a. Transient ischemic attacks of the brainstem
b. Transient global cerebral ischemia
c. Multiple sclerosis

neuromuscular junction (such as myasthenia gravis) may present with symmetric proximal weakness (Chap. 366), often associated with ptosis, diplopia, or bulbar weakness and fluctuating in severity during the day. Extreme fatigability present in some cases of myasthenia gravis may even suggest episodic weakness, but strength rarely returns fully to normal. The proximal weakness of anterior horn cell disease is most often asymmetric, but may be symmetric if familial (Chap. 353). Numbness does not occur with any of these diseases. The evaluation usually begins with determination of the serum creatine kinase level and electrophysiologic studies.

Weakness in a Restricted Distribution   In some patients, weakness does not fit any of the above patterns. Examples include weakness limited to the extraocular, hemifacial, bulbar, or respiratory muscles. If unilateral, restricted weakness is usually due to lower motor neuron or peripheral nerve disease, such as in a facial palsy (Chap. 355) or an isolated superior oblique muscle paresis (Chap. 25). Relatively symmetric weakness of extraocular or bulbar muscles is usually due to a myopathy (Chap. 367) or neuromuscular junction disorder (Chap. 366). Bilateral facial palsy with areflexia suggests Guillain-Barré syndrome (Chap. 365). Worsening of relatively symmetric weakness with fatigue is characteristic of neuromuscular junction disorders. Asymmetric bulbar weakness is usually due to motor neuron disease. Weakness limited to respiratory muscles is uncommon and is usually due to motor neuron disease, myasthenia gravis, or polymyositis/dermatomyositis (Chap. 369).

SPASMS AND CRAMPS

Spontaneous or exercise-related discomfort from muscles is usually benign. However, a number of disorders of the motor system are characteristically painful. *Myalgias* (Chap. 367) are pains that are felt in muscle; the term does not imply an involuntary contraction. *Spasms* and *cramps* refer to episodes of involuntary contraction of one or more muscles. Cramps are usually painful, whereas spasms are not necessarily uncomfortable.

Involuntary contraction of muscle may occur with disorders of the CNS, lower motor neuron, or muscle. Contractions that originate within the CNS and are associated with upper motor neuron signs are usually referred to as spasms and generally affect the flexors or extensors of one or more limbs. Those that originate within the CNS and are not associated with upper motor neuron signs include movement disorders discussed below, as well as the rare stiff-person syndrome and tetanus. Muscle rigidity from active muscle contraction can occur in the malignant hyperthermia syndrome, usually associated with general anesthesia. In the neuroleptic malignant syndrome, muscle rigidity arises from CNS overactivity. Involuntary contractions that originate in the lower motor neurons are usually cramps, occasionally tetany, or rarely neuromyotonia. Spasms that originate in muscle or muscle membrane generally manifest as delayed relaxation after voluntary contraction (myotonia or rarely a contracture). These conditions may be difficult to distinguish clinically but are often well characterized by EMG.

Stiff-Person Syndrome   This rare syndrome is characterized by slowly progressive muscle stiffness and superimposed spasms. The stiffness commonly begins in the low back and spreads over months up the spine and into the limbs but not into the jaw. The gait becomes stiff, and there is hyperlordosis of the lumbar spine. Spasms are often produced by startle. Emotional stress tends to worsen the stiffness as well as the frequency and severity of spasms. The spontaneous motor activity disappears during sleep. The syndrome is often associated with diabetes mellitus and can be paraneoplastic, accompanying Hodgkin's lymphoma, small cell cancer of the lung, and breast cancer. Most patients have a serum antibody against glutamic acid decarboxylase, an enzyme responsible for synthesis of the inhibitory neurotransmitter γ-aminobutyric acid (GABA). Stiffness results from loss of descending brainstem or segmental spinal inhibitory influences on the lower motor neurons. EMG studies reveal continuous motor unit activity that is similar to voluntary effort with preservation of the silent period to muscle stretch. Stiffness and spasms typically respond partially to treatment with baclofen or benzodiazepines.

Tetanus   This rare hyperexcitable state results from exposure to tetanus toxin in patients infected with *Clostridium tetani* (Chap. 124). Painful spasms typically begin with jaw closure (trismus) and soon become generalized. EMG studies reveal continuous motor unit activity that is similar to voluntary effort except for loss of the silent period to muscle stretch.

Cramps   These are the most common type of involuntary muscle contraction. Cramps are a painful contraction of a single muscle that produces a palpable knot within the muscle for seconds to minutes and is relieved by passive stretch of the muscle or spontaneously. EMG studies reveal motor unit activity that has too high a discharge frequency to be voluntary. If cramps are associated with weakness, the weakness is almost always lower motor neuron in origin. When strength is normal, no definable condition is usually found, although dehydration, hypothyroidism, or uremia is occasionally present. If prominent, membrane stabilizing drugs, such as carbamazepine, may provide symptomatic benefit.

Tetany   Tetany is characterized by contraction of distal muscles of the hands (carpal spasm with extension of interphalangeal joints and adduction and flexion of the metacarpophalangeal joints) and feet (pedal spasm) and is associated with tingling around the mouth and distally in the limbs. Tetany with carpopedal spasms is a common manifestation of hypocalcemia or respiratory alkalosis (even from hyperventilation). EMG studies reveal single or more often grouped motor unit discharges at low discharge frequency.

Neuromyotonia (Isaac's Syndrome)   Neuromyotonia is characterized by muscle stiffness at rest that persists during sleep and by delayed relaxation after voluntary effort. Distal limb muscles are usually affected most severely, but all skeletal muscle may be involved. Gait may be stiff, and close inspection of the muscle reveals undulation of the overlying skin due to continuous muscle fiber contractions (myokymia). The continuous muscle fiber activity generates heat, and excessive sweating is common. EMG studies commonly reveal myokymic discharges, especially in familial cases. Rarely, EMGs record high-frequency neuromyotonic discharges. Autoantibodies against voltage-gated potassium channels have been demonstrated in some cases, and plasma exchange may be effective.

Myotonia   This is a nonpainful delay in the relaxation of muscle after voluntary activity. Delay in opening the hand after a forceful grip (grip myotonia) is common. These disorders are usually familial and worsen in cold weather. EMG demonstrates a waxing and waning discharge of individual muscle fibers.

Contracture   A painful inability to relax a muscle after voluntary activity due to energy depletion characterizes certain metabolic disorders with failure of energy production, such as myophosphorylase deficiency (McArdle's disease). EMG studies reveal electrical silence.

MOVEMENT DISORDERS

In these disorders, abnormal movements (or *dyskinesias*) occur due to a disturbance of fluency and speed of voluntary movement or the presence of unintended extra movements. Because they are so distinct from the pyramidal disorders that cause upper motor neuron weakness, movement disorders are often referred to as *extrapyramidal diseases*. *Hyperkinetic movement disorders* are those in which an excessive amount of spontaneous motor activity is seen or in which abnormal involuntary movements occur. *Hypokinetic movement disorders* are characterized by *akinesia* or *bradykinesia*, in which purposeful motor activity is absent or reduced ("poverty of movement").

PATHOGENESIS   Movement disorders result from disease of the basal ganglia, paired subcortical gray matter structures consisting of the caudate and the putamen (which together are called the striatum), the internal and external segments of the globus pallidus, the subthalamic nucleus, and the substantia nigra (see Chap. 351).

Parkinson's disease the prototypic hypokinetic movement disorder, results from a loss of dopaminergic neurons in the substantia nigra pars compacta. This leads to less excitation of striatal neurons that express the D_1 type of dopamine receptors and less inhibition of D_2 striatal neurons, both contributing to reduced facilitation of cortically initiated movement. The resting tremor of Parkinson's disease is less readily explained by this model but may result from effects on cholinergic interneurons in the striatum. *Huntington's disease* (Chap. 350), a hyperkinetic movement disorder, may be explained by selective loss of D_2 striatal neurons, resulting in disinhibition of cortically initiated movements without normal feedback control. The pathogenesis of hemiballismus is similar—a direct lesion of the glutamatergic neurons in the subthalamic nucleus (usually from a stroke) leads to disinhibition of thalamocortical projections.

Hyperkinetic Movement Disorders Abnormal involuntary movements may be rhythmical or irregular. Those that are rhythmical are termed *tremors*, with the uncommon exception of *palatal and segmental myoclonus*. Tremors are divided into three types: rest, postural, and intention tremor. A *rest tremor* is maximal at rest and becomes less prominent with activity. A gradual onset is characteristic of parkinsonism and is commonly associated with bradykinesia and cogwheel rigidity (Chap. 351). A rest tremor that develops acutely is usually due to toxins [such as exposure to 1-methyl-4-phenyl-1,2,3,6-tetrahydropyridine (MPTP)] or dopamine blocking drugs (such as phenothiazines). A *postural tremor* is maximal while limb posture is actively maintained against gravity; it is lessened by rest and is not markedly enhanced during voluntary movement toward a target. A postural tremor that develops acutely is usually due to toxic or metabolic factors (for example, hyperthyroidism) or stress. The insidious onset of a postural tremor suggests a benign or familial essential tremor. An *intention tremor* is most prominent during voluntary movement toward a target and is not present during postural maintenance or at rest. It is a sign of cerebellar disease (Chap. 352). *Asterixis*, which may superficially resemble a tremor, is an intermittent inhibition of muscle contraction that occurs with metabolic encephalopathy (Chap. 257). This leads, for example, to a momentary and repetitive partial flexion of the wrists during attempted sustained wrist extension.

Irregular involuntary movements are characterized by their speed and location, and by whether they can be suppressed voluntarily. The slowest are athetosis and dystonia. *Athetosis* is a slow, writhing, sinuous movement that occurs nearly continuously in distal muscles. *Dystonia* is a slowly varying but nearly continuous deviation of posture about one or more joints; it may occur in a proximal or distal limb or in axial structures. Dystonia is a more sustained deviation of posture than athetosis, although these two phenomena overlap considerably. →*The further evaluation of athetosis and dystonia is discussed in Chap. 351.*

Among the rapid irregular movements, *tics* are controlled with voluntary effort, while the others are not. Tics often occur repetitively in a single location but are sometimes multifocal.

Chorea, hemiballismus, and myoclonus are rapid, irregular jerks that cannot be voluntarily suppressed. *Hemiballismus* manifests as a sudden and often violent flinging movement of a proximal limb, usually an arm. Hemiballismus usually develops acutely due to infarction of the contralateral subthalamic nucleus but occasionally develops subacutely or chronically due to other lesions of this nucleus.

Chorea is a rapid, jerky, irregular movement that tends to occur in the distal limbs or face but may also occur in proximal limbs and trunk. Acute or subacute onset is usually due to toxins including excess levodopa or dopamine-agonist therapy or, less often, neuroleptics, birth control pills, pregnancy (chorea gravidarum), hyperthyroidism, or the antiphospholipid syndrome. In children, it may be associated with rheumatic fever and, in such cases, is referred to as *Sydenham's chorea*. The gradual onset of chorea is typical of degenerative neurologic diseases, such as Huntington's disease.

Myoclonus is a rapid, brief, irregular movement that is usually multifocal. Myoclonus can occur spontaneously at rest, in response to sensory stimuli, or with voluntary movements. It is a symptom that occurs in a wide variety of metabolic and neurologic disorders. Posthypoxic intention myoclonus is a special myoclonic syndrome that occurs as a sequel to transient cerebral anoxia. Myoclonus may result from lipid storage disease, encephalitis, prion diseases, or metabolic encephalopathies due to respiratory failure, chronic renal failure, hepatic failure, or electrolyte imbalance. Myoclonus is also a feature of certain types of epilepsy (Chap. 348). *Palatal and segmental myoclonus* are uncommon rhythmic forms of myoclonus that may resemble tremor; they are caused by structural disease of the brainstem or spinal cord at the level of the abnormal movement.

Hypokinetic Movement Disorders These manifest as bradykinesia, with a masked, expressionless facial appearance, loss of associated limb movements during walking, and rigid en bloc turning. If bradykinesia is associated only with a rest tremor, cogwheel rigidity, or impairment of postural reflexes (especially with a tendency to fall backwards), Parkinson's disease is likely. If cognitive, language, upper motor neuron, sensory, or autonomic signs are also present, a *multisystem degenerative neurologic disease* is present. →*These disorders are discussed in Chaps. 351, 352, and 354.*

IMBALANCE AND DISORDERS OF GAIT

Imbalance is the impaired ability to maintain the intended orientation of the body in space. It is generally manifest as difficulty in maintaining an upright posture while standing or walking; a severe imbalance may also affect the ability to maintain posture while seated. Patients with imbalance commonly complain of a feeling of unsteadiness or dysequilibrium. Whereas imbalance and unsteadiness are synonymous, *dysequilibrium* implies the additional component of impaired spatial orientation even while lying down. Patients with dysequilibrium commonly also experience *vertigo*, defined as an hallucination of rotatory movement.

PATHOGENESIS ■ Imbalance and Limb Ataxia Imbalance results from disorders of the vestibular, sensory, or cerebellar systems, whereas limb ataxia is produced by disorders of the sensory or cerebellar systems. Asymmetric vestibular sensory input to the brainstem and cerebellum produces asymmetric imbalance, but not limb ataxia. Sensory ataxia is caused by lesions that affect the peripheral sensory fibers; dorsal root ganglia cells; posterior columns of the spinal cord; or lemniscal system in the brainstem, thalamus, or parietal cortex (Chap. 22). Impairment of the proprioceptive sensory feedback to the cerebellum, basal ganglia, and cortex produces sensory ataxia. Sensory ataxia results in imbalance and disturbs the fluency and integration of limb movements that can be partially alleviated by visual feedback. Imbalance with cerebellar ataxia results from disorders of proprioceptive, spinocerebellar, or vestibular sensory input; the integration of these inputs in the brainstem or midline cerebellar vermis or flocculonodular lobe; or the motor output to the spinal neurons that control muscles of the proximal limbs and trunk. Cerebellar limb ataxia results from disorders of the spinocerebellar and corticopontocerebellar inputs, the integration of these inputs in the intermediate and lateral cerebellum, or the output to the spinal neurons (via the red nucleus and rubrospinal tract) or to the cortex. These pathways ensure adequate speed, fluency, and integration of limb movements. The lateral cerebellar hemispheres coordinate a polysynaptic feedback circuit that modulates cortically initiated limb movement.

Disorders of Gait Walking is one of the most complicated motor activities. Cyclical stepping movements produced by the lumbosacral spinal cord centers are modified by cortical, basal ganglionic, brainstem, and cerebellar influences based on proprioceptive, vestibular, and visual feedback.

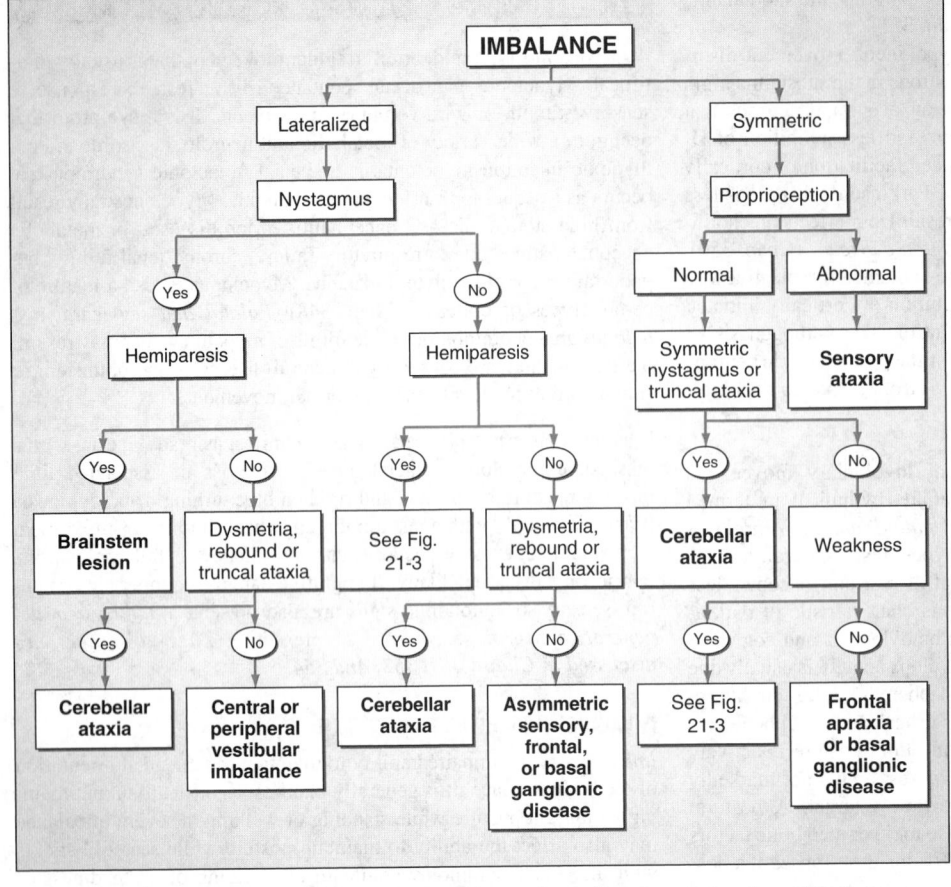

FIGURE 21-4 An algorithm for evaluation of imbalance without weakness; if weakness is present, see Fig. 21-3.

resolve if a provocative position is maintained (extinction) or repeated (habituation). Lateralized imbalance of gradual onset or persisting for >2 weeks, accompanied by nystagmus, may result from lesions of the semicircular canal or vestibular nerve, brainstem, or cerebellum.

Imbalance with sensory ataxia is characterized by marked worsening when visual feedback is removed. The patient can often assume the upright stance with feet together cautiously with eyes open. With eye closure, balance is rapidly lost (positive Romberg sign) in various directions at random. Sensory examination reveals impairment of proprioception at the toes and ankles, usually associated with an even more prominent abnormality of vibratory perception. Prompt evaluation for vitamin B_{12} deficiency is important, as this disorder is reversible if recognized early. Depression or absence of reflexes points to peripheral nerve disorders. Spasticity with extensor plantar responses suggests posterior column and spinal cord disorders. Rarely, sensory ataxia produces lateralized imbalance. In these cases, the disorder is usually in the parietal lobe or thalamus, but may also be due to an asymmetric sensory neuropathy or posterior column disease.

Sensory limb ataxia is similar to cerebellar limb ataxia but is markedly worse when the eyes are closed. Examination also reveals abnormal proprioception and vibratory perception. The approach focuses on localizing the proprioceptive impairment to the peripheral nerves, the posterior columns of the spinal cord, or rarely the parietal lobe.

Other forms of imbalance occur, but the fundamental problem is usually a primary disorder of strength, extrapyramidal function, or cortical initiation of movement, as indicated in Fig. 21-4.

Abnormal Gait Each of the disorders discussed in this chapter produces a characteristic gait disturbance. If the neurologic examination is normal except for an abnormal gait, diagnosis may be difficult even for the experienced clinician.

Hemiparetic gait characterizes spastic hemiparesis. In its most severe form, an abnormal posture of the limbs is produced by spasticity. The arm is adducted and internally rotated, with flexion of the elbow, wrist, and fingers and with extension of the hip, knee, and ankle. Forward swing of the spastic leg during walking requires abduction and circumduction at the hip, often with contralateral tilt of the trunk to prevent the toes catching on the floor as the leg is advanced. In its mildest form, the affected arm is held in a normal position, but swings less than the normal arm. The affected leg is flexed less than the normal leg during its forward swing and is more externally rotated. A hemiparetic gait is a common residual sign of a stroke.

Paraparetic gait is a walking pattern in which both legs are moved in a slow, stiff manner with circumduction, similar to the leg movement in a hemiparetic gait. In many patients, the legs tend to cross with each forward swing ("scissoring"). A paraparetic gait is a common sign of spinal cord disease and also occurs in cerebral palsy.

Steppage gait is produced by weakness of ankle dorsiflexion. Because of the partial or complete foot drop, the leg must be lifted higher than usual to avoid catching the toe on the floor during the forward swing of the leg. If unilateral, steppage gait is usually due to L5 radiculopathy, sciatic neuropathy, or peroneal neuropathy. If bilateral, it

Imbalance A guide to interpretation of imbalance without weakness is presented in Fig. 21-4.

Imbalance with cerebellar ataxia typically produces truncal ataxia, which is usually revealed during the process of rising from a chair, assuming the upright stance with the feet together, or performing some other activity while standing. Once a desired position is reached, imbalance may be surprisingly mild. As walking begins, the imbalance recurs. Patients usually learn to lessen the imbalance by walking with the legs widely separated. The imbalance is usually not lateralized; may be accompanied by symmetric nystagmus; and is caused by toxic, metabolic, inflammatory, or neurodegenerative diseases. Asymmetric cerebellar ataxia suggests structural disease from ischemia, tumor, or other mass lesion.

Cerebellar limb ataxia is characterized by dysmetria (irregular errors in amplitude and force of movements); intention tremor (accentuation as the target is approached); dysdiadochokinesia (errors in rythm, velocity or force); and excessive rebound of outstretched arms against a resistance that is suddenly removed. Muscle tone is often modestly reduced; this contributes to the abnormal rebound due to decreased activation of segmental spinal cord reflexes and also to pendular reflexes, i.e., a tendency for a tendon reflex to produce multiple swings to and fro after a single tap. If involvement is asymmetric, lateralized imbalance is common and usually associated with asymmetric nystagmus. →*For further discussion of cerebellar diseases, see Chap. 352.*

Imbalance with vestibular dysfunction is characterized by a consistent tendency to fall to one side. The patient commonly complains of vertigo rather than imbalance, especially if the onset is acute. Acute vertigo associated with lateralized imbalance but no other neurologic signs is often due to disorders of the semicircular canal (Chap. 20); the presence of other neurologic signs suggests brainstem ischemia (Chap. 349) or multiple sclerosis (Chap. 359). When the vestibular dysfunction is peripheral, positional nystagmus and vertigo tend to

is the common result of a distal polyneuropathy or lumbosacral polyradiculopathy.

Waddling gait results from proximal lower limb weakness, most often from myopathy but occasionally from neuromuscular junction disease or a proximal symmetric spinal muscular atrophy. With weakness of hip flexion, the trunk is tilted away from the leg that is being moved to lift the hip and provide extra distance between the foot and the floor, and the pelvis is rotated forward to assist with forward motion of the leg. Because pelvic girdle weakness is customarily bilateral, the pelvic lift and rotation alternate from side to side, giving the waddling appearance to the gait.

Parkinsonian gait is characterized by a forward stoop, with modest flexion at the hips and knees. The arms are flexed at the elbows and adducted at the shoulders, often with a 4- to 6-Hz resting pronation-supination tremor but little other movement, even during walking. Walking is initiated slowly by leaning forward and maintained with short rapid steps, during which the feet shuffle along the floor. The pace tends to accelerate (festination) as the upper body gradually leans further ahead of the feet, whether movement is forward (propulsion) or backward (retropulsion). The postural instability leads to falls (Chap. 351).

Apraxic gait results from bilateral frontal lobe disease with impaired ability to plan and execute sequential movements. This gait superficially resembles that of parkinsonism, in that the posture is stooped and any steps taken are short and shuffling. However, initiation and maintenance of walking are impaired in a different manner. Each movement that is required for walking can usually be performed, if tested in isolation while sitting or lying. However, when asked to step forward while standing, a long pause often occurs before any attempt is made to flex at the hip and advance, as if the patient is "glued to the ground." Once walking is initiated, it is not maintained, even in an abnormal festinating manner. Rather, after one or several steps are taken, walking is stopped for several seconds or longer. The process is then repeated. Dementia and incontinence may coexist.

Choreoathetotic gait is characterized by an intermittent, irregular movement that disrupts the smooth flow of a normal gait. Flexion or extension movements at the hip are common and unpredictable but readily observed as a pelvic lurch.

Cerebellar ataxic gait is a broad-based gait disorder in which the speed and length of stride varies irregularly from step to step. With midline cerebellar disease, as in alcoholics, posture is erect but the feet are separated; lower limb ataxia is commonly present as well. With disease of the cerebellar hemispheres, limb ataxia and nystagmus are commonly present as well.

Sensory ataxic gait may resemble a cerebellar gait, with its broad-based stance and difficulty with change in position. However, although balance may be maintained with the eyes open, loss of visual input through eye closure results in rapid loss of balance with a fall (positive Romberg sign), unless the physician assists the patient.

Vestibular gait is one in which the patient consistently tends to fall to one side, whether walking or standing. Cranial nerve examination usually demonstrates an asymmetric nystagmus. The possibilities of unilateral sensory ataxia and hemiparesis are excluded by the findings of normal proprioception and strength.

Astasia-abasia is a typical hysterical gait disorder. Although the patient usually has normal coordination of leg movements in bed or while sitting, the patient is unable to stand or walk without assistance. If distracted, stationary balance is sometimes maintained and several steps are taken normally, followed by a dramatic demonstration of imbalance with a lunge toward the examiner's arms or a nearby bed.

FURTHER READING

CAPADAY C: The special nature of human walking and its neural control. Trends Neurosci 25:370, 2002

DIETZ V: Proprioception and locomotor disorders. Nat Rev Neurosci 3:781, 2002

---

22 | NUMBNESS, TINGLING, AND SENSORY LOSS
Arthur K. Asbury

NORMAL SENSATION

Normal somatic sensation reflects a continuous day and night monitoring process that occupies considerable moment-to-moment nervous system capacity. Little of this activity reaches consciousness under ordinary conditions. In contrast, disordered sensation, particularly if experienced as painful, is alarming and dominates the sufferer's attention. Abnormalities of sensation, especially if painful, tend to make those suffering seek medical help. The physician must be able to recognize abnormal sensations by how they are described, know their type and likely site of origin, and understand their implications. →*For a consideration of pain, see Chap. 11.*

POSITIVE AND NEGATIVE PHENOMENA Abnormal sensory phenomena may be divided into two categories, positive and negative. The prototypical positive phenomenon is tingling (pins-and-needles), and the principal negative phenomenon is numbness. In addition to tingling, positive sensory phenomena include other altered sensations that are described as pricking, bandlike, lightning-like shooting feelings (lancinations), aching, knifelike, twisting, drawing, pulling, tightening, burning, searing, electrical, or raw feelings. These descriptors are frequently the actual words used by patients. Such sensations are usually experienced as painful, but not necessarily.

Positive phenomena usually result from trains of impulses generated at a site or sites of lowered threshold or heightened excitability along a sensory pathway, either peripheral or central. The nature and severity of an abnormal sensation depend on the number, rate, timing, and distribution of ectopic impulses and the type and function of nervous tissue in which they arise. Because positive phenomena represent excessive activity in sensory pathways, they are not necessarily associated with sensory deficit (loss) upon examination.

Negative phenomena represent loss of sensory function and are characterized by diminished or absent feeling, often experienced as numbness. In contrast to positive phenomena, negative phenomena are accompanied by abnormal findings on sensory examination. In disorders affecting peripheral sensation, it is estimated that at least half the afferent axons innervating a given site are lost or functionless before sensory deficit can be demonstrated by clinical examination. This threshold varies according to how rapidly sensory nerve fibers have lost function. If the rate of loss is slow and chronic, lack of cutaneous feeling may be unnoticed by the patient and difficult to demonstrate on examination, even though few sensory fibers are functioning. Rapidly evolving sensory abnormality usually evokes both positive and negative phenomena that are readily noticed. Subclinical degrees of sensory dysfunction not demonstrable on clinical sensory examination may be revealed by sensory nerve conduction studies or somatosensory evoked potentials (Chap. 359). Sensory symptoms may be either positive or negative, but sensory signs on examination are always a measure of negative phenomena.

TERMINOLOGY Words used to characterize sensory disturbance are descriptive and have been arrived at mainly by convention. Paresthesia and dysesthesia are general terms used to denote sensory symptoms (positive phenomena) and are usually stated in the plural form. *Paresthesias* usually refer to tingling or pins-and-needles sensations but may also include a wide variety of other abnormal sensations, excepting pain. Sometimes "paresthesias" carry the implication that the abnormal sensations are perceived without an apparent stimulus. *Dysesthesia* is a more general term denoting all types of abnormal sensations, even painful ones, whether a stimulus is evident or not.

While paresthesias and dysesthesias refer to sensations described by patients, another set of terms refers to sensory abnormalities found on examination. These include *hypesthesia* or *hypoesthesia* (reduction of cutaneous sensation to a specific type of testing such as pressure, light touch, and warm or cold stimuli); *anesthesia* (complete absence of skin sensation to the same stimuli plus pinprick); and *hypalgesia* (referring to reduced pain perception, i.e., nociception, such as the pricking quality elicited by a pin). *Hyperesthesia* means pain in response to touch. Similarly, *allodynia* describes the situation in which a nonpainful stimulus, once perceived, is experienced as painful, even excruciating. An example is elicitation of a painful sensation by application of a vibrating tuning fork. *Hyperalgesia* denotes severe pain in response to a mildly noxious stimulus, and *hyperpathia*, a broad term, encompasses all the phenomena described by hyperesthesia, allodynia, and hyperalgesia. With hyperpathia, the threshold for a sensory stimulus is increased and the perception is delayed, but once felt, is unduly painful.

Disorders of deep sensation, arising from muscle spindles, tendons, and joints, affect proprioception (position sense). Manifestations include imbalance (particularly with eyes closed or in the dark), clumsiness of precision movements, and unsteadiness of gait, which are referred to collectively as *sensory ataxia* (Chap. 21). Other findings on examination usually, but not invariably, include reduced or absent joint position and vibratory sensibility and absent deep tendon reflexes in the affected limbs. Romberg's sign is positive, which means that the patient sways or topples when asked to stand with feet close together and eyes closed. In severe states of deafferentation involving deep sensation, the patient cannot walk or stand unaided or even sit unsupported. Continuous, sometimes wormlike involuntary movements, called *pseudoathetosis*, of the outstretched hands and fingers occur, particularly with eyes closed. Such patients are severely disabled.

ANATOMY OF SENSATION   Cutaneous afferent innervation is conveyed by a rich variety of receptors, both naked nerve endings (nociceptors and thermoreceptors) and encapsulated terminals (mechanoreceptors). Each type of receptor has its own set of sensitivities to specific stimuli, size and distinctness of receptive fields, and adaptational qualities. Much of the knowledge about these receptors has come from the development of techniques to study single intact nerve fibers intraneurally in awake, unanesthetized human subjects. It is possible not only to record from single nerve fibers, large or small, but also to stimulate single fibers in isolation. A single impulse, whether elicited by a natural stimulus or evoked by electrical microstimulation, in a large myelinated afferent fiber may be both perceived and localized.

Afferent fibers of all sizes in peripheral nerve trunks traverse the dorsal roots and enter the dorsal horn of the spinal cord (Fig. 22-1). From there the smaller fibers take a different route to the parietal cortex than the larger fibers. The polysynaptic projections of the smaller fibers (unmyelinated and small myelinated), which subserve mainly nociception, temperature sensibility, and touch, cross and ascend in the opposite anterior and lateral columns of the spinal cord, through the brainstem, to the ventral posterolateral (VPL) nucleus of the thalamus, and ultimately project to the postcentral gyrus of the parietal cortex (Chap. 11). This is referred to as the *spinothalamic pathway*, or *anterolateral system*. The larger fibers, which subserve tactile and position sense and kinesthesia, project rostrally in the posterior column on the same side of the spinal cord and make their first synapse in the gracile or cuneate nuclei of the lower medulla. The second-order neuron decussates and ascends in the medial lemniscus located medially in the medulla and in the tegmentum of the pons and midbrain and synapses in the VPL nucleus. The third-order neuron projects to pa-

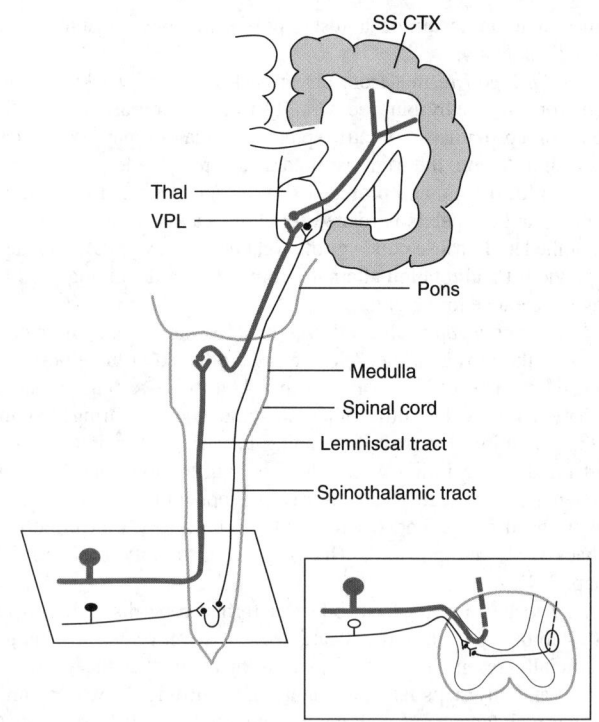

FIGURE 22-1   Schematic diagram of lemniscal and spinothalamic pathways. Note that the large fibers that subserve proprioception and discriminative touch ascend ipsilaterally as the lemniscal pathway in the posterior column of the spinal cord, and that the small fibers that subserve pain, thermal sensation, and crude touch ascend contralaterally as the spinothalamic pathway in the anterior and lateral columns of the spinal cord (insert). SS CTX, somatosensory cortex; Thal, thalamus; VPL, ventral posterolateral nucleus.

rietal cortex; this large fiber system is referred to as the *posterior column–medial lemniscal pathway* (lemniscal, for short). Note that although the lemniscal and the anterolateral pathways both project up the spinal cord to the thalamus, it is the (crossed) anterolateral pathway that is referred to as the *spinothalamic tract*, by convention.

Although the fiber types and functions that make up the spinothalamic and lemniscal systems are relatively well known, it has been found that many other fibers, particularly those associated with touch, pressure, and position sense, ascend in a diffusely distributed pattern both ipsilaterally and contralaterally in the anterolateral quadrants of the spinal cord. This explains why an individual with a complete lesion of the posterior columns of the spinal cord may have little sensory deficit on examination.

EXAMINATION OF SENSATION

The main components of the sensory examination are tests of primary sensation. These include the sense of pain, touch, vibration, joint position, and thermal sensation, both hot and cold (Table 22-1). Detailed descriptions of how to perform the various tests of the sensory examination can be found in standard texts (see "Bibliography").

Some general principles pertain. The examiner must depend on patient responses, particularly when testing cutaneous sensation (pin, touch, warm or cold). This subjective element complicates the interpretation of the sensory examination. Further, some patients are only partially examinable. In a stuporous patient, sensory examination is reduced to observing the briskness of withdrawal in response to a pinch or other noxious stimulus. Comparison of response on one side of the body to the other is essential. In the alert but uncooperative patient, cutaneous sensation may be unexaminable. However, it is usually possible to get some idea of proprioceptive function by noting the patient's best performance of movements requiring balance and precision. Frequently, patients present with sensory symptoms that do not fit an anatomic localization and that are accompanied by either no abnormalities or gross inconsistencies on examination. The examiner should then consider whether the sensory symptoms are a disguised request for help with psychological or situational problems. Discretion must be used in pursuing this possibility. Finally, sensory examination of a patient who has no neurologic complaints can be brief and consist of pin, touch, and vibration testing in the hands and feet plus evaluation of stance and gait, including the Romberg maneuver. Evaluation of stance and gait also tests the integrity of motor and cerebellar systems.

PRIMARY SENSATION (See Table 22-1)

The sense of pain is usually tested with a clean pin, asking the patient to focus on the pricking or unpleasant quality of the stimulus and not just the pressure or touch sensation elicited. Areas of hypalgesia should be mapped by proceeding radially from the most hypalgesic site (Figs. 22-2 and 22-3).

Temperature sensation, to both hot and cold, is probably best tested with water flasks filled with water of the desired temperature, using a thermometer to verify the temperature. This is impractical in most settings. An alternative way to test cold sensation is to touch a metal object, such as a tuning fork at room temperature, to the skin. For testing warm temperatures, the tuning fork or other metal object may be held under warm water of the desired temperature and then used. Both cold and warm should be tested because different receptors respond to each.

Touch is usually tested with a wisp of cotton or a fine camelhair brush. In general, it is better to avoid testing touch on hairy skin because of the profusion of sensory endings that surround each hair follicle.

Joint position testing is a measure of proprioception, one of the most important functions of the sensory system. With the patient keeping eyes closed, joint position is tested in the great toe and in the fingers. If errors are made in recognizing the direction of passive movements of the toe or the finger, more proximal joints should be tested. A test of proximal joint position sense, primarily at the shoulder, is performed by asking the patient to bring the two index fingers together with arms extended and eyes closed. Normal individuals can do this accurately, with errors of a centimeter or less.

The sense of vibration is tested with a tuning fork, preferably a large one that vibrates at 128 Hz. Vibration is usually tested at bony prominences, beginning distally at the malleoli of the ankles, and at the knuckles. If abnormalities are found, more proximal sites can be examined. Vibratory thesholds at the same site in the patient and the examiner may be compared for control purposes.

QUANTITATIVE SENSORY TESTING Effective sensory testing devices have been developed over the past two decades. Quantitative sensory testing is particularly useful for serial evaluation of cutaneous sensation in clinical trials. Threshold testing for touch and vibratory and thermal sensation is the most widely used application.

CORTICAL SENSATION The most commonly used tests of cortical function are two-point discrimination, touch localization, and bilateral simultaneous stimulation and tests for graphesthesia and stereognosis. Abnormalities of these sensory tests, in the presence of normal primary sensation in an alert cooperative patient, signify a lesion of the parietal cortex or thalamocortical projections to the parietal lobe. If primary sensation is altered, these cortical discriminative functions will usually be abnormal, too. Comparisons should always be made between analogous sites on the two sides of the body because the deficit with a specific parietal lesion is likely to be hemilateral. Side-to-side comparisons hold true for all cortical sensory testing.

Two-point discrimination is tested by special calipers, the points of which may be set from 2 mm to several centimeters apart and then applied simultaneously to the site to be tested. The pulp of the finger tips is a common site to test; a normal individual can distinguish about 3-mm separation of points there.

Touch localization is usually carried out by light pressure for an instant with the examiner's fingertip, asking the patient, whose eyes are closed, to identify the site of touch with his or her fingertip. *Bilateral simultaneous stimulation* at analogous sites (e.g., the dorsa of both hands) can be carried out to determine whether the perception of touch is extinguished consistently on one side or the other. The phenomenon is referred to as *extinction. Graphesthesia* means the capacity to recognize with eyes closed letters or numbers drawn by the examiner's fingertip on the palm of the hand. Once again, the comparison of one side with the other is of prime importance. Inability to recognize numbers or letters is termed *agraphesthesia*.

Stereognosis refers to the ability to identify common objects by palpation, recognizing their shape, texture, and size. Common standard objects are the best test objects, such as a marble, a paper clip, or coins. Patients with normal stereognosis should be able to distinguish a dime from a penny and a nickel from a quarter without looking. Patients should only be allowed to feel the object with one hand at a time. If they are unable to identify it in one hand, it should be placed in the other for comparison. Individuals unable to identify common objects and coins in one hand who can do so in the other are said to have *astereognosis* of the abnormal hand.

LOCALIZATION OF SENSORY ABNORMALITIES

Sensory symptoms and signs can result from lesions at almost any level of the nervous system, including parietal cortex, deep white matter, thalamus, brainstem, spinal cord, spinal root, peripheral nerve, and sensory receptor. Noting the distribution and nature of sensory symptoms and signs is the most important way to localize their source. The extent, configuration, symmetry, quality, and severity are the key observations.

Dysesthesias without sensory findings by examination can be difficult to interpret. To illustrate, tingling dysesthesias in an acral distribution (hands and feet) can be systemic in origin, e.g., secondary to hyperventilation, or can be induced by a medication, such as the diuretic acetazolamide. Distal dysesthesias can also be an early event in an evolving polyneuropathy or can herald a myelopathy, such as with vitamin B_{12} deficiency. Sometimes distal dysesthesias have no definable basis. In contrast, dysesthesias that correspond to a particular peripheral nerve territory denote a lesion of that nerve trunk. For instance, dysesthesias restricted to the fifth digit and the adjacent one-half of the fourth finger on one hand reliably point to disorder of the ulnar nerve, most commonly at the elbow.

NERVE AND ROOT In focal nerve trunk lesions severe enough to cause a deficit, sensory abnormalities are readily mapped and generally have discrete boundaries (Figs. 22-2 and 22-3). Root lesions, referred to as radicular, are frequently accompanied by deep, aching pain along the

---

TABLE 22-1 *Testing Primary Sensation*

Sense	Test Device	Endings Activated	Fiber Size Mediating	Central Pathway
Pain	Pinprick	Cutaneous nociceptors	Small	SpTh, also D
Temperature, heat	Warm metal object	Cutaneous thermoreceptors for hot	Small	SpTh
Temperature, cold	Cold metal object	Cutaneous thermoreceptors for cold	Small	SpTh
Touch	Cotton wisp, fine brush	Cutaneous mechanoreceptors, also naked endings	Large and small	Lem, also D and SpTh
Vibration	Tuning fork, 128 Hz	Mechanoreceptors, especially pacinian corpuscles	Large	Lem, also D
Joint position	Passive movement of specific joints	Joint capsule and tendon endings, muscle spindles	Large	Lem, also D

Note: D, diffuse ascending projections in ipsilateral and contralateral anterolateral columns; SpTh, spinothalamic projection, contralateral; Lem, posterior column and lemniscal projection, ipsilateral.

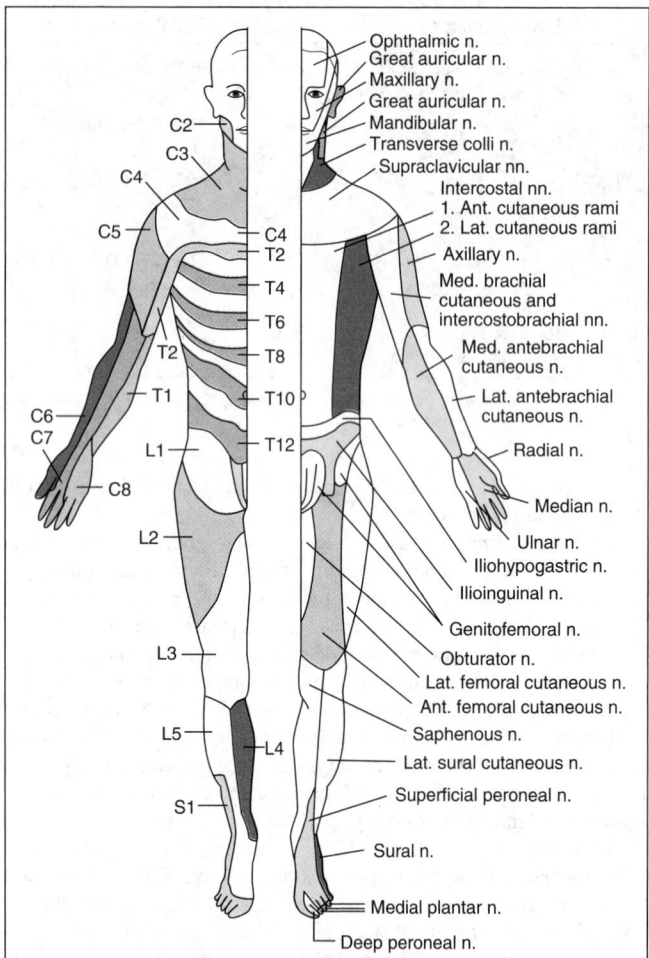

FIGURE 22-2 Anterior view of dermatomes *(left)* and cutaneous areas *(right)* supplied by individual peripheral nerves. *(Modified from MB Carpenter and J Sutin, in Human Neuroanatomy, 8th ed, Baltimore, Williams & Wilkins, 1983.)*

course of the related nerve trunk. With compression of a fifth lumbar (L5) or first sacral (S1) root, as may occur with a ruptured intervertebral disc, sciatica (radicular pain relating to the sciatic nerve trunk) is a frequent manifestation (Chap. 15). With a lesion affecting a single root, sensory deficit in the distribution of that root is often minimal or not demonstrable at all. This is because adjacent root territories overlap extensively.

Polyneuropathies are generally graded, distal, and symmetric in distribution of deficit (Chap. 363). Dysesthesias begin in the toes and ascend symmetrically, followed by numbness. When dysesthesias reach the knees, they have usually also appeared in the fingertips. The process appears to be nerve length–dependent, and the deficit is often described as "stocking-glove" in type. Although most polyneuropathies are pansensory and affect all modalities of sensation, selective sensory dysfunction according to nerve fiber size may occur. In polyneuropathies that affect small nerve fibers selectively, the hallmark is burning, painful dysesthesias with reduced pinprick and thermal sensation but with sparing of proprioception, motor function, and even deep tendon jerks. Touch is variably involved, but when spared, the sensory pattern is referred to as *sensory dissociation*. Sensory dissociation patterns can be seen with spinal cord lesions (see below) as well as with small fiber neuropathies. In contrast to small fiber polyneuropathies, large fiber polyneuropathies are characterized by position sense deficit, imbalance, absent tendon jerks, and variable motor dysfunction but preservation of most cutaneous sensation. Dysesthesias, if present at all, tend to be tingling or bandlike.

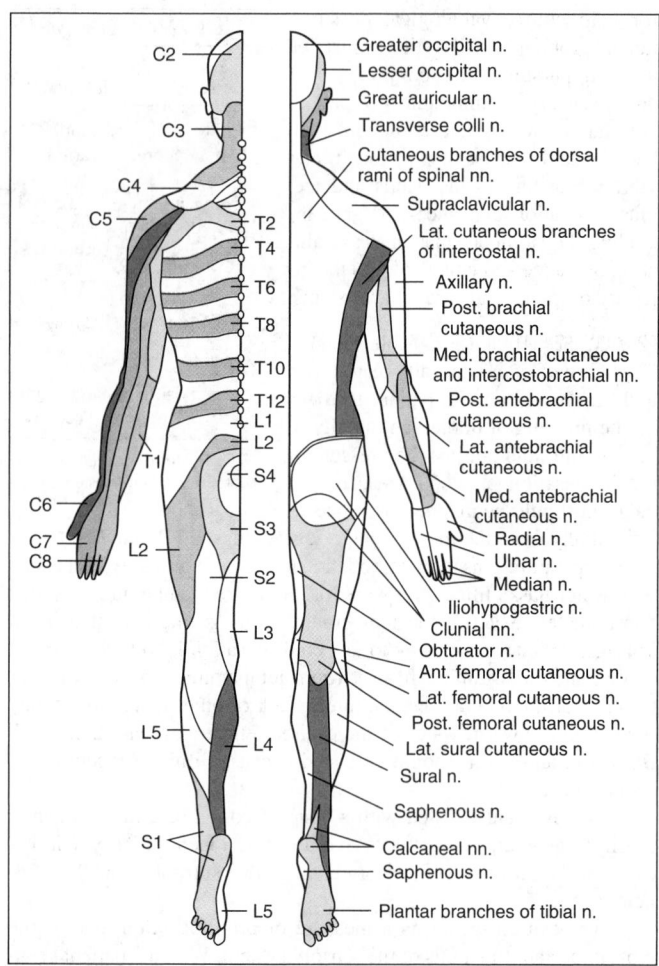

FIGURE 22-3 Posterior view of dermatomes *(left)* and cutaneous areas *(right)* supplied by individual peripheral nerves. *(Modified from MB Carpenter and J Sutin, in Human Neuroanatomy, 8th ed, Baltimore, Williams & Wilkins, 1983.)*

SPINAL CORD (See also Chap. 356)   If the spinal cord is transected, all sensation is lost below the level of transection. Bladder and bowel function are also lost, as is motor function. Hemisection of the spinal cord produces the Brown-Séquard syndrome, which involves absent pain and temperature sensation on the opposite side below the lesion, and loss of proprioceptive sensation and loss of motor power on the same side below the lesion (see Figs. 22-1 and 356-1). Dissociated sensory deficit patterns (see above) are also a sign of spinothalamic tract involvement in the spinal cord, especially if the deficit is unilateral and has an upper level on the torso. Bilateral spinothalamic tract involvement occurs with lesions affecting the center of the spinal cord, such as happens with expansion of the central canal in syringomyelia. Sensory dissociation is characteristic of syringomyelia.

BRAINSTEM   Harlequin patterns of sensory disturbance, in which one side of the face and the opposite side of the body are affected, localize to the lateral medulla. Here a small lesion may damage both the ipsilateral descending trigeminal tract and ascending spinothalamic fibers subserving the opposite arm, leg, and hemitorso (see "Lateral medullary syndrome" in Fig. 349-8). In the tegmentum of the pons and midbrain, where the lemniscal and spinothalamic tracts merge, a lesion here causes pansensory loss on the contralateral side.

THALAMUS   Hemisensory disturbance with tingling numbness from head to foot is often thalamic in origin but can also be anterior parietal. If abrupt in onset, the lesion is likely to be due to a small stroke (lacunar infarction), particularly if localized to the thalamus. Occasionally, with lesions affecting the VPL nucleus or adjacent white matter, a syndrome of thalamic pain, also called *Déjerine-Roussy syndrome*, may ensue. This persistent, unrelenting hemipainful state is often described in dramatic terms such as "like the flesh is being torn from my limbs" or "as though that side is bathed in acid."

CORTEX With lesions of the parietal lobe involving either the cortex or subjacent white matter, the most prominent symptoms are contralateral hemineglect, hemi-inattention, and a tendency not to use the affected hand and arm. On cortical sensory testing (two-point discrimination, graphesthesia, etc.), abnormalities are often found, but primary sensation is usually intact. Anterior parietal infarction may present as a pseudothalamic syndrome with crossed hemilateral loss of primary sensation from head to toe. Dysesthesias or a sense of numbness may also occur, and rarely, a painful state.

FOCAL SENSORY SEIZURES These are generally due to lesions in the area of the postcentral and/or precentral gyrus. The principal symptoms of focal sensory seizures are tingling or numbness or both, but additional, more complex sensations may occur, such as a rushing feeling, a sense of warmth, or a sense of movement without detectable motion. Likely sites of unilateral symptom origin are in the arm or hand, face, leg, or foot, and symptoms often spread as in a Jacksonian march. Duration of seizures is variable; they may be transient, lasting only seconds, or they may persist for an hour or more. Focal motor features, like clonic jerking, can supervene, and seizures often become generalized with loss of consciousness and tonic-clonic jerking. On occasion, symptoms occur in a symmetric bilateral fashion, for instance, in both hands, as a result of involvement of the second sensory area (unilaterally) located in the rolandic area at and just above the Sylvian fissure.

23 | APHASIA, MEMORY LOSS, AND OTHER FOCAL CEREBRAL DISORDERS
M.-Marsel Mesulam

The cerebral cortex of the human brain contains approximately 20 billion neurons spread over an area of 2.5 m². The *primary sensory* areas provide an obligatory portal for the entry of sensory information into cortical circuitry, whereas the *primary motor* areas provide a final common pathway for coordinating complex motor acts. The primary sensory and motor areas constitute 10% of the cerebral cortex. The rest is subsumed by unimodal, heteromodal, paralimbic, and limbic areas, collectively known as the *association cortex* (Fig. 23-1). The association cortex mediates the integrative processes that subserve cognition, emotion, and behavior. A systematic testing of these mental functions is necessary for the effective clinical assessment of the association cortex and its diseases.

According to current thinking, there are no centers for "hearing words," "perceiving space," or "storing memories." Cognitive and behavioral functions (domains) are coordinated by intersecting *large-scale neural networks* that contain interconnected cortical and subcortical components. The network approach to higher cerebral function has at least four implications of clinical relevance: (1) a single domain such as language or memory can be disrupted by damage to any one of several areas, as long as these areas belong to the same network; (2) damage confined to a single area can give rise to multiple deficits, involving the functions of all networks that intersect in that region; (3) damage to a network component may give rise to minimal or transient deficits if other parts of the network undergo compensatory reorganization; and (4) individual anatomic sites within a network display a relative (but not absolute) specialization for different behavioral aspects of the relevant function. Five anatomically defined large-scale networks are most relevant to clinical practice: a perisylvian network for language; a parietofrontal network for spatial cognition; an occipitotemporal network for face and object recognition; a limbic network for retentive memory; and a prefrontal network for attention and behavior.

THE LEFT PERISYLVIAN NETWORK FOR LANGUAGE: APHASIAS AND RELATED CONDITIONS

Language allows the communication and elaboration of thoughts and experiences by linking them to arbitrary symbols known as words. The neural substrate of language is composed of a distributed network centered in the perisylvian region of the *left* hemisphere. The posterior pole of this network is known as *Wernicke's area* and includes the posterior third of the superior temporal gyrus and a surrounding rim of inferior parietal and midtemporal cortex. An essential function of Wernicke's area is to transform sensory inputs into their neural word representations so that these can establish the distributed associations that give the word its meaning. The anterior pole of the language network, known as *Broca's area*, includes the posterior part of the inferior frontal gyrus and a surrounding rim of prefrontal heteromodal

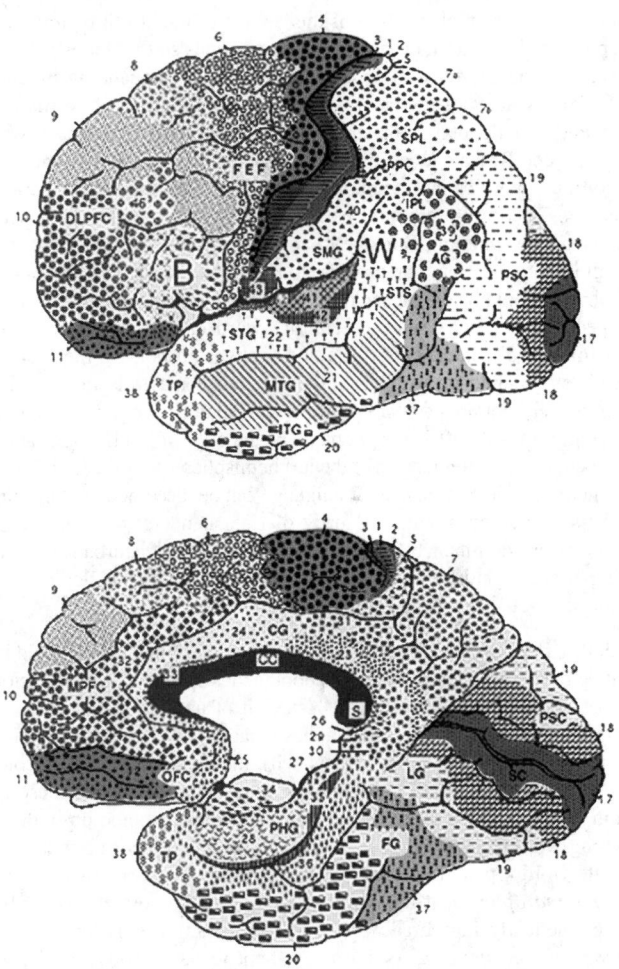

FIGURE 23-1 Lateral (*top*) and medial (*bottom*) views of the cerebral hemispheres. The numbers refer to the Brodmann cytoarchitectonic designations. Area 17 corresponds to primary visual cortex, 41–42 to primary auditory cortex, 1–3 to primary somatosensory cortex, and 4 to primary motor cortex. The rest of the cerebral cortex contains association areas. AG, angular gyrus; B, Broca's area; CC, corpus callosum; CG, cingulate cortex; DLPFC, dorsolateral prefrontal cortex; FEF, frontal eye fields (premotor cortex); FG, fusiform gyrus; IPL, inferior parietal lobule; ITG, inferior temporal gyrus; LG, lingual gyrus; MPFC, medial prefrontal cortex; MTG, middle temporal gyrus; OFC, orbitofrontal cortex; PHG, parahippocampal gyrus; PPC, posterior parietal cortex; PSC, peristriate cortex; SC, striate cortex; SMG, supramarginal gyrus; SPL, superior parietal lobule; STG, superior temporal gyrus; STS, superior temporal sulcus; TP, temporopolar cortex; W, Wernicke's area.

TABLE 23-1 *Clinical Features of Aphasias and Related Conditions*

	Comprehension	Repetition of Spoken Language	Naming	Fluency
Wernicke's	Impaired	Impaired	Impaired	Preserved or increased
Broca's	Preserved (except grammar)	Impaired	Impaired	Decreased
Global	Impaired	Impaired	Impaired	Decreased
Conduction	Preserved	Impaired	Impaired	Preserved
Nonfluent (motor) transcortical	Preserved	Preserved	Impaired	Impaired
Fluent (sensory) transcortical	Impaired	Preserved	Impaired	Preserved
Isolation	Impaired	Echolalia	Impaired	No purposeful speech
Anomic	Preserved	Preserved	Impaired	Preserved except for word-finding pauses
Pure word deafness	Impaired only for spoken language	Impaired	Preserved	Preserved
Pure alexia	Impaired only for reading	Preserved	Preserved	Preserved

cortex. An essential function of this area is to transform neural word representations into their articulatory sequences so that the words can be uttered in the form of spoken language. The sequencing function of Broca's area also appears to involve the ordering of words into sentences that contain a meaning-appropriate *syntax* (grammar). Wernicke's and Broca's areas are interconnected with each other and with additional perisylvian, temporal, prefrontal, and posterior parietal regions, making up a neural network subserving the various aspects of language function. Damage to any one of these components or to their interconnections can give rise to language disturbances (*aphasia*). Aphasia should be diagnosed only when there are deficits in the formal aspects of language such as naming, word choice, comprehension, spelling, and syntax. Dysarthria and mutism do not, by themselves, lead to a diagnosis of aphasia. The language network shows a left hemisphere dominance pattern in the vast majority of the population. In approximately 90% of right handers and 60% of left handers, aphasia occurs only after lesions of the left hemisphere. In some individuals no hemispheric dominance for language can be discerned, and in some others (including a small minority of right handers) there is a right hemisphere dominance for language. A language disturbance occurring after a right hemisphere lesion in a right hander is called *crossed aphasia*.

CLINICAL EXAMINATION The clinical examination of language should include the assessment of naming, spontaneous speech, comprehension, repetition, reading, and writing. A deficit of naming (*anomia*) is the single most common finding in aphasic patients. When asked to name common objects (pencil or wristwatch), the patient may fail to come up with the appropriate word, may provide a circumlocutious description of the object ("the thing for writing"), or may come up with the wrong word (*paraphasia*). If the patient offers an incorrect but legitimate word ("pen" for "pencil"), the naming error is known as a *semantic paraphasia*; if the word approximates the correct answer but is phonetically inaccurate ("plentil" for "pencil"), it is known as a *phonemic paraphasia*. Asking the patient to name body parts, geometric shapes, and component parts of objects (lapel of coat, cap of pen) can elicit mild forms of anomia in patients who can otherwise name common objects. In most anomias, the patient cannot retrieve the appropriate name when shown an object but can point to the appropriate object when the name is provided by the examiner. This is known as a one-way (or retrieval-based) naming deficit. A two-way naming deficit exists if the patient can neither provide nor recognize the correct name, indicating the presence of a language comprehension impairment. *Spontaneous speech* is described as "fluent" if it maintains appropriate output volume, phrase length, and melody or as "nonfluent" if it is sparse, halting, and average utterance length is below

four words. The examiner should also note if the speech is paraphasic or circumlocutious; if it shows a relative paucity of substantive nouns and action verbs versus function words (prepositions, conjunctions); and if word order, tenses, suffixes, prefixes, plurals, and possessives are appropriate. *Comprehension* can be tested by assessing the patient's ability to follow conversation, by asking yes-no questions ("Can a dog fly?", "Does it snow in summer?") or asking the patient to point to appropriate objects ("Where is the source of illumination in this room?"). Statements with embedded clauses or passive voice construction ("If a tiger is eaten by a lion, which animal stays alive?") help to assess the ability to comprehend complex syntactic structure. Commands to close or open the eyes, stand up, sit down, or roll over should not be used to assess overall comprehension since appropriate responses aimed at such axial movements can be preserved in patients who otherwise have profound comprehension deficits.

Repetition is assessed by asking the patient to repeat single words, short sentences, or strings of words such as "No ifs, ands, or buts." The testing of repetition with tongue-twisters such as "hippopotamus" or "Irish constabulary" provides a better assessment of dysarthria and pallilalia than aphasia. Aphasic patients may have little difficulty with tongue-twisters but have a particularly hard time repeating a string of function words. It is important to make sure that the number of words does not exceed the patient's attention span. Otherwise, the failure of repetition becomes a reflection of the narrowed attention span rather than an indication of an aphasic deficit. *Reading* should be assessed for deficits in reading aloud as well as comprehension. *Writing* is assessed for spelling errors, word order, and grammar. *Alexia* describes an inability to either read aloud or comprehend single words and simple sentences; *agraphia* (or dysgraphia) is used to describe an acquired deficit in the spelling or grammar of written language.

The correspondence between individual deficits of language function and lesion location does not display a rigid one-to-one relationship and should be conceptualized within the context of the distributed network model. Nonetheless, the classification of aphasic patients into specific clinical syndromes helps to determine the most likely anatomic distribution of the underlying neurologic disease and has implications for etiology and prognosis (Table 23-1). Aphasic syndromes can be divided into "central" syndromes, which result from damage to the two epicenters of the language network (Broca's and Wernicke's areas), and "disconnection" syndromes, which arise from lesions that interrupt the functional connectivity of these centers with each other and with the other components of the language network. The syndromes outlined below are idealizations; pure syndromes occur rarely.

Wernicke's Aphasia Comprehension is impaired for spoken and written language. Language output is fluent but is highly paraphasic and circumlocutious. The tendency for paraphasic errors may be so pronounced that it leads to strings of neologisms, which form the basis of what is known as "jargon aphasia." Speech contains large numbers of function words (e.g., prepositions, conjunctions) but few substantive nouns or verbs that refer to specific actions. The output is therefore voluminous but uninformative. For example, a patient attempts to describe how his wife accidentally threw away something important, perhaps his dentures: "We don't need it anymore, she says. And with it when that was downstairs was my teeth-tick . . . a . . . den . . . dentith . . . my dentist. And they happened to be in that bag . . . see? How could this have happened? How could a thing like this happen . . . So she says we won't need it anymore . . . I didn't think we'd use it. And now if I have any problems anybody coming a month from now, 4 months from now, or 6 months from now, I have a new dentist. Where my two . . . two little pieces of dentist that I use . . . that I . . . all gone. If she throws the whole thing away . . . visit some friends of hers and she can't throw them away."

Gestures and pantomime do not improve communication. The patient does not seem to realize that his or her language is incomprehensible and may appear angry and impatient when the examiner fails to decipher the meaning of a severely paraphasic statement. In some patients this type of aphasia can be associated with severe agitation and paranoid behaviors. One area of comprehension that may be preserved is the ability to follow commands aimed at axial musculature. The dissociation between the failure to understand simple questions ("What is your name") in a patient who rapidly closes his or her eyes, sits up, or rolls over when asked to do so is characteristic of Wernicke's aphasia and helps to differentiate it from deafness, psychiatric disease, or malingering. Patients with Wernicke's aphasia cannot express their thoughts in meaning-appropriate words and cannot decode the meaning of words in any modality of input. This aphasia therefore has expressive as well as receptive components. Repetition, naming, reading, and writing are also impaired.

The lesion site most commonly associated with Wernicke's aphasia is the posterior portion of the language network and tends to involve at least parts of Wernicke's area. An embolus to the inferior division of the middle cerebral artery, and to the posterior temporal or angular branches in particular, is the most common etiology (Chap. 349). Intracerebral hemorrhage, severe head trauma, or neoplasm are other causes. A coexisting right hemi- or superior quadrantanopia is common, and mild right nasolabial flattening may be found, but otherwise the examination is often unrevealing. The paraphasic, neologistic speech in an agitated patient with an otherwise unremarkable neurologic examination may lead to the suspicion of a primary psychiatric disorder such as schizophrenia or mania, but the other components characteristic of acquired aphasia and the absence of prior psychiatric disease usually settle the issue. Some patients with Wernicke's aphasia due to intracerebral hemorrhage or head trauma may improve as the hemorrhage or the injury heals. In most other patients, prognosis for recovery is guarded.

Broca's Aphasia Speech is nonfluent, labored, interrupted by many word-finding pauses, and usually dysarthric. It is impoverished in function words but enriched in meaning-appropriate nouns and verbs. Abnormal word order and the inappropriate deployment of *bound morphemes* (word endings used to denote tenses, possessives, or plurals) lead to a characteristic agrammatism. Speech is telegraphic and pithy but quite informative. In the following passage, a patient with Broca's aphasia describes his medical history: "I see . . . the dotor, dotor sent me . . . Bosson. Go to hospital. Dotor . . . kept me beside. Two, tee days, doctor send me home."

Output may be reduced to a grunt or single word ("yes" or "no"), which is emitted with different intonations in an attempt to express approval or disapproval. In addition to fluency, naming and repetition are also impaired. Comprehension of spoken language is intact, except for syntactically difficult sentences with passive voice structure or embedded clauses. Reading comprehension is also preserved, with the occasional exception of a specific inability to read small grammatical words such as conjunctions and pronouns. The last two features indicate that Broca's aphasia is not just an "expressive" or "motor" disorder and that it may also involve a comprehension deficit for function words and syntax. Patients with Broca's aphasia can be tearful, easily frustrated, and profoundly depressed. Insight into their condition is preserved, in contrast to Wernicke's aphasia. Even when spontaneous speech is severely dysarthric, the patient may be able to display a relatively normal articulation of words when singing. This dissociation has been used to develop specific therapeutic approaches (melodic intonation therapy) for Broca's aphasia. Additional neurologic deficits usually include right facial weakness, hemiparesis or hemiplegia, and a buccofacial apraxia characterized by an inability to carry out motor commands involving oropharyngeal and facial musculature (e.g., pa-

tients are unable to demonstrate how to blow out a match or suck through a straw). Visual fields are intact. The cause is most often infarction of Broca's area (the inferior frontal convolution; "B" in Fig. 23-1) and surrounding anterior perisylvian and insular cortex, due to occlusion of the superior division of the middle cerebral artery (Chap. 349). Mass lesions including tumor, intracerebral hemorrhage, or abscess may also be responsible. Small lesions confined to the posterior part of Broca's area may lead to a nonaphasic and often reversible deficit of speech articulation, usually accompanied by mild right facial weakness. When the cause of Broca's aphasia is stroke, recovery of language function generally peaks within 2 to 6 months, after which time further progress is limited.

Global Aphasia Speech output is nonfluent, and comprehension of spoken language is severely impaired. Naming, repetition, reading, and writing are also impaired. This syndrome represents the combined dysfunction of Broca's and Wernicke's areas and usually results from strokes that involve the entire middle cerebral artery distribution in the left hemisphere. Most patients are initially mute or say a few words, such as "hi" or "yes." Related signs include right hemiplegia, hemisensory loss, and homonymous hemianopia. Occasionally, a patient with a lesion in Wernicke's area will present with a global aphasia that soon resolves into Wernicke's aphasia.

Conduction Aphasia Speech output is fluent but paraphasic, comprehension of spoken language is intact, and repetition is severely impaired. Naming and writing are also impaired. Reading aloud is impaired, but reading comprehension is preserved. The lesion sites spare Broca's and Wernicke's areas but may induce a functional disconnection between the two so that neural word representations formed in Wernicke's area and adjacent regions cannot be conveyed to Broca's area for assembly into corresponding articulatory patterns. Occasionally, a Wernicke's area lesion gives rise to a transient Wernicke's aphasia that rapidly resolves into a conduction aphasia. The paraphasic output in conduction aphasia interferes with the ability to express meaning, but this deficit is not nearly as severe as the one displayed by patients with Wernicke's aphasia. Associated neurologic signs in conduction aphasia vary according to the primary lesion site.

Nonfluent Transcortical Aphasia (Transcortical Motor Aphasia) The features are similar to Broca's aphasia, but repetition is intact and agrammatism may be less pronounced. The neurologic examination may be otherwise intact, but a right hemiparesis can also exist. The lesion site disconnects the intact language network from prefrontal areas of the brain and usually involves the anterior watershed zone between anterior and middle cerebral artery territories or the supplementary motor cortex in the territory of the anterior cerebral artery.

Fluent Transcortical Aphasia (Transcortical Sensory Aphasia) Clinical features are similar to those of Wernicke's aphasia, but repetition is intact. The lesion site disconnects the intact core of the language network from other temporoparietal association areas. Associated neurologic findings may include hemianopia. Cerebrovascular lesions (e.g., infarctions in the posterior watershed zone) or neoplasms that involve the temporoparietal cortex posterior to Wernicke's area are the most common causes.

Isolation Aphasia This rare syndrome represents a combination of the two transcortical aphasias. Comprehension is severely impaired, and there is no purposeful speech output. The patient may parrot fragments of heard conversations (*echolalia*), indicating that the neural mechanisms for repetition are at least partially intact. This condition represents the pathologic function of the language network when it is isolated from other regions of the brain. Broca's and Wernicke's areas tend to be spared, but there is damage to the surrounding frontal, parietal, and temporal cortex. Lesions are patchy and can be associated with anoxia, carbon monoxide poisoning, or complete watershed zone infarctions.

Anomic Aphasia   This form of aphasia may be considered the "minimal dysfunction" syndrome of the language network. Articulation, comprehension, and repetition are intact, but confrontation naming, word finding, and spelling are impaired. Speech is enriched in function words but impoverished in substantive nouns and verbs denoting specific actions. Language output is fluent but paraphasic, circumlocutious, and uninformative. The lesion sites can be anywhere within the left hemisphere language network, including the middle and inferior temporal gyri. *Anomic aphasia is the single most common language disturbance seen in head trauma, metabolic encephalopathy, and Alzheimer's disease.* The language impairment of Alzheimer's disease almost always leads to fluent aphasias (e.g., anomic, Wernicke's, conduction, or fluent transcortical aphasia). The insidious onset and relentless progression of nonfluent language disturbances (Broca's or nonfluent transcortical aphasia) can be seen in *primary progressive aphasia,* a degenerative syndrome most commonly associated with focal nonspecific neuronal loss or Pick's disease.

Pure Word Deafness   This is not a true aphasic syndrome because the language deficit is modality-specific. The most common lesions are either bilateral or left-sided in the superior temporal gyrus. The net effect of the underlying lesion is to interrupt the flow of information from the unimodal auditory association cortex to Wernicke's area. Patients have no difficulty understanding written language and can express themselves well in spoken or written language. They have no difficulty interpreting and reacting to environmental sounds since primary auditory cortex and subcortical auditory relays are intact. Since auditory information cannot be conveyed to the language network, however, it cannot be decoded into neural word representations and the patient reacts to speech as if it were in an alien tongue that cannot be deciphered. Patients cannot repeat spoken language but have no difficulty naming objects. In time, patients with pure word deafness teach themselves lip reading and may appear to have improved. There may be no additional neurologic findings, but agitated paranoid reactions are frequent in the acute stages. Cerebrovascular lesions are the most frequent cause.

Pure Alexia without Agraphia   This is the visual equivalent of pure word deafness. The lesions (usually a combination of damage to the left occipital cortex and to a posterior sector of the corpus callosum—the splenium) interrupt the flow of visual input into the language network. There is usually a right hemianopia, but the core language network remains unaffected. The patient can understand and produce spoken language, name objects in the left visual hemifield, repeat, and write. However, the patient acts as if illiterate when asked to read even the simplest sentence because the visual information from the written words (presented to the intact left visual hemifield) cannot reach the language network. Objects in the left hemifield may be named accurately because they activate nonvisual associations in the right hemisphere, which, in turn, can access the language network through transcallosal pathways anterior to the splenium. Patients with this syndrome may also lose the ability to name colors, although they can match colors. This is known as a *color anomia.* The most common etiology of pure alexia is a vascular lesion in the territory of the posterior cerebral artery or an infiltrating neoplasm in the left occipital cortex that involves the optic radiations as well as the crossing fibers of the splenium. Since the posterior cerebral artery also supplies medial temporal components of the limbic system, the patient with pure alexia may also experience an amnesia, but this is usually transient because the limbic lesion is unilateral.

Aphemia   There is an acute onset of severely impaired fluency (often mutism), which cannot be accounted for by corticobulbar, cerebellar, or extrapyramidal dysfunction. Recovery is the rule and involves an intermediate stage of hoarse whispering. Writing, reading, and comprehension are intact, so this is not a true aphasic syndrome. Partial lesions of Broca's area or subcortical lesions that undercut its connections with other parts of the brain may be present. Occasionally, the lesion site is on the medial aspects of the frontal lobes and may involve the supplementary motor cortex of the left hemisphere.

Apraxia   This generic term designates a complex motor deficit that cannot be attributed to pyramidal, extrapyramidal, cerebellar, or sensory dysfunction and that does not arise from the patient's failure to understand the nature of the task. The form that is most frequently encountered in clinical practice is known as *ideomotor apraxia.* Commands to perform a specific motor act ("cough," "blow out a match") or to pantomime the use of a common tool (a comb, hammer, straw, or toothbrush) in the absence of the real object cannot be followed. The patient's ability to comprehend the command is ascertained by demonstrating multiple movements and establishing that the correct one can be recognized. Some patients with this type of apraxia can imitate the appropriate movement (when it is demonstrated by the examiner) and show no impairment when handed the real object, indicating that the sensorimotor mechanisms necessary for the movement are intact. Some forms of ideomotor apraxia represent a disconnection of the language network from pyramidal motor systems: commands to execute complex movements are understood but cannot be conveyed to the appropriate motor areas, even though the relevant motor mechanisms are intact. *Buccofacial apraxia* involves apraxic deficits in movements of the face and mouth. *Limb apraxia* encompasses apraxic deficits in movements of the arms and legs. Ideomotor apraxia is almost always caused by lesions in the left hemisphere and is commonly associated with aphasic syndromes, especially Broca's aphasia and conduction aphasia. Its presence cannot be ascertained in patients with language comprehension deficits. The ability to follow commands aimed at axial musculature ("close the eyes," "stand up") is subserved by different pathways and may be intact in otherwise severely aphasic and apraxic patients. Patients with lesions of the anterior corpus callosum can display a special type of ideomotor apraxia confined to the left side of the body. Since the handling of real objects is not impaired, ideomotor apraxia, by itself, causes no major limitation of daily living activities.

Ideational apraxia refers to a deficit in the execution of a goal-directed sequence of movements in patients who have no difficulty executing the individual components of the sequence. For example, when asked to pick up a pen and write, the sequence of uncapping the pen, placing the cap at the opposite end, turning the point towards the writing surface, and writing may be disrupted, and the patient may be seen trying to write with the wrong end of the pen or even with the removed cap. These motor sequencing problems are usually seen in the context of confusional states and dementias rather than focal lesions associated with aphasic conditions. *Limb-kinetic apraxia* involves a clumsiness in the actual use of tools that cannot be attributed to sensory, pyramidal, extrapyramidal, or cerebellar dysfunction. This condition can emerge in the context of focal premotor cortex lesions or *corticobasal ganglionic degeneration.*

Gerstmann's Syndrome   The combination of *acalculia* (impairment of simple arithmetic), *dysgraphia* (impaired writing), *finger anomia* (an inability to name individual fingers such as the index or thumb), and *right-left confusion* (an inability to tell whether a hand, foot, or arm of the patient or examiner is on the right or left side of the body) is known as Gerstmann's syndrome. In making this diagnosis it is important to establish that the finger and left-right naming deficits are not part of a more generalized anomia and that the patient is not otherwise aphasic. When Gerstmann's syndrome is seen in isolation, it is commonly associated with damage to the inferior parietal lobule (especially the angular gyrus) in the left hemisphere.

Aprosodia   Variations of melodic stress and intonation influence the meaning and impact of spoken language. For example, the two statements "He *is* clever." and "He is *clever*?" contain an identical word choice and syntax but convey vastly different messages because of differences in the intonation and stress with which the statements are uttered. This aspect of language is known as *prosody.* Damage to perisylvian areas in the right hemisphere can interfere with speech prosody and can lead to syndromes of aprosodia. Damage to right hemisphere regions corresponding to Wernicke's area can selectively impair decoding of speech prosody, whereas damage to right hemisphere regions corresponding to Broca's area yields a greater impairment in the ability to introduce meaning-appropriate prosody into spoken language. The latter deficit is the most common type of aprosodia identified in clinical practice—the patient produces grammatically correct language with accurate word choice but the statements are uttered in a monotone that interferes with the ability to convey the intended stress and affect. Patients with this type of aprosodia give the mistaken impression of being depressed or indifferent.

Subcortical Aphasia Damage to subcortical components of the language network (e.g., the striatum and thalamus of the left hemisphere) can also lead to aphasia. The resulting syndromes contain combinations of deficits in the various aspects of language but rarely fit the specific patterns described in Table 23-1. An anomic aphasia accompanied by dysarthria or a fluent aphasia with hemiparesis should raise the suspicion of a subcortical lesion site.

THE PARIETOFRONTAL NETWORK FOR SPATIAL ORIENTATION: NEGLECT AND RELATED CONDITIONS

HEMISPATIAL NEGLECT Adaptive orientation to significant events within the extrapersonal space is subserved by a large-scale network containing three major cortical components. The *cingulate cortex* provides access to a limbic-motivational mapping of the extrapersonal space, the *posterior parietal cortex* to a sensorimotor representation of salient extrapersonal events, and the *frontal eye fields* to motor strategies for attentional behaviors (Fig. 23-2). Subcortical components of this network include the striatum and the thalamus. Contralesional hemispatial neglect represents one outcome of damage to any of the cortical or subcortical components of this network. *The traditional view that hemispatial neglect always denotes a parietal lobe lesion is inaccurate.* In keeping with this anatomic organization, the clinical manifestations of neglect display three behavioral components: sensory events

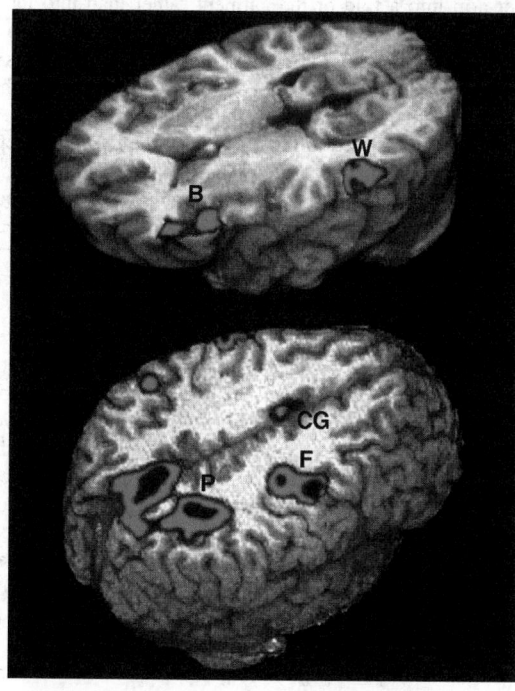

FIGURE 23-2 Functional magnetic resonance imaging of language and spatial attention in neurologically intact subjects. The dark areas show regions of task-related significant activation. (*Top*) The subjects were asked to determine if two words were synonymous. This language task led to the simultaneous activation of the two epicenters of the language network, Broca's area (B) and Wernicke's area (W). The activations are exclusively in the left hemisphere. (*Bottom*) The subjects were asked to shift spatial attention to a peripheral target. This task led to the simultaneous activation of the three epicenters of the attentional network, the posterior parietal cortex (P), the frontal eye fields (F), and the cingulate gyrus (CG). The activations are predominantly in the right hemisphere. (*Courtesy of Darren Gitelman, MD.*)

(or their mental representations) within the neglected hemispace have a lesser impact on overall awareness; there is a paucity of exploratory and orienting acts directed toward the neglected hemispace; and the patient behaves as if the neglected hemispace was motivationally devalued.

According to one model of spatial cognition, the right hemisphere directs attention within the *entire* extrapersonal space, whereas the left hemisphere directs attention mostly within the contralateral right hemisphere. Consequently, unilateral left hemisphere lesions do not give rise to much contralesional neglect since the ipsilateral attentional mechanisms of the right hemisphere can compensate for the loss of the *contralaterally* directed attentional functions of the left hemisphere. Unilateral right hemisphere lesions, however, give rise to severe contralesional left hemispatial neglect because the unaffected left hemisphere does not contain ipsilateral attentional mechanisms. This model is consistent with clinical experience, which shows that contralesional neglect is more common, severe, and lasting after damage to the right hemisphere than after damage to the left hemisphere. Severe neglect for the right hemispace is rare, even in left handers with left hemisphere lesions.

Patients with severe neglect may fail to dress, shave, or groom the left side of the body; may fail to eat food placed on the left side of the tray; and may fail to read the left half of sentences. When the examiner draws a large circle [12 to 15 cm (5 to 6 in.) in diameter] and asks the patient to place the numbers 1 to 12 as if the circle represented the face of a clock, there is a tendency to crowd the numbers on the right side and leave the left side empty. When asked to copy a simple line drawing, the patient fails to copy detail on the left; and when asked to write, there is a tendency to leave an unusually wide margin on the left.

Two bedside tests that are useful in assessing neglect are *simultaneous bilateral stimulation* and *visual target cancellation*. In the former, the examiner provides either unilateral or simultaneous bilateral stimulation in the visual, auditory, and tactile modalities. Following right hemisphere injury, patients who have no difficulty detecting unilateral stimuli on either side experience the bilaterally presented stimulus as coming only from the right. This phenomenon is known as *extinction* and is a manifestation of the sensory-representational aspect of hemispatial neglect. In the target detection task, targets (e.g., As) are interspersed with foils (e.g., other letters of the alphabet) on a 21.5 to 28.0 cm (8.5 to 11 in.) sheet of paper and the patient is asked to circle all the targets. A failure to detect targets on the left is a manifestation of the exploratory deficit in hemispatial neglect (Fig. 23-3*A*). Hemianopia, by itself, does not interfere with performance in this task since the patient is free to turn the head and eyes to the left. The normal tendency in target detection tasks is to start from the left upper quadrant and move systematically in horizontal or vertical sweeps. Some patients show a tendency to start the process from the right and proceed in a haphazard fashion. This represents a subtle manifestation of left neglect, even if the patient eventually manages to detect all the appropriate targets. Some patients with neglect may also deny the existence of hemiparesis and may even deny ownership of the paralyzed limb, a condition known as *anosognosia.*

Cerebrovascular lesions and neoplasms in the right hemisphere are the most common causes of hemispatial neglect. Depending on the site of the lesion, the patient with neglect may also have hemiparesis, hemihypesthesia, and hemianopia on the left, but these are not invariant findings. The majority of patients display considerable improvement of hemispatial neglect, usually within the first several weeks.

BÁLINT'S SYNDROME, SIMULTANAGNOSIA, DRESSING APRAXIA, AND CONSTRUCTION APRAXIA Bilateral involvement of the network for spatial attention, especially its parietal components, leads to a state of severe spatial disorientation known as *Bálint's syndrome*. Bálint's syndrome involves deficits in the orderly visuomotor scanning of the environment (*oculomotor apraxia*) and in accurate manual reaching toward visual targets (*optic ataxia*). The third and most dramatic component of Bálint's syndrome is known as *simultanagnosia* and reflects an

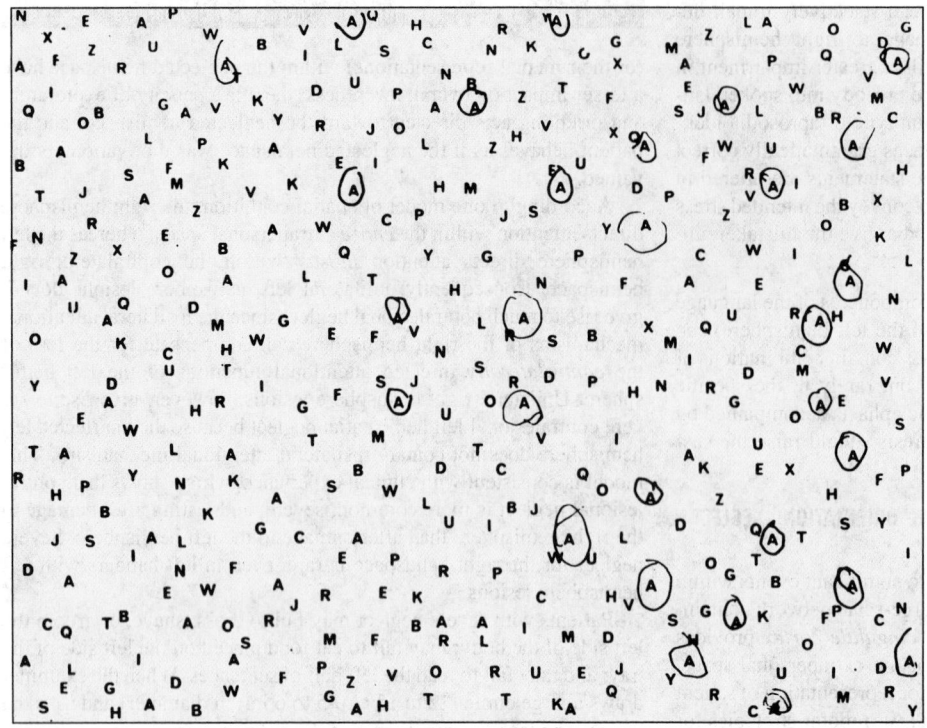

A

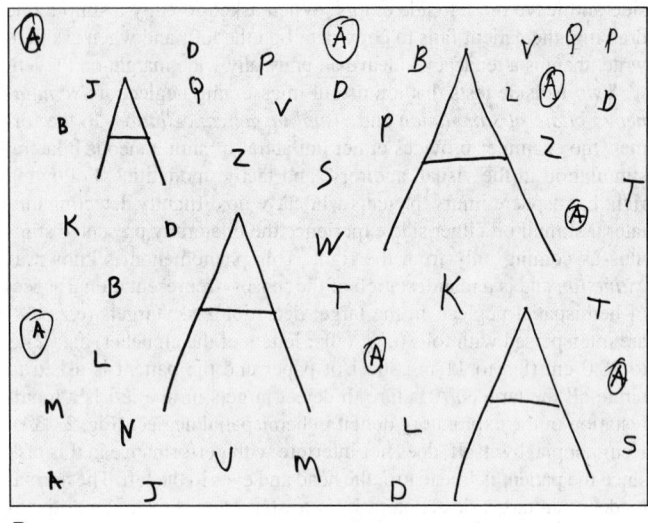

B

FIGURE 23-3 *A.* A 47-year-old man with a large frontoparietal lesion in the right hemisphere was asked to circle all the As. Only targets on the right are circled. This is a manifestation of left hemispatial neglect. *B.* A 70-year-old woman with a 2-year history of degenerative dementia was able to circle most of the small targets but ignored the larger ones. This is a manifestation of simultanagnosia.

be used for the bedside diagnosis of simultanagnosia. In this modification, some of the targets (e.g., As) are made to be much larger than the others [7.5 to 10 cm vs 2.5 cm (3 to 4 in. vs 1 in.) in height], and all targets are embedded among foils. Patients with simultanagnosia display a counterintuitive but characteristic tendency to miss the larger targets (Fig. 23-3*B*). This occurs because the information needed for the identification of the larger targets cannot be confined to the immediate line of gaze and requires the integration of visual information across a more extensive field of view. The greater difficulty in the detection of the larger targets also indicates that poor acuity is not responsible for the impairment of visual function and that the problem is central rather than peripheral. Bálint's syndrome results from bilateral dorsal parietal lesions; common settings include watershed infarction between the middle and posterior cerebral artery territories, hypoglycemia, sagittal sinus thrombosis, or atypical forms of Alzheimer's disease. In patients with Bálint's syndrome due to stroke, bilateral visual field defects (usually inferior quadrantanopias) are common.

Another manifestation of bilateral (or right-sided) dorsal parietal lobe lesions is *dressing apraxia*. The patient with this condition is unable to align the body axis with the axis of the garment and can be seen struggling as he or she holds a coat from its bottom or extends his or her arm into a fold of the garment rather than into its sleeve. Lesions that involve the posterior parietal cortex also lead to severe difficulties in copying simple line drawings. This is known as a *construction apraxia* and is much more severe if the lesion is in the right hemisphere. In some patients with right hemisphere lesions, the drawing difficulties are confined to the left side of the figure and represent a manifestation of hemispatial neglect; in others, there is a more universal deficit in reproducing contours and three-dimensional perspective. Dressing apraxia and construction apraxia represent special instances of a more general disturbance in spatial orientation.

THE OCCIPITOTEMPORAL NETWORK FOR FACE AND OBJECT RECOGNITION: PROSOPAGNOSIA AND OBJECT AGNOSIA

Perceptual information about faces and objects is initially encoded in primary (striate) visual cortex and adjacent (upstream) peristriate visual association areas. This information is subsequently relayed first to the downstream visual association areas of occipitotemporal cortex and then to other heteromodal and paralimbic areas of the cerebral cortex. Bilateral lesions in the fusiform and lingual gyri of occipitotemporal cortex disrupt this process and interfere with the ability of otherwise intact perceptual information to activate the distributed multimodal associations that lead to the recognition of faces and objects. The resultant face and object recognition deficits are known as *prosopagnosia* and *visual object agnosia*.

The patient with prosopagnosia cannot recognize familiar faces, including, sometimes, the reflection of his or her own face in the mirror. This is not a perceptual deficit since prosopagnosic patients can easily tell if two faces are identical or not. Furthermore, a prosopagnosic patient who cannot recognize a familiar face by visual inspection alone can use auditory cues to reach appropriate recognition if allowed to listen to the person's voice. The deficit in prosopagnosia is therefore modality-specific and reflects the existence of a lesion that prevents the activation of otherwise intact multimodal templates by relevant visual input. Damasio has pointed out that the deficit in prosopagnosia

inability to integrate visual information in the center of gaze with more peripheral information. The patient gets stuck on the detail that falls in the center of gaze without attempting to scan the visual environment for additional information. The patient with simultanagnosia "misses the forest for the trees." Complex visual scenes cannot be grasped in their entirety, leading to severe limitations in the visual identification of objects and scenes. For example, a patient who is shown a table lamp and asked to name the object may look at its circular base and call it an ash tray. Some patients with simultanagnosia report that objects they look at may suddenly vanish, probably indicating an inability to look back at the original point of gaze after brief saccadic displacements. Movement and distracting stimuli greatly exacerbate the difficulties of visual perception. Simultanagnosia can sometimes occur without the other two components of Bálint's syndrome.

A modification of the letter cancellation task described above canis not limited to the recognition of faces but that it can also extend to the recognition of individual members of larger generic object groups. For example, prosopagnosic patients characteristically have no difficulty with the generic identification of a face as a face or of a car as a car, but they cannot recognize the identity of an individual face or the make of an individual car. This reflects a visual recognition deficit for proprietary features that characterize individual members of an object class. When recognition problems become more generalized and extend to the generic identification of common objects, the condition is known as visual object agnosia. In contrast to prosopagnosic patients, those with object agnosia cannot recognize a face as a face or a car as a car.

It is important to distinguish visual object agnosia from anomia. The patient with anomia cannot name the object but can describe its use. In contrast, the patient with visual agnosia is unable either to name a visually presented object or to describe its use. The characteristic lesions in prosopagnosia and visual object agnosia consist of bilateral infarctions in the territory of the posterior cerebral arteries. Associated deficits can include visual field defects (especially superior quadrantanopias) or a centrally based color blindness known as achromatopsia. Rarely, the responsible lesion is unilateral. In such cases, prosopagnosia is associated with lesions in the right hemisphere and object agnosia with lesions in the left.

THE LIMBIC NETWORK FOR MEMORY: AMNESIAS

Limbic and paralimbic areas (such as the hippocampus, amygdala, and entorhinal cortex), the anterior and medial nuclei of the thalamus, the medial and basal parts of the striatum, and the hypothalamus collectively constitute a distributed network known as the *limbic system* (see Fig. 350-1). The behavioral affiliations of this network include the coordination of emotion, motivation, autonomic tone, and endocrine function. An additional area of specialization for the limbic network, and the one which is of most relevance to clinical practice, is that of declarative (conscious) memory for recent episodes and experiences. A disturbance in this function is known as an *amnestic state*. In the absence of deficits in motivation, attention, language, or visuospatial function, the clinical diagnosis of a persistent global amnestic state is always associated with bilateral damage to the limbic network, usually within the hippocampo-entorhinal complex or the thalamus.

Although the limbic network is the site of damage for amnestic states, it is almost certainly not the storage site for memories. Memories are stored in widely distributed form throughout the cerebral cortex. The role attributed to the limbic network is to bind these distributed fragments into coherent events and experiences that can sustain conscious recall. Damage to the limbic network does not necessarily destroy memories but interferes with their conscious (declarative) recall in coherent form. The individual fragments of information remain preserved despite the limbic lesions and can sustain what is known as *implicit memory*. For example, patients with amnestic states can acquire new motor or perceptual skills, even though they may have no conscious knowledge of the experiences that led to the acquisition of these skills.

The memory disturbance in the amnestic state is multimodal and includes retrograde and anterograde components. The *retrograde amnesia* involves an inability to recall experiences that occurred before the onset of the amnestic state. Relatively recent events are more vulnerable to retrograde amnesia than more remote and more extensively consolidated events. A patient who comes to the emergency room complaining that he cannot remember his identity but who can remember the events of the previous day is almost certainly not suffering from a neurologic cause of memory disturbance. The second and most important component of the amnestic state is the *anterograde amnesia*, which indicates an inability to store, retain, and recall new knowledge. Patients with amnestic states cannot remember what they ate a few minutes ago or the details of an important event they may have experienced a few hours ago. In the acute stages, there may also be a tendency to fill in memory gaps with inaccurate, fabricated, and often implausible information. This is known as *confabulation*. Patients with

the amnestic syndrome forget that they forget and tend to deny the existence of a memory problem when questioned.

The patient with an amnestic state is almost always disoriented, especially to time. Accurate temporal orientation and accurate knowledge of current news rule out a major amnestic state. The anterograde component of an amnestic state can be tested with a list of four to five words read aloud by the examiner up to five times or until the patient can immediately repeat the entire list without intervening delay. In the next phase of testing, the patient is allowed to concentrate on the words and to rehearse them internally for 1 min before being asked to recall them. Accurate performance in this phase indicates that the patient is motivated and sufficiently attentive to hold the words online for at least 1 min. The final phase of the testing involves a retention period of 5 to 10 min, during which the patient is engaged in other tasks. Adequate recall at the end of this interval requires offline storage, retention, and retrieval. Amnestic patients fail this phase of the task and may even forget that they were given a list of words to remember. Accurate recognition of the words by multiple choice in a patient who cannot recall them indicates a less severe memory disturbance that affects mostly the retrieval stage of memory. The retrograde component of an amnesia can be assessed with questions related to autobiographical or historical events. The anterograde component of amnestic states is usually much more prominent than the retrograde component. In rare instances, usually associated with temporal lobe epilepsy or benzodiazepine intake, the retrograde component may dominate.

The assessment of memory can be quite challenging. Bedside evaluations may only detect the most severe impairments. Less severe memory impairments, as in the case of patients with temporal lobe epilepsy, mild head injury or early dementia, require quantitative evaluations by neuropsychologists. Confusional states caused by toxic-metabolic encephalopathies and some types of frontal lobe damage interfere with attentional capacity and lead to secondary memory impairments, even in the absence of any limbic lesions. This sort of memory impairment can be differentiated from the amnestic state by the presence of additional impairments in the attention-related tasks described below in the section on the frontal lobes.

Many neurologic diseases can give rise to an amnestic state. These include tumors (of the sphenoid wing, posterior corpus callosum, thalamus, or medial temporal lobe), infarctions (in the territories of the anterior or posterior cerebral arteries), head trauma, herpes simplex encephalitis, Wernicke-Korsakoff encephalopathy, paraneoplastic limbic encephalitis, and degenerative dementias such as Alzheimer's or Pick's disease. The one common denominator of all these diseases is that they lead to the bilateral lesions within one or more components in the limbic network, most commonly the hippocampus, entorhinal cortex, the mammillary bodies of the hypothalamus, and the limbic thalamus. Occasionally, unilateral left-sided lesions can give rise to an amnestic state, but the memory disorder tends to be transient. Depending on the nature and distribution of the underlying neurologic disease, the patient may also have visual field deficits, eye movement limitations, or cerebellar findings.

Transient global amnesia is a distinctive syndrome usually seen in late middle age. Patients become acutely disoriented and repeatedly ask who they are, where they are, what they are doing. The spell is characterized by anterograde amnesia (inability to retain new information) and a retrograde amnesia for relatively recent events that occurred before the onset. The syndrome usually resolves within 24 to 48 h and is followed by the filling-in of the period affected by the retrograde amnesia, although there is persistent loss of memory for the events that occurred during the ictus. Recurrences are noted in approximately 20% of patients. Migraine, temporal lobe seizures, and transient ischemic events in the posterior cerebral territory have been postulated as causes of transient global amnesia. The absence of associated neurologic findings may occasionally lead to the incorrect diagnosis of a psychiatric disorder.

THE PREFRONTAL NETWORK FOR ATTENTION AND BEHAVIOR

Approximately one-third of all the cerebral cortex in the human brain is located in the frontal lobes. The frontal lobes can be subdivided into motor-premotor, dorsolateral prefrontal, medial prefrontal, and orbitofrontal components. The terms *frontal lobe syndrome* and *prefrontal cortex* refer only to the last three of these four components. These are the parts of the cerebral cortex that show the greatest phylogenetic expansion in primates and especially in humans. The dorsolateral prefrontal, medial prefrontal, and orbitofrontal areas, and the subcortical structures with which they are interconnected (i.e., the head of the caudate and the dorsomedial nucleus of the thalamus), collectively make up a large-scale network that coordinates exceedingly complex aspects of human cognition and behavior.

The prefrontal network plays an important role in behaviors that require an integration of thought with emotion and motivation. There is no simple formula for summarizing the diverse functional affiliations of the prefrontal network. Its integrity appears important for the simultaneous awareness of context, options, consequences, relevance, and emotional impact so as to allow the formulation of adaptive inferences, decisions, and actions. Damage to this part of the brain impairs mental flexibility, reasoning, hypothesis formation, abstract thinking, foresight, judgment, the online (attentive) holding of information, and the ability to inhibit inappropriate responses. Behaviors impaired by prefrontal cortex lesions, especially those related to the manipulation of mental content, are often referred to as "executive functions."

Even very large bilateral prefrontal lesions may leave all sensory, motor, and basic cognitive functions intact while leading to isolated but dramatic alterations of personality and behavior. The most common clinical manifestations of damage to the prefrontal network take the form of two relatively distinct syndromes. In the *frontal abulic syndrome*, the patient shows a loss of initiative, creativity, and curiosity and displays a pervasive emotional blandness and apathy. In the *frontal disinhibition syndrome*, the patient becomes socially disinhibited and shows severe impairments of judgment, insight, and foresight. The dissociation between intact intellectual function and a total lack of even rudimentary common sense is striking. Despite the preservation of all essential memory functions, the patient cannot learn from experience and continues to display inappropriate behaviors without appearing to feel emotional pain, guilt, or regret when such behaviors repeatedly lead to disastrous consequences. The impairments may emerge only in real-life situations when behavior is under minimal external control and may not be apparent within the structured environment of the medical office. Testing judgment by asking patients what they would do if they detected a fire in a theater or found a stamped and addressed envelope on the road is not very informative since patients who answer these questions wisely in the office may still act very foolishly in the more complex real-life setting. The physician must therefore be prepared to make a diagnosis of frontal lobe disease on the basis of historic information alone even when the office examination of mental state may be quite intact.

The abulic syndrome tends to be associated with damage to the dorsolateral prefrontal cortex, and the disinhibition syndrome with the medial prefrontal or orbitofrontal cortex. These syndromes tend to arise almost exclusively after bilateral lesions, most frequently in the setting of head trauma, stroke, ruptured aneurysms, hydrocephalus, tumors (including metastases, glioblastoma, and falx or olfactory groove meningiomas), or focal degenerative diseases. Unilateral lesions confined to the prefrontal cortex may remain silent until the pathology spreads to the other side. The emergence of developmentally primitive reflexes, also known as frontal release signs, such as grasping (elicited by stroking the palm) and sucking (elicited by stroking the lips) are seen primarily in patients with large structural lesions that extend into the premotor components of the frontal lobes or in the context of metabolic encephalopathies. The vast majority of patients

with prefrontal lesions and frontal lobe behavioral syndromes do not display these reflexes.

Damage to the frontal lobe disrupts a variety of attention-related functions including working memory (the transient online holding of information), concentration span, the scanning and retrieval of stored information, the inhibition of immediate but inappropriate responses, and mental flexibility. The capacity for focusing on a trend of thought and the ability to voluntarily shift the focus of attention from one thought or stimulus to another can become impaired. Digit span (which should be seven forward and five reverse) is decreased; the recitation of the months of the year in reverse order (which should take less than 15 s) is slowed; and the fluency in producing words starting with a, f, or s that can be generated in 1 min (normally 12 or more per letter) is diminished even in nonaphasic patients. Characteristically, there is a progressive slowing of performance as the task proceeds; e.g., the patient asked to count backwards by 3s may say "100, 97, 94, . . 91, ... 88," etc., and may not complete the task. In "go–no-go" tasks (where the instruction is to raise the finger upon hearing one tap but to keep it still upon hearing two taps), the patient shows a characteristic inability to keep still in response to the "no go" stimulus; mental flexibility (tested by the ability to shift from one criterion to another in sorting or matching tasks) is impoverished; distractibility by irrelevant stimuli is increased; and there is a pronounced tendency for impersistence and perseveration.

These attentional deficits disrupt the orderly registration and retrieval of new information and lead to *secondary* memory deficits. Such memory deficits can be differentiated from the *primary* memory impairments of the amnestic state by showing that they improve when the attentional load of the task is decreased. Working memory (also known as immediate memory) is an attentional function based on the temporary online holding of information. It is closely associated with the integrity of the prefrontal network and the ascending reticular activating system. Retentive memory, on the other hand, depends on the stable (offline) storage of information and is associated with the integrity of the limbic network. The distinction of the underlying neural mechanisms is illustrated by the observation that severely amnestic patients who cannot remember events that occurred a few minutes ago may have intact if not superior working memory capacity as shown in tests of digit span.

Lesions in the caudate nucleus or in the dorsomedial nucleus of the thalamus (subcortical components of the prefrontal network) can also produce a frontal lobe syndrome. This is one reason why the mental state changes associated with degenerative basal ganglia diseases, such as Parkinson's or Huntington's disease, may take the form of a frontal lobe syndrome. Because of its widespread connections with other regions of association cortex, one essential computational role of the prefrontal network is to function as an integrator, or "orchestrator," for other networks. Bilateral multifocal lesions of the cerebral hemispheres, none of which are individually large enough to cause specific cognitive deficits such as aphasia or neglect, can collectively interfere with the connectivity and integrating function of prefrontal cortex. A frontal lobe syndrome is the single most common behavioral profile associated with a variety of bilateral multifocal brain diseases including metabolic encephalopathy, multiple sclerosis, vitamin B_{12} deficiency, and others. In fact, the vast majority of patients with the clinical diagnosis of a frontal lobe syndrome tend to have lesions that do not involve prefrontal cortex but involve either the subcortical components of the prefrontal network or its connections with other parts of the brain. In order to avoid making a diagnosis of "frontal lobe syndrome" in a patient with no evidence of frontal cortex disease, it is advisable to use the diagnostic term *frontal network syndrome*, with the understanding that the responsible lesions can lie anywhere within this distributed network.

The patient with frontal lobe disease raises potential dilemmas in differential diagnosis: the abulia and blandness may be misinterpreted as depression, and the disinhibition as idiopathic mania or acting-out. Appropriate intervention may be delayed while a treatable tumor keeps expanding. An informed approach to frontal lobe disease and its behavioral manifestations may help to avoid such errors.

CARING FOR THE PATIENT WITH DEFICITS OF HIGHER CEREBRAL FUNCTION

Some of the deficits described in this chapter are so complex that they may bewilder not only the patient and family but also the physician. It is imperative to carry out a systematic clinical evaluation in order to characterize the nature of the deficits and explain them in lay terms to the patient and family. Such an explanation can allay at least some of the anxieties, address the mistaken impression that the deficit (e.g., social disinhibition or inability to recognize family members) is psychologically motivated, and lead to practical suggestions for daily living activities. The consultation of a skilled neuropsychologist may aid in the formulation of diagnosis and management. Patients with simultanagnosia, for example, may benefit from the counterintuitive instruction to stand back when they cannot find an item so that a greater search area falls within the immediate field of gaze. Some patients with frontal lobe disease can be extremely irritable and abusive to spouses and yet display all the appropriate social graces during the visit to the medical office. In such cases, the history may be more important than the bedside examination in charting a course of treatment.

Reactive depression is common in patients with higher cerebral dysfunction and should be treated. These patients may be sensitive to the usual doses of antidepressants or anxiolytics and deserve a careful titration of dosage. Brain damage may cause a dissociation between feeling states and their expression, so that a patient who may superficially appear jocular could still be suffering from an underlying depression that deserves to be treated. In many cases, agitation may be controlled with reassurance. In other cases, treatment with benzodiazepines or sedating antidepressants may become necessary. The use of neuroleptics for the control of agitation should be reserved for refractory cases since extrapyramidal side effects are frequent in patients with coexisting brain damage.

Spontaneous improvement of cognitive deficits due to acute neurologic lesions is common. It is most rapid in the first few weeks but may continue for up to 2 years, especially in young individuals with single brain lesions. The mechanisms for this recovery are incompletely understood. Some of the initial deficits appear to arise from remote dysfunction (diaschisis) in parts of the brain that are interconnected with the site of initial injury. Improvement in these patients may reflect, at least in part, a normalization of the remote dysfunction. Other mechanisms may involve functional reorganization in surviving neurons adjacent to the injury or the compensatory use of homologous structures, e.g., the right superior temporal gyrus with recovery from Wernicke's aphasia. In some patients with large lesions involving Broca's and Wernicke's areas, only Wernicke's area may show contralateral compensatory reorganization (or bilateral functionality), giving rise to a situation where a lesion that should have caused a global aphasia becomes associated with a residual Broca's aphasia. Prognosis

for recovery from aphasia is best when Wernicke's area is spared. Cognitive rehabilitation procedures have been used in the treatment of higher cortical deficits. There are few controlled studies, but some do show a benefit of rehabilitation in the recovery from hemispatial neglect and aphasia. Some types of deficits may be more prone to recovery than others. For example, patients with nonfluent aphasias are more likely to benefit from speech therapy than patients with fluent aphasias and comprehension deficits. In general, lesions that lead to a denial of illness (e.g., anosognosia) are associated with cognitive deficits that are more resistant to rehabilitation. The recovery of higher cortical dysfunction is rarely complete. Periodic neuropsychological assessment is necessary for quantifying the pace of the improvement and for generating specific recommendations for cognitive rehabilitation, modifications in the home environment, and the timetable for returning to school or work.

In general medical practice, most patients with deficits in higher cognitive functions will be suffering from dementia. There is a mistaken belief that dementias are anatomically diffuse and that they cause global cognitive impairments. This is only true at the terminal stages. During most of the clinical course, dementias are exquisitely selective with respect to anatomy and cognitive pattern. Alzheimer's disease, for example, causes the greatest destruction in medial temporal areas belonging to the memory network and is clinically characterized by a correspondingly severe amnesia. There are other dementias where memory is intact. Frontal lobe dementia results from a selective degeneration of the frontal lobe and leads to a gradual dissolution of behavior and complex attention. Primary progressive aphasia is characterized by a gradual atrophy of the left perisylvian language network and leads to a progressive dissolution of language that can remain isolated for up to 10 years. An enlightened approach to the differential diagnosis and treatment of these patients requires an understanding of the principles that link neural networks to higher cerebral functions.

FURTHER READING

DAMASIO AR, DAMASIO H: Aphasia and the neural basis of language, in *Principles of Behavioral and Cognitive Neurology*, 2d ed, M-M Mesulam (ed). New York, Oxford University Press, 2000

GITELMAN DR et al: A large-scale distributed network for covert spatial attention. Further anatomical delineation based on stringent behavioral and cognitive controls. Brain 122:1093, 1999

HEISS W-D et al: Differential capacity of left and right hemispheric areas for compensation of poststroke aphasia. Ann Neurol 45:430, 1999

LEIGUARDA RC, MARSDEN CD: Limb apraxias. Higher-order disorders of sensorimotor integration. Brain 123:860, 2000

MESULAM M-M: Behavioral neuroanatomy: Large-scale networks, association cortex, frontal syndromes, the limbic system and hemispheric specializations, in *Principles of Behavioral and Cognitive Neurology*, 2d ed, M-M Mesulam (ed). New York, Oxford University Press, 2000

———: The human frontal lobes: Transcending the default mode through contingent encoding, in *Principles of Frontal Lobe Function*, DT Stuss, RT Knight (eds). New York, Oxford University Press, 2002

24 SLEEP DISORDERS
Charles A. Czeisler, John W. Winkelman, Gary S. Richardson

Disturbed sleep is among the most frequent health complaints physicians encounter. More than one-half of adults in the United States experience at least intermittent sleep disturbances. For most, it is an occasional night of poor sleep or daytime sleepiness. However, at least 15 to 20% of adults report chronic sleep disturbance or misalignment of circadian timing, which can lead to serious impairment of daytime functioning. In addition, such problems may contribute to or exacerbate medical or psychiatric conditions. Thirty years ago, many such complaints were treated with hypnotic medications without further di-

agnostic evaluation. Since then, a distinct class of sleep and arousal disorders has been identified.

PHYSIOLOGY OF SLEEP AND WAKEFULNESS

Most adults sleep 7 to 8 h per night, although the timing, duration, and internal structure of sleep vary among healthy individuals and as a function of age. At the extremes, infants and the elderly have frequent interruptions of sleep. In the United States, adults of intermediate age tend to have one consolidated sleep episode per day, although in some cultures sleep may be divided into a midafternoon nap and a shortened night sleep. Two principal systems govern the sleep-wake cycle: one actively generates sleep and sleep-related processes and another times sleep within the 24-h day. Either intrinsic abnormalities in these sys-

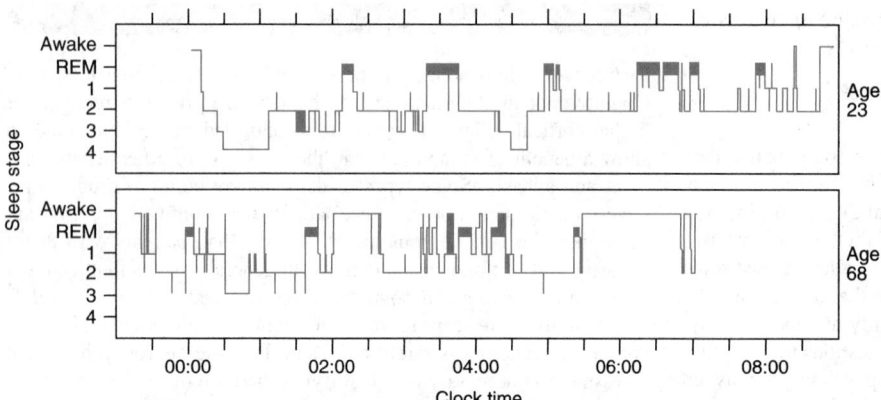

FIGURE 24-1 Stages of REM sleep (solid bars), the four stages of NREM sleep, and wakefulness over the course of the entire night for representative young and older adult men. Characteristic features of sleep in older people include reduction of slow-wave sleep, frequent spontaneous awakenings, early sleep onset, and early morning awakening. *(From the Division of Sleep Medicine, Brigham and Women's Hospital.)*

tems or extrinsic disturbances (environmental, drug- or illness-related) can lead to sleep or circadian rhythm disorders.

STATES AND STAGES OF SLEEP States and stages of human sleep are defined on the basis of characteristic patterns in the electroencephalogram (EEG), the electrooculogram (EOG—a measure of eye-movement activity), and the surface electromyogram (EMG) measured on the chin and neck. The continuous recording of this array of electrophysiologic parameters to define sleep and wakefulness is termed *polysomnography*.

Polysomnographic profiles define two states of sleep: (1) rapid-eye-movement (REM) sleep, and (2) non-rapid-eye-movement (NREM) sleep. NREM sleep is further subdivided into four stages, characterized by increasing arousal threshold and slowing of the cortical EEG. REM sleep is characterized by a low-amplitude, mixed-frequency EEG similar to that of NREM stage 1 sleep. The EOG shows bursts of REM similar to those seen during eyes-open wakefulness. Chin EMG activity is absent, reflecting the brainstem-mediated muscle atonia that is characteristic of that state.

ORGANIZATION OF HUMAN SLEEP Normal nocturnal sleep in adults displays a consistent organization from night to night (Fig. 24-1). After sleep onset, sleep usually progresses through NREM stages 1 to 4 within 45 to 60 min. Slow-wave sleep (NREM stages 3 and 4) predominates in the first third of the night and comprises 15 to 25% of total nocturnal sleep time in young adults. The percentage of slow-wave sleep is influenced by several factors, most notably age (see below). Prior sleep deprivation increases the rapidity of sleep onset and both the intensity and amount of slow-wave sleep.

The first REM sleep episode usually occurs in the second hour of sleep. More rapid onset of REM sleep in a young adult (particularly if <30 min) may suggest pathology such as endogenous depression, narcolepsy, circadian rhythm disorders, or drug withdrawal. NREM and REM alternate through the night with an average period of 90 to 110 min (the "ultradian" sleep cycle). Overall, REM sleep constitutes 20 to 25% of total sleep, and NREM stages 1 and 2 are 50 to 60%.

Age has a profound impact on sleep state organization (Fig. 24-1). Slow-wave sleep is most intense and prominent during childhood, decreasing sharply at puberty and across the second and third decades of life. After age 30, there is a progressive decline in the amount of slow-wave sleep, and the amplitude of delta EEG activity comprising slow-wave sleep is profoundly reduced. The depth of slow-wave sleep, as measured by the arousal threshold to auditory stimulation, also decreases with age. In the otherwise healthy older person, slow-wave sleep may be completely absent, particularly in males.

A different age profile exists for REM sleep than for slow-wave sleep. In infancy, REM sleep may comprise 50% of total sleep time, and the percentage is inversely proportional to developmental age. The amount of REM sleep falls off sharply over the first postnatal year as

a mature REM-NREM cycle develops; thereafter, REM sleep occupies a relatively constant percentage of total sleep time.

NEUROANATOMY OF SLEEP Experimental studies in animals have variously implicated the medullary reticular formation, the thalamus, and the basal forebrain in the generation of sleep, while the brainstem reticular formation, the midbrain, the subthalamus, the thalamus, and the basal forebrain have all been suggested to play a role in the generation of wakefulness or EEG arousal.

Current hypotheses suggest that the capacity for sleep and wakefulness generation is distributed along an axial "core" of neurons extending from the brainstem rostrally to the basal forebrain. Complex commingling of neuronal groups occurs at many points along this brainstem-forebrain axis. A cluster of γ-aminobutyric acid (GABA) and galaninergic neurons in the ventrolateral preoptic (VLPO) hypothalamus is selectively activated coincident with sleep onset. These neurons project to and inhibit histaminergic cell groups in the tuberomammilary nucleus that are important to the ascending arousal system, suggesting that the hypothalamic VLPO neurons may play a key executive role in sleep regulation.

Specific regions in the pons are associated with the neurophysiologic correlates of REM sleep. Small lesions in the dorsal pons result in the loss of the descending muscle inhibition normally associated with REM sleep; microinjections of the cholinergic agonist carbachol into the pontine reticular formation appear to produce a state with all of the features of REM sleep. These experimental manipulations are mimicked by pathologic conditions in humans and animals. In narcolepsy, for example, abrupt, complete, or partial paralysis (cataplexy) occurs in response to a variety of stimuli. In dogs with this condition, physostigmine, a central cholinesterase inhibitor, increases the frequency of cataplectic attacks, while atropine decreases their frequency. Conversely, in REM sleep behavior disorder (see below), patients suffer from incomplete motor inhibition during REM sleep, resulting in involuntary, occasionally violent movement during REM sleep.

NEUROCHEMISTRY OF SLEEP Early experimental studies that focused on the raphe nuclei of the brainstem appeared to implicate serotonin as the primary sleep-promoting neurotransmitter, while catecholamines were considered to be responsible for wakefulness. Subsequent work has demonstrated that the raphe-serotonin system may facilitate sleep but is not necessary for its expression. Pharmacologic studies of sleep and wakefulness suggest roles for other neurotransmitters as well. Pontine cholinergic neurotransmission is known to play a role in REM sleep generation. The alerting influence of caffeine implicates adenosine, whereas the hypnotic effect of benzodiazepines and barbiturates suggests a role for endogenous ligands of the GABA$_A$ receptor complex. A newly characterized neuropeptide, hypocretin (orexin), has recently been implicated in the pathophysiology of narcolepsy (see below), but its role in normal sleep regulation remains to be defined.

A variety of sleep-promoting substances have been identified, although it is not known whether or not they are involved in the endogenous sleep-wake regulatory process. These include prostaglandin D$_2$, delta sleep–inducing peptide, muramyl dipeptide, interleukin 1, fatty acid primary amides, and melatonin. The hypnotic effect of these substances is commonly limited to NREM or slow-wave sleep, although peptides that increase REM sleep have also been reported. Many putative "sleep factors," including interleukin 1 and prostaglandin D$_2$, are immunologically active as well, suggesting a link between immune function and sleep-wake states.

PHYSIOLOGY OF CIRCADIAN RHYTHMICITY The sleep-wake cycle is the most evident of the many 24-h rhythms in humans. Prominent daily variations also occur in endocrine, thermoregulatory, cardiac, pulmonary, renal, gastrointestinal, and neurobehavioral functions. At the molecular level, endogenous circadian rhythmicity is driven by self-sustaining transcriptional/translational feedback loops (Fig. 24-2). In evaluating a daily variation in humans, it is important to distinguish between those rhythmic components passively evoked by periodic environmental or behavioral changes (e.g., the increase in blood pressure and heart rate upon assumption of the upright posture) and those actively driven by an endogenous oscillatory process (e.g., the circadian variation in plasma cortisol that persists under a variety of environmental and behavioral conditions).

While it is now recognized that many peripheral tissues in mammals have circadian clocks that regulate diverse physiologic processes, these independent tissue-specific oscillations are coordinated by a central neural pacemaker located in the suprachiasmatic nuclei (SCN) of the hypothalamus. Bilateral destruction of these nuclei results in a loss of the endogenous circadian rhythm of locomotor activity, which can be restored only by transplantation of the same structure from a donor animal. The genetically determined period of this endogenous neural oscillator, which averages ~24.2 h in humans, is normally synchronized to the 24-h period of the environmental light-dark cycle. Small differences in circadian period underlie variations in diurnal preference, with the circadian period shorter in morning than in evening types. Entrainment of mammalian circadian rhythms by the light-dark cycle is mediated via the retinohypothalamic tract, a monosynaptic pathway that links specialized, photoreceptive retinal ganglion cells directly to the SCN. Humans are exquisitely sensitive to the resetting effects of light, particularly at the blue end (~460 to 480 nm) of the visible spectrum.

The timing and internal architecture of sleep are directly coupled to the output of the endogenous circadian pacemaker. Paradoxically, the endogenous circadian rhythms of sleep tendency, sleepiness, and REM sleep propensity all peak near the habitual wake time, just after the nadir of the endogenous circadian temperature cycle, whereas the circadian wake propensity rhythm peaks 1 to 3 h before the habitual bedtime. These rhythms are thus timed to oppose the homeostatic decline of sleep tendency during the habitual sleep episode and the rise

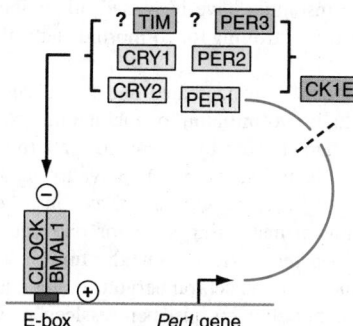

FIGURE 24-2 Model of the molecular feedback loop at the core of the mammalian circadian clock. The positive element of the feedback loop (+) is the transcriptional activation of the *Per1* gene (and probably other clock genes) by a heterodimer of the transcription factors CLOCK and BMAL1 (also called MOP3) bound to an E-box DNA regulatory element. The *Per1* transcript and its product, the clock component PER1 protein, accumulate in the cell cytoplasm. As it accumulates, the PER1 protein is recruited into a multiprotein complex thought to contain other circadian clock component proteins such as cryptochromes (CRYs), Period proteins (PERs), and others. This complex is then transported into the cell nucleus (across the dotted line), where it functions as the negative element in the feedback loop (−) by inhibiting the activity of the CLOCK-BMAL1 transcription factor heterodimer. As a consequence of this action, the concentration of PER1 and other clock proteins in the inhibitory complex falls, allowing CLOCK-BMAL1 to activate transcription of *Per1* and other genes and begin another cycle. The dynamics of the 24-h molecular cycle are controlled at several levels, including regulation of the rate of PER protein degradation by casein kinase-1 epsilon (CK1E). Additional limbs of this genetic regulatory network, omitted for the sake of clarity, are thought to contribute stability. Question marks denote putative clock proteins, such as Timeless (TIM), as yet lacking genetic proof of a role in the mammalian clock mechanism. (*Copyright © Charles J. Weitz, Ph.D., Department of Neurobiology, Harvard Medical School.*)

of sleep tendency throughout the usual waking day, respectively. Misalignment of the output of the endogenous circadian pacemaker with the desired sleep-wake cycle can, therefore, induce insomnia, decreased alertness, and impaired performance evident in night-shift workers and airline travelers.

BEHAVIORAL CORRELATES OF SLEEP STATES AND STAGES Polysomnographic staging of sleep correlates with behavioral changes during specific states and stages. During the transitional state between wakefulness and sleep (stage 1 sleep), subjects may respond to faint auditory or visual signals without "awakening." Memory incorporation is inhibited at the onset of NREM stage 1 sleep, which may explain why individuals aroused from that transitional sleep stage frequently deny having been asleep. Such transitions may intrude upon behavioral wakefulness after sleep deprivation, notwithstanding attempts to remain continuously awake (see "Shift-Work Sleep Disorder," below).

Awakenings from REM sleep are associated with recall of vivid dream imagery >80% of the time. The reliability of dream recall increases with REM sleep episodes occurring later in the night. Imagery may also be reported after NREM sleep interruptions, though these typically lack the detail and vividness of REM sleep dreams. The incidence of NREM sleep dream recall can be increased by selective REM sleep deprivation, suggesting that REM sleep and dreaming per se are not inexorably linked.

PHYSIOLOGIC CORRELATES OF SLEEP STATES AND STAGES All major physiologic systems are influenced by sleep. Changes in cardiovascular function include a decrease in blood pressure and heart rate during NREM and particularly during slow-wave sleep. During REM sleep, phasic activity (bursts of eye movements) is associated with variability in both blood pressure and heart rate mediated principally by the vagus. Cardiac dysrhythmias may occur selectively during REM sleep. Respiratory function also changes. In comparison to relaxed wakefulness, respiratory rate becomes more regular during NREM sleep (especially slow-wave sleep) and tonic REM sleep and becomes very irregular during phasic REM sleep. Minute ventilation decreases in NREM sleep out of proportion to the decrease in metabolic rate at sleep onset, resulting in a higher P_{CO_2}.

Endocrine function also varies with sleep. Slow-wave sleep is associated with secretion of growth hormone, while sleep in general is associated with augmented secretion of prolactin. Sleep has a complex effect on the secretion of luteinizing hormone (LH): during puberty, sleep is associated with increased LH secretion, whereas sleep in the mature woman inhibits LH secretion in the early follicular phase of the menstrual cycle. Sleep onset (and probably slow-wave sleep) is associated with inhibition of thyroid-stimulating hormone and of the adrenocorticotropic hormone–cortisol axis, an effect that is superimposed on the prominent circadian rhythms in the two systems.

The pineal hormone melatonin is secreted predominantly at night in both day- and night-active species, reflecting the direct modulation of pineal activity by the circadian pacemaker through a circuitous neural pathway from the SCN to the pineal gland. Melatonin secretion is not dependent upon the occurrence of sleep, persisting in individuals kept awake at night. In addition, exogenous melatonin increases sleepiness and may potentiate sleep when administered to good sleepers attempting to sleep during daylight hours at a time when endogenous melatonin levels are low. The efficacy of melatonin as a sleep-promoting therapy for patients with insomnia is currently not known.

Sleep is also accompanied by alterations of thermoregulatory function. NREM sleep is associated with an attenuation of thermoregulatory responses to either heat or cold stress, and animal studies of thermosensitive neurons in the hypothalamus document an NREM-sleep-dependent reduction of the thermoregulatory set-point. REM sleep is associated with complete absence of thermoregulatory responsiveness, effectively resulting in functional poikilothermy. However, the potential adverse impact of this failure of thermoregulation is blunted by inhibition of REM sleep by extreme ambient temperatures.

TABLE 24-1 *Evaluation of the Patient with the Complaint of Excessive Daytime Somnolence*

Findings on History and Physical Examination	Diagnostic Evaluation	Diagnosis	Therapy
Obesity, snoring, hypertension	Polysomnography with respiratory monitoring	Obstructive sleep apnea	Continuous positive airway pressure; ENT surgery (e.g., uvulopalatopharyngoplasty); dental appliance; pharmacologic therapy (e.g., protriptyline); weight loss
Cataplexy, hypnogogic hallucinations, sleep paralysis, family history	Polysomnography with multiple sleep latency testing	Narcolepsy-cataplexy syndrome	Stimulants (e.g., modafinil, methylphenidate); REM-suppressant antidepressants (e.g., protriptyline); genetic counseling
Restless legs syndrome, disturbed sleep, predisposing medical condition (e.g., anemia or renal failure)	Polysomnography with bilateral anterior tibialis EMG monitoring	Periodic limb movements of sleep	Treatment of predisposing condition, if possible; dopamine agonists (e.g., pramipexole); benzodiazepines (e.g., clonazepam)
Disturbed sleep, predisposing medical conditions (e.g., asthma) and/or predisposing medical therapies (e.g., theophylline)	Sleep-wake diary recording	Insomnias (see text)	Treatment of predisposing condition and/or change in therapy, if possible; behavioral therapy; short-acting benzodiazepine receptor agonist (e.g., zolpidem)

Note: ENT, ears, nose, throat; REM, rapid eye movement; EMG, electromyogram.

DISORDERS OF SLEEP AND WAKEFULNESS

APPROACH TO THE PATIENT

Patients may seek help from a physician because of one of several symptoms: (1) an acute or chronic inability to sleep adequately at night (insomnia); (2) chronic fatigue, sleepiness, or tiredness during the day; or (3) a behavioral manifestation associated with sleep itself. Complaints of insomnia or excessive daytime sleepiness should be viewed as symptoms (much like fever or pain) of underlying disorders. Knowledge of the differential diagnosis of these presenting complaints is essential to identify the underlying medical disorder. Only then can appropriate treatment, rather than nonspecific approaches (e.g., over-the-counter sleeping aids), be applied. Diagnoses of exclusion, such as primary insomnia, should be made only after other diagnoses have been ruled out. Table 24-1 outlines the diagnostic and therapeutic approach to the patient with a complaint of excessive daytime sleepiness.

A careful history is essential. In particular, the duration, severity, and consistency of the symptoms are important, along with the patient's estimate of the consequences of reported sleep loss on waking function. Information from a friend or family member can be invaluable; some patients may be unaware of, or will underreport, such potentially embarrassing symptoms as heavy snoring or falling asleep while driving.

Completion by the patient of a day-by-day sleep-work-drug log for at least 2 weeks can help the physician better understand the nature of the complaint. Work times and sleep times (including daytime naps and nocturnal awakenings) as well as drug and alcohol use, including caffeine and hypnotics, should be noted each day. In addition, the sleep times should be recorded.

Polysomnography is necessary for the diagnosis of specific disorders such as narcolepsy and sleep apnea and may be of utility in other settings as well. In addition to the three electrophysiologic variables used to define sleep states and stages, the standard clinical polysomnogram includes measures of respiration (respiratory effort, air flow, and oxygen saturation), anterior tibialis EMG, and electrocardiogram. Evaluation of penile tumescence during nocturnal sleep can also help determine whether the cause of erectile dysfunction in a patient is psychogenic or organic (Chap. 43).

EVALUATION OF INSOMNIA Insomnia is the complaint of inadequate sleep; it can be classified according to the nature of sleep disruption and the duration of the complaint. Insomnia is subdivided into difficulty falling asleep (*sleep onset insomnia*), frequent or sustained awakenings (*sleep maintenance insomnia*), early morning awakenings (*sleep offset insomnia*), or persistent sleepiness despite sleep of adequate duration (*nonrestorative sleep*). Similarly, the duration of the symptom influences diagnostic and therapeutic considerations. An insomnia complaint lasting one to several nights (within a single episode) is termed *transient insomnia* and is typically the result of situational stress or a change in sleep schedule or environment (e.g., jet lag). *Short-term insomnia* lasts from a few days to 3 weeks. Disruption of this duration is usually associated with more protracted stress, such as recovery from surgery or short-term illness. *Long-term insomnia*, or *chronic insomnia*, lasts for months or years and, in contrast with short-term insomnia, requires a thorough evaluation of underlying causes (see below). Chronic insomnia is often a waxing and waning disorder, with spontaneous or stressor-induced exacerbations.

An occasional night of poor sleep, typically in the setting of stress or excitement about external events, is both common and without lasting consequences. However, persistent insomnia can lead to impaired daytime function, injury due to accidents, and the development of major depression. In addition, there is emerging evidence that individuals with chronic insomnia have increased utilization of health care resources, even after controlling for co-morbid medical and psychiatric disorders.

All insomnias can be exacerbated and perpetuated by behaviors that are not conducive to initiating or maintaining sleep. *Inadequate sleep hygiene* is characterized by a behavior pattern prior to sleep or a bedroom environment that is not conducive to sleep. Noise or light in the bedroom can interfere with sleep, as can a bed partner with periodic limb movements during sleep or one who snores loudly. Clocks can heighten the anxiety about the time it has taken to fall asleep. Drugs that act on the central nervous system, large meals, vigorous exercise, or hot showers just before sleep may interfere with sleep onset. Many individuals participate in stressful work-related activities in the evening, producing a state incompatible with sleep onset. In preference to hypnotic medications, patients should be counseled to avoid stressful activities before bed, develop a soporific bedtime ritual, and to prepare and reserve the bedroom environment for sleeping. Consistent, regular rising times should be maintained daily, including weekends.

PRIMARY INSOMNIA ■ Insomnia without Identifiable Cause Many patients with chronic insomnia have no clear, single identifiable underlying cause for their difficulties with sleep. Rather, such patients often have multiple etiologies for their insomnia, which may evolve over the years. Primary insomnia is thus a diagnosis of exclusion, often without a clear underlying single cause. In addition, the chief sleep complaint may change over time, with initial insomnia predominating at one point, and multiple awakenings or nonrestorative sleep occurring at other times. Subsyndromal psychiatric disorders (e.g., anxiety and mood complaints), negative conditioning to the sleep environment (psychophysiologic insomnia, see below), amplification of the time spent awake (sleep-state misperception), physiologic hyperarousal, and poor sleep hygiene (see above) may all be present. As these processes may be both causes and consequences of chronic insomnia, many individuals will have a progressive course to their symptoms in which the severity is proportional to the chronicity, and much of the complaint may persist even after effective treatment of the initial inciting etiology. Treatment of primary insomnia is often directed to each of the putative contributing factors: behavior therapies for anxiety and negative conditioning (see below), pharmacotherapy for mood/anxiety disorders, an emphasis on maintenance of good sleep hygiene, and intermittent hypnotics for exacerbations of the insomnia.

If insomnia persists after treatment of these contributing factors, empirical pharmacotherapy is often used on a nightly or intermittent basis. A variety of sedative compounds are used for this purpose. Alcohol and antihistamines are the most commonly used nonprescription sleep aids. The former may help with sleep onset, but is associated with sleep disruption during the night and can escalate into abuse, dependence, and withdrawal in the predisposed individual. Antihistamines may be of benefit when used intermittently, but produce rapid tolerance and have multiple side effects (especially anticholinergic), which limit their use. Benzodiazepine receptor agonists are the most effective and well-tolerated class of medications for insomnia. The broad range of half-lives allows flexibility in the duration of sedative action. Zaleplon (5 to 20 mg), with a half-life of 1 to 2 h, zolpidem (5 to 10 mg) and triazolam (0.125 to 0.25 mg), with half-lives of 2 to 3 h, and temazepam (15 to 30 mg) and lorazepam (0.5 to 2 mg), with half-lives of 6 to 12 h, are the most commonly prescribed agents in this family. Generally, side effects are minimal if the dose is kept low and the serum concentration is minimized during the waking hours (by using the shortest-acting, effective agent). However, with even brief continuous use, rebound insomnia can occur upon discontinuation. There are only limited data supporting sustained efficacy of benzodiazepine receptor agonists; caution should be exercised in long-term use. The likelihood of rebound insomnia and tolerance can be minimized by short durations of treatment, intermittent use, or gradual tapering of the dose. For acute insomnia, nightly use of a benzodiazepine receptor agonist for a maximum of 2 to 4 weeks is advisable. For chronic insomnia, intermittent use is recommended. Benzodiazepine receptor agonists should be avoided, or used very judiciously, in patients with a history of substance abuse. The heterocyclic antidepressants (trazodone, amitriptyline, and doxepin) are the most commonly prescribed alternatives to benzodiazepine receptor agonists due to their lack of abuse potential and lower cost. Trazodone (25 to 100 mg) is used more commonly than the tricyclic antidepressants as it has a much shorter half-life (5 to 9 h), has much less anticholinergic activity (sparing patients, particularly the elderly, constipation, urinary retention, and tachycardia), is associated with less weight gain, and is much safer in overdose. The risk of priapism is small (~1 in 10,000).

Psychophysiologic Insomnia Persistent *psychophysiologic insomnia* is a behavioral disorder in which patients are preoccupied with a perceived inability to sleep adequately at night. The sleep disturbance is often triggered by an emotionally stressful event; however, the poor sleep habits and beliefs about sleep acquired during the stressful period persist long after the initial incident. Such patients become hyperaroused by their own persistent efforts to sleep or the sleep environment, and the insomnia is a conditioned or learned response. They may be able to fall asleep more easily at unscheduled times (when not trying) or outside the home environment. Polysomnographic recording in patients with psychophysiologic insomnia reveals an objective sleep disturbance, often with an abnormally long sleep latency; frequent nocturnal awakenings; and an increased amount of stage 1 transitional sleep. Rigorous attention should be paid to sleep hygiene and correction of counterproductive, arousing behaviors before bedtime. Behavioral therapies are the treatment modality of choice, with only intermittent use of medications. When patients are awake for >20 min, they should read or perform other relaxing activities to distract themselves from insomnia-related anxiety. In addition, bedtime and waketime should be scheduled to restrict time in bed to be equal to their perceived total sleep time. This will generally produce sleep deprivation, greater sleep drive, and, eventually, better sleep. Time in bed can then be gradually expanded.

SECONDARY INSOMNIA ■ Transient Situational Insomnia This typically develops after a change in the sleeping environment (e.g., in an unfamiliar hotel or hospital bed) or before or after a significant life event, such as a change of occupation, loss of a loved one, illness, or anxiety over a deadline or examination. Increased sleep latency, frequent awakenings from sleep, and early morning awakening can all occur. Recovery is generally rapid, usually within a few weeks. Treatment is symptomatic, with intermittent use of hypnotics and resolution of the underlying stress. *Altitude insomnia* describes a sleep disturbance that is a common consequence of exposure to high altitude. Periodic breathing of the Cheyne-Stokes type occurs during NREM sleep about half the time at high altitude, with restoration of a regular breathing pattern during REM sleep. Both hypoxia and hypocapnia are thought to be involved in the development of periodic breathing. Frequent awakenings and poor quality sleep characterize altitude insomnia, which is generally worst on the first few nights at high altitude but may persist. Treatment with acetazolamide can decrease time spent in periodic breathing and substantially reduce hypoxia during sleep.

Insomnia Associated with Mental Disorders Approximately 80% of patients with psychiatric disorders describe sleep complaints. There is considerable heterogeneity, however, in the nature of the sleep disturbance both between conditions and among patients with the same condition. *Depression* can be associated with sleep onset insomnia, sleep maintenance insomnia, or early morning wakefulness. However, hypersomnia occurs in some depressed patients, especially adolescents and those with either bipolar or seasonal (fall/winter) depression (Chap. 371). Indeed, sleep disturbance is an important vegetative sign of depression and may commence before any mood changes are perceived by the patient. Consistent polysomnographic findings in depression include decreased REM sleep latency, lengthened first REM sleep episode, and shortened first NREM sleep episode; however, these findings are not specific for depression, and the extent of these changes varies with age and symptomatology. Depressed patients also show decreased slow-wave sleep and reduced sleep continuity.

In *mania* and *hypomania*, sleep latency is increased and total sleep time can be reduced. Patients with *anxiety disorders* tend not to show the changes in REM sleep and slow-wave sleep seen in endogenously depressed patients. *Chronic alcoholics* lack slow-wave sleep, have decreased amounts of REM sleep (as an acute response to alcohol), and have frequent arousals throughout the night. This is associated with impaired daytime alertness. The sleep of chronic alcoholics may remain disturbed for years after discontinuance of alcohol usage. Sleep architecture and physiology are disturbed in *schizophrenia* (with a decreased amount of stage 4 sleep and a lack of augmentation of REM sleep following REM sleep deprivation); chronic schizophrenics often show day-night reversal, sleep fragmentation, and insomnia.

Insomnia Associated with Neurologic Disorders A variety of neurologic diseases result in sleep disruption through both indirect, nonspecific mechanisms (e.g., pain in cervical spondylosis or low back pain) or by impairment of central neural structures involved in the generation and control of sleep itself. For example, *dementia* from any cause has long been associated with disturbances in the timing of the sleep-wake cycle, often characterized by nocturnal wandering and an exacerbation of symptomatology at night (so-called sundowning).

Epilepsy may rarely present as a sleep complaint (Chap. 348). Often the history is of abnormal behavior, at times with convulsive movements during sleep, and the differential diagnosis includes REM sleep behavior disorder, sleep apnea syndrome, and periodic movements of sleep (see above). Diagnosis requires nocturnal EEG recording. Other neurologic diseases associated with abnormal movements, such as

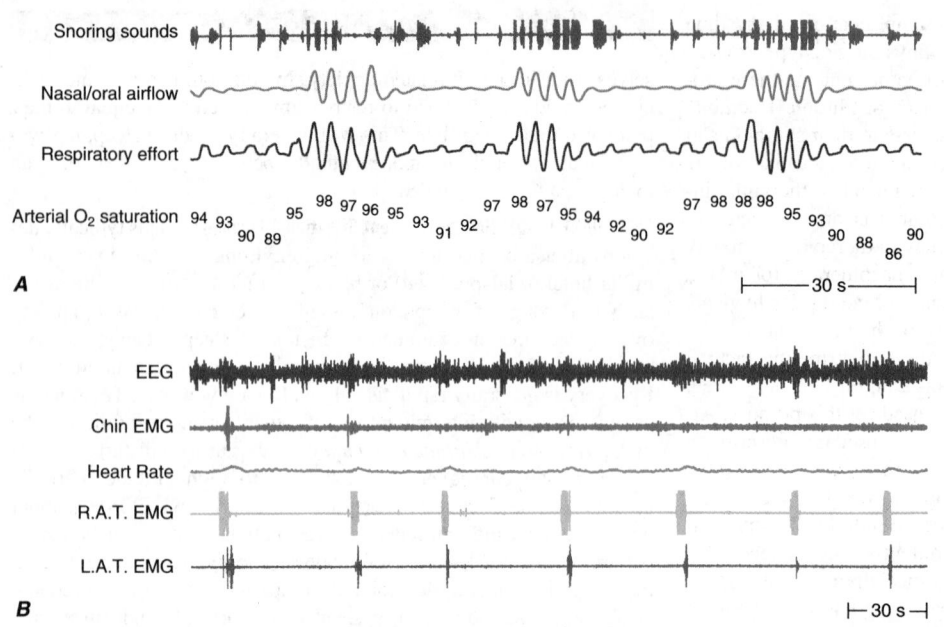

FIGURE 24-3 Polysomnographic recordings of (*A*) obstructive sleep apnea and (*B*) periodic limb movement of sleep. Note the snoring and reduction in air flow in the presence of continued respiratory effort, associated with the subsequent oxygen desaturation (upper panel). Periodic limb movements occur with a relatively constant intermovement interval and are associated with changes in the EEG and heart rates acceleration (lower panel). Abbreviations: R.A.T., right anterior tibialis; L.A.T., left anterior tibialis. (*From the Division of Sleep Medicine, Brigham and Women's Hospital.*)

Parkinson's disease, hemiballismus, Huntington's chorea, and *Gilles de la Tourette syndrome* (Chap. 351), are also associated with disrupted sleep, presumably through secondary mechanisms. However, the abnormal movements themselves are greatly reduced during sleep. Headache syndromes (*migraine* or *cluster headache*) may show sleep-associated exacerbations (Chap. 14) by unknown mechanisms.

Fatal familial insomnia is a rare hereditary disorder caused by degeneration of anterior and dorsomedial nuclei of the thalamus. Insomnia is a prominent early symptom. Progressively, the syndrome produces autonomic dysfunction, dysarthria, myoclonus, coma, and death. The pathogenesis is a mutation in the prion gene (Chap. 362).

Insomnia Associated with Other Medical Disorders A number of medical conditions are associated with disruptions of sleep. The association is frequently nonspecific, e.g., that between sleep disruption and chronic pain from rheumatologic disorders. Attention to this association is important in that sleep-associated symptoms are often the presenting complaint. Treatment of the underlying medical disorder or symptom is the most useful approach. Sleep disruption can also result from the appropriate use of drugs such as glucocorticoids (see below).

One prominent association is between sleep disruption and *asthma*. In many asthmatics there is a prominent daily variation in airway resistance that results in marked increases in asthmatic symptoms at night, especially during sleep. In addition, treatment of asthma with theophylline-based compounds, adrenergic agonists, or glucocorticoids can independently disrupt sleep. When sleep disruption is a side effect of asthma treatment, inhaled glucocorticoids (e.g., beclomethasone) that do not disrupt sleep may provide a useful alternative.

Cardiac ischemia may also be associated with sleep disruption. The ischemia itself may result from increases in sympathetic tone as a result of sleep apnea. Patients may present with complaints of nightmares or vivid, disturbing dreams, with or without awareness of the more classic symptoms of angina or of the sleep disordered breathing. Treatment of the sleep apnea may substantially improve the angina and the nocturnal sleep quality. *Paroxysmal nocturnal dyspnea* can also occur as a consequence of sleep-associated cardiac ischemia that causes pulmonary congestion exacerbated by the recumbent posture.

Chronic obstructive pulmonary disease is also associated with sleep disruption, as is *cystic fibrosis, menopause, hyperthyroidism, gastroesophageal reflux, chronic renal failure*, and *liver failure*.

Medication-, Drug-, or Alcohol-Dependent Insomnia Disturbed sleep can result from ingestion of a wide variety of agents. Caffeine is perhaps the most common pharmacologic cause of insomnia. It produces increased latency to sleep onset, more frequent arousals during sleep, and a reduction in total sleep time for up to 8 to 14 h after ingestion. As few as three to five cups of coffee can significantly disturb sleep in some patients; therefore, a 1- to 2-month trial without caffeine should be attempted in patients with these symptoms. Similarly, alcohol and nicotine can interfere with sleep, despite the fact that many patients use them to relax and promote sleep. Although alcohol can increase drowsiness and shorten sleep latency, even moderate amounts of alcohol increase awakenings in the second half of the night. In addition, alcohol ingestion prior to sleep is contraindicated in patients with sleep apnea because of the inhibitory effects of alcohol on upper airway muscle tone. Acutely, amphetamines and cocaine suppress both REM sleep and total sleep time, which return to normal with chronic use. Withdrawal leads to a REM sleep rebound. A number of prescribed medications can produce insomnia. Antidepressants, sympathomimetics, and glucocorticoids are common causes. In addition, severe rebound insomnia can result from the acute withdrawal of hypnotics, especially following the use of high doses of benzodiazepines with a short half-life. For this reason, hypnotic doses should be low to moderate, the total duration of hypnotic therapy should usually be limited to 2 to 3 weeks, and prolonged drug tapering is encouraged.

RESTLESS LEGS SYNDROME (RLS) Patients with this sensory-motor disorder report a creeping or crawling dysesthesia deep within the calves or feet, or sometimes even in the upper extemities, that is associated with an irresistible urge to move the affected limbs. For most patients with RLS, the dysesthesias and restlessness are much worse in the evening or night compared to the daytime and frequently interfere with the ability to fall asleep. The disorder is exacerbated by inactivity and temporarily relieved by movement. In contrast, paresthesias secondary to peripheral neuropathy persists with activity. The severity of this chronic disorder may wax and wane with time and can be exacerbated by sleep deprivation, caffeine, and pregnancy. The prevalence is 1 to 5% of young to middle-age adults and increases to 10 to 20% in those >60 years. There appear to be important differences in RLS prevalence among racial groups, with higher prevalence in those of Northern European ancestry. Roughly one-third of patients (particularly those with an early age of onset) will have multiple affected family members, possibly with an autosomal dominant pattern. Iron deficiency and renal failure may cause RLS, which is then considered secondary RLS. The symptoms of RLS are exquisitely sensitive to dopaminergic drugs (e.g., pramipexole 0.25 to 1.0 mg q8pm or ropinirole 0.5 to 4.0 mg q8pm), which are the treatment of choice. Narcotics, benzodiazepines, and certain anticonvulsants may also be of therapeutic value. Most patients with restless legs also experience periodic limb movements of sleep, although the reverse is not the case.

PERIODIC LIMB MOVEMENT DISORDER *Periodic limb movement disorder*, previously known as *nocturnal myoclonus*, is the principal objective polysomnographic finding in 17% of patients with insomnia and 11% of those with excessive daytime somnolence (Fig. 24-3). It is often unclear whether it is an incidental finding or the cause of disturbed sleep. Stereotyped, 0.5- to 5.0-s extensions of the great toe and dorsiflexion of the foot recur every 20 to 40 s during NREM sleep, in episodes lasting from minutes to hours. Most such episodes occur during the first half of the night. The disorder occurs in a wide variety of sleep disorders (including narcolepsy, sleep apnea, REM sleep behavior disorder, and various forms of insomnia) and may be associated with frequent arousals and an increased number of sleep-stage transitions. The incidence increases with age: 44% of people over age 65 without a sleep complaint have more than five periodic leg movements per hour of sleep. The pathophysiology is not well understood, though individuals with high spinal transections can exhibit periodic leg movements during sleep, suggesting the existence of a spinal generator. Polysomnography with bilateral surface EMG recording of the anterior tibialis is used to establish the diagnosis. Treatment options include dopaminergic medications or benzodiazepines.

EVALUATION OF DAYTIME SLEEPINESS Daytime impairment due to sleep loss may be difficult to quantify for several reasons. First, sleepiness is not necessarily proportional to subjectively assessed sleep deprivation. In obstructive sleep apnea, for example, the repeated brief interruptions of sleep associated with resumption of respiration at the end of apneic episodes result in daytime sleepiness, despite the fact that the patient may be unaware of the sleep fragmentation. Second, subjective descriptions of waking impairment vary from patient to patient. Patients may describe themselves as "sleepy," "fatigued," or "tired" and may have a clear sense of the meaning of those terms, while others may use the same terms to describe a completely different condition. Third, sleepiness, particularly when profound, may affect judgment in a manner analogous to ethanol, such that subjective awareness of the condition and the consequent cognitive and motor impairment is reduced. Finally, patients may be reluctant to admit that sleepiness is a problem, both because they are generally unaware of what constitutes normal alertness and because sleepiness is generally viewed pejoratively, ascribed more often to a deficit in motivation than to an inadequately addressed physiologic sleep need.

Specific questioning about the occurrence of sleep episodes during normal waking hours, both intentional and unintentional, can overcome the inconsistencies among subjective characterizations and help to interpret the adverse impact of sleepiness on daytime function. Specific areas to be addressed include the occurrence of inadvertent sleep episodes while driving or in other safety-related settings, sleepiness while at work or school (and the relationship of sleepiness to work and school performance), and the effect of sleepiness on social and family life. Evidence for significant daytime impairment [in association either with the diagnosis of a primary sleep disorder, such as narcolepsy or sleep apnea, or with imposed or self-selected sleep-wake schedules (see "Shift-Work Sleep Disorder," below)] raises the question of the physician's responsibility to notify motor vehicle licensing authorities of the increased risk of sleepiness-related vehicle accidents. As with epilepsy, legal requirements vary from state to state, and existing legal precedents do not provide a consistent interpretation of the balance between the physician's responsibility and the patient's right to privacy. At a minimum, physicians should document discussions with the patient regarding the increased risk of operating a vehicle, as well as a recommendation that driving be suspended until successful treatment or schedule modification can be instituted.

The distinction between fatigue and sleepiness can be useful in the differentiation of patients with complaints of fatigue or tiredness in the setting of disorders such as fibromyalgia (Chap. 315), chronic fatigue syndrome (Chap. 370), or endocrine deficiencies such as hypothyroidism (Chap. 320) or Addison's disease (Chap. 321). While patients with these disorders can typically distinguish their daytime symptoms from the sleepiness that occurs with sleep deprivation, substantial overlap can occur. This is particularly true when the primary disorder also results in chronic sleep disruption (e.g., sleep apnea in hypothyroidism) or in abnormal sleep (e.g., fibromyalgia).

While clinical evaluation of the complaint of excessive sleepiness is usually adequate, objective quantification is sometimes necessary. Assessment of daytime functioning as an index of the adequacy of

sleep can be made with the multiple sleep latency test (MSLT), which involves repeated measurement of sleep latency (time to onset of sleep) under standardized conditions during a day following quantified nocturnal sleep. The average latency across four to six tests (administered every 2 h across the waking day) provides an objective measure of daytime sleep tendency. Disorders of sleep that result in pathologic daytime somnolence can be reliably distinguished with the MSLT. In addition, the multiple measurements of sleep onset may identify direct transitions from wakefulness to REM sleep that are suggestive of specific pathologic conditions (e.g., narcolepsy).

NARCOLEPSY Narcolepsy is both a disorder of the ability to sustain wakefulness voluntarily and a disorder of REM sleep regulation (Table 24-2). The classic "narcolepsy tetrad" consists of excessive daytime somnolence plus three specific symptoms related to an intrusion of REM sleep characteristics (e.g., muscle atonia, vivid dream imagery) into the transition between wakefulness and sleep: (1) sudden weakness or loss of muscle tone without loss of consciousness, often elicited by emotion (cataplexy); (2) hallucinations at sleep onset (hypnogogic hallucinations) or upon awakening (hypnopompic hallucinations); and (3) muscular paralysis upon awakening (sleep paralysis). The severity of cataplexy varies, as patients may have two to three attacks per day or per decade. Some patients with objectively confirmed narcolepsy (see below) may show no evidence of cataplexy. In those with cataplexy, the extent and duration of an attack may also vary, from a transient sagging of the jaw lasting a few seconds to rare cases of flaccid paralysis of the entire voluntary musculature for up to 20 to 30 min. Symptoms of narcolepsy typically begin in the second decade, although the onset ranges from ages 5 to 50. Once established, the disease is chronic without remissions. Secondary forms of narcolepsy have been described (e.g., after head trauma).

Narcolepsy affects about 1 in 4000 people in the United States and appears to have a genetic basis. Recently, several convergent lines of evidence suggests that the hypothalamic neuropeptide hypocretin (orexin) is involved in the pathogenesis of narcolepsy: (1) a mutation in the hypocretin receptor 2 gene has been associated with canine narcolepsy; (2) hypocretin "knockout" mice that are genetically unable to produce this neuropeptide exhibit a phenotype, as assessed by behavioral and electrophysiologic criteria, that is similar to human narcolepsy; and (3) cerebrospinal fluid levels of hypocretin are reduced in most patients who have narcolepsy with cataplexy. The inheritance pattern of narcolepsy in humans is more complex than in the canine model. However, almost all narcoleptics with cataplexy are positive for HLA DQB1*0602 (Chap. 296), suggesting that an autoimmune process may be responsible.

Diagnosis The diagnostic criteria continue to be a matter of debate. Certainly, objective verification of excessive daytime somnolence, typically with MSLT mean sleep latencies <8 min, is an essential if nonspecific diagnostic feature. Other conditions that cause excessive sleepiness, such as sleep apnea or chronic sleep restriction, must be rigorously excluded. The other objective diagnostic feature of narcolepsy is the presence of REM sleep in at least two of the naps during the MSLT. Abnormal regulation of REM sleep is also manifested by

TABLE 24-2 *Prevalence of Symptoms in Narcolepsy*

Symptom	Prevalence, %
Excessive daytime somnolence	100
Disturbed sleep	87
Cataplexy	76
Hypnagogic hallucinations	68
Sleep paralysis	64
Memory problems	50

Source: Modified from TA Roth, L Merlotti in SA Burton et al (eds), *Narcolepsy 3rd International Symposium: Selected Symposium Proceedings*, Chicago, Matrix Communications, 1989.

the appearance of REM sleep immediately or within minutes after sleep onset in 50% of narcoleptic patients, a rarity in unaffected individuals maintaining a conventional sleep-wake schedule. The REM-related symptoms of the classic narcolepsy tetrad are variably present. There is increasing evidence that narcoleptics with cataplexy (one-half to two-thirds of patients) may represent a more homogeneous group than those without this symptom. However, a history of cataplexy can be difficult to establish reliably. Hypnogogic and hypnopompic hallucinations and sleep paralysis are often found in nonnarcoleptic individuals and may be present in only one-half of narcoleptics. Nocturnal sleep disruption is commonly observed in narcolepsy but is also a nonspecific symptom. Similarly, a history of "automatic behavior" during wakefulness (a trancelike state during which simple motor behaviors persist) is not specific for narcolepsy and serves principally to corroborate the presence of daytime somnolence.

℞ TREATMENT

The treatment of narcolepsy is symptomatic. Somnolence is treated with wake-promoting therapeutics. Modafinil is now the drug of choice, principally because it is associated with fewer side effects than older stimulants and has a long half-life; 200 to 400 mg is given as a single daily dose. Older drugs such as methylphenidate (10 mg bid to 20 mg qid or dextroamphetamine (10 mg bid) are still used as alternatives, particularly in refractory patients.

Treatment of the REM-related phenomena cataplexy, hypnogogic hallucinations, and sleep paralysis requires the potent REM sleep suppression produced by antidepressant medications. The tricyclic antidepressants [e.g., protriptyline (10 to 40 mg/d) and clomipramine (25–50 mg/d)] and the selective serotonin reuptake inhibitors (SSRIs) [e.g., fluoxetine (10 to 20 mg/d)] are commonly used for this purpose. Efficacy of the antidepressants is limited largely by anticholinergic side effects (tricyclics) and by sleep disturbance and sexual dysfunction (SSRIs). Adequate nocturnal sleep time and planned daytime naps (when possible) are important preventative measures.

SLEEP APNEA SYNDROMES Respiratory dysfunction during sleep is a common, serious cause of excessive daytime somnolence as well as of disturbed nocturnal sleep. An estimated 2 to 5 million people in the United States have a reduction or cessation of breathing for 10 to 150 s, from thirty to several hundred times every night during sleep. These episodes may be due to either an occlusion of the airway (*obstructive sleep apnea*), absence of respiratory effort (*central sleep apnea*), or a combination of these factors (*mixed sleep apnea*) (Fig. 24-3). Failure to recognize and treat these conditions appropriately may lead to impairment of daytime alertness; increased risk of sleep-related motor vehicle accidents; hypertension and other serious cardiovascular complications; and increased mortality. Sleep apnea is particularly prevalent in overweight men and in the elderly, yet it is estimated to remain undiagnosed in 80 to 90% of affected individuals. This is unfortunate since effective treatments are available. →*Readers are referred to Chap. 247 for a comprehensive review of the diagnosis and treatment of patients with these conditions.*

PARASOMNIAS The term *parasomnia* refers to abnormal behaviors that arise from or occur during sleep. A continuum of parasomnias arise from NREM sleep, from brief confusional arousals to sleepwalking and night terrors. The presenting complaint is usually related to the behavior itself, but the parasomnias can disturb sleep continuity or lead to mild impairments in daytime alertness. Only one parasomnia is known to occur in REM sleep, i.e., REM sleep behavior disorder (RBD; see below).

Sleepwalking (Somnambulism) Patients affected by this disorder carry out automatic motor activities that range from simple to complex. Individuals may leave the bed, walk, urinate inappropriately, eat, or exit from the house while remaining only partially aware. Full arousal may be difficult, and some patients may respond to attempted awakening

with agitation or even violence. Sleepwalking arises from stage 3 or 4 NREM sleep and is most common in children and adolescents, when these sleep stages are most robust. Episodes are usually isolated but may be recurrent in 1 to 6% of patients. The cause is unknown, though it has a familial basis in roughly one-third of cases.

Sleep Terrors This disorder, also called *pavor nocturnus*, occurs primarily in young children during the first several hours after sleep onset, in stages 3 and 4 of NREM sleep. The child suddenly screams, exhibiting autonomic arousal with sweating, tachycardia, and hyperventilation. The individual may be difficult to arouse and rarely recalls the episode on awakening in the morning. Recurrent attacks are rare. Parents are usually reassured to learn that the condition is self-limited and benign, and that no specific therapy is indicated. Both sleep terrors and sleepwalking represent abnormalities of arousal. In contrast, *nightmares* (dream anxiety attacks) occur during REM sleep and cause full arousal, with intact memory for the unpleasant episode.

REM Sleep Behavior Disorder RBD is a rare condition that is distinct from other parasomnias in that it occurs during REM sleep. It primarily afflicts men of middle age or older, many of whom have a history of prior neurologic disease. In fact, over one-third of patients will go on to develop Parkinson's disease (Chap. 351) within 10 to 20 years. Presenting symptoms consist of agitated or violent behavior during sleep, reported by a bed partner. In contrast to typical somnambulism, injury to patient or bed partner is not uncommon, and, upon awakening, the patient reports vivid, often unpleasant, dream imagery. The principal differential diagnosis is that of nocturnal seizures, which can be excluded with polysomnography. In RBD, seizure activity is absent on the EEG, and disinhibition of the usual motor atonia is observed in the EMG during REM sleep, at times associated with complex motor behaviors. The pathogenesis is unclear, but damage to brainstem areas mediating descending motor inhibition during REM sleep may be responsible. In support of this hypothesis are the remarkable similarities between RBD and the sleep of animals with bilateral lesions of the pontine tegmentum in areas controlling REM sleep motor inhibition. Treatment with clonazepam (0.5 to 1.0 mg qhs) provides sustained improvement in almost all reported cases.

Sleep Bruxism Bruxism is an involuntary, forceful grinding of teeth during sleep that affects 10 to 20% of the population. The patient is usually unaware of the problem. The typical age of onset is 17 to 20 years, and spontaneous remission usually occurs by age 40. Sex distribution appears to be equal. In many cases, the diagnosis is made during dental examination, damage is minor, and no treatment is indicated. In more severe cases, treatment with a rubber tooth guard is necessary to prevent disfiguring tooth injury. Stress management or, in some cases, biofeedback can be useful when bruxism is a manifestation of psychological stress. There are anecdotal reports of benefit using benzodiazepines.

Sleep Enuresis Bedwetting, like sleepwalking and night terrors, is another parasomnia that occurs during sleep in the young. Before age 5 or 6, nocturnal enuresis should probably be considered a normal feature of development. The condition usually improves spontaneously at puberty, has a prevalence in late adolescence of 1 to 3%, and is rare in adulthood. In older patients with enuresis a distinction must be made between primary and secondary enuresis, the latter being defined as bedwetting in patients who have been fully continent for 6 to 12 months. Treatment of primary enuresis is reserved for patients of appropriate age (>5 or 6 years) and consists of bladder training exercises and behavioral therapy. Urologic abnormalities are more common in primary enuresis and must be assessed by urologic examination. Important causes of secondary enuresis include emotional disturbances, urinary tract infections or malformations, cauda equina lesions, epilepsy, sleep apnea, and certain medications. Symptomatic pharmacotherapy is usually accomplished with desmopressin (0.2 mg qhs), oxybutynin chloride (5 to 10 mg qhs) or imipramine (10 to 50 mg qhs).

Miscellaneous Parasomnias Other clinical entities fulfill the definition of a parasomnia in that they occur selectively during sleep and are associated with some degree of sleep disruption. Examples include *jactatio capitis nocturna* (nocturnal headbanging), sleep talking, nocturnal paroxysmal dystonia, and nocturnal leg cramps.

CIRCADIAN RHYTHM SLEEP DISORDERS

A subset of patients presenting with either insomnia or hypersomnia may have a disorder of sleep *timing* rather than sleep *generation*. Disorders of sleep timing can be either organic (i.e., due to an intrinsic defect in the circadian pacemaker or its input from entraining stimuli) or environmental (i.e., due to a disruption of exposure to entraining stimuli from the environment). Regardless of etiology, the symptoms reflect the influence of the underlying circadian pacemaker on sleep-wake function. Thus, effective therapeutic approaches should aim to entrain the oscillator at an appropriate phase.

Rapid Time-Zone Change (Jet Lag) Syndrome More than 60 million people experience transmeridian air travel annually, which is often associated with excessive daytime sleepiness, sleep onset insomnia, and frequent arousals from sleep, particularly in the latter half of the night. Gastrointestinal discomfort is common. The syndrome is transient, typically lasting 2 to 14 d depending on the number of time zones crossed, the direction of travel, and the traveler's age and phase-shifting capacity. Travelers who spend more time outdoors reportedly adapt more quickly than those who remain in hotel rooms, presumably due to bright (outdoor) light exposure. Avoidance of antecedent sleep loss and obtaining nap sleep on the afternoon prior to overnight travel greatly reduces the difficulty of extended wakefulness. Laboratory studies suggest that submilligram doses of the pineal hormone melatonin can enhance sleep efficiency, but only if taken when endogenous melatonin concentrations are low (i.e., during biologic daytime), and furthermore that melatonin may induce phase shifts in human rhythms. A large-scale clinical trial evaluating the safety and efficacy of melatonin as a treatment for jet lag and other circadian sleep disorders is needed.

Shift-Work Sleep Disorder More than 7 million workers in the United States regularly work at night, either on a permanent or rotating schedule. In addition, each week millions elect to remain awake at night to meet deadlines, drive long distances, or participate in recreational activities, leading to both sleep loss and misalignment of their circadian rhythms with respect to their sleep-wake cycle. Chronic shift workers have higher rates of cardiac, gastrointestinal, and reproductive disorders. Studies of regular night-shift workers indicate that the circadian timing system usually fails to adapt successfully to such inverted schedules. This leads to a misalignment between the desired work-rest schedule and the output of the pacemaker and in disturbed daytime sleep. Sleep deprivation, increased length of time awake prior to work, and misalignment of circadian phase produce decreased alertness and performance, increased reaction time, and increased risk of performance lapses, thereby resulting in greater safety hazards among night workers and other sleep-deprived individuals. Sleep disturbance nearly doubles the risk of a fatal work accident.

Sleep onset is associated with marked attenuation in perception of both auditory and visual stimuli and lapses of consciousness. The sleepy individual may thus attempt to perform routine and familiar motor tasks during the transition state between wakefulness and sleep (stage 1 sleep) in the absence of adequate sensory input from the environment. Motor vehicle operators are especially vulnerable to sleep-related accidents since the sleep-deprived driver or operator often fails to heed the warning signs of fatigue. Such attempts to override the powerful biologic drive for sleep by the sheer force of will can yield a catastrophic outcome when sleep processes intrude involuntarily upon the waking brain. Such intrusions typically last only seconds but are known on occasion to persist for longer durations. These frequent brief intrusions of stage 1 sleep into behavioral wakefulness are a major component of the impaired psychomotor performance seen with sleepiness. There is a significant increase in the risk of sleep-related, fatal-to-the-driver highway crashes in the early morning and late af-

ternoon hours, coincident with bimodal peaks in the daily rhythm of sleep tendency.

Safety programs should promote education about sleep and increase awareness of the hazards associated with night work and should be aimed at minimizing both circadian disruption and sleep deprivation. The work schedule should minimize: (1) exposure to night work, (2) the frequency of shift rotation so that shifts do not rotate more than once every 2 to 3 weeks, (3) the number of consecutive night shifts, and (4) the duration of night shifts. In fact, shift durations of >18 h should be universally recognized as increasing the risk of sleep-related errors and performance lapses. Caffeine is undoubtedly the most widely used wake-promoting drug, but it cannot forestall sleep indefinitely and does not shield users from sleep-related performance lapses. Postural changes, exercise, and strategic placement of nap opportunities can sometimes temporarily reduce the risk of fatigue-related performance lapses. Properly timed exposure to bright light can facilitate rapid adaptation to night-shift work. An adequate number of safe highway rest areas, shoulder rumble strips, and strict enforcement and compliance monitoring of hours-of-service policies are needed to reduce the risk of sleep-related transportation crashes.

Delayed Sleep Phase Syndrome Delayed sleep phase syndrome is characterized by: (1) reported sleep onset and wake times intractably later than desired, (2) actual sleep times at nearly the same clock hours daily, and (3) essentially normal all-night polysomnography except for delayed sleep onset. Patients exhibit an abnormally delayed endogenous circadian phase, with the temperature minimum during the constant routine occurring later than normal. This delayed phase could be due to: (1) an abnormally long, genetically determined intrinsic period of the endogenous circadian pacemaker; (2) an abnormally reduced phase-advancing capacity of the pacemaker; or (3) an irregular prior sleep-wake schedule, characterized by frequent nights when the patient chooses to remain awake well past midnight (for social, school, or work reasons). In most cases, it is difficult to distinguish among these factors, since patients with an abnormally long intrinsic period are more likely to "choose" such late-night activities because they are unable to sleep at that time. Patients tend to be young adults. This self-perpetuating condition can persist for years and does not usually respond to attempts to reestablish normal bedtime hours. Treatment methods involving bright-light phototherapy during the morning hours or melatonin administration in the evening hours show promise in these patients, although the relapse rate is high.

Advanced Sleep Phase Syndrome Advanced sleep phase syndrome (ASPS) is the converse of the delayed sleep phase syndrome. Most commonly, this syndrome occurs in older people, 15% of whom report that they cannot sleep past 5 A.M., with twice that number complaining that they wake up too early at least several times per week. Patients with ASPS experience excessive daytime sleepiness during the evening hours, when they have great difficulty remaining awake, even in social settings. Typically, patients awaken from 3 to 5 A.M. each day, often several hours before their desired wake times. In addition to age-related ASPS, an early-onset familial variant of this condition has also been reported. In one such family, autosomal dominant ASPS was due to a missense mutation in a circadian clock component (PER2, as shown in Fig. 24-2) that altered the circardian period. Patients with ASPS may benefit from bright-light phototherapy during the evening hours, designed to reset the circadian pacemaker to a later hour.

Non-24-Hour Sleep-Wake Disorder This condition can occur when the maximal phase-advancing capacity of the circadian pacemaker is not adequate to accommodate the difference between the 24-h geophysical day and the intrinsic period of the pacemaker in the patient. Alternatively, patients' self-selected exposure to artificial light may drive the circadian pacemaker to a >24-h schedule. Affected patients are not able to maintain a stable phase relationship between the output of the pacemaker and the 24-h day. Such patients typically present with an incremental pattern of successive delays in sleep onsets and wake times, progressing in and out of phase with local time. When the patient's endogenous rhythms are out of phase with the local environment, insomnia coexists with excessive daytime sleepiness. Conversely, when the endogenous rhythms are in phase with the local environment, symptoms remit. The intervals between symptomatic periods may last several weeks to several months. Blind individuals unable to perceive light are particularly susceptible to this disorder. Nightly low-dose (0.5 mg) melatonin administration has been reported to improve sleep and, in some cases, even to induce synchronization of the circadian pacemaker.

MEDICAL IMPLICATIONS OF CIRCADIAN RHYTHMICITY Prominent circadian variations have been reported in the incidence of acute myocardial infarction, sudden cardiac death, and stroke, the leading causes of death in the United States. Platelet aggregability is increased after arising in the early morning hours, coincident with the peak incidence of these cardiovascular events. A better understanding of the possible role of circadian rhythmicity in the acute destabilization of a chronic condition such as atherosclerotic disease could improve the understanding of the pathophysiology.

Diagnostic and therapeutic procedures may also be affected by the time of day at which data are collected. Examples include blood pressure, body temperature, the dexamethasone suppression test, and plasma cortisol levels. The timing of chemotherapy administration has been reported to have an effect on the outcome of treatment. Few physicians realize the extent to which routine measures are affected by the time (or sleep/wake state) when the measurement is made.

In addition, both the toxicity and effectiveness of drugs can vary during the day. For example, more than a fivefold difference has been observed in mortality rates following administration of toxic agents to experimental animals at different times of day. Anesthetic agents are particularly sensitive to time-of-day effects. Finally, the physician must be increasingly aware of the public health risks associated with the ever-increasing demands made by the duty-rest-recreation schedules in our round-the-clock society.

FURTHER READING

FLEMONS WW: Clinical practice. Obstructive sleep apnea. N Engl J Med 347: 498, 2002

SCAMMELL TE: The neurobiology, diagnosis, and treatment of narcolepsy. Ann Neurol 53:154, 2003

SMITH MT: Comparative meta-analysis of pharmacotherapy and behavior therapy for persistent insomnia. Am J Psychiatry 159:5, 2002

Section 4   Disorders of the Eyes, Ears, Nose, and Throat

25 | DISORDERS OF THE EYE
Jonathan C. Horton

THE HUMAN VISUAL SYSTEM

The visual system provides a supremely efficient means for the rapid assimilation of information from the environment to aid in the guidance of behavior. The act of seeing begins with the capture of images focused by the cornea and lens upon a light-sensitive membrane in the back of the eye, called the *retina*. The retina is actually part of the brain, banished to the periphery to serve as a transducer for the conversion of patterns of light energy into neuronal signals. Light is absorbed by photopigment in two types of receptors: rods and cones. In the human retina there are 100 million rods and 5 million cones. The rods operate in dim (scotopic) illumination. The cones function under daylight (photopic) conditions. The cone system is specialized for color perception and high spatial resolution. The majority of cones are located within the macula, the portion of the retina serving the central 10° of vision. In the middle of the macula a small pit termed the *fovea*, packed exclusively with cones, provides best visual acuity.

Photoreceptors hyperpolarize in response to light, activating bipolar, amacrine, and horizontal cells in the inner nuclear layer. After processing of photoreceptor responses by this complex retinal circuit, the flow of sensory information ultimately converges upon a final common pathway: the ganglion cells. These cells translate the visual image impinging upon the retina into a continuously varying barrage of action potentials that propagates along the primary optic pathway to visual centers within the brain. There are a million ganglion cells in each retina, and hence a million fibers in each optic nerve.

Ganglion cell axons sweep along the inner surface of the retina in the nerve fiber layer, exit the eye at the optic disc, and travel through the optic nerve, optic chiasm, and optic tract to reach targets in the brain. The majority of fibers synapse upon cells in the lateral geniculate body, a thalamic relay station. Cells in the lateral geniculate body project in turn to the primary visual cortex. This massive afferent retinogeniculocortical sensory pathway provides the neural substrate for visual perception. Although the lateral geniculate body is the main target of the retina, separate classes of ganglion cells project to other subcortical visual nuclei involved in different functions. Ganglion cells

that mediate pupillary constriction and circadian rhythms are light sensitive, owing to a novel visual pigment, melanopsin. Pupil responses are mediated by input to the pretectal olivary nuclei in the midbrain. The pretectal nuclei send their output to the Edinger-Westphal nuclei, which in turn provide parasympathetic innervation to the iris sphincter via an interneuron in the ciliary ganglion. Circadian rhythms are timed by a retinal projection to the suprachiasmatic nucleus. Visual orientation and eye movements are served by retinal input to the superior colliculus. Gaze stabilization and optokinetic reflexes are governed by a group of small retinal targets known collectively as the *brainstem accessory optic system*.

The eyes must be rotated constantly within their orbits to place and maintain targets of visual interest upon the fovea. This activity, called *foveation*, or looking, is governed by an elaborate efferent motor system. Each eye is moved by six extraocular muscles, supplied by cranial nerves from the oculomotor (III), trochlear (IV), and abducens (VI) nuclei. Activity in these ocular motor nuclei is coordinated by pontine and midbrain mechanisms for smooth pursuit, saccades, and gaze stabilization during head and body movements. Large regions of the frontal and parietooccipital cortex control these brainstem eye movement centers by providing descending supranuclear input.

CLINICAL ASSESSMENT OF VISUAL FUNCTION

REFRACTIVE STATE In approaching the patient with reduced vision, the first step is to decide whether refractive error is responsible. In *emmetropia*, parallel rays from infinity are focused perfectly upon the retina. Sadly, this condition is enjoyed by only a minority of the population. In *myopia*, the globe is too long, and light rays come to a focal point in front of the retina. Near objects can be seen clearly, but distant objects require a diverging lens in front of the eye. In *hyperopia*, the globe is too short, and hence a converging lens is used to supplement the refractive power of the eye. In *astigmatism*, the corneal surface is not perfectly spherical, necessitating a cylindrical corrective lens. In recent years it has become possible to correct refractive error with the excimer laser by performing LASIK (laser in situ keratomileusis) to alter the curvature of the cornea.

With the onset of middle age, *presbyopia* develops as the lens within the eye becomes unable to increase its refractive power to accommodate upon near objects. To compensate for presbyopia, the emmetropic patient must use reading glasses. The patient already wearing glasses for distance correction usually switches to bifocals. The only exception is the myopic patient, who may achieve clear vision at near simply by removing glasses containing the distance prescription.

Refractive errors usually develop slowly and remain stable after adolescence, except in unusual circumstances. For example, the acute onset of diabetes mellitus can produce sudden myopia because of lens edema induced by hyperglycemia. Testing vision through a pinhole aperture is a useful way to screen quickly for refractive error. If the visual acuity is better through a pinhole than with the unaided eye, the patient needs a refraction to obtain best corrected visual acuity.

VISUAL ACUITY The Snellen chart is used to test acuity at a distance of 6 m (20 ft). For convenience, a scale version of the Snellen chart, called the Rosenbaum card, is held at 36 cm (14 in) from the patient (Fig. 25-1). All subjects should be able to read the 6/6 m (20/20 ft) line with each eye using their refractive correction, if any. Patients who need reading glasses because of presbyopia must wear them for accurate testing with the Rosenbaum card. If 6/6 (20/20) acuity is not present in each eye, the deficiency in vision must be explained. If

worse than 6/240 (20/800), acuity should be recorded in terms of counting fingers, hand motions, light perception, or no light perception. Legal blindness is defined by the Internal Revenue Service as a best corrected acuity of 6/60 (20/200) or less in the better eye, or a binocular visual field subtending 20° or less. For driving the laws vary by state, but most require a corrected acuity of 6/12 (20/40) in at least one eye. Patients with a homonymous hemianopia should not drive.

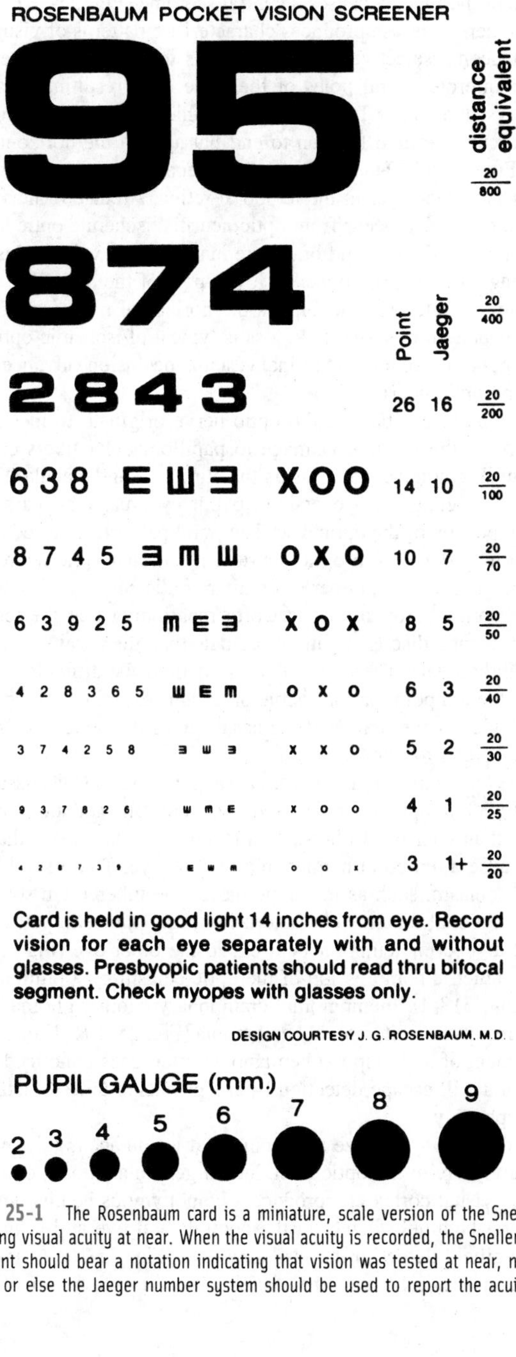

PUPILS The pupils should be tested individually in dim light with the patient fixating on a distant target. If they respond briskly to light, there is no need to check the near response, because isolated loss of constriction (miosis) to accommodation does not occur. For this reason, the ubiquitous abbreviation PERRLA (pupils equal, round, and reactive to light and accommodation) implies a wasted effort with the last step. However, it is important to test the near response if the light response is poor or absent. Light-near dissociation occurs with neurosyphilis (Argyll Robertson pupil), lesions of the dorsal midbrain (obstructive hydrocephalus, pineal region tumors), and after aberrant regeneration (oculomotor nerve palsy, Adie's tonic pupil).

An eye with no light perception has no pupillary response to direct light stimulation. If the retina or optic nerve is only partially injured, the direct pupillary response will be weaker than the consensual pupillary response evoked by shining a light into the other eye. This *relative afferent pupillary defect* (Marcus Gunn pupil) can be elicited with the swinging flashlight test. It is an extremely useful sign in retrobulbar optic neuritis and other optic nerve diseases, where it may be the sole objective evidence for disease.

Subtle inequality in pupil size, up to 0.5 mm, is a fairly common finding in normal persons. The diagnosis of essential or physiologic anisocoria is secure as long as the relative pupil asymmetry remains constant as ambient lighting varies. Anisocoria that increases in dim light indicates a sympathetic paresis of the iris dilator muscle. The triad of miosis with ipsilateral ptosis and anhidrosis constitutes Horner's syndrome, although anhidrosis is an inconstant feature. Brainstem stroke, carotid dissection, or neoplasm impinging upon the sympathetic chain are occasionally identified as the cause of Horner's syndrome, but most cases are idiopathic.

Anisocoria that increases in bright light suggests a parasympathetic palsy. The first concern is an oculomotor nerve paresis. This possibility is excluded if the eye movements are full and the patient has no ptosis or diplopia. Acute pupillary dilation (mydriasis) can occur from damage to the ciliary ganglion in the orbit. Common mechanisms are infection (herpes zoster, influenza), trauma (blunt, penetrating, surgical), or ischemia (diabetes, temporal arteritis). After denervation of the iris sphincter the pupil does not respond well to light, but the response to near is often relatively intact. When the near stimulus is removed, the pupil redilates very slowly compared with the normal pupil, hence the term *tonic pupil*. In Adie's syndrome, a tonic pupil occurs in conjunction with weak or absent tendon reflexes in the lower extremities. This benign disorder, which occurs predominantly in healthy young women, is assumed to represent a mild dysautonomia. Tonic pupils are also associated with Shy-Drager syndrome, segmental hypohidrosis, diabetes, and amyloidosis. Occasionally, a tonic pupil is discovered incidentally in an otherwise completely normal, asymptomatic individual. The diagnosis is confirmed by placing a drop of dilute (0.125%) pilocarpine into each eye. Denervation hypersensitivity produces pupillary constriction in a tonic pupil, whereas the normal pupil shows no response. Pharmacologic dilation from accidental or deliberate instillation of anticholinergic agents (atropine, scopolamine drops) into the eye can also produce pupillary mydriasis. In this situation, normal strength (1%) pilocarpine causes no constriction.

Both pupils are affected equally by systemic medications. They are small with narcotic use (morphine, heroin) and large with anticholinergics (scopolamine). Parasympathetic agents (pilocarpine, demecarium bromide) used to treat glaucoma produce miosis. In any patient with an unexplained pupillary abnormality, a slit-lamp examination is

ROSENBAUM POCKET VISION SCREENER

Card is held in good light 14 inches from eye. Record vision for each eye separately with and without glasses. Presbyopic patients should read thru bifocal segment. Check myopes with glasses only.

DESIGN COURTESY J. G. ROSENBAUM, M.D.

PUPIL GAUGE (mm.)

FIGURE 25-1 The Rosenbaum card is a miniature, scale version of the Snellen chart for testing visual acuity at near. When the visual acuity is recorded, the Snellen distance equivalent should bear a notation indicating that vision was tested at near, not at 6 m (20 ft), or else the Jaeger number system should be used to report the acuity.

helpful to exclude surgical trauma to the iris, an occult foreign body, perforating injury, intraocular inflammation, adhesions (synechia), angle-closure glaucoma, and iris sphincter rupture from blunt trauma.

EYE MOVEMENTS AND ALIGNMENT   Eye movements are tested by asking the patient with both eyes open to pursue a small target such as a penlight into the cardinal fields of gaze. Normal ocular versions are smooth, symmetric, full, and maintained in all directions without nystagmus. Saccades, or quick refixation eye movements, are assessed by having the patient look back and forth between two stationary targets. The eyes should move rapidly and accurately in a single jump to their target. Ocular alignment can be judged by holding a penlight directly in front of the patient at about 1 m. If the eyes are straight, the corneal light reflex will be centered in the middle of each pupil. To test eye alignment more precisely, the cover test is useful. The patient is instructed to gaze upon a small fixation target in the distance. One eye is covered suddenly while observing the second eye. If the second eye shifts to fixate upon the target, it was misaligned. If it does not move, the first eye is uncovered and the test is repeated on the second eye. If neither eye moves, the eyes are aligned orthotropically. If the eyes are orthotropic in primary gaze but the patient complains of diplopia, the cover test should be performed with the head tilted or turned in whatever direction elicits diplopia. With practice the examiner can detect an ocular deviation (heterotropia) as small as 1 to 2° with the cover test. Deviations can be measured by placing prisms in front of the misaligned eye to determine the power required to neutralize the fixation shift evoked by covering the other eye.

STEREOPSIS   Stereoacuity is determined by presenting targets with retinal disparity separately to each eye using polarized images. The most popular office tests measure a range of thresholds from 800 to 40 seconds of arc. Normal stereoacuity is 40 seconds of arc. If a patient achieves this level of stereoacuity, one is assured that the eyes are aligned orthotropically and that vision is intact in each eye. Random dot stereograms have no monocular depth cues and provide an excellent screening test for strabismus and amblyopia in children.

COLOR VISION   The retina contains three classes of cones, with visual pigments of differing peak spectral sensitivity: red (560 nm), green (530 nm), and blue (430 nm). The red and green cone pigments are encoded on the X chromosome; the blue cone pigment on chromosome 7. Mutations of the blue cone pigment are exceedingly rare. Mutations of the red and green pigments cause congenital X-linked color blindness in 8% of males. Affected individuals are not truly color blind; rather, they differ from normal subjects in how they perceive color and how they combine primary monochromatic lights to match a given color. Anomalous trichromats have three cone types, but a mutation in one cone pigment (usually red or green) causes a shift in peak spectral sensitivity, altering the proportion of primary colors required to achieve a color match. Dichromats have only two cone types and will therefore accept a color match based upon only two primary colors. Anomalous trichromats and dichromats have 6/6 (20/20) visual acuity, but their hue discrimination is impaired. Ishihara color plates can be used to detect red-green color blindness. The test plates contain a hidden number, visible only to subjects with color confusion from red-green color blindness. Because color blindness is almost exclusively X-linked, it is worth screening only male children.

The Ishihara plates are often used to detect acquired defects in color vision, although they are intended as a screening test for congenital color blindness. Acquired defects in color vision frequently result from disease of the macula or optic nerve. For example, patients with a history of optic neuritis often complain of color desaturation long after their visual acuity has returned to normal. Color blindness can also occur from bilateral strokes involving the ventral portion of the occipital lobe (cerebral achromatopsia). Such patients can perceive only shades of gray and may also have difficulty recognizing faces (prosopagnosia). Infarcts of the dominant occipital lobe sometimes give

rise to color anomia. Affected patients can discriminate colors, but they cannot name them.

VISUAL FIELDS   Vision can be impaired by damage to the visual system anywhere from the eyes to the occipital lobes. One can localize the site of the lesion with considerable accuracy by mapping the visual field deficit by finger confrontation and then correlating it with the topographic anatomy of the visual pathway (Fig. 25-2). Quantitative visual field mapping is performed by computer-driven perimeters (Humphrey, Octopus) that present a target of variable intensity at fixed positions in the visual field (Fig. 25-2A). By generating an automated printout of light thresholds, these static perimeters provide a sensitive means of detecting scotomas in the visual field. They are exceedingly useful for serial assessment of visual function in chronic diseases such as glaucoma or pseudotumor cerebri.

The crux of visual field analysis is to decide whether a lesion is before, at, or behind the optic chiasm. If a scotoma is confined to one eye, it must be due to a lesion anterior to the chiasm, involving either the optic nerve or retina. Retinal lesions produce scotomas that correspond optically to their location in the fundus. For example, a superior-nasal retinal detachment results in an inferior-temporal field cut. Damage to the macula causes a central scotoma (Fig. 25-2B).

Optic nerve disease produces characteristic patterns of visual field loss. Glaucoma selectively destroys axons that enter the superotemporal or inferotemporal poles of the optic disc, resulting in arcuate scotomas shaped like a Turkish scimitar, which emanate from the blind spot and curve around fixation to end flat against the horizontal meridian (Fig. 25-2C). This type of field defect mirrors the arrangement of the nerve fiber layer in the temporal retina. Arcuate or nerve fiber layer scotomas also occur from optic neuritis, ischemic optic neuropathy, optic disc drusen, and branch retinal artery or vein occlusion.

Damage to the entire upper or lower pole of the optic disc causes an altitudinal field cut that follows the horizontal meridian (Fig. 25-2D). This pattern of visual field loss is typical of ischemic optic neuropathy but also occurs from retinal vascular occlusion, advanced glaucoma, and optic neuritis.

About half the fibers in the optic nerve originate from ganglion cells serving the macula. Damage to papillomacular fibers causes a cecocentral scotoma encompassing the blind spot and macula (Fig. 25-2E). If the damage is irreversible, pallor eventually appears in the temporal portion of the optic disc. Temporal pallor from a cecocentral scotoma may develop in optic neuritis, nutritional optic neuropathy, toxic optic neuropathy, Leber's hereditary optic neuropathy, and compressive optic neuropathy. It is worth mentioning that the temporal side of the optic disc is slightly more pale than the nasal side in most normal individuals. Therefore, it can sometimes be difficult to decide whether the temporal pallor visible on fundus examination represents a pathologic change. Pallor of the nasal rim of the optic disc is a less equivocal sign of optic atrophy.

At the optic chiasm, fibers from nasal ganglion cells decussate into the contralateral optic tract. Crossed fibers are damaged more by compression than uncrossed fibers. As a result, mass lesions of the sellar region cause a temporal hemianopia in each eye. Tumors anterior to the optic chiasm, such as meningiomas of the tuberculum sella, produce a junctional scotoma characterized by an optic neuropathy in one eye and a superior temporal field cut in the other eye (Fig. 25-2G). More symmetric compression of the optic chiasm by a pituitary adenoma (Fig. 318-4), meningioma, craniopharyngioma, glioma, or aneurysm results in a bitemporal hemianopia (Fig. 25-2H). The insidious development of a bitemporal hemianopia often goes unnoticed by the patient and will escape detection by the physician unless each eye is tested separately.

It is difficult to localize a postchiasmal lesion accurately, because injury anywhere in the optic tract, lateral geniculate body, optic radiations, or visual cortex can produce a homonymous hemianopia, i.e., a temporal hemifield defect in the contralateral eye and a matching nasal hemifield defect in the ipsilateral eye (Fig. 25-2I). A unilateral postchiasmal lesion leaves the visual acuity in each eye unaffected, although the patient may read the letters on only the left or right half of the eye chart. Lesions of the optic radiations tend to cause poorly matched or incongruous field defects in each eye. Damage to the optic radiations in the temporal lobe (Meyer's loop) produces a superior quadrantic homonymous hemianopia (Fig. 25-2*J*), whereas injury to the optic radiations in the parietal lobe results in an inferior quadrantic homonymous hemianopia (Fig. 25-2*K*). Lesions of the primary visual cortex give rise to dense, congruous hemianopic field defects. Occlusion of the posterior cerebral artery supplying the occipital lobe is a frequent cause of total homonymous hemianopia. Some patients with hemianopia after occipital stroke have macular sparing, because the macular representation at the tip of the occipital lobe is supplied by collaterals from the middle cerebral artery (Fig. 25-2*L*). Destruction of both occipital lobes produces cortical blindness. This condition can be distinguished from bilateral prechiasmal visual loss by noting that the pupil responses and optic fundi remain normal.

RED OR PAINFUL EYE

Corneal Abrasions These are seen best by placing a drop of fluorescein in the eye and looking with the slit lamp using a cobalt-blue light. A penlight with a blue filter will suffice if no slit lamp is available. Damage to the corneal epithelium is revealed by yellow fluorescence of the exposed basement membrane underlying the epithelium. It is important to check for foreign bodies. To search the conjunctival fornices, the lower lid should be pulled down and the upper lid everted. A foreign body can be removed with a moistened cotton-tipped applicator after placing a drop of topical anesthetic, such as proparacaine, in the eye. Alternatively, it may be possible to flush the foreign body from the eye by irrigating copiously with saline or artificial tears. If the corneal epithelium has been abraded, antibiotic ointment and a patch should be applied to the eye. A drop of an intermediate-acting cycloplegic, such as cyclopentolate hydrochloride 1%, helps to reduce pain by relaxing the ciliary body. The eye should be reexamined the next day. Minor abrasions may not require patching and cycloplegia.

Subconjunctival Hemorrhage This results from rupture of small vessels bridging the potential space between the episclera and conjunctiva. Blood dissecting into this space can produce a spectacular red eye, but vision is not affected and the hemorrhage resolves without treatment. Subconjunctival hemorrhage is usually spontaneous but can occur from blunt trauma, eye rubbing, or vigorous coughing. Occasionally it is a clue to an underlying bleeding disorder.

Pinguecula This is a small, raised conjunctival nodule at the temporal or nasal limbus. In adults such lesions are extremely common and have little significance, unless they become inflamed (pingueculitis). A *pte-*

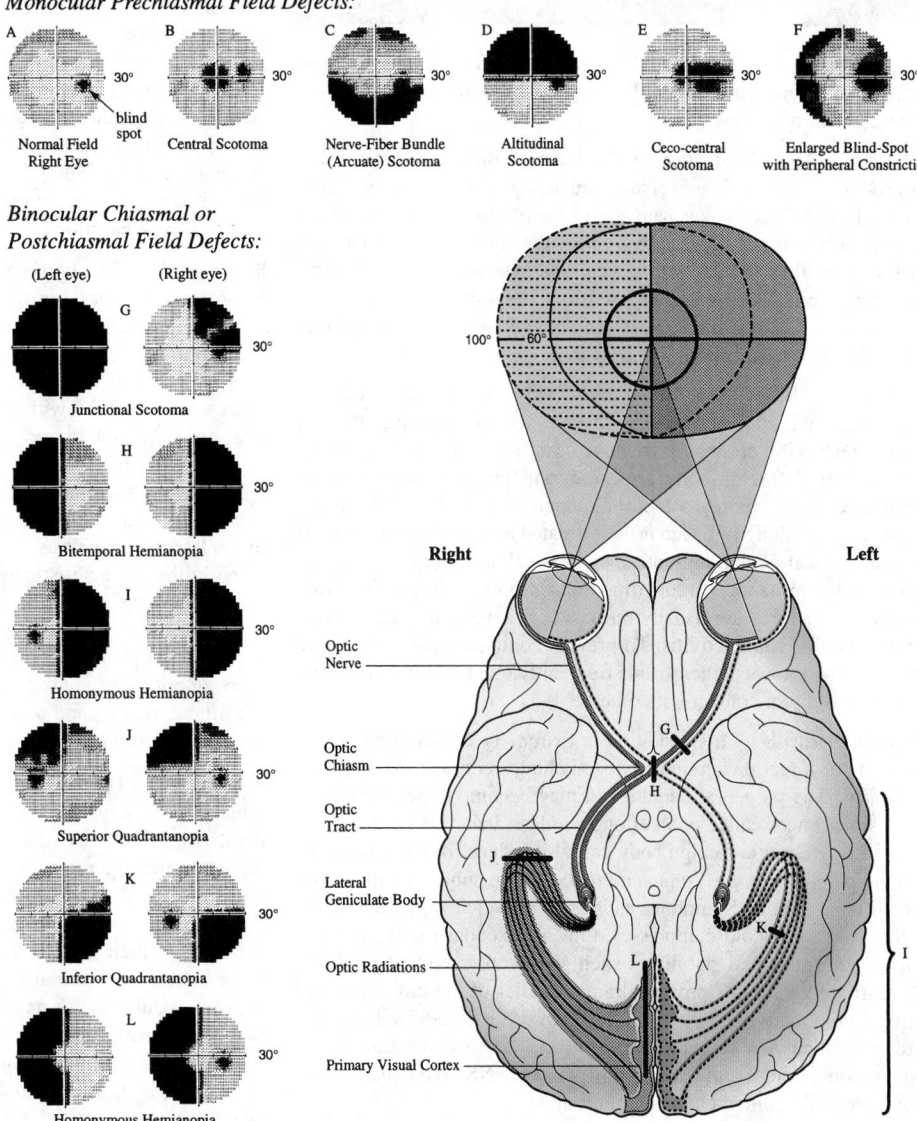

Monocular Prechiasmal Field Defects:

Normal Field Right Eye — blind spot

A 30° — Central Scotoma B 30°

Nerve-Fiber Bundle (Arcuate) Scotoma C 30°

Altitudinal Scotoma D 30°

Ceco-central Scotoma E 30°

Enlarged Blind-Spot with Peripheral Constriction F 30°

Binocular Chiasmal or Postchiasmal Field Defects:

(Left eye) (Right eye)

G — Junctional Scotoma 30°

H — Bitemporal Hemianopia 30°

I — Homonymous Hemianopia 30°

J — Superior Quadrantanopia 30°

K — Inferior Quadrantanopia 30°

L — Homonymous Hemianopia with Macular Sparing 30°

Right   Left

Optic Nerve

Optic Chiasm

Optic Tract

Lateral Geniculate Body

Optic Radiations

Primary Visual Cortex

FIGURE 25-2 Ventral view of the brain, correlating patterns of visual field loss with the sites of lesions in the visual pathway. The visual fields overlap partially, creating 120° of central binocular field flanked by a 40° monocular crescent on either side. The visual field maps in this figure were done with a computer-driven perimeter (Humphrey Instruments, Carl Zeiss, Inc.). It plots the retinal sensitivity to light in the central 30° using a gray scale format. Areas of visual field loss are shown in black. The examples of common monocular, prechiasmal field defects are all shown for the right eye. By convention, the visual fields are always recorded with the left eye's field on the left, and the right eye's field on the right, just as the patient sees the world.

rygium resembles a pinguecula but has crossed the limbus to encroach upon the corneal surface. Removal is justified when symptoms of irritation or blurring develop, but recurrence is a common problem.

Blepharitis This refers to inflammation of the eyelids. The most common form occurs in association with acne rosacea or seborrheic dermatitis. The eyelid margins are usually colonized heavily by staphylococci. Upon close inspection, they appear greasy, ulcerated, and crusted with scaling debris that clings to the lashes. Treatment consists of warm compresses, strict eyelid hygiene, and topical antibiotics such as *erythromycin*. An external *hordeolum* (sty) is caused by staphylococcal infection of the superficial accessory glands of Zeis or Moll located in the eyelid margins. An internal hordeolum occurs after suppurative infection of the oil-secreting meibomian glands within the tarsal plate of the eyelid. Systemic antibiotics, usually tetracyclines, are sometimes necessary for treatment of meibomian gland inflammation (meibomitis) or chronic, severe blepharitis. A *chalazion* is a painless, granulomatous inflammation of a meibomian gland that produces a pealike nodule within the eyelid. It can be incised and drained, or injected with glucocorticoids. Basal cell, squamous cell, or meibomian gland carcinoma should be suspected for any nonhealing, ulcerative lesion of the eyelids.

Dacrocystitis An inflammation of the lacrimal drainage system, this can produce epiphora (tearing) and ocular injection. Gentle pressure over the lacrimal sac evokes pain and reflux of mucus or pus from the tear puncta. Dacrocystitis usually occurs after obstruction of the lacrimal system. It is treated with topical and systemic antibiotics, followed by probing or surgery to reestablish patency. *Entropion* (inversion of the eyelid) or *ectropion* (sagging or eversion of the eyelid) can also lead to epiphora and ocular irritation.

Conjunctivitis This is the most common cause of a red, irritated eye. Pain is minimal, and the visual acuity is reduced only slightly. The most common viral etiology is adenovirus infection. It causes a watery discharge, mild foreign-body sensation, and photophobia. Bacterial infection tends to produce a more mucopurulent exudate. Mild cases of infectious conjunctivitis are usually treated empirically with broad-spectrum topical ocular antibiotics, such as sulfacetamide 10%, polymixin-bacitracin-neomycin, or trimethoprim-polymixin combination. Smears and cultures are usually reserved for severe, resistant, or recurrent cases of conjunctivitis. To prevent contagion, patients should be admonished to wash their hands frequently, not to touch their eyes, and to avoid direct contact with others.

Allergic Conjunctivitis This condition is extremely common and often mistaken for infectious conjunctivitis. Itching, redness, and epiphora are typical. The palpebral conjunctiva may become hypertropic with giant excrescences called cobblestone papillae. Irritation from contact lenses or any chronic foreign body can also induce formation of cobblestone papillae. *Atopic conjunctivitis* occurs in subjects with atopic dermatitis or asthma. Symptoms caused by allergic conjunctivitis can be alleviated with cold compresses, topical vasoconstrictors, antihistamines, and mast-cell stabilizers such as cromolyn sodium. Topical glucocorticoid solutions provide dramatic relief of immune-mediated forms of conjunctivitis, but their long-term use is ill-advised because of the complications of glaucoma, cataract, and secondary infection. Topical nonsteroidal anti-inflammatory agents (NSAIDs) such as ketorolac tromethamine are a better alternative.

Keratoconjunctivitis Sicca Also known as dry eye, it produces a burning, foreign-body sensation, injection, and photophobia. In mild cases the eye appears surprisingly normal, but tear production measured by wetting of a filter paper (Schirmer strip) is deficient. A variety of systemic drugs, including antihistaminic, anticholinergic, and psychotropic medications, result in dry eye by reducing lacrimal secretion. Disorders that involve the lacrimal gland directly, such as sarcoidosis or Sjögren's syndrome, also cause dry eye. Patients may develop dry eye after radiation therapy if the treatment field includes the orbits. Problems with ocular drying are also common after lesions affecting cranial nerves V or VII. Corneal anesthesia is particularly dangerous, because the absence of a normal blink reflex exposes the cornea to injury without pain to warn the patient. Dry eye is managed by frequent and liberal application of artificial tears and ocular lubricants. In severe cases the tear puncta can be plugged or cauterized to reduce lacrimal outflow.

Keratitis This is a threat to vision because of the risk of corneal clouding, scarring, and perforation. Worldwide, the two leading causes of blindness from keratitis are trachoma from chlamydial infection and vitamin A deficiency related to malnutrition. In the United States, contact lenses play a major role in corneal infection and ulceration. They should not be worn by anyone with an active eye infection. In evaluating the cornea, it is important to differentiate between a superficial infection (*keratoconjunctivitis*) and a deeper, more serious ulcerative process. The latter is accompanied by greater visual loss, pain, photophobia, redness, and discharge. Slit-lamp examination shows disruption of the corneal epithelium, a cloudy infiltrate or abscess in the

stroma, and an inflammatory cellular reaction in the anterior chamber. In severe cases, pus settles at the bottom of the anterior chamber, giving rise to a hypopyon. Immediate empirical antibiotic therapy should be initiated after corneal scrapings are obtained for Gram's stain, Giemsa stain, and cultures. Fortified topical antibiotics are most effective, supplemented with subconjunctival antibiotics as required. A fungal etiology should always be considered in the patient with keratitis. Fungal infection is common in warm humid climates, especially after penetration of the cornea by plant or vegetable material.

Herpes Simplex The *herpes viruses* are a major cause of blindness from keratitis. Most adults in the United States have serum antibodies to herpes simplex, indicating prior viral infection (Chap. 163). Primary ocular infection is generally caused by herpes simplex type 1, rather than type 2. It manifests as a unilateral follicular blepharoconjunctivitis, easily confused with adenoviral conjunctivitis unless telltale vesicles appear on the periocular skin or conjunctiva. A dendritic pattern of corneal epithelial ulceration revealed by fluorescein staining is pathognomonic for herpes infection but is seen in only a minority of primary infections. Recurrent ocular infection arises from reactivation of the latent herpes virus. Viral eruption in the corneal epithelium may result in the characteristic herpes dendrite. Involvement of the corneal stroma produces edema, vascularization, and iridocyclitis. Herpes keratitis is treated with topical antiviral agents, cycloplegics, and oral acyclovir. Topical glucocorticoids are effective in mitigating corneal scarring but must be used with extreme caution because of the danger of corneal melting and perforation. Topical glucocorticoids also carry the risk of prolonging infection and inducing glaucoma.

Herpes Zoster Herpes zoster from reactivation of latent varicella (chickenpox) virus causes a dermatomal pattern of painful vesicular dermatitis. Ocular symptoms can occur after zoster eruption in any branch of the trigeminal nerve but are particularly common when vesicles form on the nose, reflecting nasociliary (V1) nerve involvement (Hutchinson's sign). Herpes zoster ophthalmicus produces corneal dendrites, which can be difficult to distinguish from those seen in herpes simplex. Stromal keratitis, anterior uveitis, raised intraocular pressure, ocular motor nerve palsies, acute retinal necrosis, and postherpetic scarring and neuralgia are other common sequelae. Herpes zoster ophthalmicus is treated with antiviral agents and cycloplegics. In severe cases, glucocorticoids may be added to prevent permanent visual loss from corneal scarring.

Episcleritis This is an inflammation of the episclera, a thin layer of connective tissue between the conjunctiva and sclera. Episcleritis resembles conjunctivitis but is a more localized process and discharge is absent. Most cases of episcleritis are idiopathic, but some occur in the setting of an autoimmune disease. *Scleritis* refers to a deeper, more severe inflammatory process, frequently associated with a connective tissue disease such as rheumatoid arthritis, lupus erythematosus, polyarteritis nodosa, Wegener's granulomatosis, or relapsing polychondritis. The inflammation and thickening of the sclera can be diffuse or nodular. In anterior forms of scleritis, the globe assumes a violet hue and the patient complains of severe ocular tenderness and pain. With posterior scleritis the pain and redness may be less marked, but there is often proptosis, choroidal effusion, reduced motility, and visual loss. Episcleritis and scleritis should be treated with NSAIDs. If these agents fail, topical or even systemic glucocorticoid therapy may be necessary, especially if an underlying autoimmune process is active.

Uveitis Involving the anterior structures of the eye, this is also called *iritis* or *iridocyclitis*. The diagnosis requires slit-lamp examination to identify inflammatory cells floating in the aqueous humor or deposited upon the corneal endothelium (keratic precipitates). Anterior uveitis develops in sarcoidosis, ankylosing spondylitis, juvenile rheumatoid arthritis, inflammatory bowel disease, psoriasis, Reiter's syndrome, and Behçet's disease. It is also associated with herpes infections, syphilis, Lyme disease, onchocerciasis, tuberculosis, and leprosy. Although anterior uveitis can occur in conjunction with many diseases, no cause is found to explain the majority of cases. For this reason, laboratory evaluation is usually reserved for patients with recurrent or severe anterior uveitis. Treatment is aimed at reducing inflammation and scarring by judicious use of topical glucocorticoids. Dilation of the pupil reduces pain and prevents the formation of synechiae.

Posterior Uveitis This is diagnosed by observing inflammation of the vitreous, retina, or choroid on fundus examination. It is more likely than anterior uveitis to be associated with an identifiable systemic disease. Some patients have panuveitis, or inflammation of both the anterior and posterior segments of the eye. Posterior uveitis is a manifestation of autoimmune diseases such as sarcoidosis, Behçet's disease, Vogt-Koyanagi-Harada syndrome, and inflammatory bowel disease (Fig. 25-3). It also accompanies diseases such as toxoplasmosis, onchocerciasis, cysticercosis, coccidioidomycosis, toxocariasis, and histoplasmosis; infections caused by organisms such as *Candida*, *Pneumocystis carinii*, *Cryptococcus*, *Aspergillus*, herpes, and cytomegalovirus (see Fig. 166-1); and other diseases such as syphilis, Lyme disease, tuberculosis, cat-scratch disease, Whipple's disease, and brucellosis. In multiple sclerosis, chronic inflammatory changes can develop in the extreme periphery of the retina (pars planitis or intermediate uveitis).

Acute Angle-Closure Glaucoma This is a rare and frequently misdiagnosed cause of a red, painful eye. Susceptible eyes have a shallow anterior chamber, either because the eye has a short axial length (hyperopia) or a lens enlarged by the gradual development of cataract. When the pupil becomes mid-dilated, the peripheral iris blocks aqueous outflow via the anterior chamber angle and the intraocular pressure rises abruptly, producing pain, injection, corneal edema, obscurations, and blurred vision. In some patients, ocular symptoms are overshadowed by nausea, vomiting, or headache, prompting a fruitless workup for abdominal or neurologic disease. The diagnosis is made by measuring the intraocular pressure during an acute attack or by observing a narrow chamber angle by means of a specially mirrored contact lens. Acute angle closure is treated with oral or intravenous acetazolamide, topical beta blockers, prostaglandin analogues, α_2-adrenergic agonists, and pilocarpine to induce miosis. If these measures fail, a laser can be used to create a hole in the peripheral iris to relieve pupillary block. Many physicians are reluctant to dilate patients routinely for fundus examination because they fear precipitating an angle-closure glaucoma. The risk is actually remote and more than outweighed by the potential benefit to patients of discovering a hidden fundus lesion visible only through a fully dilated pupil. Moreover, a single attack of angle closure after pharmacologic dilation rarely causes any permanent damage to the eye and serves as an inadvertent provocative test to identify patients with narrow angles who would benefit from prophylactic laser iridectomy.

Endophthalmitis This occurs from bacterial, viral, fungal, or parasitic infection of the internal structures of the eye. It is usually acquired by hematogenous seeding from a remote site. Chronically ill, diabetic, or immunosuppressed patients, especially those with a history of indwelling intravenous catheters or positive blood cultures, are at greatest risk for endogenous endophthalmitis. Although most patients have ocular pain and injection, visual loss is sometimes the only symptom. Septic emboli, from a diseased heart valve or a dental abscess, that lodge in the retinal circulation can give rise to endophthalmitis. White-centered retinal hemorrhages (Roth's spots) are considered pathognomonic for subacute bacterial endocarditis, but they also appear in leukemia, diabetes, and many other conditions. Endophthalmitis also occurs as a complication of ocular surgery, occasionally months or even years after the operation. An occult penetrating foreign body or unrecognized trauma to the globe should be considered in any patient with unexplained intraocular infection or inflammation.

TRANSIENT OR SUDDEN VISUAL LOSS

Amaurosis Fugax This term refers to a transient ischemic attack of the retina (Chap. 349). Because neural tissue has a high rate of metabolism, interruption of blood flow to the retina for more than a few seconds results in *transient monocular blindness*, a term used interchangeably with amaurosis fugax. Patients describe a rapid fading of vision like a curtain descending, sometimes affecting only a portion of the visual field. Amaurosis fugax usually occurs from an embolus that becomes stuck within a retinal arteriole (Fig. 25-4). If the embolus breaks up or passes, flow is restored and vision returns quickly to normal without permanent damage. With prolonged interruption of blood flow, the inner retina suffers infarction. Ophthalmoscopy reveals zones of whitened, edematous retina following the distribution of branch retinal arterioles. Complete occlusion of the central retinal artery produces arrest of blood flow and a milky retina with a cherry-red fovea (Fig. 25-5). Emboli are composed of either cholesterol (Hollenhorst plaque), calcium, or platelet-fibrin debris. The most common source is an atherosclerotic plaque in the carotid artery or aorta, although emboli can also arise from the heart, especially in patients with diseased valves, atrial fibrillation, or wall motion abnormalities.

In rare instances, amaurosis fugax occurs from low central retinal artery perfusion pressure in a patient with a critical stenosis of the ipsilateral carotid artery and poor collateral flow via the circle of Willis. In this situation, amaurosis fugax develops when there is a dip in systemic blood pressure or a slight worsening of the carotid stenosis. Sometimes there is contralateral motor or sensory loss, indicating concomitant hemispheric cerebral ischemia.

Retinal arterial occlusion also occurs rarely in association with retinal migraine, lupus erythematosus, anticardiolipin antibodies (Fig. 25-5), anticoagulant deficiency states (protein S, protein C, and antithrombin III deficiency), pregnancy, intravenous drug abuse, blood dyscrasias, dysproteinemias, and temporal arteritis.

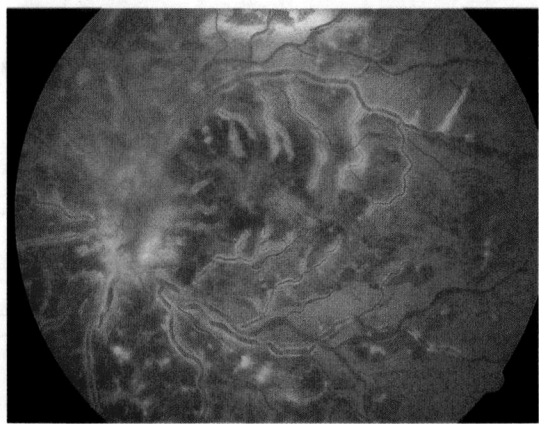

FIGURE 25-3 Retinal vasculitis, uveitis, and hemorrhage in a 32-year-old woman with Crohn's disease. Note that the veins are frosted with a white exudate. Visual acuity improved from 20/400 to 20/20 following treatment with intravenous methylprednisolone.

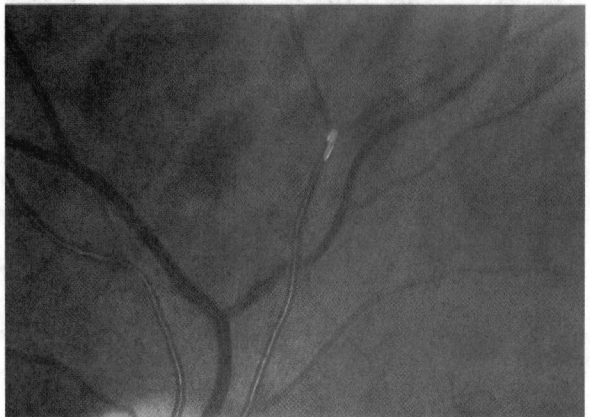

FIGURE 25-4 Hollenhorst plaque lodged at the bifurcation of a retinal arteriole proves that a patient is shedding emboli from either the carotid artery, great vessels, or heart.

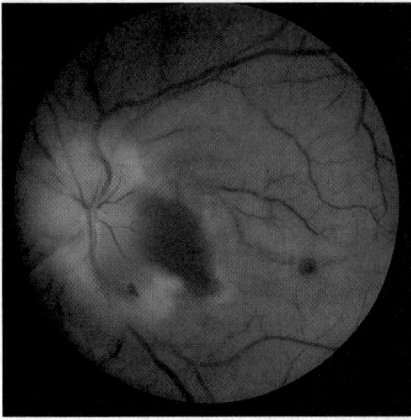

FIGURE 25-5   Central retinal artery occlusion combined with ischemic optic neuropathy in a 19-year-old woman with an elevated titer of anticardiolipin antibodies. Note the orange dot (rather than cherry red) corresponding to the fovea and the spared patch of retina just temporal to the optic disc.

Marked *systemic hypertension* causes sclerosis of retinal arterioles, splinter hemorrhages, focal infarcts of the nerve fiber layer (cotton-wool spots), and leakage of lipid and fluid (hard exudate) into the macula (Fig. 25-6). In hypertensive crisis, sudden visual loss can result from vasospasm of retinal arterioles and retinal ischemia. In addition, acute hypertension may produce visual loss from ischemic swelling of the optic disc. Patients with acute hypertensive retinopathy should be treated by lowering the blood pressure. However, the blood pressure should not be reduced precipitously, because there is a danger of optic disc infarction from sudden hypoperfusion.

Impending *branch* or *central retinal vein occlusion* can produce prolonged visual obscurations that resemble those described by patients with amaurosis fugax. The veins appear engorged and phlebitic, with numerous retinal hemorrhages (Fig. 25-7). In some patients, venous blood flow recovers spontaneously, while others evolve a frank obstruction with extensive retinal bleeding ("blood and thunder" appearance), infarction, and visual loss. Venous occlusion of the retina is often idiopathic, but hypertension, diabetes, and glaucoma are prominent risk factors. Polycythemia, thrombocythemia, or other factors leading to an underlying hypercoagulable state should be corrected; aspirin treatment may be beneficial.

Anterior Ischemic Optic Neuropathy (AION)   This is caused by insufficient blood flow through the posterior ciliary arteries supplying the optic disc. It produces painless, monocular visual loss that is usually sudden, although some patients have progressive worsening. The optic disc appears swollen and surrounded by nerve fiber layer splinter hemor-

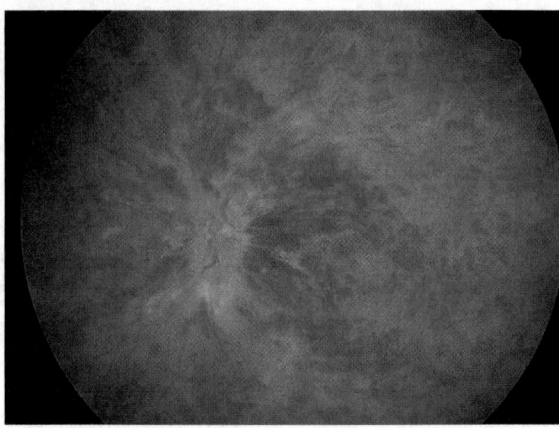

FIGURE 25-7   Central retinal vein occlusion can produce massive retinal hemorrhage ("blood and thunder"), ischemia, and vision loss.

rhages (Fig. 25-8). AION is divided into two forms: arteritic and nonarteritic. The nonarteritic form of AION is most common. No specific cause can be identified, although diabetes and hypertension are frequent risk factors. No treatment is available. About 5% of patients, especially those over age 60, develop the arteritic form of AION in conjunction with giant cell (temporal) arteritis (Chap. 306). It is urgent to recognize arteritic AION so that high doses of glucocorticoids can be instituted immediately to prevent blindness in the second eye. Symptoms of polymyalgia rheumatica may be present; the sedimentation rate and C-reactive protein level are usually elevated. In a patient with visual loss from suspected arteritic AION, temporal artery biopsy is mandatory to confirm the diagnosis. Glucocorticoids should be started immediately, without waiting for the biopsy to be completed. The diagnosis of arteritic AION is difficult to sustain in the face of a negative temporal artery biopsy, but such cases do occur.

Posterior Ischemic Optic Neuropathy   This is an infrequent cause of acute visual loss, induced by the combination of severe anemia and hypotension. Cases have been reported after major blood loss during surgery, exsanguinating trauma, gastrointestinal bleeding, and renal dialysis. The fundus usually appears normal, although optic disc swelling develops if the process extends far enough anteriorly. Vision can be salvaged in some patients by prompt blood transfusion and reversal of hypotension.

Optic Neuritis   This is a common inflammatory disease of the optic nerve. In the Optic Neuritis Treatment Trial (ONTT), the mean age of patients was 32 years, 77% were female, 92% had ocular pain (especially with eye movements), and 35% had optic disc swelling. In most patients, the demyelinating event was retrobulbar and the ocular fun-

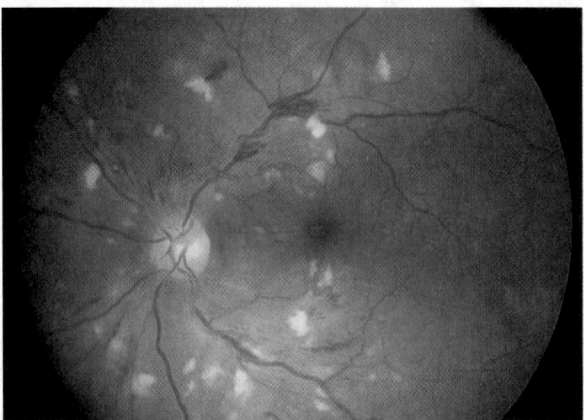

FIGURE 25-6   Hypertensive retinopathy with scattered flame (splinter) hemorrhages and cotton wool spots (nerve fiber layer infarcts) in a patient with headache and a blood pressure of 234/120.

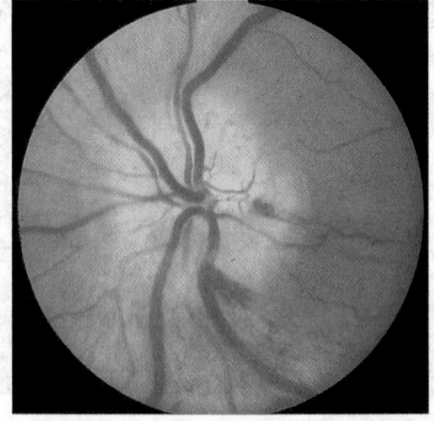

FIGURE 25-8   Anterior ischemic optic neuropathy from temporal arteritis in a 78-year-old woman with pallid disc swelling, hemorrhage, visual loss, myalgia, and an erythrocyte sedimentation rate of 86 mm/h.

dus appeared normal on initial examination (Fig. 25-9), although optic disc pallor slowly developed over subsequent months.

Virtually all patients experience a gradual recovery of vision after a single episode of optic neuritis, even without treatment. This rule is so reliable that failure of vision to improve after a first attack of optic neuritis casts doubt upon the original diagnosis. Treatment with high-dose intravenous methylprednisolone (250 mg every 6 h for 3 days) followed by oral prednisone (1 mg/kg per day for 11 days) makes no difference in final acuity (measured 6 months after the attack), but the recovery of visual function occurs more rapidly.

For some patients, optic neuritis remains an isolated event. However, the ONTT showed that the 5-year cumulative probability of developing clinically definite multiple sclerosis following optic neuritis is 30%. In patients with two or more demyelinating plaques on brain magnetic resonance (MR) imaging, treatment with interferon beta-1a can retard the development of more lesions. In summary, an MR scan is recommended in every patient with a first attack of optic neuritis. When visual loss is severe (worse than 20/100), treatment with intravenous followed by oral glucocorticoids hastens recovery. If multiple lesions are present on the MR scan, treatment with interferon beta-1a should be broached with the patient.

Leber's Hereditary Optic Neuropathy This is a disease of young men, characterized by gradual painless, severe, central visual loss in one eye, followed weeks or months later by the same process in the other eye. Acutely, the optic disc appears mildly plethoric with surface capillary telangiectases, but no vascular leakage on fluorescein angiography. Eventually optic atrophy ensues. Leber's optic neuropathy is caused by a point mutation at codon 11778 in the mitochondrial gene encoding nicotinamide adenine dinucleotide dehydrogenase (NADH) subunit 4. Additional mutations responsible for the disease have been identified, most in mitochondrial genes encoding proteins involved in electron transport. Mitochondrial mutations causing Leber's neuropathy are inherited from the mother by all her children, but usually only sons develop symptoms. There is no treatment.

Toxic Optic Neuropathy This can result in acute visual loss with bilateral optic disc swelling and central or cecocentral scotomas. Such cases have been reported to result from exposure to ethambutol, methyl alcohol (moonshine), ethylene glycol (antifreeze), or carbon monoxide. In toxic optic neuropathy, visual loss can also develop gradually and produce optic atrophy (Fig. 25-10) without a phase of acute optic disc edema. Many agents have been implicated as a cause of toxic optic neuropathy, but the evidence supporting the association for many is weak. The following is a partial list of potential offending drugs or toxins: disulfiram, ethchlorvynol, chloramphenicol, amiodarone, monoclonal anti-CD3 antibody, ciprofloxacin, digitalis, streptomycin, lead, arsenic, thallium, D-penicillamine, isoniazid, emetine, and sulfonamides. Deficiency states, induced either by starvation, malabsorption, or alcoholism, can lead to insidious visual loss. Thiamine, vitamin B_{12}, and folate levels should be checked in any patient with unexplained, bilateral central scotomas and optic pallor.

Papilledema This connotes bilateral optic disc swelling from raised intracranial pressure (Fig. 25-11). Headache is a frequent, but not in-

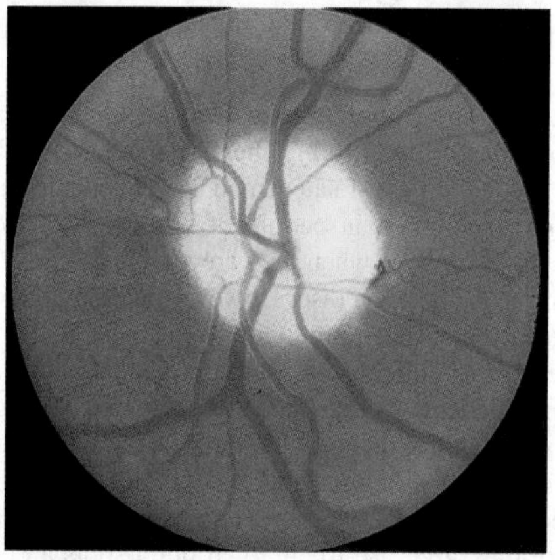

FIGURE 25-10 Optic atrophy is not a specific diagnosis, but refers to the combination of optic disc pallor, arteriolar narrowing, and nerve fiber layer destruction produced by a host of eye diseases, especially optic neuropathies.

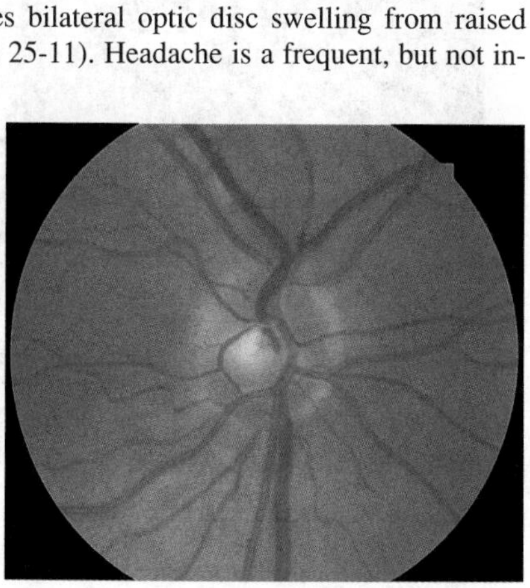

variable, accompaniment. All other forms of optic disc swelling, e.g., from optic neuritis or ischemic optic neuropathy, should be called "optic disc edema." This convention is arbitrary but serves to avoid confusion. Often it is difficult to differentiate papilledema from other forms of optic disc edema by fundus examination alone. Transient visual obscurations are a classic symptom of papilledema. They can occur in only one eye or simultaneously in both eyes. They usually last seconds but can persist longer if the papilledema is fulminant. Obscurations follow abrupt shifts in posture or happen spontaneously. When obscurations are prolonged or spontaneous, the papilledema is more threatening. Visual acuity is not affected by papilledema unless the papilledema is severe, long-standing, or accompanied by macular edema and hemorrhage. Visual field testing shows enlarged blind spots and peripheral constriction (Fig. 25-2F). With unremitting papilledema, peripheral visual field loss progresses in an insidious fashion while the optic nerve develops atrophy. In this setting, reduction of optic disc swelling is an ominous sign of a dying nerve rather than an encouraging indication of resolving papilledema.

Evaluation of papilledema requires neuroimaging to exclude an intracranial lesion. MR angiography is appropriate in selected cases to search for a dural venous sinus occlusion or an arteriovenous shunt. If neuroradiologic studies are negative, the subarachnoid opening pressure should be measured by lumbar puncture. An elevated pressure, with normal cerebrospinal fluid, points by exclusion to the diagnosis of *pseudotumor cerebri* (idiopathic intracranial hypertension). The majority of patients are young, female, and obese. Treatment with a carbonic anhydrase inhibitor such as acetazolamide lowers intracranial pressure by reducing the production of cerebrospinal fluid. Weight reduction is vital but often unsuccessful. If acetazolamide and weight loss fail, and visual field loss is progressive, a shunt should be performed without delay to prevent blindness. Occasionally, emergency

FIGURE 25-9 Retrobulbar optic neuritis is characterized by a normal fundus examination initially, hence the rubric, "the doctor sees nothing, and the patient sees nothing." Optic atrophy develops after severe or repeated attacks.

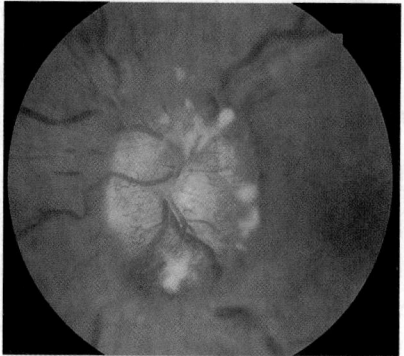

FIGURE 25-11 Papilledema means optic disc edema from raised intracranial pressure. This obese young women with pseudotumor cerebri was misdiagnosed as a migraineur until fundus examination was performed, showing optic disc elevation, hemorrhages, and cotton wool spots.

surgery is required for sudden blindness caused by fulminant papilledema.

Optic Disc Drusen These are refractile deposits within the substance of the optic nerve head (Fig. 25-12). They are unrelated to drusen of the retina, which occur in age-related macular degeneration. Optic disc drusen are most common in people of northern European descent. Their diagnosis is obvious when they are visible as glittering particles upon the surface of the optic disc. However, in many patients they are hidden beneath the surface, producing pseudo-papilledema. It is important to recognize optic disc drusen to avoid an unneccessary evaluation for papilledema. Ultrasound or computed tomography (CT) scanning is sensitive for detection of buried optic disc drusen because they contain calcium. In most patients, optic disc drusen are an incidental, innocuous finding, but they can produce visual obscurations. On perimetry they give rise to enlarged blind spots and arcuate scotomas from damage to the optic disc. With increasing age, drusen tend to become more exposed on the disc surface as optic atrophy develops. Hemorrhage, choroidal neovascular membrane, and AION are more likely to occur in patients with optic disc drusen. No treatment is available.

Vitreous Degeneration This occurs in all individuals with advancing age, leading to visual symptoms. Opacities develop in the vitreous, casting annoying shadows upon the retina. As the eye moves, these distracting "floaters" move synchronously, with a slight lag caused by inertia of the vitreous gel. Vitreous traction upon the retina causes mechanical stimulation, resulting in perception of flashing lights. This photopsia is brief and confined to one eye, in contrast to the bilateral, prolonged scintillations of cortical migraine. Contraction of the vitreous can result in sudden separation from the retina, heralded by an alarming shower of floaters and photopsia. This process, known as *vitreous detachment*, is a frequent involutional event in the elderly. It is not harmful unless it damages the retina. A careful examination of the dilated fundus is important in any patient complaining of floaters or photopsia to search for peripheral tears or holes. If such a lesion is found, laser application or cryotherapy can forestall a retinal detachment. Occasionally a tear ruptures a retinal blood vessel, causing vitreous hemorrhage and sudden loss of vision. On attempted ophthalmoscopy the fundus is hidden by a dark red haze of blood. Ultrasound is required to examine the interior of the eye for a retinal tear or detachment. If the hemorrhage does not resolve spontaneously, the vitreous can be removed surgically. Vitreous hemorrhage also occurs from the fragile neovascular vessels that proliferate on the surface of the retina in diabetes, sickle cell anemia, and other ischemic ocular diseases.

Retinal Detachment This produces symptoms of floaters, flashing lights, and a scotoma in the peripheral visual field corresponding to the detachment (Fig. 25-13). If the detachment includes the fovea, there is an afferent pupil defect and the visual acuity is reduced. In most eyes, retinal detachment starts with a hole, flap, or tear in the peripheral retina (rhegmatogenous retinal detachment). Patients with peripheral retinal thinning (lattice degeneration) are particularly vulnerable to this process. Once a break has developed in the retina, liquified vitreous is free to enter the subretinal space, separating the retina from the pigment epithelium. The combination of vitreous traction upon the retinal surface and passage of fluid behind the retina leads inexorably to detachment. Patients with a history of myopia, trauma, or prior cataract extraction are at greatest risk for retinal detachment. The diagnosis is confirmed by ophthalmoscopic examination of the dilated eye.

Classic Migraine (See also Chap. 14) This usually occurs with a visual aura lasting about 20 min. In a typical attack, a small central disturbance in the field of vision marches toward the periphery, leaving a transient scotoma in its wake. The expanding border of migraine scotoma has a scintillating, dancing, or zig-zag edge, resembling the bastions of a fortified city, hence the term *fortification spectra*. Patients' descriptions of fortification spectra vary widely and can be confused with amaurosis fugax. Migraine patterns usually last longer and are perceived in both eyes, whereas amaurosis fugax is briefer and occurs in only one eye. Migraine phenomena also remain visible in the dark or with the eyes closed. Generally they are confined to either the right or left visual hemifield, but sometimes both fields are involved simultaneously. Patients often have a long history of stereotypic attacks. After the visual symptoms recede, headache develops in most patients.

Transient Ischemic Attacks Vertebrobasilar insufficiency may result in acute homonymous visual symptoms. Many patients mistakenly describe symptoms in their left or right eye, when in fact they are occurring in the left or right hemifield of both eyes. Interruption of blood supply to the visual cortex causes a sudden fogging or graying of vision, occasionally with flashing lights or other positive phenomena that mimic migraine. Cortical ischemic attacks are briefer in duration than migraine, occur in older patients, and are not followed by headache. There may be associated signs of brainstem ischemia, such as diplopia, vertigo, numbness, weakness, or dysarthria.

Stroke This occurs when interruption of blood supply from the posterior cerebral artery to the visual cortex is prolonged. The only finding on examination is a homonymous visual field defect that stops abruptly at the vertical meridian. Occipital lobe stroke is usually due to thrombotic occlusion of the vertebrobasilar system, embolus, or dissection. Lobar hemorrhage, tumor, abscess, and arteriovenous malformation are other common causes of hemianopic cortical visual loss.

Factitious (Functional, Nonorganic) Visual Loss This is claimed by hysterics or malingerers. The latter comprise the vast majority, seeking sym-

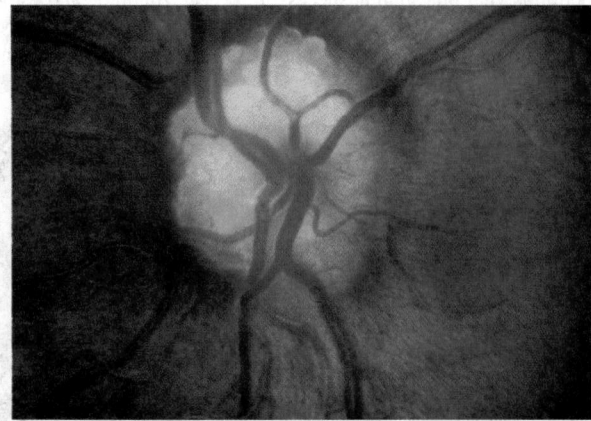

FIGURE 25-12 Optic disc drusen are calcified deposits of unknown etiology within the optic disc. They are sometimes confused with papilledema.

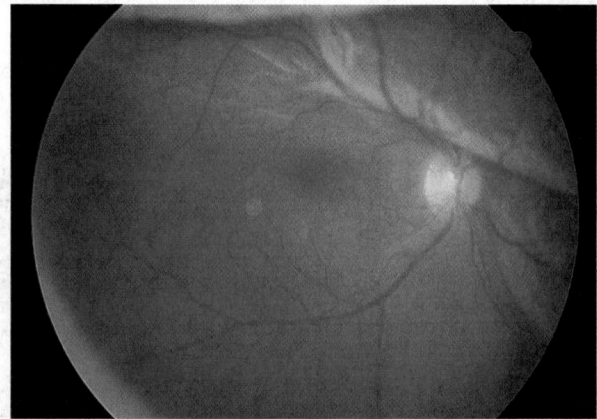

FIGURE 25-13 Retinal detachment appears as an elevated sheet of retinal tissue with folds. In this patient the fovea was spared, so acuity was normal, but a superior detachment produced an inferior scotoma.

pathy, special treatment, or financial gain by feigning loss of sight. The diagnosis is suspected when the history is atypical, physical findings are lacking or contradictory, inconsistencies emerge on testing, and a secondary motive can be identified. In our litigious society, the fraudulent pursuit of recompense has spawned an epidemic of factitious visual loss.

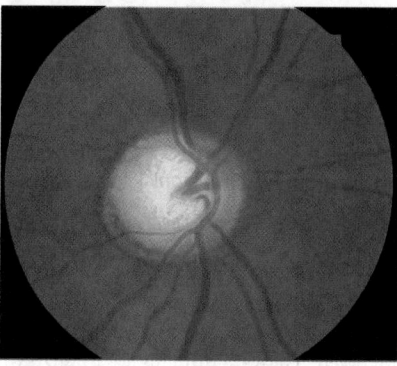

FIGURE 25-14 Glaucoma results in "cupping" as the neural rim is destroyed and the central cup becomes enlarged and excavated. The cup-to-disc ratio is about 0.7/1.0 in this patient.

CHRONIC VISUAL LOSS

Cataract This is a clouding of the lens sufficient to reduce vision. Most cataracts develop slowly as a result of aging, leading to gradual impairment of vision. The formation of cataract occurs more rapidly in patients with a history of ocular trauma, uveitis, or diabetes mellitus. Cataracts are acquired in a variety of genetic diseases, such as myotonic dystrophy, neurofibromatosis type 2, and galactosemia. Radiation therapy and glucocorticoid treatment can induce cataract as a side effect. The cataracts associated with radiation or glucocorticoids have a typical posterior subcapsular location. Cataract can be detected by noting an impaired red reflex when viewing light reflected from the fundus with an ophthalmoscope or by examining the dilated eye using the slit lamp.

The only treatment for cataract is surgical extraction of the opacified lens. Over a million cataract operations are performed each year in the United States. The operation is generally done under local anesthesia on an outpatient basis. A plastic or silicone intraocular lens is placed within the empty lens capsule in the posterior chamber, substituting for the natural lens and leading to rapid recovery of sight. More than 95% of patients who undergo cataract extraction can expect an improvement in vision. In many patients, the lens capsule remaining in the eye after cataract extraction eventually turns cloudy, causing a secondary loss of vision. A small opening is made in the lens capsule with a laser to restore clarity.

Glaucoma This is a slowly progressive, insidious optic neuropathy, usually associated with chronic elevation of intraocular pressure. In Americans of African descent it is the leading cause of blindness. The mechanism whereby raised intraocular pressure injures the optic nerve is not understood. Axons entering the inferotemporal and superotemporal aspects of the optic disc are damaged first, producing typical nerve fiber bundle or arcuate scotomas on perimetric testing. As fibers are destroyed, the neural rim of the optic disc shrinks and the physiologic cup within the optic disc enlarges (Fig. 25-14). This process is referred to as pathologic "cupping." The cup-to-disc diameter is expressed as a ratio, e.g., 0.2/1. The cup-to-disc ratio ranges widely in normal individuals, making it difficult to diagnose glaucoma reliably simply by observing an unusually large or deep optic cup. Careful documentation of serial examinations is helpful. In the patient with physiologic cupping, the large cup remains stable, whereas in the patient with glaucoma it expands relentlessly over the years. Detection of visual field loss by computerized perimetry also contributes to the diagnosis. Finally, most patients with glaucoma have raised intraocular pressure. However, many patients with typical glaucomatous cupping and visual field loss have intraocular pressures that apparently never exceed the normal limit of 20 mmHg (so-called low-tension glaucoma).

In acute angle-closure glaucoma, the eye is red and painful due to abrupt, severe elevation of intraocular pressure. Such cases account for only a handful of patients with glaucoma. Most patients with glaucoma have open, anterior chamber angles. The cause of raised intraocular pressure in open angle glaucoma is unknown but is associated with gene mutations in the heritable forms.

Glaucoma is usually painless (except in angle-closure glaucoma). Foveal acuity is spared until end-stage disease is reached. For these reasons, severe and irreversible damage can occur before either the patient or physician recognizes the diagnosis. Screening of patients for glaucoma by noting the cup-to-disc ratio on ophthalmoscopy and by measuring intraocular pressure is vital. Glaucoma is treated with topical adrenergic agonists, cholinergic agonists, beta blockers, and prostaglandin analogues. Occasionally, systemic absorption of beta blocker

from eye drops can be sufficient to cause side effects of bradycardia, hypotension, heart block, bronchospasm, or depression. Topical or oral carbonic anhydrase inhibitors are used to lower intraocular pressure by reducing aqueous production. Laser treatment of the trabecular meshwork in the anterior chamber angle improves aqueous outflow from the eye. If medical or laser treatments fail to halt optic nerve damage from glaucoma, a filter must be constructed surgically (trabeculectomy) to release aqueous from the eye in a controlled fashion.

Macular Degeneration This is a major cause of gradual, painless, bilateral central visual loss in the elderly. The old term, "senile macular degeneration," misinterpreted by many patients as an unflattering reference, has been replaced with "age-related macular degeneration." It occurs in a nonexudative (dry) form and an exudative (wet) form. The nonexudative process begins with the accumulation of extracellular deposits, called drusen, underneath the retinal pigment epithelium. On ophthalmoscopy, they are pleomorphic but generally appear as small discrete yellow lesions clustered in the macula (Fig. 25-15). With time they become larger, more numerous, and confluent. The retinal pigment epithelium becomes focally detached and atrophic, causing visual loss by interfering with photoreceptor function. Treatment with vitamins C and E, beta carotene, and zinc may retard dry macular degeneration.

Exudative macular degeneration, which develops in only a minority of patients, occurs when neovascular vessels from the choroid grow through defects in Bruch's membrane into the potential space beneath the retinal pigment epithelium. Leakage from these vessels produces elevation of the retina and pigment epithelium, with distortion (metamorphopsia) and blurring of vision. Although onset of these symptoms is usually gradual, bleeding from subretinal choroidal neovascular membranes sometimes causes acute visual loss. The neovascular membranes can be difficult to see on fundus examination because they are beneath the retina. Fluorescein or indocyanine green angiography is extremely useful for their detection. In some patients, prompt laser ablation of choroidal neovascular membranes seen on fluorescein angiography can halt the exudative process. However, the neovascular membranes frequently recur, requiring constant vigilance and repeated photocoagulation.

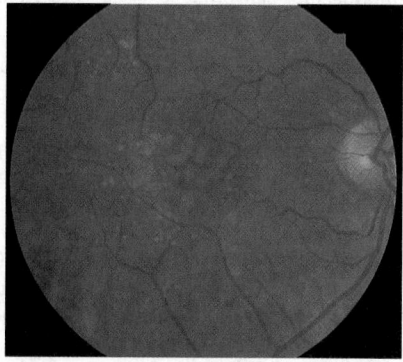

FIGURE 25-15 Age-related macular degeneration begins with the accumulation of drusen within the macula. They appear as scattered yellow subretinal deposits.

Major or repeated hemorrhage under the retina from neovascular membranes results in fibrosis, development of a round (disciform) macular scar, and permanent loss of central vision. Surgical attempts to remove subretinal membranes in age-related macular degeneration have not improved vision in most patients. However, outcomes have been more encouraging for patients with choroidal neovascular membranes from ocular histoplasmosis syndrome.

Central Serous Chorioretinopathy   This primarily affects males between the ages of 20 and 50. Leakage of serous fluid from the choroid causes small, localized detachment of the retinal pigment epithelium and the neurosensory retina. These detachments produce acute or chronic symptoms of metamorphopsia and blurred vision when the macula is involved. They are difficult to visualize with a direct ophthalmoscope because the detached retina is transparent and only slightly elevated. Diagnosis of central serous chorioretinopathy is made easily by fluorescein angiography, which shows dye streaming into the subretinal space. The cause of central serous chorioretinopathy is unknown. Symptoms may resolve spontaneously if the retina reattaches, but recurrent detachment is common. Laser photocoagulation has benefited some patients with this condition.

Diabetic Retinopathy   A rare disease until 1921, when the discovery of insulin resulted in a dramatic improvement in life expectancy for patients with diabetes mellitus, it is now a leading cause of blindness in the United States. The retinopathy of diabetes takes years to develop but eventually appears in nearly all cases. Regular surveillance of the dilated fundus is crucial for any patient with diabetes. In advanced diabetic retinopathy, the proliferation of neovascular vessels leads to blindness from vitreous hemorrhage, retinal detachment, and glaucoma (see Fig. 323-9). These complications can be avoided in most patients by administration of panretinal laser photocoagulation at the appropriate point in the evolution of the disease. →*For further discussion of the manifestations and management of diabetic retinopathy, see Chap. 323.*

Retinitis Pigmentosa   This is a general term for a disparate group of rod and cone dystrophies characterized by progressive night blindness, visual field constriction with a ring scotoma, loss of acuity, and an abnormal electroretinogram (ERG). It occurs sporadically or in an autosomal recessive, dominant, or X-linked pattern. Irregular black deposits of clumped pigment in the peripheral retina, called *bone spicules* because of their vague resemblance to the spicules of cancellous bone, give the disease its name (Fig. 25-16). The name is actually a misnomer because retinitis pigmentosa is not an inflammatory process. Most cases are due to a mutation in the gene for rhodopsin, the rod photopigment, or in the gene for peripherin, a glycoprotein located in photoreceptor outer segments. Vitamin A (15,000 IU/day) slightly retards the deterioration of the ERG in patients with retinitis pigmentosa but has no beneficial effect on visual acuity or fields. Some forms of retinitis pigmentosa occur in association with rare, hereditary systemic diseases (olivopontocerebellar degeneration, Bassen-Kornzweig disease, Kearns-Sayre syndrome, Refsum's disease). Chronic treatment with chloroquine, hydroxychloroquine, and phenothiazines (especially thioridazine) can produce visual loss from a toxic retinopathy that resembles retinitis pigmentosa.

Epiretinal Membrane   This is a fibrocellular tissue that grows across the inner surface of the retina, causing metamorphopsia and reduced visual acuity from distortion of the macula. A crinkled, cellophane-like membrane is visible on the retinal examination. Epiretinal membrane is most common in patients over 50 years of age and is usually unilateral. Most cases are idiopathic, but some occur as a result of hypertensive retinopathy, diabetes, retinal detachment, or trauma. When visual acuity is reduced to the level of about 6/24 (20/80), vitrectomy and surgical peeling of the membrane to relieve macular puckering are recommended. Contraction of an epiretinal membrane sometimes gives rise to a *macular hole*. Most macular holes, however, are caused by

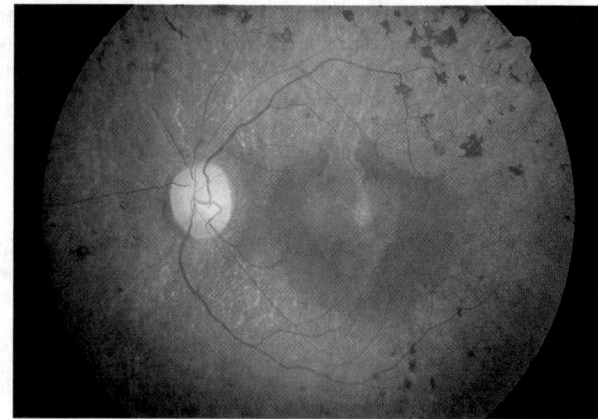

FIGURE 25-16   Retinitis pigmentosa with black clumps of pigment in the retinal periphery known as "bone spicules." There is also atrophy of the retinal pigment epithelium, making the vasculature of the choroid easily visible.

local vitreous traction within the fovea. Vitrectomy can improve acuity in selected cases.

Melanoma and Other Tumors   Melanoma is the most common primary tumor of the eye (Fig. 25-17). It causes photopsia, an enlarging scotoma, and loss of vision. A small melanoma is often difficult to differentiate from a benign choroidal nevus. Serial examinations are required to document a malignant pattern of growth. Treatment of melanoma is controversial. Options include enucleation, local resection, and irradiation. *Metastatic tumors* to the eye outnumber primary tumors. Breast and lung carcinoma have a special propensity to spread to the choroid or iris. Leukemia and lymphoma also commonly invade ocular tissues. Sometimes their only sign on eye examination is cellular debris in the vitreous, which can masquerade as a chronic posterior uveitis. *Retrobulbar tumor* of the optic nerve (meningioma, glioma) or *chiasmal tumor* (pituitary adenoma, meningioma) produces gradual visual loss with few objective findings, except for optic disc pallor. Rarely, sudden expansion of a pituitary adenoma from infarction and bleeding (*pituitary apoplexy*) causes acute retrobulbar visual loss, with headache, nausea, and ocular motor nerve palsies. In any patient with visual field loss or optic atrophy, CT or MR scanning should be considered if the cause remains unknown after careful review of the history and thorough examination of the eye.

PROPTOSIS

When the globes appear asymmetric, the clinician must first decide which eye is abnormal. Is one eye recessed within the orbit (*enophthalmos*) or is the other eye protuberant (*exophthalmos*, or *proptosis*)? A small globe or a Horner's syndrome can give the appearance of enophthalmos. True enophthalmos occurs commonly after trauma, from atrophy of retrobulbar fat, or fracture of the orbital floor. The position of the eyes within the orbits is measured using a Hertel exophthalmometer, a hand-held instrument that records the position of the anterior corneal surface relative to the lateral orbital rim. If this instrument is not available, relative eye position can be judged by

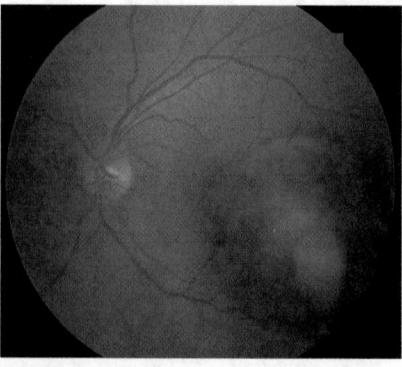

FIGURE 25-17   Melanoma of the choroid, appearing as an elevated dark mass in the inferior temporal fundus, just encroaching upon the fovea.

bending the patient's head forward and looking down upon the orbits. A proptosis of only 2 mm in one eye is detectable from this perspective. The development of proptosis implies a space-occupying lesion in the orbit, and usually warrants CT or MR imaging.

Graves' Ophthalmopathy This is the leading cause of proptosis in adults (Chap. 320). The proptosis is often asymmetric and can even appear to be unilateral. Orbital inflammation and engorgement of the extraocular muscles, particularly the medial rectus and the inferior rectus, account for the protrusion of the globe. Corneal exposure, lid retraction, conjunctival injection, restriction of gaze, diplopia, and visual loss from optic nerve compression are cardinal symptoms. Graves' ophthalmopathy is treated with oral prednisone (60 mg/d) for 1 month, followed by a taper over several months, topical lubricants, eyelid surgery, eye muscle surgery, or orbital decompression. Radiation therapy is not effective.

Orbital Pseudotumor This is an idiopathic, inflammatory orbital syndrome, frequently confused with Graves' ophthalmopathy. Symptoms are pain, limited eye movements, proptosis, and congestion. Evaluation for sarcoidosis, Wegener's granulomatosis, and other types of orbital vasculitis or collagen-vascular disease is negative. Imaging often shows swollen eye muscles (orbital myositis) with enlarged tendons. By contrast, in Graves' ophthalmopathy the tendons of the eye muscles are usually spared. The Tolosa-Hunt syndrome may be regarded as an extension of orbital pseudotumor through the superior orbital fissure into the cavernous sinus. The diagnosis of orbital pseudotumor is difficult. Biopsy of the orbit frequently yields nonspecific evidence of fat infiltration by lymphocytes, plasma cells, and eosinophils. A dramatic response to a therapeutic trial of systemic glucocorticoids indirectly provides the best confirmation of the diagnosis.

Orbital Cellulitis This causes pain, lid erythema, proptosis, conjunctival chemosis, restricted motility, decreased acuity, afferent pupillary defect, fever, and leukocytosis. It often arises from the paranasal sinuses, especially by contiguous spread of infection from the ethmoid sinus through the lamina papyracea of the medial orbit. A history of recent upper respiratory tract infection, chronic sinusitis, thick mucous secretions, or dental disease is significant in any patient with suspected orbital cellulitis. Blood cultures should be obtained, but they are usually negative. Most patients respond to empirical therapy with broad-spectrum intravenous antibiotics. Occasionally, orbital cellulitis follows an overwhelming course, with massive proptosis, blindness, septic cavernous sinus thrombosis, and meningitis. To avert this disaster, orbital cellulitis should be managed aggressively in the early stages, with immediate antibiotic therapy and imaging of the orbits. Prompt surgical drainage of an orbital abscess or paranasal sinusitis is indicated if optic nerve function deteriorates despite antibiotics.

Tumors Tumors of the orbit cause painless, progressive proptosis. The most common primary tumors are hemangioma, lymphangioma, neurofibroma, dermoid cyst, adenoid cystic carcinoma, optic nerve glioma, optic nerve meningioma, and benign mixed tumor of the lacrimal gland. Metastatic tumor to the orbit occurs frequently in breast carcinoma, lung carcinoma, and lymphoma. Diagnosis by fine-needle aspiration followed by urgent radiation therapy can sometimes preserve vision.

Carotid Cavernous Fistulas With anterior drainage through the orbit these produce proptosis, diplopia, glaucoma, and corkscrew, arterialized conjunctival vessels. Direct fistulas usually result from trauma. They are easily diagnosed because of the prominent signs produced by high-flow, high-pressure shunting. Indirect fistulas, or dural arteriovenous malformations, are more likely to occur spontaneously, especially in older women. The signs are more subtle and the diagnosis is frequently missed. The combination of slight proptosis, diplopia, enlarged muscles, and an injected eye is often mistaken for thyroid ophthalmopathy. A bruit heard upon auscultation of the head, or reported by the patient, is a valuable diagnostic clue. Imaging shows an enlarged superior ophthalmic vein in the orbits. Carotid cavernous shunts can be eliminated by intravascular embolization.

PTOSIS

Blepharoptosis This is an abnormal drooping of the eyelid. Unilateral or bilateral ptosis can be congenital, from dysgenesis of the levator palpebrae superioris, or from abnormal insertion of its aponeurosis into the eyelid. Acquired ptosis can develop so gradually that the patient is unaware of the problem. Inspection of old photographs is helpful in dating the onset. A history of prior trauma, eye surgery, contact lens use, diplopia, systemic symptoms (e.g., dysphagia or peripheral muscle weakness), or a family history of ptosis should be sought. Fluctuating ptosis that worsens late in the day is typical of myasthenia gravis. Examination should focus upon evidence for proptosis, eyelid masses or deformities, inflammation, pupil inequality, or limitation of motility. The width of the palpebral fissures is measured in primary gaze to quantitate the degree of ptosis. The ptosis will be underestimated if the patient compensates by lifting the brow with the frontalis muscle.

Mechanical Ptosis This occurs in many elderly patients from stretching and redundancy of eyelid skin and subcutaneous fat (dermatochalasis). The extra weight of these sagging tissues causes the lid to droop. Enlargement or deformation of the eyelid from infection, tumor, trauma, or inflammation also results in ptosis on a purely mechanical basis.

Aponeurotic Ptosis This is an acquired dehiscence or stretching of the aponeurotic tendon, which connects the levator muscle to the tarsal plate of the eyelid. It occurs commonly in older patients, presumably from loss of connective tissue elasticity. Aponeurotic ptosis is also a frequent sequela of eyelid swelling from infection or blunt trauma to the orbit, cataract surgery, or hard contact lens usage.

Myogenic Ptosis The causes of *myogenic ptosis* include myasthenia gravis (Chap. 366) and a number of rare myopathies that manifest with ptosis. The term *chronic progressive external ophthalmoplegia* refers to a spectrum of systemic diseases caused by mutations of mitochondrial DNA. As the name implies, the most prominent findings are symmetric, slowly progressive ptosis and limitation of eye movements. In general, diplopia is a late symptom because all eye movements are reduced equally. In the *Kearns-Sayre* variant, retinal pigmentary changes and abnormalities of cardiac conduction develop. Peripheral muscle biopsy shows characteristic "ragged-red fibers." *Oculopharyngeal dystrophy* is a distinct autosomal dominant disease with onset in middle age, characterized by ptosis, limited eye movements, and trouble swallowing. *Myotonic dystrophy*, another autosomal dominant disorder, causes ptosis, ophthalmoparesis, cataract, and pigmentary retinopathy. Patients have muscle wasting, myotonia, frontal balding, and cardiac abnormalities.

Neurogenic Ptosis This results from a lesion affecting the innervation to either of the two muscles that open the eyelid: Müller's muscle or the levator palpebrae superioris. Examination of the pupil helps to distinguish between these two possibilities. In Horner's syndrome, the eye with ptosis has a smaller pupil and the eye movements are full. In an oculomotor nerve palsy, the eye with the ptosis has a larger, or a normal, pupil. If the pupil is normal but there is limitation of adduction, elevation, and depression, a pupil-sparing oculomotor nerve palsy is likely (see next section). Rarely, a lesion affecting the small, central subnucleus of the oculomotor complex will cause bilateral ptosis with normal eye movements and pupils.

DOUBLE VISION

The first point to clarify is whether diplopia persists in either eye after covering the fellow eye. If it does, the diagnosis is monocular diplopia. The cause is usually intrinsic to the eye and therefore has no dire implications for the patient. Corneal aberrations (e.g., keratoconus, pterygium), uncorrected refractive error, cataract, or foveal traction may give rise to monocular diplopia. Occasionally it is a symptom of malingering or psychiatric disease. Diplopia alleviated by covering one eye is binocular diplopia and is caused by disruption of ocular alignment. Inquiry should be made into the nature of the double vision (purely side-by-side versus partial vertical displacement of images), mode of onset, duration, intermittency, diurnal variation, and associated neurologic or systemic symptoms. If the patient has diplopia while being examined, motility testing should reveal a deficiency corresponding to the patient's symptoms. However, subtle limitation of ocular excursions is often difficult to detect. For example, a patient with a slight left abducens nerve paresis may appear to have full eye movements, despite a complaint of horizontal diplopia upon looking to the left. In this situation, the cover test provides a more sensitive method for demonstrating the ocular misalignment. It should be conducted in primary gaze, and then with the head turned and tilted in each direction. In the above example, a cover test with the head turned to the right will maximize the fixation shift evoked by the cover test.

Occasionally, a cover test performed in an asymptomatic patient during a routine examination will reveal an ocular deviation. If the eye movements are full and the ocular misalignment is equal in all directions of gaze (concomitant deviation), the diagnosis is strabismus. In this condition, which affects about 1% of the population, fusion is disrupted in infancy or early childhood. To avoid diplopia, vision is suppressed from the nonfixating eye. In some children, this leads to impaired vision (amblyopia, or "lazy" eye) in the deviated eye.

Binocular diplopia occurs from a wide range of processes: infectious, neoplastic, metabolic, degenerative, inflammatory, and vascular. One must decide if the diplopia is neurogenic in origin or due to restriction of globe rotation by local disease in the orbit. Orbital pseudotumor, myositis, infection, tumor, thyroid disease, and muscle entrapment (e.g., from a blowout fracture) cause restrictive diplopia. The diagnosis of restriction is usually made by recognizing other associated signs and symptoms of local orbital disease in conjunction with imaging.

Myasthenia Gravis (See also Chap. 366)   This is a major cause of diplopia. The diplopia is often intermittent, variable, and not confined to any single ocular motor nerve distribution. The pupils are always normal. Fluctuating ptosis may be present. Many patients have a purely ocular form of the disease, with no evidence of systemic muscular weakness. The diagnosis can be confirmed by an intravenous edrophonium injection or by an assay for antiacetylcholine receptor antibodies. Negative results from these tests do not exclude the diagnosis. *Botulism* from food or wound poisoning can mimic ocular myasthenia.

After restrictive orbital disease and myasthenia gravis are excluded, a lesion of a cranial nerve supplying innervation to the extraocular muscles is the most likely cause of binocular diplopia.

Oculomotor Nerve   The third cranial nerve innervates the medial, inferior, and superior recti; inferior oblique; levator palpebrae superioris; and the iris sphincter. Total palsy of the oculomotor nerve causes ptosis, a dilated pupil, and leaves the eye "down and out" because of the unopposed action of the lateral rectus and superior oblique. This combination of findings is obvious. More challenging is the diagnosis of an early or partial oculomotor nerve palsy. In this setting, any combination of ptosis, pupil dilation, and weakness of the eye muscles supplied by the oculomotor nerve may be encountered. Frequent serial examinations during the evolving phase of the palsy and a high index of suspicion help ensure that the diagnosis is not missed. The advent of an oculomotor nerve palsy with any degree of pupil involvement in an otherwise healthy patient, especially when accompanied by pain, raises the specter of a circle of Willis aneurysm. If an MR imaging shows no compressive lesion, an arteriogram must be considered to rule out an aneurysm of either the posterior communicating artery or the basilar artery. If the pupil is entirely normal, with all other components of an oculomotor palsy present, aneurysm is so rare that an angiogram is seldom indicated.

A lesion of the oculomotor nucleus in the rostral midbrain produces signs that differ from those caused by a lesion of the nerve itself. There is bilateral ptosis because the levator muscle is innervated by a single central subnucleus. There is also weakness of the contralateral superior rectus, because it is supplied by the oculomotor nucleus on the other side. Occasionally both superior recti are weak. Isolated nuclear oculomotor palsy is rare. Usually neurologic examination reveals additional signs to suggest brainstem damage from infarction, hemorrhage, tumor, or infection.

Injury to structures surrounding fascicles of the oculomotor nerve descending through the midbrain has given rise to a number of classic eponymic designations. In *Nothnagel's syndrome*, injury to the superior cerebellar peduncle causes ipsilateral oculomotor palsy and contralateral cerebellar ataxia. In *Benedikt's syndrome*, injury to the red nucleus results in ipsilateral oculomotor palsy and contralateral tremor, chorea, and athetosis. *Claude's syndrome* incorporates features of both the aforementioned syndromes, by injury to both the red nucleus and the superior cerebellar peduncle. Finally, in *Weber's syndrome*, injury to the cerebral peduncle causes ipsilateral oculomotor palsy with contralateral hemiparesis.

In the subarachnoid space the oculomotor nerve is vulnerable to aneurysm, meningitis, tumor, infarction, and compression. In cerebral herniation the nerve becomes trapped between the edge of the tentorium and the uncus of the temporal lobe. Oculomotor palsy can also occur from midbrain torsion and hemorrhages during herniation. In the cavernous sinus, oculomotor palsy arises from carotid aneurysm, carotid cavernous fistula, cavernous sinus thrombosis, tumor (pituitary adenoma, meningioma, metastasis), herpes zoster infection, and the Tolosa-Hunt syndrome.

The etiology of an isolated, pupil-sparing oculomotor palsy often remains an enigma, even after neuroimaging and extensive laboratory testing. Most cases are thought to result from microvascular infarction of the nerve, somewhere along its course from the brainstem to the orbit. Usually the patient complains of pain. Diabetes, hypertension, and vascular disease are major risk factors. Spontaneous recovery over a period of months is the rule. If this fails to occur, or if new findings develop, the diagnosis of microvascular oculomotor nerve palsy should be reconsidered. Aberrant regeneration is common when the oculomotor nerve is injured by trauma or compression (tumor, aneurysm). Miswiring of sprouting fibers to the levator muscle and the rectus muscles results in elevation of the eyelid upon downgaze or adduction. The pupil also constricts upon attempted adduction, elevation, or depression of the globe. Aberrant regeneration is not seen after oculomotor palsy from microvascular infarct and hence vitiates that diagnosis.

Trochlear Nerve   The fourth cranial nerve originates in the midbrain, just caudal to the oculomotor nerve complex. Fibers exit the brainstem dorsally and cross to innervate the contralateral superior oblique. The principal actions of this muscle are to depress and to intort the globe. A palsy therefore results in hypertropia and excyclotorsion. The cyclotorsion is seldom noticed by patients. Instead, they complain of vertical diplopia, especially upon reading or looking down. The vertical diplopia is also exacerbated by tilting the head toward the side with the muscle palsy, and alleviated by tilting it away. This "head tilt test" is a cardinal diagnostic feature.

Isolated trochlear nerve palsy occurs from all the causes listed above for the oculomotor nerve, except aneurysm. The trochlear nerve is particularly apt to suffer injury after closed head trauma. The free edge of the tentorium is thought to impinge upon the nerve during a concussive blow. Most isolated trochlear nerve palsies are idiopathic and hence diagnosed by exclusion as "microvascular." Spontaneous improvement occurs over a period of months in most patients. A base-down prism (conveniently applied to the patient's glasses as a stick-on Fresnel lens) may serve as a temporary measure to alleviate diplopia. If the palsy does not resolve, the eyes can be realigned by weakening the inferior oblique muscle.

Abducens Nerve   The sixth cranial nerve innervates the lateral rectus muscle. A palsy produces horizontal diplopia, worse on gaze to the side of the lesion. A nuclear lesion has different consequences, because the abducens nucleus contains interneurons that project via the medial longitudinal fasciculus to the medial rectus subnucleus of the contralateral oculomotor complex. Therefore, an abducens nuclear lesion produces a complete lateral gaze palsy, from weakness of both the ipsilateral lateral rectus and the contralateral medial rectus. *Foville's syndrome* following dorsal pontine injury includes lateral gaze palsy, ipsilateral facial palsy, and contralateral hemiparesis incurred by damage to descending corticospinal fibers. *Millard-Gubler syndrome* from ventral pontine injury is similar, except for the eye findings. There is lateral rectus weakness only, instead of gaze palsy, because the abducens fascicle is injured rather than the nucleus. Infarct, tumor, hemorrhage, vascular malformation, and multiple sclerosis are the most common etiologies of brainstem abducens palsy.

After leaving the ventral pons, the abducens nerve runs forward along the clivus to pierce the dura at the petrous apex, where it enters the cavernous sinus. Along its subarachnoid course it is susceptible to meningitis, tumor (meningioma, chordoma, carcinomatous meningitis), subarachnoid hemorrhage, trauma, and compression by aneurysm or dolichoectatic vessels. At the petrous apex, mastoiditis can produce deafness, pain, and ipsilateral abducens palsy (*Gradenigo's syndrome*). In the cavernous sinus, the nerve can be affected by carotid aneurysm, carotid cavernous fistula, tumor (pituitary adenoma, meningioma, nasopharyngeal carcinoma), herpes infection, and Tolosa-Hunt syndrome.

Unilateral or bilateral abducens palsy is a classic sign of raised intracranial pressure. The diagnosis can be confirmed if papilledema is observed on fundus examination. The mechanism is still debated but is probably related to rostral-caudal displacement of the brainstem. The same phenomenon accounts for abducens palsy from low intracranial pressure (e.g., after lumbar puncture, spinal anesthesia, or spontaneous dural cerebrospinal fluid leak).

Treatment of abducens palsy is aimed at prompt correction of the underlying cause. However, the cause remains obscure in many instances, despite diligent evaluation. As mentioned above for isolated trochlear or oculomotor palsy, most cases are assumed to represent microvascular infarcts because they often occur in the setting of diabetes or other vascular risk factors. Some cases may develop as a postinfectious mononeuritis (e.g., following a viral flu). Patching one eye or applying a temporary prism will provide relief of diplopia until the palsy resolves. If recovery is incomplete, eye muscle surgery can nearly always realign the eyes, at least in primary position. A patient with an abducens palsy that fails to improve should be reevaluated for an occult etiology (e.g., chordoma, carcinomatous meningitis, carotid cavernous fistula, myasthenia gravis).

Multiple Ocular Motor Nerve Palsies These should not be attributed to spontaneous microvascular events affecting more than one cranial nerve at a time. This remarkable coincidence does occur, especially in diabetic patients, but the diagnosis is made only in retrospect after exhausting all other diagnostic alternatives. Neuroimaging should focus on the cavernous sinus, superior orbital fissure, and orbital apex, where all three ocular motor nerves are in close proximity. In the diabetic or compromised host, fungal infection (*Aspergillus*, Mucorales, *Cryptococcus*) is a frequent cause of multiple nerve palsies. In the patient with systemic malignancy, carcinomatous meningitis is a likely diagnosis. Cytologic examination may be negative despite repeated sampling of the cerebrospinal fluid. The cancer-associated Lambert-Eaton myasthenic syndrome can also produce ophthalmoplegia. Giant cell (temporal) arteritis occasionally manifests as diplopia from ischemic palsies of extraocular muscles. Fisher syndrome, an ocular variant of Guillain-Barré, can produce ophthalmoplegia with areflexia and ataxia. Often the ataxia is mild, and the areflexia is overlooked because the physician's attention is focused upon the eyes. Antiganglioside antibodies (GQ1b) can be detected in about 50% of cases.

Supranuclear Disorders of Gaze These are often mistaken for multiple ocular motor nerve palsies. For example, Wernicke's encephalopathy

can produce nystagmus and a partial deficit of horizontal and vertical gaze that mimics a combined abducens and oculomotor nerve palsy. The disorder occurs in malnourished or alcoholic patients and can be reversed by thiamine. Infarct, hemorrhage, tumor, multiple sclerosis, encephalitis, vasculitis, and Whipple's disease are other important causes of supranuclear gaze palsy. Disorders of vertical gaze, especially downwards saccades, are an early feature of progressive supranuclear palsy. Smooth pursuit is affected later in the course of the disease. Parkinson's disease, Huntington's chorea, and olivopontocerebellar degeneration can also affect vertical gaze.

The *frontal eye field* of the cerebral cortex is involved in generation of saccades to the contralateral side. After hemispheric stroke, the eyes usually deviate towards the lesioned side because of the unopposed action of the frontal eye field in the normal hemisphere. With time, this deficit resolves. Seizures generally have the opposite effect: the eyes deviate conjugately away from the irritative focus. *Parietal lesions* disrupt smooth pursuit of targets moving toward the side of the lesion. Bilateral parietal lesions produce *Balint's syndrome*, characterized by impaired eye-hand coordination (optic ataxia), difficulty initiating voluntary eye movements (ocular apraxia), and visuospatial disorientation (simultanagnosia).

Horizontal Gaze Descending cortical inputs mediating horizontal gaze ultimately converge at the level of the pons. Neurons in the paramedian pontine reticular formation are responsible for controlling conjugate gaze toward the same side. They project directly to the ipsilateral abducens nucleus. A lesion of either the paramedian pontine reticular formation or the abducens nucleus causes an ipsilateral conjugate gaze palsy. Lesions at either locus produce nearly identical clinical syndromes, with the following exception: vestibular stimulation (oculocephalic maneuver or caloric irrigation) will succeed in driving the eyes conjugately to the side in a patient with a lesion of the paramedian pontine reticular formation, but not in a patient with a lesion of the abducens nucleus.

INTERNUCLEAR OPHTHALMOPLEGIA This results from damage to the medial longitudinal fasciculus ascending from the abducens nucleus in the pons to the oculomotor nucleus in the midbrain (hence, "internuclear"). Damage to fibers carrying the conjugate signal from abducens interneurons to the contralateral medial rectus motoneurons results in a failure of adduction on attempted lateral gaze. For example, a patient with a left internuclear ophthalmoplegia will have slowed or absent adducting movements of the left eye. A patient with bilateral injury to the medial longitudinal fasciculus will have bilateral internuclear ophthalmoplegia. Multiple sclerosis is the most common cause, although tumor, stroke, trauma, or any brainstem process may be responsible. *One-and-a-half syndrome* is due to a combined lesion of the medial longitudinal fasciculus and the abducens nucleus on the same side. The patient's only horizontal eye movement is abduction of the eye on the other side.

Vertical Gaze This is controlled at the level of the midbrain. The neuronal circuits affected in disorders of vertical gaze are not fully elucidated, but lesions of the rostral interstitial nucleus of the medial longitudinal fasciculus and the interstitial nucleus of Cajal cause supranuclear paresis of upgaze, downgaze, or all vertical eye movements. Distal basilar artery ischemia is the most common etiology. *Skew deviation* refers to a vertical misalignment of the eyes, usually constant in all positions of gaze. The finding has poor localizing value because skew deviation has been reported after lesions in widespread regions of the brainstem and cerebellum.

PARINAUD'S SYNDROME Also known as dorsal midbrain syndrome, this is a distinct supranuclear vertical gaze disorder from damage to the posterior commissure. It is a classic sign of hydrocephalus from aqueductal stenosis. Pineal region tumors, cysticercosis, and stroke also cause Parinaud's syndrome. Features include loss of upgaze (and sometimes downgaze), convergence-retraction nystagmus on attempted upgaze, downwards ocular deviation ("setting sun" sign), lid retraction (Collier's sign), skew deviation, pseudoabducens palsy, and light-near dissociation of the pupils.

Nystagmus   This is a rhythmical oscillation of the eyes, occurring physiologically from vestibular and optokinetic stimulation or pathologically in a wide variety of diseases (Chap. 20). Abnormalities of the eyes or optic nerves, present at birth or acquired in childhood, can produce a complex, searching nystagmus with irregular pendular (sinusoidal) and jerk features. This nystagmus is commonly referred to as *congenital sensory nystagmus*. It is a poor term, because even in children with congenital lesions, the nystagmus does not appear until several months of age. *Congenital motor nystagmus*, which looks similar to congenital sensory nystagmus, develops in the absence of any abnormality of the sensory visual system. Visual acuity is also reduced in congenital motor nystagmus, probably by the nystagmus itself, but seldom below a level of 20/200.

JERK NYSTAGMUS   This is characterized by a slow drift off the target, followed by a fast corrective saccade. By convention, the nystagmus is named after the quick phase. Jerk nystagmus can be downbeat, upbeat, horizontal (left or right), and torsional. The pattern of nystagmus may vary with gaze position. Some patients will be oblivious to their nystagmus. Others will complain of blurred vision, or a subjective, to-and-fro movement of the environment (oscillopsia) corresponding to their nystagmus. Fine nystagmus may be difficult to see upon gross examination of the eyes. Observation of nystagmoid movements of the optic disc on ophthalmoscopy is a sensitive way to detect subtle nystagmus.

GAZE-EVOKED NYSTAGMUS   This is the most common form of jerk nystagmus. When the eyes are held eccentrically in the orbits, they have a natural tendency to drift back to primary position. The subject compensates by making a corrective saccade to maintain the deviated eye position. Many normal patients have mild gaze-evoked nystagmus. Exaggerated gaze-evoked nystagmus can be induced by drugs (seda-

tives, anticonvulsants, alcohol); muscle paresis; myasthenia gravis; demyelinating disease; and cerebellopontine angle, brainstem, and cerebellar lesions.

VESTIBULAR NYSTAGMUS   *Vestibular nystagmus* results from dysfunction of the labyrinth (Ménière's disease), vestibular nerve, or vestibular nucleus in the brainstem. Peripheral vestibular nystagmus often occurs in discrete attacks, with symptoms of nausea and vertigo. There may be associated tinnitus and hearing loss. Sudden shifts in head position may provoke or exacerbate symptoms.

DOWNBEAT NYSTAGMUS   *Downbeat nystagmus* occurs from lesions near the craniocervical junction (Chiari malformation, basilar invagination). It has also been reported in brainstem or cerebellar stroke, lithium or anticonvulsant intoxication, alcoholism, and multiple sclerosis. *Upbeat nystagmus* is associated with damage to the pontine tegmentum, from stroke, demyelination, or tumor.

Opsoclonus   This rare, dramatic disorder of eye movements consists of bursts of consecutive saccades (saccadomania). When the saccades are confined to the horizontal plane, the term *ocular flutter* is preferred. It can occur from viral encephalitis, trauma, or a paraneoplastic effect of neuroblastoma, breast carcinoma, and other malignancies. It has also been reported as a benign, transient phenomenon in otherwise healthy patients.

FURTHER READING

AREDS REPORT NO. 8: A randomized, placebo-controlled, clinical trial of high-dose supplementation with vitamins C and E, beta carotene, and zinc for age-related macular degeneration and vision loss. Arch Ophthalmol 119: 1417, 2001

BECK RW et al: Interferon beta-1a for early multiple sclerosis: CHAMPS trial subgroup analyses. Ann Neurol 51:481, 2002

BENAVENTE O et al: Prognosis after transient monocular blindness associated with carotid artery stenosis. N Engl J Med 345:1084, 2001

NEGI A, VERNON SA: An overview of the eye in diabetes. JR Soc Med 96: 266, 2003

SOLOMON R, DONNENFELD ED: Recent advances and future frontiers in treating age-related cataracts. JAMA 290:248, 2003

---

26   DISORDERS OF SMELL, TASTE, AND HEARING
Anil K. Lalwani, James B. Snow, Jr.

SMELL

The sense of smell determines the flavor and palatability of food and drink. It serves, along with the trigeminal system, as a monitor of inhaled chemicals, including dangerous substances such as natural gas, smoke, and air pollutants. Olfactory dysfunction affects ~1% of people under age 60 and more than half of the population beyond this age.

DEFINITIONS   *Smell* is the perception of odor by the nose. *Taste* is the perception of salty, sweet, sour, or bitter by the tongue. Related sensations during eating such as somatic sensations of coolness, warmth, and irritation are mediated through the trigeminal, glossopharyngeal, and vagal afferents in the nose, oral cavity, tongue, pharynx, and larynx. *Flavor* is the complex interaction of taste, smell, and somatic sensation. Terms relating to disorders of smell include *anosmia*, an absence of the ability to smell; *hyposmia*, a decreased ability to smell; *hyperosmia*, an increased sensitivity to an odorant; *dysosmia*, distortion in the perception of an odor; *phantosmia*, perception of an odorant where none is present; and *agnosia*, inability to classify, contrast, or identify odor sensations verbally, even though the ability to distinguish between odorants or to recognize them may be normal. An odor stimulus is referred to as an *odorant*. Each category of smell dysfunction can be further subclassified as total (applying to all odorants) or partial (dysfunction of only select odorants).

PHYSIOLOGY OF SMELL   The *olfactory neuroepithelium* is located in the superior part of the nasal cavities. It contains an orderly arrangement

of bipolar olfactory receptor cells, microvillar cells, sustentacular cells, and basal cells. The dendritic process of the bipolar cell has a bulb-shaped vesicle that projects into the mucous layer and bears six to eight cilia containing the odorant. Each bipolar cell contains 56 cm^2 (9 in.^{2}) of surface area to receive olfactory stimuli.

Microvillar cells are located adjacent to the receptor cells on the surface of the neuroepithelium. Sustentacular cells, unlike their counterparts in the respiratory epithelium, are not specialized to secrete mucus. Although they form a tight barrier separating neurons from the outside environment, their complete function is unknown. The basal cells are progenitors of other cell types in the olfactory neuroepithelium, including the bipolar receptor cells. There is a regular turnover of bipolar receptor cells, which function as the primary sensory neurons. In addition, with injury to the cell body or its axon, the receptor cell is replaced by a differentiated basal cell, which reestablishes a central neural connection. These primary sensory neurons are unique among sensory systems in that they are regularly replaced and regenerate after injury.

The unmyelinated axons of receptor cells form the fila of the olfactory nerve, pass through the cribriform plate, and terminate within spherical masses of neuropil, termed *glomeruli*, in the olfactory bulb. The glomeruli are the focus of a high degree of convergence of information, since many more fibers enter than leave them. The main second-order neurons are mitral cells. The primary dendrite of each mitral cell extends into a single glomerulus. Axons of the mitral cells project along with the axons of adjacent tufted cells to the limbic system, including the anterior olfactory nucleus and the amygdala. Cognitive awareness of smell requires stimulation of the prepiriform cortex or amygdaloid nuclei.

A secondary site of olfactory chemosensation is located in the epithelium of the vomeronasal organ, a tubular structure that opens on the ventral aspect of the nasal septum. Sensory neurons located in the vomeronasal organ detect pheromones, nonvolatile chemical signals that in lower mammals trigger innate and stereotyped reproductive and social behaviors, as well as neuroendocrine changes. Neurons from the organ project to the accessory olfactory bulbs and not the main olfactory bulb, as does the olfactory neuroepithelium. Whether humans use the vomeronasal organ to detect and respond to chemical signals from others remains controversial. Development of the olfactory and vomeronasal system appears to be required for normal sexual maturation.

The sensation of smell begins with introduction of an odorant to the cilia of the bipolar neuron. Most odorants are hydrophobic; as they move from the air phase of the nasal cavity to the aqueous phase of the olfactory mucous, they are transported toward the cilia by small water-soluble proteins called *odorant-binding proteins* and reversibly bind to receptors on the cilia surface. Binding leads to conformational changes in the receptor protein, activation of G protein–coupled second messengers, and generation of action potentials in the primary neurons. Intensity appears to be coded by the amount of firing in the afferent neurons.

Olfactory receptor proteins belong to the large family of G protein–coupled receptors that also includes rhodopsins; α- and β-adrenergic receptors; muscarinic acetylcholine receptors; and neurotransmitter receptors for dopamine, serotonin, and substance P. In humans, there are 300 to 1000 olfactory receptor genes belonging to 20 different families located in clusters at more than 25 different chromosomal locations. Each olfactory neuron seems to express only one or, at most, a few receptor genes, thus providing the molecular basis of odor discrimination. Bipolar cells that express similar receptors appear to be scattered across discrete spatial zones. These similar cells converge on a select few glomeruli in the olfactory bulb. The result is a potential spatial map of how we receive odor stimuli, much like the tonotopic organization of how we perceive sound.

DISORDERS OF THE SENSE OF SMELL These are caused by conditions that interfere with the access of the odorant to the olfactory neuroepithelium (transport loss), injure the receptor region (sensory loss), or damage central olfactory pathways (neural loss). Currently no clinical tests exist to differentiate these different types of olfactory losses. Fortunately, the history of the disease provides important clues to the cause. The leading causes of olfactory disorders are summarized in Table 26-1; the most common etiologies are head trauma in children and young adults, and viral infections in older adults.

Head trauma is followed by unilateral or bilateral impairment of smell in up to 15% of cases; anosmia is more common than hyposmia. Olfactory dysfunction is more common when trauma is associated with loss of consciousness, moderately severe head injury (grades II to V), and skull fracture. Frontal injuries and fractures disrupt the cribriform plate and olfactory axons that perforate it. Sometimes there is an associated cerebrospinal fluid (CSF) rhinorrhea resulting from a tearing of the dura overlying the cribriform plate and paranasal sinuses. Anosmia may also follow blows to the occiput. Once traumatic anosmia develops, it is usually permanent; only 10% of patients ever improve or recover. Perversion of the sense of smell may occur as a transient phase in the recovery process.

Viral infections destroy the olfactory neuroepithelium, which is replaced by respiratory epithelium. Parainfluenza virus type 3 appears to be especially detrimental to human olfaction. HIV infection is associated with subjective distortion of taste and smell, which may become more severe as the disease progresses. The loss of taste and smell may play an important role in the development and progression of HIV-associated wasting. Congenital anosmias are rare but important. Kallmann syndrome is an X-linked disorder characterized by congen-

TABLE 26-1 *Causes of Olfactory Dysfunction*

Transport Losses	**Neural Losses**
Allergic rhinitis	AIDS
Bacterial rhinitis and sinusitis	Alcoholism
Congenital abnormalities	Alzheimer's disease
Nasal neoplasms	Cigarette smoke
Nasal polyps	Depression
Nasal septal deviation	Diabetes mellitus
Nasal surgery	Drugs/Toxins
Viral infections	Huntington's chorea
Sensory Losses	Hypothyroidism
Drugs	Kallmann syndrome
Neoplasms	Malnutrition
Radiation therapy	Neoplasms
Toxin exposure	Neurosurgery
Viral infections	Parkinson's disease
	Trauma
	Vitamin B_{12} deficiency
	Zinc deficiency

ital anosmia and hypogonadotropic hypogonadism resulting from a failure of migration from the olfactory placode of olfactory receptor neurons and neurons synthesizing gonadotropin-releasing hormone (Chap. 325). Anosmia can also occur in albinos. The receptor cells are present but are hypoplastic, lack cilia, and do not project above the surrounding supporting cells.

Meningiomas of the inferior frontal region are the most frequent neoplastic cause of anosmia; loss of smell may be the only neurologic abnormality. Rarely, anosmia can occur with gliomas of the frontal lobe. Occasionally, pituitary adenomas, craniopharyngiomas, suprasellar meningiomas, and aneurysms of the anterior part of the circle of Willis extend forward and damage olfactory structures. These tumors and hamartomas may also induce seizures with olfactory hallucinations, indicating involvement of the uncus of the temporal lobe.

Dysosmia, subjective distortions of olfactory perception, may occur with intranasal diseases that partially impair smell or may represent a phase in the recovery from a neurogenic anosmia. Most dysosmic disorders consist of disagreeable odors, sometimes accompanied by distortions of taste. Dysosmia also can occur with depression.

APPROACH TO THE PATIENT

Unilateral anosmia is rarely a complaint and is only recognized by separate testing of smell in each nasal cavity. Bilateral anosmia, on the other hand, brings patients to medical attention. Anosmic patients usually complain of a loss of the sense of taste even though their taste thresholds may be within normal limits. In actuality, they are complaining of a loss of flavor detection, which is mainly an olfactory function. The physical examination should include a thorough inspection of the ears, upper respiratory tract, and head and neck. A neurologic examination emphasizing the cranial nerves and cerebellar and sensorimotor function is essential. Any signs of depression should be noted.

Sensory olfactory function can be assessed by any of several methods. The Odor Stix test uses a commercially available odor-producing magic marker–like pen held approximately 8 to 15 cm (3 to 6 in.) from the patient's nose. The 30-cm alcohol test uses a freshly opened isopropyl alcohol packet held approximately 30 cm (12 in.) from the patient's nose. There is a commercially available scratch-and-sniff card containing three odors available for testing olfaction grossly. A superior test is the University of Pennsylvania Smell Identification Test (UPSIT). This consists of a 40-item, forced choice, microencapsulated odor, scratch-and-sniff paradigm. For example, one of the items reads, "This odor smells most like (a) chocolate, (b) banana, (c) onion, or (d) fruit punch." The test is highly reliable, is sensitive to age and sex differences, and provides an accurate quantitative determination of the olfactory deficit. The average score for total anosmics is slightly higher than that expected on the basis of chance because of the inclusion of some odorants that act by trigeminal stimulation.

Following assessment of sensory olfactory function, the detection threshold for the odorant phenyl ethyl alcohol should be established using a graduated stimulus. Sensitivity for each side of the nose is determined with a detection threshold for phenyl ethyl methyl ethyl carbinol. Nasal resistance can also be measured with anterior rhinomanometry for each side of the nose.

Computed tomography (CT) or magnetic resonance imaging (MRI) of the head is required to rule out paranasal sinusitis; neoplasms of the anterior cranial fossa, nasal cavity, or paranasal sinuses; or unsuspected fractures of the anterior cranial fossa. Bone abnormalities are best seen with CT. MRI is useful in evaluating olfactory bulbs, ventricles, and other soft tissue of the brain. Coronal CT is optimal for assessing cribriform plate, anterior cranial fossa, and sinus anatomy.

Techniques have been developed to biopsy the olfactory neuroepithelium, but in view of the widespread degeneration of the olfactory neuroepithelium and intercalation of respiratory epithelium in the olfactory area of adults with no apparent olfactory dysfunction, biopsy material must be interpreted cautiously.

℞ TREATMENT

Therapy for patients with transport olfactory losses due to allergic rhinitis, bacterial rhinitis and sinusitis, polyps, neoplasms, and structural abnormalities of the nasal cavities can be undertaken with a high likelihood for improvement. Allergy management; antibiotic therapy; topical and systemic glucocorticoid therapy; and surgery for nasal polyps, deviation of the nasal septum, and chronic hyperplastic sinusitis are frequently effective in restoring the sense of smell.

There is no proven treatment for sensorineural olfactory losses. Fortunately, spontaneous recovery often occurs. Zinc and vitamin therapy (especially with vitamin A) are advocated by some. Profound zinc deficiency can produce loss and distortion of the sense of smell but is not a clinically important problem except in very limited geographic areas (Chap. 61). The epithelial degeneration associated with vitamin A deficiency can cause anosmia, but in western societies the prevalence of vitamin A deficiency is low. Exposure to cigarette smoke and other airborne toxic chemicals can cause metaplasia of the olfactory epithelium. Spontaneous recovery can occur if the insult is discontinued. Counseling of patients is therefore helpful in these cases.

More than half of people over age 60 suffer from olfactory dysfunction. No effective treatment exists for presbyosmia, but patients are often reassured to learn that this problem is common in their age group. In addition, early recognition and counseling can help patients to compensate for the loss of smell. The incidence of natural gas–related accidents is disproportionately high in the elderly, perhaps due in part to the gradual loss of smell. Mercaptan, the pungent odor in natural gas, is an olfactory stimulant and does not activate taste receptors. Many elderly with olfactory dysfunction experience a decrease in flavor sensation and find it necessary to hyperflavor food, usually by increasing the amount of salt in their diet.

TASTE

Compared with disorders of smell, gustatory disorders are uncommon. Loss of olfactory sensitivity is often accompanied by complaints of loss of the sense of taste, usually with normal detection thresholds for taste.

DEFINITIONS Disturbances of the sense of taste may be categorized as *total ageusia*, total absence of gustatory function or inability to detect the qualities of sweet, salt, bitter, or sour; *partial ageusia*, ability to detect some of but not all the qualitative gustatory sensations; *specific ageusia*, inability to detect the taste quality of certain substances; *total hypogeusia*, decreased sensitivity to all tastants; *partial hypogeusia*,

decreased sensitivity to some tastants; and *dysgeusia* or *phantogeusia*, distortion in the perception of a tastant, i.e., the perception of the wrong quality when a tastant is presented or the perception of a taste when there has been no tastant ingested. Confusions between sour and bitter, and less commonly between salty and bitter, may represent semantic misunderstandings or have true pathophysiologic bases. It may be possible to differentiate between the loss of flavor recognition in patients with olfactory losses who complain of a loss of taste as well as smell by asking if they are able to taste sweetness in sodas, saltiness in potato chips, etc.

PHYSIOLOGY OF TASTE The taste receptor cells are located in the taste buds, spherical groups of cells arranged in a pattern resembling the segments of a citrus fruit. At the surface, the taste bud has a pore into which microvilli of the receptor cells project. Unlike the olfactory system, the receptor cell is not the primary neuron. Instead, gustatory afferent nerve fibers contact individual taste receptor cells. There are at least five receptor populations. Taste buds are located in the papillae along the lateral margin and dorsum of the tongue; at the junction of the dorsum and the base of the tongue; and in the palate, epiglottis, larynx, and esophagus.

The sense of taste is mediated through the facial, glossopharyngeal, and vagal nerves. The chorda tympani branch of the facial nerve subserves taste from the anterior two-thirds of the tongue. The posterior third of the tongue is supplied by the lingual branch of the glossopharyngeal nerve. Afferents from the palate travel with the greater superficial petrosal nerve to the geniculate ganglion and then via the facial nerve to the brainstem. The internal branch of the superior laryngeal nerve of the vagus nerve contains the taste afferents from the larynx, including the epiglottis and esophagus.

The central connections of the nerves terminate in the brainstem in the nucleus of the tractus solitarius. The central pathway from the nucleus of the tractus solitarius projects to the ipsilateral parabrachial nuclei of the pons. Two divergent pathways project from the parabrachial nuclei. One ascends to the gustatory relay in the dorsal thalamus, synapses, and continues to the cortex of the insula. There is also evidence for a direct pathway from the parabrachial nuclei to the cortex. (Olfaction and gustation appear to be unique among sensory systems in that at least some fibers bypass the thalamus.) The other pathway from the parabrachial nuclei goes to the ventral forebrain, including the lateral hypothalamus, substantia innominata, central nucleus of the amygdala, and the stria terminalis.

Tastants gain access to the receptor cells through the taste pore. Four classes of taste are recognized: sweet, salt, sour, and bitter. Individual gustatory afferent fibers almost always respond to a number of different chemicals. Response patterns of gustatory afferent axons can be grouped into classes based on the stimulus chemical that produces the largest response. For example, for sucrose-best response neurons, the second-best stimulus is almost always sodium chloride. The fact that individual gustatory afferent fibers respond to a large number of different chemicals led to the *across-fiber-pattern* theory of gustatory coding, while the best-stimulus analysis led to the concept of *labeled* afferents. It appears that labeled fibers are important for establishing gross quality, but the across-fiber pattern within a best-stimulus category, and perhaps among categories, is needed for discriminating chemicals within qualities. For example, sweetness may be carried by sucrose-best neurons, but the differentiation of sucrose and fructose may require a comparison of the relative activity among sucrose-best, salt-best, and quinine-best neurons. As with olfaction and other sensory systems, intensity appears to be encoded by the quantity of neural activity.

DISORDERS OF THE SENSE OF TASTE Disorders of the sense of taste are caused by conditions that interfere with the access of the tastant to the receptor cells in the taste bud (transport loss), injure receptor cells (sensory loss), or damage gustatory afferent nerves and central gustatory pathways (neural loss) (Table 26-2). *Transport gustatory losses* result from xerostomia due to many causes, including Sjögren's syndrome, radiation therapy, heavy-metal intoxication, and bacterial col-

TABLE 26-2 Causes of Gustatory Dysfunction

Transport Gustatory Losses	Neural Gustatory Losses
Drugs	Diabetes mellitus
Heavy-metal intoxication	Hypothyroidism
Radiation therapy	Oral neoplasms
Sjögren's syndrome	Oral surgery
Xerostomia	Radiation therapy
Sensory Gustatory Losses	Renal disease
Aging	Stroke and other CNS disorders
Candidiasis	Trauma
Drugs (antithyroid and	Upper respiratory tract infections
antineoplastic)	
Endocrine disorders	
Oral neoplasms	
Pemphigus	
Radiation therapy	
Viral infections (especially with	
herpes viruses)	

onization of the taste pore. *Sensory gustatory losses* are caused by inflammatory and degenerative diseases in the oral cavity; a vast number of drugs, particularly those that interfere with cell turnover such as antithyroid and antineoplastic agents; radiation therapy to the oral cavity and pharynx; viral infections; endocrine disorders; neoplasms; and aging. *Neural gustatory losses* occur with neoplasms, trauma, and surgical procedures in which the gustatory afferents are injured. Taste buds degenerate when their gustatory afferents are transected but remain when their somatosensory afferents are severed. Patients with renal disease have increased thresholds for sweet and sour tastes, which resolves with dialysis.

A side effect of medication is the single most common cause of taste dysfunction in clinical practice. Xerostomia, regardless of the etiology, can be associated with taste dysfunction. It is associated with poor oral clearance and poor dental hygeine, and can adversely affect the oral mucosa, all leading to dysgeusia. However, severe salivary gland failure does not necessarily lead to taste complaints. Xerostomia, the use of antibiotics or glucocorticoids, or immunodeficiency can lead to overgrowth of *Candida*; overgrowth alone, without thrush or overt signs of infection, can be associated with bad taste or hypogeusia. When taste dysfunction occurs in a patient at risk for fungal overgrowth, a trial of nystatin or other antifungal medication is warranted.

Upper respiratory infections and head trauma can lead to both smell and taste dysfunction; taste is more likely to improve than smell. The mechanism of taste disturbance in these situations is not well understood. Trauma to the chorda tympani branch of the facial nerve during middle ear surgery or third molar extractions is relatively common and can cause dysgeusia. Bilateral chorda tympani injuries are usually associated with hypogeusia, whereas unilateral lesions produce only limited symptoms.

Finally, aging itself may be associated with reduced taste sensitivity. The taste dysfunction may be limited to a single compound and may be mild.

APPROACH TO THE PATIENT

Patients who complain of loss of taste should be evaluated for both gustatory and olfactory function. Clinical assessment of taste is not as well developed or standardized as that of smell. The first step is to perform suprathreshold whole-mouth taste testing for quality, intensity, and pleasantness perception of four taste qualities: sweet, salty, sour, and bitter. Most commonly used reagents for taste testing are sucrose, citric acid or hydrochloric acid, caffeine or quinine (sulfate or hydrochloride), and sodium chloride. The taste stimuli should be freshly prepared. For quantification, detection thresholds are obtained by applying graduated dilutions to the tongue quadrants or by whole-mouth sips. Electric taste testing (*electrogustometry*) is used clinically to identify taste deficits in specific quadrants of the tongue. Regional gustatory testing may also be performed to assess for the possibility of loss localized to one or

more receptor fields as a result of a peripheral or central lesion. The history of the disease and localization studies provide important clues to the reason for taste disturbance. For example, absence of taste on the anterior two-thirds of the tongue associated with a facial paralysis indicates that the lesion is proximal to the juncture of the chorda tympani branch with the facial nerve in the mastoid.

℞ TREATMENT

Treatment of gustatory disorders is limited. No effective therapies exist for the sensorineural disorders of taste. Altered taste due to surgical stretch injury of chorda tympani nerve usually improves within 3 to 4 months, while dysfunction is usually permanent with transection of the nerve. Taste dysfunction following trauma may resolve spontaneously without intervention and is more likely to do so than posttraumatic smell dysfunction. Idiopathic alterations of taste sensitivity usually remain stable or worsen; zinc and vitamin therapy are of unproven value. Directed therapy to address factors that affect taste perception can be of value. Xerostomia can be treated with artificial saliva, providing some benefits to patients with a disturbed salivary milieu. Oral pilocarpine may be beneficial for a variety of forms of xerostomia. Appropriate treatment of bacterial and fungal infections of the oral cavity can be of great help in improving taste function. Taste disturbance related to drugs can often be resolved by changing the prescribed medication.

HEARING

Hearing loss is one of the most common sensory disorders in humans and can present at any age. Nearly 10% of the adult population has some hearing loss, and one-third of individuals over the age of 65 have a hearing loss of sufficient magnitude to require a hearing aid.

PHYSIOLOGY OF HEARING (Fig. 26-1) The function of the external and middle ear is to amplify sound to facilitate mechanotransduction by hair cells in the inner ear. Sound waves enter the external auditory canal and set the tympanic membrane in motion, which in turn moves the malleus, incus, and stapes of the middle ear. Movement of the footplate of the stapes causes pressure changes in the fluid-filled inner ear eliciting a traveling wave in the basilar membrane of the cochlea. The tympanic membrane and the ossicular chain in the middle ear serve as an impedence-matching mechanism, improving the efficiency of energy transfer from air to the fluid-filled inner ear.

Stereocilia of the hair cells of the organ of Corti, which rests on the basilar membrane, are in contact with the tectorial membrane and are deformed by the traveling wave. A point of maximal displacement of the basilar membrane is determined by the frequency of the stimulating tone. High-frequency tones cause maximal displacement of the basilar membrane near the base of the cochlea. As the frequency of the stimulating tone decreases, the point of maximal displacement moves toward the apex of the cochlea.

The inner and outer hair cells of the organ of Corti have different innervation patterns, but both are mechanoreceptors. The afferent innervation relates principally to the inner hair cells, and the efferent innervation relates principally to outer hair cells. The motility of the outer hair cells alters the micromechanics of the inner hair cells creating a cochlear amplifier, which explains the exquisite sensitivity and frequency selectivity of the cochlea.

The current concept of cochlear transduction is that displacement of the tips of the stereocilia allows potassium to flow into the cell, resulting in its depolarization. The potassium influx opens calcium channels near the base of the cell, stimulating transmitter release. The neurotransmitter at the hair cell and cochlear nerve dendrite interface is thought to be glutamate. Each of the cochlear nerve neurons can be activated at a frequency and intensity specific for that cell. This specificity is maintained at each point of the central auditory pathway: dorsal and ventral cochlear nuclei, trapezoid body, superior olivary

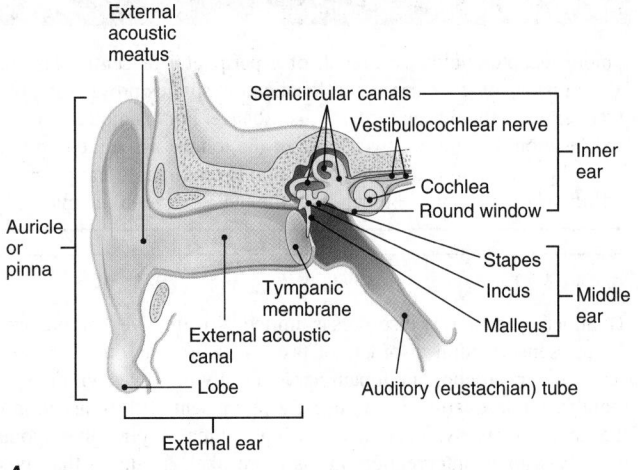

FIGURE 26-1 *A.* Drawing of modified coronal section through external ear and temporal bone, with structures of the middle and inner ear demonstrated.

B. High-resolution view of inner ear.

complex, lateral lemniscus, inferior colliculus, medial geniculate body, and auditory cortex. At low frequencies, individual auditory nerve fibers can respond more or less synchronously with the stimulating tone. At higher frequencies, phase-locking occurs so that neurons alternate in response to particular phases of the cycle of the sound wave. Intensity is encoded by the amount of neural activity in individual neurons, the number of neurons that are active, and the specific neurons that are activated.

GENETIC CAUSES OF HEARING LOSS More than half of childhood hearing impairment is thought to be hereditary; hereditary hearing impairment (HHI) can also manifest later in life. HHI may be classified as either nonsyndromic, when hearing loss is the only clinical abnormality, or syndromic, when hearing loss is associated with anomalies in other organ systems. Nearly two-thirds of HHIs are nonsyndromic, and the remaining one-third are syndromic. Between 70 and 80% of nonsyndromic HHI is inherited in an autosomal recessive manner; another 15 to 20% is autosomal dominant. Less than 5% is X-linked or maternally inherited via the mitochondria.

Over 60 loci harboring genes for nonsyndromic HHI have been mapped, with equal numbers of dominant and recessive modes of inheritance; numerous genes have now been cloned (Table 26-3). The hearing genes fall into the categories of structural proteins (MYO7A, MYO15, TECTA, DIAPH1), transcription factors (POU3F4, POU4F3), ion channels (KCNQ4, PDS), and gap junction proteins (Cx26, Cx30, Cx31). Several of these genes, including connexin 26 (Cx26), TECTA, and MYO7A, cause both autosomal dominant and recessive forms of nonsyndromic HHI. In general, the hearing loss associated with dominant genes has its onset in adolescence or adulthood and varies in severity, whereas the hearing loss associated with recessive inheritance is congenital and profound. Connexin 26 is particularly important because it is associated with nearly 20% of cases of childhood deafness; in heterozygotes the onset of hearing loss may be in adolescence or adulthood. Two frame-shift mutations, 30delG and 167delT, account for >50% of the cases, making population screening feasible. The 167delT mutation is highly prevalent in Ashkenazi Jews; it is predicted that 1 in 1765 individuals in this population will be homozygous and affected. The hearing loss can also vary among the members of the same family, suggesting that other genes or factors likely influence the auditory phenotype.

The contribution of genetics to presbycusis (see below) is also becoming better understood. In addition to connexin 26, several other nonsyndromic genes are associated with hear-

TABLE 26-3 *Nonsyndromic Genes and Loci*

Locus	Gene	Function	Inheritance
DFNB1	GBJ2 (Cx26)	Forms gap junctions, or plasma membrane channels, with connexins	AR
DFNB2	MYO7A	Moves different macromolecular structures relative to actin filaments	AR
DFNB3	MYO15	Organizes actin in hair cells	AR
DFNB4	PDS	Encodes highly hydrophobic proteins containing the sulphate transporter signature	AR
DFNB9	OTOF	Involved in trafficking of membrane vesicles	AR
DFNB21	TECTA	Includes an amino-terminal hydrophobic signal sequence for translocation across the membrane and a carboxy-terminal hydrophobic region characteristic of precursors of glycosylphosphatidylinositol-linked membrane-bound proteins	AR
DFNA1	DIAPH1	Involved in cytokinesis and establishment of cell polarity	AD
DFNA2	GJB3 (Cx31)	Forms gap junction protein	AD
	KCNQ4	Forms potassium channel	
DFNA3	GJB2 (Cx26)	Forms gap junctions, or plasma membrane channels, with connexins	AD
	GBJ6 (Cx30)		
DFNA5	DFNA5	Unknown; related to a gene that is upregulated in estrogen receptor–negative breast carcinomas	AD
DFNA8/12	TECTA	Includes an amino-terminal hydrophobic signal sequence for translocation across the membrane and a carboxy-terminal hydrophobic region characteristic of precursors of glycosylphosphatidylinositol-linked membrane-bound proteins	AD
DFNA9	COCH	Involved in hemostasis, complement system, immune system, and extracellular matrix assembly	AD
DFNA11	MYO7A	Moves different macromolecular structures relative to actin filaments	AD
DFNA15	POU4F3	Serves as a critical developmental regulator for the determination of cellular phenotypes	AD
DFN3	POU3F4	Serves as a critical developmental regulator for the determination of cellular phenotypes	X-linked

Note: AD, autosomal dominant; AR, autosomal recessive.

ing loss that progresses with age. Sensitivity to aminoglycoside oto-toxicity can be maternally transmitted through a mitochondrial mutation. Susceptibility to noise-induced hearing loss may also be genetically determined.

There are over 200 syndromic forms of hearing loss. These include Usher syndrome (retinitis pigmentosa and hearing loss), Waardenburg syndrome (pigmentary abnormality and hearing loss), Pendred syndrome (thyroid organification defect and hearing loss), Alport syndrome (renal disease and hearing loss), Jervell and Lange-Nielsen syndrome (prolonged QT interval and hearing loss), neurofibromatosis type 2 (bilateral acoustic schwannoma), and mitochondrial disorders [mitochondrial encephalopathy, lactic acidosis, and stroke-like episodes (MELAS); myoclonic epilepsy and ragged red fibers (MERRF); progressive external ophthalmoplegia (PEO)].

DISORDERS OF THE SENSE OF HEARING   Hearing loss can result from disorders of the auricle, external auditory canal, middle ear, inner ear, or central auditory pathways (Fig. 26-2). *In general, lesions in the auricle, external auditory canal, or middle ear cause conductive hearing losses, whereas lesions in the inner ear or eighth nerve cause sensorineural hearing losses.*

Conductive Hearing Loss   This results from obstruction of the external auditory canal by cerumen, debris, and foreign bodies; swelling of the lining of the canal; atresia or neoplasms of the canal; perforations of the tympanic membrane; disruption of the ossicular chain, as occurs with necrosis of the long process of the incus in trauma or infection; otosclerosis; or fluid, scarring, or neoplasms in the middle ear.

Cholesteatoma, stratified squamous epithelium in the middle ear or mastoid, occurs frequently in adults. This is a benign, slowly growing lesion that destroys bone and normal ear tissue. Theories of pathogen-

esis include traumatic implantation and invasion, immigration and invasion through a perforation, and metaplasia following chronic infection and irritation. On examination, there is often a perforation of the tympanic membrane filled with cheesy white squamous debris. A chronically draining ear that fails to respond to appropriate antibiotic therapy should raise suspicion of a cholesteatoma. Conductive hearing loss secondary to ossicular erosion is common. Surgery is required to remove this destructive process.

Conductive hearing loss with a normal ear canal and intact tympanic membrane suggests ossicular pathology. Fixation of the stapes from *otosclerosis* is a common cause of low-frequency conductive hearing loss. It occurs equally in men and women and has a simple autosomal dominant inheritance with incomplete penetrance. Hearing impairment usually presents between the late teens to the forties. In women, the hearing loss is often first noticeable during pregnancy, as the otosclerotic process is accelerated during pregnancy. A hearing aid or a simple outpatient surgical procedure (stapedectomy) can provide adequate auditory rehabilitation. Extension of otosclerosis beyond the stapes footplate to involve the cochlea (cochlear otosclerosis) can lead to mixed or sensorineural hearing loss. Fluoride therapy to prevent hearing loss associated with cochlear otosclerosis is of uncertain value.

Eustachian tube dysfunction is extremely common in adults and may predispose to acute otitis media (AOM) or serous otitis media (SOM). Trauma, AOM, or chronic otitis media are the usual factors responsible for tympanic membrane perforation. While small perforations often heal spontaneously, larger defects usually require surgical intervention. Tympanoplasty is highly effective (>90%) in the repair of tympanic membrane perforations. Otoscopy is usually sufficient to

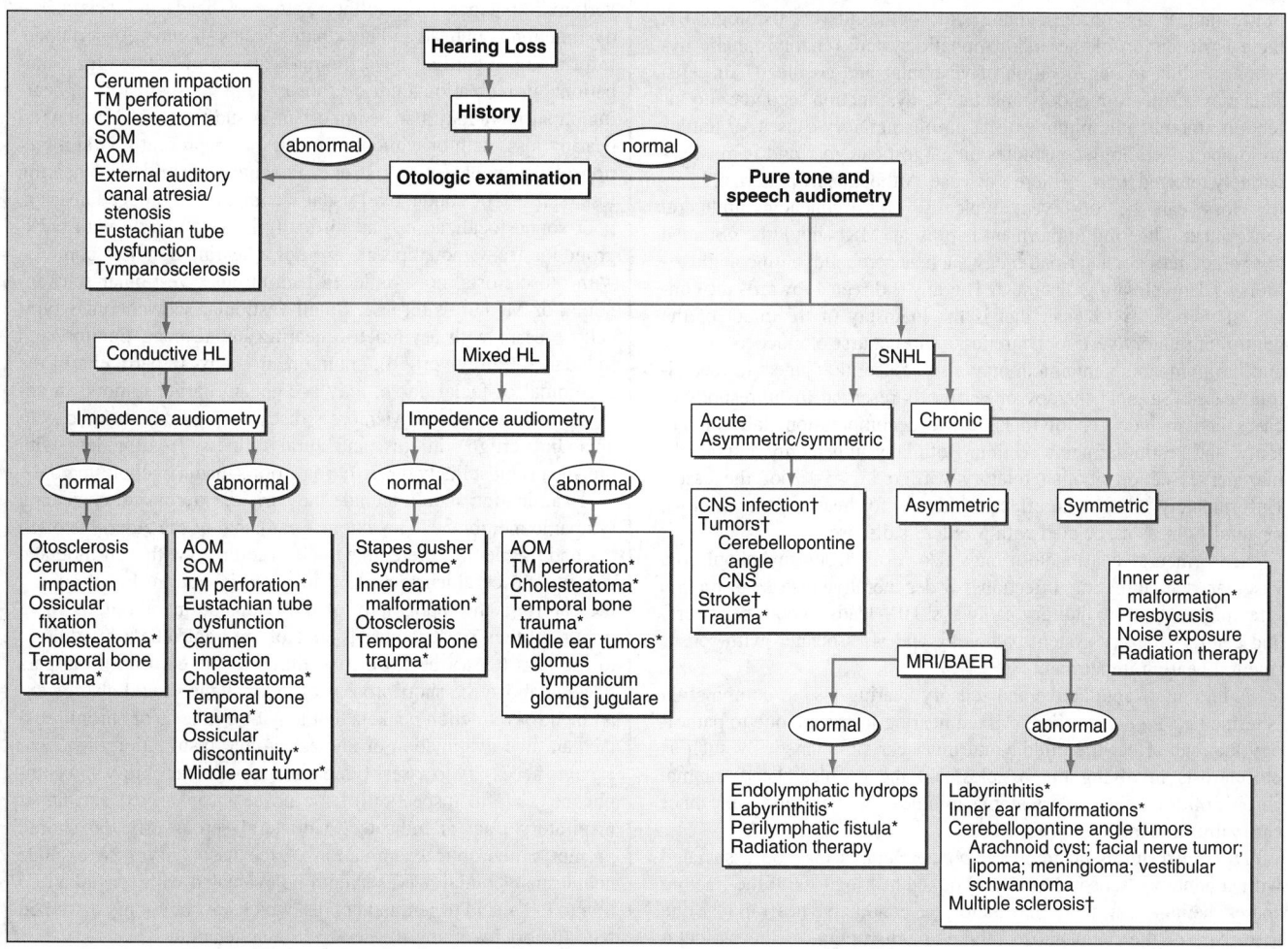

FIGURE 26-2   An algorithm for the approach to hearing loss. HL, hearing loss; SNHL, sensorineural hearing loss; TM, tympanic membrane; SOM, serous otitis media; AOM, acute otitis media; *, CT scan of temporal bone; †, MRI scan.

diagnose AOM, SOM, chronic otitis media, cerumen impaction, tympanic membrane perforation, and eustachian tube dysfunction.

Sensorineural Hearing Loss   Damage to the hair cells of the organ of Corti may be caused by intense noise, viral infections, ototoxic drugs (e.g., salicylates, quinine and its synthetic analogues, aminoglycoside antibiotics, loop diuretics such as furosemide and ethacrynic acid, and cancer chemotherapeutic agents such as cisplatin), fractures of the temporal bone, meningitis, cochlear otosclerosis (see above), Ménière's disease, and aging. Congenital malformations of the inner ear may be the cause of hearing loss in some adults. Genetic predisposition alone or in concert with environmental influences may also be responsible.

Presbycusis (age-associated hearing loss) is the most common cause of sensorineural hearing loss in adults. In the early stages, it is characterized by symmetric, gentle to sharply sloping high-frequency hearing loss. With progression, the hearing loss involves all frequencies. More importantly, the hearing impairment is associated with significant loss in clarity. There is a loss of discrimination for phonemes, recruitment (abnormal growth of loudness), and particular difficulty in understanding speech in noisy environments. Hearing aids may provide limited rehabilitation once the word recognition score deteriorates below 50%. Improvements in cochlear implants have made them the treatment of choice when hearing aids prove inadequate.

Ménière's disease is characterized by episodic vertigo, fluctuating sensorineural hearing loss, tinnitus, and aural fullness. Tinnitus and/or deafness may be absent during the initial attacks of vertigo, but they invariably appear as the disease progresses and are increased in severity during an acute attack. The annual incidence of Ménière's disease is 0.5 to 7.5 per 1000; onset is most frequently in the fifth decade of life but may also occur in young adults or the elderly. Histologically, there is distention of the endolymphatic system (endolymphatic hydrops) leading to degeneration of vestibular and cochlear hair cells. This may result from endolymphatic sac dysfunction secondary to infection, trauma, autoimmune disease, inflammatory causes, or tumor; an idiopathic etiology constitutes the largest category and is most accurately referred to as Ménière's disease. Although any pattern of hearing loss can be observed, typically, low-frequency, unilateral sensorineural hearing impairment is present. MRI should be obtained to exclude retrocochlear pathology such as cerebellopontine angle tumors or demyelinating disorders. Therapy is directed towards the control of vertigo. A low-salt diet is the mainstay of treatment for the control of rotatory vertigo. Diuretics, a short course of glucocorticoids, and intratympanic gentamicin may also be useful adjuncts in recalcitrant cases. Surgical therapy of vertigo is reserved for unresponsive cases and includes endolymphatic sac decompression, labyrinthectomy, and vestibular nerve section. Both labyrinthectomy and vestibular nerve section abolish rotatory vertigo in >90% of the cases. Unfortunately, there is no effective therapy for hearing loss, tinnitus, or aural fullness associated with Ménière's disease.

Sensorineural hearing loss may also result from any neoplastic, vascular, demyelinating, infectious, or degenerative disease or trauma affecting the central auditory pathways. HIV leads to both peripheral and central auditory system pathology and is associated with sensorineural hearing impairment.

A finding of conductive and sensory hearing loss in combination is termed *mixed hearing loss*. Mixed hearing losses are due to pathology that can affect the middle and inner ear simultaneously such as otosclerosis involving the ossicles and the cochlea, head trauma, chronic otitis media, cholesteatoma, middle ear tumors, and some inner ear malformations.

Trauma resulting in temporal bone fractures may be associated with conductive, sensorineural, and mixed hearing loss. If the fracture spares the inner ear, there may simply be conductive hearing loss due to rupture of the tympanic membrane or disruption of the ossicular chain. These abnormalities are amenable to surgical correction. Profound hearing loss and severe vertigo are associated with temporal bone fractures involving the inner ear. A perilymphatic fistula associated with leakage of inner-ear fluid into the middle ear can occur and may require surgical repair. An associated facial nerve injury is not uncommon. CT is best suited to assess fracture of the traumatized temporal bone, evaluate the ear canal, and determine the integrity of the ossicular chain and the involvement of the inner ear. CSF leaks that accompany temporal bone fractures are usually self-limited; the use of prophylactic antibiotics is controversial.

Tinnitus is defined as the perception of a sound when there is no sound in the environment. It may have a buzzing, roaring, or ringing quality and may be pulsatile (synchronous with the heartbeat). Tinnitus is often associated with either a conductive or sensorineural hearing loss. The pathophysiology of tinnitus is not well understood. The cause of the tinnitus can usually be determined by finding the cause of the associated hearing loss. Tinnitus may be the first symptom of a serious condition such as a vestibular schwannoma. Pulsatile tinnitus requires evaluation of the vascular system of the head to exclude vascular tumors such as glomus jugulare tumors, aneurysms, and stenotic arterial lesions; it may also occur with SOM.

APPROACH TO THE PATIENT

The goal in the evaluation of a patient with auditory complaints is to determine (1) the nature of the hearing impairment (conductive vs. sensorineural), (2) the severity of the impairment (mild, moderate, severe, profound), (3) the anatomy of the impairment (external ear, middle ear, inner ear, or central auditory pathway), and (4) the etiology. The history should elicit characteristics of the hearing loss, including the duration of deafness, unilateral vs. bilateral involvement, nature of onset (sudden vs. insidious), and rate of progression (rapid vs. slow). The presence or absence of tinnitus, vertigo, imbalance, aural fullness, otorrhea, headache, facial nerve dysfunction, and head and neck paresthesias should be ascertained. Information regarding head trauma, exposure to ototoxins, occupational or recreational noise exposure, and family history of hearing impairment may also be important. A sudden onset of unilateral hearing loss, with or without tinnitus, may represent a viral infection of the inner ear or a stroke. Patients with unilateral hearing loss (sensory or conductive) usually complain of reduced hearing, poor sound localization, and difficulty hearing clearly with background noise. Gradual progression of a hearing deficit is common with otosclerosis, noise-induced hearing loss, vestibular schwannoma, or Ménière's disease. Small vestibular schwannomas typically present with asymmetric hearing impairment, tinnitus, and imbalance (rarely vertigo); cranial neuropathy, in particular of the trigeminal or facial nerve, may accompany larger tumors. In addition to hearing loss, Ménière's disease may be associated with episodic vertigo, tinnitus, and aural fullness. Hearing loss with otorrhea is most likely due to chronic otitis media or cholesteatoma.

Examination should include the auricle, external ear canal, and tympanic membrane. The external ear canal of the elderly is often dry and fragile; it is preferable to clean cerumen with wall-mounted suction and cerumen loops and to avoid irrigation. In examining the eardrum, the topography of the tympanic membrane is more important than presence or absence of the light reflex. In addition to the pars tensa (the lower two-thirds of the eardrum), the pars flaccida above the short process of the malleus should also be examined for retraction pockets that may be evidence of chronic eustachian tube dysfunction or cholesteatoma. Insufflation of the ear canal is necessary to assess tympanic membrane mobility and compliance. Careful inspection of the nose, nasopharynx, and upper respiratory tract is indicated. Unilateral serous effusion should prompt a fiberoptic examination of the nasopharynx to exclude neoplasms. Cranial nerves should be evaluated with special attention to facial and trigeminal nerves, which are commonly disturbed with tumors involving the cerebellopontine angle.

The Rinne and Weber tuning fork tests, with a 256- or 512-Hz tuning fork, are used to screen for hearing loss, differentiate conductive from sensorineural hearing losses, and to confirm the findings of audiologic evaluation. Rinne's test compares the ability to hear by air conduction with the ability to hear by bone conduction. The tines of a vibrating tuning fork are held near the opening of the external auditory canal, and then the stem is placed on the mastoid process; for direct contact, it may be placed on teeth or dentures. The patient is asked to indicate whether the tone is louder by air conduction or bone conduction. Normally, and in the presence of sensorineural hearing loss, a tone is heard louder by air conduction than by bone conduction; however, with conductive hearing loss of ≥30 dB (see "Audiologic Assessment," below), the bone-conduction stimulus is perceived as louder than the air-conduction stimulus. For the Weber test, the stem of a vibrating tuning fork is placed on the head in the midline and the patient asked whether the tone is heard in both ears or better in one ear than in the other. With a unilateral conductive hearing loss, the tone is perceived in the affected ear. With a unilateral sensorineural hearing loss, the tone is perceived in the unaffected ear. A 5-dB difference in hearing between the two ears is required for lateralization.

LABORATORY ASSESSMENT OF HEARING ■ **Audiologic Assessment** The minimum audiologic assessment for hearing loss should include the measurement of pure tone air-conduction and bone-conduction thresholds, speech reception threshold, discrimination score, tympanometry, acoustic reflexes, and acoustic-reflex decay. This test battery provides a comprehensive screening evaluation of the whole auditory system and allows one to determine whether further differentiation of a sensory (cochlear) from a neural (retrocochlear) hearing loss is indicated.

Pure tone audiometry assesses hearing acuity for pure tones. The test is administered by an audiologist and is performed in a sound-attenuated chamber. The pure tone stimulus is delivered with an audiometer, an electronic device that allows the presentation of specific frequencies (generally between 250 and 8000 Hz) at specific intensities. Air and bone conduction thresholds are established for each ear. Air conduction thresholds are established by presenting the stimulus in air with the use of headphones. Bone conduction thresholds are accomplished by placing the stem of a vibrating tuning fork or an oscillator of an audiometer in contact with the head. In the presence of a hearing loss, broad-spectrum noise is presented to the nontest ear for *masking* purposes so that responses are based on perception from the ear under test.

The responses are measured in decibels. An *audiogram* is a plot of intensity in decibels of hearing threshold versus frequency. A decibel (dB) is equal to 20 times the logarithm of the ratio of the sound pressure required to achieve threshold in the patient to the sound pressure required to achieve threshold in a normal hearing person. Therefore, a change of 6 dB represents doubling of sound pressure, and a change of 20 dB represents a tenfold change in sound pressure. Loudness, which depends on the frequency, intensity, and duration of a sound, doubles with approximately each 10-dB increase in sound pressure level. Pitch, on the other hand, does not directly correlate with frequency. The perception of pitch changes slowly in the low and high frequencies. In the middle tones, which are important for human speech, pitch varies more rapidly with changes in frequency.

Pure tone audiometry establishes the presence and severity of hearing impairment, unilateral vs. bilateral involvement, and the type of hearing loss. Conductive hearing losses with a large mass component, as is often seen in middle-ear effusions, produce elevation of thresholds that predominate in the higher frequencies. Conductive hearing losses with a large stiffness component, as in fixation of the footplate of the stapes in early otosclerosis, produce threshold elevations in the lower frequencies. Often, the conductive hearing loss involves all frequencies, suggesting involvement of both stiffness and mass. In general, sensorineural hearing losses such as presbycusis affect higher frequencies more than lower frequencies. An exception is Ménière's disease, which is characteristically associated with low-frequency sen-

sorineural hearing loss. Noise-induced hearing loss has an unusual pattern of hearing impairment in which the loss at 4000 Hz is greater than at higher frequencies. Vestibular schwannomas characteristically affect the higher frequencies, but any pattern of hearing loss can be observed.

Speech recognition requires greater synchronous neural firing than is necessary for appreciation of pure tones. *Speech audiometry* tests the clarity with which one hears. The *speech reception threshold* (SRT) is defined as the intensity at which speech is recognized as a meaningful symbol and is obtained by presenting two-syllable words with an equal accent on each syllable. The intensity at which the patient can repeat 50% of the words correctly is the SRT. Once the SRT is determined, discrimination or word recognition ability is tested by presenting one-syllable words at 25 to 40 dB above the speech reception threshold. The words are phonetically balanced in that the phonemes (speech sounds) occur in the list of words at the same frequency that they occur in ordinary conversational English. An individual with normal hearing or conductive hearing loss can repeat 88 to 100% of the phonetically balanced words correctly. Patients with a sensorineural hearing loss have variable loss of discrimination. As a general rule, neural lesions are associated with more deterioration in discrimination ability than are lesions in the inner ear. For example, in a patient with mild asymmetric sensorineural hearing loss, a clue to the diagnosis of vestibular schwannoma is the presence of greater than expected deterioration in discrimination ability. Deterioration in discrimination ability at higher intensities above the SRT also suggests a lesion in the eighth nerve or central auditory pathways.

Tympanometry measures the impedance of the middle ear to sound and is useful in diagnosis of middle-ear effusions. A *tympanogram* is the graphic representation of change in impedance or compliance as the pressure in the ear canal is changed. Normally, the middle ear is most compliant at atmospheric pressure, and the compliance decreases as the pressure is increased or decreased; this pattern is seen with normal hearing or in the presence of sensorineural hearing loss. Compliance that does not change with change in pressure suggests middle-ear effusion. With a negative pressure in the middle ear, as with eustachian tube obstruction, the point of maximal compliance occurs with negative pressure in the ear canal. A tympanogram in which no point of maximal compliance can be obtained is most commonly seen with discontinuity of the ossicular chain. A reduction in the maximal compliance peak can be seen in otosclerosis.

During tympanometry, an intense tone elicits contraction of the stapedius muscle. The change in compliance of the middle ear with contraction of the stapedius muscle can be detected. The presence or absence of this *acoustic reflex* is important in the anatomic localization of facial nerve paralysis as well as hearing loss. Normal or elevated acoustic reflex thresholds in an individual with sensorineural hearing impairment suggests a cochlear hearing loss. Assessment of *acoustic reflex decay* helps differentiate sensory from neural hearing losses. In neural hearing loss, the reflex adapts or decays with time.

Otoacoustic emissions (OAE) can be measured with microphones inserted into the external auditory canal. The emissions may be spontaneous or evoked with sound stimulation. The presence of OAEs indicates that the outer hair cells of the organ of Corti are intact and can be used to assess auditory thresholds and to distinguish sensory from neural hearing losses.

Evoked Responses *Electrocochleography* measures the earliest evoked potentials generated in the cochlea and the auditory nerve. Receptor potentials recorded include the cochlear microphonic, generated by the outer hair cells of the organ of Corti, and the summating potential, generated by the inner hair cells in response to sound. The whole nerve action potential representing the composite firing of the first-order neurons can also be recorded during electrocochleography. Clinically, the test is useful in the diagnosis of Ménière's disease, where an elevation of the ratio of summating potential to action potential is seen.

Brainstem auditory evoked responses (BAERs) are useful in differentiating the site of sensorineural hearing loss. In response to sound, five distinct electrical potentials arising from different stations along the peripheral and central auditory pathway can be identified using computer averaging from scalp surface electrodes. BAERs are valuable in situations in which patients cannot or will not give reliable voluntary thresholds. They are also used to assess the integrity of the auditory nerve and brainstem in various clinical situations, including intraoperative monitoring and in determination of brain death.

Imaging Studies The choice of radiologic tests is largely determined by whether the goal is to evaluate the bony anatomy of the external, middle, and inner ear or to image the auditory nerve and brain. Axial and coronal CT of the temporal bone with fine 1-mm cuts is ideal for determining the caliber of the external auditory canal, integrity of the ossicular chain, and presence of middle-ear or mastoid disease; it can also detect inner-ear malformations. CT is also ideal for the detection of bone erosion often seen in the presence of chronic otitis media and cholesteatoma. MRI is superior to CT for imaging of retrocochlear pathology such as vestibular schwannoma, meningioma, other lesions of the cerebellopontine angle, demyelinating lesions of the brainstem, and brain tumors. Recent experience suggests that both CT and MRI are equally capable of identifying inner-ear malformations and assessing cochlear patency for preoperative evaluation of patients for cochlear implantation.

℞ TREATMENT

In general, conductive hearing losses are amenable to surgical intervention and correction, while sensorineural hearing losses are permanent. Atresia of the ear canal can be surgically repaired, often with significant improvement in hearing. Tympanic membrane perforations due to chronic otitis media or trauma can be repaired with an outpatient tympanoplasty. Likewise, conductive hearing loss associated with otosclerosis can be treated by stapedectomy, which is successful in 90 to 95% of cases. Tympanostomy tubes allow the prompt return of normal hearing in individuals with middle-ear effusions. Hearing aids are effective and well-tolerated in patients with conductive hearing losses.

Patients with mild, moderate, and severe sensorineural hearing losses are regularly rehabilitated with hearing aids of varying configuration and strength. Hearing aids have been improved to provide greater fidelity and have been miniaturized. The current generation of hearing aids can be placed entirely within the ear canal, thus reducing the stigma associated with their use. In general, the more severe the hearing impairment, the larger the hearing aid required for auditory rehabilitation. Digital hearing aids lend themselves to individual programming, and multiple and directional microphones at the ear level may be helpful in noisy surroundings. Since all hearing aids amplify noise as well as speech, the only absolute solution to the problem found thus far is to place the microphone closer to the speaker than the noise source. This arrangement is not possible with a self-contained, cosmetically acceptable device. It is cumbersome and requires a user-friendly environment.

In many situations, including lectures and the theater, hearing-impaired persons benefit from assistive devices that are based on the principle of having the speaker closer to the microphone than any source of noise. Assistive devices include infrared and frequency modulated (FM) transmission as well as an electromagnetic loop around the room for transmission to the individual's hearing aid. Hearing aids with telecoils can also be used with properly equipped telephones in the same way.

In the event that the hearing aid provides inadequate rehabilitation, cochlear implants may be appropriate. Criteria for implantation include severe to profound hearing loss with word recognition score ≤30% under best aided conditions. Worldwide, more than 20,000 deaf individuals (including 4000 children) have received cochlear implants. Cochlear implants are neural prostheses that convert sound energy to electrical energy and can be used to stimulate the auditory division of the eighth nerve directly. In most cases of profound hearing impairment, the auditory hair cells are lost but the ganglionic cells of the auditory division of the eighth nerve are preserved. Cochlear implants consist of electrodes that are inserted into the cochlea through the round window, speech processors that extract acoustical elements of speech for conversion to electrical currents, and a means of transmitting the electrical energy through the skin. Patients with implants experience sound that helps with speech reading, allows open-set word recognition, and helps in modulating the person's own voice. Usually, within 3 months after implantation, adult patients can understand speech without visual cues. With the current generation of multichannel cochlear implants, nearly 75% of patients are able to converse on the telephone. It is anticipated that improvements in the electrode design and speech processors will permit further enhancement in understanding speech, especially in the presence of background noise.

For individuals who have had both eighth nerves destroyed by trauma or bilateral vestibular schwannomas (e.g., neurofibromatosis type 2), brainstem auditory implants placed near the cochlear nucleus may provide auditory rehabilitation. It is hoped that additional advances may provide benefits similar to those with the cochlear implant.

Tinnitus often accompanies hearing loss. Tinnitus and background noise can significantly affect understanding of speech in individuals with hearing impairment. Therapy for tinnitus is usually directed towards minimizing the appreciation of tinnitus. Relief of the tinnitus may be obtained by masking it with background music. Hearing aids are also helpful in tinnitus suppression, as are tinnitus maskers, devices that present a sound to the affected ear that is more pleasant to listen to than the tinnitus. The use of a tinnitus masker is often followed by several hours of inhibition of the tinnitus. Antidepressants have also shown beneficial effect in helping patients deal with tinnitus.

Tinnitus and background noise can significantly affect understanding of speech in individuals with hearing impairment. Hard-of-hearing individuals often benefit from a reduction in unnecessary noise (e.g., radio or television) to enhance the signal-to-noise ratio. Speech comprehension is aided by lip reading; therefore the impaired listener should be seated so that the face of the speaker is well-illuminated and easily seen. Speaking directly into the ear is occasionally helpful, but usually more is lost than gained because the speaker's face can no longer be seen. Speech should be slow enough to make each word distinct, but overly slow speech is distracting and loses contextual and speech-reading benefits. Although speech should be in a loud, clear voice, one should be aware that in sensorineural hearing losses in general and in elderly hard-of-hearing persons in particular, recruitment (abnormal perception of loud sounds) may be troublesome. Above all, optimal communication cannot take place without both parties giving it their full and undivided attention.

PREVENTION Conductive hearing losses may be prevented by prompt antibiotic therapy of adequate duration for AOM and by ventilation of the middle ear with tympanostomy tubes in middle-ear effusions lasting ≥12 weeks. Loss of vestibular function and deafness due to aminoglycoside antibiotics can largely be prevented by careful monitoring of serum peak and trough levels.

Some 10 million Americans have noise-induced hearing loss, and 20 million are exposed to hazardous noise in their employment. Noise-induced hearing loss can be prevented by avoidance of exposure to loud noise or by regular use of ear plugs or fluid-filled ear muffs to attenuate intense sound. Noise-induced hearing loss results from recreational as well as occupational activities and begins in adolescence. High-risk activities for noise-induced hearing loss include wood and metal working with electrical equipment and target practice and hunting with small firearms. All internal-combustion and electric engines, including snow and leaf blowers, snowmobiles, outboard motors, and chain saws, require protection of the user with hearing protectors. Virtually all noise-induced hearing loss is preventable through education, which should begin before the teenage years. Programs of industrial conservation of hearing are required when the exposure over an 8-h period averages 85 dB. Workers in such noisy environments can be protected with preemployment audiologic assessment, the mandatory use of hearing protectors, and annual audiologic assessments.

FURTHER READING

BALLENGER JJ, SNOW JB (eds): *Ballenger's Otorhinolaryngology Head and Neck Surgery*, 16th ed. Baltimore, BC Decker, 2002

GURTLER N, LALWANI AK: Etiology of syndromic and nonsyndromic sensorineural hearing loss. Otolaryngol Clin North Am 35:891, 2002

ZADEH MH et al: Diagnosis and treatment of sudden-onset sensorineural hearing loss: A study of 51 patients. Otolaryngol Head Neck Surg 128:92, 2003

27 INFECTIONS OF THE UPPER RESPIRATORY TRACT
Michael A. Rubin, Ralph Gonzales, Merle A. Sande

Infections of the upper respiratory tract (URIs) have a tremendous impact on public health. They are among the most common reasons for visits to primary care providers, and, although the illnesses are typically mild, their high incidence and transmission rates place them among the leading causes of time lost from work or school. Even though the minority (~25%) of cases are caused by bacteria, URIs are the leading diagnoses for which antibiotics are prescribed on an outpatient basis in the United States. The enormous consumption of antibiotics for these illnesses has contributed to the rise in antibiotic resistance among common community-acquired pathogens such as *Streptococcus pneumoniae*—a trend that in itself has had a tremendous impact on public health.

Although most URIs are caused by viruses, distinguishing patients with primary viral infection from those with primary bacterial infection is difficult. Signs and symptoms of bacterial and viral URIs are, in fact, indistinguishable. Because routine, rapid testing is neither available nor practical for most syndromes, acute infections are diagnosed largely on clinical grounds. This situation makes the judicious use of antibiotics in this setting challenging.

NONSPECIFIC INFECTIONS OF THE UPPER RESPIRATORY TRACT

Nonspecific URIs are a broadly defined group of disorders that collectively constitute the leading cause of ambulatory care visits in the United States. Nonspecific URIs, by definition, have no prominent localizing features. They are identified by a variety of descriptive names, including *acute infective rhinitis*, *acute rhinopharyngitis/nasopharyngitis*, *acute coryza*, and *acute nasal catarrh*, as well as by the inclusive label *common cold*.

Etiology   The large assortment of URI classifications reflects the wide variety of causative infectious agents and the varied manifestations of common pathogens. Nearly all nonspecific URIs are caused by viruses spanning multiple virus families and large numbers of antigenic types. For instance, rhinoviruses (Chap. 170), the most common cause (~30 to 40% of cases), consist of at least 100 immunotypes; other causes include influenza virus (3 immunotypes; Chap. 171) as well as parainfluenza virus (4 immunotypes), coronavirus (at least 3 immunotypes), and adenovirus (47 immunotypes) (Chap. 170). Respiratory syncytial virus (RSV) also accounts for a small percentage of cases each year, as do some viruses not typically associated with URIs (e.g., enteroviruses, rubella virus, and varicella-zoster virus). Even with sophisticated diagnostic and culture techniques, a substantial proportion (25 to 30%) of cases have no assigned pathogen.

Manifestations   The signs and symptoms of nonspecific URI are similar to those of other URIs but lack a pronounced localization to one particular anatomic location, such as the sinuses, pharynx, or lower airway. Nonspecific URI is commonly described as an acute, mild, and self-limited catarrhal syndrome, with a median duration of ~1 week. Signs and symptoms are diverse and frequently variable across patients. The principal signs and symptoms of nonspecific URI include rhinorrhea (with or without purulence), nasal congestion, cough, and sore throat; other manifestations, such as fever, malaise, sneezing, and hoarseness, are more variable, with fever more common among infants and young children. Occasionally, clinical features reflect the underlying viral pathogen; myalgias and fatigue, for example, are sometimes seen with influenza and parainfluenza infections, while conjunctivitis may suggest infection with adenovirus or enterovirus. Findings on physical examination are frequently nonspecific and unimpressive. Between 0.5 and 2% of colds are complicated by secondary bacterial infections (e.g., rhinosinusitis, otitis media, and pneumonia), particularly in high-risk populations such as infants, elderly persons, and chronically ill patients. Secondary bacterial infections are usually associated with a prolonged course of illness, worsening of illness severity, and localization of signs and symptoms. The presence of purulent secretions from the nares or throat has often been used as an indication of sinusitis or pharyngitis. However, these secretions are also seen in nonspecific URI and, in the absence of other clinical features, are poor predictors of bacterial infection.

℞ TREATMENT

Antibiotics have no role in the treatment of uncomplicated nonspecific URI. In the absence of clinical evidence of bacterial infection, treatment remains entirely symptom-based, with use of decongestants and nonsteroidal anti-inflammatory drugs. Other therapies directed at specific symptoms are often useful, including dextromethorphan for cough and lozenges with topical anesthetic for sore throat. Clinical trials of zinc, vitamin C, echinacea, and other alternative remedies have revealed no consistent benefit for the treatment of nonspecific URI.

INFECTIONS OF THE SINUS

Sinusitis refers to an inflammatory condition involving the four paired structures surrounding the nasal cavities. Although most cases of sinusitis involve more than one sinus, the maxillary sinus is most commonly involved, followed in frequency by the ethmoid, frontal, and sphenoid sinuses. Each sinus is lined with a respiratory epithelium that produces mucus, which is transported out by ciliary action through the sinus ostium and into the nasal cavity. Normally, mucus does not accumulate in the sinuses, which remain sterile despite their adjacency to the bacterium-filled nasal passages. When the sinus ostia are obstructed, however, or when ciliary clearance is impaired or absent, the secretions can be retained, producing the typical signs and symptoms of sinusitis. The retained secretions may become infected with a variety of pathogens, including viruses, bacteria, and fungi. Sinusitis affects a tremendous proportion of the population, accounts for millions of visits to primary care physicians each year, and is the fifth leading diagnosis for which antibiotics are prescribed. It is typically classified by duration of illness (acute vs. chronic); by etiology (infectious vs. noninfectious); and, when infectious, by the offending pathogen type (viral, bacterial, or fungal).

ACUTE SINUSITIS   Acute sinusitis—defined as sinusitis of <4 weeks' duration—constitutes the vast majority of sinusitis cases. Most cases are diagnosed in the ambulatory care setting and occur primarily as a consequence of a preceding viral URI. Differentiating acute bacterial and viral sinusitis on clinical grounds is difficult. Therefore, it is perhaps unsurprising that antibiotics are prescribed frequently (in 85 to 98% of all cases) for this condition.

Etiology   A number of infectious and noninfectious factors can contribute to acute obstruction of the sinus ostia or impairment of ciliary clearance, with consequent sinusitis. Noninfectious causes include allergic rhinitis (with either mucosal edema or polyp obstruction), barotrauma (e.g., from deep-sea diving or air travel), or chemical irritants. Illnesses such as nasal and sinus tumors (e.g., squamous cell carcinoma) or granulomatous diseases (e.g., Wegener's granulomatosis or rhinoscleroma) can also produce obstruction of the sinus ostia, while conditions leading to altered mucus content (e.g., cystic fibrosis) can cause sinusitis through impaired mucus clearance. In the hospital setting, nasotracheal intubation is a major risk factor for nosocomial sinusitis in intensive care units.

Acute infectious sinusitis can be caused by a variety of organisms, including viruses, bacteria, and fungi. Viral rhinosinusitis is far more common than bacterial sinusitis, although relatively few studies have sampled sinus aspirates for the presence of different viruses. In those studies that have done so, the viruses most commonly isolated—both alone and with bacteria—have been rhinovirus, parainfluenza virus, and influenza virus. Bacterial causes of sinusitis have been better described. Among community-acquired cases, *S. pneumoniae* and nontypable *Haemophilus influenzae* are the most common pathogens, accounting for 50 to 60% of cases. *Moraxella catarrhalis* causes disease in a significant percentage (20%) of children but less often in adults. Other streptococcal species and *Staphylococcus aureus* cause a small percentage of cases. Anaerobes are occasionally found in association with infections of the roots of premolar teeth that spread into the adjacent maxillary sinuses. The role of *Chlamydia pneumoniae* and *Mycoplasma pneumoniae* in the pathogenesis of acute sinusitis is still unclear. Nosocomial cases are commonly associated with bacteria found in the hospital environment, including *S. aureus*, *Pseudomonas aeruginosa*, *Serratia marcescens*, *Klebsiella pneumoniae*, and *Enterobacter* species. Often, these infections are polymicrobial and involve organisms that are highly resistant to numerous antibiotics. Fungi are also established causes of sinusitis, although most acute cases are in immunocompromised patients and represent invasive, life-threatening infections. The best-known example is rhinocerebral mucormycosis caused by fungi of the order Mucorales, which includes *Rhizopus*, *Rhizomucor*, *Mucor*, *Absidia*, and *Cunninghamella*. These infections usually occur in diabetic patients with ketoacidosis but also develop in transplant recipients, patients with hematologic malignancies, and patients receiving chronic glucocorticoid or deferoxamine therapy. Other hyaline molds, such as *Aspergillus* and *Fusarium* species, are also occasional causes of this disease.

Manifestations   Most cases of acute sinusitis present after or in conjunction with a viral URI, and it can be difficult to discriminate the clinical features of one from the other. A large proportion of patients with colds have sinus inflammation, although bacterial sinusitis complicates only 0.2 to 2% of these viral infections. Common presenting symptoms of sinusitis include nasal drainage and congestion, facial pain or pressure, and headache. Thick, purulent or discolored nasal discharge is often thought to indicate bacterial sinusitis, but it also occurs early in viral infections such as the common cold and is not specific to bacterial infection. Other nonspecific symptoms include cough, sneezing, and fever. Tooth pain, most often involving the upper molars, is associated with bacterial sinusitis, as is halitosis.

In acute sinusitis, sinus pain or pressure often localizes to the involved sinus (particularly the maxillary sinus) and can be worse when the patient bends over or is supine. Although rare, symptoms of advanced sphenoid or ethmoid sinus infection can be profound, including severe frontal or retroorbital pain radiating to the occiput, thrombosis of the cavernous sinus, and signs of orbital cellulitis. Acute focal sinusitis is uncommon but should be considered in the patient with severe symptoms over the maxillary sinus and fever, regardless of illness duration. Similarly, advanced frontal sinusitis can present with a condition known as *Pott's puffy tumor*, with soft tissue swelling and pitting edema over the frontal bone from a communicating subperiosteal abscess. Life-threatening complications include meningitis, epidural abscess, and cerebral abscess.

Patients with acute fungal sinusitis (such as mucormycosis) often present with symptoms related to pressure effects, particularly when the infection has spread to the orbits and cavernous sinus. Signs such as orbital swelling and cellulitis, proptosis, ptosis, and decreased extraocular movement are common, as is retroorbital or periorbital pain. Nasopharyngeal ulcerations, epistaxis, and headaches are also frequent, and involvement of cranial nerves V and VII has been described in more advanced cases. Bony erosion may be evident on examination. Oftentimes, the patient does not appear seriously ill despite the rapidly progressive nature of these infections.

Patients with acute nosocomial sinusitis are often critically ill and thus do not manifest the typical clinical features of sinus disease. This diagnosis should be suspected, however, when hospitalized patients who have appropriate risk factors (e.g., nasotracheal intubation) develop fever of uncertain origin.

Diagnosis   Distinguishing viral from bacterial sinusitis in the ambulatory setting is usually difficult, given the relatively low sensitivity and specificity of the common clinical features. One clinical feature that has been used to help guide diagnostic and therapeutic decision-making is illness duration. Because acute bacterial sinusitis is uncommon in patients whose symptoms have lasted <7 days, several authorities now recommend reserving this diagnosis for patients with appropriate symptoms (e.g., facial or tooth pain in combination with purulent nasal discharge) that have persisted for >7 days (Table 27-1). Nonetheless, of the patients who meet these criteria, only 40 to 50% have true bacterial sinusitis. The use of computed tomography (CT) or sinus radiography is not recommended for routine cases, particularly early in the course of illness (i.e., at <7 days), given the high prevalence of similar abnormalities among cases of acute viral rhinosinusitis. In the evaluation of persistent, recurrent, or chronic sinusitis, CT of the sinuses is the radiographic study of choice.

The clinical history and/or setting can often identify cases of acute anaerobic bacterial sinusitis, acute fungal sinusitis, or sinusitis from noninfectious causes, such as allergic rhinosinusitis. In the case of an immunocompromised patient with acute fungal sinus infection, immediate examination by an otolaryngologist is required. Biopsies of involved areas should be examined by a pathologist for evidence of fungal hyphal elements and tissue invasion. Cases of suspected acute nosocomial sinusitis should be confirmed by a sinus CT scan. Because therapy should target the offending organism, a sinus aspirate should be obtained, if possible, for culture and susceptibility testing.

℞ TREATMENT

Most patients with a diagnosis of acute rhinosinusitis based on clinical grounds improve without antibiotic therapy. The preferred initial approach in adult patients with mild to moderate symptoms of <7 days' duration are therapies aimed at facilitating sinus drainage, such as oral and topical decongestants, nasal saline lavage, and—in patients with a history of chronic sinusitis or allergies—nasal glucocorticoids. Adult patients fulfilling the above criteria who do not improve after 7 days and those with more severe symptoms (regardless of duration) should be treated with antibiotics (Table 27-1). Empirical therapy should consist of the most narrow-spectrum agent active against the most common bacterial pathogens, including *S. pneumoniae* and *H. influenzae*—e.g., amoxicillin. No clinical trials support the use of broad-spectrum agents for routine cases of bacterial sinusitis, even in the current era of drug-resistant *S. pneumoniae*. Up to 10% of patients do not respond

TABLE 27-1 Guidelines for the Diagnosis and Treatment of Selected Upper Respiratory Tract Infections

Syndrome, Age Group	Diagnostic Criteria	Treatment Recommendations
ACUTE SINUSITIS		

Adults	Moderate symptoms (e.g., nasal purulence/congestion or cough) for >7 d *or*
	Severe symptoms (any duration), including unilateral/focal facial swelling or tooth pain
		Initial therapy:
		  Amoxicillin, 875 mg PO bid for 10 d *or*
		  TMP-SMX, 1 DS tablet PO bid for 10 d
		Exposure to antibiotics within 30 d:
		  Amoxicillin, 1000 mg PO bid for 10 d *or*
		  Amoxicillin/clavulanate, 875 mg PO bid for 10 d *or*
		  Antipneumococcal fluoroquinolone (e.g., levofloxacin, 500 mg PO qd) for 7 d
		Recent treatment failure:
		  Amoxicillin (1500 mg) *plus* clavulanate (125 mg) PO bid for 10 d *or*
		  Amoxicillin (1500 mg) *plus* clindamycin (300 mg qid) PO for 10 d *or*
		  Antipneumococcal fluoroquinolone (e.g., levofloxacin, 500 mg PO qd) for 7 d

Children	Moderate symptoms (e.g., nasal purulence/congestion or cough) for 10–14 d or longer *or*
	Severe symptoms (any duration), including fever (>102°F), unilateral/focal facial swelling or pain
		Initial therapy: 10-d course of oral treatment with:
		  Amoxicillin, 45–90 mg/kg per day (up to 2 g) in divided doses (bid or tid) *or*
		  Cefuroxime axetil, 30 mg/kg per day in divided doses (bid) *or*
		  Cefdinir, 14 mg/kg qd
		Exposure to antibiotics within 30 d or recent treatment failure: 10-d course of oral treatment with:
		  Amoxicillin, 90 mg/kg per day (up to 2 g), *plus* clavulanate, 6.4 mg/kg per day; both in divided doses (bid) *or*
		  Cefuroxime axetil, 30 mg/kg per day in divided doses (bid) *or*
		  Cefdinir, 14 mg/kg qd

ACUTE PHARYNGITIS		
Adults	Clinical suspicion of streptococcal pharyngitis (e.g., fever, tonsillar swelling, exudate, enlarged/tender anterior cervical lymph nodes, absence of cough or coryza)[a] *with* History of rheumatic fever *or* Documented household exposure *or* Positive rapid strep screen	Penicillin V, 500 mg PO bid for 10 d *or* Cephalexin, 250 mg PO qid for 10 d *or* Erythromycin, 250 mg PO qid for 10 d *or* Benzathine penicillin G, single dose of 1.2 million units IM
Children	Clinical suspicion of streptococcal pharyngitis (e.g., tonsillar swelling, exudate, enlarged/tender anterior cervical lymph nodes, absence of coryza) *with* History of rheumatic fever *or* Documented household exposure *or* Positive rapid strep screen *or* Positive throat culture (for those with negative rapid strep screen)	Amoxicillin, 45 mg/kg per day PO in divided doses (bid or tid) for 10 d *or* Penicillin VK, 50 mg/kg per day PO in divided doses (bid) for 10 d Cephalexin, 50 mg/kg per day PO in divided doses (qid) for 10 d Benzathine penicillin G, single dose of 25,000 units/kg IM
ACUTE OTITIS MEDIA		

Adults and children	Fluid in middle ear, evidenced by decreased tympanic membrane mobility, air/fluid level behind tympanic membrane, bulging tympanic membrane, purulent otorrhea *and*
	Signs and symptoms of middle-ear disease, including fever, irritability, otalgia, decreased hearing, tinnitus, vertigo
		Initial therapy[b]:
		  Amoxicillin, 90 mg/kg per day (up to 2 g) PO in divided doses (bid or tid) *or*
		  Amoxicillin, 90 mg/kg per day (up to 2 g), *plus* clavulanate, 6.4 mg/kg per day; both PO in divided doses (bid) *or*
		  Cefdinir, 14 mg/kg PO qd *or*
		  Clindamycin, 20 mg/kg per day PO in divided doses (tid), *plus* TMP-SMX, 10 mg/kg per day PO in divided doses (bid)
		Exposure to antibiotics within 30 d or recent treatment failure:
		  Amoxicillin, 90 mg/kg per day (up to 2 g), *plus* clavulanate, 6.4 mg/kg per day; both PO in divided doses (bid) for 10 d *or*
		  Cefdinir, 14 mg/kg PO qd for 10 d *or*
		  Ceftriaxone, 50 mg/kg IM qd for 3 d *or*
		  Consider myringotomy

[a] Some organizations support treating adults with these symptoms and signs without the need for rapid streptococcal antigen testing.

[b] Duration: 10 d for patients <2 years old, 5–7 d for patients 2–5 years old, and 5–7 d (with consideration of observation only in previously healthy individuals with mild disease) for patients >5 years old.

Note: DS, double-strength; TMP-SMX, trimethoprim-sulfamethoxazole.
Source: Cooper et al; Hickner et al; O'Brien et al; SF Dowell et al: Pediatrics 101:165, 1998; B Schwartz et al: Pediatrics 101:171, 1998.

to initial antimicrobial therapy, and these patients should be considered for sinus aspiration and/or lavage by an otolaryngologist. The use of prophylactic antibiotics to prevent episodes of recurrent acute bacterial sinusitis is not recommended.

Surgical intervention and intravenous antibiotics are usually reserved for patients with severe disease or those with intracranial complications, such as abscess or orbital involvement. Immunocompromised patients with acute invasive fungal sinusitis usually require extensive surgical debridement and treatment with intravenous antifungal agents active against fungal hyphal forms, such as amphotericin B. Specific therapy should be individualized according to the fungal species and the patient's attributes.

Treatment of nosocomial sinusitis should begin with broad-spectrum antibiotics to cover common pathogens such as *S. aureus* and gram-negative bacilli. Therapy should then be tailored to the results of culture and susceptibility testing of sinus aspirates.

CHRONIC SINUSITIS Chronic sinusitis is characterized by symptoms of sinus inflammation lasting >12 weeks. This illness is most commonly associated with either bacteria or fungi, and clinical cure in most cases is very difficult. Many patients have undergone treatment with repeated courses of antibacterial agents and multiple sinus surgeries, increasing their risk of colonization with antibiotic-resistant pathogens and of surgical complications. Patients often suffer significant morbidity, sometimes over many years.

In *chronic bacterial sinusitis*, infection is thought to be due to the impairment of mucociliary clearance from repeated infections rather than to persistent bacterial infection. However, the pathogenesis of this condition is poorly understood. Although certain conditions (e.g., cystic fibrosis) can predispose patients to chronic bacterial sinusitis, most patients with this infection do not have obvious underlying conditions that result in the obstruction of sinus drainage, the impairment of ciliary action, or immune dysfunction. Patients experience constant nasal congestion and sinus pressure, with intermittent periods of greater severity, which may persist for years. CT can be helpful in defining the extent of disease and the response to therapy. The management team should include an otolaryngologist to conduct endoscopic examinations and obtain tissue samples for histologic examination and culture.

Chronic fungal sinusitis is a disease of immunocompetent hosts and is usually noninvasive, although slowly progressive invasive disease is sometimes seen. Noninvasive disease, which is typically associated with hyaline molds such as *Aspergillus* species and dematiaceous molds such as *Curvularia* or *Bipolaris* species, can present as a number of different scenarios. In mild, indolent disease, which usually occurs in the setting of repeated failures of antibacterial therapy, only nonspecific mucosal changes may be seen on sinus CT. Endoscopic surgery is usually curative in these patients, with no need for antifungal therapy. Another form of disease presents with longstanding, often unilateral symptoms and opacification of a single sinus on imaging studies as a result of a mycetoma (fungus ball) within the sinus. Treatment for this condition is also surgical, although systemic antifungal therapy may be warranted in the rare case where bony erosion occurs. A third form of disease, known as *allergic fungal sinusitis*, is seen in patients with a history of nasal polyposis and asthma, who often have had multiple sinus surgeries. Patients with this condition produce a thick, eosinophilic mucus with the consistency of peanut butter that contains sparse fungal hyphae on histologic examination. Patients often present with pansinusitis.

℞ TREATMENT

Treatment of chronic bacterial sinusitis can be challenging and consists primarily of repeated culture-guided courses of antibiotics, sometimes for 3 to 4 weeks at a time; administration of intranasal glucocorticoids; and mechanical irrigation of the sinus with sterile saline solution. When this management approach fails, sinus surgery may be indicated and sometimes provides significant, albeit short-term, alleviation. Treatment of chronic fungal sinusitis consists of surgical removal of impacted mucus. Recurrence, unfortunately, is common.

INFECTIONS OF THE EAR AND MASTOID

Infections of the ear and associated structures can involve both the middle and external ear, including the skin, cartilage, periosteum, ear canal, and tympanic and mastoid cavities. Both viruses and bacteria are known causes of these infections, some of which result in significant morbidity if not treated appropriately.

INFECTIONS OF THE EXTERNAL EAR STRUCTURES ■ Auricular Cellulitis Auricular cellulitis is an infection of the skin overlying the external ear and typically follows minor local trauma. It presents with the typical signs and symptoms of a skin/soft tissue infection, with tenderness, erythema, swelling, and warmth of the external ear (particularly the lobule) but without apparent involvement of the ear canal or inner structures. Treatment consists of warm compresses and oral antibiotics such as dicloxacillin that are active against typical skin and soft tissue pathogens (specifically, *S. aureus* and streptococci). Intravenous antibiotics, such as a first-generation cephalosporin (e.g., cefazolin) or a penicillinase-resistant penicillin (e.g., nafcillin) are occasionally needed for more severe cases.

Perichondritis Perichondritis, an infection of the perichondrium of the auricular cartilage, typically follows local trauma (e.g., ear piercing, burns, or lacerations). Occasionally, when the infection spreads down to the cartilage of the pinna itself, patients may also have chondritis. The infection may closely resemble auricular cellulitis, with erythema, swelling, and extreme tenderness of the pinna, although the lobule is less often involved in perichondritis. The most common pathogens are *P. aeruginosa* and *S. aureus*, although other gram-negative and gram-positive organisms are occasionally involved. Treatment consists of systemic antibiotics active against both *P. aeruginosa* and *S. aureus*. An antipseudomonal penicillin (e.g., piperacillin) or a combination of a penicillinase-resistant penicillin plus an antipseudomonal quinolone (e.g., nafcillin plus ciprofloxacin) is typically used. Incision and drainage may be helpful for culture and for resolution of infection, which often takes weeks.

Otitis Externa The term *otitis externa* refers to a collection of diseases involving primarily the auditory meatus. Otitis externa usually results from a combination of heat, retained moisture, and desquamation and maceration of the outer canal epithelium. The disease exists in a number of forms, which are identified as localized, diffuse, chronic, or invasive. They are all predominantly bacterial in origin, with *P. aeruginosa* and *S. aureus* the most common pathogens.

Acute localized otitis externa (furunculosis) can develop in the outer third of the ear canal, where skin overlies cartilage and hair follicles are numerous. As with furunculosis elsewhere on the body, *S. aureus* is the usual pathogen, and treatment typically consists of an oral antistaphylococcal penicillin (e.g., dicloxacillin), with incision and drainage in cases of abscess formation.

Acute diffuse otitis externa is also known as "swimmer's ear," although it can develop in the absence of swimming. Heat, humidity, and the loss of protective cerumen lead to excessive moisture and elevation of the pH in the ear canal, which in turn lead to skin maceration and irritation. Infection may then occur; the predominant pathogen is *P. aeruginosa*, although other gram-negative and gram-positive organisms have been recovered from patients with this condition. The illness often starts with itching and progresses to severe pain, which is usually triggered by manipulation of the pinna or tragus. The onset of pain is usually accompanied by the development of an erythematous, swollen ear canal, often with scant white, clumpy discharge. Treatment consists of cleansing the canal to remove debris and to enhance the activity of topical therapies—usually hypertonic saline or mixtures of alcohol and acetic acid. Inflammation can also be decreased by adding glucocorticoids to the treatment regimen or by using Burow's solution (aluminum acetate in water). Antibiotics are most effective when given topically. Otic mixtures provide adequate pathogen coverage; these preparations usually combine neomycin with polymyxin, with or without glucocorticoids.

Chronic otitis externa is caused primarily by repeated local irritation, most commonly arising from persistent drainage from a chronic middle-ear infection. Other causes of repeated irritation, such as cotton swabs or other foreign objects inserted into the ear canal, can lead to this condition, as can rare chronic infections such as syphilis, tuberculosis, or leprosy. Chronic otitis externa typically presents as erythematous, scaling dermatitis in which the predominant symptom is pruritus rather than pain; this condition must be differentiated from several others that produce a similar clinical picture, such as atopic dermatitis, seborrheic dermatitis, psoriasis, and dermatomycosis. Therapy consists of identifying and treating or removing the offending process, although successful resolution is frequently difficult.

Invasive otitis externa, also known as "malignant" or "necrotizing" otitis externa, is an aggressive and potentially life-threatening disease that occurs predominantly in elderly diabetics and other immunocompromised patients. The disease begins in the external canal, progresses slowly over weeks to months, and often is difficult to distinguish from a severe case of chronic otitis externa because of the presence of purulent otorrhea and an erythematous swollen ear and external canal. Severe, deep-seated otalgia is often noted and can help differentiate invasive from chronic otitis externa. The characteristic finding on examination is granulation tissue in the posteroinferior wall of the external canal, near the junction of bone and cartilage. If left unchecked, the infection can migrate to the base of the skull (resulting in skull-base osteomyelitis) and on to the meninges and brain, with a high associated mortality rate. Cranial nerve involvement is occasionally seen, with the facial nerve usually affected first and most often. Thrombosis of the sigmoid sinus can occur if the infection extends to that area. CT, which can reveal osseous erosion of the temporal bone and skull base, can be used to help determine the extent of disease, as can gallium and technetium-99 scintigraphy studies. *P. aeruginosa* is by far the most common pathogen involved, although *S. aureus*, *Staphylococcus epidermidis*, *Aspergillus*, *Actinomyces*, and some gram-negative bacteria have been associated with this disease. Cleansing of the external canal and biopsy of the granulation tissue within the canal (or of deeper tissues) should be performed in all cases to isolate the offending organism in culture. Intravenous antibiotic therapy is directed specifically toward the recovered pathogen. For *P. aeruginosa*, the regimen typically includes an antipseudomonal penicillin or cephalosporin (e.g., piperacillin or ceftazidime) with an aminoglycoside. A fluoroquinolone antibiotic is frequently used in place of the aminoglycoside and can even be administered orally, given its excellent bioavailability. Antibiotic drops containing an agent active against *Pseudomonas* (e.g., ciprofloxacin) are also usually prescribed and are combined with glucocorticoids to reduce inflammation. Cases of invasive *Pseudomonas* otitis externa recognized in the early stages can sometimes be treated with oral and otic fluoroquinolones alone, albeit with close follow-up. Extensive surgical debridement, once an important component of the treatment approach, is now rarely indicated.

INFECTIONS OF MIDDLE-EAR STRUCTURES *Otitis media* is an inflammatory condition of the middle ear that results from dysfunction of the eustachian tube in association with a number of illnesses, including URIs and chronic rhinosinusitis. The inflammatory response to these conditions leads to the development of a sterile transudate within the middle-ear and mastoid cavities. Infection may occur if bacteria or viruses from the nasopharynx contaminate this fluid, producing an acute (or sometimes chronic) illness.

Acute Otitis Media   Acute otitis media results when pathogens from the nasopharynx are introduced into the inflammatory fluid collected in the middle ear—e.g., by nose blowing during a URI. The proliferation of these pathogens in this space leads to the development of the typical signs and symptoms of acute middle-ear infection. The diagnosis of acute otitis media requires the demonstration of fluid in the middle ear (with tympanic membrane immobility) and the accompanying signs or symptoms of local or systemic illness (Table 27-1).

ETIOLOGY   Acute otitis media typically follows a viral URI. The causative viruses (most commonly RSV, influenza virus, rhinovirus, and enterovirus) can themselves cause subsequent acute otitis media; more often, they predispose the patient to bacterial otitis media. Studies using tympanocentesis have consistently found *S. pneumoniae* to be the most important bacterial cause, isolated in up to 35% of cases. *H. influenzae* (nontypable strains) and *M. catarrhalis* are also common bacterial causes of acute otitis media. Viruses, such as those mentioned above, have been recovered either alone or with bacteria in 17 to 40% of cases.

MANIFESTATIONS   Fluid in the middle ear is typically demonstrated or confirmed with pneumatic otoscopy. In the absence of fluid, the tympanic membrane moves visibly with the application of positive and negative pressure, but this movement is dampened when fluid is present. With bacterial infection, the tympanic membrane can also be erythematous, bulging, or retracted and occasionally can spontaneously perforate. The signs and symptoms accompanying infection can be local or systemic, including otalgia, otorrhea, diminished hearing, fever, or irritability. Erythema of the tympanic membrane is often evident but is nonspecific as it is frequently seen in association with inflammation of the upper respiratory mucosa (e.g., during examination of young children). Other signs and symptoms occasionally reported include vertigo, nystagmus, and tinnitus.

℞ TREATMENT

There has been considerable debate on the usefulness of antibiotics for the treatment of acute otitis media. Although most cases resolve clinically 1 week after the onset of illness, there appears to be some benefit to the use of antibiotics, with a higher proportion of treated than of untreated patients free of illness 3 to 5 days after diagnosis. The difficulty of predicting which patients will benefit from antibiotic therapy has led to different approaches. In the Netherlands, for instance, physicians typically manage acute otitis media with initial observation and aggressive pain management with anti-inflammatory therapy, reserving antibiotics for high-risk patients, patients with complicated disease, or patients who do not improve after 48 to 72 h. In contrast, many experts in the United States continue to recommend antibiotic therapy for children <2 years old in light of the higher frequency of secondary complications in this young and functionally immunocompromised population.

Given that most studies of the etiologic agents of acute otitis media consistently document similar pathogen profiles, therapy is generally empirical except in those few cases where tympanocentesis is warranted—e.g., cases in newborns, cases refractory to therapy, or cases in patients who are severely ill or who have an immune deficiency. Despite resistance to penicillin and amoxicillin in roughly one-quarter of *S. pneumoniae* isolates, one-third of *H. influenzae* isolates, and nearly all *M. catarrhalis* isolates, outcome studies continue to find that amoxicillin is as successful as any other agent, and it remains the drug of first choice in recommendations from the Centers for Disease Control and Prevention (CDC; Table 27-1). Therapy is typically administered for 5 to 7 days for uncomplicated acute otitis media; longer courses (e.g., 10 days) have traditionally been prescribed, but evidence suggests that this duration should be reserved for complicated cases or for children <2 years old, in whom short-course therapy may be inadequate.

A switch in regimen is recommended if there is no clinical improvement by the third day of therapy, given the possibility of infection with a β-lactamase-producing strain of *H. influenzae* or *M. catarrhalis* or with a strain of penicillin-resistant *S. pneumoniae*. Decongestants and antihistamines are frequently used as adjunctive therapy to reduce congestion and relieve obstruction of the eustachian tube, but clinical trials have yielded no significant evidence of benefit with either class of agents.

Recurrent Acute Otitis Media   Recurrent acute otitis media (more than three episodes within 6 months or four episodes within 12 months) is generally due to relapse or reinfection, although data indicate that the majority of early recurrences are new infections. In general, the same pathogens responsible for acute otitis media cause recurrent disease; even so, the recommended treatment consists of antibiotics active against β-lactamase-producing organisms. Antibiotic prophylaxis for patients with recurrent acute otitis media [e.g., with trimethoprim-sulfamethoxazole (TMP-SMX) or amoxicillin] can reduce recurrences by an average of one episode per year, but this benefit is small compared with the cost of the drug and the high likelihood of colonization with antibiotic-resistant pathogens. Other approaches, including placement of tympanostomy tubes, adenoidectomy, and tonsillectomy plus adenoidectomy, are of questionable overall value, given the relatively small benefit compared with the potential for complications.

Serous Otitis Media   Serous otitis media, or otitis media with effusion, exists when fluid is present in the middle ear for an extended period and in the absence of signs and symptoms of infection. In general, acute effusions are self-limited; most resolve in 2 to 4 weeks. In some cases, however (in particular after an episode of acute otitis media), effusions can persist for months. These chronic effusions are often associated with a significant hearing loss in the affected ear. In younger children, persistent effusions and decreased hearing can be associated with impairment of language acquisition skills. The great majority of cases of otitis media with effusion resolve spontaneously within 3 months without antibiotic therapy. Antibiotic therapy or myringotomy with insertion of tympanostomy tubes is typically reserved for patients in whom bilateral effusion (1) has persisted for at least 3 months and (2) is associated with significant bilateral hearing loss. With this conservative approach and the application of strict diagnostic criteria for acute otitis media and otitis media with effusion, it is estimated that 6 to 8 million courses of antibiotics could be avoided each year.

Chronic Otitis Media   Chronic suppurative otitis media is characterized by persistent or recurrent purulent otorrhea in the setting of tympanic membrane perforation. Usually, there is also some degree of conductive hearing loss. This condition is sometimes divided into two subcategories: active and inactive. Inactive disease is characterized by a central perforation of the tympanic membrane, which allows drainage of purulent fluid from the middle ear. When the perforation is more peripheral, squamous epithelium from the auditory canal may invade the middle ear through the perforation, forming a mass of keratinaceous debris (*cholesteatoma*) at the site of invasion. This mass can enlarge and has the potential to erode bone and promote further infection, which can lead to meningitis, brain abscess, or paralysis of cranial nerve VII. Treatment of chronic active otitis media is surgical; mastoidectomy, myringoplasty, and tympanoplasty can be performed as outpatient surgical procedures, with an overall success rate of ~80%. Chronic inactive otitis media is more difficult to cure, usually requiring repeated courses of topical antibiotic drops during periods of drainage. Systemic antibiotics may offer better cure rates, but their role in the treatment of this condition remains unclear.

Mastoiditis   Acute mastoiditis was a relatively common condition in children before the introduction of antibiotics. Because the mastoid air cells connect with the middle ear, the process of fluid collection and infection in the mastoid is usually the same as in the middle ear. Early and frequent treatment of acute otitis media is most likely the reason that the incidence of acute mastoiditis has declined to only 1.2 to 2.0 cases per 100,000 person-years in countries with high prescribing rates for acute otitis media. In countries like the Netherlands, where antibiotics are used sparingly for acute otitis media, the incidence rate of acute mastoiditis is roughly twice that seen in countries like the United States. However, neighboring Denmark has a rate of acute mastoiditis similar to that in the Netherlands but an antibiotic-prescribing rate for acute otitis media more similar to that in the United States.

In typical acute mastoiditis, purulent exudate collects in the mastoid air cells, producing pressure that may result in erosion of the surrounding bone and the formation of abscess-like cavities that are usually evident on CT. Patients typically present with pain, erythema, and swelling of the mastoid process along with displacement of the pinna, usually in conjunction with the typical signs and symptoms of acute middle-ear infection. Rarely, patients can develop severe complications if the infection tracks under the periosteum of the temporal bone to cause a subperiosteal abscess, erodes through the mastoid tip to cause a deep neck abscess, or extends posteriorly to cause septic thrombosis of the lateral sinus.

Cultures of purulent fluid should be performed whenever possible to help guide antimicrobial therapy. Initial empirical therapy is usually directed against the typical organisms associated with acute otitis me-

dia, such as *S. pneumoniae, H. influenzae,* and *M. catarrhalis.* Some patients with more severe or prolonged courses of illness should be treated for infection with *S. aureus* and gram-negative bacilli (including *Pseudomonas*). Broad empirical therapy is usually narrowed once culture results become available. Most patients can be treated conservatively with intravenous antibiotics; surgery (cortical mastoidectomy) can be reserved for complicated cases and those in which conservative treatment has failed.

INFECTIONS OF THE PHARYNX AND ORAL CAVITY

Oropharyngeal infections range from mild, self-limited viral illnesses to serious, life-threatening bacterial infections. The most common presenting symptom is sore throat—one of the most frequent reasons for ambulatory care visits among adults and children. Although sore throat is a symptom in many noninfectious illnesses as well, the overwhelming majority of patients with a new sore throat have acute pharyngitis of viral or bacterial etiology.

ACUTE PHARYNGITIS   Millions of visits to primary care providers each year are for sore throat; the majority of cases of acute pharyngitis are caused by typical respiratory viruses. The most important source of concern is infection with group A β-hemolytic *Streptococcus* (*S. pyogenes*), which can progress to acute rheumatic fever and acute glomerulonephritis, the risk for both of which can be reduced by timely penicillin therapy.

Etiology   A wide variety of organisms cause acute pharyngitis. The relative importance of the different pathogens can only be estimated, since a significant proportion of cases (~30%) have no identified cause. Respiratory viruses are the most common identifiable cause of acute pharyngitis, with rhinoviruses (~20% of cases) and coronaviruses (at least 5%) accounting for a large proportion. Influenza virus, parainfluenza virus, and adenovirus also account for a measurable share of cases, the latter as part of the more clinically severe syndrome of pharyngoconjunctival fever. Other important but less common viral causes include herpes simplex virus (HSV) types 1 and 2, coxsackievirus A, cytomegalovirus (CMV), and Epstein-Barr virus (EBV). Acute HIV infection can present as acute pharyngitis and should be considered in high-risk populations.

Acute bacterial pharyngitis is typically caused by *S. pyogenes,* which accounts for ~5 to 15% of all cases of acute pharyngitis in adults; rates vary depending on the season and on health care system utilization. Group A streptococcal pharyngitis is primarily a disease of children 5 to 15 years of age; it is uncommon among children <3 years old, as is rheumatic fever. Streptococci of groups C and G account for a minority of cases, although these serogroups are nonrheumatogenic. The remaining bacterial causes of the acute pharyngitis are seen infrequently (<1% each) but should be considered in appropriate exposure groups because of the severity of illness if left untreated; these etiologic agents include *Neisseria gonorrhoeae, Corynebacterium diphtheriae, Corynebacterium ulcerans, Yersinia enterocolitica,* and *Treponema pallidum* (in secondary syphilis). Anaerobic bacteria can also cause acute pharyngitis (*Vincent's angina*) and can contribute to more serious polymicrobial infections, such as peritonsillar or retropharyngeal abscess (see below). Atypical organisms such as *M. pneumoniae* and *C. pneumoniae* have been recovered from patients with acute pharyngitis; whether these agents are commensals or causes of acute infection is debatable.

Manifestations   Although the signs and symptoms accompanying acute pharyngitis are not reliable predictors of the etiologic agent, the clinical presentation occasionally suggests that one etiology is more likely than another. Acute pharyngitis due to respiratory viruses such as rhinovirus or coronavirus is usually not severe and is typically associated with a constellation of coryzal symptoms better characterized as nonspecific URI. Findings on physical examination are uncommon; fever is rare, and tender cervical adenopathy and pharyngeal exudates are not seen. In contrast, acute pharyngitis from influenza virus can be severe and is much more likely to be associated with fever as well as with myalgias, headache, and cough. The presentation of pharyngo-conjunctival fever due to adenovirus infection is similar. Since pharyngeal exudate may be present on examination, this condition can be difficult to differentiate from streptococcal pharyngitis. However, adenoviral pharyngitis is distinguished by the presence of conjunctivitis in one-third to one-half of patients. Acute pharyngitis from primary HSV infection can also mimic streptococcal pharyngitis in some cases, with pharyngeal inflammation and exudate, but the presence of vesicles and shallow ulcers on the palate can help differentiate the two diseases. This HSV syndrome is distinct from pharyngitis caused by coxsackievirus (*herpangina*), which is associated with small vesicles that develop on the soft palate and uvula and then rupture to form shallow white ulcers. Acute exudative pharyngitis coupled with fever, fatigue, generalized lymphadenopathy, and (on occasion) splenomegaly is characteristic of infectious mononucleosis due to EBV or CMV. Acute primary infection with HIV is frequently associated with fever and acute pharyngitis as well as with myalgias, arthralgias, malaise, and occasionally a nonpruritic maculopapular rash, which later may be followed by lymphadenopathy and mucosal ulcerations without exudate.

The clinical features of acute pharyngitis caused by streptococci of groups A, C, and G are all similar, ranging from a relatively mild illness without many accompanying symptoms to clinically severe cases with profound pharyngeal pain, fever, chills, and abdominal pain. A hyperemic pharyngeal membrane with tonsillar hypertrophy and exudate is usually seen, along with tender anterior cervical adenopathy. Coryzal manifestations, including cough, are typically absent; when present, they suggest a viral etiology. Strains of *S. pyogenes* that generate erythrogenic toxin can also produce scarlet fever, characterized by an erythematous rash and strawberry tongue. The other types of acute bacterial pharyngitis (e.g., gonococcal, diphtherial, and yersinial) often present as exudative pharyngitis with or without other clinical features. Their etiologies are often suggested only by the clinical history.

Diagnosis The primary goal of diagnostic testing is to separate acute streptococcal pharyngitis from pharyngitis of other etiologies (particularly viral) so that antibiotics can be prescribed more efficiently for patients to whom they may be beneficial. The most appropriate standard for the diagnosis of streptococcal pharyngitis, however, has not been definitively established. Throat swab culture is generally regarded as such. However, this method cannot distinguish between infection and colonization, and it takes 24 to 48 h to yield results that vary according to technique and culture conditions. Rapid antigen-detection tests offer good specificity (>90%) but lower sensitivity that varies across the clinical spectrum of disease (65 to 90%). Several clinical prediction systems (see Table 27-1) can increase the sensitivity of rapid antigen-detection tests to >90% in controlled settings. Since the sensitivities achieved in routine clinical practice are often lower, several medical and professional societies continue to recommend that all negative rapid antigen-detection tests in children be confirmed by a throat culture to limit transmission and complications of illness caused by group A streptococci. The CDC, the Infectious Diseases Society of America, the American College of Physicians, and the American Academy of Family Physicians do not recommend backup culture when adults have a negative rapid antigen-detection test, however, given the lower prevalence and smaller benefit in this age group.

Cultures and rapid diagnostic tests for other causes of acute pharyngitis, such as influenza virus, adenovirus, HSV, EBV, CMV, and *M. pneumoniae*, are available in some locations and can be used when these infections are suspected. In general, the monospot test for EBV is preferable to an assay for EBV antibodies, since the latter does not distinguish antecedent from current infection. Testing is also available for HIV RNA or antigen (p24) when acute primary HIV infection is suspected. If other bacterial causes are suspected (particularly *N. gonorrhoeae*, *C. diphtheriae*, or *Y. enterocolitica*), specific cultures should be requested since these organisms may be missed on routine throat swab culture.

℞ TREATMENT

Antibiotic treatment of pharyngitis due to *S. pyogenes* confers numerous benefits, including a decrease in the risk of rheumatic fever. The magnitude of this benefit is fairly small, however, since rheumatic fever is now a rare disease, even in untreated patients. When therapy is started within 48 h of illness onset, however, symptom duration is also decreased. An additional benefit of therapy is the potential to reduce the spread of streptococcal pharyngitis, particularly in areas of overcrowding or close contact. Antibiotic therapy for acute pharyngitis is therefore recommended in cases where *S. pyogenes* is confirmed as the etiologic agent by rapid antigen-detection test or throat swab culture. Otherwise, antibiotics should be given in routine cases only when another bacterial cause has been identified. Effective therapy for streptococcal pharyngitis consists of either a single dose of intramuscular benzathine penicillin or a full 10-day course of oral penicillin (Table 27-1). Erythromycin can be used in place of penicillin, although erythromycin resistance among *S. pyogenes* strains in some parts of the world (particularly Europe) can prohibit the use of this drug. Newer (and more expensive) antibiotics are also active against streptococci but offer no greater efficacy than the above agents. Testing for cure is unnecessary and may reveal only chronic colonization. There is no evidence to support antibiotic treatment of group C or G streptococcal pharyngitis or of pharyngitis in which *Mycoplasma* or *Chlamydia* has been recovered. Penicillin prophylaxis (benzathine penicillin G, 1.2 million units intramuscularly every 3 to 4 weeks) is indicated for patients at risk of recurrent rheumatic fever.

Treatment of viral pharyngitis is entirely symptom-based except in infection with influenza virus or HSV. For influenza, a number of therapeutic agents exist, including amantadine, rimantadine, and the two newer agents oseltamivir and zanamivir. All of these agents need to be started within 36 to 48 h of symptom onset to reduce illness duration meaningfully. Of these agents, only oseltamivir and zanamivir are active against both influenza A and influenza B and therefore can be used when local infection patterns are unknown. Oropharyngeal HSV infection sometimes responds to treatment with antiviral agents such as acyclovir, although these drugs are often reserved for patients who are immunosuppressed.

Complications Although rheumatic fever is the best-known complication of acute streptococcal pharyngitis, its risk following acute infection remains quite low. Other complications include acute glomerulonephritis and numerous suppurative conditions, such as peritonsillar abscess (*quinsy*), otitis media, mastoiditis, sinusitis, bacteremia, and pneumonia—all of which occur at extremely low rates. Although antibiotic treatment of acute streptococcal pharyngitis can prevent the development of rheumatic fever, there is no evidence that it can prevent acute glomerulonephritis. Some evidence supports antibiotic use to prevent the suppurative complications of streptococcal pharyngitis, particularly peritonsillar abscess, which can also involve oral anaerobes. Abscesses are usually accompanied by severe pharyngeal pain, dysphagia, and fever, often with medial displacement of the tonsil on examination. Oral penicillin remains the recommended therapy for peritonsillar abscess, with clindamycin as an alternative. Early use of antibiotics in these cases has substantially reduced the need for surgical drainage.

ORAL INFECTIONS Aside from periodontal disease such as gingivitis, infections of the oral cavity most commonly involve HSV or *Candida* species. In addition to causing painful cold sores on the lips, HSV can infect the tongue and buccal mucosa, causing the formation of irritating vesicles. Although topical antiviral agents (such as acyclovir or penciclovir) can be used externally for cold sores, oral or intravenous acyclovir is often needed for primary infections, extensive oral infections, and infections in immunocompromised patients. Oropharyngeal candidiasis (*thrush*) is caused by a variety of *Candida* species, most often *C. albicans*. Thrush occurs predominantly in neonates, immunocompromised patients (especially those with AIDS), and patients who have received prolonged antibiotic or glucocorticoid therapy. In addition to sore throat, patients often complain of a burning tongue, and physical examination reveals friable white or gray plaques on the gingiva, tongue, and oral mucosa. Treatment usually consists of an oral antifungal suspension (nystatin or clotrimazole) or oral fluconazole. In the cases of fluconazole-refractory thrush seen occasionally in patients with AIDS, the limited therapeutic options include oral suspensions of either itraconazole or amphotericin B.

Vincent's angina, also known as *acute necrotizing ulcerative gingivitis* or *trench mouth*, is a unique and dramatic form of gingivitis characterized by painful, inflamed gingiva with ulcerations of the interdental papillae that bleed easily. Since oral anaerobes are the cause, patients typically have halitosis and frequently present with fever, malaise, and lymphadenopathy. Treatment consists of debridement and oral administration of penicillin plus metronidazole, with clindamycin alone as an alternative.

Ludwig's angina is a rapidly progressive, potentially fulminant cellulitis involving the sublingual and submandibular spaces that typically originates from an infected or recently extracted tooth, most commonly the lower second and third molars. Improved dental care has substantially reduced the incidence of this disorder. Infection in these areas leads to dysphagia, odynophagia, and "woody" edema in the sublingual region, forcing the tongue up and back with the potential for airway obstruction. Fever, dysarthria, and drooling may also be noted, and patients may speak in a "hot potato" voice. Intubation or tracheostomy may be necessary to secure the airway, as asphyxiation is the most common cause of death. Patients should be monitored closely and treated promptly with intravenous antibiotics directed against streptococci and oral anaerobes. Recommended agents include ampicillin/sulbactam and high-dose penicillin plus metronidazole.

Postanginal septicemia (Lemierre's disease) is a rare anaerobic oropharyngeal infection caused predominantly by *Fusobacterium necrophorum*. The illness typically starts as a sore throat (most commonly in adolescents and young adults), which may present as exudative tonsillitis or peritonsillar abscess. Infection of the deep pharyngeal tissue allows organisms to drain into the lateral pharyngeal space, which contains the carotid artery and internal jugular vein. Septic thrombophlebitis of the internal jugular vein can result, with associated pain, dysphagia, and neck swelling and stiffness. Sepsis usually occurs 3 to 10 days after the onset of sore throat and is often coupled with metastatic infection to the lung and other distant sites. Occasionally, the infection can extend along the carotid sheath and into the posterior mediastinum, resulting in mediastinitis, or it can erode into the carotid artery, with the early sign of repeated small bleeds into the mouth. The mortality rate from these invasive infections can be as high as 50%. Treatment consists of intravenous antibiotics (penicillin G or clindamycin) and surgical drainage of any purulent collections. The concomitant use of anticoagulants to prevent embolization remains controversial but is often advised.

INFECTIONS OF THE LARYNX AND EPIGLOTTIS

LARYNGITIS   *Laryngitis* is defined as any inflammatory process involving the larynx and can be caused by a variety of infectious and noninfectious processes. The vast majority of laryngitis cases seen in clinical practice in developed countries are acute. Acute laryngitis is a common syndrome caused predominantly by the same viruses responsible for many other URIs. In fact, most cases of acute laryngitis occur in the setting of a viral URI.

Etiology   Nearly all major respiratory viruses have been implicated in acute viral laryngitis, including rhinovirus, influenza virus, parainfluenza virus, adenovirus, coxsackievirus, coronavirus, and RSV. Acute laryngitis can also be associated with acute bacterial respiratory infections, such as those caused by group A *Streptococcus* or *C. diphtheriae* (although diphtheria has been all but eliminated in the United States).

Another bacterial pathogen thought to play a role (albeit unclear) in the pathogenesis of acute laryngitis is *M. catarrhalis*, which has been recovered on nasopharyngeal culture from a significant percentage of people with acute laryngitis. Chronic laryngitis of infectious etiology is much less common in developed than in developing countries. Laryngitis due to *Mycobacterium tuberculosis* is often difficult to distinguish from laryngeal cancer, in part because of the frequent absence of signs, symptoms, and radiographic findings typical of pulmonary disease. *Histoplasma* and *Blastomyces* may cause laryngitis, often as a complication of systemic infection. *Candida* species can cause laryngitis as well, often in association with thrush or esophagitis and particularly in immunosuppressed patients. Rare cases of chronic laryngitis are due to *Coccidioides* and *Cryptococcus*.

Manifestations   Laryngitis is characterized by hoarseness and can also be associated with reduced vocal pitch or aphonia. As acute laryngitis is caused predominantly by respiratory viruses, these symptoms usually occur in association with other symptoms and signs of URI, including rhinorrhea, nasal congestion, cough, and sore throat. Direct laryngoscopy often reveals diffuse laryngeal erythema and edema, along with vascular engorgement of the vocal folds. Chronic disease (e.g., tuberculous laryngitis), in addition, often includes mucosal nodules and ulcerations visible on laryngoscopy; these lesions are sometimes mistaken for laryngeal cancer.

℞ TREATMENT

Acute laryngitis is usually treated with humidification and voice rest alone. Antibiotics are not recommended except when group A *Streptococcus* is cultured, in which case penicillin is the drug of choice. The choice of therapy for chronic laryngitis depends on the pathogen, whose identification usually requires biopsy with culture. Patients with laryngeal tuberculosis are highly contagious because of the large number of organisms that are easily aerosolized. These patients should be managed in the same way as patients with active pulmonary disease.

CROUP   The term *croup* actually denotes a group of diseases collectively referred to as "croup syndrome," all of which are acute and predominantly viral respiratory illnesses characterized by marked swelling of the subglottic region of the larynx. Croup primarily affects children <6 years old. For a detailed discussion of this entity, the reader is referred to a text of pediatric medicine.

EPIGLOTTITIS   *Acute epiglottitis* (supraglottitis) is an acute, rapidly progressive cellulitis of the epiglottis and adjacent structures that can result in complete—and potentially fatal—airway obstruction in both children and adults. Before the widespread use of *H. influenzae* type b (Hib) vaccine, this entity was much more common among children, with a peak incidence at ~3.5 years of age. In some countries, mass vaccination against Hib has reduced the annual incidence of acute epiglottitis in children by >90%; over the same period, the annual incidence in adults has changed little. Because of the danger of airway obstruction, acute epiglottitis constitutes a medical emergency, particularly in children, and prompt diagnosis and airway protection are of utmost importance.

Etiology   After the introduction of the Hib vaccine, disease incidence among children in the United States declined dramatically. Nevertheless, lack of vaccination or vaccine failure have meant that many pediatric cases seen today are still due to Hib. In adults and (more recently) in children, a variety of other bacterial pathogens have been associated with epiglottitis, the most common being group A *Streptococcus*. Other pathogens seen less frequently include *S. pneumoniae*, *Haemophilus parainfluenzae*, and *S. aureus*. Viruses have not yet been established as a cause of acute epiglottitis.

Manifestations and Diagnosis   Epiglottitis typically presents more acutely in young children than in adolescents or adults. On presentation, most children have had symptoms for <24 h, including high fever, severe sore throat, tachycardia, systemic toxicity, and (in many cases) drooling while sitting forward. Symptoms and signs of respiratory obstruction may also be present and may progress rapidly. The somewhat milder illness in adolescents and adults often follows 1 or 2 days of severe sore throat and is commonly accompanied by dyspnea, drooling, and stridor. Physical examination of patients with acute epiglottitis may reveal moderate or severe respiratory distress, with inspiratory stridor and retractions of the chest wall. These findings *diminish* as the disease progresses and the patient tires. Conversely, oropharyngeal examination reveals injection that is much less severe than would be predicted from the symptoms—a finding that should alert the clinician to a cause of symptoms and obstruction that lies beyond the tonsils. The diagnosis is often made on clinical grounds, although direct fiberoptic laryngoscopy is frequently performed in a controlled environment (e.g., an operating room) in order to visualize and culture the typical edematous "cherry-red" epiglottis and to facilitate placement of an endotracheal tube. Direct visualization in an examination room (e.g., with a tongue blade and indirect laryngoscopy) is not recommended because of the risk of immediate laryngospasm and complete airway obstruction. Lateral neck radiographs and laboratory tests can assist in the diagnosis but may delay the critical securing of the airway and cause the patient to be excessively moved or repositioned, risking further airway compromise. Neck radiographs typically show an enlarged edematous epiglottis (the "thumbprint sign"), usually with a dilated hypopharynx and normal subglottic structures. Laboratory tests typically show mild to moderate leukocytosis with a predominance of neutrophils. Blood cultures are positive in a significant proportion of cases.

℞ TREATMENT

Security of the airway is always of primary concern in acute epiglottitis, even if the diagnosis is only suspected. Mere observation for signs of impending airway obstruction is not routinely recommended, particularly in children. Many adults have been managed in this way since the illness is perceived to be milder in this age group, but some data suggest that this approach may be risky and probably should be reserved only for adult patients who have yet to develop dyspnea or stridor. Once the airway has been secured and blood and epiglottis specimens have been obtained for culture, treatment with intravenous antibiotics should be given to cover the most likely organisms, particularly *H. influenzae*. Because rates of ampicillin resistance in this organism have risen significantly in recent years, therapy with a β-lactam/β-lactamase inhibitor combination or a second- or third-generation cephalosporin is recommended. Typically, ampicillin/sulbactam, cefuroxime, cefotaxime, or ceftriaxone is given, with clindamycin and TMP-SMX reserved for patients allergic to β-lactams. Antibiotic therapy should be continued for 7 to 10 days and should be tailored, if necessary, to the organism recovered in culture. If the household contacts of a patient with *H. influenzae* epiglottitis include an unvaccinated child under the age of 4, all members of the household (including the patient) should receive prophylactic rifampin for 4 days to eradicate *H. influenzae* carriage.

INFECTIONS OF THE DEEP NECK STRUCTURES

Deep neck infections are usually extensions of infection from other primary sites, most often within the pharynx or oral cavity. Many of these infections are life-threatening but are difficult to detect at early stages when they may be more easily managed. Three of the most clinically relevant spaces in the neck are the submandibular (and sublingual) space, the lateral pharyngeal (or parapharyngeal) space, and the retropharyngeal space. These spaces communicate with one another and with other important structures in the head, neck, and thorax, providing infections with easy access to areas including the mediastinum, carotid sheath, skull base, and meninges. Once infection reaches these sensitive areas, mortality rates can be as high as 20 to 50%.

Infection of the submandibular and/or sublingual space typically originates from an infected or recently extracted lower tooth. The result is the severe, life-threatening infection referred to as Ludwig's angina

(see under "Oral Infections," above). Lateral pharyngeal (or parapharyngeal) space infection is most often a complication of common infections of the oral cavity and upper respiratory tract, including tonsillitis, peritonsillar abscess, pharyngitis, mastoiditis, or periodontal infection. This space, located deep to the lateral wall of the pharynx, contains a number of sensitive structures, including the carotid artery, internal jugular vein, cervical sympathetic chain, and portions of cranial nerves IX through XII; at its distal end, it opens into the posterior mediastinum. Involvement of this space with infection can therefore be rapidly fatal. Examination may reveal some tonsillar displacement, trismus, and neck rigidity, but lateral pharyngeal wall swelling can easily be missed. The diagnosis can be confirmed by CT. Treatment consists of airway management, operative drainage of fluid collections, and at least a 10-day course of intravenous therapy with an antibiotic active against streptococci and oral anaerobes (e.g., ampicillin/sulbactam). A particularly severe form of this infection involving the components of the carotid sheath, called postanginal septicemia (or Lemierre's disease), is described above ("Oral Infections"). Infection of the retropharyngeal space can also be extremely dangerous, as this space runs posterior to the pharynx from the skull base to the superior mediastinum. Infections in this space are more common in children <5 years old because of the presence of several small retropharyngeal lymph nodes that typically atrophy by the age of 4 years. Infection is usually a consequence of extension from another site of infection, most commonly acute pharyngitis. Other sources include otitis media, tonsillitis, dental infections, Ludwig's angina, and anterior extension of vertebral osteomyelitis. Retropharyngeal space infection can also follow penetrating trauma to the posterior pharynx (e.g., from an endoscopic procedure). Infections are commonly polymicrobial, with a mixture of aerobes and anaerobes; group A β-hemolytic streptococci and *S. aureus* are the most common pathogens. Tuberculosis was a frequent cause in the past but now is rarely seen in the United States.

Patients with retropharyngeal abscess typically present with sore throat, fever, dysphagia, and neck pain and are often drooling because of difficulty and pain with swallowing. Examination may reveal tender cervical adenopathy, neck swelling, and diffuse erythema and edema of the posterior pharynx as well as a bulge in the posterior pharyngeal wall, although the latter may not be obvious on routine inspection. A soft tissue mass is usually demonstrable by lateral neck radiography or CT. Because of the risk of airway obstruction, treatment begins with securing of the airway, which is followed by a combination of surgical drainage and intravenous antibiotic administration. Initial empirical therapy should cover streptococci, oral anaerobes, and *S. aureus*; ampicillin/sulbactam, clindamycin alone, or clindamycin plus ceftriaxone is usually effective. Complications occur primarily as a result of extension to other areas, including rupture into the posterior pharynx, which may lead to aspiration pneumonia and empyema. Extension may also occur to the lateral pharyngeal space and mediastinum, resulting in mediastinitis and pericarditis, or into nearby major blood vessels. All these events are associated with a high mortality rate.

FURTHER READING

BISNO AL: Acute pharyngitis. N Engl J Med 344:205, 2001

COOPER RJ et al: Principles of appropriate antibiotic use for acute pharyngitis in adults: Background. Ann Intern Med 134:509, 2001

GONZALES R et al: Principles of appropriate antibiotic use for treatment of nonspecific upper respiratory tract infections in adults: Background. Ann Intern Med 134:490, 2001

——— et al: Principles of appropriate antibiotic use for treatment of uncomplicated acute bronchitis: Background. Ann Intern Med 134:521, 2001

HICKNER JM et al: Principles of appropriate antibiotic use for acute rhinosinusitis in adults: Background. Ann Intern Med 2001; 134:498, 2001

O'BRIEN KL et al: Acute sinusitis—principles of judicious use of antimicrobial agents. Pediatrics 101:174, 1998

VAN ZUIJLEN DA et al: National differences in incidence of acute mastoiditis: Relationship to prescribing patterns of antibiotics for acute otitis media? Pediatr Infect Dis J 20:140, 2001

As primary care physicians and consultants, internists are often asked to evaluate patients with disease of the oral soft tissues, teeth, and pharynx. Knowledge of the oral milieu and its unique structures is necessary to guide preventive services and recognize oral manifestations of local or systemic disease. Furthermore, internists frequently collaborate with dentists in the care of patients with a variety of medical conditions that impact oral health or who undergo dental procedures that increase the patient's risk of medical complications.

DISEASES OF THE TEETH AND PERIODONTAL STRUCTURES ■ Tooth and Periodontal Structure Tooth formation begins during the sixth week of embryonic life and continues through the first 17 years of age. Tooth development begins in utero and continues until after the tooth erupts. Normally all 20 deciduous teeth have erupted by age 3 and have been shed by age 13. Permanent teeth, eventually totaling 32, begin to erupt by age 6 and have completely erupted by age 14, though third molars (wisdom teeth) may erupt later.

The erupted tooth consists of the visible crown covered with enamel and the root submerged below the gum line and covered with bonelike cementum. *Dentin*, a material that is denser than bone and exquisitely sensitive to pain, forms the majority of the tooth substance. Dentin surrounds a core of myxomatous *pulp* containing the vascular and nerve supply. The tooth is held firmly in the alveolar socket by the *periodontium*, supporting structures that consist of the gingivae, alveolar bone, cementum, and periodontal ligament. The periodontal ligament tenaciously binds the tooth's cementum to the alveolar bone. Above this ligament is a collar of attached gingiva just below the crown. A few millimeters of unattached or free gingiva (1 to 3 mm) overlaps the base of the crown, forming a shallow sulcus along the gum-tooth margin.

Dental Caries, Pulpal and Periapical Disease, and Complications Dental caries begin asymptomatically as a destructive process of the hard surface of the tooth. *Streptococcus mutans*, principally, along with other bacteria colonize the organic buffering film on the tooth surface to produce *plaque*. If not removed by brushing or the natural cleaning action of saliva and oral soft tissues, bacterial acids demineralize the enamel. Fissures and pits on the occlusion surfaces are the most frequent sites of decay. Surfaces adjacent to tooth restorations and exposed roots are also vulnerable, particularly as teeth are retained in an aging population. Over time dental caries extend to the underlying dentin, leading to cavitation of the enamel and ultimately penetration to the tooth pulp, producing *acute pulpitis*. At this early stage when the pulp infection is limited, the tooth becomes sensitive to percussion and hot or cold, and pain resolves immediately when the irritating stimulus is removed. Should the infection spread throughout the pulp, *irreversible pulpitis* occurs leading to pulp necrosis. At this late stage pain is severe and has a sharp or throbbing visceral quality that may be worse when the patient lies down. Once pulp necrosis is complete, pain may be constant or intermittent, but cold sensitivity is lost.

Treatment of caries involves removal of the softened and infected hard tissue; sealing the exposed dentin; and restoration of the tooth structure with silver amalgam, composite plastic, gold, or porcelain. Once irreversible pulpitis occurs, root canal therapy is necessary and the contents of the pulp chamber and root canals are removed, followed by thorough cleaning, antisepsis, and filling with an inert material. Alternatively, the tooth may be extracted.

Pulpal infection, if it does not egress through the decayed enamel, leads to *periapical abscess* formation, which produces pain on chewing. If the infection is mild and chronic, a *periapical granuloma* or eventually a *periapical cyst* forms, either of which produces radiolucency at the root apex. When unchecked, a periapical abscess can erode into the alveolar bone producing osteomyelitis, penetrate and drain through the gingivae (*parulis* or *gumboil*), or track along deep fascial planes producing a virulent cellulitis (*Ludwig's angina*) involving the submandibular space and floor of the mouth (Chap. 148). Elderly patients, those with diabetes mellitus, and patients taking glucocorticoids may experience little or no pain and fever as these complications develop.

Periodontal Disease Periodontal disease accounts for more tooth loss than caries, particularly in the elderly. Like dental caries, chronic infection of the gingiva and anchoring structures of the tooth begins with formation of bacterial plaque. The process begins invisibly above the gum line and in the gingival sulcus. Plaque, including mineralized plaque (*calculus*), is preventable by appropriate dental hygiene, including periodic professional cleaning. Left undisturbed, chronic inflammation ensues and produces a painless hyperemia of the free and attached gingivae (*gingivitis*) that typically bleeds with brushing. If ignored, severe *periodontitis* occurs, leading to deepening of the physiologic sulcus and destruction of the periodontal ligament. Pockets develop around the teeth that become filled with pus and debris. As the periodontium is destroyed, teeth loosen and exfoliate. Eventually there is resorption of the alveolar bone.

Acute and aggressive forms of periodontal disease are seen less commonly than the chronic forms described above. However, if the host is stressed or exposed to a new pathogen, rapidly progressive and destructive disease of the periodontal tissue can occur. A virulent example is *acute necrotizing ulcerative gingivitis* (ANUG), or *Vincent's infection*, characterized as "trench mouth" during World War I. Stress, poor oral hygiene, and tobacco and alcohol use are risk factors. The presentation includes sudden gingival inflammation, ulceration, bleeding, interdental gingival necrosis, and fetid halitosis. *Localized juvenile periodontitis*, seen in adolescents, is particularly destructive and appears to be associated with impaired neutrophil chemotaxis. *AIDS-related periodontitis* resembles ANUG in some patients or a more destructive form of adult chronic periodontitis in others. It may also produce a gangrene-like destructive process of the oral soft tissues and bone that resembles *noma*, seen in severely malnourished children in developing nations.

Prevention of Tooth Decay and Periodontal Infection Despite the reduced prevalence of dental caries and periodontal disease in the United States due in large part to water fluoridation and improved dental care, respectively, both diseases constitute a major public health problem worldwide and for certain groups. The internist can promote prevention by including questions about dental care and hygiene as part of health maintenance. Special populations at high risk for dental caries and periodontal disease include those with xerostomia (Sjögren's syndrome, drug-induced, postirradiation head and neck), diabetics, alcoholics, tobacco users, those with Down's syndrome, and those with gingival hyperplasia. Furthermore, patients lacking dental care access (low socioeconomic status) and those with reduced ability to provide self-care (e.g., nursing-home residents, those with dementia or upper extremity disability) suffer at a disproportionate rate. It is important to provide counseling regarding regular dental hygiene and professional cleaning, use of fluoride-containing toothpaste, professional fluoride treatments, and use of electric toothbrushes for patients with limited dexterity and to give instruction to caregivers for those unable to perform self-care.

Developmental and Systemic Disease Affecting the Teeth and Periodontium Malocclusion is the most common developmental problem, which in addition to a problem with cosmesis, can interfere with mastication unless corrected through orthodontic techniques. Impacted third molars are common and occasionally become infected. Acquired prognathism due to *acromegaly* may also lead to malocclusion, as may deformity of the maxilla and mandible due to *Paget's disease* of the bone. Delayed tooth eruption, receding chin, and a protruding tongue are occasional features of *cretinism* and *hypopituitarism*. Congenital syphilis produces tapering, notched (*Hutchinson's*) incisors and finely nodular (*mulberry*) molar crowns.

Enamel hypoplasia results in crown defects ranging from pits to deep fissures of primary or permanent teeth. Intrauterine infection (syphilis, rubella), vitamin deficiency (A, C, or D), disorders of calcium metabolism (malabsorption, vitamin D–resistant rickets, hypoparathyroidism), prematurity, high fever, or rare inherited defects (*amelogenesis imperfecta*) are all causes. Tetracycline, given in sufficiently high doses during the first 8 years, may produce enamel hypoplasia and discoloration. Exposure to endogenous pigments can discolor developing teeth: *erythroblastosis fetalis* (green or bluish-black), congenital liver disease (green or yellow-brown), and porphyria (red or brown that fluoresces with ultraviolet light). *Mottled enamel* occurs if excessive fluoride is ingested during development. Worn enamel is seen with age, bruxism, or excessive acid exposure (e.g., chronic gastric reflux or bulimia).

Premature tooth loss resulting from periodontitis is seen with cyclic neutropenia, Papillon-Lefèvre syndrome, Chédiak-Higashi syndrome, and leukemia. Rapid focal tooth loosening is most often due to infection, but rarer causes include histiocytosis X, Ewing's sarcoma, osteosarcoma, or Burkitt's lymphoma. Early loss of primary teeth is a feature of *hypophosphatasia*, a rare inborn error of metabolism.

Pregnancy may produce severe gingivitis and localized *pyogenic granulomas*. Severe periodontal disease occurs with *Down's syndrome* and *diabetes mellitus*. *Gingival hyperplasia* may be caused by phenytoin, calcium channel blockers (e.g., nifedipine), and cyclosporine. *Idiopathic familial gingival fibromatosis* and several syndrome-related disorders appear similar. Removal of the medication often reverses the drug-induced form, though surgery may be needed to control both. *Linear gingival erythema* is variably seen in patients with advanced HIV infection and probably represents immune deficiency and decreased polymorphonuclear activity. Diffuse or focal gingival swelling may be a feature of early or late *acute myelomonocytic leukemia* as well as of other lymphoproliferative disorders. A rare, but pathognomonic, sign of Wegener's granulomatosis is a red-purplish, granular gingivitis (*strawberry gums*).

DISEASES OF THE ORAL MUCOSA ■ Infection Most oral mucosal diseases involve microorganisms (Table 28-1).

Pigmented Lesions See Table 28-2

Dermatologic Diseases See Tables 28-1, 28-2, and 28-3 and Chaps. 46 to 51

Diseases of the Tongue See Table 28-4

HIV Disease and AIDS See Tables 28-1, 28-2, 28-3, and 28-5; Chaps. 172 and 173; and see Figs. 165-1 and 187-1.

Ulcers Ulceration is the most common oral mucosal lesion encountered. Although there are many possible causes, the host and pattern of lesions, including the presence of systemic features, narrow the differential diagnosis (Table 28-1). Most acute ulcers are painful and self-limited. Recurrent *aphthous ulcers* and herpes simplex infection constitute the majority. Persistent and deep aphthous ulcers can be idiopathic or seen with HIV/AIDS. Aphthous lesions are often the presenting symptom in *Behçet's disease*. Similar appearing, though less painful, lesions may occur with *Reiter's syndrome*, and aphthous ulcers are occasionally present during phases of discoid or *systemic lupus erythematosus*. Aphthous-like ulcers are seen in *Crohn's disease*, but unlike the common aphthous variety, they may exhibit granulomatous inflammation histologically. Recurrent aphthae in some patients with *celiac disease* have been reported to remit with elimination of gluten.

Of major concern are chronic, relatively painless ulcers and mixed red/white patches (*erythroplakia* and *leukoplakia*) of more than 2 weeks' duration. *Squamous cell carcinoma* and *premalignant dysplasia* should be considered early and a diagnostic biopsy obtained. The importance is underscored because early-stage malignancy is vastly more treatable than late-stage disease. High-risk sites include the lower lip, floor of the mouth, ventral and lateral tongue, and soft palate–tonsillar pillar complex. Significant risk factors for oral cancer in western countries includes sun-exposure (lower lip) and tobacco and al-

cohol use. In India and some other Asian countries, smokeless tobacco mixed with betel nut, slaked lime, and spices is a common cause of oral cancer. Less common etiologies include syphilis and Plummer-Vinson syndrome.

Rarer causes of chronic ulcer such as tuberculosis, fungal infection, Wegener's granulomatosis, and midline granuloma may look identical to carcinoma. Making the correct diagnosis depends on recognizing other clinical features and biopsy of the lesion. The syphilitic *chancre* is typically painless and therefore easily missed. Regional lymphadenopathy is invariably present. Confirmation is achieved using appropriate bacterial and serologic tests.

Disorders of mucosal fragility often produce painful oral ulcers that fail to heal within 2 weeks. *Mucous membrane pemphigoid* and *pemphigus vulgaris* are the major acquired disorders. While clinical features are often distinctive, immunohistochemical examination should be performed for diagnosis and to distinguish these entities from *lichen planus* and drug reactions.

Hematologic and Nutritional Disease Internists are more likely to encounter patients with acquired, rather than congenital, bleeding disorders. Bleeding after minor trauma should stop after 15 min and within an hour of tooth extraction if local pressure is applied. Bleeding in excess of this, if not due to continued injury or rupture of a large vessel, should lead to investigation for a clotting abnormality. In addition to bleeding, petechiae and ecchymoses are prone to occur at the line of vibration between the soft and hard palates in patients with platelet dysfunction or thrombocytopenia.

All forms of leukemia, but particularly *acute myelomonocytic leukemia*, can produce gingival bleeding, ulcers, and gingival enlargement. Oral ulcers are a feature of *agranulocytosis*, and ulcers and mucositis are often severe complications of chemotherapy and radiation therapy for hematologic and other malignancies. *Plummer-Vinson syndrome* (iron deficiency, angular stomatitis, glossitis, and dysphagia) raises the risk of oral squamous cell cancer and esophageal cancer at the postcricoidal tissue web. Atrophic papillae and a red, burning tongue may occur with *pernicious anemia. B group vitamin deficiencies* produce many of these same symptoms as well as oral ulceration and cheilosis. Swollen, bleeding gums, ulcers, and loosening of the teeth are a consequence of *scurvy*.

NONDENTAL CAUSES OF ORAL PAIN Most oral pain emanates from inflamed or injured tooth pulp or periodontal tissues, and this fact often leads clinicians to overlook nonodontogenic causes. In most instances toothache is predictable and proportional to the stimulus applied and an identifiable condition (e.g., caries, abscess) is found. Local anesthesia eliminates pain originating from dental or periodontal structures, but not referred pains. The most common nondental origin is myofascial pain referred from muscles of mastication. The masticatory muscles are tender and ache with increased use. Many sufferers exhibit bruxism that is secondary to stress and anxiety. *Temporomandibular disorder* is closely related. It predominantly affects females between ages 15 and 45. Features include pain, limited mandibular movement, and temporomandibular joint sounds. The etiologies are complex, and malocclusion does not play the primary role once attributed to it. *Osteoarthritis* is a common cause of masticatory pain. Anti-inflammatory medication, jaw rest, soft foods, and heat provide relief. With treatment complete, remission of pain is the rule. The temporomandibular joint is involved in 50% of patients with *rheumatoid arthritis* and is usually a late feature of severe disease. Bilateral preauricular pain, particularly in the morning, limits range of motion.

Migrainous neuralgia is sometimes so localized to the mouth as to present a diagnostic challenge. Episodes of pain and remission without identifiable cause and absence of relief with local anesthesia are important clues. *Trigeminal neuralgia* (tic douloureaux) may involve the entire branch or part of the mandibular or maxillary branches of the fifth cranial nerve and produce pain in one or a few teeth. Pain may occur spontaneously or may be triggered by touching the lip or gin-

Condition	Usual Location	Clinical Features	Course
VIRAL DISEASES			
Primary acute herpetic gingivostomatitis [herpes simplex virus (HSV) type 1, rarely type 2]	Lip and oral mucosa (buccal, gingival, lingual mucosa)	Labial vesicles that rupture and crust, and intraoral vesicles that quickly ulcerate; extremely painful; acute gingivitis, fever, malaise, foul odor, and cervical lymphadenopathy; occurs primarily in infants, children, and young adults	Heals spontaneously in 10–14 days. Unless secondarily infected, lesions lasting >3 weeks are not due to primary HSV infection.
Recurrent herpes labialis	Mucocutaneous junction of lip, perioral skin	Eruption of groups of vesicles that may coalesce, then rupture and crust; painful to pressure or spicy foods	Lasts about 1 week, but condition may be prolonged if secondarily infected. If severe, topical or oral antiviral may reduce healing time.
Recurrent intraoral herpes simplex	Palate and gingiva	Small vesicles on keratinized epithelium that rupture and coalesce; painful	Heals spontaneously in about 1 week. If severe, topical or oral antiviral may reduce healing time.
Chickenpox (varicella-zoster virus)	Gingiva and oral mucosa	Skin lesions may be accompanied by small vesicles on oral mucosa that rupture to form shallow ulcers; may coalesce to form large bullous lesions that ulcerate; mucosa may have generalized erythema	Lesions heal spontaneously within 2 weeks.
Herpes zoster (reactivation of varicella-zoster virus)	Cheek, tongue, gingiva, or palate	Unilateral vesicular eruptions and ulceration in linear pattern following sensory distribution of trigeminal nerve or one of its branches	Gradual healing without scarring unless secondarily infected; postherpetic neuralgia is common. Oral acyclovir, famcyclovir, or valacylovir reduce healing time and postherpetic neuralgia
Infectious mononucleosis (Epstein-Barr virus)	Oral mucosa	Fatigue, sore throat, malaise, fever, and cervical lymphadenopathy; numerous small ulcers usually appear several days before lymphadenopathy; gingival bleeding and multiple petechiae at junction of hard and soft palates	Oral lesions disappear during convalescence; no treatment though glucocorticoids indicated if tonsillar swelling compromises airway
Herpangina (coxsackievirus A; also possibly coxsackie B and echovirus)	Oral mucosa, pharynx, tongue	Sudden onset of fever, sore throat, and oropharyngeal vesicles, usually in children under 4 years, during summer months; diffuse pharyngeal congestion and vesicles (1–2 mm), grayish-white surrounded by red areola; vesicles enlarge and ulcerate	Incubation period 2–9 days; fever for 1–4 days; recovery uneventful
Hand, foot, and mouth disease (coxsackievirus A16 most common)	Oral mucosa, pharynx, palms, and soles	Fever, malaise, headache with oropharyngeal vesicles that become painful, shallow ulcers; highly infectious; usually affects children under age 10	Incubation period 2–18 days; lesions heal spontaneously in 2–4 weeks
Primary HIV infection	Gingiva, palate, and pharynx	Acute gingivitis and oropharyngeal ulceration, associated with febrile illness resembling mononucleosis and including lymphadenopathy	Followed by HIV seroconversion, asymptomatic HIV infection, and usually ultimately by HIV disease
BACTERIAL OR FUNGAL DISEASES			
Acute necrotizing ulcerative gingivitis ("trench mouth," Vincent's infection)	Gingiva	Painful, bleeding gingiva characterized by necrosis and ulceration of gingival papillae and margins plus lymphadenopathy and foul odor	Debridement and diluted (1:3) peroxide lavage provide relief within 24 h; antibiotics in acutely ill patients; relapse may occur
Prenatal (congenital) syphilis	Palate, jaws, tongue, and teeth	Gummatous involvement of palate, jaws, and facial bones; Hutchinson's incisors, mulberry molars, glossitis, mucous patches, and fissures on corner of mouth	Tooth deformities in permanent dentition irreversible
Primary syphilis (chancre)	Lesion appears where organism enters body; may occur on lips, tongue, or tonsillar area	Small papule developing rapidly into a large, painless ulcer with indurated border; unilateral lymphadenopathy; chancre and lymph nodes containing spirochetes; serologic tests positive by third to fourth weeks	Healing of chancre in 1–2 months, followed by secondary syphilis in 6–8 weeks
Secondary syphilis	Oral mucosa frequently involved with mucous patches, primarily on palate, also at commissures of mouth	Maculopapular lesions of oral mucosa, 5–10 mm in diameter with central ulceration covered by grayish membrane; eruptions occurring on various mucosal surfaces and skin accompanied by fever, malaise, and sore throat	Lesions may persist from several weeks to a year
Tertiary syphilis	Palate and tongue	Gummatous infiltration of palate or tongue followed by ulceration and fibrosis; atrophy of tongue papillae produces characteristic bald tongue and glossitis	Gumma may destroy palate, causing complete perforation

(continued)

TABLE 28-1—(Continued)

Condition	Usual Location	Clinical Features	Course
Gonorrhea	Lesions may occur in mouth at site of inoculation or secondarily by hematogenous spread from a primary focus elsewhere	Most pharyngeal infection is asymptomatic; may produce burning or itching sensation; oropharynx and tonsils may be ulcerated and erythematous; saliva viscous and fetid	More difficult to eradicate than urogenital infection, though pharyngitis usually resolves with appropriate antimicrobial treatment
Tuberculosis	Tongue, tonsillar area, soft palate	A painless, solitary, 1–5 cm, irregular ulcer covered with a persistent exudate; ulcer has a firm undermined border	Autoinnoculation from pulmonary infection usual; lesions resolve with appropriate antimicrobial therapy
Cervicofacial actinomycosis	Swellings in region of face, neck, and floor of mouth	Infection may be associated with an extraction, jaw fracture, or eruption of molar tooth; in acute form resembles an acute pyogenic abscess, but contains yellow "sulfur granules" (gram-positive mycelia and their hyphae)	Typically swelling is hard and grows painlessly; multiple abscesses with draining tracks develop; penicillin first choice; surgery usually necessary
Histoplasmosis	Any area of the mouth, particularly tongue, gingiva, or palate	Nodular, verrucous, or granulomatous lesions; ulcers are indurated and painful; usual source hematogenous or pulmonary source, but may be primary	Systemic antifungal therapy necessary to treat
Candidiasis (Table 28-3)			
DERMATOLOGIC DISEASES			
Mucous membrane pemphigoid	Typically produces marked gingival erythema and ulceration; other areas of oral cavity, esophagus, and vagina may be affected	Painful, grayish-white collapsed vesicles or bullae of full-thickness epithelium with peripheral erythematous zone; gingival lesions desquamate, leaving ulcerated area	Protracted course with remissions and exacerbations; involvement of different sites occurs slowly; glucocorticoids may temporarily reduce symptoms but do not control the disease
Erythema multiforme minor and major (Stevens-Johnson syndrome)	Primarily the oral mucosa and the skin of hands and feet	Intraoral ruptured bullae surrounded by an inflammatory area; lips may show hemorrhagic crusts; the "iris," or "target," lesion on the skin is pathognomonic; patient may have severe signs of toxicity	Onset very rapid; usually idiopathic, but may be associated with trigger such as drug reaction; condition may last 3–6 weeks; mortality with EM major 5–15% if untreated
Pemphigus vulgaris	Oral mucosa and skin; sites of mechanical trauma (soft/hard palate, frenulum, lips buccal mucosa)	Usually (>70%) presents with oral lesions; fragile, ruptured bullae and ulcerated oral areas; mostly in older adults	With repeated occurrence of bullae, toxicity may lead to cachexia, infection, and death within 2 years; often controllable with oral glucocorticoids
Lichen planus	Oral mucosa and skin	White striae in mouth; purplish nodules on skin at sites of friction; occasionally causes oral mucosal ulcers and erosive gingivitis	White striae alone usually asymptomatic; erosive lesions often difficult to treat, but may respond to glucocorticoids
OTHER CONDITIONS			
Recurrent aphthous ulcers	Usually on nonkeratinized oral mucosa (buccal and labial mucosa, floor of mouth, soft palate, lateral and ventral tongue)	Single or clusters of painful ulcers with surrounding erythematous border; lesions may be 1–2 mm in diameter in crops (herpetiform), 1–5 mm (minor), or 5–15 mm (major)	Lesions heal in 1–2 weeks but may recur monthly or several times a year; protective barrier with orabase and topical steroids give symptomatic relief; systemic glucocorticoids may be needed in severe cases
Behçet's syndrome	Oral mucosa, eyes, genitalia, gut, and CNS	Multiple aphthous ulcers in mouth; inflammatory ocular changes, ulcerative lesions on genitalia; inflammatory bowel disease and CNS disease	Oral lesions often first manifestation; persist several weeks and heal without scarring
Traumatic ulcers	Anywhere on oral mucosa; dentures frequently responsible for ulcers in vestibule	Localized, discrete ulcerated lesions with red border; produced by accidental biting of mucosa, penetration by a foreign object, or chronic irritation by a denture	Lesions usually heal in 7–10 days when irritant is removed, unless secondarily infected
Squamous cell carcinoma	Any area in the mouth, most commonly on lower lip, tongue, and floor of mouth	Ulcer with elevated, indurated border; failure to heal, pain not prominent; lesions tend to arise in areas of erythro/leukoplakia or in smooth atrophic tongue	Invades and destroys underlying tissues; frequently metastasizes to regional lymph nodes
Acute myeloid leukemia (usually monocytic)	Gingiva	Gingival swelling and superficial ulceration followed by hyperplasia of gingiva with extensive necrosis and hemorrhage; deep ulcers may occur elsewhere on the mucosa complicated by secondary infection	Usually responds to systemic treatment of leukemia; occasionally requires local radiation therapy
Lymphoma	Gingiva, tongue, palate and tonsillar area	Elevated, ulcerated area that may proliferate rapidly, giving the appearance of traumatic inflammation	Fatal if untreated; may indicate underlying HIV infection
Chemical or thermal burns	Any area in mouth	White slough due to contact with corrosive agents (e.g., aspirin, hot cheese) applied locally; removal of slough leaves raw, painful surface	Lesion heals in several weeks if not secondarily infected

Note: CNS, central nervous system.

TABLE 28-2 Pigmented Lesions of the Oral Mucosa

Condition	Usual Location	Clinical Features	Course
Oral melanotic macule	Any area of the mouth	Discrete or diffuse localized, brown to black macule	Remains indefinitely; no growth
Diffuse melanin pigmentation	Any area of the mouth	Diffuse pale to dark-brown pigmentation; may be physiologic ("racial") or due to smoking	Remains indefinitely
Nevi	Any area of the mouth	Discrete, localized, brown to black pigmentation	Remains indefinitely
Malignant melanoma	Any area of the mouth	Can be flat and diffuse, painless, brown to black, or can be raised and nodular	Expands and invades early; metastasis leads to death
Addison's disease	Any area of the mouth but mostly buccal mucosa	Blotches or spots of bluish-black to dark-brown pigmentation occurring early in the disease, accompanied by diffuse pigmentation of skin; other symptoms of adrenal insufficiency	Condition controlled by steroid replacement
Peutz-Jeghers syndrome	Any area of the mouth	Dark-brown spots on lips, buccal mucosa, with characteristic distribution of pigment around lips, nose, eyes, and on hands; concomitant intestinal polyposis	Oral pigmented lesions remain indefinitely; gastrointestinal polyps may become malignant
Drug ingestion (neuroleptics, oral contraceptives, minocycline, zidovudine, quinine derivatives)	Any area of the mouth	Brown, black, or gray areas of pigmentation	Gradually disappears following cessation of drug
Amalgam tattoo	Gingiva and alveolar mucosa	Small blue-black pigmented areas associated with embedded amalgam particles in soft tissues; these may show up on radiographs as radiopaque particles in some cases	Remains indefinitely
Heavy metal pigmentation (bismuth, mercury, lead)	Gingival margin	Thin blue-black pigmented line along gingival margin; rarely seen except for children exposed to lead-based paint	Indicative of systemic absorption; no significance for oral health
Black hairy tongue	Dorsum of tongue	Elongation of filiform papillae of tongue, which become stained by coffee, tea, tobacco, or pigmented bacteria	Improves within 1–2 weeks with gentle brushing of tongue or discontinuation of antibiotic if due to bacterial overgrowth
Fordyce "spots"	Buccal and labial mucosa	Numerous small yellowish spots just beneath mucosal surface; no symptoms; due to hyperplasia of sebaceous glands	Benign; remains without apparent change
Kaposi's sarcoma	Palate most common, but may occur in any other site	Red or blue plaques of variable size and shape; often enlarge, become nodular and may ulcerate	Usually indicative of HIV infection or non-Hodgkin's lymphoma; rarely fatal, but may require treatment for comfort or cosmesis
Mucous retention cysts	Buccal and labial mucosa	Bluish-clear fluid filled cyst due to extravasated mucous from injured minor salivary gland	Benign; painless unless traumatized; may be removed surgically

giva, brushing the teeth, or chewing. *Glossopharyngeal neuralgia* produces similar acute neuropathic symptoms in the distribution of the ninth cranial nerve. Swallowing, sneezing, coughing, or pressure on the tragus of the ear triggers pain that is felt in the base of the tongue, pharynx, and soft palate and may be referred to the temporomandibular joint. *Neuritis* involving the maxillary and mandibular divisions of the trigeminal nerve (e.g., maxillary sinusitis, neuroma, and leukemic infiltrate) is distinguished from ordinary toothache by the neuropathic quality of the pain. Occasionally *phantom pain* follows tooth extraction. Often the earliest symptom of *Bell's palsy* in the day or so before facial weakness develops is pain and hyperalgesia behind the ear and side of the face. Likewise, similar symptoms may precede visible lesions of herpes zoster infecting the seventh nerve (*Ramsey-Hunt syndrome*) or trigeminal nerve. Either condition may leave *postherpetic neuralgia* in its wake. *Coronary ischemia* may produce pain exclusively in the face and jaw. Like typical angina pectoris, it is usually reproducible with increased myocardial demand. Aching in several upper molar or premolar teeth may point to *maxillary sinusitis*. Failure to relieve by anesthetizing the teeth and confirmation with appropriate radiographs support the clinical diagnosis.

Giant cell arteritis is notorious for producing headache, but it may also produce facial pain or sore throat that is mistaken for other causes. Jaw and tongue claudication with prolonged chewing or talking is relatively common. Tongue infarction is rare. Patients with *subacute thyroiditis* often experience pain referred to the face or jaw. Oral and pharyngeal causes may be sought before the tender thyroid gland and transient hyperthyroidism are appreciated.

Burning mouth syndrome (glossodynia) is present in the absence of mucosal lesions and predominantly affects women over 50. Poorly fitting dentures, anxiety, and depression are common and treatable causes. Tongue-thrusting habit is a cause in some elderly sufferers. The symptom occasionally leads to the discovery of vitamin B_{12} deficiency, iron deficiency, *Plummer-Vinson syndrome*, diabetes mellitus, low-grade *Candida* infection, food sensitivity (e.g., cinnamon), or subtle xerostomia.

DISEASES OF THE SALIVARY GLANDS Saliva is essential to oral health. Its major components, water and mucin, serve as a cleansing solvent and lubricating fluid. In addition it contains antimicrobial factors (e.g., lysozyme, lactoperoxidase, secretory IgA), epidermal growth factor, minerals, and buffering systems. The major salivary glands secrete intermittently in response to autonomic stimulation, which is high during a meal but low otherwise. The parotid secretion is serous or watery, the sublingual is mostly mucus, and the submandibular is a balance of the two elements. Hundreds of minor glands in the lips and cheeks secrete mucus continuously. It is easy to appreciate how oral function becomes impaired when salivary function is reduced. Dry mouth (*xerostomia*) is perceived when salivary flow is reduced by 50%. The most common etiology is medication, especially drugs with anticholinergic properties, but also alpha and beta blockers, calcium channel blockers, and diuretics. Other causes of chronic dryness include Sjögren's syndrome, chronic parotitis, salivary duct obstruction, diabetes mellitus, HIV/AIDS, and irradiation for head and neck cancer. Management involves eliminating or limiting drying medications, preventive dental care, and supplementing oral liquid. Sugarless mints or chewing gum may stimulate salivary secretion if dysfunction is mild. When sufficient exocrine tissue remains, pilocarpine or cevimeline has been shown to increase secretions and reduce symptoms. Commercial

TABLE 28-3 *White Lesions of Oral Mucosa*

Condition	Usual Location	Clinical Features	Course
Lichen planus	Buccal mucosa, tongue, gingiva, and lips; skin	Striae, white plaques, red areas, ulcers in mouth; purplish papules on skin; may be asymptomatic, sore, or painful; lichenoid drug reactions may look similar	Protracted; responds to topical steroids
White sponge nevus	Oral mucosa, vagina, anal mucosa	Painless white thickening of epithelium; adolescent/early adult onset; familial	Benign and permanent
Smoker's leukoplakia and smokeless tobacco lesions	Any area of oral mucosa, sometimes related to location of habit	White patch that may become firm, rough, or red-fissured and ulcerated; may become sore and painful but usually painless	May or may not resolve with cessation of habit; 2% develop squamous cell carcinoma; early biopsy essential
Erythroplakia with or without white patches	Floor of mouth common in men; tongue and buccal mucosa in women	Velvety, reddish plaque; occasionally mixed with white patches or smooth red areas	High risk of squamous cell cancer; early biopsy essential
Candidiasis	Any area mouth	*Pseudomembranous type* ("thrush"): creamy white curdlike patches that reveal a raw, bleeding surface when scraped; found in sick infants, debilitated elderly patients receiving high doses of glucocorticoids or broad-spectrum antibiotics, or in patients with AIDS	Responds favorably to antifungal therapy and correction of predisposing causes where possible
		Erythematous type: flat, red, sometimes sore areas in same groups of patients	Course same as for pseudomembranous type
		Candidal leukoplakia: nonremovable white thickening of epithelium due to *Candida*	Responds to prolonged antifungal therapy
		Angular cheilitis: sore fissures at corner of mouth	Responds to topical antifungal therapy
Hairy leukoplakia	Usually lateral tongue, rarely elsewhere on oral mucosa	White areas ranging from small and flat to extensive accentuation of vertical folds; found in HIV carriers in all risk groups for AIDS	Due to EBV; responds to high dose acyclovir but recurs; rarely causes discomfort unless secondarily infected with *Candida*
Warts (papillomavirus)	Anywhere on skin and oral mucosa	Single or multiple papillary lesions, with thick, white keratinized surfaces containing many pointed projections; cauliflower lesions covered with normal-colored mucosa or multiple pink or pale bumps (focal epithelial hyperplasia)	Lesions grow rapidly and spread; consider squamous cell carcinoma and rule out with biopsy; excision or laser therapy; may regress in HIV infected patients on antiretroviral therapy

Note: EBV, Epstein-Barr virus.

saliva substitutes or gels relieve dryness but must be supplemented with fluoride applications to prevent caries.

Sialolithiasis presents most often as painful swelling but in some instances as just swelling or pain. The obstructing stone produces spasm upon eating. Conservative therapy consists of local heat, massage, and hydration. Promotion of salivary secretion with mints or lemon drops may flush out small stones. Antibiotic treatment is necessary when bacterial infection in suspected. In adults *acute bacterial parotitis* is typically unilateral and most commonly affects postoperative patients within the first 2 weeks of surgery. *Staphylococcus aureus* is the most common bacterial agent. Dehydration is a major risk for parotitis, as is advanced age and chronic debilitating disease. *Chronic bacterial sialadenitis* is a consequence of lowered salivary secretion and recurrent bacterial infection. When suspected bacterial infection is not responsive to therapy, the differential diagnosis should be expanded to include benign and malignant neoplasms, lymphoproliferative disorders, Sjögren's syndrome, sarcoidosis, tuberculosis, lymphadenitis, actinomycosis, and Wegener's granulomatosis. Bilateral nontender parotid enlargement occurs with diabetes mellitus, cirrhosis, bulimia, HIV/AIDS, and drugs (e.g., iodide, propylthiouracil).

TABLE 28-4 *Alterations of the Tongue*

Type of Change	Clinical Features
SIZE OR MORPHOLOGY CHANGES	
Macroglossia	Enlarged tongue that may be part of a syndrome found in developmental conditions such as Down's syndrome; may be due to tumor (hemangioma or lymphangioma), metabolic disease (such as primary amyloidosis), or endocrine disturbance (such as acromegaly or cretinism)
Fissured ("scrotal") tongue	Dorsal surface and sides of tongue covered by painless shallow or deep fissures that may collect debris and become irritated
Median rhomboid glossitis	Congenital abnormality of tongue with ovoid, denuded area in median posterior portion of the tongue; may be associated with candidiasis and may respond to antifungals
COLOR CHANGES	
"Geographic" tongue (benign migratory glossitis)	Asymptomatic inflammatory condition of the tongue, with rapid loss and regrowth of filiform papillae, leading to appearance of denuded red patches "wandering" across the surface of the tongue
Hairy tongue	Elongation of filiform papillae of the medial dorsal surface area due to failure of keratin layer of the papillae to desquamate normally; brownish-black coloration may be due to staining by tobacco, food, or chromogenic organisms
"Strawberry" and "raspberry" tongue	Appearance of tongue during scarlet fever due to the hypertrophy of fungiform papillae plus changes in the filiform papillae
"Bald" tongue	Atrophy may be associated with xerostomia, pernicious anemia, iron-deficiency anemia, pellagra, or syphilis; may be accompanied by painful burning sensation; may be an expression of erythmematous candidiasis and respond to antifungals

TABLE 28-5 *Oral Lesions Associated with HIV Infection*

Lesion Morphology	Etiologies
Papules, nodules, plaques	Candidiasis (hyperplastic and pseudomembranous)[a]
	Condyloma acuminatum (human papillomavirus infection)
	Squamous cell carcinoma (preinvasive and invasive)
	Non-Hodgkin's lymphoma[a]
	Hairy leukoplakia[a]
Ulcers	Recurrent aphthous ulcers[a]
	Angular cheilitis
	Squamous cell carcinoma
	Acute necrotizing ulcerative gingivitis[a]
	Necrotizing ulcerative periodontitis[a]
	Necrotizing ulcerative stomatitis
	Non-Hodgkin's lymphoma[a]
	Viral infection (herpes simplex, herpes zoster, cytomegalovirus)
	Mycobacterium tuberculosis, mycobacterium avium-intracellulare
	Fungal infection (histoplasmosis, cryptococcosis, candidiasis, geotrichosis, aspergillosis)
	Bacterial infection (*Escherichia coli, Enterobacter cloacae, Klebsiella pneumoniae, Pseudomonas aeruginosa*)
	Drug reactions (single or multiple ulcers)
Pigmented lesions	Kaposi's sarcoma[a]
	Bacillary angiomatosis (skin and visceral lesions more common than oral)
	Zidovudine pigmentation (skin, nails, and occasionally oral mucosa)
	Addison's disease
Miscellaneous	Linear gingival erythema[a]

[a] Strongly associated with HIV infection.

Pleomorphic adenoma comprises two-thirds of all salivary neoplasms. The parotid is the principle salivary gland affected, and the tumor presents as a firm, slow-growing mass. Though benign, recurrence is common if not completely resected. Malignant tumors such as *mucoepidermoid carcinoma, adenoid cystic carcinoma,* and *adenocarcinoma* tend to grow relatively fast, depending upon grade. They may ulcerate and invade nerves, producing numbness and facial paralysis and correspondingly worsen overall prognosis; 5-year survival is about 68% for malignant salivary gland cancers.

DENTAL CARE OF MEDICALLY COMPLEX PATIENTS Procedures performed in the course of routine dental care (e.g., extraction, scaling and cleaning, tooth restoration, and root canal) are remarkably safe. The most common concerns that arise in the care of dental patients with medical disease are fear of excessive bleeding for patients on anticoagulants, infection of the heart valves and prosthetic devices from hematogenous seeding of oral flora, and cardiovascular complication resulting from vasopressors used with local anesthetic during dental treatment. Experience has confirmed that the risks of any of these complications are very low—far lower than many physicians or dentists imagine.

Patients undergoing tooth extraction or alveolar and gingival surgery rarely experience uncontrolled bleeding when warfarin anticoagulation is maintained within the therapeutic range currently recommended for prevention of venous thrombosis, atrial fibrillation, or mechanical heart valve. While the risk of bleeding is low, embolic complications and death have been reported during subtherapeutic anticoagulation. Therapeutic anticoagulation should be confirmed before and continued through the procedure. Likewise, low-dose aspirin (e.g., 81 to 325 mg) can be safely continued. Bleeding is controlled with local pressure (e.g., gauze), suturing, topical thrombin, or tranexamic acid mouthwash.

Patients at high or moderate risk for bacterial endocarditis (Chap. 109) should maintain optimal oral hygiene, including flossing, and have regular professional cleaning. Prophylactic antibiotics are recommended for all at-risk patients who undergo dental and oral procedures likely to cause significant bleeding and therefore bacteremia. Should unexpected bleeding occur, antibiotics given within 2 h following the procedure will provide effective prophylaxis.

Hematogenous bacterial seeding from oral infection can undoubtedly produce late prosthetic joint infection and therefore requires removal of the infected tissue (e.g., drainage, extraction, root canal) and appropriate antibiotic therapy. However, scientific evidence that late prosthetic joint infection occurs following routine dental procedures

is lacking. For this reason, antibiotic prophylaxis is not recommended before dental surgery in patients with orthopedic pins, screws, and plates. It is, however, advised within the first 2 years after joint replacement and for patients with prosthetic joints who have inflammatory arthropathies, immunosuppression (e.g., drug-, radiation-, or disease-induced), type 1 diabetes mellitus, previous prosthetic joint infection, hemophilia, or malnourishment.

Concern often arises regarding the use of vasoconstrictors in patients with hypertension and heart disease. Vasoconstrictors enhance the depth and duration of local anesthesia, thus reducing the anesthetic dose and potential toxicity. If caution is used to avoid intravascular injection, 2% lidocaine with 1:100,000 epinephrine (limited to a total of 0.036 mg epinephrine) can be used safely in those with controlled hypertension and stable coronary heart disease, arrhythmia, or congestive heart failure. Precaution should be taken with patients taking tricyclic antidepressants and nonselective beta blockers since these drugs may potentiate the effect of epinephrine.

Elective dental treatments should be postponed for at least 1 month after myocardial infarction. After this time the risk of reinfarction is low provided the patient is medically stable (e.g., stable rhythm, stable angina, and free of heart failure). Patients who have suffered a stroke should have elective dental care deferred until 6 months after the cerebrovascular accident. In both situations, effective stress reduction requires good pain control. This includes using the minimal amount of vasoconstrictor necessary to provide good hemostasis and local anesthesia.

HALITOSIS Halitosis, or "bad breath," typically emanates from the oral cavity or nasal passages. Volatile sulfur compounds resulting from bacterial decay of food and cellular debris account for the malodor. Periodontal disease, caries and acute forms of gingivitis, poorly fitting dentures, oral abscess, and tongue coating are usual causes. Treatment includes correcting poor hygiene, treating infection, and tongue brushing. Any cause for xerostomia can produce and exacerbate halitosis. Temporary odor due to diet (e.g., garlic) should be self-evident. Pockets of decay in the tonsillar crypts, esophageal diverticulum, esophageal stasis (e.g., achalasia, stricture), sinusitis, and lung abscess account for some instances. A few systemic diseases produce distinctive odors: renal failure (ammoniacal, urinary), hepatic (fishy), and ketoacidosis (sweet, fruity). *Helicobacter pylori* gastritis can also be associated with ammoniacal breath. Distinguishing an oral from a nasal source is accomplished by pinching the nose while exhaling through the mouth and closing the mouth while exhaling through the nose. If no odor is objectively detectable, then pseudo-halitosis or even halitophobia must be considered. These conditions represent varying degrees of psychiatric illness.

AGING AND ORAL HEALTH While tooth loss and dental disease are not normal consequences of aging, a complex array of structural and functional changes occurs with age that can impact oral heath. Subtle changes in tooth structure (e.g., diminished pulp space and volume, sclerosis of dentinal tubules, altered proportions of nerve and vascular pulp content) result in diminished or altered pain sensitivity, reduced reparative capacity, and increased tooth brittleness. In addition age-associated fatty replacement of salivary acini may reduce physiologic reserve, thus increasing the risk of xerostomia due to medication and disease.

Poor oral hygiene often results when vision fails or when patients lose manual dexterity and upper extremity flexibility. This is particularly common for nursing home residents and must be emphasized since regular oral cleaning and dental care has been shown to reduce the incidence of pneumonia. Other risks for dental decay include limited lifetime fluoride exposure and preference by some older adults for intensely sweet foods when taste and olfaction wane. These factors occur in an increasing proportion of persons over age 75 who retain teeth that have extensive restorations and exposed roots. Without assiduous personal and professional care, decay can become quite advanced, yet remain asymptomatic. The result is that much of a tooth or the entire tooth can become destroyed before the process is detected.

Periodontal disease, a leading cause of tooth loss, is indicated by loss of alveolar bone height. Over 90% of Americans have some degree of periodontal disease by age 50. Healthy adults who have not experienced significant alveolar bone loss by the sixth decade do not typically develop significant worsening with advancing age.

Complete edentulousness with advanced age is less common than in previous decades. Nevertheless, it is still present in approximately 50% of Americans age ≥85. Speech, mastication, and facial contours are dramatically affected. Dentures can improve speech articulation and restore diminished facial contours. Mastication is restored less predictably and improves chewing to no more than 15% of natural ability. Those expecting dentures to improve oral intake are often disappointed. On the other hand, more acceptable cosmetic appearance, clearer speech, and modestly improved chewing are attainable goals. Dentures require periodic adjustment to accommodate inevitable remodeling that leads to a diminished volume of the alveolar ridge. Pain can result from friction or traumatic lesions produced by loose dentures. Poor fit and poor oral hygiene may create an environment that allows candidiasis to develop. This may be asymptomatic or painful and is indicated by erythematous smooth or granular tissue conforming to an area covered by the appliance.

ACKNOWLEDGMENT

The author acknowledges the contribution to this chapter by the previous author, Dr. John S. Greenspan.

FURTHER READING

LITTLE JW et al (eds): *Dental Management of the Medically Compromised Patient*, 6th ed. St. Louis, Mosby, 2002

REGEZI JA, SCIUBBA JJ: *Oral Pathology: Clinical Pathologic Correlations*. 4th ed. Philadelphia, Saunders, 2002

SHIP JA et al: Xerostomia and the geriatric patient. J Am Geriatr Soc 50:535, 2002

SILVERMAN S et al (eds): *Essentials of Oral Medicine*. Ontario, BC Decker, 2002

TAKEYOSHI Y et al: Oral care reduces pneumonia in older patients in nursing homes. J Am Geriatr Soc 50:430, 2002

Section 5   Alterations in Circulatory and Respiratory Functions

29 DYSPNEA AND PULMONARY EDEMA
Roland H. Ingram, Jr., Eugene Braunwald

DYSPNEA

Breathing is controlled by central and peripheral mechanisms that adjust ventilation appropriate to increased metabolic demands during physical activity and increase ventilation in excess of metabolic demands in conditions such as anxiety and fear. A normal resting person is unaware of the act of breathing, and while he or she may become conscious of breathing during mild to moderate exertion, no discomfort is experienced. However, during and following exhausting exertion, an individual may become unpleasantly aware of breathing yet feel reasonably assured that the sensation will be transitory and is appropriate to the level of exercise. Therefore, as a cardinal symptom of diseases affecting the cardiorespiratory system, *dyspnea* is defined as an *abnormally uncomfortable awareness of breathing*.

Although dyspnea is not painful in the usual sense of the word, it is, like pain, involved with both the perception of a sensation and the reaction to that perception. Patients experience a number of uncomfortable sensations related to breathing and use an even larger number of verbal expressions to describe these sensations, such as "cannot get enough air," "air does not go all the way down," "smothering feeling or tightness or tiredness in the chest," and a "choking sensation." It may be necessary, therefore, to review the patient's history meticulously in order to ascertain whether the more abstruse descriptions do, in fact, represent dyspnea. Once it is established that a patient has dyspnea, it is of paramount importance to define the circumstances in which it occurs and to assess associated symptoms. There are situations in which breathing appears labored but in which dyspnea does not occur. For example, the hyperventilation associated with metabolic acidemia is rarely accompanied by dyspnea. On the other hand, patients with apparently normal breathing patterns may complain of shortness of breath.

QUANTITATION OF DYSPNEA   The gradation of dyspnea is based on the amount of physical exertion required to produce the sensation. In assessing the severity of dyspnea, it is important to obtain a clear understanding of the patient's general physical condition, work history, and recreational habits. For example, the development of dyspnea in a trained runner upon running 2 mi may signify a much more serious disturbance than a similar degree of breathlessness in a sedentary person upon running a fraction of this distance. Interindividual variation in perception must also be considered. Some patients with severe disease may complain of only mild dyspnea; others with mild disease may experience more severe shortness of breath. Some patients with lung or heart disease may have such reduced capabilities due to other disease (e.g., peripheral vascular insufficiency or severe osteoarthritis of the hips or knees) that exertional dyspnea is precluded despite serious impairment of pulmonary or cardiac function.

Some patterns of dyspnea are not directly related to physical exertion. Sudden and unexpected dyspneic episodes at rest can be associated with pulmonary emboli, spontaneous pneumothorax, hypercapnea secondary to breath holding, or anxiety. Nocturnal episodes of severe paroxysmal dyspnea are characteristic of left ventricular failure. Dyspnea upon assuming the supine posture, *orthopnea* (see below and Chap. 216), thought to be mainly characteristic of congestive heart failure, may also occur in some patients with asthma and chronic obstruction of the airways and is a regular finding in the rare occurrence of bilateral diaphragmatic paralysis. *Trepopnea* is used to describe the unusual circumstance in which dyspnea occurs only in a lateral decubitus position, most often in patients with heart disease, while *platypnea* is dyspnea that occurs only in the upright position. Positional alterations in ventilation-perfusion relationships (Chap. 234) have been invoked to explain these patterns.

MECHANISMS OF DYSPNEA (See Fig. 29-1)   Dyspnea occurs whenever the work of breathing is excessive. Increased force generation is required of the respiratory muscles to produce a given volume change if the chest wall or lungs are less compliant or if resistance to airflow is increased. Increased work of breathing also occurs when the venti-

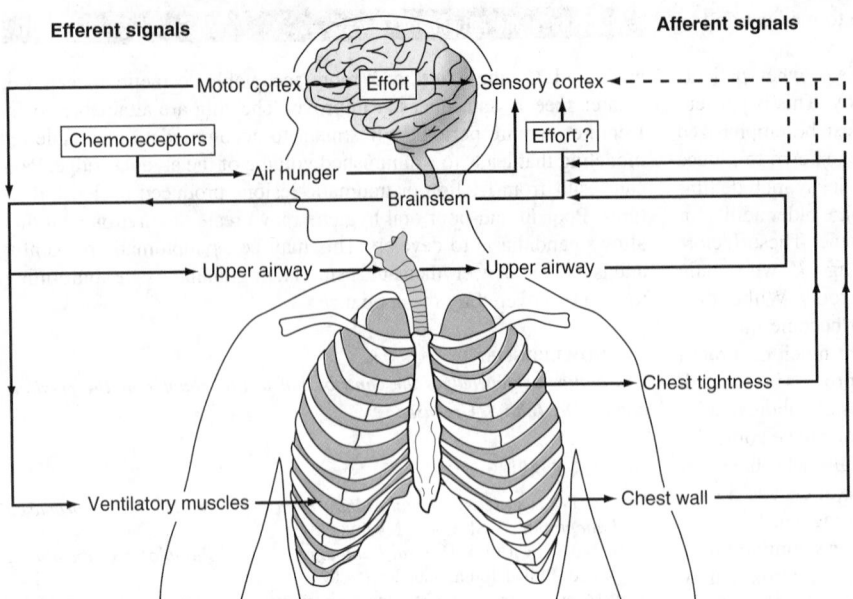

Efferent signals   **Afferent signals**

Motor cortex — Effort — Sensory cortex

Chemoreceptors

Air hunger

Brainstem

Upper airway → Upper airway

Chest tightness

Ventilatory muscles   Chest wall

Effort ?

FIGURE 29-1 Efferent and afferent signals that contribute to the sensation of dyspnea. There is evidence that the sense of respiratory effort arises from a signal transmitted from the motor cortex to the sensory cortex simultaneously with the outgoing motor command to the ventilatory muscles. The motor output of the brainstem may also contribute to the sense of effort, as shown in the arrow from the brainstem to the sensory cortex. The sense of air hunger arises, in part, from increased respiratory activity within the brainstem, and the sensation of chest tightness probably results from stimulation of vagal-irritant receptors. While afferent information from airway, lung, and chest wall receptors probably passes through the brainstem before reaching the sensory cortex, the dashed lines indicate uncertainty about whether some afferents bypass the brainstem and project directly to the sensory cortex. (*From HL Manning, RM Schwartzstein, Pathophysiology of dyspnea. N Engl J Med 333:1547, 1995, with permission.*)

lation is excessive for the level of activity. Although an individual is more apt to become dyspneic when the work of breathing is increased, the work theory does not account for the perceptual difference between a deep breath with a normal mechanical load and a normal-sized breath with an increased mechanical load. The work might be the same with both breaths, but the normal one with the increased load will be associated with discomfort. In fact, with respiratory loading, such as adding a resistance at the mouth, there is an increase in respiratory center output that is disproportionate to the increase in the work of breathing. It has been postulated that whenever the force that muscles actually generate during breathing approaches some fraction of their maximal force-generating ability, which may vary among individuals, dyspnea ensues due to transduction of mechanical to neural stimuli.

In all likelihood, several different mechanisms operate to different degrees in the various clinical situations in which dyspnea occurs. In some circumstances, dyspnea is evoked by stimulation of receptors in the upper respiratory tract; in others it may originate from receptors in the lungs, airways, respiratory muscles, chest wall, or some combination of these structures. In any event, dyspnea is characterized by an excessive or abnormal activation of the respiratory centers in the brainstem. This activation comes about from stimuli transmitted from or through a variety of structures and pathways, including (1) intrathoracic receptors via the vagal nerves; (2) afferent somatic nerves, particularly from the respiratory muscles and chest wall, but also from other skeletal muscles and joints; (3) chemoreceptors in the brain, aortic, and carotid bodies, and elsewhere in the circulation; (4) higher (cortical) centers; and perhaps (5) afferent fibers in the phrenic nerves. In general, despite the interindividual variations described above, there is a reasonable correlation between the severity of dyspnea and the magnitude of disturbances of pulmonary or cardiac function that are responsible.

The mechanisms responsible for dyspnea may vary in different conditions (Table 29-1).

DIFFERENTIAL DIAGNOSIS ■ Obstructive Disease of Airways (See also Chaps. 236 and 242)

Obstruction to airflow can be present anywhere from the extrathoracic airways out to the small airways in the periphery of the lung. Large extrathoracic airway obstruction can occur acutely, as with aspiration of food or a foreign body, or with angioedema of the glottis. An allergic history together with a few scattered hives should raise the possibility of glottic edema. Acute upper airway obstruction is a medical emergency. More chronic forms can occur with tumors or with fibrotic stenosis following tracheostomy or prolonged endotracheal intubation. Whether acute or chronic, the cardinal symptom is dyspnea, and the characteristic signs are stridor and retraction of the supraclavicular fossae with *inspiration*.

Obstruction of intrathoracic airways can occur acutely and intermittently or can be present chronically with worsening during respiratory infections. Acute intermittent obstruction with wheezing is typical of *asthma* (Chap. 236). Chronic cough with expectoration is typical of *chronic bronchitis* (Chap. 242) and *bronchiectasis* (Chap. 240). Most often there are prolongation of expiration and coarse rhonchi that are generalized in chronic bronchitis and may be localized in the case of bronchiectasis. Intercurrent infection results in worsening of the cough, increased expectoration of purulent sputum, and more severe dyspnea. During such episodes, the patient may complain of nocturnal paroxysms of dyspnea with wheezing relieved by cough and expectoration of sputum. Despite the fact that severe limitation of expiratory flow and hyperinflation of the lung are characteristic of these diseases, the sensory experience is often that of an inability to take in a sufficiently deep breath rather than difficulty in exhaling.

The patient with predominant *emphysema* is characterized by many years of exertional dyspnea progressing to dyspnea at rest (Chap. 242). Although a parenchymal disease by definition, emphysema is invariably accompanied by obstruction of airways.

Diffuse Parenchymal Lung Diseases (See also Chap. 243) This category includes a large number of diseases ranging from acute pneumonia to chronic disorders such as sarcoidosis and the various forms of *pneumoconiosis* (Chap. 238). History, physical findings, and radiographic abnormalities often provide clues to the diagnosis. The patients are often tachypneic with arterial P_{CO_2} and P_{O_2} values below normal. Exertion often further reduces the arterial P_{O_2}. Lung volumes are decreased, and the lungs are stiffer, i.e., less compliant, than normal.

Pulmonary Vascular Occlusive Diseases (See also Chap. 244) Repeated episodes of dyspnea at rest often occur with recurrent pulmonary em-

TABLE 29-1 *Likely Mechanisms of Dyspnea in Selected Conditions*

Condition	Mechanism
Asthma	Increased sense of effort
	Stimulation of irritant receptors in airways
Neuromuscular disease	Increased sense of effort
COPD	Increased sense of effort
	Hypoxia
	Hypercapnia
	Dynamic airway compression
Mechanical ventilation	Afferent mismatch
	Factors associated with the underlying condition
Pulmonary embolism	Stimulation of pressure receptors in pulmonary vasculature or right atrium (possible)

Note: COPD, chronic obstructive pulmonary disease.
Source: From HL Manning, RM Schwartzstein, Pathophysiology of dyspnea. N Engl J Med 333:1547, 1995, with permission.

boli. Near syncope on exertion is another suggestive symptom. Evidence of a source for emboli, such as phlebitis of a lower extremity or the pelvis, is quite helpful in leading the physician to suspect the diagnosis. Arterial blood gases are most often abnormal, but lung volumes are frequently normal or only minimally abnormal.

Diseases of the Chest Wall or Respiratory Muscles (See also Chap. 246) The physical examination establishes the presence of a chest wall disease such as severe kyphoscoliosis, pectus excavatum, or ankylosing spondylitis. Although all three of these deformities may be associated with dyspnea, only severe kyphoscoliosis regularly interferes with ventilation sufficiently to produce chronic cor pulmonale and respiratory failure.

Both weakness and paralysis of respiratory muscles can lead to respiratory failure and dyspnea (Chap. 246), but most often the signs and symptoms of the neurologic or muscular disorder are more prominently manifested in other systems.

Heart Disease In patients with cardiac disease, exertional dyspnea occurs most commonly as a consequence of an elevated pulmonary capillary pressure, which in turn may be due to left ventricular dysfunction (Chaps. 215 and 216), reduced left ventricular compliance, and mitral stenosis. The elevation of hydrostatic pressure in the pulmonary vascular bed tends to upset the Starling equilibrium (see "Pulmonary Edema," below) with resulting transudation of liquid into the interstitial space, reducing the compliance of the lungs and stimulating J (juxtacapillary) receptors in the alveolar interstitial space. When it is prolonged, pulmonary venous hypertension results in thickening of the walls of small pulmonary vessels and an increase in perivascular cells and fibrous tissue, causing a further reduction in compliance. The competition for space among vessels, airways, and increased fluid within the interstitial space compromises the lumina of small airways, increasing the airways' resistance. Diminution in compliance and an increase in the airways' resistance increase the work of breathing. In advanced congestive heart failure, usually involving elevation of both pulmonary and systemic venous pressures, hydrothorax may develop, interfering further with pulmonary function and intensifying dyspnea.

Orthopnea, i.e., dyspnea in the supine position, is the result of the alteration of gravitational forces when this position is assumed, which elevates pulmonary venous and capillary pressures. These, in turn, increase the pulmonary closing volume (Chap. 234) and reduce the vital capacity.

PAROXYSMAL NOCTURNAL DYSPNEA Also known as *cardiac asthma*, this condition is characterized by attacks of severe shortness of breath that generally occur at night and usually awaken the patient from sleep. The attack is precipitated by stimuli that aggravate previously existing pulmonary congestion; frequently, the total blood volume is augmented at night because of the reabsorption of edema from dependent portions of the body during recumbency. A sleeping patient can tolerate relatively severe pulmonary engorgement and may awaken only when actual pulmonary edema and bronchospasm have developed, with the feeling of suffocation and with wheezing respirations.

Two other forms of nocturnal dyspnea must be distinguished from that due to heart failure. Chronic bronchitis is characterized by mucus hypersecretion and, after a few hours sleep, secretions can accumulate and produce dyspnea and wheezing, both of which are relieved by cough and expectoration of sputum. Asthma patients have circadian variations in their degree of airway obstruction. The obstruction becomes most severe between 2 A.M. and 4 A.M. and can be sufficiently severe that the patient awakens with a sense of suffocation, extreme dyspnea, and wheezing. Although there is a prominent inflammatory component to nocturnal asthma, inhaled bronchodilators usually improve symptoms quickly.

CHEYNE-STOKES RESPIRATION See Chap. 216 ■ *Diagnosis* The diagnosis of cardiac dyspnea depends on the recognition of heart disease on the basis of the clinical examination supplemented by noninvasive testing. There may be a history of antecedent myocardial infarction; third and fourth heart sounds may be audible; and/or there may be evidence of

left ventricular enlargement, jugular neck vein distention, and/or peripheral edema. Often there are radiographic signs of heart failure, with evidence of interstitial edema, pulmonary vascular redistribution, and accumulation of liquid in the septal planes and pleural cavity. Transthoracic echocardiography is particularly useful in establishing the diagnosis of structural heart disease, which can be responsible for dyspnea. Specifically, left atrial and/or left ventricular dilatation, left ventricular hypertrophy, a reduced left ventricular ejection fraction, and disorders of left ventricular wall motion may be clues to the presence of a cardiac etiology of otherwise unexplained dyspnea.

DIFFERENTIATION BETWEEN CARDIAC AND PULMONARY DYSPNEA In most patients with dyspnea there is obvious clinical evidence of disease of the heart and/or lungs. Like patients with cardiac dyspnea, patients with chronic obstructive lung disease may also waken at night with dyspnea, but, as pointed out above, this is usually associated with sputum production; the dyspnea is relieved after these patients rid themselves of secretions. The difficulty in the distinction between cardiac and pulmonary dyspnea may be compounded by the coexistence of diseases involving both organ systems.

In patients in whom the etiology of dyspnea is not clear, it is desirable to carry out pulmonary function testing, for these tests may be helpful in determining whether dyspnea is produced by heart disease, lung disease, abnormalities of the chest wall, or anxiety (Chap. 235). In addition to the usual means of assessing patients for heart disease, determination of the ejection fraction at rest and during exercise by echocardiography or radionuclide ventriculography is helpful in the differential diagnosis of dyspnea. The left ventricular ejection fraction is depressed in left ventricular failure, while the right ventricular ejection fraction may be low at rest or may decline during exercise in patients with severe lung disease. Both left and right ventricular ejection fractions are normal at rest and during exercise in dyspnea due to anxiety or malingering. Careful observation during the performance of an exercise treadmill test will often help in the identification of the patient who is malingering or whose dyspnea is secondary to anxiety. Under these circumstances, the patient usually complains of severe shortness of breath but appears to be breathing either effortlessly or totally irregularly. Cardiopulmonary testing, in which the patient's maximal functional exercise capacity is assessed while measurements of the electrocardiogram, blood pressure, oxygen consumption, arterial saturation (oximetry), and ventilation are carried out, is useful in the differentiation between cardiac and pulmonary dyspnea (Table 29-2).

ANXIETY STATES Dyspnea experienced by a patient with anxiety alone is difficult to evaluate. The signs and symptoms of acute and chronic

---

TABLE 29-2 Patterns of Abnormality in Cardiopulmonary Exercise Testing[a]

Cardiovascular limitation
  Heart rate ≥85% of predicted maximum
  Low anaerobic threshold
  Reduced maximal oxygen consumption
  Drop in blood pressure with exercise
  Arrhythmias or ischemic changes on ECG
  Does not achieve maximal predicted ventilation
  Does not have significant desaturation
Respiratory limitation
  Achieves or exceeds maximal predicted ventilation
  Significant desaturation (<90%)
  Stable or increase dead space–to–tidal volume ratio
  Development or bronchospasm with falling FEV_1
  Does not achieve 85% of predicted maximal heart rate
  No ischemic ECG changes

[a] All features will not be present in a particular case, and there may be elements of both cardiovascular and respiratory causes of shortness of breath. One looks for the predominant pattern in assessing the etiology of the patient's exercise limitation.
Note: ECG, electrocardiogram; FEV_1, forced expiratory volume in 1 s.
Source: From RM Schwartzstein, D Feller-Kopman, in E Braunwald, L Goldman (eds): *Primary Cardiology*, 2d ed. Philadelphia, Saunders, 2003

hyperventilation do not serve to distinguish between anxiety states and other processes, such as recurrent pulmonary emboli. Another potentially confusing situation is seen when chest pain and electrocardiographic changes accompany the hyperventilation syndrome. When present and attributable to this condition, also referred to as *neurocirculatory asthenia*, the chest pain is often sharp, fleeting, and in various loci, and the electrocardiographic changes are most often seen during repolarization. Frequent sighing respirations and an irregular breathing pattern point to a psychogenic origin of the dyspnea. Anxiety and depression in association with heart or lung disease can serve to intensify dyspnea symptoms beyond what would be expected for a given degree of dysfunction.

PULMONARY EDEMA

CARDIOGENIC PULMONARY EDEMA (See Table 29-3, IA) An increase in pulmonary venous pressure, which results initially in engorgement of the pulmonary vasculature, is common in most instances of dyspnea in association with congestive heart failure. The lungs become less compliant, the resistance of small airways increases, and there is an increase in lymphatic flow that apparently serves to maintain a constant pulmonary extravascular liquid volume. Mild tachypnea is present. If the increase in intravascular pressure is sufficient both in magnitude and duration, there is a net gain of liquid in the extravascular space, i.e., *interstitial* edema. At this point symptoms worsen, tachypnea increases, gas exchange deteriorates further, and radiographic changes, such as Kerley B lines and loss of distinct vascular margins, are seen. At this stage, the capillary endothelial intercellular junctions widen and allow passage of macromolecules into the interstices.

Further elevations in intravascular pressure disrupt the tight junctions between alveolar lining cells, and *alveolar* edema ensues, with outpouring of liquid that contains both red blood cells and macromolecules. With yet more severe disruption of the alveolar-capillary membrane, edematous liquid floods the alveoli and airways. At this point, full-blown clinical pulmonary edema with bilateral wet rales and rhonchi occurs, and the chest radiograph may show diffuse haziness of the lung fields with greater density in the more proximal hilar regions. Typically, the patient is anxious and perspires freely, and the sputum is frothy and bloodtinged. Gas exchange is more severely compromised with worsening hypoxia. Without effective treatment (Chap. 255), progressive acidemia, hypercapnia, and respiratory arrest ensue.

The sequence of liquid accumulation described above follows the Starling law of capillary-interstitial liquid exchange:

$$\text{Liquid accumulation} = K[(P_c - P_{IF}) - \sigma(\pi_{pl} - \pi_{IF})] - Q_{lymph}$$

where K, hydraulic conductance (directly proportional to membrane surface area and inversely proportional to membrane thickness); P_c, mean intracapillary pressure; π_{IF}, oncotic pressure of interstitial liquid; σ, reflection coefficient of macromolecules; P_{IF}, mean interstitial liquid pressure; π_{pl}, oncotic pressure of the plasma; Q_{lymph}, lymphatic flow.

The pressures tending to move liquid out of the vessel are P_c and π_{IF}, which are normally more than offset by pressures tending to move liquid back into the vasculature, i.e., the algebraic sum of P_{IF} and π_{pl}. Implicit in the preceding equation is that lymphatic flow can increase in the case of imbalance of forces and result in no net accumulation of interstitial liquid. Further elevations in P_c not only increase the outward movement of liquid in each capillary region but also recruit more of the capillary bed, which increases K. These two effects lead to liquid filtration that exceeds clearance capability by the lymphatics, and liquid accumulates in the loose interstitial spaces of the lung. Even greater increases in P_c open first the loose endothelial intercellular junctions and later the tight alveolar intercellular junctions with an increase in permeability to macromolecules. This secondary disruption of both the function and structure of the alveolar-capillary membrane leads to alveolar flooding.

NONCARDIOGENIC PULMONARY EDEMA (See Table 29-3, IB, IC, II, III, and IV) Several clinical conditions are associated with pulmonary edema based on an imbalance of Starling forces other than through primary elevations of pulmonary capillary pressure. Although diminished plasma oncotic pressure in hypoalbuminemic states (e.g., severe liver disease, nephrotic syndrome, protein-losing enteropathy) might be expected to lead to pulmonary edema, the balance of forces normally so strongly favors resorption that even in these conditions some elevation of capillary pressure is usually necessary before interstitial edema develops. Increased negativity of interstitial pressure has been implicated in the genesis of unilateral pulmonary edema following rapid evacuation of a large pneumothorax. In this situation, the findings may be apparent only by radiography, but occasionally the patient experiences dyspnea with physical findings localized to the edematous lung. It has been proposed that large negative intrapleural pressures during acute severe asthma may be associated with the development of interstitial edema. Lymphatic blockade secondary to fibrotic and inflammatory diseases or lymphangitic carcinomatosis may lead to interstitial edema. In such instances, both clinical and radiographic manifestations are dominated by the underlying disease process.

Other conditions characterized by increases in the interstitial liquid content of the lungs appear to be associated primarily with disruption of the alveolar-capillary membranes. Any number of spontaneously occurring or environmental toxic insults, including diffuse pulmonary infections, aspiration, and shock (particularly due to sepsis, hemor-

---

TABLE 29-3 *Classification of Pulmonary Edema Based on Initiating Mechanism*

I. Imbalance of Starling forces
  A. Increased pulmonary capillary pressure
    1. Increased pulmonary venous pressure without left ventricular failure (e.g., mitral stenosis)
    2. Increased pulmonary venous pressure secondary to left ventricular failure
    3. Increased pulmonary capillary pressure secondary to increased pulmonary arterial pressure (so-called overperfusion pulmonary edema)
  B. Decreased plasma oncotic pressure
    1. Hypoalbuminemia
  C. Increased negativity of interstitial pressure
    1. Rapid removal of pneumothorax with large applied negative pressures (unilateral)
    2. Large negative pleural pressures due to acute airway obstruction alone with increased end-expiratory volumes (asthma)
II. Altered alveolar-capillary membrane permeability (acute respiratory distress syndrome)
  A. Infectious pneumonia—bacterial, viral, parasitic
  B. Inhaled toxins (e.g., phosgene, ozone, chlorine, Teflon fumes, nitrogen dioxide, smoke)
  C. Circulating foreign substances (e.g., snake venom, bacterial endotoxins)
  D. Aspiration of acidic gastric contents
  E. Acute radiation pneumonitis
  F. Endogenous vasoactive substances (e.g., histamine, kinins)
  G. Disseminated intravascular coagulation
  H. Immunologic—hypersensitivity pneumonitis, drugs (nitrofurantoin), leukoagglutinins
  I. Shock lung in association with nonthoracic trauma
  J. Acute hemorrhagic pancreatitis
III. Lymphatic insufficiency
  A. After lung transplant
  B. Lymphangitic carcinomatosis
  C. Fibrosing lymphangitis (e.g., silicosis)
IV. Unknown or incompletely understood
  A. High-altitude pulmonary edema
  B. Neurogenic pulmonary edema
  C. Narcotic overdose
  D. Pulmonary embolism
  E. Eclampsia
  F. After cardioversion
  G. After anesthesia
  H. After cardiopulmonary bypass

Source: From Braunwald et al., with permission.

rhagic pancreatitis, and following cardiopulmonary bypass), are associated with diffuse pulmonary edema that clearly does not have a hemodynamic origin. →*These conditions, which may lead to the acute respiratory distress syndrome, are discussed in Chap. 251.*

Other Forms of Pulmonary Edema There are three forms of pulmonary edema whose precise mechanism remains unexplained. *Narcotic overdose* is a well-recognized antecedent to pulmonary edema. Although illicit use of parenteral heroin is the most frequent cause, parenteral and oral overdoses of legitimate preparations of morphine, methadone, and dextropropoxyphene have also been associated with pulmonary edema. The earlier idea that injected impurities lead to the disorder is untenable. Available evidence suggests that there are alterations in the permeability of alveolar and capillary membranes rather than an elevation of pulmonary capillary pressure.

Exposure to high altitude in association with severe physical exertion is a well-recognized setting for pulmonary edema in unacclimatized yet otherwise healthy persons. Acclimatized high-altitude natives also develop this syndrome upon return to high altitude after a relatively brief sojourn at low altitudes. The syndrome is far more common in persons under the age of 25 years. The mechanism for high-altitude pulmonary edema (HAPE) remains obscure, and studies have been conflicting, some suggesting pulmonary venous constriction and others indicating pulmonary arteriolar constriction as the prime mechanisms. A role for hypoxia at high altitude is suggested by the fact that patients respond to the administration of oxygen and/or return to lower altitudes. Hypoxia per se does not alter permeability of the alveolar-capillary membrane. Hence increased cardiac output and pulmonary arterial pressures with exercise combined with hypoxic pulmonary arteriolar constriction, which is more prominent in young persons, may combine to make this an example of prearteriolar, high-pressure pulmonary edema. HAPE has also been attributed to a defect in the absorption of liquid driven by active alveolar transepithelial sodium transport. Prophylactic inhalation of the β_2 agonist salmeterol has been shown to reduce the incidence of this condition.

Neurogenic pulmonary edema has been described in patients with central nervous system disorders and without apparent preexisting left ventricular dysfunction. Although most experimental studies have implicated sympathetic nervous system activity, the mechanism whereby sympathetic efferent activity leads to pulmonary edema is a matter of speculation. It is known that a massive adrenergic nerve discharge leads to peripheral vasoconstriction with elevation of blood pressure and shifts of blood to the central circulation. In addition, it is probable that a reduction in left ventricular compliance also occurs, and both factors serve to increase left atrial pressures sufficiently to induce pulmonary edema on a hemodynamic basis. Some experimental evidence suggests that stimulation of adrenergic receptors increases capillary permeability directly, but this effect is relatively minor as compared with the imbalance of Starling forces.

TREATMENT OF PULMONARY EDEMA See Chap. 255

FURTHER READING

GIVERTZ ME et al: Clinical aspects of heart failure; high-output heart failure; pulmonary edema, in D Zipes et al (eds), *Braunwald's Heart Disease*, 7th ed, Philadelphia, Saunders, 2005

MANNING HL, SCHWARTZSTEIN RM: Respiratory symptoms in asthma: Physiological and clinical implications. J Asthma 38:447, 2001

MANNING HL, MAHLER DA: Pathophysiology of dyspnea. Monaldi Arch Chest Dis 56:325, 2001

SCHWARTZSTEIN RM, FELLER-KOPMAN D: Approach to the patient with dyspnea, in E Braunwald, L Goldman (eds), *Primary Cardiology*, 2d ed, Philadelphia, Elsevier, 2003

30 COUGH AND HEMOPTYSIS
Steven E. Weinberger

COUGH

Cough is an explosive expiration that provides a normal protective mechanism for clearing the tracheobronchial tree of secretions and foreign material. When excessive or bothersome, it is also one of the most common symptoms for which medical attention is sought. Reasons for the latter include discomfort from the cough itself, interference with normal lifestyle, and concern for the cause of the cough, especially fear of cancer.

MECHANISM

Coughing may be initiated either voluntarily or reflexively. As a defensive reflex it has both afferent and efferent pathways. The *afferent limb* includes receptors within the sensory distribution of the trigeminal, glossopharyngeal, superior laryngeal, and vagus nerves. The *efferent limb* includes the recurrent laryngeal nerve and the spinal nerves. The cough starts with a deep inspiration followed by glottic closure, relaxation of the diaphragm, and muscle contraction against a closed glottis. The resulting markedly positive intrathoracic pressure causes narrowing of the trachea. Once the glottis opens, the large pressure differential between the airways and the atmosphere coupled with tracheal narrowing produces rapid flow rates through the trachea. The shearing forces that develop aid in the elimination of mucus and foreign materials.

ETIOLOGY

Cough can be initiated by a variety of irritant triggers either from an exogenous source (smoke, dust, fumes, foreign bodies) or from an endogenous origin (upper airway secretions, gastric contents). These stimuli may affect receptors in the upper airway (especially the pharynx and larynx) or in the lower respiratory tract, following access to the tracheobronchial tree by inhalation or by aspiration. When cough is triggered by upper airway secretions (as with postnasal drip) or gastric contents (as with gastroesophageal reflux), the initiating factor may go unrecognized and the cough can be persistent. Additionally, prolonged exposure to such irritants may initiate airway inflammation, which can itself precipitate cough and sensitize the airway to other irritants. Cough associated with gastroesophageal reflux is due only in part to irritation of upper airway receptors or to aspiration of gastric contents, as a vagally mediated reflex mechanism secondary to acid in the distal esophagus may also contribute.

Any disorder resulting in inflammation, constriction, infiltration, or compression of airways can be associated with cough. Inflammation commonly results from airway infections, ranging from viral or bacterial bronchitis to bronchiectasis. In viral bronchitis, airway inflammation sometimes persists long after resolution of the typical acute symptoms, thereby producing a prolonged cough, lasting for weeks. Pertussis infection is also a possible cause of persistent cough in adults; however, diagnosis is generally made on clinical grounds (Chap. 133). Asthma is a common cause of cough. Although the clinical setting commonly suggests when a cough is secondary to asthma, some patients present with cough in the absence of wheezing or dyspnea, thus making the diagnosis more subtle ("cough variant asthma"). A neoplasm infiltrating the airway wall, such as bronchogenic carcinoma or a carcinoid tumor, is commonly associated with cough. Airway infiltration with granulomas may also trigger a cough, as seen with endobronchial sarcoidosis or tuberculosis. Compression of airways results from extrinsic masses, including lymph nodes, mediastinal tumors, and aortic aneurysms.

Examples of parenchymal lung disease potentially producing cough include interstitial lung disease, pneumonia, and lung abscess.

Congestive heart failure may be associated with cough, probably as a consequence of interstitial as well as peribronchial edema. A nonproductive cough complicates the use of angiotensin-converting enzyme (ACE) inhibitors in 5 to 20% of patients taking these agents. Onset is usually within 1 week of starting the drug but can be delayed up to 6 months. Although the mechanism is not known with certainty, it may relate to accumulation of bradykinin or substance P, both of which are degraded by ACE.

The most common causes of cough can be categorized according to the duration of the cough. Acute cough (<3 weeks) is most often due to upper respiratory infection (especially the common cold, acute bacterial sinusitis, and pertussis), but more serious disorders, such as pneumonia, pulmonary embolus, and congestive heart failure, can also present in this fashion. Chronic cough (>3 weeks) in a smoker raises the possibilities of chronic obstructive lung disease or bronchogenic carcinoma. In a nonsmoker who has a normal chest radiograph and is not taking an ACE inhibitor, the most common causes of chronic cough are postnasal drip, asthma, and gastroesophageal reflux. Eosinophilic bronchitis in the absence of asthma has also been recognized as a potential cause of chronic cough.

APPROACH TO THE PATIENT

A detailed *history* frequently provides the most valuable clues for etiology of the cough. Particularly important questions include:

1. Is the cough acute or chronic?
2. At its onset, were there associated symptoms suggestive of a respiratory infection?
3. Is it seasonal or associated with wheezing?
4. Is it associated with symptoms suggestive of postnasal drip (nasal discharge, frequent throat clearing, a "tickle in the throat") or gastroesophageal reflux (heartburn or sensation of regurgitation)? (The absence of such suggestive symptoms does not exclude either of these diagnoses, particularly in the case of gastroesophageal reflux.)
5. Is it associated with fever or sputum? If sputum is present, what is its character?
6. Does the patient have any associated diseases or risk factors for disease (e.g., cigarette smoking, risk factors for infection with HIV, environmental exposures)?
7. Is the patient taking an ACE inhibitor?

The general *physical examination* may point to a systemic or nonpulmonary cause of cough, such as heart failure, primary nonpulmonary neoplasm, or AIDS. Examination of the oropharynx may provide suggestive evidence for postnasal drip, including oropharyngeal mucus or erythema, or a "cobblestone" appearance to the mucosa. Auscultation of the chest may demonstrate inspiratory stridor (indicative of upper airway disease), rhonchi or expiratory wheezing (indicative of lower airway disease), or inspiratory crackles (suggestive of a process involving the pulmonary parenchyma, such as interstitial lung disease, pneumonia, or pulmonary edema).

Chest radiography may be particularly helpful in suggesting or confirming the cause of the cough. Important potential findings include the presence of an intrathoracic mass lesion, a localized pulmonary parenchymal infiltrate, or diffuse interstitial or alveolar disease. An area of honeycombing or cyst formation may suggest bronchiectasis, while symmetric bilateral hilar adenopathy may suggest sarcoidosis.

Pulmonary function testing (Chap. 234) is useful for assessing the functional abnormalities that accompany certain disorders producing cough. Measurement of forced expiratory flow rates can demonstrate reversible airflow obstruction characteristic of asthma. When asthma is considered but flow rates are normal, broncho-provocation testing with methacholine or cold-air inhalation can demonstrate hyperreactivity of the airways to a bronchoconstrictive stimulus. Measurement of lung volumes and diffusing capacity is useful primarily for demonstration of a restrictive pattern, often seen with any of the diffuse interstitial lung diseases.

If *sputum* is produced, gross and microscopic examination may provide useful information. Purulent sputum suggests chronic bronchitis, bronchiectasis, pneumonia, or lung abscess. Blood in the sputum may be seen in the same disorders, but its presence also raises the question of an endobronchial tumor. Greater than 3% eosinophils seen on staining of induced sputum in a patient without asthma suggests the possibility of eosinophilic bronchitis. Gram and acid-fast stains and cultures may demonstrate a particular infectious pathogen, while sputum cytology may provide a diagnosis of a pulmonary malignancy.

More specialized studies are helpful in specific circumstances. *Fiberoptic bronchoscopy* is the procedure of choice for visualizing an endobronchial tumor and collecting cytologic and histologic specimens. Inspection of the tracheobronchial mucosa can demonstrate endobronchial granulomas often seen in sarcoidosis, and endobronchial biopsy of such lesions or transbronchial biopsy of the lung interstitium can confirm the diagnosis. Inspection of the airway mucosa by bronchoscopy can also demonstrate the characteristic appearance of endobronchial Kaposi's sarcoma in patients with AIDS. *High-resolution computed tomography* (HRCT) can confirm the presence of interstitial disease and frequently suggests a diagnosis based on the pattern of disease. It is the procedure of choice for demonstrating dilated airways and confirming the diagnosis of bronchiectasis.

A diagnostic algorithm for evaluation of chronic cough is presented in Fig. 30-1.

COMPLICATIONS

Common complications of coughing include chest and abdominal wall soreness, urinary incontinence, and exhaustion. On occasion, paroxysms of coughing may precipitate syncope (cough syncope; Chap. 20), consequent to markedly positive intrathoracic and alveolar pressures, diminished venous return, and decreased cardiac output. Although cough fractures of the ribs may occur in otherwise normal patients, their occurrence should at least raise the possibility of pathologic fractures, which are seen with multiple myeloma, osteoporosis, and osteolytic metastases.

℞ TREATMENT

Definitive treatment of cough depends on determining the underlying cause and then initiating specific therapy. Elimination of an exogenous inciting agent (cigarette smoke, ACE inhibitors) or an endogenous trigger (postnasal drip, gastroesophageal reflux) is usually effective when such a precipitant can be identified. Other important management considerations are treatment of specific respiratory tract infections, bronchodilators for potentially reversible airflow obstruction, inhaled glucocorticoids for eosinophilic bronchitis, chest physiotherapy and other methods to enhance clearance of secretions in patients with bronchiectasis, and treatment of endobronchial tumors or interstitial lung disease when such therapy is available and appropriate. In patients with chronic, unexplained cough, an empirical approach to treatment is often used for both diagnostic and therapeutic purposes, starting with an antihistamine-decongestant combination or nasal ipratropium spray to treat unrecognized postnasal drip. If ineffective, this may be followed sequentially by treatment for asthma and for gastroesophageal reflux.

Symptomatic or nonspecific therapy of cough should be considered when: (1) the cause of the cough is not known or specific treatment is not possible, and (2) the cough performs no useful function or causes marked discomfort. An irritative, nonproductive cough may be suppressed by an antitussive agent, which increases the latency or threshold of the cough center. Such agents include codeine (15 mg qid) or nonnarcotics such as dextromethorphan (15 mg qid). These drugs provide symptomatic relief by interrupting prolonged, self-perpetuating paroxysms. However, a cough productive of significant quantities of sputum should usually not be suppressed, since retention of sputum in the tracheobronchial tree may interfere with the distribution of ventilation, alveolar aeration, and the ability of the lung to resist infection.

Other agents working by a variety of mechanisms have also been used to control cough, but objective information assessing their benefit is meager. For example, the inhaled anticholinergic agent, ipratropium bromide (2 to 4 puffs qid), has been used with the rationale of inhibiting the efferent limb of the cough reflex.

HEMOPTYSIS

Hemoptysis is defined as the expectoration of blood from the respiratory tract, a spectrum that varies from blood-streaking of sputum to coughing up large amounts of pure blood. *Massive hemoptysis* is variably defined as the expectoration of >100 to >600 mL over a 24-h period, although the patient's estimation of the amount of blood is notoriously unreliable. Expectoration of even relatively small amounts of blood is a frightening symptom and can be a marker for potentially serious disease, such as bronchogenic carcinoma. Massive hemoptysis, on the other hand, can represent an acutely life-threatening problem. Large amounts of blood can fill the airways and the alveolar spaces, not only seriously disturbing gas exchange but potentially causing the patient to suffocate.

ETIOLOGY

Because blood originating from the nasopharynx or the gastrointestinal tract can mimic blood coming from the lower respiratory tract, it is important to determine initially that the blood is not coming from one of these alternative sites. Clues that the blood is originating from the gastrointestinal tract include a dark red appearance and an acidic pH, in contrast to the typical bright red appearance and alkaline pH of true hemoptysis.

An etiologic classification of hemoptysis can be based on the site of origin within the lungs (Table 30-1). The most common site of bleeding is the airways, i.e., the tracheobronchial tree, which can be affected by inflammation (acute or chronic bronchitis, bronchiectasis) or by neoplasm (bronchogenic carcinoma, endobronchial metastatic carcinoma, or bronchial carcinoid tumor). The bronchial arteries, which originate either from the aorta or from intercostal arteries and are therefore part of the high-pressure systemic circulation, are the source of bleeding in bronchitis or bronchiectasis or with endobronchial tumors. Blood originating from the pulmonary parenchyma can be either from a localized source, such as an infection (pneumonia, lung abscess, tuberculosis), or from a process diffusely affecting the parenchyma (as with a coagulopathy or with an autoimmune process such as Goodpasture's syndrome). Disorders primarily affecting the pulmonary vasculature include pulmonary embolic disease and those conditions associated with elevated pulmonary venous and capillary pressures, such as mitral stenosis or left ventricular failure.

Although the relative frequency of the different etiologies of hemoptysis varies from series to series, most recent studies indicate that bronchitis and bronchogenic carcinoma are the two most common causes. Despite the lower frequency of tuberculosis and bronchiectasis seen in recent compared to older series, these two disorders still represent the most common causes of massive hemoptysis in several series. Even after extensive evaluation, a sizable proportion of patients (up to 30% in some series) have no identifiable etiology for their hemoptysis. These patients are classified as having idiopathic or cryptogenic hemoptysis, and subtle airway or parenchymal disease is presumably responsible for the bleeding.

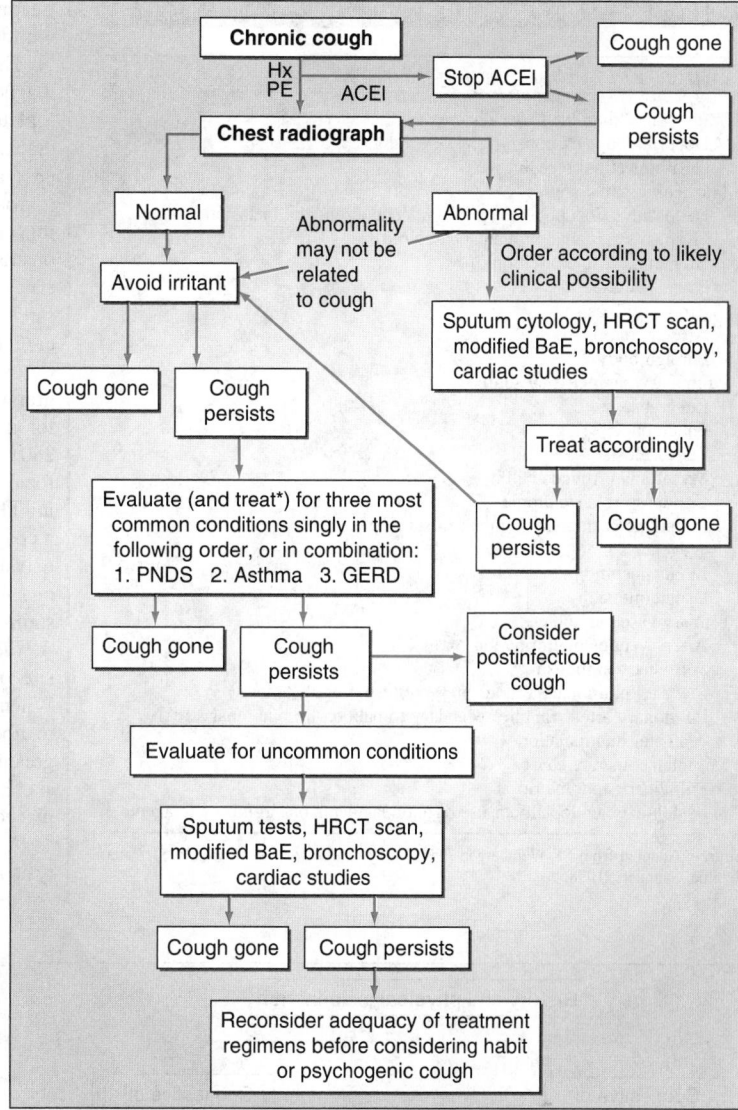

FIGURE 30-1 An algorithm for the evaluation of chronic cough. ACEI, angiotensin-converting enzyme inhibitor; BaE, barium esophagography; GERD, gastroesophageal reflux disease; HRCT, high-resolution computed tomography; Hx, history; PE, physical examination; PNDS, postnasal drip syndrome. *Treatment is either targeted to a presumptive diagnosis or given empirically. [Adapted from RS Irwin: Chest 114(Suppl):133S, 1998, with permission.]

APPROACH TO THE PATIENT

The *history* is extremely valuable. Hemoptysis that is described as blood-streaking of mucopurulent or purulent sputum often suggests bronchitis. Chronic production of sputum with a recent change in quantity or appearance favors an acute exacerbation of chronic bronchitis. Fever or chills accompanying blood-streaked purulent sputum suggests pneumonia, whereas a putrid smell to the sputum raises the possibility of lung abscess. When sputum production has been chronic and copious, the diagnosis of bronchiectasis should be considered. Hemoptysis following the acute onset of pleuritic chest pain and dyspnea is suggestive of pulmonary embolism.

A history of previous or coexisting disorders should be sought, such as renal disease (seen with Goodpasture's syndrome or Wegener's granulomatosis), lupus erythematosus (with associated pulmonary hemorrhage from lupus pneumonitis), or a previous malignancy (either recurrent lung cancer or endobronchial metastasis from a nonpulmonary primary tumor). In a patient with AIDS, endobronchial or pulmonary parenchymal Kaposi's sarcoma should be considered. Risk factors for bronchogenic carcinoma, particularly smoking and asbestos exposure, should be sought. Patients should be questioned about previous bleeding disorders,

TABLE 30-1 *Differential Diagnosis of Hemoptysis*

Source other than the lower respiratory tract
    Upper airway (nasopharyngeal) bleeding
    Gastrointestinal bleeding
Tracheobronchial source
    Neoplasm (bronchogenic carcinoma, endobronchial metastatic tumor,
     Kaposi's sarcoma, bronchial carcinoid)
    Bronchitis (acute or chronic)
    Bronchiectasis
    Broncholithiasis
    Airway trauma
    Foreign body
Pulmonary parenchymal source
    Lung abscess
    Pneumonia
    Tuberculosis
    Mycetoma ("fungus ball")
    Goodpasture's syndrome
    Idiopathic pulmonary hemosiderosis
    Wegener's granulomatosis
    Lupus pneumonitis
    Lung contusion
Primary vascular source
    Arteriovenous malformation
    Pulmonary embolism
    Elevated pulmonary venous pressure (esp. mitral stenosis)
    Pulmonary artery rupture secondary to balloon-tip pulmonary artery
     catheter manipulation
Miscellaneous/rare causes
    Pulmonary endometriosis
    Systemic coagulopathy or use of anticoagulants or thrombolytic agents

Source: Adapted from SE Weinberger, *Principles of Pulmonary Medicine*, 3d ed, Philadelphia, Saunders, 1998.

treatment with anticoagulants, or use of drugs that can be associated with thrombocytopenia.

The *physical examination* may also provide helpful clues to the diagnosis. For example, examination of the lungs may demonstrate a pleural friction rub (pulmonary embolism), localized or diffuse crackles (parenchymal bleeding or an underlying parenchymal process associated with bleeding), evidence of airflow obstruction (chronic bronchitis), or prominent rhonchi, with or without wheezing or crackles (bronchiectasis). Cardiac examination may demonstrate findings of pulmonary arterial hypertension, mitral stenosis, or heart failure. Skin examination may reveal Kaposi's sarcoma, arteriovenous malformations of Osler-Rendu-Weber disease, or lesions suggestive of systemic lupus erythematosus.

Diagnostic evaluation of hemoptysis starts with a chest radiograph (often followed by a computed tomographic scan) to look for a mass lesion, findings suggestive of bronchiectasis (Chap. 240), or focal or diffuse parenchymal disease (representing either focal or diffuse bleeding or a focal area of pneumonitis). Additional initial screening evaluation often includes a complete blood count, a coagulation profile, and assessment for renal disease with a urinalysis and measurement of blood urea nitrogen and creatinine levels. When sputum is present, examination by Gram and acid-fast stains (along with the corresponding cultures) is indicated.

Fiberoptic bronchoscopy is particularly useful for localizing the site of bleeding and for visualization of endobronchial lesions. When bleeding is massive, rigid bronchoscopy is often preferable to fiberoptic bronchoscopy because of better airway control and greater suction capability. In patients with suspected bronchiectasis, HRCT is now the diagnostic procedure of choice, having replaced bronchography.

A diagnostic algorithm for evaluation of nonmassive hemoptysis is presented in Fig. 30-2.

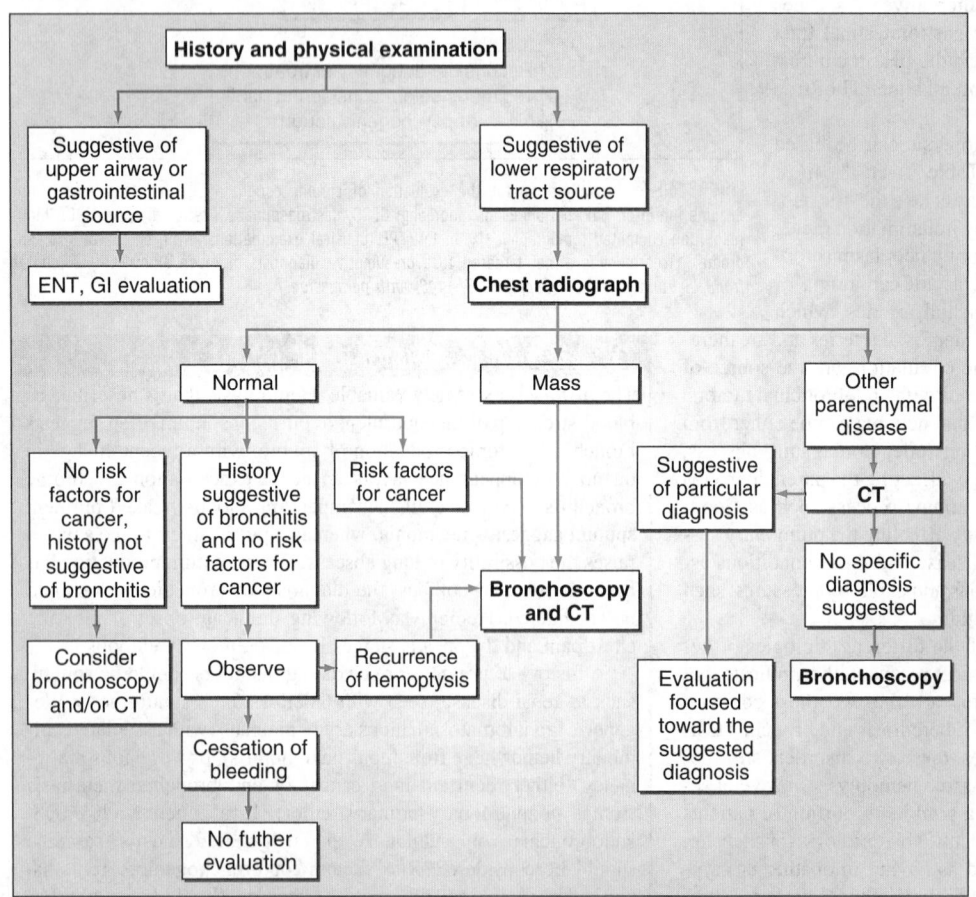

FIGURE 30-2 An algorithm for the evaluation of non-massive hemoptysis. CT, computed tomography.

Rx TREATMENT

The rapidity of bleeding and its effect on gas exchange determine the urgency of management. When the bleeding is confined to either blood-streaking of sputum or production of small amounts of pure blood, gas exchange is usually preserved; establishing a diagnosis is the first priority. When hemoptysis is massive, maintaining adequate gas exchange, preventing blood from spilling into unaffected areas of lung, and avoiding asphyxiation are the highest priorities. Keeping the patient at rest and partially suppressing cough may help the bleeding to subside. If the origin of the blood is known and is limited to one lung, the bleeding lung should be placed in the dependent position, so that blood is not aspirated into the unaffected lung.

With massive bleeding, the need to control the airway and maintain adequate gas exchange may necessitate endotracheal intubation and mechanical ventilation. In patients in danger of flooding the lung contralateral to the side of hemorrhage despite proper positioning, isolation of the right and left mainstem bronchi from each other can be achieved by selectively intubating the nonbleeding lung (often with bronchoscopic guidance) or by using specially designed double-lumen endotracheal tubes. Another option involves inserting a balloon catheter through a bronchoscope by direct visualization and inflating the balloon to occlude the bronchus leading to the bleeding site. This technique not only prevents aspiration of blood into unaffected areas but also may promote tamponade of the bleeding site and cessation of bleeding.

Other available techniques for control of significant bleeding include laser phototherapy, electrocautery, embolotherapy, and surgical resection of the involved area of lung. With bleeding from an endobronchial tumor, the neodymium:yttrium-aluminum-garnet (Nd:YAG) laser can often achieve at least temporary hemostasis by coagulating the bleeding site. Electrocautery, which uses an electric current for thermal destruction of tissue, can be used similarly for management of bleeding from an endobronchial tumor. Embolotherapy involves an arteriographic procedure in which a vessel proximal to the bleeding site is cannulated, and a material such as Gelfoam is injected to occlude the bleeding vessel. Surgical resection is a therapeutic option either for the emergent therapy of life-threatening hemoptysis that fails to respond to other measures or for the elective but definitive management of localized disease subject to recurrent bleeding.

FURTHER READING

GIBSON PG et al: Eosinophilic bronchitis: Clinical manifestations and implications for treatment. Thorax 57:178, 2002

HIRSHBERG B et al: Hemoptysis: Etiology, evaluation, and outcome in a tertiary referral hospital. Chest 112:440, 1997

IRWIN RS, MADISON JM: The diagnosis and treatment of cough. N Engl J Med 343:1715, 2000

———, WIDDICOMBE J: Cough, in *Textbook of Respiratory Medicine*, 3d ed JF Murray, JA Nadel (eds). Philadelphia, Saunders, 2000, pp 553–566

ISRAILI ZH, HALL WD: Cough and angioneurotic edema associated with angiotensin-converting enzyme inhibitor therapy. Ann Intern Med 117:234, 1992

JEAN-BAPTISTE E: Clinical assessment and management of massive hemoptysis. Crit Care Med 28:1642, 2000

31 HYPOXIA AND CYANOSIS
Eugene Braunwald

HYPOXIA

The fundamental purpose of the cardiorespiratory system is to deliver O_2 (and substrates) to the cells and to remove CO_2 (and other metabolic products) from them. Proper maintenance of this function depends on intact cardiovascular and respiratory systems and a supply of inspired gas containing adequate O_2. When hypoxia occurs consequent to respiratory failure, Pa_{O_2} declines, Pa_{CO_2} usually rises (Chap. 234), and the hemoglobin-oxygen (Hb-O_2) dissociation curve (see Fig. 91-2) is displaced to the right, with greater quantities of O_2 released at any level of tissue P_{O_2}. Arterial hypoxemia, i.e., a reduction of O_2 saturation of arterial blood (Sa_{O_2}), and consequent cyanosis are likely to be more marked when such depression of Pa_{O_2} results from pulmonary disease than when the depression occurs as the result of a decline in the fraction of oxygen in inspired air (FI_{O_2}). In this situation Pa_{CO_2} falls secondary to anoxia-induced hyperventilation and the Hb-O_2 dissociation curve is displaced to the left, limiting the decline in Sa_{O_2} at any level of Pa_{O_2}.

CAUSES OF HYPOXIA

ANEMIC HYPOXIA A reduction in the hemoglobin concentration of the blood is attended by a corresponding decline in the O_2-carrying capacity of the blood. In anemic hypoxia, the Pa_{O_2} is normal; but as a consequence of the reduction of the hemoglobin concentration, the absolute quantity of O_2 transported per unit volume of blood is diminished. As the anemic blood passes through the capillaries and the usual quantity of O_2 is removed from it, the P_{O_2} in the venous blood declines to a greater degree than would normally be the case.

CARBON MONOXIDE INTOXICATION (See also Chap. 377) Hemoglobin that is combined with carbon monoxide (carboxyhemoglobin, COHb) is unavailable for O_2 transport. In addition, the presence of COHb shifts the Hb-O_2 dissociation curve to the left (see Fig. 91-2) so that O_2 is unloaded only at lower tensions. By such formation of COHb, a given degree of reduction in O_2-carrying power produces a far greater degree of tissue hypoxia than the equivalent reduction in hemoglobin due to simple anemia.

RESPIRATORY HYPOXIA Arterial unsaturation is a common finding in advanced pulmonary disease. The most common cause of respiratory hypoxia is ventilation-perfusion mismatch, which results from perfusion of poorly ventilated alveoli. As discussed in Chap. 234, it may also be caused by hypoventilation, and it is then associated with an elevation of Pa_{CO_2}. These two forms of respiratory hypoxia may be recognized because they are usually correctable by inspiring 100% O_2 for several minutes. A third cause is shunting of blood across the lung from right to left by perfusion of nonventilated portions of the lung, as in pulmonary atelectasis or through arteriovenous connections in the lung. The low Pa_{O_2} in this situation is correctable only in part by an FI_{O_2} of 100%.

HYPOXIA SECONDARY TO HIGH ALTITUDE As one ascends rapidly to 3000 m (approximately 10,000 ft), the alveolar P_{O_2} declines to about 60 mmHg, and impaired memory and other cerebral symptoms of hypoxia may develop. At higher altitudes, arterial saturation declines rapidly and symptoms become more serious; and at 5000 m (approximately 15,000 ft) unacclimatized individuals usually cease to be able to function normally.

HYPOXIA SECONDARY TO RIGHT-TO-LEFT EXTRAPULMONARY SHUNTING From a physiologic viewpoint, this cause of hypoxia resembles intrapulmonary right-to-left shunting but is caused by congenital cardiac malformations such as tetralogy of Fallot, transposition of the great arteries, and Eisenmenger's syndrome (Chap. 218). As in pulmonary right-to-left shunting, the Pa_{O_2} cannot be restored to normal with inspiration of 100% O_2.

CIRCULATORY HYPOXIA As in anemic hypoxia, the Pa_{O_2} is usually normal, but venous and tissue P_{O_2} values are reduced as a consequence of reduced tissue perfusion and greater tissue O_2 extraction. Generalized circulatory hypoxia occurs in heart failure (Chap. 216) and in most forms of shock (Chap. 253).

SPECIFIC ORGAN HYPOXIA Decreased perfusion of any organ resulting in localized circulatory hypoxia may occur secondary to organic arterial obstruction, as in atherosclerosis, or as a consequence of vasoconstriction (Chap. 232), as observed in Raynaud's phenomenon. Localized hypoxia may also result from venous obstruction and the resultant congestion and reduced arterial inflow. Edema, which increases the distance through which O_2 diffuses before it reaches cells, also can cause localized hypoxia. In an attempt to maintain adequate perfusion to more vital organs, vasoconstriction may reduce perfusion in the limbs and skin, causing hypoxia of these regions in patients with heart failure or hypovolemic shock.

INCREASED O_2 REQUIREMENTS If the O_2 consumption of the tissues is elevated without a corresponding increase in perfusion, tissue hypoxia ensues and the P_{O_2} in venous blood becomes reduced. Ordinarily, the clinical picture of patients with hypoxia due to an elevated metabolic rate is quite different from that in other types of hypoxia; the skin is warm and flushed, owing to increased cutaneous blood flow that dissipates the excessive heat produced, and cyanosis is usually absent.

Exercise is a classic example of increased tissue O_2 requirements. These increased demands are normally met by several mechanisms operating simultaneously: (1) increasing the cardiac output and ventilation and thus O_2 delivery to the tissues; (2) preferentially directing the blood to the exercising muscles by changing vascular resistances in various circulatory beds, directly and/or reflexly; (3) increasing O_2 extraction from the delivered blood and widening the arteriovenous O_2 difference; and (4) reducing the pH of the tissues and capillary blood, shifting the Hb-O_2 curve to the right and unloading more O_2 from hemoglobin. If the capacity of these mechanisms is exceeded, then hypoxia, especially of the exercising muscles, will result.

IMPROPER OXYGEN UTILIZATION   Cyanide (Chap. 377) and several other similarly acting poisons cause cellular hypoxia. The tissues are unable to utilize O_2, and as a consequence, the venous blood tends to have a high O_2 tension. This condition has been termed *histotoxic hypoxia*.

EFFECTS OF HYPOXIA

Changes in the central nervous system, particularly the higher centers, are especially important consequences of hypoxia. Acute hypoxia causes impaired judgment, motor incoordination, and a clinical picture closely resembling that of acute alcoholism. When hypoxia is long-standing, fatigue, drowsiness, apathy, inattentiveness, delayed reaction time, and reduced work capacity occur. As hypoxia becomes more severe, the centers of the brainstem are affected, and death usually results from respiratory failure. With the reduction of Pa_{O_2}, cerebro-vascular resistance decreases and cerebral blood flow increases, in an attempt to maintain O_2 delivery to the brain. However, when the reduction of Pa_{O_2} is accompanied by hyperventilation and a reduction of Pa_{CO_2}, cerebrovascular resistance rises, cerebral blood flow falls, and hypoxia is intensified. Hypoxia also causes pulmonary arterial constriction, which shunts blood away from poorly ventilated toward better-ventilated portions of the lung. However, it also increases pulmonary vascular resistance and right ventricular afterload.

Glucose is normally broken down to pyruvic acid. However, the further breakdown of pyruvate and the generation of adenosine triphosphate (ATP) consequent to it require O_2, and in the presence of hypoxia increasing proportions of pyruvate are reduced to lactic acid, which cannot be broken down further, causing metabolic acidosis. Under these circumstances, the total energy obtained from the breakdown of carbohydrate is greatly reduced, and the quantity of energy available for the production of ATP becomes inadequate.

An important component of the respiratory response to hypoxia originates in special chemosensitive cells in the carotid and aortic bodies and in the respiratory center in the brainstem. The stimulation of these cells by hypoxia increases ventilation, with a loss of CO_2, and leads to respiratory alkalosis. When combined with the metabolic acidosis resulting from the production of lactic acid, the serum bicarbonate level declines (Chap. 42).

Diminished P_{O_2} in any tissue results in local vasodilatation, and the diffuse vasodilatation that occurs in generalized hypoxia raises the cardiac output. In patients with underlying heart disease, the requirements of the peripheral tissues for an increase of cardiac output with hypoxia may precipitate congestive heart failure. In patients with ischemic heart disease, a reduced Pa_{O_2} may intensify myocardial ischemia and further impair left ventricular function.

One of the important mechanisms of compensation for chronic hypoxia is an increase in the hemoglobin concentration and in the number of red blood cells in the circulating blood, i.e., the development of polycythemia secondary to erythropoietin production (Chap. 95). →*The approach to the patient with hypoxia is presented in Chap. 234.*

CYANOSIS

Cyanosis refers to a bluish color of the skin and mucous membranes resulting from an increased quantity of reduced hemoglobin, or of hemoglobin derivatives, in the small blood vessels of those areas. It is usually most marked in the lips, nail beds, ears, and malar eminences. Cyanosis, especially if developed recently, is more commonly detected by a family member than the patient. The florid skin characteristic of polycythemia vera (Chap. 95) must be distinguished from the true cyanosis discussed here. A cherry-colored flush, rather than cyanosis, is caused by COHb (Chap. 377). The degree of cyanosis is modified by the color of the cutaneous pigment and the thickness of the skin, as well as by the state of the cutaneous capillaries. The accurate clinical detection of the presence and degree of cyanosis is difficult, as proved by oximetric studies. In some instances, central cyanosis can be detected reliably when the Sa_{O_2} has fallen to 85%; in others, particularly in dark-skinned persons, it may not be detected until it has declined to 75%. In the latter case, examination of the mucous membranes in the oral cavity and the conjunctivae rather than examination of the skin is more helpful in the detection of cyanosis.

The increase in the quantity of reduced hemoglobin in the mucocutaneous vessels that produces cyanosis may be brought about either by an increase in the quantity of venous blood as the result of dilatation of the venules and venous ends of the capillaries or by a reduction in the Sa_{O_2} in the capillary blood. In general, cyanosis becomes apparent when the mean capillary concentration of reduced hemoglobin exceeds 40 g/L (4 g/dL). It is the *absolute* rather than the *relative* quantity of reduced hemoglobin that is important in producing cyanosis. Thus, in a patient with severe anemia, the relative amount of reduced hemoglobin in the venous blood may be very large when considered in relation to the total amount of hemoglobin in the blood. However, since the concentration of the latter is markedly reduced, the *absolute* quantity of reduced hemoglobin may still be small, and therefore patients with severe anemia and even *marked* arterial desaturation may not display cyanosis. Conversely, the higher the total hemoglobin content, the greater is the tendency toward cyanosis; thus, patients with marked polycythemia tend to be cyanotic at higher levels of Sa_{O_2} than patients with normal hematocrit values. Likewise, local passive congestion, which causes an increase in the total amount of reduced hemoglobin in the vessels in a given area, may cause cyanosis. Cyanosis is also observed when nonfunctional hemoglobin such as methemoglobin or sulfhemoglobin (Chap. 91) is present in blood.

Cyanosis may be subdivided into central and peripheral types. In the *central* type, the Sa_{O_2} is reduced or an abnormal hemoglobin derivative is present, and the mucous membranes and skin are both affected. *Peripheral* cyanosis is due to a slowing of blood flow and abnormally great extraction of O_2 from normally saturated arterial blood. It results from vasoconstriction and diminished peripheral blood flow, such as occurs in cold exposure, shock, congestive failure, and peripheral vascular disease. Often in these conditions the mucous membranes of the oral cavity or those beneath the tongue may be spared. Clinical differentiation between central and peripheral cyanosis may not always be simple, and in conditions such as cardiogenic shock with pulmonary edema there may be a mixture of both types.

DIFFERENTIAL DIAGNOSIS

CENTRAL CYANOSIS (Table 31-1)   Decreased Sa_{O_2} results from a marked reduction in the Pa_{O_2}. This reduction may be brought about by a decline in the FI_{O_2} without sufficient compensatory alveolar hyperventilation to maintain alveolar P_{O_2}. Cyanosis does not occur to a significant degree in an ascent to an altitude of 2500 m (8000 ft) but is marked in a further ascent to 5000 m (16,000 ft). The reason for this difference becomes clear on studying the *S* shape of the Hb-O_2 dissociation curve (see Fig. 91-2). At 2500 m (8000 ft) the FI_{O_2} is about 120 mmHg, the alveolar P_{O_2} is approximately 80 mmHg, and the Sa_{O_2} is nearly normal. However, at 5000 m (16,000 ft) the FI_{O_2} and alveolar P_{O_2} are about 85 and 50 mmHg, respectively, and the Sa_{O_2} is only about 75%. This leaves 25% of the hemoglobin in the arterial blood in the reduced form, an amount likely to be associated with cyanosis in the absence of anemia. Similarly, a mutant hemoglobin with a low affinity for O_2 (e.g., Hb Kansas) causes lowered Sa_{O_2} saturation and resultant central cyanosis (Chap. 91).

TABLE 31-1 *Causes of Cyanosis*

CENTRAL CYANOSIS

Decreased arterial oxygen saturation
   Decreased atmospheric pressure—high altitude
   Impaired pulmonary function
      Alveolar hypoventilation
      Uneven relationships between pulmonary ventilation and perfusion
        (perfusion of hypoventilated alveoli)
      Impaired oxygen diffusion
   Anatomic shunts
      Certain types of congenital heart disease
      Pulmonary arteriovenous fistulas
      Multiple small intrapulmonary shunts
   Hemoglobin with low affinity for oxygen
Hemoglobin abnormalities
   Methemoglobinemia—hereditary, acquired
   Sulfhemoglobinemia—acquired
   Carboxyhemoglobinemia (not true cyanosis)

PERIPHERAL CYANOSIS

Reduced cardiac output
Cold exposure
Redistribution of blood flow from extremities
Arterial obstruction
Venous obstruction

Seriously *impaired pulmonary function*, through perfusion of unventilated or poorly ventilated areas of the lung or alveolar hypoventilation, is a common cause of central cyanosis (Chap. 234). This condition may occur acutely, as in extensive pneumonia or pulmonary edema, or chronically with chronic pulmonary diseases (e.g., emphysema). In the latter situation, secondary polycythemia is generally present and clubbing of the fingers may occur. However, in many types of chronic pulmonary disease with fibrosis and obliteration of the capillary vascular bed, cyanosis does not occur because there is relatively little perfusion of underventilated areas.

Another cause of reduced Sa_{O_2} is *shunting of systemic venous blood into the arterial circuit*. Certain forms of congenital heart disease are associated with cyanosis (Chap. 218). Since blood flows from a higher-pressure to a lower-pressure region, for a cardiac defect to result in a right-to-left shunt, it must ordinarily be combined with an obstructive lesion distal (downstream) to the defect or with elevated pulmonary vascular resistance. The most common congenital cardiac lesion associated with cyanosis in the adult is the combination of ventricular septal defect and pulmonary outflow tract obstruction (*tetralogy of Fallot*). The more severe the obstruction, the greater the degree of right-to-left shunting and resultant cyanosis. In patients with patent ductus arteriosus, pulmonary hypertension, and right-to-left shunt, *differential cyanosis* results; that is, cyanosis occurs in the lower but not in the upper extremities. →*The mechanisms for the elevated pulmonary vascular resistance that may produce cyanosis in the presence of intra- and extracardiac communications without pulmonic stenosis (Eisenmenger syndrome) are discussed in Chap. 218.*

Pulmonary arteriovenous fistulae (Chap. 48) may be congenital or acquired, solitary or multiple, microscopic or massive. The severity of cyanosis produced by these fistulae depends on their size and number. They occur with some frequency in hereditary hemorrhagic telangiectasia. Sa_{O_2} reduction and cyanosis may also occur in some patients with cirrhosis, presumably as a consequence of pulmonary arteriovenous fistulas or portal vein–pulmonary vein anastomoses.

In patients with cardiac or pulmonary right-to-left shunts, the presence and severity of cyanosis depend on the size of the shunt relative to the systemic flow as well as on the Hb-O_2 saturation of the venous blood. With increased extraction of O_2 from the blood by the exercising muscles, the venous blood returning to the right side of the heart is more unsaturated than at rest, and shunting of this blood intensifies the cyanosis. Also, since the systemic vascular resistance falls with exercise, the right-to-left shunt is augmented by exercise in patients with congenital heart disease and communications between the two

sides of the heart. Secondary polycythemia occurs frequently in patients with arterial O_2 unsaturation and contributes to the cyanosis.

Cyanosis can be caused by small amounts of circulating methemoglobin and by even smaller amounts of sulfhemoglobin (Chap. 91). Although they are uncommon causes of cyanosis, these abnormal hemoglobin pigments should be sought by spectroscopy when cyanosis is not readily explained by malfunction of the circulatory or respiratory systems. Generally, digital clubbing does not occur with them. The diagnosis of methemoglobinemia can be suspected if the patient's blood remains brown after being mixed in a test tube and exposed to air.

PERIPHERAL CYANOSIS Probably the most common cause of peripheral cyanosis is the normal vasoconstriction resulting from exposure to cold air or water. When cardiac output is reduced, cutaneous vasoconstriction occurs as a compensatory mechanism so that blood is diverted from the skin to more vital areas such as the central nervous system and heart, and cyanosis of the extremities may result, even though the arterial blood is normally saturated.

Arterial obstruction to an extremity, as with an embolus, or arteriolar constriction, as in cold-induced vasospasm (Raynaud's phenomenon, Chap. 232), generally results in pallor and coldness, but there may be associated cyanosis. Venous obstruction, as in thrombophlebitis, dilates the subpapillary venous plexuses and thereby intensifies cyanosis.

APPROACH TO THE PATIENT

Certain features are important in arriving at the cause of cyanosis:

1. A careful history must be obtained, particularly timing of the onset of cyanosis. Cyanosis present since birth or infancy is usually due to congenital heart disease.

2. Central and peripheral cyanosis must be differentiated. Evidence of disorders of the respiratory or cardiovascular systems are helpful. Massage or gentle warming of a cyanotic extremity will increase peripheral blood flow and abolish peripheral but not central cyanosis.

3. The presence or absence of clubbing of the digits (see below) should be ascertained. Clubbing *without* cyanosis is frequent in patients with infective endocarditis and inflammatory bowel disease; it may occasionally occur in healthy persons, and in some instances it may be occupational, e.g., in jackhammer operators. The combination of cyanosis and clubbing is frequent in patients with congenital heart disease and right-to-left shunting and is seen occasionally in patients with pulmonary disease such as lung abscess or pulmonary arteriovenous fistulae. In contrast, peripheral cyanosis or acutely developing central cyanosis is *not* associated with clubbed digits.

4. Pa_{O_2} and Sa_{O_2} should be ascertained and in patients in whom the mechanism of cyanosis is obscure spectroscopic and other examinations of the blood performed to look for abnormal types of hemoglobin (critical in the differential diagnosis of cyanosis).

CLUBBING

The selective bullous enlargement of the distal segments of the fingers and toes due to proliferation of connective tissue, particularly on the dorsal surface, is termed *clubbing*; there is increased sponginess of the soft tissue at the base of the nail. Clubbing may be hereditary, idiopathic, or acquired and associated with a variety of disorders, including cyanotic congenital heart disease, infective endocarditis, and a variety of pulmonary conditions (among them primary and metastatic lung cancer, bronchiectasis, lung abscess, cystic fibrosis, and mesothelioma), as well as with some gastrointestinal diseases (including inflammatory bowel disease and hepatic cirrhosis).

Clubbing in patients with primary and metastatic lung cancer, mesothelioma, bronchiectasis, and hepatic cirrhosis may be associated with *hypertrophic osteoarthropathy*. In this condition, the subperiosteal formation of new bone in the distal diaphyses of the long bones of the extremities causes pain and symmetric arthritis-like changes in the shoulders, knees, ankles, wrists, and elbows. The diagnosis of hypertrophic osteoarthropathy may be confirmed by bone radiographs. Although the mechanism of clubbing is unclear, it appears to be secondary to a humoral substance that causes dilation of the vessels of the fingertip.

FURTHER READING

BEALL CM: Tibetan and Andean patterns of adaptation to high-altitude hypoxia. Hum Biol 72:201, 2000

FISHMAN AP: Approach to the patient with respiratory symptoms: Cyanosis and clubbing, in *Fishman's Pulmonary Diseases and Disorders*, 3d ed, Fishman AP et al (eds). Philadelphia, Saunders, 1998, pp 382–383

GRIFFEY RT et al: Cyanosis. J Emerg Med 18:369, 2000

GRIFKA RG: Cyanotic congenital heart disease with increased pulmonary blood flow. Pediatr Clin North Am 46:405, 1999

HACKETT PH, ROACH RC: Current concepts: High altitude illness. N Engl J Med 345:107, 2001

MYERS KA, FARQUHAR DR: The rational clinical examination. Does the patient have clubbing? JAMA 286:341, 2001

WALDMAN JD, WERNLY JA. Cyanotic congenital heart disease with decreased pulmonary blood flow in children. Pediatr Clin North Am 46:385, 1999

32 EDEMA
Eugene Braunwald

Edema is defined as a clinically apparent increase in the interstitial fluid volume, which may expand by several liters before the abnormality is evident. Therefore, a weight gain of several kilograms usually precedes overt manifestations of edema, and a similar weight loss from diuresis can be induced in a slightly edematous patient before "dry weight" is achieved. *Anasarca* refers to gross, generalized edema. *Ascites* (Chap. 39) and *hydrothorax* refer to accumulation of excess fluid in the peritoneal and pleural cavities, respectively, and are considered to be special forms of edema.

Depending on its cause and mechanism, edema may be localized or have a generalized distribution; it is recognized in its generalized form by puffiness of the face, which is most readily apparent in the periorbital areas, and by the persistence of an indentation of the skin following pressure; this is known as "pitting" edema. In its more subtle form, edema may be detected by noting that after the stethoscope is removed from the chest wall, the rim of the bell leaves an indentation on the skin of the chest for a few minutes. When the ring on a finger fits more snugly than in the past or when a patient complains of difficulty in putting on shoes, particularly in the evening, edema may be present.

PATHOGENESIS

About one-third of the total-body water is confined to the extracellular space. Approximately 25% of the latter, in turn, is composed of the plasma volume, and the remainder is interstitial fluid.

STARLING FORCES   The forces that regulate the disposition of fluid between these two components of the extracellular compartment are frequently referred to as the *Starling forces* (see p. 204). The hydrostatic pressure within the vascular system and the colloid oncotic pressure in the interstitial fluid tend to promote movement of fluid from the vascular to the extravascular space. On the other hand, the colloid oncotic pressure contributed by the plasma proteins and the hydrostatic pressure within the interstitial fluid, referred to as the *tissue tension*, promote the movement of fluid into the vascular compartment. Consequently there is a movement of water and diffusible solutes from the vascular space at the arteriolar end of the capillaries. Fluid is returned from the interstitial space into the vascular system at the venous end of the capillary and by way of the lymphatics. Unless these channels are obstructed, lymph flow rises with increases in net movement of fluid from the vascular compartment to the interstitium. These flows are usually balanced so that a steady state exists in the sizes of the intravascular and interstitial compartments, and yet a large exchange between them occurs. However, should any one of the hydrostatic or oncotic pressure gradients be altered significantly, a further net movement of fluid between the two components of the extracellular space will take place. The development of edema then depends on one or more alterations in the Starling forces so that there is increased flow of fluid from the vascular system into the interstitium or into a body cavity.

Edema due to increase in capillary pressure may result from an elevation of venous pressure due to obstruction in venous drainage. This increase in capillary pressure may be generalized, as occurs in congestive heart failure. The Starling forces may be imbalanced when the colloid oncotic pressure of the plasma is reduced, owing to any factor that may induce hypoalbuminemia, such as saline expansion, malnutrition, liver disease, loss of protein into the urine or into the gastrointestinal tract, or a severe catabolic state.

CAPILLARY DAMAGE   Edema may also result from damage to the capillary endothelium, which increases its permeability and permits the transfer of protein into the interstitial compartment. Injury to the capillary wall can result from drugs, viral or bacterial agents, and thermal or mechanical trauma. Increased capillary permeability may also be a consequence of a hypersensitivity reaction and is characteristic of immune injury. Damage to the capillary endothelium is presumably responsible for inflammatory edema, which is usually nonpitting, localized, and accompanied by other signs of inflammation—redness, heat, and tenderness.

REDUCTION OF EFFECTIVE ARTERIAL VOLUME   In many forms of edema the *effective arterial blood volume*, an as yet poorly defined parameter of the filling of the arterial tree, is reduced, and as a consequence a series of physiologic responses designed to restore it to normal are set into motion. A key element of these responses is the retention of salt and therefore of water, principally by the renal proximal tubule, ultimately leading to edema.

REDUCED CARDIAC OUTPUT   A reduction of cardiac output, whatever the cause, is associated with a lowering of the effective arterial blood volume as well as of renal blood flow, constriction of the efferent renal arterioles, and an elevation of the filtration fraction, i.e., the ratio of glomerular filtration rate to renal plasma flow. In severe heart failure there is a reduction in the glomerular filtration rate. Activation of the sympathetic nervous system and of the renin-angiotensin systems is responsible for renal vasoconstriction. The finding that α-adrenergic blocking agents and/or angiotensin-converting enzyme (ACE) inhibitors augment renal blood flow and induce diuresis supports the role of these two systems in elevating renal vascular resistance and salt and water retention when cardiac output is reduced.

RENAL FACTORS   Heart failure and other conditions, such as nephrotic syndrome and cirrhosis that reduce effective arterial blood volume, cause renal efferent arteriolar constriction. This, in turn, reduces the hydrostatic pressure while the increased filtration fraction raises the colloid osmotic pressure in the peritubular capillaries, thus enhancing salt and water reabsorption in the proximal tubule as well as in the ascending limb of the loop of Henle.

In addition, the diminished renal blood flow characteristic of states in which the effective arterial blood volume is reduced is translated by the renal juxtaglomerular cells into a signal for increased renin release (Chap. 321). The mechanisms responsible for this release include: (1) a baroreceptor response in which reduced renal perfusion results in incomplete filling of the renal arterioles and diminished stretch of the juxtaglomerular cells, a signal that provides for the elaboration and/or release of renin (see below); (2) reduced glomerular filtration which lowers the sodium chloride load reaching the distal renal tubules; this is sensed by the macula densa, which signals the neighboring juxtaglomerular cells to secrete renin; (3) activation of the β-adrenergic receptors in the juxtaglomerular cells by the sympathetic nervous system and circulating catecholamines stimulates renin release. These three mechanisms generally act in concert.

THE RENIN-ANGIOTENSIN-ALDOSTERONE (RAA) SYSTEM (See also Chap. 321)

Renin, an enzyme with a molecular weight of about 40,000, acts on its substrate, angiotensinogen, an α_2 globulin synthesized by the liver, to release angiotensin I, a decapeptide, which is broken down to angiotensin II (AII), an octapeptide. AII has generalized vasoconstrictor properties; it is especially active on the efferent arterioles and independently increases Na$^+$ reabsorption in the proximal tubule. The RAA system has long been recognized as a hormone system. However, it also operates locally. Both circulating and intrarenally produced AII contribute to renal vasoconstriction and to salt and water retention. These renal effects of AII are mediated by activation of AII type 1 receptors, which can be blocked by specific antagonists (angiotensin receptor blockers) such as losartan. AII also enters the circulation and stimulates the production of aldosterone by the zona glomerulosa of the adrenal cortex. In patients with heart failure, not only is aldosterone secretion elevated but the biologic half-life of aldosterone is prolonged, which further increases the plasma level of the hormone. A depression of hepatic blood flow, particularly during exercise, secondary to a reduction in cardiac output, is responsible for the reduced hepatic catabolism of aldosterone. Aldosterone, in turn, enhances Na$^+$ reabsorption (and K$^+$ excretion) by the collecting tubule. The activation of the RAA system is most striking in the early phase of acute, severe heart failure and is less intense in patients with chronic, stable, compensated heart failure.

Although increased quantities of aldosterone are secreted in heart failure and in other edematous states and although blockade of the action of aldosterone by spironolactone (an aldosterone antagonist) or amiloride (a blocker of epithelial Na$^+$ channels) often induces a moderate diuresis in edematous states, persistent augmented levels of aldosterone (or other mineralocorticoids) alone do not always promote accumulation of edema, as witnessed by the lack of striking fluid retention in most instances of primary aldosteronism (Chap. 321). Furthermore, although normal individuals retain some salt and water with the administration of potent mineralocorticoids, such as deoxycorticosterone acetate or fludrocortisone, this accumulation is self-limiting, despite continued exposure to the steroid, a phenomenon known as *mineralocorticoid escape*. The failure of normal individuals who receive large doses of mineralocorticoids to accumulate large quantities of extracellular fluid and to develop edema is probably a consequence of an increase in glomerular filtration rate (pressure natriuresis) and through the action of natriuretic substance(s) (see below). The continued secretion of aldosterone may be more important in the accumulation of fluid in edematous states because patients with edema secondary to heart failure, nephrotic syndrome, and cirrhosis are generally unable to repair the deficit in effective arterial blood volume. As a consequence they do not develop pressure natriuresis.

ARGININE VASOPRESSIN (AVP) (See also Chap. 319) The secretion of

AVP occurs in response to increased intracellular osmolar concentration and by stimulating V_2 receptors increases the reabsorption of free water in the renal distal tubule and collecting duct, thereby increasing total-body water. Circulating AVP is elevated in many patients with heart failure secondary to a nonosmotic stimulus associated with decreased effective arterial volume. Such patients fail to show the normal reduction of AVP with a reduction of osmolality, contributing to hyponatremia and edema formation.

ENDOTHELIN This is a potent peptide vasoconstrictor released by endothelial cells; its concentration is elevated in heart failure and contributes to renal vasoconstriction, Na$^+$ retention, and edema in heart failure.

NATRIURETIC PEPTIDES (See also Chap. 215) Atrial distention and/or a

sodium load cause release into the circulation of atrial natriuretic peptide (ANP), a polypeptide; a high-molecular-weight precursor of ANP is stored in secretory granules within atrial myocytes. Release of ANP causes (1) excretion of sodium and water by augmenting glomerular filtration rate, inhibiting sodium reabsorption in the proximal tubule, and inhibiting release of renin and aldosterone; and (2) arteriolar and venous dilatation by antagonizing the vasoconstrictor actions of AII, AVP, and sympathetic stimulation. Thus, ANP has the capacity to oppose sodium retention and arterial pressure elevation in hypervolemic states.

The closely related brain natriuretic peptide (BNP) is stored primarily in cardiac ventricular myocardium and is released when ventricular diastolic pressure rises. Its actions are similar to those of ANP. Circulating levels of ANP and BNP are elevated in congestive heart failure but obviously not sufficiently to prevent edema formation. In addition, in edematous states (particularly heart failure), there is abnormal resistance to the actions of natriuretic peptides.

CLINICAL CAUSES OF EDEMA

OBSTRUCTION OF VENOUS (AND LYMPHATIC) DRAINAGE OF A LIMB In this

condition the hydrostatic pressure in the capillary bed upstream (proximal) to the obstruction increases so that an abnormal quantity of fluid is transferred from the vascular to the interstitial space. Since the alternative route (i.e., the lymphatic channels) may also be obstructed, an increased volume of interstitial fluid in the limb develops, i.e., there is trapping of fluid in the extremity, causing local edema at the expense of the blood volume in the remainder of the body, thereby reducing effective arterial blood volume and leading to the retention of salt and water until the deficit in plasma volume has been corrected. Tissue tension rises in the affected limb until it counterbalances the primary alterations in the Starling forces, at which time no further fluid accumulates. The net effect is a local increase in the volume of interstitial fluid. This same sequence occurs in ascites and hydrothorax, in which fluid is trapped or accumulates in the cavitary space, depleting the intravascular volume and leading to secondary salt and fluid retention, as already described.

CONGESTIVE HEART FAILURE (See also Chap. 216) In this disorder, the

impaired systolic emptying of the ventricle(s) and/or the impairment of ventricular relaxation promotes an accumulation of blood in the venous circulation at the expense of the effective arterial volume, and the aforementioned sequence of events (Fig. 32-1) is initiated. In mild heart failure, a small increment of total blood volume may repair the deficit of arterial volume and establish a new steady state. Through the operation of Starling's law of the heart, an increase in ventricular diastolic volume promotes a more forceful contraction and may thereby restore the cardiac output (Fig. 216-1). However, if the cardiac disorder is more severe, fluid retention continues, and the increment in blood volume accumulates in the venous circulation. With reduction in cardiac output, a decrease in baroreflex-mediated inhibition of the vasomotor center activates renal vasoconstrictor nerves and the RAA system, causing sodium and water retention.

Incomplete ventricular emptying (systolic heart failure) and/or inadequate ventricular relaxation (diastolic heart failure) both lead to an elevation of ventricular diastolic pressure. If the impairment of cardiac function primarily involves the right ventricle, pressures in the systemic veins and capillaries rise, augmenting the transudation of fluid into the interstitial space and enhancing the likelihood of peripheral edema. The elevated systemic venous pressure is transmitted to the thoracic duct with consequent reduction of lymph drainage, further increasing the accumulation of edema.

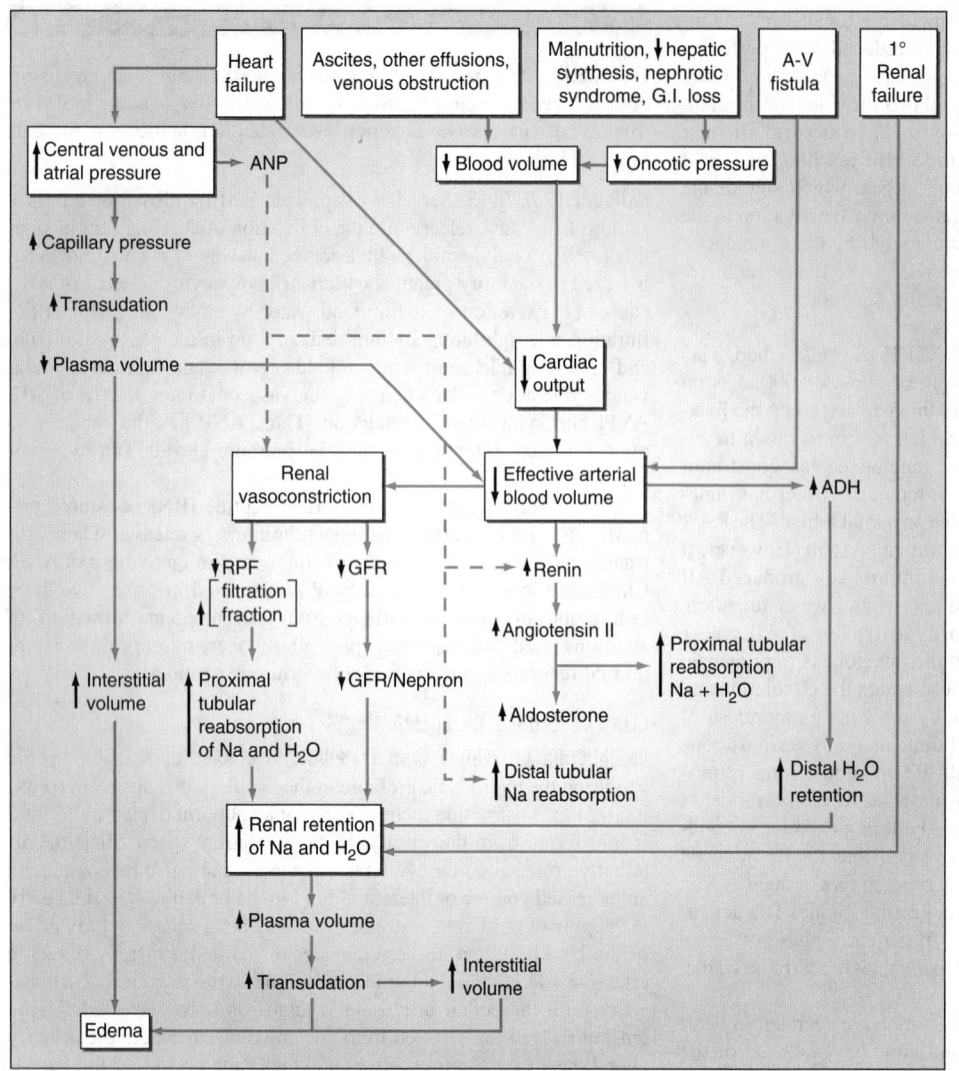

FIGURE 32-1 Sequence of events leading to the formation and retention of salt and water and the development of edema. ANP, atrial natriuretic peptide; RPF, renal plasma flow; GFR, glomerular filtration rate. Inhibitory influences are shown by broken lines. ADH, antidiuretic hormone.

CIRRHOSIS (See also Chap. 39 and Chap. 289) This condition is characterized by hepatic venous outflow blockade, which in turn expands the splanchnic blood volume and increases hepatic lymph formation. Intrahepatic hypertension acts as a potent stimulus for renal Na^+ retention and a reduction of effective arterial blood volume. These alterations are frequently complicated by hypoalbuminemia secondary to reduced hepatic synthesis, which reduce the effective arterial blood volume further, leading to activation of the RAA system, of renal sympathetic nerves, and other salt- and water-retaining mechanisms. The concentration of circulating aldosterone is elevated by the liver's failure to metabolize this hormone. Initially, the excess interstitial fluid is localized preferentially proximal (upstream) to the congested portal venous system and obstructed hepatic lymphatics, i.e., in the peritoneal cavity. In later stages, particularly when there is severe hypoalbuminemia, peripheral edema may develop. The excess production of prostaglandins (PGE_2 and PGI_2) in cirrhosis attenuates renal Na^+ retention. When the synthesis of these substances is inhibited by nonsteroidal anti-inflammatory agents, renal function deteriorates and Na^+ retention increases.

DRUG-INDUCED EDEMA A large number of widely used drugs can cause edema (Table 32-1). Mechanisms include renal vasoconstriction (nonsteroidal anti-inflammatory agents and cyclosporine), arteriolar dilatation (vasodilators), augmented renal sodium reabsorption (steroid hormones), and capillary damage (interleukin 2).

IDIOPATHIC EDEMA This syndrome, which occurs almost exclusively in women, is characterized by periodic episodes of edema (unrelated to

If the impairment of cardiac function (incomplete ventricular emptying and/or inadequate relaxation) involves the left ventricle primarily, then pulmonary venous and capillary pressures rise. Pulmonary artery pressure rises and this in turn interferes with the emptying of the right ventricle, leading to an elevation of right ventricular diastolic and of central and systemic venous pressures, thereby enhancing the likelihood of the formation of peripheral edema. The elevation of pulmonary capillary pressure may cause pulmonary edema, which impairs gas exchange. The resultant hypoxemia may impair cardiac function further, sometimes causing a vicious circle.

NEPHROTIC SYNDROME AND OTHER HYPOALBUMINEMIC STATES (See also Chap. 264) The primary alteration in this disorder is a diminished colloid oncotic pressure due to losses of large quantities of protein into the urine. This promotes a net movement of fluid into the interstitium, causes hypovolemia, and initiates the edema-forming sequence of events described above, including activation of the RAA system. With severe hypoalbuminemia and the consequent reduced colloid osmotic pressure, the salt and water that are retained cannot be restrained within the vascular compartment, total and effective arterial blood volumes decline, and hence the stimuli to retain salt and water are not abated. A similar sequence of events occurs in other conditions that lead to *severe* hypoalbuminemia, including severe nutritional deficiency states, severe, chronic liver disease, and protein-losing enteropathy. In the nephrotic syndrome, impaired renal Na^+ excretion contributes to edema, even in the absence of severe hypoalbuminemia.

TABLE 32-1 *Drugs Associated with Edema Formation*

Nonsteroidal anti-inflammatory drugs
Antihypertensive agents
   Direct arterial/arteriolar vasodilators
      Minoxidil
      Hydralazine
      Clonidine
      Methyldopa
      Guanethidine
   Calcium channel antagonists
   α-Adrenergic antagonists
Steroid hormones
   Glucocorticoids
   Anabolic steroids
   Estrogens
   Progestins
Cyclosporine
Growth hormone
Immunotherapies
   Interleukin 2
   OKT3 monoclonal antibody

Source: From Chertow.

the menstrual cycle), frequently accompanied by abdominal distention. Diurnal alterations in weight occur with orthostatic retention of sodium and water, so that the patient may weigh several pounds more after having been in the upright posture for several hours. Such large diurnal weight changes suggest an increase in capillary permeability that appears to fluctuate in severity and to be aggravated by hot weather. There is some evidence that a reduction in plasma volume occurs in this condition with secondary activation of the RAA system and impaired suppression of AVP release. Idiopathic edema should be distinguished from cyclical or premenstrual edema, in which the sodium and water retention may be secondary to excessive estrogen stimulation. There are also some cases in which the edema appears to be diuretic-induced. It has been postulated that in these patients, chronic diuretic administration leads to mild blood volume depletion, which causes chronic hyperreninemia and juxtaglomerular hyperplasia. Salt-retaining mechanisms appear to overcompensate for the direct effects of the diuretics. *Acute* withdrawal of diuretics can then leave the sodium-retaining forces unopposed, leading to fluid retention and edema. Decreased dopaminergic activity and reduced urinary kallikrein and kinin excretion have been reported in this condition and may also be of pathogenetic importance.

℞ TREATMENT

The treatment of idiopathic cyclic edema includes a reduction in salt intake, rest in the supine position for several hours each day, the wearing of elastic stockings (which should be put on before arising in the morning), and an attempt to understand any underlying emotional problems. A variety of pharmacologic agents including ACE inhibitors, progesterone, the dopamine receptor agonist bromocriptine, and the sympathomimetic amine dextroamphetamine have all been reported to be useful when administered to patients who do not respond to simpler measures. Diuretics may be helpful initially but may lose their effectiveness with continuous administration; accordingly, they should be employed sparingly, if at all. Discontinuation of diuretics paradoxically leads to diuresis in diuretic-induced edema, described above.

DIFFERENTIAL DIAGNOSIS

LOCALIZED EDEMA (See also Chap. 232)

Edema originating from inflammation or hypersensitivity is usually readily identified. Localized edema due to venous or lymphatic obstruction may be caused by thrombophlebitis, chronic lymphangitis, resection of regional lymph nodes, filariasis, etc. Lymphedema is particularly intractable because restriction of lymphatic flow results in increased protein concentration in the interstitial fluid, a circumstance that aggravates retention of fluid.

GENERALIZED EDEMA

The differences between the three major causes of generalized edema are shown in Table 32-2.

The great majority of patients with generalized edema suffer from advanced cardiac, renal, hepatic, or nutritional disorders. Consequently, the differential diagnosis of generalized edema should be directed toward identifying or excluding these several conditions.

EDEMA OF HEART FAILURE (See also Chap. 216) The presence of heart disease, as manifested by cardiac enlargement and gallop rhythm, together with evidence of cardiac failure, such as dyspnea, basilar rales, venous distention, and hepatomegaly, usually indicate that edema results from heart failure. Noninvasive tests such as echocardiography and radionuclide angiography may be helpful in establishing the diagnosis of heart failure.

EDEMA OF THE NEPHROTIC SYNDROME (See also Chap. 264) Marked proteinuria (>3.5 g/d), hypoalbuminemia (<35 g/L), and in some instances hypercholesterolemia are present. This syndrome may occur during the course of a variety of kidney diseases, which include glomerulonephritis, diabetic glomerulosclerosis, and hypersensitivity reactions. A history of previous renal disease may or may not be elicited.

EDEMA OF ACUTE GLOMERULONEPHRITIS AND OTHER FORMS OF RENAL FAILURE
The edema occurring during the acute phases of glomerulonephritis is characteristically associated with hematuria, proteinuria, and hypertension. Although some evidence supports the view that the fluid retention is due to increased capillary permeability, in most instances the edema results from primary retention of sodium and water by the kidneys owing to renal insufficiency. This state differs from congestive heart failure in that it is characterized by a normal (or sometimes even increased) cardiac output and a normal arterial–mixed venous oxygen difference. Patients with edema due to renal failure commonly have evidence of pulmonary congestion on chest roentgenograms before cardiac enlargement is significant, but they may not develop orthopnea. Patients with *chronic* renal failure may also develop edema due to primary renal retention of sodium and water.

TABLE 32-2 *Principal Causes of Generalized Edema: History, Physical Examination, and Laboratory Findings*

Organ System	History	Physical Examination	Laboratory Findings
Cardiac	Dyspnea with exertion prominent—often associated with orthopnea—or paroxysmal nocturnal dyspnea	Elevated jugular venous pressure, ventricular (S_3) gallop; occasionally with displaced or dyskinetic apical pulse; peripheral cyanosis, cool extremities, small pulse pressure when severe	Elevated urea nitrogen-to-creatinine ratio common; elevated uric acid; serum sodium often diminished; liver enzymes occasionally elevated with hepatic congestion
Hepatic	Dyspnea infrequent, except if associated with significant degree of ascites; most often a history of ethanol abuse	Frequently associated with ascites; jugular venous pressure normal or low; blood pressure lower than in renal or cardiac disease; one or more additional signs of chronic liver disease (jaundice, palmar erythema, Dupuytren's contracture, spider angiomata, male gynecomastia; asterixis and other signs of encephalopathy) may be present	If severe, reductions in serum albumin, cholesterol, other hepatic proteins (transferrin, fibrinogen); liver enzymes elevated, depending on the cause and acuity of liver injury; tendency toward hypokalemia, respiratory alkalosis; macrocytosis from folate deficiency
Renal	Usually chronic: may be associated with uremic signs and symptoms, including decreased appetite, altered (metallic or fishy) taste, altered sleep pattern, difficulty concentrating, restless legs or myoclonus: dyspnea can be present, but generally less prominent than in heart failure	Blood pressure may be elevated; hypertensive or diabetic retinopathy in selected cases; nitrogenous fetor; periorbital edema may predominate; pericardial friction rub in advanced cases with uremia	Albuminuria, hypoalbuminemia; sometimes, elevation of serum creatinine and urea nitrogen; hyperkalemia, metabolic acidosis, hyperphosphatemia, hypocalcemia, anemia (usually normocytic)

Source: From Chertow.
Note: S$_3$, third heart sound.

EDEMA OF CIRRHOSIS (See also Chap. 289)   Ascites and biochemical and clinical evidence of hepatic disease (collateral venous channels, jaundice, and spider angiomas) characterize edema of hepatic origin. The ascites (Chap. 39) is frequently refractory to treatment because it collects as a result of a combination of obstruction of hepatic lymphatic drainage, portal hypertension, and hypoalbuminemia. Edema may also occur in other parts of the body in these patients as a result of hypoalbuminemia. Furthermore, a sizable accumulation of ascitic fluid may increase intraabdominal pressure and impede venous return from the lower extremities; hence, it tends to promote accumulation of edema in this region as well.

EDEMA OF NUTRITIONAL ORIGIN   A diet grossly deficient in protein over a prolonged period may produce hypoproteinemia and edema. The latter may be intensified by the development of beriberi heart disease (Chap. 223), also of nutritional origin, in which multiple peripheral arteriovenous fistulae result in reduced effective systemic perfusion and effective arterial blood volume, thereby enhancing edema formation (Chap. 61). Edema may actually become intensified when famished subjects are first provided with an adequate diet. The ingestion of more food may increase the quantity of NaCl ingested, which is then retained along with water. So-called refeeding edema may also be linked to increased release of insulin, which directly increases tubular sodium reabsorption. In addition to hypoalbuminemia, hypokalemia and caloric deficits may be involved in the edema of starvation.

OTHER CAUSES OF EDEMA   These include hypothyroidism, in which the edema (myxedema) is located typically in the pretibial region and which may also be associated with periorbital puffiness. Exogenous hyperadrenocortism, pregnancy, and administration of estrogens and vasodilators, particularly dihydropyridines such as nifedipine, may also all cause edema.

DISTRIBUTION OF EDEMA

The distribution of edema is an important guide to the cause. Thus, edema limited to one leg or to one or both arms is usually the result of venous and/or lymphatic obstruction. Edema resulting from hypoproteinemia characteristically is generalized, but it is especially evident in the very soft tissues of the eyelids and face and tends to be most pronounced in the morning because of the recumbent posture assumed during the night. Less common causes of facial edema include trichinosis, allergic reactions, and myxedema. Edema associated with heart failure, on the other hand, tends to be more extensive in the legs and to be accentuated in the evening, a feature also determined largely by posture. When patients with heart failure have been confined to bed, edema may be most prominent in the presacral region. Paralysis reduces lymphatic and venous drainage on the affected side and may be responsible for unilateral edema.

ADDITIONAL FACTORS IN DIAGNOSIS

The color, thickness, and sensitivity of the skin are significant. Local tenderness and warmth suggest inflammation. Local cyanosis may signify a venous obstruction. In individuals who have had repeated episodes of prolonged edema, the skin over the involved areas may be thickened, indurated, and often red.

Measurement or estimation of the venous pressure is of importance in evaluating edema. Elevation in an isolated part of the body usually reflects localized venous obstruction. Generalized elevation of systemic venous pressure usually indicates the presence of congestive heart failure. Ordinarily, a significant generalized increase in venous pressure can be recognized by the level at which cervical veins collapse (Chap. 209). In patients with obstruction of the superior vena cava, edema is confined to the face, neck, and upper extremities, where the venous pressure is elevated compared with that in the lower extremities. Measurement of venous pressure in the upper extremities is also useful in patients with massive edema of the lower extremities and ascites; it is elevated in the upper extremities when the edema is on a cardiac basis (e.g., advanced heart failure, constrictive pericarditis, or tricuspid stenosis) but is normal when it is secondary to cirrhosis. Severe heart failure may cause ascites that may be distinguished from the ascites caused by hepatic cirrhosis by the jugular venous pressure, which usually is elevated in heart failure and normal in cirrhosis.

Determination of the concentration of serum albumin aids importantly in identifying those patients in whom edema is due, at least in part, to diminished intravascular colloid oncotic pressure. The presence of proteinuria also affords useful clues. The absence of proteinuria excludes nephrotic syndrome but cannot exclude nonproteinuric causes of renal failure. Slight to moderate proteinuria is the rule in patients with heart failure.

APPROACH TO THE PATIENT

An important first question is whether the edema is localized or generalized. If it is localized, those phenomena that may be responsible should be concentrated upon. If the edema is generalized, it should be determined, first, if there is serious hypoalbuminemia, e.g., serum albumin <25 g/L. If so, the history, physical examination, urinalysis, and other laboratory data will help evaluate the question of cirrhosis, severe malnutrition, protein-losing gastroenteropathy, or the nephrotic syndrome as the underlying disorder. If hypoalbuminemia is not present, it should be determined if there is evidence of congestive heart failure of a severity to promote generalized edema. Finally, it should be determined whether the patient has an adequate urine output, or if there is significant oliguria or even anuria. →*These abnormalities are discussed in Chaps. 40, 260, and 261.*

FURTHER READING

ABASSI ZA et al: Control of extracellular fluid volume and the pathophysiology of edema formation, in *The Kidney*, 7th ed, BM Brenner (ed). Philadelphia, Saunders, 2004, pp 777–856

CHERTOW GM: Approach to the patient with edema, in E Braunwald, L Goldman (eds): *Cardiology for the Primary Care Physician,* 2nd ed, Philadelphia, Saunders, 2003, p 117–128

DISKIN CJ et al: Edema, oncotic pressure, and free entropy: Novel considerations for treatment of edema through attention to thermodynamics. Nephron 78:131, 1998

MCCULLOUGH JC: Renal disorders and heart disease, in Zipes D et al (eds): *Braunwald's Heart Disease,* 7th ed, Philadelphia, Saunders, 2005

SCHRIER RW, FASSETT RG: A critique of the overfill hypothesis of sodium and water retention in the nephrotic syndrome. Kidney Int 53:1111, 1998

33 | DYSPHAGIA
Raj K. Goyal

Dysphagia is defined as a sensation of "sticking" or obstruction of the passage of food through the mouth, pharynx, or esophagus. It should be distinguished from other symptoms related to swallowing. *Aphagia* signifies complete esophageal obstruction, which is usually due to bolus impaction and represents a medical emergency. *Difficulty in initiating a swallow* occurs in disorders of the voluntary phase of swallowing. However, once initiated, swallowing is completed normally. *Odynophagia* means painful swallowing. Frequently, odynophagia and dysphagia occur together. *Globus pharyngeous* is the sensation of a lump lodged in the throat. However, no difficulty is encountered when swallowing is performed. *Misdirection of food*, resulting in nasal regurgitation and laryngeal and pulmonary aspiration of food during swallowing, is characteristic of oropharyngeal dysphagia. *Phagophobia*, meaning fear of swallowing, and *refusal to swallow* may occur in hysteria, rabies, tetanus, and pharyngeal paralysis due to fear of aspiration. Painful inflammatory lesions that cause odynophagia may also cause refusal to swallow. Some patients may feel the food as it goes down the esophagus. This esophageal sensitivity is not associated with either food sticking or obstruction, however. Similarly, the *feeling of fullness in the epigastrium* that occurs after a meal or after swallowing air should not be confused with dysphagia.

PHYSIOLOGY OF SWALLOWING The process of swallowing begins with a voluntary (oral) phase during which a bolus of food is pushed into the pharynx by the contraction of the tongue. The bolus then activates oropharyngeal sensory receptors that initiate the involuntary (pharyngeal and esophageal) phase, or deglutition reflex. The deglutition reflex is a complex series of events and serves both to propel food through the pharynx and the esophagus and to prevent its entry into the airway. When the bolus is propelled backward by the tongue, the larynx moves forward and the upper esophageal sphincter opens. As the bolus moves into the pharynx, contraction of the superior pharyngeal constrictor against the contracted soft palate initiates a peristaltic contraction that proceeds rapidly downward to move the bolus through the pharynx and the esophagus. The lower esophageal sphincter opens as the food enters the esophagus and remains open until the peristaltic contraction has swept the bolus into the stomach. Peristaltic contraction in response to a swallow is called *primary peristalsis*. It involves inhibition followed by sequential contraction of muscles along the entire swallowing passage. The inhibition that precedes the peristaltic contraction is called *deglutitive inhibition*. Local distention of the esophagus from food activates intramural reflexes in the smooth muscle and results in *secondary peristalsis*, which is limited to the thoracic esophagus. *Tertiary contractions* are nonperistaltic because they occur simultaneously over a long segment of the esophagus. Tertiary contractions may occur in response to a swallow or esophageal distention, or they may occur spontaneously.

PATHOPHYSIOLOGY OF DYSPHAGIA The normal transport of an ingested bolus through the swallowing passage depends on the size of the ingested bolus; the luminal diameter of the swallowing passage; the force of peristaltic contraction; and deglutitive inhibition, including normal relaxation of upper and lower esophageal sphincters during swallowing. Dysphagia caused by a large bolus or luminal narrowing is called *mechanical dysphagia*, whereas dysphagia due to weakness of peristaltic contractions or to impaired deglutitive inhibition causing nonperistaltic contractions and impaired sphincter relaxation is called *motor dysphagia*.

Mechanical Dysphagia Mechanical dysphagia can be caused by a very large food bolus, intrinsic narrowing, or extrinsic compression of the lumen. In an adult, the esophageal lumen can distend up to 4 cm in diameter. When the esophagus cannot dilate beyond 2.5 cm in diam-

eter, dysphagia to normal solid food can occur. Dysphagia is always present when the esophagus cannot distend beyond 1.3 cm. Circumferential lesions produce dysphagia more consistently than do lesions that involve only a portion of circumferences of the esophageal wall, as uninvolved segments retain their distensibility. The causes of mechanical dysphagia are listed in Table 33-1. Common causes include carcinoma, peptic and other benign strictures, and lower esophageal ring.

Motor Dysphagia Motor dysphagia may result from difficulty in initiating a swallow or from abnormalities in peristalsis and deglutitive inhibition due to diseases of the esophageal striated or smooth muscle.

Diseases of the striated muscle involve the pharynx, upper esophageal sphincter, and cervical esophagus. The striated muscle is innervated by a somatic component of the vagus with cell bodies of the lower motor neurons located in the nucleus ambiguus. These neurons are cholinergic and excitatory and are the sole determinant of the muscle activity. Peristalsis in the striated muscle segment is due to sequential central activation of neurons innervating muscles at different levels along the esophagus. Motor dysphagia of the pharynx results from neuromuscular disorders causing muscle paralysis, simultaneous nonperistaltic contraction, or loss of opening of the upper esophageal sphincter. Loss of opening of the upper sphincter is caused by paralysis of geniohyoid and other suprahyoid muscles or loss of deglutitive inhibition of the cricopharyngeus muscle. Because each side of the pharynx is innervated by ipsilateral nerves, a unilateral lesion of motor neurons leads to unilateral pharyngeal paralysis. Although lesions of striated muscle also involve the cervical part of the esophagus, the clinical manifestations of pharyngeal dysfunction usually overshadow those due to esophageal involvement.

Diseases of the smooth-muscle segment involve the thoracic part of the esophagus and the lower esophageal sphincter. The smooth muscle is innervated by the parasympathetic component of the vagal preganglionic fibers and postganglionic neurons in the myenteric ganglia. The vagal pathway consists of parallel excitatory and inhibitory pathways that use acetylcholine and nitric oxide as neurotransmitters, respectively. The activation of inhibitory nerves causes inhibition that is followed by rebound contraction. These pathways are involved in the resting tone of the lower esophageal sphincter, swallow-induced lower esophageal sphincter opening, and inhibition followed by peristaltic contractions in the esophageal body. Dysphagia results when the peristaltic contractions are weak or nonperistaltic or when the lower sphincter fails to relax normally. Loss of contractile power occurs due to muscle weakness, as in scleroderma. The nonperistaltic contractions and impaired relaxation of the lower esophageal sphincter result from a defect in inhibitory vagal innervation and account for dysphagia in achalasia.

The causes of motor dysphagia are also listed in Table 33-1. Important causes are pharyngeal paralysis, cricopharyngeal achalasia, scleroderma of the esophagus, achalasia, and diffuse esophageal spasm and related motor disorders.

APPROACH TO THE PATIENT

History The history can provide a presumptive diagnosis in >80% of patients. The type of food causing dysphagia provides useful information. Difficulty only with solids implies mechanical dysphagia with a lumen that is not severely narrowed. In advanced obstruction, dysphagia occurs with liquids as well as solids. In contrast, motor dysphagia due to achalasia and diffuse esophageal spasm is equally affected by solids and liquids from the very onset. Patients with scleroderma have dysphagia to solids that is unrelated to posture and to liquids while recumbent but not upright. When peptic stricture develops in patients with scleroderma, dysphagia becomes more persistent.

The duration and course of dysphagia are helpful in diagnosis. Transient dysphagia may be due to an inflammatory process. Pro-

TABLE 33-1 *Causes of Dysphagia*

MECHANICAL DYSPHAGIA

I. Luminal
   A. Large bolus
   B. Foreign body
II. Intrinsic narrowing
   A. Inflammatory condition causing edema and swelling
      1. Stomatitis
      2. Pharyngitis, epiglottitis
      3. Esophagitis
         a. Viral (herpes simplex, varicella-zoster, cytomegalovirus)
         b. Bacterial
         c. Fungal (candidal)
         d. Mucocutaneous bullous diseases
         e. Caustic, chemical, thermal injury
   B. Webs and rings
      1. Pharyngeal (Plummer-Vinson syndrome)
      2. Esophageal (congenital, inflammatory)
      3. Lower esophageal mucosal ring (Schatzki ring)
   C. Benign strictures
      1. Peptic
      2. Caustic and pill-induced
      3. Inflammatory (Crohn's disease, candidal, mucocutaneous lesions)
      4. Ischemic
      5. Postoperative, postirradiation
      6. Congenital
   D. Malignant tumors
      1. Primary carcinoma
         a. Squamous cell carcinoma
         b. Adenocarcinoma
         c. Carcinosarcoma
         d. Pseudosarcoma
         e. Lymphoma
         f. Melanoma
         g. Kaposi's sarcoma
      2. Metastatic carcinoma
   E. Benign tumors
      1. Leiomyoma
      2. Lipoma
      3. Angioma
      4. Inflammatory fibroid polyp
      5. Epithelial papilloma
III. Extrinsic compression
   A. Cervical spondylitis
   B. Vertebral osteophytes
   C. Retropharyngeal abscess and masses
   D. Enlarged thyroid gland
   E. Zenker's diverticulum
   F. Vascular compression
      1. Aberrant right subclavian artery
      2. Right-sided aorta
      3. Left atrial enlargement
      4. Aortic aneurysm
   G. Posterior mediastinal masses
   H. Pancreatic tumor, pancreatitis
   I. Postvagotomy hematoma and fibrosis

MOTOR (NEUROMUSCULAR) DYSPHAGIA

I. Difficulty in initiating swallowing reflex
   A. Paralysis of the tongue
   B. Oropharyngeal anesthesia
   C. Lack of saliva (e.g., Sjögren's syndrome)
   D. Lesions of sensory components of vagus and glossopharyngeal nerves
   E. Lesions of swallowing center
II. Disorders of pharyngeal and esophageal striated muscle
   A. Muscle weakness
      1. Lower motor neuron lesion (bulbar paralysis)
         a. Cerebrovascular accident
         b. Motor neuron disease
         c. Poliomyelitis, postpolio syndrome
         d. Polyneuritis
         e. Amyotrophic lateral sclerosis
         f. Familial dysautonomia
      2. Neuromuscular
         a. Myasthenia gravis
      3. Muscle disorders
         a. Polymyositis
         b. Dermatomyositis
         c. Myopathies (myotonic dystrophy, oculopharyngeal myopathy)
   B. Nonperistaltic contractions or impaired deglutitive inhibition
      1. Pharynx and upper esophagus
         a. Rabies
         b. Tetanus
         c. Extrapyramidal tract disease
         d. Upper motor neuron lesions (pseudobulbar paralysis)
      2. Upper esophageal sphincter (UES)
         a. Paralysis of suprahyoid muscles (causes same as paralysis of pharyngeal musculature)
         b. Cricopharyngeal achalasia
III. Disorders of esophageal smooth muscle
   A. Paralysis of esophageal body causing weak contractions
      1. Scleroderma and related collagen vascular diseases
      2. Hollow visceral myopathy
      3. Myotonic dystrophy
      4. Metabolic neuromyopathy (amyloid, alcohol?, diabetes?)
      5. Achalasia (classical)
   B. Nonperistaltic contractions or impaired deglutitive inhibition
      1. Esophageal body
         a. Diffuse esophageal spasm
         b. Achalasia (vigorous)
         c. Variants of diffuse esophageal spasm
      2. Lower esophageal sphincter
         a. Achalasia
            (1) Primary
            (2) Secondary
               (a) Chagas' disease
               (b) Carcinoma
               (c) Lymphoma
               (d) Neuropathic intestinal pseudoobstruction syndrome
               (e) Toxins and drugs
         b. Lower esophageal muscular (contractile) ring

gressive dysphagia lasting a few weeks to a few months is suggestive of carcinoma of the esophagus. Episodic dysphagia to solids lasting several years indicates a benign disease characteristic of a lower esophageal ring.

The site of dysphagia described by the patient helps to determine the site of esophageal obstruction; the lesion is at or below the perceived location of dysphagia.

Associated symptoms provide important diagnostic clues. Nasal regurgitation and tracheobronchial aspiration with swallowing are hallmarks of pharyngeal paralysis or a tracheoesophageal fistula. Tracheobronchial aspiration unrelated to swallowing may be secondary to achalasia, Zenker's diverticulum, or gastroesophageal reflux.

Severe weight loss that is out of proportion to the degree of dysphagia is highly suggestive of carcinoma. When hoarseness precedes dysphagia, the primary lesion is usually in the larynx.

Hoarseness following dysphagia may suggest involvement of the recurrent laryngeal nerve by extension of esophageal carcinoma. Sometimes hoarseness may be due to laryngitis secondary to gastroesophageal reflux. Association of laryngeal symptoms and dysphagia also occurs in various neuromuscular disorders. Hiccups may rarely occur with a lesion in the distal portion of the esophagus. Unilateral wheezing with dysphagia indicates a mediastinal mass involving the esophagus and a large bronchus.

Chest pain with dysphagia occurs in diffuse esophageal spasm and related motor disorders. Chest pain resembling diffuse esophageal spasms may occur in esophageal obstruction due to a large bolus. A prolonged history of heartburn and reflux preceding dysphagia indicates peptic stricture. A history of prolonged nasogastric intubation, ingestion of caustic agents, ingestion of pills without water, previous radiation therapy, or associated mucocutaneous diseases may provide the cause of esophageal stricture. If odynophagia is present, candidal or herpes esophagitis or pill-induced esophagitis should be suspected.

In patients with AIDS or other immunodeficiency states, esophagitis due to opportunistic infections such as *Candida*, herpes simplex virus, or cytomegalovirus and tumors such as Kaposi's sarcoma and lymphoma should be suspected.

Physical Examination Physical examination is important in motor dysphagia due to skeletal muscle, neurologic, and oropharyngeal diseases. Signs of bulbar or pseudobulbar palsy, including dysarthria, dysphonia, ptosis, tongue atrophy, and hyperactive jaw jerk, in addition to evidence of generalized neuromuscular disease, should be sought. The neck should be examined for thyromegaly or a spinal abnormality. A careful inspection of the mouth and pharynx should disclose lesions that may interfere with passage of food because of pain or obstruction. Changes in the skin and extremities may suggest a diagnosis of scleroderma and other collagen vascular diseases or mucocutaneous diseases such as pemphigoid or epidermolysis bullosa, which may involve the esophagus. Cancer spread to lymph nodes and liver may be evident. Pulmonary complications of acute aspiration pneumonia or chronic aspiration may be present.

Diagnostic Procedures Dysphagia is nearly always a symptom of organic disease rather than a functional complaint. If oropharyngeal

dysphagia is suspected, videofluoroscopy of oropharyngeal swallowing should be obtained. If mechanical dysphagia is suspected on clinical history, barium swallow, esophagogastroscopy and endoscopic biopsies are the diagnostic procedures of choice. Barium swallow and esophageal motility studies are diagnostic tests for motor dysphagia. Esophagogastroscopy may be needed in patients with motor dysphagia to exclude an associated structural abnormality (Chap. 273).

FURTHER READING

GOYAL RK, HIRANO I: Mechanisms of disease: The enteric nervous system. N Engl J Med 334:110, 1996

HENDRIX TR: Art and science of history taking in the patient with difficulty swallowing. Dysphagia 8:69, 1993

KOCH WM: Swallowing disorders. Diagnosis and therapy. Med Clin North Am 77:571, 1993

MORTON RE et al: Videofluoroscopy in the assessment of feeding disorders of children with neurological problems. J Dev Med Child Neurol 35:388, 1993

SPIEKER MR: Evaluating dysphagia. Am Fam Physician 61:3639, 2000

34 NAUSEA, VOMITING, AND INDIGESTION
William L. Hasler

Nausea is the subjective feeling of a need to vomit. *Vomiting* (emesis) is the oral expulsion of upper gastrointestinal contents resulting from contractions of gut and thoracoabdominal wall musculature. Vomiting is contrasted with *regurgitation*, the effortless passage of gastric contents into the mouth. *Rumination* is the repeated regurgitation of stomach contents, which are often rechewed and then reswallowed. In contrast to vomiting, these phenomena often exhibit some volitional control. *Indigestion* is a nonspecific term that encompasses a variety of upper abdominal complaints including nausea, vomiting, heartburn, regurgitation, and dyspepsia (upper abdominal discomfort or pain). Some individuals with dyspepsia report ulcer-like symptoms such as epigastric burning or gnawing discomfort. Others experience symptoms of gastric dysmotility such as postprandial fullness, bloating, eructation (belching), anorexia (loss of appetite), and early satiety (an inability to complete a meal due to premature fullness).

NAUSEA AND VOMITING

MECHANISMS Vomiting is coordinated by the brainstem and is effected by neuromuscular responses in the gut, pharynx, and thoracoabdominal wall. The mechanisms underlying nausea are poorly understood but likely involve the cerebral cortex, as nausea requires conscious perception. Electroencephalographic studies show activation of temporofrontal cortical regions with induction of nausea.

Coordination of Emesis Several brainstem nuclei initiate emesis, including the nucleus tractus solitarius, the dorsal vagal and phrenic nuclei, and medullary nuclei that regulate respiration; nuclei that control pharyngeal, facial, and tongue movements coordinate the initiation of emesis. The neurotransmitters involved in this coordination are uncertain; however, roles for neurokinin NK_1, serotonin, and vasopressin pathways are postulated.

Somatic and visceral muscles exhibit stereotypic responses during emesis. Inspiratory thoracic and abdominal wall muscles contract, producing high intrathoracic and intraabdominal pressures that facilitate expulsion of gastric contents. The gastric cardia herniates across the diaphragm, and the larynx moves upward to promote oral propulsion of the vomitus. Under normal conditions, distally migrating gut contractions are regulated by an electrical phenomenon, the slow wave,

which cycles at 3 cycles/min in the stomach and 11 cycles/min in the duodenum. With emesis, slow waves are replaced by orally propagating spike activity, which induces retrograde contractions that assist in the oral expulsion of small-intestinal contents.

Activators of Emesis Emetic stimuli act at several anatomic sites. Emesis provoked by noxious thoughts or smells originates in the cerebral cortex, whereas cranial nerves mediate vomiting after gag reflex activation. Motion sickness and inner ear disorders act on the labyrinthine apparatus, while gastric irritants and emetogenic anticancer agents such as cisplatin stimulate gastroduodenal vagal afferent nerves. Nongastric visceral afferents are activated by small intestinal and colonic obstruction and mesenteric ischemia. The area postrema, a medullary nucleus, responds to bloodborne emetic stimuli and is termed the *chemoreceptor trigger zone*. Many emetic drugs act on the area postrema as do bacterial toxins and metabolic disorders such as uremia, hypoxia, and ketoacidosis.

Neurotransmitters that mediate induction of vomiting are selective for these anatomic sites. Labyrinthine disorders stimulate vestibular cholinergic muscarinic M_1 and histaminergic H_1 receptors, whereas gastroduodenal vagal afferent stimuli activate serotonin $5-HT_3$ receptors. The area postrema is richly served by nerve fibers acting on $5-HT_3$, M_1, H_1, and dopamine D_2 receptor subtypes. Optimal pharmacologic management requires an understanding of these pathways.

DIFFERENTIAL DIAGNOSIS Nausea and vomiting are caused by conditions within and outside the gut as well as by drugs and circulating toxins (Table 34-1).

Intraperitoneal Disorders Visceral obstruction and inflammation of hollow and solid viscera may produce vomiting as the main symptom. Gastric obstruction results from ulcer disease and malignancy, whereas small-bowel and colonic obstructions occur as a consequence of adhesions, benign or malignant tumors, volvulus, intussusception, or inflammatory diseases such as Crohn's disease. The superior mesenteric artery syndrome, occurring after weight loss or prolonged bed rest, results when the duodenum is compressed by the overlying superior mesenteric artery. Abdominal irradiation impairs intestinal contractile function and induces strictures. Biliary colic causes nausea by action

TABLE 34-1 *Causes of Nausea and Vomiting*

Intraperitoneal	Extraperitoneal	Medications/Metabolic Disorders
Obstructing disorders	Cardiopulmonary disease	Drugs
Pyloric obstruction	Cardiomyopathy	Cancer chemotherapy
Small bowel obstruction	Myocardial infarction	Antibiotics
Colonic obstruction	Labyrinthine disease	Cardiac antiarrhythmics
Superior mesenteric artery	Motion sickness	Digoxin
syndrome	Labyrinthitis	Oral hypoglycemics
Enteric infections	Malignancy	Oral contraceptives
Viral	Intracerebral disorders	Endocrine/metabolic disease
Bacterial	Malignancy	Pregnancy
Inflammatory diseases	Hemorrhage	Uremia
Cholecystitis	Abscess	Ketoacidosis
Pancreatitis	Hydrocephalus	Thyroid and parathyroid disease
Appendicitis	Psychiatric illness	Adrenal insufficiency
Hepatitis	Anorexia and bulimia nervosa	Toxins
Impaired motor function	Depression	Liver failure
Gastroparesis	Psychogenic vomiting	Ethanol
Intestinal	Postoperative vomiting	
pseudoobstruction	Cyclic vomiting syndrome	
Functional dyspepsia		
Gastroesophageal reflux		
Biliary colic		
Abdominal irradiation		

on visceral afferent nerves. Vomiting with pancreatitis, cholecystitis, and appendicitis is due to localized visceral irritation and induction of ileus. Enteric infections with viruses or bacteria such as *Staphylococcus aureus* and *Bacillus cereus* are among the most common causes of acute vomiting, especially in children. Opportunistic infections such as cytomegalovirus or herpes simplex induce emesis in immunocompromised individuals.

Disordered gut motor function also commonly causes nausea and vomiting. *Gastroparesis* is defined as a delay in emptying of food from the stomach and occurs after vagotomy for peptic ulcer; with pancreatic adenocarcinoma; with mesenteric vascular insufficiency; or in systemic diseases such as diabetes, scleroderma, and amyloidosis. Idiopathic gastroparesis occurring in the absence of systemic illness may follow a viral prodrome suggesting an infectious etiology. *Intestinal pseudoobstruction* is characterized by disrupted intestinal and colonic motor activity and leads to intestinal retention of food residue and secretions; bacterial overgrowth; nutrient malabsorption; and symptoms of nausea, vomiting, bloating, pain, and altered defecation. Intestinal pseudoobstruction may be idiopathic, inherited as a familial visceral myopathy or neuropathy, or result from systemic disease or as a paraneoplastic consequence of malignancy (especially small-cell lung carcinoma). Patients with functional dyspepsia and irritable bowel syndrome may report prominent nausea and vomiting, as do some individuals with gastroesophageal reflux.

Extraperitoneal Disorders Myocardial infarction and congestive heart failure are cardiac causes of nausea and vomiting. Emesis occurs after 25% of surgical operations, most commonly laparotomy and orthopedic surgery, and is more prevalent in women. Increased intracranial pressure from tumors, bleeding, abscess, or obstruction to cerebrospinal fluid outflow produces prominent vomiting with or without nausea. Motion sickness, labyrinthitis, and Ménière's disease evoke symptoms via labyrinthine pathways. Cyclic vomiting syndrome is a rare disorder of unknown etiology that produces episodes of intractable nausea and vomiting, usually in children. The syndrome shows a strong association with migraine headaches, suggesting that some cases may be migraine variants. Patients with psychiatric illnesses, including anorexia nervosa, bulimia, anxiety, and depression, may report significant nausea. Psychogenic vomiting occurs most commonly in women with other emotional problems.

Medications and Metabolic Disorders Drugs evoke vomiting by action on the stomach (analgesics, erythromycin) or area postrema (digoxin, opiates, anti-parkinsonian drugs). Emetogenic agents include antibiotics, antiarrhythmics, antihypertensives, oral hypoglycemics, and contra-

ceptives. Cancer chemotherapy causes vomiting that is acute (within hours of administration), delayed (after 1 or more days), or anticipatory. Acute emesis resulting from highly emetogenic agents such as cisplatin is mediated by 5-HT$_3$ pathways, whereas delayed emesis is 5-HT$_3$ independent. Anticipatory nausea often responds better to anxiolytic therapy than to antiemetics.

Metabolic disorders elicit nausea and vomiting in certain settings. Pregnancy is the most prevalent endocrinologic cause of nausea, occurring in 70% of women in the first trimester. Hyperemesis gravidarum is a severe form of nausea of pregnancy that can produce significant fluid loss and electrolyte disturbances. Uremia, ketoacidosis, adrenal insufficiency, as well as parathyroid and thyroid disease are other metabolic causes of emesis.

Circulating toxins evoke symptoms through effects on the area postrema. Endogenous toxins are generated in fulminant liver failure, whereas exogenous enterotoxins may be produced by enteric bacterial infection. Ethanol intoxication is a common toxic cause of nausea and vomiting.

APPROACH TO THE PATIENT

History and Physical Examination The history helps define the etiology of unexplained nausea and vomiting. Drugs, toxins, and gastrointestinal infections often cause acute symptoms, while established illnesses evoke chronic complaints. Pyloric obstruction and gastroparesis produce vomiting within 1 h of eating, whereas emesis from intestinal obstruction occurs later. In severe cases of gastroparesis, the vomitus may contain food residue ingested hours or days previously. Hematemesis raises suspicion of an ulcer or malignancy or a Mallory-Weiss tear, whereas feculent emesis is noted with distal intestinal or colonic obstruction. Bilious vomiting excludes gastric obstruction, whereas emesis of undigested food is consistent with a Zenker's diverticulum or achalasia. Relief of abdominal pain by emesis characterizes small-bowel obstruction, but vomiting has no effect on pancreatitis or cholecystitis pain. Pronounced weight loss raises concern about malignancy or obstruction. Fevers suggest inflammation, while an intracranial source is considered if there are headaches or visual field changes. Vertigo or tinnitus indicates labyrinthine disease.

The physical examination complements the history. Orthostatic hypotension and poor skin turgor indicate intravascular fluid depletion. Pulmonary abnormalities raise concern that vomitus was aspirated. Abdominal auscultation may reveal absent bowel sounds with ileus. High-pitched rushes suggest bowel obstruction, while a succession splash on abrupt lateral movement of the patient is found with gastroparesis or pyloric obstruction. Tenderness or involuntary guarding raises suspicion of inflammation, whereas fecal blood suggests mucosal injury from ulcer, ischemia, or tumor. Neurologic etiologies present with papilledema, visual field loss, or focal neural abnormalities. Neoplasm is suggested by palpable masses or adenopathy.

Diagnostic Testing With intractable symptoms or an elusive diagnosis, selected diagnostic tests can direct clinical management. Electrolyte replenishment is indicated for hypokalemia or metabolic alkalosis. Detection of iron-deficiency anemia mandates a search for mucosal injury. Pancreaticobiliary disease is suggested by abnormal pancreatic enzymes or liver biochemistries, whereas endocrinologic, rheumatologic, or paraneoplastic etiologies are diagnosed by specific hormone or serologic testing. If luminal obstruction is suspected, supine and upright abdominal radiographs may show intestinal air-fluid levels with reduced colonic air. Ileus is characterized by diffusely dilated air-filled bowel loops.

Anatomic studies may be indicated if initial testing is nondiagnostic. Upper endoscopy detects ulcer or malignancy, and small-bowel barium radiography diagnoses partial small-bowel obstruction. Colonoscopy or contrast barium enema can detect colonic obstruction. Abdominal ultrasound or computed tomography (CT) defines intraperitoneal inflammatory processes, while CT or magnetic resonance imaging (MRI) of the head can delineate intracranial sources of nausea and vomiting. Mesenteric angiography or MRI is useful when ischemia is considered.

TABLE 34-2   Treatment of Nausea and Vomiting

Treatment	Mechanism	Examples	Clinical Indications
Antiemetic agents	Antihistaminergic	Dimenhydrinate, meclizine	Motion sickness, inner ear disease
	Anticholinergic	Scopolamine	Motion sickness, inner ear disease
	Antidopaminergic	Prochlorperazine, droperidol	Medication-, toxin-, or metabolic-induced emesis
	5-HT$_3$ antagonist	Ondansetron, granisetron	Chemotherapy- and radiation-induced emesis, postoperative emesis
	Tricyclic antidepressant	Amitriptyline, nortriptyline	Functional nausea
Prokinetic agents	5-HT$_4$ agonist	Cisapride	Gastroparesis, functional dyspepsia, gastroesophageal reflux disease, intestinal pseudoobstruction
	5-HT$_4$ agonist and antidopaminergic	Metoclopramide	Gastroparesis, functional dyspepsia
	Motilin agonist	Erythromycin	Gastroparesis, ?Intestinal pseudoobstruction
	Peripheral antidopaminergic	Domperidone	Gastroparesis, functional dyspepsia
Special settings	Somatostatin analogue	Octreotide	Intestinal pseudoobstruction
	Benzodiazepines	Lorazepam	Anticipatory nausea and vomiting with chemotherapy
	Glucocorticoids	Methylprednisolone, dexamethasone	Chemotherapy-induced emesis
	Cannabinoids	Tetrahydrocannabinol	?Chemotherapy-induced emesis

Gastrointestinal motility testing may detect a motor disorder that contributes to symptoms when anatomic abnormalities are absent. Gastroparesis is most commonly diagnosed with gastric scintigraphy, by which emptying of a radiolabeled meal is measured. Electrogastrography, a noninvasive method to test gastric slow-wave activity using cutaneous electrodes placed over the stomach, has been proposed as an alternative means of diagnosing gastroparesis. The diagnosis of intestinal pseudoobstruction is suggested by abnormal barium transit on small-bowel contrast radiography. Small-intestinal manometry may provide confirmation of the diagnosis and further characterize the motor abnormality as neuropathic or myopathic based on contractile patterns. Such investigation can obviate the need for open intestinal biopsy to evaluate for smooth-muscle or neuronal degeneration.

Rx TREATMENT

General Principles   Therapy of vomiting is tailored to correction of medically or surgically remediable abnormalities, if possible. Hospitalization is considered for severe dehydration, especially if oral fluid replenishment cannot be sustained. Once oral intake is tolerated, nutrients are restarted with liquids that are low in fat, as lipids delay gastric emptying. Foods high in indigestible residues are avoided because these also prolong gastric retention.

Antiemetic Medications   The most commonly used antiemetic agents act on the central nervous system (Table 34-2). Antihistamines such as meclizine and dimenhydrinate and anticholinergic drugs such as scopolamine act on labyrinthine-activated pathways and are useful in motion sickness and inner ear disorders. Phenothiazine and butyrophenone dopamine D$_2$ antagonists are used to treat emesis evoked by area postrema stimuli and are effective for medication, toxic, and metabolic etiologies. Dopamine antagonists freely cross the blood-brain barrier and may cause anxiety, dystonic reactions, hyperprolactinemic effects (galactorrhea and sexual dysfunction), and irreversible tardive dyskinesia.

Other drug classes have antiemetic properties. Serotonin 5-HT$_3$ antagonists such as ondansetron and granisetron are useful in the treatment of postoperative vomiting, after radiation therapy, and in the prevention of cancer chemotherapy–induced emesis. The usefulness of 5-HT$_3$ antagonists for other causes of emesis is less well established. Low-dose tricyclic antidepressants provide symptomatic benefit in patients with unexplained nausea of a functional nature, as well as in diabetic patients with nausea and vomiting whose disease is of long standing.

Gastrointestinal Motor Stimulants   Drugs that stimulate gastric emptying are indicated for gastroparesis (Table 34-2). Metoclopramide, a combined 5-HT$_4$ agonist and D$_2$ antagonist, is effective in gastroparesis, but antidopaminergic side effects limit its use in 20% of patients. Erythromycin, a macrolide antibiotic, potently increases gastroduodenal motility by action on receptors for motilin, an endogenous stimulant of fasting motor activity. Intravenous erythromycin is useful in patients with refractory gastroparesis; however, oral forms of the drug also have some effect. Domperidone, a D$_2$ antagonist not available in the United States, has prokinetic and antiemetic effects but does not cross into most other brain regions; thus, anxiety and dystonic reactions are rare. The main side effects of domperidone are induction of hyperprolactinemia through effects on pituitary regions served by a porous blood-brain barrier.

Patients with refractory upper gut motility disorders pose significant challenges. Liquid suspensions of prokinetic drugs may be beneficial as liquids empty from the stomach more rapidly than pills. Metoclopramide can be administered subcutaneously in patients who do not respond to oral drugs. Intestinal pseudoobstruction may respond to the somatostatin analogue octreotide, which induces propagative small-intestinal motor complexes. Pyloric injections of botulinum toxin are reported in uncontrolled studies to benefit patients with idiopathic or diabetic gastroparesis. Placement of a feeding jejunostomy reduces hospitalizations and improves overall health in some patients with gastroparesis who do not respond to drug therapy. Surgical options are limited for refractory cases, but postvagotomy gastroparesis may improve with near-total resection of the stomach. Implanted gastric electrical pacemakers and neurostimulators may reduce symptoms, improve quality-of-life, and decrease health care expenditures in patients with medication-refractory gastroparesis.

Selected Clinical Settings   Cancer chemotherapeutic agents such as cisplatin are intensely emetogenic. Given prophylactically, 5-HT$_3$ antagonists prevent chemotherapy-induced acute vomiting in most cases (Table 34-2). Optimal antiemetic effects are often obtained with a 5-HT$_3$ antagonist in combination with a glucocorticoid. High-dose metoclopramide is also effective in chemotherapy-evoked emesis, whereas benzodiazepines such as lorazepam are useful in reducing anticipatory nausea and vomiting. Delayed emesis 1 to 5 days after chemotherapy is more refractory to treatment. Novel neurokinin NK$_1$ antagonists may be potent antiemetic and antinausea drugs during both the acute and the delayed periods after chemotherapy. Cannabinoids such as tetrahydrocannabinol, long advocated for cancer-associated emesis, produce significant side effects and are no more effective than antidopaminergic agents. Most current drug regimens are more effective at controlling emesis than nausea.

The clinician should exercise caution in managing the pregnant patient with nausea. Studies of the teratogenic effects of available antiemetic agents provide conflicting results. Few controlled trials have been performed in the nausea of pregnancy, although antihistamines such as meclizine and antidopaminergics such as prochlorperazine are more effective than placebo. Alternative therapies such as pyridoxine, acupressure, or ginger are being tested.

Controlling emesis in children with cyclic vomiting syndrome is a challenge. 5-HT$_3$ antagonists are a mainstay of treatment. Considering the possible link to migraine headaches, anti-migraine therapy with antidepressants and the serotonin 5-HT$_1$ agonist, sumatriptan, may be tried.

INDIGESTION

MECHANISMS The most common causes of indigestion are gastroesophageal acid reflux and functional dyspepsia. Other cases are a consequence of a more serious organic illness.

Gastroesophageal Acid Reflux Acid reflux can result from a variety of physiologic defects. Reduced lower esophageal sphincter (LES) tone is an important cause of reflux in scleroderma and pregnancy and may also be a factor in patients without other systemic conditions. Many individuals show frequent transient LES relaxations, during which acid bathes the esophagus. Overeating and aerophagia can transiently override the barrier function of the LES, whereas impaired esophageal body motility and reduced salivary secretion prolong acid exposure. The role of hiatal hernias is controversial—although most reflux patients exhibit hiatal hernias, most individuals with hiatal hernias do not have excess heartburn.

Gastric Motor Dysfunction Disturbed gastric motility is purported to cause acid reflux in some cases of indigestion. Delayed gastric emptying also is found in 25 to 50% of functional dyspeptics. The relation of these defects to symptom induction is uncertain; many studies show poor correlation between symptom severity and the degree of motor dysfunction. Abnormal gastric fundic relaxation after eating may cause selected dyspeptic symptoms such as bloating, fullness, nausea, and early satiety. A current focus of investigation is developing drugs that enhance fundic relaxation.

Visceral Afferent Hypersensitivity Disturbed gastric sensory function may also cause functional dyspepsia. Visceral afferent hypersensitivity was first demonstrated in patients with irritable bowel syndrome who had heightened perception of rectal balloon inflation without changes in rectal compliance. Patients with dyspepsia may experience discomfort with fundic distention to lower pressures than healthy control subjects.

Other Factors *Helicobacter pylori* has a clear etiologic role in peptic ulcer disease, but ulcers cause only a minority of cases of dyspepsia. The importance of *H. pylori* in the genesis of functional dyspepsia is controversial, but most investigators believe it is of minor importance. In contrast, functional dyspepsia is associated with a reduced sense of physical and mental well-being and is exacerbated by stress, suggesting an important role for psychological factors. Analgesics cause dys-

pepsia; nitrates, calcium channel blockers, theophylline, and progesterone promote acid reflux. Other exogenous factors that induce acid reflux include ethanol, tobacco, and caffeine via LES relaxation. Genetic factors may contribute to development of acid reflux.

DIFFERENTIAL DIAGNOSIS ■ Gastroesophageal Reflux Disease Gastroesophageal reflux disease (GERD) is prevalent in Western society. Heartburn is reported once monthly by 40% of Americans and daily by 7 to 10%. Most cases of heartburn occur because of excess acid reflux; however, some patients exhibit heightened sensitivity to normal amounts of acid exposure.

Functional Dyspepsia Functional dyspepsia, defined as ≥3 months of dyspepsia without an organic cause, is also common. Nearly 25% of the populace has abdominal discomfort at least six times yearly, but only 10 to 20% consult physicians. Functional dyspepsia accounts for 60% of cases of dyspepsia. Most patients with functional dyspepsia follow a benign course, but a small number with *H. pylori* infection or on nonsteroidal anti-inflammatory drugs (NSAIDs) progress to ulcer formation. As with idiopathic gastroparesis, some cases of functional dyspepsia appear to result from prior gastrointestinal infection.

Ulcer Disease In most cases of GERD, the esophagus is not damaged. However, 5% of patients develop esophageal ulcers, and some form strictures. Symptoms do not reliably distinguish nonerosive from erosive or ulcerative esophagitis. From 15 to 25% of cases of dyspepsia stem from ulcers of the stomach or duodenum. The most common causes of ulcer disease are gastric infection with *H. pylori* and use of NSAIDs. Other rare causes of gastroduodenal ulcer include Crohn's disease and Zollinger-Ellison syndrome, a condition resulting from gastrin overproduction by an endocrine tumor (Chap. 274).

Malignancy Dyspeptic patients often seek care because of fear of cancer. However, <2% of cases result from gastroesophageal malignancy. Esophageal squamous cell carcinoma occurs most often in those patients with histories of tobacco or ethanol intake. Other risk factors include prior caustic ingestion, achalasia, and the hereditary disorder tylosis. Esophageal adenocarcinoma usually complicates long-standing acid reflux. Between 8 and 20% of GERD patients exhibit glandular mucosal (intestinal) metaplasia of the squamous epithelium in the lower esophagus, termed *Barrett's metaplasia*. This condition predisposes to esophageal adenocarcinoma. Gastric malignancies include adenocarcinoma, which is more prevalent in certain Asian societies, and lymphoma (Chap. 77).

Other Causes Alkaline reflux esophagitis produces GERD-like symptoms in patients who have had surgery for peptic ulcer disease. Opportunistic fungal or viral esophageal infections may produce heartburn or chest discomfort but more often cause odynophagia. Biliary colic is in the differential diagnosis of dyspepsia, but most patients with true biliary colic report discrete episodes of right upper quadrant or epigastric pain rather than chronic burning discomfort, nausea, and bloating. Intestinal lactase deficiency produces gas, bloating, discomfort, and diarrhea after lactose ingestion; it occurs in 15% of Caucasians of northern European descent but is more common in African Americans and Asians. Other carbohydrate intolerance syndromes (e.g., fructose, sorbitol) produce similar symptoms. Pancreatic disease (chronic pancreatitis and malignancy), hepatocellular carcinoma, celiac sprue, Ménétrier's disease, infiltrative diseases (sarcoidosis and eosinophilic gastroenteritis), mesenteric ischemia, thyroid and parathyroid disease, and abdominal wall strain cause dyspepsia. Extraperitoneal etiologies of indigestion include congestive heart failure and tuberculosis.

APPROACH TO THE PATIENT

History and Physical Examination GERD classically produces heartburn, a substernal warmth beginning in the epigastrium that moves toward the neck. Heartburn is often exacerbated by meals and may awaken the patient. Associated symptoms include regurgitation of acid and water brash, the reflex release of salty salivary secretions into the mouth. Atypical symptoms include pharyngitis, asthma, cough, bronchitis, hoarseness, and chest pain that mimics angina. Some patients with acid reflux on esophageal pH testing do not report heartburn and instead note abdominal pain or other symptoms.

Some individuals with dyspepsia report ulcer-like symptoms including epigastric gnawing or burning that is relieved by meals or acid suppression. Others experience dysmotility-like fullness or pain that is aggravated by eating and associated with nausea, eructation, and early satiety. There is overlap of functional dyspepsia with other functional disorders such as irritable bowel syndrome.

The physical examination of individuals with GERD and functional dyspepsia is usually normal. In atypical GERD, pharyngeal erythema and wheezing may be present. Poor dentition may occur with prolonged acid regurgitation. Patients with functional dyspepsia may have epigastric tenderness or abdominal distention.

Discrimination between functional and organic causes of indigestion mandates exclusion of selected historic and examination features. Odynophagia suggests esophageal infection; dysphagia promotes concern about a benign or malignant esophageal blockage. Other features that raise alarm include unexplained weight loss, recurrent vomiting, occult or gross gastrointestinal bleeding, jaundice, and a palpable mass or adenopathy.

Diagnostic Testing Because indigestion is prevalent and because most cases result from GERD or functional dyspepsia, a general principle of diagnostic testing is to perform only limited and directed testing of selected individuals.

Once alarm factors are excluded, patients with typical GERD do not need further evaluation and are treated empirically. Upper endoscopy is indicated to exclude mucosal injury in patients with atypical symptoms, symptoms unresponsive to acid-suppressing drugs, or alarm factors. For heartburn >5 years in duration, especially in patients >50 years old, endoscopy is recommended by some experts to screen for Barrett's metaplasia. However, the benefits of this approach have not been validated in controlled studies. Ambulatory esophageal pH testing is considered for drug-refractory symptoms and atypical symptoms such as unexplained chest pain. Esophageal manometry is most commonly ordered when surgical treatment of GERD is considered. A low LES pressure may predict failure with drug therapy and identify patients who may require surgery. Demonstration of disordered esophageal body peristalsis may affect the decision to operate or modify the type of operation chosen. Manometry with provocative testing may clarify the diagnosis in patients with atypical symptoms. Blinded perfusion of saline then acid into the esophagus, known as the *Bernstein test*, can delineate whether unexplained chest discomfort results from acid reflux.

Upper endoscopy is performed as the initial diagnostic test in patients with unexplained dyspepsia who are >45 years old, have alarm factors, or are on NSAIDs because of the elevated risk of malignancy and ulcer in these groups. For younger patients without alarm factors not on NSAIDs, the "test and treat" approach is commonly applied. Determination of *H. pylori* status is made with urea breath testing, stool antigen measurement, or blood serology testing. Those who are *H. pylori* positive are treated to eradicate the infection. For those with negative tests, an acid suppressive regimen is offered empirically. If symptoms resolve on these regimens, no further intervention is required. Endoscopy is reserved for those who fail to respond to treatment of *H. pylori*–positive or –negative dyspepsia. Some clinicians advocate an alternative approach in which those with *H. pylori* undergo endoscopy before treatment. Eradication therapy is then offered only to those with proven ulcer disease. This approach may be preferred where gastric cancer is prevalent and endoscopy less costly.

Further testing is indicated if other factors are present. If bleeding is reported, a blood count is obtained to exclude anemia. Thyroid chemistries or calcium levels are done to screen for metabolic

disease. For suspected pancreaticobiliary causes, pancreatic and liver chemistry are obtained. If abnormalities are found, abdominal ultrasound or CT may give important information. Gastric emptying scintigraphy is considered for patients with dysmotility-like dyspepsia when drug treatment fails. Hydrogen breath testing after lactose ingestion may be performed for suspected lactase deficiency.

Rx TREATMENT

General Principles In mild indigestion, reassurance that a careful evaluation revealed no serious organic disease may be the only intervention required. Drugs that cause acid reflux or dyspepsia should be stopped if possible. Patients with GERD should limit ethanol, caffeine, chocolate, and tobacco use because of their effects on the LES. Other measures in GERD include ingestion of a low-fat diet, avoidance of snacks before bedtime, and elevation of the head of the bed.

Specific therapies for organic disease should be offered when possible. Surgery is appropriate in biliary colic, while diet changes are indicated for lactase deficiency and celiac sprue. Some illnesses such as peptic ulcer disease may be cured by specific medical regimens. However, as most indigestion is caused by GERD or functional dyspepsia, medications that reduce gastric acid, stimulate motility, or blunt gastric sensitivity are indicated.

Acid Suppressing or Neutralizing Medications Drugs that reduce or neutralize gastric acid are the most prescribed agents for GERD. Histamine H_2 receptor antagonists such as cimetidine, ranitidine, famotidine, and nizatidine are useful in mild to moderate GERD. For uncomplicated heartburn, H_2 receptor antagonists are given for 4 weeks before considering endoscopy. For severe symptoms or for many cases of erosive or ulcerative esophagitis, proton pump inhibitors such as omeprazole, lansoprazole, rabeparzole, pantoprazole, or esomeprazole are needed. These drugs, which inhibit gastric H^+, K^+-ATPase, are more potent than H_2 receptor antagonists. Acid suppressants may be taken continuously or as needed, depending on symptom severity. Many patients initially started on a proton pump inhibitor can be stepped down to an H_2 antagonist. The role of combined therapy with a proton pump inhibitor and an H_2 antagonist is undefined. Liquid antacids are useful for short-term control of mild GERD but are less effective for severe disease unless given at high doses that produce side effects (diarrhea with magnesium-containing agents and constipation with aluminum-containing agents). Sucralfate is a salt of aluminum hydroxide and sucrose octasulfate and buffers acid and binds pepsin and bile salts. Its efficacy in GERD and functional dyspepsia is unproven.

Acid-suppressing drugs are advocated for first-line therapy of *H. pylori*–negative dyspepsia, especially with ulcer-like symptoms. Ranitidine is of benefit in the treatment of functional dyspepsia versus placebo. In young patients without alarm symptoms, a 4-week trial of an H_2 receptor antagonist or proton pump inhibitor is given. Endoscopy is performed only if symptoms do not improve.

Helicobacter pylori Eradication *H. pylori* eradication is indicated only for peptic ulcer and gastric mucosa–associated lymphoid tissue lymphoma. The usefulness of *H. pylori* eradication in patients with functional dyspepsia is unproven, but evidence suggests that <15% of cases relate to *H. pylori*. Patients with ulcer-like symptoms may respond. *H. pylori* eradication is not useful in the treatment of GERD; some reports suggest that elimination of the organism increases the risk of developing GERD and others show no effect. Several drug combinations show efficacy; most include 10 to 14 days of a proton pump inhibitor or bismuth subsalicylate in concert with two antibiotics.

Gastrointestinal Motor Stimulants Motor stimulants such as metoclopramide, erythromycin, and domperidone have limited utility in GERD.

The γ-aminobutyric acid B (GABA-B) agonist baclofen reduces esophageal acid exposure by inhibiting transient LES relaxations; the clinical role of the drug is being studied. Domperidone may be useful in functional dyspepsia and may be given instead of acid suppressants as initial empirical therapy of young patients without alarm symptoms and without *H. pylori* infection. Patients with dysmotility-like dyspepsia may respond preferentially to motor-stimulating drugs.

Other Options Antireflux surgery may be offered to GERD patients with poorly controlled symptoms, disease complications, or unbearable life-style impairments. Fundoplication can be performed laparoscopically; the Nissen and Toupet procedures involve wrapping the proximal stomach around the LES to increase LES pressure. Dysphagia may be a long-term complication of these procedures. Endoscopic interventions at the gastroesophageal junction including radiofrequency energy delivery, suturing, biopolymer implantation, and gastroplication have been used in refractory GERD; their efficacy is being assessed.

Some patients with functional dyspepsia are refractory to acid suppressants or prokinetic drugs but may respond to low-dose tricyclic antidepressant therapy. The mechanism of action in functional dyspepsia is unknown but may involve blunting of visceral pain processing in the brain. Gas and bloating may be the most troubling symptoms in some patients with indigestion and can be difficult to treat. Dietary exclusion of gas-producing foods such as legumes and use of simethicone or activated charcoal benefit some patients. Psychological treatments may be offered for refractory functional dyspepsia, but no convincing data suggest efficacy.

FURTHER READING

HAUG TT et al: The prevalence of nausea in the community: Psychological, social and somatic factors. Gen Hosp Psych 24:81, 2002

HESKETH PJ: Potential role of the NK$_1$ receptor antagonists in chemotherapy-induced nausea and vomiting. Support Care Cancer 9:350, 2001

McCOLL KE et al: Randomised trial of endoscopy with testing for *Helicobacter pylori* compared with non-invasive *H. pylori* testing alone in the management of dyspepsia. BMJ 324:999, 2002

RABENECK L et al: A double blind, randomized, placebo-controlled trial of proton pump inhibitor therapy in patients with uninvestigated dyspepsia. Am J Gastroenterol 97:3045, 2002

TACK J et al: Clinical and pathophysiological characteristics of acute-onset functional dyspepsia. Gastroenterology 122:1738, 2002

TALLEY NJ: Dyspepsia: Management guidelines for the millennium. Gut 50 (Suppl 4):iv72, 2002

35 DIARRHEA AND CONSTIPATION
David A. Ahlquist, Michael Camilleri

Diarrhea and constipation are exceedingly common and together exact an enormous toll in terms of morbidity, loss of work productivity, and consumption of medical resources. Worldwide, more than 1 billion people suffer one or more episodes of acute diarrhea each year. Among the 100 million persons affected annually by acute diarrhea in the United States, nearly half must restrict activities, 10% consult physicians, 250,000 require hospitalization, and roughly 3000 die (primarily the elderly). The annual economic burden to society is estimated at >$20 billion. Because of poor sanitation and more limited access to health care, acute infectious diarrhea remains one of the most common causes of mortality in developing countries, particularly among children, accounting for 5 to 8 million deaths per year. Population statistics on chronic diarrhea and constipation are more uncertain, perhaps due to variable definitions and reporting, but the frequency of these conditions is also high. Based on United States population surveys, prevalence rates for chronic diarrhea range from 2 to 7% and for chronic constipation from 3 to 17%. Diarrhea and constipation are among the most common patient complaints faced by internists and primary care physicians, and they account for nearly 50% of referrals to gastroenterologists.

Although diarrhea and constipation may present as mere nuisance symptoms at one extreme, they can be severe or life-threatening at the other. Even mild symptoms may signal a serious underlying gastrointestinal lesion, such as colorectal cancer, or systemic disorder, such as thyroid disease. Given the heterogeneous causes and potential severity of these common complaints, it is imperative for clinicians to appreciate the pathophysiology, etiologic classification, diagnostic strategies, and therapeutic principles of diarrhea and constipation so that rational and cost-effective care can be delivered.

NORMAL PHYSIOLOGY

The human small intestine and colon perform important functions including the secretion and absorption of water and electrolytes, the storage and subsequent transport of intraluminal contents aborally, and the salvage of some nutrients after bacterial metabolism of carbohydrate that are not absorbed in the small intestine. The main motor functions are summarized in Table 35-1. Alterations in fluid and electrolyte handling contribute significantly to diarrhea. Alterations in motor and sensory functions of the human colon result in highly prevalent syndromes such as irritable bowel syndrome, chronic diarrhea, and chronic constipation.

NEURAL CONTROL The small intestine and colon have intrinsic and extrinsic innervation. The *intrinsic innervation*, also called the enteric nervous system, comprises myenteric, submucosal, and mucosal neuronal layers. The function of these layers is modulated by interneurons through the actions of neurotransmitter amines or peptides, including acetylcholine, opioids, norepinephrine, serotonin, ATP, and nitric oxide. The myenteric plexus regulates smooth-muscle function, and the submucosal plexus affects secretion and absorption.

The *extrinsic innervations* of the small intestine and colon are part of the autonomic nervous system and also modulate both motor and secretory functions. The parasympathetic nerve supply conveys both visceral sensory as well as excitatory pathways to the motor components of the colon. Parasympathetic fibers via the vagus nerve reach the small intestine and proximal colon along the branches of the superior mesenteric artery. The distal colon is supplied by sacral parasympathetic nerves (S$_{2-4}$) via the pelvic plexus; these fibers course through the wall of the colon as ascending intracolonic fibers as far as, and in some instances including, the proximal colon. The chief excitatory neurotransmitters controlling motor function are acetylcholine and the tachykinins, such as substance P. The sympathetic nerve supply modulates motor functions and reaches the small intestine and colon alongside the arterial arcades of the superior and inferior mesenteric vessels. Sympathetic input to the gut is generally excitatory to sphincters and inhibitory to nonsphincteric muscle. Visceral afferents convey sensation from the gut to the central nervous system; initially, they course along sympathetic fibers, but as they approach the spinal cord they separate, have cell bodies in the dorsal root ganglion, and enter the dorsal horn of the spinal cord. Afferent signals are conveyed

TABLE 35-1 *Normal Gastrointestinal Motility: Functions at Different Anatomic Levels*

Stomach and small bowel	Colon: Irregular mixing, absorption,
Synchronized MMCs in fasting	transit
Accommodation, trituration,	Ascending, transverse: reservoirs
mixing, transit	Descending: conduit
Stomach, ~3 h	Sigmoid/rectum: volitional reservoir
Small bowel, ~3 h	
Ileal reservoir empties boluses	

Note: MMC, migrating motor complex.

to the brain along the lateral spinothalamic tract and the nociceptive dorsal column pathway and are then perceived. Other afferent fibers synapse in the prevertebral ganglia and reflexly modulate intestinal motility.

INTESTINAL FLUID ABSORPTION AND SECRETION On an average day, 9 L of fluid enters the gastrointestinal tract; approximately 1 L of residual fluid reaches the colon; the stool excretion of fluid constitutes about 0.2 L/d. The colon has a large capacitance and functional reserve and may recover up to four times its usual volume of 0.8 L/d, provided the rate of flow permits reabsorption to occur. Thus, the colon can partially compensate for intestinal absorptive or secretory disorders.

In the colon, sodium absorption is predominantly electrogenic, and uptake takes place at the apical membrane; it is compensated for by the export functions of the basolateral sodium pump. A variety of neural and non-neural mediators regulate colonic fluid and electrolyte balance, including cholinergic, adrenergic, and serotonergic mediators. Angiotensin and aldosterone also influence colonic absorption, reflecting the common embryologic development of the distal colonic epithelium and the renal tubules.

SMALL INTESTINAL MOTILITY During fasting, the motility of the small intestine is characterized by a cyclical event called the migrating motor complex (MMC), which serves to clear nondigestible residue from the small intestine. This organized, propagated series of contractions lasts on average 4 min, occurs every 60 to 90 min, and usually involves the entire small intestine. After food ingestion, the small intestine produces irregular, mixing contractions of relatively low amplitude, except in the distal ileum where more powerful contractions occur intermittently and empty the ileum by bolus transfers.

ILEOCOLONIC STORAGE AND SALVAGE The distal ileum acts as a reservoir, emptying intermittently by bolus movements. This action allows time for salvage of fluids, electrolytes, and nutrients. Segmentation by haustra compartmentalizes the colon and facilitates mixing, retention of residue, and formation of solid stools. In health, the ascending and transverse regions of colon function as reservoirs (average transit, 15 h), and the descending colon acts as a conduit (average transit, 3 h). The colon is efficient at conserving sodium and water, a function that is particularly important in sodium-depleted patients in whom the small intestine alone is unable to maintain sodium balance. Diarrhea or constipation may result from alteration in the reservoir function of the proximal colon or the propulsive function of the left colon. Constipation may also result from disturbances of the rectal or sigmoid reservoir, typically as a result of dysfunction of the pelvic floor or the coordination of defecation.

COLONIC MOTILITY AND TONE The small intestinal MMC only rarely continues into the colon. However, short duration or phasic contractions mix colonic contents, and high-amplitude propagated contractions (HAPCs) are sometimes associated with mass movements through the colon and occur approximately five times per day, usually on awakening in the morning and postprandially. Increased frequency of HAPCs may result in diarrhea. The predominant phasic contractions are irregular and nonpropagated and serve as a "mixing" function.

Colonic tone refers to the background contractility upon which phasic contractile activity (typically contractions lasting <15 s) is superimposed. It is an important cofactor in the colon's capacitance (volume accommodation) and sensation.

COLONIC MOTILITY AFTER MEAL INGESTION After meal ingestion, colonic phasic and tonic contractility increase for a period of approximately 2 h. The initial phase (about 10 min) is mediated by the vagus nerve in response to mechanical distention of the stomach. The subsequent response of the colon requires caloric stimulation and is at least in part mediated by hormones, e.g., gastrin and serotonin.

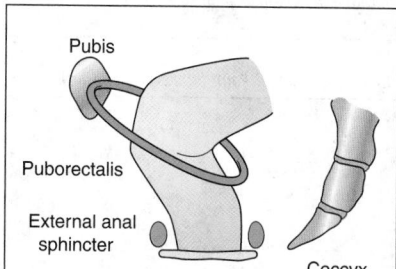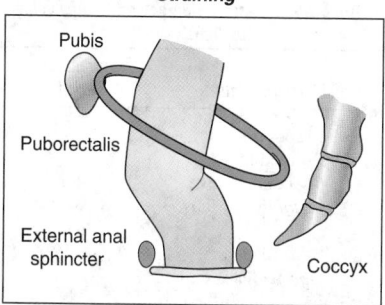

FIGURE 35-1 Mechanisms involved in continence and defecation. Note the importance of pelvic floor and anal sphincter functions. Continence requires: contraction of puborectalis, maintenance of anorectal angle, normal rectal sensation, and contraction of sphincter. Defecation requires: relaxation of puborectalis, straightening of anorectal angle, and relaxation of sphincter.

DEFECATION Tonic contraction of the puborectalis muscle, which forms a sling around the rectoanal junction, is important to maintain continence; during defecation, sacral parasympathetic nerves relax this muscle, facilitating the straightening of the rectoanal angle (Fig. 35-1). Distention of the rectum results in transient relaxation of the internal anal sphincter via intrinsic and reflex sympathetic innervation. As sigmoid and rectal contractions increase the pressure within the rectum, the rectosigmoid angle opens by >15°. Voluntary relaxation of the external anal sphincter (striated muscle innervated by the pudendal nerve) permits the evacuation of feces; this evacuation process can be augmented by an increase in intraabdominal pressure created by the Valsalva maneuver.

DIARRHEA

DEFINITION Diarrhea is loosely defined as passage of abnormally liquid or unformed stools at an increased frequency. For adults on a typical Western diet, stool weight >200 g/d can generally be considered diarrheal. Because of the fundamental importance of duration to diagnostic considerations, diarrhea may be further defined as *acute* if <2 weeks, *persistent* if 2 to 4 weeks, and *chronic* if >4 weeks in duration.

Two common conditions, usually associated with the passage of stool totaling <200 g/d, must be distinguished from diarrhea, as diagnostic and therapeutic algorithms differ. *Pseudodiarrhea*, or the frequent passage of small volumes of stool, is often associated with rectal urgency and accompanies the irritable bowel syndrome or anorectal disorders such as proctitis. *Fecal incontinence* is the involuntary discharge of rectal contents and is most often caused by neuromuscular disorders or structural anorectal problems. Diarrhea and urgency, especially if severe, may aggravate or cause incontinence. Pseudodiarrhea and fecal incontinence occur at prevalence rates comparable to or higher than that of chronic diarrhea and should always be considered in patients complaining of "diarrhea." A careful history and physical examination generally allow these conditions to be discriminated from true diarrhea.

ACUTE DIARRHEA More than 90% of cases of acute diarrhea are caused by infectious agents; these cases are often accompanied by vomiting, fever, and abdominal pain. The remaining 10% or so are caused by medications, toxic ingestions, ischemia, and other conditions.

Infectious Agents Most infectious diarrheas are acquired by fecal-oral transmission via direct personal contact or, more commonly, via ingestion of food or water contaminated with pathogens from human or animal feces. In the immunologically competent person, the resident fecal microflora, containing >500 taxonomically distinct species, are rarely the source of diarrhea and may actually play a role in suppressing the growth of ingested pathogens. Acute infection or injury occurs when the ingested agent overwhelms the host's mucosal immune and nonimmune (gastric acid, digestive enzymes, mucus secretion, peristalsis, and suppressive resident flora) defenses. Established clinical associations with specific enteropathogens may offer diagnostic clues.

TABLE 35-2 *Association between Pathobiology of Causative Agents and Clinical Features in Acute Infectious Diarrhea*

Pathobiology/Agents	Incubation Period	Vomiting	Abdominal Pain	Fever	Diarrhea
Toxin producers					
Preformed toxin					
Bacillus cereus,	1–8 h	3–4+	1–2+	0–1+	3–4+, watery
Staphylococcus aureus,	8–24 h				
Clostridium perfringens					
Enterotoxin					
Vibrio cholerae,	8–72 h	2–4+	1–2+	0–1+	3–4+, watery
enterotoxigenic *Escherichia coli,* *Klebsiella pneumoniae,* *Aeromonas* species					
Enteroadherent					
Enteropathogenic and enteroadherent, *E. coli, Giardia* organisms, cryptosporidiosis, helminths	1–8 d	0–1+	1–3+	1–2+	1–2+, watery
Cytotoxin-producers					
Clostridium difficile	1–3 d	0–1+	3–4+	1–2+	1–3+, usually watery, occasionally bloody
Hemorrhagic *E. coli*	12–72 h	0–1+	3–4+	1–2+	1–3+, initially watery, quickly bloody
Invasive organisms					
Minimal inflammation					
Rotavirus and Norwalk agent	1–3 d	1–2+	2–3+	3–4+	1–3+, watery
Variable inflammation					
Salmonella, Campylobacter, and *Aeromonas* species, *Vibrio parahaemolyticus, Yersinia*	12 h–11 d	0–3+	2–4+	3–4+	1–4+, watery or bloody
Severe inflammation					
Shigella species, enteroinvasive *E. coli, Entamoeba histolytica*	12 h–8 d	0–1+	3–4+	3–4+	1–2+, bloody

Source: Adapted from DW Powell, in T Yamada (ed): *Textbook of Gastroenterology and Hepatology,* 4th ed. Philadelphia, Lippincott, Williams & Wilkins, 2003; and DR Syndman, in SL Gorbach (ed): *Infectious Diarrhea.* London, Blackwell, 1986.

In the United States, high risk groups are recognized:

1. *Travelers.* Nearly 40% of tourists to endemic regions of Latin America, Africa, and Asia develop so-called traveler's diarrhea, most commonly due to enterotoxigenic *Escherichia coli* as well as to *Campylobacter, Shigella,* and *Salmonella.* Visitors to Russia (especially St. Petersburg) may have increased risk of *Giardia*-associated diarrhea; visitors to Nepal may acquire *Cyclospora.* Campers, backpackers, and swimmers in wilderness areas may become infected with *Giardia.*

2. *Consumers of certain foods.* Diarrhea closely following food consumption at a picnic, banquet, or restaurant may suggest infection with *Salmonella, Campylobacter,* or *Shigella* from chicken; enterohemorrhagic *E. coli* (O157:H7) from undercooked hamburger; *Bacillus aureus* from fried rice; *Staphylococcus aureus* or *Salmonella* from mayonnaise or creams; *Salmonella* from eggs; and *Vibrio* species, *Salmonella,* or acute hepatitis A or B from seafood, especially if raw.

3. *Immunodeficient persons.* Individuals at risk for diarrhea include those with either primary immunodeficiency (e.g., IgA deficiency, common variable hypogammaglobulinemia, chronic granulomatous disease) or the much more common secondary immunodeficiency states (e.g., AIDS, senescence, pharmacologic suppression). Common enteropathogens often cause a more severe and protracted diarrheal illness, and, particularly in persons with AIDS, opportunistic infections, such as by *Mycobacterium* species, certain viruses (cytomegalovirus, adenovirus, and herpes simplex), and protozoa (*Cryptosporidium, Isospora belli,* Microsporidia, and *Blastocystis hominis*) may also play a role (Chap. 173). In patients with AIDS, agents transmitted venereally per rectum (e.g., *Neisseria gonorrhoeae, Treponema pallidum, Chlamydia*) may contribute to proctocolitis.

4. *Daycare participants and their family members.* Infections with *Shigella, Giardia, Cryptosporidium,* rotavirus, and other agents are very common and should be considered.

5. *Institutionalized persons.* Infectious diarrhea is one of the most frequent categories of nosocomial infections in many hospitals and long-term care facilities; the causes are a variety of microorganisms but most commonly *Clostridium difficile.*

The pathophysiology underlying acute diarrhea by infectious agents produces specific clinical features that may also be helpful in diagnosis (Table 35-2). Profuse watery diarrhea secondary to small bowel hypersecretion occurs with ingestion of preformed bacterial toxins, enterotoxin-producing bacteria, and enteroadherent pathogens. Diarrhea associated with marked vomiting and minimal or no fever may occur abruptly within a few hours after ingestion of the former two types; vomiting is usually less, and abdominal cramping or bloating is greater; fever is higher with the latter. Cytotoxin-producing and invasive microorganisms all cause high fever and abdominal pain. Invasive bacteria and *Entamoeba histolytica* often cause bloody diarrhea (referred to as *dysentery*). *Yersinia* invades the terminal ileal and proximal colon mucosa and may cause especially severe abdominal pain with tenderness mimicking acute appendicitis.

Finally, infectious diarrhea may be associated with systemic manifestations. Reiter's syndrome (arthritis, urethritis, and conjunctivitis) may accompany or follow infections by *Salmonella, Campylobacter, Shigella,* and *Yersinia.* Yersiniosis may also lead to an autoimmune-type thyroiditis, pericarditis, and glomerulonephritis. Both enterohemorrhagic *E. coli* (O157:H7) and *Shigella* can lead to the *hemolytic-uremic syndrome* with an attendant high mortality rate. Acute diarrhea can also be a major symptom of several systemic infections including *viral hepatitis, listeriosis, legionellosis,* and *toxic shock syndrome.*

Other Causes Side effects from medications are probably the most common noninfectious cause of acute diarrhea, and etiology may be suggested by a temporal association between use and symptom onset. Although innumerable medications may produce diarrhea, some of the more frequently incriminated include antibiotics, cardiac antidysrhythmics, antihypertensives, nonsteroidal anti-inflammatory drugs (NSAIDs), certain antidepressants, chemotherapeutic agents, bronchodilators, antacids, and laxatives. Occlusive or nonocclusive *ischemic colitis* typically occurs in persons >50 years, often presents as acute lower abdominal pain preceding watery, then bloody diarrhea, and generally results in acute inflammatory changes in the sigmoid or left colon while sparing the rectum. Acute diarrhea may accompany colonic *diverticulitis* and *graft-versus-host disease.* Acute diarrhea, often associated with systemic compromise, can follow ingestion of toxins including organophosphate insecticides, amanita and other mushrooms, arsenic, and preformed environmental toxins in seafoods, such as ciguatera and scombroid. The conditions causing chronic diarrhea can also be confused with acute diarrhea early in their course. This confusion may occur with inflammatory bowel disease and some of the other inflammatory chronic diarrheas that may have an abrupt rather than insidious onset and exhibit features that mimic infection.

APPROACH TO THE PATIENT

The decision to evaluate acute diarrhea depends on its severity and duration and on various host factors (Fig. 35-2). Most episodes of acute diarrhea are mild and self-limited and do not justify the cost and potential morbidity of diagnostic or pharmacologic interventions. Indications for evaluation include profuse diarrhea with dehydration, grossly bloody stools, fever ≥38.5° C, duration >48 h without improvement, new community outbreaks, associated severe abdominal pain in patients >50 years, and elderly (≥70 years) or immunocompromised patients. In some cases of moderately severe febrile diarrhea associated with fecal leukocytes (or increased fecal levels of the leukocyte proteins) or with gross blood, a diagnostic evaluation might be avoided in favor of an empirical antibiotic trial (see below).

The cornerstone of diagnosis in those suspected of severe acute infectious diarrhea is microbiologic analysis of the stool. Workup includes cultures for bacterial and viral pathogens, direct inspection for ova and parasites, and immunoassays for certain bacterial toxins (*C. difficile*), viral antigens (rotavirus), and protozoal antigens (*Giardia, E. histolytica*). The aforementioned clinical and epidemiologic associations may assist in focusing the evaluation. If a particular pathogen or set of possible pathogens is so implicated, then either the whole panel of routine studies may not be necessary or, in some instances, special cultures may be appropriate as for enterohemorrhagic and other types of *E. coli, Vibrio* species, and *Yersinia.* Molecular diagnosis of pathogens in stool can be made by identification of unique DNA sequences; and evolving microarray technologies could lead to a more rapid, sensitive, specific, and cost-effective diagnostic approach in the future.

Persistent diarrhea is commonly due to *Giardia,* but additional causative organisms that should be considered include *C. difficile* (especially if antibiotics had been administered), *E. histolytica, Cryptosporidium, Campylobacter,* and others. If stool studies are unrevealing, then flexible sigmoidoscopy with biopsies and upper endoscopy with duodenal aspirates and biopsies may be indicated.

Structural examination by sigmoidoscopy, colonoscopy, or abdominal computed tomographic scanning (or other imaging approaches) may be appropriate in patients with uncharacterized persistent diarrhea to exclude inflammatory bowel disease, or as an initial approach in patients with suspected noninfectious acute diarrhea such as might be caused by ischemic colitis, diverticulitis, or partial bowel obstruction.

℞ TREATMENT

Fluid and electrolyte replacement are of central importance to all forms of acute diarrhea. Fluid replacement alone may suffice for mild cases. Oral sugar-electrolyte solutions (sport drinks or designed formulations) should be instituted promptly with severe diarrhea to limit dehydration, which is the major cause of death. Profoundly dehydrated patients, especially infants and the elderly, require intravenous rehydration.

In moderately severe nonfebrile and nonbloody diarrhea, antimotility antisecretory agents such as loperamide can be useful adjuncts to control symptoms. Such agents should be avoided with febrile dysentery, which may be exacerbated or prolonged by them. Bismuth subsalicylate may reduce symptoms of vomiting and diarrhea but should not be used to treat immunocompromised patients because of the risk of bismuth encephalopathy.

Judicious use of antibiotics is appropriate in selected instances of acute diarrhea and may reduce its severity and duration (Fig. 35-2). Many physicians treat moderately to severely ill patients with febrile dysentery empirically without diagnostic evaluation using a quinolone, such as ciprofloxacin (500 mg bid for 3 to 5 d). Empirical treatment can also be considered for suspected giardiasis with metronidazole (250 mg qid for 7 d). Selection of antibiotics and dosage regimens are otherwise dictated by specific pathogens and conditions found (Chaps. 113, 134, 137–143). Antibiotic coverage is indicated whether or not a causative organism is discovered in patients who are immunocompromised, have mechanical heart valves or recent vascular grafts, or are elderly. Antibiotic prophylaxis is indicated for certain patients traveling to high-risk countries in whom the likelihood or seriousness of acquired diarrhea would be especially high, including those with immunocompromise, inflammatory bowel disease, or gastric achlorhydria. Use of trimethoprim/sulfamethoxazole or ciprofloxacin may reduce bacterial diarrhea in such travelers by 90%.

CHRONIC DIARRHEA Diarrhea lasting >4 weeks warrants evaluation to exclude serious underlying pathology. In contrast to acute diarrhea, most of the many causes of chronic diarrhea are noninfectious. The classification of chronic diarrhea by pathophysiologic mechanism facilitates a rational approach to management (Table 35-3).

Secretory Causes Secretory diarrheas are due to derangements in fluid and electrolyte transport across the enterocolic mucosa. They are char-

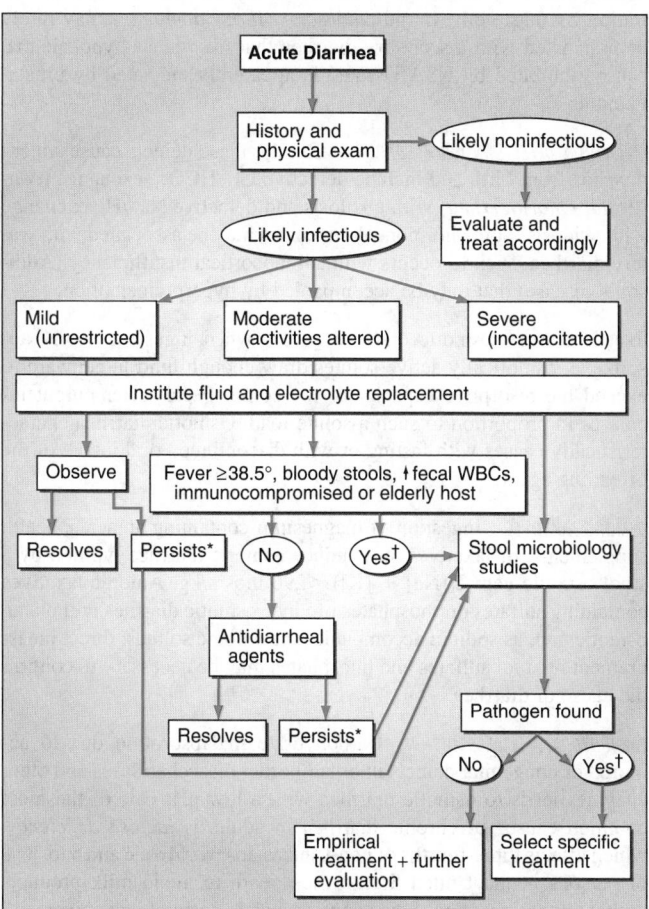

FIGURE 35-2 Algorithm for the management of acute diarrhea. Consider empirical Rx before evaluation with (*) metronidazole and (†) with quinolone.

TABLE 35-3 *Major Causes of Chronic Diarrhea According to Predominant Pathophysiologic Mechanism*

Secretory causes	**Inflammatory causes**
Exogenous stimulant laxatives	Idiopathic inflammatory bowel
Chronic ethanol ingestion	disease (Crohn's chronic
Other drugs and toxins	ulcerative colitis)
Endogenous laxatives (dihydroxy	Microscopic and collagenous
bile acids)	colitis
Idiopathic secretory diarrhea	Immune-related mucosal disease
Certain bacterial infections	(1° or 2° immunodeficiencies,
Bowel resection, disease, or	food allergy, eosinophilic
fistula (↓ absorption)	gastroenteritis, graft-vs-host
Partial bowel obstruction or fecal	disease)
impaction	Infections (invasive bacteria,
Hormone-producing tumors	viruses, and parasites)
(carcinoid, VIPoma, medullary	Radiation injury
cancer of thyroid, mastocytosis,	Gastrointestinal malignancies
gastrinoma, colorectal villous	**Dysmotile causes**
adenoma)	Visceral neuromyopathies
Addison's disease	Hyperthyroidism
Congenital electrolyte absorption	Drugs (prokinetic agents)
defects	**Factitial causes**
Osmotic causes	Munchausen
Osmotic laxatives (Mg²⁺, PO₄³⁻,	Bulimia
SO₄²⁻)	
Lactase and other disaccharide	
deficiencies	
Nonabsorbable carbohydrates	
(sorbitol, lactulose,	
polyethylene glycol)	
Steatorrheal causes	
Intraluminal maldigestion	
(pancreatic exocrine	
insufficiency, bacterial	
overgrowth, liver disease)	
Mucosal malabsorption (celiac	
sprue, Whipple's disease,	
infections,	
abetalipoproteinemia, ischemia)	
Postmucosal obstruction (1° or 2°	
lymphatic obstruction)	

acterized clinically by watery, large-volume fecal outputs that are typically painless and persist with fasting. Because there is no malabsorbed solute, stool osmolality is accounted for by normal endogenous electrolytes with no fecal osmotic gap.

MEDICATIONS Side effects from regular ingestion of drugs and toxins are the most common secretory causes of chronic diarrhea. Hundreds of prescription and over-the-counter medications (see "Other Causes of Acute Diarrhea," above) may produce unwanted diarrhea. Surreptitious or habitual use of stimulant laxatives [e.g., senna, cascara, bisacodyl, ricinoleic acid (castor oil)] must also be considered. Chronic ethanol consumption may cause a secretory-type diarrhea due to enterocyte injury with impaired sodium and water absorption as well as to rapid transit and other alterations. Inadvertent ingestion of certain environmental toxins (e.g., arsenic) may lead to chronic rather than acute forms of diarrhea. Certain bacterial infections may occasionally persist and be associated with a secretory-type diarrhea.

BOWEL RESECTION, MUCOSAL DISEASE, OR ENTEROCOLIC FISTULA These conditions may result in a secretory-type diarrhea because of inadequate surface for resorption of secreted fluids and electrolytes. Unlike other secretory diarrheas, this subset of conditions tends to worsen with eating. With disease (e.g., Crohn's ileitis) or resection of <100 cm of terminal ileum, dihydroxy bile acids may escape absorption and stimulate colonic secretion (cholorrheic diarrhea). This mechanism may contribute to so-called *idiopathic secretory diarrhea*, in which bile acids are functionally malabsorbed from a normal-appearing terminal ileum. Partial bowel obstruction, ostomy stricture, or fecal impaction may paradoxically lead to increased fecal output due to hypersecretion.

HORMONES Although uncommon, the classic examples of secretory diarrhea are those mediated by hormones. *Metastatic gastrointestinal carcinoid tumors* or, rarely, *primary bronchial carcinoids* may produce watery diarrhea alone or as part of the carcinoid syndrome that comprises episodic flushing, wheezing, dyspnea, and right-sided valvular heart disease. Diarrhea is due to the release into the circulation of potent intestinal secretagogues including serotonin, histamine, prostaglandins, and various kinins. Pellagra-like skin lesions may rarely occur as the result of serotonin overproduction with niacin depletion. *Gastrinoma*, one of the most common neuroendocrine tumors, most typically presents with refractory peptic ulcers, but diarrhea occurs in up to one-third of cases and may be the only clinical manifestation in 10%. While various secretagogues released with gastrin may play a role, the diarrhea most often results from fat maldigestion owing to pancreatic enzyme inactivation by low intraduodenal pH. The watery diarrhea hypokalemia achlorhydria syndrome, also called *pancreatic cholera*, is due to a non-β cell pancreatic adenoma, referred to as a *VIPoma*, that secretes vasoactive intestinal peptide (VIP) and a host of other peptide hormones including pancreatic polypeptide, secretin, gastrin, gastrin-inhibitory polypeptide, neurotensin, calcitonin, and prostaglandins. The secretory diarrhea is often massive with stool volumes >3 L/d; daily volumes as high as 20 L have been reported. Life-threatening dehydration; neuromuscular dysfunction from associated hypokalemia, hypomagnesemia, or hypercalcemia; flushing; and hyperglycemia may accompany a VIPoma. *Medullary carcinoma of the thyroid* may present with watery diarrhea caused by calcitonin, other secretory peptides, or prostaglandins. This tumor occurs sporadically or, in 25 to 50% of cases, as a feature of multiple endocrine neoplasia type IIa with pheochromocytomas and hyperparathyroidism. Prominent diarrhea is often associated with metastatic disease and poor prognosis. *Systemic mastocytosis*, which may be associated with the skin lesion urticaria pigmentosa, may cause diarrhea that is either secretory and mediated by histamine or inflammatory and due to intestinal filtration by mast cells. Large *colorectal villous adenomas* may rarely be associated with a secretory diarrhea that may cause hypokalemia, can be inhibited by NSAIDs, and is apparently mediated by prostaglandins.

CONGENITAL DEFECTS IN ION ABSORPTION Rarely, these defects cause watery diarrhea from birth and include defective Cl⁻/HCO₃⁻ exchange (*congenital chloridorrhea*) with alkalosis and defective Na⁺/H⁺ exchange with acidosis. Some hormone deficiencies may be associated with watery diarrhea, such as occurs with adrenocortical insufficiency (Addison's disease) that may be accompanied by hyperpigmentation.

Osmotic Causes Osmotic diarrhea occurs when ingested, poorly absorbable, osmotically active solutes draw enough fluid lumenward to exceed the resorptive capacity of the colon. Fecal water output increases in proportion to such a solute load. Osmotic diarrhea characteristically ceases with fasting or with discontinued oral intake of the offending agent.

OSMOTIC LAXATIVES Ingestion of magnesium-containing antacids, health supplements, or laxatives may induce osmotic diarrhea typified by a stool osmotic gap: 2([Na] + [K]) <290 mosm/kg. Anionic laxatives containing sulfates or phosphates produce osmotic diarrhea without an osmotic gap, as sodium accompanies the anionic solutes; direct measurement of stool sulfates and phosphates may be necessary to confirm the cause of diarrhea.

CARBOHYDRATE MALABSORPTION Carbohydrate malabsorption due to acquired or congenital defects in brush-border disaccharidases and other enzymes leads to osmotic diarrhea with a low pH. One of the most common causes of chronic diarrhea in adults is *lactase deficiency*, which affects three-fourths of non-Caucasians worldwide and 5 to 30% of persons in the United States; most learn to avoid milk products without an intervention. Some sugars, such as sorbitol, are universally malabsorbed, and diarrhea ensues with ingestion of ample medications, gum, or candies sweetened with these nonabsorbable sugars.

Lactulose, used to acidify stools in patients with hepatic failure, also causes diarrhea on this basis.

Steatorrheal Causes Fat malabsorption may lead to greasy, foul-smelling, difficult-to-flush diarrhea often associated with weight loss and nutritional deficiencies due to concomitant malabsorption of amino acids and vitamins. Increased fecal output is caused by the osmotic effects of fatty acids, especially after bacterial hydroxylation, and, to a lesser extent, by the burden of neutral fat. Quantitatively, steatorrhea is defined as stool fat exceeding the normal 7 g/d; daily fecal fat averages 15 to 25 g with small intestinal diseases and is often >40 g with pancreatic exocrine insufficiency. Intraluminal maldigestion, mucosal malabsorption, or lymphatic obstruction may produce steatorrhea.

INTRALUMINAL MALDIGESTION This condition most commonly results from pancreatic exocrine insufficiency, which occurs when >90% of pancreatic secretory function is lost. *Chronic pancreatitis*, usually a sequela of ethanol abuse, most frequently causes pancreatic insufficiency. Other causes include *cystic fibrosis*, *pancreatic duct obstruction*, and rarely, *somatostatinoma*. Bacterial overgrowth in the small intestine may deconjugate bile acids and alter micelle formation that impairs fat digestion; it occurs with stasis from a blind-loop, small bowel diverticulum or dysmotility and is especially likely in the elderly. Finally, cirrhosis or biliary obstruction may lead to mild steatorrhea due to deficient intraluminal bile acid concentration.

MUCOSAL MALABSORPTION Mucosal malabsorption occurs from a variety of enteropathies but most prototypically and perhaps most commonly from *celiac sprue*. This gluten-sensitive enteropathy characterized by villous atrophy and crypt hyperplasia in the proximal small bowel often presents with fatty diarrhea associated with multiple nutritional deficiencies of varying severity and affects all ages. *Tropical sprue* may produce a similar histologic and clinical syndrome but occurs in residents of or travelers to tropical climates; its often abrupt onset and response to antibiotics suggest an infectious etiology. *Whipple's disease*, due to the actinomycete *Treponema whippleii* and histiocytic infiltration of the small bowel mucosa, is a less common cause of steatorrhea that most typically occurs in young or middle-aged men; it is frequently associated with arthralgias, fever, lymphadenopathy, and extreme fatigue and may affect the central nervous system and endocardium. A similar clinical and histologic picture results from *Mycobacterium avium-intracellulare* infection in patients with AIDS. *Abetalipoproteinemia* is a rare defect of chylomicron formation and fat malabsorption in children associated with acanthocytic erythrocytes, ataxia, and retinitis pigmentosa. Several other conditions may cause mucosal malabsorption including infections, especially with protozoa such as *Giardia*, numerous medications (e.g., colchicine, cholestyramine, neomycin), and chronic ischemia.

POSTMUCOSAL LYMPHATIC OBSTRUCTION The pathophysiology of this condition, which is due to the rare *congenital intestinal lymphangiectasia* or to *acquired lymphatic obstruction* secondary to trauma, tumor, or infection, leads to the unique constellation of fat malabsorption with enteric losses of protein (often causing edema) and lymphocytes (with resultant lymphocytopenia) that enter the portal circulation directly. Carbohydrate and amino acid absorption are preserved.

Inflammatory Causes Inflammatory diarrheas are generally accompanied by pain, fever, bleeding, or other manifestations of inflammation. The mechanism of diarrhea may not only be exudation but, depending on lesion site, may include fat malabsorption, disrupted fluid/electrolyte absorption, and hypersecretion or hypermotility from release of cytokines and other inflammatory mediators. The unifying feature on stool analysis is the presence of leukocytes or leukocyte-derived proteins such as calprotectin. With severe inflammation, exudative protein loss can lead to anasarca (generalized edema). Any middle-aged or older person with chronic inflammatory-type diarrhea, especially with blood, should be carefully evaluated to exclude a colorectal or large enteric tumor.

IDIOPATHIC INFLAMMATORY BOWEL DISEASE The illnesses in this category, which include *Crohn's disease* and *chronic ulcerative colitis*, are among the most common organic causes of chronic diarrhea in adults and range in severity from mild to fulminant and life-threatening. They may be associated with uveitis, polyarthralgias, cholestatic liver disease (primary sclerosing cholangitis), and various skin lesions (erythema nodosum, pyoderma gangrenosum). *Microscopic colitis*, including *collagenous colitis*, is an increasingly recognized cause of chronic watery diarrhea; biopsy of a normal appearing colorectum is required for histologic diagnosis.

PRIMARY OR SECONDARY FORMS OF IMMUNODEFICIENCY Immunodeficiency may lead to prolonged infectious diarrhea. With common, variable *hypogammaglobulinemia*, diarrhea is particularly prevalent and often the result of giardiasis.

EOSINOPHILIC GASTROENTERITIS Eosinophil infiltration of the mucosa, muscularis, or serosa at any level of the gastrointestinal tract may cause diarrhea, pain, vomiting, or ascites. Affected patients often have an atopic history, Charcot-Leyden crystals due to extruded eosinophil contents may be seen on microscopic inspection of stool, and peripheral eosinophilia is present in 50 to 75% of patients. While hypersensitivity to certain foods occurs in adults, true food allergy causing chronic diarrhea is rare.

OTHER CAUSES Chronic inflammatory diarrhea may be caused by *radiation enterocolitis*, *chronic graft-versus-host disease*, *Behçet's syndrome*, and *Cronkite-Canada syndrome*, among others.

Dysmotile Causes Rapid transit may accompany many diarrheas as a secondary or contributing phenomenon, but primary dysmotility is an unusual etiology of true diarrhea. Stool features often suggest a secretory diarrhea, but mild steatorrhea of up to 14 g of fat per day can be produced by maldigestion from rapid transit alone. *Hyperthyroidism*, *carcinoid syndrome*, and certain drugs (e.g., prostaglandins, prokinetic agents) may produce hypermotility with resultant diarrhea. Primary visceral neuromyopathies or idiopathic acquired intestinal pseudo-obstruction may lead to stasis with secondary bacterial overgrowth causing diarrhea. *Diabetic diarrhea*, often accompanied by peripheral and generalized autonomic neuropathies, may occur in part because of intestinal dysmotility.

The exceedingly common *irritable bowel syndrome* (10% point prevalence, 1 to 2% per year incidence) is characterized by disturbed intestinal and colonic motor and sensory responses to various stimuli. Symptoms of stool frequency typically cease at night, alternate with periods of constipation, are accompanied by abdominal pain relieved with defecation, and rarely result in weight loss or true diarrhea.

Factitial Causes Factitial diarrhea accounts for up to 15% of unexplained diarrheas referred to tertiary care centers. Either as a form of *Munchausen syndrome* (deception or self-injury for secondary gain) or *bulimia*, some patients covertly self-administer laxatives alone or in combination with other medications (e.g., diuretics) or surreptitiously add water or urine to stool sent for analysis. Such patients are typically women, often with histories of psychiatric illness, and disproportionately from careers in health care. Hypotension and hypokalemia are common co-presenting features. Such patients often deny this possibility when confronted, but they do benefit from psychiatric counseling when they acknowledge their behavior.

APPROACH TO THE PATIENT

The laboratory tools available to evaluate the very common problem of chronic diarrhea are extensive, and many are costly and invasive. As such, the diagnostic evaluation must be rationally directed by a careful history and physical examination, and simple triage tests are often warranted before complex investigations are launched (Fig. 35-3). The history, physical examination, and routine blood studies should attempt to characterize the mechanism of diarrhea, identify diagnostically helpful associations, and assess the

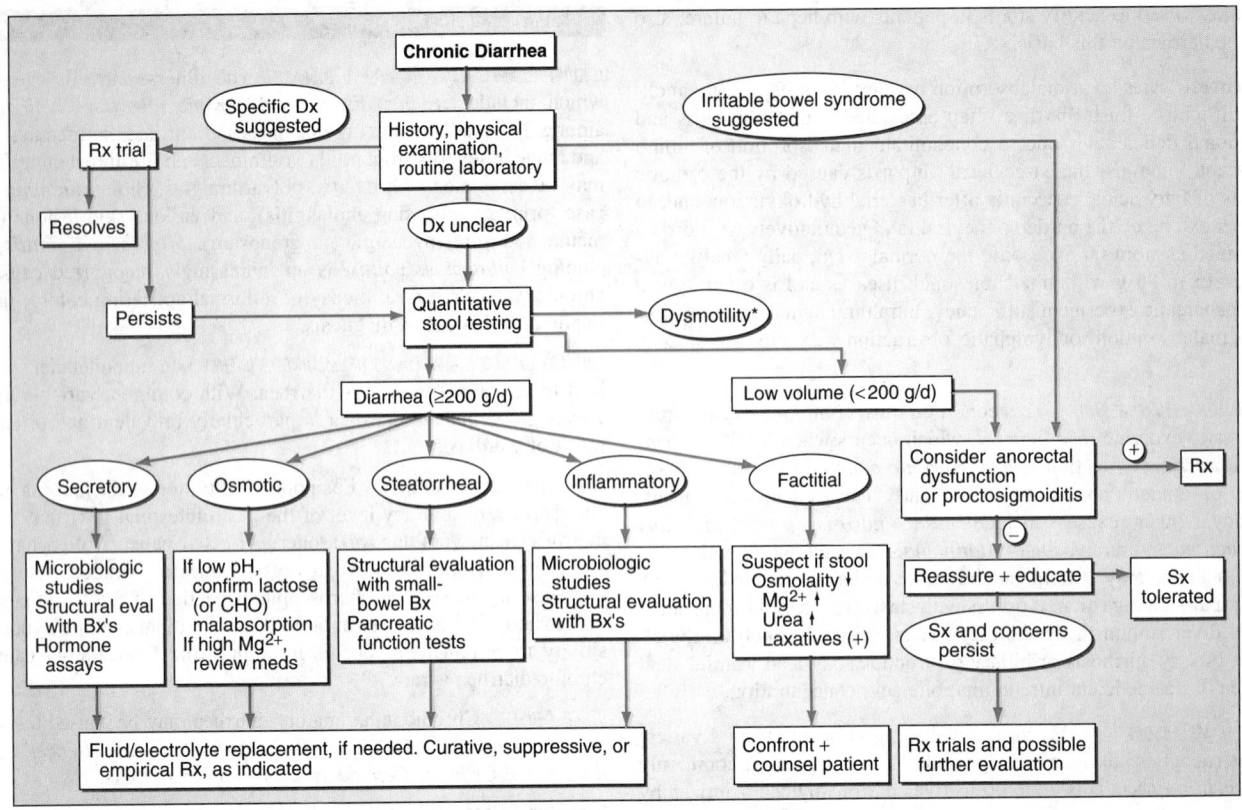

FIGURE 35-3 Algorithm for the management of chronic diarrhea.* Dysmotility presents variable stool profile.

patient's fluid/electrolyte and nutritional status. Patients should be questioned about the onset, duration, pattern, aggravating (especially diet) and relieving factors, and stool characteristics of their diarrhea. The presence or absence of fecal incontinence, fever, weight loss, pain, certain exposures (travel, medications, contacts with diarrhea), and common extraintestinal manifestations (skin changes, arthralgias, oral aphtha) should be noted. Physical findings may offer clues such as a thyroid mass, wheezing, heart murmurs, edema, hepatomegaly, abdominal masses, lymphadenopathy, mucocutaneous abnormalities, perianal fistulae, or anal sphincter laxity. Peripheral blood counts may reveal leukocytosis that suggests inflammation; anemia that reflects blood loss or nutritional deficiencies; or eosinophilia that may occur with parasitoses, neoplasia, collagen-vascular disease, allergy, or eosinophilic gastroenteritis. Blood chemistries may demonstrate electrolyte, hepatic, or other metabolic disturbances.

A therapeutic trial is often appropriate, definitive, and highly cost effective when a specific diagnosis is suggested on the initial physician encounter. For example, chronic watery diarrhea, which ceases with fasting in an otherwise healthy young adult, may justify a trial of a lactose-restricted diet; bloating and diarrhea persisting since a mountain backpacking trip may warrant a trial of metronidazole for likely giardiasis; and postprandial diarrhea persisting since an ileal resection might be due to bile acid malabsorption and be treated with cholestyramine before further evaluation. Persistent symptoms require additional investigation.

Certain diagnoses may be suggested on the initial encounter, e.g., idiopathic inflammatory bowel disease; however, additional focused evaluations may be necessary to confirm the diagnosis and characterize the severity or extent of disease so that treatment can be best guided. Patients suspected of having irritable bowel syndrome should be initially evaluated with proctosigmoidoscopy and mucosal biopsies; those with normal findings might be reassured and, as indicated, treated empirically with antispasmodics, antidiarrheals, bulk agents, anxiolytics, or antidepressants. Any patient who presents with chronic diarrhea and hematochezia should be evaluated with stool microbiologic studies and colonoscopy.

In an estimated two-thirds of cases, the cause for chronic diarrhea remains unclear after the initial encounter, and further testing is required. Quantitative stool collection and analyses can yield important objective data that may establish a diagnosis or characterize the type of diarrhea as a triage for focused additional studies (Fig. 35-3). If stool weight is >200 g/d, additional stool analyses should be performed that might include electrolyte concentration, pH, occult blood testing, leukocyte inspection (or leukocyte protein assay), fat quantitation, and laxative screens.

For secretory diarrheas (watery, normal osmotic gap), possible medication-related side effects or surreptitious laxative use should be reconsidered. Microbiologic studies should be done including fecal bacterial cultures (including media for *Aeromonas* and *Pleisiomonas*), inspection for ova and parasites, and *Giardia* antigen assay (the most sensitive test for giardiasis). Small bowel bacterial overgrowth can be excluded by intestinal aspirates with quantitative cultures or with glucose or xylose breath tests involving measurement of breath hydrogen or other metabolite (e.g., $^{14}CO_2$). However, interpretation of these breath tests may be confounded by disturbances of intestinal transit. When suggested by history or other findings, screens for peptide hormones should be pursued (e.g., serum gastrin, VIP, calcitonin, and thyroid hormone/thyroid stimulating hormone, or urinary 5-hydroxyindolacetic acid and histamine). Upper endoscopy and colonoscopy with biopsies and small-bowel barium x-rays are helpful to rule out structural or occult inflammatory disease.

Further evaluation of osmotic diarrhea should include tests for lactose intolerance and magnesium ingestion, the two most common causes. Low fecal pH suggests carbohydrate malabsorption; lactose malabsorption can be confirmed by lactose breath testing or by a therapeutic trial with lactose exclusion and observation of the effect of lactose challenge (e.g., a quart of milk). Lactase determination on small-bowel biopsy is generally not available. If fecal Mg^{2+} or laxative levels are elevated, then inadvertent or surreptitious ingestion should be considered and psychiatric help should be sought.

For those with proven fatty diarrhea, endoscopy with small-bowel biopsy (including aspiration for *Giardia* and quantitative cultures) should be performed; if this procedure is unrevealing, a small-bowel radiograph is often an appropriate next step. If small-bowel studies are negative or if pancreatic disease is suspected, pancreatic exocrine insufficiency should be excluded with direct tests, such as the secretin-cholecystokinin stimulation test, or by indirect tests, such as assay of fecal chymotrypsin activity or a bentiromide test.

Chronic inflammatory-type diarrheas should be suspected by the presence of blood or leukocytes in the stool. Such findings warrant stool cultures, inspection for ova and parasites, *C. difficile* toxin assay, colonoscopy with biopsies, and, if indicated, small-bowel oral contrast studies.

℞ TREATMENT

Treatment of chronic diarrhea depends on the specific etiology and may be curative, suppressive, or empirical. If the cause can be eradicated, treatment is curative as with resection of a colorectal cancer, antibiotic administration for Whipple's disease, or discontinuation of an offending drug. For many chronic conditions, diarrhea can be controlled by suppression of the underlying mechanism. Examples include elimination of dietary lactose for lactase deficiency or gluten for celiac sprue, use of glucocorticoids or other anti-inflammatory agents for idiopathic inflammatory bowel diseases, adsorptive agents such as cholestyramine for ileal bile acid malabsorption, proton pump inhibitors such as omeprazole for the gastric hypersecretion of gastrinomas, somatostatin analogues such as octreotide for malignant carcinoid, prostaglandin inhibitors such as indomethacin for medullary carcinoma of the thyroid, and pancreatic enzyme replacement for pancreatic insufficiency. When the specific cause or mechanism of chronic diarrhea evades diagnosis, empirical therapy may be beneficial. Mild opiates such as diphenoxylate or loperamide are often helpful in mild or moderate watery diarrhea. For those with more severe diarrhea, codeine or tincture of opium may be beneficial. Such antimotility agents should be avoided with inflammatory bowel disease, as toxic megacolon may be precipitated. Clonidine, an α_2-adrenergic agonist, may allow control of diabetic diarrhea. For all patients with chronic diarrhea, fluid and electrolyte repletion is an important component of management (see "Acute Diarrhea," above). Replacement of fat-soluble vitamins may also be necessary in patients with chronic steatorrhea.

CONSTIPATION

DEFINITION Constipation is a common complaint in clinical practice and usually refers to persistent, difficult, infrequent, or seemingly incomplete defecation. Because of the wide range of normal bowel habits, constipation is difficult to define precisely. Most persons have at least three bowel movements per week; however, stool frequency alone is not a sufficient criterion for the diagnosis of constipation because many constipated patients describe a normal frequency of defecation but subjective complaints of excessive straining, hard stools, lower abdominal fullness, and a sense of incomplete evacuation. The individual patient's symptoms must be analyzed in detail to ascertain what is meant by "constipation" or "difficulty" with defecation.

Stool form and consistency are well correlated with the time elapsed from the preceding defecation. Hard, pelletly stools occur with slow transit, while loose watery stools are associated with rapid transit. Small, pelletly stools are more difficult to expel than large ones.

The perception of hard stools or excessive straining is more difficult to assess objectively, and the need for enemas or digital disimpaction is a clinically useful way to corroborate the patient's perceptions of difficult defecation.

Psychosocial factors may also be important. A person whose parents attached great importance to daily defecation will become greatly concerned when he or she misses a daily bowel movement; some children withhold stool to gain attention; and some adults are simply too busy or too embarrassed to interrupt their work when the call to have a bowel movement is sensed.

CAUSES Pathophysiologically, chronic constipation generally results from inadequate fiber intake or from disordered colonic transit or anorectal function as a result of a neurogastroenterologic disturbance, certain drugs, or in association with a large number of systemic diseases that affect the gastrointestinal tract (Table 35-4). Constipation of recent onset may be a symptom of significant organic disease such as tumor or stricture. In *idiopathic constipation*, a subset of patients exhibit delayed emptying of the ascending and transverse colon with prolongation of transit (often in the proximal colon) and a reduced frequency of propulsive colonic contractions (HAPCs). *Outlet obstruction to defecation* (also called *evacuation disorders*) may cause delayed colonic transit, which is usually corrected by biofeedback retraining of the disordered defecation. Constipation of any cause may be exacerbated by chronic illnesses that lead to physical or mental impairment and result in inactivity or physical immobility.

APPROACH TO THE PATIENT

A careful history should explore the patient's symptoms and confirm whether he or she is indeed constipated based on frequency (e.g., fewer than three bowel movements per week), consistency (lumpy/hard), excessive straining, prolonged defecation time, or need to support the perineum or digitate the anorectum. In the vast majority of cases (probably >90%), there is no underlying cause (e.g., cancer, depression, or hypothyroidism), and constipation responds to ample hydration, exercise, and supplementation of dietary fiber (15 to 25 g/d). A good diet and medication history and attention to psychosocial issues are key. Physical examination and, particularly, a rectal examination should exclude most of the important diseases that present with constipation and possibly indicate features suggesting an evacuation disorder (e.g., high anal sphincter tone).

There is broad consensus on the selection of patients for further investigation. The presence of weight loss, rectal bleeding, or anemia with constipation mandates either sigmoidoscopy plus barium enema or colonoscopy alone, particularly in patients >40 years, to exclude structural diseases such as cancer or strictures. Colonoscopy alone is most cost effective in this setting since it provides an opportunity to biopsy mucosal lesions, perform polypectomy, or dilate strictures. Barium enema has advantages over colonoscopy in the patient with isolated constipation, since it is less costly and identifies colonic dilatation and all significant mucosal lesions or strictures that are likely to present with constipation. Melanosis coli, or pigmentation of the colon mucosa, indicates the use of

TABLE 35-4 *Causes of Constipation in Adults*

Types of Constipation and Causes	Examples
Recent onset	
Colonic obstruction	Neoplasm: stricture: ischemic, diverticular, inflammatory
Anal sphincter spasm	Anal fissure, painful hemorrhoids
Medications	
Chronic	
Irritable bowel syndrome	Constipation–predominant, alternating
Medications	Ca^{2+} blockers, antidepressants
Colonic pseudo-obstruction	Slow transit constipation, megacolon (rare Hirschsprung's, Chagas)
Disorders of rectal evacuation	Pelvic floor dysfunction, anismus, descending perineum syndrome, rectal mucosal prolapse, rectocele
Endocrinopathies	Hypothyroidism, hypercalcemia, pregnancy
Psychiatric disorders	Depression, eating disorders, drugs
Neurologic disease	Parkinsonism, multiple sclerosis, spinal cord injury
Generalized muscle disease	Progressive systemic sclerosis

anthraquinone laxatives such as cascara or senna; however, this is usually apparent from a careful history. An unexpected disorder such as megacolon or cathartic colon may also be detected by colonic radiographs. Measurement of serum calcium and thyroid stimulating hormone levels will identify rare patients with metabolic disorders.

Patients with more troublesome constipation may not respond to fiber alone and may be helped by a bowel training regimen: taking an osmotic laxative and evacuating with enema or glycerine suppository as needed. After breakfast, a distraction-free 15 to 20 min on the toilet without straining is encouraged. Excessive straining may lead to development of hemorrhoids, and, if there is weakness of the pelvic floor or injury to the pudendal nerve, may result in obstructed defecation from descending perineum syndrome several years later. Those few who do not benefit from the simple measures delineated above or require long-term treatment with stimulant laxatives with the attendant risk of developing laxative abuse syndrome are assumed to have severe or intractable constipation and should have further investigation (Fig. 35-4).

INVESTIGATION OF SEVERE CONSTIPATION A small minority (probably <5%) of all patients with constipation have cases that are considered severe or "intractable"; these are the patients most likely to be seen by gastroenterologists or in referral centers. Further observation of the patient may occasionally reveal a previously unrecognized cause, such as an evacuation disorder, laxative abuse, malingering, or psychiatric disorder. In these patients, recent studies suggest that evaluations of the physiologic function of the colon and pelvic floor and of psychological status aid in the rational choice of treatment. Even among these highly selected patients with severe constipation, a cause can be identified in only about 30% (see below).

Measurement of Colonic Transit Radiopaque marker transit tests are easy, repeatable, generally safe, inexpensive, reliable, and highly applicable in evaluating constipated patients in clinical practice. There are several validated methods that are very simple. For example, radiopaque

markers are ingested, and an abdominal flat film taken 5 d later should indicate passage of 80% of the markers out of the colon. This test does not provide useful information about the transit profile of the stomach and small bowel, and avoidance of laxatives or enemas during the testing period is essential.

Radioscintigraphy with a delayed-release capsule containing radio-labeled particles has been used to noninvasively characterize normal, accelerated, or delayed colonic function over 24 to 48 h with low radiation exposure. This approach simultaneously assesses gastric, small-bowel, and colonic transit. The disadvantages are the greater cost and the need for specific materials prepared in a nuclear medicine laboratory.

Anorectal and Pelvic Floor Tests Pelvic floor dysfunction is suggested by the inability to evacuate the rectum, a feeling of persistent rectal fullness, rectal pain, the need to extract stool from the rectum digitally, application of pressure on the posterior wall of the vagina, support of the perineum during straining, and excessive straining. These significant symptoms should be contrasted with the sense of incomplete rectal evacuation, which is common in irritable bowel syndrome.

Patients with clinically suspected obstruction of defecation should also be evaluated by a psychologist to identify eating disorders or a "need to control," to provide stress management or relaxation training, and to identify depression.

A simple clinical test in the office to document a nonrelaxing puborectalis muscle is to have the patient strain to expel the index finger during a digital rectal examination. Motion of the puborectalis posteriorly during straining indicates proper coordination of the pelvic floor muscles.

Measurement of perineal descent is relatively easy to gauge clinically by placing the patient in the left decubitus position and watching the perineum to assess either paucity or lack of descent (<1.5 cm, a sign of pelvic floor dysfunction) or perineal ballooning during straining relative to bony landmarks (>4 cm, suggesting excessive perineal descent).

A useful overall test of evacuation is the balloon expulsion test. A urinary catheter is placed in the rectum, the balloon is inflated to 50 mL with water, and a determination is made about whether the patient can expel it while seated on a toilet or in the left lateral decubitus position. In the lateral position, the weight needed to facilitate expulsion of the balloon (normal, 0 to 200 g) is determined.

Anorectal manometry is not often contributory in the evaluation of patients presenting with severe constipation, except when an excessively high resting or squeeze anal sphincter tone suggests anismus (anal sphincter spasm). This test also identifies rare syndromes, such as adult Hirschsprung's disease, by the absence of the rectoanal inhibitory reflex or the presence of occult incontinence.

Defecography (a dynamic barium enema including lateral views obtained during barium expulsion) reveals "soft abnormalities" in many patients; the most relevant findings are the measured changes in rectoanal angle, anatomic defects of the rectum, and enteroceles or rectoceles. In a very small proportion of patients, significant anatomic defects associated with intractable constipation respond best to surgical treatment. These defects include severe intussusception with complete outlet obstruction due to funnel-shaped plugging at the anal canal or an extremely large rectocele that is preferentially filled during attempts at defecation instead of expulsion of the barium through the anus. In summary, defecography requires an interested and experienced radiologist, and abnormalities are not pathognomonic for pelvic floor dysfunction. More commonly, outlet obstruction results from a nonrelaxing puborectalis muscle, which impedes rectal emptying, rather than from defects identified by defecography.

Dynamic imaging studies such as proctography during defecation or scintigraphic expulsion of artificial stool help measure perineal descent and the rectoanal angle during rest, squeezing, and straining, and scintigraphic expulsion quantitates the amount of "artificial stool" emptied. Failure of the rectoanal angle to increase significantly (~15°) during straining confirms pelvic floor dysfunction.

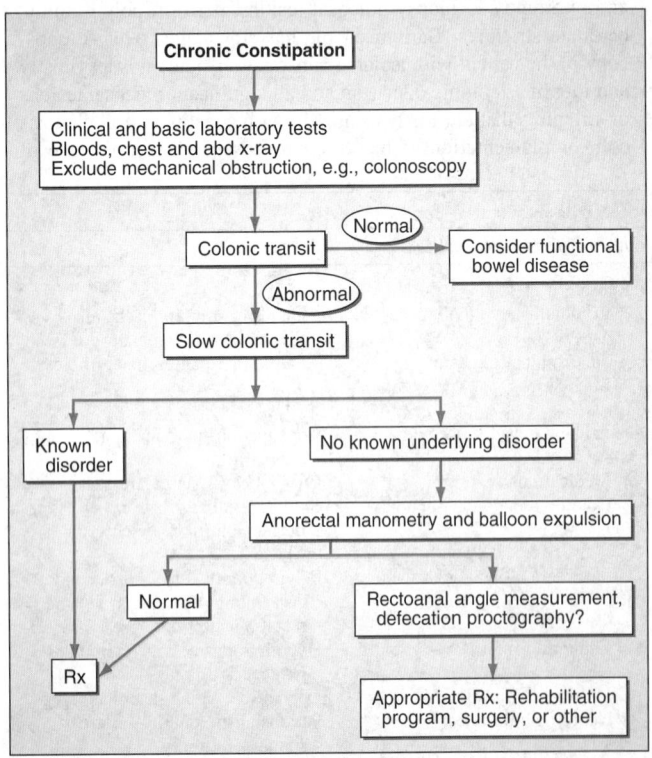

FIGURE 35-4 Algorithm for the management of constipation.

Neurologic testing (electromyography) is more helpful in the evaluation of patients with incontinence than of those with symptoms suggesting obstructed defecation. The absence of neurologic signs in the lower extremities suggests that any documented denervation of the puborectalis results from pelvic (e.g., obstetric) injury or from stretching of the pudendal nerve by chronic, long-standing straining.

Ultrasonography identifies sphincter or rectal wall defects and may help select patients for surgical correction. Spinal-evoked responses during electrical rectal stimulation or stimulation of external anal sphincter contraction by applying magnetic stimulation over the lumbosacral cord identify patients with limited sacral neuropathies with sufficient residual nerve conduction to attempt biofeedback training.

In summary, a balloon expulsion test is an important screening test for anorectal dysfunction. If positive, an anatomic evaluation of the rectum or anal sphincters and an assessment of pelvic floor relaxation are the tools for evaluating patients in whom obstructed defecation is suspected.

℞ TREATMENT

After the cause of constipation is characterized, a treatment decision can be made. Slow transit constipation requires aggressive medical or surgical treatment; anismus or pelvic floor dysfunction usually responds to biofeedback management (Fig. 35-4). However, only about 30% of patients with severe constipation are found to have such a physiologic disorder.

Patients with slow transit constipation are treated with bulk, osmotic, and stimulant laxatives, including fiber, psyllium, milk of magnesia, lactulose, polyethylene glycol (colonic lavage solution), and bisacodyl. If a 2- to 3-month trial of medical therapy fails and patients continue to have documented slow transit constipation unassociated with obstructed defecation, colectomy with ileorectostomy is indicated. The decision to resort to surgery is facilitated in the presence

of megacolon and megarectum. The complications after surgery include small-bowel obstruction (11%) and fecal soiling, particularly at night during the first postoperative year.

Patients who have a combined disorder should pursue pelvic floor retraining (biofeedback and muscle relaxation), psychological counseling, and dietetic advice first, followed by colectomy and ileorectosomy if colonic transit studies do not normalize with biofeedback alone. In patients with pelvic floor dysfunction alone, biofeedback training has a 70 to 80% success rate, measured by the acquisition of comfortable stool habits. Attempts to manage pelvic floor dysfunction with operations (internal anal sphincter or puborectalis muscle division) have achieved only mediocre success and have been largely abandoned.

FURTHER READING

AMERICAN GASTROENTEROLOGICAL ASSOCIATION: Medical Position Statement: Guidelines for the evaluation and management of chronic diarrhea. Gastroenterology 116:1461, 1991

BRANDT LJ et al: Systematic review on the management of irritable bowel syndrome in North America. Am J Gastroenterol 97 (Suppl):S1, 2002

CAMILLERI M et al: Clinical management of intractable constipation. Ann Intern Med 121:520, 1994

DUPONT HL and Practice Parameters Committee of the American College of Gastroenterology: Guidelines on acute infectious diarrhea in adults. Am J Gastroenterol 92:1962, 1997

FINE KD, SCHILLER LR: AGA technical review on the evaluation and management of chronic diarrhea. Gastroenterology 116:1461, 1999

LOCKE GR et al: AGA Medical Position Statement: Guidelines on constipation. Gastroenterology 119:1761, 2000

ROHNER P et al: Etiological agents of infectious diarrhea: Implications for requests for microbial culture. J Clin Microbiol 35:1427, 1997

36 | WEIGHT LOSS
Carol M. Reife

Significant unintentional weight loss in a previously healthy individual is often a harbinger of underlying systemic disease. During the routine medical history, inquiry should always be made about changes in weight; loss of 5% of body weight over 6 to 12 months should prompt further evaluation.

PHYSIOLOGY OF WEIGHT REGULATION

The normal individual maintains body weight at a remarkably stable "set point," given the wide variation in daily caloric intake and level of activity. Because of the physiologic importance of maintaining energy stores, voluntary weight loss is difficult to achieve and sustain.

Appetite and metabolism are regulated by an intricate network of neural and hormonal factors. The hypothalamic feeding and satiety centers play a central role in these processes (Chap. 64). Neuropeptides such as corticotropin-releasing hormone (CRH), α-melanocyte stimulating hormone (α-MSH), and cocaine- and amphetamine-related transcript (CART) induce anorexia by acting centrally on satiety centers. The gastrointestinal peptides ghrelin, glucagon, somatostatin, and cholecystokinin signal satiety and thus decrease food intake. Hypoglycemia suppresses insulin, reducing glucose utilization and inhibiting the satiety center.

Leptin is produced by adipose tissue, and it plays a central role in the long-term maintenance of weight homeostasis by acting on the hypothalamus to decrease food intake and increase energy expenditure (Chap. 64). Leptin suppresses expression of hypothalamic neuropeptide Y, a potent appetite stimulatory peptide, and it increases the expression of α-MSH, which acts through the MC4R melanocortin receptor to decrease appetite. Thus, leptin activates a series of downstream neural pathways that alter food-seeking behavior and metabolism.

However, leptin deficiency, which occurs in conjunction with the loss of adipose tissue, stimulates appetite and induces adaptive responses including inhibition of hypothalamic thyrotropin-releasing hormone (TRH) and gonadotropin-releasing hormone (GnRH).

A variety of cytokines, including tumor necrosis factor α (TNF-α), interleukin (IL) 6 (IL-6), IL-1, interferon γ (IFN-γ), ciliary neurotrophic factor (CNTF), and leukemia inhibitory factor (LIF), can induce cachexia (Chap. 16). In addition to causing anorexia, these factors may stimulate fever, depress myocardial function, modulate immune and inflammatory responses, and induce a variety of specific metabolic alterations. TNF-α, for example, preferentially mobilizes fat but spares skeletal muscle. Levels of one or more of these cytokines may be increased in patients with cancer, sepsis, chronic inflammatory conditions, AIDS, and congestive heart failure.

Weight loss occurs when energy expenditure exceeds calories available for energy utilization (Chap. 62). In most individuals, approximately half of food energy is utilized for basal processes such as maintenance of body temperature. In a 70-kg person, basal activity consumes about 1800 kcal/d. About 40% of caloric intake is used for physical activity, although athletes may use more than 50% during vigorous exercise. About 10% of caloric intake is used for dietary thermogenesis, the energy expended for digestion, absorption, and metabolism of food.

Mechanisms of weight loss include decreased food intake, malabsorption, loss of calories, and increased energy requirements (Fig. 36-1). Changes in weight may involve loss of tissue mass or body fluid content. A deficit of 3500 kcal generally correlates with the loss of 0.45 kg (1 lb) of body fat, but one must also consider water weight [1 kg/L (2.2 lb/L)] gained or lost. Weight loss that persists over weeks to months reflects the loss of tissue mass.

Food intake may be influenced by a wide variety of visual, olfactory, and gustatory stimuli as well as by genetic, psychological, and social factors. Absorption may be impaired because of pancreatic in-

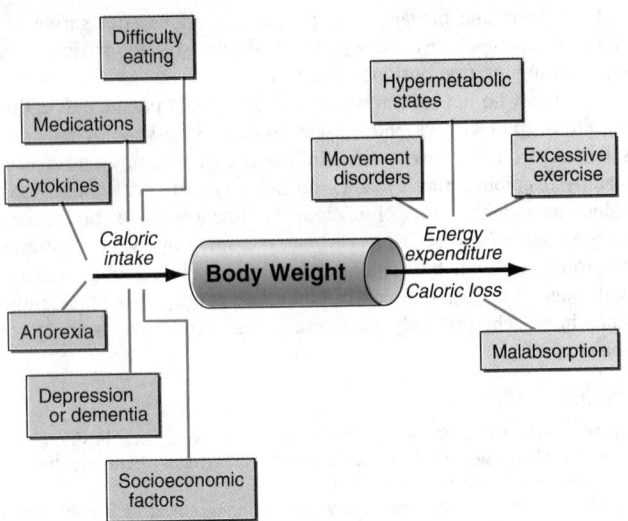

FIGURE 36-1 Energy balance and pathophysiology of weight loss.

TABLE 36-1 *Causes of Weight Loss*

Cancer	Medications
Endocrine and metabolic	Antibiotics
Hyperthyroidism	Nonsteroidal anti-inflammatory drugs
Diabetes mellitus	Serotonin reuptake inhibitors
Pheochromocytoma	Metformin
Adrenal insufficiency	Levodopa
Gastrointestinal disorders	ACE inhibitors
Malabsorption	Other drugs
Obstruction	Disorders of the mouth and teeth
Pernicious anemia	Age-related factors
Cardiac disorders	Physiologic changes
Chronic ischemia	Decreased taste and smell
Chronic congestive heart	Functional disabilities
failure	Neurologic
Respiratory disorders	Stroke
Emphysema	Parkinson's disease
Chronic obstructive	Neuromuscular disorders
pulmonary disease	Dementia
Renal insufficiency	Social
Rheumatologic disease	Isolation
Infections	Economic hardship
HIV	Psychiatric and behavioral
Tuberculosis	Depression
Parasitic infection	Anxiety
Subacute bacterial	Bereavement
endocarditis	Alcoholism
	Eating disorders
	Increased activity or exercise
	Idiopathic

sufficiency, cholestasis, celiac sprue, intestinal tumors, radiation injury, inflammatory bowel disease, infection, or medication effect. These disease processes may be manifest as changes in stool frequency and consistency. Calories may also be lost due to vomiting or diarrhea, glucosuria in diabetes mellitus, or fistulous drainage. Resting energy expenditure decreases with age and can be affected by thyroid status. Beginning at about age 60, body weight declines by an average of 0.5% per year. Body composition is also affected by aging; adipose tissue increases and lean muscle mass decreases with age.

SIGNIFICANCE OF WEIGHT LOSS

Unintentional weight loss, especially in the elderly, is not uncommon and is associated with increased morbidity and mortality rates, even after comorbid conditions have been taken into account. Prospective studies indicate that significant involuntary weight loss is associated with a mortality rate of 25% over the next 18 months. Retrospective studies of significant weight loss in the elderly document mortality rates of 9 to 38% over a 2- to 3-year period.

Cancer patients with weight loss have decreased performance status, impaired responses to chemotherapy, and reduced median survival (Chap. 66). Marked weight loss also predisposes to infection. Patients undergoing elective surgery, who have lost >4.5 kg (>10 lb) in 6 months, have higher surgical mortality rates. Vitamin and nutrient deficiencies also can accompany significant weight loss (Chap. 61).

CAUSES OF WEIGHT LOSS

The list of possible causes of weight loss is extensive (Table 36-1). In the elderly, the most common causes of weight loss are depression, cancer, and benign gastrointestinal disease. Lung and gastrointestinal cancer are the most common malignancies in patients presenting with weight loss. In younger individuals, diabetes mellitus, hyperthyroidism, psychiatric disturbances including eating disorders, and infection, especially with HIV, should be considered.

The cause of involuntary weight loss is rarely occult. Careful history and physical examination, in association with directed diagnostic testing, will identify the cause of weight loss in 75% of patients. The etiology of weight loss may not be found in the remaining patients, despite extensive testing. Patients with negative evaluations tend to have lower mortality rates than those found to have organic disease.

Patients with medical causes of weight loss usually have signs or symptoms that suggest involvement of a particular organ system. Gastrointestinal tumors, including those of the pancreas and liver, may affect food intake early in the course of illness, causing weight loss before other symptoms are apparent. Lung cancer may present with post-obstructive pneumonia, dyspnea, or cough and hemoptysis; how-

ever, it may be silent and should be considered even in those without a history of cigarette smoking. Depression and isolation can cause profound weight loss, especially in the elderly. Chronic pulmonary disease and congestive heart failure can produce anorexia, and they also increase resting energy expenditure. Weight loss may be the presenting sign of infectious diseases such as HIV infection, tuberculosis, endocarditis, and fungal or parasitic infections. Hyperthyroidism or pheochromocytoma increases metabolism. Elderly patients with apathetic hyperthyroidism may present with weight loss and weakness, with few other manifestations of thyrotoxicosis. New-onset diabetes mellitus is often accompanied by weight loss, reflecting glucosuria and loss of the anabolic actions of insulin. Adrenal insufficiency may be suggested by increased pigmentation, hyponatremia, and hyperkalemia.

APPROACH TO THE PATIENT

Before extensive evaluation is undertaken, it is important to confirm weight loss and to determine the time interval over which it has occurred. Almost half of patients who claim significant weight loss have no actual change when body weight is measured objectively. In the absence of documentation, changes in belt notch size or the fit of clothing may be confirmatory. Not infrequently, patients who have actually sustained significant weight loss are unaware that it has occurred. Routine documentation of weight during office visits is therefore important.

The review of systems should focus on signs or symptoms that are associated with disorders that commonly cause weight loss. These include fever, pain, shortness of breath or cough, palpitations, and evidence of neurologic disease. Gastrointestinal disturbances, including difficulty eating, dysphagia, anorexia, nausea, and change in bowel habits, should be sought. Travel history, use of cigarettes and alcohol, and all medications should be reviewed, and patients should be questioned about previous illness or surgery as well as diseases in family members. Risk factors for HIV infection should be assessed. Signs of depression, evidence of dementia, and social factors, including financial issues that might affect food intake, should be considered.

Physical examination should begin with weight determination and documentation of vital signs. The skin should be examined for

TABLE 36-2 Screening Tests for Evaluation of Involuntary Weight Loss

Initial testing	Additional testing
CBC	HIV test
Electrolytes, calcium, glucose	Upper and/or lower gastrointestinal endoscopy
Renal and liver function tests	Abdominal CT scan or MRI
Urinalysis	Chest CT scan
TSH	
Chest x-ray	
Recommended cancer screening	

pallor, jaundice, turgor, scars from prior surgery, and stigmata of systemic disease. The search for oral thrush or dental disease, thyroid gland enlargement, adenopathy, and respiratory or cardiac abnormalities and a detailed examination of the abdomen often lead to clues for further evaluation. Rectal examination, including prostate examination and testing of stool for occult blood, should be performed in men; and all women should have a pelvic examination, even if they have had a hysterectomy. Neurologic examination should include mental status assessment and screening for depression.

Laboratory testing should confirm or exclude possible diagnoses elicited from the history and physical examination (Table 36-2). An initial phase of testing should include a complete blood

count with differential, serum chemistry tests including glucose, electrolytes, renal and liver tests, calcium, thyroid-stimulating hormone (TSH), urinalysis, and chest x-ray. Patients at risk for HIV infection should have HIV antibody testing. In all cases, recommended cancer screening tests appropriate for the gender and age group, such as mammograms and Pap smears, should be updated (Chap. 67). If gastrointestinal signs or symptoms are present, upper and/or lower endoscopy and abdominal imaging with either computed tomography (CT) or magnetic resonance imaging (MRI) have a relatively high yield, consistent with the high prevalence of gastrointestinal disorders in patients with weight loss. If an etiology of weight loss is not found, careful clinical follow-up, rather than persistent undirected testing, is reasonable.

FURTHER READING

BOURAS EP, LANGE SM: Rational approach to patients with unintentional weight loss. Mayo Clinic Proc 76:923, 2001

INUI A: Cancer anorexia-cachexia syndrome: Current issues in research and management. Cancer J Clinicians 52:72, 2002

REIFE CM: Involuntary weight loss. Med Clin North Am 79:299, 1995

SCHWARTZ MW: Brain pathways controlling food intake and body weight. Exp Biol Med 226:978, 2001

WALLACE JI: Involuntary weight loss in elderly outpatients: Recognition, etiologies, and treatment. Clin Geriatr Med 13:717, 1997

37 GASTROINTESTINAL BLEEDING
Loren Laine

Bleeding from the gastrointestinal (GI) tract may present in five ways. *Hematemesis* is vomitus of red blood or "coffee-grounds" material. *Melena* is black, tarry, foul-smelling stool. *Hematochezia* is the passage of bright red or maroon blood from the rectum. *Occult GI bleeding* (GIB) may be identified in the absence of overt bleeding by special examination of the stool (e.g., guaiac testing). Finally, patients may present only with *symptoms of blood loss or anemia* such as lightheadedness, syncope, angina, or dyspnea.

SOURCES OF GASTROINTESTINAL BLEEDING

UPPER GASTROINTESTINAL SOURCES OF BLEEDING (Table 37-1)   The annual incidence of hospital admissions for upper GIB (UGIB) in the United States and Europe is approximately 0.1%, with a mortality rate of ~5 to 10%. Patients rarely die from exsanguination; rather, they die due to decompensation from other underlying illnesses. The mortality rate for patients under 60 years of age in the absence of malignancy or organ failure is <1%. The three independent clinical predictors of death in patients hospitalized with UGIB are increasing age, comorbidities, and hemodynamic compromise (tachycardia or hypotension).

Peptic ulcers are the most common cause of UGIB, accounting for about 50% of cases. Mallory-Weiss tears account for 5 to 15% of cases. The proportion of patients bleeding from varices varies widely from

TABLE 37-1 Sources of Bleeding in Patients Hospitalized for Acute UGIB

Sources of Bleeding	Proportion of Patients (%)
Ulcers	35–62
Varices	4–31
Mallory-Weiss tears	4–13
Gastroduodenal erosions	3–11
Erosive esophagitis	2–8
Malignancy	1–4
No source identified	7–25

Source: Data from Rockall et al; GF Longstreth: Am J Gastroenterol 90:206, 1995; EM Vreeburg et al: Am J Gastroenterol 92:236, 1997; and L Laine: West J Med 155:274, 1991.

~5 to 30%, depending on the population. Hemorrhagic or erosive gastropathy [e.g., due to nonsteroidal anti-inflammatory drugs (NSAIDs) or alcohol] and erosive esophagitis often cause mild UGIB, but major bleeding is rare.

Peptic Ulcers   In addition to clinical features, characteristics of an ulcer at endoscopy provide important prognostic information. One-third of patients with active bleeding or a nonbleeding visible vessel have further bleeding that requires urgent surgery if they are treated conservatively. These patients clearly benefit from endoscopic therapy with bipolar electrocoagulation, heater probe, or injection therapy (e.g., absolute alcohol, 1:10,000 epinephrine), with reductions in bleeding, hospital stay, mortality rate, and costs. In contrast, patients with clean-based ulcers have rates of recurrent bleeding approaching zero. If there is no other reason for hospitalization, such patients may be discharged on the first hospital day, following stabilization. Patients without clean-based ulcers should usually remain in the hospital for 3 days, since most episodes of recurrent bleeding occur within 3 days.

Randomized controlled trials document that high-dose constant infusion intravenous omeprazole (80-mg bolus and 8-mg/h infusion), used to raise intragastric pH to between 6 and 7 and enhance clot stability, decreases further bleeding (but not mortality), even after the use of appropriate endoscopic therapy in patients with high-risk ulcers (active bleeding, nonbleeding visible vessel, and perhaps adherent clot). In the United States, the same dose of the only available intravenous proton pump inhibitor, pantoprazole, is used after endoscopic confirmation of an ulcer with high-risk findings.

Approximately one-third of patients with a bleeding ulcer will rebleed within the next 1 to 2 years. Prevention of recurrent bleeding focuses on the three main factors in ulcer pathogenesis, *Helicobacter pylori*, NSAIDs, and acid. Eradication of *H. pylori* in patients with bleeding ulcers decreases rates of rebleeding to <5%. If a bleeding ulcer develops in a patient taking NSAIDs, the NSAIDs should be discontinued if possible. If NSAIDs must be continued, initial treatment should be with a proton pump inhibitor. Subsequently patients should either switch from a nonselective NSAID to a cyclooxygenase 2 (COX-2) specific inhibitor or add GI co-therapy. Proton pump inhibitors and misoprostol are effective co-therapies, but proton pump inhibitors are preferred due to less frequent dosing (once daily) and fewer side effects (e.g., diarrhea). Patients at very high risk (e.g., elderly with prior bleeding ulcer) should probably take a COX-2 specific inhibitor and a proton pump inhibitor. Patients with bleeding ulcers unrelated to *H. pylori* or NSAIDs should remain on full-dose antisecretory therapy indefinitely. →*Peptic ulcers are discussed in Chap. 274.*

Mallory-Weiss Tears The classic history is vomiting, retching, or coughing preceding hematemesis, especially in an alcoholic patient. Bleeding from these tears, which are usually on the gastric side of the gastroesophageal junction, stops spontaneously in 80 to 90% of patients and recurs in only 0 to 5%. Endoscopic therapy is indicated for actively bleeding Mallory-Weiss tears. Angiographic therapy with intraarterial infusion of vasopressin or embolization and operative therapy with oversewing of the tear are rarely required. →*Mallory-Weiss tears are discussed in Chap. 273.*

Esophageal Varices Patients with variceal hemorrhage have poorer outcomes than patients with other sources of UGIB. Endoscopic therapy for acute bleeding and repeated sessions of endoscopic therapy to eradicate esophageal varices significantly reduces rebleeding and mortality. Ligation is the endoscopic therapy of choice for esophageal varices because it has less rebleeding, a lower mortality rate, fewer local complications, and requires fewer treatment sessions to achieve variceal eradication as compared to sclerotherapy.

Acute treatment with octreotide (50-μg bolus and 50-μg/h intravenous infusion for 2 to 5 days) may help in the control of acute bleeding, and this has replaced vasopressin as the medical therapy of choice for acute variceal bleeding in the United States. Agents such as somatostatin and terlipressin, available outside the United States, are also effective. Over the long term, treatment with nonselective beta blockers decreases recurrent bleeding from esophageal varices. Beta blockers are commonly given along with chronic endoscopic therapy.

In patients who have persistent or recurrent bleeding despite endoscopic and medical therapy, more invasive therapy is warranted. Transjugular intrahepatic portosystemic shunt (TIPS) decreases rebleeding more effectively than endoscopic therapy, although hepatic encephalopathy is more common and the mortality rates are comparable. Most patients with TIPS have shunt stenosis within 1 to 2 years and require reinstrumentation. Therefore, TIPS is most appropriate for patients with more severe liver disease and those in whom transplant is anticipated. Patients with milder, well-compensated cirrhosis should probably undergo decompressive surgery (e.g., distal splenorenal shunt).

Portal hypertension is also responsible for bleeding from gastric varices, varices in the small and large intestine, and portal hypertensive gastropathy and enterocolopathy.

Hemorrhagic and Erosive Gastropathy ("Gastritis") Hemorrhagic and erosive gastropathy, or gastritis, refers to endoscopically visualized subepithelial hemorrhages and erosions. These are mucosal lesions and thus do not cause major bleeding. They develop in various clinical settings, the most important of which are NSAID use, alcohol intake, and stress. Half of patients who chronically ingest NSAIDs have erosions (15 to 30% have ulcers), while up to 20% of actively drinking alcoholic patients with symptoms of UGIB have evidence of subepithelial hemorrhages or erosions.

Stress-related gastric mucosal injury occurs only in extremely sick patients: those who have experienced serious trauma, major surgery, burns covering more than one-third of the body surface area, major intracranial disease, and severe medical illness (i.e., ventilator dependence, coagulopathy). Significant bleeding probably does not develop unless ulceration occurs. The mortality rate in these patients is quite high because of their serious underlying illnesses.

The incidence of bleeding from stress-related gastric mucosal injury or ulceration has decreased dramatically in recent years, most likely due to better care of critically ill patients. Pharmacologic prophylaxis for bleeding may be considered in the high-risk patients mentioned above. The best data suggest that intravenous H$_2$-receptor an-

tagonist therapy is the treatment of choice, although sucralfate is also effective. Prophylactic therapy decreases bleeding but does not lower the mortality rate.

Other Causes Other, less frequent causes of UGIB include erosive duodenitis, neoplasms, aortoenteric fistulas, vascular lesions [including hereditary hemorrhagic telengectasias (Osler-Weber-Rendu) and gastric antral vascular ectasia ("watermelon stomach")], Dieulafoy's lesion (in which an aberrant vessel in the mucosa bleeds from a pinpoint mucosal defect), prolapse gastropathy (prolapse of proximal stomach into esophagus with retching, especially in alcoholics), and hemobilia and hemosuccus pancreaticus (bleeding from the bile duct or pancreatic duct).

SMALL-INTESTINAL SOURCES OF BLEEDING Small-intestinal sources of bleeding (bleeding from sites beyond the reach of the standard upper endoscope) are difficult to diagnose and are responsible for the majority of cases of obscure GIB. Fortunately, small-intestinal bleeding is uncommon. The most common causes are vascular ectasias and tumors (e.g., adenocarcinoma, leiomyoma, lymphoma, benign polyps, carcinoid, metastases, and lipoma). Other less common causes include Crohn's disease, infection, ischemia, vasculitis, small-bowel varices, diverticula, Meckel's diverticulum, duplication cysts, and intussusception. NSAIDs induce small-intestinal erosions and ulcers and may be a relatively common cause of chronic, obscure GIB.

Meckel's diverticulum is the most common cause of significant lower GIB (LGIB) in children, decreasing in frequency as a cause of bleeding with age. In adults <40 to 50 years, small-bowel tumors often account for obscure GIB; in patients >50 to 60 years, vascular ectasias are usually responsible.

Vascular ectasias should be treated with endoscopic therapy if possible. Surgical therapy can be used for vascular ectasias isolated to a segment of the small intestine when endoscopic therapy is unsuccessful. Although estrogen/progesterone compounds have been used for vascular ectasias, a double-blind trial found no benefit in prevention of recurrent bleeding. Isolated lesions, such as tumors, diverticula, or duplications, are generally treated with surgical resection.

COLONIC SOURCES OF BLEEDING The incidence of hospitalizations for LGIB is about one-fifth that for UGIB. Hemorrhoids are probably the most common cause of LGIB; anal fissures also cause minor bleeding and pain. If these local anal processes, which rarely require hospitalization, are excluded, the most common causes of LGIB in adults are diverticula, vascular ectasias (especially in the proximal colon of patients >70 years), neoplasms (primarily adenocarcinoma), and colitis—most commonly infectious or idiopathic inflammatory bowel disease, but occasionally ischemic or radiation-induced. Uncommon causes include post-polypectomy bleeding, solitary rectal ulcer syndrome, NSAID-induced ulcers or colitis, trauma, varices (most commonly rectal), lymphoid nodular hyperplasia, vasculitis, and aortocolic fistulas. In children and adolescents, the most common colonic causes of significant GIB are inflammatory bowel disease and juvenile polyps.

Diverticular bleeding is abrupt in onset, usually painless, sometimes massive, and often from the right colon; minor and occult bleeding is not characteristic. Clinical reports suggest that bleeding colonic diverticula stop bleeding spontaneously in approximately 80% of patients and rebleed in about 20 to 25% of patients. Intraarterial vasopressin may halt the bleeding, at least temporarily. If bleeding persists or recurs, segmental surgical resection is indicated.

Bleeding from right colonic vascular ectasias in the elderly may be overt or occult; it tends to be chronic and only occasionally is hemodynamically significant. Endoscopic hemostatic therapy may be useful in the treatment of vascular ectasias, as well as discrete bleeding ulcers and post-polypectomy bleeding, while endoscopic polypectomy, if possible, is used for bleeding colonic polyps. Surgical therapy is generally required for major, persistent, or recurrent bleeding from the wide variety of colonic sources of GIB that cannot be treated medically or endoscopically.

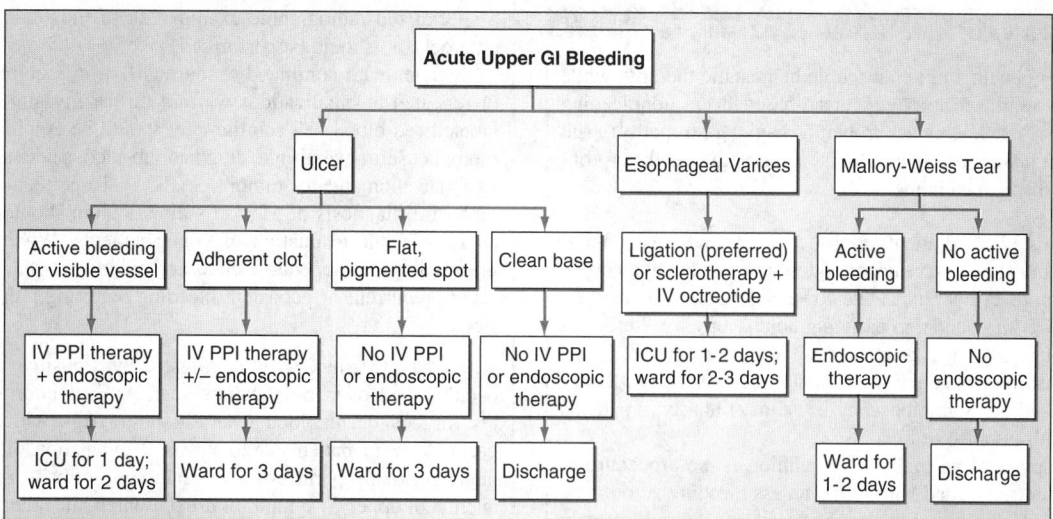

FIGURE 37-1 Suggested algorithm for patients with acute upper gastrointestinal bleeding. Recommendations on level of care and time of discharge assume patient is stabilized without further bleeding or other concomitant medical problems. PPI, proton pump inhibitor; ICU, intensive care unit.

APPROACH TO THE PATIENT

Measurement of the heart rate and blood pressure is the best way to assess a patient with GIB. Clinically significant bleeding leads to postural changes in heart rate or blood pressure, tachycardia, and, finally, recumbent hypotension. In contrast, the hemoglobin does not fall immediately with acute GIB, due to proportionate reductions in plasma and red cell volumes (i.e., "people bleed whole blood"). Thus, hemoglobin may be normal or only minimally decreased at the initial presentation of a severe bleeding episode. As extravascular fluid enters the vascular space to restore volume, the hemoglobin falls, but this process may take up to 72 h. Patients with slow, chronic GIB may have very low hemoglobin values despite normal blood pressure and heart rate. With the development of iron-deficiency anemia, the mean corpuscular volume will be low and red blood cell distribution width will be increased.

Differentiation of Upper from Lower GIB Hematemesis indicates an upper GI source of bleeding (above the ligament of Treitz). Melena indicates that blood has been present in the GI tract for at least 14 h. Thus, the more proximal the bleeding site, the more likely melena will occur. Hematochezia usually represents a lower GI source of bleeding, although an upper GI lesion may bleed so briskly that blood does not remain in the bowel long enough for melena to develop. When hematochezia is the presenting symptom of UGIB, it is associated with hemodynamic instability and dropping hemoglobin. Bleeding lesions of the small bowel may present as melena or hematochezia. Other clues to UGIB include hyperactive bowel sounds and an elevated blood urea nitrogen level (due to volume depletion and blood proteins absorbed in the small intestine).

A nonbloody nasogastric aspirate may be seen in up to 16% of patients with UGIB—usually from a duodenal source. Even a bile-stained appearance does not exclude a bleeding postpyloric lesion since reports of bile in the aspirate are incorrect in about 50% of cases. Testing of aspirates that are not grossly bloody for occult blood is not useful.

Diagnostic Evaluation of the Patient with GIB ■ UPPER GIB (Fig. 37-1) History and physical examination are

not usually diagnostic of the source of GIB. Upper endoscopy is the test of choice in patients with UGIB and should be performed urgently in patients with hemodynamic instability (hypotension, tachycardia, or postural changes in heart rate or blood pressure). Early endoscopy is also beneficial in cases of milder bleeding for management decisions. Patients with major bleeding and high-risk endoscopic findings (e.g., varices, ulcers with active bleeding or a

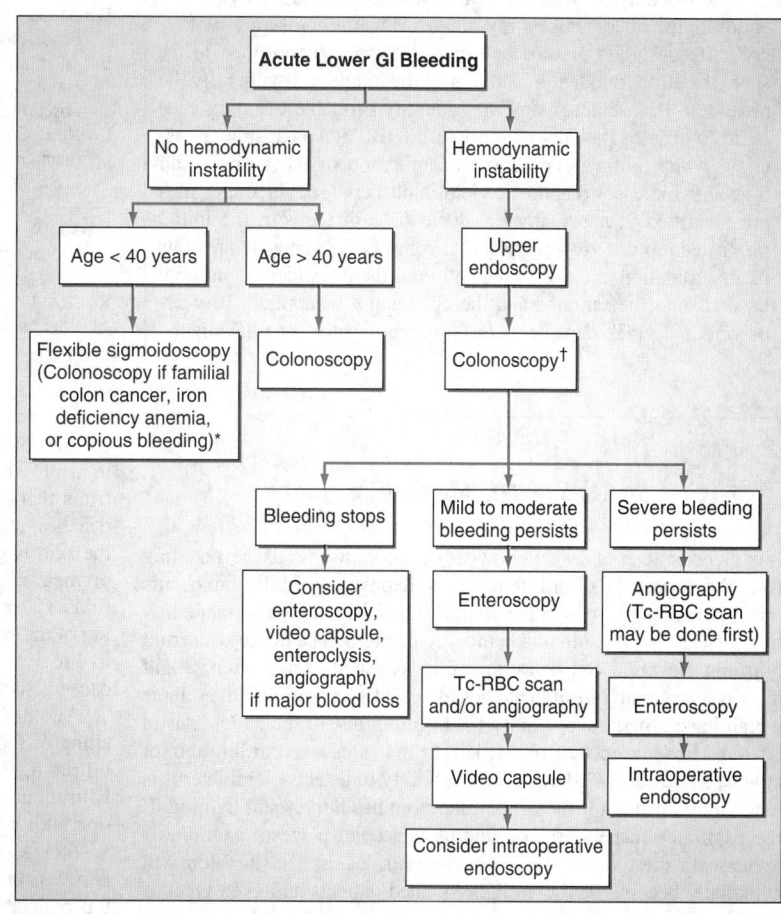

FIGURE 37-2 Suggested algorithm for patients with acute lower gastrointestinal bleeding. Sequential recommendations under "Hemodynamic instability" assume a test is found to be nondiagnostic before next test is performed. *Some suggest colonoscopy for any degree of rectal bleeding in patients <40 years old as well. †If massive bleeding does not allow time for colonic lavage, proceed to angiography. Tc-RBC, 99mtechnetium-labeled red blood cell.

visible vessel) benefit from endoscopic hemostatic therapy, while patients with low-risk lesions (e.g., clean-based ulcers, nonbleeding Mallory-Weiss tears, erosive or hemorrhagic gastropathy) who have stable vital signs and hemoglobin, and no other medical problems, can be discharged home.

LOWER GIB (Fig. 37-2)   Patients with hematochezia and hemodynamic instability should have upper endoscopy to rule out an upper GI source before evaluation of the lower GI tract. Patients with presumed LGIB may undergo early sigmoidoscopy for the detection of obvious, low-lying lesions. However, the procedure is difficult with brisk bleeding, and it is usually not possible to identify the area of bleeding. Sigmoidoscopy is useful primarily in patients <40 years with minor bleeding.

Colonoscopy after an oral lavage solution is the procedure of choice in patients admitted with LGIB unless bleeding is too massive or unless sigmoidoscopy has disclosed an obvious actively bleeding lesion. ^{99M}Tc-labeled red cell scan allows repeated imaging for up to 24 h and may identify the general location of bleeding. However, radionuclide scans should be interpreted with caution because results, especially from later images, are highly variable. In active LGIB, angiography can detect the site of bleeding (extravasation of contrast into the gut) and permits treatment with intraarterial infusion of vasopressin or embolization. Even after bleeding has stopped, angiography may identify lesions with abnormal vasculature, such as vascular ectasias or tumors.

GIB OF OBSCURE ORIGIN   Obscure GIB is defined as recurrent acute or chronic bleeding for which no source has been identified by routine endoscopic and contrast x-ray studies. Push enteroscopy, with a specially designed enteroscope or a pediatric colonoscope to inspect the entire duodenum and part of the jejunum, is generally the next step. Push enteroscopy may identify probable bleeding sites in 20 to 40% of patients with obscure GIB. Video capsule endoscopy, which allows endoscopic examination of the entire small intestine, increases diagnostic yield in obscure GIB: bleeding sites are identified in approximately 30 to 65% of cases in the initial published reports. However, lack of control of the capsule prevents its manipulation and full visualization of the intestine; in addition, tissue cannot be sampled and therapy cannot be applied. If enteroscopy and video capsule endoscopy are negative or unavailable, a specialized radiographic examination of the small bowel (e.g., enteroclysis) should be performed.

Patients with continued obscure GIB who require transfusions or repeated hospitalizations warrant further investigations. ^{99M}Tc-labeled red blood cell scintigraphy should be employed. Angiography is useful even if bleeding has subsided, since it may disclose vascular anomalies or tumor vessels. ^{99M}Tc-pertechnetate scintigraphy for diagnosis of Meckel's diverticulum should be done, especially in the evaluation of young patients. When all tests are unrevealing, intraoperative endoscopy is indicated in patients with severe recurrent or persistent bleeding requiring repeated transfusions.

OCCULT GIB   Occult GIB is manifested by a positive test for fecal occult blood or iron-deficiency anemia. Evaluation of a positive test for fecal occult blood generally should begin with colonoscopy, particularly in patients >40 years. If evaluation of the colon is negative, many perform upper endoscopy only if iron-deficiency anemia or upper GI symptoms are present, while others recommend upper endoscopy in all patients since up to 25 to 40% of these patients may have some abnormality noted on upper endoscopy. If standard endoscopic tests are unrevealing, enteroscopy, video capsule endoscopy, and/or enteroclysis may be considered in patients with iron-deficiency anemia.

FURTHER READING

CHAN FK et al: Celecoxib versus diclofenac and omeprazole in reducing the risk of recurrent ulcer bleeding in patients with arthritis. N Engl J Med 347: 2104, 2002

CIPOLLETTA L et al: Outpatient management for low-risk nonvariceal upper GI bleeding: A randomized controlled trial. Gastrointest Endosc 55:1, 2002

D'AMICO G et al: Pharmacological treatment of portal hypertension: An evidence-based approach. Semin Liver Dis 19:475, 1999

ELL C et al: The first prospective controlled trial comparing wireless capsule endoscopy with push enteroscopy in chronic gastrointestinal bleeding. Endoscopy 34:685, 2002

LAINE L, COOK D: Endoscopic ligation compared with sclerotherapy for treatment of esophageal variceal bleeding: A meta-analysis. Ann Intern Med 123:280, 1995

——, PETERSON WL: Bleeding peptic ulcer. N Engl J Med 331:717, 1994

LAU JYW et al: Effect of intravenous omeprazole on recurrent bleeding after endoscopic treatment of bleeding peptic ulcers. N Engl J Med 343:310, 2000

ROCKALL TA et al: Incidence of and mortality from acute upper gastrointestinal haemorrhage in the United Kingdom. BMJ 311:222, 1995

38 JAUNDICE
Daniel S. Pratt, Marshall M. Kaplan

Jaundice, or icterus, is a yellowish discoloration of tissue resulting from the deposition of bilirubin. Tissue deposition of bilirubin occurs only in the presence of serum hyperbilirubinemia and is a sign of either liver disease or, less often, a hemolytic disorder. The degree of serum bilirubin elevation can be estimated by physical examination. Slight increases in serum bilirubin are best detected by examining the sclerae which have a particular affinity for bilirubin due to their high elastin content. The presence of scleral icterus indicates a serum bilirubin of at least 51 μmol/L (3.0 mg/dL). The ability to detect scleral icterus is made more difficult if the examining room has fluorescent lighting. If the examiner suspects scleral icterus, a second place to examine is underneath the tongue. As serum bilirubin levels rise, the skin will eventually become yellow in light-skinned patients and even green if the process is long-standing; the green color is produced by oxidation of bilirubin to biliverdin.

The differential diagnosis for yellowing of the skin is limited. In addition to jaundice, it includes carotenoderma, the use of the drug quinacrine, and excessive exposure to phenols. Carotenoderma is the yellow color imparted to the skin by the presence of carotene; it occurs in healthy individuals who ingest excessive amounts of vegetables and fruits that contain carotene, such as carrots, leafy vegetables, squash, peaches, and oranges. Unlike jaundice, where the yellow coloration of the skin is uniformly distributed over the body, in carotenoderma the pigment is concentrated on the palms, soles, forehead, and nasolabial folds. Carotenoderma can be distinguished from jaundice by the sparing of the sclerae. Quinacrine causes a yellow discoloration of the skin in 4 to 37% of patients treated with it. Unlike carotene, quinacrine can cause discoloration of the sclerae.

Another sensitive indicator of increased serum bilirubin is darkening of the urine, which is due to the renal excretion of conjugated bilirubin. Patients often describe their urine as tea or cola colored. Bilirubinuria indicates an elevation of the direct serum bilirubin fraction and therefore the presence of liver disease.

Increased serum bilirubin levels occur when an imbalance exists between bilirubin production and clearance. A logical evaluation of the patient who is jaundiced requires an understanding of bilirubin production and metabolism.

PRODUCTION AND METABOLISM OF BILIRUBIN (See also Chap. 284)   Bilirubin, a tetrapyrrole pigment, is a breakdown product of heme (ferroprotoporphyrin IX). About 70 to 80% of the 250 to 300 mg of bilirubin produced each day is derived from the breakdown of hemoglobin in senescent red blood cells. The remainder comes from prematurely destroyed erythroid cells in bone marrow and from the turnover of hemoproteins such as myoglobin and cytochromes found in tissues throughout the body.

The formation of bilirubin occurs in reticuloendothelial cells, primarily in the spleen and liver. The first reaction, catalyzed by the microsomal enzyme heme oxygenase, oxidatively cleaves the α bridge of the porphyrin group and opens the heme ring. The end products of this reaction are biliverdin, carbon monoxide, and iron. The second reaction, catalyzed by the cytosolic enzyme biliverdin reductase, reduces the central methylene bridge of biliverdin and converts it to bilirubin. Bilirubin formed in the reticuloendothelial cells is virtually insoluble in water. This is due to tight internal hydrogen bonding between the water-soluble moieties of bilirubin, proprionic acid carboxyl groups of one dipyrrolic half of the molecule with the imino and lactam groups of the opposite half. This configuration blocks solvent access to the polar residues of bilirubin and places the hydrophobic residues on the outside. To be transported in blood, bilirubin must be solubilized. This is accomplished by its reversible, noncovalent binding to albumin. Unconjugated bilirubin bound to albumin is transported to the liver, where it, but not the albumin, is taken up by hepatocytes via a process that at least partly involves carrier-mediated membrane transport. No specific bilirubin transporter has yet been identified (Chap. 284, Fig. 284-1).

After entering the hepatocyte, unconjugated bilirubin is bound to the cytosolic protein ligandin, or glutathione S-transferase B. Whereas ligandin was initially thought to be a transport protein, responsible for delivering unconjugated bilirubin from the plasma membrane to the endoplasmic reticulum, it now appears that its role may in fact be to reduce bilirubin efflux back into the plasma. Studies suggest that unconjugated bilirubin may well rapidly diffuse unaided through the aqueous cytosol between membranes. In the endoplasmic reticulum, bilirubin is solubilized by conjugation to glucuronic acid, a process that disrupts the internal hydrogen bonds and yields bilirubin monoglucuronide and diglucuronide. The conjugation of glucuronic acid to bilirubin is catalyzed by bilirubin uridine-diphosphate (UDP) glucuronosyltransferase. The now hydrophilic bilirubin conjugates diffuse from the endoplasmic reticulum to the canalicular membrane, where bilirubin monoglucuronide and diglucuronide are actively transported into canalicular bile by an energy-dependent mechanism involving the multiple drug resistance protein 2.

The conjugated bilirubin excreted into bile drains into the duodenum and passes unchanged through the proximal small bowel. Conjugated bilirubin is not taken up by the intestinal mucosa. When the conjugated bilirubin reaches the distal ileum and colon, it is hydrolyzed to unconjugated bilirubin by bacterial β-glucuronidases. The unconjugated bilirubin is reduced by normal gut bacteria to form a group of colorless tetrapyrroles called urobilinogens. About 80 to 90% of these products are excreted in feces, either unchanged or oxidized to orange derivatives called urobilins. The remaining 10 to 20% of the urobilinogens are passively absorbed, enter the portal venous blood, and are reexcreted by the liver. A small fraction (usually <3 mg/dL) escapes hepatic uptake, filters across the renal glomerulus, and is excreted in urine.

MEASUREMENT OF SERUM BILIRUBIN The terms direct- and indirect-reacting bilirubin are based on the original van den Bergh reaction. This assay, or a variation of it, is still used in most clinical chemistry laboratories to determine the serum bilirubin level. In this assay, bilirubin is exposed to diazotized sulfanilic acid, splitting into two relatively stable dipyrrylmethene azopigments that absorb maximally at 540 nm, allowing for photometric analysis. The direct fraction is that which reacts with diazotized sulfanilic acid in the absence of an accelerator substance such as alcohol. The direct fraction provides an approximate determination of the conjugated bilirubin in serum. The total serum bilirubin is the amount that reacts after the addition of alcohol. The indirect fraction is the difference between the total and the direct

bilirubin and provides an estimate of the unconjugated bilirubin in serum.

With the van den Bergh method, the normal serum bilirubin concentration usually is 17 μmol/L (<1 mg/dL). Up to 30%, or 5.1 μmol/L (0.3 mg/dL), of the total may be direct-reacting (conjugated) bilirubin. Total serum bilirubin concentrations are between 3.4 and 15.4 μmol/L (0.2 and 0.9 mg/dL) in 95% of a normal population.

Several new techniques, although less convenient to perform, have added considerably to our understanding of bilirubin metabolism. First, they demonstrate that in normal persons or those with Gilbert's syndrome, almost 100% of the serum bilirubin is unconjugated; <3% is monoconjugated bilirubin. Second, in jaundiced patients with hepatobiliary disease, the total serum bilirubin concentration measured by these new, more accurate methods is lower than the values found with diazo methods. This suggests that there are diazo-positive compounds distinct from bilirubin in the serum of patients with hepatobiliary disease. Third, these studies indicate that in jaundiced patients with hepatobiliary disease, monoglucuronides of bilirubin predominate over the diglucuronides. Fourth, part of the direct-reacting bilirubin fraction includes conjugated bilirubin that is covalently linked to albumin. This albumin-linked bilirubin fraction (*delta fraction* or *biliprotein*) represents an important fraction of total serum bilirubin in patients with cholestasis and hepatobiliary disorders. Albumin-bound conjugated bilirubin is formed in serum when hepatic excretion of bilirubin glucuronides is impaired and the glucuronides are present in serum in increasing amounts. By virtue of its tight binding to albumin, the clearance rate of albumin-bound bilirubin from serum approximates the half-life of albumin, 12 to 14 days, rather than the short half-life of bilirubin, about 4 h.

The prolonged half-life of albumin-bound conjugated bilirubin explains two previously unexplained enigmas in jaundiced patients with liver disease: (1) that some patients with conjugated hyperbilirubinemia do not exhibit bilirubinuria during the recovery phase of their disease because the bilirubin is bound to albumin and therefore not filtered by the renal glomeruli and (2) that the elevated serum bilirubin level declines more slowly than expected in some patients who otherwise appear to be recovering satisfactorily. Late in the recovery phase of hepatobiliary disorders, all the conjugated bilirubin may be in the albumin-linked form. Its value in serum falls slowly because of the long half-life of albumin.

MEASUREMENT OF URINE BILIRUBIN Unconjugated bilirubin is always bound to albumin in the serum, is not filtered by the kidney, and is not found in the urine. Conjugated bilirubin is filtered at the glomerulus and the majority is reabsorbed by the proximal tubules; a small fraction is excreted in the urine. Any bilirubin found in the urine is conjugated bilirubin. The presence of bilirubinuria implies the presence of liver disease. A urine dipstick test (Ictotest) gives the same information as fractionation of the serum bilirubin. This test is very accurate. A false-negative test is possible in patients with prolonged cholestasis due to the predominance of conjugated bilirubin covalently bound to albumin.

APPROACH TO THE PATIENT

The bilirubin present in serum represents a balance between input from production of bilirubin and hepatic/biliary removal of the pigment. Hyperbilirubinemia may result from (1) overproduction of bilirubin; (2) impaired uptake, conjugation, or excretion of bilirubin; or (3) regurgitation of unconjugated or conjugated bilirubin from damaged hepatocytes or bile ducts. An increase in unconjugated bilirubin in serum results from either overproduction, impairment of uptake, or conjugation of bilirubin. An increase in conjugated bilirubin is due to decreased excretion into the bile ductules or backward leakage of the pigment. The initial steps in evaluating the patient with jaundice are to determine (1) whether the hyperbilirubinemia is predominantly conjugated or unconjugated in na-

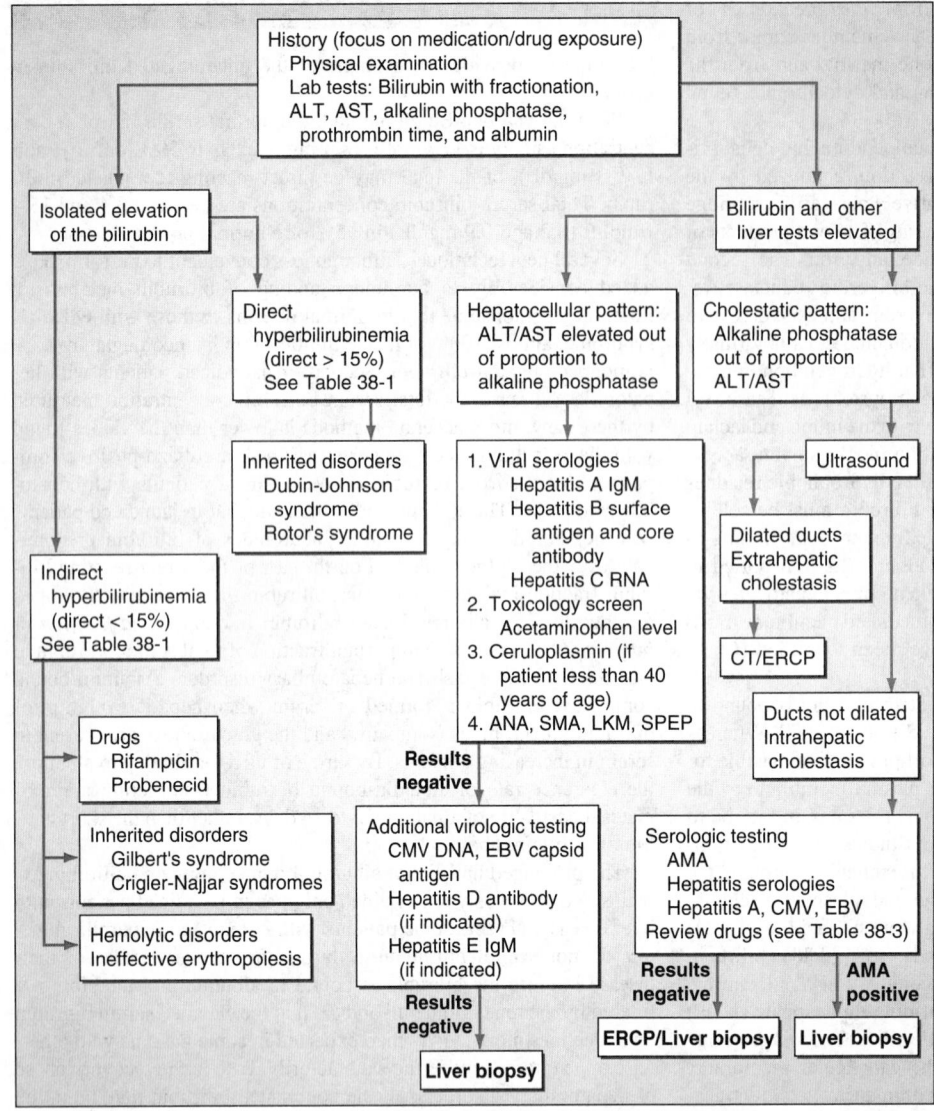

FIGURE 38-1 Evaluation of the patient with jaundice. ERCP, endoscopic retrograde cholangiopancreatography; CT, computed tomography; ALT, alanine aminotransferase; AST, aspartate aminotransferase; SMA, smooth-muscle antibody; AMA, antimitochondrial antibody; LKM, liver-kidney microsomal antibody; SPEP, serum protein electrophoresis; CMV, cytomegalovirus; EBV, Epstein-Barr virus.

ture, and (2) whether other biochemical liver tests are abnormal. The thoughtful interpretation of limited data will allow for a rational evaluation of the patient (Fig. 38-1). This discussion will focus solely on the evaluation of the adult patient with jaundice.

Isolated Elevation of Serum Bilirubin ■ *UNCONJUGATED HYPERBILIRUBINEMIA*

The differential diagnosis of an isolated unconjugated hyperbilirubinemia is limited (Table 38-1). The critical determination is whether the patient is suffering from a hemolytic process resulting in an overproduction of bilirubin (hemolytic disorders and ineffective erythropoiesis) or from impaired hepatic uptake/conjugation of bilirubin (drug effect or genetic disorders).

Hemolytic disorders that cause excessive heme production may be either inherited or acquired. Inherited disorders include spherocytosis, sickle cell anemia, and deficiency of red cell enzymes such as pyruvate kinase and glucose-6-phosphate dehydrogenase. In these conditions, the serum bilirubin rarely exceeds 86 μmol/L (5 mg/dL). Higher levels may occur when there is coexistent renal or hepatocellular dysfunction, or in acute hemolysis such as a sickle cell crisis. In evaluating jaundice in patients with chronic hemolysis, it is important to remember the high incidence of pigmented (calcium bilirubinate) gallstones found in these patients, which increases the likelihood of choledocholithiasis as an alternative explanation for hyperbilirubinemia.

Acquired hemolytic disorders include microangiopathic hemolytic anemia (e.g., hemolytic-uremic syndrome), paroxysmal nocturnal hemoglobinuria, and immune hemolysis. Ineffective erythropoiesis occurs in cobalamin, folate, and iron deficiencies.

In the absence of hemolysis, the physician should consider a problem with the hepatic uptake or conjugation of bilirubin. Certain drugs, including rifampicin and probenecid, may cause unconjugated hyperbilirubinemia by diminishing hepatic uptake of bilirubin. Impaired bilirubin conjugation occurs in three genetic conditions: Crigler-Najjar syndrome, types I and II, and Gilbert's syndrome. *Crigler-Najjar type I* is an exceptionally rare condition found in neonates and characterized by severe jaundice [bilirubin >342 μmol/L (> 20 mg/dL)] and neurologic impairment due to kernicterus, frequently leading to death in infancy or childhood. These patients have a complete absence of bilirubin UDP glucuronosyltransferase activity, usually due to mutations in the critical 3′ domain of the UDP glucuronosyltransferase gene, and are totally unable to conjugate, hence cannot excrete bilirubin. The only effective treatment is orthotopic liver transplantation. Use of gene therapy and allogeneic hepatocyte infusion are experimental approaches of future promise for this devastating disease.

Crigler-Najjar type II is somewhat more common than type I. Patients live into adulthood with serum bilirubin levels that range from 103 to 428 μmol/L (6 to 25 mg/dL). In these patients, mutations in the bili-

TABLE 38-1 *Causes of Isolated Hyperbilirubinemia*

I. Indirect hyperbilirubinemia
  A. Hemolytic disorders
    1. Inherited
      a. Spherocytosis, elliptocytosis
         Glucose-6-phosphate dehydrogenase and pyruvate kinase deficiencies
      b. Sickle cell anemia
    2. Acquired
      a. Microangiopathic hemolytic anemias
      b. Paroxysmal nocturnal hemoglobinuria
      c. Immune hemolysis
  B. Ineffective erythropoiesis
    1. Cobalamin, folate, thalassemia, and severe iron deficiencies
  C. Drugs
    1. Rifampicin, probenecid, ribavirin
  D. Inherited conditions
    1. Crigler-Najjar types I and II
    2. Gilbert's syndrome
II. Direct hyperbilirubinemia
  A. Inherited conditions
    1. Dubin-Johnson syndrome
    2. Rotor's syndrome

rubin UDP glucuronosyltransferase gene cause reduced but not completely absent activity of the enzyme. Bilirubin UDP glucuronosyltransferase activity can be induced by the administration of phenobarbital, which can reduce serum bilirubin levels in these patients. Despite marked jaundice, these patients usually survive into adulthood, although they may be susceptible to kernicterus under the stress of intercurrent illness or surgery.

Gilbert's syndrome is also marked by the impaired conjugation of bilirubin due to reduced bilirubin UDP glucuronosyltransferase activity. Patients with Gilbert's syndrome have a mild unconjugated hyperbilirubinemia with serum levels almost always <103 μmol/L (6 mg/dL). The serum levels may fluctuate, and jaundice is often identified only during periods of fasting. One molecular defect that has been identified in patients with Gilbert's syndrome is in the TATAA element in the 5' promoter region of the bilirubin UDP glucuronosyltransferase gene upstream of exon 1. This defect alone is not necessarily sufficient for producing the clinical syndrome of Gilbert's as there are patients who are homozygous for this defect yet do not have the levels of hyperbilirubinemia typically seen in Gilbert's syndrome. Unlike both Crigler-Najjar syndromes, Gilbert's syndrome is very common. The reported incidence is 3 to 7% of the population with males predominating over females by a ratio of 2–7:1.

CONJUGATED HYPERBILIRUBINEMIA Elevated conjugated hyperbilirubinemia is found in two rare inherited conditions: *Dubin-Johnson syndrome* and *Rotor's syndrome* (Table 38-1). Patients with both conditions present with asymptomatic jaundice, typically in the second generation of life. The defect in Dubin-Johnson syndrome is mutations in the gene for multiple drug resistance protein 2. These patients have altered excretion of bilirubin into the bile ducts. Rotor's syndrome seems to be a problem with the hepatic storage of bilirubin. Differentiating between these syndromes is possible, but clinically unnecessary, due to their benign nature.

Elevation of Serum Bilirubin with Other Liver Test Abnormalities The remainder of this chapter will focus on the evaluation of the patient with a conjugated hyperbilirubinemia in the setting of other liver test abnormalities. This group of patients can be divided into those with a primary hepatocellular process and those with intra- or extrahepatic cholestasis. Being able to make this differentiation will guide the physician's evaluation (Fig. 38-1). This differentiation is made on the basis of the history and physical examination as well as the pattern of liver test abnormalities.

HISTORY A complete medical history is perhaps the single most important part of the evaluation of the patient with unexplained jaundice. Important considerations include the use of or exposure to any chemical or medication, either physician-prescribed or over-the-counter, such as herbal and vitamin preparations and other drugs such as anabolic steroids. The patient should be carefully questioned about possible parenteral exposures, including transfusions, intravenous and intranasal drug use, tattoos, and sexual activity. Other important questions include recent travel history, exposure to people with jaundice, exposure to possibly contaminated foods, occupational exposure to hepatotoxins, alcohol consumption, the duration of jaundice, and the presence of any accompanying symptoms such as arthralgias, myalgias, rash, anorexia, weight loss, abdominal pain, fever, pruritus, and changes in the urine and stool. While none of these latter symptoms are specific for any one condition, they can suggest a particular diagnosis. A history of arthralgias and myalgias predating jaundice suggests hepatitis, either viral or drug-related. Jaundice associated with the sudden onset of severe right upper quadrant pain and shaking chills suggests choledocholithiasis and ascending cholangitis.

PHYSICAL EXAMINATION The general assessment should include assessment of the patient's nutritional status. Temporal and proximal muscle wasting suggests long-standing diseases such as pancreatic cancer or cirrhosis. Stigmata of chronic liver disease, including

spider nevi, palmar erythema, gynecomastia, caput medusae, Dupuytren's contractures, parotid gland enlargement, and testicular atrophy are commonly seen in advanced alcoholic (Laennec's) cirrhosis and occasionally in other types of cirrhosis. An enlarged left supraclavicular node (Virchow's node) or periumbilical nodule (Sister Mary Joseph's nodule) suggests an abdominal malignancy. Jugular venous distention, a sign of right-sided heart failure, suggests hepatic congestion. Right pleural effusion, in the absence of clinically apparent ascites, may be seen in advanced cirrhosis.

The abdominal examination should focus on the size and consistency of the liver, whether the spleen is palpable and hence enlarged, and whether there is ascites present. Patients with cirrhosis may have an enlarged left lobe of the liver which is felt below the xiphoid and an enlarged spleen. A grossly enlarged nodular liver or an obvious abdominal mass suggests malignancy. An enlarged tender liver could be viral or alcoholic hepatitis or, less often, an acutely congested liver secondary to right-sided heart failure. Severe right upper quadrant tenderness with respiratory arrest on inspiration (Murphy's sign) suggests cholecystitis or, occasionally, ascending cholangitis. Ascites in the presence of jaundice suggests either cirrhosis or malignancy with peritoneal spread.

LABORATORY TESTS When the physician encounters a patient with unexplained jaundice, there are a battery of tests that are helpful in the initial evaluation. These include total and direct serum bilirubin with fractionation, aminotransferases, alkaline phosphatase, albumin, and prothrombin time tests. Enzyme tests [alanine aminotransferase (ALT), aspartate aminotransferase (AST), and alkaline phosphatase] are helpful in differentiating between a hepatocellular process and a cholestatic process (Table 283-1; Fig. 38-1), a critical step in determining what additional workup is indicated. Patients with a hepatocellular process generally have a disproportionate rise in the aminotransferases compared to the alkaline phosphatase. Patients with a cholestatic process have a disproportionate rise in the alkaline phosphatase compared to the aminotransferases. The bilirubin can be prominently elevated in both hepatocellular and cholestatic conditions and therefore is not necessarily helpful in differentiating between the two.

In addition to the enzyme tests, all jaundiced patients should have additional blood tests, specifically an albumin level and a prothrombin time, to assess liver function. A low albumin suggests a chronic process such as cirrhosis or cancer. A normal albumin is suggestive of a more acute process such as viral hepatitis or choledocholithiasis. An elevated prothrombin time indicates either vitamin K deficiency due to prolonged jaundice and malabsorption of vitamin K or significant hepatocellular dysfunction. The failure of the prothrombin time to correct with parenteral administration of vitamin K indicates severe hepatocellular injury.

The results of the bilirubin, enzyme, albumin, and prothrombin time tests will usually indicate whether a jaundiced patient has a hepatocellular or a cholestatic disease. The causes and evaluation of each of these are quite different.

HEPATOCELLULAR CONDITIONS Hepatocellular diseases that can cause jaundice include viral hepatitis, drug or environmental toxicity, alcohol, and end-stage cirrhosis from any cause (Table 38-2). Wilson's disease should be considered in young adults. Autoimmune hepatitis is typically seen in young to middle-aged women but may affect men and women of any age. Alcoholic hepatitis can be differentiated from viral and toxin-related hepatitis by the pattern of the aminotransferases. Patients with alcoholic hepatitis typically have an AST:ALT ratio of at least 2:1. The AST rarely exceeds 300 U/L. Patients with acute viral hepatitis and toxin-related injury severe enough to produce jaundice typically have aminotransferases greater than 500 U/L, with the ALT greater than or equal to the AST. The degree of aminotransferase elevation can occasionally help in differentiating between hepatocellular and cholestatic

TABLE 38-2   *Hepatocellular Conditions That May Produce Jaundice*

Viral hepatitis
  Hepatitis A, B, C, D, and E
  Epstein-Barr virus
  Cytomegalovirus
  Herpes simplex
Alcohol
Drug toxicity
  Predictable, dose-dependent, e.g., acetaminophen
  Unpredictable, idiosyncratic, e.g., isoniazid
Environmental toxins
  Vinyl chloride
  Jamaica bush tea—pyrrolizidine alkaloids
  Kava Kava
  Wild mushrooms—*Amanita phalloides* or *A. verna*
Wilson's disease
Autoimmune hepatitis

processes. While ALT and AST values less than 8 times normal may be seen in either hepatocellular or cholestatic liver disease, values 25 times normal or higher are seen primarily in acute hepatocellular diseases. Patients with jaundice from cirrhosis can have normal or only slight elevations of the aminotransferases.

When the physician determines that the patient has a hepatocellular disease, appropriate testing for acute viral hepatitis includes a hepatitis A IgM antibody, a hepatitis B surface antigen and core IgM antibody, and a hepatitis C viral RNA test. It can take many weeks for the hepatitis C antibody to become detectable, making it an unreliable test if acute hepatitis C is suspected. Depending on circumstances, studies for hepatitis D, E, Epstein-Barr virus (EBV), and cytomegalovirus (CMV) may be indicated. Ceruloplasmin is the initial screening test for Wilson's disease. Testing for autoimmune hepatitis usually includes an antinuclear antibody and measurement of specific immunoglobulins.

Drug-induced hepatocellular injury can be classified either as predictable or unpredictable. Predictable drug reactions are dose-dependent and affect all patients who ingest a toxic dose of the drug in question. The classic example is acetaminophen hepatotoxicity. Unpredictable or idiosyncratic drug reactions are not dose-dependent and occur in a minority of patients. A great number of drugs can cause idiosyncratic hepatic injury. Environmental toxins are also an important cause of hepatocellular injury. Examples include industrial chemicals such as vinyl chloride, herbal preparations containing pyrrolizidine alkaloids (Jamaica bush tea) and Kava Kava, and the mushrooms *Amanita phalloides* or *A. verna* that contain highly hepatotoxic amatoxins.

CHOLESTATIC CONDITIONS   When the pattern of the liver tests suggests a cholestatic disorder, the next step is to determine whether it is intra- or extrahepatic cholestasis (Fig. 38-1). Distinguishing intrahepatic from extrahepatic cholestasis may be difficult. History, physical examination, and laboratory tests are often not helpful. The next appropriate test is an ultrasound. The ultrasound is inexpensive, does not expose the patient to ionizing radiation, and can detect dilation of the intra- and extrahepatic biliary tree with a high degree of sensitivity and specificity. The absence of biliary dilatation suggests intrahepatic cholestasis, while the presence of biliary dilatation indicates extrahepatic cholestasis. False-negative results occur in patients with partial obstruction of the common bile duct or in patients with cirrhosis or primary sclerosing cholangitis (PSC) where scarring prevents the intrahepatic ducts from dilating.

Although ultrasonography may indicate extrahepatic cholestasis, it rarely identifies the site or cause of obstruction. The distal common bile duct is a particularly difficult area to visualize by ultrasound because of overlying bowel gas. Appropriate next tests include computed tomography (CT) and endoscopic retrograde

cholangiopancreatography (ERCP). CT scanning is better than ultrasonography for assessing the head of the pancreas and for identifying choledocholithiasis in the distal common bile duct, particularly when the ducts are not dilated. ERCP is the "gold standard" for identifying choledocholithiasis. It is performed by introducing a side-viewing endoscope perorally into the duodenum. The ampulla of Vater is visualized and a catheter is advanced through the ampulla. Injection of dye allows for the visualization of the common bile duct and the pancreatic duct. The success rate for cannulation of the common bile duct ranges from 80 to 95%, depending on the operator's experience. Beyond its diagnostic capabilities, ERCP allows for therapeutic interventions, including the removal of common bile duct stones and the placement of stents. In patients in whom ERCP is unsuccessful, transhepatic cholangiography can provide the same information. Magnetic resonance cholangiopancreatography is a rapidly developing, noninvasive technique for imaging the bile and pancreatic ducts; this may replace ERCP as the initial diagnostic test in cases where the need for intervention is felt to be small.

In patients with apparent *intrahepatic cholestasis*, the diagnosis is often made by serologic testing in combination with percutaneous liver biopsy. The list of possible causes of intrahepatic cholestasis is long and varied (Table 38-3). A number of conditions that typically cause a hepatocellular pattern of injury can also present as a cholestatic variant. Both hepatitis B and C can cause a cholestatic hepatitis (fibrosing cholestatic hepatitis) that has histologic features that mimic large duct obstruction. This disease variant has been reported in patients who have undergone solid organ transplantation. Hepatitis A, alcoholic hepatitis, EBV, and CMV may also present as cholestatic liver disease.

Drugs may cause intrahepatic cholestasis, a variant of drug-induced hepatitis. Drug-induced cholestasis is usually reversible after eliminating the offending drug, although it may take many

TABLE 38-3   *Cholestatic Conditions That May Produce Jaundice*

I. Intrahepatic
  A. Viral hepatitis
    1. Fibrosing cholestatic hepatitis—hepatitis B and C
    2. Hepatitis A, Epstein-Barr virus, cytomegalovirus
  B. Alcoholic hepatitis
  C. Drug toxicity
    1. Pure cholestasis—anabolic and contraceptive steroids
    2. Cholestatic hepatitis—chlorpromazine, erythromycin estolate
    3. Chronic cholestasis—chlorpromazine and prochlorperazine
  D. Primary biliary cirrhosis
  E. Primary sclerosing cholangitis
  F. Vanishing bile duct syndrome
    1. Chronic rejection of liver transplants
    2. Sarcoidosis
    3. Drugs
  G. Inherited
    1. Benign recurrent cholestasis
  H. Cholestasis of pregnancy
  I. Total parenteral nutrition
  J. Nonhepatobiliary sepsis
  K. Benign postoperative cholestasis
  L. Paraneoplastic syndrome
  M. Venoocclusive disease
  N. Graft-versus-host disease
II. Extrahepatic
  A. Malignant
    1. Cholangiocarcinoma
    2. Pancreatic cancer
    3. Gallbladder cancer
    4. Ampullary cancer
    5. Malignant involvement of the porta hepatis lymph nodes
  B. Benign
    1. Choledocholithiasis
    2. Primary sclerosing cholangitis
    3. Chronic pancreatitis
    4. AIDS cholangiopathy

months for cholestasis to resolve. Drugs most commonly associated with cholestasis are the anabolic and contraceptive steroids. Cholestatic hepatitis has been reported with chlorpromazine, imipramine, tolbutamide, sulindac, cimetidine, and erythromycin estolate. It also occurs in patients taking trimethoprim, sulfamethoxazole, and penicillin-based antibiotics such as ampicillin, dicloxacillin, and clavulinic acid. Rarely, cholestasis may be chronic and associated with progressive fibrosis despite early discontinuation of the drug. Chronic cholestasis has been associated with chlorpromazine and prochlorperazine.

Primary biliary cirrhosis is a disease predominantly of middle-aged women in which there is a progressive destruction of interlobular bile ducts. The diagnosis is made by the presence of the antimitochondrial antibody that is found in 95% of patients. *Primary sclerosing cholangitis* is characterized by the destruction and fibrosis of larger bile ducts. The disease may involve only the intrahepatic ducts and present as intrahepatic cholestasis. However, in 95% of patients with PSC, both intra- and extrahepatic ducts are involved. The diagnosis of PSC is made by ERCP. The pathognomonic findings are multiple strictures of bile ducts with dilatations proximal to the strictures. Approximately 75% of patients with PSC have inflammatory bowel disease.

The *vanishing bile duct syndrome* and *adult bile ductopenia* are rare conditions in which there are a decreased number of bile ducts seen in liver biopsy specimens. The histologic picture is similar to that found in primary biliary cirrhosis. This picture is seen in patients who develop chronic rejection after liver transplantation and in those who develop graft-versus-host disease after bone marrow transplantation. Vanishing bile duct syndrome also occurs in rare cases of sarcoidosis, in patients taking certain drugs including chlorpromazine, and idiopathically. There are also familial forms of intrahepatic cholestasis, including the *familial intrahepatic cholestatic syndromes, I–III*. Benign recurrent cholestasis is an autosomal recessive disease that appears to be due to mutations in a P type ATPase, which probably acts as a bile acid transporter. The disease is marked by recurrent episodes of jaundice and pruritus; the episodes are self-limited but can be debilitating. *Cholestasis of pregnancy* occurs in the second and third trimesters and resolves after delivery. Its cause is unknown, but the condition is probably inherited and cholestasis can be triggered by estrogen administration.

Other causes of intrahepatic cholestasis include total parenteral nutrition (TPN), nonhepatobiliary sepsis, benign postoperative cholestasis, and a paraneoplastic syndrome associated with a number of different malignancies, including Hodgkin's disease, medullary thyroid cancer, hypernephroma, renal sarcoma, T cell lymphoma, prostate cancer, and several gastrointestinal malignancies. In patients developing cholestasis in the intensive care unit, the major considerations should be sepsis, shock liver, and TPN jaundice. Jaundice occurring after bone marrow transplantation is most likely due to venoocclusive disease or graft-versus-host disease.

Causes of *extrahepatic cholestasis* can be split into malignant

and benign (Table 38-3). Malignant causes include pancreatic, gallbladder, ampullary, and cholangiocarcinoma. The latter is most commonly associated with PSC and is exceptionally difficult to diagnose because its appearance is often identical to PSC. Pancreatic and gallbladder tumors, as well as cholangiocarcinoma, are rarely resectable and have poor prognoses. Ampullary carcinoma has the highest surgical cure rate of all the tumors that present as painless jaundice. Hilar lymphadenopathy due to metastases from other cancers may cause obstruction of the extrahepatic biliary tree.

Choledocholithiasis is the most common cause of extrahepatic cholestasis. The clinical presentation can range from mild right upper quadrant discomfort with only minimal elevations of the enzyme tests to ascending cholangitis with jaundice, sepsis, and circulatory collapse. PSC may occur with clinically important strictures limited to the extrahepatic biliary tree. In cases where there is a dominant stricture, patients can be effectively managed with serial endoscopic dilatations. Chronic pancreatitis rarely causes strictures of the distal common bile duct, where it passes through the head of the pancreas. AIDS cholangiopathy is a condition, usually due to infection of the bile duct epithelium with CMV or cryptosporidia, which has a cholangiographic appearance similar to that of PSC. These patients usually present with greatly elevated serum alkaline phosphatase levels, mean of 800 IU/L, but the bilirubin is often near normal. These patients do not typically present with jaundice.

SUMMARY The goal of this chapter is not to provide an encyclopedic review of all of the conditions that can cause jaundice. Rather, it is intended to provide a framework that helps a physician to evaluate the patient with jaundice in a logical way (Fig. 38-1).

Simply stated, the initial step is to obtain appropriate blood tests to determine if the patient has an isolated elevation of serum bilirubin. If so, is the bilirubin elevation due to an increased unconjugated or conjugated fraction? If the hyperbilirubinemia is accompanied by other liver test abnormalities, is the disorder hepatocellular or cholestatic? If cholestatic, is it intra- or extrahepatic? All of these questions can be answered with a thoughtful history, physical examination, and interpretation of laboratory and radiologic tests and procedures.

FURTHER READING

BERG CL et al: Bilirubin metabolism and the pathophysiology of jaundice, in *Schiff's Diseases of the Liver*, 8th ed, ER Schiff et al (eds). Philadelphia, Lippincott Williams & Wilkins, 1999

Fox IJ et al: Treatment of the Crigler-Najjar syndrome type I with hepatocyte transplantation. N Engl J Med 338:1422, 1998

GLASOVA H, BEUERS U: Extrahepatic manifestations of cholestasis. J Gastroenterol Hepatol 9:938, 2002

PRATT DS, KAPLAN MM: Laboratory tests, in *Schiff's Diseases of the Liver*, 8th ed, ER Schiff et al (eds). Philadelphia, Lippincott Williams & Wilkins, 1999

TRAUNER M et al: Molecular pathogenesis of cholestasis. N Engl J Med 339:1217, 1998

39 ABDOMINAL SWELLING AND ASCITES
Robert M. Glickman

ABDOMINAL SWELLING

Abdominal swelling or distention is a common problem in clinical medicine and may be the initial manifestation of a systemic disease or of otherwise unsuspected abdominal disease. *Subjective* abdominal enlargement, often described as a sensation of fullness or bloating, is usually transient and is often related to a functional gastrointestinal disorder when it is not accompanied by objective physical findings of

increased abdominal girth or local swelling. *Obesity* and lumbar lordosis, which may be associated with prominence of the abdomen, may usually be distinguished from true increases in the volume of the peritoneal cavity by history and careful physical examination.

CLINICAL HISTORY Abdominal swelling may first be noticed by the patient because of a progressive increase in belt or clothing size, the appearance of abdominal or inguinal hernias, or the development of a localized swelling. Often, considerable abdominal enlargement has gone unnoticed for weeks or months, either because of coexistent obesity or because the ascites formation has been insidious, without pain or localizing symptoms. Progressive abdominal distention may be associated with a sensation of "pulling" or "stretching" of the flanks or groins and vague low back pain. Localized pain usually results from involvement of an abdominal organ (e.g., a passively congested liver, large spleen, or colonic tumor). Pain is uncommon in cirrhosis with ascites, and when it is present, pancreatitis, hepatocellular carcinoma, or peritonitis should be considered. Tense ascites or abdominal tumors may produce increased intraabdominal pressure, resulting in indigestion and heartburn due to gastroesophageal reflux or dyspnea, abdominal wall hernias (inguinal and umbilical) orthopnea, and tachypnea from elevation of the diaphragm. A coexistent pleural effusion, more commonly on the right, presumably due to leakage of ascitic fluid through lymphatic channels in the diaphragm, may also contribute to respiratory embarrassment. A large pleural effusion, obscuring most of the lung is known as a *hepatic hydrothorax*. The patient with diffuse abdominal swelling should be questioned about increased alcohol intake, a prior episode of jaundice or hematuria, or a change in bowel habits. Such historic information may provide the clues that will lead one to suspect an occult cirrhosis, a colonic tumor with peritoneal seeding, congestive heart failure, or nephrosis.

PHYSICAL EXAMINATION   A carefully executed general physical examination can yield valuable clues concerning the etiology of abdominal swelling. Thus palmar erythema and spider angiomas suggest an underlying cirrhosis, while supraclavicular adenopathy (Virchow's node) should raise the question of an underlying gastrointestinal malignancy.

Inspection of the abdomen is important. By noting the abdominal contour, one may be able to distinguish localized from generalized swelling. The tensely distended abdomen with tightly stretched skin, bulging flanks, and everted umbilicus is characteristic of ascites. A prominent abdominal venous pattern with the direction of flow away from the umbilicus is often a reflection of portal hypertension; venous collaterals with flow from the lower part of the abdomen toward the umbilicus suggest obstruction of the inferior vena cava; flow downward toward the umbilicus suggests superior vena cava obstruction. "Doming" of the abdomen with visible ridges from underlying intestinal loops is usually due to intestinal obstruction or distention. An epigastric mass, with evident peristalsis proceeding from left to right, usually indicates underlying pyloric obstruction. A liver with metastatic deposits may be visible as a nodular right upper quadrant mass moving with respiration.

Auscultation may reveal the high-pitched, rushing sounds of early intestinal obstruction or a succussion sound due to increased fluid and gas in a dilated hollow viscus. Careful auscultation over an enlarged liver occasionally reveals the harsh bruit of a vascular tumor, especially a hepatocellular carcinoma, or the leathery friction rub of a surface nodule. A venous hum at the umbilicus may signify portal hypertension and an increased collateral blood flow around the liver. A fluid wave and flank dullness that shifts with change in position of the patient are important signs that indicate the presence of peritoneal fluid. In obese patients, small amounts of fluid may be difficult to demonstrate; on occasion, the fluid may be detected by abdominal percussion with patients on their hands and knees. Small amounts of ascites often can only be detected by ultrasound examination of the abdomen, which can detect as little as 100 mL of fluid. Careful percussion should serve to distinguish generalized abdominal enlargement from localized swelling due to an enlarged uterus, ovarian cyst, or distended bladder. Percussion can also outline an abnormally small or large liver. Loss of normal liver dullness may result from massive hepatic necrosis; it also may be a clue to free gas in the peritoneal cavity, as from perforation of a hollow viscus.

Palpation is often difficult with massive ascites, and ballottement of overlying fluid may be the only method of palpating the liver or spleen. A slightly enlarged spleen in association with ascites may be the only evidence of an occult cirrhosis. When there is evidence of portal hypertension, a soft liver suggests that obstruction to portal flow is extrahepatic; a firm liver suggests cirrhosis as the likely cause of

the portal hypertension. A very hard or nodular liver is a clue that the liver is infiltrated with tumor, and when accompanied by ascites, it suggests that the latter is due to peritoneal seeding. The presence of a hard periumbilical nodule (Sister Mary Joseph's nodule) suggests metastatic disease from a pelvic or gastrointestinal primary tumor. A pulsatile liver and ascites may be found in tricuspid insufficiency.

An attempt should be made to determine whether a mass is solid or cystic, smooth or irregular, and whether it moves with respiration. The liver, spleen, and gallbladder should descend with respiration unless they are fixed by adhesions or extension of tumor beyond the organ. A fixed mass not descending with respiration may indicate that it is retroperitoneal. Tenderness, especially if localized, may indicate an inflammatory process such as an abscess; it also may be due to stretching of the visceral peritoneum or tumor necrosis. Rectal and pelvic examinations are mandatory; they may reveal otherwise undetected masses due to tumor or infection.

Radiographic and laboratory examinations are essential for confirming or extending the impressions gained on physical examination. Upright and recumbent films of the abdomen may demonstrate the dilated loops of intestine with fluid levels characteristic of intestinal obstruction or the diffuse abdominal haziness and loss of psoas margins suggestive of ascites. Ultrasonography is often of value in detecting ascites, determining the presence of a mass, or evaluating the size of the liver and spleen. Computed tomography (CT) scanning provides similar information. CT scanning is often necessary to visualize the retroperitoneum, pancreas, and lymph nodes. A plain film of the abdomen may reveal the distended colon of otherwise unsuspected ulcerative colitis and give valuable information as to the size of the liver and spleen. An irregular and elevated right side of the diaphragm may be a clue to a liver abscess or hepatocellular carcinoma. Studies of the gastrointestinal tract with barium or other contrast media are usually necessary in the search for a primary tumor.

ASCITES

The evaluation of a patient with ascites requires that the cause of the ascites be established. In most cases ascites appears as part of a well-recognized illness, that is, cirrhosis, congestive heart failure, nephrosis, or disseminated carcinomatosis. In these situations, the physician should determine that the development of ascites is indeed a consequence of the basic underlying disease and not due to the presence of a separate or related disease process. This distinction is necessary even when the cause of ascites seems obvious. For example, when the patient with compensated cirrhosis and minimal ascites develops progressive ascites that is increasingly difficult to control with sodium restriction or diuretics, the temptation is to attribute the worsening of the clinical picture to progressive liver disease. However, an occult hepatocellular carcinoma, portal vein thrombosis, spontaneous bacterial peritonitis, or even tuberculosis may be responsible for the decompensation. The disappointingly low success in diagnosing tuberculous peritonitis or hepatocullar carcinoma in the patient with cirrhosis and ascites reflects the too-low index of suspicion for the development of such superimposed conditions. Similarly, the patient with congestive heart failure may develop ascites from a disseminated carcinoma with peritoneal seeding.

Diagnostic paracentesis (50 to 100 mL) should be part of the routine evaluation of the patient with ascites. The fluid should be examined for its gross appearance; protein content, cell count, and differential cell count should be determined; and Gram's and acid-fast stains and culture should be performed. Cytologic and cell-block examination may disclose an otherwise unsuspected carcinoma. Table 39-1 presents some of the features of ascitic fluid typically found in various disease states. In some disorders, such as cirrhosis, the fluid has the characteristics of a transudate (<25 g protein per liter and a specific gravity of <1.016); in others, such as peritonitis, the features are those of an exudate. Rather than the total protein content of ascites, many authors prefer the use of a *serum-ascites albumin gradient* (SAG) to characterize ascites. The gradient correlates directly with portal pressure. A gradient >1.1 g/dL (high gradient) is characteristic

TABLE 39-1 *Characteristics of Ascitic Fluid in Various Disease States*

Condition	Gross Appearance	Protein, g/L	Serum-Ascites Albumin Gradient, g/dL	Cell Count		Other Tests
				Red Blood Cells, >10,000/μL	White Blood Cells, per μL	
Cirrhosis	Straw-colored or bile-stained	<25 (95%)	>1.1	1%	<250 (90%);[a] predominantly mesothelial	
Neoplasm	Straw-colored, hemorrhagic, mucinous, or chylous	>25 (75%)	<1.1	20%	>1000 (50%); variable cell types	Cytology, cell block, peritoneal biopsy
Tuberculous peritonitis	Clear, turbid, hemorrhagic, chylous	>25 (50%)	<1.1	7%	>1000 (70%); usually >70% lymphocytes	Peritoneal biopsy, stain and culture for acid-fast bacilli
Pyogenic peritonitis	Turbid or purulent	If purulent, >25	<1.1	Unusual	Predominantly polymorphonuclear leukocytes	Positive Gram's stain, culture
Congestive heart failure	Straw-colored	Variable, 15–53	>1.1	10%	<1000 (90%); usually mesothelial, mononuclear	
Nephrosis	Straw-colored or chylous	<25 (100%)	<1.1	Unusual	<250; mesothelial, mononuclear	If chylous, ether extraction, Sudan staining
Pancreatic ascites (pancreatitis, pseudocyst)	Turbid, hemorrhagic, or chylous	Variable, often >25	<1.1	Variable, may be blood-stained	Variable	Increased amylase in ascitic fluid and serum

[a] Because the conditions of examining fluid and selecting patients were not identical in each series, the percentage figures (in parentheses) should be taken as an indication of the order of magnitude rather than as the precise incidence of any abnormal finding.

of uncomplicated cirrhotic ascites and differentiates ascites due to portal hypertension from ascites not due to portal hypertension >95% of the time. A gradient <1.1 g/dL (low gradient) suggests that the ascites is not due to portal hypertension with >95% accuracy and mandates a search for other causes (Table 39-1). Although there is variability of the ascitic fluid in any given disease state, some features are sufficiently characteristic to suggest certain diagnostic possibilities. For example, blood-stained fluid with >25 g protein per liter is unusual in uncomplicated cirrhosis but is consistent with tuberculous peritonitis or neoplasm. Cloudy fluid with a predominance of polymorphonuclear cells and a positive Gram's stain are characteristic of bacterial peritonitis; if most cells are lymphocytes, tuberculosis should be suspected. The complete examination of each fluid is most important, for occasionally only one finding may be abnormal. For example, if the fluid is a typical transudate but contains >250 white blood cells per microliter, the finding should be recognized as atypical for cirrhosis and should warrant a search for tumor or infection. This is especially true in the evaluation of cirrhotic ascites where occult peritoneal infection may be present with only minor elevations in the white blood cell count of the peritoneal fluid (300 to 500 cells/μL). Since Gram's stain of the fluid may be negative in a high proportion of such cases, careful culture of the peritoneal fluid is mandatory. Bedside innoculation of blood culture flasks with ascitic fluid results in a dramatically increased incidence of positive cultures when bacterial infection is present (90 versus 40% positivity with conventional cultures done by the laboratory). Direct visualization of the peritoneum (laparoscopy) may disclose peritoneal deposits of tumor, tuberculosis, or metastatic disease of the liver. Biopsies are taken under direct vision, often adding to the diagnostic accuracy of the procedure.

Chylous ascites refers to a turbid, milky, or creamy peritoneal fluid due to the presence of thoracic or intestinal lymph. Such a fluid shows Sudan-staining fat globules microscopically and an increased triglyceride content by chemical examination. Opaque milky fluid usually has a triglyceride concentration of >11.3 μmol/L (>1000 mg/dL). A turbid fluid due to leukocytes or tumor cells may be confused with chylous fluid (pseudochylous), and it is often helpful to carry out alkalinization and ether extraction of the specimen. Alkali tend to dissolve cellular proteins and thereby reduce turbidity; ether extraction leads to clearing if the turbidity of the fluid is due to lipid. Chylous ascites is most often the result of lymphatic obstruction from trauma, tumor, tuberculosis, filariasis (Chap. 202), or congenital abnormalities. It may also be seen in the nephrotic syndrome.

Rarely, ascitic fluid may be *mucinous* in character, suggesting either pseudomyxoma peritonei (Chap. 279) or rarely a colloid carcinoma of the stomach or colon with peritoneal implants.

On occasion, ascites may develop as a seemingly isolated finding in the absence of a clinically evident underlying disease. Then, a careful analysis of ascitic fluid may indicate the direction the evaluation should take. A useful framework for the workup starts with an analysis of whether the fluid is classified as a high (transudate) or low (exudate) gradient fluid. *High gradient (transudative) ascites* of unclear etiology is most often due to occult cirrhosis, right-sided venous hypertension raising hepatic sinusoidal pressure, or hypoalbuminemic states such as nephrosis or protein-losing enteropathy. Cirrhosis with well-preserved liver function (normal albumin) resulting in ascites is invariably associated with significant portal hypertension (Chap. 288). Evaluation should include liver function tests, liver-spleen scan, or other hepatic imaging procedure (i.e., CT or ultrasound) to detect nodular changes in the liver or a colloid shift of isotope to suggest portal hypertension. On occasion, a wedged hepatic venous pressure can be useful to document portal hypertension. Finally, if clinically indicated, a liver biopsy will confirm the diagnosis of cirrhosis and perhaps suggest its etiology. Other etiologies may result in hepatic venous congestion and resultant ascites. Right-sided cardiac valvular disease and particularly constrictive pericarditis should raise a high index of suspicion and may require cardiac imaging and cardiac catheterization for definitive diagnosis. Hepatic vein thrombosis is evaluated by visualizing the hepatic veins with imaging techniques (Doppler ultrasound, angiography, CT scans, magnetic resonance imaging) to demonstrate obliteration, thrombosis, or obstruction by tumor. Uncommonly, transudative ascites may be associated with benign tumors of the ovary, particularly fibroma (Meigs' syndrome) with ascites and hydrothorax.

Low gradient (exudative) ascites should initiate an evaluation for primary peritoneal processes, most importantly infection and tumor. Routine bacteriologic culture of ascitic fluid often yields a specific organism causing infectious peritonitis. Tuberculous peritonitis (Table 39-1) is best diagnosed by peritoneal biopsy, either percutaneously or via laparoscopy. Histologic examination invariably shows granulomata that may contain acid-fast bacilli. Since cultures of peritoneal fluid and biopsies for tuberculosis may require 6 weeks, characteristic histology with appropriate stains allows antituberculosis therapy to be started promptly. Similarly, the diagnosis of peritoneal seeding by tumor can usually be made by cytologic analysis of peritoneal fluid or by peritoneal biopsy if cytology is negative. Appropriate diagnostic studies can then be undertaken to determine the nature and site of the primary tumor. Pancreatic ascites (Table 39-1) is invariably associated with an extravasation of pancreatic fluid from the pancreatic ductal system, most commonly from a leaking pseudocyst. Ultrasound or CT examination of the pancreas followed by visualization of the pancreatic

duct by direct cannulation [viz., endoscopic retrograde cholangiopancreatography (ERCP)] usually discloses the site of leakage and permits resective surgery to be carried out.

An analysis of the physiologic and metabolic factors involved in the production of ascites (detailed in Chap. 288), coupled with a complete evaluation of the nature of the ascitic fluid, invariably discloses the etiology of the ascites and permits appropriate therapy to be instituted.

ACKNOWLEDGMENT
Dr. Kurt J. Isselbacher was the co-author of this chapter in previous editions.

FURTHER READING

LIPSKY MS, STERNBACH MR: Evaluation and initial management of patients with ascites. Am Fam Physician 54:1327, 1996

McHUTCHISON JG: Differential diagnosis of ascites. Semin Liver Dis 17:191, 1997

PARSONS SL et al: Malignant ascites. Br J Surg 83:6, 1996

PINTO PC et al: Large volume paracentesis in nonedematous patients with tense ascites: Its effect on intravascular volume. Hepatology 8:207, 1988

RUNYON BA: Management of adult patients with ascites caused by cirrhosis. Hepatology 27:264, 1998

———— et al: The serum-ascites albumin gradient in the differential diagnosis of ascites. Ann Intern Med 117:215, 1992

Section 7   Alterations in Renal and Urinary Tract Function

---

40 | AZOTEMIA AND URINARY ABNORMALITIES
Bradley M. Denker, Barry M. Brenner

Body homeostasis is maintained predominantly through the cellular processes that together comprise normal kidney function. Disturbances to any of these functions can lead to a constellation of abnormalities that may be detrimental to survival. The clinical manifestations of these diseases will depend upon the pathophysiology of the renal injury and will often be initially identified as a complex of symptoms, abnormal physical findings, and laboratory changes that will allow the identification of specific syndromes. These renal syndromes (summarized in Table 40-1) may arise as the consequence of a systemic illness or can occur as a primary renal disease. Nephrologic syndromes usually consist of several elements that reflect the underlying pathologic processes and the duration of the disease and typically include one or more of the following features: (1) disturbances in urine volume (oliguria, anuria, polyuria); (2) abnormalities of urine sediment [red blood cells (RBC); white blood cells, casts, and crystals]; (3) abnormal excretion of serum proteins (proteinuria); (4) reduction in glomerular filtration rate (GFR) (azotemia); (5) presence of hypertension and/or expanded total body volume (edema); (6) electrolyte abnormalities; or (7) in some syndromes, fever/pain. The combination of these findings should permit identification of one of the major nephrologic syndromes (Table 40-1) and will allow the differential diagnoses to be narrowed and the appropriate diagnostic evaluation and therapeutic course to be determined. Each of these syndromes and their associated diseases are discussed in more detail in subsequent chapters. This chapter will focus on several aspects of renal abnormalities that are critically important to distinguishing these processes: (1) reduction in GFR leading to azotemia, (2) alterations of the urinary sediment and/or protein excretion, and (3) abnormalities of urinary volume.

AZOTEMIA

ASSESSMENT OF GLOMERULAR FILTRATION RATE

Monitoring the GFR is important in both the hospital and outpatient settings, and several different methodologies are available (discussed below). In most acute clinical circumstances a measured GFR is not available, and it is necessary to estimate the GFR from the serum

creatinine level in order to provide appropriate doses of drugs that are excreted into the urine. Serum creatinine is the most widely used marker for GFR, and the GFR is related directly to the urine creatinine excretion and inversely to the serum creatinine (U_{Cr}/P_{Cr}). Based upon this relationship and some important caveats (discussed below), the GFR will fall proportionately with the increase in P_{Cr}. Failure to account for GFR reductions in drug dosing can lead to significant morbidity and mortality from drug toxicities (e.g., digoxin, aminoglycosides). In the outpatient setting, the serum creatinine is often used as a surrogate for GFR (although much less accurate; see below). In patients with chronic progressive renal failure there is an approximately linear relationship between $1/P_{Cr}$ and time. The slope of this line will remain constant for an individual patient, and when values are obtained that do not fall on this line, an investigation for a superimposed acute process (e.g., volume depletion, drug reaction) should be initiated. It should be emphasized that the signs and symptoms of uremia will develop at significantly different levels of serum creatinine depending upon the patient (size, age, and sex), the underlying renal disease, existence of concurrent diseases, and true GFR. In general, patients do not develop symptomatic uremia until renal insufficiency is usually quite severe (GFR < 15 mL/min).

A reduced GFR leads to retention of nitrogenous waste products (azotemia) such as serum urea nitrogen and creatinine. Azotemia may result from reduced renal perfusion, intrinsic renal disease, or postrenal processes (ureteral obstruction; see below and Fig. 40-1). Precise determination of GFR is problematic as both commonly used markers (urea and creatinine) have characteristics that affect their accuracy as markers of clearance. Urea clearance is generally an underestimate of GFR because of tubule urea reabsorption and may be as low as one-half of GFR measured by other techniques.

Creatinine is a small, freely filtered solute that varies little from day to day (since it is derived from muscle metabolism of creatine). However, serum creatinine can increase acutely from dietary ingestion of cooked meat. Creatinine can be secreted by the proximal tubule through an organic cation pathway. There are many clinical settings where a creatinine clearance is not available, and decisions concerning

Syndromes	Important Clues to Diagnosis	Findings That Are Common	Location of Discussion of Diseases-Causing Syndrome
Acute or rapidly progressive renal failure	Anuria Oliguria Documented recent decline in GFR	Hypertension, hematuria Proteinuria, pyuria Casts, edema	Chaps. 260, 264, 266, 270
Acute nephritis	Hematuria, RBC casts Azotemia, oliguria Edema, hypertension	Proteinuria Pyuria Circulatory congestion	Chap. 264
Chronic renal failure	Azotemia for >3 months Prolonged symptoms or signs of uremia Symptoms or signs of renal osteodystrophy Kidneys reduced in size bilaterally Broad casts in urinary sediment	Hematuria, proteinuria Casts, oliguria Polyuria, nocturia Edema, hypertension Electrolyte disorders	Chaps. 259, 261
Nephrotic syndrome	Proteinuria >3.5 g per 1.73 m² per 24 h Hypoalbuminemia Hyperlipidemia Lipiduria	Casts Edema	Chap. 264
Asymptomatic urinary abnormalities	Hematuria Proteinuria (below nephrotic range) Sterile pyuria, casts		Chap. 264
Urinary tract infection	Bacteriuria >10⁵ colonies per milliliter Other infectious agent documented in urine Pyuria, leukocyte casts Frequency, urgency Bladder tenderness, flank tenderness	Hematuria Mild azotemia Mild proteinuria Fever	Chap. 269
Renal tubule defects	Electrolyte disorders Polyuria, nocturia Symptoms or signs of renal osteodystrophy Large kidneys Renal transport defects	Hematuria "Tubular" proteinuria Enuresis	Chaps. 265, 266
Hypertension	Systolic/diastolic hypertension	Proteinuria Casts Azotemia	Chaps. 230, 267
Nephrolithiasis	Previous history of stone passage or removal Previous history of stone seen by x-ray Renal colic	Hematuria Pyuria Frequency, urgency	Chap. 268
Urinary tract obstruction	Azotemia, oliguria, anuria Polyuria, nocturia, urinary retention Slowing of urinary stream Large prostate, large kidneys Flank tenderness, full bladder after voiding	Hematuria Pyuria Enuresis, dysuria	Chap. 270

Note: GFR; glomerular filtration rate; RBC, red blood cell.

drug dosing must be made based on the serum creatinine. A formula that allows an estimate of creatinine clearance in men that accounts for age-related decreases in GFR, body weight, and sex has been derived by Cockcroft-Gault:

$$\text{Creatinine clearance (mL/min)} = \frac{(140 - \text{age}) \times \text{lean body weight (kg)}}{\text{plasma creatinine (mg/dL)} \times 72}$$

This value should be multiplied 0.85 for women, since a lower fraction of the body weight is composed of muscle. The gradual loss of muscle from chronic illness, chronic use of glucocorticoids, or malnutrition can mask significant changes in GFR with small or imperceptible changes in serum creatinine. More accurate determinations of GFR are available using inulin clearance or radionuclide-labeled markers such as ¹²⁵I-iothalamate or EDTA. These methods are highly accurate due to precise quantitation and the absence of any renal reabsorption/secretion and should be used to follow GFR in patients in whom creatinine is not likely to be a reliable indicator (patients with decreased muscle mass secondary to age, malnutrition, concurrent illnesses). (See also Table 261-2.)

APPROACH TO THE PATIENT

Once it has been established that GFR is reduced, the physician must decide if this represents acute or chronic renal failure. The clinical situation, history, and laboratory data often make this an easy distinction. However, the laboratory abnormalities characteristic of chronic renal failure, including anemia, hypocalcemia, and hyperphosphatemia, are often also present in patients presenting with acute renal failure. Radiographic evidence of renal osteodystrophy (Chap. 261) would be seen only in chronic renal failure but is a very late finding, and these patients are usually on dialysis. The urinalysis and renal ultrasound can occasionally facilitate distinguishing acute from chronic renal failure. An approach to the evaluation of azotemic patients is shown in Fig. 40-1. Patients with advanced chronic renal insufficiency often have some proteinuria, nonconcentrated urine (isosthenuria), and small kidneys on ultrasound characterized by increased echogenicity and cortical thinning. Treatment should be directed toward slowing the progression of renal disease and providing symptomatic relief for edema, acidosis, anemia, and hyperphosphatemia, as discussed in Chap. 261. Acute renal failure (Chap. 260) can result from processes affecting renal blood flow (prerenal azotemia), intrinsic renal diseases (affecting vessels, glomeruli, or tubules), or postrenal processes (obstruction to urine flow in ureters, bladder, or urethra) (Chap. 270).

PRERENAL FAILURE Decreased renal perfusion accounts for 40 to 80% of acute renal failure and, if appropriately treated, is readily reversible. The etiologies of prerenal azotemia include any cause of decreased circulating blood volume such as volume loss (gastrointestinal hemorrhage, burns, diarrhea, diuretics), volume sequestration (pancreatitis, peritonitis, rhabdomyolysis), or decreased effective circulating volume (cardiogenic shock, sepsis). Renal perfusion can also be affected by reductions in cardiac output from peripheral vasodilatation (sepsis, drugs) or profound renal vasoconstriction [severe heart failure, hepatorenal syndrome, drugs such as nonsteroidal anti-inflammatory drugs (NSAIDs)]. True, or "ef-

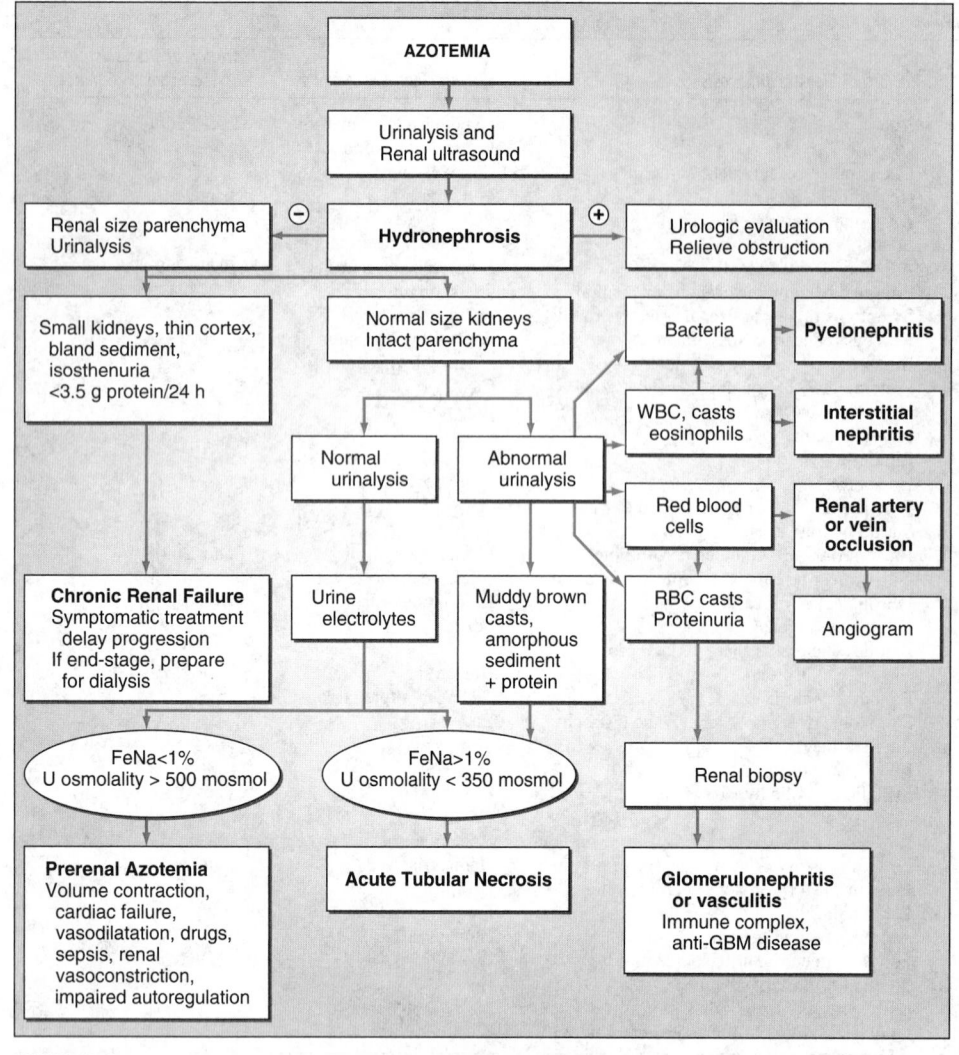

FIGURE 40-1 Approach to the patient with azotemia. WBC, white blood cell; RBC, red blood cell; GBM, glomerular basement membrane.

Figure content:

AZOTEMIA → Urinalysis and Renal ultrasound → Hydronephrosis

Hydronephrosis (−) → Renal size parenchyma Urinalysis

Hydronephrosis (+) → Urologic evaluation Relieve obstruction

→ Small kidneys, thin cortex, bland sediment, isosthenuria <3.5 g protein/24 h → Chronic Renal Failure: Symptomatic treatment delay progression If end-stage, prepare for dialysis

→ Normal size kidneys Intact parenchyma → Normal urinalysis / Abnormal urinalysis

Normal urinalysis → Urine electrolytes → FeNa<1% U osmolality > 500 mosmol → Prenatal Azotemia: Volume contraction, cardiac failure, vasodilatation, drugs, sepsis, renal vasoconstriction, impaired autoregulation

Abnormal urinalysis → Muddy brown casts, amorphous sediment + protein → FeNa>1% U osmolality < 350 mosmol → Acute Tubular Necrosis

Bacteria → Pyelonephritis
WBC, casts eosinophils → Interstitial nephritis
Red blood cells → Renal artery or vein occlusion → Angiogram
RBC casts Proteinuria → Renal biopsy → Glomerulonephritis or vasculitis: Immune complex, anti-GBM disease

fective," hypovolemia leads to a fall in mean arterial pressure, which in turn triggers a series of neural and humoral responses that include activation of the sympathetic nervous and renin-angiotensin-aldosterone systems and ADH release. GFR is maintained by prostaglandin-mediated relaxation of afferent arterioles and angiotensin II–mediated constriction of efferent arterioles. Once the mean arterial pressure falls below 80 mmHg, there is a steep decline in GFR.

Blockade of prostaglandin production by NSAIDs can result in severe vasoconstriction and acute renal failure under these circumstances. Angiotensin-converting enzyme (ACE) inhibitors decrease efferent arteriolar tone and can decrease glomerular capillary perfusion pressure. Patients on NSAIDs and/or ACE inhibitors are most susceptible to hemodynamically mediated acute renal failure when blood volume is reduced for any reason. Patients with renal artery stenosis are dependent upon efferent arteriolar vasoconstriction for maintenance of glomerular filtration pressure and are particularly susceptible to precipitous decline in GFR when given ACE inhibitors.

Prolonged renal hypoperfusion can lead to acute tubular necrosis (ATN; an intrinsic renal disease discussed below). The urinalysis and urinary electrolytes can be useful in distinguishing prerenal azotemia from ATN (Table 40-2). The urine of patients with prerenal azotemia can be predicted from the stimulatory actions of norepinephrine, angiotensin II, ADH, and low tubule fluid flow on salt and water reabsorption. In prerenal conditions the tubules are intact, leading to a concentrated urine (>500 mosm), avid Na re-

tention (urine Na concentration <20 mM/L; fractional excretion of Na <1%), and $U_{Cr}/P_{Cr} > 40$ (Table 40-2). The prerenal urine sediment is usually normal or has occasional hyaline and granular casts, while the sediment of ATN is usually filled with cellular debris and muddy brown granular casts.

INTRINSIC RENAL DISEASE When prerenal and postrenal azotemia have been excluded as etiologies of renal failure, an intrinsic parenchymal renal disease is present. Intrinsic renal disease can arise from processes involving large renal vessels, microvasculature and glomeruli, or tubulointerstitium. Ischemic and toxic ATN account for about 90% of acute intrinsic renal failure. As outlined in Fig. 40-1, the clinical setting and urinalysis are helpful in separating the possible etiologies of acute intrinsic renal failure. Prerenal azotemia and ATN are part of a spectrum of renal hypoperfusion; evidence of structural tubule injury is present in ATN, whereas prompt reversibility occurs with prerenal azotemia upon restoration of adequate renal perfusion. Thus, ATN can often be distinguished from prerenal azotemia by urinalysis and urine electrolyte composition (Table 40-2 and Fig. 40-1). Ischemic ATN is observed most frequently in patients who have undergone major surgery, trauma, severe hypovolemia, overwhelming sepsis, or extensive burns. Nephrotoxic ATN complicates the administration of many common medications, usually by inducing a combination of intrarenal vasoconstriction, direct tubule toxicity, and/or tubular obstruction. The kidney is vulnerable to toxic injury by virtue of its rich blood supply (25% of cardiac output) and its ability to concentrate and metabolize toxins. A diligent search for hypotension and nephrotoxins will usually uncover the specific etiology of ATN. Discontinuation of nephrotoxins and stabilizing blood pressure will often suffice without the need for dialysis while the tubules recover. *→An extensive list of potential drugs and toxins implicated in ATN can be found in Chap. 260.*

Processes that involve the tubules and interstitium can lead to acute renal failure. These include drug-induced interstitial nephritis

TABLE 40-2 *Laboratory Findings in Acute Renal Failure*

Index	Prerenal Azotemia	Oliguric Acute Renal Failure
BUN/P_{Cr} Ratio	>20:1	10–15:1
Urine sodium (U_{Na}), meq/L	<20	>40
Urine osmolality, mosmol/L H_2O	>500	<350
Fractional excretion of sodium $FE_{Na} = \dfrac{U_{Na} \times P_{Cr} \times 100}{P_{Na} \times U_{Cr}}$	<1%	>2%
Urine/plasma creatinine (U_{Cr}/P_{Cr})	>40	<20

Note: BUN, Blood urea nitrogen; P_{Cr}, plasma creatinine; U_{Na}, urine sodium concentration; P_{Na}, plasma sodium concentration; U_{Cr}, urine creatinine concentration.

(especially antibiotics, NSAIDs, and diuretics), severe infections (both bacterial and viral), systemic diseases (e.g., systemic lupus erythematosus), or infiltrative disorders (e.g., sarcoid, lymphoma, or leukemia). A list of drugs associated with allergic interstitial nephritis can be found in Chap. 266. The urinalysis usually shows mild to moderate proteinuria, hematuria, and pyuria (approximately 75% of cases) and occasionally white blood cell casts. The finding of RBC casts in interstitial nephritis has been reported but should prompt a search for glomerular diseases. Occasionally renal biopsy will be needed to distinguish among these possibilities. The finding of eosinophils in the urine is suggestive of allergic interstitial nephritis and is optimally observed by using a Hansel stain. The absence of eosinophiluria, however, does not exclude the possibility of acute interstitial nephritis.

Occlusion of large renal vessels including arteries and veins is an uncommon cause of acute renal failure. A significant reduction in GFR by this mechanism suggests bilateral processes or a unilateral process in a patient with a single functioning kidney. Renal arteries can be occluded with atheroemboli, thromboemboli, in situ thrombosis, aortic dissection, or vasculitis. Atheroembolic renal failure can occur spontaneously but is most often associated with recent aortic instrumentation. The emboli are cholesterol-rich and lodge in medium and small renal arteries, leading to an eosinophil-rich inflammatory reaction. Patients with atheroembolic acute renal failure often have a normal urinalysis, but the urine may contain eosinophils and casts. The diagnosis can be confirmed by renal biopsy, but this is often unnecessary when other stigmata of atheroemboli are present (livedo reticularis, distal peripheral infarcts, eosinophilia). Renal artery thrombosis may lead to mild proteinuria and hematuria, whereas renal vein thrombosis typically induces heavy proteinuria and hematuria. →*These vascular complications often require angiography for confirmation and are discussed in Chap. 267.*

Diseases of glomeruli (glomerulonephritis or vasculitis) and the renal microvasculature (hemolytic uremic syndromes, thrombotic thrombocytopenic purpura, or malignant hypertension) usually present with various combinations of glomerular injury: proteinuria, hematuria, reduced GFR, and alterations of Na excretion leading to hypertension, edema, and circulatory congestion (acute nephritic syndrome). These findings may occur as primary renal diseases or as renal manifestations of systemic diseases. The clinical setting and other laboratory data will help distinguish primary renal from systemic diseases. The finding of RBC casts in the urine is an indication for early renal biopsy (Fig. 40-1) as the pathologic pattern has important implications for diagnosis, prognosis, and treatment. Hematuria without RBC casts can also be an indication of glomerular disease, and this evaluation is summarized in Fig. 40-2. →*A detailed discussion of glomerulonephritis and diseases of the microvasculature can be found in Chap. 264.*

POSTRENAL AZOTEMIA Urinary tract obstruction accounts for fewer than 5% of cases of acute renal failure, but it is usually reversible and must be ruled out early in the evaluation (Fig. 40-1). Since a single kidney is capable of adequate clearance, acute renal failure from obstruction requires obstruction at the urethra or bladder outlet, bilateral ureteral obstruction, or unilateral obstruction in a patient with a single functioning kidney. Obstruction is usually diagnosed by the presence of ureteral dilatation on renal ultrasound. However, early in the course of obstruction or if the ureters are unable to dilate (such as encasement by pelvic tumors), the ultrasound examination may be negative. →*The specific urologic conditions that cause obstruction are discussed in Chap. 270.*

OLIGURIA AND ANURIA *Oliguria* refers to a 24-h urine output of <500 mL, and *anuria* is the complete absence of urine formation. Anuria can be caused by total urinary tract obstruction, total renal artery or vein occlusion, and shock (manifested by severe hypotension and intense renal vasoconstriction). Cortical necrosis, ATN, and rapidly progressive glomerulonephritis can occasionally cause

anuria. Oliguria can accompany any cause of acute renal failure and carries a more serious prognosis for renal recovery in all conditions except prerenal azotemia. *Nonoliguria* refers to urine output in excess of 500 mL/day in patients with acute or chronic azotemia. With nonoliguric ATN, disturbances of potassium and hydrogen balance are less severe than in oliguric patients and recovery to normal renal function is usually more rapid.

ABNORMALITIES OF THE URINE

PROTEINURIA

The evaluation of proteinuria is shown schematically in Fig. 40-3 and is typically initiated after colorimetric detection of proteinuria by dipstick examination. The dipstick measurement detects mostly albumin and gives false-positive results when pH > 7.0 and the urine is very concentrated or contaminated with blood. A very dilute urine may obscure significant proteinuria on dipstick examination, and proteinuria that is not predominantly albumin will be missed. This is particularly important for the detection of Bence Jones proteins in the urine of patients with multiple myeloma. Tests to measure total urine concentration accurately rely on precipitation with sulfosalicylic or trichloracetic acids. Currently, ultrasensitive dipsticks are available to measure microalbuminuria (30 to 300 mg/d), an early marker of glomerular disease that has been shown to predict glomerular injury in early diabetic nephropathy (Fig. 40-3).

The magnitude of proteinuria and the protein composition in the urine depend upon the mechanism of renal injury leading to protein losses. Both charge and size selectivity normally prevent virtually all

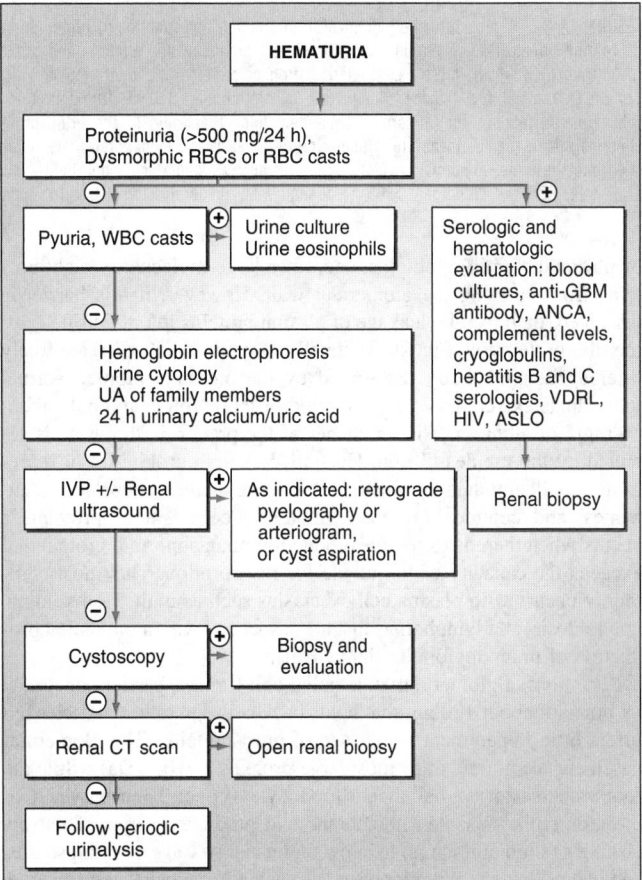

FIGURE 40-2 Approach to the patient with hematuria. RBC, red blood cell; WBC, white blood cell; GBM, glomerular basement membrane; ANCA, antineutrophil cytoplasmic antibody; VDRL, venereal disease research laboratory; ASLO, antistreptolysin O; UA, urinalysis; IVP, intravenous pyelography; CT, computed tomography.

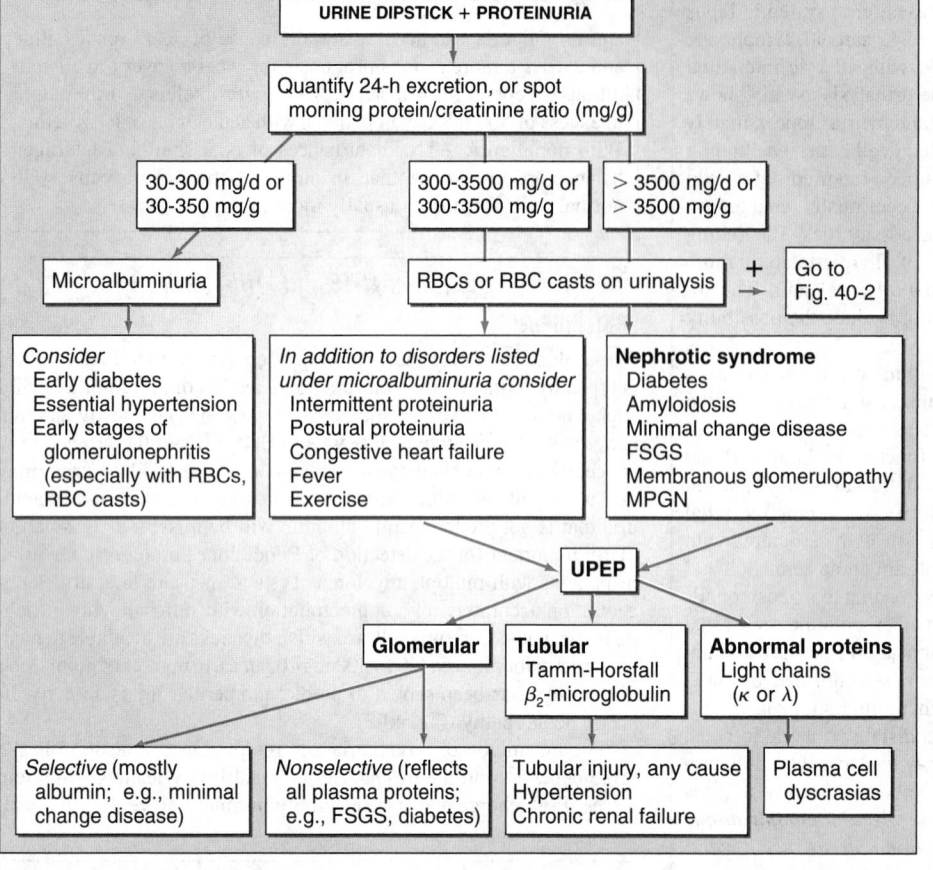

FIGURE 40-3 Approach to the patient with proteinuria. Investigation of proteinuria is often initiated by a positive dipstick on routine urinalysis. Conventional dipsticks detect predominantly albumin and cannot detect urinary albumin levels of 30 to 300 mg/d. However, more exact determination of proteinuria should employ a 24-h urine collection or a spot morning protein/creatinine ratio (mg/g). The pattern of proteinuria on UPEP (urine protein electrophoresis) can be classified as "glomerular," "tubular," or "abnormal" depending upon the origin of the urine proteins. Glomerular proteinuria is due to abnormal glomerular permeability. "Tubular proteins" such as Tamm-Horsfall are normally produced by the renal tubule and shed into the urine. Abnormal circulating proteins such as kappa or lambda light chains are readily filtered because of their small size. RBC, red blood cell; FSGS, focal segmental glomerulosclerosis; MPGN, membranoproliferative glomerulonephritis.

of plasma albumin, globulins, and other large-molecular-weight proteins from crossing the glomerular wall. However, if this barrier is disrupted, there can be leakage of plasma proteins into the urine (glomerular proteinuria; Fig. 40-3). Smaller proteins (<20 kDa) are freely filtered but are readily reabsorbed by the proximal tubule. Normal individuals excrete less than 150 mg/d of total protein and only about 30 mg/d of albumin. The remainder of the protein in the urine is secreted by the tubules (Tamm-Horsfall, IgA, and urokinase) or represents small amounts of filtered β_2-microglobulin, apoproteins, enzymes, and peptide hormones. Another mechanism of proteinuria occurs when there is excessive production of an abnormal protein that exceeds the capacity of the tubule for reabsorption. This most commonly occurs with plasma cell dyscrasias such as multiple myeloma, amyloidosis, and lymphomas that are associated with monoclonal production of immunoglobulin light chains.

The normal glomerular endothelial cell forms a barrier penetrated by pores of about 100 nm that holds back cells and other particles but offers little impediment to passage of most proteins. The glomerular basement membrane traps most large proteins (>100 kDa), while the foot processes of epithelial cells (podocytes) cover the urinary side of the glomerular basement membrane and produce a series of narrow channels (slit diaphragms) to allow molecular passage of small solutes and water. Some glomerular diseases, such as minimal change disease, cause fusion of glomerular epithelial cell foot processes, resulting in predominantly "selective" (Fig. 40-3) loss of albumin. Other glomerular diseases can present with disruption of the basement membrane and slit diaphragms (e.g., by immune complex deposition), resulting

in large amounts of protein losses that include albumin and other plasma proteins. The fusion of foot processes causes increased pressure across the capillary basement membrane, resulting in areas with larger pore sizes. The combination of increased pressure and larger pores results in significant proteinuria ("nonselective"; Fig. 40-3).

When the total daily excretion of protein exceeds 3.5 g, there is often associated hypoalbuminemia, hyperlipidemia, and edema (nephrotic syndrome; Table 40-1). However, total daily urinary protein excretion greater than 3.5 g can occur without the other features of the nephrotic syndrome in a variety of other renal diseases (Fig. 40-3). Plasma cell dyscrasias (multiple myeloma) can be associated with large amounts of excreted light chains in the urine, which may not be detected by dipstick (which detects mostly albumin). The light chains produced from these disorders are filtered by the glomerulus and overwhelm the reabsorptive capacity of the proximal tubule. A sulfosalicylic acid precipitate that is out of proportion to the dipstick estimate is suggestive of light chains (Bence Jones protein), and light chains typically redissolve upon warming of the precipitate. Renal failure from these disorders occurs through a variety of mechanisms including tubule obstruction (cast nephropathy) and light chain deposition.

Hypoalbuminemia in nephrotic syndrome occurs through excessive urinary losses, and increased proximal tubule catabolism of filtered albumin. Hepatic rates of albumin synthesis are increased. Edema forms from primary renal sodium retention and from reduced plasma oncotic pressure, which favors fluid movement from capillaries to interstitium. The mechanisms designed to correct the decrease in effective intravascular volume contribute to edema formation in some patients. These mechanisms include activation of the renin-angiotensin system, antidiuretic hormone, and the sympathetic nervous system, which contribute to excessive renal salt and water reabsorption.

The severity of edema correlates with the degree of hypoalbuminemia and is modified by other factors such as heart disease or peripheral vascular disease. The diminished plasma oncotic pressure and urinary losses of regulatory proteins appear to stimulate hepatic lipoprotein synthesis. The resulting hyperlipidemia results in lipid bodies (fatty casts, oval fat bodies) in the urine. Other proteins are lost in the urine, leading to a variety of metabolic disturbances. These include thyroxine-binding globulin, cholecalciferol-binding protein, transferrin, and metal-binding proteins. A hypercoagulable state frequently accompanies severe nephrotic syndrome due to urinary losses of antithrombin III, reduced serum levels of proteins S and C, hyperfibrinogenemia, and enhanced platelet aggregation. Some patients develop severe IgG deficiency with resulting defects in immunity. Many diseases (some listed in Fig. 40-3) and drugs can cause the nephrotic syndrome, and a complete list can be found in Chap. 264.

HEMATURIA, PYURIA, AND CASTS

Isolated hematuria without proteinuria, other cells, or casts is often indicative of bleeding from the urinary tract. Normal red blood cell excretion is up to 2 million RBCs per day. Hematuria is defined as two to five RBCs per high-power field (HPF) and can be detected by dipstick. Common causes of isolated hematuria include stones, neoplasms, tuberculosis, trauma, and prostatitis. Gross hematuria with blood clots is almost never indicative of glomerular bleeding; rather, it suggests a postrenal source in the urinary collecting system. Evaluation of patients presenting with microscopic hematuria is outlined in Fig. 40-2. A single urinalysis with hematuria is common and can result from menstruation, viral illness, allergy, exercise, or mild trauma. Annual urinalysis of servicemen over a 10-year period showed an incidence of 38%. However, persistent or significant hematuria (>three RBCs/HPF on three urinalyses, or a single urinalysis with >100 RBCs, or gross hematuria) identified significant renal or urologic lesions in 9.1% of over 1000 patients. Even patients who are chronically anticoagulated should be investigated as outlined in Fig. 40-2. The suspicion for urogenital neoplasms in patients with isolated painless hematuria (nondysmorphic RBCs) increases with age. Neoplasms are rare in the pediatric population, and isolated hematuria is more likely to be "idiopathic" or associated with a congenital anomaly. Hematuria with pyuria and bacteriuria is typical of infection and should be treated with antibiotics after appropriate cultures. Acute cystitis or urethritis in women can cause gross hematuria. Hypercalciuria and hyperuricosuria are also risk factors for unexplained isolated hematuria in both children and adults. In some of these patients (50 to 60%), reducing calcium and uric acid excretion through dietary interventions can eliminate the microscopic hematuria.

Isolated microscopic hematuria can be a manifestation of glomerular diseases. The RBCs of glomerular origin are often dysmorphic when examined by phase-contrast microscopy. Irregular shapes of RBCs may also occur due to pH and osmolarity changes found in the distal tubule. There is, however, significant observer variability in detecting dysmorphic RBCs, especially if a phase-contrast microscope is not available. The most common etiologies of isolated glomerular hematuria are IgA nephropathy, hereditary nephritis, and thin basement membrane disease. IgA nephropathy and hereditary nephritis can have episodic gross hematuria. A family history of renal failure is often present in patients with hereditary nephritis, and patients with thin basement membrane disease often have other family members with microscopic hematuria. A renal biopsy is needed for the definitive diagnosis of these disorders, which are discussed in more detail in Chap. 264. Hematuria with dysmorphic RBCs, RBC casts, and protein excretion >500 mg/d is virtually diagnostic of glomerulonephritis. RBC casts form as RBCs that enter the tubular fluid become trapped in a cylindrical mold of gelled Tamm-Horsfall protein. Even in the absence of azotemia, these patients should undergo serologic evaluation and renal biopsy as outlined in Fig. 40-2.

Isolated pyuria is unusual since inflammatory reactions in the kidney or collecting system are also associated with hematuria. The presence of bacteria suggests infection, and white blood cell casts with bacteria are indicative of pyelonephritis. White blood cells and/or white blood cell casts may also be seen in tubulointerstitial processes such as interstitial nephritis, systemic lupus erythematosus, and transplant rejection. In chronic renal diseases, degenerated cellular casts called *waxy casts* can be seen in the urine. *Broad casts* are thought to arise in the dilated tubules of enlarged nephrons that have undergone compensatory hypertrophy in response to reduced renal mass (i.e., chronic renal failure). A mixture of broad casts typically seen with chronic renal failure together with cellular casts and RBCs may be seen in smoldering processes such as chronic glomerulonephritis with active glomerulitis.

ABNORMALITIES OF URINE VOLUME

The volume of urine produced varies depending upon the fluid intake, renal function, and physiologic demands of the individual. See "Azotemia," above, for discussion of decreased (oliguria) or absent urine production (anuria). →*The physiology of water formation and renal water conservation are discussed in Chap. 259.*

POLYURIA

By history, it is often difficult for patients to distinguish urinary frequency (often of small volumes) from polyuria, and a 24-h urine collection is needed for evaluation (Fig. 40-4). It is necessary to determine if the polyuria represents a solute or water diuresis and if the diuresis is appropriate for the clinical circumstances. The average person excretes between 600 and 800 mosmol of solutes per day, primarily as urea and electrolytes. The urine osmolality can help distinguish a solute from water diuresis. If the urine output is >3 L/d (arbitrarily defined as polyuria) and the urine is dilute (<250 mosmol/L), then total mosmol excretion is normal and a water diuresis is present. This circumstance could arise from polydipsia, inadequate secretion of vasopressin (central diabetes insipidus), or failure of renal tubules to respond to vasopressin (nephrogenic diabetes insipidus). If the urine volume is >3 L/d and urine osmolality is >300 mosmol/L, then a solute diuresis is clearly present and a search for the responsible solute(s) is mandatory.

Excessive filtration of a poorly reabsorbed solute such as glucose, mannitol, or urea can depress reabsorption of NaCl and water in the proximal tubule and lead to enhanced excretion in the urine. Poorly controlled diabetes mellitus is the most common cause of a solute diuresis, leading to volume depletion and serum hypertonicity. Since the urine Na concentration is less than that of blood, more water than Na is lost, causing hypernatremia and hypertonicity. Common iatrogenic solute diuresis occurs from mannitol administration, radiocontrast media, and high-protein feedings (enterally or parenterally), leading to increased urea production and excretion. Less commonly, excessive Na loss may occur from cystic renal diseases, Bartter's syndrome, or during the course of a tubulointerstitial process (such as

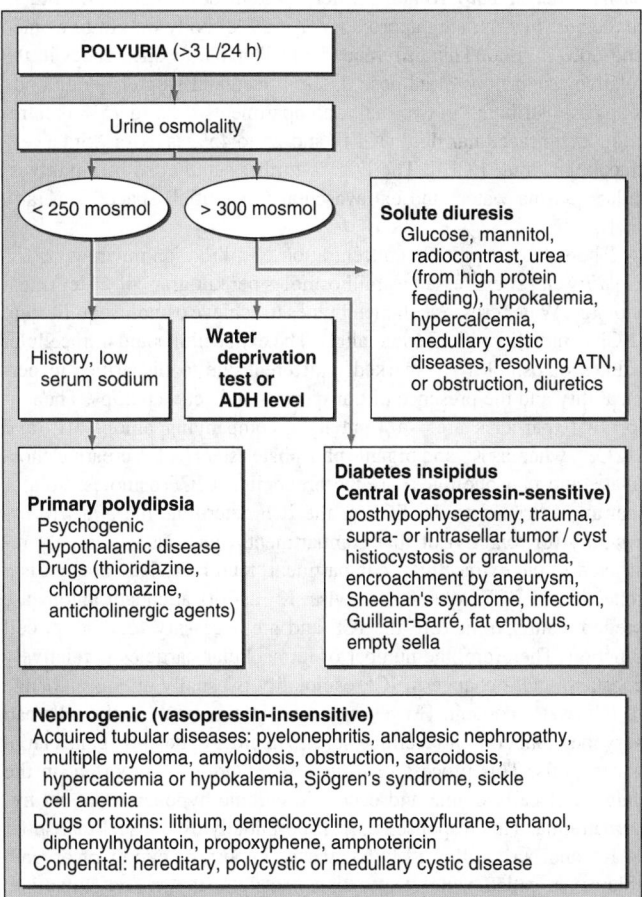

FIGURE 40-4 Approach to the patient with polyuria. ATN, acute tubular necrosis; ADH, antidiuretic hormone.

resolving ATN). In these so-called salt-wasting disorders, the tubule damage results in direct impairment of Na reabsorption and indirectly reduces the responsiveness of the tubule to aldosterone. Usually, the Na losses are mild, and the obligatory urine output is less than 2 L/d (resolving ATN and postobstructive diuresis are exceptions and may be associated with significant natriuresis and polyuria.)

Formation of large volumes of dilute urine represent polydipsic states or diabetes insipidus. Primary polydipsia can result from habit, psychiatric disorders, neurologic lesions, or medications. During deliberate polydipsia, extracellular fluid volume is normal or expanded and vasopressin levels are reduced because serum osmolality tends to be near the lower limits of normal.

Central diabetes insipidus may be idiopathic in origin or secondary to a variety of hypothalamic conditions including posthypophysectomy or trauma or neoplastic, inflammatory, vascular, or infectious hypothalamic diseases. Idiopathic central diabetes insipidus is associated with selective destruction of the vasopressin-secreting neurons in the supraoptic and paraventricular nuclei and can be inherited as an autosomal dominant trait or occur spontaneously. Nephrogenic diabetes insipidus can occur in a variety of clinical situations as summarized in Fig. 40-4.

A plasma vasopressin level is recommended as the best method for distinguishing between central and nephrogenic diabetes insipidus. Alternatively, a water deprivation test plus exogenous vasopressin may also distinguish primary polydipsia from central and nephrogenic diabetes insipidus. →*For a detailed discussion, see Chap. 319.*

FURTHER READING

ANDERSON S et al: Renal and systemic manifestations of glomerular disease, in BM Brenner (ed): *Brenner & Rector's The Kidney*, 7th ed. Philadelphia, Saunders, 2004, pp 1927–1954

BERL T, VERBALIS J: Pathophysiology of water metabolism, in BM Brenner (ed): *Brenner & Rector's The Kidney*, 7th ed. Philadelphia, Saunders, 2004, pp 857–920

BICHET DG: Nephrogenic diabetes insipidus. Am J Med 105(5):431, 1998

BOUTE N et al: NPHS2, encoding the glomerular protein podocin, is mutated in autosomal recessive steroid-resistant nephrotic syndrome. Nat Genet 24: 349, 2000

GROSSFELD GD, CARROLL PR: Evaluation of asymptomatic microscopic hematuria. Urol Clin North Am 25:661, 1998

LAMIERE N, VANHOLDER R: Pathophysiologic features and prevention of human and experimental acute tubulonecrosis. J Am Soc Nephrol 12:S20, 2001

MARIANI AJ et al: The significance of adult hematuria: 1000 hematuria evaluations including a risk-benefit and cost-effectiveness analysis. J Urol 141: 350, 1989

41 FLUID AND ELECTROLYTE DISTURBANCES
Gary G. Singer, Barry M. Brenner

SODIUM AND WATER

COMPOSITION OF BODY FLUIDS Water is the most abundant constituent in the body, comprising approximately 50% of body weight in women and 60% in men. This difference is attributable to differences in the relative proportions of adipose tissue in men and women. Total body water is distributed in two major compartments—55 to 75% is intracellular [intracellular fluid (ICF)], and 25 to 45% is extracellular [extracellular fluid (ECF)]. The ECF is further subdivided into intravascular (plasma water) and extravascular (interstitial) spaces in a ratio of 1:3.

The solute or particle concentration of a fluid is known as its *osmolality* and is expressed as milliosmoles per kilogram of water (mosmol/kg). Water crosses cell membranes to achieve osmotic equilibrium (ECF osmolality = ICF osmolality). The extracellular and intracellular solutes or osmoles are markedly different due to disparities in permeability and the presence of transporters and active pumps. The major ECF particles are Na^+ and its accompanying anions Cl^- and HCO_3^-, whereas K^+ and organic phosphate esters (ATP, creatine phosphate, and phospholipids) are the predominant ICF osmoles. Solutes that are restricted to the ECF or the ICF determine the *effective osmolality* (or *tonicity*) of that compartment. Since Na^+ is largely restricted to the extracellular compartment, total body Na^+ content is a reflection of ECF volume. Likewise, K^+ and its attendant anions are predominantly limited to the ICF and are necessary for normal cell function. Therefore, the number of intracellular particles is relatively constant, and a change in ICF osmolality is usually due to a change in ICF water content. However, in certain situations, brain cells can vary the number of intracellular solutes in order to defend against large water shifts. This process of *osmotic adaptation* is important in the defense of cell volume and occurs in chronic hyponatremia and hypernatremia. This response is mediated initially by transcellular shifts of K^+ and Na^+, followed by synthesis, import, or export of organic solutes (so-called osmolytes) such as inositol, betaine, and glutamine. During chronic hyponatremia, brain cells lose solutes, thereby defending cell volume and diminishing neurologic symptoms. The converse occurs during chronic hypernatremia. Certain solutes, such as urea, do not contribute to water shift across cell membranes and are known as *ineffective osmoles*.

Fluid movement between the intravascular and interstitial spaces occurs across the capillary wall and is determined by the Starling forces—capillary hydraulic pressure and colloid osmotic pressure. The transcapillary hydraulic pressure gradient exceeds the corresponding oncotic pressure gradient, thereby favoring the movement of plasma ultrafiltrate into the extravascular space. The return of fluid into the intravascular compartment occurs via lymphatic flow.

WATER BALANCE (See also Chap. 259) The normal plasma osmolality is 275 to 290 mosmol/kg and is kept within a narrow range by mechanisms capable of sensing a 1 to 2% change in tonicity. To maintain a steady state, water intake must equal water excretion. Disorders of water homeostasis result in hypo- or hypernatremia. Normal individuals have an obligate water loss consisting of urine, stool, and evaporation from the skin and respiratory tract. Gastrointestinal excretion is usually a minor component of total water output, except in patients with vomiting, diarrhea, or high enterostomy output states. Evaporative or insensitive water losses are important in the regulation of core body temperature. Obligatory renal water loss is mandated by the minimum solute excretion required to maintain a steady state. Normally, about 600 mosmols must be excreted per day, and since the maximal urine osmolality is 1200 mosmol/kg a minimum urine output of 500 mL/d is required for neutral solute balance.

Water Intake The primary stimulus for water ingestion is *thirst*, mediated either by an increase in effective osmolality or a decrease in ECF volume or blood pressure. *Osmoreceptors*, located in the anterolateral hypothalamus, are stimulated by a rise in tonicity. Ineffective osmoles, such as urea and glucose, do not play a role in stimulating thirst. The average osmotic threshold for thirst is approximately 295 mosmol/kg and varies among individuals. Under normal circumstances, daily water intake exceeds physiologic requirements.

Water Excretion In contrast to the ingestion of water, its excretion is tightly regulated by physiologic factors. The principal determinant of renal water excretion is *arginine vasopressin* (AVP; formerly antidiuretic hormone), a polypeptide synthesized in the supraoptic and paraventricular nuclei of the hypothalamus and secreted by the posterior pituitary gland. The binding of AVP to V_2 receptors on the basolateral membrane of principal cells in the collecting duct activates adenylyl cyclase and initiates a sequence of events that leads to the insertion of water channels into the luminal membrane. These water channels that are specifically activated by AVP are encoded by the *aquaporin-2* gene (Chap. 319). The net effect is passive water reabsorption along an osmotic gradient from the lumen of the collecting duct to the hypertonic medullary interstitium. The major stimulus for AVP secretion is hypertonicity. Since the major ECF solutes are Na^+ salts, effective osmolality is primarily determined by the plasma Na^+ concentration. An increase or decrease in tonicity is sensed by hypothalamic osmoreceptors as a decrease or increase in cell volume, respectively, leading to enhancement or suppression of AVP secretion. The osmotic threshold for AVP release is 280 to 290 mosmol/kg, and the system is sufficiently sensitive that plasma osmolality varies by no more than 1 to 2%.

Nonosmotic factors that regulate AVP secretion include *effective circulating (arterial) volume*, nausea, pain, stress, hypoglycemia, pregnancy, and numerous drugs. The hemodynamic response is mediated by baroreceptors in the carotid sinus. The sensitivity of these receptors is significantly lower than that of the osmoreceptors. In fact, depletion of blood volume sufficient to result in a decreased mean arterial pressure is necessary to stimulate AVP release, whereas small changes in effective circulating volume have little effect.

To maintain homeostasis and a normal plasma Na^+ concentration, the ingestion of solute-free water must eventually lead to the loss of the same volume of electrolyte-free water. Three steps are required for the kidney to excrete a water load: (1) filtration and delivery of water (and electrolytes) to the diluting sites of the nephron; (2) active reabsorption of Na^+ and Cl^- without water in the thick ascending limb of the loop of Henle and, to a lesser extent, in the distal nephron; and (3) maintenance of a dilute urine due to impermeability of the collecting duct to water in the absence of AVP. Abnormalities of any of these steps can result in impaired free water excretion, and eventual hyponatremia.

SODIUM BALANCE Sodium is actively pumped out of cells by the Na^+, K^+-ATPase pump. As a result, 85 to 90% of all Na^+ is extracellular, and the ECF volume is a reflection of total body Na^+ content. Normal volume regulatory mechanisms ensure that Na^+ loss balances Na^+ gain. If this does not occur, conditions of Na^+ excess or deficit ensue and are manifest as edematous or hypovolemic states, respectively. It is important to distinguish between disorders of osmoregulation and disorders of volume regulation since water and Na^+ balance are regulated independently. Changes in Na^+ concentration generally reflect disturbed water homeostasis, whereas alterations in Na^+ content are manifest as ECF volume contraction or expansion and imply abnormal Na^+ balance.

Sodium Intake Individuals eating a typical western diet consume approximately 150 mmol of NaCl daily. This normally exceeds basal requirements. As noted above, sodium is the principal extracellular cation. Therefore, dietary intake of Na^+ results in ECF volume expansion, which in turn promotes enhanced renal Na^+ excretion to maintain steady state Na^+ balance.

Sodium Excretion (See also Chap. 259) The regulation of Na^+ excretion is multifactorial and is the major determinant of Na^+ balance. A Na^+ deficit or excess is manifest as a decreased or increased effective circulating volume, respectively. Changes in effective circulating volume tend to lead to parallel changes in glomerular filtration rate (GFR). However, tubule Na^+ reabsorption, and not GFR, is the major regulatory mechanism controlling Na^+ excretion. Almost two-thirds of filtered Na^+ is reabsorbed in the proximal convoluted tubule—this process is electroneutral and isoosmotic. Further reabsorption (25 to 30%) occurs in the thick ascending limb of the loop of Henle via the apical $Na^+-K^+-2Cl^-$ *cotransporter*—this is an active process and is also electroneutral. Distal convoluted tubule reabsorption of Na^+ (5%) is mediated by the *thiazide-sensitive* Na^+-Cl^- *cotransporter*. Final Na^+

reabsorption occurs in the cortical and medullary collecting ducts, the amount excreted being reasonably equivalent to the amount ingested per day.

HYPOVOLEMIA

ETIOLOGY True volume depletion, or hypovolemia, generally refers to a state of combined salt and water loss exceeding intake, leading to ECF volume contraction. The loss of Na^+ may be renal or extrarenal (Table 41-1).

Renal Many conditions are associated with excessive urinary NaCl and water losses, including diuretics. Pharmacologic diuretics inhibit specific pathways of Na^+ reabsorption along the nephron with a consequent increase in urinary Na^+ excretion. Enhanced filtration of nonreabsorbed solutes, such as glucose or urea, can also impair tubular reabsorption of Na^+ and water, leading to an osmotic or solute diuresis. This often occurs in poorly controlled diabetes mellitus and in patients receiving high-protein hyperalimentation. Mannitol is a diuretic that produces an osmotic diuresis because the renal tubule is impermeable to mannitol. Many tubule and interstitial renal disorders are associated with Na^+ wasting. Excessive renal losses of Na^+ and water may also occur during the diuretic phase of acute tubular necrosis (Chap. 260) and following the relief of bilateral urinary tract obstruction. Finally, mineralocorticoid deficiency (hypoaldosteronism) causes salt wasting in the presence of normal intrinsic renal function.

Massive renal water excretion can also lead to hypovolemia. The ECF volume contraction is usually less severe since two-thirds of the volume lost is intracellular. Conditions associated with excessive urinary water loss include *central diabetes insipidus* (CDI) and *nephrogenic diabetes insipidus* (NDI). These two disorders are due to impaired secretion of and renal unresponsiveness to AVP, respectively, and are discussed below.

Extrarenal Nonrenal causes of hypovolemia include fluid loss from the gastrointestinal tract, skin, and respiratory system and third-space accumulations (burns, pancreatitis, peritonitis). Approximately 9 L of fluid enters the gastrointestinal tract daily, 2 L by ingestion and 7 L by secretion. Almost 98% of this volume is reabsorbed so that fecal fluid loss is only 100 to 200 mL/d. Impaired gastrointestinal reabsorption or enhanced secretion leads to volume depletion. Since gastric secretions have a low pH (high H^+ concentration) and biliary, pancreatic, and intestinal secretions are alkaline (high HCO_3^- concentration),

---

TABLE 41-1 *Causes of Hypovolemia*

I. ECF volume contracted
  A. Extrarenal Na^+ loss
    1. Gastrointestinal
       (vomiting, nasogastric suction, drainage, fistula, diarrhea)
    2. Skin/respiratory
       (insensible losses, sweat, burns)
    3. Hemorrhage
  B. Renal Na^+ and water loss
    1. Diuretics
    2. Osmotic diuresis
    3. Hypoaldosteronism
    4. Salt-wasting nephropathies
  C. Renal water loss
    1. Diabetes insipidus (central or nephrogenic)
II. ECF volume normal or expanded
  A. Decreased cardiac output
    1. Myocardial, valvular, or pericardial disease
  B. Redistribution
    1. Hypoalbuminemia
       (hepatic cirrhosis, nephrotic syndrome)
    2. Capillary leak
       (acute pancreatitis, ischemic bowel, rhabdomyolysis)
  C. Increased venous capacitance
    1. Sepsis

Note: ECF, extracellular fluid.

vomiting and diarrhea are often accompanied by metabolic alkalosis and acidosis, respectively.

Water evaporation from the skin and respiratory tract contributes to thermoregulation. These *insensible losses* amount to 500 mL/d. During febrile illnesses, prolonged heat exposure, exercise, or increased salt and water loss from skin, in the form of sweat, can be significant and lead to volume depletion. The Na^+ concentration of sweat is normally 20 to 50 mmol/L and decreases with profuse sweating due to the action of aldosterone. Since sweat is hypotonic, the loss of water exceeds that of Na^+. The water deficit is minimized by enhanced thirst. Nevertheless, ongoing Na^+ loss is manifest as hypovolemia. Enhanced evaporative water loss from the respiratory tract may be associated with hyperventilation, especially in mechanically ventilated febrile patients.

Certain conditions lead to fluid sequestration in a *third space*. This compartment is extracellular but is not in equilibrium with either the ECF or the ICF. The fluid is effectively lost from the ECF and can result in hypovolemia. Examples include the bowel lumen in gastrointestinal obstruction, subcutaneous tissues in severe burns, retroperitoneal space in acute pancreatitis, and peritoneal cavity in peritonitis. Finally, severe hemorrhage from any source can result in volume depletion.

PATHOPHYSIOLOGY ECF volume contraction is manifest as a decreased plasma volume and hypotension. Hypotension is due to decreased venous return (preload) and diminished cardiac output; it triggers baroreceptors in the carotid sinus and aortic arch and leads to activation of the sympathetic nervous system and the renin-angiotensin system. The net effect is to maintain mean arterial pressure and cerebral and coronary perfusion. In contrast to the cardiovascular response, the renal response is aimed at restoring the ECF volume by decreasing the GFR and filtered load of Na^+ and, most importantly, by promoting tubular reabsorption of Na^+. Increased sympathetic tone increases proximal tubular Na^+ reabsorption and decreases GFR by causing preferential afferent arteriolar vasoconstriction. Sodium is also reabsorbed in the proximal convoluted tubule in response to increased angiotensin II and altered peritubular capillary hemodynamics (decreased hydraulic and increased oncotic pressure). Enhanced reabsorption of Na^+ by the collecting duct is an important component of the renal adaptation to ECF volume contraction. This occurs in response to increased *aldosterone* and AVP secretion, and suppressed *atrial natriuretic peptide* secretion.

CLINICAL FEATURES A careful history is often helpful in determining the etiology of ECF volume contraction (e.g., vomiting, diarrhea, polyuria, diaphoresis). Most symptoms are nonspecific and secondary to electrolyte imbalances and tissue hypoperfusion and include fatigue, weakness, muscle cramps, thirst, and postural dizziness. More severe degrees of volume contraction can lead to end-organ ischemia manifest as oliguria, cyanosis, abdominal and chest pain, and confusion or obtundation. Diminished skin turgor and dry oral mucous membranes are poor markers of decreased interstitial fluid. Signs of intravascular volume contraction include decreased jugular venous pressure, postural hypotension, and postural tachycardia. Larger and more acute fluid losses lead to hypovolemic shock, manifest as hypotension, tachycardia, peripheral vasoconstriction, and hypoperfusion—cyanosis, cold and clammy extremities, oliguria, and altered mental status.

DIAGNOSIS A thorough history and physical examination are generally sufficient to diagnose the etiology of hypovolemia. Laboratory data usually confirm and support the clinical diagnosis. The blood urea nitrogen (BUN) and plasma creatinine concentrations tend to be elevated, reflecting a decreased GFR. Normally, the BUN:creatinine ratio is about 10:1. However, in *prerenal azotemia*, hypovolemia leads to increased urea reabsorption and a proportionately greater elevation in BUN than plasma creatinine, and a BUN:creatinine ratio of 20:1 or higher. An increased BUN (relative to creatinine) may also be due to increased urea production that occurs with hyperalimentation (high-protein), glucocorticoid therapy, and gastrointestinal bleeding.

The appropriate response to hypovolemia is enhanced renal Na^+ and water reabsorption, which is reflected in the urine composition. Therefore, the urine Na^+ concentration should usually be <20 mmol/L except in conditions associated with impaired Na^+ reabsorption, as in acute tubular necrosis (Chap. 260). Another exception is hypovolemia due to vomiting, since the associated metabolic alkalosis and increased filtered HCO_3^- impair proximal Na^+ reabsorption. In this case, the urine Cl^- is low (<20 mmol/L). The urine osmolality and specific gravity in hypovolemic subjects are generally >450 mosmol/kg and 1.015, respectively, reflecting the presence of enhanced AVP secretion. However, in hypovolemia due to diabetes insipidus, urine osmolality and specific gravity are indicative of inappropriately dilute urine.

℞ TREATMENT

The therapeutic goals are to restore normovolemia with fluid similar in composition to that lost and to replace ongoing losses. Symptoms and signs, including weight loss, can help estimate the degree of volume contraction and should also be monitored to assess response to treatment. Mild volume contraction can usually be corrected via the oral route. More severe hypovolemia requires intravenous therapy. Isotonic or normal saline (0.9% NaCl or 154 mmol/L Na^+) is the solution of choice in normonatremic and mildly hyponatremic individuals and should be administered initially in patients with hypotension or shock. Severe hyponatremia may require hypertonic saline (3.0% NaCl or 513 mmol/L Na^+). Hypernatremia reflects a proportionally greater deficit of water than Na^+, and its correction will therefore require a hypotonic solution such as half-normal saline (0.45% NaCl or 77 mmol/L Na^+) or 5% dextrose in water. Patients with significant hemorrhage, anemia, or intravascular volume depletion may require blood transfusion or colloid-containing solutions (albumin, dextran). Hypokalemia may be present initially or may ensue as a result of increased urinary K^+ excretion; it should be corrected by adding appropriate amounts of KCl to replacement solutions.

HYPONATREMIA

ETIOLOGY A plasma Na^+ concentration less than 135 mmol/L usually reflects a hypotonic state. However, plasma osmolality may be normal or increased in some cases of hyponatremia. Isotonic or slightly hypotonic hyponatremia may complicate transurethral resection of the prostate or bladder because large volumes of isoosmotic (mannitol) or hypoosmotic (sorbital or glycine) bladder irrigation solution can be absorbed and result in a dilutional hyponatremia. The metabolism of sorbitol and glycine to CO_2 and water may lead to hypotonicity if the accumulated fluid and solutes are not rapidly excreted. Hypertonic hyponatremia is usually due to hyperglycemia or, occasionally, intravenous administration of mannitol. Relative insulin deficiency causes myocytes to become impermeable to glucose. Therefore, during poorly controlled diabetes mellitus, glucose is an effective osmole and draws water from muscle cells, resulting in hyponatremia. Plasma Na^+ concentration falls by 1.4 mmol/L for every 100 mg/dL rise in the plasma glucose concentration.

Most causes of hyponatremia are associated with a low plasma osmolality (Table 41-2). In general, hypotonic hyponatremia is due either to a primary water gain (and secondary Na^+ loss) or a primary Na^+ loss (and secondary water gain). In the absence of water intake or hypotonic fluid replacement, hyponatremia is usually associated with hypovolemic shock due to a profound sodium deficit and transcellular water shift. Contraction of the ECF volume stimulates thirst and AVP secretion. The increased water ingestion and impaired renal excretion result in hyponatremia. It is important to note that *diuretic-induced hyponatremia* is almost always due to thiazide diuretics. Loop diuretics decrease the tonicity of the medullary interstitium and impair maximal urinary concentrating capacity. This limits the ability of AVP to promote water retention. In contrast, thiazide diuretics lead to Na^+ and K^+ depletion and AVP-mediated water retention. Hyponatremia can also occur by a process of *desalination*. This occurs when the urine

TABLE 41-2 *Causes of Hyponatremia*

I. Pseudohyponatremia
    A. Normal plasma osmolality
        1. Hyperlipidemia
        2. Hyperproteinemia
        3. Posttransurethral resection of prostate/bladder tumor
    B. Increased plasma osmolality
        1. Hyperglycemia
        2. Mannitol
II. Hypoosmolal hyponatremia
    A. Primary Na^+ loss (secondary water gain)
        1. Integumentary loss: sweating, burns
        2. Gastrointestinal loss: vomiting, tube drainage, fistula, obstruction, diarrhea
        3. Renal loss: diuretics, osmotic diuresis, hypoaldosteronism, salt-wasting nephropathy, postobstructive diuresis, nonoliguric acute tubular necrosis
    B. Primary water gain (secondary Na^+ loss)
        1. Primary polydipsia
        2. Decreased solute intake (e.g., beer potomania)
        3. AVP release due to pain, nausea, drugs
        4. Syndrome of inappropriate AVP secretion
        5. Glucocorticoid deficiency
        6. Hypothyroidism
        7. Chronic renal insufficiency
    C. Primary Na^+ gain (exceeded by secondary water gain)
        1. Heart failure
        2. Hepatic cirrhosis
        3. Nephrotic syndrome

tonicity (the sum of the concentrations of Na^+ and K^+) exceeds that of administered intravenous fluids (including isotonic saline). This accounts for some cases of acute postoperative hyponatremia and cerebral salt wasting after neurosurgery.

Hyponatremia in the setting of ECF volume expansion is usually associated with edematous states, such as congestive heart failure, hepatic cirrhosis, and the nephrotic syndrome. These disorders all have in common a decreased effective circulating arterial volume, leading to increased thirst and increased AVP levels. Additional factors impairing the excretion of solute-free water include a reduced GFR, decreased delivery of ultrafiltrate to the diluting site (due to increased proximal fractional reabsorption of Na^+ and water), and diuretic therapy. The degree of hyponatremia often correlates with the severity of the underlying condition and is an important prognostic factor. Oliguric acute and chronic renal failure may be associated with hyponatremia if water intake exceeds the ability to excrete equivalent volumes.

Hyponatremia in the absence of ECF volume contraction, decreased effective circulating arterial volume, or renal insufficiency is usually due to increased AVP secretion resulting in impaired water excretion. Ingestion or administration of water is also required since high levels of AVP alone are usually insufficient to produce hyponatremia. This disorder, commonly termed the *syndrome of inappropriate antidiuretic hormone secretion* (SIADH), is the most common cause of normovolemic hyponatremia and is due to the nonphysiologic release of AVP from the posterior pituitary or an ectopic source (Chap. 319). Renal free water excretion is impaired while the regulation of Na^+ balance is unaffected. The most common causes of SIADH include neuropsychiatric and pulmonary diseases, malignant tumors, major surgery (postoperative pain), and pharmacologic agents. Severe pain and nausea are physiologic stimuli of AVP secretion; these stimuli are inappropriate in the absence of hypovolemia or hyperosmolality. The pattern of AVP secretion can be used to classify SIADH into four subtypes: (1) erratic autonomous AVP secretion (ectopic production); (2) normal regulation of AVP release around a lower osmolality set point or *reset osmostat* (cachexia, malnutrition); (3) normal AVP response to hypertonicity with failure to suppress completely at low osmolality (incomplete pituitary stalk section); and (4) normal AVP secretion with increased sensitivity to its actions or secretion of some other antidiuretic factor (rare).

Hormonal excess or deficiency may cause hyponatremia. Adrenal insufficiency (Chap. 321) and hypothyroidism (Chap. 320) may present with hyponatremia and should not be confused with SIADH. Although decreased mineralocorticoids may contribute to the hyponatremia of adrenal insufficiency, it is the cortisol deficiency that leads to hypersecretion of AVP both indirectly (secondary to volume depletion) and directly (cosecreted with corticotropin-releasing factor). The mechanisms by which hypothyroidism leads to hyponatremia include decreased cardiac output and GFR and increased AVP secretion in response to hemodynamic stimuli.

Finally, hyponatremia may occur in the absence of AVP or renal failure if the kidney is unable to excrete the dietary water load. In psychogenic or primary polydipsia, compulsive water consumption may overwhelm the normally large renal excretory capacity of 12 L/d (Chap. 319). These patients often have psychiatric illnesses and may be taking medications, such as phenothiazines, that enhance the sensation of thirst by causing a dry mouth. The maximal urine output is a function of the minimum urine osmolality achievable and the mandatory solute excretion. Metabolism of a normal diet generates about 600 mosmol/d, and the minimum urine osmolality in humans is 50 mosmol/kg. Therefore, the maximum daily urine output will be about 12 L (600 ÷ 50 = 12). A solute excretion rate of greater than ~750 mosmol/d is, by definition, an *osmotic diuresis*. A low-protein diet may yield as few as 250 mosmol/d, which translates into a maximal urine output of 5 L/d at a minimum urine tonicity of 50 mosmol/kg. Beer drinkers typically have a poor dietary intake of protein and electrolytes and consume large volumes (of beer), which may exceed the renal excretory capacity and result in hyponatremia. This phenomenon is referred to as *beer potomania*.

CLINICAL FEATURES The clinical manifestations of hyponatremia are related to osmotic water shift leading to increased ICF volume, specifically brain cell swelling or cerebral edema. Therefore, the symptoms are primarily neurologic, and their severity is dependent on the rapidity of onset and absolute decrease in plasma Na^+ concentration. Patients may be asymptomatic or complain of nausea and malaise. As the plasma Na^+ concentration falls, the symptoms progress to include headache, lethargy, confusion, and obtundation. Stupor, seizures, and coma do not usually occur unless the plasma Na^+ concentration falls acutely below 120 mmol/L or decreases rapidly. As described above, adaptive mechanisms designed to protect cell volume occur in chronic hyponatremia. Loss of Na^+ and K^+, followed by organic osmolytes, from brain cells decreases brain swelling due to secondary transcellular water shifts (from ICF to ECF). The net effect is to minimize cerebral edema and its symptoms.

DIAGNOSIS (Fig. 41-1) Hyponatremia is not a disease but a manifestation of a variety of disorders. The underlying cause can often be ascertained from an accurate history and physical examination, including an assessment of ECF volume status and effective circulating arterial volume. The differential diagnosis of hyponatremia, an expanded ECF volume, and decreased effective circulating volume includes congestive heart failure, hepatic cirrhosis, and the nephrotic syndrome. Hypothyroidism and adrenal insufficiency tend to present with a near-normal ECF volume and decreased effective circulating arterial volume. All of these diseases have characteristic signs and symptoms. Patients with SIADH are usually euvolemic.

Four laboratory findings often provide useful information and can narrow the differential diagnosis of hyponatremia: (1) the plasma osmolality, (2) the urine osmolality, (3) the urine Na^+ concentration, and (4) the urine K^+ concentration. Since ECF tonicity is determined primarily by the Na^+ concentration, most patients with hyponatremia have a decreased plasma osmolality. The appropriate renal response to hypoosmolality is to excrete the maximum volume of dilute urine, i.e., urine osmolality and specific gravity of less than 100 mosmol/kg and 1.003, respectively. This occurs in patients with primary polydipsia. If this is not present, it suggests impaired free water excretion due

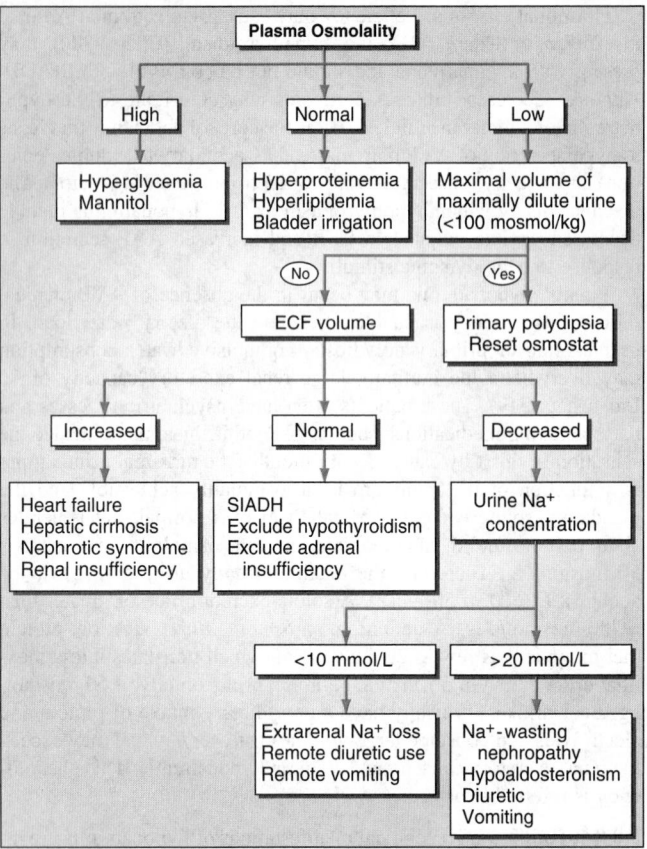

FIGURE 41-1 Algorithm depicting clinical approach to hyponatremia. ECF, extracellular fluid; SIADH, syndrome of inappropriate antidiuretic hormone secretion.

to the action of AVP on the kidney. The secretion of AVP may be a physiologic response to hemodynamic stimuli or it may be inappropriate in the presence of hyponatremia and euvolemia. Since Na^+ is the major ECF cation and is largely restricted to this compartment, ECF volume contraction represents a deficit in total body Na^+ content. Therefore, volume depletion in patients with normal underlying renal function results in enhanced tubule Na^+ reabsorption and a urine Na^+ concentration less than 20 mmol/L. The finding of a urine Na^+ concentration greater than 20 mmol/L in hypovolemic hyponatremia implies a salt-wasting nephropathy, diuretic therapy, hypoaldosteronism, or occasionally vomiting. Both the urine osmolality and the urine Na^+ concentration can be followed serially when assessing response to therapy.

SIADH is characterized by hypoosmotic hyponatremia in the setting of an inappropriately concentrated urine (urine osmolality greater than 100 mosmol/kg). Patients are typically normovolemic and have normal Na^+ balance. They tend to be mildly volume expanded secondary to water retention and have a urine Na^+ excretion rate equal to intake (urine Na^+ concentration usually greater than 40 mmol/L). By definition, they have normal renal, adrenal, and thyroid function and usually have normal K^+ and acid-base balance. SIADH is often associated with hypouricemia due to the uricosuric state induced by volume expansion. In contrast, hypovolemic patients tend to be hyperuricemic secondary to increased proximal urate reabsorption.

℞ TREATMENT

The goals of therapy are twofold: (1) to raise the plasma Na^+ concentration by restricting water intake and promoting water loss; and (2) to correct the underlying disorder. Mild asymptomatic hyponatremia is generally of little clinical significance and requires no treatment. The management of asymptomatic hyponatremia associated with ECF volume contraction should include Na^+ repletion, generally in the form

of isotonic saline. The direct effect of the administered NaCl on the plasma Na^+ concentration is trivial. However, restoration of euvolemia removes the hemodynamic stimulus for AVP release, allowing the excess free water to be excreted. The hyponatremia associated with edematous states tends to reflect the severity of the underlying disease and is usually asymptomatic. These patients have increased total body water that exceeds the increase in total body Na^+ content. Treatment should include restriction of Na^+ and water intake, correction of hypokalemia, and promotion of water loss in excess of Na^+. The latter may require the use of loop diuretics with replacement of a proportion of the urinary Na^+ loss to ensure net free water excretion. Dietary water restriction should be less than the urine output. Correction of the K^+ deficit may raise the plasma Na^+ concentration by favoring a shift of Na^+ out of cells as K^+ moves in. Water restriction is also a component of the therapeutic approach to hyponatremia associated with primary polydipsia, renal failure, and SIADH (Chap. 319).

The rate of correction of hyponatremia depends on the absence or presence of neurologic dysfunction. This, in turn, is related to the rapidity of onset and magnitude of the fall in plasma Na^+ concentration. In asymptomatic patients, the plasma Na^+ concentration should be raised by no more than 0.5 to 1.0 mmol/L per h and by less than 10 to 12 mmol/L over the first 24 h. Acute or severe hyponatremia (plasma Na^+ concentration <110 to 115 mmol/L) tends to present with altered mental status and/or seizures and requires more rapid correction. Severe symptomatic hyponatremia should be treated with hypertonic saline, and the plasma Na^+ concentration should be raised by 1 to 2 mmol/L per hour for the first 3 to 4 h or until the seizures subside. Once again, the plasma Na^+ concentration should probably be raised by no more than 12 mmol/L during the first 24 h. The quantity of Na^+ required to increase the plasma Na^+ concentration by a given amount can be estimated by multiplying the deficit in plasma Na^+ concentration by the total body water.

Under normal conditions, total body water is 50 or 60% of lean body weight in women or men, respectively. Therefore, to raise the plasma Na^+ concentration from 105 to 115 mmol/L in a 70-kg man requires 420 mmol [(115 − 105) × 70 × 0.6] of Na^+. The risk of correcting hyponatremia too rapidly is the development of the *osmotic demyelination syndrome* (ODS). This is a neurologic disorder characterized by flaccid paralysis, dysarthria, and dysphagia. The diagnosis is usually suspected clinically and can be confirmed by appropriate neuroimaging studies. There is no specific treatment for the disorder, which is associated with significant morbidity and mortality. Patients with chronic hyponatremia are most susceptible to the development of ODS, since their brain cell volume has returned to near normal as a result of the osmotic adaptive mechanisms described above. Therefore, administration of hypertonic saline to these individuals can cause sudden osmotic shrinkage of brain cells. In addition to rapid or overcorrection of hyponatremia, risk factors for ODS include prior cerebral anoxic injury, hypokalemia, and malnutrition, especially secondary to alcoholism. Water restriction in primary polydipsia and intravenous saline therapy in ECF volume–contracted patients may also lead to overly rapid correction of hyponatremia as a result of AVP suppression and a brisk water diuresis. This can be prevented by administration of water or use of an AVP analogue to slow down the rate of free water excretion. →*For further discussion, see Chap. 319.*

HYPERNATREMIA

ETIOLOGY Hypernatremia is defined as a plasma Na^+ concentration greater than 145 mmol/L. Since Na^+ and its accompanying anions are the major effective ECF osmoles, hypernatremia is a state of hyperosmolality. As a result of the fixed number of ICF particles, maintenance of osmotic equilibrium in hypernatremia results in ICF volume contraction. Hypernatremia may be due to primary Na^+ gain or water deficit. The two components of an appropriate response to hypernatremia are increased water intake stimulated by thirst and the excretion of the minimum volume of maximally concentrated urine reflecting AVP secretion in response to an osmotic stimulus.

In practice, the majority of cases of hypernatremia result from the loss of water. Since water is distributed between the ICF and the ECF in a 2:1 ratio, a given amount of solute-free water loss will result in a twofold greater reduction in the ICF compartment than the ECF compartment. For example, consider three scenarios: the loss of 1 L of water, isotonic NaCl, or half-isotonic NaCl. If 1 L of water is lost, the ICF volume will decrease by 667 mL, whereas the ECF volume will fall by only 333 mL. Due to the fact that Na+ is largely restricted to the ECF, this compartment will decrease by 1 L if the fluid lost is isoosmotic. One liter of half-isotonic NaCl is equivalent to 500 mL of water (one-third ECF, two-thirds ICF) plus 500 mL of isotonic saline (all ECF). Therefore, the loss of 1 L of half-isotonic saline decreases the ECF and ICF volumes by 667 mL and 333 mL, respectively.

The degree of hyperosmolality is typically mild unless the thirst mechanism is abnormal or access to water is limited. The latter occurs in infants, the physically handicapped, patients with impaired mental status, in the postoperative state, and in intubated patients in the intensive care unit. On rare occasions, impaired thirst may be due to *primary hypodipsia*. This usually occurs as a result of damage to the hypothalamic osmoreceptors that control thirst and tends to be associated with abnormal osmotic regulation of AVP secretion. Primary hypodipsia may be due to a variety of pathologic changes including granulomatous disease, vascular occlusion, and tumors. A subset of hypodipsic hypernatremia, referred to as *essential hypernatremia*, does not respond to forced water intake. This appears to be due to a specific osmoreceptor defect resulting in nonosmotic regulation of AVP release. Thus, the hemodynamic effects of water loading lead to AVP suppression and excretion of dilute urine.

The source of free water loss is either renal or extrarenal. Nonrenal loss of water may be due to evaporation from the skin and respiratory tract (insensible losses) or loss from the gastrointestinal tract. Insensible losses are increased with fever, exercise, heat exposure, and severe burns and in mechanically ventilated patients. Furthermore, the Na+ concentration of sweat decreases with profuse perspiration, thereby increasing solute-free water loss. Diarrhea is the most common gastrointestinal cause of hypernatremia. Specifically, osmotic diarrheas (induced by lactulose, sorbitol, or malabsorption of carbohydrate) and viral gastroenteritides result in water loss exceeding that of Na+ and K+. In contrast, secretory diarrheas (e.g., cholera, carcinoid, VIPoma) have a fecal osmolality (twice the sum of the concentrations of Na+ and K+) similar to that of plasma and present with ECF volume contraction and a normal plasma Na+ concentration or hyponatremia.

Renal water loss is the most common cause of hypernatremia and is due to drug-induced or osmotic diuresis or diabetes insipidus (Chap. 319). Loop diuretics interfere with the countercurrent mechanism and produce an isoosmotic solute diuresis. This results in a decreased medullary interstitial tonicity and impaired renal concentrating ability. The presence of non-reabsorbed organic solutes in the tubule lumen impairs the osmotic reabsorption of water. This leads to water loss in excess of Na+ and K+, known as an osmotic diuresis. The most frequent cause of an osmotic diuresis is hyperglycemia and glucosuria in poorly controlled diabetes mellitus. Intravenous administration of mannitol and increased endogenous production of urea (high-protein diet) can also result in an osmotic diuresis.

Hypernatremia secondary to nonosmotic urinary water loss is usually due to: (1) Central diabetes insipidus (CDI) characterized by impaired AVP secretion, or (2) NDI resulting from end-organ (renal) resistance to the actions of AVP. The most common cause of CDI is destruction of the neurohypophysis. This may occur as a result of trauma, neurosurgery, granulomatous disease, neoplasms, vascular accidents, or infection. In many cases, CDI is idiopathic and may occasionally be hereditary. The familial form of the disease is inherited in an autosomal dominant fashion and has been attributed to mutations in the propressophysin (AVP precursor) gene. Nephrogenic diabetes insipidus (NDI) may be either inherited or acquired. Congenital NDI is an X-linked recessive trait due to mutations in the V2 receptor gene. Mutations in the autosomal *aquaporin-2* gene may also result in NDI. The *aquaporin-2* gene encodes the water channel protein whose membrane insertion is stimulated by AVP. The causes of sporadic NDI are numerous and include drugs (especially lithium), hypercalcemia, hypokalemia, and conditions that impair medullary hypertonicity (e.g., papillary necrosis or osmotic diuresis). Pregnant women, in the second or third trimester, may develop NDI as a result of excessive elaboration of vasopressinase by the placenta.

Finally, although infrequent, a primary Na+ gain may cause hypernatremia. For example, inadvertent administration of hypertonic NaCl or NaHCO3 or replacing sugar with salt in infant formula can produce this complication.

CLINICAL FEATURES As a consequence of hypertonicity, water shifts out of cells, leading to a contracted ICF volume. A decreased brain cell volume is associated with an increased risk of subarachnoid or intracerebral hemorrhage. Hence, the major symptoms of hypernatremia are neurologic and include altered mental status, weakness, neuromuscular irritability, focal neurologic deficits, and occasionally coma or seizures. Patients may also complain of polyuria or thirst. For unknown reasons, patients with polydipsia from CDI tend to prefer ice-cold water. The signs and symptoms of volume depletion are often present in patients with a history of excessive sweating, diarrhea, or an osmotic diuresis. As with hyponatremia, the severity of the clinical manifestations is related to the acuity and magnitude of the rise in plasma Na+ concentration. Chronic hypernatremia is generally less symptomatic as a result of adaptive mechanisms designed to defend cell volume. Brain cells initially take up Na+ and K+ salts, later followed by accumulation of organic osmolytes such as inositol. This serves to restore the brain ICF volume towards normal.

DIAGNOSIS (Fig. 41-2) A complete history and physical examination will often provide clues as to the underlying cause of hypernatremia. Relevant symptoms and signs include the absence or presence of thirst, diaphoresis, diarrhea, polyuria, and the features of ECF volume contraction. The history should include a list of current and recent medications, and the physical examination is incomplete without a thorough mental status and neurologic assessment. Measurement of urine volume and osmolality are essential in the evaluation of hyperosmolality. The appropriate renal response to hypernatremia is the excretion of the minimum volume (500 mL/d) of maximally concentrated urine (urine osmolality >800 mosmol/kg). These findings suggest extrarenal

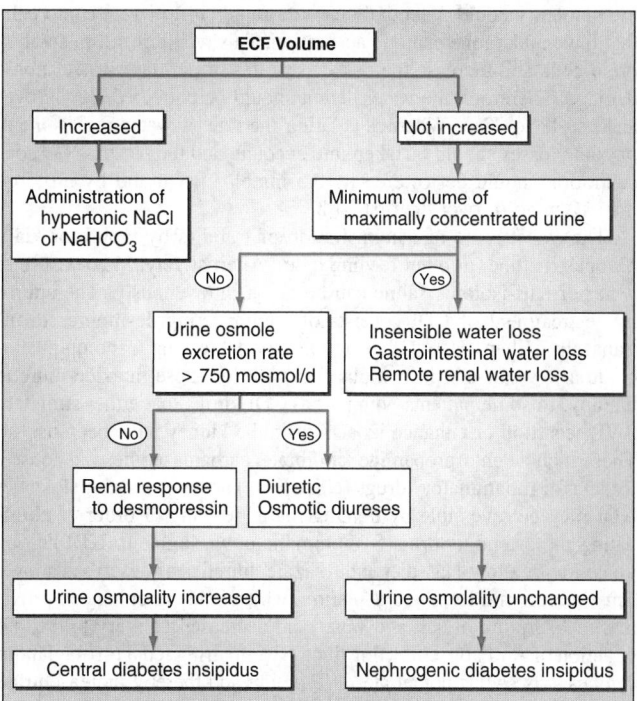

FIGURE 41-2 Algorithm depicting clinical approach to hypernatremia.

or remote renal water loss or administration of hypertonic Na$^+$ salt solutions. The presence of a primary Na$^+$ excess can be confirmed by the presence of ECF volume expansion and natriuresis (urine Na$^+$ concentration usually >100 mmol/L).

Many causes of hypernatremia are associated with polyuria and a submaximal urine osmolality. The product of the urine volume and osmolality, i.e., the solute excretion rate, is helpful in determining the basis of the polyuria (see above). To maintain a steady state, total solute excretion must equal solute production. As stated above, individuals eating a normal diet generate ~600 mosmol/d. Therefore, daily solute excretion in excess of 750 mosmol defines an osmotic diuresis. This can be confirmed by measuring the urine glucose and urea. In general, both CDI and NDI present with polyuria and hypotonic urine (urine osmolality <250 mosmol/kg). The degree of hypernatremia is usually mild unless there is an associated thirst abnormality. The clinical history, physical examination, and pertinent laboratory data can often rule out causes of acquired NDI. CDI and NDI can generally be distinguished by administering the AVP analogue desmopressin (10 μg intranasally) after careful water restriction. The urine osmolality should increase by at least 50% in CDI and will not change in NDI. Unfortunately, the diagnosis may sometimes be difficult due to partial defects in AVP secretion and action.

℞ TREATMENT

The therapeutic goals are to stop ongoing water loss by treating the underlying cause and to correct the water deficit. The ECF volume should be restored in hypovolemic patients. The quantity of water required to correct the deficit can be calculated from the following equation:

$$\text{Water deficit} = \frac{\text{Plasma Na}^+ \text{ concentration} - 140}{140} \times \text{Total body water}$$

In hypernatremia due to water loss, total body water is approximately 50 and 40% of lean body weight in men and women, respectively. For example, a 50-kg woman with a plasma Na$^+$ concentration of 160 mmol/L has an estimated free water deficit of 2.9 L {[(160 − 140) ÷ 140] × (0.4 × 50)}. As in hyponatremia, rapid correction of hypernatremia is potentially dangerous. In this case, a sudden decrease in osmolality could potentially cause a rapid shift of water into cells that have undergone osmotic adaptation. This would result in swollen brain cells and increase the risk of seizures or permanent neurologic damage. Therefore, the water deficit should be corrected slowly over at least 48 to 72 h. When calculating the rate of water replacement, ongoing losses should be taken into account, and the plasma Na$^+$ concentration should be lowered by 0.5 mmol/L per h and by no more than 12 mmol/L over the first 24 h.

The safest route of administration of water is by mouth or via a nasogastric tube (or other feeding tube). Alternatively, 5% dextrose in water or half-isotonic saline can be given intravenously. The appropriate treatment of CDI consists of administering desmopressin intranasally (Chap. 319). Other options for decreasing urine output include a low-salt diet in combination with low-dose thiazide diuretic therapy. In some patients with partial CDI, drugs that either stimulate AVP secretion or enhance its action on the kidney have been useful. These include chlorpropamide, clofibrate, carbamazepine, and nonsteroidal anti-inflammatory drugs (NSAIDs). The concentrating defect in NDI may be reversible by treating the underlying disorder or eliminating the offending drug. Symptomatic polyuria due to NDI can be treated with a low-Na$^+$ diet and thiazide diuretics as described above. This induces mild volume depletion, which leads to enhanced proximal reabsorption of salt and water and decreased delivery to the site of action of AVP, the collecting duct. By impairing renal prostaglandin synthesis, NSAIDs potentiate AVP action and thereby increase urine osmolality and decrease urine volume. Amiloride may be useful in patients with NDI who need to be on lithium. The nephrotoxicity of

lithium requires the drug to be taken up into collecting duct cells via the amiloride-sensitive Na$^+$ channel.

POTASSIUM

POTASSIUM BALANCE Potassium is the major intracellular cation. The normal plasma K$^+$ concentration is 3.5 to 5.0 mmol/L, whereas that inside cells is about 150 mmol/L. Therefore, the amount of K$^+$ in the ECF (30 to 70 mmol) constitutes less than 2% of the total body K$^+$ content (2500 to 4500 mmol). The ratio of ICF to ECF K$^+$ concentration (normally 38:1) is the principal result of the resting membrane potential and is crucial for normal neuromuscular function. The basolateral Na$^+$, K$^+$-ATPase pump actively transports K$^+$ in and Na$^+$ out of the cell in a 2:3 ratio, and the passive outward diffusion of K$^+$ is quantitatively the most important factor that generates the resting membrane potential. The activity of the electrogenic Na$^+$, K$^+$-ATPase pump may be stimulated as a result of an increased intracellular Na$^+$ concentration and inhibited in the setting of digoxin toxicity or chronic illness such as heart failure or renal failure.

The K$^+$ intake of individuals on an average western diet is 40 to 120 mmol/d or approximately 1 mmol/kg per day, 90% of which is absorbed by the gastrointestinal tract. Maintenance of the steady state necessitates matching K$^+$ ingestion with excretion. Initially, extrarenal adaptive mechanisms, followed later by urinary excretion, prevent a doubling of the plasma K$^+$ concentration that would occur if the dietary K$^+$ load remained in the ECF compartment. Immediately following a meal, most of the absorbed K$^+$ enters cells as a result of the initial elevation in the plasma K$^+$ concentration and facilitated by insulin release and basal catecholamine levels. Eventually, however, the excess K$^+$ is excreted in the urine (see below). The regulation of gastrointestinal K$^+$ handling is not well understood. The amount of K$^+$ lost in the stool can increase from 10 to 50 or 60% (of dietary intake) in chronic renal insufficiency. In addition, colonic secretion of K$^+$ is stimulated in patients with large volumes of diarrhea, resulting in potentially severe K$^+$ depletion.

POTASSIUM EXCRETION (See also Chap. 259)   Renal excretion is the major route of elimination of dietary and other sources of excess K$^+$. The filtered load of K$^+$ (GFR × plasma K$^+$ concentration = 180 L/d × 4 mmol/L = 720 mmol/d) is 10- to 20-fold greater than the ECF K$^+$ content. Some 90% of filtered K$^+$ is reabsorbed by the proximal convoluted tubule and loop of Henle. Proximally, K$^+$ is reabsorbed passively with Na$^+$ and water, whereas the luminal Na$^+$-K$^+$-2Cl$^-$ cotransporter mediates K$^+$ uptake in the thick ascending limb of the loop of Henle. Therefore, K$^+$ delivery to the distal nephron [distal convoluted tubule and cortical collecting duct (CCD)] approximates dietary intake. Net distal K$^+$ secretion or reabsorption occurs in the setting of K$^+$ excess or depletion, respectively. The cell responsible for K$^+$ secretion in the late distal convoluted tubule (or connecting tubule) and CCD is the principal cell. Virtually all regulation of renal K$^+$ excretion and total body K$^+$ balance occurs in the distal nephron. Potassium secretion is regulated by two physiologic stimuli—aldosterone and hyperkalemia. Aldosterone is secreted by the zona glomerulosa cells of the adrenal cortex in response to high renin and angiotensin II or hyperkalemia. The plasma K$^+$ concentration, independent of aldosterone, can directly affect K$^+$ secretion. In addition to the K$^+$ concentration in the lumen of the CCD, renal K$^+$ loss depends on the urine flow rate, a function of daily solute excretion (see above). Since excretion is equal to the product of concentration and volume, increased distal flow rate can significantly enhance urinary K$^+$ output. Finally, in severe K$^+$ depletion, secretion of K$^+$ is reduced and reabsorption in the cortical and medullary collecting ducts is upregulated.

HYPOKALEMIA

ETIOLOGY (See Table 41-3)   Hypokalemia, defined as a plasma K$^+$ concentration <3.5 mmol/L, may result from one (or more) of the following: decreased net intake, shift into cells, or increased net loss. Diminished intake is seldom the sole cause of K$^+$ depletion since urinary excretion can be effectively decreased to less than 15 mmol/d as a

TABLE 41-3 *Causes of Hypokalemia*

I. Decreased intake
  A. Starvation
  B. Clay ingestion
II. Redistribution into cells
  A. Acid-base
    1. Metabolic alkalosis
  B. Hormonal
    1. Insulin
    2. β_2-Adrenergic agonists (endogenous or exogenous)
    3. α-Adrenergic antagonists
  C. Anabolic state
    1. Vitamin B_{12} or folic acid (red blood cell production)
    2. Granulocyte-macrophage colony stimulating factor (white blood cell production)
    3. Total parenteral nutrition
  D. Other
    1. Pseudohypokalemia
    2. Hypothermia
    3. Hypokalemic periodic paralysis
    4. Barium toxicity
III. Increased loss
  A. Nonrenal
    1. Gastrointestinal loss (diarrhea)
    2. Integumentary loss (sweat)
  B. Renal
    1. Increased distal flow: diuretics, osmotic diuresis, salt-wasting nephropathies
    2. Increased secretion of potassium
      a. Mineralocorticoid excess: primary hyperaldosteronism, secondary hyperaldosteronism (malignant hypertension, renin-secreting tumors, renal artery stenosis, hypovolemia), apparent mineralocorticoid excess (licorice, chewing tobacco, carbenoxolone), congenital adrenal hyperplasia, Cushing's syndrome, Bartter's syndrome
      b. Distal delivery of non-reabsorbed anions: vomiting, nasogastric suction, proximal (type 2) renal tubular acidosis, diabetic ketoacidosis, glue-sniffing (toluene abuse), penicillin derivatives
      c. Other: amphotericin B, Liddle's syndrome, hypomagnesemia

---

result of net K^+ reabsorption in the distal nephron. With the exception of the urban poor and certain cultural groups, the amount of K^+ in the diet almost always exceeds that excreted in the urine. However, dietary K^+ restriction may exacerbate the hypokalemia secondary to increased gastrointestinal or renal loss. An unusual cause of decreased K^+ intake is ingestion of clay (geophagia), which binds dietary K^+ and iron. This custom was previously common among African Americans in the American South.

Redistribution into Cells Movement of K^+ into cells may transiently decrease the plasma K^+ concentration without altering total body K^+ content. For any given cause, the magnitude of the change is relatively small, often less than 1 mmol/L. However, a combination of factors may lead to a significant fall in the plasma K^+ concentration and may amplify the hypokalemia due to K^+ wasting. Metabolic alkalosis is often associated with hypokalemia. This occurs as a result of K^+ redistribution as well as excessive renal K^+ loss. Treatment of diabetic ketoacidosis with insulin may lead to hypokalemia due to stimulation of the Na^+-H^+ antiporter and (secondarily) the Na^+, K^+-ATPase pump. Furthermore, uncontrolled hyperglycemia often leads to K^+ depletion from an osmotic diuresis (see below). Stress-induced catecholamine release and administration of β_2-adrenergic agonists directly induce cellular uptake of K^+ and promote insulin secretion by pancreatic islet β cells. *Hypokalemic periodic paralysis* is a rare condition characterized by recurrent episodic weakness or paralysis (Chap. 367). Since K^+ is the major ICF cation, anabolic states can potentially result in hypokalemia due to a K^+ shift into cells. This may occur following rapid cell growth seen in patients with pernicious anemia treated with vitamin B_{12} or with neutropenia after treatment with granulocyte-macrophage colony stimulating factor. Massive transfusion with thawed washed red blood cells (RBCs) could cause hypokalemia since frozen RBCs lose up to half of their K^+ during storage.

Nonrenal Loss of Potassium Excessive sweating may result in K^+ depletion from increased integumentary and renal K^+ loss. Hyperaldosteronism, secondary to ECF volume contraction, enhances K^+ excretion in the urine (Chap. 321). Normally, K^+ lost in the stool amounts to 5 to 10 mmol/d in a volume of 100 to 200 mL. Hypokalemia subsequent to increased gastrointestinal loss can occur in patients with profuse diarrhea (usually secretory), villous adenomas, VIPomas, or laxative abuse. However, the loss of gastric secretions does not account for the moderate to severe K^+ depletion often associated with vomiting or nasogastric suction. Since the K^+ concentration of gastric fluid is 5 to 10 mmol/L, it would take 30 to 80 L of vomitus to achieve a K^+ deficit of 300 to 400 mmol typically seen in these patients. In fact, the hypokalemia is primarily due to increased renal K^+ excretion. Loss of gastric contents results in volume depletion and metabolic alkalosis, both of which promote kaliuresis. Hypovolemia stimulates aldosterone release, which augments K^+ secretion by the principal cells. In addition, the filtered load of HCO_3^- exceeds the reabsorptive capacity of the proximal convoluted tubule, thereby increasing distal delivery of $NaHCO_3$, which enhances the electrochemical gradient favoring K^+ loss in the urine.

Renal Loss of Potassium (See also Chap. 321) In general, most cases of chronic hypokalemia are due to renal K^+ wasting. This may be due to factors that increase the K^+ concentration in the lumen of the CCD or augment distal flow rate. Mineralocorticoid excess commonly results in hypokalemia. *Primary hyperaldosteronism* is due to dysregulated aldosterone secretion by an adrenal adenoma (Conn's syndrome) or carcinoma or to adrenocortical hyperplasia. In a rare subset of patients, the disorder is familial (autosomal dominant) and aldosterone levels can be suppressed by administering low doses of exogenous glucocorticoid. The molecular defect responsible for *glucocorticoid-remediable hyperaldosteronism* is a rearranged gene (due to a chromosomal crossover), containing the 5'-regulatory region of the 11β-hydroxylase gene and the coding sequence of the aldosterone synthase gene. Consequently, mineralocorticoid is synthesized in the zona fasciculata and regulated by corticotropin. A number of conditions associated with hyperreninemia result in secondary hyperaldosteronism and renal K^+ wasting. High renin levels are commonly seen in both renovascular and malignant hypertension. Renin-secreting tumors of the juxtaglomerular apparatus are a rare cause of hypokalemia. Other tumors that have been reported to produce renin include renal cell carcinoma, ovarian carcinoma, and Wilms' tumor. Hyperreninemia may also occur secondary to decreased effective circulating arterial volume.

In the absence of elevated renin or aldosterone levels, enhanced distal nephron secretion of K^+ may result from increased production of non-aldosterone mineralocorticoids in *congenital adrenal hyperplasia*. Glucocorticoid-stimulated kaliuresis does not normally occur due to the conversion of cortisol to cortisone by 11β-hydroxysteroid dehydrogenase (11β-HSDH). Therefore, 11β-HSDH deficiency or suppression allows cortisol to bind to the aldosterone receptor and leads to the *syndrome of apparent mineralocorticoid excess*. Drugs that inhibit the activity of 11β-HSDH include glycyrrhetinic acid, present in licorice, chewing tobacco, and carbenoxolone. The presentation of Cushing's syndrome may include hypokalemia if the capacity of 11β-HSDH to inactivate cortisol is overwhelmed by persistently elevated glucocorticoid levels.

Liddle's syndrome is a rare familial (autosomal dominant) disease characterized by hypertension, hypokalemic metabolic alkalosis, renal K^+ wasting, and suppressed renin and aldosterone secretion. Increased distal delivery of Na^+ with a non-reabsorbable anion (not Cl^-) enhances K^+ secretion. Classically, this is seen with *proximal (type 2) renal tubular acidosis* (RTA) and vomiting, associated with bicarbonaturia. Diabetic ketoacidosis and toluene abuse (glue-sniffing) can lead to increased delivery of β-hydroxybutyrate and hippurate, respectively, to the CCD and to renal K^+ loss. High doses of penicillin derivatives administered to volume-depleted patients may likewise promote renal K^+ secretion as well as an osmotic diuresis. *Classic distal (type 1) RTA* is associated with hypokalemia due to increased renal K^+ loss, the mechanism of which is uncertain. Amphotericin B causes hypokalemia due to increased distal nephron permeability to Na^+ and K^+ and to renal K^+ wasting.

Bartter's syndrome is a disorder characterized by hypokalemia, metabolic alkalosis, hyperreninemic hyperaldosteronism secondary to ECF volume contraction, and juxtaglomerular apparatus hyperplasia. Finally, diuretic use and abuse are common causes of K^+ depletion. Carbonic anhydrase inhibitors, loop diuretics, and thiazides are all kaliuretic. The degree of hypokalemia tends to be greater with long-acting agents and is dose-dependent. Increased renal K^+ excretion is due primarily to increased distal solute delivery and secondary hyperaldosteronism (due to volume depletion).

CLINICAL FEATURES   The clinical manifestations of K^+ depletion vary greatly between individual patients, and their severity depends on the degree of hypokalemia. Symptoms seldom occur unless the plasma K^+ concentration is less than 3 mmol/L. Fatigue, myalgia, and muscular weakness of the lower extremities are common complaints and are due to a lower (more negative) resting membrane potential. More severe hypokalemia may lead to progressive weakness, hypoventilation (due to respiratory muscle involvement), and eventually complete paralysis. Impaired muscle metabolism and the blunted hyperemic response to exercise associated with profound K^+ depletion increase the risk of rhabdomyolysis. Smooth-muscle function may also be affected and manifest as paralytic ileus.

The electrocardiographic changes of hypokalemia (Fig. 210-17) are due to delayed ventricular repolarization and do not correlate well with the plasma K^+ concentration. Early changes include flattening or inversion of the T wave, a prominent U wave, ST-segment depression, and a prolonged QU interval. Severe K^+ depletion may result in a prolonged PR interval, decreased voltage and widening of the QRS complex, and an increased risk of ventricular arrhythmias, especially in patients with myocardial ischemia or left ventricular hypertrophy. Hypokalemia may also predispose to digitalis toxicity. Hypokalemia is often associated with acid-base disturbances related to the underlying disorder. In addition, K^+ depletion results in intracellular acidification and an increase in net acid excretion or new HCO_3^- production. This is a consequence of enhanced proximal HCO_3^- reabsorption, increased renal ammoniagenesis, and increased distal H^+ secretion. This contributes to the generation of metabolic alkalosis frequently present in hypokalemic patients. NDI (see above) is not uncommonly seen in K^+ depletion and is manifest as polydipsia and polyuria. Glucose intolerance may also occur with hypokalemia and has been attributed to either impaired insulin secretion or peripheral insulin resistance.

DIAGNOSIS (Fig. 41-3)   In most cases, the etiology of K^+ depletion can be determined by a careful history. Diuretic and laxative abuse as well as surreptitious vomiting may be difficult to identify but should be excluded. Rarely, patients with a marked leukocytosis (e.g., acute myeloid leukemia) and normokalemia may have a low measured plasma K^+ concentration due to white blood cell uptake of K^+ at room temperature. This *pseudohypokalemia* can be avoided by storing the blood sample on ice or rapidly separating the plasma (or serum) from the cells.

After eliminating decreased intake and intracellular shift as potential causes of hypokalemia, examination of the renal response can help to clarify the source of K^+ loss. The appropriate response to K^+ depletion is to excrete less than 15 mmol/d of K^+ in the urine, due to increased reabsorption and decreased distal secretion. Hypokalemia with minimal renal K^+ excretion suggests that K^+ was lost via the skin or gastrointestinal tract or that there is a remote history of vomiting or diuretic use. As described above, renal K^+ wasting may be due to factors that either increase the K^+ concentration in the CCD or increase the distal flow rate (or both). The ECF volume status, blood pressure,

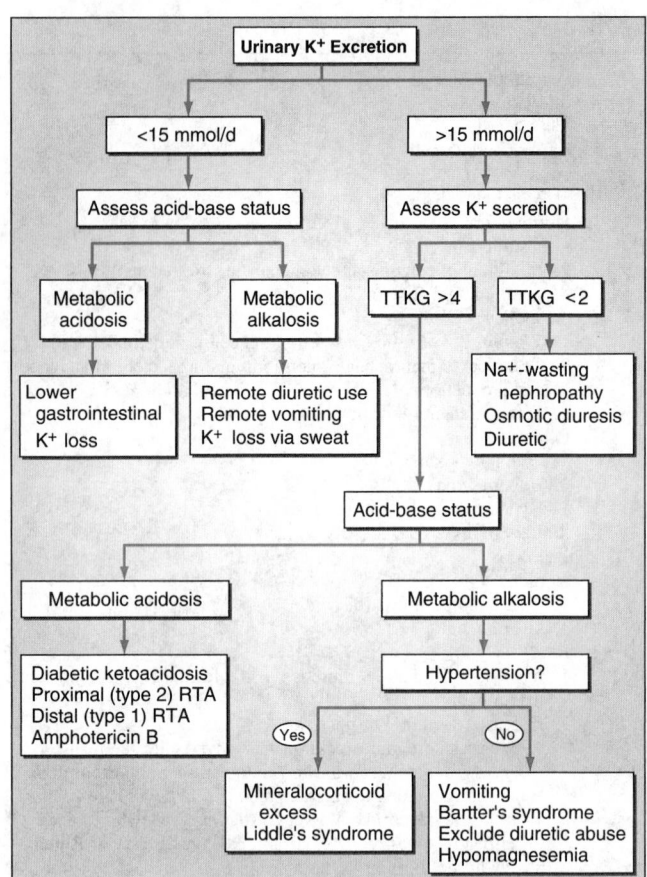

FIGURE 41-3   Algorithm depicting clinical approach to hypokalemia. TTKG, transtubular K^+ concentration gradient; RTA, renal tubular acidosis.

and associated acid-base disorder may help to differentiate the causes of excessive renal K^+ loss. A rapid and simple test designed to evaluate the driving force for net K^+ secretion is the *transtubular K^+ concentration gradient* (TTKG). The TTKG is the ratio of the K^+ concentration in the lumen of the CCD ($[K^+]_{CCD}$) to that in peritubular capillaries or plasma ($[K^+]_P$). The validity of this measurement depends on three assumptions: (1) few solutes are reabsorbed in the medullary collecting duct (MCD), (2) K^+ is neither secreted nor reabsorbed in the MCD, and (3) the osmolality of the fluid in the terminal CCD is known. Significant reabsorption or secretion of K^+ in the MCD seldom occurs, except in profound K^+ depletion or excess, respectively. When AVP is acting ($OSM_U \geq OSM_P$), the osmolality in the terminal CCD is the same as that of plasma, and the K^+ concentration in the lumen of the distal nephron can be estimated by dividing the urine K^+ concentration ($[K^+]_U$) by the ratio of the urine to plasma osmolality (OSM_U/OSM_P):

$$[K^+]_{CCD} = [K^+]_U \div (OSM_U/OSM_P)$$

$$TTKG = \frac{[K^+]_{CCD}}{[K^+]_P} = \frac{[K^+]_U \div (OSM_U/OSM_P)}{[K^+]_P}$$

Hypokalemia with a TTKG greater than 4 suggests renal K^+ loss due to increased distal K^+ secretion. Plasma renin and aldosterone levels are often helpful in differentiating the various causes of hyperaldosteronism. Bicarbonaturia and the presence of other non-reabsorbed anions also increase the TTKG and lead to renal K^+-wasting.

℞ **TREATMENT**

The therapeutic goals are to correct the K^+ deficit and to minimize ongoing losses. With the exception of periodic paralysis, hypokalemia resulting from transcellular shifts rarely requires intravenous K^+ supplementation, which can lead to rebound hyperkalemia. It is generally safer to correct hypokalemia via the oral route. The degree of K^+ depletion does not correlate well with the plasma K^+ concentration. A decrement of 1 mmol/L in the plasma K^+ concentration (from 4.0 to 3.0 mmol/L) may represent a total body K^+ deficit of 200 to 400 mmol, and patients with plasma levels under 3.0 mmol/L often require in excess of 600 mmol of K^+ to correct the deficit. Furthermore, factors promoting K^+ shift out of cells (e.g., insulin deficiency in diabetic ketoacidosis) may result in underestimation of the K^+ deficit. Therefore, the plasma K^+ concentration should be monitored frequently when assessing the response to treatment. Potassium chloride is usually the preparation of choice and will promote more rapid correction of hypokalemia and metabolic alkalosis. Potassium bicarbonate and citrate (metabolized to HCO_3^-) tend to alkalinize the patient and would be more appropriate for hypokalemia associated with chronic diarrhea or RTA.

Patients with severe hypokalemia or those unable to take anything by mouth require intravenous replacement therapy with KCl. The maximum concentration of administered K^+ should be no more than 40 mmol/L via a peripheral vein or 60 mmol/L via a central vein. The rate of infusion should not exceed 20 mmol/h unless paralysis or malignant ventricular arrhythmias are present. Ideally, KCl should be mixed in normal saline since dextrose solutions may initially exacerbate hypokalemia due to insulin-mediated movement of K^+ into cells. Rapid intravenous administration of K^+ should be used judiciously and requires close observation of the clinical manifestations of hypokalemia (electrocardiogram and neuromuscular examination).

HYPERKALEMIA

ETIOLOGY Hyperkalemia, defined as a plasma K^+ concentration >5.0 mmol/L, occurs as a result of either K^+ release from cells or decreased renal loss. Increased K^+ intake is rarely the sole cause of hyperkalemia since the phenomenon of *potassium adaptation* ensures rapid K^+ excretion in response to increases in dietary consumption. Iatrogenic hyperkalemia may result from overzealous parenteral K^+ replacement or in patients with renal insufficiency. *Pseudohyperkalemia* represents an artificially elevated plasma K^+ concentration due to K^+ movement out of cells immediately prior to or following venipuncture. Contributing factors include prolonged use of a tourniquet with or without repeated fist clenching, hemolysis, and marked leukocytosis or thrombocytosis. The latter two result in an elevated serum K^+ concentration due to release of intracellular K^+ following clot formation. Pseudohyperkalemia should be suspected in an otherwise asymptomatic patient with no obvious underlying cause. If proper venipuncture technique is used and a plasma (not serum) K^+ concentration is measured, it should be normal. Intravascular hemolysis, tumor lysis syndrome, and rhabdomyolysis all lead to K^+ release from cells as a result of tissue breakdown.

Metabolic acidoses, with the exception of those due to the accumulation of organic anions, can be associated with mild hyperkalemia resulting from intracellular buffering of H^+ (see above). Insulin deficiency and hypertonicity (e.g., hyperglycemia) promote K^+ shift from the ICF to the ECF. The severity of exercise-induced hyperkalemia is related to the degree of exertion. It is due to release of K^+ from muscles and is usually rapidly reversible, often associated with rebound hypokalemia. Treatment with beta blockers rarely causes hyperkalemia but may contribute to the elevation in plasma K^+ concentration seen with other conditions. *Hyperkalemic periodic paralysis* (Chap. 367) is a rare autosomal dominant disorder characterized by episodic weakness or paralysis, precipitated by stimuli that normally lead to mild hyperkalemia (e.g., exercise). The genetic defect appears to be a single amino acid substitution due to a mutation in the gene for the skeletal muscle Na^+ channel. Hyperkalemia may occur with severe digitalis toxicity due to inhibition of the Na^+,K^+-ATPase pump. Depolarizing muscle relaxants such as succinylcholine can increase the plasma K^+ concentration, especially in patients with massive trauma, burns, or neuromuscular disease.

Chronic hyperkalemia is virtually always associated with decreased renal K^+ excretion due to either impaired secretion or diminished distal solute delivery (Table 41-4). The latter is seldom the only cause of impaired K^+ excretion but may significantly contribute to hyperkale-

TABLE 41-4 *Causes of Hyperkalemia*

  I. Renal failure
 II. Decreased distal flow (i.e., decreased effective circulating arterial volume)
III. Decreased K^+ secretion
   A. Impaired Na^+ reabsorption
     1. Primary hypoaldosteronism: adrenal insufficiency, adrenal enzyme deficiency (21-hydroxylase, 3β-hydroxysteroid dehydrogenase, corticosterone methyl oxidase)
     2. Secondary hypoaldosteronism: hyporeninemia, drugs (ACE inhibitors, NSAIDs, heparin)
     3. Resistance to aldosterone: pseudohypoaldosteronism, tubulointerstitial disease, drugs (K^+-sparing diuretics, trimethoprim, pentamidine)
   B. Enhanced Cl^- reabsorption (chloride shunt)
     1. Gordon's syndrome
     2. Cyclosporine

Note: ACE, angiotensin-converting enzyme; NSAIDs, nonsteroidal anti-inflammatory drugs.

mia in protein-malnourished (low urea excretion) and ECF volume–contracted (decreased distal NaCl delivery) patients. Decreased K^+ secretion by the principal cells results from either impaired Na^+ reabsorption or increased Cl^- reabsorption.

Hyporeninemic hypoaldosteronism is a syndrome characterized by euvolemia or ECF volume expansion and suppressed renin and aldosterone levels (Chaps. 321 and 323). This disorder is commonly seen in mild renal insufficiency, diabetic nephropathy, or chronic tubulointerstitial disease. Patients frequently have an impaired kaliuretic response to exogenous mineralocorticoid administration, suggesting that enhanced distal Cl^- reabsorption (electroneutral Na^+ reabsorption) may account for many of the findings of hyporeninemic hypoaldosteronism. NSAIDs inhibit renin secretion and the synthesis of vasodilatory renal prostaglandins. The resultant decrease in GFR and K^+ secretion is often manifest as hyperkalemia. As a rule, the degree of hyperkalemia due to hypoaldosteronism is mild in the absence of increased K^+ intake or renal dysfunction.

Angiotensin-converting enzyme (ACE) inhibitors block the conversion of angiotensin I to angiotensin II. Angiotensin receptor antagonists directly inhibit the actions of angiotensin II on AT1 angiotensin II receptors. The actions of both of these classes of drugs result in impaired aldosterone release. Patients at increased risk of ACE inhibitor or angiotensin receptor antagonist–induced hyperkalemia include those with diabetes mellitus, renal insufficiency, decreased effective circulating arterial volume, bilateral renal artery stenosis, or concurrent use of K^+-sparing diuretics or NSAIDs.

Decreased aldosterone synthesis may be due to *primary adrenal insufficiency* (Addison's disease) or congenital adrenal enzyme deficiency (Chap. 321). Heparin (including low-molecular-weight heparin) inhibits production of aldosterone by the cells of the zona glomerulosa and can lead to severe hyperkalemia in a subset of patients with underlying renal disease, diabetes mellitus, or those receiving K^+-sparing diuretics, ACE inhibitors, or NSAIDs. *Pseudohypoaldosteronism* is a rare familial disorder characterized by hyperkalemia, metabolic acidosis, renal Na^+ wasting, hypotension, high renin and aldosterone levels, and end-organ resistance to aldosterone. The gene encoding the mineralocorticoid receptor is normal in these patients, and the electrolyte abnormalities can be reversed with suprapharmacologic doses of an exogenous mineralocorticoid (e.g., 9α-fludrocortisone) or an inhibitor of 11β-HSDH (e.g., carbenoxolone). The kaliuretic response to aldosterone is impaired by K^+-sparing diuretics. Spironolactone is a competitive mineralocorticoid antagonist, whereas amiloride and triamterene block the apical Na^+ channel of the principal cell. Two other drugs that impair K^+ secretion by blocking distal nephron Na^+ reabsorption are trimethoprim and pentamidine. These antimicrobial agents may contribute to the hyperkalemia often seen in patients infected with HIV who are being treated for *Pneumocystis carinii* pneumonia.

Hyperkalemia frequently complicates acute oliguric renal failure due to increased K^+ release from cells (acidosis, catabolism) and decreased excretion. Increased distal flow rate and K^+ secretion per nephron compensate for decreased renal mass in chronic renal insufficiency. However, these adaptive mechanisms eventually fail to maintain K^+ balance when the GFR falls below 10 to 15 mL/min or oliguria ensues. Otherwise asymptomatic urinary tract obstruction is an often overlooked cause of hyperkalemia. Other nephropathies associated with impaired K^+ excretion include drug-induced interstitial nephritis, lupus nephritis, sickle cell disease, and diabetic nephropathy.

Gordon's syndrome is a rare condition characterized by hyperkalemia, metabolic acidosis, and a normal GFR. These patients are usually volume-expanded with suppressed renin and aldosterone levels as well as refractory to the kaliuretic effect of exogenous mineralocorticoids. It has been suggested that these findings could all be accounted for by increased distal Cl^- reabsorption (electroneutral Na^+ reabsorption), also referred to as a *Cl^- shunt*. A similar mechanism may be partially responsible for the hyperkalemia associated with cyclosporine nephrotoxicity. *Hyperkalemic distal (type 4) RTA* may be due to either hypoaldosteronism or a Cl^- shunt (aldosterone-resistant).

CLINICAL FEATURES Since the resting membrane potential is related to the ratio of the ICF to ECF K^+ concentration, hyperkalemia partially depolarizes the cell membrane. Prolonged depolarization impairs membrane excitability and is manifest as weakness, which may progress to flaccid paralysis and hypoventilation if the respiratory muscles are involved. Hyperkalemia also inhibits renal ammoniagenesis and reabsorption of NH_4^+ in the thick ascending limb of the loop of Henle. Thus, net acid excretion is impaired and results in metabolic acidosis, which may further exacerbate the hyperkalemia due to K^+ movement out of cells.

The most serious effect of hyperkalemia is cardiac toxicity, which does not correlate well with the plasma K^+ concentration. The earliest electrocardiographic changes include increased T-wave amplitude, or peaked T waves. More severe degrees of hyperkalemia result in a prolonged PR interval and QRS duration, atrioventricular conduction delay, and loss of P waves. Progressive widening of the QRS complex and merging with the T wave produces a sine wave pattern. The terminal event is usually ventricular fibrillation or asystole.

DIAGNOSIS (Fig. 41-4) With rare exceptions, chronic hyperkalemia is always due to impaired K^+ excretion. If the etiology is not readily apparent and the patient is asymptomatic, pseudohyperkalemia should be excluded, as described above. Oliguric acute renal failure and severe chronic renal insufficiency should also be ruled out. The history should focus on medications that impair K^+ handling and potential sources of K^+ intake. Evaluation of the ECF compartment, effective circulating volume, and urine output are essential components of the physical examination. The severity of hyperkalemia is determined by the symptoms, plasma K^+ concentration, and electrocardiographic abnormalities.

The appropriate renal response to hyperkalemia is to excrete at least 200 mmol of K^+ daily. In most cases, diminished renal K^+ loss is due to impaired K^+ secretion, which can be assessed by measuring the transtubular K^+ concentration gradient (TTKG). A TTKG <10 implies a decreased driving force for K^+ secretion due to either hypoaldosteronism or resistance to the renal effects of mineralocorticoid. This can be determined by evaluating the kaliuretic response to administration of mineralocorticoid (e.g., 9α-fludrocortisone). Primary adrenal insufficiency can be differentiated from hyporeninemic hypoaldosteronism by examining the renin-aldosterone axis. Renin and aldosterone levels should be measured in the supine and upright positions, following three days of Na^+ restriction (Na^+ intake <10 mmol/d) in combination with a loop diuretic to induce mild volume contraction. Aldosterone-resistant hyperkalemia can result from the various causes of impaired distal Na^+ reabsorption or from a Cl^- shunt. The former leads to salt wasting, ECF volume contraction, and high renin

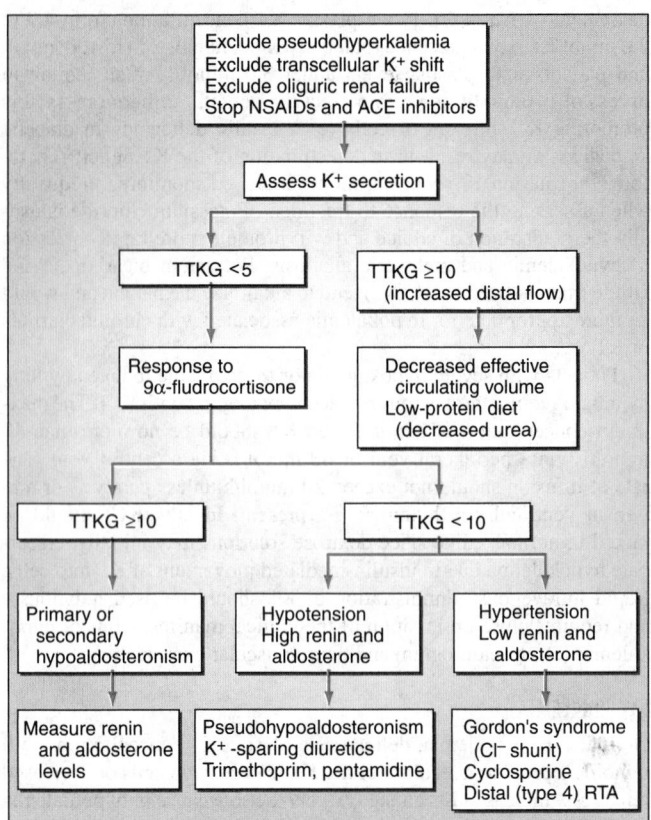

FIGURE 41-4 Algorithm depicting clinical approach to hyperkalemia. NSAID, nonsteroidal anti-inflammatory drug; ACE, angiotensin-converting enzyme; RTA, renal tubular acidosis; TTKG, transtubular K^+ concentration gradient.

and aldosterone levels. In contrast, enhanced distal Cl^- reabsorption is associated with volume expansion and suppressed renin and aldosterone secretion. As mentioned above, hypoaldosteronism seldom causes severe hyperkalemia in the absence of increased dietary K^+ intake, renal insufficiency, transcellular K^+ shifts, or antikaliuretic drugs.

TREATMENT

The approach to therapy depends on the degree of hyperkalemia as determined by the plasma K^+ concentration, associated muscular weakness, and changes on the electrocardiogram. Potentially fatal hyperkalemia rarely occurs unless the plasma K^+ concentration exceeds 7.5 mmol/L and is usually associated with profound weakness and absent P waves, QRS widening, or ventricular arrhythmias on the electrocardiogram.

Severe hyperkalemia requires emergent treatment directed at minimizing membrane depolarization, shifting K^+ into cells, and promoting K^+ loss. In addition, exogenous K^+ intake and antikaliuretic drugs should be discontinued. Administration of calcium gluconate decreases membrane excitability. The usual dose is 10 mL of a 10% solution infused over 2 to 3 min. The effect begins within minutes but is short-lived (30 to 60 min), and the dose can be repeated if no change in the electrocardiogram is seen after 5 to 10 min. Insulin causes K^+ to shift into cells by mechanisms described previously and will temporarily lower the plasma K^+ concentration. Although glucose alone will stimulate insulin release from normal pancreatic β cells, a more rapid response generally occurs when exogenous insulin is administered (with glucose to prevent hypoglycemia). A commonly recommended combination is 10 to 20 units of regular insulin and 25 to 50 g of glucose. Obviously, hyperglycemic patients should not be given glucose. If effective, the plasma K^+ concentration will fall by 0.5 to 1.5 mmol/L in 15 to 30 min and the effect will last for several hours. Alkali therapy with intravenous $NaHCO_3$ can also shift K^+ into cells. This is safest when administered as an isotonic solution of 3 ampules per liter (134 mmol/L NaHCO₃) and ideally should be reserved for severe hyperkalemia associated with metabolic acidosis. Patients with end-stage renal disease seldom respond to this intervention and may not tolerate the Na^+ load and resultant volume expansion. When administered parenterally or in nebulized form, β_2-adrenergic agonists promote cellular uptake of K^+ (see above). The onset of action is 30 min, lowering the plasma K^+ concentration by 0.5 to 1.5 mmol/L, and the effect lasts 2 to 4 h.

Removal of K^+ can be achieved using diuretics, cation-exchange resin, or dialysis. Loop and thiazide diuretics, often in combination, may enhance K^+ excretion if renal function is adequate. Sodium polystyrene sulfonate is a cation-exchange resin that promotes the exchange of Na^+ for K^+ in the gastrointestinal tract. Each gram binds 1 mmol of K^+ and releases 2 to 3 mmol of Na^+. When given by mouth, the usual dose is 25 to 50 g mixed with 100 mL of 20% sorbitol to prevent constipation. This will generally lower the plasma K^+ concentration by 0.5 to 1.0 mmol/L within 1 to 2 h and last for 4 to 6 h. Sodium polystyrene sulfonate can also be administered as a retention enema consisting of 50 g of resin and 50 mL of 70% sorbitol mixed in 150 mL of tap water. The sorbitol should be omitted from the enema in postoperative patients due to the increased incidence of sorbitol-induced colonic necrosis, especially following renal transplantation. The most rapid and effective way of lowering the plasma K^+ concentration is hemodialysis. This should be reserved for patients with renal failure and those with severe life-threatening hyperkalemia unresponsive to more conservative measures. Peritoneal dialysis also removes K^+ but is only 15 to 20% as effective as hemodialysis. Finally, the underlying cause of the hyperkalemia should be treated. This may involve dietary modification, correction of metabolic acidosis, cautious volume expansion, and administration of exogenous mineralocorticoid.

FURTHER READING

ADROGUE HJ, MADIAS NE: Hypernatremia. N Engl J Med 342:1493, 2000

ADROGUE HJ, MADIAS NE: Hyponatremia. N Engl J Med 342:1581, 2000

BERL T, VERBALIS J: Pathophysiology of water metabolism, in BM Brenner (ed): *Brenner & Rector's The Kidney*, 7th ed. Philadelphia, Saunders, 2004, pp 857–920

COHN JN et al: New guidelines for potassium replacement in clinical practice: A contemporary review by the National Council on Potassium in Clinical Practice. Arch Intern Med 160:2429, 2000

GOLDSZMIDT MA, ILIESCU EA: DDAVP to prevent rapid correction in hyponatremia. Clin Nephrol 53:226, 2000

GROSS P: Treatment of severe hyponatremia. Kidney Int 60:2417, 2001

HARRIGAN MR: Cerebral salt wasting syndrome. Crit Care Clin 17:125, 2001

MOUNT DB: Disorders of potassium balance, in BM Brenner (ed): *Brenner & Rector's The Kidney*, 7th ed. Philadelphia, Saunders, 2004, pp 997–1040

NIELSEN S et al: Aquaporins in the kidney: From molecules to medicine. Physiol Rev 82:205, 2002

WARNOCK DG: Genetic forms of renal potassium and magnesium wasting. Am J Med 112:235, 2002

42 ACIDOSIS AND ALKALOSIS
Thomas D. DuBose, Jr.

NORMAL ACID-BASE HOMEOSTASIS

Systemic arterial pH is maintained between 7.35 and 7.45 by extracellular and intracellular chemical buffering together with respiratory and renal regulatory mechanisms. The control of arterial CO_2 tension (Pa_{CO_2}) by the central nervous system and respiratory systems and the control of the plasma bicarbonate by the kidneys stabilize the arterial pH by excretion or retention of acid or alkali. The metabolic and respiratory components that regulate systemic pH are described by the Henderson-Hasselbalch equation:

$$pH = 6.1 + \log \frac{HCO_3^-}{Pa_{CO_2} \times 0.0301}$$

Under most circumstances, CO_2 production and excretion are matched, and the usual steady-state Pa_{CO_2} is maintained at 40 mmHg. Underexcretion of CO_2 produces hypercapnia, and overexcretion causes hypocapnia. Nevertheless, production and excretion are again matched at a new steady-state Pa_{CO_2}. Therefore, the Pa_{CO_2} is regulated primarily by neural respiratory factors (Chap. 246) and is not subject to regulation by the rate of CO_2 production. Hypercapnia is usually the result of hypoventilation rather than of increased CO_2 production. Increases or decreases in Pa_{CO_2} represent derangements of neural respiratory control or are due to compensatory changes in response to a primary alteration in the plasma $[HCO_3^-]$.

Primary changes in Pa_{CO_2} can cause acidosis or alkalosis, depending on whether Pa_{CO_2} is above or below the normal value of 40 mmHg (respiratory acidosis or alkalosis, respectively). Primary alteration of Pa_{CO_2} evokes cellular buffering and renal adaptation, a slow process that becomes more efficient with time. A primary change in the plasma $[HCO_3^-]$ as a result of metabolic or renal factors results in compensatory changes in ventilation that blunt the changes in blood pH that would occur otherwise. Such respiratory alterations are referred to as *secondary*, or compensatory, changes, since they occur in response to primary metabolic changes.

The kidneys regulate plasma $[HCO_3^-]$ through three main processes: (1) "reabsorption" of filtered HCO_3^-, (2) formation of titratable acid, and (3) excretion of NH_4^+ in the urine. The kidney filters approximately 4000 mmol of HCO_3^- per day. To reabsorb the filtered load of HCO_3^-, the renal tubules must therefore secrete 4000 mmol of hydrogen ions. Between 80 and 90% of HCO_3^- is reabsorbed in the proximal tubule. The distal nephron reabsorbs the remainder and secretes protons, as generated from metabolism, to defend systemic pH. While this quantity of protons, 40 to 60 mmol/d, is small, it must be secreted to prevent chronic positive H^+ balance and metabolic acidosis. This quantity of secreted protons is represented in the urine as titratable acid and NH_4^+. Metabolic acidosis in the face of normal renal function increases NH_4^+ production and excretion. NH_4^+ production and excretion are impaired in chronic renal failure, hyperkalemia, and renal tubular acidosis.

In sum, these regulatory responses, including chemical buffering, the regulation of Pa_{CO_2} by the respiratory system, and the regulation of $[HCO_3^-]$ by the kidneys, act in concert to maintain a systemic arterial pH between 7.35 and 7.45.

DIAGNOSIS OF GENERAL TYPES OF DISTURBANCES

The most common clinical disturbances are simple acid-base disorders, i.e., metabolic acidosis or alkalosis or respiratory acidosis or alkalosis. Since compensation is not complete, the pH is abnormal in simple disturbances. More complicated clinical situations can give rise to mixed acid-base disturbances.

SIMPLE ACID-BASE DISORDERS Primary respiratory disturbances (primary changes in Pa_{CO_2}) invoke compensatory metabolic responses (secondary changes in $[HCO_3^-]$), and primary metabolic disturbances elicit predictable compensatory respiratory responses. Physiologic compensation can be predicted from the relationships displayed in Table 42-1. Primary changes in Pa_{CO_2} or $[HCO_3^-]$ alter systemic pH and cause acidosis or alkalosis. To illustrate, metabolic acidosis due to an increase in endogenous acids (e.g., ketoacidosis) lowers extracellular fluid $[HCO_3^-]$ and decreases extracellular pH. This stimulates the medullary chemoreceptors to increase ventilation and to return the ratio of $[HCO_3^-]$ to Pa_{CO_2}, and thus pH, toward normal, although not to normal. The degree of respiratory compensation expected in a simple form of metabolic acidosis can be predicted from the relationship: $Pa_{CO_2} = (1.5 \times [HCO_3^-]) + 8$, i.e., the Pa_{CO_2} is expected to decrease 1.25 mmHg for each mmol per liter decrease in $[HCO_3^-]$. Thus, a patient

TABLE 42-1 *Prediction of Compensatory Responses on Simple Acid-Base Disturbances*

Disorder	Prediction of Compensation
Metabolic acidosis	$Pa_{CO_2} = (1.5 \times HCO_3^-) + 8$
	or
	Pa_{CO_2} will $\downarrow$ 1.25 mmHg per mmol/L $\downarrow$ in $[HCO_3^-]$
	or
	$Pa_{CO_2} = [HCO_3^-] + 15$
Metabolic alkalosis	Pa_{CO_2} will $\uparrow$ 0.75 mmHg per mmol/L $\uparrow$ in $[HCO_3^-]$
	or
	Pa_{CO_2} will $\uparrow$ 6 mmHg per 10 mmol/L $\uparrow$ in $[HCO_3^-]$
	or
	$Pa_{CO_2} = [HCO_3^-] + 15$
Respiratory alkalosis	
Acute	$[HCO_3^-]$ will $\downarrow$ 2 mmol/L per 10 mmHg $\downarrow$ in Pa_{CO_2}
Chronic	$[HCO_3^-]$ will $\downarrow$ 4 mmol/L per 10 mmHg $\downarrow$ in Pa_{CO_2}
Respiratory acidosis	
Acute	$[HCO_3^-]$ will $\uparrow$ 1 mmol/L per 10 mmHg $\uparrow$ in Pa_{CO_2}
Chronic	$[HCO_3^-]$ will $\uparrow$ 4 mmol/L per 10 mmHg $\uparrow$ in Pa_{CO_2}

with metabolic acidosis and $[HCO_3^-]$ of 12 mmol/L would be expected to have a Pa_{CO_2} between 24 and 28 mmHg. Values for Pa_{CO_2} below 24 or greater than 28 mmHg define a mixed disturbance (metabolic acidosis and respiratory alkalosis or metabolic alkalosis and respiratory acidosis, respectively). Another way to judge the appropriateness of the response in $[HCO_3^-]$ or Pa_{CO_2} is to use an acid-base nomogram (Fig. 42-1). While the shaded areas of the nomogram show the 95% confidence limits for normal compensation in simple disturbances, finding acid-base values within the shaded area does not necessarily rule out a mixed disturbance. Imposition of one disorder over another may result in values lying within the area of a third. Thus, the nomogram, while convenient, is not a substitute for the equations in Table 42-1.

MIXED ACID-BASE DISORDERS Mixed acid-base disorders—defined as independently coexisting disorders, not merely compensatory responses—are often seen in patients in critical care units and can lead to dangerous extremes of pH. A patient with diabetic ketoacidosis (metabolic acidosis) may develop an independent respiratory problem leading to respiratory acidosis or alkalosis. Patients with underlying

pulmonary disease may not respond to metabolic acidosis with an appropriate ventilatory response because of insufficient respiratory reserve. Such imposition of respiratory acidosis on metabolic acidosis can lead to severe acidemia and a poor outcome. When metabolic acidosis and metabolic alkalosis coexist in the same patient, the pH may be normal or near normal. When the pH is normal, an elevated anion gap (see below) denotes the presence of a metabolic acidosis. A diabetic patient with ketoacidosis may have renal dysfunction resulting in simultaneous metabolic acidosis. Patients who have ingested an overdose of drug combinations such as sedatives and salicylates may have mixed disturbances as a result of the acid-base response to the individual drugs (metabolic acidosis mixed with respiratory acidosis or respiratory alkalosis, respectively). Even more complex are triple acid-base disturbances. For example, patients with metabolic acidosis due to alcoholic ketoacidosis may develop metabolic alkalosis due to vomiting and superimposed respiratory alkalosis due to the hyperventilation of hepatic dysfunction or alcohol withdrawal.

DIAGNOSIS OF ACID-BASE DISORDERS A stepwise approach to the diagnosis of acid-base disorders follows and is summarized in Table 42-2. Care should be taken when measuring blood gases to obtain the arterial blood sample without using excessive heparin. In the determination of arterial blood gases by the clinical laboratory, both pH and Pa_{CO_2} are measured, and the $[HCO_3^-]$ is calculated from the Henderson-Hasselbalch equation. This calculated value should be compared with the measured $[HCO_3^-]$ (total CO_2) on the electrolyte panel. These two values should agree within 2 mmol/L. If they do not, the values may not have been drawn simultaneously, a laboratory error may be present, or an error could have been made in calculating the $[HCO_3^-]$. After verifying the blood acid-base values, one can then identify the precise acid-base disorder.

The most common causes of acid-base disorders should be kept in mind while probing the history for clues about the etiology. For example, established chronic renal failure is expected to cause a metabolic acidosis, and chronic vomiting frequently causes metabolic alkalosis. Patients with pneumonia, sepsis, or cardiac failure frequently have respiratory alkalosis, and patients with chronic obstructive pulmonary disease or a sedative drug overdose often display a respiratory acidosis. The drug history is important since loop or thiazide diuretics may cause metabolic alkalosis, and the carbonic anhydrase inhibitor acetazolamide can result in metabolic acidosis.

Blood for electrolytes and arterial blood gases should be drawn simultaneously prior to therapy, since an increase in $[HCO_3^-]$ occurs with metabolic alkalosis and respiratory acidosis. Conversely, a decrease in $[HCO_3^-]$ occurs in metabolic acidosis and respiratory alkalosis.

Metabolic acidosis leads to hyperkalemia as a result of cellular shifts in which H^+ is exchanged for K^+ or Na^+. For each decrease in blood pH of 0.10, the plasma $[K^+]$ should rise by 0.6 mmol/L. This relationship is not invariable. Diabetic ketoacidosis, lactic acidosis, diarrhea, and renal tubular acidosis (RTA) are often associated with potassium depletion because of urinary K^+ wasting.

Anion Gap All evaluations of acid-base disorders should include a simple calculation of the anion gap (AG); it represents those unmeasured anions in plasma (normally 10 to 12 mmol/L) and is calculated as

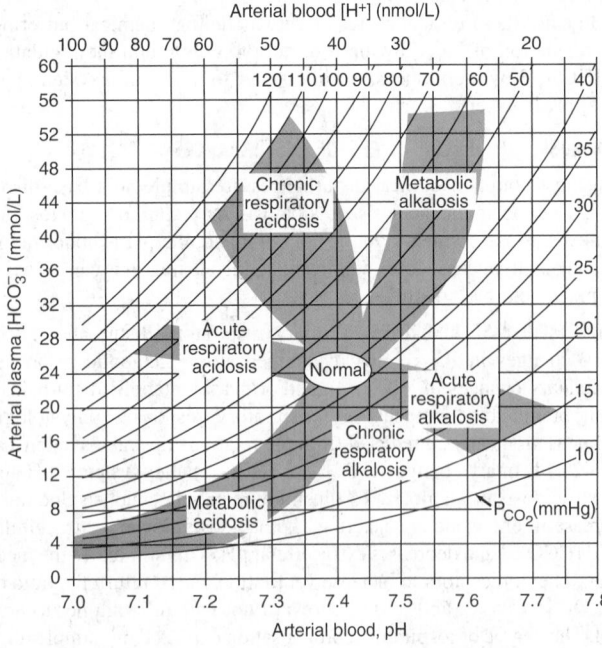

Arterial blood $[H^+]$ (nmol/L)

FIGURE 42-1 Acid-base nomogram. Shown are the 90% confidence limits of the normal respiratory and metabolic compensations for primary acid-base disturbances. *(From DuBose, used with permission.)*

TABLE 42-2 *Steps in Acid-Base Diagnosis*

1. Obtain arterial blood gases (ABGs) and electrolytes (lytes) simultaneously.
2. Compare $[HCO_3]$ on ABG and lytes to verify accuracy.
3. Calculate anion gap (AG).
4. Know four causes of high AG acidosis (ketoacidosis, lactic acid acidosis, renal failure, and toxins).
5. Know two causes of high hyperchloremic or nongap acidosis (bicarbonate loss from GI tract, renal tubular acidosis).
6. Estimate compensatory response (Table 42-1).
7. Compare ΔAG and ΔHCO_3^-.
8. Compare change in $[Cl^-]$ with change in $[Na^+]$.

follows: $AG = Na^+ - (Cl^- + HCO_3^-)$. The unmeasured anions include anionic proteins, phosphate, sulfate, and organic anions. When acid anions, such as acetoacetate and lactate, accumulate in extracellular fluid, the AG increases, causing a high-AG acidosis. An increase in the AG is most often due to an increase in unmeasured anions and less commonly is due to a decrease in unmeasured cations (calcium, magnesium, potassium). In addition, the AG may increase with an increase in anionic albumin, either because of increased albumin concentration or alkalosis, which alters albumin charge. A decrease in the AG can be due to (1) an increase in unmeasured cations; (2) the addition to the blood of abnormal cations, such as lithium (lithium intoxication) or cationic immunoglobulins (plasma cell dyscrasias); (3) a reduction in the major plasma anion albumin concentration (nephrotic syndrome); (4) a decrease in the effective anionic charge on albumin by acidosis; or (5) hyperviscosity and severe hyperlipidemia, which can lead to an underestimation of sodium and chloride concentrations. A fall in serum albumin by 1 g/dL from the normal value (4.5 g/dL) decreases the anion gap by 2.5 meq/L.

In the face of a normal serum albumin, a high AG is usually due to non-chloride-containing acids that contain inorganic (phosphate, sulfate), organic (ketoacids, lactate, uremic organic anions), exogenous (salicylate or ingested toxins with organic acid production), or unidentified anions. By definition, therefore, a high-AG acidosis has two identifying features: a low [HCO_3^-] and an elevated AG. The latter is present even if an additional acid-base disorder is superimposed to modify the [HCO_3^-] independently. Simultaneous metabolic acidosis of the high-AG variety plus either chronic respiratory acidosis or metabolic alkalosis represents such a situation in which [HCO_3^-] may be normal or even high. However, the AG is elevated, and [Cl^-] is depressed.

Similarly, normal values for [HCO_3^-], Pa_{CO_2}, and pH do not ensure the absence of an acid-base disturbance. For instance, an alcoholic who has been vomiting may develop a metabolic alkalosis with a pH of 7.55, Pa_{CO_2} of 48 mmHg, [HCO_3^-] of 40 mmol/L, [Na^+] of 135, [Cl^-] of 80, and [K^+] of 2.8. If such a patient were then to develop a superimposed alcoholic ketoacidosis with a β-hydroxybutyrate concentration of 15 mM, arterial pH would fall to 7.40, [HCO_3^-] to 25 mmol/L, and the Pa_{CO_2} to 40 mmHg. Although these blood gases are normal, the AG is elevated at 30 mmol/L, indicating a mixed metabolic alkalosis and metabolic acidosis.

METABOLIC ACIDOSIS

Metabolic acidosis can occur because of an increase in endogenous acid production (such as lactate and ketoacids), loss of bicarbonate (as in diarrhea), or accumulation of endogenous acids (as in renal failure). Metabolic acidosis has profound effects on the respiratory, cardiac, and nervous systems. The fall in blood pH is accompanied by a characteristic increase in ventilation, especially the tidal volume (Kussmaul respiration). Intrinsic cardiac contractility may be depressed, but inotropic function can be normal because of catecholamine release. Both peripheral arterial vasodilation and central venoconstriction can be present; the decrease in central and pulmonary vascular compliance predisposes to pulmonary edema with even minimal volume overload. Central nervous system function is depressed, with headache, lethargy, stupor, and, in some cases, even coma. Glucose intolerance may also occur.

There are two major categories of clinical metabolic acidosis: high-anion-gap (AG) and normal-AG, or hyperchloremic acidosis (Table 42-3 and Table 42-4).

TABLE 42-3 *Causes of High-Anion-Gap Metabolic Acidosis*

Lactic acidosis	Toxins
Ketoacidosis	Ethylene glycol
Diabetic	Methanol
Alcoholic	Salicylates
Starvation	Renal failure (acute and chronic)

TABLE 42-4 *Causes of Non-Anion-Gap Acidosis*

I. Gastrointestinal bicarbonate loss
  A. Diarrhea
  B. External pancreatic or small-bowel drainage
  C. Ureterosigmoidostomy, jejunal loop, ileal loop
  D. Drugs
    1. Calcium chloride (acidifying agent)
    2. Magnesium sulfate (diarrhea)
    3. Cholestyramine (bile acid diarrhea)
II. Renal acidosis
  A. Hypokalemia
    1. Proximal RTA (type 2)
    2. Distal (classic) RTA (type 1)
  B. Hyperkalemia
    1. Generalized distal nephron dysfunction (type 4 RTA)
      a. Mineralocorticoid deficiency
      b. Mineralocorticoid resistance
      c. ↓Na^+ delivery to distal nephron
      d. Tubulointerstitial disease
      e. Ammonium excretion defect
III. Drug-induced hyperkalemia (with renal insufficiency)
  A. Potassium-sparing diuretics (amiloride, triamterene, spironolactone)
  B. Trimethoprim
  C. Pentamidine
  D. Angiotensin-converting enzyme inhibitors and AT-II receptor blockers
  E. Nonsteroidal anti-inflammatory drugs
  F. Cyclosporine
IV. Other
  A. Acid loads (ammonium chloride, hyperalimentation)
  B. Loss of potential bicarbonate: ketosis with ketone excretion
  C. Expansion acidosis (rapid saline administration)
  D. Hippurate
  E. Cation exchange resins

Note: RTA, renal tubular acidosis; AT-II, angiotensin-II receptor blockers.

℞ TREATMENT

Treatment of metabolic acidosis with alkali should be reserved for severe acidemia except when the patient has no "potential HCO_3^-" in plasma. Potential [HCO_3^-] can be estimated from the increment (Δ) in the AG (ΔAG = patient's AG − 10). It must be determined if the acid anion in plasma is metabolizable (i.e., β-hydroxybutyrate, acetoacetate, and lactate) or nonmetabolizable (anions that accumulate in chronic renal failure and after toxin ingestion). The latter requires return of renal function to replenish the [HCO_3^-] deficit, a slow and often unpredictable process. Consequently, patients with a normal AG acidosis (hyperchloremic acidosis), a slightly elevated AG (mixed hyperchloremic and AG acidosis), or an AG attributable to a nonmetabolizable anion in the face of renal failure should receive alkali therapy, either orally ($NaHCO_3$ or Shohl's solution) or intravenously ($NaHCO_3$), in an amount necessary to slowly increase the plasma [HCO_3^-] into the 20 to 22 mmol/L range.

Controversy exists, however, in regard to the use of alkali in patients with a pure AG acidosis owing to accumulation of a metabolizable organic acid anion (ketoacidosis or lactic acidosis). In general, severe acidosis (pH <7.20) warrants the intravenous administration of 50 to 100 meq of $NaHCO_3$, over 30 to 45 min, during the initial 1 to 2 h of therapy. Provision of such modest quantities of alkali in this situation seems to provide an added measure of safety, but it is essential to monitor plasma electrolytes during the course of therapy, since the [K^+] may decline as pH rises. The goal is to increase the [HCO_3^-] to 10 meq/L and the pH to 7.15, not to increase these values to normal.

HIGH-ANION-GAP ACIDOSES There are four principal causes of a high-AG acidosis: (1) lactic acidosis, (2) ketoacidosis, (3) ingested toxins, and (4) acute and chronic renal failure (Table 42-3). Initial screening to differentiate the high-AG acidoses should include (1) a probe of the history for evidence of drug and toxin ingestion and measurement of arterial blood gas to detect coexistent respiratory alkalosis (salicylates); (2) determination of whether diabetes mellitus is present (diabetic ketoacidosis); (3) a search for evidence of alcoholism or increased levels of β-hydroxybutyrate (alcoholic ketoacidosis); (4) observation for clinical signs of uremia and determination of the blood urea nitrogen (BUN) and creatinine (uremic acidosis); (5) inspection of the urine for oxalate crystals (ethylene glycol); and (6) recognition of the numerous clinical settings in which lactate levels may be increased (hypotension, shock, cardiac failure, leukemia, cancer, and drug or toxin ingestion).

Lactic Acidosis   An increase in plasma L-lactate may be secondary to poor tissue perfusion (type A)—circulatory insufficiency (shock, circulatory failure), severe anemia, mitochondrial enzyme defects, and inhibitors (carbon monoxide, cyanide)—or to aerobic disorders (type B)—malignancies, diabetes mellitus, renal or hepatic failure, severe infections (cholera, malaria), seizures, AIDS, or drugs/toxins (biguanides, ethanol, methanol, isoniazid, AZT analogues, and fructose). Unrecognized bowel ischemia or infarction in a patient with severe atherosclerosis or cardiac decompensation receiving vasopressors is a common cause of lactic acidosis. D-Lactic acid acidosis, which may be associated with jejunoileal bypass or intestinal obstruction and is due to formation of D-lactate by gut bacteria, may cause both an increased AG and hyperchloremia.

Rx TREATMENT

The underlying condition that disrupts lactate metabolism must first be corrected; tissue perfusion must be restored when it is inadequate. Vasoconstrictors should be avoided, if possible, since they may worsen tissue perfusion. Alkali therapy is generally advocated for acute, severe acidemia (pH <7.15) to improve cardiac function and lactate utilization. However, $NaHCO_3$ therapy may paradoxically depress cardiac performance and exacerbate acidosis by enhancing lactate production (HCO_3^- stimulates phosphofructokinase). While the use of alkali in moderate lactic acidosis is controversial, it is generally agreed that attempts to return the pH or $[HCO_3^-]$ to normal by administration of exogenous $NaHCO_3$ are deleterious. A reasonable approach is to infuse sufficient $NaHCO_3$ to raise the arterial pH to no more than 7.2 over 30 to 40 min.

    $NaHCO_3$ therapy can cause fluid overload and hypertension because the amount required can be massive when accumulation of lactic acid is relentless. Fluid administration is poorly tolerated because of central venoconstriction, especially in the oliguric patient. If the underlying cause of the lactic acidosis can be remedied, blood lactate will be converted to HCO_3^- and may result in an overshoot alkalosis.

Ketoacidosis ■ *DIABETIC KETOACIDOSIS*   This condition is caused by increased fatty acid metabolism and the accumulation of ketoacids (acetoacetate and β-hydroxybutyrate). Diabetic ketoacidosis usually occurs in insulin-dependent diabetes mellitus in association with cessation of insulin or an intercurrent illness, such as an infection, gastroenteritis, pancreatitis, or myocardial infarction, which increases insulin requirements temporarily and acutely. The accumulation of ketoacids accounts for the increment in the AG and is accompanied most often by hyperglycemia [glucose >17 mmol/L (300 mg/dL)]. It should be noted that since insulin prevents production of ketones, bicarbonate therapy is rarely needed except with extreme acidemia (pH <7.1), and then in only limited amounts (see "Treatment" for lactic acidosis). →*The management of this condition is described in Chap. 323.*

ALCOHOLIC KETOACIDOSIS   Chronic alcoholics can develop ketoacidosis when alcohol consumption is abruptly curtailed; it is usually associated with binge drinking, vomiting, abdominal pain, starvation, and volume depletion. The glucose concentration is low or normal, and acidosis may be severe because of elevated ketones, predominantly β-hydrox-

ybutyrate. Mild lactic acidosis may coexist because of alteration in the redox state. The nitroprusside ketone reaction (Acetest) can detect acetoacetic acid but not β-hydroxybutyrate, so that the degree of ketosis and ketonuria can be underestimated. Typically, insulin levels are low, and concentrations of triglyceride, cortisol, glucagon, and growth hormone are increased.

Rx TREATMENT

Extracellular fluid deficits should be repleted by intravenous administration of saline and glucose (5% dextrose in 0.9% NaCl). Hypophosphatemia, hypokalemia, and hypomagnesemia may coexist and should be corrected. Hypophosphatemia usually emerges 12 to 24 h after admission, may be exacerbated by glucose infusion, and, if severe, may induce rhabdomyolysis. Upper gastrointestinal hemorrhage, pancreatitis, and pneumonia may accompany this disorder.

Drug- and Toxin-Induced Acidosis ■ *SALICYLATES* (See also Chap. 377.) Salicylate intoxication in adults usually causes respiratory alkalosis, mixed metabolic acidosis–respiratory alkalosis, or a pure high-AG metabolic acidosis. In the latter example, which is less common, only a portion of the AG is due to the salicylates. Lactic acid production is also often increased.

Rx TREATMENT

This should begin with vigorous gastric lavage with isotonic saline (not $NaHCO_3$) followed by administration of activated charcoal. In the acidotic patient, to facilitate removal of salicylate, intravenous $NaHCO_3$ is administered in amounts adequate to alkalinize the urine and to maintain urine output (urine pH >7.5). While this form of therapy is straightforward in acidotic patients, a coexisting respiratory alkalosis may make this approach hazardous. Acetazolamide may be administered when an alkaline diuresis cannot be achieved, but this drug can cause systemic metabolic acidosis if HCO_3^- is not replaced. Hypokalemia may occur with an alkaline diuresis from $NaHCO_3$ and should be treated promptly and aggressively. Glucose-containing fluids should be administered because of the danger of hypoglycemia. Excessive insensible fluid losses may cause severe volume depletion and hypernatremia. If renal failure prevents rapid clearance of salicylate, hemodialysis can be performed against a bicarbonate dialysate.

ALCOHOLS   Under most physiologic conditions, sodium, urea, and glucose generate the osmotic pressure of blood. Plasma osmolality is calculated according to the following expression: $P_{osm} = 2Na^+ + Glu + BUN$ (all in mmol/L), or, using conventional laboratory values in which glucose and BUN are expressed in milligrams per deciliter: $P_{osm} = 2Na^+ + Glu/18 + BUN/2.8$. The calculated and determined osmolality should agree within 10 to 15 mmol/kg H_2O. When the measured osmolality exceeds the calculated osmolality by more than 15 to 20 mmol/kg H_2O, one of two circumstances prevails. Either the serum sodium is spuriously low, as with hyperlipidemia or hyperproteinemia (pseudohyponatremia), or osmolytes other than sodium salts, glucose, or urea have accumulated in plasma. Examples include mannitol, radiocontrast media, isopropyl alcohol, ethylene glycol, ethanol, methanol, and acetone. In this situation, the difference between the calculated osmolality and the measured osmolality (*osmolar gap*) is proportional to the concentration of the unmeasured solute. With an appropriate clinical history and index of suspicion, identification of an osmolar gap is helpful in identifying the presence of poison-associated AG acidosis.

ETHYLENE GLYCOL (See also Chap. 377.)   Ingestion of ethylene glycol (commonly used in antifreeze) leads to a metabolic acidosis and severe damage to the central nervous system, heart, lungs, and kidneys. The increased AG and osmolar gap are attributable to ethylene glycol and its metabolites, oxalic acid, glycolic acid, and other organic acids. Lactic acid production increases secondary to inhibition of the tricarboxylic acid cycle and altered intracellular redox state. Diagnosis is facilitated by recognizing oxalate crystals in the urine, the presence of an osmolar gap in serum, and a high-AG acidosis. Treatment should not be delayed while awaiting measurement of ethylene glycol levels in this setting.

℞ TREATMENT

This includes the prompt institution of a saline or osmotic diuresis, thiamine and pyridoxine supplements, fomepizole or ethanol, and hemodialysis. The intravenous administration of the alcohol dehydrogenase inhibitor fomepizole (4-methylpyrazole; 7 mg/kg as a loading dose) or ethanol intravenously to achieve a level of 22 mmol/L (100 mg/dL) serves to lessen toxicity because they compete with ethylene glycol for metabolism by alcohol dehydrogenase. Fomepizole, although expensive, offers the advantages of a predictable decline in ethylene glycol levels without the adverse effects, such as excessive obtundation, associated with ethyl alcohol infusion.

METHANOL (See also Chap. 377.) The ingestion of methanol (wood alcohol) causes metabolic acidosis, and its metabolites formaldehyde and formic acid cause severe optic nerve and cental nervous system damage. Lactic acid, ketoacids, and other unidentified organic acids may contribute to the acidosis. Due to its low molecular weight (32 Da), an osmolar gap is usually present.

℞ TREATMENT

This is similar to that for ethylene glycol intoxication, including general supportive measures, fomepizole or ethanol administration, and hemodialysis.

RENAL FAILURE (See also Chaps. 260 and 261) The hyperchloremic acidosis of moderate renal insufficiency is eventually converted to the high-AG acidosis of advanced renal failure. Poor filtration and reabsorption of organic anions contribute to the pathogenesis. As renal disease progresses, the number of functioning nephrons eventually becomes insufficient to keep pace with net acid production. Uremic acidosis is characterized, therefore, by a reduced rate of NH_4^+ production and excretion, primarily due to decreased renal mass. $[HCO_3^-]$ rarely falls below 15 mmol/L, and the AG rarely exceeds 20 mmol/L. The acid retained in chronic renal disease is buffered by alkaline salts from bone. Despite significant retention of acid (up to 20 mmol/d), the serum $[HCO_3^-]$ does not decrease further, indicating participation of buffers outside the extracellular compartment. Chronic metabolic acidosis results in significant loss of bone mass due to reduction in bone calcium carbonate. Chronic acidosis also increases urinary calcium excretion, proportional to cumulative acid retention.

℞ TREATMENT

Both uremic acidosis and the hyperchloremic acidosis of renal failure require oral alkali replacement to maintain the $[HCO_3^-]$ between 20 and 24 mmol/L. This can be accomplished with relatively modest amounts of alkali (1.0 to 1.5 mmol/kg body weight per day). It is assumed that alkali replacement prevents the harmful effects of H^+ balance on bone and prevents or retards muscle catabolism. Sodium citrate (Shohl's solution) or $NaHCO_3$ tablets are equally effective alkalinizing salts. Citrate enhances the absorption of aluminum from the gastrointestinal tract and should never be given together with aluminum-containing antacids because of the risk of aluminum intoxication. When hyperkalemia is present, furosemide (60 to 80 mg/d) should be added.

HYPERCHLOREMIC (NONGAP) METABOLIC ACIDOSES

Alkali can be lost from the gastrointestinal tract in diarrhea or from the kidneys (renal tubular acidosis, RTA). In these disorders (Table 42-4), reciprocal changes in $[Cl^-]$ and $[HCO_3^-]$ result in a normal AG. In pure hyperchloremic acidosis, therefore, the increase in $[Cl^-]$ above the normal value approximates the decrease in $[HCO_3^-]$. The absence of such a relationship suggests a mixed disturbance.

In diarrhea, stools contain a higher $[HCO_3^-]$ and decomposed HCO_3^- than plasma so that metabolic acidosis develops along with

volume depletion. Instead of an acid urine pH (as anticipated with systemic acidosis), urine pH is usually around 6 because metabolic acidosis and hypokalemia increase renal synthesis and excretion of NH_4^+, thus providing a urinary buffer that increases urine pH. Metabolic acidosis due to gastrointestinal losses with a high urine pH can be differentiated from RTA (Chap. 265) because urinary NH_4^+ excretion is typically low in RTA and high with diarrhea. Urinary NH_4^+ levels can be estimated by calculating the urine anion gap (UAG): UAG = $[Na^+ + K^+]_u - [Cl^-]_u$. When $[Cl^-]_u > [Na^+ + K^+]$, and the urine gap is negative, the urine ammonium level is appropriately increased, suggesting an extrarenal cause of the acidosis. Conversely, when the urine anion gap is positive, the urine ammonium level is low, suggesting a renal cause of the acidosis.

Loss of functioning renal parenchyma by progressive renal disease leads to hyperchloremic acidosis when the glomerular filtration rate (GFR) is between 20 and 50 mL/min and to uremic acidosis with a high AG when the GFR falls to <20 mL/min. Such a progression occurs commonly with tubulointerstitial forms of renal disease, but hyperchloremic metabolic acidosis can persist with advanced glomerular disease. In advanced renal failure, ammoniagenesis is reduced in proportion to the loss of functional renal mass, and ammonium accumulation and trapping in the outer medullary collecting tubule may also be impaired. Because of adaptive increases in K^+ secretion by the collecting duct and colon, the acidosis of chronic renal insufficiency is typically normokalemic.

Proximal RTA (type 2 RTA) (Chap. 265) is most often due to generalized proximal tubular dysfunction manifested by glycosuria, generalized aminoaciduria, and phosphaturia (Fanconi syndrome). With a low plasma $[HCO_3^-]$, the urine pH is acid (pH <5.5). The fractional excretion of $[HCO_3^-]$ may exceed 10 to 15% when the serum $HCO_3^- > 20$ mmol/L. Since HCO_3^- is not reabsorbed normally in the proximal tubule, therapy with $NaHCO_3$ will enhance renal potassium wasting and hypokalemia.

The typical findings in classic distal RTA (type 1 RTA) include hypokalemia, hyperchloremic acidosis, low urinary NH_4^+ excretion (positive UAG, low urine $[NH_4^+]$), and inappropriately high urine pH (pH >5.5). Such patients are unable to acidify the urine below a pH of 5.5. Most patients have hypocitraturia and hypercalciuria, so nephrolithiasis, nephrocalcinosis, and bone disease are common. In type 4 RTA, hyperkalemia is disproportionate to the reduction in GFR because of coexisting dysfunction of potassium and acid secretion. Urinary ammonium excretion is invariably depressed, and renal function may be compromised, for example, due to diabetic nephropathy, amyloidosis, or tubulointerstital disease. →*See Chap. 265 for the pathophysiology, diagnosis, and treatment of RTA.*

Hyporeninemic Hypoaldosteronism (See also Chap. 321) This condition typically causes hyperchloremic metabolic acidosis, most commonly in older adults with diabetes mellitus or tubulointerstitial disease and renal insufficiency. Patients usually have mild to moderate renal insufficiency and acidosis, with elevation in serum $[K^+]$ (5.2 to 6.0 mmol/L), concurrent hypertension, and congestive heart failure. Both the metabolic acidosis and the hyperkalemia are out of proportion to impairment in GFR. Nonsteroidal anti-inflammatory drugs trimethoprim, pentamidine, and angiotensin-converting enzyme (ACE) inhibitors can also cause hyperkalemia with hyperchloremic metabolic acidosis in patients with renal insufficiency (Table 42-4).

METABOLIC ALKALOSIS

Metabolic alkalosis is manifested by an elevated arterial pH, an increase in the serum $[HCO_3^-]$, and an increase in Pa_{CO_2} as a result of compensatory alveolar hypoventilation. It is often accompanied by hypochloremia and hypokalemia. The patient with a high $[HCO_3^-]$ and a low $[Cl^-]$ has either metabolic alkalosis or chronic respiratory acidosis. As shown in Table 42-1, the Pa_{CO_2} increases 6 mmHg for each 10-mmol/L increase in the $[HCO_3^-]$ above normal. Stated differently, in the range of $[HCO_3^-]$ from 10 to 40 mmol/L, the predicted Pa_{CO_2}

is approximately equal to the $[HCO_3^-] + 15$. The arterial pH establishes the diagnosis, since it is increased in metabolic alkalosis and decreased or normal in respiratory acidosis. Metabolic alkalosis frequently occurs in association with other disorders such as respiratory acidosis or alkalosis or metabolic acidosis.

PATHOGENESIS Metabolic alkalosis occurs as a result of net gain of $[HCO_3^-]$ or loss of nonvolatile acid (usually HCl by vomiting) from the extracellular fluid. Since it is unusual for alkali to be added to the body, the disorder involves a generative stage, in which the loss of acid usually causes alkalosis, and a maintenance stage, in which the kidneys fail to compensate by excreting HCO_3^- because of volume contraction, a low GFR, or depletion of Cl^- or K^+.

Under normal circumstances, the kidneys have an impressive capacity to excrete HCO_3^-. Continuation of metabolic alkalosis represents a failure of the kidneys to eliminate HCO_3^- in the usual manner. For HCO_3^- to be added to the extracellular fluid, it must be administered exogenously or synthesized endogenously, in part or entirely by the kidneys. The kidneys will retain, rather than excrete, the excess alkali and maintain the alkalosis if (1) volume deficiency, chloride deficiency, and K^+ deficiency exist in combination with a reduced GFR, which augments distal tubule H^+ secretion; or (2) hypokalemia exists because of autonomous hyperaldosteronism. In the first example, alkalosis is corrected by administration of NaCl and KCl, whereas in the latter it is necessary to repair the alkalosis by pharmacologic or surgical intervention, not with saline administration.

DIFFERENTIAL DIAGNOSIS To establish the cause of metabolic alkalosis (Table 42-5), it is necessary to assess the status of the extracellular fluid volume (ECFV), the recumbent and upright blood pressure, the serum $[K^+]$, and the renin-aldosterone system. For example, the presence of chronic hypertension and chronic hypokalemia in an alkalotic patient suggests either mineralocorticoid excess or that the hypertensive patient is receiving diuretics. Low plasma renin activity and normal urine $[Na^+]$ and $[Cl^-]$ in a patient who is not taking diuretics indicate a primary mineralocorticoid excess syndrome. The combination of hypokalemia and alkalosis in a normotensive, nonedematous patient can be due to Bartter's or Gitelman's syndrome, magnesium deficiency, vomiting, exogenous alkali, or diuretic ingestion. Determination of urine electrolytes (especially the urine $[Cl^-]$) and screening of the urine for diuretics may be helpful. If the urine is alkaline, with an elevated $[Na^+]$ and $[K^+]$ but low $[Cl^-]$, the diagnosis is usually either vomiting (overt or surreptitious) or alkali ingestion. If the urine is relatively acid and has low concentrations of Na^+, K^+, and Cl^-, the most likely possibilities are prior vomiting, the posthypercapnic state, or prior diuretic ingestion. If, on the other hand, neither the urine sodium, potassium, nor chloride concentrations are depressed, magnesium deficiency, Bartter's or Gitelman's syndrome, or current diuretic ingestion should be considered. Bartter's syndrome is distinguished from Gitelman's syndrome because of hypocalciuria and hypomagnesemia in the latter disorder. The genetic and molecular basis of these two disorders has been elucidated recently (Chap. 265).

Alkali Administration Chronic administration of alkali to individuals with normal renal function rarely, if ever causes alkalosis. However, in patients with coexistent hemodynamic disturbances, alkalosis can develop because the normal capacity to excrete HCO_3^- may be exceeded or there may be enhanced reabsorption of HCO_3^-. Such patients include those who receive oral or intravenous HCO_3^-, acetate loads (parenteral hyperalimentation solutions), citrate loads (transfusions), or antacids plus cation-exchange resins (aluminum hydroxide and sodium polystyrene sulfonate).

METABOLIC ALKALOSIS ASSOCIATED WITH ECFV CONTRACTION, K^+ DEPLETION, AND SECONDARY HYPERRENINEMIC HYPERALDOSTERONISM ■ **Gastrointestinal Origin**
Gastrointestinal loss of H^+ from vomiting or gastric aspiration results in retention of HCO_3^-. The loss of fluid and NaCl in vomitus or na-

TABLE 42-5 Causes of Metabolic Alkalosis

I. Exogenous HCO_3^- loads
  A. Acute alkali administration
  B. Milk-alkali syndrome
II. Effective ECFV contraction, normotension, K^+ deficiency, and secondary hyperreninemic hyperaldosteronism
  A. Gastrointestinal origin
    1. Vomiting
    2. Gastric aspiration
    3. Congenital chloridorrhea
    4. Villous adenoma
    5. Combined administration of sodium polystyrene sulfonate (Kayexalate) and aluminum hydroxide
  B. Renal origin
    1. Diuretics
    2. Edematous states
    3. Posthypercapnic state
    4. Hypercalcemia/hypoparathyroidism
    5. Recovery from lactic acidosis or ketoacidosis
    6. Nonreabsorbable anions including penicillin, carbenicillin
    7. Mg^{2+} deficiency
    8. K^+ depletion
    9. Bartter's syndrome (loss of function mutations in TALH)
    10. Gitelman's syndrome (loss of function mutation in Na^+-Cl^- cotransporter in DCT)
III. ECFV expansion, hypertension, K^+ deficiency, and mineralocorticoid excess
  A. High renin
    1. Renal artery stenosis
    2. Accelerated hypertension
    3. Renin-secreting tumor
    4. Estrogen therapy
  B. Low renin
    1. Primary aldosteronism
      a. Adenoma
      b. Hyperplasia
      c. Carcinoma
    2. Adrenal enzyme defects
      a. 11β-Hydroxylase deficiency
      b. 17α-Hydroxylase deficiency
    3. Cushing's syndrome or disease
    4. Other
      a. Licorice
      b. Carbenoxolone
      c. Chewer's tobacco
      d. Lydia Pinkam tablets
IV. Gain of function mutation of renal sodium channel with ECFV expansion, hypertension, K^+ deficiency, and hyporeninemic-hypoaldosteronism
  A. Liddle's syndrome

Note: ECFV, extracellular fluid volume; TALH, thick ascending limb of Henle's loop; DCT, distal convoluted tubule.

sogastric suction results in contraction of the ECFV and an increase in the secretion of renin and aldosterone. Volume contraction causes a reduction in GFR and an enhanced capacity of the renal tubule to reabsorb HCO_3^-. During active vomiting, there is continued addition of HCO_3^- to plasma in exchange for Cl^-, and the plasma $[HCO_3^-]$ exceeds the reabsorptive capacity of the proximal tubule. The excess $NaHCO_3$ reaches the distal tubule, where secretion is enhanced by an aldosterone and the delivery of the poorly reabsorbed anion, HCO_3^-. Because of contraction of the ECFV and hypochloremia, Cl^- is avidly conserved by the kidney. Correction of the contracted ECFV with NaCl and repair of K^+ deficits corrects the acid-base disorder.

Renal Origin ■ *DIURETICS* (See also Chap. 216) Drugs that induce chloruresis, such as thiazides and loop diuretics (furosemide, bumetanide, torsemide, and ethracrynic acid), acutely diminish the ECFV without altering the total body bicarbonate content. The serum $[HCO_3^-]$ increases. The chronic administration of diuretics tends to generate an alkalosis by increasing distal salt delivery, so that K^+ and H^+ secretion are stimulated. The alkalosis is maintained by persistence of the contraction of the ECFV, secondary hyperaldosteronism, K^+ deficiency, and the direct effect of the diuretic (as long as diuretic administration continues). Repair of the alkalosis is achieved by providing isotonic saline to correct the ECFV deficit.

BARTTER'S SYNDROME AND GITELMAN'S SYNDROME   See Chap. 265.

NONREABSORBABLE ANIONS AND MAGNESIUM DEFICIENCY   Administration of large quantities of nonreabsorbable anions, such as penicillin or carbenicillin, can enhance distal acidification and K^+ secretion by increasing the transepithelial potential difference (lumen negative). Mg^{2+} deficiency results in hypokalemic alkalosis by enhancing distal acidification through stimulation of renin and hence aldosterone secretion.

POTASSIUM DEPLETION   Chronic K^+ depletion may cause metabolic alkalosis by increasing urinary acid excretion. Both NH_4^+ production and absorption are enhanced and HCO_3^- reabsorption is stimulated. Chronic K^+ deficiency upregulates the renal H^+, K^+-ATPase to increase K^+ absorption at the expense of enhanced H^+ secretion. Alkalosis associated with severe K^+ depletion is resistant to salt administration, but repair of the K^+ deficiency corrects the alkalosis.

AFTER TREATMENT OF LACTIC ACIDOSIS OR KETOACIDOSIS   When an underlying stimulus for the generation of lactic acid or ketoacid is removed rapidly, as with repair of circulatory insufficiency or with insulin therapy, the lactate or ketones are metabolized to yield an equivalent amount of HCO_3^-. Other sources of new HCO_3^- are additive with the original amount generated by organic anion metabolism to create a surfeit of HCO_3^-. Such sources include (1) new HCO_3^- added to the blood by the kidneys as a result of enhanced acid excretion during the preexisting period of acidosis, and (2) alkali therapy during the treatment phase of the acidosis. Acidosis-induced contraction of the ECFV and K^+ deficiency act to sustain the alkalosis.

POSTHYPERCAPNIA   Prolonged CO_2 retention with chronic respiratory acidosis enhances renal HCO_3^- absorption and the generation of new HCO_3^- (increased net acid excretion). If the Pa_{CO_2} is returned to normal, metabolic alkalosis results from the persistently elevated $[HCO_3^-]$. Alkalosis develops if the elevated Pa_{CO_2} is abruptly returned toward normal by a change in mechanically controlled ventilation. Associated ECFV contraction does not allow complete repair of the alkalosis by correction of the Pa_{CO_2} alone, and alkalosis persists until Cl^- supplementation is provided.

METABOLIC ALKALOSIS ASSOCIATED WITH ECFV EXPANSION, HYPERTENSION, AND HYPERALDOSTERONISM

Mineralocorticoid administration or excess production [primary aldosteronism of Cushing's syndrome and adrenal cortical enzyme defects (Chap. 321)] increases net acid excretion and may result in metabolic alkalosis, which may be worsened by associated K^+ deficiency. ECFV expansion from salt retention causes hypertension and antagonizes the reduction in GFR and/or increases tubule acidification induced by aldosterone and by K^+ deficiency. The kaliuresis persists and causes continued K^+ depletion with polydipsia, inability to concentrate the urine, and polyuria. Increased aldosterone levels may be the result of autonomous primary adrenal overproduction or of secondary aldosterone release due to renal overproduction of renin. In both situations, the normal feedback of ECFV on net aldosterone production is disrupted, and hypertension from volume retention can result.

Liddle's syndrome (Chap. 265) results from increased activity of the collecting duct Na^+ channel (ENaC) and is a rare inherited disorder associated with hypertension due to volume expansion manifested as hypokalemic alkalosis and normal aldosterone levels.

Symptoms   With metabolic alkalosis, changes in central and peripheral nervous system function are similar to those of hypocalcemia (Chap. 331); symptoms include mental confusion, obtundation, and a predisposition to seizures, paresthesia, muscular cramping, tetany, aggravation of arrhythmias, and hypoxemia in chronic obstructive pulmonary disease. Related electrolyte abnormalities include hypokalemia and hypophosphatemia.

℞ TREATMENT

This is primarily directed at correcting the underlying stimulus for HCO_3^- generation. If primary aldosteronism is present, correction of the underlying cause will reverse the alkalosis. $[H^+]$ loss by the stomach or kidneys can be mitigated by the use of H_2 receptor blockers, H^+, K^+-ATPase inhibitors, or the discontinuation of diuretics. The second aspect of treatment is to remove the factors that sustain HCO_3^- reabsorption, such as ECFV contraction or K^+ deficiency. Although K^+ deficits should be repaired, NaCl therapy is usually sufficient to reverse the alkalosis if ECFV contraction is present, as indicated by a low urine $[Cl^-]$.

If associated conditions preclude infusion of saline, renal HCO_3^- loss can be accelerated by administration of acetazolamide, a carbonic anhydrase inhibitor, which is usually effective in patients with adequate renal function but can worsen K^+ losses. Dilute hydrochloric acid (0.1 N HCl) is also effective but can cause hemolysis. Alternatively, acidification can also be achieved with oral NH_4Cl, which should be avoided in the presence of liver disease. Hemodialysis against a dialysate low in $[HCO_3^-]$ and high in $[Cl^-]$ can be effective when renal function is impaired.

RESPIRATORY ACIDOSIS

Respiratory acidosis can be due to severe pulmonary disease, respiratory muscle fatigue, or abnormalities in ventilatory control and is recognized by an increase in Pa_{CO_2} and decrease in pH (Table 42-6). In acute respiratory acidosis, there is an immediate compensatory elevation (due to cellular buffering mechanisms) in HCO_3^-, which increases 1 mmol/L for every 10-mmHg increase in Pa_{CO_2}. In chronic respiratory acidosis (>24 h), renal adaptation increases the $[HCO_3^-]$ by 4 mmol/L for every 10-mmHg increase in Pa_{CO_2}. The serum HCO_3^- usually does not increase above 38 mmol/L.

The clinical features vary according to the severity and duration of the respiratory acidosis, the underlying disease, and whether there is

TABLE 42-6   *Respiratory Acid-Base Disorders*

I. Alkalosis	II. Acidosis
A. Central nervous system stimulation	A. Central
1. Pain	1. Drugs (anesthetics, morphine, sedatives)
2. Anxiety, psychosis	2. Stroke
3. Fever	3. Infection
4. Cerebrovascular accident	B. Airway
5. Meningitis, encephalitis	1. Obstruction
6. Tumor	2. Asthma
7. Trauma	C. Parenchyma
B. Hypoxemia or Tissue hypoxia	1. Emphysema
1. High altitude, $\downarrow Pa_{CO_2}$	2. Pneumoconiosis
2. Pneumonia, pulmonary edema	3. Bronchitis
3. Aspiration	4. Adult respiratory distress syndrome
4. Severe anemia	5. Barotrauma
C. Drugs or hormones	D. Neuromuscular
1. Pregnancy, progesterone	1. Poliomyelitis
2. Salicylates	2. Kyphoscoliosis
3. Nikethamide	3. Myasthenia
D. Stimulation of chest receptors	4. Muscular dystrophies
1. Hemothorax	E. Miscellaneous
2. Flail chest	1. Obesity
3. Cardiac failure	2. Hypoventilation
4. Pulmonary embolism	3. Permissive hypercapnia
E. Miscellaneous	
1. Septicemia	
2. Hepatic failure	
3. Mechanical hyperventilation	
4. Heat exposure	
5. Recovery from metabolic acidosis	

accompanying hypoxemia. A rapid increase in Pa_{CO_2} may cause anxiety, dyspnea, confusion, psychosis, and hallucinations and may progress to coma. Lesser degrees of dysfunction in chronic hypercapnia include sleep disturbances, loss of memory, daytime somnolence, personality changes, impairment of coordination, and motor disturbances such as tremor, myoclonic jerks, and asterixis. Headaches and other signs that mimic raised intracranial pressure, such as papilledema, abnormal reflexes, and focal muscle weakness, are due to vasoconstriction secondary to loss of the vasodilator effects of CO_2.

Depression of the respiratory center by a variety of drugs, injury, or disease can produce respiratory acidosis. This may occur acutely with general anesthetics, sedatives, and head trauma or chronically with sedatives, alcohol, intracranial tumors, and the syndromes of sleep-disordered breathing, including the primary alveolar and obesity-hypoventilation syndromes (Chaps. 246 and 247). Abnormalities or disease in the motor neurons, neuromuscular junction, and skeletal muscle can cause hypoventilation via respiratory muscle fatigue. Mechanical ventilation, when not properly adjusted and supervised, may result in respiratory acidosis, particularly if CO_2 production suddenly rises (because of fever, agitation, sepsis, or overfeeding) or alveolar ventilation falls because of worsening pulmonary function. High levels of positive end-expiratory pressure in the presence of reduced cardiac output may cause hypercapnia as a result of large increases in alveolar dead space (Chap. 234). Permissive hypercapnia is being used with increasing frequency because of studies suggesting lower mortality rates than with conventional mechanical ventilation, especially with severe central nervous system or heart disease. Although the potential beneficial effects of permissive hypercapnia may be mitigated by correction of the acidemia, it seems prudent, nevertheless, to keep the pH in the range of 7.2 to 7.3 by administration of $NaHCO_3$.

Acute hypercapnia follows sudden occlusion of the upper airway or generalized bronchospasm as in severe asthma, anaphylaxis, inhalational burn, or toxin injury. Chronic hypercapnia and respiratory acidosis occur in end-stage obstructive lung disease. Restrictive disorders involving both the chest wall and the lungs can cause respiratory acidosis because the high metabolic cost of respiration causes ventilatory muscle fatigue. Advanced stages of intrapulmonary and extrapulmonary restrictive defects present as chronic respiratory acidosis.

The diagnosis of respiratory acidosis requires, by definition, the measurement of Pa_{CO_2} and arterial pH. A detailed history and physical examination often indicate the cause. Pulmonary function studies (Chap. 234), including spirometry, diffusion capacity for carbon monoxide, lung volumes, and arterial Pa_{CO_2} and O_2 saturation, usually make it possible to determine if respiratory acidosis is secondary to lung disease. The workup for nonpulmonary causes should include a detailed drug history, measurement of hematocrit, and assessment of upper airway, chest wall, pleura, and neuromuscular function.

Rx TREATMENT

The management of respiratory acidosis depends on its severity and rate of onset. Acute respiratory acidosis can be life-threatening, and measures to reverse the underlying cause should be undertaken simultaneously with restoration of adequate alveolar ventilation. This may necessitate tracheal intubation and assisted mechanical ventilation. Oxygen administration should be titrated carefully in patients with severe obstructive pulmonary disease and chronic CO_2 retention who are breathing spontaneously (Chap. 242). When oxygen is used injudiciously, these patients may experience progression of the respiratory acidosis. Aggressive and rapid correction of hypercapnia should be avoided, because the falling Pa_{CO_2} may provoke the same complications noted with acute respiratory alkalosis (i.e., cardiac arrhythmias, reduced cerebral perfusion, and seizures). The Pa_{CO_2} should be lowered gradually in chronic respiratory acidosis, aiming to restore the Pa_{CO_2} to baseline levels and to provide sufficient Cl^- and K^+ to enhance the renal excretion of HCO_3^-.

Chronic respiratory acidosis is frequently difficult to correct, but measures aimed at improving lung function (Chap. 242) can help some patients and forestall further deterioration in most.

RESPIRATORY ALKALOSIS

Alveolar hyperventilation decreases Pa_{CO_2} and increases the HCO_3^-/Pa_{CO_2} ratio, thus increasing pH (Table 42-6). Nonbicarbonate cellular buffers respond by consuming HCO_3^-. Hypocapnia develops when a sufficiently strong ventilatory stimulus causes CO_2 output in the lungs to exceed its metabolic production by tissues. Plasma pH and $[HCO_3^-]$ appear to vary proportionally with Pa_{CO_2} over a range from 40 to 15 mmHg. The relationship between arterial $[H^+]$ concentration and Pa_{CO_2} is about 0.7 mmol/L per mmHg (or 0.01 pH unit/mmHg), and that for plasma $[HCO_3^-]$ is 0.2 mmol/L per mmHg. Hypocapnia sustained longer than 2 to 6 h is further compensated by a decrease in renal ammonium and titratable acid excretion and a reduction in filtered HCO_3^- reabsorption. Full renal adaptation to respiratory alkalosis may take several days and requires normal volume status and renal function. The kidneys appear to respond directly to the lowered Pa_{CO_2} rather than to alkalosis per se. In chronic respiratory alkalosis a 1-mmHg fall in Pa_{CO_2} causes a 0.4- to 0.5-mmol/L drop in $[HCO_3^-]$ and a 0.3-mmol/L fall (or 0.003 rise in pH) in $[H^+]$.

The effects of respiratory alkalosis vary according to duration and severity but are primarily those of the underlying disease. Reduced cerebral blood flow as a consequence of a rapid decline in Pa_{CO_2} may cause dizziness, mental confusion, and seizures, even in the absence of hypoxemia. The cardiovascular effects of acute hypocapnia in the conscious human are generally minimal, but in the anesthetized or mechanically ventilated patient, cardiac output and blood pressure may fall because of the depressant effects of anesthesia and positive-pressure ventilation on heart rate, systemic resistance, and venous return. Cardiac arrhythmias may occur in patients with heart disease as a result of changes in oxygen unloading by blood from a left shift in the hemoglobin-oxygen dissociation curve (Bohr effect). Acute respiratory alkalosis causes intracellular shifts of Na^+, K^+, and PO_4^- and reduces free $[Ca^{2+}]$ by increasing the protein-bound fraction. Hypocapnia-induced hypokalemia is usually minor.

Chronic respiratory alkalosis is the most common acid-base disturbance in critically ill patients and, when severe, portends a poor prognosis. Many cardiopulmonary disorders manifest respiratory alkalosis in their early to intermediate stages, and the finding of normocapnia and hypoxemia in a patient with hyperventilation may herald the onset of rapid respiratory failure and should prompt an assessment to determine if the patient is becoming fatigued. Respiratory alkalosis is common during mechanical ventilation.

The hyperventilation syndrome may be disabling. Paresthesia, circumoral numbness, chest wall tightness or pain, dizziness, inability to take an adequate breath, and, rarely, tetany may themselves be sufficiently stressful to perpetuate the disorder. Arterial blood-gas analysis demonstrates an acute or chronic respiratory alkalosis, often with hypocapnia in the range of 15 to 30 mmHg and no hypoxemia. Central nervous system diseases or injury can produce several patterns of hyperventilation and sustained Pa_{CO_2} levels of 20 to 30 mmHg. Hyperthyroidism, high caloric loads, and exercise raise the basal metabolic rate, but ventilation usually rises in proportion so that arterial blood gases are unchanged and respiratory alkalosis does not develop. Salicylates are the most common cause of drug-induced respiratory alkalosis as a result of direct stimulation of the medullary chemoreceptor (Chap. 377). The methylxanthines, theophylline, and aminophylline stimulate ventilation and increase the ventilatory response to CO_2. Progesterone increases ventilation and lowers arterial Pa_{CO_2} by as much as 5 to 10 mmHg. Therefore, chronic respiratory alkalosis is a common feature of pregnancy. Respiratory alkalosis is also prominent in liver failure, and the severity correlates with the degree of hepatic insufficiency. Respiratory alkalosis is often an early finding in gram-negative septicemia, before fever, hypoxemia, or hypotension develop.

The diagnosis of respiratory alkalosis depends on measurement of arterial pH and Pa_{CO_2}. The plasma $[K^+]$ is often reduced and the $[Cl^-]$ increased. In the acute phase, respiratory alkalosis is not associated with increased renal HCO_3^- excretion, but within hours net acid excretion is reduced. In general, the HCO_3^- concentration falls by 2.0 mmol/L for each 10-mmHg decrease in Pa_{CO_2}. Chronic hypocapnia reduces the serum $[HCO_3^-]$ by 5.0 mmol/L for each 10-mmHg decrease in Pa_{CO_2}. It is unusual to observe a plasma $HCO_3^- <12$ mmol/L as a result of a pure respiratory alkalosis.

When a diagnosis of respiratory alkalosis is made, its cause should be investigated. The diagnosis of hyperventilation syndrome is made by exclusion. In difficult cases, it may be important to rule out other conditions such as pulmonary embolism, coronary artery disease, and hyperthyroidism.

℞ TREATMENT

The management of respiratory alkalosis is directed toward alleviation of the underlying disorder. If respiratory alkalosis complicates ventilator management, changes in dead space, tidal volume, and frequency can minimize the hypocapnia. Patients with the hyperventilation syndrome may benefit from reassurance, rebreathing from a paper bag during symptomatic attacks, and attention to underlying psychological

stress. Antidepressants and sedatives are not recommended. β-Adrenergic blockers may ameliorate peripheral manifestations of the hyperadrenergic state.

FURTHER READING

DuBose TD Jr: Acid-base disorders, in BM Brenner (ed): *Brenner and Rector's The Kidney*, 7th ed. Philadelphia, Saunders, 2004, pp 921–996
———, Alpern RJ: Renal tubular acidosis, in CR Scriver et al (eds): *The Metabolic and Molecular Bases of Inherited Disease*, 8th ed. New York, McGraw-Hill, 2001
Fall PJ: A stepwise approach to acid-base disorders: Practical patient evaluation for metabolic acidosis and other conditions. Postgrad Med 107:249, 253, 257, 2000
Galla JH: Metabolic alkalosis. J Am Soc Nephrol 11:369, 2000
Madias NE, Cohen JJ: Respiratory alkalosis and acidosis, in DW Seldin, G Giebisch (eds): *The Kidney: Physiology and Pathophysiology*, 2d ed. New York, Raven, 1992, pp 2733–2758
Wesson DE et al: Clinical syndromes of metabolic alkalosis, in DW Seldin, G Giebisch (eds): *The Kidney: Physiology and Pathophysiology*, 3d ed. Philadelphia: Lippincott Williams and Wilkins, 2000, pp 2055–2072

Section 8   Alterations in Sexual Function and Reproduction

43 SEXUAL DYSFUNCTION
Kevin T. McVary

Male sexual dysfunction affects 10 to 25% of middle-aged and elderly men. Female sexual dysfunction occurs with a similar frequency. Demographic changes, the popularity of newer treatments, and greater awareness of sexual dysfunction by patients and society have led to increased diagnosis and associated health care expenditures for the management of this common disorder. Because many patients are reluctant to initiate discussion of their sex lives, the physician should address this topic directly to elicit a history of sexual dysfunction.

PHYSIOLOGY OF MALE SEXUAL RESPONSE

Normal male sexual function requires (1) an intact libido; (2) the ability to achieve and maintain penile erection; (3) ejaculation; and (4) detumescence. *Libido* refers to sexual desire and is influenced by a variety of visual, olfactory, tactile, auditory, imaginative, and hormonal stimuli. Sex steroids, particularly testosterone, act to increase libido. Libido can be diminished by hormonal or psychiatric disorders or by medications.

Penile tumescence leading to erection depends on the increased flow of blood into the lacunar network after complete relaxation of the arteries and corporal smooth muscle. The microarchitecture of the corpora is composed of a mass of smooth muscle (trabecula) which contains a network of endothelial-lined vessels (lacunar spaces). Subsequent compression of the trabecular smooth muscle against the fibroelastic tunica albuginea causes a passive closure of the emissary veins and accumulation of blood in the corpora. In the presence of a full erection and a competent valve mechanism, the corpora become noncompressible cylinders from which blood does not escape.

The central nervous system exerts an important influence by either stimulating or antagonizing spinal pathways that mediate erectile function and ejaculation. The erectile response is mediated by a combination of central (psychogenic) and peripheral (reflexogenic) innervation. Sensory nerves that originate from receptors in the penile skin and glans converge to form the dorsal nerve of the penis, which travels to the S2-S4 dorsal root ganglia via the pudendal nerve. Parasympathetic nerve fibers to the penis arise from neurons in the intermediolateral columns of S2-S4 sacral spinal segments. Sympathetic inner-

vation originates from the T-11 to the L-2 spinal segments and descends through the hypogastric plexus.

Neural input to smooth muscle tone is crucial to the initiation and maintenance of an erection. There is also an intricate interaction between the corporal smooth muscle cell and its overlying endothelial cell lining (Fig. 43-1A). Nitric oxide, which induces vascular relaxation, promotes erection and is opposed by endothelin-1 (ET-1), which mediates vascular contraction. Nitric oxide is synthesized from L-arginine by nitric oxide synthase, and is released from the nonadrenergic, noncholinergic (NANC) autonomic nerve supply to act postjunctionally on smooth muscle cells. Nitric oxide increases the production of cyclic $3',5'$-guanosine monophosphate (cyclic GMP), which induces relaxation of the smooth muscle (Fig. 43-1B). Cyclic GMP is gradually broken down by phosphodiesterase type 5 (PDE-5). Inhibitors of PDE-5, such as the oral medication sildenafil, maintain erections by reducing the breakdown of cyclic GMP. However, if nitric oxide is not produced at some level, the addition of PDE-5 inhibitor is not effective, as the drug facilitates but does not initiate the initial enzyme cascade. In addition to nitric oxide, vasoactive prostaglandins (PGE_1, $PGF_{2\alpha}$) are synthesized within the cavernosal tissue and increase cyclic AMP levels, also leading to relaxation of cavernosal smooth muscle cells.

Ejaculation is stimulated by the sympathetic nervous system, which results in contraction of the epididymis, vas deferens, seminal vesicles, and prostate, causing seminal fluid to enter the urethra. Seminal fluid emission is followed by rhythmic contractions of the bulbocavernosus and ischiocavernosus muscles, leading to ejaculation. *Premature ejaculation* is usually related to anxiety or a learned behavior and is amenable to behavioral therapy or treatment with medications such as selective serotonin reuptake inhibitors (SSRIs). *Retrograde ejaculation* results when the internal urethral sphincter does not close, and it may occur in men with diabetes or after surgery involving the bladder neck.

Detumescence is mediated by released norepinephrine from the sympathetic nerves, release of endothelin from the vascular surface, and contraction of smooth muscle induced by activation of postsynaptic α-adrenergic receptors. These events increase venous outflow and restore the flaccid state. Venous leak can cause premature detumescence and is thought to be caused by insufficient relaxation of the corporal smooth muscle rather than a specific anatomic defect. *Pria-*

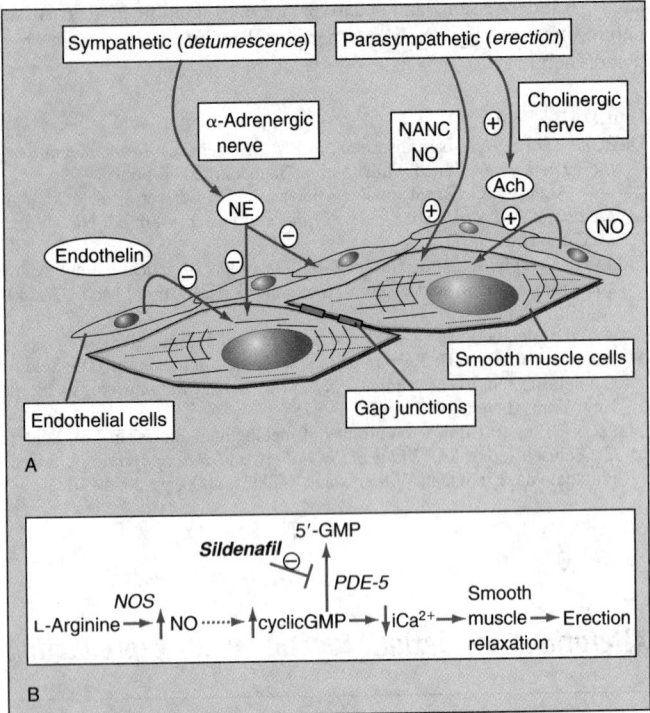

FIGURE 43-1 Pathways that control erection and detumescence. *A.* Erection is mediated by cholinergic parasympathetic pathways, and nonadrenergic, noncholinergic (NANC) pathways, which release nitric oxide (NO). Endothelial cells also release NO, which induces vascular smooth muscle cell relaxation, allowing enhanced blood flow, and leading to erection. Detumescence is mediated by sympathetic pathways that release norepinephrine and stimulate α-adrenergic pathways, leading to contraction of vascular smooth muscle cells. Endothelin, released from endothelial cells, also induces contraction. *B.* Biochemical pathways of NO synthesis and action. Sildenafil enhances erectile function by inhibiting phosphodiesterase type 5 (PDE-5), thereby maintaining high levels of cyclic 3',5'-guanosine monophosphate (cyclic GMP). NOS, nitric oxide synthase; iCa²⁺, intracellular calcium.

pism refers to a persistent and painful erection and may be associated with sickle cell anemia, hypercoagulable states, spinal cord injury, or injection of vasodilator agents into the penis.

ERECTILE DYSFUNCTION

EPIDEMIOLOGY Erectile dysfunction (ED) is not considered a normal part of the aging process. Nonetheless, it is associated with certain physiologic and psychological changes related to age. In the Massachusetts Male Aging Study (MMAS), a community-based survey of men between the ages of 40 and 70, 52% of responders reported some degree of ED. Complete ED occurred in 10% of respondents, moderate ED occurred in 25%, and minimal ED in 17%. The incidence of moderate or severe ED more than doubled between the ages of 40 and 70. In the National Health and Social Life Survey (NHSLS), which was a nationally representative sample of men and women age 18 to 59 years, 10% of men reported being unable to maintain an erection (corresponding to the proportion of men in the MMAS reporting severe ED). Incidence was highest among men in the 50 to 59 age group (21%) and among men who were poor (14%), divorced (14%), and less educated (13%).

The incidence of ED is also higher among men with certain medical disorders such as diabetes mellitus, heart disease, hypertension, and decreased HDL levels. Smoking is a significant risk factor in the development of ED. Medications used to treat diabetes or cardiovascular disease are additional risk factors (see below). There is a higher incidence of ED among men who have undergone radiation or surgery for prostate cancer and in those with a lower spinal cord injury. Psychological causes of ED include depression, anger, or stress from unemployment or other causes.

PATHOPHYSIOLOGY ED may result from three basic mechanisms: (1) failure to initiate (psychogenic, endocrinologic, or neurogenic); (2) failure to fill (arteriogenic); or (3) failure to store (venoocclusive dysfunction) adequate blood volume within the lacunar network. These categories are not mutually exclusive, and multiple factors contribute to ED in many patients. For example, diminished filling pressure can lead secondarily to venous leak. Psychogenic factor frequently coexist with other etiologic factors and should be considered in all cases. Diabetic, atherosclerotic, and drug-related causes account for >80% of cases of ED in older men.

Vasculogenic The most frequent organic cause of ED is a disturbance of blood flow to and from the penis. Atherosclerotic or traumatic arterial disease can decrease flow to the lacunar spaces, resulting in decreased rigidity and an increased time to full erection. Excessive outflow through the veins, despite adequate inflow, may also contribute to ED. This situation may be due to insufficient relaxation of trabecular smooth muscle and may occur in anxious individuals with excessive adrenergic tone or in those with damaged parasympathetic outflow. Structural alterations to the fibroelastic components of the corpora may cause a loss of compliance and an inability to compress the tunical veins. This condition may result from aging, increased cross-linking of collagen fibers induced by nonenzymatic glycosylation, hypoxia, or altered synthesis of collagen associated with hypercholesterolemia.

Neurogenic Disorders that affect the sacral spinal cord or the autonomic fibers to the penis preclude nervous system relaxation of penile smooth muscle, thus leading to ED. In patients with spinal cord injury, the degree of ED depends on the completeness and level of the lesion. Patients with incomplete lesions or injuries to the upper part of the spinal cord are more likely to retain erectile capabilities than those with complete lesions or injuries to the lower part. Although 75% of patients with spinal cord injuries have some erectile capability, only 25% have erections sufficient for penetration. Other neurologic disorders commonly associated with ED include multiple sclerosis and peripheral neuropathy. The latter is often due to either diabetes or alcoholism. Pelvic surgery may cause ED through disruption of the autonomic nerve supply.

Endocrinologic Androgens increase libido, but their exact role in erectile function remains unclear. Individuals with castrate levels of testosterone can achieve erections from visual or sexual stimuli. Nonetheless, normal levels of testosterone appear to be important for erectile function, particularly in older males. Androgen replacement therapy can improve depressed erectile function when it is secondary to hypogonadism; it is not useful for ED when endogenous testosterone levels are normal. Increased prolactin may decrease libido by suppressing gonadotropin-releasing hormone (GnRH), and it also leads to decreased testosterone levels. Treatment of hyperprolactinemia with dopamine agonists can restore libido and testosterone.

Diabetic ED occurs in 35 to 75% of men with diabetes mellitus. Pathologic mechanisms are primarily related to diabetes-associated vascular and neurologic complications. Diabetic macrovascular complications are mainly related to age, whereas microvascular complications correlate with the duration of diabetes and the degree of glycemic control (Chap. 323). Individuals with diabetes also have reduced amounts of nitric oxide synthase in both endothelial and neural tissues.

Psychogenic Two mechanisms contribute to the inhibition of erections in psychogenic ED. First, psychogenic stimuli to the sacral cord may inhibit reflexogenic responses, thereby blocking activation of vasodilator outflow to the penis. Second, excess sympathetic stimulation in an anxious man may increase penile smooth muscle tone. The most common causes of psychogenic ED are performance anxiety, depression, relationship conflict, loss of attraction, sexual inhibition, conflicts over sexual preference, sexual abuse in childhood, and fear of pregnancy or sexually transmitted disease. Almost all patients with ED, even when it has a clear-cut organic basis, develop a psychogenic component as a reaction to ED.

Medication-Related Medication-induced ED (Table 43-1) is estimated to occur in 25% of men seen in general medical outpatient clinics. Among the antihypertensive agents, the thiazide diuretics and beta blockers have been implicated most frequently. Calcium channel blockers and angiotensin-converting enzyme inhibitors are less frequently cited. These drugs may act directly at the corporal level (e.g., calcium channel blockers) or indirectly by reducing pelvic blood pressure, which is important in the development of penile rigidity. α Adrenergic blockers are less likely to cause ED. Estrogens, GnRH agonists, H_2 antagonists, and spironolactone cause ED by suppressing gonadotropin production or by blocking androgen action. Antidepressant and antipsychotic agents—particularly neuroleptics, tricyclics, and SSRIs—are associated with erectile, ejaculatory, orgasmic, and sexual desire difficulties.

Although many medications can cause ED, patients frequently have concomitant risk factors that confound the clinical picture. If there is a strong association between the institution of a drug and the onset of ED, alternative medications should be considered. Otherwise, it is often practical to treat the ED without attempting multiple changes in medications, as it may be difficult to establish a causal role for the drug.

CLINICAL EVALUATION A good physician-patient relationship helps to unravel the possible causes of ED, many of which require discussion of personal and sometimes embarrassing topics. For this reason, a primary care provider is often ideally suited to initiate the evaluation. A complete medical and sexual history should be taken in an effort to assess whether the cause of ED is organic, psychogenic, or multifactorial (Fig. 43-2). Initial questions should focus on the onset of symptoms, the presence and duration of partial erections, and the progression of ED. A history of nocturnal or early morning erections is useful for distinguishing physiologic from psychogenic ED. Nocturnal erections occur during rapid eye movement (REM) sleep and require intact neurologic and circulatory systems. Organic causes of ED are generally characterized by a gradual and persistent change in rigidity or the

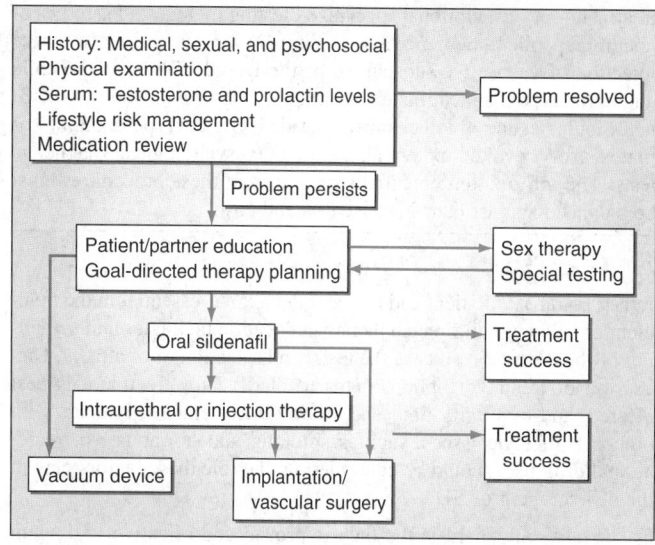

FIGURE 43-2 Algorithm for the evaluation and management of patients with ED.

inability to sustain nocturnal, coital, or self-stimulated erections. The patient should also be questioned about the presence of penile curvature or pain with coitus. It is also important to address libido, as decreased sexual drive and ED are sometimes the earliest signs of endocrine abnormalities (e.g., increased prolactin, decreased testosterone levels). It is useful to ask whether the problem is confined to coitus with one or other partners; ED arises not uncommonly in association with new or extramarital sexual relationships. Situational ED, as opposed to consistent ED, suggests psychogenic causes. Ejaculation is much less commonly affected than erection, but questions should be asked about whether ejaculation is normal, premature, delayed, or absent. Relevant risk factors should be identified, such as diabetes mellitus, coronary artery disease, lipid disorders, hypertension, peripheral vascular disease, smoking, alcoholism, and endocrine or neurologic disorders. The patient's surgical history should be explored with an emphasis on bowel, bladder, prostate, or vascular procedures. A complete drug history is also important. Social changes that may precipitate ED are also crucial to the evaluation, including health worries, spousal death, divorce, relationship difficulties, and financial concerns.

The physical examination is an essential element in the assessment of ED. Signs of hypertension as well as evidence of thyroid, hepatic, hematologic, cardiovascular, or renal diseases should be sought. An assessment should be made of the endocrine and vascular systems, the external genitalia, and the prostate gland. The penis should be carefully palpated along the corpora to detect fibrotic plaques. Reduced testicular size and loss of secondary sexual characteristics are suggestive of hypogonadism. Neurologic examination should include assessment of anal sphincter tone, the bulbocavernosus reflex, and testing for peripheral neuropathy.

Although hyperprolactinemia is uncommon, a serum prolactin level should be measured, as decreased libido and/or erectile dysfunction may be the presenting symptoms of a prolactinoma or other mass lesions of the sella (Chap. 318). The serum testosterone level should be measured and, if low, gonadotropins should be measured to determine whether hypogonadism is primary (testicular) or secondary (hypothalamic-pituitary) in origin (Chap. 325). Serum chemistries, CBC, and lipid profiles may be of value, if not performed recently, as they can yield evidence of anemia, diabetes, hyperlipidemia, or other systemic diseases associated with ED. Determination of serum PSA should be conducted according to recommended clinical guidelines (Chap. 81).

Additional diagnostic testing is rarely necessary in the evaluation of ED. However, in selected patients, specialized testing may provide insight into pathologic mechanisms of ED and aid in the selection of

TABLE 43-1 *Drugs Associated with Erectile Dysfunction*

Classification	Drugs
Diuretics	Thiazides
	Spironolactone
Antihypertensives	Calcium channel blockers
	Methyldopa
	Clonidine
	Reserpine
	β-Blockers
	Guanethidine
Cardiac/anti-hyperlipidemics	Digoxin
	Gemfibrozil
	Clofibrate
Antidepressants	Selective serotonin reuptake inhibitors
	Tricyclic antidepressants
	Lithium
	Monoamine oxidase inhibitors
Tranquilizers	Butyrophenones
	Phenothiazines
H_2 antagonists	Ranitidine
	Cimetidine
Hormones	Progesterone
	Estrogens
	Corticosteroids
	GnRH agonists
	5α-Reductase inhibitors
	Cyproterone acetate
Cytotoxic agents	Cyclophosphamide
	Methotrexate
	Roferon-A
Anticholinergics	Disopyramide
	Anticonvulsants
Recreational	Ethanol
	Cocaine
	Marijuana

treatment options. Optional specialized testing includes: (1) studies of nocturnal penile tumescence and rigidity; (2) vascular testing (in-office injection of vasoactive substances, penile Doppler ultrasound, penile angiography, dynamic infusion cavernosography/cavernosometry); (3) neurologic testing (biothesiometry-graded vibratory perception; somatosensory evoked potentials); and (4) psychological diagnostic tests. The information potentially gained from these procedures must be balanced against their invasiveness and cost.

℞ TREATMENT

Patient Education   Patient and partner education is essential in the treatment of ED. In goal-directed therapy, education facilitates understanding of the disease, results of the tests, and selection of treatment. Discussion of treatment options helps to clarify how treatment is best offered, and to stratify first- and second-line therapies. Patients with high-risk lifestyle issues, such as smoking, alcohol abuse, or recreational drug use, should be counseled on the role these factors play in the development of ED.

Oral Agents   Sildenafil is the only approved and effective oral agent for the treatment of ED. Sildenafil has markedly improved the management of ED because it is effective for the treatment of a broad range of causes of ED, including psychogenic, diabetic, vasculogenic, post-radical prostatectomy (nerve-sparing procedures), and spinal cord injury. Sildenafil is a selective and potent inhibitor of PDE-5, the predominant phosphodiesterase isoform found in the penis. It is administered in doses of 25, 50, or 100 mg, and enhances erections after sexual stimulation. The onset of action is approximately 60 to 90 min. Reduced initial doses should be considered for patients who are elderly, have renal insufficiency, or are taking medications that inhibit the CYP3A4 metabolic pathway in the liver (e.g., erythromycin, cimetidine, ketoconazole, and, possibly, itraconazole and mibefradil), as they may increase the serum concentration of sildenafil. The drug does not affect ejaculation, orgasm, or sexual drive. Side effects associated with sildenafil include headaches (19%), facial flushing (9%), dyspepsia (6%) and nasal congestion (4%). Approximately 7% of men may experience transient altered color vision (blue halo effect). Sildenafil is contraindicated in men receiving nitrate therapy for cardiovascular disease, including agents delivered by oral, sublingual, transnasal, or topical routes. These agents can potentiate its hypotensive effect and may result in profound shock. Likewise, amyl/butyl nitrates "poppers" may have a fatal synergistic effect on blood pressure. Sildenafil should also be avoided in patients with congestive heart failure and cardiomyopathy because of the risk of vascular collapse. Because sexual activity leads to an increase in physiologic expenditure [5 to 6 metabolic equivalents (METS)], physicians have been advised to exercise caution in prescribing any drug for sexual activity to those with active coronary disease, heart failure, borderline hypotension, hypovolemia, and to those on complex antihypertensive regimens.

Androgen Therapy   Testosterone replacement is used to treat both primary and secondary causes of hypogonadism (Chap. 325). Androgen supplementation in the setting of normal testosterone is rarely efficacious and is discouraged. Methods of androgen replacement include parenteral administration of long-acting testosterone esters (enanthate and cypionate), oral preparations (17 α-alkylated derivatives), and transdermal patches, and gels (Chap. 325). The long-acting 17 β-hydroxy esters of testosterone are the safest, most cost-effective, and practical preparations available. The administration of 200 to 300 mg intramuscularly every 2 to 3 weeks provides a practical option but is far from an ideal physiologic replacement. Oral androgen preparations have the potential for hepatotoxicity and should be avoided. Transdermal delivery of testosterone using patches or gels more closely mimics physiologic testosterone levels, but it is unclear whether this translates into improved sexual function. Testosterone therapy is contraindicated in men with androgen-sensitive cancers and may be inappropriate for men with bladder neck obstruction. It is generally advisable to measure PSA before giving androgen. Hepatic function should be tested before and during testosterone therapy.

Vacuum Constriction Devices   Vacuum constriction devices (VCD) are a well-established, noninvasive therapy. They are a reasonable treatment alternative for select patients who cannot take sildenafil or do not desire other interventions. VCD draw venous blood into the penis and use a constriction ring to restrict venous return and maintain tumescence. Adverse events with VCD include pain, numbness, bruising, and altered ejaculation. Additionally, many patients complain that the devices are cumbersome and that the induced erections have a non-physiologic appearance.

Intraurethral Alprostadil   If a patient fails to respond to oral agents, a reasonable next choice is intraurethral or self-injection of vasoactive substances. Intraurethral prostaglandin E$_1$ (alprostadil), in the form of a semisolid pellet (doses of 125 to 1000 μg), is delivered with an applicator. Approximately 65% of men receiving intraurethral alprostadil respond with an erection when tested in the office, but only 50% of those achieve successful coitus at home. Intraurethral insertion is associated with a markedly reduced incidence of priapism in comparison to intracavernosal injection.

Intracavernosal Self-Injection   Injection of synthetic formulations of alprostadil is effective in 70 to 80% of patients with ED, but discontinuation rates are high because of the invasive nature of administration. Doses range between 1 and 40 μg. Injection therapy is contraindicated in men with a history of hypersensitivity to the drug and in men at risk for priapism (hypercoagulable states, sickle cell disease). Side effects include local adverse events, prolonged erections, pain, and fibrosis with chronic use. Various combinations of alprostadil, phentolamine, and/or papaverine are sometimes used.

Surgery   A less frequently used form of therapy for ED involves the surgical implantation of a semi-rigid or inflatable penile prosthesis. These surgical treatments are invasive, associated with potential complications, and generally reserved for treatment of refractory ED. Despite their high cost and invasiveness, penile prostheses are associated with high rates of patient satisfaction.

SEX THERAPY   A course of sex therapy may be useful for addressing specific interpersonal factors that may affect sexual functioning. Sex therapy generally consists of in-session discussion and at-home exercises specific to the person and the relationship. It is preferable if therapy includes both partners, provided the patient is involved in an ongoing relationship.

FEMALE SEXUAL DYSFUNCTION

Female sexual dysfunction (FSD) has traditionally included disorders of desire, arousal, pain, and muted orgasm. The associated risk factors for FSD are similar to those in males: cardiovascular disease, endocrine disorders, hypertension, neurologic disorders, and smoking (Table 43-2).

TABLE 43-2   *Risk Factors for Female Sexual Dysfunction*

Neurologic disease: stroke, spinal cord injury, Parkinsonism
Trauma, genital surgery, radiation
Endocrinopathies: diabetes, hyperprolactinemia
Liver and/or renal failure
Cardiovascular disease
Psychological factors and interpersonal relationship disorders: sexual abuse, life stressors
Medications
    Antiandrogens: Cimetidine, spironolactone
    Antidepressants, Alcohol, hypnotics, sedatives
    Antiestrogens or GnRH antagonists
    Antihistamines, sympathomimetic amines
    Antihypertensives: Diuretics, calcium channel blockers
    Alkylating agents
    Anticholinergics

EPIDEMIOLOGY   Epidemiologic data are limited but the available estimates suggest that as many as 43% of women complain of at least one sexual problem. Despite the recent interest in organic causes of FSD, desire and arousal phase disorders (including lubrication complaints) remain the most common presenting problems when surveyed in a community-based population.

PHYSIOLOGY OF THE FEMALE SEXUAL RESPONSE   Although there are the obvious anatomic differences as well as variation in the density of vascular and neural beds in males and females, the primary effectors of sexual response are strikingly similar. Intact sensation is important for arousal. Thus, reduced levels of sexual functioning are more common in women with peripheral neuropathies (e.g., diabetes). Vaginal lubrication is a transudate of serum that results from the increased pelvic blood flow associated with arousal. Vascular insufficiency from a variety of causes may compromise adequate lubrication and result in dyspareunia. Similar to the male response, cavernosal and arteriole smooth muscle relaxation occurs via increased NOS activity and produces engorgement in the clitoris and surrounding vestibule. Orgasm requires an intact sympathetic outflow tract; hence, orgasmic disorders are common in female patients with spinal cord injuries.

CLINICAL EVALUATION   The evaluation of FSD previously occurred mainly in a psychosocial context. However, inconsistencies between diagnostic categories based on only psychosocial considerations, and the emerging recognition of organic etiologies, has led to a new classification of FSD. This diagnostic scheme is based on four components that are not mutually exclusive: (1) *Hypoactive sexual desire*—the persistent or recurrent lack of sexual thoughts and/or receptivity to sexual activity, which causes personal distress. Hypoactive sexual desire may result from endocrine failure or may be associated with psychological or emotional disorders; (2) *Sexual arousal disorder*—the persistent or recurrent inability to attain or maintain sexual excitement, which causes personal distress; (3) *Orgasmic disorder*—the persistent or recurrent loss of orgasmic potential after sufficient sexual stimulation and arousal, which causes personal distress; (4) *Sexual pain disorder*—persistent or recurrent genital pain associated with noncoital sexual stimulation, which causes personal distress. This newer classification emphasizes "personal distress" as a requirement for dysfunction and provides clinicians an organized framework for evaluation prior to or in conjunction with more traditional counseling methods.

TREATMENT

Patient Education   Patient and partner education is essential in the treatment of FSD. Educating the couple about normal anatomy and physiologic responses is often necessary. Physiologic changes associated with aging and/or disease should be explained. Maximizing physical health and avoiding lifestyles (e.g., smoking, alcohol abuse) and medications likely to produce FSD are prudent (Table 43-2).

Hormonal Therapy   In postmenopausal women, estrogen replacement therapy may be helpful in treating vaginal atrophy, decreasing coital pain, and improving clitoral sensitivity (Chap. 327). Estrogen replacement in the form of local cream is the preferred method, as it avoids systemic side effects. Androgen levels in women decline substantially before menopause. However, low levels of testosterone or dehydroepiandrosterone (DHEA) are not effective predictors of a positive therapeutic outcome with androgen therapy. The widespread use of exogenous androgens is not supported by the literature except in select circumstances (premature ovarian failure or menopausal states) and in secondary arousal disorders.

Oral Agents   The efficacy of PDE-5 inhibitors in FDS has been a marked disappointment given the proposed role of nitric oxide-dependent physiology in the normal female sexual response. The use of sildenafil for FSD should be discouraged pending proof that it is effective.

Clitoral Vacuum Device   In patients with arousal and orgasmic difficulties, the option of using a clitoral vacuum device may be explored. This handheld battery-operated device has a small soft plastic cup that applies a vacuum over the stimulated clitoris. This causes increased cavernosal blood flow, engorgement, and vaginal lubrication.

FURTHER READING

BERMAN JR et al: Female sexual dysfunction: Incidence, pathophysiology, evaluation, and treatment options. Urology 54:385–391, 1999

DAVIS SR. The clinical use of androgens in female sexual disorders. J Sex Marital Ther 24:153, 1998

FELDMAN HA et al: Impotence and its medical and psychosocial correlates: Results of the Massachusetts Male Aging Study. J Urol 151:54, 1994

LAUMANN EO et al: Sexual dysfunction in the United States. JAMA 81:553, 1999

LUE TF: Drug therapy: Erectile dysfunction. N Engl J Med 342:1802, 2000

44 HIRSUTISM AND VIRILIZATION
David A. Ehrmann

Hirsutism, defined as excessive male-pattern hair growth, affects approximately 10% of women. If often represents a variation of normal hair growth, but rarely it is a harbinger of a serious underlying condition. Hirsutism is often idiopathic but may be caused by conditions associated with androgen excess, such as polycystic ovarian syndrome (PCOS) or congenital adrenal hyperplasia (CAH) (Table 44-1). Cutaneous manifestations commonly associated with hirsutism include acne and male-pattern balding (androgenic alopecia). *Virilization* refers to the state in which androgen levels are sufficiently high to cause additional signs and symptoms such as deepening of the voice, breast atrophy, increased muscle bulk, clitoromegaly, and increased libido; virilization is an ominous sign that suggests the possibility of an ovarian or adrenal neoplasm.

HAIR FOLLICLE GROWTH AND DIFFERENTIATION

Hair can be categorized as either *vellus* (fine, soft, and not pigmented) or *terminal* (long, coarse, and pigmented). The number of hair follicles does not change over an individual's lifetime, but the follicle size and type of hair can change in response to numerous factors, particularly androgens. Androgens are necessary for terminal hair and sebaceous gland-development and mediate differentiation of pilosebaceous units (PSUs) into either a terminal hair follicle or a sebaceous gland. In the former case, androgens transform the vellus hair into a terminal hair; in the latter, the sebaceous component proliferates and the hair remains vellus.

There are three phases in the cycle of hair growth: (1) *anagen* (growth phase), (2) *catagen* (involution phase), and (3) *telogen* (rest phase). Depending on the body site, hormonal regulation may play an important role in the hair growth cycle. For example, the eyebrows, eyelashes, and vellus hairs are androgen-insensitive, whereas the axillary and pubic areas are sensitive to low levels of androgens. Hair growth on the face, chest, upper abdomen, and back requires greater levels of androgens and is therefore more characteristic of the pattern typically seen in males. Androgen excess in women leads to increased hair growth in most androgen-sensitive sites except in the scalp region, where hair loss occurs because androgens cause scalp hairs to spend less time in the anagen phase.

Although androgen excess underlies most cases of hirsutism, there is only a modest correlation between androgen levels and the quantity of hair growth. This is due to the fact that hair growth from the follicle also depends on local growth factors, and there is variability in end-

TABLE 44-1 *Causes of Hirsutism*

Gonadal hyperandrogenism
    Ovarian hyperandrogenism
    Polycystic ovary syndrome/functional ovarian hyperandrogenism
    Ovarian steroidogenic blocks
    Syndromes of extreme insulin resistance
    Ovarian neoplasms
Adrenal hyperandrogenism
    Premature adrenarche
    Functional adrenal hyperandrogenism
    Congenital adrenal hyperplasia (nonclassic and classic)
    Abnormal cortisol action/metabolism
    Adrenal neoplasms
Other endocrine disorders
    Cushing's syndrome
    Hyperprolactinemia
    Acromegaly
Peripheral androgen overproduction
    Obesity
    Idiopathic
Pregnancy-related hyperandrogenism
    Hyperreactio luteinalis
    Thecoma of pregnancy
Drugs
    Androgens
    Oral contraceptives containing androgenic progestins
    Minoxidil
    Phenytoin
    Diazoxide
    Cyclosporine
True hermaphroditism

organ sensitivity. Genetic factors and ethnic background also influence hair growth. In general, dark-haired individuals tend to be more hirsute than blonde or fair individuals. Asians and Native Americans have relatively sparse hair in regions sensitive to high androgen levels, whereas people of Mediterranean descent are more hirsute.

CLINICAL ASSESSMENT

Historic elements relevant to the assessment of hirsutism include the age of onset and rate of progression of hair growth and associated symptoms or signs (e.g., acne). Depending on the cause, excess hair growth is typically first noted during the second and third decades. The growth is usually slow but progressive. Sudden development and rapid progression of hirsutism suggests the possibility of an androgen-secreting neoplasm, in which case virilization may also be present.

The age of onset of menstrual cycles (menarche) and the pattern of the menstrual cycle should be ascertained; irregular cycles from the time of menarche onward are more likely to result from ovarian rather than adrenal androgen excess. Associated symptoms such as galactorrhea should prompt evaluation for hyperprolactinemia (Chap. 318) and possibly hypothyroidism (Chap. 320). Hypertension, striae, easy bruising, centripetal weight gain, and weakness suggest hypercortisolism (Cushing's syndrome; Chap. 321). Rarely, patients with growth hormone excess (i.e., acromegaly) will present with hirsutism. Use of medications such as phenytoin, minoxidil, or cyclosporine may be associated with androgen-independent causes of excess hair growth (i.e., hypertrichosis). A family history of infertility and/or hirsutism may indicate disorders such as nonclassic CAH (Chap. 321).

Physical examination should include measurement of height, weight, and calculation of body mass index (BMI). A BMI >25 kg/m² is indicative of excess weight for height, and values >30 kg/m² are often seen in association with hirsutism. Notation should be made of blood pressure, as adrenal causes may be associated with hypertension. Cutaneous signs sometimes associated with androgen excess and insulin resistance include acanthosis nigricans and skin tags.

An objective clinical assessment of hair distribution and quantity is central to the evaluation in any woman presenting with hirsutism. This assessment permits the distinction between hirsutism and hypertrichosis and provides a baseline reference point to gauge the response to treatment. A simple and commonly used method to grade hair growth is the modified scale of Ferriman and Gallwey (Fig. 44-1), where each of nine androgen-sensitive sites is graded from 0 to 4. Approximately 95% of Caucasian women have a score below 8 on this scale; thus, it is normal for most women to have some hair growth in androgen-sensitive sites. Scores above 8 suggest excess androgen-mediated hair growth, a finding that should be assessed further by hormonal evaluation (see below). In racial/ethnic groups that are less likely to manifest hirsutism (e.g., Asian women), additional cutaneous

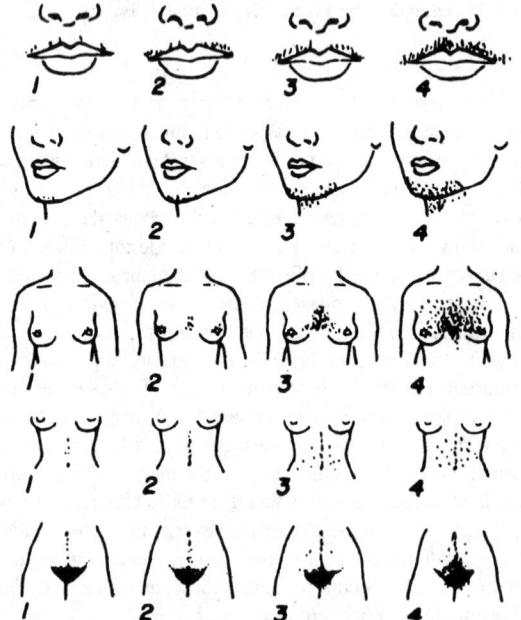
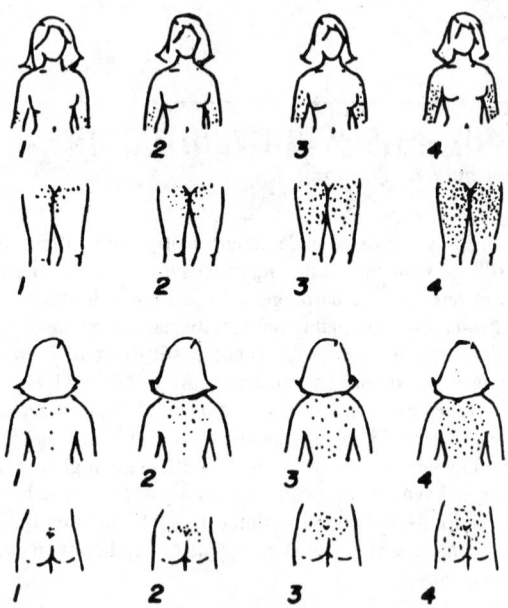

FIGURE 44-1 Hirsutism scoring scale of Ferriman and Gallwey. The nine body areas possessing androgen-sensitive areas are graded from 0 (no terminal hair) to 4 (frankly virile) to obtain a total score. A normal hirsutism score is less than 8. *[Reproduced from DA Ehrmann et al: Hyperandrogenism, hirsutism, and polycystic ovarian syndrome, in LJ DeGroot et al (eds), Endocrinology, 4th ed. Philadelphia, Saunders, 2000; with permission.]*

evidence of androgen excess should be sought, including pustular acne or thinning hair.

HORMONAL EVALUATION

Androgens are secreted by the ovaries and adrenal glands in response to their respective tropic hormones, luteinizing hormone (LH) and adrenocorticotropic hormone (ACTH). The principal circulating steroids involved in the etiology of hirsutism are testosterone, androstenedione, dehydroepiandrosterone (DHEA) and its sulfated form (DHEAS). The ovaries and adrenal glands normally contribute about equally to testosterone production. Approximately half of the total testosterone originates from direct glandular secretion, and the remainder is derived from the peripheral conversion of androstenedione and DHEA (Chap. 325).

Although it is the most important circulating androgen, testosterone is, in effect, the penultimate androgen in mediating hirsutism; it is converted to the more potent dihydrotestosterone (DHT) by the enzyme 5α-reductase, which is located in the PSU. DHT has a higher affinity for, and slower dissociation from, the androgen receptor. The local production of DHT allows it to serve as the primary mediator of androgen action at the level of the pilosebaceous unit. There are two isoenzymes of 5α-reductase: type 2 is found in the prostate gland and in hair follicles, whereas type 1 is found primarily in sebaceous glands.

One approach to testing for hyperandrogenemia is depicted in Fig. 44-2. In addition to measuring blood levels of testosterone and DHEAS, it is also important to measure the level of free (or unbound) testosterone. The fraction of testosterone that is not bound to its carrier protein, sex-hormone binding globulin (SHBG), is biologically available for conversion to DHT and for binding to androgen receptors. Hyperinsulinemia and/or androgen excess decrease hepatic production of SHBG, resulting in levels of total testosterone within the high-normal range, whereas the unbound hormone is more substantially elevated. Although there is a decline in ovarian testosterone production after menopause, ovarian estrogen production decreases to an even greater extent, and the concentration of SHBG is reduced. Consequently, there is an increase in the relative proportion of unbound testosterone, and it may exacerbate hirsutism after menopause.

Because adrenal androgens are readily suppressed by low doses of glucocorticoids, the dexamethasone androgen-suppression test may broadly distinguish ovarian from adrenal androgen overproduction. A blood sample is obtained before and after administering dexamethasone (0.5 mg orally every 6 h for 4 days). An adrenal source is suggested by suppression of unbound testosterone into the normal range; incomplete suppression suggests ovarian androgen excess.

A baseline plasma total testosterone level >12 nmol/L (>3.5 ng/mL) usually indicates a virilizing tumor, whereas a level >7 nmol/L (>2 ng/mL) is suggestive. A basal DHEAS level >18.5 μmol/L (>7000 μg/L) suggests an adrenal tumor. Although DHEAS has been proposed as a "marker" of predominant adrenal androgen excess, it is not unusual to find modest elevations in DHEAS among women with PCOS. Computed tomography (CT) or magnetic resonance imaging (MRI) should be used to localize an adrenal mass, and ultrasound will usually suffice to identify an ovarian mass, if clinical evaluation and hormonal levels suggest these possibilities.

PCOS is the most common cause of ovarian androgen excess (Chap. 326). However, the increased ratio of LH to follicle-stimu-

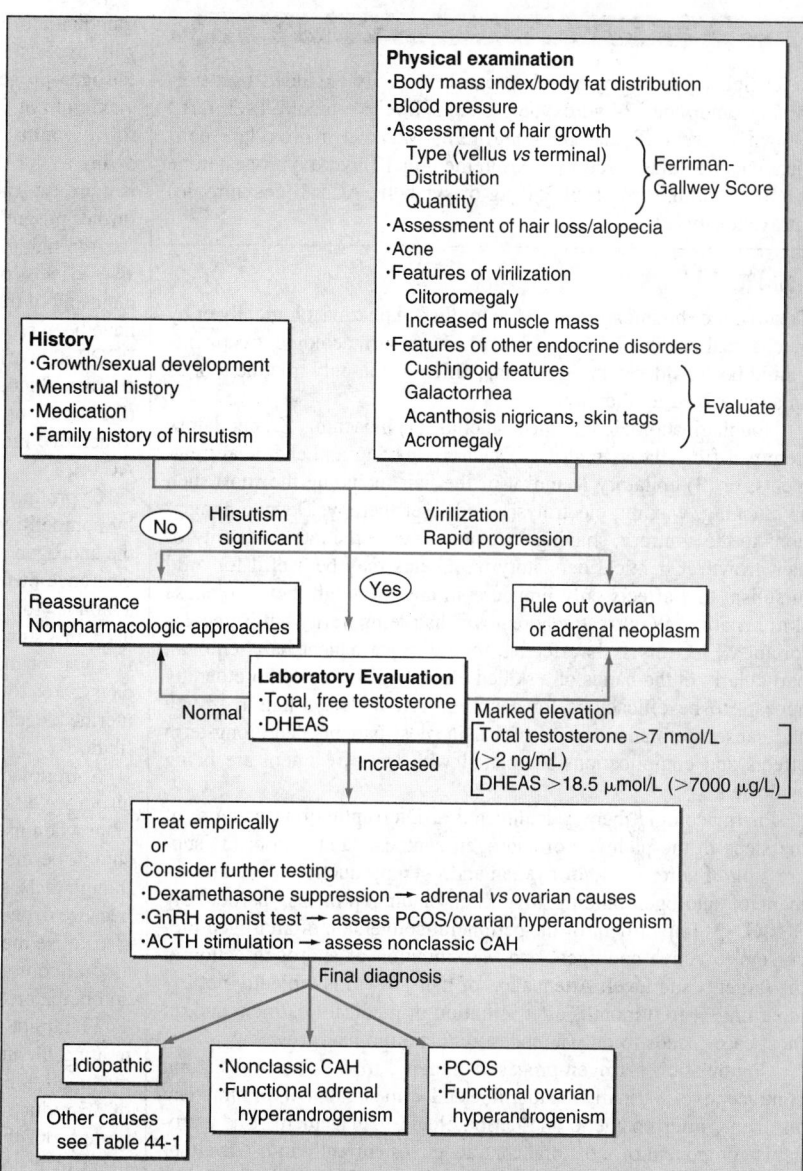

FIGURE 44-2 Algorithm for the evaluation and differential diagnosis of hirsutism. ACTH, adrenocorticotropic hormone; CAH, congenital adrenal hyperplasia; DHEAS, sulfated form of dehydroepiandrosterone; GnRH, gonadotropin-releasing hormone; PCOS, polycystic ovarian syndrome.

lating hormone that is characteristic of carefully studied patients with PCOS is not seen in up to half of these women due to the pulsatility of gonadotropins. If performed, ultrasound shows enlarged ovaries and increased stroma in many women with PCOS. However, polycystic ovaries may also be found in women without clinical or laboratory features of PCOS. Therefore, polycystic ovaries are a relatively insensitive and nonspecific finding for the diagnosis of ovarian hyperandrogenism. Gonadotropin-releasing hormone agonist testing can be used to make a specific diagnosis of ovarian hyperandrogenism. A peak 17-hydroxyprogesterone level ≥7.8 nmol/L (≥2.6 μg/L), after the administration of 100 μg nafarelin (or 10 μg/kg leuprolide) subcutaneously, is virtually diagnostic of ovarian hyperandrogenism.

Nonclassic CAH is most commonly due to 21-hydroxylase deficiency but can also be caused by autosomal recessive defects in other steroidogenic enzymes necessary for adrenal corticosteroid synthesis (Chap. 321). Because of the enzyme defect, the adrenal gland cannot secrete glucocorticoids efficiently (especially cortisol). This results in diminished negative feedback inhibition of ACTH, leading to compensatory adrenal hyperplasia and the accumulation of steroid precursors that are subsequently converted to androgen.

Deficiency of 21-hydroxylase can be reliably excluded by determining a morning 17-hydroxyprogesterone level <6 nmol/L (<2 μg/L) (drawn in the follicular phase). Alternatively, 21-hydroxylase deficiency can be diagnosed by measurement of 17-hydroxyprogesterone 1 h after administration of 250 μg of synthetic ACTH (cosyntropin) intravenously.

℞ TREATMENT

Treatment of hirsutism may be accomplished pharmacologically or by mechanical means of hair removal. Nonpharmacologic treatments should be considered in all patients, either as the only treatment or as an adjunct to drug therapy.

Nonpharmacologic treatments include (1) bleaching; (2) depilatory (removal from the skin surface) such as shaving and chemical treatments; or (3) epilatory (removal of the hair including the root) such as plucking, waxing, electrolysis, and laser therapy. Despite perceptions to the contrary, shaving does not increase the rate or density of hair growth. Chemical depilatory treatments may be useful for mild hirsutism that affects only limited skin areas, though they can cause skin irritation. Wax treatment removes hair temporarily but is uncomfortable. Electrolysis is effective for more permanent hair removal, particularly in the hands of a skilled electrologist. Laser phototherapy appears to be efficacious for hair removal. It delays hair regrowth and causes permanent hair removal in most patients. The long-term effects and complications associated with laser treatment are being evaluated.

Pharmacologic therapy is directed at interrupting one or more of the steps in the pathway of androgen synthesis and action: (1) suppression of adrenal and/or ovarian androgen production; (2) enhancement of androgen-binding to plasma-binding proteins, particularly SHBG; (3) impairment of the peripheral conversion of androgen precursors to active androgen; and (4) inhibition of androgen action at the target tissue level. Attenuation of hair growth is typically not evident until 4 to 6 months after initiation of medical treatment and, in most cases, leads to only a modest reduction in hair growth.

Combination estrogen-progestin therapy, in the form of an oral contraceptive, is usually the first-line endocrine treatment for hirsutism and acne, after cosmetic and dermatologic management. The estrogenic component of most oral contraceptives currently in use is either ethinyl estradiol or mestranol. The suppression of LH leads to reduced production of ovarian androgens. The reduced androgen levels also result in a dose-related increase in SHBG, thereby lowering the fraction of unbound plasma testosterone. Combination therapy has also been demonstrated to decrease DHEAS, perhaps by reducing ACTH levels. Estrogens also have a direct, dose-dependent suppressive effect on sebaceous cell function.

The choice of a specific oral contraceptive should be predicated on the progestational component, as progestins vary in their suppressive effect on SHBG levels and in their androgenic potential. Ethynodiol diacetate has relatively low androgenic potential, whereas progestins such as norgestrel and levonorgestrel are pargenic, as judged from their attenuation of the estrogen-induced increase in SHBG. Norgestimate exemplifies the newer generation of progestins that are virtually nonandrogenic. Drospirenone, an analogue of spironolactone that has both antimineralocorticoid and antiandrogenic activities, has been approved for use as a progestational agent in combination with ethinyl estradiol. Its properties suggest that it should be the preferred choice for the treatment of hirsutism.

Oral contraceptives are contraindicated in women with a history of thromboembolic disease or in women with increased risk of breast or other estrogen-dependent cancers (Chap. 327). There is a relative contraindication to the use of oral contraceptives in smokers or in those with hypertension or a history of migraine headaches. In most trials, estrogen-progestin therapy alone improves the extent of acne by a maximum of 50 to 70%. The effect on hair growth may not be evident for 6 months, and the maximum effect may require 9 to 12 months owing to the length of the hair growth cycle. Improvements in hirsutism are typically in the range of 20%, but there may be an arrest of further progression of hair growth.

Adrenal androgens are more sensitive than cortisol to the suppressive effects of glucocorticoids. Therefore, glucocorticoids are the mainstay of treatment in patients with CAH. Although glucocorticoids have been reported to restore ovulatory function in some women with PCOS, this effect is highly variable. Because of side effects from excessive glucocorticoids, low doses should be used. Dexamethasone (0.2 to 0.5 mg) or prednisone (5 to 10 mg) should be taken at bedtime to achieve maximal suppression by inhibiting the nocturnal surge of ACTH.

Cyproterone acetate is the prototypic antiandrogen. It acts mainly by competitive inhibition of the binding of testosterone and DHT to the androgen receptor. In addition, it may act to enhance the metabolic clearance of testosterone by inducing hepatic enzymes. Although not available for use in the United States, cyproterone acetate is widely used in Canada, Mexico, and Europe. Cyproterone (50 to 100 mg) is given on days 1 to 15 and ethinyl estradiol (50 μg) is given on days 5 to 26 of the menstrual cycle. Side effects include irregular uterine bleeding, nausea, headache, fatigue, weight gain, and decreased libido.

Spironolactone, usually used as a mineralocorticoid antagonist, is also a weak antiandrogen. It is almost as effective as cyproterone acetate when used at high enough doses (100 to 200 mg daily). Patients should be monitored intermittently for hyperkalemia or hypotension, though these side effects are uncommon. Pregnancy should be avoided because of the risk of feminization of a male fetus. Spironolactone can also cause menstrual irregularity. It is often used in combination with an oral contraceptive, which suppresses ovarian androgen production and helps prevent pregnancy.

Flutamide is a potent nonsteroidal antiandrogen that is effective in treating hirsutism, but concerns about the induction of hepatocellular dysfunction have limited its use. Finasteride is a competitive inhibitor of 5α-reductase type 2. Beneficial effects on hirsutism have been reported, but the predominance of 5α-reductase type 1 in the PSU appears to account for its limited efficacy. Finasteride would also be expected to impair sexual differentiation in a male fetus, and it should not be used in women who may become pregnant.

Eflornithine cream (Vaniqa) has been approved as a novel treatment for unwanted facial hair in women, but long-term efficacy remains to be established. It can cause skin irritation under exaggerated conditions of use. Ultimately, the choice of any specific agent(s) must be tailored to the unique needs of the patient being treated. As noted previously, pharmacologic treatments for hirsutism should be used in conjunction with nonpharmacologic approaches. It is also helpful to review the pattern of female hair distribution in the normal population to dispel unrealistic expectations.

FURTHER READING

CARMINA E: Antiandrogens for the treatment of hirsutism. Expert Opin Investig Drugs 11:357, 2002

FALSETTI L et al: Management of hirsutism. Am J Clin Dermatol 1:89, 2000

HORDINSKY M et al: Hair loss and hirsutism in the elderly. Clin Geriatr Med 18:121, 2002

LANIGAN SW: Management of unwanted hair in females. Clin Exp Dermatol 26:644, 2001

SANCHEZ LA et al: Laser hair reduction in the hirsute patient: A critical assessment. Hum Reprod Update 8:169, 2002

The concept of reproductive choice is now firmly entrenched in developed countries and has dramatically altered reproductive behavior. The availability of effective contraceptive methods prevents unintended pregnancies and has important economic and social implications. Infertility, on the other hand, can be accompanied by substantial stress and disappointment. Fortunately, the ability to diagnose and to treat various causes of infertility now provides an array of effective new approaches to this condition.

INFERTILITY

DEFINITION AND PREVALENCE *Infertility* is defined as the inability to conceive after 12 months of unprotected sexual intercourse. In a study of 5574 English and American women who ultimately conceived, pregnancy occurred in 50% within 3 months, 72% within 6 months, and 85% within 12 months. These findings are consistent with predictions based on *fecundability*, the probability of achieving pregnancy in one menstrual cycle (approximately 20 to 25% in healthy young couples). Assuming a fecundability of 0.25, 98% of couples should conceive within 13 months. Based on this definition, the National Survey of Family Growth reports a 14% rate of infertility in the United States in married women aged 15 to 44. The infertility rate has remained relatively stable over the past 30 years, although the proportion of couples without children has risen, reflecting a trend to delay childbearing. This trend has important implications because of an age-related decrease in fecundability, which begins at age 35 and is exacerbated after age 40.

CAUSES OF INFERTILITY The spectrum of infertility ranges from reduced conception rates or the need for medical intervention to irreversible causes of infertility (*sterility*). Infertility can be attributed primarily to male factors in 25%, female factors in 58%, and is unexplained in about 17% of couples (Fig. 45-1). Not uncommonly, both male and female factors contribute to infertility.

APPROACH TO THE PATIENT

Initial Evaluation In all couples presenting with infertility, the initial evaluation includes discussion of the appropriate timing of intercourse and discussion of modifiable risk factors such as smoking, alcohol, caffeine, and obesity. A description of the range of investigations that may be required and a brief description of infertility treatment options, including adoption, should be reviewed. Initial investigations are focused on determining whether the primary cause of the infertility is male, female, or both. These investigations include a semen analysis in the male, confirmation of ovulation in the female, and, in the majority of situations, documentation of tubal patency in the female. Although frequently used in the past, recent studies have not supported the efficacy of postcoital testing of sperm interaction with cervical mucus as a routine component of initial testing. Strategies for further evaluation are described below and in Chaps. 325 and 326. In some cases, after an extensive evaluation has excluded identifiable male or female causes of infertility, the disorder is classified as unexplained infertility.

Psychological Aspects of Infertility Infertility is invariably associated with psychological stress. In addition to the diagnostic and therapeutic procedures, stress may result from repeated cycles of hope and loss associated with each new procedure or cycle of treatment that does not result in the birth of a child. These feelings are often combined with a sense of isolation from friends and family. Counseling and stress-management techniques should be introduced early in the evaluation of infertility. When extreme, stress can contribute to infertility; for example, stress may impair hypothalamic

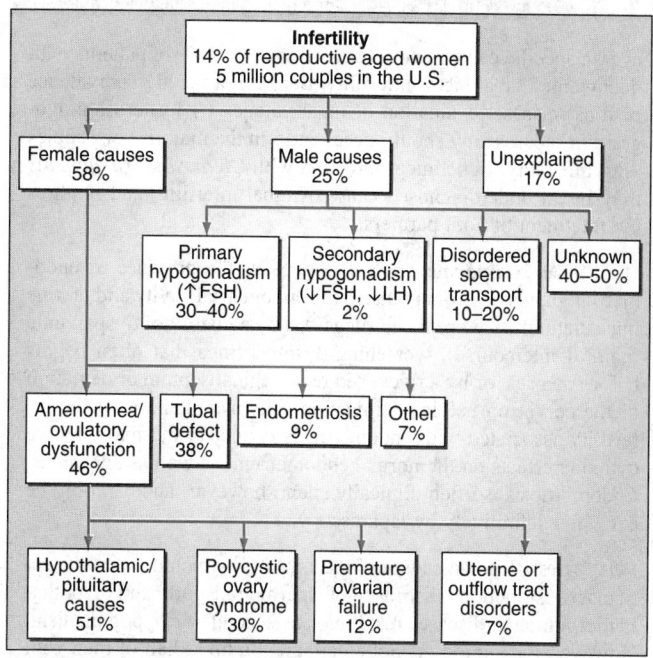

FIGURE 45-1 *Causes of infertility. FSH, follicle-stimulating hormone; LH, luteinizing hormone.*

control of ovulation. Infertility and its treatment do not appear to be associated with long-term psychological sequelae.

Female Causes Abnormalities in menstrual function constitute the most common cause of female infertility. These disorders, which include ovulatory dysfunction and abnormalities of the uterus or outflow tract, may present as amenorrhea (absence of menses) or as irregular or short menstrual cycles. A careful history and physical examination and a limited number of laboratory tests will help to determine whether the abnormality is (1) hypothalamic or pituitary [low follicle-stimulating hormone (FSH), luteinizing hormone (LH), and estradiol with or without an increase in prolactin]; (2) polycystic ovarian syndrome (PCOS; irregular cycles and hyperandrogenism in the absence of other causes of androgen excess); (3) ovarian (low estradiol with increased FSH); or (4) uterine or outflow tract abnormality. The frequency of these diagnoses depends on whether the amenorrhea is primary or occurs after normal puberty and menarche (Fig. 45-1). →*The approach to further evaluation of these disorders is described in detail in Chap. 326.*

OVULATORY DYSFUNCTION In women with a history of regular menstrual cycles, *evidence of ovulation* should be sought by using urinary ovulation predictor kits (they reflect the preovulatory gonadotropin surge but do not confirm ovulation), basal body temperature charts, or a mid-luteal phase progesterone level. The mid-luteal phase progesterone increase (usually >3 ng/mL) confirms ovulation and corpus luteum function and is responsible for the rise in basal body temperature [>0.3°C (>0.6°F) for 10 days]. An endometrial biopsy to exclude luteal phase insufficiency is no longer considered an essential part of the infertility workup for most patients. Even in the presence of ovulatory cycles, evaluation of *ovarian reserve* is recommended for women over 35 by measurement of FSH on day 3 of the cycle or in response to clomiphene, an estrogen antagonist (see below). An FSH level <10 IU/mL on cycle day 3 predicts adequate ovarian oocyte reserve. Inhibin B, an ovarian hormone that selectively suppresses FSH, is not of additional benefit in assessment of ovarian reserve.

TUBAL DISEASE Tubal disease may result from pelvic inflammatory disease (PID), appendicitis, endometriosis, pelvic adhesions, tubal surgery, and previous use of an intrauterine device (IUD). However, a specific cause is not identified in up to 50% of patients with documented tubal factor infertility. Because of the high prevalence of tubal disease, evaluation of tubal patency by hysterosalpingo-gram or laparoscopy should occur early in the majority of couples with infertility. Subclinical infection with *Chlamydia trachomatis* may be an underdiagnosed cause of tubal infertility and requires the treatment of both partners.

ENDOMETRIOSIS *Endometriosis* is defined as the presence of endo-metrial glands or stroma outside the endometrial cavity and uterine musculature. Its presence is suggested by a history of dyspareunia (painful intercourse), worsening dysmenorrhea that often begins before menses, or by a thickened rectovaginal septum or deviation of the cervix on pelvic examination. The pathogenesis of the in-fertility associated with endometriosis is unclear but may involve cytokine effects on the normal endometrium as well as adhesions. Endometriosis is often clinically silent, however, and can only be excluded definitively by laparoscopy.

Male Causes Known causes of male infertility include primary tes-ticular dysfunction, disorders of sperm transport, and hypotha-lamic-pituitary disease resulting in secondary hypogonadism. However, the etiology is not ascertained in up to half of men with suspected male factor infertility (Fig. 45-1). The key initial diag-nostic test is a *semen analysis*. Although 95% confidence limits can be used to define normal semen parameters, data relating sperm counts to fecundability are more useful. Such studies suggest that normal fertility is associated with sperm counts of >48 million/mL, with a motility of >63%, with >12% exhibiting normal morphology, whereas subfertility is seen with sperm counts of <13 million/mL, motility of <32%, and <9% normal morphology. Abnormalities of spermatogenesis may have a genetic component. Y chromosome microdeletions and *POLG* variants are increasingly recognized as a cause of *azoospermia* (absence of sperm) or *oligospermia* (low sperm count). Y chromosome microdeletions have also been iden-tified in a subset of men with elevated FSH levels and idiopathic infertility. Testosterone levels should be measured if the sperm count is low on repeated examination or if there is clinical evidence of hypogonadism. A low testosterone level may result from *pri-mary gonadal deficiency*; in this condition, levels of LH and FSH will be elevated. Less commonly, low testosterone and decreased spermatogenesis result from hypothalamic or pituitary disease, in which case the LH and FSH levels will be low (Chap. 325).

Acquired disorders of the testes are often associated with im-paired spermatogenesis with relatively preserved Leydig cell func-tion; thus, testosterone levels may be normal. Such abnormalities include viral orchitis (especially mumps) and other infectious causes such as tuberculosis or sexually transmitted diseases (STDs), chemotherapy (especially the alkylating agents cyclophos-phamide and chlorambucil), ionizing radiation, and drugs that may impair fertility directly or through inhibition of testicular androgen production or action. Anabolic androgen abuse should be consid-ered in a well-androgenized man with low gonadotropins and tes-tosterone but a suppressed sperm count. Prolonged elevation of testicular temperature may impair spermatogenesis, e.g., cryptor-chidism, after an acute febrile illness or in association with vari-cocele. A potential role for environmental toxins as a cause of impaired spermatogenesis has been suggested based on an apparent decrease in sperm counts over the past several decades, but a direct cause-and-effect relationship has not been established.

SECONDARY HYPOGONADISM Low gonadotropin levels, associated with low testosterone, may signal the presence of a pituitary macroad-enoma or hypothalamic tumor (in both cases prolactin levels may be elevated; Chap. 318) or may be the first presentation of hemo-chromatosis (Chap. 336) or other systemic illness. Recent studies have identified several genetic causes of gonadotropin-releasing

hormone (GnRH) deficiency (*KAL* and *DAX-1*), as well as muta-tions that lead to isolated gonadotropin deficiency (GnRH receptor, LHβ, FSHβ mutations) (Chap. 318).

DISORDERED SPERM TRANSPORT Patients with low sperm counts and normal hormonal levels may be found to have obstructive abnor-malities of the vas deferens or epididymis. The most common causes of vas deferens obstruction are previous vasectomy or ac-cidental ligation during inguinal surgery. Congenital absence of the vas deferens can be diagnosed by a deficiency of fructose in the ejaculate and is often associated with an abnormality of the cystic fibrosis transmembrane regulator (*CFTR*) gene. Young's syn-drome, characterized by inspissated secretions, can also preclude normal sperm transport.

℞ TREATMENT

The treatment of infertility should be tailored to the problems unique to each couple. In many situations, including unexplained infertility, mild to moderate endometriosis, and/or borderline semen parameters, a stepwise approach to infertility is optimal, beginning with low-risk interventions and moving to more invasive, higher risk interventions only if necessary. After determination of all infertility factors and their correction, if possible, this approach might include, in increasing order of complexity: (1) expectant management, (2) clomiphene citrate (see below) with or without intrauterine insemination (IUI), (3) gonadotro-pins with or without IUI, and (4) in vitro fertilization (IVF). The time used to complete the evaluation, correction, and expectant manage-ment can be longer in women <30, but this process should be ad-vanced rapidly in women >35. In some situations, expectant manage-ment will not be appropriate.

Ovulatory Dysfunction Treatment of ovulatory dysfunction should first be directed at identification of the etiology of the disorder to allow specific management when possible. Dopamine agonists, for example, may be indicated in patients with hyperprolactinemia (Chap. 318); life-style modification may be successful in women with low body weight or a history of intensive exercise (Chap. 65).

Medications used for ovulation induction include clomiphene cit-rate, gonadotropins, and pulsatile GnRH. *Clomiphene citrate* is a non-steroidal estrogen antagonist that increases FSH and LH levels by blocking estrogen negative feedback at the hypothalamus. The efficacy of clomiphene for ovulation induction is highly dependent on patient selection. It induces ovulation in 70 to 80% of women with PCOS and is the initial treatment of choice in these patients, particularly in con-junction with the use of insulin-sensitizing agents, such as metformin. Clomiphene citrate is less successful in patients with hypogonadotro-pic hypogonadism.

Gonadotropins are highly effective for ovulation induction in women with hypogonadotropic hypogonadism and PCOS and are used to induce multiple follicular recruitment in unexplained infertility and in older reproductive-aged women. Disadvantages include a significant risk of multiple gestation and the risk of ovarian hyperstimulation, but careful monitoring and a conservative approach to ovarian stimulation reduce these risks. Currently available gonadotropins include urinary preparations of LH and FSH, highly purified FSH, and recombinant FSH. Though FSH is the key component, the addition of some LH (or human chorionic gonadotropin) may improve results, particularly in hypogonadotropic patients.

Pulsatile GnRH is highly effective for restoring ovulation in pa-tients with hypothalamic amenorrhea but is not widely available in the United States. Pregnancy rates are similar to those following the use of gonadotropins, but rates of multiple gestation are lower and there is virtually no risk of ovarian hyperstimulation.

None of these methods are effective in women with premature ovarian failure in whom donor oocyte or adoption are the methods of choice.

Tubal Disease If hysterosalpingography suggests a tubal or uterine cavity abnormality, or if a patient is ≥35 at the time of initial evaluation, laparoscopy with tubal lavage is recommended, often with a hysteroscopy. Although tubal reconstruction may be attempted if tubal disease is identified, IVF is often used instead, as these patients are at increased risk of developing an ectopic pregnancy.

Endometriosis Though 60% of women with minimal or mild endometriosis may conceive within 1 year without treatment, laparoscopic resection or ablation appears to improve conception rates. Medical management of advanced stages of endometriosis is widely used for symptom control but has not been shown to enhance fertility (Chap. 326). In moderate to severe endometriosis, conservative surgery is associated with pregnancy rates of 50 and 39% respectively, compared with rates of 25 and 5% with expectant management alone. In some patients, IVF may be the treatment of choice.

Male Factor Infertility Treatment options for male factor infertility have expanded greatly in recent years. Secondary hypogonadism is highly amenable to treatment with pulsatile GnRH or gonadotropins (Chap. 325). In vitro techniques have provided new opportunities for patients with primary testicular failure and disorders of sperm transport. Choice of initial treatment options depends on sperm concentration and motility. Expectant management should be attempted initially in men with mild male factor infertility (sperm count of 15 to 20 × 10^6/mL and normal motility). Moderate male factor infertility (10 to 15 × 10^6/mL and 20 to 40% motility) should begin with IUI alone or in combination with treatment of the female partner with clomiphene or gonadotropins, but it may require IVF with or without intracytoplasmic sperm injection (ICSI). For men with a severe defect (sperm count of <10 × 10^6/mL, 10% motility), IVF with ICSI or donor sperm should be used.

Assisted Reproductive Technologies The development of assisted reproductive technologies (ART) has dramatically altered the treatment of male and female infertility. IVF is indicated for patients with many causes of infertility that have not been successfully managed with more conservative approaches. IVF or ICSI is often the treatment of choice in couples with a significant male factor or tubal disease, whereas IVF using donor oocytes is used in patients with premature ovarian failure and in women of advanced reproductive age. Success rates depend on the age of the woman and the cause of the infertility and are generally 18 to 24% per cycle when initiated in women <40. In women >40, there is a marked decrease in both the number of oocytes retrieved and their ability to be fertilized. Though often effective, IVF is expensive and requires careful monitoring of ovulation induction and invasive techniques, including the aspiration of multiple follicles. IVF is associated with a significant risk of multiple gestation (31% twins, 6% triplets, and 0.2% higher order multiples).

CONTRACEPTION

Though various forms of contraception are widely available, approximately 30% of births in the United States are the result of unintended pregnancy. Teenage pregnancies continue to represent a serious public health problem in the United States, with >1 million unintended pregnancies each year—a significantly greater incidence than in other industrialized nations.

Contraceptive methods are widely used (Table 45-1). Only 15% of couples report having unprotected sexual intercourse in the past 3

TABLE 45-1 *Effectiveness of Different Forms of Contraception*

Method of Contraception	Theoretical Effectiveness, %[a]	Actual Effectiveness, %[a]	% Continuing Use at 1 Year[b]	Contraceptive Methods Used by U.S. Women[c]
Barrier methods				
Condoms	98	88	63	20
Diaphragm	94	82	58	2
Cervical cap	94	82	50	<1
Spermicides	97	79	43	1
Sterilization				
Male	99.9	99.9	100	11
Female	99.8	99.6	100	28
Intrauterine device				1
Copper T380	99	97	78	
Progestasert	98	97	81	
Mirena	99.9	99.8		
Oral contraceptive pill			72	27
Combination	99.9	97		
Progestin only	99.5	97		
Long-acting progestins				
Depo-Provera	99.7	99.7	70	<1
Norplant	99.7	99.7	85	1

[a] Adapted from Trussell J et al, Obstet Gynecol 76:558, 1990.
[b] Adapted from Contraceptive Technology Update. Contraceptive Technology, Feb. 1996, vol 17, No 1, pp 13–24.
[c] Adapted from Piccinino LJ and Mosher WD, Fam Plan Perspective 30:4, 1998.

months. A reversible form of contraception is used by >50% of couples. Sterilization (in either the male or female) has been employed as a permanent form of contraception by over a third of couples. Pregnancy termination is relatively safe when directed by health care professionals but is rarely the option of choice.

No single contraceptive method is ideal, although all are safer than carrying a pregnancy to term. The effectiveness of a given method of contraception is dependent on the efficacy of the method itself, compliance, and appropriate use. Knowledge of the advantages and disadvantages of each contraceptive is essential for counseling an individual about the methods that are safest and most consistent with his or her lifestyle. Discrepancies between theoretical and actual effectiveness emphasize the importance of patient education and compliance when considering various forms of contraception (Table 45-1).

BARRIER METHODS Barrier contraceptives (such as condoms, diaphragms, and cervical caps) and spermicides are easily available, reversible, and have fewer side effects than hormonal methods. However, their effectiveness is highly dependent on compliance and proper use (Table 45-1). A major advantage of barrier contraceptives is the protection provided against STDs (Chap. 115). Consistent use is associated with a decreased risk of gonorrhea, nongonococcal urethritis, and genital herpes, probably due in part to the concomitant use of spermicides. Condom use also reduces the transmission of HIV infection. Natural membrane condoms may be less effective than latex condoms, and petroleum-based lubricants can degrade condoms and decrease their efficacy for preventing HIV infection. A highly effective female condom, which also provides protection against STDs, was approved in 1994 but has not achieved widespread use.

STERILIZATION Sterilization is the method of birth control most frequently chosen by fertile men and multiparous women >30 (Table 45-1). Sterilization prevents fertilization by surgical interruption of the fallopian tubes in women or the vas deferens in men. Although tubal ligation and vasectomy are potentially reversible, these procedures should be considered permanent and should not be undertaken without careful patient counseling.

Several methods of *tubal ligation* have been developed, all of which are highly effective with a 10-year cumulative pregnancy rate of 1.85 per 100 women. However, when pregnancy does occur, the risk of ectopic pregnancy may be as high as 30%. In addition to prevention of pregnancy, tubal ligation reduces the risk of ovarian cancer, possibly by limiting the upward migration of potential carcinogens.

Vasectomy is an outpatient surgical procedure that has little risk and is highly effective. The development of azoospermia may be delayed for 2 to 6 months, and other forms of contraception must be used until two sperm-free ejaculations provide proof of sterility.

INTRAUTERINE DEVICES IUDs inhibit pregnancy primarily through a spermicidal effect caused by a sterile inflammatory reaction produced by the presence of a foreign body in the uterine cavity (copper IUDs) or by the release of progestins (Progestasert, Mirena). IUDs provide a high level of efficacy in the absence of systemic metabolic effects, and ongoing motivation is not required to ensure efficacy once the device has been placed. However, only 1% of women in the United States use this method compared to a utilization rate of 15 to 30% in much of Europe and Canada. This relatively low utilization rate continues despite evidence that the newer devices are not associated with increased rates of pelvic infection and infertility, as occurred with earlier devices. Screening for STDs should be performed prior to insertion, and an IUD should not be used in women at high risk for development of STDs or in women at high risk for bacterial endocarditis.

HORMONAL METHODS ▪ Oral Contraceptive Pills Because of their ease of use and efficacy, oral contraceptive pills are the most widely used form of hormonal contraception. They act by suppressing ovulation, changing cervical mucus, and altering the endometrium. The current formulations are made from synthetic estrogens and progestins. The estrogen component of the pill consists of ethinyl estradiol or mestranol, which is metabolized to ethinyl estradiol. Multiple synthetic progestins are available. Norethindrone and its derivatives are used in many formulations. Low-dose norgestimate and the more recently developed progestins (desogestrel, gestodene, drospirenone) have a less androgenic profile; levonorgestrel appears to be the most androgenic of the progestins and should be avoided in patients with hyperandrogenic features. The three major formulations of oral contraceptives are: (1) fixed-dose estrogen-progestin combination, (2) phasic estrogen-progestin combination, and (3) progestin only. Combination formulations are administered daily for 3 weeks followed by a week of no medication during which menstrual bleeding generally occurs. Progestin-only pills are administered continuously. There has been recent interest in the development of extended oral contraceptives, reducing the number of episodes of withdrawal bleeding. An oral, trimonthly regimen is currently under investigation in the United States. Preliminary studies indicate that headache is reduced, although there is an early incidence of breakthrough bleeding.

Current doses of ethinyl estradiol range from 20 to 50 μg. However, indications for the 50-μg dose are rare, and the majority of formulations contain 35 μg of ethinyl estradiol. The reduced estrogen and progesterone content in the second- and third-generation pills has decreased both side effects and risks associated with oral contraceptive use (Table 45-2). At the currently used doses, patients must be cautioned not to miss pills due to the potential for ovulation. Side effects, including break-through bleeding, amenorrhea, breast tenderness, and weight gain, are often responsive to a change in formulation.

The microdose progestin-only minipill is less effective as a contraceptive, having a pregnancy rate of 2 to 7 per 100 women-years. However, it may be appropriate for women with cardiovascular disease or for women who cannot tolerate synthetic estrogens.

New Methods A *weekly contraceptive patch* (Ortho Evra) is now available. It has similar efficacy to oral contraceptives and may be associated with less breakthrough bleeding. Approximately 2% of patches fail to adhere, and a similar percentage of women have skin reactions. Efficacy is lower in women >90 kg. A *monthly contraceptive injection* (Lunelle) is also available. This estrogen/progestin combination is highly effective, with a first-year failure rate of <0.2%, but it may be less effective in obese women. Its use is associated with bleeding irregularities that diminish over time. Fertility returns rapidly after discontinuation. A *monthly vaginal ring* (NuvaRing) is now approved for contraceptive use. It is highly effective, with a 12-month failure rate of 0.7%. The device is intended to be left in place during intercourse.

TABLE 45-2 *Oral Contraceptives: Contraindications and Disease Risk*

I. Contraindications
  A. Absolute
    1. Previous thromboembolic event or stroke
    2. History of an estrogen-dependent tumor
    3. Active liver disease
    4. Pregnancy
    5. Undiagnosed abnormal uterine bleeding
    6. Hypertriglyceridemia
    7. Women over age 35 who smoke heavily (>15 cigarettes per day)
  B. Relative
    1. Hypertension
    2. Women receiving anticonvulsant drug therapy
II. Disease risks
  A. Increased
    1. Coronary heart disease—increased only in smokers > 35; no relation to progestin type
    2. Hypertension—relative risk 1.8 (current users) and 1.2 (previous users)
    3. Venous thrombosis—relative risk ~4; markedly increased with factor V Leiden or prothrombin-gene mutations
    4. Stroke—increased only in combination with hypertension; unclear relation to migraine headache
    5. Cerebral vein thrombosis—relative risk ~13–15; synergistic with prothrombin-gene mutation
    6. Cervical cancer—relative risk 2–4
  B. Decreased
    1. Ovarian cancer—50% reduction in risk
    2. Endometrial cancer—40% reduction in risk
  C. No effect
    1. Breast cancer

If removed during intercourse, it must be reinserted within 3 h. Ovulation returns within the first recovery cycle after discontinuation.

Long-Term Contraceptives Long-term progestin administration in the form of Depo-Provera and Norplant (Table 45-1) act primarily by inhibiting ovulation and causing changes in the endometrium and cervical mucus that result in decreased implantation and sperm transport. Depo-Provera requires an intramuscular injection and is effective for 3 months, but return of fertility after discontinuation may be delayed for up to 12 to 18 months. Norplant requires surgical insertion but is effective for up to 5 years afer insertion; fertility is possible shortly after its removal. Amenorrhea, irregular bleeding, and weight gain are the most common adverse effects associated with both injectable forms of contraception. A major advantage of the injectable progestin-based contraceptives is the apparent lack of increased arterial and venous thromboembolic events, but increased gallbladder disease and decreased bone density may result.

POSTCOITAL CONTRACEPTION Postcoital contraceptive methods prevent implantation or cause regression of the corpus luteum and are highly efficacious if used appropriately. Unprotected intercourse without regard to the time of the month carries an 8% incidence of pregnancy, an incidence that can be reduced to 2% by the use of emergency contraceptives within 72 h of unprotected intercourse. Certain oral contraceptive pills can be used within 72 h of unprotected intercourse [Ovral (2 tablets, 12 h apart) and Lo/Ovral (4 tablets, 12 h apart)]. Preven (50 mg ethinyl estradiol and 0.25 mg levonorgestrel) and Plan B (0.75 mg levonorgestrel) are now approved for postcoital contraception. Side effects are common with these high doses of hormones and include nausea, vomiting, and breast soreness. Recent studies suggest that 600 mg mifepristone (RU486), a progesterone receptor antagonist, may be equally as effective or more effective than hormonal regimens, with fewer side effects.

MALE HORMONAL CONTRACEPTION An effective and reversible male contraceptive has long been sought, and surveys indicate that a "male pill" would be acceptable to both men and women. Complete suppression of spermatogenesis is required for acceptable contraception but is not achieved reliably with testosterone alone. However, the combination of a long-acting testosterone preparation with a GnRH antagonist or a progestin such as norgestral, desonorgestrel, or norethisterone results in effective contraception, suggesting that a male contraceptive may be forthcoming.

FURTHER READING

ABMA JC et al and the National Center for Health Statistics: Fertility, family planning, and women's health: New data from the 1995 Survey of Family Growth. Vital Health Stat 23, no. 10

ANDERSON RA et al: Male contraception. Endocr Rev 23:735, 2002

GUZIK DS et al: Sperm morphology, motility and concentration in fertile and infertile men. N Engl J Med 345:1388, 2001

KURODA-KAWAGUCHI T et al: The AZFc region of the Y chromosome features massive palindromes and uniform recurrent deletions in infertile men. Nat Genet 29:279, 2001

MARCHBANKS PA et al. Oral contraceptives and the risk of breast cancer. N Engl J Med 346:2025, 2002

TRUSSELL J, VAUGHAN B: Contraceptive failure, method-related discontinuation and resumption of use: Results from the 1995 National Survey of Family Growth. Fam Plan Perspect 31:64, 1999

Section 9   Alterations in the Skin

46 APPROACH TO THE PATIENT WITH A SKIN DISORDER
Thomas J. Lawley, Kim B. Yancey

The challenge of examining the skin lies in distinguishing normal from abnormal, significant findings from trivial ones, and in integrating pertinent signs and symptoms into an appropriate differential diagnosis. The fact that the largest organ in the body is visible is both an advantage and a disadvantage to those who examine it. It is advantageous because no special instrumentation is necessary and because the skin can be biopsied with little morbidity. However, the casual observer can be misled by a variety of stimuli and overlook important, subtle signs of skin or systemic disease. For instance, the sometimes minor differences in color and shape that distinguish a malignant melanoma (Fig. 46-1) from a benign pigmented nevus (Fig. 46-2) can be difficult to recognize. To aid in the interpretation of skin lesions, a variety of descriptive terms have been developed to characterize cutaneous lesions (Tables 46-1 and 46-2 and Fig. 46-3) and to formulate a differential diagnosis (Table 46-3). For instance, the finding of large numbers of scaling papules, usually indicative of a primary skin disease, places the patient in a different diagnostic category than would hemorrhagic papules, which may indicate vasculitis or sepsis (Figs. 46-4 and 46-5, respectively). It is important to differentiate primary skin lesions from secondary skin changes. If the examiner focuses on linear erosions overlying an area of erythema and scaling, he or she may incorrectly assume that the erosion is the primary lesion and the redness and scale are secondary, while the correct interpretation would be that the patient has a pruritic eczematous dermatitis with erosions caused by scratching.

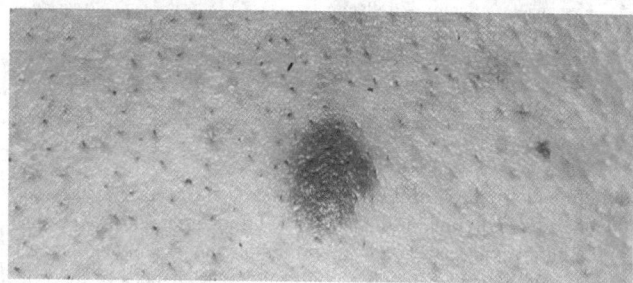

FIGURE 46-2   Nevi are benign proliferations of nevomelanocytes characterized by regularly shaped hyperpigmented macules or papules of a uniform color.

APPROACH TO THE PATIENT

In examining the skin it is usually advisable to assess the patient before taking an extensive history. This way, the entire cutaneous surface is sure to be evaluated, and objective findings can be integrated with relevant historic data. Four basic features of any cutaneous lesion must be noted and considered in the examination of

TABLE 46-1   Descriptions of Primary Skin Lesions

Macule: A flat, colored lesion, <2 cm in diameter, not raised above the surface of the surrounding skin. A "freckle," or ephelid, is a prototype pigmented macule.

Patch: A large (>2 cm), flat lesion with a color different from the surrounding skin. This differs from a macule only in size.

Papule: A small, solid lesion, <0.5 cm in diameter, raised above the surface of the surrounding skin and hence palpable (e.g., a closed comedone, or whitehead, in acne).

Nodule: A larger (0.5–5.0 cm), firm lesion raised above the surface of the surrounding skin. This differs from a papule only in size (e.g., dermal nevus).

Tumor: A solid, raised growth >5 cm in diameter.

Plaque: A large (>1 cm), flat-topped, raised lesion; edges may either be distinct (e.g., in psoriasis) or gradually blend with surrounding skin (e.g., in eczematous dermatitis).

Vesicle: A small, fluid-filled lesion, <0.5 cm in diameter, raised above the plane of surrounding skin. Fluid is often visible, and the lesions are often translucent [e.g., vesicles in allergic contact dermatitis caused by *Toxicodendron* (poison ivy)].

Pustule: A vesicle filled with leukocytes. Note: The presence of pustules does not necessarily signify the existence of an infection.

Bulla: A fluid-filled, raised, often translucent lesion >0.5 cm in diameter.

Cyst: A soft, raised, encapsulated lesion filled with semisolid or liquid contents.

Wheal: A raised, erythematous papule or plaque, usually representing short-lived dermal edema.

Telangiectasia: Dilated, superficial blood vessels.

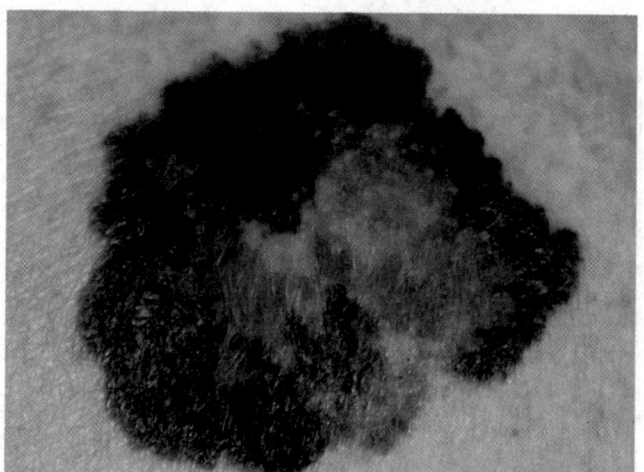

FIGURE 46-1   Superficial spreading melanoma is the most common type of malignant melanoma and demonstrates color variegation (black, blue, brown, pink, and white) and irregular borders.

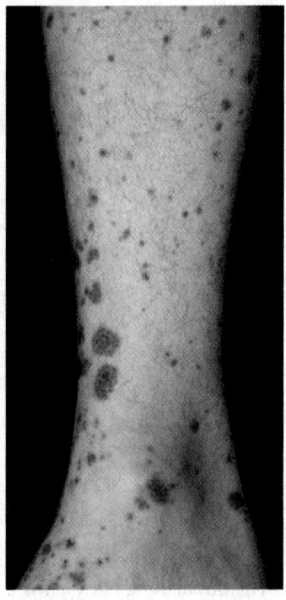

FIGURE 46-4   Palpable purpuric papules on the lower legs are seen in this patient with cutaneous small vessel vasculitis. (*Courtesy of Robert Swerlick, MD.*)

skin: the distribution of the eruption, the type(s) of primary lesion, the shape of individual lesions, and the arrangement of the lesions. In the initial examination it is important that the patient be disrobed as completely as possible. This will minimize chances of missing important individual skin lesions and make it possible to assess the distribution of the eruption accurately. The patient should first be viewed from a distance of about 1.5 to 2 m (4 to 6 ft) so that the general character of the skin and the distribution of lesions can be evaluated. Indeed, distribution of lesions often correlates highly with diagnosis (Fig. 46-6). For example, a hospitalized patient with a generalized erythematous exanthem is more likely to have a drug eruption than is a patient with a similar rash limited to the sun-exposed portions of the face. The presence or absence of lesions on mucosal surfaces should also be determined. Once the distribution of the lesions has been established, the nature of the primary

lesion must be determined. Thus, when lesions are distributed on elbows, knees, and scalp, the most likely possibility based solely on distribution is psoriasis or dermatitis herpetiformis (Figs. 46-7 and 46-8, respectively). The primary lesion in psoriasis is a scaly papule that soon forms erythematous plaques covered with a white scale, whereas that of dermatitis herpetiformis is an urticarial papule that quickly becomes a small vesicle. In this manner, identification of the primary lesion directs the examiner toward the proper diagnosis. Secondary changes in skin can also be quite helpful. For example, scale represents excessive epidermis, while crust is the result of a discontinuous epithelial cell layer. Palpation of skin lesions can also yield insight into the character of an eruption. Thus red papules on the lower extremities that blanch with pressure can be a manifestation of many different diseases, but hemorrhagic red papules that do not blanch with pressure indicate palpable purpura characteristic of necrotizing vasculitis (Fig. 46-4).

The shape of lesions is also an important feature. Flat, round, erythematous papules and plaques are common in many cutaneous diseases. However, target-shaped lesions that consist in part of erythematous plaques are specific for erythema multiforme (Fig. 46-9). In the same way, the arrangement of individual lesions is important. Erythematous papules and vesicles can occur in many conditions, but their arrangement in a specific linear array suggests an external etiology such as allergic contact (Fig. 46-10) or primary

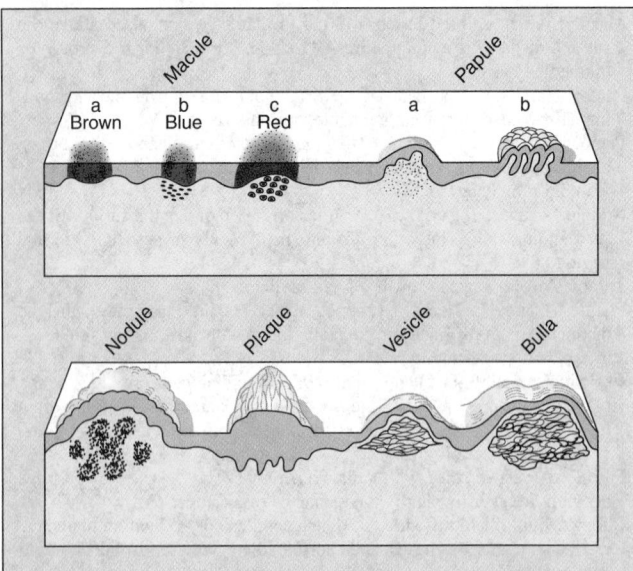

FIGURE 46-3   A schematic representation of several common primary skin lesions (see Table 46-1).

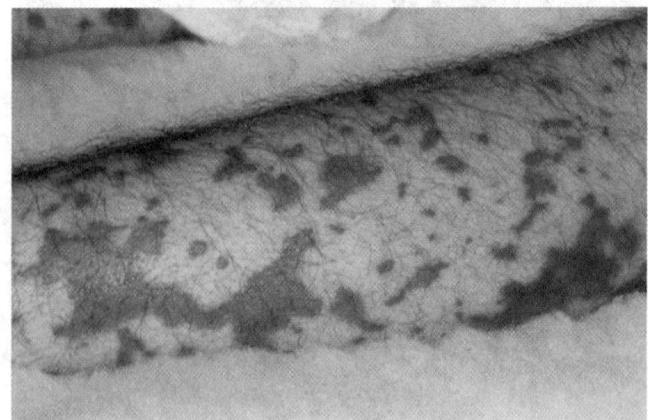

FIGURE 46-5   Fulminant meningococcemia with extensive angular purpuric patches. (*Courtesy of Stephen E. Gellis, MD.*)

TABLE 46-3 *Selected Common Dermatologic Conditions*

Diagnosis	Common Distribution	Usual Morphology	Diagnosis	Common Distribution	Usual Morphology
Acne vulgaris	Face, upper back	Open and closed comedones, erythematous papules, pustules, cysts	Seborrheic keratosis	Trunk, face	Brown plaques with adherent, greasy scale; "stuck on" appearance
Rosacea	Blush area of cheeks, nose, forehead, chin	Erythema, telangiectasias, papules, pustules	Folliculitis	Any hair-bearing area	Follicular pustules
Seborrheic dermatitis	Scalp, eyebrows, perinasal areas	Erythema with greasy yellow-brown scale	Impetigo	Anywhere	Papules, vesicles, pustules, often with honey-colored crusts
Atopic dermatitis	Antecubital and popliteal fossae; may be widespread	Patches and plaques of erythema, scaling, and lichenification; pruritus	Herpes simplex	Lips, genitalia	Grouped vesicles progressing to crusted erosions
Stasis dermatitis	Ankles, lower legs	Patches of erythema and scaling on background of hyperpigmentation associated with signs of venous insufficiency	Herpes zoster	Dermatomal, usually trunk but may be anywhere	Vesicles limited to a dermatome (often painful)
Dyshidrotic eczema	Palms, soles, sides of fingers and toes	Deep vesicles	Varicella	Face, trunk, relative sparing of extremities	Lesions arise in crops and quickly progress from erythematous macules to papules to vesicles to pustules to crusts
Allergic contact dermatitis	Anywhere	Localized erythema, vesicles, scale, and pruritus (e.g., fingers, earlobes—nickel; dorsal aspect of foot—shoe; exposed surfaces—poison ivy)	Pityriasis rosea	Trunk (Christmas tree pattern); herald patch followed by multiple smaller lesions	Symmetric erythematous patches with a collarette of scale
Psoriasis	Elbows, knees, scalp, lower back, fingernails (may be generalized)	Papules and plaques covered with silvery scale; nails have pits	Tinea versicolor	Chest, back, abdomen, proximal extremities	Scaly hyper- or hypopigmented macules
Lichen planus	Wrists, ankles, mouth (may be widespread)	Violaceous flat-topped papules and plaques	Candidiasis	Groin, beneath breasts, vagina, oral cavity	Erythematous macerated areas with satellite pustules; white, friable patches on mucous membranes
Keratosis pilaris	Extensor surfaces of arms and thighs, buttocks	Keratotic follicular papules with surrounding erythema	Dermatophytosis	Feet, groin, beard, or scalp	Varies with site, (e.g., tinea corporis—scaly annular patch)
Melasma	Forehead, cheeks, temples, upper lip	Tan to brown patches	Scabies	Groin, axillae, between fingers and toes, beneath breasts	Excoriated papules, burrows, pruritus
Vitiligo	Periorificial, trunk, extensor surfaces of extremities, flexor wrists, axillae	Chalk-white macules	Insect bites	Anywhere	Erythematous papules with central puncta
Actinic keratosis	Sun-exposed areas	Skin-colored or red-brown macule or papule with dry, rough, adherent scale	Cherry angioma	Trunk	Red, blood-filled papules
			Keloid	Anywhere (site of previous injury)	Firm tumor, pink, purple, or brown
Basal cell carcinoma	Face	Papule with pearly, telangiectatic border on sun-damaged skin	Dermatofibroma	Anywhere	Firm red to brown nodule that shows dimpling of overlying skin with lateral compression
Squamous cell carcinoma	Face, especially lower lip, ears	Indurated and possibly hyperkeratotic lesions often showing ulceration and/or crusting	Acrochordons (skin tags)	Groin, axilla, neck	Fleshy papules
			Urticaria	Anywhere	Wheals, sometimes with surrounding flare; pruritus
			Transient acantholytic dermatosis	Trunk, especially anterior chest	Erythematous papules
			Xerosis	Extensor extremities, especially legs	Dry, erythematous, scaling patches; pruritus

irritant dermatitis. In contrast, lesions with a generalized arrangement are common and suggest a systemic etiology.

As in other branches of medicine, a complete history should be obtained to emphasize the following features:

1. Evolution of lesions
   a. Site of onset
   b. Manner in which the eruption progressed or spread
   c. Duration
   d. Periods of resolution or improvement in chronic eruptions
2. Symptoms associated with the eruption
   a. Itching, burning, pain, numbness
   b. What, if anything, has relieved symptoms
   c. Time of day when symptoms are most severe
3. Current or recent medications (prescribed as well as over-the-counter)
4. Associated systemic symptoms (e.g., malaise, fever, arthralgias)
5. Ongoing or previous illnesses
6. History of allergies
7. Presence of photosensitivity
8. Review of systems

DIAGNOSTIC TECHNIQUES Many skin diseases can be diagnosed on gross clinical appearance, but sometimes relatively simple diagnostic procedures can yield valuable information. In most instances, they can be performed at the bedside with a minimum of equipment.

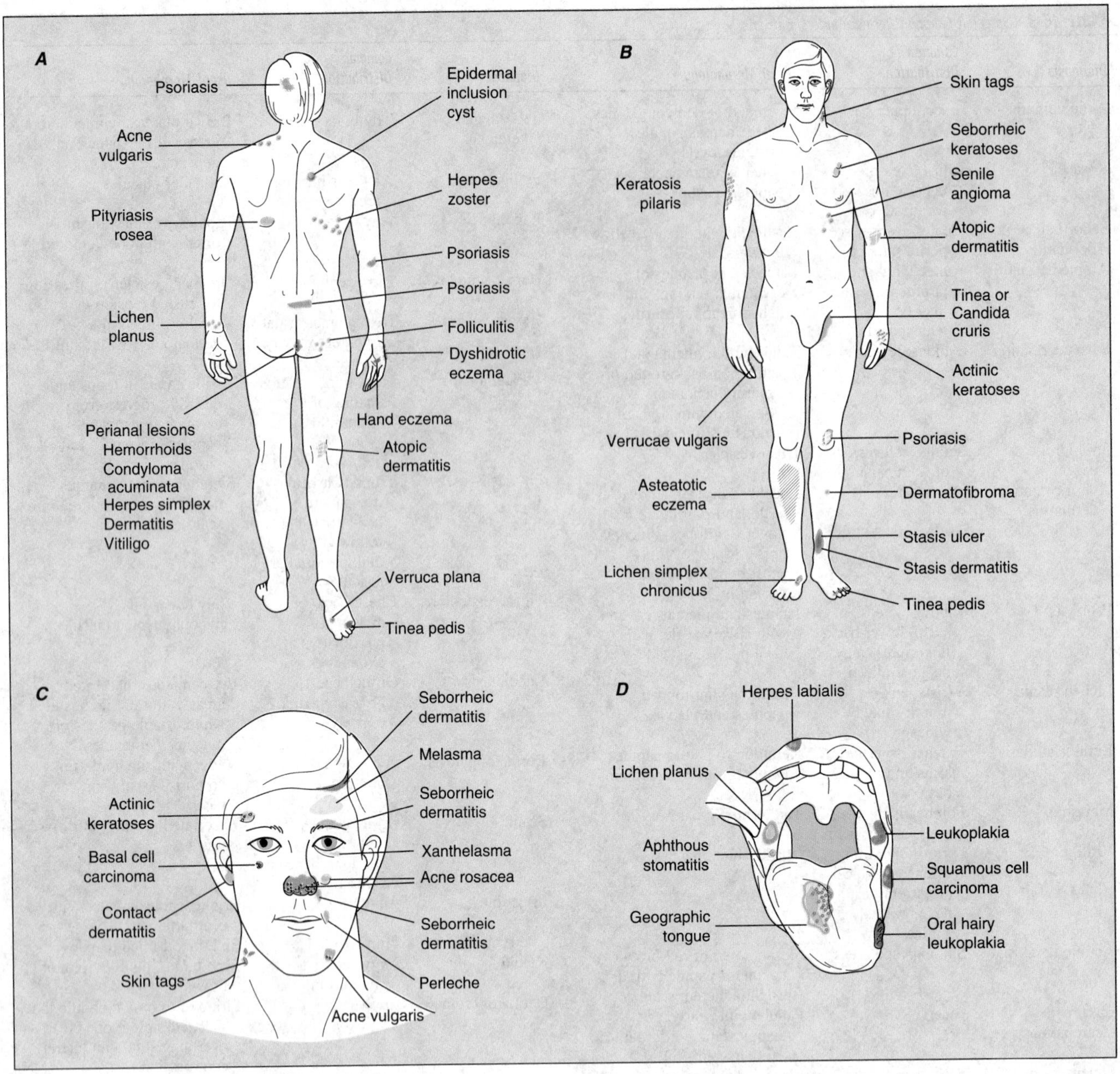

A

Psoriasis
Acne vulgaris
Pityriasis rosea
Lichen planus
Perianal lesions
 Hemorrhoids
 Condyloma acuminata
 Herpes simplex
 Dermatitis
 Vitiligo
Epidermal inclusion cyst
Herpes zoster
Psoriasis
Psoriasis
Folliculitis
Dyshidrotic eczema
Hand eczema
Atopic dermatitis
Verruca plana
Tinea pedis

B

Keratosis pilaris
Verrucae vulgaris
Asteatotic eczema
Lichen simplex chronicus
Skin tags
Seborrheic keratoses
Senile angioma
Atopic dermatitis
Tinea or Candida cruris
Actinic keratoses
Psoriasis
Dermatofibroma
Stasis ulcer
Stasis dermatitis
Tinea pedis

C

Actinic keratoses
Basal cell carcinoma
Contact dermatitis
Skin tags
Seborrheic dermatitis
Melasma
Seborrheic dermatitis
Xanthelasma
Acne rosacea
Seborrheic dermatitis
Perleche
Acne vulgaris

D

Lichen planus
Aphthous stomatitis
Geographic tongue
Herpes labialis
Leukoplakia
Squamous cell carcinoma
Oral hairy leukoplakia

FIGURE 46-6   *A–D.* The distribution of some common dermatologic diseases and lesions.

Skin Biopsy   A skin biopsy is a straightforward minor surgical procedure; however, it is important to biopsy a lesion that is most likely to yield diagnostic findings. This decision may require expertise in skin diseases and knowledge of superficial anatomic structures in selected areas of the body. In this procedure, a small area of skin is anesthetized with 1% lidocaine with or without epinephrine. The skin lesion in question can be excised with a scalpel or removed by punch biopsy. In the latter technique, a punch is pressed against the surface of the skin and rotated with downward pressure until it penetrates to the subcutaneous tissue. The circular biopsy is then lifted with forceps, and the bottom is cut with iris scissors. Biopsy sites may or may not need suture closure, depending on size and location.

KOH Preparation   A potassium hydroxide (KOH) preparation is performed on scaling skin lesions where a fungal etiology is a possibility. The edge of such a lesion is scraped gently with a scalpel blade, and the removed scale is collected on a glass microscope slide and treated with 1 to 2 drops of a solution of 10 to 20% KOH. KOH dissolves keratin and allows easier visualization of fungal elements. Brief heating of the slide accelerates dissolution of keratin. When the preparation

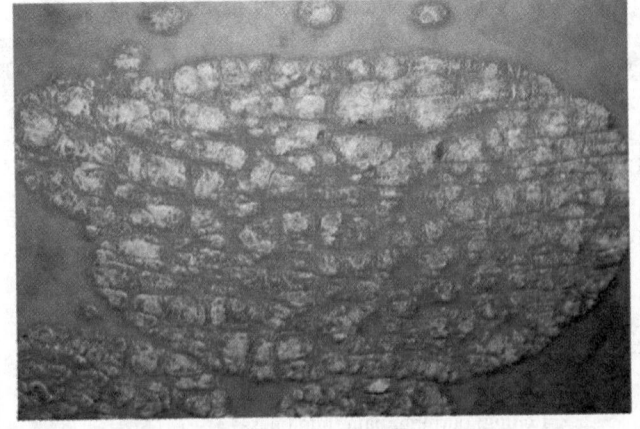

FIGURE 46-7   Psoriasis is characterized by small and large erythematous plaques with adherent silvery scale.

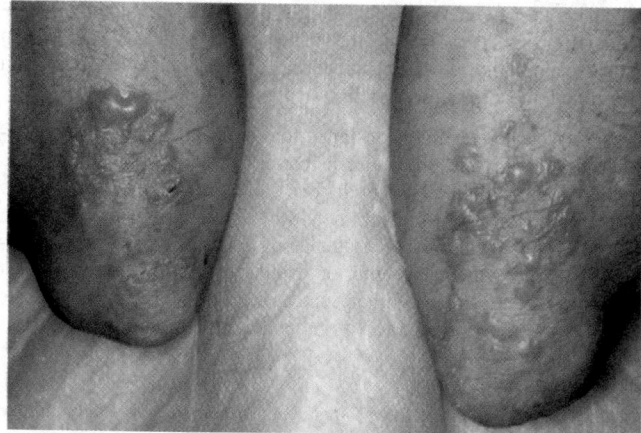

FIGURE 46-8 Dermatitis herpetiformis manifested by pruritic, grouped vesicles in a typical location. The vesicles are often excoriated and may occur on knees, buttocks, and posterior scalp.

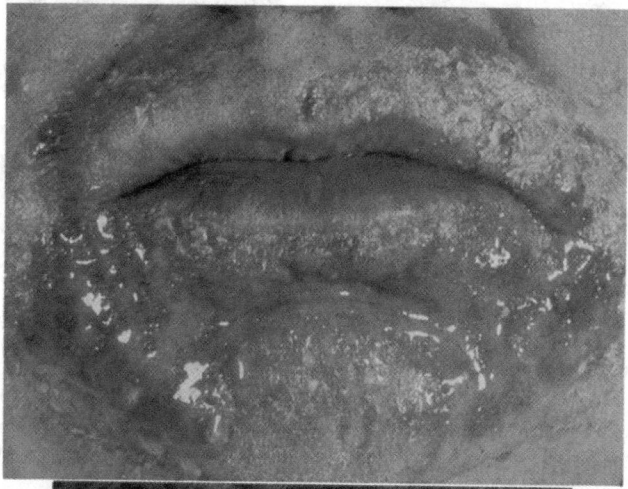

A

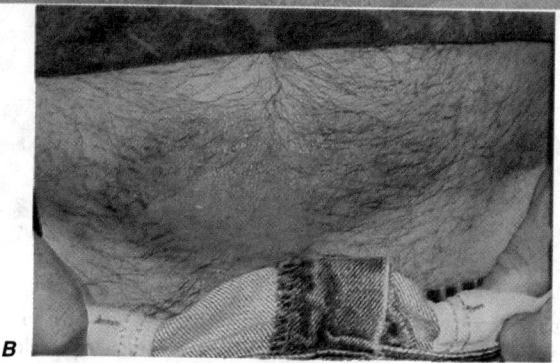

B

FIGURE 46-10 *A.* Allergic contact dermatitis, acute phase, with sharply demarcated, weeping, eczematous plaques in a perioral distribution. *B.* Allergic contact dermatitis to nickel, chronic phase demonstrating an erythematous, lichenified, weeping plaque on skin chronically exposed to a metal snap. (*B, Courtesy of Robert Swerlick, MD.*)

is viewed under the microscope, the refractile hyphae will be seen more easily when the light intensity is reduced and the condenser is lowered. This technique can be utilized to identify hyphae in dermatophyte infections (see Fig. 190-1), pseudohyphae and budding yeast in *Candida* infections (see Fig. 187-1), and fragmented hyphae and spores in tinea versicolor. The same sampling technique can be used to obtain scale for culture of selected pathogenic organisms.

Tzanck Smear A Tzanck smear is a cytologic technique most often used in the diagnosis of herpesvirus infections [simplex or varicella-zoster (see Figs. 164-1 and 164-3). An early vesicle, not a pustule or crusted lesion, is unroofed, and the base of the lesion is scraped gently with a scalpel blade. The material is placed on a glass slide, air-dried, and stained with Giemsa or Wright's stain. Multinucleated epithelial giant cells suggest the presence of herpes, but culture or immunofluorescence testing must be performed to identify the specific virus.

Diascopy Diascopy is designed to assess whether a skin lesion will blanch with pressure as, for example, in determining whether a red lesion is hemorrhagic or simply blood-filled. For instance, urticaria (Fig. 46-11) will blanch with pressure, whereas a purpuric lesion caused by necrotizing vasculitis (Fig. 46-4) will not. Diascopy is performed by pressing a microscope slide or magnifying lens against a lesion and noting the amount of blanching that occurs. Granulomas often have an "apple jelly" appearance on diascopy.

Wood's Light A Wood's lamp generates 360-nm ultraviolet (or "black") light that can be used to aid the evaluation of certain skin disorders. For example, a Wood's lamp will cause erythrasma (a superficial, intertriginous infection caused by *Corynebacterium minutissimum*) to show a characteristic coral red color, and wounds colonized by *Pseudomonas* to appear pale blue. Tinea capitis caused by certain dermatophytes such as *Microsporum canis* or *M. audouini* exhibits a yellow fluorescence. Pigmented lesions of the epidermis such as freckles are accentuated, while dermal pigment such as postinflammatory hyperpigmentation fades under a Wood's light. Vitiligo (Fig. 46-12)

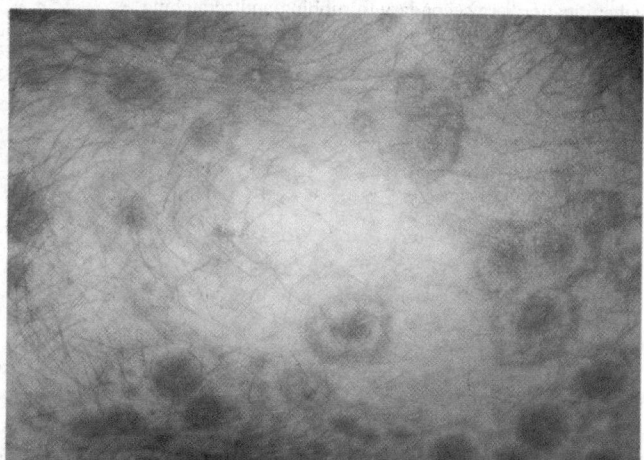

FIGURE 46-9 Erythema multiforme is characterized by multiple erythematous plaques with a target or iris morphology and usually represents a hypersensitivity reaction to drugs or infections (especially herpes simplex virus). (*Courtesy of the Yale Resident's Slide Collection.*)

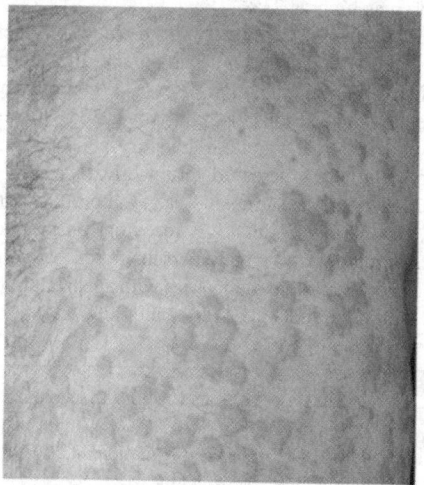

FIGURE 46-11 Urticaria showing characteristic discrete and confluent, edematous, erythematous papules and plaques.

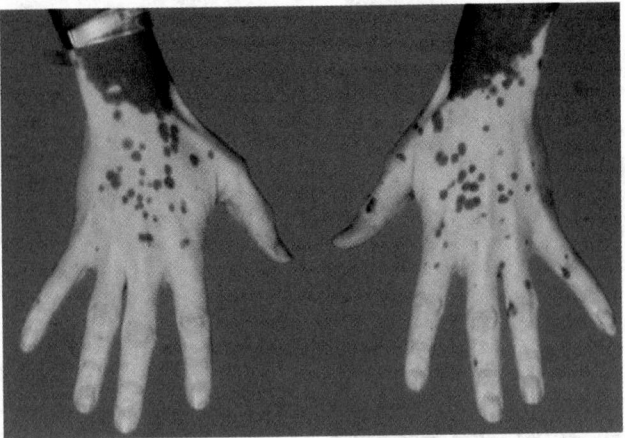

FIGURE 46-12   Vitiligo in a typical acral distribution demonstrating striking cutaneous depigmentation, as a result of loss of melanocytes.

appears totally white under a Wood's lamp, and previously unsuspected areas of involvement often become apparent. A Wood's lamp may also aid in the demonstration of tinea versicolor and in recognition of ash leaf spots in patients with tuberous sclerosis.

Patch Tests   Patch testing is designed to document sensitivity to a specific antigen. In this procedure, a battery of suspected allergens is applied to the patient's back under occlusive dressings and allowed to remain in contact with the skin for 48 h. The dressings are removed, and the area is examined for evidence of delayed hypersensitivity reactions (e.g., erythema, edema, or papulovesicles). This test is best performed by physicians with special expertise in patch testing and is often helpful in the evaluation of patients with chronic dermatitis.

FURTHER READING

ARNDT KA et al (eds): *Cutaneous Medicine and Surgery, An Integrated Program in Dermatology.* Philadelphia, Saunders, 1996
CHAMPION RH et al (eds): *Textbook of Dermatology*, 6th ed. Oxford, Blackwell Scientific, 1999
DERMATOLOGY LEXICON PROJECT: www.dermatology lexicon.org
FREEDBERG IM et al (eds): *Fitzpatrick's Dermatology in General Medicine*, 5th ed. New York, McGraw-Hill, 1999

47   ECZEMA, PSORIASIS, CUTANEOUS INFECTIONS, ACNE, AND OTHER COMMON SKIN DISORDERS
Calvin O. McCall, Thomas J. Lawley

ECZEMA AND DERMATITIS

Eczema, or dermatitis, is a reaction pattern that presents with variable clinical and histologic findings and is the final common expression for a number of disorders, including atopic dermatitis, allergic contact and irritant contact dermatitis, dyshidrotic eczema, nummular eczema, lichen simplex chronicus, asteatotic eczema, and seborrheic dermatitis. Primary lesions may include papules, erythematous macules, and vesicles, which can coalesce to form patches and plaques. In severe eczema, secondary lesions from infection or excoriation, marked by weeping and crusting, may predominate. Long-standing dermatitis is often dry and is characterized by thickened, scaling skin (*lichenification*).

ATOPIC DERMATITIS   Atopic dermatitis (AD) is the cutaneous expression of the atopic state, characterized by a family history of asthma, hay fever, or dermatitis in up to 70% of patients. Some of the features of atopic eczema are shown in Table 47-1. The prevalence of atopic dermatitis is increasing worldwide, with a point prevalence in Norwegian school children as high as 23%.

The etiology of AD is only partially defined, but there is a clear genetic predisposition. When both parents are affected by AD, over 80% of their children manifest the disease. When only one parent is affected, the prevalence drops to slightly over 50%. Patients with AD may display a variety of immunoregulatory abnormalities including increased IgE synthesis; increased serum IgE; increased specific IgE to foods, aeroallergens, bacteria, and bacterial products; increased expression of CD23 (low-affinity IgE receptor) on monocytes and B cells; and impaired delayed type hypersensitivity reactions.

The clinical presentation often varies with age. Half of patients with AD present within the first year of life, and 80% present by 5 years of age. About 80% ultimately coexpress allergic rhinitis or asthma. The infantile pattern is characterized by weeping inflammatory patches and crusted plaques that occur on the face, neck, and extensor surfaces. The childhood and adolescent pattern is marked by dermatitis of flexural skin, particularly in the antecubital and popliteal fossae (Fig. 47-1). AD may resolve spontaneously, but over half of all individuals affected as children will have dermatitis in adult life. The distribution of lesions may be similar to those seen in childhood. However, adults frequently have localized disease, manifesting as hand eczema or lichen simplex chronicus (see below). In patients with localized disease, AD may be suspected because of a typical personal history, family history, or the presence of cutaneous stigmata of AD such as perioral pallor, an extra fold of skin beneath the lower eyelid (Dennie's line), increased palmar skin markings, and an increased incidence of cutaneous infections, particularly with *Staphylococcus aureus*. Regardless of other manifestations, pruritus is a prominent characteristic of AD and is exacerbated by dry skin. Many of the cutaneous findings in affected patients, such as lichenification, are secondary to rubbing and scratching.

TABLE 47-1   *Clinical Features of Atopic Dermatitis*

1. Pruritus and scratching
2. Course marked by exacerbations and remissions
3. Lesions typical of eczematous dermatitis
4. Personal or family history of atopy (asthma, allergic rhinitis, food allergies, or eczema)
5. Clinical course lasting longer than 6 weeks

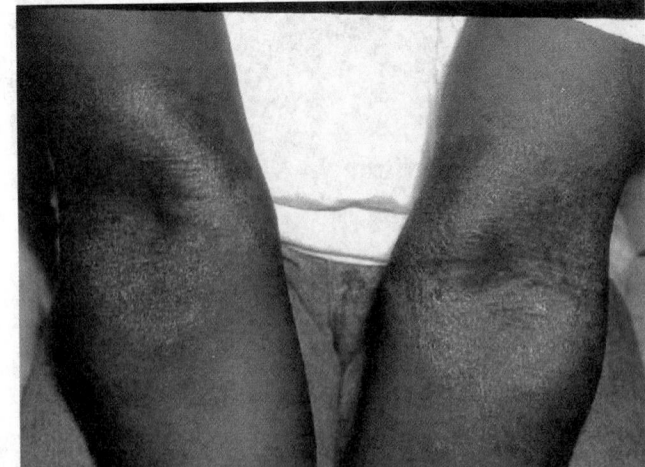

FIGURE 47-1   Atopic dermatitis with hyperpigmentation, lichenification, and scaling in the antecubital fossae. (Courtesy of Robert Swerlick, MD.)

Histologic examination of the skin affected by AD may demonstrate features of acute or chronic dermatitis. Immunopathology shows activated, memory T helper cells. AD skin lesions may also demonstrate IgE-bearing CD1a+ Langerhans cells, and these cells have been implicated in AD disease pathophysiology through mediation of hypersensitivity responses to environmental antigens.

℞ TREATMENT

Therapy of AD should include avoidance of cutaneous irritants, adequate moisturizing, judicious use of topical anti-inflammatory agents, and prompt treatment of secondary infection. Patients should be instructed to bathe using warm, but not hot, water and to limit their use of soap. Immediately after bathing while the skin is still moist, a topical anti-inflammatory agent in a cream or ointment base should be applied to areas of dermatitis, and all other skin areas should be lubricated with a moisturizer. Approximately 30 g of a topical agent is required to cover the entire body surface of an average adult.

Until recently, low- to midpotency topical glucocorticoids were employed in most treatment regimens for AD. Skin atrophy and the potential for systemic absorption, especially with more potent agents, were constant concerns. Two non-glucocorticoid anti-inflammatory agents are now available, tacrolimus ointment and pimecrolimus cream. These agents are macrolide immunosuppressants derived from soil fungi and are approved for use in AD. Reports of broader effectiveness appear in the literature. These agents do not cause skin atrophy and do not suppress the hypothalamic-pituitary-adrenal axis. They may replace topical glucocorticoids in some patients, but they are more costly than generic topical glucocorticoids. The non-steroid agents or low-potency topical glucocorticoids should be selected for use on the face or intertriginous areas to minimize the risk of skin atrophy.

Crusted and weeping skin lesions should be treated with systemic antibiotics with activity against *S. aureus* since secondary infection often exacerbates eczema. The frequency of macrolide-resistant organisms makes the use of penicillinase-resistant penicillins or cephalosporins preferable. Dicloxacillin or cephalexin (250 mg four times daily for 7 to 10 days) is generally adequate to decrease heavy colonization. As an adjunct, the use of triclosan-containing antibacterial washes and intermittent nasal mupirocin may be useful as prophylactic measures. The role of dietary allergens in atopic dermatitis is controversial, and there is little evidence that they play any role outside of infancy.

Control of pruritus is essential for treatment, since AD often represents "an itch that rashes." Antihistamines are most often used to control pruritus, and mild sedation may be responsible for their antipruritic action. Sedation may also limit their usefulness. Unlike their effects in urticaria, nonsedating antihistamines and selective H$_2$ blockers are of little use in controlling the pruritus of AD.

Treatment with systemic glucocorticoids should be limited to severe exacerbations unresponsive to conservative topical therapy. In the patient with chronic AD, therapy with systemic glucocorticoids will generally clear the skin only briefly, but cessation of the systemic therapy will invariably be accompanied by return, if not worsening, of the dermatitis. Patients who do not respond to conventional therapies should be considered for patch testing to rule out allergic contact dermatitis. Immunotherapy with aeroallergens has not proven useful in AD, unlike its effect in allergic rhinitis and extrinsic asthma.

CONTACT DERMATITIS Contact dermatitis is an inflammatory process in skin caused by an exogenous agent or agents that directly or indirectly injure the skin. This injury may be caused by an inherent characteristic of a compound—irritant contact dermatitis (ICD). An example of ICD would be dermatitis induced by a concentrated acid or base. Agents that cause allergic contact dermatitis (ACD) induce an antigen-specific immune response. The clinical lesions of contact dermatitis may be acute (wet and edematous) or chronic (dry, thickened, and scaly), depending on the persistence of the insult (see Fig. 46-10). The most common presentation of contact dermatitis is hand eczema, and it is frequently related to occupational exposures. Occupation-related

contact dermatitis represents a significant proportion of occupation-induced injury, affecting over 60,000 persons annually.

ICD is generally strictly demarcated and often localized to areas of thin skin (eyelids, intertriginous areas) or to areas where the irritant was occluded. Lesions may range from minimal skin erythema to areas of marked edema, vesicles, and ulcers. Chronic low-grade irritant dermatitis is the most common type of ICD, and the most common area of involvement is the hands (see below). The most common irritants encountered are chronic wet work, soaps, and detergents. Treatment should be directed to avoidance of irritants and use of protective gloves or clothing.

ACD is a manifestation of delayed-type hypersensitivity mediated by memory T lymphocytes in the skin. The most common cause of ACD is exposure to plants, especially to members of the family Anacardiaceae, including the genus *Toxicodendrun*. Poison ivy, poison oak, and poison sumac are members of this genus and cause an allergic reaction marked by erythema, vesiculation, and severe pruritus. The eruption is often linear, corresponding to areas where plants have touched the skin. The sensitizing antigen common to these plants is urushiol, an oleoresin containing the active ingredient pentadecylcatechol. The oleoresin may adhere to skin, clothing, tools, and pets, and contaminated articles may cause dermatitis even after prolonged storage. Blister fluid does not contain urushiol and is not capable of inducing skin eruption in exposed subjects. Other allergens may be more difficult to identify, especially if the exposure is chronic and the skin becomes thickened and scaly.

℞ TREATMENT

If ACD is suspected and an offending agent is identified and removed, the eruption will resolve. Usually, treatment with high-potency fluorinated topical glucocorticoids is enough to relieve symptoms while the ACD runs its course. For those patients who require systemic therapy, daily oral prednisone beginning at 1 mg/kg, but usually not exceeding 60 mg/d, is sufficient. It should be tapered over 2 to 3 weeks, and each daily dose given in the morning with food.

Identification of a contact allergen can be a difficult and time-consuming task. Patients with dermatitis unresponsive to conventional therapy or with an unusual and patterned distribution should be suspected of having ACD. They should be questioned carefully regarding occupational exposures, topical medicaments, and oral medications. Common sensitizers include preservatives in topical preparations, nickel sulfate, potassium dichromate, thimerosal, neomycin sulfate, fragrances, formaldehyde, and rubber-curing agents. Patch testing is helpful in identifying these agents, but should not be attempted on patients with widespread active dermatitis or on those taking systemic glucocorticoids.

HAND ECZEMA Hand eczema is a very common, chronic skin disorder. It represents a large proportion of occupation-associated skin disease. It may be associated with other cutaneous disorders such as AD or may occur by itself. Similar to other forms of dermatitis, both exogenous and endogenous factors play important roles in the expression of hand dermatitis. Chronic, excessive exposure to water and detergents may initiate or aggravate this disorder. It may present with dryness and cracking of the skin of the hands as well as with variable amounts of erythema and edema. Often, the dermatitis will begin under rings where water and irritants are trapped. A variant of hand dermatitis, dyshidrotic eczema, presents with multiple, intensely pruritic, small papules and vesicles occurring on the thenar and hypothenar eminences and the sides of the fingers (Fig. 47-2). Lesions tend to occur in crops that slowly form crusts and heal.

The evaluation of a patient with hand eczema should include an assessment of potential occupation-associated exposures. Predominant involvement of the dorsal surface of the hands with sparing of the palmar surface suggests a possible contact dermatitis. The history

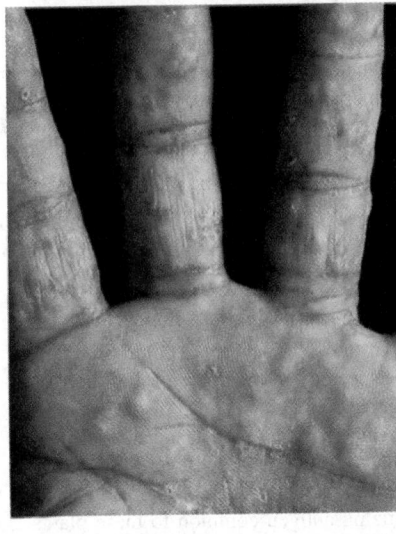

FIGURE 47-2 Dyshidrotic eczema, characterized by deep-seated vesicles and scaling on palms and lateral fingers, is often associated with an atopic diathesis.

should be directed to identifying possible irritant or allergen exposures. The use of rubber gloves to protect dermatitic skin is sometimes associated with the development of delayed-type hypersensitivity reactions to agents used for cross-linking rubber. Such reactions can be detected by patch testing. Less commonly, patients may manifest hand dermatitis as a consequence of developing immediate-type hypersensitivity reactions to latex. These are of particular concern since these patients are at risk for anaphylactic reactions. The most sensitive method of detection is the use of scratch testing with latex extract. However, this should be done with extreme caution only in a setting where an anaphylactic reaction can be treated. A latex radioallergosorbent test is available but is only about 60% sensitive.

℞ TREATMENT

Therapy of hand dermatitis is directed toward avoidance of irritants, identification of possible contact allergens, treatment of coexistent infection, and application of topical glucocorticoids. Whenever possible, the hands should be protected by gloves, preferably vinyl. Most patients can be treated with cool moist compresses (dressings) to dry and debride acute inflammatory lesions and to decrease swelling, followed by application of a mid- to high-potency topical glucocorticoid in a cream or ointment base. As with atopic dermatitis, treatment of secondary infection by staphylococci or streptococci is essential for good control. Additionally, patients with hand dermatitis should be examined for dermatophyte infection by KOH preparation and culture (see below).

NUMMULAR ECZEMA Nummular eczema is characterized by circular or oval "coinlike" lesions. Initially, this eruption consists of small edematous papules that become crusted and scaly. The most common locations are on the trunk or the extensor surfaces of the extremities, particularly on the pretibial areas or dorsum of the hands. It occurs more frequently in men and is most commonly seen in middle age. The etiology of nummular eczema is unknown. The treatment of nummular eczema is similar to that for other forms of dermatitis.

LICHEN SIMPLEX CHRONICUS Lichen simplex chronicus may represent the end stage of a variety of pruritic and eczematous disorders. It consists of a well-circumscribed plaque or plaques with lichenified or thickened skin due to chronic scratching or rubbing. Common areas involved include the posterior nuchal region, dorsum of the feet, or ankles. Treatment of lichen simplex chronicus centers around breaking the cycle of chronic itching and scratching, which often occur during sleep. High-potency topical glucocorticoids are helpful in alleviating pruritus in most cases, but in recalcitrant cases, application of topical glucocorticoids under occlusion or intralesional injection of glucocor-

ticoids may be required. Oral antihistamines such as hydroxyzine (10 to 25 mg every 6 h) or tricyclic antidepressants with antihistaminic activity such as doxepin (10 to 25 mg at bedtime) are useful as antipruritics primarily due to their sedating action. Higher doses of these agents may be required, but sedation can become bothersome. Patients need to be counseled regarding driving or operating heavy equipment after taking these medications due to their potentially potent sedative activity.

ASTEATOTIC ECZEMA Asteatotic eczema, also known as *xerotic eczema* or *"winter itch,"* is a mildly inflammatory dermatitis that develops in areas of extremely dry skin, especially during the dry winter months. This form of eczema accounts for a large number of physician visits because of the associated pruritus. Fine cracks and scale, with or without erythema, characteristically develop in areas of dry skin, especially on the anterior surfaces of the lower extremities in elderly patients. Asteatotic eczema responds well to topical moisturizers and the avoidance of cutaneous irritants. Overbathing and the use of harsh soaps exacerbate asteatotic eczema. Moisturizers should be applied to dry skin areas twice daily and always applied to damp skin after bathing. Prescription emollients containing ammonium lactate or urea are useful in patients with extremely dry skin, but they may be associated with skin irritation. Emollients should be applied after leaving the bath or shower to avoid increasing the risk of falling.

STASIS DERMATITIS AND STASIS ULCERATION Stasis dermatitis develops on the lower extremities secondary to venous incompetence and chronic edema. Early findings in stasis dermatitis consist of mild erythema and scaling associated with pruritus. The typical initial site of involvement is the medial aspect of the ankle, often over a distended vein (Fig. 47-3). As the disorder progresses, the dermatitis becomes progressively pigmented, due to chronic erythrocyte extravasation leading to cutaneous hemosiderin deposition. As with other forms of dermatitis, stasis dermatitis may become acutely inflamed, with crusting and exudate. Chronic stasis dermatitis is often associated with dermal fibrosis that is recognized clinically as brawny edema of the skin. Stasis dermatitis is often complicated by secondary infection and contact dermatitis. Severe stasis dermatitis may precede the development of stasis ulcers.

℞ TREATMENT

Patients with stasis dermatitis and stasis ulceration benefit greatly from leg elevation and the routine use of compression stockings with a gradient of at least 30 to 40 mmHg. Stockings providing less compression, such as antiembolism hose, are poor substitutes. Use of emollients and/or midpotency topical glucocorticoids and avoidance of irritants are also helpful in treating stasis dermatitis. Protecting the legs from injury, including scratching, and control of chronic edema are essential to prevent ulcers.

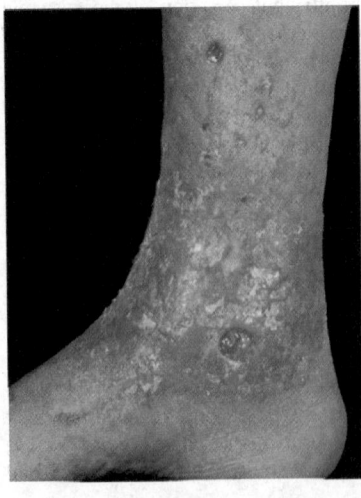

FIGURE 47-3 Stasis dermatitis showing erythematous, scaly, and oozing patches over the lower leg. Several stasis ulcers are also seen in this patient.

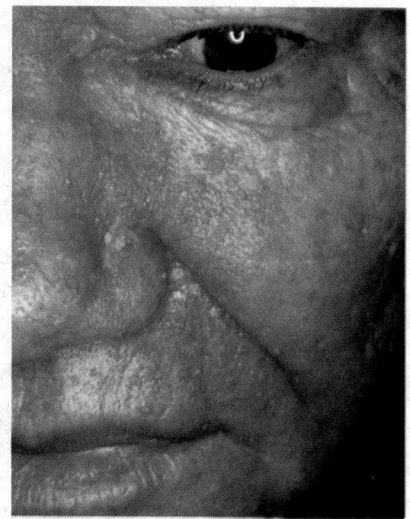

FIGURE 47-4 Seborrheic dermatitis showing central facial erythema with overlying greasy, yellowish scale. (Courtesy of Jean Bolognia, MD.)

Stasis ulcers are difficult to treat, and resolution of these lesions is slow. It is extremely important to elevate the affected limb as much as possible. The ulcer should be kept clear of necrotic material by gentle debridement and covered with a semipermeable dressing under pressure. Glucocorticoids should not be applied to ulcers, since they may retard healing. Secondarily infected lesions should be treated with appropriate oral antibiotics, but it should be noted that all ulcers will become colonized with bacteria, and the purpose of antibiotic therapy should not be to clear all bacterial growth. Care must be taken to exclude treatable causes of leg ulcers (hypercoagulation, vasculitis) before beginning the chronic management outlined above.

SEBORRHEIC DERMATITIS Seborrheic dermatitis is a common, chronic disorder, characterized by greasy scales overlying erythematous patches or plaques. The most common location is in the scalp where it may be recognized as severe dandruff. On the face, seborrheic dermatitis affects the eyebrows, eyelids, glabella, and nasolabial folds (Fig. 47-4). Scaling of the external auditory canal is common in seborrheic dermatitis and may be mistaken for a fungal infection (otomycosis). The postauricular areas often become macerated and tender. Additionally, seborrheic dermatitis may develop in the central chest, axilla, groin, submammary folds, and gluteal cleft. Rarely, it may cause a widespread generalized dermatitis.

Seborrheic dermatitis may be evident within the first few weeks of life, and within this context it occurs in the scalp ("cradle cap"), face, or groin. It is rarely seen in children beyond infancy but becomes evident again during adult life. Although it is frequently seen in patients with Parkinson's disease, in those who have had cerebrovascular accidents, and in those with HIV infection, the overwhelming majority of individuals with seborrheic dermatitis have no underlying disorder.

TREATMENT

Treatment with low-potency topical glucocorticoids in conjunction with a topical antifungal agent, such as ketoconazole cream or ciclopirox cream, is often effective. The scalp and beard areas may benefit from shampoos containing coal tar and/or salicylic acid. Shampoos should be left in place 3 to 5 min before rinsing. High-potency topical glucocorticoid solutions (betamethasone or fluocinonide) are effective for control of severe scalp involvement. Fluorinated topical glucocorticoids should not be used on the face since this is often associated with the development of rebound worsening and steroid-induced rosacea or atrophy.

PAPULOSQUAMOUS DISORDERS (Table 47-2)

PSORIASIS Psoriasis is one of the most common dermatologic diseases, affecting up to 2.5% of the world's population. It is a chronic inflammatory skin disorder clinically characterized by erythematous, sharply demarcated papules and rounded plaques, covered by silvery micaceous scale. The skin lesions of psoriasis are variably pruritic. Traumatized areas often develop lesions of psoriasis (Koebner or isomorphic phenomenon). Additionally, other external factors may exacerbate psoriasis including infections, stress, and medications (lithium, beta blockers, and antimalarials).

The most common variety of psoriasis is called *plaque type*. Patients with plaque-type psoriasis will have stable, slowly enlarging plaques, which remain basically unchanged for long periods of time. The most common areas for plaque psoriasis to occur are the elbows, knees, gluteal cleft, and the scalp. Involvement tends to be symmetric. *Inverse psoriasis* affects the intertriginous regions including the axilla, groin, submammary region, and navel; it also tends to affect the scalp, palms, and soles. The individual lesions are sharply demarcated plaques (see Fig. 46-7) but may be moist due to their location. Plaque psoriasis generally develops slowly and runs an indolent course. It rarely remits spontaneously.

Eruptive psoriasis (guttate psoriasis) is most common in children and young adults. It develops acutely in individuals without psoriasis or in those with chronic plaque psoriasis. Patients present with many small erythematous, scaling papules, frequently after upper respiratory tract infection with β-hemolytic streptococci. The differential diagnosis should include pityriasis rosea and secondary syphilis. *Pustular psoriasis* is another variant. Patients may have disease localized to the palms and soles or generalized and associated with fever, malaise, diarrhea, and arthralgias.

About half of all patients with psoriasis have fingernail involvement, appearing as punctate pitting, nail thickening, or subungual hyperkeratosis. About 5 to 10% of patients with psoriasis have associated joint complaints, and these are most often found in patients with fingernail involvement. Although some have the coincident occurrence

TABLE 47-2	*Papulosquamous Disorders*		
	Clinical Features	**Other Notable Features**	**Histologic Features**
Psoriasis	Sharply demarcated, erythematous plaques with mica-like scale; predominantly elbows, knees, and scalp; atypical forms may localize to intertriginous areas; eruptive forms may be associated with infection (Reiter's syndrome)	May be aggravated by certain drugs, infection; severe forms seen associated with HIV	Acanthosis, vascular proliferation
Lichen planus	Purple polygonal papules marked by severe pruritus; lacy white markings, especially associated with mucous membrane lesions	Certain drugs may induce: thiazides, antimalarial drugs	Interface dermatitis
Pityriasis rosea	Rash often preceded by herald patch; oval to round plaques with trailing scale; most often affects the trunk, and eruption lines up in skin folds giving a "fir tree"-like appearance; generally spares palms and soles	Variable pruritus; self-limited resolving in 2–8 weeks; may be imitated by secondary syphilis	Pathologic features often nonspecific
Dermatophytosis	Polymorphous appearance depending on dermatophyte, body site, and host response; sharply defined to ill-demarcated scaly plaques with or without inflammation; may be associated with hair loss	KOH preparation may show branching hyphae; culture helpful	Hyphae and neutrophils in stratum corneum

of classic rheumatoid arthritis (Chap. 301), many have joint disease that falls into one of three types associated with psoriasis: (1) asymmetric inflammatory arthritis most commonly involving the distal and proximal interphalangeal joints and less commonly the knees, hips, ankles, and wrists; (2) a seronegative rheumatoid arthritis–like disease; a significant portion of these patients go on to develop a severe destructive arthritis; or (3) disease limited to the spine (psoriatic spondylitis).

The etiology of psoriasis is still poorly understood, but there is clearly a genetic component to the disease. Over 50% of patients with psoriasis report a positive family history. Psoriasis has been linked to HLA-Cw6 and, to a lesser extent, to HLA-DR7. Psoriatic lesions are characterized by infiltration of skin with activated T cells, which appear to have a role in the pathophysiology of psoriasis. Presumably, cytokines from activated T cells elaborate growth factors that stimulate keratinocyte hyperproliferation. Agents that inhibit T cell activation, clonal expansion, or release of proinflammatory cytokines are often effective for the treatment of severe psoriasis.

℞ TREATMENT

Treatment of psoriasis depends on the type, location, and extent of disease. All patients should be instructed to avoid excess drying or irritation of their skin and to maintain adequate cutaneous hydration. Most patients with localized, plaque-type psoriasis can be managed with midpotency topical glucocorticoids, although their long-term use is often accompanied by loss of effectiveness (tachyphylaxis) and atrophy of the skin. A topical vitamin D analogue (calcipotriene) and a retinoid (tazarotene) are also efficacious in the treatment of psoriasis and have largely replaced other topical agents such as coal tar, salicylic acid, and anthralin.

Ultraviolet light, natural or artificial, is an effective therapy for patients with widespread psoriasis. Ultraviolet B (UV-B) light is effective alone, or may be combined with coal tar or anthralin. The combination of the ultraviolet A (UV-A) spectrum with either oral or topical psoralens (PUVA) is also extremely effective for the treatment of psoriasis, but long-term use may be associated with an increased incidence of squamous cell cancer and melanoma of the skin.

Various other agents can be used for severe, widespread psoriatic disease. Oral glucocorticoids should not be used for the treatment of psoriasis due to the potential for developing life-threatening pustular psoriasis when therapy is discontinued. Methotrexate is an effective agent, especially in patients with psoriatic arthritis; however, liver toxicity and bone marrow suppression limit its use. The synthetic retinoid, acitretin, is effective in some patients with severe psoriasis. It is a potent teratogen and should not be used in women of childbearing potential. The evidence implicating psoriasis as a T cell–mediated disorder has directed therapeutic efforts to immunoregulation. Cyclosporine is highly effective in selected patients with severe disease, but nephrotoxicity and hypertension complicate its use. Much attention is currently directed toward the development of biologic agents with more selective immunosuppressive properties and better safety profiles. Etanercept, a tumor necrosis factor α (TNF-α) inhibitor, is now approved for psoriatic arthritis and is in clinical trials for psoriasis. Other agents in clinical trials target TNF-α and other proinflammatory cytokines, T cell activation, and lymphocyte trafficking in an attempt to suppress the inflammation characteristic of psoriasis.

LICHEN PLANUS Lichen planus (LP) is a papulosquamous disorder in which the primary lesions are pruritic, polygonal, flat-topped, violaceous papules. Close examination of the surface of these papules often reveals a network of gray lines (Wickham's striae). The skin lesions may occur anywhere but have a predilection for the wrists, shins, lower back, and genitalia (Fig. 47-5). Involvement of the scalp may lead to hair loss. LP commonly involves mucous membranes, particularly the buccal mucosa, where it can present as a white netlike eruption. Its etiology is unknown, but cutaneous eruptions clinically resembling LP

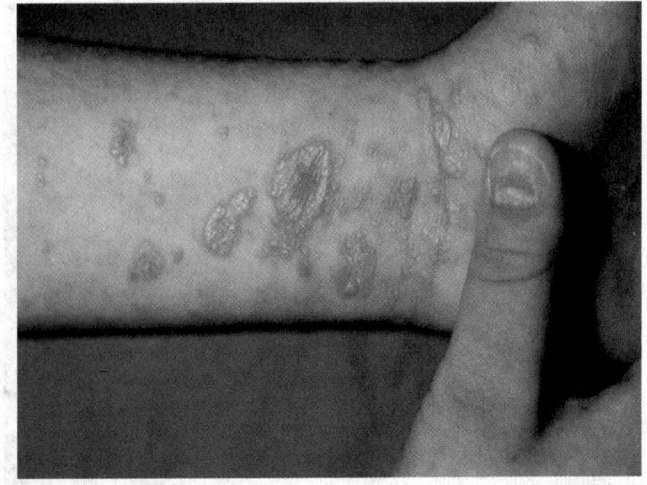

FIGURE 47-5 Lichen planus showing multiple flat-topped, violaceous papules and plaques. Nail dystrophy as seen in this patient's thumbnail may also be a feature. (Courtesy of Robert Swerlick, MD.)

have been observed after administration of numerous drugs, including thiazide diuretics, gold, antimalarials, penicillamine, and phenothiazines, and in patients with skin lesions of chronic graft-versus-host disease. Additionally, LP may be associated with hepatitis C infection. The course of LP is variable, but most patients have spontaneous remissions 6 months to 2 years after the onset of disease. Topical glucocorticoids are the mainstay of therapy.

PITYRIASIS ROSEA Pityriasis rosea (PR) is a papulosquamous eruption of unknown etiology that occurs more commonly in the spring and fall. Its first manifestation is the development of a 2- to 6-cm annular lesion (the herald patch). This is followed in a few days to a few weeks by the appearance of many smaller annular or papular lesions with a predilection to occur on the trunk (Fig. 47-6). The lesions are generally oval, with their long axis parallel to the skin-fold lines. Individual lesions may range in color from red to brown and have a trailing scale. PR shares many clinical features with the eruption of secondary syphilis, but palm and sole lesions are extremely rare in PR and common in secondary syphilis. The eruption tends to be moderately pruritic and lasts 3 to 8 weeks. Treatment is generally directed at alleviating pruritus and consists of oral antihistamines, midpotency topical glucocorticoids, and, in some cases, the use of UV-B phototherapy.

CUTANEOUS INFECTIONS (Table 47-3)

IMPETIGO AND ECTHYMA Impetigo is a common superficial bacterial infection of skin caused by group A β-hemolytic streptococci (Chap.

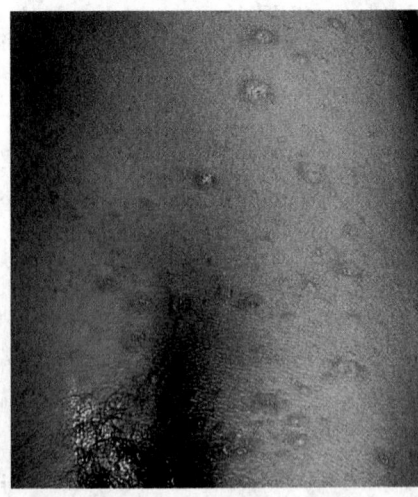

FIGURE 47-6 Pityriasis rosea in which multiple round to oval erythematous patches with fine central scale are distributed along the skin tension lines on the trunk.

TABLE 47-3 *Common Skin Infections*

	Clinical Features	Etiologic Agent	Treatment
Impetigo	Honey-colored crusted papules, plaques, or bullae	Group A *Streptococcus* and *Staphylococcus aureus*	Systemic or topical antistaphylococcal antibiotics
Dermatophytosis	Inflammatory or noninflammatory annular scaly plaques; may have hair loss; groin involvement spares scrotum; hyphae on KOH preparation	*Trichophyton, Epidermophyton,* or *Microsporum* sp.	Topical azoles, systemic griseofulvin, terbinafine, or azoles
Candidiasis	Inflammatory papules and plaques with satellite pustules, frequently in intertriginous areas; may involve scrotum; pseudohyphae on KOH preparation	*Candida albicans* and other *Candida* species	Topical nystatin or azoles; systemic azoles for resistant disease
Tinea versicolor	Hyperpigmented or hypopigmented scaly patches on the trunk; characteristic mixture of hyphae and spores on KOH preparation ("spaghetti and meatballs")	*Malassezia furfur*	Topical selenium sulfide lotion or azoles

121) or *S. aureus* (Chap. 120). The primary lesion is a superficial pustule that ruptures and forms a characteristic yellow-brown honey-colored crust (see Fig. 121-1). Lesions caused by staphylococci may be tense, clear bullae, and this less common form of the disease is called *bullous impetigo*. Lesions may occur on normal skin or in areas already affected by another skin disease. Ecthyma is a variant of impetigo that generally occurs on the lower extremities and causes punched-out ulcerative lesions. Treatment of both ecthyma and impetigo involves gentle debridement of adherent crusts, which is facilitated by the use of soaks and topical antibiotics, in conjunction with appropriate oral antibiotics.

ERYSIPELAS AND CELLULITIS →*See Chap. 110*

DERMATOPHYTOSIS Dermatophytes are fungi that infect skin, hair, and nails and include members of the genera *Trichophyton, Microsporum,* and *Epidermophyton*. Tinea corporis, or infection of the relatively hairless skin of the body (glabrous skin), may have a variable appearance depending on the extent of the associated inflammatory reaction (see Fig. 46-11). It may have the typical annular appearance of "ringworm" or appear as deep inflammatory nodules or granulomas. Involvement of the groin (tinea cruris) is more common in males than females. It presents as a scaling, erythematous eruption that spares the scrotum. Infection of the foot (tinea pedis) is the most common dermatophyte infection and is often chronic; it is characterized by variable erythema, edema, scaling, pruritus, and occasionally vesiculation. Involvement may be widespread or localized, but almost invariably involves the web space between the fourth and fifth toes. Infection of the nails (tinea unguium or onychomycosis) occurs in many patients with tinea pedis and is characterized by opacified, thickened nails and subungual debris. Dermatophyte infection of the scalp (tinea capitis) has returned in epidemic proportions, particularly affecting inner-city children, but it also affects adults. The predominant organism is *T. tonsurans*, which can produce a relatively noninflammatory infection with mild scale and hair loss that is diffuse or localized. Localized disease may be well defined or irregular. *T. tonsurans* can also cause a markedly inflammatory dermatosis with edema and nodules. This latter presentation is a kerion.

The diagnosis of tinea can be made from skin scrapings, nail scrapings, or hair by culture or direct microscopic examination with potassium hydroxide (KOH). Hair, nail scrapings, and scrapings from markedly inflamed skin may fail to show hyphae on direct examination.

℞ TREATMENT

Both topical and systemic therapies may be used to treat dermatophyte infections. Treatment depends on the site involved and the type of infection. Topical therapy is generally effective for uncomplicated tinea corporis, tinea cruris, and limited tinea pedis. It is not effective as a monotherapy for tinea capitis or onychomycosis. Topical imidazoles, triazoles, and allylamines may all be effective topical therapies for dermatophyte infections. Haloprogin, undecylenic acid, ciclopirox olamine, and tolnaftate are also effective, but nystatin is not active against dermatophytes. Topicals are generally applied twice daily, and treatment should continue 1 week beyond clinical resolution of the infection. Tinea pedis often requires longer treatment courses and frequently relapses. Oral antifungal agents may be required for recalcitrant tinea pedis or tinea corporis with a nodular (granulomatous) component.

Oral antifungal agents are required for dermatophyte infections involving the hair and nails and for other infections unresponsive to topical therapy. A fungal etiology should be confirmed by direct microscopic examination or by culture prior to prescribing oral antifungal agents. All of the oral agents may cause hepatotoxicity and should not be used in women who are pregnant or breast-feeding.

Griseofulvin is the only oral agent approved in the United States for dermatophyte infections involving the skin, hair, or nails. Itraconazole and terbinafine are approved for onychomycosis; however, the literature cites multiple examples of their effective use in other dermatophyte infections. When griseofulvin is used, a daily dose of 500 mg of microsized or 350 mg of ultramicrosized griseofulvin administered with a fatty meal is an adequate dose for most dermatophyte infections. Higher doses are required for tinea pedis and onychomycosis. The duration of therapy may be 2 weeks for uncomplicated tinea corporis or as long as 6 to 18 months for nail infections. Due to high relapse rates, griseofulvin is seldom used for nail infections. The usual adult dose of griseofulvin for tinea capitis is 1 g of microsized or 0.5 g of ultramicrosized given daily for 6 to 8 weeks or until cultures are negative. The adjunctive use of topical antifungal agents may be useful, but topical therapy alone is not adequate for tinea capitis. Markedly inflammatory tinea capitis may result in scarring and hair loss, and systemic or topical glucocorticoids may be helpful in preventing these sequelae. Common side effects of griseofulvin include gastrointestinal distress, headache, and urticaria.

Oral itraconazole and terbinafine are approved for onychomycosis. Itraconazole is given as either continuous daily therapy (200 mg/d) or pulses (200 mg twice daily for 1 week per month) administered with food. Fingernails require 2 months of continuous therapy or two pulses. Toenails require 3 months of continuous therapy or three pulses. Itraconazole has the potential for serious interactions with other drugs requiring the P450 enzyme system for metabolism. Terbinafine (250 mg/d) is also effective for onychomycosis. Therapy with terbinafine is continued for 6 weeks for fingernail infections and 12 weeks for toenail infections. Terbinafine has fewer drug-drug interactions, but caution should be used when patients are on multiple medications.

TINEA VERSICOLOR Tinea versicolor is caused by a non-dermatophyte, dimorphic fungus, *Malassezia furfur*, a normal inhabitant of the skin. As the yeast form, it generally does not cause disease (except for folliculitis in certain individuals). However, in some individuals, it converts to the hyphal form and causes characteristic lesions. The expression of infection is promoted by heat and humidity. The typical lesions consist of oval scaly macules, papules, and patches concentrated on the chest, shoulders, and back but only rarely on the face or distal extremities. On dark skin, they often appear as hypopigmented areas, while on light skin, they are slightly erythematous or hyperpigmented. In some darkly pigmented individuals, they may only appear as scaling patches. A KOH preparation from scaling lesions will demonstrate a confluence of short hyphae and round spores (so-called spaghetti and meatballs). Solutions containing sulfur, salicylic acid, or selenium sulfide will clear the infection if used daily for a week and then intermittently thereafter. Treatment with a single 400-mg oral dose of ketoconazole is also effective.

CANDIDIASIS Candidiasis is a fungal infection caused by a related group of yeasts, whose manifestations may be localized to the skin, or rarely, may be systemic and life-threatening. The causative organism is usually *Candida albicans*, but may also be *C. tropicalis*, *C. parapsilosis*, or *C. krusei*. These organisms are normal saprophytic inhabitants of the gastrointestinal tract but may overgrow (usually due to broad-spectrum antibiotic therapy) and cause disease at a number of cutaneous sites. Other predisposing factors include diabetes mellitus, chronic intertrigo, oral contraceptive use, and cellular immune deficiency. Candidiasis is a very common infection in HIV-infected individuals (Chap. 173). The oral cavity is commonly involved. Lesions may occur on the tongue or buccal mucosa (thrush) and appear as white plaques (see Fig. 46-12). Microscopic examination of scrapings demonstrate both pseudohyphae and yeast forms. Fissured, macerated lesions at the corners of the mouth (perlèche) are often seen in individuals with poorly fitting dentures and may also be associated with candidal infection. Additionally, candidal infections have an affinity for sites that are chronically wet and macerated and may occur around nails (onycholysis and paronychia) and in intertriginous areas. Intertriginous lesions are characteristically edematous, erythematous, and scaly, with scattered "satellite pustules." In males, there is often involvement of the penis and scrotum as well as the inner aspect of the thighs. In contrast to dermatophyte infections, candidal infections are frequently painful and accompanied by a marked inflammatory response. Diagnosis of candidal infection is based upon the clinical pattern and demonstration of yeast on KOH preparation or culture.

TREATMENT

Treatment routinely involves removing any predisposing factors such as antibiotic therapy or chronic wetness and the use of appropriate topical or systemic antifungal therapy. Effective topical agents include nystatin or topical azoles (miconazole, clotrimazole, econazole, or ketoconazole). These agents are generally effective in clearing mucous membrane or glabrous skin involvement in nonimmunosuppressed patients. The associated inflammatory response that often accompanies candidal infection on glabrous skin can be treated with a mild glucocorticoid lotion or cream (2.5% hydrocortisone). Systemic therapy is generally reserved for immunosuppressed patients or individuals with chronic or recurrent disease who fail to respond to or tolerate appropriate topical therapy.

WARTS Warts are cutaneous neoplasms that are caused by papilloma viruses. Approximately 80 different human papilloma viruses (HPV) have been described, and this number will likely increase. Typical verruca vulgaris lesions are sessile, dome-shaped, usually about a centimeter in diameter, and their surface is hyperkeratotic consisting of many small filamentous projections. The HPV that cause typical verruca vulgaris also cause typical plantar warts, flat warts (or verruca plana), and filiform warts in intertriginous areas. Plantar warts are endophytic and are covered by thick keratin. Paring of the wart will generally demonstrate a central core of keratinized debris and punctate

bleeding points. Filiform warts are most commonly seen on the face, neck, and skin folds and present as papillomatous lesions on a narrow base. Flat warts are only slightly elevated and have a velvety, nonverrucous surface. They have a propensity for the face, arms, and legs and are often spread by shaving.

Genital warts generally begin as small papillomas that may grow to form large fungating lesions. In women, they may involve either the labia, perineum, or perianal skin. Additionally, the mucosa of the vagina, urethra, and anus can be involved, as well as the cervical epithelium. In men, the lesions often occur initially in the coronal sulcus, but may be seen on the shaft of the penis, the scrotum, perianal skin, or in the urethra.

Within the past decade, appreciable evidence has accumulated that suggests HPV plays a role in the development of neoplasia of the uterine cervix and external genitalia (Chap. 83). HPV types 16 and 18 have been most intensely studied, while recent evidence also implicates other types. Lesions may initially appear as small, flat, velvety, hyperpigmented papules occurring on the genitalia or perianal skin. Histologic examination of biopsies from affected sites may reveal changes associated with typical warts and/or features typical of intraepidermal carcinoma (Bowen's disease). Squamous cell carcinomas associated with HPV infections have also been observed in extragenital skin (Chap. 73). This is most commonly seen in patients immunosuppressed after organ transplantation.

TREATMENT

There are many modalities available to treat warts, but no single therapy is universally effective. Factors that influence the choice of therapy include the location of the wart, extent of disease, the age and immunologic status of the patient, and the patient's desire for therapy. Perhaps the most useful and convenient method for treating warts in almost any location is cryotherapy with liquid nitrogen. Equally effective, but requiring much more patient compliance, is the use of keratolytic agents such as salicylic acid plasters or solutions. For genital warts, in-office application of a podophyllin solution is moderately effective but may be associated with marked local reactions. Prescription preparations of dilute, purified podophyllin are available for home use. Topical imiquimod, a potent inducer of local cytokine release, has also been approved for use in genital warts. Conventional and laser surgical procedures may be required for recalcitrant warts. Recurrence of warts appears to be common to all these modalities.

Treatment of warts, other than anogenital warts, should be tempered by the observation that a majority of warts in normal individuals resolve spontaneously within 1 to 2 years. Also, very few warts are associated with malignancy, and those are usually located in the anogenital region.

HERPES SIMPLEX →*See Chap. 163*

HERPES ZOSTER →*See Chap. 164*

ACNE

ACNE VULGARIS Acne vulgaris is a self-limited disorder primarily of teenagers and young adults, although perhaps 10 to 20% of adults may continue to experience some form of the disorder. The permissive factor for the expression of the disease in adolescence is the increase in sebum production by sebaceous glands after puberty. Small cysts, called *comedones*, form in hair follicles due to blockage of the follicular orifice by retention of sebum and keratinous material. The activity of bacteria (*Proprionobacterium acnes*) within the comedones releases free fatty acids from sebum, causes inflammation within the cyst, and results in rupture of the cyst wall. An inflammatory foreign-body reaction develops as a result of extrusion of oily and keratinous debris from the cyst.

The clinical hallmark of acne vulgaris is the comedone, which may be closed (whitehead) or open (blackhead). Closed comedones appear as 1- to 2-mm pebbly white papules, which are accentuated when the

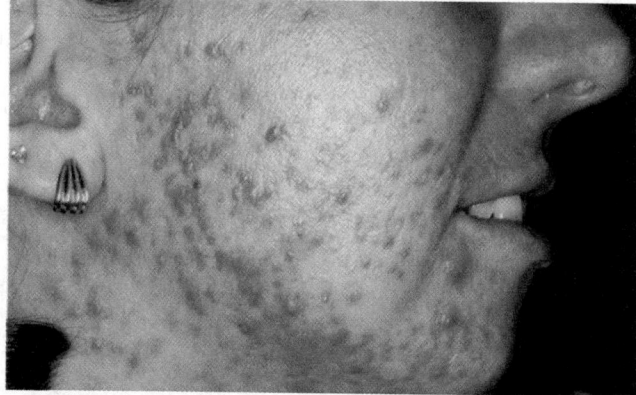

FIGURE 47-7 Acne vulgaris with inflammatory papules, pustules, and comedones. (Courtesy of Kalman Watsky, MD.)

skin is stretched. They are the precursors of inflammatory lesions of acne vulgaris. The contents of closed comedones are not easily expressed. Open comedones, which rarely result in inflammatory acne lesions, have a large dilated follicular orifice and are filled with easily expressible oxidized, darkened, oily debris. Comedones are usually accompanied by inflammatory lesions: papules, pustules, or nodules.

The earliest lesions seen in early adolescence are generally mildly inflamed or noninflammatory comedones on the forehead. Subsequently, more typical inflammatory lesions develop on the cheeks, nose, and chin (Fig. 47-7). The most common location for acne is the face, but involvement of the chest and back is not uncommon. Most disease remains mild and does not lead to scarring. However, a small number of patients develop large inflammatory cysts and nodules, which may drain and result in significant scarring.

Exogenous and endogenous factors can alter the expression of acne vulgaris. Friction and trauma may rupture preexisting microcomedones and elicit inflammatory acne lesions. This is commonly seen with headbands or chin straps of athletic helmets. Application of comedogenic topical agents in cosmetics or hair preparations or chronic topical exposure to certain industrial compounds that are comedogenic may elicit or aggravate acne. Glucocorticoids, applied topically or administered systemically in high doses, may also elicit acne. Other systemic medications such as lithium, isoniazid, halogens, phenytoin, and phenobarbital may produce acneiform eruptions, or aggravate preexisting acne.

℞ TREATMENT

Treatment of acne vulgaris is directed toward elimination of comedones by normalization of follicular keratinization, decreasing sebaceous gland activity, decreasing the population of *P. acnes*, and decreasing inflammation. Acne vulgaris may be treated with either local or systemic medications. Minimal to moderate, pauci-inflammatory disease may respond adequately to local therapy alone. Although areas affected with acne should be kept clean, there is little evidence to suggest that removal of surface oils plays an important role in therapy. Overly vigorous scrubbing may aggravate acne due to mechanical rupture of comedones. Topical agents such as retinoic acid, benzoyl peroxide, or salicylic acid may alter the pattern of epidermal desquamation, preventing the formation of comedones and aiding in the resolution of preexisting cysts. Topical antibacterial agents such as benzoyl peroxide, azelaic acid, topical erythromycin (with or without zinc), or clindamycin are also useful adjuncts to therapy.

Patients with moderate to severe acne with a prominent inflammatory component will benefit from the addition of systemic therapy, such as tetracycline or erythromycin, in doses of 250 to 1000 mg/d. Such antibiotics appear to have an anti-inflammatory effect independent of their antibacterial effect. Female patients who do not respond to oral antibiotics may benefit from hormonal therapy. Women placed on oral contraceptives containing ethinyl estradiol and norgestimate

have demonstrated improvement in their acne when compared to a placebo control.

Patients with severe nodulocystic acne unresponsive to the therapies discussed above may benefit from treatment with the synthetic retinoid, isotretinoin. Its use is highly regulated due to its potential for severe adverse events, primarily teratogenicity. Recently there have also been concerns that it is associated with severe depression in some patients. The latter has not been proved. At present, prescribers must receive from the manufacturer training, certification, and stickers to affix to each prescription. These measures are imposed to ensure that all prescribers are familiar with the risks of isotretinoin; that all female patients have two negative pregnancy tests prior to initiating therapy and a negative pregnancy test prior to each refill; and that all patients have been warned about the risks associated with isotretinoin, including depression. Additionally, patients receiving this medication develop extremely dry skin and cheilitis and must be followed for development of hypertriglyceridemia.

ACNE ROSACEA Acne rosacea is an inflammatory disorder predominantly affecting the central face. It is seen almost exclusively in adults, only rarely affecting patients under 30 years of age. Rosacea is seen more often in women, but those most severely affected are men. It is characterized by the presence of erythema, telangiectases, and superficial pustules (Fig. 47-8), but is not associated with the presence of comedones. Rosacea only rarely involves the chest or back.

There is a relationship between the tendency for pronounced facial flushing and the subsequent development of acne rosacea. Often, individuals with rosacea initially demonstrate a pronounced flushing reaction. This may be in response to heat, emotional stimuli, alcohol, hot drinks, or spicy foods. As the disease progresses, the flush persists longer and longer and may eventually become permanent. Papules, pustules, and telangiectases can become superimposed on the persistent flush. Rosacea of very long standing may lead to connective tissue overgrowth, particularly of the nose (rhinophyma). Rosacea may also be complicated by various inflammatory disorders of the eye, including keratitis, blepharitis, iritis, and recurrent chalazion. These ocular problems are potentially sight-threatening and warrant ophthalmologic evaluation.

℞ TREATMENT

Acne rosacea can be treated topically or systemically. Mild disease often responds to topical metronidazole or sodium sulfacetamide. More severe disease requires oral tetracycline in doses ranging from 250 to 1000 mg/d. Residual telangiectasia may respond to laser therapy. Topical glucocorticoids, especially potent agents, should be avoided since chronic use of these preparations may elicit rosacea. Topical therapy of the skin is not effective treatment for ocular disease.

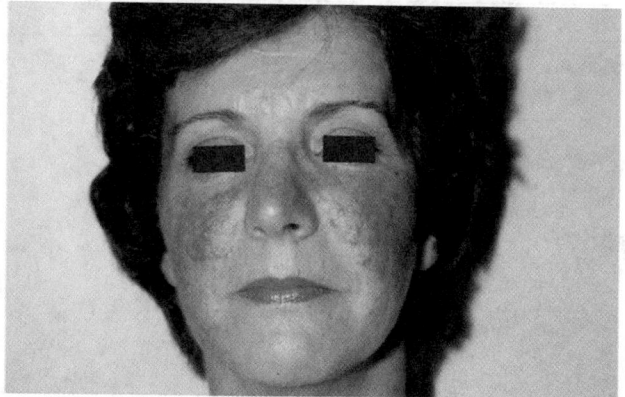

FIGURE 47-8 Acne rosacea with prominent facial erythema, telangiectasia, scattered papules, and small pustules. (Courtesy of Robert Swerlick, MD.)

SKIN DISEASES AND SMALLPOX VACCINATION

Given the potential threat of a bioterrorism attack with smallpox, vaccinations against smallpox are available to the general public, although they are not recommended. Because of a higher incidence of adverse events associated with smallpox vaccination in patients with a history of certain skin diseases, including atopic dermatitis, eczema, severe acne, and psoriasis, such vaccination is contraindicated in patients with these conditions in the absence of a bioterrorism attack and a real or potential exposure to smallpox. In the case of such exposure, the risk of smallpox infection outweighs the risk of adverse events from the vaccine (Chap. 205).

FURTHER READING

BOS JD, DERIE MA: The pathogenesis of psoriasis: Immunological facts and speculations. Immunol Today 20:40, 1999

COHEN DE: Occupational dermatoses, in *Handbook of Occupational Safety and Health*, 2d ed, LJ DiBerardinis (ed). New York, Wiley, 1999, p 697

FREEDBURG IM et al (eds): *Fitzpatrick's Dermatology in General Medicine*, 5th ed. New York, McGraw-Hill, 1999

HENGGE UR et al: Topical immunomodulators—progress towards treating inflammation, infection, and cancer. Lancet Infect Dis 1:189, 2001

KRUEGER JG: The immunologic basis for the treatment of psoriasis with new biologic agents. J Am Acad Dermatol 46:1, 2002

48 SKIN MANIFESTATIONS OF INTERNAL DISEASE
Jean L. Bolognia, Irwin M. Braverman

It is now a generally accepted concept in medicine that the skin can show signs of internal disease. Therefore, in textbooks of medicine one finds a chapter describing in detail the major systemic disorders that can be identified by cutaneous signs. The underlying assumption of such a chapter is that the clinician has been able to identify the disorder in the patient and needs only to read about it in the textbook. In reality, concise differential diagnoses and the identification of these disorders are actually difficult for the nondermatologist because he or she is not well versed in the recognition of cutaneous lesions or their spectrum of presentations. Therefore, the authors of this chapter have decided to cover this particular topic of cutaneous medicine not by discussing individual disorders but by describing and discussing the various presenting clinical signs and symptoms that indicate the presence of these disorders. Concise differential diagnoses will be generated in which the significant diseases will be briefly discussed and distinguished from the more common disorders that have no significance for internal diseases. The latter disorders are reviewed in table form and always need to be excluded when considering the former. For a detailed description of individual diseases, the reader should consult a dermatologic text.

PAPULOSQUAMOUS SKIN LESIONS (Table 48-1)   When an eruption is characterized by elevated lesions, papules (<1 cm), or plaques (>1 cm), in association with scale, it is referred to as a *papulosquamous lesion*. The most common papulosquamous diseases—*psoriasis, tinea, pityriasis rosea*, and *lichen planus*—are primary cutaneous disorders (Chap. 47). When psoriatic lesions are accompanied by arthritis, the possibility of psoriatic arthritis or *Reiter's disease* should be considered. A history of oral ulcers, conjunctivitis, uveitis, and/or urethritis points to the latter diagnosis. In *guttate psoriasis* there is an acute onset of small, widely scattered, uniform lesions, often in association with a streptococcal infection. Lithium, beta blockers, HIV infection, and a rapid taper of systemic glucocorticoids are also known to exacerbate psoriasis.

Whenever the diagnosis of pityriasis rosea or lichen planus is made, it is important to review the patient's medications because the eruption can be treated by simply discontinuing the offending agent. Pityriasis rosea–like drug eruptions are seen most commonly with beta blockers, angiotensin-converting enzyme (ACE) inhibitors, gold, and metronidazole, while the drugs that can produce a lichenoid eruption include gold, antimalarials, thiazides, quinidine, phenothiazines, sulfonylureas, and ACE inhibitors. Lichen planus–like lesions are also observed in chronic graft-versus-host disease.

In its early stages, *cutaneous T cell lymphoma* (CTCL) may be confused with eczema or psoriasis, but it often fails to respond to the appropriate therapy for those inflammatory diseases. CTCL can develop within lesions of large-plaque parapsoriasis and is suggested by an increase in the thickness of the lesions. The diagnosis of CTCL is established by skin biopsy in which collections of atypical T lymphocytes are found in the epidermis and dermis. As the disease progresses, cutaneous tumors and lymph node involvement may appear.

In *secondary syphilis* there are scattered red-brown papules with thin scale. The eruption often involves the palms and soles and can resemble pityriasis rosea. Associated findings are helpful in making the diagnosis and include annular plaques on the face, nonscarring alopecia, condyloma lata (broad-based and moist), and mucous patches as well as lymphadenopathy, malaise, fever, headache, and myalgias. The interval between the primary chancre and the secondary stage is usually 4 to 8 weeks, and spontaneous resolution without appropriate therapy is seen.

ERYTHRODERMA (Table 48-2)   *Erythroderma* is the term used when the majority of the skin surface is erythematous (red in color). There may be associated scale, erosions, or pustules as well as shedding of the hair and nails. Potential systemic manifestations include fever, chills, hypothermia, reactive lymphadenopathy, peripheral edema, hypoal-

---

TABLE 48-1   *Selected Causes of Papulosquamous Skin Lesions*

1. Primary cutaneous disorders
   a. Psoriasis[a]
   b. Tinea[a]
   c. Pityriasis rosea[a]
   d. Lichen planus[a]
   e. Parapsoriasis
   f. Bowen's disease (squamous cell carcinoma in situ)[b]
2. Drugs
3. Systemic diseases
   a. Lupus erythematosus[c]
   b. Cutaneous T cell lymphoma
   c. Secondary syphilis
   d. Reiter's disease
   e. Sarcoidosis[d]

[a] Discussed in detail in Chap. 47.
[b] Associated with chronic sun exposure and exposure to arsenic.
[c] See also "Red Lesions" in "Papulonodular Skin Lesions."
[d] See also "Red-Brown Lesions" in "Papulonodular Skin Lesions."

TABLE 48-2   *Causes of Erythroderma*

1. Primary cutaneous disorders
   a. Psoriasis[a]
   b. Dermatitis (atopic, stasis, contact, seborrheic)[a]
   c. Pityriasis rubra pilaris
2. Drugs
3. Systemic diseases
   a. Cutaneous T cell lymphoma
   b. Lymphoma
4. Idiopathic

[a] Discussed in detail in Chap. 47.

TABLE 48-3 Erythroderma (Primary Cutaneous Disorders)

	Initial Lesions	Location of Initial Lesions	Other Findings	Diagnostic Aids	Treatment
Psoriasis[a]	Pink-red, silvery scale, sharply demarcated	Elbows, knees, scalp, presacral area	Nail dystrophy, arthritis, pustules	Skin biopsy	Oral retinoid ± PUVA; UV-B; methotrexate; cyclosporine; monoclonal antibodies
Dermatitis[a]					
Atopic	Acute: Erythema, fine scale, crust, indistinct borders Chronic: Lichenification (increased skin markings)	Antecubital and popliteal fossae, neck, hands	Pruritus Family history of atopy, including asthma, allergic rhinitis or conjunctivitis, and atopic dermatitis Rule out secondary infection with *S. aureus* Rule out superimposed irritant contact dermatitis	Skin biopsy	Topical glucocorticoids, tacrolimus, pimecrolimus, tar, and antipruritics; oral antihistamines; open wet dressings; UV-B + UV-A; PUVA; oral/IM glucocorticoids; cyclosporine Topical or oral antibiotics
Stasis	Erythema, crusting, excoriations	Lower extremities	Pruritus, lower extremity edema History of venous ulcers, thrombophlebitis, and/or cellulitis Rule out cellulitis Rule out superimposed contact dermatitis, e.g., topical neomycin	Skin biopsy	Topical glucocorticoids; open; wet dressings; leg elevation; pressure stockings
Contact	Local: Erythema, crusting, vesicles, and bullae	Depends on offending agent	Irritant—onset often within hours Allergic—delayed-type hypersensitivity; lag time of 48 h	Patch testing	Remove irritant or allergen; topical glucocorticoids; oral antihistamines; oral/IM glucocorticoids
	Systemic: Erythema, fine scale, crust	Generalized	Patient has history of allergic contact dermatitis to topical agent and then receives systemic medication that is structurally related, e.g., ethylenediamine, (topical) aminophylline (IV)	Patch testing	Same as local
Seborrheic	Pink-red, greasy scale	Scalp, nasolabial folds, eyebrows, intertriginous zones	Flares with stress, HIV infection Associated with Parkinson's disease	Skin biopsy	Topical glucocorticoids and imidazoles
Pityriasis rubra pilaris	Orange-red, perifollicular papules	Generalized, but characteristic "skip" areas of normal skin	Wax-like keratoderma Rule out cutaneous T cell lymphoma	Skin biopsy	Isotretinoin or acitretin; methotrexate

[a] Discussed in detail in Chap. 47.

Note: PUVA, psoralens + ultraviolet A irradiation; UV-B, ultraviolet B; UV-A, ultraviolet A; IM, intramuscular; IV, intravenous.

buminemia, and high-output cardiac failure. The major etiologies of erythroderma are (1) cutaneous diseases such as psoriasis and dermatitis (Table 48-3); (2) drugs; (3) systemic diseases, most commonly CTCL; and (4) idiopathic. In the first three groups, the location and description of the initial lesions, prior to the development of the erythroderma, aid in the diagnosis. For example, a history of red scaly plaques on the elbows and knees would point to psoriasis. It is also important to examine the skin carefully for a migration of the erythema and associated secondary changes such as pustules or erosions. Migratory waves of erythema studded with superficial pustules are seen in *pustular psoriasis*.

Drug-induced erythroderma (exfoliative dermatitis) may begin as a morbilliform eruption (Chap. 50) or may arise as diffuse erythema. Fever and peripheral eosinophilia often accompany the eruption, and occasionally there is an associated allergic interstitial nephritis. A number of drugs can produce an erythroderma, including penicillins, sulfonamides, carbamazepine, phenytoin, gold, allopurinol, and captopril. While reactions to anticonvulsants can lead to a pseudolymphoma syndrome (with adenopathy, hepatitis, and circulating atypical lymphocytes), reactions to allopurinol may be accompanied by hepatitis, gastrointestinal bleeding, and nephropathy.

The most common malignancy that is associated with erythroderma is CTCL; in some series, up to 25% of the cases of erythroderma were

due to CTCL. The patient may progress from isolated plaques and tumors, but more commonly the erythroderma is present throughout the course of the disease (Sézary syndrome). In the Sézary syndrome, there are circulating atypical T lymphocytes, pruritus, and lymphadenopathy. In cases of erythroderma where there is no apparent cause (idiopathic), longitudinal follow-up is mandatory to monitor for the possible development of CTCL. There have been isolated case reports of erythroderma secondary to some solid tumors—lung, liver, prostate, thyroid, and colon—but it is usually in a late stage of the disease.

ALOPECIA (Table 48-4) The two major forms of alopecia are scarring and nonscarring. In *scarring alopecia* there are associated fibrosis, inflammation, and loss of hair follicles. A smooth scalp with a decreased number of follicular openings is usually observed clinically, but in some cases the changes are seen only in biopsy specimens from the affected areas. In *nonscarring alopecia* the hair shafts are gone, but the hair follicles are preserved, explaining the reversible nature of nonscarring alopecia.

The most common causes of nonscarring alopecia include *telogen effluvium*, *androgenetic alopecia*, *alopecia areata*, *tinea capitis*, and *traumatic alopecia* (Table 48-5). In women with androgenetic alopecia, an elevation in circulating levels of androgens may be seen as a result of ovarian or adrenal gland dysfunction. When there are

TABLE 48-4   Causes of Alopecia

I. Nonscarring alopecia	II. Scarring alopecia
A. Primary cutaneous disorders	A. Primary cutaneous disorders
1. Telogen effluvium	1. Cutaneous lupus
2. Androgenetic alopecia	2. Lichen planus
3. Alopecia areata	3. Folliculitis decalvans
4. Tinea capitis	4. Linear scleroderma
5. Traumatic alopecia	(morphea)
B. Drugs	5. Traumatic alopecia[a]
C. Systemic diseases	B. Systemic diseases
1. Lupus erythematosus	1. Lupus erythematosus
2. Secondary syphilis	2. Sarcoidosis
3. Hypothryoidism	3. Cutaneous metastases
4. Hyperthyroidism	
5. Hypopituitarism	
6. Deficiencies of protein,	
iron, biotin, and zinc	

[a] Also referred to as follicular degeneration.

signs of virilization, such as a deepened voice and enlarged clitoris, the possibility of an ovarian or adrenal gland tumor should be considered.

Exposure to various drugs can also cause diffuse hair loss, usually by inducing a telogen effluvium. An exception is the anagen effluvium observed with antimitotic agents such as daunorubicin. Alopecia is a side effect of the following drugs: warfarin, heparin, propylthiouracil, carbimazole, vitamin A, isotretinoin, acitretin, lithium, beta blockers, colchicine, and amphetamines. Fortunately, spontaneous regrowth usually follows discontinuation of the offending agent.

Less commonly, nonscarring alopecia is associated with *lupus erythematosus* and *secondary syphilis*. In systemic lupus there are two forms of alopecia—one is scarring secondary to discoid lesions (see below) and the other is nonscarring. The latter form may be diffuse and involve the entire scalp, or it may be localized to the frontal scalp and result in multiple short hairs ("lupus hairs"). Scattered, poorly circumscribed patches of alopecia with a "moth-eaten" appearance are a manifestation of the secondary stage of syphilis. Diffuse thinning of the hair is also associated with hypothyroidism and hyperthyroidism (Table 48-4).

Scarring alopecia is more frequently the result of a primary cutaneous disorder such as *lichen planus, folliculitis decalvans, cutaneous lupus,* or *linear scleroderma (morphea)* than it is a sign of systemic disease. Although the scarring lesions of *discoid lupus* can be seen in patients with systemic lupus, in the majority of cases the disease process is limited to the skin. Less common causes of scarring alopecia include *sarcoidosis* (see "Papulonodular Skin Lesions," below) and *cutaneous metastases.*

In the early phases of discoid lupus, lichen planus, and folliculitis decalvans, there are circumscribed areas of alopecia. Fibrosis and subsequent loss of follicles are observed primarily in the center of the individual lesions, while the inflammatory process is most prominent at the periphery. The areas of active inflammation in discoid lupus are erythematous with scale, whereas the areas of previous inflammation are often hypopigmented with a rim of hyperpigmentation. In lichen planus the peripheral perifollicular macules are usually violet-colored. Complete examination of the skin and oral mucosa combined with a biopsy and direct immunofluorescence microscopy will aid in distinguishing these two entities. The peripheral active lesions in folliculitis decalvans are follicular pustules; these patients can develop a reactive arthritis.

FIGURATE SKIN LESIONS (Table 48-6)   In *figurate eruptions,* the lesions form rings and arcs that are usually erythematous but can be skin-colored to brown. Most commonly, they are due to primary cutaneous diseases such as *tinea, urticaria, erythema annulare centrifugum,* and *granuloma annulare* (Chaps. 47 and 49). An underlying systemic illness is found in a second, less common group of migratory annular erythemas. It includes *erythema gyratum repens, erythema migrans, erythema marginatum,* and *necrolytic migratory erythema.*

In erythema gyratum repens, one sees hundreds of mobile concentric arcs and wavefronts that resemble the grain in wood. A search for an underlying malignancy is mandatory in a patient with this eruption. Erythema migrans is the cutaneous manifestation of Lyme disease, which is caused by the spirochete *Borrelia burgdorferi.* In the initial stage (3 to 30 days after tick bite), a single annular lesion is usually seen, which can expand to ≥ 10 cm in diameter. Within several days, approximately half the patients develop multiple smaller erythematous lesions at sites distant from the bite. Associated symptoms include fever, headache, photophobia, myalgias, arthralgias, and malar rash. Erythema marginatum is seen in patients with rheumatic fever, primarily on the trunk. Lesions are pink-red in color, flat to mildly elevated, and transient.

There are additional cutaneous diseases that present as annular eruptions but lack an obvious migratory component. Examples include *CTCL, annular cutaneous lupus* (also referred to as *subacute lupus*), *secondary syphilis,* and *sarcoidosis* (see "Papulonodular Skin Lesions," below).

ACNE (Table 48-7)   In addition to *acne vulgaris* and *acne rosacea,* the two major forms of acne (Chap. 47), there are drugs and systemic diseases that can lead to acneiform eruptions (Table 48-7).

Patients with the *carcinoid syndrome* have episodes of flushing of the head, neck, and sometimes the trunk. Resultant skin changes of the face, in particular telangiectasias, may mimic the clinical appearance of acne rosacea.

PUSTULAR LESIONS   *Acneiform eruptions* (see "Acne," above) and *folliculitis* represent the most common pustular dermatoses. An important consideration in the evaluation of follicular pustules is a determination of the associated pathogen, e.g., normal flora, *Staphylococcus aureus, Pityrosporum.* Noninfectious forms of folliculitis include HIV-associated eosinophilic folliculitis and folliculitis secondary to drugs such as glucocorticoids and lithium. Administration of high-dose oral glucocorticoids can result in a widespread eruption of follicular pustules on the trunk, characterized by lesions in the same stage of development. With regard to underlying systemic diseases, nonfollicular-based pustules are a characteristic component of pustular psoriasis and can be seen in septic emboli of bacterial or fungal origin (see "Purpura," below).

TELANGIECTASIAS (Table 48-8)   In order to distinguish the various types of telangiectasias, it is important to examine the shape and configuration of the dilated blood vessels. *Linear telangiectasias* are seen on the face of patients with *actinically damaged skin* and *acne rosacea* and they are found on the legs of patients with *venous hypertension* and *essential telangiectasia.* Patients with an unusual form of *mastocytosis* (telangiectasia macularis eruptiva perstans) and the *carcinoid syndrome* (see "Acne," above) also have linear telangiectasias. Lastly, linear telangiectasias are found in areas of cutaneous inflammation. For example, lesions of discoid lupus frequently have telangiectasias within them.

Poikiloderma is a term used to describe a patch of skin with (1) reticulated hypo- and hyperpigmentation, (2) wrinkling secondary to epidermal atrophy, and (3) telangiectasias. Poikiloderma does not imply a single disease entity—although becoming less common, it is seen in skin damaged by *ionizing radiation,* as well as in patients with autoimmune connective tissue diseases, primarily *dermatomyositis* (DM).

In *scleroderma,* the dilated blood vessels have a unique configuration and are known as *mat telangiectasias.* The lesions are broad macules that usually measure 2 to 7 mm in diameter but occasionally are larger. Mats have a polygonal or oval shape, and their erythematous color may be uniform or the result of delicate telangiectasias. The most common locations for mat telangiectasias are the face, oral mucosa, and hands—peripheral sites that are prone to intermittent ischemia. The CREST (calcinosis cutis, Raynaud's phenomenon, esophageal dysmotility, sclerodactyly, and telangiectasia) variant of scleroderma

(Chap. 303) is associated with a chronic course and anticentromere antibodies. Mat telangiectasias are an important clue to the diagnosis of the CREST syndrome as well as systemic scleroderma, for they may be the only cutaneous finding.

Periungual telangiectasias are pathognomonic signs of the three major autoimmune connective tissue diseases—*lupus erythematosus, scleroderma*, and *DM*. They are easily visualized by the naked eye and occur in at least two-thirds of these patients. In both DM and lupus there is associated nailfold erythema, and in DM the erythema is often accompanied by "ragged" cuticles and fingertip tenderness. Under 10× magnification, the blood vessels in the nailfolds of lupus patients are tortuous and resemble "glomeruli," whereas in scleroderma and DM there is a loss of capillary loops and those that remain are markedly dilated.

In *hereditary hemorrhagic telangiectasia* (Osler-Rendu-Weber disease), the lesions usually appear during adulthood and are most commonly seen on the mucous membranes, face, and distal extremities, including under the nails. They represent arteriovenous (AV) malformations of the dermal microvasculature, are dark red in color, and are usually slightly elevated. When the skin is stretched over an individual lesion, an eccentric punctum with radiating legs is seen. Although the degree of systemic involvement varies in this autosomal dominant disease (due to mutations in either the endoglin or activin receptor–like kinase gene), the major symptoms are recurrent epistaxis and gastrointestinal bleeding. The fact that these mucosal telangiectasias are actually AV communications helps to explain their tendency to bleed.

TABLE 48-5 *Nonscarring Alopecia (Primary Cutaneous Disorders)*

	Clinical Characteristics	Pathogenesis	Treatment
Telogen effluvium	Diffuse shedding of normal hairs Follows either major stress (high fever, severe infection) or change in hormones (post partum) Reversible without treatment	Stress causes the normally asynchronous growth cycles of individual hairs to become synchronous; therefore, large numbers of growing (anagen) hairs simultaneously enter the dying (telogen) phase	Observation; discontinue any drugs that have alopecia as a side effect; must exclude underlying metabolic causes, e.g., hypothyroidism, hyperthyroidism
Androgenetic alopecia	Miniaturization of hairs along the midline of the scalp Recession of the anterior scalp line in men and some women	Increased sensitivity of affected hairs to the effects of testosterone Increased levels of circulating androgens (ovarian or adrenal source in women)	If no evidence of hyperandrogen state, then topical minoxidil ± tretinoin; finasteride[a]; hair transplant
Alopecia areata	Well-circumscribed, circular areas of hair loss, 2–5 cm in diameter In extensive cases, coalescence of lesions and/or involvement of other hair-bearing surfaces of the body Pitting of the nails	The germinative zones of the hair follicles are surrounded by T lymphocytes Occasional associated diseases: hyperthyroidism, hypothyroidism, vitiligo, Down's syndrome	Topical anthralin; intralesional glucocorticoids; topical contact sensitizers
Tinea	Varies from scaling with minimal hair loss to discrete patches with "black dots" (broken hairs) to boggy plaque with pustules (kerion)	Invasion of hairs by dermatophytes, most commonly *Trichophyton tonsurans*	Oral griseofulvin or terbinafine plus 2.5% selenium sulfide or ketoconazole shampoo; examine family members
Traumatic alopecia	Broken hairs Irregular outline	Traction with curlers, rubber bands, braiding Exposure to heat or chemicals Mechanical pulling (trichotillomania)	Discontinuation of offending hair style or chemical treatments; trichotillomania may require hair clipping and observation of shaved hairs or biopsy for diagnosis, followed by psychotherapy

[a] To date, FDA-approved for men.

HYPOPIGMENTATION (Table 48-9)

Disorders of hypopigmentation are classified as either diffuse or localized. The classic example of *diffuse hypopigmentation* is *oculocutaneous albinism* (OCA). The most common forms are due to mutations in the tyrosinase gene (type I) or the *P* gene (type II); patients with type IA OCA have a total lack of enzyme activity. At birth, different forms of OCA can appear similar—white hair, gray-blue eyes, and pink-white skin. However, the patients with no tyrosinase activity maintain this phenotype, whereas those with decreased activity or *P* gene mutations will acquire some pigmentation of the eyes, hair, and skin as they age. The degree of pigment formation is also a function of racial background, and the pigmentary dilution is readily apparent when patients are compared to their first-degree relatives. The ocular findings in OCA correlate with the degree of hypopigmentation and include decreased visual acuity, nystagmus, photophobia, and monocular vision.

The differential diagnosis of *localized hypomelanosis* includes the following primary cutaneous disorders: *idiopathic guttate hypomelanosis, postinflammatory hypopigmentation, tinea (pityriasis) versicolor, vitiligo, chemical leukoderma, nevus depigmentosus* (see below), and *piebaldism* (Table 48-9). In this group of diseases, the areas of involvement are macules or patches with a decrease or absence of

pigmentation. Patients with vitiligo also have an increased incidence of several autoimmune disorders, including hypothyroidism, Graves' disease, pernicious anemia, Addison's disease, uveitis, alopecia areata, chronic mucocutaneous candidiasis, and the polyglandular autoimmune syndromes (types I and II). Diseases of the thyroid gland are the most frequently associated disorders, occurring in up to 30% of patients with vitiligo. Circulating autoantibodies are often found, and the most common ones are antithyroglobulin, antimicrosomal, and antiparietal cell antibodies.

There are three systemic diseases that should be considered in a patient with skin findings suggestive of vitiligo—*Vogt-Koyanagi-Harada syndrome, scleroderma*, and *melanoma-associated leukoderma*. A history of aseptic meningitis, nontraumatic uveitis, tinnitus, hearing loss, and/or dysacousis points to the diagnosis of the Vogt-Koyanagi-Harada syndrome. In these patients, the face and scalp are the most common locations of pigment loss. The vitiligo-like leukoderma seen in patients with scleroderma has a clinical resemblance to idiopathic vitiligo that has begun to repigment as a result of treatment; that is, perifollicular macules of normal pigmentation are seen within areas of depigmentation. The basis of this leukoderma is unknown;

TABLE 48-6   Causes of Figurate Skin Lesions

I. Primary cutaneous disorders
  A. Tinea
  B. Urticaria (≥90%)
  C. Erythema annulare centrifugum
  D. Granuloma annulare
  E. Psoriasis
II. Systemic diseases
  A. Migratory
    1. Erythema migrans
    2. Urticaria (≤10%)
    3. Erythema gyratum repens
    4. Erythema marginatum
    5. Pustular psoriasis
    6. Necrolytic migratory erythema (glucagonoma syndrome)[a]
  B. Nonmigratory
    1. Sarcoidosis
    2. Subacute lupus erythematosus
    3. Secondary syphilis
    4. Cutaneous T cell lymphoma (e.g., mycosis fungoides)

[a] Migratory erythema with erosions; favors lower extremities and girdle area.

TABLE 48-7   Causes of Acneiform Eruptions

I. Primary cutaneous disorders
  A. Acne vulgaris
  B. Acne rosacea
II. Drugs, e.g., anabolic steroids, glucocorticoids, lithium, iodides
III. Systemic diseases
  A. Increased androgen production
    1. Adrenal origin, e.g., Cushing's disease, 21-hydroxylase deficiency
    2. Ovarian origin, e.g., polycystic ovary disease
  B. Cryptococcosis, disseminated
  C. Dimorphic fungi
  D. Behçet's disease

TABLE 48-8   Causes of Telangiectasias

I. Primary cutaneous disorders
  A. Linear
    1. Acne rosacea
    2. Actinically damaged skin
    3. Venous hypertension
    4. Essential telangiectasia
    5. Within basal cell carcinomas
  B. Poikiloderma
    1. Ionizing radiation[a]
    2. Poikiloderma vasculare atrophicans
  C. Spider angioma
    1. Idiopathic
    2. Pregnancy
II. Systemic diseases
  A. Linear
    1. Carcinoid
    2. Ataxia-telangiectasia
    3. Mastocytosis
  B. Poikiloderma
    1. Dermatomyositis
    2. Cutaneous T cell lymphoma
    3. Xeroderma pigmentosum
  C. Mat
    1. Scleroderma
  D. Periungual
    1. Lupus erythematosus
    2. Scleroderma
    3. Dermatomyositis
  E. Papular
    1. Hereditary hemorrhagic telangiectasia
  F. Spider angioma
    1. Cirrhosis

[a] Becoming less common.

TABLE 48-9   Causes of Hypopigmentation

I. Primary cutaneous disorders
  A. Diffuse
    1. Generalized vitiligo[a]
  B. Localized
    1. Idiopathic guttate hypomelanosis
    2. Postinflammatory
    3. Tinea (pityriasis) versicolor
    4. Vitiligo
    5. Chemical leukoderma
    6. Nevus depigmentosus
    7. Piebaldism
II. Systemic diseases
  A. Diffuse
    1. Oculocutaneous albinism[b]
      a. Hermansky-Pudlak syndrome[c]
      b. Chédiak-Higashi syndrome[d]
    2. Phenylketonuria
    3. Homocystinuria
  B. Localized
    1. Vogt-Koyanagi-Harada
    2. Scleroderma
    3. Melanoma-associated leukoderma
    4. Tuberous sclerosis
    5. Hypomelanosis of Ito/mosaicism
    6. Incontinentia pigmenti (stage IV)
    7. Sarcoidosis
    8. Tuberculoid and indeterminate leprosy
    9. Cutaneous T cell lymphoma

[a] Absence of melanocytes.
[b] Normal number of melanocytes.
[c] Platelet storage defect and restrictive lung disease secondary to deposits of ceroid-like material; one form due to mutations in β subunit of adaptor protein.
[d] Giant lysosomal granules and recurrent infections.

there is no evidence of inflammation in areas of involvement, but it can resolve if the underlying connective tissue disease becomes inactive. In contrast to idiopathic vitiligo, melanoma-associated leukoderma often begins on the trunk, and its appearance should prompt a search for metastatic disease. The possibility exists that the destruction of normal melanocytes is the result of an immune response against malignant melanocytes.

There are two systemic disorders that may have the cutaneous findings of piebaldism (Table 48-10). They are *Hirschsprung's disease* and *Waardenburg's syndrome*. A possible explanation for both disorders is an abnormal embryonic migration or survival of two neural crest–derived elements, one of them being melanocytes and the other myenteric ganglion cells (Hirschsprung's disease) or auditory nerve cells (Waardenburg's syndrome). The latter syndrome is characterized by congenital sensorineural hearing loss, dystopia canthorum (lateral displacement of the inner canthi but normal interpupillary distance), heterochromic irises, and a broad nasal root, in addition to the piebaldism. Patients with Waardenburg's syndrome have been shown to have mutations in two genes that encode DNA-binding proteins, *PAX-3* and *MITF*, while patients with Hirschsprung's disease and white spotting have mutations in one of three genes—endothelin 3, endothelin B receptor, and *SOX-10*.

In *tuberous sclerosis*, the earliest cutaneous sign is an ash leaf spot. These lesions are often present at birth and are usually multiple; however, detection may require Wood's lamp examination, especially in fair-skinned individuals. The pigment within them is reduced but not absent. The average size is 1 to 3 cm, and the common shapes are polygonal and lance-ovate. Examination of the patient for additional cutaneous signs such as adenoma sebaceum (multiple angiofibromas of the face), ungual and gingival fibromas, fibrous plaques of the forehead, and connective tissue nevi (shagreen patches) is re-

commended. It is important to remember that an ash leaf spot on the scalp will result in *poliosis*, which is a circumscribed patch of gray-white hair. Internal manifestations include seizures, mental retardation, central nervous system (CNS) and retinal hamartomas, renal angiomyolipomas, and cardiac rhabdomyomas. The latter can be detected in up to 60% of children (<18 years) with tuberous sclerosis by echocardiography.

Nevus depigmentosus is a stable, well-circumscribed hypomelanosis that is present at birth. There is usually a single circular or rectangular lesion, but occasionally the nevus has a segmental or whorled pattern. It is important to distinguish this more common entity from ash leaf spots especially when there are multiple lesions. In *hypomelanosis of Ito*, swirls and streaks of hypopigmentation run parallel to one another in a pattern that resembles a marble cake. Lesions may progress or regress with time, and in up to a third of patients, associated abnormalities are found including in the musculoskeletal system (asymmetry), the CNS (seizures and mental retardation), and the eyes (strabismus and hypertelorism). Chromosomal mosaicism has been de-

TABLE 48-10 *Hypopigmentation (Primary Cutaneous Disorders, Localized)*

	Clinical Characteristics	Wood's Lamp Examination (UV-A; Peak = 365 nm)	Skin Biopsy Specimen	Pathogenesis	Treatment
Idiopathic guttate hypomelanosis	Common; acquired; 1 to 4 mm in diameter Shins and extensor forearms	Less enhancement than vitiligo	Abrupt decrease in epidermal melanin content	Possible somatic mutations as a reflection of aging; UV exposure	None
Postinflammatory hypopigmentation	Can develop within active lesions, as in subacute lupus, or after the lesion fades, as in dermatitis	Depends on particular disease Usually less enhancement than in vitiligo	Type of inflammatory infiltrate depends on specific disease	Block in transfer of melanin from melanocytes to keratinocytes could be secondary to edema or decrease in contact time Destruction of melanocytes if inflammatory cells attack basal layer	Treat underlying inflammatory disease
Tinea (pityriasis) versicolor	Common disorder Upper trunk and neck Shawl-like distribution Young adults Macules have fine white scale when scratched	Golden fluorescence	Hyphae and budding yeast in stratum corneum	Invasion of stratum corneum by the yeast *Pityrosporum* Yeast is lipophilic and produces C_9 and C_{11} dicarboxylic acids, which in vitro inhibit tyrosinase	Selenium sulfide 2.5%; topical imidazoles; oral imidazoles or triazoles
Vitiligo	Acquired; progressive Symmetric areas of complete pigment loss Periorificial—around mouth, nose, eyes, nipples, umbilicus, anus Other areas—flexor wrists, extensor distal extremities Segmental form is less common—unilateral, dermatomal-like	More apparent Chalk-white	Absence of melanocytes Mild inflammation	Possible autoimmune phenomenon that results in destruction of melanocytes—humoral and/or cellular Alternative hypothesis is self-destruction of melanocytes and circulating antibodies or cytotoxic T cells as a secondary phenomenon	Topical glucocorticoids; UV-B; PUVA; transplants; depigmentation if widespread
Chemical leukoderma	Similar appearance to vitiligo Often begins on hands Satellite lesions in areas not exposed to chemicals	More apparent Chalk-white	Decreased number or absence of melanocytes	Exposure to chemicals that selectively destroy melanocytes, in particular phenols and catechols (germicides; adhesives) Release of cellular antigens and activation of circulating lymphocytes may explain satellite phenomenon	Avoid exposure to offending agent, then treat as vitiligo
Piebaldism	Autosomal dominant Congenital, stable White forelock Areas of hypomelanosis contain normally pigmented and hyperpigmented macules of various sizes Symmetric involvement of central forehead, ventral trunk, and mid regions of upper and lower extremities	Enhancement of leukoderma and hyperpigmented macules	Hypomelanotic areas—few to no melanocytes	Defect in migration of melanoblasts from neural crest to ventral skin or failure of melanoblasts to survive or differentiate in these areas Mutations within the c-*kit* proto-oncogene that encodes the tyrosine kinase receptor for mast/stem cell growth factor	None; occasionally transplants

Note: PUVA, *p*soralens + *u*ltraviolet *A* irradiation; UV-B, *u*ltraviolet B.

tected in these patients; this lends support to the hypothesis that the pattern is the result of the migration of two clones of primordial melanocytes, each with a different pigment potential.

Localized areas of decreased pigmentation are commonly seen as a result of cutaneous inflammation (Table 48-10) and have been observed in the skin overlying active lesions of sarcoidosis (see "Papulonodular Skin Lesions," below) as well as in CTCL. Cutaneous infections also present as disorders of hypopigmentation, and in *tuberculoid leprosy* there are a few asymmetric patches of hypomelanosis that have associated anesthesia, anhidrosis, and alopecia. Biopsy specimens of the palpable border show dermal granulomas that contain rare, if any, *Mycobacterium leprae* organisms.

HYPERPIGMENTATION (Table 48-11) Disorders of hyperpigmentation are also divided into two groups—localized and diffuse. The localized forms are due to an epidermal alteration, a proliferation of melanocytes, or an increase in pigment production. Both seborrheic keratoses and acanthosis nigricans belong to the first group. *Seborrheic keratoses* are common lesions, but in one clinical setting they are a sign of systemic disease, and that setting is the sudden appearance of multiple lesions, often with an inflammatory base and in association with acrochordons (skin tags) and acanthosis nigricans. This is termed the *sign of Leser-Trélat* and signifies an internal malignancy. *Acanthosis nigricans* can also be a reflection of an internal malignancy, most commonly of the gastrointestinal tract, and it appears as velvety hy-

TABLE 48-11   *Causes of Hyperpigmentation*

I. Primary cutaneous disorders
  A. Localized
    1. Epidermal alteration
      a. Seborrheic keratosis
      b. Acanthosis nigricans (obesity)
      c. Pigmented actinic keratosis
    2. Proliferation of melanocytes
      a. Lentigo
      b. Nevus
      c. Melanoma
    3. Increased pigment production
      a. Ephelides (freckles)
      b. Café au lait macule
  B. Localized and diffuse
    1. Drugs
II. Systemic diseases
  A. Localized
    1. Epidermal alteration
      a. Seborrheic keratoses (sign of Leser-Trélat)
      b. Acanthosis nigricans (endocrine disorders, paraneoplastic)
    2. Proliferation of melanocytes
      a. Lentigines (Peutz-Jeghers and LEOPARD syndromes; xero-
        derma pigmentosum)
      b. Nevi [Carney complex (LAMB and NAME syndromes)][a]
    3. Increased pigment production
      a. Café au lait macules (neurofibromatosis, McCune-Albright
        syndrome[b])
      b. Urticaria pigmentosa[c]
    4. Dermal pigmentation
      a. Incontinentia pigmenti (stage III)
      b. Dyskeratosis congenita
  B. Diffuse
    1. Endocrinopathies
      a. Addison's disease
      b. Nelson syndrome
      c. Ectopic ACTH syndrome
    2. Metabolic
      a. Porphyria cutanea tarda
      b. Hemochromatosis
      c. Vitamin B_{12}, folate deficiency
      d. Pellagra
      e. Malabsorption, Whipple's disease
    3. Melanosis secondary to metastatic melanoma
    4. Autoimmune
      a. Biliary cirrhosis
      b. Scleroderma
      c. POEMS syndrome
      d. Eosinophilia-myalgia syndrome[d]
    5. Drugs and metals

[a] Also lentigines.
[b] Polyostotic fibrous dysplasia.
[c] See also "Papulonodular Skin Lesions."
[d] Late 1980s.

perpigmentation, primarily in flexural areas. In the majority of patients, acanthosis nigricans is associated with obesity and insulin resistance, but it may be a reflection of an endocrinopathy such as acromegaly, Cushing's syndrome, the Stein-Leventhal syndrome, or insulin-resistant diabetes mellitus (type A, type B, and lipoatrophic forms).

A proliferation of melanocytes results in the following pigmented lesions: *lentigo, melanocytic nevus,* and *melanoma* (Chap. 73). In an adult, the majority of lentigines are related to sun exposure, which explains their distribution. However, in the Peutz-Jeghers and LEOPARD [*l*entigines; *E*CG abnormalities, primarily conduction defects; *o*cular hypertelorism; *p*ulmonary stenosis and subaortic valvular stenosis; *a*bnormal genitalia (cryptorchidism, hypospadias); *r*etardation of growth; and *d*eafness (sensorineural)] syndromes, lentigines do serve as a clue to systemic disease. In *LEOPARD syndrome,* hundreds of lentigines develop during childhood and are scattered over the entire surface of the body. The lentigines in patients with *Peutz-Jeghers syndrome* are located primarily around the nose and mouth, on the hands

and feet, and within the oral cavity. While the pigmented macules on the face may fade with age, the oral lesions persist. However, similar intraoral lesions are also seen in Addison's disease and as a normal finding in darkly pigmented individuals. Patients with this autosomal dominant syndrome (due to mutations in a novel serine threonine kinase gene) have multiple benign polyps of the gastrointestinal tract, testicular tumors, and an increased risk of developing gastrointestinal (primarily colon), breast, and gynecologic cancers.

Lentigines are also seen in association with cardiac myxomas and have been described in two syndromes whose findings overlap: *LAMB* (*l*entigines, *a*trial myxomas, *m*ucocutaneous myxomas, and *b*lue nevi) *syndrome* and *NAME* [*n*evi, *a*trial myxoma, *m*yxoid neurofibroma, and *e*phelides (freckles)] *syndrome*. These patients can also have evidence of endocrine overactivity in the form of Cushing's syndrome, acromegaly, or sexual precocity (Carney complex).

The third type of localized hyperpigmentation is due to a local increase in pigment production, and it includes *ephelides* and café au lait macules (CALM). The latter are most commonly associated with two disorders—neurofibromatosis (NF) and McCune-Albright syndrome. *CALM* are flat, uniformly light brown in color, and can vary in size from 0.5 to 12 cm. Approximately 80% of adult patients with *type I NF* will have six or more CALM measuring ≥1.5 cm in diameter. Additional findings are discussed in the section on neurofibromas (see "Papulonodular Skin Lesions," below). In comparison with NF, the CALM in patients with *McCune-Albright syndrome* [polyostotic fibrous dysplasia with precocious puberty in females due to mosaicism for an activating mutation in a G protein ($G_s\alpha$) gene] are usually larger, more irregular in outline, and tend to respect the midline. CALM have also been associated with pulmonary stenosis (Watson syndrome), tuberous sclerosis, the LEOPARD syndrome, and multiple endocrine neoplasia (MEN), but a few such lesions can be found in normal individuals.

In incontinentia pigmenti, dyskeratosis congenita, and bleomycin pigmentation, the areas of localized hyperpigmentation form a pattern—swirled in the first, reticulated in the second, and flagellate in the third. In *dyskeratosis congenita,* atrophic reticulated hyperpigmentation is seen on the neck, thighs, and trunk and is accompanied by nail dystrophy, pancytopenia, and leukoplakia of the oral and anal mucosa. The latter often develops into squamous cell carcinoma. In addition to the flagellate pigmentation (linear streaks) on the trunk, patients receiving bleomycin often have hyperpigmentation on the elbows, knees, and small joints of the hand.

Localized hyperpigmentation is seen as a side effect of several other *systemic medications,* including those that produce fixed drug reactions [phenolphthalein, nonsteroidal anti-inflammatory drugs (NSAIDs), sulfonamides, and barbiturates] and those that can complex with melanin (antimalarials). Fixed drug eruptions recur in the same location as circular areas of erythema that can become bullous and then resolve as brown macules. The eruption usually appears within hours of administration of the offending agent, and common locations include the genitalia, extremities, and perioral region. Chloroquine and hydroxychloroquine produce gray-brown to blue-black discoloration of the shins, hard palate, and face, while blue macules can be seen on the lower extremities and in sites of inflammation with prolonged minocycline administration. Estrogen in oral contraceptives can induce melasma—symmetric brown patches on the face, especially the cheeks, upper lip, and forehead. Similar changes are seen in pregnancy, in patients receiving phenytoin, and in the adult form of Gaucher's disease. In the latter group there is also hyperpigmentation of the distal lower extremities.

In the diffuse forms of hyperpigmentation, the darkening of the skin may be of equal intensity over the entire body or may be accentuated in sun-exposed areas. The causes of diffuse hyperpigmentation can be divided into four groups—endocrine, metabolic, autoimmune, and drugs. The endocrinopathies that frequently have associated hyperpigmentation include *Addison's disease, Nelson syndrome,* and *ectopic ACTH syndrome.* In these diseases, the increased pigmentation is diffuse but is accentuated in the palmar creases, sites of friction, scars, and the oral mucosa. An overproduction of the pituitary hormones α-MSH (melanocyte-stimulating hormone) and ACTH can lead to an increase in melanocyte activity. These peptides are products of the proopiomelanocortin gene and exhibit homology; e.g., α-MSH and ACTH share 13 amino acids. A minority of the patients with Cushing's disease or hyperthyroidism have generalized hyperpigmentation.

The metabolic causes of hyperpigmentation include *porphyria cutanea tarda* (PCT), *hemochromatosis, vitamin B₁₂ deficiency, folic acid deficiency, pellagra, malabsorption*, and *Whipple's disease*. In patients with PCT (see "Vesicles/Bullae," below), the skin darkening is seen in sun-exposed areas and is a reflection of the photoreactive properties of porphyrins. The increased level of iron in the skin of patients with hemochromatosis stimulates melanin pigment production and leads to the classic bronze color. Patients with pellagra have a brown discoloration of the skin, especially in sun-exposed areas, as a result of nicotinic acid (niacin) deficiency. In the areas of increased pigmentation, there is a thin varnish-like scale. These changes are also seen in patients who are vitamin B₆ deficient, have functioning carcinoid tumors (increased consumption of niacin), or take isoniazid. Approximately 50% of the patients with Whipple's disease have an associated generalized hyperpigmentation in association with diarrhea, weight loss, arthritis, and lymphadenopathy. A diffuse slate-blue color is seen in patients with melanosis secondary to metastatic melanoma. Although there is a debate as to whether the color is due to single-cell metastases in the dermis or to a widespread deposition of melanin resulting from the high concentration of circulating melanin precursors, there is more evidence to support the latter.

Of the autoimmune diseases associated with diffuse hyperpigmentation, *biliary cirrhosis* and *scleroderma* are the most common, and occasionally both disorders are seen in the same patient. The skin is dark brown in color, especially in sun-exposed areas. In biliary cirrhosis the hyperpigmentation is accompanied by pruritus, jaundice, and xanthomas, whereas in scleroderma it is accompanied by sclerosis of the extremities, face, and, less commonly, the trunk. Additional clues to the diagnosis of scleroderma are telangiectasias, calcinosis cutis, Raynaud's phenomenon, and distal ulcerations (see "Telangiectasias," above). The differential diagnosis of cutaneous sclerosis with hyperpigmentation includes the POEMS [*p*olyneuropathy; *o*rganomegaly (liver, spleen, lymph nodes); *e*ndocrinopathies (impotence, gynecomastia); *M*-protein; and *s*kin changes] syndrome. The skin changes include hyperpigmentation, skin thickening, hypertrichosis, and angiomas.

Diffuse hyperpigmentation that is due to drugs or metals can result from one of several mechanisms—induction of melanin pigment formation, complexing of the drug or its metabolites to melanin, and deposits of the drug in the dermis. Busulfan; cyclophosphamide; long-term, high-dose ACTH; and inorganic arsenic induce pigment production. Complexes containing melanin or hemosiderin plus the drug or its metabolites are seen in patients receiving chlorpromazine and minocycline. The sun-exposed skin as well as the conjunctivae of patients on long-term, high-dose chlorpromazine can become blue-gray in color. Patients taking minocycline may develop a diffuse blue-gray, muddy appearance in sun-exposed areas in addition to pigmentation of the mucous membranes, teeth, nails, bones, and thyroid. Administration of amiodarone can result in both a phototoxic eruption (exaggerated sunburn) and/or a brown or blue-gray discoloration of sun-exposed skin. Biopsy specimens of the latter show yellow-brown granules in dermal macrophages, which represent intralysosomal accumulations of lipids, amiodarone, and its metabolites. Actual deposits of a particular drug or metal in the skin are seen with silver (argyria), where the skin appears blue-gray in color; gold (chrysiasis), where the skin has a brown to blue-gray color; and clofazimine, where the skin appears reddish brown. The associated hyperpigmentation is accentuated in sun-exposed areas, and discoloration of the eye is seen with gold (sclerae) and clofazimine (conjunctivae).

VESICLES/BULLAE

(Table 48-12) Depending on their size, cutaneous blisters are referred to as *vesicles* (<0.5 cm) or *bullae* (>0.5 cm). The

TABLE 48-12 Causes of Vesicles/Bullae

I. Primary cutaneous diseases	II. Systemic diseases
A. Primary blistering diseases (autoimmune)	A. Autoimmune
1. Pemphigus[a]	1. Paraneoplastic pemphigus[a]
2. Bullous pemphigoid[b]	B. Infections
3. Gestational pemphigoid[b]	1. Cutaneous emboli[b]
4. Cicatricial pemphigoid[b]	C. Metabolic
5. Dermatitis herpetiformis[b,c]	1. Diabetic bullae[a,b]
6. Linear IgA disease[b]	2. Porphyria cutanea tarda[b]
7. Epidermolysis bullosa acquisita[b,d]	3. Porphyria variegata[b]
B. Secondary blistering diseases	4. Pseudoporphyria[b]
1. Contact dermatitis[a]	5. Bullous dermatosis of hemodialysis[b]
2. Erythema multiforme[a,b]	D. Ischemia
3. Toxic epidermal necrolysis[b]	1. Coma bullae
C. Infections	
1. Varicella/zoster virus[a,e]	
2. Herpes simplex virus[a,e]	
3. Enteroviruses, e.g., hand-foot-and-mouth disease	
4. Staphylococcal scalded-skin syndrome[a,f]	
5. Bullous impetigo[a]	

[a] Intraepidermal.
[b] Subepidermal.
[c] Associated with gluten enteropathy.
[d] Associated with inflammatory bowel disease.
[e] Also systemic.
[f] In adults, associated with renal failure and immunocompromised state.

primary blistering disorders include *pemphigus vulgaris, pemphigus foliaceus, pemphigus erythematosus, paraneoplastic pemphigus, bullous pemphigoid, gestational pemphigoid, cicatricial pemphigoid, epidermolysis bullosa acquisita, linear IgA disease*, and *dermatitis herpetiformis* (Chap. 49).

Vesicles and bullae are also seen in *contact dermatitis*, both allergic and irritant forms (Chap. 47). When there is a linear arrangement of vesicular lesions, an exogenous cause should be suspected. Bullous disease secondary to the ingestion of drugs can take one of several forms, including phototoxic eruptions, isolated bullae, toxic epidermal necrolysis (TEN), and erythema multiforme major (Chap. 50). Clinically, phototoxic eruptions resemble an exaggerated sunburn with diffuse erythema and bullae in sun-exposed areas. The most commonly associated drugs are thiazides, doxycycline, sulfonamides, NSAIDs, and psoralens. The development of a phototoxic eruption is dependent on the doses of both the drug and ultraviolet (UV)-A irradiation.

Toxic epidermal necrolysis is characterized by bullae that arise on widespread areas of erythema and then slough. This results in large areas of denuded skin. The associated morbidity, such as sepsis, and mortality are relatively high and are a function of the extent of epidermal necrosis. In addition, these patients may also have involvement of the mucous membranes and intestinal tract. Drugs are the primary cause of TEN, and the most common offenders are phenytoin, barbiturates, sulfonamides, penicillins, and NSAIDs. Severe acute graft-versus-host disease (grade 4) can also resemble TEN.

In *erythema multiforme* (EM), the primary lesions are pink-red macules and edematous papules, the centers of which may become vesicular. The clue to the diagnosis of EM, as opposed to a drug-induced morbilliform exanthem, is the development of a "dusky" violet color or petechiae in the center of the lesions. Target or iris lesions are also characteristic of EM and arise as a result of active centers and borders in combination with centrifugal spread. However, iris lesions need not be present to make the diagnosis of EM.

EM has been subdivided into two major groups: (1) herpes simplex virus (HSV)-associated and (2) EM major due to drugs or *Mycoplasma pneumoniae*. Involvement of the mucous membranes (oral, nasal, ocular, and genital) is seen more commonly in the latter form. Hemorrhagic crusts of the lips are characteristic of EM major as well as herpes simplex, pemphigus vulgaris, and paraneoplastic pemphigus. Fever, malaise, myalgias, sore throat, and cough may precede or accompany the eruption. The lesions of EM usually resolve over 3 to 6 weeks but may be recurrent, especially when due to HSV.

Induction of EM major is most often due to drugs, especially sulfonamides, phenytoin, barbiturates, penicillins, and carbamazepine. In addition to HSV (in which lesions appear 7 to 12 days after the viral eruption), EM can also follow vaccinations, radiation therapy, and exposure to environmental toxins.

In addition to primary blistering disorders and hypersensitivity reactions, bacterial and viral infections can lead to vesicles and bullae. The most common infectious agents are herpes simplex (Chap. 163), herpes varicella-zoster (Chap. 164), and staphylococci (Chap. 120).

Staphylococcal scalded-skin syndrome (SSSS) and *bullous impetigo* are two blistering disorders associated with staphylococcal (phage group II) infection. In SSSS, the initial findings are redness and tenderness of the central face, neck, trunk, and intertriginous zones. This is followed by short-lived flaccid bullae and a slough or exfoliation of the superficial epidermis. Crusted areas then develop, characteristically around the mouth. SSSS is distinguished from TEN by the following features: younger age group, more superficial site of blister formation, no oral lesions, shorter course, less morbidity and mortality, and an association with staphylococcal exfoliative toxin ("exfoliatin"), not drugs. A rapid diagnosis of SSSS versus TEN can be made by a frozen section of the blister roof or exfoliative cytology of the blister contents. In SSSS the site of staphylococcal infection is usually extracutaneous (conjunctivitis, rhinorrhea, otitis media, pharyngitis, tonsillitis), and the cutaneous lesions are sterile, whereas in bullous impetigo the skin lesions are the site of infection. Impetigo is more localized than SSSS and usually presents with honey-colored crusts. Occasionally, superficial purulent blisters also form. *Cutaneous emboli* from gram-negative infections may present as isolated bullae, but the base of the lesion is purpuric or necrotic, and it may develop into an ulcer (see "Purpura," below).

Several metabolic disorders are associated with blister formation, including diabetes mellitus, renal failure, and porphyria. Local hypoxia secondary to decreased cutaneous blood flow can also produce blisters, which explains the presence of bullae over pressure points in comatose patients (coma bullae). In *diabetes mellitus*, tense bullae with clear viscous fluid arise on normal skin. The lesions can be as large as 6 cm in diameter and are located on the distal extremities. There are several types of porphyria, but the most common form with cutaneous findings is *PCT*. In sun-exposed areas (primarily the face and hands), the skin is very fragile, and trauma leads to erosions and tense vesicles. These lesions then heal with scarring and formation of milia; the latter are firm, 1- to 2-mm white or yellow papules that represent epidermoid inclusion cysts. Associated findings can include hypertrichosis of the lateral malar region (men) or face (women) and, in sun-exposed areas, hyperpigmentation and firm sclerotic plaques. An elevated level of urinary uroporphyrins confirms the diagnosis and is due to a decrease in uroporphyrinogen decarboxylase activity. Precipitating agents include alcohol, iron, chlorinated hydrocarbons, hepatitis C infection, and hepatomas.

The differential diagnosis of PCT includes (1) *porphyria variegata*—the skin signs of PCT plus the systemic findings of acute intermittent porphyria; it has a diagnostic plasma porphyrin fluorescence emission at 626 nm; (2) *drug-induced bullous photosensitivity* (pseudoporphyria)—the clinical and histologic findings are similar to PCT, but porphyrins are normal; etiologic agents include naproxen, furosemide, tetracycline, and nalidixic acid; (3) *bullous dermatosis of hemodialysis*—the same appearance as PCT, but porphyrins are usually normal or occasionally borderline elevated; patients have chronic renal failure and are on hemodialysis; (4) PCT associated with hepatomas,

hepatic carcinomas, and hemodialysis; and (5) *epidermolysis bullosa acquisita* (Chap. 49).

EXANTHEMS (Table 48-13)   Exanthems are characterized by an acute generalized eruption. The two most common presentations are erythematous macules and papules (morbilliform) and confluent blanching erythema (scarlatiniform). *Morbilliform* eruptions are usually due to either drugs or viral infections. For example, up to 5% of the patients receiving penicillins, sulfonamides, phenytoin, or gold will develop a maculopapular eruption. Accompanying signs may include pruritus, fever, eosinophilia, and transient lymphadenopathy. Similar maculopapular eruptions are seen in the classic childhood viral exanthems, including (1) *rubeola* (measles)—a prodrome of coryza, cough, and conjunctivitis followed by Koplik's spots on the buccal mucosa; the eruption begins behind the ears, at the hairline, and on the forehead and then spreads down the body, often becoming confluent; (2) *rubella*—it begins on the forehead and face and then spreads down the body; it resolves in the same order and is associated with retroauricular and suboccipital lymphadenopathy; and (3) *erythema infectiosum* (fifth disease)—erythema of the cheeks is followed by a reticulated pattern on extremities; it is secondary to a parvovirus B19 infection, and an associated arthritis is seen in adults.

Both measles and rubella are seen in unvaccinated young adults, and an atypical form of measles is seen in adults immunized with either killed measles vaccine or killed vaccine followed in time by live vaccine. In contrast to classic measles, the eruption of atypical measles begins on the palms, soles, wrists, and knuckles, and the lesions may become purpuric. The patient with atypical measles can have pulmonary involvement and be quite ill. Rubelliform and roseoliform eruptions are also associated with *Epstein-Barr virus* (5 to 15% of patients), *echovirus*, *coxsackievirus*, and *adenovirus* infections. Detection of specific IgM antibodies or fourfold elevations in IgG antibodies allows the proper diagnosis. Occasionally, a maculopapular drug eruption is a reflection of an underlying viral infection. For example, about 95% of the patients with infectious mononucleosis who are given ampicillin will develop a rash.

Of note, early in the course of infections with *Rickettsia* and meningococcus, prior to the development of purpura, the lesions may be erythematous macules and papules. This is also the case in chickenpox prior to the development of vesicles. Maculopapular eruptions are associated with early *HIV infection*, early secondary *syphilis*, *typhoid fever*, and *acute graft-versus-host disease*. In the last, lesions frequently begin on the palms and soles; the macular rose spots of typhoid fever involve primarily the anterior trunk.

The prototypic *scarlatiniform* eruption is seen in *scarlet fever* and is due to an erythrotoxin produced by group A β-hemolytic streptococcal infections, most commonly pharyngitis. This eruption is characterized by diffuse erythema, which begins on the neck and upper trunk, and red follicular puncta. Additional findings include a white

TABLE 48-13   *Causes of Exanthems*
I. Morbilliform
A. Drugs
B. Viral
1. Rubeola (measles)
2. Rubella
3. Erythema infectiosum
4. Epstein-Barr virus, echovirus, coxsackievirus, and adenovirus
5. Early HIV (plus mucosal ulcerations)
C. Bacterial
1. Typhoid fever
2. Early secondary syphilis
3. Early *Rickettsia*
4. Early meningococcemia
D. Acute graft-versus-host disease
E. Kawasaki's disease
II. Scarlatiniform
A. Scarlet fever
B. Toxic shock syndrome
C. Kawasaki's disease

strawberry tongue (white coating with red papillae) followed by a red strawberry tongue (red tongue with red papillae); petechiae of the palate; a facial flush with circumoral pallor; linear petechiae in the antecubital fossae; and desquamation of the involved skin, palms, and soles 5 to 20 days after onset of the eruption. A similar desquamation of the palms and soles is seen in toxic shock syndrome (TSS), Kawasaki's disease, and after severe febrile illnesses. Certain strains of staphylococci also produce an erythrotoxin that leads to the same clinical findings as in streptococcal scarlet fever, except that the antistreptolysin O titers are not elevated.

In *toxic shock syndrome*, staphylococcal (phage group I) infections produce an exotoxin (TSST-1) that causes the fever and rash, as well as enterotoxins. Initially, the majority of cases were reported in menstruating women who were using tampons. However, other sites of infection, including wounds and vaginitis, can lead to TSS. The diagnosis of TSS is based on clinical criteria (Chap. 120), and three of these involve mucocutaneous sites (diffuse erythema of the skin, desquamation of the palms and soles 1 to 2 weeks after onset of illness, and involvement of the mucous membranes). The latter is characterized as hyperemia of the vagina, oropharynx, or conjunctivae. Similar systemic findings have been described in *streptococcal toxic shock–like syndrome* (Chap. 121), and although an exanthem is seen less often than in TSS due to a staphylococcal infection, the underlying infection is often in the soft tissue.

The cutaneous eruption in *Kawasaki's disease* (mucocutaneous lymph node syndrome) (Chap. 121) is polymorphous, but the two most common forms are morbilliform and scarlatiniform. Additional mucocutaneous findings include bilateral conjunctival injection; erythema and edema of the hands and feet followed by desquamation; and diffuse erythema of the oropharynx, red strawberry tongue, and erosions with crusting on the lips. This clinical picture can resemble TSS and scarlet fever, but clues to the diagnosis of Kawasaki's disease are cervical lymphadenopathy, lip erosions, and thrombocytosis. The most serious associated systemic finding in this disease is coronary aneurysm secondary to arteritis. Aneurysms may lead to sudden death, primarily within the first 30 days of the illness. Scarlatiniform eruptions are also seen in the early phase of SSSS (see "Vesicles/Bullae," above) and as reactions to drugs.

URTICARIA (Table 48-14)   *Urticaria* (hives) are transient lesions that are composed of a central wheal surrounded by an erythematous halo. Individual lesions are round, oval, or figurate and are often pruritic. Acute and chronic urticaria have a wide variety of allergic etiologies and reflect edema in the dermis. Urticarial lesions can also be seen in patients with mastocytosis (urticaria pigmentosa), hyperthyroidism, and juvenile rheumatoid arthritis (JRA). In JRA, the lesions coincide with the fever spike, are transient, and are due to dermal infiltrates of neutrophils.

The common *physical urticarias* include dermographism, solar urticaria, cold urticaria, and cholinergic urticaria. Patients with *dermographism* exhibit linear wheals following minor pressure or scratching of the skin. It is a common disorder, affecting ~5% of the population.

TABLE 48-14   *Causes of Urticaria*

I. Primary cutaneous disorders
   A. Acute and chronic urticaria[a]
   B. Physical urticaria
      1. Dermatographism
      2. Solar urticaria[b]
      3. Cold urticaria[b]
      4. Cholinergic urticaria[b]
   C. Angioedema (hereditary and acquired)[b]
II. Systemic diseases
   A. Urticarial vasculitis
   B. Hepatitis B or C infection
   C. Serum sickness
   D. Angioedema (hereditary and acquired)

[a] A small minority develop anaphylaxis.
[b] Also systemic.

Solar urticaria characteristically occurs within minutes of sun exposure and is a skin sign of one systemic disease—erythropoietic protoporphyria. In addition to the urticaria, these patients have subtle pitted scarring of the nose and hands. *Cold urticaria* is precipitated by exposure to the cold, and therefore exposed areas are usually affected. In some cases, the disease is associated with abnormal circulating proteins—more commonly cryoglobulins and less commonly cryofibrinogens and cold agglutinins. Additional systemic symptoms include wheezing and syncope, thus explaining the need for these patients to avoid swimming in cold water. *Cholinergic urticaria* is precipitated by heat, exercise, or emotion and are characterized by small wheals with relatively large flares. They are occasionally associated with wheezing.

Whereas urticaria are the result of dermal edema, subcutaneous edema leads to the clinical picture of *angioedema*. Sites of involvement include the eyelids, lips, tongue, larynx, and gastrointestinal tract as well as the subcutaneous tissue. Angioedema occurs alone or in combination with urticaria, including urticarial vasculitis and the physical urticarias. Both acquired and hereditary (autosomal dominant) forms of angioedema occur (Chap. 298), and in the latter, urticaria is rarely, if ever, seen.

Urticarial vasculitis is an immune complex disease that may be confused with simple urticaria. In contrast to simple urticaria, individual lesions tend to last longer than 24 h and usually develop central petechiae that can be observed even after the urticarial phase has resolved. The patient may also complain of burning rather than pruritus. On biopsy, there is a leukocytoclastic vasculitis of the small blood vessels. Although many cases of urticarial vasculitis are idiopathic in origin, it can be a reflection of an underlying systemic illness such as lupus erythematosus, Sjögren's syndrome, or hereditary complement deficiency. There is a spectrum of urticarial vasculitis that ranges from purely cutaneous to multisystem involvement. The most common systemic signs and symptoms are arthralgias and/or arthritis, nephritis, and crampy abdominal pain, with asthma and chronic obstructive lung disease seen less often. Hypocomplementemia occurs in one- to two-thirds of patients, even in the idiopathic cases. Urticarial vasculitis can also be seen in patients with *hepatitis B* and *hepatitis C* infections, *serum sickness*, and *serum sickness–like illnesses*.

PAPULONODULAR SKIN LESIONS (Table 48-15)   In the *papulonodular diseases*, the lesions are elevated above the surface of the skin and may coalesce to form plaques. The location, consistency, and color of the lesions are the keys to their diagnosis; this section is organized on the basis of color.

White Lesions   In *calcinosis cutis* there are firm white to white-yellow papules with an irregular surface. When the contents are expressed, a chalky white material is seen. *Dystrophic calcification* is seen at sites of previous inflammation or damage to the skin. It develops in acne scars as well as on the distal extremities of patients with scleroderma and in the subcutaneous tissue and intermuscular fascial planes in DM. The latter is more extensive and is more commonly seen in children. An elevated calcium phosphate product, most commonly due to secondary hyperparathyroidism in the setting of renal failure, can lead to nodules of *metastatic calcinosis cutis*, which tend to be subcutaneous and periarticular. These patients can also develop calcification of muscular arteries and subsequent ischemic necrosis (calciphylaxis).

Skin-Colored Lesions   There are several types of skin-colored lesions, including epidermoid inclusion cysts, lipomas, rheumatoid nodules, neurofibromas, angiofibromas, neuromas, and adnexal tumors such as tricholemmomas. Both *epidermoid inclusion cysts* and *lipomas* are very common mobile subcutaneous nodules—the former are rubbery and compressible and drain cheeselike material (sebum and keratin) if incised. Lipomas are firm and somewhat lobulated on palpation. When extensive facial epidermoid inclusion cysts develop in childhood or there is a family history of such lesions, the patient should be examined for other signs of Gardner syndrome, including osteomas and desmoid

TABLE 48-15 *Papulonodular Skin Lesions According to Color Groups*

I. White
  A. Calcinosis cutis
II. Skin-colored
  A. Rheumatoid nodules
  B. Neurofibromas (von Recklinghausen's disease)
  C. Angiofibromas (tuberous sclerosis, MEN syndrome, type 1)
  D. Neuromas (MEN syndrome, type 2b)
  E. Adnexal tumors
    1. Basal cell carcinomas (nevoid basal cell carcinoma syndrome)
    2. Tricholemmomas (Cowden's disease)
  F. Osteomas (Gardner syndrome)
  G. Primary cutaneous disorders
    1. Epidermal inclusion cysts
    2. Lipomas
III. Pink/translucent[a]
  A. Amyloidosis
  B. Papular mucinosis
IV. Yellow
  A. Xanthomas
  B. Tophi
  C. Necrobiosis lipoidica
  D. Pseudoxanthoma elasticum
  E. Sebaceous adenomas (Torre syndrome)
V. Red[a]
  A. Papules
    1. Angiokeratomas (Fabry's disease)
    2. Bacillary angiomatosis (primarily in AIDS)
  B. Papules/plaques
    1. Cutaneous lupus
    2. Lymphoma cutis
    3. Leukemia cutis

  C. Nodules
    1. Panniculitis
    2. Cutaneous polyarteritis nodosa
    3. Systemic vasculitis
  D. Primary cutaneous disorders
    1. Arthropod bites
    2. Cherry hemangiomas
    3. Infections, e.g., erysipelas, sporotrichosis
    4. Polymorphous light eruption
    5. Lymphocytoma cutis (pseudolymphoma)
VI. Red-brown[a]
  A. Sarcoidosis
  B. Sweet's syndrome
  C. Urticaria pigmentosa
  D. Erythema elevatum diutinum (chronic leukocytoclastic vasculitis)
  E. Lupus vulgaris
VII. Blue[a]
  A. Venous malformations (blue rubber bleb syndrome)
  B. Primary cutaneous disorders
    1. Venous lake
    2. Blue nevus
VIII. Violaceous
  A. Lupus pernio (sarcoidosis)
  B. Lymphoma cutis
  C. Cutaneous lupus
IX. Purple
  A. Kaposi's sarcoma
  B. Angiosarcoma
  C. Palpable purpura
X. Brown-black[b]
XI. Any color
  A. Metastases

[a] May have darker hue in more darkly pigmented individuals.
[b] See also "Hyperpigmentation."
Note: MEN, multiple endocrine neoplasia.

glands or remain undifferentiated. *Basal cell carcinomas* (BCCs) are examples of adnexal tumors that have little or no evidence of differentiation. Clinically, they are translucent papules with rolled borders, telangiectasias, and central erosion. BCCs commonly arise in sun-damaged skin of the head and neck. When a patient has multiple BCCs, especially prior to age 30, the possibility of the nevoid basal cell carcinoma syndrome should be raised. It is inherited as an autosomal dominant trait and is associated with jaw cysts, palmar and plantar pits, frontal bossing, medulloblastomas, and calcification of the falx cerebri and diaphragma sellae. *Tricholemmomas* are also skin-colored adnexal tumors but differentiate toward hair follicles and can have a wartlike appearance. The presence of multiple tricholemmomas on the face and cobblestoning of the oral mucosa points to the diagnosis of Cowden's disease (multiple hamartoma syndrome) due to mutations in the *PTEN* gene. Internal organ involvement (in decreasing order of frequency) includes fibrocystic disease and carcinoma of the breast, adenomas and carcinomas of the thyroid, and gastrointestinal polyposis. Keratoses of the palms, soles, and dorsa of the hands are also seen.

tumors. *Rheumatoid nodules* are firm, 0.5- to 4-cm nodules that tend to localize around pressure points, especially the elbows. They are seen in approximately 20% of patients with rheumatoid arthritis and 6% of patients with Still's disease. Biopsies of the nodules show palisading granulomas. Similar lesions that are smaller and shorter-lived are seen in rheumatic fever.

Neurofibromas (benign Schwann cell tumors) are soft papules or nodules that exhibit the "button-hole" sign, that is, they invaginate into the skin with pressure in a manner similar to a hernia. Single lesions are seen in normal individuals, but multiple neurofibromas, usually in combination with six or more CALM measuring >1.5 cm (see "Hyperpigmentation," above), axillary freckling, and multiple Lisch nodules, are seen in von Recklinghausen's disease (NF type I; Chap. 359). In some patients the neurofibromas are localized and unilateral due to somatic mosaicism.

Angiofibromas are firm, pink to skin-colored papules that measure from 3 mm to several centimeters in diameter. When they are located on the central cheeks (adenoma sebaceum), the patient has tuberous sclerosis or MEN syndrome, type 1. The former is an autosomal disorder due to mutations in two different genes, and the associated findings are discussed in the section on ash leaf spots as well as in Chap. 359.

Neuromas (benign proliferations of nerve fibers) are also firm, skin-colored papules. They are more commonly found at sites of amputation and as rudimentary supernumerary digits. However, when there are multiple neuromas on the eyelids, lips, distal tongue, and/or oral mucosa, the patient should be investigated for other signs of the MEN syndrome, type 2b. Associated findings include marfanoid habitus, protuberant lips, intestinal ganglioneuromas, and medullary thyroid carcinoma (>75% of patients; Chap. 330).

Adnexal tumors are derived from pluripotential cells of the epidermis that can differentiate toward hair, sebaceous, apocrine, or eccrine

Pink Lesions The cutaneous lesions associated with primary systemic *amyloidosis* are pink in color and translucent. Common locations are the face, especially the periorbital and perioral regions, and flexural areas. On biopsy, homogeneous deposits of amyloid are seen in the dermis and in the walls of blood vessels; the latter lead to an increase in vessel wall fragility. As a result, petechiae and purpura develop in clinically normal skin as well as in lesional skin following minor trauma, hence the term *pinch purpura*. Amyloid deposits are also seen in the striated muscle of the tongue and result in macroglossia.

Even though specific mucocutaneous lesions are rarely seen in secondary amyloidosis and are present in only about 30% of the patients with primary amyloidosis, a rapid diagnosis of systemic amyloidosis can be made by an examination of abdominal subcutaneous fat. By special staining, deposits are seen around blood vessels or individual fat cells in 40 to 50% of patients. There are also three forms of amyloidosis that are limited to the skin and that should not be construed as cutaneous lesions of systemic amyloidosis. They are macular amyloidosis (upper back), lichenoid amyloidosis (usually lower extremities), and nodular amyloidosis. In macular and lichenoid amyloidosis, the deposits are composed of altered epidermal keratin. Recently, macular and lichenoid amyloidosis have been associated with MEN syndrome, type 2a.

Patients with *multicentric reticulohistiocytosis* also have pink-colored papules and nodules on the face and mucous membranes as well as on the extensor surface of the hands and forearms. They have a polyarthritis that can mimic rheumatoid arthritis clinically. On histologic examination, the papules have characteristic giant cells that are not seen in biopsies of rheumatoid nodules. Pink to skin-colored papules that are firm, 2 to 5 mm in diameter, and often in a linear arrangement are seen in patients with *papular mucinosis*. This disease is also referred to as *lichen myxedematosus* or *scleromyxedema*. The latter name comes from the brawny induration of the face and extremities that may accompany the papular eruption. Biopsy specimens of the papules show localized mucin deposition, and serum protein electrophoresis demonstrates a monoclonal spike of IgG, usually with a λ light chain.

Yellow Lesions Several systemic disorders are characterized by yellow-colored cutaneous papules or plaques—hyperlipidemia (xanthomas), gout (tophi), diabetes (necrobiosis lipoidica), pseudoxanthoma elasticum, and Torre syndrome (sebaceous tumors). Eruptive xanthomas are the most common form of *xanthomas*, and are associated with hypertriglyceridemia (types I, III, IV, and V). Crops of yellow papules with erythematous halos occur primarily on the extensor surfaces of the extremities and the buttocks, and they spontaneously involute with a fall in serum triglycerides. Increased β-lipoproteins (primarily types II and III) result in one or more of the following types of xanthoma: xanthelasma, tendon xanthomas, and plane xanthomas. Xanthelasma are found on the eyelids, whereas tendon xanthomas are frequently associated with the Achilles and extensor finger tendons; plane xanthomas are flat and favor the palmar creases, face, upper trunk, and scars. Tuberous xanthomas are frequently associated with hypertriglyceridemia, but they are also seen in patients with hypercholesterolemia (type II) and are found most frequently over the large joints or hand. Biopsy specimens of xanthomas show collections of lipid-containing macrophages (foam cells).

Patients with several disorders, including biliary cirrhosis, can have a secondary form of hyperlipidemia with associated tuberous and planar xanthomas. However, patients with myeloma have *normolipemic flat xanthomas*. This latter form of xanthoma may be ≥12 cm in diameter and is most frequently seen on the upper trunk or side of the neck. It is important to note that the most common setting for eruptive xanthomas is uncontrolled diabetes mellitus. The least specific sign for hyperlipidemia is xanthelasma, because at least 50% of the patients with this finding have normal lipid profiles.

In *tophaceous gout* there are deposits of monosodium urate in the skin around the joints, particularly those of the hands and feet. Additional sites of *tophi* formation include the helix of the ear and the olecranon and prepatellar bursae. The lesions are firm, yellow in color, and occasionally discharge a chalky material. Their size varies from 1 mm to 7 cm, and the diagnosis can be established by polarization of the aspirated contents of a lesion. Lesions of *necrobiosis lipoidica* are found primarily on the shins (90%), and patients can have diabetes mellitus or develop it subsequently. Characteristic findings include a central yellow color, atrophy (transparency), telangiectasias, and an erythematous border. Ulcerations can also develop within the plaques. Biopsy specimens show necrobiosis of collagen, granulomatous inflammation, and obliterative endarteritis.

In *pseudoxanthoma elasticum* (PXE) there is an abnormal deposition of calcium on the elastic fibers of the skin, eye, and blood vessels. In the skin, the flexural areas such as the neck, axillae, antecubital fossae, and inguinal area are the primary sites of involvement. Yellow papules coalesce to form reticulated plaques that have an appearance similar to that of plucked chicken skin. In severely affected skin, hanging, redundant folds develop. Biopsy specimens of involved skin show swollen and irregularly clumped elastic fibers with deposits of calcium. In the eye, the calcium deposits in Bruch's membrane lead to angioid streaks and choroiditis; in the arteries of the heart, kidney, gastrointestinal tract, and extremities, the deposits lead to angina, hypertension, gastrointestinal bleeding, and claudication, respectively. Long-term administration of D-penicillamine can lead to PXE-like skin changes as well as elastic fiber alterations in internal organs.

Adnexal tumors that have differentiated toward sebaceous glands include sebaceous adenoma, sebaceous carcinoma, and sebaceous hyperplasia. Except for sebaceous hyperplasia, which is commonly seen on the face, these tumors are fairly rare. Patients with Torre syndrome have one or more *sebaceous adenoma(s)*, and they can also have sebaceous carcinomas and sebaceous hyperplasia as well as keratoacanthomas. The internal manifestations of Torre syndrome include *multiple* carcinomas of the gastrointestinal tract (primarily colon) as well as cancers of the larynx, genitourinary tract, and endometrium.

Red Lesions Cutaneous lesions that are red in color have a wide variety of etiologies; in an attempt to simplify their identification, they will be subdivided into papules, papules/plaques, and subcutaneous nodules. Common red papules include *arthropod bites* and *cherry hemangiomas*; the latter are small, bright-red, dome-shaped papules that represent benign proliferation of capillaries. In patients with AIDS, the development of multiple red hemangioma-like lesions points to bacillary angiomatosis, and biopsy specimens show clusters of bacilli that stain positive with the Warthin-Starry stain; the pathogens have been identified as *Bartonella henselae* and *B. quintana*. Disseminated visceral disease is seen primarily in immunocompromised hosts but can occur in immunocompetent individuals.

Multiple *angiokeratomas* are seen in Fabry's disease, an X-linked recessive lysosomal storage disease that is due to a deficiency of α-galactosidase A. The lesions are red to red-blue in color and can be quite small in size (1 to 3 mm), with the most common location being the lower trunk. Associated findings include chronic renal failure, peripheral neuropathy, and corneal opacities (cornea verticillata). Electron photomicrographs of angiokeratomas and clinically normal skin demonstrate lamellar lipid deposits in fibroblasts, pericytes, and endothelial cells that are diagnostic of this disease. Widespread acute eruptions of erythematous papules are discussed in the section on exanthems.

There are several infectious diseases that present as erythematous papules or nodules in a sporotrichoid pattern, that is, in a linear arrangement along the lymphatic channels. The two most common etiologies are *Sporothrix schenckii* (sporotrichosis) and *M. marinum* (atypical mycobacteria). The organisms are introduced as a result of trauma, and a primary inoculation site is often seen in addition to the lymphatic nodules. Additional causes include *Nocardia*, *Leishmania*, and other dimorphic fungi; culture of lesional tissue will aid in the diagnosis.

The diseases that are characterized by erythematous plaques with scale are reviewed in the papulosquamous section, and the various forms of dermatitis are discussed in the section on erythroderma. Additional disorders in the differential diagnosis of red papules/plaques include *erysipelas*, *polymorphous light eruption* (PMLE), *lymphocytoma cutis*, *cutaneous lupus*, *lymphoma cutis*, and *leukemia cutis*. The first three diseases represent primary cutaneous disorders. PMLE is characterized by erythematous papules and plaques in a primarily sun-exposed distribution—dorsum of the hand, extensor forearm, and face. Lesions follow exposure to UV-B and/or UV-A, and in northern latitudes PMLE is most severe in the late spring and early summer. A process referred to as "hardening" occurs with continued UV exposure, and the eruption fades, but in temperate climates it will recur in the spring. PMLE must be differentiated from cutaneous lupus, and this is accomplished by histologic examination and direct immunofluorescence of the lesions. Lymphocytoma cutis (pseudolymphoma) is a *benign* polyclonal proliferation of lymphocytes in the skin that presents as infiltrated pink-red to red-purple papules and plaques; it must be distinguished from lymphoma cutis.

Several types of red plaques are seen in patients with systemic *lupus*, including (1) erythematous urticarial plaques across the cheeks and nose in the classic butterfly rash; (2) erythematous discoid lesions with fine or "carpet-tack" scale, telangiectasias, central hypopigmentation, peripheral hyperpigmentation, follicular plugging, and atrophy located on the face, scalp, external ears, arms, and upper trunk; and (3) psoriasiform or annular lesions of subacute lupus with hypopigmented centers located on the face, extensor arms, and upper trunk. Additional cutaneous findings include (1) a violaceous flush on the face and V of the neck; (2) urticarial vasculitis (see "Urticaria," above); (3) lupus panniculitis (see below); (4) diffuse alopecia; (5) alopecia secondary to discoid lesions; (6) periungual telangiectasias and erythema; (7) EM-like lesions that may become bullous; and (8) distal ulcerations secondary to Raynaud's phenomenon, vasculitis, or livedoid vasculopathy. Patients with only discoid lesions usually have the form of lupus that is limited to the skin. However, 2 to 10% of these patients eventually develop systemic lupus. Direct immunofluorescence of involved skin shows deposits of IgG or IgM and C3 in a granular distribution along the dermal-epidermal junction.

In *lymphoma cutis* there is a proliferation of malignant lymphocytes or histiocytes in the skin, and the clinical appearance resembles that of lymphocytoma cutis—infiltrated pink-red to red-purple papules and plaques. Lymphoma cutis can occur anywhere on the surface of the skin, whereas the sites of predilection for lymphocytomas include the malar ridge, tip of the nose, and earlobes. Patients with non-Hodgkin's lymphomas have specific cutaneous lesions more often than those with Hodgkin's disease, and occasionally, the skin nodules precede the development of extracutaneous non-Hodgkin's lymphoma or represent the only site of involvement. Arcuate lesions are sometimes seen in lymphoma and lymphocytoma cutis as well as in CTCL. *Leukemia cutis* has the same appearance as lymphoma cutis, and specific lesions are seen more commonly in monocytic leukemias than in lymphocytic or granulocytic leukemias. Cutaneous chloromas (granulocytic sarcomas) may precede the appearance of circulating blasts in acute nonlymphocytic leukemia and, as such, represent a form of aleukemic leukemia cutis.

Common causes of erythematous subcutaneous nodules include inflamed epidermoid inclusion cysts, acne cysts, and furuncles. *Panniculitis*, an inflammation of the fat, also presents as subcutaneous nodules and is frequently a sign of systemic disease. There are several forms of panniculitis, including erythema nodosum, erythema induratum/nodular vasculitis, lupus profundus, lipomembranous lipodermatosclerosis, α_1-antitrypsin deficiency, facticial, and fat necrosis secondary to pancreatic disease. Except for erythema nodosum, these lesions may break down and ulcerate or heal with a scar. The shin is the most common location for the nodules of erythema nodosum, whereas the calf is the most common location for lesions of erythema induratum. In erythema nodosum the nodules are initially red but then develop a blue color as they resolve. Patients with erythema nodosum but no underlying systemic illness can still have fever, malaise, leukocytosis, arthralgias, and/or arthritis. However, the possibility of an underlying illness should be excluded, and the most common associations are streptococcal infections, upper respiratory infections, sarcoidosis, and inflammatory bowel disease. The less common associations include tuberculosis, histoplasmosis, coccidioidomycosis, psittacosis, drugs (oral contraceptives, sulfonamides, aspartame, bromides, iodides), cat-scratch fever, and infections with *Yersinia*, *Salmonella*, and *Chlamydia*.

Erythema induratum and nodular vasculitis share a similar histology and were thought to represent the clinical spectrum of a single entity; subsequently they have been separated, with the latter idiopathic and the former associated with the presence of *M. tuberculosis* DNA by polymerase chain reaction (PCR) in 25 to 70% of patients. The lesions of lupus profundus are found primarily on the upper arms and buttocks (sites of abundant fat) and are seen in both the cutaneous and systemic forms of lupus. The overlying skin may be normal, erythematous, or have the changes of discoid lupus. The subcutaneous fat necrosis that is associated with pancreatic disease is presumably secondary to circulating lipases and is seen in patients with pancreatic carcinoma as well as in patients with acute and chronic pancreatitis. In this disorder there may be an associated arthritis, fever, and inflammation of visceral fat. Histologic examination of deep incisional biopsy specimens will aid in the diagnosis of the particular type of panniculitis.

Subcutaneous erythematous nodules are also seen in *cutaneous polyarteritis nodosa* (PAN) and as a manifestation of *systemic vasculitis*, e.g., systemic PAN, allergic granulomatosis, or Wegener's granulomatosis (Chap. 306). Cutaneous PAN presents with painful subcutaneous nodules and ulcers within a red-purple, netlike pattern of livedo reticularis. The latter is due to slowed blood flow through the superficial horizontal venous plexus. The majority of lesions are found on the lower extremity, and while arthralgias and myalgias may accompany cutaneous PAN, there is no evidence of systemic involvement. In both the cutaneous and systemic forms of vasculitis, skin biopsy specimens of the associated nodules will show the changes characteristic of a vasculitis; the size of the vessel involved will depend on the particular disease.

Red-Brown Lesions The cutaneous lesions in *sarcoidosis* (Chap. 309) are classically red to red-brown in color, and with diascopy (pressure with a glass slide) a yellow-brown residual color is observed that is secondary to the granulomatous infiltrate. The waxy papules and plaques may be found anywhere on the skin, but the face is the most common location. Usually there are no surface changes, but occasionally the lesions will have scale. Biopsy specimens of the papules show "naked" granulomas in the dermis, i.e., granulomas surrounded by a minimal number of lymphocytes. Other cutaneous findings in sarcoidosis include annular lesions with an atrophic or scaly center, papules within scars, hypopigmented macules and papules, alopecia, acquired ichthyosis, erythema nodosum, and lupus pernio (see below).

The differential diagnosis of sarcoidosis includes foreign-body granulomas produced by chemicals such as beryllium and zirconium, late secondary syphilis, and *lupus vulgaris*. Lupus vulgaris is a form of cutaneous tuberculosis that is seen in previously infected and sensitized individuals. There is often underlying active tuberculosis elsewhere, usually in the lungs or lymph nodes. At least 90% of the lesions occur in the head and neck area and are red-brown plaques with a yellow-brown color on diascopy. Secondary scarring and squamous cell carcinomas can develop within the plaques. Cultures or PCR analysis of the lesions should be done because it is rare for the acid-fast stain to show bacilli within the dermal granulomas.

Sweet's syndrome is characterized by red to red-brown plaques and nodules that are frequently painful and occur primarily on the head, neck, and upper extremities. The patients also have fever, neutrophilia, and a dense dermal infiltrate of neutrophils in the lesions. In approximately 10% of the patients there is an associated malignancy, most commonly acute nonlymphocytic leukemia. Sweet's syndrome has also been reported with lymphoma, chronic leukemia, myeloma, myelodysplastic syndromes, and solid tumors (primarily of the genitourinary tract). The differential diagnosis includes neutrophilic eccrine hidradenitis and atypical forms of pyoderma gangrenosum. Extracutaneous sites of involvement include joints, muscles, eye, kidney (proteinuria, occasionally glomerulonephritis), and lung (neutrophilic infiltrates). The idiopathic form of Sweet's syndrome is seen more often in women, following a respiratory tract infection.

A generalized distribution of red-brown macules and papules is seen in the form of mastocytosis known as *urticaria pigmentosa* (Chap. 298). Each lesion represents a collection of mast cells in the dermis, with hyperpigmentation of the overlying epidermis. Stimuli such as rubbing cause these mast cells to degranulate, and this leads to the formation of localized urticaria (Darier's sign). Additional symptoms can result from mast cell degranulation and include headache, flushing, diarrhea, and pruritus. Mast cells also infiltrate various organs such as the liver, spleen, and gastrointestinal tract in up to 30 to 50% of patients with urticaria pigmentosa, and accumulations of mast cells in the bones may produce either osteosclerotic or osteolytic shadows on radiographs. In the majority of these patients, however, the internal involvement remains fairly static. A subtype of chronic leukocytoclastic vasculitis, *erythema elevatum diutinum* (EED), also presents with papules that are red-brown in color. The papules coalesce into plaques on the extensor surfaces of knees, elbows, and the small joints of the hand. Flares of EED have been associated with streptococcal infections.

Blue Lesions Lesions that are blue in color are the result of either vascular ectasias and tumors or melanin pigment in the dermis. *Venous lakes* (ectasias) are compressible dark-blue lesions that are found commonly in the head and neck region. *Venous malformations* are also compressible blue papules and nodules that can occur anywhere on the body, including the oral mucosa. When there are multiple rather than single congenital lesions, the patient may have the blue rubber bleb syndrome or Mafucci's syndrome. Patients with the blue rubber bleb syndrome also have vascular anomalies of the gastrointestinal tract that may bleed, whereas patients with Mafucci's syndrome have associated dyschondroplasia and osteochondromas. *Blue nevi* (moles) are seen when there are collections of pigment-producing nevus cells in the dermis. These benign papular lesions are dome-shaped and occur most commonly on the dorsum of the hand or foot.

Violaceous Lesions Violaceous papules and plaques are seen in *lupus pernio, lymphoma cutis,* and *cutaneous lupus.* Lupus pernio is a particular type of sarcoidosis that involves the tip of the nose and the earlobes, with lesions that are violaceous in color rather than red-brown. This form of sarcoidosis is associated with involvement of the upper respiratory tract. The plaques of lymphoma cutis and cutaneous lupus may be red or violaceous in color and were discussed above.

Purple Lesions Purple-colored papules and plaques are seen in vascular tumors, such as *Kaposi's sarcoma* (Chap. 173) and *angiosarcoma,* and when there is extravasation of red blood cells into the skin in association with inflammation, as in *palpable purpura* (see "Purpura," below). Patients with congenital or acquired AV fistulas and venous hypertension can develop purple papules on the lower extremities that can resemble Kaposi's sarcoma clinically and histologically; this condition is referred to as pseudo-Kaposi sarcoma (acral angiodermatitis). Angiosarcoma is found most commonly on the scalp and face of elderly patients or within areas of chronic lymphedema and presents as purple papules and plaques. In the head and neck region the tumor often extends beyond the clinically defined borders and may be accompanied by facial edema.

Brown and Black Lesions Brown- and black-colored papules are reviewed in "Hyperpigmentation," above.

Cutaneous Metastases These are discussed last because they can have a wide range of colors. Most commonly they present as either firm, skin-colored subcutaneous nodules or firm, red to red-brown papulonodules. The lesions of lymphoma cutis range from pink-red to plum in color, whereas metastatic melanoma can be pink, blue, or black in color. Cutaneous metastases develop from hematogenous or lymphatic spread and are most often due to the following primary carcinomas: in men, lung, colon, melanoma, and oral cavity; and in women, breast, colon, and lung. These metastatic lesions may be the initial presentation of the carcinoma, especially when the primary site is the lung, kidney, or ovary.

PURPURA (Table 48-16) *Purpura* are seen when there is an extravasation of red blood cells into the dermis and, as a result, the lesions do not blanch with pressure. This is in contrast to those erythematous or violet-colored lesions that are due to localized vasodilatation—they do blanch with pressure. Purpura ($\geq$3 mm) and petechiae ($\leq$2 mm) are divided into two major groups, palpable and nonpalpable. The most frequent causes of *nonpalpable* petechiae and purpura are primary cutaneous disorders such as *trauma, solar purpura,* and *capillaritis.* Less common causes are *steroid purpura* and *livedoid vasculitis* (see "Ulcers," below). Solar purpura are seen primarily on the extensor forearms, while glucocorticoid purpura secondary to potent topical steroids or endogenous or exogenous Cushing's syndrome can be more widespread. In both cases there is alteration of the supporting connective tissue that surrounds the dermal blood vessels. In contrast, the petechiae that result from capillaritis are found primarily on the lower extremities. In capillaritis there is an extravasation of erythrocytes as a result of perivascular lymphocytic inflammation. The petechiae are bright red, 1 to 2 mm in size, and scattered within annular or coin-shaped yellow-brown macules. The yellow-brown color is caused by hemosiderin deposits within the dermis.

Systemic causes of nonpalpable purpura fall into several categories, and those secondary to clotting disturbances and vascular fragility will be discussed first. The former group includes *thrombocytopenia* (Chap. 101), *abnormal platelet function* as is seen in uremia, and *clotting factor defects.* The initial site of presentation for thrombocytopenia-

TABLE 48-16 Causes of Purpura

I. Primary cutaneous disorders	c. Thrombotic thrombocytopenic purpura
A. Nonpalpable	d. Warfarin reaction
1. Trauma	4. Emboli
2. Solar purpura	a. Cholesterol
3. Steroid purpura	b. Fat
4. Capillaritis	5. Possible immune complex
5. Livedoid vasculitis[a]	a. Gardner-Diamond syndrome (autoerythrocyte sensitivity)
II. Systemic diseases	b. Waldenström's hypergammaglobulinemic purpura
A. Nonpalpable	B. Palpable
1. Clotting disturbances	1. Vasculitis
a. Thrombocytopenia (including ITP)	a. Leukocytoclastic vasculitis
b. Abnormal platelet function	b. Polyarteritis nodosa
c. Clotting factor defects	2. Emboli[b]
2. Vascular fragility	a. Acute meningococcemia
a. Amyloidosis	b. Disseminated gonococcal infection
b. Ehlers-Danlos syndrome	c. Rocky Mountain spotted fever
c. Scurvy	d. Ecthyma gangrenosum
3. Thrombi	
a. Disseminated intravascular coagulation	
b. Monoclonal cryoglobulinemia	

[a] Also associated with systemic diseases.
[b] Bacterial, fungal, or parasitic.
Note: ITP, idiopathic thrombocytopenic purpura.

induced petechiae is the distal lower extremity. Capillary fragility leads to nonpalpable purpura in patients with systemic *amyloidosis* (see "Papulonodular Skin Lesions," above), disorders of collagen production such as *Ehlers-Danlos syndrome,* and *scurvy.* In scurvy there are flattened corkscrew hairs with surrounding hemorrhage on the lower extremities, in addition to gingivitis. Vitamin C is a cofactor for lysyl hydroxylase, an enzyme involved in the posttranslational modification of procollagen that is necessary for cross-link formation.

In contrast to the previous group of disorders, the purpura seen in the following group of diseases are associated with thrombi formation within vessels. It is important to note that these thrombi are demonstrable in skin biopsy specimens. This group of disorders includes disseminated intravascular coagulation (DIC), monoclonal cryoglobulinemia, thrombotic thrombocytopenic purpura, and reactions to warfarin. DIC is triggered by several types of infection (gram-negative, gram-positive, viral, and rickettsial) as well as by tissue injury and neoplasms. Widespread purpura and hemorrhagic infarcts of the distal extremities are seen. Similar lesions are found in purpura fulminans, which is a form of DIC associated with fever and hypotension that occurs more commonly in children following an infectious illness such as varicella, scarlet fever, or an upper respiratory tract infection. In both disorders, hemorrhagic bullae can develop in involved skin.

Monoclonal cryoglobulinemia is associated with multiple myeloma, Waldenström's macroglobulinemia, lymphocytic leukemia, and lymphoma. Purpura, primarily of the lower extremities, and hemorrhagic infarcts of the fingers and toes are seen in these patients. Exacerbations of disease activity can follow cold exposure or an increase in serum viscosity. Biopsy specimens show precipitates of the cryoglobulin within dermal vessels. Similar deposits have been found in the lung, brain, and renal glomeruli. Patients with *thrombotic thrombocytopenic purpura* can also have hemorrhagic infarcts as a result of intravascular thromboses. Additional signs include thrombocytopenic purpura, fever, and microangiopathic hemolytic anemia (Chap. 93).

Administration of *warfarin* can result in painful areas of erythema that become purpuric and then necrotic with an adherent black eschar. This reaction is seen more often in women and in areas with abundant subcutaneous fat—breasts, abdomen, buttocks, thighs, and calves. The erythema and purpura develop between the third and tenth day of therapy, most likely as a result of a transient imbalance in the levels of anticoagulant and procoagulant vitamin K–dependent factors. Continued therapy does not exacerbate preexisting lesions, and patients with an inherited or acquired deficiency of protein C are at increased risk for this particular reaction as well as for purpura fulminans.

Purpura secondary to *cholesterol emboli* are usually seen on the lower extremities of patients with atherosclerotic vascular disease. They often follow anticoagulant therapy or an invasive vascular procedure such as an arteriogram but also occur spontaneously from disintegration of atheromatous plaques. Associated findings include livedo reticularis, gangrene, cyanosis, subcutaneous nodules, and ischemic ulcerations. Multiple step sections of the biopsy specimen may be necessary to demonstrate the cholesterol clefts with the vessels. Petechiae are also an important sign of *fat embolism* and occur primarily on the upper body 2 to 3 days after a major injury. By using special fixatives, the emboli can be demonstrated in biopsy specimens of the petechiae. Emboli of tumor or thrombus are seen in patients with atrial myxomas and marantic endocarditis.

In the *Gardner-Diamond syndrome* (autoerythrocyte sensitivity), female patients develop large ecchymoses within areas of painful, warm erythema. Intradermal injections of autologous erythrocytes or phosphatidyl serine derived from the red cell membrane can reproduce the lesions in some patients; however, there are instances where a reaction is seen at an injection site of the forearm but not in the midback region. The latter has led some observers to view Gardner-Diamond syndrome as a cutaneous manifestation of severe emotional stress. *Waldenström's hypergammaglobulinemic purpura* is a chronic disorder characterized by petechiae on the lower extremities. There are circulating complexes of IgG–anti-IgG molecules, and exacerbations are associated with prolonged standing or walking.

Palpable purpura are further subdivided into vasculitic and embolic. In the group of vasculitic disorders, *leukocytoclastic vasculitis* (LCV), also known as *allergic* or *small-vessel vasculitis*, is the one most commonly associated with palpable purpura (Chap. 306). Underlying etiologies include drugs (e.g., antibiotics), infections (e.g., hepatitis C), and connective tissue diseases. *Henoch-Schönlein purpura* is a subtype of acute LCV that is seen primarily in children and adolescents following an upper respiratory infection. The majority of lesions are found on the lower extremities and buttocks. Systemic manifestations include fever, arthralgias (primarily of the knees and ankles), abdominal pain, gastrointestinal bleeding, and nephritis. Direct immunofluorescence examination shows deposits of IgA within dermal blood vessel walls. In *polyarteritis nodosa*, specific cutaneous lesions result from a vasculitis of arterial vessels rather than postcapillary venules as in LCV. The arteritis leads to ischemia of the skin, and this explains the irregular outline of the purpura (see below).

Several types of infectious emboli can give rise to palpable purpura. These embolic lesions are usually *irregular* in outline as opposed to the lesions of LCV, which are *circular* in outline. The irregular outline is indicative of a cutaneous infarct, and the size corresponds to the area of skin that received its blood supply from that particular arteriole or artery. The palpable purpura in LCV are circular because the erythrocytes simply diffuse out evenly from the postcapillary venules as a result of inflammation. Infectious emboli are most commonly due to gram-negative cocci (meningococcus, gonococcus), gram-negative rods (Enterobacteriaceae), and gram-positive cocci (*Staphylococcus*). Additional causes include *Rickettsia* and, in immunocompromised patients, *Candida* and opportunistic fungi.

The embolic lesions in *acute meningococcemia* are found primarily on the trunk, lower extremities, and sites of pressure, and a gunmetal-gray color often develops within them. Their size varies from 1 mm to several centimeters, and the organisms can be cultured from the lesions. Associated findings include a preceding upper respiratory tract infection, fever, meningitis, DIC, and, in some patients, a deficiency of the terminal components of complement. In *disseminated gonococcal infection* (arthritis-dermatitis syndrome), a small number of papules and vesicopustules with central purpura or hemorrhagic necrosis

are found on the distal extremities. Additional symptoms include arthralgias, tenosynovitis, and fever. To establish the diagnosis, a Gram stain of these lesions should be performed. *Rocky Mountain spotted fever* is a tick-borne disease that is caused by *R. rickettsii*. A several-day history of fever, chills, severe headache, and photophobia precedes the onset of the cutaneous eruption. The initial lesions are erythematous macules and papules on the wrists, ankles, palms, and soles. With time, the lesions spread centripetally and become purpuric.

Lesions of *ecthyma gangrenosum* begin as edematous, erythematous papules or plaques and then develop central purpura and necrosis. Bullae formation also occurs in these lesions, and they are frequently found in the girdle region. The organism that is classically associated with ecthyma gangrenosum is *Pseudomonas aeruginosa*, but other gram-negative rods such as *Klebsiella*, *Escherichia coli*, and *Serratia* can produce similar lesions. In immunocompromised hosts, the list of potential pathogens is expanded to include *Candida* and opportunistic fungi.

ULCERS The approach to the patient with a cutaneous ulcer is outlined in Table 48-17. →*Peripheral vascular diseases of the extremities are reviewed in Chap. 232, as is Raynaud's phenomenon.*

Livedoid vasculitis (atrophie blanche) represents a combination of a vasculopathy with intravascular thrombosis. Purpuric lesions and livedo reticularis are found in association with painful ulcerations of the lower extremities. These ulcers are often slow to heal, but when they do, irregularly shaped white scars are formed. The majority of cases are secondary to venous hypertension, but possible underlying illnesses include cryofibrinogenemia and disorders of hypercoagulability, e.g., the antiphospholipid syndrome (Chaps. 102 and 300).

In *pyoderma gangrenosum*, the border of the ulcers has a characteristic appearance of an undermined necrotic violaceous edge and a peripheral erythematous halo. The ulcers often begin as pustules that then expand rather rapidly to a size as large as 20 cm. Although these lesions are most commonly found on the lower extremities, they can arise anywhere on the surface of the body, including sites of trauma (pathergy). An estimated 30 to 50% of cases are idiopathic, and the

TABLE 48-17 *Causes of Cutaneous Ulcers*

I. Primary cutaneous disorders
  A. Peripheral vascular disease (Chap. 232)
    1. Venous
    2. Arterial
  B. Livedoid vasculopathy[a]
  C. Squamous cell carcinoma, e.g., within scars
  D. Infections, e.g., ecthyma caused by *Streptococcus* (Chap. 121)
II. Systemic diseases
  A. Lower legs
    1. Leukocytoclastic vasculitis[b]
    2. Hemoglobinopathies (Chap. 91)
    3. Cryoglobulinemia,[b] cryofibrinogenemia
    4. Cholesterol emboli[b]
    5. Necrobiosis lipoidica[c]
    6. Antiphospholipid syndrome (Chap. 102)
    7. Neuropathic[d] (Chap. 323)
    8. Panniculitis
  B. Hands and feet
    1. Raynaud's phenomenon (Chap. 232)
  C. Generalized
    1. Pyoderma gangrenosum
    2. Calciphylaxis (Chap. 332)
    3. Infections, e.g., dimorphic fungi, chronic herpes varicella–zoster
    4. Lymphoma
  D. Mucosal
    1. Behçet's syndrome (Chap. 307)
    2. Erythema multiforme
    3. Primary blistering disorders (Chap. 49)
    4. Lupus erythematosus
    5. Inflammatory bowel disease

[a] Also associated with systemic diseases.
[b] Reviewed in section on "Purpura."
[c] Reviewed in section on "Papulonodular Skin Lesions."
[d] Favors plantar surface of the foot.

most common associated disorders are ulcerative colitis and Crohn's disease. Less commonly, it is associated with chronic active hepatitis, seropositive rheumatoid arthritis, acute and chronic granulocytic leukemia, polycythemia vera, and myeloma. Additional findings in these patients, even those with idiopathic disease, are cutaneous anergy and a benign monoclonal gammopathy. Because the histology of pyoderma gangrenosum is nonspecific, the diagnosis is made clinically by excluding less common causes of similar-appearing ulcers such as necrotizing vasculitis, Meleney's ulcer (synergistic infection at a site of trauma or surgery), dimorphic fungi, cutaneous amebiasis, spider bites, and facticial. In the myeloproliferative disorders, the ulcers may be more superficial with a pustulobullous border, and these lesions provide a connection between classic pyoderma gangrenosum and acute febrile neutrophilic dermatosis (Sweet's syndrome).

FEVER AND RASH The major considerations in a patient with a fever and a rash are inflammatory diseases versus infectious diseases. In the hospital setting, the most common scenario is a patient who has a drug rash plus a fever secondary to an underlying infection. However, it should be emphasized that a drug reaction can lead to both a cutaneous eruption and a fever ("drug fever"). Additional inflammatory diseases that are often associated with a fever include pustular psoriasis, erythroderma, and Sweet's syndrome. Lyme disease, secondary syphilis, and viral and bacterial exanthems (see "Exanthems," above) are examples of infectious diseases that produce a rash and a fever. Lastly, it is important to determine whether or not the cutaneous lesions represent septic emboli (see "Purpura," above). Such lesions usually have evidence of ischemia in the form of purpura, necrosis, or impending necrosis (gunmetal-gray color). In the patient with thrombocytopenia, however, purpura can be seen in inflammatory reactions such as morbilliform drug eruptions and infectious lesions.

FURTHER READING

BOLOGNIA JL et al: *Dermatology*. Philadelphia, Mosby, 2003

BRAVERMAN IM: *Skin Signs of Systemic Disease*, 3d ed. Philadelphia, Saunders, 1998

CALLEN JP et al: *Dermatological Signs of Internal Disease*, 3d ed. Philadelphia, Saunders, 2003

SYBERT VP: *Genetic Skin Disorders*. New York, Oxford University Press, 1997

WEEDON D: *Skin Pathology*. 2d ed. London, Churchill Livingstone, 2002

49 IMMUNOLOGICALLY MEDIATED SKIN DISEASES
Kim B. Yancey, Thomas J. Lawley

A number of immunologically mediated skin diseases and immunologically mediated systemic disorders with cutaneous manifestations are now recognized as distinct entities with consistent clinical, histologic, and immunopathologic findings. Many of these disorders are due to autoimmune mechanisms. Clinically, they are characterized by morbidity (pain, pruritus, disfigurement) and in some instances by mortality (largely due to loss of epidermal barrier function and/or secondary infection). The major features of the more common immunologically mediated skin diseases are summarized in this chapter (Table 49-1).

PEMPHIGUS VULGARIS Pemphigus vulgaris (PV) is a blistering skin disease seen predominantly in elderly patients. Patients with PV have an increased incidence of the HLA-DR4 and -DRw6 serologically defined haplotypes. This disorder is characterized by the loss of cohesion between epidermal cells (a process termed *acantholysis*) with the resultant formation of intraepidermal blisters. Clinical lesions of PV typically consist of flaccid blisters on either normal-appearing or erythematous skin. These blisters rupture easily, leaving denuded areas that may crust and enlarge peripherally (Fig. 49-1). Substantial portions of the body surface may be denuded in severe cases. Manual pressure to the skin of these patients may elicit the separation of the epidermis (Nikolsky's sign). This finding, while characteristic of PV, is not specific to this disorder and is also seen in toxic epidermal necrolysis, Stevens-Johnson syndrome, and a few other skin diseases. Lesions in PV typically present on the oral mucosa, scalp, face, neck, axilla, and trunk. In most patients, lesions begin in the mouth; involvement of other mucosal surfaces (e.g., pharyngeal, laryngeal, esophageal, conjunctival, vulval, or rectal) can occur in severe disease. Pruritus may be a feature of early pemphigus lesions; extensive denudation may be associated with severe pain. Lesions usually heal without scarring, except at sites complicated by secondary infection or mechanically induced dermal wounds. Nonetheless, postinflammatory hyperpigmentation is usually present at sites of healed lesions for some time.

Biopsies of early lesions demonstrate intraepidermal vesicle formation secondary to loss of cohesion between epidermal cells (i.e., acantholytic blisters). Blister cavities contain acantholytic epidermal cells, which appear as round homogeneous cells containing hyperchromatic nuclei. Basal keratinocytes remain attached to the epidermal basement membrane, hence blister formation is within the suprabasal portion of the epidermis. Lesional skin may contain focal collections of intraepidermal eosinophils within blister cavities; dermal alterations are slight, often limited to an eosinophil-predominant leukocytic infiltrate. Direct immunofluorescence microscopy of lesional or intact patient skin shows deposits of IgG on the surface of keratinocytes; in contrast, deposits of complement components are typically found in lesional but not uninvolved skin. Deposits of IgG on keratinocytes are derived from circulating autoantibodies directed against cell-surface antigens. Circulating autoantibodies can be demonstrated in 80 to 90% of PV patients by indirect immunofluorescence microscopy; monkey esophagus is the optimal substrate for these studies. Patients with PV have IgG autoantibodies directed against *desmogleins* (Dsgs), transmembrane desmosomal glycoproteins that belong to the cadherin supergene family of calcium-dependent adhesion molecules. Such autoantibodies can now be precisely quantitated by enzyme-linked immunosorbent assay (ELISA). Most patients with early PV (i.e., only mucosal involvement) have only anti-Dsg3 autoantibodies; most patients with advanced disease (i.e., involvement of skin and mucosa) have both anti-Dsg3 and anti-Dsg1 autoantibodies. Recent studies have shown that the anti-Dsg autoantibody profile in these patients' sera as well as the tissue distribution of Dsg3 and Dsg1 determine the site of blister formation in patients with pemphigus. Experimental studies have also shown that these autoantibodies are pathogenic (i.e., responsible for blister formation) and that their titer correlates with disease activity.

PV can be life-threatening. Prior to the availability of glucocorticoids, the mortality ranged from 60 to 90%; the current mortality is approximately 5%. Common causes of morbidity and mortality are infection and complications of treatment with glucocorticoids. Bad prognostic factors include advanced age, widespread involvement, and the requirement for high doses of glucocorticoids (with or without other immunosuppressive agents) for control of disease. The course of PV in individual patients is variable and difficult to predict. Some patients achieve remission (40% of patients in some series), but others may require long-term treatment or succumb to complications of their disease or its treatment. The mainstay of treatment is systemic glucocorticoids. Patients with moderate to severe disease are usually started on prednisone, 60 to 80 mg/d. If new lesions continue to appear

TABLE 49-1   *Immunologically Mediated Blistering Diseases*

Disease	Clinical	Histology	Immunopathology	Autoantigens[a]
Pemphigus foliaceus	Crusts and shallow erosions on scalp, central face, upper chest, and back	Acantholytic blister formed in superficial layer of epidermis	Cell surface deposits of IgG on keratinocytes	Dsg1
Pemphigus vulgaris	Flaccid blisters, denuded skin, oromucosal lesions	Acantholytic blister formed in suprabasal layer of epidermis	Cell surface deposits of IgG on keratinocytes	Dsg3 (plus Dsg1 in patients with skin involvement)
Bullous pemphigoid	Large tense blisters on flexor surfaces and trunk	Blister formed in subepidermal region; usually eosinophil-rich infiltrate	Linear band of IgG and/or C3 in epidermal BMZ[a]	BPAG1, BPAG2
Pemphigoid gestationis	Pruritic, urticarial plaques, rimmed by vesicles and bullae on the trunk and extremities	Teardrop-shaped, subepidermal blisters in dermal papillae; eosinophil-rich infiltrate	Linear band of C3 in epidermal BMZ	BPAG2 (plus BPAG1 in some patients)
Linear IgA disease	Pruritic small papules on extensor surfaces; occasionally larger, arciform blisters	Subepidermal blister with neutrophils in dermal papillae	Linear band of IgA in epidermal BMZ	BPAG2 (see text for specific details)
Cicatricial pemphigoid	Erosive and/or blistering lesions of mucous membranes and possibly the skin; scarring of some sites	Subepidermal blister that may or may not include a leukocytic infiltrate	Linear band of IgG, IgA, and/or C3 in epidermal BMZ	BPAG2, laminin 5, or others
Epidermolysis bullosa acquisita	Blisters, erosions, scars, and milia on sites exposed to trauma; widespread, inflammatory, tense blisters may be seen initially	Subepidermal blister that may or may not include a leukocytic infiltrate	Linear band of IgG and/or C3 in epidermal BMZ	Type VII collagen
Dermatitis herpetiformis	Extremely pruritic small papules and vesicles on elbows, knees, buttocks, and posterior neck	Subepidermal blister with neutrophils in dermal papillae	Granular deposits of IgA in dermal papillae	Epidermal transglutaminase

[a] Autoantigens bound by these patients' autoantibodies are defined as follows: Dsg1, desmoglein 1; Dsg3, desmoglein 3; BPAG1, bullous pemphigoid antigen 1; BPAG2, bullous pemphigoid antigen 2; BMZ, basement membrane zone.

after 1 to 2 weeks of treatment, the dose may need to be increased. Many regimens combine an immunosuppressive agent with systemic glucocorticoids for control of PV. The most frequently used are either azathioprine (1 to 2 mg/kg per day), or mycophenolate mofetil (20 to 35 mg/kg per day), cyclophosphamide (1 to 2 mg/kg per day). It is important to bring severe or progressive disease under control quickly to lessen the severity and/or duration of this disorder.

PEMPHIGUS FOLIACEUS   Pemphigus foliaceus (PF) is distinguished from PV by several features. In PF, acantholytic blisters are located high within the epidermis, usually just beneath the stratum corneum. Hence PF is a more superficial blistering disease than PV. The distribution of lesions in the two disorders is much the same, except that in PF mucous membranes are almost always spared. Patients with PF rarely demonstrate intact blisters but rather exhibit shallow erosions associated with erythema, scale, and crust formation. Mild cases of PF resemble severe seborrheic dermatitis; severe PF may cause extensive exfoliation. Sun exposure (ultraviolet irradiation) may be an aggravating factor. A blistering skin disease endemic to south central Brazil known as *fogo selvagem*, or *Brazilian pemphigus*, is clinically, histologically, and immunopathologically indistinguishable from PF.

Patients with PF have immunopathologic features in common with PV. Specifically, direct immunofluorescence microscopy of perilesional skin demonstrates IgG on the surface of keratinocytes. As in PV, patients with PF frequently have circulating IgG autoantibodies against keratinocyte cell surface antigens. Guinea pig esophagus is the optimal substrate for indirect immunofluorescence microscopy studies of sera from patients with PF. In PF, autoantibodies are directed against Dsg1, a 160-kDa desmosomal cadherin. As noted for PV, the autoantibody profile in patients with PF (i.e., anti-Dsg1) and the normal tissue distribution of this autoantigen (i.e., low expression in oral mucosa) is thought to account for the distribution of lesions in this disease.

Although pemphigus has been associated with several autoimmune diseases, its association with thymoma and/or myasthenia gravis is particularly notable. To date, more than 30 cases of thymoma and/or myasthenia gravis have been reported in association with pemphigus, usually with PF. Patients may also develop pemphigus as a consequence of drug exposure. The most frequently implicated agent is penicillamine; other offenders include captopril, rifampin, piroxicam, penicillin, and phenobarbital. Drug-induced pemphigus usually resembles PF rather than PV; autoantibodies in these patients have the same antigenic specificity as they do in other pemphigus patients. In most patients, lesions resolve following discontinuation of the drug; however, some patients require treatment with systemic glucocorticoids and/or immunosuppressive agents.

PF is generally a far less severe disease than PV and carries a better prognosis. Localized disease can be treated conservatively with topical or intralesional glucocorticoids; more active cases can usually be controlled with systemic glucocorticoids.

PARANEOPLASTIC PEMPHIGUS   Paraneoplastic pemphigus (PNP) is an autoimmune acantholytic mucocutaneous disease associated with an occult or confirmed neoplasm. Patients with PNP typically show painful mucosal erosive lesions in association with papulosquamous eruptions that often progress to blisters. Palm and sole involvement is common in these patients and raises the possibility that prior reports of neoplasia-associated erythema multiforme actually may have represented unrecognized cases of PNP. Biopsies of lesional skin from these patients show varying combinations of acantholysis, keratinocyte necrosis, and vacuolar-interface dermatitis. Direct immunofluorescence microscopy of patient skin shows deposits of IgG and complement on the surface

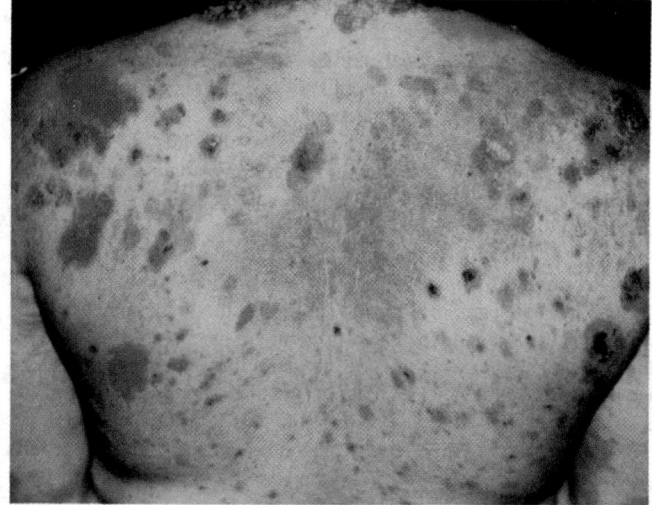

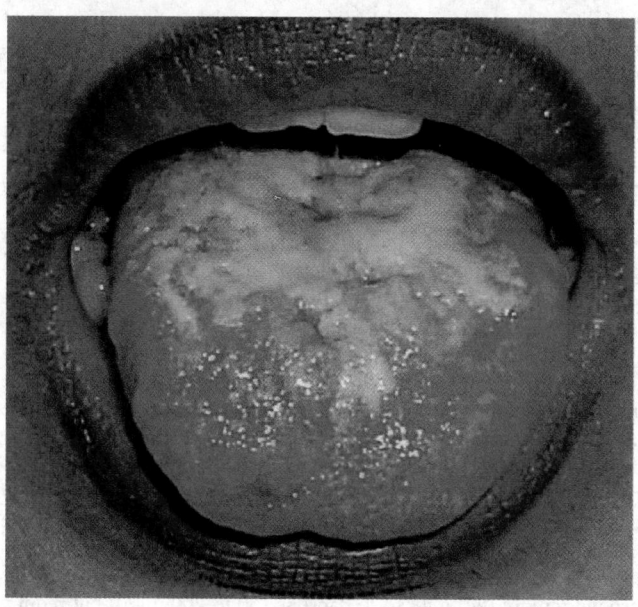

FIGURE 49-1 *A.* Pemphigus vulgaris demonstrating flaccid bullae that are easily ruptured, resulting in multiple erosions and crusted plaques. *B.* Pemphigus vulgaris almost invariably involves the oral mucosa and may present with erosions involving the gingiva, buccal mucosa, palate, posterior pharynx, or the tongue. (*B*, Courtesy of Robert Swerlick, MD.)

of keratinocytes and (variably) similar immunoreactants in the epidermal basement membrane zone. Patients with PNP have IgG autoantibodies against cytoplasmic proteins that are members of the plakin family (e.g., desmoplakins I and II, bullous pemphigoid antigen 1, envoplakin, periplakin, and plectin) and cell-surface proteins that are members of the cadherin family (e.g., Dsg3). Because immunoadsorption of anti-Dsg3 IgG is sufficient to eliminate the ability of PNP sera to induce blisters in an experimental passive transfer animal model, these particular autoantibodies are thought to play the key pathogenic role in blister formation in these patients.

Although PNP is generally resistant to conventional therapies (i.e., those used to treat PV), patients may improve (or even remit) following resection of underlying neoplasms. The predominant neoplasms associated with this disorder are non-Hodgkin's lymphoma, chronic lymphocytic leukemia, Castleman's disease, thymoma, and spindle cell tumors.

BULLOUS PEMPHIGOID Bullous pemphigoid (BP) is an autoimmune subepidermal blistering disease usually seen in the elderly. Lesions typically consist of tense blisters on either normal-appearing or erythematous skin (Fig. 49-2). The lesions are usually distributed over the lower abdomen, groin, and flexor surface of the extremities; oral mu-

cosal lesions are found in 10 to 40% of patients. Pruritus may be nonexistent or severe. As lesions evolve, tense blisters tend to rupture and be replaced by flaccid lesions or erosions with or without surmounting crust. Nontraumatized blisters heal without scarring. The major histocompatibility complex class II allele HLA-DQβ1*0301 is prevalent in patients with BP. Despite isolated reports, several studies have shown that patients with BP do not have an increased incidence of malignancy in comparison with appropriately age- and gender-matched controls.

While biopsies of early lesional skin demonstrate subepidermal blisters, the histologic features depend on the character of the particular lesion. Lesions on normal-appearing skin generally show a sparse perivascular leukocytic infiltrate with some eosinophils; conversely, biopsies of inflammatory lesions typically show an eosinophil-rich infiltrate within the papillary dermis at sites of vesicle formation and in perivascular areas. In addition to eosinophils, cell-rich lesions also contain mononuclear cells and neutrophils. It is not always possible to distinguish BP from other subepidermal blistering diseases by routine histologic techniques.

Immunopathologic studies have broadened our understanding of this disease and aided its diagnosis. Direct immunofluorescence microscopy of normal-appearing perilesional skin shows linear deposits of IgG and/or C3 in the epidermal basement membrane. The sera of approximately 70% of these patients contain circulating IgG autoantibodies that bind the epidermal basement membrane of normal human skin in indirect immunofluorescence microscopy. An even higher percentage of patients shows reactivity to the epidermal side of 1 *M* NaCl split skin [an alternative immunofluorescence microscopy test substrate that is commonly used to distinguish circulating IgG anti-basement membrane autoantibodies in patients with BP from those in patients with similar, yet different, subepidermal blistering diseases (e.g., epidermolysis bullosa acquisita, see below)]. No correlation exists between the titer of these autoantibodies and disease activity. In BP, circulating autoantibodies recognize 230- and 180-kDa hemidesmosome-associated proteins in basal keratinocytes [i.e., bullous pemphigoid antigen (BPAG)1 and BPAG2, respectively]. Autoantibodies are thought to develop against these antigens (more specifically, initially against BPAG2), deposit in situ, and activate complement that subsequently produces dermal mast cell degranulation and granulocyte-rich infiltrates that cause tissue damage and blister formation.

BP may persist for months to years, with exacerbations or remissions. Although extensive involvement may result in widespread erosions and compromise cutaneous integrity, the mortality rate is rela-

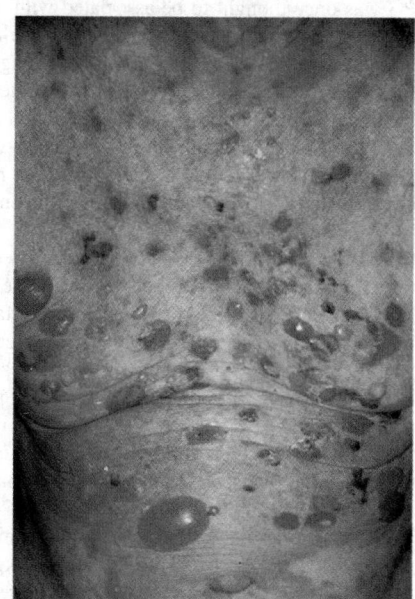

FIGURE 49-2 Bullous pemphigoid with tense vesicles and bullae on erythematous, urticarial bases. (Courtesy of the Yale Resident's Slide Collection.)

tively low. Nonetheless, deaths may occur in elderly and/or debilitated patients. The mainstay of treatment is systemic glucocorticoids. Patients with local or minimal disease can sometimes be controlled with topical glucocorticoids alone; patients with more extensive lesions generally respond to systemic glucocorticoids either alone or in combination with immunosuppressive agents. Patients will usually respond to prednisone, 40 to 60 mg/d. In some instances, azathioprine (1 to 2 mg/kg per day), mycophenolate mofetil (20 to 35 mg/kg per day), or cyclophosphamide (1 to 2 mg/kg per day) are necessary adjuncts.

PEMPHIGOID GESTATIONIS Pemphigoid gestationis (PG), also known as *herpes gestationis*, is a rare, nonviral, subepidermal blistering disease of pregnancy and the puerperium. PG may begin during any trimester of pregnancy or present shortly after delivery. Lesions are usually distributed over the abdomen, trunk, and extremities; mucous membrane lesions are rare. Skin lesions in these patients may be quite polymorphic and consist of erythematous urticarial papules and plaques, vesiculopapules, and/or frank bullae. Lesions are almost always very pruritic. Severe exacerbations of PG frequently occur after delivery, typically within 24 to 48 h. PG tends to recur in subsequent pregnancies, often beginning earlier during such gestations. Brief flare-ups of disease may occur with resumption of menses and may develop in patients later exposed to oral contraceptives. Occasionally, infants of affected mothers demonstrate transient skin lesions.

Biopsies of early lesional skin show teardrop-shaped subepidermal vesicles forming in dermal papillae in association with an eosinophil-rich leukocytic infiltrate. Differentiation of PG from other subepidermal bullous diseases by light microscopy is often difficult. However, direct immunofluorescence microscopy of perilesional skin from PG patients reveals the immunopathologic hallmark of this disorder—linear deposits of C3 in the epidermal basement membrane zone. These deposits develop as a consequence of complement activation produced by low titer IgG anti-basement membrane zone autoantibodies. Recent studies have shown that the majority of PG sera contain autoantibodies that recognize BPAG2, the same 180-kDa hemidesmosome-associated protein that is targeted by autoantibodies in patients with BP—a subepidermal bullous disease that resembles PG morphologically, histologically, and immunopathologically.

The goals of therapy in patients with PG are to prevent the development of new lesions, relieve intense pruritus, and care for erosions at sites of blister formation. Most patients require treatment with moderate doses of daily glucocorticoids (i.e., 20 to 40 mg of prednisone) at some point in their course. Mild cases (or brief flare-ups) may be controlled by vigorous use of potent topical glucocorticoids. Although PG was once thought to be associated with an increased risk of fetal morbidity and mortality, the best evidence now suggests that these infants are only at increased risk of being slightly premature or "small for dates." Current evidence suggests that there is no difference in the incidence of uncomplicated live births in PG patients treated with systemic glucocorticoids and in those managed more conservatively. If systemic glucocorticoids are administered, newborns are at risk for development of reversible adrenal insufficiency.

DERMATITIS HERPETIFORMIS Dermatitis herpetiformis (DH) is an intensely pruritic, papulovesicular skin disease characterized by lesions symmetrically distributed over extensor surfaces (i.e., elbows, knees, buttocks, back, scalp, and posterior neck) (see Fig. 46-8). The primary lesion in this disorder is a papule, papulovesicle, or urticarial plaque. Because pruritus is prominent, patients may present with excoriations and crusted papules but no observable primary lesions. Patients sometimes report that their pruritus has a distinctive burning or stinging component; the onset of such local symptoms reliably heralds the development of distinct clinical lesions 12 to 24 h later. Almost all DH patients have an associated, usually subclinical, gluten-sensitive enteropathy (Chap. 275), and more than 90% express the HLA-B8/DRw3 and HLA-DQw2 haplotypes. DH may present at any age, including childhood; onset in the second to fourth decades is most common. The disease is typically chronic.

Biopsy of early lesional skin reveals neutrophil-rich infiltrates within dermal papillae. Neutrophils, fibrin, edema, and microvesicle formation at these sites are characteristic of early disease. Older lesions may demonstrate nonspecific features of a subepidermal bulla or an excoriated papule. Because the clinical and histologic features of this disease can be variable and resemble other subepidermal blistering disorders, the diagnosis is confirmed by direct immunofluorescence microscopy of normal-appearing perilesional skin. Such studies demonstrate granular deposits of IgA (with or without complement components) in the papillary dermis and along the epidermal basement membrane zone. IgA deposits in the skin are unaffected by control of disease with medication; however, these immunoreactants may diminish in intensity or disappear in patients maintained for long periods on a strict gluten-free diet (see below). Patients with DH have granular deposits of IgA in their epidermal basement membrane zone and should be distinguished from individuals with linear IgA deposits at this site (see below).

Although most DH patients do not report overt gastrointestinal symptoms or have laboratory evidence of malabsorption, biopsies of small bowel usually reveal blunting of intestinal villi and a lymphocytic infiltrate in the lamina propria. As is true for patients with celiac disease, this gastrointestinal abnormality can be reversed by a gluten-free diet. Moreover, if maintained, this diet alone may control the skin disease and eventuate in clearance of IgA deposits from these patients' epidermal basement membrane zone. Subsequent gluten exposure in such patients alters the morphology of their small bowel, elicits a flare-up of their skin disease, and is associated with the reappearance of IgA in their epidermal basement membrane zone. As in patients with celiac disease, dietary gluten sensitivity in patients with DH is associated with IgA anti-endomysial autoantibodies that target tissue transglutaminase. Recent studies suggest that patients with DH also have high-avidity IgA autoantibodies against epidermal transglutaminase and that the latter is co-localized with granular deposits of IgA in the papillary dermis of DH patients. Patients with DH also have an increased incidence of thyroid abnormalities, achlorhydria, atrophic gastritis, and antigastric parietal cell antibodies. These associations likely relate to the high frequency of the HLA-B8/DRw3 haplotype in these patients, since this marker is commonly linked to autoimmune disorders. The mainstay of treatment of DH is dapsone, a sulfone. Patients respond rapidly (24 to 48 h) to dapsone (50 to 200 mg/d) but require careful pretreatment evaluation and close follow-up to ensure that complications are avoided or controlled. All patients on more than 100 mg/d dapsone will have some hemolysis and methemoglobinemia. These are expected pharmacologic side effects of this agent. Gluten restriction can control DH and lessen dapsone requirements; this diet must rigidly exclude gluten to be of maximal benefit. Many months of dietary restriction may be necessary before a beneficial result is achieved. Good dietary counselling by a trained dietitian is essential.

LINEAR IGA DISEASE Linear IgA disease, once considered a variant form of dermatitis herpetiformis, is actually a separate and distinct entity. Clinically, these patients may resemble patients with typical cases of DH, BP, or other subepidermal blistering diseases. Lesions typically consist of papulovesicles, bullae, and/or urticarial plaques, predominantly on extensor (as seen in "classic" DH), central, or flexural sites. Oral mucosal involvement occurs in some patients. Severe pruritus resembles that in patients with DH. Patients with linear IgA disease do not have an increased frequency of the HLA-B8/DRw3 haplotype or an associated enteropathy and hence are not candidates for a gluten-free diet.

The histologic alterations in early lesions may be virtually indistinguishable from those in DH. However, direct immunofluorescence microscopy of normal-appearing perilesional skin reveals linear deposits of IgA (and often C3) in the epidermal basement membrane zone. Most patients with linear IgA disease demonstrate circulating IgA anti-basement membrane autoantibodies against epitopes in the extracellular domain of BPAG2, a transmembrane protein found in hemidesmosomes of basal keratinocytes. These patients generally respond to treatment with dapsone, 50 to 200 mg/d.

EPIDERMOLYSIS BULLOSA ACQUISITA
EBA is a rare, noninherited, polymorphic, chronic, subepidermal blistering disease. (The inherited form is discussed in Chap. 342.) Patients with classic or noninflammatory EBA have blisters on noninflamed skin, atrophic scars, milia, nail dystrophy, and oral lesions. Because lesions generally occur at sites exposed to minor trauma, classic EBA is considered to be a mechanobullous disease. Other patients with EBA have widespread inflammatory, scarring, and bullous lesions that resemble severe BP. Inflammatory EBA may evolve into the classic, noninflammatory form of this disease. Rare patients present with lesions that predominate on mucous membranes. The HLA-DR2 haplotype is found with increased frequency in EBA patients. Recent studies suggest that EBA is often associated with inflammatory bowel disease (especially Crohn's disease).

The histology of lesional skin varies depending on the character of the lesion being studied. Noninflammatory bullae show subepidermal blisters with a sparse leukocytic infiltrate and resemble those in patients with porphyria cutanea tarda. Inflammatory lesions consist of a subepidermal blister and neutrophil-rich leukocytic infiltrates in the superficial dermis. EBA patients have continuous deposits of IgG (and frequently C3 as well as other complement components) in a linear pattern within the epidermal basement membrane zone. Ultrastructurally, these immunoreactants are found in the sublamina densa region in association with anchoring fibrils, wheat stack–like structures that extend from the lamina densa into the underlying papillary dermis. Approximately 50% of EBA patients have circulating IgG anti-basement membrane autoantibodies directed against type VII collagen—the collagen species that comprises anchoring fibrils. Such IgG autoantibodies bind the dermal side of 1 M NaCl split skin (in contrast to IgG autoantibodies in patients with BP that bind either epidermal or both sides of this indirect immunofluorescence microscopy test substrate).

Treatment of EBA is generally unsatisfactory. Some patients with inflammatory EBA may respond to systemic glucocorticoids, either alone or in combination with immunosuppressive agents. Other patients (especially those with neutrophil-rich inflammatory lesions) may respond to dapsone. The chronic, noninflammatory form of this disease is largely resistant to treatment, although some patients may respond to cyclosporine or intravenous immunoglobulin.

CICATRICIAL PEMPHIGOID
Cicatricial pemphigoid (CP) is a rare, acquired, subepithelial blistering disease characterized by erosive lesions of mucous membranes and skin that result in scarring of at least some sites of involvement. Immunopathologically, perilesional mucosa and skin of patients with CP demonstrate in situ deposits of immunoreactants in epithelial basement membranes. Common sites of involvement include the oral mucosa (especially the gingiva) and conjunctiva; other sites that may be affected include the nasopharyngeal, laryngeal, esophageal, urogenital, and rectal mucosa. Skin lesions (present in about one-third of patients) tend to predominate on the scalp, face, and upper trunk and generally consist of a few scattered erosions or tense blisters on an erythematous or urticarial base. CP is typically a chronic and progressive disorder. Serious complications may arise as a consequence of ocular, laryngeal, esophageal, or urogenital lesions. Erosive conjunctivitis may result in shortened fornices, symblephara, ankyloblepharon, entropion, corneal opacities, and (in severe cases) blindness. Similarly, erosive lesions of the larynx may cause hoarseness, pain, and tissue loss that if unrecognized and untreated may eventuate in complete destruction of the airway. Esophageal lesions may result in stenosis and/or strictures that may place patients at risk for aspiration. Strictures may also complicate urogenital involvement.

Biopsies of lesional tissue generally demonstrate subepithelial vesiculobullae and a mononuclear leukocytic infiltrate. Neutrophils and eosinophils may be seen in biopsies of early lesions; older lesions may demonstrate a scant leukocytic infiltrate and fibrosis. Direct immu-

nofluorescence microscopy of perilesional tissue typically demonstrates deposits of IgG, IgA, and/or C3 in these patients' epithelial basement membranes. Because many of these patients show no evidence of circulating anti-basement membrane autoantibodies, testing of perilesional skin is important diagnostically. Although CP was once thought to be a single nosologic entity, it is now largely regarded as a disease phenotype that may develop as a consequence of an autoimmune reaction against a variety of different molecules in epithelial basement membranes (e.g., BPAG2, laminin 5, type VII collagen, and other antigens yet to be completely defined). Treatment of CP is largely dependent upon sites of involvement. Due to potentially severe complications, ocular, laryngeal, esophageal, and/or urogenital involvement require aggressive systemic treatment with dapsone, prednisone, or the latter in combination with another immunosuppressive agent (e.g., azathioprine, mycophenolate mofetil, or cyclophosphamide) or intravenous immunoglobulin. Less threatening forms of the disease may be managed with topical or intralesional glucocorticoids.

AUTOIMMUNE SYSTEMIC DISEASES WITH PROMINENT CUTANEOUS FEATURES

DERMATOMYOSITIS
The cutaneous manifestations of dermatomyositis (Chap. 369) are often distinctive but at times may resemble those of systemic lupus erythematosus (SLE) (Chap. 300), scleroderma (Chap. 303), or other overlapping connective tissue diseases (Chap. 303). The extent and severity of cutaneous disease may or may not correlate with the extent and severity of the myositis. The cutaneous manifestations of dermatomyositis are similar whether the disease appears in childhood or old age, except that calcification of subcutaneous tissue is a common late sequela in childhood dermatomyositis.

The cutaneous signs of dermatomyositis may precede or follow the development of myositis by weeks to years. Cases lacking muscle involvement (i.e., dermatomyositis sine myositis) have also been reported. The most common manifestation is a purple-red discoloration of the upper eyelids, sometimes associated with scaling ("heliotrope" erythema; Fig. 49-3) and periorbital edema. Erythema on the cheeks and nose in a "butterfly" distribution may resemble the eruption in SLE. Erythematous or violaceous scaling patches are common on the upper anterior chest, posterior neck, scalp, and the extensor surfaces of the arms, legs, and hands. Erythema and scaling may be particularly prominent over the elbows, knees, and the dorsal interphalangeal joints. Approximately one-third of patients have violaceous, flat-topped papules over the dorsal interphalangeal joints that are pathognomonic of dermatomyositis (Gottron's sign or Gottron's papules; Fig. 49-4). These lesions can be contrasted with the erythema and scaling

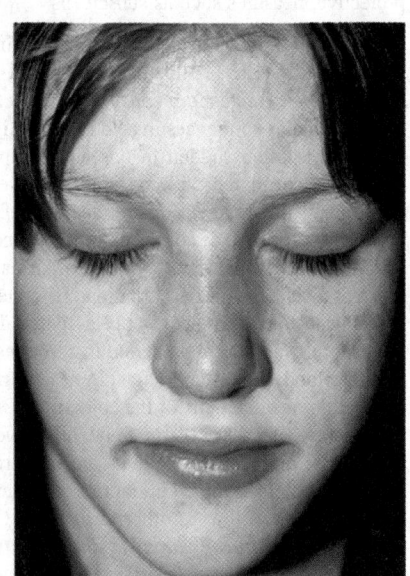

FIGURE 49-3 Dermatomyositis Periorbital violaceous erythema characterizes the classic heliotrope rash. (Courtesy of James Krell, MD.)

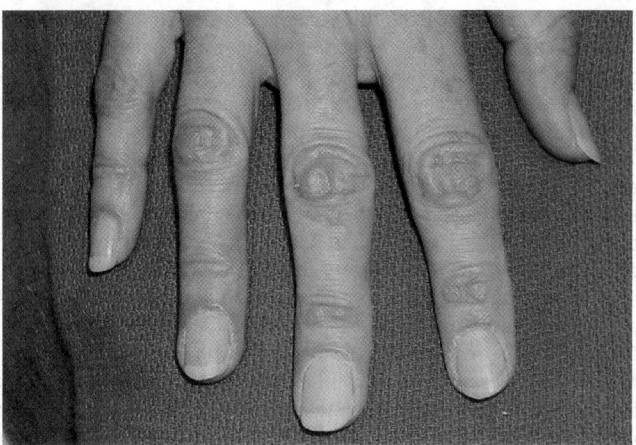

FIGURE 49-4 Dermatomyositis often involves the hands as erythematous flat-topped papules over the knuckles (Gottron's sign) and periungual telangiectasias.

on the dorsum of the fingers in some patients with SLE, which spares the skin over the interphalangeal joints. Periungual telangiectasia may be prominent, and a lacy or reticulated erythema may be associated with fine scaling on the extensor surfaces of the thighs and upper arms. Other patients, particularly those with long-standing disease, develop areas of hypopigmentation, hyperpigmentation, mild atrophy, and telangiectasia known as *poikiloderma*. Poikiloderma is rare in both SLE and scleroderma and thus can serve as a clinical sign that distinguishes dermatomyositis from these two diseases. Cutaneous changes may be similar in scleroderma and dermatomyositis and may include thickening and binding down of the skin of the hands (sclerodactyly) as well as Raynaud's phenomenon. However, the presence of severe muscle disease, Gottron's papules, heliotrope erythema, and poikiloderma serve to distinguish patients with dermatomyositis. Skin biopsy of erythematous, scaling lesions of dermatomyositis may reveal only mild nonspecific inflammation but sometimes may show changes indistinguishable from those found in SLE, including epidermal atrophy, hydropic degeneration of basal keratinocytes, edema of the upper dermis, and a mild mononuclear cell infiltrate. Direct immunofluorescence microscopy of lesional skin is usually negative, although granular deposits of immunoglobulin(s) and complement in the epidermal basement membrane zone have been described in some patients. Treatment should be directed at the systemic disease. In the few instances where adjunctive cutaneous therapy is desirable, topical glucocorticoids are sometimes useful. These patients should avoid exposure to ultraviolet irradiation and use photoprotective measures such as sunscreens.

LUPUS ERYTHEMATOSUS   The cutaneous manifestations of lupus erythematosus (LE) (Chap. 300) can be divided into acute, subacute, and chronic types. *Acute cutaneous LE* is characterized by erythema of the nose and malar eminences in a "butterfly" distribution (Fig. 49-5). The erythema is often sudden in onset, accompanied by edema and fine scale, and correlated with systemic involvement. Patients may have widespread involvement of the face as well as erythema and scaling of the extensor surfaces of the extremities and upper chest. These acute lesions, while sometimes evanescent, usually last for days and are often associated with exacerbations of systemic disease. Skin biopsy of acute lesions may show only a sparse dermal infiltrate of mononuclear cells and dermal edema. In some instances, cellular infiltrates around blood vessels and hair follicles are notable, as is hydropic degeneration of basal cells of the epidermis. Direct immunofluorescence microscopy of lesional skin frequently reveals deposits of immunoglobulin(s) and complement in the epidermal basement membrane zone. Treatment is aimed at control of systemic disease; photoprotection in this, as well as in other forms of LE, is very important.

Subacute cutaneous lupus erythematosus (SCLE) is characterized by a widespread photosensitive, nonscarring eruption. About half of

these patients have SLE in which severe renal and central nervous system involvement is uncommon. SCLE may present as a papulosquamous eruption that resembles psoriasis or annular lesions that resemble those seen in erythema multiforme. In the papulosquamous form, discrete erythematous papules arise on the back, chest, shoulders, extensor surfaces of the arms, and the dorsum of the hands; lesions are uncommon on the face, flexor surfaces of the arms, and below the waist. The slightly scaling papules tend to merge into large plaques, some with a reticulate appearance. The annular form involves the same areas and presents with erythematous papules that evolve into oval, circular, or polycyclic lesions. The lesions of SCLE are more widespread but have less tendency for scarring than do lesions of discoid LE. Skin biopsy reveals a dense mononuclear cell infiltrate around hair follicles and blood vessels in the superficial dermis, combined with hydropic degeneration of basal cells in the epidermis. Direct immunofluorescence microscopy of lesional skin reveals deposits of immunoglobulin(s) in the epidermal basement membrane zone in about half these cases. A particulate pattern of IgG deposition around basal keratinocytes has recently been associated with SCLE. Most SCLE patients have anti-Ro antibodies. Local therapy is usually unsuccessful, and most patients require treatment with aminoquinoline antimalarials. Low-dose therapy with oral glucocorticoids is sometimes necessary; photoprotective measures against both ultraviolet B and A wavelengths are very important.

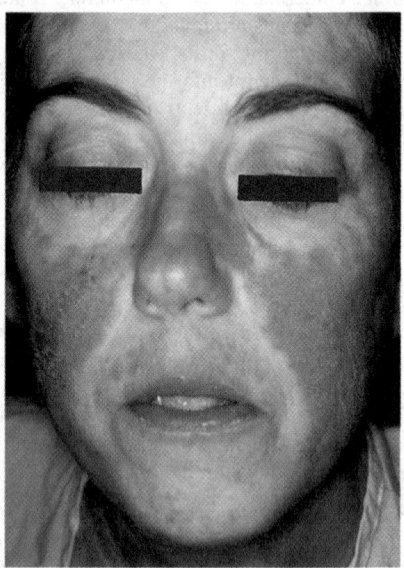

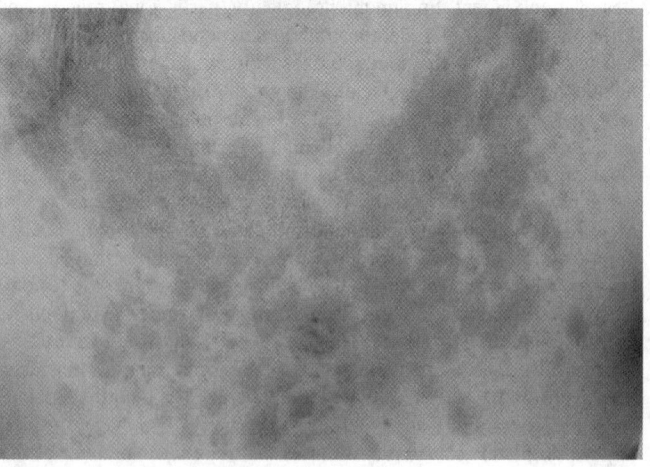

FIGURE 49-5   *A.* Systemic lupus erythematosus showing prominent, scaly, malar erythema. Involvement of other sun-exposed sites is also common. *B.* Acute LE on the upper chest demonstrating brightly erythematous and slightly edematous papules and plaques. (*B*, Courtesy of Robert Swerlick, MD.)

Discoid lupus erythematosus (DLE) is characterized by discrete lesions, most often on the face, scalp, or external ears. The lesions are erythematous papules or plaques with a thick, adherent scale that occludes hair follicles (follicular plugging). When the scale is removed, its underside will show small excrescences that correlate with the openings of hair follicles and is termed a "carpet tack" appearance. This finding is relatively specific for DLE. Long-standing lesions develop central atrophy, scarring, and hypopigmentation but frequently have erythematous, sometimes raised borders at the periphery (Fig. 49-6). These lesions persist for years and tend to expand slowly. Only 5 to 10% of patients with DLE meet the American Rheumatism Association criteria for SLE. However, typical discoid lesions are frequently seen in patients with SLE. Biopsy of DLE lesions shows hyperkeratosis, follicular plugging, and atrophy of the epidermis; hydropic degeneration of basal keratinocytes; and a mononuclear cell infiltrate adjacent to epidermal, adnexal, and microvascular basement membranes. Direct immunofluorescence microscopy demonstrates immunoglobulin(s) and complement deposits at the basement membrane zone in about 90% of cases. Treatment is focused on control of local cutaneous disease and consists mainly of photoprotection and topical or intralesional glucocorticoids. If local therapy is ineffective, use of aminoquinoline antimalarials may be indicated.

SCLERODERMA AND MORPHEA The skin changes of scleroderma (Chap. 303) usually begin on the hands, feet, and face, with episodes of recurrent nonpitting edema. Sclerosis of the skin begins distally on the fingers (sclerodactyly) and spreads proximally, usually accompanied by resorption of bone of the fingertips, which may have punched out ulcers, stellate scars, or areas of hemorrhage (Fig. 49-7). The fingers may actually shrink in size and become sausage-shaped, and since the fingernails are usually unaffected, the nails may curve over the end of the fingertips. Periungual telangiectasias are usually present, but periungual erythema is rare. In advanced cases, the extremities show contractures and calcinosis cutis. Facial involvement includes a smooth, unwrinkled brow, taut skin over the nose, shrinkage of tissue around the mouth, and perioral radial furrowing (Fig. 49-8). Matlike telangiectasias are often present, particularly on the face and hands. Involved skin feels indurated, smooth, and bound to underlying structures; hyperpigmentation and hypopigmentation are also often present. Raynaud's phenomenon, i.e., cold-induced blanching, cyanosis, and reactive hyperemia, is present in almost all patients and can precede development of scleroderma by many years. The combination of calcinosis cutis, Raynaud's phenomenon, esophageal dysmotility, sclerodactyly, and telangiectasia has been termed the *CREST syndrome*. Anticentromere antibodies have been reported in a very high percentage of patients with the CREST syndrome but in only a small minority of patients with scleroderma. Skin biopsy reveals

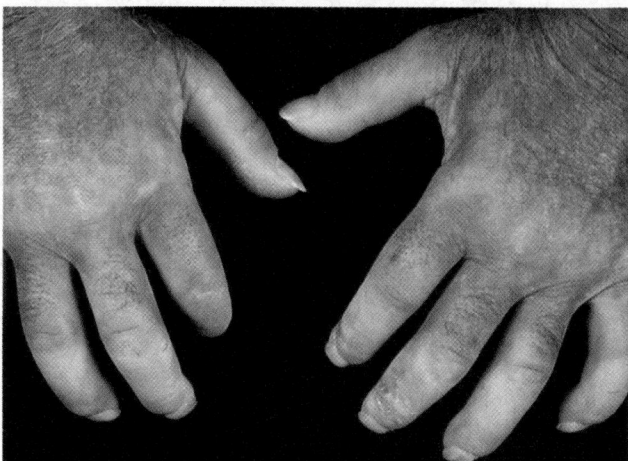

FIGURE 49-7 Scleroderma showing acral sclerosis and focal digital ulcers.

thickening of the dermis and homogenization of collagen bundles. Direct immunofluorescence microscopy of lesional skin is usually negative.

Morphea, which has been called *localized scleroderma*, is characterized by localized thickening and sclerosis of skin, usually affecting young adults or children. Morphea begins as erythematous or flesh-colored plaques that become sclerotic, develop central hypopigmentation, and demonstrate an erythematous border. In most cases, patients have one or a few lesions, and the disease is termed *localized morphea*. In some patients, widespread cutaneous lesions may occur, without systemic involvement. This form is called *generalized morphea*. Most patients with morphea do not have autoantibodies. Skin biopsy of morphea is indistinguishable from that of scleroderma. Linear scleroderma is a limited form of disease that presents in a linear, bandlike distribution and tends to involve deep as well as superficial layers of skin. Scleroderma and morphea are usually quite resistant to therapy. For this reason, physical therapy to prevent joint contractures and to maintain function is employed and is often helpful.

Diffuse fasciitis with eosinophilia is a clinical entity that can sometimes be confused with scleroderma. There is usually the sudden onset of swelling, induration, and erythema of the extremities frequently following significant physical exertion. The proximal portions of extremities (arms, forearms, thighs, legs) are more often involved than are the hands and feet. While the skin is indurated, it is usually not bound down as in scleroderma; contractures may occur early second-

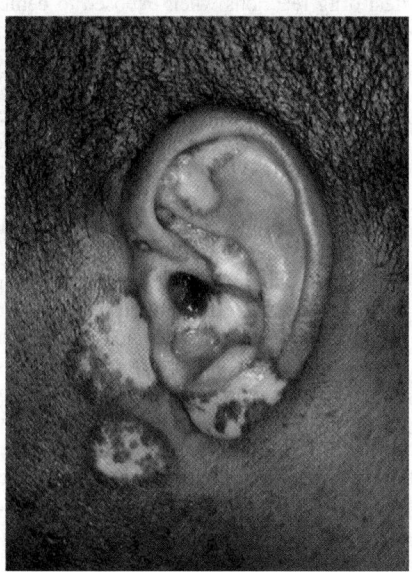

FIGURE 49-6 Violaceous, hyperpigmented, atrophic plaques, often with evidence of follicular plugging, which may result in scarring, are characteristic of discoid lupus erythematosus.

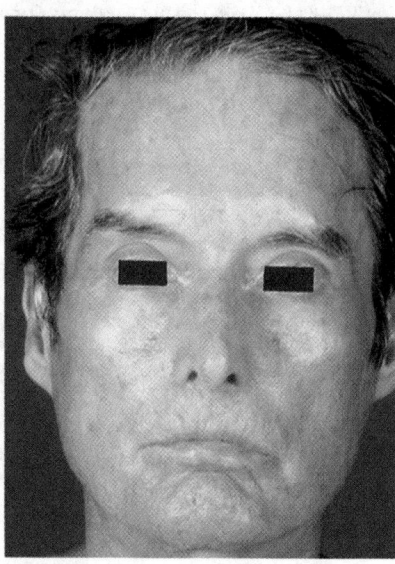

FIGURE 49-8 Scleroderma characterized by typical expressionless, mask-like facies.

ary to fascial involvement. The latter may also cause muscle groups to be separated (i.e., the "groove sign") and veins to appear depressed (i.e., sunken veins). These skin findings are accompanied by peripheral blood eosinophilia, increased erythrocyte sedimentation rate, and sometimes hypergammaglobulinemia. Deep biopsy of affected areas of skin reveals inflammation and thickening of the deep fascia overlying muscle. An inflammatory infiltrate composed of eosinophils and mononuclear cells is usually found. Patients with eosinophilic fasciitis appear to be at increased risk to develop bone marrow failure or other hematologic abnormalities. While the ultimate course of eosinophilic fasciitis is uncertain, many patients respond favorably to treatment with prednisone in doses ranging from 40 to 60 mg/d.

The *eosinophilia-myalgia syndrome*, a disorder reported in epidemic numbers in 1989 and linked to ingestion of L-tryptophan manufactured by a single company in Japan, is a multisystem disorder characterized by debilitating myalgias and absolute eosinophilia in association with varying combinations of arthralgias, pulmonary symp-

toms, and peripheral edema. In a later phase (i.e., 3 to 6 months after initial symptoms), these patients often develop localized sclerodermatous skin changes, weight loss, and/or neuropathy (Chap. 303). The precise cause of this syndrome, which may resemble other sclerotic skin conditions, is unknown. However, the implicated lots of L-tryptophan contained the contaminant 1,1-ethylidene bis[tryptophan]. This contaminant may be pathogenic or a marker for another substance that provokes the disorder.

FURTHER READING

AMAGAI M: Pemphigus: Autoimmunity to epidermal cell adhesion molecules. Adv Dermatol 11:319, 1996

ANHALT GJ et al: Paraneoplastic pemphigus. Adv Dermatol 12:77, 1997

SCHMIDT E, ZILLIKENS D: Autoimmune and inherited subepidermal blistering diseases: Advances in the clinic and the laboratory. Adv Dermatol 16:113, 2000

UDEY MC, STANLEY JR: Pemphigus—diseases of antidesmosomal autoimmunity. JAMA 282:572, 1999

YANCEY KB, EGAN CA: Pemphigoid: Clinical, histologic, immunopathologic, and therapeutic considerations. JAMA 284:350, 2000

50 CUTANEOUS DRUG REACTIONS
Olivier M. Chosidow, Robert S. Stern, Bruce U. Wintroub

Cutaneous reactions are among the most frequent adverse reactions to drugs. Prompt recognition of these reactions, drug withdrawal, and appropriate therapeutic interventions can minimize toxicity. This chapter focuses on adverse cutaneous reactions to drugs other than topical agents and reviews the incidence, patterns, and pathogenesis of cutaneous reactions to drugs and other therapeutic agents.

USE OF PRESCRIPTION DRUGS IN THE UNITED STATES More than 1.5 billion prescriptions for 60,000 drug products, which include over 2000 different active agents, are dispensed each year in the United States. Hospital inpatients alone annually receive about 120 million courses of drug therapy, and half of adult Americans receive prescription drugs on a regular outpatient basis. Many additional patients use over-the-counter medicines that may cause adverse cutaneous reactions.

INCIDENCE OF CUTANEOUS REACTIONS Although adverse drug reactions are common, it is difficult to ascertain their incidence, seriousness, and ultimate health effects. Available information comes from evaluations of hospitalized patients, epidemiologic surveys, premarketing studies, and voluntary reporting, most notably to the U.S. Food and Drug Administration's Medwatch System. In a systematic literature review of cutaneous reactions to drugs, the reaction rates varied from 0 to 8% and were highest for antibiotics (Table 50-1). In a series of 48,005 inpatients over a 20-year period, morbilliform rash (91%) and urticaria (6%) were the most frequent skin reactions.

The relative risk of Stevens-Johnson syndrome (SJS) and toxic

epidermal necrolysis (TEN), perhaps the most important severe cutaneous reactions, has been quantified in an international case control study and case series. Sulfonamide antibiotics, allopurinol, amine antiepileptic drugs (phenytoin and carbamazepine), lamotrigine, and the oxicam nonsteroidal anti-inflammatory drugs (NSAIDs) are associated with the highest risk of these reactions.

PATHOGENESIS OF DRUG REACTIONS

Untoward cutaneous responses to drugs can arise as a result of immunologic or nonimmunologic mechanisms. Immunologic reactions require activation of host immunologic pathways and are designated *drug allergy*. Drug reactions occurring through nonimmunologic mechanisms may be due to activation of effector pathways, overdosage, cumulative toxicity, side effects, ecologic disturbance, interactions between drugs, metabolic alterations, exacerbation of preexisting dermatologic conditions, or inherited protein or enzyme deficiencies. It is often not possible to specify the responsible drug or pathogenic mechanism because the skin responds to a variety of stimuli through a limited number of reaction patterns. The mechanism of many drug reactions is unknown.

IMMUNOLOGIC DRUG REACTIONS Drugs frequently elicit an immune response, but only a small number of individuals experience clinical hypersensitivity reactions. For example, most patients exposed to penicillin develop demonstrable antibodies to penicillin but do not manifest drug reactions when exposed to penicillin. Multiple factors determine the capacity of a drug to elicit an immune response, including the molecular characteristics of the drug and host effects.

Increases in *molecular* size and complexity are associated with increased immunogenicity, and macromolecular drugs such as protein or peptide hormones are highly antigenic. Most drugs are small organic molecules <1000 Da in size, and the capacity of such small molecules to elicit an immune response depends on their ability to act as haptens, i.e., to form stable, usually covalent, bonds with tissue macromolecules, an extremely rare event.

Route of administration of a drug or simple chemical can influence the nature of the *host* immune response. For example, topical application of antigens tends to induce delayed hypersensitivity, and exposure to antigens via oral or nasal cavities stimulates production of secretory immunoglobins, IgA and IgE, and occasionally IgM. Frequency of sensitization through intravenous administration of drugs varies, but anaphylaxis is a more likely consequence with this route of exposure than following oral administration.

The degree of drug exposure and individual variability in absorption and metabolism of a given agent may alter immunogenic load. The variable degree of in vivo acetylation of hydralazine provides a

TABLE 50-1 *Cutaneous Reactions to Drugs Received by at Least 1000 Patients (BCDSP)[a]*

Drug	Reactions, No.	Recipients, No.	Rate, %	95% Confidence Interval
Amoxicillin	63	1225	5.1	3.9–6.4
Ampicillin	215	4763	4.5	3.9–5.1
Co-trimoxazole	46	1235	3.7	2.7–4.8
Semisynthetic penicillins	41	1436	2.9	2.0–3.7
Red blood cells	67	3386	2.0	1.5–2.4
Penicillin G	68	4204	1.6	1.2–2.0
Cephalosporins	27	1781	1.5	0.9–2.1
Gentamicin	13	1277	1.0	0.5–1.6

[a] BCDSP, Boston Collaborative Drug Surveillance Program.
Source: Adapted from Bigby.

clinical example of this phenomenon. Hydralazine produces a lupus-like syndrome associated with antinuclear antibody formation more frequently in patients who acetylate the drug slowly. Frequent high-dose and interrupted courses of therapy are also important risk factors for development of drug allergy.

Pathogenesis of Allergic Drug Reactions ■ *IGE-DEPENDENT REACTIONS* IgE-dependent drug reactions are usually manifest in the skin and gastrointestinal, respiratory, and cardiovascular systems (Chap. 298). Primary symptoms and signs include pruritus, urticaria, nausea, vomiting, cramps, bronchospasm, and laryngeal edema and, on occasion, anaphylactic shock with hypotension and death. Immediate reactions may occur within minutes of drug exposure, and accelerated reactions occur hours or days after drug administration. Accelerated reactions are usually urticarial and may include laryngeal edema. Penicillin and related drugs are the most frequent causes of IgE-dependent reactions. Release of chemical mediators such as histamine, adenosine, leukotrienes, prostaglandins, platelet-activating factor, enzymes, and proteoglycans from sensitized tissue, mast cells, or circulating basophilic leukocytes results in vasodilation and edema. Release is triggered when polyvalent drug protein conjugates cross-link IgE molecules fixed to sensitized cells. The clinical manifestations are determined by interaction of the released chemical mediator with its target organ, i.e., skin, respiratory, gastrointestinal, and/or cardiovascular systems. Certain routes of administration favor different clinical patterns (i.e., oral route: gastrointestinal effects; intravenous route: circulatory effects).

IMMUNE-COMPLEX–DEPENDENT REACTIONS Serum sickness is produced by circulating immune complexes and is characterized by fever, arthritis, nephritis, neuritis, edema, and an urticarial, papular, or purpuric rash (Chap. 306). The syndrome requires an antigen that remains in the circulation for prolonged periods so that when antibody is synthesized, circulating antigen-antibody complexes are formed. Serum sickness was first described following administration of foreign sera, but drugs are now the usual cause. Drugs that produce serum sickness include the penicillins, sulfonamides, thiouracils, cholecystographic dyes, phenytoin, aminosalicylic acid, heparin, and antilymphocyte globulin. Cephalosporin administration in febrile children is associated with a high risk of a clinically similar reaction, but the mechanism of this reaction is unknown. In classic serum sickness, symptoms develop 6 days or more after exposure to a drug, the latent period representing the time needed to synthesize antibody. The antibodies responsible for immune-complex–dependent drug reactions are largely of the IgG or IgM class. Vasculitis, a relatively rare cutaneous complication of drugs, may also be a result of immune complex deposition (Chap. 306).

CYTOTOXICITY AND DELAYED HYPERSENSITIVITY Cytotoxicity and delayed hypersensitivity mechanisms may be important in the etiology of morbilliform exanthema, hypersensitivity syndrome, SJS, or TEN, but this is not proven. Systemic manifestations occur frequently. The antigen may be the drug or its metabolites, and it is likely that different T lymphocyte populations are activated. T_H1 type cells will lead to the production of interleukin (IL)-2 and interferon (IFN)-γ and subsequent activation of cytotoxic T cells. In early lesions of morbilliform exanthema or TEN, histopathologic studies have shown expression of HLA-DR and intercellular adhesion molecule (ICAM)-1 by keratinocytes, CD4 cells (in the dermis), and CD8 T cells (in the epidermis) and apoptosis of keratinocytes (facilitated by tumor necrosis factor α, perforin, and granzyme secretion, and *fas*-ligand expression). T_H2 type cells produce cytokines such as IL-5 and eotaxin, which may be involved in hypersensitivity syndrome (see below).

NONIMMUNOLOGIC DRUG REACTIONS Nonimmunologic mechanisms are responsible for the majority of drug reactions; however, only the most important mechanisms will be discussed.

Nonimmunologic Activation of Effector Pathways Drug reactions may result from nonimmunologic activation of effector pathways by three mechanisms: First, drugs may release mediators directly from mast cells and basophils and present as anaphylaxis, urticaria, and/or angio-edema. Urticarial anaphylactic reactions induced by opiates, polymyxin B, tubocurarine, radiocontrast media, and dextrans may occur by this mechanism. Second, drugs may activate complement in the absence of antibody. This is an additional mechanism through which radiocontrast media may act. Third, drugs such as aspirin and other NSAIDs may alter pathways of arachidonic acid metabolism and induce urticaria.

Phototoxicity Phototoxic reactions may be drug-induced or may occur in metabolic disorders in which a photosensitizing chemical is overproduced. A phototoxic reaction occurs when enough chromophore (drug or metabolic product) absorbs sufficient radiation to cause a reaction or interaction with target tissue. Drug-induced phototoxic reactions can occur on first exposure. Phototoxic injury is usually manifest as a photodistributed dermatitis.

Exacerbation of Preexisting Diseases A variety of agents can exacerbate preexisting diseases. For example, lithium can exacerbate acne and psoriasis in a dose-dependent manner. Beta-blocking agents and IFN-α may induce psoriasis. Withdrawal of glucocorticoids can exacerbate psoriasis or atopic dermatitis.

Inherited Enzyme or Protein Deficiencies Specific genetically determined defects in the ability of an individual to detoxify toxic reactive drug metabolites may predispose such individuals to the development of severe drug reactions, especially hypersensitivity syndrome, and perhaps TEN associated with use of sulfonamides and anticonvulsants. However, in a prospective cohort of 136 HIV-infected patients treated with sulfonamides, no association of drug eruption with acetylation genotype or glutathione levels was found.

Alterations of Immunologic Status Alterations in patients' immunologic status may also modify the risk of cutaneous reactions. Bone marrow transplant patients, HIV-infected persons, and persons with Epstein-Barr virus infection are at higher risk of developing cutaneous reactions to drugs. Skin reactions to trimethoprim-sulfamethoxazole are seen in about a third of HIV-infected users of this drug, but desensitization can be accomplished. Dapsone, trimethoprim alone, and amoxicillin-clavulanate are also frequent causes of drug eruptions in HIV-infected patients. The advent of highly active antiretroviral therapy (HAART) may have decreased the risk of cutaneous reactions in HIV patients (Chap. 173).

A CLINICAL CLASSIFICATION OF CUTANEOUS DRUG REACTIONS

URTICARIA/ANGIOEDEMA *Urticaria* is a skin reaction characterized by pruritic, red wheals. Lesions may vary from a small point to a large area. Individual lesions rarely last more than 24 h. When deep dermal and subcutaneous tissues are also swollen, this reaction is known as *angioedema*. Angioedema may involve mucous membranes and may be part of a life-threatening anaphylactic reaction. Urticarial lesions, along with pruritus and morbilliform (or maculopapular) eruptions, are among the most frequent types of cutaneous reactions to drugs.

Drug-induced urticaria may be caused by three mechanisms: an IgE-dependent mechanism, circulating immune complexes (serum sickness), and nonimmunologic activation of effector pathways. IgE-dependent urticarial reactions usually occur within 36 h but can occur within minutes. Reactions occurring within minutes to hours of drug exposure are termed *immediate reactions*, whereas those that occur 12 to 36 h after drug exposure are designated *accelerated reactions*. Immune-complex–induced urticaria associated with serum sickness usually occurs from 6 to 12 days after first exposure. In this syndrome, the urticarial eruption may be accompanied by fever, hematuria, arthralgias, hepatic dysfunction, and neurologic symptoms.

Certain drugs, such as NSAIDs, angiotensin-converting enzyme (ACE) inhibitors, and radiographic dyes, may induce urticarial reactions, angioedema, and anaphylaxis in the absence of drug-specific antibody. Although ACE inhibitors, aspirin, penicillin, and blood products are the most frequent causes of urticarial eruptions, urticaria has been observed in association with nearly all drugs. Drugs may also cause chronic urticaria, which lasts more than 6 weeks. Aspirin frequently exacerbates this problem.

The treatment of urticaria or angioedema depends on the severity of the reaction and the rate at which it is evolving. In severe cases, especially with respiratory or cardiovascular compromise, epinephrine is the mainstay of therapy, but its effect is reduced in patients using beta blockers. For more seriously affected patients, treatment with systemic glucocorticoids, sometimes intravenously administered, are helpful. In addition to drug withdrawal, for patients with only cutaneous symptoms and without symptoms of angioedema or anaphylaxis, oral antihistamines are usually sufficient.

PHOTOSENSITIVITY ERUPTIONS Photosensitivity eruptions are usually most marked in sun-exposed areas but may extend to sun-protected areas. The mechanism of photosensitivity eruptions is almost always phototoxicity. Phototoxic reactions are also most marked in sun-exposed areas, resemble sunburn, and can occur with first exposure to a drug. Their severity depends on the tissue level of the drug, the extent of exposure to light, and the efficiency of the photosensitizer (Chap. 51).

Common orally administered photosensitizing drugs include many fluoroquinolones and doxycycline. Other drugs less frequently encountered are chlorpromazine, other tetracyclines, thiazides, and at least two NSAIDs (ibuprofen and naproxen). The majority of the common photosensitizing drugs have action spectrums in the long-wave ultraviolet A (UV-A) range. Photosensitive reactions abate with removal of either the drug or ultraviolet radiation. Because UV-A and visible light, which trigger these reactions, are not easily absorbed by nonopaque sunscreens and are transmitted through window glass, these reactions may be difficult to block.

Photosensitivity reactions are treated by avoiding exposure to ultraviolet light (sunlight), use of high-potency sunscreens which block UV-A light, and treating the reaction as one would a sunburn. Rarely, individuals develop persistent reactivity to light, necessitating long-term avoidance of sun exposure.

PIGMENTATION CHANGES Drugs, either systemic or topical, may cause a variety of pigmentary changes in the skin. Oral contraceptives may induce melasma. Long-term minocycline or perfloxacin may cause blue-gray pigmentation, while amiodarone causes a more purple coloration. Long-term high-dose phenothiazine results in gray-brown pigmentation of sun-exposed areas. Numerous cancer chemotherapeutic agents may be associated with pigmentation. Bleomycin, busulphan, daunorubicin, cyclophosphamide, hydroxyurea, and methotrexate pigmentation changes may also occur in mucous membranes (busulphan), nails (zidovudine), hair, and teeth. Gold may cause blue-gray pigmentation in light-exposed areas.

VASCULITIS Cutaneous necrotizing vasculitis often presents as palpable purpuric lesions that may be generalized or limited to the lower extremities or other dependent areas (Chap. 306). Urticarial lesions, ulcers, and hemorrhagic blisters also occur. Vasculitis may involve other organs, including the liver, kidney, brain, and joints. Drugs are only one cause of vasculitis, with infection and collagen vascular disease responsible for the majority of cases.

Propylthiouracil induces a cutaneous vasculitis that is accompanied by leukopenia and splenomegaly. Direct immunofluorescent changes in these lesions suggest immune-complex deposition. Drugs implicated in vasculitic eruptions include allopurinol, thiazides, sulfonamides, penicillin, and some NSAIDs.

HYPERSENSITIVITY SYNDROME Initially described with phenytoin, hypersensitivity syndrome presents as an erythematous eruption that may become purpuric or lichenoid and is accompanied by many of the following features: fever, facial and periorbital edema, tender generalized lymphadenopathy, leukocytosis (often with atypical lymphocytes and eosinophils), hepatitis, and sometimes nephritis or pneu-

monitis. The cutaneous reaction usually begins 2 to 8 weeks after the drug is begun and may resolve with drug cessation. However, symptoms may persist for several weeks, especially hepatitis. With phenytoin, an increased risk of this syndrome is associated with an inherited deficiency of epoxide hydrolase, an enzyme required for metabolism of a toxic intermediate arene oxide that is formed during metabolism of phenytoin by the cytochrome P450 system. This explains why the eruption recurs with rechallenge, and cross-reactions among aromatic anticonvulsants, including phenytoin, carbamazepine, and barbiturates, are frequent. The role of human herpes virus (HHV)-6 infection is still unclear. Other drugs causing this syndrome include lamotrigine, minocycline, dapsone, allopurinol, sulfonamides, and abacavir and zalcitabine in HIV-infected patients. Mortality as high as 10% has been reported. In life-threatening situations such as hepatitis, systemic glucocorticoids (prednisone, 0.5 to 1.0 mg/kg) seems to reduce symptoms. Topical high-potency glucocorticoids may be helpful too. In all cases, urgent withdrawal of the suspected drug is required.

WARFARIN NECROSIS OF THE SKIN This rare reaction occurs usually between the third and tenth days of therapy with warfarin derivatives, usually in women. Lesions are sharply demarcated, erythematous, indurated, and purpuric and may resolve or progress to form large, irregular, hemorrhagic bullae with eventual necrosis and slow-healing eschar formation.

Development of the syndrome is unrelated to drug dose or underlying condition. Favored sites are breasts, thighs, and buttocks. The course is not altered by discontinuation of the drug after onset of the eruption. Similar reactions have been associated with heparin. Warfarin reactions are associated with protein C deficiency. Protein C is a vitamin K–dependent protein with a shorter half-life than other clotting proteins and is in part responsible for control of fibrinolysis. Since warfarin inhibits synthesis of vitamin K–dependent coagulation factors, warfarin anticoagulation in heterozygotes for protein C deficiency causes a precipitous fall in circulating levels of protein C, permitting hypercoagulability and thrombosis in the cutaneous microvasculature, with consequent areas of necrosis. Heparin-induced necrosis may have clinically similar features but is probably due to heparin-induced platelet aggregation with subsequent occlusion of blood vessels.

Warfarin-induced cutaneous necrosis is treated with vitamin K and heparin. Vitamin K reverses the effects of warfarin, and heparin acts as an anticoagulant. Treatment with protein C concentrates may also be helpful in individuals with deficiencies of protein C, the predisposing factor for development of these reactions.

MORBILLIFORM REACTIONS Morbilliform or maculopapular eruptions are the most common of all drug-induced reactions, often start on the trunk or areas of pressure or trauma, and consist of erythematous macules and papules that are frequently symmetric and may become confluent. Involvement of mucous membranes, palms, and soles is variable; the eruption may be associated with moderate to severe pruritus and fever.

The pathogenesis is unclear. A hypersensitivity mechanism has been suggested, although these reactions do not always recur following drug rechallenge. Diagnosis is rarely assisted by laboratory or patch testing; differentiation from viral exanthem is the principal differential diagnostic consideration. Unless the suspect drug is essential it should be discontinued. Occasionally these eruptions may decrease or fade with continued use of the responsible drug.

Morbilliform reactions usually develop within 1 week of initiation of therapy and last 1 to 2 weeks; however, reactions to some drugs, especially penicillin and drugs with long half-lives, may begin more than 2 weeks after therapy has begun and last as long as 2 weeks after therapy has ceased.

Morbilliform eruptions are usually treated by discontinuing the suspect medications symptomatically. Oral antihistamines, emollients, and soothing baths are useful for treatment of pruritus. Short courses of potent topical glucocorticoids can reduce inflammation and symptoms and are probably helpful. Systemic glucocorticoid treatment is rarely indicated.

FIXED DRUG REACTIONS These reactions are characterized by one or more sharply demarcated, erythematous lesions in which hyperpigmentation results after resolution of the acute inflammation; with rechallenge, the lesion recurs in the same (i.e., "fixed") location. Lesions often involve the lips, hands, legs, face, genitalia, and oral mucosa and cause burning. Most patients have multiple lesions. Patch testing is useful to establish the etiology. Fixed drug eruptions have been associated with phenolphthalein, sulfonamides, tetracyclines, phenylbutazone, NSAIDs, and barbiturates. Although cross-sensitivity appears to occur between different tetracycline compounds, cross-sensitivity was not elicited when different sulfonamide compounds were administered to patients as part of provocation testing.

LICHENOID DRUG ERUPTIONS A lichenoid cutaneous reaction, clinically and morphologically indistinguishable from lichen planus, is associated with a variety of drugs and chemicals. Eosinophils are more common when the reaction is drug-induced. Gold and antimalarials are most often associated with this eruption. Sulfomamides, thiazides, and antihypertensive agents, including beta blockers and captopril, have also been reported to cause lichenoid reactions.

PUSTULAR ERUPTIONS Acute generalized exanthematous pustulosis (AGEP) is often associated with exposure to drugs, most notably antibiotics. Usually beginning on the face or intertriginous areas, small nonfollicular pustules overlying erythematous and edematous skin may coalesce and lead to superficial ulceration. Fever is present, and differentiating this eruption from TEN in its initial stages may be difficult. AGEP often begins within a few days of initiating drug treatment.

STEVENS-JOHNSON SYNDROME AND TOXIC EPIDERMAL NECROLYSIS SJS and TEN are terms that, most believe, describe the same drug-induced disorder, which is characterized by blisters and epidermal detachment resulting from epidermal necrosis in the absence of substantial dermal inflammation. The term *SJS* is now used to describe patients with blisters developing on dusky or purpuric macules in which total percent body surface area blistering and eventual detachment is <10%. The term *SJS/TEN* is used to describe patients with 10 to 30% detachment, and *TEN* is used to describe patients with >30% detachment. Erythema multiforme (EM) is a third term which, in the past, was used to describe patients now designated as having SJS. EM is now used by most to describe patients with typical "target" lesions resulting as a reaction to infection, most commonly from herpes simplex virus.

SJS, SJS/TEN, and TEN patients initially present with acute symptoms, painful skin lesions, fever >39°C (102.2°F), sore throat, and visual impairment resulting from mucous membrane and ocular lesions. Intestinal and pulmonary involvement are associated with a poor prognosis, as are a greater extent of epidermal detachment and older age. About 5% of SJS and 30% of TEN affected persons die from their disease. Drugs that most commonly cause SJS, SJS/TEN, or TEN are sulfonamides, lamotrigine, aromatic anticonvulsants, and oxicam NSAIDs. Many treatments affecting immune responses or cytokines have been advocated, but none have been shown to be efficacious in well-controlled trials. Because drug-induced epidermal apoptosis has been proposed as a possible pathogenesis, intravenous immunoglobulin (IVIG) has been used recently by some with success in the absence of side effects or additional toxicity. At this time, the best results come from early diagnosis, immediate discontinuation of any suspected drug, and supportive therapy, paying close attention to ocular complications, often in burn units or intensive care units.

DRUGS OF SPECIAL INTEREST

PENICILLIN The incidence of cutaneous reactions to penicillin is about 1%. About 85% of cutaneous reactions to penicillin are morbilliform, and about 10% are urticaria or angioedema.

IgG, IgM, and IgE antibodies can be produced; IgG and IgM antipenicillin antibodies play a role in the development of hemolytic anemia, whereas anaphylaxis and serum sickness appear to be due to IgE antibodies in serum.

In patients with suspected IgE-mediated reactions to penicillin for whom future treatment is anticipated, accurate tests for sensitization are available. Current practice is to perform skin testing with a commercially available penicilloyl determinant preparation (Pre-pen, Kremers-Urban) and with fresh penicillin and, if possible, with another source of minor (nonpenicilloyl) determinants such as aged or base-treated penicillin. Antibodies to minor determinants are common in patients experiencing anaphylaxis, but testing with major determinants alone detects most patients at risk for anaphylaxis.

About one-fourth of patients with positive history of penicillin allergy have a positive skin test, while 6% (3 to 10%) with no history of penicillin sensitivity demonstrate a positive skin response to penicillin. Administering penicillin to those patients with a positive skin test produces reactions in a high proportion (50 to 100%); conversely, only a few patients (0.5%) with a negative skin test react to the drug, and reactions tend to be mild and to occur late. Since a false-negative skin test may occur during or just after an acute reaction, testing should be performed either prospectively or several months after a suspected reaction. As many as 80% of patients lose anaphylactic sensitivity and IgE antibody after several years. Radioallergosorbent tests and other in vitro tests offer no advantage over properly performed skin testing. Some cross-reactivity between penicillin and nonpenicillin β-lactam antibiotics (e.g., cephalosporins) occurs, but the majority of penicillin-allergic patients will tolerate cephalosporins. Persons who have negative skin tests to penicillin rarely develop reactions to cephalosporins.

In the face of a positive clinical history of penicillin reaction, another drug should be chosen. If this is not feasible or prudent (e.g., in a pregnant patient with syphilis or with enterococcal endocarditis), skin testing with penicillin is warranted. If skin tests are negative, cautious administration of penicillin is acceptable, although some recommend desensitization of such patients if the reaction was likely to be IgE-mediated. In those with positive skin tests, desensitization is mandatory if therapeutic use of β-lactam antibiotics is to be undertaken. Various protocols are available, including oral and parenteral approaches. Oral desensitization appears to have lower risk of serious anaphylactic reactions during desensitization. However, desensitization carries the risk of anaphylaxis regardless of how it is performed. After desensitization, many patients experience non-life-threatening IgE-mediated untoward reactions to penicillin during their course of therapy. Desensitization is not effective in those with exfoliative dermatitis or morbilliform reactions due to penicillin.

NONSTEROIDAL ANTI-INFLAMMATORY DRUGS NSAIDs, including aspirin and indomethacin (indometacin), cause two broad categories of allergic-like symptoms in susceptible individuals: (1) approximately 1% of persons experience urticaria or angioedema, and (2) about half as many (0.5%) experience rhinosinusitis and asthma; however, about 10% of adults with asthma and one-third of individuals with nasal polyposis and sinusitis may respond adversely to aspirin.

Urticaria/angioedema may be delayed up to 24 h and may occur at any age. The rhinosinusitis-asthma syndrome generally develops within 1 h of drug administration. In young patients, the reaction pattern often begins as watery rhinorrhea, which can be complicated by nasal and sinus infection, and polyposis, bloody discharge, and nasal eosinophilia. In many individuals with this syndrome, asthma that can be life-threatening eventually ensues whenever NSAIDs are subsequently ingested, and symptoms may persist despite avoidance of these drugs. Proof of the association of symptoms and NSAID use requires either clear-cut history of symptoms following drug ingestion or an oral challenge. For the latter to be performed with relative safety, (1) asthma must be under good control, (2) the procedure must be conducted in a hospital setting by experienced personnel capable of recognizing and treating acute respiratory responses, and (3) the challenge should begin with very low doses (i.e., not >30 mg) of aspirin and increase every 1 to 2 h in doubling doses as tolerated to 650 mg.

While cross-reactivity between NSAIDs is common, it is not immunologic, and patients who are sensitive to NSAIDs cannot be identified by assessment of IgE antibody to aspirin, lymphocyte sensitization, or in vitro immunologic testing.

RADIOCONTRAST MEDIA Large numbers of patients are exposed to radiocontrast agents. High-osmolality radiocontrast media are about five times more likely to induce urticaria (1%) or anaphylaxis than newer low-osmolality media. Severe reactions are rare with either type of contrast media. About one-third of those with mild reactions to previous exposure reereact on reexposure. In most cases, these reactions are probably not immunologic. Pretreatment with prednisone and diphenhydramine reduces reaction rates. Persons with a reaction to a high-osmolality contrast media should be given low-osmolality media if later contrast studies are required.

ANTICONVULSANTS Of the anticonvulsants, the single orally administered agent with the highest risk of severe adverse cutaneous reactions is the antiseizure medicine lamotrigine. Older anticonvulsants, including phenytoin and carbamazepine, are also associated with many types of severe reactions and a high incidence of less severe reactions, particularly in children. In addition to SJS, TEN, and the hypersensitivity syndrome discussed above, the aromatic anticonvulsants can induce a pseudolymphoma syndrome and induce gingival hyperplasia.

SULFONAMIDES Sulfonamides have perhaps the highest risk of causing cutaneous eruptions and are the drugs most frequently implicated in SJS and TEN. The combination of sulfamethoxazole and trimethoprim frequently induces adverse cutaneous reactions in patients with AIDS (Chap. 173). Desensitization is often successful in AIDS patients with morbilliform eruptions but does not work in AIDS patients who manifest erythroderma, fever, or a bullous reaction in response to their earlier sulfonamide exposure.

VANCOMYCIN Vancomycin causes two unusual but recognizable cutaneous reactions: Linear IgA bullous dermatosis and "red man syndrome." The first is an autoimmune disorder characterized by pruritic vesiculobullous skin lesions favoring the trunk, proximal extremities, and acral region. When the syndrome is drug-induced, most cases have been associated with vancomycin, but a variety of other drugs have been reported to cause the same clinical picture.

The red man syndrome occurs during rapid intravenous infusion of vancomycin. This is thought to be a histamine-related anaphylactoid reaction characterized by flushing, diffuse maculopapular eruption, hypotension, and, in rare cases, cardiac arrest.

AGENTS USED IN CANCER CHEMOTHERAPY Since many agents used in cancer chemotherapy inhibit cell division, rapidly proliferating elements of the skin, including hair, mucous membranes, and appendages, are sensitive to their effects; as a result, stomatitis and alopecia are among the most frequent dose-dependent side effects of chemotherapy. Various nail abnormalities have been described: onycholysis, dystrophy, Beau's lines, white lines, and pigmentation. Sterile cellulitis and phlebitis and ulceration of pressure areas occur with many of these agents. Also reported is acral erythema, which begins with dysesthesia followed by redness and a painful edematous eruption of the palms and soles; it is caused by cytarabin, doxorubicin, methotrexate, and 5-fluorouracil. Urticaria, angioedema, and exfoliative dermatitis have also been seen, as has local and diffuse hyperpigmentation.

GLUCOCORTICOIDS Both systemic and topical glucocorticoids cause a variety of skin changes, including acneiform eruptions, atrophy, striae, and other stigmata of Cushing's syndrome, and in sufficiently high doses can retard wound healing. Patients using glucocorticoids are at higher risk for bacterial, yeast, and fungal skin infections that may be misinterpreted as drug eruptions but are instead drug side effects.

CYTOKINE THERAPY Alopecia is a common complication of IFN-α. Induction or exacerbation of various immune-mediated disorders (psoriasis, lichen planus, lupus erythematosus) has been also reported with this agent. IFN-β injection has been associated with local necrosis of the skin. Granulocyte colony-stimulating factor may induce various neutrophilic dermatosis, including Sweet's syndrome, pyoderma gangrenosum, neutrophilic eccrine hidradenitis, and vasculitis, and can exacerbate psoriasis.

IL-2 is associated with frequent cutaneous reactions including exanthema, facial edema, xerosis, and pruritus. Cases of pemphigus vulgaris, linear IgA disease, psoriasis, and vitiligo have also been described in association with this drug.

ANTIMALARIAL AGENTS Antimalarial agents are used as therapy for several skin diseases, including the skin manifestations of lupus and polymorphous light eruption, but they can also induce cutaneous reactions. Although also used to treat porphyria cutanea tarda at low doses, in patients with asymptomatic porphyria cutanea tarda, higher doses of chloroquine increase porphyrin levels to such an extent that they may exacerbate the disease.

Pigmentation disturbances, including black pigmentation of the face, mucous membranes, and pretibial and subungual areas, occur with antimalarials. Quinacrine (mepacrine) causes generalized, cutaneous yellow discoloration.

GOLD Chrysotherapy has been associated with a variety of dose-related dermatologic reactions (including maculopapular eruptions), which can develop as long as 2 years after initiation of therapy and require months to resolve. Erythema nodosum, psoriasiform dermatitis, vaginal pruritus, eruptions similar to those of pityriasis rosea, hyperpigmentation, and lichenoid eruptions resembling those seen with antimalarial agents have been reported. After a cutaneous reaction, it is sometimes possible to reinstitute gold therapy at lower doses without recurrence of the dermatitis.

DIAGNOSIS OF DRUG REACTIONS

Possible causes of an adverse reaction can be assessed as definite, probable, possible, or unlikely based on six variables: (1) previous experience with the drug in the general population, (2) alternative etiologic candidates, (3) timing of events, (4) drug levels or evidence of overdose, (5) patient reaction to drug discontinuation, and (6) patient reaction to rechallenge.

PREVIOUS EXPERIENCE Tables of relative reaction rates are available and are useful to assess the likelihood that a given drug is responsible for a given cutaneous reaction. The specific morphologic pattern of a drug reaction, however, may modify these reaction rates by increasing or decreasing the likelihood that a given drug is responsible for a given reaction. For example, since fixed eruptions due to drugs are more often seen with barbiturates than with penicillin, a fixed drug reaction in a patient taking both types of agents is more likely to be due to the barbiturate, even though penicillins have a higher overall drug reaction rate.

ALTERNATIVE ETIOLOGIC CANDIDATES A cutaneous eruption may be due to exacerbation of preexisting disease or to development of new disease unrelated to drugs. For example, a patient with psoriasis may have a flare-up of disease coincidental with administration of penicillin for streptococcal infection; in this case, infection is a more likely cause for the flare-up than drug reaction.

TIMING OF EVENTS Most drug reactions of the skin occur within 1 to 2 weeks of initiation of therapy. Hypersensitivity syndrome may occur later (up to 8 weeks) after initiating drug therapy. Fixed drug reactions and generalized exanthematous pustulosis often occur earlier (within 48 h), as do reactions of all types in persons with prior sensitization to that drug or a cross-sensitizing agent.

DRUG LEVELS Some cutaneous reactions are dependent on dosage or cumulative toxicity. For example, lichenoid dermatoses due to gold administration appear more often in patients taking high doses.

DISCONTINUATION Most adverse cutaneous reactions to drugs remit with discontinuation of the suspected agent. A reaction is considered unlikely to be drug-related if improvement occurs while the drug is

TABLE 50-2 *Clinical and Laboratory Findings Associated with More Serious Drug-Induced Cutaneous Clinical Findings*

Cutaneous
Confluent erythema
Facial edema or central facial involvement
Skin pain
Palpable purpura
Skin necrosis
Blisters or epidermal detachment
Positive Nikolsky's sign
Mucous membrane erosions
Urticaria
Swelling of tongue

General
High fever [temperature >40°C (>104°F)]
Enlarged lymph nodes
Arthralgias or arthritis
Shortness of breath, wheezing, hypotension

Laboratory results
Eosinophil count >1000/μL
Lymphocytosis with atypical lymphocytes
Abnormal liver function tests

Source: Adapted from Roujeau and Stern.

continued or if a patient fails to improve after stopping the drug and appropriate therapy.

RECHALLENGE Rechallenge provides the most definitive information concerning adverse cutaneous reactions to drugs, since a reaction failing to recur on rechallenge with a drug is unlikely to be due to that agent. Rechallenge is usually impractical, however, because the need to ensure patient safety and comfort outweighs the value of the possible information derived from rechallenge.

Of special importance is the rapid recognition of reactions that may become serious or life-threatening. Table 50-2 lists clinical and laboratory features that, if present, suggest the reaction may be serious. Table 50-3 provides key features of the most serious adverse cutaneous reactions.

DIAGNOSIS OF DRUG ALLERGY

Tests for IgE responses include in vivo and in vitro methods, but such tests are available for only a limited number of drugs, including penicillins and cephalosporins, some peptide and protein drugs (insulin, xenogeneic sera), and some agents used for general anesthesia. In vivo testing is accomplished by prick puncture and/or by intradermal skin testing. A wheal-and-flare response 2×2 mm greater than that seen with a saline control within 20 min is considered indicative of IgE-mediated mast cell degranulation, provided (1) the patient is not dermographic, (2) the drug does not nonspecifically degranulate mast cells, (3) the drug concentration is not high enough to be irritating, and (4) the buffer itself does not cause wheal-and-flare responses.

Skin testing with major and minor determinants of penicillins or cephalosporins has proved useful for identifying patients at risk of anaphylactic reactions to these agents. However, skin tests themselves carry a small risk of anaphylaxis. Negative skin tests do not rule out IgE-mediated reactivity, and the risk of anaphylaxis in response to

TABLE 50-3 *Clinical Features of Selected Severe Cutaneous Reactions Often Induced by Drugs*

Diagnosis	Mucosal Lesions	Typical Skin Lesions	Frequent Signs and Symptoms	Alternative Causes not Related to Drugs
Stevens-Johnson syndrome	Erosions usually at ≥two sites	Small blisters on dusky purpuric macules or atypical targets; rare areas of confluence; detachment ≤10% of body surface area	10–30% of cases involve fever	
Toxic epidermal necrolysis[a]	Erosions usually at ≥two sites	Individual lesions like those seen in Stevens-Johnson syndrome; confluent erythema; outer layer of epidermis separates readily from basal layer with lateral pressure; large sheet of necrotic epidermis; total detachment of >30% of body surface area	Nearly all cases involve fever, "acute skin failure," leukopenia	
Hypersensitivity syndrome	Infrequent	Severe exanthematous rash (may become purpuric), exfoliative dermatitis	30–50% of cases involve fever, lymphadenopathy, hepatitis, nephritis, carditis, eosinophilia, atypical lymphocytes	Cutaneous lymphoma
Acute generalized exanthematous pustulosis	About 50% erosions mouth, tongue	Initially nonfollicular small pustules overlying edematous erythema, sometimes leading to superficial ulcers	Fever, burning, pruritus, facial swelling, leukocytosis, hypocalcemia	Infection
Serum sickness or reactions resembling serum sickness	Absent	Morbilliform lesions, sometimes with urticaria	Fever, arthralgias	Infection
Anticoagulant-induced necrosis	Infrequent	Erythema then purpura and necrosis, especially of fatty areas	Pain in affected areas	Disseminated intravascular coagulopathy, septicemia
Angioedema	Often involved	Urticaria or swelling of central part of face	Respiratory distress, cardiovascular collapse	Insect stings, foods

[a] Overlap of Stevens-Johnson syndrome and toxic epidermal necrolysis with features of both and attachment of 10 to 30% of body surface area may occur.

Source: Adapted from Roujeau and Stern.

penicillin administration in patients with negative skin tests is about 1%; about two-thirds of patients with a positive skin test and history of a previous adverse reaction to penicillin experience an allergic response on rechallenge. Skin tests may be negative in allergic patients receiving antihistamines or in those whose allergy is to determinants not present in the test reagent. Although less well studied, similar techniques can identify patients who are sensitive to protein drugs and to agents such as gallamine and succinylcholine. Most other drugs are small molecules, and skin testing with them is unreliable.

There are no generally available and reliable tests for assessing causality of non-IgE-mediated reactions, except possibly patch tests for assessment of fixed drug reactions. Therefore, diagnosis usually relies on clinical factors rather than test results.

FURTHER READING

BIGBY M: Rates of cutaneous reactions to drugs. Arch Dermatol 137:765, 2001

BREATHNACH SM: Adverse cutaneous reactions to drugs. Clin Med 2:15, 2002

ROUJEAU JC, STERN RS: Severe adverse cutaneous reactions to drugs. N Engl J Med 331:1272, 1994

———— et al: Medication use and the risk of Stevens-Johnson syndrome or toxic epidermal necrolysis. N Engl J Med 333:1600, 1995

VAN DER LINDEN PD et al: Skin reactions to antibacterial agents in general practice. J Clin Epidemiol 51:703, 1998

WARD HA et al: Cutaneous manifestations of antiretroviral therapy. J Am Acad Dermatol 46:284, 2002

51 PHOTOSENSITIVITY AND OTHER REACTIONS TO LIGHT
David R. Bickers

SOLAR RADIATION   Sunlight is the most visible and obvious source of comfort in the environment. The sun provides the beneficial effects of warmth and vitamin D synthesis; however, acute and chronic sun exposure also have pathologic consequences. Few effects of sun exposure beyond those affecting the skin have been identified, but cutaneous exposure to sunlight is the major cause of human skin cancer and can exert immunosuppressive effects as well.

The sun's energy reaching the earth's surface is limited to components of the ultraviolet (UV), the visible, and portions of the infrared spectra. The cutoff at the short end of the UV is at approximately 290 nm; this is due primarily to stratospheric ozone formed by highly energetic ionizing radiation, thereby preventing penetration to the earth's surface of the shorter, more energetic, potentially more harmful wavelengths of solar radiation. Indeed, concern about destruction of the ozone layer by chlorofluorocarbons released into the atmosphere has led to international agreements to reduce production of these chemicals.

Measurements of solar flux indicate that there is a twentyfold regional variation in the amount of energy at 300 nm that reaches the earth's surface. This variability relates to seasonal effects; the path of sunlight transmission through ozone and air; the altitude (4% increase for each 300 m of elevation); the latitude (increasing intensity with decreasing latitude); and the amount of cloud cover, fog, and pollution.

The major components of the photobiologic action spectrum capable of affecting human skin include the UV and visible wavelengths between 290 and 700 nm. In addition, the wavelengths beyond 700 nm in the infrared spectrum primarily emit heat and under certain circumstances may exacerbate the pathologic effects of energy in the UV and visible spectra.

The UV spectrum reaching the earth represents <10% of total incident solar energy and is arbitrarily divided into two major segments: UV-B, and UV-A. This includes the wavelengths between 290 and 400 nm. UV-B consists of wavelengths between 290 and 320 nm. This portion of the photobiologic action spectrum is the most efficient in producing redness or erythema in human skin and hence is sometimes known as the "sunburn spectrum." UV-A represents those wavelengths between 320 and 400 nm and is approximately 1000-fold less efficient in producing skin redness than is UV-B.

The wavelengths between 400 and 700 nm are visible to the human eye. The photon energy in the visible spectrum is not capable of damaging human skin in the absence of a photosensitizing chemical. Without the absorption of energy by a molecule there can be no photosensitivity. Thus the *absorption spectrum* of a molecule is defined as the range of wavelengths absorbed by it, whereas the *action spectrum* for an effect of incident radiation is defined as the range of wavelengths that evoke the response.

Photosensitivity occurs when a photon-absorbing chemical (chromophore) present in the skin absorbs incident energy, becomes excited, and transfers the absorbed energy to various structures or to oxygen.

UV RADIATION (UVR) AND SKIN STRUCTURE AND FUNCTION   Skin consists of two major compartments: the outer epidermis, a stratified squamous epithelium, and the underlying dermis rich in matrix proteins such as collagen and elastin. Both of these compartments are susceptible to damage from sun exposure. The epidermis and the dermis contain several chromophores capable of absorbing incident solar energy including nucleic acids, proteins, and lipids. The outermost epidermal layer, the stratum corneum, is a major absorber of UV-B, and <10% of incident UV-B wavelengths penetrate through the epidermis to the dermis. Approximately 3% of radiation below 300 nm, 20% of radiation below 360 nm, and 33% of short visible radiation reaches the basal cell layer in untanned human skin. In contrast, UV-A readily penetrates to the dermis and is capable of altering structural and matrix proteins that contribute to the aged appearance of chronically sun-exposed skin, particularly in individuals of light complexion.

Epidermal DNA, predominantly in keratinocytes, absorbs UV-B and undergoes structural changes including the formation of cyclobutane dimers and 6,4-photoproducts. These structural changes are potentially mutagenic and can be repaired by mechanisms that result in their recognition and excision and the reestablishment of normal base sequences. The efficient repair of these structural aberrations is crucial, since individuals with defective DNA repair are at high risk for the development of cutaneous cancer. For example, patients with xeroderma pigmentosum (XP), an autosomal recessive disorder, are characterized by variably deficient repair of UV-induced photoproducts, and their skin phenotype often manifests the dry, leathery appearance of prematurely photoaged skin as well as basal cell and squamous cell carcinomas and melanoma in the first two decades of life. Studies in mice using knockout gene technology have verified the importance of functional genes regulating these repair pathways in preventing the development of UV-induced cancer. Furthermore, incorporation of a bacterial DNA repair enzyme, T4N5 endonuclease, into liposomes in a product applied to skin of patients with XP selectively removes cyclobutane pyrimidine dimers and reduces the degree of solar damage and skin cancer.

Cutaneous Optics and Chromophores   Chromophores are endogenous or exogenous chemical components that can absorb physical energy. Endogenous chromophores are of two types: (1) chemicals that are normal components of skin, including nucleic acids, proteins, lipids, and 7-dehydrocholesterol, the precursor of vitamin D; and (2) chemicals, such as porphyrins, synthesized elsewhere in the body that circulate in the bloodstream and diffuse into the skin. Normally, only trace amounts of porphyrins are present in the skin, but in selected diseases known as the porphyrias (Chap. 337), increased amounts are released into the circulation from the bone marrow and the liver and are transported to the skin, where they absorb incident energy both in the Soret band, around 400 nm (short visible), and to a lesser extent in the red portion of the visible spectrum (580 to 660 nm). This results in the generation of reactive oxygen species that can mediate structural damage to the skin, manifest as erythema, edema, urticaria, or blister formation.

Acute Effects of Sun Exposure The acute effects of skin exposure to sunlight include sunburn and vitamin D synthesis.

SUNBURN This painful skin condition is caused predominantly by UV-B. Generally speaking, an individual's ability to tolerate sunlight is inversely proportional to the degree of melanin pigmentation. Melanin, a complex tyrosine polymer, is synthesized in specialized epidermal dendritic cells known as melanocytes and is packaged into *melanosomes* that are transferred via dendritic process into *keratinocytes*, thereby providing photoprotection and simultaneously darkening the skin. Sun-induced melanogenesis is a consequence of increased tyrosinase activity in melanocytes that in turn may be due to a combination of eicosanoid and endothelin-1 release. The Fitzpatrick classification of human skin is a function of the efficiency of the epidermal-melanin unit and can usually be ascertained by asking an individual two questions: (1) Do you burn after sun exposure? and (2) Do you tan after sun exposure? The answers to these questions permit division of the population into six skin types varying from type I (always burn, never tan) to type VI (never burn, always tan) (Table 51-1).

Sunburn is due to vasodilatation of dermal blood vessels. There is a lag in time between skin exposure to sunlight and the development of visible redness (usually 4 to 12 h), suggesting that an epidermal chromophore causes delayed production and/or release of vasoactive mediator(s), or cytokines, that diffuse to the dermal vasculature to evoke vasodilatation.

The action spectrum for sunburn erythema includes the UV-B and UV-A. Photons in the UV-B are at least 1000-fold more efficient than photons in the UV-A in evoking the response. However, UV-A may contribute to sunburn erythema at midday when much more UV-A than UV-B is present in the solar spectrum. UV-induced activation of nuclear factor-κB (NF-κB)-dependent gene transactivation can augment release of several proinflammatory cytokines including interleukin (IL) 1B, 1L-6, vascular endothelial growth factor, and tumor necrosis factor α. Local accumulation of these cytokines occurs in sunburned skin. It is of interest that nonsteroidal anti-inflammatory drugs can reduce sunburn erythema, perhaps by blocking I-κB kinase 2, the enzyme essential for nuclear translocation of cytosolic NF-κB.

VITAMIN D PHOTOCHEMISTRY Cutaneous exposure to UV-B causes photolysis of epidermal 7-dehydrocholesterol converting it to pre-vitamin D$_3$, which then undergoes a temperature-dependent isomerization to form the stable hormone vitamin D$_3$. This compound then diffuses to the dermal vasculature and circulates systemically where it is converted to the functional hormone 1,25-dihydroxy vitamin D$_3$ [1,25(OH)$_2$D$_3$]. Vitamin D metabolites from the circulation or those produced in the skin itself can augment epidermal differentiation signaling. Aging substantially decreases the ability of human skin to photocatalytically produce vitamin D$_3$. This, coupled with the widespread use of sunscreens that filter out UV-B, has led to concern that vitamin D deficiency may become a significant clinical problem in the elderly. Nonetheless, at least one double-blind placebo-controlled trial has

shown that a broad-spectrum sunscreen applied topically for several months has no significant effect on measured plasma vitamin D metabolites.

Chronic Effects of Sun Exposure: Nonmalignant The clinical features of photodamaged sun-exposed skin consist of wrinkling, blotchiness, and telangiectasia and a roughened, irregular, "weather-beaten" leathery appearance. Whether this photoaging represents accelerated chronologic aging or a separate and distinct process is not clear.

Within chronically sun-exposed epidermis, there is thickening (acanthosis) and morphologic heterogeneity within the basal cell layer. Higher but irregular melanosome content may be present in some keratinocytes, indicating prolonged residence of the cells in the basal cell layer. These structural changes may help to explain the leathery texture and the blotchy discoloration of sun-damaged skin.

The dermis and its connective tissue matrix are the major site for sun-associated chronic damage, manifest as solar elastosis, a massive increase in thickened irregular masses of abnormal elastic fibers. Collagen fibers are also abnormally clumped in the deeper dermis of sun-damaged skin. The chromophore(s), the action spectra, and the specific biochemical events orchestrating these changes are only partially understood. Chronologically aged, sun-protected skin and photoaged skin share important molecular features including connective tissue damage, elevated matrix metalloproteinase levels, and reduced collagen production.

Chronic Effects of Sun Exposure: Malignant One of the major known consequences of chronic skin exposure to sunlight is nonmelanoma skin cancer. The two types of nonmelanoma skin cancer are *basal cell carcinoma* and *squamous cell carcinoma* (Chap. 73). There are three major steps for cancer induction: initiation, promotion, and progression. Exposure of human skin to sunlight results in *initiation*, a step whereby structural (mutagenic) changes in DNA evoke an irreversible alteration in the target cell (*keratinocyte*) that begins the tumorigenic process. Exposure to a tumor initiator such as UV-B is believed to be a necessary but not sufficient step in the malignant process, since initiated skin cells not exposed to tumor promoters do not generally develop tumors. The second stage in tumor development is *promotion*, a multistep process whereby chronic exposure to sunlight evokes epigenetic changes that culminate in the clonal expansion of initiated cells and cause the development, over many years, of premalignant growths known as *actinic keratoses*, a minority of which may progress to form skin cancer. Based on extensive studies it seems clear that UV-B is a *complete carcinogen*, meaning that it can act as both a tumor initiator and a promoter.

The third and final step in the malignant process is *malignant conversion* of benign precursors into malignant lesions, a process thought to require additional genetic alterations in already transformed cells. Skin carcinogenesis is thought to be caused by the accumulation of mutations in the tumor suppressor gene p53 as a result of UV-induced DNA damage. Indeed both human and murine UV-induced skin cancers have unique p53 mutations (C $\rightarrow$ T and CC $\rightarrow$ TT transitions) that are present in the majority of these lesions. Studies have shown that sunscreens can substantially reduce the frequency of these signature mutations in p53 and can dramatically inhibit the induction of tumors. The p53 mutations are present in normal human skin, in actinic keratoses, and in nonmelanoma skin cancers including basal cell and squamous cell carcinomas.

Basal cell carcinomas also manifest mutations in the tumor-suppressor gene known as *patched*, which results in activation of hedgehog signaling, and enhanced activity of *smoothened*, which in turn causes downstream activation of transcription factors that augment cell proliferation. Thus, these tumors can manifest mutations in both p53 and in *patched*.

Sun exposure causes nonmelanoma and melanoma cancers of the skin, although the evidence is far more direct for its role in nonmelanoma (basal cell and squamous cell carcinoma) than in melanoma.

TABLE 51-1 *Skin Type and Sunburn Sensitivity (Fitzpatrick Classification)*

Type	Description
I	Always burn, never tan
II	Always burn, sometimes tan
III	Sometimes burn, sometimes tan
IV	Sometimes burn, always tan
V	Never burn, sometimes tan
VI	Never burn, always tan

Approximately 80% of nonmelanoma skin cancers develop on exposed body area, including the face, the neck, and the hands. Major risk factors include male sex, childhood sun exposures, older age, fair skin, and residence at latitudes closer to the equator. Whites of darker complexions (e.g., Hispanics) have one-tenth the risk of developing such cancers compared to fair-skinned individuals. Blacks are at substantially reduced risk for all forms of skin cancer. One million individuals in the United States develop nonmelanoma skin cancer annually, and the lifetime risk for a fair-skinned individual to develop such a neoplasm is estimated at approximately 15%. A consensus exists that the incidence of nonmelanoma skin cancer in the population is increasing at the rate of 2 to 3% per year, for unknown reasons.

The relationship of sun exposure to melanoma development is less clear-cut, but suggestive evidence supports an association. Melanomas occasionally develop by the teenage years, indicating that the latent period for tumor growth is less than that of nonmelanoma skin cancer. Melanomas are among the most rapidly increasing of all human malignancies (Chap. 73). Epidemiologic studies of immigrant populations of similar ethnic stock indicate that individuals born in one area or who migrate to the same locale before age 10 have higher age-specific melanoma rates than individuals arriving later. It is thus reasonable to conclude that life in a sunny climate from birth or early childhood increases the risk of melanoma. In general, risk does not correlate with cumulative sun exposure but may relate to the duration and extent of exposure in childhood.

Meta-analysis of 17 case-control studies in patients with melanoma concluded that the protective effect of sunscreens against this type of tumor could not be substantiated. Since no prospective studies are available to address this issue, it seems reasonable to recommend that patients at risk for melanoma utilize photoprotection such as sun avoidance, high sun protective factor (SPF) sunscreens, and protective clothing.

Immunologic Effects Exposure to solar radiation suppresses both local and systemic immune responses. The action spectrum for UV-induced immunosuppression closely mimics the absorption spectrum of urocanic acid. UV-induced *trans-cis* isomerization of urocanic acid in the stratum corneum leads to its systemic absorption and consequent immunosuppressive effects. Furthermore administration of modest doses of UV-B to human skin reduces the degree of allergic sensitization to the potent contact allergen, dinitrochlorobenzene. This is associated with depletion of epidermal Langerhans cells.

Higher doses of UV-radiation evoke diminished immunologic responses to antigens introduced either epicutaneously or intracutaneously at sites distant from the irradiated site. These suppressed responses are also associated with the induction of antigen-specific suppressor T lymphocytes and may be mediated by as yet undefined factors that are released from epidermal cells at the irradiated site. One important consequence of chronic sun exposure and the concomitant immunosuppression is enhanced risk of skin cancer. Perhaps the most graphic demonstration of the role of immunosuppression in enhancing the risk of nonmelanoma skin cancer has come from studies of patients receiving organ transplantation who are on chronic immunosuppressive antirejection drug regimens. More than 50% of transplant patients develop basal and squamous cell carcinomas, and these cancers are the most common malignancy arising in renal transplant recipients. These patients require close periodic monitoring and rigorous photoprotection using sunscreens, protective clothing, and sun avoidance.

PHOTOSENSITIVITY DISEASES The diagnosis of photosensitivity requires a careful history to define the duration of the signs and symptoms, the length of time between exposure to sunlight and the development of subjective complaints, and visible changes in the skin. The age of onset can also be a helpful clue; for example, the acute photosensitivity of erythropoietic protoporphyria almost always begins in childhood, whereas the chronic photosensitivity of porphyria cutanea tarda (PCT) typically begins in the fourth and fifth decades. A history of exposure

to topical and systemic drugs and chemicals may provide important clues. Many classes of drugs can cause photosensitivity on the basis of either phototoxicity or photoallergy. Fragrances such as musk ambrette that were previously present in numerous cosmetic products are also potent photosensitizers.

Examination of the skin may also offer important clues. Anatomic areas that are naturally protected from direct sunlight such as the hairy scalp, the upper eyelids, the retroauricular areas, and the infranasal and submental regions may be spared, whereas exposed areas show characteristic features of the pathologic process. These anatomic localization patterns are often helpful, but not infallible, in making the diagnosis. For example, airborne contact sensitizers that are blown onto the skin may produce dermatitis that can be difficult to distinguish from photosensitivity, despite the fact that such material may trigger skin reactivity in areas shielded from direct sunlight.

Many dermatologic conditions may be caused or aggravated by sunlight (Table 51-2). The role of light in evoking these responses may be dependent on genetic abnormalities ranging from well-described defects in DNA repair that occur in XP to the inherited abnormalities in heme synthesis that characterize the porphyrias. In certain photosensitivity diseases, the chromophore has been identified, whereas in the majority, the energy-absorbing agent is unknown.

Polymorphous Light Eruption After sunburn, the most common type of photosensitivity disease is *polymorphous light eruption* (PLE), the mechanism of which is unknown. Many affected individuals never seek medical attention because the condition is often transient, becoming manifest each spring with initial sun exposure but then subsiding spontaneously with continuing exposure, a phenomenon known as "hardening." The major manifestations of PLE include pruritic (often intensely so) erythematous papules that may coalesce into plaques in

TABLE 51-2 *Classification of Photosensitivity Diseases*

Type	Disease
Genetic	Erythropoietic porphyria
	Erythropoietic protoporphyria
	Porphyria cutanea tarda—familial
	Variegate porphyria
	Hepatoerythropoietic porphyria
	Albinism
	Xeroderma pigmentosum
	Rothmund-Thompson disease
	Bloom syndrome
	Cockayne's disease
	Phenylketonuria
Metabolic	Porphyria cutanea tarda—sporadic
	Hartnup disease
	Kwashiorkor
	Pellagra
	Carcinoid syndrome
Phototoxic	
Internal	Drugs
External	Drugs, plants, food
Photoallergic	
Immediate	Solar urticaria
Delayed	Drug photoallergy
	Persistent light reaction/chronic actinic dermatitis
Neoplastic and	Photoaging
degenerative	Actinic keratosis
	Melanoma and nonmelanoma skin cancer
Idiopathic	Polymorphous light eruption
	Hydroa aestivale
	Actinic prurigo
Photoaggravated	Lupus erythematosus
	Systemic
	Subacute cutaneous
	Discoid
	Dermatomyositis
	Herpes simplex
	Lichen planus actinicus
	Acne vulgaris (aestivale)

a patchy distribution on exposed areas of the trunk and forearms. The face is usually less seriously involved.

The diagnosis can be confirmed by skin biopsy and by performing phototest procedures in which skin is exposed to multiple erythema doses of UV-A and UV-B. The action spectrum for PLE is usually within these portions of the solar spectrum.

Treatment of this PLE includes the use of sunscreens and the induction of hardening by the cautious administration of artificial UV-B and/or UV-A radiation for 2 to 3 weeks in the spring.

Phototoxicity and Photoallergy These photosensitivity disorders are related to the topical or systemic administration of drugs and other chemicals. Both reactions require the absorption of energy by a drug or chemical resulting in the production of an excited-state photosensitizer that can transfer its absorbed energy to a bystander molecule or to molecular oxygen, thereby generating tissue-destructive chemical species.

Phototoxicity is a nonimmunologic reaction caused by drugs and chemicals, a few of which are listed in Table 51-3. The usual clinical manifestations include erythema resembling a sunburn reaction that quickly desquamates, or "peels," within several days. In addition, edema, vesicles, and bullae may occur.

Photoallergy is much less common and is distinct in that the immune system participates in the pathologic process. The excited-state photosensitizer may create highly unstable haptenic free radicals that bind covalently to macromolecules to form a functional antigen capable of evoking a delayed hypersensitivity response. Some of the drugs and chemicals that produce photoallergy are listed in Table 51-4. The clinical manifestations typically differ from those of phototoxicity in that an intensely pruritic eczematous dermatitis tends to predominate and evolves into lichenified, thickened, "leathery" changes in sun-exposed areas. A small subset (perhaps 5 to 10%) of patients with photoallergy may develop a persistent exquisite hypersensitivity to light even when the offending drug or chemical is identified and eliminated, a condition known as *persistent light reaction*.

A very uncommon type of persistent photosensitivity is known as *chronic actinic dermatitis*. These patients are typically elderly men with a long history of preexisting allergic contact dermatitis or photosensitivity. They are usually exquisitely sensitive to UV-B, UV-A, and visible wavelengths.

Diagnostic confirmation of phototoxicity and photoallergy can often be obtained using phototest procedures. In patients with suspected phototoxicity, determining the minimal erythema dose (MED) while the patient is exposed to a suspected agent and then repeating the MED after discontinuation of the agent may provide a clue to the causative drug or chemical. Photopatch testing can be performed to confirm the diagnosis of photoallergy. This is a simple variant of ordinary patch testing in which a series of known photoallergens is applied to the skin in duplicate and one set is irradiated with a suberythema dose of UV-A. Development of eczematous changes at sites exposed to sensitizer and light is a positive result. The characteristic abnormality in patients

TABLE 51-4 *Photoallergic Drugs*

	Topical	Systemic
6-Methylcoumarin	+	
Aminobenzoic acid and esters	+	
Bithionol	+	
Chlorpromazine		+
Diclofenac		+
Fluoroquinolones		+
Halogenated salicylanilides	+	
Hypericin (St John's Wort)	+	+
Musk ambrette	+	
Piroxicam		+
Promethazine		+
Sulfonamides		+
Sulfonylureas		+

with persistent light reaction is a diminished threshold to erythema evoked by UV-B. Patients with chronic actinic dermatitis usually manifest a broad spectrum of UV hyperresponsiveness and require rigorous photoprotection for relief of their symptoms.

The management of drug photosensitivity involves first and foremost the elimination of exposure to the chemical agents responsible for the reaction and minimization sun exposure. The acute symptoms of phototoxicity may be ameliorated by cool, moist compresses, topical glucocorticoids, and systemically administered NSAIDs. In severely affected individuals, a rapidly tapered course of systemic glucocorticoids may be useful. Judicious use of analgesics may be necessary.

Photoallergic reactions require a similar management approach. Furthermore, patients with persistent light reaction and chronic actinic dermatitis must be meticulously protected against light exposure. In selected patients in whom chronic systemic high-dose glucocorticoids pose unacceptable risks, it may be necessary to employ cytotoxic agents such as azathioprine or cyclophosphamide.

Porphyria The porphyrias (Chap. 337) are a group of diseases that have in common inherited or acquired derangements in the synthesis of heme. Heme is an iron-chelated tetrapyrrole or porphyrin, and the nonmetal chelated porphyrins are potent photosensitizers that absorb light intensely in both the short (400 to 410 nm) and the long (580 to 650 nm) portions of the visible spectrum.

Heme cannot be reutilized and must be continuously synthesized, and the two body compartments with the largest capacity for its production are the bone marrow and the liver. Accordingly, the porphyrias originate in one or the other of these organs, with the end result of excessive endogenous production of potent photosensitizing porphyrins. The porphyrins circulate in the bloodstream and diffuse into the skin, where they absorb solar energy, become photoexcited, generate reactive oxygen species, and evoke cutaneous photosensitivity. The mechanism of porphyrin photosensitization is known to be photodynamic, or oxygen-dependent, and is mediated by reactive oxygen species such as singlet oxygen and superoxide anions.

Porphyria cutanea tarda is the most common type of human porphyria and is associated with decreased activity of the enzyme uroporphyrinogen decarboxylase associated with a number of gene mutations. There are two basic types of PCT: (1) the sporadic or acquired type, generally seen in individuals ingesting ethanol or receiving estrogens; and (2) the inherited type, in which there is autosomal dominant transmission of deficient enzyme activity. Both forms are associated with increased hepatic iron stores.

In both types of PCT, the predominant feature is a chronic photosensitivity characterized by increased fragility of sun-exposed skin, particularly areas subject to repeated trauma such as the dorsa of the hands, the forearms, the face, and the ears. The predominant skin lesions are vesicles and bullae that rupture, producing moist erosions, often with a hemorrhagic base, that heal slowly with crusting and

TABLE 51-3 *Phototoxic Drugs*

	Topical	Systemic
Amiodarone		+
Dacarbazine		+
Fluoroquinolones		+
5-Fluorouracil	+	+
Furosemide		+
Nalidixic acid		+
Phenothiazines		+
Psoralens	+	+
Retinoids	+/−	+
Sulfonamides		+
Sulfonylureas		+
Tetracyclines		+
Thiazides		+
Vinblastine		+

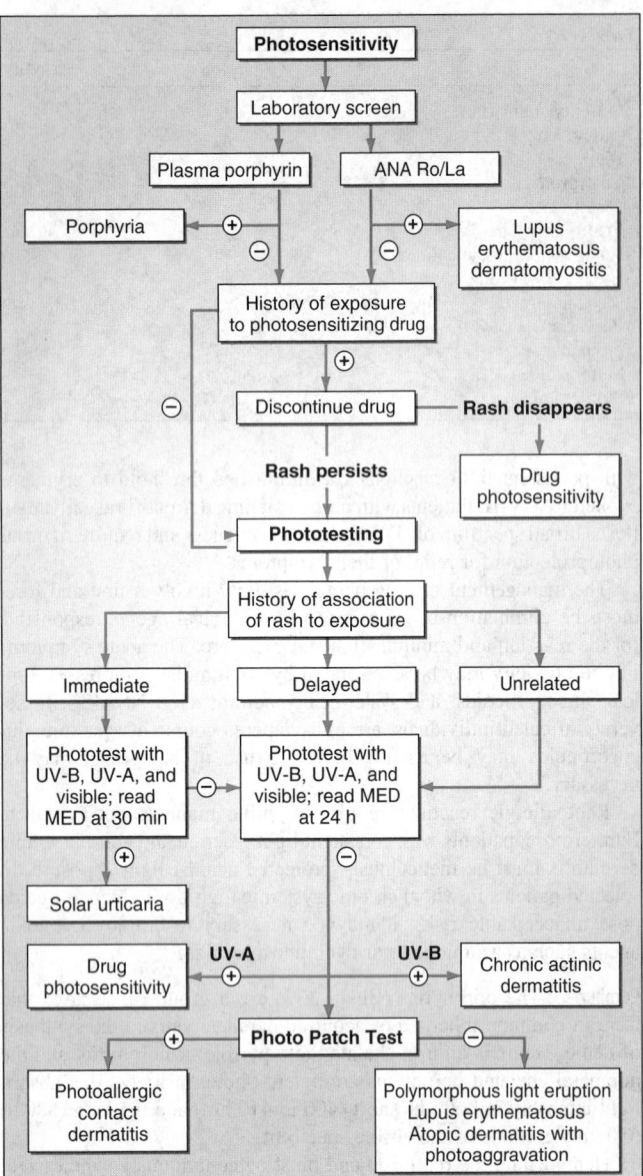

FIGURE 51-1 An algorithm for the diagnosis of a patient with photosensitivity.

purplish discoloration of the affected skin. Hypertrichosis, mottled pigmentary change, and scleroderma-like induration are associated features. Biochemical confirmation of the diagnosis can be obtained by measurement of urinary porphyrin excretion, plasma porphyrin assay, and by assay of erythrocyte and/or hepatic uroporphyrinogen decarboxylase. Multiple mutations of the uroporphyrinogen decarboxylase gene have been identified in human populations, including exon skipping and base substitutions. Some patients with PCT have associated mutations in the *HFE* gene linked to hemochromatosis. This could contribute to the iron overload seen in PCT, although iron status as measured by serum ferritin, iron levels, and transferrin saturation is no different from that in PCT patients without *HFE* mutations. Prior hepatitis C infection appears to be an independent risk factor for PCT.

Treatment of PCT consists of repeated phlebotomies to diminish the excessive hepatic iron stores and/or intermittent low doses of the antimalarial drugs chloroquine and hydroxychloroquine. Long-term remission of the disease can be achieved if the patient eliminates exposure to porphyrinogenic agents.

Erythropoietic protoporphyria originates in the bone marrow and is due to a decrease in the mitochondrial enzyme ferrochelatase secondary to numerous gene mutations. The major clinical features include an acute photosensitivity characterized by subjective burning and stinging of exposed skin that often develops during or just after exposure. There may be associated skin swelling and, after repeated episodes, a waxlike scarring.

The diagnosis is confirmed by demonstration of elevated levels of free erythrocyte protoporphyrin. Detection of increased plasma protoporphyrin helps to differentiate lead poisoning and iron-deficiency anemia, in both of which elevated erythrocyte protoporphyrin levels occur in the absence of cutaneous photosensitivity and of elevated plasma protoporphyrin levels.

Treatment consists of reducing sun exposure and the oral administration of the carotenoid β-carotene, which is an effective scavenger of free radicals. This drug increases tolerance to sun exposure in many affected individuals, although it has no effect on deficient ferrochelatase.

An algorithm for managing patients with photosensitivity is illustrated in Fig. 51-1.

PHOTOPROTECTION Since photosensitivity of the skin results from exposure to sunlight, it follows that absolute avoidance of the sun would eliminate these disorders. Unfortunately, contemporary life-styles make this an impractical alternative for most individuals, and this has led to a search for better approaches to photoprotection.

Natural photoprotection is provided by structural proteins in the epidermis, particularly keratins and melanin. The amount of melanin and its distribution in cells is genetically regulated, and individuals of darker complexion (skin types IV to VI) are at decreased risk for the development of acute sunburn and cutaneous malignancy.

Other forms of photoprotection include clothing and sunscreens. Clothing constructed of tightly woven sun-protective fabrics, irrespective of color, affords substantial protection. Wide-brimmed hats, long sleeves, and trousers all reduce direct exposure. Sunscreens are now considered to be over-the-counter drugs and category I ingredients are recognized by the U.S. Food and Drug Administration (FDA) as monographed and safe and effective. These are listed in Table 51-5. Sunscreens are rated for their photoprotective effect by their SPF. The SPF is simply a ratio of the time required to produce sunburn erythema with and without sunscreen application. The monograph stipulates that sunscreens must be rated on a scale ranging from minimal (SPF $\nless$2 and $\not>$12) to moderate (SPF $\nless$12 and $\not>$30) to high (SPF ≥30, labeled as 30+). No SPF number >30 can be placed on the label.

In addition to light absorption, a critical determinant of the sustained photoprotective effect of sunscreens is their water-resistance. The FDA monograph has also defined strict testing criteria for sunscreens making this claim.

Some degree of photoprotection can also be achieved by limiting the time of exposure during the day. Since the majority of an individual's total lifetime sun exposure may occur by the age of 18, it is important to educate parents and young children about the hazards of

TABLE 51-5 *FDA Category 1 Monographed Sunscreen Ingredients[a]*

Ingredients	Maximum Concentration, %
p-Aminobenzoic acid (PABA)	15
Avobenzone	3
Cinoxate	3
Dioxybenzone (benzophenone-8)	3
Homosalate	15
Menthyl anthranilate	5
Octocrylene	10
Octyl methoxycinnamate	7.5
Octyl salicylate	5
Oxybenzone (benzophenone-3)	6
Padimate (octyl dimethyl PABA)	8
Phenylbenzimidazole sulfonic acid	4
Sulisobenzone (benzophenone-4)	10
Titanium dioxide	25
Trolamine salicylate	12
Zinc oxide	25

[a] FDA, U.S. Food and Drug Administration.

sunlight. Simply eliminating exposure at midday will substantially reduce lifetime UV-B exposure.

PHOTOTHERAPY AND PHOTOCHEMOTHERAPY UV can also be used therapeutically. The administration of UV-B alone or in combination with topically applied agents can induce remissions of psoriasis and atopic dermatitis.

Photochemotherapy in which topically applied or systemically administered psoralens are combined with UV-A (PUVA) is also effective in treating psoriasis and in the early stages of cutaneous T cell lymphoma and vitiligo. Psoralens are tricyclic furocoumarins that, when intercalated into DNA and exposed to UV-A, form adducts with pyrimidine bases and eventually form DNA cross-links. These structural changes are thought to decrease DNA synthesis and relate to the improvement that occurs in psoriasis. The reason that PUVA photochemotherapy is effective in cutaneous T cell lymphoma is not clear.

In addition to its effects on DNA, PUVA photochemotherapy also stimulates melanin synthesis, and this provides the rationale for its use in the depigmenting disease vitiligo. Oral 8-methoxypsoralen and UV-A appear to be most effective in this regard, but as many as 100 treatments extending over 12 to 18 months may be required to promote satisfactory repigmentation.

Not surprisingly the major side effects of long-term UV-B phototherapy and PUVA photochemotherapy mimic those seen in individuals with chronic sun exposure and include skin dryness, actinic keratoses, and an increased risk of melanoma and nonmelanoma skin cancer. Despite these risks, the therapeutic index of these modalities continues to be excellent.

FURTHER READING

ANANTHASWAMY HN et al: Inhibition of UVB-induced p53 mutations and skin cancer by sunscreens: Implications for skin cancer prevention. Exp Dermatol 11(Suppl 1):40, 2002

DRAELOS ZD: A dermatologist's perspective on the final sunscreen monograph. J Am Acad Dermatol 44:109, 2001

MARKS R et al: The effect of regular sunscreen use on vitamin D levels in an Australian population. Results of a randomized clinical trial. Arch Dermatol 131:1337, 1995

MATSUMURA Y, ANANTHASWAMY NH: Molecular mechanisms of photocarcinogenesis. Front Biosci 7:765, 2002

ROELANDTS R: The diagnosis of photosensitivity. Arch Dermatol 136:1152, 2000

Section 10   Hematologic Alterations

52 ANEMIA AND POLYCYTHEMIA
John W. Adamson, Dan L. Longo

HEMATOPOIESIS AND THE PHYSIOLOGIC BASIS OF RED CELL PRODUCTION *Hematopoiesis* is the process by which the formed elements of the blood are produced. The process is regulated through a series of steps beginning with the pluripotent hematopoietic stem cell. Stem cells are capable of producing red cells, all classes of granulocytes, monocytes, platelets, and the cells of the immune system. Commitment of the stem cell to the specific cell lineages appears not to be regulated by known exogenous growth factors or cytokines. Rather, stem cells develop into differentiated cell types through incompletely defined molecular events that are intrinsic to the stem cell itself. Following lineage commitment (or differentiation), hematopoietic progenitor and precursor cells come increasingly under the regulatory influence of growth factors and hormones. For red cell production, erythropoietin (EPO) is the regulatory hormone. EPO is required for the maintenance of committed erythroid progenitor cells that, in the absence of the hormone, undergo programmed cell death (*apoptosis*). The regulated process of red cell production is *erythropoiesis*, and its key elements are illustrated in Fig. 52-1.

In the bone marrow, the first morphologically recognizable erythroid precursor is the pronormoblast. This cell can undergo 4 to 5 cell divisions that result in the production of 16 to 32 mature red cells. With increased EPO production, or the administration of EPO as a drug, early progenitor cell numbers are amplified and, in turn, give rise to increased numbers of erythrocytes. The regulation of EPO production itself is linked to O_2 transport.

In mammals, O_2 is transported to tissues bound to the hemoglobin contained within circulating red cells. The mature red cell is 8 μm in diameter, anucleate, discoid in shape, and extremely pliable in order to traverse the microcirculation successfully; its membrane integrity is maintained by the intracellular generation of ATP. Normal red cell production results in the daily replacement of 0.8 to 1% of all circulating red cells in the body. The average red cell lives 100 to 120 days. The machinery responsible for red cell production is called the *erythron*. The erythron is a dynamic organ made up of a rapidly proliferating pool of marrow erythroid precursor cells and a large mass of mature circulating red blood cells. The size of the red cell mass reflects the balance of red cell production and destruction. The physiologic basis of red cell production and destruction provides an understanding of the mechanisms that can lead to anemia.

The physiologic regulator of red cell production, the glycoprotein hormone EPO, is produced and released by peritubular capillary lining cells within the kidney. These cells are highly specialized epithelial-like cells. A small amount of EPO is produced by hepatocytes. The fundamental stimulus for EPO production is the availability of O_2 for tissue metabolic needs. Impaired O_2 delivery to the kidney can result from a decreased red cell mass (*anemia*), impaired O_2 loading of the hemoglobin molecule (*hypoxemia*), or, rarely, impaired blood flow to the kidney (renal artery stenosis). EPO governs the day-to-day production of red cells, and ambient levels of the hormone can be measured in the plasma by sensitive immunoassays—the normal level being 10 to 25 U/L. When the hemoglobin concentration falls below 100 to 120 g/L (10 to 12 g/dL), plasma EPO levels increase in proportion to the severity of the anemia. In circulation, EPO has a half-clearance time of 6 to 9 h. EPO acts by binding to specific receptors on the surface of marrow erythroid precursors, inducing them to proliferate and to mature. Under the stimulus of EPO, red cell production

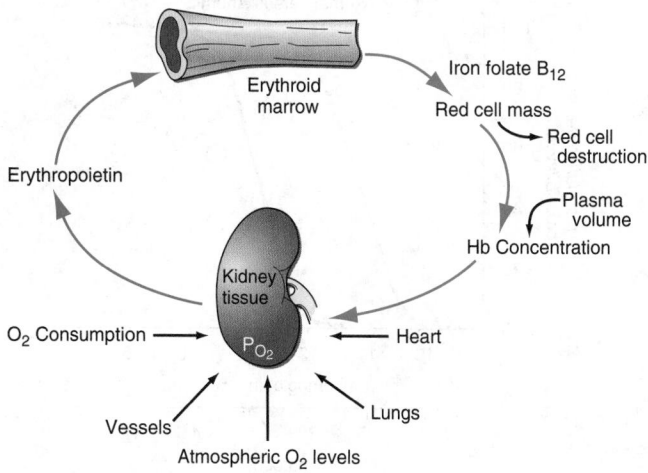

FIGURE 52-1 The physiologic regulation of red cell production by tissue oxygen tension. Hb, hemoglobin.

can increase four- to fivefold within a 1- to 2-week period but only in the presence of adequate nutrients, especially iron. The functional capacity of the erythron, therefore, requires normal renal production of EPO, a functioning erythroid marrow, and an adequate supply of substrates for hemoglobin synthesis. A defect in any of these key components can lead to anemia. Generally, anemia is recognized in the laboratory when a patient's hemoglobin level or hematocrit is reduced below an expected value (the normal range). The likelihood and severity of anemia are defined based on the deviation of the patient's hemoglobin/hematocrit from values expected for age- and sex-matched normal subjects. The lower ranges of distribution of hemoglobin/hematocrit values for adult males and females are shown in Fig. 52-2. The hemoglobin concentration in adults has a Gaussian distribution. The mean hematocrit value for adult males is 47% (± SD 7) and that for adult females is 42% (± 5). Any single hematocrit or hemoglobin value carries with it a likelihood of associated anemia. Thus, a hematocrit of ≤39% in an adult male or <35% in an adult female has only about a 25% chance of being normal. Suspected low hemoglobin or hematocrit values are more easily interpreted if there are historic values for the same patient for comparison.

The critical elements of erythropoiesis—EPO production, iron availability, the proliferative capacity of the bone marrow, and effective maturation of red cell precursors—are used for the initial classification of anemia (see below).

ANEMIA

CLINICAL PRESENTATION OF ANEMIA ■ **Signs and Symptoms** Anemia is most often recognized by abnormal screening laboratory tests. Patients less commonly present with advanced anemia and its attendant signs and symptoms. Acute anemia is nearly always due to blood loss or hemolysis. If blood loss is mild, enhanced O_2 delivery is achieved through changes in the O_2-hemoglobin dissociation curve mediated by a decreased pH or increased CO_2 (*Bohr effect*). With acute blood loss, hypovolemia dominates the clinical picture and the hematocrit and hemoglobin levels do not reflect the volume of blood lost. Signs of vascular instability appear with acute losses of 10 to 15% of the total blood volume. In such patients, the issue is not anemia but hypotension and decreased organ perfusion. When >30% of the blood volume is lost suddenly, patients are unable to compensate with the usual mechanisms of vascular contraction and changes in regional blood flow. The patient prefers to remain supine and will show postural hypotension and tachycardia if upright. If the volume of blood lost is >40% (i.e., >2 L in the average-sized adult), signs of hypovolemic shock including confusion, dyspnea, diaphoresis, hypotension, and tachycardia appear (Chap. 93). Such patients have significant deficits in vital organ perfusion and require immediate volume replacement.

With acute hemolytic disease, the signs and symptoms depend on the mechanism that leads to red cell destruction. Intravascular hemolysis with release of free hemoglobin may be associated with acute back pain, free hemoglobin in the plasma and urine, and renal failure. Symptoms associated with more chronic or progressive anemia depend on the age of the patient and the adequacy of blood supply to critical organs. Symptoms associated with moderate anemia include fatigue, loss of stamina, breathlessness, and tachycardia (particularly with physical exertion). However, because of the intrinsic compensatory mechanisms that govern the O_2-hemoglobin dissociation curve, the gradual onset of anemia—particularly in young patients—may not be associated with signs or symptoms until the anemia is severe [hemoglobin <70 to 80 g/L (7 to 8 g/dL)]. When anemia develops over a period of days or weeks, the total blood volume is normal to slightly increased and changes in cardiac output and regional blood flow help compensate for the overall loss in O_2-carrying capacity. Changes in the position of the O_2-hemoglobin dissociation curve account for some of the compensatory response to anemia. With chronic anemia, intracellular levels of 2,3-bisphosphoglycerate rise, shifting the dissociation curve to the right and facilitating O_2 unloading. This compensatory mechanism can only maintain normal tissue O_2 delivery in the face of a 20 to 30 g/L (2 to 3 g/dL) deficit in hemoglobin concentration. Finally, further protection of O_2 delivery to vital organs is achieved by the shunting of blood away from organs that are relatively rich in blood supply, particularly the kidney, gut, and skin.

Certain disorders are commonly associated with anemia. Chronic inflammatory states (e.g., infection, rheumatoid arthritis) are associated with mild to moderate anemia, whereas lymphoproliferative disorders, such as chronic lymphocytic leukemia and certain other B cell neoplasms, may be associated with autoimmune hemolysis.

APPROACH TO THE PATIENT

The evaluation of the patient with anemia requires a careful history and physical examination. Nutritional history related to drugs or alcohol intake and family history of anemia should always be assessed. Certain geographic backgrounds and ethnic origins are associated with an increased likelihood of an inherited disorder of the hemoglobin molecule or intermediary metabolism. Glucose-6-phosphate dehydrogenase deficiency and certain hemoglobinopathies are seen more commonly in those of Middle Eastern or African origin. Other information that may be useful includes exposure to certain toxic agents or drugs and symptoms related to other disorders commonly associated with anemia. These include

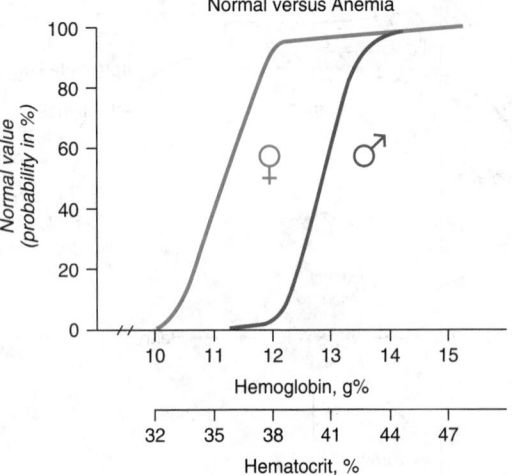

Normal versus Anemia

FIGURE 52-2 The probability that a particular hemoglobin or hematocrit value is abnormal is different in men and women.

TABLE 52-1 *Laboratory Tests in Anemia Diagnosis*

I. Complete blood count (CBC)	II. Iron supply studies
A. Red blood cell count	A. Serum iron
1. Hemoglobin	B. Total iron-binding
2. Hematocrit	capacity
3. Reticulocyte count	C. Serum ferritin, marrow
B. Red blood cell indices	iron stain
1. Mean cell volume (MCV)	III. Marrow examination
2. Mean cell hemoglobin (MCH)	A. Aspirate
3. Mean cell hemoglobin	1. M/E ratio[a]
concentration (MCHC)	2. Cell morphology
4. Red cell distribution width	3. Iron stain
(RDW)	B. Biopsy
C. White blood cell count	1. Cellularity
1. Cell differential	2. Morphology
2. Nuclear segmentation of	
neutrophils	
D. Platelet count	
E. Cell morphology	
1. Cell size	
2. Hemoglobin content	
3. Anisocytosis	
4. Poikilocytosis	
5. Polychromasia	

[a] M/E ratio, ratio of myeloid to erythroid precursors.

TABLE 52-2   *Red Blood Cell Indices*

Index	Normal Value
Mean cell volume (MCV) = (hematocrit × 10)/(red cell count × 10⁶)	90 ± 8 fL
Mean cell hemoglobin (MCH) = (hemoglobin × 10)/(red cell count × 10⁶)	30 ± 3 pg
Mean cell hemoglobin concentration = (hemoglobin × 10)/hematocrit, or MCH/MCV	33 ± 2%

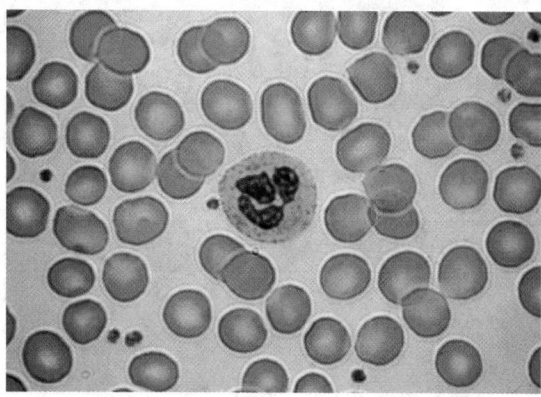

FIGURE 52-3   Normal blood smear (Wright's stain). High-power field showing normal red cells, a neutrophil, and a few platelets. (*From Hillman and Ault.*)

symptoms and signs such as bleeding, fatigue, malaise, fever, weight loss, night sweats, and other systemic symptoms. Clues to the mechanisms of anemia may be provided on physical examination by findings of infection, blood in the stool, lymphadenopathy, splenomegaly, or petechiae. Splenomegaly and lymphadenopathy suggest an underlying lymphoproliferative disease, while petechiae suggest platelet dysfunction. Past laboratory measurements may be helpful to determine a time of onset.

In the anemic patient, physical examination may demonstrate a forceful heartbeat, strong peripheral pulses, and a systolic "flow" murmur. The skin and mucous membranes may be pale if the hemoglobin is <80 to 100 g/L (8 to 10 g/dL). This part of the physical examination should focus on areas where vessels are close to the surface such as the mucous membranes, nail beds, and palmar creases. If the palmar creases are lighter in color than the surrounding skin when the hand is hyperextended, the hemoglobin level is usually <80 g/L (8 g/dL).

Laboratory Evaluation   Table 52-1 lists the tests used in the initial workup of anemia. A routine complete blood count (CBC) is required as part of the evaluation and includes the hemoglobin, hematocrit, and red cell indices: the mean cell volume (MCV) in femtoliters, mean cell hemoglobin (MCH) in picograms per cell, and mean concentration of hemoglobin per volume of red cells (MCHC) in grams per liter (non-SI: grams per deciliter). The red cell indices are calculated as shown in Table 52-2, and the normal variations in the hemoglobin and hematocrit with age are shown in Table 52-3. A number of physiologic factors affect the normal CBC values including age, gender, pregnancy, smoking, and altitude. High-normal hemoglobin values may be seen in men and women who live at altitude or smoke heavily. Hemoglobin elevations due to smoking reflect normal compensation due to the displacement of O_2 by CO in hemoglobin binding. Other important information is provided by the reticulocyte count and measurements of iron supply including *serum iron, total iron-binding capacity* (TIBC; an indirect measure of the transferrin level), and *serum ferritin.* Marked alterations in the red cell indices usually reflect disorders of maturation or iron deficiency. Clinical laboratories also provide a description of both the red and white cells, a white cell differential count, and the platelet count. In patients with severe anemia and abnormalities in red blood cell morphology, a bone marrow aspirate or biopsy may be important to assist in the diagnosis. Other tests of value in the diagnosis of specific anemias are discussed in chapters on specific disease states.

The components of the CBC also help in the classification of anemia. *Microcytosis* is reflected by a lower than normal MCV

(<80), whereas high values (>100) reflect *macrocytosis*. The MCH and MCHC reflect defects in hemoglobin synthesis (*hypochromia*). Automated cell counters describe the red cell volume distribution width (RDW). The MCV (representing the peak of the distribution curve) is insensitive to the appearance of small populations of macrocytes or microcytes. An experienced laboratory technician will be able to identify minor populations of large or small cells or hypochromic cells before the red cell indices change.

PERIPHERAL BLOOD SMEAR   The peripheral blood smear provides important information about defects in red cell production. As a complement to the red cell indices, the blood smear also reveals variations in cell size (*anisocytosis*) and shape (*poikilocytosis*). The degree of anisocytosis usually correlates with increases in the RDW or the range of cell sizes. Poikilocytosis suggests a defect in the maturation of red cell precursors in the bone marrow or fragmentation of circulating red cells. The blood smear may also reveal *polychromasia*—red cells that are slightly larger than normal and grayish blue in color on the Wright-Giemsa stain. These cells are reticulocytes that have been prematurely released from the bone marrow, and their color represents residual amounts of ribosomal RNA. These cells appear in circulation in response to EPO stimulation or to architectural damage of the bone marrow (fibrosis, infiltration of the marrow by malignant cells, etc.) that results in their disordered release from the marrow. The appearance of nucleated red cells, Howell-Jolly bodies, target cells, sickle cells, and others may provide clues to specific disorders (see Figs. 52-3 to 52-11).

RETICULOCYTE COUNT   An accurate reticulocyte count is key to the initial classification of anemia. Normally, reticulocytes are red cells

TABLE 52-3   *Changes in Normal Hemoglobin/Hematocrit Values with Age and Pregnancy*

Age/Sex	Hemoglobin g/dL	Hematocrit %
At birth	17	52
Childhood	12	36
Adolescence	13	40
Adult man	16 (±2)	47 (±6)
Adult woman (menstruating)	13 (±2)	40 (±6)
Adult woman (postmenopausal)	14 (±2)	42 (±6)
During pregnancy	12 (±2)	37 (±6)

Source: From Hillman and Ault.

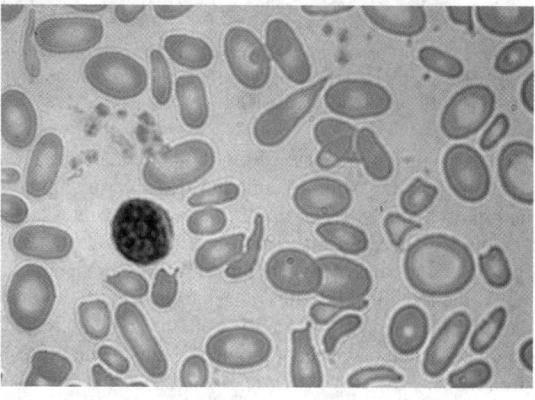

FIGURE 52-4   Severe iron-deficiency anemia. Microcytic and hypochromic red cells smaller than the nucleus of a lymphocyte associated with marked variation in size (anisocytosis) and shape (poikilocytosis). (*From Hillman and Ault.*)

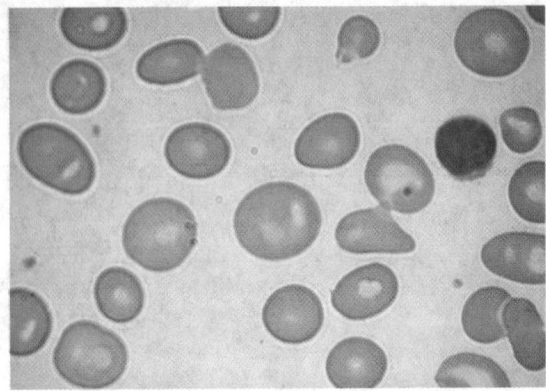

FIGURE 52-5   Macrocytosis. Red cells are larger than a small lymphocyte and well hemoglobinized. Often macrocytes are oval-shaped, so-called macroovalocytes.

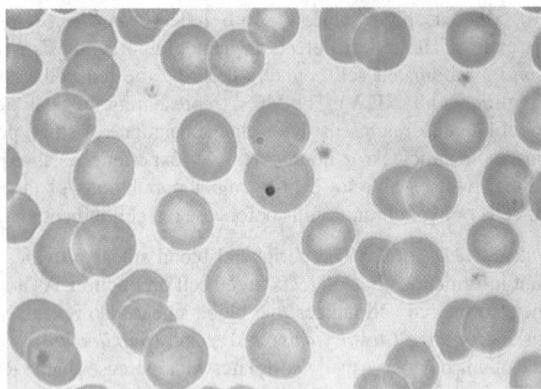

FIGURE 52-6   Howell-Jolly bodies. In the absence of a functional spleen, nuclear remnants are not culled from the red cells and remain as small homogeneously staining blue inclusions on Wright stain. (*From Hillman and Ault.*)

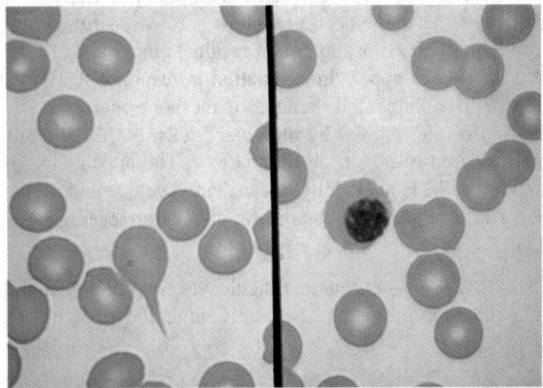

FIGURE 52-7   Red cell changes in myelofibrosis. The left panel shows a teardrop-shaped cell. The right panel shows a nucleated red cell. These forms are seen in myelofibrosis with extramedullary hematopoiesis.

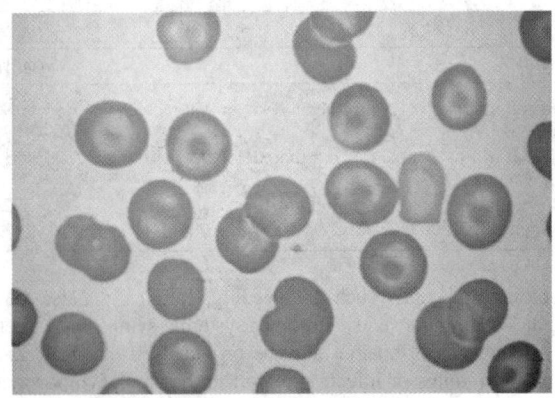

FIGURE 52-8   Target cells. Target cells have a bull's-eye appearance and are seen in thalassemia and in liver disease. (*From Hillman and Ault.*)

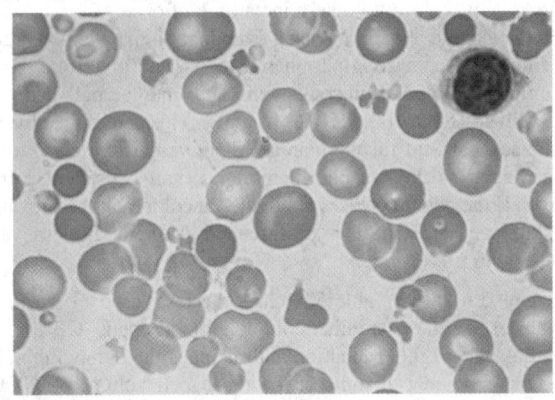

FIGURE 52-9   Red cell fragmentation. Red cells may become fragmented in the presence of foreign bodies in the circulation such as mechanical heart valves or in the setting of thermal injury. (*From Hillman and Ault.*)

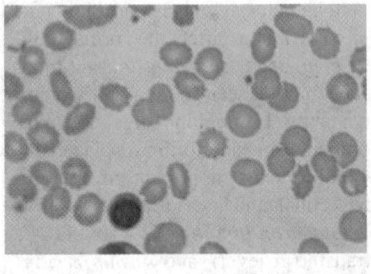

FIGURE 52-10   Uremia. The red cells in uremia may acquire numerous, regularly spaced, small spiny projections. Such cells, called burr cells or echinocytes, are readily distinguishable from irregularly spiculated acanthocytes shown in Fig. 52-11.

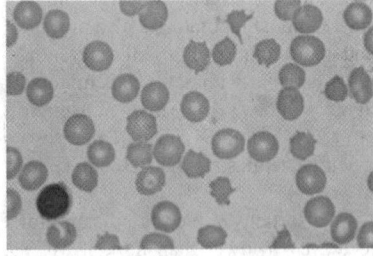

FIGURE 52-11   Spur cells. Spur cells are recognized as distorted red cells containing several irregularly distributed thornlike projections. Cells with this morphologic abnormality are also called acanthocytes. (*Courtesy of Elaine Jaffe, MD.*)

that have been recently released from the bone marrow. They are identified by staining with a supravital dye that precipitates the residual ribosomal RNA (Fig. 52-12). These precipitates appear as blue or black punctate spots. This residual RNA is metabolized over the first 24 to 36 h of the reticulocyte's lifespan in circulation. Normally, the reticulocyte count ranges from 1 to 2% and reflects the daily replacement of 0.8 to 1.0% of the circulating red cell population. A reticulocyte count provides a reliable measure of red cell production.

In the initial classification of anemia, the patient's reticulocyte count is compared with the expected reticulocyte response. In general, if the EPO and erythroid marrow responses to moderate ane-

mia [hemoglobin <100 g/L (10 g/dL)] are intact, the red cell production rate increases to two to three times normal within 10 days following the onset of anemia. In the face of established anemia, a reticulocyte response less than two to three times normal indicates an inadequate marrow response.

In order to use the reticulocyte count to estimate marrow response, two corrections are necessary. The first correction adjusts the reticulocyte count based on the reduced number of circulating red cells. With anemia, the percentage of reticulocytes may be increased while the absolute number is unchanged. To correct for this effect, the reticulocyte percentage is multiplied by the ratio of the patient's hemoglobin or hematocrit to the expected hemoglobin/

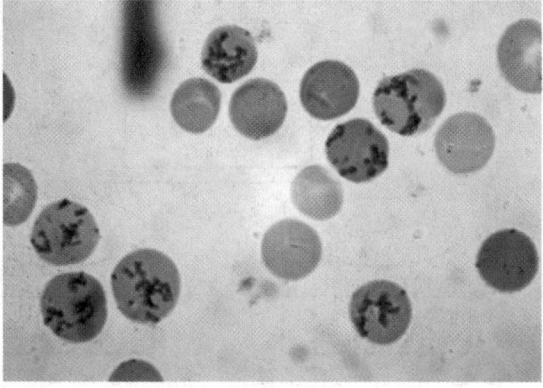

FIGURE 52-12 Reticulocytes. Methylene blue stain demonstrates residual RNA in newly made red cells. (*Courtesy of Elaine Jaffe, MD.*)

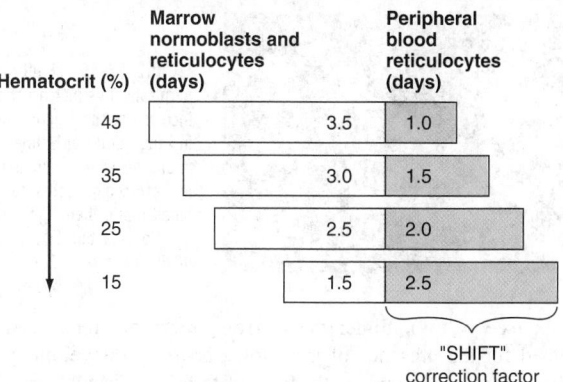

FIGURE 52-13 Correction of reticulocyte count based on level of anemia and the circulatory life span of prematurely released reticulocytes. Erythroid cells take about 4.5 days to mature. At normal hematocrit levels, they are released to the circulation with about 1 day left as reticulocytes. However, with different levels of anemia, erythroid cells are released from the marrow prematurely. Most patients come to clinical attention with hematocrits in the mid-20s and thus, a correction factor of 2 is commonly used because the observed reticulocytes will live for 2 days in the circulation before losing their RNA.

hematocrit for the age and gender of the patient (Table 52-4). This provides an estimate of the reticulocyte count corrected for anemia. In order to convert the corrected reticulocyte count to an index of marrow production, a further correction is required, depending on whether some of the reticulocytes in circulation have been released from the marrow prematurely. For this second correction, the peripheral blood smear is examined to see if there are polychromatophilic macrocytes present. These cells, representing prematurely released reticulocytes, are referred to as "shift" cells, and the relationship between the degree of shift and the necessary shift correction factor is shown in Fig. 52-13. The correction is necessary because these prematurely released cells survive as reticulocytes in circulation for >1 day, thereby providing a falsely high estimate of daily red cell production. If polychromasia is increased, the reticulocyte count, already corrected for anemia, should be divided again by a factor of 2 to account for the prolonged reticulocyte maturation time. The second correction factor varies from 1 to 3 depending on the severity of anemia. In general, a correction of 2 is commonly used. An appropriate correction is shown in Table 52-4. If polychromatophilic cells are not seen on the blood smear, the second correction is not required. The now doubly corrected reticulocyte count is the *reticulocyte production index*, and it provides an estimate of marrow production relative to normal.

Premature release of reticulocytes is normally due to increased EPO stimulation. However, if the integrity of the bone marrow release process is lost through tumor infiltration, fibrosis, or other disorders, the appearance of nucleated red cells or polychromatophilic macrocytes should still invoke the second reticulocyte correction. The shift correction should always be applied to a patient with anemia and a very high reticulocyte count to provide a true index of effective red cell production. Patients with severe chronic hemolytic anemia may increase red cell production as much as six- to sevenfold. This measure alone, therefore, confirms the fact that the patient has an appropriate EPO response, a normally functioning bone marrow, and sufficient iron available to meet the demands for new red cell formation. If the reticulocyte production index is

<2 in the face of established anemia, a defect in erythroid marrow proliferation or maturation must be present.

TESTS OF IRON SUPPLY AND STORAGE The laboratory measurements that reflect the availability of iron for hemoglobin synthesis include the serum iron, the TIBC, and the percent transferrin saturation. The percent transferrin saturation is derived by dividing the serum iron level (× 100) by the TIBC. The normal serum iron ranges from 9 to 27 μmol/L (50 to 150 μg/dL), while the normal TIBC is 54 to 64 μmol/L (300 to 360 μg/dL); the transferrin saturation ranges from 25 to 50%. A diurnal variation in the serum iron leads to a variation in the percent transferrin saturation. The serum ferritin is used to evaluate total-body iron stores. Adult males have serum ferritin levels that average about 100 μg/L, corresponding to iron stores of about 1 g. Adult females have lower serum ferritin levels averaging 30 μg/L, reflecting lower iron stores. A serum ferritin level of 10 to 15 μg/L represents depletion of body iron stores. However, ferritin is also an acute-phase reactant and, in the presence of acute or chronic inflammation, may rise severalfold above baseline levels. As a rule, a serum ferritin >200 μg/L means there is at least some iron in tissue stores.

BONE MARROW EXAMINATION A bone marrow aspirate and smear or a needle biopsy may be useful in the diagnosis of a marrow disorder such as myelofibrosis, a red cell maturation defect, or an infiltrative disease (Figs. 52-14 to 52-16). The increase or decrease of one cell lineage (myeloid vs. erythroid) compared to another is obtained by a differential count of nucleated cells in a bone marrow smear [the myeloid/erythroid (M/E) ratio]. A patient with a hypoproliferative anemia (see below) and a reticulocyte production index <2 will demonstrate an M/E ratio of 2 or 3:1. In contrast, patients with hemolytic disease and a production index >3 will have an M/E ratio of at least 1:1. Maturation disorders are identified from the discrepancy between the M/E ratio and the reticulocyte production

---

TABLE 52-4 *Calculation of Reticulocyte Production Index*

Correction #1 for anemia:
  This correction produces the corrected reticulocyte count
  In a person whose reticulocyte count is 9%, hemoglobin 7.5 g/dL, hematocrit 23%, the absolute reticulocyte count = 9 × (7.5/15)[or ×(23/45)] = 4.5%
Correction #2 for longer life of prematurely released reticulocytes in the blood:
  This correction produces the reticulocyte production index
  In a person whose reticulocyte count is 9%, hemoglobin 7.5 gm/dL, hematocrit 23%, the reticulocyte production index =

$$9 \times \frac{(7.5/15)(\text{hemoglobin correction})}{2 \text{ (maturation time correction)}} = 2.25$$

FIGURE 52-14 Normal bone marrow. This is a low-power view of a section of normal marrow stained with hematoxylin and eosin (H&E). Note that the nucleated cellular elements account for about 40 to 50% and the fat (clear areas) accounts for about 50 to 60% of the area. (*Courtesy of Elaine Jaffe, MD.*)

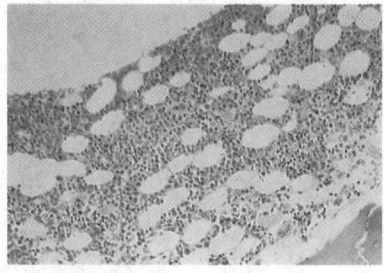

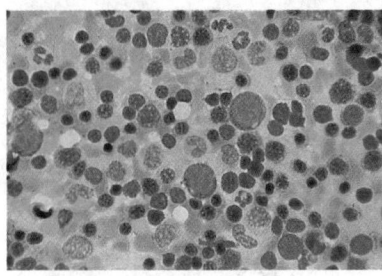

FIGURE 52-15 Erythroid hyperplasia. This marrow shows an increase in the fraction of cells in the erythroid lineage as might be seen when a normal marrow compensates for acute blood loss or hemolysis. The M/E ratio is about 1:1. (*Courtesy of Elaine Jaffe, MD.*)

index (see below). Either the marrow smear or biopsy can be stained for the presence of iron stores or iron in developing red cells. The storage iron is in the form of ferritin or *hemosiderin*. On carefully prepared bone marrow smears, small ferritin granules can normally be seen in 20 to 40% of developing erythroblasts. Such cells are called *sideroblasts*.

Other Laboratory Measurements Additional laboratory tests may be of value in confirming specific diagnoses. →*For details of these tests and how they are applied in individual disorders, see Chaps. 90 to 94.*

DEFINITION AND CLASSIFICATION OF ANEMIA ■ Initial Classification of Anemia
Classifying an anemia according to the functional defect in red cell production helps organize the subsequent use of laboratory studies. The three major classes of anemia are: (1) marrow production defects (*hypoproliferation*), (2) red cell maturation defects (*ineffective erythropoiesis*), and (3) decreased red cell survival (*blood loss/hemolysis*). This functional classification of anemia then guides the selection of specific clinical and laboratory studies designed to complete the differential diagnosis and to plan appropriate therapy. The classification is shown in Fig. 52-17. A hypoproliferative anemia is typically seen with a low reticulocyte production index together with little or no change in red cell morphology (a normocytic, normochromic anemia) (Chap. 90). Maturation disorders typically have a slight to moderately elevated reticulocyte production index that is accompanied by either macrocytic (Chap. 92) or microcytic (Chaps. 90, 91) red cell indices. Increased red blood cell destruction secondary to hemolysis results in an increase in the reticulocyte production index to at least three times normal (Chap. 93), provided sufficient iron is available for hemoglobin synthesis. Hemorrhagic anemia does not typically result in production indices of more than 2.5 times normal because of the limitations placed on expansion of the erythroid marrow by iron availability.

In the first branch point of the classification of anemia, a reticulocyte production index >2.5 indicates that hemolysis is most likely. A reticulocyte production index <2 indicates either a hypoproliferative anemia or maturation disorder. The latter two possibilities can often be distinguished by the red cell indices, by examination of the peripheral blood smear, or by a marrow examination. If the red cell indices are normal, the anemia is almost certainly hypoproliferative in nature. Maturation disorders are characterized by ineffective red cell production and a low reticulocyte production index. Bizarre red cell shapes—macrocytes or hypochromic microcytes—are seen on the peripheral blood smear. With a hypoproliferative anemia, no erythroid hyperpla-

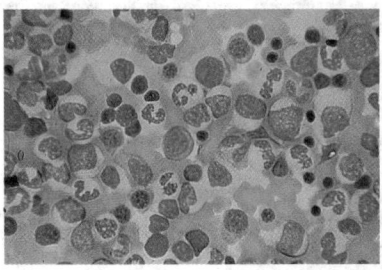

FIGURE 52-16 Myeloid hyperplasia. This marrow shows an increase in the fraction of cells in the myeloid or granulocytic lineage as might be seen in a normal marrow responding to infection. The M/E ratio is >3:1. (*Courtesy of Elaine Jaffe, MD.*)

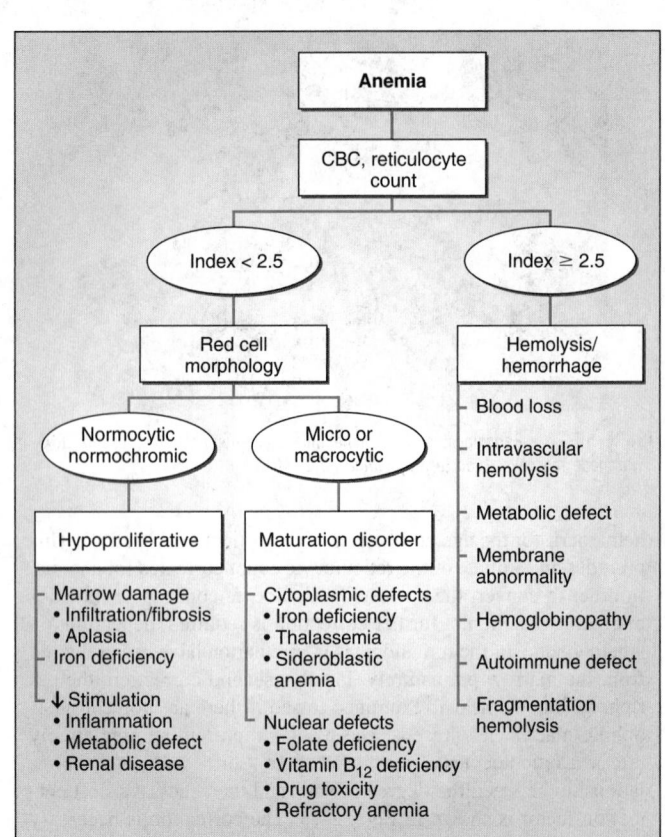

FIGURE 52-17 The physiologic classification of anemia. CBC, complete blood count.

sia is noted in the marrow, whereas patients with ineffective red cell production have erythroid hyperplasia and an M/E ratio <1:1.

Hypoproliferative Anemias At least 75% of all cases of anemia are hypoproliferative in nature. A hypoproliferative anemia reflects absolute or relative marrow failure in which the erythroid marrow has not proliferated appropriately for the degree of anemia. The majority of hypoproliferative anemias are due to mild to moderate iron deficiency or inflammation. A hypoproliferative anemia can result from marrow damage, iron deficiency, or inadequate EPO stimulation. The last may reflect impaired renal function, suppression of EPO production by inflammatory cytokines such as interleukin 1, or reduced tissue needs for O_2 from metabolic disease such as hypothyroidism. Only occasionally is the marrow unable to produce red cells at a normal rate, and this is most prevalent in patients with renal failure. In general, hypoproliferative anemias are characterized by normocytic, normochromic red cells, although microcytic, hypochromic cells may be observed with mild iron deficiency or long-standing chronic inflammatory disease. The key laboratory tests in distinguishing between the various forms of hypoproliferative anemia include the serum iron and iron-binding capacity, evaluation of renal and thyroid function, a marrow biopsy or aspirate to detect marrow damage or infiltrative disease, and serum ferritin to assess iron stores. Occasionally, an iron stain of the marrow will be needed to determine the pattern of iron distribution. Patients with the anemia of acute or chronic inflammation show a distinctive pattern of serum iron (low), TIBC (normal or low), percent transferrin saturation (low), and serum ferritin (normal or high). A distinct pattern of results is noted in mild to moderate iron deficiency (low serum iron, high TIBC, low percent transferrin saturation, low serum ferritin) (Chap. 90). Marrow damage by a drug, infiltrative disease such as leukemia or lymphoma, or marrow aplasia can usually be diagnosed from the peripheral blood and bone marrow morphology. With infiltrative disease or fibrosis, a marrow biopsy will likely be required.

Maturation Disorders The presence of anemia with an inappropriately low reticulocyte production index, macro- or microcytosis on smear, and abnormal red cell indices suggests a maturation disorder. Maturation disorders are divided into two categories: nuclear maturation defects, associated with macrocytosis and abnormal marrow development, and cytoplasmic maturation defects, associated with microcytosis and hypochromia usually from defects in hemoglobin synthesis. The low reticulocyte production index is a reflection of the ineffective erythropoiesis that results from the destruction within the marrow of developing erythroblasts. Marrow morphology shows an M/E ratio of <1:1, diagnostic of erythroid hyperplasia.

Nuclear maturation defects result from vitamin B_{12} or folic acid deficiency, drug damage, or myelodysplasia. Drugs that interfere with cellular DNA metabolism, such as methotrexate or alkylating agents, can produce a nuclear maturation defect. Alcohol, alone, is also capable of producing macrocytosis and a variable degree of anemia, but this is usually associated with coincident folic acid deficiency. Measurements of folic acid and vitamin B_{12} are key not only in identifying the specific vitamin deficiency but also because they reflect different pathogenetic mechanisms.

Cytoplasmic maturation defects result from severe iron deficiency or abnormalities in globin or heme synthesis. Iron deficiency occupies an unusual position in the classification of anemia. If the iron-deficiency anemia is mild to moderate, erythroid marrow proliferation is decreased and the anemia is classified as hypoproliferative. However, if the anemia is severe and prolonged, the erythroid marrow will become hyperplastic despite the inadequate iron supply, and the anemia will be classified as ineffective erythropoiesis with a cytoplasmic maturation defect. In either case, a reduced reticulocyte production index, microcytosis, and a classic pattern of iron values make the diagnosis clear and easily distinguish iron deficiency from other cytoplasmic maturation defects such as the thalassemias. Defects in heme synthesis, in contrast to globin synthesis, are less common and may be acquired or inherited (Chap. 337). Acquired abnormalities are usually associated with myelodysplasia, may lead to either a macro- or microcytic anemia, and are frequently associated with mitochondrial iron loading. In these cases, iron is taken up by the mitochondria of the developing erythroid cell but not incorporated into heme. The iron-encrusted mitochondria surround the nucleus of the erythroid cell, forming a ring. Based on the distinctive finding of so-called ringed sideroblasts on the marrow iron stain, patients are diagnosed as having a sideroblastic anemia—almost always reflecting myelodysplasia. Again, studies of iron parameters are helpful in the differential diagnosis and management of these patients.

Blood Loss/Hemolytic Anemia   In contrast to anemias associated with an inappropriately low reticulocyte production index, blood loss or hemolysis is associated with red cell production indices ≥2.5 times normal. The stimulated erythropoiesis is reflected in the blood smear by the appearance of increased numbers of polychromatophilic macrocytes. A marrow examination is rarely indicated if the reticulocyte production index is increased appropriately. The red cell indices are typically normocytic or slightly macrocytic, reflecting the increased number of reticulocytes. Acute blood loss is not associated with an increased reticulocyte production index because of the time required to increase EPO production and, subsequently, marrow proliferation. Subacute blood loss may be associated with modest reticulocytosis. Anemia from chronic blood loss presents more often as iron deficiency than with the picture of increased red cell production.

The evaluation of blood loss anemia is usually not difficult. Most problems arise when a patient presents with an increased red cell production index from an episode of acute blood loss that went unrecognized. The cause of the anemia and increased red cell production may not be obvious. The confirmation of a recovering state may require observations over a period of 2 to 3 weeks, during which the hemoglobin concentration will be seen to rise and the reticulocyte production index fall.

Hemolytic disease, while dramatic, is among the least common forms of anemia. The ability to sustain a high reticulocyte production index reflects the ability of the erythroid marrow to compensate for hemolysis and the efficient recycling of iron from the destroyed red cells to support new hemoglobin synthesis. The level of response will depend on the severity of the anemia and the nature of the underlying disease process.

Hemoglobinopathies, such as sickle cell disease and the thalassemias, present a mixed picture. The reticulocyte index may be high but is inappropriately low for the degree of marrow erythroid hyperplasia (Chap. 91).

Hemolytic anemias present in different ways. Some appear suddenly as an acute, self-limited episode of intravascular or extravascular hemolysis, a presentation pattern often seen in patients with autoimmune hemolysis or with inherited defects of the Embden-Meyerhof pathway or the glutathione reductase pathway. Patients with inherited disorders of the hemoglobin molecule or red cell membrane generally have a lifelong clinical history typical of the disease process. Those with chronic hemolytic disease, such as hereditary spherocytosis, may actually present not with anemia but with a complication stemming from the prolonged increase in red cell destruction such as aplastic crisis, symptomatic bilirubin gallstones, or splenomegaly.

The differential diagnosis of an acute or chronic hemolytic event requires the careful integration of family history, pattern of clinical presentation, and a number of highly specific laboratory studies (Chap. 93). Some of the more common congenital hemolytic anemias may be identified from the red cell morphology, a routine laboratory test such as hemoglobin electrophoresis, or a screen for red cell enzymes. Acquired defects in red cell survival are often immunologically mediated and require a direct or indirect antiglobulin test or a cold agglutinin titer to detect the presence of hemolytic antibodies or complement-mediated red cell destruction.

℞ TREATMENT

An overriding principle is to initiate treatment of mild to moderate anemia only when a specific diagnosis is made. Rarely, in the acute setting, anemia may be so severe that red cell transfusions are required before a specific diagnosis is made. Whether the anemia is of acute or gradual onset, the selection of the appropriate treatment is determined by the documented cause(s) of the anemia. Often, the cause of the anemia may be multifactorial. For example, a patient with severe rheumatoid arthritis who has been taking anti-inflammatory drugs may have a hypoproliferative anemia associated with chronic inflammation as well as chronic blood loss associated with intermittent gastrointestinal bleeding. In every circumstance, it is important to evaluate the patient's iron status fully before and during the treatment of any anemia. →*Transfusion is discussed in Chap. 99; iron therapy is discussed in Chap. 90; treatment of megaloblastic anemia is discussed in Chap. 92; treatment of other entities is discussed in their respective chapters (sickle cell anemia, Chap. 91; hemolytic anemias, Chap. 93; aplastic anemia and myelodysplasia, Chap. 94).*

Therapeutic options for the treatment of anemias have expanded dramatically during the past 25 years. Blood component therapy is available and safe. Recombinant EPO as an adjunct to anemia management has transformed the lives of patients with chronic renal failure on dialysis. Improvements in the management of sickle cell crises and sickle cell anemia also have occurred. Eventually, patients with inherited disorders of globin synthesis or mutations in the globin gene, such as sickle cell disease, may benefit from the successful introduction of targeted genetic therapy (Chap. 59).

POLYCYTHEMIA

Polycythemia is defined as an increase in circulating red blood cells above normal. This increase may be real or only apparent because of a decrease in plasma volume (spurious or relative). The term *erythrocytosis* may be used interchangeably with polycythemia, but some draw a distinction between them; erythrocytosis implies documentation of increased red cell mass, whereas polycythemia refers to any increase in red cells. Often patients with polycythemia are detected through an incidental finding of elevated hemoglobin or hematocrit levels. Concern that the hemoglobin level may be abnormally high is usually triggered at 170 g/L (17 g/dL) for men and 150 g/L (15 g/dL) for women. Hematocrit levels >50% in men or >45% in women may be abnormal. Hematocrits >60% in men and >55% in women are almost invariably associated with increased red cell mass.

Historic features useful in the differential diagnosis include smoking history; living at high altitude; or a history of congenital heart disease, peptic ulcer disease, sleep apnea, chronic lung disease, or renal disease.

Patients with polycythemia may be asymptomatic or experience symptoms related to the increased red cell mass or an underlying disease process that leads to increased red cell production. The dominant symptoms from increased red cell mass are related to hyperviscosity and thrombosis (both venous and arterial), because the blood viscosity increases logarithmically at hematocrits >55%. Manifestations range from digital ischemia to Budd-Chiari syndrome with hepatic vein thrombosis. Abdominal thromboses are particularly common. Neurologic symptoms such as vertigo, tinnitus, headache, and visual disturbances may occur. Hypertension is often present. Patients with *polycythemia vera* may have aquagenic pruritus and symptoms related to hepatosplenomegaly. Patients may have easy bruising, epistaxis, or bleeding from the gastrointestinal tract. Patients with hypoxemia may develop cyanosis on minimal exertion or have headache, impaired mental acuity, and fatigue.

The physical examination usually reveals a ruddy complexion. Splenomegaly favors polycythemia vera as the diagnosis (Chap. 95). The presence of cyanosis or evidence of a right-to-left shunt suggests congenital heart disease presenting in the adult, particularly tetralogy of Fallot or Eisenmenger syndrome (Chap. 218). Increased blood viscosity raises pulmonary artery pressure; hypoxemia can lead to increased pulmonary vascular resistance. Together these factors can produce cor pulmonale.

Polycythemia can be spurious (related to a decrease in plasma volume; Gaisbock's syndrome), primary, or secondary in origin. The secondary causes are all associated with increases in EPO levels: either a physiologically adapted appropriate elevation based on tissue hypoxia (lung disease, high altitude, CO poisoning, high-affinity hemoglobinopathy) or an abnormal overproduction (renal cysts, renal artery stenosis, tumors with ectopic EPO production). A rare familial form of polycythemia is associated with normal EPO levels but hyperresponsive EPO receptors due to mutations.

APPROACH TO THE PATIENT

As shown in Fig. 52-18, the first step is to document the presence of an increased red cell mass using the principle of isotope dilution by administering ^{51}Cr-labeled autologous red blood cells to the patient and sampling blood radioactivity over a 2-h period. If the red cell mass is normal (<36 mL/kg in men, <32 mL/kg in women), the patient has spurious polycythemia. If the red cell mass is increased (>36 mL/kg in men, >32 mL/kg in women), serum EPO levels should be measured. If EPO levels are low or unmeasurable, the patient most likely has polycythemia vera. Ancillary tests that support this diagnosis include elevated white blood cell count, increased absolute basophil count, thrombocytosis, elevated leukocyte alkaline phosphatase levels, and elevated serum vitamin B_{12} and vitamin B_{12}–binding protein levels.

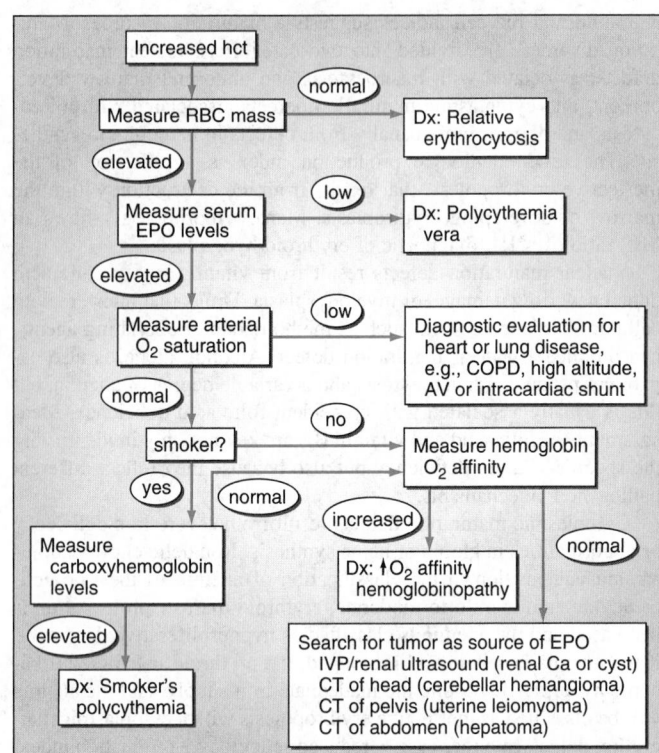

FIGURE 52-18 An approach to diagnosing patients with polycythemia. RBC, red blood cell; EPO, erythropoietin; COPD, chronic obstructive pulmonary disease; AV, atrioventricular; IVP, intravenous pyelogram; CT, computed tomography.

If serum EPO levels are elevated, one attempts to distinguish whether the elevation is a physiologic response to hypoxia or is related to autonomous production. Patients with low arterial O_2 saturation (<92%) should be further evaluated for the presence of heart or lung disease, if they are not living at high altitude. Patients with normal O_2 saturation who are smokers may have elevated EPO levels because of CO displacement of O_2. If carboxyhemoglobin (COHb) levels are high, the diagnosis is smoker's polycythemia. Such patients should be urged to stop smoking. Those who cannot stop smoking require phlebotomy to control their polycythemia. Patients with normal O_2 saturation who do not smoke either have an abnormal hemoglobin that does not deliver O_2 to the tissues (evaluated by finding elevated O_2-hemoglobin affinity) or have a source of EPO production that is not responding to the normal feedback inhibition. Further workup is dictated by the differential diagnosis of EPO-producing neoplasms. Hepatoma, uterine leiomyoma, and renal cancer or cysts are all detectable with abdominopelvic computed tomography scans. Cerebellar hemangiomas may produce EPO, but they nearly always present with localizing neurologic signs and symptoms rather than polycythemia-related symptoms.

ACKNOWLEDGMENT
Dr. Robert S. Hillman wrote this chapter in the 14th edition, and elements of his chapter were retained here.

FURTHER READING

HILLMAN RS, AULT KA: *Hematology in Clinical Practice.* New York, McGraw-Hill, 2002

53 BLEEDING AND THROMBOSIS
Robert I. Handin

Hemorrhage, intravascular thrombosis, and embolism are common clinical manifestations of many diseases. The normal hemostatic system limits blood loss by precisely regulated interactions between components of the vessel wall, blood platelets, and plasma proteins. However, when disease or trauma damages large arteries and veins, excessive bleeding may occur, despite a normal hemostatic system. Less frequently, hemorrhage is caused by an inherited or acquired disorder of the hemostatic machinery itself. A large number of bleeding disorders have been identified.

In addition, unregulated activation of the hemostatic system may cause thrombosis and embolism, which can reduce blood flow to critical organs such as the brain and myocardium. Although we understand less about the pathophysiology of thrombosis than of hemostatic failure, certain patient groups have been identified that are particularly prone to thrombosis and embolism. These include patients who (1) are immobilized after surgery, (2) have chronic congestive heart failure, (3) have atherosclerotic vascular disease, (4) have a malignancy, or (5) are pregnant. Most of these "thrombosis-prone" patients have inherited or acquired "hypercoagulable" or "prethrombotic" disorders.

Certain information in the patient's history, such as the mode of onset and sites of bleeding, a family bleeding tendency, and a record of drug ingestion, helps establish the correct diagnosis. Physical examination can identify bleeding in the skin or joint deformities due to previous hemarthroses. Ultimately, however, bleeding disorders are diagnosed by laboratory tests. General screening tests are used first, to document a systemic disorder, and are then supplemented by specific tests of coagulation protein or platelet function to arrive at an accurate diagnosis.

The hypercoagulable or prethrombotic patient can also be identified by a careful history. Three important clues to this diagnosis are: (1) repeated episodes of thromboembolism without an obvious predisposing condition, (2) a family history of thrombosis, and (3) well-documented thromboembolism in adolescents and young adults. All of the known inherited prethrombotic disorders can be diagnosed with specific immunologic, functional, or genetic tests.

NORMAL HEMOSTASIS

Accurate diagnosis and treatment of patients with either bleeding or thrombosis require knowledge of the pathophysiology of hemostasis. The process can be divided into primary and secondary components and is initiated when trauma, surgery, or disease disrupts the vascular endothelial lining and blood is exposed to subendothelial connective tissue. *Primary hemostasis* is the name given to the process of platelet plug formation at sites of injury. It occurs within seconds of injury and is of prime importance in stopping blood loss from capillaries, small arterioles, and venules (Fig. 53-1). *Secondary hemostasis* consists of the reactions of the plasma coagulation system that result in fibrin formation. It requires several minutes for completion. The fibrin strands that are produced strengthen the primary hemostatic plug. This reaction is particularly important in larger vessels and prevents bleeding from recurring hours or days after the injury. Although presented here as separate events, primary and secondary hemostasis are closely linked. For example, activated platelets accelerate plasma coagulation, and products of the plasma coagulation reaction, such as thrombin, induce platelet activation.

Effective primary hemostasis requires three critical events—platelet adhesion, granule release, and platelet aggregation. Within a few seconds of injury, platelets adhere to collagen fibrils in vascular subendothelium by at least two collagen receptors, glycoprotein (Gp) Ia/IIa, a member of the integrin family, and GpVI. GpVI binding of collagen transduces signals that activate platelets through the Fc receptor (FcRγ). As shown in Fig. 53-2, this interaction with collagen is stabilized by the von Willebrand factor (vWF), an adhesive glyco-

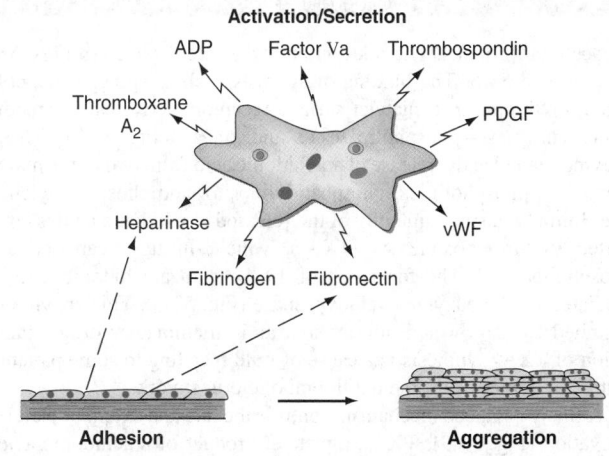

FIGURE 53-1 Schematic presentation of the major events in primary hemostasis. The first event is platelet adhesion, the interaction of platelets with a nonplatelet surface such as vascular subendothelium. This is followed by platelet activation and secretion. Some of the products secreted by platelets are depicted. Abbreviations: ADP, adenosine diphosphate; PDGF, platelet-derived growth factor; vWF, von Willebrand factor. The final event is the binding of activated platelets to the adherent monolayer in the process of platelet aggregation.

protein that allows platelets to remain attached to the vessel wall despite the high shear forces generated within the vascular lumen. The vWF accomplishes this task by forming a link between a platelet receptor site on Gp Ib/IX and collagen fibrils. The adherent, activated platelets then release preformed granule constituents and generate de novo mediators like those depicted in Fig. 53-1.

As in other cells, platelet activation and secretion are regulated by changes in the level of cyclic nucleotides, the influx of calcium, hydrolysis of membrane phospholipids, and phosphorylation of critical

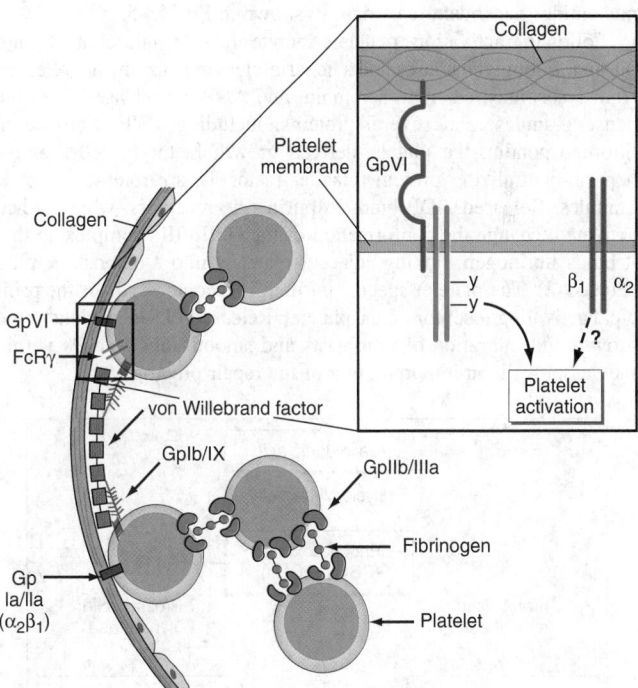

FIGURE 53-2 The molecular basis of platelet adhesion and aggregation. Adhesion of platelets to vascular subendothelium is facilitated by the interaction of two platelet collagen receptors, GpIa/IIa ($\alpha_2\beta_1$) integrin and GpVI with collagen. The binding of collagen to GpVI causes it to interact with FcRγ, which is phosphorylated and transduces activation signals in the platelet. Adhesion is stabilized by the von Willebrand factor, which forms a bridge between collagen fibrils in the vessel wall and receptors on platelet glycoprotein Ib/IX (GpIb/IX). In a similar manner, platelet aggregation is mediated by fibrinogen, which links adjacent platelets via receptors on the platelet glycoprotein IIb/IIIa complex (GpIIb/IIIa, α_{IIb}/β_3).

337

intracellular proteins. The relevant pathways are depicted in Figs. 53-3, 53-4, and 53-5. The binding of agonists such as epinephrine, collagen, or thrombin to platelet surface receptors activates two membrane enzymes—phospholipase C and phospholipase A_2. These enzymes catalyze the release of arachidonic acid from two of the major membrane phospholipids, phosphatidylinositol and phosphatidylcholine. Initially, a small quantity of the released arachidonic acid is converted to thromboxane A_2 (TXA_2), which, in turn, can activate phospholipase C. The formation of TXA_2 from arachidonic acid is mediated by the enzyme cyclooxygenase (Fig. 53-3). This enzyme is inhibited by aspirin and nonsteroidal anti-inflammatory drugs. Inhibition of TXA_2 synthesis is a cause of mild bleeding in some patients and is the same way some antithrombotic drugs work.

A finely balanced mechanism controls the rate and extent of platelet activation (Fig. 53-3). TXA_2, a platelet product of arachidonic acid, stimulates platelet activation and secretion. In contrast, prostacyclin, an endothelial cell product of arachidonic acid metabolism, inhibits platelet activation by raising intraplatelet levels of cyclic adenosine monophosphate. In addition, endothelial cells have an ecto-ADPase on their surface that hydrolyzes the platelet agonist adenosine diphosphate (ADP) and limits its effects.

Platelet signal transduction pathways are complex (Fig. 53-4). Potential platelet-activating agents bind to a surface receptor that initiates a cascade of signaling events. The four major classes of receptors are: (1) GpIb/IX complex that binds vWF; (2) integrin family receptors [GpIIB/IIIa ($\alpha IIb\beta_3$) binds fibrinogen; GpIa/IIa ($\alpha_2\beta_1$) binds collagen]; (3) seven membrane-spanning "serpentine" receptors that bind thrombin (PAR1) or TXA_2; and (4) GpVI/FcγRIIa that binds collagen. Signaling induces calcium flux and leads to remodeling of the cytoskeleton, change in shape, formation of filopodia, and granule release. These changes allow the platelet to adhere to substrata and form intravascular aggregates in concert with platelet and matrix glycoproteins such as collagen, vWF, and fibrinogen. The details of the guanine nucleotide–dependent reactions are shown in Fig. 53-5.

Following activation, platelets secrete their granule contents into plasma. Endoglycosidases and a heparin-cleaving enzyme are released from lysosomes; calcium, serotonin, and ADP are released from the dense granules; and several proteins, including vWF, fibronectin, thrombospondin, the platelet-derived growth factor (PDGF), and a heparin-neutralizing protein (platelet factor 4), are released from α granules. Released ADP binds to purinergic receptors, which, when activated, change the conformation of the GpIIb/IIIa complex so that it binds fibrinogen, linking adjacent platelets into a hemostatic plug (Fig. 53-2). The platelet-specific purinergic receptor P_2Y_{12} is the principal activating receptor on the platelet. Released PDGF stimulates the growth and migration of fibroblasts and smooth-muscle cells within the vessel wall, an important part of the repair process.

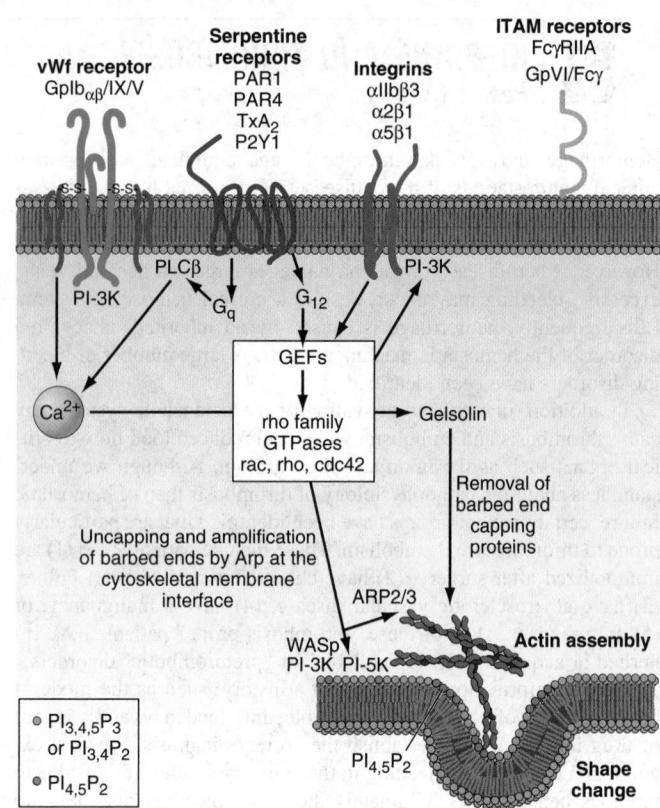

FIGURE 53-4   Platelet signal transduction overview. Actin assembly, platelet shape change, granule secretion, and the activation of some receptors are regulated by the level of intracellular calcium, the activity of guanosine triphosphatases (GTPases), and the synthesis of polyphosphoinositides. The best understood signal transduction pathway involves the multimembrane-spanning or serpentine receptors that include as agonists thrombin and thromboxane A_2. As shown, the receptors couple to downstream signaling molecules via heterotrimeric G proteins. For example, thrombin binding to PAR1 leads to the phosphorylation and dissociation of the Gq trimer complex, the activation of phospholipase $C\beta$ (PLCβ), the hydrolysis of membrane phosphatidylinositol 4,5-bisphosphate ($PI_{4,5}P_2$) to inositol 1,4,5-triphosphate (IP_3), and diacylglycerol (DAG). IP_3 binds to receptors on the smooth endoplasmic reticulum to release calcium into the cytosol. Calcium then activates gelsolin, which fragments actin filaments and mediates the activation of myosin II by myosin light chain kinase (MLCK). At the same time trimeric guanosine triphosphatase (GTPase) G_{12} is activated, leading to the stimulation of guanine exchange factors (GEFs) that activate small GTPases of the rhoA family. GTP-rac activates downstream effectors including the lipid kinases phosphoinositide 5-kinase (PI-5K) and phosphoinositide 3-kinase (PI-3K). Activation of other receptors, as shown in the figure, induces other signal transduction pathways with parallel but distinct effects. Stimulation of receptors such as GpVI and FcγRIIA, which contain an immunoreceptor tyrosine-based activation motif (ITAM), increases tyrosine phosphorylation of these receptors, the tyrosine kinase Syk, the adaptor SLP76, and PLCγ. Phosphorylation activates PLCγ to hydrolyze lipids, which, in turn, promote calcium release and actin assembly. These are two of the complex signaling pathways leading to platelet activation. [*From JH Hartwig, JE Italiano, Jr, in RI Handin et al (eds), Blood: Principles and Practice of Hematology, 2d ed. Philadelphia, Lippincott Williams & Wilkins, 2003, pp 1062–1079; with permission.*]

As the primary hemostatic plug is being formed, plasma coagulation proteins are activated to initiate secondary hemostasis. An overall picture of the coagulation scheme, including the role of various inhibitors, is shown in Fig. 53-6. In the classic view of coagulation, four reactions have been defined (Fig. 53-7) that culminate in the production of enough thrombin to convert a small amount of plasma fibrinogen to fibrin. Each of the reactions requires the formation of a surface-bound complex and the conversion of inactive precursor proteins into active proteases by limited proteolysis, and each is regulated by both plasma and cellular cofactors and calcium.

In *reaction 1*, the intrinsic, or contact, phase of coagulation, three plasma proteins, Hageman factor (factor XII), high-molecular-weight kininogen (HMWK), and prekallikrein (PK), form a complex on vascular subendothelial collagen. After binding to HMWK, factor XII is slowly converted to an active protease (XIIa), which then activates PK to kallikrein and factor XI to XIa. Kallikrein accelerates the conversion

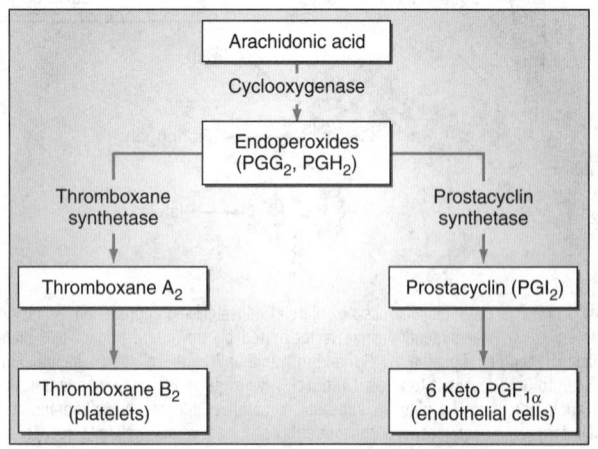

FIGURE 53-3   Generation of thromboxane A_2 in platelets and prostacyclin (PGI_2) in endothelial cells.

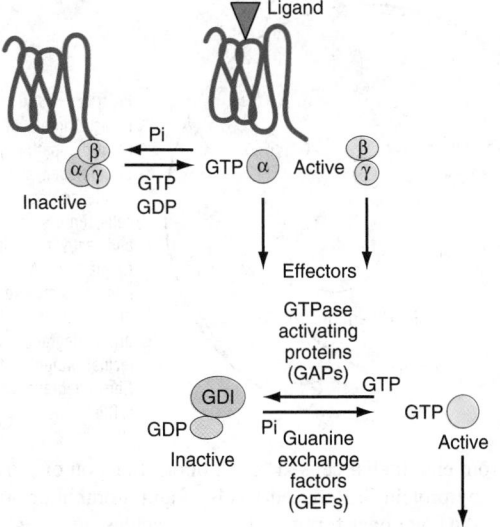

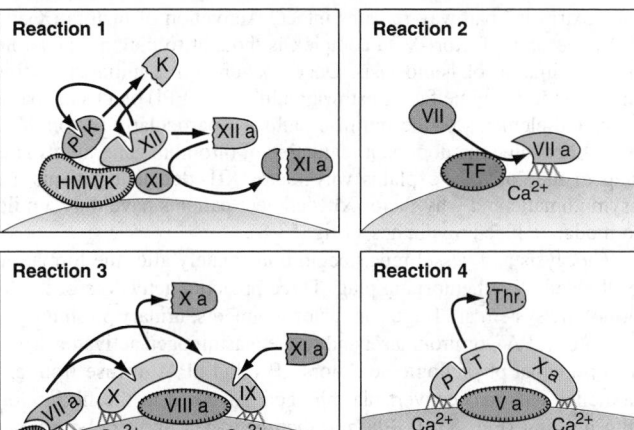

FIGURE 53-5   A more detailed look at G protein activation and inactivation—a key step in platelet and other cellular signal transduction pathways. G proteins exist as inactive membrane-bound heterotrimeric (α, β, γ) complexes. Binding of ligand to one of the multimembrane-spanning (usually 7 passes through the membrane) receptors leads to the conversion of the inactive guanosine diphosphate (GDP) form of the G protein complex to the active guanosine triphosphate (GTP) form that then dissociates into the GTP-α and the β, γ subunits. The dissociated subunits go on to mediate downstream events as shown in Fig. 53-4. GTP-activating proteins (GAPs) convert GTP to GDP, which then favors reassociation of the subunits to form the inactive heterotrimer. GDP dissociation inhibitors (GDI) maintain the α-GDP complex in an inactive state. The released Pi is then added to the low-molecular-weight small G proteins in the cytosol by the guanine nucleotide exchange factors (GEFs). The active forms of these low-molecular-weight G proteins also effect downstream events shown in Fig. 53-4. [From JH Hartwig, JE Italiano, Jr, in RI Handin et al (eds), Blood: Principles and Practice of Hematology, 2d ed. Philadelphia, Lippincott William & Wilkins, 2003, pp 1062–1079; with permission.]

FIGURE 53-7   The major coagulation reactions are subdivided and depicted in schematic form to emphasize their similarity. They all rely on the formation of surface-bound enzyme-cofactor complexes. Abbreviations: PK, prekallikrein; K, kallikrein; HMWK, high-molecular-weight kininogen; TF, tissue factor; Ca²⁺, calcium; PT, prothrombin; Thr, thrombin. By convention, other coagulation factors are indicated by roman numerals, with a lowercase "a" appended to indicate their active form. The ^^^ is used to indicate the Gla (di-γ-carboxyglutamic acid)–containing domains of factors VII, IX, X, Xa, and PT, which bind calcium and phospholipid. Hatching is used to indicate proteins that adhere to surfaces by hydrophobic interaction.

of XII to XIIa, while XIa participates in subsequent coagulation reactions. An alternative mechanism for the activation of factor XI may exist, as patients who are deficient in either factor XII, HMWK, or PK have apparently normal hemostasis and no clinical bleeding.

Reaction 2 provides a second pathway to initiate coagulation by activating factor VII to a protease. In this extrinsic, or tissue factor–dependent, pathway, a complex is formed between factor VII, calcium, and tissue factor, a ubiquitous lipoprotein present in cellular membranes and exposed by cellular injury. The tissue factor–VII pathway

is continuously active and makes a major contribution to basal coagulation; indeed, it seems to be the major way to initiate coagulation. Factor VII and three other coagulation proteins—factors II (prothrombin), IX, and X—require calcium and vitamin K for biologic activity. These proteins are synthesized in the liver, where a vitamin K–dependent carboxylase catalyzes a unique posttranslational modification that adds a second carboxyl group to certain glutamic acid residues. Pairs of these di-γ-carboxyglutamic acid (Gla) residues bind calcium, which alters protein comformation for binding to phospholipid surfaces and confers biologic activity. Inhibition of this modification by vitamin K antagonists (e.g., warfarin) is the basis of one of the most common forms of anticoagulant therapy.

In *reaction 3*, factor X is activated by the proteases generated in the two previous reactions. In one reaction, a calcium- and lipid-dependent complex is formed between factors VIII, IX, and X. Within this complex, factor IX is first converted to IXa by factor XIa that was generated within the intrinsic pathway (reaction 1). Factor X is then activated by factor IXa in concert with factor VIII. Alternatively, both factors IX and X can be activated more directly by factor VIIa, generated via the extrinsic pathway (reaction 2). Activation of factors IX and X provides a link between the intrinsic and extrinsic coagulation pathways (Fig. 53-6).

Reaction 4, the final step, converts prothrombin to thrombin in the presence of factor V, calcium, and phospholipid. Although prothrombin conversion can take place on various natural and artificial phospholipid-rich surfaces, it proceeds several thousand times faster on the surface of activated platelets or endothelial cells. Thrombin has multiple functions in hemostasis. Although its principal role in hemostasis is the conversion of fibrinogen to fibrin, it also activates factors V, VIII, and XIII and stimulates platelet aggregation and secretion. Following the release of fibrinopeptides A and B from the α and β chains of fibrinogen, the modified molecule, now called *fibrin monomer*, polymerizes into an insoluble gel. The fibrin polymer is then stabilized by the cross-linking of individual chains by factor XIIIa, a plasma transglutaminase (Fig. 53-6).

Although the classic view of coagulation had clinical utility, it left several important questions unanswered: (1) Why does factor XII deficiency dramatically prolong partial thromboplastin time (PTT) but not cause bleeding? (2) Why is there heterogeneity in the bleeding symptoms of patients with factor XI deficiency? (3) Why do deficiencies in factors VIII or IX produce such dramatic bleeding even though

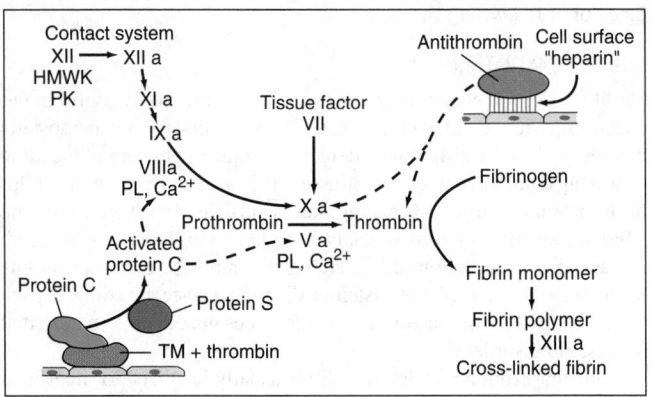

FIGURE 53-6   A schematic diagram of some of the clinically important coagulation reactions. The unactivated or precursor proteins are indicated by roman numerals, and the active form by the addition of a lowercase "a"—a standard convention. Other abbreviations: HMWK, high-molecular-weight kininogen; PK, prekallikrein; PL, phospholipid; TM, thrombomodulin; Ca²⁺, calcium. There are two independent activation pathways, the contact system and the tissue factor–mediated, or extrinsic, system. They merge at the point of factor X activation and lead to the generation of thrombin, which converts fibrinogen into fibrin. These reactions are regulated by antithrombin, which forms complexes with all of the coagulation protein serine proteases except factor VII, and by the protein C–protein S system, which inactivates factors V and VIII.

the "extrinsic" pathway remains intact? Activation of factors IX and X by the tissue factor–VIIa complex is thought to play a major role in the initiation of hemostasis. Once coagulation is initiated by this interaction, the tissue factor pathway inhibitor (TFPI) blocks the pathway, and elements of the intrinsic pathway, particularly factors VIII and IX, become the dominant regulators of thrombin generation. This step in the pathway explains why factor XII–deficient patients are asymptomatic and why factor XI–deficient patients have only a mild to moderate bleeding diathesis (Fig. 53-8).

Clot lysis and vessel repair begin immediately after the formation of the definitive hemostatic plug. Three potential activators of the fibrinolytic system are Hageman factor fragments; urinary plasminogen activator (uPA), or urokinase; and tissue plasminogen activator (tPA). The principal physiologic activators, tPA and uPA, diffuse from endothelial cells and convert plasminogen, adsorbed to the fibrin clot, into plasmin (Fig. 53-9). Plasmin then degrades fibrin polymer into small fragments, which are cleared by the monocyte-macrophage scavenger system. Although plasmin can also degrade fibrinogen, the reaction remains localized because (1) tPA and some forms of uPA activate plasminogen more effectively when it is adsorbed to fibrin clots; (2) any plasmin that enters the circulation is rapidly bound and neutralized by the α_2 plasmin inhibitor (patients who lack this factor have unchecked fibrinolysis and bleed); and (3) endothelial cells release a plasminogen activator inhibitor (PAI) 1, which blocks the action of tPA.

Only a small quantity of each coagulation enzyme is converted to its active form. As a consequence, the hemostatic plug does not propagate beyond the site of injury. Precise regulation is important, since each milliliter of blood contains enough clotting material to clot all the fibrinogen in the body in 10 to 15 s. Blood fluidity is maintained by the flow of blood, the adsorption of coagulation factors to surfaces and their trapping in the emerging clot, and by multiple inhibitors in plasma. These factors reduce the concentration of these potent enzymes and cofactors and reduce reaction rates. Antithrombin, proteins C and S, and TFPI are important inhibitors that maintain blood fluidity.

These inhibitors have distinct modes of action. Antithrombin forms complexes with all serine protease coagulation factors except factor VII (Fig. 53-6). Rates of complex formation are accelerated by heparin and heparin-like molecules on the surface of the endothelial cells. Heparin's ability to accelerate antithrombin activity is the basis for its anticoagulant action. Protein C is converted to an active protease by thrombin after it is bound to an endothelial cell protein called *thrombomodulin*. Activated protein C then inactivates the two plasma cofactors V and VIII by limited proteolysis, which slows down two critical coagulation reactions. Protein C may also stimulate the release

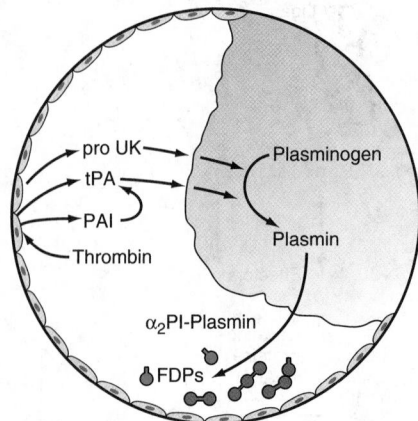

FIGURE 53-9 A schematic diagram of the fibrinolytic pathway. Tissue plasminogen activator (tPA) is released from endothelial cells, enters the fibrin clot, and activates plasminogen to plasmin. Any free plasmin is complexed with α_2 plasmin inhibitor (α_2PI). Fibrin is degraded to low-molecular-weight fragments, fibrin degradation products (FDPs).

of tPA from endothelial cells. The inhibitory function of protein C is enhanced by protein S. Reduced levels of antithrombin or proteins C and S, or dysfunctional forms of these molecules, result in a hypercoagulable or prethrombotic state. In addition, a particularly common heritable defect associated with a hypercoagulable state is the presence of a form of factor V (factor V Leiden) that is resistant to protein C inhibition. Between 20 and 50% of patients with unexplained venous thromboembolism have this defect.

Blood coagulation is not uniform throughout the body. The composition of the blood clot varies with the site of injury. Hemostatic plugs or thrombi that form in veins where blood flow is slow are rich in fibrin and trapped red blood cells and contain relatively few platelets. They are often called *red thrombi* because of their appearance in surgical and pathologic specimens. The friable ends of these red thrombi, which most often form in leg veins, can break off and embolize to the pulmonary circulation. Conversely, clots that form in arteries under conditions of high flow are predominantly composed of platelets and have little fibrin. These *white thrombi* may readily dislodge from the arterial wall and embolize to distant sites, causing temporary or permanent ischemia. These clots are a particularly common cause of embolism in the cerebral and retinal circulation, where they may lead to transient neurologic dysfunction (transient ischemic attacks), including temporary monocular blindness (amaurosis fugax), or to strokes. In addition, most episodes of myocardial infarction are due to thrombi that form after the rupture of atherosclerotic plaques within diseased coronary arteries. Hemostatic plugs, which are a physiologic response to injury, are very similar to pathologic thrombi. Thrombosis has been described as coagulation occurring in the wrong place or at the wrong time.

CLINICAL EVALUATION

HISTORY Certain elements of the history are particularly useful in determining whether bleeding is caused by an underlying hemostatic disorder or by a local anatomic defect. One clue is a history of bleeding following common hemostatic stresses such as dental extraction, childbirth, or minor surgery. Bleeding that is sufficiently severe to require a blood transfusion merits special attention. A family history of bleeding and bleeding from multiple sites that cannot be linked to trauma or surgery also suggest a systemic disorder. Since bleeding can be mild, lack of a family history of bleeding does not exclude an inherited hemostatic disorder.

Bleeding from a platelet disorder is usually localized to superficial sites such as the skin and mucous membranes, comes on immediately after trauma or surgery, and is readily controlled by local measures (Table 53-1). In contrast, bleeding from plasma coagulation defects occurs hours or days after injury and is unaffected by local therapy. Such bleeding most often occurs in deep subcutaneous tissues, muscles, joints, or body cavities. A thorough history may establish the presence of a hemostatic disorder and guide initial laboratory testing.

PHYSICAL EXAMINATION The most common site to observe bleeding is in the skin and mucous membranes. Collections of blood in the skin

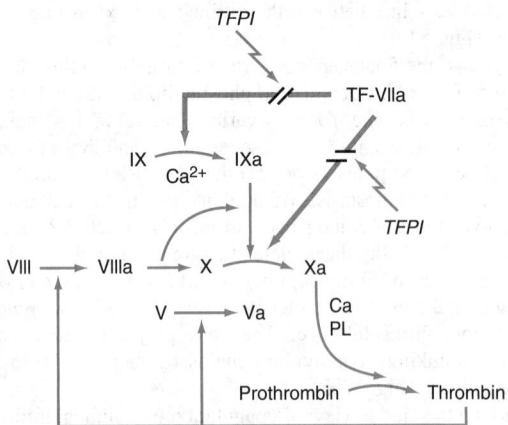

FIGURE 53-8 The contribution of the tissue factor–VIIa complex (TF-VIIa) and tissue factor pathway inhibitor (TFPI) to coagulation. Initial activation of factor IX by TF-VIIa compensates for deficiencies in the early factors, e.g., factors XII and XI. The subsequent inhibition of TF-VIIa by TFPI makes sustained activation of factor X by IXa and VIIIa critical for normal hemostasis. PL, phospholipid.

TABLE 53-1 *Differences in the Clinical Manifestations of Disorders of Primary and Secondary Hemostasis*

Manifestations	Defects of Primary Hemostasis (Platelet Defects)	Defects of Secondary Hemostasis (Plasma Protein Defects)
Onset of bleeding after trauma	Immediate	Delayed—hours or days
Sites of bleeding	Superficial—skin, mucous membranes, nose, gastrointestinal and genitourinary tracts	Deep—joints, muscle, retroperitoneum
Physical findings	Petechiae, ecchymoses	Hematomas, hemarthroses
Family history	Autosomal dominant	Autosomal or X-linked recessive
Response to therapy	Immediate; local measures effective	Requires sustained systemic therapy

are called *purpura* and may be subdivided on the basis of the site of bleeding in the skin. Small pinpoint hemorrhages into the dermis due to the leakage of red cells through capillaries are called *petechiae* and are characteristic of platelet disorders—in particular, severe thrombocytopenia. Larger subcutaneous collections of blood due to leakage of blood from small arterioles and venules are called *ecchymoses* (common bruises) or, if somewhat deeper and palpable, *hematomas*. They are also common in patients with platelet defects and result from minor trauma. Dilated capillaries, or *telangiectasia*, may cause bleeding without any hemostatic defect. In addition, the loss of connective tissue support for capillaries and small veins that accompanies aging increases the fragility of superficial vessels, such as those on the dorsum of the hand, leading to extravasation of blood into subcutaneous tissue—*senile purpura*. Menorrhagia is sometimes a serious problem in women with severe thrombocytopenia or platelet dysfunction. Some patients with primary hemostatic defects, especially von Willebrand's disease, may have recurrent gastrointestinal hemorrhage, often associated with angiodysplasia, a common vascular malformation in the gastrointestinal tract.

Bleeding into body cavities, the retroperitoneum, or joints is a common manifestation of plasma coagulation defects. Repeated joint bleeding may cause synovial thickening, chronic inflammation, and fluid collections and may erode articular cartilage and lead to chronic joint deformity and limited mobility. Joint deformities are particularly common in patients with deficiencies of factors VIII and IX, the two sex-linked coagulation disorders referred to as the *hemophilias*. For unclear reasons, hemarthroses are much less common in patients with other plasma coagulation defects. Blood collections in various body cavities or soft tissues can cause secondary necrosis of tissues or nerve compression. Retroperitoneal hematomas can cause femoral nerve compression, and large collections of poorly coagulated blood in soft tissues occasionally mimic malignant growths—the *pseudotumor syndrome*. Two of the most life-threatening sites of bleeding are in the oropharynx, where bleeding can compromise the airway, and in the central nervous system. Intracerebral hemorrhage is one of the leading causes of death in patients with severe coagulation disorders. Because of their need for plasma and factor concentrates derived from multiple donors, many patients with hemophilia were infected with HIV before effective testing of donors was in place. HIV infection can induce thrombocytopenia and exacerbate bleeding in hemophilia patients.

LABORATORY TESTS The most important screening tests of the primary hemostatic system are (1) a bleeding time (a sensitive measure of platelet function), and (2) a platelet count. The latter correlates well with the propensity to bleed. The normal platelet count is 150,000 to 450,000/μL of blood. As long as the count is >100,000/μL, patients are usually asymptomatic and the bleeding time remains normal. Platelet counts of 50,000 to 100,000/μL cause mild prolongation of the bleeding time; bleeding occurs only from severe trauma or other stress. Patients with platelet counts <50,000/μL have easy bruising, mani-

TABLE 53-2 *Causes of Thrombocytopenia*

Decreased marrow production of megakaryocytes
  Marrow infiltration with tumor, fibrosis
  Marrow failure—aplastic, hypoplastic anemias, drug effects
Splenic sequestration of circulating platelets
  Splenic enlargement due to tumor infiltration
  Splenic congestion due to portal hypertension
Increased destruction of circulating platelets
  Nonimmune destruction
    Vascular prostheses, cardiac valves
    Disseminated intravascular coagulation
    Sepsis
    Vasculitis
  Immune destruction
    Autoantibodies to platelet antigens
    Drug-associated antibodies
    Circulating immune complexes (systemic lupus erythematosus, viral agents, bacterial sepsis)

fested by skin purpura after minor trauma and bleeding after mucous membrane surgery. Patients with a platelet count <20,000/μL have an appreciable incidence of spontaneous bleeding, usually have petechiae, and may have intracranial or other spontaneous internal bleeding. The major causes of thrombocytopenia are outlined in Table 53-2.

Patients with qualitative platelet abnormalities have a normal platelet count and a prolonged bleeding time (Table 53-3). The bleeding time is ascertained by making a small, superficial skin incision and timing the duration of blood flow from the wounded area. With careful standardization, bleeding time is a reliable and sensitive test of platelet function. A template or an automated scalpel controls the length and depth of the incision (usually 1 mm deep by 9 mm long), and a sphygmomanometer inflated to 40 mmHg distends the capillary bed of the forearm uniformly. The bleeding time test must be performed by an experienced technician, as small differences in technique have a big effect on outcome. Any patient with a bleeding time >10 min has an increased risk of bleeding, but the risk does not become great until the bleeding time is >15 or 20 min. As shown in Fig. 53-10, the relationship between the platelet count and the bleeding time is roughly linear. When a defect in primary hemostasis is uncovered, specialized testing is needed to determine the cause of the platelet dysfunction (Table 53-3). A precise diagnosis is important in determining the proper treatment. Occasional patients with a strong history of bleeding, particularly those with mild von Willebrand's disease, may have a normal bleeding time when initially tested, owing to cyclical variations in the level of the vWF. Repeated testing may be necessary to establish an accurate diagnosis. Bleeding time is not an effective screening test for preoperative patients.

Plasma coagulation function is readily assessed with the PTT, pro-

TABLE 53-3 *Primary Hemostatic (Platelet) Disorders*

Defects of platelet adhesion
  von Willebrand's disease
  Bernard-Soulier syndrome (absence or dysfunction of GpIb/IX)
Defects of platelet aggregation
  Glanzmann's thrombasthenia (absence or dysfunction of GpIIb/IIIa)
Defects of platelet release
  Decreased cyclooxygenase activity
    Drug-induced—aspirin, nonsteroidal anti-inflammatory agents
    Congenital
  Granule storage pool defects
    Congenital
    Acquired
  Uremia
  Platelet coating (e.g., penicillin or paraproteins)
Defect of platelet coagulant activity
  Scott's syndrome

Abbreviation: Gp, glycoprotein.

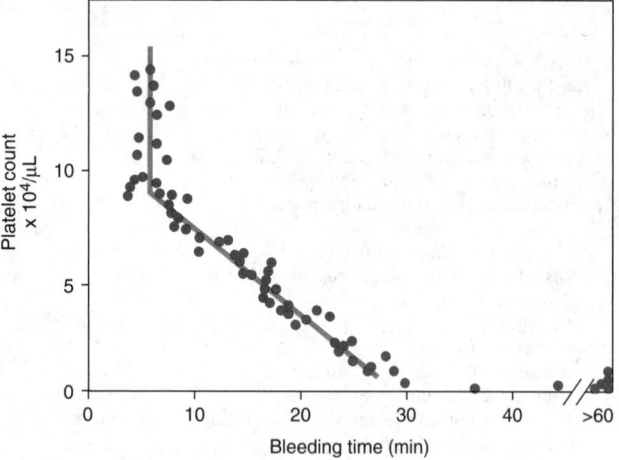

FIGURE 53-10   The relationship between the platelet count and the bleeding time. *(From LA Harker, Hemostasis Manual, 2d ed. Philadelphia, FA Davis Company, 1974.)*

thrombin time (PT), thrombin time (TT), and quantitative fibrinogen determination (Fig. 53-6, Table 53-4). The PTT screens the intrinsic limb of the coagulation system and tests for the adequacy of factors XII, HMWK, PK, XI, IX, and VIII. The PT screens the extrinsic or tissue factor–dependent pathway. Both tests also evaluate the common coagulation pathway involving all the reactions that occur after the activation of factor X. Prolongation of the PT and PTT that does not resolve after the addition of normal plasma suggests a coagulation inhibitor. A specific test for the conversion of fibrinogen to fibrin is needed when both the PTT and PT are prolonged—either a TT or a clottable fibrinogen level can be employed. When abnormalities are noted in any of the screening tests, more specific coagulation factor assays can be ordered to determine the nature of the defect.

Several rare coagulation abnormalities may be missed as they do not affect these screening tests: factor XIII deficiency, α_2 plasmin inhibitor deficiency, PAI-1 deficiency (PAI-1 is the major inhibitor of plasminogen activators), and Scott's syndrome, a platelet coagulant defect. A test for factor XIII–dependent fibrin cross-linking, like clot solubility in 5 M urea, should be ordered when the PT and PTT are both normal but the history of bleeding is strong. The fibrinolytic

system can be assessed by measuring the rate of clot lysis with the euglobulin lysis or whole blood clot lysis tests and by measuring the levels of α_2 plasmin inhibitor and PAI-1. Scott's syndrome can be detected by measuring the serum PT, which assesses the amount of residual prothrombin.

Conditions associated with thrombosis are listed in Table 53-5. Patients suspected of having a hypercoagulable or prethrombotic disorder on the basis of clinical information should be tested with specific assays to screen for the known defects. Currently available tests can identify 50 to 60% of the cases of familial or recurrent venous thrombosis.

Inhibitor syndromes or circulating anticoagulants are usually due to antibodies that impair coagulation factor activity. They are an infrequent cause of bleeding and require specialized diagnostic testing. Inhibitors are likely when screening test abnormalities cannot be reversed by adding normal plasma to patient plasma. Antibodies against specific coagulation factors may develop in: (1) postpartum women, (2) patients with autoimmune disorders such as systemic lupus erythematosus (SLE), (3) patients taking drugs such as penicillin and streptomycin, and (4) otherwise healthy elderly individuals. In addition, between 10 to 20% of patients with severe hemophilia who have received multiple plasma infusions develop inhibitory antibodies. Some patients, especially those with SLE, may also have a nonspecific form of anticoagulant antibody that interferes with phospholipid binding of coagulation factors and prolongs the PT and PTT but does not cause clinical bleeding. The presence of the lupus anticoagulant may increase the risk of thromboembolism and may cause placental infarction, recurrent midtrimester abortion, and venous and arterial thrombosis. The lupus-like anticoagulant is one manifestation of the anticardiolipin antibody syndrome. Patients may have anticardiolipin antibodies that do not prolong the PTT, but they still have an increased risk of thrombosis. Occasionally, patients develop inhibitors that are not antibodies. For example, several patients with clinical bleeding have been found to have circulating mucopolysaccharides that have heparin-like activity.

TABLE 53-4   *Relationship between Secondary Hemostatic Disorders and Coagulation Test Abnormalities*

Prolonged partial thromboplastin time (PTT)
  No clinical bleeding—factors XII, HMWK, PK
  Mild or rare bleeding—factor XI
  Frequent, severe bleeding—factors VIII and IX
Prolonged prothrombin time (PT)
  Factor VII deficiency
  Vitamin K deficiency—early
  Warfarin anticoagulant ingestion
Prolonged PTT and PT
  Factor II, V, or X deficiency
  Vitamin K deficiency—late
  Warfarin anticoagulant ingestion
Prolonged thrombin time (TT)
  Mild or rare bleeding—afibrinogenemia
  Frequent, severe bleeding—dysfibrinogenemia
  Heparin-like inhibitors or heparin administration
Prolonged PT and/or PTT not corrected with normal plasma
  Specific or nonspecific inhibitor syndromes
Clot solubility in 5 M urea
  Factor XIII deficiency
  Inhibitors or defective cross-linking
Rapid clot lysis
  α_2 plasmin inhibitor

Abbreviations: HMWK, high-molecular-weight kininogen; PK, prekallikrein.

TABLE 53-5   *Thrombotic Disorders*

Inherited
  Defective inhibition of coagulation factors
    Factor V Leiden (resistant to inhibition by activated protein C)
    Antithrombin III deficiency
    Protein C deficiency
    Protein S deficiency
    Prothrombin gene mutation (G20210A)
  Impaired clot lysis
    Dysfibrinogenemia
    Plasminogen deficiency
    tPA deficiency
    PAI-1 excess
  Uncertain mechanism
    Homocystinuria - ? endothelial damage
Acquired
  Diseases or syndromes
    Lupus anticoagulant/anticardiolipin antibody syndrome
    Malignancy
    Myeloproliferative disorder
    Thrombotic thrombocytopenic purpura
    Estrogen treatment
    Hyperlipidemia
    Diabetes mellitus
    Hyperviscosity
    Nephrotic syndrome
    Congestive heart failure
    Paroxysmal nocturnal hemoglobinuria
  Physiologic states
    Pregnancy (especially postpartum)
    Obesity
    Postoperative state
    Immobilization
    Old age

FURTHER READING

CROWTHER MA, KELTON JG: Congenital thrombophilic states associated with venous thrombosis: A qualitative overview and proposed classification. Ann Intern Med 138:128, 2003

GEORGE JN et al: Platelets: Thrombotic thrombocytopenic purpura. Hematology 2002 (American Society of Hematology Education Program book). 315:2002

HARTWIG JH, ITALIANO JE JR: Life of the blood platelet, in *Blood: Principles and Practice of Hematology*, 2nd ed, RI Handin et al (eds). Philadelpia, Lippincott Williams & Wilkins, 2003

MANN KG et al: The dynamics of thrombin formation. Arterioscler Thromb Vasc Biol 1:17, 2003

54 ENLARGEMENT OF LYMPH NODES AND SPLEEN
Patrick H. Henry, Dan L. Longo

This chapter is intended to serve as a guide to the evaluation of patients who present with enlargement of the lymph nodes (*lymphadenopathy*) or the spleen (*splenomegaly*). Lymphadenopathy is a rather common clinical finding in primary care settings, whereas palpable splenomegaly is less so.

LYMPHADENOPATHY

Lymphadenopathy may be an incidental finding in patients being examined for various reasons or it may be a presenting sign or symptom of the patient's illness. The physician must eventually decide whether the lymphadenopathy is a normal finding or one that requires further study, up to and including biopsy. Soft, flat, submandibular nodes (<1 cm) are often palpable in healthy children and young adults, and healthy adults may have palpable inguinal nodes of up to 2 cm, which are considered normal. Further evaluation of these normal nodes is not warranted. In contrast, if the physician believes the node(s) to be abnormal, then pursuit of a more precise diagnosis is needed.

APPROACH TO THE PATIENT

Lymphadenopathy may be a primary or secondary manifestation of numerous disorders, as shown in Table 54-1. Many of these disorders are infrequent causes of lymphadenopathy. Analysis of lymphadenopathy in primary care practice has shown that more than two-thirds of patients have nonspecific causes or upper respiratory illnesses (viral or bacterial), and <1% have a malignancy. In one study, researchers reported that 186 of 220 patients (84%) referred for evaluation of lymphadenopathy had a "benign" diagnosis. The remaining 34 patients (16%) had a malignancy (lymphoma or metastatic adenocarcinoma). Of the 186 patients with benign lymphadenopathy, 63% (112) had a nonspecific or reactive etiology (no causative agent found), and the remainder had a specific cause demonstrated, most commonly infectious mononucleosis, toxoplasmosis, or tuberculosis. Thus, the vast majority of patients with lymphadenopathy will have a nonspecific etiology requiring few diagnostic tests.

Clinical Assessment The physician will be aided in the pursuit of an explanation for the lymphadenopathy by a careful medical history, physical examination, selected laboratory tests, and perhaps an excisional lymph node biopsy.

The *medical history* should reveal the setting in which lymphadenopathy is occurring. Symptoms such as sore throat, cough, fever, night sweats, fatigue, weight loss, or pain in the nodes should be sought. The patient's age, sex, occupation, exposure to pets, sexual behavior, and use of drugs such as diphenylhydantoin are other important historic points. For example, children and young adults usually have benign (i.e., nonmalignant) disorders, such as viral or bacterial upper respiratory infections, infectious mononucleosis, toxoplasmosis, and, in some countries, tuberculosis, which account for the observed lymphadenopathy. In contrast, after age 50 the incidence of malignant disorders increases and that of benign disorders decreases.

The *physical examination* can provide useful clues such as the extent of lymphadenopathy (localized or generalized), size of nodes, texture, presence or absence of nodal tenderness, signs of

inflammation over the node, skin lesions, and splenomegaly. A thorough ear, nose, and throat (ENT) examination is indicated in adult patients with cervical adenopathy and a history of tobacco use. Localized or regional adenopathy implies involvement of a single anatomic area. Generalized adenopathy has been defined as involvement of three or more noncontiguous lymph node areas. Many of the causes of lymphadenopathy (Table 54-1) can produce localized *or* generalized adenopathy, so this distinction is of limited

TABLE 54-1 *Diseases Associated with Lymphadenopathy*

1. Infectious diseases
   a. Viral—infectious mononucleosis syndromes (EBV, CMV), infectious hepatitis, herpes simplex, herpesvirus-6, varicella-zoster virus, rubella, measles, adenovirus, HIV, epidemic keratoconjunctivitis, vaccinia, herpesvirus-8
   b. Bacterial—streptococci, staphylococci, cat-scratch disease, brucellosis, tularemia, plague, chancroid, melioidosis, glanders, tuberculosis, atypical mycobacterial infection, primary and secondary syphilis, diphtheria, leprosy
   c. Fungal—histoplasmosis, coccidioidomycosis, paracoccidioidomycosis
   d. Chlamydial—lymphogranuloma venereum, trachoma
   e. Parasitic—toxoplasmosis, leishmaniasis, trypanosomiasis, filariasis
   f. Rickettsial—scrub typhus, rickettsialpox
2. Immunologic diseases
   a. Rheumatoid arthritis
   b. Juvenile rheumatoid arthritis
   c. Mixed connective tissue disease
   d. Systemic lupus erythematosus
   e. Dermatomyositis
   f. Sjögren's syndrome
   g. Serum sickness
   h. Drug hypersensitivity—diphenylhydantoin, hydralazine, allopurinol, primidone, gold, carbamazepine, etc.
   i. Angioimmunoblastic lymphadenopathy
   j. Primary biliary cirrhosis
   k. Graft-vs.-host disease
   l. Silicone-associated
3. Malignant diseases
   a. Hematologic—Hodgkin's disease, non-Hodgkin's lymphomas, acute or chronic lymphocytic leukemia, hairy cell leukemia, malignant histiocytosis, amyloidosis
   b. Metastatic—from numerous primary sites
4. Lipid storage diseases—Gaucher's, Niemann-Pick, Fabry, Tangier
5. Endocrine diseases—hyperthyroidism
6. Other disorders
   a. Castleman's disease (giant lymph node hyperplasia)
   b. Sarcoidosis
   c. Dermatopathic lymphadenitis
   d. Lymphomatoid granulomatosis
   e. Histiocytic necrotizing lymphadenitis (Kikuchi's disease)
   f. Sinus histiocytosis with massive lymphadenopathy (Rosai-Dorfman disease)
   g. Mucocutaneous lymph node syndrome (Kawasaki's disease)
   h. Histiocytosis X
   i. Familial mediterranean fever
   j. Severe hypertriglyceridemia
   k. Vascular transformation of sinuses
   l. Inflammatory pseudotumor of lymph node

Note: EBV, Epstein-Barr virus; CMV, cytomegalovirus.

utility in the differential diagnosis. Nevertheless, generalized lymphadenopathy is frequently associated with nonmalignant disorders such as infectious mononucleosis [Epstein-Barr virus (EBV) or cytomegalovirus (CMV)], toxoplasmosis, AIDS, other viral infections, systemic lupus erythematosus (SLE), and mixed connective tissue disease. Acute and chronic lymphocytic leukemias and malignant lymphomas also produce generalized adenopathy in adults.

The site of localized or regional adenopathy may provide a useful clue about the cause. Occipital adenopathy often reflects an infection of the scalp, and preauricular adenopathy accompanies conjunctival infections and cat-scratch disease. The most frequent site of regional adenopathy is the neck, and most of the causes are benign—upper respiratory infections, oral and dental lesions, infectious mononucleosis, other viral illnesses. The chief malignant causes include metastatic cancer from head and neck, breast, lung, and thyroid primaries. Enlargement of supraclavicular and scalene nodes is always abnormal. Because these nodes drain regions of the lung and retroperitoneal space, they can reflect either lymphomas, other cancers, or infectious processes arising in these areas. Virchow's node is an enlarged left supraclavicular node infiltrated with metastatic cancer from a gastrointestinal primary. Metastases to supraclavicular nodes also occur from lung, breast, testis, or ovarian cancers. Tuberculosis, sarcoidosis, and toxoplasmosis are nonneoplastic causes of supraclavicular adenopathy. Axillary adenopathy is usually due to injuries or localized infections of the ipsilateral upper extremity. Malignant causes include melanoma or lymphoma and, in women, breast cancer. Inguinal lymphadenopathy is usually secondary to infections or trauma of the lower extremities and may accompany sexually transmitted diseases such as lymphogranuloma venereum, primary syphilis, genital herpes, or chancroid. These nodes may also be involved by lymphomas and metastatic cancer from primary lesions of the rectum, genitalia, or lower extremities (melanoma).

The size and texture of the lymph node(s) and the presence of pain are useful parameters in evaluating a patient with lymphadenopathy. Nodes <1.0 cm² in area (1.0 × 1.0 cm or less) are almost always secondary to benign, nonspecific reactive causes. In one retrospective analysis of younger patients (9 to 25 years) who had a lymph node biopsy, a maximum diameter of >2 cm served as one discriminant for predicting that the biopsy would reveal malignant or granulomatous disease. Another study showed that a lymph node size of 2.25 cm² (1.5 cm × 1.5 cm) was the best discriminating limit for distinguishing malignant or granulomatous lymphadenopathy from other causes of lymphadenopathy. Patients with node(s) ≤1.0 cm² should be observed after excluding infectious mononucleosis and/or toxoplasmosis unless there are symptoms and signs of an underlying systemic illness.

The texture of lymph nodes may be described as soft, firm, rubbery, hard, discrete, matted, tender, movable, or fixed. Tenderness is found when the capsule is stretched during rapid enlargement, usually secondary to an inflammatory process. Some malignant diseases such as acute leukemia may produce rapid enlargement and pain in the nodes. Nodes involved by lymphoma tend to be large, discrete, symmetric, rubbery, firm, mobile, and nontender. Nodes containing metastatic cancer are often hard, nontender, and nonmovable because of fixation to surrounding tissues. The coexistence of splenomegaly in the patient with lymphadenopathy implies a systemic illness such as infectious mononucleosis, lymphoma, acute or chronic leukemia, SLE, sarcoidosis, toxoplasmosis, cat-scratch disease, or other less common hematologic disorders. The patient's story should provide helpful clues about the underlying systemic illness.

Nonsuperficial presentations (thoracic or abdominal) of adenopathy are usually detected as the result of a symptom-directed diagnostic workup. Thoracic adenopathy may be detected by routine chest roentgenography or during the workup for superficial adenopathy. It may also be found because the patient complains of a cough or wheezing from airway compression; hoarseness from recurrent laryngeal nerve involvement; dysphagia from esophageal compression; or swelling of the neck, face, or arms secondary to compression of the superior vena cava or subclavian vein. The differential diagnosis of mediastinal and hilar adenopathy includes primary lung disorders and systemic illnesses that characteristically involve mediastinal or hilar nodes. In the young, mediastinal adenopathy is associated with infectious mononucleosis and sarcoidosis. In endemic regions, histoplasmosis can cause unilateral paratracheal lymph node involvement that mimics lymphoma. Tuberculosis can also cause unilateral adenopathy. In older patients, the differential diagnosis includes primary lung cancer (especially among smokers), lymphomas, metastatic carcinoma (usually lung), tuberculosis, fungal infection, and sarcoidosis.

Enlarged intraabdominal or retroperitoneal nodes are usually malignant. Although tuberculosis may present as mesenteric lymphadenitis, these masses usually contain lymphomas or, in young men, germ cell tumors.

Laboratory Investigation The laboratory investigation of patients with lymphadenopathy must be tailored to elucidate the etiology suspected from the patient's history and physical findings. One study from a family practice clinic evaluated 249 younger patients with "enlarged lymph nodes, not infected" or "lymphadenitis." No laboratory studies were obtained in 51%. When studies were performed, the most common were a complete blood count (33%), throat culture (16%), chest x-ray (12%), or monospot test (10%). Only eight patients (3%) had a node biopsy, and half of those were normal or reactive. The complete blood count can provide useful data for the diagnosis of acute or chronic leukemias, EBV or CMV mononucleosis, lymphoma with a leukemic component, pyogenic infections, or immune cytopenias in illnesses such as SLE. Serologic studies may demonstrate antibodies specific to components of EBV, CMV, HIV, and other viruses; *Toxoplasma gondii*; *Brucella*; etc. If SLE is suspected, then antinuclear and anti-DNA antibody studies are warranted.

The chest x-ray is usually negative, but the presence of a pulmonary infiltrate or mediastinal lymphadenopathy would suggest tuberculosis, histoplasmosis, sarcoidosis, lymphoma, primary lung cancer, or metastatic cancer and demands further investigation.

A variety of imaging techniques [computed tomography (CT), magnetic resonance imaging (MRI), ultrasound, color Doppler ultrasonography] have been employed to differentiate benign from malignant lymph nodes, especially in patients with head and neck cancer. CT and MRI are comparably accurate (65 to 90%) in the diagnosis of metastases to cervical lymph nodes. Ultrasonography has been used to determine the long (L) axis, short (S) axis, and a ratio of long to short axis in cervical nodes. An L/S ratio of <2.0 has a sensitivity and a specificity of 95% for distinguishing benign and malignant nodes in patients with head and neck cancer. This ratio has greater specificity and sensitivity than palpation or measurement of either the long or the short axis alone.

The indications for lymph node biopsy are imprecise, yet it is a valuable diagnostic tool. The decision to biopsy may be made early in a patient's evaluation or delayed for up to 2 weeks. Prompt biopsy should occur if the patient's history and physical findings suggest a malignancy; examples include a solitary, hard, nontender cervical node in an older patient who is a chronic user of tobacco; supraclavicular adenopathy; and solitary or generalized adenopathy that is firm, movable, and suggestive of lymphoma. If a primary head and neck cancer is suspected as the basis of a solitary, hard cervical node, then a careful ENT examination should be performed. Any mucosal lesion that is suspicious for a primary neoplastic process should be biopsied first. If no mucosal lesion is detected, an excisional biopsy of the largest node should be performed. Fine-needle aspiration should not be performed as the first diagnostic procedure. Most diagnoses require more tissue than such aspiration can provide, and it often delays a definitive diagnosis. Fine-needle aspiration should be reserved for thyroid nodules and for confirmation of relapse in patients whose primary diagnosis is known. If the primary physician is uncertain about whether to proceed to biopsy, consultation with a hematologist or medical oncologist should be helpful. In primary care practices, <5% of lymphadenopathy patients will require a biopsy. That percentage will be considerably larger in referral practices, i.e., hematology, oncology, or otolaryngology (ENT).

Two groups have reported algorithms that they claim will identify more precisely those lymphadenopathy patients who should have a biopsy. Both reports were retrospective analyses in referral practices. The first study involved patients 9 to 25 years of age who had a node biopsy performed. Three variables were identified that predicted those young patients with peripheral lymphadenopathy who should undergo biopsy; lymph node size >2 cm in diameter and abnormal chest x-ray had positive predictive value, whereas recent ENT symptoms had negative predictive values. The second study evaluated 220 lymphadenopathy patients in a hematology unit and identified five variables [lymph node size, location (supraclavicular or nonsupraclavicular), age (>40 years or <40 years), texture (nonhard or hard), and tenderness] that were utilized in a mathematical model to identify those patients requiring a biopsy. Positive predictive value was found for age >40 years, supraclavicular location, node size >2.25 cm², hard texture, and lack of pain or tenderness. Negative predictive value was evident for age <40 years, node size <1.0 cm², nonhard texture, and tender or painful nodes. Ninety-one percent of those who required biopsy were correctly classified by this model. Since both of these studies were retrospective analyses and one was limited to young patients, it is not known how useful these models would be if applied prospectively in a primary care setting.

Most lymphadenopathy patients do not require a biopsy, and at least half require no laboratory studies. If the patient's history and physical findings point to a benign cause for lymphadenopathy, then careful follow-up at a 2- to 4-week interval can be employed. The patient should be instructed to return for reevaluation if the node(s) increase in size. Antibiotics are not indicated for lymphadenopathy unless there is strong evidence of a bacterial infection. Glucocorticoids should not be used to treat lymphadenopathy because their lympholytic effect obscures some diagnoses (lymphoma, leukemia, Castleman's disease) and they contribute to delayed healing or activation of underlying infections. An exception to this statement is the life-threatening pharyngeal obstruction by enlarged lymphoid tissue in Waldeyer's ring that is occasionally seen in infectious mononucleosis.

SPLENOMEGALY

STRUCTURE AND FUNCTION OF THE SPLEEN   The spleen is a reticuloendothelial organ that has its embryologic origin in the dorsal mesogastrium at about 5 weeks' gestation. It arises in a series of hillocks, migrates to its normal adult location in the left upper quadrant (LUQ), and is attached to the stomach via the gastrolienal ligament and to the kidney via the lienorenal ligament. When the hillocks fail to unify into a single tissue mass, accessory spleens may develop in around 20% of persons. The function of the spleen has been elusive. Galen believed it was the source of "black bile" or melancholia, and the word *hypochondria* (literally, beneath the ribs) and the idiom "to vent one's spleen" attest to the beliefs that the spleen had an important influence on the psyche and emotions. In humans, its normal physiologic roles seem to be the following:

1. Maintenance of quality control over erythrocytes in the red pulp by removal of senescent and defective red blood cells. The spleen accomplishes this function through a unique organization of its parenchyma and vasculature (Fig. 54-1).
2. Synthesis of antibodies in the white pulp.

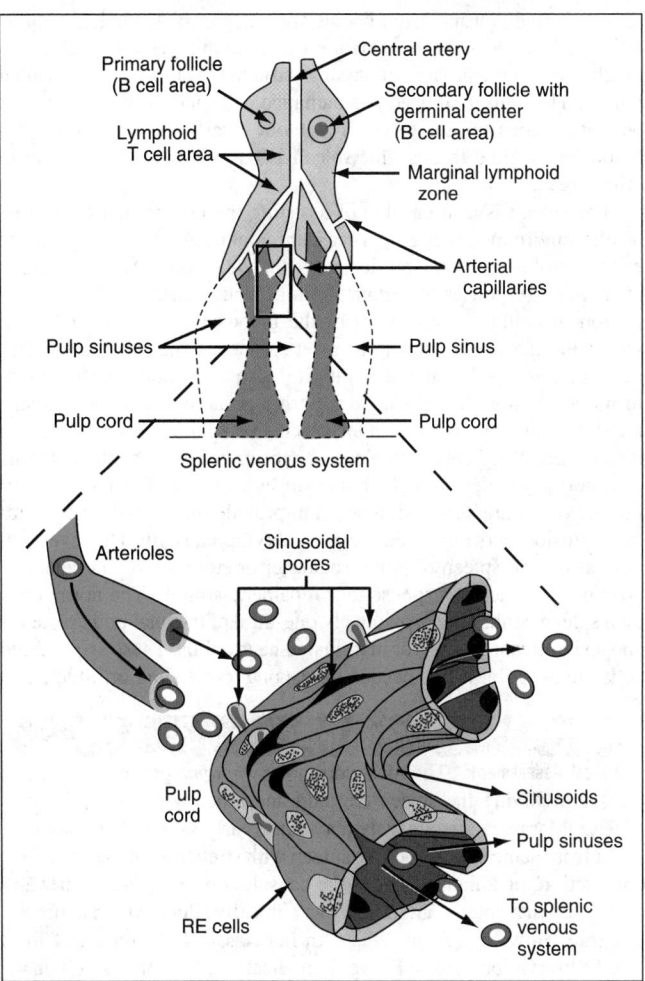

FIGURE 54-1   Schematic spleen structure. The spleen comprises many units of red and white pulp centered around small branches of the splenic artery, called central arteries. White pulp is lymphoid in nature and contains B cell follicles, a marginal zone around the follicles, and T cell–rich areas sheathing arterioles. The red pulp areas include pulp sinuses and pulp cords. The cords are dead ends. In order to regain access to the circulation, red blood cells must traverse tiny openings in the sinusoidal lining. Stiff, damaged, or old red cells cannot enter the sinuses. (*Top portion of figure from CA Janeway et al: Immunobiology, 5th edition, New York, Garland, 2001; Bottom portion of figure from RS Hillman, KA Ault: Hematology in Clinical Practice. New York, McGraw-Hill, 1995.*)

3. The removal of antibody-coated bacteria and antibody-coated blood cells from the circulation.

An increase in these normal functions may result in splenomegaly.

The spleen is composed of red pulp and white pulp, which are Malpighi's terms for the red blood–filled sinuses and reticuloendothelial cell–lined cords and the white lymphoid follicles arrayed within the red pulp matrix. The spleen is in the portal circulation. The reason for this is unknown but may relate to the fact that lower blood pressure allows less rapid flow and minimizes damage to normal erythrocytes. Blood flows into the spleen at a rate of about 150 mL/min through the splenic artery, which ultimately ramifies into central arterioles. Some blood goes from the arterioles to capillaries and then to splenic veins and out of the spleen, but the majority of blood from central arterioles flows into the macrophage-lined sinuses and cords. The blood entering the sinuses reenters the circulation through the splenic venules, but the blood entering the cords is subjected to an inspection of sorts. In order to return to the circulation, the blood cells in the cords must squeeze through slits in the cord lining to enter the sinuses that lead to the venules. Old and damaged erythrocytes are less deformable and are retained in the cords, where they are destroyed and their components recycled. Red cell inclusion bodies such as parasites, nuclear residua (Howell-Jolly bodies), or denatured hemoglobin (Heinz bodies) are pinched off in the process of passing through the slits, a process called *pitting*. The culling of dead and damaged cells and the pitting of cells with inclusions appear to occur without significant delay since the blood transit time through the spleen is only slightly slower than in other organs.

The spleen is also capable of assisting the host in adapting to its hostile environment. It has at least three adaptational functions: (1) clearance of bacteria and particulates from the blood, (2) the generation of immune responses to certain invading pathogens, and (3) the generation of cellular components of the blood under circumstances in which the marrow is unable to meet the needs (i.e., extramedullary hematopoiesis). The latter adaptation is a recapitulation of the blood-forming function the spleen plays during gestation. In some animals, the spleen also serves a role in the vascular adaptation to stress because it stores red blood cells (often hemoconcentrated to higher hematocrits than normal) under normal circumstances and contracts under the influence of β-adrenergic stimulation to provide the animal with an autotransfusion and improved oxygen-carrying capacity. However, the normal human spleen does not sequester or store red blood cells and does not contract in response to sympathetic stimuli. The normal human spleen contains approximately one-third of the total body platelets and a significant number of marginated neutrophils. These sequestered cells are available when needed to respond to bleeding or infection.

APPROACH TO THE PATIENT

Clinical Assessment   The most common *symptoms* produced by diseases involving the spleen are pain and a heavy sensation in the LUQ. Massive splenomegaly may cause early satiety.Pain may result from acute swelling of the spleen with stretching of the capsule, infarction, or inflammation of the capsule. For many years, it was believed that splenic infarction was clinically silent, which at times is true. However, Soma Weiss, in his classic 1942 report of the self-observations by a Harvard medical student on the clinical course of subacute bacterial endocarditis, documented that severe LUQ and pleuritic chest pain may accompany thromboembolic occlusion of splenic blood flow. Vascular occlusion, with infarction and pain, is commonly seen in children with sickle cell crises. Rupture of the spleen, either from trauma or infiltrative disease that breaks the capsule, may result in intraperitoneal bleeding, shock, and death. The rupture itself may be painless.

A palpable spleen is the major *physical sign* produced by diseases affecting the spleen and suggests enlargement of the organ. The normal spleen is said to weigh <250 g, decreases in size with age, normally lies entirely within the rib cage, has a maximum cephalocaudad diameter of 13 cm by ultrasonography or maximum length of 12 cm and/or width of 7 cm by radionuclide scan, and is usually not palpable. However, a palpable spleen was found in 3% of 2200 asymptomatic, male, freshman college students. Follow-up at 3 years revealed that 30% of those students still had a palpable spleen without any increase in disease prevalence. Ten-year follow-up found no evidence for lymphoid malignancies. Furthermore, in some tropical countries (e.g., New Guinea) the incidence of splenomegaly may reach 60%. Thus, the presence of a palpable spleen does not always equate with presence of disease. Even when disease is present, splenomegaly may not reflect the primary disease but rather a reaction to it. For example, in patients with Hodgkin's disease, only two-thirds of the palpable spleens show involvement by the cancer.

Physical examination of the spleen utilizes primarily the techniques of palpation and percussion. Inspection may reveal a fullness in the LUQ that descends on inspiration, a finding associated with a massively enlarged spleen. Auscultation may reveal a venous hum or a friction rub.

Palpation can be accomplished by bimanual palpation, ballot-

ment, and palpation from above (Middleton maneuver). For bimanual palpation, which is at least as reliable as the other techniques, the patient is supine with flexed knees. The examiner's left hand is placed on the lower rib cage and pulls the skin toward the costal margin, allowing the fingertips of the right hand to feel the tip of the spleen as it descends while the patient inspires slowly, smoothly, and deeply. Palpation is begun with the right hand in the left lower quadrant with gradual movement toward the left costal margin, thereby identifying the lower edge of a massively enlarged spleen. When the spleen tip is felt, the finding is recorded as centimeters below the left costal margin at some arbitrary point, i.e., 10 to 15 cm, from the midpoint of the umbilicus or the xiphisternal junction. This allows other examiners to compare findings or the initial examiner to determine changes in size over time. Bimanual palpation in the right lateral decubitus position adds nothing to the supine examination.

Percussion for splenic dullness is accomplished with any of three techniques described by Nixon, Castell, or Barkun:

1. *Nixon's method*: The patient is placed on the right side so that the spleen lies above the colon and stomach. Percussion begins at the lower level of pulmonary resonance in the posterior axillary line and proceeds diagonally along a perpendicular line toward the lower midanterior costal margin. The upper border of dullness is normally 6 to 8 cm above the costal margin. Dullness >8 cm in an adult is presumed to indicate splenic enlargement.

2. *Castell's method*: With the patient supine, percussion in the lowest intercostal space in the anterior axillary line (8th or 9th) produces a resonant note if the spleen is normal in size. This is true during expiration or full inspiration. A dull percussion note on full inspiration suggests splenomegaly.

3. *Percussion of Traube's semilunar space*: The borders of Traube's space are the sixth rib superiorly, the left midaxillary line laterally, and the left costal margin inferiorly. The patient is supine with the left arm slightly abducted. During normal breathing, this space is percussed from medial to lateral margins, yielding a normal resonant sound. A dull percussion note suggests splenomegaly.

Studies comparing methods of percussion and palpation with a standard of ultrasonography or scintigraphy have revealed sensitivity of 56 to 71% for palpation and 59 to 82% for percussion. Reproducibility among examiners is better for palpation than percussion. Both techniques are less reliable in obese patients or patients who have just eaten. Thus, the physical examination techniques of palpation and percussion are imprecise at best. It has been suggested that the examiner perform percussion first and, if positive, proceed to palpation; if the spleen is palpable, then one can be reasonably confident that splenomegaly exists. However, not all LUQ masses are enlarged spleens; gastric or colon tumors and pancreatic or renal cysts or tumors can mimic splenomegaly.

The presence of an enlarged spleen can be more precisely determined, if necessary, by liver-spleen radionuclide scan, CT, MRI, or ultrasonography. The latter technique is the current procedure of choice for routine assessment of spleen size (normal = a maximum cephalocaudad diameter of 13 cm) because it has high sensitivity and specificity and is safe, noninvasive, quick, mobile, and less costly. Nuclear medicine scans are accurate, sensitive, and reliable but are costly, require greater time to generate data, and utilize immobile equipment. They have the advantage of demonstrating accessory splenic tissue. CT and MRI provide accurate determination of spleen size, but the equipment is immobile and the procedures are expensive. MRI appears to offer no advantage over CT. Changes in spleen structure such as mass lesions, infarcts, inhomogeneous infiltrates, and cysts are more readily assessed by CT, MRI, or ultrasonography. None of these techniques is very reliable in the detection of patchy infiltration (e.g., Hodgkin's disease).

Differential Diagnosis   Many of the diseases associated with splenomegaly are listed in Table 54-2. They are grouped according to the presumed basic mechanisms responsible for organ enlargement:

1. Hyperplasia or hypertrophy related to a particular splenic function such as reticuloendothelial hyperplasia (work hypertrophy) in diseases such as hereditary spherocytosis or thalassemia syndromes that require removal of large numbers of defective red blood cells; immune hyperplasia in response to systemic infection (infectious mononucleosis, subacute bacterial endocarditis) or to immunologic diseases (immune thrombocytopenia, SLE, Felty's syndrome).

2. Passive congestion due to decreased blood flow from the spleen in conditions that produce portal hypertension (cirrhosis, Budd-Chiari syndrome, congestive heart failure).

3. Infiltrative diseases of the spleen (lymphomas, metastatic cancer, amyloidosis, Gaucher's disease, myeloproliferative disorders with extramedullary hematopoiesis).

The differential diagnostic possibilities are much fewer when the spleen is "massively enlarged," that is, it is palpable more than 8 cm below the left costal margin or its drained weight is ≥1000 g (Table 54-3). The vast majority of such patients will have non-Hodgkin's lymphoma, chronic lymphocytic leukemia, hairy cell leukemia, chronic myelogenous leukemia, myelofibrosis with myeloid metaplasia, or polycythemia vera.

Laboratory Assessment The major laboratory abnormalities accompanying splenomegaly are determined by the underlying systemic illness. Erythrocyte counts may be normal, decreased (thalassemia major syndromes, SLE, cirrhosis with portal hypertension), or increased (polycythemia vera). Granulocyte counts may be normal, decreased (Felty's syndrome, congestive splenomegaly, leukemias), or increased (infections or inflammatory disease, myeloproliferative disorders). Similarly, the platelet count may be normal, decreased when there is enhanced sequestration or destruction of platelets in an enlarged spleen (congestive splenomegaly, Gaucher's disease, immune thrombocytopenia), or increased in the myeloproliferative disorders such as polycythemia vera.

The complete blood count may reveal cytopenia of one or more blood cell types, which should suggest *hypersplenism*. This condition is characterized by splenomegaly, cytopenia(s), normal or hyperplastic bone marrow, and a response to splenectomy. The latter characteristic is less precise because reversal of cytopenia, particularly granulocytopenia, is sometimes not sustained after splenectomy. The cytopenias result from increased destruction of the cellular elements secondary to reduced flow of blood through enlarged and congested cords (congestive splenomegaly) or to immune-mediated mechanisms. In hypersplenism, various cell types usually have normal morphology on the peripheral blood smear, although the red cells may be spherocytic due to loss of surface area during their longer transit through the enlarged spleen. The increased marrow production of red cells should be reflected as an increased reticulocyte production index, although the value may be less than expected due to increased sequestration of reticulocytes in the spleen.

The need for additional laboratory studies is dictated by the differential diagnosis of the underlying illness of which splenomegaly is a manifestation.

SPLENECTOMY Splenectomy is infrequently performed for diagnostic purposes, especially in the absence of clinical illness or other diagnostic tests that suggest underlying disease. More often splenectomy is performed for staging the extent of disease in patients with Hodgkin's disease, for symptom control in patients with massive splenomegaly, for disease control in patients with traumatic splenic rupture, or for correction of cytopenias in patients with hypersplenism or immune-mediated destruction of one or more cellular blood elements.

TABLE 54-2 *Diseases Associated with Splenomegaly Grouped by Pathogenic Mechanism*

ENLARGEMENT DUE TO INCREASED DEMAND FOR SPLENIC FUNCTION	ENLARGEMENT DUE TO ABNORMAL SPLENIC OR PORTAL BLOOD FLOW
Reticuloendothelial system hyperplasia (for removal of defective erythrocytes)	Cirrhosis
Spherocytosis	Hepatic vein obstruction
Early sickle cell anemia	Portal vein obstruction, intrahepatic or extrahepatic
Ovalocytosis	Cavernous transformation of the portal vein
Thalassemia major	Splenic vein obstruction
Hemoglobinopathies	Splenic artery aneurysm
Paroxysmal nocturnal hemoglobinuria	Hepatic schistosomiasis
Nutritional anemias	Congestive heart failure
Immune hyperplasia	Hepatic echinococcosis
Response to infection (viral, bacterial, fungal, parasitic)	Portal hypertension (any cause including the above): "Banti's disease"
Infectious mononucleosis	**INFILTRATION OF THE SPLEEN**
AIDS	
Viral hepatitis	*Intracellular or extracellular depositions*
Cytomegalovirus	Amyloidosis
Subacute bacterial endocarditis	Gaucher's disease
Bacterial septicemia	Niemann-Pick disease
Congenital syphilis	Tangier disease
Splenic abscess	Hurler's syndrome and other mucopolysaccharidoses
Tuberculosis	Hyperlipidemias
Histoplasmosis	*Benign and malignant cellular infiltrations*
Malaria	Leukemias (acute, chronic, lymphoid, myeloid, monocytic)
Leishmaniasis	Lymphomas
Trypanosomiasis	Hodgkin's disease
Ehrlichiosis	Myeloproliferative syndromes (e.g., polycythemia vera)
Disordered immunoregulation	Angiosarcomas
Rheumatoid arthritis (Felty's syndrome)	Metastatic tumors (melanoma is most common)
Systemic lupus erythematosus	Eosinophilic granuloma
Collagen vascular diseases	Histiocytosis X
Serum sickness	Hamartomas
Immune hemolytic anemias	Hemangiomas, fibromas, lymphangiomas
Immune thrombocytopenias	Splenic cysts
Immune neutropenias	**UNKNOWN ETIOLOGY**
Drug reactions	
Angioimmunoblastic lymphadenopathy	Idiopathic splenomegaly
Sarcoidosis	Berylliosis
Thyrotoxicosis (benign lymphoid hypertrophy)	Iron-deficiency anemia
Interleukin 2 therapy	
Extramedullary hematopoiesis	
Myelofibrosis	
Marrow damage by toxins, radiation, strontium	
Marrow infiltration by tumors, leukemias, Gaucher's disease	

TABLE 54-3 *Diseases Associated with Massive Splenomegaly*[a]

Chronic myelogenous leukemia	Gaucher's disease
Lymphomas	Chronic lymphocytic leukemia
Hairy cell leukemia	Sarcoidosis
Myelofibrosis with myeloid metaplasia	Autoimmune hemolytic anemia
Polycythemia vera	Diffuse splenic hemangiomatosis

[a] The spleen extends greater than 8 cm below left costal margin and/or weighs more than 1000 g.

Splenectomy is necessary for routine staging of patients with Hodgkin's disease only in those with clinical stage I or II disease in whom radiation therapy alone is contemplated as the treatment. Noninvasive staging of the spleen in Hodgkin's disease is not a sufficiently reliable basis for treatment decisions because one-third of normal-sized spleens will be involved with Hodgkin's disease and one-third of enlarged spleens will be tumor-free. Although splenectomy in chronic myelogenous leukemia does not affect the natural history of disease, removal of the massive spleen usually makes patients significantly more comfortable and simplifies their management by significantly reducing transfusion requirements. Splenectomy is an effective secondary or tertiary treatment for two chronic B cell leukemias, hairy cell leukemia and prolymphocytic leukemia, and for the very rare splenic mantle cell or marginal zone lymphoma. Splenectomy in these diseases may be associated with significant tumor regression in bone marrow and other sites of disease. Similar regressions of systemic disease have been noted after splenic irradiation in some types of lymphoproliferative disease, especially chronic lymphocytic leukemia and prolymphocytic leukemia. This has been termed the *abscopal effect*. Such systemic tumor responses to local therapy directed at the spleen suggest that there may be some hormone or growth factor produced by the spleen that affects tumor cell proliferation, but this conjecture is not yet substantiated. A common therapeutic indication for splenectomy is traumatic or iatrogenic splenic rupture. In a fraction of patients with splenic rupture, peritoneal seeding of splenic fragments can lead to *splenosis*—the presence of multiple rests of spleen tissue not connected to the portal circulation. This ectopic spleen tissue may cause pain or gastrointestinal obstruction, as in endometriosis. A large number of hematologic, immunologic, and congestive causes of splenomegaly can lead to destruction of one or more cellular blood elements. In the majority of such cases, splenectomy can correct the cytopenias, particularly anemia and thrombocytopenia. In a large series of patients seen in two tertiary care centers, the indication for splenectomy was diagnostic in 10% of the patients, therapeutic in 44%, staging for Hodgkin's disease in 20%, and incidental to another procedure in 26%. Perhaps the only contraindication to splenectomy is the presence of marrow failure, in which the enlarged spleen is the only source of hematopoietic tissue.

The absence of the spleen has minimal long-term effects on the hematologic profile. In the immediate postsplenectomy period, there may be some leukocytosis (up to $25,000/\mu L$) and thrombocytosis (up to $1 \times 10^6/\mu L$), but within 2 to 3 weeks, blood cell counts and survival of each cell lineage are usually normal. The chronic manifestations of splenectomy are marked variation in size and shape of erythrocytes (anisocytosis, poikilocytosis) and the presence of Howell-Jolly bodies (nuclear remnants), Heinz bodies (denatured hemoglobin), basophilic stippling, and an occasional nucleated erythrocyte in the peripheral blood. When such erythrocyte abnormalities appear in a patient whose spleen has not been removed, one should suspect splenic infiltration by tumor that has interfered with its normal culling and pitting function.

The most serious consequence of splenectomy is increased susceptibility to bacterial infections, particularly those with capsules such as *Streptococcus pneumoniae*, *Haemophilus influenzae*, and some gram-negative enteric organisms. Patients under age 20 years are particularly susceptible to overwhelming sepsis with *S. pneumoniae*, and the overall actuarial risk of sepsis in patients who have had their spleens removed is about 7% in 10 years. The case-fatality rate for pneumococcal sepsis in splenectomized patients is 50 to 80%. About 25% of patients without spleens will develop a serious infection at some time in their life. The frequency is highest within the first 3 years after splenectomy. About 15% of the infections are polymicrobial, and lung, skin, and blood are the most common sites. No increased risk of viral infection has been noted in patients who have no spleen. The susceptibility to bacterial infections relates to the inability to remove opsonized bacteria from the bloodstream and a defect in making antibodies to T cell–independent antigens such as the polysaccharide components of bacterial capsules. Pneumococcal vaccine (23-valent polysaccharide vaccine) should be administered to all patients 2 weeks before elective splenectomy. The Advisory Committee on Immunization Practices recommends that even splenectomized patients receive pneumococcal vaccine with a repeat vaccination 5 years later. Efficacy has not been proven in this setting, and the recommendation discounts the possibility that administration of the vaccine may actually lower the titer of specific pneumococcal antibodies. A more effective pneumococcal vaccine that involves T cells in the response is in development. The vaccine to *Neisseria meningitidis* should also be given to patients in whom elective splenectomy is planned. No other vaccines are routinely recommended in this setting.

Splenectomized patients should be educated to consider any unexplained fever as a medical emergency. Prompt medical attention with evaluation and treatment of suspected bacteremia may be lifesaving. Routine chemoprophylaxis with oral penicillin can result in the emergence of drug-resistant strains and is not recommended.

In addition to an increased susceptibility to bacterial infections, splenectomized patients are also more susceptible to the parasitic disease babesiosis. The splenectomized patient should avoid areas where the parasite *Babesia* is endemic (e.g., Cape Cod, MA).

Surgical removal of the spleen is an obvious cause of hyposplenism. Patients with sickle cell disease often suffer from autosplenectomy as a result of splenic destruction by the numerous infarcts associated with sickle cell crises during childhood. Indeed, the presence of a palpable spleen in a patient with sickle cell disease after age 5 suggests a coexisting hemoglobinopathy, e.g., thalassemia or hemoglobin C. In addition, patients who receive splenic irradiation for a neoplastic or autoimmune disease are also functionally hyposplenic. The term *hyposplenism* is preferred to *asplenism* in referring to the physiologic consequences of splenectomy because asplenia is a rare, specific, and fatal congenital abnormality in which there is a failure of the left side of the coelomic cavity (which includes the splenic anlagen) to develop normally. Infants with asplenia have no spleens, but that is the least of their problems. The right side of the developing embryo is duplicated on the left so there is liver where the spleen should be, there are two right lungs, and the heart comprises two right atria and two right ventricles.

FURTHER READING

BARKUN AN et al: The bedside assessment of splenic enlargement. Am J Med 91:512, 1991

GRAVES SA et al: Does this patient have splenomegaly? JAMA 270:2218, 1993

KRAUS MD et al: The spleen as a diagnostic specimen: A review of ten years' experience at two tertiary care institutions. Cancer 91:2001, 2001

MCINTYRE OR, EBAUGH FG JR: Palpable spleens: Ten year follow-up. Ann Intern Med 90:130, 1979

PANGALIS GA et al: Clinical approach to lymphadenopathy. Semin Oncol 20: 570, 1993

PREVENTION OF PNEUMOCOCCAL DISEASE: Recommendations of the Advisory Committee on Immunization Practices. MMWR 46(RR-8):1, 1997

WILLIAMSON HA JR: Lymphadenopathy in a family practice: A descriptive study of 240 cases. J Fam Pract 20:449, 1985

Leukocytes are the major cells comprising inflammatory and immune responses and include neutrophils, T and B lymphocytes, natural killer (NK) cells, monocytes, eosinophils, and basophils. These cells have specific functions, such as antibody production by B lymphocytes or destruction of bacteria by neutrophils, but in no single infectious disease is the exact role of the cell types completely established. Thus, whereas neutrophils are classically thought to be critical to host defense against bacteria, they may also play important roles in defense against viral infections.

The blood delivers leukocytes to the various tissues from the bone marrow, where they are produced. Normal blood leukocyte counts are 4.3 to 10.8×10^9/L with neutrophils representing 45 to 74% of the cells, bands 0 to 4%, lymphocytes 16 to 45%, monocytes 4 to 10%, eosinophils 0 to 7%, and basophils 0 to 2%. The various leukocytes are derived from a common stem cell in the bone marrow. Three-fourths of the nucleated cells of bone marrow are committed to the production of leukocytes. Leukocyte maturation in the marrow is under the regulatory control of a number of different factors, known as colony-stimulating factors and interleukins (ILs). Because an alteration in the number and type of leukocytes is often associated with disease processes, total white blood count (WBC) (cells per microliter) and differential counts are informative. The lymphocytes and basophils are discussed in Chaps. 295 and 298, respectively. This chapter focuses on the neutrophils, monocytes, and eosinophils.

NEUTROPHILS

MATURATION Important events in neutrophil life are summarized in Fig. 55-1. In normal humans, neutrophils are produced only in the bone marrow. The minimum number of stem cells necessary to support hematopoiesis is estimated to be 400 to 500. Human blood monocytes, tissue macrophages, and stromal cells produce colony-stimulating factors, hormones required for the growth of monocytes and neutrophils in the bone marrow. The hematopoietic system not only produces enough neutrophils ($\sim 1.3 \times 10^{11}$ cells per 80-kg person per day) to carry out physiologic functions but also has a large reserve stored in the marrow, which can be mobilized in response to inflammation or infection. An increase in the number of blood neutrophils is called *neutrophilia*, and the presence of immature cells is termed a *shift to the left*. A decrease in the number of blood neutrophils is called *neutropenia*.

Neutrophils and monocytes evolve from pluripotent stem cells under the influence of cytokines and colony-stimulating factors (Fig. 55-2). The proliferation phase through the metamyelocyte takes about 1 week, while the maturation phase from metamyelocyte to mature neutrophil takes another week. The myeloblast is the first recognizable precursor cell and is followed by the *promyelocyte*. The promyelocyte evolves when the classic lysosomal granules, called the *primary*, or *azurophil*, *granules*, are produced. The primary granules contain hydrolases, elastase, myeloperoxidase, cathepsin G, cationic proteins, and bactericidal/permeability-increasing protein, which is important for killing gram-negative bacteria. Azurophil granules also contain *defensins*, a family of cysteine-rich polypeptides with broad antimicrobial activity against bacteria, fungi, and certain enveloped viruses. The promyelocyte divides to produce the *myelocyte*, a cell responsible for the synthesis of the spe-

cific, or *secondary*, *granules*, which contain unique (specific) constituents such as lactoferrin, vitamin B_{12}–binding protein, membrane components of the nicotinamide-adenine dinucleotide phosphate (NADPH) oxidase required for hydrogen peroxide production, histaminase, and receptors for certain chemoattractants and adherence-promoting factors (CR3) as well as receptors for the basement membrane component, laminin. The secondary granules do not contain acid hydrolases and therefore are not classic lysosomes. Packaging of secondary granule contents during myelopoiesis is controlled by CCAAT/enhancer binding protein-ε. Secondary granule contents are readily released extracellularly, and their mobilization is important in modulating inflammation. During the final stages of maturation no cell division occurs, and the cell passes through the metamyelocyte stage and then to the band neutrophil with a sausage-shaped nucleus (Fig. 55-3). As the band cell matures, the nucleus assumes a lobulated configuration. The nucleus of neutrophils normally contains up to four segments (Fig. 55-4). Excessive segmentation (more than five nuclear lobes) may be a manifestation of folate or vitamin B_{12} deficiency (Fig. 92-4). The Pelger-Hüet anomaly (Fig. 55-5), an infrequent dominant benign inherited trait, results in neutrophils with distinctive bilobed nuclei that must be distinguished from band forms. The physiologic role of the multilobed nucleus of neutrophils is unknown, but it may allow great deformation of neutrophils during migration into tissues at sites of inflammation.

In severe acute bacterial infection, prominent neutrophil cytoplasmic granules, called *toxic granulations*, are occasionally seen. Toxic granulations are immature or abnormally staining azurophil granules. Cytoplasmic inclusions, also called *Döhle bodies* (Fig. 55-3), can be seen during infection and are fragments of ribosome-rich endoplasmic reticulum. Large neutrophil vacuoles are often present in acute bacterial infection and probably represent pinocytosed (internalized) membrane.

Neutrophils are heterogeneous in function. Monoclonal antibodies have been developed that recognize only a subset of mature neutrophils. The meaning of neutrophil heterogeneity is not known.

The morphology of eosinophils and basophils is shown in Fig. 55-6.

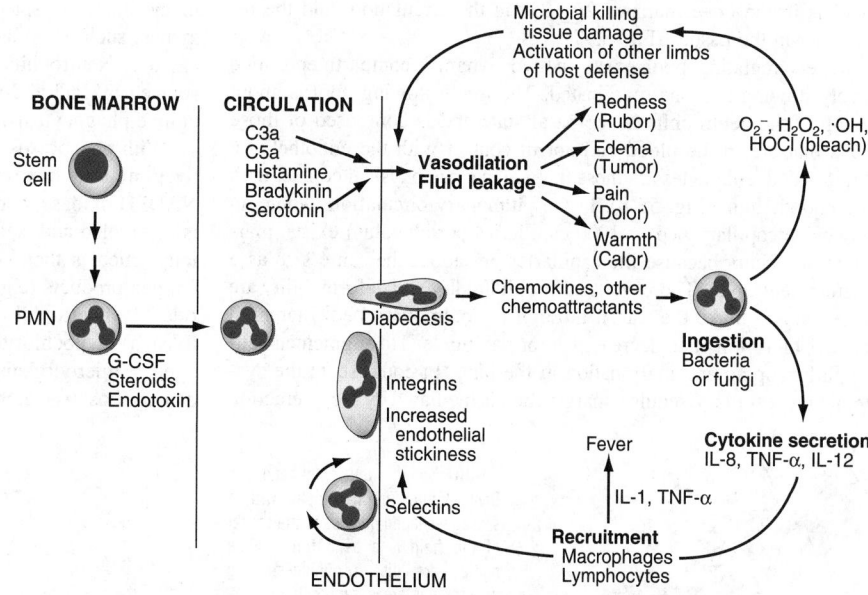

FIGURE 55-1 Schematic events in neutrophil production, recruitment, and inflammation. The four cardinal signs of inflammation (rubor, tumor, calor, dolor) are indicated, as are the interactions of neutrophils with other cells and cytokines. PMN, polymorphonuclear leukocytes; G-CSF, granulocyte colony-stimulating factor; IL, interleukin; TNF-α, tumor necrosis factor.

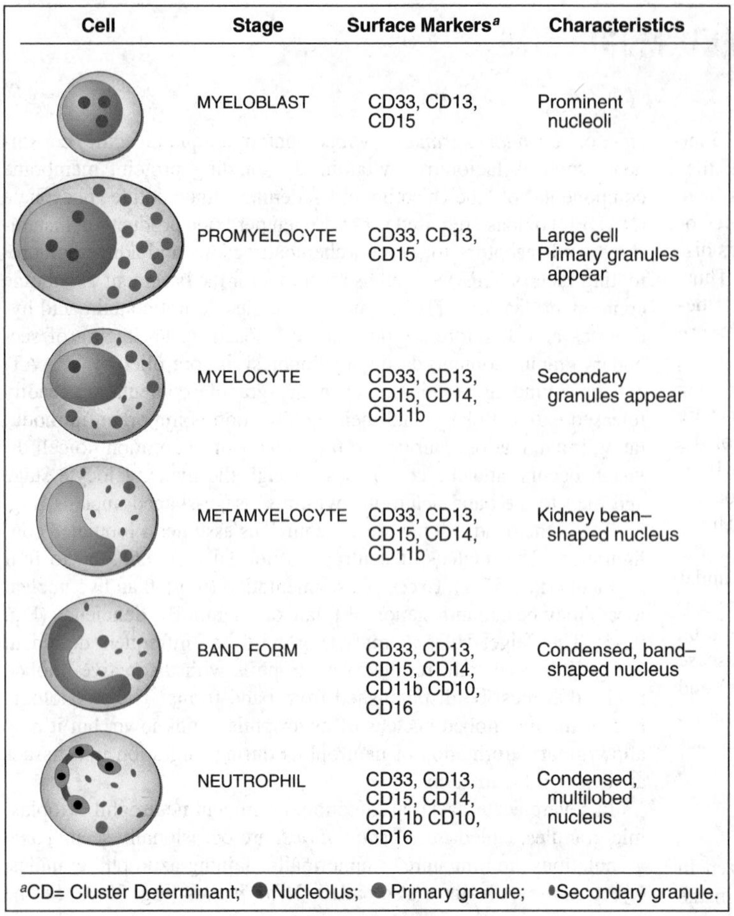

Cell	Stage	Surface Markers[a]	Characteristics
	MYELOBLAST	CD33, CD13, CD15	Prominent nucleoli
	PROMYELOCYTE	CD33, CD13, CD15	Large cell Primary granules appear
	MYELOCYTE	CD33, CD13, CD15, CD14, CD11b	Secondary granules appear
	METAMYELOCYTE	CD33, CD13, CD15, CD14, CD11b	Kidney bean–shaped nucleus
	BAND FORM	CD33, CD13, CD15, CD14, CD11b CD10, CD16	Condensed, band–shaped nucleus
	NEUTROPHIL	CD33, CD13, CD15, CD14, CD11b CD10, CD16	Condensed, multilobed nucleus

[a]CD= Cluster Determinant; ● Nucleolus; ● Primary granule; ● Secondary granule.

FIGURE 55-2 Stages of neutrophil development are schematically shown. G-CSF and GM-CSF are critical to this process. Identifying cellular characteristics and specific cell-surface markers are listed for each maturational stage.

MARROW RELEASE AND CIRCULATING COMPARTMENTS Specific signals, including IL -1, tumor necrosis factor-α (TNF-α), the colony-stimulating factors, complement fragments, and perhaps other cytokines, mobilize leukocytes from the bone marrow and deliver them to the blood in an unstimulated state. Under normal conditions, ~90% of the neutrophil pool is in the bone marrow, 2 to 3% in the circulation, and the remainder in the tissues (Fig. 55-7).

The circulating pool exists in two dynamic compartments: one freely flowing and one marginated. The freely flowing pool is about one-half the neutrophils in the basal state and is composed of those cells that are in the blood and not in contact with the endothelium. Marginated leukocytes are those that are in close physical contact with the endothelium (Fig. 55-8). In the pulmonary circulation, where an extensive capillary bed (~1000 capillaries per alveolus) exists, margination occurs because the capillaries are about the same size as a mature neutrophil. Therefore, neutrophil fluidity and deformability are necessary to make the transit through the pulmonary bed. Increased neutrophil rigidity and decreased deformability lead to augmented neutrophil trapping and margination in the lung. In contrast, in the systemic postcapillary venules, margination is mediated by the interaction of specific cell-surface molecules. *Selectins* are glycoproteins expressed on neutrophils and endothelial cells, among others, that cause a low-affinity interaction, resulting in "rolling" of the neutrophil along the endothelial surface. On neutrophils, the molecule L-selectin [cluster determinant (CD) 62L] binds to glycosylated proteins on endothelial cells [e.g., glycosylation-dependent cell adhesion molecule (GlyCAM1) and CD34]. Glycoproteins on neutrophils, most importantly sialyl-Lewis^x (SLe^x, CD15s), are targets for binding of selectins expressed on endothelial cells [E-selectin (CD62E) and P-selectin (CD62P)] and other leukocytes. In response to chemotactic stimuli from injured tissues (e.g., complement product C5a, leukotriene B$_4$, IL-8) or bacterial products [e.g., *N*-formylmethionylleucylphenylalanine (f-metleuphe)], neutrophil adhesiveness increases, and the cells "stick" to the endothelium through *integrins*. The integrins are leukocyte glycoproteins that exist as complexes of a common CD18 β chain with CD11a (LFA-1), CD11b (also called either Mac-1, CR3, or the C3bi receptor), and CD11c (p150,95). CD11a/CD18 and CD11b/CD18 bind to specific endothelial receptors [intercellular adhesion molecules (ICAM) 1 and 2.]

On cell stimulation, L-selectin is shed; receptors for chemoattractants and opsonins are mobilized; and the phagocytes orient toward the chemoattractant source in the extravascular space, increase their motile activity (chemokinesis), and migrate directionally (chemotaxis) into tissues. The process of migration into tissues is called *diapedesis* and involves the crawling of neutrophils between postcapillary endothelial cells that open junctions between adjacent cells to permit leukocyte passage. Diapedesis involves platelet/endothelial cell adhesion molecule (PECAM) 1 (CD31), which is expressed on both the emigrating leukocyte and the endothelial cells. The endothelial responses (increased blood flow from increased vasodilation and permeability) are mediated by anaphylatoxins (e.g., C3a and C5a) as well as vasodilators such as histamine, bradykinin, serotonin, nitric oxide, vascular endothelial growth factor (VEGF), and prostaglandins E and I. Cytokines regulate some of these processes [e.g., TNF-α induction of VEGF, interferon (IFN) γ inhibition of prostaglandin E.

In the healthy adult, most neutrophils leave the body by migration through the mucous membrane of the gastrointestinal tract. Normally, neutrophils spend a short time in the circulation (half-life, 6 to 7 h). Senescent neutrophils are cleared from the circulation by macrophages in the lung and spleen. Once in the tissues, neutrophils release enzymes, such as collagenase and elastase, that help establish abscess cavities. Neutrophils ingest pathogenic materials that have been opsonized by IgG and C3b. Fibronectin and the tetrapeptide tuftsin facilitate phagocytosis.

With phagocytosis comes a burst of oxygen consumption and activation of the hexose-monophosphate shunt. A membrane-associated NADPH oxidase, consisting of membrane and cytosolic components, is assembled and catalyzes the reduction of oxygen to superoxide anion, which is then converted to hydrogen peroxide and other toxic oxygen products (e.g., hydroxyl radical). Hydrogen peroxide + chloride + neutrophil myeloperoxidase generate hypochlorous acid (bleach), hypochlorite, and chlorine. These products oxidize and halogenate microorganisms and tumor cells and, when uncontrolled, can damage host tissue. Strongly cationic proteins, defensins, and probably

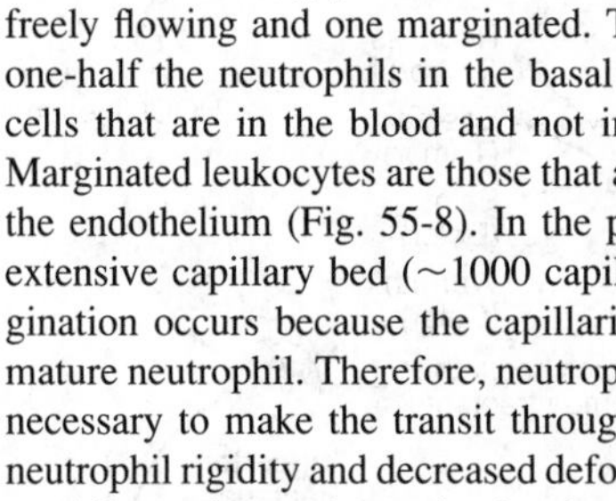

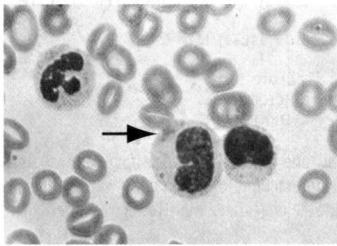

FIGURE 55-3 Neutrophil band with Döhle body. The neutrophil with a sausage-shaped nucleus in the center of the field is a band form. Döhle bodies are discrete, blue-staining nongranular areas found in the periphery of the cytoplasm of the neutrophil in infections and other toxic states. They represent aggregates of rough endoplasmic reticulum.

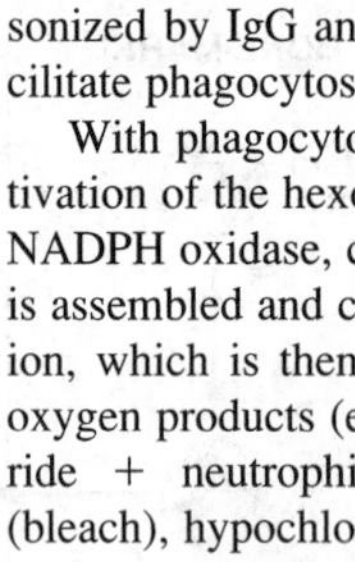

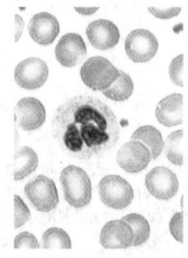

FIGURE 55-4 Normal granulocyte. The normal granulocyte has a segmented nucleus with heavy, clumped chromatin; fine neutrophilic granules are dispersed throughout the cytoplasm.

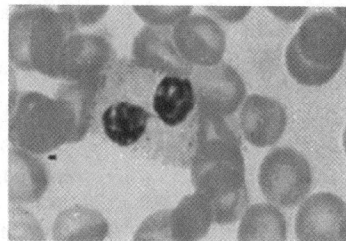

FIGURE 55-5 Pelger-Hüet anomaly. In this benign disorder, the majority of granulocytes are bilobed. The nucleus frequently has a spectacle-like, or "pince-nez," configuration.

nitric oxide also participate in microbial killing. Other enzymes, such as lysozyme and acid proteases, help digest microbial debris. After 1 to 4 days in tissues neutrophils die. The apoptosis of neutrophils is also cytokine-regulated; granulocyte colony-stimulating factor (G-CSF) and IFN-γ prevent their death. Under certain conditions, such as in delayed-type hypersensitivity, monocyte accumulation occurs within 6 to 12 h of initiation of inflammation. Neutrophils, monocytes, microorganisms in various states of digestion, and altered local tissue cells make up the inflammatory exudate, pus. Myeloperoxidase confers the characteristic green color to pus and may participate in turning off the inflammatory process by inactivating chemoattractants and immobilizing phagocytic cells.

Neutrophils respond to certain cytokines [IFN-γ, granulocyte-macrophage colony-stimulating factor (GM-CSF), IL-8] and produce cytokines and chemotactic signals [TNF-α, IL-8, macrophage inflammatory protein (MIP) 1] that modulate the inflammatory response. In the presence of fibrinogen, f-metleuphe or leukotriene B_4 induces IL-8 production by neutrophils, providing autocrine amplification of inflammation. *Chemokines* (chemoattractant cytokines) are small proteins produced by many different cell types, including endothelial cells, fibroblasts, epithelial cells, neutrophils, and monocytes, that regulate neutrophil and monocyte recruitment and activation. The chemokines transduce their signals through heterotrimeric G protein–linked receptors that have seven cell membrane–spanning domains, the same type of cell-surface receptor that mediates the response to the classic chemoattractants f-metleuphe and C5a. Four major groups of chemokines are recognized based on the cysteine structure near the N terminus: C, CC, CXC, and CXXXC. The CXC cytokines such as IL-8 mainly attract neutrophils; CC chemokines such as MIP-1 attract lymphocytes, monocytes, eosinophils, and basophils; the C chemokine lymphotactin is T cell tropic; the CXXXC chemokine fractalkine attracts neutrophils, monocytes, and T cells. These molecules and their receptors not only regulate the trafficking and activation of inflammatory cells, but chemokine receptors serve as co-receptors for HIV infection (Chap. 173) and have a role in atherogenesis.

NEUTROPHIL ABNORMALITIES A defect in the neutrophil life cycle can lead to dysfunction and compromised host defenses. Inflammation is often depressed, and the clinical result is often recurrent and severe bacterial and fungal infections. Aphthous ulcers of mucous membranes (gray ulcers without pus) and gingivitis and periodontal disease suggest a phagocytic cell disorder. Patients with congenital phagocyte defects can have infections within the first few days of life. Skin, ear, upper and lower respiratory tract, and bone infections are common. Sepsis and meningitis are rare. In some disorders the frequency of infection is variable, and patients can go for months or even years without major infection. Aggressive management of these congenital diseases has extended the life span of patients well beyond 30 years.

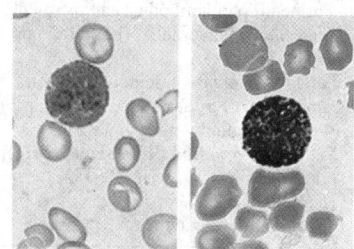

FIGURE 55-6 Normal eosinophil and basophil. The eosinophil contains large, bright orange granules and usually a bilobed nucleus. The basophil contains large purple-black granules that fill the cell and obscure the nucleus.

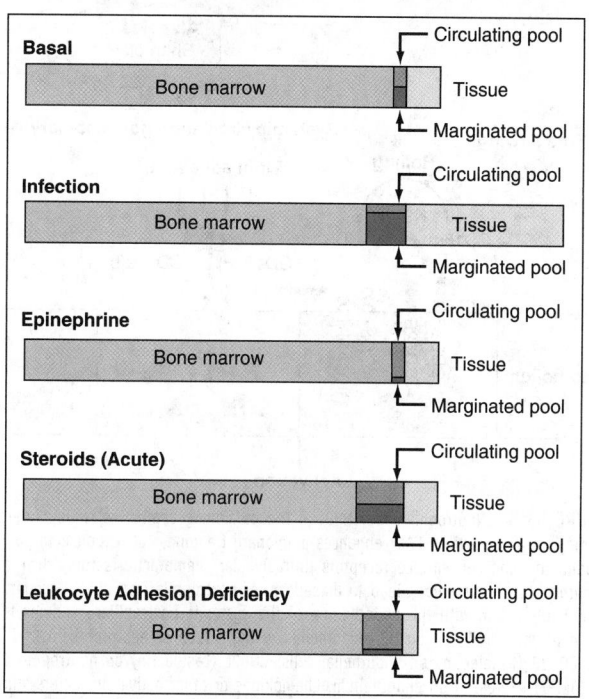

FIGURE 55-7 Schematic neutrophil distribution and kinetics between the different anatomic and functional pools.

Neutropenia The consequences of absent neutrophils are dramatic. Susceptibility to infectious diseases increases sharply when neutrophil counts fall below 1000 cells/μL. When the absolute neutrophil count (ANC; band forms and mature neutrophils combined) falls to <500 cells/μL, control of endogenous microbial flora (e.g., mouth, gut) is impaired; when the ANC is <200/μL, the inflammatory process is absent. Neutropenia can be due to depressed production, increased peripheral destruction, or excessive peripheral pooling. A falling neutrophil count or a significant decrease in the number of neutrophils below steady-state levels, together with a failure to increase neutrophil counts in the setting of infection or other challenge, requires investigation. Acute neutropenia, such as that caused by cancer chemotherapy, is more likely to be associated with increased risk of infection than neutropenia of long duration (months to years) that reverses in response to infection or carefully controlled administration of endotoxin (see "Laboratory Diagnosis," below).

Some causes of inherited and acquired neutropenia are listed in Table 55-1. The most common neutropenias are iatrogenic, resulting from the use of cytotoxic or immunosuppressive therapies for malignancy or control of autoimmune disorders. These drugs cause neutropenia because they result in decreased production of rapidly growing progenitor (stem) cells of the marrow. Certain antibiotics such as chloramphenicol, trimethoprim-sulfamethoxazole, flucytosine, vidarabine, and the antiretroviral drug zidovudine may cause neutropenia by inhibiting proliferation of myeloid precursors. The marrow suppression is generally dose-related and dependent on continued administration of the drug. Recombinant human G-CSF usually reverses this form of neutropenia.

Another important mechanism for iatrogenic neutropenia is the effect of drugs that serve as immune haptens and sensitize neutrophils or neutrophil precursors to immune-mediated peripheral destruction. This form of drug-induced neutropenia can be seen within 7 days of exposure to the drug; with previous drug exposure, resulting in pre-existing antibodies, neutropenia may occur a few hours after administration of the drug. Although any drug can cause this form of neutropenia, the most frequent causes are commonly used antibiotics, such as sulfa-containing compounds, penicillins, and cephalosporins. Fever and eosinophilia may also be associated with drug reactions, but

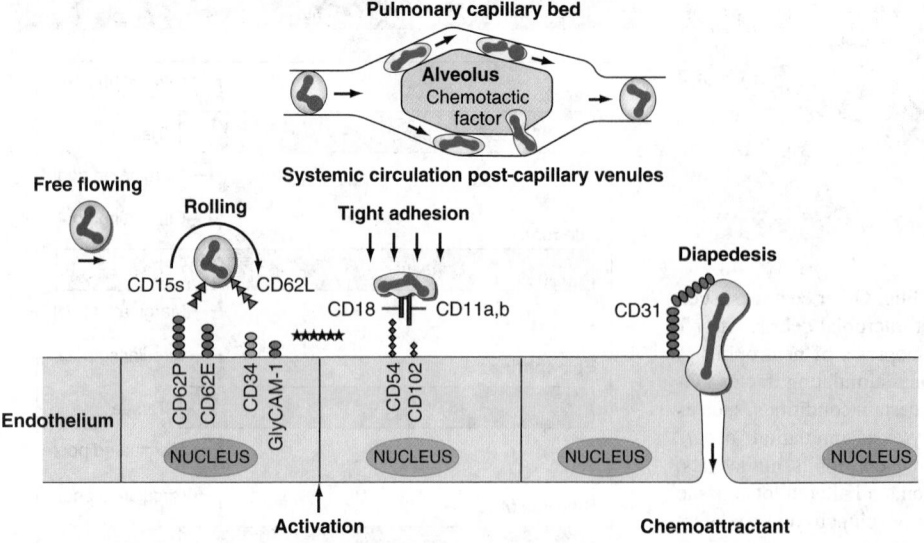

FIGURE 55-8 Neutrophil travel through the pulmonary capillaries is dependent on neutrophil deformability. Neutrophil rigidity (e.g., caused by C5a) enhances pulmonary trapping and response to pulmonary pathogens in a way that is not so dependent upon cell-surface receptors. Intraalveolar chemotactic factors, such as those caused by certain bacteria (e.g., *Streptococcus pneumoniae*) lead to diapedesis of neutrophils from the pulmonary capillaries into the alveolar space. Neutrophil interaction with the endothelium of the systemic postcapillary venules is dependent on molecules of attachment. The neutrophil "rolls" along the endothelium using selectins: neutrophil CD15s (sialyl-Lewis^x) binds to CD62E (E-selectin) and CD62P (P-selectin) on endothelial cells; CD62L (L-selectin) on neutrophils binds to CD34 and other molecules (e.g., GlyCAM-1) expressed on endothelium. Chemokines or other activation factors stimulate integrin-mediated "tight adhesion": CD11a/CD18 (LFA-1) and CD11b/CD18 (Mac-1, CR3) bind to CD54 (ICAM-1) and CD102(ICAM-2) on the endothelium. Diapedesis occurs between endothelial cells: CD31 (PECAM-1) expressed by the emigrating neutrophil interacts with CD31 expressed at the endothelial cell-cell junction.

often these signs are not present. Drug-induced neutropenia can be severe, but discontinuation of the sensitizing drug is sufficient for recovery, which is usually seen within 5 to 7 days and is complete by 10 days. Readministration of the sensitizing drug should be avoided, since abrupt neutropenia will often result. For this reason, diagnostic challenge should be avoided.

Autoimmune neutropenias caused by circulating antineutrophil antibodies are another form of acquired neutropenia that results in increased destruction of neutrophils. Acquired neutropenia may also be seen with viral infections, including infection with HIV. Acquired neutropenia may be cyclic in nature, occurring at intervals of several weeks. Acquired cyclic or stable neutropenia may be associated with an expansion of large granular lymphocytes (LGL), which may be T cells, NK cells, or NK-like cells. Patients with LGL lymphocytosis may have moderate blood and bone marrow lymphocytosis, neutropenia, polyclonal hypergammaglobulinemia, splenomegaly, rheumatoid arthritis, and absence of lymphadenopathy. Such patients may have a chronic and relatively stable course. Recurrent bacterial infections are frequent. Benign and malignant forms of this syndrome occur. In some patients, a spontaneous regression has occurred even after 11 years, suggesting an immunoregulatory defect as the basis for at least one form of the disorder. Glucocorticoids, cyclosporine, IFN-α, and nucleosides such as 2-chlorodeoxyadenosine each have induced remission.

Hereditary Neutropenias Hereditary neutropenias are rare and may manifest in early childhood as a profound constant neutropenia or agranulocytosis. Congenital forms of neutropenia include Kostmann's syndrome (neutrophil count < 100/μL), which is often fatal; more benign severe chronic neutropenia (neutrophil count of 300 to 1500/μL) due to mutations in neutrophil elastase; the cartilage-hair hypoplasia syndrome due to mutations in the mitochondrial RNA-processing endoribonuclease, RMRP; Shwachman-Diamond syndrome associated with pancreatic insufficiency due to mutations in the Shwachman-Bodian-Diamond syndrome gene, *SBDS*; myelokathexis, a congenital disorder characterized by neutrophil degeneration, hypersegmentation, and myeloid hyperplasia in the marrow associated with decreased expression of bcl-X$_L$ in myeloid precursors and accel-

erated apoptosis due to mutations in the chemokine receptor CXCR4; and neutropenias associated with other immune defects (X-linked agammaglobulinemia, ataxia telangiectasia, IgA deficiency). Mutations in the G-CSF receptor on chromosome 1 associated with poor response to G-CSF can develop in severe congenital neutropenia and are linked to myeloid malignancy. Hereditary cyclic neutropenia, an autosomal dominant trait, is typically diagnosed in infancy and is characterized by a remarkably regular 3-week cycle. Hereditary cyclic neutropenia actually is cyclic hematopoiesis, also due to mutations in the neutrophil elastase gene. Glucocorticoids and G-CSF blunt the cycling in some patients.

Maternal factors can be associated with neutropenia in the newborn. Transplacental transfer of IgG directed against antigens on fetal neutrophils can result in peripheral destruction. Drugs (e.g., thiazides) ingested during pregnancy can cause neutropenia in the newborn by either depressed production or peripheral destruction.

The presence of immunoglobulin directed toward neutrophils is seen in Felty's syndrome—a triad of rheumatoid arthritis, splenomegaly, and neutropenia (Chap. 301). Patients with Felty's syndrome who respond to splenectomy with an increase in their neutrophil count also have lower postoperative serum neutrophil-binding IgG. Some of these patients have neutropenia associated with an increased number of LGL. Splenomegaly with peripheral trapping and destruction of neutrophils is also seen in lysosomal storage diseases and in portal hypertension.

Neutrophilia Neutrophilia results from increased neutrophil production, increased marrow release, or defective margination (Table 55-2). The most important acute cause of neutrophilia is infection. Neutrophilia from acute infection represents both increased production and increased marrow release. Increased production is also associated with chronic inflammation and certain myeloproliferative diseases. In-

TABLE 55-1 *Causes of Neutropenia*

Decreased Production

Drug-induced—alkylating agents (nitrogen mustard, busulfan, chlorambucil, cyclophosphamide); antimetabolites (methotrexate, 6-mercaptopurine, 5-flucytosine); noncytotoxic agents [antibiotics (chloramphenicol, penicillins, sulfonamides), phenothiazines, tranquilizers (meprobamate), anticonvulsants (carbamazepine), antipsychotics (clozapine), certain diuretics, anti-inflammatory agents, antithyroid drugs, many others]

Hematologic diseases—idiopathic, cyclic neutropenia, Chédiak-Higashi syndrome, aplastic anemia, infantile genetic disorders (see text)

Tumor invasion, myelofibrosis

Nutritional deficiency—vitamin B$_{12}$, folate (especially alcoholics)

Infection—tuberculosis, typhoid fever, brucellosis, tularemia, measles, infectious mononucleosis, malaria, viral hepatitis, leishmaniasis, AIDS

Peripheral Destruction

Antineutrophil antibodies and/or splenic or lung trapping

Autoimmune disorders—Felty's syndrome, rheumatoid arthritis, lupus erythematosus

Drugs as haptens—aminopyrine, α-methyldopa, phenylbutazone, mercurial diuretics, some phenothiazines

Wegener's granulomatosis

Peripheral Pooling (Transient Neutropenia)

Overwhelming bacterial infection (acute endotoxemia)

Hemodialysis

Cardiopulmonary bypass

TABLE 55-2 Causes of Neutrophilia

Increased Production
 Idiopathic
 Drug-induced—glucocorticoids
 Infection—bacterial, fungal, sometimes viral
 Inflammation—thermal injury, tissue necrosis, myocardial and pulmonary
  infarction, hypersensitivity states, collagen vascular diseases
 Myeloproliferative diseases—myelocytic leukemia, myeloid
  metaplasia, polycythemia vera
Increased Marrow Release
 Glucocorticoids
 Acute infection (endotoxin)
 Inflammation—thermal injury
Decreased or Defective Margination
 Drugs—epinephrine, glucocorticoids, nonsteroidal anti-inflammatory
  agents
 Stress, excitement, vigorous exercise
 Leukocyte adhesion deficiency type 1 (integrin β chain, CD18);
  leukocyte adhesion deficiency type 2 (selectin ligand, CD15s, sialyl-
  Lewis^x)
Miscellaneous
 Metabolic disorders—ketoacidosis, acute renal failure, eclampsia,
  acute poisoning
 Drugs—lithium
 Other—metastatic carcinoma, acute hemorrhage or hemolysis

creased marrow release and mobilization of the marginated leukocyte pool are induced by glucocorticoids. Release of epinephrine, as with vigorous exercise, excitement, or stress, will demarginate neutrophils in the spleen and lungs and double the neutrophil count in minutes. Leukocytosis with cell counts of 10,000 to 25,000/μL occurs in response to infection and other forms of acute inflammation and results from both release of the marginated pool and mobilization of marrow reserves. Persistent neutrophilia with cell counts of ≥30,000 to 50,000/μL is called a *leukemoid reaction*, a term often used to distinguish this degree of neutrophilia from leukemia. In a leukemoid reaction, the circulating neutrophils are usually mature and not clonally derived.

Abnormal Neutrophil Function Inherited and acquired abnormalities of phagocyte function are listed in Table 55-3. The resulting diseases are best considered in terms of the functional defects of adherence, chemotaxis, and microbicidal activity. The distinguishing features of the important inherited disorders of phagocyte function are shown in Table 55-4.

DISORDERS OF ADHESION Two types of leukocyte adhesion deficiency (LAD) have been described. Both are autosomal recessive traits and result in the inability of neutrophils to exit the circulation to sites of

infection, leading to leukocytosis and increased susceptibility to infection (Fig. 55-8). Patients with LAD 1 have mutations in CD18, the common component of the integrins LFA-1, Mac-1, and p150,95, leading to a defect in tight adhesion between neutrophils and the endothelium. The heterodimer formed by CD18/CD11b (Mac-1) is also the receptor for the complement-derived opsonin C3bi (CR3). The CD18 gene is located on distal chromosome 21q. Variable expression of the defect determines the severity of clinical disease. Complete lack of expression of the leukocyte integrins results in severe phenotype in which inflammatory stimuli do not increase the expression of leukocyte integrins on neutrophils or activated T and B cells. Neutrophils (and monocytes) from patients with LAD 1 adhere poorly to endothelial cells and protein-coated surfaces and exhibit defective spreading, aggregation, and chemotaxis. Patients with LAD 1 have recurrent bacterial and fungal infections involving skin, oral and genital mucosa, and respiratory and intestinal tracts; persistent leukocytosis (neutrophil counts of 15,000 to 20,000/μL because cells do not marginate; and, in severe cases, a history of delayed separation of the umbilical stump. Infections, especially of the skin, may become necrotic with progressively enlarging borders, slow healing, and development of dysplastic scars. The most common bacteria are *Staphylococcus aureus* and enteric gram-negative bacteria. LAD 2 is caused by an abnormality of fucosylation of SLe^x(CD15s), the ligand on neutrophils that interacts with selectins on endothelial cells. It is now also known as *congenital disorder of glycosylation IIc* (CDGIIc).

DISORDERS OF NEUTROPHIL GRANULES The most common neutrophil defect is myeloperoxidase deficiency, a primary granule defect inherited as an autosomal recessive trait; the incidence is ~1 in 2000 persons. Isolated myeloperoxidase deficiency is not associated with clinically compromised defenses, presumably because other defense systems such as hydrogen peroxide generation are amplified. Microbicidal activity of neutrophils is delayed but not absent. Myeloperoxidase deficiency may make other acquired host defense defects more serious. An acquired form of myeloperoxidase deficiency occurs in myelomonocytic leukemia and acute myeloid leukemia.

Chédiak-Higashi syndrome (CHS) is a rare disease with autosomal recessive inheritance due to defects in the lysosomal transport protein LYST, encoded by the gene *CHS1* at 1q42. This protein is required for normal packaging and disbursement of granules. Neutrophils (and all cells containing lysosomes) from patients with CHS characteristically have large granules (Fig. 55-9). Patients with CHS have an increased number of infections resulting from many bacterial agents. CHS neutrophils and monocytes have impaired chemotaxis and abnormal rates of microbial killing due to slow rates of fusion of the lysosomal granules with phagosomes. NK cell function is also impaired.

TABLE 55-3 Types of Granulocyte and Monocyte Disorders

Function	Cause of Indicated Dysfunction		
	Drug-Induced	Acquired	Inherited
Adherence-aggregation	Aspirin, colchicine, alcohol, glucocorticoids, ibuprofen, piroxicam	Neonatal state, hemodialysis	Leukoctye adhesion deficiency types 1 and 2
Deformability		Leukemia, neonatal state, diabetes mellitus, immature neutrophils	
Chemokinesis-chemotaxis	Glucocorticoids (high dose), auranofin, colchicine (weak effect), phenylbutazone, naproxen, indomethacin, interleukin 2	Thermal injury, malignancy, malnutrition, periodontal disease, neonatal state, systemic lupus erythematosus, rheumatoid arthritis, diabetes mellitus, sepsis, influenza virus infection, herpes simplex virus infection, acrodermatitis enteropathica, AIDS	Chédiak-Higashi syndrome, neutrophil-specific granule deficiency, hyper IgE–recurrent infection (Job's) syndrome (in some patients), Down syndrome, α-mannosidase deficiency, severe combined immunodeficiency, Wiskott-Aldrich syndrome
Microbicidal activity	Colchicine, cyclophosphamide, glucocorticoids (high dose), TNF-α blocking antibodies	Leukemia, aplastic anemia, certain neutropenias, tuftsin deficiency, thermal injury, sepsis, neonatal state, diabetes mellitus, malnutrition, AIDS	Chédiak-Higashi syndrome, neutrophil-specific granule deficiency, chronic granulomatous disease, defects in IFN-γ/IL-12 axis

Clinical Manifestations	Cellular or Molecular Defects	Diagnosis
CHRONIC GRANULOMATOUS DISEASES (70% X-LINKED, 30% AUTOSOMAL RECESSIVE)		
Severe infections of skin, ears, lungs, liver, and bone with catalase-positive microorganisms such as *S. aureus*, *Burkholderia cepacia*, *Aspergillus* spp., *Chromobacterium violaceum*; often hard to culture organism; excessive inflammation with granulomas, frequent lymph node suppuration; granulomas can obstruct GI or GU tracts; gingivitis, aphthous ulcers, seborrheic dermatitis	No respiratory burst due to the lack of one of four NADPH oxidase subunits in neutrophils, monocytes, and eosinophils	NBT or DHR test; no superoxide and H_2O_2 production by neutrophils; immunoblot for NADPH oxidase components; genetic detection
CHÉDIAK-HIGASHI SYNDROME (AUTOSOMAL RECESSIVE)		
Recurrent pyogenic infections, especially with *S. aureus*; many patients get lymphoma-like illness during adolescence; periodontal disease; partial oculocutaneous albinism, nystagmus, progressive peripheral neuropathy, mental retardation in some patients	Reduced chemotaxis and phagolysosome fusion, increased respiratory burst activity, defective egress from marrow, abnormal skin window; defect in LYST	Giant primary granules in neutrophils and other granule-bearing cells (Wright's stain); genetic detection
SPECIFIC GRANULE DEFICIENCY (AUTOSOMAL RECESSIVE?)		
Recurrent infections of skin, ears, and sinopulmonary tract; delayed wound healing; decreased inflammation; bleeding diathesis	Abnormal chemotaxis, impaired respiratory burst and bacterial killing, failure to upregulate chemotactic and adhesion receptors with stimulation, defect in transcription of granule proteins; defect in cEPB-ε	Lack of secondary (specific) granules in neutrophils (Wright's stain), no neutrophil-specific granule contents (i.e., lactoferrin), no defensins, platelet α granule abnormality; genetic detection
MYELOPEROXIDASE DEFICIENCY (AUTOSOMAL RECESSIVE)		
Clinically normal except in patients with underlying disease such as diabetes mellitus; then candidiasis or other fungal infections	No myeloperoxidase due to pre- and posttranslational defects	No peroxidase in neutrophils; genetic detection
LEUKOCYTE ADHESION DEFICIENCY (AUTOSOMAL RECESSIVE)		
Type 1: Delayed separation of umbilical cord, sustained neutrophilia, recurrent infections of skin and mucosa, gingivitis, periodontal disease	Impaired phagocyte adherence, aggregation, spreading, chemotaxis, phagocytosis of C3bi-coated particles; defective production of CD18 subunit common to leukocyte integrins	Reduced phagocyte surface expression of the CD18-containing integrins with monoclonal antibodies against LFA-1 (CD18/CD11a), Mac-1 or CR3 (CD18/CD11b), p150,95 (CD18/CD11c); genetic detection
Type 2: Mental retardation, short stature, Bombay (hh) blood phenotype, recurrent infections, neutrophilia	Impaired phagocyte rolling along endothelium	Reduced phagocyte surface expression of Sialyl-Lewis^x, with monoclonal antibodies against CD15s; genetic detection
PHACOCYTE ACTIVATION DEFECTS (X-LINKED AND AUTOSOMAL RECESSIVE)		
NEMO deficiency: mild hypohidrotic ectodermal dysplasia; broad based immune defect: pyogenic and encapsulated bacteria, viruses, *Pneumocystis*, mycobacteria; X-linked	Impaired phagocyte activiation by IL-1, IL-18, TLR, CD40, TNF-α leading to problems with inflammation and antibody production	Poor in vitro response to endotoxin; lack of NF-κB activation; genetic detection
IRAK4 deficiency: susceptibility to pyogenic bacteria such as staphylococci, streptococci, clostridia; resistant to mycobacteria; autosomal recessive	Impaired phagocyte activation by endotoxin through TLR and other pathways; TNF-α signaling preserved	Poor in vitro response to endotoxin; lack of NF-κB activation by endotoxin; genetic detection
HYPER IGE–RECURRENT INFECTION SYNDROME (AUTOSOMAL DOMINANT) (JOB'S SYNDROME)		
Eczematoid or pruritic dermatitis, "cold" skin abscesses, recurrent pneumonias with *S. aureus* with bronchopleural fistulae and cyst formation, mild eosinophilia, mucocutaneous candidiasis, characteristic facies, restrictive lung disease, scoliosis, delayed primary dental deciduation	Reduced chemotaxis in some patients, reduced suppressor T cell activity	Clinical features, involving lungs, skeleton, and immune system; serum IgE > 2000 IU/mL
MYCOBACTERIA SUSCEPTIBILITY (AUTOSOMAL DOMINANT AND RECESSIVE FORMS)		
Severe local or disseminated infections with bacille Calmette-Guérin (BCG), nontuberculous mycobacteria, salmonella, histoplasmosis, poor granuloma formation	Inability to kill intracellular organisms due to low IFN-γ production; mutations in IFN-γ receptors, IL-12 receptor, IL-12 p40, STAT-1, NEMO	Low or very high levels of IFN-γ receptor 1; functional assays of cytokine production and response; genetic detection

Abbreviations: GI, gastrointestinal; GU, genitourinary; NADPH, nicotinamide-adenine dinucleotide phosphate, NBT, nitroblue tetrazolium (dye test), DHR, dihydrorhodamine (oxidation test); LYST, lysosomal transport protein; cEBP-ε, CCAAT/enhancer binding protein-ε; NEMO, NF-κB essential modulator; TLR, Toll-like receptor; IL, interleukin; TNF, tumor necrosis factor; IRAK4, IL-1 receptor–associated kinase protein-ε, NEMO 4; IFN, interferon.

Specific granule deficiency is a rare autosomal recessive disease in which the production of secondary granules and their contents, as well as the primary granule component defensins, is defective. The defect in bacterial killing leads to severe bacterial infections. One type of specific granule deficiency is due to a mutation in the CCAAT/enhancer binding protein-ε, a regulator of expression of granule components.

CHRONIC GRANULOMATOUS DISEASE Chronic granulomatous disease (CGD) is a group of disorders of granulocyte and monocyte oxidative metab-

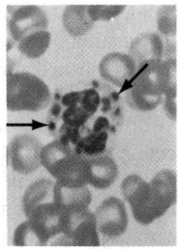

FIGURE 55-9 Chédiak-Higashi syndrome. In this disorder, the granulocytes contain huge cytoplasmic granules formed from aggregation and fusion of azurophilic and specific granules. Large abnormal granules are found in other granule-containing cells throughout the body.

olism. Although CGD is rare, with an incidence of 1 in 200,000 individuals, it is an important model of defective neutrophil oxidative metabolism. Most often CGD is inherited as an X-linked recessive trait; 30% of patients inherit the disease in an autosomal recessive pattern. Mutations in the genes for the four proteins that assemble at the plasma membrane account for all patients with CGD. Two proteins (a 91-kDa protein, abnormal in X-linked CGD, and a 22-kDa protein, absent in one form of autosomal recessive CGD) form the heterodimer cytochrome b-558 in the plasma membrane. Two other proteins (47 and 67 kDa, abnormal in the other autosomal recessive forms of CGD) are cytoplasmic in origin and interact with the cytochrome after cell activation to form NADPH oxidase, required for hydrogen peroxide production. Leukocytes from patients with CGD have severely diminished hydrogen peroxide production. The genes involved in each of the defects have been cloned and sequenced and the chromosome locations identified. Patients with CGD characteristically have increased numbers of infections due to catalase-positive microorganisms (organisms that destroy their own hydrogen peroxide). When patients with CGD become infected, they often have extensive inflammatory reactions, and lymph node suppuration is common despite the administration of appropriate antibiotics. Aphthous ulcers and chronic inflammation of the nares are often present. Granulomas are frequent and can obstruct the gastrointestinal or genitourinary tracts. The excessive inflammation probably reflects failure to degrade chemoattractants and antigens, leading to persistent neutrophil accumulation. Impaired killing of intracellular microorganisms by macrophages may lead to persistent cell-mediated immune activation and granuloma formation. Autoimmune complications such as immune thrombocytopenic purpura (ITP) and juvenile rheumatoid arthritis (JRA) are also increased in CGD. In addition, discoid lupus is more common in X-linked carriers.

DISORDERS OF PHAGOCYTE ACTIVATION Phagocytes depend on cell-surface stimulation to induce signals that evoke multiple levels of the inflammatory response, including cytokine synthesis, chemotaxis, and antigen presentation. Mutations affecting the major pathway that signals through NF-κB have been noted in patients with a variety of infection susceptibility syndromes. If the defects are at a very late stage of signal transduction, in the protein critical for NF-κB activation known as the NF-κB essential modulator (NEMO), then affected males develop ectodermal dysplasia and severe immune deficiency with susceptibility to bacteria, fungi, mycobacteria, and viruses. If the defect in NF-κB activation is closer to the signaling source, in the IL-1 receptor–associated kinase 4 (IRAK4), then children have a marked suceptibility to pyogenic infections early in life but develop resistance to infection later.

MONONUCLEAR PHAGOCYTES

The mononuclear phagocyte system is composed of monoblasts, promonocytes, and monocytes in addition to the structurally diverse tissue macrophages that make up what was previously referred to as the reticuloendothelial system. Macrophages are long-lived phagocytic cells capable of many of the functions of neutrophils. They are also secretory cells that participate in many immunologic and inflammatory processes distinct from neutrophils. Monocytes leave the circulation by diapedesis more slowly than neutrophils and have a half-life in the blood of 12 to 24 h.

After blood monocytes arrive in the tissues, they differentiate into macrophages ("big eaters") with specialized functions suited for specific anatomic locations. Macrophages are particularly abundant in capillary walls of the lung, spleen, liver, and bone marrow, where they function to remove microorganisms and other noxious elements from the blood. Alveolar macrophages, liver Kupffer cells, splenic macrophages, peritoneal macrophages, bone marrow macrophages, lymphatic macrophages, brain microglial cells, and dendritic macrophages all have specialized functions. Macrophage-secreted products include lysozyme, neutral proteases, acid hydrolases, arginase, complement components, enzyme inhibitors (plasmin, α_2-macroglobulin), binding proteins (transferrin, fibronectin, transcobalamin II), nucleosides, and cytokines (TNF-α; IL-1, -8, -12, and -18). IL-1 (Chaps. 16 and 295) has many functions, including initiating fever in the hypothalamus, mobilizing leukocytes from the bone marrow, and activating lymphocytes and neutrophils. TNF-α is a pyrogen that duplicates many of the actions of IL-1 and plays an important role in the pathogenesis of gram-negative shock (Chap. 254). TNF-α stimulates production of hydrogen peroxide and related toxic oxygen species by macrophages and neutrophils. In addition, TNF-α induces catabolic changes that contribute to the profound wasting (cachexia) associated with many chronic diseases.

Other macrophage-secreted products include reactive oxygen and nitrogen metabolites, bioactive lipids (arachidonic acid metabolites and platelet-activating factors), chemokines, colony-stimulating factors, and factors stimulating fibroblast and vessel proliferation. Macrophages help regulate the replication of lymphocytes and participate in the killing of tumors, viruses, and certain bacteria (*Mycobacterium tuberculosis* and *Listeria monocytogenes*). Macrophages are key effector cells in the elimination of intracellular microorganisms. Their ability to fuse to form giant cells that coalesce into granulomas in response to some inflammatory stimuli is important in the elimination of intracellular microbes and is under the control of IFN-γ. Nitric oxide induced by IFN-γ is an important effector against intracellular parasites, including tuberculosis and *Leishmania*.

Macrophages play an important role in the immune response (Chap. 295). They process and present antigen to lymphocytes and secrete cytokines that modulate and direct lymphocyte development and function. Macrophages participate in autoimmune phenomena by removing immune complexes and other substances from the circulation. Polymorphisms in macrophage receptors for immunoglobulin (FcγRII) determine suceptibility to some infections and autoimmune diseases. In wound healing, they dispose of senescent cells, and they contribute to atheroma development. Macrophage elastase mediates development of emphysema from cigarette smoking.

DISORDERS OF THE MONONUCLEAR PHAGOCYTE SYSTEM Many disorders of neutrophils extend to mononuclear phagocytes. Thus, drugs that suppress neutrophil production in the bone marrow can cause monocytopenia. Transient monocytopenia occurs after stress or glucocorticoid administration. Monocytosis is associated with tuberculosis, brucellosis, subacute bacterial endocarditis, Rocky Mountain spotted fever, malaria, and visceral leishmaniasis (kala azar). Monocytosis also occurs with malignancies, leukemias, myeloproliferative syndromes, hemolytic anemias, chronic idiopathic neutropenias, and granulomatous diseases such as sarcoidosis, regional enteritis, and some collagen vascular diseases. Patients with LAD, hyperimmunoglobulin E–recurrent infection (Job's) syndrome, CHS, and CGD all have defects in the mononuclear phagocyte system.

Monocyte cytokine production or response is impaired in some patients with disseminated nontuberculous mycobacterial infection who are not infected with HIV. Genetic defects in the pathways regulated by IFN-γ and IL-12 lead to impaired killing of intracellular bacteria, mycobacteria, salmonellae, and certain viruses (Fig. 55-10).

Certain viral infections impair mononuclear phagocyte function. For example, influenza virus infection causes abnormal monocyte chemotaxis. Mononuclear phagocytes can be infected by HIV using

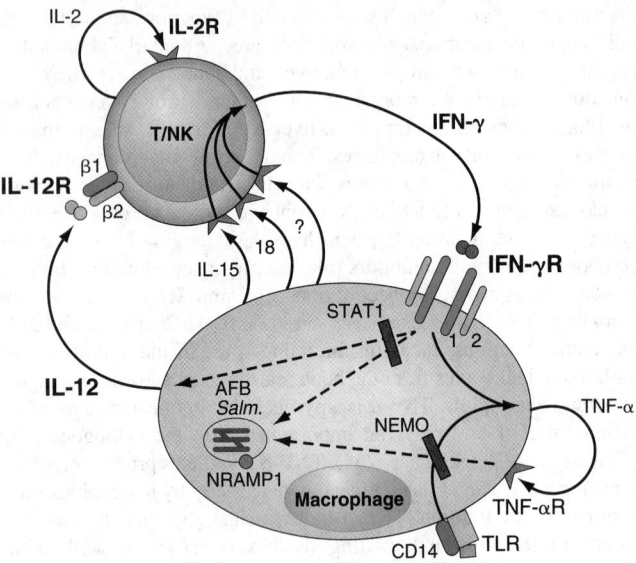

FIGURE 55-10 Lymphocyte-macrophage interactions underlying resistance to mycobacteria and other intracellular parasites such as *Salmonella. Mycobacteria* infect macrophages, leading to the production of IL-12, which activates T or NK cells through its receptor, leading to production of IL-2 and IFN-γ. IFN-γ acts through its receptor on macrophages to upregulate TNF-α and IL-12 and kill intracellular parasites. Mutant forms of the cytokines and receptors shown in large type have been found in severe cases of nontuberculous mycobacterial infection and salmonellosis.

CCR5, the chemokine receptor that acts as a co-receptor with CD4 for HIV. T lymphocytes produce IFN-γ, which induces FcR expression and phagocytosis and stimulates hydrogen peroxide production by mononuclear phagocytes and neutrophils. In certain diseases, such as AIDS, IFN-γ production may be deficient, while in other diseases, such as T cell lymphomas, excessive release of IFN-γ may be associated with erythrophagocytosis by splenic macrophages.

Gain-of-function mutations in the TNF-α receptor cause TNF-α receptor–associated periodic syndromes (TRAPS) that are characterized by recurrent fever in the absence of infection, due to persistent stimulation of the TNF-α receptor. Administration of the TNF-α antagonists infliximab, etanercept, and adalimumab has been associated with severe infections such as tuberculosis.

Monocytopenia occurs with acute infections, with stress, and after treatment with glucocorticoids. Monocytopenia also occurs in aplastic anemia, hairy cell leukemia, acute myeloid leukemia, and as a direct result of myelotoxic drugs.

EOSINOPHILS

Eosinophils and neutrophils share similar morphology, many lysosomal constituents, phagocytic capacity, and oxidative metabolism. Eosinophils express a specific chemoattractant receptor and respond to a specific chemokine, eotaxin. Little is known about the role of eosinophils. Eosinophils are much longer lived than neutrophils, and unlike neutrophils, tissue eosinophils can recirculate. During most infections, eosinophils are not important. However, in invasive helminthic infections, such as hookworm, schistosomiasis, strongyloidiasis, toxocariasis, trichinosis, filariasis, echinococcosis, and cysticercosis, the eosinophil plays a central role in host defense. Eosinophils are associated with bronchial asthma, cutaneous allergic reactions, and other hypersensitivity states.

The distinctive feature of the red-staining (Wright's stain) eosinophil granule is its crystalline core consisting of an arginine-rich protein (major basic protein) with histaminase activity, important in host defense against parasites. Eosinophil granules also contain a unique eosinophil peroxidase that catalyzes the oxidation of many substances by hydrogen peroxide and may facilitate killing of microorganisms.

Eosinophil peroxidase, in the presence of hydrogen peroxide and halide, initiates mast cell secretion in vitro and thereby promotes inflammation. Eosinophils contain cationic proteins, some of which bind to heparin and reduce its anticoagulant activity. Eosinophil-derived neurotoxin and eosinophil cationic protein are ribonucleases that can kill respiratory syncytial virus. Eosinophil cytoplasm contains Charcot-Leyden crystal protein, a hexagonal bipyramidal crystal first observed in a patient with leukemia and then in sputum of patients with asthma; this protein is lysophospholipase and may function to detoxify certain lysophospholipids.

Several factors enhance the eosinophil's function in host defense. T cell–derived factors enhance the ability of eosinophils to kill parasites. Mast cell–derived eosinophil chemotactic factor of anaphylaxis (ECFa) increases the number of eosinophil complement receptors and enhances eosinophil killing of parasites. Eosinophil colony-stimulating factors (e.g., IL-5) produced by macrophages increase eosinophil production in the bone marrow and activate eosinophils to kill parasites.

EOSINOPHILIA Eosinophilia is the presence of >500 eosinophils per microliter of blood and is common in many settings besides parasite infection. Significant tissue eosinophilia can occur without an elevated blood count. A common cause of eosinophilia is allergic reaction to drugs (iodides, aspirin, sulfonamides, nitrofurantoin, penicillins, and cephalosporins). Allergies such as hay fever, asthma, eczema, serum sickness, allergic vasculitis, and pemphigus are associated with eosinophilia. Eosinophilia also occurs in collagen vascular diseases (e.g., rheumatoid arthritis, eosinophilic fasciitis, allergic angiitis, and periarteritis nodosa) and malignancies (e.g., Hodgkin's disease; mycosis fungoides; chronic myelogenous leukemia; and cancer of the lung, stomach, pancreas, ovary, or uterus), as well as in Job's syndrome and CGD. Eosinophilia is commonly present in the helminthic infections. IL-5 is the dominant eosinophil growth factor. Therapeutic administration of the cytokines IL-2 and GM-CSF frequently leads to transient eosinophilia. The most dramatic hypereosinophilic syndromes are Loeffler's syndrome, tropical pulmonary eosinophilia, Loeffler's endocarditis, eosinophilic leukemia, and idiopathic hypereosinophilic syndrome (50,000 to 100,000/μL).

The idiopathic hypereosinophilic syndrome represents a heterogeneous group of disorders with the common feature of prolonged eosinophilia of unknown cause and organ system dysfunction, including the heart, central nervous system, kidneys, lungs, gastrointestinal tract, and skin. The bone marrow is involved in all affected individuals, but the most severe complications involve the heart and central nervous system. Clinical manifestations and organ dysfunction are highly variable. Eosinophils are found in the involved tissues and likely cause tissue damage by local deposition of toxic eosinophil proteins such as eosinophil cationic protein and major basic protein. In the heart, the pathologic changes lead to thrombosis, endocardial fibrosis, and restrictive endomyocardiopathy. The damage to tissues in other organ systems is similar. Some cases are due to mutations involving the platelet derived growth factor receptor and these are extremely sensitive to the tyrosine kinase inhibitor imatinib. Glucocorticoids may also induce remission. In patients who do not respond to glucocorticoids, a cytotoxic agent such as hydroxyurea has been used successfully to lower the peripheral blood eosinophil counts and to improve the prognosis markedly. IFN-α is also effective in some patients, including those unresponsive to hydroxyurea. Aggressive medical and surgical approaches are used to manage patients with cardiovascular complications.

The *eosinophilia-myalgia syndrome* is a multisystem disease with prominent cutaneous, hematologic, and visceral manifestations that frequently evolves into a chronic course and can occasionally be fatal. The syndrome is characterized by eosinophilia (eosinophil count > 1000/μL) and generalized disabling myalgias without other recognized causes. Eosinophilic fasciitis, pneumonitis, and myocarditis; neuropathy culminating in respiratory failure; and encephalopathy may occur. The disease is caused by ingesting contaminants in L-tryptophan–containing products. Eosinophils, lymphocytes, macrophages, and fibroblasts accumulate in the affected tissues, but their role in pathogenesis is unclear. Activation of eosinophils and fibroblasts and the deposition of eosinophil-derived toxic proteins in affected tissues may contribute. IL-5 and transforming growth factor β have been implicated as potential mediators. Treatment is withdrawal of products containing L-tryptophan and the administration of glucocorticoids. Most patients recover fully, remain stable, or show slow recovery, but the disease can be fatal in up to 5% of patients.

EOSINOPENIA Eosinopenia occurs with stress, such as acute bacterial infection, and after treatment with glucocorticoids. The mechanism of eosinopenia of acute bacterial infection is unknown but is independent of endogenous glucocorticoids, since it occurs in animals after total adrenalectomy. There is no known adverse effect of eosinopenia.

HYPERIMMUNOGLOBULIN E-RECURRENT INFECTION SYNDROME

The hyperimmunoglobulin E–recurrent infection (HIE) syndrome, or Job's syndrome, is a rare multisystem disease in which the immune system, bone, teeth, lung, and skin are affected. Abnormal chemotaxis is a variable feature. The molecular basis for this syndrome is not known, but some cases show autosomal dominant transmission with linkage to 4q. Patients with this syndrome have characteristic facies with broad nose, kyphoscoliosis and osteoporosis, and eczema. The primary teeth erupt normally but do not deciduate, often requiring extraction. Patients develop recurrent sinopulmonary and cutaneous infections that tend to be much less inflamed than appropriate for the degree of infection and have been referred to as "cold abscesses." A high degree of suspicion is required to diagnose infections in these patients, who may appear well despite extensive disease. The cold abscesses have been considered a reflection of too few phagocytes arriving too late, perhaps due to a lymphocyte factor inhibiting chemotaxis. However, the chemotactic defect in these patients is variable, and the fundamental basis for the impaired defenses is complex and poorly defined.

LABORATORY DIAGNOSIS AND MANAGEMENT

Initial studies of WBC and differential and often a bone marrow examination may be followed by assessment of bone marrow reserves (steroid challenge test), marginated circulating pool of cells (epinephrine challenge test), and marginating ability (endotoxin challenge test) (Fig. 55-7). In vivo assessment of inflammation is possible with a Rebuck skin window test or an in vivo blister assay, which measures the ability of leukocytes and inflammatory mediators to accumulate locally in the skin. In vitro tests of phagocyte aggregation, adherence, chemotaxis, phagocytosis, degranulation, and microbicidal activity (for *S. aureus*) may help pinpoint cellular or humoral lesions. Deficiencies of oxidative metabolism are detected with either the nitroblue tetrazolium (NBT) dye test or the dihydrorhodamine (DHR) oxidation test. These tests are based on the ability of products of oxidative metabolism to alter the oxidation states of reporter molecules so that they can be detected microscopically (NBT) or by flow cytometry (DHR). Qualitative studies of superoxide and hydrogen peroxide production may further define neutrophil oxidative function.

Patients with leukopenias or leukocyte dysfunction often have delayed inflammatory responses. Therefore, clinical manifestations may be minimal despite overwhelming infection, and unusual infections must always be suspected. Early signs of infection demand prompt, aggressive culturing for microorganisms, use of antibiotics, and surgical drainage of abscesses. Prolonged courses of antibiotics are often required. In patients with CGD, prophylactic antibiotics (trimethoprim-sulfamethoxazole) and antifungals (itraconazole) markedly diminish the frequency of life-threatening infections. Short courses of glucocorticoids may relieve gastrointestinal or genitourinary tract obstruction by granulomas in patients with CGD. Recombinant human IFN-γ, which nonspecifically stimulates phagocytic cell function, reduces the frequency of infections in patients with CGD by 70% and reduces the severity of infection. This effect of IFN-γ in CGD is additive to the effect of prophylactic antibiotics. The recommended dose is 50 $\mu g/m^2$ subcutaneously three times weekly. IFN-γ has also been used successfully in the treatment of leprosy, nontuberculous mycobacteria, and visceral leishmaniasis.

Rigorous oral hygiene reduces but does not eliminate the discomfort of gingivitis, periodontal disease, and aphthous ulcers; chlorhexidine mouthwash and tooth brushing with a hydrogen peroxide–sodium bicarbonate paste helps many patients. Oral antifungal agents (fluconazole) have reduced mucocutaneous candidiasis in patients with Job's syndrome. Androgens, glucocorticoids, lithium, and immunosuppressive therapy have been used to restore myelopoiesis in patients with neutropenia due to impaired production. Recombinant G-CSF is useful in the management of certain forms of neutropenia due to depressed neutrophil production, especially those related to cancer chemotherapy. Patients with chronic neutropenia with evidence of a good bone marrow reserve need not receive prophylactic antibiotics. Patients with chronic or cyclic neutrophil counts < 500/μL may benefit from prophylactic antibiotics and G-CSF during periods of neutropenia. Oral trimethoprim-sulfamethoxazole (160/800 mg) twice daily can prevent infection. Increased numbers of fungal infections are not seen in patients with CGD on this regimen. Oral quinolones such as levofloxacin and ciprofloxacin are alternatives.

In the setting of cytotoxic chemotherapy with severe, persistent neutropenia, trimethoprim-sulfamethoxazole prevents *Pneumocystis carinii* pneumonia. These patients, and patients with phagocytic cell dysfunction, should avoid heavy exposure to airborne soil, dust, or decaying matter (mulch, manure), which are often rich in *Nocardia* and the spores of *Aspergillus* and other fungi. Restriction of activities or social contact has no proven role in reducing risk of infection.

Cure of some congenital phagocyte defects is possible by bone marrow transplantation (Chap. 100). However, complications of bone marrow transplantation are still serious, and with rigorous medical care many patients with phagocytic disorders can go for years without a life-threatening infection. The identification of specific gene defects in patients with LAD 1, CGD, and other immunodeficiencies has led to gene therapy trials in a number of genetic white cell disorders.

FURTHER READING

Dale DC et al: Cyclic neutropenia. Semin Hematol 39:89, 2002

Lekstrom-Himes JA, Gallin JI: Immunodeficiency diseases caused by defects in phagocytes. N Engl J Med 343:1703, 2000

Nathan C: Points of control in inflammation. Nature 420:846, 2002

Picard C et al: Pyogenic bacterial infections in humans with IRAK-4 deficiency. Science 299:2076, 2003

Rosenberg HF, Domachowske JB: Eosinophils, eosinophil ribonucleases, and their role in host defense against respiratory virus pathogens. J Leukoc Biol 70:691; 2001

Segal BH et al: Genetic, biochemical, and clinical features of chronic granulomatous disease. Medicine (Baltimore) 79:170, 2000

56 | PRINCIPLES OF HUMAN GENETICS
J. Larry Jameson, Peter Kopp

IMPACT OF GENETICS ON MEDICAL PRACTICE

The beginning of the new millennium was marked by the announcement that the vast majority of the human genome has been sequenced. This milestone in the exploration of the human genome was preceded by numerous conceptual and technological advances. They include, among others, the elucidation of the DNA double-helix structure, the discovery of restriction enzymes and the polymerase chain reaction (PCR), the development and automatization of DNA sequencing, and the generation of genetic and physical maps by the Human Genome Project (HGP). The consequences of this wealth of knowledge for the practice of medicine are profound, but the integration of genetics into the everyday practice of medicine remains challenging. To date, the most significant impact of genetics has been to enhance our understanding of disease etiology and pathogenesis. In the near term, we can expect an increasing role for genetics in the diagnosis, prevention, and treatment of disease (Chaps. 58 and 59).

Genetics has traditionally been viewed through the window of relatively rare single-gene diseases. Taken together, these rare disorders account for up to 10% of pediatric admissions and childhood mortality. It is, however, increasingly apparent that virtually every medical condition with the exception of simple trauma has a genetic component. As is often evident from a patient's family history, many common disorders such as hypertension, heart disease, asthma, diabetes mellitus, and mental illnesses are significantly influenced by the genetic background. These polygenic or multifactorial disorders involve the contributions of many different genes, as well as environmental factors, that can modify disease risk (Chap. 58). Cancer has a genetic basis since it results from acquired somatic mutations in genes controlling growth and differentiation (Chap. 68). In addition, the development of many cancers is associated with a hereditary predisposition. The prevalence of genetic diseases, combined with their severity and chronic nature, imposes a great financial, social, and emotional burden on society.

Genetics has historically focused on chromosomal and metabolic disorders, reflecting the long-standing availability of techniques to diagnose these conditions. For example, conditions such as trisomy 21 (Down syndrome) or monosomy X (Turner syndrome) can be diagnosed using cytogenetics (Chap. 57). Likewise, many metabolic disorders (e.g., phenylketonuria, familial hypercholesterolemia) are diagnosed using biochemical analyses. Recent advances in DNA diagnostics have extended the field of genetics to include virtually all medical specialties. In cardiology, for example, the molecular basis of inherited cardiomyopathies and ion channel defects that predispose to arrhythmias is being defined (Chaps. 214 and 221). In neurology, genetics has unmasked the pathophysiology of a startling number of neurodegenerative disorders (Chap. 345). Hematology has evolved dramatically, from its incipient genetic descriptions of hemoglobinopathies to the current understanding of the molecular basis of red cell membrane defects, clotting disorders, and thrombotic disorders (Chaps. 91 and 102). It is now abundantly clear that neoplasia and the acquisition of metastatic potential can be described in genetic terms (Chaps. 68 and 69).

New concepts derived from genetic studies can sometimes clarify the pathogenesis of disorders that were previously opaque. For example, although many different genetic defects can cause peripheral neuropathies, disruption of the normal folding of the myelin sheaths is frequently a common final pathway (Chap. 364). Several genetic causes of obesity appear to converge on a physiologic pathway that involves products of the proopiomelanocortin polypeptide and the MC4R receptor, thus identifying a key mechanism for appetite control (Chap. 64). A similar situation is emerging for genetically distinct forms of Alzheimer's disease, several of which lead to the formation of neurofibrillary tangles (Chap. 350). Increasingly, the identification of defective genes can pinpoint cellular pathways involved in key physiologic processes. Examples include identification of the cystic fibrosis conductance regulator (CFTR) gene, the Duchenne muscular dystrophy (DMD) gene, which encodes dystrophin, and the fibroblast growth factor receptor-3 (FGFR3) gene, which is responsible for achondroplastic dwarfism. Similarly, transgenic (over)expression, and targeted gene "knockout" and "knockin" models help to unravel the physiologic function of genes. Genetic approaches have proven invaluable for the detection of infectious pathogens and are used clinically to identify agents that are difficult to culture such as mycobacteria, viruses, and parasites. In many cases, molecular genetics has improved the feasibility and accuracy of diagnostic testing, enhanced our understanding of pathophysiology, and is beginning to open new avenues for therapy, including gene and cellular therapy (Chap. 59).

The astounding rate at which new genetic information is being generated creates a major challenge for physicians, health care providers, and basic investigators. The terminology and techniques used for discovery evolve continuously. Much genetic information presently resides in computer databases or is being published in basic science journals. Databases provide easy access to the expanding information about the human genome, genetic disease, and genetic testing (Table 56-1). For example, several thousand monogenic disorders are summarized in a large, continuously evolving compendium, referred to as the *Online Mendelian Inheritance in Man* (OMIM) catalog (Table 56-1). The ongoing refinement of bioinformatics is simplifying the access to this seemingly daunting onslaught of new information.

APPROACH TO THE PATIENT

For the practicing clinician, the family history remains an essential step in recognizing the possibility of a hereditary component. When taking the history, it is useful to draw a detailed pedigree of the first-degree relatives (e.g., parents, siblings, and children), since they share 50% of genes with the patient. Standard symbols for pedigrees are depicted in Fig. 56-1. The family history should include information about ethnic background, age, health status, and (infant) deaths. Next, the physician should explore whether there is a family history of the same or related illnesses to the current problem. An inquiry focused on commonly occurring disorders such as cancers, heart disease, and diabetes mellitus should follow. Because of the possibility of age-dependent expressivity and penetrance, the family history may need updating. If the findings suggest a genetic disorder, the clinician will have to assess whether some of the patient's relatives may be at risk of carrying or transmitting the disease. In this circumstance, it is useful to confirm and extend the pedigree based on input from several family members. This information may form the basis for carrier detection, genetic counseling, early intervention, and prevention of a disease in relatives of the index patient (Chap. 59).

In instances where a diagnosis at the molecular level may be relevant, the physician will have to identify an appropriate laboratory that can perform the test. If a disease-causing mutation is expected in all cells due to germline transmission, DNA can be collected from any tissue, most commonly nucleated blood cells. In the case of somatic mutations, which are limited to a neoplastic

TABLE 56-1 *Selected Databases Relevant for Genomics and Genetic Disorders*

Site	URL	Comment
National Center for Biotechnology Information (NCBI)	http://www.ncbi.nlm.nih.gov/	Molecular biology information, public databases, computational biology
		Software for analyzing genome data
		Extensive links to other databases, genome resources, and educational primers
National Human Genome Research Institute	http://www.genome.gov/	Web links providing information about the human genome sequence, genomes of other organisms, and genomic research
Ensembl Genome browser	http://www.ensembl.org/	Maps and sequence information of eukaryotic genomes
Online Mendelian Inheritance in Man (OMIM)	http://www.ncbi.nlm.nih.gov/omim/	Online compendium of Mendelian disorders and human genes causing genetic disorders
Office of Biotechnology Activities National Institutes of Health	www4.od.nih.gov/oba/	Information about recombinant DNA and gene transfer
		Medical, ethical, legal, and social issues raised by genetic testing
		Medical, ethical, legal, and social issues raised by xenotransplantation
American College of Medical Genetics	http://www.acmg.net/	Extensive links to other databases relevant for the diagnosis, treatment and prevention of genetic disease
Cancer Genome Anatomy Project (CGAP)	http://cgap.nci.nih.gov/	Information about gene expression profiles of normal, precancer, and cancer cells
GenLink	http://www.genlink.wustl.edu	Multimedia database resource for human genetics and telomere research
GeneTests-GeneClinics	http://www.genetests.org/	International directory of genetic testing laboratories and prenatal diagnosis clinics
		Reviews and educational materials
Dolan DNA Learning Center, Cold Spring Harbor Laboratories	http://www.dnalc.org	Educational material about selected genetic disorders, DNA, eugenics, and genetic origin
HUGO Gene Nomenclature	http://www.gene.ucl.ac.uk/nomenclature	Gene names and symbols
MITOMAP, a human mitochondrial genome database	http://www.mitomap.org	A compendium of polymorphisms and mutations of the human mitochondrial DNA
Mitochondrial disorders	http://www.neuro.wustl.edu/neuromuscular/mitosyn.html	Overview on clinical syndromes associated with mtDNA mutations
DNA repeat sequences & disease	http://www.neuro.wustl.edu/neuromuscular/mother/dnarep.htm	Overview on clinical syndromes associated with DNA repeats
Online Mendelian Inheritance in Animals (OMIA)	http://www.angis.su.oz.au/Databases/BIRX/omia	Online compendium of Mendelian disorders in animals
The Jackson Laboratory	http://www.jax.org/	Information about murine models and the mouse genome

Note: Databases are evolving constantly. Pertinent information may be found by using links listed in the few selected databases.
Instructions for the use of genome-related databases have been published [Nat Genet 32 (Suppl):1–79, 2002].

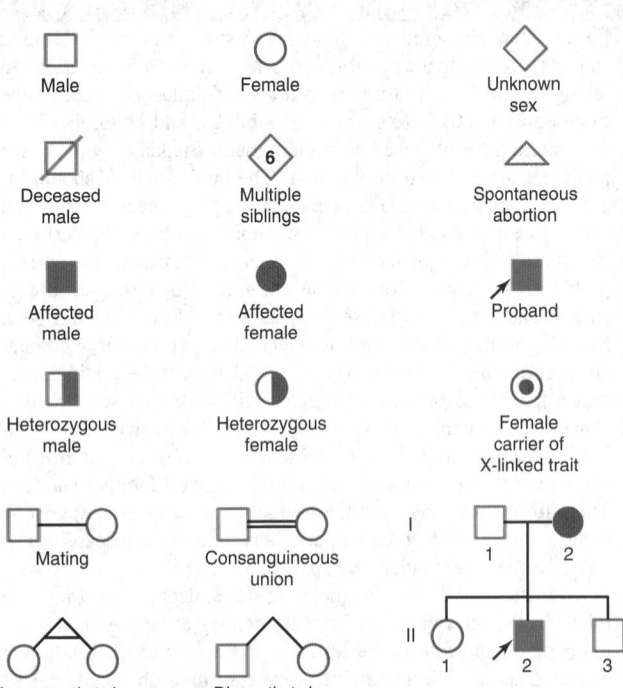

FIGURE 56-1 *Standard pedigree symbols.*

tissue, an adequate sample of this lesion is used for extraction of DNA or RNA. For the detection of pathogens, the material to be analyzed will vary and may include blood, cerebrospinal fluid, solid tissues, sputum, or fluid obtained through bronchioalveolar lavage.

CHROMOSOMES AND DNA REPLICATION

ORGANIZATION OF DNA INTO CHROMOSOMES ■ Size of the Human Genome
The human genome is divided into 23 different chromosomes, including 22 autosomes (numbered 1 to 22) and the X and Y sex chromosomes. Adult cells are diploid, meaning they contain two homologous sets of 22 autosomes and a pair of sex chromosomes. Females have two X chromosomes (XX), whereas males have one X and one Y chromosome (XY). As a consequence of meiosis, germ cells (sperm or oocytes) are haploid and contain one set of 22 autosomes and one of the sex chromosomes. At the time of fertilization, the diploid genome is reconstituted by pairing of the homologous chromosomes from the mother and father. With each cell division (mitosis), chromosomes are replicated, paired, segregated, and divided into two daughter cells (Chap. 57).

The human genome is estimated to contain about 30,000 to 40,000 genes, a smaller number than initially predicted, that are divided among the 23 chromosomes. A *gene* is a functional unit that is regulated by transcription (see below) and encodes a product, either RNA or protein, that exerts activity within or outside the cell. Historically, genes were identified because they conferred specific traits that are transmitted from one generation to the next. Increasingly, they are characterized based on expression in various tissues. The number of genes greatly underestimates the complexity of genetic expression, as single genes can generate multiple spliced mRNA products, which are translated into proteins that are subject to complex posttranslational modification, such as phosphorylation. *Proteomics* is an emerging field focused on protein variation and function.

Human DNA consists of about 3 billion base pairs (bp) of DNA per haploid genome. DNA length is normally measured in units of 1000 bp (kilobases, kb) or 1,000,000 bp (megabases, Mb). Not all DNA encodes genes. In fact, genes account for only about 10 to 15% of DNA. Much of the remaining DNA consists of highly repetitive sequences, the function of which is poorly understood. These repetitive DNA regions, along with nonrepetitive sequences that do not encode genes, may serve a structural role in the packaging of DNA into chromatin (DNA bound to histone proteins) and chromosomes (Fig. 56-2). If only 10% of DNA is expressed and there are 30,000 genes, the average gene site would be about 10 kb in length. Although many genes are about this size, the range is quite broad. For example, some genes are only a few hundred bp, whereas others, like the *DMD* gene, are extraordinarily large (2 Mb).

Structure of DNA   Each gene is composed of a linear polymer of DNA. DNA is a double-stranded helix composed of four different bases: adenine (A), thymidine (T), guanine (G), and cytosine (C). Adenine is paired to thymidine, and guanine is paired to cytosine, by hydrogen bond interactions that span the double helix. DNA has several remarkable features that make it ideal for the transmission of genetic information. It is relatively stable, at least in comparison to RNA or proteins. The double-stranded nature of DNA and its feature of strict base-pair complementarity permit faithful replication during cell division. As described below, complementarity also allows the trans-

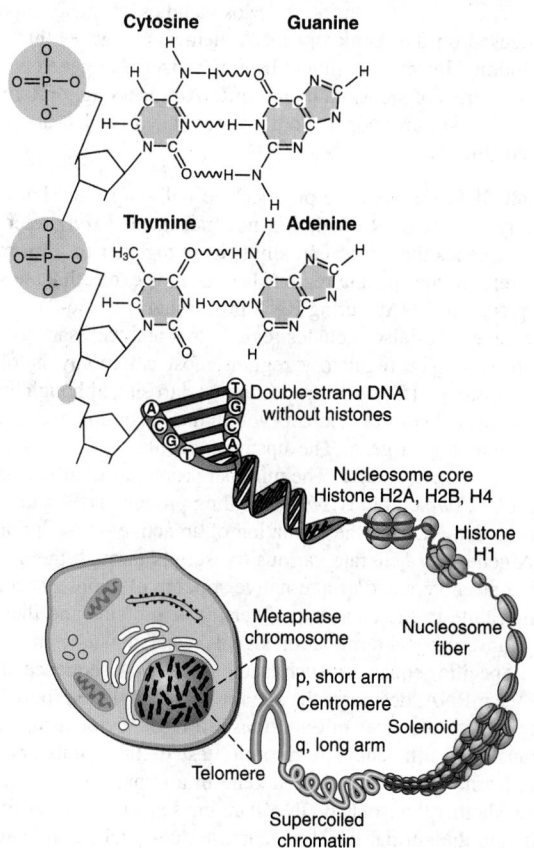

FIGURE 56-2   Structure of chromatin and chromosomes. Chromatin is composed of double-strand DNA that is wrapped around histone and nonhistone proteins forming nucleosomes. The nucleosomes are further organized into solenoid structures. Chromosomes assume their characteristic structure, with short (p) and long (q) arms at the metaphase stage of the cell cycle.

mission of genetic information from DNA → RNA → protein (Fig. 56-3). Messenger RNA (mRNA) is encoded by the so-called sense or coding strand of the DNA double helix and is translated into proteins by ribosomes.

The presence of four different bases provides surprising genetic diversity. In the protein-coding regions of genes, the DNA bases are arranged into codons, a triplet of bases that specifies a particular amino acid. It is possible to arrange the four bases into 64 different triplet codons (4^3). Each codon specifies 1 of the 20 different amino acids, or a regulatory signal, such as initiation and stop of translation. Because there are more codons than amino acids, the genetic code is degenerate; that is, most amino acids can be specified by several different codons. By arranging the codons in different combinations and in various lengths, it is possible to generate the tremendous diversity of primary protein structure.

REPLICATION OF DNA AND MITOSIS   Genetic information in DNA is transmitted to daughter cells under two different circumstances: (1) somatic cells divide by mitosis, allowing the diploid ($2n$) genome to replicate itself completely in conjunction with cell division; and (2) germ cells (sperm and ova) undergo meiosis, a process that enables the reduction of the diploid ($2n$) set of chromosomes to the haploid state ($1n$) (Chap. 57).

Prior to mitosis, cells exit the resting, or G_0 state, and enter the cell cycle (Chap. 69). After traversing a critical checkpoint in G_1, cells undergo DNA synthesis (S phase), during which the DNA in each chromosome is replicated, yielding two pairs of sister chromatids ($2n \rightarrow 4n$). The process of DNA synthesis requires stringent fidelity in order to avoid transmitting errors to subsequent generations of cells. Genetic abnormalities of DNA mismatch/repair include xeroderma pigmentosum, Bloom syndrome, ataxia telangiectasia, and hereditary nonpolyposis colon cancer (HNPCC), among others. Many of these disorders strongly predispose to neoplasia because of the rapid acquisition of additional mutations (Chap. 68). After completion of DNA synthesis, cells enter G_2 and progress through a second checkpoint before entering mitosis. At this stage, the chromosomes condense and are aligned along the equatorial plate at metaphase. The two identical sister chromatids, held together at the centromere, divide and migrate to opposite poles of the cell (see Fig. 57-3). After formation of a nuclear membrane around the two separated sets of chromatids, the cell divides and two daughter cells are formed, thus restoring the diploid ($2n$) state.

ASSORTMENT AND SEGREGATION OF GENES DURING MEIOSIS   Meiosis occurs only in germ cells of the gonads. It shares certain features with mitosis but involves two distinct steps of cell division that reduce the chromosome number to the haploid state. In addition, there is active recombination that generates genetic diversity. During the first cell division, two sister chromatids ($2n \rightarrow 4n$) are formed for each chromosome pair and there is an exchange of DNA between homologous paternal and maternal chromosomes. This process involves the formation of *chiasmata*, structures that correspond to the DNA segments that cross over between the maternal and paternal homologues (Fig. 56-4). Usually there is at least one crossover on each chromosomal arm; recombination occurs more frequently in female meiosis than in male meiosis. Subsequently, the chromosomes segregate randomly. Because there are 23 chromosomes, there exist 2^{23} (>8 million) possible combinations of chromosomes. Together with the genetic exchanges that occur during recombination, chromosomal segregation generates tremendous diversity, and each gamete is genetically unique. The process of recombination, and the independent segregation of chromosomes, provide the foundation for performing linkage analyses, whereby one attempts to correlate the inheritance of certain chromosomal regions (or linked genes) with the presence of a disease or genetic trait (see below).

After the first meiotic division, which results in two daughter cells ($2n$), the two chromatids of each chromosome separate during a second

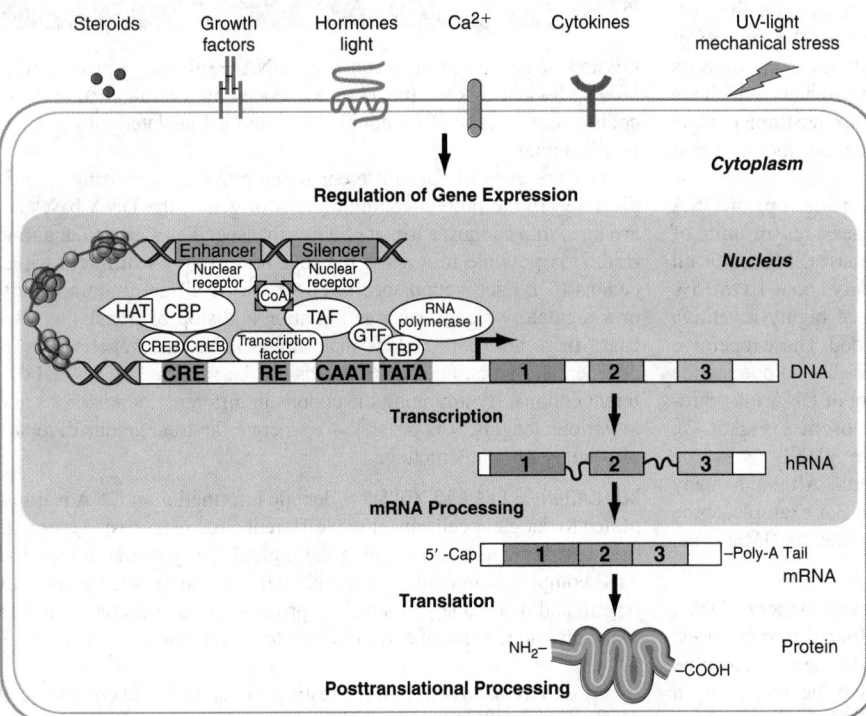

FIGURE 56-3 Flow of genetic information. Multiple extracellular signals activate intracellular signal cascades that result in altered regulation of gene expression through the interaction of transcription factors with regulatory regions of genes. RNA polymerase transcribes DNA into RNA that is processed to mRNA by excision of intronic sequences. The mRNA is translated into a polypeptide chain to form the mature protein after undergoing posttranslational processing. HAT, histone acetyl transferase; CBP, CREB-binding protein; CREB, cyclic AMP response element–binding protein; CRE, cyclic AMP responsive element; CoA, Co activator; TAF, TBP-associated factors; GTF, general transcription factors; TBP, TATA-binding protein; TATA, TATA box; RE, response element; NH_2, aminoterminus; COOH, carboxyterminus.

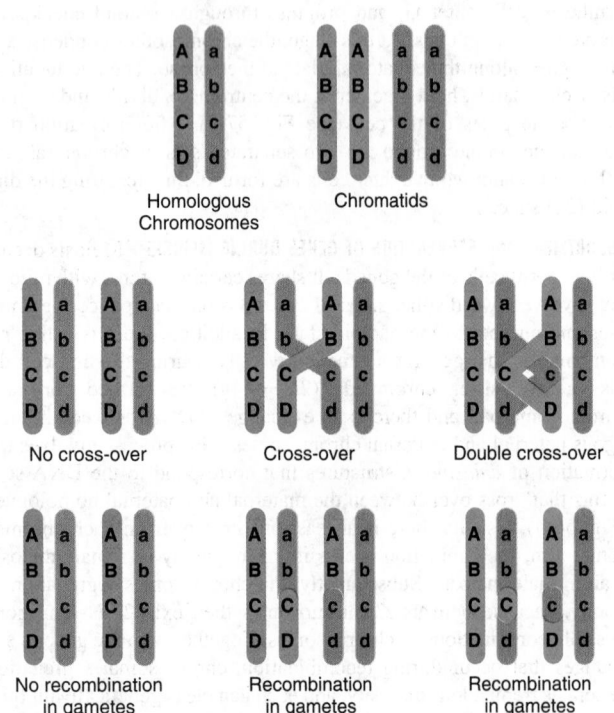

FIGURE 56-4 Crossing-over and genetic recombination. During chiasma formation, either of the two sister chromatids on one chromosome pairs with one of the chromatids of the homologous chromosome. Genetic recombination occurs through crossing-over and results in recombinant and nonrecombinant chromosome segments in the gametes. Together with the random segregation of the maternal and paternal chromosomes, recombination contributes to genetic diversity and forms the basis of the concept of linkage.

meiotic division to yield four gametes with a haploid state (1*n*). When the egg is fertilized by sperm, the two haploid sets are combined, thereby restoring the diploid state (2*n*) in the zygote.

REGULATION OF GENE EXPRESSION

Mechanisms that regulate gene expression play a critical role in the function of genes. The new field of *functional genomics* is based on the concept that understanding gene regulation and function will provide a better understanding of physiology and offer novel therapeutic opportunities. The transcription of genes is controlled primarily by *transcription factors* that bind to DNA sequences in the regulatory regions of genes. As described below, mutations in transcription factors cause a significant number of genetic disorders. Gene expression is also influenced by *epigenetic events*, such as X-inactivation and imprinting, processes in which DNA methylation is associated with the silencing (i.e., suppression) of expression. Several genetic disorders, such as Prader-Willi syndrome (neonatal hypotonia, developmental delay, obesity, short stature, and hypogonadism) and Albright hereditary osteodystrophy (resistance to parathyroid hormone, short stature, brachydactyly, resistance to other hormones in certain subtypes), exhibit the consequences of genomic imprinting. Most studies of gene expression have focused on the regulatory DNA elements of genes that control transcription. However, it should be emphasized that gene expression requires a series of steps, including mRNA processing, protein translation, and posttranslational modifications, all of which are actively regulated (Fig. 56-3).

STRUCTURE OF GENES A gene product is usually a protein but can occasionally consist of RNA that is not translated. *Exons* refer to the portion of genes that are eventually spliced together to form mRNA. *Introns* refer to the spacing regions between the exons that are spliced out of precursor RNAs during RNA processing (Fig. 56-3).

The gene locus also includes regions that are necessary to control its expression. The regulatory regions most commonly involve sequences upstream (5′) of the transcription start site, although there are also examples of control elements within introns or downstream of the coding regions of a gene. The upstream regulatory regions are also referred to as the *promoter*. The minimal promoter usually consists of a TATA box (which binds TATA-binding protein, TBP) and initiator sequences that enhance the formation of an active transcription complex. A gene may generate various transcripts through the use of alternative promoters and/or alternative splicing of exons, mechanisms that contribute to the enormous diversity of proteins and their functions. Transcriptional termination signals reside downstream, or 3′, of a gene. Specific sequences, such as the AAUAAA sequence at the 3′ end of the mRNA, designate the site for polyadenylation (poly-A tail), a process that influences mRNA transport to the cytoplasm, stability, and translation efficiency. A rigorous test of the regulatory region boundaries involves expressing a gene in a transgenic animal to determine whether the isolated DNA flanking sequences are sufficient to recapitulate the normal developmental, tissue-specific, and signal-responsive features of the endogenous gene. This has been accomplished for only a few genes; there are many examples in which large genomic fragments only partially reconstitute normal gene regulation in vivo, implying the presence of distant regulatory sequences. This approach is critical to our understanding of mechanisms that regulate genes and is also relevant for gene therapy strategies that require normal gene regulation (Chap. 59).

As genes are dissected with greater resolution, the number of DNA sequences and transcription factors that regulate transcription is much greater than originally anticipated. Most genes contain at least 15 to 20 discrete regulatory elements within 300 bp of the transcription start site. This densely packed promoter region often contains binding sites for ubiquitous transcription factors such as CAAT box/enhancer binding protein (C/EBP), cyclic AMP response element–binding (CREB) protein, selective promoter factor 1 (Sp-1), or activator protein 1 (AP-1). However, factors involved in cell-specific expression may also bind to these sequences. For example, basic helix-loop-helix (bHLH) proteins bind to E-boxes in the promoters of myogenic genes, and steroidogenic factor 1 (SF-1) binds to a specific recognition site in the regulatory region of multiple steroidogenic enzyme genes. Key regulatory elements may also reside at some distance from the proximal promoter. The globin and the immunoglobulin genes, for example, contain *locus control regions* that are several kilobases away from the structural sequences of the gene. Specific groups of transcription factors that bind to these promoter and enhancer sequences provide a combinatorial code for regulating transcription. In this manner, relatively ubiquitous factors interact with more restricted factors to allow each gene to be expressed and regulated in a unique manner that is dependent on developmental state, cell type, and numerous extracellular stimuli. As described below, the transcription factors that bind to DNA actually represent only the first level of regulatory control. Other proteins—*coactivators* and *co-repressors*—interact with the DNA-binding transcription factors to generate large regulatory complexes. These complexes are subject to control by numerous cell-signaling pathways, including phosphorylation and acetylation. Ultimately, the recruited transcription factors interact with, and stabilize, components of the basal transcription complex that assembles at the site of the TATA box and initiator region. This basal transcription factor complex consists of >30 different proteins. Gene transcription occurs when RNA polymerase begins to synthesize RNA from the DNA template.

Mutations can occur in all domains of a gene (Fig. 56-5). A point mutation occurring within the coding region leads to an amino acid substitution if the codon is altered. Point mutations that introduce a premature stop codon result in a truncated protein. Large deletions may affect a portion of a gene or an entire gene, whereas small deletions and insertions alter the reading frame if they do not represent a multiple of three bases. These "frameshift" mutations lead to an entirely altered carboxy terminus. Mutations occurring in regulatory or intronic regions may result in altered expression or splicing of genes. Examples are shown in Fig. 56-6.

TRANSCRIPTIONAL ACTIVATION AND REPRESSION

Every gene is controlled uniquely, whether in its spatial or temporal pattern of expression or in its response to extracellular signals. It is estimated that transcription factors account for about 30% of expressed genes. A growing number of identified genetic diseases involve

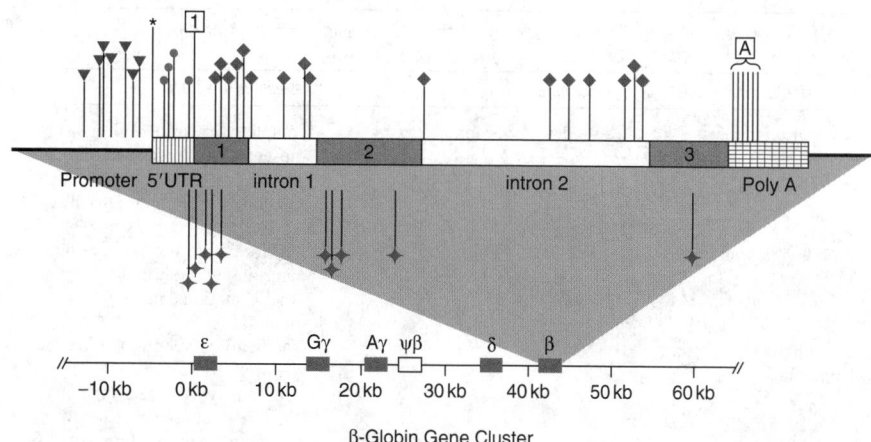

FIGURE 56-5   Point mutations causing β-thalassemia as example of allelic heterogeneity. The β-globin gene is located in the globin gene cluster. Point mutations can be located in the promoter, the CAP site, the 5′-untranslated region, the initiation codon, each of the three exons, the introns, or the polyadenylation signal. Many mutations introduce missense or nonsense mutations, whereas others cause defective RNA splicing. Not shown here are deletion mutations of the β-globin gene or larger deletions of the globin locus that can also result in thalassemia. ▼, Promoter mutations; *, CAP site; ●, 5′UTR; ⬚1, Initiation codon; ◆, Defective RNA processing; ✦, Missense and nonsense mutations; Ⓐ, Poly A signal.

transcription factors (Table 56-2). The MODY (maturity-onset diabetes of the young) disorders are representative of this group of diseases; mutations in several different islet cell–specific transcription factors cause various forms of MODY (Chap. 323).

Transcriptional activation can be divided into three main mechanisms:

1. Events that alter chromatin structure can enhance the access of transcription factors to DNA. For example, histone acetylation opens chromatin structure and is correlated with transcriptional activation.

2. Posttranslational modifications of transcription factors, such as phosphorylation, can induce the assembly of active transcription complexes. As an example, phosphorylation of CREB protein on serine 133 induces a conformational change that allows the recruitment of CREB-binding protein (CBP), a factor that integrates the actions of many transcription factors, including proteins, with histone acetyltransferase activity.

3. Transcriptional activators can displace a repressor protein. This mechanism is particularly common during development when the pattern of transcription factor expression changes dynamically.

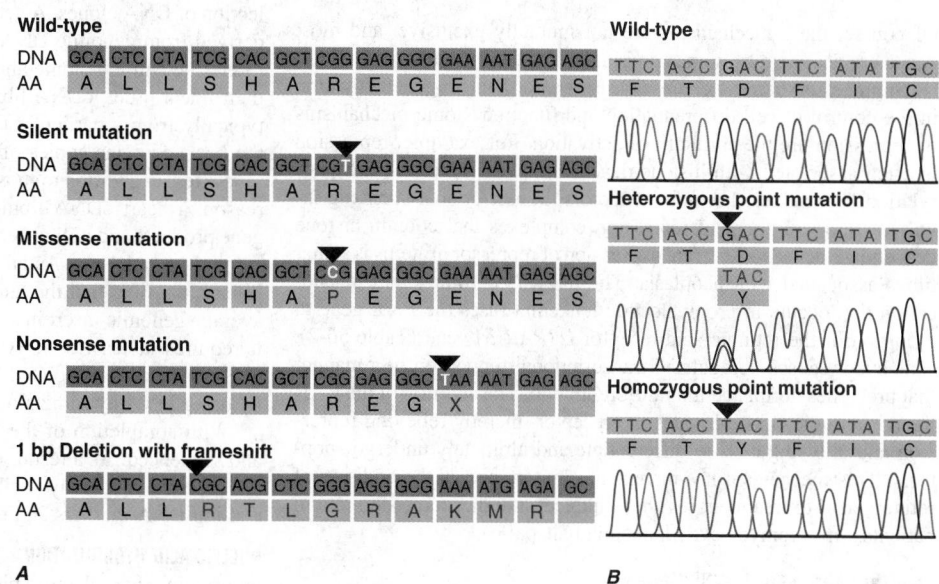

FIGURE 56-6   A. Examples of mutations. The coding strand is shown with the encoded amino acid sequence. B. Chromatograms of sequence analyses after amplification of genomic DNA by polymerase chain reaction.

TABLE 56-2 *Selected Examples of Diseases Caused by Mutations and Rearrangements in Transcription Factor Classes*

Transcription Factor Class	Example	Associated Disorder
Nuclear receptors	Androgen receptor	Complete or partial androgen insensitivity (recessive missense mutations)
		Spinobulbar muscular atrophy (CAG repeat expansion)
Zinc finger proteins	WT-1	WAGR syndrome: Wilm's tumor, aniridia, genitourinary malformations, mental retardation
Basic helix-loop-helix	MITF	Waardenburg syndrome type 2A
Homeobox	IPF1	Maturity onset of diabetes mellitus type 4 (heterozygous mutation/haploinsufficiency)
		Pancreatic agenesis (homozygous mutation)
Leucine zipper	Retina leucine zipper (NRL)	Autosomal dominant retinitis pigmentosa
High- mobility group (HMG) proteins	SRY	Sex-reversal
Forkhead	HNF4α, HNF1α, HNF1β	Maturity-onset of diabetes mellitus types 1, 3, 5
Paired box	PAX-3	Waardenburg syndrome types 1 and 3
T-box	TBX-5	Holt-Oram syndrome (thumb anomalies, atrial or ventricular septum defects, phocomelia)
Cell cycle control proteins	P53	Li-Fraumeni syndrome, other cancers
Coactivators	CREB binding protein (CBP)	Rubenstein-Taybi syndrome
General transcription factors	TATA-binding protein (TBP)	Spinocerebellar ataxia 17 (CAG expansion)
Transcription elongation factor	VHL	von Hippel-Lindau syndrome (renal cell carcinoma, pheochromocytoma, pancreatic tumors, hemangioblastomas)
		Autosomal dominant inheritance, somatic inactivation of second allele
Runt	CBFA2	Familial thrombocytopenia with propensity to acute myelogenous leukemia
Chimeric proteins due to translocations	PML—RAR	Acute promyelocytic leukemia t(15;17)(q22;q11.2-q12) translocation

Abbreviations: SRY, sex determining region Y; HNF, hepatocyte nuclear factor; CREB (cAMP responsive element binding) binding protein; VHL, von Hippel-Lindau; PML, promyelocytic leukemia; RAR, retinoic acid receptor.

Of course, these mechanisms are not mutually exclusive, and most genes are activated by some combination of these events.

Suppression of gene expression is as important as gene activation in the control of cell differentiation and function. Some mechanisms of repression are the corollary of activation. For example, repression is often associated with histone deacetylation or protein dephosphorylation. For nuclear hormone receptors, transcriptional silencing involves the recruitment of repression complexes that contain histone deacetylase activity. Aberrant expression of repressor proteins is sometimes associated with neoplasia. The t(15;17) chromosomal translocation that occurs in promyelocytic leukemia fuses the *PML* gene to a portion of the retinoic acid receptor α (*RAR* α) gene (Table 56-2). This event causes unregulated transcriptional repression in a manner that precludes normal cellular differentiation. The addition of the RAR ligand, retinoic acid, activates the receptor, thereby relieving repression and allowing cells to differentiate and ultimately undergo apoptosis. This mechanism has therapeutic importance as the addition of retinoic acid to treatment regimens induces a higher remission rate in patients with promyelocytic leukemia (Chap. 96).

CLONING AND SEQUENCING DNA

Since the mid-1970s, eight Nobel prizes have been awarded for research that led, directly or indirectly, to major methodological advances and to profound insights into genetics. Examples include the discoveries of reverse transcriptase, restriction enzymes, plasmid cloning vectors, DNA sequencing, and PCR. A description of recombinant DNA techniques, the methodology used for the manipulation, analysis, and characterization of DNA segments, is beyond the scope of this chapter. As these methods are widely used in genetics and molecular diagnostics, however, it is useful to review briefly some of the fundamental principles of cloning and DNA sequencing.

CLONING OF GENES *Cloning* refers to the creation of a recombinant DNA molecule that can be propagated indefinitely. The ability to clone genes and cDNAs therefore provides a permanent and renewable source of these reagents. Cloning is essential for DNA sequencing, nucleic acid hybridization studies, expression of recombinant proteins, and other recombinant DNA procedures.

The cloning of DNA involves the insertion of a DNA fragment into a cloning vector, followed by the propagation of the recombinant DNA in a host cell. The most straightforward cloning strategy involves inserting a DNA fragment into bacterial plasmids. Plasmids are small, autonomously replicating, circular DNA molecules that propagate separately from the chromosome in bacterial cells. The process of DNA insertion relies heavily on the use of restriction enzymes, which cleave DNA at highly specific sequences (usually 4 to 6 bp in length). Restriction enzymes generate complementary, cohesive sequences at the ends of the DNA fragment, which allow them to be efficiently ligated to the plasmid vector. Because plasmids contain genes that confer resistance to antibiotics, their presence in the host cell can be used for selection and DNA amplification.

A variety of vectors (e.g., plasmids, phage, bacterial, or yeast artificial chromosomes) are used for cloning. Many of these are used for creating *libraries*, a term that refers to a collection of DNA clones. A genomic library represents an array of clones derived from genomic DNA. These overlapping DNA fragments represent the entire genome and can ultimately be arranged according to their linear order. cDNA libraries reflect clones derived from mRNA, typically from a particular tissue source. Thus, a cDNA library from the heart contains copies of mRNA expressed specifically in cardiac myocytes, in addition to those that are expressed ubiquitously. For this reason, a heart cDNA library will be enriched with cardiac-specific gene products and will differ from cDNA libraries generated from liver or pituitary mRNAs. As an example of the complexity of a genomic library, consider that the human genome contains 3×10^9 bp and the average genomic insert in a λ phage library is about 10^4 bp. Therefore, it requires at least 3×10^5 clones to represent all genomic DNA. Specific clones are isolated from the several hundred thousand clones by using DNA hybridization.

With completion of the HGP, all human genes have been cloned and sequenced. As a result, many of these cloning procedures are now unnecessary or greatly facilitated by the extensive information concerning DNA markers and the sequence of DNA (see below).

NUCLEIC ACID HYBRIDIZATION Nucleic acid *hybridization* is a fundamental principle in molecular biology that takes advantage of the fact that the two complementary strands of nucleic acids bind, or *hybridize*, to one another with very high specificity. The goal of hybridization is to detect specific nucleic acid (DNA or RNA) sequences in a complex background of other sequences. This technique is used for Southern blotting, Northern blotting, and for screening libraries (see above). Further adaptation of hybridization techniques has led to the development of microarray DNA chips.

Southern Blot Southern blotting is used to analyze whether genes have been deleted or rearranged. It is also used to detect restriction fragment length polymorphisms (RFLPs). Genomic DNA is digested with restriction endonucleases and separated by gel electrophoresis. Individual fragments can then be transferred to a membrane and detected after hybridization with specific radioactive DNA probes. Because single base-pair mismatches can disrupt the hybridization of short DNA probes (oligonucleotides), a variation of the Southern blot, termed *oligonucleotide-specific hybridization* (OSH), uses short oligonucleotides to distinguish normal from mutant genes.

Northern Blot Northern blots are used to analyze patterns and levels of gene expression in different tissues. In a northern blot, mRNA is separated on a gel and transferred to a membrane, and specific transcripts are detected using radiolabeled DNA as a probe. This technique is rapidly being supplanted by more sensitive and comprehensive methods such as reverse transcriptase (RT)–PCR and gene expression arrays on DNA chips (see below).

Microarray Technology A rapidly evolving approach to genome-scale studies consists of *microarrays*, or *DNA chips*. These approaches consist of thousands of synthetic nucleic acid sequences aligned on thin glass or silicon surfaces. Fluorescently labeled test sample DNA or RNA is hybridized to the chip, and a computerized scanner detects sequence matches. Microarrays allow the detection of variations in DNA sequence and are used for mutational analysis and genotyping. Alternatively, the expression pattern of large numbers of mRNA transcripts can be determined by hybridization of RNA samples to cDNA or genomic microarrays. This method has tremendous potential in the era of functional genomics (e.g., a comprehensive analysis of gene expression profiles). As one example, microarrays can be used to develop genetic fingerprints of different types of malignancies, providing information useful for classification, pathophysiology, prognosis, and treatment.

THE POLYMERASE CHAIN REACTION The PCR, introduced in 1985, has revolutionized the way DNA analyses are performed and has become a cornerstone of molecular biology and genetic analysis. In essence, PCR provides a rapid way of cloning (amplifying) specific DNA fragments in vitro (Fig. 56-7). Exquisite specificity is conferred by the use of PCR primers, which are designed for a given DNA sequence. The geometric amplification of the DNA after multiple cycles yields remarkable sensitivity. As a result, PCR can be used to amplify DNA from very small samples, including single cells. These properties also allow DNA amplification from a variety of tissue sources including blood samples, biopsies, surgical or autopsy specimens, or cells from hair or saliva. PCR can also be used to study mRNA. In this case, the enzyme RT is first used to convert the RNA to DNA, which can then be amplified by PCR. This procedure, commonly known as *RT-PCR*, is useful as a quantitative measure of gene expression.

PCR provides a key component of molecular diagnostics. It provides a strategy for the rapid amplification of DNA (or mRNA) to search for mutations by a wide array of techniques, including DNA sequencing. PCR is also used for the amplification of highly polymorphic di- or trinucleotide repeat sequences, which allow various polymorphic alleles to be traced in genetic linkage or association studies. PCR is increasingly used to diagnose various microbial pathogens.

DNA SEQUENCING DNA sequencing is now an automated procedure. Although many protocols exist, the most commonly used strategy is based on the Sanger method in which dideoxynucleotides are used to randomly terminate DNA polymerization at each of the four bases (A,G,T,C). After separating the array of terminated DNA fragments using high-resolution gel or capillary electrophoresis, it is possible to deduce the DNA sequence by examining the progression of fragment

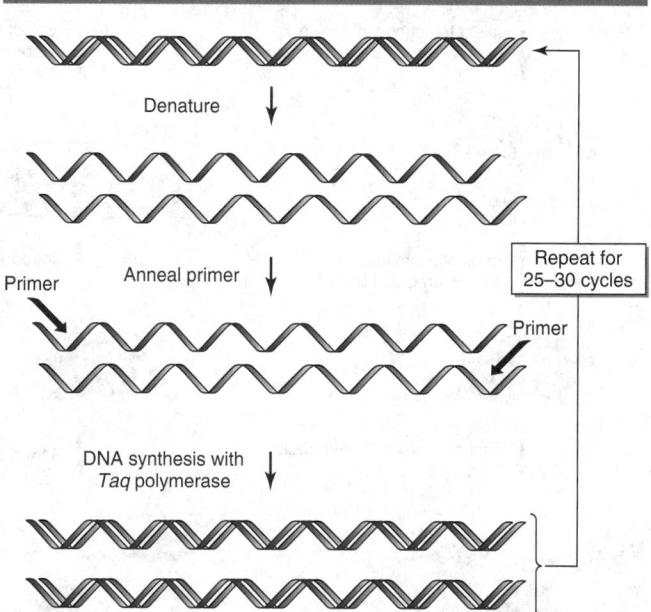

FIGURE 56-7 Polymerase chain reaction. The polymerase chain reaction (PCR) generates multiple copies of a DNA segment. After denaturing the double-stranded (ds) DNA, complementary synthetic oligonucleotide primers of about 20 bp are annealed on each side of the fragment of interest. A heat-stable polymerase then extends the oligonucleotides and synthesizes the complementary strand. This cycle is repeated 25 to 30 times. The number of DNA-amplified DNA segments is thus doubled after every PCR cycle.

lengths generated in each of the four nucleotide reactions. The use of fluorescently labeled dideoxynucleotides allows automated detection of the different bases and direct computer analysis of the DNA sequence (Fig. 56-6). Efforts are underway to develop faster, more cost-effective DNA sequencing technologies. These include the use of mass spectrometry; detection of fluorescently labeled bases in flow cytometry; direct reading of the DNA sequence by scanning, tunneling, or atomic force microscopy; and sequence analysis using DNA chips.

TRANSGENIC MICE AS MODELS OF GENETIC DISEASE

Several organisms have been studied extensively as genetic models, including *Mus musculus* (mouse), *Drosophila melanogaster* (fruit fly), *Caenorhabditis elegans* (nematode), *Saccharomyces cerevisiae* (baker's yeast), and *Escherichia coli* (colonic bacterium). The ability to use these evolutionarily distant organisms as genetic models that are relevant to human physiology reflects a surprising conservation of genetic pathways and gene function. Transgenic mouse models have been particularly valuable, because many human and mouse genes exhibit similar structure and function, and because manipulation of the mouse genome is relatively straightforward compared to those of other mammalian species.

Transgenic strategies in mice can be divided into two main approaches: (1) expression of a gene by random insertion into the genome, and (2) deletion or targeted mutagenesis of a gene by homologous recombination with the native endogenous gene (knockout, knockin) (Fig. 56-8; Table 56-3). Transgenic mice are generated by pronuclear injection of foreign DNA into fertilized mouse oocytes and subsequent transfer into the oviduct of pseudopregnant foster mothers.

Transgenic expression of genes can be useful for studying disorders that are sensitive to gene dosage. Overexpression of *PMP22*, for example, mimics a common duplication of this gene in type IA Charcot-Marie-Tooth disease (Chap. 364). Duplication of the *PMP22* gene results in high levels of expression of peripheral myelin protein 22, and this dosage effect is responsible for the demyelinating neuropathy. Expression of the Y chromosome–specific gene, *SRY*, in XX females demonstrates that *SRY* is sufficient to induce the formation of testes. This finding confirms the pathogenic role of *SRY* translocations to the

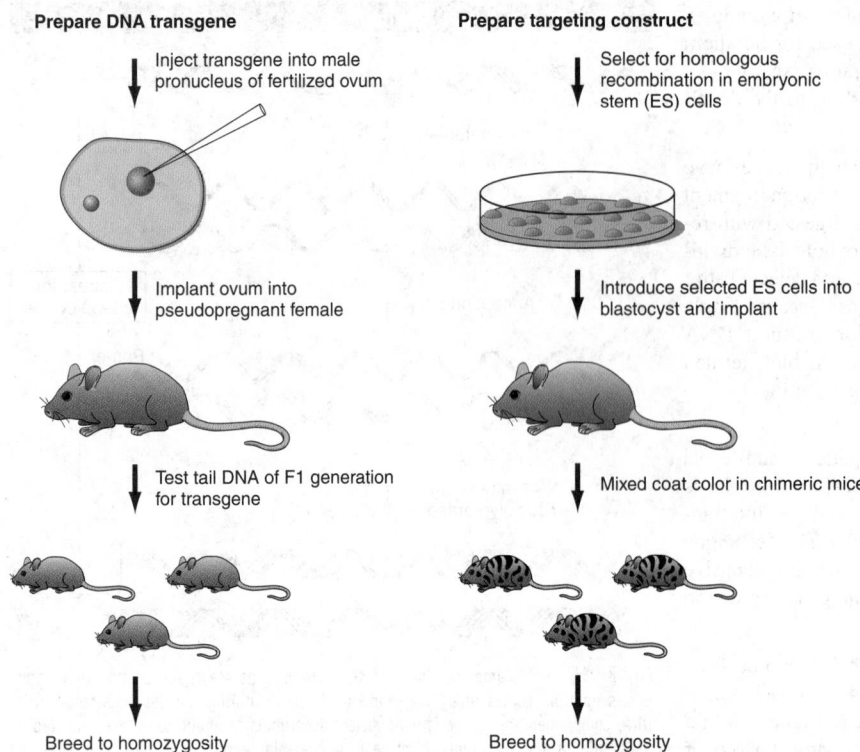

Prepare DNA transgene

Inject transgene into male pronucleus of fertilized ovum

Implant ovum into pseudopregnant female

Test tail DNA of F1 generation for transgene

Breed to homozygosity

Prepare targeting construct

Select for homologous recombination in embryonic stem (ES) cells

Introduce selected ES cells into blastocyst and implant

Mixed coat color in chimeric mice

Breed to homozygosity

FIGURE 56-8   Transgenic mouse models. *Left.* Transgenic mice are generated by pronuclear injection of foreign DNA into fertilized mouse oocytes and subsequent transfer into the oviduct of pseudopregnant foster mothers. *Right.* For targeted mutagenesis (gene knockout/knockin), embryonic stem (ES) cells are transfected with the targeted (mutagenized) transgene. The transgene undergoes homologous recombination with the wild-type gene. After selection, positive ES cells are introduced into blastocysts and implanted into foster mothers. Chimeric mice can be identified based on the mixed coat color of the offspring. Heterozygous mice are bred to obtain mice homozygous for the mutant allele.

X chromosome in sex-reversed XX females. Huntington disease is an autosomal dominant disorder caused by expansion of a CAG trinucleotide repeat that encodes a polyglutamine tract. Targeted deletion of the Huntington disease (*HD*) gene does not induce the neurologic disorder. On the other hand, transgenic expression of the entire gene or of the first exon containing the expanded polyGlu repeat is sufficient to cause many features of the neurologic disorder, indicating a gain-of-function property for the expanded polyGlu-containing protein. Transgenic strategies can also be used as a precursor to gene therapy. Expression of dystrophin, the protein that is deleted in Duchenne muscular dystrophy, partially corrects the disorder in a mouse model of Duchenne's. Targeted expression of oncogenes has been valuable to study mechanisms of neoplasia and to generate immortalized cell lines. For example, expression of the simian virus 40 (SV40) large T antigen under the direction of the insulin promoter induces the formation of islet cell tumors.

The creation of gene knockout and knockin models takes advantage of the fact that a segment of DNA can be substituted by another that is identical (homologous), or nearly identical, by recombination. This permits integration of deletions that disrupt the gene (knockout) or selected mutations (knockin) into the target gene of choice. The transgene is introduced into embryonic stem (ES) cells by transfection and, after selection of cells with an integrated transgene, the positive ES cells are introduced into blastocysts and implanted into foster mothers. Chimeric mice can be identified based on the mixed coat color of the offspring. Heterozygous mice are bred to obtain mice homozygous for the mutant allele. This is particularly useful for genes that would be lethal if deleted universally or during early development. The list of genes that have been modified by this approach is very large.

Many of these knockouts do not have an apparent phenotype, either because of redundant functions of the other genes or because the phenotype is subtle. For example, deletion of the hypoxanthine phosphoribosyltransferase (HPRT) gene (*Hprt*) does not cause characteristic features of Lesch-Nyhan syndrome in mice because of their reliance on adenine phosphoribosyltransferase (APRT) in the purine salvage pathway. Deletion of the retinoblastoma (*Rb*) gene does not lead to retinoblastoma or other tumors that characterize the human syndrome. These examples underscore the fact that the functions of genes, and their interactions with genetic background and the environment, are not necessarily identical in mice and humans. On the other hand, the deletion of many genes provides a remarkably faithful model of human disorders. In addition to clarifying pathophysiology, these models facilitate the development of therapies, both genetic and pharmaceutical.

Many variations of these basic approaches now exist that allow genes to be expressed or deleted in specific cell types, at different times during development, or at varying levels. Consequently, transgenic technology has emerged as a powerful strategy for defining the physiologic effects of deleting or overexpressing a gene, as well as providing unique genetic models for dissecting pathophysiology or testing therapies. In addition to transgenic animal models, naturally occurring mutations in mice and other species continue to provide fundamental insights into human disease. A compendium of natural and transgenic animal models is provided in continuously evolving databases (Table 56-1).

Human pluripotential *stem cells* have recently been developed, and, consistent with their potential for self-renewal, these cell lines express high levels of telomerase, an enzyme that is essential for allowing repeated replication of the ends of eukaryotic chromosomes. Although much remains to be learned about the properties of pluripotential stem cells, they may prove useful for transplantation, drug testing, or for other purposes (Chap. 59).

IMPLICATIONS OF THE HUMAN GENOME PROJECT

The HGP was initiated in the mid-1980s as an ambitious effort to characterize the human genome, culminating in a complete DNA sequence. The initial main goals were (1) creation of genetic maps, (2) development of physical maps, and (3) determination of the complete human DNA sequence. Some analogies help in appreciating the scope of the HGP. The 23 pairs of human chromosomes encode approximately 30,000 to 40,000 genes. The total length of DNA is about 3 billion bp, which is nearly 1000-fold greater than that of the *E. coli* genome. If the human DNA sequence were printed out, it would correspond to about 120 volumes of *Harrison's Principles of Internal Medicine.*

THE GENETIC MAP   Given the size and complexity of the human genome, initial efforts aimed at developing genetic maps to provide orientation and to delimit where a gene of interest may be located. A *genetic map* describes the order of genes and defines the position of a gene relative to other loci on the same chromosome. It is constructed by assessing how frequently two markers are inherited together (e.g., *linked*) by association studies. Distances of the genetic map are expressed in recombination units, or centimorgans (cM). One cM corresponds to a recombination frequency of 1% between two polymorphic markers; 1 cM corresponds to approximately 1 Mb of DNA (Fig. 56-4). Any polymorphic sequence variation can be useful for mapping purposes. Examples of polymorphic markers include variable number of tandem repeats (VNTRs), RFLPs, microsatellite repeats, and single nucleotide polymorphisms (SNPs); the latter two methods are now used predominantly because of the high density of markers and because they are amenable to automated procedures. Current efforts aim at creating high quality, dense SNP maps and haplotype maps (e.g., linear arrangements of alleles) of the human genome through the identification of as many as 500,000 SNPs. These variations, which are amenable to automated analysis with DNA chips, will greatly facilitate association and linkage studies for the elucidation of the complex interactions among multiple genes and life-style factors in multifactorial disorders. SNP patterns may ultimately become useful for the prediction of disease predisposition and pharmacogenomics.

THE PHYSICAL MAP Cytogenetics and chromosomal banding techniques provide a relatively low-resolution microscopic view of genetic loci. Physical maps indicate the position of a locus or gene in absolute values. Sequence-tagged sites (STSs) are used as a standard unit for physical mapping and serve as sequence-specific landmarks for arranging overlapping cloned fragments in the same order as they occur in the genome. These overlapping clones allow the characterization of contiguous DNA sequences, commonly referred to as *contigs*. This approach led to high-resolution physical maps by cloning the whole genome into overlapping fragments and has been essential for the identification of disease-causing genes by positional cloning. The complete DNA sequence of each chromosome, now already complete for several chromosomes and as draft for the whole genome, provides the highest resolution physical map.

STATUS OF DNA SEQUENCING The primary focus of the HGP was to obtain DNA sequence for the entire human genome as well as model organisms. Although the prospect of determining the complete sequence of the human genome seemed daunting several years ago, technical advances in DNA sequencing and bioinformatics led to the completion of a draft human sequence in June 2000, well in advance of the original goal year of 2003. The whole genomes of more than 800 organisms have been sequenced partially or completely. They include, among others, eukaryotes such as man and mouse; *S. cerevisiae*, *C. elegans*, and *D. melanogaster*; bacteria (e.g., *E. coli*); and archeae, viruses, organelles (mitochondriae, chloroplasts), and plants (e.g., *Arabidopsis thaliana*). For the human genome, the current goal is now to achieve 99.99% (1 error in 10,000 bp) accuracy. This level of accuracy is important for many reasons, including efforts to determine the degree of DNA sequence variation in the population. Comparisons of the DNA sequence from multiple individuals or populations will allow assessments of genetic variance in the human population. Another goal is to develop a complete set of full-length human cDNAs and to define their locations on the physical map.

CURRENT DIRECTIONS ARISING FROM THE HGP The primary goals of the HGP have been achieved, but there are numerous remaining challenges, including (1) refining the sequence information and solving ambiguities, (2) establishing catalogs of sequence variations and SNPs, (3) characterizing the expression pattern of thousands of genes simultaneously in order to detect differences between various tissues in health and disease (*functional genomics*), (4) identifying the genes that play critical roles in the development of polygenic and multifactorial disorders, and (5) developing large-scale analyses of protein expression (*proteomics*).

ETHICAL ISSUES Implicit in the HGP is the idea and hope that identifying disease-causing genes can lead to improvements in diagnosis,

TABLE 56-3 *Genetic Modified Animals*

Commonly Used Description	Technical Principle	Remarks
Transgenic	Pronuclear injection of transgene	Commonly used
		Genomic DNA or cDNA constructs
		Random integration of transgene
		Variable copy numbers of transgene
		Variable expression in each individual founder
		Gain of function models due to overexpression using tissue-specific promoters
		Loss of function models using anti-sense and dominant negative transgenes
		Inducible expression possible (Tetracycline, ecdysone)
		Applicable to several species
(Targeted) Knockout	Substitution of functional gene with inactive gene by homologous recombination in embryonic stem cells	Predominantly used in mice
		Tissue-specific knockout possible (Cre/lox)
		Absence of phenotype possible due to redundancy
(Targeted) Knockin	Introduction of subtle mutation(s) into gene by substitution of endogenous gene with gene carrying a specific mutation. Homologous recombination in embryonic stem cells	Predominantly used in mice
		Can accurately model human disease
Forward genetics	Mutations created randomly by ENU (N-ethyl-N-nitrourea)	Selection of phenotype followed by genetic characterization
		Useful for cloning of novel genes
Cloning	Introduction of nucleus into enucleated eggs (nuclear transfer)	Successful in several mammalian species including sheep (Dolly), mice, cows, monkeys
		Cloning of genetically identical individuals
		May affect life span
		Ethical concerns

prognosis, and treatment. It is estimated that most individuals harbor several serious recessive genes. However, completion of the human genome sequence, determination of the association of genetic defects with disease, and studies of genetic variation raise many new issues with implications for the individual and mankind. The controversies concerning the cloning of mammals and the establishment of human embryonic stem cells underscore the relevance of these questions. Moreover, the information gleaned from genotypic results can have quite different impacts, depending on the availability of strategies to modify the course of disease. For example, the identification of mutations that cause multiple endocrine neoplasia (MEN) type 2 or hemochromatosis allows specific interventions for affected family members. On the other hand, at present, the identification of an Alzheimer or Huntington disease gene does not alter therapy. Genetic test results can generate anxiety in affected individuals and family members, and there is the possibility of discrimination on the basis of the test results. Most genetic disorders are likely to fall into an intermediate category where the opportunity for prevention or treatment is significant but limited (Chap. 58). For these reasons, the scientific components of the HGP have been paralleled by efforts to examine ethical and legal implications as new issues arise. About 5% of the HGP budget had been allocated to studies addressing the ethical, legal, and social implications associated with the increasing knowledge about the human genome and the genetic basis of disease.

Many issues raised by the genome project are familiar, in principle, to medical practitioners. For example, an asymptomatic patient with increased low-density lipoprotein (LDL) cholesterol, high blood pressure, or a strong family history of early myocardial infarction is known to be at increased risk of coronary heart disease. In such cases, it is clear that the identification of risk factors and an appropriate intervention are beneficial. Likewise, patients with phenylketonuria, cystic fibrosis, or sickle cell anemia are often identified as having a genetic disease early in life. These precedents can be helpful for adapting policies that relate to genetic information. We can anticipate similar efforts, whether based on genotypes or other markers of genetic predisposition, to be applied to many disorders. One confounding aspect of the rapid expansion of information is that our ability to make clinical predictions often lags behind genetic advances. For example, when genes that predispose to breast cancer, such as *BRCA1*, are described, they generate tremendous public interest in the potential to predict disease, but many years of clinical research are still required to rigorously establish genotype and phenotype correlations.

Whether related to informed consent, participation in research, or the management of a genetic disorder that affects an individual or their families, there is a great need for more information about fundamental principles of genetics. The pervasive nature of the role of genetics in medicine makes it imperative for physicians and other health care professionals to become more informed about genetics, and to provide advice and counseling in conjunction with trained genetic counselors (Chap. 58). The application of screening and prevention strategies will therefore require intensive patient and physician education, changes in health care financing, and legislation to protect patient's rights.

TRANSMISSION OF GENETIC DISEASE

ORIGINS AND TYPES OF MUTATIONS A *mutation* can be defined as any change in the primary nucleotide sequence of DNA regardless of its functional consequences. Some mutations may be lethal, others are less deleterious, and some may confer an evolutionary advantage. Mutations can occur in the germline (sperm or oocytes); these can be transmitted to progeny. Alternatively, mutations can occur during embryogenesis or in somatic tissues. Mutations that occur during development lead to *mosaicism*, a situation in which tissues are composed of cells with different genetic constitutions. If the germline is mosaic, a mutation can be transmitted to some progeny but not others, which sometimes leads to confusion in assessing the pattern of inheritance. Somatic mutations that do not affect cell survival can sometimes be detected because of variable phenotypic effects in tissues (e.g., pigmented lesions in McCune-Albright syndrome). Other somatic mutations are associated with neoplasia because they confer a growth advantage to cells. Epigenetic events, heritable changes that do not involve changes in gene sequence (e.g., altered DNA methylation), may influence gene expression or facilitate genetic damage. With the exception of triplet nucleotide repeats, which can expand (see below), mutations are usually stable.

Mutations are structurally diverse—they can involve the entire genome, as in triploidy (one extra set of chromosomes), or gross numerical or structural alterations in chromosomes or individual genes (Chap. 57). Large deletions may affect a portion of a gene or an entire gene, or, if several genes are involved, they may lead to a *contiguous gene syndrome*. Unequal crossing-over between homologous genes can result in fusion gene mutations, as illustrated by color blindness (Chap. 25). Mutations involving single nucleotides are referred to as *point mutations* (Fig. 56-6). Substitutions are called *transitions* if a purine is replaced by another purine base (A $\leftrightarrow$ G) or if a pyrimidine is replaced by another pyrimidine (C $\leftrightarrow$ T). Changes from a purine to a pyrimidine, or vice versa, are referred to as *transversions*. If the DNA sequence change occurs in a coding region and alters an amino acid, it is called a *missense mutation*. Depending on the functional consequences of such a missense mutation, amino acid substitutions in different regions of the protein can lead to distinct phenotypes. *Polymorphisms* are sequence variations that have a frequency of at least 1%. Usually, they do not result in a perceptible phenotype. Often they consist of single base-pair substitutions that do not alter the protein coding sequence because of the degenerate nature of the genetic code, although it is possible that some might alter mRNA stability, translation, or the amino acid sequence. These types of silent base substitutions and SNPs are encountered frequently during genetic testing

and must be distinguished from true mutations that alter protein expression or function. Small nucleotide deletions or insertions cause a shift of the codon reading frame (*frameshift*). Most commonly, reading frame alterations result in an abnormal protein segment of variable length before termination of translation occurs at a stop codon (*nonsense mutation*) (Fig. 56-6). Mutations in intronic sequences or in exon junctions may destroy or create splice donor or splice acceptor sites. Mutations may also be found in the regulatory sequences of genes, resulting in reduced gene transcription.

Mutation Rates As noted before, mutations represent an important cause of genetic diversity as well as disease. Mutation rates are difficult to determine in humans because many mutations are silent and because testing is often not adequate to detect the phenotypic consequences. Mutation rates vary in different genes but are estimated to occur at a rate of about 10^{-10}/bp per cell division. Germline mutation rates (as opposed to somatic mutations) are relevant in the transmission of genetic disease. Because the population of oocytes is established very early in development, only about 20 cell divisions are required for completed oogenesis, whereas spermatogenesis involves about 30 divisions by the time of puberty and 20 cell divisions each year thereafter. Consequently, the probability of acquiring new point mutations is much greater in the male germline than the female germline, in which rates of aneuploidy are increased (Chap. 57). Thus, the incidence of new point mutations in spermatogonia increases with paternal age (e.g., achondrodysplasia, Marfan syndrome, neurofibromatosis). It is estimated that about 1 in 10 sperm carries a new deleterious mutation. The rates for new mutations are calculated most readily for autosomal dominant and X-linked disorders and are $\sim 10^{-5}$ to 10^{-6}/locus per generation. Because most monogenic diseases are relatively rare, new mutations account for a significant fraction of cases. This is important in the context of genetic counseling, as a new mutation can be transmitted to the affected individual but does not necessarily imply that the parents are at risk to transmit the disease to other children. An exception to this is when the new mutation occurs early in germline development, leading to *gonadal mosaicism*.

Unequal Crossing-Over Normally, DNA recombination in germ cells occurs with remarkable fidelity to maintain the precise junction sites for the exchanged DNA sequences (Fig. 56-4). However, mispairing of homologous sequences leads to unequal crossover, with gene duplication on one of the chromosomes and gene deletion on the other chromosome. A significant fraction of growth hormone (*GH*) gene deletions, for example, involve unequal crossing-over (Chap. 318). The *GH* gene is a member of a large gene cluster that includes a growth hormone variant gene as well as several structurally related chorionic somatomammotropin genes and pseudogenes (highly homologous but functionally inactive relatives of a normal gene). Because such gene clusters contain multiple homologous DNA sequences arranged in tandem, they are particularly prone to undergo recombination and, consequently, gene duplication or deletion. On the other hand, duplication of the *PMP22* gene because of unequal crossing-over results in increased gene dosage and type IA Charcot-Marie-Tooth disease (Chap. 364). Unequal crossing-over resulting in deletion of *PMP22* causes a distinct neuropathy called *hereditary liability to pressure palsy* (Chap. 364).

Glucocorticoid-remediable aldosteronism (GRA) is caused by a rearrangement involving the genes that encode aldosterone synthase (*CYP11B2*) and steroid 11β-hydroxylase (*CYP11B1*), normally arranged in tandem on chromosome 8q. These two genes are 95% identical, predisposing to gene duplication and deletion by unequal crossing-over. The rearranged gene product contains the regulatory regions of 11β-hydroxylase fused to the coding sequence of aldosterone synthase. Consequently, the latter enzyme is expressed in the adrenocorticotropic hormone (ACTH)-dependent zona fasciculata of the adrenal gland, resulting in overproduction of mineralocorticoids and hypertension (Chap. 321).

Gene conversion refers to a nonreciprocal exchange of homologous genetic information; it is probably more common than generally recognized. In human genetics, gene conversion has been used to explain how an internal portion of a gene is replaced by a homologous segment copied from another allele or locus; these genetic alterations may range from a few nucleotides to a few thousand nucleotides. As a result of gene conversion, it is possible for short DNA segments of two chromosomes to be identical, even though these sequences are distinct in the parents. A practical consequence of this phenomenon is that nucleotide substitutions can occur during gene conversion between related genes, often altering the function of the gene. In disease states, gene conversion often involves intergenic exchange of DNA between a gene and a related pseudogene. For example, the 21-hydroxylase gene (*CYP21A*) is adjacent to a nonfunctional pseudogene. Many of the nucleotide substitutions that are found in the *CYP21A* gene in patients with congenital adrenal hyperplasia correspond to sequences that are present in the pseudogene, suggesting gene conversion as a mechanism of mutagenesis. In addition, mitotic gene conversion has been suggested as a mechanism to explain revertant mosaicism in which an inherited mutation is "corrected" in certain cells. For example, patients with autosomal recessive generalized atrophic benign epidermolysis bullosa have acquired reverse mutations in one of the two mutated *COL17A1* alleles, leading to clinically unaffected patches of skin.

Insertions and Deletions   Though many instances of insertions and deletions occur as a consequence of unequal crossing-over, there is also evidence for internal duplication, inversion, or deletion of DNA sequences. The fact that certain deletions or insertions appear to occur repeatedly as independent events suggests that specific regions within the DNA sequence predispose to these errors. For example, certain regions of the *DMD* gene appear to be hot spots for deletions.

Errors in DNA Repair   Because mutations caused by defects in DNA repair accumulate as somatic cells divide, these types of mutations are particularly important in the context of neoplastic disorders (Chap. 69). Several genetic disorders involving DNA repair enzymes underscore their importance. Patients with xeroderma pigmentosum have defects in DNA damage recognition or in the nucleotide excision and repair pathway (Chap. 73). Exposed skin is dry and pigmented and is extraordinarily sensitive to the mutagenic effects of ultraviolet irradiation. More than 10 different genes have been shown to cause the different forms of xeroderma pigmentosum. This finding is consistent with the earlier classification of this disease into different complementation groups in which normal function is rescued by the fusion of cells derived from two different forms of xeroderma pigmentosum.

Ataxia telangiectasia causes large telangiectatic lesions of the face, cerebellar ataxia, immunologic defects, and hypersensitivity to ionizing radiation (Chap. 352). The discovery of the ataxia telangiectasia mutated (*ATM*) gene reveals that it is homologous to genes involved in DNA repair and control of cell cycle checkpoints. Mutations in the *ATM* gene give rise to defects in meiosis as well as increasing susceptibility to damage from ionizing radiation. Fanconi's anemia is also associated with an increased risk of multiple acquired genetic abnormalities. It is characterized by diverse congenital anomalies and a strong predisposition to develop aplastic anemia and acute myelogenous leukemia (Chap. 96). Cells from these patients are susceptible to chromosomal breaks caused by a defect in genetic recombination. At least eight different complementation groups have been identified, and several loci and genes associated with Fanconi's anemia have been mapped or cloned.

HNPCC is caused by mutations in one of several different mismatch repair (MMR) genes including MutS homologue 2 (*MSH2*) and MutL homologue 1 (*MLH1*) (Chap. 77). These enzymes are involved in the detection of nucleotide mismatches and in the recognition of slipped-strand trinucleotide repeats. Germline mutations in these genes lead to microsatellite instability and a high mutation rate in colon cancer. This syndrome is characterized by autosomal dominant transmission of colon cancer, young age (<50 years) of presentation, predisposition to lesions in the proximal large bowel, and associated malignancies such as uterine cancer and ovarian cancer. Genetic screening

tests for this disorder are now being used for families considered to be at risk (Chap. 58). Recognition of HNPCC allows early screening with colonoscopy and the implementation of prevention strategies using nonsteroidal anti-inflammatory drugs.

CpG and Dipyrimidine Sequences   Certain DNA sequences are particularly susceptible to mutagenesis. Successive pyrimidine residues (e.g., T-T or C-C) are subject to the formation of ultraviolet light–induced photoadducts. If these pyrimidine dimers are not repaired by the nucleotide excision repair pathway, mutations will be introduced after DNA synthesis. The dinucleotide C-G, or CpG, is also a hot spot for a specific type of mutation. In this case, methylation of the cytosine is associated with an enhanced rate of deamination to uracil, which is then replaced with thymine. This $C \rightarrow T$ transition (or $G \rightarrow A$ on the opposite strand) accounts for at least one-third of point mutations associated with polymorphisms and mutations. Many of the *MSH2* mutations in HNPCC, for example, involve CpG sequences. In addition to the fact that certain types of mutations ($C \rightarrow T$ or $G \rightarrow A$) are relatively common, the nature of the genetic code also results in overrepresentation of certain amino acid substitutions.

Unstable DNA Sequences   *Trinucleotide repeats* may be unstable and expand beyond a critical number. Mechanistically, the expansion is thought to be caused by unequal recombination and slipped mispairing. A premutation represents a small increase in trinucleotide copy number. In subsequent generations, the expanded repeat may increase further in length and result in an increasingly severe phenotype, a process called *dynamic mutation* (see below for discussion of anticipation). Trinucleotide expansion was first recognized as a cause of the fragile X syndrome, one of the most common causes of mental retardation. Other disorders arising from a similar mechanism include Huntington disease (Chap. 350), X-linked spinobulbar muscular atrophy (Chap. 353), and myotonic dystrophy (Chap. 368) (Table 56-4). Malignant cells are also characterized by genetic instability, indicating a breakdown in mechanisms that regulate DNA repair and the cell cycle.

FUNCTIONAL CONSEQUENCES OF MUTATIONS   Functionally, mutations can be broadly classified as gain-of-function and loss-of-function mutations. Gain-of-function mutations are typically dominant, i.e., they result in phenotypic alterations when a single allele is affected. Inactivating mutations are usually recessive, and an affected individual is homozygous or compound heterozygous (e.g., carrying two different mutant alleles) for the disease-causing mutations. Alternatively, mutation in a single allele can result in *haploinsufficiency*, a situation in which one normal allele is not sufficient to maintain a normal phenotype. Haploinsufficiency is a commonly observed mechanism in diseases associated with mutations in transcription factors (Table 56-2). Remarkably, the clinical features among patients with an identical mutation in a transcription factor often vary significantly. One mechanism underlying this variability consists in the influence of modifying genes. Haploinsufficiency can also affect the expression of rate-limiting enzymes. For example, haploinsufficiency in enzymes involved in heme synthesis can cause porphyrias (Chap. 337).

An increase in dosage of a gene product may also result in disease, as illustrated by the duplication of the *DAX1* gene in dosage-sensitive sex-reversal (Chap. 328). Mutation in a single allele can also result in loss of function due to a dominant-negative effect. In this case, the mutated allele interferes with the function of the normal gene product by one of several different mechanisms: (1) a mutant protein may interfere with the function of a multimeric protein complex, as illustrated by mutations in type 1 collagen (*COL1A1*, *COL1A2*) genes in osteogenesis imperfecta (Chap. 342); (2) a mutant protein may occupy binding sites on proteins or promoter response elements, as illustrated by thyroid hormone resistance, a disorder in which inactivated thyroid hormone receptor binds to target genes and functions as an antagonist of normal receptors (Chap. 320); or (3) a mutant protein can be cytotoxic as in α_1 antitrypsin deficiency (Chap. 242) or autosomal dominant neurohypophyseal diabetes insipidus (Chap. 319), in which the

TABLE 56-4 Selected Trinucleotide Repeat Disorders

Disease	Locus	Repeat	Triplet Length Normal/Disease	Inheritance	Gene Product
X-Chromosomal spinobulbar muscular atrophy (SBMA)	Xq11-q12	CAG	11–34/40–62	XR	Androgen receptor
Fragile X-syndrome (FRAXA)	Xq27.3	CGG	6–50/200–300	XR	FMR-1 protein
Fragile X-syndrome (FRAXE)	Xq28	GCC	6–25/>200	XR	FMR-2 protein
Dystrophia myotonica (DM)	19q13.2-q13.3	CTG	5–30/200–1000	AD, variable penetrance	Myotonin protein kinase
Huntington disease (HD)	4p16.3	CAG	11–34/37–121	AD	Huntington
Spinocerebellar ataxia type 1 (SCA1)	6p21.3-21.2	CAG	19–36/39–83	AD	Ataxin 1
Spinocerebellar ataxia type 2 (SCA2)	12q24.1	CAG	15–31/34–400	AD	Ataxin 2
Spinocerebellar ataxia type 3 (SCA3); Machado Joseph disease (MD)	14q21	CAG	13–36/55–86	AD	SC3/MJD1
Spinocerebellar ataxia type 6 (SCA6, CACNAIA)	19p13.1-13.2	CAG	4–16/20–33	AD	Alpha 1A voltage-dependent calcium channel
Spinocerebellar ataxia type 7 (SCA7)	3p21.1-p12	CAG	4–19/37 ≥ 300	AD	Ataxin 7
Spinocerebellar ataxia type 12 (SCA12)	5q31	CAG	6–26/66–78	AD	Protein phosphatase 2A
Dentorubral pallidoluysiane atrophy (DRPLA)	12p	CAG	7–23/49–75	AD	Atrophin
Friedreich ataxia (FRDA1)	9q13-21	GAA	7–22/200–900	AR	Frataxin

Abbreviations: AD, autosomal dominant; AR, autosomal recessive; XR, X-linked recessive.

abnormally folded proteins are trapped within the endoplasmic reticulum and ultimately cause cellular damage.

GENOTYPE AND PHENOTYPE ■ Alleles, Genotypes, and Haplotypes

An observed trait is referred to as a *phenotype*; the genetic information defining the phenotype is called the *genotype*. Alternative forms of a gene or a genetic marker are referred to as *alleles*. Alleles may be polymorphic variants of nucleic acids that have no apparent effect on gene expression or function. In other instances, these variants may have subtle effects on gene expression, thereby conferring the adaptive advantages associated with genetic diversity. On the other hand, allelic variants may reflect mutations in a gene that clearly alter its function. The common Glu → Val sickle cell mutation (E6V) in the *β-globin* gene and the δF508 deletion of phenylalanine (F) in the *CFTR* gene are examples of allelic variants of these genes. Because each individual has two copies of each chromosome (one inherited from the mother and one inherited from the father), he or she can have only two alleles at a given locus. However, there can be many different alleles in the population. The normal or common allele is usually referred to as *wild type*. When alleles at a given locus are identical, the individual is *homozygous*. Inheriting such identical copies of a mutant allele occurs in many autosomal recessive disorders, particularly in circumstances of consanguinity. If the alleles are different, the individual is *heterozygous* at this locus (Fig. 56-6). If two different mutant alleles are inherited at a given locus, the individual is said to be a *compound heterozygote*. *Hemizygous* is used to describe males with a mutation in an X chromosomal gene or a female with a loss of one X chromosomal locus.

Genotypes describe the specific alleles at a particular locus. For example, there are three common alleles (E2, E3, E4) of the apolipoprotein E (*APOE*) gene. The genotype of an individual can therefore be described as *APOE3/4* or *APOE4/4* or any other variant. These designations indicate which alleles are present on the two chromosomes in the *APOE* gene at locus 19q13.2. In other cases, the genotype might be assigned arbitrary numbers (e.g., 1/2) or letters (e.g., B/b) to distinguish different alleles.

A *haplotype* refers to a group of alleles that are closely linked together at a genomic locus. Haplotypes are useful for tracking the transmission of genomic segments within families and for detecting evidence of genetic recombination, if the crossover event occurs between the alleles (Fig. 56-4). As an example, various alleles at the histocompatibility locus antigen (HLA) on chromosome 6p are used to establish haplotypes associated with certain disease states. For example, 21-hydroxylase deficiency, complement deficiency, and hemochromatosis are each associated with specific HLA haplotypes. It is now recognized that these genes lie in close vicinity to the HLA locus, which explains why HLA associations were identified even before the disease genes were cloned and localized. In other cases, specific HLA associations with diseases such as ankylosing spondylitis (HLA-B27) or type 1 diabetes mellitus (HLA-DR4) reflect the role of specific HLA allelic variants in susceptibility to these autoimmune diseases.

Allelic Heterogeneity *Allelic heterogeneity* refers to the fact that different mutations in the same genetic locus can cause an identical or similar phenotype. For example, many different mutations of the *β-globin* locus can cause *β*-thalassemia (Fig. 56-5). In essence, allelic heterogeneity reflects the fact that many different mutations are capable of altering protein structure and function. For this reason, maps of inactivating mutations in genes usually show a near-random distribution. Exceptions include: (1) a founder effect, in which a particular mutation that does not affect reproductive capacity can be traced to a single individual; (2) "hot spots" for mutations, in which the nature of the DNA sequence predisposes to a recurring mutation; and (3) localization of mutations to certain domains that are particularly critical for protein function. Allelic heterogeneity creates a practical problem for genetic testing because one must often examine the entire genetic locus for mutations, as these can differ in each patient.

Phenotypic Heterogeneity *Phenotypic heterogeneity* occurs when more than one phenotype is caused by allelic mutations (e.g., different mutations in the same gene). For example, mutations in the *myosin VIIIA* gene can result in four distinct clinical disorders: (1) autosomal recessive deafness DFNB2, (2) autosomal dominant nonsyndromic deafness DFNA11, (3) Usher 1B syndrome [congenital deafness, retinitis pigmentosa (Fig. 56-9)], and (4) an atypical variant of Usher's syndrome.

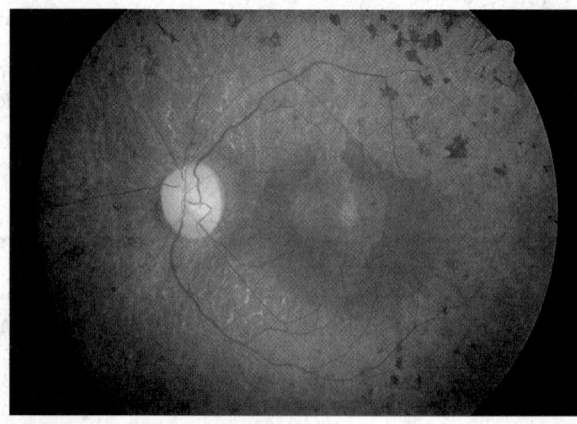

FIGURE 56-9 Retinitis pigmentosa with black clumps of pigment in the retinal periphery, known as "bone spicules." There is also atrophy of the retinal pigment epithelium, making the vasculature of the choroid easily visible.

Similarly, identical mutations in the *FGFR2* gene can result in very distinct phenotypes: Crouzon syndrome (craniofacial synostosis), or Pfeiffer syndrome (acrocephalopolysyndactyly).

Locus or Nonallelic Heterogeneity and Phenocopies

Nonallelic or locus heterogeneity refers to the situation in which a similar disease phenotype results from mutations at different genetic loci (Table 56-5). This often occurs when more than one gene product produces different subunits of an interacting complex or when different genes are involved in the same genetic cascade or physiologic pathway. For example, osteogenesis imperfecta can arise from mutations in two different procollagen genes (*COL1A1* or *COL1A2*) that are located on different chromosomes (Chap. 342). The effects of inactivating mutations in these two genes are similar because the protein products comprise different subunits of the helical collagen fiber. Similarly, muscular dystrophy syndromes can be caused by mutations in various genes, consistent with the fact that it can be transmitted in an X-linked (Duchenne or Becker), autosomal dominant (limb-girdle muscular dystrophy type 1), or autosomal recessive (limb-girdle muscular dystrophy type 2) manner (Chap. 368). Mutations in the X-linked *DMD* gene, which encodes dystrophin, are the most common cause of muscular dystrophy. This feature reflects the large size of the gene as well as the fact that the phenotype is expressed in hemizygous males because they have only a single copy of the X chromosome. Dystrophin is associated with a large group of additional proteins that form the membrane-associated cytoskeleton in muscle. Mutations in several components of this protein complex can also cause muscular dystrophy syndromes. Although the phenotypic features of some of these disorders are distinct, the phenotypic spectrum caused by mutations in different genes overlaps, thereby leading to nonallelic heterogeneity. It should be noted that mutations in dystrophin also cause allelic heterogeneity. For example, mutations in the *DMD* gene can cause either Duchenne or the less severe Becker muscular dystrophy, depending on the severity of the protein defect.

Recognition of nonallelic heterogeneity is important for several reasons: (1) the ability to identify disease loci in linkage studies is reduced by including patients with similar phenotypes but different genetic disorders; (2) genetic testing is more complex because several different genes need to be considered along with the possibility of different mutations in each of the candidate genes; and (3) novel information is gained about how genes or proteins interact, providing unique insights into molecular physiology.

Phenocopies refer to circumstances in which nongenetic conditions mimic a genetic disorder. For example, features of toxin- or drug-induced neurologic syndromes can resemble those seen in Huntington disease, and vascular causes of dementia share phenotypic features with familial forms of Alzheimer dementia (Chap. 350). Children born with activating mutations of the thyroid-stimulating hormone receptor (TSH-R) exhibit goiter and thyrotoxicosis similar to that seen in neonatal Graves' disease, which is caused by the transfer of maternal autoantibodies to the fetus (Chap. 320). As in nonallelic heterogeneity, the presence of phenocopies has the potential to confound linkage studies and genetic testing. Patient history and subtle differences in phenotype can often provide clues that distinguish these disorders from related genetic conditions.

Variable Expressivity and Incomplete Penetrance

It is not uncommon for the same genetic mutation to cause a phenotypic spectrum illustrating the phenomenon of *variable expressivity*. This may include different

TABLE 56-5 *Selected Examples of Locus Heterogeneity*

Phenotype	Gene	Chromosomal Location	Protein
Familial hypertrophic cardiomyopathy			
Genes encoding for sarcomeric proteins	*MYH7*	14q12	Myosin heavy chain beta
	TNNT2	1q2	Troponin-T2
	TPM1	15q22.1	Tropomyosin α
	MYBPC3	11p11q	Myosin binding protein C
	TNN13	19q13.4	Troponin 1
	MYL3	3p	Myosin light chain 3
	MYL2	12q23-24.3	Myosin light chain 2
	TTN	2q24.3	Cardiac titin
	ACTC	15q11	Cardiac alpha actin
	MYH6	14q1	Myosin heavy chain alpha
	TNNC1	3p21.3-3p14.3	Cardiac troponin C
Nonsarcomeric proteins	*MTT1*	Mitochondrial	tRNA isoleucine and tRNA glycine
	PRKAG2	7q35-q36	AMP-activated protein kinase γ2 subunit
	DMPK	19q13	Myotonin protein kinase (myotonic dystrophy)
	FRDA	9q13	Frataxin (Friedreich ataxia)
Polycystic kidney disease			
	PKD1	16p13.3-13.12	Polycystin 1 (AD)
	PKD2	4q21.-23	Polycystin 2 (AD)
	PKHD1	6p21.1-p12	Fibrocystin (AR)
Familial breast cancer			
BRCA1	*BRCA1*	17q21	BRCA1 (RNA polymerase II component)
BRCA2	*BRCA2*	13q12.3	BRCA2

manifestations of a complex disorder (e.g., MEN), the severity of the disorder (e.g., sickle cell anemia), or the age of disease onset (e.g., Alzheimer dementia). MEN-1 illustrates several of these features. Families with this autosomal dominant disorder develop tumors of the parathyroid gland, endocrine pancreas, and the pituitary gland (Chap. 330). However, the pattern of tumors in the different glands, the age at which tumors develop, and the types of hormones produced vary among affected individuals, even within a given family. In this example, the phenotypic variability arises, in part, because of the requirement for a second mutation in the normal copy of the *MEN1* gene, as well as the large array of different cell types that are susceptible to the effects of *MEN1* gene mutations. In part, variable expression reflects the influence of modifier genes, or genetic background, on the effects of a particular mutation. Even in identical twins, in whom the genetic constitution is the same, one can occasionally see variable expression of a genetic disease.

Interactions with the environment can also influence the course of a disease. For example, the manifestations and severity of hemochromatosis can be influenced by iron intake (Chap. 336), and the course of phenylketonuria is affected by exposure to phenylalanine in the diet (Chap. 343). Other metabolic disorders, such as hyperlipidemias and porphyria, also fall into this category. Many mechanisms, including genetic effects and environmental influences, can therefore lead to variable expressivity. In genetic counseling, it is particularly important to recognize this variability, as one cannot always predict the course of disease, even when the mutation is known.

Penetrance refers to the proportion of individuals with a mutant genotype that express the phenotype. If all carriers of a mutant express the phenotype, penetrance is complete, whereas it is said to be *incomplete* or *reduced* if some individuals do not have any features of the phenotype. Dominant conditions with incomplete penetrance are characterized by skipping of generations with unaffected carriers transmitting the mutant gene. For example, hypertrophic obstructive cardiomyopathy (HCM) caused by mutations in the *myosin-binding protein C* gene is a dominant disorder with clinical features in only a subset of patients who carry the mutation (Chap. 221). Patients who have the mutation but no evidence of the disease can still transmit the disorder to subsequent generations. In many conditions with postnatal onset, the proportion of gene carriers who are affected varies with age. When describing penetrance, one has to therefore specify age. For

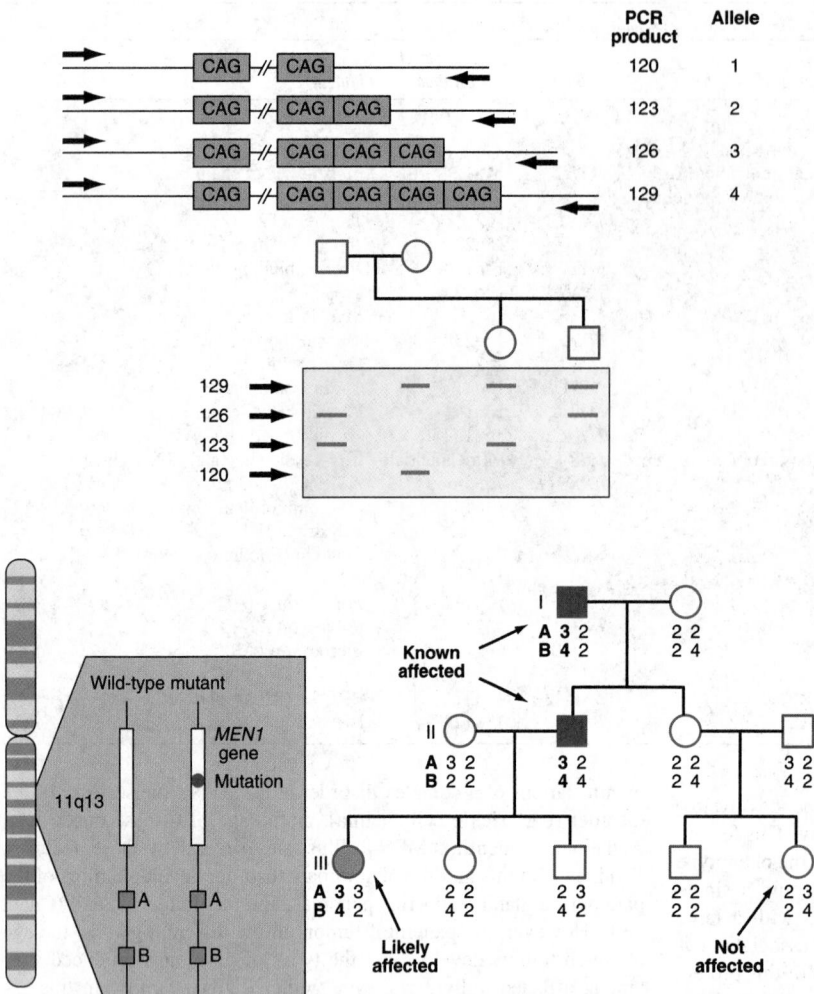

PCR product	Allele
120	1
123	2
126	3
129	4

FIGURE 56-10 CAG repeat length and linkage analysis in multiple endocrine neoplasia type 1. *Upper panel.* Detection of different alleles using polymorphic microsatellite markers. The example depicts a CAG trinucleotide repeat. PCR with primers flanking the polymorphic region results in products of variable length, depending on the number of CAG repeats. After characterization of the alleles in the parents, transmission of the paternal and maternal alleles can be determined. *Lower panel.* Genotype analysis using microsatellite markers in a family with multiple endocrine neoplasia type 1. Two microsatellite markers, A and B, are located in close proximity to the *MEN1* gene on chromosome 11q13. For each individual, the A and B alleles have been determined. Based on this analysis, the genotype A3,B4 is linked to the disease because it occurs in the two affected individuals I-1 and II-1 but not in unaffected siblings. Because the disease allele is linked to A3,B4 within the affected family, it is likely that the individual III-1 is a carrier of the mutated *MEN1* gene. Although III-5 also has the A3,B4 genotype, she has inherited the allele from her unaffected father (II-4), who is not related to the original family. The A3,B4 genotype is only associated with MEN-1 in the original family, but not in the general population. Therefore, individual III-5 is not at risk for developing the disease.

example, for disorders such as Huntington disease or familial amyotrophic lateral sclerosis, which present late in life, the rate of penetrance is influenced by the age at which the clinical assessment is performed. *Imprinting* can also modify the penetrance of a disease (see below). For example, in patients with Albright hereditary osteodystrophy, mutations in the Gsα subunit (*GNAS1* gene) are expressed clinically only in individuals who inherit the mutation from their mother (Chap. 334).

Sex-Influenced Phenotypes Certain mutations affect males and females quite differently. In some instances, this is because the gene resides on the X or Y sex chromosomes (X-linked disorders and Y-linked disorders). As a result, the phenotype of mutated X-linked genes will be expressed fully in males but variably in heterozygous females, depending on the degree of X-inactivation and the function of the gene. For example, most heterozygous female carriers of factor VIII deficiency (hemophilia A) are asymptomatic because sufficient factor VIII is produced to prevent a defect in coagulation (Chap. 102). On the other hand, some females heterozygous for the X-linked lipid storage

defect caused by α-galactosidase A deficiency (Fabry disease) experience mild manifestations of painful neuropathy, as well as other features of the disease (Chap. 340). Because only males have a Y chromosome, mutations in genes such as *SRY*, which causes male-to-female sex-reversal, or *DAZ* (deleted in azoospermia), which causes abnormalities of spermatogenesis, are unique to males (Chap. 328).

Other diseases are expressed in a sex-limited manner because of the differential function of the gene product in males and females. Activating mutations in the luteinizing hormone receptor cause dominant male-limited precocious puberty in boys (Chap. 325). The phenotype is unique to males because activation of the receptor induces testosterone production in the testis, whereas it is functionally silent in the immature ovary. Homozygous inactivating mutations of the follicle-stimulating hormone (FSH) receptor cause primary ovarian failure in females because the follicles do not develop in the absence of FSH action. In contrast, affected males have a more subtle phenotype, because testosterone production is preserved (allowing sexual maturation) and spermatogenesis is only partially impaired (Chap. 325). In congenital adrenal hyperplasia, most commonly caused by 21-hydroxylase deficiency, cortisol production is impaired and ACTH stimulation of the adrenal gland leads to increased production of androgenic precursors (Chap. 321). In females, the increased androgen level causes ambiguous genitalia, which can be recognized at the time of birth. In males, the diagnosis may be made on the basis of adrenal insufficiency at birth, because the increased adrenal androgen level does not alter sexual differentiation, or later in childhood, because of the development of precocious puberty. Hemochromatosis is more common in males than in females, presumably because of differences in dietary iron intake and losses associated with menstruation and pregnancy in females (Chap. 336).

GENETIC LINKAGE *Genetic linkage* refers to the fact that genes are physically connected, or linked, to one another along the chromosomes. Two fundamental principles are essential for understanding the concept of linkage: (1) when two genes are close together on a chromosome, they are usually transmitted together, unless a recombination event separates them (Fig. 56-4); and (2) the odds of a crossover, or recombination event, between two linked genes is proportional to the distance that separates them. Thus, genes that are further apart are more likely to undergo a recombination event than genes that are very close together. The detection of chromosomal loci that segregate with a disease by linkage can be used to identify the gene responsible for the disease (*positional cloning*) and to predict the odds of disease gene transmission in genetic counseling.

Polymorphisms are essential for linkage studies because they provide a means to distinguish the maternal and paternal chromosomes in an individual. On average, 1 out of every 1000 bp varies from one person to the next. Although this degree of variation seems low (99.9% identical), it means that >3 million sequence differences exist between any two unrelated individuals and the probability that the sequence at such loci will differ on the two homologous chromosomes is high (often >70 to 90%). These sequence variations include VNTRs, short tandem repeats (STRs), and SNPs. Most STRs, also called *polymorphic microsatellite markers*, consist of di-, tri-, or tetranucleotide repeats that can be measured readily using PCR (Fig. 56-10). Characterization of SNPs, using DNA chips, provides a promising means for rapid analysis of genetic variation and linkage. Although this sequence variation usually has no apparent functional consequence, it provides much of the basis for variation in genetic traits.

In order to identify a chromosomal locus that segregates with a disease, it is necessary to determine the genotype or haplotype of DNA samples from one or several pedigrees. One can then assess whether certain marker alleles cosegregate with the disease. Markers that are closest to the disease gene are less likely to undergo recombination events and therefore receive a higher linkage score. Linkage is expressed as a lod (logarithm of odds) score—the ratio of the probability that the disease and marker loci are linked rather than unlinked. Lod scores of +3 (1000:1) are generally accepted as supporting linkage, whereas a score of −2 is consistent with the absence of linkage.

An example of the use of linkage analysis is shown in Fig. 56-10. In this case, the gene for the autosomal dominant disorder, MEN-1, is known to be located on chromosome 11q13. Using positional cloning, the *MEN1* gene was identified and shown to encode menin, a tumor suppressor. Affected individuals inherit a mutant form of the *MEN1* gene, predisposing them to certain types of tumors (parathyroid, pituitary, pancreatic islet) (Chap. 330). In the tissues that develop a tumor, a "second hit" occurs in the normal copy of the *MEN1* gene. This somatic mutation may be a point mutation, a microdeletion, or loss of a chromosomal fragment (detected as loss of heterozygosity, LOH). Within a given family, linkage to the *MEN1* gene locus can be assessed without necessarily knowing the specific mutation in the *MEN1* gene. Using polymorphic STRs that are close to the *MEN1* gene, one can assess transmission of the different *MEN1* alleles and compare this pattern to development of the disorder to determine which allele is associated with risk of MEN-1. In the pedigree shown, the affected grandfather in generation I carries alleles 3 and 4 on the chromosome with the mutated *MEN1* gene and alleles 2 and 2 on his other chromosome 11. Consistent with linkage of the 3/4 genotype to the *MEN1* locus, his son in generation II is affected, whereas his daughter (who inherits the 2/2 genotype from her father) is unaffected. In the third generation, transmission of the 3/4 genotype indicates risk of developing MEN-1, assuming that no genetic recombination between the 3/4 alleles and the *MEN1* gene has occurred. After a specific mutation in the *MEN1* gene is identified within a family, it is possible to track transmission of the mutation itself, thereby eliminating uncertainty caused by recombination.

CHROMOSOMAL DISORDERS Chromosomal or cytogenetic disorders are caused by numerical or structural aberrations in chromosomes. Deviations in chromosome number are common causes of abortions, developmental disorders, and malformations. *Contiguous gene syndromes*, i.e., large deletions affecting several genes, have been useful for identifying the location of new disease-causing genes. Because of the variable size of gene deletions in different patients, a systematic comparison of phenotypes and locations of deletion breakpoints allows positions of particular genes to be mapped within the critical genomic region. →*For discussion of disorders of chromosome number and structure, see Chap. 57.*

MONOGENIC MENDELIAN DISORDERS Monogenic human diseases are frequently referred to as *Mendelian disorders* because they obey the principles of genetic transmission originally set forth in Gregor Mendel's classic work. The continuously updated OMIM catalog lists several thousand of these disorders and provides information about the clinical phenotype, molecular basis, allelic variants, and pertinent animal models (Table 56-1). The mode of inheritance for a given phenotypic trait or disease is determined by pedigree analysis. All affected and unaffected individuals in the family are recorded in a pedigree using standard symbols (Fig. 56-1). The principles of allelic segregation, and the transmission of alleles from parents to children, are illustrated in Fig. 56-11. One dominant (A) allele and one recessive (a) allele can display three Mendelian modes of inheritance: autosomal dominant, autosomal recessive, and X-chromosomal. About 65% of human monogenic disorders are autosomal dominant, 25% are autosomal recessive, and 5%

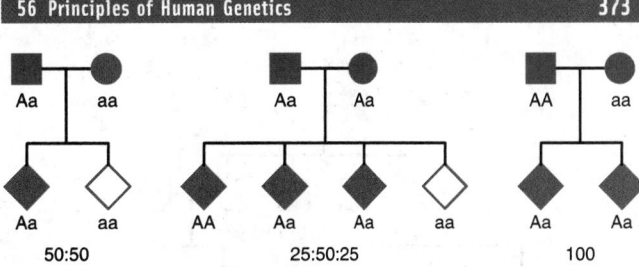

FIGURE 56-11   Segregation of alleles. Segregation of genotypes in the offspring of parents with one dominant (A) and one recessive (a) allele. The distribution of the parental alleles to their offspring depends on the combination present in the parents.

are X-linked. Genetic testing is now available for many of these disorders and plays an increasingly important role in clinical medicine (Chap. 58).

Autosomal Dominant Disorders Autosomal dominant disorders assume particular relevance because mutations in a single allele are sufficient to cause the disease. In contrast to recessive disorders, in which disease pathogenesis is relatively straightforward because there is loss of gene function, in dominant disorders there are various disease mechanisms, many of which are unique to the function of the genetic pathway involved.

In autosomal dominant disorders, individuals are affected in successive generations; the disease does not occur in the offspring of unaffected individuals. Males and females are affected with equal frequency because the defective gene resides on one of the 22 autosomes (Fig. 56-12A). Autosomal dominant mutations alter one of the two alleles at a given locus. Because the alleles segregate randomly at meiosis, the probability that an offspring will be affected is 50%. Unless there is a new germline mutation, an affected individual has an affected parent. Children with a normal genotype do not transmit the disorder. Due to differences in penetrance or expressivity (see above), the clinical manifestations of autosomal dominant disorders may be variable. Because of these variations, it is sometimes challenging to determine the pattern of inheritance.

It should be recognized, however, that some individuals acquire a mutated gene from an unaffected parent. De novo germline mutations occur more frequently during later cell divisions in gametogenesis, which explains why siblings are rarely affected. As noted before, new germline mutations occur more frequently in fathers of advanced age. For example, the average age of fathers with new germline mutations that cause Marfan's syndrome is approximately 37 years, whereas fathers who transmit the disease by inheritance have an average age of about 30 years.

Autosomal Recessive Disorders The clinical expression of autosomal recessive disorders is more uniform than in autosomal dominant disorders. Most mutated alleles lead to a complete or partial loss of function. They frequently involve enzymes in metabolic pathways, receptors, or proteins in signaling cascades. In an autosomal recessive disease, the affected individual, who can be of either sex, is a homozygote or compound heterozygote for a single-gene defect. With a few important exceptions, autosomal recessive diseases are rare and often occur in the context of parental consanguinity. The relatively high frequency of certain recessive disorders, such as sickle cell anemia, cystic fibrosis, and thalassemia, is partially explained by a selective biologic advantage for the heterozygous state (see below). Though heterozygous carriers of a defective allele are usually clinically normal, they may display subtle differences in phenotype that only become apparent with more precise testing or in the context of certain environmental influences. In sickle cell anemia, for example, heterozygotes are normally asymptomatic. However, in situations of dehydration or diminished oxygen pressure, sickle cell crises can also occur in heterozygotes (Chap. 91).

In most instances, an affected individual is the offspring of heterozygous parents. In this situation, there is a 25% chance that the off-

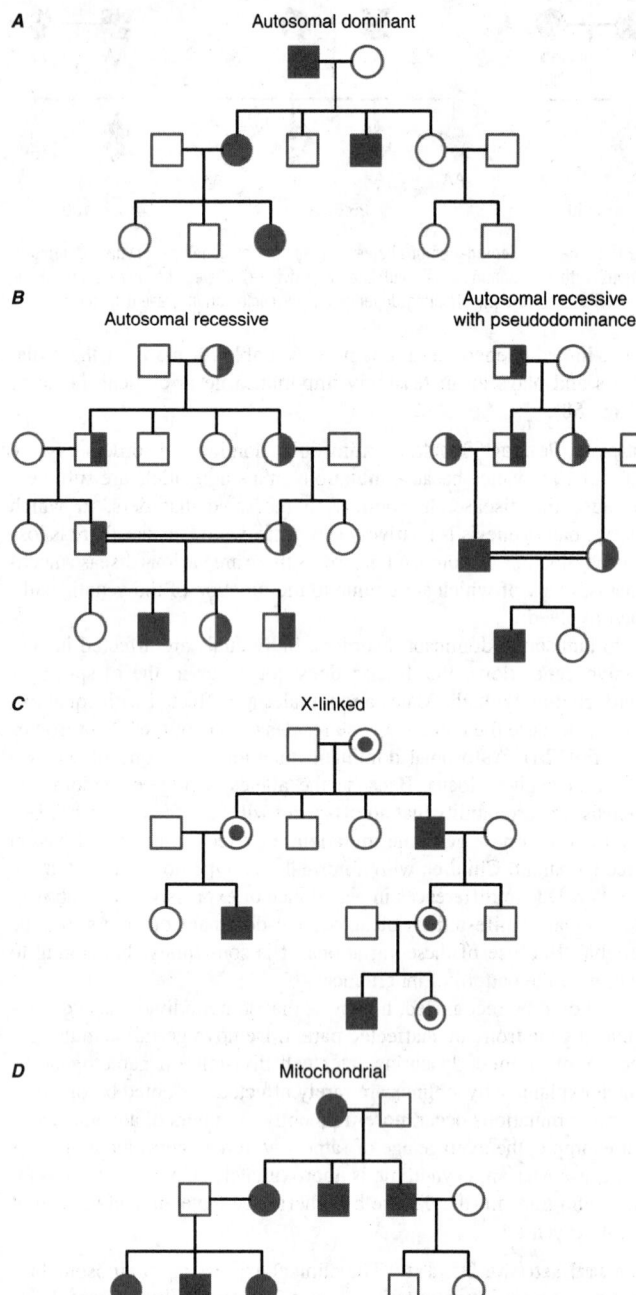

FIGURE 56-12   Dominant, recessive, X-linked, and mitochondrial (matrilinear) inheritance.

spring will have a normal genotype, a 50% probability of a heterozygous state, and a 25% risk of homozygosity for the recessive alleles (Fig. 56-12*B*). In the case of one unaffected heterozygous and one affected homozygous parent, the probability of disease increases to 50% for each child. In this instance, the pedigree analysis mimics an autosomal dominant mode of inheritance (*pseudodominance*). In contrast to autosomal dominant disorders, new mutations in recessive alleles are rarely manifest because they usually result in an asymptomatic carrier state.

X-Linked Disorders   Males have only one X chromosome; consequently, a daughter always inherits her father's X chromosome in addition to one of her mother's two X chromosomes. A son inherits the Y chromosome from his father and one maternal X chromosome. Thus, the characteristic features of X-linked inheritance are (1) the absence of father-to-son transmission, and (2) the fact that all daughters of an

affected male are obligate carriers of the mutant allele (Fig. 56-12*C*). The risk of developing disease due to a mutant X-chromosomal gene differs in the two sexes. Because males have only one X chromosome, they are hemizygous for the mutant allele; thus, they are more likely to develop the mutant phenotype, regardless of whether the mutation is dominant or recessive. A female may be either heterozygous or homozygous for the mutant allele, which may be dominant or recessive. The terms *X-linked dominant* or *X-linked recessive* are therefore only applicable to expression of the mutant phenotype in women. In addition, the expression of X-chromosomal genes is influenced by X chromosome inactivation (see below).

Y-Linked Disorders   Only a few genes are known on the Y chromosome. One such gene, the sex-region determining Y factor (*SRY*), or testis-determining factor (*TDF*), is crucial for normal male development. Normally there is infrequent exchange of sequences on the Y chromosome with the X chromosome. Because the *SRY* region is closely adjacent to the pseudoautosomal region, a chromosomal segment on the X and Y chromosomes with a high degree of homology, a crossing-over occasionally involves the *SRY* region. Translocations can result in XY females with the Y chromosome lacking the *SRY* gene or XX males harboring the *SRY* gene on one of the X chromosomes (Chap. 328). Point mutations in the *SRY* gene may also result in individuals with an XY genotype and an incomplete female phenotype. Most of these mutations occur de novo. Men with oligospermia/azoospermia frequently have microdeletions on the long arm of the Y chromosome that involve one or more of the azoospermia factor (*AZF*) genes.

EXCEPTIONS TO SIMPLE MENDELIAN INHERITANCE PATTERNS ▪ Mitochondrial Disorders   Mendelian inheritance refers to the transmission of genes encoded by DNA contained in the nuclear chromosomes. In addition, each mitochondrion contains several copies of a circular chromosome. The mitochondrial DNA (mtDNA) is small (16.5 kb) and encodes transfer and ribosomal RNAs, and 13 proteins that are components of the respiratory chain involved in oxidative phosphorylation and ATP generation. The mitochondrial genome does not recombine and is inherited through the maternal line because sperm does not contribute significant cytoplasmic components to the zygote. A noncoding region of the mitochondrial chromosome, referred to as D-loop, is highly polymorphic. This property, together with the absence of mtDNA recombination, makes it a valuable tool for studies tracing human migration and evolution, and it is also used for specific forensic applications.

Inherited mitochondrial disorders are transmitted in a matrilineal fashion; all children from an affected mother will inherit the disease, but it will not be transmitted from an affected father to his children (Fig. 56-12*D*). Alterations in the mtDNA affecting enzymes required for oxidative phosphorylation lead to reduction of ATP supply, generation of free radicals, and induction of apoptosis. Several syndromic disorders arising from mutations in the mitochondrial genome are known in humans and they affect both protein-coding and tRNA genes (Tables 56-1 and 56-6). The broad clinical spectrum often involves (cardio)myopathies and encephalopathies because of the high dependence of these tissues on oxidative phosphorylation. The age of onset and the clinical course are highly variable because of the unusual mechanisms of mtDNA, which replicates independently from nuclear DNA. During cell replication, the proportion of wild-type and mutant mitochondria can drift among different cells and tissues. The resulting heterogeneity in the proportion of mitochondria with and without a mutation is referred to as *heteroplasmia* and underlies the phenotypic variability that is characteristic of mitochondrial diseases.

Acquired somatic mutations in mitochondria are thought to be involved in several age-dependent degenerative disorders affecting predominantly muscle and the peripheral and central nervous system (e.g., Alzheimer's and Parkinson's disease). Establishing that a mtDNA alteration is causal for a clinical phenotype is challenging because of the high degree of polymorphism in mtDNA and the phenotypic variability characteristic of these disorders. Certain pharmacologic treatments may have an impact on mitochondria and/or their function. For

TABLE 56-6 *Selected Mitochondrial Diseases*

Disease/Syndrome	MIM #
MELAS syndrome: mitochondrial myopathy with encephalopathy, lactic acidosis, and stroke	540000 540050
Leber's optic atrophy: hereditary optical neuropathy	535000
Kearns-Sayre syndrome (KSS): ophthalmoplegia, pigmental degeneration of the retina, cardiomyopathy	530000
MERRF syndrome: myoclonic epilepsy and ragged red fibers	545030
Maternally inherited myopathy and cardiomyopathy (MMC)	590050
Neurogenic muscular weakness with ataxia and retinitis pigmentosa (NARP)	551500
Progressive external ophthalmoplegia (CEOP)	258470
Pearson syndrome (PEAR): bone marrow and pancreatic failure	557000
Autosomal dominant inherited mitochondrial myopathy with mitochondrial deletion (ADMIMY)	157640
Somatic mutations in cytochrome *b* gene: exercise intolerance, lactic acidosis, complex III deficiency, muscle pain, ragged-red fibers	

example, treatment with the antiretroviral compound azidothymidine (AZT) causes an acquired mitochondrial myopathy through depletion of muscular mtDNA.

Mosaicism Mosaicism refers to the presence of two or more genetically distinct cell lines in the tissues of an individual. It results from a mutation that occurs during embryonic, fetal, or extrauterine development. The developmental stage at which the mutation arises will determine whether germ cells and/or somatic cells are involved. Chromosomal mosaicism results from non-disjunction at an early embryonic mitotic division, leading to the persistence of more than one cell line, as exemplified by some patients with Turner syndrome (Chap. 328). Somatic mosaicism is characterized by a patchy distribution of genetically altered somatic cells. The McCune-Albright syndrome, for example, is caused by activating mutations in the stimulatory G protein α ($G_s\alpha$) that occur early in development (Chap. 334). The clinical phenotype varies depending on the tissue distribution of the mutation; manifestations include ovarian cysts that secrete sex steroids and cause precocious puberty, polyostotic fibrous dysplasia, café-au-lait skin pigmentation, growth hormone–secreting pituitary adenomas, and hypersecreting autonomous thyroid nodules (Chap. 326).

X-Inactivation, Imprinting, and Uniparental Disomy According to traditional Mendelian principles, the parental origin of a mutant gene is irrelevant for the expression of the phenotype. Nonetheless, there are important exceptions to this rule. X-inactivation prevents the expression of most genes on one of the two X-chromosomes in every cell of a female. Gene inactivation also occurs on selected chromosomal regions of autosomes. This phenomenon, referred to as *genomic imprinting*, leads to preferential expression of an allele depending on its parental origin. It is of pathophysiologic importance in disorders where the transmission of disease is dependent on the sex of the transmitting parent and, thus, plays an important role in the expression of certain genetic disorders. Two classic examples are the Prader-Willi syndrome and Angelman syndrome (Chap. 57). Prader-Willi syndrome is characterized by diminished fetal activity, obesity, hypotonia, mental retardation, short stature, and hypogonadotropic hypogonadism. Deletions in the Prader-Willi syndrome occur exclusively on the paternal chromosome 15. In contrast, patients with Angelman syndrome, characterized by mental retardation, seizures, ataxia, and hypotonia, have deletions at the same site of chromosome 15; however, they are located on the maternal chromosome 15. These two syndromes may also result from *uniparental disomy*. In this case, the syndromes are not caused by deletions on chromosome 15 but by the inheritance of either two maternal chromosomes (Prader-Willi syndrome) or two paternal chromosomes (Angelman syndrome).

Imprinting and the related phenomenon of allelic exclusion may be more common than currently documented, as it is difficult to examine levels of mRNA expression from the maternal and paternal alleles in specific tissues or in individual cells. Genomic imprinting, or uniparental disomy, is involved in the pathogenesis of several other disorders and malignancies (Chap. 57). Hydatidiform mole contains a normal number of diploid chromosomes, but they are all of paternal origin. The opposite situation occurs in ovarian teratomata, with 46 chromosomes of maternal origin. Expression of the imprinted gene for insulin-like growth factor II (IGF-II) is involved in the pathogenesis of the cancer-predisposing Beckwith-Wiedemann syndrome (BWS) (Chap. 68). These children show somatic overgrowth with organomegalies and hemihypertrophy, and they have an increased risk of embryonal malignancies such as Wilm's tumor. Normally, only the paternally derived copy of the *IGF-II* gene is active and the maternal copy is inactive. Imprinting of the *IGF-II* gene is regulated by *H19*, which encodes an RNA transcript that is not translated into protein. Disruption or lack of *H19* methylation leads to a relaxation of *IGF-II* imprinting and expression of both alleles. Heritable changes in gene expression not associated with DNA sequence alterations are referred to as *epigenetic effects*; these changes are increasingly recognized to play a role in human diseases and possibly in aging as well.

Somatic Mutations Cancer can be defined as a genetic disease at the cellular level (Chap. 68). Cancers are monoclonal in origin, indicating that they have arisen from a single precursor cell with one or several mutations in genes controlling growth and/or differentiation. These acquired somatic mutations are restricted to the tumor and its metastases and are not found in the surrounding normal tissue. The molecular alterations include dominant gain-of-function mutations in oncogenes, recessive loss-of-function mutations in tumor supressor genes and DNA repair genes, gene amplification, and chromosome rearrangements. Rarely, a single mutation in certain genes may be sufficient to transform a normal cell into a malignant cell. In most cancers, however, the development of a malignant phenotype requires several genetic alterations for the gradual progression from a normal cell to a cancerous cell, a phenomenon termed *multistep carcinogenesis* (Chaps. 68 and 69).

In many cancer syndromes, there is an inherited *predisposition* to tumor formation. In these instances, a germline mutation is inherited in an autosomal dominant fashion. This germline alteration affects one allele of an autosomal tumor suppressor gene. If the second allele is inactivated by a somatic mutation in a given cell, this will lead to neoplastic growth (two-hit model, or Knudson hypothesis). Thus, the defective allele in the germline is transmitted in a dominant pattern, though tumorigenesis results from a recessive loss of the tumor suppressor gene in an affected tissue. The classic example to illustrate this phenomenon is retinoblastoma, which can occur as a sporadic or hereditary tumor. In sporadic retinoblastoma, both copies of the retinoblastoma (*RB*) gene are inactivated through two somatic events. In hereditary retinoblastoma, one mutated or deleted *RB* allele is inherited in an autosomal dominant manner and the second allele is inactivated by a subsequent somatic mutation. This two-hit model applies to other inherited cancer syndromes such as MEN-1 (Chap. 330) and neurofibromatosis type 2 (Chap. 358).

Nucleotide Repeat Expansion Disorders Several diseases are associated with an increase in the number of nucleotide repeats above a certain threshold (Table 56-4). The repeats are sometimes located within the coding region of the genes, as in Huntington disease or the X-linked form of spinal and bulbar muscular atrophy (SBMA, Kennedy syndrome). In other instances, the repeats probably alter gene regulatory sequences. If an expansion is present, the DNA fragment is unstable and tends to expand further during cell division. The length of the nucleotide repeat often correlates with the severity of the disease. When repeat length increases from one generation to the next, disease manifestations may worsen or be observed at an earlier age; this phenomenon is referred to as *anticipation*. In Huntington disease, for example, there is a correlation between age of onset and length of the triplet codon expansion (Chap. 350). Anticipation has also been doc-

TABLE 56-7 *Genetic Approaches for Identifying Disease Genes*

Method	Indications and Advantages	Limitations
Linkage analysis	Analysis of monogenic traits Suitable for genome scan Control population not required Useful for multifactorial disorders in isolated populations	Difficult to collect large informative pedigrees Difficult to obtain sufficient statistical power for complex traits

Allele-sharing methods
  Affected sib and relative pair analyses
 	
  Sib pair analysis
	Suitable for identification of susceptibility genes in polygenic and multifactorial disorders
	Suitable for genome scan
	Control population not required if allele frequencies are known
	Statistical power can be increased by including parents and relatives
		Difficult to collect sufficient number of subjects
		Difficult to obtain sufficient statistical power for complex traits

Association studies
  Case-control studies
  Linkage disequilibrium
  Transmission distortion test
	Suitable for identification of susceptibility genes in polygenic and multifactorial disorders
	Suitable for testing specific allelic variants of known candidate loci
	Does not necessarily need relatives
		Requires large sample size and matched control population
		False-positive results in the absence of suitable control population

umented in other diseases caused by dynamic mutations in trinucleotide repeats (Table 56-4). The repeat number may also vary in a tissue-specific manner. In myotonic dystrophy, the CTG repeat may be tenfold greater in muscle tissue than in lymphocytes (Chap. 368).

POPULATION GENETICS AND ASSOCIATION STUDIES ■ Overview of Population Genetics In population genetics, the focus changes from alterations in an individual's genome to the distribution pattern of different genotypes of alleles in the population. In a case where there are only two alleles, A and a, the frequency of the genotypes will be $p^2 + 2pq + q^2 = 1$, with p^2 corresponding to the frequency of AA, $2pq$ to the frequency of Aa, and q^2 to aa. When the frequency of an allele is known, the frequency of the genotype can be calculated. Alternatively, one can determine an allele frequency, if the genotype frequency has been determined.

Allele frequencies vary among ethnic groups and geographical regions. For example, heterozygous mutations in the *CFTR* gene are relatively common in populations of European origin but are rare in the African population. Allele frequencies may vary because certain allelic variants confer a selective advantage. For example, heterozygotes for the sickle cell mutation, which is particularly common in West Africa, are more resistant to malarial infection because the erythrocytes of heterozygotes provide a less favorable environment for *Plasmodium* parasites. Though homozygosity for the sickle cell gene is associated with severe anemia and sickle crises (Chap. 91), heterozygotes have a higher probability of survival because of the reduced morbidity and mortality from malaria; this phenomenon has led to an increased frequency of the mutant allele. Recessive conditions are more prevalent in geographically isolated populations because of the more restricted gene pool.

Allelic Association and Linkage Disequilibrium There are two primary strategies for mapping genes that cause or increase susceptibility to human disease: (1) classic linkage can be performed based on a known genetic model (see above) or, when the model is unknown, by studying pairs of affected relatives; or (2) disease genes can be mapped using allelic association studies (Table 56-7). *Allelic association* refers to a situation in which the frequency of an allele is significantly increased or decreased in a particular disease. Linkage and association differ in several aspects. Genetic linkage is demonstrable in families or sibships. Association studies, on the other hand, compare a population of affected individuals with a control population. Association studies can be performed as case-control studies that include unrelated affected individuals and matched controls, or as family-based studies that compare the frequencies of alleles transmitted or not transmitted to affected children.

Allelic association studies are particularly useful for identifying susceptibility genes in complex diseases. When alleles at two loci occur more frequently in combination than would be predicted (based on known allele frequencies and recombination fractions), they are said to be in *linkage disequilibrium*. In Fig. 56-13, a mutation, Z, has occurred at a susceptibility locus where the normal allele is Y. The mutation is in close proximity to a genetic polymorphism with allele A or B. With time, the chromosomes carrying the A and Z alleles accumulate and represent 10% of the chromosomes in the population. The fact that the disease susceptibility gene, Z, is found preferentially, or exclusively, in association with the A allele illustrates linkage disequilibrium. Though not all chromosomes carrying the A allele carry the disease gene, the A allele is associated with an increased risk because of its possible association with the Z allele. This model implies that it may be possible in the future to identify Z directly to provide a more accurate prediction of disease susceptibility. Evidence for linkage disequilibrium can be helpful in mapping disease genes because it suggests that the two loci, in this case A and Z, are tightly linked.

POLYGENIC DISEASE AND COMPLEX GENETIC TRAITS ■ Approach to Polygenic and Multifactorial Disease The expression of many common diseases such as cardiovascular disease, hypertension, diabetes, asthma, psychiatric disorders, and certain cancers is determined by genetic background, environmental factors, and lifestyle (Table 56-8). A trait is called *polygenic* if multiple genes are thought to contribute to the phenotype or *multifactorial* if multiple genes are assumed to interact with environmental factors. Genetic models for complex traits need to account for genetic heterogeneity and interactions with other genes and the environment. Complex genetic traits may be influenced by modifying genes that are not linked to the main gene involved in the pathogenesis of the trait. This type of gene-gene interaction, or *epistasis*, plays an important role in polygenic traits that require the simultaneous presence of variations in multiple genes in order to result in a pathologic phenotype. Gene-environment interactions are relevant for many monogenic and polygenic disorders. In phenylketonuria, the phenotypic expression of the disease depends not only on the presence

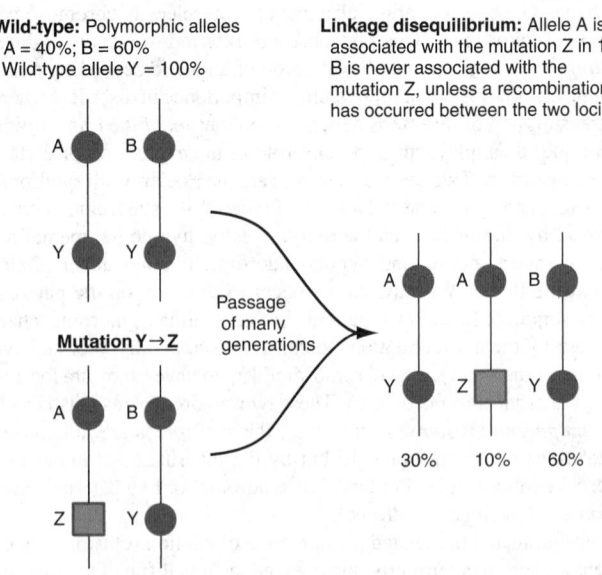

FIGURE 56-13 Linkage disequilibrium.

Disorder	Genes or Susceptibility Locus	Chromosomal Location	Other Factors
DIABETES MELLITUS			
Monogenic forms of diabetes			
MODY 1	HNF4α (hepatocyte nuclear factor 4α)	20q12-q13.1	
MODY 1	GCK (glucokinase)	7p15-p13	
MODY 1	HNF1α (hepatocyte nuclear factor 1α)	12q24.2	
MODY 1	IPF1 (insulin promoter factor 1)	13q12.1	
MODY 5 (Renal cysts, diabetes)	HNF1β (hepatocyte nuclear factor 1β)	17cen-q21.3	
MODY 6	NeuroD1 (neurogenic differention factor 1)	2q32	
Loci and genes associated with susceptibility	Genes and loci identified by linkage/association studies		Diet
for diabetes mellitus type 2	CPN10 (Calpain-10)	2q37.3	Energy expenditure
	1q, 3q, 8p, 12q, 20q	1q, 3q, 8p, 12q, 20q	Obesity
	"Candidate genes" with possible contribution		
	Peroxisome proliferator receptor gamma	3p25	
	Insulin	11p15	
	Sulfonylurea receptor	11p15.1	
	IPF1 (insulin promoter factor 1)	13q12.1	
	IRS-1 (insulin receptor substrate)	2q36	
	KCNJ11 (ATP-sensitive K channel Kir6.2)	11p15.1	
	AMP1 (adiponectin)	3q27	
	PGC-1	6p21.3-p21.1	
HYPERTENSION			
Monogenic forms			
Apparent mineralocorticoid excess	11-Ketoreductase		
Glucocorticoid-remediable HTN	CYP11B1 (unequal crossover with CYP11B2)		
Glucocorticoid-remediable HTN	CYP11B2 (unequal crossover with CYP11B1)		
17-alpha hydroxylase deficiency	17α hydroxylase		
Liddle's syndrome	SCNN1B		
Liddle's syndrome	SCNN1G		
Pseudohypoaldosteronism type II	WNK1		
Pseudohypoaldosteronism type II	WNK4		
Early onset HTN (AD)	MR		
Early onset HTN (AD)	BBS2		
Bardet-Biedl syndrome type 2	BBS4		
Loci and genes associated with susceptibility	Loci identified by linkage/association studies		Salt intake
for essential hypertension	1p, 2p, 2q, 3, 5p, 5q, 6p, 6q, 7q, 8q, 11q, 15q, 16q, 17, 18q, 19p, 22q, Xp		
	"Candidate genes" with possible contribution		
	Angiotensinogen	1q42-43	
	Angiotensin converting enzyme	17q23	
	Angiotensin receptor 1	3q21-25	
	G-protein subunit 3	12p13	

of the mutation in the phenylalanine hydroxylase gene but also on the exposure to the amino acid phenylalanine (Chap. 343). Type 2 diabetes mellitus provides a paradigm for considering a multifactorial disorder, as genetic, nutritional, and lifestyle factors are intimately interrelated in disease pathogenesis (Chap. 323). The identification of genetic variations and environmental factors that either predispose or protect against disease is essential for predicting disease risk, designing preventive strategies, and developing novel therapeutic approaches (Chap. 58). The study of rare monogenic diseases may provide insight into genetic and molecular mechanisms that are subsequently of importance for the understanding of complex diseases. For example, the identification of the insulin promoter factor 1 in maturity-onset of diabetes type 4 defined it as a *candidate gene* in the pathogenesis of diabetes mellitus type 2 (Tables 56-2 and 56-8). Genome scans have identified various loci that may be associated with susceptibility to development of diabetes mellitus in certain populations. Efforts to identify susceptibility genes require very large sample sizes, and positive results may depend on ethnicity, ascertainment criteria, and statistical analysis. Association studies analyzing the potential influence of (biologically functional) SNPs and SNP haplotypes on a particular phenotype are a promising approach for the detection of involved genes.

APPROACH TO THE PATIENT

Identifying the Disease-Causing Gene *Genomic medicine* aims to enhance the quality of medical care through the use of genotypic analysis (DNA testing) to identify genetic predisposition to disease, to select more specific pharmacotherapy, and to design individu-

alized medical care based on genotype. Genotype can be deduced by analysis of protein (e.g., hemoglobin, apoprotein E), mRNA, or DNA. However, technological advances have made DNA analysis particularly useful because it can be readily applied to all but the largest genes (Fig. 56-14).

DNA testing is performed by mutational analysis or linkage studies in individuals at risk for a genetic disorder known to be present in a family. Mass screening programs require tests of high sensitivity and specificity to be cost-effective. Prerequisites for the success of genetic screening programs include the following: that the disorder is potentially serious; that it can be influenced at a presymptomatic stage by changes in behavior, diet, and/or pharmaceutical manipulations; and that the screening does not result in any harm or discrimination. Screening in Jewish populations for the autosomal recessive neurodegenerative storage disease Tay-Sachs has reduced the number of affected individuals. In contrast, screening for sickle cell trait/disease in African Americans has led to unanticipated problems of discrimination by health insurers and employers. Mass screening programs harbor additional potential problems. For example, screening for the most common genetic alteration in cystic fibrosis, the ΔF508 mutation with a frequency of ~70% in northern Europe, is feasible and seems to be effective. One has to keep in mind, however, that there is pronounced allelic heterogeneity and that the disease can be caused by >600 other mutations. The search for these less common mutations would substantially increase costs but not the effectiveness of the screening program as a whole. Occupational screening programs aim to detect

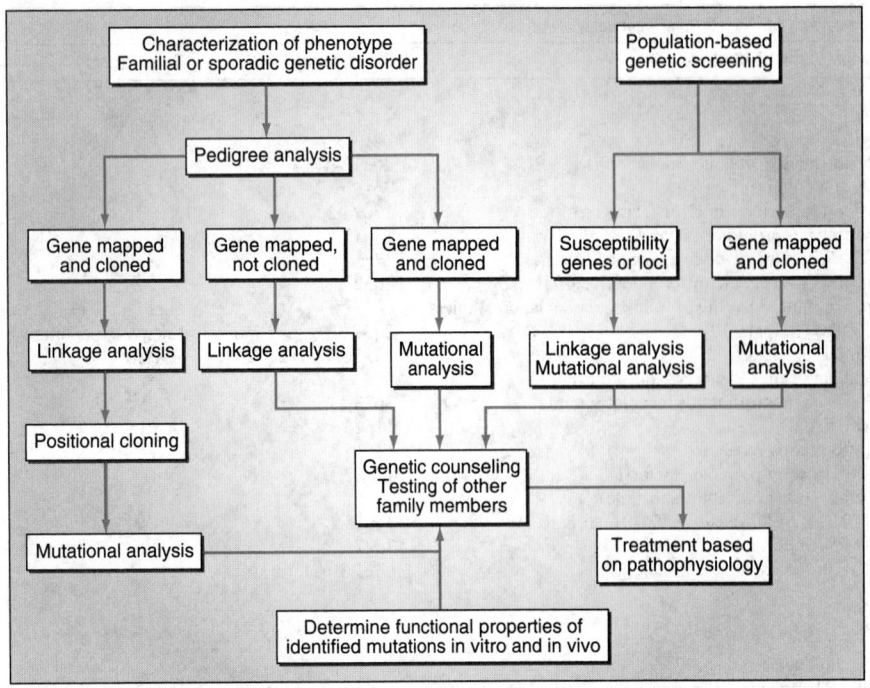

FIGURE 56-14 Approach to genetic disease.

individuals with increased risk for certain professional activities (e.g., α_1 antitrypsin deficiency and smoke or dust exposure).

MUTATIONAL ANALYSES DNA sequence analysis is increasingly used as a diagnostic tool and has significantly enhanced diagnostic accuracy. It is used for determining carrier status and for prenatal testing in monogenic disorders (Chap. 58). Numerous techniques are available for the detection of mutations (Table 56-9). In a very broad sense, one can distinguish between techniques that allow for screening the absence or presence of known mutations (screening mode) or techniques that definitively characterize mutations. Analyses of large alterations in the genome are possible using cytogenetics, fluorescent in situ hybridization (FISH), and Southern blotting (Chap. 57).

More discrete sequence alterations rely heavily on the use of the PCR, which allows rapid gene amplification and analysis. Moreover, PCR makes it possible to perform genetic testing and mutational analysis with small amounts of DNA extracted from leukocytes or even from single cells, buccal cells, or hair roots. Screening for point mutations can be performed by numerous methods (Table 56-9); most are based on the recognition of mismatches between nucleic acid duplexes, electrophoretic separation of single- or double-stranded DNA, or sequencing of DNA fragments amplified by PCR. DNA sequencing can be performed directly on PCR products or on fragments cloned into plasmid vectors amplified in bacterial host cells.

RT-PCR may be useful to detect absent or reduced levels of mRNA expression due to a mutated allele. Protein truncation tests (PTT) can be used to detect the broad array of mutations that result in premature termination of a polypeptide during its synthesis. The isolated cDNA is transcribed and translated in vitro, and the proteins are analyzed by gel electrophoresis. Comparison of electrophoretic mobility with the wild-type protein allows detection of truncated mutants.

The majority of traditional diagnostic methods are gel-based. Novel technologies for the analysis of mutations, genetic mapping, and mRNA expression profiles are in rapid development. DNA chip technologies allow hybridization of DNA or RNA to hundreds of thousands of probes simultaneously. Microarrays are being used clinically for mutational analysis of several human disease genes, as well as for the identification of viral sequence variations. Together with the knowledge gained from the HGP, these technologies provide the foundation to expand from a focus on single genes to analyses at the scale of the genome.

TABLE 56-9 *Methods Used for the Detection of Mutations*

Method	Principle	Type of Mutation Detected
COMMONLY USED TECHNIQUES		
Cytogenic analysis	Unique visual appearance of various chromosomes	Numerical or structural abnormalities in chromosomes
Fluorescent in situ hybridization (FISH)	Hybridization to chromosomes with fluorescently labeled probes	Numerical or structural abnormalities in chromosomes
Southern blot	Hybridization with genomic probe or cDNA probe after digestion of high molecular DNA	Large deletion, insertion, rearrangement, expansions of triplet repeat, amplification
Polymerase chain reaction (PCR)	Amplification of DNA segment	Expansion of triplet repeats, variable number of tandem repeats (VNTR), gene rearrangements, translocations; prepare DNA for other mutation methods
Reverse transcriptase PCR (RT-PCR)	Reverse transcription, amplification of DNA segment → absence or reduction of mRNA transcription	Analyze expressed mRNA (cDNA) sequence; detect loss of expression
DNA sequencing	Direct sequencing of PCR products Sequencing of DNA segments cloned into plasmid vectors	Point mutations, small deletions, and insertions
Restriction fragment polymorphism (RFLP)	Detection of altered restriction pattern of genomic DNA (Southern blot) or PCR products	Point mutations, small deletions, and insertions
OTHER TECHNIQUES		
Single-strand conformational polymorphism (SSCP)	PCR of DNA segment: Mutations result in conformational change and altered mobility	Point mutations, small deletions, and insertions
Denaturing gradient gel electrophoresis (DGGE)	PCR of DNA segment: Mutations result in conformational change and altered mobility	Point mutations, small deletions, and insertions
RNAse cleavage	Cleavage of mismatch between mutated and wild type sequence	Point mutations, small deletions, and insertions
Oligonucleotide specific hybridization (OSH)	Hybridization of PCR products to wild type or mutated oligonucleotides immobilized on chips or slides	Point mutations, small deletions, and insertions
Microarrays	Hybridization of PCR products to wild type or mutated oligonucleotides	Point mutations, small deletions, and insertions
Protein truncation test (PTT)	Transcription/translation of cDNA isolated from tissue sample	Mutations leading to premature truncations

A general algorithm for the approach to mutational analysis is outlined in Fig. 56-14. The importance of a detailed clinical phenotype cannot be overemphasized. This is the step where one should also consider the possibility of genetic heterogeneity and phenocopies. If obvious candidate genes are suggested by the phenotype, they can be analyzed directly. After identification of a mutation, it is essential to demonstrate that it segregates with the phenotype. The functional characterization of novel mutations is labor intensive and may require analyses in vitro or in transgenic models in order to document the relevance of the genetic alteration.

Prenatal diagnosis of numerous genetic diseases in instances with a high risk for certain disorders is now possible by direct DNA analysis. *Amniocentesis* involves the removal of a small amount of amniotic fluid, usually at 16 weeks of gestation. Cells can be collected and submitted for karyotype analyses, FISH, and mutational analysis of selected genes. The main indications for amniocentesis include advanced maternal age above age 35, abnormal serum triple marker test (α-fetoprotein, β human chorionic gonadotropin, pregnancy-associated plasma protein A, or unconjugated estriol), a family history of chromosomal abnormalities, or a Mendelian disorder amenable to genetic testing. Prenatal diagnosis can also be performed by *chorionic villus sampling* (CVS), in which a small amount of the chorion is removed by a transcervical or transabdominal biopsy. Chromosomes and DNA obtained from these cells can be submitted for cytogenetic and mutational analyses. CVS can be performed earlier in gestation (weeks 9 to 12) than amniocentesis, an aspect that may be of relevance when termination of pregnancy is a consideration. Later in pregnancy, beginning at about 18 weeks of gestation, percutaneous umbilical blood sampling (PUBS) permits collection of fetal blood for lymphocyte culture and analysis. In combination with in vitro fertilization (IVF) techniques, it is even possible to perform genetic diagnoses in a single cell removed from the four- to eight-cell embryo or to analyze the first polar body from an oocyte. Preconceptual diagnosis thereby avoids therapeutic abortions but is extremely costly and labor intensive. Lastly, it has to be emphasized that excluding a specific disorder by any of these approaches is never equivalent to the assurance of having a normal child.

Mutations in certain cancer susceptibility genes, such as *BRCA1* and *BRCA2*, may identify individuals with an increased risk for the development of malignancies and result in risk-reducing interventions. The detection of mutations is an important diagnostic and prognostic tool in leukemias and lymphomas. The demonstration of the presence or absence of mutations and polymorphisms is also relevant for the rapidly evolving field of pharmacogenomics, including the identification of differences in drug treatment response or metabolism as a function of genetic background. For example, the thiopurine drugs 6-mercaptopurine and azathioprine are commonly used cytotoxic and immunosuppressive agents. They are metabolized by thiopurine methyltransferase (TPMT), an enzyme with variable activity associated with genetic polymorphisms in 10% of Caucasians and complete deficiency in about 1/300 individuals. Patients with intermediate or deficient TPMT activity are at risk for excessive toxicity, including fatal myelosuppression. Characterization of these polymorphisms allows mercaptopurine doses to be modified based on TPMT genotype. Pharmacogenomics may increasingly permit individualized drug therapy, improve drug effectiveness, reduce adverse side effects, and provide cost-effective pharmaceutical care.

FURTHER READING

BROWN PO, BOTSTEIN D: Exploring the new world of the genome with DNA microarrays. Nat Genet (Suppl) 21:33, 1999

COLLINS FS, MCKUSICK V: Implications of the Human Genome Project for medical science. JAMA 285:540, 2001

COTTON RGH, KAZAZIAN HH JR: The HUGO mutation database initiative: Issues, databases, and perspectives for the new millenium. Hum Mutat 15: 1, 2000

Instructions for the use of genome-related databases. Nat Genet 32 (Suppl):1, 2002

ROSES AD: Pharmacogenomics and the practice of medicine. Nature 405:857, 2000

57 | CHROMOSOME DISORDERS
Terry Hassold, Stuart Schwartz

In humans, the normal diploid number of chromosomes is 46, consisting of 22 pairs of autosomal chromosomes (numbered 1 to 22 in decreasing size) and one pair of sex chromosomes (XX in females and XY in males). The genome is estimated to contain between 30,000 and 40,000 genes. Even the smallest autosome contains between 200 and 300 genes. Not surprisingly, duplications or deletions of chromosomes, or even small chromosome segments, have profound consequences on normal gene expression, leading to severe developmental and physiologic abnormalities.

Deviations in number or structure of the 46 human chromosomes are astonishingly common, despite severe deleterious consequences. Chromosomal disorders occur in an estimated 10 to 25% of all pregnancies. They are the leading cause of fetal loss and, among pregnancies surviving to term, the leading known cause of birth defects and mental retardation.

In recent years, the practice of cytogenetics has shifted from conventional cytogenetic methodology to a union of cytogenetic and molecular techniques. Formerly the province of research laboratories, fluorescence in situ hybridization (FISH) and related molecular cytogenetic technologies have been incorporated into everyday practice in clinical laboratories. As a result, there is an increased appreciation of the importance of "subtle" constitutional cytogenetic abnormalities,

such as microdeletions and imprinting disorders, as well as previously recognized translocations and disorders of chromosome number.

VISUALIZING CHROMOSOMES

CONVENTIONAL CYTOGENETIC ANALYSIS In theory, chromosome preparations can be obtained from any actively dividing tissue by causing the cells to arrest in metaphase, the stage of the cell cycle when chromosomes are maximally condensed. In practice, only a small number of tissues are used for routine chromosome analysis: amniocytes or chorionic villi for prenatal testing, and blood, bone marrow, or skin fibroblasts for postnatal studies. Samples of blood, bone marrow, and chorionic villi can be processed using short-term culture techniques that yield results in 1 to 3 days. Analysis of other tissue types typically involves long-term cell culture, requiring 1 to 3 weeks of processing before cytogenetic analysis is possible.

Cells are isolated at metaphase or prometaphase, and treated chemically or enzymatically to reveal chromosome "bands" (Fig. 57-1). Analysis of the number of chromosomes in the cell, and the distribution of bands on individual chromosomes, allows the identification of numerical or structural abnormalities. This strategy is useful for characterizing the normal chromosome complement and determining the incidence and types of major chromosome abnormalities.

Each human chromosome contains two specialized structures: a centromere and two telomeres. The centromere, or primary constriction, divides the chromosome into short (p) and long (q) arms and is responsible for the segregation of chromosomes during cell division.

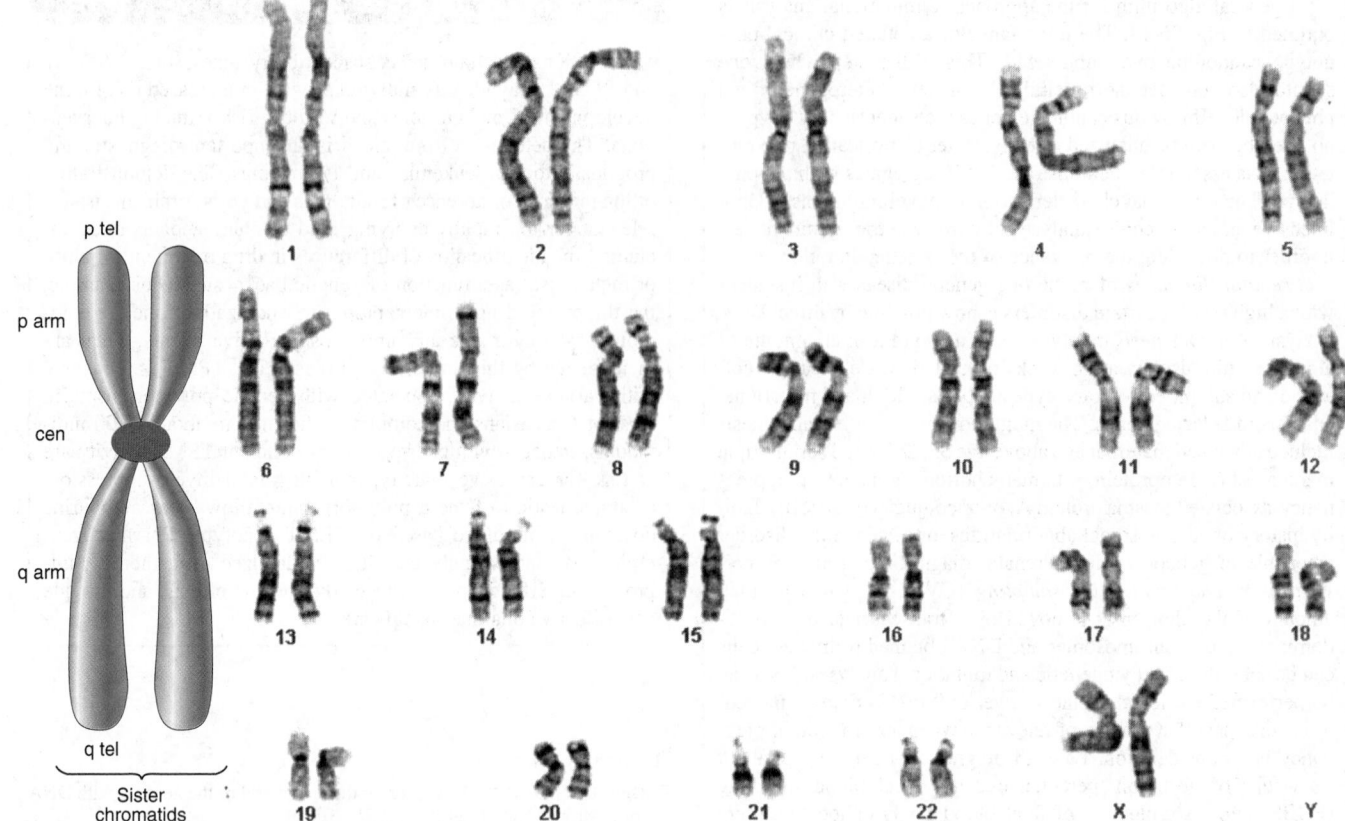

FIGURE 57-1 *A.* An idealized human chromosome, showing the centromere (cen), long (q) and short (p) arms, and telomeres (tel). *B.* A G-banded human karyotype from a normal (46,XX) female.

The telomeres, or chromosome ends, "cap" the p and q arms and are important for allowing DNA replication at the ends of the chromosomes. Prior to DNA replication, each chromosome consists of a single chromatid copy of the DNA double helix. After DNA replication and continuing until the time of cell division (including metaphase, when chromosomes are typically visualized), each chromosome consists of two identical sister chromatids (Fig. 57-1).

MOLECULAR CYTOGENETICS The introduction of FISH methodologies in the late 1980s revolutionized the field of cytogenetics. In principle, FISH is similar to other DNA-DNA hybridization methodologies. The probe is labeled with a hapten, such as biotin or digoxigenin, to allow detection with a fluorophore (e.g., FITC or rhodamine). After the hybridization step, the specimen is counter-stained and the preparations are visualized with a fluorescence microscope.

Types of FISH Probes A variety of probes are available for use with FISH, including chromosome-specific paints (chromosome libraries), repetitive probes, and single-copy probes (Fig. 57-2). Chromosome libraries hybridize to sequences that span the entirety of the chromosome from which they are derived and, as a result, they can be used to "paint" individual chromosomes.

Repetitive probes recognize amplified DNA sequences present in chromosomes. The most common are α-satellite DNA probes that are complementary to DNA sequences found at the centromeric regions of all human chromosomes. A vast number of *single-copy probes* are now available as a result of the human genome project. These probes can be as small as 1 kb, though normally they are much larger and are packaged into cosmids (40 kb), bacterial artificial chromosomes (BACs) or P1 clones (100 to 200 kb), or yeast artificial chromosomes (YACs) (1 to 2 Mb). Many are available commercially, including probes for a variety of microdeletion syndromes and for subtelomeric regions of individual chromosomes.

Applications of FISH The majority of FISH applications involve hybridization of one or two probes of interest as an adjunctive procedure

to conventional chromosomal banding techniques. In this regard, FISH can be utilized to identify specific chromosomes, characterize de novo duplications or deletions, and clarify subtle chromosomal rearrangements. Its greatest utilization, however, is in the detection of microdeletions (see below). Though conventional cytogenetic studies can detect some microdeletions, initial detection and/or confirmation with FISH is essential. In fact, since appropriate FISH probes have become available, detection of microdeletion syndromes has increased significantly.

In addition to metaphase FISH, cells can be analyzed at a variety of stages. Interphase analysis, for example, can be used to make a rapid diagnosis in instances when metaphase chromosome preparations are not yet available (e.g., amniotic fluid interphase analysis). Interphase analysis also increases the number of cells available for examination, allows for investigation of nuclear organization, and provides results when cells do not progress to metaphase. One specialized type of interphase analysis involves the application of FISH to paraffin-embedded sections, thereby preserving the architecture of the tissue.

The use of interphase FISH has increased recently, especially for analyses of amniocentesis samples. These studies are performed on uncultured amniotic fluid, typically using DNA probes specific for the chromosomes most commonly identified in trisomies (chromosomes 13, 18, 21, and the X and Y). These studies can be performed rapidly (24 to 72 h) and will ascertain about 60% of the abnormalities detected prenatally. Another area in which interphase analysis is routinely utilized is cancer cytogenetics (Chap. 68). Many site-specific translocations are associated with specific types of malignancies. For example, there are probes available for both the Abelson (Abl) oncogene and breakpoint cluster region (bcr) involved in chronic myelogenous leukemia (CML); these probes are labeled in red and green, respectively; the fusion of these genes in CML combines the fluorescent colors and appears as a yellow hybridization signal.

In addition to standard metaphase and interphase FISH analyses, a number of enhanced techniques have been developed for specific types of analysis, including multicolor FISH techniques, reverse painting, comparative genomic hybridization, and fiber FISH. *Spectral karyotyping* (SKY) and multicolor FISH (m-FISH) techniques use combinatorially labeled probes that create a unique color for individual chromosomes. This technology is useful in the identification of unknown chromosome material (such as markers of duplications) but is most commonly used with the complex rearrangements seen in cancer specimens.

Comparative genomic hybridization (CGH) is a method that can be used only when DNA is available from a specimen of interest. The entire DNA specimen from the sample of interest is labeled in one color (e.g., green), and the normal control DNA specimen is indicated by another color (e.g., red). These are mixed in equal amounts and hybridized to normal metaphase chromosomes. The red-to-green ratio is analyzed by a computer program, which determines where the DNA of interest may have gains or losses of material. This technique is useful in the analysis of tumors, particularly in those cases where cytogenetic analysis is not possible.

Fiber FISH is a technique in which chromosomes are mechanically stretched, using one of a variety of different methods. It provides a higher resolution of analysis than conventional FISH.

INDICATIONS FOR CYTOGENETIC ANALYSIS

Primary indications for karyotypic analysis vary according to the developmental stage/age of the conceptus/individual under investigation. One especially important application is in prenatal diagnosis (particularly for pregnancies involving older women), assaying for chromosomal abnormalities in either chorionic villi of first-trimester fetuses or amniotic fluid of second-trimester fetuses. Tissue specimens from spontaneously aborted fetuses or stillbirths can also be examined for chromosome abnormalities. Interphase cytogenetics (using FISH) is increasingly being used to study individual blastomeres of preimplantation embryos (with in vitro fertilization-derived pregnancies). This makes it possible to detect aneuploid or structurally unbalanced embryos or, in the case of sex-linked disorders, to identify male conceptuses; such embryos would not be used to initiate pregnancies.

Among infants and children, peripheral blood is examined, most often in individuals with specific phenotypic abnormalities. For example, karotypic analysis can be used for the confirmation or exclusion of a specific chromosomal syndrome (e.g., trisomy 21); in patients with unexplained psychomotor retardation with or without dysmorphic features; in cases of monogenic disorders associated with mental retardation and/or dysmorphic features; and with abnormalities of sexual differentiation and development.

In adults, peripheral blood can be examined in patients with infertility or recurrent miscarriages, since chromosome abnormalities can lead to meiotic arrest or to genetically unbalanced gametes. An important branch of cytogenetics is concerned with analyses of bone marrow, unstimulated peripheral blood, and lymph nodes of tumors, as chromosomal abnormalities are a common correlate of leukemia, lymphoma, and solid tumors (Chap. 68).

CYTOGENETIC TESTING IN PRENATAL DIAGNOSIS The vast majority of prenatal diagnostic studies are performed to rule out a chromosomal ab-

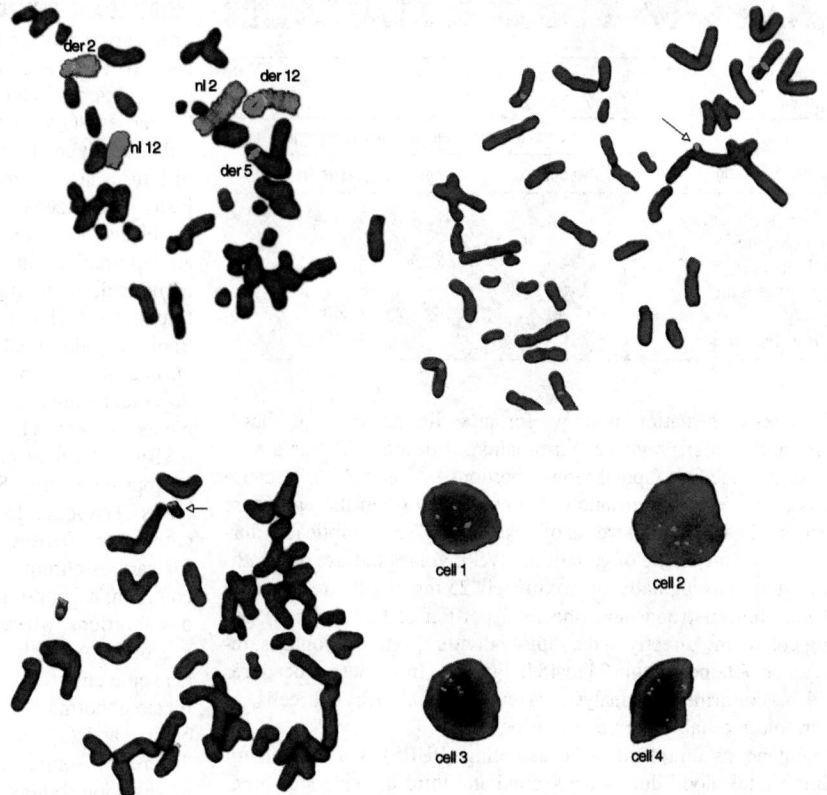

FIGURE 57-2 Examples of different applications of fluorescence in situ hybridization (FISH) to human metaphase and interphase preparations. Top left, chromosome-specific "paint" probes demonstrating hybridization to normal chromosomes 2 (red) and 12 (green), as well as indicating a translocation between the short arm of chromosome 12 and the long arm of chromosome 2. This hybridization also demonstrates that some of the short arm of chromosome 12 has been inserted into the short arm of chromosome 5. Top right, a repetitive DNA probe specific for centromeric α-satellite sequences on chromosome 7 (red) and chromosome 10 (green) hybridizes to the centromeric region of the appropriate chromosomes, as well as to a marker chromosome derived from chromosome 10. Bottom left, two-color FISH used to detect a microdeletion of chromosome 22 associated with velocardiofacial (VCF) syndrome. A probe for ARSA (a locus on the distal portion of chromosome 22, visualized as a green signal) is observed on both chromosomes. However, a probe for TUPLE1 (a locus within the VCF region of chromosome 22, visualized in red) hybridizes only to the normal chromosome. The arrow points to the deleted chromosome. Bottom right, interphase FISH using chromosome 13 (green) and chromosome 21 (red) unique sequence probes on interphase cells from direct amniotic fluid preparations. In each of the four interphase cells, three chromosome 21 signals are observed, indicating the presence of trisomy 21 in the fetus.

normality, but cells may also be propagated for biochemical studies or molecular analyses of DNA. Three procedures are used to obtain samples for prenatal diagnosis: amniocentesis, chorionic villus sampling (CVS), and fetal blood sampling. Amniocentesis is the most common procedure and is routinely performed at 15 to 17 weeks of gestation. On some occasions, early amniocentesis at 12 to 14 weeks is performed to expedite results, although less fluid is obtained at this time. Early amniocentesis carries a greater risk of spontaneous abortion or fetal injury but provides results at an earlier stage of pregnancy.

The vast majority of amniocenteses are performed in the context of advanced maternal age, the best-known correlate of trisomy (see below). Additional reasons for amniocentesis referral include an abnormal "triple- or quad-marker assay" and/or detection of ultrasound abnormalities. In this assay, levels of human chorionic gonadotropin, α-fetoprotein, and unconjugated estriol (and, in the quad assay, inhibin) in the maternal serum are quantified and used to adjust the maternal age-predicted risk of a trisomy 21 or trisomy 18 fetus. Specific ultrasound abnormalities, when detected at midtrimester, can also be associated with chromosomal defects. When a nonspecific ultrasound abnormality is present, the estimated risk of a chromosomal defect is approximately 16%. Associations of chromosomal abnormalities and specific types of abnormal ultrasound findings are listed in Table 57-1.

CVS is the second most common procedure for genetic prenatal diagnosis. Because this procedure is routinely performed at about 10

TABLE 57-1 *Frequency of Chromosome Abnormalities, Identified on the Basis of Abnormal Ultrasound Findings*

Ultrasound Finding	Chromosomal Abnormalities (Frequency)	
	Average, %	Range in Different Studies, %
Abnormal ultrasound (nonspecific)	16	13–35
Omphalocele	39	26–54
Cystic hygroma	68	46–78
Congenital heart disease	30	8–40
Choroid plexus cyst	5	4–10

to 12 weeks of gestation, it allows for an earlier detection of abnormalities and a safer pregnancy termination, if desired. CVS is a relatively safe procedure (spontaneous abortions, <0.5 to 1%). Because there is an increased association of limb defects when the procedure is performed earlier (<10 weeks of gestation), CVS is applicable during a narrow time frame of gestation. CVS involves the use of a catheter inserted transvaginally; approximately 25 mg of villi are aspirated from the chorion frondosum (the fetal portion of the placenta). By adding colchicine directly to the rapidly dividing cytotrophoblasts, results can be obtained within 24 to 48 h. Findings from these procedures should be confirmed by analyses of cultured mesenchymal cells, as they are more reliably derived from the fetus.

Percutaneous umbilical blood sampling (PUBS) is a method for obtaining fetal blood during the second and third trimesters of pregnancy. PUBS is usually performed when ultrasound abnormalities are detected late in the second trimester. PUBS is also used when cytogenetic results from amniocentesis need clarification, such as in the detection of mosaicism.

CHROMOSOME ABNORMALITIES

CHROMOSOMES IN CELL DIVISION To understand the etiology of chromosome abnormalities, it is important to review the movement of chromosomes during cell division. In somatic tissues, chromosomes are replicated during the S-phase of the cell cycle, so that each replicated chromosome consists of two identical sister chromatids. When the cell enters mitosis, each of the 46 chromosomes align on the metaphase plate, with the centomeres co-oriented toward opposite spindle poles (Fig. 57-3). At anaphase the sister chromatids separate, with each of the daughter cells receiving one sister chromatid from each of the 46 chromosomes.

Chromosome segregation is more complicated in germ cell division, since the number of chromosomes must be reduced from 46 to 23 in the mature sperm and eggs. This is accomplished by two rounds of division—meiosis I and meiosis II (Fig. 57-3). In meiosis I, homologous chromosomes pair and exchange genetic material, then align on the metaphase plate, and finally separate from one another. Thus, by the end of meiosis I, only 23 of the original 46 chromosomes are represented in each of the two daughter cells. Meiosis II quickly follows meiosis I and is essentially a "haploid mitosis," involving separation of the sister chromatids in each of the 23 chromosomes.

Although the fundamentals of meiosis are the same in males and females, there are important distinctions, particularly in the timing of meiotic divisions. In males, meiosis begins with puberty and continues throughout the individual's lifetime. In females, meiosis begins prenatally, with oocytes proceeding through the first stages of meiosis I but arresting at mid-prophase. At the time of birth, the first meiotic division is suspended in oocytes. Only after ovulation many years later do oocytes complete meiosis I and proceed to the metaphase stage of meiosis II; if fertilized, the oocyte then completes the second meiotic division. Thus, in females, the first meiotic division takes at least 10 to 15 years and as many as 40 to 45 years to complete. Maternal age-related increases in the incidence of trisomy are likely the consequence of this protracted process of cell division.

INCIDENCE AND TYPES OF CHROMOSOME ABNORMALITIES Errors in meiosis, or in early cleavage divisions, occur with extraordinary frequency. At least 10 to 25% of all pregnancies, for example, involve chromosomally abnormal conceptions. A large proportion of these terminate in the earliest stages of pregnancy, many of which go unrecognized. Nevertheless, even among clinically recognized pregnancies, nearly 10% of fetuses are chromosomally unbalanced. For the three types of clinically recognized pregnancies—spontaneous abortions, stillbirths, and livebirths—the frequencies of different chromosomal abnormalities are summarized in Table 57-2. The most common abnormalities are numerical, involving fetuses with additional (trisomy) or missing (monosomy) chromosomes, or those with one (triploidy) or two (tetraploidy) additional sets of chromosomes. Structural chromosome abnormalities are much less common, although several of the most important clinical chromosomal disorders involve structural rearrangements (see below).

By far the most common abnormality is trisomy, which is identified in approximately 25% of spontaneous abortions and 0.3% of newborns. Trisomies for all chromosomes have now been identified in embryos or fetuses, but there is considerable variation in frequency for various chromosomes. For example, trisomy 16 is extraordinarily common, accounting for about one-third of all trisomies in spontaneous abortions, whereas trisomies 1, 5, 11, and 19 have been identified less often. Available evidence suggests two reasons for this variation: (1) some chromosomes (e.g., chromosome 16) are more likely to segregate abnormally or undergo nondisjunction during meiosis than are others; and (2) the potential for development varies widely among different trisomic conditions, with some being eliminated very early in gestation, others surviving to the time of clinical pregnancy recognition, and some (e.g., trisomies 13, 18, and 21 and sex chromosome trisomies) being compatible with survival to term.

CHROMOSOMAL SYNDROMES

While most chromosomally abnormal conceptions perish in utero, several conditions are compatible with survival to term. The best-char-

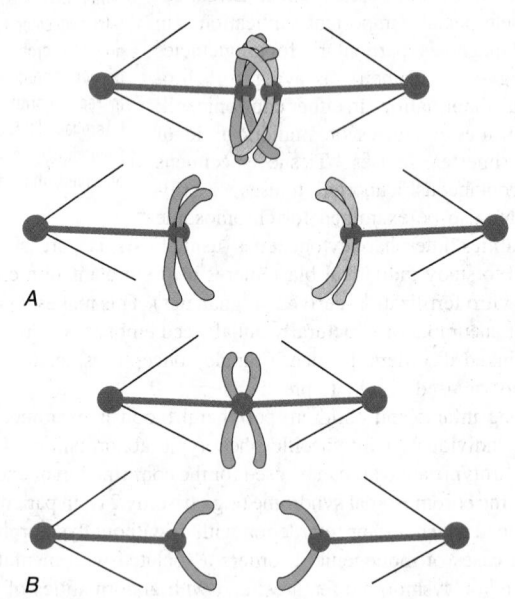

FIGURE 57-3 Chromosome segregation in meiosis. *A.* In meiosis I, each of the 23 pairs of chromosomes finds its "partner," or homologue, and exchanges genetic material (recombines) with it. At metaphase, each homologous pair aligns on the equatorial plate; at anaphase, each member of the homologous pair segregates from its partner. Thus, at the end of meiosis I, each daughter cell contains 23 chromosomes, with each chromosome consisting of two sister chromatids. *B.* In meiosis II, each chromosome aligns on the metaphase plate, and at anaphase, each of the two sister chromatids divide from one another. Thus, at the end of meiosis II, each daughter cell (e.g., the oocyte or spermatocyte) contains 23 chromosomes, with each chromosome consisting of one sister chromatid. In mitosis, the chromosomes behave exactly as they do in meiosis II, except that somatically dividing cells contain 46 chromosomes, not the 23 that are present in the meiosis II cell.

acterized of these are numerical abnormalities involving loss or gain of individual chromosomes, and abnormalities resulting from unbalanced translocations. FISH and other molecular studies have led to the identification of two "new" types of chromosome abnormalities, commonly referred to as microdeletion syndromes and imprinting syndromes.

NUMERICAL ABNORMALITIES Virtually all types of numerical abnormalities are eliminated prenatally, so that only those involving small, gene-poor autosomes or the sex chromosomes are identified with any frequency among liveborns. Clinically, the most important of these is trisomy 21, the most frequent cause of Down syndrome. Depending on the maternal age structure of the population and the utilization of prenatal testing, the incidence of trisomy 21 ranges from 1/600 to 1/1000 live births, making it the most common chromosome abnormality in live-born individuals. Like most trisomies, the incidence of trisomy 21 is highly correlated with maternal age, increasing from about 1/1500 live births for women 20 years of age to 1/30 for women 45 years of age and older.

In addition to trisomy 21, only two other autosomal trisomies, 13 and 18, occur with any frequency in livebirths. Incidence rates for trisomies 13 and 18 in livebirths are 1/20,000 and 1/10,000, respectively. Unlike trisomy 21, which is associated with near-normal life expectancy, both trisomies 13 and 18 are associated with death in infancy, typically occurring during the first year of life.

Three sex chromosome trisomies—the 47,XXX, 47,XXY (Klinefelter syndrome), and 47,XYY conditions—are quite common, with each occurring in about 1/2000 newborns. Of all the trisomic conditions, these three have the fewest phenotypic complications. In fact, with the exception of infertility in Klinefelter syndrome (Chap. 328), it is likely that most individuals with such trisomic conditions would go undetected. The additional Y chromosome in the 47,XYY condition is small and contains only a few genes. Most Y-linked genes are involved in testicular development or spermatogenesis. Thus, dosage imbalance of Y-linked genes has relatively little effect on other developmental processes. The 47,XYY genotype is associated with increased height. Its role in antisocial behavior, postulated initially because of an increased prevalence among some penalized populations, is unclear.

For the 47,XXX and 47,XXY conditions, the situation is different—the X chromosome contains over 1000 genes, many of them essential for normal development. How, then, are 47,XXX and 47,XXY individuals spared from the catastrophic consequences of dosage imbalance? The answer lies in the biology of X chromosome gene expression. In normal females, one of the chromosomes undergoes *X inactivation* in somatic cells. The inactivation of the paternal or maternal X chromosome occurs randomly in each somatic cell and thereby serves as a mechanism of dosage compensation, ensuring that males and females have equal expression of most X-linked genes. The inactivation process occurs at the blastocyst stage of development; prior to this, both X chromosomes are active. In addition, not all X-linked genes are inactivated. Some genes on the X chromosome "escape" the inactivating mechanism and are expressed from both X chromosomes. In disorders such as Klinefelter syndrome, some genes may be expressed from both X chromosomes, resulting in its phenotypic features.

As a rule, monosomic conditions are incompatible with fetal development and, consequently, autosomal monosomies are only rarely identified in spontaneous abortions and are not found among live-born individuals. In fact, the only monosomy compatible with live birth is the 45,X condition, which causes Turner syndrome. The 45,X chromosome constitution occurs with surprisingly high frequency, present in at least 1 to 2% of all pregnancies. More than 99% of all 45,X conceptions are spontaneously aborted. Thus, live-born individuals with a 45,X chromosome constitution represent a rare group of survivors. The 45,X phenotype is mild, presumably because the second copy of many X chromosomal genes is normally inactivated. Nonetheless, Turner syndrome causes gonadal dysgenesis, resulting in infertility and failure to undergo secondary sexual development, along with a number of other phenotypic features (Chap. 328). Several other structural abnormalities of the X chromosome such as deletions, isochromosome X, or ring chromosomes can cause Turner syndrome. Mosaicism, including 45,X/45,XX, 45X/45,XXX, 45,X/45,XY, and others, also occurs (see below) and contributes to the phenotypic spectrum in Turner syndrome.

Because numerical abnormalities originate in meiosis (Table 57-3), affected individuals have missing or extra chromosomes in all cells. In a small proportion of cases, a mitotic nondisjunctional event occurs at an early stage in an individual with an initially normal chromosome constitution. Alternatively, a "normalizing" mitotic nondisjunctional event may result in a normal chromosome complement in some cells of an embryo. In either case, the embryo is a mosaic, with some cells bearing a normal chromosome constitution and others an aneuploid number of chromosomes. The phenotypic consequences are difficult to predict because they depend on the timing of nondisjunction and the distribution of normal and abnormal cells in different tissues. Nevertheless, mosaicism may lead to clinical abnormalities indistinguishable from those of nonmosaic individuals; for example, nearly 5% of all cases of Down syndrome involve individuals with mosaic trisomy 21, and about 15% of individuals with Turner syndrome are mosaic for various sex chromosomal constitutions as described above.

The Origin and Etiology of Numerical Abnormalities Over the past decade, a number of studies have used DNA polymorphisms to investigate the

TABLE 57-2 Frequency and Distribution of Chromosome Abnormalities in Different Types of Clinically Recognizable Pregnancies

Chromosome Abnormality	Frequency of Abnormality			Probability of Surviving to Term, %
	Spontaneous Abortion	Stillbirth	Livebirth	
Trisomy, all	25.1	4.0	0.3	5
+13, 18, 21	4.5	2.7	0.14	15
+16	7.5	—	—	0
Sex chromosome monosomy (45,X)	8.7	0.1	0.01	1
Triploidy	6.4	0.2	—	0
Tetraploidy	2.4	—	—	0
Structural abnormality	2.0	0.8	0.3	45
Total abnormalities	50.0	5.1	0.6	5

TABLE 57-3 Studies of the Parent and Meiotic/Mitotic Stage of Origin of Human Trisomies and Sex Chromosome Monosomy

	Origin, %				
	Paternal		Maternal		
	I	II	I	II	Mitotic
TRISOMY					
2	28	—	54	13	6
7	—	—	17	26	57
15	—	15	76	9	—
16	—	1	96	3	—
18	—	—	33	56	11
21	3	5	67	22	2
22	3	—	94	3	—
XXY	46	—	38	14	3
XXX	—	6	60	16	18
MONOSOMY					
X[a]	80		20		

[a] Results pertain to nonmosaic 45,X individuals.

origin of different types of chromosome abnormalities (Fig. 57-4). The most thoroughly investigated types have been numerical abnormalities (Table 57-3). Sex chromosome monosomy usually results from loss of the paternal sex chromosome, regardless of whether the conception is live-born or spontaneously aborted.

Trisomies show remarkable variation in parental origin. For example, paternal nondisjunction is responsible for nearly 50% of 47,XXY but only 5 to 10% of cases of trisomies 13, 14, 15, 21, and 22; it is rarely, if ever, the source of the additional chromosome in trisomy 16. Similarly, there is considerable variability in the meiotic stage of origin. For example, all cases of trisomy 16 may be due to meiosis I errors, whereas for trisomy 21, one-third of cases are associated with meiosis II errors, and for trisomy 18, the majority of cases are apparently due to meiosis II nondisjunction. In spite of this variation in parental and meiotic origin, nondisjunction at maternal meiosis I appears to be the most common source of trisomy.

Maternal Age and Trisomy   The association between increasing maternal age and trisomy is the most important etiologic factor in congenital chromosomal disorders. Among women under the age of 25, approximately 2% of all clinically recognized pregnancies are trisomic; by the age of 36, however, this figure increases to 10% and by the age of 42, to over 33% (Fig. 57-5). This association between maternal age and trisomy is exerted without respect to race, geography, or socioeconomic factors and likely affects segregation of all chromosomes.

Despite the importance of increasing age, little is known about the mechanism by which aging leads to abnormal chromosomal segregation. As noted above, it is thought to originate in maternal meiosis I

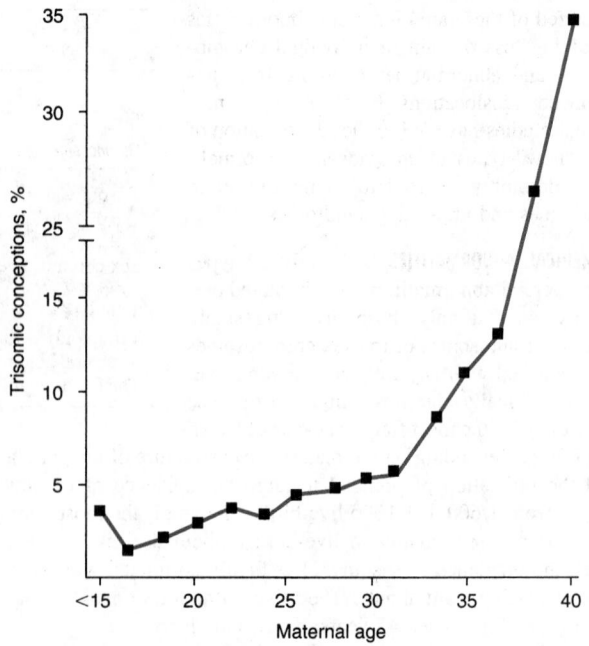

FIGURE 57-5   Estimated maternal age-adjusted rates of trisomy among all clinically recognized pregnancies (e.g., spontaneous abortions, stillbirths, and livebirths). Among women in their forties, over 25% of all pregnancies are estimated to involve a trisomic conception; the vast majority of these spontaneously abort, with only trisomies 13, 18, and 21 and sex chromosome trisomies surviving to term with any appreciable frequency.

owing to the protracted time to completion (often ≥40 years) in females, and recent studies suggest that it may be associated with alterations in meiotic crossing-over. In trisomy 21, for example, crossover patterns appear to be similarly abnormal in younger and older mothers of trisomic conceptions. Thus, it has been suggested that two distinct steps, or "hits," may be involved in maternal age-related nondisjunction. The first hit, which is age independent, involves the establishment of a "vulnerable" crossover configuration in the fetal oocyte; the second hit, which is age dependent, involves abnormal processing of the vulnerable bivalent structure at metaphase I. If this model is correct, it suggests that the nondisjunctional process is the same in younger and older women, but it occurs more frequently with aging, possibly because of age-dependent degradation of meiotic proteins.

STRUCTURAL CHROMOSOME ABNORMALITIES   Structural rearrangements involve breakage and reunion of chromosomes. Although less common than numerical abnormalities, they present additional challenges from a genetic counseling standpoint. This is because structural abnormalities, unlike numerical abnormalities, can be present in "balanced" form in clinically normal individuals but transmitted in "unbalanced" form to progeny, thereby resulting in a hereditary form of chromosome abnormality.

Rearrangements may involve exchanges of material between different chromosomes (translocations) or loss, gain, or rearrangements of individual chromosomes (e.g., deletions, duplications, inversions, rings, or isochromosomes). Of particular clinical importance are *translocations*, which involve two basic types: Robertsonian and reciprocal. Robertsonian rearrangements are a special class of translocation, in which the long arms of two acrocentric chromosomes (chromosomes 13, 14, 15, 21, and 22) join together, generating a fusion chromosome that contains virtually all of the genetic material of the original two chromosomes. If the Robertsonian translocation is present in unbalanced form, a monosomic or trisomic conception ensues. For example, approximately 3% of Down syndrome cases are attributable to unbalanced Robertsonian translocations, most often involving chromosomes 14 and 21. In this instance, the affected individual has 46 chromosomes, including one structurally normal chromosome 14, two structurally normal chromosomes 21, and one fusion 14/21 chromosome. This effect leads to a normal diploid dosage for chromosome 14 and to

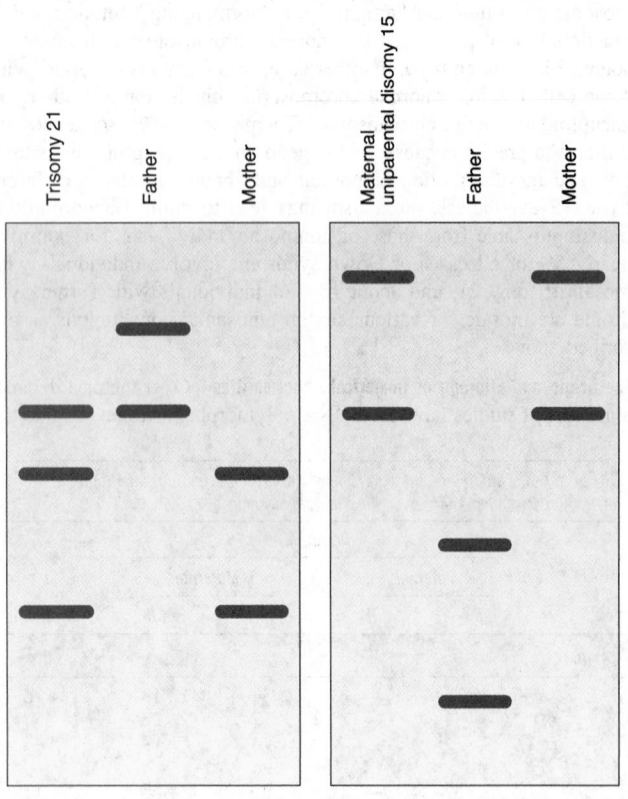

A. Parental origin of trisomy 21   B. Parental origin of PWS

FIGURE 57-4   Use of DNA technology to determine the origin of chromosome abnormalities. A. Analysis of a chromosome 21–specific DNA polymorphism demonstrates that the trisomic individual received two chromosomes 21 from his mother and one from his father; thus, the extra chromosome 21 resulted from an error in oogenesis. B. Inheritance of a chromosome 15–specific DNA polymorphism in an individual with Prader-Willi syndrome (PWS). The affected individual has received two maternal, but no paternal, chromosomes 15; thus, the individual is said to have maternal uniparental disomy 15, a common cause of PWS.

a triplication of chromosome 21, thus resulting in Down syndrome. Similarly, a small proportion of individuals with trisomy 13 syndrome are clinically affected because of an unbalanced Robertsonian translocation.

Reciprocal translocations involve mutual exchanges between any two chromosomes. In this circumstance, the phenotypic consequences associated with unbalanced translocations depend on the location of the breakpoints, which dictate the amount of material that has been "exchanged" between the two chromosomes. Because most reciprocal translocations involve unique sets of breakpoints, it is difficult to predict the phenotypic consequences in any one situation. In general, severity is determined by the amount of excess or missing chromosome material in individuals with unbalanced translocations.

In addition to rearrangements between chromosomes, there are several examples of intrachromosome structural abnormalities. The most common and deleterious of these involve loss of chromosome material due to deletions. The two best-characterized deletion syndromes, Wolf-Hirschhorn syndrome and cri-du-chat syndrome, result from loss of relatively small chromosomal segments on chromosomes 4p and 5p, respectively. Nonetheless, each is associated with multiple congenital anomalies, developmental delays, profound retardation, and reduced lifespan.

Microdeletion Syndromes The term *contiguous gene syndrome* refers to genetic disorders that mimic a combination of single gene disorders. They result from the deletion of a small number of tightly clustered genes. Because some are too small to be detected cytogenetically, they are termed microdeletions. The application of molecular techniques has led to the identification of at least 18 of these microdeletion syndromes (Table 57-4). Some of the more common ones include the Wilms' tumor–aniridia complex (WAGR), Miller Dieker syndrome (MDS), and velocardiofacial (VCF) syndrome. WAGR is characterized by mental retardation and involvement of multiple organs, including kidney (Wilm's tumor), eye (aniridia), and the genitourinary system. The cytogenetic abnormality involves a deletion of a part of the short arm of chromosome 11 (11p13), which typically is detectable on well-banded chromosome preparations. In MDS, a disorder characterized by mental retardation, dysmorphic faces, and lissencephaly, the deletion involves chromosome 17 (17p13). Using FISH, 17p deletions have been detected in over 90% of patients with MDS as well as in 20% of cases of isolated lissencephaly.

Deletions involving the long arm of chromosome 22 (22q11) are the most common microdeletions identified to date, present in approximately 1/3000 newborns. VCF syndrome, the most commonly associated syndrome, consists of learning disabilities or mild mental retardation, palatal defects, a hypoplastic aloe nasi and long nose, and congenital heart defects (conotruncal defect). Some individuals with 22q11 deletion are more severely affected and present with DiGeorge syndrome, which involves abnormalities in the development of the third and fourth branchial arches leading to thymic hypoplasia, parathyroid hypoplasia, and conotruncal heart defects. In approximately 30% of these cases, a deletion at 22q11 can be detected with high-resolution banding; by combing conventional cytogenetics, FISH, and molecular detection techniques (i.e., Southern blotting or polymerase chain reaction analyses), these rates improve to over 90%. Additional studies have demonstrated a surprisingly high frequency of 22q11 de-

TABLE 57-4 *Some Commonly Identified Microdeletion and Microduplication Syndromes*			
Syndrome	Cytogenetic Location	Principal Features	Imprinting Effects
Langer-Giedion syndrome	8q24.1 (del)	Sparse hair, bulbous nose, variable mental retardation	No
WAGR complex	11p13 (del)	Wilms' tumor, aniridia, genitourinary disorders, mental retardation	No
Beckwith-Wiedemann syndrome	11p15 (dup)	Macrosomia, macroglossia, omphalocoele	Yes, occasionally associated with "paternal uniparental disomy" (see text)
Retinoblastoma	13q14.11 (del)	Retinoblastoma due to homozygous loss of functional RB allele	No obvious effect, although abnormal RB allele more likely to be paternal
Prader-Willi syndrome	15q11-13 (del)	Obesity, hypogonadism, mental retardation	Yes; prototypic imprinting disorder (see text)
Angelman syndrome	15q11-13 (del)	Ataxic gait	With Prader-Willi syndrome, prototypic imprinting disorder (see text)
α-Thalassemia and mental retardation	16p13.3 (del)	α-thalassemia and mental retardation, due to deletion of distal 16p, including α-globin locus	No
Smith-Magenis syndrome	17p11.2 (del)	Brachycephaly, midface hypoplasia, mental retardation	No
Miller-Dieker syndrome	17p13 (del)	Dysmorphic facies, lissencephaly	No
Charcot-Marie-Tooth syndrome type 1A	17p11.2 (dup)	Progressive neuropathy due to micro-duplication	No
DiGeorge syndrome/velocardiofacial syndrome	22q11 (del)	Abnormalities of third and fourth branchial arches	No

letions in individuals with nonsyndromic conotruncal defects. Approximately 10% of individuals with a 22q11 deletion inherited it from a parent with a similar deletion.

Smith-Magenis syndrome involves a microdeletion localized to the proximal region of the short arm of chromosome 17 (17p11.2). Affected individuals have mental retardation, dysmorphic facial features, delayed speech, peripheral neuropathy, and behavior abnormalities. Most of these deletions can be detected with cytogenetic analysis, although FISH is available to confirm these findings. In contrast, William syndrome, a chromosome 7 (7q11.23) microdeletion, cannot be diagnosed with standard or high-resolution analysis; it is only detectable utilizing FISH or other molecular methods. William syndrome involves a deletion of the elastin gene and is characterized by mental retardation, dysmorphic features, a gregarious personality, premature aging, and congenital heart disease (usually supravalvular aortic stenosis).

In addition to microdeletion syndromes, there is now at least one well-described microduplication syndrome, Charcot-Marie-Tooth type 1A (CMT1A). This is a nerve conduction disease previously thought to be transmitted as a simple autosomal dominant disorder. Recent molecular studies have demonstrated that affected individuals are heterozygous for duplication of a small region of chromosome 17 (17p11.2-12). Although it is not yet clear why increased gene dosage would result in CMT1A, the inheritance pattern is explained by the fact that one-half of the offspring of affected individuals inherit the duplication-carrying chromosome.

IMPRINTING DISORDERS Two other microdeletion syndromes, Prader-Willi syndrome (PWS) and Angelman syndrome (AS), exhibit parent-of-origin, or "imprinting," effects. For many years, it has been known that cytogenetically detectable deletions of chromosome 15 occur in a proportion of patients with PWS, as well as in those with AS. This seemed curious, as the clinical manifestations of the two syndromes are very dissimilar. PWS is characterized by obesity, hypogonadism, and mild to moderate mental retardation, whereas AS is associated with microcephaly, ataxic gait, seizures, inappropriate laughter, and severe mental retardation. New insight into the pathogenesis of these disorders has been provided by the recognition that parental origin of the deletion determines which phenotype ensues: if the deletion is paternal, the result is PWS, whereas if the deletion is maternal, the result is AS (Fig. 57-2).

This scenario is complicated further by the recognition that not all individuals with PWS or AS carry the chromosome 15 deletion. For such individuals, the parental origin of the chromosome 15 region is again the important determinant. In PWS, for example, nondeletion patients invariably have two maternal and no paternal chromosomes 15 [maternal uniparental disomy (UPD)], whereas for some nondeletion AS patients the reverse is true (paternal UPD). This indicates that at least some genes on chromosome 15 are differently expressed, depending on which parent contributed the chromosome. Additionally, this means that normal fetal development requires the presence of one maternal and one paternal copy of chromosome 15.

Approximately 70% of PWS cases are due to paternal deletions of 15q11-q13, whereas 25% are due to maternal UPD, and about 5% are caused by mutations in a chromosome 15 imprinting center. In AS, 75% of cases are due to maternal deletions, and only 2% are due to paternal UPD. The remaining cases are presumably caused by imprinting mutations (5%), or mutations in the *UBE3A* gene, which is associated with AS. The UPD cases are mostly caused by meiotic nondisjunction resulting in trisomy 15, subsequently followed by a normalizing mitotic nondisjunction event ("trisomy rescue") resulting in two normal chromosomes 15, both from the same parent. *UBE3A* is the only maternally imprinted gene known in the critical region of chromosome 15. However, several paternally imprinted genes, or expressed-sequence tags (ESTs), have been identified, including *ZNF127*, *IPW*, *SNRPN*, *SNURF*, *PAR1*, and *PAR5*.

Chromosomal regions that behave in the manner observed in PWS and AS are said to be *imprinted*. This phenomenon is involved in differential expression of certain genes on different chromosomes. Chromosome 11 is one of these with an imprinted region, since it is known that a small proportion of individuals with the Beckwith-Wiedemann overgrowth syndrome have two paternal but no maternal copies of this chromosome.

ACQUIRED CHROMOSOME ABNORMALITIES IN CANCER (See also Chap. 68 for detailed discussion of cancer genetics)

In addition to the constitutional cytogenetic chromosomal abnormalities that are present at birth, somatic chromosomal changes can be acquired later in life and are often associated with malignant conditions. As with constitutional abnormalities, somatic changes can include the net loss of chromosomal material (due to a deletion or loss of a chromosome), net gain of material (duplication or gain of a chromosome), and relocation of DNA sequences (translocation). Cytogenetic changes have been particularly well studied in (1) leukemias, e.g., Philadelphia chromosome translocation in CML [t(9;22)(q34.1; q11.2)]; and (2) lymphomas, e.g., translocations of *MYC* in Burkitt's [t(8;14)(q24;q32)]. These and other translocations are useful for diagnosis, classification, and prognosis. Analyses of cytogenetic changes are also useful in certain solid tumors. For example, a complex karyotype with Wilms' tumor, diploidy in medulloblastoma, and Her-2/ neu amplification in breast cancer are poor prognostic signs.

FURTHER READING

JIANG F, KATZ RL: Use of interphase fluorescence in situ hybridization as a powerful diagnostic tool in cytology. Diagn Mol Pathol 11:47, 2002

NASMYTH K: Segregating sister genomes: the molecular biology of chromosome separation. Science 297:559, 2002

NICHOLLS RD et al: Imprinting in Prader-Willi and Angelman syndromes. Trends Genet 14:194, 1998

STUMM M et al: Molecular cytogenetic techniques for the diagnosis of chromosomal abnormalities in childhood disease. Eur J Pediatr 158:531, 1999

58   THE PRACTICE OF GENETICS IN CLINICAL MEDICINE
Susan Miesfeldt, J. Larry Jameson

IMPLICATIONS OF MOLECULAR GENETICS FOR INTERNAL MEDICINE

The field of medical genetics has traditionally focused on chromosomal abnormalities (Chap. 57) and Mendelian disorders (Chap. 56). However, there is genetic susceptibility to many common adult-onset diseases including atherosclerosis, hypertension, autoimmune diseases, diabetes mellitus, Alzheimer disease, psychiatric disorders, and many forms of cancer. Genetic contributions to these common disorders involve more than the ultimate expression of an illness; these genes can also influence the severity of infirmity, response to treatment, and progression of disease.

The primary care clinician is now faced with the role of recognizing and counseling patients at risk for a number of genetically influenced illnesses. Among the greater than 30,000 genes in the human genome, it is estimated that each of us harbors several potentially deleterious mutations. Fortunately, many of these alterations are recessive and clinically silent. An even greater number, however, represent genetic variants that alter disease susceptibility or severity. Genetic medicine is changing the way diseases are classified, enhancing our understanding of pathophysiology, providing practical information concerning drug metabolism and therapeutic responses, and allowing for individualized screening and health care management programs. In view of these changes, the physician must integrate personal medical history, family history, and diagnostic molecular testing into the overall care of individual patients and their families. In addition, the internist has

an important role in educating patients about the indications, benefits, risks, and limitations of genetic testing in the management of a number of diverse diseases. This is a difficult task as scientific advances in genetic medicine, and media attention to these advances, have outpaced the translation of these discoveries into standards of clinical care.

COMMON ADULT-ONSET GENETIC DISORDERS

MULTIFACTORIAL INHERITANCE The risk for many adult-onset disorders reflects the combined effects of genetic factors at multiple loci that may function independently, or in combination with other genes or environmental factors. Our understanding of the genetic basis of these disorders is incomplete, despite the clear recognition of genetic susceptibility. In type 2 diabetes mellitus, for example, the concordance rate in monozygotic twins ranges between 50 and 90%. Diabetes or impaired glucose tolerance occurs in 40% of siblings and in 30% of the offspring of an affected individual. Despite the fact that diabetes affects 5% of the population and exhibits a high degree of heritability, there are only a few examples of genetic mutations (most of which are rare) that might account for the familial nature of the disease. They include certain mitochondrial DNA disorders (Chap. 56), mutations in a cascade of genes that control pancreatic islet cell development and function (*HNF4α*, *HNF1α*, *IPF1*, *glucokinase*), insulin receptor mutations, and others (Chap. 323). Obesity and other factors that contribute to insulin resistance represent major risk factors for type 2 diabetes.

Current models for the genetic basis of type 2 diabetes propose the involvement of more than a dozen genes: some genes influence pancreatic islet cell development or function; others modulate glucose sensing; and an important group determine insulin sensitivity, either directly by affecting insulin signaling or indirectly by regulating body weight or composition. Superimposed on this genetic background are environmental influences such as diet, exercise, pregnancy, and medications.

Identifying these susceptibility genes is a formidable task. Nonetheless, a reasonable goal for this type of disease is to identify genes that increase (or decrease) disease risk by a factor of two or more. For common diseases such as diabetes or heart disease, this level of risk has important implications for health. Much the same way that cholesterol is currently used as a biochemical marker of cardiovascular risk, we can anticipate the development of genetic panels with similar predictive power. Tests for a large number of genetic disorders are available; a website (www.genetests.org) lists various laboratories that perform specific tests. The advent of DNA-sequencing chips represents an important technical advance that promises to make large-scale testing more feasible (Chap. 56). The decision whether or not to perform a genetic test for a particular inherited adult-onset disorder, such as hemochromatosis, multiple endocrine neoplasia (MEN) type 1, prolonged QT syndrome, or Huntington disease, is complex; it depends on the clinical features of the disorder, the desires of the patient and family, and whether the results of genetic testing will alter medical decision-making or treatment (see below).

THE FAMILY HISTORY Pending further advances in genetic testing, the key to assessing the inherited risk for common adult-onset diseases rests in the collection and interpretation of a detailed personal and family medical history in conjunction with a directed physical examination. For example, a history of multiple family members with early-onset coronary artery disease, glucose intolerance, and hypertension should suggest increased risk for genetic, and perhaps environmental, predisposition to insulin resistance (Chap. 323). Individual patients with this family history should be monitored for the possible development of hypertension, diabetes, and hyperlipidemia. They should be counseled about the importance of avoiding additional risk factors such as obesity and cigarette smoking.

Family history should be recorded in the form of a pedigree which greatly assists the assessment of risk in the individual patient (Chap. 56). At a minimum, pedigrees should convey health-related data on all first-degree relatives and selected second-degree relatives, including grandparents. When pedigrees appear to suggest an inherited disease, they should be extended to include additional family members. The determination of risk for an asymptomatic individual will vary depending on the size of the pedigree, the number of unaffected relatives, and the types of diagnoses within the family. For example, a woman with two first-degree relatives with breast cancer is at greater risk for a Mendelian disorder if she has a total of three female first-degree relatives than if she has a total of ten female first-degree relatives. Additional variables that should be documented in the pedigree include the age at diagnosis of each affected family member, present age of all family members, the presence or absence of nonhereditary risk factors among those affected with diseases, and the finding of multiple diseases in an individual patient. For instance, a woman with a history of both colon cancer and endometrial cancer is at risk for hereditary nonpolyposis colon cancer (HNPCC) regardless of her family history.

When assessing the personal and family history, the physician should be alert to a younger age of disease onset than is usually seen in the general population. A 30-year-old with acute myocardial infarction should be considered at risk for a hereditary trait, even if there is no family history of premature coronary artery disease (Chap. 224). The absence of the nonhereditary risk factors typically associated with a disease also raises the prospect of genetic risk factors. A personal or family history of deep-vein thrombosis, in the absence of known nongenetic risk factors, suggests a hereditary thrombotic disorder (Chap.

102). The physical examination may also provide important clues concerning the risk for a specific inherited disorder. A patient with xanthomas at a young age should prompt consideration of familial hypercholesterolemia. Some adult-onset disease-causing mutations are more prevalent in certain ethnic groups. For instance, >2% of the Ashkenazi population carry one of three specific mutations in the BRCA1 or BRCA2 genes. The prevalence of the factor V Leiden allele ranges from 3 to 7% in Caucasians but is much less common in Africans or Asians.

Recall of family history is sometimes inaccurate. This is especially so when the history is remote and families become more dispersed. It can be helpful to ask patients to fill out family history forms before or after their visits, as this provides them with an opportunity to contact relatives. Attempts should be made to confirm the illnesses reported in the family history before making important, and in certain circumstances, irreversible management decisions. This process is often labor intensive and ideally involves interviews of additional family members or reviewing medical records, autopsy reports, and death certificates.

Nongenetic factors associated with disease risk should also be reviewed in full, including occupation, diet, living conditions, and social habits. For example, patients at hereditary risk for heart disease should be questioned about tobacco use, diet, exercise, and lipid levels. Patients should also be asked about their health screening and prevention behaviors, as well as medication use. These nonhereditary factors contribute to the assessment of overall risk and represent an important focus for disease prevention.

Although many inherited disorders will be suggested by the clustering of relatives with the same or related conditions, it is important to note that *disease penetrance* is incomplete for most multifactorial genetic disorders. As a result, the pedigree obtained in such families may not exhibit a clear Mendelian pattern of inheritance, as not all family members carrying the disease-associated alleles will manifest a clinical disorder. Furthermore, genes associated with some of these disorders often exhibit *variable expression* of disease. For example, the breast cancer–associated gene BRCA1 can predispose to several different malignancies in the same family, including cancers of the breast, ovary, and prostate (Chap. 68). For common diseases such as breast cancer, some family members without the disease-causing mutation may also develop breast cancer, representing another confounding variable in the pedigree analysis.

Some of the aforementioned features of the family history are illustrated in Fig. 58-1. In this example, the proband, a 36-year-old woman, has a strong history of breast and ovarian cancer on the paternal side of her family. The early age of onset, as well as the co-occurrence of breast and ovarian cancer in this family, suggests the possibility of an inherited alteration in BRCA1 or BRCA2. It is unclear though—without genetic testing—whether her father inherited such a mutation and transmitted it to her. After appropriate genetic counseling of the proband and her family, one approach to DNA analysis in this family is to test the potentially affected 42-year-old living cousin for the presence of a BRCA1 or BRCA2 mutation. If a mutation is found, then it is possible to test for this particular alteration in the proband and other family members, if they so desire. In the example shown, if the proband's father has the BRCA1 mutation, there is a 50:50 probability that the mutation has been transmitted to her, and genetic testing can be used to establish the absence or presence of this particular risk factor.

GENETIC TESTING FOR ADULT-ONSET DISORDERS

A critical first step before initiating genetic testing is to assure that the correct clinical diagnosis has been made, whether based on family history, characteristic physical findings, or biochemical testing. Careful clinical assessment can define the *phenotype*, thereby preventing unnecessary testing and directing testing towards the most probable candidate genes. Many disorders exhibit the feature of *locus heterogeneity*, which refers to the fact that mutations in different genes can

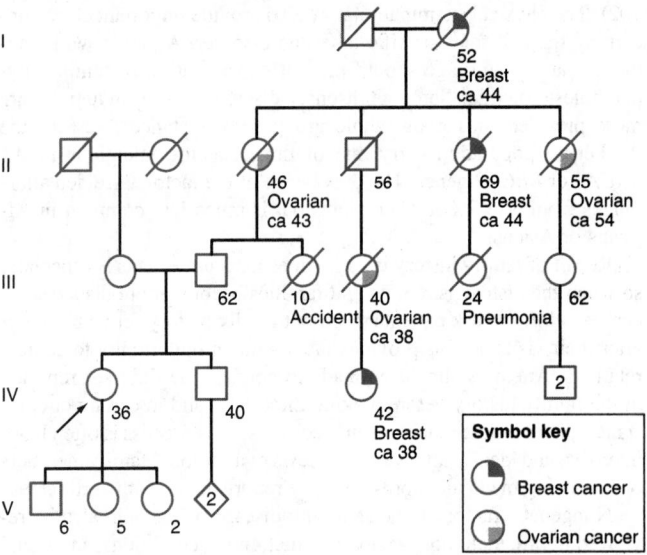

FIGURE 58-1 A 36-year-old woman (arrow) seeks consultation because of her family history of cancer. The patient expresses concern that the multiple cancers in her relatives imply an inherited predisposition to develop cancer. The family history is recorded and records of the patient's relatives confirm the reported diagnoses.

cause phenotypically similar disorders. For example, osteogenesis imperfecta (Chap. 342), long QT syndrome (Chap. 214), muscular dystrophy (Chap. 368), homocystinuria (Chap. 343), retinitis pigmentosa (Chap. 25) and hereditary predisposition to colon cancer (Chap. 77) or breast cancer (Chap. 76) can each be caused by mutations in distinct genes. The pattern of disease transmission, clinical course, and treatment may differ significantly, depending on which gene is affected. In these cases, the choice of which genes to test is often determined by unique clinical features, the relative prevalence of mutations in various genes, or test availability.

Like all laboratory tests, there are limitations to the accuracy and interpretation of genetic tests. In addition to technical errors, genetic tests are often designed to detect only the most common mutations. In this case, a negative result must be qualified by the possibility that the individual may have a mutation that is not included in the test.

In addition to molecular testing for established disease, genetic testing for susceptibility to chronic disease is being increasingly integrated into the practice of medicine. In most cases, however, the discovery of disease-associated genes has greatly outpaced studies that assess clinical outcomes and the impact of interventions. Until such evidence-based studies are available, predictive molecular testing must be approached with caution and should be offered only to patients who have been adequately counseled and have provided informed consent (Fig. 58-2). In the majority of cases, genetic testing should be offered only to individuals with a suggestive personal or family medical history or in the context of a clinical trial.

Predictive genetic testing falls into two distinct categories. *Presymptomatic testing* applies to diseases where a specific genetic alteration is associated with a near 100% likelihood of developing disease. In contrast, *predisposition testing* predicts a risk for disease that is less than 100%. For example, presymptomatic testing is available for those at risk for Huntington's disease, whereas predisposition testing is considered for those at risk for hereditary breast cancer. It is important to note that, for the majority of adult-onset, multifactorial genetic disorders, testing is purely predictive. Test results cannot reveal with confidence whether, when, or how the disease will manifest itself. For example, not everyone with the apolipoprotein E allele (ε4) will develop Alzheimer's disease, and individuals without this genetic marker can still develop the disorder (Chap. 350).

Molecular analysis is generally more informative if testing is initiated in a symptomatic family member, since the identification of a

mutation can direct the testing of other at-risk family members (whether they are symptomatic or not). In the absence of additional familial or environmental risk factors, individuals who test negative for the mutation found in the affected family member can be informed that they are at general population risk for that particular disease. Furthermore, they can be reassured that they are not at risk for passing on the mutation to their children. On the other hand, asymptomatic family members who test positive for the known mutation must be informed that they are at increased risk for disease development and for transmitting the mutation to their children.

A negative test result is interpreted differently when no genetic mutation is found in a symptomatic family member. In this difficult circumstance, the test performed on a given gene may not detect all mutations in that gene (false negative) or the individual may have a mutation in a different disease-associated gene that was not tested.

Clinicians providing pretest counseling and education should assess the patient's ability to cope with test results. Individuals who demonstrate signs and symptoms of emotional distress should have their psychosocial needs addressed before proceeding with molecular testing. Generally, genetic testing should not be offered at a time of personal crisis or acute illness within the family. Patients will derive more benefit from test results if they are emotionally able to comprehend and absorb the information. It is important to assess patients' preconceived notions of their personal likelihood of disease in preparing pretest educational strategies. Often, patients harbor unwarranted fear or denial of their likelihood of genetic risk.

Genetic testing has the potential of affecting the way individual family members relate to one another, both negatively and positively. As a result, patients addressing the option of molecular testing must consider how test results might impact their relationships with rela-

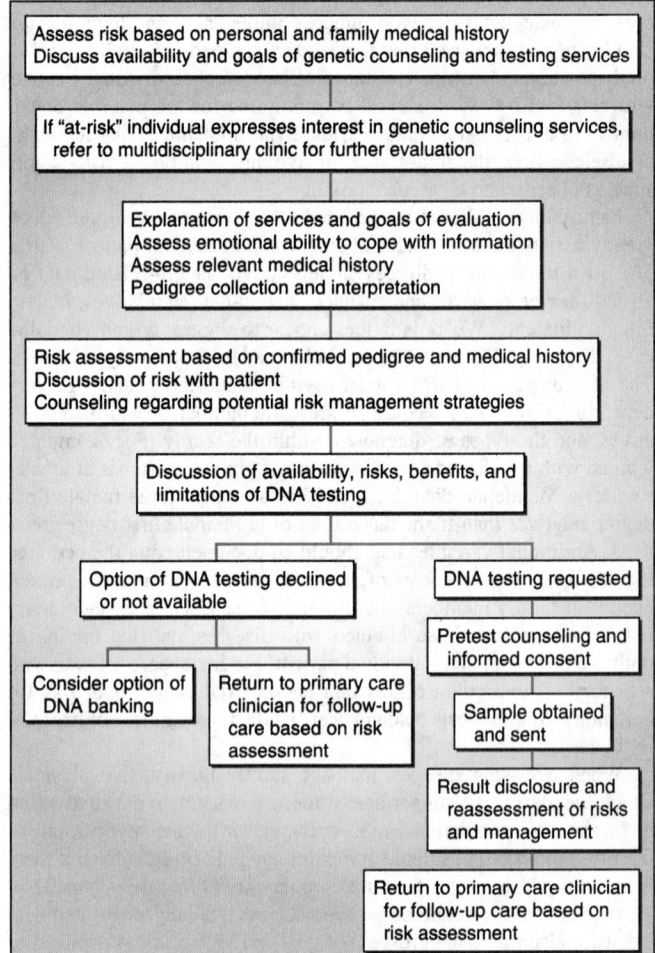

FIGURE 58-2 Algorithm for genetic counseling and testing.

tives, spouses, and friends. In families with a known genetic mutation, those who test positive must consider the impact of their carrier status on their present and future lifestyles; those who test negative may manifest *survivor guilt*. Family members are likely to differ in their emotional and social responses to the same information. Counseling should also address the potential consequences of test results on relationships with a spouse or child. Parents who are found to have a disease-associated mutation often express considerable anxiety and despair as they address the issue of risk to their children.

When a condition does not manifest until adulthood, clinicians will be faced with the question of whether at-risk children should be offered molecular testing and, if so, at what age. Although the matter is debated, several professional organizations have cautioned that genetic testing for adult-onset disorders should not be offered to children. Many of these conditions are not preventable and, consequently, such information can pose significant psychosocial risk to the child. In addition, there is concern that testing during childhood violates a child's right to make an informed decision regarding testing upon reaching adulthood. On the other hand, testing should be offered in childhood for disorders that may manifest early in life, especially when management options are available. For example, children at risk for familial adenomatous polyposis (FAP), associated with alterations in the *APC* gene, may develop polyps as early as their teens, and progression to an invasive cancer can occur by their twenties. Likewise, children at risk for MEN type 2, which is caused by mutations in the *RET* proto-oncogene, may develop medullary thyroid cancer early in childhood, and the issue of prophylactic thyroidectomy should be addressed with the parents of children with documented mutations (Chap. 330).

INFORMED CONSENT When the issue of testing is addressed, patients should be strongly encouraged to involve other relatives in the decision-making process, as molecular diagnostics will likely have an impact on the entire family. Informed consent for molecular testing begins with detailed education and counseling. The patient must fully understand the risks, benefits, and limitations of undergoing the analysis. Informed consent should include a written document, drafted clearly and concisely in a language and format that is comprehensible to the patient, who should be made aware of the disposition of test results. Informed consent should also include a discussion of the mechanics of testing. Most molecular testing for hereditary disease involves DNA-based analysis of peripheral blood. In the majority of circumstances, test results should be given only to the individual, in person, and with a support person in the room.

Because molecular testing of an asymptomatic individual often allows prediction of future risk, the patient should understand any potential long-term medical, psychological, and social implications of this decision. In the United States, legislation affecting this area is still evolving, and it is important to explore with the patient the potential impact that test results may have on employment, as well as future health, and disability and life insurance coverage.

Patients should understand that alternatives to molecular analysis remain available if they decide not to proceed with this option. They should also be notified that testing is available in the future if they are not currently prepared to undergo analysis. The option of DNA banking should be presented so that samples are readily available for future use by family members, if needed. DNA banking is a particularly valuable option for those individuals who are not expected to survive their illness and cannot immediately proceed with testing.

FOLLOW-UP CARE AFTER TESTING Depending on the nature of the genetic disorder, posttest interventions may include (1) cautious surveillance and appropriate health care screening, (2) specific medical interventions, (3) chemoprevention, (4) risk avoidance, and (5) referral to support services. For example, patients with known pathologic mutations in *BRCA1* or *BRCA2* are offered intensive screening as well as the option of prophylactic mastectomy and/or oophorectomy. In addition, such women may be eligible for preventive treatment with tamoxifen, or enrollment in a chemoprevention clinical trial. In contrast, those at known risk for Huntington's disease are offered continued follow-up

and supportive services, including physical and occupational therapy, and social services or support groups, as indicated. Specific interventions will change as translational research continues to enhance our understanding of these genetic diseases and as more is learned about the functions of the proteins involved.

Individuals who test negative for a mutation in a disease-associated gene identified in an affected family member must be reminded that they may still be at risk for the disease. This is of particular importance for common diseases such as diabetes mellitus, cancer, and coronary artery disease. For example, a woman who finds that she does not carry the disease-associated mutation in *BRCA2* previously discovered in her family must be reminded that she still requires the same breast cancer screening recommended for the general population.

GENETIC COUNSELING AND EDUCATION

Genetic counseling should be distinguished from genetic testing and screening, even though genetic counselors are often involved in issues related to testing. Genetic counseling refers to *a communication process that deals with human problems associated with the occurrence or risk of a genetic disorder in a family*. Genetic risk assessment is complex and often involves elements of uncertainty. Counseling therefore includes genetic education as well as psychosocial counseling. Genetic counselors may be called upon by other health care professionals (or by individual patients and families) to address a broad range of issues directly and indirectly involved with genetic disease (Table 58-1). The role of the genetic counselor includes the following:

- Gather and document a detailed family history
- Educate the patient about general genetic principles related to disease risk, both for themselves and others in their family
- Assess and enhance the patient's ability to cope with the genetic information offered
- Discuss how nongenetic factors may relate to the ultimate expression of disease
- Address medical management issues
- Assist in determining the role of genetic testing for the individual and family
- Ensure that the patient is aware of the risks, benefits, and limitations of the various genetic testing options
- Assist the patient, family and referring physician in the interpretation of the test results
- Refer the patient and other at-risk family members for additional medical and support services, if necessary.

The complexity of genetic counseling and the broad scope of genetic diseases have led to the development of specialized, multidisciplinary clinics designed to provide broad-based support and medical care for those at risk and their family members. Such specialty clinics are well established in the areas of cancer and neurodegenerative disorders. The multidisciplinary teams are often composed of medical geneticists, specialist physicians, genetic counselors, nurses, psychologists, social workers, and biomedical ethicists who work together to consider difficult diagnostic, treatment, and testing decisions. Such a format also provides primary care physicians with invaluable support and assistance as they follow and treat at-risk patients.

The approach to genetic counseling has important ethical, social, and financial implications. Philosophies related to genetic counseling vary widely by country and center. In North American centers, for

TABLE 58-1 *Indications for Genetic Counseling*

Advanced maternal (>35) or paternal (>50) age
Consanguinity
Previous history of a child with birth defects or a genetic disorder
Personal or family history suggestive of a genetic disorder
High-risk ethnic groups; known carriers of genetic alterations
Documented genetic alteration in a family member
Ultrasound or prenatal testing suggesting a genetic disorder

TABLE 58-2 *Examples of Genetic Testing and Possible Interventions*

Genetic Disorder	Inheritance	Genes	Interventions
ONCOLOGY			
Hereditary nonpolyposis colon cancer	AD	MSH2, MLH1, MSH6, PMS1, PMS2	Early cancer screening
Familial adenomatous polyposis	AD	APC	Nonsteroidal anti-inflammatory drugs
			Early endoscopic screening
			Colectomy
Familial breast and ovarian cancer	AD	BRCA1, BRCA2	Estrogen receptor antagonists
			Early screening by exams and mammography
			Consider prophylactic surgery
Familial melanoma	AD	CDKN2A	Avoid UV light
			Screening and biopsies
Basal cell nevus syndrome	AD	PTCH	Avoid UV light
			Screening and biopsies
HEMATOLOGY			
Factor V Leiden	AD	F5	Avoid thrombogenic risk factors and oral contraceptives
Hemophilia A	XL	F8C	Factor VIII replacement
Hemophilia B	XL	F9	Factor IX replacement
			Possible gene therapy
Glucose-6-PO4 dehydrogenase deficiency	XL	G6PD	Avoid oxidant drugs
CARDIOVASCULAR			
Hypertrophic cardiomyopathy	AD	MYH7, MYBPC3, TNNT2, TPM1	Echocardiographic screening
			Early pharmacologic intervention
Long QT syndrome	AD	KCNQ1, KCNH2, SCN5A, LQT4, KCNE1, KCNE2	Electrocardiographic screening and electrophysiologic testing
			Early pharmacologic intervention
			Possible implantable cardioverter defibrillator
Marfan syndrome	AD	FBN1	Echocardiographic screening
			Prophylactic beta blockers
GASTROINTESTINAL			
Familial Mediterranean fever	AR	MEFV	Colchicine treatment
Hemochromatosis	AR	HFE	Phlebotomy
PULMONARY			
α-1 Antitrypsin deficiency	AR	PI	Avoid smoking
			Avoid occupational and environmental toxins
Primary pulmonary hypertension	AD	BMPR2	Treatment with pulmonary vasodilators
RENAL			
Polycystic kidney disease	AD	PKD1	Prevent hypertension
			Prevent urinary tract infections
			Kidney transplantation
Nephrogenic diabetes insipidus	XL, AR	AVPR2, AQP2	Fluid replacement
			Thiazides, amiloride
ENDOCRINE			
Neurohypophyseal diabetes insipidus	AD	AVP	Replace vasopressin
Maturity onset diabetes of the young	AD	Multiple genes	Screen and treat for diabetes
Familial hypocalciuric hypercalcemia	AD	CASR	Avoid parathyroidectomy
Kallmann syndrome	XL	KAL	Induce puberty with hormone replacement
Multiple endocrine neoplasia type 2	AD	RET	Prophylactic thyroidectomy
			Screen for pheochromocytoma and hyperparathyroidism
21-Hydroxylase deficiency	AR	CYP21	Glucocorticoid and mineralocorticoid treatment
NEUROLOGIC			
Malignant hyperthermia	AD	RYR1	Avoid precipitating anesthetics
Hyperkalemic periodic paralysis	AD	SCN4A	Acetazolamide
Adrenoleukodystrophy	XL	ABCD1	Possible bone marrow transplant for severe childhood CNS form
Duchenne and Becker muscular dystrophy	XL	DMD	Glucocorticoids
			Possible future myoblast transfer
Familial Parkinson's disease	AD	SNCA, PARK2	Amantadine, anticholinergics, levodopa, monoamine oxidase B inhibitors
Wilson's disease	AR	ATP7B	D-Penicillamine treatment

Abbreviations: AD, autosomal dominant; AR, autosomal recessive: CNS, central nervous system; XL, X-linked

example, counseling is generally offered in a nondirective manner, wherein patients learn to understand how their values factor into a particular medical decision. Nondirective counseling is particularly appropriate when there are no data demonstrating a clear benefit associated with a particular intervention or when an intervention is considered experimental. For example, nondirective genetic counseling is employed when a person is deciding whether or not to undergo genetic testing for Huntington's disease (Chap. 350). At this time, there is no clear benefit (in terms of medical outcome) to an at-risk individual undergoing genetic testing for this disease, as its course cannot be altered by therapeutic interventions. However, testing can have an important impact on this individual's perception of the future and his or her interpersonal relationships and plans for reproduction. Therefore, the decision to pursue testing rests on the individual's belief system and values. On the other hand, a more directive approach is appropriate when a condition can be treated. In a family with FAP, colon cancer screening and prophylactic colectomy should be recommended for known *APC* mutation carriers. The counselor and clinician following this family must ensure that the at-risk family members have access to the resources necessary to adhere to these recommendations.

Genetic education is central to an individual's ability to make an informed decision regarding testing options and treatment. Although genetic counselors represent one source of genetic education, other health care providers also need to contribute to patient education. Patients at risk for genetic disease should understand fundamental medical genetic principles and terminology relevant to their situation. This includes the concept of genes, how they are transmitted, and how they confer hereditary disease risk. An adequate knowledge of patterns of inheritance will allow patients to understand the probability of disease risk for themselves and other family members. It is also important to impart the concepts of disease penetrance and expression. For most complex adult-onset genetic disorders, asymptomatic patients should be advised that a positive test result does not always translate into future disease development. In addition, the role of nongenetic factors, such as environmental exposures, must be discussed in the context of multifactorial disease risk and disease prevention. Finally, patients should understand the natural history of the disease as well as the potential options for intervention, including screening, prevention, and—in certain circumstances—pharmacologic treatment or prophylactic surgery.

THERAPEUTIC INTERVENTIONS BASED ON GENETIC RISK FOR DISEASE

Specific treatments are now available for an increasing number of genetic disorders, whether identified through population-based screening or directed testing (Table 58-2). Although the strategies for therapeutic interventions are best developed for childhood hereditary metabolic diseases, these principles are making their way into the diagnosis and management of adult-onset disorders. Hereditary hemochromatosis illustrates many of the issues raised by the availability of genetic screening in the adult population. For instance, it is relatively common (approximately 1 in 200 individuals of northern European descent are homozygous), and its complications are potentially preventable through phlebotomy (Chap. 336). The identification of the *HFE* gene, mutations of which are associated with this syndrome, has sparked interest in the use of DNA-based testing for presymptomatic diagnosis of the disorder. However, up to one-third of individuals who are homozygous for the *HFE* mutation do not have evidence of iron overload. Consequently, in the absence of a positive family history, current recommendations include phenotypic screening for evidence of iron overload followed by genetic testing. Whether genetic screening for hemochromatosis will someday be coupled to assessment of phenotypic expression awaits further studies. In contrast to the issue of population screening, it is important to test and counsel other family members when the diagnosis of hemochromatosis has been made in a proband. Testing allows the physician to exclude family members who are not at risk. It also permits presymptomatic detection of iron overload and the institution of treatment (phlebotomy) before the development of organ damage.

Preventive measures and therapeutic interventions are not restricted to metabolic disorders. Identification of familial forms of long QT

syndrome, associated with ventricular arrythmias, allows early electrocardiographic testing and the use of prophylactic antiarrythmic therapy, overdrive pacemakers, or defibrillators (Chap. 214). Individuals with familial hypertrophic cardiomyopathy can be screened by ultrasound, treated with beta blockers or other drugs, and counseled about the importance of avoiding strenuous exercise and dehydration (Chap. 221). Likewise, individuals with Marfan syndrome can be treated with beta blockers and monitored for the development of aortic aneurysms (Chap. 231). Individuals with α_1 antitrypsin deficiency can be strongly counseled to avoid cigarette smoking and exposure to environmental pulmonary and hepatotoxins. Various host genes influence the pathogenesis of certain infectious diseases in humans, including HIV (Chap. 173). The factor V Leiden allele increases risk of thrombosis (Chap. 53). Approximately 3% of the worldwide population is heterozygous for this mutation. Moreover, it is found in up to 25% of patients with recurrent deep-vein thrombosis or pulmonary embolism. Women who are heterozygous or homozygous for this allele should therefore avoid the use of oral contraceptives and receive heparin prophylaxis after surgery or trauma.

The field of pharmacogenomics seeks to identify genes that alter drug metabolism or confer susceptibility to toxic drug reactions. Examples include succinylcholine sensitivity, malignant hyperthermia, dihydropyrimidine dehydrogenase deficiency, the porphyrias, and glucose-6-phosphate dehydrogenase (G6PD) deficiency.

As noted above, the identification of genes that increase the risk of specific types of neoplasia is rapidly changing the management of many cancers. Identifying family members with mutations that predispose to FAP or hereditary nonpolyposis colon cancer (HNPCC) can lead to recommendations of early cancer screening or prophylactic surgery (Chap. 77). Similar principles apply to familial forms of melanoma, basal cell carcinoma, and cancers of the breast, ovary, and thyroid gland. It should be recognized, however, that most cancers harbor several distinct genetic abnormalities by the time they acquire invasive or metastatic potential (Chaps. 68 and 69). Consequently, the major impact of genetic testing in these cases is to allow more intensive clinical screening, as it remains very challenging to predict disease penetrance, expression, or the clinical course of these diseases.

Although genetic diagnosis of these and other disorders is only beginning to be used in the clinical setting, predictive testing holds the promise of allowing earlier and more targeted interventions that can reduce the morbidity and mortality associated with these disorders. We can expect the availability of genetic tests to expand rapidly. A critical challenge for physicians and other health care providers is to keep pace with these advances in genetic medicine and to implement testing judiciously. Meeting this goal will enhance patient care through adequate counseling, directed testing, and appropriate interventions, with the ultimate objective being the reduction of morbidity and mortality from genetic diseases.

FURTHER READING

BIESECKER BB, MARTEAU TM: Future of genetic counselling: An international perspective. Nat Genet 22:133, 1999

HARPER PS: *Practical Genetic Counselling*, 5th ed. Oxford, Butterworth Heinmann, 1998

MCKINNON WC et al: Predisposition genetic testing for late-onset disorders in adults: Position paper of the National Society of Genetic Counselors. JAMA 278:1217, 1997

PATENAUDE AF et al: Genetic testing and psychology. New roles, new responsibilities. Am Psychol 57:271, 2002

THE AMERICAN COLLEGE OF MEDICAL GENETICS: Points to consider: Ethical, legal and psychosocial implications of genetic testing in children and adolescents. Am J Hum Genet 57:1233, 1995

Gene therapy uses gene replacement to repair or treat disease. *Stem cell replacement* involves the administration of pluripotent, renewable cells to organs irreversibly damaged by disease. The disciplines of gene and cell therapy are now converging, offering unique opportunities to translate new knowledge of genetics and stem cell biology into the clinical setting. The technical, safety, and ethical challenges of these new treatment approaches are substantial, but their enormous promise provides strong incentive for ongoing research.

GENE TRANSFER IN CLINICAL MEDICINE

METHODS OF GENE TRANSFER Approaches to gene transfer can be divided broadly into: (1) ex vivo, in which genes are transferred into cells that are subsequently introduced into the patient; or (2) in vivo, in which genes are introduced directly into tissues, some of which are not readily accessible for ex vivo approaches. Ex vivo approaches are amenable to combining gene transfer with stem cell replacement (see below). In vivo gene transfer approaches have found relatively few clinical applications because of problems with targeting and regulating gene expression, maintaining gene expression, and avoiding toxicity.

Techniques for transferring genes include viral vectors and nonviral methods. *Viral vectors* take advantage of the fact that viruses enter cells efficiently and already contain genes that facilitate expression in host cells. In addition, some viruses such as retroviruses, lentiviruses, and adeno-associated viruses (AAVs) integrate genes into the host genome, facilitating long-term expression. However, technical limitations with viral production, the carrying capacity for the transferred gene, and the requirement for cell replication for effective integration (e.g., retroviruses) have hampered applications using these viruses. Nonetheless, viruses currently provide the best approach for long-lasting genetic modifications, as might be applied to stem cells or somatic cells. Adenoviruses have been widely used because they are easily produced in high titer, infect both quiescent and dividing cells, and can accommodate up to 10 kb of DNA. However, DNA transferred by adenoviruses is episomal (does not integrate into the host genome), resulting in relatively short-term gene expression over several weeks. The current generation of adenoviruses induces variable cytotoxicity and elicits immune responses—features that are useful for cytotoxic gene therapy but not for gene replacement.

Nonviral gene transfer includes the use of liposomes, electroporation, particle-mediated uptake, and direct uptake of naked DNA or oligonucleotides. Although these methods are relatively simple to perform and introduce minimal toxicity, they are much less efficient than viral-mediated approaches.

CHALLENGES ASSOCIATED WITH GENE THERAPY Gene therapy can be defined as the introduction of genes into cells or tissues with the goal of modifying the function of the tissue or producing a protein product beneficial for normal physiology. Potential applications of gene therapy are summarized in Table 59-1. Progress in gene therapy has been slow, reflecting substantial hurdles as investigators move closer to clinical applications. A few examples of potential applications highlight the status of this field and illustrate the requirements for successful gene therapy.

Significant therapeutic benefit can be achieved by the delivery of a single protein—insulin—to the patient with *diabetes mellitus*. In this case, the protein is secreted and can therefore be delivered extracellularly. The ability to produce recombinant human insulin has been a major advance. However, effective intensive insulin therapy remains difficult to achieve because of the exquisite regulation needed for dynamic metabolic responses to meals, exercise, and environmental stresses (Chap. 323). Clearly, much benefit would be gained if the insulin gene could be replaced and regulated normally. Although the gene has been cloned, and its regulatory elements have been characterized, insulin regulation requires multiple features of the normal pancreatic islet beta cell, including metabolic sensing mechanisms, an array of specific transcription factors that regulate the insulin gene, specialized protein-processing enzymes and secretory granules, and various channels that depolarize in response to metabolic signals. Thus, insulin gene therapy will not be successful in the absence of critical cellular features that recapitulate the function of the beta cell.

In contrast to insulin, where the goal is to secrete the protein for actions elsewhere in the body, many proteins function within a particular cell type, significantly complicating the delivery problem. For example, patients with *sickle cell anemia* or *β-thalassemia* have mutations in their β-globin genes (Chap. 91). In this case, one must introduce the replacement genes into specific cells and ensure regulated and sustained expression. The initial delivery and the long-term expression of the introduced gene are two distinct problems. Even if β-hemoglobin is expressed and regulated successfully in a red cell, the cell itself will only last for several weeks. Successful treatment there-

TABLE 59-1 *Examples of Disorders Potentially Amenable to Gene Therapy*

Disease	Gene Therapy Strategy
Inherited disorders	**Gene addition**
Cystic fibrosis	Express CFTR in pulmonary system and/or GI tract
Familial hypercholesterolemia	Express LDL receptor in liver
Hemophilias A and B	Express factor VIII or IX and secrete in circulation
Thalassemia	Express normal globin in red blood cells
Immunodeficiencies	Express deficient genes, such as adenosine deaminase
Metabolic disorders	Express missing enzymes or transporters
Duchenne's muscular dystrophy	Express mutant dystrophin protein in muscle cells
Retinitis pigmentosa (recessive)	Express normal protein in retina
	Gene correction
Lesch-Nyhan	Modify hypoxanthine phosphoribosyl transferase locus
Retinitis pigmentosa (dominant)	Correct missense mutation
Sickle cell disease	Correct β-globin mutation
Cystic fibrosis	Correct ΔF508 mutation in pulmonary system
Cardiovascular diseases	**Modify vascular biology**
Coronary artery restenosis	Block cell proliferation in vessel wall
Peripheral vascular disease	Induce angiogenesis
Hypertension	Express genes (e.g., tissue kallikrein) to induce vasodilation
Cancer	**Multiples approaches**
Many types	Express immunostimulants in or near malignant cells
	Express toxic genes in tumor cells (e.g., HSV-TK)
	Express genes to protect from chemotherapy in normal cells
Infectious diseases	
Viral diseases	Express genes that block viral replication or function, including ribozymes, decoys, dominant negative proteins
Many	Express antigens as recombinant vaccines
Miscellaneous	
Rheumatoid arthritis	Express anti-inflammatory cytokines in joints
Parkinson's disease	Express genes required for L-dopa synthesis in striatum
Neurodegenerative disease	Express neurotrophic factors

Note: CFTR, cystic fibrous transmembrane regulator; GI, gastrointestinal; LDL, low-density lipoprotein; HSV, herpes simplex virus; TK, thymidine kinase.

fore requires that the therapeutic genes be introduced into long-lived cells that can be renewed continuously to restore normal erythrocytes. Again, it is important to combine gene replacement or correction in the context of the normal host cell, in this case, an erythroblast.

Cystic fibrosis is caused by mutations in the cystic fibrosis transmembrane regulator (CFTR), a protein that regulates epithelial cell transport of Na^+ and Cl^- in the lung, gastrointestinal tract, sweat glands, and genitourinary system (Chap. 241). Gene delivery of the CFTR is more straightforward, in principle, as regulation of its expression level is less critical. The first attempt at gene therapy for cystic fibrosis was performed in 1993 using adenovirus-mediated transfer of the CFTR. This vector provides high level expression and is particularly effective for delivery to the lung. However, adenoviral expression is transient and induces immune responses that can limit subsequent viral administration. No clinical efficacy was demonstrated in the initial trials. Other viral delivery approaches are under investigation, but the challenge remains to target expression to particular tissues and to introduce the gene into a renewable population of cells.

The delivery of toxic, or suicide, genes to cancer cells is one of the most active areas of gene therapy research. Particularly for localized tumors, such as brain tumors or endocrine tumors, it may be possible to deliver highly toxic genes such as diphtheria toxin to tumor cells. For some tumor types, specific promoters can be used to express the toxic gene selectively in the cancer cell. Viruses have also been designed to replicate selectively in cells that lack certain tumor-suppressor genes, such as p53. An advantage of gene therapy for cancer cells is that long-term expression is not required. On the other hand, like chemotherapy or radiotherapy, gene therapy approaches must kill tumor cells with high efficacy without introducing significant toxicity. One novel approach is designed to increase the immunogenicity of tumors by expressing foreign antigens or cytokines that might increase endogenous immune responses.

FACTOR IX REPLACEMENT IN HEMOPHILIA B: POTENTIAL PARADIGM FOR GENE REPLACEMENT

An excellent candidate for somatic gene therapy is hemophilia B, an X-linked blood clotting disorder caused by a deficiency of factor IX (Chap. 102). Factor IX is normally produced in the liver and secreted into the circulation. Clotting times can be corrected with <5% of the normal levels of factor IX; thus, low levels of factor IX should be sufficient for clinical benefit. The factor IX gene has been inserted into AAV vectors and introduced into muscle and liver cells. AAVs can be produced at high enough titers that the factor IX gene can be transferred to relatively large numbers of cells. Wild-type AAV has no known pathology, and the AAV particle does not provoke significant inflammatory or immune responses. Studies of AAV-mediated factor IX gene transfer in canine and murine models lacking factor IX have shown efficacy, although correction of the clotting abnormality is transient because inhibitory antibodies against human factor IX are generated in these species.

In an initial human clinical trial, AAV–factor IX was injected at multiple sites in a skeletal muscle that could be excised in the event of an unanticipated adverse event. At moderate doses of vector, factor IX expression and low levels of circulating factor IX were detected. The patients had decreased need for supplemental factor IX injections, but no significant decrease in clotting time was observed.

A different strategy has been employed to express factor VIII in dermal fibroblasts of patients with hemophilia A. Factor VIII was expressed under control of the fibronectin promoter and transferred ex vivo to dermal fibroblasts. The genetically modified cells were injected into the omentum. In four of six patients, plasma levels of factor VIII increased but then declined, probably because the cells were not renewable. This ex vivo approach represents a combination of gene transfer and cellular therapy.

CHARACTERISTICS OF STEM CELLS

The use of stem cell therapy addresses several of the shortcomings of gene therapy, including the need to express genes in specific types of host cells, such as erythrocytes or neurons, and the need to regulate gene expression in response to physiologic signals. Recent advances in stem cell biology greatly enhance the prospects for applying cell therapy (Table 59-2).

Although murine embryonic stem cells (ESCs) have been studied for many years, human ESCs were successfully cultured in vitro only in 1998. *Stem cells* are the undifferentiated progenitors that can develop into highly specialized cells that form the various organs. Stem cells vary in their replicative capacity and in their differentiation potential. A convenient classification of stem cells is as follows:

1. *Totipotent stem cells* can form a placenta and can develop into a complete embryo. These features are characteristic of the cells derived from the first few divisions of the fertilized oocyte.
2. *Pluripotent stem cells* are capable of forming tissues derived from all three major germline layers—endoderm, mesoderm, and ectoderm. These features are exhibited by making chimeras in which ESCs are injected into a blastocyst to become integrated into all tissues in the animal. Cells derived from the inner cell mass of the blastocyst will divide in culture indefinitely, retain a stable genome, and maintain the potential to contribute to all tissues. Common use of the term *embryonic stem cells* refers to lines with these characteristics.
3. *Multipotent stem cells* are the progenitors of cells in particular tissues. Tissues such as bone marrow, skin, intestinal tract, and liver have tremendous regenerative potential and continuously renew their cell populations. In these cases, the multipotent stem cells give rise to multiple cell types characteristic of a particular tissue.

Embryonic germ cells (EGCs) can be derived from the precursors of the germ line. Unlike totipotent ESCs, EGCs cannot be incorporated into the inner cell mass. However, cell lines established from the developing germ cells form chimeras and, like ESCs, contribute to all tissue lines of the embryo.

Stem cells are self-renewing while at the same time generating daughter cells that are more differentiated. The expression of telomerase, an enzyme critical for maintaining the telomeres, is consistent with the self-renewing feature of stem cells. Microarray studies, which examine patterns of gene expression, have identified several hundred genes that are shared by various types of stem cells. For continuous

TABLE 59-2 *Potential Applications of Stem Cell Therapy*

Disease	Stem Cell Therapy Goal
Hematologic disorders	
Leukemias	Replace marrow; graft vs tumor
Multiple myeloma	Replace marrow; graft vs tumor
Sickle cell anemia	Replace or correct erythrocytes
Autoimmune diseases	
Systemic lupus erythematosus	Reconstitute immune system
Crohn disease	Reconstitute immune system
Immune deficiency disorders	
Severe combined immune deficiency	Gene correction in immune cells
Wiscott-Aldrich	Gene correction in immune cells
Cardiovascular diseases	
Myocardial ischemia	Replace ischemic cardiomyocytes
Hepatic disease	
Hepatic failure	Replace or regenerate hepatocytes
Metabolic disorders	
Diabetes	Replace pancreatic islets or induce beta cell differentiation
Osteoporosis	Regenerate bone
Gaucher disease	Express glucocerebrosidase in macrophages
Musculoskeletal disorders	
Duchenne muscular dystrophy	Replace myoblasts
Neurologic disorders	
Parkinson's disease	Replace dopamine-producing neurons

renewal, some daughter cells must remain undifferentiated, while others become committed and generate more differentiated cells (Fig. 59-1).

The ability of ESCs to become incorporated into the germ line has allowed the genome of mouse ESCs to be manipulated in culture before being introduced into blastocysts to form chimeric mice (Chap. 56). Because these mice contain germ cells derived from the cultured ESCs, some animals born in the second generation are derived entirely from the cultured and manipulated ESCs. The genetic manipulation of ESCs has made the mouse a very useful model organism for studying the effects of targeted mutagenesis (gene knock-out or knock-in). Access to cultured ESCs offers the potential for differentiation into multiple tissue types, including cells of the blood, brain, and other tissues.

Emerging evidence indicates that adult tissues previously thought to have little or no plasticity, such as the central nervous system (CNS) and heart, do have some regenerative potential, implying the presence of stem cells, or the ability to attract and adopt circulating stem cells (Fig. 59-2). Thus, most adult tissues appear to contain stem cells, but the characteristics of these so-called adult stem cells are highly variable and appear to depend on the tissue of origin as well as on the mesenchymal niche in which the cells are located. The hematopoietic system, gastrointestinal tract, and skin exemplify highly regenerative tissues in which stem cell populations have been partially characterized.

HEMATOPOIETIC STEM CELLS (See also Chap. 100)

Hematopoietic stem cells (HSCs) provide a relatively well-studied model of adult stem cells. Although HSCs are used routinely for bone marrow transplantation, the technology is complex to implement in part because the stem cells do not grow in culture. An additional difficulty is that the stem cell property is not a stable feature but is dependent on signals derived from other cells that provide a *stem cell niche*. Adherent mesenchymal cells in the bone marrow contain a second class of stem cell, called a *stromal stem cell* or a *mesenchymal stem cell*, which is capable of generating mesodermal cells such as connective tissue or muscle. Adherent cells from the bone marrow can be expanded for long periods to generate yet another stem cell with the potential to form many other cell types, including liver, endothelial, and neural cells. This *mesenchymal adult progenitor cell* may also

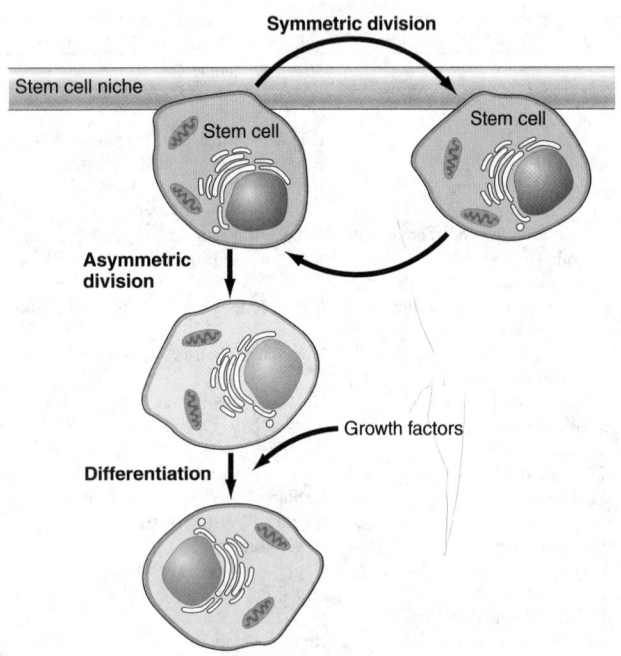

Symmetric division

Stem cell niche

Stem cell

Stem cell

Asymmetric division

Growth factors

Differentiation

FIGURE 59-1 Stem cells have the capacity for self-renewal through symmetric division or they can generate daughter cells that enter specific differentiation pathways, usually in response to extrinsic cell contacts or growth factor signals.

have the potential to form the various cell types of the blood. The implication is that the bone marrow mesenchyme can generate a pluripotent stem cell that is similar to ESCs, at least in some ways.

All blood cells, as well as vascular endothelial cells, are derived from a common progenitor termed the *hemangioblast*. Adoptive transfer of these cells demonstrates that the myeloid and lymphoid cells of a recipient are derived from the donor. Moreover, bone marrow from primary recipients can be transplanted into secondary and tertiary recipients, demonstrating that HSCs can self-renew.

HEMATOPOIETIC STEM CELL DIFFERENTIATION Bone marrow cells cultured in semi-solid medium give rise to colonies of a specific hematopoietic lineage, such as red cells [the colony forming unit (CFU) erythroid (CFU-E)], granulocytes (CFU-G), monocytes (CFU-M), or B cells (CFU-B). Less common are cells that give rise to multiple different cell types such as the colony-forming unit granulocyte, erythroid, macrophage (CFU-GEM). Current models predict that as pluripotent stem cells proliferate, they become progressively committed to fewer hematopoietic lineages and eventually to a single lineage. The differentiation of stem cells appears to involve the ordered sequential expression of transcription factors that dictate lineage. For example, the Gata-1 transcription factor is required for the terminal differentiation of erythroid and megakaryocytic cells, whereas the Gata-2 factor is required for proliferation of the most primitive multilineage hematopoietic cells. Interleukin (IL) receptor signaling (IL-7Rα and the common chain, γc) and the JAK3 kinase are critical for the production of both T and B cells.

HEMATOPOIETIC STEM CELL ENRICHMENT Repopulation assays with limiting numbers of mouse bone marrow cells have shown that the number of HSCs is at least 100-fold lower than the frequency of colony-forming cells. Fluorescence-activated cell sorting using monoclonal antibodies against cell surface proteins has allowed the separation of HSCs from cells that cannot repopulate irradiated mice. Most methods begin with the removal of bone marrow cells expressing markers associated with a specific lineage of peripheral blood cells. Lineage negative (Lin−) cells, which comprise <5% of bone marrow cells, are enriched for colony-forming cells and can repopulate irradiated mice, whereas Lin+ cells have no colony-forming cells. HSCs among the Lin− cells are positively identified by the expression of the c-kit receptor and the Ly-6 antigen known as Sca-1. Lin− c-*kit*+ Sca-1+ cells are highly enriched for HSCs as well as for cells capable of generating T and B cells (common lymphoid progenitors). The common lymphoid progenitors express the IL-7 receptor α-chain, whereas HSCs are IL-7Rα−. Lin− c-*kit*+ Sca-1+ IL-7Rα− cells represent the most highly enriched population of mouse HSCs.

Surrogate assays have been developed for the study of human HSCs. The long term culture initiating cell assay is an in vitro system in which single human bone marrow cells are placed on a layer of bone marrow–derived fibroblasts and endothelial cells. Some of these cells can be placed onto new feeder cells where they continue to produce colony-forming cells, indicating both proliferation and self-renewal.

The most widely used in vivo surrogate assays for human HSCs involve the injection of human hematopoietic cells into genetically immune-deficient mice. The simplest model uses mice homozygous for the severe combined immune deficiency (*scid*) mutation, a deletion of the p350 DNA-dependent kinase gene that causes a failure of T and B cell development. The NOD strain of mice is deficient in natural killer cells, and NOD mice homozygous for the *scid* mutation (NOD/SCID) are good hosts for human hematopoietic cells. Human cells engraft in these animals, and their progeny can be detected in the bone marrow for ≥12 weeks after transplantation. Using these and other models, human HSCs have been shown to be Lin− and express the CD34 antigen. Lin− CD34+ cells can be further enriched for HSCs by sorting for cells that express Thy-1 and do not express CD38. Lin− CD34+ Thy-1+ CD38− cells are highly enriched for HSCs and are present at a frequency of <0.02% in human bone marrow.

Human and mouse HSCs share the ability to export the vital dyes

Hoechst 33342 and/or Rhodamine 123 efficiently. Dye export from HSCs is controlled by Bcrp, a member of the ATP-binding cassette transporter protein family that is expressed at high levels in HSCs. The ability to export Hoechst 33342 and Rhodamine 123 is shared by stem cells in other adult tissues, suggesting a common behavior of stem cells.

GENETIC MODIFICATION OF STEM CELLS

Stem cells are the ideal targets for gene therapy approaches. Because stem cells are able to self-renew, gene insertion into stem cells followed by engraftment into the patient should lead to a lifetime supply of corrected cells. In organs where cells are constantly lost and replaced, such as the hematopoietic and epithelial systems, introduction of a gene into a cell that cannot self-renew would require repeated treatments. The ability of stem cells to proliferate and differentiate into different types of mature cells ensures that the correct cell type will have the transferred gene. A problem is that most genes whose function needs to be replaced in disease states are expressed mainly in terminally differentiated cells and are not normally expressed in stem cells.

A variety of methods have been developed to transfer new genetic material into cells, including direct injection of DNA and gene transfer by viruses such as adenovirus, AAV or various RNA tumor viruses. Because RNA tumor viruses integrate into the genome of the target cell, they are currently the method of choice for stem cell gene transfer. The retroviruses have been modified such that most viral proteins are deleted, leaving only sequences important for viral integration. Recombinant virus vectors replace the protein-encoding sequences with a gene of interest. Because packaging sequences are deleted, the viruses do not replicate. The first recombinant RNA viral vectors were based on the Moloney murine leukemia viruses (MMuLV) but transduction efficiencies were very low (<1% of human cells). Although strategies to enhance MMuLV titers, attachment, and integration are ongoing, other retroviruses, such as vesicular stomatitis virus (VSV) and lentivirus, appear more promising. After the RNA virus genome enters the cell, it is converted into DNA by reverse transcriptase packaged with the RNA genome. Integration into the host genome occurs only during cell division. Thus, strategies to recruit cells into the cell cycle (e.g., transforming growth factor β antibodies) or to extend the G_1 to S-phase transition (e.g., antisense p27KIP-1 oligonucleotides) appear to enhance viral integration into stem cells.

HEMATOPOIETIC STEM CELL GENE THERAPY ■ Bone Marrow Transplantation

This is used in thousands of patients yearly and is an example of cell therapy (Chap. 100). The success of bone marrow transplantation reflects the fact that the many cell types of the blood are derived from progenitor stem cells. Bone marrow transplantation is used to treat numerous acquired (aplastic anemia, myelodysplasia, leukemia, and lymphoma) and inherited (immune deficiencies, thalassemia, and sickle cell disease) hematologic and immunologic diseases. Ongoing studies are examining its applicability in selected autoimmune disorders such as refractory systemic lupus erythematosus and Crohn disease. Genetic modification of HSCs may achieve certain therapeutic goals (e.g., resistance to chemotherapy) or allow correction of a genetic defect.

Severe Combined Immune Deficiencies (SCID) This causes defects in both T and B lymphocyte production. Patients with SCID do not have cell-mediated or humoral immune responses and are subject to chronic life-threatening infections. The two most common forms of SCID are adenosine deaminase (ADA) deficiency (ADA-SCID) and deficiency of the X-linked IL-2 receptor γ-chain (γc, X-SCID) (Chap. 297). Bone

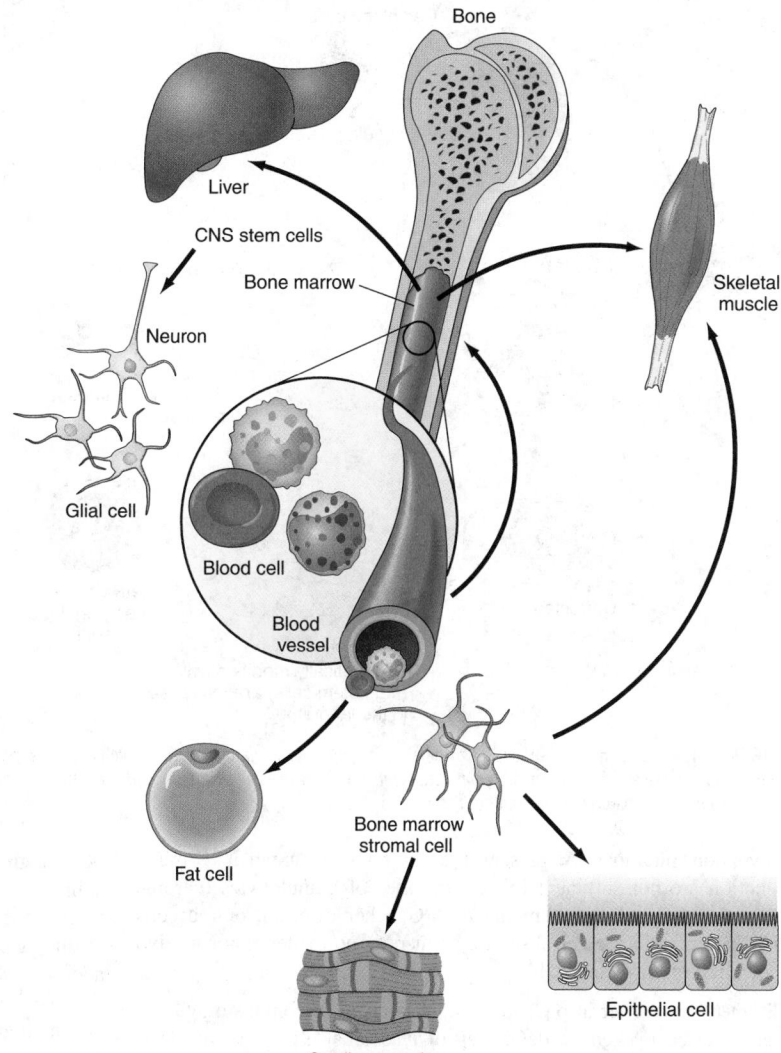

FIGURE 59-2 Plasticity of adult stem cells. CNS, central nervous system. [*Adapted from NIH Guide on Stem Cells: Scientific Promise and Future, 2001 (http://www.nih.gov/news/stemcell/scireport.htm.)*]

marrow transplantation from an MHC-matched related donor is the treatment of choice and is effective in about 70 to 80% of patients.

Because the gene defects are known, ADA-SCID and X-SCID patients without a matched donor are excellent candidates for stem cell gene therapy. The first human gene therapy trial was performed in 1991. T lymphocytes from two ADA-deficient patients receiving ADA enzyme therapy were expanded and transduced with a retrovirus vector containing the ADA gene. Between 2 and 10% of the transduced T cells expressed the transferred gene and were reinfused into the patients. Clinical improvements, including positive responses to vaccinations, were documented in both patients despite the gradual disappearance of transduced cells to background levels over the next 5 years. In 2000, the first successful stem cell gene therapy was reported. Cord blood CD34+ cells from X-SCID newborns transduced with a γc retrovirus vector were reinfused into the patients. Approximately 98% of circulating T lymphocytes and 1% of circulating B lymphocytes contained the γc vector, compared to <0.1% of myeloid cells, demonstrating in vivo selection. The patients responded to clinical vaccinations and have been living at home without supportive care. Unfortunately, two recipients of marrow transduced with a γc retrovirus vector have developed a clinical disorder that resembles leukemia, and further studies have been suspended.

Wiscott-Aldrich Syndrome (WAS) This is an X-linked T lymphocyte disorder that can be accompanied by platelet dysfunction. Bone marrow transplantation can cure WAS, and in vivo selection for corrected cells has been demonstrated in several clinically normal WAS patients with

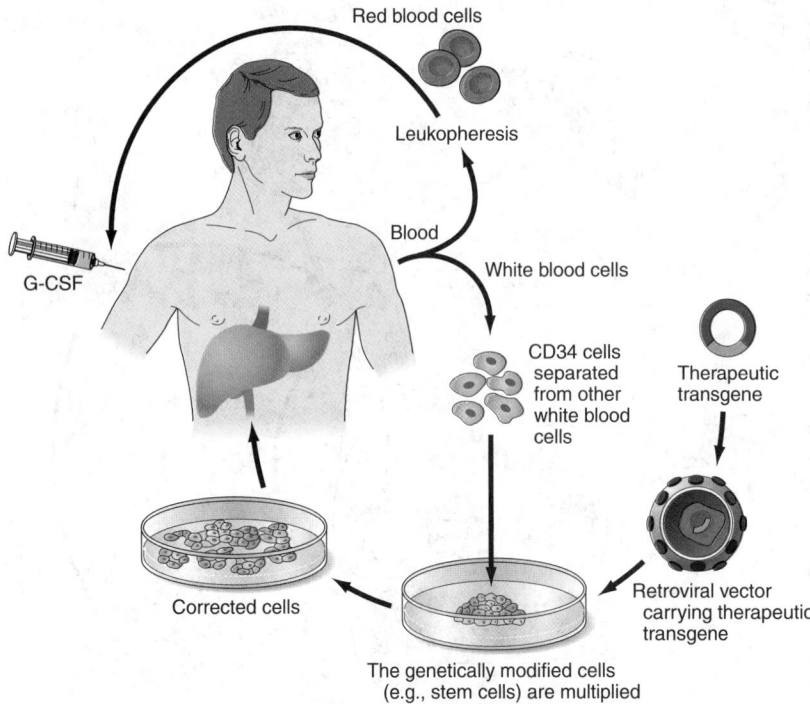

FIGURE 59-3 Strategy for introducing a therapeutic gene into hematopoietic stem cells to be used for autologous transplantation. [*Adapted from Pittsburgh Gaucher Disease Diagnosis and Treatment Program (http://gaucher.mgh.harvard.edu/centers/Pitt.html.)*]

reversion mutations. At present, the low rates of human HSC transduction are not sufficient to treat diseases of granulocytes (chronic granulomatous disease), monocytes (Gaucher disease), or red cells (thalassemia, sickle cell disease), as there is no evidence for in vivo selection of corrected cells.

Gaucher Disease (See also Chap. 340) This is a lysosomal storage disease caused by genetic deficiency of lysosomal glucocerebrosidase. Clinical manifestations reflect the accumulation of lipid-laden macrophages, referred to as *Gaucher cells*, in bone, liver, spleen, and other viscera. Macrophage-targeted enzyme replacement therapy has proven highly effective in Gaucher disease. Trials are currently underway to harvest a patient's HSCs, insert a normal copy of the gene encoding glucocerebrosidase using retroviruses, and return the modified cells to the patient (Fig. 59-3). This strategy represents a potential paradigm for disorders in which stem cells can be modified and reconstituted into normal tissues.

EMBRYONIC AND SOMATIC STEM CELL TECHNOLOGY IN MEDICINE

CARDIOVASCULAR SYSTEM The high incidence of cardiac disease has made regeneration of damaged cardiac muscle of great interest. Skeletal myoblasts can improve function in the damaged heart, but it is not clear if these cells confer long-term benefit. Myocardium has some regenerative capacity; pluripotent cells hone into areas of damaged myocardium. In men who receive heart transplants from female donors, XY-derived host cells are found in the donor tissue, particularly in regions of injury. Stem cells with the potential to generate cardiac tissue have been isolated from the bone marrow. In mouse models, labeled ESCs are incorporated into ischemic regions of the heart and reconstitute vascular and connective tissue as well as cardiac myocytes, and they express a number of highly specific cardiac markers. These findings imply that local factors, perhaps produced in response to injury, induce specific patterns of cellular differentiation.

LIVER The liver is capable of extensive regeneration. In most cases, regeneration is not caused by rare stem cells but rather by the rapid division of differentiated hepatocytes. Hepatocytes can be transplanted serially from one animal to another, demonstrating their extensive proliferative potential in vivo. It has been difficult, however, to establish conditions for long-term growth in vitro. When hepatocytes are inadequate for regeneration, less abundant stem cells in the liver become activated. The term *oval cell* is often used to refer to stem cells in the liver, but other pluripotent cells also appear capable of liver regeneration. For example, hepatocytes may be generated from cell populations enriched for HSCs as demonstrated by engraftment into animals with an otherwise fatal deficiency in liver function. Pluripotent cells derived from the bone marrow and capable of long-term culture can differentiate into liver cells in vitro. There is also evidence that HSCs can fuse with hepatocytes to generate new liver cells. ESCs can also generate liver cells.

PANCREATIC ISLETS The liver and pancreas share a number of developmental transcription factors and growth factors but ultimately diverge into distinct organs containing highly specialized cells. The pancreas is composed of two distinct cell types, the exocrine and endocrine cells. The islets of Langerhans contain the beta cells, which secrete insulin. Improvements in islet transplantation and immunosuppression regimens have resulted in some patients being free of exogenous insulin administration. However, the number of donor islets is very limited. Expansion of the beta cell population in vivo or in vitro would be useful. Stem cells in the adult pancreas reside near the pancreatic ducts and are competent to differentiate into the endocrine cell types. Self-assembling structures similar to pancreatic islets can be derived from ESCs. These embryonic stem–derived cells secrete insulin in response to glucose. An alternative approach involves attempts to alter the differentiation program of hepatic progenitor cells by introducing pancreas-specific transcription factors, such as PDX-1, using adenoviruses. In mouse models, PDX-1 induces a small fraction of liver cells to produce insulin and some of these cells appear to cycle and maintain a beta cell–like phenotype. Although much work remains to characterize and improve these models, early findings suggest that stem cell plasticity may offer a means to increase the population of insulin-producing cells.

NERVOUS SYSTEM The peripheral nervous system (PNS) is generated by an epithelial to mesenchymal transition that occurs in the neural crest. The precursor cells of the PNS are flexible and can give rise to progeny with multiple fates. *PNS stem cells* with somewhat different properties can be found in adult as well as fetal animals.

The many complex cell types of the CNS are generated from epithelial precursors that are not committed to specific fates. *CNS stem cells* can be expanded in tissue culture and generate the three major cell types of the brain: neurons, astrocytes, and oligodendrocytes. Multipotent cells can be obtained in large numbers from both the developing and adult brain. Neurons generated by fetal and adult CNS stem cells form functional excitatory and inhibitory synapses.

Although many types of neurons exist in the brain, the idea that the brain is derived from stem cells has stimulated attempts to exploit the regenerative potential of stem cell therapy to treat neurologic disease in the adult brain.

Parkinson's Disease Transplantation of fetal brain tissue may provide benefit to patients with Parkinson's disease. Dopamine neurons that are functional and long lasting can be obtained by grafting the tissue of the ventral fetal midbrain into the dorsal striatum. Raclopride is a drug that binds to dopamine receptors and radioactive raclopride can be imaged in the human brain using position emission tomography scanning. The displacement of raclopride has been used to show that grafted midbrain neurons release dopamine. This is one of several types of data supporting the idea of transplantation in Parkinson's disease.

The current procedures also have limitations. For optimal effects, the tissue from several fetal brains must be used; as the tissue must be at a specific stage in development, the logistics are difficult. Unexplained adverse reactions have been noted, and efficacy is hard to predict. ESCs offer a potential solution to the problem of variable tissue sources as they expand for long periods in tissue culture and can differentiate through midbrain precursors into dopamine secreting neurons. *Nuclear transfer* represents another approach in which an ESC can be generated from an oocyte after replacing its nucleus with one from a host somatic cell. Preliminary studies show that these ntESCs also readily form dopamine neurons.

Both ESC-derived and normal midbrain neurons express receptors for glial derived neurotrophic factor (GDNF). Gene therapy data in monkeys suggest that GDNF delivery may provide clinical benefit in Parkinson's patients. Clinical trials with GDNF are now underway.

ESCs can also be differentiated into cells similar to motor neurons, which degenerate in amyotrophic lateral sclerosis. ESCs can also be used as a source for large numbers of oligodendrocytes, a cell type that is lost in multiple sclerosis.

New neurons are not normally produced in most regions of the adult CNS. However, large numbers of new neurons are produced in the adult dentate gyrus of the hippocampus and the olfactory bulb. Pyramidal neurons can be regenerated in the CA1 region of the hippocampus and the cerebral cortex. New neurons are also generated in the adult striatum. Thus, endogenous precursors may be capable of regenerating neurons after injury to the adult nervous system.

ETHICAL ISSUES

Gene and stem cell therapies raise ethical and socially contentious issues that must be addressed in parallel with the scientific and medical opportunities. Our society has great diversity with respect to religious beliefs, concepts of individual rights, tolerance for uncertainty and risk, and boundaries for how scientific interventions should be used to alter the outcome of disease. In the United States, the federal government has authorized research using existing human ESC lines but has restricted the use of federal funds for developing new human ESC lines. Studies of the characteristics of these existing lines, including whether they are stable over time, are ongoing.

In considering ethical issues associated with the use of stem cells, it is helpful to draw from experience with other scientific advances, such as organ transplantation, recombinant DNA technology, implantation of mechanical devices, neuroscience and cognitive research, in vitro fertilization, and prenatal genetic testing. From these and other precedents, we learn the importance of understanding and testing fundamental biology in the laboratory setting and in animal models before applying new techniques in carefully controlled clinical trials. When these trials occur, they must include full informed consent and have careful oversight by external review groups.

Ultimately, there will be medical interventions that are scientifically feasible but ethically or socially unacceptable to some members of a society. Since genetic research raises fundamentally difficult questions of identity, it has raised deep fears about our ability to assure justice, access, and safety in genetic medicine. Health care providers and experts with backgrounds in ethics, law, and sociology must help guard against the premature or inappropriate application of gene or stem cell therapies, and the inappropriate use of vulnerable population groups. On the other hand, these therapies offer important new strategies for the treatment of otherwise irreversible disorders. An open dialogue between the scientific community, physicians, patients and their advocates, lawmakers, and the lay population is critically important to raise and address important ethical issues and to balance the benefits and risks associated with gene and stem cell transfer.

FURTHER READING

BISHOP AE et al: Embryonic stem cells. J Pathol 197:424, 2002

IVANOVA NB et al: A stem cell molecular signature. Science 298:601, 2002

JIANG Y et al: Pluripotency of mesenchymal stem cells derived from adult marrow. Nature 418:41, 2002

KARBLING M, ESTROV Z: Adult stem cells for tissue repair—a new therapeutic concept? N Engl J Med 349:570, 2003

WAKAYAMA T et al: Differentiation of embryonic stem cell lines generated from adult somatic cells by nuclear transfer. Science 292:740, 2001

60 | NUTRITIONAL REQUIREMENTS AND DIETARY ASSESSMENT
Johanna Dwyer

Nutrients are substances that are not synthesized in the body in sufficient amounts and therefore must be supplied by the diet. Nutrient requirements for groups of healthy persons have been defined on the basis of experimental evidence. For good health we require energy-providing nutrients (protein, fat, and carbohydrate), vitamins, minerals, and water. Specific nutrient requirements include 9 essential amino acids, several fatty acids, 4 fat-soluble vitamins, 10 water-soluble vitamins, and choline. Several inorganic substances, including 4 minerals, 7 trace minerals, 3 electrolytes, and the ultratrace elements, must also be supplied in the diet.

The required amounts of the essential nutrients differ by age and physiologic state. Conditionally essential nutrients are not required in the diet but must be supplied to individuals who do not synthesize them in adequate amounts, such as those with genetic defects, those having pathologic states with nutritional implications, and developmentally immature infants. Many organic phytochemicals and zoochemicals present in foods have various health effects. For example, dietary fiber has beneficial effects on gastrointestinal function.

ESSENTIAL NUTRIENT REQUIREMENTS

ENERGY For weight to remain stable, energy intake must match energy output. The major components of energy output are resting energy expenditure (REE) and physical activity; minor sources include the energy cost of metabolizing food (thermic effect of food or specific dynamic action) and shivering thermogenesis (e.g., cold-induced thermogenesis). The average energy intake is about 2800 kcal/d for American men and about 1800 kcal/d for American women, though these estimates vary with body size and activity level. Formulas for estimating REE are useful for assessing the energy needs of an individual whose weight is stable. Thus, for males, REE = 900 + 10w, and for females, REE = 700 + 7w, where w is weight in kilograms. The calculated REE is then adjusted for physical activity level by multiplying by 1.2 for sedentary, 1.4 for moderately active, or 1.8 for very active individuals. The final figure provides an estimate of total caloric needs in a state of energy balance. →*For further discussion of energy balance in health and disease, see Chap. 62.*

PROTEIN Dietary protein consists of both essential and nonessential amino acids that are required for protein synthesis, whereas certain amino acids can also be used for energy and gluconeogenesis. The nine essential amino acids are histidine, isoleucine, leucine, lysine, methionine/cystine, phenylalanine/tyrosine, threonine, tryptophan, and valine. When energy intake is inadequate, protein intake must be increased, since ingested amino acids are diverted into pathways of glucose synthesis and oxidation. In extreme energy deprivation, protein-calorie malnutrition may ensue (Chap. 62).

For adults, the recommended dietary allowance (RDA) for protein is about 0.6 g/kg desirable body weight per day, assuming that energy needs are met and that the protein is of relatively high biologic value. Current recommendations for a healthy diet call for at least 10 to 14% of calories from protein. Biologic value tends to be highest for animal proteins, followed by proteins from legumes (beans), cereals (rice, wheat, corn), and roots. Combinations of plant proteins that complement one another in biologic value or combinations of animal and plant proteins can increase biologic value and lower total protein requirements.

Protein needs increase during growth, pregnancy, lactation, and rehabilitation during treatment of malnutrition. The tolerance to dietary protein is decreased in renal insufficiency and liver failure. Normal protein intake can precipitate encephalopathy in patients with cirrhosis of the liver or worsen uremia in those with renal failure.

FAT AND CARBOHYDRATE Fats are a concentrated source of energy and constitute on average 34% of calories in U.S. diets. However, for optimal health, fat intake should total no more than 30% of calories. Saturated fat and trans-fat should be limited to <10% of calories, and polyunsaturated fats to <10% of calories, with monounsaturated fats comprising the remainder of fat intake. At least 55% of total calories should be derived from carbohydrates. The brain requires about 100 g/d of glucose for fuel; other tissues use about 50 g/d. Over time, adaptations in carbohydrate needs are possible in hypocaloric states. For example, reduced insulin levels lead to adipose tissue breakdown and cause the body to burn more fatty acids. However, some tissues (e.g., brain and red blood cells) rely on glucose supplied either exogenously or from muscle proteolysis (Chap. 324).

WATER For adults, 1 to 1.5 mL water per kcal of energy expenditure is sufficient under usual conditions to allow for normal variations in physical activity, sweating, and solute load of the diet. Water losses include 50 to 100 mL/d in the feces, 500 to 1000 mL/d by evaporation or exhalation, and, depending on the renal solute load, ≥1000 mL/d in the urine. If external losses increase, intakes must increase accordingly to avoid underhydration. Fever increases water losses by approximately 200 mL/d per °C; diarrheal losses vary but may be as great as 5 L/d in severe diarrhea. Heavy sweating and vomiting also increase water losses. When renal function is normal and solute intakes are adequate, the kidneys can adjust to increased water intake by excreting up to 18 L/d of excess water (Chap. 319). However, obligatory urine outputs can compromise hydration status when there is inadequate intake or when losses increase in disease or kidney damage.

Infants have high requirements for water because of their large ratio of surface area to volume, the limited capacity of the immature kidney to handle high renal solute loads, and their inability to communicate their thirst. Increased water needs during pregnancy are low, perhaps an additional 30 mL/d. During lactation, milk production increases water requirements so that approximately 1000 mL/d of additional water is needed, or 1 mL for each mL of milk produced. Special attention must be paid to the water needs of the elderly, who have reduced total body water and blunted thirst sensation, and may be taking diuretics.

OTHER NUTRIENTS See Chap. 61 for detailed description of vitamins and trace minerals.

DIETARY REFERENCE INTAKES AND RECOMMENDED DIETARY ALLOWANCES

Fortunately, human life and well-being can be maintained within a fairly wide range for most nutrients. However, the capacity for adaptation is not infinite—too much, as well as too little, intake of a nutrient may have adverse effects or alter the health benefits conferred by another nutrient. Therefore, benchmark recommendations on nutrient intakes have been developed to guide clinical practice. These quantitative estimates of nutrient intakes are collectively referred to as the *dietary reference intakes* (DRIs). The DRIs supplant the *recommended daily allowances* (RDAs), the single reference values used in the United States since 1989. DRIs include the *estimated average requirement* (EAR) for nutrients, as well as three other reference values used for dietary planning for individuals: the RDA, the *adequate intake*

(AI), and the tolerable *upper level* (UL). The current DRIs for vitamins and elements are provided in Tables 60-1 and 60-2, respectively.

ESTIMATED AVERAGE REQUIREMENT When florid dietary deficiency diseases such as rickets, scurvy, xerophthalmia, and protein-calorie malnutrition were common, nutrient adequacy was assumed by the absence of clinical signs of a dietary deficiency disease. Later, it was determined that biochemical and other changes were evident long before the clinical deficiency became apparent. Consequently, criteria of adequacy are now based on biologic markers when they are available. Current efforts focus on the amount of a nutrient that reduces the risk of chronic degenerative diseases. Priority is given to sensitive biochemical, physiologic, or behavioral tests that reflect early changes in regulatory processes or maintenance of body stores of nutrients.

The EAR is the amount of a nutrient estimated to be adequate for half of the healthy individuals of a specific age and sex. The types of evidence and criteria used to establish nutrient requirements vary by nutrient, age, and physiologic group. The EAR is not an effective estimate of nutrient adequacy in individuals because it is a median requirement for a group; 50% of individuals in a group fall below the requirement and 50% fall above it. Thus, a person with a usual intake at the EAR has a 50% risk of an inadequate intake. For these reasons, other standards, described below, are more useful for clinical purposes.

RECOMMENDED DIETARY ALLOWANCES The RDA is the average daily dietary intake level that meets the nutrient requirements of nearly all healthy persons of a specific sex, age, life stage, or physiologic condition (such as pregnancy or lactation). The RDA is the nutrient-intake goal for planning diets of individuals.

The RDA is defined statistically as 2 standard deviations (SD) above the EAR to ensure that the needs of any given individual are met. The RDAs are used to formulate food guides such as the U.S. Department of Agriculture (USDA) Food Guide Pyramid for individuals, to create food exchange lists for therapeutic diet planning, and as a standard for describing the nutritional content of processed foods and nutrient supplements. The nutrient content in a food is stated by weight or as a percent of the daily value (DV), a variant of the RDA

TABLE 60-1   *Dietary Reference Intakes: Recommended Intakes for Individuals—Vitamins*

Life-Stage Group	Vitamin A, $\mu g/d^a$	Vitamin C, mg/d	Vitamin D, $\mu g/d^{b,c}$	Vitamin E, mg/d^d	Vitamin K, $\mu g/d$	Thiamine, mg/d	Riboflavin, mg/d	Niacin, mg/d^e	Vitamin B_6, mg/d	Folate, $\mu g/d^f$	Vitamin B_{12}, $\mu g/d$	Pantothenic Acid, mg/d	Biotin, $\mu g/d$	Choline, mg/d^g
Infants														
0–6 mo	400	40	5	4	2.0	0.2	0.3	2	0.1	65	0.4	1.7	5	125
7–12 mo	500	50	5	5	2.5	0.3	0.4	4	0.3	80	0.5	1.8	6	150
Children														
1–3 y	**300**	**15**	5	**6**	30	**0.5**	**0.5**	**6**	**0.5**	**150**	**0.9**	2	8	200
4–8 y	**400**	**25**	5	**7**	55	**0.6**	**0.6**	**8**	**0.6**	**200**	**1.2**	3	12	250
Males														
9–13 y	**600**	**45**	5	**11**	60	**0.9**	**0.9**	**12**	**1.0**	**300**	**1.8**	4	20	375
14–18 y	**900**	**75**	5	**15**	75	**1.2**	**1.3**	**16**	**1.3**	**400**	**2.4**	5	25	550
19–30 y	**900**	**90**	5	**15**	120	**1.2**	**1.3**	**16**	**1.3**	**400**	**2.4**	5	30	550
31–50 y	**900**	**90**	5	**15**	120	**1.2**	**1.3**	**16**	**1.3**	**400**	**2.4**	5	30	550
51–70 y	**900**	**90**	10	**15**	120	**1.2**	**1.3**	**16**	**1.7**	**400**	**2.4**[h]	5	30	550
>70 y	**900**	**90**	15	**15**	120	**1.2**	**1.3**	**16**	**1.7**	**400**	**2.4**[h]	5	30	550
Females														
9–13 y	**600**	**45**	5	**11**	60	**0.9**	**0.9**	**12**	**1.0**	**300**	**1.8**	4	20	375
14–18 y	**700**	**65**	5	**15**	75	**1.0**	**1.0**	**14**	**1.2**	**400**[i]	**2.4**	5	25	400
19–30 y	**700**	**75**	5	**15**	90	**1.1**	**1.1**	**14**	**1.3**	**400**[i]	**2.4**	5	30	425
31–50 y	**700**	**75**	5	**15**	90	**1.1**	**1.1**	**14**	**1.3**	**400**[i]	**2.4**	5	30	425
51–70 y	**700**	**75**	10	**15**	90	**1.1**	**1.1**	**14**	**1.5**	**400**	**2.4**[h]	5	30	425
>70 y	**700**	**75**	15	**15**	90	**1.1**	**1.1**	**14**	**1.5**	**400**	**2.4**[h]	5	30	425
Pregnancy														
≤18 y	**750**	**80**	5	**15**	75	**1.4**	**1.4**	**18**	**1.6**	**600**[i]	**2.6**	6	30	450
19–30 y	**770**	**85**	5	**15**	90	**1.4**	**1.4**	**18**	**1.9**	**600**[i]	**2.6**	6	30	450
31–50 y	**770**	**85**	5	**15**	90	**1.4**	**1.4**	**18**	**1.9**	**600**[i]	**2.6**	6	30	450
Lactation														
≤18 y	**1200**	**115**	5	**19**	75	**1.4**	**1.6**	**17**	**2.0**	**500**	**2.8**	7	35	550
19–30 y	**1300**	**120**	5	**19**	90	**1.4**	**1.6**	**17**	**2.0**	**500**	**2.8**	7	35	550
31–50 y	**1300**	**120**	5	**19**	90	**1.4**	**1.6**	**17**	**2.0**	**500**	**2.8**	7	35	550

Note: This table presents recommended dietary allowances (RDAs) in **bold type** and adequate intakes (AIs) in ordinary type. RDAs and AIs may both be used as goals for individual intake. RDAs are set to meet the needs of almost all individuals (97 to 98%) in a group. For healthy breastfed infants, the AI is the mean intake. The AI for other life stage and gender groups is believed to cover needs of all individuals in the group, but lack of data or uncertainty in the data prevent being able to specify with confidence the percentage of individuals covered by this intake.

[a] As retinol activity equivalents (RAEs). 1 RAE = 1 μg retinol, 12 μg β-carotene, 24 μg α-carotene, or 24 μg β-cryptoxanthin. To calculate RAEs from retinol equivalents (REs) of provitamin A carotenoids in foods, divide the REs by 2. For preformed vitamin A in foods or supplements and for provitamin A carotenoids in supplements, 1 RE = 1 RAE.

[b] As calciferol. 1 μg calciferol = 40 IU vitamin D.

[c] In the absence of adequate exposure to sunlight.

[d] As α-tocopherol. α-Tocopherol includes *RRR*-α-tocopherol, the only form of α-tocopherol that occurs naturally in foods, and the *2R*-stereoisomeric forms of α-tocopherol (*RRR*-, *RSR*-, *RRS*-, and *RSS*-α-tocopherol) that occur in fortified foods and supplements. It does not include the *2S*-stereoisomeric forms of α-tocopherol (*SRR*-, *SSR*-, *SRS*-, and *SSS*-α-tocopherol), also found in fortified foods and supplements.

[e] As niacin equivalents (NE). 1 mg of niacin = 60 mg of tryptophan; 0–6 months = preformed niacin (not NE).

[f] As dietary folate equivalents (DFEs). 1 DFE = 1 μg food folate = 0.6 μg of folic acid from fortified food or as a supplement consumed with food = 0.5 μg of a supplement taken on an empty stomach.

[g] Although AIs have been set for choline, there are few data to assess whether a dietary supply of choline is needed at all stages of the life cycle, and it may be that the choline requirement can be met by endogenous synthesis at some of these stages.

[h] Because 10 to 30% of older people may malabsorb food-bound B_{12}, it is advisable for those >50 years to meet their RDA mainly by consuming foods fortified with B_{12} or a supplement containing B_{12}.

[i] In view of evidence linking inadequate folate intake with neural tube defects in the fetus, it is recommended that all women capable of becoming pregnant consume 400 μg from supplements or fortified foods in addition to intake of food folate from a varied diet.

[j] It is assumed that women will continue consuming 400 μg from supplements or fortified food until their pregnancy is confirmed and they enter prenatal care, which ordinarily occurs after the end of the periconceptional period—the critical time for formation of the neural tube.

Source: Food and Nutrition Board, Institute of Medicine—National Academy of Sciences Dietary Reference Intakes, 2000, 2002, reprinted with permission. Courtesy of the National Academy Press, Washington, DC. www.nap.edu

Life-Stage Group	Calcium, mg/d[a]	Chromium, μg/d	Copper, μg/d	Fluoride, mg/d	Iodine, μg/d	Iron, mg/d	Magnesium, mg/d	Manganese, mg/d	Molybdenum, μg/d	Phosphorus, mg/d	Selenium, μg/d	Zinc, mg/d
Infants												
0–6 mo	210	0.2	200	0.01	110	0.27	30	0.003	2	100	15	2
7–12 mo	270	5.5	220	0.5	130	**11**	75	0.6	3	275	20	**3**
Children												
1–3 y	500	11	**340**	0.7	**90**	**7**	**80**	1.2	**17**	**460**	**20**	**3**
4–8 y	800	15	**440**	1	**90**	**10**	**130**	1.5	**22**	**500**	**30**	**5**
Males												
9–13 y	1300	25	**700**	2	**120**	**8**	**240**	1.9	**34**	**1250**	**40**	**8**
14–18 y	1300	35	**890**	3	**150**	**11**	**410**	2.2	**43**	**1250**	**55**	**11**
19–30 y	1000	35	**900**	4	**150**	**8**	**400**	2.3	**45**	**700**	**55**	**11**
31–50 y	1000	35	**900**	4	**150**	**8**	**420**	2.3	**45**	**700**	**55**	**11**
51–70 y	1200	30	**900**	4	**150**	**8**	**420**	2.3	**45**	**700**	**55**	**11**
>70 y	1200	30	**900**	4	**150**	**8**	**420**	2.3	**45**	**700**	**55**	**11**
Females												
9–13 y	1300	21	**700**	2	**120**	**8**	**240**	1.6	**34**	**1250**	**40**	**8**
14–18 y	1300	24	**890**	3	**150**	**15**	**360**	1.6	**43**	**1250**	**55**	**9**
19–30 y	1000	25	**900**	3	**150**	**18**	**310**	1.8	**45**	**700**	**55**	**8**
31–50 y	1000	25	**900**	3	**150**	**18**	**320**	1.8	**45**	**700**	**55**	**8**
51–70 y	1200	20	**900**	3	**150**	**8**	**320**	1.8	**45**	**700**	**55**	**8**
>70 y	1200	20	**900**	3	**150**	**8**	**320**	1.8	**45**	**700**	**55**	**8**
Pregnancy												
≤18 y	1300	29	**1000**	3	**220**	**27**	**400**	2.0	**50**	**1250**	**60**	**12**
19–30 y	1000	30	**1000**	3	**220**	**27**	**350**	2.0	**50**	**700**	**60**	**11**
31–50 y	1000	30	**1000**	3	**220**	**27**	**360**	2.0	**50**	**700**	**60**	**11**
Lactation												
≤18 y	1300	44	**1300**	3	**290**	**10**	**360**	2.6	**50**	**1250**	**70**	**13**
19–30 y	1000	45	**1300**	3	**290**	**9**	**310**	2.6	**50**	**700**	**70**	**12**
31–50 y	1000	45	**1300**	3	**290**	**9**	**320**	2.6	**50**	**700**	**70**	**12**

Note: This table presents recommended dietary allowances (RDAs) in **bold type** and adequate intakes (AIs) in ordinary type. RDAs and AIs may both be used as goals for individual intake. RDAs are set to meet the needs of almost all individuals (97 to 98%) in a group. For healthy breastfed infants, the AI is the mean intake. The AI for other life stage and gender groups is believed to cover needs of all individuals in the group, but lack of data or uncertainty in the data prevent being able to specify with confidence the percentage of individuals covered by this intake.

Source: Food and Nutrition Board, Institute of Medicine—National Academy of Sciences Dietary Reference Intakes, 2000, 2002, reprinted with permission. Courtesy of the National Academy Press, Washington, DC. www.nap.edu

that, for an adult, represents the highest RDA for an adult consuming 2000 kcal/d.

The risk of dietary inadequacy increases as intake falls further below the RDA. However, the RDA is an overly generous criterion for evaluating nutrient adequacy. For example, by definition the RDA exceeds the actual requirements of all but about 2 to 3% of the population. Therefore, many people whose intake falls below the RDA may still be getting enough of the nutrient.

ADEQUATE INTAKE It is not possible to set an RDA for some nutrients that do not have an established EAR. In this circumstance, the AI is based on observed, or experimentally determined, approximations of nutrient intakes in healthy people. In the DRIs established to date, AIs rather than RDAs are proposed for infants up to age 1 year, as well as for calcium, chromium, vitamin D, fluoride, manganese, pantothenic acid, biotin, and choline for persons of all ages.

TOLERABLE UPPER LEVELS OF NUTRIENT INTAKE Excessive nutrient intake can disturb body functions and cause acute, progressive, or permanent disabilities. The tolerable UL is the highest level of chronic nutrient intake (usually daily) that is unlikely to pose a risk of adverse health effects for most of the population. Data on the adverse effects of large amounts of many nutrients are unavailable or too limited to establish a UL. Therefore, the lack of a UL does *not* mean that the risk of adverse effects from high intake is nonexistent. Healthy individuals derive no established benefit from consuming nutrient levels above the RDA or AI. Individual nutrients in foods that most people eat rarely reach levels that exceed the UL. However, nutritional supplements provide more concentrated amounts of nutrients per dose and, as a result, pose a potential risk of toxicity. Nutrient supplements are labeled with "supplement facts" that express the amount of nutrient in absolute units or as the percent of the DV provided per recommended serving size. Total nutrient consumption, including both food and supplements, should not exceed RDA levels.

FACTORS ALTERING NUTRIENT NEEDS

The DRIs are affected by age, sex, rate of growth, pregnancy, lactation, physical activity, composition of diet, concomitant diseases, and drugs. When only slight differences exist between the requirements for nutrient sufficiency and excess, dietary planning becomes more difficult.

PHYSIOLOGIC FACTORS Growth, strenuous physical activity, pregnancy, and lactation increase needs for energy and several essential nutrients. Energy needs rise during pregnancy, due to the demands of fetal growth, and during lactation, because of the increased energy required for milk production. Energy needs decrease with loss of lean body mass, the major determinant of REE. Because both health and physical activity tend to decline with age, energy needs in older persons, especially those over 70, tend to be less than those of younger persons.

DIETARY COMPOSITION Dietary composition affects the biologic availability and utilization of nutrients. For example, the absorption of iron may be impaired by high amounts of calcium or lead; non-heme iron uptake may be impaired by the lack of ascorbic acid and amino acids in the meal. Protein utilization by the body may be decreased when essential amino acids are not present in sufficient amounts. Animal foods, such as milk, eggs, and meat, have high biologic values with most of the needed amino acids present in adequate amounts. Plant proteins in corn (maize), soy, and wheat have lower biologic values and must be combined with other plant or animal proteins to achieve optimal utilization by the body.

ROUTE OF ADMINISTRATION The RDAs apply only to oral intakes. When nutrients are administered parenterally, similar values can sometimes be used for amino acids, carbohydrates, fats, sodium, chloride, potassium, and most of the vitamins, since their intestinal absorption is nearly 100%. However, the oral bioavailability of most mineral elements may be only half that obtained by parenteral administration. For

TABLE 60-3 *The USDA Food Guide Pyramid for Healthy Persons*

Servings and Examples of Standard Portion Sizes	Lower: 1600 kcal	Moderate: ~2200 kcal	Higher: ~2800 kcal
Bread group			
1 slice bread; 1 oz. ready-to-eat cereal; ½ cup cooked cereal, rice, or pasta	6	9	22
Vegetable group			
1 cup raw leafy vegetables; ½ cup other vegetables, cooked or chopped raw; ¾ cup vegetable juice	3	4	5
Fruit group			
1 medium banana, apple, or orange; ½ cup chopped, cooked, or canned fruit; ¾ cup fruit juice	2	3	4
Milk group			
1 cup milk or yogurt, 1.5 oz natural cheese, 1 oz processed cheese	2–3[a]	2–3[a]	1–3[a]
Meat group			
2–3 oz cooked lean meat, poultry or fish; ½ cup cooked dry beans; 1 egg or 2 Tbsp. peanut butter count as 1 oz lean meat	5	5	7
Total fat, g	53	73	93
Total added sugars, tsp	6	12	18

[a] Women who are pregnant or breastfeeding, teenagers, and young adults to age 24 need 3 servings.
Source: US Department of Agriculture, Human Nutrition Information Service. *The Food Guide Pyramid*, Home and Garden Bulletin Number 252, US Department of Agriculture, Washington DC, August 1992.

some nutrients that are not readily stored in the body, or cannot be stored in large amounts, timing of administration may also be important. For example, amino acids cannot be used for protein synthesis if they are not supplied together; instead they will be used for energy production.

DISEASE Specific dietary deficiency diseases include protein-calorie malnutrition; iron, iodine, and vitamin A deficiency; megaloblastic anemia due to vitamin B_{12} or folic acid deficiency; vitamin D–deficiency rickets; and scurvy, beriberi, and pellagra (Chaps. 61 and 62). Each deficiency disease is characterized by imbalances at the cellular level between the supply of nutrients or energy and the body's nutritional needs for growth, maintenance, and other functions. Imbalances in nutrient intakes are recognized as risk factors for certain chronic degenerative diseases, such as saturated fat and cholesterol in coronary artery disease; sodium in hypertension; obesity in hormone-dependent endometrial and breast cancers; and ethanol in alcoholism. Since the etiology and pathogenesis of these disorders are multifactorial, diet is only one of many risk factors. Osteoporosis, for example, is associated with calcium deficiency, as well as risk factors related to environment (e.g., smoking, sedentary lifestyle), physiology (e.g., estrogen deficiency), genetic determinants (e.g., defects in collagen metabolism), and drug use (chronic steroids) (Chap. 333).

DIETARY ASSESSMENT

In clinical situations, nutritional assessment is an iterative process that involves: (1) screening for malnutrition, (2) assessing the diet and other data to establish either the absence or presence of malnutrition and its possible causes, and (3) planning for the most appropriate nutritional therapy. Some disease states affect the bioavailability, requirements, utilization, or excretion of specific nutrients. In these circumstances, specific measurements of various nutrients may be required to ensure adequate replacement (Chap. 62).

Most health care facilities have a nutrition screening process in place for identifying possible malnutrition after hospital admission. Nutritional screening is required by the Joint Commission on Accreditation of Healthcare Organizations (JCAHO), but there are no universally recognized or validated standards. The factors that are usually assessed include abnormal weight for height or body mass index (e.g., BMI <19 or >25); reported weight change (involuntary loss or gain of >5 kg in the past 6 months) (Chap. 36); diagnoses with known nutritional implications (metabolic disease, any disease affecting the gastrointestinal tract, alcoholism, and others); present therapeutic dietary prescription; chronic poor appetite; presence of chewing and swallowing problems or major food intolerances; need for assistance with preparing or shopping for food, eating, or other aspects of self care; and social isolation. Reassessment of nutrition status should occur periodically in hospitalized patients—at least once every week.

A more complete dietary assessment is indicated for patients who exhibit a high risk of malnutrition on nutrition screening. The type of assessment varies based on the clinical setting, severity of the patient's illness, and stability of his or her condition.

ACUTE CARE SETTINGS In acute care settings, anorexia, various diseases, test procedures, and medications can compromise dietary intake. Under such circumstances, the goal is to identify and avoid inadequate intake and assure appropriate alimentation. Dietary assessment focuses on what patients are currently eating, whether they are able and willing to eat, and whether they experience any problems with eating. Dietary intake assessment is based on information from observed intakes; medical record; history; clinical examination; and anthropometric, biochemical, and functional status. The objective is to gather enough information to establish the likelihood of malnutrition due to poor dietary intake or other causes to assess whether nutritional therapy is indicated.

Simple observations may suffice to suggest inadequate oral intake. These include dietitians' and nurses' notes, the amount of food eaten on trays, frequent tests and procedures that are likely to cause meals to be skipped, nutritionally inadequate diet orders such as clear liquids or full liquids for more than a few days, fever, gastrointestinal distress, vomiting, diarrhea, a comatose state, and diseases or treatments that involve any part of the alimentary tract. Acutely ill patients with diet-related diseases such as diabetes need assessment because an inappropriate diet may exacerbate these conditions and adversely affect other therapies. Abnormal biochemical values [serum albumin levels <35 g/L (<3.5 mg/dL); serum cholesterol levels <3.9 mmol/L (<150 mg/dL)] are nonspecific but may also indicate a need for further nutritional assessment.

Most therapeutic diets offered in hospitals are calculated to meet individual nutrient requirements and the RDA. Exceptions include clear liquids, some full liquid diets, and test diets, which are inadequate for several nutrients and should not be used, if possible, for more than 24 h. As much as half of the food served to hospitalized patients is not eaten, and so it cannot be assumed that the intakes of hospitalized patients are adequate. Dietary assessment should compare how much and what food the patient has consumed with the diet that has been provided. Major deviations in intakes of energy, protein, fluids, or other nutrients of special concern for the patient's illness should be noted and corrected.

Nutritional monitoring is especially important for patients who are very ill and who have extended lengths of stay. Patients who are fed by special enteral and parenteral routes also require special nutritional assessment and monitoring by physicians with training in nutrition support and/or dietitians with certification in nutrition support (Chap. 63).

AMBULATORY SETTINGS The aim of dietary assessment in the outpatient setting is to determine whether the patient's usual diet is a health risk in itself or if it contributes to existing chronic disease-related problems. Dietary assessment also provides the basis for planning a diet that fulfills therapeutic goals while ensuring patient adherence. The outpatient dietary assessment should review the adequacy of present and usual food intakes, including vitamin and mineral supplements, medications, and alcohol, as all of these may affect the patient's nutritional status. The assessment should focus on the dietary constituents that are most likely to be involved or compromised by a specific diagnosis, as well as any comorbidities that are present. More than one day's intake should be reviewed to provide a better representation of the usual diet.

There are many ways to assess the adequacy of the patient's habitual diet. These include a food guide, a food exchange list, a diet history, or a food frequency questionnaire. A commonly used food guide for healthy persons is the USDA's food pyramid, which is useful as a basis for identifying inadequate intakes of essential nutrients, as well as likely excesses in fat, saturated fat, sodium, sugar, and alcohol (Table 60-3). The guide can be adjusted by varying the number of servings to provide for the needs of persons of different ages and life cycle stages. Those who follow ethnic or unusual dietary patterns may need extra instruction on how foods should be categorized, as well as the appropriate portion sizes that constitute a serving. The process of reviewing the guide with patients helps them transition to healthier dietary patterns and identifies food groups eaten in excess of recommendations or in insufficient quantities. For those on therapeutic diets, assessment against food exchange lists may be useful. These include, for example, the American Diabetes Association food exchange lists for diabetes, or the American Dietetic Association food exchange lists for renal disease.

NUTRITIONAL STATUS ASSESSMENT Full nutritional status assessment is reserved for seriously ill patients and those at very high nutritional risk when the cause of malnutrition is still uncertain after initial clinical evaluation and dietary assessment. It involves multiple dimensions, including documentation of dietary intake, anthropometric measurements, biochemical measurements of blood and urine, clinical examination, health history, and functional status. →*For further discussion of nutritional assessment, see Chap. 62.*

FURTHER READING

OWEN OE et al: A reappraisal of the caloric requirements of men. Am J Clin Nutr 46:875, 1987
——: A reappraisal of caloric requirements in healthy women. Am J Clin Nutr 44:1, 1986
STANDING COMMITTEE ON THE SCIENTIFIC EVALUATION OF DIETARY REFERENCE INTAKES, FOOD AND NUTRITION BOARD, INSTITUTE OF MEDICINE: *Dietary Reference Intakes for Vitamin A, Vitamin K, Arsenic, Boron, Chromium, Copper, Iodine, Iron, Manganese, Molybdenum, Nickel, Silicon, Vanadium, and Zinc.* Washington, National Academy Press, 2001
——: *Dietary Reference Intakes: Applications in Dietary Assessment.* Washington, National Academy Press, 2000
——: *Dietary Reference Intakes for Calcium, Phosphorus, Magnesium, Vitamin D, and Fluoride.* Washington, National Academy Press, 1997

61 VITAMIN AND TRACE MINERAL DEFICIENCY AND EXCESS
Robert M. Russell

Vitamins and trace minerals are required constituents of the human diet since they are either inadequately synthesized or not synthesized in the human body. Only small amounts of these substances are needed for carrying out essential biochemical reactions (e.g., acting as coenzymes or prosthetic groups). Overt vitamin or trace mineral deficiencies are rare in western countries due to a plentiful, varied, and inexpensive food supply; however, multiple nutrient deficiencies may appear together in persons who are ill or alcoholic. Moreover, subclinical vitamin and trace mineral deficiencies, as diagnosed by laboratory testing, are quite common in the normal population—especially in the geriatric age group.

Body stores of vitamins and minerals vary tremendously. For example, vitamin B_{12} and vitamin A stores are large, and an adult may not become deficient for 1 or more years after being on a depleted diet. However, folate and thiamine may become depleted within weeks when eating a deficient diet. Therapeutic modalities can deplete essential nutrients from the body; for example, hemodialysis removes water-soluble vitamins, which must be replaced by supplementation.

There are several roles for vitamins and trace minerals in diseases: (1) deficiencies of vitamins and minerals may be caused by disease states such as malabsorption; (2) both deficiency and excess of vitamins and minerals can cause disease in and of themselves (e.g., vitamin A intoxication and liver disease); and (3) vitamins and minerals in high doses may be used as drugs (e.g., niacin for hypercholesterolemia). The hematologic-related vitamins and minerals (Chaps. 90, 92) are considered only briefly in this chapter, as are the bone-related vitamins and minerals (vitamin D, calcium, phosphorus; Chap. 331), since they are covered elsewhere (see Tables 61-1, 61-2, and Fig. 61-1).

VITAMINS

THIAMINE (VITAMIN B₁)

Thiamine was the first B vitamin to be identified and is therefore also referred to as vitamin B_1. Thiamine functions in the decarboxylation of α-ketoacids, such as pyruvate α-ketoglutarate, and branched-chain amino acids and thus is a source of energy generation. In addition, thiamine pyrophosphate acts as a coenzyme for a transketolase reaction that mediates the conversion of hexose and pentose phosphates. It has also been postulated that thiamine plays a role in peripheral nerve conduction, although the exact chemical reactions underlying this function are unknown.

FOOD SOURCES The median intake of thiamine in the United States from food alone is 2 mg/d. Primary food sources for thiamine include yeast, pork, legumes, beef, whole grains, and nuts. Milled and polished rice contain little thiamine, if any. Thiamine deficiency is therefore more common in cultures that rely heavily on a rice-based diet. Tea, coffee (caffeinated and decaffeinated), raw fish, and shellfish contain thiamineases, which can destroy the vitamin. Thus, drinking large amounts of tea or coffee can theoretically lower thiamine body stores.

DEFICIENCY Most dietary deficiency of thiamine worldwide is the result of poor dietary intake. In western countries, the primary causes of thiamine deficiency are alcoholism and chronic illness, such as cancer. Alcohol is known to interfere directly with the absorption of thiamine and with the synthesis of thiamine pyrophosphate. Thiamine should always be replenished when refeeding a patient with alcoholism, as carbohydrate repletion without adequate thiamine can precipitate acute thiamine deficiency.

Thiamine deficiency in its early stage induces anorexia and nonspecific symptoms (e.g., irritability). Prolonged thiamine deficiency causes beriberi, which is classically categorized as wet or dry, although there is considerable overlap. In either form of beriberi, patients may complain of pain and parathesia. *Wet beriberi* presents primarily with cardiovascular symptoms, due to impaired myocardial energy metabolism and dysautonomia, and can occur after 3 months of a thiamine-deficient diet. Patients present with an enlarged heart, tachycardia, high-output congestive heart failure, peripheral edema, and peripheral neuritis. Patients with *dry beriberi* present with a symmetric peripheral neuropathy of the motor and sensory systems with diminished reflexes. The neuropathy affects the legs most markedly, and patients have difficulty rising from a squatting position.

Alcoholic patients with chronic thiamine deficiency may also have central nervous system manifestations known as *Wernicke's enceph-*

TABLE 61-1 *Principal Clinical Findings of Vitamin Malnutrition*

Nutrient	Clinical Finding	Dietary Level per Day Associated with Overt Deficiency in Adults	Contributing Factors to Deficiency
Thiamine	Beriberi: neuropathy, muscle weakness and wasting, cardiomegaly, edema, ophthalmoplegia, confabulation	<0.3 mg/1000 kcal	Alcoholism
Riboflavin	Magenta tongue, angular stomatitis, seborrhea, cheilosis	<0.6 mg	—
Niacin	Pellagra: pigmented rash of sun-exposed areas, bright red tongue, diarrhea, apathy, memory loss, disorientation	<9.0 niacin equivalents	Alcoholism, vitamin B_6 deficiency, riboflavin deficiency
Vitamin B_6	Seborrhea, glossitis convulsions, neuropathy, depression, confusion, microcytic anemia	<0.2 mg	Alcoholism, isoniazid
Folate	Megaloblastic anemia, atrophic glossitis, depression, ↑ homocysteine,	<100 μg/d	Alcoholism, sulfasalazine, pyrimethamine, triamterene
Vitamin B_{12}	Megaloblastic anemia, loss of vibratory and position sense, abnormal gait, dementia, impotence, loss of bladder and bowel control, ↑ homocysteine, ↑ methylmalonic acid	<1.0 μg/d	Gastric atrophy (pernicious anemia), terminal ileal disease, strict vegetarianism
Vitamin C	Scurvy: petechiae, ecchymosis, coiled hairs, inflamed and bleeding gums, joint effusion, poor wound healing	<10 mg/d	Smoking, alcoholism
Vitamin A	Xerophthalmia, nightblindness, Bitôt spots, follicular hyperkeratosis, impaired embryonic development, immune dysfunction	<300 μg/d	Fat malabsorption, infection, measles, alcoholism, protein-energy malnutrition
Vitamin D	Rickets: skeletal deformation, rachitic rosary, bowed legs; osteomalacia	<2.0 μg/d	Aging, lack of sunlight exposure, fat malabsorption
Vitamin E	Peripheral neuropathy, spinocerebellar ataxia, skeletal muscle atrophy, retinopathy	Not described unless underlying contributing factor is present	Occurs only with fat malabsorption, or genetic abnormalities of vitamin E metabolism/transport
Vitamin K	Elevated prothrombin time, bleeding	<10 μg/d	Fat malabsorption, liver disease, antibiotic use

alopathy, consisting of horizontal nystagmus, ophthalmoplegia (due to weakness of one or more extraocular muscles), cerebellar ataxia, and mental impairment (Chap. 372). When there is an additional loss of memory and a confabulatory psychosis, the syndrome is known as *Wernicke-Korsakoff syndrome*.

The laboratory diagnosis of thiamine deficiency is usually made by a functional enzymatic assay of transketolase activity measured before and after the addition of thiamine pyrophosphate. A >25% stimulation by the addition of thiamine pyrophosphate (an activity coefficient of 1.25) is taken as abnormal. Thiamine or the phosphorylated esters of thiamine in serum or blood can also be measured by high-performance liquid chromatography (HPLC) to detect deficiency.

℞ **TREATMENT**

In acute thiamine deficiency with either cardiovascular or neurologic signs, 100 mg/d of thiamine should be given parenterally for 7 days, followed by 10 mg/d orally until there is complete recovery. Cardiovascular improvement occurs in ≤12 h, and ophthalmoplegic improvement occurs within 24 h. Other manifestations gradually clear, although psychosis in the Wernicke-Korsakoff syndrome may be permanent or persist for several months.

TOXICITY Although anaphylaxis has been reported after high doses of thiamine, no adverse effects have been recorded from either food or supplements at high doses. Thiamine supplements may be bought over the counter in doses of up to 50 mg/d.

RIBOFLAVIN (VITAMIN B_2)

Riboflavin is important for the metabolism of fat, carbohydrate, and protein, reflecting its role as a respiratory coenzyme and an electron donor. Enzymes that contain flavin adenine dinucleotide (FAD) or flavin-mononucleotide (FMN) as prosthetic groups are known as *flavoenzymes* (e.g., succinic acid dehydrogenase, monoamine oxidase, glutathione reductase).

Although much is known about the chemical and enzymatic reactions of riboflavin, the clinical manifestations of riboflavin deficiency are nonspecific and similar to those of other B vitamin deficiencies.

Riboflavin deficiency is manifested principally by lesions of the mucocutaneous surfaces of the mouth and skin (Table 61-1). In addition to the mucocutaneous lesions, corneal vascularization, anemia, and personality changes have been described with riboflavin deficiency.

DEFICIENCY AND EXCESS Riboflavin deficiency is almost always due to dietary deficiency. Milk, other dairy products, and enriched breads and cereals are the most important dietary sources of riboflavin in the United States, although lean meat, fish, eggs, broccoli, and legumes are also good sources. Riboflavin is extremely sensitive to light, and milk should be stored in containers that protect against photodegradation. Laboratory diagnosis of riboflavin deficiency can be made by measurement of red blood cell or urinary riboflavin concentrations or by measurement of erythrocyte glutathione reductase activity, with and without added FAD. Because the capacity of the gastrointestinal tract to absorb riboflavin is limited (~20 mg if given in one oral dose), riboflavin toxicity has not been described.

NIACIN (VITAMIN B_3)

The term *niacin* refers to nicotinic acid and nicotinamide and their biologically active derivatives. Nicotinic acid and nicotinamide serve as precursors of two coenzymes, nicotinamide adenine dinucleotide (NAD) and NAD phosphate (NADP), which are important in numerous oxidation and reduction reactions in the body. In addition, NAD and NADP are active in adenine diphosphate–ribose transfer reactions involved in DNA repair and calcium mobilization.

METABOLISM AND REQUIREMENTS Nicotinic acid and nicotinamide are absorbed well from the stomach and small intestine. Niacin bioavailability is high from beans, milk, meat, and eggs; bioavailability from cereal grains is lower. Since flour is enriched with the "free" niacin (i.e., non-coenzyme form), bioavailability is excellent. Median intakes of niacin in the United States considerably exceed the recommended dietary allowance (RDA).

The amino acid tryptophan can be converted to niacin with an efficiency of 60:1 by weight. Thus, the RDA for niacin is expressed in niacin equivalents. A lower conversion of tryptophan to niacin occurs if a patient is vitamin B_6- or riboflavin-deficient or in the presence of isoniazid. The urinary excretion products of niacin include 2-pyridone and 2-methyl nicotinamide, measurements of which are used in diagnosis of niacin deficiency.

DEFICIENCY Niacin deficiency causes *pellagra*, which is mostly found among people eating corn-based diets in parts of China, Africa, and India. Pellagra in North America is found mainly among alcoholics; in patients with congenital defects of intestinal and kidney absorption of tryptophan (Hartnup's disease; Chap. 343); and in patients with carcinoid syndrome (Chap. 329), where there is increased conversion of tryptophan to serotonin. The early symptoms of pellagra include loss of appetite, generalized weakness and irritability, abdominal pain, and vomiting. Bright-red glossitis then ensues, followed by a characteristic skin rash that is pigmented and scaling, particularly in skin areas exposed to sunlight. This rash is known as "Casal's necklace" because it forms a ring around the neck; it is seen in advanced cases. Vaginitis and esophagitis may also occur. Diarrhea (in part due to proctitis and in part due to malabsorption), depression, seizures, and dementia are also part of the pellagra syndrome—the four D's: *d*ermatitis, *di*arrhea, and *d*ementia leading to *d*eath.

Treatment of pellagra consists of oral supplementation of 100 to 200 mg of nicotinamide or nicotinic acid three times daily for 5 days. High doses of nicotinic acid (≥ 3 g nicotinic acid per day) are used for the treatment of elevated cholesterol levels and in the treatment of types 2, 4, and 5 hyperlipidemias (Chap. 335).

TOXICITY Prostaglandin-mediated flushing has been observed at daily doses as low as 50 mg of niacin when taken as a supplement or as therapy for hypertriglyceridemia. There is no evidence of toxicity from niacin derived from food sources. Flushing may be accompanied by skin dryness, itching, and headache. Premedication with aspirin may alleviate these symptoms. Nausea, vomiting, and abdominal pain also occur at similar doses of niacin. Hepatic toxicity is the most serious toxic reaction due to niacin and may present as jaundice with elevated aspartate aminotransferase (AST) and alanine aminotranferase (ALT) levels. A few cases of fulminant hepatitis requiring liver transplantation have been reported at doses of 3 to 9 g/d. Other toxic reactions include glucose intolerance, macular edema, and macular cysts. The upper limit for daily niacin intake has been set at 35 mg. However, this upper limit does not pertain to the therapeutic use of niacin.

PYRIDOXINE (VITAMIN B₆)

Vitamin B_6 refers to a family of compounds including pyridoxine, pyridoxal, pyridoxamine, and their 5′-phosphate derivatives. 5′-Pyridoxal phosphate (PLP) is a cofactor for more than 100 enzymes involved in amino acid metabolism. Vitamin B_6 is also involved in heme and neurotransmitter synthesis and in the metabolism of glycogen, lipids, steroids, sphingoid bases, and several vitamins, including the conversion of tryptophan to niacin.

DIETARY SOURCES Plants contain vitamin B_6 in the form of pyridoxine, whereas animal tissues contain PLP and pyridoxamine phosphate. The

Vitamin	Active derivative or cofactor form	Principal function
Thiamine (B₁)	Thiamine pyrophosphate	Coenzyme for cleavage of carbon-carbon bonds; amino acid and carbohydrate metabolism
Riboflavin (B₂)	Flavin mononucleotide (FMN) and flavin adenine dinucleotide (FAD)	Cofactor for oxidation, reduction reactions, and covalently attached prosthetic groups for some enzymes
Niacin 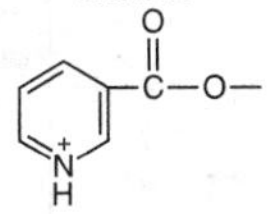	Nicotinamide adenine dinucleotide phosphate (NADP) and nicotinamide adenine dinucleotide (NAD)	Coenzymes for oxidation and reduction reactions
Vitamin B₆	Pyridoxal phosphate	Cofactor for enzymes of amino acid metabolism
Folate 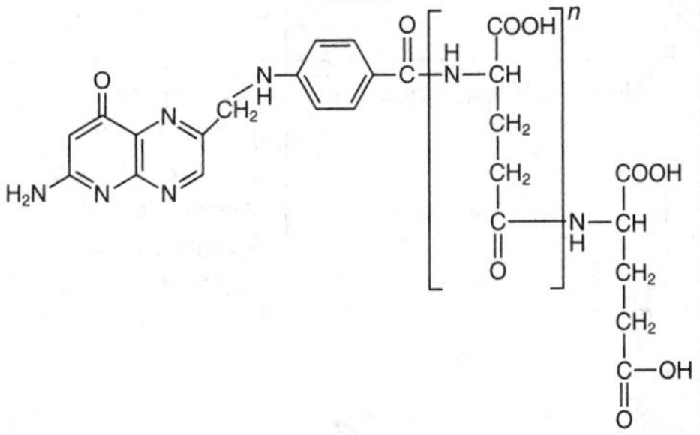	Polyglutamate forms of (5, 6, 7, 8) tetrahydrofolate with carbon unit attachments	Coenzyme for one carbon transfer in nucleic acid and amino acid metabolism
Vitamin B₁₂	Methylcobalamine Adenosylcobalamin	Coenzyme for methionine synthase and L-methylmalonyl-CoA mutase

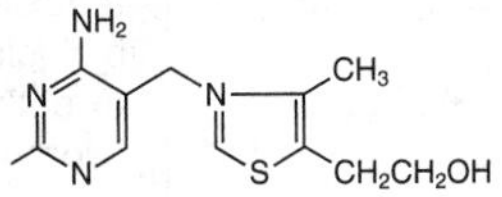

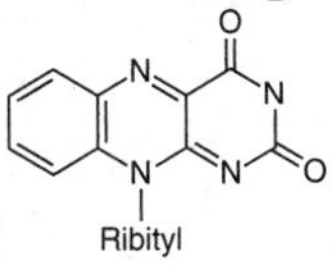

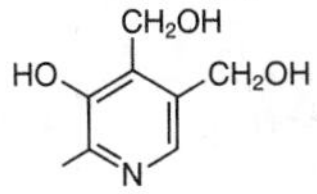

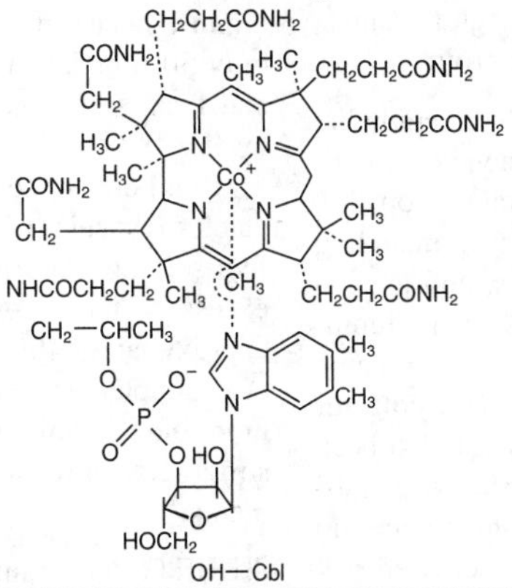

FIGURE 61-1 The structures and principal functions of vitamins associated with human disorders.

405

Vitamin	Active derivative or cofactor form	Principal function
Vitamin C 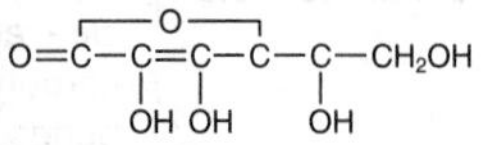 O=C—C=C—C—C—CH₂OH OH OH OH	Ascorbic acid and dehydrascorbic acid	Participation as a redox ion in many biological oxidation and hydrogen transfer reactions
Vitamin A 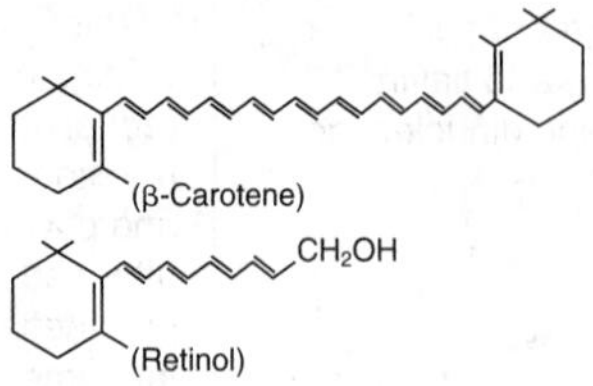 (β-Carotene) CH₂OH (Retinol)	Retinol, retinaldehyde, and retinoic acid	Formation of rhodopsin (vision) and glycoproteins (epithelial cell function); also regulates gene transcription
Vitamin D 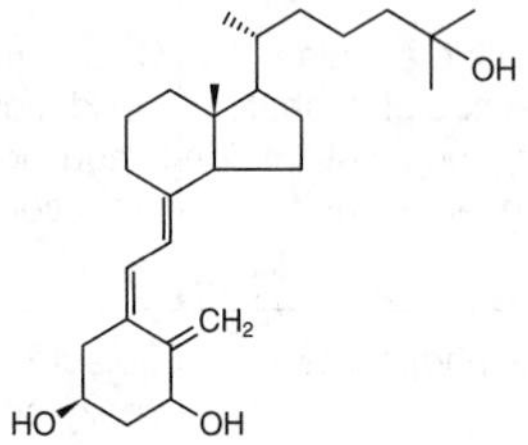 OH CH₂ HO OH	1, 25-Dihyroxy vitamin	Maintenance of blood calcium and phosphorous levels; antiproliferative hormone
Vitamin E 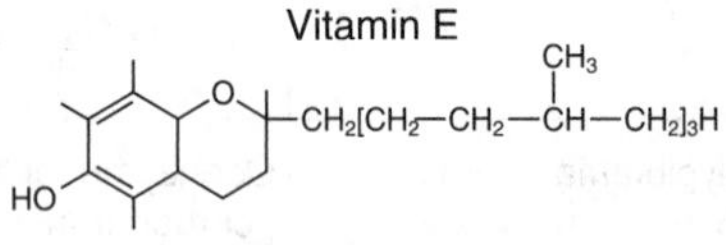 CH₃ CH₂[CH₂—CH₂—CH—CH₂]₃H HO	Tocopherols and tocotrienols	Antioxidants
Vitamin K 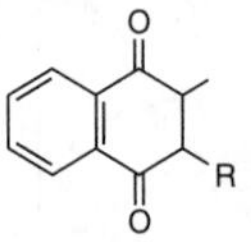 R	Vitamin K hydroquinone	Cofactor for posttranslation carboxylation of many proteins including essential clotting factors

FIGURE 61-1—(continued)

vitamin B_6 contained in plants is less bioavailable than that from animal tissues. Rich food sources of vitamin B_6 include legumes, nuts, wheat bran, and meat, although it is present in all food groups.

DEFICIENCY Symptoms of vitamin B_6 deficiency include epithelial changes, as seen frequently with other B vitamin deficiencies. In addition, severe vitamin B_6 deficiency can lead to peripheral neuropathy, abnormal electroencephalograms, and personality changes including depression and confusion. In infants, diarrhea, seizures, and anemia have been reported. Microcytic, hypochromic anemia is due to diminished hemoglobin synthesis, since the first enzyme involved in heme biosynthesis (amino-levulinate synthase) requires PLP as a cofactor (Chap. 90). In some case reports, platelet dysfunction has also been reported. Since vitamin B_6 is necessary for the conversion of homocysteine to cystathionine, it is possible that chronic low-grade vitamin B_6 deficiency may result in hyperhomocystinemia and increased risk of cardiovascular disease (Chaps. 225 and 343).

Certain medications such as isoniazid, L-dopa, penicillamine, and cycloserine interact with PLP due to a reaction with carbonyl groups. The increased ratio of AST (or SGOT) to ALT (or SGPT) seen in alcoholic liver disease reflects the relative vitamin B_6 dependence of ALT. Vitamin B_6 dependency syndromes that require pharmacologic doses of vitamin B_6 are rare, but include cystathionine β-synthase deficiency, pyridoxine-responsive (primarily sideroblastic) anemias, and gyrate atrophy with chorioretinal degeneration due to decreased activity of the mitochondrial enzyme ornithine aminotransferase. In these situations, 100 to 200 mg/d of oral vitamin B_6 are required for treatment.

High doses of vitamin B_6 have been used to treat carpal tunnel syndrome, premenstrual syndrome, schizophrenia, autism, and diabetic neuropathy but have not been found to be effective.

The laboratory diagnosis of vitamin B_6 deficiency is generally made on the basis of low plasma PLP values (<20 nmol/L). Treatment of vitamin B_6 deficiency is 50 mg/d; higher doses of 100 to 200 mg/d are given if vitamin B_6 deficiency is related to medication use. Vitamin B_6 should not be given with L-dopa, since the vitamin interferes with the action of this drug.

TOXICITY The safe upper limit for vitamin B_6 has been set at 100 mg/d, although no adverse effects have been associated with high intakes of vitamin B_6 from food sources only. When toxicity occurs, it causes a severe sensory neuropathy, leaving patients unable to walk. Some cases of photosensitivity and dermatitis have also been reported.

FOLATE, VITAMIN B_{12} See Chap. 90.

VITAMIN C

Both ascorbic acid and its oxidized product dehydroascorbic acid are biologically active. Actions of vitamin C include antioxidant activity, promotion of nonheme iron absorption, carnitine biosynthesis, and the conversion of dopamine to norepinephrine. Vitamin C is also important for connective tissue metabolism and cross-linking, and it is a component of many drug-metabolizing enzyme systems, particularly the mixed-function oxidase systems.

ABSORPTION AND DIETARY SOURCES Almost complete absorption of vitamin C occurs if <100 mg is administered in a single dose; however, only 50% or less is absorbed at doses >1 g. Enhanced degradation and fecal and urinary excretion of vitamin C occur at higher intake levels.

Good dietary sources of vitamin C include citrus fruits, green vegetables (especially broccoli), tomatoes, and potatoes. Consumption of five servings of fruits and vegetables a day provides vitamin C in excess of the RDA, 60 mg/d for males and females. In addition, approximately 40% of the U.S. population takes vitamin C as a dietary supplement in which "natural forms" of vitamin C are no more bioavailable than synthetic forms. Smoking, hemodialysis, and stress (e.g., infection, trauma) appear to increase vitamin C requirements.

DEFICIENCY Vitamin C deficiency causes scurvy; in the United States, this is seen primarily among the poor and elderly and in alcoholics who consume <10 mg/d of vitamin C. Vitamin C deficiency has also been described among individuals consuming macrobiotic diets. Symptoms of scurvy primarily reflect impaired formation of mature connective tissue and include bleeding into skin (petechiae, ecchymoses, perifollicular hemorrhages); inflamed and bleeding gums; and manifestations of bleeding into joints, the peritoneal cavity, pericardium, and the adrenal glands. In children, vitamin C deficiency may cause impaired bone growth. Laboratory diagnosis of vitamin C deficiency is made on the basis of low plasma or leukocyte levels.

Administration of vitamin C (200 mg/d) improves the symptoms of scurvy within a matter of several days. High-dose vitamin C supplementation (e.g., 1 to 2 g/d) may slightly decrease the symptoms and duration of upper respiratory tract infections. Vitamin C supplementation has also been reported to be useful in Chédiak-Higashi syndrome (Chap. 55) and osteogenesis imperfecta (Chap. 342). Diets high in vitamin C have been claimed to lower the incidence of certain cancers, particularly esophageal and gastric cancers. If proven, this effect may be due to the fact that vitamin C can prevent the conversion of nitrites and secondary amines to carcinogenic nitrosomines. However, one intervention study from China did not show vitamin C to be protective.

TOXICITY   Taking >2 g of vitamin C in a single dose may result in abdominal pain, diarrhea, and nausea; doses >3 g have been reported to elevate blood levels of ALT, lactic acid dehydrogenase, and uric acid. Since vitamin C may be metabolized to oxalate, it is feared that chronic, high-dose vitamin C supplementation could result in an increased prevalence of kidney stones. However, this has not been borne out in several trials, except in patients with preexisting renal disease. Thus, it is reasonable to advise patients with a past history of kidney stones to not take large doses of vitamin C. There is also an unproven, but possible, risk that chronic high doses of vitamin C could promote iron overload in patients taking supplemental iron. High doses of vitamin C can induce hemolysis in patients with glucose-6-phosphate dehydrogenase deficiency, and doses >1 g/d can cause false-negative guaiac reactions as well as interfere with tests for urinary glucose.

BIOTIN

Biotin is a water-soluble vitamin that plays a role in gluconeogenesis and fatty acid synthesis and serves as a CO_2 carrier on the surface of both cytosolic and mitochondrial carboxylase enzymes. The vitamin also functions in the catabolism of specific amino acids (e.g., leucine). Excellent food sources of biotin include liver, soy, beans, yeast, and egg yolks; however, egg white contains the protein avidin, which strongly binds the vitamin and reduces its bioavailability.

Biotin deficiency has been induced by experimental feeding of egg white diets and in patients with short bowels who received biotin-free parenteral nutrition. In the adult, biotin deficiency results in mental changes (depression, hallucinations), paresthesia, anorexia, and nausea. A scaling, seborrheic, and erythematous rash may occur around the eyes, nose, and mouth as well as on the extremities. In infants, biotin deficiency presents as hypotonia, lethargy, and apathy. In addition, the infant may develop alopecia and a characteristic rash that includes the ears. The laboratory diagnosis of biotin deficiency can be established based on a decreased urinary concentration. Treatment requires pharmacologic doses of biotin, using up to 10 mg/d.

PANTOTHENIC ACID

Pantothenic acid is a component of coenzyme A and phosphopantetheine, which are involved in fatty acid metabolism and the synthesis of cholesterol, steroid hormones, and all compounds formed from isoprenoid units. In addition, pantothenic acid is involved in the acetylation of proteins. The vitamin is excreted in the urine, and the laboratory diagnosis of deficiency is made on the basis of low urinary vitamin levels.

The vitamin is ubiquitous in the food supply. Liver, yeast, egg yolks, and vegetables are particularly good sources. Human pantothenic acid deficiency has only been demonstrated in experimental feeding of diets low in pantothenic acid or by giving a specific pantothenic acid antagonist. The symptoms of pantothenic acid deficiency are nonspecific and include gastrointestinal disturbance, depression, muscle cramps, paresthesia, ataxia, and hypoglycemia. Pantothenic acid deficiency is believed to have caused the burning feet syndrome seen in prisoners of war during World War II. No toxicity of this vitamin has been reported.

CHOLINE

Choline is a precursor for acetylcholine, phospholipids, and betaine. Choline is necessary for the structural integrity of cell membranes, cholinergic neurotransmission, lipid and cholesterol metabolism, and transmembrane signaling. Recently, a recommended adequate intake was set at 550 mg/d for adult males and 425 mg/d for adult females. Choline is thought to be a "conditionally essential" nutrient, in that de novo synthesis occurs in the liver and is less than the vitamin's utilization only under certain stress conditions. Choline deficiency has occurred in patients receiving parenteral nutrition devoid of choline. Deficiency results in fatty liver and elevated transaminase levels. The diagnosis of choline deficiency is made on the basis of low plasma levels.

Toxicity from choline results in hypotension, cholinergic sweating, diarrhea, salivation, and a fishy body odor. The upper limit for choline has been set at 3.5 g/d. Therapeutically, choline has been suggested for patients with dementia and for patients at high risk of cardiovascular disease, due to its ability to lower cholesterol and homocysteine levels. However, such benefits have yet to be documented.

VITAMIN A

Vitamin A, in the strictest sense, refers to retinol. However, the oxidized metabolites, retinaldehyde and retinoic acid, are also biologically active compounds. The term *retinoids* includes synthetic molecules that are chemically related to retinol. Retinaldehyde (11-*cis*) is the essential form of vitamin A that is required for normal vision, whereas retinoic acid is necessary for normal morphogenesis, growth, and cell differentiation. Retinoic acid does not function in vision and, in contrast to retinol, is not involved in reproduction. Vitamin A also plays a role in iron utilization, humoral immunity, T cell–mediated immunity, natural killer cell activity, and phagocytosis. Vitamin A is commercially available in esterified forms (e.g., acetate, palmitate) since it is more stable as an ester.

There are over 600 carotenoids in nature, and approximately 50 of these can be metabolized to vitamin A. β-Carotene is the most prevalent carotenoid in the food supply that has provitamin A activity. It is estimated that 12 μg or greater of dietary β-carotene is equivalent to 1 μg of retinol, whereas 24 μg or greater of other dietary provitamin A carotenoids (e.g., cryptoxanthin, α-carotene) is equivalent to 1 μg of retinol.

METABOLISM   The liver contains approximately 90% of the vitamin A reserves and secretes vitamin A in the form of retinol, which is bound to retinol-binding protein. Once this has occurred, the retinol-binding protein complex interacts with a second protein, transthyretin. This trimolecular complex functions to prevent vitamin A from being filtered by the kidney glomerulus, to protect the body against the toxicity of retinol and to allow retinol to be taken up by specific cell-surface receptors that recognize retinol-binding protein. A certain amount of vitamin A enters peripheral cells even if it is not bound to retinol-binding protein. After retinol is internalized by the cell, it becomes bound to a series of cellular retinol-binding proteins, which function as sequestering and transporting agents as well as coligands for enzymatic reactions. Certain cells also contain retinoic acid–binding proteins, which have the same sequestering functions as well as enabling retinoic acid metabolism.

Retinoic acid is a ligand for certain nuclear receptors that act as transcription factors. Two families of receptors (RAR and RXR receptors) are active in retinoid-mediated gene transcription. Retinoid receptors regulate transcription by binding as dimeric complexes to specific DNA sites, the retinoic acid response elements, in target genes (Chap. 317). The receptors can either stimulate or repress gene expression in response to their ligands. RAR binds all-*trans* retinoic acid and 9-*cis* retinoic acid, whereas RXR binds only 9-*cis* retinoic acid.

The retinoid receptors play an important role in controlling cell proliferation and differentiation. Retinoic acid is useful in the treatment of promyeolcytic leukemia (Chap. 96) and is also used in the treatment of cystic acne because it inhibits keratinization, decreases sebum secretion, and possibly alters the inflammatory reaction (Chap. 47). RXRs dimerize with other nuclear receptors to function as coregulators of genes responsive to retinoids, thyroid hormone, and calcitriol. RXR agonists induce insulin sensitivity experimentally, perhaps because RXR is a cofactor for the peroxisome-proliferator-activated receptors (PPARs), which are targets for the thiazolidinedione drugs such as rosiglitazone and troglitazone (Chap. 323).

DIETARY SOURCES The retinol activity equivalent (RAE) is used to express the vitamin A value of food. One RAE is defined as 1 μg of retinol (0.003491 mmol), 12 μg of β-carotene, and 24 μg of other provitamin A carotenoids. In older literature, vitamin A was often expressed in international units (IU), with 1 RAE being equal to 3.33 IU of retinol and 20 IU of β-carotene, but these units are no longer in current scientific use.

Liver and fish are excellent food sources for preformed vitamin A; vegetable sources of provitamin A carotenoids include dark-green and -colored fruits and vegetables. Children are particularly susceptible to vitamin A deficiency because neither breast nor cow's milk supplies enough vitamin A to prevent deficiency. Areas of the world where vitamin A deficiency is particularly prevalent include parts of Africa, South America, and Southeast Asia. Vitamin A deficiency occurs in more than 250,000 children each year, resulting in blindness and a 50% mortality rate within the year. In western countries, vitamin A deficiency is seen primarily among patients with diseases associated with fat malabsorption (e.g., celiac sprue, short-bowel syndrome). Concurrent zinc deficiency can interfere with the mobilization of vitamin A from liver stores. Alcohol interferes with the conversion of retinol to retinaldehyde in the eye by competing for alcohol (retinol) dehydrogenase. Drugs that interfere with the absorption of vitamin A include mineral oil, neomycin, and cholestyramine.

DEFICIENCY Symptoms of vitamin A deficiency include hyperkeratotic skin lesions, and xerophthalmia (e.g., Bitôt spots, which are white patches of keratinized epithelium appearing on the sclera). Aggressive xerophthalmia can result in corneal ulceration. If untreated, proteolytic destruction and rupture of the cornea ensues with permanent blindness, although vitamin A treatment of patients with corneal ulcers can also result in blindness due to permanent corneal scarring. Children with vitamin A deficiency have increased mortality, primarily from infectious diseases, measles, respiratory diseases, and diarrhea. Extremely low birth weight infants (<1000 g) should be treated parenterally with 1500 μg (or RAE) of vitamin A three times a week for 4 weeks.

There are no specific deficiency signs or symptoms that result from carotenoid deficiency. It was postulated that β-carotene would be an effective chemopreventive for cancer because numerous epidemiologic studies had shown that diets high in β-carotene were associated with lower incidences of cancers of the respiratory and digestive system. However, intervention studies using high doses of β-carotene actually resulted in more lung cancers than in placebo-treated groups. Non-provitamin A carotenoids, such as lutein and zeaxanthin, have been suggested to protect against macular degeneration. The non-provitamin A carotenoid lycopene has been proposed to protect against prostate cancer. However, the effectiveness of these agents has not been proven by intervention studies, and the mechanisms underlying these purported biologic actions are unknown.

The diagnosis of vitamin A deficiency is made by measurement of serum retinol (normal range, 30 to 65 μg/dL), tests of dark adaptation, impression cytology of the conjunctiva (decreased numbers of mucous-secreting cells), or measurement of body storage pools, either directly by liver biopsy or by isotopic dilution after administering a stable isotope of vitamin A.

Vitamin A deficiency with ocular changes should be treated by administering 30 mg of vitamin A intramuscularly, or 60 mg orally. In areas of endemic vitamin A deficiency, this is followed by 60 mg vitamin A capsules at 6-month intervals. Vitamin A deficiency in patients with malabsorptive diseases, who have abnormal dark adaptation or symptoms of night blindness without ocular changes, should be treated for 1 month with 15 mg/d orally of a water micelle preparation of vitamin A. This is followed by lower maintenance doses with the exact amount determined by monitoring serum retinol.

TOXICITY Acute toxicity of vitamin A was first noted in Arctic explorers who ate polar bear liver and has also been seen after administration of 150 mg in adults or 100 mg in children. Acute toxicity is manifested by increased intracranial pressure, vertigo, diplopia, bulging fontanels in children, seizures, and exfoliative dermatitis; it may result in death. Chronic vitamin A intoxication has been seen in normal adults who ingest 15 mg/d of vitamin A for a period of several months and in children who ingest 6 mg/d. Manifestations include dry skin, cheilosis, glossitis, vomiting, alopecia, bone pain, hypercalcemia, lymph node enlargement, hyperlipidemia, amenorrhea, and features of pseudotumor cerebri with increased intracranial pressure and papilledema. Liver fibrosis with portal hypertension and bone demineralization may also result from chronic vitamin A intoxication. When vitamin A is provided in excess to pregnant women, congenital malformations have included spontaneous abortions, craniofacial abnormalities, and valvular heart disease. In pregnancy, the daily dose of vitamin A should not exceed 3 mg. Commercially available retinoid derivatives are also toxic, including 13-cis-retinoic acid, which has been associated with birth defects. As a result, contraception should be continued for at least 1 year, and possibly longer, in women who have taken 13-cis retinoic acid.

High doses of carotenoids do not result in toxic symptoms. However, carotenemia, which is characterized by a yellowing of the skin (creases of the palms and soles) but not the sclerae, may be present after ingestion of >30 mg of β-carotene on a daily basis. Hypothyroid patients are particularly susceptible to the development of carotenemia due to impaired breakdown of carotene to vitamin A. Reduction of carotenes from the diet results in the disappearance of skin yellowing and carotenemia over a period of 30 to 60 days.

VITAMIN D See Chap. 331, Fig. 61-1, and Table 61-1.

VITAMIN E

Vitamin E is a collective name for the 2R stereoisomers of α tocopherol. Vitamin E acts as a chain-breaking antioxidant and is an efficient pyroxyl radical scavenger, which protects low-density lipoproteins (LDLs) and polyunsaturated fats in membranes from oxidation. A network of other antioxidants (e.g., vitamin C, glutathione) and enzymes maintains vitamin E in a reduced state. Vitamin E also inhibits prostaglandin synthesis and the activities of protein kinase C and phospholipase A_2.

ABSORPTION AND METABOLISM After absorption, vitamin E is taken up from chylomicrons by the liver, and an hepatic α tocopherol transport protein mediates intracellular vitamin E transport and incorporation into very low density lipoprotein (VLDL). The transport protein has particular affinity for the RRR isomeric form of α tocopherol; thus this natural isomer has the most biologic activity.

REQUIREMENT Vitamin E is widely distributed in the food supply and is particularly high in sunflower oil, safflower oil, and wheat germ oil; γ tocotrionols are notably present in soybean and corn oils. Vitamin E is also found in meats, nuts, and cereal grains, and small amounts are present in fruits and vegetables. Vitamin E pills containing doses of 50 to 1000 mg are ingested by a large fraction of the U.S. population. Diets high in polyunsaturated fats may necessitate a slightly higher requirement for vitamin E.

Dietary deficiency of vitamin E does not exist. Vitamin E deficiency is seen in only severe and prolonged malabsorptive diseases, such as celiac disease, or after small-intestinal resection. Children with cystic fibrosis or prolonged cholestasis may develop vitamin E deficiency characterized by areflexia and hemolytic anemia. Children with abetalipoproteinemia cannot absorb or transport vitamin E and become deficient quite rapidly. A familial form of isolated vitamin E deficiency also exists, which is due to a defect in the α tocopherol transport protein. Vitamin E deficiency causes axonal degeneration of the large myelinated axons and results in posterior column and spinocerebellar symptoms. Peripheral neuropathy is initially characterized by areflexia, with progression to an ataxic gait, and by decreased vibration and position sensations. Ophthalmoplegia, skeletal myopathy, and pigmented retinopathy may also be features of vitamin E deficiency. The laboratory diagnosis of vitamin E deficiency is made on the basis of low blood levels of α tocopherol (<5 μg/mL, or <0.8 mg of α tocopherol per gram of total lipids).

Rx TREATMENT

Symptomatic vitamin E deficiency should be treated with 800 to 1200 mg of α tocopherol per day. Patients with abetalipoproteinemia may need as much as 5000 to 7000 mg/d. Children with symptomatic vitamin E deficiency should be treated with 400 mg/d orally of water-miscible esters; alternatively, 2 mg/kg per day may be administered intramuscularly. Vitamin E in high doses may protect against oxygen-induced retrolental fibroplasia and bronchopulmonary dysplasia, as well as intraventricular hemorrhage of prematurity. Vitamin E has been suggested to increase sexual performance, to treat intermittent claudication, and to slow the aging process, but evidence for these properties is lacking. High doses (60 to 800 mg/d) of vitamin E have been shown in controlled trials to improve parameters of immune function, but intervention studies using vitamin E to prevent cardiovascular disease have not shown efficacy.

TOXICITY High doses of vitamin E (>800 mg/d) may reduce platelet aggregation and interfere with vitamin K metabolism and are therefore contraindicated in patients taking warfarin. Nausea, flatulence, and diarrhea have been reported at doses >1 g/d.

VITAMIN K

There are two natural forms of vitamin K: vitamin K I, also known as *phylloquinone*, from vegetable and animal sources, and vitamin K II, or *menaquinone*, which is synthesized by bacterial flora and found in hepatic tissue. *Menadione*, or vitamin K III, is a chemically synthesized pro-vitamin that can be converted to menaquinone by the liver.

Vitamin K is required for the posttranslational carboxylation of glutamic acid, which is necessary for calcium binding to γ-carboxylated proteins such as prothrombin (factor II); factors VII, IX, and X; protein C; protein S; and proteins found in bone (bone gla, matrix gla protein, and osteocalcin). However, the importance of vitamin K for bone mineralization is not known. Warfarin-type drugs inhibit γ carboxylation by preventing the conversion of vitamin K to its active hydroquinone form.

DIETARY SOURCES Vitamin K is found in green leafy vegetables such as kale and spinach, but appreciable amounts are also present in butter, margarine, liver, milk, ground beef, coffee, and pears. Vitamin K is present in vegetable oils and is particularly rich in olive oil and soybean oil. The average daily intake by Americans is estimated to be approximately 100 μg/d.

DEFICIENCY The symptoms of vitamin K deficiency are due to hemorrhage, and newborns are particularly susceptible because of low fat stores, low breast milk levels of vitamin K, sterility of the infantile intestinal tract, liver immaturity, and poor placental transport. Intracranial bleeding, as well as gastrointestinal and skin bleeding, can occur in vitamin K–deficient infants 1 to 7 days after birth. Thus, vitamin K (1 mg intramuscularly) is given prophylactically at the time of delivery.

Vitamin K deficiency in adults may be seen in patients with chronic small-intestinal disease (e.g., celiac disease, Crohn's disease), obstructed biliary tracts, or after small-bowel resection. Broad-spectrum antibiotic treatment can precipitate vitamin K deficiency by reducing gut bacteria, which synthesize menaquinones, and by inhibiting the

metabolism of vitamin K. The diagnosis of vitamin K deficiency is usually made on the basis of an elevated prothrombin time or reduced clotting factors, although vitamin K may also be measured directly by HPLC. Vitamin K deficiency is treated using a parenteral dose of 10 mg. For patients with chronic malabsorption, 1 to 2 mg/d of vitamin K should be given orally, or 1 to 2 mg/week can be taken parenterally. Patients with liver disease may have an elevated prothrombin time because of liver cell destruction as well as vitamin K deficiency. If an elevated prothrombin time does not improve on vitamin K therapy, it can be deduced that it is not the result of vitamin K deficiency.

TOXICITY Parenteral doses of the water-soluble vitamin K derivative (menadione) have been reported to cause hemolytic anemia and hypobilirubinemia in infants. Toxicity from dietary phylloquinones and menaquinones has not been described. High doses of vitamin K can impair the actions of oral anticoagulants.

MINERALS See Table 61-2.

CALCIUM See Chap. 331.

ZINC

Zinc is an integral component of many metalloenzymes in the body; it is involved in the synthesis and stabilization of proteins, DNA, and RNA and plays a structural role in ribosomes and membranes. Zinc is necessary for the binding of steroid hormone receptors and several other transcription factors to DNA. Zinc is absolutely required for normal spermatogenesis, fetal growth, and embryonic development.

ABSORPTION The absorption of zinc from the diet is inhibited by dietary phytate, fiber, oxalate, iron, and copper, as well as by certain drugs including penicillamine, sodium valproate, and ethambutol. Meat, shellfish, nuts, and legumes are good sources of bioavailable zinc, whereas zinc in grains is less available for absorption.

DEFICIENCY Mild zinc deficiency has been described in many diseases including diabetes mellitus, AIDS, cirrhosis, alcoholism, inflammatory bowel disease, malabsorption syndromes, and sickle cell anemia. In these diseases, mild chronic zinc deficiency can cause stunted growth in children, decreased taste sensation (hypogusia), and impaired immune function. Severe chronic zinc deficiency has been described as a cause of hypogonadism and dwarfism in several Middle Eastern countries. In these children, hypopigmented hair is also part of the syndrome. Acrodermatitis enteropathica is a rare autosomal recessive disorder characterized by abnormalities in zinc absorption. Clinical manifestations include diarrhea, alopecia, muscle wasting, depression, irritability, and a rash involving the extremities, face, and perineum. The rash is characterized by vesicular and pustular crusting with scaling and erythema. Occasional patients with Wilson's disease have developed zinc deficiency as a consequence of penicillamine therapy (Chap. 339).

The diagnosis of zinc deficiency is usually made by a serum zinc level of <12 μmol/L (<70 μg/dL). Pregnancy and birth control pills may cause a slight depression in serum zinc levels, and hypoalbuminemia from any cause can result in hypozincemia. In acute stress situations, zinc may be redistributed from serum into tissues. Zinc deficiency may be treated with 60 mg elemental zinc, orally twice a day. Zinc gluconate lozenges (13 mg elemental Zn every 2 h while awake) have been reported to reduce the duration and symptoms of the common cold in adults, but studies are conflicting.

TOXICITY Acute zinc toxicity after oral ingestion causes nausea, vomiting, and fever. Zinc fumes from welding may also be toxic and cause fever, respiratory distress, excessive salivation, sweating, and headache. Chronic large doses of zinc may depress immune function and cause hypochromic anemia as a result of copper deficiency.

COPPER

Copper is an integral part of numerous enzyme systems including amine oxidases, ferrooxidase (ceruloplasmin), cytochrome-c oxidase,

TABLE 61-2 *Deficiencies and Toxicities of Metals*

Element	Deficiency	Toxicity	Tolerable Upper (Dietary) Intake Level
Boron	No biologic function determined	Developmental defects, male sterility, testicular atrophy	20 mg/d (extrapolated from animal data)
Calcium	Reduced bone mass, osteoporosis	Renal insufficiency (milk-alkalai syndrome), nephrolithiasis, impaired iron absorption	2500 mg/d (milk-alkalai)
Copper	Anemia, growth retardation, defective keratinization and pigmentation of hair, hypothermia, degenerative changes in aortic elastin, osteopenia, mental deterioration	Nausea, vomiting, diarrhea, hepatic failure, tremor, mental deterioration, hemolytic anemia, renal dysfunction	10 mg/d (liver toxicity)
Chromium	Impaired glucose tolerance	Occupational: renal failure, dermatitis, pulmonary cancer	ND
Fluoride	↑ Dental caries	Dental and skeletal fluorosis, osteoscleroisis	10 mg/d (fluorosis)
Iodine	Thyroid enlargement, ↓ T$_4$	Thyroid dysfunction, acne-like eruptions	1100 µg/d (thyroid dysfunction)
Iron	Muscle abnormalities, kilonychia, pica, anemia, ↓ work performance, impaired cognitive development, premature labor, ↑ perinatal maternal mortality	Gastrointestinal effects (nausea, vomiting, diarrhea, constipation), iron overload with organ damage, acute systemic toxicity	45 mg/d of elemental iron (GI side effects)
Manganese	Impaired growth and skeletal development, reproduction, lipid and carbohydrate metabolism; upper body rash	General: Neurotoxicity, Parkinson-like symptoms Occupational: Encephalitis-like syndrome, Parkinson-like syndrome, psychosis, pneumoconiosis	11 mg/d (neurotoxicity)
Molybdenum	Severe neurologic abnormalities	Reproductive and fetal abnormalities	2 mg/d extrapolated from animal data
Selenium	Cardiomyopathy, heart failure, striated muscle degeneration	General: Alopecia, nausea, vomiting, abnormal nails, emotional lability, peripheral neuropathy, lassitude, garlic odor to breath, dermatitis Occupational: Lung and nasal carcinomas, liver necrosis, pulmonary inflammation	400 µg/d (hair, nail changes)
Phosphorous	Rickets (osteomalacia), proximal muscle weakness, rhabdomyolysis, paresthesia, ataxia, seizure, confusion, heart failure, hemolysis, acidosis	Hyperphosphatemia	4000 mg/d
Zinc	Growth retardation, ↓ taste and smell, alopecia, dermatitis, diarrhea, immune dysfunction, failure to thrive, gonadal atrophy, congenital malformations	General: Reduced copper absorption, gastritis, sweating, fever, nausea, vomiting. Occupational: Respiratory distress, pulmonary fibrosis	40 mg/d (impaired copper metabolism)

Note: ND, not determined; GI, gastrointestinal.

superoxide dismutase, and dopamine hydroxylase. As such, copper plays a role in iron metabolism, melanin synthesis, and central nervous system function; the synthesis and cross-linking of elastin and collagen; and the scavenging of superoxide radicals. Dietary sources of copper include shellfish, liver, nuts, legumes, bran, and organ meats.

DEFICIENCY Dietary copper deficiency is relatively rare, although it has been described in premature infants who are fed milk diets and in infants with malabsorption (Table 61-2). Copper deficiency anemia has been reported in patients with malabsorptive diseases and nephrotic syndrome and in patients treated for Wilson's disease with chronic high doses of oral zinc, which can interfere with copper absorption. Menkes kinky hair syndrome is an X-linked metabolic disturbance of copper metabolism characterized by mental retardation, hypocupremia, and decreased circulating ceruloplasmin (Chap. 342). It is caused by mutations in a copper-transporting *ATP7A* gene. Children with this disease often die within 5 years because of dissecting aneurysms or cardiac rupture.

The diagnosis of copper deficiency is usually made on the basis of low serum levels of copper (<65 µg/dL) and low ceruloplasmin levels (<18 mg/dL). Serum levels of copper may be elevated in pregnancy or stress conditions since ceruloplasmin is an acute-phase reactant and 90% of circulating copper is bound to ceruloplasmin.

TOXICITY Copper toxicity is usually accidental (Table 61-2). In severe cases, kidney failure, liver failure, and coma may ensue. In Wilson's disease, mutations in the copper-transporting *ATP7B* gene lead to accumulation of copper in the liver and brain, with low blood levels due to decreased ceruloplasmin (Chap. 339).

SELENIUM

Selenium, in the form of selenocysteine, is a component of the enzyme glutathione peroxidase, which serves to protect proteins, cell membranes, lipids, and nucleic acids from oxidant molecules. Selenocysteine is also found in the deiodinase enzymes, which mediate the deiodination of thyroxine to triiodothyronine (Chap. 320). Rich dietary sources of selenium include seafood, muscle meat, and cereals, although the selenium content of cereal is determined by the soil concentration. Countries with low soil concentrations include parts of Scandinavia, China, and New Zealand. *Keshan disease* is an endemic cardiomyopathy found in children and young women residing in regions of China where dietary intake of selenium is low (<20 µg/d). Concomitant deficiencies of iodine and selenium may worsen the clinical manifestations of cretinism.

CHROMIUM

Chromium potentiates the action of insulin in patients with impaired glucose tolerance, presumably by increasing insulin receptor–mediated signaling. In addition, in some patients, improvement in blood lipid profiles has been reported. The usefulness of chromium supplements in muscle building are not substantiated. Rich food sources of chromium include yeast, meat, and grain products. Chromium in the trivalent state is found in supplements and is largely nontoxic; however, chromium-6 is a product of stainless steel welding and is a known pulmonary carcinogen, as well as causing liver, kidney, and central nervous system damage.

MAGNESIUM See Chap. 331.

FLUORIDE, MANGANESE, AND ULTRATRACE ELEMENTS

An essential function for *fluoride* in humans has not been described, although it is useful for the maintenance of structure in teeth and bone. Adult fluorosis results in mottled and pitted defects in tooth enamel as well as brittle bone (skeletal fluorosis).

Manganese and molybdenum deficiencies have been reported in patients with rare genetic abnormalities and in a few patients receiving prolonged total parenteral nutrition. Several manganese-specific enzymes have been identified (e.g., manganese superoxide dismutase). Deficiencies of manganese have been reported to result in bone demineralization, poor growth, ataxia, and convulsions.

Ultratrace elements are defined as those needed in amounts <1 mg/d. Essentiality has not been established for most ultratrace elements, although *iodine* is clearly essential (Chap. 320). *Molybdenum* is necessary for the activity of sulfite and xanthine oxidase, and molybdenum deficiency may result in skeletal and brain lesions.

FURTHER READING

PANEL ON MICRONUTRIENTS, FOOD AND NUTRITION BOARD, INSTITUTE OF MEDICINE: *Dietary Reference Intakes for Calcium, Phosphorus, Magnesium, Vitamin D, and Fluoride: Standing Committee on the Scientific Evaluation of Dietary Reference Intakes.* Washington, DC, National Academy Press, 1997

————: *Dietary Reference Intakes for Thiamin, Riboflavin, Niacin, Vitamin B6, Folate, Vitamin B12, Pantothenic Acid, Biotin, and Choline: A Report of the Standing Committee on the Scientific Evaluation of Dietary Reference Intakes and its Panel on Folate, Other B Vitamins, and Choline and Subcommittee on Upper Reference Levels of Nutrients.* Washington, DC, National Academy Press, 2000

————: *Dietary Reference Intakes for Vitamin C, Vitamin E, Selenium, and Carotenoids: A Report of the Panel on Dietary Antioxidants and Related Compounds, Subcommittees on Upper Intakes, and the Standing Committee on the Scientific Evaluation of Dietary Reference Intakes.* Washington, DC, National Academy Press, 2000

————: *Dietary Reference Intakes for Vitamin A, Vitamin K, Arsenic, Boron, Chromium, Copper, Iodine, Iron, Manganese, Molybdenum, Nickel, Silicon, Vanadium, and Zinc: A Report of the Subcommittees on Upper Reference Levels of Nutrients and of Interpretation and Uses of Dietary Reference Intakes, and the Standing Committee on the Scientific Evaluation of Dietary Reference Intakes.* Washington, DC, National Academy Press, 2001

62 MALNUTRITION AND NUTRITIONAL ASSESSMENT
Charles H. Halsted

Malnutrition is a frequent component of acute and chronic illness and is found in ~50% of all hospitalized adults. It contributes to increased in-hospital morbidity and mortality in both medical and surgical patients, and leads to more frequent hospital admissions among the elderly. Malnutrition results from various combinations of starvation, abnormal assimilation of the diet, the stress response of illness, and abnormal nutrient metabolism. Nutritional assessment should be considered an integral part of the clinical evaluation and used as a basis for nutritional support in the overall therapeutic plan.

Two forms of severe malnutrition are recognized under conditions of inadequate food supply or distribution: *marasmus* refers to generalized starvation with loss of body fat and protein, whereas *kwashiorkor* refers to selective protein malnutrition with edema and fatty liver. These distinctions, however, seldom apply to malnourished patients in more developed societies where features of combined protein-calorie malnutrition (PCM) are seen in acute and chronic illnesses. The potential medical consequences of unrecognized malnutrition are depicted in Fig. 62-1.

Patients lose weight when the intake or gastrointestinal assimilation of dietary calories is insufficient to meet normal energy expenditure, the expenditure of body energy stores is greater than energy assimilated by the body, or the metabolism of energy is significantly impaired by the intrinsic disease process. The etiologies of malnutrition can be categorized according to decreased intake or assimilation of diet, increased loss of nutrients from the body, and mixed mechanisms that reflect abnormal nutrient metabolism, as summarized in Table 62-1.

ENERGY BALANCE AND BODY COMPOSITION IN HEALTH AND DISEASE

Energy balance and body weight are sustained in health by the consumption of dietary energy (calories) in an amount equal to the daily expenditure of energy. Simply put, undernutrition results from the intake or absorption of fewer calories than energy spent, and overnutrition represents less expenditure of energy than calories consumed. In healthy individuals, daily total energy expenditure (TEE) is composed of basal or resting energy expenditure (REE, about 60% of total), the thermic cost of digestion (about 10% of total), and modest physical activity (about 30% of total). The REE represents the cost of all intrinsic metabolic reactions and is directly related to the fat-free mass (FFM) of the body. As depicted in Fig. 62-2, the human body stores 15 to 25% of its energy as fat (greater in women than men), which is available for the release of stored fatty acids during starvation. The remaining FFM is composed of extracellular and intracellular water, the bony skeleton, glycogen, and skeletal and visceral protein. Aside from body fat, energy reserves are also provided by intracellular glycogen and protein, which, together with intracellular water, constitute the body cell mass (BCM). Thus, in addition to the enzymes that support the normal metabolic machinery of the body, the BCM provides reserve protein for energy production by gluconeogenesis during the stress response.

The energy stores in a healthy 70-kg man include about 15 kg as fat, 6 kg as protein, and 0.4 kg as glycogen. During a 24-h fast, energy needs are met by the consumption of liver glycogen stores and the conversion by gluconeogenesis of up to 75 g of body protein to glucose. During longer fasting, the REE decreases by as much as 25%

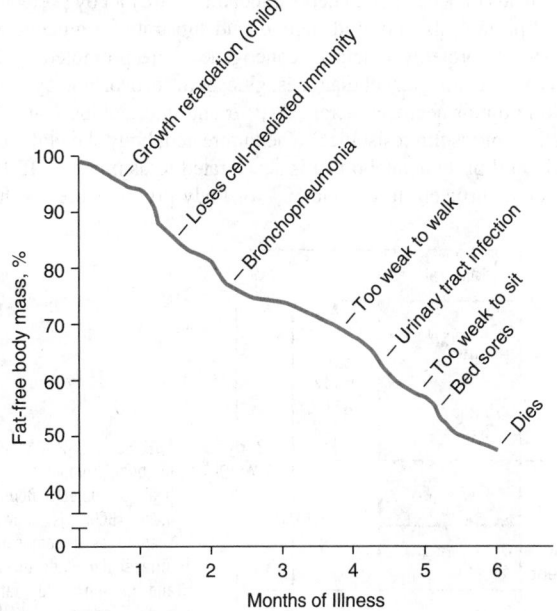

FIGURE 62-1 Hypothetical history of progressive protein-calorie malnutrition in a patient with wasting illness. (*Reproduced with permission from Heymsfield et al.*)

TABLE 62-1 *Etiologies of Protein-Calorie Malnutrition*

I. Starvation (hypometabolism with reliance on body fat stores)
  A. Decreased diet intake
    1. Social and economic: poverty, chronic alcoholism
    2. Psychiatric: anorexia nervosa, severe depression
    3. Neurodegenerative dementias of aging
    4. Anorexia associated with AIDS, disseminated cancer, renal failure
    5. Abdominal pain triggered by food intake: pancreatitis, intestinal ischemia
  B. Decreased assimilation of the diet
    1. Impaired transit of diet, e.g., benign or malignant esophageal, gastric, or intestinal obstruction
    2. Impaired digestion of diet, e.g., pancreatic insufficiency, short bowel syndrome
    3. Intestinal malabsorption of dietary constituents, e.g., celiac disease
II. Stress (hypermetabolism with reliance on protein stores for gluconeogenesis)
  A. Acute trauma, e.g., accident, burns, major surgery
  B. Acute sepsis
  C. Acute or chronic inflammation: pancreatitis, collagen diseases, chronic infectious disease, e.g., tuberculosis, AIDS opportunistic infections
III. Mixed mechanisms
  A. Futile metabolic cycles and anorexia, e.g., AIDS, disseminated cancer
  B. Increased energy demands, e.g., chronic obstructive pulmonary disease
  C. Abnormal metabolism and decreased biliary digestion, e.g., chronic liver disease
  D. Protein-losing enteropathy and chronic inflammation, e.g., Crohn's disease, ulcerative colitis

and the decreased energy needs are supplied by gluconeogenesis, derived from stores of body fat (about 150 g/d), which provides ketones, and muscle, which provides protein (about 20 g/d). While normal-weight individuals can sustain total fasting for about 2 months, obese individuals can fast for periods >12 months, depending on the size of their fat stores.

The metabolic responses to the stress of acute critical illness (e.g., following accidental or surgical trauma or sepsis) significantly modify energy balance. In contrast to the hypometabolism of starvation, the acute stress response is characterized by hypermetabolism, in which the demands of accelerated energy expenditure are met by skeletal and visceral proteolysis to provide amino acid substrate for gluconeogenesis. Muscle proteolysis and gluconeogenesis are promoted by high levels of circulating catecholamines, glucagon, cortisol, and cytokines, including tumor necrosis factor (TNF) α and interleukins 1 and 6, in the setting of insulin resistance. When untreated, body skeletal muscle and visceral protein catabolism is accelerated to as much as 150 g/d, an amount sufficient to deplete 50% of body protein stores within 3

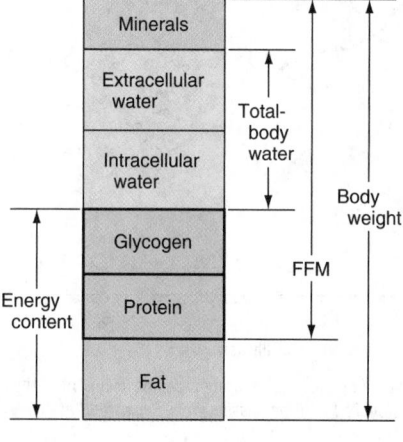

FIGURE 62-2 Schematic of body composition of a healthy subject. Body cell mass (BCM) is shown by shading as a composite of intracellular water, glycogen, and protein. FFM, fat-free mass. (*Adapted with permission from Heymsfield et al.*)

weeks. In the malnourished patient with chronic illness in whom acute trauma or sepsis superimposes cytokine-mediated proteolysis, progressive PCM is associated with decreased cardiac and renal function, fluid retention, muscle and intestinal mucosal atrophy, loss of intracellular minerals (zinc, magnesium, and phosphorus), diminished cell-mediated immune functions, increased risk of infection, and eventual death (Fig. 62-1).

CLINICAL EVALUATION OF THE MALNOURISHED PATIENT

Both outpatients and inpatients are at risk for malnutrition if they meet one or more of the following criteria: (1) unintentional loss of ~10% of usual body weight in the preceding 3 months, (2) body weight <90% of ideal for height, or (3) body mass index [BMI; the weight (kg) divided by the height (m²)] <18.5. With regard to varying levels of severity, body weight <90% of ideal for height represents risk of malnutrition, body weight <85% of ideal constitutes *malnutrition*, <70% of ideal represents *severe malnutrition*, and <60% of ideal is usually incompatible with survival. An overview of the evaluation of malnutrition in the sick adult is depicted in Fig. 62-3.

THE PATIENT HISTORY The clinical nutritional history is based on understanding the etiologies and pathophysiology of malnutrition and should focus on changes in diet and body weight, socioeconomic conditions, and symptoms unique to each clinical setting (Table 62-2). Social and economic conditions that may lead to poverty and malnutrition include inadequate income, homelessness, drug abuse, or chronic alcoholism. During binge drinking in chronic alcoholics, ethanol typically contributes more than half of daily food calories; ethanol catabolism consumes energy and promotes unbalanced metabolism of fat and carbohydrates. Depending on the severity of injury or illness, critically ill surgical and medical patients predictably develop stress-related PCM if increased nutritional needs are not met after 5 to 10 days. The malnourished patient with digestive disease etiology may complain of dysphagia or recurrent vomiting, chronic diarrhea, or recurrent abdominal pain that is exacerbated by eating. On the general medical service, PCM may be an integral part of the clinical presentation of chronic recurrent pancreatitis, renal failure, chronic liver disease, chronic obstructive pulmonary disease, disseminated cancer, or chronic infections such as AIDS or tuberculosis.

THE PHYSICAL EXAMINATION A careful physical examination can characterize the extent of malnutrition. Measurements of unclothed weight and height are essential for establishing the severity of malnutrition in all patients but may be confounded by the effects of fluid overload as a result of edema and ascites. Normal values of weight for height are shown in Table 62-3. Without recourse to a table, a simplified approach for estimating ideal body weight is to assume 106 lb for 5 ft plus 6 lb per additional inch for men, or 105 lb for 5 ft plus 5 lb per additional inch for women, assuming a range of ±10%.

Specific Physical Findings of Malnutrition During the conventional physical examination, the observant and experienced clinician can identify multiple and specific findings of PCM and its associated micronutrient deficiencies (Chap. 61). A variety of nutritional deficiencies can be identified by examination of the patient's general appearance, including skin, hair, nails, mucus membranes, and neurologic system (Table 62-4). Initially, a pinch of the posterior upper arm may reveal loss of subcutaneous fat in the malnourished patient. Hollowing of the temporal muscles, wasting of upper arms and thigh muscles, easily plucked hair, and peripheral edema are all consistent with protein deficiency. Examination of the skin may reveal the papular keratitis ("goose bump rash") of vitamin A deficiency, perifollicular hemorrhages of vitamin C deficiency, ecchymoses of vitamin K deficiency, the "flaky paint" lower extremity rash of zinc deficiency, hyperpigmentation of skin-exposed areas from niacin deficiency, seborrhea of essential fatty acid deficiency, spooning of nails in iron deficiency, and transverse nail pigmentation in protein deficiency. The eye examination yields conjunctival pallor of anemia, pericorneal and corneal opacities of severe vitamin A deficiency ("Bitot spots"), and nystagmus and isolated ocular muscle paresis of thiamine deficiency. The oral examination may reveal angular stomatitis and cheilosis of either riboflavin or niacin deficiency; glossitis with smooth and red tongue of riboflavin, niacin, vitamin B_{12}, or pyridoxine deficiency; and hypertrophied bleeding gums of vitamin C deficiency. Examination of the neurologic system, particularly in the setting of chronic alcohol abuse, may detect memory loss with confabulation, a wide-based gait, and past pointing, which, together with ophthalmoplegia and peripheral neuropathy, constitute the Wernicke-Korsakoff syndrome of thiamine deficiency. Other neurologic causes of dementia include pellagra due to niacin and/or tryptophan deficiency. Additional causes of peripheral neuropathy include deficiencies of pyridoxine or vitamin E; loss of distal vibratory and position sense is characteristic of the subacute combined degeneration of vitamin B_{12} deficiency.

Anthropometry Measurements of subcutaneous fat and skeletal muscle are important to determine the severity of PCM. Using specialized calipers and a tape measure, anthropometry estimates body fat from the thickness of the skin fold of the posterior mid-upper arm. Anthropometric measurements in healthy and malnourished adults are shown in Table 62-5. Mid-arm muscle circumference is estimated by using the equation:

$$\text{Mid-arm muscle circumference} = \text{mid-upper circumference (cm)}$$
$$- (\pi \times \text{triceps skin-fold thickness}) \text{ (cm)}$$

LABORATORY ASSESSMENT Selected use of laboratory tests, most of which are widely available, is essential for characterizing and quantifying malnutrition. Laboratory findings that are often attributed to chronic disease may, in actuality, reflect the response to PCM or selected micronutrient deficiencies in the setting of chronic illness.

Serum Visceral Proteins Serum albumin, which has a 2- to 3-week half-life, is a sensitive but nonspecific measure of PCM. A normal serum albumin level in a well-hydrated patient is inconsistent with PCM. In contrast, a low serum albumin level could reflect PCM, but can also occur because of increased plasma volume in an overhydrated patient, or because of chronic liver, renal, or cardiopulmonary failure. The serum albumin level falls during the acute stress of surgery, sepsis, or other acute inflammatory illness because of a combination of increased circulating extracellular volume and TNF-α-mediated inhibition of albumin synthesis. Several shorter-lived visceral proteins can also be measured to estimate the severity of PCM. These include transferrin (1-week half-life), prealbumin or retinol-binding protein complex (2-day half-life), and fibronectin (1-day half-life).

Vitamins and Minerals Assays (see also Chap. 61) PCM is typically associated with low serum levels of vitamin A, zinc, and magnesium. Abnormal digestion and absorption of dietary fat are associated with deficiencies of fat-soluble vitamins A, D, and E, whereas intestinal mucosal malabsorption (as in celiac disease) is commonly associated with additional deficiencies of iron and folic acid. Chronic alcoholism is frequently associated with thiamine, folate, vitamin A, and zinc deficiencies. Normal ranges for vitamins are listed in the Appendix.

Assessment of Immune Function PCM is associated with atrophy of thymic-dependent lymphoid structures and reduced T cell–mediated immunity. Conversely, B cell–mediated production of immunoglobulins is usually unaffected. Total lymphocyte count (total white cell count × fraction as lymphocytes) is often <1000/μL in PCM and may be accompanied by anergy to common skin test antigens.

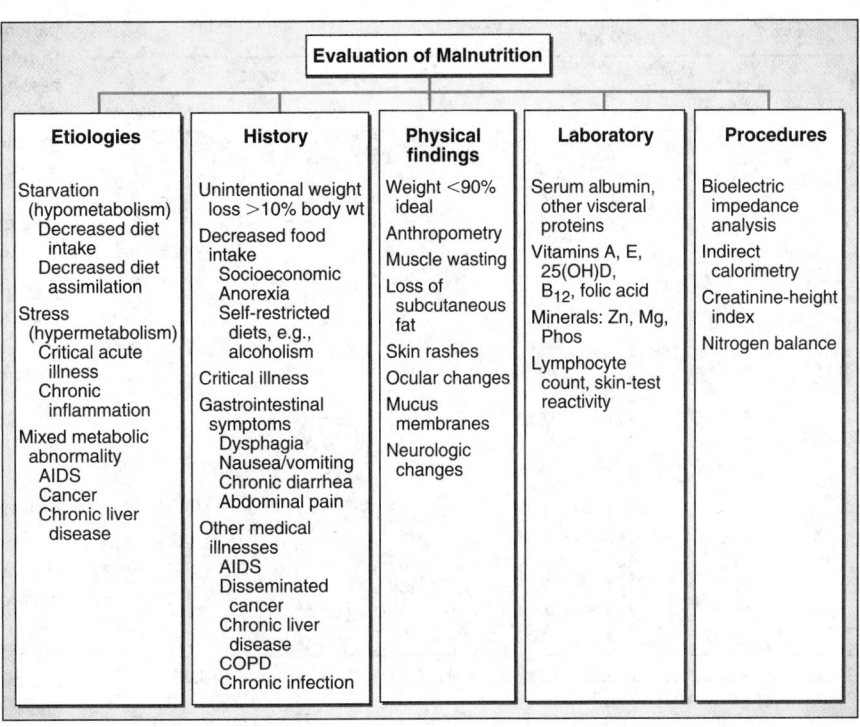

FIGURE 62-3 Conceptual framework for the nutritional assessment of sick patients. COPD, chronic obstructive pulmonary disease.

SPECIALIZED PROCEDURES FOR NUTRITIONAL ASSESSMENT Several specialized procedures are used to assess energy and protein stores and energy expenditure in malnourished patients. These procedures may be employed during the initial nutritional assessment or may serve as an index of the efficacy of nutritional support during the treatment of malnourished patients.

Bioelectric Impedance Analysis Bioelectric impedance analysis (BIA) is a simplified and portable method for measurement of body fat, FFM,

TABLE 62-2 *The Patient History of Weight Loss and Malnutrition*

Finding	Example/Interpretation
Involuntary diet restriction	Poverty due to inadequate income
Anorexia	Anorexia nervosa, severe depression, dementia, AIDS, cancer, chronic renal disease
Inadequate diet selection	Chronic alcoholism, fad diets, strict vegetarianism
Critical illness	Untreated stress response to trauma, burn, major surgery, sepsis
Gastrointestinal symptoms	
Dysphagia	Esophageal obstruction impairs diet transit
Nausea, vomiting	Gastric or intestinal obstruction impairs diet transit
Chronic diarrhea	Pancreatic, biliary, or intestinal mucosal disease impairs digestion and absorption
	Protein-losing enteropathy in inflammatory bowel disease
Chronic abdominal pain	Self-limited food intake reduces pain: e.g., pancreatitis, intestinal ischemia, inflammatory bowel disease
Other chronic medical diseases	Combinations of anorexia, increased energy demands, and abnormal nutrient metabolism: e.g., recurrent pancreatitis, AIDS, disseminated cancer, chronic liver disease, chronic obstructive pulmonary disease, chronic infectious illness

TABLE 62-3 Ideal Weight for Height

Men				Women			
Height[a]	Weight[a]	Height	Weight	Height	Weight	Height	Weight
145	51.9	166	64.0	140	44.9	161	56.9
146	52.4	167	64.6	141	45.4	162	57.6
147	52.9	168	65.2	142	45.9	163	58.3
148	53.5	169	65.9	143	46.4	164	58.9
149	54.0	170	66.6	144	47.0	165	59.5
150	54.5	171	67.3	145	47.5	166	60.1
151	55.0	172	68.0	146	48.0	167	60.7
152	55.6	173	68.7	147	48.6	168	61.4
153	56.1	174	69.4	148	49.2	169	62.1
154	56.6	175	70.1	149	49.8		
155	57.2	176	70.8	150	50.4		
156	57.9	177	71.6	151	51.0		
157	58.6	178	72.4	152	51.5		
158	59.3	179	73.3	153	52.0		
159	59.9	180	74.2	154	52.5		
160	60.5	181	75.0	155	53.1		
161	61.1	182	75.8	156	53.7		
162	61.7	183	76.5	157	54.3		
163	62.3	184	77.3	158	54.9		
164	62.9	185	78.1	159	55.5		
165	63.5	186	78.9	160	56.2		

[a] Values are expressed in cm for height and kg for weight. To obtain height in inches, divide by 2.54. To obtain weight in pounds, multiply by 2.2.

Source: Adapted from GL Blackburn et al: J Parenter Enteral Nutr 1:11, 1977; with permission.

and total-body water. BIA is performed by measuring the electric conductivity of a weak current between electrodes placed on the dorsal surfaces of the hands and feet. The measurement reflects differences in the impedance to electric current, which is greatest through fat and least through water. Lean body mass can be calculated by subtracting fat mass from body weight or by dividing total-body water by 0.73.

Overall, BIA is most useful in assessing body fat and FFM in stable

TABLE 62-4 Physical Findings of Malnutrition

Finding	Deficiency/Interpretation
General appearance	
Weight loss	Malnutrition <90% of ideal body weight
	Severe <70% of ideal body weight
Decreased temporal and proximal extremity muscle mass	Decreased skeletal protein
Decreased skin-fold thickness by "pinch test"	Decreased body fat stores
Skin, nails, and hair	
Easily plucked hair	Protein
Easy bruising, perifollicular hemorrhages	Vitamin C
"Flaky paint" rash of lower extremities	Zinc
Coarse skin, "goose bumps"	Vitamin A
Hyperpigmentation of sun-exposed areas	Niacin, tryptophan
Spooning of nails	Iron
Eyes	
Conjunctival pallor	Anemia (nonspecific)
Bitot spot	Vitamin A
Ophthalmoplegia	Thiamine
Mouth and mucus membranes	
Nasolabial seborrhea	Essential fatty acids
Glossitis (smooth, red tongue) and/or cheilosis	Riboflavin, niacin, vitamin B_{12}, pyridoxine, folate
Diminished taste	Zinc
Neurologic system	
Disorientation	Niacin, phosphorus
Confabulation	Thiamine
Cerebellar gait, past pointing	Thiamine
Peripheral neuropathy	Thiamine, pyridoxine, vitamin E
Lost vibratory, position sense	Vitamin B_{12}

patients and in those who suffer from conditions leading to relative starvation. However, BIA can also be used to assess critically ill patients with decreased intracellular water space and BCM and expanded extracellular compartment size. Reduced BCM correlates inversely with increased metabolic rate. BIA may be confounded in AIDS patients receiving protease-inhibitor therapy, if they exhibit lipodystrophy with associated redistribution of interscapular, abdominal, and breast fat (Chap. 173).

Energy Expenditure The REE is directly proportional to both FFM and BCM and can be estimated in healthy individuals by the Harris and Benedict formula on the basis of weight in kg (W), height in cm (H), and age in years (A):

$$\text{REE (men)} = 66.473 + 13.751(W) + 5.0033\ (H) - 6.7550\ (A)\ \text{kcal/d}$$

$$\text{REE (women)} = 655.0955 + 9.4634(W) + 1.8496\ (H) - 4.6756\ (A)\ \text{kcal/d}$$

However, this equation tends to overestimate REE in obese individuals, and it is unreliable in estimating energy requirements in sick patients who may be hypo- or hypermetabolic. For estimating TEE, i.e., requirements, the REE in the nonexercising sick patient can be calculated by the Harrison and Benedict formula or estimated at 25% kcal/kg of ideal body weight for height, then modified by adding another 10% for digestion and metabolism of intravenous or enteral feeding and an additional 12.5% for each degree of fever over 37°C, as well as an additional multiplier commensurate with the severity of illness (e.g., 25% for general surgery, 50% for sepsis, and 100% for extensive third-degree burns). TEE can be measured at the bedside more precisely by the gas-exchange method of indirect calorimetry using a mobile metabolic cart. This procedure is applicable to ventilator-independent and -dependent patients whose fractional intake of oxygen is <0.45. Because the goal is to reach an accurate approximation of the 24-h energy requirement, measurements must be taken at intervals during the day and must account for several variables, including food intake and activity. To calculate the energy cost of metabolism by indirect calorimetry, the volumes (V) of oxygen consumed and carbon dioxide produced are measured over a given period of time, according to the modified Weir equation where

$$\text{REE} = 3.9\ V_{O_2} + 1.1\ V_{CO_2}$$

Indirect calorimetry also provides the respiratory quotient (RQ), which is the ratio of carbon dioxide produced to oxygen consumed during the process of gas collection. The RQ decreases when fat is the predominant substrate for metabolism (as in starvation) and increases when the contribution of carbohydrate increases (as during stress with gluconeogenesis). In healthy individuals, the RQ usually falls between 0.80 and 0.90. An RQ <0.7 is consistent with active ketogenesis from endogenous fatty acid metabolism with limited generation of carbon dioxide. An RQ >1.0 indicates net lipogenesis, or the conversion of substrate carbohydrate to fat—a situation that occurs with overfeed-

TABLE 62-5 Anthropometric Measurements in Adults

% Standard	Men	Women	Interpretation
TRICEPS SKIN-FOLD, MM			
100	12.5	16.5	Adequate
50	6.0	8.0	Borderline
20	2.5	3.0	Severe depletion
MID-ARM MUSCLE CIRCUMFERENCE, CM			
100	25.5	23.0	Adequate
80	20.0	18.5	Borderline
60	15.0	14.0	Depletion
40	10.0	9.0	Severe depletion

Source: Adapted from SL Morgan, Weinsier RL: *Fundamentals of Clinical Nutrition*, St. Louis, Mosby, 1998, p 167; with permission.

ing. Values that fall outside the range of 0.65 to 1.25 suggest an error in measurement technique.

Creatinine Excretion in the 24-h Urine Creatinine, the metabolic product of skeletal muscle creatine, is produced at a constant rate and in an amount directly proportional to skeletal muscle mass. With steady-state day-to-day renal function, each gram of creatinine in the 24-h urine collection represents 18.5 g of fat-free skeletal muscle. Since skeletal muscle is the major component of FFM, measurement of creatinine in the 24-h urine collection can be used as a relative measure of this body compartment during the initial assessment or to assess the efficacy of nutritional support. The *creatinine coefficient* represents the amount of creatinine excreted per kilogram of body weight; it is equal to 23 mg/kg of ideal body weight in men and 18 mg/kg of ideal body weight in women. The *creatinine-height index* represents the ratio of the measured 24-h urine creatinine excretion to the value predicted by the creatinine coefficient for the patient's ideal body weight. These values can be calculated from estimation of the patient's ideal body weight according to height (Table 62-3). The constancy of creatinine excretion depends on steady-state renal function and the accuracy of the measurements depends on the reliability of the urine collection. Unpredictable creatinine excretion may occur through feces or skin in patients with serum creatinine levels >530 μmol/L (>6 mg/dL). The presence of ascites does not compromise the accuracy of the 24-h urine creatinine as a reflection of FFM or BCM in patients with chronic liver disease.

Urine Nitrogen Excretion and Nitrogen Balance Nitrogen balance provides an index of protein gain or loss: 1 g nitrogen is equivalent to 6.25 g protein. Nitrogen balance can be assessed by measuring the difference between nitrogen consumed through the mouth, enteral tube, or intravenous sources and nitrogen excreted in the urine, feces, and other intestinal sources. Accurate measurement of nitrogen balance requires complete measurement of nitrogen losses from all possible excretory routes. In most cases, total urine nitrogen can be calculated by dividing 24-h urinary urea nitrogen by 0.85 and assuming approximately 2 g/d for nitrogen losses in feces and sweat. On the other hand, when the clinical condition includes extensive diarrhea and/or protein losses from pancreatic or enterocutaneous fistulas, the accuracy of nitrogen balance requires measurement of total nitrogen by the modified Kjeldahl technique in both urine and enteric sources. Total nitrogen measurements are also advisable in patients with liver failure, where urinary ammonia becomes a major and alternative source of nitrogen.

INTEGRATED BEDSIDE NUTRITIONAL ASSESSMENT Several different approaches have been developed to simplify the process of nutritional assessment by using selective measurements that relate malnutrition to the specific medical condition and the severity of the underlying disease process.

Subjective Global Assessment This approach incorporates historic and physical findings as a basis for nutrition assessment by the trained physician. Major components in the history include evaluation of the extent of recent weight loss, changes in dietary intake, presence of significant gastrointestinal symptoms persisting more than 2 weeks, alterations in functional status, and the metabolic demand of the patient's underlying disease. During the physical examination, emphasis is placed on findings of depletion of subcutaneous body fat; skeletal muscle wasting; typical changes in skin, mucus membranes, and neurologic examination; as well as the presence of edema. Integration of the historic and physical data permits ranking of patients according to the following categories: adequate nutrition, moderate malnutrition, or severe malnutrition. Though the developers of the subjective global assessment have reported good sensitivity and specificity, the approach is still highly dependent on the training and experience of the clinician.

Prognostic Nutritional Assessment Several paradigms have been developed to link different parameters of nutritional assessment with clinical prognosis. Each approach links specific features of malnutrition with certain measurements of cell-mediated immunity, since abnormal immune function is a common pathway for increased risk in the malnourished patient. A surgical prognostic nutritional index predicts morbidity based on preoperative measurements of serum albumin, transferrin, triceps skin-fold thickness, and delayed hypersensitivity to skin-test antigens. Another PCM score links survival in alcoholic liver disease to both skin-fold and mid-arm muscle measurements; the creatinine-height index; values for serum albumin, transferrin, prealbumin, and retinol-binding protein; the total lymphocyte count; and the skin-test response to a series of antigens. The Maastricht index predicts survival in patients with serious gastrointestinal diseases on the basis of factors related to serum albumin, retinol-binding protein, lymphocyte count, and deviation from the patient's ideal body weight.

FURTHER READING

BAKER JP et al: Nutritional assessment: A comparison of clinical judgment and objective measurements. N Engl J Med 306:969, 1982

GUIGOZ Y, VELLAS B: Assessing the nutritional status of the elderly: The Mini Nutritional Assessment as part of the geriatric evaluation. Nutr Rev 54:S59, 1998

HALSTED CH: Clinical nutrition education—relevance and role models. Am J Clin Nutr 67:192, 1998

HEYMSFIELD SB et al: Nutritional assessment of malnutrition by anthropomorphic methods, in *Modern Nutrition in Health and Disease*, 9th ed, ME Shils et al (eds). Philadelphia, Lea & Febiger, 1999, p 903

KLIPSTEIN-GROBUSCH K, REILLY J: Energy intake and expenditure in elderly patients admitted to the hospital with acute illness. Br J Nutr 73:323, 1995

MENDENHALL C et al: Relationship of protein calorie malnutrition to alcoholic liver disease: A reexamination of data from two Veterans Administration Cooperative Studies. Alcohol Clin Exp Res 19:635, 1995

NABER THJ et al: Prevalence of malnutrition in nonsurgical hospitalized patients and its association with disease complications. Am J Clin Nutr 66:1232, 1997

UNDERWOOD BA: Health and nutrition in women, infants, and children: Overview of the global situation and the Asian enigma. Nutr Rev 2002 60:S7, 2002

YANOVSKI SZ et al: Bioelectrical impedance analysis in body composition measurement: National Institutes of Health technology assessment conference statement. Am J Clin Nutr 64:524S, 1996

63 ENTERAL AND PARENTERAL NUTRITION THERAPY
Lyn Howard

Parenteral and enteral nutrition provide life-sustaining therapy for patients who cannot take adequate food by mouth and who consequently are at risk for malnutrition and its effects, including susceptibility to infection, weakness, and immobility; these features predispose the patient to aspiration pneumonia, pulmonary embolism, and pressure sores, all of which delay recovery from illness and increase mortality.

The term *enteral* refers to feeding via the gut and hence includes normal eating, but in the present context implies the infusion of formulas, via a tube, into the upper gastrointestinal tract. *Parenteral* refers to the infusion of nutrient solutions into the bloodstream. Although these are different approaches to nutritional support, their goals are the same.

Where feasible, enteral nutrition (EN) is the preferred route because it sustains the digestive, absorptive, and immunologic barrier functions of the gastrointestinal tract. Several developments have made tube feeding easier and more acceptable to patients. Small-bore pliable tubes have largely replaced large-bore rubber tubes, and double-lumen

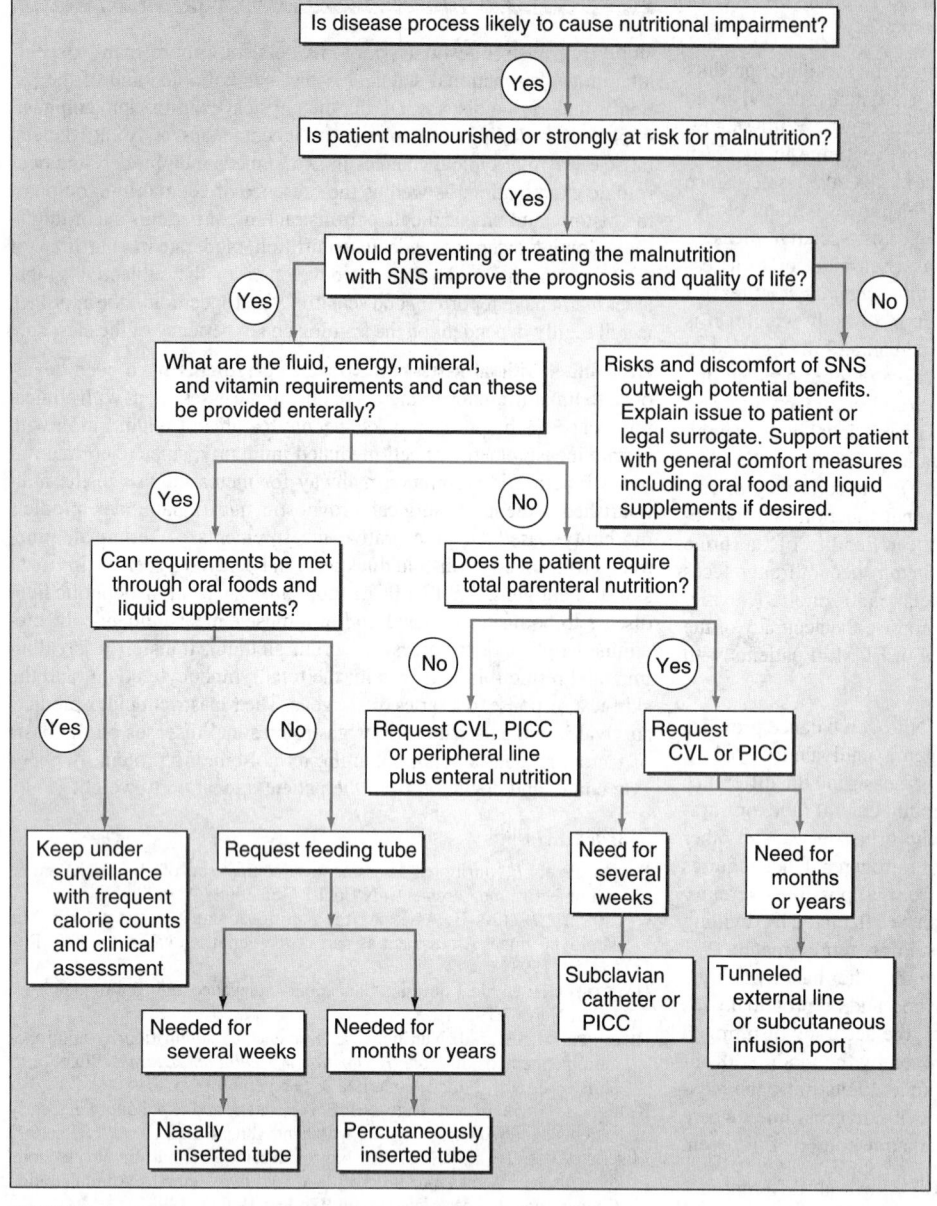

FIGURE 63-1 Should specialized nutrition support (SNS) be undertaken and, if so, how? An algorithm. PICC, peripherally inserted central catheter; CVL, central venous line.

Flow diagram elements:

- Is disease process likely to cause nutritional impairment? → Yes
- Is patient malnourished or strongly at risk for malnutrition? → Yes
- Would preventing or treating the malnutrition with SNS improve the prognosis and quality of life?
  - Yes → What are the fluid, energy, mineral, and vitamin requirements and can these be provided enterally?
  - No → Risks and discomfort of SNS outweigh potential benefits. Explain issue to patient or legal surrogate. Support patient with general comfort measures including oral food and liquid supplements if desired.
- What are the fluid, energy, mineral, and vitamin requirements and can these be provided enterally?
  - Yes → Can requirements be met through oral foods and liquid supplements?
    - Yes → Keep under surveillance with frequent calorie counts and clinical assessment
    - No → Request feeding tube
      - Needed for several weeks → Nasally inserted tube
      - Needed for months or years → Percutaneously inserted tube
  - No → Does the patient require total parenteral nutrition?
    - No → Request CVL, PICC or peripheral line plus enteral nutrition
    - Yes → Request CVL or PICC
      - Need for several weeks → Subclavian catheter or PICC
      - Need for months or years → Tunneled external line or subcutaneous infusion port

tubes are now available for simultaneous gastric suction and jejunal feeding when there is concern about gastric retention and aspiration. Enteral tubes can be inserted into the stomach or jejunum through the nose or, for long-term use, directly through the abdominal wall, using endoscopic, radiologic, or surgical techniques. Once the enterocutaneous tract is established, a "button" entry port can replace the protruding tube.

Complete nutrition by vein with sufficient calories, amino acids, minerals, and vitamins to permit wound healing, restoration of normal body composition of a cachectic patient, and growth in children became feasible with the development of high-flow central vein catheters. Parental nutrition (PN) is now available in all large hospitals and for some patients at home.

THE DECISION PROCESS FOR USING PARENTERAL OR ENTERAL NUTRITION

The decision to use specialized nutrition support (SNS) should be based on the likelihood that averting or redressing malnutrition will improve the quality of life, or the ability to recover from a serious illness. Approximately 15 to 20% of hospitalized patients have evidence of malnutrition. Some malnourished patients benefit from SNS;

for others, wasting is an inevitable component of a terminal disease. A flow diagram of the steps involved in deciding whether SNS should be undertaken and, if so, how, is depicted in Fig. 63-1.

The first step requires consideration of the nutritional implications of the disease process. Is the condition or its treatment likely to impair appetite or food ingestion and absorption for a prolonged period of time? The second step is to determine whether the patient is already sufficiently malnourished that lean body mass is decreased and critical functions such as healing and ventilation are impaired. The presence or absence of metabolic stress should be noted, since injury or infection evokes the secretion of hormonal and cytokine factors that reduce the efficiency of nutrition repletion.

Weight loss without physiologic impairment is probably of no consequence. Physiologic impairment usually develops when more than 20% of body protein is lost and is more likely if key organ systems, such as the gut or liver, are directly affected by disease. Once it is recognized that the patient is malnourished or at major risk, the next question is whether SNS will impact positively on the patient's response to the disease, improving quality of life. While the provision of food and water is part of basic medical care, nutrition delivered by tube, enteral or parenteral, is associated with risk and discomfort and should be recommended only when potential benefit exceeds risk, and undertaken with the consent of the patient. Like all life support measures, these therapies are difficult to withdraw, once started.

If preventing or treating malnutrition with SNS is appropriate, then nutritional requirements must be determined and the route of nutrient delivery should be selected. The route depends primarily on the degree of gut function but somewhat on the technical resources available.

RISKS AND BENEFITS OF SPECIALIZED NUTRITION SUPPORT

The risks are determined primarily by patient factors such as state of alertness and swallowing competence, the route of delivery, and the experience of the supervising clinical team. The safest and least costly approach is to avoid SNS, if possible, by close attention to oral food intake, by adding an oral liquid supplement, or by using medications to stimulate appetite. Nutrient intake is monitored with frequent calorie counts. This more physiologic approach is the most metabolically efficient since normal eating initiates the cephalic phase of digestion. Tube-fed infants grow better if the cephalic phase is stimulated by having the infant suck on a pacifier.

Anorexia, impairment of swallowing, or bowel disease can limit intake and absorption of oral nutrients, in which case tube EN is considered next. The bowel and its associated digestive organs derive 70% of their required nutrients directly from food in the lumen. Glutamine, short-chain fatty acids, and nucleotides may have particular importance in maintaining gut integrity. Enteral feeding also supports gut function by stimulating splanchnic blood flow, neuronal activity, IgA antibody release, and secretion of gastrointestinal hormones such as epidermal growth factor that stimulate gut trophic activity. All these factors support the gut as an immunologic barrier against enteric pathogens. For these reasons, some luminal nutrition should always be provided, if possible, even when PN is required to provide most of the support. In the past, bowel rest through PN was thought to be the cornerstone of treatment for many severe gastrointestinal disorders, but the value of some EN is now widely accepted, and strict bowel rest is rarely appropriate. PN alone is necessary in severe hemorrhagic pancreatitis, necrotizing enterocolitis, prolonged ileus, and distal bowel obstruction.

SNS is expensive, accounting for >1% of all health care dollars. Consequently, in assessing effectiveness, hard clinical end points, such as mortality rate, incidence of major complications, and duration of hospital stay are required for risk-benefit studies. Better nitrogen balance, increased levels of serum albumin, and improved delayed hypersensitivity are softer end points. Table 63-1 summarizes the current evidence-based evaluation of SNS treatment in disease states. The data are strictly from randomized controlled trials, in many instances combined into meta-analyses. This analysis emphasized that SNS is beneficial primarily for conditions associated with severe protein-calorie malnutrition or when oral intake is interrupted for prolonged periods of time (e.g., >9 days).

A practical consideration is the availability of tube or line placement expertise, especially in critically ill patients. Placement of a central venous catheter is a widely available bedside technique and can be done by specially trained personnel using a peripherally inserted central catheter. While inserting a nasogastric tube is a bedside pro-

TABLE 63-1 Evidence-Based Evaluation of SNS in Different Disease States[a]

Disease State	Type of SNS	Comment
Perioperative		
Preoperative	PN	Only beneficial in severe PCM
		↓ Postoperative complications 10%
	EN	↓ Postoperative complications ≥25%
Postoperative	PN	↓ Complications and MR if oral intake not resumed in 9 days
	Early EN vs PN	↓ Septic complications with EN if PN calories higher
	EN with CEN	↓ Postoperative complications and hospital stay (CEN: arginine, W₃FA, nucleotides)
Critical illness	PN	Only beneficial in severe PCM
		↓ Complications if lipid not used
	Early EN vs PN	↓ Septic complications with EN if PN calories higher
	EN with CEN	Risk ≥ benefit if CEN arginine
Cancer		
Cachexia	PN	Risk ≥ benefit with CXT/RXT; beneficial in cancer surgery in severe PCM
	EN	No clear benefit
BMT	PN/EN	Better long-term survival
	PN with CEN	↓ Early MR, ↓ hospital stay (CEN: glutamine)
	Home PN vs IV hydration	Outcome same; PN associated with less weight loss but delayed oral intake
Liver failure	PN/EN with CEN	Beneficial if encephalopathy prevents adequate protein intake (CEN: ↑ BCAA, ↓ AAA)
Renal failure		
Acute	PN with AA vs PN without AA	PN with AA: ↓ septic complications; EAA or EAA and NEAA equally good
Chronic	Low-protein diet	Did not reduce rate of GFR deterioration
	IDPN	No benefit on MR shown
Pancreatitis		
Acute	PN	Risk > benefit except in severe pancreatitis
	Early PN vs late PN	Early PN, ↓ MR in severe pancreatitis
	EN vs PN	↓ Septic complications with EN if PN calories higher
Inflammatory bowel disease		
Crohn's	PN vs EN	No benefit from bowel rest
	EN polymeric vs elemental	No difference
	EN vs steroids	EN: slower improvement, shorter remissions
	Exclusion vs regular oral diet	Elimination of foods that induce GI distress prolongs remission
Ulcerative colitis	PN vs oral diet/steroids	No difference
Short bowel syndrome	PN with CEN	hGH and glutamine supplements did not ↑ bowel adaption
Pulmonary disease		
Acute, ventilated	PN/EN	↓ CHO, ↑ fat calories aided weaning process
	EN intermittent vs continuous	No difference in gastric colonization
Chronic	EN gastric vs jejunal	↓ Aspiration, better intake with jejunal
	EN gastric vs postpyloric	No difference in risk of aspiration
HIV disease	PN vs EN	Gain in body cell mass same but PN ↑ fat and water gain; EN led to better physical functioning
	PN vs dietary counseling	No difference in survival after 2 months, but PN led to better functioning

Note: SNS, specialized nutrition support; PN, parenteral nutrition; PCM, protein-calorie malnutrition; MR, mortality rate; Early EN, tube feeding started within 48 h of onset of acute condition; EN, tube feeding; CEN, conditionally essential nutrients; W₃FA, omega 3 fatty acids; CXT, chemotherapy; RXT, radiation therapy; BMT, bone marrow transplant; BCAA, branch chain amino acids; AAA, aromatic amino acids; EAA, essential amino acids; NEAA, nonessential amino acids; IDPN, intradialytic parenteral nutrition; GFR, glomerular filtration rate; hGH, human growth hormone; CHO, carbohydrate.

Diagnosis	Number in Group	Age in Years	% Survival[a] on Therapy	Therapy Status, % at 1 year[b]			Rehabilitation[c] Status, % in 1st year			Complications[d] per Patient-Year	
				Full Oral Nutrition	Continued on HPEN Rx	Died	C	P	M	HPEN	NonHPEN
HOME PARENTERAL NUTRITION											
Crohn's disease	562	36	96	70	25	2	60	38	2	0.9	1.1
Ischemic bowel disease	331	49	87	27	48	19	53	41	6	1.4	1.1
Motility disorder	299	45	87	31	44	21	49	39	12	1.3	1.1
Congenital bowel defect	172	5	94	42	47	9	63	27	11	2.1	1.0
Hyperemesis gravidarum	112	28	100	100	0	0	83	16	1	1.5	3.5
Chronic pancreatitis	156	42	90	82	10	5	60	38	2	1.2	2.5
Radiation enteritis	145	58	87	28	49	22	42	49	9	0.8	1.1
Chronic adhesive obstructions	120	53	83	47	34	13	23	68	10	1.7	1.4
Cystic fibrosis	51	17	50	38	13	36	24	66	16	0.8	3.7
Cancer	2122	44	20	26	8	63	29	57	14	1.1	3.3
AIDS	280	33	10	13	6	73	8	63	29	1.6	3.3
HOME ENTERAL NUTRITION											
Neurologic disorders of swallowing	1134	65	55	19	25	48	5	24	71	0.3	0.9
Cancer	1644	61	30	30	6	59	21	59	21	0.4	2.7

[a] Survival rates on therapy are values at 1 year, calculated by the life table method. This will differ from the percentage listed as died under Therapy Status, since all patients with known end points are considered in this latter measure. The ratio of observed versus expected deaths is equivalent to a Standard Mortality Ratio.
[b] Not shown are those patients who were back in hospital or who had changed therapy type by 12 months.
[c] Rehabilitation is designated complete (C), partial (P), or minimal (M), relative to the patient's ability to sustain normal age-related activity.
[d] Complications refer only to those complications that resulted in rehospitalization.
Source: Derived from North American HPEN Registry.

cedure, many sick patients have impaired gastric emptying, and intragastric feeding increases risk of aspiration pneumonia. Obtaining enteral access to the jejunum usually requires fluoroscopy in an endoscopic or radiologic unit. If a surgical laparotomy is required, a jejunal feeding tube can be placed simultaneously. Studies have shown that such tubes must be beyond the ligament of Treitz to avoid aspiration; an intraduodenal tube is no safer than an intragastric tube.

While most SNS is delivered in hospitals, some patients require SNS on a long-term basis. If they have a safe environment and a willingness to learn the self-care techniques, SNS can be administered at home. The clinical outcome of patients with severe intestinal disorders that use home PN or EN are summarized in Table 63-2. PN infused at home is usually cycled overnight to give greater daytime freedom. Cycling requires a 1-h taper up and down to avoid sudden changes in blood sugar. SNS is not usually appropriate in terminally ill patients but is an option if the patient and family request treatment and quality survival for several months is predicted.

THE DESIGN OF INDIVIDUAL REGIMENS

FLUID REQUIREMENTS These can be determined by adding the normal daily requirement (120 mL/kg of body weight for infants, 35 mL/kg of body weight for adults) to any abnormal loss. If the patient is on PN or EN, any oral intake should be subtracted from the estimate (Table 63-3). Since abnormal loss of enteric fluid implies significant mineral losses, extra amounts of these nutrients, as well as fluid (Table 63-4), must be added to the SNS formula.

ENERGY REQUIREMENTS (See also Chap. 62) Ultimately, energy expenditure dictates energy requirements, but in the early phase of nutrition repletion, requirements may not reflect expenditure. For example, malnourished patients are hypometabolic and may expend only 85 kJ/kg (20 kcal/kg) per day, but more calories are needed both for tissue repletion and because the metabolic rate increases with refeeding. Conversely, a highly stressed patient (sepsis, trauma) may expend 165 kJ/kg (40 kcal/kg) per day with a significant proportion of the calories coming from protein breakdown and gluconeogenesis and

---

TABLE 63-3 *Estimation of Daily Fluid Requirements*

NORMAL 70-KG MAN

Intake	Output
Normal requirement: $35 \times 70 =$ ~2500 mL/d (derived from oral liquids of 1200 mL, or 5 glasses/cups per day and solid food providing 1300 mL, 1000 mL from water in food, 300 mL from water generated by metabolism of foods)	Urine: 1600 mL/d Insensible loss: 800 mL/d Stool: 100 mL/d [sweat loss can be up to 2 L/d; each degree of fever (C) = 200 mL/d]

TUBE ENTERAL PATIENT

58-kg woman recovering from total gastrectomy for gastric cancer and supported by jejunostomy feedings, taking nothing by mouth or intravenously but experiencing 600 mL of diarrheal losses/day:
  Normal requirement $35 \times 58 =$ ~2000 mL/d
  Abnormal gastrointestinal loss $600 - 100 = 500$ mL/d
  Total per tube requirement = 2500 mL/d

PARENTERAL PATIENT

66-kg man with a high jejunostomy following massive bowel resection for Crohn's disease with oral intake of 2000 mL/day and jejunostomy loss of 4000 mL/day:
  Normal requirement $35 \times 66 = 2300$ mL/d
  Abnormal gastrointestinal loss $(4000 - 100)$ minus oral intake (2000) = 1900 mL/d
  Total parenteral requirement = 4200 mL/d

TABLE 63-4 *Enteric Fluid Volumes and Their Sodium, Potassium, Chloride, and Bicarbonate Content[a]*

	L/d[b]	Na, mmol/L	K,[c] mmol/L	Cl, mmol/L	HCO_3,[d] mmol/L
Oral intake	2–3				
Enteric secretions					
Saliva	1–2	10	30	10	30
Gastric juice	2	60	9	90	0
Bile	2–3	150	10	90	70
Small bowel	1	100	5	100	20
Colon	Variable	40	100	15	60

[a] Enteric secretions are also rich in divalent cations (Ca, Mg, Zn, Cu), and their loss is increased by steatorrhea, a high bowel fistula, or prolonged suction.
[b] Of the 9 L/d of oral and enteric fluid presented to the upper small bowel, normally 50% is absorbed in the jejunum, 40% in the ileum, and 10% in the colon. In short bowel patients, the colon may absorb greater amounts, up to 3 L/d.
[c] Potassium losses are small except in secretions distal to the ileocecal valve. The colon ion exchange is partly controlled by aldosterone, and therefore, Na^+ depletion increases K^+ loss in the stool.
[d] Bicarbonate losses must be replaced in parenteral solutions as acetane or lactate because of potential precipitation of bicarbonate with ingredients such as calcium.

from catecholamine-induced lipolysis. Oxidation of exogenous glucose plateaus at 100 kJ/kg (25 kcal/kg) per day, and administering a higher glucose load induces hepatic steatosis. Providing such patients with additional calories as exogenous fat does not suppress endogenous lipolysis. Furthermore, lipid solutions are made from vegetable oil and egg phospholipid and lack apoproteins, which they acquire from endogenous lipoproteins. Initially, the artificial chylomicron is taken up by the reticuloendothelial system, causing potential blockade. For all these reasons, modest hypocaloric glucose feeding with minimal parenteral fat is safer in the acutely stressed subject.

Parenteral lipid solutions are available as 10 or 20% isotonic solutions and are infused separately from amino acids and glucose or as a combined "three-in-one solution," obviating the need for an extra pump. Three-in-one PN solutions are less stable, and destabilized fat particles may coalesce into larger droplets, becoming fat emboli. For this reason, three-in-one solutions have a shorter storage life and must be mixed by a pharmacist who is knowledgeable about correct mixing sequence and safe levels of electrolytes and trace elements. Iron, for example, cannot be added to this solution.

Polyunsaturated vegetable oils are used in most enteral formulas because a diseased gastrointestinal tract absorbs them better than animal fat. Median-chain triglycerides (c8–12) may be added because of their simpler absorption. Though fat must supply the long-chain essential fatty acids (1 to 4% of energy from linoleic and linolenic acid) (Table 63-5), larger amounts (30% of energy) are safe in relatively stable patients and avoid the hazard of providing large amounts of carbohydrate calories (e.g., hyperglycemia and hepatic steatosis). Substituting omega-3 polyunsaturated fish oils for polyunsaturated vegetable fats may blunt the catabolic response to burn injury, trauma, and radiation by reducing the synthesis of prostaglandins that enhance the inflammatory response. Such fats are currently available in enteral formulas and are being tested in parenteral formulas.

Carbohydrate usually provides 60 to 70% of all calories and is provided as glucose [monohydrous dextrose, 14 kJ/g (3.4 kcal/g)] in parenteral solutions and as disaccharides (sucrose) and oligosaccharides (starch fragments) in enteral formulas to maximize absorption while limiting the intraluminal osmolar load. Fructooligosaccharides have been shown to promote normal gut flora.

PROTEIN OR AMINO ACID REQUIREMENTS The recommended dietary protein allowance of 0.8 g/kg per day is adequate for nonstressed patients, such as a starved patient with a high-grade esophageal stricture. Catabolic patients, in contrast, may require up to 1.5 g/kg per day of protein to induce positive nitrogen balance and reconstitute normal lean body mass. Early studies showed that recombinant human growth hormone increases lean body mass. However, subsequent trials have

---

TABLE 63-6 *Central Venous Access for Parenteral Nutrition*

Type of Catheters	Advantages	Disadvantages

Peripherally inserted central catheter
  Single lumen
  Double lumen
	Insertion cost low; can be done at bedside or by vascular radiology using Doppler guidance; especially advantageous for patients with neck wounds such as tracheostomies	High incidence of skin site irritation; tendency to break at hub; home patient requires assistance with weekly dressing change

Centrally inserted externalized catheter (subclavian, jugular, femoral)
  Single lumen
  Multilumen
	Can be inserted at bedside; relatively low cost; can be changed over a guidewire if clinically indicated: best site subclavian > jugular > femoral vein	10% incidence of mechanical complication with insertion, higher if physician inexperienced; need dedicated nutrition line; multiple-lumen catheters have increased sepsis rate

Centrally inserted, tunneled catheter or subcutaneous port	More stable for long-term use; when needle out, patients with ports have less disturbance of body image and can shower and swim without risk	More expensive device requiring operating room insertion; ports require needle stick.

TABLE 63-5 *Daily Enteral and Parenteral Requirements of Essential Fatty Acids, Minerals, and Vitamins*

Nutrient	Daily Requirement, Adult Range	
	Enteral	Parenteral
Essential fatty acids, % kcal	1–2	2–4
Calcium, g	0.8–1.2	0.2–0.4 (10–20 mmol)
Phosphorus, g	0.8–1.2	0.4–0.8
Potassium, g	2–5	3–4 (75–100 mmol)
Sodium, g	1–3	1–3 (50–150 mmol)
Chloride, g	2.5–5	3–4[a] (100–130 mmol)
Magnesium, g	0.3	0.3 (20 mmol)
Iron, mg	10	1–2
Zinc, mg	15	3–12
Copper, mg	2–3	0.3–0.5
Iodine, mg	0.15	0.15
Manganese, mg	2–5	2–5
Chromium, μg	50–200	15–30
Molybdenum, μg	150–300	20–120
Selenium, μg	50–200	50–100
Ascorbic acid, mg	60	100
Thiamine, mg	1.4	3.0
Riboflavin, mg	1.6	3.6
Niacin, mg	18	40
Biotin, μg	60	60
Pantothenic acid, mg	5	15
Pyridoxine, mg	2.0	4.0
Folic acid, μg	400	400
Cobalamin, μg	3.0	5
Vitamin A, μg	1000	1000
Vitamin D, μg	10	5–10
Vitamin E, mg	8–10	10–15
Vitamin K, μg	70–140	200

[a] In addition to chloride anions there is a parenteral requirement for bicarbonate equivalents to protect normal acid-base balance. These are provided as 100 mmol or more per day of acetate or lactate because of potential precipitation of bicarbonate with ingredients such as calcium.

TABLE 63-7 *Monitoring the Patient on Total Parenteral Nutrition*

CLINICAL DATA MONITORED DAILY

Sense of well-being: symptoms suggesting fluid overload, high or low blood glucose, electrolyte imbalance, etc.
Strength as judged by graded activity: getting out of bed, walking, stair climbing
Vital signs: temperature, blood pressure, pulse rate, and respiratory rate
Fluid balance: weight; fluid input (intravenous +/− enteral) vs fluid output (urine, stool, gastric suction, etc.)
Delivery equipment for parenteral nutrition: tubing, pump, filter, catheter, dressing (skin checked for local infection at time of dressing change)
Composition of nutrient solution

LABORATORY DATA

Finger stick glucose	Three times daily until patient stable
Blood glucose Na, K, Cl, HCO₃ Blood urea nitrogen	Daily until glucose infusion load and patient stable, then twice weekly
Liver function studies Serum creatinine, albumin PO₄, Ca, Mg Hb/Hct, WBC	Baseline, then twice weekly
INR	Baseline, then weekly
Micronutrient tests	As indicated

Note: Hb, hemoglobin; Hct, hematocrit; WBC, white blood cell (count); INR, international normalized ratio.

TABLE 63-8 *Complications of Total Parenteral Nutrition (TPN)*

First 48 h	First 2 Weeks	3 Months Onward
MECHANICAL		

Complications from catheter insertion:
  Cephalad displacement
  Pneumothorax
  Hemothorax
Detachment of line at catheter hub with blood loss or air embolism
	Catheter coming out of vein, more common if Silastic
	Detachment of line at catheter hub with blood loss or air embolism
	Thrombosis
		Detachment of line at catheter hub with blood loss or air embolism
		Fractures or tears in catheter
		Catheter embedded in vein wall

METABOLIC		
Fluid overload Hyperglycemia Hypophosphatemia Hypokalemia	Cardiopulmonary failure Refeeding edema Hyperosmolar nonketotic hyperglycemic coma Acid-base imbalance Electrolyte imbalance	Essentially fatty acid deficiency Iron deficiency Vitamin deficiencies TPN metabolic bone disease TPN liver disease Zinc, copper, chromium, selenium, molybdenum, deficiency
INFECTIOUS		
	Catheter-induced sepsis Exit site infection	Catheter-induced sepsis Tunnel infections Exit site infection

TABLE 63-9 *Enteral Feeding Tubes*

Type/Insertion Technique	Clinical Uses	Potential Complications
NASOGASTRIC TUBE		
External measurement: nostril, ear, xiphisternum; tube stiffened by ice water or stylet; position verified by injecting air and auscultating, aspirating gastric acid, or by x-ray	Short-term clinical situation (weeks) or longer periods with intermittent insertion; bolus feeding simpler, but continuous drip with pump better tolerated	Aspiration; ulceration of nasal and esophageal tissues, leading to stricture
NASOJEJUNAL TUBE		
External measurement: nostril, ear, anterior superior iliac spine (medical malleolus in infants); tube stiffened by stylet and passed through pylorus under fluoroscopy or with endoscopic loop	Short-term clinical situations where gastric emptying impaired or proximal leak suspected; requires continuous drip with pump	Spontaneous pulling back into stomach (position verified by aspirating content, pH > 6); diarrhea common, fiber-containing formula may help
GASTROSTOMY TUBE		
Percutaneous placement endoscopically, radiologically, or surgically: after tract established, can be converted to a gastric "button"	Long-term clinical situations, swallowing disorders, or impaired small-bowel absorption requiring continuous drip	Aspiration; irritation around tube exit site; peritoneal leak; balloon migration and obstruction of pylorus
JEJUNOSTOMY TUBE		
Percutaneous placement endoscopically or radiologically via pylorus or endoscopically or surgically directly into the jejunum	Long-term clinical situations where gastric emptying impaired; requires continuous drip with pump; direct endoscopic placement (PEJ) is the most comfortable for the patient	Clogging or displacement of tube; jejunal fistula if large-bore tube used; diarrhea from dumping; irritation of surgical anchoring suture
COMBINED GASTROJEJUNOSTOMY TUBE		
Percutaneous placement endoscopically, radiologically, or surgically; intragastric arm for continuous or intermittent gastric suction; jejunal arm for enteral feeding	Used for patients with impaired gastric emptying and at high risk for aspiration or patients with acute pancreatitis or proximal leaks	Clogging: especially of small bore jejunal tube

Note: All small tubes are at risk for clogging, especially if used for crushed medications. In long-term enteral nutrition patients, gastrostomy and jejunostomy tubes can be exchanged for a low-profile "button" once the tract is established.

shown an association with increased mortality in critically ill patients.

In a stable patient the adequacy of protein support can be assessed acutely by analyzing protein balance:

Protein balance

$$= \text{protein intake} - \text{protein loss}$$

where protein loss = [(24-h urine urea nitrogen (g) + 4) × 6.25]. Over a long period, protein balance is assessed by documenting wound healing, restoration of normal body composition, or resumption of longitudinal growth. In states of disturbed protein utilization (e.g., renal and hepatic failure), azotemia and abnormal plasma amino acid patterns develop. The benefit of special enteral and parenteral solutions that correct these aberrations is only established in hepatic encephalopathy (Table 63-1).

When amino acids are infused systemically, rather than via the more physiologic portal vein, methionine, the only sulfur-containing amino acid in most parenteral solutions, is transaminated in peripheral tissues rather than transulfurated in the liver. As a result, downstream sulfur products such as carnitine, taurine, and glutathione become relatively deficient. Preliminary studies suggest that the addition of an intermediate compound, *S*-adenosyl methionine, to parenteral solutions reduces cholestasis. In enteral formulas, protein is provided either as a complete protein with high biologic value and low immunogenicity, such as egg albumin or casein, or as partially hydrolysed short oligopeptides. Studies have shown that while amino acid transport mechanisms are defective with inflamed gastrointestinal mucosa, peptide absorption remains normal.

MINERAL AND VITAMIN REQUIREMENTS

Parenteral and enteral mineral and vitamin requirements are summarized in Table 63-5. Electrolyte modifications are necessary if the patient has significant gastrointestinal losses (Table 63-4) or renal failure. Requirements of some minerals and vitamins are higher when administered parenterally rather than enterally for several reasons: (1) many micronutrients delivered into the systemic rather than the portal circulation are not captured by the liver and instead pass directly into the urine; (2) patients with bowel disease often have increased enteric loss of sodium, potassium, chloride, and bicarbonate and malabsorption of divalent cations, fat-soluble vitamins, and vitamin B_{12}; and (3) nutrients may adhere to the tubing and delivery bags, and exposure to oxygen and light may destroy vitamins (particularly vitamin A).

INFUSION TECHNIQUE AND PATIENT MONITORING

Partial and short-term PN can be provided via a peripheral vein if the majority of the energy is supplied by isotonic fat solutions; long-term PN using glucose as the chief energy source requires administration via a central vein catheter so the hypertonic solution is rapidly diluted in a high-flow system. The preferred site for central vein infusion is the superior vena cava. Access sites and catheter choices are summarized in Table 63-6. Peripherally inserted central catheters are the most economical option for short-term PN. Tunneled catheters and implanted subcutaneous ports require operating room insertion but are more stable for long-term use. Central catheters should be changed when clinically indicated; routine changes are costly and hazardous. Chlorhexidine solution is a more effective local antiseptic than iodophor or alcohol. Although transparent dressings are helpful in stabilizing catheters and allow easy observation of the skin site, the incidence of catheter-related sepsis is higher than with traditional dry gauze dressings; newer transparent dressings that trap less moisture are under investigation. Catheters made from Silastic material or polyurethane are associated with lower complications than polyvinylchloride catheters. Several types of needleless systems use hub valves, and while inadvertent needle sticks are prevented, contamination rates are higher with these devices used for long-term PN. Appropriate clinical and laboratory monitoring for patients on parenteral nutrition is summarized in Table 63-7.

COMPLICATIONS ■ Mechanical

The insertion of a central venous catheter should be performed only by trained personnel, using an aseptic technique. The correct catheter position must be confirmed by x-ray before hypertonic nutrient solution is infused. Insertion complications are listed in Table 63-8. Catheter thrombosis may occur, especially if the catheter is used for withdrawing blood samples, and extension of the thrombosis to the central vein is frequently coincident with infection. Thrombosed catheters can sometimes be unblocked by thrombolytic agents. The addition of heparin (1000 U/L) to the PN solution to prevent thrombosis is controversial; no randomized, controlled studies demonstrate benefit, and heparin can contribute to loss of bone mineral, which is already a problem with long-term PN. Low-dose oral warfarin (1 mg/d), which does not alter prothrombin time, has been shown to reduce catheter thrombosis.

Metabolic

Fluid overload can cause congestive heart failure, particularly in elderly and debilitated patients. Glucose overload can cause an osmotic diuresis or stimulate insulin secretion, which in turn promotes extracellular to intracellular shifts of potassium and phosphorous. Such shifts are most dangerous in cachectic patients with depletion of potassium and phosphorus stores and can cause arrhythmias, cardiopulmonary dysfunction, and neurologic symptoms. To avoid these problems, PN should be started slowly and monitored carefully. Glucose content is increased gradually as the patient demonstrates tolerance of the high glucose load. Late metabolic complications include cholestatic liver disease, with bile sludging and gallstone formation. The exact cause of the liver disease is not understood, but lack of enteral stimulation to bile flow and defective sulfur amino acid metabolism and cholesterol solubilization appear to play a role. Chole-

TABLE 63-10 Enteral Formulas

Composition Characteristics	Clinical Indications
STANDARD ENTERAL FORMULA	
1. Complete dietary products (+)[a]	Suitable for most patients requiring tube feeding; flavors available for oral use
a. Caloric density 1 kcal/mL	
b. Protein ~14% cals, caseinates, soy, lactalbumin	
c. Fat ~30% cals, corn, soy, safflower oils	
d. CHO ~60% cals, hydrolysed corn starch, maltodextrin, sucrose	
e. Recommended daily intake of all minerals and vitamins in >1500 kcal/d	
f. Osmolality (mosmol/kg): ~300	
MODIFIED ENTERAL FORMULAS	
1. Caloric density 1.5–2 kcal/mL (+)	Fluid-restricted patients
2. a. High protein ~20% cals (+)	Protein malnutrition and ↓ wound healing
b. Hydrolysed protein to small peptides (++)	↓ Protein digestion/absorption or allergy
c. ↑ Glutamine, arginine, S-containing amino acids, nucleotides (+++)	Severely immunocompromised patients
d. ↑ Branch-chain amino acids, ↓ aromatic amino acids (+++)	Liver failure patients intolerant of 0.8 g/kg per day of regular protein
e. Low protein of high biologic value	Renal failure patients
3. a. Low fat, partial MCT substitution (+)	Fat malabsorption
b. ↑ Fat >40% cals (++)	Pulmonary failure with ↑ P_{CO_2} on standard formulas
c. ↑ Fat from MUFA (++)	Poorly controlled diabetes mellitus
d. Fat ↑ in w3 (fish oil) and ↓ w6 (+++)	Immunocompromised and autoimmune disorder
4. a. Fiber provided as soy polysaccharide (+)	Diarrhea/constipation
b. Fiber provided as blenderized fruits and vegetables (++)	↓ Binding of dilantin
5. ↑ Minerals (Zn) and vitamins (A and C) (++)	Decubitus ulcers

[a] Cost: + inexpensive; ++ moderately expensive; +++ very expensive.
Note: CHO, carbohydrate; MCT, medium-chain triglyceride; MUFA, monounsaturated fatty acids; w3 or w6, polyunsatuated fat with first double bond at carbon 3 (fish oils) or carbon 6 (vegetable oils).

stasis is less likely to occur if some enteral feeding is maintained. PN induces hypercalciuria and can result in negative calcium balance and osteopenia. Once patients on long-term PN change to sustained anabolism, deficiencies of micronutrients such as essential fatty acids, trace minerals, and vitamins may develop unless they are supplied in adequate amounts (Table 63-5).

Infectious

Infection of the access line rarely occurs in the first 72 h, and fever during this period is usually due to infection elsewhere or some other cause. Infection of the access line should be suspected if the fever defervesces when the infusion of the parenteral formula is tapered.

Positive central line and peripheral blood cultures suggest catheter sepsis, if no other infectious source is identified. *Staphylococcus epidermidis* infection can often be cleared (80 to 90% of the time) without catheter removal. To improve the chances of clearing the line, the biofilm from the internal surface is removed by thrombolytic treatment and antibiotics are given through the catheter and left as a "lock" in the catheter for several hours. *S. aureus* or fungal infections require catheter removal to prevent life-threatening metastatic spread. Catheter sepsis rates are similar in single-lumen central lines dedicated to PN whether inserted peripherally, via the subclavian vein, or tunneled; multiple-lumen catheters are associated with a greater incidence of sepsis. Although there is no evidence to support the use of prophylactic antibiotics, recurrent catheter sepsis may be avoided if small amounts of an antibiotic solution are left in the line, along with a heparin lock.

ENTERAL NUTRITION

TUBE PLACEMENT AND PATIENT MONITORING

The types of enteral feeding tubes, methods of insertion, their clinical uses, and potential complications are outlined in Table 63-9. The different types of enteral formulas are listed in Table 63-10. Patients on enteral feeding are at risk for many of the same metabolic complications as those who receive PN and should be monitored in the same manner (Table 63-7). Since small-bore tubes are easily displaced, tube position should be checked at intervals by aspirating and measuring the pH of the gut fluid (<4 in stomach, >6 in jejunum).

COMPLICATIONS ■ Aspiration The debilitated patient with poor gastric emptying and impairment of swallowing and cough mechanisms is at risk for aspiration; this is particularly so for those who are on respirators. Tracheal suctioning induces coughing and gastric regurgitation, and cuffs on endotracheal or tracheostomy tubes seldom protect against aspiration. Under these circumstances, it may be safer to institute jejunal feeding. A continuous gastric drip is better tolerated in sick patients than intermittent bolus feeding; a drip is essential for intrajejunal feeding.

Diarrhea Enteral feeding often causes diarrhea, especially if bowel function is compromised by disease or drugs, particularly broadspectrum antibiotics. Diarrhea may be controlled by the use of a continuous drip, with a fiber-containing formula or by adding an anticholinergic medication to the formula. Diarrhea associated with enteral feeding does not necessarily imply inadequate absorption of nutrients, other than water and electrolytes. Since luminal nutrients exert trophic effects on the gut mucosa and enhance the enteric immunologic barrier, it is often appropriate to persist with tube feeding, despite the diarrhea, even when this necessitates supplemental parenteral fluid support.

THE SCOPE AND COST OF NUTRITION SUPPORT

As many as 25% of patients entering tertiary care hospitals have central catheters placed, and 20 to 30% of these catheters are used for parenteral nutrition. The incidence of catheter-related infection reflects the severity of the underlying medical condition and varies from 2 to 30 per thousand catheter days, depending on the type of patients involved. In critically ill patients, catheter sepsis is associated with a 35% mortality rate and a high cost per survivor. Most catheter-related complications derive from faulty insertion and management of the catheter rather than defects in the device. In large tertiary care hospitals, the insertion and management of these lines by specially trained teams can reduce complications by 80%, impacting significantly on outcome and costs. The growing shift from parenteral to enteral nutrition may produce cost savings, but the true cost of complex enteral feeding is not known. Home PN costs approximately half as much as similar treatment in the hospital, and home EN costs significantly less.

FURTHER READING

BOZZETTI F et al: Perioperative total parenteral nutrition in malnourished, gastrointestinal cancer patient, a randomized, clinical trial. JPEN 24:7, 2000

HEYLAND DK et al: Should immunonutrition become routine in critically ill patients? A systematic review of the evidence. JAMA 286(8):22, 2001

HOWARD L et al: Current use and clinical outcome of home parenteral and enteral nutrition therapies in the United States. Gastroenterology 109:335, 1995

KORETZ RL et al: AGA technical review on parenteral nutrition. Gastroenterology 121:970, 2001

WOODCOCK NP et al: Enteral versus parenteral nutrition: A pragmatic study. Nutrition 17:1, 2000

64 OBESITY
Jeffrey S. Flier, Eleftheria Maratos-Flier

In a world where food supplies are intermittent, the ability to store energy in excess of what is required for immediate use is essential for survival. Fat cells, residing within widely distributed adipose tissue depots, are adapted to store excess energy efficiently as triglyceride and, when needed, to release stored energy as free fatty acids for use at other sites. This physiologic system, orchestrated through endocrine and neural pathways, permits humans to survive starvation for as long as several months. However, in the presence of nutritional abundance and a sedentary lifestyle, and influenced importantly by genetic endowment, this system increases adipose energy stores and produces adverse health consequences.

DEFINITION AND MEASUREMENT *Obesity* is a state of excess adipose tissue mass. Although often viewed as equivalent to increased body weight, this need not be the case—lean but very muscular individuals may be overweight by arbitrary standards without having increased adiposity. Body weights are distributed continuously in populations, so that a medically meaningful distinction between lean and obese is somewhat arbitrary. Obesity is therefore more effectively defined by assessing its linkage to morbidity or mortality.

Although not a direct measure of adiposity, the most widely used method to gauge obesity is the *body mass index* (BMI), which is equal to weight/height^2 (in kg/m^2) (Fig. 64-1). Other approaches to quantifying obesity include anthropometry (skin-fold thickness), densitometry (underwater weighing), computed tomography (CT) or magnetic resonance imaging (MRI), and electrical impedance. Using data from the Metropolitan Life Tables, BMIs for the midpoint of all heights and frames among both men and women range from 19 to 26 kg/m^2; at a similar BMI, women have more body fat than men. Based on unequivocal data of substantial morbidity, a BMI of 30 is most commonly used as a threshold for obesity in both men and women. Large-scale epidemiologic studies suggest that all-cause, metabolic, cancer, and cardiovascular morbidity begin to rise (albeit at a slow rate) when BMIs are ≥ 25, suggesting that the cut-off for obesity should be lowered. Some authorities use the term *overweight* (rather than obese) to describe individuals with BMIs between 25 and 30. A BMI between 25 and 30 should be viewed as medically significant and worthy of therapeutic intervention, especially in the presence of risk factors that are influenced by adiposity, such as hypertension and glucose intolerance.

The distribution of adipose tissue in different anatomic depots also has substantial implications for morbidity. Specifically, intraabdominal and abdominal subcutaneous fat have more significance than subcutaneous fat present in the buttocks and lower extremities. This distinction is most easily made by determining the waist-to-hip ratio, with a ratio >0.9 in women and >1.0 in men being abnormal. Many of the most important complications of obesity, such as insulin resistance, diabetes, hypertension, and hyperlipidemia, and hyperandrogenism in women, are linked more strongly to intraabdominal and/or upper body fat than to overall adiposity. The mechanism underlying this association is unknown but may relate to the fact that intraabdominal adipocytes are more lipolytically active than those from other depots. Release of free fatty acids into the portal circulation has adverse metabolic actions, especially on the liver.

PREVALENCE Data from the National Health and Nutrition Examination Surveys (NHANES) show that the percent of the American adult population with obesity (BMI > 30) has increased from 14.5% (between 1976 and 1980) to 30.5% (between 1999 and 2000). As many as 64% of U.S. adults ≥20 years of age were overweight (defined as BMI > 25) between the years of 1999 and 2000. Extreme obesity (BMI ≥ 40) has also increased and affects 4.7% of the population. The increasing prevalence of medically significant obesity raises great concern. Obesity is more common among women and in the poor; the prevalence in children is also rising at a worrisome rate.

PHYSIOLOGIC REGULATION OF ENERGY BALANCE Substantial evidence suggests that body weight is regulated by both endocrine and neural components that ultimately influence the effector arms of energy intake and expenditure. This complex regulatory system is necessary because even small imbalances between energy intake and expenditure will ultimately have large effects on body weight. For example, a 0.3%

positive imbalance over 30 years would result in a 9-kg (20-lb) weight gain. This exquisite regulation of energy balance cannot be monitored easily by calorie-counting in relation to physical activity. Rather, body weight regulation or dysregulation depends on a complex interplay of hormonal and neural signals. Alterations in stable weight by forced overeeding or food deprivation induce physiologic changes that resist these perturbations: with weight loss, appetite increases and energy expenditure falls; with overeeding, appetite falls and energy expenditure increases. This latter compensatory mechanism frequently fails, however, permitting obesity to develop when food is abundant and physical activity is limited. A major regulator of these adaptive responses is the adipocyte-derived hormone leptin, which acts through brain circuits (predominantly in the hypothalamus) to influence appetite, energy expenditure, and neuroendocrine function (see below).

Appetite is influenced by many factors that are integrated by the brain, most importantly within the hypothalamus (Fig. 64-2). Signals that impinge on the hypothalamic center include neural afferents, hormones, and metabolites. Vagal inputs are particularly important, bringing information from viscera, such as gut distention. Hormonal signals include leptin, insulin, cortisol, and gut peptides such as ghrelin, peptide YY (PYY), and cholecystokinin, which signal to the brain through direct action on hypothalamic control centers and/or via the vagus nerve. Metabolites, including glucose, can influence appetite, as seen by the effect of hypoglycemia to induce hunger; however, glucose is not normally a major regulator of appetite. These diverse hormonal, metabolic, and neural signals act by influencing the expression and release of various hypothalamic peptides [e.g., neuropeptide Y (NPY), Agouti-related peptide (AgRP), α melanocyte-stimulating hormone (α-MSH), and melanin-concentrating hormone (MCH)] that are integrated with serotonergic, catecholaminergic, and opioid signaling pathways (see below). Psychological and cultural factors also appear to play a role in the final expression of appetite. Apart from rare syndromes involving leptin, its receptor, and the melanocortin system, specific defects in this complex appetite control network that influence common causes of obesity are not well understood.

Energy expenditure includes the following components: (1) resting or basal metabolic rate; (2) the energy cost of metabolizing and storing food; (3) the thermic effect of exercise; and (4) adaptive thermogenesis, which varies in response to chronic caloric intake (rising with increased intake). Basal metabolic rate accounts for about 70% of daily energy expenditure, whereas active physical activity contributes 5 to 10%. Thus, a significant component of daily energy consumption is fixed.

Genetic models in mice indicate that mutations in certain genes (e.g., targeted deletion of the insulin receptor in adipose tissue) protect against obesity, apparently by increasing energy expenditure. Adaptive thermogenesis occurs in *brown adipose tissue* (BAT), which plays an important role in energy metabolism in many mammals. In contrast to white adipose tissue, which is used to store energy in the form of lipids, BAT expends stored energy as heat. A mitochondrial *uncoupling pro-*

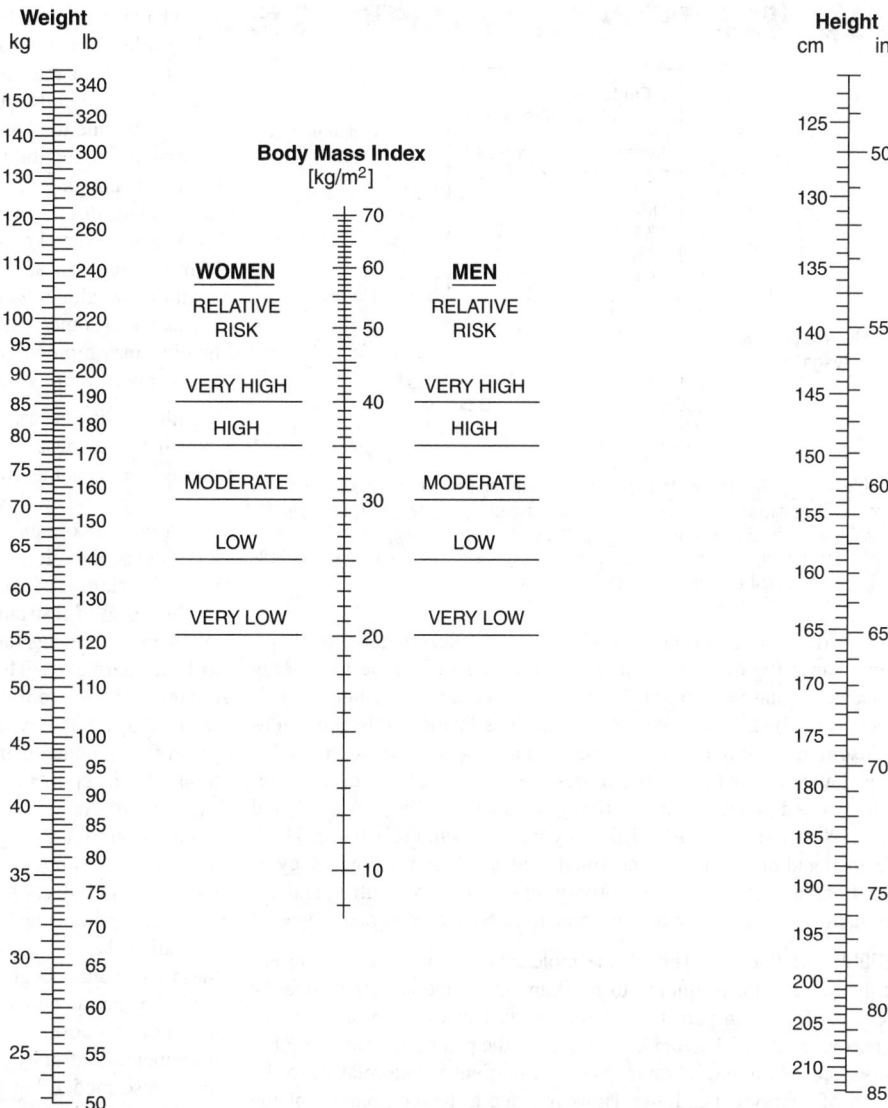

FIGURE 64-1 Nomogram for determining body mass index. To use this nomogram, place a ruler or other straight edge between the body weight (without clothes) in kilograms or pounds located on the left-hand line and the height (without shoes) in centimeters or inches located on the right-hand line. The body mass index is read from the middle of the scale and is in metric units. (*Copyright 1979, George A. Bray, M.D. Used with permission.*)

tein (UCP-1) in BAT dissipates the hydrogen ion gradient in the oxidative respiration chain and releases energy as heat. The metabolic activity of BAT is increased by a central action of leptin, acting through the sympathetic nervous system, which heavily innervates this tissue. In rodents, BAT deficiency causes obesity and diabetes; stimulation of BAT with a specific adrenergic agonist (β_3 agonist) protects against diabetes and obesity. Although BAT exists in humans (especially in neonates), its physiologic role is not yet established. Homologues of UCP-1 may mediate uncoupled mitochondrial respiration in other tissues.

THE ADIPOCYTE AND ADIPOSE TISSUE Adipose tissue is composed of the lipid-storing adipose cell and a stromal/vascular compartment in which preadipocytes reside. Adipose mass increases by enlargement of adipose cells through lipid deposition, as well as by an increase in the number of adipocytes. The process by which adipose cells are derived from a mesenchymal preadipocyte involves an orchestrated series of differentiation steps mediated by a cascade of specific transcription factors. One of the key transcription factors is *peroxisome proliferator-activated receptor* γ (PPARγ), a nuclear receptor that binds the thiazolidinedione class of insulin-sensitizing drugs used in the treatment of type 2 diabetes (Chap. 323).

Although the adipocyte has generally been regarded as a storage

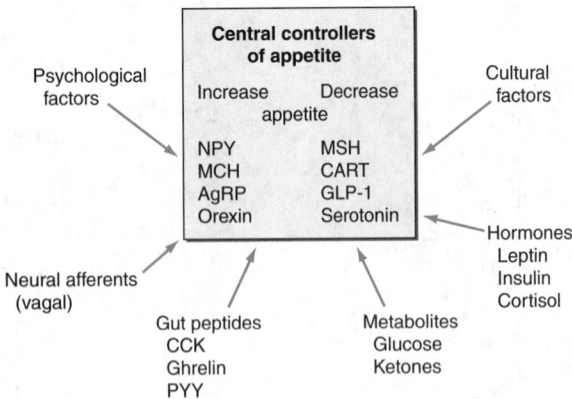

FIGURE 64-2 The factors that regulate appetite through effects on central neural circuits. Some factors that increase or decrease appetite are listed. NPY, neuropeptide Y; MCH, melanin-concentrating hormone; AgRP, Agouti-related peptide; MSH, melanocyte-stimulating hormone; CART, cocaine- and amphetamine-related transcript; GLP-1, glucagon-related peptide-1; CCK, cholecystokinin.

depot for fat, it is also an endocrine cell that releases numerous molecules in a regulated fashion (Fig. 64-3). These include the energy balance-regulating hormone leptin, cytokines such as tumor necrosis factor (TNF) α, complement factors such as factor D (also known as *adipsin*), prothrombotic agents such as plasminogen activator inhibitor I, and a component of the blood pressure regulating system, angiotensinogen. Adiponectin (or ACRP30) enhances insulin sensitivity and lipid oxidation, whereas resistin may induce insulin resistance. These factors, and others not yet identified, play a role in the physiology of lipid homeostasis, insulin sensitivity, blood pressure control, and coagulation and are likely to contribute to obesity-related pathologies.

ETIOLOGY OF OBESITY Though the molecular pathways regulating energy balance are beginning to be illuminated, the causes of obesity remain elusive. In part, this reflects the fact that obesity is a heterogeneous group of disorders. At one level, the pathophysiology of obesity seems simple: a chronic excess of nutrient intake relative to the level of energy expenditure. However, due to the complexity of the neuroendocrine and metabolic systems that regulate energy intake, storage, and expenditure, it has been difficult to quantitate all the relevant parameters (e.g., food intake and energy expenditure) over time in human subjects.

Role of Genes versus Environment Obesity is commonly seen in families, and the heredibility of body weight is similar to that for height. Inheritance is usually not Mendelian, however, and it is difficult to distinguish the role of genes and environmental factors. Adoptees usually resemble their biologic rather than adoptive parents with respect to obesity, providing strong support for genetic influences. Likewise, identical twins have very similar BMIs whether reared together or apart, and their BMIs are much more strongly correlated than those of dizygotic twins. These genetic effects appear to relate to both energy intake and expenditure.

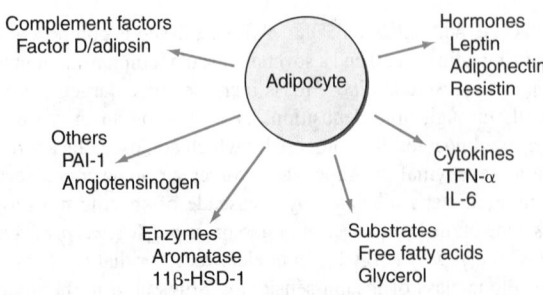

FIGURE 64-3 Factors released by the adipocyte that can affect peripheral tissues. PAI, plasminogen activator inhibitor; TNF, tumor necrosis factor.

Whatever the role of genes, it is clear that the environment plays a key role in obesity, as evidenced by the fact that famine prevents obesity in even the most obesity-prone individual. In addition, the recent increase in the prevalence of obesity in the United States is too rapid to be due to changes in the gene pool. Undoubtedly, genes influence the susceptibility to obesity when confronted with specific diets and availability of nutrition. Cultural factors are also important—these relate to both availability and composition of the diet and to changes in the level of physical activity. In industrial societies, obesity is more common among poor women, whereas in underdeveloped countries, wealthier women are more often obese. In children, obesity correlates to some degree with time spent watching television. High-fat diets may promote obesity, as may diets rich in simple (as opposed to complex) carbohydrates.

Specific Genetic Syndromes For many years obesity in rodents has been known to be caused by a number of distinct mutations distributed through the genome. Most of these single-gene mutations cause both hyperphagia and diminished energy expenditure, suggesting a link between these two parameters of energy homeostasis. Identification of the *ob* gene mutation in genetically obese (ob/ob) mice represented a major breakthrough in the field. The ob/ob mouse develops severe obesity, insulin resistance, and hyperphagia, as well as efficient metabolism (e.g., it gets fat even when given the same number of calories as lean littermates). The product of the *ob* gene is the peptide leptin, a name derived from the Greek root *leptos*, meaning thin. Leptin is secreted by adipose cells and acts primarily through the hypothalamus. Its level of production provides an index of adipose energy stores (Fig. 64-4). High leptin levels decrease food intake and increase energy expenditure. Another mouse mutant, db/db, which is resistant to leptin, has a mutation in the leptin receptor and develops a similar syndrome. The *OB* gene is present in humans and expressed in fat. Several families with morbid, early-onset obesity caused by inactivating mutations in either leptin or the leptin receptor have been described, thus demonstrating the biologic relevance of leptin in humans. The obesity in these individuals begins shortly after birth, is severe, and is accompanied by neuroendocrine abnormalities. The most prominent of these is hypogonadotropic hypogonadism, which is reversed by leptin replacement. Central hypothyroidism and growth retardation are seen in the mouse model, but their occurrence in leptin-deficient humans is less clear. To date, there is no evidence to suggest that mutations or polymorphisms in the leptin or leptin receptor genes play a prominent role in common forms of obesity.

Mutations in several other genes cause severe obesity in humans (Table 64-1); each of these syndromes is rare. Mutations in the gene encoding proopiomelanocortin (POMC) cause severe obesity through failure to synthesize α-MSH, a key neuropeptide that inhibits appetite in the hypothalamus. The absence of POMC also causes secondary

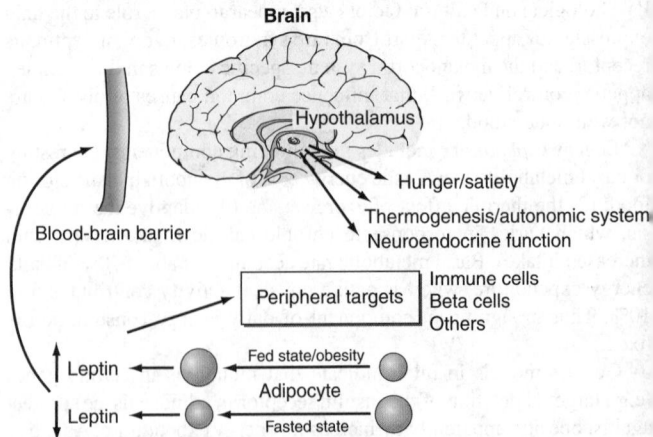

FIGURE 64-4 The physiologic system regulated by leptin. Rising or falling leptin levels act through the hypothalamus to influence appetite, energy expenditure, and neuroendocrine function and through peripheral sites to influence systems such as the immune system.

adrenal insufficiency due to absence of adrenocorticotropic hormone (ACTH), as well as pale skin and red hair due to absence of MSH. Proenzyme convertase 1 (PC-1) mutations are thought to cause obesity by preventing synthesis of α-MSH from its precursor peptide, POMC. α-MSH binds to the type 4 melanocortin receptor (MC4R), a key hypothalamic receptor that inhibits eating. Heterozygous mutations of this receptor appear to account for as much as 5% of severe obesity. These five genetic defects define a pathway through which leptin (by stimulating POMC and increasing MSH) restricts food intake and limits weight (Fig. 64-5).

In addition to these human obesity genes, studies in rodents reveal several other molecular candidates for hypothalamic mediators of human obesity or leanness. The *tub* gene encodes a hypothalamic peptide of unknown function; mutation of this gene causes late-onset obesity. The *fat* gene encodes carboxypeptidase E, a peptide-processing enzyme; mutation of this gene is thought to cause obesity by disrupting production of one or more neuropeptides. AgRP is coexpressed with NPY in arcuate nucleus neurons. AgRP antagonizes α-MSH action at MC4 receptors, and its overexpression induces obesity. In contrast, a mouse deficient in the peptide MCH, whose administration causes feeding, is lean.

A number of complex human syndromes with defined inheritance are associated with obesity (Table 64-2). Although specific genes are undefined at present, their identification will likely enhance our understanding of more common forms of human obesity. In the Prader-Willi syndrome, obesity coexists with short stature, mental retardation, hypogonadotropic hypogonadism, hypotonia, small hands and feet, fish-shaped mouth, and hyperphagia. Most patients have a chromosome 15 deletion (Chap. 57). Laurence-Moon-Biedl syndrome is characterized by obesity, mental retardation, retinitis pigmentosa, polydactyly, and hypogonadotropic hypogonadism.

Other Specific Syndromes Associated with Obesity ■ *CUSHING'S SYNDROME*
Although obese patients commonly have central obesity, hypertension, and glucose intolerance, they lack other specific stigmata of Cushing's syndrome (Chap. 321). Nonetheless, a potential diagnosis of Cushing's syndrome is often entertained. Cortisol production and urinary metabolites (17OH steroids) may be increased in simple obesity. Unlike in Cushing's syndrome, however, cortisol levels in blood and urine in the basal state and in response to corticotropin-releasing hormone (CRH) or ACTH are normal; the overnight 1-mg dexamethasone suppression test is normal in 90%, with the remainder being normal on a standard 2-day low-dose dexamethasone suppression test. Obesity may be associated with local reactivation of cortisol in fat by 11β hydroxysteroid dehydrogenase 1, an enzyme that converts cortisone to cortisol.

HYPOTHYROIDISM The possibility of hypothyroidism should be considered, but it is an uncommon cause of obesity; hypothyroidism is easily ruled out by measuring thyroid-stimulating hormone (TSH). Much of the weight gain that occurs in hypothyroidism is due to myxedema (Chap. 320).

INSULINOMA Patients with insulinoma often gain weight as a result of overeating to avoid hypoglycemia symptoms (Chap. 324). The increased substrate plus high insulin levels promote energy storage in fat. This can be marked in some individuals but is modest in most.

CRANIOPHARYNGIOMA AND OTHER DISORDERS INVOLVING THE HYPOTHALAMUS
Whether through tumors, trauma, or inflammation, hypothalamic dysfunction of systems controlling satiety, hunger, and energy expenditure can cause varying degrees of obesity (Chap. 318). It is uncommon to identify a discrete anatomic basis for these disorders. Subtle hypothalamic dysfunction is probably a more common cause of obesity than can be documented using currently available imaging techniques. Growth hormone (GH), which exerts lipolytic activity, is diminished in obesity and is increased with weight loss. Despite low GH levels, insulin-like growth factor (IGF) I (somatomedin) production is normal, suggesting that GH suppression is a compensatory response to increased nutritional supply.

Pathogenesis of Common Obesity Obesity can result from increased energy intake, decreased energy expenditure, or a combination of the two. Thus, identifying the etiology of obesity should involve measurements of both parameters. However, it is nearly impossible to perform direct and accurate measurements of energy intake in free-living individuals. Obese people, in particular, often underreport intake. Measurements of chronic energy expenditure have only recently become available using doubly labeled water or metabolic chamber/rooms. In subjects at stable weight and body composition, energy intake equals expenditure. Consequently, these techniques allow determination of energy intake in free-living individuals. The level of energy expenditure differs in established obesity, during periods of weight gain or loss, and in the pre- or postobese state. Studies that fail to take note of this phenomenon are not easily interpreted.

There is increased interest in the concept of a body weight "set point." This idea is supported by physiologic mechanisms centered around a sensing system in adipose tissue that reflects fat stores and a receptor, or "adipostat," that is in the hypothalamic centers. When fat

Gene	Gene Product	Mechanism of Obesity	In Human	In Rodent
Lep (ob)	Leptin, a fat-derived hormone	Mutation prevents leptin from delivering satiety signal; brain perceives starvation	Yes	Yes
LepR (db)	Leptin receptor	Same as above	Yes	Yes
POMC	Proopiomelanocortin, a precursor of several hormones and neuropeptides	Mutation prevents synthesis of melanocyte-stimulating hormone (MSH), a satiety signal	Yes	Yes
MC4R	Type 4 receptor for MSH	Mutation prevents reception of satiety signal from MSH	Yes	Yes
AgRP	Agouti-related peptide, a neuropeptide expressed in the hypothalamus	Overexpression inhibits signal through MC4R	No	Yes
PC-1	Prohormone convertase 1, a processing enzyme	Mutation prevents synthesis of neuropeptide, probably MSH	Yes	No
Fat	Carboxypeptidase E, a processing enzyme	Same as above	No	Yes
Tub	Tub, a hypothalamic protein of unknown function	Hypothalamic dysfunction	No	Yes

TABLE 64-1 *Some Obesity Genes in Humans and Mice*

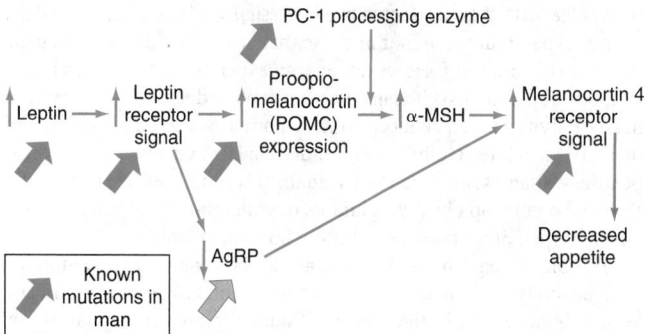

FIGURE 64-5 A central pathway through which leptin acts to regulate appetite and body weight. Leptin signals through proopiomelanocortin (POMC) neurons in the hypothalamus to induce increased production of α melanocyte-stimulating hormone (α-MSH), requiring the processing enzyme PC-1 (proenzyme convertase 1). α-MSH acts as an agonist on melanocortin-4 receptors to inhibit appetite, and the neuropeptide AgRp (Agouti-related peptide) acts as an antagonist of this receptor. Mutations that cause obesity in humans are indicated by the solid green arrows.

TABLE 64-2 *A Comparison of Syndromes of Obesity—Hypogonadism and Mental Retardation*

Feature	Syndrome				
	Prader-Willi	Laurence-Moon-Biedl	Ahlstrom	Cohen	Carpenter
Inheritance	Sporadic; two-thirds have defect	Autosomal recessive	Autosomal recessive	Probably autosomal recessive	Autosomal recessive
Stature	Short	Normal; infrequently short	Normal; infrequently short	Short or tall	Normal
Obesity	Generalized Moderate to severe Onset 1–3 yrs	Generalized Early onset, 1–2 yrs	Truncal Early onset, 2–5 yrs	Truncal Mid-childhood, age 5	Truncal, gluteal
Craniofacies	Narrow bifrontal diameter Almond-shaped eyes Strabismus V-shaped mouth High-arched palate	Not distinctive	Not distinctive	High nasal bridge Arched palate Open mouth Short philtrum	Acrocephaly Flat nasal bridge High-arched palate
Limbs	Small hands and feet Hypotonia	Polydactyly	No abnormalities	Hypotonia Narrow hands and feet	Polydactyly Syndactyly Genu valgum
Reproductive status	1° Hypogonadism	1° Hypogonadism	Hypogonadism in males but not in females	Normal gonadal function or hypogonadotrophic hypogonadism	2° Hypogonadism
Other features	Enamel hypoplasia Hyperphagia Temper tantrums Nasal speech			Dysplastic ears Delayed puberty	
Mental retardation	Mild to moderate		Normal intelligence	Mild	Slight

stores are depleted, the adipostat signal is low, and the hypothalamus responds by stimulating hunger and decreasing energy expenditure to conserve energy. Conversely, when fat stores are abundant, the signal is increased, and the hypothalamus responds by decreasing hunger and increasing energy expenditure. The recent discovery of the *ob* gene, and its product leptin, provides a molecular basis for this physiologic concept (see above).

What Is the Status of Food Intake in Obesity? (Do the Obese Eat More Than the Lean?) This question has stimulated much debate, due in part to the methodologic difficulties inherent in determining food intake. Many obese individuals believe that they eat small quantities of food, and this claim has often been supported by the results of food intake questionnaires. However, it is now established that average energy expenditure increases as people get more obese, due primarily to the fact that metabolically active lean tissue mass increases with obesity. Given the laws of thermodynamics, the obese person must therefore eat more than the average lean person to maintain their increased weight. It may be the case, however, that a subset of individuals who are predisposed to obesity have the capacity to become obese initially without an absolute increase in caloric consumption.

What Is the State of Energy Expenditure in Obesity? The average total daily energy expenditure is higher in obese than lean individuals when measured at stable weight. However, energy expenditure falls as weight is lost, due in part to loss of lean body mass and to decreased sympathetic nerve activity. When reduced to near-normal weight and maintained there for a while, (some) obese individuals have lower energy expenditure than (some) lean individuals. There is also a tendency for those who develop obesity as infants or children to have lower resting energy expenditure rates than those who remain lean.

The physiologic basis for variable rates of energy expenditure (at a given body weight and level of energy intake) is essentially unknown. A mutation in the human β_3 adrenergic receptor may be associated with increased risk of obesity and/or insulin resistance in certain (but not all) populations. Homologues of the BAT uncoupling protein, named UCP-2 and UCP-3, have been identified in both rodents and humans. UCP-2 is expressed widely, whereas UCP-3 is primarily expressed in skeletal muscle. These proteins may play a role in disordered energy balance.

One newly described component of thermogenesis, called *nonex-ercise activity thermogenesis* (NEAT), has been linked to obesity. It is the thermogenesis that accompanies physical activities other than volitional exercise, such as the activities of daily living, fidgeting, spontaneous muscle contraction, and maintaining posture. NEAT accounts for about two-thirds of the increased daily energy expenditure induced by overfeeding. The wide variation in fat storage seen in overfed individuals is predicted by the degree to which NEAT is induced. The molecular basis for NEAT and its regulation are unknown.

Leptin in Typical Obesity The vast majority of obese people have increased leptin levels but do not have mutations of either leptin or its receptor. They appear, therefore, to have a form of functional "leptin resistance." Data suggesting that some individuals produce less leptin per unit fat mass than others or have a form of relative leptin deficiency that predisposes to obesity are at present contradictory and unsettled. The mechanism for leptin resistance, and whether it can be overcome by raising leptin levels, is not yet established. Some data suggest that leptin may not effectively cross the blood-brain barrier as levels rise. It is also possible that leptin signaling inhibitors are involved in the leptin-resistant state.

PATHOLOGIC CONSEQUENCES OF OBESITY Obesity has major adverse effects on health. Morbidly obese individuals (>200% ideal body weight) have as much as a twelvefold increase in mortality. Mortality rates rise as obesity increases, particularly when obesity is associated with increased intraabdominal fat (see above). It is also apparent that the degree to which obesity affects particular organ systems is influenced by susceptibility genes that vary in the population.

Insulin Resistance and Type 2 Diabetes Mellitus Hyperinsulinemia and insulin resistance are pervasive features of obesity, increasing with weight gain and diminishing with weight loss. Insulin resistance is more strongly linked to intraabdominal fat than to fat in other depots. The molecular link between obesity and insulin resistance in tissues such as fat, muscle, and liver has been sought for many years. Major factors under investigation include: (1) insulin itself, by inducing receptor downregulation; (2) free fatty acids, known to be increased and capable of impairing insulin action; (3) intracellular lipid accumulation; and (4) various circulating peptides produced by adipocytes, including the cytokines TNF-α and interleukin (IL) 6 , and the "adipokines" adiponectin and resistin, which are produced by adipocytes, have altered expression in obese adipocytes, and are capable of modifying insulin action. Despite nearly universal insulin resistance, most obese individuals do not develop diabetes, suggesting that the onset of diabetes requires an interaction between obesity-induced insulin resistance and other factors that predispose to diabetes, such as impaired insulin secretion (Chap. 323). Obesity, however, is a major risk factor for diabetes, and as many as 80% of patients with type 2 diabetes mellitus are obese. Weight loss and exercise, even of modest degree, are associated with increased insulin sensitivity and often improve glucose control in diabetes.

Reproductive Disorders Disorders that affect the reproductive axis are associated with obesity in both men and women. Male hypogonadism is associated with increased adipose tissue, often distributed in a pattern more typical of females. In men >160% ideal body weight, plasma testosterone and sex hormone–binding globulin (SHBG) are often reduced, and estrogen levels (derived from conversion of adrenal androgens in adipose tissue) are increased (Chap. 325). Gynecomastia may be seen. However, masculinization, libido, potency, and spermatogenesis are preserved in most of these individuals. Free testosterone may be decreased in morbidly obese men whose weight exceeds 200% ideal body weight.

Obesity has long been associated with menstrual abnormalities in women, particularly in women with upper body obesity (Chap. 326). Common findings are increased androgen production, decreased SHBG, and increased peripheral conversion of androgen to estrogen. Most obese women with oligomenorrhea have the polycystic ovarian syndrome (PCOS), with its associated anovulation and ovarian hyperandrogenism; 40% of women with PCOS are obese. Most nonobese women with PCOS are also insulin-resistant, suggesting that insulin resistance, hyperinsulinemia, or the combination of the two are causative or contribute to the ovarian pathophysiology in PCOS in both obese and lean individuals. In obese women with PCOS, weight loss or treatment with insulin-sensitizing drugs often restores normal menses. The increased conversion of androstenedione to estrogen, which occurs to a greater degree in women with lower body obesity, may contribute to the increased incidence of uterine cancer in postmenopausal women with obesity.

Cardiovascular Disease The Framingham Study revealed that obesity was an independent risk factor for the 26-year incidence of cardiovascular disease in men and women [including coronary disease, stroke, and congestive heart failure (CHF)]. The waist/hip ratio may be the best predictor of these risks. When the additional effects of hypertension and glucose intolerance associated with obesity are included, the adverse impact of obesity is even more evident. The effect of obesity on cardiovascular mortality in women may be seen at BMIs as low as 25. Obesity, especially abdominal obesity, is associated with an atherogenic lipid profile, with increased low-density lipoprotein (LDL) cholesterol, very low density lipoprotein, and triglyceride, and decreased high-density lipoprotein cholesterol (Chap. 335). Obesity is also associated with hypertension. Measurement of blood pressure in the obese requires use of a larger cuff size to avoid artifactual increases. Obesity-induced hypertension is associated with increased peripheral resistance and cardiac output, increased sympathetic nervous system tone, increased salt sensitivity, and insulin-mediated salt retention; it is often responsive to modest weight loss.

Pulmonary Disease Obesity may be associated with a number of pulmonary abnormalities. These include reduced chest wall compliance, increased work of breathing, increased minute ventilation due to increased metabolic rate, and decreased total lung capacity and functional residual capacity (Chap. 234). Severe obesity may be associated with obstructive sleep apnea and the "obesity hypoventilation syndrome" (Chap. 246). Sleep apnea can be obstructive (most common), central, or mixed. Weight loss (10 to 20 kg) can bring substantial improvement, as can major weight loss following gastric bypass or restrictive surgery. Continuous positive airway pressure has been used with some success.

Gallstones Obesity is associated with enhanced biliary secretion of cholesterol, supersaturation of bile, and a higher incidence of gallstones, particularly cholesterol gallstones (Chap. 292). A person 50% above ideal body weight has about a sixfold increased incidence of symptomatic gallstones. Paradoxically, fasting increases supersaturation of bile by decreasing the phospholipid component. Fasting-induced cholecystitis is a complication of extreme diets.

Cancer Obesity in males is associated with higher mortality from cancer, including cancer of the esophagus, colon, rectum, pancreas, liver, and prostate; obesity in females is associated with higher mortality from cancer of the gallbladder, bile ducts, breasts, endometrium, cervix, and ovaries. Some of the latter may be due to increased rates of conversion of androstenedione to estrone in adipose tissue of obese individuals. It was recently estimated that obesity accounts for 14% of cancer deaths in men, and 20% in women in the United States.

Bone, Joint, and Cutaneous Disease Obesity is associated with an increased risk of osteoarthritis, no doubt partly due to the trauma of added weight bearing and joint malalignment. The prevalence of gout may also be increased (Chap. 313). Among the skin problems associated with obesity is acanthosis nigricans, manifested by darkening and thickening of the skin folds on the neck, elbows, and dorsal interphalangeal spaces. Acanthosis reflects the severity of underlying insulin resistance and diminishes with weight loss. Friability of skin may be increased, especially in skin folds, enhancing the risk of fungal and yeast infections. Finally, venous stasis is increased in the obese.

℞ TREATMENT

Obesity is a chronic medical condition. Successful treatment, defined as the sustained attainment of normal body weight without producing unacceptable treatment-induced morbidity, is rarely achieved in clinical practice. Many approaches produce short-term weight loss, and this has clear benefits for associated morbidities such as hypertension and diabetes. Although enormous resources are expended in pursuit of obesity therapies, most patients are unsuccessful at achieving and sustaining weight loss over time.

Treatment goals should be guided by the health risks of obesity in any given individual (Fig. 64-6). The clinician should always consider

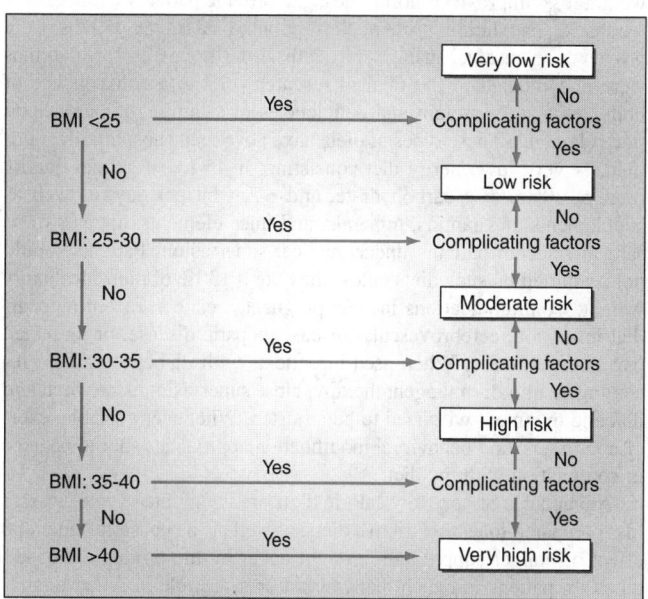

FIGURE 64-6 Risk classification algorithm. The patient is first placed into a category based on body mass index. The presence or absence of complicating factors determines the degree of health risk. Complicating factors include elevated abdominal-gluteal ratio (male: 1.0, female: 0.9), diabetes mellitus, hypertension, hyperlipidemia, male sex, and age <40. (*Copyright 1987, George A. Bray, MD. Used with permission.*)

the possibility that an individual has an identified cause of obesity, such as hypothyroidism, hypercortisolism, male hypogonadism, insulinoma, or central nervous system disease that affects hypothalamic function. Although they are infrequent causes of obesity, specific therapy may be available.

Behavior Modification   The principles of behavior modification provide the underpinnings for many current programs of weight reduction. Typically, the patient is requested to monitor and record the circumstances related to eating, and rewards are designed to modify maladaptive behaviors. Patients may benefit from counseling offered in a stable group setting for extended periods of time, including after weight loss.

Diet   Reduced caloric intake is the cornerstone of obesity treatment. The fundamental goal is the sustained reduction of energy intake below that of energy expenditure. The difficulty in achieving this goal has led to a wide array of suggested diets that vary in recommended calorie content (from total fasting to mild reductions), as well as specific food content and form (e.g., liquid vs. solid). There is no scientific evidence to validate the utility of specific "fad diets." The main diet regimens in use follow several general facts relevant to food intake and weight loss. First, a deficit of 7500 kcal will produce a weight loss of ~1 kg. Therefore, eating 100 kcal/d less for a year should cause a 5-kg weight loss, and a deficit of 1000 kcal/d should cause a loss of ~1 kg per week. The rate of weight loss on a given caloric intake is related to the rate of energy expenditure. Because obese individuals have a higher metabolic rate than lean individuals, and because men have a higher metabolic rate than women (due to their greater lean body mass), the rate of weight loss is greater among the more obese and among men (relative to women). With chronic caloric restriction, metabolic rate diminishes because of reduced lean body mass (along with much greater loss in fat mass) and possibly because of other adaptations. This fall in metabolic rate with food restriction slows the rate of weight loss on a constant diet. With total starvation or diets restricted to <600 kcal/d, initial weight loss over the first week results predominantly from natriuresis and the loss of fluids.

Very low energy diets (e.g., 400 to 600 kcal/d) may be appropriate for short-term treatment of obesity in selected patients. They are most commonly used for periods of 1 to 2 months to initiate more rapid weight loss, improve comorbidities, and provide patients with positive feedback. The liquid protein diets popularized in the 1970s were proved to be unsafe, causing >60 deaths. Life-threatening arrhythmias were documented in the clinical research setting, a consequence of both low-quality protein and deficiencies of vitamins, minerals, and trace elements. These types of diets have now been substantially modified. A very low energy diet consisting of 45 to 70 g high-quality protein, 30 to 50 g carbohydrate, and ~2 g fat per day, as well as supplements of vitamins, minerals, and trace elements, appears to be safe in selected patients under medical supervision. Patients should not be started on such diets unless they are >130% of their ideal body weight. Contraindications include pregnancy, cancer, recent myocardial infarction, cerebrovascular disease, hepatic disease, or untreated psychiatric disease. When used in patients with diabetes who are receiving insulin or oral agent therapy, close supervision is required and diabetic treatment will need to be adjusted. Whenever possible, exercise regimens and behavioral modification approaches should be used in conjunction with the diet.

Advantages of very low calorie diets are the greater rate of weight loss compared to less restrictive diets, as well as the possible beneficial effect of hunger suppression brought about by the production of ketones. In patients on such diets, blood pressure, blood glucose, cholesterol, and triglyceride levels fall, and pulmonary function and exercise tolerance improve. Sleep apnea may improve within a few weeks. Complications of these very low energy diets are usually minor and include fatigue, constipation or diarrhea, dry skin, hair loss, menstrual irregularities, orthostatic dizziness, and difficulty concentrating.

Cholelithiasis and pancreatitis may occur when such diets are interrupted by binge eating; gallstones have been shown to develop in as many as 25% of patients while on the diet.

Low-calorie diets, >800 kcal/d, are applicable to most patients and have fewer restrictions than the very low calorie diets. Considerable controversy has attended the question of which diet composition is most appropriate for promoting weight loss. Though commonly recommended, benefits resulting from very low fat diets are modest at best. Nonetheless, the health effects of low-fat diets—apart from curbing obesity—may be important. A diet rich in fruits, vegetables, whole grains, and other low–glycemic index carbohydrates may promote weight loss and is preferable to low-fat diets in which large amounts of simple carbohydrates are substituted for fats. The latter may actually promote obesity. Some have advocated diets with protein replacement of simple carbohydrates in an effort to minimize insulin production. The efficacy of this strategy, aside from overall calorie reduction, is unknown. Recent data suggest that very low carbohydrate "Atkins" style diets are more effective for short-term weight loss when compared to standard caloric restriction. Weight loss on such diets is not associated with adverse effects on such indices as lipid profile, glycemic control, or blood pressure. However, these diets have not been shown to be more effective in maintaining weight loss, and the possible long-term consequences of maintaining a lower body weight at the expense of consuming more saturated fat are unknown.

An important aspect of diet therapy should include education aimed at preventing weight gain. Knowledge of the caloric and nutritional content of foods is generally poor. In the absence of studies demonstrating convincingly that one type of diet is more effective and safe than another, an emphasis on helping patients understand the caloric content of specific portions is a helpful aid to weight loss and weight maintenance in many individuals.

Exercise   Exercise is an important component of the overall approach to treating obesity. Increased energy expenditure is the most obvious mechanism for an effect of exercise. The impact of an exercise regimen as a sole therapy of obesity has been difficult to document. On the other hand, exercise appears to be a valuable means to sustain diet therapy (Fig. 64-7). Even if exercise had no such salutary effect, it would be valuable in the obese individual for its effects on cardiovascular tone and blood pressure. Because many obese individuals have not engaged in exercise on a regular basis and may have cardiovascular risk factors, it should be introduced gradually and under medical supervision, especially in the most obese individuals.

Drugs   Despite modest short-term benefits from several agents, medication-induced weight loss is not a cure and is often associated with rebound weight gain after the cessation of drug use. Substantial side effects from several anti-obesity medications, and the potential for drug abuse, have combined to create a wariness about this approach. On the other hand, there is a great medical need for safe and effective

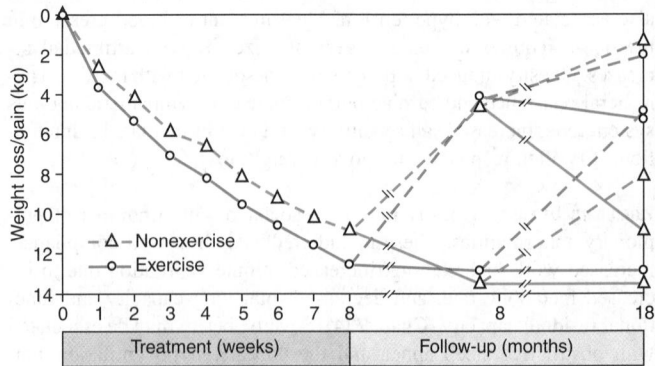

FIGURE 64-7   Weight loss and exercise. During the first 8 weeks, subjects were divided into two groups, one treated with diet and the other with diet plus exercise, with no difference in weight loss. Thereafter the subjects who exercised maintained better weight loss than those that did not. (*After KN Pavlou et al: Am J Clin Nutr 49: 1115, 1989.*)

therapies, so many possible compounds have been evaluated. On the basis of placebo-controlled trials, the U.S. Food and Drug Administration (FDA) approved several amphetamine-like agents for short-term use. Phentermine is an amphetamine-like drug with low addictive potential that showed modest efficacy (10 vs. 4.4 kg of weight loss over a 24-week period in a well-controlled study). This class of drugs is thought to act centrally by reducing appetite. The over-the-counter drug phenylpropanolamine HCl, had similar efficacy to prescription appetite suppressants in short-term studies but was withdrawn from the market in 2001 because of an association with cerebral hemorrhage. Drugs that promote serotonin release or inhibit serotonin reuptake, such as fenfluramine, have had modest efficacy as single agents. When fenfluramine was administered together with phentermine, as "fen-phen," the combination gained wide use for several years based on controlled trials that demonstrated modest but definite efficacy and reduction of comorbidities. However, the risk of primary pulmonary hypertension was increased up to 20-fold in association with this treatment. The FDA withdrew approval of the fen-phen combination in 1997 when reports demonstrated an association with right- and left-sided valvular heart disease. The histopathologic features of the valvular disease are similar to those seen in carcinoid syndrome and are thought to result from fenfluramine. The occurrence of this complication has been verified in multiple studies, and fenfluramine has been removed from the market.

Sibutramine is a central reuptake inhibitor of both norepinephrine and serotonin that was originally developed as an antidepressant. Using a once-daily dose over 24 weeks, it produced a 7% weight loss in a double-blind, placebo-controlled trial. It lowered cholesterol and triglyceride levels and exhibited similar clinical efficacy to fenfluramine. Sibutramine increases pulse by an average of 4 to 5 beats per minute and blood pressure by 1 to 3 mmHg, and this plus modest efficacy has limited its broad adoption. Orlistat is an inhibitor of intestinal lipase with no systemic availability that causes modest weight loss due to drug-induced fat malabsorption. A randomized, double-blind trial over 2 years revealed modest weight loss (8.7 kg for 120 mg orlistat versus 5.8 kg from diet alone) during the first year and better maintenance of weight loss in a second year compared to the placebo-treated group (3.2 kg regained vs. 5.6 kg regained for placebo). LDL cholesterol and insulin levels were also reduced. Gastrointestinal side effects include oily stools, flatulence, and fecal urgency and usually diminish as patients choose to limit fat intake to avoid the symptoms. Absorption of fat-soluble vitamins is decreased. In patients with obesity and type 2 diabetes mellitus, the antidiabetic medication metformin tends to decrease body weight. The mechanism appears to involve inhibition of appetite. Thyroid hormone has little place in the treatment of obesity, as the vast majority of obese individuals are euthyroid. It promotes loss of lean body mass and raises the risk of complications from the hyperthyroid state.

In the rare cases of leptin deficiency caused by mutations of the leptin gene, the administration of recombinant leptin is highly effective for regulating hunger and inducing loss of fat mass while preserving lean body mass. The response to leptin is limited or absent in common obesity, which is associated with hyperleptinemia and leptin resistance. New drugs are also being developed based on recent insights into central pathways that regulate body weight. These include antagonists for NPY receptors (subtypes Y1, Y5) and MCH receptors and agonists for melanocortin 4 receptors.

Surgery Morbid obesity, commonly defined as a BMI > 40, is estimated to increase mortality by as much as twelvefold in men between 25 and 34 years of age and sixfold between 35 and 45 years of age. Deaths from cardiovascular disease, diabetes, and accidents have been documented. In response to typically ineffective treatment using diet, exercise, and available drugs, surgical approaches are increasingly be-

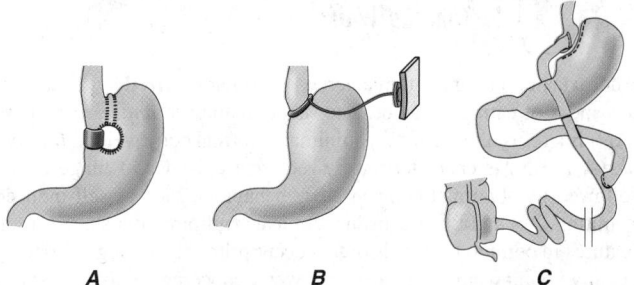

FIGURE 64-8 Examples of operative interventions used for surgical manipulation of the gastrointestinal tract. *A.* Vertical banded gastroplasty; *B.* adjustable gastric banding; *C.* Roux-en-Y gastric bypass.

ing employed. The potential benefits of surgery include major weight loss and improvement in hypertension, diabetes, sleep apnea, CHF, angina, hyperlipidemia, and venous disease. Several different approaches have been used, sometimes without adequate long-term assessment of efficacy and complications. Jejunoileal bypass surgery has been abandoned because of complications, which included electrolyte disturbances, nephrolithiasis, gallstones, gastric ulcers, arthritis, and hepatic dysfunction, with cirrhosis occurring in as many as 7% of patients. Two procedures in common use today are the vertical-banded gastroplasty and the Roux-en-Y gastric bypass (Fig. 64-8). The former is a purely restrictive procedure, while the latter combines restriction with slight malabsorption and may also reduce appetite via suppression of the gastric hormone ghrelin, which stimulates appetite. Gastric bypass is most often performed by laparotomy but may be performed laparascopically in some patients. A third procedure, laparoscopic adjustable gastric banding, is widely used in Europe and Australia and is being introduced in the United States. This procedure may be viewed as "less drastic" than gastric bypass but appears capable of producing substantial weight loss, albeit with shorter periods of follow-up.

Following the National Institutes of Health Consensus Conference on Gastrointestinal Surgery for Severe Obesity in 1991, it was recommended that suitable patients be selected using the following criteria: (1) a BMI > 35 with an associated comorbidity or a BMI > 40; (2) repeated failures of other therapeutic approaches; (3) at eligible weight for 3 to 5 years; (4) capability of tolerating surgery; (5) absence of alcoholism, other addictions, or major psychopathology; and (6) prior clearance by a psychiatrist. It is recommended that an appropriately experienced surgeon work together with nutritionists and other support personnel; evaluation and follow-up programs should be monitored closely.

ACKNOWLEDGMENT

The authors acknowledge the contributions of Dr. George A. Bray, who wrote this chapter in the 14th edition.

FURTHER READING

CROWLEY VE et al: Obesity therapy: Altering the energy intake and expenditure balance sheet. Nat Rev Drug Disc 1:276, 2002

FAROOQI IS et al: Clinical spectrum of obesity and mutations of the melanocortin 4 receptor gene. N Engl J Med 348:1160, 2003

FLEGAL KM et al: Prevalence and trends in obesity among US adults, 1999–2000. JAMA 288:1723, 2002

FLIER JS, MARATOS-FLIER E Editorial: The stomach speaks—ghrelin and weight reduction. N Engl J Med 346:1662, 2002

FONTAINE KR et al: Years of life lost due to obesity. JAMA:289, 2003

SPIEGELMAN BM, FLIER JS et al: Obesity and the regulation of energy balance. Cell 104:531, 2001

Anorexia nervosa and bulimia nervosa are characterized by severe disturbances of eating behavior. The salient feature of *anorexia nervosa* (AN) is a refusal to maintain a minimally normal body weight. *Bulimia nervosa* (BN) is characterized by recurrent episodes of binge eating followed by abnormal compensatory behaviors, such as self-induced vomiting. AN and BN are distinct clinical syndromes but share certain features in common. Both disorders occur primarily among previously healthy young women who become overly concerned with body shape and weight. Many patients with BN have past histories of anorexia nervosa, and many patients with anorexia nervosa engage in binge eating and purging behavior. In the current diagnostic system, the critical distinction between AN and BN depends on body weight: patients with AN are, by definition, significantly underweight, whereas patients with BN have body weights in the normal range or above.

Binge eating disorder (BED) is a more recently described syndrome characterized by repeated episodes of binge eating, similar to those of BN, in the absence of inappropriate compensatory behavior. Patients with BED are typically middle-aged men or women with significant obesity. They have an increased frequency of anxiety and depression compared to similarly obese patients without BED. It is not known whether patients with BED are at increased risk for medical complications or what treatment strategies are indicated.

ANOREXIA NERVOSA

EPIDEMIOLOGY Among women, the lifetime prevalence of the full syndrome of AN is approximately 0.5%. AN is much less common in males. AN is more prevalent in cultures where food is plentiful and in which being thin is associated with attractiveness. Individuals who pursue interests that place a premium on thinness, such as ballet and modeling, are at greater risk. The incidence of AN appears to have increased in recent decades.

ETIOLOGY The etiology of AN is unknown but appears to involve a combination of psychological, biologic, and cultural risk factors. Risk factors, such as sexual or physical abuse and a family history of mood disturbance, are best viewed as nonspecific risk factors that increase vulnerability to a range of psychiatric disorders, including AN.

Patients who develop AN are inclined to be more obsessional and perfectionist than their peers. The disorder often begins as a diet not distinguishable at the outset from those undertaken by many adolescents and young women. As weight loss progresses, the fear of gaining weight grows; dieting becomes stricter; and psychological, behavioral, and medical aberrations increase. Eating disorders, including AN, may develop among individuals with type 1 diabetes mellitus, and are associated with poorer glycemic control and an increased frequency of complications (Chap. 323).

Numerous physiologic disturbances, including abnormalities in a variety of neurotransmitter systems, have been described in AN (see below). It is difficult to distinguish neurochemical, metabolic, and hormonal changes that may have a role in the initiation or perpetuation of the syndrome from those that are secondary to the disorder. The resolution of most of these abnormalities with weight restoration argues against their having a critical etiologic role.

Genetic factors contribute to the risk of development of AN, as its incidence is greater in families with one affected member and the concordance in monozygotic twins is greater than in dizygotic twins. However, specific genes have not been identified.

CLINICAL FEATURES (Table 65-1) AN typically begins in mid to late adolescence, sometimes in association with a stressful life event such as leaving home for school. The disorder occasionally develops in early puberty, before menarche, but seldom begins after age 40. Despite being underweight, patients with AN are irrationally afraid of gaining weight, often out of a concern that weight gain will get "out

of control." They also exhibit a distortion of body image, which may express itself in several ways. For example, despite being emaciated, patients with AN may believe that their body as a whole, or some part of their body, is too fat. Further weight loss is viewed by the patient as a fulfilling accomplishment, while weight gain is seen as a personal failure. Patients with AN rarely complain of hunger or fatigue and often exercise extensively. Despite the denial of hunger, one-quarter to one-half of patients with AN engage in eating binges. Patients tend to become socially withdrawn and increasingly committed to work or study, dieting, and exercise. As weight loss progresses, thoughts of food dominate mental life and idiosyncratic rules develop around eating. Patients with AN may obsessively collect cookbooks and recipes and be drawn to food-related occupations.

Physical Features Patients with AN typically have few physical complaints but may note cold intolerance. Gastrointestinal motility is diminished, leading to reduced gastric emptying and constipation. Some women who develop AN after menarche report that their menses ceased before significant weight loss occurred. Weight and height should be measured to allow calculation of body mass index (BMI; kg/m^2). Vital signs may reveal bradycardia, hypotension, and mild hypothermia. Soft, downy hair growth (lanugo) sometimes occurs, and alopecia may be seen. Salivary gland enlargement, which is associated with starvation as well as with binge eating and vomiting, may make the face appear surprisingly full in contrast to the marked general wasting. Acrocyanosis of the digits is common, and peripheral edema can be seen in the absence of hypoalbuminemia, particularly when the patient begins to regain weight. Some patients who consume large amounts of vegetables containing vitamin A develop a yellow tint to the skin (*hypercarotenemia*), which is especially notable on the palms.

Laboratory Abnormalities Mild normochromic, normocytic anemia is frequent, as is mild to moderate leukopenia, with a disproportionate reduction of polymorphonuclear leukocytes. Dehydration may result in slightly increased levels of blood urea nitrogen and creatinine. Serum transaminase levels may increase, especially during the early phases of refeeding. The level of serum proteins is usually normal. Blood sugar is often low and serum cholesterol may be moderately elevated. Hypokalemic alkalosis suggests self-induced vomiting or the use of diuretics. Hyponatremia is common and may result from excess fluid intake and disturbances in the secretion of antidiuretic hormone.

Endocrine Abnormalities The regulation of virtually every endocrine system is altered in AN, but the most striking changes occur in the reproductive system. Amenorrhea is hypothalamic in origin and reflects diminished production of gonadotropin-releasing hormone (GnRH). When exogenous GnRH is administered in a pulsatile manner, pituitary responses of luteinizing hormone (LH) and follicle stimulating hormone (FSH) are normalized, indicating the absence of a primary pituitary abnormality. The resulting gonadotropin deficiency causes low plasma estrogen in women and reduced testosterone in men. The hypothalamic GnRH pulse generator is exquisitely sensitive, particularly in women, to body weight, stress, and exercise, each of which may contribute to *hypothalamic amenorrhea* in AN (Chap. 326). Although the mechanisms underlying these effects are unknown, the decreased adipose tissue associated with weight loss leads to a marked reduction in leptin, a hormone that plays a permissive role in GnRH production (Chap. 64).

Serum cortisol and 24-h urine free cortisol levels are generally elevated but without characteristic clinical signs of cortisol excess. Thyroid function tests resemble the pattern seen in euthyroid sick syndrome (Chap. 320). Thyroxine (T$_4$) and free T$_4$ levels are usually in the low-normal range, triiodothyronine (T$_3$) levels are reduced, and reverse T$_3$ (rT$_3$) is elevated. The level of thyroid stimulating hormone (TSH) is normally or partially suppressed. Growth hormone is increased, but insulin-like growth factor 1 (IGF-1), which is produced mainly by the liver, is reduced, as in other conditions of starvation. Diminished bone density is routinely observed in AN and reflects the effects of multiple nutritional deficiencies, reduced gonadal steroids, and increased cortisol. The degree of bone density reduction is proportional to the length of the illness, and patients are at risk for the development of symptomatic fractures. The occurrence of AN during adolescence may lead to the premature cessation of linear bone growth and a failure to achieve expected adult height.

Cardiac Abnormalities Cardiac output is reduced, and congestive heart failure occurs rarely during rapid refeeding. The electrocardiogram usually shows sinus bradycardia, reduced QRS voltage, and nonspecific ST-T-wave abnormalities. Some patients develop a prolonged QT_c interval, which may predispose to serious arrhythmias, particularly when electrolyte abnormalities are also present.

DIAGNOSIS The diagnosis of AN is based on the presence of characteristic behavioral, psychological, and physical attributes (Table 65-2). Widely accepted diagnostic criteria are provided by the American Psychiatric Association's *Diagnostic and Statistical Manual of Mental Disorders* (DSM-IV). These criteria include weight <85% of that expected for age and height, which is roughly equivalent to a BMI of 18.5 kg/m² for adult women. This weight criterion is somewhat arbitrary, so that a patient who meets all other diagnostic criteria but weighs between 85 and 90% of expected would still merit the diagnosis of AN. The current diagnostic criteria require that women with AN not have spontaneous menses, but occasional patients with the characteristics and complications of AN describe regular menstruation. Two mutually exclusive subtypes of AN are specified in DSM-IV. Patients whose weight loss is maintained primarily by caloric restriction, perhaps augmented by excessive exercise, are considered to have the "restricting" subtype of AN. The "binge eating/purging" subtype is characterized by binge eating, self-induced vomiting and/or laxative abuse. Patients with the binge/purge subtype are more prone to develop electrolyte imbalances, are more emotionally labile, and are more likely to have other problems with impulse control, such as drug abuse.

The diagnosis of AN can usually be made confidently on the basis of history when significant weight loss is accomplished by restrictive dieting and excessive exercise and is accompanied by a marked reluctance to gain weight. Patients with AN often deny that they have a serious problem and may be brought to medical attention by concerned family or friends. In atypical presentations, other causes of significant weight loss in previously healthy young people should be considered, including inflammatory bowel disease, gastric outlet obstruction, diabetes mellitus, central nervous system (CNS) tumors, and neoplasm (Chap. 36).

PROGNOSIS The course and outcome of AN are highly variable. One-quarter to one-half of patients eventually recover fully, with few psychological or physical sequelae. However, many patients have persistent difficulties with weight maintenance, depression, and eating disturbances, including BN. The development of obesity following AN is rare. The long-term mortality of AN is among the highest associated with any psychiatric disorder. Approximately 5% of patients die per decade of follow-up, primarily due to the physical effects of chronic starvation or by suicide.

Virtually all of the physiologic abnormalities associated with AN are observed in other forms of starvation and markedly improve or disappear with weight gain. A worrisome exception is the reduction in bone mass, which may not recover fully, particularly when AN occurs during adolescence when peak bone mass is normally achieved.

℞ TREATMENT

Because of the profound physiologic and psychological effects of starvation, there is a broad consensus that weight restoration to 90% of predicted weight is the primary goal in the treatment of AN. Unfortunately, because most patients resist this goal, the management of AN is often accompanied by frustration for the patient, the family, and the physician. Patients typically exaggerate their food intake and minimize their symptoms. Some patients resort to subterfuge to make their weights appear higher, for example, by water-loading before they are weighed. In attempting to engage the patient in treatment, it may be useful for the physician to elicit the patient's physical concerns (e.g., about osteoporosis, weakness, or fertility) and, if possible, educate the patient regarding the importance of normalizing nutritional status in order to address those concerns. The physician should attempt to reassure the patient that weight gain will not be permitted to get "out of control" but simultaneously emphasize that weight restoration is medically and psychologically imperative.

TABLE 65-1 *Common Characteristics of Anorexia Nervosa and Bulimia Nervosa*

	Anorexia Nervosa[a]	Bulimia Nervosa
CLINICAL CHARACTERISTICS		
Onset	Mid-adolescence	Late adolescence/early adulthood
Female:male	10:1	10:1
Prevalence in women	0.5%	1–3%
Weight	Markedly decreased	Usually normal
Menstruation	Absent	Usually normal
Binge eating	25–50%	Required for diagnosis
Mortality	~5% Per decade	Low
PHYSICAL AND LABORATORY FINDINGS[A]		
Skin/extremities	Lanugo	
	Acrocyanosis	
	Edema	
Cardiovascular	Bradycardia	
	Hypotension	
Gastrointestinal	Salivary gland enlargement	Salivary gland enlargement
	Slow gastric emptying	Dental erosion
	Constipation	
	Elevated liver enzymes	
Hematopoietic	Normochromic, normocyctic anemia	
	Leukopenia	
Fluid/Electrolyte	Increased BUN, creatinine	Hypokalemia
	Hyponatremia	Hypochloremia
		Alkalosis
Endocrine	Hypoglycemia	
	Low estrogen or testosterone	
	Low LH and FSH	
	Low-normal thyroxine	
	Normal TSH	
	Increased cortisol	
Bone	Osteopenia	

[a] Patients with the binge-eating/purging subtype of anorexia nervosa may also exhibit the physical and laboratory findings associated with bulimia nervosa.

Abbreviations: BUN, blood urea nitrogen; LH, luteinizing hormone; FSH, follicle stimulating hormone; TSH, thyroid stimulating hormone.

TABLE 65-2 *Diagnostic Features of Anorexia Nervosa*

Refusal to maintain body weight at or above a minimally normal weight for age and height. (This includes a failure to achieve weight gain expected during a period of growth leading to an abnormally low body weight.)

Intense fear of weight gain or becoming fat.

Distortion of body image (e.g., feeling fat despite an objectively low weight or minimizing the seriousness of low weight).

Amenorrhea. (This criterion is met if menstrual periods occur only following hormone—e.g., estrogen—administration.)

The intensity of the initial treatment, including the need for hospitalization, is determined by the patient's current weight, the rapidity of recent weight loss, and the severity of medical and psychological complications (Fig. 65-1). Hospitalization should be strongly considered for patients weighing <75% of expected, even if the results of routine blood studies are within normal limits. Acute medical problems, such as severe electrolyte imbalances, should be identified and addressed. Nutritional restoration can almost always be successfully accomplished by oral feeding, and parenteral methods are rarely required. For severely underweight patients, sufficient calories (approximately 1500 to 1800 kcal/d) should be provided initially in divided meals as food or liquid supplements to maintain weight and to permit stabilization of fluid and electrolyte balance. Calories can then be gradually increased to achieve a weight gain of 1 to 2 kg (2 to 4 lb) per week, typically requiring an intake of 3000 to 4000 kcal/d. Meals must be supervised, ideally by personnel who are firm regarding the necessity of food consumption, empathic regarding the challenges entailed, and reassuring regarding the patient's eventual recovery. Patients have great psychological difficulty complying with the need for increased caloric consumption, and the assistance of psychiatrists or psychologists experienced in the treatment of AN is usually necessary.

Less severely affected patients may be treated in a partial hospitalization program where medical and psychiatric supervision is available and several meals can be monitored each day. Outpatient treatment may suffice for mildly ill patients. Weight must be monitored at frequent intervals, and explicit goals agreed on for weight gain, with the understanding that more intensive treatment will be required if the level of care initially employed is not successful. For younger patients, the active involvement of the family in treatment is crucial regardless of the treatment venue.

Psychiatric treatment focuses primarily on two issues. First, patients require much emotional support during the period of weight gain. Patients often intellectually agree with the need to gain weight, but strenuously resist increases in caloric intake, and often surreptitiously discard food that is provided. Second, patients must learn to base their self-esteem not on the achievement of an inappropriately low weight, but on the development of satisfying personal relationships and the attainment of reasonable academic and occupational goals. While this is often possible, some patients with AN develop other serious emotional and behavioral symptoms such as depression, self-mutilation, obsessive-compulsive behavior, and suicidal ideation. These symptoms may require additional therapeutic interventions, in the form of psychotherapy, medication, or hospitalization.

Medical complications occasionally occur during refeeding. As in other forms of malnutrition, fluid retention and peripheral edema may occur, but generally do not require specific treatment in the absence of cardiac, renal, or hepatic dysfunction. Acute gastric dilatation has been described when refeeding has been rapid. Transient modest elevations in serum levels of liver enzymes occasionally occur. Low levels of magnesium and phosphate should be repleted. Multivitamins should be given, and it is important to ensure adequate intake of vitamin D (400 IU/d) and calcium (1500 mg/d) to minimize bone loss.

No psychotropic medications are of established value in the treatment of AN; tricyclic antidepressants are contraindicated when there is prolongation of the QT_c interval. The alterations of cortisol and thyroid hormone metabolism do not require specific treatment and are corrected by weight gain. Estrogen treatment appears to have minimal impact on bone density in underweight patients but may be helpful to relieve symptoms of estrogen deficiency.

BULIMIA NERVOSA

EPIDEMIOLOGY   In women, the full syndrome of BN occurs with a lifetime prevalence of 1 to 3%. Variants of the disorder, such as occasional binge eating or purging, are much more common and occur in 5 to 10% of young women. The frequency of BN among men is less than one-tenth of that among women. The prevalence of BN increased dra-

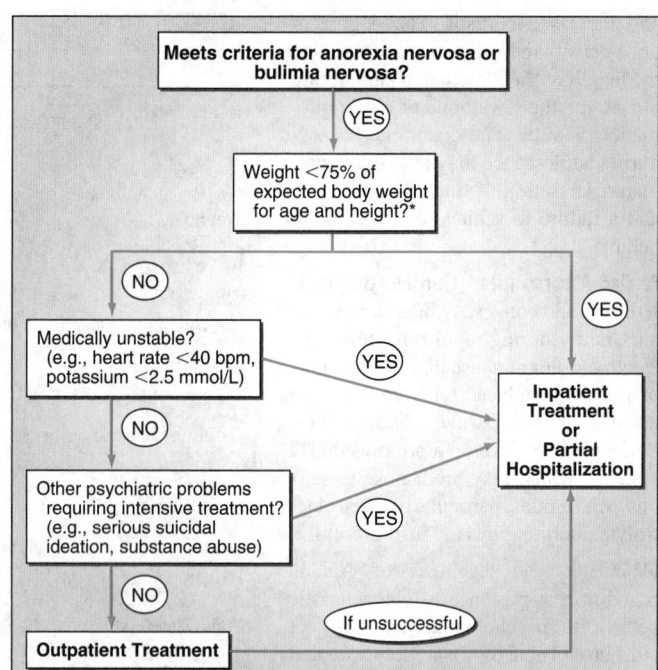

FIGURE 65-1   An algorithm for basic treatment decisions regarding patients with anorexia nervosa or bulimia nervosa. Based on the American Psychiatric Association's practice guidelines for the treatment of patients with eating disorders. *Although outpatient management may be considered for patients with anorexia nervosa weighing more than 75% of expected, there should be a low threshold for using more intensive interventions if the weight loss has been rapid or if current weight is <80% of expected.

matically in the early 1970s and 1980s but may have leveled off or declined somewhat in recent years.

ETIOLOGY   As with AN, the etiology of BN is likely to be multifactorial. Patients who develop BN describe a higher-than-expected prevalence of childhood and parental obesity, suggesting that a predisposition towards obesity may increase vulnerability to this eating disorder. The marked increase in the number of cases of BN during the past 25 years and the rarity of BN in underdeveloped countries suggest that cultural factors are important. Several biologic abnormalities in patients with BN may perpetuate this disorder once it has begun. These include abnormalities of CNS serotonergic function, which is involved in the regulation of eating behavior, and disruption of peripheral satiety mechanisms, including the release of cholecystokinin (CCK) from the small intestine.

CLINICAL FEATURES   (Table 65-3)   The typical patient presenting for treatment of BN is a woman of normal weight in her mid-twenties who reports binge eating and purging 5 to 10 times a week for 5 to 10 years. The disorder usually begins in late adolescence or early adulthood during or following a diet, often in association with depressed mood. The self-imposed caloric restriction leads to increased hunger and to overeating. In an attempt to avoid weight gain, the patient induces vomiting, takes laxatives or diuretics, or engages in some other form of compensatory behavior. During binges, patients with this dis-

TABLE 65-3   *Diagnostic Features of Bulimia Nervosa*

Recurrent episodes of binge eating, which is characterized by the consumption of a large amount of food in a short period of time and a feeling that the eating is out of control.
Recurrent inappropriate behavior to compensate for the binge eating, such as self-induced vomiting.
The occurrence of both the binge eating and the inappropriate compensatory behavior at least twice weekly, on average, for 3 months.
Overconcern with body shape and weight.

Note: If the diagnostic criteria for anorexia nervosa are simultaneously met, only the diagnosis of anorexia nervosa is given.

order tend to consume large amounts of sweet foods with a high fat content, such as dessert items. The most frequent compensatory behaviors are self-induced vomiting and laxative abuse, but a wide variety of techniques have been described, including the omission of insulin injections by individuals with type 1 diabetes mellitus. Initially, patients may experience a sense of satisfaction that appealing food can be eaten without weight gain. However, as the disorder progresses, patients perceive diminished control over eating. Binges increase in size and frequency and are provoked by a variety of stimuli, such as transient depression, anxiety, or a sense that too much food has been consumed in a normal meal. Between binges, patients attempt to restrict caloric intake, which increases hunger and sets the stage for the next binge. Typically, patients with BN are ashamed of their behavior and endeavor to keep their disorder hidden from family and friends. Like patients with AN, those with BN place an unusual emphasis on weight and shape as a basis for their self-esteem. Many patients with BN have mild symptoms of depression. Some patients exhibit serious mood and behavioral disturbances, such as suicide attempts, sexual promiscuity, and drug and alcohol abuse. Although vomiting may be triggered initially by manual stimulation of the gag reflex, most patients with BN develop the ability to induce vomiting at will. Rarely, patients resort to the regular use of syrup of ipecac. Laxatives and diuretics are frequently taken in impressive quantities, such as 30 or 60 laxative pills on a single occasion. The resulting fluid loss produces dehydration and a feeling of emptiness but has little impact on caloric balance.

The physical abnormalities associated with BN primarily result from the purging behavior. Painless bilateral salivary gland hypertrophy (sialadenosis) may be noted. A scar or callus on the dorsum of the hand may develop due to repeated trauma from the teeth among patients who manually stimulate the gag reflex. Recurrent vomiting and the exposure of the lingual surfaces of the teeth to stomach acid lead to loss of dental enamel and eventually to chipping and erosion of the front teeth. Laboratory abnormalities are surprisingly infrequent, but hypokalemia, hypochloremia, and hyponatremia are observed occasionally. Repeated vomiting may lead to alkalosis, whereas repeated laxative abuse may produce a mild metabolic acidosis. Serum amylase may be mildly elevated due to an increase in the salivary isoenzyme.

Serious physical complications resulting from BN are rare. Oligomenorrhea and amenorrhea are more frequent than among women without eating disorders. Arrhythmias occasionally occur secondary to electrolyte disturbances. Tearing of the esophagus and rupture of the stomach have been reported, and constitute life-threatening events. Some patients who have chronically abused laxatives or diuretics develop transient peripheral edema when this behavior ceases, presumably due to high levels of aldosterone secondary to persistent fluid and electrolyte depletion.

DIAGNOSIS The critical diagnostic features of BN are repeated episodes of binge eating followed by inappropriate and abnormal behaviors aimed at avoiding weight gain (Table 65-3). The diagnosis of BN requires a candid history from the patient detailing frequent, large eating binges followed by the purposeful use of inappropriate mechanisms to avoid weight gain. Most patients with BN who present for treatment are distressed by their inability to control their eating behavior but are able to provide such details if queried in a supportive and nonjudgmental fashion.

As in AN, there are two mutually exclusive subtypes of BN. Patients with the "purging" subtype utilize compensatory behaviors that directly rid the body of calories or fluids (e.g., self-induced vomiting, laxative or diuretic abuse), whereas those with the "nonpurging" subtype attempt to compensate for binges by fasting or by excessive exercise. Patients with the nonpurging subtype tend to be heavier and are less prone to fluid and electrolyte disturbances.

PROGNOSIS The prognosis of BN is much more favorable than that of AN. Mortality is low, and full recovery occurs in approximately 50% of patients within 10 years. Approximately 25% of patients have persistent symptoms of BN over many years. Few patients progress from BN to AN.

℞ TREATMENT

BN can usually be treated on an outpatient basis (Figure 65-1). Cognitive behavioral therapy (CBT) is a short-term (4 to 6 months) psychological treatment that focuses on the intense concern with shape and weight, the persistent dieting, and the binge eating and purging that characterize this disorder. Patients are directed to monitor the circumstances, thoughts, and emotions associated with binge/purge episodes, to eat regularly, and to challenge their assumptions linking weight to self-esteem. CBT produces symptomatic remission in 25 to 50% of patients.

Numerous double-bind, placebo-controlled trials have documented that antidepressant medications are useful in the treatment of BN but are probably somewhat less effective than CBT. Although efficacy has been established for virtually all chemical classes of antidepressants, only the selective serotonin reuptake inhibitor fluoxetine (Prozac) has been approved for use in BN by the U.S. Food and Drug Administration. Antidepressant medications are helpful even for patients with BN who are not depressed, and the dose of fluoxetine recommended for BN (60 mg/d) is higher than that typically used to treat depression. These observations suggest that different mechanisms may underlie the utility of these medications in BN and in depression.

A subset of patients with BN does not respond adequately to CBT, antidepressant medication, or their combination. More intensive forms of treatment, including hospitalization, may be required for such patients.

FURTHER READING

AMERICAN PSYCHIATRIC ASSOCIATION: Practice guideline for the treatment of patients with eating disorders (revision). Am J Psychiatry 157(Suppl 1): 1, 2000.

BECKER AE et al: Eating disorders. N Engl J Med 340:1092, 1999

KAYE WH et al: Anorexia and bulimia nervosa. Annu Rev Med 51:299, 2000

MEHLER PS: Diagnosis and care of patients with anorexia nervosa in primary care settings. Ann Intern Med 134:1048, 2001

WALSH BT, DEVLIN MJ: Eating disorders: Progress and problems. Science 280:1387, 1998

66 APPROACH TO THE PATIENT WITH CANCER
Dan L. Longo

The application of current treatment techniques (surgery, radiation therapy, chemotherapy, and biological therapy) results in the cure of >50% of patients diagnosed with cancer. Nevertheless, patients experience the diagnosis of cancer as one of the most traumatic and revolutionary events that has ever happened to them. Independent of prognosis, the diagnosis brings with it a change in a person's self-image and in his or her role in the home and workplace. The prognosis of a person who has just been found to have pancreatic cancer is the same as the prognosis of the person with aortic stenosis who develops the first symptoms of congestive heart failure (median survival, about 8 months). However, the patient with heart disease may remain functional and maintain a self-image as a fully intact person with just a malfunctioning part, a diseased organ ("a bum ticker"). By contrast, the patient with pancreatic cancer has a completely altered self-image and is viewed differently by family and anyone who knows the diagnosis. He or she is being attacked and invaded by a disease that could be anywhere in the body. Every ache or pain takes on desperate significance. Cancer is an exception to the coordinated interaction among cells and organs. In general, the cells of a multicellular organism are programmed for collaboration. Many diseases occur because the specialized cells fail to perform their assigned task. Cancer takes this malfunction one step further. Not only is there a failure of the cancer cell to maintain its specialized function, but it also strikes out on its own; the cancer cell competes to survive using natural mutability and natural selection to seek advantage over normal cells in a recapitulation of evolution. One consequence of the traitorous behavior of cancer cells is that the patient feels betrayed by his or her body. The cancer patient feels that he or she, and not just a body part, is diseased.

THE MAGNITUDE OF THE PROBLEM

No nationwide cancer registry exists; therefore, the incidence of cancer is estimated on the basis of the National Cancer Institute's Surveillance, Epidemiology, and End Results (SEER) database, which tabulates cancer incidence and death figures from nine sites, accounting for about 10% of the U.S. population, and from population data from the Bureau of the Census. In 2004, 1.36 million new cases of invasive cancer (699,560 men, 668,470 women) were diagnosed and 563,700 persons (290,890 men, 272,810 women) died from cancer. The percent distribution of new cancer cases and cancer deaths by site for men and women are shown in Table 66-1. Cancer incidence has been declining by about 2% each year since 1992.

The most significant risk factor for cancer overall is age; two-thirds of all cases were in those over age 65. Cancer incidence increases as the third, fourth, or fifth power of age in different sites. For the interval between birth and age 39, 1 in 72 men and 1 in 51 women will develop cancer; for the interval between ages 40 and 59, 1 in 12 men and 1 in 11 women will develop cancer; and for the interval between ages 60 and 79, 1 in 3 men and 1 in 5 women will develop cancer.

Cancer is the second leading cause of death behind heart disease. Deaths from heart disease have declined 45% in the United States since 1950 and continue to decline. After a 70-year period of increases, cancer deaths began to decline in 1997 (Fig. 66-1). The five leading causes of cancer deaths are shown for various populations in Table 66-2. Along with the decrease in incidence has come an increase in survival for cancer patients. The 5-year survival for white patients was 39% in 1960–1963 and 64% in 1992–1998. Cancers are more often deadly in blacks; the 5-year survival was 53% for the 1992–1998

TABLE 66-1 *Distribution of Cancer Incidence and Deaths for 2004[a]*

Male			Female		
Sites	%	Number	Sites	%	Number
CANCER INCIDENCE					
Prostate	33	230,110	Breast	32	215,990
Lung and bronchus	13	93,110	Lung and bronchus	12	80,660
Colon and rectum	11	73,620	Colon and rectum	11	73,380
Bladder	6	44,640	Endometrium	6	40,320
Melanoma	4	29,900	Ovary	4	25,580
Lymphoma	4	28,850	Lymphoma	4	25,520
Kidney	3	22,080	Melanoma	4	25,200
Leukemia	3	19,020	Thyroid	3	17,640
Oral cavity	3	18,550	Pancreas	2	16,120
Pancreas	2	15,740	Bladder	2	15,600
All other	18	123,940	All other	20	132,460
CANCER DEATHS					
Lung and bronchus	32	91,930	Lung and bronchus	25	68,510
Prostate	10	29,900	Breast	15	40,110
Colon and rectum	10	28,320	Colon and rectum	10	28,410
Pancreas	5	15,440	Ovary	6	16,090
Leukemia	5	12,990	Pancreas	6	15,830
Lymphoma	4	11,090	Leukemia	6	10,310
Esophagus	4	10,250	Lymphoma	4	9,020
Liver and bile duct	3	9,450	Endometrium	3	7,090
Bladder	3	8,780	Myeloma	2	5,640
Kidney	3	7,870	Brain	2	5,490
All other	21	64,870	All other	24	66,310

[a] Data exclude basal and squamous cell skin cancers and carcinoma in situ except the bladder.
Source: From Jemal et al, with permission.

interval. Incidence and mortality vary among racial and ethnic groups (Table 66-3). The basis for these differences is unclear.

PATIENT MANAGEMENT

Important information is obtained from every portion of the routine history and physical examination. The duration of symptoms may reveal the chronicity of disease. The past medical history may alert the physician to the presence of underlying diseases that may affect the choice of therapy or the side effects of treatment. The social history may reveal occupational exposure to carcinogens or habits, such as smoking or alcohol consumption, that may influence the course of disease and its treatment. The family history may suggest an underlying familial cancer predisposition and point out the need to begin surveillance or other preventive therapy for unaffected siblings of the patient. The review of systems may suggest early symptoms of metastatic disease or a paraneoplastic syndrome.

DIAGNOSIS The diagnosis of cancer relies most heavily on invasive tissue biopsy and should never be made without obtaining tissue; no noninvasive diagnostic test is sufficient to define a disease process as cancer. Although in rare clinical settings (e.g., thyroid nodules) fine-needle aspiration is an acceptable diagnostic procedure, the diagnosis generally depends on obtaining adequate tissue to permit careful eval-

435

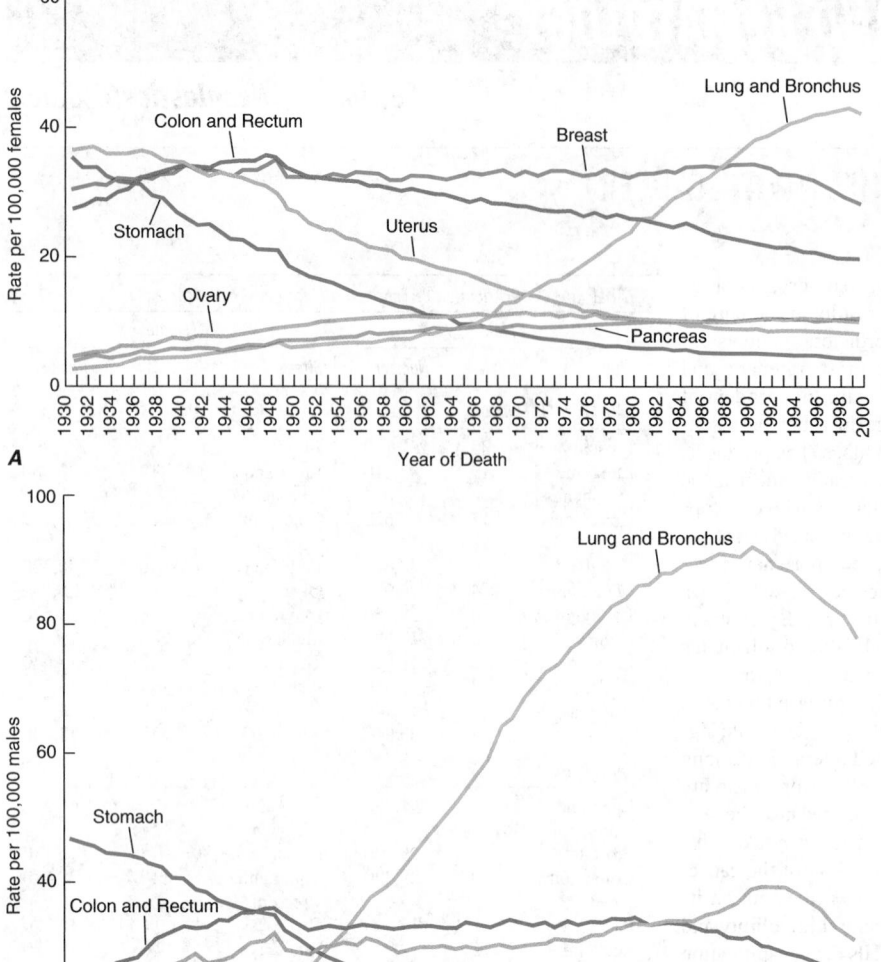

FIGURE 66-1 Sixty-year trend in cancer death rates for (*A*) women and (*B*) men, by site in the United States, 1930–1999. Rates are per 100,000 age-adjusted to the 2000 U.S. standard population. (*From Jemal et al.*)

t(8;14) translocation of Burkitt's lymphoma. Increasing evidence links the expression of certain genes with the prognosis and response to therapy (Chaps. 68, 69).

Occasionally a patient will present with a metastatic disease process that is defined as cancer on biopsy but has no apparent primary site of disease. Efforts should be made to define the primary site based on age, sex, sites of involvement, histology and tumor markers, and personal and family history. Particular attention should be focused on ruling out the most treatable causes (Chap. 85).

Once the diagnosis of cancer is made, the management of the patient is best undertaken as a multidisciplinary collaboration among the primary care physician, medical oncologists, surgical oncologists, radiation oncologists, oncology nurse specialists, pharmacists, social workers, rehabilitation medicine specialists, and a number of other consulting professionals working closely with each other and with the patient and family.

DEFINING THE EXTENT OF DISEASE AND THE PROGNOSIS The first priority in patient management after the diagnosis of cancer is established and shared with the patient is to determine the extent of disease. The curability of a tumor usually is inversely proportional to the tumor burden. Ideally, the tumor will be diagnosed before symptoms develop or as a consequence of screening efforts (Chap. 67). A very high proportion of such patients can be cured. However, most patients with cancer present with symptoms related to the cancer, caused either by mass effects of the tumor or by alterations associated with the production of cytokines or hormones by the tumor.

For most cancers, the extent of disease is evaluated by a variety of noninvasive and invasive diagnostic tests and procedures. This process is called *staging*. There are two types. *Clinical staging* is based on physical examination, radiographs, isotopic scans, computed tomography, and other imaging procedures; *pathologic staging* takes into account information obtained during a surgical procedure, which might include intraoperative palpation, resection of regional lymph nodes and/or tissue adjacent to the tumor, and inspection and biopsy of organs commonly involved in disease spread. Pathologic staging includes histologic examination of all tissues removed during the surgical procedure. Surgical procedures performed may include a simple lymph node biopsy or more extensive procedures such as thoracotomy, mediastinoscopy, or laparotomy. Surgical staging may occur in a separate procedure or may be done at the time of definitive surgical resection of the primary tumor.

Knowledge of the predilection of particular tumors for spread to adjacent or distant organs helps direct the staging evaluation.

Information obtained from staging is used to define the extent of disease either as localized, as exhibiting spread

uation of the histology of the tumor, its grade, and its invasiveness and to yield further molecular diagnostic information, such as the expression of cell-surface markers or intracellular proteins that typify a particular cancer, or the presence of a molecular marker, such as the

TABLE 66-2 *The Five Leading Primary Tumor Sites for Patients Dying of Cancer Based on Age and Sex in 2001*

Rank	All Ages	Under 20	20–39	40–59	60–79	>80
			Age			
1	M,F: lung	M,F: leukemia	M: leukemia F: breast	M: lung F: breast	M,F: lung	M,F: lung
2	M: prostate F: breast	M,F: brain	M: brain F: cervix	M: colorectal F: lung	M: colorectal F: breast	M: prostate F: colorectal
3	M,F: colorectal	M: bone sarcoma F: endocrine	M: colorectal F: leukemia	M: pancreas F: colorectal	M: prostate F: colorectal	M,F: colorectal F: breast
4	M,F: pancreas	M: endocrine F: bone sarcoma	M: lymphoma F: lung	M: liver F: ovary	M,F: pancreas	M: bladder F: pancreas
5	M: leukemia F: ovary	M, F: soft tissue sarcoma	M: lung F: brain	M: esophagus F: pancreas	M: leukemia F: ovary	M: leukemia F: lymphoma

Note: M, male; F, female.

outside of the organ of origin to regional but not distant sites, or as metastatic to distant sites. The most widely used system of staging is the TNM (tumor, node, metastasis) system codified by the International Union Against Cancer and the American Joint Committee on Cancer (AJCC).[1] The TNM classification is an anatomically based system that categorizes the tumor on the basis of the size of the primary tumor lesion (T1–4, where a higher number indicates a tumor of larger size), the presence of nodal involvement (usually N0 and N1 for the absence and presence, respectively, of involved nodes, although some tumors have more elaborate systems of nodal grading), and the presence of metastatic disease (M0 and M1 for the absence and presence, respectively, of metastases). The various permutations of T, N, and M scores (sometimes including tumor

TABLE 66-3 Cancer Incidence and Mortality in Racial and Ethnic Groups 1992–1999

Site	White	Black	Asian/Pacific Islander	American Indian	Hispanic
INCIDENCE PER 100,000 POPULATION					
All	M: 568.2	M: 703.6	M: 408.9	M: 277.7	M: 393.1
	F: 424.4	F: 404.8	F: 306.5	F: 224.2	F: 290.5
Breast (F)	137	120.7	93.4	59.4	82.6
Colon/rectum	M: 64.4	M: 70.7	M: 58.7	M: 40.7	M: 43.9
	F: 46.1	F: 55.8	F: 39.5	F: 30.8	F: 29.7
Lung	M: 82.9	M: 124.1	M: 63.8	M: 51.4	M: 44.1
	F: 51.1	F: 53.2	F: 28.5	F: 23.3	F: 22.8
Prostate (M)	172.9	275.3	107.2	60.7	127.6
MORTALITY PER 100,000 POPULATION					
All	M: 258.1	M: 369	M: 160.6	M: 154.5	M: 163.7
	F: 171.2	F: 204.5	F: 104.4	F: 110.4	F: 105.7
Breast (F)	29.3	37.3	13.1	14.8	17.5
Colon	M: 26.1	M: 34.8	M: 16.5	M: 14.6	M: 16.6
	F: 18.4	F: 25.4	F: 11.6	F: 11.3	F: 10.6
Lung	M: 81.7	M: 113	M: 42.3	M: 49.3	M: 38.2
	F: 41.1	F: 39.6	F: 19.3	F: 24.9	F: 13.8
Prostate (M)	32.9	75.1	15.1	18.8	22.6

Note: M, male; F, female.

histologic grade G) are then broken into stages, usually designated by the roman numerals I through IV. Tumor burden increases and curability decreases with increasing stage. Other anatomic staging systems are used for some tumors, e.g., the Dukes classification for colorectal cancers, the International Federation of Gynecologists and Obstetricians (FIGO) classification for gynecologic cancers, and the Ann Arbor classification for Hodgkin's disease.

Certain tumors cannot be grouped on the basis of anatomic considerations. For example, hematopoietic tumors such as leukemia, myeloma, and lymphoma are often disseminated at presentation and do not spread like solid tumors. For these tumors, other prognostic factors have been identified (Chaps. 96, 97, 98).

In addition to tumor burden, a second major determinant of treatment outcome is the physiologic reserve of the patient. Patients who are bedridden before developing cancer are likely to fare worse, stage for stage, than fully active patients. Physiologic reserve is a determinant of how a patient is likely to cope with the physiologic stresses imposed by the cancer and its treatment. This factor is difficult to assess directly. Instead, surrogate markers for physiologic reserve are used, such as the patient's age or Karnofsky performance status (Table 66-4). Older patients and those with a Karnofsky performance status <70 have a poor prognosis unless the poor performance is a reversible consequence of the tumor.

Increasingly, biologic features of the tumor are being related to prognosis. The expression of particular oncogenes, drug-resistance genes, apoptosis-related genes, and genes involved in metastasis are being found to influence response to therapy and prognosis. The presence of selected cytogenetic abnormalities may influence survival. Tumors with higher growth fractions, as assessed by expression of proliferation-related markers such as proliferating cell nuclear antigen (PCNA), behave more aggressively than tumors with lower growth fractions. Information obtained from studying the tumor itself will increasingly be used to influence treatment decisions.

MAKING A TREATMENT PLAN From information on the extent of disease and the prognosis and in conjunction with the patient's wishes, it is determined whether the treatment approach should be curative or palliative in intent. Cooperation among the various professionals involved in cancer treatment is of the utmost importance in treatment planning. For some cancers, chemotherapy or chemotherapy plus radiation therapy delivered before the use of definitive surgical treatment (so-called neoadjuvant therapy) may improve the outcome, as seems to be the

case for locally advanced breast cancer and head and neck cancers. In certain settings in which combined modality therapy is intended, coordination among the medical oncologist, radiation oncologist, and surgeon is crucial to achieving optimal results. Sometimes the chemotherapy and radiation therapy need to be delivered sequentially, and other times concurrently. Surgical procedures may precede or follow other treatment approaches. It is best for the treatment plan either to follow a standard protocol precisely or else to be part of an ongoing clinical research protocol evaluating new treatments. Ad hoc modifications of standard protocols are likely to compromise treatment results.

The choice of treatment approaches was formerly dominated by the local culture in both the university and the practice settings. However, it is now possible to gain access electronically to standard treatment protocols and to every approved clinical research study in North America through a personal computer interface with the Internet.[2]

The skilled physician also has much to offer the patient for whom curative therapy is no longer an option. Often a combination of guilt and frustration over the inability to cure the patient and the pressure of a busy schedule greatly limit the time a physician spends with a patient who is receiving only palliative care. Resist these forces. In addition to the medicines administered to alleviate symptoms (see below), it is important to remember the comfort that is provided by holding the patient's hand, continuing regular examinations, and taking time to talk.

MANAGEMENT OF DISEASE AND TREATMENT COMPLICATIONS Because cancer therapies are toxic (Chaps. 70, 71), patient management involves addressing complications of both the disease and its treatment as well as the complex psychosocial problems associated with cancer. In the short term during a course of curative therapy, the patient's functional status may decline. Treatment-induced toxicity is less acceptable if the goal of therapy is palliation. The most common side effects of treatment are nausea and vomiting (see below), febrile neutropenia (Chap. 72), and myelosuppression (Chap. 70). Therapeutic tools are now available to minimize the acute toxicity of cancer treatment.

New symptoms developing in the course of cancer treatment should

---

[1] The AJCC *Manual for Staging Cancer*, 5th edition, can be obtained from the AJCC at 55 East Erie Street, Chicago, IL, 60611.

[2] The National Cancer Institute maintains a database called PDQ (Physician Data Query) that is accessible on the Internet under the name CancerNet at *wwwicic.nci.nih.gov/health.htm*. Information can be obtained through a facsimile machine using CancerFax by dialing 301-402-5874. Patient information is also provided by the National Cancer Institute in at least three formats: on the Internet via CancerNet at *wwwicic.nci.nih.gov/patient.htm*, through the CancerFax number listed above, or by calling 1-800-4-CANCER. The quality control for the information provided through these services is rigorous.

TABLE 66-4 *Karnofsky Performance Index*

Performance Status	Functional Capability of the Patient
100	Normal; no complaints; no evidence of disease
90	Able to carry on normal activity; minor signs or symptoms of disease
80	Normal activity with effort; some signs or symptoms of disease
70	Cares for self; unable to carry on normal activity or do active work
60	Requires occasional assistance but is able to care for most needs
50	Requires considerable assistance and frequent medical care
40	Disabled; requires special care and assistance
30	Severely disabled; hospitalization is indicated although death is not imminent
20	Very sick; hospitalization necessary; active supportive treatment is necessary
10	Moribund, fatal processes progressing rapidly
0	Dead

always be assumed to be reversible until proven otherwise. The fatalistic attribution of anorexia, weight loss, and jaundice to recurrent or progressive tumor could result in a patient dying from a reversible intercurrent cholecystitis. Intestinal obstruction may be due to reversible adhesions rather than progressive tumor. Systemic infections, sometimes with unusual pathogens, may be a consequence of the immunosuppression associated with cancer therapy. Some drugs used to treat cancer or its complications (e.g., nausea) may produce central nervous system symptoms that look like metastatic disease or may mimic paraneoplastic syndromes such as the syndrome of inappropriate antidiuretic hormone. A definitive diagnosis should be pursued and may even require a repeat biopsy.

A critical component of cancer management is assessing the response to treatment. In addition to a careful physical examination in which all sites of disease are physically measured and recorded in a flow chart by date, response assessment usually requires periodic repeating of imaging tests that were abnormal at the time of staging. If imaging tests have become normal, repeat biopsy of previously involved tissue is performed to document complete response by pathologic criteria. Biopsies are not usually required if there is macroscopic residual disease. A *complete response* is defined as disappearance of all evidence of disease, and a *partial response* as >50% reduction in the sum of the products of the perpendicular diameters of all measureable lesions. *Progressive disease* is defined as the appearance of any new lesion or an increase of >25% in the sum of the products of the perpendicular diameters of all measurable lesions. Tumor shrinkage or growth that does not meet any of these criteria is considered *stable disease*. Some sites of involvement (e.g., bone) or patterns of involvement (e.g., lymphangitic lung or diffuse pulmonary infiltrates) are considered unmeasurable. No response is complete without biopsy documentation of their resolution, but partial responses may exclude their assessment unless clear objective (though unmeasurable) progression has occurred.

Tumor markers may be useful in patient management in certain tumors. Response to therapy may be difficult to gauge with certainty. However, some tumors produce or elicit the production of markers that can be measured in the serum or urine and, in a particular patient, rising and falling levels of the marker are usually associated with increasing or decreasing tumor burden, respectively. Some clinically useful tumor markers are shown in Table 66-5. Tumor markers are not in themselves specific enough to permit a diagnosis of malignancy to be made, but once a malignancy has been diagnosed and shown to be associated with elevated levels of a tumor marker, the marker can be used to assess response to treatment.

The recognition and treatment of depression are important com-

ponents of management. The incidence of depression in cancer patients is ~25% overall and may be greater in patients with greater debility. This diagnosis is likely in a patient with a depressed mood (dysphoria) and/or a loss of interest in pleasure (anhedonia) for at least 2 weeks. In addition, three or more of the following symptoms are usually present: appetite change, sleep problems, psychomotor retardation or agitation, fatigue, feelings of guilt or worthlessness, inability to concentrate, and suicidal ideation. Patients with these symptoms should receive therapy. Medical therapy with a serotonin reuptake inhibitor such as fluoxetine (10 to 20 mg/d), sertraline (50 to 150 mg/d), or paroxetine (10 to 20 mg/d) or a tricyclic antidepressant such as amitriptyline (50 to 100 mg/d) or desipramine (75 to 150 mg/d) should be tried, allowing 4 to 6 weeks for response. Effective therapy should be continued at least 6 months after resolution of symptoms. If therapy is unsuccessful, other classes of antidepressants may be used. In addition to medication, psychosocial interventions such as support groups, psychotherapy, and guided imagery may be of benefit.

Many patients opt for unproven or unsound approaches to treatment when it appears that conventional medicine is unlikely to be curative. Those seeking such alternatives are often well educated and may be early in the course of their disease. Unsound approaches are usually hawked on the basis of unsubstantiated anecdotes and not only cannot help the patient but may be harmful. Physicians should strive to keep communications open and nonjudgmental, so that patients are more likely to discuss with the physician what they are actually doing. The appearance of unexpected toxicity may be an indication that a supplemental therapy is being taken.[3]

LONG-TERM FOLLOW-UP/LATE COMPLICATIONS At the completion of treatment, sites originally involved with tumor are reassessed, usually by radiography or imaging techniques, and any persistent abnormality is biopsied. If disease persists, the multidisciplinary team discusses a new salvage treatment plan. If the patient has been rendered disease-free by the original treatment, the patient is followed regularly for disease recurrence. The optimal guidelines for follow-up care are not known. For many years, a routine practice has been to follow the patient monthly for 6 to 12 months, then every other month for a year, every 3 months for a year, every 4 months for a year, every 6 months for a year, and then annually. At each visit, a battery of laboratory and radiographic and imaging tests were obtained on the assumption that it is best to detect recurrent disease before it becomes symptomatic. However, where follow-up procedures have been examined, this assumption has been found to be untrue. Studies of breast cancer, melanoma, lung cancer, colon cancer, and lymphoma have all failed to support the notion that asymptomatic relapses are more readily cured by salvage therapy than symptomatic relapses. In view of the enormous cost of a full battery of diagnostic tests and their manifest lack of impact on survival, new guidelines are emerging for less frequent follow-up visits, during which the history and physical examination are the major investigations performed.

As time passes, the likelihood of recurrence of the primary cancer diminishes. For many types of cancer, survival for 5 years without recurrence is tantamount to cure. However, important medical problems can occur in patients treated for cancer and must be examined (Chap. 89). Some problems emerge as a consequence of the disease and some as a consequence of the treatment. An understanding of these disease- and treatment-related problems may help in their detection and management.

Despite these concerns, most patients who are cured of cancer return to normal lives.

SUPPORTIVE CARE In many ways, the success of cancer therapy depends on the success of the supportive care. Failure to control the symptoms

---

[3]Information about unsound methods may be obtained from the National Council Against Health Fraud, Box 1276, Loma Linda, CA 92354, or from the Center for Medical Consumers and Health Care Information, 237 Thompson Street, New York, NY 10012.

of cancer and its treatment may lead patients to abandon curative therapy. Of equal importance, supportive care is a major determinant of quality of life. Even when life cannot be prolonged, the physician must strive to preserve its quality. Quality-of-life measurements have become common end-points of clinical research studies. Furthermore, palliative care has been shown to be cost-effective when approached in an organized fashion. A credo for oncology could be to cure sometimes, to extend life often, and to comfort always.

Pain Pain occurs with variable frequency in the cancer patient: 25 to 50% of patients present with pain at diagnosis, 33% have pain associated with treatment, and 75% have pain with progressive disease. The pain may have several causes. In about 70% of cases, pain is caused by the tumor itself—by invasion of bone, nerves, blood vessels, or mucous membranes or obstruction of a hollow viscus or duct. In about 20% of cases, pain is related to a surgical or invasive medical procedure, to radiation injury (mucositis, enteritis, or plexus or spinal cord injury), or to chemotherapy injury (mucositis, peripheral neuropathy, phlebitis, steroid-induced aseptic necrosis of the femoral head). In 10% of cases, pain is unrelated to cancer or its treatment.

Assessment of pain requires the methodical investigation of the history of the pain, its location, character, temporal features, provocative and palliative factors, and intensity (Chap. 11); a review of the oncologic history and past medical history as well as personal and social history; and a thorough physical examination. The patient should be given a 10-division visual analogue scale on which to indicate the severity of the pain. The clinical condition is often dynamic, making it necessary to reassess the patient frequently. Pain therapy should not be withheld while the cause of pain is being sought.

A variety of tools are available with which to address cancer pain. About 85% of patients will have pain relief from pharmacologic intervention. However, other modalities, including antitumor therapy (such as surgical relief of obstruction, radiation therapy, and strontium-89 or samarium-153 treatment for bone pain), neurostimulatory techniques, regional analgesia, or neuroablative procedures are effective in an additional 12% or so. Thus, very few patients will have inadequate pain relief if appropriate measures are taken. →*A specific approach to pain relief is detailed in Chap. 9.*

Nausea Emesis in the cancer patient is usually caused by chemotherapy (Chap. 70). Its severity can be predicted from the drugs used to treat the cancer. Three forms of emesis are recognized on the basis of their timing with regard to the noxious insult. *Acute emesis*, the most common variety, occurs within 24 h of treatment. *Delayed emesis* occurs 1 to 7 days after treatment; it is rare, but, when present, usually follows cisplatin administration. *Anticipatory emesis* occurs before administration of chemotherapy and represents a conditioned response to visual and olfactory stimuli previously associated with chemotherapy delivery.

Acute emesis is the best understood form. Stimuli that activate signals in the chemoreceptor trigger zone in the medulla, the cerebral cortex, and peripherally in the intestinal tract lead to stimulation of the vomiting center in the medulla, the motor center responsible for coordinating the secretory and muscle contraction activity that leads to emesis. Diverse receptor types participate in the process, including

TABLE 66-5 Tumor Markers		
Tumor Markers	Cancer	Non-Neoplastic Conditions
HORMONES		
Human chorionic gonadotropin	Gestational trophoblastic disease, gonadal germ cell tumor	Pregnancy
Calcitonin	Medullary cancer of the thyroid	
Catecholamines	Pheochromocytoma	
ONCOFETAL ANTIGENS		
Alphafetoprotein	Hepatocellular carcinoma, gonadal germ cell tumor	Cirrhosis, hepatitis
Carcinoembryonic antigen	Adenocarcinomas of the colon, pancreas, lung, breast, ovary	Pancreatitis, hepatitis, inflammatory bowel disease, smoking
ENZYMES		
Prostatic acid phosphatase	Prostate cancer	Prostatitis, prostatic hypertrophy
Neuron-specific enolase	Small cell cancer of the lung, neuroblastoma	
Lactate dehydrogenase	Lymphoma, Ewing's sarcoma	Hepatitis, hemolytic anemia, many others
TUMOR-ASSOCIATED PROTEINS		
Prostate-specific antigen	Prostate cancer	Prostatitis, prostatic hypertrophy
Monoclonal immunoglobulin	Myeloma	Infection, MGUS[a]
CA-125	Ovarian cancer, some lymphomas	Menstruation, peritonitis, pregnancy
CA 19-9	Colon, pancreatic, breast cancer	Pancreatitis, ulcerative colitis
CD30	Hodgkin's disease, anaplastic large cell lymphoma	—
CD25	Hairy cell leukemia, adult T cell leukemia/lymphoma	—

[a] MGUS, monoclonal gammopathy of uncertain significance.

dopamine, serotonin, histamine, opioid, and acetylcholine receptors. The serotonin receptor antagonists ondansetron and granisetron are the most effective drugs against highly emetogenic agents, but they are expensive.

As with the analgesia ladder, emesis therapy should be tailored to the situation. For mildly and moderately emetogenic agents, prochlorperazine, 5 to 10 mg orally or 25 mg rectally, is effective. Its efficacy may be enhanced by administering the drug before the chemotherapy is delivered. Dexamethasone, 10 to 20 mg intravenously, is also effective and may enhance the efficacy of prochlorperazine. For highly emetogenic agents such as cisplatin, mechlorethamine, dacarbazine, and streptozocin, combinations of agents work best and administration should begin 6 to 24 h before treatment. Ondansetron, 8 mg orally every 6 h the day before therapy and intravenously on the day of therapy, plus dexamethasone, 20 mg intravenously before treatment, is an effective regimen. Addition of oral aprepitant (a substance P/neurokinin 1 receptor antagonist) to this regimen (125 mg on day 1, 80 mg on days 2 and 3) further decreases the risk of both acute and delayed vomiting. Like pain, emesis is easier to prevent than to alleviate.

Delayed emesis may be related to bowel inflammation from the therapy and can be controlled with oral dexamethasone and oral metoclopramide, a dopamine receptor antagonist that also blocks serotonin receptors at high dosages. The best strategy for preventing anticipatory emesis is to control emesis in the early cycles of therapy to prevent the conditioning from taking place. If this is unsuccessful, prophylactic antiemetics the day before treatment may help. Experimental studies are evaluating behavior modification.

Effusions Fluid may accumulate abnormally in the pleural cavity, pericardium, or peritoneum. Asymptomatic malignant effusions may not require treatment. Symptomatic effusions occurring in tumors responsive to systemic therapy usually do not require local treatment but respond to the treatment for the underlying tumor. Symptomatic effusions occurring in tumors unresponsive to systemic therapy may require local treatment in patients with a life expectancy of at least 6 months.

Pleural effusions due to tumors may or may not contain malignant cells. Lung cancer, breast cancer, and lymphomas account for about 75% of malignant pleural effusions. Their exudative nature is usually gauged by an effusion/serum protein ratio of ≥ 0.5 or an effusion/serum lactate dehydrogenase ratio of ≥ 0.6. When the condition is symptomatic, thoracentesis is usually performed first. In most cases, symptomatic improvement occurs for <1 month. Chest tube drainage is required if symptoms recur within 2 weeks. Fluid is aspirated until the flow rate is <100 mL in 24 h. Then either 60 units of bleomycin or 1 g of doxycycline is infused into the chest tube in 50 mL of 5% dextrose in water; the tube is clamped; the patient is rotated on four sides, spending 15 min in each position; and, after 1 to 2 h, the tube is again attached to suction for another 24 h. The tube is then disconnected from suction and allowed to drain by gravity. If <100 mL drains over the next 24 h, the chest tube is pulled, and a radiograph taken 24 h later. If the chest tube continues to drain fluid at an unacceptably high rate, sclerosis can be repeated. Bleomycin may be somewhat more effective than doxycycline but is very expensive. Doxycycline is usually the drug of first choice. If neither doxycycline nor bleomycin is effective, talc can be used.

Symptomatic pericardial effusions are usually treated by creating a pericardial window or by stripping the pericardium. If the patient's condition does not permit a surgical procedure, sclerosis can be attempted with doxycycline and/or bleomycin.

Malignant ascites is usually treated with repeated paracentesis of small volumes of fluid. If the underlying malignancy is unresponsive to systemic therapy, peritoneovenous shunts may be inserted. Despite the fear of disseminating tumor cells into the circulation, widespread metastases are an unusual complication. The major complications are occlusion, leakage, and fluid overload. Patients with severe liver disease may develop disseminated intravascular coagulation.

Nutrition   Cancer and its treatment may lead to a decrease in nutrient intake of sufficient magnitude to cause weight loss and alteration of intermediary metabolism. The prevalence of this problem is difficult to estimate because of variations in the definition of cancer cachexia, but most patients with advanced cancer experience weight loss and decreased appetite. A variety of both tumor-derived factors (e.g., bombesin, adrenocorticotropic hormone) and host-derived factors (e.g., tumor necrosis factor, interleukins 1 and 6, growth hormone) contribute to the altered metabolism, and a vicious cycle is established in which protein catabolism, glucose intolerance, and lipolysis cannot be reversed by the provision of calories.

It remains controversial how to assess nutritional status and when and how to intervene. Efforts to make the assessment objective have included the use of a prognostic nutritional index based on albumin levels, triceps skin fold thickness, transferrin levels, and delayed-type hypersensitivity skin testing. However, a simpler approach has been to define the threshold for nutritional intervention as >10% unexplained body weight loss, serum transferrin level <1500 mg/L (150 mg/dL), and serum albumin <34 g/L (3.4 g/dL).

The decision is important, because it appears that cancer therapy is substantially more toxic and less effective in the face of malnutrition. Nevertheless, it remains unclear whether nutritional intervention can alter the natural history. Unless some pathology is affecting the absorptive function of the gastrointestinal tract, enteral nutrition provided orally or by tube feeding is preferred over parenteral supplementation. However, the risks associated with the tube may outweigh the benefits. Megestrol acetate, a progestational agent, has been advocated as a pharmacologic intervention to improve nutritional status. Research in this area may provide more tools in the future as cytokine-mediated mechanisms are further elucidated.

Psychosocial Support   The psychosocial needs of patients vary with their situation. Patients undergoing treatment experience fear, anxiety, and depression. Self-image is often seriously compromised by deforming surgery and loss of hair. Women who receive cosmetic advice that enables them to look better also feel better. Loss of control over how one spends time can contribute to the sense of vulnerability. Juggling the demands of work and family with the demands of treatment may create enormous stresses. Sexual dysfunction is highly prevalent and needs to be discussed openly with the patient. An empathetic health care team is sensitive to the individual patient's needs and permits negotiation where such flexibility will not adversely affect the course of treatment.

Cancer survivors have other sets of difficulties. Patients may have fears associated with the termination of a treatment they associate with their continued survival. Adjustments are required to physical losses and handicaps, real and perceived. Patients may be preoccupied with minor physical problems. They perceive a decline in their job mobility and view themselves as less desirable workers. They may be victims of job and/or insurance discrimination. Patients may experience difficulty reentering their normal past life. They may feel guilty for having survived and may carry a sense of vulnerability to colds and other illnesses. Perhaps the most pervasive and threatening concern is the ever-present fear of relapse (the Damocles syndrome).

Patients in whom therapy has been unsuccessful have other problems related to the end of life.

Death and Dying   The most common causes of death in patients with cancer are infection (leading to circulatory failure), respiratory failure, hepatic failure, and renal failure. Intestinal blockage may lead to inanition and starvation. Central nervous system disease may lead to seizures, coma, and central hypoventilation. About 70% of patients develop dyspnea preterminally. However, many months usually pass between the diagnosis of cancer and the occurrence of these complications, and during this period the patient is severely affected by the possibility of death. The path of unsuccessful cancer treatment usually occurs in three phases. First, there is optimism at the hope of cure; when the tumor recurs, there is the acknowledgment of an incurable disease, and the goal of palliative therapy is embraced in the hope of being able to live with disease; finally, at the disclosure of imminent death, another adjustment in outlook takes place. The patient imagines the worst in preparation for the end of life and may go through stages of adjustment to the diagnosis. These stages include denial, isolation, anger, bargaining, depression, acceptance, and hope. Of course, patients do not all progress through all the stages or proceed through them in the same order or at the same rate. Nevertheless, developing an understanding of how the patient has been affected by the diagnosis and is coping with it is an important goal of patient management.

It is best to speak frankly with the patient and the family regarding the likely course of disease. These discussions can be difficult for the physician as well as for the patient and family. The critical features of the interaction are to reassure the patient and family that everything that can be done to provide comfort will be done. They will not be abandoned. Many patients prefer to be cared for in their homes or in a hospice setting rather than a hospital. The American College of Physicians has published a book called *Home Care Guide for Cancer: How to Care for Family and Friends at Home* that teaches an approach to successful problem-solving in home care. With appropriate planning, it should be possible to provide the patient with the necessary medical care as well as the psychological and spiritual support that will prevent the isolation and depersonalization that can attend inhospital death.

The care of dying patients may take a toll on the physician. A "burnout" syndrome has been described that is characterized by fatigue, disengagement from patients and colleagues, and a loss of self-fulfillment. Efforts at stress reduction, maintenance of a balanced life, and setting realistic goals may combat this disorder.

End-of-Life Decisions   Unfortunately, a smooth transition in treatment goals from curative to palliative may not be possible in all cases because of the occurrence of serious treatment-related complications or rapid disease progression. Vigorous and invasive medical support for a reversible disease or treatment complication is assumed to be justified. However, if the reversibility of the condition is in doubt, the patient's wishes determine the level of medical care. These wishes should be elicited before the terminal phase of illness and reviewed periodically. Information about advance directives can be obtained from the American Association of Retired Persons, 601 E Street, NW, Washington, DC 20049, 202-434-2277 or Choice in Dying, 250 West 57th Street, New York, NY 10107, 212-366-5540. →*A full discussion of end-of-life management is in Chap. 9.*

FURTHER READING

CLINICAL PRACTICE GUIDELINE NUMBER 9, MANAGEMENT OF CANCER PAIN. U.S. Department of Health and Human Services, Agency for Health Care Policy and Research publication no. 94-0592, 1994

GRUNBERG SM, HESKETH PJ: Control of chemotherapy-induced emesis. N Engl J Med 329:1790, 1993

JEMAL A, JIWARI RC, MURRAY T et al: Cancer statistics, 2004. CA Cancer J Clin 54:8, 2004

LEVY MH: Pharmacologic treatment of cancer pain. N Engl J Med 335:1124, 1996

THERASSE P et al: New guidelines to evaluate response to treatment in solid tumors. J Natl Cancer Inst 92:205, 2000

WALSH D et al: The symptoms of advanced cancer: Relationship to age, gender, and performance status in 1000 patients. Support Care Cancer 8:175, 2000

67 PREVENTION AND EARLY DETECTION OF CANCER
Otis W. Brawley, Barnett S. Kramer

Cancer prevention and control is a burgeoning field because of advances in understanding the biology of carcinogenesis. The field has expanded beyond the identification and avoidance of carcinogens to include studies of specific interventions to lower cancer risk, as well as screening for early detection of cancer.

Central to cancer prevention and control is the concept that carcinogenesis is not an event but a process, a series of discrete cellular changes that result in progressively more autonomous cellular processes. *Primary prevention* concerns the identification and manipulation of the genetic, biologic, and environmental factors in the causal pathway. Smoking cessation, diet modification, and chemoprevention are primary prevention activities. *Secondary prevention* concerns the identification of asymptomatic neoplastic lesions combined with effective therapy. Screening is a form of secondary prevention.

EDUCATION AND HEALTHFUL HABITS Public education on the avoidance of identified risk factors for cancer and encouraging healthy habits were among early efforts in cancer prevention and control. Many educational messages have come to the public through commercials in the print and electronic media and through school health courses. The physician is a potentially powerful messenger in this education campaign about the hazards of smoking, the benefits of a healthful diet and exercise, use of proven screening methods, and sun avoidance.

Smoking Cessation Tobacco use through cigarettes and other means is the most avoidable risk factor for cardiovascular disease and cancer. The degree of smoke exposure, meaning the number of cigarettes smoked per day as well as the level of inhalation of cigarette smoke, is correlated with risk of lung cancer mortality. Light and low-tar cigarettes are not safer because smokers tend to inhale them more frequently and deeply. Those who stop smoking have a lower lung cancer mortality rate than those who continue smoking, despite the fact that some carcinogen-induced genetic mutations persist for years. In addition to lung cancer, cigarette smoking is a causative agent in cancers of the larynx, oropharynx, esophagus, bladder, and pancreas.

Smoking cessation and avoidance have the potential to save and extend more lives than any other public health activity. A smoker has a one in three lifetime risk of dying prematurely of a smoking-related cancer or cardiovascular or pulmonary disease. Indeed, more human lives are lost due to cardiovascular disease caused by smoking than from smoking-related cancer. The risk of tobacco smoke is not necessarily limited to the smoker. Epidemiologic studies suggest that environmental tobacco smoke may cause lung cancer and other pulmonary diseases in nonsmokers.

Nonsmoking persons should be encouraged not to start smoking, and persons who smoke should be encouraged to stop. Tobacco prevention is a pediatric issue. Over 80% of American smokers begin smoking before the age of 18. Nearly 20% of Americans aged 12 to 18 have smoked a cigarette in the past month. Counseling of adolescents and young adults is critical to prevent smoking. A physician's simple advice to not start smoking or to quit smoking can be of benefit. Physicians should query patients on tobacco use on every office visit, record the answer with the vital signs, and ask smokers if they would like assistance in quitting.

Current approaches to smoking cessation recognize that smoking is an addiction (Chap. 375). The smoker who is quitting goes through a process with identifiable stages that include contemplation of quitting, an action phase in which the smoker quits, and a maintenance phase. Smokers who quit completely are more likely to be successful than those who gradually reduce the number of cigarettes smoked or change to lower tar or nicotine cigarettes. More than 90% of the Americans who have successfully quit smoking did so on their own without participation in an organized cessation program, but cessation programs are helpful for some smokers. The Community Intervention Trial for Smoking Cessation (COMMIT) was a community-based 4-year program. COMMIT demonstrated that light smokers (<25 cigarettes per day) can benefit from simple cessation messages and cessation programs. The quit rate (fraction of the subjects followed who achieved and maintained cessation at the end of the trial) was 30.6% in the intervention communities and 27.5% in the control communities. This finding is statistically significant, but modest. The control communities enjoyed a substantial decrease in smoking through study participation. The COMMIT interventions were not successful for heavy smokers (>25 cigarettes per day). Heavy smokers need an intensive, broad-based cessation program that includes counseling, behavioral strategies, and pharmacologic adjuncts such as nicotine replacement and bupropion.

Cigar smoking has increased in the past 10 years, especially in younger adults. The health risks of cigars are similar to those of cigarettes. Smoking two cigars per day doubles the risk for oral and esophageal cancer; three to four cigars per day increases the risk of oral cancer eight-fold and esophageal cancer four-fold. The risks of occasional cigar smoking are unknown.

Smokeless tobacco is the fastest growing part of the tobacco industry and represents a significant health risk. Chewing tobacco is a carcinogen linked to dental caries, gingivitis, oral leukoplakia, and oral cancer. The systemic effects of smokeless tobacco may increase risks for other cancers.

Diet Modification Dietary modification may have significant potential for lowering cancer risk in western culture. Studies of international dietary patterns and animal studies suggest that diets high in fat increase the risk for cancers of the breast, colon, prostate, and endometrium. These cancers have their highest incidence and mortalities in western countries, where fat comprises an average of 40 to 45% of the total calories consumed. In populations at low risk for these cancers, fat accounts for <20% of calories.

Despite correlations, dietary fat has not been proven to cause cancer. Case-control and cohort epidemiologic studies give conflicting results. In addition, diet is a highly complex exposure to many nutrients and chemicals. Low-fat diets may render some protection through anticarcinogens found in vegetables, fruits, legumes, nuts, and grains. Protective substances found in these foods include phenols, sulfur-containing compounds, flavones, and fiber.

In observational studies, dietary fiber appears protective against colonic polyps and invasive cancer of the colon. The mechanisms involved are complex and speculative. They involve binding of oxidized bile acids and generation of soluble fiber products, such as butyrate, that may have differentiating properties. Transit time is not greatly affected. High-fiber diets may also protect against breast and prostate cancer by absorbing and inactivating dietary estrogenic and androgenic cancer promoters. Protective effects of fiber have not been proved in a prospective clinical trial.

The Polyp Prevention Trial randomly assigned 2000 elderly persons to a low-fat, high-fiber diet versus routine diet for 4 years. No differences were noted in polyp formation.

The U.S. National Institutes of Health Women's Health Initiative, launched in 1994, is a long-term clinical trial enrolling more than 100,000 women aged 45 to 69. It studies the potential cancer-preventing effects of a low-fat diet and vitamin supplementation. Results are not yet available. Scientific evidence does not currently establish the anticarcinogenic value of vitamin, mineral, or nutritional supplements in amounts greater than that provided by a good diet. However, consuming at least five servings of fruits and vegetables a day decreases dietary fat and increases fiber; such a diet may lower the risk of cardiovascular disease.

Sun Avoidance Nonmelanoma skin cancers (basal cell and squamous cell) are induced by cumulative exposure to ultraviolet radiation. Intermittent acute sun exposure and sun damage have been linked to melanoma. Sunburns, especially in childhood and adolescence, are associated with an increased risk of melanoma in adulthood. Reduction of sun exposure through use of protective clothing and changes in the pattern of outdoor activities can reduce skin cancer risk. Sunscreens decrease the risk of actinic keratoses, the precursor to squamous cell skin cancer, but melanoma risk may be increased. Sunscreens prevent burning and may encourage more prolonged exposure to the sun; yet they may not filter out wavelengths of energy that cause melanoma.

Educational interventions to help people assess their risk of developing skin cancer accurately have some impact. Self-examination for skin pigment characteristics associated with melanoma, such as freckling, may be useful in identifying people at high risk. People who recognize themselves as being at risk tend to be more compliant with sun-avoidance recommendations. Possible risk factors for melanoma include a propensity to sunburn, a large number of benign melanocytic nevi, and atypical nevi.

CANCER CHEMOPREVENTION Chemoprevention of cancer involves the use of specific natural or synthetic chemical agents to reverse, suppress, or prevent carcinogenesis before the development of invasive malignancy.

Cancer develops through an accumulation of genetic changes that are potential points of intervention to prevent cancer. The initial genetic changes are termed *initiation*. The alteration can be inherited or acquired through the action of physical, infectious, or chemical carcinogens. Like most human diseases, cancer arises through an interaction between genetics and environmental exposures (Table 67-1). Influences that cause the initiated cell to progress through the carcinogenic process and to change phenotypically are termed *promoters*. Promoters include hormones such as androgens, linked to prostate cancer, and estrogen, linked to breast and endometrial cancer. The distinction between an initiator and a promoter is sometimes arbitrary; some components of cigarette smoke are "complete carcinogens," acting as both initiators and promoters. Cancer can be prevented or controlled through interference with the factors that cause initiation, promotion, or progression. Compounds of interest in chemoprevention

TABLE 67-1 Carcinogens and Associated Cancers or Neoplasms

Carcinogens[a]	Associated Cancer or Neoplasm
Alkylating agents	Acute myelocytic leukemia, bladder cancer
Androgens	Prostate cancer
Aromatic amines (dyes)	Bladder cancer
Arsenic	Cancer of the lung, skin
Asbestos	Cancer of the lung, pleura, peritoneum
Benzene	Acute myelocytic leukemia
Chromium	Lung cancer
Diethylstilbestrol (prenatal)	Vaginal cancer (clear cell)
Epstein-Barr virus	Burkitt's lymphoma, nasal T cell lymphoma
Estrogens	Cancer of the endometrium, liver, breast
Ethyl alcohol	Cancer of the liver, esophagus, head and neck
Helicobacter pylori	Gastric cancer
Hepatitis B or C virus	Liver cancer
Human immunodeficiency virus	Non-Hodgkin's lymphoma, Kaposi's sarcoma, squamous cell carcinomas (especially of the urogenital tract)
	Human papilloma virus
Human T cell lymphotropic virus type I (HTLV-I)	Adult T cell leukemia/lymphoma
Immunosuppressive agents (azathioprine, cyclosporine, glucocorticoids)	Non-Hodgkin's lymphoma
Nitrogen mustard gas	Cancer of the lung, head and neck, nasal sinuses
Nickel dust	Cancer of the lung, nasal sinuses
Phenacetin	Cancer of the renal pelvis and bladder
Polycyclic hydrocarbons	Cancer of the lung, skin (especially squamous cell carcinoma of scrotal skin)
Schistosomiasis	Bladder cancer (squamous cell)
Sunlight (ultraviolet)	Skin cancer (squamous cell and melanoma)
Tobacco (including smokeless)	Cancer of the upper aerodigestive tract, bladder
Vinyl chloride	Liver cancer (angiosarcoma)

[a] Agents that are thought to act as cancer initiators and/or promoters.

often have antimutagenic, antioxidant, antiproliferative, or pro-apoptotic activity.

A number of chemoprevention strategies are undergoing clinical trials. However, tamoxifen is the only chemoprevention currently approved by the U.S. Food and Drug Administration; it lowers risk of breast cancer in high-risk women.

Multiple Cancer Site Prevention Trials The Physicians' Health Trial involves 22,071 American male physicians. Participants were randomly assigned to receive β-carotene, aspirin, and/or placebo in a 2 $\times$ 2 factorial design. All major medical events were recorded. In 1988, the aspirin arm was unblinded after the trial demonstrated that aspirin therapy causes a significant reduction in cardiovascular mortality. β-Carotene was not associated with a decreased cancer risk compared to placebo.

The Women's Health Study, launched in 1992, is a 10-year trial involving 44,000 female nurses. Subjects are randomly assigned to β-carotene, α-tocopherol, aspirin, and/or placebo in a factorial design yielding eight different treatment groups. The end points are total epithelial cancers, breast cancer, lung cancer, colon cancer, and vascular disease.

The Women's Health Initiative uses a partial factorial design that places women in 22 intervention groups. Participants can receive calcium and vitamin D supplementation, hormone replacement therapy, and counseling to increase exercise and cease smoking. Prevention of a number of cancers, cardiovascular disease, osteoporosis, and other diseases will be assessed. The portion of the trial comparing combined estrogen plus progestin replacement therapy to placebo in women with an intact uterus was halted in 2002 due to an excess of cardiovascular events and breast cancer in the hormone therapy arm. Colon cancer was decreased in the hormone therapy arm. Prior epidemiologic studies had consistently shown a decrease in cardiovascular disease in women taking hormone replacement therapy. The risk of developing Alzheimer's disease was doubled in the combined hormone therapy arm, and quality of life was not improved compared to placebo. Therefore the strength of evidence from prospective randomized, controlled trials is considered to outweigh the prior evidence of benefit. At present combined estrogen plus progestin therapy is not recommended for disease prevention because of the results of this study. The estrogen-only portion of the trial (in women with prior hysterectomy) is still in progress.

Chemoprevention of Cancers of the Upper Aerodigestive Tract Smoking causes diffuse epithelial injury in the head, neck, esophagus, and lung. Patients cured of squamous cell cancers of the lung, esophagus, head, and neck are at risk (as high as 5% per year) of developing a second cancer of the upper aerodigestive tract. Cessation of cigarette smoking does not markedly decrease the cured cancer patient's risk of second malignancy, even though it does lower the cancer risk in those who have never developed a malignancy. Smoking cessation may halt the early stages of the carcinogenic process (such as metaplasia), but it may have no effect on late stages of carcinogenesis. This "field carcinogenesis" hypothesis for cancer of the upper aerodigestive tract has made "cured" patients an important population for chemoprevention of second malignancies. A randomized, placebo-controlled clinical trial has demonstrated that adjuvant isoretinoin (13-*cis*-retinoic acid) can reduce the incidence of second primary tumors in patients treated with local therapy for head and neck cancer. However, overall survival was not improved due to mortality from recurrences of the primary tumor.

Oral leukoplakia, a premalignant lesion commonly found in smokers, has been used as an intermediate marker allowing the demonstration of chemopreventive activity in smaller, shorter-duration, randomized, placebo-controlled trials. Response was associated with upregulation of retinoic acid receptor β. Therapy with isoretinoin causes regression of oral leukoplakia. However, the lesions recur when the agent is withdrawn, suggesting the need for chronic administration of retinoids. Premalignant lesions in the oropharyngeal area have also responded to β-carotene, retinol, α-tocopherol (vitamin E), and selenium. Further study to improve the definition of the activity of these drugs is ongoing. Isoretinoin was shown not to prevent second malignancies in patients cured of early-stage non-small cell lung cancer, and those who were current smokers had higher lung cancer mortality rates than those not taking isoretinoin.

Several large-scale trials have assessed agents in the chemoprevention of lung cancer in patients at high risk. In the Alpha-Tocopherol/Beta-Carotene (ATBC) Lung Cancer Prevention Trial, participants were male smokers, aged 50 to 69 at entry. At entry, participants had smoked an average of one pack of cigarettes per day for 35.9 years. Participants received α-tocopherol, β-carotene, and/or placebo in a randomized, 2×2 factorial design. After a median follow-up of 6.1 years, lung cancer incidence and mortality were statistically significantly *increased* in those receiving β-carotene. α-Tocopherol had no effect on lung cancer mortality, and no evidence suggested interaction between the two drugs. Patients receiving α-tocopherol had a higher incidence of hemorrhagic stroke.

The Beta-Carotene and Retinol Efficacy Trial (CARET) involved 17,000 American smokers and workers with asbestos exposure. Entrants were randomly assigned to one of four arms and received β-carotene, retinol, and/or placebo in a 2×2 factorial design. This trial demonstrated harm from β-carotene: a lung cancer rate of 5 per 1000 subjects per year for those taking placebo and of 6 per 1000 subjects per year for those taking β-carotene. The difference was statistically significant.

These ATBC and CARET results demonstrate the importance of testing chemoprevention hypotheses before implementing them widely, because the results stand in contrast to a number of observational epidemiologic studies. In the ATBC trial, participants taking α-tocopherol had a one-third reduction in the incidence of prostate cancer, compared to those not taking α-tocopherol. The Physicians' Health Trial showed neither an increased nor a decreased risk of lung cancer in those using β-carotene; fewer of its participants were smokers than those in the ATBC and CARET studies.

Chemoprevention of Colon Cancer Many of the current colon cancer prevention trials are based on the premise that most colorectal cancers develop from adenomatous polyps. These trials use adenoma recurrence or disappearance as a surrogate end point to assess colon cancer prevention. Early clinical trial results suggest that nonsteroidal anti-inflammatory drugs (NSAIDs), such as piroxicam, sulindac, and aspirin, may prevent adenoma formation or cause regression of adenomatous polyps. The mechanism of action of NSAIDs is unknown, but they are presumed to work through the cyclooxygenase pathway. In the Physicians' Health Trial, aspirin had no effect on colon cancer incidence, although the 6-year assessment period may not have been long enough to evaluate this end point definitively. Studies evaluating NSAIDs as colon cancer chemopreventive agents have not yet been completed.

Cyclooxygenase 2 inhibitors may be even more effective at colon cancer prevention. High-dose celecoxib reduces the number of colorectal polyps in patients with familial adenomatous polyposis and is under study for prevention of sporadic colorectal cancer.

Epidemiologic studies suggest that diets high in calcium lower colon cancer risk. Calcium binds bile and fatty acids, which cause hyperproliferation of colonic epithelium. It is hypothesized that this effect reduces intraluminal exposure to these compounds. Early data from randomized studies suggest that calcium supplementation decreases the risk of adenomatous polyp recurrence by about 20%, even though it does not decrease the proliferative rate of the colonic epithelium. Epithelial proliferative rate may not be an adequate surrogate marker in colon cancer prevention trials. Trials of calcium with cancer incidence end points are underway.

The Women's Health Initiative demonstrated a significant reduction in colon cancer among women taking combined hormone replacement therapy. However, the increased risk of cardiovascular events and breast cancer probably outweighs the benefit.

Prevention of Hormonally Driven Cancers Hormonal manipulation is being tested in the primary prevention of breast and prostate cancer. Tamoxifen is an antiestrogen with partial estrogen agonistic activity in some tissues, such as endometrium and bone. One of its actions is to upregulate transforming growth factor β, which decreases breast cell proliferation. In randomized placebo-controlled trials to assess tamoxifen as an adjuvant in breast cancer treatment, this drug reduced the number of new breast cancers in the uninvolved breast by more than a third. In a randomized placebo-controlled trial involving >13,000 women at high risk, tamoxifen decreased the risk of developing cancer by 49% compared to placebo. Tamoxifen also reduced the risk of bone fractures; a small increase in risk of endometrial cancer, stroke, pulmonary emboli, and deep vein thrombosis was noted. A trial to compare tamoxifen with another selective estrogen receptor modulator, raloxifene, is ongoing. Raloxifene may have less risk of endometrial cancer.

Finasteride is a 5α-reductase inhibitor. It inhibits the conversion of testosterone to dihydrotestosterone, a more potent stimulator of prostate cell proliferation than testosterone. In an F344 rat model of carcinogen-induced prostate cancer, finasteride decreased the incidence of cancers. Finasteride produced a 20% decrease in overall prostate cancer, but a slight increase in high-grade (Gleason score 7–10) prostate cancer in men over age 55 years.

Selenium is being tested as a prostate cancer preventive agent based on laboratory studies and a small clinical trial aimed at prevention of skin cancer. Men taking selenium to prevent skin cancer were found to have a significantly reduced incidence of prostate cancer (16 on placebo arm; 4 on selenium arm). The ATBC study cited above showed that risk of prostate cancer was reduced in those taking vitamin E (99 prostate cancers on vitamin E; 151 cases on placebo). The findings on selenium and vitamin E were serendipitous and based on secondary analysis. A prospective study is underway.

Vaccines and Cancer Prevention   A number of infectious agents have been linked to the development of cancer, leading to interest in developing vaccines to protect against these agents. The hepatitis B vaccine is quite effective in preventing hepatitis and hepatomas due to chronic hepatitis B infection. Public health officials are encouraging widespread administration of this vaccine, especially in Asia, where the disease is epidemic. Human papilloma virus (HPV) vaccines are being developed to prevent cervical cancer, and *Helicobacter pylori* vaccines are aimed at gastric cancer. Antibiotic eradication of *H. pylori* may also be a cancer prevention strategy.

SURGICAL PREVENTION OF CANCER   Some organs in some people are at such high risk of developing cancer that surgical removal of the organ at risk is recommended. Women with severe cervical dysplasia are treated with conization and occasionally even hysterectomy. Colectomy is used to prevent colon cancer in people with familial polyposis and those with ulcerative colitis. Based on a study in 139 women with *BRCA1* and *BRCA2* mutations, many women with a genetic predisposition to breast cancer opt to have bilateral mastectomy rather than close surveillance. Of the 139 women, 76 chose mastectomy and 63 chose surveillance; none of the 76 who underwent mastectomy developed breast cancer, but 8 of the 63 women under careful surveillance developed breast cancer. A randomized study is unlikely to be done, and assessment of the effects of prophylactic mastectomy on mortality is also unlikely to be done.

CANCER SCREENING   Screening is a means of detecting disease early in asymptomatic individuals, with the goal of decreasing morbidity and mortality. While screening can potentially save lives and has clearly been shown to do so in the case of cervical, colon, and probably breast cancer, it is also subject to a number of biases, which can suggest a benefit when actually there is none. Bias can even mask net harm. Early detection does not in itself confer benefit. To be of value, screening must detect disease earlier, and treatment of earlier disease must yield a better outcome than treatment at the onset of symptoms. Cause-specific mortality, rather than survival after diagnosis, is the preferred end point (see below).

Because screening is done on asymptomatic, healthy persons, it should offer substantial likelihood of benefit that outweighs harm. Screening tests and their appropriate use should be carefully evaluated before their use is widely encouraged in screening programs as a matter of public policy.

Screening examinations, tests, or procedures are usually not diagnostic of cancer but instead indicate that a cancer may be present. The diagnosis is then made following a workup that includes a biopsy and pathologic confirmation.

A number of genes have been identified that predispose for a disease, and many more will be identified in the near future. Testing for these genes can define a high-risk population. The ability to predict the development of a particular cancer may some day present therapeutic options as well as ethical dilemmas. It may eventually allow for early intervention to prevent a cancer or limit its severity. People at high risk will be ideal candidates for chemoprevention and screening; however, efficacy of these interventions in the high-risk population should be investigated. Currently, persons at high risk for a particular cancer can engage in intensive screening. While this course is clinically prudent, it is not known if it saves lives in these populations.

TABLE 67-2   Definition of Terms

Term	Definition
Sensitivity	The proportion of persons with the condition who test positive: $a/(a + c)$
Specificity	The proportion of persons without the condition who test negative: $d/(b + d)$
Positive predictive value	The proportion of persons with a positive test who have the condition: $a/(a + b)$
Negative predictive value	The proportion of persons with a negative test who do not have the condition: $d/(c + d)$

		Condition present	Condition absent
a = true positive			
b = false positive	Positive test	a	b
c = false negative			
d = true negative	Negative test	c	d

The Accuracy of Screening   A screening test's accuracy or ability to discriminate disease is described by four indices: sensitivity, specificity, positive predictive value, and negative predictive value (Table 67-2). *Sensitivity* is the proportion of persons with the disease who test positive in the screen (i.e., the ability of the test to detect disease when it is present). *Specificity* is the proportion of persons who do not have the disease and test negative in the screening test (i.e., the ability of a test to tell that the disease is not present). The *positive predictive value* is the proportion of persons who test positive who actually have the disease. Similarly, *negative predictive value* is the proportion of who test negative and do not have the disease. The sensitivity and specificity of a test are relatively independent of the underlying prevalence (or risk) of the disease in the population screened, but the predictive values depend strongly on the prevalence of the disease (Table 67-3).

Screening is most beneficial, efficient, and economical when the target disease is common in the population being screened. To be valuable, the screening test should have a high specificity; sensitivity need not be very high, as demonstrated in Table 67-3.

Potential Biases of Screening Tests   The common biases of screening are lead time, length, and selection. These biases can make a screening test seem beneficial when actually it is not (or even causes net harm). Whether beneficial or not, screening can create the false impression of an epidemic by increasing the number of cancers diagnosed. It can also produce a shift in proportion of patients diagnosed at an early stage that improves survival statistics without reducing mortality (i.e., the number of deaths from a given cancer relative to the number of people at risk for the cancer). In such a case, the *apparent* duration of

TABLE 67-3   Predictive Value Relationships[a]

Positive predictive value (PPV) is a function of sensitivity, specificity, and prevalence:

$$PPV = \frac{\text{prevalence} \times \text{sensitivity}}{(\text{prevalence} \times \text{sensitivity}) + (1 - \text{prevalence})(1 - \text{specificity})}$$

PPV for a prevalence of 5 per 1000:

	PPV for a Sensitivity of, %	
Specificity	0.8	0.95
0.95	7	9
0.999	80	83

PPV for a prevalence of 1 per 10,000:

	PPV for a Sensitivity of, %	
Specificity	0.8	0.95
0.95	0.2	0.2
0.999	7	9

[a] The positive predictive value is expressed as a percentage. It is influenced by the sensitivity and specificity of the screening test and the prevalence of the disease being screened for. As shown here, for relatively uncommon diseases, such as cancer, the positive predictive value is influenced particularly strongly by the specificity of the screening test at a given prevalence.

survival increases without lives being saved or life expectancy changed.

Lead-time bias occurs when a test does not influence the natural history of the disease; the patient is merely diagnosed at an earlier date. When lead-time bias occurs, survival *appears* increased, but life is not really prolonged. The screening test only prolongs the time the subject is aware of the disease and spends as a patient.

Length bias occurs when slow-growing, less aggressive cancers are detected during screening. Cancers diagnosed due to the onset of symptoms between scheduled screenings are on average more aggressive, and treatment outcomes are not as favorable. An extreme form of length bias is termed *overdiagnosis*, the detection of "pseudodisease." The reservoir of some undetected slow-growing tumors is large. Many of these tumors fulfill the histologic criteria of cancer but will never become clinically significant or cause death. This problem is compounded by the fact that the most common cancers appear most frequently at ages when competing causes of death are more frequent.

Selection bias must be considered in assessing the results of any screening effort. The population most likely to seek screening may differ from the general population to which the screening test might be applied. The individuals screened may have volunteered because of a particular risk factor not found in the general population, such as a strong family history. In general, volunteers for studies may be more health conscious and likely to have a better prognosis or lower mortality rate, irrespective of the screening result. This is termed the *healthy volunteer effect*.

Potential Drawbacks of Screening Risks associated with screening include harm caused by the screening intervention itself, harm due to the further investigation of persons with positive test results (both true and false positives), and harm from the treatment of persons with a true-positive result, even if life is extended by treatment. The diagnosis and treatment of cancers that would never have caused medical problems can lead to the harm of unnecessary treatment and give patients the anxiety of a cancer diagnosis. The psychosocial impact of cancer screening, whether the result is positive or negative, can also be substantial when applied to the entire population.

Assessment of Screening Tests Good clinical trial design can offset some biases of screening and demonstrate the relative risks and benefits of a screening test. A randomized, controlled screening trial with cause-specific mortality as the end point provides the strongest support for a screening intervention. In a randomized trial, two like populations are randomly established. One is given the medical standard of care (which may be no screening at all), and the other receives the screening intervention being assessed. The two populations are compared over time. Efficacy for the population studied is established when the group receiving the screening test has a better cause-specific mortality rate than the control group. Studies showing a reduction in the incidence of advanced-stage disease, an improved survival, or a stage shift are weaker (and possibly misleading) evidence of benefit. These latter criteria are necessary but not sufficient to establish the value of a screening test.

Although a randomized, controlled screening trial provides the strongest evidence to support the usefulness of a screening test, it is not perfect. Unless the trial is population-based, it does not remove the issue of generalizability to the target population. Screening trials generally involve thousands of persons and last for years. Less definitive study designs are therefore often used to estimate the effectiveness of screening practices. After a randomized controlled clinical trial, in descending order of strength, evidence may be derived from:

The findings of internally controlled trials using intervention allocation methods other than randomization (e.g., allocation determined by birth date, date of clinic visit);

The findings of cohort or case-control analytic observational studies;

The results of multiple time series studies with or without the intervention;

The opinions of respected authorities based on clinical experience, descriptive studies, or consensus reports of experts (the weakest evidence because even experts can be misled by the biases described above).

Screening for Specific Cancers Widespread screening for cervical, colon, and probably breast cancer is beneficial for certain age groups. Special surveillance of those at high risk for a specific cancer because of a family history or a genetic risk factor may be prudent, but few studies have been carried out to assess the impact of this practice on mortality in specific high-risk populations. A number of organizations have considered whether or not to endorse routine use of certain screening tests. Because these groups have not used the same criteria to judge whether a screening test should be endorsed, they have arrived at different recommendations. The screening guidelines of the U.S. Preventive Services Task Force, the Canadian Task Force on Preventive Health Care, and the American Cancer Society are often quoted and show a range of recommendations (Table 67-4).

BREAST CANCER Breast self-examination, clinical breast examination by a care giver, and mammography have been advocated as useful screening tools. Only breast self-examination, screening mammography alone, and screening mammography with clinical examination have been evaluated in randomized controlled trials. Magnetic resonance

TABLE 67-4 *Screening Recommendations for Asymptomatic Normal-Risk Subjects[a]*

Test or Procedure	USPSTF	ACS	CTFPHC
Sigmoidoscopy	>50, periodically <50, not recommended	≥50, every 3–5 years	Insufficient evidence
Fecal occult blood testing	≥50, every year	≥50, every year	Insufficient evidence
Digital rectal examination	No recommendation	≥40, every year	Poor evidence to include or exclude
Prostate-specific antigen	Insufficient evidence to recommend	M: ≥50, every year	Recommendation against
Pap test	F: 18–65, every 1–3 years	F with uterine cervix, beginning 3 years after first intercourse or by age 21. Yearly for standard Pap; every 2 years with liquid test.	Fair evidence to include in examination of sexually active women
Pelvic examination	Do not recommend, advise adnexal palpation during exam for other reasons	F: 18–40, every 1–3 years with Pap test; >40, every year	Not considered
Endometrial tissue sampling	Not considered	At menopause if obese or a history of unopposed estrogen use	Not considered
Breast self-examination	No recommendation	≥20, monthly	Insufficient evidence to make a recommendation
Breast clinical examination	F: >50, every year	F: 20–40, every 3 years; >40, yearly	F: >50, every year
Mammography	F: 40–75, every 1–2 years	F: ≥40, every year	F: 50–69, every year
Complete skin examination	Not recommended	20–39, every 3 years	Poor evidence to include or exclude

[a] Summary of the screening procedures recommended for the general population by U.S. Preventive Services Task Force (USPSTF), the American Cancer Society (ACS), and the Canadian Task Force on Prevention Health Care (CTFPHC). These recommendations refer to asymptomatic persons who have no risk factors, other than age or gender, for the targeted condition. *Note*: F, female; M, male.

imaging is being assessed and may be more accurate than mammography in women at high risk.

A number of trials have suggested that annual or biennial screening with mammography or mammography plus clinical breast examination in women over the age of 50 saves lives. Each trial has been criticized for design flaws. In most trials, the breast cancer mortality rate is decreased by 20 to 30%. Experts disagree on whether average-risk women aged 40 to 49 should receive regular screening (Table 67-4). The significance of the screening effect in women aged 40 to 49 depends on the statistical test used. An analysis of eight large randomized trials showed no benefit from mammographic screening for women aged 40 to 49 when assessed 5 to 7 years after trial entry. However, a small benefit emerged 10 to 12 years after study entry. What proportion of this benefit is due to screening after these women turned 50 is not known. In randomized screening studies of women aged 50 to 69, the decline in mortality begins about 5 years after initiation of screening. Nearly half of women aged 40 to 49 years screened annually will have false-positive mammograms necessitating further evaluation, often including biopsy. The risk of false-positive testing should be discussed with the patient.

While no study has shown breast self-examination to decrease mortality, it is recommended as prudent by many organizations. A substantial fraction of breast cancers are first detected by patients. Self-examination leads to increased biopsy rate without reducing breast cancer mortality.

Genetic screening for *BRCA1* and *BRCA2* mutations and other markers of breast cancer risk has identified a group of women at high risk for breast cancer. Unfortunately, when to begin and the optimal frequency of screening have not been defined. Mammography is less sensitive at detecting breast cancers in women carrying *BRCA* mutations, possibly because such cancers occur in younger women, in whom mammography is known to be less sensitive.

CERVICAL CANCER   Screening with Papanicolaou smears decreases cervical cancer mortality. The cervical cancer mortality rate has fallen substantially since the widespread use of the Pap smear, although this trend actually began earlier. Most screening guidelines recommend regular Pap testing for all women who are or have been sexually active for 3 years or have reached the age of 21. With the onset of sexual activity comes the risk of sexual transmission of HPV, the most common etiologic factor for cervical cancer. The recommended interval for Pap screening varies from 1 to 3 years. At age 30, women who have had three normal test results in a row may get screened every 2 to 3 years. An upper age limit at which screening ceases to be effective is not known, but women age ≥70 years who have had no abnormal results in the previous 10 years may choose to stop screening.

COLORECTAL CANCER   Fecal occult blood testing, digital rectal examination, rigid and flexible sigmoidoscopy, radiographic barium contrast studies, and colonoscopy have been considered for colorectal cancer screening. Annual fecal occult blood testing using hydrated specimens could reduce colorectal cancer mortality by a third. The sensitivity for fecal occult blood is increased if specimens are rehydrated before testing, but at the cost of lower specificity. The false-positive rate for rehydrated fecal occult blood testing is high; 1 to 5% of persons tested have a positive result. About 2 to 10% of those with occult blood in the stool have cancer, and 20 to 30% have adenomas. The high false-positive rate of fecal occult blood testing dramatically increases the number of colonoscopies performed.

Two case-control studies suggest that regular screening of people over 50 with sigmoidoscopy decreases mortality. These types of studies are prone to selection biases. A quarter to a third of polyps can be discovered with the rigid sigmoidoscope; half are found with a 35-cm flexible scope, and two-thirds to three-quarters are found with a 60-cm scope. Diagnosis of polyposis by sigmoidoscopy should lead to evaluation of the entire colon with colonoscopy and/or barium enema. The most efficient interval for screening sigmoidoscopy is unknown.

Case-control studies suggest that testing at intervals of up to 15 years may confer benefit.

One-time colonoscopy detects about 25% more advanced lesions (polyps > 10 mm, villous adenomas, polyps with high-grade dysplasia, invasive cancer) than does one-time fecal occult blood testing with sigmoidoscopy. Colonoscopy is well suited to screening subjects at high risk, such as those with ulcerative colitis or family predisposition. Perforation rates are 3/1000 for colonoscopy and 1/1000 for sigmoidoscopy. Debate continues on whether full colonoscopy is too expensive and invasive for widespread use as a screening tool in standard-risk populations. Data are not available on digital rectal examination or barium enema as colon cancer screening tools, but both are insensitive.

LUNG CANCER   Chest radiographs and sputum cytology have been evaluated as methods for lung cancer screening. No reduction in lung cancer mortality has been found in these studies, although all the controlled trials performed have had low statistical power. Even screening of high-risk subjects (smokers) has not been proved to be beneficial. Spiral computed tomography (CT) can diagnose lung cancers at early stages; however, false-positive rates are high. Spiral CT screening increases the number of lesions detected and increases the number of diagnostic and therapeutic procedures. However, its capacity to save lives is being tested.

OVARIAN CANCER   Adnexal palpation, transvaginal ultrasound, and serum CA-125 determination have been considered for ovarian cancer screening. Adnexal palpation is too insensitive to detect ovarian cancer at an early enough stage to affect mortality substantially. Neither transvaginal ultrasound nor CA-125 screening has been tested in a completed randomized prospective trial. Ovarian cancer screening can lead to an invasive diagnostic workup, which may include laparotomy. In a clinical study, 0.6% of 900 adult women had a serum CA-125 level >35 U/mL. Thus, if 100,000 adult women were screened, 600 would be identified as having a high CA-125 level. The prevalence of ovarian cancer in the female adult population is ~20 per 100,000. Thus, the screening test would identify 600 women who would undergo further evaluation to identify 20 cases of ovarian cancer. Some of these 600 would only be inconvenienced by an ultrasound examination. Others would undergo an exploratory laparotomy. A large proportion of the 20 women identified as having ovarian cancer would have advanced, incurable disease and thus not benefit from screening. A National Institutes of Health consensus conference in 1994 concluded that routine screening for ovarian cancer was not indicated for standard-risk women or those with a single affected family member, but that it might be worthwhile in families with genetic ovarian cancer syndromes.

PROSTATE CANCER   The most common prostate cancer screening modalities are digital rectal examination and assays for serum prostate-specific antigen (PSA). Newer serum tests, such as measurement of the ratio of bound to free serum PSA, have yet to be fully evaluated. An emphasis on PSA screening has caused prostate cancer to become the most common non-skin cancer diagnosed in American males. Screening for this disease is very prone to lead-time bias, length bias, and overdiagnosis, and substantial debate rages among experts on whether it is effective. Some experts are concerned that prostate cancer screening, more than screening for other cancers, may cause net harm. Prostate cancer screening clearly detects many asymptomatic cancers, but the ability to distinguish tumors that are lethal but still curable from those that pose little or no threat to health is limited. Men over age 50 have a very high prevalence of indolent, clinically insignificant prostate cancers. No well-designed trial has demonstrated the benefit of prostate cancer screening and treatment.

The placebo arm of the Prostate Cancer Prevention Trial showed that rigorous screening of low-risk men for 7 years leads to the diagnosis of prostate cancer in >12% of patients. However, >12% of patients with normal annual DREs and PSAs biopsied after 7 years were found to have cancer. Thus, prostate cancer screening had moderate success in early detection, but screening missed half the prostate cancers.

The effectiveness of radical prostatectomy, radiation therapy, and other treatments for low-stage prostate cancer is also under study in randomized trials. Definitive treatment of cancers detected by screening may cause morbidity for some men, such as impotence and urinary incontinence, and carries a low but finite risk of death. Comparison of radical prostatectomy to "watchful waiting" in clinically diagnosed (not screening PSA-detected) prostate cancers showed a decreased rate of death from prostate cancer for those undergoing surgery, but overall mortality was not different in the two arms. Patients undergoing surgery had a higher rate of impotence and urinary incontinence.

Ongoing randomized trials are comparing usual care to prostate screening and comparing definitive therapy to "watchful waiting." The American Cancer Society and the American Urologic Association recommend that men be offered screening after being informed of the potential risks and benefits. A man should have a life expectancy of at least 10 years to be eligible for screening. The U.S. Preventive Services Task Force finds insufficient evidence to recommend prostate cancer screening (Table 67-4).

ENDOMETRIAL CANCER   Transvaginal ultrasound and endometrial sampling have been advocated as screening tests for endometrial cancer. Benefit from routine screening has not been shown. Transvaginal ultrasound and endometrial sampling are indicated for workup of vaginal bleeding in postmenopausal women but are not considered as screening tests in symptomatic women.

SKIN CANCER   Visual examination of all skin surfaces by the patient or by a health care provider is used in screening for basal and squamous cell cancers and melanoma. No prospective randomized study has been performed to look for a mortality decrease. Observational epidemiologic evidence from Scotland and Australia suggests that screening programs have caused a stage shift in melanomas diagnosed. Screening may reinforce sun avoidance and other skin cancer prevention behaviors.

FURTHER READING

THE CANADIAN TASKFORCE ON PREVENTIVE HEALTH CARE: www.ctfphc.org/

HUMPHREY LL et al: Breast cancer screening: A summary of the evidence for the U.S. Preventive Services Task Force. Ann Intern Med 137:347, 2002

KIM ES et al: Chemoprevention of aerodigestive tract cancers. Annu Rev Med 53:223, 2002

THE NATIONAL CANCER INSTITUTE CANCERNET: cancernet.nci.nih.gov/

NATIONAL INSTITUTES OF HEALTH CONSENSUS DEVELOPMENT PANEL: Breast cancer screening for women ages 40–49. J Natl Cancer Inst 89: 1015, 1997

SCREENING FOR PROSTATE CANCER: Recommendation and rationale. Ann Intern Med 137:915, 2002

SMITH RA et al: American Cancer Society guidelines for the early detection of cancer, 2003. CA Cancer J Clin 53:27, 2003

STOUTJESDIJK M: Magnetic resonance imaging and mammography in women with a hereditary risk of breast cancer. J Natl Cancer Inst 93:1095, 2001

68 CANCER GENETICS
Pat J. Morin, Jeffrey M. Trent, Francis S. Collins, Bert Vogelstein

CANCER IS A GENETIC DISEASE   Cancer arises through a series of somatic alterations in DNA that results in unrestrained cellular proliferation. Most of these alterations involve actual sequence changes in DNA (i.e., mutations). They may arise as a consequence of random replication errors, exposure to carcinogens (e.g., radiation), or faulty DNA repair processes. While most cancers arise sporadically, familial clustering of cancers occurs in certain families who carry a germline mutation in a cancer gene.

HISTORIC PERSPECTIVE   The concept of cancer genetics is relatively new. The idea that cancer progression is driven by sequential somatic mutations in specific genes has only gained general acceptance in the last 25 years. Before the advent of the microscope, cancer was believed to be composed of aggregates of mucus or other noncellular matter. By the middle of the nineteenth century, it became clear that tumors were masses of cells and that these cells arose from the normal cells of the tissue in which the cancer originated. However, the molecular basis for the uncontrolled proliferation of cancer cells was to remain a mystery for another century. During that time, a number of theories for the origin of cancer were postulated. The great biochemist Otto Warburg proposed the combustion theory of cancer, which stipulated that cancer was due to abnormal oxygen metabolism: while normal cells required oxygen, cancer cells could survive in its absence. In addition, some believed that all cancers were caused by viruses, and that cancer was in fact a contagious disease.

In the end, observations of cancer occurring in chimney sweeps, studies of x-rays, and the overwhelming data demonstrating cigarette smoke as a causative agent in lung cancer, together with Ames's work on chemical mutagenesis, were sufficient to convince many that cancer originated through changes in DNA. Although the viral theory of cancer did not prove to be generally accurate, the study of retroviruses led to the discovery of the first human *oncogenes* in the mid to late 1970s. Soon after, the study of families with genetic predisposition to cancer was instrumental in the discovery of *tumor suppressor genes*. The field that studies the type of mutations, as well as the consequence of these mutations in tumor cells, is now known as cancer genetics.

THE CLONAL ORIGIN AND MULTISTEP NATURE OF CANCER   Nearly all cancers originate from a single cell; this clonal origin is a critical discriminating feature between neoplasia and hyperplasia. Multiple cumulative mutational events are invariably required for the progression from normal to fully malignant phenotype. The process can be seen as Darwinian microevolution in which, at each successive step, the mutated cells gain a growth advantage resulting in an increased representation relative to their neighbors (Fig. 68-1). It is believed that five to ten accumulated mutations are necessary for a cell to progress from the normal to the fully malignant phenotype.

We are beginning to understand the precise nature of the genetic alterations responsible for some malignancies and to get a sense of the order in which they occur. The best studied example is colon cancer, in which analyses of DNA from tissues extending from normal colon epithelium through adenoma to carcinoma have identified some of the genes mutated in the process (Fig. 68-2). Similar progression models are being elucidated for other malignancies.

GENERAL CLASSES OF CANCER GENES   There are two major classes of cancer genes. The first class comprises genes that directly affect cell growth either positively (*oncogenes*) or negatively (*tumor suppressor*

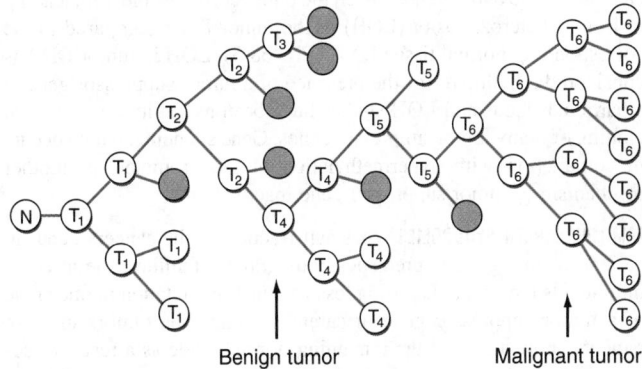

FIGURE 68-1   Multistep clonal development of malignancy. In this diagram a series of five cumulative mutations (T1, T2, T4, T5, T6), each with a modest growth advantage acting alone, eventually results in a malignant tumor. Note that not all such alterations result in progression; for example, the T3 clone is a dead end. The actual number of cumulative mutations necessary to transform from the normal to the malignant state is unknown in most tumors. (*After P Nowell, Science 194:23, 1976, with permission.*)

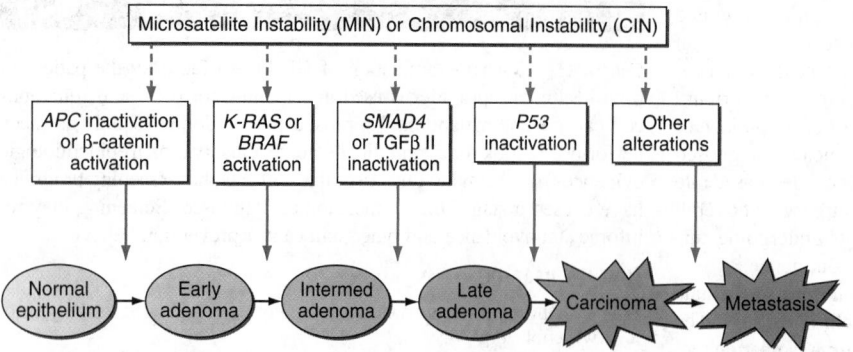

FIGURE 68-2 Progressive somatic mutational steps in the development of colon carcinoma. The accumulation of alterations in a number of different genes results in the progression from normal epithelium through adenoma to full-blown carcinoma. Genetic instability (microsatellite or chromosomal) accelerates the progression by increasing the likelihood of mutation at each step. Patients with familial polyposis are already one step into this pathway, since they inherit a germline alteration of the *APC* gene. TGF, transforming growth factor.

genes). These genes exert their effects on tumor growth through their ability to control cell division (cell birth) or cell death (apoptosis). Oncogenes are tightly regulated in normal cells. In cancer cells, oncogenes acquire mutations that relieve this control and lead to increased activity of the gene product. This mutational event typically occurs in a single allele of the oncogene and acts in a dominant fashion. In contrast, the normal function of tumor suppressor genes is to restrain cell growth and this function is lost in cancer. Because of the diploid nature of mammalian cells, both alleles must be inactivated to completely lose the function of a tumor suppressor gene, leading to a recessive mechanism at the cellular level. From these ideas and studies on the inherited form of retinoblastoma, Knudson and others formulated the *two-hit hypothesis*, which in its modern version states that both copies of a tumor suppressor gene must be inactivated in cancer.

The second class of cancer genes, the *caretakers*, do not directly affect cell growth but rather affect the ability of the cell to maintain the integrity of its genome. Cells with deficiency in these genes have an increased rate of mutations in all the genes, including oncogenes and tumor suppressor genes. This "mutator" phenotype was first hypothesized by Loeb to explain how the multiple mutational events required for tumorigenesis can occur in the lifetime of an individual. A mutation phenotype has now been observed in cancer at both the nucleotide sequence and chromosomal levels.

MECHANISMS OF TUMOR SUPPRESSOR INACTIVATION The two major types of somatic lesions observed in tumor suppressor genes during tumor development are *point mutations* and *large deletions*. Point mutations in the coding region of tumor suppressor genes will frequently lead to truncated protein products or otherwise nonfunctional proteins. Similarly, deletions lead to the loss of a functional product and sometimes encompass the entire gene or even the entire chromosome arm, leading to loss of heterozygosity (LOH) in the tumor DNA compared to the corresponding normal tissue DNA (Fig. 68-3). LOH in tumor DNA is considered a hallmark for the presence of a tumor suppressor gene at a particular locus and LOH studies have been useful in the positional cloning of many tumor suppressor genes. Gene silencing, which occurs in conjunction with hypermethylation of the promoter, is another mechanism of tumor suppressor gene inactivation.

FAMILIAL CANCER SYNDROMES A small fraction of the cancers occur in patients with a genetic predisposition. In these families, the affected individuals have a predisposing loss-of-function mutation in one allele of a tumor suppressor gene or caretaker gene. The tumors in these patients show a loss of the remaining normal allele as a result of somatic events (point mutations or deletions), in agreement with the Knudson hypothesis (Fig. 68-3). Thus, most cells of an individual with an inherited loss-of-function mutation in a tumor suppressor gene are functionally normal and only the rare cells that develop a mutation in the remaining normal allele will exhibit uncontrolled growth. The normal function of tumor suppressors is to restrain growth, to promote

differentiation (gatekeeper genes), or to preserve genome integrity (caretaker genes).

Roughly 100 syndromes of familial cancer have been reported, although many are rare. The majority are inherited as autosomal dominant traits although some of those associated with DNA repair abnormalities (xeroderma pigmentosum, Fanconi's anemia, ataxia telangiectasia) are autosomal recessive. Table 68-1 shows a number of cancer predisposition syndromes and the responsible genes. The current paradigm states that the genes mutated in familial syndromes can also be targets for somatic mutations in sporadic (noninherited) tumors. The study of cancer syndromes has thus provided invaluable insights into the mechanisms of progression for many tumor types. This section examines the case of inherited colon cancer in detail, but the same general lessons can be applied to all the cancer syndromes listed in Table 68-1.

Familial adenomatous polyposis (FAP) is a dominantly inherited colon cancer syndrome due to germline mutations in the adenomatous polyposis coli (*APC*) tumor suppressor gene on chromosome 5. Patients with this syndrome develop hundreds to thousands of adenomas in the colon. Each of these adenomas has lost the normal remaining allele of *APC* but has not yet accumulated the required additional mutations to generate fully malignant cells (Fig. 68-2). However, out of these thousands of benign adenomas, several will invariably acquire further abnormalities and a subset will even develop into fully malignant cancers. *APC* is thus considered to be a gatekeeper for colon tumorigenesis; Fig. 68-4 shows germline and somatic mutations found in the *APC* gene. The function of the APC protein is still not completely understood but likely provides differentiation and apoptotic cues to colonic cells as they migrate up the crypts. Defects in this process may lead to abnormal accumulation of cells that should normally undergo apoptosis and slough off.

In contrast to FAP, patients with hereditary nonpolyposis colon cancer (HNPCC or Lynch syndrome) do not develop multiple polyposis but instead develop only one or a small number of adenomas that rapidly progress to cancer. HNPCC is commonly defined by family

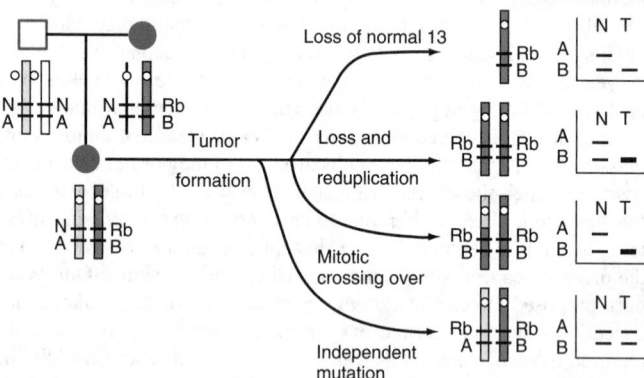

FIGURE 68-3 Diagram of possible mechanisms for tumor formation in an individual with hereditary (familial) retinoblastoma. On the left is shown the pedigree of an affected individual who has inherited the abnormal (Rb) allele from her affected mother. The four chromosomes of her two parents are drawn to indicate their origin. Just below the retinoblastoma locus a polymorphic marker is also analyzed in this family. The patient is AB at this locus, like her mother, whereas her father is AA. Thus the B allele must be on the chromosome carrying the retinoblastoma disease gene. Tumor formation results when the normal allele (N), which this patient inherited from her father, is inactivated. On the right are shown four possible ways in which this could occur. In each case, the resulting chromosome 13 arrangement is shown, as well as the results of a Southern blot comparing normal tissue with tumor tissue. Note that in the first three situations the normal allele (A) has been lost in the tumor tissue, which is referred to as loss of heterozygosity (LOH). (*From TD Gelehrter and FS Collins, in Principles of Medical Genetics, Baltimore, Williams and Wilkins, 1990, with permission.*)

history, with at least three individuals over at least two generations developing colon or endometrial cancer, and with at least one individual diagnosed before the age of 50. Most HNPCC is due to mutations in one of four DNA mismatch repair genes (Table 68-1), which are components of a repair system that is normally responsible for correcting errors in freshly replicated DNA. Germline mutations in *MSH2* and *MLH1* account for more than 60% of HNPCC cases, while mutations in *MSH6* and *PMS2* are much less frequent. When a somatic mutation inactivates the remaining wild-type allele of a mismatch repair gene, the cell develops a hypermutable phenotype characterized by profound genomic instability, especially for the short repeated sequences called *microsatellites*. This microsatellite instability (MIN) favors the development of cancer by increasing the rate of mutations in many genes, including oncogenes and tumor suppressor genes (Fig. 68-2). These genes can thus be considered caretakers. Figure 68-5 shows an example of the instability in allele sizes for dinucleotide repeats in the cancers of HNPCC patients.

While most autosomal dominant inherited cancer syndromes are due to mutations in tumor suppressor genes (Table 68-1), there are a few interesting exceptions. Multiple endocrine neoplasia type II, a dominant disorder characterized by pituitary adenomas, medullary carcinoma of the thyroid, and (in some pedigrees) pheochromocytoma, is due to gain-of-function mutations in the protooncogene *RET* on chromosome 10. Similarly, gain-of-function mutations in the tyrosine kinase domain of the *MET* oncogene lead to hereditary papillary renal carcinoma. Interestingly, loss-of-function mutations in the *RET* gene cause a completely different disease, Hirschsprung's disease [aganglionic megacolon (Chaps. 279 and 330)].

Although the Mendelian forms of cancer described above have taught us much about the mechanisms of growth control, most forms of cancer do not follow simple patterns of inheritance. In many instances (e.g., lung cancer), a strong environmental contribution is at work. Even in such circumstances, however, some individuals may be more genetically susceptible to developing cancer, given the appropriate exposure, due to the presence of modifier alleles.

GENETIC TESTING FOR FAMILIAL CANCER The discovery of cancer susceptibility genes raises the possibility of DNA testing to predict the risk of cancer in individuals of affected families. An algorithm for cancer risk assessment and decision-making in high-risk families using genetic testing is shown in Fig. 68-6. Once a mutation is discovered in a family, subsequent testing of asymptomatic family members can be crucial in patient management. A negative gene test in these individuals can prevent years of anxiety in the knowledge that their cancer risk is no higher than that of the general population. On the other hand, a positive test may lead to alteration of clinical management, such as increased frequency of cancer screening and, when feasible and appropriate, prophylactic surgery. Potential negative consequences of a positive test result include psychological distress (anxiety, depression) and discrimination (insurance, employment). Testing should therefore not be conducted without counseling before and after disclosure of the test result. In addition, the decision to test should depend on whether effective interventions exist for the particular type of cancer to be tested. Despite these caveats, genetic cancer testing for some cancer syndromes already appears to have greater benefits than risks and many companies now offer testing for various genes associated with the predisposition to breast cancer (*BRCA1* and *BRCA2*), melanoma (*p16INK4*), and colon cancer (*APC* and the HNPCC genes).

Because of the inherent problems of genetic testing such as cost,

TABLE 68-1 *Cancer Syndromes and Associated Genes*

Syndrome	Gene	Chromosome	Inheritance	Tumors
Ataxia telangiectasia	*ATM*	11q22-q23	AR	Breast cancer
Bloom syndrome	*BLM*	15q26.1	AR	Cancer of all types
Familial adenomatous polyposis	*APC*	5q21	AD	Intestinal adenoma, colorectal cancer
Familial melanoma	*p16INK4*	9p21	AD	Melanoma, pancreatic cancer
Familial Wilms' tumor	*WT1*	11p13	AD	Pediatric kidney cancer
Hereditary breast/ovarian cancer	*BRCA1* *BRCA2*	17q21 13q12.3	AD	Breast, ovarian, colon, prostate
Hereditary multiple exostoses	*EXT1* *EXT2*	8q24 11p11-12	AD	Exostoses, chondrosarcoma
Hereditary prostate cancer	*HPC1*	1q24-25	AD	Prostate carcinoma
Hereditary retinobastoma	*RB1*	13q14.2	AD	Retinoblastoma, osteosarcoma
Hereditary nonpolyposis colon cancer (HNPCC)	*MSH2* *MLH1* *MSH6* *PMS2*	2p16 3p21.3 2p16 7p22	AD	Colon, endometrial, ovarian, stomach, small bowel, ureter carcinoma
Hereditary papillary renal carcinoma	*MET*	7q31	AD	Papillary renal tumor
Li-Fraumeni	*TP53*	17p13.1	AD	Sarcoma, breast cancer
Multiple endocrine neoplasia type 1	*MEN1*	11q13	AD	Parathyroid, endocrine, pancreas, pituitary
Multiple endocrine neoplasia type 2a	*RET*	10q11.2	AD	Medullary thyroid carcinoma, pheochromocytoma
Neurofibromatosis type 1	*NF1*	17q11.2	AD	Neurofibroma, neurofibrosarcoma, brain tumor
Neurofibromatosis type 2	*NF2*	22q12.2	AD	Vestibular schwannoma, meningioma, spine
Nevoid basal cell carcinoma syndrome (Gorlin syndrome)	*PTCH*	9q22.3	AD	Basal cell carcinoma, medulloblastoma, jaw cysts
Tuberous sclerosis	*TSC1* *TSC2*	9q34 16p13.3	AD	Angiofibroma, renal angiomyolipoma
Von Hippel–Lindau	*VHL*	3p25-26	AD	Kidney, cerebellum, pheochromocytoma

Note: AD, autosomal dominant; AR, autosomal recessive.

specificity, and sensitivity, it is not yet appropriate to offer these tests to the general population. However, testing may be appropriate in some subpopulations with a known increased risk, even without a defined family history. For example, two mutations in the breast cancer susceptibility gene *BRCA1*, 185delAG and 5382insC, exhibit a sufficiently high frequency in the Ashkenazi Jewish population that genetic testing of an individual of this ethnic group may be warranted.

It is important that genetic test results be communicated to families by trained genetic counselors. To ensure that the families clearly understand its advantages and disadvantages and the impact it may have on their management and psyche, genetic testing should never be done before counseling. Significant expertise is needed to communicate the results of genetic testing to families. For example, one common mistake is to misinterpret the result of negative genetic tests. For many cancer predisposition genes, the sensitivity of genetic testing is only 70% or less (i.e., of 100 kindreds tested, disease-causing mutations can be identified in only 70). Therefore, such testing should in general begin with an affected member of the kindred (the youngest family member still alive who has had the cancer of interest). If a mutation is not identified in this individual, then the test should be reported as noninformative (Fig. 68-6) rather than negative (because it is possible that the mutation in this individual is not detectable by standard genetic assays for purely technical reasons). On the other hand, if a mutation can be identified in this individual, then testing of other family mem-

449

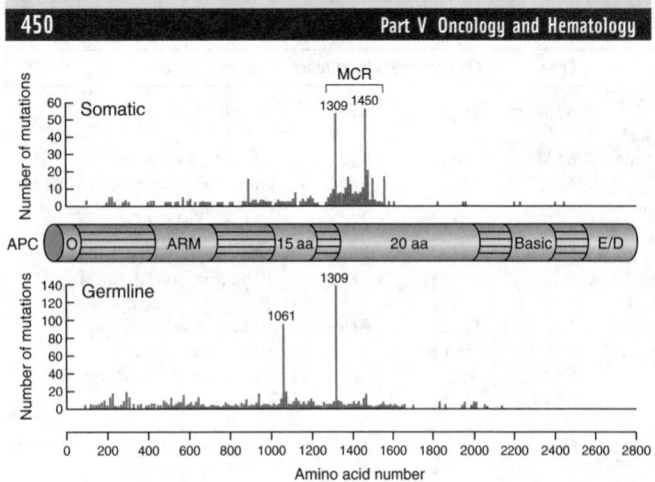

FIGURE 68-4   Germline and somatic mutations in the tumor suppressor gene *APC*. *APC* encodes a 2843-amino-acid protein with 6 major domains: an oligomerization region (O), armadillo repeats (ARM), 15-amino-acid repeats (15 AA), 20-amino-acid repeats (20 AA), a basic region, and a domain involved in binding EB1 and the *Drosophila* discs large homologue (E/D). Shown are the positions within the *APC* gene of a total of 650 somatic and 826 germline mutations (from the APC database at http://p53.curie.fr/). The vast majority of these mutations result in the truncation of the APC protein. Germline mutations are found to be relatively evenly distributed up to codon 1600 except for 2 mutation hotspots at amino acids 1061 and 1309, which together account for one-third of the mutations found in familial adenomatous polyposis (FAP) families. Somatic *APC* mutations in colon tumors cluster in an area of the gene known as the *mutation cluster region* (MCR). The location of the MCR suggests that the 20-amino-acid domain plays a crucial role in tumor suppression. Note that loss of the second functional *APC* allele in tumors from FAP families often occurs through loss of heterozygosity.

bers can be performed, and the sensitivity of such subsequent tests will be 100% (because the mutation in the family is in this case known to be detectable by the assay methods used).

ONCOGENES IN HUMAN CANCER   Oncogenes of the kind found in human cancers were initially discovered through their presence in the genome of retroviruses capable of causing cancers in chickens, mice, and rats. The cellular homologues of these viral genes are often targets of mutation or aberrant regulation in human cancer. Whereas many oncogenes were discovered because of their presence in retroviruses, other oncogenes, particularly those involved in translocations characteristic of particular leukemias and lymphomas, were isolated through genomic approaches. Investigators cloned the sequences surrounding the chromosomal translocations observed cytogenetically and then de-

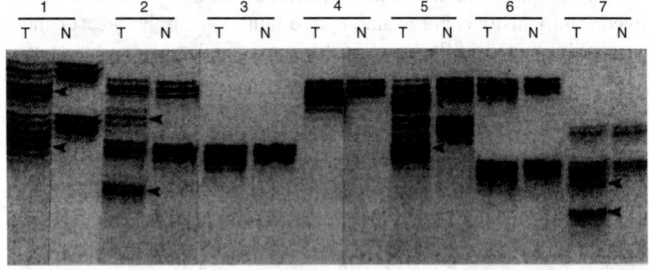

FIGURE 68-5   Demonstration of microsatellite instability in normal and tumor tissue from hereditary nonpolyposis colon cancer (HNPCC) patients. In each case the lane marked T contains DNA from a tumor, and the lane marked N contains DNA from normal tissue of the same patient. The marker (*D2S123*, located on chromosome 2) is a microsatellite composed of a tandem repeat of the dinucleotide CA, which varies in length from chromosome to chromosome. Normally, however, the length of the repeat is stable in somatic tissues. In this example, a polymerase chain reaction analysis has been applied to genomic DNA, and new alleles for the marker are apparent in tumors 1, 2, 5, and 7. Because the tumor tissue is defective in DNA mismatch repair, clonal abnormalities in copying of the CA repeat have arisen. Errors are also occurring in functional genes, eventually resulting in the malignant phenotype. (*From LA Aaltonen et al, Clues to the pathogenesis of familial colorectal cancer. Science 260:812, 1993 with permission; Copyright 1993 AAAS.*)

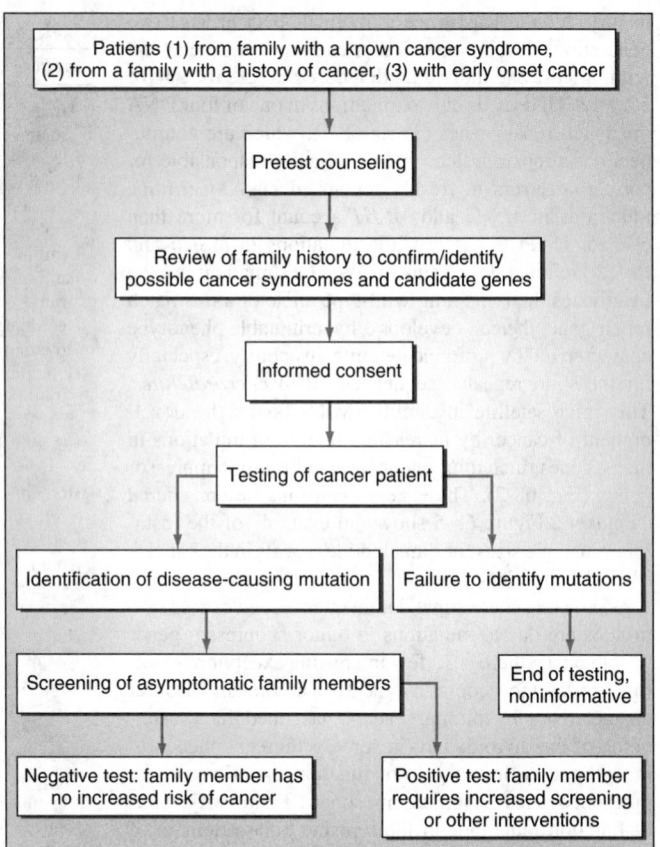

FIGURE 68-6   Algorithm for genetic testing in a family with cancer predisposition. The key step is the identification of a mutation in a cancer patient, which allows testing of asymptomatic family members. Asymptomatic family members who test positive may require increased screening or surgery, whereas others are at no greater risk for cancer than the general population.

duced the nature of the genes that were the targets of these translocations (see below). Some of these were oncogenes known from retroviruses [like *ABL*, involved in chronic myelogenous leukemia (CML)], while others were new (like *BCL2*, involved in B cell lymphoma). In the normal cellular environment, protooncogenes have crucial roles in cell proliferation and differentiation. Table 68-2 is a partial list of oncogenes known to be involved in human cancer.

The normal growth and differentiation of cells is controlled by growth factors, which bind to receptors on the surface of the cell. The signals generated by the membrane receptors are transmitted inside the cells through signaling cascades involving kinases, G proteins, and other regulatory proteins. Ultimately, these signals affect the activity of transcription factors in the nucleus, which regulate the expression of genes crucial in cell proliferation, cell differentiation, and cell death. Oncogene products have been found to function at critical steps in these pathways (Chap. 69), and inappropriate activation of these pathways can lead to tumorigenesis.

MECHANISMS OF ONCOGENE ACTIVATION   Mechanisms that upregulate (or activate) cellular oncogenes fall into three broad categories: point mutation, DNA amplification, and chromosomal rearrangement.

Point Mutation   Point mutation is a common mechanism of oncogene activation. For example, mutations in one of the *RAS* genes (*HRAS*, *KRAS*, or *NRAS*) are present in up to 85% of pancreatic cancers and 50% of colon cancers but are relatively uncommon in other cancer types. Remarkably—and in contrast to the diversity of mutations found in tumor suppressor genes (Fig. 68-4)—most of the activated *RAS* genes contain point mutations in codons 12, 13, or 61 (which convey resistance to GAP, a protein that interacts with RAS and inactivates it through substitution of the GTP cofactor with GDP). The restricted pattern of mutation compared to tumor suppressor genes reflects the fact that gain-of-function mutations of on-cogenes are more difficult to attain than simple inactivation. Indeed, inactivation of a gene can be attained through the introduction of a stop codon anywhere in the coding sequence, whereas activations require precise substitutions at residues that normally downregulate the activity of the encoded protein. The specificity of oncogene mutations provides specific diagnostic opportunities, as it is much simpler to find mutations at specified positions than it is when mutations can be scattered throughout the gene (as in tumor suppressor genes).

DNA Amplification The second mechanism for activation of oncogenes is DNA sequence amplification, leading to overexpression of the gene product. This increase in DNA copy number may cause cytologically recognizable chromosome alterations referred to as *homogeneous staining regions* (HSRs), if integrated within chromosomes or *double minutes* (dmins), if extrachromosomal in nature. The recognition of DNA amplification is accomplished through various cytogenetic techniques such as comparative genomic hybridization (CGH) and fluorescence in situ hybridization (FISH), which allow the visualization of chromosomal aberrations using fluorescent dyes. With these techniques, the entire genome can be surveyed for gains and losses of DNA sequences, thus pinpointing chromosomal regions likely to contain genes important in the development or progression of cancer. Noncytogenetic, molecular techniques for identifying amplifications have more recently become available.

Numerous genes have been reported to be amplified in cancer. Several genes, including *NMYC* and *LMYC*, were identified through their presence within the amplified DNA sequences of a tumor and had homology to known oncogenes. Because the region amplified often extends to hundreds of thousands of base pairs, more than one oncogene may be amplified in some cancers (particularly sarcomas). Genes simultaneously amplified in many cases include *MDM2*, *GLI*, *CDK4*, and *SAS*. Demonstration of amplification of a cellular gene is often a predictor of poor prognosis. For example, *ERBB2/HER2* and *NMYC* are often amplified in aggressive breast cancers and neuroblastoma, respectively.

Chromosomal Rearrangement Chromosomal alterations provide important clues to the genetic changes in cancer. The chromosomal alterations in human solid tumors such as carcinomas are heterogeneous and complex and likely reflect selection for the loss of tumor suppressor genes on the involved chromosome. In contrast, the chromosome alterations in liquid tumors (leukemias and lymphomas) are often simple translocations, i.e., reciprocal transfers of chromosome arms from one chromosome to another. Consequently, many detailed and informative chromosome analyses have been performed on hematopoietic cancers. The breakpoints of recurring chromosome abnormalities usually occur at the site of cellular oncogenes. Table 68-3 lists representative examples of recurring chromosome alterations in malignancy and the associated gene(s) rearranged or deregulated by the chromosomal rearrangement. Translocations are particularly common in lymphoid tumors, probably because these cell types normally rearrange their DNA to generate antigen receptors. Indeed, antigen receptor genes are commonly involved in the translocations, implying that an imperfect regulation of receptor gene rearrangement may be involved in the pathogenesis. An example is Burkitt's lymphoma, a B cell tumor characterized by a reciprocal translocation between chromosomes 8 and 14. Molecular analysis of Burkitt's lymphomas demonstrated that the breakpoints occurred within or near the *MYC* locus on chromosome 8 and within the immunoglobulin heavy chain locus on chromosome 14, resulting in the transcriptional activation of *MYC*. Enhancer activation by translocation, although not universal, appears to play an important role in malignant progression. In addition to transcription factors and signal transduction molecules, translocation may result in the overexpression of cell cycle regulatory proteins such as cyclins and of proteins that regulate cell death such as bcl-2.

The first reproducible chromosome abnormality detected in human malignancy was the Philadelphia chromosome detected in CML. This cytogenetic abnormality is generated by reciprocal translocation involving the *ABL* oncogene, a tyrosine kinase on chromosome 9, being placed in proximity to the *BCR* (breakpoint cluster region) on chromosome 22. Figure 68-7 illustrates the generation of the translocation and its protein product. The consequence of expression of the *BCR-ABL* gene product is the activation of signal transduction pathways leading to cell growth independent of normal external signals. Interestingly, a compound (gleevec) that specifically blocks the activity of *BCR-ABL* was synthesized and shown to exhibit remarkable efficacy with little toxicity in patients with CML. Knowledge of genetic alterations in cancer can lead to mechanism-based design and development of a new generation of cancer drugs.

TABLE 68-2 Common Oncogenes Altered in Human Cancers

Oncogene	Function	Alteration in Cancer	Neoplasm
AKT1	Serine/threonine kinase	Amplification	Gastric carcinoma
AKT2	Serine/threonine kinase	Amplification	Ovarian, breast, pancreas
CTNNB1	Signal transduction	Point mutation	Colon, prostate, melanoma, skin, others
FOS	Transcription factor	Overexpression	Osteosarcomas
ERBB2	Receptor tyrosine kinase	Point mutation, amplification	Breast, ovary, stomach, neuroblastoma
JUN	Transcription factor	Overexpression	Lung
MET	Receptor tyrosine kinase	Point mutation, rearrangement	Osteocarcinoma, kidney, glioma
MYB	Transcription factor	Amplification	AML, CML, colon, melanoma
MYC	Transcription factor	Amplification	Breast, colon, gastric, lung
LMYC	Transcription factor	Amplification	Lung carcinoma, bladder
NMYC	Transcription factor	Amplification	Neuroblastoma, lung cancer
HRAS	GTPase	Point mutation	Colon, lung, pancreas
KRAS	GTPase	Point mutation	Melanoma, colorectal cancer, AML
NRAS	GTPase	Point mutation	Various carcinomas, melanoma
REL	Transcription factor	Rearrangement, amplification	Lymphomas
WNT1	Growth factor	Amplification	Retinoblastoma

Note: AML, acute myelogenous leukemia; CML, chronic myelogenous leukemia.

TABLE 68-3 Representative Oncogenes at Chromosomal Translocations

Gene (Chromosome)	Translocation	Malignancy
ABL (9q34.1)–BCR (22q11)	(9;22)(q34;q11)	Chronic myelogenous leukemia
ATF1 (12q13)–EWS (22q12)	(12;22)(q13;q12)	Malignant melanoma of soft parts (MMSP)
BCL1 (11q13.3)–IgH (14q32)	(11;14)(q13;q32)	Mantle cell lymphoma
BCL2 (18q21.3)–IgH (14q32)	(14;18)(q32;q21)	Follicular lymphoma
FLI1 (11q24)–EWS (22q12)	(11;22)(q24;q12)	Ewing's sarcoma
LCK (1p34)–TCRB (7q35)	(1;7)(p34;q35)	T cell acute lymphocytic leukemia (ALL)
MYC (8q24)–IgH (14q32)	(8;14)(q24;q32)	Burkitt's lymphoma, B cell ALL
WT1 (11p13)–EWS (22q12)	(11;22)(p13;q12)	Desmoplastic small round cell tumor (DSRCT)
PAX3 (2q35)–FKHR/ALV(13q14)	(2;13)(q35;q14)	Alveolar rhabdomyosarcoma
PAX7 (1p36)–KHR/ALV(13q14)	(1;13)(p36;q14)	Alveolar rhabdomyosarcoma
RET (10q11.2)	(10;17)(q11.2;q23)	Papillary thyroid carcinomas

Source: From R Hesketh: *The Oncogene and Tumour Suppressor Gene Facts Book*, 2d ed. San Diego, Academic Press, 1997; with permission.

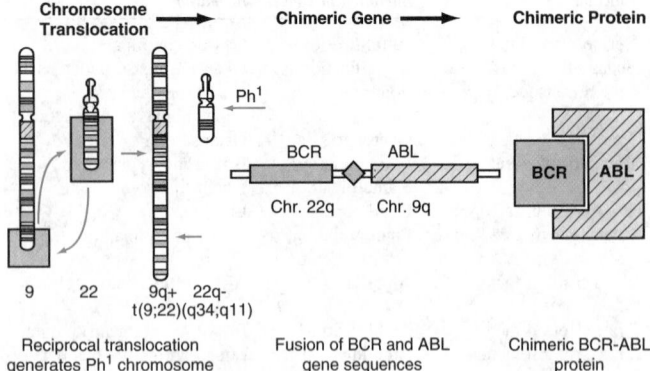

FIGURE 68-7 Specific translocation seen in chronic myelogenous leukemia (CML). The Philadelphia chromosome (Ph) is derived from a reciprocal translocation between chromosomes 9 and 22 with the breakpoint joining the sequences of the *ABL* oncogene with the *BCR* gene. The fusion of these DNA sequences allows the generation of an entirely novel fusion protein with modified function. (*Courtesy of ER Fearon and KR Cho.*)

CHROMOSOMAL INSTABILITY IN SOLID TUMORS Solid tumors are generally highly aneuploid, containing an abnormal number of chromosomes; these chromosomes also exhibit structural alterations such as translocations, deletions, and amplifications. Again, colon cancer has proven to be a particularly useful model for the study of chromosomal instability (CIN). As described above, some familial cases are characterized by the presence of MIN. Interestingly, MIN and CIN appear to be mutually exclusive in colon cancer, suggesting that they represent alternative mechanisms for the generation of a mutator phenotype in this cancer (Fig. 68-2). Other cancer types rarely exhibit MIN but almost always exhibit CIN. Normal cells possess several cell cycle checkpoints, often defined as quality control requirements that have to be met before subsequent events are allowed to take place. The spindle checkpoint, which ensures proper chromosome attachment to the mitotic spindle before allowing the sister chromatid to separate, has been shown to be deficient in certain cancers. The genes that, when mutated, may cause CIN have in general not yet been identified, although a few candidates mutated in a small number of tumors have been discovered. The identification of the cause of CIN in tumors will likely be a formidable task, considering that several hundred genes are thought to control the mitotic checkpoint and other cellular processes assuring proper chromosome segregation. Regardless of the mechanisms underlying CIN, the measurement of the number of chromosomal alterations present in tumors is now possible with both cytogenetic and molecular techniques, and several studies have shown that this information can be useful for prognostic purposes.

VIRUSES IN HUMAN CANCER Certain human malignancies are associated with viruses. Examples include Burkitt's lymphoma (Epstein-Barr virus), hepatocellular carcinoma (hepatitis virus), cervical cancer [human papillomavirus (HPV)], and T cell leukemia (retroviruses). The mechanisms of action of these viruses are varied but always involve activation of growth-promoting pathways or inhibition of tumor suppressor products in the infected cells. For example, HPV proteins E6 and E7 bind and inactivate cellular tumor suppressors p53 and pRB, respectively. Viruses are not sufficient for cancer development but constitute one alteration in the multistep process of cancer.

EPIGENETIC REGULATION OF GENE EXPRESSION IN CANCER An *epigenetic modification* refers to a change in the genome, heritable by cell progeny, that does not involve a change in the DNA sequence. The inactivation of the second X chromosome in female cells is an example of an epigenetic mechanism that prevents gene expression from the inactivated chromosome. During embryologic development, regions of chromosomes from one parent are silenced and gene expression proceeds from the chromosome of the other parent. For most genes, expression occurs from both alleles or randomly from one allele or the other. The preferential expression of a particular gene exclusively from the allele contributed by one parent is called *parental imprinting* and is thought to be regulated by covalent modifications of chromatin protein and DNA (particularly methylation) of the silenced llele.

The role of epigenetic control mechanisms in the development of human cancer is unclear. However, a general decrease in the level of DNA methylation has been noted as a common change in cancer. In addition, numerous genes, including some tumor suppressor genes, appear to become hypermethylated and silenced during tumorigenesis. *VHL* and *p16INK4* are well-studied examples of tumor suppressor genes that are silenced through methylation in human cancers. Overall, epigenetic mechanisms may be responsible for reprogramming the expression of a large number of genes in cancer and, together with the mutation of specific genes, are likely to be crucial in the development of human malignancies.

GENE EXPRESSION PROFILING IN CANCER The tumorigenesis process, driven by alterations in tumor suppressors, oncogenes, and epigenetic regulation, is accompanied by changes in gene expression. The advent of powerful new techniques such as microarrays and serial analysis of gene expression (SAGE) has allowed the study of gene expression in neoplastic cells on a scale never before accomplished. Indeed, it is now possible to identify expression levels of thousands of genes expressed in normal and cancer tissues. Figure 68-8 shows a typical cDNA array experiment examining gene expression in cancer. This global knowledge of gene expression allows the identification of differentially expressed genes and, in principle, the understanding of the complex molecular circuitry regulating normal and neoplastic behaviors. Such studies have led to molecular profiling of tumors, which has suggested general methods for distinguishing tumors of various biologic behaviors (molecular classification), elucidating pathways relevant to the development of tumors and identifying molecular targets for the detection and therapy of cancer. The first practical applications of this technology have suggested that global gene expression profiling can provide prognostic information not evident from other clinical or

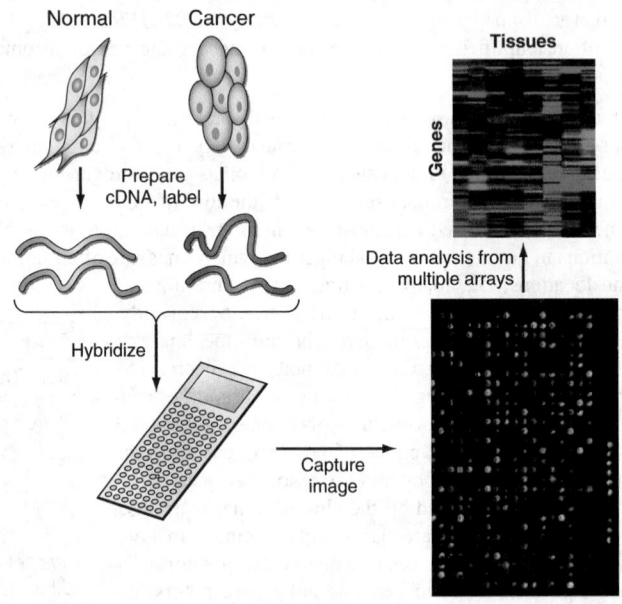

FIGURE 68-8 A cDNA array experiment. RNA is prepared from cells, reverse transcribed to cDNA, and labeled with fluorescent dyes (typically green for normal cells and red for cancer cells). The fluorescent probes are mixed and hybridized to the cDNA array. Each spot on the array is a cDNA fragment that represents a different gene. The image is then captured with a fluorescence camera; red spots indicate higher expression in tumor compared with reference while green spots represent the opposite. Yellow signals indicate equal expression levels in normal and tumor specimens. After clustering analysis of multiple arrays, the results are typically represented graphically using Treeview software, which shows, for each sample, a color-coded representation of gene expression for every gene on the array.

laboratory tests. The National Cancer Institute, in conjunction with the National Center for Biotechnology Information, has undertaken the Cancer Genome Anatomy Project (CGAP) (*www.ncbi.nlm.nih.gov/ncicgap/*) to collect data on gene expression in normal and malignant tissues and make it available on the Internet.

THE FUTURE   It is clear that there has been a revolution in cancer genetics in the past 20 years. Identification of cancer genes has led to a better understanding of the tumorigenesis process and has had important repercussions on all fields of biology. In spite of these spectacular advances, however, there has been little overall improvement in cancer death rates. It is hoped that, as the molecular mechanisms of cancer initiation and development continue to be elucidated, novel therapies based on pathophysiology rather than empiricism will emerge. Time will tell whether these strategies will rely on novel combinations or dosing schedules of conventional drugs or will be based on new approaches such as those involving gene therapy or immunotherapy. In addition, a better understanding of the molecular pathways and genetic alterations in cancer cells may lead to the development of sensitive strategies for early detection of cancer.

FURTHER READING

EMERY J: Common hereditary cancers and implications for primary care. Lancet 358:56, 2001

GOLUB TR et al: Molecular classification of cancer: Class discovery and class prediction by gene expression monitoring. Science 286:531, 1999

JALLEPALLI PV, LENGAUER C: Chromosome segregation and cancer: Cutting through the mystery. Nat Rev Cancer 1:109, 2001

LOEB LA: Mutator phenotype may be required for multistage carcinogenesis. Cancer Res 51:3075, 1991

MUNGER K: Disruption of oncogene/tumor suppressor networks during human carcinogenesis. Cancer Invest 20:71, 2002

STRAUSBERG RL et al: In silico analysis of cancer through the Cancer Genome Anatomy Project. Trends Cell Biol 11:S66, 2001

VOGELSTEIN B, KINZLER KW: The multistep nature of cancer. Trends Genet 9:138, 1993

YAN et al: Genetic testing—present and future. Science 289:1890, 2000

69   CANCER CELL BIOLOGY AND ANGIOGENESIS
Robert G. Fenton, Dan L. Longo

Two characteristic features define a cancer: unregulated cell growth and tissue invasion/metastasis. Unregulated cell growth without invasion is a feature of *benign neoplasms*, or new growths. Cancer is a synonym for *malignant neoplasm*. Cancers of epithelial tissues are called *carcinomas*; cancers of nonepithelial (mesenchymal) tissues are called *sarcomas*.

Cancer is a genetic disease. The malignant phenotype often requires mutations in several different genes. Cancer cells generally retain the capacity to proliferate by acquiring mutations in cell cycle regulatory genes (particularly those regulating the G_1 checkpoint). Often mutations activate cell pathways leading to proliferation and block pathways of differentiation. The normal cell has protective mechanisms that lead to the repair of cell damage; these repair pathways are often abnormal in cancer cells. When a normal cell has sustained too much damage to repair, the cell activates a suicide pathway to prevent damage to the organ. These cell death pathways are also commonly altered in cancer cells, leading to the survival of damaged cells that would normally die.

The accumulation of genetic lesions may lead through an identifiable progression of altered phenotypes as is noted in colon cancer: hyperplasia $\rightarrow$ adenoma $\rightarrow$ dysplasia $\rightarrow$ carcinoma in situ $\rightarrow$ invasive carcinoma. However, in many tissues, premalignant changes cannot be readily identified. Genetic changes lead to both loss and acquisition of properties: a loss of the differentiated function of the cell but the acquisition of novel characteristics that facilitate metastasis, such as the ability to break through basement membranes, migrate through the extracellular matrix and into the vascular tree, and generate new blood vessels to support colonization in remote sites.

CANCER CELL BIOLOGY

The treatment of most human cancers with conventional cytoreductive agents has been unsuccessful due to the Gompertzian-like growth kinetics of solid tumors and the genetic instability that predisposes to the development of intrinsic and acquired drug resistance. Rationally designed, target-based therapeutic agents directed against the specific molecular derangements that distinguish malignant from nonmalignant cells have become possible with advances in the understanding of oncogene and tumor-suppressor pathways. New agents can be classified by their specific molecular targets, such as tyrosine kinase inhibitors or farnesyltransferase inhibitors, or by their general mechanism of action, such as inhibition of cell cycle progression or angiogenesis.

Novel therapeutics include small molecules, peptides, oligonucleotides, and monoclonal antibodies. This chapter describes the convergence of scientific, pharmacologic, and medical knowledge that has led to the targeted therapy of cancer.

THERAPEUTIC APPROACHES TO CELL CYCLE ABNORMALITIES IN CANCER   The mechanism of cell division is substantially the same in all dividing cells and has been conserved throughout evolution. The process assures that the cell accurately duplicates its contents, especially its chromosomes. The cell cycle is divided into four phases. During M-phase, the replicated chromosomes are separated and packaged into two new nuclei by mitosis and the cytoplasm is divided between the two daughter cells by cytokinesis. The other three phases of the cell cycle are called *interphase*: G_1 (gap 1), during which the cell determines its readiness to commit to DNA synthesis; S (DNA synthesis), during which the genetic material is replicated and no re-replication is permitted; and G_2 (gap 2), during which the fidelity of DNA replication is assessed and errors are corrected.

Deregulation of the molecular mechanisms controlling cell cycle progression is a hallmark of cancer. Progression from one phase of the cell cycle to the next is controlled by the orderly activation of cyclin-dependent kinases (CDKs) that are regulated by signaling events that couple a cell's physiologic response to its extracellular milieu. The transition through G_1 into S-phase is a critical regulator of cell proliferation, and the phosphorylation state of the retinoblastoma tumor-suppressor protein (pRB) at the restriction point determines whether a cell will enter S-phase (where DNA synthesis occurs). The complex of CDK4 or CDK6 with D type cyclins forms a G_1-specific kinase whose activity is regulated by growth factors, nutrients, and cell-cell and cell-matrix interactions. Subsequent formation of an active CDK2/cyclin E complex results in full phosphorylation of pRB, relieving its inhibitory effects on the S-phase-regulating transcription factor E2F/DP1, and permitting the activation of genes required for S-phase (such as dihydrofolate reductase, thymidine kinase, and DNA polymerase). The activity of CDK/cyclin complexes can be blocked by CDK-inhibitors including $p21^{Cip1/Waf1}$, $p16^{Ink4a}$, and $p27^{Kip1}$, which block S-phase progression by preventing the phosphorylation of pRB.

Genetic lesions that render the retinoblastoma pathway nonfunctional are thought to occur in almost all human cancers. The result of these lesions is loss of the function of pRB as guardian of the G_1 restriction point, enabling cancer cells to enter a mitotic cycle without the normal input from external signals. Current therapeutic efforts to reverse the derangements of the retinoblastoma pathway have taken two main approaches. All kinases require the binding of ATP (and substrate) to the enzyme active site, followed by transfer of the γ-phosphate to serine, threonine, or tyrosine residues of the substrate. One of the first kinase inhibitors to reach clinical trial was UCN-01, a staurosporine analogue, which had broad activity against many serine/threonine kinases and hence lacked specificity. Flavopiridol was the first relatively selective CDK inhibitor identified, with Ki or IC_{50}s in the 40- to 400-nM range. Although flavopiridol was initially thought to inhibit tumor cell proliferation by inhibition of cell cycle CDKs, it is now clear that non-cell cycle functions of the CDK7/cyclin H and CDK9/cyclin T1 complexes may be critical for flavopiridol's antitumor activity due to inhibition of transcription of cellular mRNA. Phase II clinical trials of flavopiridol are in progress. Laboratory efforts are focused on the development of novel classes of CDK inhibitors capable of specifically targeting individual CDK/cyclin complexes. This may prove difficult given the great structural similarity of the active sites of these kinases. A second therapeutic endeavor to regain control of pRB function involves reversing the epigenetic silencing of p16^{Ink4a} gene and is discussed below.

p53, the "guardian of the genome," is a sequence-specific transcription factor whose activity is regulated through tight control of p53 protein levels. Normally, levels of p53 are kept low by its association with the mdm2 oncogene product, which binds p53 and shuttles it out of the nucleus for proteolytic degradation. In response to noxious stimuli that induce DNA damage, such as gamma irradiation or chemotherapy, p53 is phosphorylated by several kinases that regulate the DNA damage checkpoint. This causes dissociation of p53 from mdm2, leading to increased p53 protein levels. This activates transcription of genes leading to cell cycle arrest (p21$^{Cip1/Waf1}$) or apoptosis (pro-apoptotic Bcl-2 family members, genes regulating metabolism of reactive oxygen species, and death receptors such as DR5). Inducers of p53 include hypoxia, DNA damage (caused by ultraviolet radiation, gamma irradiation, or chemotherapy), ribonucleotide depletion, and telomere shortening. Further, deregulated activity of oncogenes such as *Myc*, which promote aberrant G_1/S transition, results in p53-induced apoptosis. This is mediated by a second product of the Ink4a locus, p14^{ARF}, which is encoded by an *a*lternative *r*eading *f*rame from p16^{Ink4a}. Levels of ARF are upregulated by *Myc* and E2F, and ARF binds to mdm2 and rescues p53 from its inhibitory effect. This oncogene checkpoint leads to the death of renegade cells that attempt to transverse the restriction point without appropriate physiologic signals.

Acquired mutation in p53 is the most common genetic alteration found in human cancer (>50%); germline mutation in p53 is the causative genetic lesion of the Li-Fraumeni familial cancer syndrome. In many tumors, one p53 allele on chromosome 17p is deleted and the other is mutated. The mutations often abrogate the DNA binding function of p53 that is required for its transcription factor activity and tumor-suppressor functions. Inactivation of the p53 pathway compromises cell cycle arrest, attenuates apoptosis induced by DNA damage or other stimuli, and predisposes cells to chromosome instability. This genomic instability greatly increases the probability that p53 null cells will acquire additional mutations and become malignant. Almost all human cancers have genetic alterations that bypass the Rb and p53 tumor-suppressor pathways.

Therapies directed at p53 are based on the observations that tumors expressing mutant p53 are often more resistant to chemotherapy than tumors with wild-type p53, and that mutant p53 proteins accumulate to high levels in tumor cells. If the transcriptional functions of the mutant p53 could be reestablished in tumor cells, massive apoptosis might ensue, whereas normal cells would be protected because they express very low levels of wild-type 53. Investigators have screened chemical libraries for compounds that inhibit tumor cell growth in a mutant p53-dependent manner. One compound entered cells and induced mutant p53 to adopt an active conformation such that p53-de-

pendent transcriptional activation was restored and apoptosis was selectively induced. This compound also had anti-tumor activity in murine xenograft models. These experiments constitute a proof of principle for targeting mutant p53 in human cancer through the novel mechanism of restoring an active conformation to a mutant tumor-suppressor protein. Clinical development is planned.

Compounds have been identified that act through a p53-dependent mechanism to protect normal cells from genotoxic damage. Selenium has been known as a cancer preventative for many years, but its mechanism of action is unknown. Selenomethionine, the main form of selenium in our diets, participates in a redox reaction resulting in the reduction of two cysteine residues within p53, leading to an induction of p53 DNA-binding activity. However, this form of p53 activates DNA repair pathways without affecting cell growth; the repair of genetic lesions may explain the cancer-preventative activity of selenomethionine. Other investigators have identified a low-molecular-weight, cell-permeable compound that inhibits the apoptotic functions of wild-type p53. This compound protected mice from the toxic effects of radiation therapy and chemotherapy, including bone marrow suppression, gastrointestinal dysfunction, and hair loss.

Knowledge of the molecular events governing cell cycle regulation has led to the development of viruses that replicate selectively in tumor cells with defined genetic lesions. Such "oncolytic" viruses include adenoviruses designed to replicate in tumor cells that lack functional p53 or have defects in the pRB pathway, in which replication of the mutant virus is dependent on deregulated E2F transcription factor activity. The former group includes an adenovirus mutant lacking the viral p55 protein (which binds and inhibits p53 in normal cells). This virus has demonstrated efficacy in phase II clinical trials of head and neck tumors, especially when combined with 5-fluorouracil and cisplatin (50% partial or complete response). The complexities of virus-host interactions (i.e., the immune response against replicating virus) will require further refinements of this novel technology before the clinical utility of this approach can be fully realized.

TELOMERASE DNA polymerase is unable to replicate the end of chromosomes, resulting in the loss of DNA at the specialized ends of chromosomes (called *telomeres*) with each replication cycle. At birth, human telomeres are 15- to 20-kilobase pairs long and are composed of tandem repeats of a six-nucleotide sequence (TTAGGG) that associate with specialized telomere-binding proteins to form a T-loop structure that protects the ends of chromosomes from being recognized as broken or damaged DNA. The loss of telomeric repeats with each cell division cycle causes gradual telomere shortening, leading to growth arrest (called *replicative senescence*) when one or more critically short telomeres triggers a p53-regulated DNA-damage checkpoint response. Cells can bypass this growth arrest if pRB and p53 are nonfunctional, but cell death ensues when the unprotected ends of chromosomes precipitate chromosome fusions or other catastrophic DNA rearrangements (termed *crisis*). The ability to bypass telomere-based growth limitations is thought to be a critical step in the evolution of most malignancies. This occurs by the reactivation of telomerase expression in cancer cells. Telomerase is an enzyme that adds TTAGGG repeats onto the 3' ends of chromosomes. It contains a catalytic subunit with reverse transcriptase activity (hTERT) and an RNA component that provides the template for telomere extension. Most normal somatic cells do not express sufficient telomerase to prevent telomere attrition with each cell division. Exceptions include stem cells (including those found in hematopoietic tissues, gut and skin epithelium, and germ cells) that require extensive cell division to maintain tissue homeostasis. More than 90% of human cancers express high levels of telomerase that prevent telomere exhaustion and allow indefinite cell proliferation. In vitro experiments indicate that inhibition of telomerase enzymatic activity leads to tumor cell apoptosis. Major efforts are underway to develop methods to inhibit telomerase activity in cancer cells. The reverse transcriptase activity of telomerase is a prime target for small-molecule pharmaceuticals that will enter clinical trials. The protein component of telomerase (hTERT) can act as a tumor-associated antigen that could be recognized by antigen-specific cytotoxic T lymphocytes (CTL) that lyse human melanoma, prostate, lung, breast, and colon cancer cells in vitro. Phase I clinical studies of telomerase vaccines are underway.

SIGNAL TRANSDUCTION PATHWAYS AS THERAPEUTIC TARGETS IN CANCER CELLS

Since the discovery that the v-*src* oncogene has protein tyrosine kinase activity, the central role of tyrosine phosphorylation in the regulation of cell proliferation in response to growth factors has become apparent. Many tyrosine kinases act at the apex of signaling pathways and are transmembrane proteins (receptor tyrosine kinases, RTK) or are associated with structures at the plasma membrane (*Src*-, Janus-, and *Fak*-family kinases). Tyrosine kinases are normally activated by specific ligands, and their activity is short-lived and reversed by protein tyrosine phosphatases (PTP). Phosphotyrosine and adjacent amino acid residues serve as docking sites for signal transduction proteins including those with protein-kinase, lipid-kinase, nucleotide exchange, lipase, and other enzymatic activities (Fig. 69-1). The unregulated activity of specific tyrosine kinases characterizes a number of human cancers, and their important roles in cancer cell proliferation and survival has validated these enzymes as targets for drug development efforts. Tyrosine kinases become constitutively activated and lead to the development of neoplastic diseases in three ways: chromosomal translocation, overexpression, and point mutation (Table 69-1). More than 30 different tyrosine kinases have been implicated in human cancer.

TARGETING Bcr-Abl WITH IMATINIB: PROOF OF PRINCIPLE

The protein product of the Philadelphia chromosome occurs in all patients with chronic myeloid leukemia (CML) and in about 30% of patients with adult acute lymphoid leukemia (ALL) and encodes the fusion protein Bcr-Abl. Although the c-*Abl* protooncogene is a nuclear protein whose kinase activity is tightly regulated as a part of the DNA damage response pathway (and actually induces growth arrest), the Bcr-Abl fusion protein is largely cytoplasmic with a constitutively activated tyrosine kinase domain. The deregulated tyrosine kinase activity of Bcr-Abl is required for its transforming activity. The Abl tyrosine kinase inhibitor, imatinib mesylate (Gleevec), has validated the concept of a molecularly targeted approach to cancer treatment.

Imatinib is a low-molecular-weight competitive inhibitor of the ATP binding site of Bcr-Abl, c-Abl, platelet-derived growth factor receptor (PDGFR), and c-Kit; hence it is not absolutely specific for the *Bcr-Abl* oncogene product. Clinical studies have demonstrated remarkable activity of this agent in CML. In Phase II studies of 532 chronic phase CML patients in whom interferon treatment had failed, 95% obtained a hematologic complete response, with only 9% relapse after a median follow-up of 18 months. Imatinib was also active in CML blast crisis with a 52% response rate, although the responses were short lived (78% relapse within 1 year). Relapse during treatment with imatinib was associated with reactivation of the tyrosine kinase either by amplification of the *Bcr-Abl* locus leading to increased levels of Bcr-Abl protein or, more commonly, by point mutations within the Bcr-Abl kinase domain that decreased imatinib binding without loss of Bcr-Abl kinase activity. These data constitute genetic proof that the

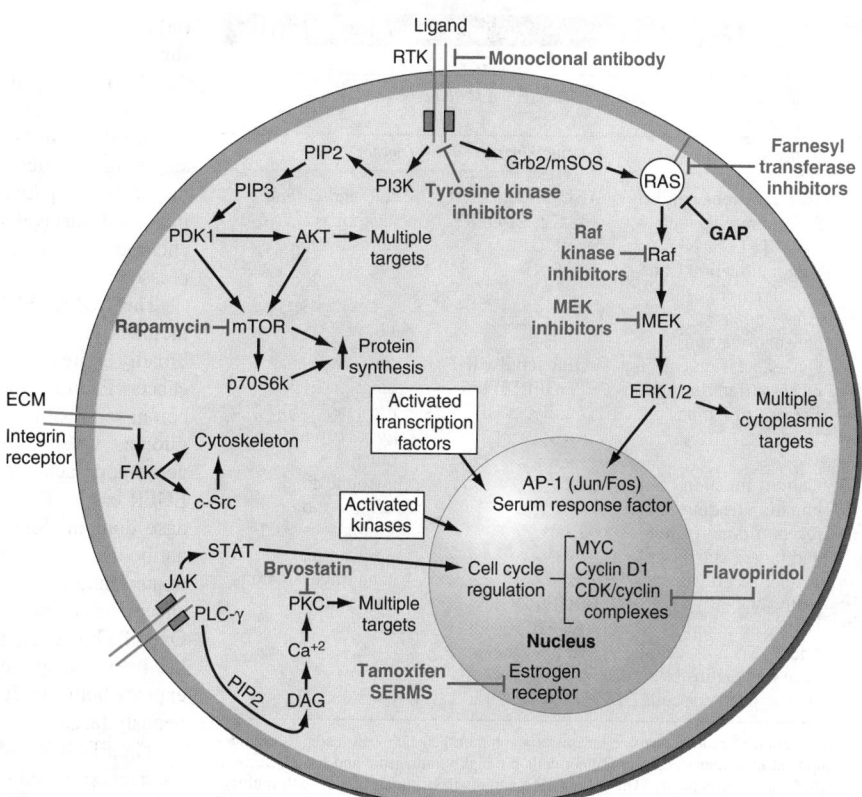

FIGURE 69-1 Therapeutic targeting of signal transduction pathways in cancer cells. Three major signal transduction pathways are activated by receptor tyrosine kinases (RTK). 1. The protooncogene Ras is activated by the Grb2/mSOS guanine nucleotide exchange factor, which induces an association with Raf and activation of downstream kinases (MEK and ERK1/2). 2. Activated PI3K phosphorylates the membrane lipid PIP2 to generate PIP3, which acts as a membrane-docking site for a number of cellular proteins including the serine/threonine kinases PDK1 and Akt. PDK1 has numerous cellular targets including Akt and mTOR. Akt phosphorylates target proteins that promote resistance to apoptosis and cell cycle progression, while mTOR and its target p70S6K upregulate protein synthesis to potentiate cell growth. 3. Activation of PLC-γ leads the formation of diacylglycerol (DAG) and increased intracellular calcium, with activation of multiple isoforms of PKC and other enzymes regulated by the calcium/calmodulin system. Other important signaling pathways involve non-RTKs that are activated by cytokine or integrin receptors. Janus kinases (JAK) phosphorylate STAT (signal transducer and activator of transcription) transcription factors, which translocate to the nucleus and activate target genes. Integrin receptors mediate cellular interactions with the extracellular matrix (ECM), inducing activation of FAK (focal adhesion kinase) and c-Src, which activate multiple downstream pathways, including modulation of the cell cytoskeleton. Many activated kinases and transcription factors migrate into the nucleus where they regulate gene transcription, thus completing the path from extracellular signals, such as growth factors, to a change in cell phenotype, such as induction of differentiation or cell proliferation. The nuclear targets of these processes include transcription factors (e.g., Myc, AP-1, and serum response factor) and the cell cycle machinery (CDKs and cyclins). Inhibitors of many of these pathways have been developed for the treatment of human cancers. Examples of inhibitors that are currently being evaluated in clinical trials are shown in blue.

target of imatinib is the Bcr-Abl tyrosine kinase, and that Bcr-Abl kinase activity is still required by imatinib-resistant cells. Computer modeling of the x-ray crystal structure of Bcr-Abl and its mutant forms is being used to guide the synthesis of the next generation of kinase inhibitors that may be able to overcome this acquired drug resistance.

Imatinib has also demonstrated targeted activity against gastrointestinal stromal tumors (GIST), rare mesenchymal tumors of the gastrointestinal tract (stomach and small intestine). The pathogenic molecular event in this disease is mutation of the proto-oncogene c-*Kit*, leading to the constitutive activation of this receptor tyrosine kinase. This prevents the normal differentiation of gut stem cells into interstitial cells of Cajal and induces proliferation and survival of tumor cells. Imatinib, which inhibits the c-Kit kinase domain, has demonstrated significant activity (>50% partial responses, many of long duration) in this chemotherapy-refractory tumor. Patients with chronic myelomonocytic leukemia (CMML, a myeloproliferative disorder) often harbor a Tel-PDGFR translocation that results in constitutive activation of the PDGFR kinase domain exclusively in the leukemic cells. Imatinib inhibits this kinase and has demonstrated significant activity in this disease. It may have activity in glioblastomas, which often express a PDGFR/PDGF autocrine growth loop.

TABLE 69-1 *Tyrosine Kinases Are Activated by Multiple Genetic Events in Human Cancers*[a]

Mechanisms	Tyrosine Kinases	Cancers
1. Translocations generate fusion proteins with BCR, TEL, or NPM. Oligomerization leads to activation of the kinase by cross-phosphorylation.	ABL, ALK, FGFR, JAK2, PDGFR, TRKC	Acute and chronic leukemias, fibrosarcoma
2. Overexpression causing receptor dimerization in absence of ligand.	EGFR family, IGFR PDGFR, FGFR family, c-MET	Breast, ovarian, lung, gastric, prostate, glioblastoma, others
3. Gain-of-function point mutation leading to receptor dimerization and kinase activation	c-KIT c-RET	Gastrointestinal stromal tumors Medullary thyroid CA
4. Autocrine growth pathway	MET/HGF PDGF/PDGFR	Rhabdomyosarcomas Glioblastoma
5. Overexpression of ligands such as VEGF or angiopoietins by stroma or tumor cells	VEGFR TIE2	Many tumors

[a] Deregulation of protein tyrosine kinases is a common genetic event leading to the development of human neoplasia. Tumor cells are highly mutagenic and have defects in DNA-damage checkpoints. This permits the outgrowth of tumor clones with multiple genetic anomalies, some of which promote tumor progression by increasing proliferation, enhancing resistance to apoptosis, and promoting angiogenesis.
Abbreviations: BCR, breakpoint cluster region; TEL, Ets-family transcription factor; NPM, nucleophosmin; ABL, Abelson tyrosine kinase; ALK, anaplastic lymphoma kinase; FGFR, fibroblast growth factor receptor; JAK2, Janus kinase 2; PDGFR, platelet-derived growth factor receptor; TRKC, neurotropin tyrosine receptor kinase C; EGFR, epidermal growth factor receptor; IGFR, insulin-like growth factor receptor; c-MET, receptor for hepatocyte growth factor (HGF); c-KIT, receptor for stem cell factor; c-RET, receptor for glial-derived neurotrophic factors; VEGFR, vascular endothelial growth factor receptor; TIE2, angiopoietin receptor.

These examples extend the proof of principle that selective targeting of signaling pathways in cancer cells can be highly efficacious with minimal toxicity. Imatinib has become the paradigm of targeted drug development in other diseases. For instance, 30% of acute myeloid leukemias (AML) encode mutations in the Fms-like tyrosine kinase FLT-3. Internal tandem duplications of the juxtamembrane domain of this RTK, or point mutations in the activation loop of the kinase domain, lead to constitutive activation of the kinase and confer a poor prognosis. Four chemically distinct inhibitors of FLT-3 are currently in clinical trials. These differ in potency of inhibition of the FLT-3 kinase and in the spectrum of cross-reactivity against other tyrosine kinases. Differences in toxicity are expected, as is the development of drug resistance. However, if multiple clinically active inhibitors can be developed, drug resistance may be avoided by combination therapy.

RECEPTOR TYROSINE KINASES RTKs are transmembrane glycoproteins that undergo dimerization upon ligand binding, with activation of their cytoplasmic tyrosine kinase domains by proximity-induced transphosphorylation of the activation loop. Tyrosine residues of the receptor or adaptor proteins (such as IRS-1 or Shc) are phosphorylated and act as docking sites for proteins containing SH2 (Src-homology 2) or PTB (phosphotyrosine binding) domains, thus initiating multiple signal transduction pathways (Fig. 69-1). These pathways regulate the proliferation, survival, migration, and angiogenesis of many solid tumors and are therefore viewed as attractive potential targets for cancer therapy. HER2/*neu* is a target in human breast cancer.

The gene encoding HER2/*neu* [a member of the epidermal growth factor receptor (EGFR) family] is amplified in ~30% of breast cancers. Tumors that overexpress HER2/*neu* are less responsive to chemotherapy, and patients with these tumors have a reduced survival compared with patients with normal levels of HER2/*neu*. Trastuzumab (Hercep-

tin) is a humanized monoclonal antibody that binds HER2/*neu* on the surface of tumor cells and induces internalization of the receptor, thereby reducing the level of surface expression. This leads to inhibition of cell cycle progression and renders cancer cells more susceptible to the induction of apoptosis. In clinical trials, trastuzumab as a single agent induced 15% responses in previously treated metastatic breast cancer patients. In phase III studies, a statistically significant increased survival occurred when trastuzumab was combined with chemotherapy in breast cancers in which HER-2/*neu* was overexpressed.

The EGFR (ERBB1) is another member of the RTK family that includes ERBB2 (HER2/*neu*), ERBB3, and ERB4. The EGFR is broadly expressed in normal cells and is overexpressed in many human cancers including head and neck, lung, esophageal, gastric, pancreatic, colon, renal cell, breast, ovarian, cervical, and prostate cancers, and gliomas. Overexpression correlates with poor clinical outcome. Targeted approaches include the use of antibodies directed against the EGFR extracellular domain and small-molecule inhibitors of the kinase domain. Single-agent clinical trials of anti-EGFR monoclonal antibodies or tyrosine kinase inhibitors in patients with previously treated lung and colon cancer demonstrated some antitumor activity, and studies combining these agents with chemotherapy are in progress. Overall, however, the therapeutic efficacy of EGFR-targeted agents has been disappointing. Of interest is that some breast cancers overexpress both the EGFR and HER2/*neu*, and clinical trials to simultaneously target both RTKs are under consideration.

The PDGFR and its ligand platelet-derived growth factor (PDGF), are overexpressed in many glioblastomas and in subsets of melanoma, ovarian, pancreatic, gastric, lung, and prostate cancers. Overexpression of the hepatocyte growth factor receptor MET has been observed in many human cancers and correlates with a poor prognosis, perhaps due to its role in invasion and metastasis. Small-molecular inhibitors of these RTKs are being developed for clinical use. As described below, the vascular endothelial growth factor receptor (VEGFR), TIE, and EPH RTK families have been identified as important therapeutic targets for inhibition of angiogenesis.

Signaling Pathways Downstream of RTKs: Ras and PI3K Several oncogene and tumor-suppressor gene products are components of signal transduction pathways that emanate from RTK activation (Fig. 69-1). The most extensively studied are the Ras/mitogen-activated protein (MAP) kinase pathway and the phosphatidylinositol-3-kinase (PI3K) pathway, both of which regulate multiple processes in cancer cells, including cell cycle progression, resistance to apoptotic signals, and cell motility. The development of inhibitors of these pathways constitutes an important avenue of anticancer drug development.

Mutations of the *Ras* protooncogene occur in 20% of human cancers and result in loss of the response of oncogenic Ras to GTPase-activating proteins (GAPs). The constitutively activated, GTP-bound Ras activates downstream effectors including the Ras/MAP kinase and PI3K/Akt pathways. Cancers of the pancreas, colon, and lung and AML harbor frequent *Ras* mutations, with the K-*Ras* allele affected more commonly (85%) than N-*Ras* (15%); H-*Ras* mutations are uncommon in human cancers. In addition, *Ras* activity in tumor cells can be aberrantly increased by other mechanisms, including upregulation of RTK activity and mutation of GAP proteins (e.g., *NF1* mutations in type I neurofibromatosis). Ras proteins localize to the inner plasma membrane and require posttranslational modifications, including addition of a farnesyl lipid moiety to the cysteine residue of the carboxy-terminal CAAX-box motif. Inhibition of RAS farnesylation by rationally designed farnesyltransferase inhibitors (FTIs) demonstrated encouraging efficacy in preclinical models, most of which utilized oncogenic forms of H-Ras. Despite this, clinical trials of FTIs in patients whose tumors harbor *Ras* mutations have been disappointing. Lack of efficacy has been shown in pancreatic, colon, and bladder carcinomas, while some activity has been seen in AML and CML. Upon further study, it appears that in the presence of FTIs, lipid modification of the K- and N-Ras proteins occurs by addition of a distinct lipid (geranylgeranyl) by the action of geranylgeranyl transferase (GGT), which results in restoration of Ras function. Thus, while FTIs are likely to have antitumor activity in select human cancers, their mechanism of action appears to occur by inhibition of farnesylation of proteins other than Ras, perhaps RhoB.

Effector pathways downstream of Ras are also targets of anticancer drug efforts. Activation of the Raf serine/threonine kinase is induced by binding to Ras and leads to activation of the MAP kinase pathway (Fig. 69-1). Two-thirds of melanomas and 10% of colon cancers harbor activating mutations in the *BRAF* gene, leading to constitutive activation of the downstream MAP/ERK kinase (MEK) and extracellular signal-regulated kinases (ERK1/2). This results in the phosphorylation of ERK's cytoplasmic and nuclear targets and alters the pattern of normal cellular gene expression. Inhibitors of Raf kinases have entered phase I clinical trials; their activity against tumors expressing mutant *BRAF* will be of special interest. MEK inhibitors are also demonstrating activity in phase I clinical trials.

PI3K is a heterodimeric lipid kinase that catalyses the conversion of phosphatidylinositol bisphosphate (PIP_2) to phosphatidylinositol trisphosphate (PIP_3), which acts as a plasma membrane docking site for proteins that contain a pleckstrin homology (PH) domain. These include the serine/threonine kinases Akt and PDK1 that are key downstream effectors of PI3K action (Fig. 69-1). The PI3K pathway is activated in 30 to 40% of human cancers and is thought to play a critical role in tumor cell survival, as well as promoting proliferation and migration. Amplification of the gene encoding the catalytic subunit of PI3K (p110) is observed in ovarian cancer, and amplification of the *Akt2* gene occurs in breast, ovarian, and pancreatic cancers. The tumor suppressor PTEN (phosphatase with tensin homology), a lipid phosphatase that acts as an off signal for PI3K by dephosphorylating PIP_3, is mutated in many human cancers, leading to unchecked activity of the PI3K pathway. Akt promotes cell survival by inhibiting apoptosis-promoting proteins and through activation of the transcription factor nuclear factor of κB (NFκB); it also enhances cell cycle progression by inhibition of glycogen synthetase kinase 3 (GSK3), which prevents cyclin D1 degradation. Furthermore, the growth of cancer cells requires the activation of two downstream kinases, mammalian target of rapamycin (mTOR) and p70S6K, whose activities promote the translation of cellular mRNAs. Targeted interruption of the PI3K pathway is being attempted at multiple levels. Inhibitors of mTOR, including rapamycin and its more soluble ester derivative CCI-779, selectively kill human tumor cell lines with PTEN mutations and upregulated PI3K pathway activity. Clinical trials of CCI-779 are under way. Because of the great sequence homology between kinase domains, it is unclear if isoform-specific drugs can be developed and whether these will enable tumor targeting without undue toxicity.

RTKs activate other signaling pathways. Activation of phospholipase C-γ(PLC) results in the hydrolysis of PIP_2 into diacylglycerol (DAG) and IP_3. DAG together with calcium ion (Ca^{2+}) activates protein kinase C (PKC), a family of serine/threonine-specific protein kinases with different activation requirements, subcellular locations, and substrates in different cell types. PKC is the target of tumor-promoting phorbol esters, and its activation can modulate cell proliferation, differentiation, and tumorigenesis. The PKC inhibitor bryostatin 1 has reached phase II clinical trials and thus far has demonstrated only minimal antitumor activity. However, an antisense oligonucleotide directed against PKC and a number of small molecule inhibitors that demonstrate greater selectivity for PKC isoforms are undergoing clinical evaluation.

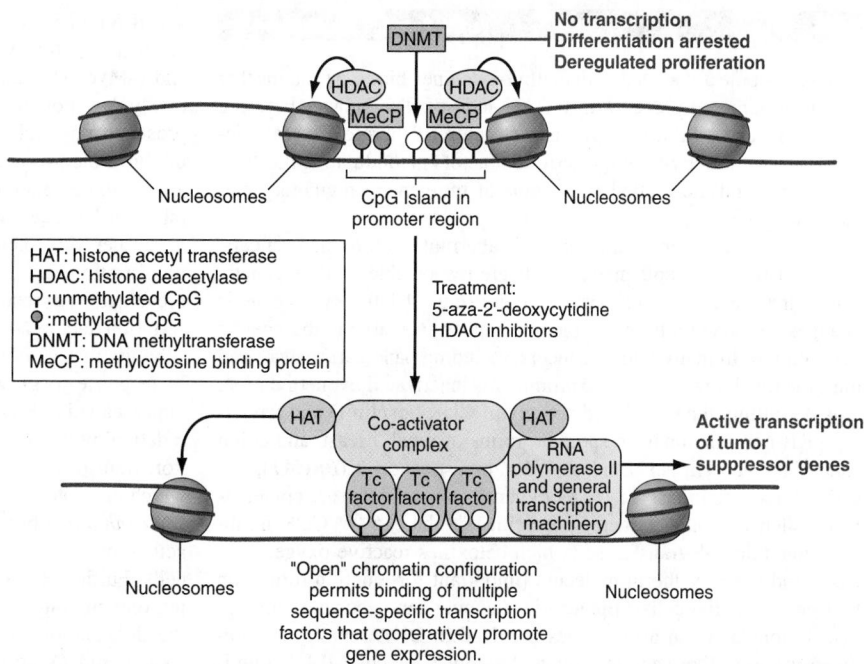

FIGURE 69-2 Epigenetic regulation of gene expression in cancer cells. Tumor-suppressor genes are often epigenetically silenced in cancer cells. In the upper panel, a CpG island within the promoter and enhancer regions of the gene has been methylated, resulting in the recruitment of methyl-cytosine binding proteins and complexes with histone deacetylase (HDAC) activity. Chromatin is in a condensed, nonpermissive conformation that inhibits transcription. Clinical trials are under way utilizing the combination of demethylating agents such as 5-aza-2'-deoxycytidine plus HDAC inhibitors, which together confer an open, permissive chromatin structure (*lower panel*). Transcription factors bind to specific DNA sequences in promoter regions and, through protein-protein interactions, recruit coactivator complexes containing histone acetyl transferase (HAT) activity. This enhances transcription initiation by RNA polymerase II and associated general transcription factors. The expression of the tumor-suppressor gene commences, with phenotypic changes that may include growth arrest, differentiation, or apoptosis.

ALTERATIONS IN GENE TRANSCRIPTION IN CANCER CELLS: ROLE OF EPIGENETIC CHANGES

Chromatin structure regulates the hierarchical order of sequential gene transcription that governs differentiation and tissue homeostasis. Disruption of chromatin remodeling leads to aberrant gene expression and can induce proliferation of undifferentiated cells, leading to cancer. *Epigenetics* is defined as changes that alter the pattern of gene expression that persist across at least one cell division, but are not caused by changes in the DNA code. Epigenetic changes include alterations of chromatin structure mediated by methylation of cytosine residues in CpG dinucleotides, modification of histones by acetylation or methylation, or changes in higher-order chromosome structure (Fig. 69-2). The transcriptional regulatory regions of active genes often contain a high frequency of CpG dinucleotides (referred to as *CpG islands*), which under normal circumstances remain unmethylated. Expression of these genes is regulated by transient association with repressor or activator proteins. However, hypermethylation of promoter regions is a common mechanism by which tumor-suppressor loci are epigenetically silenced in cancer cells. Thus one allele may be inactivated by mutation or deletion (as occurs in loss of heterozygosity), while expression of the other allele is epigenetically silenced. The mechanisms that target suppressor oncogenes for this form of gene silencing are unknown.

Acetylation of the amino terminus of the core histones H3 and H4 induces an open chromatin conformation that promotes transcription initiation. Histone acetylases are components of coactivator complexes recruited to promoter/enhancer regions by sequence-specific transcription factors during the activation of genes (Fig. 69-2). Histone deacetylases (HDACs; at least 17 encoded in the human genome) are recruited to genes by transcriptional repressors and prevent the initiation of gene transcription. Methylated cytosine residues in promoter regions become associated with methyl-cytosine–binding proteins that recruit protein complexes with HDAC activity. The balance between permissive and inhibitory chromatin structure is therefore largely determined by the activity of transcription factors in modulating the "histone code" and the methylation status of the genetic regulatory elements of genes.

The pattern of gene transcription is aberrant in all human cancers, and in many cases, epigenetic events are responsible. Unlike genetic events that alter DNA primary structure (e.g., deletions), epigenetic changes are potentially reversible and appear amenable to therapeutic intervention. In many human cancers, including pancreatic cancer and multiple myeloma, the p16^{Ink4a} promoter is inactivated by methylation, thus permitting the unchecked activity of CDK4/cyclin D and rendering pRB nonfunctional. In sporadic forms of renal, breast, and colon cancer, the von Hippel–Lindau (*VHL*), breast cancer 1 (*BRCA1*), and serine/threonine kinase 11 (*STK11*) genes, respectively, are epigenetically silenced. Other targeted genes include the p15^{Ink4b} CDK inhibitor, glutathione-S-transferase (which detoxifies reactive oxygen species), and the E-cadherin molecule (important for junction formation between epithelial cells). Epigenetic silencing can occur in premalignant lesions and can affect genes involved in DNA repair, thus predisposing to further genetic damage. Examples include MLH1 (mut L homologue) in hereditary nonpolyposis colon cancer (HNPCC), which is critical for repair of mismatched bases that occur during DNA synthesis, and 0^6-methylguanine-DNA methyltransferase, which removes alkylated guanine adducts from DNA and is often silenced in colon, lung, and lymphoid tumors.

Many human leukemias have chromosomal translocations that code for novel fusion proteins with enzymatic activities that alter chromatin structure. The PML-RARα fusion protein, generated by the t(15;17) observed in most cases of acute promyelocytic leukemia (APL), binds to promoters containing retinoic acid response elements and recruits HDAC to these promoters, effectively inhibiting gene expression. This arrests differentiation at the promyelocyte stage and promotes tumor cell proliferation and survival. Treatment with pharmacologic doses of all-*trans* retinoic acid (ATRA), the ligand for RARα, results in the release of HDAC activity and the recruitment of coactivators, which overcomes the differentiation block. This induced differentiation of APL cells has greatly improved treatment of these patients and has provided a treatment paradigm for the reversal of epigenetic changes in cancer. However, for other leukemia-associated fusion proteins, such as AML-ETO and the MLL fusion proteins seen in AML and ALL, no ligand is known. Therefore, efforts are ongoing to determine the structural basis for interactions between translocation fusion proteins and chromatin remodeling proteins, and to use this information to rationally design small molecules that will disrupt specific protein-protein associations. Drugs that block the enzymatic activity of HDAC are being developed. A number of different chemical classes of HDAC inhibitors have demonstrated antitumor activity in phase I studies. The next generation of such agents may have specific activity against a subset of HDAC proteins, permitting selective activation of genes in different types of cancers.

Major therapeutic efforts are also under way to reverse the hypermethylation of CpG islands that characterizes many solid tumors. Drugs that induce DNA demethylation, such as 5-aza-2'-deoxycytidine, can lead to reexpression of silenced genes in cancer cells with restoration of function. However, 5-aza-2'-deoxycytidine has limited aqueous solubility and is myelosuppressive. Other inhibitors of DNA methyltransferases are in development. In ongoing clinical trials, inhibitors of DNA methylation are being combined with HDAC inhibitors. The hope is that by reversing coexisting epigenetic changes, the deregulated patterns of gene transcription in cancer cells will be at least partially reversed.

Aberrant signal transduction pathways activate a number of transcription factors that promote tumor cell proliferation and survival. These include signal transducer and activator of transcription (STAT)-

3 and STAT5, NFκB, β-catenin (a component of the APC tumor-suppressor pathway), the heterodimer of c-Jun and Fos known as AP1, and c-Myc. The ability to target these transcription factors therapeutically does not currently exist. However, structural and molecular approaches may make it possible to identify small molecules that would inhibit protein-protein interactions needed for transcription factor dimerization or interaction with coactivator proteins. A small-molecule inhibitor has been developed that blocks the association of Myc with its partner Max, thereby inhibiting Myc-induced transformation. Many transcription factors are activated by phosphorylation, which can be prevented by tyrosine- or serine/threonine kinase inhibitors. The transcription factor NFκB is a heterodimer composed of p65 and p50 subunits that associate with an inhibitor, IκB, in the cell cytoplasm. In response to growth factor or cytokine signaling, a multi-subunit kinase called IKK (IκB-kinase) phosphorylates IκB and directs its degradation by the ubiquitin/proteasome system. NFκB, free of its inhibitor, translocates to the nucleus and activates target genes, many of which promote the survival of tumor cells. Novel drugs called *proteasome inhibitors* block the proteolysis of IκB, thereby preventing NFκB activation. For unexplained reasons, this is selectively toxic to tumor cells. Further studies have indicated that the antitumor effects of proteasome inhibitors are more complicated and involve the inhibition of the degradation of multiple cellular proteins. Proteasome inhibitors [bortezomib (Velcade)] have shown very significant activity in patients with multiple myeloma, including partial and complete remissions. Inhibitors of IKK are also in development, with the hope of more selectively blocking the degradation of IκB, thus "locking" NFκB in an inhibitory complex and rendering the cancer cell more susceptible to apoptosis-inducing agents.

Estrogen receptors (ERs) and androgen receptors, members of the steroid hormone family of nuclear receptors, are targets of inhibition by drugs used to treat breast and prostate cancers, respectively. Tamoxifen, a partial agonist and antagonist of ER function, can mediate tumor regression in metastatic breast cancer and can prevent disease recurrence in the adjuvant setting, saving thousands of lives each year. Tamoxifen binds to the ER and modulates its transcriptional activity, inhibiting activity in the breast but promoting activity in bone and uterine epithelium. Selective estrogen receptor modulators (SERMs) have been developed with the hope of a more beneficial modulation of ER activity, i.e., antiestrogenic activity in the breast, uterus, and ovary, but estrogenic for bone, brain, and cardiovascular tissues. Aromatase inhibitors, which block the conversion of androgens to estrogens in breast and subcutaneous fat tissues, have significant antitumor activity in postmenopausal breast cancer patients. However, deleterious effects may occur in other tissues due to estrogen deprivation, such as loss of bone density. The development of agents that modulate the activity of transcription factors in defined ways will yield important new agents for the treatment of cancer and other diseases.

APOPTOSIS

The homeostasis of adult organisms requires a balance between the death of aged, terminally differentiated cells and their renewal by proliferation of committed stem cell progenitors. Genetic damage to growth-regulating genes of stem cells could lead to catastrophic results for the host as a whole. However, genetic events such as activation of Myc expression or loss of the Rb checkpoint, which would be predicted to lead to unregulated cell proliferation, instead lead to the death of that cell. Metazoans have evolved a genetic program that induces the programmed death of cells that lose normal growth regulation; this process is referred to as *apoptosis*. Much as a panoply of intra- and extracellular signals impinge upon the core cell cycle machinery to regulate cell division, so too these signals regulate a core enzymatic machinery that regulates cell death and survival.

Programmed cell death is induced by two main pathways (Fig. 69-3). The extrinsic pathway of apoptosis is activated by cross-linking members of the tumor necrosis factor (TNF) receptor superfamily, such as CD95 (Fas) by its ligand (CD95L), or the binding to death receptors DR4 and DR5 by their ligand TRAIL (TNF-related apoptosis-inducing ligand). This induces the association of FADD (Fas-associated death domain) and procaspase-8 to death domain motifs of the receptors. Caspase-8 is activated by proximity-induced proteolysis and then cleaves and activates effector caspases-3 and -7, which then target cellular constituents (including DNA, cytoskeletal proteins, and a variety of regulatory proteins), inducing the morphologic appearance characteristic of apoptosis. The intrinsic pathway of apoptosis is initiated by the release of cytochrome c and SMAC (second mitochondrial activator of caspases) from the mitochondrial intermembrane space in response to a variety of noxious stimuli, including DNA damage, loss of adherence to the extracellular matrix (ECM), oncogene-induced proliferation, and growth factor deprivation. Upon release into the cytoplasm, cytochrome c associates with dATP, procaspase-9, and the adaptor protein APAF-1, leading to the sequential activation of caspase-9 and effector caspases. SMAC binds to and blocks the function of inhibitor of apoptosis proteins (IAPs), negative regulators of caspase activation. The release of apoptosis-inducing proteins from the mitochondria is regulated by pro- and antiapoptotic members of the Bcl-2 family. Antiapoptotic members (e.g., Bcl-2, Bcl-XL, and Mcl-1) associate with the mitochondrial outer membrane via their carboxy termini, exposing to the cytoplasm a hydrophobic binding pocket composed of Bcl-2 homology (BH) domains 1, 2, and 3 that is crucial for their activity. Perturbations of normal physiologic processes in specific cellular compartments lead to the activation of BH3-only proapoptotic family members (such as Bad, Bik, Bid, Puma, and others) that can induce pore formation in the mitochondrial outer membrane by altering the conformation of the outer-membrane proteins Bax and Bak. If BH3-only proteins are sequestered by Bcl-2, Bcl-XL, or Mcl-1, pores do not form and apoptosis-inducing proteins are not released from the mitochondrion. The relative levels of expression of antiapoptotic Bcl-2 family members compared to the levels of proapoptotic BH3-only proteins at the mitochondrial membrane determines the activation state of the intrinsic pathway. The mitochondrion must therefore be recognized not only as an organelle with vital roles in intermediary metabolism and oxidative phosphorylation but also as a central regulatory structure of the apoptotic process.

The evolution of tumor cells to a more malignant phenotype requires the acquisition of a broad range of genetic changes that subvert apoptosis pathways and permit the cancer cells to survive. Resistance to apoptosis predisposes not only to the development of cancer but also to resistance to anticancer therapies, including radiation and chemotherapy. However, because of their deranged physiology, cancer cells may be more vulnerable than normal cells to therapeutic interventions that target apoptosis pathways. For instance, overexpression of Bcl-2 occurs in non-Hodgkin lymphoma; prostate, breast, and lung cancers; and melanoma. Genasense is phosphorothioate antisense oligonucleotide directed at the first six codons of the Bcl-2 open reading frame, which mediates the destruction of Bcl-2 mRNA and subsequent downmodulation of Bcl-2 protein levels. Genasense has demonstrated activity in phase I and phase II clinical trials. Targeting of antiapoptotic Bcl-2 family members has also been accomplished by the identification of several low-molecular-weight compounds that bind to the hydrophobic pockets of either Bcl-2 or Bcl-XL and block their ability to associate with death-inducing BH3-only proteins. These first-generation compounds inhibit the antiapoptotic activities of Bcl-2 and Bcl-XL at micromolar concentrations, and higher-affinity derivatives with better pharmacokinetic properties should soon enter clinical testing. Of note is that the chemotherapeutic drug, paclitaxel, binds to and stabilizes microtubules. This induces the

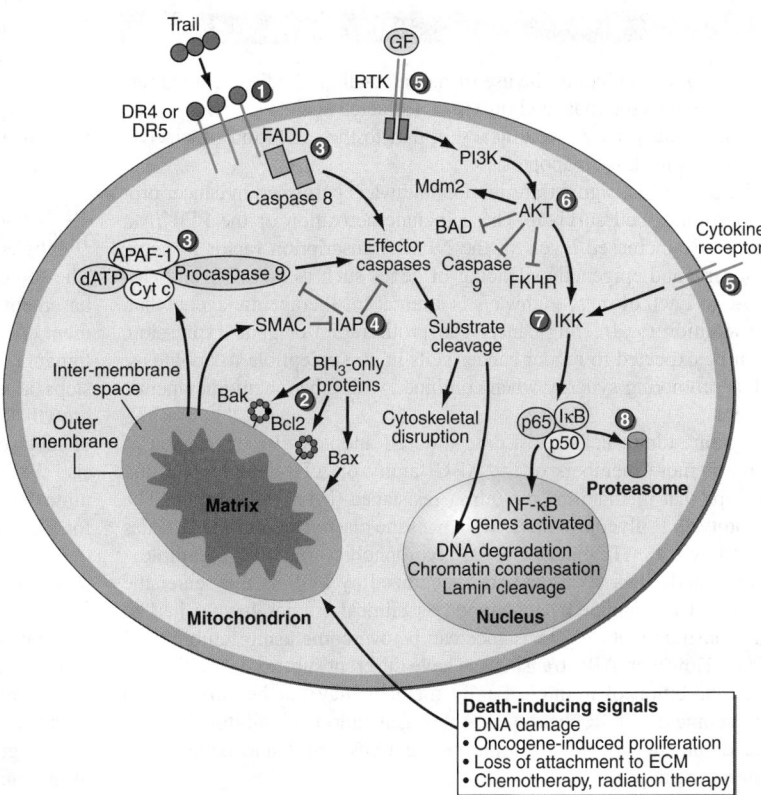

FIGURE 69-3 Therapeutic strategies to overcome aberrant survival pathways in cancer cells. 1. The extrinsic pathway of apoptosis can be selectively induced in cancer cells by TRAIL (the ligand for death receptors 4 and 5) or by agonistic monoclonal antibodies. 2. Inhibition of antiapoptotic Bcl-2 family members with antisense oligonucleotides or inhibitors of the BH3-binding pocket will promote formation of Bak- or Bax-induced pores in the mitochondrial outer membrane. 3. Epigenetic silencing of APAF-1, caspase-8, and other proteins can be overcome using demethylating agents and inhibitors of histone deacetylases. 4. Inhibitor of apoptosis proteins (IAP) block activation of caspases; small-molecule inhibitors of IAP function (mimicking SMAC action) should lower the threshold for apoptosis. 5. Signal transduction pathways originating with activation of receptor tyrosine kinase receptors (RTKs) or cytokine receptors promote survival of cancer cells by a number of mechanisms. Inhibiting receptor function with monoclonal antibodies, such as trastuzumab, or inhibition of receptor-associated tyrosine kinase activity can inhibit the pathway. 6. The Akt kinase phosphorylates many regulators of apoptosis to promote cell survival; inhibitors of Akt may render tumor cells more sensitive to apoptosis-inducing signals; however, the possibility of toxicity to normal cells may limit the therapeutic value of these agents. 7 and 8. Activation of the transcription factor NFκB (composed of p65 and p50 subunits) occurs when its inhibitor, IκB, is phosphorylated by IκB-kinase (IKK), with subsequent degradation of IκB by the proteasome. Inhibition of IKK activity should selectively block the activation of NFκB target genes, many of which promote cell survival. Inhibitors of proteasome function have entered clinical trials and may work in part by preventing destruction of IκB, thus blocking NFκB nuclear localization. NFκB is unlikely to be the only target for proteasome inhibitors.

phosphorylation and inactivation of Bcl-2, thus enhancing its activity against resistant tumor cells.

The IAP family member, survivin, is highly expressed in many human cancers but is undetectable in most adult tissues, suggesting that tumor-specific modalities can be found to inhibit its antiapoptotic functions. Small-molecule inhibitors are in development that will block the caspase-inhibitory functions of survivin and other IAP family members. Preclinical studies targeting death receptors DR4 and DR5 have demonstrated that recombinant, soluble, human TRAIL or humanized monoclonal antibodies with agonist activity against DR4 or DR5 can induce apoptosis of tumor cells while sparing normal cells. The mechanisms for this selectivity may include expression of decoy receptors or elevated levels of intracellular inhibitors (such as FLIP, which competes with caspase-8 for FADD) by normal cells but not tumor cells. Synergy has been shown between TRAIL-induced apoptosis and chemotherapeutic agents. For instance, some colon cancers encode mutated Bax protein as the result of mismatch repair (MMR) defects and are resistant to TRAIL. However, upregulation of Bak by chemotherapy restores the ability of TRAIL to activate the mitochondrial pathway of apoptosis (by death receptor–mediated cleavage of the BH3-only protein Bid, which activates Bak). Other protein-based therapeutics, including the use of monoclonal antibodies trastuzumab (see previous sections) and rituximab (directed against CD20 on B cell malignancies), may owe efficacy in part to the inhibition of survival pathways leading to apoptosis.

Many of the signal transduction pathways perturbed in cancer promote tumor cell survival. These include activation of the PI3K/Akt pathway, increased levels of the NFκB transcription factor in many cancers, and epigenetic silencing of genes such as APAF-1 and caspase-8. Each of these pathways is a target for therapeutic agents that, in addition to affecting cancer cell proliferation or gene expression, can be expected to render cancer cells more susceptible to apoptosis, thus promoting synergy when combined with other chemotherapeutic agents.

Some tumor cells resist drug-induced apoptosis by expression of one or more members of the ABC family of ATP-dependent efflux pumps that mediate the multidrug resistance (MDR) phenotype. The prototype, P-glycoprotein (PGP), spans the plasma membrane 12 times and has two ATP-binding sites. Hydrophobic drugs (e.g., anthracyclines and vinca alkaloids) are recognized by PGP as they enter the cell and are pumped out. Numerous clinical studies have failed to demonstrate that drug resistance can be overcome using inhibitors of PGP. However, ABC transporters have different substrate specificities, and inhibition of a single family member may not be sufficient to overcome the MDR phenotype. A new generation of inhibitors is under development with higher affinities for transporters and better pharmacokinetic profiles.

OTHER THERAPEUTIC TARGETS

The geldanamycin derivative 17-AAG (17-allylaminogeldanamycin) has entered clinical trials as a selective inhibitor of heat-shock protein (Hsp)90. Hsp90 functions as a chaperone by binding to and promoting the proper folding of many cellular proteins including steroid hormone receptors, HER2/*neu*, Raf, Cdk4 and -6, Bcr-Abl, and mutant forms of p53. Inhibition of Hsp90 function results in the unfolding and subsequent degradation of its target proteins, leading to an inhibition of cell proliferation. Hsp90 inhibitors have activity against CML cells that are resistant to imatinib, perhaps by destabilizing mutant Bcr-Abl proteins. The growth of a wide range of human cancer cells was inhibited by 17AAG, often with rapid decrease in the levels of Raf and loss of MAP kinase signaling activity. Promising synergy was noted with a number of chemotherapeutic agents, including paclitaxel and doxorubicin. Inhibition of Hsp90 also blocks signaling via the androgen and estrogen receptors, thus making it an attractive therapeutic target in prostate and breast cancers. The fact that tumor cells express high levels of Hsp90 supports an important role in tumor cell survival. Phase I clinical trials of 17AAG did not demonstrate dramatic single-agent activity, but studies of 17AAG in combination with other chemotherapeutic agents are planned.

Cyclooxygenase 2 (COX-2) catalyzes the rate-limiting step in prostaglandin biosynthesis. Prostaglandins bind to G protein–coupled receptors and have pleiotropic biologic effects, promoting proliferation, enhanced survival, migration, and angiogenesis. Prostaglandins are pro-inflammatory and some can directly damage DNA. Tumor cell expression of COX-2 and the synthesis of prostaglandins such as PGE$_2$ are upregulated by cytokines and growth factors and by tumor-associated inflammatory cells. Chronic inflammation is etiologic in some cases of stomach cancers (*Helicobacter pylori*), colon cancer (ulcerative colitis), hepatic cancer (chronic hepatitis), and bladder cancer (schistosomiasis). COX-2 levels are upregulated in many premalignant lesions including oral leukoplakia, actinic keratosis, and carcinoma in situ of the bladder, breast, and prostate. Its overexpression in many cancers correlates with invasiveness and decreased survival. COX-2 upregulation in HER2/*neu*-expressing breast cancer is associated with induction of aromatase expression, leading to increased production of estrogen and enhanced tumor growth. In a number of animal models, COX-2 inhibitors prevented the development of tumors, including the

Min mouse model of adenomatous polyposis. Clinical data indicate that patients taking cyclooxygenase inhibitors have decreased risk of cancer, especially colon cancers. Studies are in progress to define the cyclooxygenase products and their downstream targets that promote tumorigenesis in efforts to further enhance chemoprevention of human cancers.

METASTASIS: DETERMINING RISK AND DEVELOPING THERAPEUTIC STRATEGIES

The three major features of tissue invasion are cell adhesion to the basement membrane, local proteolysis of the membrane, and movement of the cell through the rent in the membrane and the ECM. Malignant cells that gain access to the circulation must then repeat those steps at a remote site and generate blood vessels to support local growth. There are currently few drugs that directly target the process of metastasis. Metalloproteinase inhibitors (see "Tumor Angiogenesis," below) represent an initial attempt to inhibit the migration of tumor cells into blood and lymphatic vessels. The rate-limiting step for metastasis is the ability for tumor cells to survive and expand in the novel microenvironment of the metastatic site, and multiple host-tumor interactions determine the ultimate outcome.

Analysis of gene expression patterns of primary tumors by microarray technology may predict the likelihood of metastasis. It remains unclear if the metastatic phenotype is a characteristic of most cells constituting the primary tumor, or if clonal variants with this capacity evolve during tumor progression. About eight metastasis-suppressor genes have been identified that normally suppress the growth of micrometastases in their new environment. The loss of function of these genes enhances metastasis, although the molecular mechanisms remain to be determined. It may soon be possible to predict which primary tumors are at greatest risk to metastasize and to block tumor spread using specific inhibitors of the metastatic process.

Bone metastases are extremely painful, cause fractures of weight-bearing bones, can lead to hypercalcemia, and are a major cause of morbidity for cancer patients. Osteoclasts and their bone marrow–derived precursors express the surface receptor RANK (receptor activator of NFκB), which is required for terminal differentiation and activation of osteoclasts. Osteoblasts and other stromal cells express RANK ligand, as both a membrane-bound and soluble ligand. Osteoprotegerin (OPG), a soluble receptor for RANK ligand produced by stromal cells, acts as a decoy receptor to inhibit RANK activation. The relative balance of RANK ligand and OPG determines the activation state of RANK on osteoclasts. Many tumors increase osteoclast activity by secretion of substances such as parathyroid hormone (PTH), PTH-related peptide, interleukin (IL) 1, or Mip1, that perturb the homeostatic balance of bone remodeling by increasing RANK signaling. One example is multiple myeloma, where tumor cell–stromal cell interactions activate osteoclasts and inhibit osteoblasts, leading to the development of multiple lytic lesions. Inhibition of RANK ligand by intravenous administration of recombinant OPG or the extracellular domain of RANK linked to an immunoglobulin Fc-receptor (RANK-Fc) can prevent further bone destruction. Bisphosphonates are also effective inhibitors of osteoclast function. Better understanding of signaling pathways downstream of RANK and the mechanisms that regulate the formation of blastic bone lesions should lead to novel therapies to prevent bone destruction, induce bone healing, and may even alter the bone microenvironment in ways that induce the death of metastatic tumor cells.

TUMOR ANGIOGENESIS

The growth of primary and metastatic tumors to larger than a few millimeters requires the recruitment of neighboring blood vessels and vascular endothelial cells to support their metabolic requirements. This is because the diffusion limit for oxygen in tissues is ~100 μM. This is true of solid tumors and hematologic malignancies such as lymphomas, acute leukemia, and multiple myeloma, where increased numbers of blood vessels are observed in the pathologic bone marrow. A critical element in the growth of primary tumors and formation of metastatic sites is the *angiogenic switch*: the ability of the tumor to promote the formation of new capillaries from preexisting host vessels. The angiogenic switch is a phase in tumor development when the dynamic balance of pro- and antiangiogenic factors is tipped in favor of vessel formation by the effects of the tumor on its immediate environment. Stimuli for tumor angiogenesis include hypoxia, inflammation, and genetic lesions in oncogenes or tumor suppressors that alter tumor cell gene expression. Angiogenesis consists of several steps, including the stimulation of endothelial cells (ECs) by growth factors, the degradation of the ECM by proteases, proliferation of ECs and migration into the tumor, and the eventual formation of new capillary tubes.

Tumor blood vessels are not normal; they have chaotic architecture and blood flow. Due to an imbalance of angiogenic regulators such as vascular endothelial growth factor (VEGF) and angiopoietins (see below), tumor vessels are tortuous and dilated with an uneven diameter, excessive branching, and shunting. Tumor blood flow is variable, with areas of hypoxia and acidosis leading to the selection of variants that are resistant to hypoxia-induced apoptosis (often due to the loss of p53 expression). Tumor vessel walls have numerous openings, widened interendothelial junctions, and discontinuous or absent basement membrane; this contributes to the high vascular permeability of these vessels and, together with lack of functional intratumoral lymphatics, causes interstitial hypertension within the tumor (which also interferes with the delivery of therapeutics to the tumor). Tumor blood vessels lack perivascular cells such as pericytes and smooth muscle cells that normally regulate vasoactive control in response to tissue metabolic needs.

Unlike normal blood vessels, the vascular lining of tumor vessels is not a homogenous layer of ECs but often consists of a mosaic of ECs and tumor cells; the concept of cancer cell–derived vascular channels, which may be lined by ECM secreted by the tumor cells, is referred to as *vascular mimickry*. It is unclear whether tumor cells actually form structural elements of vascular channels or represent tumor cells in transit into or out of the vessel. However, the former is supported by evidence that in some human colon cancers, tumor cells can comprise up to 15% of vessel walls. The ECs of angiogenic blood vessels are unlike quiescent ECs found in adult vessels, where only 0.01% of ECs are dividing. During tumor angiogenesis, ECs are highly proliferative and express a number of plasma membrane proteins that are characteristic of activated endothelium, including growth factor receptors and adhesion molecules such as integrins.

MECHANISMS OF TUMOR VESSEL FORMATION   Tumors utilize a number of mechanisms to promote their vascularization, and in each case they subvert normal angiogenic processes to suit this purpose (Fig. 69-4). Primary or metastatic tumor cells sometimes arise in proximity to host blood vessels and grow around these vessels, parasitizing nutrients by coopting the local blood supply. However, most tumor blood vessels arise by the process of *sprouting*, in which tumors secrete trophic angiogenic molecules, the most potent being VEGF, that induce the proliferation and migration of host ECs into the tumor. Sprouting in normal and pathogenic angiogenesis is regulated by three families of transmembrane RTKs expressed on ECs and their ligands (VEGFs, angiopoietins, ephrins), which are produced by tumor cells, inflammatory cells, or stromal cells in the tumor microenvironment.

When tumor cells arise in or metastasize to an avascular area, they grow to a size limited by hypoxia and nutrient deprivation. Hypoxia, a key regulator of tumor angiogenesis, causes the transcriptional induction of the gene encoding VEGF by a process that involves stabilization of the transcription factor hypoxia-inducible factor (HIF)1. Under normoxic conditions, EC HIF-1 levels are maintained at a low level by proteasome-mediated destruction regulated by a ubiquitin E3-ligase encoded by the VHL tumor-suppressor locus. However, under hypoxic conditions, the HIF-1 protein is not hydroxylated and association with VHL does not occur; therefore HIF-1 levels increase, and target genes including VEGF, nitric oxide synthetase (NOS), and Ang2 are induced. Loss of the *VHL* genes, as occurs in familial and sporadic renal cell carcinomas, also results in HIF-1 stabilization and induction

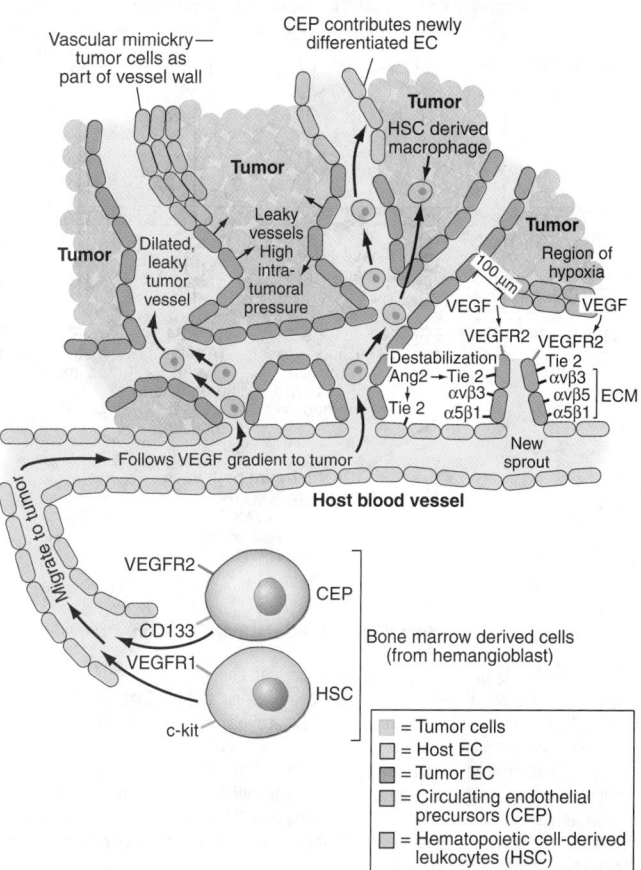

FIGURE 69-4 Tumor angiogenesis is a complex process involving many different cell types that must proliferate, migrate, invade, and differentiate in response to signals from the tumor microenvironment. Endothelial cells (ECs) sprout from host vessels in response to VEGF, bFGF, Ang2, and other proangiogenic stimuli. Sprouting is stimulated by VEGF/VEGFR2, Ang2/Tie-2, and integrin/extracellular matrix (ECM) interactions. Bone marrow–derived circulating endothelial precursors (CEPs) migrate to the tumor in response to VEGF and differentiate into ECs, while hematopoietic stem cells differentiate into leukocytes, including tumor-associated macrophages that secrete angiogenic growth factors and produce MMPs that remodel the ECM and release bound growth factors. Tumor cells themselves may directly form parts of vascular channels within tumors. The pattern of vessel formation is haphazard: vessels are tortuous, dilated, leaky, and branch in random ways. This leads to uneven blood flow within the tumor, with areas of acidosis and hypoxia (which stimulate release of angiogenic factors) and high intratumoral pressures that inhibit delivery of therapeutic agents.

of VEGF. Most tumors have hypoxic regions due to poor blood flow, and tumor cells in these areas stain positive for HIF-1 expression; in renal cancers with *VHL* deletion, all of the tumor cells express high levels of HIF-1, and VEGF-induced angiogenesis leads to high microvascular density (hence the term *hypernephroma*).

VEGF and its receptors are required for *vasculogenesis* (the de novo formation of blood vessels from differentiating endothelial cells, as occurs during embryonic development) and angiogenesis under normal (wound healing, corpus luteum formation) and pathologic processes (tumor angiogenesis, inflammatory conditions such as rheumatoid arthritis). VEGF-A is a heparin-binding glycoprotein with at least four isoforms (splice variants) that regulates blood vessel formation by binding to the RTKs VEGFR1 and VEGFR2, which are expressed on all ECs in addition to a subset of hematopoietic cells (Fig. 69-5). VEGFR2 regulates EC proliferation, migration, and survival, while VEGFR1 may act as an antagonist of R1 in ECs but is probably also important for angioblast differentiation during embryogenesis. Tumor vessels appear to be more dependent on VEGFR signaling for growth and survival than normal ECs. While VEGF signaling is a critical initiator of angiogenesis, this is a complex process regulated by additional signaling pathways. The angiopoietin, Ang1,

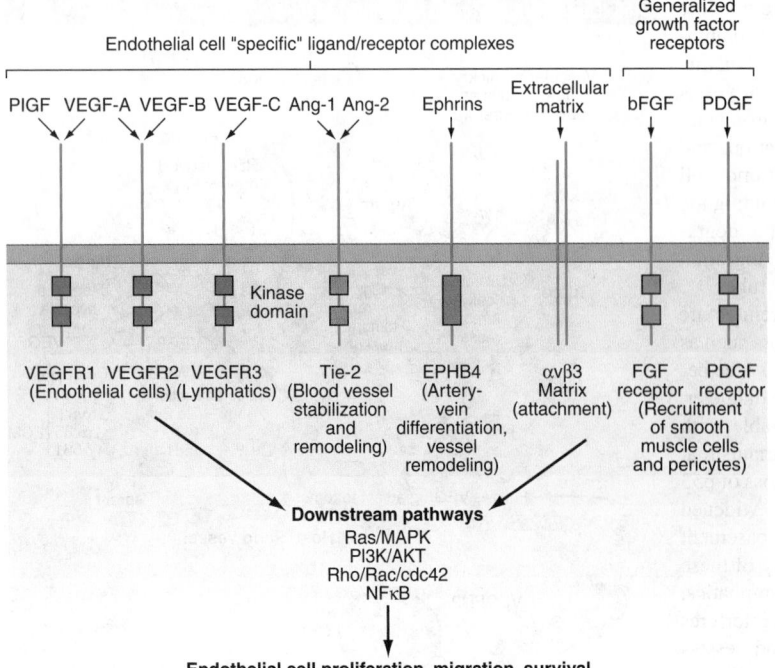

Endothelial cell "specific" ligand/receptor complexes

Generalized growth factor receptors

PlGF VEGF-A VEGF-B VEGF-C Ang-1 Ang-2 Ephrins Extracellular matrix bFGF PDGF

Kinase domain

VEGFR1 (Endothelial cells) VEGFR2 (Lymphatics) VEGFR3 Tie-2 (Blood vessel stabilization and remodeling) EPHB4 (Artery-vein differentiation, vessel remodeling) αvβ3 Matrix (attachment) FGF receptor PDGF receptor (Recruitment of smooth muscle cells and pericytes)

Downstream pathways
Ras/MAPK
PI3K/AKT
Rho/Rac/cdc42
NFκB

Endothelial cell proliferation, migration, survival

FIGURE 69-5 Critical molecular determinants of endothelial cell biology. Angiogenic endothelium expresses a number of receptors not found on resting endothelium. These include receptor tyrosine kinases (RTK) and integrins that bind to the extracellular matrix and mediate endothelial cells adhesion, migration, and invasion. Endothelial cells (ECs) also express RTK (i.e., the FGF and PDGF receptors) that are found on many other cell types. Critical functions mediated by activated RTK include proliferation, migration, and enhanced survival of endothelial cells, as well as regulation of the recruitment of perivascular cells and bloodborne circulating endothelial precursors and hematopoietic stem cells to the tumor. Intracellular signaling via EC-specific RTK utilizes molecular pathways that may be targets for future antiangiogenic therapies.

produced by stromal cells, binds to the EC RTK Tie-2 and promotes the interaction of ECs with the ECM and perivascular cells, such as pericytes and smooth muscle cells, to form tight, non-leaky vessels. PDGF and basic fibroblast growth factor (bFGF) help to recruit these perivascular cells. Ang1 is required for maintaining the quiescence and stability of mature blood vessels and prevents the vascular permeability normally induced by VEGF and inflammatory cytokines.

For tumor cell–derived VEGF to initiate sprouting from host vessels, the stability conferred by the Ang1/Tie2 pathway must be perturbed; this occurs by the secretion of Ang2 by ECs that are undergoing active remodeling. Ang2 binds to Tie2 and is a competitive inhibitor of Ang1 action: under the influence of Ang2, preexisting blood vessels become more responsive to remodeling signals, with less adherence of ECs to stroma and associated perivascular cells and more responsiveness to VEGF. Therefore, Ang2 is required at early stages of tumor angiogenesis for destabilizing the vasculature by making host ECs more sensitive to angiogenic signals. Since tumor ECs are blocked by Ang2, there is no stabilization by the Ang1/Tie2 interaction, and tumor blood vessels are leaky, hemorrhagic, and have poor association of ECs with underlying stroma. Sprouting tumor ECs express high levels of the transmembrane protein Ephrin-B2 and its receptor, the RTK EPH whose signaling appears to work with the angiopoietins during vessel remodeling. During embryogenesis, EPH receptors are expressed on the endothelium of primordial venous vessels while the transmembrane ligand ephrin-B2 is expressed by cells of primordial arteries; the reciprocal expression may regulate differentiation and patterning of the vasculature.

A number of ubiquitously expressed host molecules play critical roles in normal and pathologic angiogenesis. Proangiogenic cytokines, chemokines, and growth factors secreted by stromal cells or inflammatory cells make important contributions to neovascularization, including bFGF, transforming growth factor-α (TGF-α), TNF-α, and IL-8. In contrast to normal endothelium, angiogenic endothelium overexpresses specific members of the integrin family of ECM-binding

proteins that mediate EC adhesion, migration, and survival. Specifically, expression of integrins $\alpha_v\beta_3$, $\alpha_v\beta_5$, and $\alpha_5\beta_1$ mediate spreading and migration of ECs and are required for angiogenesis induced by VEGF and bFGF, which in turn can upregulate EC integrin expression. The $\alpha_v\beta_3$ integrin physically associates with VEGFR2 in the plasma membrane and promotes signal transduction from each receptor to promote EC proliferation (via focal adhesion kinase, src, PI3K, and other pathways) and survival (by inhibition of p53 and increasing the Bcl2/Bax expression ratio). In addition, $\alpha_v\beta_3$ forms cell surface complexes with matrix metalloproteinases (MMPs), zinc-requiring proteases that cleave ECM proteins, leading to enhanced EC migration and the release of heparin-binding growth factors including VEGF and bFGF. EC adhesion molecules can be upregulated (i.e., by VEGF, TNF-α) or downregulated (by TGF-β); this, together with chaotic blood flow explains poor leukocyte-endothelial interactions in tumor blood vessels and may help tumor cells avoid immune surveillance.

In addition to sprouting, the architecture of the tumor vasculature is influenced by two other mechanisms. One process, called *intussuception*, occurs when tumor cells grow into a vessel, functionally dividing it into two branches. More recently, it was discovered that cells derived from hematopoietic progenitors in the host bone marrow contribute to tumor angiogenesis in a process linked to the secretion of VEGF, and PlGF (placenta-derived growth factor) by tumor cells and their surrounding stroma. VEGF promotes the mobilization and recruitment of circulating endothelial cell precursors (CEPs) and hematopoietic stem cells (HSCs) to tumors where they colocalize and appear to cooperate in neovessel formation. CEPs express VEGFR2, while HSCs express VEGFR1, a receptor, or VEGF and PlGF. Both CEPs and HSCs are derived from a common precursor, the hemangioblast. CEPs are thought to differentiate into ECs, whereas the role of HSC-derived cells (such as tumor-associated macrophages) may be to secrete angiogenic factors required for sprouting and stabilization of ECs (VEGF, bFGF, angiopoietins) and to activate MMPs, resulting in ECM remodeling and growth factor release. In mouse tumor models and in human cancers, increased numbers of CEPs and subsets of VEGFR1+ or VEGFR-expressing HSCs can be detected in the circulation, which may correlate with increased levels of serum VEGF. It is not yet known whether levels of these cells have prognostic value or if changes during treatment correlate with inhibition of tumor angiogenesis. Whether CEPs and VEGFR1-expressing HSCs are required to maintain the long-term integrity of established tumor vessels is also unknown.

Lymphatic vessels also exist within tumors. Development of tumor lymphatics is associated with expression of VEGFR3 and its ligands VEGF-C and VEGF-D. The role of these vessels in tumor cell metastasis to regional lymph nodes remains to be determined, since, as discussed above, interstitial pressures within tumors are high and most lymphatic vessels may exit in a collapsed and nonfunctional state. However, VEGF-C levels in primary human tumors, including lung, prostate, and colorectal cancers, correlate significantly with metastasis to regional lymph nodes.

ANTIANGIOGENIC THERAPY Understanding the molecular mechanisms that regulate tumor angiogenesis may provide unique opportunities for cancer treatment. Acquired drug resistance of tumor cells due to their high intrinsic mutation rate is a major cause of treatment failure in human cancers. ECs comprising the tumor vasculature are genetically stable and do not share genetic changes with tumor cells; the EC apoptosis pathways are therefore intact. Each EC of a tumor vessel helps provide nourishment to many tumor cells, and although tumor angiogenesis can be driven by a number of exogenous proangiogenic stimuli, experimental data indicate that blockade of a single growth factor (e.g., VEGF) may inhibit tumor-induced vascular growth. Because tumor blood vessels are distinct from normal ones, they may be selectively destroyed without affecting normal vessels. Angiogenesis inhibitors function by targeting the critical molecular pathways involved in EC proliferation, migration, and/or survival, many of which are unique to the activated endothelium in tumors. Inhibition of growth factor and adhesion-dependent signaling pathways can induce EC apoptosis with concomitant inhibition of tumor growth. Different types of tumors use distinct molecular mechanisms to activate the angiogenic switch. Therefore, it is doubtful that a single antiangiogenic strategy will suffice for all human cancers; rather, a number of therapeutics will need to be developed, each responding to distinct programs of angiogenesis that have been developed by specific human cancers.

A number of strategies have been developed to selectively target tumor vasculature (Table 69-2, Fig. 69-6), and many novel antiangiogenic agents are currently in clinical trials. Inhibition of VEGF function blunts angiogenesis and tumor growth in a variety of tumor models by selectively inducing the apoptosis of immature ECs that are not associated with pericytes or smooth muscle cells, but spares normal host vessels. Humanized anti-VEGF monoclonal antibodies are active in colon cancer. A number of small, cell-permeable chemicals that inhibit the tyrosine kinase activity of VEGFR2 or VEGFR1 are being tested. The latter drugs may synergize in their antiangiogenic effects, since VEGFR2 inhibitors should block EC proliferation, migration, and survival, while VEGFR1 inhibitors are predicted to inhibit VEGF and PlGF-mediated recruitment of CEPs, HSCs, and inflammatory cells to the tumor bed. The relative efficacy of these agents may vary since some tumors may be dependent on VEGFR2-induced sprouting while others are more dependent on the bone marrow–derived EC precursors. Angiogenesis induced by bFGF can be blocked by inhibitors of the VEGF pathway, demonstrating a linkage between these pathways. Inhibitors of the Ang/Tie2 and Ephrin/EPH pathways are in development.

Blocking antibodies or antagonistic peptides to $\alpha_v\beta_3$ integrin, which interrupt the $\alpha_v\beta_3$- mediated adhesion to matrix proteins, leads to the inhibition of tumor and growth factor–induced angiogenesis in vivo by selectively inducing apoptosis of ECs in newly formed vessels. This indicates that ligation of the $\alpha_v\beta_3$ receptor is required for the survival of ECs of the angiogenic phenotype. Integrins are also required for EC migration and are important regulators of MMP activity, which modulates movement through and the release of growth factors from the ECM. Humanized monoclonal antibodies directed against $\alpha_v\beta_3$ are currently in clinical trial, as are small-molecule inhibitors of $\alpha_v\beta_3$, such as circular peptides containing the arg-gly-asp (RGD) integrin binding site. A number of clinical trials are testing the ability of MMP inhibitors to block tumor metastasis as well as angiogenesis. The discovery that ECs from various normal tissues encode unique surface markers suggests that tumors arising in different tissues may also express unique "vascular addressins," which could be targeted.

A number of endogenous, physiologic inhibitors of angiogenesis have been discovered. *Angiostatin* is a 38-kDa kringle domain–containing polypeptide fragment of plasminogen generated in the tumor microenvironment by proteases derived from tumor and stromal cells (including MMPs secreted by tumor-associated macrophages). Angiostatin inhibits in vivo tumor angiogenesis and induces tumor dormancy in murine models, and its antiangiogenic effects are mediated in part by induction of EC apoptosis. *Endostatin* is a C-terminal cleavage product of collagen XVIII generated by cathepsin or elastase-like proteolytic activities. It inhibits EC migration and promotes apoptosis by binding to $\alpha_v\beta_3$ and -β_5 integrins and downregulating expression of survival factors such as Bcl-2 and Bcl-XL. Antiangiogenic peptide domains of other normal host proteins have also been defined. Purified angiostatin and endostatin are highly specific inhibitors of activated ECs in vitro and in murine models and have entered clinical trials. Although tumor responses have been disappointingly rare, pharmacokinetic data indicate bolus administration of recombinant endostatin

TABLE 69-2 *Antiangiogenic Treatments Currently in Clinical Trials: Molecular Pathways as Targets*

I. Receptor tyrosine kinase pathways		
A. Endothelial cell (EC) specific		
1. VEGFR1 kinase inhibitors		Decreased recruitment of CEPs, HSCs to tumor vessels
2. VEGFR2 kinase inhibitors		Inhibition of EC proliferation, migration, survival
3. Anti-VEGF monoclonal antibody		Inhibition of VEGF signaling to EC, CEPs, HSCs
B. Non-EC specific		
1. FGFR, PDGF kinase inhibitors		Inhibition of EC functions; decreased recruitment of perivascular cells
2. Anti-ERB-B2 monoclonal antibody		Inhibition of tumor VEGF production; increased thrombospondin-1
II. Integrin receptors/ extracellular matrix		
A. Integrin inhibitors		
1. RGD circular pentapeptides		Inhibition of integrin-mediated attachment to ECM with induction of EC apoptosis
2. Anti-$\alpha_v\beta_3$ monoclonal antibodies		Detachment of EC from matrix with induction of apoptosis
B. Matrix metalloproteinase inhibitors		Inhibition of EC and tumor invasion; decreased release of GF from matrix binding sites
III. Endogenous angiogenesis inhibitors		
A. Peptides derived from host proteins		
1. Angiostatin (plasminogen fragment)		Mechanisms of action unclear; may inhibit EC cell surface ATP synthase activity; binds to $\alpha_v\beta_3$ and other integrins
2. Endostatin (collagen XVIII fragment)		Mechanisms unclear; binds to EC integrins; may block GF binding to heparin sulfate; inhibits EC migration and induces apoptosis
B. Hormones		Inhibits EC microtubules
1. 2-methoxy-estradiol (2-ME)		
IV. Other agents		
A. Chemokines/cytokines		
1. IL-12		Induction of IFN-γ, IP-10, and MiG
2. IFN-α		Inhibition of bFGF production by tumor
B. Synthetic compounds		
1. TNP-490 (fumagillan analogue)		Inhibition of EC methionine aminopeptidase (required for EC proliferation)
2. Thalidomide		In vitro evidence for antiangiogenic activity; proven therapeutic activity in human multiple myeloma

Abbreviations: VEGFR, vascular endothelial growth factor receptor; CEP, circulating endothelial cell precursors; HSC, hematopoietic stem cells; FGFR, fibroblast growth factor receptor; PDGF, platelet-derived growth factor; RGD, arg-gly-asp; ECM, extracellular matrix; GF, growth factor; IL, interleukin; IFN, interferon; IP-10, interferon-inducible protein-10; MiG, monokine induced by IFN-γ; bFGF, basic fibroblast growth factor.

does not maintain sufficient serum concentrations of the inhibitor for antiangiogenic activity to occur.

A number of more general signaling pathways are also important for EC function and can be targeted. Trastuzumab, a monoclonal antibody that inhibits signaling from the ERB-B2 tyrosine kinase receptor expressed by some breast and ovarian cancers, decreases expression of VEGF and upregulates expression of thrombospondin-1 (an angiogenic inhibitor), by tumor cells. Inhibition of fibroblast growth

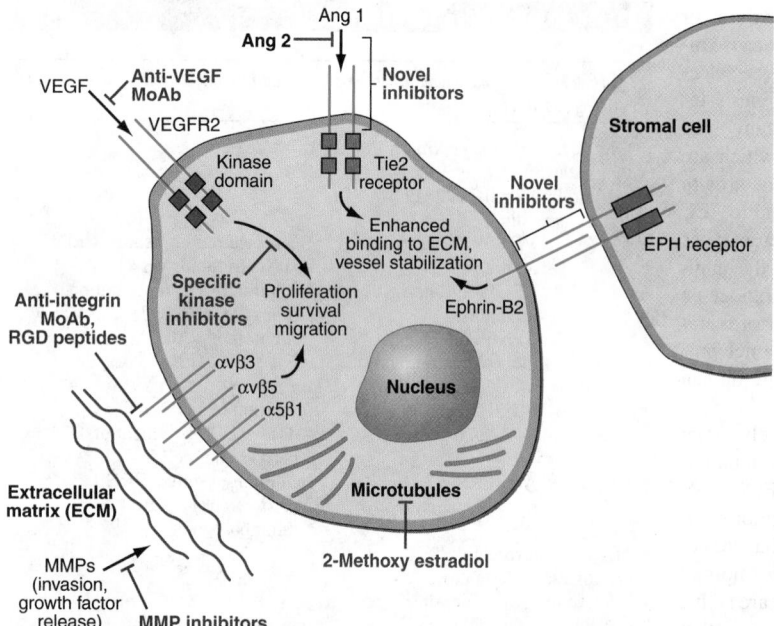

FIGURE 69-6 Knowledge of the molecular events governing tumor angiogenesis has led to a number of therapeutic strategies to block tumor blood vessel formation. Multiple inhibitors of the VEGF/VEGFR pathway are in clinical trial, and other endothelial cell–specific receptor tyrosine kinase pathways (e.g., angiopoietin/Tie2 and ephrin/EPH) are likely targets for the future. Inhibition of integrin binding to the ECM, and ECM breakdown by matrix-metalloproteinase inhibitors (MMPs), should lead to EC apoptosis and inhibition of EC migration and invasion. Other targets include intracellular signaling pathways, inhibition of cytoskeletal elements (i.e., by 2-methoxy estradiol, 2-ME), and compounds whose mechanisms of antiangiogenic activity are unknown, such as thalidomide and the endogenous inhibitors (endostatin, angiostatin).

factor (FGF) and PDGF receptor signaling by kinase inhibitors may block EC proliferation and recruitment of supporting stromal cells into the tumor milieu. Signal transduction pathways downstream of RTK and integrin signaling, such as the Ras/MAP kinase, PI3K/Akt, and Src family kinase pathways, are important antitumor therapeutic targets that are also important for angiogenesis. FTIs have been shown to block VEGF expression by tumor cells. EC survival requires the activity of the serine/threonine kinase Akt, and inhibitors of this kinase may have potent antiangiogenic activity. Src kinases integrate VEGF/integrin signaling associated with focal adhesion kinase (FAK) activation and dynamic remodeling of the cell cytoskeleton; Src inhibitors should block EC motility as well as survival. Arachidonic acid metabolism may be important for $\alpha_v\beta_3$-induced proliferation and migration of EC; COX-2 inhibitors may inhibit $\alpha_v\beta_3$-mediated EC activities. Giant cell tumors of bone and angioblastomas that occur in young children, and can be severely debilitating or life-threatening, appear to depend uniquely on bFGF as their main angiogenic factor. Low daily doses of interferon block tumor cell production of bFGF and after 1 to 2 years of treatment can mediate the complete eradication of these tumors.

The conceptual design of antiangiogenic clinical trials may require a paradigm shift from conventional chemotherapy. In tumor models,

the combination of low daily doses of standard chemotherapy agents combined with antiangiogenic agents can synergize to induce apoptosis of the tumor vasculature, even when the tumor cells are resistant to high doses of the same agents. The initial response to successful antiangiogenic treatment is a decrease in vascular permeability and lower intratumoral pressure; this results in an initial increase in tumor blood flow that can transiently increase tumor growth (but could also provide increased delivery of chemotherapeutic drugs to the tumor). Clinicians will need to be prepared to weather this initial "tumor flare" without stopping antiangiogenic treatment. Inhibition of new vessel formation in human cancers may induce stable disease rather than tumor regression, and progression-free survival may be a more appropriate endpoint than a reduction of tumor volume. This implies a need for chronic, daily administration to prevent regrowth of blood vessels between doses, and will require orally administered drugs that can be tolerated for prolonged times. Surrogate markers will therefore be needed to evaluate the clinical effectiveness of antiangiogenic therapies. Circulating factors may not be useful, since tumors and their stroma produce a number of positive and negative regulators of angiogenesis. The circulating levels of CEPs might be a marker of response, but this remains speculative. The promise of the antiangiogenic approach to cancer treatment depends on tumor selectivity, which may not always be predictable. Phase I clinical trial testing of a VEGFR2 kinase inhibitor demonstrated no serious toxicity. Yet when it was combined with cisplatin and gemcitabine for the treatment of solid tumors, 8 of 19 patients experienced serious thrombotic events, including pulmonary embolism and stroke. Antiangiogenic agents may sensitize normal ECs to apoptosis induction by chemotherapeutic agents, with exposure of tissue factor in subendothelial vessel wall. This underscores the potential toxicity of targeting ECs in vivo.

FURTHER READING

BYKOV VJN et al: Restoration of the tumor suppressor function of mutant p53 by a low-molecular-weight compound. Nat Med 8:282, 2002

CRISTOFANILLI M et al: Angiogenesis modulation in cancer research: Novel clinical approaches. Nat Rev Drug Discovery 1:415, 2002

DANCEY J, SAUSVILLE EA: Issues and progress with protein kinase inhibitors for cancer treatment. Nat Rev Drug Discovery 2:296, 2003

DRUKER BJ: Inhibition of the Bcr-Abl tyrosine kinase as a therapeutic strategy for CML. Oncogene 21:8541, 2002

HANAHAN D, WEINBERG RA: The hallmarks of cancer. Cell 100:57, 2000

JOHNSTONE RW: Histone-deacetylase inhibitors: Novel drugs for the treatment of cancer. Nat Rev Drug Discovery 1:287, 2002

JONES PA, BAYLIN SB: The fundamental role of epigenetic events in cancer. Nat Rev Genetics 3:415, 2002

REED JC: Apoptosis-based therapies. Nat Rev Drug Discovery 1:111, 2002

RODEN DM, GEORGE AL: The genetic basis of variability in drug responses. Nat Rev Drug Discovery 1:37, 2002

SAUSVILLE EA: Complexities in the development of cyclin-dependent kinase inhibitor drugs. Trends Mol Med 8:S32, 2002

---

70 PRINCIPLES OF CANCER TREATMENT: SURGERY, CHEMOTHERAPY, AND BIOLOGIC THERAPY
Edward A. Sausville, Dan L. Longo

The goal of cancer treatment is first to eradicate the cancer. If this primary goal cannot be accomplished, the goal of cancer treatment shifts to palliation, the amelioration of symptoms, and preservation of quality of life while striving to extend life. The dictum *primum non nocere* is not necessarily the guiding principle of cancer therapy. When cure of cancer is possible, cancer treatments may be undertaken despite

the certainty of severe and perhaps life-threatening toxicities. Every cancer treatment has the potential to cause harm, and treatment may be given that produces toxicity with no benefit. The therapeutic index of many interventions is quite narrow, and most treatments are given to the point of toxicity. Conversely, when the clinical goal is palliation, careful attention to minimizing the toxicity of potentially toxic treatments becomes a significant goal. Irrespective of the clinical scenario, the guiding principle of cancer treatment should be *primum succerrere*, "first hasten to help." Radical surgical procedures, large-field hyperfractionated radiation therapy, high-dose chemotherapy, and maximum tolerable doses of cytokines such as interleukin (IL) 2 are all used in certain settings where 100% of the patients will experience toxicity and side effects from the intervention, and only a fraction of the patients will experience benefit. One of the challenges of cancer treatment is to use the various treatment modalities alone and together in a fashion that maximizes the chances for patient benefit.

Cancer treatments are divided into four main types: surgery, radiation therapy (including photodynamic therapy), chemotherapy (including hormonal therapy and molecularly targeted therapy), and biologic therapy (including immunotherapy and gene therapy). The modalities are often used in combination, and agents in one category can act by several mechanisms. For example, cancer chemotherapy agents can induce differentiation, and antibodies (a form of immunotherapy) can be used to deliver radiation therapy. Surgery and radiation therapy are considered local treatments, though their effects can influence the behavior of tumor at remote sites. Chemotherapy and biologic therapy are usually systemic treatments. *Oncology*, the study of tumors including treatment approaches, is a multidisciplinary effort with surgical-, radiotherapy-, and internal medicine–related areas of expertise. Treatments for patients with hematologic malignancies are often shared by hematologists and medical oncologists. →*Principles of radiation therapy are discussed in Chap. 71.*

Cancer behaves in many ways as an organ that attempts to regulate its own growth. However, cancers have not set an appropriate limit on how much growth should be permitted. Normal organs and cancers share the property of having a population of cells in cycle and actively renewing and a population of cells not in cycle. In cancers, cells that are not dividing are heterogeneous; some have sustained too much genetic damage to replicate but have defects in their death pathways that permit their survival; some are starving for nutrients and oxygen; and some are reversibly out of cycle poised to be recruited back into cycle and expand if needed. Severely damaged and starving cells are unlikely to kill the patient. The problem is that the cells that are reversibly not in cycle are capable of replenishing tumor cells physically removed or damaged by radiation and chemotherapy.

Tumors follow a Gompertzian growth curve (Fig. 70-1); the growth

fraction of a neoplasm starts at 100% with the first transformed cell and declines exponentially over time until by the time of diagnosis at a tumor burden of 1 to 5×10^9 tumor cells, the growth fraction is usually 1 to 4%. Thus, peak growth rate may actually occur before the tumor is detectable. A key aspect of a successful tumor is the ability to stimulate the development of a new supporting stroma through angiogenesis and production of proteases to allow invasion through basement membranes and normal tissue barriers (Chap. 69). Specific cellular mechanisms promote entry or withdrawal of tumor cells from the cell cycle. For example, when a tumor recurs after surgery or chemotherapy, frequently its growth is accelerated and the growth fraction of the tumor is increased. This pattern is similar to that seen in regenerating organs. Partial resection of the liver results in the recruitment of cells into the cell cycle, and the resected liver volume is replaced. Similarly, chemotherapy-damaged bone marrow increases its growth to replace cells killed by chemotherapy. However, cancers do not recognize a limit on their expansion. Monoclonal gammopathy of uncertain significance may be an example of a clonal neoplasm with intrinsic features that stop its growth before a lethal tumor burden is reached. A fraction of patients with this disorder go on to develop fatal multiple myeloma, but probably this occurs because of the accumulation of additional genetic lesions. Elucidation of the mechanisms that regulate this "organ-like" behavior of tumors may provide additional clues to cancer control and treatment.

PRINCIPLES OF CANCER SURGERY

Surgery is used in cancer prevention, diagnosis, staging, treatment (for both localized and metastatic disease), palliation, and rehabilitation.

PREVENTION Cancer can be prevented by surgery in people who have premalignant lesions resected (e.g., premalignant lesions of skin, colon, cervix) and in those who are at increased risk of cancer from either an underlying disease (colectomy in those with pancolonic involvement with ulcerative colitis), the presence of genetic lesions (colectomy for familial polyposis; thyroidectomy for multiple endocrine neoplasia type 2; bilateral mastectomy or oophorectomy for familial breast or ovarian cancer syndromes), or a developmental anomaly (orchiectomy in those with an undescended testis). In some cases, prophylactic surgery is more radical than the surgical procedures used to treat the cancer after it develops. The assessment of risk involves many factors and should be undertaken with care before advising a patient to undergo such a major procedure. For breast cancer prevention, many experts use a 20% risk of developing breast cancer over the next 5 years as a threshold. However, patient fears play a major role in defining candidates for cancer prevention surgery. Counseling and education may not be enough to allay the fears of someone who has lost close family members to a malignancy.

DIAGNOSIS The ideal diagnostic procedure varies with the type of cancer, its anatomical location, and the medical condition of the patient. However, the underlying principle is to obtain as much tissue as safely possible. Tumors may be heterogeneous in appearance. Pathologists are better able to make the diagnosis when they have more tissue to examine. In addition to light-microscopic inspection of a tumor for pattern of growth, degree of cellular atypia, invasiveness, and morphologic features that aid in the differential diagnosis, sufficient tissue is of value in searching for genetic abnormalities and protein expression patterns that may aid in differential diagnosis or to provide information about prognosis or likely response to treatment. Histologically similar tumors may have very different gene expression patterns when assessed by such techniques as microarray analysis using gene chips, with important differences in response to treatment. Such testing requires that the tissue be handled properly (e.g., immunologic detection of proteins is more effective in fresh-frozen tissue rather than in formalin-fixed tissue); thus, coordination among the surgeon, pathologist, and primary care physician is essential to ensure that the amount of information learned from the biopsy material is maximized.

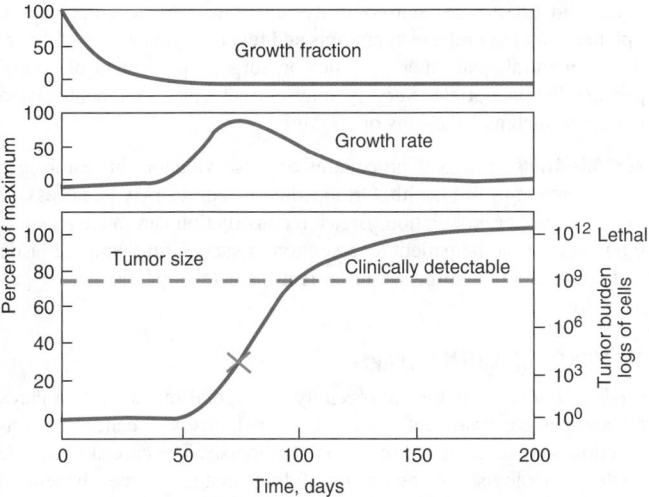

FIGURE 70-1 Gompertzian tumor growth. The growth fraction of a tumor declines exponentially over time (*top*). The growth rate of a tumor peaks before it is clinically detectable (*middle*). Tumor size increases slowly, goes through an exponential phase, and slows again as the tumor reaches the size at which limitation of nutrients or autoor host regulatory influences can occur. The maximum growth rate occurs at 1/e, the point at which the tumor is about 37% of its maximum size (marked with an X). Tumor becomes detectable at a burden of about 10^9 (1 cm³) and kills the patient at a tumor burden of about 10^{12} (1 kg). Efforts to treat the tumor and reduce its size can result in an increase in the growth fraction and an increase in growth rate.

These goals are best met by an *excisional biopsy* in which the entire tumor mass is removed with a small margin of normal tissue surrounding it. If an excisional biopsy cannot be performed, *incisional biopsy* is the procedure of second choice. A wedge of tissue is removed, and an effort is made to include the majority of the cross-sectional diameter of the tumor in the biopsy to minimize sampling error. When the diagnosis is being made through an endoscope or via fluoroscopy, it may be necessary to obtain a *core-needle biopsy* of the mass; considerably less tissue is obtained and the diagnosis may be less certain. However, this procedure often provides enough information to plan a definitive surgical procedure. Least reliable in diagnosis of primary cancer is *fine-needle aspiration*. This technique generally obtains only a suspension of cells from within a mass. This approach (with stereotactic guidance of the needle) is the procedure of choice in the diagnosis of brain tumors and may be useful in diagnosing thyroid nodules and in confirming persistent or recurrent disease in a patient with known cancer, but the procedure is overutilized in primary diagnosis. It would be preferable to perform a larger open operation to obtain more tissue in most sites. The biopsy techniques that involve cutting into tumor carry with them a risk of facilitating the spread of the tumor.

STAGING   As noted in Chap. 66, an important component of patient management is defining the extent of disease. Radiographic and other imaging tests can be helpful in defining the clinical stage; however, pathologic staging requires defining the extent of involvement by documenting the histologic presence of tumor in tissue biopsies obtained through a surgical procedure. Axillary lymph node sampling in breast cancer and lymph node sampling at laparotomy for lymphomas and testicular, colon, and other intraabdominal cancers provide crucial information for treatment planning and may determine the extent and nature of primary cancer treatment.

TREATMENT   Surgery is the most effective means of treating cancer. About 40% of cancer patients are cured today by surgery. Unfortunately, a large fraction of patients with solid tumors (perhaps 60%) have metastatic disease that is not accessible for removal. However, even when the disease is not curable by surgery alone, the removal of tumor can obtain important benefits, including local control of tumor, preservation of organ function, debulking that permits subsequent therapy to work better, and staging information on extent of involvement. Cancer surgery aiming for cure is usually planned to excise the tumor completely with an adequate margin of normal tissue (the margin varies with the tumor and the anatomy), touching the tumor as little as possible to prevent vascular and lymphatic spread, and minimizing operative risk. Extending the procedure to resect draining lymph nodes obtains prognostic information, but such resections alone generally do not improve survival.

Increasingly, laparoscopic approaches are being used to address primary abdominal and pelvic tumors. Lymph node spread may be assessed using the sentinel node approach, in which the first draining lymph node a spreading tumor would encounter is defined by injecting a dye at operation and then resecting the first node to turn blue. The sentinel node assessment is continuing to undergo clinical evaluation but appears to provide reliable information without the risks (lymphedema, lymphangiosarcoma) associated with resection of all the regional nodes. Advances in adjuvant chemotherapy and radiation therapy following surgery have permitted a substantial decrease in the extent of primary surgery necessary to obtain the best outcomes. Thus, lumpectomy with radiation therapy is as effective as modified radical mastectomy for breast cancer, and limb-sparing surgery followed by adjuvant radiation therapy and chemotherapy has replaced radical primary surgical procedures involving amputation and disarticulation for childhood rhabdomyosarcomas. More limited surgery is also being employed to spare organ function, as in larynx and bladder cancer. The magnitude of operations necessary to optimally control and cure cancer has also been diminished by technical advances; for example, the circular anastomotic stapler has allowed narrower (<2 cm) margins

in colon cancer without compromise of local control rates, and many patients who would have had colostomies are able to maintain normal anatomy.

In some settings, e.g., bulky testicular cancer or stage III breast cancer, surgery is not the first treatment modality employed. After an initial diagnostic biopsy, chemotherapy and/or radiation therapy are delivered to reduce the size of the tumor and control clinically undetected metastatic disease, and such therapy is followed by a surgical procedure to remove residual masses. This is called *neoadjuvant therapy*. Because the sequence of treatment is critical to success and is different from the standard surgery-first approach, coordination among the surgical oncologist, radiation oncologist, and medical oncologist is crucial.

Surgery may be curative in a subset of patients with metastatic disease. Patients with lung metastases from osteosarcoma may be cured by resection of the lung lesions. In patients with colon cancer who have fewer than five liver metastases restricted to one lobe and no extrahepatic metastases, hepatic lobectomy may produce long-term disease-free survival in 25% of selected patients. Surgery can also be associated with systemic antitumor effects. In the setting of hormonally responsive tumors, oophorectomy and/or adrenalectomy may control estrogen production and orchiectomy may reduce androgen production, both with effects on metastatic tumor growth. If resection of the primary lesion takes place in the presence of metastases, the noted change in tumor behavior is most often acceleration of growth, perhaps based on the removal of a source of angiogenesis inhibitors and mass-related growth regulators in the tumor. However, on rare occasions (certain renal cancers), primary tumor resection is accompanied by regression of metastatic lesions. Similarly, splenectomy in some cases of lymphoma may be associated with regression of disease at remote sites. This phenomenon, called the *abscopal effect*, is attributed to the removal of a source of growth or angiogenic factors upon which the remote sites depend for growth.

PALLIATION   Surgery is employed in a number of ways for supportive care: insertion of central venous catheters, diagnostic evaluation of pulmonary infiltrates, control of pleural and pericardial effusions and ascites, caval interruption for recurrent pulmonary emboli, stabilization of cancer-weakened weight-bearing bones, and control of hemorrhage, among others. Surgical bypass of gastrointestinal, urinary tract, or biliary tree obstruction can alleviate symptoms and prolong survival. Surgical procedures may provide relief of otherwise intractable pain or reverse neurologic dysfunction (cord decompression). Splenectomy may relieve symptoms and reverse hypersplenism. Intrathecal or intrahepatic therapy relies on surgical placement of appropriate infusion portals. Surgery may correct other treatment-related toxicities such as adhesions or strictures.

REHABILITATION   Surgical procedures are also valuable in restoring a cancer patient to full health. Orthopedic procedures may be necessary to assure proper ambulation. Breast reconstruction can make an enormous impact on the patient's perception of successful therapy. Plastic and reconstructive surgery can correct the effects of disfiguring primary treatment.

PRINCIPLES OF CHEMOTHERAPY

Medical oncology is the subspecialty of internal medicine that cares for and designs treatment approaches to patients with cancer, in conjunction with surgical and radiation oncologists. The core skills of the medical oncologist include the use of drugs that may have a beneficial effect on the natural history of the patient's illness or favorably influence the patient's quality of life.

HISTORIC BACKGROUND   The treatment of patients with cancer using chemicals, in the hope of causing regressions of established tumors or to slow the rate of tumor growth, arose by analogy to the proposition of Ehrlich that bacteria might be killed selectively by compounds with intrinsic affinity for bacteria, in effect acting as "magic bullets." Candidate compounds that might have selectivity for cancer cells were suggested by the marrow-toxic effects of sulfur and nitrogen mustards, first noted in their use in chemical warfare. These observations led in the 1940s to the first clinical experiments where notable regressions of hematopoietic tumors followed use of these compounds by Gilman and colleagues. As these compounds caused covalent modification of DNA, the structure of DNA was thereby identified as a potential target for drug design efforts to produce antineoplastic agents. Biochemical studies demonstrating the requirement of growing tumor cells for precursors of nucleic acids led to nearly contemporaneous studies by Farber of folate analogues. The cure of patients with advanced choriocarcinoma by methotrexate in the 1950s provided further impetus to define the value of chemotherapeutic agents in many different tumor types. This resulted in efforts to understand unique metabolic requirements for biosynthesis of nucleic acids and led to the design, rational for the time, of compounds that might selectively inhibit DNA synthesis in proliferating cancer cells. The capacity of hormonal manipulations including oophorectomy and orchiectomy to cause regressions of breast and prostate cancers, respectively, provided a rationale for efforts to interdict various aspects of hormone function in hormone-dependent tumors. The serendipitous finding that certain poisons derived from bacteria or plants could affect normal DNA or mitotic spindle function allowed completion of the classic armamentarium of drugs with proven efficacy and a relative margin of safety in the treatment of certain cancers.

END POINTS OF DRUG ACTION Chemotherapy agents may be used for the treatment of active, clinically apparent cancer. Table 70-1,**A** lists those

---

TABLE 70-1 *Curability of Cancers with Chemotherapy*

A. Advanced cancers with possible cure
Acute lymphoid and acute myeloid leukemia (pediatric/adult)
Hodgkin's disease (pediatric/adult)
Lymphomas—certain types (pediatric/adult)
Germ cell neoplasms
  Embryonal carcinoma
  Teratocarcinoma
  Seminoma or dysgerminoma
  Choriocarcinoma
Gestational trophoblastic neoplasia
Pediatric neoplasms
  Wilm's tumor
  Embryonal rhabdomyosarcoma
  Ewing's sarcoma
  Peripheral neuroepithelioma
  Neuroblastoma
Small-cell lung carcinoma
Ovarian carcinoma

B. Advanced cancers possibly cured by chemotherapy and radiation
Squamous carcinoma (head and neck)
Squamous carcinoma (anus)
Breast carcinoma
Carcinoma of the uterine cervix
Non-small cell lung carcinoma (stage III)
Small-cell lung carcinoma

C. Cancers possibly cured with chemotherapy as adjuvant to surgery
Breast carcinoma
Colorectal carcinoma[a]
Osteogenic sarcoma
Soft tissue sarcoma

D. Cancers possibly cured with "high-dose" chemotherapy with stem cell support
Relapsed leukemias, lymphoid and myeloid
Relapsed lymphomas, Hodgkin's and non-Hodgkin's
Chronic myeloid leukemia
Multiple myeloma

E. Cancers responsive with useful palliation, but not cure, by chemotherapy
Bladder carcinoma
Chronic myeloid leukemia
Hairy cell leukemia
Chronic lymphocytic leukemia
Lymphoma—certain types
Multiple myeloma
Gastric carcinoma
Cervix carcinoma
Endometrial carcinoma
Soft tissue sarcoma
Head and neck cancer
Adrenocortical carcinoma
Islet-cell neoplasms
Breast carcinoma
Colorectal carcinoma

F. Tumor poorly responsive in advanced stages to chemotherapy
Pancreatic carcinoma
Biliary-tract neoplasms
Renal carcinoma
Thyroid carcinoma
Carcinoma of the vulva
Non-small cell lung carcinoma
Prostate carcinoma
Melanoma
Hepatocellular carcinoma

[a] Rectum also receives radiation therapy.

---

tumors considered curable by conventionally available chemotherapeutic agents when used to address disseminated or metastatic cancers. If a tumor is localized to a single site, serious consideration of surgery or primary radiation therapy should be given, as these treatment modalities may be curative as local treatments. Chemotherapy may be employed after the failure of these modalities to eradicate a local tumor or as part of multimodality approaches to offer primary treatment to a clinically localized tumor. In this event, it can allow organ preservation when given with radiation, as in larynx or other upper airway sites; or sensitize tumors to radiation when given, for example, to patients concurrently receiving radiation for lung or cervix cancer (Table 70-1,**B**). Chemotherapy can be administered as an adjuvant, i.e., in addition to surgery (Table 70-1,**C**) or radiation, after all clinically apparent disease has been removed. This use of chemotherapy may have curative potential in breast and colorectal neoplasms, as it attempts to eliminate clinically unapparent tumor that may have already disseminated. As noted above, small tumors frequently have high growth fractions and therefore may be intrinsically more susceptible to the action of antiproliferative agents. Chemotherapy is routinely used in "conventional" dose regimens. In general, these doses produce reversible acute side effects primarily consisting of transient myelosuppression with or without gastrointestinal toxicity (usually nausea), which are readily managed. High-dose chemotherapy regimens are predicated on the observation that the concentration-effect curve for many anticancer agents is rather steep, and increased dose can produce markedly increased therapeutic effect, although at the cost of potentially life-threatening complications that require intensive support, usually in the form of hematopoietic stem cell support from the patient (*autologous*) or from donors matched for histocompatibility loci (*allogeneic*). High-dose regimens nonetheless have definite curative potential in defined clinical settings (Table 70-1,**D**).

Karnofsky was among the first to champion the evaluation of a chemotherapeutic agent's benefit by carefully quantitating its effect on tumor size and using these measurements to decide objectively the basis for further treatment of a particular patient or further clinical evaluation of a drug's potential. A partial response (PR) is defined conventionally as a decrease by at least 50% in a tumor's bi-dimensional area; a complete response (CR) connotes disappearance of all tumor; progression of disease signifies an increase in size of existing lesions by >25% from baseline or best response or development of new lesions; and "stable" disease fits into none of the above categories. More recently proposed evaluation systems utilize unidimensional measurement, but the intent is similar in rigorously defining evidence for the activity of the agent in assessing its value to the patient.

If cure is not possible, chemotherapy may be undertaken with the goal of palliating some aspect of the tumor's effect on the host. Common tumors that may be meaningfully addressed with palliative intent are listed in Table 70-1,**E**. Usually tumor-related symptoms may manifest as pain, weight loss, or some local symptom related to the tumor's effect on normal structures. Patients treated with palliative intent should be aware of their diagnosis and the limitations of the proposed treatments, have access to supportive care, and have suitable "performance status," according to assessment algorithms such as the one developed by Karnofsky or by the Eastern Cooperative Oncology Group (ECOG). ECOG performance status 0 (PS0) patients are without symptoms; PS1 patients have mild symptoms not requiring treatment; PS2, symptoms requiring some treatment; PS3, disabling symptoms, but allowing ambulation for >50% of the day; PS4, ambulation <50% of the day. Only PS0 to PS2 patients are generally considered suitable for palliative (noncurative) treatment. If there is curative potential, even poor performance status patients may be treated, but their prognosis is usually inferior to that of good performance patients treated with similar regimens.

PATH FOR NEW CANCER DRUG DISCOVERY AND DEVELOPMENT The usefulness of any drug is governed by the extent to which a given dose causes a useful result (therapeutic effect; in the case of anticancer agents, toxicity to tumor cells) as opposed to a toxic effect, reflecting injury to the host. The *therapeutic index* is the degree of separation between toxic and therapeutic doses. Really useful drugs have large therapeutic indices, and this usually occurs when the drug target is expressed in the disease-causing compartment as opposed to the normal compartment. Classically, selective toxicity of an agent for an organ is governed by the expression of an agent's target; or differential accumulation into or elimination from compartments where toxicity is experienced or ameliorated, respectively. Current "conventional cytotoxic" antineoplastic agents have the unfortunate property that their targets are present in both normal and tumor tissues. In the main they therefore have relatively narrow therapeutic indices.

Agents with promise for the treatment of cancer have in the past been detected empirically through screening for antiproliferative effects in animal or human tumors, usually in rodent hosts or through inhibition of tumor cells growing in tissue culture. An optimal schedule for demonstrating antitumor activity in animals is defined in further preclinical studies, as is the optimal drug formulation for a given route and schedule. Safety testing in two species on an analogous schedule of administration defines the starting dose for a phase I trial in humans. This is established as a fraction, usually one-sixth to one-tenth, of the dose just causing easily reversible toxicity in the more sensitive animal species. Escalating doses of the drug are then given during the human phase I trial until reversible toxicity is observed. Dose-limiting toxicity (DLT) defines a dose that conveys greater toxicity than would be acceptable in routine practice, allowing definition of a lower maximal tolerated dose (MTD). The occurrence of toxicity is correlated if possible with plasma drug concentrations. The MTD or a dose just lower than the MTD is usually the dose suitable for phase II trials, where a fixed dose is administered to a relatively homogeneous set of patients in an effort to define whether the drug causes regression of tumors. An "active" agent conventionally has PR rates of at least 20 to 25% with reversible non-life-threatening side effects, and it may then be suitable for study in phase III trials to assess efficacy in comparison to standard or no therapy. Response is but the most immediate indicator of drug effect. To be clinically valuable, responses must translate into clinical benefit. This is conventionally established by a beneficial effect on overall survival, or at least an increased time to further progression of disease. Active efforts are being made to quantitate effects of anticancer agents on quality of life. Cancer drug clinical trials conventionally use a toxicity grading scale where grade I toxicities do not require treatment; grade II often require symptomatic treatment but are not life-threatening; grade III toxicities are potentially life-threatening if untreated; grade IV toxicities are actually life-threatening; and grade V toxicities are those that result in the patient's death.

The process of cancer drug development is likely to evolve in significant ways in the near future as (1) the molecular analysis of human tumors defines more precisely the molecular targets that can be the focus of drug discovery efforts, and (2) clinical trials are undertaken only after means of assessing the behavior of the drug in relation to its target have been developed. The basis for optimism and anticipated change in clinical trials methodology extends from emerging understanding of the basis for cancer incidence and progression. Cancer arises from genetic lesions that cause an excess of cell growth or division, with inadequate cell death (Chap. 68). In addition, failure of cellular differentiation results in altered cellular position and capacity to proliferate while cut off from normal cell regulatory signals. An overall schema for understanding cancer progression can be seen in Fig. 70-2. Normally, cells in a differentiated state are stimulated to enter the cell cycle from a quiescent state, or G_0, or continue after completion of a prior cell division cycle in response to environmental cues including growth factor and hormonal signals. Cells progress through G_1 and enter S-phase after passing through "checkpoints," which are biochemically regulated transition points, to assure that the genome is "ready" for replication. The cyclin-dependent kinases

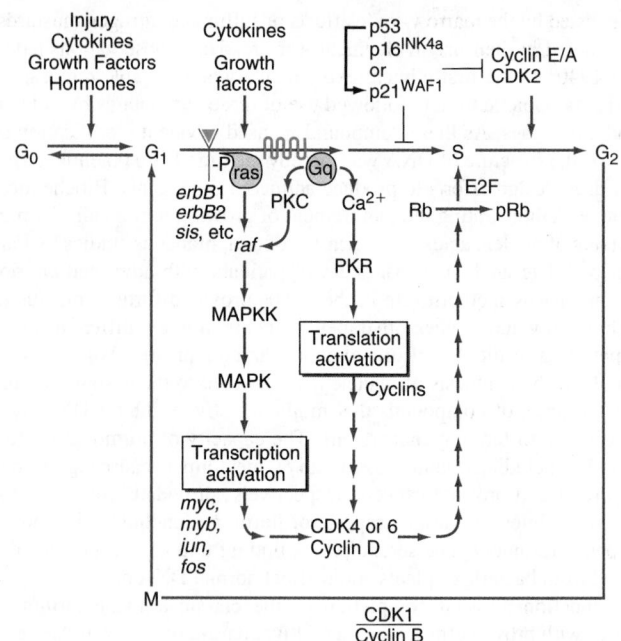

FIGURE 70-2 Basis for neoplastic growth and progression. Normally cells are stimulated to enter a proliferating state through the action of growth factors, positional signals, or cytokines. Cells enter G_1 under the influence of normal signaling pathways including tyrosine kinase receptors coupled to ras protooncogenes or seven-transmembrane receptors coupled through heterotrimeric guanine nucleotide binding (0) proteins, especially Gq linked to calcium- and lipid-mediated signaling pathways through protein kinase C (PKC). Cells activate transcription and translation of key regulatory molecules such as the cyclins, which activate cyclin-dependent kinases (CDKs) 4 or 6. Phosphorylation of the retinoblastoma susceptibility protein (pRb) causes release of E2F transcription factors to an active state, promoting the transcription of multiple genes allowing progression through S-phase, where DNA is replicated. Tumor cells possess activated oncogenes such as *erbB*1, *erbB*2, and *sis* or mutated *ras* gene products that are tonically activated, thus driving proliferation autonomously. *Raf* and the mitogen-activated kinases, MAPKK and MAPK, amplify the growth signal in a kinase cascade. "Brakes" to cell cycle progression include the p53-mediated G_1 to S-phase checkpoint, mediated by the CDK inhibitors p16[INK4a] and p21[WAF1]. Progression through S-phase is also promoted by CDK2 acting in concert with cyclins E and A, and initiation of cell division is governed by the action of CDK1 acting in concert with cyclin B.

(CDKs) are enzymes that critically regulate cell cycle progression from one phase to the next. One important checkpoint is mediated by the p53 tumor-suppressor gene product, acting through its upregulation of the p21[WAF1] inhibitor of CDK function, acting on CDKs 4 or 6. These kinase molecules can also be inhibited by the p16[INK4A] and p27[KIP1] CDK inhibitors, but in turn are activated by cyclins of the D family (which appear during G_1) and the proper sequence of regulatory phosphorylations. Activated CDKs 4 or 6 phosphorylate, and thus inactivate, the product of the retinoblastoma susceptibility gene, *pRb*, which in its nonphosphorylated state complexes with transcription factors of the E2F family. Phosphorylated *pRb* releases E2Fs, which activate genes important in completing DNA replication during S-phase, progression through which is promoted by CDK2 acting in concert with cylins A and E. During G_2, another checkpoint occurs, in which the cell assures the completion of correct DNA synthesis. Cells then progress into M-phase under the influence of CDK1 and cyclin B. Cells may then go on to a subsequent division cycle or enter into a quiescent, differentiated state.

Also shown in Fig. 70-2 are the sites of action of protooncogenes, regulators of cellular proliferation that, in an active state, promote cell growth, and whose deregulation produces oncogenes, originally discovered as the genes encoded by tumor-forming viruses in animals. Oncogenes can be divided into two families: (1) those that act in the cytoplasm to disrupt normal growth factor–related signaling, including *ras*, *raf*, and the tyrosine kinases of the *src* and *erbB* or *sis* families; and (2) nuclear oncogenes, including *jun*, *fos*, *myc*, and *myb*, that act to alter transcriptional control of cassettes of genes. In contrast, tumor-suppressor genes, including *p53* and *pRb*, act as cellular "brakes" whose normal function is to inhibit or prevent unregulated cellular growth. The capacity to divide indefinitely is provided by activation of telomerase, which allows continued replication of chromosomes by addressing the unique need of chromosome ends to be continually renewed to a proper length to allow normal mitosis. The capacity to invade and metastasize is conveyed by elaboration of matrix metalloproteases and plasminogen activators and the capacity to recruit host stromal cells at the site of invasion through tumor-induced angiogenesis.

Currently used drugs for the treatment of cancer focus principally on the proximate biochemistry of nucleic acid and mitotic spindle structure or function. Drugs of the future may seek to replace lost function of tumor-suppressor genes; counter the action of activated oncogenes; influence the capacity of cells to die; prevent normal chromosomal end replication; actually infect cells with viruses designed to replicate in the milieu of the cancer but not the normal cell; cause differentiation of cells with exit from the cell cycle by activating the appropriate genes; and use immunologic strategies, including antibodies and engineered cells to be directed at targets expressed on the surface of cancer cells.

BIOLOGIC BASIS FOR CANCER CHEMOTHERAPY The classic view of how cancer chemotherapeutic agents cause regressions of tumors focused on animal models such as the L1210 murine leukemia system, where cancer cells grow exponentially after inoculation into the peritoneal cavity of an isogenic mouse. The interaction of drug with its biochemical target in the cancer cell was proposed to result in "unbalanced growth" that was not sustainable and therefore resulted in cell death, directly as a result of interacting with the drug's proximal target. Agents could be categorized (Fig. 70-3) as cell cycle–active, phase-specific (e.g., antimetabolites, purines, and pyrimidines in S-phase; vinca alkaloids in M), and phase-nonspecific agents [e.g., alkylators, and antitumor antibiotics including the anthracyclines, dactinomycin (formerly actinomycin D), and mitomycin], which can injure DNA at any phase of the cell cycle but appear to then block in S-phase or G_2 at a checkpoint in the cell cycle before cell division. Cells arrested at a checkpoint may repair DNA lesions. Checkpoints have been defined at the G_1 to S transition, mediated by the tumor-suppressor gene *p53* (giving rise to the characterization of *p53* as a "guardian of the genome"); at the G_2 to M transition, mediated by the *chk1* kinase and additional p53-related pathways influencing the function of CDK1; and during M-phase, to ensure the integrity of the mitotic spindle. The importance of the concept of checkpoints extends from the hypothesis that repair of chemotherapy-mediated damage can occur while cells are stopped at a checkpoint; therefore, manipulation of checkpoint function emerges as an important basis of affecting resistance to chemotherapeutic agents.

Resistance to drugs was postulated to arise either from cells not being in the appropriate phase of the cell cycle or from decreased uptake, increased efflux, metabolism of the drug, or alteration of the target, e.g., by mutation or overexpression. Indeed, p170PGP (p170 P-glycoprotein; *mdr* gene product) was recognized from experiments with cells growing in tissue culture as mediating the efflux of chemotherapeutic agents in resistant cells. Certain neoplasms, particularly hematopoietic tumors, have an adverse prognosis if they express high levels of p170PGP, and modulation of this protein's function has been attempted by a variety of strategies.

Combinations of agents were proposed to afford the opportunity to affect many different targets or portions of the cell cycle at once, particularly if the toxic effects for the host of the different components of the combination were distinct. Combinations of agents were actually more effective in animal model systems than single agents, particularly if the tumor cell inoculum was high. This thinking led to the design of "combination chemotherapy" regimens, where drugs acting by different mechanisms (e.g., an alkylating agent plus an antimetabolite plus a mitotic spindle blocker) were combined. Particular combinations were chosen to emphasize drugs whose individual toxicities to the host were, if possible, distinct.

This view of cancer drug action is grossly oversimplified. Most tumors do not grow in an exponential pattern but rather follow Gompertzian kinetics, where the rate of tumor growth decreases as tumor mass increases (Fig. 70-1). Thus, a tumor has quiescent, differentiated compartments; proliferating compartments; and both well-vascularized and necrotic regions. Also, cell death is itself a closely regulated process. *Necrosis* refers to cell death induced, for example, by physical damage with the hallmarks of cell swelling and membrane disruption. *Apoptosis*, or programmed cell death, refers to a highly ordered process whereby cells respond to defined stimuli by dying, and it recapitulates the necessary cell death observed during the ontogeny of the organism. *Anoikis* refers to death of epithelial cells after removal from the normal milieu of substrate, particularly from cell-to-cell contact. Cancer chemotherapeutic agents can cause both necrosis and apoptosis. Apoptosis is characterized by chromatin condensation (giving rise to "apoptotic bodies"); cell shrinkage; and, in living animals, phagocytosis by surrounding stromal cells without evidence of inflammation. This process is regulated either by signal transduction systems that promote a cell's demise after a certain level of insult is achieved, or in response to specific cell-surface receptors that mediate cell death signals. Modulation of apoptosis by manipulation of signal transduction pathways has emerged as a basis for understanding the actions of currently used drugs and designing new strategies to improve their use.

The current view envisions that the interaction of a chemotherapeutic drug with its target, e.g., of an alkylating agent with DNA, causes or is itself a signal that initiates a "cascade" of further signaling steps to trigger an "execution phase" where proteases, nucleases, and endogenous regulators of the cell death pathway are activated. Effective cancer chemotherapeutic agents are efficient activators of apoptosis through signal transduction pathways (Fig. 70-4). For example, in the cytokine-mediated pathway, exogenous ligands such as the Fas ligand (FasL) bind to cell-surface receptors (CD95; Fas), or tumor necrosis factor (TNF) or its homologue Apo2L binds to its cognate receptors and directly recruits accessory molecules to activate a protease cascade (utilizing members of the caspase family of *cys*teine *asp*artyl prote*ases*), resulting in apoptosis. In a second pathway, growth factor deprivation elicits poorly defined signals that result in protease activation. Chemotherapeutic agents create molecular lesions (in DNA or cellular membranes) as a consequence of combining with their respective molecular targets. These lesions are sensed by a cellular "damage sensor," whose molecular nature is unclear, which leads to mitochondrial damage. Release of mitochondrial factors (e.g.,

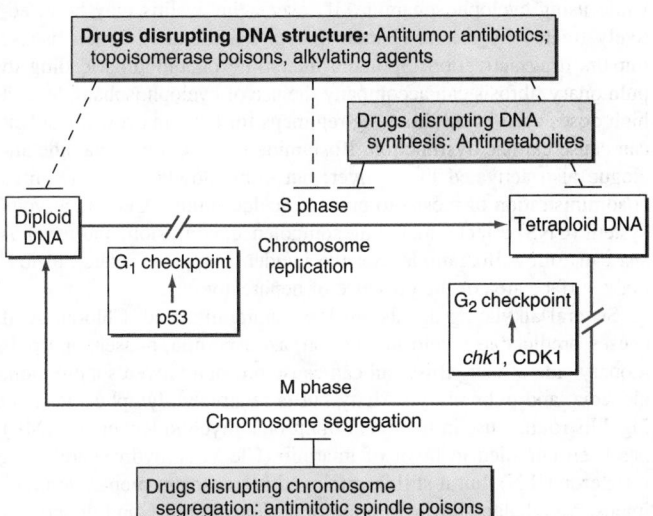

FIGURE 70-3 Location of drug action in the cell cycle. Cancer chemotherapy agents can be broadly described as phase-specific agents acting in S-(antimetabolites) and M-(spindle poisons) phase, respectively, and phase-nonspecific agents that injure their targets throughout the cycle but cause arrest of cell cycle progression at checkpoints. The G_1 checkpoint is mediated through p53 acting on CDKs 4,6, and 2, and the G_2 checkpoint is mediated in part by the *chk1* kinase acting on CDK1.

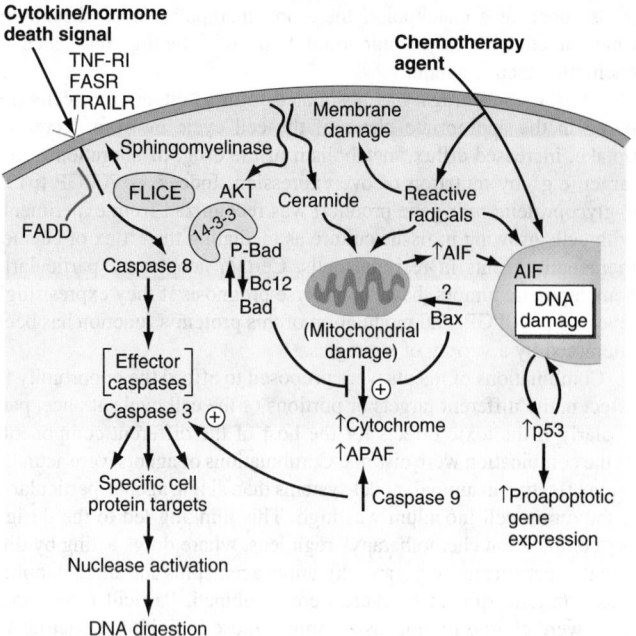

FIGURE 70-4 Integration of cell death responses. Cell death through an apoptotic mechanism requires active participation of the cell. In response to hormonal or cytokine death signals, receptors activate "upstream" cysteine aspartyl proteases (caspases), which then directly digest cytoplasmic and nuclear proteins, resulting in activation of "downstream" caspases; these cause activation of nucleases resulting in the characteristic DNA fragmentation that is a hallmark of apoptosis. Chemotherapy agents that create lesions in DNA seem to activate aspects of this process through a pathway that appears to result in damage to mitochondria, perhaps by activating the transcription of genes whose products can produce or modulate the toxicity of free radicals. In addition, membrane damage with activation of sphingomyelinases results in the production of ceramides that can have a direct action at mitochondria. The antiapoptotic protein bcl2 attenuates mitochondrial toxicity, while proapoptotic gene products such as bax antagonize the action of bcl2. Damaged mitochondria release cytochrome C and "apoptosis activating factor," which can directly activate caspase 9, resulting in propagation of a direct signal to other downstream caspases through protease activation. Apoptosis-inducing factor (AIF) is also released from the mitochondrion and then can translocate to the nucleus, bind to DNA, and generate free radicals to further damage DNA. An additional proapoptotic stimulus is the bad protein, which can heterodimerize with bcl2 gene family members to antagonize apoptosis. Importantly, though, bad protein function can be retarded by its sequestration as phospho-bad through the 14-3-3 adapter proteins. The phosphorylation of bad is mediated by the action of the AKT kinase in a way that defines how growth factors that activate this kinase can retard apoptosis and promote cell survival.

APAF1, cytochrome c) promotes the activation of another set of caspases. Apoptosis-inducing factor (AIF) is another mitochondrial factor that upon release can translocate to the nucleus and promote DNA damage in its own right, without necessarily activating caspases. Damage to the plasma membrane, e.g., from free radicals generated by certain chemotherapeutic agents, leads to activation of acid sphingomyelinase to release lipid components including ceramides, which then promote apoptosis through a variety of pathways including direct mitochondrial damage.

While apoptotic mechanisms are important in regulating cellular proliferation and the behavior of tumor cells in vitro, in vivo it is unclear whether all of the actions of chemotherapeutic agents to cause cell death can be attributed to apoptotic mechanisms. Loss of clonogenic survival (conventionally detecting the capacity of a few cells to survive) may predict clinical value more reliably than detection of apoptotic changes in the majority of tumor cells. However, changes in molecules that regulate apoptosis are clearly correlated with clinical outcomes (e.g., bcl$_2$ overexpression in certain lymphomas conveys poor prognosis; proapoptotic bax expression is associated with a better outcome in ovarian carcinoma). A better understanding of the relationship of cell death and cell survival mechanisms is needed.

CHEMOTHERAPEUTIC AGENTS USED FOR CANCER TREATMENT Table 70-2 lists commonly used cancer chemotherapy agents and pertinent clinical aspects of their use. The drugs and schedules listed are examples of regimens that have proved tolerable and useful; the specific doses that may be used in a particular patient may vary somewhat with the particular treatment protocol, or plan, of treatment. Significant variation from these dose ranges should be carefully verified to avoid or anticipate toxicity. Not included in Table 70-2 are hormone receptor–directed agents, as the side effects are generally those expected from the interruption or augmentation of hormonal effect, and doses used in most cases are those that adequately saturate the intended hormone receptor. The drugs listed may be usefully grouped into three general categories: those affecting DNA, those affecting microtubules, and molecularly targeted agents.

Direct DNA-Interactive Agents ■ *FORMATION OF COVALENT DNA ADDUCTS* Alkylating agents as a class break down, either spontaneously or after normal organ or tumor cell metabolism, to reactive intermediates that covalently modify bases in DNA. This leads to cross-linkage of DNA strands or the appearance of breaks in DNA as a result of repair efforts. "Broken" or cross-linked DNA is intrinsically unable to complete normal replication or cell division; in addition, it is a potent activator of cell cycle checkpoints and signaling pathways that can activate apoptosis. As a class, alkylating agents share similar toxicities: myelosuppression, alopecia, gonadal dysfunction, mucositis, and pulmonary fibrosis. They differ greatly in a spectrum of normal organ toxicities. As a class they share the capacity to cause "second" neoplasms, particularly leukemia, many years after use, particularly when used in low doses for protracted periods.

Nitrogen mustard (mechlorethamine) is the prototypic agent of this class, decomposing rapidly in aqueous solution to yield potentially a bifunctional carbonium ion. It must be administered shortly after preparation into a rapidly flowing intravenous line. It is a powerful vesicant, and infiltration may be symptomatically ameliorated by infiltration of the affected site with 1/6 *M* thiosulfate. Even without infiltration, aseptic thrombophlebitis is frequent. It can be used topically as a dilute solution in cutaneous lymphomas, with a notable incidence of hypersensitivity reactions. It causes moderate nausea after intravenous administration.

Cyclophosphamide is inactive unless metabolized by the liver to 4-hydroxy-cyclophosphamide, which decomposes into alkylating species, as well as to chloroacetaldehyde and acrolein. The latter causes chemical cystitis; therefore excellent hydration must be maintained while using cyclophosphamide. If severe, the cystitis may be effectively treated by mesna (2-mercaptoethanesulfonate). Liver disease impairs drug activation. Sporadic interstitial pneumonitis leading to pulmonary fibrosis can accompany the use of cyclophosphamide, and high doses used in conditioning regimens for bone marrow transplant can cause cardiac dysfunction. Ifosfamide is a cyclophosphamide analogue also activated in the liver, but more slowly, and it requires coadministration of mesna to prevent bladder injury. Central nervous system (CNS) effects, including somnolence, confusion, and psychosis, can follow ifosfamide use; the incidence appears related to low body surface area or the presence of nephrectomy.

Several alkylating agents are less commonly used. Chlorambucil causes predictable myelosuppression, azoospermia, nausea, and pulmonary side effects. Busulfan can cause profound myelosuppression, alopecia, and pulmonary toxicity but is relatively "lymphocyte sparing." Its routine use in treatment of chronic myeloid leukemia (CML) has been curtailed in favor of imatinib (Gleevec), hydroxyurea, and interferon (IFN), but it still is employed in transplant preparation regimens. Melphalan shows variable oral bioavailability and undergoes extensive binding to albumin and α_1-acidic glycoprotein. Mucositis appears more prominently.

Nitrosoureas break down to carbamoylating species that not only cause a distinct pattern of DNA base pair–directed toxicity but also can covalently modify proteins. They share the feature of causing relatively delayed bone marrow toxicity, which can be cumulative and

TABLE 70-2 *Commonly Used Cancer Chemotherapy Agents*

Drug	Examples of Usual Doses	Toxicity	Interactions, Issues
DIRECT DNA-INTERACTING AGENTS			
Alkylators			
Cyclophosphamide	400–2000 mg/m² IV 100 mg/m² PO qd	Marrow (relative platelet sparing) Cystitis Common alkylator[a] Cardiac (high dose)	Liver metabolism required to activate to phosphoramide mustard + acrolein Mesna protects against "high-dose" bladder damage
Mechlorethamine	6 mg/m² IV day 1 and day 8	Marrow Vesicant Nausea	Topical use in cutaneous lymphoma
Chlorambucil	1–3 mg/m² qd PO	Marrow Common alkylator[a]	
Melphalan	8 mg/m² qd × 5, PO	Marrow (delayed nadir) GI (high dose)	Decreased renal function delays clearance
Carmustine (BCNU)	200 mg/m² IV 150 mg/m² PO	Marrow (delayed nadir) GI, liver (high dose) Renal	
Lomustine (CCNU)	100–300 mg/m² PO	Marrow (delayed nadir)	
Ifosfamide	1.2 g/m² per day qd × 5 + mesna	Myelosuppressive Bladder Neurologic Metabolic acidosis Neuropathy	Isomeric analogue of cyclophosphamide More lipid soluble Greater activity vs testicular neoplasms and sarcomas Must use mesna
Procarbazine	100 mg/m² per day qd ×14	Marrow Nausea Neurologic Common alkylator[a]	Liver and tissue metabolism required Disulfiran-like effect with ethanol Acts as MAOI HBP after tyrosinase-rich foods
Dacarbazine (DTIC)	375 mg/m² IV day 1 & day 15	Marrow Nausea Flulike	Metabolic activation
Temozolomide	150–200 mg/m² qd × 5 q28d *or* 75 mg/m² qd × 6–7 weeks	Nausea/vomiting Headache/fatigue Constipation	Infrequent myelosuppression
Altretamine (formerly hexamethylmelamine)	260 mg/m² per day qd ×14–21 as 4 divided oral doses	Nausea Neurologic (mood swing) Neuropathy Marrow (less)	Liver activation Barbiturates enchance/cimetidine diminishes
Cisplatin	20 mg/m² qd ×5 IV 1 q3–4 weeks *or* 100–200 mg/m² per dose IV q3–4 weeks	Nausea Neuropathy Auditory Marrow platelets > WBCs Renal Mg²⁺, Ca²⁺	Maintain high urine flow; osmotic diuresis, monitor intake/output K⁺, Mg²⁺ Emetogenic—prophylaxis needed Full dose if CrCl > 60 mL/min and tolerate fluid push
Carboplatin	365 mg/m² IV q3–4 weeks as adjusted for CrCl	Marrow platelets > WBCs Nausea Renal (high dose)	Reduce dose according to CrCl: to AUC of 5–7 mg/mL per min [AUC = dose/(CrCl + 25)]
Oxaliplatin	130 mg/m² q3 weeks over 2 h *or* 85 mg/m² q2 weeks	Nausea Anemia	Acute reversible neurotoxicity; chronic sensory neurotox cumulative with dose; reversible laryngopharyngeal spasm
Antitumor antibiotics			
Bleomycin	15–25 mg/d qd ×5 IV bolus or continuous IV	Pulmonary Skin effects Raynaud's Hypersensitivity	Inactivate by bleomycin hydrolase (decreased in lung/skin) O₂ enhances pulmonary toxicity Cisplatin-induced decrease in CrCl may increase skin/lung toxicity Reduce dose if CrCl < 60 mL/min
Actinomycin D	10–15 μg/kg per day qd ×5 IV bolus	Marrow Nausea Mucositis Vesicant Alopecia	Radiation recall

(continued)

TABLE 70-2 *Commonly Used Cancer Chemotherapy Agents*—(Continued)

Drug	Examples of Usual Doses	Toxicity	Interactions, Issues
Mithramycin	15–20 µg/kg qd ×4–7 (hypercalcemia) *or* 50 µg/kg qod ×3–8 (antineoplastic)	Marrow Liver Renal Mucositis Hypocalcemia Nausea Vesicant	Acute hemorrhagic syndrome
Mitomycin C	6–10 mg/m² q6 weeks	Marrow Vesicant Hemolytic-uremic syndrome Lung CV—heart failure	Treat superficial bladder cancers by intravesical infusion Delayed marrow toxicity Cumulative marrow toxicity
Etoposide (VP16-213)	100–150 mg/m² IV qd ×3–5d *or* 50 mg/m² PO qd ×21d *or* up to 1500 mg/m² per dose (high dose with stem cell support)	Marrow (WBCs > platelet) Alopecia Hypotension Hypersensitivity (rapid IV) Nausea Mucositis (high dose)	Hepatic metabolism—renal 30% Reduce doses with renal failure Schedule-dependant (5 day better than 1 day) Late leukemogenic Accentuate antimetabolite action
Teniposide (VM-26)	150–200 mg/m² twice per week for 4 weeks	Marrow Alopecia	
Amsacrine	100–150 mg/m² IV qd ×5	Marrow Mucositis Nausea CV—arrhythmia (avoid hypokalemia)	Decrease dose by 30% if liver or renal failure
Topotecan	20 mg/m² IV q3–4 weeks over 30 min *or* 1.5–3 mg/m² q3–4 weeks over 24 h *or* 0.5 mg/m² per day over 21 days	Marrow Mucositis Nausea Mild alopecia	Reduce dose with renal failure No liver toxicity
Irinotecan (CPT II)	100–150 mg/m² IV over 90 min q3–4 weeks *or* 30 mg/m² per day over 120 h	Diarrhea: "early onset" with cramping, flushing, vomiting; "late onset" after several doses Marrow Alopecia Nausea Vomiting Pulmonary	Prodrug requires enzymatic clearance to active drug "SN 38" Early diarrhea likely due to biliary excretion Late diarrhea, use "high-dose" loperamide (2 mg q2–4 h)
Doxorubicin and daunorubicin	45–60 mg/m² dose q3–4 weeks *or* 10–30 mg/m² dose q week *or* continuous-infusion regimen	Marrow Mucositis Alopecia Cardiovascular acute/chronic Vesicant	Heparin aggregate; coadministration increases clearance Acetaminophen, BCNU increase liver toxicity Radiation recall
Idarubicin	10–15 mg/m² IV q 3 weeks *or* 10 mg/m² IV qd ×3	Marrow Cardiac (less than doxorubicin)	None established
Epirubicin	150 mg/m² IV q3 weeks	Marrow Cardiac	None established
Mitoxantrone	12 mg/m² qd ×3 *or* 12–14 mg/m² q3 weeks	Marrow Cardiac (less than doxorubicin) Vesicant (mild) Blue urine, sclerae, nails	Interacts with heparin Less alopecia, nausea than doxorubicin Radiation recall

INDIRECT DNA-INTERACTING AGENTS

Antimetabolites Deoxycoformycin	4 mg/m² IV every other week	Nausea Immunosuppression Neurologic Renal	Excretes in urine Reduce dose for renal failure Inhibits adenosine deaminase
6-Mercaptopurine	75 mg/m² PO *or* up 500 mg/m² PO (high dose)	Marrow Liver Nausea	Variable bioavailability Metabolize by xanthine oxidase Decrease dose with allopurinol Increased toxicity with thiopurine methyltransferase deficiency

TABLE 70-2— (Continued)

Drug	Examples of Usual Doses	Toxicity	Interactions, Issues
6-Thioguanine	2–3 mg/kg per day for up to 3–4 weeks	Marrow Liver Nausea	Variable bioavailability Increased toxicity with thiopurine methyltransferase deficiency

Azathioprine	1–5 mg/kg per day	Marrow
		Nausea
		Liver
			Metabolizes to 6MP, therefore reduce dose
			  with allopurinol
			Increased toxicity with thiopurine
			  methyltransferase deficiency

2-Chlorodeoxyadenosine	0.09 mg/kg per day qd ×7 as continuous infusion	Marrow Renal Fever	Notable use in hairy cell leukemia
Hydroxyurea	20–50 mg/kg (lean body weight) PO qd or 1–3 g/d	Marrow Nausea Mucositis Skin changes Rare renal, liver, lung, CNS	Decrease dose with renal failure Augments antimetabolite effect
Methotrexate	15–30 mg PO or IM qd ×3–5 or 30 mg IV days 1 and 8 or 1.5–12 g/m² per day (with leucovorin)	Marrow Liver/lung Renal tubular Mucositis	Rescue with leucovorin Excreted in urine Decrease dose in renal failure NSAIDs increase renal toxicity
5-Fluorouracil	375 mg/m² IV qd ×5 or 600 mg/m² IV days 1 and 8	Marrow Mucositis Neurologic Skin changes	Toxicity enhanced by leucovorin Dihydropyrimidine dehydrogenase deficiency increases toxicity Metabolizes in tissues

Capecitabine	665 mg/m² bid continuous; 1250 mg/m² bid
	  2 weeks on/ 1 off; 829 mg/m² bid 2
	  weeks on/ 1 off + 60 mg/d leucovorin
		Diarrhea
		Hand-foot syndrome
			Prodrug of 5FU due to intratumoral
			  metabolism

Cytosine arabinoside	100 mg/m² per day qd ×7 by continuous
	  infusion
	or 1–3 g/m² dose IV bolus
		Marrow
		Mucositis
		Neurologic (high dose)
		Conjunctivitis (high dose)
		Noncardiogenic pulmonary
		  edema
			Enhances activity of alkylating agents
			Metabolizes in tissues by deamination

Azacytidine	750 mg/m² per week
	or 150–200 mg/m² per day ×5–10 (bolus)
	  or (continuous IV)
		Marrow
		Nausea
		Liver
		Neurologic
		Myalgia
			Use limited to leukemia
			Altered methylation of DNA alters gene
			  expression

Gemcitabine	1000 mg/m² IV weekly ×7	Marrow Nausea Hepatic Fever/"flu syndrome"	
Fludarabine phosphate	25 mg/m² IV qd ×5	Marrow Neurologic Lung	Dose reduction with renal failure Metabolized to F-ara converted to F-ara ATP in cells by deoxycytidine kinase
Asparaginase	25,000 IU/m² q3–4 weeks or 6000 IU/m² per day qod for 3–4 weeks or 1000–2000 IU/m² for 10–20 days	Protein synthesis Clotting factors Glucose Albumin Hypersensitivity CNS Pancreatitis Hepatic	Blocks methotrexate action

Antimitotic agents
Vincristine
	1–1.4 mg/m² per week	Vesicant
		Marrow
		Neurologic
		GI: ileus/constipation; bladder
		  hypotoxicity; SIADH
		Cardiovascular
			Hepatic clearance
			Dose reduction for bilirubin
			  >1.5 mg/dL
			Prophylactic bowel regimen

(continued)

TABLE 70-2 *Commonly Used Cancer Chemotherapy Agents—(Continued)*

Drug	Examples of Usual Doses	Toxicity	Interactions, Issues
Vinblastine	6–8 mg/m² per week	Vesicant Marrow Neurologic (less common but similar spectrum to other vincas) Hypertension Raynaud's	Hepatic clearance Dose reduction as with vincristine
Vinorelbine	15–30 mg/m² per week	Vesicant Marrow Allergic/bronchospasm (immediate) Dyspnea/cough (subacute) Neurologic (less prominent but similar spectrum to other vincas)	Hepatic clearance
Paclitaxel	135–175 mg/m² per 24-h infusion *or* 175 mg/m² per 3-h infusion *or* 140 mg/m² per 96-h infusion *or* 250 mg/m² per 24-h infusion plus G-CSF	Hypersensitivity Marrow Mucositis Alopecia Sensory neuropathy CV conduction disturbance Nausea—infrequent	Premedicate with steroids, H₁ and H₂ blockers Hepatic clearance Dose reduction as with vincas
Docetaxel	100 mg/m² per 1-h infusion q3 weeks	Hypersensitivity Fluid retention syndrome Marrow Dermatologic Sensory neuropathy Nausea infrequent Some stomatitis	Premedicate with steroids, H₁ and H₂ blockers
Estramustine phosphate	14 mg/kg per day in 3–4 divided doses with water >2 h after meals Avoid Ca²⁺-rich foods	Nausea Vomiting Diarrhea CHF Thrombosis Gynecomastia	

MOLECULARLY TARGETED AGENTS

Drug	Examples of Usual Doses	Toxicity	Interactions, Issues
Imatinib	400 mg/d, continuous	Nausea Periorbital edema	Myelosuppression not frequent in solid tumor indications
Tretinoin	45 mg/m² per day until complete response + anthrocycline-based regimen in APL	Teratogenic Cutaneous	APL differentiation syndrome: pulmonary dysfunction/infiltrate, pleural/pericardial effusion, fever
Bexarotene	300–400 mg/m² per day, continuous	Hypercholesterolemia Hypertriglyceridemia Cutaneous Teratogenic	Central hypothyroidism
Gemtuzumab ogomicin	9 mg/m² over 2 h q2 weeks, usually followed by chemotherapy or marrow transplant	Neutropenia Thrombosytopenia Hepatic	Postinfusion syndrome: fever, chills, hypotension Rare hepatic venoocclusive disease Mucositis uncommon
Denileukin deftitox	9–18 μg/kg per day × 5 d q 3 wk	Nausea/vomiting Chills/fever Asthenia Hepatic	Acute hypersensitivity: hypotension, vasodilation, rash, chest tightness Vascular leak: hypotension, edema, hypoalbuminemia, thrombotic events (MI, DVT, CVA)

MISCELLANEOUS

Drug	Examples of Usual Doses	Toxicity	Interactions, Issues
Arsenic trioxide	0.16 mg/kg per day up to 50 days in APL	↑QT_c Peripheral neuropathy Musculoskeletal pain Hyperglycemia	APL differentiation syndrome (see under tretinoin)

[a] Common alkylator: alopecia, pulmonary, infertility, plus teratogenesis.
Note: APL, acute promyelocytic leukemia; AUC, area under the curve; CHF, congestive heart failure; CNS, central nervous system; CrCl, creatinine clearance; CV, cardiovascular; CVA, cerebrovascular accident; DVT, deep venous thrombosis; G-CSF, granulocyte col- ony-stimulating factor; GI, gastrointestinal; HBP, high blood pressure; MAOI, monoamine oxidase inhibitors; MI, myocardial infarction; 6MP, 6-mercaptopurine; NSAIDs, nonsteroidal anti-inflammatory drugs; SIADH, syndrome of inappropriate antidiuretic hormone; WBCs, white blood cells.

long-lasting. Streptozotocin is unique in that its glucose-like structure conveys specific toxicity to the islet cells of the pancreas (for whose derivative tumor types it is prominently indicated) as well as causing renal toxicity in the form of Fanconi's syndrome, including amino aciduria, glycosuria, and renal tubular acidosis. Methyl CCNU (lomustine) causes direct glomerular as well as tubular damage, cumulatively related to dose and time of exposure.

Procarbazine is metabolized in the liver and possibly in tumor cells to yield a variety of free radical and alkylating species. In addition to myelosuppression, it causes hypnotic and other CNS effects, including vivid nightmares. It can cause a disulfiram-like syndrome on ingestion of ethanol. Altretamine (formerly hexamethylmelamine) and thiotepa can chemically give rise to alkylating species, although the nature of the DNA damage has not been well characterized in either case. Thiotepa can be used for intrathecal treatment of neoplastic meningitis. Dacarbazine (DTIC) is activated in the liver to yield the highly reactive methyl diazonium cation. It causes only modest myelosuppression 21 to 25 days after a dose but causes prominent nausea on day 1. Temozolomide is structurally related to dacarbazine but was designed to be activated by nonenzymatic hydrolysis in tumors, and is orally bioavailable.

Cisplatin was discovered fortuitously by observing that bacteria present in electrolysis solutions could not divide. Only the *cis* diamine configuration is active as an antitumor agent. It is hypothesized that in the intracellular environment, a chloride is lost from each position, being replaced by a water molecule. The resulting positively charged species is an efficient bifunctional interactor with DNA, forming Pt-based cross-links. Cisplatin requires administration with adequate hydration, including forced diuresis with mannitol to prevent kidney damage; even with the use of hydration, gradual decrease in kidney function is common, along with noteworthy anemia. Hypomagnesemia frequently attends cisplatin use and can lead to hypocalcemia and tetany. Other common toxicities include neurotoxocity with stocking and glove sensorimotor neuropathy. Hearing loss occurs in 50% of patients treated with conventional doses. Cisplatin is intensely emetogenic, requiring prophylactic antiemetics. Myelosuppression is less evident than with other alkylating agents. Chronic vascular toxicity (Raynaud's syndrome, coronary artery disease) is a more unusual toxicity. Carboplatin displays less nephro-, oto-, and neurotoxicity. However, myelosuppression is more frequent, and as the drug is exclusively cleared through the kidney, adjustment of dose for creatinine clearance must be accomplished through use of various dosing nomograms. Oxaliplatin is used in colon cancers refractory to other treatments. Its place in the primary and adjuvant treatment of colon tumors is being defined, along with tests of activity in other tumors. It is prominently neurotoxic.

ANTITUMOR ANTIBIOTICS AND TOPOISOMERASE POISONS Antitumor antibiotics are substances produced by bacteria that in nature appear to provide chemical defense against other hostile microorganisms. As a class they bind to DNA directly and can frequently undergo electron transfer reactions to generate free radicals in close proximity to DNA, leading to DNA damage in the form of single strand breaks or cross-links. Topoisomerase poisons include natural products or semi-synthetic species derived ultimately from plants, and they modify enzymes that regulate the capacity of DNA to unwind to allow normal replication or transcription. DNA damage from these agents can occur in any cell cycle phase, but cells tend to arrest in S-phase or G_2 of the cell cycle in cells with p53 and Rb pathway lesions as the result of defective checkpoint mechanisms in cancer cells.

Doxorubicin is the most widely active and frequently used antineoplastic agent. It can intercalate into DNA, thereby altering DNA structure, replication, and topoisomerase function. It can also undergo redox cycling by accepting electrons into its quinone ring system. It causes predictable myelosuppression, alopecia, nausea, and mucositis. In addition, it causes acute cardiotoxicity in the form of atrial and ventricular dysrhythmias, but these are rarely of clinical significance. In contrast, cumulative doses >550 mg/m^2 are associated with a 10% incidence of chronic cardiomyopathy. The incidence of cardiomyopathy appears to be related to schedule (peak serum concentration), with low dose, frequent treatment, or continuous infusions better tolerated than intermittent higher dose exposures. Its cardiotoxicity is increased when given together with trastuzumab (Herceptin), the anti-HER2/*neu* antibody. Radiation recall or interaction with concomitantly administered radiation to cause local site complications is frequent. The drug is a powerful vesicant, with necrosis of tissue apparent 4 to 7 days after an extravasation; therefore it should be administered into a rapidly flowing intravenous line. The drug is metabolized by the liver, so doses must be reduced by 50 to 75% in the presence of liver dysfunction. Daunorubicin is closely related to doxorubicin and was actually introduced first into leukemia treament, where it remains part of curative regimens and has been shown preferable to doxorubicin owing to less mucositis and colonic damage. Idarubicin is an orally acting doxorubicin analogue whose ultimate place in therapy is uncertain. Encapsulation of daunorubicin into a liposome has been accomplished, with attenuation of cardiac toxicity and noteworthy activity in Kaposi's sarcoma. Liposome-encapsulated doxorubicin may have activity in prostate cancer.

Bleomycin refers to a mixture of glycopeptides that have the unique feature of forming complexes with Fe^{2+} while also bound to DNA. Oxidation of Fe^{2+} gives rise to superoxide and hydroxyl radicals. The drug causes little, if any, myelosuppression. The drug is cleared rapidly, but augmented skin and pulmonary toxicity in the presence of renal failure has led to the recommendation that doses be reduced by 50 to 75% in the face of a creatinine clearance <25 mL/min. Bleomycin is not a vesicant and can be administered intravenously, intramuscularly, or subcutaneously. Common side effects include fever and chills, facial flush, and Raynaud's syndrome. Hypertension can follow rapid intravenous administration, and the incidence of anaphylaxis with early preparations of the drug has led to the practice of administering a test dose of 0.5 to 1 unit before the rest of the dose. The most feared complication of bleomycin treatment is pulmonary fibrosis, which increases in incidence at >300 cumulative units administered and is minimally responsive to treatment (e.g., glucocorticoids). The earliest indicator of an adverse effect is a decline in the DL_{CO}, although cessation of drug immediately upon documentation of a decrease in DL_{CO} may not prevent further decline in pulmonary function. Bleomycin is inactivated by a bleomycin hydrolase, whose concentration is diminished in skin and lung. Because bleomycin-dependent electron transport is dependent on O_2, bleomycin toxicity may become apparent after exposure to transient very high PI_{O_2}. Thus, during surgical procedures, patients with prior exposure to bleomycin should be maintained on the lowest PI_{O_2} consistent with maintaining adequate tissue oxygenation.

Dactinomycin intercalates into DNA and appears to have less, but not absent, capacity to undergo electron transfer reactions. It causes severe myelosuppression, nausea, alopecia, and mucositis. It is a notable vesicant. Mithramycin historically was used against testicular and other neoplasms; however, in addition to causing nausea, myelosuppression, and vesicant properties, it causes an acute hemorrhagic syndrome consisting of platelet function defects in association with indicators of disseminated intravascular coagulation. It is used in current practice to control hypercalcemia. In addition, renal and hepatic dysfunction may complicate its use.

Mitomycin C undergoes reduction of its quinone function to generate a bifunctional DNA alkylating agent. It is a broadly active antineoplastic agent with a number of unpredictable toxicities, including delayed bronchospasm 12 to 14 h after dosing and a chronic pulmonary fibrosis syndrome more frequent at doses of 50 to 60 mg/m^2. Cardiomyopathy has been described, particularly in a setting of prior radiation therapy. A hemolytic/uremic syndrome carries an ultimate mortality rate of 25 to 50% and is poorly treated by conventional component support and exchange transfusion. Mitomycin is a notable vesicant and causes substantial nausea and vomiting. It can be used for intravesical instillation for curative treatment of superficial transitional bladder carcinomas and, with radiation therapy, for curative treatment of anal carcinoma.

Mitoxantrone is a synthetic compound that was designed to recapitulate features of doxorubicin but with less cardiotoxicity. It is quantitatively less cardiotoxic (comparing the ratio of cardiotoxic to therapeutically effective doses), but its status in therapy is unclear as doses of 150 mg/m^2 have produced evidence of 10% incidence of cardiotoxicity; it also causes alopecia.

Etoposide was synthetically derived from the plant product podophyllotoxin; it binds directly to topoisomerase II and DNA in a reversible ternary complex. It stabilizes the covalent intermediate in the enzyme's action where the enzyme is covalently linked to DNA. This "alkali-labile" DNA bond was historically a first hint that an enzyme such as a topoisomerase might exist. The drug therefore causes a prominent G$_2$ arrest, reflecting the action of a DNA damage checkpoint. Prominent clinical effects include myelosuppression, nausea, and transient hypotension related to the speed of administration of the agent. Etoposide is a mild vesicant but is relatively free from other large-organ toxicities. Teniposide is a structural relative with unique activity in childhood acute lymphoid leukemia. When given at high doses or very frequently, topoisomerase inhibitors may cause acute leukemia associated with chromosome 11q23 abnormalities in up to 1% of exposed patients.

Camptothecin was isolated from extracts of a Chinese tree and had notable antileukemia activity. Early clinical studies with the sodium salt of the hydrolyzed camptothecin lactone showed evidence of toxicity with little antitumor activity. Identification of topoisomerase I as the target of camptothecins and the need to preserve lactone structure allowed additional efforts to identify active members of this series. Topoisomerase I is responsible for unwinding the DNA strand by introducing single strand breaks and allowing rotation of one strand about the other. In S-phase, topoisomerase I–induced breaks that are not promptly resealed lead to progress of the replication fork off the end of a DNA strand. The DNA damage is a potent signal for induction of apoptosis. Camptothecins promote the stabilization of the DNA linked to the enzyme in a so-called cleavable complex, analogous to the action of etoposide with topoisomerase II. Topotecan is a camptothecin derivative approved for use in ovarian tumors. Toxicity is limited to myelosuppression and mucositis. CPT-11, or irinotecan, is a camptothecin with evidence of activity in colon carcinoma. In addition to myelosuppression, it causes a secretory diarrhea, which can be treated effectively with loperamide or octreotide.

Indirect Effectors of DNA Function: Antimetabolites A broad definition of antimetabolites would include compounds with structural similarity to precursors of purines or pyrimidines or that interfere with purine or pyrimidine synthesis. Antimetabolites can cause DNA damage indirectly, through misincorporation into DNA, abnormal timing or progression through DNA synthesis, or altered function of pyrimidine and purine biosynthetic enzymes. They tend to convey greatest toxicity to cells in S-phase, and the degree of toxicity increases with duration of exposure. Common toxic manifestations include stomatitis, diarrhea, and myelosuppression. Second malignancies are not associated with their use.

Methotrexate inhibits dihydrofolate reductase, which regenerates reduced folates from the oxidized folates produced when thymidine monophosphate is formed from deoxyuridine monophosphate. Without reduced folates, cells die a "thymineless" death. N-5 tetrahydrofolate or N-5 formyltetrahydrofolate (leucovorin) can bypass this block and rescue cells from methotrexate, which is maintained in cells by polyglutamylation. The drug and other reduced folates are transported into cells by the folate carrier, and high concentrations of drug can bypass this carrier and allow diffusion of drug directly into cells. These properties have suggested the design of "high-dose" methotrexate regimens with leucovorin rescue of normal marrow and mucosa as part of curative approaches to osteosarcoma in the adjuvant setting and hematopoietic neoplasms of children and adults. Methotrexate is cleared by the kidney by both glomerular filtration and tubular secretion, and toxicity is augmented by renal dysfunction and drugs such as salicylates, probenecid, and nonsteroidal anti-inflammatory agents that undergo tubular secretion. With normal renal function, 15 mg/m^2 leucovorin will rescue 10^{-8} to 10^{-6} M methotrexate in three to four doses. However, with decreased creatinine clearance, doses of 50 to 100 mg/m^2 are continued until methotrexate levels are $<5 \times 10^{-8}$ M. In addition to bone marrow suppression and mucosal irritation, methotrexate can cause renal failure itself at high doses owing to crystallization in renal tubules; therefore high-dose regimens require alkalinization of urine with increased flow by hydration. Methotrexate can be sequestered in third space collections and leech back into the general circulation, causing prolonged myelosuppression. Less frequent adverse effects include reversible increases in transaminases and hypersensitivity-like pulmonary syndrome. Chronic low-dose methotrexate can cause hepatic fibrosis. When administered to the intrathecal space, methotrexate can cause chemical arachnoiditis and CNS dysfunction. Trimetrexate is a methotrexate derivative that is not polyglutamylated and does not use the reduced folate carrier.

5-Fluorouracil (5FU) represents an early example of "rational" drug design in that it originated from the observation that tumor cells incorporate radiolabeled uracil more efficiently into DNA than normal cells, especially gut. 5FU is metabolized in cells to 5′FdUMP, which inhibits thymidylate synthetase (TS). In addition, misincorporation can lead to single strand breaks, and RNA can aberrantly incorporate FUMP. 5FU is metabolized by dihydropyrimidine dehydrogenase, and deficiency of this enzyme can lead to excessive toxicity from 5FU. Oral bioavailability varies unreliably, but orally administered analogues of 5FU such as capecitabine have been developed that allow at least equivalent activity to many parenteral 5FU-based approaches to refractory cancers. Intravenous administration of 5FU leads to bone marrow suppression after short infusions but to stomatitis after prolonged infusions. Leucovorin augments the activity of 5FU by promoting formation of the ternary covalent complex of 5FU, the reduced folate, and TS. Less frequent toxicities include CNS dysfunction, with prominent cerebellar signs, and endothelial toxicity manifested by thrombosis, including pulmonary embolus and myocardial infarction.

Cytosine arabinoside (ara-C) is incorporated into DNA after formation of ara-CTP, resulting in S-phase-related toxicity. Continuous infusion schedules allow maximal efficiency, with uptake maximal at 5 to 7 μM. Ara-C can be administered intrathecally. Adverse effects include nausea, diarrhea, stomatitis, chemical conjunctivitis, and cerebellar ataxia. Gemcitabine is a cytosine derivative that is similar to ara-C in that it is incorporated into DNA after anabolism to the triphosphate, rendering DNA susceptible to breakage and repair synthesis, which differs from that in ara-C in that gemcitabine-induced lesions are very inefficiently removed. In contrast to ara-C, gemcitabine appears to have useful activity in a variety of solid tumors, with limited nonmyelosuppressive toxicities. 6-Thioguanine and 6-mercaptopurine (6MP) are used in the treatment of acute lymphoid leukemia. Although administered orally, they display variable bioavailability. 6MP is metabolized by xanthine oxidase and therefore requires dose reduction when used with allopurinol.

Fludarabine phosphate is a prodrug of F-adenine arabinoside (F-ara-A), which in turn was designed to diminish the susceptibility of ara-A to adenosine deaminase. F-ara-A is incorporated into DNA and can cause delayed cytotoxicity even in cells with low growth fraction, including chronic lymphocytic leukemia and follicular B cell lymphoma. CNS dysfunction and T cell depletion leading to opportunistic infections can occur in addition to myelosuppression. 2-Chlorodeoxyadenosine is a similar compound with activity in hairy cell leukemia. 2-Deoxycoformycin inhibits adenosine deaminase, with resulting increase in dATP levels. This causes inhibition of ribonucleotide reductase as well as augmented susceptibility to apoptosis, particularly in T cells. Renal failure and CNS dysfunction are notable toxicities in addition to immunosuppression.

Hydroxyurea inhibits ribonucleotide reductase, resulting in S-phase block. It is orally bioavailable and the drug of choice for the acute management of myeloproliferative states. Asparaginase is not classically considered an antimetabolite as it causes breakdown of extracellular asparagine required for protein synthesis in certain leukemic cells. However, it effectively stops DNA synthesis by preventing the requisite concurrent protein synthesis, and therefore it has a similar functional outcome as the classic antimetabolites. As asparaginase is a foreign protein, hypersensitivity reactions are common, as are effects on organs such as pancreas and liver that require continuing protein synthesis. This results in decreased insulin secretion with hyperglycemia, with or without hyperamylasemia and clotting function abnormalities. The latter may be associated with CNS and dural vein thrombosis.

Mitotic Spindle Inhibitors Microtubules are cellular structures that form the mitotic spindle and in interphase cells are responsible for the cellular "scaffolding" along which various motile and secretory processes occur. Microtubules are composed of repeating noncovalent multimers of a heterodimer of α and β subunits of the protein tubulin. Vincristine binds to the tubulin dimer with the result that microtubules are disaggregated. This results in the block of growing cells in M-phase; however, toxic effects in G_1 and S-phase are also evident. The drug is bound to blood-formed elements, leading to its occasional use as vinca-loaded platelets to treat autoimmune thrombocytopenia. The drug is metabolized by the liver, and dose adjustment in the presence of hepatic dysfunction is required. It is a powerful vesicant, and infiltration can be treated by local heat and infiltration of hyaluronidase. At clinically used intravenous doses, neurotoxicity in the form of glove-and-stocking neuropathy is frequent. Children tolerate 2 mg/m², but adult doses may be capped at 2 mg total to lower the incidence of disabling chronic neuropathy; whether this compromises needed dose intensity in curative regimens is uncertain. Acute neuropathic effects include jaw pain, paralytic ileus, urinary retention, and the syndrome of inappropriate antidiuretic hormone secretion. Myelosuppression is not seen. Vinblastine is similar to vincristine, except that it tends to be more myelotoxic, with more frequent thrombocytopenia and also mucositis and stomatitis. Vinorelbine is a vinca alkaloid that appears to have differences in resistance patterns in comparison to vincristine and vinblastine; it may be administered orally.

The taxanes include paclitaxel and docetaxel. These agents differ from the vinca alkaloids in that the taxanes stabilize microtubules against depolymerization. The "stabilized" microtubules function abnormally and are not able to undergo the normal dynamic changes of microtubule function necessary for cell cycle completion. Taxanes are among the most broadly active antineoplastic agents for use in solid tumors, with evidence of activity in ovarian cancer, breast cancer, Kaposi's sarcoma, and lung tumors. They are administered intravenously, and paclitaxel requires use of a cremophore-containing vehicle that can cause hypersensitivity reactions. Premedication with regimens including dexamethasone (20 mg orally or intravenously 12 and 6 h before treatment) and diphenhydramine (50 mg) and cimetidine (300 mg), both 30 min before treatment, decreases but does not eliminate the risk of hypersensitivity reactions to the paclitaxel vehicle. Docetaxel uses a polysorbate 80 formulation, which can cause fluid retention in addition to hypersensitivity reactions, and dexamethasone premedication with or without antihistamines is frequently used. Paclitaxel causes hypersensitivity reactions, myelosuppression, neurotoxicity in the form of glove-and-stocking numbness, and paresthesia. Cardiac rhythm disturbances were observed in phase I and II trials, most commonly asymptomatic bradycardia but also, much more rarely, varying degrees of heart block. These have not emerged as clinically significant in the majority of patients. Infrequently occurring evidence of myocardial ischemia during paclitaxel administration cannot yet be clearly related to the drug. Docetaxel causes comparable degrees of myelosuppression and neuropathy. Hypersensitivity reactions, including bronchospasm, dyspnea, and hypotension, are less frequent but occur to some degree in up to 25% of patients. Fluid reten-

tion appears to result from a vascular leak syndrome that can aggravate preexisting effusions. Rash can complicate docetaxel administration, appearing prominently as a pruritic maculopapular rash affecting the forearms, but it has also been associated with fingernail ridging, breakdown, and skin discoloration. Stomatitis appears to be somewhat more frequent than with paclitaxel.

Estramustine was originally synthesized as a mustard derivative that might be useful in neoplasms that possessed estrogen receptor sites. However, no evidence of interaction with DNA was observed. Surprisingly, the drug caused metaphase arrest, and subsequent study revealed that it binds to microtubule-associated proteins, resulting in abnormal microtubule function. Estramustine binds to estramustine-binding proteins (EMBP), which are notably present in prostate tumor tissue. The drug is used as an oral formulation in patients with prostate cancer. Gastrointestinal and cardiovascular adverse effects related to the estrogen moiety occur in up to 10% of patients, including worsened heart failure and thromboembolic phenomena. Gynecomastia and nipple tenderness can also occur.

Hormonal Agents The family of steroid hormone receptor–related molecules have emerged as prominent targets for small molecules useful in cancer treatment. When bound to their cognate ligands, these receptors can alter gene transcription and, in certain tissues, induce apoptosis. The pharmacologic effect is a mirror or parody of the normal effects of the agent acting in nontransformed tissue, although the effects on tumors are mediated by indirect effects in some cases.

Glucocorticoids are generally given in "pulsed" high-dose exposure in leukemias and lymphomas, where they induce apoptosis in tumor cells. Cushing's syndrome or inadvertent adrenal suppression on withdrawal from high-dose glucocorticoids can be significant complications, along with infections common in immunosuppressed patients, in particular *Pneumocystis* pneumonia, which classically appears a few days after completing a course of high-dose steroids. Tamoxifen is a partial estrogen receptor antagonist; it has a tenfold greater degree of antitumor activity in breast cancer patients whose tumors express estrogen receptors than in those who have low or no levels of expression. Side effects include a somewhat increased risk of estrogen-related cardiovascular complications, such as thromboembolic phenomena, and a small increased incidence of endometrial carcinoma, which appears after chronic use. Progestational agents including medroxyprogesterone acetate, androgens including fluoxymesterone (Halotestin), and, paradoxically, estrogens have approximately the same degeree of activity in primary hormonal treatment of breast cancers that have elevated expression of estrogen receptor protein. Estrogen is not used often owing to prominent cardiovascular and uterotropic activity.

Prostate cancer is classically treated by diethylstilbesterol (DES) acting as an estrogen at the level of the hypothalamus to downregulate hypothalamic luteinizing hormone (LH) production, resulting in decreased elaboration of testosterone by the testicle. For this reason, orchiectomy is equally as effective as moderate-dose DES, inducing responses in 80% of previously untreated patients with prostate cancer but without the prominent cardiovascular side effects of DES, including thrombosis and exacerbation of coronary artery disease. In the event that orchiectomy is not accepted by the patient, testicular androgen suppression can also be effected by luteinizing hormone–releasing hormone (LHRH) agonists such as leuprolide and goserelin. These agents cause tonic stimulation of the LHRH receptor, with the loss of its normal pulsatile activation resulting in its desensitization and decreased output of LH by the anterior pituitary. Therefore, as primary hormonal manipulation in prostate cancer one can choose orchiectomy or leuprolide, not both. The addition of actual antagonists of androgens acting at the androgen receptor, including flutamide or bicalutamide, is of uncertain additional benefit in extending overall response duration, but it clearly prevents the activation of androgen receptors by adrenal androgens, and the combined use of orchiectomy or leuprolide plus flutamide is referred to as "total androgen blockade."

Tumors that respond to a primary hormonal manipulation may frequently respond to second and third hormonal manipulations. Thus, breast tumors that had previously responded to tamoxifen have, on relapse, notable response rates to withdrawal of tamoxifen itself or to subsequent addition of a progestin. Likewise, initial treatment of prostate cancers with leuprolide plus flutamide may be followed after disease progression by response to withrawal of flutamide. These responses may result from the removal of antagonists from mutant steroid hormone receptors that have come to depend on the presence of the antagonist as a growth-promoting influence.

Additional strategies to treat refractory breast and prostate cancers that possess steroid hormone receptors may also address adrenal capacity to produce androgens and estrogens, even after orchiectomy or oophorectomy, respectively. Thus, aminoglutethimide or ketoconazole can be used to block adrenal synthesis by interfering with the enzymes of steroid hormone metabolism. Administration of these agents requires concomitant hydrocortisone replacement and additional glucocorticoid doses administered in the event of physiologic stress. Steroid hormone–inducing "aromatase" activity may be present in tumor tissue, and second- or third-line approaches to inhibition of aromatase activity may also be affected by such agents as anastrazole and letrozole. The toxicity profile and activity of the aromatase inhibitors make them candidates for first-line therapy for breast cancer.

Humoral mechanisms can also result in complications of an underlying malignancy. Adrenocortical carcinomas can cause Cushing's syndrome as well as syndromes of androgen or estrogen excess. Mitotane can counteract these by decreasing synthesis of steroid hormones. Islet cell neoplasms can cause debilitating diarrhea, treated with the somatostatin analogue octreotide. Prolactin-secreting tumors can be effectively managed by the dopaminergic agononist bromocriptine.

MOLECULARLY TARGETED THERAPIES A better understanding of cancer cell biology has suggested many new targets for cancer drug discovery and development. These include the products of oncogenes and tumor-suppressor genes; regulators of cell death pathways; mediators of cellular immortality such as telomerase; and molecules responsible for microenvironmental molding such as proteases or angiogenic factors. The essential difference in the development of agents that would target these processes is that the basis for discovery of the candidate drug is the a priori importance of the target in the biology of the tumor, rather than the initial detection of drug candidates based on the phenomenon of tumor cell regression in tissue culture or in animals.

The most successful example of this class is imatinib mesylate (Gleevec). This protein kinase antagonist was selected as an inhibitor of the platelet-derived growth factor receptor (PDGFR) tyrosine kinase and was subsequently found to inhibit the bcr-abl kinase present in CML cells and reflecting the pathogenic t(9;22) chromosomal translocation in that tumor. It is also a potent inhibitor of the kit kinase originally defined as the stem cell factor receptor, a hematopoetic growth factor. Outstanding activity of imatinib has been noted in IFN-refractory CML with minimal toxicity, and it is also active in neoplasms driven by kit, such as gastrointestinal stromal sarcomas (GISTs), and by PDGFR, such as dermatofibrosarcoma protuberans. In each of these cases a clear link of the biology of the successfully treated neoplasm to the activity of the drug-susceptible target was a key factor in identifying patients who derived benefit from the drug.

Many classes of molecularly targeted small-molecule cancer therapeutics are under development or are in active clinical trials, including various protein kinase antagonists, farnesyltransferase antagonists originally designed to counter ras oncogene function, and protease inhibitors (Chap. 69). Many of these agents have not had evidence of frequent antitumor activity as single drugs in phase II trials. Their future use will likely depend on the evolution of more refined strategies to diagnose with accuracy the dependence of the tumor's biology on the presence of the drugs' targets. Alternatively, combinations of molecularly targeted agents with chemotherapeutic agents or with each other may evolve to address the multiplicity of genetic lesions present in solid tumors. These combinations will differ strategically from the approach used to evolve combinations of cytotoxic agents, which frequently combined agents with the same target, but which possessed differing toxicity. In contrast, combinations of molecularly targeted agents may address different pathways governing tumor biology in a manner more conceptually analogous to highly active antiretroviral therapy, where optimal disease suppression results from addressing two different gene products upon which successful viral replication depends.

An additional example related conceptually to molecularly targeted strategies is the use of retinoids, including tretinoin, the all-*trans*-isomer of retinoic acid, or isotretinoin, the 13-*cis* isomer of retinoic acid, to cause "differentiation" by acting on the retinoid receptor, a member of the steroid hormone receptor family. Leukemias and certain squamous neoplasms, including those of the skin and cervix, appear to be uniquely responsive in certain cases to retinoids. In particular, tretinoin is part of curative regimens for acute promyelocytic leukemia (APL) and appears to act by causing accelerated degradation of the fusion protein created by the t(15; 17) translocation that fuses the retinoic acid receptor α and the promyelocytic leukemia (PML) transcription factor. Acute side effects related to differentiation of promyelocytes to mature granulocytes may result in pulmonary symptoms related to granulocyte sequestration in the pulmonary vasculature; these are treated by respiratory support and glucocorticoids. This example also illustrates the important role of defining the molecular basis of empirical observations to refine a treatment strategy. Long before the definition of the t(15; 17)-derived fusion protein transcription factor now known to be the target of tretinoin, the growth and differentiation of certain leukemia cells including APL cells were known to be greatly influenced by retinoids. Empirical clinical trials of retinoids in China confirmed evidence of clinical activity of the agent before trials in the west. In this case, understanding the action of a drug led to the definition of the target. Another retinoid with activity in empirically driven clinical trials is the synthetic retinoid X receptor ligand bexarotene, which has noteworthy activity in cutaneous T cell lymphoma.

Whether derived by design a priori or through the explication of antiproliferative activity on the part of novel agents, the future will evolve additional classes of molecules whose targets are known to be causally related to neoplastic behavior. How to evaluate these agents efficiently and thoroughly is a current challenge. Empirical strategies treat a series of diseases with the novel agents without reference to the expression or activity of the target. Clinical utility dictates which agents move forward in development. While potentially inefficient, this approach has nonetheless yielded curative regimens in leukemias, lymphomas, germ cell neoplasms, and breast and colon tumors; e.g., when the latter two diseases are treated with chemotherapy after primary treatment of the local tumor with surgery and/or radiation therapy. Rigorously applied molecularly targeted development strategies, exemplified by imatinib's initial studies, would restrict drug use only to tumors with known activity or presence of the target. The former strategy risks inefficiency but is open to clinical observations that importantly influence development strategies. In all likelihood, a mix of empirical and targeted strategies will be of value in defining new, useful treatments for cancer. Examples of encouraging results of the empirical type include preliminary evidence of activity of bortezomib (Velcade), a proteosome inhibitor, in refractory multiple myeloma, and the epidermal growth factor receptor (EGFR) antagonist gefitinib (Iressa) in refractory lung cancer. Bortezomib was rationally designed to inhibit the proteosome, the multicomponent subcellular complex that degrades cell proteins as part of their normal turnover processes. The observation of activity in myeloma was an empirical outcome of a clinical trial. Likewise, simple expression of EGFR does not appear to uniquely correlate with gefitinib activity in patients with lung cancer. These examples highlight a difficulty in the more general use of molecularly targeted agents; specifically, how to select patients likely to respond to such agents. In many cases it is not obvious, as the relation of their target's action to the biologic success of the tumors in which they might be used is not clear. This is in contrast to conventional chemotherapeutic agents, where successful tumor growth obviously depends on DNA synthesis and microtubule function. These issues are very much a matter for current clinical and basic research.

An alternative way of thinking about molecularly targeted cancer therapeutics might recognize that there are actually many classes of cancer molecular targets. *Pathogenic targets* address the important events in the incidence and spread of a tumor; *differentiation-related targets* might reflect the tissue of origin; *pharmacological targets* would capitalize on intratumoral capacity to metabolize potentially active agents; *microenvironmental targets* would define processes important in molding stroma to allow successful blood supply and invasive properties. Drugs addressing all of these types of targets are in development. Certain "targeted toxins" exemplify some of these approaches. Targeted toxins utilize molecules with high affinity for defined tumor cell surface molecules, such as a leukemia differentiation antigen, to which a therapeutic antibody can deliver a covalently linked potent cytotoxin (e.g., gemtuzumab ozogamicin, a drug linked to anti-CD33), or a growth factor such as IL-2 to deliver a toxin (in the form of diphtheria toxin in denileukin diftitox) to cells bearing the IL-2 receptor. The value of such targeted approaches is that in addition to maximizing the therapeutic index by differential expression of the target in tumor (as opposed to nonrenewable normal cells), selection of patients for clinical trial and (perhaps eventually for routine clinical use) can capitalize on assessing the target in the tumor. The tools to accomplish this goal will include newer strategies to categorize tumors based on their biology rather than simply tissue of origin or histologic features.

ACUTE COMPLICATIONS OF CANCER CHEMOTHERAPY ■ Myelosuppression The
common cytotoxic chemotherapeutic agents almost invariably affect bone marrow function. Titration of this effect determines in many cases the MTD of the agent on a given schedule. The normal kinetics of blood cell turnover influence the sequence and sensitivity of each of the formed elements. Polymorphonuclear leukocytes (PMNs; $t_{1/2} =$ 6 to 8 h), platelets ($t_{1/2} =$ 5 to 7 days), and red blood cells (RBCs; $t_{1/2} =$ 120 days) have respectively most, less, and least susceptibility to usually administered cytotoxic agents. The nadir count of each cell type in response to classes of agents is characteristic. Maximal neutropenia occurs 6 to 14 days after conventional doses of anthracyclines, antifolates, and antimetabolites. Alkylating agents differ from each other in the timing of cytopenias. Nitrosoureas, DTIC, and procarbazine can display delayed marrow toxicity, first appearing 6 weeks after dosing.

Complications of myelosuppression result from the predictable sequelae of the missing cells' function. *Febrile neutropenia* refers to the clinical presentation of fever (one temperature ≥38.5°C or three readings ≥38°C but ≤38.5°C per 24 h) in a neutropenic patient with an uncontrolled neoplasm involving the bone marrow or, more usually, in a patient undergoing treatment with cytotoxic agents. Mortality from uncontrolled infection varies inversely with the neutrophil count. If the nadir neutrophil count is >1000/μL, there is little risk; if <500/μL, risk of death is markedly increased. Management of febrile neutropenia has conventionally included empirical coverage with antibiotics for the duration of neutropenia (Chap. 72). Selection of antibiotics is governed by the expected association of infections with certain underlying neoplasms; careful physical examination (with scrutiny of catheter sites, dentition, mucosal surfaces, and perirectal and genital orifices by gentle palpation); chest x-ray; and Gram stain and culture of blood, urine, and sputum (if any) to define a putative site of infection. In the absence of any originating site, a broadly acting β-lactam with anti-*Pseudomonas* activity, such as ceftazidime, is begun empirically. The addition of vancomycin to cover potential cutaneous sites of origin (until these are ruled out or shown to originate from methicillin-sensitive organisms) or metronidazole or imipenem for abdominal or other sites favoring anaerobes reflects modifications tailored to individual patient presentations. The coexistence of pulmo-

nary compromise raises a distinct set of potential pathogens, including *Legionella*, *Pneumocystis*, and fungal agents that may require further diagnostic evaluations such as bronchoscopy with bronchoalveolar lavage. Febrile neutropenic patients can be stratified broadly into two prognostic groups. The first, with expected short duration of neutropenia and no evidence of hypotension or abdominal or other localizing symptoms, may be expected to do well even with less complex, oral regimens, e.g., ciprofloxacin or amoxicillin and clavulinic acid. Detailed evaluation of such simple oral programs and intravenous regimens is ongoing. A less favorable prognostic group are patients with expected prolonged neutropenia, evidence of sepsis, and end-organ compromise, particularly pneumonia. These patients clearly require tailoring of their antibiotic regimen to their underlying presentation, with frequent empirical addition of antifungal agents if fever persists for 7 days without identification of an adequately treated organism or site.

Transfusion of granulocytes has no role in the management of febrile neutropenia, owing to their exceedingly short half-life, mechanical fragility, and clinical syndromes of pulmonary compromise with leukostasis after their use. Instead, colony-stimulating factors (CSFs) are used to augment bone marrow production of PMNs. These include early-acting factors such as IL-1, IL-3, and stem cell factor, which act on multiple lineages, and late-acting lineage-specific factors such as G-CSF (granulocyte colony-stimulating factor) or GM-CSF (granulocyte-macrophage colony-stimulating factor), erythropoietin, thrombopoietin, IL-6, and IL-11. CSFs are overused in oncology practice. The settings in which their use has been proved effective are limited. G-CSF, GM-CSF, erythropoietin, and IL-11 are currently approved for use. The American Society of Clinical Oncology has developed practice guidelines for the use of G-CSF and GM-CSF (Table 70-3). Primary administration (i.e., shortly after completing chemotherapy to reduce the nadir) of G-CSF to patients receiving cytotoxic regimens associated with a 40% incidence of febrile neutropenia has reduced the incidence of febrile neutropenia in several studies by about 50%. Most patients, however, receive regimens that do not have such a high risk of expected febrile neutropenia, and therefore most patients initially should not receive G-CSF or GM-CSF. Special circumstances such as a documented history of febrile neutropenia with the regimen in a particular patient; extensive compromise of marrow by prior radiation or chemotherapy; or active, open wounds or deep-seated infection may support primary treatment with G-CSF or GM-CSF. Administration of G-CSF or GM-CSF to afebrile neutropenic patients or to patients with low-risk febrile neutropenia as defined above is not recommended, although administration to high-risk patients with febrile neutropenia and evidence of organ compromise is reasonable. G-CSF or GM-CSF is conventionally started 24 to 72 h after completion of chemotherapy and continued until a PMN count of 10,000/μL is achieved. Also, patients with myeloid leukemias undergoing induction therapy may have a slight reduction in the duration of neutropenia if G-CSF (not GM-CSF) is commenced after completion of therapy and may be of particular value in elderly patients, but the influence on long-term outcome has not been defined. GM-CSF probably has a more restricted utility than G-CSF, with its use currently limited to patients after autologous bone marrow transplants, although proper head-to-head comparisons with G-CSF have not been conducted in most instances. GM-CSF may be associated with more systemic side effects.

Dangerous degrees of thrombocytopenia do not frequently complicate the management of patients with solid tumors receiving cytotoxic chemotherapy (with the possible exception of certain carboplatin-containing regimens), but they are frequent in patients with certain hematologic neoplasms where marrow is infiltrated with tumor. Severe bleeding related to thrombocytopenia occurs with increased frequency at platelet counts <20,000/μL and is very prevalent at counts <5000/μL. Prophylactic transfusions to keep platelets >20,000/μL are warranted in patients with leukemia (the threshold for transfusion is

TABLE 70-3   *Indications for the Clinical Use of G-CSF or GM-CSF*

Preventive Uses

With the first cycle of chemotherapy (so-called primary CSF administration)

  Not needed on a routine basis

  Use if the probability of febrile neutropenia is ≥40%

  Use if patient has preexisting neutropenia or active infection

With subsequent cycles if febrile neutropenia has previously occurred (so-called secondary CSF administration)

  Not needed after short duration neutropenia without fever

  Use if patient had febrile neutropenia in previous cycle

  Use if prolonged neutropenia (even without fever) delays therapy

Therapeutic Uses

Afebrile neutropenic patients

  No evidence of benefit

Febrile neutropenic patients

  No evidence of benefit

  May feel compelled to use in the face of clinical deterioration from sepsis, pneumonia, or fungal infection, but benefit unclear

To augment dose-intensity of chemotherapy in patients with curable malignancies

  No evidence of benefit

In bone marrow or peripheral blood stem cell transplantation

  Use to mobilize stem cells from marrow

  Use to hasten myeloid recovery

In acute myeloid leukemia

  G-CSF of minor or no benefit

  GM-CSF of no benefit and may be harmful

In myelodysplastic syndromes

  Not routinely beneficial

  Use intermittently in subset with neutropenia and recurrent infection

What Dose and Schedule Should Be Used?

G-CSF: 5 μg/kg per day subcutaneously

GM-CSF: 250 μg/m² per day subcutaneously

When Should Therapy Begin and End?

When indicated, start 24–72 h after chemotherapy

Continue until absolute neutrophil count is 10,000/μL

Do not use concurrently with chemotherapy or radiation therapy

Note: G-CSF, granulocyte colony-stimulating factor; GM-CSF, granulocyte-macrophage colony-stimulating factor.
Source: From the American Society of Clinical Oncology.

10,000/μL in patients with solid tumors and no other bleeding diathesis or physiologic stressors such as fever or hypotension). Careful review of medication lists to prevent exposure to nonsteroidal anti-inflammatory agents and maintenance of clotting factor levels adequate to support near-normal prothrombin and partial thromboplastin time tests are of import in minimizing the risk of bleeding in the thrombocytopenic patient. Certain cytokines in clinical investigation have shown ability to increase platelets (e.g., IL-6, IL-1, thrombopoietin), but clinical benefit and safety are not yet proven. IL-11 (oprelvekin) is approved for use in the setting of expected thrombocytopenia, but its effects on platelet counts are small and it is associated with side effects such as headache, fever, malaise, syncope, cardiac arrhythmias, and fluid retention.

Anemia associated with chemotherapy can be managed by transfusion of packed RBCs. Transfusion is not undertaken until the hemoglobin falls to <80 g/L (8 g/dL) or if compromise of end-organ function occurs or an underlying condition (e.g., coronary artery disease) calls for maintenance of hemoglobin >90 g/L (9 g/dL). Patients who are to receive therapy for >2 months on a "stable" regimen and who are likely to require continuing transfusions are also candidates for erythropoietin to maintain hemoglobin of 90 to 100 g/L (9 to 10 g/dL). In the setting of adequate iron stores and serum erythropoietin levels <100 ng/mL, erythropoietin, 150 U three times a week, can produce a slow increase in hemoglobin over about 2 months of administration. Depot formulations can be administered less frequently. It is unclear whether higher hemoglobin levels, up to 110 to 120 g/L (11 to 12 g/dL) are associated with improved quality of life to a degree that justifies the more intensive erythropoietin use. In addition, certain

treatment regimens, e.g., chemoradiation of cervix and head and neck neoplasms, may have enhanced likelihood of response in association with improved delivery of O_2. Evidence is emerging that erythropoietin may have undesirable effects in that it can rescue hypoxic cells from death. This may be a disadvantage in cancer but a great advantage in the setting of heart attacks and strokes.

Nausea and Vomiting   The most common side effect of chemotherapy administration is nausea, with or without vomiting. Antineoplastic agents vary in their capacity to cause nausea and vomiting. Mechlorethamine, nitrosoureas, streptozotocin, DTIC, cisplatin, and actinomycin are highly emetogenic and produce vomiting in virtually all patients. Doxorubicin, daunorubicin, and conventional-dose cyclophosphamide are moderately emetogenic. Antimetabolites are dose- and schedule-dependent, with single doses of methotrexate and fluorouracil producing at worst anorexia; while 5-day regimens of 5FU and high-dose methotrexate produce nausea in ~50% of patients. Other agents such as chlorambucil, melphalan, and busulfan in conventional doses produce little tendency to emesis.

Emesis is a reflex caused by stimulation of the vomiting center in the medulla. Input to the vomiting center comes from the chemoreceptor trigger zone (CTZ) and afferents from the peripheral gastrointestinal tract, cerebral cortex, and heart. In addition, a conditioned reflex may contribute to anticipatory nausea arising after repeated cycles of chemotherapy. Accordingly, antiemesis agents differ in their locus of action. Combining agents from different classes or the sequential use of different classes of agent is the cornerstone of successful management of chemotherapy-induced nausea and vomiting. Of great importance are the prophylactic administration of agents and such psychological techniques as the maintenance of a supportive milieu, counseling, and relaxation to augment the action of antiemetic agents.

Antidopaminergic phenothiazines act directly at the CTZ and include prochlorperazine (Compazine), 10 mg intramuscularly or intravenously, 10 to 25 mg orally, or 25 mg per rectum every 4 to 6 h for up to four doses; and thiethylperazine (Torecan), 10 mg by potentially all the above routes every 6 h. Haloperidol (Haldol) is a butyrophenone dopamine antagonist given at 0.5 to 1.0 mg intramuscularly or orally every 8 h. Antihistamines such as diphenhydramine (Benadryl) have little intrinsic antiemetic capacity but are frequently given to prevent or treat dystonic reactions that can complicate use of the antidopaminergic agents. Lorazepam (Ativan) is a short-acting benzodiazepine that provides an anxiolytic effect to augment the effectiveness of a variety of agents when used at 1 to 2 mg intramuscularly, intravenously, or orally every 4 to 6 h. Dexamethasone (Decadron) likewise augments the action of a variety of agents when used at 4 to 40 mg intravenously or orally, given before treatment and repeated up to 10 mg orally every 6 h four times. Metoclopramide (Reglan) acts on peripheral dopamine receptors to augment gastric emptying and is used in high doses for highly emetogenic regimens (1 to 2 mg/kg intravenously 30 min before chemotherapy and every 2 h for up to three additional doses as needed); intravenous doses of 10 to 20 mg every 4 to 6 h as needed or 50 mg orally 4 h before and 8 and 12 h after chemotherapy are used for moderately emetogenic regimens. Serotonin antagonists are useful in moderately to severely emetogenic regimens; ondansetron (Zofran) is given as 0.15 mg/kg intravenously for three doses just before and at 4 and 8 h after chemotherapy, and granisetron (Kytril) is given as a single dose of 0.01 mg/kg just before chemotherapy. 5-9-Tetrahydrocannabinol (Marinol) is a rather weak antiemetic compared to other available agents, but it may be useful for persisting nausea and is used orally at 10 mg every 3 to 4 h as needed. Aprepitant is the first of a novel class of drugs, neurokinin receptor blockers; its addition to serotonin antagonists improves control of emesis against strongly emetogenic agents such as cisplatin. The usual dose is 125 mg orally on day 1, 80 mg orally on days 2 and 3.

Alopecia   Chemotherapeutic agents vary widely in causing alopecia, with anthracyclines, alkylating agents, and topoisomerase inhibitors reliably causing near total alopecia when given at therapeutic doses. Antimetabolites are more variably associated with alopecia. Psychological support and the use of cosmetic resources are to be encouraged, and "chemo caps" that reduce scalp temperature to decrease the degree of alopecia should be discouraged, particularly during the treatment with curative intent of neoplasms such as leukemia, lymphoma, or in adjuvant breast cancer therapy. The richly vascularized scalp can certainly harbor micrometastatic or disseminated disease.

Gonadal Dysfunction and Pregnancy Cessation of ovulation and azoospermia reliably result from alkylating agent– and topoisomerase poison–containing regimens. The duration of these effects varies with age and sex. Males treated for Hodgkin's disease with mechlorethamine- and procarbazine-containing regimens are effectively sterile, whereas fertility usually returns after regimens including cisplatin, vinblastine, or etoposide and after bleomycin for testicular cancer. Sperm banking before treatment may be considered to support patients likely to be sterilized by treatment. Females experience amenorrhea with anovulation after alkylating agent therapy but are likely to recover normal menses if treatment is completed before age 30 and unlikely to recover menses after age 35. Even those who regain menses usually experience premature menopause. As the magnitude and extent of decreased fertility can be difficult to predict, patients should be counseled to maintain effective contraception, preferably by barrier means, during and after therapy. Resumption of efforts to conceive should be considered in the context of the likely prognosis of the patient. Hormone-replacement therapy should be undertaken in women who do not have a hormonally responsive tumor. For those patients who have had a hormone-sensitive tumor primarily treated by a local modality, conventional practice would counsel against hormone replacement, but this issue is very much a matter for current clinical investigations.

Chemotherapy agents have variable effects on the success of pregnancy (Chap. 6). All agents tend to have increased risk of adverse outcomes when administered during the first trimester, and strategies to delay chemotherapy, if possible, until after this milestone should be considered if the pregnancy is to continue to term. Patients in their second or third trimester can be treated with most regimens for the common neoplasms afflicting women in their child-bearing years with the exception of antimetabolites, particularly antifolates, which have notable teratogenic or fetotoxic effects throughout pregnancy. The need for anticancer chemotherapy per se is infrequently a clear basis to recommend termination of a concurrent pregnancy, although each treatment strategy in this circumstance must be tailored to the individual needs of the patient. →*Chronic effects of cancer treatment are reviewed in Chap. 89.*

BIOLOGIC THERAPY

No postulates resembling principles have emerged from efforts to develop biologic approaches to cancer treatment. The goal of biologic therapy is to manipulate the host-tumor interaction in favor of the host. Theoretically, biologic approaches should reflect a bell-shaped dose-response curve where the maximum biologic effect is less than the MTD. Empirical trial and error has led to the discovery that a number of biologic treatment approaches may produce antitumor effects, but nearly all of them are most active at their MTD. As a class, biologic therapies may be distinguished from molecularly targeted agents in that biologic therapies require an active response (e.g., reexpression of silenced genes) on the part of the tumor cell or on the part of the host (e.g., immunologic effects) to allow therapeutic effect. This may be contrasted with the antiproliferative or apoptotic response that is the ultimate goal of molecularly targeted agents discussed above. However, there is much commonality in the strategies to evaluate and use molecularly targeted and biologic therapies.

IMMUNE MEDIATORS OF ANTITUMOR EFFECTS The very existence of a cancer in a person is testimony to the failure of the immune system to deal effectively with the cancer. Tumors have a variety of means of avoiding the immune system: (1) they are often only subtly different from their normal counterparts; (2) they are capable of downregulating their major histocompatibility complex antigens, effectively masking them from recognition by T cells; (3) they are inefficient at presenting antigens to the immune system; (4) they can cloak themselves in a protective shell of fibrin to minimize contact with surveillance mechanisms; and (5) they can produce a range of soluble molecules, including potential immune targets, that can distract the immune system from recognizing the tumor cell. Some of the cell products initially polarize the immune response away from cellular immunity (shifting from T_H1 to T_H2 responses; Chap. 295) and ultimately lead to defects in T cells that prevent their activation and cytotoxic activity. Cancer treatment further suppresses host immunity. A variety of strategies are being tested to overcome these barriers.

Cell-Mediated Immunity The strongest evidence that the immune system can exert clinically meaningful antitumor effects comes from allogeneic bone marrow transplantation. Adoptively transferred T cells from the donor expand in the tumor-bearing host, recognize the tumor as being foreign, and can mediate impressive antitumor effects (graft-versus-tumor effects). Three types of experimental interventions are being developed to take advantage of the ability of T cells to kill tumor cells.

1. Allogeneic T cells are being transferred to cancer-bearing hosts in three major settings: in the form of allogeneic bone marrow transplantation, as pure lymphocyte transfusions following bone marrow recovery after allogeneic bone marrow transplantation, and as pure lymphocyte transfusions following immunosuppressive (but not myeloablative) therapy (so-called minitransplants). In each of these settings, the effector cells are donor T cells that recognize the tumor as being foreign, probably through minor histocompatibility differences. The main risk of such therapy is the development of graft-versus-host disease because of the minimal difference between the cancer and the normal host cells. This approach has been highly effective in certain hematologic cancers.

2. Autologous T cells are being removed from the tumor-bearing host, manipulated in several ways in vitro, and given back to the patient. The two major classes of autologous T cell manipulation are (1) to develop tumor antigen–specific T cells and expand them to large numbers over many weeks ex vivo before administration, and (2) to activate the cells with polyclonal stimulators such as anti-CD3 and anti-CD28 after a short period ex vivo and try to expand them in the host after adoptive transfer with stimulation by IL-2, for example. Short periods removed from the patient permit the cells to overcome the tumor-induced T cell defects, and such cells traffic and home to sites of disease better than cells that have been in culture for many weeks. Individual centers have successful experiences with one or the other approach but not both, and whether one is superior to the other is not known.

3. Tumor vaccines are aimed at boosting T cell immunity. The finding that mutant oncogenes that are expressed only intracellularly can be recognized as targets of T cell killing greatly expanded the possibilities for tumor vaccine development. No longer is it difficult to find something different about tumor cells. However, major difficulties remain in getting the tumor-specific peptides presented in a fashion to prime the T cells. Tumors themselves are very poor at presenting their own antigens to T cells at the first antigen exposure (*priming*). Priming is best accomplished by professional antigen-presenting cells (dendritic cells). Thus, a number of experimental strategies are aimed at priming host T cells against tumor-associated peptides. Vaccine adjuvants such as GM-CSF appear capable of attracting antigen-presenting cells to a skin site containing a tumor antigen. Such an approach has been documented to eradicate microscopic residual disease in follicular lymphoma and give rise to tumor-specific T cells. Purified antigen-presenting cells can be pulsed with tumor, its membranes, or particular tumor antigens and delivered as a vaccine. Tumor cells can be transfected with genes that attract antigen-presenting cells. Other ideas are also being tested. In a variation on the theme of adop-

tive transfer, the tumor vaccine may be given to the normal bone marrow and lymphoid cell donor of an allogeneic transplant so that the donor immune system has more cells capable of recognizing the tumor specifically. Vaccines against viral cancers (papilloma virus in cervical cancer), lymphomas, and melanomas have had modest clinical success.

Antibodies In general, antibodies are not very effective at killing cancer cells. Because the tumor seems to influence the host toward making antibodies rather than generating cellular immunity, it is inferred that antibodies are easier for the tumor to fend off. Many patients can be shown to have serum antibodies directed at their tumors, but these do not appear to influence disease progression. However, the ability to grow very large quantities of high-affinity antibody directed at a tumor by the hybridoma technique has led to the application of antibodies to the treatment of cancer. The first study of a monoclonal antibody in cancer was published in 1980 and demonstrated many hurdles that needed to be overcome to make the approach successful. It seemed best to attack a determinant that was not shed or modulated by the tumor. A target that was involved in an important function for the tumor cells might be superior to a physiologically irrelevant target. Murine antibodies were not very effective because they did not mediate human effector mechanisms well and the host nearly always made antibodies against the therapeutic antibody that prevented it from finding the target.

The lessons were learned; humanized antibodies against the CD20 molecule expressed on B cell lymphomas (rituximab) and against the HER-2/*neu* receptor overexpressed on epithelial cancers, especially breast cancer (trastuzumab), have become reliable tools in the oncologists armamentarium. Each used alone can cause tumor regression (rituximab > trastuzumab), and both appear to potentiate the effects of combination chemotherapy given just after antibody administration. Antibodies to CD52 and vascular endothelial growth factor are active in chronic lymphoid leukemia and colon cancer, respectively. Conjugation of antibodies to drugs and toxins was discussed above, and conjugates of antibodies with isotopes, photodynamic agents, and other killing moieties may also be effective. Radioconjugates targeting CD20 on lymphomas have been approved for use [ibritumomab tiuxetan (Zevalin), using yttrium-90)]. Other conjugates are associated with problems that have not yet been solved (e.g., antigenicity, instability, poor tumor penetration).

Cytokines There are >70 separate proteins and glycoproteins with biologic effects in humans: IFN-α, -β, -γ; IL-1 through -29 (so far); the TFN family [including lymphotoxin, TFN-related apoptosis-inducing ligand (TRAIL), CD40 ligand, and others]; and the chemokine family. Only a fraction of these has been tested against cancer; only IFN-α and IL-2 are in routine clinical use.

About 20 different genes encode IFN-α, and their biologic effects are indistinguishable. Interferon induces the expression of many genes,

inhibits protein synthesis, and exerts a number of different effects on diverse cellular processes. Its antitumor effects appear to be antagonized in vitro by thymidine, suggesting that de novo thymidylate synthesis is also affected. The two recombinant forms that are commercially available are IFN-α2a and -α2b. In general, interferon antitumor effects are dose-related, and IFN is most effective at its MTD. Interferon is not curative for any tumor but can induce partial responses in follicular lymphoma, hairy cell leukemia, CML, melanoma, and Kaposi's sarcoma. It has been used in the adjuvant setting in stage II melanoma, multiple myeloma, and follicular lymphoma, with uncertain effects on survival. It produces fever, fatigue, a flulike syndrome, malaise, myelosuppression, and depression and can induce clinically significant autoimmune disease.

IL-2 must exert its antitumor effects indirectly through augmentation of immune function. Its biologic activity is to promote the growth and activity of T cells and natural killer (NK) cells. High doses of IL-2 can produce tumor regressions in certain patients with metastatic melanoma and renal cell cancer. About 2 to 5% of patients may experience complete remissions that are durable, unlike any other treatment for these tumors. IL-2 is associated with myriad clinical side effects: intravascular volume depletion, capillary leak syndrome, adult respiratory distress syndrome, hypotension, fever, chills, skin rash, and impaired renal and liver function. Patients may require blood pressure support and intensive care to manage the toxicity. However, once the agent is stopped, most of the toxicities reverse completely within 3 to 6 days.

GENE THERAPIES

No gene therapy has been approved for routine clinical use. Several strategies are under evaluation, including the use of viruses that cannot replicate to express genes that can allow the action of drugs or directly inhibit cancer cell growth; viruses that can actually replicate but only in the context of the tumor cell; or viruses that can express antigens in the context of the tumor and therefore provoke a host-mediated immune response. Key issues in the success of these approaches will be in defining safe viral vector systems that escape host immune function and effectively target the tumor or tumor cell milieu. Other gene therapy strategies would utilize therapeutic oligonucleoides to target the expression of genes important in the maintenance of tumor cell viability.

FURTHER READING

AMERICAN SOCIETY OF CLINICAL ONCOLOGY: Update of recommendations for use of hematopoietic colony-stimulating factors: Evidence-based clinical practice guidelines. J Clin Oncol 14:1957, 1996

CHABNER BA, LONGO DL (eds): *Cancer Chemotherapy and Biotherapy: Principles and Practice*, 3d ed. Philadelphia, Lippincott Williams & Wilkins, 2001

SAUSVILLE E et al: Signal transduction-directed cancer treatments. Annu Rev Pharmacol Toxicol 43:199, 2003

71 PRINCIPLES OF RADIATION THERAPY
Stephen M. Hahn, Eli Glatstein

All human beings are constantly exposed to ionizing radiation. Environmental sources include the cosmic radiation from space and radiation from the ground and from inhaled and ingested materials. Airline travel and mining both increase exposure to the background radiation. For example, air travel at 30,000 ft exposes individuals to a dose equivalent of 0.5 mrem/h. Radiation originating in the body comes mainly from radioactive potassium, which emits beta and gamma rays. Lungs are exposed to radiation from inhaled air, which contains small amounts of radioactive radon. Cosmic exposure contributes ~28 mrem per year. The ground and internal sources contribute ~26 and 27 mrem

per year, respectively. The most prominent man-made sources of radiation include x-ray equipment, nuclear weapons, and radioactive medications.

TERMINOLOGY AND DEFINITIONS

The first major unit of radiation exposure was the roentgen (R), defined as an amount of x-rays or gamma rays that produces a specific amount of ionization in a unit of air under standard temperature and pressure (Table 71-1); this quantity can be measured directly in an ionization chamber. The rad (*r*adiation *a*bsorbed *d*ose) is defined as 100 ergs/g of tissue. Thus, the rad represents a net deposition of energy in a three-dimensional volume, because x-rays attenuate as they traverse tissue. The rad has been replaced by the Système Internationale (SI) unit of the gray (Gy), which represents 100 rad. Roentgens and rads can be

TABLE 71-1 Units and Definitions

Unit	Quantity Measured	Definition
Roentgen (R)	Exposure	Amount of x-rays or gamma rays that produces a specific amount of ionization in a given volume of air
Rad	Dose	100 ergs deposited per gram of tissue
Gray (Gy)	Dose	SI unit of dose; equals 100 rad
Rem	Dose equivalence	Unit that reflects the biologic response. It is used to compare various types of radiation
Sievert (Sv)	Dose equivalence	SI unit of dose equivalence; equals 100 rem

converted by means of various tables; the relation between them depends on photon energy.

The above definitions reflect physical variables. The unit that reflects the biologic response and that can be used to compare the effects of various types of radiation is the unit of dose equivalence, the rem (*roentgen* *equivalent* in *man*). The rem has been replaced by the SI unit, the sievert (Sv), which equals 100 rem. These units reflect the exposure or absorption dose multiplied by a biologic factor that represents the biologic effectiveness of the specific type of radiation (see below).

TYPES OF IONIZING RADIATION

The absorption of energy from radiation in tissue often leads to excitation or ionization. Excitation involves elevation of an electron in an atom or molecule to a higher energy state without actual ejection of the electron. Ionization involves actual ejection of one or more electrons from the atom. Ionizing radiation is subclassified as electromagnetic (photon) or particulate radiation (Table 71-2). X-rays and gamma rays are examples of electromagnetic photon radiation; they differ only in their source. X-rays are produced mechanically, by making electrons strike a target, which causes the electrons to give up their kinetic energy as x-rays, while gamma rays are produced by nuclear disintegration of radioactive isotopes.

X-rays can be thought of as packets of energy, or photons. X-rays have no mass or charge, travel in straight lines, and attenuate continuously as they traverse tissue. Gamma rays have similar properties. Each photon contains an amount of energy equal to $h\nu$, where h is Planck's constant and ν is the radiation frequency. The critical difference between nonionizing and ionizing radiation is the energy of individual photons, not the energy of the total dose.

Types of *particulate radiation* include electrons, protons, alpha particles, neutrons, negative pi-mesons, and heavy charged ions; these have discrete mass and charge (except for neutrons, which lack charge;

TABLE 71-2 Common Types of Ionizing Radiation

Type	Mass	Charge	Comment
Electromagnetic			
X-ray	0	0	X-rays and gamma rays do not differ except in the source. Gamma rays are produced intranuclearly, and x-rays are produced extranuclearly (i.e., mechanically).
Gamma ray	0	0	
Particulate			
Electron (e)	9.1×10^{-31} kg	-1	—
Proton (p)	$2000 \times e$	$+1$	Exhibits a Bragg peak
Neutron (n)	$2000 \times e$	0	Cannot be accelerated by an electrical field
Alpha particle	$2p + 2n$ $\sim 8000 \times e$	$+2$	Helium nucleus

Table 71-2). *Electrons*, or *beta particles*, are small and negatively charged and can be accelerated to close to the speed of light. They decelerate fairly rapidly in tissue and penetrate it to only a limited depth. Thus, electron beams are often used to treat superficial problems. *Protons* are positively charged and have a mass about 2000 times that of an electron. Protons stop abruptly, depending on their energy; in the process of sudden deceleration, most of their energy is given up, which tends to cause ionization just before the proton stops. This region of enhanced ionization, sometimes called the Bragg peak, means that proton beams exert their effects in a relatively compact region. Therefore, protons may have advantages over other types of particulate radiation with respect to conforming the dose to the treatment volume. *Alpha particles* are helium nuclei, consisting of two protons and two neutrons. The mass and charge are great enough that these particles do not penetrate far through matter unless they have tremendous energy; even a piece of paper is enough to protect against most alpha particles. Because these particles are charged, they can be accelerated in electrical fields.

Neutrons are similar in mass to protons (having an atomic mass of 1), but they are not charged and therefore cannot be accelerated in an electrical field. Neutron beams are produced by colliding charged particles into a suitable target or are emitted as a fission product of heavy radioactive atoms. *Heavy charged ions* are nuclei of heavier elements that have a positive charge owing to the stripping away of some or all of the orbiting electrons.

Equal doses of different types of radiation do not necessarily produce equal biologic effects; thus 1 Gy of neutrons produces a greater biologic effect than 1 Gy of x-rays. The biologic effects produced by a given dose of radiation can be quantified by the relative biologic effectiveness (RBE) value, which relates them to the effects produced by 250-keV photon radiation as a standard. In general, the greater the RBE value for a given type of radiation, the greater the biologic effect. The RBE value will be greater for more densely ionizing radiation, such as neutrons. The RBE value depends on the linear energy transfer (see below), the dose, the dose rate, and the nature of the biologic system.

The linear energy transfer (LET) is the amount of ionization occurring per unit length of the radiation track. It is usually expressed as kilovolts per micron and increases with the square of the charge of the incident particle. High-LET radiation is biologically different from low-LET (i.e., conventional) radiation: Hypoxic and oxygenated cells respond similarly to high-LET irradiation, whereas it takes about three times as much low-LET radiation to produce a given killing effect in hypoxic cells as in oxygenated cells. It is thought that low-LET radiation must produce multiple hits on DNA to destroy a cell, whereas high-LET radiation need produce only a single hit on DNA to kill a cell. Representative values of LET and RBE are given in Table 71-3.

Radiation, especially x-rays, is absorbed and causes ionization in three major ways: the *photoelectric effect*, the *Compton effect*, and *pair production*. At low energies (30 to 100 keV), as in diagnostic radiology, the photoelectric effect is important. In this process, the incident photon interacts with an electron in one of the outer shells of an atom (typically K, L, or M). If the energy of the photon is greater than the

TABLE 71-3 Linear Energy Transfer and Relative Biologic Effectiveness Values

Type of Radiation	LET Values, keV/μm
Cobalt-60 gamma rays	0.2
250-keV x-rays	2.0
10 MeV protons	4.7

Type of Radiation	RBE Values (Quality Factors)
X-rays, gamma rays, and electrons	1
Neutrons	3–20
Heavy particles	1–20

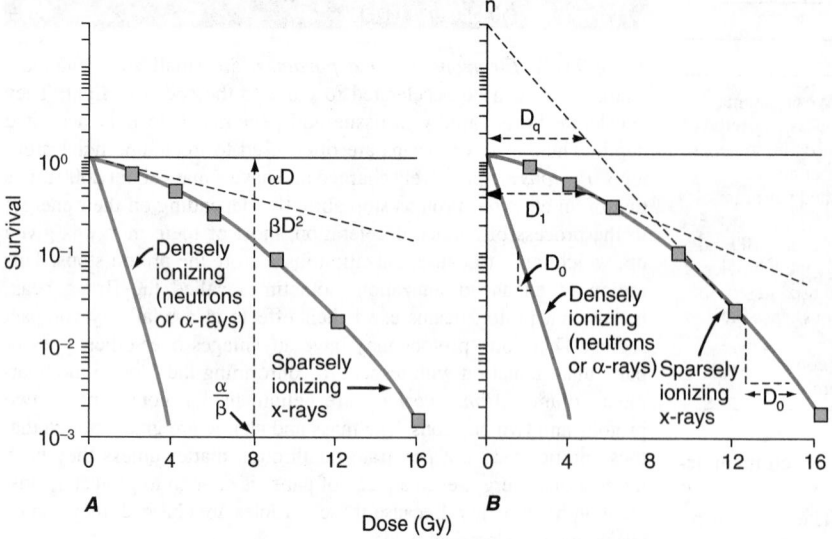

FIGURE 71-1 Shape of survival curve for mammalian cells exposed to radiation. The fraction of cells surviving is plotted on a logarithmic scale against dose on a linear scale. For alpha particles or low-energy neutrons (said to be densely ionizing), the dose-response curve is a straight line from the origin (i.e., survival is an exponential function of dose). The survival curve can be described by just one parameter, the slope. For x-rays or gamma rays (said to be sparsely ionizing), the dose-response curve has an initial linear slope, followed by a shoulder; at higher doses the curve tends to become straight again. *A.* The experimental data are fitted to a linear-quadratic function. There are two components of cell killing: one is proportional to dose (αD), while the other is proportional to the square of the dose (βD^2). The dose at which the linear and quadratic components are equal is the ratio α/β. The linear-quadratic curve bends continuously but is a good fit to experimental data for the first few decades of survival. *B.* The curve is described by the initial slope (D_1), the final slope (D_0), and a parameter that represents the width of the shoulder, either n or D_q. *(From Hall, with permission.)*

binding energy of the electron, then the electron is expelled from the orbit with a kinetic energy that is equal to the energy of the incident photon minus the binding energy of the electron. The photoelectric effect varies as a function of the cube of the atomic number of the material exposed (Z^3); this fact explains why bone is visualized much better than soft tissue on radiographs.

At higher energies, as used in therapeutic radiology, the Compton effect dominates. In this process, the incident photon interacts with an electron in an orbital shell. Part of the incident photon energy appears as kinetic energy of electrons, and the residual energy continues as a less energetic deflected photon.

At energy levels >1.02 MeV, the photons may be absorbed through pair production. In this process, both a positron and an electron are produced in the absorbing material. A positron has the same mass as an electron but has a positive instead of a negative charge. The positron travels a very short distance in the absorbing medium before it interacts with another electron. When that happens, the entire mass of both particles is converted to energy, with the emission of two photons in exactly opposite directions.

BIOLOGIC EFFECTS OF RADIATION

Radiation must produce double-strand breaks in DNA to kill a cell, owing partly to the high capacity of mammalian cells for repairing single-strand damage. Radiation can also produce effects indirectly by interacting with water (which makes up ~80% of a cell's volume) to generate free radicals, which can damage the cell. Free radicals are highly reactive chemical entities that lack a stable number of outer-shell electrons. A free radical is not stable and has a life span of a fraction of a second. It is estimated that most x-ray-induced cell damage is due to the formation of hydroxyl radicals, as follows:

$$\text{Ionizing radiation} + H_2O \rightarrow H_2O^+ + e^-$$
$$H_2O^+ + H_2O \rightarrow H_3O^+ + OH\bullet$$
$$OH\bullet \rightarrow \text{Cell damage}$$

The usual end result of radiation damage is cell death. The biologic effects on epithelial cell reproduction are typically expressed only when the damaged cells attempt to divide. Another biologic effect is the induction of cancerous growth by mutation many years after radiation exposure. Patients who receive radiation have a significant risk of neoplasm for at least two to three decades after their exposure; this risk is significantly higher than that of the population as a whole.

RADIATION-INDUCED CHROMOSOME ABERRATIONS

Chromosome breaks can occur when cells are irradiated. The broken ends of chromosomes can combine with broken ends of different chromosomes. These abnormal combinations are most readily seen during mitosis. Chromosome abnormalities typically occur in cells irradiated in the G_1 phase of the cell cycle, before the doubling of genetic material. If cells are irradiated in the G_2 phase, chromatid aberrations may result. The frequency of chromosomal aberrations in peripheral circulating lymphocytes can be used to correlate with the total body dose received. The dose can be estimated by comparing the chromosomal changes to in vitro cultures exposed to controlled doses of irradiation. The minimum dose that can be detected by peripheral lymphocyte analysis is about 0.1 to 0.2 Sv (10 to 20 rem). Lymphocyte analysis may provide evidence of recent total-body exposure.

CELL SURVIVAL CURVE The dose-response curve for all mammalian cells appears to have a linear-quadratic relationship. In simple terms, the mathematical model that explains the relationship between the dose and the fraction of surviving cells has both linear and exponential components. The linear component results from double-stranded chromosomal breaks produced by single hits. The exponential component represents breaks produced by multiple hits. Figure 71-1 shows the shape of a typical survival curve for mammalian cells exposed to radiation. The fraction of cells surviving is plotted on a semilogarithmic scale. For x-rays or gamma rays, the dose-response curve has a shoulder that is followed by a straight line curve as the dose is increased. The shoulder appears to represent the cell's ability to repair sublethal injury. For alpha particles or lower energy neutrons, the dose-response curve is a straight line from the origin. Thus, the survival rate is an exponential function of the dose.

In all mammalian cell lines studied, increases in the radiation dose decrease the survival rate of cells. However, a number of factors may contribute to a reduced sensitivity to radiation in human tumors in vivo, including extrinsic factors such as hypoxia and intrinsic factors such as expression of particular oncogenes, including *ras*. The biologic basis for this altered sensitivity to radiation has not been fully defined.

Four important processes that occur after radiation exposure can be summarized as the "four R's" of radiobiology. The first is *repair*. Repair is temperature dependent and is thought to represent the enzymatic mechanisms for healing intracellular injury. The second R is *reoxygenation*, a process whereby oxygen (and other nutrients) are actually better distributed to viable cells following radiation injury and cell killing. The third R is *repopulation*, the ability of the cell population to continue to divide and to replace dying and dead cells. The fourth R is *redistribution*, which reflects the variability of a cell's radiosensitivity over the cell cycle. Radiosensitivity can vary through the cell cycle by as much as a factor of 3. The G_1 phase has the most variable length of all the phases of the cell cycle. For most cell lines, cells that have a short G_1 period are most sensitive at the G_2/mitosis interface, less sensitive in G_1, and most resistant toward the end of the synthesis (S) period.

Radiation therapy is effective in cancer treatment when it exerts greater cytotoxic effects on tumor cells than on normal tissues (i.e., improving the therapeutic index). A major determinant of the therapeutic index is exploiting differences in the four R's between tumor cells and normal tissues. Fractionated radiation exploits differences in the four R's between tumor and normal tissues, thereby improving the therapeutic index.

NORMAL TISSUE EFFECTS OF RADIATION Therapeutic radiation leads to acute effects that typically manifest during treatment and resolve a few weeks after the completion of therapy. Late effects are also produced by radiotherapy and typically do not occur until several months or years after treatment is delivered. The clinical response to radiation may be related to the interactions of various growth factors and cytokines. For example, radiation can induce growth factors and cytokines such as tumor necrosis factor (TNF) and interleukin (IL) 1. TNF can induce proliferation of fibroblasts and enhance the inflammatory response. TNF and IL-1 have been shown to radioprotect hematopoietic cells in vitro by increasing the D_0 of the cell survival curve (Fig. 71-1). TNF also enhances killing of a human tumor cell line by irradiation. TNF may produce radioprotection or radiosensitization, depending on the cell type. Efforts to modulate radiation effects with TNF remain experimental. Other factors implicated in the radiation response are basic fibroblast growth factor and platelet-derived growth factor β, which may be associated with late effects of radiation on vessels.

The degree and the duration of functional recovery of normal tissues are related to the number of stem cells surviving after irradiation. If the stem cells are destroyed in the irradiated volume and replacement from adjacent tissues is inadequate, radiation injury will persist, causing late toxic effects. True late effects develop independent of early reactions; they may also occur despite recovery from acute radiation injury.

Table 71-4 shows the frequency of radiation tolerance seen with fractionated radiotherapy at 5 years of follow-up. These numbers are rough estimates at best. The clinical manifestations of irradiation will depend on the volume of the organ irradiated, the total dose, the dose per fraction, and the length of time taken to deliver the dose, and probably genetic/biologic factors. Dose per fraction is the most important factor determining normal tissue effects. This is why daily fractionation doses of 180 cGy to 200 cGy are used in most curative treatment situations. In addition, the cellular consequences of treatment can be progressive over time. Thus, length of follow-up is also crucial in judging late clinical sequelae from radiation.

THERAPEUTIC RADIATION Radiation therapy is a physical form of treatment that damages any tissue in its path. In the target tissue, radiation damages DNA (usually single-strand breaks) and generates free radi-

cals from cell water that are capable of damaging cell membranes, proteins, and organelles. Radiation damage is dependent on oxygen; hypoxic cells are more resistant. Augmentation of oxygen is the basis for radiation sensitization. Sulfhydryl compounds interfere with free radical generation and may act as radiation protectors. The challenge for radiation treatment planning is to deliver the radiation to the tumor volume with as little normal tissue in the field as possible.

Therapeutic radiation is delivered in three ways: *teletherapy*, with beams of radiation generated at a distance and aimed at the tumor within the patient; *brachytherapy*, with encapsulated sources of radiation implanted directly into or adjacent to tumor tissues; and *systemic therapy*, with radionuclides targeted in some fashion to a site of tumor. Teletherapy is the most commonly used form of radiation therapy.

Radiation from any source decreases in intensity as a function of the square of the distance from the source (inverse square law). Thus, if the radiation source is 5 cm above the skin surface and the tumor is 5 cm below the skin surface, the intensity of radiation in the tumor will be $5^2/10^2$, or 25% of the intensity at the skin. By contrast, if the radiation source is moved to 100 cm from the patient, the intensity of radiation in the tumor will be $100^2/105^2$, or 91% of the intensity at the skin. Teletherapy maintains intensity over a larger volume of target tissue by increasing the source-to-surface distance. In brachytherapy, the source-to-surface distance is small; thus, the effective treatment volume is small.

X-rays and gamma rays are the forms of radiation most commonly used to treat cancer. They are both electromagnetic, nonparticulate waves that cause the ejection of an orbital electron when absorbed. This orbital electron ejection is called *ionization*. X-rays are generated by linear accelerators; gamma rays are generated from decay of atomic nuclei in radioisotopes such as cobalt and radium. These waves behave biologically as packets of energy, called *photons*. Particulate forms of radiation are also used in certain circumstances. Electron beams have a very low tissue penetrance and are used to treat skin conditions such as mycosis fungoides. Neutron beams may be somewhat more effective than x-rays in treating salivary gland tumors. However, aside from these specialized uses, particulate forms of radiation such as neutrons, protons, and negative mesons, which should do more tissue damage because of their higher LET and be less dependent on oxygen, have not yet found wide applicability to cancer treatment.

A number of parameters influence the damage done to tissue by radiation. Hypoxic cells are relatively resistant. Nondividing cells are more resistant than dividing cells. In addition to these biologic parameters, physical parameters of the radiation are also crucial. The energy of the radiation determines its ability to penetrate tissue. Low-energy orthovoltage beams (150 to 400 kV) scatter when they strike the body, much like light diffuses when it strikes particles in the air. Such beams result in more damage to adjacent normal tissues and less radiation delivered to the tumor. Megavoltage radiation (>1 MeV) has very low lateral scatter; this produces a skin-sparing effect, more homogeneous distribution of the radiation energy, and greater deposit of the energy in the tumor, or *target volume*. The tissues that the beam passes through to get to the tumor are called the *transit volume*. The maximum dose in the target volume is often the cause of complications to tissues in the transit volume, and the minimum dose in the target volume influences the likelihood of tumor recurrence. Dose homogeneity in the target volume is the goal.

Radiation is quantitated on the basis of the amount of radiation absorbed in the patient, not based upon the amount of radiation generated by the machine. Radiation dose is measured by placing detectors at the body surface or calculating the dose based on radiating phantoms that resemble human form and substance. Radiation dose has three determinants: total absorbed dose, number of fractions, and time. A frequent error is to omit the number of fractions and the duration of treatment. This is analogous to saying that a runner completed a race in 20 s; without knowing how far he or she ran, the result is difficult to interpret. The time could be very good for a 200-m race or very

TABLE 71-4 *Class 1 Organs: Fatal or Severe Morbidity Following Cumulative Doses of Radiation Delivered with Standard Fractionation*

Organ	Injury	$TD_{5/5}$[a]	$TD_{50/5}$[b]	Whole or Partial Organ (Field Size or Length)
Bone marrow	Aplasia, pancytopenia	250	450	Whole
		3000	4000	Segmental
Liver	Acute and chronic hepatitis	2500	4000	Whole
		1500	2000	Whole (strip)
Stomach	Perforation, ulcer, hemorrhage	4500	5500	100 cm
Intestine	Ulcer, perforation, hemorrhage	4500	5500	400 cm
		5000	6500	100 cm
Brain	Infarction, necrosis	5000	6000	Whole
Spinal cord	Infarction, necrosis	4500	5500	10 cm
Heart	Pericarditis, pancarditis	4500	5500	60%
		7000	8000	25%
Lung	Acute and chronic pneumonitis	3000	3500	100 cm
		1500	2500	Whole
Kidney	Acute and chronic nephrosclerosis	1500	2000	Whole (strip)
		2000	2500	Whole
Fetus	Death	200	400	Whole

[a] $TD_{5/5}$ is the minimal tolerance dose—the dose that, when administered to a given patient population under a standard set of treatment conditions, results in a rate of severe complications of 5% or less within 5 years of treatment.

[b] $TD_{50/5}$ is the maximal tolerance dose—the dose that, when administered to a given population under a standard set of treatment conditions, results in a rate of severe complications of 50% within 5 years of treatment.

Source: From P Rubin et al (eds): *Radiation Biology and Radiation Pathology Syllabus*, set RT 1: *Radiation Oncology*. Chicago, American College of Radiology, 1975.

poor for a 100-m race. Thus, a typical course of radiation therapy should be described as 4500 cGy delivered to a particular target (e.g., mediastinum) over 5 weeks in 180-cGy fractions. Most curative radiation treatment programs are delivered once a day, 5 days a week in 150- to 200-cGy fractions.

Although radiation can interfere with many cellular processes, many experts feel that a cell must undergo a double-strand DNA break from radiation in order to be killed. The factors that influence tumor cell killing include the D_0 of the tumor (the dose required to deliver an average of one lethal hit to all the cells in a population), the D_q of the tumor (the threshold dose—a measure of the cell's ability to repair sublethal damage), hypoxia, tumor mass, growth fraction, and cell cycle time and phase (cells in late G_1 and S are more resistant). Rate of clinical response is not predictive; some cells do not die after radiation exposure until they attempt to replicate.

Compounds that incorporate into DNA and alter its stereochemistry (e.g., halogenated pyrimidines, cisplatin) augment radiation effects. Hydroxyurea, another DNA synthesis inhibitor, also potentiates radiation effects. Compounds that deplete thiols (e.g., buthionine sulfoximine) can also augment radiation effects. Hypoxia is a major factor that interferes with radiation effects.

APPLICATION TO PATIENTS ■ Teletherapy Radiation therapy can be used alone or together with chemotherapy to produce cure of localized tumors and control of the primary site of disease in tumors that have disseminated. Therapy is planned based on the use of a simulator with the treatment field or fields designed to accommodate an individual patient's anatomic features. Individualized treatment planning employs lead shielding tailored to shape the field and limit the radiation exposure of normal tissue. Often the radiation is delivered from two or three different positions. Conformal three-dimensional treatment planning permits the delivery of higher doses of radiation to the target volume without increasing complications in the transit volume.

Radiation therapy is a component of curative therapy for a number of diseases including breast cancer, Hodgkin's disease, head and neck cancer, prostate cancer, and gynecologic cancers. Radiation therapy can also palliate disease symptoms in a variety of settings: relief of bone pain from metastatic disease, control of brain metastases, reversal of spinal cord compression and superior vena caval obstruction, shrinkage of painful masses, and opening threatened airways. In high-risk settings, radiation therapy can prevent the development of leptomeningeal disease and brain metastases in acute leukemia and lung cancer.

Brachytherapy Brachytherapy involves placing a sealed source of radiation into or adjacent to the tumor and withdrawing the radiation source after a period of time precisely calculated to deliver a chosen dose of radiation to the tumor. This approach is often used to treat brain tumors and cervical cancer. The difficulty with brachytherapy is the short range of radiation effects (the inverse square law) and the inability to shape the radiation to fit the target volume. Normal tissue may receive substantial exposure to the radiation, with attendant radiation enteritis or cystitis in cervix cancer or brain injury in brain tumors.

Radionuclides and Radioimmunotherapy Nuclear medicine physicians or radiation oncologists may administer radionuclides with therapeutic effects. Iodine 131 is used to treat thyroid cancer as iodine is naturally taken up preferentially by the thyroid. It emits gamma rays that destroy the normal thyroid as well as the tumor. Strontium 89 and samarium 153 are two radionuclides that are preferentially taken up in bone, particularly sites of new bone formation. Both are capable of controlling bone metastases and the pain associated with them, but the dose-limiting toxicity is myelosuppression.

Monoclonal antibodies and other ligands can be attached to radioisotopes by conjugation (for nonmetal isotopes) or by chelation (for metal isotopes), and the targeting moiety can result in the accumulation of the radionuclide preferentially in tumor. Iodine 131–labeled anti-CD20 and yttrium 90–labeled anti-CD20 are active in B cell lymphoma, and other labeled antibodies are being evaluated. Thyroid uptake of labeled iodine is blocked by cold iodine. Dose-limiting toxicity is myelosuppression.

Photodynamic Therapy Some chemical structures (porphyrins, phthalocyanines) are selectively taken up by cancer cells by mechanisms not fully defined. When light, usually delivered by a laser, is shone on cells containing these compounds, free radicals are generated and the cells die. Hematoporphyrins and light are being used with increasing frequency to treat skin cancer; ovarian cancer; and cancers of the lung, colon, rectum, and esophagus. Palliation of recurrent locally advanced disease can sometimes be dramatic and last many months.

TOXICITY Though radiation therapy is most often administered to a local region, systemic effects, including fatigue, anorexia, nausea, and vomiting, may develop related in part to the volume of tissue irradiated, dose fractionation, radiation fields, and individual susceptibility. Bone is among the most radioresistant organs, radiation effects being manifested mainly in children through premature fusion of the epiphyseal growth plate. By contrast, the male testis, female ovary, and bone marrow are the most sensitive organs. Any bone marrow in a radiation field will be eradicated by therapeutic irradiation. Organs with less need for cell renewal, such as heart, skeletal muscle, and nerves, are more resistant to radiation effects. In radiation-resistant organs, the vascular endothelium is the most sensitive component. Organs with more self-renewal as a part of normal homeostasis, such as the hematopoietic system and mucosal lining of the intestinal tract, are more sensitive. Acute toxicities include mucositis, skin erythema (ulceration in severe cases), and bone marrow toxicity. Often these can be alleviated by interruption of treatment.

Chronic toxicities are more serious. Radiation of the head and neck region often produces thyroid failure. Cataracts and retinal damage can lead to blindness. Salivary glands stop making saliva, which leads to dental caries and poor dentition. Taste and smell can be affected. Mediastinal irradiation leads to a threefold increased risk of fatal myocardial infarction. Other late vascular effects include chronic constrictive pericarditis, lung fibrosis, viscus stricture, spinal cord transection, and radiation enteritis. A serious late toxicity is the development of second solid tumors in or adjacent to the radiation fields. Such tumors can develop in any organ or tissue and occur at a rate of about 1% per year beginning in the second decade after treatment. Some organs vary in susceptibility to radiation carcinogenesis. Women under age 30 experience a ≥ 100-fold increase in the incidence of breast cancer after chest or mantle-field radiation; women treated after age 30 have little or no increased risk of breast cancer. No data suggest that a threshold dose of therapeutic radiation exists below which the incidence of second cancers is decreased. High rates of second tumors have been documented in people who receive as little as 1000 cGy.

Central Nervous System Traditionally, the central nervous system (CNS) has been described as relatively resistant to radiation-induced changes. When the human brain is treated with standard fractionation (180 to 200 cGy/d), acute reactions are seldom observed.

Subacute CNS reactions to radiation treatment are more common. The clinical manifestations may include *Lhermitte's sign*, which is a self-limited paresthesia occurring with flexion of the neck. It is believed to be due to transient demyelination of the spinal cord following significant radiation exposure. It can be seen 1 to 3 months after completion of radiation treatment to the spinal cord. The frequency of Lhermitte's sign varies according to the type of radiation therapy and has been reported to be as high as 15% after mantle-field radiation. Mild encephalopathy and focal neurologic changes can also occur after irradiation limited to the cranium. If radiation treatments to the brain are given at the same time that chemotherapeutic agents are administered, the effects can be more severe, presumably reflecting altered permeability to the drugs. The effect of cranial irradiation is believed to be secondary to radiation effects on the replicating oligodendrocytes and possibly on the microvasculature. Both clinical and radiologic changes may simulate tumor progression and can often pose diagnostic and treatment dilemmas. A typical example of this kind of conundrum would be attempting to distinguish clinically between radionecrosis and recurrent tumor in patients with gliomas after radiotherapy.

Postirradiation pathology and associated clinical symptoms typically begin 6 to 36 months after radiation therapy and are related to the total dose and volume treated. Fraction size appears to be the most important variable affecting the rate of postirradiation brain necrosis. Neurocognitive changes can also be seen in children after cranial irradiation. The important pretreatment factors that predict the degree of late CNS effects include the age of the patient when cranial irradiation was given and neurocognitive functional level at the time of treatment.

A unique late effect of cranial irradiation combined with chemotherapy, known as *leukoencephalopathy*, has been described in some patients. Leukoencephalopathy is a necrotizing reaction usually noted 4 to 12 months after combined treatment with methotrexate and cranial irradiation. Dementia and dysarthria are often observed and may progress to seizures, ataxia, or death.

Transverse myelitis after radiation treatment is a spinal cord reaction similar to cerebral necrosis. This syndrome consists of progressive and irreversible leg weakness and loss of bladder function and sensation referrable to a single spinal cord level. Flaccid paralysis eventually occurs. Symptoms can occur as early as 6 months after radiation treatment, but the usual time to onset is 12 to 24 months. Lhermitte's sign does not correlate with transverse myelitis.

Skin   Skin reaction can be seen within 2 weeks of fractionated radiotherapy, a delay that correlates with the time required for cells to move from the basal to the keratinized layer of skin. The severity of the reaction depends on the skin dose per fraction and the total dose delivered to an area of skin. Erythema is observed, soon followed by dry desquamation. The skin at this time can be erythematous, warm, and sometimes edematous. The vessels in the upper dermis are dilated, and inflammatory infiltration with granulocytes, macrophages, eosinophils, plasma cells, and lymphocytes is noted.

When a severe skin reaction occurs, it is usually located where the beam strikes the skin tangentially. *Moist desquamation* consists of eruption of the epidermal layer. Healing is through reepithelialization from cells of less affected basal layers. When skin reactions are severe, treatment interruptions are needed to permit healing.

Dry desquamation is treated conservatively. Symptoms of dryness can be alleviated by advising the patient to wear only cotton fabric next to the affected skin and to refrain from the use of irritants of any kind. If treatment becomes necessary, hydrophilic agents that do not contain heavy metals are recommended. Moist desquamation is best managed by leaving the affected area dry and open to air.

A chronic reaction to radiation can be seen starting 6 to 12 months after irradiation. The epidermis may become atrophic and may be more easily injured than normal skin. Interstitial fibrosis and telangiectasia may also be increased. Hyperpigmentation of irradiated skin outlining the treatment field can be seen within a couple of months after completion of irradiation. This will fade gradually. The skin becomes thin, and hair loss may be permanent. Radiation therapy can induce second malignancies, which tend to be more aggressive than cancers arising in patients without significant radiation exposure.

Heart and Blood Vessels   When cardiac disease appears after radiation treatment, it is often difficult to tell to what extent the radiation treatment was causative. The pathogenesis of atherosclerotic heart disease is multifactorial. Exposure of a large heart volume to high-dose radiation therapy accelerates the development of coronary artery disease. Acute "pericarditis" may result from cardiac irradiation. The symptoms may include chest pain and fever, with or without pericardial effusion. This syndrome is usually self-limited and typically manifests itself a few months after treatment. Asymptomatic pericardial effusion may be the most common manifestation of radiation-induced heart

disease. It is usually detected by chest x-ray and confirmed by an echocardiogram.

Most patients with symptomatic radiation-induced constrictive pericarditis will have received >40 Gy to a large portion of the heart. The risk increases significantly with cardiac doses >50 Gy.

Chronic cardiac changes may have their onset from 6 months to several years after irradiation. The clinical symptoms may indicate chronic constrictive disease due to pericardial, myocardial, and endocardial fibrosis—a pancarditis. The clinical signs may include dyspnea, chest pain, venous distention, pleural effusion, and paradoxical pulse.

Lung   The clinical symptoms of radiation pneumonitis can be separated into early and late phases. During the early phase, clinical manifestations may include dyspnea, cough, and fever. Shortness of breath is relatively infrequent. It is more common to observe only the radiologic changes on a chest x-ray, without clinical symptoms. The clinical signs and symptoms of radiation pneumonitis may appear in 3 to 6 weeks if a large region of lung is irradiated to a dose >25 Gy. An infiltrate outlining the treatment field may become evident on the chest x-ray. Radiation changes rarely occur outside the treated field. Computed tomography can often help in distinguishing radiation pneumonitis from other causes of the infiltrate. The frequency of radiation pneumonitis can be reduced with careful treatment planning designed to lower the total dose given to the treated lung volume. Permanent scarring that results in respiratory compromise may develop if the dose and the volume of lung irradiated are excessive. Dyspnea and cough may be severe and debilitating.

Patients with symptoms of radiation pneumonitis may respond rapidly to glucocorticoids, but the medication has little effect on fibrotic changes. Glucocorticoids must be tapered very slowly to avoid rebound exacerbation of symptoms, which can prove lethal for some patients. Prophylactic administration of glucocorticoids is of no proven merit. Supportive care includes bronchodilators and oxygen at the lowest possible FI_{O_2}.

Digestive Tract   Pathologic changes of the epithelial layer occur early during radiation treatments. The underlying submucosa may become edematous, with dilation of capillaries. Recovery from radiation damage can be expected within a few weeks after completion of radiation therapy, provided that sufficient numbers of stem cells are left. The radioresponsiveness of the aerodigestive tract, like that of other structures, is not uniform but varies according to the location.

Patients often have symptoms from radiation exposure that are similar to other forms of acute gastritis. The clinical signs include epigastric pain, loss of appetite, nausea, and vomiting. Decreased gastric acidity is observed after 15 to 20 Gy of fractionated radiation therapy. The tolerance of the stomach to radiation is also aggravated by addition of systemic chemotherapy, such as 5-fluorouracil.

The germinal centers of the bowel mucosa are in the crypts of Lieberkühn. Newly formed cells move upward along the walls of the crypts as transitional cells, undergoing maturation. The epithelial lining of the small bowel is the most rapidly renewed system in the human body and is completely renewed in 3 to 6 days. Within 12 to 24 h after the first dose of radiation therapy, pathologic evidence of dead cells are seen in the mucosal lining. Complete denudation of the mucosal surface rarely occurs during a regular course of radiation treatment because of the high capacity of the mucosa for regeneration. However, a focal area of erosion may be seen. The histologic appearance may be nearly normal within 2 to 3 weeks after radiation therapy.

Clinical manifestations of acute radiation enteropathy are nausea and vomiting, diarrhea, and cramping pain. Relevant factors contributing to the pathogenesis of diarrhea include malabsorption and alterations in the intestinal bacterial flora. The severity of symptoms, as in other anatomic areas, is proportional to the irradiated volume and the total dose.

Symptoms of chronic radiation enteropathy include diarrhea, abdominal cramping, nausea, malabsorption, vomiting, and obstruction. Progressive fibrosis, perforation, fistula formation, and stenosis of the irradiated portion of the bowel can occur during the chronic phase of radiation enteropathy. Most clinical manifestations of chronic changes occur between 6 months and 5 years after radiation therapy.

Conservative noninvasive treatment can frequently control gastrointestinal symptoms. A low-residue or elemental diet may be beneficial. When nonsurgical treatment fails to relieve severe symptoms, surgical intervention is often indicated.

Bladder Radiation injury to the bladder generally becomes symptomatic 3 to 6 weeks after the start of treatment, and symptoms usually subside 3 to 4 weeks after completion of radiation therapy. Patients often complain of increased frequency and dysuria. Cystoscopy often shows diffuse mucosal changes similar to those of acute cystitis. Sometimes desquamation and ulceration can be seen. Without infection, urinary symptoms are managed symptomatically. Concurrent chemotherapy with cytotoxic agents such as cyclophosphamide increases the severity of the acute bladder reaction.

The late effects of high radiation doses to the bladder may include contracture in size, interstitial fibrosis, telangiectasia, and ulceration. The blood vessels may be dilated and prone to rupture, resulting in painless hematuria. These changes are often difficult to distinguish from tumor recurrence and progression. A contracted bladder may result from doses >60 Gy.

Testes and Ovaries In general, type B spermatogonia are exquisitely sensitive to the effects of radiation. The type A spermatogonia are thought to be more resistant because their longer cell cycle time allows considerable variation in radiosensitivity among different phases of the cell cycle. Sertoli cells and Leydig cells are less radiosensitive than the spermatogonia. Elevated levels of follicle-stimulating hormone (FSH) and luteinizing hormone (LH) have been observed after as little as 75 cGy. Doses as low as 10 cGy to the testicles may result in injury to the type B spermatogonia. The single dose required for permanent sterilization on normal human males is believed to be between 6 and 10 Gy. In normal human males, sperm count recovery requires 9 to 18 months after a fractionated dose of 8 to 100 cGy.

The radiation dose necessary to induce ovarian failure is age-dependent. A single dose of 3 to 4 Gy can induce amenorrhea in almost all women over 40 years of age. In young women, oogenesis is much less sensitive to radiation than is spermatogenesis in men.

ACUTE TOTAL-BODY IRRADIATION The data regarding the acute effects of total-body irradiation on humans come primarily from Japanese survivors of the atomic bomb, Marshallese exposed to radioactive fallout in 1954, and persons exposed to radiation from the Chernobyl nuclear accident. Early symptoms of acute total-body irradiation, known as the *prodromal radiation syndrome*, may last for a limited time. Clinical manifestations depend on the total-body dose. At doses >100 Gy, death usually occurs 24 to 48 h later from neurologic and cardiovascular failure. This is known as the *cerebrovascular syndrome*. Because cerebrovascular damage causes death very quickly, the failures of other systems do not have time to develop.

At doses between 5 and 12 Gy, death may occur in a matter of days as a result of the *gastrointestinal syndrome*. The symptoms during this period may include nausea, vomiting, and prolonged diarrhea for several days leading to dehydration, sepsis, and death. A total-body dose >10 Gy is uniformly fatal unless supportive therapy (fluid, electrolytes, blood products, and antibiotics) is given. The process of intestinal denudation depends on the dose and may take between 3 and 120 days. Death from intestinal denudation usually occurs before the full effects of radiation on the blood-forming elements are seen.

At total-body doses between 2 and 8 Gy, death may occur 2 to 4 weeks after exposure from bone marrow failure, the *hematopoietic syndrome*. The full effect of radiation is not apparent until the mature hematopoietic cells are depleted. Clinical symptoms during this period may include chills, fatigue, and petechial hemorrhage. Peripheral blood lymphopenia develops during the first 12 to 48 h after any significant exposure. Beyond 5 to 6 Gy, the rate and magnitude of the drop are not well correlated to radiation exposure. Some stem cells may survive acute exposure to ≥10 Gy. Death is from infection or bleeding and usually occurs before anemia can develop (red blood cell half-life is 100 to 120 days).

The LD$_{50/60}$ (the dose at which 50% of the population is dead by 60 days) is around 3.25 Gy if support is not given. There is considerable variability in the total-body dose tolerated. The very young and the old are more radiosensitive than middle-aged and young adults. Females in general appear to be more tolerant of radiation than males. Persons exposed to <2 Gy will require little or no therapy but should probably be observed closely with daily blood counts for a few days.

The role of bone marrow transplantation for patients exposed to acute total-body irradiation is debated. At doses <8 Gy, the patient is likely to survive with supportive care. Most people exposed to doses >10 Gy will die from the gastrointestinal syndrome. Therefore, 8 to 10 Gy may be the dose range in which bone marrow transplantation could have a role, although the Chernobyl experience did not confirm this prediction. Estimating the dose received by a given patient after radiation exposure is difficult. However, exposure estimation must be done quickly because bone marrow transplantation is most effective if it is performed within the first 3 to 5 days after exposure.

RADIATION AND CANCER INDUCTION Some nonlethal changes in DNA sequences caused by irradiation may cause malignant transformations. Thus, it is not surprising that second neoplasms can be caused by exposure to ionizing radiation. However, paradoxically, this risk decreases with doses above a certain level. Whether there is a "safe" dose that will not induce any cancer is not likely. Estimates of the risk of developing cancer after low-level exposure to ionizing radiation are often derived by extrapolation from the risks for higher doses and acute exposures. Predicted risks of cancer are, therefore, prone to modification depending on the assumptions made about the data available for analysis.

Throughout the history of human exposure to ionizing radiation, increased rates of cancer have been noted after exposure to radiation. The populations studied include survivors of the atomic bomb during World War II; radium watch-dial painters who shaped their brush tips with their tongues; patients who underwent multiple fluoroscopic examinations for tuberculosis, received spinal irradiation for ankylosing spondylitis, and received breast irradiation for postpartum mastitis; and others. Exposure to ionizing radiation at an earlier age appears to increase the chance of developing radiation-induced carcinomas. However, the radiation-induced cancers have an age of onset similar to that of the native cancers, and the available data argue against radiation as the only cause of the increased incidence of cancers seen after exposure to radiation. Table 71-5 shows examples of cancer observed in specific situations.

Because a safe dose of radiation is unknown at present, it is prudent to avoid routine exposures to ionizing irradiation.

TABLE 71-5 *Examples of Radiation-Induced Cancers*

Types of Exposure	Types of Cancer Observed
Neck irradiation during infancy for benign conditions	Thyroid carcinoma
Radiation therapy for other malignant tumors	Thyroid carcinoma
	Breast cancer
	Gastric cancer
	Melanoma
	Lung cancer
	Sarcomas in the field
Cranial irradiation	Central nervous system tumors
Breast irradiation for postpartum mastitis	Breast cancer
Brush-licking by radium dial painters	Bone sarcomas
Uranium mining	Lung cancer
In utero exposure	Leukemia

FURTHER READING

HALL EJ: *Radiobiology for the Radiologist*, 5th ed. Philadelphia, Lippincott Williams & Wilkins, 2000

HEVEZI JM: Emerging technology in cancer treatment: Radiotherapy modalities. Oncology 17:1445, 2003

METTLER FA JR, UPTON AC: *Medical Effects of Ionizing Radiation*, 2d ed, Philadelphia, Saunders, 1995

MOSS WT, COX JD: *Moss' Radiation Oncology: Rationale, Technique, Results*, 7th ed. St. Louis, Mosby, 1994

PEREZ CP, BRADY LW: *Principles and Practice of Radiation Oncology*, 3d ed. Philadelphia, Lippincott Williams & Wilkins, 1998

RUBIN P: Late effects of normal tissues consensus conference. Int J Radiat Oncol Biol Phys 31:5, 1995

RUIFROK ACC, MCBRIDE WH: Growth factors: Biological and clinical aspects. Int J Radiat Oncol Biol Phys 43:877, 1999

72 INFECTIONS IN PATIENTS WITH CANCER
Robert Finberg

Infections are a common cause of death and an even more common cause of morbidity in patients with a wide variety of neoplasms. Autopsy studies show that most deaths from acute leukemia and half of deaths from lymphoma are caused directly by infection. With more intensive chemotherapy, patients with solid tumors have also become more likely to die of infection.

A physical predisposition to infection (Table 72-1) can be a result of the neoplasm's production of a break in the skin; for example, a squamous cell carcinoma may cause local invasion of the epidermis, which allows bacteria to gain access to the subcutaneous tissue and permits the development of cellulitis. The artificial closing of a normally patent orifice can also predispose to infection: Obstruction of a ureter by a tumor can cause urinary tract infection, and obstruction of the bile duct can cause cholangitis. Part of the host's normal defense against infection depends on the continuous emptying of a viscus; without emptying, a few bacteria present as a result of bacteremia or local transit can multiply and cause disease.

A similar problem can affect patients whose lymph node integrity has been disrupted by radical surgery, particularly patients who have had radical node dissections. A common clinical problem following radical mastectomy is the development of cellulitis (usually caused by streptococci or staphylococci) because of lymphedema and/or inadequate lymph drainage. In most cases, this problem can be addressed by local measures designed to prevent fluid accumulation and breaks in the skin, but antibiotic prophylaxis has been necessary in refractory cases.

A life-threatening problem common to many cancer patients is the loss of the reticuloendothelial capacity to clear microorganisms after splenectomy. Splenectomy may be performed as part of the management of hairy cell leukemia, chronic lymphocytic leukemia (CLL), and chronic myelocytic leukemia (CML) and in Hodgkin's disease. Even after curative therapy for the underlying disease, the lack of a spleen predisposes such patients to rapidly fatal infections. The loss of the spleen through trauma similarly predisposes the normal host to overwhelming infection for as long as 25 years after splenectomy. The splenectomized patient should be counseled about the risks of infection with certain organisms, such as the protozoan *Babesia* (Chap. 195) and *Capnocytophaga canimorsus* (formerly dysgonic fermenter 2, or DF-2), a bacterium carried in the mouths of animals (Chap. 131). Since encapsulated bacteria (*Streptococcus pneumoniae*, *Haemophilus influenzae*, and *Neisseria meningitidis*) are the organisms most commonly associated with postsplenectomy sepsis, splenectomized persons should be vaccinated (and revaccinated; Table 72-2) against the capsular polysaccharides of these organisms. Many clinicians recommend giving splenectomized patients a small supply of antibiotics effective against *S. pneumoniae*, *N. meningitidis*, and *H. influenzae* to avert rapid, overwhelming sepsis in the event that they cannot present for medical attention immediately after the onset of fever or other symptoms of bacterial infection.

The level of suspicion of infections with certain organisms should depend on the type of cancer diagnosed (Table 72-3). Diagnosis of multiple myeloma or CLL should alert the clinician to the possibility of hypogammaglobulinemia. While immunoglobulin replacement therapy can be effective, in most cases prophylactic antibiotics are a cheaper, more convenient method of eliminating bacterial infections in CLL patients with hypogammaglobulinemia. Patients with acute lymphocytic leukemia (ALL), patients with non-Hodgkin's lymphoma, and all cancer patients treated with high-dose glucocorticoids (or glucocorticoid-containing chemotherapy regimens) should receive antibiotic prophylaxis for *Pneumocystis* infection (Table 72-3) for the duration of their chemotherapy. In addition to exhibiting susceptibility to certain infectious organisms, patients with cancer are likely to manifest their infections in characteristic ways.

TABLE 72-1 *Normal Barriers to Infections*

Type of Defense	Specific Lesion	Cells Involved	Organism	Cancer Association	Disease
Physical barrier	Breaks in skin	Skin epithelial cells	Staphylococci, streptococci	Head and neck, squamous cell carcinoma	Cellulitis, extensive skin infection
Emptying of fluid collections	Occlusion of orifices: ureters, bile duct, colon	Luminal epithelial cells	Gram-negative bacilli	Renal, ovarian, biliary tree, metastatic diseases of many cancers	Rapid, overwhelming bacteremia, urinary tract infection
Lymphatic disease	Node dissection	Lymph nodes	Staphylococci, streptococci	Breast cancer surgery	Cellulitis
Splenic clearance of microorganisms	Splenectomy	Splenic reticuloendothelial cells	*Streptococcus pneumoniae*, *Haemophilus influenzae*, *Neisseria meningitidis*, *Babesia*, *Capnocytophaga canimorsus*	Hodgkin's disease, leukemia, idiopathic thrombocytopenic purpura	Rapid, overwhelming sepsis
Phagocytosis	Lack of granulocytes	Granulocytes (neutrophils)	Staphylococci, streptococci, enteric organisms, fungi	Hairy cell, acute myelocytic, and acute lymphocytic leukemias	Bacteremia
Humoral immunity	Lack of antibody	B cells	*S. pneumoniae*, *H. influenzae*, *N. meningitidis*	Chronic lymphocytic leukemia, multiple myeloma	Infections with encapsulated organisms, sinusitis, pneumonia
Cellular immunity	Lack of T cells	T cells and macrophages	*Mycobacterium tuberculosis*, *Listeria*, herpesviruses, fungi, other intracellular parasites	Hodgkin's disease, leukemia, T cell lymphoma	Infections with intracellular bacteria, fungi, parasites

TABLE 72-2 Vaccination of Cancer Patients Receiving Chemotherapy

Vaccine	Use in Indicated Patients		
	Intensive Chemotherapy	Hodgkin's Disease	Bone Marrow Transplantation
Diphtheria-tetanus (diphtheria, pertussis, tetanus; DPT) for children <7 years old	Primary series and boosters as necessary	No special recommendation	12, 14, and 24 months after transplantation
Poliomyelitis[a]	Complete primary series and boosters	No special recommendation	12, 14, and 24 months after transplantation
Haemophilus influenzae type b conjugate	Primary series and booster for children	Immunization before treatment and booster 3 months afterward	12, 14, and 24 months after transplantation
Hepatitis A	Not routinely recommended	Not routinely recommended	Not routinely recommended
Hepatitis B	Complete series	No special recommendation	12, 14, and 24 months after transplantation
23-Valent pneumococcal	Every 5 years	Immunization before treatment and booster 3 months afterward	12 and 24 months after transplantation
4-Valent meningococcal	Should be administered to splenectomized patients and patients living in endemic areas, including college students in dormitories	Should be administered to splenectomized patients and patients living in endemic areas, including college students in dormitories	Should be administered to splenectomized patients and patients living in endemic areas, including college students in dormitories
Influenza	Seasonal immunization	Seasonal immunization	Seasonal immunization
Measles/mumps/rubella	Contraindicated	Contraindicated	After 24 months in patients without graft-versus-host disease
Varicella-zoster virus	Contraindicated[b]	Contraindicated	Contraindicated

[a] Live-virus vaccine is contraindicated; inactivated vaccine should be used.
[b] Contact the manufacturer for more information on use in children with acute lymphocytic leukemia.

SYSTEM-SPECIFIC SYNDROMES

SKIN-SPECIFIC SYNDROMES Skin lesions are common in cancer patients, and their appearance may permit the diagnosis of systemic bacterial or fungal infection. While cellulitis caused by skin organisms such as *Streptococcus* or *Staphylococcus* is common, neutropenic patients [those with fewer than 500 functional polymorphonuclear leukocytes (PMNs) per microliter] and patients with impaired blood or lymphatic drainage may develop infections with unusual organisms. Innocent-looking macules or papules may be the first sign of bacterial or fungal sepsis in immunocompromised patients (Fig. 72-1). In the neutropenic host, a macule progresses rapidly to ecthyma gangrenosum, a usually painless, round, necrotic lesion consisting of a central black or gray-black eschar with surrounding erythema. Ecthyma gangrenosum is located in nonpressure areas (as distinguished from necrotic lesions associated with lack of circulation) and is often associated with *Pseudomonas aeruginosa* bacteremia (Chap. 136) but may be caused by other bacteria.

Candidemia (Chap. 187) is also associated with a variety of skin conditions and commonly presents as a maculopapular rash. Punch biopsy of the skin may be the best method for diagnosis.

Cellulitis, an acute spreading inflammation of the skin, is most often caused by infection with group A *Streptococcus* or *Staphylococcus aureus*, virulent organisms normally found on the skin (Chap. 110). Although cellulitis tends to be circumscribed in normal hosts, it may spread rapidly in neutropenic patients. A tiny break in the skin may lead to spreading cellulitis, which is characterized by pain and erythema; in such patients, signs of infection (e.g., purulence) are often lacking. What might be a furuncle in a normal host may require amputation because of uncontrolled infection in a patient presenting with leukemia. A dramatic response to an infection that might be trivial in a normal host can mark the first sign of leukemia. Fortunately, granulocytopenic patients are likely to be infected with certain types of organisms (Table 72-4); thus the selection of an antibiotic regimen is somewhat easier than it might otherwise be. (See discussion below on the selection of antibiotics for use in neutropenic patients.) It is essential to recognize cellulitis early and to treat it aggressively. Patients who are neutropenic or have previously received antibiotics for other reasons may develop cellulitis with unusual organisms (e.g., *Escherichia coli*, *Pseudomonas*, or fungi). Early treatment, even of innocent-looking lesions, is essential to prevent necrosis and loss of tissue. Debridement to prevent spread may sometimes be necessary early in the course of disease, but it can often be performed after chemotherapy, when the PMN count increases.

Sweet's syndrome, or *febrile neutrophilic dermatosis*, was originally described in women with elevated white blood cell counts. The disease is characterized by the presence of leukocytes in the lower dermis, with edema of the papillary body. Ironically, this disease now is usually seen in neutropenic patients with cancer, most often in association with acute leukemia but also in association with a variety of other malignancies. Sweet's syndrome usually presents as red or bluish-red papules or nodules that may coalesce and form sharply bordered plaques. The edema may suggest vesicles, but on palpation the lesions are solid, and vesicles probably never arise in this disease. The lesions are most common on the face, neck, and arms. On the legs, they may

TABLE 72-3 Infections and Cancer

Cancer	Underlying Immune Abnormality	Organisms Causing Infection
Multiple myeloma	Hypogammaglobulinemia	Streptococcus pneumoniae, Haemophilus influenzae, Neisseria meningitidis
Chronic lymphocytic leukemia	Hypogammaglobulinemia	S. pneumoniae, H. influenzae, N. meningitidis
Acute myelocytic or lymphocytic leukemia	Granulocytopenia, skin and mucous-membrane lesions	Extracellular gram-positive and gram-negative bacteria, fungi
Hodgkin's disease	Abnormal T cell function	Intracellular pathogens (Mycobacterium tuberculosis, Listeria, Salmonella, Cryptococcus, Mycobacterium avium)
Non-Hodgkin's lymphoma and acute lymphocytic leukemia	Glucocorticoid chemotherapy, T and B cell dysfunction	Pneumocystis
Colon and rectal tumors	Local abnormalities[a]	Streptococcus bovis (bacteremia)
Hairy cell leukemia	Abnormal T cell function	Intracellular pathogens (M. tuberculosis, Listeria, Cryptococcus, M. avium)

[a] The reason for this association is not well defined.

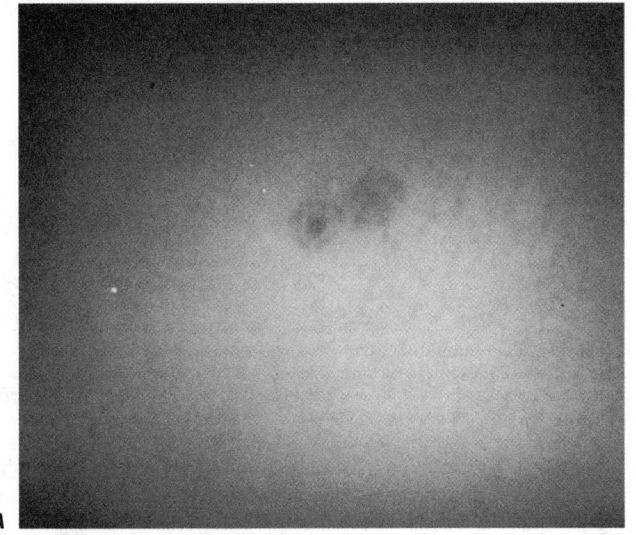
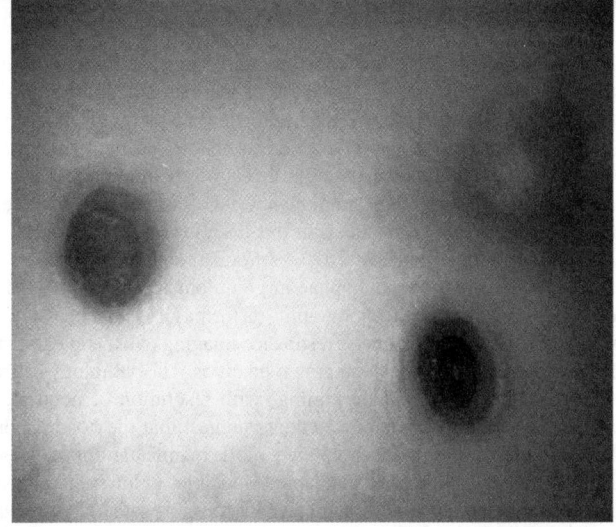

FIGURE 72-1 *A.* Papules related to *Escherichia coli* bacteremia in a neutropenic patient with acute lymphocytic leukemia. *B.* The same lesion the following day.

be confused with erythema nodosum. The development of lesions is often accompanied by high fevers and an elevated erythrocyte sedimentation rate. Both the lesions and the temperature elevation respond dramatically to glucocorticoids. Treatment begins with high doses of glucocorticoids (60 mg/d of prednisone) followed by tapered doses over the next 2 to 3 weeks.

Data indicate that *erythema multiforme* with mucous membrane involvement is often associated with herpes simplex virus (HSV) infection and is distinct from Stevens-Johnson syndrome, which is associated with drugs and tends to have a more widespread distribution. Since cancer patients are both immunosuppressed (and therefore susceptible to herpes infections) and heavily treated with drugs (and therefore subject to Stevens-Johnson syndrome), both of these conditions are common in this population.

Cytokines, which are used as adjuvants or primary treatments for cancer, can themselves cause characteristic rashes, further complicating the differential diagnosis. This phenomenon is a particular problem in bone marrow transplant recipients (Chap. 117), who, in addition to having the usual chemotherapy-, antibiotic-, and cytokine-induced rashes, are plagued by graft-versus-host disease.

CATHETER-RELATED INFECTIONS Because intravenous catheters are commonly used in cancer chemotherapy and are prone to infection (Chap. 116), they pose a major problem in the care of patients with cancer. Some catheter-associated infections can be treated with antibiotics, while in others the catheter must be removed. If the patient has a "tunneled" catheter (which consists of an entrance site, a subcutaneous tunnel, and an exit site), a red streak over the subcutaneous part of the line (the tunnel) is grounds for immediate removal of the catheter. Failure to remove catheters under these circumstances may result in extensive cellulitis and tissue necrosis.

More common than tunnel infections are exit-site infections, often with erythema around the area where the line penetrates the skin. Most

authorities (Chap. 120) recommend treatment (usually with vancomycin) for an exit-site infection caused by a coagulase-negative *Staphylococcus*. Treatment of coagulase-positive staphylococcal infection is associated with a poorer outcome, and it is advisable to remove the catheter if possible. Similarly, many clinicians remove catheters associated with infections due to *P. aeruginosa* and *Candida* species, since such infections are difficult to treat and bloodstream infections with these organisms are likely to be deadly. Catheter infections caused by *Burkholderia cepacia*, *Stenotrophomonas* spp., *Agrobacterium* spp., and *Acinetobacter baumannii* as well as *Pseudomonas* spp. other than *aeruginosa* are likely to be very difficult to eradicate with antibiotics alone. Similarly, isolation of *Bacillus*, *Corynebacterium*, and *Mycobacterium* spp. should prompt removal of the catheter.

GASTROINTESTINAL TRACT–SPECIFIC SYNDROMES ■ Upper Gastrointestinal Tract Disease ■ *INFECTIONS OF THE MOUTH* The oral cavity is rich in aerobic and anaerobic bacteria (Chap. 148) that normally live in a commensal relationship with the host. The antimetabolic effects of chemotherapy cause a breakdown of host defenses, leading to ulceration of the mouth and the potential for invasion by resident bacteria. Mouth ulcerations afflict most patients receiving chemotherapy and have been associated with viridans streptococcal bacteremia. A variety of topical rinses and elixirs have been proposed to treat these ulcerations. Although some may have a local anesthetic effect, the efficacy of any of these therapies in the prevention of disease is unproven. Similarly, the efficacy of mouthwashes in the prevention of esophagitis or invasive candidiasis is doubtful. Fluconazole, on the other hand, is clearly effective in the treatment of both local infections (thrush) and systemic infections (esophagitis) due to *Candida albicans*. Newer azoles (such as voriconazole) are similarly effective.

Noma (*cancrum oris*), commonly seen in malnourished children, is a penetrating disease of the soft and hard tissues of the mouth and adjacent sites, with resulting necrosis and gangrene. It has a counterpart in immunocompromised patients and is thought to be due to invasion of the tissues by *Bacteroides*, *Fusobacterium*, and other normal inhabitants of the mouth. Noma is associated with debility, poor oral hygiene, and immunosuppression.

Viruses, particularly HSV, are a prominent cause of morbidity in immunocompromised patients, in whom they are associated with severe mucositis. The use of acyclovir, either prophylactically or therapeutically, is of value.

ESOPHAGEAL INFECTIONS The differential diagnosis of esophagitis (usually presenting as substernal chest pain upon swallowing) includes herpes simplex and candidiasis, both of which are readily treatable.

Lower Gastrointestinal Tract Disease Hepatic candidiasis (Chap. 187) results from seeding of the liver (usually from a gastrointestinal source)

TABLE 72-4 *Organisms Likely to Cause Infections in Granulocytopenic Patients*

Gram-positive cocci	*Enterobacter* spp.
Staphylococcus epidermidis	*Serratia* spp.
Staphylococcus aureus	*Acinetobacter* spp.[a]
Viridans *Streptococcus*	*Citrobacter* spp.
Enterococcus faecalis	Gram-positive bacilli
Streptococcus pneumoniae	Diphtheroids
Gram-negative bacilli	JK bacillus[a]
Escherichia coli	Fungi
Klebsiella spp.	*Candida* spp.
Pseudomonas aeruginosa	*Aspergillus* spp.
Non-*aeruginosa Pseudomonas* spp.[a]	

[a] Often associated with intravenous catheters.

in neutropenic patients. It is most common in patients being treated for acute leukemia and usually presents symptomatically around the time the neutropenia resolves. The characteristic picture is that of persistent fever unresponsive to antibiotics; abdominal pain and tenderness or nausea; and elevated serum levels of alkaline phosphatase in a patient with hematologic malignancy who has recently recovered from neutropenia. The diagnosis of this disease (which may present in an indolent manner and persist for several months) is based on the finding of yeasts or pseudohyphae in granulomatous lesions. Hepatic ultrasound or computed tomography (CT) may reveal bull's-eye lesions. In some cases, magnetic resonance imaging (MRI) reveals small lesions not visible by other imaging modalities. The pathology (a granulomatous response) and the timing (with resolution of neutropenia and an elevation in granulocyte count) suggest that the host response to *Candida* is an important component of the manifestations of disease. In many cases, although organisms are visible, cultures of biopsied material may be negative. The designation *hepatosplenic candidiasis* or *hepatic candidiasis* is a misnomer because the disease often involves the kidneys and other tissues; the term *chronic disseminated candidiasis* may be more appropriate. Because of the risk of bleeding with liver biopsy, diagnosis is often based on imaging studies (MRI, CT). Amphotericin B is traditionally used for therapy (often for several months, until all manifestations of disease have disappeared), but fluconazole may be useful for outpatient therapy. The use of other antifungal agents and combination therapy is less well studied.

Typhlitis *Typhlitis*, sometimes referred to as necrotizing colitis, neutropenic colitis, necrotizing enteropathy, ileocecal syndrome, or cecitis, is a clinical syndrome of fever and right-lower-quadrant tenderness in an immunosuppressed host. This syndrome is classically seen in neutropenic patients after chemotherapy with cytotoxic drugs. It may be more common among children than among adults and appears to be much more common among patients with acute myelocytic leukemia (AML) or ALL than among those with other types of cancer. Physical examination reveals right-lower-quadrant tenderness, with or without rebound tenderness. Associated diarrhea (often bloody) is common, and the diagnosis can be confirmed by the finding of a thickened cecal wall on CT or ultrasonography. Plain films may reveal a right-lower-quadrant mass, but CT with contrast or MRI is a much more sensitive means of making the diagnosis. Although surgery is sometimes attempted to avoid perforation from ischemia, most cases resolve with medical therapy alone. The disease is sometimes associated with positive blood cultures (usually for aerobic gram-negative bacilli), and therapy is recommended for a broad spectrum of bacteria (particularly gram-negative bacilli, likely bowel flora).

Clostridium difficile–Induced Diarrhea Cancer patients are predisposed to the development of *C. difficile* diarrhea (Chap. 114) as a consequence of chemotherapy alone. Thus, they may have positive toxin tests before receiving antibiotics. Obviously, such patients are also subject to *C. difficile*–induced diarrhea as a result of antibiotic pressure. *C. difficile* should always be considered as a possible cause of diarrhea in cancer patients who have received antibiotics.

CENTRAL NERVOUS SYSTEM–SPECIFIC SYNDROMES ■ Meningitis The presentation of meningitis in patients with lymphoma or CLL, patients receiving chemotherapy (particularly with glucocorticoids) for solid tumors, and patients who have received bone marrow transplants suggests a diagnosis of cryptococcal or listerial infection. As noted previously, splenectomized patients are susceptible to rapid, overwhelming infection with encapsulated bacteria (including *S. pneumoniae*, *H. influenzae*, and *N. meningitidis*). Similarly, patients who are antibody-deficient (such as patients with CLL, those who have received intensive chemotherapy, or those who have undergone bone marrow transplantation) are likely to have infections caused by these bacteria. Other cancer patients, however, because of their defective cellular immunity, are likely to be infected with other pathogens (Table 72-3).

TABLE 72-5 Differential Diagnosis of Central Nervous System Infections in Patients with Cancer

Findings on CT or MRI	Underlying Predisposition	
	Prolonged Neutropenia	Defects in Cellular Immunity[a]
Mass lesions	*Aspergillus* brain abscess *Nocardia* brain abscess *Cryptococcus* brain abscess	Toxoplasmosis EBV-LPD
Diffuse encephalitis	PML (J-C virus)	Infection with VZV, CMV, HSV, HHV-6, J-C virus (PML), *Listeria*

[a] High-dose glucocorticoid therapy, cytotoxic chemotherapy.
Abbreviations: CMV, cytomegalovirus; CT, computed tomography; EBV-LPD, Epstein-Barr virus lymphoproliferative disease; HHV-6, human herpesvirus type 6; HSV, herpes simplex virus; PML, progressive multifocal leukoencephalopathy.

Encephalitis The spectrum of disease resulting from viral encephalitis is expanded in immunocompromised patients. Cancer patients receiving high-dose cytotoxic chemotherapy or any chemotherapy that affects T cell function (e.g., fludarabine) or antibodies that eliminate T cells (e.g., anti-CD3) or cytokine activity are predisposed to infections with intracellular organisms similar to those encountered in patients with AIDS (Chap. 173). Infection with varicella-zoster virus (VZV) has been associated with encephalitis that may be caused by VZV-related vasculitis. Chronic viral infections may also be associated with dementia and encephalitic presentations, and a diagnosis of progressive multifocal leukoencephalopathy should be considered when a patient who has received chemotherapy presents with dementia (Table 72-5). Other abnormalities of the central nervous system (CNS) that may be confused with infection include normal-pressure hydrocephalus and vasculitis resulting from CNS irradiation. It may be possible to differentiate these conditions by MRI.

Brain Masses Mass lesions of the brain most often present as headache with or without fever or neurologic abnormalities. Infections associated with mass lesions may be caused by bacteria (particularly *Nocardia*), fungi (particularly *Cryptococcus* or *Aspergillus*), or parasites (*Toxoplasma*). Epstein-Barr virus (EBV)–associated lymphoproliferative disease may also present as single or multiple mass lesions of the brain. A biopsy may be required for a definitive diagnosis.

PULMONARY INFECTIONS Pneumonia (Chap. 239) in immunocompromised patients may be difficult to diagnose because conventional methods of diagnosis depend on the presence of neutrophils. Bacterial pneumonia in neutropenic patients may present without purulent sputum—or, in fact, without any sputum at all—and may not produce physical findings suggestive of chest consolidation (rales or egophony).

In granulocytopenic patients with persistent or recurrent fever, the chest x-ray pattern may help to localize an infection and thus to determine which investigative tests and procedures should be undertaken and which therapeutic options should be considered (Table 72-6). The difficulties encountered in the management of pulmonary infiltrates relate in part to the difficulties of performing diagnostic procedures on

TABLE 72-6 Differential Diagnosis of Chest Infiltrates in Immunocompromised Patients

Infiltrate	Cause of Pneumonia	
	Infectious	Noninfectious
Localized	Bacteria, *Legionella*, mycobacteria	Local hemorrhage or embolism, tumor
Nodular	Fungi (e.g., *Aspergillus* or *Mucor*), *Nocardia*	Recurrent tumor
Diffuse	Viruses (especially CMV), *Chlamydia*, *Pneumocystis*, *Toxoplasma gondii*, mycobacteria	Congestive heart failure, radiation pneumonitis, drug-induced lung injury, diffuse alveolar hemorrhage (described after BMT)

Abbreviations: BMT, bone marrow transplantation; CMV, cytomegalovirus.

the patients involved. When platelet counts can be increased to adequate levels by transfusion, microscopic and microbiologic evaluation of the fluid obtained by endoscopic bronchial lavage is often diagnostic. Lavage fluid should be cultured for *Mycoplasma*, *Chlamydia*, *Legionella*, *Nocardia*, fungi, and more common bacterial pathogens. In addition, the possibility of *Pneumocystis* pneumonia should be considered, especially in patients with ALL or lymphoma who have not received prophylactic trimethoprim-sulfamethoxazole (TMP-SMX). The characteristics of the infiltrate may be helpful in decisions about further diagnostic and therapeutic maneuvers. Nodular infiltrates suggest fungal pneumonia (e.g., that caused by *Aspergillus* or *Mucor*). Such lesions may best be approached by visualized biopsy procedures.

Aspergillus spp. (Chap. 188) can colonize the skin and respiratory tract or cause fatal systemic illness. Although *Aspergillus* may cause aspergillomas in a previously existing cavity or may produce allergic bronchopulmonary aspergillosis, the major problem posed by this genus in neutropenic patients is invasive disease due to *A. fumigatus* or *A. flavus*. The organisms enter the host following colonization of the respiratory tract, with subsequent invasion of the blood vessels. The disease is likely to present as a thrombotic or embolic event because of the ability of the organisms to invade blood vessels. The risk of infection with *Aspergillus* correlates directly with the duration of neutropenia. In prolonged neutropenia, positive surveillance cultures for colonization of the nasopharynx with *Aspergillus* may predict the development of disease.

Patients with *Aspergillus* infection often present with pleuritic chest pain and fever, which are sometimes accompanied by cough. Hemoptysis may be an ominous sign. Chest x-rays may reveal new focal infiltrates or nodules. Chest CT may reveal a characteristic halo consisting of a mass-like infiltrate surrounded by an area of low attenuation. The presence of a "crescent sign" on a chest x-ray or a chest CT scan, in which the mass progresses to central cavitation, is characteristic of invasive *Aspergillus* infection but may develop as the lesions are resolving.

In addition to causing pulmonary disease, *Aspergillus* may invade through the nose or palate, with deep sinus penetration. The appearance of a discolored area in the nasal passages or on the hard palate should prompt a search for invasive *Aspergillus*. This situation is likely to require surgical debridement. Treatment (Chap. 188) with high doses of amphotericin B has been successful in curing granulocytopenic patients of invasive *Aspergillus* infection after the return of granulocytes. Catheter infections with *Aspergillus* usually require both removal of the catheter and antifungal therapy.

Diffuse interstitial infiltrates suggest viral, parasitic, or *Pneumocystis* pneumonia. If the patient has a diffuse interstitial pattern on chest x-ray, it may be reasonable to institute empirical treatment with TMP-SMX (for *Pneumocystis*) and a quinolone (for *Chlamydia*, *Mycoplasma*, and *Legionella*) or an erythromycin derivative (e.g., azithromycin) while considering invasive diagnostic procedures. Noninvasive procedures, such as staining of sputum smears for *Pneumocystis*, serum cryptococcal antigen tests, and urine testing for *Legionella* only, may be helpful. In transplant recipients who are seropositive for cytomegalovirus (CMV), a determination of CMV load in the serum should be considered. The availability of viral load studies (which allow physicians to quantitate viruses) has superseded simple measurement of serum IgG, which merely documents prior exposure to virus. Infections with viruses that cause only upper respiratory symptoms in immunocompetent hosts, such as respiratory syncytial virus, influenza viruses, and parainfluenza viruses, may be associated with fatal pneumonitis in immunocompromised hosts. An attempt at early diagnosis by nasopharyngeal aspiration should be considered so that appropriate treatment can be instituted.

While bleomycin is the most common cause of chemotherapy-induced lung disease, other causes include alkylating agents (such as cyclophosphamide, chlorambucil, and melphalan), nitrosoureas [carmustine (BCNU), lomustine (CCNU), and methyl-CCNU], busulfan, procarbazine, methotrexate, and hydroxyurea. Both infectious and noninfectious (drug- and/or radiation-induced) pneumonitis can cause fever and abnormalities on chest x-ray; thus, the differential diagnosis of an infiltrate in a patient receiving chemotherapy encompasses a broad range of conditions (Table 72-6). Since the treatment of radiation pneumonitis (which may respond dramatically to glucocorticoids) or drug-induced pneumonitis is different from that of infectious pneumonia, a biopsy may be important in the diagnosis. Unfortunately, no definitive diagnosis can be made in ~30% of cases, even after bronchoscopy.

Open-lung biopsy is the "gold standard" of diagnostic techniques. Biopsy via a visualized thoracostomy can replace an open procedure in many cases. When a biopsy cannot be performed, empirical treatment can be undertaken with a quinolone or erythromycin (or an erythromycin derivative such as azithromycin) and TMP-SMX (in the case of diffuse infiltrates) or with amphotericin B or other antifungal agents (in the case of nodular infiltrates). The risks should be weighed carefully in these cases. If inappropriate drugs are administered, empirical treatment may prove toxic or ineffective; either of these outcomes may be riskier than biopsy.

CARDIOVASCULAR INFECTIONS Patients with Hodgkin's disease are prone to persistent infections by *Salmonella*, sometimes (and particularly often in elderly patients) affecting a vascular site. The use of intravenous catheters deliberately lodged in the right atrium is associated with a high incidence of bacterial endocarditis (presumably related to valve damage followed by bacteremia). Nonbacterial thrombotic endocarditis has been described in association with a variety of malignancies (most often solid tumors) and may follow bone marrow transplantation as well. The presentation of an embolic event with a new cardiac murmur suggests this diagnosis. Blood cultures are negative in this disease of unknown pathogenesis.

ENDOCRINE SYNDROMES In addition to infections of the skin, gastrointestinal tract, and pulmonary and cardiovascular systems, infections of the endocrine system have been described in immunocompromised patients. *Candida* infection of the thyroid during neutropenia can be defined by indium-labeled white cell scans or gallium scans after neutrophil counts increase. CMV infection can cause adrenalitis with or without resulting adrenal insufficiency. The presentation of a sudden endocrine anomaly in an immunocompromised patient may be a sign of infection in the involved end organ.

MUSCULOSKELETAL INFECTIONS Infection that is a consequence of vascular compromise (resulting in gangrene) can occur when a tumor restricts the blood supply to muscles, bones, or joints. The process of diagnosis and treatment of such infection is similar to that in normal hosts, with the following caveats: (1) In terms of diagnosis, a lack of physical findings resulting from a lack of granulocytes in the granulocytopenic patient should make the clinician more aggressive in obtaining tissue rather than relying on physical signs. (2) In terms of therapy, aggressive debridement of infected tissues may be required, but it is usually difficult to operate on patients who have recently received chemotherapy, both because of a lack of platelets (which results in bleeding complications) and because of a lack of white blood cells (which may lead to secondary infection). A blood culture positive for *Clostridium perfringens* (an organism commonly associated with gas gangrene) can have a number of meanings (Chap. 126). Bloodstream infections with intestinal organisms like *Streptococcus bovis* and *C. perfringens* may arise spontaneously from lower gastrointestinal lesions (tumor or polyps); alternatively, these lesions may be harbingers of invasive disease. The clinical setting must be considered in order to define the appropriate treatment for each case.

RENAL AND URETERAL INFECTIONS Infections of the urinary tract are common among patients whose ureteral excretion is compromised (Table 72-1). *Candida*, which has a predilection for the kidney, can invade either from the bloodstream or in a retrograde manner (via the ureters or bladder) in immunocompromised patients. The presence of "fungus balls" or persistent candiduria suggests invasive disease. Persistent funguria (with *Aspergillus* as well as *Candida*) should prompt a search for a nidus of infection in the kidney.

Certain viruses are typically seen only in immunosuppressed patients. BK virus (polyomavirus hominis 1) has been documented in the urine of bone marrow transplant recipients and, like adenovirus, may be associated with hemorrhagic cystitis. BK-induced cystitis usually remits with decreasing immunosuppression. Anecdotal reports have described the treatment of infections due to adenovirus and BK virus with cidofovir (see below).

ABNORMALITIES THAT PREDISPOSE TO INFECTION

THE LYMPHOID SYSTEM It is beyond the scope of this chapter to detail how all the immunologic abnormalities that result from cancer or from chemotherapy for cancer lead to infections. Disorders of the immune system are discussed in other sections of this book. As has been noted, patients with antibody deficiency are predisposed to overwhelming infection with encapsulated bacteria (including *S. pneumoniae, H. influenzae,* and *N. meningitidis*). Infections that result from the lack of a functional cellular immune system are described in Chap. 173. It is worth mentioning, however, that patients undergoing intensive chemotherapy for any form of cancer will have not only defects due to granulocytopenia but also lymphocyte dysfunction, which may be profound. Thus, these patients—especially those receiving glucocorticoid-containing regimens or drugs that inhibit T cell activation or cytokine induction—should be given prophylaxis for *Pneumocystis* pneumonia.

THE HEMATOPOIETIC SYSTEM Initial studies in the 1960s revealed a dramatic increase in the incidence of infections (fatal and nonfatal) among cancer patients with a granulocyte count of <500/μL. Recent studies have cited a figure of 48.3 infections per 100 neutropenic patients (<1000 granulocytes per microliter) with hematologic malignancies and solid tumors, or 46.3 infections per 1000 days at risk.

Neutropenic patients are unusually susceptible to infection with a wide variety of bacteria; thus, antibiotic therapy should be initiated promptly to cover likely pathogens if infection is suspected. Indeed, early initiation of antibacterial agents is mandatory to prevent deaths. These patients are susceptible to gram-positive and gram-negative organisms found commonly on the skin and in the bowel (Table 72-4). Because treatment with narrow-spectrum agents leads to infection with organisms not covered by the antibiotics used, the initial regimen should target pathogens likely to be initial causes of bacterial infection in neutropenic hosts (Fig. 72-2).

℞ TREATMENT

Antibacterial Therapy Hundreds of antibacterial regimens have been tested for use in patients with cancer. The major risk of infection is related to the degree of neutropenia seen as a consequence of either the disease or therapy. Many of the relevant studies involved small populations in which the outcomes were generally good, and most lacked the statistical power to detect differences among the regimens studied. Each febrile neutropenic patient should be approached as a unique problem, with particular attention given to previous infections and recent exposures to antibiotics. Several general guidelines are useful in the initial treatment of neutropenic patients with fever (Fig. 72-2):

1. It is necessary to use antibiotics active against both gram-negative and gram-positive bacteria (Table 72-4) in the initial regimen.
2. An aminoglycoside or an antibiotic without good activity against gram-positive organisms (e.g., ciprofloxacin or aztreonam) alone is not adequate in this setting.
3. The agents used should reflect both the epidemiology and the antibiotic resistance pattern of the hospital. For example, in hospitals where there is gentamicin resistance, amikacin-containing regimens should be considered; in hospitals with frequent *P. aeruginosa* infections, a regimen with the highest level of activity against

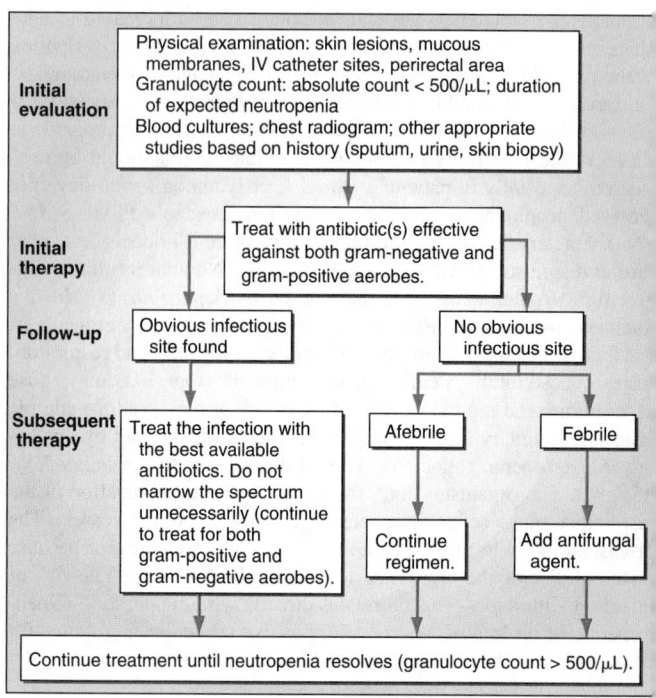

FIGURE 72-2 Algorithm for the diagnosis and treatment of febrile neutropenic patients.

this pathogen (such as tobramycin plus a semisynthetic penicillin) would be reasonable for initial therapy.
4. A single third-generation cephalosporin constitutes an appropriate initial regimen in many hospitals (if the pattern of resistance justifies its use).
5. Most standard regimens are designed for patients who have not previously received prophylactic antibiotics. The development of fever in a patient receiving antibiotics affects the choice of subsequent therapy (which should target resistant organisms and organisms known to cause infections in patients being treated with the antibiotics already administered).
6. Randomized trials have indicated that it is safe to use oral antibiotic regimens to treat "low-risk" patients with fever and neutropenia. Outpatients who are expected to remain neutropenic for <10 days and who have no concurrent medical problems (such as hypotension, pulmonary compromise, or abdominal pain) can be classified as low risk and treated with a broad-spectrum oral regimen. On the basis of large studies, it can be concluded that this therapy is safe and effective, at least when delivered in the inpatient setting. Outpatient treatment has been assessed in small studies, but data from large randomized trials demonstrating the safety of outpatient treatment of fever and neutropenia are not yet available.

The initial antibacterial regimen should be refined on the basis of culture results (Fig. 72-2). Blood cultures are the most relevant on which to base therapy; surface cultures of skin and mucous membranes may be misleading. In the case of gram-positive bacteremia or another gram-positive infection, it is important that the antibiotic be optimal for the organism isolated. If the infection is caused by certain gram-negative pathogens (such as *P. aeruginosa*), a synergistic combination of antibiotics (usually a semisynthetic penicillin, such as piperacillin, plus an aminoglycoside) may be appropriate. Although it is not desirable to leave the patient unprotected, the addition of more and more antibacterial agents to the regimen is not appropriate unless there is a clinical or microbiologic reason to do so. Planned progressive therapy (the serial, empirical addition of one drug after another without culture data) is not efficacious in most settings and may have unfortunate consequences. Simply adding another antibiotic for fear that a gram-negative infection is present is a dubious practice. The synergy exhibited by β-lactams and aminoglycosides against certain gram-negative organisms (especially *P. aeruginosa*) provides the rationale for using two antibiotics in this setting. Mere addition of a quinolone or another antibiotic not likely to exhibit synergy for "double coverage" has not been shown to be of benefit and may cause additional toxicities and side effects. Cephalosporins can cause bone marrow suppression, and vancomycin is associated with neutropenia in some healthy people (Chap. 118). Furthermore, the addition of multiple cephalosporins may induce β-lactamase production by some organisms; cephalosporins and double β-lactam combinations should probably be avoided altogether in *Enterobacter* infections.

Antifungal Therapy Fungal infections in cancer patients are most often associated with neutropenia. Neutropenic patients are predisposed to the development of invasive fungal infections, most commonly those due to *Candida* and *Aspergillus* species and occasionally those caused by *Fusarium, Trichosporon,* and *Bipolaris.* Cryptococcal infection, which is common among patients taking immunosuppressive agents, is uncommon among neutropenic patients receiving chemotherapy for AML. Invasive candidal disease is usually caused by *C. albicans* or *C. tropicalis* but can be caused by *C. krusei, C. parapsilosis,* and *C. glabrata.*

For decades it has been common clinical practice to add amphotericin B to antibacterial regimens if a neutropenic patient remains febrile despite 4 to 7 days of treatment with antibacterial agents. The rationale for the empirical addition of amphotericin B is that it is difficult to culture fungi before they cause disseminated disease and that mortality from disseminated fungal infections in granulocytopenic patients is high. Prior to the introduction of newer azoles into clinical practice, amphotericin B was the mainstay of antifungal therapy. The insolubility of amphotericin B has resulted in the marketing of several amphotericin B–lipid formulations. Lipid preparations have been shown to be less toxic than the amphotericin B deoxycholate complex. However, because of the high cost of the lipid preparations, at many centers their use is reserved for patients who fail to respond to standard amphotericin B. Since the side effects of the formulations differ, unnecessary switching from one to another is not recommended.

Although fluconazole has been demonstrated to be efficacious in the treatment of infections due to many *Candida* spp., its use against serious fungal infections in immunocompromised patients has been limited by its narrow spectrum: it has no activity against *Aspergillus* or against several non-*albicans Candida* spp. The release of newer broad-spectrum azoles (such as voriconazole) has provided another option for the treatment of *Aspergillus* infection (including CNS infection, in which amphotericin B has usually failed). In fact, experience indicates that these drugs may well supplant amphotericin B as the mainstay of treatment because of their lesser toxicity and better penetration into cerebrospinal fluid and other sites. Clinicians should be aware that the spectrum of each azole is somewhat different and that no drug can be assumed to be efficacious against all fungi. For example, while voriconazole is active against *Pseudallescheria boydii,*

amphotericin B is not; however, voriconazole has no activity against *Mucor.* →*For a full discussion of antifungal therapy, see Chap. 182.*

The introduction of new antifungal agents with different mechanisms of activity (e.g., the echinocandins) has opened the door to combination antifungal therapy. Studies in progress are assessing the use of these agents in cancer patients.

Antiviral Therapy The availability of a variety of agents with activity against herpes group viruses (and of some new agents with a broader spectrum of activity) has resulted in a greater focus on the treatment of viral infections, which pose a major problem in cancer patients. Among the viral diseases that affect cancer patients, those caused by the herpes group viruses are prominent. Serious (and sometimes fatal) infections due to HSV and CMV are well documented, and VZV infections may be fatal to patients receiving chemotherapy. The roles of human herpesvirus (HHV) 6, HHV-7, and HHV-8 (also known as Kaposi's sarcoma herpesvirus) in cancer patients are currently being defined (Chap. 166). While most clinical experience is with acyclovir, which can be used therapeutically or prophylactically, a number of derivative drugs offer advantages over this agent (Table 72-7).

In addition to the herpes group viruses, several respiratory viruses (especially respiratory syncytial virus) may cause serious disease in cancer patients. While vaccination with influenza vaccine is recommended (see below), it may be ineffective in this patient population. The availability of antiviral drugs with activity against influenza viruses gives the clinician additional options for the treatment of these patients (Table 72-8).

Other Therapeutic Modalities Another way to address the problems of the febrile neutropenic patient is to replenish the neutrophil population. Although granulocyte transfusions are efficacious in the treatment of refractory gram-negative bacteremia, they do not have a documented role in prophylaxis. Because of the expense, the risk of leukoagglutinin reactions (which has probably been decreased by improved cell-separation procedures), and the risk of transmission of CMV from unscreened donors (which has been reduced by the use of filters),

TABLE 72-7 *Antiviral Agents Active against Herpesviruses*

Agent	Description	Spectrum	Toxicity	Other Issues
Acyclovir	Inhibits HSV polymerase	HSV, VZV ($\pm$ CMV, EBV)	Rarely has side effects; crystalluria can occur at high doses	Long history of safety; original antiviral agent
Famciclovir	Prodrug of penciclovir (a guanosine analogue)	HSV, VZV ($\pm$ CMV)	Associated with cancer in rats	Longer effective half-life than acyclovir
Valacyclovir	Prodrug of acyclovir; better absorption	HSV, VZV ($\pm$ CMV)	Associated with thrombotic microangiopathy in one study of immunocompromised patients	Better oral absorption and longer effective half-life than acyclovir; can be given as a single daily dose for prophylaxis
Ganciclovir	More potent polymerase inhibitor; more toxic than acyclovir	HSV, VZV, CMV, HHV-6	Bone marrow suppression	Neutropenia may respond to G-CSF or GM-CSF
Valganciclovir	Prodrug of ganciclovir; better absorption	HSV, VZV, CMV, HHV-6	Bone marrow suppression	—
Cidofovir	Nucleotide analogue of cytosine	HSV, VZV, CMV; has good in vitro activity against adenovirus and others	Nephrotoxic marrow suppression	Given IV once a week
Foscarnet	Phosphonoformic acid; inhibits viral DNA polymerase	HSV, VZV, CMV, HHV-6	Nephrotoxic; electrolyte abnormalities common	IV only

Abbreviations: $\pm$, agent has some activity but not enough for the treatment of infections; CMV, cytomegalovirus; EBV, Epstein-Barr virus; G-CSF, granulocyte colony-stimulating factor; GM-CSF, granulocyte-macrophage colony-stimulating factor; HHV, human herpesvirus; HSV, herpes simplex virus; VZV, varicella-zoster virus.

TABLE 72-8 *Other Antiviral Agents Useful in the Treatment of Infections in Cancer Patients*

Agent	Description	Spectrum	Toxicity	Other Issues
Amantadine Rimantadine	Interferes with uncoating	Influenza A only	5–10% fewer CNS effects with rimantadine	May be given prophylactically
Zanamivir	Neuraminidase inhibitor	Influenza A and B	Usually well tolerated	Inhalation only
Oseltamivir	Neuraminidase inhibitor	Influenza A and B	Usually well tolerated	PO dosing
Pleconaril	Blocks enterovirus binding and uncoating	90% of enteroviruses, 80% of rhinoviruses	Generally well tolerated	Decreases duration of meningitis; available for compassionate use only
Interferons	Cytokines with broad spectrum of activity	Used locally for warts, systemically for hepatitis	Fever, myalgias, bone marrow suppression	Not shown to be helpful in CMV infection; use limited by toxicity
Ribavirin	Purine analogue (precise mechanism of action unknown)	Broad theoretical spectrum; documented use against RSV, Lassa fever virus, and hepatitis viruses (with interferon)	IV form causes anemia	Given by aerosol for RSV infection (efficacy in doubt); approved for use in children with heart/ lung disease

Abbreviations: CMV, cytomegalovirus; CNS, central nervous system; RSV, respiratory syncytial virus.

granulocyte transfusion is reserved for patients unresponsive to antibiotics. This modality is efficacious for documented gram-negative bacteremia refractory to antibiotics, particularly in situations where granulocyte numbers will be depressed for only a short period. The demonstrated usefulness of granulocyte colony-stimulating factor (G-CSF) in mobilizing neutrophils and advances in preservation techniques may make this option more useful than in the past.

A variety of cytokines, including G-CSF and granulocyte-macrophage colony-stimulating factor, enhance granulocyte recovery after chemotherapy and consequently shorten the period of maximal vulnerability to fatal infections. The role of these cytokines in routine practice is still a matter of some debate. Most authorities recommend their use only when neutropenia is both severe and prolonged. The cytokines themselves may have adverse effects, including fever, hypoxemia, and pleural effusions or serositis in other areas (Chap. 295). Since there is little evidence that their routine administration lessens the risk of death and since they are still expensive, the use of these cytokines has not become the standard of care in all centers. The role of other cytokines (such as macrophage colony-stimulating factor for monocytes or interferon-γ) in preventing or treating infections in granulocytopenic patients is under investigation.

Once neutropenia has resolved, patients are not at increased risk of infection. However, depending on what drugs they receive, patients who continue on chemotherapeutic protocols remain at high risk for certain diseases. Any patient receiving more than a maintenance dose of glucocorticoids (including many treatment regimens for diffuse lymphoma) should also receive prophylactic TMP-SMX because of the risk of *Pneumocystis* infection; those with ALL should receive such prophylaxis for the duration of chemotherapy.

PREVENTION OF INFECTION IN CANCER PATIENTS

EFFECT OF THE ENVIRONMENT Outbreaks of fatal *Aspergillus* infection have been associated with construction projects and materials in several hospitals. The association between spore counts and risk of infection suggests the need for a high-efficiency air-handling system in hospitals that care for large numbers of neutropenic patients. The use of laminar-flow rooms and prophylactic antibiotics has decreased the number of infectious episodes in severely neutropenic patients. However, because of the expense of such a program and the failure to show that it dramatically affects mortality, most centers do not routinely use laminar flow to care for neutropenic patients. Some centers use "reverse isolation," in which health care providers and visitors to a patient who is neutropenic wear gowns and gloves. Since most of the infec-

tions these patients develop are due to organisms that colonize the patients' own skin and bowel, the validity of such schemes is dubious, and limited clinical data do not support their use. Hand washing by all staff caring for neutropenic patients should be required to prevent the spread of resistant organisms.

The presence of large numbers of bacteria (particularly *P. aeruginosa*) in certain foods, especially fresh vegetables, has led some authorities to recommend a special "low-bacteria" diet. A diet consisting of cooked and canned food is satisfactory to most neutropenic patients and does not involve elaborate disinfection or sterilization protocols. However, there are no studies to support even this type of dietary restriction. Counseling of patients to avoid leftovers, deli foods, and unpasteurized dairy products is recommended.

PHYSICAL MEASURES Although few studies address this issue, patients with cancer are predisposed to infections resulting from anatomic compromise (e.g., lymphedema resulting from node dissections after radical mastectomy). Surgeons who specialize in cancer surgery can provide specific guidelines for the care of such patients, and patients benefit from common-sense advice about how to prevent infections in vulnerable areas.

IMMUNOGLOBULIN REPLACEMENT Many patients with multiple myeloma or CLL have immunoglobulin deficiencies as a result of their disease, and all allogeneic bone marrow transplant recipients are hypogammaglobinemic for a period after transplantation. However, current recommendations reserve intravenous immunoglobulin (IVIg) replacement therapy for those patients with severe (<400 mg/dL), prolonged hypogammaglobulinemia. Antibiotic prophylaxis has been shown to be cheaper and efficacious in preventing infections in most CLL patients with hypogammaglobulinemia. Routine use of IVIg replacement is not recommended.

SEX The use of condoms is recommended for severely immunocompromised patients. Any sexual practice that results in oral exposure to feces is not recommended. Neutropenic patients should be advised to avoid any practice that results in trauma, as even microscopic cuts may result in bacterial invasion and fatal sepsis.

ANTIBIOTIC PROPHYLAXIS There is no consensus on the use of prophylactic antibiotics in neutropenic patients. The incidence of infection is lower among patients who receive broad-spectrum antibiotic prophylaxis than among those who do not. Because of the prolongation of neutropenia associated with the use of TMP-SMX, some clinicians use broad-spectrum agents such as quinolones (e.g., levofloxacin). Either regimen can be given orally, and both have the advantage of inactivity against anaerobic organisms; thus, neither is likely to disrupt the bowel flora and permit colonization with new aerobes or *Candida*. However, all antibiotic regimens have adverse effects and can lead to the selection of resistant organisms in a hospital. For these reasons, many clinicians reserve their use for patients with the longest periods of neutropenia (e.g., bone marrow transplant recipients). The same issues apply to the use of antifungal agents. While agents such as fluconazole may prevent infections with susceptible organisms (e.g., *C. albicans*), they can cause a concomitant increase in infections due to resistant fungi (e.g., *C. krusei*). Thus, the decision to use antifungal prophylaxis may vary with the fungi endemic in a given hospital. Prophylaxis for

Pneumocystis is mandatory for patients with ALL and for all cancer patients receiving glucocorticoid-containing chemotherapy regimens.

VACCINATION OF CANCER PATIENTS In general, patients undergoing chemotherapy respond less well to vaccines than normal hosts. Their greater need for vaccines thus leads to a dilemma in their management. Purified proteins and inactivated vaccines are almost never contraindicated and should be given to patients even during chemotherapy. For example, all adults should receive diphtheria-tetanus toxoid boosters at the indicated times as well as seasonal influenza vaccine. However, if possible, vaccination should not be undertaken concurrent with cytotoxic chemotherapy. If patients are expected to be receiving chemotherapy for several months and vaccination is indicated (for example, influenza vaccination in the fall), the vaccine should be given midcycle—as far apart in time as possible from the antimetabolic agents that will prevent an immune response. The meningococcal and pneumococcal polysaccharide vaccines should be given to patients before splenectomy, if possible. The *H. influenzae* type b conjugate vaccine should be administered to all splenectomized patients.

In general, live virus (or live bacterial) vaccines should not be given

to patients during intensive chemotherapy because of the risk of disseminated infection. Recommendations on vaccination are summarized in Table 72-2.

FURTHER READING

BERGHMANS T et al: Therapeutic use of granulocyte and granulocyte-macrophage colony-stimulating factors in febrile neutropenic cancer patients. A systematic review of the literature with meta-analysis. Support Care Cancer 10:181, 2002

CENTERS FOR DISEASE CONTROL AND PREVENTION: Guidelines for preventing opportunistic infections among hematopoietic stem cell transplant recipients. MMWR Recomm Rep 49:1, 2000

HUGHES WT et al: 2002 guidelines for the use of antimicrobial agents in neutropenic patients with cancer. Clin Infect Dis 34:730, 2002

MERMEL LA et al: Guidelines for the management of intravascular catheter–related infections. Clin Infect Dis 32:1249, 2001

WALSH TJ et al: Voriconazole compared with liposomal amphotericin B for empirical antifungal therapy in patients with neutropenia and persistent fever. N Engl J Med 346:225, 2002

73 CANCER OF THE SKIN
Katarina G. Chiller, Carl Washington, Arthur J. Sober, Howard K. Koh

NONMELANOMA SKIN CANCER

Nonmelanoma skin cancer (NMSC) is the most common cancer in the United States, with an estimated annual incidence of >1.3 million cases. Basal cell carcinomas (BCCs) account for 70 to 80% of NMSCs. Squamous cell carcinomas (SCCs), while representing only ~20% of NMSC, are more significant because of their ability to metastasize; they account for most of the 2300 deaths annually. Incidence rates have risen dramatically over the past decade.

ETIOLOGY The cause of BCC and SCC is multifactorial. Cumulative exposure to sunlight, principally the ultraviolet B (UV-B) spectrum, is the most significant factor. Other factors associated with a higher incidence of skin cancer are male sex, older age, Celtic descent, a fair complexion, a tendency to sunburn easily, and an outdoor occupation. The incidence of these tumors increases with decreasing latitude. Most tumors develop on sun-exposed areas of the head and neck. Tumors are more common on the left side of the body in the United States but on the right side in England, presumably owing to asymmetric exposure during driving. As the earth's protective ozone shield continues to thin, further increases in the incidence of skin cancer can be anticipated. In certain geographic areas, exposure to arsenic in well water or from industrial sources may significantly increase the risk of BCC and SCC. Skin cancer in affected individuals may be seen with or without other cutaneous markers of chronic arsenism (e.g., arsenical keratoses). Less common is exposure to the cyclic aromatic hydrocarbons in tar, soot, or shale. The risk of lip or oral SCC is increased with cigarette smoking. Human papillomaviruses and UV radiation may act as cocarcinogens.

Host factors associated with a high risk of skin cancer include immunosuppression induced by disease or drugs. Transplant recipients receiving chronic immunosuppressive therapy are particularly prone to SCC. The frequency of skin cancer is proportional to the duration of immunosuppression and the extent of sun exposure. Skin cancer is not uncommon in patients infected with HlV, and it may be more aggressive in this setting. Other factors include ionizing radiation, thermal burn scars, and chronic ulcerations. Several heritable conditions are associated with skin cancer (e.g., albinism, xeroderma pigmentosum, and basal cell nevus syndrome). Mutations in the tumor suppressor *patch* gene have been implicated in the development of BCC.

CLINICAL PRESENTATION NMSCs are often asymptomatic, but nonhealing ulceration, bleeding, or pain can occur in advanced lesions.

Basal Cell Carcinoma BCC is a malignancy arising from epidermal basal cells. The least invasive of BCC subtypes, *superficial BCC*, classically consists of truncal erythematous, scaling plaques that slowly enlarge. This BCC subtype may be confused with benign inflammatory dermatoses, especially nummular eczema and psoriasis. BCC can also present as a small, slow growing pearly nodule, often with small telangiectatic vessels on its surface (*nodular BCC*). The occasional presence of melanin in this variant of nodular BCC (*pigmented BCC*) may lead to the erroneous diagnosis of malignant melanoma. *Morpheaform (fibrosing) BCC*, the most invasive subtype, manifests itself as a solitary, flat or slightly depressed, indurated, whitish or yellowish plaque. Borders are typically indistinct, a feature associated with a greater potential for extensive subclinical spread.

Squamous Cell Carcinoma Primary *cutaneous SCC* is a malignant neoplasm of keratinizing epidermal cells. SCC can grow rapidly and metastasize. The clinical features of SCC vary widely. Commonly, SCC appears as an ulcerated erythematous nodule or superficial erosion on the skin or lower lip, but it may present as a verrucous papule or plaque. Overlying telangiectasias are uncommon. The margins of this tumor may be ill defined, and fixation to underlying structures may occur. Cutaneous SCC may develop anywhere on the body but usually arises on sun-damaged skin. A related neoplasm, keratoacanthoma, typically appears as a dome-shaped papule with a central keratotic crater, expands rapidly, and commonly regresses without therapy. This lesion can be difficult to differentiate from SCC.

Actinic keratoses and *cheilitis*, both premalignant forms of SCC, present as hyperkeratotic papules on sun-exposed areas. The potential for malignant degeneration in untreated lesions ranges from 0.25 to 20%. *Bowen's disease*, the in situ form of SCC, presents as a scaling, erythematous plaque. Treatment of premalignant and in situ lesions reduces the subsequent risk of invasive disease.

NATURAL HISTORY ■ **Basal Cell Carcinoma** The natural history of BCC is that of a slowly enlarging, locally invasive neoplasm. The degree of local destruction and risk of recurrence vary with the size, duration, location, and histologic subtype of the tumor; presence of recurrent disease; and various patient characteristics. Location on the central face, ears, or the scalp may portend a higher risk. Small nodular, pigmented, cystic, or superficial BCCs respond well to most treatments. Large lesions or morpheaform subtype may be more aggressive. The metastatic potential of BCC has been estimated to be 0.0028 to 0.1%. Persons with either BCC or SCC have an increased risk of developing subsequent skin cancers, estimated to be up to 40% in 5 years.

Squamous Cell Carcinoma The natural history of SCC depends on both tumor and host characteristics. Tumors arising on actinically damaged skin have a lower metastatic potential than those on protected surfaces. The metastatic frequency of cutaneous SCC, reported at 0.3 to 5.2%, occurs most frequently in regional draining lymph nodes. Tumors occurring on the lower lip and ear have metastatic potentials approaching 13 and 11%, respectively. The metastatic potential of SCC arising in scars, chronic ulcerations, and genital or mucosal surfaces is higher. The overall metastatic rate for recurrent tumors may approach 30%. Large, poorly differentiated, deep tumors, with perineural or lymphatic invasion, often behave aggressively. Multiple tumors with rapid growth and aggressive behavior can be a therapeutic challenge in immunosuppressed patients.

Rx TREATMENT

Basal Cell Carcinoma The most frequently used treatment modalities for BCC include electrodesiccation and curettage (ED&C), excision, cryosurgery, radiation therapy, laser therapy, Mohs micrographic surgery (MMS), topical 5-fluorouracil, and topical immunomodulators. The mode of therapy chosen depends on tumor characteristics, patient age, medical status, preferences of the patient, and other factors. ED&C remains the method most commonly employed by dermatologists. This method is selected for low-risk tumors (e.g., a small primary tumor of a less aggressive subtype in a favorable location). Excision, which offers the advantage of histologic control, is usually selected for more aggressive tumors or those in high-risk locations or, in many instances, for aesthetic reasons. Cryosurgery using liquid nitrogen may be used in certain low-risk tumors, but it requires specialized equipment (cryoprobes) to be effective for advanced neoplasms. Radiation therapy, while not employed as often as surgical modalities, offers an excellent chance for cure in many cases of BCC. It is useful in patients not considered surgical candidates and as a surgical adjunct in high-risk tumors. Younger patients may not be good candidates for radiation therapy because of the risks of long-term carcinogenesis and radiodermatitis. Despite rapidly advancing technology in laser development, their long-term efficacy in treating infiltrative or recurrent lesions is still unknown. On the other hand, MMS, a specialized type of surgical excision that permits the best histologic control and preservation of uninvolved tissue, is associated with cure rates >98%. It is the preferred modality for lesions that are recurrent, in a high-risk location, or large and ill-defined and where maximal tissue conservation is critical (e.g., the eyelids). Topical 5-fluorouracil therapy should be limited to superficial BCC. New lines of topicals, the immunomodulators, show promise in their efficacy at treating superficial and even nodular BCCs. Imiquimod, a relatively well-tolerated cream, has successfully undergone phase III clinical trials. Intralesional chemotherapy (5-fluorouracil and interferon) and photodynamic therapy (which employs selective activation of a photoactive drug by visible light) have been used successfully in patients with numerous tumors.

Squamous Cell Carcinoma The therapy of cutaneous SCC should be based on an analysis of risk factors influencing the biologic behavior of the tumor. These include the size, location, and degree of histologic differentiation of the tumor as well as the age and physical condition of the patient. Surgical excision, MMS, and radiation therapy are standard methods of treatment. Cryosurgery and ED&C have been used successfully for premalignant lesions and small primary tumors. Metastases are treated with lymph node dissection, irradiation, or both. 13-*cis*-retinoic acid (1 mg orally every day) plus interferon α (3 million units subcutaneously or intramuscularly every day) may produce a partial response in most patients. Systemic chemotherapy combinations that include cisplatin may also be palliative in some patients.

PREVENTION As the vast majority of skin cancers are related to chronic UV radiation exposure, patient and physician education could dramatically reduce their incidence. Emphasis should be placed on pre-

ventive measures beginning early in life. Patients must understand that damage from UV-B begins early, despite the fact that cancers develop years later. Regular use of sunscreens and protective clothing should be encouraged. Avoidance of tanning salons and midday (10 A.M. to 2 P.M.) sun exposure is recommended. Precancerous and in situ lesions should be treated early. Early detection of small tumors affords simpler treatment modalities with higher cure rates and lower morbidity. In patients with a history of skin cancer, long-term follow-up for the detection of recurrence, metastasis, and new skin cancers should be emphasized. Chemoprophylaxis using synthetic retinoids is useful in controlling new lesions in some patients with multiple tumors.

OTHER NONMELANOMA CUTANEOUS MALIGNANCIES Neoplasms of cutaneous adnexa and sarcomas of fibrous, mesenchymal, fatty, and vascular tissues make up 1 to 2% of NMSC (Table 73-1). Some can portend a poor prognosis such as *Merkel cell carcinoma*, which is a neural crest–derived, highly aggressive malignancy that exhibits a metastatic rate of 75%, and a 5-year survival rate of 30 to 40%. Others, such as the human herpes virus 8–induced, HIV-related *Kaposi's sarcoma*, exhibit a more indolent course. The recent marked decrease in incidence of this tumor parallels the institution of the highly active antiretroviral therapy.

MELANOMA

Pigmented skin lesions are among the most common findings on physical examination. The challenge is to distinguish cutaneous melanomas, which may be lethal, from the remainder, which with rare exceptions are benign. Cutaneous neoplasms are depicted in Fig. 73-1; benign and malignant pigmented lesions are shown in Fig. 73-2.

EPIDEMIOLOGY Melanomas originate from neural crest–derived melanocytes, pigment cells present normally in the epidermis and sometimes in the dermis. This tumor will affect approximately 54,200 individuals per year in the United States, resulting in >8,200 deaths. The tumor can affect adults of all ages, even young individuals (starting in the mid-teens); it has distinct clinical features that make it detectable at a time when cure by surgical excision is possible; and it is located on the skin surface, where it is visible. The incidence has increased dramatically (a 300% increase in the past 40 years). If the incidence continues to increase at the present rate, within a decade, lifetime risk of melanoma will be ≥1%. The reason for this increase is uncertain but may involve increased recreational sun exposure, especially early in life. Individuals of similar ethnic background who immigrate after childhood to areas of high sun exposure (e.g., Israel and Australia) have lower melanoma rates than individuals of similar age who were either born in those countries or immigrated before age 10. The individuals most susceptible to development of melanoma are those with fair complexions, red or blond hair, blue eyes, and freckles and who tan poorly and sunburn easily. In one literature survey, 9 of 11 studies linked increased melanoma risk to history of sunburn. Other factors associated with increased risk include a family history of melanoma (~1 in 10 melanoma patients have a family member with mel-

TABLE 73-1 *Other Nonmelanoma Cutaneous Malignancies*

Tumor Type	Most Common Location	Recurrence Rate,[a] %	Metastatic Rate, %
Atypical fibroxanthoma	Head and neck	21	4
Merkel cell carcinoma	Head and neck	40	75
Dermatofibrosarcoma protuberans	Trunk	50	1
Sebaceous carcinoma	Eyelid	12	30
Microcystic adnexal carcinoma	Face	50	1 case
Porocarcinoma	Extremity	20	10
Eccrine carcinoma	Head and neck	36	11
Angiosarcoma	Head and neck	75	75

[a] Recurrence rates are the highest reported and were established prior to widespread use of Mohs micrographic surgery.

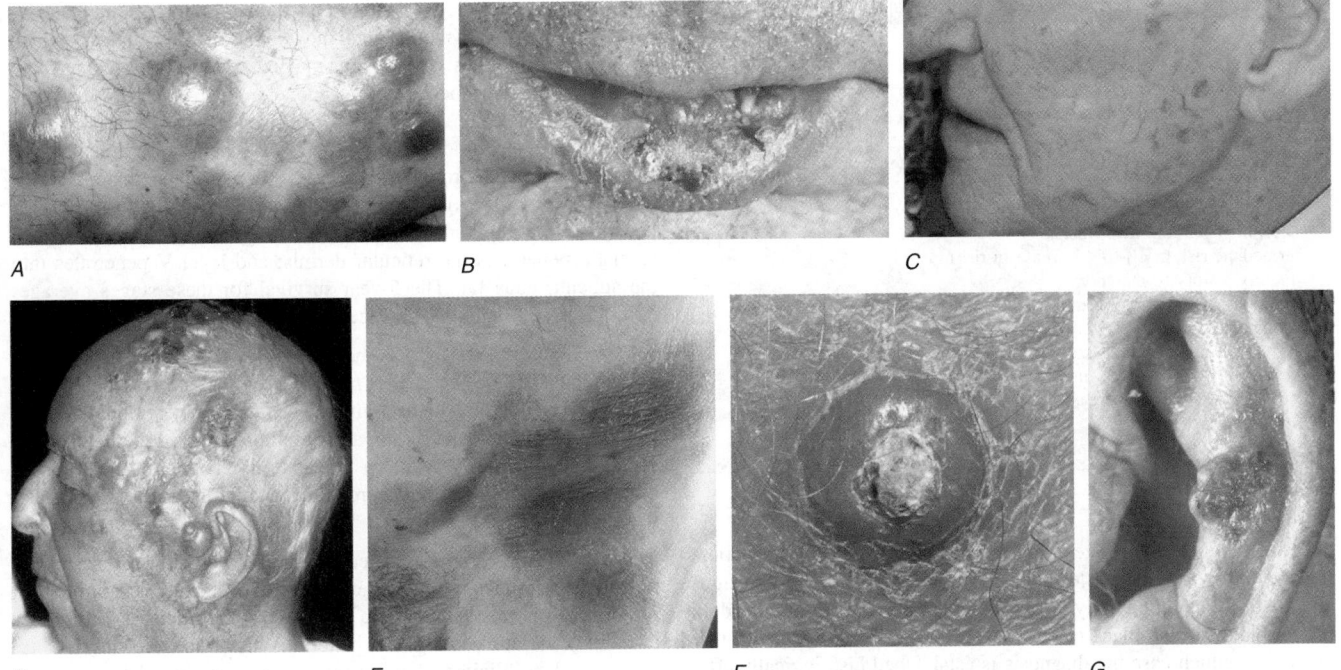

FIGURE 73-1 *A.* Non-Hodgkin's lymphoma involves the skin with typical violaceous, "plum-colored" nodules. *B.* Squamous cell carcinoma is seen here as a hyperkeratotic crusted and somewhat eroded plaque on the lower lip. Sun-exposed skin such as the head, neck, hands, and arms are other typical sites of involvement. *C.* Actinic keratoses consists of hyperkeratotic erythematous papules and patches on sun-exposed skin. They arise in middle-aged to older adults and have some potential for malignant transfor- mation. *D.* Metastatic carcinoma to the skin is characterized by inflammatory, often ulcerated dermal nodules. *E.* Mycosis fungoides is a cutaneous T cell lymphoma, and plaque stage lesions are seen in this patient. *F.* Keratoacanthoma is a low-grade squa- mous cell carcinoma that presents as an exophytic nodule with central keratinous debris. *G.* This basal cell carcinoma shows central ulceration and a pearly, rolled, telangiectatic tumor border.

anoma); the presence of a clinically atypical mole (dysplastic nevus), a giant congenital melanocytic nevus, or a small to medium-sized con- genital melanocytic nevus (see below); the presence of a higher than average number of ordinary melanocytic nevi; and immunosuppres- sion (Table 73-2). A 64-fold increased risk for individuals with 50 or more moles ≥2 mm in size has been reported. About 30% of mela- nomas arise in a nevus. Melanoma is relatively rare in heavily pig- mented peoples. Dark-skinned populations (such as those of India and Puerto Rico), blacks, and East Asians have rates 10 to 20 times lower than lighter-skinned whites. In keeping with the role of sun exposure, the incidence is inversely correlated with the latitude of residence; at any latitude, darker-skinned persons have the lowest incidence.

CLINICAL CHARACTERISTICS There are four types of cutaneous melanoma (Table 73-3). In three of these—*superficial spreading melanoma, len- tigo maligna melanoma,* and *acral lentiginous melanoma*—the lesion has a period of superficial (so-called radial) growth during which it increases in size but does not penetrate deeply. It is during this period that the melanoma is most capable of being cured by surgical excision. The fourth type—*nodular melanoma*—does not have a recognizable radial growth phase and usually presents as a deeply invasive lesion, capable of early metastasis. When tumors begin to penetrate deeply into the skin, they are in the so-called vertical growth phase. Mela- nomas with a radial growth phase are characterized by irregular and sometimes notched borders, variation in pigment pattern, and variation

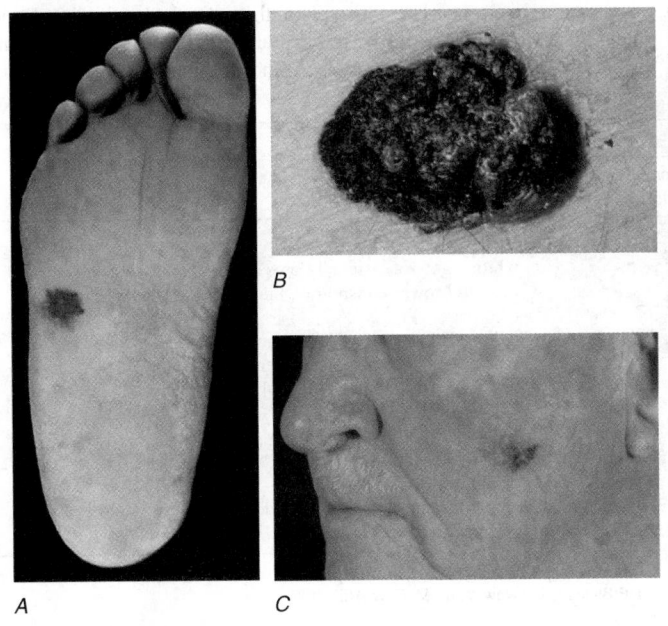

FIGURE 73-2 *A.* Acral lentiginous melanoma is more common in blacks, Asians, and Hispanics and occurs as an enlarging hyperpigmented macule or plaque on the palms and soles. Lateral pigment diffusion is present. *B.* Nodular melanoma most commonly manifests itself as a rapidly growing, often ulcerated or crusted black nodule. *C.* Lentigo maligna melanoma occurs on sun-exposed skin as a large, hyperpigmented macule or plaque with irregular borders and variable pigmentation. *D.* Dysplastic nevi are irreg- ularly pigmented and shaped nevomelanocytic lesions which may be associated with familial melanoma.

TABLE 73-2   Risk Factors for Cutaneous Melanoma

High risk (>50-fold increase in risk)
  Persistently changing mole
  Clinically atypical moles in patient with two family members with
    melanoma
  Adulthood (vs. childhood)
  >50 nevi ≥2 mm in diameter
Intermediate risk (~10-fold increase in risk)
  Family history of melanoma
  Sporadic clinically atypical moles
  Congenital nevi (?)
  White ethnicity (vs. black or East Asian ethnicity)
  Personal history of prior melanoma
Low risk (2- to 4-fold increase in risk)
  Immunosuppression
  Sun sensitivity or excess exposure to sun

Source: Adapted from AR Rhodes et al: JAMA 258:3146, 1987.

in color. An increase in size or change in color is noted by the patient in 70% of early lesions. Bleeding, ulceration, and pain are late signs and are of little help in early recognition. Nodular melanomas are dark brown-black to blue-black nodules. Melanomas occasionally are amelanotic, in which case the diagnosis is established histologically after biopsy of a new or changing skin nodule. Lentigo maligna melanoma is usually confined to chronically sun-damaged, sun-exposed sites (face, neck, back of hands) in older individuals. Acral lentiginous melanoma occurs on the palms, soles, nail beds, and mucous membranes. While this type occurs in whites, it is most frequent (along with nodular melanoma) in blacks and East Asians. Superficial spreading melanoma is most frequent in whites. Melanomas arising in dysplastic nevi (see below) are usually of this type. The back is the most common site for melanoma in men. In women, the back and the lower leg (from knee to ankle) are frequent sites.

PROGNOSTIC FACTORS   The most important prognostic factor is the stage at the time of presentation. Fortunately, most melanomas are diagnosed in clinical stages I and II. The revised staging system for melanoma is based on microscopic primary tumor depth (Breslow's thickness), presence of ulceration, evidence of nodal involvement, presence of microscopic satellites, and presence of metastatic disease (Table 73-4). Certain anatomic sites may affect the prognosis. The favorable sites appear to be the forearm and leg (excluding feet), while unfavorable sites include scalp, hands, feet, and mucous membranes. In general, women with stage I or II disease have a better survival than men, perhaps in part because of earlier diagnosis; women frequently have melanomas on the lower leg, where self-recognition is more likely and prognosis is better. Older individuals, in general, have poorer prognoses. This finding has been explained in part by a ten-

dency toward later diagnosis (and thus thicker tumors) in men and by a higher proportion in men of acral melanomas (palmar-plantar), which have a poorer prognosis. Melanoma may recur after many years. About 10 to 15% of first-time recurrences develop >5 years after treatment of the original lesion. The time to recurrence varies inversely with tumor thickness. An alternative prognostic scheme for clinical stages I and II melanoma, proposed by Clark, is based on the anatomic level of invasion in the skin. Level I is intraepidermal (in situ); level II penetrates the papillary dermis; level III spans the papillary dermis; level IV penetrates the reticular dermis; and level V penetrates into the subcutaneous fat. The 5-year survival for these stages averages 100, 95, 82, 71, and 49%, respectively.

NATURAL HISTORY   Melanomas may spread by the lymphatic channels or the bloodstream. The earliest metastases are often to regional lymph nodes. Surgical lymphadenectomy may control early regional disease. Liver, lung, bone, and brain are common sites of hematogenous spread, but unusual sites, such as the anterior chamber of the eye, may also be involved. Once widespread metastatic disease is established, the likelihood of cure is low.

MANAGEMENT   The entire cutaneous surface, including the scalp and mucous membranes, should be examined in each patient. Bright room illumination is important, and a 7× to 10× hand lens is helpful for evaluating variation in pigment pattern. A history of relevant risk factors should be elicited. Any suspicious lesions should be biopsied, evaluated by a specialist, or recorded by chart and/or photography for follow-up. Examination of the lymph nodes and palpation of the abdominal viscera are part of the staging examination for suspected melanoma. The patient should be advised to have other family members screened if either melanoma or clinically atypical moles (dysplastic nevi) are present. The detection of early melanoma in relatives on screening has been reported. Melanoma prevention is based on protection from the sun. Routine use of a sunblock with sun protection factor ≥15, use of protective clothing, and avoiding intense midday ultraviolet exposure should be recommended. The patient should be educated in the clinical features of melanoma and advised to report any growth or other change in a pigmented lesion. Patient education brochures are available from the American Cancer Society, the American Academy of Dermatology, the National Cancer Institute, and the Skin Cancer Foundation. Self-examination at 6- to 8-week intervals may enhance the likelihood of detecting change. The importance of routine follow-up visits for melanoma patients and patients with clinically atypical moles (dysplastic nevi) should be emphasized, as these visits may facilitate early detection of new tumors.

Precursor Lesions   Clinically atypical moles, also termed *dysplastic nevi*, occur in certain families affected by melanoma. In some families, melanomas occur nearly exclusively in the individuals with dysplastic nevi. These nevi appear to be transmitted as an autosomal dominant trait that involves chromosome 9p16. In other families, the nevi may

TABLE 73-3   Clinical Features of Malignant Melanoma

Type	Site	Average Age at Diagnosis, Years	Duration of Known Existence, Years	Color
Lentigo maligna melanoma	Sun-exposed surfaces, particularly malar region of cheek and temple	70	5–20[a] or longer	In flat portions, shades of brown and tan predominant, but whitish gray occasionally present; in nodules, shades of reddish brown, bluish gray, bluish black
Superficial spreading melanoma	Any site (more common on upper back and, in women, on lower legs)	40–50	1–7	Shades of brown mixed with bluish red (violaceous), bluish black, reddish brown, and often whitish pink, and the border of lesion is at least in part visibly and/or palpably elevated
Nodular melanoma	Any site	40–50	Months to less than 5 years	Reddish blue (purple) or bluish black; either uniform in color or mixed with brown or black
Acral lentiginous melanoma	Palm, sole, nail bed, mucous membrane	60	1–10	In flat portions, dark brown predominantly; in raised lesions (plaques) brown-black or blue-black predominantly

[a] During much of this time, the precursor stage, lentigo maligna, is confined to the epidermis.

Source: Adapted from AJ Sober, in *Pathophysiology of Dermatologic Diseases*, NA Soter, HP Baden (eds). New York, McGraw-Hill, 1984.

not be present in all individuals with an increased risk of melanoma. The melanomas may arise in clinically atypical moles or in normal skin (in the latter situation the mole acts as a marker of increased risk). Individuals with clinically atypical moles and two family members with melanoma have been reported to have a >50% lifetime risk for developing melanoma. Table 73-5 lists the features that are characteristic of clinically atypical moles and that differentiate them from benign acquired nevi. The number of clinically atypical moles may vary from one to several hundred. Clinically atypical moles usually differ from each other in appearance. The borders are often hazy and indistinct, and the pigment pattern is more highly varied than that in benign acquired nevi. Of the 90% of melanoma patients whose disease is regarded as sporadic (i.e., who lack a family history of melanoma), ~40% have clinically atypical moles, as compared with an estimated 5 to 10% of the population at large. Further studies to determine the background frequency of clinically atypical moles are required, once greater unanimity exists regarding their clinical and histopathologic features. The observation that at least 20% of sporadic melanomas arise in association with a clinically atypical mole makes this the most important precursor for melanoma. Less frequent precursors include the giant congenital melanocytic nevus and the small congenital melanocytic nevus (although the latter relationship is disputed by some). Congenital melanocytic nevi are present at birth or appear in the neonatal period (tardive form). The *giant melanocytic nevus*, also called the bathing trunk, cape, or garment nevus, is a rare malformation that affects perhaps 1 in 30,000 to 1 in 100,000 individuals. These nevi are usually >20 cm in diameter and may cover more than half the body surface. Giant nevi often occur in association with multiple small congenital nevi. The borders are sharp, and hair may be present. The lesions are usually dark brown and may have darker and lighter areas. Pigment is haphazardly displayed. The surface is smooth to rugose or cerebriform and may vary from one portion of the lesion to another. A lifetime risk of melanoma development of 6% has been estimated. The risk is greatest before age 5 and next greatest between ages 5 and 10. Early detection of melanoma is difficult in these lesions because of the deep dermal or subcutaneous origin of primary melanoma and because of the large and varied surface of the nevus. Prophylactic excision early in life can be accomplished by staged removal with coverage by split-thickness skin grafts. The use of cultured keratinocytes for coverage appears promising. At present, there are no uniform management guidelines for giant congenital nevi. The *small-to medium-sized congenital melanocytic nevus*, which affects approximately 1% of persons, presents usually as a raised dark- to medium-brown lesion with a smooth or papillomatous surface. The border is sharp, and lesions may be oriented along lines of skin cleavage. Follicular hyper- and hypopigmentation may coexist in a salt-and-pepper configuration. The lesion may have an excess of thick, coarse hairs. The risk of melanoma developing in these lesions is not known; however, melanomas can arise in these lesions. Considerations of body surface area suggest that the incidence of melanomas arising in small congenital melanocytic nevi is probably higher than would be expected by chance. The remnants of a nevus with histopathologic features of a congenital nevus have been observed in 2 to 6% of melanomas. The management of small- to medium-sized congenital melanocytic nevi remains controversial; prophylactic removal under local anesthesia in the early teen years is appropriate. Melanomas in small congenital melanocytic nevi appear to occur after this period of life.

Differential Diagnosis The aim of differential diagnosis is to distinguish benign pigmented lesions from melanoma and its precursor. If melanoma is a consideration, then biopsy is appropriate. Some benign look-

alikes may be removed in the process of trying to detect authentic melanoma. Table 73-6 summarizes the distinguishing features of benign lesions that may be confused with melanoma. Early detection of melanoma may be facilitated by applying the "ABCD rules": A—asymmetry, benign lesions are usually symmetric; B—border irregularity, most nevi have clear-cut borders; C—color variegation, benign lesions usually have uniform light or dark pigment; D—diameter >6 mm (the size of a pencil eraser). Consideration may be given for ev-

TABLE 73-4 Prognosis of Melanoma by Thickness (Breslow) and Revised AJCC Stages: 5-Year Survival Rates

AJCC Stage	Thickness, mm	Ulceration	Nodal Disease	Distant Metastases
0	In situ	N/A	No	No
IA	<1	No	No	No
IB	<1	Yes	No	No
	1.01–2.0	No	No	No
IIA	1.01–2.0	Yes	No	No
	2.01–4.0	No	No	No
IIB	2.01–4.0	Yes	No	No
	>4.0	No	No	No
IIC	>4.0	Yes	No	No
IIIA	Any	No	Yes	
			1 node w/microscopic disease	No
			2–3 nodes w/microscopic disease	No
IIIB	Any	Yes	1 node w/microscopic disease	No
	Any	Yes	2–3 nodes w/microscopic disease	No
	Any	No	1 node w/macroscopic disease	No
	Any	No	2–3 nodes w/macroscopic disease	No
	Any	Any	In transit or satellite disease w/out nodal disease	No
	Any			
IIIC	Any	Yes	1 node w/macroscopic disease	No
		Yes	2–3 nodes w/macroscopic disease	No
		Any	≥4 metastatic or matted nodes, or in transit mets/satellites or metastatic nodes	No
IV	Any	Any	Any	Yes

Note: AJCC, American Joint Commission for Cancer.

TABLE 73-5 Clinical Features Distinguishing Atypical Moles from Benign Acquired Nevi

Clinical Feature	Clinically Atypical Moles	Benign Acquired Nevi
Color	Variable mixtures of tan, brown, black, or red/pink within a single nevus; nevi may look very different from each other	Uniformly tan or brown
Shape	Irregular borders; pigment may fade off into surrounding skin; macular portion at the edge of the nevus	Round; sharp, clear-cut borders between the nevus and the surrounding skin; may be flat or elevated
Size	Usually >6 mm in diameter; may be >10 mm; occasionally <6 mm	Usually <6 mm in diameter
Number	Often very many (>100), but occasionally may be only one	In a typical adult, 10 to 40 are scattered over the body; perhaps 15% of patients have no nevi
Location	Sun-exposed areas; the back is the most common site, but dysplastic nevi may also be seen on the scalp, breasts, and buttocks	Generally on the sun-exposed surfaces of the skin above the waist; the scalp, breasts, and buttocks are rarely involved

Source: Modified from RI Friedman et al (eds): *Cancer of the Skin*. Philadelphia, Saunders, 1991.

TABLE 73-6 *Pigmented Lesions that Must Be Distinguished from Cutaneous Melanoma and Its Precursors*

Blue nevus	Gunmetal or cerulean blue, blue-gray. Stable over time. One-half occur on dorsa of hands and feet. Lesions are usually single, small, 3 mm to <1 cm. Must be distinguished from nodular melanoma.
Compound nevus	Round or oval shape, well-demarcated, smooth-bordered. May be dome-shaped or papillomatous; colors range from flesh colored to very dark brown, with individual nevi being relatively homogeneous in color.
Hemangioma	Dome-shaped reddish, purple, blue nodule. Compression with a glass microscope slide may result in blanching. Must be distinguished from nodular melanoma.
Junctional nevus	Flat to barely raised brown lesion. Sharp border. Fine pigmentary stippling visible, especially upon magnification.
Lentigo Juvenile Solar	Flat, uniformly medium or dark brown lesion with sharp border. Solar lentigines are acquired lesions on sites of chronic solar exposure (face and backs of hands). Lesions are 2 mm to ≥1 cm. Solar lentigines have reticulate pigmentation upon magnification.
Pigmented basal cell carcinoma	Papular border. May have central ulceration. Usually on a sun-exposed surface in an older patient. Patient usually has dark brown eyes and dark brown or black hair.
Pigmented dermatofibroma	Lesion is not well demarcated visually, is firm, and dimples downward when compressed laterally. Usually on extremities. Usually <6 mm.
Seborrheic keratosis	Rough, sharp-bordered lesions that feel waxy and "stuck on"; range in color from flesh to tan, to dark brown. Presence of keratin plugs in surface is helpful for discriminating especially dark lesions from melanoma.
Subungual hematoma	Maroon (red-brown) coloration. As lesion grows out from nail fold, a curving clear area is seen.
Tattoo (medical or traumatic)	In medical tattoo, lesions are small pigmentary dots, often blue or green, which make a regular pattern (rectangle). Traumatic tattoos are irregular, and pigmentation may appear black.

olution ("E"), as any of the other features become more significant as the lesion is changing.

Biopsy Any pigmented cutaneous lesion that has changed in size or shape or has other features suggestive of malignant melanoma is a candidate for biopsy. The recommended technique is a full-thickness excisional biopsy, as that facilitates pathologic assessment of the lesion, permits accurate measurement of thickness if the lesion is melanoma, and constitutes treatment if the lesion is benign. Shave biopsy or curettage of a suspected melanoma is contraindicated. For large lesions or lesions on anatomic sites where excisional biopsy may not be feasible (such as the face, hands, or feet), an incisional biopsy through the most nodular or darkest area of the lesion is acceptable; this should include the vertical growth phase of the primary tumor, if present. Data from prospective studies do not indicate that an incisional biopsy facilitates the spread of melanoma.

Staging Once the diagnosis of malignant melanoma has been confirmed, the tumor must be staged to determine prognosis and treatment. The history should probe for evidence of metastatic disease, such as malaise, weight loss, headaches, visual difficulty, or bone pain. The physical examination should be directed especially to the skin, regional draining lymph nodes, central nervous system, liver, and spleen. In the absence of signs or symptoms of metastasis, few laboratory or radiologic tests are indicated for staging purposes. Aside from a chest radiograph and, possibly, liver function tests, no other tests or scans

are routinely indicated unless the history or physical examination suggests metastasis to a specific organ. Specifically, liver-spleen scans and computed tomography have a low yield and are not cost-effective. However, once signs of metastasis exist, favored sites of spread, such as the liver, lungs, bone, and brain, should be scanned. Appropriate evaluations place patients into four clinical stages (Table 73-4).

℞ TREATMENT

Surgical Management For a newly diagnosed cutaneous melanoma, wide surgical excision of the lesion with a margin of normal skin is necessary to remove all malignant cells and minimize local recurrence. The appropriate width of the margin is a source of controversy. A World Health Organization trial prospectively randomized between 1- and 3-cm margins in 612 patients with thin malignant melanomas (≤2 mm thick) reported that the narrower margin resulted in higher rates of local recurrence but no difference in rates of nodal or distant metastases, disease-free survival, or overall survival after 7.5 years of follow-up. Another large randomized trial comparing 2- or 4-cm surgical margins for intermediate-thickness lesions (1 to 4 mm thick) also found no significant differences in overall survival. The following margins can be recommended for primary melanoma: in situ: 0.5 cm; invasive up to 1 mm thick: 1.0 cm; 1 to 4 mm thick: 2.0 cm; >4 mm thick: 2.5 to 3.0 cm. For lesions on the face, hands, and feet, strict adherence to these margins must give way to individual considerations about the constraints of surgery and minimization of morbidity. In all instances, however, inclusion of subcutaneous fat in the surgical specimen facilitates adequate thickness measurement and assessment of surgical margins by the pathologist.

ELECTIVE REGIONAL NODE DISSECTION Elective regional node dissection in the American Joint Commission for Cancer (AJCC) stage II disease (without palpable adenopathy) has been advocated, based on the hypothesis that melanoma metastasizes in an orderly fashion from the skin to regional lymph nodes and finally to distant sites. If that is the case, surgical excision of nodal micrometastasis could theoretically provide definitive treatment at a time of relatively low tumor burden and perhaps improve survival. The efficacy of this procedure remains controversial; while some retrospective series suggest a survival benefit, two randomized studies examining this question in patients with limb melanomas and clinical stage I disease showed no survival advantage for wide local excision followed by immediate elective regional node dissection compared with wide local excision followed by delayed dissection (only if nodes became palpable). Furthermore, the procedure has associated morbidity, and some lesions, especially those on the trunk, have ambiguous nodal draining sites, making it difficult to decide which area to dissect. Sentinel lymph node examination has been shown to be a valuable staging tool and, in instances of a negative sentinel lymph node, may obviate the need for elective regional nodal dissection. Patients with lesions <0.75 mm thick have an excellent prognosis and need no node dissection; at the other extreme, patients with lesions 3.5 mm thick have such a high risk for distant metastases that elective node dissection may not alter the ultimate clinical outcome. A subset of patients with AJCC stage II lesions of intermediate thickness may benefit from elective regional node dissection, but there is no consensus about which patients should undergo this procedure. An ongoing randomized surgical trial may resolve this issue.

Adjuvant Therapy For patients who are free of disease but at high risk for metastases, adjuvant therapy that complements surgery is needed to destroy occult micrometastases, prolong disease-free survival, and improve the cure rate. Many strategies have been tried unsuccessfully. However, adjuvant interferon α (either 2a or 2b) may be capable of improving disease-free and overall survival in some, particularly in patients with nodal metastases (stage III disease). The U.S. Food and Drug Administration has approved a high-dose interferon adjuvant protocol consisting of 20 million units per square meter intravenously 5 days a week for 4 weeks followed by 10 million units per square meter subcutaneously three times a week for 11 months. Ongoing studies are attempting to define the minimal effective dose, because, in nearly half of patients, these doses of interferon are associated with severe toxicity, including flulike illness and decline in performance status. The toxicity reverses promptly with lower doses and when therapy is stopped.

Treatment of Metastatic Disease Melanoma can metastasize to any organ, the brain being a particularly common site. Metastatic melanoma is generally incurable, with survival in patients with visceral metastases generally <1 year. Thus, the goal of treatment is usually palliation. Patients with soft tissue and node metastases fare better than those with liver and brain metastases. Metastases limited to regional nodes (AJCC stage III disease) warrant a therapeutic lymph node dissection. Surgical excision of a single metastasis to the lung or to a surgically accessible brain site can prolong survival. Trials of stereotactic radiosurgery will determine its future role in the treatment of brain metastases. More often, however, patients have multiple brain metastases that require radiation therapy and glucocorticoids. Radiation therapy can provide local palliation for recurrent tumors or metastases. Patients who have advanced regional disease limited to a limb may benefit from hyperthermic limb perfusion with melphalan and tumor necrosis factor. Complete response rates >90% have been reported; responses are associated with significant palliation of symptoms.

A number of drugs and biologicals have minimal antitumor activity (15 to 20% partial response rates) in metastatic melanoma, including dacarbazine (DTIC); the nitrosoureas carmustine (BCNU), lomustine (CCNU), and semustine (methyl-CCNU); platinum analogues such as cisplatin and carboplatin; vinca alkyloids such as vincristine, vinblastine, and vindesine; the taxanes paclitaxel and docetaxel; interferon α; and interleukin 2 (IL-2). Single-agent dacarbazine is considered the standard treatment. This agent has been given at a number of different doses and schedules; 250 mg/m^2 intravenously every day for 5 days every 3 weeks is a standard schedule. Dacarbazine-based combination regimens are probably more effective. Ongoing trials are attempting to define superior combinations. Interferon and IL-2 produce response rates similar to those seen with cytotoxic agents; however, at active doses, they usually cause greater toxicity than chemotherapy.

Melanoma can express cell surface antigens that may be recognized by host immune cells. Melanoma antigens (MAGEs)-1, -2, and -3 (endogenous proteins controlled by genes on the X chromosome; there may be up to 12 of these genes) and tyrosinase, an enzyme involved in melanin synthesis, are antigens that are processed into peptides and presented to T cells via HLA-A antigens on the tumor, particularly the HLA-A1 and A2 alleles, which are expressed in about 85% of patients with melanoma. In addition, a melanoma antigen called MART is recognized in the context of class II MHC antigens. These melanoma-associated antigens alone or in combination may make it possible to develop vaccination strategies against melanoma. Such strategies include the use of purified proteins as immunogens and the use of genetically altered tumor cells to elicit a T cell response. Alternative experimental approaches include efforts to expand tumor-specific T cells (obtained either from the tumor as tumor-infiltrating lymphocytes or harvested from the peripheral blood after vaccination) in vitro and transfer them into patients in large numbers. In addition, monoclonal antibodies to tumor antigens are being tested, with some early indication of efficacy in ~15% of patients. All of these experimental approaches will need considerable further development before being applicable on a wide scale. Advances in treating metastatic disease may be applicable in the adjuvant setting.

The absence of curative therapy for patients with metastatic melanoma underscores the importance of early detection and prevention as strategies to decrease melanoma mortality.

FURTHER READING

BALCH CM et al: Prognostic factors analysis of 17,600 melanoma patients: Validation of the AJCC staging system. J Clin Oncol 19:2001

CREAGAN ET et al: Randomized surgical adjuvant clinical trial of recombinant interferon-alfa-2a in selected patients with malignant melanoma. J Clin Oncol 13:2776, 1995

DRAKE LA et al: Guidelines of care of basal cell carcinoma. J Am Acad Dermatol 26:117, 1992

———— et al: Guidelines of care for cutaneous squamous cell carcinoma. J Am Acad Dermatol 28:628, 1993

GEISSE JK et al: Imiquimod 5% cream for the treatment of superficial basal cell carcinoma: A double-blind, randomized, vehicle-controlled study. J Am Acad Dermatol 47:390, 2002

JOHNSON TM et al: Staging workup, sentinel node biopsy, and follow-up tests for melanoma: Update of current concepts, 140:107, 2004

74 HEAD AND NECK CANCER
Everett E. Vokes

Epithelial carcinomas of the head and neck arise from the mucosal surfaces in the head and neck area and typically are squamous cell in origin. This category includes tumors of the paranasal sinuses, the oral cavity, and the nasopharynx, oropharynx, hypopharynx, and larynx. Tumors of the salivary glands differ from the more common carcinomas of the head and neck in etiology, histopathology, clinical presentation, and therapy. Thyroid malignancies are described in Chap. 320.

INCIDENCE AND EPIDEMIOLOGY The number of new cases of head and neck cancers in the United States was 38,530 in 2004, accounting for about 3% of adult malignancies. The worldwide incidence exceeds half a million cases annually. In North America and Europe, the tumors usually arise from the oral cavity, oropharynx, or larynx, whereas nasopharyngeal cancer is more common in the Mediterranean countries and in the Far East.

ETIOLOGY AND GENETICS Alcohol and tobacco use are the most common risk factors for head and neck cancer in the United States. Smokeless tobacco is an etiologic agent for oral cancers. Other potential carcinogens include marijuana and occupational exposures such as nickel refining, exposure to textile fibers, and woodworking.

Dietary factors may contribute. The incidence of head and neck cancer is highest in people with the lowest consumption of fruits and vegetables. Certain vitamins, including dietary carotenoids, may be protective; retinoids are being tested for prevention.

Some head and neck cancers may have a viral etiology. The DNA of human papillomavirus has been detected in the tissue of oral and tonsil cancers, and may predispose to oral cancer in the absence of tobacco and alcohol use. Epstein-Barr virus (EBV) infection is associated with nasopharyngeal cancer. Nasopharyngeal cancer occurs endemically in some countries of the Mediterranean and Far East, where EBV antibody titers can be measured to screen high-risk populations. Nasopharyngeal cancer has also been associated with consumption of salted fish.

No specific risk factors or environmental carcinogens have been identified for salivary gland tumors.

HISTOPATHOLOGY, CARCINOGENESIS, AND MOLECULAR BIOLOGY Squamous cell head and neck cancers can be divided into well-differentiated, moderately well-differentiated, and poorly differentiated categories. Patients with poorly differentiated tumors have a worse prognosis than those with well-differentiated tumors. For nasopharyngeal cancers, the less common differentiated squamous cell carcinoma is distinguished from nonkeratinizing and undifferentiated carcinoma (lymphoepithelioma) that contains infiltrating (bystander) lymphocytes.

Salivary gland tumors can arise from the major (parotid, submandibular, sublingual) or minor salivary glands (located in the submucosa of the upper aerodigestive tract). Most parotid tumors are benign, but half of submandibular and sublingual gland tumors and most minor salivary gland tumors are malignant. Malignant tumors include mucoepidermoid and adenoidcystic carcinomas and adenocarcinomas.

The mucosal surface of the entire pharynx is exposed to alcohol- and tobacco-related carcinogens and is at risk for the development of a premalignant or malignant lesion, such as erythroplakia or leukoplakia (hyperplasia, dysplasia), that can progress to invasive carcinoma. Alternatively, multiple synchronous or metachronous cancers can develop. In fact, patients with early-stage head and neck cancer are at greater risk of dying of a second malignancy than of dying from a recurrence of the primary disease.

Second head and neck malignancies are not therapy-induced; they reflect the exposure of the upper aerodigestive mucosa to the same carcinogens that caused the first cancer. These second primaries develop in the head and neck area, the lung, or the esophagus.

Chromosomal deletions and other alterations, most frequently involving chromosomes 3p, 9p, 17p, and 13q, have been identified in both premalignant and malignant head and neck lesions, as have mutations in tumor suppressor genes, commonly the p53 gene. Amplification of oncogenes is less common, but overexpression of PRAD-1/bcl-1 (cyclin D1), bcl-2, transforming growth factor β, and the epidermal growth factor receptor have been described. The latter finding correlates positively with tumor size and poor outcome and is a target for experimental treatments.

Resected tumor specimens with histopathologically negative margins ("complete resection") can have undetectable residual tumor cells with persistent p53 mutations at the margins. Thus, a tumor-specific p53 mutation can be detected in some phenotypically "normal" surgical margins, indicating residual disease. Patients with such submicroscopic marginal involvement may have a worse prognosis than patients with negative margins.

CLINICAL PRESENTATION AND DIFFERENTIAL DIAGNOSIS Most head and neck cancers occur after age 50, although these cancers can appear in younger patients, including those without known risk factors. The manifestations vary according to the stage and primary site of the tumor. Patients with nonspecific signs and symptoms in the head and neck area should be evaluated with a thorough otolaryngologic exam, particularly if symptoms persist longer than 2 to 4 weeks.

Cancer of the nasopharynx typically does not cause early symptoms. However, on occasion it may cause unilateral serous otitis media due to obstruction of the eustachian tube, unilateral or bilateral nasal obstruction, or epistaxis. Advanced nasopharyngeal carcinoma causes neuropathies of the cranial nerves.

Carcinomas of the oral cavity present as nonhealing ulcers, changes in the fit of dentures, or painful lesions. Tumors of the tongue base or oropharynx can cause decreased tongue mobility and alterations in speech. Cancers of the oropharynx or hypopharynx rarely cause early symptoms, but they may cause sore throat and/or otalgia.

Hoarseness may be an early symptom of laryngeal cancer, and persistent hoarseness requires referral to a specialist for indirect laryngoscopy and/or radiographic studies. If a head and neck lesion treated initially with antibiotics does not resolve in a short period, further workup is indicated; to simply continue the antibiotic treatment may be to lose the chance of early diagnosis of a malignancy.

Advanced head and neck cancers in any location can cause severe pain, otalgia, airway obstruction, cranial neuropathies, trismus, odynophagia, dysphagia, decreased tongue mobility, fistulas, skin involvement, and massive cervical lymphadenopathy, which may be unilateral or bilateral. Some patients have enlarged lymph nodes even though no primary lesion can be detected by endoscopy or biopsy; these patients are considered to have carcinoma of unknown primary (Fig. 74-1). If the enlarged nodes are located in the upper neck and the tumor cells are of squamous cell histology, the malignancy probably arose from a mucosal surface in the head or neck. Tumor cells in supraclavicular

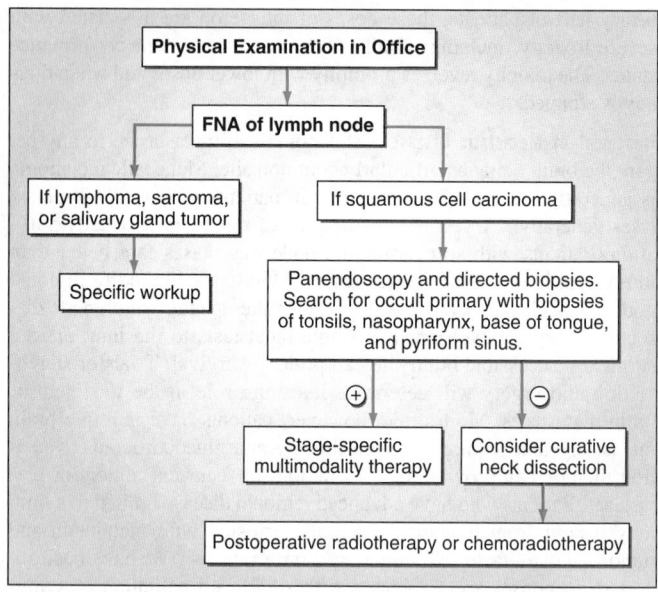

FIGURE 74-1 Evaluation of a patient with cervical adenopathy without a primary mucosal lesion; a diagnostic workup. FNA, fine-needle aspiration.

lymph nodes may also arise from a primary site in the chest or abdomen.

The physical examination should include inspection of all visible mucosal surfaces and palpation of the floor of mouth and tongue and of the neck. In addition to tumors themselves, leukoplakia, a white mucosal patch, or erythroplakia, a red mucosal patch, may be observed; these "premalignant" lesions can represent hyperplasia, dysplasia, or carcinoma in situ. All visible or palpable lesions should be biopsied. Further examination should be performed by a specialist. Additional staging procedures include computed tomography of the head and neck to identify the extent of the disease. Patients with lymph node involvement should have chest radiography and a bone scan to screen for distant metastases. The definitive staging procedure is an endoscopic examination under anesthesia, which may include laryngoscopy, esophagoscopy, and bronchoscopy; during this procedure, multiple biopsy samples are obtained to establish a primary diagnosis, define the extent of primary disease, and identify any additional premalignant lesions or second primaries.

Head and neck tumors are classified according to the TNM system of the American Joint Committee on Cancer. This classification varies according to the specific anatomic subsite (Tables 74-1 and 74-2). Distant metastases are found in <10% of patients at initial diagnosis, but in autopsy series, microscopic involvement of the lungs, bones, or liver is more common, particularly in patients with advanced neck lymph node disease.

In patients with lymph node involvement and no visible primary, the diagnosis should be made by lymph node excision. If the results indicate squamous cell carcinoma, a panendoscopy should be performed, with biopsy of all suspicious-appearing areas and directed biopsies of common primary sites, such as the nasopharynx, tonsil, tongue base, and pyriform sinus.

℞ TREATMENT

Patients with head and neck cancer can be categorized into three clinical groups: those with localized disease, those with locally or regionally advanced disease, and those with recurrent and/or metastatic disease. Comorbidities associated with tobacco and alcohol abuse can affect treatment outcome.

Localized Disease Nearly one-third of patients have localized disease; that is, T1 or T2 (stage I or stage II) lesions without detectable lymph node involvement or distant metastases. These lesions are treated with curative intent by surgery or radiation therapy. The choice of modality differs according to institutional expertise. Radiation therapy is often preferred for laryngeal cancer to preserve voice function, and surgery is preferred for small lesions in the oral cavity to avoid the long-term complications of radiation, such as xerostomia and dental decay. Overall 5-year survival is 60 to 90%.

Locally or Regionally Advanced Disease Locally or regionally advanced disease—disease with a large primary tumor and/or lymph node metastases—can also be treated with curative intent, but not with surgery or radiation therapy alone. Combined modality therapy including surgery, radiation therapy, and chemotherapy is most successful. Concomitant chemotherapy and radiation therapy appears to be most effective.

INDUCTION CHEMOTHERAPY In this strategy, patients receive chemotherapy [usually cisplatin and fluorouracil (5FU)] before surgery and radiation therapy. Most patients who receive three cycles show tumor reduction, and the response is clinically "complete" in up to half. This "sequential" multimodality therapy does not cure more patients than surgery plus radiation therapy alone. However, induction chemotherapy allows for organ preservation in patients with laryngeal and hypopharyngeal cancer.

CONCOMITANT CHEMORADIOTHERAPY With the concomitant strategy, chemotherapy and radiation therapy are given simultaneously rather than sequentially. Because most patients with head and neck cancer develop recurrent disease in the head and neck area, this approach is aimed at killing radiation-resistant cancer cells with chemotherapy. In addition, chemotherapy can enhance cell killing by radiation therapy. Toxicity (mucositis) is increased with concomitant chemoradiotherapy; however, meta-analysis of randomized trials documents an improvement in 5-year survival of 8% with concomitant 5FU and radiation therapy. Results seem even better with 5FU and cisplatin plus radiation therapy. Five-year survival is 34 to 50%. In addition, concomitant chemoradiotherapy produces better laryngectomy-free survival (organ preservation) than induction chemotherapy in patients with advanced larynx cancer. The use of radiation therapy together with cisplatin has produced markedly improved survival in patients with advanced nasopharyngeal cancer. The success of concomitant chemoradiotherapy in patients with unresectable disease has led to the testing of a similar approach in patients with resected disease as a postoperative therapy, but results to date have not convincingly shown improvement over postoperative radiation therapy alone.

Recurrent and/or Metastatic Disease Patients with recurrent and/or

TABLE 74-1 *TNM Classification for Head and Neck Cancer (Except Nasopharyngeal)*

PRIMARY TUMOR SITE

T Grade	Oropharynx	Hypopharynx
T1	0–2 cm	0–2 cm
T2	2.1–4 cm	>1 site, 2–4 cm
T3	>4 cm	>4 cm
T4a	Larynx, muscle of tongue, medial pterygoid, hard palate, mandible invasion	Thyroid/cricoid cartilage, hyoid bone, thyroid gland, esophagus, or central compartment soft tissue invasion
T4b	Lateral pterygoid muscle, pterygoid plates, lateral nasopharynx, or skull base or encases carotid artery invasion	Invasion of prevertebral fascia, encases carotid artery, or involves mediastinal structures

REGIONAL LYMPH NODES (N)

NX	Regional lymph nodes cannot be assessed
N0	No regional lymph node metastasis
N1	Unilateral metastasis in lymph node(s), ≤6 cm in greatest dimension, above the supraclavicular fossa
N2	Bilateral metastasis in lymph node(s), ≤6 cm in greatest dimension, above the supraclavicular fossa
N3	Metastasis in a lymph node(s) >6 cm and/or to supraclavicular fossa
	N3a > 6 cm
	N3b Extension to the supraclavicular fossa
MX	Distant metastasis cannot be assessed
M0	No distant metastasis
M1	Distant metastasis

STAGE GROUPING

Stage 0	Tis	N0	M0
Stage I	T1	N0	M0
Stage II	T2	N0	M0
Stage III	T3	N0	M0
	T1	N1	M0
	T2	N1	M0
	T3	N1	M0
Stage IVA	T4a	N0	M0
	T4a	N1	M0
	T1	N2	M0
	T2	N2	M0
	T3	N2	M0
	T4a	N2	M0
Stage IVB	T4b	Any N	M0
	Any T	N3	M0
Stage IVC	Any T	Any N	M1

TABLE 74-2 *Definition of TNM–Nasopharynx*

Primary Tumor (T)		Stage Grouping			
TX	Cannot be assessed	Stage 0	Tis	N0	M0
T0	No evidence	Stage I	T1	N0	M0
Tis	Carcinoma in situ	Stage IIA	T2a	N0	M0
T1	Tumor confined to the nasopharynx	Stage IIB	T1	N1	M0
T2	Tumor extends to soft tissues		T2	N1	M0
	T2a Tumor extends to the oropharynx and/or nasal cavity w/o parapharyngeal extension		T2a	N1	M0
	T2b Any tumor with parapharyngeal extension		T2b	N1	M0
T3	Tumor involves bony structures and/or paranasal sinuses		T2b	N2	M0
T4	Tumor with intracranial extension and/or involvement of cranial nerves, infratemporal fossa, hypopharynx, orbit, or masticator space	Stage III	T1	N2	M0
			T2a	N2	M0
Regional Lymph Nodes (N)			T2b	N2	M0
The distribution and the prognostic impact of regional lymph node spread from nasopharynx cancer, particularly of the undifferentiated type, are different from those of other head and neck mucosal cancers and justify the use of a different N classification scheme.			T3	N0	M0
NX Regional lymph nodes cannot be assessed			T3	N1	M0
N0 No regional lymph node metastasis			T3	N2	M0
N1 Unilateral metastasis in lymph node(s), ≤6 cm in greatest dimension, above the supraclavicular fossa			T4	N0	M0
N2 Bilateral metastasis in lymph node(s), ≤6 cm in greatest dimension, above the supraclavicular fossa			T4	N1	M0
N3 Metastasis in lymph node(s), >6 cm and/or to supraclavicular fossa			T4	N2	M0
N3a Greater than 6 cm in dimension			Any T	N3	M0
N3b Extension to the supraclavicular fossa			Any T	Any N	M1

metastatic disease are, with few exceptions, treated with palliative intent. Some patients may require local or regional radiation therapy for pain control, but most are given chemotherapy. Response rates to chemotherapy average only 30 to 50%; the duration of response averages only 3 months, and the median survival time is 6 to 8 months. Therefore, chemotherapy provides transient symptomatic benefit. Drugs with single-agent activity in this setting include methotrexate, 5FU, cisplatin, paclitaxel, and docetaxel. Combinations of cisplatin and 5FU, carboplatin and 5FU, and cisplatin or carboplatin and paclitaxel or docetaxel are frequently used.

CHEMOPREVENTION β-Carotene and *cis*-retinoic acid can lead to the regression of leukoplakia. However, *cis*-retinoic acid does not reduce the incidence of second primaries.

TREATMENT COMPLICATIONS Complications from treatment of head and neck cancer are usually related to the extent of surgery. Several attempts have been made to limit the extent of surgery or to replace it with chemotherapy and radiation therapy. Acute complications of radiation include mucositis and dysphagia. Long-term complications include xerostomia, loss of taste, decreased tongue mobility, second malignancies, dysphagia, and neck fibrosis. The complications of chemotherapy vary with the regimen used but usually include mye-

losuppression, mucositis, nausea and vomiting, and nephrotoxicity (with cisplatin).

SALIVARY GLAND TUMORS Most benign salivary gland tumors are treated with surgical excision, and patients with invasive salivary gland tumors are treated with surgery and radiation therapy. Neutron radiation may be particularly effective. These tumors may recur regionally; adenoidcystic carcinoma has a tendency to recur along the nerve tracks. Distant metastases may occur as late as 10 to 20 years after the initial diagnosis. For metastatic disease, therapy is given with palliative intent, usually chemotherapy with doxorubicin and/or cisplatin.

FURTHER READING

CALIFANO J et al: Genetic progression model for head and neck cancer: Implications for field cancerization. Cancer Res 56:2488, 1996
FORASTIERE A et al: Head and neck cancer. N Engl J Med 345:1890, 2001
LAMONT EB, VOKES EE: Chemotherapy in the management of squamous-cell carcinoma of the head and neck. Lancet Oncol 2:261, 2001
LICITRA L, VERMORKEN JB: Is there still a role for neoadjuvant chemotherapy in head and neck cancer? Ann Oncol 15:7, 2004
RICE DH: Salivary gland disorders. Neoplastic and nonneoplastic. Med Clin North Am 83:197, 1999
VOKES E et al: Weekly carboplatin and paclitaxel followed by concomitant TFHX chemoradiotherapy: Curative and organ preserving therapy for advanced head and neck cancer. J Clin Oncol 21:320, 2003

75 NEOPLASMS OF THE LUNG
John D. Minna

Each year, primary carcinoma of the lung affects 93,000 males and 80,000 females in the United States, 86% of whom die within 5 years of diagnosis, making it the leading cause of cancer death in both men and women. The incidence of lung cancer peaks between ages 55 and 65 years. Lung cancer accounts for 28% of all cancer deaths (32% in men, 25% in women). The smoking cessation efforts begun 30 years ago have lowered the age-adjusted lung cancer death rate in males (~70 per 100,000 male population); but, unfortunately, the rate in females is still increasing (~35 per 100,000 female population). The 5-year overall lung cancer survival rate (14%) has nearly doubled in the past 30 years. The improvement is due to advances in combined-modality treatment with surgery, radiotherapy, and chemotherapy. Thus, primary carcinoma of the lung is a major health problem with a generally grim prognosis.

PATHOLOGY

The term *lung cancer* is used for tumors arising from the respiratory epithelium (bronchi, bronchioles, and alveoli). Mesotheliomas, lymphomas, and stromal tumors (sarcomas) are distinct from epithelial lung cancer. Four major cell types make up 88% of all primary lung neoplasms according to the World Health Organization classification (Table 75-1). These are *squamous* or *epidermoid carcinoma, small cell* (also called *oat cell) carcinoma, adenocarcinoma* (including bronchoalveolar), and *large cell* (also called *large cell anaplastic) carcinoma*. The remainder include undifferentiated carcinomas, carcinoids, bronchial gland tumors (including adenoid cystic carcinomas and mucoepidermoid tumors), and rarer tumor types. The various cell types have different natural histories and responses to therapy, and thus a correct histologic diagnosis by an experienced pathologist is the first step to correct treatment. In the past 25 years, for unknown reasons, adenocarcinoma has replaced squamous cell carcinoma as the most frequent histologic subtype (Table 75-1).

Major treatment decisions are made on the basis of whether a tumor is classified as a small cell carcinoma or as one of the non-small cell varieties (squamous, adenocarcinoma, large cell carcinoma, bronchoalveolar carcinoma, and mixed versions of these). Some of the distinctions are summarized in Tables 75-1 and 75-2. At presentation, small cell carcinomas usually have already spread such that surgery is unlikely to be curative, and they are managed primarily by chemotherapy with or without radiotherapy. In contrast, non-small cell cancers that are localized at the time of presentation may be cured with either surgery or radiotherapy. Non-small cell cancers do not respond as well to chemotherapy as small cell cancers.

Ninety percent of patients with lung cancer of all histologic types are current or former cigarette smokers. Of the an-

TABLE 75-1 *Frequency, Age-Adjusted Incidence, and Survival Rates for Different Histologic Types of Lung Cancer[a]*

Histologic Type of Thoracic Malignancy	Frequency, %	Age-Adjusted Rate	5-Year Survival Rate (All Stages)
Adenocarcinoma (and all subtypes)	32	17	17
Bronchioloalveolar carcinoma	3	1.4	42
Squamous cell (epidermoid) carcinoma	29	15	15
Small cell carcinoma	18	9	5
Large cell carcinoma	9	5	11
Carcinoid	1.0	0.5	83
Mucoepidermoid carcinoma	0.1	<0.1	39
Adenoid cystic carcinoma	<0.1	<0.1	48
Sarcoma and other soft tissue tumors	0.1	0.1	30
All others and unspecified carcinomas	11.0	6	NA
Total	100	52	14

[a] Data on histology frequency and age-adjusted incidence rates per 100,000 U.S. population are from 60,514 cases of invasive lung cancer involving all races and both sexes obtained from the data for 1983–1987 of the Surveillance, Epidemiology, and End Results (SEER) Program of the National Cancer Institute; 5-year relative survival rates for all stages, all races, and both sexes are from the SEER data on 87,128 carcinomas, 1978–1986. NA, not available.
Source: Summarized from Travis et al: Cancer 75:191, 1995.

nual 171,900 new cases of lung cancer, ~50% develop in former smokers. With increased success in smoking cessation efforts, the number of former smokers will grow, and these individuals will be important candidates for early detection and chemoprevention efforts. By far the most common form of lung cancer arising in lifetime nonsmokers, in women, and in young patients (<45 years) is adenocarcinoma. However, in nonsmokers with adenocarcinoma involving the lung, the possibility of other primary sites should be considered. Squamous and small cell cancers usually present as central masses with endobronchial growth, while adenocarcinomas and large cell cancers tend to present as peripheral nodules or masses, frequently with pleural involvement. Squamous and large cell cancers cavitate in ~10 to 20% of cases. Bronchoalveolar carcinoma, a form of adenocarcinoma arising from peripheral airways, can present radiographically as a single mass; as a diffuse, multinodular lesion; or as a fluffy infiltrate.

ETIOLOGY

Most lung cancers are caused by carcinogens and tumor promoters ingested via cigarette smoking. The prevalence of smoking in the United States is 28% for males and 25% for females, age 18 years or older; 38% of high school seniors smoke. The relative risk of developing lung cancer is increased about 13-fold by active smoking and about 1.5-fold by long-term passive exposure to cigarette smoke. Chronic obstructive pulmonary disease, which is also smoking-related, further increases the risk of developing lung cancer. The lung cancer death rate is related to the total amount (often expressed in "cigarette pack-years") of cigarettes smoked, such that the risk is increased 60- to 70-fold for a man smoking two packs a day for 20 years as compared with a nonsmoker. Conversely, the chance of developing lung cancer decreases with cessation of smoking but may never return to the nonsmoker level. The increase in lung cancer rate in women is also associated with a rise in cigarette smoking. Women have a higher relative risk per given exposure than men (~1.5 fold higher), and women with lung cancer are more likely than men to have never smoked. This sex difference is likely due to a higher susceptibility to tobacco carcinogens in women.

Efforts to get people to stop smoking are mandatory. However, smoking cessation is extremely difficult, because the smoking habit represents a powerful addiction to nicotine (Chap. 375). Smoking addiction is both biologic and psychosocial. Different methods are available to help motivated smokers give up the habit including counseling, behavioral therapy, nicotine replacement (gum, patch, sublingual spray, inhaler), and antidepressants (buproprion). However, these methods are successful in only 20 to 25% of individuals at 1 year. Preventing people from starting to smoke may be more effective, an effort that needs to be targeted to children.

Molecular genetic studies have shown the acquisition by lung cancer cells of a number of genetic lesions, including activation of dominant oncogenes and inactivation of tumor suppressor or recessive oncogenes (Chaps. 68 and 69). In fact, lung cancer cells may have to accumulate a large number (perhaps ≥20) of such lesions. For the

TABLE 75-2 *Comparison of Small Cell and Non-Small Cell Lung Cancers*

Feature	Small Cell	Non-Small Cell
Histology	Scant cytoplasm; small, hyperchromatic nuclei with fine chromatin pattern; nucleoli indistinct; diffuse sheets of cells	Abundant cytoplasm; pleomorphic nuclei with coarse chromatin pattern; nucleoli often prominent; glandular or squamous architecture
GENERAL NEUROENDOCRINE PROPERTIES		
Dense-core granules	Present	Absent
Chromogranin	Present	Absent
Synaptophysin	Present	Absent
CD56 and CD57 antigens	Present	Absent
PEPTIDE HORMONE PRODUCTION		
Gastrin-releasing peptide gene products	Present	Absent
Other neuropeptides	ACTH, AVP, calcitonin, ANF	PTH
Autocrine loops	GRP/GRP receptor	HGF/MET
	SCF/KIT	NDF/ERBB2
OTHER MARKERS		
HLA, β_2-microglobulin	Absent/low	Present
Intermediate filament pattern	"SCLC"	"Non-SCLC"
Neurofilaments	Present	Absent
Opioid receptors	Present	Present
Nicotine receptors	Present	Present
EGF receptors	Low or absent	Present
Mucin	Absent	Present in adenocarcinomas
Surfactant-associated proteins	Absent	Often present
Carcinoembryonic antigen	Present	Present
RECESSIVE ONCOGENE (TUMOR SUPPRESSOR GENE) AND ALLELOTYPE ABNORMALITIES		
3p allele loss	100%	>90%
RASSF1A methylation	90%	40%
rb mutations	~90%	~20%
p16/CDKN2 mutations/absent expression	~10%	~50%
p53 mutations/abnormal expression	>90%	>50%
Promoter hypermethylation overall (*p16*, DAP Kinase, GSTP1, MGMT, *FHIT*, *RARβ*, *APC*, *ECAD*, *HCAD*, *RASSF1A*)	>80%	>80%
4p, 4q, 5q, 8p, 11p and other allele losses	Present	Present
Microsatellite alterations	Present	Present
DOMINANT ONCOGENE ABNORMALITIES		
ras mutations	<1%	~30%
myc family overexpression	>50%	10–35%
bcl-2 overexpression	>75%	>50%
Her-2/neu overexpression	<10%	~30%
Telomerase overexpression	>90%	>90%
RESPONSE		
Radiotherapy	Objective shrinkage in 80–90%; often complete response	Objective shrinkage in 30–50%; response uncommonly complete
Combination chemotherapy		
Overall regression rate	90%	40–60%
Rate of complete regression	30%	5%

dominant oncogenes, these include point mutations in the coding regions of the *ras* family of oncogenes (particularly in the K-*ras* gene in adenocarcinoma of the lung); amplification, rearrangement, and/or loss of transcriptional control of *myc* family oncogenes (c-, N-, and L-*myc*; changes in c-*myc* are found in non-small cell cancers, while changes in all *myc* family members are found in small cell lung cancer); and overexpression of *bcl-2*, *Her-2/neu*, and the telomerase gene (Table 75-2). Tumor mutations in *ras* genes are associated with a poor prognosis in non-small cell lung cancer, while tumor amplification of c-*myc* is associated with a poor prognosis in small cell lung cancer.

For the recessive oncogenes (*tumor suppressor genes*), allele loss occurs at chromosome regions 1p, 1q, 3p12-13, 3p14 (*FHIT* gene), 3p21 (*RASSF1A* gene), 3p24-25 (*RARβ* gene), 4p, 4q, 5q, 8p, 9p (*p16/CDKN2, p15,p14ARF* gene cluster), 11p13, 11p15, 13q14 (retinoblastoma, *rb*, gene), 16q, and 17p13 (*p53* gene), as well as other sites. Several candidate recessive oncogenes on chromosome 3p appear to be involved in nearly all lung cancers and may be affected early in preneoplastic lesions. The *p53* and *rb* genes are both mutated in >90% of small cell lung cancers, while *p53* is mutated in >50% and *rb* in 20% of non-small cell lung cancers. *p16/CDKN2* is abnormal in 10% of small cell and >50% of non-small cell lung cancers. The *rb* and *p16/CDKN2* genes are part of the same G_1-to-S cell cycle regulatory pathway. Either one or the other of these elements appears to be mutated or to have its expression turned off (e.g., by hypermethylation of the promoter) in the large majority of lung cancers. Tumor acquired promoter methylation may be the most frequent method of inactivating tumor-suppressor genes in lung cancer (>10 such genes commonly affected). These methylation changes inhibit gene expression and can be detected in tumor cells, preneoplastic lesions, and DNA in the sputum; their detection may improve early diagnosis and follow-up of the disease. Preneoplastic lesions found in the respiratory epithelium of lung cancer patients and smokers include hyperplasia, dysplasia (progressively severe), and carcinoma in situ. 3p allele loss (hyperplasia) followed by 9p (*p16/CDKN2*) allele loss (hyperplasia) are the earliest events; 17p (*p53*) abnormalities and then *ras* mutations are usually found only in carcinoma in situ and invasive cancer. Thus, molecular changes can be found in the earliest preneoplastic lesions and potentially even before any histologic changes are noted. Clinical trials of early diagnosis are needed to prove the usefulness of these molecular markers in the identification of very early lung cancer and in the monitoring of treatment and chemoprevention.

The large number of genetic and epigenetic lesions shows that lung cancer, like other common epithelial malignancies, is a multistep process that is likely to involve both carcinogens and tumor promoters. Prevention can be directed at both processes. Lung cancer cells produce many peptide hormones and express receptors for these hormones, which can act to stimulate tumor cell growth in an "autocrine" fashion. Highly carcinogenic derivatives of nicotine are formed in cigarette smoke. Lung cancer cells of all histologic types (and the cells from which they are derived) express nicotinic acetylcholine receptors. Nicotine activates signaling pathways in tumor and normal cells that block apoptosis. Thus, nicotine itself could be directly involved in lung cancer pathogenesis.

While lung cancer does not have a clear pattern of Mendelian inheritance, several features suggest a potential for familial association. Inherited mutations in *rb* (patients with retinoblastomas living to adulthood) and *p53* (Li-Fraumeni syndrome) genes may develop lung cancer. First-degree relatives of lung cancer probands have a two- to threefold excess risk of lung cancer or other cancers, many of which are not smoking-related. Certain alleles of the P450 enzyme system (which metabolizes carcinogens) or chromosome fragility (*mutagen sensitivity*) genotypes are associated with the development of lung cancer. The use of these polymorphisms to identify persons at very high risk of developing lung cancer would be useful in early detection and prevention efforts.

CLINICAL MANIFESTATIONS

Lung cancer gives rise to signs and symptoms caused by local tumor growth, invasion or obstruction of adjacent structures, growth in regional nodes through lymphatic spread, growth in distant metastatic sites after hematogenous dissemination, and remote effects of tumor products (paraneoplastic syndromes) (Chaps. 86 and 87).

Although 5 to 15% of patients with lung cancer are identified while they are asymptomatic, usually as a result of a routine chest radiograph, most patients present with some sign or symptom. Central or endobronchial growth of the primary tumor may cause cough, hemoptysis, wheeze and stridor, dyspnea, and postobstructive pneumonitis (fever and productive cough). Peripheral growth of the primary tumor may cause pain from pleural or chest wall involvement, cough, dyspnea on a restrictive basis, and symptoms of lung abscess resulting from tumor cavitation. Regional spread of tumor in the thorax (by contiguous growth or by metastasis to regional lymph nodes) may cause tracheal obstruction, esophageal compression with dysphagia, recurrent laryngeal nerve paralysis with hoarseness, phrenic nerve paralysis with elevation of the hemidiaphragm and dyspnea, and sympathetic nerve paralysis with Horner's syndrome (enophthalmos, ptosis, miosis, and ipsilateral loss of sweating). Malignant pleural effusion often leads to dyspnea. *Pancoast's* (or *superior sulcus tumor*) *syndrome* results from local extension of a tumor growing in the apex of the lung with involvement of the eighth cervical and first and second thoracic nerves, with shoulder pain that characteristically radiates in the ulnar distribution of the arm, often with radiologic destruction of the first and second ribs. Often Horner's syndrome and Pancoast's syndrome coexist. Other problems of regional spread include *superior vena cava syndrome* from vascular obstruction; pericardial and cardiac extension with resultant tamponade, arrhythmia, or cardiac failure; lymphatic obstruction with resultant pleural effusion; and lymphangitic spread through the lungs with hypoxemia and dyspnea. In addition, bronchoalveolar carcinoma can spread transbronchially, producing tumor growing along multiple alveolar surfaces with impairment of gas exchange, respiratory insufficiency, dyspnea, hypoxemia, and sputum production.

Extrathoracic metastatic disease is found at autopsy in >50% of patients with squamous carcinoma, 80% of patients with adenocarcinoma and large cell carcinoma, and >95% of patients with small cell cancer. Lung cancer metastases may occur in virtually every organ system. Common clinical problems related to metastatic lung cancer include brain metastases with neurologic deficits; bone metastases with pain and pathologic fractures; bone marrow invasion with cytopenias or leukoerythroblastosis; liver metastases causing liver dysfunction, biliary obstruction, and pain; lymph node metastases in the supraclavicular region and occasionally in the axilla and groin; and spinal cord compression syndromes from epidural or bone metastases. Adrenal metastases are common but rarely cause adrenal insufficiency.

Paraneoplastic syndromes are common in patients with lung cancer and may be the presenting finding or first sign of recurrence. In addition, paraneoplastic syndromes may mimic metastatic disease and, unless detected, lead to inappropriate palliative rather than curative treatment. Often the paraneoplastic syndrome may be relieved with successful treatment of the tumor. In some cases, the pathophysiology of the paraneoplastic syndrome is known, particularly when a hormone with biologic activity is secreted by a tumor (Chap. 86). However, in many cases the pathophysiology is unknown. Systemic symptoms of anorexia, cachexia, weight loss (seen in 30% of patients), fever, and suppressed immunity are paraneoplastic syndromes of unknown etiology. *Endocrine syndromes* are seen in 12% of patients: hypercalcemia and hypophosphatemia resulting from the ectopic production by squamous tumors of parathyroid hormone (PTH) or, more commonly, PTH-related peptide; hyponatremia with the syndrome of inappropriate secretion of antidiuretic hormone or possibly atrial natriuretic factor by small cell cancer; and ectopic secretion by small cell cancer of adrenocorticotropic hormone (ACTH). ACTH secretion usually results in additional electrolyte disturbances, especially hypokalemia, rather than the changes in body habitus that occur in Cushing's syndrome from a pituitary adenoma.

Skeletal–connective tissue syndromes include clubbing in 30% of cases (usually non-small cell carcinomas) and hypertrophic pulmonary osteoarthropathy in 1 to 10% of cases (usually adenocarcinomas) with periostitis and clubbing causing pain, tenderness, and swelling over the affected bones and a positive bone scan. *Neurologic-myopathic syndromes* are seen in only 1% of patients but are dramatic and include the myasthenic *Eaton-Lambert syndrome* and retinal blindness with small cell cancer, while peripheral neuropathies, subacute cerebellar degeneration, cortical degeneration, and polymyositis are seen with all lung cancer types. Many of these are caused by autoimmune responses such as the development of anti-voltage-gated calcium channel antibodies in the Eaton-Lambert syndrome (Chap. 87). Coagulation, thrombotic, or other hematologic manifestations occur in 1 to 8% of patients and include migratory venous thrombophlebitis (*Trousseau's syndrome*), nonbacterial thrombotic (marantic) endocarditis with arterial emboli, disseminated intravascular coagulation with hemorrhage, and anemia, granulocytosis, and leukoerythroblastosis. Thrombotic disease complicating cancer is usually a poor prognostic sign. Cutaneous manifestations such as dermatomyositis and acanthosis nigricans are uncommon ($\leq$1%), as are the renal manifestations of nephrotic syndrome or glomerulonephritis ($\leq$1%).

DIAGNOSIS AND STAGING

EARLY DIAGNOSIS The screening of asymptomatic persons at high risk (men >45 years who smoke $\geq$40 cigarettes per day) by means of sputum cytology and chest radiographs has not improved the survival rate. Although 90% of patients whose lung cancer was detected by screening were asymptomatic, no difference was found in the survival rates of the screened and nonscreened groups. Women have not been studied. The use of low-dose spiral computed tomography (CT) lung scanning may be more sensitive, particularly for peripheral lesions. However, false-positive rates are high (25% have abnormal tests, only 10% of which are cancers), and survival benefit for screening has not yet been shown (Chap. 67).

ESTABLISHING A TISSUE DIAGNOSIS OF LUNG CANCER Once signs, symptoms, or screening studies suggest lung cancer, a tissue diagnosis must be established. Tumor tissue can be obtained by a bronchial or transbronchial biopsy during fiberoptic bronchoscopy; by node biopsy during mediastinoscopy; from the operative specimen at the time of definitive surgical resection; by percutaneous biopsy of an enlarged lymph node, soft tissue mass, lytic bone lesion, bone marrow, or pleural lesion; by fine-needle aspiration of thoracic or extrathoracic tumor masses using CT guidance; or from an adequate cell block obtained from a malignant pleural effusion. In most cases, the pathologist should be able to make a definite diagnosis of epithelial malignancy and distinguish small cell from non-small cell lung cancer.

STAGING PATIENTS WITH LUNG CANCER Lung cancer staging consists of two parts: first, a determination of the location of tumor (anatomic staging) and, second, an assessment of a patient's ability to withstand various antitumor treatments (physiologic staging). In a patient with non-small cell lung cancer, *resectability* (whether the tumor can be entirely removed by a standard surgical procedure such as a lobectomy or pneumonectomy), which depends on the anatomic stage of the tumor, and *operability* (whether the patient can tolerate such a surgical procedure), which depends on the cardiopulmonary function of the patient, are determined.

Non-Small Cell Lung Cancer The TNM International Staging System should be used for cases of non-small cell lung cancer, particularly in preparing patients for curative attempts with surgery or radiotherapy (Table 75-3). The various T (tumor size), N (regional node involvement), and M (presence or absence of distant metastasis) factors are combined to form different stage groups. At presentation, approximately one-third of patients have disease localized enough for a curative attempt with surgery or radiotherapy (patients with stage I or II

TABLE 75-3 *Tumor, Node, Metastasis International Staging System for Lung Cancer*

		5-Year Survival Rate, %	
Stage	TNM Descriptors	Clinical Stage	Surgical-Pathologic Stage
IA	T1 N0 M0	61	67
IB	T2 N0 M0	38	57
IIA	T1 N1 M0	34	55
IIB	T2 N1 M0	24	39
IIB	T3 N0 M0	22	38
IIIA	T3 N1 M0	9	25
	T1–2–3 N2 M0	13	23
IIIB	T4 N0–1–2 M0	7	<5
	T1–2–3–4 N3 M0	3	<3
IV	Any T any N M1	1	<1

TUMOR (T) STATUS DESCRIPTOR

T0	No evidence of a primary tumor
TX	Primary tumor cannot be assessed, or tumor proven by the presence of malignant cells in sputum or bronchial washings but not visualized by imaging or bronchoscopy
TIS	Carcinoma in situ
T1	Tumor <3 cm in greatest dimension, surrounded by lung or visceral pleura, without bronchoscopic evidence of invasion more proximal than lobar bronchus (i.e., not in main bronchus)
T2	Tumor with any of following: >3 cm in greatest dimension; involves main bronchus, $\geq$2 cm distal to the carcina; invades visceral pleura; associated with atelectasis or obstructive pneumonitis extending to hilum but does not involve entire lung
T3	Tumor of any size that directly invades any of the following: chest wall (including superior sulcus tumors), diaphragm, mediastinal pleura, parietal pericardium; or tumor in main bronchus <2 cm distal to carina but without involvement of carina; or associated atelectasis or obstructive pneumonitis of entire lung
T4	Tumor of any size that invades any of the following: mediastinum, heart, great vessels, trachea, esophagus, vertebral body, carina; or tumor with a malignant pleural or pericardial effusion[a], or with satellite tumor nodule(s) within the ipsilateral primary-tumor lobe of the lung.

LYMPH NODE (N) INVOLVEMENT DESCRIPTOR

NX	Regional lymph nodes cannot be assessed
N0	No regional lymph node metastasis
N1	Metastasis to ipsilateral peribronchial and/or ipsilateral hilar lymph nodes, and intrapulmonary nodes involved by direct extension of the primary tumor
N2	Metastasis to ipsilateral mediastinal and/or subcarinal lymph nodes(s)
N3	Metastasis to contralateral mediastinal, contralateral hilar, ipsilateral or contralateral scalene, or supraclavicular lymph node(s)

DISTANT METASTASIS (M) DESCRIPTOR

MX	Presence of distant metastasis cannot be assessed
M0	No distant metastasis
M1	Distant metastasis present[b]

[a] Most pleural effusions associated with lung cancer are due to tumor. However, in a few patients with multiple negative cytopathologic exams of a non-bloody, non-exudative pleural or pericardial effusion that clinical judgment dictates is not related to the tumor, the effusion should be excluded as a staging element and the patient's disease staged as T1, T2, or T3.
[b] Separate metastatic pulmonary tumor nodule(s) in the ipsilateral nonprimary tumor lobe(s) of the lung are classified as M1.
Source: Adapted from CF Mountain. Revisions in the International System for Staging of Lung Cancer. Chest 111:1710, 1997; with permission.

disease and some with stage IIIA disease), one-third have distant metastatic disease (stage IV disease), and one-third have local or regional disease that may or may not be amenable to a curative attempt (some patients with stage IIIA disease and others with stage IIIB disease) (see below). This staging system provides useful prognostic information.

Small Cell Lung Cancer   A simple two-stage system is used. In this system, limited-stage disease (seen in about 30% of all patients with small cell lung cancer) is defined as disease confined to one hemithorax and regional lymph nodes (including mediastinal, contralateral hilar, and usually ipsilateral supraclavicular nodes), while extensive-stage disease (seen in about 70% of patients) is defined as disease exceeding those boundaries. Clinical studies such as physical examination, x-rays, CT and bone scans, and bone marrow examination are used in staging. In part, the definition of limited-stage disease relates to whether the known tumor can be encompassed within a tolerable radiation therapy port. Thus, contralateral supraclavicular nodes, recurrent laryngeal nerve involvement, and superior vena caval obstruction can all be part of limited-stage disease. However, cardiac tamponade, malignant pleural effusion, and bilateral pulmonary parenchymal involvement generally qualify disease as extensive-stage because the organs within a curative radiation therapy port cannot safely tolerate curative radiation doses.

GENERAL STAGING PROCEDURES (Table 75-4)   All patients with lung cancer should have a complete history and physical examination, with evaluation of all other medical problems, determination of performance status and history of weight loss, and a CT scan of the chest and abdomen with contrast. Positron emission tomography (PET) scans are sensitive in detecting both intrathoracic and metastatic disease. PET is useful in assessing the mediastinum and solitary pulmonary nodules. A Standardized Uptake Value (SUV) of >2.5 is highly suspicious for malignancy. False negatives can be seen in diabetes, slow-growing tumors such as bronchoalveolar carcinoma, concurrent infection such as tuberculosis, and in lesions <1 cm. Fiberoptic bronchoscopy obtains material for pathologic examination and information on tumor size, location, degree of bronchial obstruction (i.e., assesses resectability), and recurrence.

Chest radiographs and CT scans are needed to evaluate tumor size and nodal involvement; old radiographs are useful for comparison. CT scans of the thorax and upper abdomen are of use in the preoperative staging of non-small cell lung cancer to detect mediastinal nodes and pleural extension and occult abdominal disease (e.g., liver, adrenal), and in planning curative radiation therapy. However, mediastinal nodal involvement should be documented histologically if the findings will influence therapeutic decisions. Thus, sampling of lymph nodes via mediastinoscopy or thoracotomy to establish the presence or absence of N2 or N3 nodal involvement is crucial in considering a curative surgical approach for patients with non-small cell lung cancer with clinical stage I, II, or III disease. A standard nomenclature for referring to the location of lymph nodes involved with cancer has evolved (Fig. 75-1). Likewise, unless the CT-detected abnormalities are unequivocal, histology of suspicious abdominal lesions should be confirmed by procedures such as fine-needle aspiration if the patient would otherwise be considered for curative treatment. In small cell lung cancer, CT scans are used in the planning of chest radiation treatment and in the assessment of the response to chemotherapy and radiation therapy. Surgery or radiotherapy can make interpretation of conventional chest x-rays difficult; after treatment, CT scans can provide good evidence of tumor recurrence.

If signs or symptoms suggest involvement by tumor, brain CT or bone scans are performed, as well as radiography of any suspicious bony lesions. Any accessible lesions suspicious for cancer should be biopsied if involvement would influence treatment.

In patients presenting with a mass lesion on chest x-ray or CT scan and no obvious contraindications to a curative approach after the initial evaluation, the mediastinum must be investigated. Approaches vary among centers and include performing chest CT scan and mediastinoscopy (for right-sided tumors) or mediastinotomy (for left-sided lesions) on all patients and proceeding directly to thoracotomy for staging of the mediastinum. In patients presenting with disease that is confined to the chest but not resectable, and who thus are candidates for neoadjuvant chemotherapy plus surgery or for curative radiother-

---

TABLE 75-4   *Pretreatment Staging Procedures for Patients with Lung Cancer*

ALL PATIENTS

Complete history and physical examination
    Determination of performance status and weight loss
Complete blood count with platelet determination
Measurement of serum electrolytes, glucose, calcium, and phosphorus; renal and liver function tests
Electrocardiogram
Skin test for tuberculosis
Chest x-ray
CT scan of chest and abdomen
CT scan of brain and radionuclide scan of bone if any finding suggests the presence of tumor metastasis in these organs
Fiberoptic bronchoscopy with washings, brushings, and biopsy of suspicious lesions unless medically contraindicated or if it would not alter therapy (e.g., very late stage patient)
X-rays of suspicious bony lesions detected by scan or symptom
Barium-swallow radiographic examination if esophageal symptoms exist
Pulmonary function studies and arterial blood gas measurements if signs or symptoms of respiratory insufficiency are present
Biopsy of accessible lesions suspicious for cancer if a histologic diagnosis is not yet made or if treatment or staging decisions would be based on whether or not a lesion contained cancer

PATIENTS WITH NON-SMALL CELL LUNG CANCER WHO HAVE NO CONTRAINDICATION[a] TO CURATIVE SURGERY OR RADIOTHERAPY WITH OR WITHOUT CHEMOTHERAPY

All the above procedures, plus the following:
PET scan to evaluate mediastinum and detect metastatic disease
Pulmonary function tests and arterial blood gas measurements
Coagulation tests
CT scan of brain if symptoms suggestive
Cardiopulmonary excercise testing if performance status or pulmonary function tests are borderline
    If surgical resection is planned: surgical evaluation of the mediastinum at mediastinoscopy or at thoracotomy
    If the patient is a poor surgical risk or a candidate for curative radiotherapy: transthoracic fine-needle aspiration biopsy or transbronchial forceps biopsy of peripheral lesions if material from routine fiberoptic bronchoscopy is negative

PATIENTS PRESENTING WITH SMALL CELL OR ADVANCED NON-SMALL CELL LUNG CANCER

For proven small cell lung cancer, all the procedures under "All Patients," plus the following:
    CT scan of brain
    Bone marrow aspiration and biopsy (if peripheral blood counts abnormal)
For non-small cell lung cancer or cancer of unknown histology, all the procedures under "All Patients," plus the following:
    Fiberoptic bronchoscopy if indicated by hemoptysis, obstruction, pneumonitis, or no histologic diagnosis of cancer
    Biopsy of accessible lesions suspicious for tumor to obtain a histologic diagnosis or if therapy would be altered by finding of tumor
    Transthoracic fine-needle aspiration biopsy or transbronchial forceps biopsy of peripheral lesions if fiberoptic bronchoscopy is negative and no other material exists for a histologic diagnosis
    Diagnostic and therapeutic thoracentesis if a pleural effusion is present

---

[a] Patients with non-small cell lung cancer and extrathoracic metastatic disease, malignant pleural effusion, or intrathoracic disease beyond the bounds of a tolerable radiotherapy port.
Note: CT, computed tomography; PET, positron emission tomography.

---

apy with or without chemotherapy, other tests are done as indicated to evaluate specific symptoms. In patients presenting with non-small cell cancer that is not curable, all the general staging procedures are done, plus fiberoptic bronchoscopy as indicated to evaluate hemoptysis, obstruction, or pneumonitis, as well as thoracentesis with cytologic examination (and chest tube drainage as indicated) if fluid is present. As a rule, a radiographic finding of an isolated lesion (such as an enlarged adrenal gland) should be confirmed as cancer by fine-needle aspiration before a curative attempt is rejected.

STAGING OF SMALL CELL LUNG CANCER   Pretreatment staging for patients with small cell lung cancer includes the initial general lung cancer evaluation with chest and abdominal CT scans (because of the high frequency of hepatic and adrenal involvement) as well as fiberoptic bronchoscopy with washings and biopsies to determine the tumor extent before therapy; brain CT scan (10% of patients have metastases); bone marrow biopsy and aspiration (20 to 30% of patients have tumor in the bone marrow); and radionuclide scans (bone) if symptoms or other findings suggest disease involvement in these areas. Chest and abdominal CT scans are very useful to evaluate and follow tumor response to therapy, and chest CT scans are helpful in planning chest radiotherapy ports.

If signs or symptoms of spinal cord compression or leptomeningitis develop at any time in lung cancer patients with disease of any histologic type, a spinal CT scan or magnetic resonance imaging (MRI) scan and examination of the cerebrospinal fluid cytology are performed. If malignant cells are detected, radiotherapy to the site of compression and intrathecal chemotherapy (usually with methotrexate) are given. In addition, a brain CT or MRI scan is performed to search for brain metastases, which often are associated with spinal cord or leptomeningeal metastases.

DETERMINATION OF RESECTABILITY AND OPERABILITY
In patients with non-small cell lung cancer, the following are major contraindications to curative surgery or radiotherapy alone: extrathoracic metastases; superior vena cava syndrome; vocal cord and, in most cases, phrenic nerve paralysis; malignant pleural effusion; cardiac tamponade; tumor within 2 cm of the carina (not curable by surgery but potentially curable by radiotherapy); metastasis to the contralateral lung; bilateral endobronchial tumor (potentially curable by radiotherapy); metastasis to the supraclavicular lymph nodes; contralateral mediastinal node metastases (potentially curable by radiotherapy); and involvement of the main pulmonary artery. Most patients with small cell lung cancer have unresectable disease; however, if clinical findings suggest the potential for resection (most common with peripheral lesions), that option should be considered.

PHYSIOLOGIC STAGING Patients with lung cancer often have cardiopulmonary and other problems related to chronic obstructive pulmonary disease as well as other medical problems. To improve their preoperative condition, correctable problems (e.g., anemia, electrolyte and fluid disorders, infections, and arrhythmias) should be addressed, smoking stopped, and appropriate chest therapy instituted. Since it is not always possible to predict whether a lobectomy or pneumonectomy will be required until the time of operation, a conservative approach is to restrict resectional surgery to patients who could potentially tolerate a pneumonectomy. In addition to nonambulatory performance status, a myocardial infarction within the past 3 months is a contraindication to thoracic surgery because 20% of patients will die of reinfarction, while an infarction in the past 6 months is a relative contraindication. Other major contraindications include uncontrolled major arrhythmias, an FEV_1 (forced expiratory volume in 1 s) <1 L, CO_2 retention (resting PCO_2 > 45 mmHg), DLCO < 40%, and severe pulmonary hypertension. Recommending surgery when the FEV_1 is 1.1 to 2.0 L or <80% predicted requires careful judgment, while an FEV_1 > 2.5 L or >80% predicted usually permits a pneumonectomy. In patients with borderline lung function but a resectable tumor, cardiopulmonary exercise testing could be performed as part of the physiologic evaluation. This test allows an estimate of the maximal oxygen consumption ($\dot{V}max_{O_2}$). A $\dot{V}max_{O_2}$ < 15 mL/kg per min predicts for high risk of postoperative complications.

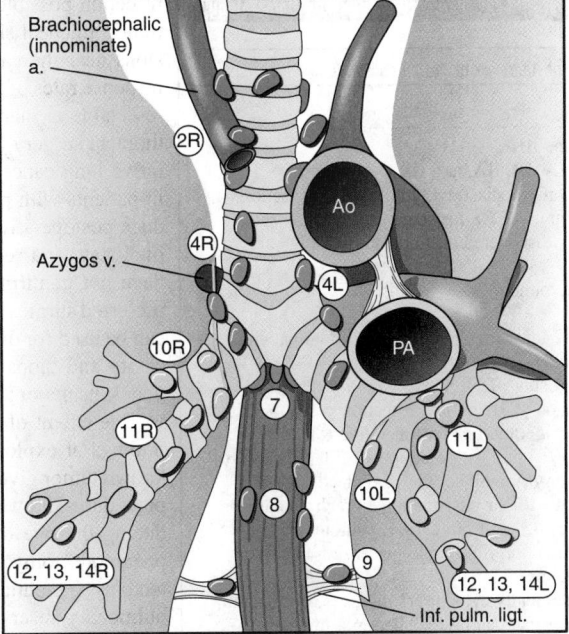

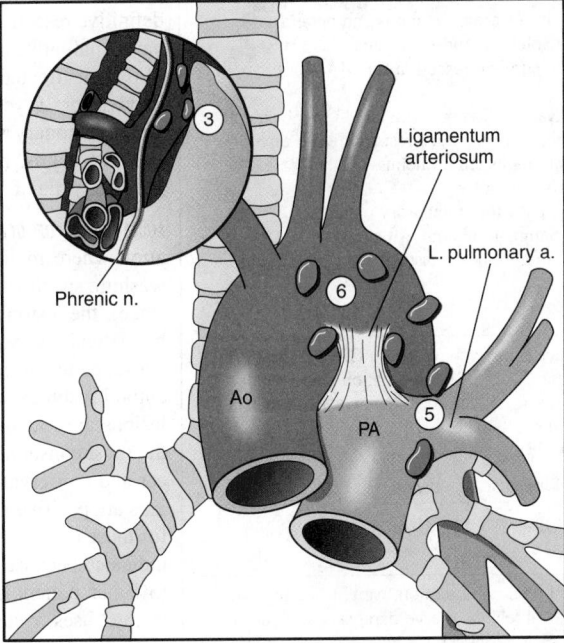

FIGURE 75-1 Regional lymph node stations for lung cancer staging. (*Used by permission from CF Mountain, C Dresler: Chest 111:1718, 1997.*)

Superior Mediastinal Nodes
- 1 Highest mediastinal
- 2 Upper paratracheal
- 3 Prevascular and retrotracheal
- 4 Lower paratracheal (including azygos nodes)

N2 = single digit, ipsilateral
N3 = single digit, contralateral or supraclavicular

Aortic Nodes
- 5 Subaortic (A-P window)
- 6 Para-aortic (ascending aorta or phrenic)

Inferior Mediastinal Nodes
- 7 Subcarinal
- 8 Paraesophageal (below carina)
- 9 Pulmonary ligament

N1 Nodes
- 10 Hilar
- 11 Interlobar
- 12 Lobar
- 13 Segmental
- 14 Subsegmental

R̶x TREATMENT
The overall treatment approach to patients with lung cancer is shown in Table 75-5. Patients should be encouraged to stop smoking. Those who do fare better than those who continue to smoke.

Non-Small Cell Lung Cancer: Localized Disease ■ *SURGERY* In patients with non-small cell lung cancer of stages IA, IB, IIA and IIB (Table 75-3) who can tolerate operation, the treatment of choice is pulmonary resection. In stage IIIA cases where the patient's age, cardiopulmonary function, and anatomy are favorable, a team approach (involving pulmonary medicine, thoracic surgery, medical and radiation oncology) is useful. Neoadjuvant chemotherapy with or without radiotherapy

TABLE 75-5 *Summary of Treatment Approach to Patients with Lung Cancer*

NON-SMALL CELL LUNG CANCER

Stages IA, IB, IIA, IIB, and some IIIA:
  Surgical resection for stages IA, IB, IIA, and IIB
  Surgical resection with complete-mediastinal lymph node dissection
    and consideration of neoadjuvant CRx for stage IIIA disease with
    "minimal N2 involvement" (discovered at thoracotomy or
    mediastinoscopy)
  Postoperative RT for patients found to have N2 disease if no
    neoadjuvant CRx given
  Discussion of risks/benefits of adjuvant CRx with individual patients
  Curative potential RT for "nonoperable" patients
Stage IIIA with selected types of stage T3 tumors:
  Tumors with chest wall invasion (T3): en bloc resection of tumor with
    involved chest wall and consideration of postoperative RT
  Superior sulcus (Pancoast's) (T3) tumors: preoperative RT (30–45 Gy)
    followed by en bloc resection of involved lung and chest wall with
    consideration of postoperative RT or intraoperative brachytherapy
  Proximal airway involvement (<2 cm from carina) without
    mediastinal nodes: sleeve resection if possible preserving distal
    normal lung or pneumonectomy
Stages IIIA "advanced, bulky, clinically evident N2 disease" (discovered
  preoperatively) and IIIB disease that can be included in a tolerable RT
  port:
  Curative potential RT + CRx if performance status and general
    medical condition are reasonable; otherwise, RT alone
  Consider neoadjuvant CRx and surgical resection for IIIA disease with
    advanced N2 involvement
Stage IIIB disease with carinal invasion (T4) but without N2 involvement:
  Consider pneumonectomy with tracheal sleeve resection with direct
    reanastomosis to contralateral mainstem bronchus
Stage IV and more advanced IIIB disease:
  RT to symptomatic local sites; CRx for ambulatory patients
  Chest tube drainage of large malignant pleural effusions
  Consider resection of primary tumor and metastasis for isolated brain
    or adrenal metastases

SMALL CELL LUNG CANCER

Limited stage (good performance status): combination CRx + chest RT
Extensive stage (good performance status): combination CRx
Complete tumor responders (all stages): consider prophylactic cranial RT
Poor-performance-status patients (all stages):
  Modified-dose combination CRx; palliative RT

BRONCHOALVEOLAR CARCINOMA (EGF receptor mutations)

Gefitinib, inhibitor of EGF receptor kinase activity

ALL PATIENTS

RT for brain metastases, spinal cord compression, weight-bearing lytic
  bony lesions, symptomatic local lesions (nerve paralyses, obstructed
  airway, hemoptysis, intrathoracic large venous obstruction, in non-
  small cell lung cancer and in small cell cancer not responding to CRx)
Appropriate diagnosis and treatment of other medical problems and
  supportive care during CRx
Encouragement to stop smoking
Entrance into clinical trial, if eligible

Abbreviations: CRx, chemotherapy; RT, radiotherapy.

may shrink the local tumor, treat micrometastases, and make surgical resection safer and more effective in selected patients. If a complete resection is possible, the 5-year survival rate for N1 disease is about 50%, while it is about 20% for N2 disease. However, only 20% of cases of N2 disease are technically resectable, and most of these are discovered to be N2 only at thoracotomy. Surgery for N2 disease is the most controversial area in the surgical management of lung cancer. Patients with N2 disease can be divided into "minimal" disease (involvement of only one node with microscopic foci, usually discovered at thoracotomy or mediastinoscopy) and the more common "advanced," bulky disease, clinically obvious on CT scans and discovered preoperatively. Patients with contralateral or bilateral positive mediastinal (N3) nodes, extracapsular nodal involvement, or fixed nodes are not considered candidates for resection. Approaches that may make

resection possible include chest wall resection for direct extension of tumor, tracheal sleeve pneumonectomy, and sleeve lobectomy for lesions near the carina. Neoadjuvant (preoperative) chemotherapy has response rates of 50 to 60% and causes unresectable disease to become resectable in many patients who respond (see below). Video-assisted thoracic surgery (VATS) via thoracoscopy is not usually used for curative lung cancer resection but may be useful for peripheral lesions in patients with poor lung function. VATS has been advocated to reduce postoperative impairment of lung function, pain, length of hospital stay, and recovery time. However, randomized controlled trials have not confirmed the advantages. Open thoracotomy remains the preferred surgical approach to curative resection of lung cancer. VATS can be used for diagnostic purposes to examine the pleural surface and cavity and biopsy peripheral lung nodules or accessible mediastinal nodes; its major therapeutic use is resection of peripheral lung nodules.

The extent of resection is a matter of surgical judgment based on findings at exploration. Conservative resection that encompasses all known tumor gives survival equal to that obtained with more extensive procedures. However, lobectomy is superior to wedge resection in reducing the rate of local recurrence. Thus, lobectomy is preferred to pneumonectomy and wedge resection. Wedge resection and segmentectomy (potentially by VATS) are reserved for patients with poor pulmonary reserve and small peripheral lesions. About 40% of all patients with lung cancer undergo thoracotomy. Of these, 75% have a definitive resection, 12% are explored only for disease extent, and 12% have a palliative procedure with known disease left behind. About 30% of patients treated with resection for cure survive for 5 years, and 15% survive for 10 years (Table 75-3). The 30-day hospital mortality rate after pulmonary resection is 3% for lobectomy and 6% for pneumonectomy. Thus, most patients thought to have a "curative" resection ultimately die of metastatic disease (usually within 5 years of surgery).

MANAGEMENT OF OCCULT AND STAGE 0 CARCINOMAS In the uncommon situation where malignant cells are identified in a sputum or bronchial washing specimen but the chest radiograph appears normal (TX tumor stage), the lesion must be localized. More than 90% can be localized by meticulous examination of the bronchial tree with a fiberoptic bronchoscope under general anesthesia and collection of a series of differential brushings and biopsies. Often, carcinoma in situ or multicentric lesions are found in these patients. Current recommendations are for the most conservative surgical resection, allowing removal of the cancer and conservation of lung parenchyma, even if the bronchial margins are positive for carcinoma in situ. The 5-year overall survival rate for these occult cancers is ~60%. Close follow-up of these patients is indicated because of the high incidence of second primary lung cancers (5% per patient per year). One approach to in situ or multicentric lesions uses systemically administered hematoporphyrin (which localizes to tumors and sensitizes them to light) followed by bronchoscopic phototherapy.

SOLITARY PULMONARY NODULE When a patient presents with an asymptomatic, solitary pulmonary nodule (defined as an x-ray density completely surrounded by normal aerated lung, with circumscribed margins, of any shape, usually 1 to 6 cm in greatest diameter), a decision to resect or follow the nodule must be made. Approximately 35% of all such lesions in adults are malignant, most being primary lung cancer, while <1% are malignant in nonsmokers under 35 years of age. A complete history, including a smoking history, physical examination, routine laboratory tests, chest CT scan, fiberoptic bronchoscopy, and old chest x-rays are obtained. PET scans are useful in detecting lung cancers >1 cm in diameter. If no diagnosis is immediately apparent, the following risk factors would all argue strongly in favor of proceeding with resection to establish a histologic diagnosis: a history of cigarette smoking; age ≥ 35 years; a relatively large lesion; lack of calcification; chest symptoms; associated atelectasis, pneumonitis, or adenopathy; growth of the lesion revealed by comparison with old x-rays; or positive PET scan. At present, only two radiographic criteria are reliable predictors of the benign nature of a solitary pulmonary nodule: lack of growth over a period >2 years and certain characteristic patterns of calcification. Calcification alone does not exclude malignancy. However, a dense central nidus, multiple punctate foci, and "bull's eye" (granuloma) and "popcorn ball" (hamartoma) calcifications are all highly suggestive of a benign lesion. An algorithm for evaluating a solitary pulmonary nodule is shown in Fig. 75-2.

When old x-rays are not available and the characteristic calcification patterns are absent, the following approach is reasonable: Nonsmoking patients <35 years can be followed with serial CT every 3 months for 1 year and then yearly. If any significant growth is found, a histologic diagnosis is needed. For patients >35 years and all patients with a smoking history, a histologic diagnosis must be made. The sample for histologic diagnosis can be obtained either at the time of nodule resection or, if the patient is a poor operative risk, via VATS or transthoracic fine-needle biopsy. Some institutions use preoperative fine-needle aspiration on all such lesions; however, all positive lesions have to be resected, and negative cytologic findings in most cases have to be confirmed by histology on a resected specimen. While much has been made of sparing patients an operation, the high probability of finding a malignancy (particularly in smokers >35 years) and the excellent chance for surgical cure when the tumor is small both suggest an aggressive approach to these lesions.

The application of low-dose spiral CT scanning to high-risk populations is under investigation. The test identifies a large number of asymptomatic pulmonary nodules that require evaluation. Approximately 23% of screened high-risk patients have an abnormality, and ~12% of the detected abnormalities are lung cancer. The American College of Radiology has developed scoring of CT-detected lesions as "benign," "indeterminate," or "abnormal." Lesions > 1 cm are usually resected; those ≤1 cm are followed for change at 3 to 6-month intervals. Although a number of early lung cancers are detected in this way, it is not yet clear that survival is improved.

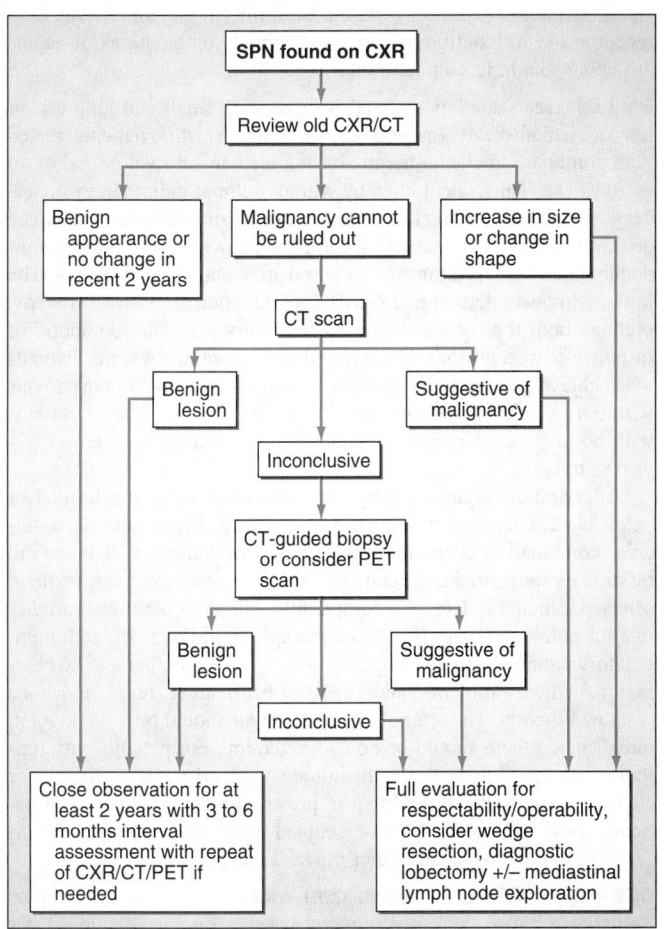

FIGURE 75-2 Algorithm for evaluation of a solitary pulmonary nodule (SPN). (CXR, chest x-ray; CT, computed tomography scan; PET, positron emission tomography.)

RADIOTHERAPY WITH CURATIVE INTENT Patients with stage III disease, as well as patients with stage I or II disease who refuse surgery or are not candidates for pulmonary resection, should be considered for radiation therapy with curative intent. The decision to administer high-dose radiotherapy is based on the extent of disease and the volume of the chest that requires irradiation. Patients with distant metastases, malignant pleural effusion, or cardiac involvement are generally not considered for curative radiation treatment. The median survival period for patients with unresectable non-small cell lung cancer localized to the chest who undergo primary radiotherapy with curative intent is <1 year. However, 6% of these patients are alive at 5 years and are cured by radiotherapy alone. In addition to being potentially curative, radiotherapy, by controlling the primary tumor, may increase the quality and length of life of noncured patients. Treatment usually involves midplane doses of 55 to 60 Gy, and the major concern is the amount of lung parenchyma and other organs in the thorax included in the treatment plan, including the spinal cord, heart, and esophagus. In patients with a major degree of underlying pulmonary disease, the treatment plan may have to be compromised because of the deleterious effect of radiation on pulmonary function. The risk of radiation pneumonitis is proportional to the radiation dose and the volume of lung in the field. The full clinical syndrome (dyspnea, fever, and radiographic infiltrate corresponding to the treatment port) occurs in 5% of cases. Acute radiation esophagitis occurs during treatment but is usually self-limited, while spinal cord injury should be avoided by careful treatment planning. Continuous hyperfractionated accelerated radiation therapy (CHART) involves delivery of 36 treatments of 1.5 Gy given 3 times a day for 12 consecutive days to a total dose of 54 Gy. The 2-year survival rate increased from 20 to 29% with CHART, although more esophagitis occurred. Brachytherapy (local radiotherapy delivered by placing radioactive "seeds" in a catheter in the tumor bed) provides a way to give a high local dose while sparing surrounding normal tissue.

COMBINED-MODALITY THERAPY WITH CURATIVE INTENT After apparently complete resection, adjuvant radiation therapy does not improve survival and may be detrimental in N0 and N1 disease.

Carcinomas of the superior pulmonary sulcus producing *Pancoast's syndrome* are usually treated with combined radiotherapy and surgery. Patients with these carcinomas should have the usual preoperative staging procedures, including mediastinoscopy and CT and PET scans, to determine tumor extent and a neurologic examination (and sometimes nerve conduction studies) to document neurologic findings. Sometimes a histologic diagnosis is not made, but the combination of tumor location and pain distribution permit a diagnostic accuracy for cancer of >90%. If mediastinoscopy is negative, curative approaches may be used in treating a Pancoast's syndrome tumor. Preoperative irradiation [30 Gy in 10 treatments] is given to the area, followed by an en bloc resection of the tumor and involved chest wall 3 to 6 weeks later. The 3-year survival rate is 40% for squamous and 20% for adeno- and large cell carcinomas. Another approach involves radiotherapy alone in curative doses and standard fractionation, which leads to survival rates similar to those from combined-modality therapy. Chemotherapy with etoposide and cisplatin plus radiotherapy to the area produces high rates of tumor resectability and >50% survival at 4 years.

A meta-analysis of chemotherapy in non-small cell lung cancer used updated data on 9387 individual patients from 52 randomized trials, both published and unpublished, with the main outcome measure being survival. Regimens containing cisplatin were significantly more effective than no treatment. Trials in early-stage disease comparing surgery with surgery plus chemotherapy gave a hazard ratio of 0.87 (13% reduction in risk of death at 5 years) in favor of chemotherapy. Confidence intervals of these data are wide. Ongoing randomized trials of adjuvant chemotherapy for stage I and II disease appear to show benefit.

The most impressive benefits were obtained when chemotherapy was added to radiotherapy for locally advanced disease (stage IIIB and some stage IIIA disease) and when chemotherapy was given preoperatively in a neoadjuvant fashion in stage IIIA disease. Preoperative neoadjuvant chemotherapy is widely used for stage IIIA disease. Preoperative combined modality therapy followed by surgical resection has given promising early results. Whether the surgery adds benefit after chemoradiotherapy has not been defined. Provided the risk/benefit ratio of using chemotherapy is discussed appropriately with patients, such therapy can be given in a noninvestigational setting. For stage IIIA disease, resection followed by postoperative radiation plus chemotherapy for N2 disease, neoadjuvant chemotherapy followed by surgical resection, or neoadjuvant chemoradiotherapy followed by resection are options. For stage IIIB and bulky IIIA disease, neoadjuvant chemotherapy (two or three cycles of a cisplatin-based combination) followed by chest radiation therapy (60 Gy) has improved median survival time from 10 to 14 months and the 5-year survival rate from 7 to 17% compared to results with radiation therapy alone. Administration of radiation and chemotherapy concurrently is being tested; myelotoxicity and esophagitis are increased, but survival improvement is not yet proven. Randomized clinical trials are also needed to evaluate the usefulness of the new agents with activity against non-small cell lung cancer, including the taxanes (paclitaxel and docetaxel), vinorelbine, gemcitabine, and the camptothecins (topotecan and irinotecan) in both adjuvant and neoadjuvant settings.

Disseminated Non-Small Cell Lung Cancer   The 70% of patients who have unresectable non-small cell cancer have a poor prognosis. Patients with performance status scores of 0 (asymptomatic), 1 (symptomatic, fully ambulatory), 2 (in bed <50% of the time), 3 (in bed >50% of the time), and 4 (bedridden) have median survival times of 34, 25, 17, 8, and 4 weeks, respectively. Standard medical management, the judicious use of pain medications, the appropriate use of radiotherapy, and outpatient chemotherapy form the cornerstone of management. Patients whose primary tumor is causing symptoms such as bronchial obstruction with pneumonitis, hemoptysis, or upper airway or superior vena cava obstruction should have radiotherapy to the primary tumor. The case for prophylactic treatment of the asymptomatic patient is to prevent major symptoms from occurring in the thorax. Usually a course of 30 to 40 Gy over 2 to 4 weeks is given to the tumor. Radiation therapy provides relief of intrathoracic symptoms with the following frequencies: hemoptysis, 84%; superior vena cava syndrome, 80%; dyspnea, 60%; cough, 60%; atelectasis, 23%; and vocal cord paralysis, 6%. Cardiac tamponade (treated with pericardiocentesis and radiation therapy to the heart), painful bony metastases (with relief in 66%), brain or spinal cord compression, and brachial plexus involvement may also be palliated with radiotherapy. Usually, with brain metastases and cord compression, dexamethasone (25 to 100 mg/d in four divided doses) is also given and then rapidly tapered to the lowest dosage that relieves symptoms.

Brain metastases are often isolated instances of relapse in patients with adenocarcinoma of the lung otherwise controlled by surgery or radiotherapy. However, there is no proven value for prophylactic cranial irradiation or for CT scans of the head in asymptomatic patients.

Pleural effusions are common and are usually treated with thoracentesis. If they recur and are symptomatic, chest tube drainage with a sclerosing agent such as intrapleural talc is used. First, the chest cavity is completely drained. Xylocaine 1% is instilled (15 mL), followed by 50 mL normal saline. Then, 10 g sterile talc is dissolved in 100 mL normal saline, and this solution is injected through the chest tube. The chest tube is clamped for 4 h if tolerated, and the patient is rotated onto different sides to distribute the sclerosing agent. The chest tube is removed 24 to 48 h later, after drainage has become slight (usually <100 mL/24 h). VATS has been used to drain and treat large malignant effusions. An indwelling pleurex catheter is equivalent to chest tube drainage and better tolerated by the patient. Symptomatic

endobronchial lesions that recur after surgery or radiotherapy or that develop in patients with severely compromised pulmonary function are difficult to treat with conventional therapy. Neodynium-YAG (yttrium-aluminum-garnet) laser therapy administered through a flexible fiberoptic bronchoscope (usually under general anesthesia) can provide palliation in 80 to 90% of patients even when the tumor has relapsed after radiotherapy. Local radiotherapy delivered by brachytherapy, photodynamic therapy using a photosensitizing agent, and endobronchial stents are other measures that can relieve airway obstruction from tumor.

CHEMOTHERAPY   The use of chemotherapy for non-small cell lung cancer requires careful judgment to balance potential benefits and toxicity. Modest survival benefits (of 1 to 2 months), symptom palliation, and improved quality of life may accrue from combination chemotherapy. Randomized trials in advanced disease comparing supportive care with supportive care plus chemotherapy gave a hazard ratio of 0.73 (27% reduction in risk of death at 1 year) in favor of including chemotherapy. Economic analysis has found chemotherapy to be cost-effective palliation. Combination chemotherapy produces an objective tumor response in ~20 to 30% of patients; the response is complete in <5%. Median survival for chemotherapy-treated patients is 9 to 10 months, and the 1-year survival rate is 40%. Thus, in patients with non-small cell lung cancer who desire chemotherapy, it is reasonable to give chemotherapy if the patient is ambulatory and is able to understand and accept the risk/benefit ratio from such therapy. The chemotherapy should be one of the published standard regimens, such as paclitaxel plus carboplatin, paclitaxel plus cisplatin, or vinorelbine plus cisplatin. Improved antiemetics have made treatment tolerable on an outpatient basis. New drugs with proven activity in non-small cell lung cancer include docetaxel, irinotecan, and gemcitabine. Docetaxel may provide a survival benefit after relapse from initial chemotherapy. Furthermore, novel agents aimed at growth factor and angiogenesis receptors and signaling pathways are being tested. Gefitinib (Iressa) inhibits the EGF receptor and has antitumor activity. Optimal combinations of agents are being sought in clinical trials.

Small Cell Lung Cancer   Untreated patients with small cell lung cancer have a median survival period of 6 to 17 weeks, while patients treated with combination chemotherapy have a median survival period of 40 to 70 weeks. Thus, chemotherapy with or without radiotherapy or surgery can prolong survival in patients with small cell lung cancer. The goal of treatment is to achieve a complete clinical regression of tumor documented by repeating the initial positive staging procedures. The initial response, determined 6 to 12 weeks after the start of therapy, predicts both the median and long-term survivals, the likelihood of response to second line therapy, and the potential for cure. Patients who achieve a complete clinical regression survive longer than patients with only partial regression, who in turn survive longer than patients with no response. Complete response is required for long-term (>3-year) survival.

After initial staging, patients are classified as having limited or extensive disease and as being physiologically able or not able to tolerate combination chemotherapy or chemoradiotherapy. The overall mortality rate from initial combination chemotherapy even in these selected patients is 1 to 5%, comparable with the operative mortality rate for pulmonary resection. Such therapy should be reserved for ambulatory patients with no prior chemotherapy or radiotherapy; no other major medical problems; and adequate heart, liver, renal, and bone marrow function. The arterial P_{O_2} on room air should be >6.6 kPa (50 mmHg), and there should be no CO_2 retention. For patients with limitations in any of these areas, the initial combined-modality therapy or chemotherapy must be modified to prevent undue toxicity. In all patients, these treatments must be coupled with supportive care for infectious, hemorrhagic, and other medical complications.

CHEMOTHERAPY   The combination most widely used is etoposide plus cisplatin or carboplatin, given every 3 weeks on an outpatient basis for 4 to 6 cycles. Other active regimens are etopside, cisplatin, and paclitaxel or the combination of irinotecan and etoposide, which conveys a longer median survival but is more toxic than etoposide plus cisplatin. Increased dose intensity of chemotherapy adds toxicity without clear survival benefit. Appropriate supportive care (antiemetic therapy, administration of fluid and saline boluses with cisplatin, monitoring of blood counts and blood chemistries, monitoring for signs of bleeding or infection, and, as required, administration of erythropoietin and granulocyte colony-stimulating factor) and adjustment of chemotherapy doses on the basis of nadir granulocyte counts are essential. The initial combination chemotherapy may result in moderate to severe granulocytopenia (e.g., granulocyte counts <500 to 1500/μL) and thrombocytopenia (platelet counts <50,000 to 100,000/μL). After the initial 4 to 6 cycles of therapy, patients should be restaged to determine if they have entered a complete clinical remission, indicated by complete disappearance of all clinically evident lesions and paraneoplastic syndromes; a partial remission; or have no response or tumor progression (seen in 10 to 20% of patients). Chemotherapy is then stopped in responding patients. More prolonged chemotherapy has not been shown to be of value. Patients whose tumors are progressing or not responding should be switched to a new, experimental chemotherapy regimen. Topotecan alone or combined with paclitaxel is active in such second-line therapy. Oral etoposide, as a single agent, has been shown to be of clinical benefit in the initial treatment of patients who are elderly or have a very poor performance status.

RADIOTHERAPY High-dose (40-Gy) radiotherapy to the whole brain should be given to patients with documented brain metastases. Prophylactic cranial irradiation (PCI) may be given to patients with complete responses, since it significantly decreases the development of brain metastases (which occur in 60 to 80% of patients living $\geq$2 years who do not receive PCI), but survival benefit is small (5%). Because some studies indicate possible deficits in cognitive ability that could be related to PCI, the long-term quality of life after PCI needs to be further studied. The patient needs to be informed of the risks and benefits of PCI. In the case of symptomatic, progressive lesions in the chest or at other critical sites, if radiotherapy has not yet been given to these areas, it may be administered in full doses (e.g., 40 Gy to the chest tumor mass).

COMBINED-MODALITY THERAPY Most patients with limited-stage small cell lung cancer should receive combined-modality therapy with etoposide plus cisplatin (or other platinum-containing regimen) and concurrent chest radiotherapy encompassing sites of known disease in the chest. Acute and chronic toxicities are expected with chemoradiotherapy, particularly when the chemotherapy and radiotherapy are given concurrently. However, the addition of chest radiation therapy to chemotherapy reduces the local failure rate and improves survival. Patients should be selected (limited-stage disease, a performance status of 0 to 1, and initial good pulmonary function) such that radiotherapy can be given in full doses and in a manner that does not sacrifice too much lung function. Some studies show twice-daily radiation fractions produce less toxicity and improve survival compared to once-daily treatments.

For extensive-stage disease, initial chest radiotherapy is usually not advocated. However, for favorable patients (e.g., those with a performance status of 0 to 1, good pulmonary function, and only one site of extensive disease), the addition of chest radiotherapy to chemotherapy can be considered. In patients who are in a chemotherapy-induced complete remission, radiotherapy appears to increase survival. For all patients, if chemotherapy is inadequate to relieve local tumor symptoms, a course of radiotherapy can be added.

About 20 to 30% of patients with limited-stage disease and 1 to 5% of patients with extensive-stage disease are cured. About 50% of patients with limited-stage and 30% of patients with extensive-stage disease enter complete remission, and 90 to 95% of all patients have complete or partial responses. These responses increase the median survival period to 10 to 12 months for patients with extensive-stage disease and to 14 to 18 months for patients with limited-stage disease, as compared with 2 to 4 months for untreated patients. In addition, most patients have relief of their tumor-related symptoms and im-

provement of performance status. However, the maintenance of good performance status in a patient receiving outpatient chemotherapy requires judgment and skill to avoid undue therapeutic toxicity. New treatments, such as new drug combinations, very intensive initial or "reinduction" therapy with autologous bone marrow infusion, and novel ways of combining chemotherapy, radiotherapy, and surgery should be given only in the context of an approved clinical protocol.

Although surgical resection is not routinely recommended for small cell lung cancer, occasional patients meet the usual requirements for resectability (stage I or II disease with negative mediastinal nodes). Moreover, this histologic diagnosis is made in some patients only on review of the resected surgical specimen. Such patients have been reported to have high cure rates (>25%) if adjuvant chemotherapy is used.

LUNG CANCER PREVENTION

Deterring children from taking up smoking and helping young adults stop smoking is likely to be the most effective lung cancer prevention. Smoking cessation programs are successful in 5 to 20% of volunteers; the poor efficacy is because of the nature of nicotine addiction.

Chemoprevention is an experimental approach to reduce lung cancer risk; at present, no benefit has been proven for chemoprevention intervention, and at least two putative chemoprevention agents, vitamin E and β-carotene, actually increase the risk of lung cancer in heavy smokers.

BENIGN LUNG NEOPLASMS

The benign neoplasms of the lung, representing <5% of all primary tumors, include bronchial adenomas and hamartomas (90% of such lesions) and a group of very uncommon benign neoplasms (epithelial tumors such as bronchial papillomas, fibroepithelial polyps; mesenchymal tumors such as chondromas, fibromas, lipomas, hemangiomas, leiomyomas, pseudolymphomas; tumors of mixed origin such as teratomas; and other diseases such as endometriosis). The diagnostic and primary-treatment approach (surgery) is basically the same for all these neoplasms. They can present as central masses causing airway obstruction, cough, hemoptysis, and pneumonitis. The masses may or may not be visible on radiographs but are usually accessible to fiberoptic bronchoscopy. Alternatively, they can present without symptoms as solitary pulmonary nodules and thus will be evaluated as part of a solitary pulmonary nodule workup. In all cases, the extent of surgery must be determined at operation, and a conservative procedure with appropriate reconstructions is usually performed.

BRONCHIAL ADENOMAS Bronchial adenomas (80% are central) are slow-growing, endobronchial lesions; they represent 50% of all benign pulmonary neoplasms. About 80 to 90% are carcinoids, 10 to 15% are adenocystic tumors (or cylindromas), and 2 to 3% are mucoepidermoid tumors. Adenomas present in patients 15 to 60 years old (average age, 45) as endobronchial lesions and are often symptomatic for several years. Patients may have a chronic cough, recurrent hemoptysis, or obstruction with atelectasis, lobar collapse, or pneumonitis and abscess formation. Bronchial carcinoids, which usually follow a benign course, and small cell lung cancers, which are highly malignant, both express a neuroendocrine phenotype. Carcinoids, like small cell lung cancers, may secrete other hormones, such as ACTH or arginine vasopressin, and can cause paraneoplastic syndromes that resolve on resection. Uncommonly, bronchial carcinoid metastases (usually to the liver) may produce the carcinoid syndrome, with cutaneous flush, bronchoconstriction, diarrhea, and cardiac valvular lesions (Chap. 329), which small cell lung cancer does not. Occasionally, pathologists may have difficulty distinguishing carcinoids from small cell lung cancers. Carcinoid tumors that have an unusually aggressive histologic appearance (referred to as *atypical carcinoids*) metastasize in 70% of cases to regional nodes, liver, or bone, compared with only a 5% rate of metastasis for carcinoids with typical histology.

Bronchial adenomas of all types, because of their endobronchial and often central location, are usually visible by fiberoptic bronchoscopy, and tissue for histologic diagnosis is obtained in this manner. Because they are hypervascular, they can bleed profusely after bronchoscopic biopsy, and this problem should be anticipated. Bronchial adenomas must be dealt with as potentially malignant and thus require removal not only for symptom relief but also because they can be locally invasive or recurrent, potentially can metastasize, and may produce paraneoplastic syndromes. Surgical excision is the primary treatment for all types of bronchial adenomas. The extent of surgery is determined at operation and should be as conservative as possible. Often bronchotomy with local excision, sleeve resection, segmental resection, or lobectomy is sufficient. Five-year survival rates after surgical resection are 95%, decreasing to 70% if regional nodes are involved. The treatment of metastatic pulmonary carcinoids is unclear because they can either be indolent or behave more like small cell lung carcinoma. Assessment of the tempo and histology of the disease in the individual patient is necessary to determine if and when chemotherapy or radiotherapy is indicated.

HAMARTOMAS Pulmonary hamartomas have a peak incidence at age 60 and are more frequent in men than in women. Histologically, they contain normal pulmonary tissue components (smooth muscle and collagen) in a disorganized fashion. They are usually peripheral, clinically silent, and benign in their behavior. Unless the radiographic findings are pathognomonic for hamartoma, with "popcorn" calcification, the lesions usually have to be resected for diagnosis, particularly if the patient is a smoker. VATS may minimize the surgical complications.

METASTATIC PULMONARY TUMORS

The lung is a frequent site of metastases from primary cancers outside the lung. Usually such metastatic disease is considered incurable. However, two special situations should be borne in mind. The first is the development of a solitary pulmonary shadow on a chest x-ray in a patient known to have an extrathoracic neoplasm. This shadow may represent a metastasis or a new primary lung cancer. Because the natural history of lung cancer is often worse than that of other primary tumors, a single pulmonary nodule in a patient with a known extrathoracic tumor is approached as though the nodule is a primary lung cancer, particularly if the patient is older than 35 years and a smoker. If a vigorous search for other sites of active cancer proves negative, the nodule is surgically resected. Second, in some cases, multiple pulmonary nodules can be resected with curative intent. This tactic is usually recommended if, after careful staging, it is found that (1) the patient can tolerate the contemplated pulmonary resection, (2) the primary tumor has been definitively and successfully treated (disease-free for >1 year), and (3) all known metastatic disease can be encompassed by the projected pulmonary resection. The key is selection and screening of patients to exclude those with uncontrolled primary tumors and other extrapulmonary metastases. Primary tumors whose pulmonary metastases have been successfully resected for cure include osteogenic and soft tissue sarcomas; colon, rectal, uterine, cervix, and corpus tumors; head and neck, breast, testis, and salivary gland cancer; melanoma; and bladder and kidney tumors. Five-year survival rates of 20 to 30% have been found in carefully selected patients, and dramatic results have been achieved in patients with osteogenic sarcomas, where resection of pulmonary metastases (sometimes requiring several thoracotomies) is becoming a standard curative treatment approach.

FURTHER READING

AMERICAN COLLEGE OF CHEST PHYSICIANS: Diagnosis and management of lung cancer: ACCP evidence-based guidelines. Chest, 123:1S, 2003

KARNATH B: Smoking cessation. Am J Med 112:399, 2002

MOUNTAIN CF: Revisions in the international system for staging lung cancer. Chest 111:1710, 1997

PAO W et al: Targeting the epidermal growth factor receptor tyrosine kinase with gefitinib in non–small–cell lung cancer. Semin Cancer Biol 14:33, 2004

SEKIDO Y et al: Molecular genetics of lung cancer. Annu Rev Med 54:73, 2003

SPECIAL ISSUE DEALING WITH ALL ASPECTS OF THE DIAGNOSIS AND TREATMENT OF SMALL CELL LUNG CANCER. Semin Oncol 30:3, 2003

SPIRA A, ETTINGER DS: Drug therapy: Multidisciplinary management of lung cancer. N Engl J Med 350:379, 2004

76 BREAST CANCER
Marc E. Lippman

Breast cancer is a malignant proliferation of epithelial cells lining the ducts or lobules of the breast. In the year 2004, about 216,000 cases of invasive breast cancer and 40,000 deaths occurred in the United States. Epithelial malignancies of the breast are the most common cause of cancer in women (excluding skin cancer), accounting for about one-third of all cancer in women. As a result of improved treatment and earlier detection, mortality from breast cancer has begun to decrease substantially in the United States. This chapter will not consider rare malignancies of the breast, such as sarcomas and lymphomas, but will focus on the epithelial cancers. Human breast cancer is a clonal disease; a single transformed cell—the product of a series of somatic (acquired) or germline mutations—is eventually able to express full malignant potential. Thus, breast cancer may exist for a long period as either a noninvasive disease or an invasive but nonmetastatic disease. These facts have very significant clinical ramifications.

GENETIC CONSIDERATIONS Not more than 10% of human breast cancers can be linked directly to germline mutations. Several genes have been implicated in familial cases. The Li-Fraumeni syndrome is characterized by inherited mutations in the p53 tumor-suppressor gene, which lead to an increased incidence of breast cancer, osteogenic sarcomas, and other malignancies. Inherited mutations in *PTEN* have also been reported.

Another tumor-suppressor gene, *BRCA-1*, has been identified at the chromosomal locus 17q21; this gene encodes a zinc finger protein, and the product therefore may function as a transcriptional factor. The gene appears to be involved in gene repair. Women who inherit a mutated allele of this gene from either parent have at least a 60 to 80% lifetime chance of developing breast cancer and about a 33% chance of developing ovarian cancer. The risk is higher among women born after 1940, presumably due to promotional effects of hormonal factors. Men who carry a mutant allele of the gene have an increased incidence of prostate cancer and breast cancer. A fourth gene, termed *BRCA-2*, which has been localized to chromosome 13q12, is also associated with an increased incidence of breast cancer in men and women.

BRCA-1 and *BRCA-2* can now be sequenced readily and germline mutations detected; patients with these mutations can be counseled appropriately. All women with strong family histories for breast cancer should be referred to genetic screening programs whenever possible, particularly women of Ashkenazi Jewish descent who have a high likelihood of a specific *BRCA-1* mutation (deletion of adenine and guanine at position 185).

Even more important than the role these genes play in inherited forms of breast cancer may be their role in sporadic breast cancer. The p53 mutation is present in approximately 40% of human breast cancers as an acquired defect. Acquired mutations in *PTEN* occur in about 10% of the cases. *BRCA-1* mutation in primary breast cancer has not been reported. However, decreased expression of *BRCA-1* mRNA (possibly via gene methylation) and abnormal cellular location of the *BRCA-1* protein have been found in some breast cancers. Loss of heterozygosity of *BRCA-1* and *BRCA-2* suggests that tumor-suppressor activity may be inactivated in sporadic cases of human breast cancer.

Finally, increased expression of a dominant oncogene plays a role in about a quarter of human breast cancer cases. The product of this gene, a member of the epidermal growth factor receptor superfamily, is called *erbB2* (HER-2, neu) and is overexpressed in these breast cancers due to gene amplification; this overexpression can contribute to transformation of human breast epithelium.

EPIDEMIOLOGY Breast cancer is a hormone-dependent disease. Women without functioning ovaries who never receive estrogen-replacement therapy do not develop breast cancer. The female to male ratio is about 150:1. For most epithelial malignancies, a log-log plot of incidence versus age shows a single-component straight-line increase with every year of life. A similar plot for breast cancer shows two components: a straight-line increase with age but with a decrease in slope beginning at the age of menopause. The three dates in a woman's life that have a major impact on breast cancer incidence are age at menarche, age at first full-term pregnancy, and age at menopause. Women who experience menarche at age 16 have only 50 to 60% of the breast cancer risk of a woman having menarche at age 12; the lower risk persists throughout life. Similarly, menopause occurring 10 years before the median age of menopause (52 years), whether natural or surgically induced, reduces lifetime breast cancer risk by about 35%. Women who have a first full-term pregnancy by age 18 have a 30 to 40% lower risk of breast cancer compared with nulliparous women. Thus, length of menstrual life—particularly the fraction occurring before first full-term pregnancy—is a substantial component of the total risk of breast cancer. These three factors (menarche, age of first full-term pregnancy, and menopause) can account for 70 to 80% of the variation in breast cancer frequency in different countries. A meta-analysis has shown that duration of maternal nursing correlates with substantial risk reduction independent of either parity or age at first full-term pregnancy.

International variation in incidence has provided some of the most important clues on hormonal carcinogenesis. A woman living to age 80 in North America has one chance in nine of developing invasive breast cancer. Asian women have one-fifth to one-tenth the risk of breast cancer of women in North America or Western Europe. Asian women have substantially lower concentrations of estrogens and progesterone. These differences cannot be explained on a genetic basis because Asian women living in a western environment have sex steroid hormone concentrations and risks identical to those of their western counterparts. These migrant women and more notably their daughters also differ markedly in height and weight from Asian women in Asia; height and weight are critical regulators of age of menarche and have substantial effects on plasma concentrations of estrogens.

The role of diet in breast cancer etiology is controversial. While there are associative links between total caloric and fat intake and breast cancer risk, the exact role of fat in the diet is unproven. Increased caloric intake contributes to breast cancer risk in multiple ways: earlier menarche, later age at menopause, and increased postmenopausal estrogen concentrations reflecting enhanced aromatase activities in fatty tissues. Moderate alcohol intake also increases the risk by an unknown mechanism. Recommendations favoring abstinence from alcohol must be weighed against other social pressures and the possible cardioprotective effect of moderate alcohol intake.

Understanding the potential role of exogenous hormones in breast cancer is of extraordinary importance because millions of American women regularly use oral contraceptives and postmenopausal hormone replacement therapy (HT). The most credible meta-analyses of oral contraceptive use suggest that these agents cause little if any increased risk of breast cancer. By contrast, oral contraceptives offer a substantial protective effect against ovarian epithelial tumors and endometrial cancers. Far more controversial are the data surrounding HT in postmenopausal women. Data from the Women's Health Initiative (WHI) trial showed in a prospectively randomized design that conjugated equine estrogens plus progestins increased the risk of breast cancer and adverse cardiovascular events but with decreases in bone fractures and colorectal cancer. On balance there were more negative events

with HT. A parallel WHI trial with >12,000 women enrolled testing conjugated estrogens alone (in women who have had hysterectomies) continues. A meta-analysis of nonrandomized HT studies suggests that most of the previously attributed benefit of HT can be accounted for by higher socioeconomic status among users, which is presumably associated with better access to health care and healthier behaviors. Certain potential benefits of HT, such as a putative protective effect on cognition with age, were not assessed in WHI. HT is an area of rapid reevaluation, but it would appear (at least from breast cancer and cardiovascular disease vantage points) that there are serious grounds for concern about long-term HT use.

In addition to the other factors, radiation may be a risk factor in younger women. Women who have been exposed before age 30 to radiation in the form of multiple fluoroscopies (200 to 300 cGy) or treatment for Hodgkin's disease (>3600 cGy) have a substantial increase in risk of breast cancer, whereas radiation exposure after age 30 appears to have a minimal carcinogenic effect on the breast.

EVALUATION OF BREAST MASSES IN MEN AND WOMEN Because the breasts are a common site of potentially fatal malignancy in women and because they frequently provide clues to underlying systemic diseases in both men and women, examination of the breast is an essential part of the physical examination. Unfortunately, internists frequently do not examine breasts in men, and, in women, they are apt to defer this evaluation to gynecologists. Because of the plausible association between early detection and improved outcome, it is the duty of every physician to distinguish breast abnormalities at the earliest possible stage and to institute a definite diagnostic workup. It is for this reason that all women should be trained in breast self-examination (BSE). Although breast cancer in men is unusual, unilateral lesions should be evaluated in the same manner as in women, with the recognition that gynecomastia in men can sometimes begin unilaterally and is often asymmetric.

Virtually all breast cancer is diagnosed by biopsy of a nodule detected either on a mammogram or by palpation. Algorithms have been developed to enhance the likelihood of diagnosing breast cancer and reduce the frequency of unnecessary biopsy (Fig. 76-1).

The Palpable Breast Mass Women should be strongly encouraged to examine their breasts monthly. A flawed study from China has sug-

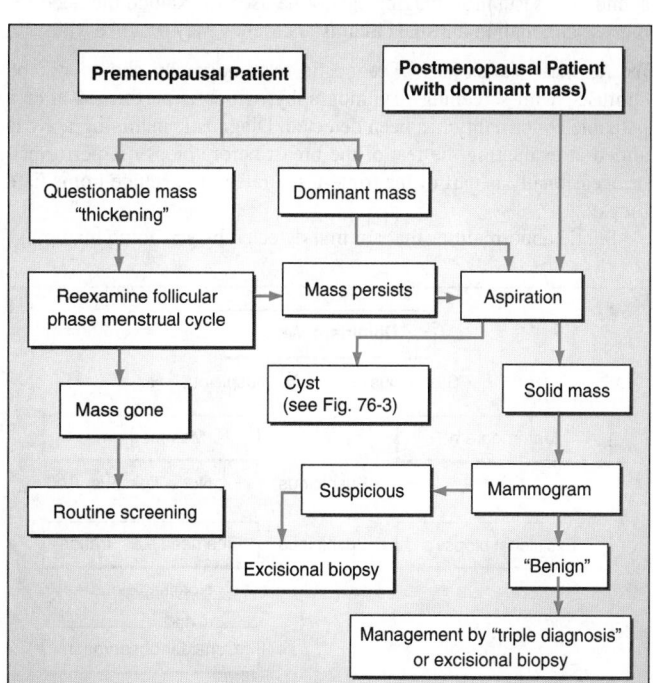

FIGURE 76-1 Approach to a palpable breast mass.

gested that BSE does not alter survival, but given its safety, the procedure should still be encouraged. The minimum benefit of this practice is the greater likelihood of detecting a mass at a smaller size when it can be treated with more limited surgery. Breast examination by the physician should be performed in good light so as to see retractions and other skin changes. The nipple and areolae should be inspected, and an attempt should be made to elicit nipple discharge. All regional lymph node groups should be examined, and any lesions should be measured. While lesions with certain features are more likely to be cancerous (hard, irregular, tethered or fixed, or painless lesions), physical examination alone cannot exclude malignancy. Furthermore, a negative mammogram in the presence of a persistent lump in the breast does not exclude malignancy.

In premenopausal women, lesions that are either equivocal or nonsuspicious on physical examination should be reexamined in 2 to 4 weeks, during the follicular phase of the menstrual cycle. Days 5 to 7 of the cycle are the best time for breast examination. A dominant mass in a postmenopausal woman or a dominant mass that persists through a menstrual cycle in a premenopausal woman should be aspirated by fine-needle biopsy or referred to a surgeon. If nonbloody fluid is aspirated and the lesion is thereby cured, the diagnosis (cyst) and therapy have been accomplished together. Solid lesions that are persistent, recurrent, complex, or bloody cysts require mammography and biopsy, although in selected patients the so-called triple diagnostic techniques (palpation, mammography, aspiration) can be used to avoid biopsy (Figs. 76-1 to 76-3). Ultrasound can be used in place of fine-needle aspiration to distinguish cysts from solid lesions. Not all solid masses are detected by ultrasound; thus, a palpable mass that is not visualized on ultrasound must be presumed to be solid.

Several points are essential in pursuing these management decision trees. First, risk factor analysis is not part of the decision structure. No constellation of risk factors, by their presence or absence, can be used to exclude biopsy. Second, fine-needle aspiration should be used only in centers that have proven skill in obtaining such specimens and analyzing them. Although the likelihood of cancer is low in the setting of a "triple negative" (benign-feeling lump, negative mammogram, and negative fine-needle aspiration), it is not zero, and the patient and physician must be aware of an 1% risk of false negativity. Third, additional technologies such as magnetic resonance imaging, ultrasound, and sestamibi imaging cannot be used to exclude the need for biopsy, although in unusual circumstances they may provoke a biopsy.

The Abnormal Mammogram Diagnostic mammography should not be confused with screening mammography, which is performed after a palpable abnormality has been detected. Diagnostic mammography is aimed at evaluating the rest of the breast before biopsy is performed or occasionally is part of the triple-test strategy to exclude immediate biopsy.

Subtle abnormalities that are first detected by screening mammog-

raphy should be evaluated carefully by compression or magnified views. These abnormalities include clustered microcalcifications, densities (especially if spiculated), and new or enlarging architectural distortion. For some nonpalpable lesions ultrasound may be helpful either to identify cysts or to guide biopsy. If there is no palpable lesion and detailed mammographic studies are unequivocally benign, the patient should have routine follow-up appropriate to the patient's age.

If a nonpalpable mammographic lesion has a low index of suspicion, mammographic follow-up in 3 to 6 months is reasonable. Workup of indeterminate and suspicious lesions has been rendered more complex by the advent of stereotactic biopsies. Morrow and colleagues have suggested that these procedures are indicated for lesions that require biopsy but are likely to be benign—that is, for cases in which the procedure probably will eliminate additional surgery. When a lesion is more probably malignant, open excisional biopsy should be performed with a needle localization technique. Others have proposed more widespread use of stereotactic core biopsies for nonpalpable lesions, on economic grounds and because diagnosis leads to earlier treatment planning. However, stereotactic diagnosis of a malignant lesion does not eliminate the need for definitive surgical procedures, particularly if breast conservation is attempted. For example after a breast biopsy with needle localization (i.e., local excision) of a stereotactically diagnosed malignancy, reexcision may still be necessary to achieve negative margins. To some extent, these issues are decided on the basis of referral pattern and the availability of the resources for stereotactic core biopsies. A reasonable approach is shown in Fig. 76-4.

Breast Masses in the Pregnant or Lactating Woman During pregnancy, the breast grows under the influence of estrogen, progesterone, prolactin, and human placental lactogen. Lactation is suppressed by progester-

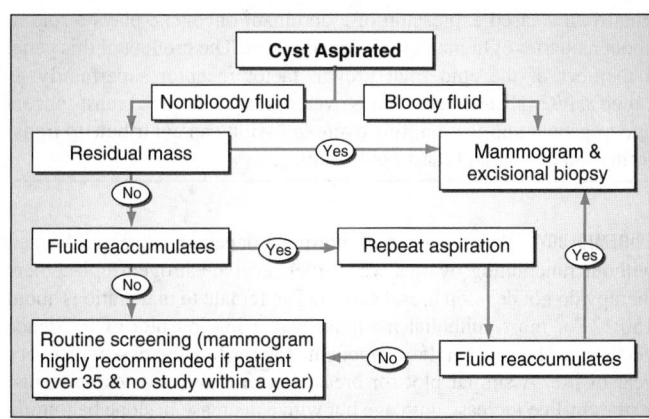

FIGURE 76-3 Management of a breast cyst.

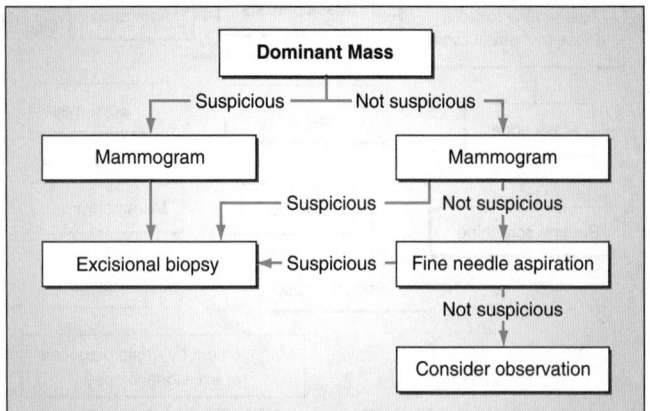

FIGURE 76-2 The "triple diagnosis" technique.

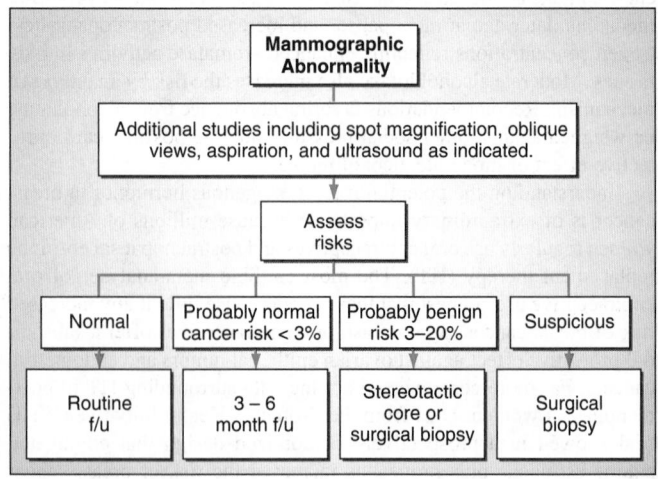

FIGURE 76-4 Approaches to abnormalities detected by mammogram. Note: f/u, follow-up; bx, biopsy.

TABLE 76-1 *Staging of Breast Cancer*

PRIMARY TUMOR (T)

T0	No evidence of primary tumor
TIS	Carcinoma in situ
T1	Tumor ≤2 cm
T2	Tumor >2 cm but ≤5 cm
T3	Tumor >5 cm
T4	Extension to chest wall, inflammation, satellite lesions, ulcerations

REGIONAL LYMPH NODES (N)

N0	No regional lymph nodes
N1	Metastasis to movable ipsilateral nodes
N2	Metastasis to matted or fixed ipsilateral nodes
N3	Metastasis to ipsilateral internal mammary nodes

DISTANT METASTASIS (M)

M0	No distant metastasis
M1	Distant metastasis (includes spread to ipsilateral supraclavicular nodes)

STAGE GROUPING

Stage 0	TIS	N0	M0
Stage I	T1	N0	M0
Stage IIA	T0	N1	M0
	T1	N1	M0
	T2	N0	M0
Stage IIB	T2	N1	M0
	T3	N0	M0
Stage IIIA	T0	N2	M0
	T1	N2	M0
	T2	N2	M0
	T3	N1, N2	M0
Stage IIIB	T4	Any N	M0
	Any T	N3	M0
Stage IV	Any T	Any N	M1

Source: Modified from the American Joint Committee on Cancer, 1992.

one, which blocks the effects of prolactin. After delivery, lactation is promoted by the fall in progesterone levels, which leaves the effects of prolactin unopposed. The development of a dominant mass during pregnancy or lactation should never be attributed to hormonal changes, and biopsy should never be performed under local anesthesia. Breast cancer develops in 1 in every 3000 to 4000 pregnancies. Stage for stage, breast cancer in pregnant patients is no different from premenopausal breast cancer in nonpregnant patients. However, pregnant women often have more advanced disease because the significance of a breast mass was not fully considered. Persistent lumps in the breast of pregnant or lactating women *can not* be attributed to benign changes based on physical findings; such patients should be promptly referred for diagnostic evaluation.

Benign Breast Masses Only about 1 in every 5 to 10 breast biopsies leads to a diagnosis of cancer, although the rate of positive biopsies varies in different countries. (These differences may be related to interpretation, medicolegal considerations, and availability of mammograms.) The vast majority of benign breast masses are due to "fibrocystic" disease, a descriptive term for small fluid-filled cysts and modest epithelial cell and fibrous tissue hyperplasia. However, fibrocystic disease is a histologic, not a clinical, diagnosis, and women who have had a biopsy with benign findings are at greater risk of developing breast cancer than those who have not had a biopsy. The subset of women with ductal or lobular cell proliferation (about 30% of patients), particularly the small fraction (3%) with atypical hyperplasia, have a fourfold greater risk of developing breast cancer than unbiopsied women, and the increase in the risk is about ninefold for women in this category who also have an affected first-degree relative. Thus, careful follow-up of these patients is required. By contrast, patients with a benign biopsy without atypical hyperplasia are at little risk and may be followed routinely.

SCREENING Breast cancer is virtually unique among the epithelial tumors in adults in that screening (in the form of annual mammography) has been proven to improve survival. Meta-analysis examining outcomes from every randomized trial of mammography conclusively shows a 25 to 30% reduction in the chance of dying from breast cancer with annual screening after age 50; the data for women between ages 40 and 50 are almost as positive. While controversy continues to surround the assessment of screening mammography, the preponderance of data as well as this author's evaluation of the literature continue to strongly support the positive benefits of screening mammography. New analyses of older randomized studies have suggested that screening may not work. While the defects in some studies cannot be corrected, most experts, including panels of the American Society of Clinical Oncology and the American Cancer Society, continue to believe that screening conveys substantial benefit. Furthermore, the profound drop in breast cancer mortality seen over the past decade is unlikely to be solely attributable to improvements in therapy. It seems prudent to recommend annual mammography for women past the age of 40. Although no randomized study of BSE has ever shown any improvement in survival, its major benefit appears to be identification of tumors appropriate for conservative local therapy. Better mammographic technology, including digitized mammography, routine use of magnified views, and greater skill in mammographic interpretation, combined with newer diagnostic techniques (magnetic resonance imaging, magnetic resonance spectroscopy, positron emission tomography, etc.) may make it possible to identify breast cancers even more reliably and earlier.

STAGING Correct staging of breast cancer patients is of extraordinary importance. Not only does it permit an accurate prognosis, but in many cases therapeutic decision-making is based largely on the TNM classification (Table 76-1). Comparison with historic series should be undertaken with caution, as the staging has changed several times in the past 20 years.

℞ TREATMENT

PRIMARY BREAST CANCER A series of randomized clinical trials both in the United States and abroad have shown that breast-conserving treatments, consisting of the removal of the primary tumor by some form of lumpectomy with or without irradiating the breast, results in a survival that is as good as that after extensive procedures, such as mastectomy or modified radical mastectomy, with or without further irradiation. Postlumpectomy breast irradiation greatly reduces the risk of recurrence in the breast. While breast conservation is associated with a possibility of recurrence in the breast, 10-year survival is at least as good as that after more radical surgery. Postoperative radiation to regional nodes following mastectomy is also associated with an improvement in survival. Since radiation therapy can also reduce the rate of local or regional recurrence, it should be strongly considered following mastectomy for women with high-risk primary tumors (i.e., T2 in size, positive margins, positive nodes). At present, approximately one-third of women in the United States are managed by lumpectomy. Breast-conserving surgery is not suitable for all patients: it is not generally suitable for tumors >5 cm (or for smaller tumors if the breast is small), for tumors involving the nipple areola complex, for tumors with extensive intraductal disease involving multiple quadrants of the breast, for women with a history of collagen-vascular disease, and for women who either do not have the motivation for breast conservation or do not have convenient access to radiation therapy. However, these groups probably do not account for more than one-third of patients who are treated with mastectomy. Thus, a great many women still undergo mastectomy who could safely avoid this procedure and probably would if appropriately counseled.

An extensive intraductal component is a predictor of recurrence in the breast, and so are several clinical variables. Both axillary lymph node involvement and involvement of vascular or lymphatic channels by metastatic tumor in the breast are associated with a higher risk of relapse in the breast but are not contraindications to breast-conserving treatment. When these patients are excluded, and when lumpectomy with negative tumor margins is achieved, breast conservation is associated with a recurrence rate in the breast of substantially <10%. The survival of patients who have recurrence in the breast is somewhat worse than that of women who do not. Thus, recurrence in the breast is a negative prognostic variable for long-term survival. However, recurrence in the breast is not the *cause* of distant metastasis. If recurrence in the breast caused metastatic disease, then women treated with lumpectomy, who have a higher rate of recurrence in the breast, should have poorer survival than women treated with mastectomy and they do not. Most patients should consult with a radiation oncologist before making a final decision concerning local therapy. However, a multimodality clinic in which the surgeon, radiation oncologist, medical oncologist, and other caregivers cooperate to evaluate the patient and develop a treatment is usually considered a major advantage by patients.

Adjuvant Therapy   The use of systemic therapy after local management of breast cancer improves survival. More than one-third of the women who would otherwise die of metastatic breast cancer remain disease-free when treated with the appropriate systemic regimen.

PROGNOSTIC VARIABLES   The most important prognostic variables are provided by *tumor staging*. The size of the tumor and the status of the axillary lymph nodes provide reasonably accurate information on the likelihood of tumor relapse. The relation of pathologic stage to 5-year survival is shown in Table 76-2. For most women, the need for adjuvant therapy can be readily defined on this basis alone. In the absence of lymph node involvement, involvement of microvessels (either capillaries or lymphatic channels) in tumors is nearly equivalent to lymph node involvement. The greatest controversy concerns women with intermediate prognoses. *There is rarely justification for adjuvant chemotherapy in most women with tumors <1 cm in size whose axillary lymph nodes are negative.* The most exciting development in this area is the use of gene expression arrays to analyze patterns of tumor gene expression.

Other prognostic variables have been sought, and some appear to influence disease-free and overall survival. What is less clear is whether they add to the information from pathologic staging.

Estrogen and progesterone receptor status are of prognostic significance. Tumors that lack either or both of these receptors are more likely to recur than tumors that have them.

Several *measures of tumor growth rate* correlate with early relapse. S-phase analysis using flow cytometry is the most accurate measure. Indirect S-phase assessments using antigens associated with the cell cycle, such as PCNA (Ki67), are also valuable. Several studies suggest that tumors with a high proportion (more than the median) of cells in the S phase pose a greater risk of relapse and that chemotherapy offers the greatest survival benefit for these tumors. For this reason, some clinicians use S-phase assessment as a deciding factor for instituting adjuvant therapy when other pathologic features are unclear. Assessment of DNA content in the form of ploidy is of modest value, with nondiploid tumors having a somewhat worse prognosis.

Histologic classification of the tumor has also been used as a prognostic factor. Tumors with a poor nuclear grade have a higher risk of recurrence than tumors with a good nuclear grade. Semiquantitative measures such as the Elston score improve the reproducibility of this measurement.

Molecular changes in the tumor are also useful. Tumors that overexpress *erbB2* (HER-2/neu) or have a mutated p53 gene have a worse prognosis. Particular interest has centered on *erbB2* overexpression as measured by histochemistry or by fluorescence in situ hybridization. In experienced hands either methodology is acceptable. Tumors that overexpress *erbB2* are more likely to respond to higher doses of doxorubicin-containing regimens. For this reason, *erbB2* expression is usually worth measuring as a means of deciding on therapy. Results of ongoing adjuvant therapy trials evaluating the role of monoclonal HER-2/neu antibodies (trastuzumab) are awaited with great interest.

To grow, a tumor must generate a neovasculature (Chap. 69). The presence of more microvessels, particularly when localized in so-called "hot spots," in a tumor is associated with a worse prognosis.

Other variables that have also been used to evaluate prognosis include proteins associated with invasiveness, such as type IV collagenase, cathepsin D, plasminogen activator, plasminogen activator receptor, and the metastasis-suppressor gene, *nm23*. None of these has been widely accepted as a prognostic variable for therapeutic decision-making. One problem in interpreting these prognostic variables is that most of them have not been examined in a study using a large cohort of patients.

ADJUVANT REGIMENS   Adjuvant therapy is the use of systemic therapies in patients whose known disease has received local therapy but who are at risk of relapse. Selection of appropriate adjuvant chemotherapy or hormone therapy is highly controversial in some situations. Meta-analyses have helped to define broad limits for therapy but do not help in choosing optimal regimens or in choosing a regimen for certain subgroups of patients. A summary of recommendations is shown in Table 76-3. In general, premenopausal women for whom any form of adjuvant systemic therapy is indicated should receive multidrug chemotherapy. The antiestrogen (tamoxifen) improves survival in premenopausal patients with positive estrogen receptor values and should be added following completion of chemotherapy. Prophylactic castration may also be associated with a substantial survival benefit (primarily in estrogen receptor–positive patients) but is not widely used in this country.

Data on postmenopausal women are also controversial. The impact of adjuvant chemotherapy is quantitatively less clear-cut than in premenopausal patients, although some survival advantage has been shown. The first decision is whether chemotherapy or tamoxifen should be used. While adjuvant tamoxifen improves survival regardless of axillary lymph node status, the improvement in survival is modest for patients in whom multiple lymph nodes are involved. For this reason, it has been usual to give chemotherapy to postmenopausal patients who have no medical contraindications and who have more than one positive lymph node; tamoxifen is commonly given simultaneously or subsequently. For postmenopausal women for whom systemic therapy is warranted but who have a more favorable prognosis, tamoxifen may be used as a single agent. Data from the ATAC trial in which >9000 women were randomly assigned to tamoxifen, anastrazole (an aromatase inhibitor), or the combination showed that anastrazole was superior to tamoxifen or the combination in preventing recurrence at 32 months of follow-up. Whether these observations will persist with longer follow-up and/or other effects on cardiovascular disease will become issues awaits further follow-up.

Most comparisons of adjuvant chemotherapy regimens show little difference among them, although slight advantages for doxorubicin-containing regimens are usually seen.

One approach—so-called neoadjuvant chemotherapy—involves the administration of adjuvant therapy before definitive surgery and radiation therapy. Because the objective response rates of patients with breast cancer to systemic therapy in this setting exceed 75%, many

TABLE 76-2   *5-Year Survival Rate for Breast Cancer by Stage*

Stage	5-Year Survival, %
0	99
I	92
IIA	82
IIB	65
IIIA	47
IIIB	44
IV	14

Source: Modified from data of the National Cancer Institute—Surveillance, Epidemiology, and End Results (SEER).

patients will be "downstaged" and may become candidates for breast-conserving therapy. At least one large randomized study has failed to show any difference in survival using this approach.

Other adjuvant treatments under investigation include the use of new drugs, such as paclitaxel and docetaxel, and therapy based on alternative kinetic and biologic models. In such approaches, high doses of single agents are used separately in relatively dose-intensive cycling regimens. One large randomized trial for node-positive patients suggests that patients treated with doxorubicin-cyclophosphamide for four cycles followed by four cycles of paclitaxel have a substantial additional gain in survival as compared with women receiving doxorubicin-cyclophosphamide alone, an outcome not validated in another large trial. Taxane use remains controversial. Very high dose therapy with stem cell transplantation in the adjuvant setting has not proved superior to standard dose therapy and should not be routinely used.

Systemic Therapy of Metastatic Disease   Nearly half of patients treated for apparently localized breast cancer develop metastatic disease. Although a very small number of these patients can enjoy long remissions when treated with combinations of systemic and local therapy, most eventually succumb. Soft tissue, bony, and visceral (lung and liver) metastases each account for approximately one-third of sites of initial relapses. However, by the time of death, most patients will have bony involvement. Recurrences can appear at any time after primary therapy. Half of all initial cancer recurrences occur >5 years after initial therapy.

Because the diagnosis of metastatic disease alters the outlook for the patient so drastically, it should not be made without biopsy. Every oncologist has seen patients with tuberculosis, gallstones, primary hyperparathyroidism, or other nonmalignant diseases misdiagnosed and treated as though they had metastatic breast cancer. This is a catastrophic mistake and justifies biopsy for virtually every patient at the time of initial suspicion of metastatic disease.

The choice of therapy requires consideration of local therapy needs, the overall medical condition of the patient, and the hormone receptor status of the tumor, as well as the exercise of clinical judgment. Because therapy of systemic disease is palliative, the potential toxicities of therapies should be balanced against the response rates. Several variables influence the response to systemic therapy. For example, the presence of estrogen and progesterone receptors is a strong indication for endocrine therapy, since the response rates for tumors that express both receptors may approach 70%. On the other hand, patients with short disease-free intervals, rapidly progressive visceral disease, lymphangitic pulmonary disease, or intracranial disease are unlikely to respond to endocrine therapy.

In many cases, systemic therapy can be withheld while the patient is managed with appropriate local therapy. Radiation therapy and occasionally surgery are effective at relieving the symptoms of metastatic disease, particularly when bony sites are involved. Many patients with bone-only or bone-dominant disease have a relatively indolent course. Under such circumstances, systemic chemotherapy has a modest effect, whereas radiation therapy may be effective for long periods. Other systemic treatments, such as strontium 89 and/or bisphosphonates, may provide a palliative benefit without inducing objective responses. Most patients with metastatic disease and certainly all who have bone involvement should receive concurrent bisphosphonates. Since the goal of therapy is to maintain well-being for as long as possible, emphasis should be placed on avoiding the most hazardous complications of metastatic disease, including pathologic fracture of the axial skeleton and spinal cord compression. New back pain in patients with cancer should be explored aggressively on an emergent basis; to wait for neurologic symptoms is a potentially catastrophic error. Metastatic involvement of endocrine organs can cause profound dysfunction, including adrenal insufficiency and hypopituitarism. Similarly, obstruction of the biliary tree or other impaired organ function may be better managed with a local therapy than with a systemic approach.

Endocrine Therapy   Normal breast tissue is estrogen-dependent. Both primary and metastatic breast cancer may retain this phenotype. The best means of ascertaining whether a breast cancer is hormone-dependent is through analysis of estrogen and progesterone receptor levels on the tumor. Tumors that are positive for the estrogen receptor and negative for the progesterone receptor have a response rate of ~30%. Tumors that have both receptors have a response rate approaching 70%. If neither receptor is present, the objective response rates are <10%. Receptor analyses provide information as to the correct ordering of endocrine therapies as opposed to chemotherapy. Because of their lack of toxicity and because some patients whose receptor analyses are reported as negative respond to endocrine therapy, an endocrine treatment should be attempted in virtually every patient with metastatic breast cancer. Potential endocrine therapies are summarized in Table 76-4. The choice of endocrine therapy is usually determined

TABLE 76-3   *Suggested Approaches to Adjuvant Therapy*

Age Group	Lymph Node Status[a]	Endocrine Receptor (ER) Status	Tumor	Recommendation
Premenopausal	Positive	Any	Any	Multidrug chemotherapy + tamoxifen if ER-positive
Premenopausal	Negative	Any	>2 cm, or 1–2 cm with other poor prognostic variables	Multidrug chemotherapy + tamoxifen if ER-positive
Postmenopausal	Positive	Negative	Any	Multidrug chemotherapy
Postmenopausal	Positive	Positive	Any	Tamoxifen with or without chemotherapy
Postmenopausal	Negative	Positive	>2 cm, or 1–2 cm with other poor prognostic variables	Tamoxifen
Postmenopausal	Negative	Negative	>2 cm, or 1–2 cm with other poor prognostic variables	Consider multidrug chemotherapy

[a] As determined by pathologic examination.

TABLE 76-4   *Endocrine Therapies for Breast Cancer*

Therapy	Comments

Castration
  Surgical
  LHRH agonists
	For premenopausal women

Antiestrogens Tamoxifen	Useful in pre- and postmenopausal women
"Pure" antiestrogens	Promising early clinical data; responses in tamoxifen-resistant patients
Surgical adrenalectomy	Rarely employed second-line choice
Aromatase inhibitors	Low toxicity and superiority to additive hormone therapy; now first choice for metastatic disease
High-dose progestogens	Common third-line choice
Hypophysectomy	Rarely used
Additive androgens or estrogens	Plausible third-line therapies; potentially toxic

Note: LHRH, luteinizing hormone–releasing hormone.

by toxicity profile and availability. In most patients, the initial endocrine therapy should now be an aromatase inhibitor rather than tamoxifen. Newer "pure" antiestrogens that are free of agonistic effects are also in clinical trial. Cases in which tumors shrink in response to tamoxifen withdrawal (as well as withdrawal of pharmacologic doses of estrogens) have been reported. Endogenous estrogen formation may be blocked by analogues of luteinizing hormone–releasing hormone in premenopausal women. Additive endocrine therapies, including treatment with progestogens, estrogens, and androgens, may also be tried in patients who respond to initial endocrine therapy; the mechanism of action of these latter therapies is unknown. Patients who respond to one endocrine therapy have at least a 50% chance of responding to a second endocrine therapy. It is not uncommon for patients to respond to two or three sequential endocrine therapies; however, combination endocrine therapies do not appear to be superior to individual agents, and combinations of chemotherapy with endocrine therapy are not useful. The median survival of patients with metastatic disease is approximately 2 years, and many patients, particularly older persons and those with hormone-dependent disease, may respond to endocrine therapy for 3 to 5 years or longer.

Chemotherapy Unlike many other epithelial malignancies, breast cancer responds to several chemotherapeutic agents, including anthracyclines, alkylating agents, taxanes, and antimetabolites. Multiple combinations of these agents have been found to improve response rates somewhat, but they have had little effect on duration of response or survival. The choice among multidrug combinations frequently depends on whether adjuvant chemotherapy was administered and, if so, what type. While patients treated with adjuvant regimens such as cyclophosphamide, methotrexate, and fluorouracil (CMF regimens) may subsequently respond to the same combination in the metastatic disease setting, most oncologists use drugs to which the patients have not been previously exposed. Once patients have progressed after combination drug therapy, it is most common to treat them with single agents. Given the significant toxicity of most drugs, the use of a single effective agent will minimize toxicity by sparing the patient exposure to drugs that would be of little value. Unfortunately, no form of in vitro drug sensitivity testing to select the drugs most efficacious for a given patient has been demonstrated to be useful.

Most oncologists use either an anthracycline or paclitaxel following failure with the initial regimen. However, the choice has to be balanced with individual needs.

The use of a humanized antibody to *erbB2* [trastuzumab (Herceptin)] combined with paclitaxel can improve response rate and survival for women whose metastatic tumors overexpress *erbB2*. The magnitude of the survival extension is modest in patients with metastatic disease. Application to adjuvant therapy may prove even more beneficial. In the past few years a series of newer agents has emerged as useful in inducing objective responses in previously treated patients, including gemcitabine, capecitabine, navelbine, and oral etoposide.

HIGH-DOSE CHEMOTHERAPY INCLUDING AUTOLOGOUS BONE MARROW TRANSPLANTATION Autologous bone marrow transplantation combined with high doses of single agents can produce improvement even in heavily pretreated patients. However, such responses are rarely, if ever, durable and are unlikely to substantially alter the clinical course for most patients with advanced metastatic disease. Randomized trials have not been encouraging, and these approaches cannot be recommended as part of clinical care outside of research settings.

STAGE III BREAST CANCER Between 10 and 25% of patients present with so-called locally advanced, or stage III, breast cancer at diagnosis. Many of these cancers are technically operable, whereas others, particularly cancers with chest wall involvement, inflammatory breast cancers, or cancers with large matted axillary lymph nodes, cannot be managed with surgery initially. Although no randomized trials have proved the efficacy of induction chemotherapy, this approach has gained widespread use. More than 90% of patients with locally advanced breast cancer show a partial or better response to multidrug chemotherapy regimens that include an anthracycline. Early administration of this treatment reduces the bulk of the disease and frequently makes the patient a suitable candidate for salvage surgery and/or radiation therapy. These patients should be managed in multimodality clinics to coordinate surgery, radiation therapy, and systemic chemotherapy. Such approaches produce long-term disease-free survival in about 30 to 50% of patients.

BREAST CANCER PREVENTION Women who have one breast cancer are at risk of developing a contralateral breast cancer at a rate of approximately 0.5% per year. When adjuvant tamoxifen is administered to these patients, the rate of development of contralateral breast cancers is reduced. In other tissues of the body, tamoxifen has estrogen-like effects that are beneficial: preservation of bone mineral density and long-term lowering of cholesterol. However, tamoxifen has estrogen-like effects on the uterus, leading to an increased risk of uterine cancer (0.75% incidence after 5 years on tamoxifen). Tamoxifen also increases the risk of cataract formation. The Breast Cancer Prevention Trial (BCPT) revealed a >49% reduction in breast cancer among women with a risk of at least 1.66% taking the drug for 5 years. Raloxifene has shown similar breast cancer prevention potency but may have different effects on bone and heart. The two agents are being compared in a prospective randomized prevention trial (the STAR trial).

NONINVASIVE BREAST CANCER Breast cancer develops as a series of molecular changes in the epithelial cells that lead to ever more malignant behavior. Increased use of mammography has led to more frequent diagnosis of noninvasive breast cancer. These lesions fall into two groups: ductal carcinoma in situ (DCIS) and lobular carcinoma in situ (lobular neoplasia). The management of both entities is controversial.

Ductal Carcinoma in Situ Proliferation of cytologically malignant breast epithelial cells within the ducts is termed *DCIS*. Significant disagreement can occur in differentiating atypical hyperplasia from DCIS. At least one-third of the cases of untreated DCIS progress to invasive breast cancer within 5 years. For many years, the standard treatment for this disease was mastectomy. However, since treatment of this condition by lumpectomy and radiation therapy gives survival that is as good as the survival for invasive breast cancer by mastectomy, it appears paradoxical to recommend more aggressive therapy for a "less" malignant disease. In one randomized trial, the combination of wide excision plus irradiation for DCIS caused a substantial reduction in the local recurrence rate as compared with wide excision alone with negative margins, though survival was identical in the two arms. No studies have compared either of these regimens to mastectomy. Addition of tamoxifen to any DCIS surgical/radiation therapy regimen further improves local control.

Several prognostic features may help to identify patients at high risk for local recurrence after either lumpectomy alone or lumpectomy with radiation therapy. These include extensive disease; age < 40; and cytologic features such as necrosis, poor nuclear grade, and comedo subtype with overexpression of *erbB2*. Some data suggest that adequate excision with careful determination of pathologically clear margins is associated with a low recurrence rates. When surgery is combined with radiation therapy, recurrence (which is usually in the same quadrant) occurs with a frequency of ≤10%. Given the fact that half of these recurrences will be invasive, about 5% of the initial cohort will eventually develop invasive breast cancer. A reasonable expectation of mortality for these patients is about 1%, a figure that approximates the mortality rate for DCIS managed by mastectomy. Although this train of reasoning has not formally been proved valid, it is reasonable at present to recommend that patients who desire breast preservation, and in whom DCIS appears to be reasonably localized, be managed by adequate surgery with meticulous pathologic evaluation, followed by breast irradiation and tamoxifen. For patients with localized DCIS, axillary lymph node dissection is unnecessary. More controversial is the question of what management is optimal when there is any degree of invasion. Because of a significant likelihood (10 to

TABLE 76-5 *Breast Cancer Surveillance Guidelines*

Test	Frequency
RECOMMENDED	
History; eliciting symptoms; physical examination	q3–6 months × 3 years; q6–12 months × 2 years; then annually
Breast self-examination	Monthly
Mammography	Annually
Pelvic examination	Annually
Patient education about symptoms of recurrence	Ongoing
Coordination of care	Ongoing
NOT RECOMMENDED	
Complete blood count	
Serum chemistry studies	
Chest radiographs	
Bone scans	
Ultrasound examination of the liver	
Computed tomography of chest, abdomen, or pelvis	
Tumor marker CA 15-3	
Tumor marker CEA	

Source: *Recommended Breast Cancer Surveillance Guidelines*, ASCO Education Book, Fall, 1997.

15%) of axillary lymph node involvement even when the primary lesion shows only microscopic invasion, it is prudent to do at least a level 1 and 2 axillary lymph node dissection for all patients with any degree of invasion; sentinel node biopsy may be substituted. Further management is dictated by the presence of nodal spread.

Lobular Neoplasia Proliferation of cytologically malignant cells within the lobules is termed *lobular neoplasia*. Nearly 30% of patients who have had adequate local excision of the lesion develop breast cancer (usually infiltrating ductal cell carcinoma) over the next 15 to 20 years. Ipsilateral and contralateral disease are equally common. Therefore, lobular neoplasia may be a premalignant lesion that suggests an elevated risk of subsequent breast cancer, rather than a form of malignancy itself, and aggressive local management seems unreasonable. Most patients should be treated with tamoxifen for 5 years and followed with careful annual mammography and semiannual physical examinations. Additional molecular analysis of these lesions may make it possible to discriminate between patients who are at risk of further progression and who require additional therapy and those in whom simple follow-up is adequate.

MALE BREAST CANCER Breast cancer is about 1/150th as frequent in men as in women. It usually presents as a unilateral lump in the breast and is frequently not diagnosed promptly. Given the small amount of soft tissue and the unexpected nature of the problem, locally advanced presentations are somewhat more common. When male breast cancer is matched to female breast cancer by age and stage, its overall prognosis is identical. Although gynecomastia may initially be unilateral or asymmetric, any unilateral mass in a man over the age of 40 should receive a careful workup all the way through biopsy. On the other hand, bilateral symmetric breast development rarely represents breast cancer and is almost invariably due to endocrine disease or a drug effect. It should be kept in mind, nevertheless, that the risk of cancer is much greater in men with gynecomastia; in such men, gross asymmetry of the breasts should arouse suspicion of cancer. Male breast cancer is best managed by mastectomy and axillary lymph node dissection (modified radical mastectomy). Patients with locally advanced disease or positive nodes should also be treated with irradiation. Approximately 90% of male breast cancers contain estrogen receptors, and approximately 60% of cases with metastatic disease respond to endocrine therapy. No randomized studies have evaluated adjuvant therapy for male breast cancer. Two historic experiences suggest that the disease responds well to adjuvant systemic therapy, and, if not medically contraindicated, the same criteria for the use of adjuvant therapy in women should be applied to men.

The sites of relapse and spectrum of response to chemotherapeutic drugs are virtually identical for breast cancers in the two sexes.

FOLLOW-UP OF BREAST CANCER PATIENTS Despite the availability of sophisticated and expensive imaging techniques and a wide range of serum tumor marker tests, no studies document that survival is influenced by early diagnosis of relapse. Surveillance guidelines are given in Table 76-5.

FURTHER READING

BENICHOU J et al: Graphs to estimate an individualized risk of breast cancer. J Clin Oncol 14:103, 1996

FISHER B et al: Twenty-year follow-up of a randomized trial comparing total mastectomy, lumpectomy, and lumpectomy plus irradiation for the treatment of invasive breast cancer. N Engl J Med 347:1233, 2002

GIORDANO S et al: Breast cancer in men. Ann Intern Med 137:678, 2002

ROUSSOUW JE et al: Risks and benefits of estrogen plus progestin in healthy postmenopausal women. JAMA 288:321, 2002

SHAPIRO CL, WINER EL (eds): Late effects of treatment and survivorship issues in early-stage breast cancer. Sem Oncol 30:729, 2003

STOCKLER M et al: Systematic reviews of chemotherapy and endocrine therapy for metastatic breast cancer. Cancer Treat Rev 26:151, 2000

VAN DE VIJVER M et al: A gene-expression signature as a predictor of survival in breast cancer. N Engl J Med 347:1999, 2002

WONG ZW, ELLIS MJ: First-line endocrine treatment of breast cancer: Aromatase inhibitor or antiestrogen? Br J Cancer 90:20, 2004

77 | GASTROINTESTINAL TRACT CANCER
Robert J. Mayer

The gastrointestinal tract is the second most common noncutaneous site for cancer and the second major cause of cancer-related mortality in the United States.

ESOPHAGEAL CANCER

INCIDENCE AND ETIOLOGY Cancer of the esophagus is a relatively uncommon but extremely lethal malignancy. The diagnosis was made in 14,250 Americans in 2004 and led to 13,300 deaths. Worldwide, the incidence of esophageal cancer varies strikingly. It occurs frequently within a geographic region extending from the southern shore of the Caspian Sea on the west to northern China on the east and encompassing parts of Iran, Central Asia, Afghanistan, Siberia, and Mongolia. High-incidence "pockets" of the disease are also present in such disparate locations as Finland, Iceland, Curaçao, southeastern Africa, and northwestern France. In North America and western Europe, the disease is more common in blacks than whites and in males than females; it appears most often after age 50 and seems to be associated with a lower socioeconomic status.

A variety of causative factors have been implicated in the development of the disease (Table 77-1). In the United States, esophageal cancer cases are either squamous cell carcinomas or adenocarcinomas. The etiology of squamous cell esophageal cancer is related to excess alcohol consumption and/or cigarette smoking. The relative risk increases with the amount of tobacco smoked or alcohol consumed, with these factors acting synergistically. The consumption of whiskey is linked to a higher incidence than the consumption of wine or beer. Squamous cell esophageal carcinoma has also been associated with the ingestion of nitrites, smoked opiates, and fungal toxins in pickled vegetables, as well as mucosal damage caused by such physical insults as long-term exposure to extremely hot tea, the ingestion of lye, radiation-induced strictures, and chronic achalasia. The presence of an esophageal web in association with glossitis and iron deficiency (i.e.,

TABLE 77-1   *Some Etiologic Factors Believed to Be Associated with Esophageal Cancer*

Excess alcohol consumption
Cigarette smoking
Other ingested carcinogens
  Nitrates (converted to nitrites)
  Smoked opiates
  Fungal toxins in pickled vegetables
Mucosal damage from physical agents
  Hot tea
  Lye ingestion
  Radiation-induced strictures
  Chronic achalasia
Host susceptibility
  Esophageal web with glossitis and iron deficiency (i.e., Plummer-
    Vinson or Paterson-Kelly syndrome)
  Congenital hyperkeratosis and pitting of the palms and soles (i.e.,
    tylosis palmaris et plantaris)
  ? Dietary deficiencies molybdenum, zinc, vitamin A
  ? Celiac sprue
  Chronic gastric reflux (i.e., Barrett's esophagus) for adenocarcinoma

Plummer-Vinson or Paterson-Kelly syndrome) and congenital hyperkeratosis and pitting of the palms and soles (i.e., tylosis palmaris et plantaris) have each been linked with squamous cell esophageal cancer, as have dietary deficiencies of molybdenum, zinc, and vitamin A.

For unclear reasons, the incidence of squamous cell esophageal cancer has decreased somewhat in both the black and white population in the United States over the past 25 years, while the rate of adenocarcinoma has risen dramatically, particularly in white males. Adenocarcinomas arise in the distal esophagus in the presence of chronic gastric reflux and gastric metaplasia of the epithelium (Barrett's esophagus), which is more common in obese persons. Adenocarcinomas arise within dysplastic columnar epithelium in the distal esophagus. Even before frank neoplasia is detectable, aneuploidy and p53 mutations are found in the dysplastic epithelium. These adenocarcinomas behave clinically like gastric adenocarcinoma and now account for >50% of esophageal cancers.

CLINICAL FEATURES   About 15% of esophageal cancers occur in the upper third of the esophagus (cervical esophagus), 35% in the middle third, and 50% in the lower third. Squamous cell carcinomas and adenocarcinomas of the esophagus cannot be distinguished radiographically or endoscopically.

Progressive dysphagia and weight loss of short duration are the initial symptoms in the vast majority of patients. Dysphagia initially occurs with solid foods and gradually progresses to include semisolids and liquids. By the time these symptoms develop, the disease is usually incurable, since difficulty in swallowing does not occur until >60% of the esophageal circumference is infiltrated with cancer. Dysphagia may be associated with pain on swallowing (odynophagia), pain radiating to the chest and/or back, regurgitation or vomiting, and aspiration pneumonia. The disease most commonly spreads to adjacent and supraclavicular lymph nodes, liver, lungs, and pleura. Tracheoesophageal fistulas may develop as the disease advances, leading to severe suffering. As with other squamous cell carcinomas, hypercalcemia may occur in the absence of osseous metastases, probably from parathormone-related peptide secreted by tumor cells (Chap. 86).

DIAGNOSIS   Attempts at endoscopic and cytologic screening for carcinoma in patients with Barrett's esophagus, while effective as a means of detecting high-grade dysplasia, have not yet been shown to improve the prognosis in individuals found to have a carcinoma. Routine contrast radiographs effectively identify esophageal lesions large enough to cause symptoms. In contrast to benign esophageal leiomyomas, which result in esophageal narrowing with preservation of a normal mucosal pattern, esophageal carcinomas characteristically cause ragged, ulcerating changes in the mucosa in association with deeper infiltration, producing a picture resembling achalasia. Smaller, potentially resectable tumors are often poorly visualized despite technically adequate esophagograms. Because of this, esophagoscopy should be performed in all patients suspected of having an esophageal abnormality, to visualize the tumor and to obtain histopathologic confirmation of the diagnosis. Because the population of persons at risk for squamous cell carcinoma of the esophagus (i.e., smokers and drinkers) also has a high rate of cancers of the lung and the head and neck region, endoscopic inspection of the larynx, trachea, and bronchi should also be done. A thorough examination of the fundus of the stomach (by retroflexing the endoscope) is imperative as well. Endoscopic biopsies of esophageal tumors fail to recover malignant tissue in one-third of cases because the biopsy forceps cannot penetrate deeply enough through normal mucosa pushed in front of the carcinoma. Cytologic examination of tumor brushings frequently complements standard biopsies and should be performed routinely. The extent of tumor spread to the mediastinum and paraaortic lymph nodes should also be assessed by computed tomography (CT) scans of the chest and abdomen and by endoscopic ultrasound. Positron emission tomography (PET) scanning may also provide useful assessment of resectability.

R_x TREATMENT

The prognosis for patients with esophageal carcinoma is poor. Fewer than 5% of patients are alive 5 years after the diagnosis; thus, management focuses on symptom control. Surgical resection of all gross tumor (i.e., total resection) is feasible in only 45% of cases, with residual tumor cells frequently present at the resection margins. Such esophagectomies have been associated with a postoperative mortality rate of 5 to 10% due to anastomotic fistulas, subphrenic abscesses, and respiratory complications. About 20% of patients who survive a total resection live 5 years. The outcome of primary radiation therapy (5500 to 6000 cGy) for squamous cell carcinomas is similar to that of radical surgery, sparing patients perioperative morbidity but often resulting in less satisfactory palliation of obstructive symptoms. The evaluation of chemotherapeutic agents in patients with esophageal carcinoma has been hampered by ambiguity in the definition of "response" (i.e., benefit) and the debilitated physical condition of many treated individuals. Nonetheless, significant reductions in the size of measurable tumor masses have been reported in 15 to 25% of patients given single-agent treatment and in 30 to 60% of patients treated with drug combinations that include cisplatin. Combination chemotherapy and radiation therapy as the initial therapeutic approach, either alone or followed by an attempt at operative resection, may be of benefit. When administered along with radiation therapy, chemotherapy produces a better survival outcome than radiation therapy alone. The use of preoperative chemotherapy and radiation therapy followed by esophageal resection appears to prolong survival as compared with historic controls, but randomized trials have produced inconsistent results.

For the incurable, surgically unresectable patient with esophageal cancer, dysphagia, malnutrition, and the management of tracheoesophageal fistulas loom as major issues. Approaches to palliation include repeated endoscopic dilatation, the surgical placement of a gastrostomy or jejunostomy for hydration and feeding, and endoscopic placement of an expansive metal stent to bypass the tumor. Endoscopic fulguration of the obstructing tumor with lasers appears to be the most promising of these techniques.

TUMORS OF THE STOMACH

GASTRIC ADENOCARCINOMA ■ **Incidence and Epidemiology**   For unclear reasons, the incidence and mortality rates for gastric cancer have decreased markedly during the past 65 years. The mortality rate from gastric cancer in the United States has dropped in men from 28 to 5.0 per 100,000 population, while in women, the rate has decreased from 27 to 2.3 per 100,000. Nonetheless, 22,710 new cases of stomach cancer were diagnosed in the United States and 11,780 Americans died of the disease in 2004. Gastric cancer incidence has decreased worldwide but remains high in Japan, China, Chile, and Ireland.

The risk of gastric cancer is greater among lower socioeconomic classes. Migrants from high- to low-incidence nations maintain their susceptibility to gastric cancer, while the risk for their offspring approximates that of the new homeland. These findings suggest that an environmental exposure, probably beginning early in life, is related to the development of gastric cancer, with dietary carcinogens considered the most likely factor(s).

Pathology About 85% of stomach cancers are adenocarcinomas, with 15% due to lymphomas and gastrointestinal stromal tumors (GIST, formerly called *leiomyosarcomas*). Gastric adenocarcinomas may be subdivided into two categories: a *diffuse type* in which cell cohesion is absent, so that individual cells infiltrate and thicken the stomach wall without forming a discrete mass; and an *intestinal type* characterized by cohesive neoplastic cells that form glandlike tubular structures. The diffuse carcinomas occur more often in younger patients, develop throughout the stomach (including the cardia), result in a loss of distensibility of the gastric wall (so-called linitis plastica or "leather bottle" appearance), and carry a poorer prognosis. Intestinal-type lesions are frequently ulcerative, more commonly appear in the antrum and lesser curvature of the stomach, and are often preceded by a prolonged precancerous process. While the incidence of diffuse carcinomas is similar in most populations, the intestinal type tends to predominate in the high-risk geographic regions and is less likely to be found in areas where the frequency of gastric cancer is declining. Thus, different etiologic factor(s) may be involved in these two subtypes. In the United States, the distal stomach is the site of origin of ~30% of gastric cancers, ~20% arise in the midportion of the stomach, and ~37% originate in the proximal third of the stomach. The remaining 13% involve the entire stomach.

Etiology The long-term ingestion of high concentrations of nitrates in dried, smoked, and salted foods appears to be associated with a higher risk. The nitrates are thought to be converted to carcinogenic nitrites by bacteria (Table 77-2). Such bacteria may be introduced exogenously through the ingestion of partially decayed foods, which are consumed in abundance worldwide by the lower socioeconomic classes. Bacteria such as *Helicobacter pylori* may also contribute to this effect by causing chronic gastritis, loss of gastric acidity, and bacterial growth in the stomach. The effect of *H. pylori* eradication on the subsequent risk for gastric cancer in high-incidence areas is under investigation. Loss of acidity may occur when acid-producing cells of the gastric antrum have been removed surgically to control benign peptic ulcer disease or when achlorhydria, atrophic gastritis, and even pernicious anemia develop in the elderly. Serial endoscopic examinations of the stomach in patients with atrophic gastritis have documented replacement of the usual gastric mucosa by intestinal-type cells. This process of intestinal metaplasia may lead to cellular atypia and eventual neoplasia. Since the declining incidence of gastric cancer in the United States primarily reflects a decline in distal, ulcerating, intestinal-type lesions, it is conceivable that better food preservation and the availability of refrigeration to all socioeconomic classes have decreased the dietary ingestion of exogenous bacteria.

Several additional etiologic factors have been associated with gastric carcinoma. Gastric ulcers and adenomatous polyps have occasionally been so linked, but data regarding a cause-and-effect relationship are unconvincing. The inadequate clinical distinction between benign gastric ulcers and small ulcerating carcinomas may, in part, account for this presumed association. The presence of extreme hypertrophy of gastric rugal folds (i.e., Ménétrier's disease), giving the impression of polypoid lesions, has been associated with a striking frequency of malignant transformation; such hypertrophy, however, does not represent the presence of true adenomatous polyps. Individuals with blood group A have a higher incidence of gastric cancer than persons with blood group O; this observation may be related to differences in the mucous secretion leading to altered mucosal protection from carcinogens. A germline mutation in the E-cadherin gene, inherited in an autosomal dominant pattern and coding for a cell adhesion protein, has been linked to a high incidence of occult gastric cancers in young asymptomatic carriers. Duodenal ulcers are not associated with gastric cancer.

Clinical Features Gastric cancers, when superficial and surgically curable, usually produce no symptoms. As the tumor becomes more extensive, patients may complain of an insidious upper abdominal discomfort varying in intensity from a vague, postprandial fullness to a severe, steady pain. Anorexia, often with slight nausea, is very common but is not the usual presenting complaint. Weight loss may eventually be observed, and nausea and vomiting are particularly prominent with tumors of the pylorus; dysphagia may be the major symptom caused by lesions of the cardia. There are no early physical signs. A palpable abdominal mass indicates long-standing growth and predicts regional extension.

Gastric carcinomas spread by direct extension through the gastric wall to the perigastric tissues, occasionally adhering to adjacent organs such as the pancreas, colon, or liver. The disease also spreads via lymphatics or by seeding of peritoneal surfaces. Metastases to intra-abdominal and supraclavicular lymph nodes occur frequently, as do metastatic nodules to the ovary (Krukenberg's tumor), periumbilical region ("Sister Mary Joseph node"), or peritoneal cul-de-sac (Blumer's shelf palpable on rectal or vaginal examination); malignant ascites may also develop. The liver is the most common site for hematogenous spread of tumor.

The presence of iron-deficiency anemia in men and of occult blood in the stool in both sexes mandates a search for an occult gastrointestinal tract lesion. A careful assessment is of particular importance in patients with atrophic gastritis or pernicious anemia. Unusual clinical features associated with gastric adenocarcinomas include migratory thrombophlebitis, microangiopathic hemolytic anemia, and acanthosis nigricans.

Diagnosis A double-contrast radiographic examination is the simplest diagnostic procedure for the evaluation of a patient with epigastric complaints. The use of double-contrast techniques helps to detect small lesions by improving mucosal detail. The stomach should be distended at some time during every radiographic examination, since decreased distensibility may be the only indication of a diffuse infiltrative carcinoma. Although gastric ulcers can be detected fairly early, distinguishing benign from malignant lesions is difficult. The anatomic location of an ulcer is not in itself an indication of the presence or absence of a cancer.

Gastric ulcers that appear benign by radiography present special problems. Some physicians believe that gastroscopy is not mandatory if the radiographic features are typically benign, if complete healing can be visualized by x-ray within 6 weeks, and if a follow-up contrast radiograph obtained several months later shows a normal appearance. However, we recommend gastroscopic biopsy and brush cytology for all patients with a gastric ulcer in order to exclude a malignancy. Malignant gastric ulcers must be recognized before they penetrate into surrounding tissues, because the rate of cure of early lesions limited to the mucosa or submucosa is >80%. Since gastric carcinomas are

TABLE 77-2 *Nitrate-Converting Bacteria as a Factor in the Causation of Gastric Carcinoma*[a]

Exogenous sources of nitrate-converting bacteria:
  Bacterially contaminated food (common in lower socioeconomic classes, who have a higher incidence of the disease; diminished by improved food preservation and refrigeration)
  ? *Helicobacter pylori* infection
Endogenous factors favoring growth of nitrate-converting bacteria in the stomach:
  Decreased gastric acidity
  Prior gastric surgery (antrectomy) (15- to 20-year latency period)
  Atrophic gastritis and/or pernicious anemia
  ? Prolonged exposure to histamine H_2-receptor antagonists

[a] Hypothesis: Dietary nitrates are converted to carcinogenic nitrites by bacteria.

TABLE 77-3 *Staging System for Gastric Carcinoma*

Stage	TNM	Features	Data from ACS	
			No. of Cases, %	5-Year Survival, %
0	TisN0M0	Node negative; limited to mucosa	1	90
IA	T1N0M0	Node negative; invasion of lamina propria or submucosa	7	59
IB	T2N0M0	Node negative; invasion of muscularis propria	10	44
II	T1N2M0	Node positive; invasion beyond mucosa but within		
	T2N1M0	wall		
		or	17	29
	T3N0M0	Node negative; extension through wall		
IIIA	T2N2M0	Node positive; invasion of muscularis propria	21	15
	T3N1-2M0	or through wall		
IIIB	T4N0-1M0	Node negative; adherence to surrounding tissue	14	9
IV	T4N2M0	Node positive; adherence to surrounding tissue		
		or	30	3
	T1-4N0-2M1	Distant metastases		

difficult to distinguish clinically or radiographically from gastric lymphomas, endoscopic biopsies should be made as deeply as possible, due to the submucosal location of lymphoid tumors.

The staging system for gastric carcinoma is shown in Table 77-3.

℞ TREATMENT

Complete surgical removal of the tumor with resection of adjacent lymph nodes offers the only chance for cure. However, this is possible in fewer than a third of patients. A subtotal gastrectomy is the treatment of choice for patients with distal carcinomas, while total or near-total gastrectomies are required for more proximal tumors. The inclusion of extended lymph node dissection to these procedures appears to confer an added risk for complications without enhancing survival. The prognosis following complete surgical resection depends on the degree of tumor penetration into the stomach wall and is adversely influenced by regional lymph node involvement, vascular invasion, and abnormal DNA content (i.e., aneuploidy), characteristics found in the vast majority of American patients. As a result, the probability of survival after 5 years for the 25 to 30% of patients able to undergo complete resection is ~20% for distal tumors and <10% for proximal tumors, with recurrences continuing to occur for at least 8 years after surgery. In the absence of ascites or extensive hepatic or peritoneal metastases, even patients whose disease is believed to be incurable by surgery should be offered resection of the primary lesion. Reduction of tumor bulk is the best form of palliation and may enhance the probability of benefit from chemotherapy and/or radiation therapy.

Gastric adenocarcinoma is a relatively radioresistant tumor, and adequate control of the primary tumor requires doses of external beam irradiation that exceed the tolerance of surrounding structures, such as bowel mucosa and spinal cord. As a result, the major role of radiation therapy in patients has been palliation of pain. Radiation therapy alone after a complete resection does not prolong survival. In the setting of surgically unresectable disease limited to the epigastrium, patients treated with 3500 to 4000 cGy did not live longer than similar patients not receiving radiotherapy; however, survival was prolonged slightly when 5-fluorouracil (5-FU) was given in combination with radiation therapy. In this clinical setting, the 5-FU may well be functioning as a radiosensitizer.

The administration of combinations of cytotoxic drugs to patients with advanced gastric carcinoma has been associated with partial responses in 30 to 50% of cases, providing significant benefit to individuals who respond to treatment. Such drug combinations have generally included 5-FU and doxorubicin together with either mitomycin-C or cisplatin. Despite this encouraging response rate, complete remissions are uncommon, the partial responses are transient, and the overall influence of multidrug therapy on survival has been a source of debate. The use of adjuvant chemotherapy alone following the complete resection of a gastric cancer has only minimally improved sur-

vival. However, postoperative chemotherapy combined with radiation therapy has been shown to reduce the recurrence rate and prolong survival.

PRIMARY GASTRIC LYMPHOMA Primary lymphoma of the stomach is relatively uncommon, accounting for <15% of gastric malignancies and about 2% of all lymphomas. The stomach is, however, the most frequent extranodal site for lymphoma, and gastric lymphoma has increased in frequency during the past 25 years. The disease is difficult to distinguish clinically from gastric adenocarcinoma; both tumors are most often detected during the sixth decade of life; present with epigastric pain, early satiety, and generalized fatigue; and are usually characterized by ulcerations with a ragged, thickened mucosal pattern demonstrated by contrast radiographs. The diagnosis of lymphoma of the stomach may occasionally be made through cytologic brushings of the gastric mucosa but usually requires a biopsy at gastroscopy or laparotomy. Failure of gastroscopic biopsies to detect lymphoma in a given case should not be interpreted as being conclusive, since superficial biopsies may miss the deeper lymphoid infiltrate. The macroscopic pathology of gastric lymphoma may also mimic adenocarcinoma, consisting of either a bulky ulcerated lesion localized in the corpus or antrum or a diffuse process spreading throughout the entire gastric submucosa and even extending into the duodenum. Microscopically, the vast majority of gastric lymphoid tumors are non-Hodgkin's lymphomas of B cell origin; Hodgkin's disease involving the stomach is extremely uncommon. Histologically, these tumors may range from well-differentiated, superficial processes [mucosa-associated lymphoid tissue (MALT)] to high-grade, large-cell lymphomas. Infection with *H. pylori*, the same bacterium associated with the development of gastric adenocarcinoma, appears to increase the risk for gastric lymphoma in general and MALT lymphomas in particular. Gastric lymphomas spread initially to regional lymph nodes (often to Waldeyer's ring) and may then disseminate. Gastric lymphomas are staged like other lymphomas (Chap. 97).

℞ TREATMENT

Primary gastric lymphoma is a far more treatable disease than adenocarcinoma of the stomach, a fact that underscores the need for making the correct diagnosis. Antibiotic treatment to eradicate *H. pylori* infection has led to regression of about 75% of gastric MALT lymphomas and should be considered before surgery, radiation therapy, or chemotherapy are undertaken in patients having such tumors. A lack of response to such antimicrobial treatment has been linked to a specific chromosomal abnormality, i.e., t(11;18). Responding patients should undergo periodic endoscopic surveillance because it remains unclear whether the neoplastic clone is eliminated or merely suppressed. Subtotal gastrectomy, usually followed by combination chemotherapy, has led to 5-year survival rates of 40 to 60% in patients with localized high-grade lymphomas. The need for a major surgical procedure is not clear, particularly in patients with preoperative radiographic evidence of nodal involvement, for whom chemotherapy alone [CHOP (cyclophosphamide, doxorubicin, vincristine, and prednisone) plus rituximab] is effective therapy. A role for radiation therapy is not defined because most recurrences develop at sites distant from the epigastrium. If widespread disease is discovered at the time of laparotomy, combination chemotherapy should be used.

GASTRIC (NONLYMPHOID) SARCOMA Leiomyosarcomas and GISTs make up 1 to 3% of gastric neoplasms. They most frequently involve the anterior and posterior walls of the gastric fundus and often ulcerate and bleed. Even those lesions that appear benign on histologic examination may behave in a malignant fashion. These tumors rarely invade adjacent viscera and characteristically do not metastasize to lymph nodes, but they may spread to the liver and lungs. The treatment of choice is surgical resection. Combination chemotherapy should be reserved for patients with metastatic disease. All such tumors should be analyzed for a mutation in the c-*kit* receptor. GISTs are unresponsive to conventional chemotherapy; ~50% of patients with such tumors, however, experience objective response when treated with imatinib mesylate (Gleevec), a selective inhibitor of the c-*kit* tyrosine kinase.

COLORECTAL CANCER

INCIDENCE Cancer of the large bowel is second only to lung cancer as a cause of cancer death in the United States; 146,940 new cases occurred in 2004, and 56,730 deaths were due to colorectal cancer. The incidence rate has remained relatively unchanged during the past 30 years while the mortality rate has decreased, particularly in females. Colorectal cancer generally occurs in individuals ≥50 years.

POLYPS AND MOLECULAR PATHOGENESIS Most colorectal cancers, regardless of etiology, arise from adenomatous polyps. A polyp is a grossly visible protrusion from the mucosal surface and may be classified pathologically as a nonneoplastic hamartoma (*juvenile polyp*), a hyperplastic mucosal proliferation (*hyperplastic polyp*), or an adenomatous polyp. Only adenomas are clearly premalignant, and only a minority of such lesions ever develop into cancer. Population-screening studies and autopsy surveys have revealed that adenomatous polyps may be found in the colons of >30% of middle-aged or elderly people; however, <1% of polyps ever become malignant. Most polyps produce no symptoms and remain clinically undetected. Occult blood in the stool may be found in <5% of patients with such lesions.

A number of molecular changes have been described in DNA obtained from adenomatous polyps, dysplastic lesions, and polyps containing microscopic foci of tumor cells (carcinoma in situ), which are thought to represent a multistep process in the evolution of normal colonic mucosa to life-threatening invasive carcinoma. These developmental steps towards carcinogenesis include, but are not restricted to, point mutations in the K-*ras* protooncogene; hypomethylation of DNA, leading to gene activation; loss of DNA ("allelic loss") at the site of a tumor-suppressor gene [the adenomatous polyposis coli (*APC*) gene] on the long arm of chromosome 5 (5q21); allelic loss at the site of a tumor-suppressor gene located on chromosome 18q [the deleted in colorectal cancer (*DCC*) gene]; and allelic loss at chromosome 17p, associated with mutations in the p53 tumor-suppressor gene (Fig. 68-2). Thus, the altered proliferative pattern of the colonic mucosa, which results in progression to a polyp and then to carcinoma, may involve the mutational activation of an oncogene followed by and coupled with the loss of genes that normally suppress tumorigenesis. It remains uncertain whether the genetic aberrations always occur in a defined order. Based on this model, however, cancer is believed to develop only in those polyps in which all of these mutational events take place.

Clinically, the probability of an adenomatous polyp becoming a cancer depends on the gross appearance of the lesion, its histologic features, and its size. Adenomatous polyps may be pedunculated (stalked) or sessile (flat-based). Cancers develop more frequently in sessile polyps. Histologically, adenomatous polyps may be tubular, villous (i.e., papillary), or tubulovillous. Villous adenomas, most of which are sessile, become malignant more than three times as often as tubular adenomas. The likelihood that any polypoid lesion in the large bowel contains invasive cancer is related to the size of the polyp, being negligible (<2%) in lesions <1.5 cm, intermediate (2 to 10%) in lesions 1.5 to 2.5 cm in size, and substantial (10%) in lesions >2.5 cm.

Following the detection of an adenomatous polyp, the entire large bowel should be visualized endoscopically or radiographically, since synchronous lesions are present in about one-third of cases. Colonoscopy should then be repeated periodically, even in the absence of a previously documented malignancy, since such patients have a 30 to 50% probability of developing another adenoma and are at a higher-than-average risk for developing a colorectal carcinoma. Adenomatous

polyps are thought to require >5 years of growth before becoming clinically significant; colonoscopy need not be carried out more frequently than every 3 years.

ETIOLOGY AND RISK FACTORS Risk factors for the development of colorectal cancer are listed in Table 77-4.

Diet The etiology for most cases of large-bowel cancer appears to be related to environmental factors. The disease occurs more often in upper socioeconomic populations who live in urban areas. Mortality from colorectal cancer is directly correlated with per capita consumption of calories, meat protein, and dietary fat and oil as well as elevations in the serum cholesterol concentration and mortality from coronary artery disease. Geographic variations in incidence are unrelated to genetic differences, since migrant groups tend to assume the large-bowel cancer incidence rates of their adopted countries. Furthermore, population groups such as Mormons and Seventh Day Adventists, whose lifestyle and dietary habits differ somewhat from those of their neighbors, have significantly lower-than-expected incidence and mortality rates for colorectal cancer. Colorectal cancer has increased in Japan since that nation has adopted a more "western" diet. At least two hypotheses have been proposed to explain the relationship to diet, neither of which is fully satisfactory.

ANIMAL FATS One hypothesis is that the ingestion of animal fats such as are found in red meats and processed meat leads to an increased proportion of anaerobes in the gut microflora, resulting in the conversion of normal bile acids into carcinogens. This provocative hypothesis is supported by several reports of increased amounts of fecal anaerobes in the stools of patients with colorectal cancer. Diets high in animal (but not vegetable) fats are also associated with high serum cholesterol, which is also associated with enhanced risk for the development of colorectal adenomas and carcinomas.

INSULIN RESISTANCE The enhanced number of calories inherent in "western" diets coupled with physical inactivity have been associated with a higher prevalence of obesity. Persons with such excess weight gain develop insulin resistance with increased circulating levels of insulin, leading to higher circulating concentrations of insulin-like growth factor type I (IGF-I). This growth factor appears to stimulate proliferation of the intestinal mucosa.

FIBER Contrary to one hypothesis, the results of randomized trials and case-controlled studies have failed to show any value for dietary fiber or diets high in fruits and vegatables in preventing the recurrence of colorectal adenomas or the development of colorectal cancer. The weight of epidemiologic evidence, however, implicates diet as being the major etiologic factor for colorectal cancer, particularly diets high in animal fat and in calories.

HEREDITARY FACTORS AND SYNDROMES As many as 25% of patients with colorectal cancer have a family history of the disease, suggesting a hereditary predisposition. Inherited large-bowel cancers can be divided into two main groups: the well-studied but uncommon polyposis syndromes and the more common nonpolyposis syndromes (Table 77-5).

Polyposis Coli Polyposis coli (familial polyposis of the colon) is a rare condition characterized by the appearance of thousands of adenomatous polyps throughout the large bowel. It is transmitted as an autosomal dominant trait; the occasional patients with no family history

TABLE 77-4 Risk Factors for the Development of Colorectal Cancer

Diet: Animal fat
Hereditary syndromes (autosomal dominant inheritance)
Polyposis coli
Nonpolyposis syndrome (Lynch syndrome)
Inflammatory bowel disease
Streptococcus bovis bacteremia
Ureterosigmoidostomy
? Tobacco use

Syndrome	Distribution of Polyps	Histologic Type	Malignant Potential	Associated Lesions
Familial adenomatous polyposis	Large intestine	Adenoma	Common	None
Gardner's syndrome	Large and small intestines	Adenoma	Common	Osteomas, fibromas, lipomas, epidermoid cysts, ampullary cancers, congenital hypertrophy of retinal pigment epithelium
Turcot's syndrome	Large intestine	Adenoma	Common	Brain tumors
Nonpolyposis syndrome (Lynch syndrome)	Large intestine (often proximal)	Adenoma	Common	Endometrial and ovarian tumors
Peutz-Jeghers syndrome	Small and large intestines, stomach	Hamartoma	Rare	Mucocutaneous pigmentation; tumors of the ovary, breast, pancreas, endometrium
Juvenile polyposis	Large and small intestines, stomach	Hamartoma, rarely progressing to adenoma	Rare	Various congenital abnormalities

probably developed the condition due to a spontaneous mutation. Polyposis coli is associated with a deletion in the long arm of chromosome 5 (including the *APC* gene) in both neoplastic (somatic mutation) and normal (germline mutation) cells. The loss of this genetic material (i.e., allelic loss) results in the absence of tumor-suppressor genes whose protein products would normally inhibit neoplastic growth. The presence of soft tissue and bony tumors, congenital hypertrophy of the retinal pigment epithelium, mesenteric desmoid tumors, and of ampullary cancers in addition to the colonic polyps characterizes a subset of polyposis coli known as *Gardner's syndrome*. The appearance of malignant tumors of the central nervous system accompanying polyposis coli defines *Turcot's syndrome*. The colonic polyps in all these conditions are rarely present before puberty but are generally evident in affected individuals by age 25. If the polyposis is not treated surgically, colorectal cancer will develop in almost all patients before age 40. Polyposis coli results from a defect in the colonic mucosa leading to an abnormal proliferative pattern and an impaired DNA repair following exposure to radiation or ultraviolet light. Once the multiple polyps that constitute polyposis coli are detected, patients should undergo a total colectomy. The ileoanal anastomotic technique allows removal of the entire bowel while retaining the anal sphincter; this appears to be the best treatment. Medical therapy with nonsteroidal anti-inflammatory drugs (NSAIDs) such as sulindac and cyclooxygenase-2 inhibitors such as celecoxib can decrease the number and size of polyps in patients with polyposis coli; however, this effect on polyps is only temporary. Colectomy remains the primary therapy. The offspring of patients with polyposis coli, who often are prepubertal when the diagnosis is made in the parent, have a 50% risk for the development of this premalignant disorder and should be carefully screened by annual flexible sigmoidoscopy until age 35. Proctosigmoidoscopy is a sufficient screening procedure because polyps tend to be evenly distributed from cecum to anus, making more-invasive and expensive techniques such as colonoscopy or barium enema unnecessary. Testing for occult blood in the stool is an inadequate screening maneuver. An alternative method for identifying carriers is testing DNA from peripheral blood mononuclear cells for the presence of a mutated *APC* gene. The detection of such a germline mutation can lead to a definitive diagnosis before the development of polyps.

Hereditary Nonpolyposis Colon Cancer Hereditary nonpolyposis colon cancer (HNPCC), also known as *Lynch syndrome*, is another autosomal dominant trait. It is characterized by the presence of three or more relatives with histologically documented colorectal cancer, one of whom is a first-degree relative of the other two; one or more cases of colorectal cancer diagnosed before age 50 in the family; and colorectal cancer involving at least two generations. In contrast to polyposis coli, HNPCC is associated with an unusually high frequency of cancer arising in the proximal large bowel. The median age for the appearance of an adenocarcinoma is <50 years, 10 to 15 years younger than the median age for the general population. Despite having a poorly differentiated histologic appearance, the proximal colon tumors in HNPCC have a better prognosis than sporadic tumors from patients of similar age. Families with HNPCC often include individuals with multiple primary cancers; the association of colorectal cancer with either ovarian or endometrial carcinomas is especially strong in women. It has been recommended that members of such families undergo biennial colonoscopy beginning at age 25 years, with intermittent pelvic ultrasonography and endometrial biopsy offered for potentially afflicted women; such a screening strategy has not yet been validated. HNPCC is associated with germline mutations of several genes, particularly *hMSH2* on chromosome 2 and *hMLH1* on chromosome 3. These mutations lead to errors in DNA replication and are thought to result in DNA instability because of defective repair of DNA mismatches, resulting in abnormal cell growth and tumor development. Testing tumor cells for "microsatellite instability" (sequence changes reflecting defective mismatch repair) in patients under age 50 with colorectal cancer and a positive family history for colorectal or endometrial cancer may identify probands with HNPCC.

INFLAMMATORY BOWEL DISEASE (See also Chap. 276) Large-bowel cancer is increased in incidence in patients with long-standing inflammatory bowel disease (IBD). Cancers develop more commonly in patients with ulcerative colitis than in those with granulomatous colitis, but this impression may result in part from the occasional difficulty of differentiating these two conditions. The risk of colorectal cancer in a patient with IBD is relatively small during the initial 10 years of the disease, but then it appears to increase at a rate of ~0.5 to 1% per year. Cancer may develop in 8 to 30% of patients after 25 years. The risk is higher in younger patients with pancolitis.

Cancer surveillance in patients with IBD is unsatisfactory. Symptoms such as bloody diarrhea, abdominal cramping, and obstruction, which may signal the appearance of a tumor, are similar to the complaints caused by a flare-up of the underlying disease. In patients with a history of IBD lasting ≥15 years who continue to experience exacerbations, the surgical removal of the colon can significantly reduce the risk for cancer and also eliminate the target organ for the underlying chronic gastrointestinal disorder. The value of such surveillance techniques as colonoscopy with mucosal biopsies and brushings for less symptomatic individuals with chronic IBD is uncertain. The lack of uniformity regarding the pathologic criteria that characterize dysplasia and the absence of data that such surveillance reduces the development of lethal cancers have made this costly practice an area of controversy.

OTHER HIGH-RISK CONDITIONS ■ *Streptococcus bovis* Bacteremia For unknown reasons, individuals who develop endocarditis or septicemia from this fecal bacteria have a high incidence of occult colorectal tumors and, possibly, upper gastrointestinal cancers as well. Endoscopic or radiographic screening appears advisable.

Ureterosigmoidostomy Colon cancer develops in 5 to 10% of people 15 to 30 years after ureterosigmoidostomy to correct congenital extrophy of the bladder. Neoplasms characteristically are found at a site distal to the ureteral implant where colonic mucosa is chronically exposed to both urine and feces.

Tobacco Use Cigarette smoking is linked to the development of colorectal adenomas, particularly after >35 years of tobacco use. No biologic explanation for this association has yet been proposed.

PRIMARY PREVENTION Several orally administered compounds have been assessed as possible inhibitors of colon cancer. The most effective class of these chemopreventive agents is aspirin and other NSAIDs, which are thought to suppress cell proliferation by inhibiting prostaglandin synthesis. Regular aspirin use reduces the risk for colonic adenomas and carcinomas as well as for death from large-bowel cancer; such use also appears to diminish the likelihood for developing additional premalignant adenomas following treatment for a prior colon carcinoma. This inhibiting effect of aspirin on colon carcinogenesis appears to increase with the duration of drug use. Oral folic acid supplements and oral calcium supplements reduce the risk of adenomatous polyps and colorectal cancers in case-controlled studies. While antioxidant vitamins such as ascorbic acid, tocopherols, and β-carotene are present in diets rich in fruits and vegetables, which have been associated with lower rates of colorectal cancer, they are ineffective at reducing the incidence of subsequent adenomas in patients who have undergone the removal of a colon adenoma. Estrogen-replacement therapy has been associated with a reduction in the risk of colorectal cancer in women, conceivably by an effect on bile acid synthesis and composition or by decreasing synthesis of IGF-I. The otherwise unexplained reduction in colorectal cancer mortality in women may be a result of the widespread use of estrogen replacement in postmenopausal individuals.

SCREENING The rationale for colorectal cancer screening programs is that the earlier detection of localized, superficial cancers in asymptomatic individuals will increase the surgical cure rate. Such screening programs are important for individuals having a family history of the disease in first-degree relatives. The relative risk for developing colorectal cancer increases to 1.75 in such individuals and may be even higher if the relative was afflicted before age 60. The prior use of proctosigmoidoscopy as a screening tool was based on the observation that 60% of early lesions are located in the rectosigmoid. For unexplained reasons, however, the proportion of large-bowel cancers arising in the rectum has been decreasing during the past several decades, with a corresponding increase in the proportion of cancers in the more proximal descending colon. As such, the potential for rigid proctosigmoidoscopy to detect a sufficient number of occult neoplasms to make the procedure cost-effective has been questioned. Flexible, fiberoptic sigmoidoscopes permit trained operators to visualize the colon for up to 60 cm, which enhances the capability for cancer detection. However, this technique still leaves the proximal half of the large bowel unscreened.

Most programs directed at the early detection of colorectal cancers have focused on digital rectal examinations and fecal occult blood testing. The digital examination should be part of any routine physical evaluation in adults older than age 40, serving as a screening test for prostate cancer in men, a component of the pelvic examination in women, and an inexpensive maneuver for the detection of masses in the rectum. The development of the Hemoccult test has greatly facilitated the detection of occult fecal blood. Unfortunately, even when performed optimally, the Hemoccult test has major limitations as a screening technique. About 50% of patients with documented colorectal cancers have a negative fecal Hemoccult test, consistent with the intermittent bleeding pattern of these tumors. When random cohorts of asymptomatic persons have been tested, 2 to 4% have Hemoccult-positive stools. Colorectal cancers have been found in <10% of these "test-positive" cases, with benign polyps being detected in an additional 20 to 30%. Thus, a colorectal neoplasm will not be found in most asymptomatic individuals with occult blood in their stool. Nonetheless, persons found to have Hemoccult-positive stool routinely undergo further medical evaluation, including sigmoidoscopy, barium

enema, and/or colonoscopy—procedures that are not only uncomfortable and expensive but also associated with a small risk for significant complications. The added cost of these studies would appear justifiable if the small number of patients found to have occult neoplasms because of Hemoccult screening could be shown to have an improved prognosis and prolonged survival. Prospectively controlled trials showed a statistically significant reduction in mortality from colorectal cancer for individuals undergoing annual screening. However, this benefit only emerged after >13 years of follow-up and was extremely expensive to achieve, since all positive tests (most of which were false-positive) were followed by colonoscopy. Moreover, these colonoscopic examinations quite likely provided the opportunity for cancer prevention through the removal of potentially premalignant adenomatous polyps since the eventual development of cancer was reduced by 20% in the cohort undergoing annual screening.

Screening techniques for large-bowel cancer in asymptomatic persons remain unsatisfactory. Compliance with any screening strategy within the general population is poor. At present, the American Cancer Society suggests fecal Hemoccult screening annually and flexible sigmoidoscopy every 5 years beginning at age 50 for asymptomatic individuals having no colorectal cancer risk factors. The American Cancer Society has proposed a "total colon examination" (i.e., colonoscopy or double-contrast barium enema) every 10 years as an alternative to Hemoccult testing with periodic flexible sigmoidoscopy. Colonoscopy has been shown to be superior to double-contrast barium enema and also to have a higher sensitivity for detecting villous or dysplastic adenomas or cancers than the strategy employing occult fecal blood testing and flexible sigmoidoscopy. Whether colonoscopy performed every 10 years beginning after age 50 will prove to be cost-effective and whether it may be supplanted as a screening maneuver by sophisticated radiographic techniques ("virtual colonoscopy") remains unclear. More effective techniques for screening are needed, perhaps taking advantage of the molecular changes that have been described in these tumors. Analysis of stool for mutation in the *APC* tumor-suppressor gene is being tested.

CLINICAL FEATURES ■ Presenting Symptoms Symptoms vary with the anatomic location of the tumor. Since stool is relatively liquid as it passes through the ileocecal valve into the right colon, cancers arising in the cecum and ascending colon may become quite large without resulting in any obstructive symptoms or noticeable alterations in bowel habits. Lesions of the right colon commonly ulcerate, leading to chronic, insidious blood loss without a change in the appearance of the stool. Consequently, patients with tumors of the ascending colon often present with symptoms such as fatigue, palpitations, and even angina pectoris and are found to have a hypochromic, microcytic anemia indicative of iron deficiency. Since the cancer may bleed intermittently, a random fecal occult blood test may be negative. As a result, the unexplained presence of iron-deficiency anemia in any adult (with the possible exception of a premenopausal, multiparous woman) mandates a thorough endoscopic and/or radiographic visualization of the entire large bowel (Fig. 77-1).

Since stool becomes more concentrated as it passes into the transverse and descending colon, tumors arising there tend to impede the passage of stool, resulting in the development of abdominal cramping, occasional obstruction, and even perforation. Radiographs of the abdomen often reveal characteristic annular, constricting lesions ("apple-core" or "napkin-ring") (Fig. 77-2).

Cancers arising in the rectosigmoid are often associated with hematochezia, tenesmus, and narrowing of the caliber of stool; anemia is an infrequent finding. While these symptoms may lead patients and their physicians to suspect the presence of hemorrhoids, the development of rectal bleeding and/or altered bowel habits demands a prompt digital rectal examination and proctosigmoidoscopy.

Staging, Prognostic Factors, and Patterns of Spread The prognosis for individuals having colorectal cancer is related to the depth of tumor

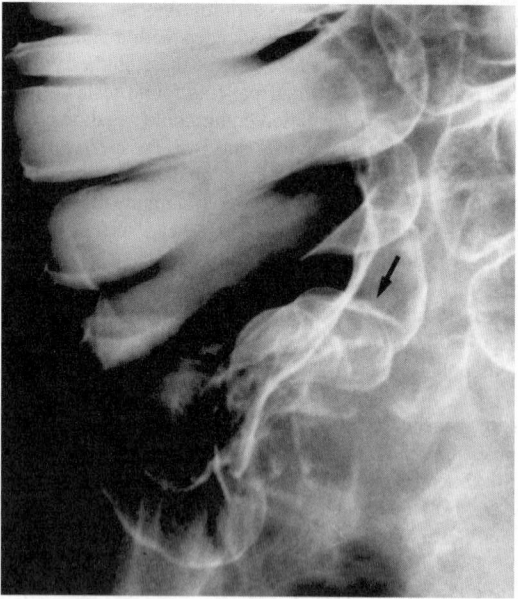

FIGURE 77-1   Double-contrast air-barium enema revealing a sessile tumor of the cecum in a patient with iron-deficiency anemia and guaiac-positive stool. The lesion at surgery was a stage B adenocarcinoma.

penetration into the bowel wall and the presence of both regional lymph node involvement and distant metastases. These variables are incorporated into the staging system introduced by Dukes and applied to a TNM classification method, in which T represents the depth of tumor penetration, N the presence of lymph node involvement, and M the presence or absence of distant metastases (Table 77-6). Superficial lesions that do not penetrate into the muscularis or involve regional lymph nodes are designated as *stage A* (T1N0M0) disease; tumors that penetrate more deeply but have not spread to lymph nodes are *stage B* disease [subclassified as stage B_1 (T2N0M0) if lesions are restricted to the muscularis and as stage B_2 (T3N0M0) if lesions involve or

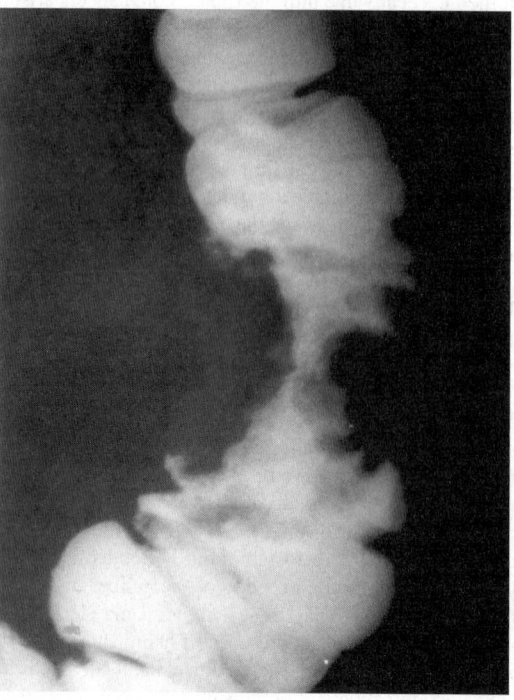

FIGURE 77-2   Annular, constricting adenocarcinoma of the descending colon. This radiographic appearance is referred to as an "apple-core" lesion and is always highly suggestive of malignancy.

TABLE 77-6   *Staging of and Prognosis for Colorectal Cancer*

Stage				Approximate 5-Year Survival, %
Dukes	TNM	Numerical	Pathologic Description	
A	T1N0M0	I	Cancer limited to mucosa and submucosa	>90
B_1	T2N0M0	I	Cancer extends into muscularis	85
B_2	T3N0M0	II	Cancer extends into or through serosa	70–80
C	TxN1M0	III	Cancer involves regional lymph nodes	35–65
D	TxNxM1	IV	Distant metastases (i.e., liver, lung)	5

penetrate the serosa]; regional lymph node involvement defines *stage C* (TxN1M0) disease; and metastatic spread to sites such as liver, lung, or bone indicates *stage D* (TxNxM1) disease. Unless gross evidence of metastatic disease is present, disease stage cannot be determined accurately before surgical resection and pathologic analysis of the operative specimens. It is not clear whether the detection of nodal metastases by special immunohistochemical molecular techniques has the same prognostic implications as disease detected by routine light microscopy.

Most recurrences after a surgical resection of a large-bowel cancer occur within the first 4 years, making 5-year survival a fairly reliable indicator of cure. The likelihood for 5-year survival in patients with colorectal cancer is stage-related (Table 77-6). That likelihood has improved during the past several decades when similar surgical stages have been compared. The most plausible explanation for this improvement appears to be more thorough intraoperative and pathologic staging. In particular, more exacting attention to pathologic detail has revealed that the prognosis following the resection of a colorectal cancer is not related merely to the presence or absence of regional lymph node involvement. Prognosis may be more precisely gauged by the number of involved lymph nodes (one to four lymph nodes versus five or more lymph nodes). Other predictors of a poor prognosis after a total surgical resection include tumor penetration through the bowel wall into pericolic fat, poorly differentiated histology, perforation and/or tumor adherence to adjacent organs (increasing the risk for an anatomically adjacent recurrence), and venous invasion by tumor (Table 77-7). Regardless of the clinicopathologic stage, a preoperative elevation of the plasma carcinoembryonic antigen (CEA) level predicts eventual tumor recurrence. The presence of aneuploidy and specific chromosomal deletions, such as allelic loss in chromosome 18q (involving the *DCC* gene) in tumor cells, appears to predict a higher risk for metastatic spread, particularly in patients with stage B_2 (T3N0M0) disease. Conversely, the detection of microsatellite instability in tumor tissue has been associated with a more favorable outcome. In contrast to most other cancers, the prognosis in colorectal cancer is not influenced by the size of the primary lesion when adjusted for nodal involvement and histologic differentiation.

TABLE 77-7   *Predictors of Poor Outcome Following Total Surgical Resection of Colorectal Cancer*

Tumor spread to regional lymph nodes
Number of regional lymph nodes involved
Tumor penetration through the bowel wall
Poorly differentiated histology
Perforation
Tumor adherence to adjacent organs
Venous invasion
Preoperative elevation of CEA titer (>5.0 ng/mL)
Aneuploidy
Specific chromosomal deletion (e.g., allelic loss on chromosome 18q)

Note: CEA, carcinoembryonic antigen.

Cancers of the large bowel generally spread to regional lymph nodes or to the liver via the portal venous circulation. The liver represents the most frequent visceral site of metastatic dissemination; it is the initial site of distant spread in one-third of recurring colorectal cancers and is involved in more than two-thirds of such patients at the time of death. In general, colorectal cancer rarely metastasizes to the lungs, supraclavicular lymph nodes, bone, or brain without prior spread to the liver. A major exception to this rule occurs in patients having primary tumors in the distal rectum, from which tumor cells may spread through the paravertebral venous plexus, escaping the portal venous system and thereby reaching the lungs or supraclavicular lymph nodes without hepatic involvement. The median survival after the detection of distant metastases is 6 to 9 months (hepatomegaly, abnormal liver chemistries) to 24 to 30 months (small liver nodule initially identified by elevated CEA level and subsequent CT scan).

℞ TREATMENT

Total resection of tumor is the optimal treatment when a malignant lesion is detected endoscopically or radiographically in the large bowel. An evaluation for the presence of metastatic disease, including a thorough physical examination, chest radiograph, biochemical assessment of liver function, and measurement of the plasma CEA level, should be performed before surgery. When possible, a colonoscopy of the entire large bowel should be performed to identify synchronous neoplasms and/or polyps. The detection of metastases should not preclude surgery in patients with tumor-related symptoms such as gastrointestinal bleeding or obstruction, but it often prompts the use of a less radical operative procedure. At the time of laparotomy, the entire peritoneal cavity should be examined, with thorough inspection of the liver, pelvis, and hemidiaphragm and careful palpation of the full length of the large bowel. Following recovery from a complete resection, patients should be observed carefully for 5 years by semiannual physical examinations and yearly blood chemistry measurements. If a complete colonoscopy was not performed preoperatively, it should be carried out within the first several postoperative months. Some authorities favor measuring plasma CEA levels at 3-month intervals because of the sensitivity of this test as a marker for otherwise undetectable tumor recurrence. Subsequent endoscopic or radiographic surveillance of the large bowel, probably at triennial intervals, is indicated, since patients who have been cured of one colorectal cancer have a 3 to 5% probability of developing an additional bowel cancer during their lifetime and a >15% risk for the development of adenomatous polyps. Anastomotic ("suture-line") recurrences are infrequent in colorectal cancer patients provided the surgical resection margins were adequate and free of tumor. Periodic CT screening, chest radiographs, or more frequent colonoscopic examinations do not affect prognosis and add unnecessary costs to postoperative surveillance.

Radiation therapy to the pelvis is recommended for patients with rectal cancer because it reduces the 20 to 25% probability of regional recurrences following complete surgical resection of stage B_2 or C tumors, especially if they have penetrated through the serosa. This alarmingly high rate of local disease recurrence is believed to be due to the fact that the contained anatomic space within the pelvis limits the extent of the resection and because the rich lymphatic network of the pelvic side wall immediately adjacent to the rectum facilitates the early spread of malignant cells into surgically inaccessible tissue. The use of sharp rather than blunt dissection of rectal cancers ("total mesorectal excision") appears to reduce the likelihood of local disease recurrence to ~10%. Radiation therapy, either pre- or postoperatively, reduces the likelihood of pelvic recurrences but does not appear to prolong survival. Preoperative radiotherapy is indicated for patients with large, potentially unresectable rectal cancers; such lesions may shrink enough to permit subsequent surgical removal. Radiation therapy is not effective in the primary treatment of colon cancer.

Chemotherapy in patients with advanced colorectal cancer has proven to be of only marginal benefit. 5-FU is the most effective single agent for this disease. Partial responses are obtained in 15 to 20% of patients. The probability of tumor response appears to be somewhat greater for patients with liver metastases when chemotherapy is infused directly into the hepatic artery, but intraarterial treatment is costly and toxic and does not appear to prolong survival. The concomitant administration of folinic acid (leucovorin) improves the efficacy of 5-FU in patients with advanced colorectal cancer, presumably by enhancing the binding of 5-FU to its target enzyme, thymidylate synthase. A threefold improvement in the partial response rate is noted when folinic acid is combined with 5-FU; however, the effect on survival is marginal, and the optimal dose schedule remains to be defined. 5-FU is generally administered intravenously but may also be given orally in the form of capecitabine with seemingly similar efficacy.

Irinotecan (CPT-11), a topoisomerase 1 inhibitor, prolongs survival when compared to supportive care in patients whose disease has progressed on 5-FU. Furthermore, the addition of irinotecan to 5-FU and leucovorin (LV) improves response rates and survival of patients with metastatic disease. The *FOLFIRI regimen* is as follows: irinotecan, 180 mg/m² as a 90-min infusion day 1; LV, 400 mg/m² as a 2-h infusion during irinotecan, immediately followed by 5-FU bolus, 400 mg/m² and 46-h continuous infusion of 2.4 to 3 g/m² every 2 weeks. Oxaliplatin, a platinum analogue, also improves the response rate when added to 5-FU and LV as initial treatment of patients with metastatic disease. The *FOLFOX regimen* is the following: 2-h infusion of LV (200 mg/m² per day) followed by a 5-FU bolus (400 mg/m² per day) and 22-h infusion (600 mg/m² per day) for 2 consecutive days every 2 weeks, together with oxaliplatin, 85 mg/m² as a 2-h infusion on day 1.

Patients with solitary hepatic metastases without clinical or radiographic evidence of additional tumor involvement should be considered for partial liver resection, because such procedures are associated with 5-year survival rates of 25 to 30% when performed on selected individuals by experienced surgeons.

The administration of 5-FU and LV for 6 months after resection of tumor in patients with stage C disease leads to a 40% decrease in recurrence rates and 30% improvement in survival. Patients with stage B_2 tumors do not appear to benefit from adjuvant therapy. In rectal cancer, the delivery of postoperative (and probably preoperative) combined modality therapy (5-FU plus radiation therapy) reduces the risk of recurrence and increases the chance of cure for patients with stages B_2 and C tumors. The 5-FU acts as a radiosensitizer when delivered together with radiation therapy. A surprising lack of use of life-extending adjuvant therapy has been documented in patients over age 65 years. This age bias is completely inappropriate as the benefits of adjuvant therapy have been documented in patients over age 65 years.

TUMORS OF THE SMALL INTESTINE

Small-bowel tumors comprise <5% of gastrointestinal neoplasms. Because of their rarity, a correct diagnosis is often delayed. Abdominal symptoms are usually vague and poorly defined, and conventional radiographic studies of the upper and lower intestinal tract often appear normal. Small-bowel tumors should be considered in the differential diagnosis in the following situations: (1) recurrent, unexplained episodes of crampy abdominal pain; (2) intermittent bouts of intestinal obstruction, especially in the absence of IBD or prior abdominal surgery; (3) intussusception in the adult; and (4) evidence of chronic intestinal bleeding in the presence of negative conventional contrast radiographs. A careful small-bowel barium study is the diagnostic procedure of choice; the diagnostic accuracy may be improved by infusing barium through a nasogastric tube placed into the duodenum (enteroclysis).

BENIGN TUMORS The histology of benign small-bowel tumors is difficult to predict on clinical and radiologic grounds alone. The symptomatology of benign tumors is not distinctive, with pain, obstruction, and hemorrhage being the most frequent symptoms. These tumors are usually discovered during the fifth and sixth decades of life, more often in the distal rather than the proximal small intestine. The most common benign tumors are adenomas, leiomyomas, lipomas, and angiomas.

Adenomas   These tumors include those of the islet cells and Brunner's glands as well as polypoid adenomas. *Islet cell adenomas* are occasionally located outside the pancreas; the associated syndromes are discussed in Chap. 329. *Brunner's gland adenomas* are not truly neoplastic but represent a hypertrophy or hyperplasia of submucosal duodenal glands. These appear as small nodules in the duodenal mucosa that secrete a highly viscous alkaline mucus. Most often, this is an incidental radiographic finding not associated with any specific clinical disorder.

Polypoid Adenomas   About 25% of benign small-bowel tumors are polypoid adenomas (Table 77-5). They may present as single polypoid lesions or, less commonly, as papillary villous adenomas. As in the colon, the sessile or papillary form of the tumor is sometimes associated with a coexisting carcinoma. Occasionally, patients with Gardner's syndrome develop premalignant adenomas in the small bowel; such lesions are generally in the duodenum. Multiple polypoid tumors may occur throughout the small bowel (and occasionally the stomach and colorectum) in the Peutz-Jeghers syndrome. The polyps are usually hamartomas (juvenile polyps) having a low potential for malignant degeneration. Mucocutaneous melanin deposits as well as tumors of the ovary, breast, pancreas, and endometrium are also associated with this autosomal dominant condition.

Leiomyomas   These neoplasms arise from smooth-muscle components of the intestine and are usually intramural, affecting the overlying mucosa. Ulceration of the mucosa may cause gastrointestinal hemorrhage of varying severity. Cramping, intermittent abdominal pain is frequently encountered.

Lipomas   These tumors occur with greatest frequency in the distal ileum and at the ileocecal valve. They have a characteristic radiolucent appearance, are usually intramural and asymptomatic, but on occasion cause bleeding.

Angiomas   While not true neoplasms, these lesions are important because they frequently cause intestinal bleeding. They may take the form of telangiectasia or hemangiomas. Multiple intestinal telangiectasias occur in a nonhereditary form confined to the gastrointestinal tract or as part of the hereditary Osler-Rendu-Weber syndrome. Vascular tumors may also take the form of isolated hemangiomas, most commonly in the jejunum. Angiography, especially during bleeding, is the best procedure for evaluating these lesions.

MALIGNANT TUMORS   While rare, small-bowel malignancies occur in patients with long-standing regional enteritis and celiac sprue as well as in individuals with AIDS. Malignant tumors of the small bowel are frequently associated with fever, weight loss, anorexia, bleeding, and a palpable abdominal mass. After ampullary carcinomas (many of which arise from biliary or pancreatic ducts), the most frequently occurring small-bowel malignancies are adenocarcinomas, lymphomas, carcinoid tumors, and leiomyosarcomas.

Adenocarcinomas   The most common primary cancers of the small bowel are adenocarcinomas, accounting for ~50% of malignant tumors. These cancers occur most often in the distal duodenum and proximal jejunum, where they tend to ulcerate and cause hemorrhage or obstruction. Radiologically, they may be confused with chronic duodenal ulcer disease or with Crohn's disease if the patient has long-standing regional enteritis. The diagnosis is best made by endoscopy and biopsy under direct vision. Surgical resection is the treatment of choice.

Lymphomas   Lymphoma in the small bowel may be primary or secondary. A diagnosis of a primary intestinal lymphoma requires histologic confirmation in a clinical setting in which palpable adenopathy and hepatosplenomegaly are absent and no evidence of lymphoma is seen on chest radiograph, CT scan, or peripheral blood smear or on bone marrow aspiration and biopsy. Symptoms referable to the small bowel are present, usually accompanied by an anatomically discernible

lesion. Secondary lymphoma of the small bowel consists of involvement of the intestine by a lymphoid malignancy extending from involved retroperitoneal or mesenteric lymph nodes (Chap. 97).

Primary intestinal lymphoma accounts for ~20% of malignancies of the small bowel. These neoplasms are non-Hodgkin's lymphomas; they usually have a diffuse, large-cell histology and are of T cell origin. Intestinal lymphoma involves the ileum, jejunum, and duodenum, in decreasing frequency, a pattern that mirrors the relative amount of normal lymphoid cells in these anatomic areas. The risk of small-bowel lymphoma is increased in patients with a prior history of malabsorptive conditions (e.g., celiac sprue), regional enteritis, and depressed immune function due to congenital immunodeficiency syndromes, prior organ transplantation, autoimmune disorders, or AIDS.

The development of localized or nodular masses that narrow the lumen results in periumbilical pain (made worse by eating) as well as weight loss, vomiting, and occasional intestinal obstruction. The diagnosis of small-bowel lymphoma may be suspected from the appearance on contrast radiographs of patterns such as infiltration and thickening of mucosal folds, mucosal nodules, areas of irregular ulceration, or stasis of contrast material. The diagnosis can be confirmed by surgical exploration and resection of involved segments. Intestinal lymphoma can occasionally be diagnosed by peroral intestinal mucosal biopsy, but since the disease mainly involves the lamina propria, full-thickness surgical biopsies are usually required.

Resection of the tumor constitutes the initial treatment modality. While postoperative radiation therapy has been given to some patients following a total resection, most authorities favor short-term (three cycles) systemic treatment with combination chemotherapy. The frequent presence of widespread intraabdominal disease at the time of diagnosis and the occasional multicentricity of the tumor often make a total resection impossible. The probability of sustained remission or cure is ~75% in patients with localized disease but is ~25% in individuals with unresectable lymphoma. In patients whose tumors are not resected, chemotherapy may lead to bowel perforation.

A unique form of small-bowel lymphoma, diffusely involving the entire intestine, was first described in oriental Jews and Arabs and is referred to as *immunoproliferative small intestinal disease* (IPSID), *Mediterranean lymphoma,* or α-heavy chain disease. This is a B cell tumor. The typical presentation includes chronic diarrhea and steatorrhea associated with vomiting and abdominal cramps; clubbing of the digits may be observed. A curious feature in many patients with IPSID is the presence in the blood and intestinal secretions of an abnormal IgA that contains a shortened α-heavy chain and is devoid of light chains. It is suspected that the abnormal α chains are produced by plasma cells infiltrating the small bowel. The clinical course of patients with IPSID is generally one of exacerbations and remissions, with death frequently resulting from either progressive malnutrition and wasting or the development of an aggressive lymphoma. The use of oral antibiotics such as tetracycline appears to be beneficial in the early phases of the disorder, suggesting a possible infectious etiology. Combination chemotherapy has been administered during later stages of the disease, with variable results. Results are better when antibiotics and chemotherapy are combined.

Carcinoid Tumors   Carcinoid tumors arise from argentaffin cells of the crypts of Lieberkühn and are found from the distal duodenum to the ascending colon, areas embryologically derived from the midgut. More than 50% of intestinal carcinoids are found in the distal ileum, with most congregating close to the ileocecal valve. Most intestinal carcinoids are asymptomatic and of low malignant potential, but invasion and metastases may occur, leading to the carcinoid syndrome (Chap. 329).

Leiomyosarcomas   Leiomyosarcomas often are >5 cm in diameter and may be palpable on abdominal examination. Bleeding, obstruction, and perforation are common. Such tumors should be analyzed for the expression of mutant c-*kit* receptor (defining GIST), and in the presence of metastatic disease, justifying treatment with imatinib mesylate (Gleevec).

CANCERS OF THE ANUS

Cancers of the anus account for 1 to 2% of the malignant tumors of the large bowel. Most such lesions arise in the anal canal, the anatomic area extending from the anorectal ring to a zone approximately halfway between the pectinate (or dentate) line and the anal verge. Carcinomas arising proximal to the pectinate line (i.e., in the transitional zone between the glandular mucosa of the rectum and the squamous epithelium of the distal anus) are known as basaloid, cuboidal, or cloacogenic tumors; about one-third of anal cancers have this histologic pattern. Malignancies arising distal to the pectinate line have a squamous cell histology, ulcerate more frequently, and constitute ~55% of anal cancers. The prognosis for patients with basaloid and squamous cell cancers of the anus is identical when corrected for tumor size and the presence or absence of nodal spread.

The development of anal cancer is associated with infection by human papillomavirus, the same organism etiologically linked to cervical cancer. The virus is sexually transmitted. The infection may lead to anal warts (condyloma accuminata), which may progress to anal intraepithelial neoplasia and on to squamous cell carcinoma. The risk for anal cancer is increased among homosexual males, presumably related to anal intercourse. Anal cancer risk is increased in both men and women with AIDS, possibly because their immunosuppressed state permits more severe papillomavirus infection. Anal cancers occur most commonly in middle-aged persons and are more frequent in women than men. At diagnosis, patients may experience bleeding, pain, sensation of a perianal mass, and pruritus.

Radical surgery (abdominal-perineal resection with lymph node sampling and a permanent colostomy) used to be the treatment of choice for this tumor type. The 5-year survival rate after such a procedure was 55 to 70% in the absence of spread to regional lymph nodes and <20% if nodal involvement was present. An alternative therapeutic approach combining external beam radiation therapy with concomitant chemotherapy has resulted in biopsy-proven disappearance of all tumor in >80% of patients whose initial lesion was <3 cm in size. Tumor has recurred in <10% of these patients, and ~70% of patients with anal cancers can be cured with nonoperative treatment. Surgery should be reserved for the minority of individuals who are found to have residual tumor after being managed initially with radiation therapy combined with chemotherapy.

FURTHER READING

BARON JA et al: A randomized trial of aspirin to prevent colorectal adenomas. N Engl J Med 348:391, 2003

CRUMP W et al: Lymphoma of the gastrointestinal tract. Semin Oncol 26:324, 1999

DEMETRI GD et al: Efficacy and safety of imatinib mesylate in advanced gastrointestinal stromal tumors. N Engl J Med 347:472, 2002

ENZINGER PC, MAYER RJ: Esophageal cancer. N Engl J Med 349:2241, 2003

FUCHS CS, MAYER RJ: Gastric carcinoma. N Engl J Med 333:32, 1995

LYNCH HT, DE LA CHAPELLE A: Hereditary colorectal cancer. N Engl J Med 348:919, 2003

MACDONALD JS, ASTROW AB: Adjuvant therapy of colon cancer. Semin Oncol 28:30, 2001

RYAN DP et al: Carcinoma of the anal canal. N Engl J Med 342:792, 2000

SPECHLER SJ: Barrett's esophagus. N Engl J Med 346:836, 2002

UEMURA N et al: *Helicobacter pylori* infection and the development of gastric cancer. N Engl J Med 345:784, 2001

WALSH JME, TERDIMAN JP: Colorectal cancer screening. JAMA 289:1288, 2003

78 TUMORS OF THE LIVER AND BILIARY TRACT
Jules L. Dienstag, Kurt J. Isselbacher

BENIGN LIVER TUMORS

HEPATOCELLULAR ADENOMAS Hepatocellular adenomas are benign tumors of the liver found predominantly in women in their third and fourth decades. Their preponderance in women suggests a hormonal influence in their pathogenesis, and oral contraceptives are thought to contribute. The risk of liver adenomas is increased among those who take anabolic steroids and exogenous androgens. Multiple hepatic adenomas have been associated with glycogen storage disease type I.

Hepatic adenomas occur predominantly in the right lobe of the liver, may be multiple, and are often quite large (>10 cm). Microscopically, they consist of normal or slightly atypical hepatocytes. These cells contain increased glycogen, making them appear paler and larger than normal. Clinical features include pain and the presence of a palpable mass or features of intratumor hemorrhage (pain and circulatory collapse). The diagnosis is usually made by a combination of techniques: sonography, computed tomography (CT), magnetic resonance imaging (MRI), selective hepatic arteriography, and radionuclide scans. The angiographic appearance is typically hypervascular but often also includes hypovascular regions. Technetium 99m scans usually show a defect, because phagocytosing Kupffer cells are absent. Like hepatocellular carcinomas, adenomas have a T_1-intense MRI appearance. The risk of malignant change is small; the risk is higher for large (>10 cm) and multiple adenomas.

Management involves imaging surveillance for small tumors. If the lesion is large (8 to 10 cm), near the surface, and resectable, surgical removal is appropriate. A patient with liver adenoma should stop taking oral contraceptives. Surgical resection may be required for tumors that do not shrink after oral contraceptives are stopped. Pregnancy increases the risk of hemorrhage and should be avoided in women with large adenomas. Patients with multiple large adenomas (e.g., those with glycogen-storage disease) may benefit from liver transplantation.

FOCAL NODULAR HYPERPLASIA Focal nodular hyperplasia is a benign tumor often identified incidentally on imaging studies or at laparoscopy done for other reasons. Like hepatic adenomas, it occurs predominantly in women; however, oral contraceptives are not implicated, and hemorrhage and necrosis are rare. The risk of hemorrhage, however, appears to be higher in women taking oral contraceptives. Typically, the lesion is a solid tumor, often in the right lobe, with a fibrous core and stellate projections. The fibrous projections contain atypical hepatocytes, biliary epithelium, Kupffer cells, and inflammatory cells. A technetium scan will usually show a hot spot because of the presence of Kupffer cells. The lesion appears vascular on angiography, and septations may be detectable by angiography, helical CT scan, and, most reliably, MRI, but only rarely by ultrasound. Surgery is indicated only for symptomatic lesions.

HEMANGIOMA AND OTHER BENIGN TUMORS *Hemangiomas* are the most common benign liver tumors, occurring predominantly in women and usually detected incidentally. The prevalence in the general population is in the range of 0.5 to 7.0%. These asymptomatic vascular lesions can be identified by MRI, contrast-enhanced CT, labeled red blood cell nuclide scans, or hepatic angiography. They do not need to be removed unless they are large and are producing a mass effect. Hemorrhage is rare, and malignant change does not occur.

Nodular regenerative hyperplasia consists of multiple hepatic nodules resulting from periportal hepatocyte regeneration with surrounding atrophy. It may be associated with an underlying condition such as malignancy or connective tissue disease. Portal hypertension (in the absence of cirrhosis) is the most common clinical manifestation. Other less common benign hepatic lesions include *bile duct adenomas* and *cystadenomas*.

CARCINOMAS OF THE LIVER

HEPATOCELLULAR CARCINOMA ■ **Epidemiology and Etiology** Primary hepatocellular carcinoma (HCC) is one of the most common tumors in the world and the third most frequent cause of cancer mortality. It is especially prevalent in regions of Asia and sub-Saharan Africa, where the annual incidence is up to 500 cases per 100,000 population. In the United States and western Europe, it is much less common; however, the annual incidence in the United States has increased from 1.4 per 100,000 during 1976 to 1980 to 2.4 per 100,000 in the 1990s. HCC is up to 4 times more common in men than in women and usually arises in a cirrhotic liver. The incidence peaks in the fifth to sixth decades of life in western countries but 1 to 2 decades earlier in regions of Asia and Africa with a high prevalence of liver carcinoma.

The principal reason for the high incidence of HCC in parts of Asia and Africa is the frequency of chronic infection with *hepatitis B virus* (HBV) and *hepatitis C virus* (HCV). These chronic infections frequently lead to cirrhosis, which itself is an important risk factor for HCC (the risk of liver cancer in a cirrhotic liver is ~3% per year); 60 to 90% of these tumors occur in patients with macronodular cirrhosis. Studies in regions of Asia where HCC and HBV infection are prevalent have shown that the incidence of this cancer is about 100-fold higher in individuals with evidence of HBV infection than in noninfected controls, particularly in those with markers of high-level HBV replication, e.g., hepatitis B e antigen (HBeAg) (Chap. 285). In China, the lifetime risk of HCC in patients with chronic hepatitis B approaches 40%. In patients with HBV infection and HCC, HBV DNA may be integrated into host genomic DNA, both in the tumor cells and in adjacent, uninvolved hepatocytes. In addition, modifications of cellular gene expression occur by insertional mutagenesis, chromosomal rearrangements, or the transcriptional transactivating activity of the X and the pre-S2 regions of the HBV genome.

HCV also leads to HCC. HCV genetic material does not become integrated into host genomic DNA. Therefore, the mechanism of HCV carcinogenesis is unclear. Whether the ability of the HCV NS3 domain or the core protein to transform cells in vitro contributes to HCC in humans remains conjectural; alternatively, repeated cycles of liver regeneration and repair common in cirrhosis may permit the emergence of a malignant clone. In Europe and Japan, HCV appears to be substantially more prevalent than HBV in cases of HCC. Both HBV and HCV can be demonstrated in some patients, but the clinical course of liver malignancy in these patients does not appear to differ from that when only one virus is implicated. One distinction in high-prevalence areas between HCC associated with HBV infection and that associated with HCV infection is in the timing of onset. In Asia, HBV is acquired at birth via perinatal transmission, whereas HCV infection is acquired primarily during adulthood from transfused blood and injections. Correspondingly, the onset of HCC occurs one to two decades earlier in those with lifelong hepatitis B than in persons with adult-acquired hepatitis C. Retrospective analysis indicates that HCC occurs on average approximately 30 years after HCV infection and almost exclusively in patients with cirrhosis. The annual incidence of HCC in cirrhotic patients with chronic hepatitis C is 1.5 to 4%. Over the last decade, the frequency of HCC in Japan has increased substantially, primarily in patients with cirrhosis associated with chronic hepatitis C. The same trend is beginning to emerge in the United States and Europe; based on the known frequency of HCV-associated cirrhosis in these populations, the incidence of new HCC cases is expected to increase more than 250-fold over the next decade.

Any agent or factor that contributes to chronic, low-grade liver cell damage and mitosis makes hepatocyte DNA more susceptible to genetic alterations. Thus, as indicated above, *chronic liver disease* of any type is a risk factor and predisposes to the development of HCC. These conditions include alcoholic liver disease, α_1-antitrypsin deficiency, hemochromatosis, tyrosinemia, primary biliary cirrhosis, and even cirrhosis associated with nonalcoholic steatohepatitis. In Africa and southern China, *aflatoxin B_1* is an important public health hazard. This mycotoxin appears to induce a very specific G-to-T mutation at codon 249 in the tumor suppressor gene p53.

The loss, inactivation, or mutation of the p53 gene has been implicated in tumorigenesis and is the most common genetic derangement present in human cancers. Thus HBV and aflatoxin B_1 have been implicated in the pathogenesis of HCC in regions of Africa and southern China where both agents are prevalent.

In view of the male predominance of HCC, hormonal factors may also play a role. HCC may occur with long-term androgenic steroid administration, with exposure to thorium dioxide or vinyl chloride (see below), and possibly with exposure to estrogens in the form of oral contraceptives.

Clinical and Laboratory Features   HCC initially may escape clinical recognition because it occurs in patients with underlying cirrhosis, and the symptoms and signs may suggest progression of the underlying disease. The most common presenting features are abdominal *pain* with detection of an abdominal mass in the right upper quadrant. A *friction rub* or *bruit* may be heard over the liver. Blood-tinged ascites occurs in about 20% of cases. Jaundice is rare, unless significant deterioration of liver function or mechanical obstruction of the bile ducts occurs. Serum elevations of alkaline phosphatase and α fetoprotein (AFP) are common (see below). An abnormal type of prothrombin, des-γ-carboxy prothrombin, is made and correlates with AFP elevations.

A small percentage of patients with HCC have a *paraneoplastic syndrome*; erythrocytosis may result from erythropoietin-like activity produced by the tumor; hypercalcemia may result from secretion of a parathyroid-like hormone. Other manifestations may include hypercholesterolemia, hypoglycemia, polymyositis, acquired porphyria, dysfibrinogenemia, cryofibrinogenemia, and vasoactive peptide-associated diarrhea.

Imaging procedures to detect liver tumors include ultrasound, CT, MRI, and hepatic artery angiography (Chap. 271). Ultrasound is frequently used to screen high-risk populations and should be the first test if HCC is suspected; it is less costly than scans, is relatively sensitive, and can detect most tumors >3 cm. Helical CT and MRI (hyperintense T2-weighted imaging) scans are being used with increasing frequency and have higher sensitivities.

AFP levels >500 μg/L are found in about 70 to 80% of patients with HCC. Lower levels may be found in patients with large metastases from gastric or colonic tumors and in some patients with acute or chronic hepatitis. High levels of serum AFP (>500 to 1000 μg/L) in an adult with liver disease and without an obvious gastrointestinal tumor strongly suggest HCC. A rising level suggests progression of the tumor or recurrence after hepatic resection or therapeutic approaches such as ablation or chemoembolization (see below). The presence of an arterially enhancing liver mass >2 cm documented with two imaging procedures or with one imaging technique together with an AFP >400 ng/mL is highly suggestive of HCC.

Percutaneous *liver biopsy* can be diagnostic if the sample is taken from an area localized by ultrasound or CT. Because these tumors tend to be vascular, percutaneous biopsies should be done with caution. Another possible risk of liver biopsy is seeding the needle track with tumor; however, despite anecdotal reports, the likelihood of needle-track seeding is estimated to be as low as 0.006% and as high as 1%. Cytologic examination of ascitic fluid is invariably negative for tumor cells. Occasionally, *laparoscopy* or *minilaparotomy*, to permit liver biopsy under direct vision, may be used. This approach has the additional advantage of sometimes identifying patients who have a localized resectable tumor suitable for partial hepatectomy.

℞ TREATMENT

Staging of HCC is based on four criteria: tumor size (< or > 50% of the liver), ascites (absent or present), bilirubin (< or > 3 mg/dL), and albumin (< or >3 g/dL) to establish Okuda stages I (no positive criteria), II (1 or 2 positives), and III (3 or 4 positives). The Okuda system predicts clinical course better than the American Joint Cancer Commission TNM system. The natural history of each stage without treatment is as follows: stage I, 8 months; stage II, 2 months; stage III, less than 1 month. Several newly proposed staging systems take additional variables into account; however, none of the new systems has been validated. As screening for HCC has detected earlier tumors, survival has increased. Surgery alone can produce survivals of 54% at 1 year, 40% at 2 years, and 28% at 3 years when cancers are detected before symptoms appear.

The course of *clinically apparent* disease is rapid; if untreated, most patients die within 3 to 6 months of diagnosis. When HCC is detected very early by serial screening of AFP and ultrasound, survival is 1 to 2 years after resection. In selected cases, therapy may prolong life. *Surgical resection* offers a chance for cure; however, few patients have a resectable tumor at the time of presentation, because of underlying cirrhosis, involvement of both hepatic lobes, or distant metastases (common sites are lung, brain, bone, and adrenal), and the 5-year survival is low. Even after successful "curative" resection of HCC, the predisposing primary liver disorder (e.g., cirrhosis, hepatitis B) persists and new cancers can arise in the residual liver.

Screening for HCC in High-risk Patients Because 20 to 30% of patients with early HCC do not have elevated levels of circulating AFP, ultrasonographic screening is recommended along with AFP determination. In a study in the Far East, persons positive for hepatitis B surface antigen, with or without liver disease, were screened serially; a number of patients with small, subclinical tumors were identified and surgical resection was performed. Follow-up observation revealed a 5-year survival rate of 70% in this group and a 10-year survival rate of 50%. These Asian patients, however, were unusual in that they had minimal or no liver disease, and their tumors tended to be unifocal or encapsulated. In another study, AFP screening every 6 months (without ultrasound) among remote Native Alaskan populations of noncirrhotic patients with chronic hepatitis B led to improved survival rates compared with historic outcomes. These findings are in contrast with those of a study in a large population of Italian patients with cirrhosis, associated in most cases with chronic HBV and/or HCV infections. Screening every 3 to 12 months permitted the detection of a 3% annual incidence of cancer in this cohort but in most cases failed to achieve the goal of early detection of surgically treatable disease. No randomized study has yet shown a survival benefit for screening patients at high risk of HCC, but most clinicians screen high-risk patients with twice-annual AFP and ultrasound.

Liver transplantation may be considered as a therapeutic option; tumor recurrence or metastases are the major problems. Patients who have a single lesion ≤5 cm or three or fewer lesions ≤3 cm have survival after liver transplantation that is the same as survival after transplantation for nonmalignant liver disease (Chap. 291). Other approaches are primarily palliative and include (1) hepatic artery embolization and chemotherapy (chemoembolization), (2) alcohol or radiofrequency ablation via ultrasound-guided percutaneous injection, and (3) ultrasound-guided cryoablation. Radiofrequency ablation and surgical resection have been equally effective for potentially resectable HCC in some studies; 5-year survival >50% has been seen. Thus, some consider radiofrequency ablation as potentially curative. Unresectable HCC is usually managed by chemoembolization ("transcatheter arterial embolization"), but results have been mixed. Some randomized trials have shown no survival advantage. Two studies (from Hong Kong and Spain) showed >20% improvement in survival with chemoembolization compared to supportive care. The Hong Kong study mainly involved patients with hepatitis B given cisplatin chemotherapy. Survival at 1 (57%), 2 (31%), and 3 years (26%) was better than that seen in the supportive care group (32, 11, and 3%, respectively). The Spanish study mainly involved patients with hepatitis C given doxorubicin chemotherapy. Survival at 1 (82%) and 2 years (63%) in the chemoembolization group was superior to survival for supportive care (63 and 27%, respectively). Outcome is related to the experience of the treating institution; highly specialized centers obtain better results than those doing fewer procedures and those using less stringent criteria for intervention. The procedure may be complicated by a postembolization syndrome (fever, chills, abdominal pain, nausea, vomiting, leukocytosis) and transient (but occasionally irreversible) hepatic decompensation.

Treatment options for unresectable disease are limited. The liver cannot tolerate high doses of radiation and the disease is not responsive to chemotherapy. Investigative immunotherapy and gene therapy techniques have not yet been successful. Based on the presence of hormone receptors on the tumor, tamoxifen has been tested, but without success, and octreotide has shown some modest activity. In patients with resectable tumors, polyprenoic acid (a retinoic acid formulation) and intra-arterial ^{131}I-labeled lipiodol have been reported to reduce the rate of recurrence.

Prevention is the preferred strategy. Hepatitis B vaccine can prevent infection and its sequelae, and a reduction in HCC has been seen in Taiwan with the introduction of universal vaccination of children. Interferon treatment reduces the incidence of hepatic failure, death, and HCC in HBV-infected patients. Whether antiviral therapy with lamivudine, adefovir, or other agents (Chap. 287) will reduce the risk of HCC in HBV-infected cirrhotic patients is unknown. Interferon may lower the risk of HCC in patients with hepatitis C–related cirrhosis, but the evidence is mainly from retrospective studies that are confounded by lead-time bias. Prospective trials have produced conflicting results. Interferon may also reduce the risk of HCV-associated HCC recurrence after resection or percutaneous ablation.

OTHER MALIGNANT LIVER TUMORS

Fibrolamellar carcinoma differs from typical HCC in that it tends to occur in young adults without underlying cirrhosis. This tumor is nonencapsulated but well circumscribed and contains fibrous lamellae; it grows slowly and is associated with a longer survival if treated. Surgical resection has resulted in 5-year survivals >50%; if the lesion is nonresectable, liver transplantation is an option, and the outcome far exceeds that observed in the nonfibrolamellar variety of HCC. *Hepatoblastoma* is a tumor of infancy that typically is associated with very high serum AFP levels. The lesions are usually solitary, may be resectable, and have a better 5-year survival than that of HCC. *Angiosarcoma* consists of vascular spaces lined by malignant endothelial cells. Etiologic factors include prior exposure to thorium dioxide, polyvinyl chloride, arsenic, and androgenic anabolic steroids. *Epithelioid hemangioendothelioma* is of borderline malignancy; most cases are benign, but bone and lung metastases occur. This tumor occurs in early adulthood, presents with right upper quadrant pain, and is heterogeneous on sonography, hypodense on CT, and without neovascularity on angiography. Immunohistochemical staining reveals expression of factor VIII antigen. In the absence of extrahepatic metastases, these lesions can be treated by surgical resection or liver transplantation.

METASTATIC TUMORS Metastatic tumors of the liver are common, ranking second only to cirrhosis as a cause of fatal liver disease. In the United States, the incidence of metastatic carcinoma is at least 20 times greater than that of primary carcinoma. At autopsy, hepatic metastases occur in 30 to 50% of patients dying from malignant disease.

Pathogenesis The liver is uniquely vulnerable to invasion by tumor cells. Its size, high rate of blood flow, double perfusion by the hepatic artery and portal vein, and Kupffer cell filtration function combine to make it the next most common site of metastases after the lymph nodes. In addition, local tissue factors or endothelial membrane characteristics appear to enhance metastatic implants. Virtually all types of neoplasms except those primary in the brain may metastasize to the liver. The most common primary tumors are those of the gastrointestinal tract, lung, and breast, as well as melanomas. Less common are metastases from tumors of the thyroid, prostate, and skin.

Clinical Features Most patients with metastases to the liver present with symptoms referable only to the primary tumor, and the asymptomatic hepatic involvement is discovered in the course of clinical evaluation. Sometimes hepatic involvement is reflected by nonspecific symptoms of weakness, weight loss, fever, sweating, and loss of appetite. Rarely, features indicating active hepatic disease, especially abdominal pain, hepatomegaly, or ascites, are present. Patients with widespread metastatic liver involvement usually have clinical signs suggestive of cancer and hepatic enlargement. Some have localized induration or tenderness, and, occasionally, a friction rub may be found over tender areas of the liver.

Results of liver biochemical tests are often abnormal, but the elevations in marker levels are often only mild and nonspecific. These signs reflect the effects of fever and wasting as well as those of the infiltrating neoplastic process itself. An increase in serum alkaline phosphatase is the most common and frequently the only abnormality. Hypoalbuminemia, anemia, and occasionally a mild elevation of aminotransferase levels may also be found with more widespread disease. Substantially elevated serum levels of carcinoembryonic antigen are usually found when the metastases are from primary malignancies in the gastrointestinal tract, breast, or lung.

Diagnosis Evidence of metastatic invasion of the liver should be sought actively in any patient with a primary malignancy, especially of the lung, gastrointestinal tract, or breast, before resection of the primary lesion. An elevated level of alkaline phosphatase or a mass apparent on ultrasound, CT, or MRI examination of the liver may provide a presumptive diagnosis. Blind percutaneous needle biopsy of the liver will result in a positive diagnosis of metastatic disease in only 60 to 80% of cases with hepatomegaly and elevated alkaline phosphatase levels. Serial sectioning of specimens, two or three repeated biopsies, or cytologic examination of biopsy smears may increase the diagnostic yield by 10 to 15%. The yield is increased when biopsies are directed by ultrasound or CT or obtained during laparoscopy.

Rx TREATMENT

Most metastatic carcinomas respond poorly to all forms of treatment, which is usually only palliative. Rarely a single, large metastasis can be removed surgically. Systemic chemotherapy may slow tumor growth and reduce symptoms, but it does not alter the prognosis. Chemoembolization, intrahepatic chemotherapy, and alcohol or radiofrequency ablation may provide palliation.

CHOLANGIOCARCINOMA Benign tumors of the extrahepatic bile ducts are extremely rare causes of mechanical biliary obstruction. Most of these are papillomas, adenomas, or cystadenomas and present with obstructive jaundice or hemobilia. Adenocarcinoma of the extrahepatic ducts is more common. There is a slight male preponderance (60%), and the incidence peaks in the fifth to seventh decades. Apparent predisposing factors include (1) some chronic hepatobiliary parasitic infestations, (2) congenital anomalies with ectactic ducts, (3) sclerosing cholangitis and chronic ulcerative colitis, and (4) occupational exposure to possible biliary tract carcinogens (employment in rubber or automotive plants). Cholelithiasis is not clearly a predisposing factor for cholangiocarcinoma. The lesions of cholangiocarcinoma may be diffuse or nodular. Nodular lesions often arise at the bifurcation of the common bile duct (Klatskin tumors) and are usually associated with a *collapsed gallbladder*, a finding that mandates cholangiography to view proximal hepatic ducts.

Patients with cholangiocarcinoma usually present with biliary obstruction, painless jaundice, pruritus, weight loss, and acholic stools. A deep-seated, vaguely localized right upper quadrant pain may be noted. Hepatomegaly and a palpable, distended gallbladder (unless the lesion is high in the duct) are frequent accompanying signs. Fever is unusual unless associated with ascending cholangitis. Because the obstructing process is gradual, the cholangiocarcinoma is often far advanced by the time it presents clinically. The diagnosis is most frequently made by cholangiography following ultrasound demonstration of dilated intrahepatic bile ducts. Any focal strictures of the bile ducts should be considered malignant until proven otherwise. Endoscopic cholangiography permits obtaining specimens for cytology (sensitivity ~60%) and insertion of stents for biliary drainage. Survival of 1 to 2 years is possible in some cases. Perhaps 20% of patients have surgically resectable tumors, but 5-year survival is only 10 to 30%. The high recurrence rate limits the value of liver transplantation. Photodynamic therapy (intravenous hematoporphyrin with cholangioscopically delivered light) has been used with promising early results.

CARCINOMA OF THE PAPILLA OF VATER The ampulla of Vater may be involved by extension of tumor arising elsewhere in the duodenum or may itself be the site of origin of a sarcoma, carcinoid tumor, or adenocarcinoma. Papillary adenocarcinomas are associated with slow growth and a more favorable clinical prognosis than diffuse, infiltrative cancers of the ampulla, which are more frequently widely invasive. The presenting clinical manifestation is usually obstructive jaundice. Endoscopic retrograde cannulation of the pancreatic duct is the preferred diagnostic technique when ampullary carcinoma is suspected, because it allows for direct endoscopic inspection and biopsy of the ampulla and for pancreatography to exclude a pancreatic malignancy. Cancer of the papilla is usually treated by wide surgical excision. Lymph node or other metastases are present at the time of surgery in approximately 20% of cases, and the 5-year survival rate following surgical therapy in this group is only 5 to 10%. In the absence of metastases, radical pancreaticoduodenectomy (the Whipple procedure) is associated with 5-year survival rates as high as 40%.

CANCER OF THE GALLBLADDER Most cancers of the gallbladder develop in conjunction with stones rather than polyps. In patients with gallstones, the risk for developing gallbladder cancer, while increased, is still quite low. In one study, gallbladder cancer developed in only 5 of 2583 patients with gallstones followed for a median of 13 years. In the United States, adenocarcinomas make up the vast majority of the estimated 6500 new cases of gallbladder cancer diagnosed each year. The female/male ratio is 4:1, and the mean age at diagnosis is approximately 70 years. The clinical presentation is most often one of unremitting right upper quadrant pain associated with weight loss, jaundice, and a palpable right upper quadrant mass. Cholangitis may supervene. The preoperative diagnosis of the condition has been facilitated by ultrasound and CT, which are also useful in guiding fine-needle aspiration and biopsy. The presence on imaging of a calcified ("porcelain") gallbladder can suggest gallbladder carcinoma; however, cancer is associated with <25% of patients with porcelain gallbladder.

Once symptoms have appeared, spread of the tumor outside the gallbladder by direct extension or by lymphatic or hematogenous routes is almost invariable. Over 75% of gallbladder carcinomas are unresectable at the time of surgery, the exceptions being tumors discovered incidentally at laparotomy. If the tumor is found by the pathologist, no additional therapy is required. If the tumor is noted by the surgeon on routine cholecystectomy, a second operation is generally performed to resect the adjacent liver, bile duct, and local lymph nodes. Incidental resectable gallbladder tumors have a 50% 5-year survival. The 1-year mortality rate for unresectable disease is about 95%, and <5% of patients survive 5 years. Radical operative resection does not appear to improve survival. Trials of radiation and chemotherapy in patients with gallbladder cancer have been disappointing.

FURTHER READING

BEFELER AS, DI BISCEGLIE AM: Hepatocellular carcinoma: Diagnosis and treatment. Gastroenterology 122:1609, 2002

BRUIX J, LLOVET JM: Clinical management of hepatocellular carcinoma. Conclusions of the Barcelona-2000 EASL conference. J Hepatology 35:421, 2001

CHANG MH: Decreasing incidence of hepatocellular carcinoma among children following universal hepatitis B immunization. Liver Int 23:309, 2003

HASSOUN Z, GORES GJ: Treatment of hepatocellular carcinoma. Clin Gastroenterol Hepatol 1:10, 2003

LLOVET JM et al: Hepatocellular carcinoma. Lancet 362:1907, 2003

———— et al: Arterial embolisation of chemoembolisation versus symptomatic treatment in patients with unresectable hepatocellular carcinoma. A randomised controlled trial. Lancet 359:1734, 2002

YANG H-I et al: Hepatitis B e antigen and the risk of hepatocellular carcinoma. N Engl J Med 347:168, 2002

79 | PANCREATIC CANCER
Robert J. Mayer

INCIDENCE AND ETIOLOGY The incidence of pancreatic carcinoma in the United States has increased as the median life expectancy of the American population has lengthened. The tumor results in the death of >98% of afflicted patients. In 2004, 31,270 individuals died of pancreatic cancer making it the fourth most common cause of cancer-related mortality. The disease is more common in males than in females and in blacks than in whites. It rarely develops before the age of 50.

Little is known about the causes of pancreatic cancer. Cigarette smoking is the most consistent risk factor, with the disease being two to three times more common in heavy smokers than in nonsmokers. Whether this association is due to a direct carcinogenic effect of tobacco metabolites on the pancreas or an as yet undefined exposure that occurs more frequently in cigarette smokers is uncertain. Patients with chronic pancreatitis are at increased risk of pancreatic cancer, as are persons with long-standing diabetes mellitus. Obesity is a risk factor for pancreatic cancer; risk is directly related to increased calorie intake. Alcohol abuse or cholelithiasis are not risk factors for pancreatic cancer. Nor is pancreatic cancer associated with coffee consumption. Mutations in K-*ras* genes have been found in >85% of specimens of human pancreatic cancer. Pancreatic cancer has been associated with mutation of the $p16^{INK4}$ gene located on chromosome 9p21, a gene also implicated in the pathogenesis of malignant melanoma, as well as mutations of the *p53*, *DPC4*, and *BRCA2* tumor suppressor genes. A series of molecular events involving a sequence of these mutations has been proposed to occur as the normal pancreatic duct progresses through dysplasia to infiltrating carcinoma.

CLINICAL FEATURES More than 90% of pancreatic cancers are ductal adenocarcinomas, with islet cell tumors constituting the remaining 5 to 10%. Pancreatic cancers occur twice as frequently in the pancreatic head (70% of cases) as in the body (20%) or tail (10%) of the gland.

With the exception of jaundice, the initial symptoms associated with pancreatic cancer are often insidious and are usually present for >2 months before the cancer is diagnosed (Table 79-1). Pain and weight loss are present in >75% of patients. The pain typically has a gnawing, visceral quality, occasionally radiating from the epigastrium to the back. Pain is often a more severe problem in lesions arising in the body or tail of the gland, as such tumors may become quite large before being detected. Characteristically, the pain improves somewhat when the patient bends forward. The development of significant pain suggests retroperitoneal invasion and infiltration of the splanchnic nerves, indicating that the primary lesion is advanced and is not surgically resectable. Rarely, such pain may be transient and associated with hyperamylasemia, indicative of acute pancreatitis caused by ductal obstruction by tumor. The weight loss observed in most patients is primarily the result of anorexia, although in the initial period of the disease, subclinical malabsorption may also be a contributing factor.

Jaundice due to biliary obstruction is found in >80% of patients having tumors in the pancreatic head and is typically accompanied by dark urine, a claylike appearance of stool, and pruritus. In contrast to the "painless jaundice" sometimes observed in patients having carcinomas of the bile ducts, duodenum, or periampullary regions, most icteric individuals with ductal carcinomas of the pancreatic head will complain of significant abdominal discomfort. Although the gallbladder is usually enlarged in patients with carcinoma of the head of the pancreas, it is palpable in <50% (Courvoisier's sign). However, the presence of an enlarged gallbladder in a jaundiced patient without biliary colic should suggest malignant obstruction of the extrahepatic biliary tree.

Glucose intolerance, presumably a direct consequence of the tumor, often develops within 2 years of the clinical diagnosis. Other initial manifestations include venous thrombosis and migratory thrombophlebitis (Trousseau's syndrome), gastrointestinal hemorrhage from varices due to compression of the portal venous system by tumor, and splenomegaly caused by cancerous encasement of the splenic vein.

DIAGNOSTIC PROCEDURES (Fig. 79-1) Despite the availability of serologic tests for tumor-associated antigens such as the carcinoembryonic antigen (CEA) and CA 19-9 and noninvasive imaging techniques such as computed tomography (CT) and ultrasonography, the early diagnosis of a potentially resectable pancreatic carcinoma remains extremely difficult. The nonspecificity of the initial symptoms and the poor sensitivity of both serologic assays and noninvasive techniques have frustrated the development of effective screening procedures. When the disease is clinically suspected in a patient having vague, persistent abdominal complaints, ultrasound should be performed to visualize the gallbladder and the pancreas, as should upper gastrointestinal contrast radiographs to rule out a hiatal hernia or a peptic ulcer. If these studies fail to provide an explanation for the symptoms, a CT scan should be considered. It should encompass not only the pancreas but also the liver, retroperitoneal lymph nodes, and pelvis, as pancreatic cancer frequently spreads within the abdomen. While more costly than ultrasonography, CT is technically simpler and more reproducible, provides better definition of the body and tail of the pancreas, and requires less interpretive skill. CT generally detects a malignant pancreatic lesion in >80% of cases; in 5 to 15% of patients with proven pancreatic carcinoma, the CT scan shows only generalized pancreatic enlargement suggesting pancreatitis rather than malignancy. False-positive results occur in about 5 to 10% of cases in which no tumor was found on laparotomy. Magnetic resonance imaging (MRI), while not superior to CT in the evaluation of pancreatic lesions, may occasionally distinguish benign from malignant neoplasms. The value of positron emission tomography (PET) has not been determined. When clinical circumstances dictate additional diagnostic evaluation, endoscopic retrograde cholangiopancreatography (ERCP) with endoscopic ultrasonography (EUS) may clarify the cause of ambiguous CT or ultrasound findings. The characteristic findings are stenosis or obstruction of either the pancreatic or the common bile duct; both duct systems are abnormal in over half of cases. Carcinoma and chronic pancreatitis can be difficult to distinguish by ERCP, particularly if both diseases are present. False-negative results with ERCP are infrequent (<5%) and usually occur in the setting of islet cell, rather than ductal, carcinomas.

Angiography, once a commonly utilized means of detecting carcinomas in the body and tail of the pancreas, has been largely replaced as a diagnostic and staging procedure by spiral CT scanning with contrast imaging. This high-resolution technology predicts the resectability of the tumor if no disease is found outside the pancreas, obstruction of the superior mesenteric-portal vein confluence is absent, or tumor extension to the celiac axis and superior mesenteric arteries is not found. Radiographic staging criteria are shown in Table 79-2.

Regardless of the results of the above diagnostic studies, a histologic confirmation of pancreatic cancer is mandatory; similar radiographic and endoscopic findings can result from other neoplasms such as islet cell tumor or lymphoma, for which the therapeutic approach and prognosis differ from those for ductal carcinoma. In patients with unresectable disease or medical contraindications to surgical resection, tissue may be obtained through a percutaneous needle aspiration biopsy of the pancreas with CT or ultrasonographic guidance.

Unfortunately, however, even laparotomy may not provide a definitive diagnosis, because chronic pancreatitis may also produce a hard mass in the head of the pancreas indistinguishable from carcinoma by

---

TABLE 79-1 *Presenting Signs and Symptoms of Pancreatic Carcinoma*

Frequent	Infrequent
Abdominal pain	Glucose intolerance
Weight loss	Palpable gallbladder
Jaundice (lesions of pancreatic head only)	Migratory thrombophlebitis
	Gastrointestinal hemorrhage
	Splenomegaly

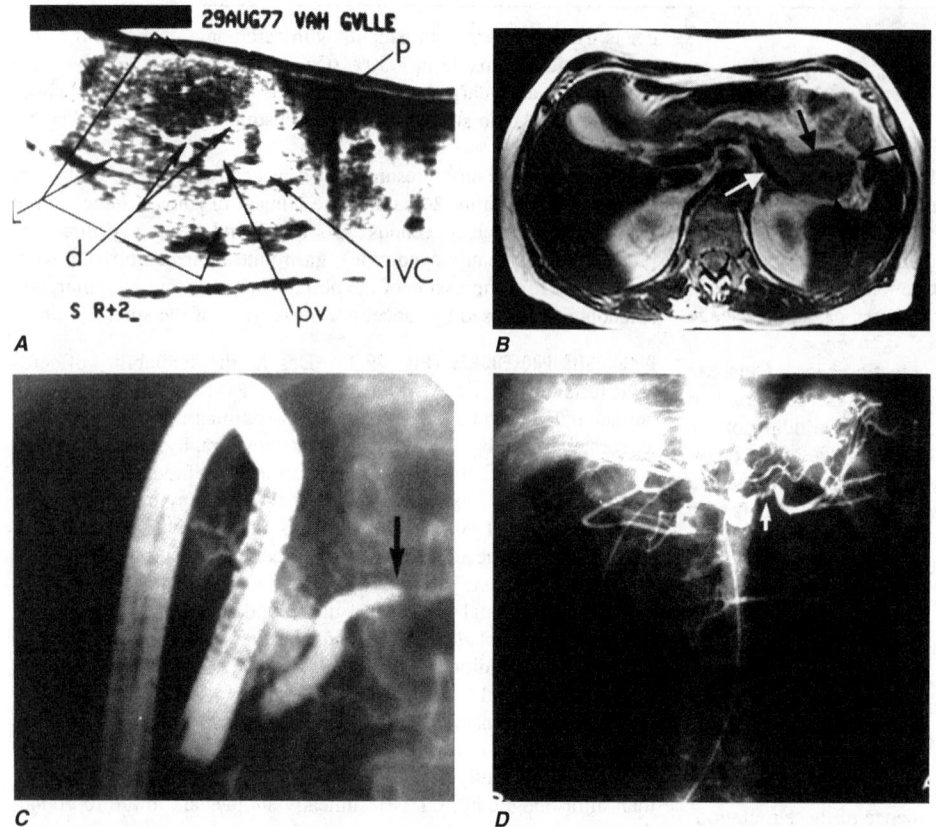

FIGURE 79-1 Carcinoma of the pancreas. *A.* Sonogram showing pancreatic carcinoma (P), dilated intrahepatic bile ducts (d), dilated portal vein (pv), and inferior vena cava (IVC). *B.* Computed tomography scan showing pancreatic carcinoma (*dark arrows*). *C.* Endoscopic retrograde showing abrupt cutoff of the duct of Wirsung (*arrow*). *D.* Arteriogram showing sheathing of splenic artery by tumor encasement (*arrow*).

palpation. Furthermore, a superficial biopsy of such a mass may not show neoplastic tissue, revealing only evidence of pancreatitis, as the cancer is often surrounded by edematous, inflamed, and fibrotic tissue (i.e., chronic pancreatitis).

℞ TREATMENT

Complete surgical resection of pancreatic tumors offers the only effective treatment for this disease. Unfortunately, such "curative" operations are only possible in 10 to 15% of patients with pancreatic cancer, usually those individuals with a tumor in the pancreatic head in whom jaundice was the initial symptom. Patients considered for such a procedure should have no evidence of metastatic spread on a chest radiograph and abdominal-pelvic CT scan and should be oper-

TABLE 79-2 *Clinical (Radiographic) Staging of Pancreatic Cancer*

Stage	Clinical/Radiographic Criteria
I	Resectable (T1–T2, selected T3,[a] NX, M0) No encasement of celiac axis or SMA Patent SMPV confluence No extrapancreatic disease
II	Locally advanced (T3, NX–1, M0) Arterial encasement (celiac axis or SMA) or venous occlusion (SMV or portal vein) No extrapancreatic disease
III	Metastatic (T1–3, NX–1, M1) Metastases typically to liver, peritoneum, and occasionally lung

[a] Resectable T3 lesions include those with isolated involvement of the SMV, portal vein, or hepatic artery without encasement of the celiac axis or SMA.

Note: T1, restricted to pancreas; T2, extension to duodenum, bile duct, or peripancreatic tissues; T3, extension to stomach, spleen, colon, or adjacent large vessels; NX, nodal status unknown; N0, regional nodes uninvolved; N1, regional nodes involved; M0, metastases absent; M1, metastases present; SMA, superior mesenteric artery; SMPV, superior mesenteric vein confluence with portal vein; SMV, superior mesenteric vein

ated on by an experienced surgeon, as mortality rates of >15% have been associated with this procedure. Curative resection is usually preceded by laparoscopic inspection of the abdomen to confirm absence of occult disease spread to the omentum, peritoneum, or liver, which would preclude curative resection. Although the potential for cure in patients with pancreatic cancer is restricted to the few who are able to undergo a complete surgical resection, the 5-year survival rate following such operations is only 10%. Nonetheless, the procedure is worth attempting, particularly for lesions in the pancreatic head, since ductal carcinomas often cannot be distinguished preoperatively from ampullary, duodenal, and distal bile duct tumors or pancreatic cyst adenocarcinomas, all of which have far higher rates of resectability and cure. Furthermore, patients who undergo resection and eventually experience disease recurrence survive three to four times longer than those whose tumor is not excised, indicating that such operations have a palliative effect. The risk for tumor recurrence is not affected by the type of operative procedure—i.e., total pancreatectomy versus pancreaticoduodenectomy ("Whipple resection")—but it is increased by the presence of lymph node metastases or tumor invasion into adjacent viscera. As a rule, pancreaticoduodenectomy or distal pancreatectomy seems preferable to total pancreatectomy because of the retention of exocrine function and avoidance of brittle diabetes.

The median survival for patients whose pancreatic cancers are surgically unresectable is 6 months. Management is directed at palliation of symptoms. Ambulatory patients having tumors in the pancreatic head should be considered for surgical diversion of the biliary system. If jaundice has already developed, therapeutic options include either nonoperative biliary decompression by endoscopic or percutaneous, transhepatic biliary drainage or surgical biliary bypass. External beam radiation in patients with unresectable tumors that have not spread beyond the pancreas does not appear to prolong survival, although a sufficient reduction in tumor size may lead to palliation of pain. However, the addition of chemotherapy with fluorouracil (5-FU) or gemcitabine to external beam irradiation has increased the survival time for these patients, presumably because the drugs act as radiosensitizing agents. In a small patient population, a combination of radiation therapy and 5-FU prolonged the survival and increased the cure rate compared to an untreated control group who had a complete surgical resection of their pancreatic cancer. Attempts at confirming this observation have resulted in controversial outcomes. The possibility of administering such chemoradiation therapy at diagnosis and before surgery (neoadjuvant treatment) to increase the potential for resectability is under investigation. Intraoperative radiation therapy has the potential to deliver higher doses of radiation to the tumor while sparing neighboring tissues but does not give better results than external beam treatment.

Chemotherapy in the management of patients with widely metastatic pancreatic cancer has been disappointing. Gemcitabine, a deoxycytidine analogue, produces improvement in the quality of life for patients with advanced pancreatic cancer. However, duration of survival is only modestly improved. Newer forms of treatment, including combining gemcitabine with other cytotoxic agents or therapies directed at specific molecular targets, such as the epidermal growth factor receptor or the vascular endothelial growth factor receptor are being evaluated. Experimental therapy should constitute the initial treatment for consenting, ambulatory patients. →*Pancreatic endocrine tumors are discussed in Chap. 329.*

FURTHER READING

ADAMEK HE et al: Pancreatic cancer detection with magnetic resonance cholangiopancreatography and endoscopic retrograde cholangiopancreatography: A prognostic controlled study. Lancet 356:190, 2000

BURRIS HA et al: Improvements in survival and clinical benefit with gemcitabine as first-line therapy for patients with advanced pancreatic cancer. A randomized trial. J Clin Oncol 15:2403, 1997

CONLON KC et al: Long-term survival after curative resection for pancreatic ductal adenocarcinoma. Clinicopathologic analysis of 5-year survivors. Ann Surg 223:273, 1996

HALLER DG: New perspectives in the management of pancreas cancer. Semin Oncol 30(suppl 11):3, 2003

HANSEL DE et al: Molecular pathogenesis of pancreatic cancer. Annu Rev Genomics Hum Genet 4:237, 2003

NEOPTOLEMOS JP et al: Adjuvant chemoradiotherapy and chemotherapy in resectable pancreatic cancer: A randomised controlled trial. Lancet 358: 1576, 2001

80 BLADDER AND RENAL CELL CARCINOMAS
Howard I. Scher, Robert J. Motzer

BLADDER CANCER

A transitional cell epithelium lines the urinary tract from the renal pelvis to the ureter, urinary bladder, and the proximal two-thirds of the urethra. Cancers can occur at any point: 90% of malignancies develop in the bladder, 8% develop in the renal pelvis, and the remaining 2% develop in the ureter or urethra. Bladder cancer is the fourth most common cancer in men and the tenth in women, with an estimated 60,240 new cases and 12,710 deaths predicted for the year 2004. The almost 5:1 ratio of incidence to mortality reflects the higher frequency of the less lethal superficial variants compared to the more lethal invasive and metastatic variants. The incidence is four times higher in men than in women, and twofold higher in whites than blacks, with a median age at diagnosis of 65 years. Once diagnosed, urothelial tumors exhibit polychronotropism—the tendency to recur over time and in new locations in the urothelial tract. As long as urothelium is present, continuous monitoring of the tract is required.

EPIDEMIOLOGY Cigarette smoking is believed to contribute to up to 50% of the diagnosed urothelial cancers in men and up to 40% in women. The risk of developing a urothelial malignancy in male smokers is increased two- to fourfold relative to nonsmokers and continues for 10 years or longer after cessation. Other implicated agents include the aniline dyes, the drugs phenacetin and chlornaphazine, and external beam radiation. Chronic cyclophosphamide exposure may also increase risk, whereas vitamin A supplements appear to be protective. Exposure to *Schistosoma haematobium*, a parasite found in many developing countries, is associated with an increase in both squamous and transitional cell carcinomas of the bladder.

PATHOLOGY More than 95% of urothelial tumors in the United States are transitional cell in origin. Pure squamous cancers with keratinization constitute 3%, adenocarcinomas 2%, and small cell tumors (with paraneoplastic syndromes) <1%. Adenocarcinomas develop primarily in the urachal remnant in the dome of the bladder or in the periurethral tissues; some assume a signet cell histology. Lymphomas or melanomas are rare. Clinical subtypes are grouped into three categories: 75% are superficial, 20% invade muscle, and 5% present with de novo metastatic disease. Of the transitional cell tumors, low-grade papillary lesions that grow on a central stalk are most common. These tumors are very friable, have a tendency to bleed, are at high risk for recurrence, and yet rarely progress to the more lethal invasive variety. About half of all invasive tumors progressed from a superficial stage. In contrast, carcinoma in situ (CIS) is a high-grade tumor that is considered a precursor of the more lethal muscle-infiltrating cancers. Tumors are rated by histologic type and grade. Grade I lesions (highly differentiated tumors) rarely progress to a higher stage, whereas grade III tumors do.

PATHOGENESIS The multicentric nature of the disease and high rate of recurrence has led to the hypothesis of a field defect in the urothelium. Molecular genetic analyses suggest that the superficial and invasive lesions develop along distinct pathways in which primary tumorigenic aberrations precede secondary changes associated with progression to a more advanced stage. Deletions of 9q are an early event; 3p and 5q deletions occur more frequently in invasive lesions. Deletions at the *TP53* locus on 17p, the *DCC* locus on 18q, and the *RB* locus on 13q24 have been seen only in invasive disease. Deletions of 3p and 11p occur in both superficial and invasive tumors. Within all clinical stages, including Tis, T1, and T2 or greater lesions, tumors with altered *TP53* have a higher risk of metastasis and death from disease.

CLINICAL PRESENTATION, DIAGNOSIS, AND STAGING Hematuria occurs in 80 to 90% of patients and often reflects exophytic tumors. Irritative symptoms are the next most common presentation and may reflect in situ disease. The bladder is the most common source of gross hematuria (40%), but benign cystitis (22%) is a more common cause than bladder cancer (15%) (Chap. 40). Microscopic hematuria is more commonly of prostate origin (25%); only 2% of bladder cancers produce microscopic hematuria. Once hematuria is documented, a urinary cytology, visualization of the urothelial tract by computed tomography (CT) or intravenous pyelogram (IVP), and cystoscopy are recommended, if no other etiology is found. Screening asymptomatic individuals for hematuria increases the diagnosis of tumors at an early stage but has not been shown to prolong life. Obstruction of the ureters may cause flank pain. Symptoms of metastatic disease are rarely the first presenting sign.

The endoscopic evaluation includes an examination under anesthesia to determine whether a palpable mass is present. A flexible endoscope is inserted into the bladder, and a bladder barbotage is performed. The visual inspection includes mapping the location, size, and number of lesions, as well as a description of the growth pattern (solid vs papillary). An intraoperative video is often recorded. All visible tumors should be resected, and a sample of the muscle underlying the tumor should be obtained to assess the depth of invasion. Normal mucosal areas are biopsied at random to ensure no field defect. A notation is made as to whether a tumor was completely or incompletely resected. Selective catheterization and visualization of the upper tracts should be performed if the cytology is positive and no disease is visible in the bladder. Ultrasonography, CT, and/or magnetic resonance imaging (MRI) may help to determine whether a tumor extends to perivesical fat (T3), and to document nodal spread. Distant metastases are assessed by CT of the chest and abdomen, MRI, or radionuclide imaging of the skeleton. Ta lesions grow as exophytic lesions; CIS lesions start on the surface and tend to invade. The revised tumor, node, metastasis (TNM) staging system is illustrated in Fig. 80-1.

℞ TREATMENT

Management depends on whether the tumor invades muscle and whether there is spread to the regional lymph nodes and beyond. The probability of spread increases with increasing T stage. At a minimum, the management of a superficial tumor is a complete endoscopic re-

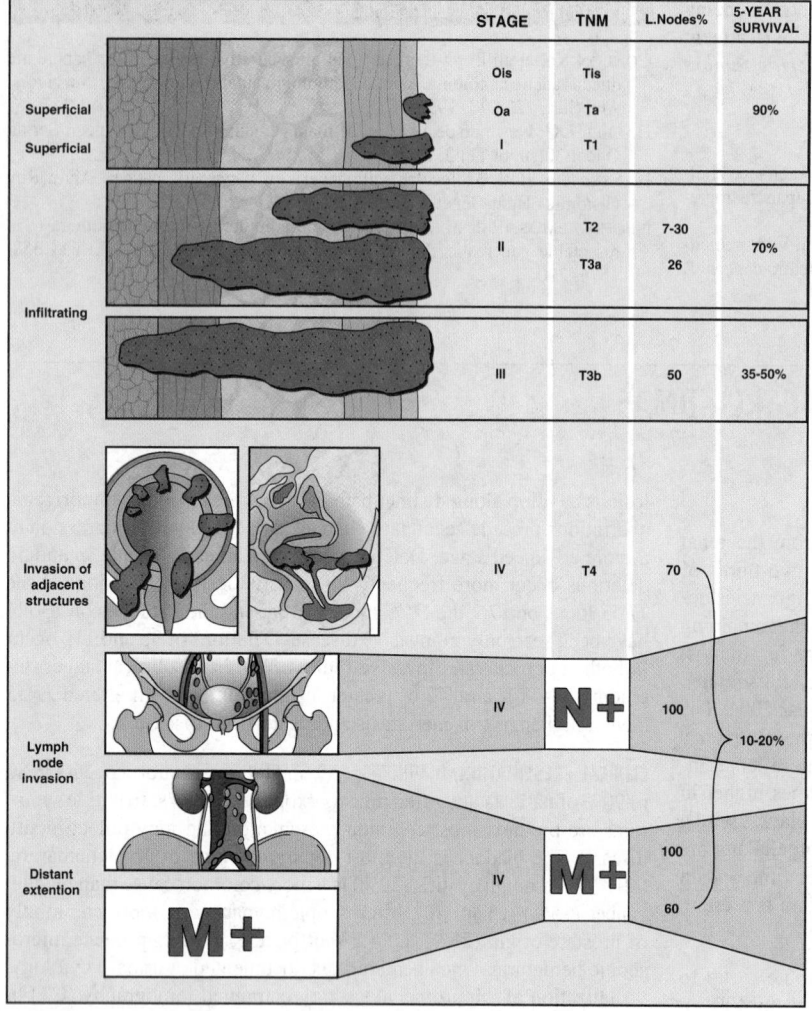

	STAGE	TNM	L.Nodes%	5-YEAR SURVIVAL
Superficial	Ois	Tis		90%
	Oa	Ta		
Superficial	I	T1		
Infiltrating	II	T2	7–30	70%
		T3a	26	
	III	T3b	50	35–50%
Invasion of adjacent structures	IV	T4	70	
Lymph node invasion	IV	N+	100	10–20%
Distant extention	IV	M+	100	
			60	

FIGURE 80-1 Bladder staging. TNM, tumor, node, metastasis.

section with or without intravesical therapy. The decision to recommend intravesical therapy depends on the histologic subtype, number of lesions, depth of invasion, and presence or absence of CIS. Recurrences develop in upwards of 50% of cases, and 5 to 20% progress to a more advanced stage. Solitary papillary lesions are generally managed by transurethral surgery alone. CIS and recurrent disease are treated by transurethral surgery followed by intravesical therapy. Radical cystectomy is the standard treatment for a tumor that has invaded muscle, either at the time of diagnosis or following treatment for superficial disease. The decision to administer systemic therapy is then based on the pathologic findings.

Superficial Disease Intravesical therapies are used in two general contexts: as an adjuvant to a complete endoscopic resection to prevent recurrence or, less commonly, to eliminate disease that cannot be controlled by endoscopic resection alone. Intravesical treatments are advised for patients with recurrent disease, >40% involvement of the bladder surface by tumor, the presence of diffuse CIS, or T1 disease. Bacillus Calmette-Guerin (BCG) in six weekly instillations, followed by maintenance, is considered standard based on randomized comparisons. Other agents with activity include mitomycin-C and interferon (IFN). The side effects include dysuria, urinary frequency, and, depending on the drug, myelosuppression or a contact dermatitis. Rarely, intravesical BCG may produce a systemic illness associated with granulomatous infections in multiple sites that requires antituberculin therapy.

Following the endoscopic resection, patients are monitored for recurrence at 3-month intervals during the first year. Those with persistent disease or new tumors are generally considered for a second course of BCG or for intravesical chemotherapy with valrubicin or gemcitabine. In some cases cystectomy is recommended, although the specific indications vary. Recurrence may develop anywhere along the urothelial tract including the renal pelvis, ureter, or urethra. A consequence of the "successful" treatment of tumors in the bladder is an increase in the frequency of extravesical recurrences. Tumors in the ureter or renal pelvis are typically managed by resection during retrograde examination or, in some cases, by instillation through the renal pelvis. Tumors of the prostatic urethra may require cystectomy if a complete resection cannot be achieved.

Invasive Disease The treatment of a tumor that has invaded muscle can be separated into control of the primary tumor and, depending on the pathologic findings at surgery, systemic chemotherapy. Radical cystectomy is the standard, although in selected cases a bladder-sparing approach that includes a complete endoscopic resection, partial cystectomy, or a combination of resection, systemic chemotherapy, and external beam radiation therapy is used. Indications for cystectomy include muscle-invading tumors not suitable for segmental resection, low-stage tumors unsuitable for conservative management (e.g., due to multicentric and frequent recurrences resistant to intravesical instillations), high-grade tumors (T1G3) associated with CIS, and bladder symptoms such as frequency or hemorrhage that impair quality of life. In some countries, external beam radiation therapy is considered standard. In the United States, its role is limited to those patients deemed unfit for cystectomy and those with unresectable local disease, and as part of an experimental approach that seeks to spare the bladder.

Radical cystectomy is major surgery that requires appropriate preoperative evaluation and management. The procedure involves removal of the bladder and pelvic lymph nodes, and creation of a conduit or reservoir for urinary flow. Grossly abnormal lymph nodes are evaluated by frozen section. If metastases are confirmed, the procedure is often aborted. In males, radical cystectomy involves the removal of the bladder, prostate and seminal vesicles, and proximal urethra. Impotence is universal unless the nerves responsible for erectile function are preserved. In females, the procedure includes removal of the bladder, urethra, uterus, fallopian tubes, ovaries, anterior vaginal wall, and surrounding fascia. Previously, urine flow was managed by directing the ureters to the abdominal wall, where it was collected in an external appliance. Currently, most patients receive a continent cutaneous reservoir that is constituted from detubularized bowel, or an orthotopic neobladder. Some 70% of men receive a neobladder. With a continent reservoir, 65 to 85% of men will be continent at night and 85 to 90% during the day. Cutaneous reservoirs are drained by intermittent catheterization; orthotopic neobladders are drained more naturally. Contraindications to a neobladder include renal insufficiency, an inability to self-catheterize, or the presence of an exophytic tumor or CIS in the urethra. Diffuse CIS in the bladder is a relative contraindication based on the risk of a urethral recurrence. Concurrent diseases in the bowel such as ulcerative colitis or Crohn's disease may hinder the use of resected bowel.

A partial cystectomy may be considered when the disease is limited to the dome of the bladder, a minimum of a 2-cm margin can be achieved, there is no CIS in other sites, and the bladder capacity is adequate after the tumor has been removed. This occurs in 5 to 10% of cases. Carcinomas in the ureter or in the renal pelvis are treated with nephroureterectomy with a bladder cuff to remove the tumor.

The probability of recurrence following surgery is predicted on the basis of pathologic stage, presence or absence of lymphatic or vascular invasion, and nodal spread. Among those who recur, the recurrence develops in a median of 1 year (range, 0.04 to 11.1 years). Long-term outcomes vary by pathologic stage and histology (Table 80-1). The number of lymph nodes removed is also prognostic whether or not tumor was in the nodes.

Metastatic Disease The primary goal of treatment for metastatic disease is to achieve a complete remission with chemotherapy alone, or with a combined-modality approach of chemotherapy followed by surgical resection of residual disease, as is done routinely for the treatment of germ cell tumors. One can define a goal in terms of cure or palliation on the basis of the probability of achieving a complete response to chemotherapy using prognostic factors, such as Karnofsky Performance Status (<80%), and whether the pattern of spread is nodal or visceral (liver, lung, or bone). For those with zero, 1, or 2 risk factors, the probability of a complete remission is 38, 25, and 5%, respectively, and median survival is 33, 13.4, and 9.3 months, respectively. Toxicities also vary as a function of risk. Treatment-related mortality has been reported in 3 to 4% of cases using some combinations. Patients with a compromised performance status, visceral disease, or bone metastases are rarely cured with chemotherapy alone; in these cases, median survivals rarely exceed 6 months.

A number of chemotherapeutic drugs have shown activity as single agents; cisplatin, paclitaxel, and gemcitabine are considered most active. Standard therapy consists of two-, three-, or four-drug combinations. Overall response rates of >50% have been reported using combinations such as methotrexate, vinblastine, doxorubicin, and cisplatin (M-VAC); cisplatin and paclitaxel (PT); gemcitabine and cisplatin (GC); or gemcitabine, paclitaxel, and cisplatin (GTC). M-VAC was considered standard, but the toxicities of neutropenia and fever, mucositis, diminished renal and auditory function, and peripheral neuropathy led to the development of alternative regimens. A comparative trial of M-VAC versus GC showed less neutropenia and fever, less mucositis, and more anemia and thrombocytopenia with the two-drug regimen.

Chemotherapy has also been evaluated in the neoadjuvant and adjuvant settings. In a randomized trial, patients receiving three cycles of neoadjuvant M-VAC followed by cystectomy had significantly better median (6.2 years) and 5-year survival (57%) compared to cystectomy alone (median survival, 3.8 years; 5-year survival, 42%). Adjuvant therapy with cisplatin, methotrexate, and vinblastine (CMV) (three cycles) appears to reduce the risk of recurrence by 15%. Additional trials are studying taxane- and gemcitabine-based combinations.

Chemotherapy has a role in invasive disease; however, for the majority of patients, chemotherapy alone is inadequate to clear the bladder of disease. Experimental studies are evaluating combined-modality approaches using chemotherapy and radiation therapy together in patients whose tumors were endoscopically removed.

The recommendation to administer adjuvant therapy is based on the risk of recurrence following cystectomy. Indications include the presence of nodal disease, extravesical tumor extension, or vascular invasion in the resected specimen. Adjuvant therapy (four cycles of combination chemotherapy) delays recurrence, although an effect on survival is less clear.

The management of bladder cancer is summarized in Table 80-2.

RENAL CELL CARCINOMA

Renal cell carcinomas account for 90 to 95% of malignant neoplasms arising from the kidney. Notable features include refractoriness to cy-

TABLE 80-2 *Management of Bladder Cancer*

Nature of Lesion	Management Approach
Superficial	Endoscopic removal, usually with intravesical therapy
Invasive disease	Cystectomy ± systemic chemotherapy (before or after surgery)
Metastatic disease	Curative or palliative chemotherapy (based on prognostic factors) ± surgery

totoxic agents, infrequent but reproducible responses to biologic response modifiers such as IFN-α and interleukin 2 (IL-2), and a variable clinical course for patients with metastatic disease, including anecdotal reports of spontaneous regression.

EPIDEMIOLOGY AND ETIOLOGY The annual incidence of renal cell carcinoma continues to rise and now includes nearly 36,000 cases annually in the United States resulting in 12,500 deaths. The male:female ratio is 2:1. Incidence peaks between the ages of 50 to 70, although this malignancy may be diagnosed at any age. Many environmental factors have been investigated as possible contributing causes; the strongest association is with cigarette smoking (accounting for 20 to 30% of cases) and obesity. Risk is also increased for patients who have acquired cystic disease of the kidney associated with end-stage renal disease, and for those with tuberous sclerosis. Most cases are sporadic, although familial forms have been reported. One is associated with von Hippel-Lindau (VHL) syndrome, which predisposes to renal cell carcinomas, retinal hemangioma, hemangioblastoma of the spinal cord and cerebellum, and pheochromocytoma. Roughly 35% of individuals with VHL disease develop renal cell cancer. An increased incidence has also been reported for first-degree relatives. Most renal cancers arise from the epithelial cells of the proximal tubules. A number of genetic alterations have been described; 97% show allelic loss at 3p. Deletions of 3p21–26 (where the *VHL* gene maps) have been identified in familial as well as sporadic tumors.

PATHOLOGY Renal cell neoplasia represents a heterogeneous group of tumors with distinct histopathologic, genetic, and clinical features ranging from benign to high-grade malignant (Table 80-3). They are classified on the basis of morphology and histology. Categories include clear cell carcinoma (60% of cases), papillary (5 to 15%), chromophobic tumors (5 to 10%), oncocytomas (5 to 10%), and collecting or Bellini duct tumors (<1%). Clear cell tumors have clear cytoplasm and usually show chromosome 3p deletions. Papillary tumors tend to be bilateral and multifocal and show trisomy 7 or 17. Chromophobic tumors are characterized by multiple chromosomal losses but do not exhibit 3p deletions and have a more indolent clinical course. Oncocytomas have a characteristic morphology including a deeply eosinophilic cytoplasm, do not exhibit 3p deletions or trisomy 7 or 17, and are considered benign neoplasms. In contrast, Bellini duct carcinomas are very rare and are thought to arise from the collecting ducts within the renal medulla. They tend to affect younger patients and are very aggressive tumors.

TABLE 80-1 *Survival Following Surgery for Bladder Cancer*

Pathologic Stage	5-Year Survival, %	10-Year Survival, %
T2,N0	89	87
T3a,N0	78	76
T3b,N0	62	61
T4,N0	50	45
Any T,N1	35	34

TABLE 80-3 *Classification of Epithelial Neoplasms Arising from the Kidney*

Carcinoma Type	Growth Pattern	Cell of Origin	Cytogenetics
Clear cell	Acinar or sarcomatoid	Proximal tubule	3p−
Papillary	Papillary or sarcomatoid	Proximal tubule	+7, +17, −Y
Chromophobic	Solid, tubular, or sarcomatoid	Cortical collecting duct	Hypodiploid
Oncocytic	Tumor nests	Cortical collecting duct	Undetermined
Collecting duct	Papillary or sarcomatoid	Medullary collecting duct	Undetermined

CLINICAL PRESENTATION The presenting signs and symptoms include hematuria, abdominal pain, and a flank or abdominal mass. This classic triad occurs in 10 to 20% of patients. Other symptoms are fever, weight loss, anemia, and a varicocele (Table 80-4). The tumor can also be found incidentally on a radiograph. Widespread use of radiologic cross-sectional imaging procedures (CT, ultrasound, MRI) contributes to earlier detection, including incidental renal masses detected during evaluation for other medical conditions. The increasing number of incidentally discovered low-stage tumors contributes to an improved 5-year survival for patients with renal cell carcinoma and increased use of nephron-sparing surgery (partial nephrectomy).

A spectrum of paraneoplastic syndromes has been associated with these malignancies, including erythrocytosis, hypercalcemia, non-metastatic hepatic dysfunction (Stauffer syndrome), and acquired dysfibrinogenemia. Erythrocytosis is noted at presentation in only about 3% of patients. Anemia, a sign of advanced disease, is more common.

The standard evaluation of patients with suspected renal cell tumors includes a CT scan of the abdomen and pelvis, a chest radiograph, urine analysis, and urine cytology. A CT of the chest is warranted if metastatic disease is suspected from the chest radiograph, as it will detect significantly smaller lesions, and their presence may influence the approach to the primary tumor. MRI is useful in evaluating the inferior vena cava in cases of suspected tumor involvement or invasion by thrombus, as well as for patients in whom contrast cannot be administered owing to either allergy or renal dysfunction. In clinical practice, any solid renal masses should be considered malignant until proven otherwise; a definitive diagnosis is required. If no metastases are demonstrated, surgery is indicated, even if the renal vein is invaded. The differential diagnosis of a renal mass includes cysts, benign neoplasms (adenoma, angiomyolipoma, oncocytoma), inflammatory lesions (pyelonephritis or abscesses), and other primary or metastatic malignant neoplasms. Other malignancies that may involve the kidney include transitional cell carcinoma of the renal pelvis, sarcoma, lymphoma, Wilms' tumor, and metastatic disease, especially from melanoma. All of these are less common causes of renal masses than is renal cell cancer.

STAGING AND PROGNOSIS Two staging systems used commonly are the Robson classification and the American Joint Committee on Cancer (AJCC) staging system. According to the Robson system, stage I tumors are confined to the kidney; stage II tumors extend through the renal capsule but are confined to Gerota's fascia; stage III tumors involve the renal vein or vena cava (stage III A) or the hilar lymph nodes (stage III B); and stage IV disease includes tumors that are locally invasive to adjacent organs (excluding the adrenal gland) or distant metastases. The rate of 5-year survival varies by stage: 66% for stage I, 64% for stage II, 42% for stage III, and 11% for stage IV. The prognosis for patients with stage IIIA lesions is similar to that of stage II disease; 5-year survival for patients with stage IIIB disease is only 20%, closer to that of stage IV.

TABLE 80-4   *Signs and Symptoms in Patients with Renal Cell Cancer*

Presenting Sign or Symptom	Incidence, %
Classic triad: hematuria, flank pain, flank mass	10–20
Hematuria	40
Flank pain	40
Palpable mass	25
Weight loss	33
Anemia	33
Fever	20
Hypertension	20
Abnormal liver function	15
Hypercalcemia	5
Erythrocytosis	3
Neuromyopathy	3
Amyloidosis	2
Increased erythrocyte sedimentation rate	55

℞ TREATMENT

Localized Tumors The standard management for stage I or II tumors and selected cases of stage III disease is radical nephrectomy. This procedure involves en bloc removal of Gerota's fascia and its contents including the kidney, the ipsilateral adrenal gland, and adjacent hilar lymph nodes. The role of a regional lymphadenectomy is controversial. Extension into the renal vein or inferior vena cava, stage III disease, does not preclude resection even if cardiopulmonary bypass is required. Half of these patients have prolonged survival if the tumor is resected. Stauffer syndrome describes the rare patient with no detectable metastatic disease who has hepatic dysfunction. These patients are also candidates for renal resection because the hepatopathy is often reversible after the primary is removed.

In selected patients who have only one kidney—depending on the size and location of the lesion—nephron-sparing approaches may be used via an open or laparoscopic approach. A nephron-sparing approach can also be used for patients with bilateral tumors, accompanied by a radical nephrectomy on the opposite side. Partial nephrectomy techniques are being applied electively to resect small masses for patients with a normal contralateral kidney. Adjuvant chemotherapy, immunotherapy, and radiation therapy are not useful following surgery, even in cases with a poor prognosis.

Advanced Disease Investigational therapy is first-line treatment for metastatic disease as no immune approach or chemotherapeutic agent has shown significant antitumor activity. The prognosis is highly variable; in one analysis, no prior nephrectomy, a Karnofsky performance status <80, low hemoglobin, high corrected calcium, and abnormal lactate dehydrogenase (LDH) were poor prognostic factors. Patients with zero, one or two, and three or more factors had a median survival of 24, 12, and 5 months, respectively. These tumors often follow an unpredictable and protracted clinical course. In one study, 10% of patients with established metastatic disease did not progress after 1 year of observation. It may be best to document progression before considering potentially toxic treatment approaches.

Surgery has a limited role for patients with metastatic disease. One indication for nephrectomy is to alleviate pain or hemorrhage of a primary tumor. Nephrectomy is not indicated to induce tumor regression (occurs in <1% of cases) or to increase sensitivity to cytokine therapy. However, long-term survival may occur in patients who relapse after nephrectomy in a solitary site that can be removed.

IFN-α and IL-2 produce regressions in 10 to 20% of patients but these are rarely durable. IL-2 was approved on the observation of durable complete remission in a small proportion of cases. IFN has also been evaluated as an adjuvant to cytoreductive surgery. In one study, patients were randomized to surgery plus IFN (5×10^6 IU/m^2, 3 times per week) versus IFN alone. The median time to progression was 5 versus 3 months, and median survival was 17 versus 7 months (hazard ratio, .54) in favor of the combined-modality approach. A second trial with a similar design showed a 3-month difference in median survival (11.1 versus 8.1 months) in favor of the combined approach. Newer cytokines and novel biologic agents are under investigation, and promising results have been reported using an inhibitor of vascular endothelial growth factor.

CARCINOMA OF THE RENAL PELVIS AND URETER

About 2500 cases of renal pelvis and ureter cancer occur each year; nearly all are transitional cell carcinomas similar to bladder cancer in biology and appearance. This tumor also is associated with chronic phenacetin abuse and with Balkan nephropathy, a chronic interstitial nephritis endemic in Bulgaria, Greece, Bosnia-Herzegovina, and Romania.

The most common symptom is painless gross hematuria, and the disease usually is detected on IVP during the workup for hematuria. Patterns of spread are like those in bladder cancer. For disease localized to the renal pelvis and ureter, nephroureterectomy (including excision of the distal ureter with a portion of the bladder) is associated with a 5-year survival of 80 to 90% for low-grade lesions. More invasive or histologically poorly differentiated tumors are more likely to recur locally and metastasize. Metastatic disease is treated with the chemotherapy used in bladder cancer, and the outcome is similar to that of metastatic transitional cell cancer of bladder origin.

FURTHER READING

ADVANCED BLADDER CANCER META-ANALYSIS COLLABORATION: Neoadjuvant chemotherapy in invasive bladder cancer: A systematic review and meta-analysis. Lancet 361:1927, 2003

BORDEN LS JR et al: Bladder cancer. Curr Opin Oncol 15:227, 2003

LINEBAN WM et al: The genetic basis of cancer of the kidney. J Urol 170:2163, 2003

MEJEAN A et al: Prognostic factors of renal cell carcinoma. J Urol 169:821, 2003

WHANG YE, GODLEY PA: Renal cell carcinoma. Curr Opin Oncol 15:213, 2003

WINQUIST E et al: Neoadjuvant chemotherapy for transitional cell carcinoma of the bladder: A systematic review and meta-analysis. J Urol 171:561, 2004

81 HYPERPLASTIC AND MALIGNANT DISEASES OF THE PROSTATE
Howard I. Scher

The frequency of both benign and malignant changes in the prostate increase with age. Autopsies of men in the eighth decade of life show hyperplastic changes in >90% and malignant changes in >70% of individuals. The high prevalence of these diseases in an elderly population with competing causes of morbidity and mortality mandates a risk-adapted approach to diagnosis and treatment. This can be achieved by considering these diseases as a series of states. Each state represents a distinct clinical milestone for which intervention(s) may be recommended based on the presence or risk of developing symptoms or death from disease in a given time frame (Fig. 81-1). For benign proliferative disorders, symptoms of urinary frequency, infection, and potential for obstruction are weighed against the side effects and complications of medical or surgical therapy. For prostate malignancies, the risk of developing the disease, symptoms, or death from cancer are balanced against the morbidities of interventions recommended and preexisting comorbid conditions.

In 2004, around 230,000 prostate cancer cases were diagnosed, of whom 29,900 succumbed. The absolute number of prostate cancer deaths has decreased in the past 5 years; this has been attributed by some to the widespread use of detection strategies based on monitoring prostate-specific antigen (PSA). However, screening has not been proven to improve survival in prospective randomized trials. The paradox of management is that although the disease remains the second leading cause of cancer deaths in men, the almost 8:1 ratio in incidence to prostate cancer–specific mortality shows that the majority of men do not die of their disease.

ANATOMY AND PATHOLOGY

The prostate is located in the pelvis and is surrounded by the rectum, the bladder, the periprostatic and dorsal vein complexes that are responsible for erectile function, and the urinary sphincter that is responsible for passive urinary control. The prostate is composed of branching tubuloalveolar glands arranged in lobules and surrounded by a stroma. The acinal unit includes an epithelial compartment made up of epithelial, basal, and neuroendocrine cells and a stromal compartment that includes fibroblasts and smooth-muscle cells. The compartments are separated by a basement membrane. PSA and acid phosphatase (ACP) are produced in the epithelial cells. Both cell types express androgen receptors and depend on androgens for growth. Testosterone, the major circulating androgen, is converted by the enzyme 5-α reductase to dihydrotestosterone in the gland. Changes in prostate size occur during puberty and after the age of 55 in the periurethral portion of the gland. Most cancers develop in the peripheral zone, which can often be palpated by a digital rectal examination (DRE).

Nonmalignant growth occurs predominantly in the transition zone around the urethra.

EPIDEMIOLOGY

The development of a prostate cancer involves a multistep process. Hypermethylation of the GSTP1 gene promoter, leading to a loss of function of a gene that detoxifies carcinogens, is one early change. Epidemiologic studies show that the risk of being diagnosed with prostate cancer increases by a factor of 2 if one first-degree relative is affected and by 4 if two or more are affected. Current estimates are that 40% of early-onset and 5 to 10% of all cancers are hereditary and follow a Mendelian inheritance pattern. Prostate cancer affects ethnic groups differently. Matched for age, the prostates of African-American males have both a greater number of precursor prostatic intraepithelial neoplasia (PIN) lesions and larger tumors than white males, possibly related to the higher levels of testosterone seen in African-American males. These lesions are highly unstable, and typically multifocal. Polymorphic variants of the androgen receptor gene, the cytochrome P450 C17 gene, and the steroid 5α-reductase type II (*SRD5A2*) gene have also been implicated in the variations in incidence. The incidence of autopsy-detected cancers is similar around the world, while the incidence of the clinical disease varies. Thus, environmental factors may play a role. High consumption of dietary fats, such as α-linoleic acid, or polycyclic aromatic hydrocarbons that form when red meats are cooked is believed to increase risk. Similar to breast cancer in Asian women, the risk of prostate cancer in Asian males increases when they move to western environments. Protective factors include the isoflavinoid genistein (which inhibits 5α-reductase), cruciferous vegetables that contain isothiocyanate sulfuraphane, retinoids such as lycopene (in pizza and tomatoes), and inhibitors of cholesterol biosynthesis. The antioxidant α-tocopherol (vitamin E) and selenium may also reduce risk.

DIAGNOSIS AND TREATMENT BY CLINICAL STATE

The clinical states framework considers the risk of morbidity from an enlarging but nonmalignant gland; the probability that a clinically significant cancer is present in an individual with or without urinary symptoms; or, for those with a prostate cancer diagnosis; the probability of developing symptoms or dying from disease. At any point in time, a patient resides in one state and remains there until the disease has progressed to the next state. Applying this paradigm, a patient with localized prostate cancer who has had all cancer removed surgically remains in the state of localized disease as long as the PSA remains undetectable. The time within a state becomes a measure of the impact of an intervention on the natural history of disease, be it benign or malignant in etiology, recognizing that the impact may not be assessable for years. It also allows a distinction between *cure*—the elimination of all cancer cells, the primary therapeutic objective when treating most cancers—and *cancer control*, in which the tempo of the illness is modulated and symptoms controlled until the patient dies of other causes. It is the concept of cancer control that makes the man-

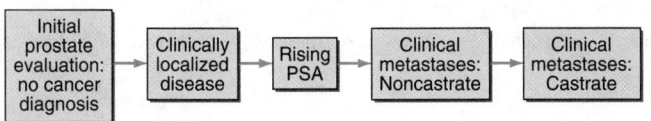

FIGURE 81-1 Clinical states of prostate cancer. PSA, prostate-specific antigen.

agement of prostate cancer unique. Even when a recurrence is documented, immediate therapy is not always necessary. Rather, as at the time of diagnosis, the need for intervention is based on the tempo of the illness as it unfolds in the individual, relative to the risk:reward ratio of the therapy being considered.

NO CANCER DIAGNOSIS ■ Symptoms The need to pursue a diagnosis of prostate cancer is based on symptoms, an abnormal DRE, or an elevated serum PSA. The urologic history should focus on symptoms of outlet obstruction, continence, potency, or a change in ejaculatory pattern. Benign proliferative disease may produce hesitancy, intermittent voiding, a diminished stream, incomplete emptying, and postvoid leakage. The severity of these symptoms can be quantitated with the self-administered American Urological Association (AUA) *Symptom Index* (Table 81-1) recognizing that the degree of symptoms does not always relate to gland size. Resistance to urine flow reduces bladder compliance, leading to nocturia, urgency, and, ultimately, to retention. Infection, tranquilizing drugs, antihistamines, or alcohol can precipitate urinary retention. Prostatitis often produces pain or induration. Symptoms of metastatic disease include pain secondary to osseous metastases, although many are asymptomatic despite extensive spread. Less common are symptoms related to marrow compromise (myelophthisis), a coagulopathy, or spinal cord compression.

Physical Examination The DRE focuses on the size, consistency, and abnormalities within or beyond the gland. Many cancers occur in the peripheral zone and can be palpated on DRE. Carcinomas are characteristically hard, nodular, and irregular, while induration may be due to benign prostatic hypertrophy (BPH) or to calculi or tumor. Overall, 20 to 25% of men with an abnormal DRE have cancer.

PROSTATE-SPECIFIC ANTIGEN

PSA is a kallikrein-like serine protease that causes liquefaction of seminal coagulum. It is produced by both nonmalignant and malignant epithelial cells. PSA is prostate specific, not prostate cancer specific, and increases may occur from prostatitis, nonmalignant enlargement of the gland (BPH), prostate cancer, and prostate biopsies. The level is not affected by the performance of a DRE. It circulates in the blood as an inactive complex with the protease inhibitors α_{-1}-antichymotrypsin and β_2-macroglobulin and has an estimated half-life in the serum of 2 to 3 days. Levels should be undetectable if the prostate has been removed. PSA immunostaining is used to establish a prostate cancer diagnosis.

PSA testing was approved for early detection in 1994. It is recommend on an annual basis along with a DRE for men over age 50

(with an anticipated survival of >10 years; this includes men up to age 76 years). For African Americans and men with a family history, testing is advised to begin at age 40. The normal range of PSA is 0 to 4 ng/mL. For values >4, the sensitivity for prostate cancer detection is 57 to 79%, the specificity is 59 to 68%, and the positive predictive value is 40 to 49%.

The PSA-based criteria used to recommend a diagnostic prostate biopsy have evolved over time. PSA values may fluctuate for no apparent reason; thus, an isolated abnormal value should be confirmed before proceeding with further testing. These evolving criteria aim to increase the sensitivity of the test for younger men more likely to die of the disease and to reduce the frequency of detecting cancers of low malignant potential in elderly men more likely to die of other causes. Age-specific reference ranges apply a lower "upper" limit of normal for younger males and higher "upper" limit for older individuals. Different thresholds alter sensitivity and specificity of detection. The threshold for performance of a biopsy is now 2.6 ng/mL for men under age 60. Prostate-specific antigen density (PSAD) measurements were developed to correct for the contribution of BPH to the total PSA level. PSAD is calculated by dividing the serum PSA by the estimated prostate weight calculated by transrectal ultrasound (TRUS). Values <0.10 are consistent with BPH, while those >0.15 suggest cancer. *PSA velocity* is the rate of change in PSA levels over time. It is particularly useful for men with values that are rising in the seemingly "normal" range. Rates of rise >0.75 ng/mL per year suggest cancer. As an example, an increase from 2.5 to 3.9 in a 1-year period would warrant further testing. Free and complexed PSA measurements are used when levels are between 4 and 10 ng/mL to decide who needs a biopsy. In cancer, the level of free PSA is lower. The ratios of free to total, complexed to total, and free to complexed PSA have also been used. In one series, specificity improved by 20% using a normal range of free/total >0.15; complexed/total <0.70; and free/complexed >0.25. A diagnostic algorithm based on the DRE and PSA findings is illustrated in Fig. 81-2. In general, a biopsy is recommended if the DRE or PSA are abnormal.

Prostate Biopsy A diagnosis of cancer is established by a TRUS-guided needle biopsy. Direct visualization assures that all areas of gland are sampled. A minimum of six separate cores, three from the right and three from the left, are advised, as is a separate biopsy of the transition zone, if clinically indicated. Performance of a biopsy is not advised in a patient with prostatitis until a course of antibiotics has been administered. The positive predictive value of an abnormal DRE is 21%, while 25% of men with a PSA > 4 ng/mL and an abnormal DRE, and 17% of men with a PSA of 2.5 to 4.0 ng/mL and normal DRE, have cancer. Those with an abnormal PSA and negative biopsy are advised to undergo a repeat biopsy.

TABLE 81-1   *AUA System Index*

Questions to Be Answered	AUA Symptom Score (Circle 1 Number on Each Line)					
	Not at All	Less than 1 Time in 5	Less than Half the Time	About Half the Time	More than Half the time	Almost Always
Over the past month, how often you have had a sensation of not emptying your bladder completely after you finished urinating?	0	1	2	3	4	5
Over the past month, how often have you had to urinate again less than 2 h after you finished urinating?	0	1	2	3	4	5
Over the past month, how often have you found you stopped and started again several times when you urinated?	0	1	2	3	4	5
Over the past month, how often have you found it difficult to postpone urination?	0	1	2	3	4	5
Over the past month, how often have you had a weak urinary stream?	0	1	2	3	4	5
Over the past month, how often have you had to push or strain to begin urination?	0	1	2	3	4	5
Over the past month, how many times did you most typically get up to urinate from the time you went to bed at night until the time you got up in the morning?	(None)	(1 time)	(2 times)	(3 times)	(4 times)	(5 times)
Sum of 7 circled numbers (AUA Symptom Score): ———						

Note: AUA, American Urological Association.   *Source*: Barry MJ et al: J Urol 148:1549, 1992. Used with permission.

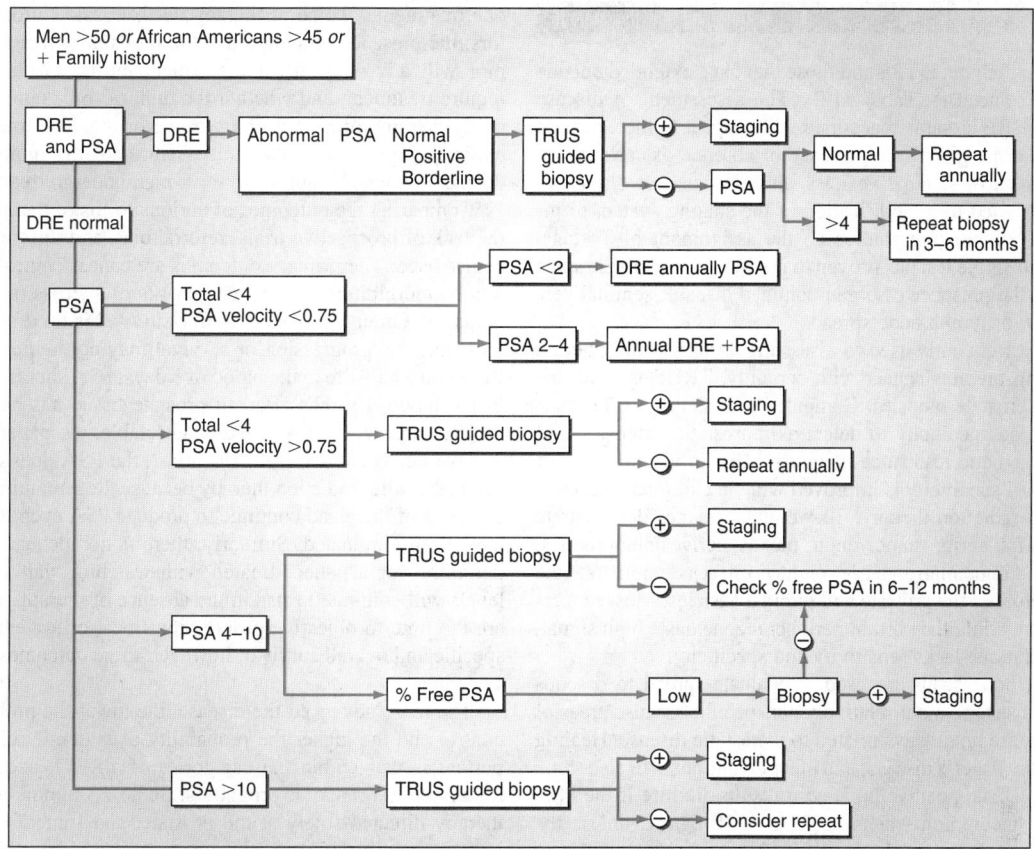

FIGURE 81-2 Algorithm for diagnostic evaluation of men based on digital rectal examination and prostate-specific antigen levels.

Pathology The noninvasive proliferation of epithelial cells within ducts is termed *prostatic intraepithelial neoplasia*. PIN is a precursor of cancer, but not all PIN lesions develop into invasive cancers. Of the cancers identified, >95% are adenocarcinomas; the remaining are squamous, transitional cell tumors, and rarely, carcinosarcomas. Metastases to the prostate are rare, but in some cases, transitional cell tumors of the bladder or colon cancers invade the gland by direct extension. Each core of the biopsy is examined for the presence of cancer, and the amount of cancer present is quantified. A measure of histologic aggressiveness is also assigned using the *Gleason grading system*, in which the dominant and secondary glandular histologic patterns are scored from 1 (well differentiated) to 5 (undifferentiated) and summed to give a total score of 2 to 10 for each tumor. The most poorly differentiated area of tumor (i.e., the area with the highest histologic grade) often determines biologic behavior. The presence or absence of perineural invasion and extracapsular spread are also recorded.

PSA-based detection strategies have changed the clinical spectrum of the disease. Now, 95 to 99% of newly diagnosed cancers are clinically localized, 40% are not palpable, and, of these, 70% are pathologically organ-confined. The downside of widespread use is the detection and treatment of cancers with such a low malignant potential that they would not have shortened survival or produced symptoms during the patient's lifetime. The side effects of treatment, including impotence, incontinence, and bowel dysfunction, are unacceptable for these cases. Formal clinical trials to assess the value of screening on prostate cancer morbidity and mortality are ongoing. Until the results of these studies are available, men are advised to make an informed decision about whether to undergo testing.

Prevention It is difficult to identify individuals who are at risk for developing a cancer that is clinically significant. The Prostate Cancer Prevention Trial is a double-blinded, randomized multicenter trial designed to investigate the ability of finasteride, a 5α-reductase inhibitor, to prevent the development of prostate cancer in men age ≥55 years.

The prostate cancer detection rate was 18.4% (803 of 4364) for finasteride and 24.4% (1147 of 4692) for placebo-treated men. However, more of the cancers detected in the finasteride group were high-grade [37% (280 of 757) vs. 22% (237 of 1068 cancers) for the placebo]. No effect on survival was detected. Vitamin E and selenium (the SELECT study) are also being tested as preventive agents.

Treatment of Benign Disease Asymptomatic patients do not require treatment regardless of the size of the gland, while those with an inability to urinate, gross hematuria, recurrent infection, or bladder stones may require surgery. Typically, obstruction does not occur and the symptoms remain stable over time. In these cases, uroflowmetry can identify patients with normal flow rates who are unlikely to benefit from treatment and those with high postvoid residuals who may need other interventions. Pressure-flow studies detect primary bladder dysfunction. Cystoscopy is recommended if hematuria is documented and to assess the urinary outflow tract before surgery. Imaging of the upper tracts is advised for patients with hematuria, a history of calculi, or prior urinary tract problems. Therapies such as finasteride, which blocks the conversion of testosterone to dihydrotestosterone, have been shown to decrease prostate size, increase urine flow rates, and improve symptoms. They will also lower baseline PSA levels by 50%, an important consideration when using PSA to guide biopsy recommendations. α-Adrenergic blockers such as terazosin act by relaxing the smooth muscle of the bladder neck and increasing peak urinary flow rates. No data show that these agents influence the progression of the disease. Surgical approaches include a transurethral resection of the prostate (TURP), transurethral incision, or removal of the gland via a retropubic, suprapubic or perineal approach. TULIP (transurethral ultrasound-guided laser-induced prostatectomy), coils, stents, and hyperthermia are also utilized.

PROSTATE CANCER STAGING The TNM staging system includes categories for cancers that are palpable on DRE, those identified solely on the basis of an abnormal PSA (T1c), those that are palpable but clinically confined to the gland (T2), and those that have extended outside of the gland (T3 and T4) (Table 81-2). The assessment of disease extent based on DRE alone is inaccurate with respect to the extent of the disease within the gland, the presence or absence of capsular invasion, involvement of seminal vesicles, and extension of disease to lymph nodes. This led to a modification of the staging system to include the results of imaging studies on the assignment of T stage. Unfortunately, no single test has proven to predict the pathologic stage accurately, be it the presence of organ-confined disease, seminal vesical involvement, or lymph node spread.

TRUS is most frequently used to assess the primary tumor, but no consistent finding predicts cancer with certainty. TRUS is used primarily to direct prostate biopsies. Computed tomography (CT) scans lack sensitivity and specificity to detect extraprostatic extension and are inferior to magnetic resonance imaging (MRI) in visualization of lymph nodes. MRI specificity is improved with an endorectal coil and aids in planning radiation therapy. T1-weighted images demonstrate the periprostatic fat, periprostatic venous plexus, perivesicular tissues, lymph nodes, and bone marrow. T2-weighted images demonstrate the internal architecture of the prostate and seminal vesicles. Most cancers have a low signal, while the normal peripheral zone has a high signal, although the technique lacks sensitivity and specificity.

Radionuclide bone scans are used to evaluate spread to osseous sites. This test is sensitive but relatively nonspecific because areas of increased uptake are not always related to metastatic disease. Healing fractures, arthritis, Paget's disease, and other conditions will also show abnormal uptake. True-positive bone scan results are rare if the PSA <8 ng/mL and uncommon when the PSA < 10 ng/mL unless the tumor is high grade. When the PSA <10 ng/mL, a positive bone scan is usually falsely positive, which in turn, leads to additional low-yield testing.

CLINICALLY LOCALIZED DISEASE Localized prostate cancers are clinically confined to the prostate. Patients with localized disease are managed by radical surgery, radiation therapy, or watchful waiting. Data from the literature do not provide clear evidence for the superiority of any

one treatment. Choice of therapy needs consideration of several factors: the presence of symptoms, the probability that the untreated tumor will adversely affect the patient during his lifetime and thus require treatment, and whether the tumor can be cured by single-modality therapy directed at the prostate or requires both local and systemic therapy to achieve cure. As most of the tumors detected are deemed clinically significant, most men undergo treatment.

Comparing the outcomes of various forms of therapy is limited by the lack of prospective trials, referral bias, and differences in the outcomes used. The primary outcomes are cancer control and treatment-related morbidities. These benchmarks of success or failure vary by modality. Often, PSA relapse–free survival is used because an effect on metastatic progression or survival may not be apparent for years. Based on a half-life in the blood of 3 days, PSA should be undetectable in the blood 4 weeks after all prostate tissue has been removed by radical surgery. If PSA remains detectable, the patient is considered to have persistent disease. In contrast, the PSA does not become undetectable after radiation therapy because the remaining nonmalignant elements of the gland continue to produce PSA even if all cancer cells have been eliminated. Similarly, there is no adequate cancer control definition for a patient treated with watchful waiting because PSA levels will continue to rise in the absence of therapy. Other outcomes are the time to objective progression (local or systemic) and cancer-specific and overall survival; however, these outcomes may take years to define.

The more advanced the disease, the lower the probability of local control and the higher the probability of systemic relapse. More important is that within the categories of T1, T2, and T3 disease are tumors with a range of prognoses. Some T3 tumors are curable with therapy directed solely at the prostate, and some T1 lesions have a high probability of systemic relapse that requires the integration of local and systemic therapy to achieve cure. T1c tumors particularly require the use of other factors to predict outcomes and select treatment. Many groups have developed prognostic models based on a combination of the initial T stage, Gleason score, and baseline PSA. Some are based on discrete cut points (PSA <10 or ≥ 10; Gleason score of ≤6, 7, or ≥8). Others are nomograms that use PSA and Gleason score as continuous variables. These algorithms are used to predict disease extent: organ confined vs. nonorgan confined, node negative or positive, and the probability of success using a PSA-based definition of failure specific to the local therapy under consideration. Exactly what cut-off value would lead a patient to accept one form of therapy vs. another is an area of active debate. Specific nomograms have been developed for radical prostatectomy, external-beam radiation therapy, and brachytherapy (seed implantation). These are being refined continually to incorporate other clinical parameters and biologic determinants. Surgical technique, radiation therapy delivery, and criteria for watchful waiting continue to be refined and improved; the year treatment was given affects outcomes independent of other factors. The improvements make treatment decisions a dynamic process.

The frequency of adverse events for the different modalities is highly variable. Of greatest concern to patients are the effects on continence, sexual potency, and bowel function. Part of the variability relates to the definition used for a specific complication and whether the patient or physician is reporting the event. Incontinence figures range from 2% to 47% and impotence rates range from 25% to 89% following radical prostatectomy. The time of the assessment is also important. After surgery, impotence is immediate but may reverse over time, while with radiation therapy, impotence is not immediate but may develop over time.

Radical Retropubic Prostatectomy (RRP) The goal of radical prostatectomy is to excise the cancer completely with a clear margin, to maintain continence by preserving the external sphincter, and to preserve potency by sparing the autonomic nerves in the neurovascular bundle. RRP is advised for patients with a life expectancy of >10 years and is performed using a retropubic, perineal, or laparoscopic approach.

TABLE 81-2 *Comparison of Clinical Stage by the TNM Classification System and the Whitmore-Jewett Staging System*

TNM Stage	Description	Whitmore-Jewett Stage	Description
T1a	Nonpalpable, with 5% or less of resected tissue with cancer	A1	Well differentiated tumor on few chips from 1 lobe
T1b	Nonpalpable, with >5% of resected tissue with cancer	A2	Involvement more diffuse
T1c	Nonpalpable, detected due to elevated serum PSA		
T2a	Palpable, half of one lobe or less	BIN	Palpable, < one lobe, surrounded by normal tissue
T2b	Palpable, > half of one lobe but not both lobes	B1	Palpable, < one lobe
T2c	Palpable, involves both lobes	B2	Palpable, one entire lobe or both lobes
T3a	Palpable, unilateral extracapsular extension	C1	Palpable, outside capsule, not into seminal vesicles
T3b	Palpable, bilateral extracapsular extension		
T3c	Tumor invades seminal vesicle(s)	C2	Palpable, seminal vesicle involved
MI	Distant metastases	D	Metastatic disease

Source: Adapted from FF Schroder et al: TNM classification of prostate cancer. Prostate (Suppl) 4:129, 1992; and American Joint Committee on Cancer, 1992.

Outcomes can be predicted using postoperative nomograms that consider pretreatment factors and the pathologic findings at surgery. PSA failure is defined as a detectable value of 0.2 or 0.4 ng/mL, although the exact definition varies among series. The techniques continue to improve as the ability to localize the tumor within or beyond the prostate are refined with different biopsy algorithms and with imaging. The result is better case selection and surgical planning, which in turn have led to more rapid recovery and higher rates of continence and potency. Factors associated with incontinence include older age, shorter urethra length, surgical technique, preservation of neurovascular bundles, and development of an anastomotic stricture. Surgical experience is also a factor. In one series, 6% of patients had mild stress urinary incontinence (SUI) (requiring 1 pad/day), 2% moderate SUI (>1 pad/day), and 0.3% severe SUI (requiring an artificial urinary sphincter). At 1 year, 92% were completely continent. In contrast, the results in a Medicare population treated at multiple centers showed that at 3, 12, and 24 months following surgery, 58, 35, and 42% wore pads in their underwear, and 24, 11, and 15% reported "a lot" of urine leakage. Factors associated with recovery of erectile function include younger age, quality erections before surgery, and the absence of damage to the neurovascular bundles. Erectile function returns in a median of 4 to 6 months if both bundles are preserved. Potency is reduced by half if at least one nerve bundle is sacrificed. In cases where cancer control requires the removal of both bundles, sural nerve grafts are being explored. Overall, with the availability of drugs such as sildenafil, intraurethral inserts of alprostadil, and intracavernosal injections of vasodilators, many patients recover satisfactory sexual function.

High-risk patients are those with a predicted high probability of failure with surgery alone based on pretreatment factors. In these situations, nomograms and predictive models can only go so far. Exactly what probability of success or failure would lead a physician to recommend and a patient to seek alternative approaches is controversial. For example, it may be appropriate to recommend radical surgery for a younger patient with a low probability of cure. To improve the outcomes of surgery for high-risk patients, neoadjuvant hormonal therapy has been explored. The results of several large trials testing 3 or 8 months of androgen ablation before surgery showed that serum PSA levels decreased by 96%, prostate volumes reduced by 34%, and margin positivity rates declined from 41 to 17%. Unfortunately, hormones did not produce an improvement in PSA relapse–free survival. Thus, neoadjuvant hormonal therapy is not recommended.

Radiation Therapy Radiation therapy is given by external beam, the implantation of radioactive sources into the gland, or a combination of both. Contemporary external beam radiation techniques now use three-dimensional conformal treatment plans to maximize the administered dose to the tumor and to minimize the exposure of the surrounding normal structures. The addition of intensity modulation (IMRT) has allowed further shaping of the isodose curves and the delivery of higher doses to the tumor and a further reduction in normal tissue exposure. These advances have allowed the safe administration of doses >80 Gy, higher local control rates, and fewer side effects. Overall, radiation therapy is associated with a higher frequency of bowel complications (mainly diarrhea) than surgery. Measures of cancer control include the proportion of patients who show a decline in PSA to <0.5 or 1 ng/mL, the proportion with "nonrising" PSA values, or the proportion with a negative biopsy of the prostate 2 years after completion of treatment. PSA relapse is defined as three consecutive rising PSA values from the nadir value, with the time to failure as the midpoint between the nadir and first rising value.

Radiation dose is important. A PSA nadir of <1.0 ng/mL was observed in 90% of patients receiving 75.6 or 81.0 Gy vs. 76 and 56% for those receiving 70.2 Gy and 64.8 Gy, respectively. The positive biopsy rates at 2.5 years were 4% for those treated with 81 Gy, vs. 36 and 27% for those receiving 70.2 or 75.6 Gy. The frequency of rectal complications relates directly to the volume of the anterior rectal wall receiving full-dose treatment. Grade 3 rectal or urinary toxicities were seen in 2.1% of cases at a median dose of 75.6 Gy. Grade 3 urethral

strictures requiring dilatation developed in 1% of cases, all of whom had undergone a TURP. Pooled data show that the frequency of grade 3 to 4 toxicities is 6.9 and 3.5%, respectively, for patients who received >70 Gy. The frequency of erectile dysfunction is related to the quality of erections pretreatment, the dose administered, and the time of assessment. The etiology is related to a disruption of the vascular supply and not the nerve fibers.

Neoadjuvant hormone therapy has also been studied in combination with radiation therapy to increase local control rates, decrease the size of the prostate so that the exposure of normal tissues to full-dose radiation is reduced, and decrease the rate of systemic failure. Short-term hormone exposures can reduce toxicities and improve local control rates, but long-term (2 to 3 years) treatment is needed to prolong the time to PSA failure and the development of metastatic disease. The impact on survival has been less clear.

Brachytherapy involves the direct implantation of the prostate with radioactive sources. It is based on the principle that the deposition of radiation energy in tissues decreases exponentially as a function of the square of the distance from the source. The goal is to deliver intensive irradiation to the prostate, minimizing the exposure of the surrounding tissues. Techniques have evolved from intraoperative manual insertion methods to the current standard, in which customized templates based on CT and ultrasonographic assessment of the tumor are used for seed placement based on computer-optimized dosimetry to achieve more homogeneous dose distributions. The implants themselves are now performed transperineally, without an open procedure, with real-time imaging. The result is a marked reduction in local failure rates with fewer complications. In a series of 197 patients followed for a median of 3 years, 5-year actuarial PSA relapse–free survival for patients with pretherapy PSA levels of 0 to 4, 4 to 10, and >10 μg/mL were 98, 90 and 89%, respectively. In a separate report of 201 patients who underwent posttreatment biopsies, 80% were negative, 17% indeterminate, and 3% were positive. The results did not change with longer follow-up. Nevertheless, many physicians feel that implantation is best reserved for patients with good or intermediate prognostic features. The procedure is well tolerated, although most patients experience urinary frequency and urgency that can persist for several months. Incontinence has been seen in 2 to 4% of cases. Higher complication rates are observed in patients who have undergone a prior TURP or who have obstructive symptoms at baseline. Proctitis has been reported in <2% of patients.

Watchful waiting, or deferred therapy, is a policy of no therapeutic intervention(s) until the tumor progresses. Progression can be based on PSA changes, local tumor growth, the development of symptoms, or metastatic disease. The practice evolved from studies of predominantly elderly men with well-differentiated tumors in whom clinically significant progression could not be demonstrated for protracted periods, during which a significant proportion died of intercurrent disease. In a structured literature review of patients treated by radical surgery, a deferred approach, or external beam radiation, the 10-year mean survivals were 93% for radical prostatectomy, 84% for deferred treatment, and 74% for external beam radiation. Risk of progression was related to grade. Men with grade 1 or 2 tumors had a 13% risk of death and 19% risk of metastases at 10 years; those with grade 3 tumors had 63 and 74% risks, respectively.

Case selection is critical, and the criteria to select those to whom watchful waiting can be applied safely are under intense study. In a recent prostatectomy series, it was estimated that 10 to 15% of patients had "insignificant" cancers. Given the multifocality of the disease, a concern is the limited ability to predict pathologic findings on the basis of a needle biopsy, even when multiple cores are obtained. Arguing against this approach is the result of a randomized trial of radical prostatectomy vs. watchful waiting from Sweden. With a median follow-up of 6.2 years, men treated by radical surgery had a lower risk of prostate cancer death relative to watchful waiting patients (4.6 vs. 8.9%) and a lower risk of metastatic progression, hazard ratio .63.

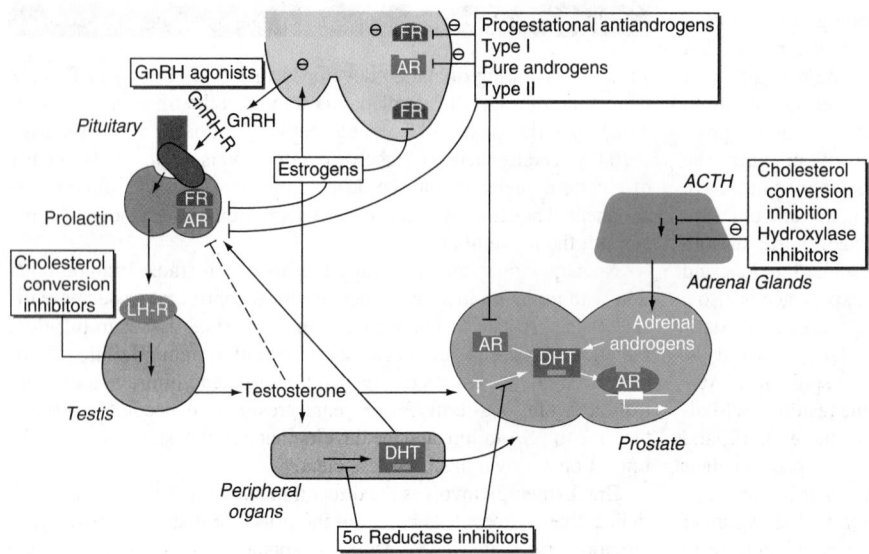

FIGURE 81-3 Sites of action of different hormone therapies.

Nevertheless, it can be anticipated that more patients may be candidates for a deferred approach as PSA testing is applied more widely and earlier.

RISING PSA This state includes patients in whom the sole manifestation of disease is a rising PSA after surgery and/or radiation therapy. By definition, no evidence of disease is found on scan. For these patients the central issue is whether the rise in PSA is the result of persistent disease in the primary site, a systemic recurrence, or both. In theory, disease that persists or has recurred in the primary site may be curable by additional local treatment. For patients who had undergone surgery, the question is whether external beam radiation therapy to the prostate bed can eliminate the disease and lead to an undetectable PSA. For radiation therapy–treated patients, the question is whether a prostatectomy would achieve cure.

The decision to recommend radiation therapy is often made on clinical grounds, as imaging studies such as CT and bone scan are typically uninformative. Some recommend a Prostascint scan: imaging with a radiolabeled antibody to prostate-specific membrane antigen (PSMA), which is highly expressed on prostate epithelial cells. Antibody localization to the prostatic fossa suggests local recurrence; localization to extrapelvic sites predicts failure of radiation therapy. Others recommend that a biopsy of the urethrovesical anastamosis be obtained before considering radiation. Factors that predict for response to salvage radiation are a positive surgical margin, a lower Gleason grade, a long interval from surgery to PSA failure, a slow PSA doubling time, and a low (<0.5 to 1.0 ng/mL) PSA value at the time of treatment. Radiation is generally not recommended if the PSA was persistently elevated after surgery (indicating that disease-free status was not achieved).

For patients with a rising PSA after radiation therapy, a salvage prostatectomy can be considered if the disease was "curable" at the onset, persistent disease has been documented by a biopsy of the prostate, and no metastatic disease is seen on imaging studies. Unfortunately, case selection is poorly defined in most series, and morbidities are significant. As currently performed, virtually all patients are impotent, and ~45% have either total urinary incontinence or stress incontinence. Major bleeding, bladder neck contractures, and rectal injury are not uncommon.

In the majority of cases, the rise in PSA indicates systemic disease. In these cases, the need for treatment should consider the probability of developing clinically detectable disease on scan and in what time frame. That immediate therapy is not required was shown in a series where patients did not receive systemic therapy until metastatic disease was documented. Overall, the median time to metastatic progression was 8 years and 63% of the patients with rising PSA values remained free of metastases at 5 years. Factors associated with progression include Gleason grade, time to recurrence, and PSA doubling times. For those with Gleason grade ≥8 tumors, the probability of metastatic progression was 37, 51, and 71% at 3, 5, and 7 years, respectively. If the time to recurrence was <2 years and PSA doubling time was long (> 10 months), the proportion with metastatic disease was 23, 32, and 53% vs. 47, 69, and 79% if the doubling time was short (< 10 months) during the same time intervals. These models continue to be refined. A difficulty making these predictions is that most patients with a rising PSA receive some form of therapy before the development of metastases.

METASTATIC DISEASE: NONCASTRATE *Metastatic disease noncastrate* refers to patients with tumors visible on an imaging study and noncastrate levels of testosterone. The patient may be newly diagnosed or have recurrent disease after treatment for localized disease. Standard treatment is to block androgen action or decrease androgen production by medical or surgical means. Over 90% of male hormones originate in the testes; <10% are synthesized in the adrenal gland. Surgical orchiectomy is the "gold standard" approach but is least acceptable by patients. Medical therapies can be divided into those that lower testosterone levels, e.g., gonadotropin-releasing hormone (GnRH) agonists and antagonists, estrogens and progestational agents, and the antiandrogens that bind to the androgen receptor but do not signal (Fig. 81-3). Ketoconazole inhibits adrenal androgen synthesis and is used after first-line castration is no longer effective. In this setting, the adrenal glands may contribute up to 40% of the active androgens in the prostate.

GnRH analogues (leuprolide acetate and goserelin acetate) initially produce a rise in luteinizing hormone and follicle-stimulating hormone (FSH), followed by a downregulation of receptors in the pituitary gland, which effects a chemical castration. They were approved on the basis of randomized comparisons showing an improved safety profile (specifically, reduced cardiovascular toxicities) relative to diethylstilbestrol (DES), with equivalent potency. The initial rise in testosterone may result in a clinical flare of the disease. As such, these agents are contraindicated in men with significant obstructive symptoms, cancer-related pain, or spinal cord compromise. Estrogens such as DES also lower testosterone levels but have fallen out of favor due to the risk of vascular complications such as fluid retention, phlebitis, emboli, and stroke.

In contrast, nonsteroidal antiandrogens such as flutamide, bicalutamide, or nilutamide block the binding of androgens to the receptor. Given alone, testosterone levels remain the same or increase. These agents were approved initially to block the flare associated with the initial rise in testosterone that results following GnRH administration. They have also been studied as part of a combined androgen blockade (CAB) or maximal androgen blockade (MAB) and as monotherapy. The concept of CAB was developed to inhibit testicular and adrenal androgens at the outset, and it preoccupied the field for many years. It is achieved clinically by combining an antiandrogen with a GnRH agonist or surgical orchiectomy. Cumulative results of randomized comparisons involving thousands of patients showed no advantage for combining an antiandrogen with surgical orchiectomy, while separate analyses of trials combining an antiandrogen with a GnRH analogue have shown a modest (<10%) survival advantage. Meta-analysis of all combined androgen blockade trials concluded that there was no benefit to the approach. In practice, most patients treated with GnRH analogue therapy receive an antiandrogen for the first 2 to 4 weeks of treatment.

The anti–prostate cancer effects of agents that lower serum testosterone levels are similar, and the clinical course is predictable: an initial response, a period of stability in which the cells are dormant and not proliferating, followed by regrowth after a variable period of time as a hormone-independent tumor. Androgen ablation is not curative. Cells that survive castration are present when the disease is first diagnosed. Considered by disease manifestation, PSA levels return to normal in 60 to 70% of cases and measurable disease regression occurs in 50%; while improvements in bone scan occur in 25% of cases, the majority remain stable. Survival is inversely proportional to disease extent. Agents that lower testosterone are associated with an androgen-deprivation syndrome that includes hot flushes, weakness, fatigue, impotence, loss of muscle mass, changes in personality, anemia, depression, and a reduction in bone density. The bone changes can be prevented by treatment with bisphosphonates along with vitamin D and calcium supplementation.

A question often asked is whether antiandrogens, which are associated with fewer hot flashes, less of an effect on libido, less muscle wasting, fewer personality changes, and less bone loss, can be used alone without compromising outcomes. Gynecomastia remains a significant problem but can be alleviated in part with the addition of tamoxifen. Most reported randomized trials suggest that the cancer-specific outcomes are inferior. Even a comparison of bicalutamide, 150 mg (three times the recommended dose of 50 mg), versus surgical castration showed a shorter time to progression and inferior survival for patients with established metastatic disease. Nevertheless, some men may accept the trade-off of a potentially inferior cancer outcome for an improved quality of life.

Another question is whether hormones should be given early, in the adjuvant setting or at the time recurrence is first documented, or late, when metastatic disease or symptoms are manifest. Trials in support of early therapy have often been underpowered relative to the "net benefit" reported or have been criticized on methodologic grounds. In one, although a survival benefit was shown for patients treated with radiation therapy and 3 years of androgen ablation relative to radiation alone, the trial was criticized for the poor outcomes for the control group. Another showing a survival benefit for patients with positive nodes randomized to medical or surgical castration compared to observation ($p = .02$) was criticized because the confidence intervals around the 5- and 8-year survival distributions overlapped between the two groups. A large randomized study comparing early to late hormone treatment (orchiectomy or GnRH analogue) in patients with locally advanced or asymptomatic metastatic disease showed that patients treated early were less likely to progress from M0 to M1 disease, develop pain, and die of prostate cancer. This trial was criticized because therapy was delayed "too long" in the late-treatment group. When patients treated by radical surgery, radiation therapy, or watchful waiting were randomly assigned to receive bicalutamide, 150 mg, or placebo, hormone treatment produced a significant reduction in the proportion of patients who developed osseous metastases at 2 years (9% for bicalutamide; 13.8% for placebo). This result has not gained acceptance in part because too many "good-risk" patients were treated and because no effect on survival was demonstrated. These criticisms are valid; however, the net influence on survival from early hormone intervention is similar to that observed in patients with breast cancer where adjuvant hormonal therapy is routinely given.

Another way to reduce the side effects of androgen ablation is to administer hormones on an intermittent basis. This was proposed as a way to prevent the emergence of castration-resistant cells by "forcing" the cells that survive androgen ablation into a normal differentiation pathway by repleting testosterone. Theoretically, surviving cells that are allowed to proliferate in the presence of androgen will retain sensitivity to androgen ablation. The duration of treatment varies from 2 to 6 months beyond the point of maximal response. Once therapy is stopped, endogenous testosterone levels increase, and the symptoms associated with androgen ablation abate. PSA levels also begin to rise, and, at some level, androgen ablation is restarted. Using this approach, multiple cycles of regression and proliferation have been documented in individual patients. It is unknown whether the intermittent approach

increases, decreases, or does not change the overall duration of sensitivity to androgen ablation. A trial to address this question is ongoing.

METASTATIC DISEASE: CASTRATE Castration-resistant disease can be manifest in many ways. For some it is a rise in PSA with no change in radiographs and no new symptoms. In others, it is a rising PSA and progression in bone, with or without symptoms of disease. Still others will show soft tissue disease with or without osseous metastases, and others have a pattern of visceral spread. The prognosis, highly variable, can also be predicted using nomograms designed for this cohort. The important distinction is that despite the failure of first-line hormone treatment, the majority of these tumors remain sensitive to second- and third-line hormonal treatments. Castration resistance does not indicate hormonal resistance. The rising PSA is an indication of continued signaling through the androgen receptor axis.

The manifestations of disease in this patient group hinder the development of drugs and treatment standards because the traditional measures of outcome such as tumor regression do not apply. No PSA-based outcomes are true surrogates for a survival benefit, and assessing changes in osseous disease using bone scans is notoriously inaccurate. It is essential to define therapeutic objectives before initiating treatment, as standards of care have changed on the basis of randomized comparisons that provide clinical benefits without prolonging life. These endpoints include the relief of symptoms and delaying metastases or the time to the development of new symptoms of disease.

The management of these patients requires first that the castrate status be documented. Patients receiving an antiandrogen alone who have elevated levels of serum testosterone should be treated first with a GnRH analogue or orchiectomy and observed for response. Patients on an anti-androgen in combination with a GnRH analogue should have the antiandrogen discontinued, as ~30% will respond to the withdrawal of the antiandrogen. Any response occurs within weeks of stopping flutamide, but may take 8 to 12 weeks with nilutamide and bicalutamide (they have a long terminal half-life). At the time of progression, a different antiandrogen can be given as these agents are not cross-resistant. Other hormones that may be active include estrogens, progestins, ketoconazole, and glucocorticoids. Those who respond to estrogens or progestins should also be evaluated for a withdrawal response at the time of progression. Cytotoxic agents are considered when hormone responses stop.

No chemotherapy regimen has been proven to prolong life in these patients. However, responses to chemotherapy that improve symptom control are not uncommon. Drugs directed at the tumor cell cytoskeleton such estramustine (Emcyt) and a taxane such as paclitaxel or docetaxel can induce responses in ≥50% using measurable disease regression as the endpoint. Seventy percent will show a >50% decline in PSA from baseline. Studies evaluating survival effects are nearly done.

Management of pain is a critical part of therapy. Optimal palliation requires assessing whether the symptoms and metastases are focal or diffuse and whether disease threatens the spinal cord, the cauda equina, or the base of the skull. Neurologic symptoms require emergent evaluation because loss of function may be permanent if not addressed in a timely manner. Single sites of pain or areas of neurologic involvement are best treated with external beam radiation. As the disease is often diffuse, palliation at one site often leads to the emergence of symptoms at another. An important principle of management was established in two randomized trials of mitoxantrone and prednisone vs. prednisone alone. In both studies, mitoxantrone-treated patients had a greater reduction in pain, used fewer narcotics, were more mobile, and had less fatigue. No survival benefit was shown.

Given the bone-dominant nature of prostate cancer spread, bone-directed therapies may be useful in patients with diffuse disease. Two bone-seeking radioisotopes, ^{89}Sr (metastron) and ^{153}Sm-EDTMP (quadramet), are approved for palliation of pain although they have no effect on PSA or on survival. Fewer patients treated with an isotope developed new areas of pain or required additional radiation therapy compared to patients receiving external beam radiation therapy alone. Addition of zoledronate to "standard therapy" in patients with castration-resistant disease resulted in fewer skeletal events relative to placebo-treated patients. The bone events included development of new pain, need for radiation therapy, and microfractures. Finally, patients randomly assigned to a combination of ^{89}Sr and doxorubicin after induction chemotherapy had fewer skeletal events and longer survival than patients treated with doxorubicin alone. Confirmatory studies are ongoing.

FURTHER READING

GONZALGO ML, ISAACS WB: Molecular pathways to prostate cancer. J Urol 170:2444, 2003

KHAN MA, PARTIN AW: Partin tables: Past and present. BJU Int 92:7, 2003

NELSON WG et al: Prostate cancer. N Engl J Med 349:366, 2003

SCHAFFER DR, SCHER HI: Prostate cancer: A dynamic illness with shifting targets. Lancet Oncol 4:407, 2003

THOMPSON IM et al: The influence of finasteride on the development of prostate cancer. N Engl J Med 349:215, 2003

THORPE A, NEAL D: Benign prostatic hyperplasia. Lancet 366:1359, 2003

YAO SL, DIPAOLA RS: evidence-based approach to prostate cancer follow-up. Semin Oncol 30:390, 2003

82 TESTICULAR CANCER
Robert J. Motzer, George J. Bosl

Primary germ cell tumors (GCTs) of the testis, arising by the malignant transformation of primordial germ cells, constitute 95% of all testicular neoplasms. Infrequently, GCTs arise from an extragonadal site, including the mediastinum, retroperitoneum, and, very rarely, the pineal gland. This disease is notable for the young age of the afflicted patients, the totipotent capacity for differentiation of the tumor cells, and its curability; about 95% of all newly diagnosed patients will be cured. Experience in the management of GCTs leads to improved outcome.

INCIDENCE AND EPIDEMIOLOGY Nearly 9000 new cases of testicular GCT were diagnosed in the United States in 2004; the incidence of this malignancy has increased slowly over the past 40 years. The tumor occurs most frequently in men between the ages of 20 and 40. A testicular mass in a man ≥50 years should be regarded as a lymphoma until proved otherwise. GCT is at least four to five times more common in white than in African-American males, and a higher incidence has been observed in Scandinavia and New Zealand than in the United States.

ETIOLOGY AND GENETICS Cryptorchidism is associated with a severalfold higher risk of GCT. Abdominal cryptorchid testes are at a higher risk than inguinal cryptorchid testes. Orchiopexy should be performed before puberty, if possible. Early orchiopexy reduces the risk of GCT and improves the ability to save the testis. An abdominal cryptorchid testis that cannot be brought into the scrotum should be removed. About 2% of men with GCTs of one testis will develop a primary tumor in the other testis. Testicular feminization syndromes increase the risk of testicular GCT, and Klinefelter's syndrome is associated with mediastinal GCT.

An isochromosome of the short arm of chromosome 12 [i(12p)] is pathognomonic for GCT of all histologic types. Excess 12p copy number either in the form of i(12p) or as increased 12p on aberrantly banded marker chromosomes occurs in nearly all GCTs, but the gene(s) on 12p involved in the pathogenesis are not yet defined.

CLINICAL PRESENTATION A painless testicular mass is pathognomonic for a testicular malignancy. More commonly, patients present with testicular discomfort or swelling suggestive of epididymitis and/or orchitis. In this circumstance, a trial of antibiotics is reasonable. However, if symptoms persist or a residual abnormality remains, then testicular ultrasound examination is indicated.

Ultrasound of the testis is indicated whenever a testicular malignancy is considered and for persistent or painful testicular swelling. If a testicular mass is detected, a radical inguinal orchiectomy should be performed. Because the testis develops from the gonadal ridge, its blood supply and lymphatic drainage originate in the abdomen and descend with the testis into the scrotum. An inguinal approach is taken to avoid breaching anatomic barriers and permitting additional pathways of spread.

Back pain from retroperitoneal metastases is common and must be distinguished from musculoskeletal pain. Dyspnea from pulmonary metastases occurs infrequently. Patients with increased serum levels of human chorionic gonadotropin (hCG) may present with gynecomastia. A delay in diagnosis is associated with a more advanced stage and possibly worse survival.

The staging evaluation for GCT includes a determination of serum levels of α fetoprotein (AFP), hCG, and lactate dehydrogenase (LDH). After orchiectomy, a chest radiograph and a computed tomography (CT) scan of the abdomen and pelvis should be performed. A chest CT scan is required if pulmonary nodules or mediastinal or hilar disease is suspected. Stage I disease is limited to the testis, epididymis, or spermatic cord. Stage II disease is limited to retroperitoneal (regional) lymph nodes. Stage III disease is disease outside the retroperitoneum, involving supradiaphragmatic nodal sites or viscera. The staging may be "clinical"—defined solely by physical examination, blood marker evaluation, and radiographs—or "pathologic"—defined by an operative procedure.

The regional draining lymph nodes for the testis are in the retroperitoneum, and the vascular supply originates from the great vessels (for the right testis) or the renal vessels (for the left testis). As a result, the lymph nodes that are involved first by a right testicular tumor are the interaortocaval lymph nodes just below the renal vessels. For a left testicular tumor, the first involved lymph nodes are lateral to the aorta (para-aortic) and below the left renal vessels. In both cases, further nodal spread is inferior and contralateral and, less commonly, above the renal hilum. Lymphatic involvement can extend cephalad to the retrocrural, posterior mediastinal, and supraclavicular lymph nodes. Treatment is determined by tumor histology (seminoma versus nonseminoma) and clinical stage (Table 82-1).

PATHOLOGY GCTs are divided into nonseminoma and seminoma subtypes. Nonseminomatous GCTs are most frequent in the third decade of life and can display the full spectrum of embryonic and adult cellular differentiation. This entity comprises four histologies: embryonal carcinoma, teratoma, choriocarcinoma, and endodermal sinus (yolk sac) tumor. Choriocarcinoma, consisting of both cytotrophoblasts and syncytiotrophoblasts, represents malignant trophoblastic differentiation and is invariably associated with secretion of hCG. Endodermal sinus tumor is the malignant counterpart of the fetal yolk sac and is associated with secretion of AFP. Pure embryonal carcinoma may secrete AFP or hCG, or both; this pattern is biochemical evidence of differentiation. Teratoma is composed of somatic cell types derived from two or more germ layers (ectoderm, mesoderm, or endoderm). Each of these histologies may be present alone or in combination with others. Nonseminomatous GCTs tend to metastasize early to sites such as the retroperitoneal lymph nodes and lung parenchyma. One-third of patients present with disease limited to the testis (stage I), one-third with retroperitoneal metastases (stage II), and one-third with more extensive supradiaphragmatic nodal or visceral metastases (stage III).

Seminoma represents about 50% of all GCTs, has a median age in the fourth decade, and generally follows a more indolent clinical course. Most patients (70%) present with stage I disease, about 20% with stage II disease, and 10% with stage III disease; lung or other visceral metastases are rare. Radiation therapy is the treatment of choice in patients with stage I disease and stage II disease where the nodes are <5 cm in maximum diameter. When a tumor contains both seminoma and nonseminoma components, patient management is directed by the more aggressive nonseminoma component.

TUMOR MARKERS Careful monitoring of the serum tumor markers AFP and hCG is essential in the management of patients with GCT, as these markers are important for diagnosis, as prognostic indicators, in monitoring treatment response, and in the detection of early relapse. Approximately 70% of patients presenting with disseminated nonseminomatous GCT have increased serum concentrations of AFP and/or hCG. While hCG concentrations may be increased in patients with either nonseminoma or seminoma histology, the AFP concentration is increased only in patients with nonseminoma. The presence of an increased AFP level in a patient whose tumor showed only seminoma indicates that an occult nonseminomatous component exists and the patient should be treated for nonseminomatous GCT. LDH levels are not as specific as AFP or hCG, but are increased in 50 to 60% patients with metastatic nonseminoma and in up to 80% of patients with advanced seminoma.

AFP, hCG, and LDH levels should be determined before and after orchiectomy. Increased serum AFP and hCG concentrations decay according to first-order kinetics; the half-life is 24 to 36 h for hCG and 5 to 7 days for AFP. AFP and hCG should be assayed serially during and after treatment. The reappearance of hCG and/or AFP or the failure of these markers to decline according to the predicted half-life is an indicator of persistent or recurrent tumor.

Rx TREATMENT

Stage I Nonseminoma If, after an orchiectomy (for clinical stage I disease), radiographs and physical examination show no evidence of disease, and serum AFP and hCG concentrations are either normal or declining to normal according to the known half-life, patients may be managed by either a nerve-sparing retroperitoneal lymph node dissection (RPLND) or surveillance. The retroperitoneal lymph nodes are involved by GCT (pathologic stage II) in 20 to 50% of these patients. The choice of surveillance or RPLND is based on the pathology of the primary tumor. If the primary tumor shows no evidence for lymphatic or vascular invasion and is limited to the testis (T1), then either option is reasonable. If lymphatic or vascular invasion is present or the tumor extends into the tunica, spermatic cord, or scrotum (T2 through T4), then surveillance should not be offered. Either approach should cure >95% of patients.

A RPLND is the standard operation for removal of the regional lymph nodes of the testis (retroperitoneal nodes). The operation removes the lymph nodes ipsilateral to the primary site and the nodal groups adjacent to the primary landing zone. The standard (modified bilateral) RPLND removes all node-bearing tissue down to the bifurcation of the great vessels, including the ipsilateral iliac nodes. The major long-term effect of this operation is retrograde ejaculation and infertility. A nerve-sparing RPLND, usually accomplished by identification and dissection of individual nerve fibers, may avoid injury to the sympathetic nerves responsible for ejaculation. Normal ejaculation is preserved in ~90% of patients. Patients with pathologic stage I disease are observed, and only the <10% who relapse require additional therapy. If retroperitoneal nodes are found to be involved at RPLND, then a decision regarding adjuvant chemotherapy is made on the basis of the extent of retroperitoneal disease (see below).

Surveillance is an option in the management of clinical stage I disease when no vascular/lymphatic invasion is found (T1). Only 20 to 30% of patients have pathologic stage II disease, implying that most

		Treatment	
Stage	Extent of Disease	Seminoma	Nonseminoma
IA	Testis only, no vascular/lymphatic invasion (T1)	Radiation therapy	RPLND or observation
IB	Testis only, with vascular/lymphatic invasion (T2), or extension through tunica albuginea (T2), or involvement of spermatic cord (T3) or scrotum (T4)	Radiation therapy	RPLND
IIA	Nodes < 2 cm	Radiation therapy	RPLND or chemotherapy often followed by RPLND
IIB	Nodes 2–5 cm	Radiation therapy	RPLND +/− adjuvant chemotherapy or chemotherapy followed by RPLND
IIC	Nodes > 5 cm	Chemotherapy	Chemotherapy, often followed by RPLND
III	Distant metastases	Chemotherapy	Chemotherapy, often followed by surgery (biopsy or resection)

TABLE 82-1 *Germ Cell Tumor Staging and Treatment*

Note: RPLND, retroperitoneal lymph node dissection.

RPLNDs in this situation are not therapeutic. Although surveillance has not been compared to RPLND in a randomized trial, all large studies show that surveillance and RPLND lead to equivalent long-term survival rates. Patient compliance is essential if surveillance is to be successful. Patients must be carefully followed with periodic chest radiography, physical examination, CT scan of the abdomen, and serum tumor marker determinations. The median time to relapse is about 7 months, and late relapses (>2 years) are rare. The 70 to 80% of patients who do not relapse require no intervention after orchiectomy; treatment is reserved for those who do relapse. When the primary tumor is classified as T2 through T4 (extension beyond testis and epididymis or lymphatic/vascular invasion is identified), nerve-sparing RPLND is preferred. About 50% of these patients have pathologic stage II disease and are destined to relapse without the RPLND.

Stage II Nonseminoma Patients with limited, ipsilateral retroperitoneal adenopathy (nodes usually ≤3 cm in largest diameter) and normal levels of AFP and hCG generally undergo a modified bilateral RPLND as primary management. Increased levels of either AFP or hCG or both imply metastatic disease outside the retroperitoneum; chemotherapy is used in this setting. The local recurrence rate after a properly performed RPLND is very low. Depending on the extent of disease, the postoperative management options include either surveillance or two cycles of adjuvant chemotherapy. Surveillance is the preferred approach for patients with resected "low-volume" metastases (tumor nodes ≤2 cm in diameter *and* <6 nodes involved) because the probability of relapse is one-third or less. For those who relapse, risk-directed chemotherapy is indicated (see below). Because relapse occurs in ≥50% of patients with "high-volume" metastases (>6 nodes involved, *or* any involved node >2 cm in largest diameter, *or* extranodal tumor extension), two cycles of adjuvant chemotherapy should be considered, as it results in cure in ≥98% of patients. Regimens consisting of etoposide (100 mg/m^2 daily on days 1 through 5) plus cisplatin (20 mg/m^2 daily on days 1 through 5) with or without bleomycin (30 units per day on days 2, 9, and 16) given at 3-week intervals are effective and well tolerated.

Stages I and II Seminoma Inguinal orchiectomy followed by retroperitoneal radiation therapy cures ~98% of patients with stage I seminoma. The dose of radiation therapy (2500 to 3000 cGy) is low and well tolerated, and the in-field recurrence rate is negligible. About 2% of patients relapse with supradiaphragmatic or systemic disease. Surveillance has been proposed as an option, and studies have shown that about 15% of patients relapse. The median time to relapse is 12 to 15 months, and late relapses (>5 years) may be more frequent than with nonseminoma. The relapse is usually treated with chemotherapy. Surveillance for clinical stage I seminoma is generally not recommended.

Nonbulky retroperitoneal disease (stage IIA and IIB) is also treated with radiation therapy. Prophylactic supradiaphragmatic fields are not used. Relapses in the anterior mediastinum are unusual. Approximately 90% of patients achieve relapse-free survival with retroperitoneal masses <5 cm in diameter. Because at least one-third of patients with bulkier disease relapse, initial chemotherapy is preferred for stage IIC disease.

Chemotherapy for Advanced GCT   Regardless of histology, patients with stage IIC and stage III GCT are treated with chemotherapy. Combination chemotherapy programs based on cisplatin at doses of 100 mg/m² plus etoposide at doses of 500 mg/m² per cycle cure 70 to 80% of such patients, with or without bleomycin, depending on risk stratification (see below). A complete response (the complete disappearance of all clinical evidence of tumor on physical examination and radiography plus normal serum levels of AFP and hCG for ≥1 month) occurs after chemotherapy alone in ~60% of patients, and another 10 to 20% become disease-free with surgical resection of residual masses containing viable GCT. Lower doses of cisplatin result in inferior survival rates.

The toxicity of four cycles of the cisplatin/bleomycin/etoposide (BEP) regimen is substantial. Nausea, vomiting, and hair loss occur in most patients, although nausea and vomiting have been markedly ameliorated by modern antiemetic regimens. Myelosuppression is frequent, and symptomatic bleomycin pulmonary toxicity occurs in ~5% of patients. Treatment-induced mortality due to neutropenia with septicemia or bleomycin-induced pulmonary failure occurs in 1 to 3% of patients. Dose reductions for myelosuppression are rarely indicated. Long-term permanent toxicities include nephrotoxicity (reduced glomerular filtration and persistent magnesium wasting), ototoxicity, and peripheral neuropathy. When bleomycin is administered by weekly bolus injection, Raynaud's phenomenon appears in 5 to 10% of patients. Other evidence of small blood vessel damage is seen less often, including transient ischemic attacks and myocardial infarction.

Risk-Directed Chemotherapy   Because not all patients are cured and treatment may cause significant toxicities, patients are stratified into "good-risk" and "poor-risk" groups according to pretreatment clinical features. For good-risk patients, the goal is to achieve maximum efficacy with minimal toxicity. For poor-risk patients, the goal is to identify more effective therapy with tolerable toxicity.

The International Germ Cell Cancer Consensus Group (IGCCCG) developed criteria to assign patients to three risk groups (good, intermediate, poor) (Table 82-2). The marker cut-offs have been incorporated into the revised TNM staging of GCT. Hence, TNM stage groupings are now based on both anatomy (site and extent of disease) and biology (marker status and histology). Seminoma is either good or intermediate risk based on the absence or presence of nonpulmonary visceral metastases. No poor-risk category exists for seminoma. Marker levels play no role in defining risk for seminoma. Nonseminomas have good-, intermediate-, and poor-risk categories based on the site of the primary tumor, the presence or absence of nonpulmonary visceral metastases, and marker levels.

For ~90% of patients with good-risk GCTs, four cycles of etoposide plus cisplatin (EP) or three cycles of BEP produce durable complete responses, with minimal acute and chronic toxicity. Pulmonary toxicity is absent when bleomycin is not used and is rare when therapy is limited to 9 weeks; myelosuppression with neutropenic fever is less frequent; and the treatment mortality rate is negligible. About 75% of intermediate-risk patients and 45% of poor-risk patients achieve durable complete remission with four cycles of BEP, and no regimen has proved superior. More effective therapy is needed.

Postchemotherapy Surgery   Resection of residual metastases after the completion of chemotherapy is an integral part of therapy. If the initial histology is nonseminoma and the marker values have normalized, all

TABLE 82-2   IGCCCG Risk Classification for Advanced Germ Cell Tumors

Risk	Nonseminoma	Seminoma
Good	Gonadal or retroperitoneal primary site	Any primary site
	Absent nonpulmonary visceral metastases	Absent nonpulmonary visceral metastases
	AFP < 1000 ng/mL	Any LDH, hCG
	Beta-hCG < 5000 mIU/mL	
	LDH < 1.5 × upper limit or normal (ULN)	
Intermediate	Gonadal or retroperitoneal primary site	Any primary site
	Absent nonpulmonary visceral metastases	Presence of nonpulmonary visceral metastases
	AFP 1000–10,000 ng/mL	Any LDH, hCG
	Beta-hCG 5000–50,000 mIU/mL	
	LDH 1.5–10 × ULN	
Poor	Mediastinal primary site	No patients classified as poor prognosis
	Presence of nonpulmonary visceral metastases	
	AFP ≥ 10,000 ng/ML	
	Beta-hCG > 50,000 mIU/mL	
	LDH > 10 × ULN	

Note: AFP, α fetoprotein; hCG, human chorionic gonadotropin; LDH, lactate dehydrogenase.
Source: From International Germ Cell Cancer Consensus Group.

sites of residual disease should be resected. In general, residual retroperitoneal disease requires a modified bilateral RPLND. Thoracotomy (unilateral or bilateral) and neck dissection are less frequently required to remove residual mediastinal, pulmonary parenchymal, or cervical nodal disease. Viable tumor (seminoma, embryonal carcinoma, yolk sac tumor, or choriocarcinoma) will be present in 15%, mature teratoma in 40%, and necrotic debris and fibrosis in 45% of resected specimens. The frequency of teratoma or viable disease is highest in residual mediastinal tumors. If necrotic debris or mature teratoma is present, no further chemotherapy is necessary. If viable tumor is present but is completely excised, two additional cycles of chemotherapy are given.

If the initial histology is pure seminoma, mature teratoma is rarely present, and the most frequent finding is necrotic debris. For residual retroperitoneal disease, a complete RPLND is technically difficult owing to extensive postchemotherapy fibrosis. Observation is recommended when no radiographic abnormality exists or a residual mass <3 cm is present. Controversy exists over what to do when the residual mass exceeds 3 cm in diameter. About 25% of such masses contain viable GCT. Some investigators prefer excision or biopsy, but radiation therapy and surveillance are alternatives.

Salvage Chemotherapy   Of patients with advanced GCT, 20 to 30% fail to achieve a durable complete response to first-line chemotherapy. A combination of cisplatin, ifosfamide and vinblastine (VeIP) will cure about 25% of patients as a second-line therapy. Substitution of paclitaxel for vinblastine may be more effective in this setting. Patients are more likely to achieve a durable complete response if they had a testicular primary tumor and relapsed from a prior complete remission to first-line cisplatin-containing chemotherapy. In contrast, if the patient failed to achieve a complete response or has a primary mediastinal nonseminoma, then standard-dose salvage therapy is rarely beneficial. Treatment options for such patients include dose-intensive treatment, experimental therapies, and surgical resection.

Chemotherapy consisting of dose-intensive, high-dose carboplatin (≥1500 mg/m²) plus etoposide (≥1200 mg/m²), with or without cyclophosphamide or ifosfamide, with peripheral blood stem cell support induces a complete response in 25 to 40% of patients who have progressed after ifosfamide-containing salvage chemotherapy. About one-half of the complete responses will be durable. High-dose therapy is the treatment of choice and standard of care for this patient population. Paclitaxel is also active in previously treated patients and shows promise in high-dose combination programs. Cure is still possible in some relapsed patients.

EXTRAGONADAL GCT AND MIDLINE CARCINOMA OF UNCERTAIN HISTOGENESIS

The prognosis and management of patients with extragonadal GCTs depends on the tumor histology and site of origin. All patients with a diagnosis of extragonadal GCT should have a testicular ultrasound examination. Nearly all patients with retroperitoneal or mediastinal seminoma achieve a durable complete response to BEP or EP. The clinical features of patients with primary retroperitoneal nonseminoma GCT are similar to those of patients with a primary of testis origin, and careful evaluation will find evidence of a primary testicular GCT in about two-thirds of cases. In contrast, a primary mediastinal nonseminomatous GCT is associated with a poor prognosis; one-third of patients are cured with standard therapy (four cycles of BEP). Patients with newly diagnosed mediastinal nonseminoma are considered to have poor-risk disease and should be considered for clinical trials testing regimens of possibly greater efficacy. In addition, mediastinal nonseminoma is associated with hematologic disorders, including acute myelogenous leukemia, myelodysplastic syndrome, and essential thrombocytosis unrelated to previous chemotherapy. These hematologic disorders are very refractory to treatment. Nonseminoma of any primary site may change into other malignant histologies such as embryonal rhabdomyosarcoma or adenocarcinoma. This is called malignant transformation. i(12p) has been identified in the transformed cell type, indicating GCT clonal origin.

A group of patients with poorly differentiated tumors of unknown histogenesis, midline in distribution, and not associated with secretion of AFP or hCG has been described; a few (10 to 20%) are cured by standard cisplatin-containing chemotherapy. i(12p) is present in ~25% of such tumors (the fraction that are cisplatin-responsive), confirming their origin from primitive germ cells. This finding is also predictive of the response to cisplatin-based chemotherapy and resulting long-

term survival. These tumors are heterogeneous; neuroepithelial tumors and lymphoma may also present in this fashion.

FERTILITY Infertility is an important consequence of the treatment of GCTs. Preexisting infertility or impaired fertility is often present. Azoospermia and/or oligospermia are present at diagnosis in at least 50% of patients with testicular GCTs. Ejaculatory dysfunction is associated with RPLND, and germ cell damage may result from cisplatin-containing chemotherapy. Nerve-sparing techniques to preserve the retroperitoneal sympathetic nerves have made retrograde ejaculation less likely in the subgroups of patients who are candidates for this operation. Spermatogenesis does recur in some patients after chemotherapy. However, because of the significant risk of impaired reproductive capacity, semen analysis and cryopreservation of sperm in a sperm bank should be recommended to all patients before treatment.

FURTHER READING

BOSL GJ et al: Testicular germ-cell cancer. N Engl J Med 337:242, 1997

CHAGANTI RSK, HOULDSWORTH J: Genetics and biology of human male germ cell tumors. Cancer Res 60:1475, 2000

INTERNATIONAL GERM CELL CANCER CONSENSUS GROUP: International Germ Cell Consensus Classification: A prognostic factor-based staging system for metastatic germ cell cancers. J Clin Oncol 15:594, 1997

KONDAGUNTA GV, MOTZER R: Adjuvant chemotherapy for stage II nonseminomatous germ cell tumors. Semin Urol 20:239, 2002

MCGLYNN KA et al: Trends in the incidence of testicular germ cell tumors in the United States. Cancer 97:63, 2003

MCGUIRE MS et al: The role of thoracotomy in managing postchemotherapy residual thoracic masses in patients with nonseminomatous germ cell tumors. BJU Int 91:469, 2003

MOTZER R et al: Sequential dose-intensive paclitaxel, ifosfamide, carboplatin, and etoposide salvage therapy for germ cell tumor patients. J Clin Oncol 18:1173, 2000

83 GYNECOLOGIC MALIGNANCIES
Robert C. Young

OVARIAN CANCER

Incidence and Epidemiology Epithelial ovarian cancer is the leading cause of death from gynecologic cancer in the United States. In 2004, 25,580 new cases were diagnosed and 16,090 women died from ovarian cancer. The disease accounts for 5% of all cancer deaths in women in the United States; more women die of this disease than from cervical and endometrial cancer combined.

The age-specific incidence of the common epithelial type of ovarian cancer increases progressively and peaks in the eighth decade. Epithelial tumors, unlike germ cell and stromal tumors, are uncommon before the age of 40. Epidemiologic studies suggest higher incidences in industrialized nations and an association with disordered ovarian function, including infertility, nulliparity, frequent miscarriages, and use of ovulation-inducing drugs such as clomiphene. Each pregnancy reduces the ovarian cancer risk by about 10%, and breast-feeding and tubal ligation also appear to reduce the risk. Oral contraceptives reduce the risk of ovarian cancer in patients with a familial history of cancer and in the general population. Many of these risk-reduction factors support the "incessant ovulation" hypothesis for ovarian cancer etiology, which implies that an aberrant repair process of the surface epithelium is central to ovarian cancer development. Estrogen replacement after menopause does not appear to increase the risk of ovarian cancer, although one study showed a modest increase in risk with >11 years of use.

Familial cases account for about 5% of all ovarian cancer, and a family history of ovarian cancer is a major risk factor. Compared to a lifetime risk of 1.6% in the general population, women with one affected first-degree relative have a 5% risk. In families with two or more affected first-degree relatives, the risk may exceed 50%. Three types of autosomal dominant familial cancer are recognized: (1) site-specific, in which only ovarian cancer is seen; (2) families with cancer of the ovary and breast; and (3) the Lynch type II cancer family syndrome with nonpolyposis colorectal cancer, endometrial cancer, and ovarian cancer.

Etiology and Genetics In women with hereditary breast/ovarian cancer, two susceptibility loci have been identified: *BRCA1*, located on chromosome 17q12-21, and *BRCA2*, on 13q12-13. Both are tumor-suppressor genes, and their protein products act as inhibitors of tumor growth. Both genes are large, and numerous mutations have been described; most are frameshift or nonsense mutations, and 86% produce truncated protein products. The implications of the many other mutations including many missense mutations are not known. The cumulative risk of ovarian cancer with critical mutations of *BRCA1* or *-2* is 25%, compared to the lifetime risk of 50% for breast cancer for similar mutations. Men in such families have an increased risk of prostate cancer.

Cytogenetic analysis of sporadic epithelial ovarian cancers generally reveals complex karyotypic rearrangements. Structural abnormalities frequently appear on chromosomes 1 and 11, and loss of heterozygosity is common on 3q, 6q, 11q, 13q, and 17. Abnormalities of oncogenes are frequently found in ovarian cancer and include c-*myc*, H-*ras*, K-*ras*, and *neu*.

Ovarian tumors (usually not epithelial) are sometimes components of complex genetic syndromes. Peutz-Jeghers syndrome (mucocutaneous pigmentation and intestinal polyps) is associated with ovarian sex cord stromal tumors and Sertoli cell tumors in men. Patients with gonadal dysgenesis (46XY genotype or mosaic for Y-containing cell lines) develop gonadoblastomas, and women with nevoid basal cell carcinomas have an increased risk of ovarian fibromas.

Clinical Presentation and Differential Diagnosis Most patients with ovarian cancer are first diagnosed when the disease has already spread beyond the true pelvis. The occurrence of abdominal pain, bloating, and urinary symptoms usually indicates advanced disease. Localized ovarian cancer is generally asymptomatic. However, progressive enlargement of a localized ovarian tumor can produce urinary frequency or constipation, and rarely torsion of an ovarian mass causes acute abdominal pain or a surgical abdomen. In contrast to cervical or endometrial cancer, vaginal bleeding or discharge is rarely seen with early ovarian cancer. The diagnosis of early disease usually occurs with palpation of an asymptomatic adnexal mass during routine pelvic examination. However, most ovarian enlargements discovered this way, especially in premenopausal women, are benign functional cysts that characteristically resolve over one to three menstrual cycles. Adnexal masses in premenarchal or postmenopausal women are more likely to be pathologic. A solid, irregular, fixed pelvic mass is usually ovarian cancer. Other causes of adnexal masses include pedunculated uterine fibroids, endometriosis, benign ovarian neoplasms, and inflammatory lesions of the bowel.

Evaluation of patients with suspected ovarian cancer should include measurement of serum levels of the tumor marker CA-125. CA-125 determinants are glycoproteins with molecular masses from 220 to 1000 kDa, and a radioimmunoassay is used to determine circulating CA-125 antigen levels. Between 80 and 85% of patients with epithelial ovarian cancer have levels of CA-125 $\geq$ 35 U/mL. Other malignant tumors can also elevate CA-125 levels, including cancers of the endometrium, cervix, fallopian tubes, pancreas, breast, lung, and colon. Certain nonmalignant conditions that can produce moderate elevations of CA-125 levels include pregnancy, endometriosis, pelvic inflammatory disease, and uterine fibroids. About 1% of normal females have serum CA-125 levels >35 U/mL. However, in postmenopausal women with an asymptomatic pelvic mass and CA-125 levels $\geq$65 U/mL, the test has a sensitivity of 97% and a specificity of 78%.

Screening In contrast to patients who present with advanced disease, patients with early ovarian cancers (stages I and II) are commonly curable with conventional therapy. Thus, effective screening procedures would improve the cure rate in this disease. Although pelvic examination can occasionally detect early disease, it is a relatively insensitive screening procedure. Transvaginal sonography is often useful, but significant false-positive results are noted, particularly in premenopausal women. In one study, 67 laparotomies were required to diagnose 1 primary ovarian cancer. Doppler flow imaging coupled with transvaginal ultrasound may improve accuracy and reduce the high rate of false positives.

CA-125 has been studied as a screening tool. Unfortunately, half of women with stages I and II ovarian cancer have CA-125 levels <65 U/mL. Attempts have been made to improve the sensitivity and specificity by combinations of procedures, commonly transvaginal ultrasound and CA-125 levels. In a screening study of 22,000 women, 42 had a positive screen and 11 had ovarian cancer (7 with advanced disease). In addition, eight women with a negative screen developed ovarian cancer. Thus, the false-positive rate would lead to a large number of unnecessary (i.e., negative) laparotomies if each positive screen resulted in a surgical exploration. The National Institutes of Health Consensus Conference recommended against screening for ovarian cancer among the general population without known risk factors for the disease. Although no evidence shows that screening saves lives, many physicians use annual pelvic examinations, transvaginal ultrasound, and CA-125 levels to screen women with a family history of ovarian cancer or breast/ovarian cancer syndromes.

In one study, proteomic spectra in the serum analyzed by an iterative searching algorithm were used to identify women with ovarian cancer. Preliminary studies have identified all 50 stage I patients with a sensitivity of 100%, a specificity of 95%, and a positive predictive value of 94%. The procedure can be automated, requires a pinprick of blood, and has many characteristics of an ideal screening test. However, difficulty in consistency of replicate samples, variation in spectroscopy equipment, and the tendency of the artificial intelligence algorithms to overfit the data makes conformation studies necessary before widespread application to screening is warranted.

Pathology Common epithelial tumors comprise most (85%) of the ovarian neoplasms. These may be benign (50%), frankly malignant (33%), or tumors of low malignant potential (16%) (tumors of borderline malignancy). Epithelial tumors of low malignant potential have the cytologic features of malignancy but do not invade the ovarian stroma. More than 75% of borderline malignancies present in early stage and generally occur in younger women. They have a much better natural history than their malignant counterpart.

There are five major subtypes of common epithelial tumors: serous (50%), mucinous (25%), endometroid (15%), clear cell (5%), and Brenner tumors (1%), the latter derived from the urothelium. Benign common epithelial tumors are almost always serous or mucinous and develop in women ages 20 to 60. They are frequently large (20 to 30 cm), bilateral, and cystic.

Malignant epithelial tumors are usually seen in women over 40. They present as solid masses, with areas of necrosis and hemorrhage. Masses >10 to 15 cm have usually already spread into the intraabdominal space. Spread eventually results in intraabdominal carcinomatosis, which leads to bowel and renal obstruction and cachexia.

Although most ovarian tumors are epithelial, two other important ovarian tumor types exist—stromal and germ cell tumors. These tumors are distinct in their cell of origin but also have different clinical presentations and natural histories and are often managed differently (see below).

Metastasis to the ovary can occur from breast, colon, gastric, and pancreatic cancers, and the Krukenberg tumor was classically described as bilateral ovarian masses from metastatic mucin-secreting gastrointestinal cancers.

Staging and Prognostic Factors Laparotomy is often the primary procedure used to establish the diagnosis. Less invasive studies useful in defining the extent of spread include chest x-rays, abdominal computed tomography scans, and abdominal and pelvic sonography. If the woman has specific gastrointestinal symptoms, a barium enema or gastrointestinal series can be performed. Symptoms of bladder or renal dysfunction can be evaluated by cystoscopy or intravenous pyelography.

A careful staging laparotomy will establish the stage and extent of disease and allow for the cytoreduction of tumor masses in patients with advanced disease. Proper laparotomy requires a vertical incision of sufficient length to ensure adequate examination of the abdominal contents. The presence, amount, and cytology of any ascites fluid should be noted. The primary tumor should be evaluated for rupture, excrescences, or dense adherence. Careful visual and manual inspection of the diaphragm and peritoneal surfaces is required. In addition to total abdominal hysterectomy and bilateral salpingo-oophorectomy, a partial omentectomy should be performed and the paracolic gutters inspected. Pelvic lymph nodes as well as para-aortic nodes in the region of the renal hilus should be biopsied. Since this surgical procedure defines stage, establishes prognosis, and determines the necessity for subsequent therapy, it should be performed by a surgeon with special expertise in ovarian cancer staging. Studies have shown that patients operated upon by gynecologic oncologists were properly staged 97% of the time, compared to 52% and 35% of cases staged by obstetricians/gynecologists and general surgeons, respectively. At the end of staging, 23% of women have stage I disease (cancer confined to the ovary or ovaries); 13% have stage II (disease confined to the true pelvis); 47% have stage III (disease spread into but confined to the abdomen); and 16% have stage IV disease (spread outside the pelvis and abdomen). The 5-year survival correlates with stage of disease: stage I—90%, stage II—70%, stage III—15 to 20%, and stage IV—1 to 5% (Table 83-1).

Prognosis in ovarian cancer is dependent not only upon stage but on the extent of residual disease and histologic grade. Patients presenting with advanced disease but left without significant residual disease after surgery have a median survival of 39 months, compared to 17 months for those with suboptimal tumor resection.

Prognosis of epithelial tumors is also highly influenced by histologic grade but less so by histologic type. Although grading systems differ among pathologists, all grading systems show a better prognosis for well- or moderately differentiated tumors and a poorer prognosis for poorly differentiated histologies. Typical 5-year survivals for patients with all stages of disease are: well-differentiated—88%, moderately differentiated—58%, poorly differentiated—27%.

The prognostic significance of pre- and postoperative CA-125 levels is uncertain. Serum levels generally reflect volume of disease, and high levels usually indicate unresectability and a poorer survival. Postoperative levels, if elevated, usually indicate residual disease. The rate of decline of CA-125 levels during initial therapy or the absolute level after one to three cycles of chemotherapy correlates with prognosis but is not sufficiently accurate to guide individual treatment decisions. Even when the CA-125 level falls to normal after surgery or chemotherapy, "second-look" laparotomy identifies residual disease in 60% of women.

Genetic and biologic factors may influence prognosis. Increased tumor levels of p53 are associated with a worse prognosis in advanced disease. Epidermal growth factor receptors in ovarian cancer are associated with a high risk of progression, but the increased expression of HER-2/neu has given conflicting prognostic results, and expression of Mdr-1 has not been of prognostic value. HER-2/neu is highly expressed in 20% of ovarian cancers, and responses have been seen to trastuzumab in this subset of patients.

TABLE 83-1 Staging and Survival in Gynecologic Malignancies

Stage	Ovarian	5-Year Survival, %	Endometrial	5-Year Survival, %	Cervix	5-Year Survival, %
0	—		—		Carcinoma in situ	100
I	Confined to ovary	90	Confined to corpus	89	Confined to uterus	85
II	Confined to pelvis	70	Involves corpus and cervix	80	Invades beyond uterus but not to pelvic wall	60
III	Intraabdominal spread	15–20	Extends outside the uterus but not outside the true pelvis	30	Extends to pelvic wall and/or lower third of vagina, or hydronephrosis	33
IV	Spread outside abdomen	1–5	Extends outside the true pelvis or involves the bladder or rectum	9	Invades mucosa of bladder or rectum or extends beyond the true pelvis	7

Rx TREATMENT

The selection of therapy for patients with epithelial ovarian cancer depends upon the stage, extent of residual tumor, and histologic grade. In general, patients are considered in three separate treatment groups: (1) those with early (stages I and II) ovarian cancer and microscopic or no residual disease; (2) patients with advanced (stage III) disease but minimal residual tumor (<1 cm) after initial surgery; and (3) patients with bulky residual tumor and advanced (stage III or IV) disease.

Patients with stage I disease, no residual tumor, and well or moderately differentiated tumors need no adjuvant therapy after definitive surgery, and 5-year survival exceeds 95%. For all other patients with early disease and those stage I patients with poor prognosis histologic grade, adjuvant therapy is probably warranted, and single-agent cisplatin or platinum-containing drug combinations improve survival by 8% (82% vs 76%, $p = .08$).

For the patients with advanced (stage III) disease but with limited or no residual disease after definitive cytoreductive surgery (about half of all stage III patients), the primary therapy is platinum-based combination chemotherapy. Approximately 70% of women respond to initial combination chemotherapy, and 40 to 50% have a complete regression of disease. Only about half of these patients are free of disease if surgically restaged. Although a variety of combinations are active, a randomized prospective trial of paclitaxel and cisplatin compared to paclitaxel and carboplatin in patients with optimally resected advanced disease demonstrated equivalent results (median time to progression 20.7 months vs 19.4 months, median survival 57.4 months vs 48.7 months) but with significantly reduced toxicity using carboplatin. This regimen of paclitaxel, 175 mg/m^2 by 3-h infusion, and carboplatin, dosed to an AUC (area under the curve) of 7.5 is the treatment of choice for patients with previously untreated advanced-stage disease.

Patients with advanced disease (stages III and IV) and bulky residual tumor are generally treated with a paclitaxel-platinum combination regimen as well and, while the overall prognosis is poorer, 5-year survival may reach 10 to 15%.

Historically, patients who had an excellent initial response to chemotherapy and no clinical evidence of disease have had a second-look laparotomy. For patients with stage I ovarian cancer or for germ cell tumors, the operation rarely detects residual tumor and has been largely abandoned. Even for those with stages II and III epithelial tumors, the second-look surgical procedure itself does not prolong overall survival. Its routine use cannot be recommended. Maintenance therapy (12 cycles of paclitaxel every 28 days) may extend progression-free survival among patients who achieve a complete response; an effect on overall survival has not yet been shown.

Patients with advanced disease whose disease recurs after initial treatment are usually not curable but may benefit significantly from limited surgery to relieve intestinal obstruction, localized radiation therapy to relieve pressure or pain from mass lesions or metastasis, or palliative chemotherapy. The selection of chemotherapy for palliation depends upon the initial regimen and evidence of drug resistance. Patients who have a complete regression of disease that lasts ≥6 months often respond to reinduction with the same agents. Patients relapsing within the first 6 months of initial therapy rarely do. Chemotherapeutic agents with >15% response rates in patients relapsing after initial combination chemotherapy include gemcitabine, topotecan, liposomal doxorubicin, and vinorelbine. Intraperitoneal chemotherapy (usually cisplatin) may be used if a small residual volume (<1 cm^3) of tumor exists. Progestational agents and antiestrogens produce responses in 5 to 15% of patients and have minimal side effects.

Patients with tumor of low malignant potential, even with advanced-stage disease, have longer survivals when managed with surgery alone. The added value of radiation and chemotherapy has not been shown.

OVARIAN GERM CELL TUMORS Fewer than 5% of all ovarian tumors are germ cell in origin. They include teratoma, dysgerminoma, endodermal sinus tumor, and embryonal carcinoma. Germ cell tumors of the ovary generally occur in younger women (75% of ovarian malignancies in women <30), display an unusually aggressive natural history, and are commonly cured with less extensive nonsterilizing surgery and chemotherapy. Women cured of these malignancies are able to conceive and have normal children.

These neoplasms can be divided into three major groups: (1) benign tumors (usually dermoid cysts); (2) malignant tumors that arise from dermoid cysts; and (3) primitive malignant germ cell tumors including dysgerminoma, yolk sac tumors, immature teratomas, embryonal carcinomas, and choriocarcinoma.

Dermoid cysts are teratomatous cysts usually lined by epidermis and skin appendages. They often contain hair, and calcified bone or teeth can sometimes be seen on conventional pelvic x-ray. They are almost always curable by surgical resection. Approximately 1% of these tumors have malignant elements, usually squamous cell carcinoma.

Malignant germ cell tumors are usually large (median—16 cm). Bilateral disease is rare except in dysgerminoma (10 to 15% bilaterality). Abdominal or pelvic pain in young women is the usual presenting symptom. Serum human chorionic gonadotropin (β-hCG) and α fetoprotein levels are useful in the diagnosis and management of these patients. Before the advent of chemotherapy, extensive surgery was routine, but it has now been replaced by careful evaluation of extent of spread followed by resection of bulky disease and preservation of one ovary, uterus, and cervix, if feasible. This allows many affected women to preserve fertility. After surgical staging, 60 to 75% of women have stage I disease and 25 to 30% have stage III disease. Stages II and IV are infrequent.

Most of the malignant germ cell tumors are managed with chemotherapy after surgery. Regimens used in testicular cancer such as PVB (cisplatin, vinblastine, bleomycin) and BEP (bleomycin, 30 units IV weekly; etoposide, 100 mg/m^2 days 1 to 5; and cisplatin, 20 mg/m^2 days 1 to 5), with three or four courses given at 21-day intervals, have produced 95% long-term survival in patients with stages I to III disease. This regimen is the treatment of choice for all malignant germ cell tumors except grade I, stage I immature teratoma, where surgery alone is adequate, and perhaps early-stage dysgerminoma, where surgery and radiation therapy are used.

Dysgerminoma is the ovarian counterpart of testicular seminoma. The tumor is very sensitive to radiation therapy. The 5-year disease-free survival is 100% in early-stage patients and 61% in stage III disease. Unfortunately, the use of radiation therapy makes many patients infertile. BEP chemotherapy is equally or more effective and does not cause infertility. In incompletely resected patients with dysgerminoma, the 2-year disease-free survival is 95% and infertility is not observed. Combination chemotherapy (BEP) has replaced postoperative radiation therapy as the treatment of choice in women with ovarian dysgerminoma.

OVARIAN STROMAL TUMORS   Stromal tumors make up <10% of ovarian tumors. They are named for the stromal tissue involved: granulosa, theca, Sertoli, Leydig, and collagen-producing stromal cells. The granulosa and theca cell stromal cell tumors occur most frequently in the first three decades of life. Granulosa cell tumors frequently produce estrogen and cause menstrual abnormalities, bleeding, and precocious puberty. Endometrial carcinoma can be seen in 5% of these women, perhaps related to the persistent hyperestrogenism. Sertoli and Leydig cell tumors, when functional, produce androgens with resultant virilization or hirsutism. Some 75% of these stromal cell tumors present in stage I and can be cured with total abdominal hysterectomy and bilateral salpingo-oophorectomy. Stromal tumors generally grow slowly, and recurrences can occur 5 to 10 years after initial surgery. Neither radiation therapy nor chemotherapy have been documented to be consistently effective, and surgical management remains the primary treatment.

CARCINOMA OF THE FALLOPIAN TUBE

The fallopian tube is the least common site of cancer in the female genital tract, although its epithelial surface far exceeds that of the ovary, where epithelial cancer is 20 times more common. Approximately 300 new cases occur yearly; 90% are papillary serous adenocarcinomas, with the remainder being mixed mesodermal, endometroid, and transitional cell tumors. *BRCA1* and *-2* mutations are found in 7% of cases. The gross and microscopic characteristics and the spread of the tumor are similar to those of ovarian cancer but can be distinguished if the tumor arises from the endosalpinx where the tubal epithelium shows a transition between benign and malignant, and the ovaries and endometrium are normal or minimally involved.

The differential diagnosis includes primary or metastatic ovarian cancer, chronic salpingitis, tuberculous salpingitis, salpingitis isthmica nodosa, and cautery artifact.

Unlike patients with ovarian cancer, patients often present with early symptoms, usually postmenopausal vaginal bleeding, pain, and leukorrhea. Surgical staging is similar to that used for ovarian cancer, and prognosis is related to stage and extent of residual disease. Patients with stages I and II disease are generally treated with surgery alone or with surgery and pelvic radiation therapy, although radiation therapy does not clearly improve 5-year survival (5-year survival stage I: 74 versus 75%, stage II: 43 versus 48%). Patients with stages III and IV disease are treated with the same chemotherapy regimens used in advanced ovarian carcinoma, and 5-year survival is similar (stage III—20%, stage IV—5%).

UTERINE CANCER

Carcinoma of the endometrium is the most common female pelvic malignancy. Approximately 40,300 new cases are diagnosed yearly, although in most (75%), tumor is confined to the uterine corpus at diagnosis and therefore most can be cured. The 7,000 deaths yearly make uterine cancer only the eighth leading cause of cancer death in females. It is primarily a disease of postmenopausal women, although 25% of cases occur in women <age 50 and 5% <age 40. The disease is common in Eastern Europe and the United States and uncommon in Asia.

Phenotypic characteristics and risk factors common in patients with endometrial cancer include obesity, altered menstruation, low fertility index, late menopause, anovulation, and postmenopausal bleeding. Exposure to unopposed estrogen from either endogenous or exogenous sources may play a central etiologic role. Women taking tamoxifen for breast cancer treatment or prevention have a twofold increased risk.

Endometrial carcinoma occurs most often in the sixth and seventh decades of life. Symptoms often include abnormal vaginal discharge (90%); abnormal bleeding (80%), which is usually postmenopausal; and leukorrhea (10%). Evaluation of such patients should include a history and physical and pelvic examinations followed by an endometrial biopsy or a fractional dilation and curettage. Outpatient procedures such as endometrial biopsy or aspiration curettage can be used but are definitive only when positive.

Between 75 and 80% of all endometrial carcinomas are adenocarcinomas, and the prognosis depends upon stage, histologic grade, and extent of myometrial invasion. Grade I tumors are highly differentiated adenocarcinomas, grade II contain some solid areas, and grade III tumors are largely solid or undifferentiated. Adenocarcinoma with squamous differentiation is seen in 10% of patients; the most differentiated form is known as *adenoacanthoma*, and the poorly differentiated form is called *adenosquamous carcinoma*. Other less common pathologies include mucinous carcinoma (5%) and papillary serous carcinoma (<10%). This latter type has a natural history similar to ovarian carcinoma and should be managed as an ovarian cancer. Rarer histologies include secretory (2%), ciliated, clear cell, and undifferentiated carcinomas.

The staging of endometrial cancer requires surgery to establish the extent of disease and the depth of myometrial invasion. Peritoneal fluid should be sampled; the abdomen and pelvis explored; and pelvic and para-aortic lymphadenectomy performed depending upon the histology, grade, and depth of invasion in the uterine specimen on frozen section. After evaluation and staging, 74% of patients are stage I, 13% are stage II, 9% are stage III, and 3% are stage IV. Five-year survival by stage is as follows: stage I—89%, stage II—80%, stage III—30%, and stage IV—9% (Table 83-1).

Patients with uncomplicated endometrial carcinoma are effectively managed with total abdominal hysterectomy and bilateral salpingo-oophorectomy. Pre- or postoperative irradiation has been used, and although vaginal cuff recurrence is reduced, survival is not altered. In women with poor histologic grade, deep myometrial invasion, or extensive involvement of the lower uterine segment or cervix, intracavitary or external beam irradiation is warranted.

About 15% of women have endometrial carcinoma with extension to the cervix only (stage II), and management depends upon the extent of cervical invasion. Superficial cervical invasion can be managed like stage I disease, but extensive cervical invasion requires radical hysterectomy or preoperative radiotherapy followed by extrafascial hysterectomy. Once disease is outside the uterus but still confined to the true pelvis (stage III), management generally includes surgery and irradiation. Patients who have involvement only of the ovary or fallopian tubes generally do well with such therapy (5-year survivals of 80%). Other stage III patients with disease extending beyond the adnexa or those with serous carcinomas of the endometrium have a significantly poorer prognosis (5-year survival of 15%).

Patients with stage IV disease (outside the abdomen or invading the bladder or rectum) are treated palliatively with irradiation, surgery, and/or progestational agents. Progestational agents produce responses in about 25% of patients. Well-differentiated tumors respond most frequently, and response can be correlated with the level of progesterone receptor expression in the tumor. The commonly used progestational agents hydroxyprogesterone (Dilalutin), megastrol (Megace), and deoxyprogesterone (Provera) all produce similar response rates, and the antiestrogen tamoxifen (Nolvadex) produces responses in 10 to 25% of patients in a salvage setting.

Chemotherapy is not very successful in advanced endometrial carcinoma. The most active single agents with consistent response rates of ≥20% include cisplatin, carboplatin, doxorubicin, epirubicin, and paclitaxel. Combinations of drugs with or without progestational agents have generally produced response rates similar to single agents.

CERVIX CANCER Carcinoma of the cervix was once the most common cause of cancer death in women, but over the past 30 years, the mortality rate has decreased by 50% due to widespread screening with the Pap smear. In 2004, ~10,500 new cases of invasive cervix cancer occurred, and >50,000 cases of carcinoma in situ were detected. There were 3,900 deaths from the disease, and of those patients, ~85% had never had a Pap smear. It remains the major gynecologic cancer in underdeveloped countries. It is more common in lower socioeconomic groups, in women with early initial sexual activity and/or multiple sexual partners, and in smokers. Venereal transmission of human papilloma virus (HPV) has an important etiologic role. Over 66 types of HPVs have been isolated, and many are associated with genital warts. Those types associated with cervical carcinoma are 16, 18, 31, 45, and 51 to 53. These, along with many other types, are also associated with cervical intraepithelial neoplasia (CIN). The protein product of HPV-16, the E7 protein, binds and inactivates the tumor-suppressor gene Rb, and the E6 protein of HPV-18 has sequence homology to the SV40 large T antigen and has the capacity to bind and inactivate the tumor-suppressor gene p53. E6 and E7 are both necessary and sufficient to cause cell transformation in vitro. These binding and inactivation events may explain the carcinogenic effects of the viruses (Chap. 169).

Vaccination against pathologic HPV appears quite promising as a cervix cancer prevention strategy. The administration of HPV-16 vaccine in a double-blind study of 2392 women completely prevented infection with the virus, and no cases of HPV-16-related CIN were seen in vaccinated women. Although this vaccine is promising, polyvalent vaccines incorporating the known pathologic HPV virus types may ultimately be required.

Uncomplicated HPV lower genital tract infection and condylomatous atypia of the cervix can progress to CIN. This lesion precedes invasive cervical carcinoma and is classified as low-grade squamous intraepithelial lesion (SIL), high-grade SIL, and carcinoma in situ. Carcinoma in situ demonstrates cytologic evidence of neoplasia without invasion through the basement membrane, can persist unchanged for 10 to 20 years, but eventually progresses to invasive carcinoma.

The Pap smear is 90 to 95% accurate in detecting early lesions such as CIN but is less sensitive in detecting cancer when frankly invasive cancer or fungating masses are present. Inflammation, necrosis, and hemorrhage may produce false-positive smears, and colposcopic-directed biopsy is required when any lesion is visible on the cervix, regardless of Pap smear findings. The American Cancer Society recommends that women after onset of sexual activity, or >age 20, have two consecutive yearly smears. If negative, smears should be repeated every 3 years. The American College of Obstetrics and Gynecology recommends yearly Pap smears with routine annual pelvic and breast examinations. The Pap smear can be reported as normal (includes benign, reactive, or reparative changes); atypical squamous cells of undetermined significance (ASCUS) or cannot exclude high-grade SIL (ASC-H); low- or high-grade CIN; or frankly malignant. Women with ASCUS, ASC-H, or low-grade CIN should have repeat smears in 3 to 6 months and be tested for HPV. Women with high-grade CIN or frankly malignant Pap smears should have colposcopic-directed cervical biopsy. Colposcopy is a technique using a binocular microscope and 3% acetic acid applied to the cervix in which abnormal areas appear white and can be biopsied directly. Cone biopsy is still required when endocervical tumor is suspected, colposcopy is inadequate, the biopsy shows microinvasive carcinoma, or when a discrepancy is noted between the Pap smear and the colposcopic findings. Cone biopsy alone is therapeutic for CIN in many patients, although a less radical electrocautery excision may be sufficient.

Approximately 80% of invasive cervix cancers are squamous cell tumors, 10 to 15% are adenocarcinomas, 2 to 5% are adenosquamous with epithelial and glandular structures, and 1 to 2% are clear cell mesonephric tumors.

Patients with cervix cancer generally present with abnormal bleeding or postcoital spotting that may increase to intermenstrual or prominent menstrual bleeding. Yellowish vaginal discharge, lumbosacral back pain, and urinary symptoms can also be seen.

The staging of cervical carcinoma is clinical and generally completed with a pelvic examination under anesthesia with cystoscopy and proctoscopy. Chest x-rays, intravenous pyelograms, and computed tomography are generally required, and magnetic resonance imaging (MRI) may be used to assess extracervical extension. Stage 0 is carcinoma in situ, stage I is disease confined to the cervix, stage II disease invades beyond the cervix but not to the pelvic wall or lower third of the vagina, stage III disease extends to the pelvic wall or lower third of the vagina or causes hydronephrosis, stage IV is present when the tumor invades the mucosa of bladder or rectum or extends beyond the true pelvis. Five-year survivals are as follows: stage I—85%, stage II—60%, stage III—33%, and stage IV—7% (Table 83-1).

Carcinoma in situ (stage 0) can be managed successfully by cone biopsy or by abdominal hysterectomy. For stage I disease, results appear equivalent for either radical hysterectomy or radiation therapy. Patients with stages II to IV disease are primarily managed with radical radiation therapy or combined modality therapy. Retroperitoneal lymphadenectomy has no proven therapeutic role. Pelvic exenterations, although uncommon, are performed for centrally recurrent or persistent disease. Reconstruction of the vagina, bladder, and rectum can often be done following this operation.

In women with locally advanced disease (stages IIB to IVA), platinum-based chemotherapy given concomitantly with radiation therapy improves survival compared to radiation therapy alone. Cisplatin, 75 mg/m² over 4 h, followed by 5-fluorouracil (5-FU), 4 g given by 96-h infusion on days 1 to 5 of radiation therapy, is a common regimen. Two additional cycles of chemotherapy are given at 3-week intervals. Concurrent chemoradiotherapy reduced the risk of recurrence by 30 to 50% across a wide spectrum of stages and presentations and is the treatment of choice in stages IIB to IV cervix cancer.

Chemotherapy has been used in patients with unresectable advanced disease or recurrent disease. Active agents with ≥20% response rates include cisplatin, 5-FU, ifosfamide, and irinotecan. No combination of agents has proved better than single agents. Intraarterial chemotherapy has been studied, either pre- or postoperatively, but is associated with substantial local toxicity and response rates of 20%.

GESTATIONAL TROPHOBLASTIC NEOPLASIA

Gestational trophoblastic diseases are a group of interrelated diseases that form a spectrum from benign hydatidiform mole to trophoblastic malignancy (placental-site trophoblastic tumor and choriocarcinoma). Malignant forms account for <1% of female gynecologic malignancies and can be cured with appropriate chemotherapy. Deaths from this disease have become rare in the United States.

Epidemiology   The incidence is about 1 per 1500 pregnancies in the United States and is nearly tenfold higher in Asia. Maternal age >45 years is a risk factor for hydatidiform mole. A prior history of molar pregnancy is also a risk factor. Choriocarcinoma occurs in ~1 in 25,000 pregnancies or 1 in 20,000 live births. Prior history of hydatidiform mole is a risk factor for choriocarcinoma. A woman with a molar pregnancy is 1000 times more likely to develop choriocarcinoma than a woman with a prior normal-term pregnancy.

Pathology and Etiology   The trophoblastic neoplasms have been divided by morphology into complete or partial hydatidiform mole, invasive mole, placental-site trophoblastomas, and choriocarcinomas. Hydatidiform moles contain clusters of villi with hydropic changes, hyperplasia of the trophoblast, and the absence of fetal vessels. Invasive moles differ only by invasion into the uterine myometrium. Placental-site trophoblastic tumors are predominately made up of cytotrophoblast cells arising from the placental implantation site. Choriocarcinomas consist of anaplastic trophoblastic tissue with both cytotrophoblastic and syncytiotrophoblastic elements and no identifiable villi.

Complete moles result from uniparental disomy in which loss of the maternal genes (23 autosomes plus X) occurs by unknown mechanisms and is followed by duplication of the paternal haploid genome (23 autosomes plus X). Uncommonly (5%), moles result from dispermic fertilization of an empty egg, resulting in either 46XY or 46XX genotype. Partial moles result from dispermic fertilization of an egg with retention of the maternal haploid set of chromosomes, resulting in diandric triploidy (Chap. 56).

Clinical Presentation   Molar pregnancies are generally associated with first-trimester bleeding, ectopic pregnancies, or threatened abortions. The uterus is inappropriately large for the length of gestation, and β-hCG levels are higher than expected. Fetal parts and heart sounds are not present. The diagnosis is generally made by the passage of grape-like clusters from the uterus, but ultrasound demonstration of the hydropic mole can be diagnostic. Patients suspected of a molar pregnancy require a chest film, careful pelvic examinations, and weekly serial monitoring of β-hCG levels.

℞ TREATMENT

Patients with hydatidiform moles require suction curettage coupled with postevacuation monitoring of β-hCG levels. In most women (80%), the β-hCG titer progressively declines within 8 to 10 days of evacuation (serum half-life is 24 to 36 h). Patients should be monitored on a monthly basis and should not become pregnant for at least a year.

Patients found to have invasive mole at curettage are generally treated with hysterectomy and chemotherapy. Approximately half of patients with choriocarcinoma develop the malignancy after a molar pregnancy, and the other half develop the malignancy after abortion, ectopic pregnancy, or occasionally after a normal full-term pregnancy.

Chemotherapy is generally used for gestational trophoblastic neoplasia and is often used in hydatidiform mole if β-hCG levels rise or plateau or if metastases develop. Patients with invasive mole or choriocarcinoma require chemotherapy. Several regimens are effective, including methotrexate at 30 mg/m^2 intramuscularly on a weekly basis until β-hCG titers are normal. However, methotrexate (1 mg/kg) every other day for 4 days followed by leukovorin (0.1 mg/kg) intravenously 24 h after methotrexate is associated with a cure rate of ≥90% and low toxicity. Intermittent courses are continued until the β-hCG titer becomes undetectable for 3 consecutive weeks, and then patients are monitored monthly for a year.

Patients with high-risk tumors (high β-hCG levels, disease presenting ≥4 months after antecedent pregnancy, brain or liver metastasis, or failure of single-agent methotrexate) are initially treated with combination chemotherapy. EMA-CO (a cyclic non-cross-resistant combination of etoposide, methotrexate, and dactinomycin alternating with cyclophosphamide and vincristine); cisplatin, bleomycin, and vinblastine; and cisplatin, etoposide, and bleomycin are effective regimens. EMA-CO is now the regimen of choice for patients with high-risk disease because of excellent survival rates (>80%) and less toxicity. The use of etoposide carries a 1.5% lifetime risk of acute myeloid leukemia (16-fold relative risk). Because of this problem, etoposide-containing regimens should be reserved for patients with high-risk features. Patients with brain or liver metastases are usually treated with local irradiation to metastatic sites in conjunction with chemotherapy. Long-term studies of patients cured of trophoblastic disease have not demonstrated an increased risk of maternal complications or fetal abnormalities with subsequent pregnancies.

FURTHER READING

JACOBS IJ: Screening for ovarian cancer: A pilot randomized trial. Lancet 353: 1207, 1999

KOUTSKY LA: A controlled trial of a human papilloma virus type 16 vaccine. N Engl J Med 347:1645, 2002

MARKMAN M et al: Phase III randomized trial of 12 versus 3 months of maintenance paclitaxel in patients with advanced ovarian cancer after complete response to platinum and paclitaxel-based chemotherapy: A Southwest Oncology Group and Gynecologic Oncology Group Trial. J Clin Oncol 21: 2460, 2003

MORRIS M et al: Pelvic radiation with concurrent chemotherapy compared with pelvic and para-aortic radiation for high-risk cervical cancer. N Engl J Med 340:1137, 1999

PETRICOIN EF et al: Use of proteomic patterns in serum to identify ovarian cancer. Lancet 359:572, 2002

SOLOMON D et al: The 2001 Bethesda System. JAMA 287:2114, 2002

STEHMAN FB et al: Innovations in the treatment of invasive cervical cancer. Cancer 98:2052, 2003

WRIGHT JD, MUTCH DG: Treatment of high-risk gestational trophoblastic tumors. Clin Obstet Gynecol 46:593, 2003

---

84 | SOFT TISSUE AND BONE SARCOMAS AND BONE METASTASES
Shreyaskumar R. Patel, Robert S. Benjamin

Sarcomas are rare (<1% of all malignancies) mesenchymal neoplasms that arise in bone and soft tissues. These tumors are usually of mesodermal origin, although a few are derived from neuroectoderm, and they are biologically distinct from the more common epithelial malignancies. Sarcomas affect all age groups; 15% are found in children <15 years and 40% occur after age 55. Sarcomas are one of the most common solid tumors of childhood and are the fifth most common cause of cancer deaths in children. Sarcomas may be divided into two groups, those derived from bone and those derived from soft tissues.

SOFT TISSUE SARCOMAS

Soft tissues include muscles, tendons, fat, fibrous tissue, synovial tissue, vessels, and nerves. Approximately 60% of soft tissue sarcomas arise in the extremities, with the lower extremities involved three times as often as the upper extremities. Thirty percent arise in the trunk, the retroperitoneum accounting for 40% of all trunk lesions. The remaining 10% arise in the head and neck.

INCIDENCE Approximately 8680 new cases of soft tissue sarcomas occurred in the United States in 2004. The annual age-adjusted incidence is ~2 per 100,000 population, but the incidence varies with age. Soft tissue sarcomas constitute 0.7% of all cancers in the general population and 6.5% of all cancers in children.

EPIDEMIOLOGY Malignant transformation of a benign soft tissue tumor is extremely rare, with the exception that malignant peripheral nerve sheath tumors (neurofibrosarcoma, malignant schwannoma) can arise from neurofibromas in patients with neurofibromatosis. Several etiologic factors have been implicated in soft tissue sarcomas.

Environmental Factors Trauma or previous injury is rarely involved, but sarcomas can arise in scar tissue resulting from a prior operation, burn, fracture, or foreign body implantation. Chemical carcinogens such as polycyclic hydrocarbons, asbestos, and dioxin may be involved in the pathogenesis.

Iatrogenic Factors Sarcomas in bone or soft tissues occur in patients who are treated with radiation therapy. The tumor nearly always arises in the irradiated field. The risk increases with time.

Viruses Kaposi's sarcoma (KS) in patients with HIV type 1, classic KS, and KS in HIV-negative homosexual men is caused by human herpes virus (HHV) 8 (Chap. 166). No other sarcomas are associated with viruses.

Immunologic Factors Congenital or acquired immunodeficiency, including therapeutic immunosuppression, increases the risk of sarcoma.

Genetic Factors Li-Fraumeni syndrome is a familial cancer syndrome in which affected individuals have germ-line abnormalities of the tumor-suppressor gene p53 and an increased incidence of soft tissue sarcomas and other malignancies, including breast cancer, osteosarcoma, brain tumor, leukemia, and adrenal carcinoma (Chap. 68). Neurofibromatosis 1 (NF-1, peripheral form, von Recklinghausen's disease) is characterized by multiple neurofibromas and café au lait spots. Neurofibromas occasionally undergo malignant degeneration to become malignant peripheral nerve sheath tumors. The gene for NF-1 is located in the pericentromeric region of chromosome 17 and encodes neurofibromin, a tumor-suppressor protein with GTPase-activating activity that inhibits Ras function (Chap. 358). Germ-line mutation of the *Rb-1* locus (chromosome 13q14) in patients with inherited retinoblastoma is associated with the development of osteosarcoma in those who survive the retinoblastoma and of soft tissue sarcomas unrelated to radiation therapy. Other soft tissue tumors, including desmoid tumors, lipomas, leiomyomas, neuroblastomas, and paragangliomas, occasionally show a familial predisposition.

Ninety percent of synovial sarcomas contain a characteristic chromosomal translocation t(X;18) (p11;q11) involving a nuclear transcription factor on chromosome 18 called *SYT* and two breakpoints on X. Patients with translocations to the second X breakpoint (*SSX2*) may have longer survival than those with translocations involving *SSX1*.

Insulin-like growth factor (IGF) type 2 is produced by some sarcomas and may act as an autocrine growth factor and as a motility factor that promotes metastatic spread. IGF-2 stimulates growth through IGF-1 receptors but its effects on motility are through different receptors. If secreted in large amounts, IGF-2 may produce hypoglycemia (Chaps. 86 and 324).

CLASSIFICATION Approximately 20 different groups of sarcomas are recognized on the basis of the pattern of differentiation toward normal tissue. For example, rhabdomyosarcoma shows evidence of skeletal muscle fibers with cross-striations; leiomyosarcomas contain interlacing fascicles of spindle cells resembling smooth muscle; and liposarcomas contain adipocytes. When precise characterization of the group is not possible, the tumors are called *unclassified sarcomas*. All of the primary bone sarcomas can also arise from soft tissues (e.g., extraskeletal osteosarcoma). The entity *malignant fibrous histiocytoma* in-

cludes many tumors previously classified as fibrosarcomas or as pleomorphic variants of other sarcomas and is characterized by a mixture of spindle (fibrous) cells and round (histiocytic) cells arranged in a storiform pattern with frequent giant cells and areas of pleomorphism.

For purposes of treatment, most soft tissue sarcomas can be considered together. However, some specific tumors have distinct features. For example, *liposarcoma* can have a spectrum of behaviors. Pleomorphic liposarcomas and dedifferentiated liposarcomas behave like other high-grade sarcomas; in contrast, well-differentiated liposarcomas (better termed *atypical lipomatous tumors*) lack metastatic potential, and myxoid liposarcomas metastasize infrequently but, when they do, have a predilection for unusual metastatic sites containing fat, such as the retroperitoneum, mediastinum, and subcutaneous tissue. Rhabdomyosarcomas, Ewing's sarcoma, and other small-cell sarcomas tend to be more aggressive and are more responsive to chemotherapy than other soft tissue sarcomas.

Gastrointestinal stromal cell tumors (GISTs), previously classified as gastrointestinal leiomyosarcomas, are now recognized as a distinct entity within soft tissue sarcomas. Its cell of origin resembles the interstitial cell of Cajal, which controls peristalsis. The majority of malignant GISTs have activating mutations of the c-*kit* gene that result in ligand-independent phosphorylation and activation of the KIT receptor tyrosine kinase, leading to tumorigenesis.

DIAGNOSIS The most common presentation is an asymptomatic mass. Mechanical symptoms referable to pressure, traction, or entrapment of nerves or muscles may be present. All new and persistent or growing masses should be biopsied, either by a cutting needle (core-needle biopsy) or by a small incision, placed so that it can be encompassed in the subsequent excision without compromising a definitive resection. Lymph node metastases occur in 5%, except in synovial and epithelioid sarcomas, clear-cell sarcoma (melanoma of the soft parts), angiosarcoma, and rhabdomyosarcoma, where nodal spread may be seen in 17%. The pulmonary parenchyma is the most common site of metastases. Exceptions are GISTs, which metastasize to the liver; myxoid liposarcomas, which seek fatty tissue: and clear-cell sarcomas, which may metastasize to bones. Central nervous system metastases are rare, except in alveolar soft part sarcoma.

Radiographic Evaluation Imaging of the primary tumor is best with plain radiographs and magnetic resonance imaging (MRI) for tumors of the extremities or head and neck and by computed tomography (CT) for tumors of the chest, abdomen, or retroperitoneal cavity. A radiograph and CT scan of the chest are important for the detection of lung metastases. Other imaging studies may be indicated, depending on the symptoms, signs, or histology.

STAGING AND PROGNOSIS The histologic grade, relationship to fascial planes, and size of the primary tumor are the most important prognostic factors. The current American Joint Commission on Cancer (AJCC) staging system is shown in Table 84-1. Prognosis is related to the stage. Cure is common in the absence of metastatic disease, but a small number of patients with metastases can also be cured. Most patients with stage IV disease die within 12 months, but some patients may live with slowly progressive disease for many years.

℞ **TREATMENT**

AJCC stage I patients are adequately treated with surgery alone. Stage II patients are considered for adjuvant radiation therapy. Stage III patients may benefit from adjuvant chemotherapy. Stage IV patients are managed primarily with chemotherapy with or without other modalities.

Surgery Soft tissue sarcomas tend to grow along fascial planes, with the surrounding soft tissues compressed to form a pseudocapsule that gives the sarcoma the appearance of a well-encapsulated lesion. This is invariably deceptive, because "shelling out" or marginal excision of

TABLE 84-1 AJCC Staging System for Sarcomas

Histologic Grade (G)	Tumor Size (T)	Node Status (N)	Metastases (M)
Well differentiated (G1)	≤5 cm (T1)	Not involved (N0)	Absent (M0)
Moderately differentiated (G2)	>5 cm (T2)	Involved (N1)	Present (M1)
Poorly differentiated (G3)	Superficial fascial involvement (Ta)		
Undifferentiated (G4)	Deep fascial involvement (Tb)		

Disease Stage	5-Year Survival, %
Stage I	98.8
A: G1,2; T1a,b; N0; M0	
B: G1,2; T2a; N0; M0	
Stage II	81.8
A: G1,2; T2b; N0; M0	
B: G3,4; T1; N0; M0	
C: G3,4; T2a; N0; M0	
Stage III G3,4; T2b; N0; M0	51.7
Stage IV	<20
A: any G; any T; N1; M0	
B: any G; any T; any N; M1	

such lesions results in a 50 to 90% probability of local recurrence. Wide excision with a negative margin, incorporating the biopsy site, is the standard surgical procedure for local disease. The adjuvant use of radiation therapy and/or chemotherapy improves the local control rate and permits the use of limb-sparing surgery with a local control rate (85 to 90%) comparable to that achieved by radical excisions and amputations. Limb-sparing approaches are indicated except when negative margins are not obtainable, when the risks of radiation are prohibitive, or when neurovascular structures are involved so that resection will result in serious functional consequences to the limb.

Radiation Therapy External beam radiation therapy is an adjuvant to limb-sparing surgery for improved local control. Preoperative radiation therapy allows the use of smaller fields and smaller doses but results in a higher rate of wound complications. Postoperative radiation therapy must be given to larger fields, as the entire surgical bed must be encompassed, and in higher doses to compensate for hypoxia in the operated field. Brachytherapy or interstitial therapy, in which the radiation source is inserted into the tumor bed, is comparable in efficacy (except in low-grade lesions), less time consuming, and less expensive.

Adjuvant Chemotherapy Chemotherapy is the mainstay of treatment for Ewing's primitive neuroectodermal tumors (PNET) and rhabdomyosarcomas. Meta-analysis of 14 randomized trials revealed a highly significant improvement in local control and disease-free survival in favor of doxorubicin-based chemotherapy. Overall survival is improved only for extremity sarcomas, however. A chemotherapy regimen including an anthracycline and ifosfamide with growth factor support improved overall survival for high-risk (high-grade, ≥5 cm primary, or locally recurrent) extremity soft tissue sarcomas.

Advanced Disease Metastatic soft tissue sarcomas are largely incurable, but up to 20% of patients who achieve a complete response become long-term survivors. The therapeutic intent, therefore, is to produce a complete remission with chemotherapy and/or surgery. Surgical resection of metastases, whenever possible, is an integral part of the management. Some patients benefit from repeated surgical excision of metastases. The two most active chemotherapeutic agents are doxorubicin and ifosfamide. These drugs show a steep dose-response relationship in sarcomas. Gemcitabine and dacarbazine also have some activity. Taxanes have selective activity in angiosarcomas, and vincristine, etoposide, and irinotecan are effective in rhadomyosarcomas and Ewing's sarcomas. Imatinib mesylate targets the KIT tyrosine kinase activity and is standard therapy for advanced/metastatic GISTs.

BONE SARCOMAS

INCIDENCE AND EPIDEMIOLOGY Bone sarcomas are rarer than soft tissue sarcomas; they accounted for only 0.2% of all new malignancies and ~2400 new cases in the United States in 2004. Several benign bone lesions have the potential for malignant transformation. Enchondromas and osteochondromas can transform into chondrosarcoma; fibrous dysplasia, bone infarcts, and Paget's disease of bone can transform into either malignant fibrous histiocytoma or osteosarcoma.

CLASSIFICATION ■ Benign Tumors The common benign bone tumors include enchondroma, osteochondroma, chondroblastoma, and chondromyxoid fibroma, of cartilage origin; osteoid osteoma and osteoblastoma, of bone origin; fibroma and desmoplastic fibroma, of fibrous tissue origin; hemangioma, of vascular origin; and giant cell tumor, of unknown origin.

Malignant Tumors The most common malignant tumors of bone are plasma cell tumors (Chap. 98). The four most common malignant nonhematopoietic bone tumors are osteosarcoma, chondrosarcoma, Ewing's sarcoma, and malignant fibrous histiocytoma. Rare malignant tumors include chordoma (of notochordal origin), malignant giant cell tumor and adamantinoma (of unknown origin), and hemangioendothelioma (of vascular origin).

Musculoskeletal Tumor Society Staging System Sarcomas of bone are staged according to the Musculoskeletal Tumor Society staging system based on grade and compartmental localization. A Roman numeral reflects the tumor grade: stage I is low-grade, stage II is high-grade, and stage III includes tumors of any grade that have lymph node or distant metastases. In addition, the tumor is given a letter reflecting its compartmental localization. Tumors designated A are intracompartmental (i.e., confined to the same soft tissue compartment as the initial tumor), and tumors designated B are extracompartmental (i.e., extending into the adjacent soft tissue compartment or into bone). The tumor node metastasis (TNM) staging system is shown in Table 84-2.

TABLE 84-2 Staging System for Bone Sarcomas

Primary tumor (T)	TX	Primary tumor cannot be assessed	
	T0	No evidence of primary tumor	
	T1	Tumor ≤8 cm in greatest dimension	
	T2	Tumor >8 cm in greatest dimension	
	T3	Discontinuous tumors in the primary bone site	
Regional lymph nodes (N)	NX	Regional lymph nodes cannot be assessed	
	N0	No regional lymph node metastasis	
	N1	Regional lymph node metastasis	
Distant metastasis (M)	MX	Distant metastasis cannot be assessed	
	M0	No distant metastasis	
	M1	Distant metastasis	
	M1a	Lung	
	M1b	Other distant sites	
Histologic grade (G)	GX	Grade cannot be assessed	
	G1	Well differentiated—low grade	
	G2	Moderately differentiated—low grade	
	G3	Poorly differentiated—high grade	
	G4	Undifferentiated—high grade (Ewing's is always classed G4)	

STAGE GROUPING

Stage IA	T1	N0	M0	G1,2 low grade
Stage IB	T2	N0	M0	G1,2 low grade
Stage IIA	T1	N0	M0	G3,4 high grade
Stage IIB	T2	N0	M0	G3,4 high grade
Stage III	T3	N0	M0	Any G
Stage IVA	Any T	N0	M1a	Any G
Stage IVB	Any T	N1	Any M	Any G
	Any T	Any N	M1b	Any G

OSTEOSARCOMA Osteosarcoma, accounting for almost 45% of all bone sarcomas, is a spindle cell neoplasm that produces osteoid (unmineralized bone) or bone. About 60% of all osteosarcomas occur in children and adolescents in the second decade of life, and about 10% occur in the third decade of life. Osteosarcomas in the fifth and sixth decades of life are frequently secondary to either radiation therapy or transformation in a preexisting benign condition, such as Paget's disease. Males are affected 1.5 to 2 times as often as females. Osteosarcoma has a predilection for metaphyses of long bones; the most common sites of involvement are the distal femur, proximal tibia, and proximal humerus. The classification of osteosarcoma is complex, but 75% of osteosarcomas fall in the "classic" category, which include osteoblastic, chondroblastic, and fibroblastic osteosarcomas. The remaining 25% are classified as "variants" on the basis of (1) clinical characteristics, as in the case of osteosarcoma of the jaw, postradiation osteosarcoma, or Paget's osteosarcoma; (2) morphologic characteristics, as in the case of telangiectatic osteosarcoma, small-cell osteosarcoma, or epithelioid osteosarcoma; or (3) location, as in parosteal or periosteal osteosarcoma. Diagnosis usually requires a synthesis of clinical, radiologic, and pathologic features. Patients typically present with pain and swelling of the affected area. A plain radiograph reveals a destructive lesion with a moth-eaten appearance, a spiculated periosteal reaction (sunburst appearance), and a cuff of periosteal new bone formation at the margin of the soft tissue mass (Codman's triangle). A CT scan of the primary tumor is best for defining bone destruction and the pattern of calcification, whereas MRI is better for defining intramedullary and soft tissue extension. A chest radiograph and CT scan are used to detect lung metastases. Metastases to the bony skeleton should be imaged by a bone scan. Almost all osteosarcomas are hypervascular. Angiography is not helpful for diagnosis, but it is the most sensitive test for assessing the response to preoperative chemotherapy. Pathologic diagnosis is established either with a core-needle biopsy, where feasible, or with an open biopsy with an appropriately placed incision that does not compromise future limb-sparing resection. Most osteosarcomas are high-grade. The most important prognostic factor for long-term survival is response to chemotherapy. Preoperative chemotherapy followed by limb-sparing surgery (which can be accomplished in >80% of patients) followed by postoperative chemotherapy is standard management. The effective drugs are doxorubicin, ifosfamide, cisplatin, and high-dose methotrexate with leucovorin rescue. The various combinations of these agents that have been used have all been about equally successful. Long-term survival rates in extremity osteosarcoma range from 60 to 80%. Osteosarcoma is radioresistant; radiation therapy has no role in the routine management. Malignant fibrous histiocytoma is considered a part of the spectrum of osteosarcoma and is managed similarly.

CHONDROSARCOMA Chondrosarcoma, which constitutes ~20 to 25% of all bone sarcomas, is a tumor of adulthood and old age with a peak incidence in the fourth to sixth decades of life. It has a predilection for the flat bones, especially the shoulder and pelvic girdles, but can also affect the diaphyseal portions of long bones. Chondrosarcomas can arise de novo or as a malignant transformation of an enchondroma or, rarely, of the cartilaginous cap of an osteochondroma. Chondrosarcomas have an indolent natural history and typically present as pain and swelling. Radiographically, the lesion may have a lobular appearance with mottled or punctate or annular calcification of the cartilaginous matrix. It is difficult to distinguish low-grade chondrosarcoma from benign lesions by x-ray or histologic examination. The diagnosis is therefore influenced by clinical history and physical examination. A new onset of pain, signs of inflammation, and progressive increase in the size of the mass suggest malignancy. The histologic classification is complex, but most tumors fall within the classic category. Like other bone sarcomas, high-grade chondrosarcomas spread to the lungs. Most chondrosarcomas are resistant to chemotherapy, and surgical resection of primary or recurrent tumors, including pulmonary metastases, is the mainstay of therapy. There are two histologic variants for which this rule does not hold, however. Dedifferentiated chondrosarcoma has a

high-grade osteosarcoma or a malignant fibrous histiocytoma component that responds to chemotherapy. Mesenchymal chondrosarcoma, a rare variant composed of a small cell element, also is responsive to systemic chemotherapy and is treated like Ewing's sarcoma.

EWING'S SARCOMA Ewing's sarcoma, which constitutes ~10 to 15% of all bone sarcomas, is common in adolescence and has a peak incidence in the second decade of life. It typically involves the diaphyseal region of long bones and also has an affinity for flat bones. The plain radiograph may show a characteristic "onion peel" periosteal reaction with a generous soft tissue mass, which is better demonstrated by CT or MRI. This mass is composed of sheets of monotonous, small, round, blue cells and can be confused with lymphoma, embryonal rhabdomyosarcoma, and small-cell carcinoma. The presence of p30/32, the product of the *mic-2* gene (which maps to the pseudoautosomal region of the X and Y chromosomes) is a cell-surface marker for Ewing's sarcoma (and other members of a family of tumors called PNETs). Most PNETs arise in soft tissues; they include peripheral neuroepithelioma, Askin's tumor (chest wall), and esthesioneuroblastoma. Glycogen-filled cytoplasm detected by staining with periodic acid–Schiff is also characteristic of Ewing's sarcoma cells. The classic cytogenetic abnormality associated with this disease (and other PNETs) is a reciprocal translocation of the long arms of chromosomes 11 and 22, t(11;22), which creates a chimeric gene product of unknown function with components from the *fli-1* gene on chromosome 11 and *ews* on 22. This disease is very aggressive, and it is therefore considered a systemic disease. Common sites of metastases are lung, bones, and bone marrow. Systemic chemotherapy is the mainstay of therapy, often being used before surgery. Doxorubicin, cyclophosphamide or ifosfamide, etoposide, vincristine, and dactinomycin are active drugs. Local treatment for the primary tumor includes surgical resection, usually with limb salvage or radiation therapy. Patients with lesions below the elbow and below the mid-calf have a 5-year survival rate of 80% with effective treatment. Ewing's sarcoma is a curable tumor, even in the presence of obvious metastatic disease, especially in children <11 years old.

TUMORS METASTATIC TO BONE

Bone is a common site of metastasis for carcinomas of the prostate, breast, lung, kidney, bladder, and thyroid and for lymphomas and sarcomas. Prostate, breast, and lung primaries account for 80% of all bone metastases. Metastatic tumors of bone are more common than primary bone tumors. Tumors usually spread to bone hematogenously, but local invasion from soft tissue masses also occurs. In descending order of frequency, the sites most often involved are the vertebrae, proximal femur, pelvis, ribs, sternum, proximal humerus, and skull. Bone metastases may be asymptomatic or may produce pain, swelling, nerve root or spinal cord compression, pathologic fracture, or myelophthisis (replacement of the marrow). Symptoms of hypercalcemia may be noted in cases of bony destruction.

Pain is the most frequent symptom. It usually develops gradually over weeks, is usually localized, and often is more severe at night. When patients with back pain develop neurologic signs or symptoms, emergency evaluation for spinal cord compression is indicated (Chap. 88). Bone metastases exert a major adverse effect on quality of life in cancer patients.

Cancer in the bone may produce osteolysis, osteogenesis, or both. Osteolytic lesions result when the tumor produces substances that can directly elicit bone resorption (vitamin D–like steroids, prostaglandins, or parathyroid hormone–related peptide) or cytokines that can induce the formation of osteoclasts (interleukin 1 and tumor necrosis factor). Osteoblastic lesions result when the tumor produces cytokines that activate osteoblasts. In general, purely osteolytic lesions are best detected by plain radiography, but they may not be apparent until they are >1 cm. These lesions are more commonly associated with hypercalcemia and with the excretion of hydroxyproline-containing peptides indicative of matrix destruction. When osteoblastic activity is prominent, the lesions may be readily detected using radionuclide bone scanning (which is sensitive to new bone formation), and the radiographic appearance may show increased bone density or sclerosis. Osteoblastic lesions are associated with higher serum levels of alkaline phosphatase, and, if extensive, may produce hypocalcemia. Although some tumors may produce mainly osteolytic lesions (e.g., kidney cancer) and others mainly osteoblastic lesions (e.g., prostate cancer), most metastatic lesions produce both types of lesion and may go through stages where one or the other predominates.

In older patients, particularly women, it may be necessary to distinguish metastatic disease of the spine from osteoporosis. In osteoporosis, the cortical bone may be preserved, whereas cortical bone destruction is usually noted with metastatic cancer.

Rx TREATMENT

Treatment of metastatic bone disease depends on the underlying malignancy and the symptoms. Some metastatic bone tumors are curable (lymphoma, Hodgkin's disease), and others are treated with palliative intent. Pain may be relieved by local radiation therapy. Hormonally responsive tumors are responsive to hormone inhibition (antiandro-

gens for prostate cancer, antiestrogens for breast cancer). Strontium 89 and samarium 153 are bone-seeking radionuclides that can exert antitumor effects and relieve symptoms. Bisphosphonates such as pamidronate may relieve pain and inhibit bone resorption. Monthly administration prevents bone-related clinical events and may reduce the incidence of bone metastases in women with breast cancer. When the integrity of a weight-bearing bone is threatened by an expanding metastatic lesion that is refractory to radiation therapy, prophylactic internal fixation is indicated. Overall survival is related to the prognosis of the underlying tumor. Bone pain at the end of life is particularly common; an adequate pain relief regimen including sufficient amounts of narcotic analgesics is required. →*The management of hypercalcemia is discussed in Chap. 332.*

FURTHER READING

BORDEN EC et al: Soft tissue sarcomas of adults: State of the translational science. Clin Cancer Res 9:1941, 2003

DEMETRI GD et al: Efficacy and safety of imatinib mesylate in advanced gastrointestinal stromal tumors. N Engl J Med 347:472, 2002

FRUSTACI S et al: Adjuvant chemotherapy for adult soft tissue sarcomas of the extremities and girdles: Results of the Italian Randomized Cooperative Group trial. J Clin Oncol 19:1238, 2001

HELMAN LJ, MELTZER P: Mechanisms of sarcoma development. Nat Rev Cancer 3:685, 2003

WITTIG JC et al: Osteosarcoma: A multidisciplinary approach to diagnosis and treatment. Am Fam Physician 65:1123, 2002

85 METASTATIC CANCER OF UNKNOWN PRIMARY SITE
Richard M. Stone

INCIDENCE AND EPIDEMIOLOGY

The presenting findings in a patient with a newly discovered malignancy may not reveal its site of origin. Patients with cancer of unknown primary site (CUPS) present difficult diagnostic and therapeutic dilemmas. First, as additional studies may be many, costly, and/or uncomfortable for the patient, the strategy used in searching for the primary must assess what, if any, result the identification of the site of origin would have on the patient's treatment and survival. Second, while individuals with CUPS fare poorly overall (median survival is 4 to 11 months), certain subgroups of patients are more likely to benefit from treatment and, in some cases, to enjoy long disease-free survival. Population-based analysis shows that two-thirds receive only supportive treatment and that only 15% are alive 1 year after diagnosis, suggesting the selection bias inherent in the more typically reported studies from tertiary care centers.

No universally accepted definition of the CUPS syndrome exists. An occult neoplasm should fulfill all of the following criteria: (1) biopsy-proven malignancy; (2) unrevealing history, physical examination, chest film, abdominal and pelvic computed tomography (CT) scans, complete blood counts, chemistry survey, mammography (women), β human chorionic gonadotropin (βhCG) levels (men), α fetoprotein (AFP) levels (men), and prostate-specific antigen (PSA) levels (men); (3) histologic evaluation not consistent with a primary tumor at the biopsy site; and (4) failure of additional diagnostic studies (based only on findings from the laboratory and pathologic review) to identify the primary site. Such additional diagnostic tests could include, for example, colonoscopy in a patient whose rectal examination discloses guaiac-positive stool or a meticulous otolaryngologic examination in a patient who presents with squamous cell carcinoma in a cervical node. Many cases that fulfill the definition of CUPS offer clues that a given organ is the probable site of origin. Epidemiologic data suggest that the incidence of cancers for which the primary site is unknown is decreasing. CUPS accounts for about 2% of all cancer diagnoses—about 24,400 cases in the year 2000. Most patients with CUPS are over age 60.

BIOLOGIC CONSIDERATIONS The biologic behavior of CUPS is unique. In ~25% of patients, the primary site becomes apparent during the course of the illness; in about 57% of patients, the primary site can be diagnosed at autopsy; but in almost 20%, the primary site remains obscure even at autopsy. Cancers presenting as CUPS often display unusual patterns of metastatic spread (e.g., pancreatic cancer presenting with bony metastases). The fact that more tumor bulk is present at distant sites than in the tissue of origin suggests that the genetic lesions underlying cases of CUPS produce a distinctly aggressive phenotype. Microsatellite DNA analysis has shown that the same pattern of genetic alterations that appears in a cervical lymph node metastasis can be found in seemingly morphologically normal aerodigestive tissue. Such data imply that clinically evident metastases may be able to arise from microscopic primary lesions. Tumors in 11% of CUPS patients, almost all with poorly differentiated adenocarcinoma, express the HER2/neu protein. Although physiologic and genetic data that might account for the distinctive natural history of CUPS neoplasms are scant, cell lines derived from such tumors may have abnormalities of chromosome 1, a finding generally associated with advanced malignancy. In some patients, the primary tumor spontaneously regresses (perhaps under immunologic attack) or necroses. In some, a primary lesion was resected years before presentation (e.g., melanoma).

CLINICAL PRESENTATION, DIAGNOSTIC EVALUATION, AND PATHOLOGY ■ History and Physical Examination Patients present with a variety of symptoms and signs, including fatigue, weight loss, other systemic symptoms, pain, abnormal bleeding, abdominal swelling, subcutaneous masses, and lymphadenopathy. Once CUPS is considered, the physician's approach must involve reasonable efforts to identify the primary site or to determine the histology or subcategory of the metastatic tumor to decide on the optimal therapy. Though usually unrevealing, a thorough history and physical examination should be carried out to elicit easily obtainable clues regarding the primary site. The patient should be questioned concerning epigastric pain, which, if present, would mandate careful exclusion of pancreatic carcinoma as well as other gastrointestinal malignancies. Symptoms referable to a given location (e.g., new cough, hematochezia, hemoptysis, change in bowel habits, unusual vaginal bleeding, nipple discharge) should prompt an aggressive specific diagnostic approach. Occupational exposure to asbestos, for example, would raise the suspicion of mesothelioma. The absence of prior smoking reduces the likelihood of lung cancer but does not exclude it. A history of fulguration of a skin lesion, colonic polypectomy, dilatation and curettage, or prostate biopsy should prompt a review of the original histology.

Pathology Review The most important aspect of the workup of a patient with CUPS is the thorough evaluation of the tissue obtained at biopsy by light microscopy, immunohistochemistry, ultrastructural studies, immunophenotyping, and karyotypic and molecular biologic analysis. First, if the original biopsy sample is inadequate for either confirmation of malignancy or the performance of additional specialized studies, rebiopsy is mandatory. The clinician must have a close working relationship with a pathologist skilled in the evaluation of tumor specimens, especially when the organ of origin is uncertain. Plans may be made to process the tissue for (1) routine light-microscopic, histochemical, and immunohistochemical analysis; (2) freezing for DNA and RNA isolation or for in situ genetic and immunologic evaluation; and (3) special fixation for ultrastructural analysis. Single-cell tumor suspensions in short-term culture permit cytogenetic analysis.

If routine histologic analysis fails to suggest the tissue of origin (e.g., gland formation in adenocarcinoma, psammoma bodies in ovarian or thyroid cancer, or spindle architecture in sarcomas), special histochemical studies may be helpful. For example, mucin positivity is helpful in recognizing a poorly differentiated adenocarcinoma. Light-microscopic analysis will show ~60% of CUPS tumors to be well or moderately differentiated adenocarcinomas, 30% poorly differentiated carcinomas/adenocarcinomas, and 5% poorly differentiated malignant neoplasms not further classifiable. In the poorly differentiated neoplasms, immunohistochemical, cytogenetic, and molecular biologic studies can be extremely useful in identifying sarcomas, germ cell carcinomas, lymphomas, neuroendocrine neoplasms (including melanoma), and other tumors whose diagnosis would suggest a more specific therapeutic approach.

Immunohistochemical Analysis Antibodies to specific cell components make it possible to characterize tumors that are not identified by standard techniques. Table 85-1 provides a list of antigens that may be assessed in undifferentiated or poorly differentiated specimens. A diagnosis of lymphoma should be excluded by employing antibodies reactive to the leukocyte common antigen (LCA, CD45). LCA-positive tumors are lymphomas and have the same chances of responding to therapy as if the diagnosis were unambiguous. About half of patients with aggressive-histology lymphoma can be cured with combination chemotherapy (Chap. 97). The immunohistochemical detection of specific types of filament proteins is helpful in the identification of carcinomas and sarcomas. The presence of keratin suggests carcinoma; all epithelial tumors contain this protein. Specific types of cytokeratins (CKs) may aid in diagnosis. For example, ovarian and lung cancers are CK20−/CK7+, colorectal cancers are CK20+/CK7−, and pancreaticobiliary tumors and transitional cell cancers are CK20+/CK7+. However, certain sarcomas, mesotheliomas, and germ cell tumors are also keratin-positive. Sarcomas may react with antibodies to desmin. Coexpression of p53 and CK5/6 is suggestive of a squamous cell primary. Sarcoma subgroups may be identified by expression of myoglobin (rhabdomyosarcoma) or factor VIII (angiosarcoma or Kaposi's sarcoma). Prostate, breast, and thyroid carcinomas express, respectively, PSA, gross cystic fluid protein, or thyroglobulin. The finding of AFP, βhCG, or placental alkaline phosphatase staining is very helpful in assigning a germ cell origin. The S-100 protein is present in virtually all primary and metastatic melanomas, including the amelanotic variety. However, S-100 positivity is also found in other tumors of neuroendocrine origin (e.g., small cell lung cancer, carcinoid, neuroepithelioma); a more specific marker for melanomas is the HMB45 (human melanoma black) antigen.

TABLE 85-1 *Possible Pathologic Evaluation of Biopsy Specimens from Patients with Metastatic Cancer of Unknown Primary Site*

Evaluation/Findings	Suggested Primary Site or Neoplasm
HISTOLOGY (HEMATOXYLIN AND EOSIN STAINING)	
Psammoma bodies, papillary configuration	Ovary, thyroid
Signet ring cells	Stomach
IMMUNOHISTOLOGY	
Leukocyte common antigen (LCA, CD45)	Lymphoid neoplasm
Leu-M1	Hodgkin's disease
Epithelial membrane antigen	Carcinoma
Cytokeratin	Carcinoma[a]
CEA	Carcinoma
HMB45	Melanoma
Desmin	Sarcoma
Thyroglobulin	Thyroid carcinoma
Calcitonin	Medullary carcinoma of the thyroid
Myoglobin	Rhabdomyosarcoma
PSA/prostatic acid phosphatase	Prostate
AFP	Liver, stomach, germ cell
Placental alkaline phosphatase	Germ cell
B, T cell markers	Lymphoid neoplasm
S-100 protein	Neuroendocrine tumor, melanoma
Gross cystic fluid protein	Breast, sweat gland
Factor VIII	Kaposi's sarcoma, angiosarcoma
Thyroid transcription factor-1 (TTF-1)	Lung adenocarcinoma, thyroid
FLOW CYTOMETRY	
B, T cell markers	Lymphoid neoplasm
ULTRASTRUCTURE	
Actin-myosin filaments	Rhabdomyosarcoma
Secretory granules	Neuroendocrine tumors
Desmosomes	Carcinoma
Premelanosomes	Melanoma
CYTOGENETICS	
Isochromosome 12p; 12q(−)	Germ cell
t(11;22)	Ewing's sarcoma, primitive neuroectodermal tumor
t(8;14)[b]	Lymphoid neoplasm
3p(−)	Small cell lung carcinoma; renal cell carcinoma, mesothelioma
t(X;18)	Synovial sarcoma
t(12;16)	Myxoid liposarcoma
t(12;22)	Clear cell sarcoma (melanoma of soft parts)
t(2;13)	Alveolar rhabdomyosarcoma
1p(−)	Neuroblastoma
RECEPTOR ANALYSIS	
Estrogen/progesterone receptor	Breast
MOLECULAR BIOLOGIC STUDIES	
Immunoglobulin, *bcl*-2, T-cell receptor gene rearrangement	Lymphoid neoplasm

[a] See text for discussion of cytokeratins.
[b] Or any other rearrangement involving an antigen-receptor gene.
Note: CEA, carcinoembryonic antigen; PSA, prostate-specific antigen; AFP, α fetoprotein.

Other Diagnostic Approaches Electron microscopy can identify cell junctions (i.e., desmosomes, typical of epithelial cancers), neuroendocrine granules, melanosomes, and muscle filaments. Cytogenetic analysis may identify tumors with specific chromosomal translocations or other genetic abnormalities (Table 85-1). Cytogenetic abnormalities can also be determined by fluorescence in situ hybridization with chromosome-specific probes, a technique that does not require cells to divide, as is the case with traditional karyotype analysis. Fresh tissue may be required for detection of estrogen or progesterone receptors (to assess breast cancer) or antigens that are sensitive to fixation. Lineage can be assigned by analysis of DNA for signature gene rearrangements, such as those of immunoglobulin (B cell) or T cell receptor (T cell). Technological advances promise to influence the diagnosis of cancer. Isolation of mRNA from tumor specimens may permit the molecular profiling of tumors by microarray analysis of gene expression. This could lead to novel classifications of tumors based on molecular characteristics that may predict clinical behavior and/or response to specific therapies.

Additional Studies If the pathologist does not identify the likely tissue of origin, it is unlikely that additional expensive diagnostic tests will benefit the patient. In females with metastatic adenocarcinoma or poorly differentiated carcinoma, mammography should be performed, although the diagnostic yield will be quite low except in patients with axillary metastases. Magnetic resonance imaging, positron-emission tomography (PET), or indium 111-pentreotide scanning can identify occult primary lesions but are expensive. The use of abdominal/pelvic CT scans leads to the identification of the primary site (often the pancreas) in up to 35% of patients but has little effect on natural history. While more sensitive than CT in detection of a primary site, the now frequently employed PET scan does not clearly lead to better outcomes. Whether to measure serum tumor markers such as AFP, βhCG, carcinoembryonic antigen (CEA), CA-125 (associated with ovarian cancer), and PSA is controversial; value has not been proved. Numerous studies have shown a lack of benefit of contrast studies (upper gastrointestinal series, barium enema, or intravenous pyelogram) in patients with CUPS who have no specific symptoms and no findings referable to the gastrointestinal or urinary tract. Moreover, autopsy series reveal that the most likely primary site of origin includes epithelial tissues such as lung, stomach, colon, and kidney, which give rise to tumors that respond poorly to chemotherapy, minimizing the therapeutic impact of such a diagnosis.

Additional invasive diagnostic studies are indicated if the presentation strongly suggests a particular primary site. For example, radiographic evidence of lung or mediastinal involvement would mandate fiberoptic bronchoscopy to exclude lung cancer. In the relatively unusual case of metastatic squamous cell cancer presenting in an inguinal lymph node, anoscopy and colposcopy should be performed to detect carcinoma of the vulva, cervix, vagina, penis, or anus, all of which may be cured even with lymph node spread. A reasonable diagnostic approach is provided in Table 85-2.

℞ TREATMENT

Prognostic Subgroups The exclusion of treatable and potentially curable neoplasms is important. Patients with squamous cell carcinoma have a somewhat longer median survival (9 months) than do those with adenocarcinoma or unclassifiable neoplasms (4 to 6 months). If laboratory studies indicate a significant likelihood that the neoplasm is a lymphoma, germ cell tumor, sarcoma, neuroendocrine tumor, or breast or prostate cancer, then disease-appropriate therapy should be administered. Patients with lymphoma or a germ cell neoplasm may be cured with combination chemotherapy. In other malignancies, effective palliative chemotherapy (for sarcoma or a breast or neuroendocrine tumor) or hormonal therapy (for breast or prostate cancer) should be strongly considered. Although often requiring electron microscopy for diagnosis, neuroendocrine tumors (especially if anaplastic) often respond to cisplatin-based chemotherapy.

Patients in whom the primary site can be identified fare somewhat better than those in whom it remains undefined. A validated prognostic model based on a multivariate analysis of clinical parameters suggested those with a good performance status without liver metastases had a median survival of 10.8 months compared with 2.4 months for patients who were more symptomatic and who had spread to the liver. Elevated serum lactate dehydrogenase alone predicted a median sur-

TABLE 85-2 *Suggested Clinical Evaluation of Patients with Metastatic Cancer of Unknown Primary Site*

History: smoking history, asbestos exposure, abdominal pain
Physical examination: lymph nodes, thyroid, skin;
  Men: prostate
  Women: breasts, pelvic examination
Laboratory evaluation: stool evaluation for occult blood; urinalysis; complete blood count; liver function tests; calcium, electrolytes, creatine; measurement of serum levels of βhCG, AFP, CEA, and CA-125 (women); chest x-ray; abdominal and pelvic CT; mammography
Pathologic evaluation: see Table 85-1

Note: PSA, prostate-specific antigen; βhCG, β-human chorionic gonadotropin; AFP, α fetoprotein; CEA, carcinoembryonic antigen; CT, computed tomography.

vival of 3.9 months (Table 85-3). Forty percent of CUPS patients may be found to have one of several clinical syndromes for which a specific therapeutic approach may be useful:

SYNDROME OF UNRECOGNIZED EXTRAGONADAL GERM CELL CANCER Some patients with poorly differentiated CUPS are responsive to chemotherapy. These patients display one or more of the following features: age <50; tumor involving midline structures, lung parenchyma, or lymph nodes; an elevated serum AFP or βhCG level; evidence of rapid tumor growth; or tumor responsiveness to previously administered radiotherapy or chemotherapy. Platinum-based chemotherapy has led to long-term survival in a fraction of patients with these features, especially those who have a favorable performance status at diagnosis, suggesting that their tumors behaved like germ cell neoplasms. If all patients with poorly differentiated carcinoma (including poorly differentiated adenocarcinoma) are treated with a chemotherapy regimen designed for germ cell cancer (e.g., cisplatin plus etoposide or vinblastine, often also with bleomycin) (Chap. 82), about 25% will respond completely and 33% will have a partial response. Patients whose disease does not respond to two cycles of therapy should not continue

TABLE 85-3 *Presentations That Dictate Specific Therapies in Patients with CUPS*

Clinicopathologic Features	Suspected Primary Site	Suggested Therapy
Squamous cell carcinoma, cervical node	Head and neck cancer	Radical neck dissection; radiotherapy ± chemotherapy
Carcinoma, axillary nodes (female)	Breast cancer	Breast radiotherapy or mastectomy, systemic adjuvant therapy
Peritoneal carcinomatosis (female)	Ovarian cancer	Debulking surgery, cisplatin-based chemotherapy
Pleural effusion, adenocarcinoma cells estrogen and/or progesterone receptor positive	Breast cancer	Systemic therapy for metastatic breast cancer
Poorly differentiated cancer, age <50, lung or retroperitoneal or mediastinal mass or lymph nodes, elevated serum βhCG or AFP levels	Germ cell tumor (extragonadal)	Cisplatin/VP-16-based chemotherapy
Bony metastases (male)	Prostate cancer	Androgen blockade (leuprolide plus flutamide)
Adenocarcinoma, liver metastases, elevated CEA level	Gastrointestinal malignancy	Surgical resection of liver lesion feasible; colonoscopy with resection (if appropriate) of tumors; 5-fluorouracil/leucovorin

Note: βhCG, β-human chorionic gonadotropin; AFP, α fetoprotein; CEA, carcinoembryonic antigen.

therapy. One in six patients survives >5 years without evidence of disease. Patients with poorly differentiated carcinoma or adenocarcinoma whose tumors have abnormalities of chromosome 12 similar to those described in patients with proven germ cell cancer are more likely to respond to platinum-based chemotherapy than are patients with a similar presentation whose tumors lack this cytogenetic abnormality.

PERITONEAL CARCINOMATOSIS IN WOMEN Women who present with increased abdominal girth and a pelvic mass or pain and who are found to have adenocarcinoma throughout the peritoneal cavity without a clear site of origin may also benefit from platinum-based chemotherapy. This syndrome has been termed *primary peritoneal papillary serous carcinoma* or *multifocal extraovarian serous carcinoma*. While breast cancer or a gastrointestinal malignancy can produce these findings, peritoneal carcinomatosis is most commonly ascribed to ovarian cancer, even in patients with apparently normal ovaries at the time of laparotomy. Especially if psammoma bodies or a papillary configuration is noted in the pathology examination or if the CA-125 level is elevated, women with adenocarcinoma of the peritoneal cavity without a defined primary should receive maximum surgical cytoreduction followed by cisplatin (or carboplatin) plus paclitaxel. The stage-specific response to such therapy appears to be comparable to that for patients with proven ovarian cancer. About 10% of patients who present in this fashion may remain free of disease 2 years after diagnosis.

CARCINOMA IN AN AXILLARY LYMPH NODE IN A FEMALE Women with adenocarcinoma or poorly differentiated carcinoma in an axillary mass should receive treatment for stage II breast cancer whether or not a careful breast examination or mammography suggests the diagnosis of primary breast cancer and whether or not estrogen or progesterone receptors are detectable in the node. Even if no lesion is found in the breast, a breast recurrence will develop in one-half of these patients if no mastectomy is performed. Modified radical mastectomy or breast irradiation may be equivalent in reducing the risk of local recurrence. In addition, adjuvant systemic therapy (chemotherapy and/or tamoxifen, depending on menopausal and estrogen receptor status) should be given to reduce the risk of developing evident metastatic breast cancer (Chap. 76). Adjuvant systemic therapy may be administered before definitive local radiation treatment. Women with axillary metastases without an obvious breast primary appear to have the same likelihood of prolonged disease-free survival as patients with typical stage II breast cancer.

BONE METASTASES IN MALES Particularly if the lesions are osteoblastic, the serum PSA level should be measured, as the probability of prostate carcinoma is high. Empirical hormonal therapy (e.g., leuprolide and flutamide) should be strongly considered.

CERVICAL LYMPH NODE METASTASES Patients who present with a neck mass should be considered to have a primary tumor of the upper aerodigestive tract (head and neck cancer) until a different source is proven. Especially if the pathologist diagnoses squamous histology and the node is located in a high or midcervical area, a careful ear, nose, and throat examination including direct laryngoscopy, nasopharyngoscopy, and random blind biopsies should be undertaken. A thyroid examination and scan should be performed to rule out a primary thyroid tumor, especially if the histology is not definitely squamous. Definitive local therapy (external beam radiation or radical neck dissection) combined with platinum-based chemotherapy may lead to prolonged survival in those with head and neck primaries (Chap. 74).

ADENOCARCINOMA AND LIVER METASTASES Liver metastases from an adenocarcinoma are not as well characterized as a syndrome as the unrecognized germ cell cancer syndrome (nor as responsive to therapy). However, such patients may have a primary stomach, biliary, or colorectal tumor. Tumors with limited hepatic involvement may be amenable to resection. A flexible sigmoidoscopy or colonoscopy may detect a potentially obstructive colon lesion. If a tumor is found, resection

may be beneficial, depending on the tumor's size; even if none is found, treatment with a combination of 5-fluorouracil plus leucovorin, with or without irinotecan, is palliative for some patients with presumed metastatic gastrointestinal malignancy. Given the severe diarrhea that may be a consequence of this regimen and the relative resistance of gastrointestinal tumors to chemotherapy, patients should be informed of the risks before treatment.

Other Patients Patients not falling into one of the preceding categories should be treated palliatively. In some patients, observation is appropriate. For example, individuals without evidence of additional metastatic disease who have undergone resection of a solitary pulmonary nodule containing malignant cells may actually have undergone definitive therapy for a small primary lung tumor. Patients presenting with a solitary brain metastasis from an unknown primary source who undergo resection of the lesion followed by whole-brain radiation therapy have a median survival of 13 months, suggesting benefit for aggressive local therapy. Radiation therapy may relieve symptoms in patients with bony pain or neurologic compromise. The largest and most poorly responsive subgroup are those with moderate to well-differentiated adenocarcinomas. Combination chemotherapy is frequently employed in such patients; however, response rates to "all-purpose" regimens [e.g., FACP (5-fluorouracil, doxorubicin, cyclophosphamide, cisplatin)] or to ICE (ifosfamide, carboplatin, etoposide) are generally well under 50%, especially if patients with poorly differentiated adenocarcinoma, who have a higher response rate, are excluded; complete responses are rare. The addition of a taxane (taxotere or paclitaxel) to such regimens has been associated with a higher response rate, albeit in selected patients. High-dose chemotherapy is not beneficial. In some series, patients with a good performance status whose disease is limited to soft tissue sites or extends only above the diaphragm have shown a better rate of response to therapy. While patients whose disease responds to treatment seem to have better survival than those whose disease does not respond, the difference may be related to inherent characteristics of the tumor rather than to a beneficial effect of chemotherapy.

Before combination chemotherapy is attempted in a patient with CUPS, the potential benefits must be weighed carefully against the certainty of toxicity. While some randomized studies have reported a benefit of one form of therapy over another, these reports are generally plagued by small numbers of patients and inadequate control of potential prognostic variables. Depending on motivation, eligibility, and availability, patients with CUPS may be candidates for evaluation of new (phase I) therapies.

FURTHER READING

CULINE S et al: Development and validation of a prognostic model to predict the length of survival in patients with carcinomas of an unknown primary. J Clin Oncol 20:4679, 2002

DENNIS JL et al: Identification from public data of molecular markers of adenocarcinoma characteristic of the site of origin. Cancer Res 62:5999, 2002

ETTINGER DS et al: NCCN practice guidelines for occult primary tumors. Oncology 12:226, 1998

FOGARTY GB et al: The usefulness of fluorine 18-labelled deoxyglucose positron emission tomography in the investigation of patients with cervical lymphadenopathy from an unknown primary tumor. Head Neck 25:138, 2002

HAINSWORTH JD, GRECO FA: Management of patients with cancer of an unknown primary site. Oncology 14:563, 2000

PAVLIDIS N et al: Diagnostic and therapeutic management of cancer of an unknown primary. Eur J Cancer 39:1990, 2003

SAAD ED, ABBRUZZESE JL: Prognostic stratification in UPC: A role for assessing the value of conventional-dose and high-dose chemotherapy for unknown primary carcinoma. Crit Rev Oncol Hematol 41:205, 2002

VAN DE WOUW AJ et al: Epidemiology of unknown primary tumours: Incidence and population-based survival of 1285 patients in Southeast Netherlands, 1984–1992. Eur J Cancer 38:409, 2002

In addition to local tissue invasion and metastasis, neoplastic cells can produce a variety of peptides that exert biologic actions at local and distant sites and can elicit responses that cause a variety of hormonal, hematologic, dermatologic, and neurologic symptoms. *Paraneoplastic syndromes* refer to the disorders that accompany benign or malignant tumors but are not directly related to mass effects or invasion by the primary tumor or its metastases. Tumors of neuroendocrine origin, such as small cell lung carcinoma (SCLC) and carcinoids, produce a wide array of peptide hormones and are common causes of paraneoplastic syndromes. However, almost every type of malignancy has the potential to produce hormones or cytokines or to induce immunologic responses. Careful studies of the prevalence of paraneoplastic syndromes indicate that they are more common than is generally appreciated. The signs, symptoms, and metabolic alterations associated with paraneoplastic disorders may be overlooked in the context of a malignancy and its treatment. Consequently, atypical clinical manifestations in a patient with cancer should prompt consideration of a paraneoplastic syndrome. In this chapter, we review the most common endocrinologic, hematologic, and dermatologic syndromes associated with underlying neoplasia.

ENDOCRINE PARANEOPLASTIC SYNDROMES

ETIOLOGY Hormones can be produced from eutopic or ectopic sources. *Eutopic* refers to the expression of a hormone from its normal tissue of origin, whereas *ectopic* refers to hormone production from an atypical tissue source. For example, adrenocorticotropic hormone (ACTH) is expressed eutopically by the corticotrope cells of the anterior pituitary but it can be expressed ectopically in SCLC. As assay methodologies have become more sensitive, it is now apparent that many hormones are produced at low levels from a wide array of tissues, in addition to the classic endocrine source. Thus, ectopic expression is often a quantitative change rather than an absolute change in tissue expression. Nevertheless, the term *ectopic expression* is firmly entrenched and conveys the abnormal physiology associated with neoplastic hormone production. In addition to high levels of hormones, ectopic expression is typically characterized by abnormal regulation of hormone production (e.g., defective feedback control) and peptide processing (resulting in large, unprocessed precursors).

A diverse array of molecular mechanisms has been suggested to cause ectopic hormone production, but this process remains incompletely understood. In rare instances, genetic rearrangements explain aberrant hormone expression. For example, translocation of the *parathyroid hormone (PTH)* gene resulted in high levels of PTH expression in an ovarian carcinoma, presumably because the genetic rearrangement brings the *PTH* gene under the control of ovary-specific regulatory elements. A related phenomenon is well documented in many forms of leukemia and lymphoma, in which somatic genetic rearrangements confer a growth advantage and frequently alter cellular differentiation and function (see Chap. 97). Although genetic rearrangements may cause selected cases of ectopic hormone production, this mechanism is probably unusual, as many tumors are associated with excessive production of a wide variety of peptides. It is likely that cellular dedifferentiation underlies most cases of ectopic hormone production. In support of this idea, many cancers are poorly differentiated histologically, and certain tumor products, such as human chorionic gonadotropin (hCG), parathyroid hormone–related protein (PTHrP), and α fetoprotein, are characteristic of gene expression at earlier developmental stages. On the other hand, the propensity of certain cancers to produce particular hormones (e.g., squamous cell carcinomas produce PTHrP) suggests that dedifferentiation is partial or that selective pathways are derepressed. These expression profiles are likely to be driven by alterations in transcriptional repression, changes in DNA methylation, or other factors that govern cell differ-

entiation. In SCLC, the pathway of differentiation has been relatively well defined. The neuroendocrine phenotype is dictated in part by the basic-helix-loop-helix (bHLH) transcription factor human achaete-scute homologue-1 (hASH1), which is expressed at abnormally high levels in SCLC associated with ectopic ACTH. The activity of hASH-1 is inhibited by hairy enhancer of split-1 (HES-1) and by Notch proteins, which are also capable of inducing growth arrest. Thus, abnormal expression of these developmental transcription factors appears to provide a link between cell proliferation and differentiation.

Ectopic hormone production would only be an epiphenomenon associated with cancer if it did not sometimes result in clinical manifestations. Excessive and unregulated production of hormones such as ACTH, PTHrP, or vasopressin can lead to substantial morbidity and can complicate the cancer treatment plan. Moreover, the paraneoplastic endocrinopathies are sometimes the presenting feature of underlying malignancy and may prompt the search for an unrecognized tumor.

A large number of paraneoplastic endocrine syndromes have been described, linking overproduction of particular hormones with specific types of tumors. However, certain recurring syndromes emerge from this large group (Table 86-1). The most common paraneoplastic endocrine syndromes include hypercalcemia from overproduction of PTHrP and other factors, hyponatremia from excess vasopressin, and Cushing's syndrome from ectopic ACTH.

SELECTED PARANEOPLASTIC ENDOCRINE SYNDROMES

HYPERCALCEMIA CAUSED BY ECTOPIC PRODUCTION OF PTHrP (See also Chap. 332) ■ **Etiology** Humoral hypercalcemia of malignancy (HHM) occurs in up to 5% of patients with cancer. HHM is most common in cancers of the lung, breast, head and neck, genitourinary tract, esophagus, and skin, and in multiple myeloma and lymphomas. There are several humoral causes of HHM but it is most often associated with overproduction of PTHrP. In addition to acting as a circulating humoral factor, many bone metastases (e.g., breast, multiple myeloma) produce PTHrP, leading to local osteolysis and hypercalcemia.

PTHrP is structurally related to PTH and it binds to the PTH receptor, explaining the similar biochemical features of HHM and hyperparathyroidism. PTHrP plays a key role in skeletal development and regulates cellular proliferation and differentiation in other tissues including skin, bone marrow, breast, and hair follicles. The mechanism of PTHrP induction in malignancy is incompletely understood but it is notable that tumor-bearing tissues commonly associated with HHM normally produce PTHrP during development or cellular renewal. Mutations in certain oncogenes, such as *Ras*, can activate PTHrP expression. In adult T cell lymphoma, the transactivating Tax protein produced by human T-cell lymphotropic virus-1 (HTLV-1) stimulates PTHrP promoter activity. Metastatic lesions to bone are more likely to produce PTHrP than are metastases in other tissues, suggesting that bone produces factors that enhance PTHrP production, or that PTHrP-producing metastases have a selective growth advantage in bone. Thus, PTHrP production can be stimulated by mutations in oncogenes, by altered expression of viral or cellular transcription factors, and by local growth factors.

Another relatively common cause of HHM is excess production of 1,25-dihydroxyvitamin D. Like granulomatous disorders associated with hypercalcemia, lymphomas can produce an enzyme that converts 25-hydroxyvitamin D to the more active 1,25-dihydroxyvitamin D, leading to enhanced gastrointestinal calcium absorption. Other causes of HHM include tumor-mediated production of osteolytic cytokines and inflammatory mediators.

Clinical Manifestations The typical presentation of HHM is a patient with a known malignancy who is found to be hypercalcemic on routine laboratory tests. Less often, hypercalcemia is the initial presenting feature of malignancy. Particularly when calcium levels are markedly increased (>14 mg/dL), patients may experience fatigue, mental status changes, dehydration, or symptoms of nephrolithiasis.

Diagnosis Features that favor HHM as opposed to primary hyperparathyroidism include known malignancy, recent onset of hypercalcemia, and very high serum calcium levels. Like hyperparathyroidism, hypercalcemia caused by PTHrP is accompanied by hypercalciuria and hypophosphatemia. Measurement of PTH is useful to exclude primary hyperparathyroidism; the PTH level should be suppressed in HHM. An elevated PTHrP level confirms the diagnosis, and it is increased in about 80% of hypercalcemic patients with cancer. 1,25-Dihydroxyvitamin D levels may be increased in patients with lymphoma.

℞ TREATMENT

The management of HHM begins with saline rehydration to dilute serum calcium and promote calciuresis. Forced diuresis with furosemide or other loop diuretics can enhance calcium excretion but provides relatively little value except in life-threatening hypercalcemia. When used, loop diuretics should be administered only after complete rehydration and with careful monitoring of fluid balance. Bisphosphonates such as pamidronate (30 to 90 mg IV) or zoledronate (4 to 8 mg IV) can reduce serum calcium within 1 to 2 days and suppress calcium release for several weeks. Oral bisphosphonates can also be used for chronic treatment. Previously used agents, such as calcitonin and mithramycin, have little utility now that bisphosphonates are available. Calcitonin (2 to 8 U/kg SC every 6 to 12 h) should be considered when rapid correction of severe hypercalcemia is needed. Hypercalcemia associated with lymphomas, multiple myeloma, or leukemia may respond to glucocorticoid treatment (e.g., prednisone 40 to 100 mg PO in four divided doses).

TABLE 86-1 *Paraneoplastic Syndromes Caused by Ectopic Hormone Production*		
Paraneoplastic Syndrome	*Ectopic Hormone*	*Typical Tumor Types*[a]
COMMON		
Hypercalcemia of malignancy	Parathyroid hormone-related protein (PTHrP)	Squamous cell (head and neck, lung, skin), breast, genitourinary, gastrointestinal
	1,25 dihydroxyvitamin D	Lymphomas
	Parathyroid hormone (PTH) (rare)	Lung, ovary
	Prostaglandin E2 (PGE2) (rare)	Renal, lung
Syndrome of inappropriate antidiuretic hormone secretion (SIADH)	Vasopressin	Lung (squamous, small cell), gastrointestinal, genitourinary, ovary
Cushing's syndrome	Adrenocorticotropic hormone (ACTH)	Lung (small cell, bronchial carcinoid, adenocarcinoma, squamous), thymus, pancreatic islet, medullary thyroid carcinoma
	Corticotropin-releasing hormone (CRH) (rare)	Pancreatic islet, carcinoid, lung, prostate
	Ectopic expression of gastric inhibitory peptide (GIP), luteinizing hormone (LH)/ human chorionic gonadotropin (hCG), other G protein–coupled receptors (rare)	Macronodular adrenal hyperplasia
LESS COMMON		
Non-islet cell hypoglycemia	Insulin-like growth factor (IGF-II)	Mesenchymal tumors, sarcomas, adrenal, hepatic, gastrointestinal, kidney, prostate
	Insulin (rare)	Cervix (small cell carcinoma)
Male feminization	hCG[b]	Testis (embryonal, seminomas), germinomas, choriocarcinoma, lung, hepatic, pancreatic islet
Diarrhea or intestinal hypermotility	Calcitonin[c]	Lung, colon, breast, medullary thyroid carcinoma
	Vasoactive intestinal peptide (VIP)	Pancreas, pheochromocytoma, esophagus
RARE		
Oncogenic osteomalacia	Phosphatonin [Fibroblast growth factor 23 (FGF23)]	Hemangiopericytomas, osteoblastomas, fibromas, sarcomas, giant cell tumors, prostate, lung
Acromegaly	Growth hormone–releasing hormone (GHRH)	Pancreatic islet, bronchial and other carcinoids
	Growth hormone (GH)	Lung, pancreatic islet
Hyperthyroidism	Thyroid-stimulating hormone (TSH)	Hydatidiform mole, embryonal tumors, struma ovarii
Hypertension	Renin	Juxtaglomerula tumors, kidney, lung, pancreas, ovary

[a] Only the most common tumor types are listed. For most ectopic hormone syndromes, an extensive list of tumors has been reported to produce one or more hormones.
[b] hCG is produced eutopically by trophoblastic tumors. Certain tumors produce disproportionate amounts of the hCG α or hCG β subunits. High levels of hCG rarely cause hyperthyroidism because of weak binding to the TSH receptor.
[c] Calcitonin is produced eutopically by medullary thyroid carcinoma and is used as a tumor marker.

ECTOPIC VASOPRESSIN: TUMOR-ASSOCIATED SIADH (See also Chap. 41) ■
Etiology Vasopressin is an antidiuretic hormone normally produced by the posterior pituitary gland. Ectopic vasopressin production by tumors is a common cause of the syndrome of inappropriate antidiuretic hormone (SIADH), occurring in at least half of patients with SCLC. Compensatory mechanisms, such as decreased thirst, suppression of aldosterone, and production of atrial natriuretic peptide (ANP), may mitigate the development of hyponatremia in patients who produce excessive vasopressin. Tumors with neuroendocrine features, such as SCLC and carcinoids, are the most common sources of ectopic vasopressin production, but it also occurs in other forms of lung cancer and with CNS lesions, head and neck cancer, and genitourinary, gastrointestinal, and ovarian cancers. The mechanism of activation of the vasopressin gene in these tumors is unknown but often involves concomitant expression of the adjacent oxytocin gene, suggesting derepression of this locus.

Clinical Manifestations Most patients with ectopic vasopressin secretion are asymptomatic and are identified because of the presence of hyponatremia on routine chemistry testing. Symptoms may include weakness, lethargy, nausea, confusion, depressed mental status, and seizures. The severity of symptoms reflects the rapidity of onset as well as the extent of hyponatremia. In most cases, hyponatremia develops slowly but may be exacerbated by the administration of intravenous fluids or the institution of new medications. Thirst is typically suppressed.

Diagnosis The diagnostic features of ectopic vasopressin production are the same as those of other causes of SIADH (see Chaps. 41 and 318). Hyponatremia and reduced serum osmolality occur in the setting of an inappropriately normal or increased urine osmolality. Unless there is concomitant volume depletion, urine sodium excretion is normal or increased. Other causes of hyponatremia should be excluded, including renal, adrenal, or thyroid insufficiency. Physiologic sources of vasopressin stimulation (CNS lesions, pulmonary disease, nausea) and adaptive circulatory mechanisms (hypotension, heart failure, hepatic cirrhosis), as well as medications, including many chemotherapeutic agents, should also be considered as possible causes of hyponatremia. Measurement of vasopressin is not usually necessary to make the diagnosis.

Rx TREATMENT

Most patients with ectopic vasopressin production develop hyponatremia over several weeks or months and it is reasonable to correct the disorder gradually unless mental status is altered or there is risk of seizures. Treatment of the underlying malignancy may reduce ectopic vasopressin production but this response is slow, if it occurs at all. Fluid restriction to less than urine output, plus insensible losses, is often sufficient to partially correct hyponatremia. However, strict monitoring of the amount and types of liquids consumed or administered intravenously is required for fluid restriction to be effective. Salt tablets or saline are not helpful unless there is concomitant volume depletion. Demeclocycline (150 to 300 mg orally three to four times daily) can be used to inhibit vasopressin action on the renal distal tubule but its onset of action is relatively slow (1 to 2 weeks). Other vasopressin antagonists are under investigation. Severe hyponatremia (Na <115 mEq/L) or mental status changes may require treatment with hypertonic (3%) or normal saline infusion together with furosemide, to enhance free water clearance. The rate of sodium correction should be slow (0.5 to 1 mEq/L per h) to prevent rapid fluid shifts and the possible development of central pontine myelinolysis.

CUSHING'S SYNDROME CAUSED BY ECTOPIC ACTH PRODUCTION (See also Chap. 321) ■ **Etiology** Ectopic production of ACTH accounts for 10 to 20% of Cushing's syndrome. The syndrome is particularly common in neuroendocrine tumors. SCLC (>50%) is by far the most common cause of ectopic ACTH, followed by thymic carcinoid (15%), islet cell tumors (10%), bronchial carcinoid (10%), other carcinoids (5%), and pheochromocytomas (2%). As noted above, the mechanism of ectopic ACTH production in neuroendocrine tumors appears to be linked to the expression of transcription factors that dictate pathways of cell differentiation. Ectopic ACTH production is caused by increased expression of the proopiomelanocortin (POMC) gene, which encodes ACTH, along with melanocyte-stimulating hormone (MSH), β lipotropin, and several other peptides. In many tumors, there is abundant but aberrant expression of the POMC gene from an internal promoter, proximal to the third exon, which encodes ACTH. However, because this product lacks the signal sequence necessary for protein processing, it is not secreted. Increased production of ACTH arises instead from less abundant, but unregulated, POMC expression from the same promoter site used in the pituitary. However, because the tumors lack many of the enzymes needed to process the POMC polypeptide, it is typically released as multiple large, biologically inactive fragments along with relatively small amounts of fully processed, active ACTH.

Rarely, corticotropin-releasing hormone (CRH) is produced by pancreatic islet tumors, SCLC, medullary thyroid cancer, carcinoids, or prostate cancer. When levels are high enough, CRH can cause pituitary corticotrope hyperplasia and Cushing's syndrome. Tumors that produce CRH sometimes also produce ACTH, raising the possibility of a paracrine mechanism for ACTH production.

A distinct mechanism for ACTH-independent Cushing's syndrome involves ectopic expression of various G protein–coupled receptors in the adrenal nodules. Ectopic expression of the gastric inhibitory peptide (GIP) receptor is the best-characterized example of this mechanism. In this case, meals induce GIP secretion, which inappropriately stimulates adrenal growth and glucocorticoid production.

Clinical Manifestations The clinical features of hypercortisolemia are detected in only a small fraction of patients with documented ectopic ACTH production. However, the ectopic ACTH syndrome is associated with several clinical features that distinguish it from other causes

of Cushing's syndrome (e.g., pituitary adenomas, adrenal adenomas, iatrogenic glucocorticoid excess). The metabolic manifestations of ectopic ACTH syndrome are dominated by fluid retention and hypertension, hypokalemia, metabolic alkalosis, glucose intolerance, and, often, steroid psychosis. Patients with ectopic ACTH syndrome generally exhibit less marked weight gain and centripetal fat redistribution, probably because the exposure to excess steroids is relatively short and because cachexia reduces the propensity for weight gain and fat deposition. The very high levels of ACTH often cause increased pigmentation, and melanotrope-stimulating hormone (MSH) activity derived from the POMC precursor peptide is also increased. The extraordinarily high glucocorticoid levels in patients with ectopic sources of ACTH can lead to marked skin fragility and easy bruising. In addition, the high cortisol levels often overwhelm the renal 11β-hydroxysteroid dehydrogenase type II enzyme, which normally inactivates cortisol and prevents it from binding to renal mineralocorticoid receptors. Consequently, in addition to the excess mineralocorticoids produced by ACTH stimulation of the adrenal gland, high levels of cortisol exert activity through the mineralocorticoid receptor, leading to severe hypokalemia.

Diagnosis The diagnosis of ectopic ACTH syndrome is usually not difficult in the setting of a known malignancy. Urine free cortisol levels fluctuate but are typically greater than 2 to 4 times normal and the plasma ACTH level is usually >100 pg/mL. A suppressed ACTH level excludes this diagnosis and indicates an ACTH-independent cause of Cushing's syndrome (e.g., adrenal or exogenous glucocorticoid). In contrast to pituitary sources of ACTH, most ectopic sources of ACTH do not respond to glucocorticoid suppression. Therefore, high-dose dexamethasone (8 mg PO) suppresses 8:00 A.M. serum cortisol (50% decrease from baseline) in about 80% of pituitary ACTH-producing adenomas but fails to suppress ectopic ACTH in about 90% of cases. Bronchial and other carcinoids are well-documented exceptions to these general guidelines, as these ectopic sources of ACTH may exhibit feedback regulation indistinguishable from pituitary adenomas, including suppression by high-dose dexamethasone, and ACTH responsiveness to adrenal blockade with metyrapone. If necessary, petrosal sinus catheterization can be used to evaluate a patient with ACTH-dependent Cushing's syndrome when the source of ACTH is unclear. After CRH stimulation, a 3:1 petrosal sinus:peripheral ACTH ratio strongly suggests a pituitary ACTH source. Imaging studies are also useful in the evaluation of suspected carcinoid lesions, allowing biopsy and characterization of hormone production using special stains.

Rx TREATMENT

The morbidity associated with the ectopic ACTH syndrome can be substantial. Patients may experience depression or personality changes because of extreme cortisol excess. Metabolic derangements including diabetes mellitus and hypokalemia can worsen fatigue. Poor wound healing and predisposition to infections can complicate the surgical management of tumors, and opportunistic infections, caused by organisms such as *Pneumocystis carinii* and mycoses, are often the cause of death in patients with ectopic ACTH production. Depending on prognosis and treatment plans for the underlying malignancy, measures to reduce cortisol levels are often indicated. Treatment of the underlying malignancy may reduce ACTH levels but is rarely sufficient to reduce cortisol levels to normal. Adrenalectomy is not practical for most of these patients but should be considered if the underlying tumor is not resectable and the prognosis is otherwise favorable (e.g., carcinoid). Medical therapy with ketoconazole (200 to 400 mg PO twice daily), metyrapone (250 to 500 mg PO every 6 h), mitotane (3 to 6 g PO in four divided doses, tapered to maintain low cortisol production), or other agents that block steroid synthesis or action is often the most practical strategy for managing the hypercortisolism associated with ectopic ACTH production (see Chap. 318). Glucocorticoid replacement should be provided to avoid adrenal insufficiency. Unfortunately, many patients will eventually escape from medical blockade.

TUMOR-INDUCED HYPOGLYCEMIA CAUSED BY EXCESS PRODUCTION OF IGF-II (See also Chap. 324) Mesenchymal tumors, hemangiopericytomas, hepatocellular tumors, adrenal carcinomas, and a variety of other large tumors have been reported to produce excessive amounts of insulin-like growth factor type II (IGF-II) precursor, which binds weakly to insulin receptors and strongly to IGF-I receptors, leading to insulin-like actions. The IGF-II gene resides on a locus on chromosome 11p15 that is normally imprinted (that is, expression is exclusively from a single parental allele). There is mounting evidence for biallelic expression of the IGF-II gene in a subset of tumors, suggesting loss of methylation and loss of imprinting as a mechanism for gene induction. In addition to increased IGF-II production, IGF-II bioavailability is increased due to complex alterations in circulating binding proteins. Increased IGF-II suppresses growth hormone (GH) and insulin, resulting in reduced IGF binding protein-3 (IGFBP-3), IGF-I, and acid-labile subunit (ALS). The reduction in ALS and IGFBP-3, which normally sequester IGF-II, causes it to be displaced to a small circulating complex that has greater access to insulin target tissues. For this reason, circulating IGF-II levels may not be markedly increased, despite causing hypoglycemia. In addition to IGF-II–mediated hypoglycemia, tumors may occupy enough of the liver to impair gluconeogenesis.

In most cases, the tumor causing hypoglycemia is clinically apparent and hypoglycemia develops in association with fasting. The diagnosis is made by documenting low serum glucose and suppressed insulin levels in association with symptoms of hypoglycemia. Serum IGF-II levels may not be increased (IGF-II assays may not detect IGF-II precursors). Increased IGF-II mRNA expression is found in most tumors. Any medications associated with hypoglycemia should be eliminated. Treatment of the underlying malignancy, if possible, may reduce the predisposition to hypoglycemia. Frequent meals and intravenous glucose, especially during sleep or fasting, are often necessary to prevent hypoglycemia. Glucagon, GH, and glucocorticoids have also been used to enhance glucose production.

HUMAN CHORIONIC GONADOTROPIN hCG is composed of α and β subunits and can be produced as intact hormone, which is biologically active, or as uncombined biologically inert subunits. Ectopic production of intact hCG occurs most often in association with testicular embryonal tumors, germ cell tumors, extragonadal germinomas, lung cancer, hepatoma, and pancreatic islet tumors. Eutopic production of hCG occurs with trophoblastic malignancies. Low levels of hCG or its uncombined α or β subunits have been reported in a wide range of tumors. hCG α subunit production is particularly common in lung cancer and pancreatic islet cancer. In men, high hCG levels stimulate steroidogenesis and aromatase activity in testicular Leydig cells, resulting in increased estrogen production and the development of gynecomastia. Precocious puberty in boys or gynecomastia in men should prompt measurement of hCG and consideration of a testicular tumor or another source of ectopic hCG production. Most women are asymptomatic. hCG is easily measured using sensitive immunoradiometric assays. Treatment should be directed at the underlying malignancy.

ONCOGENIC OSTEOMALACIA Hypophosphatemic oncogenic osteomalacia is characterized by markedly reduced serum phosphorus and renal phosphate wasting, leading to muscle weakness and osteomalacia. Serum calcium and PTH levels are normal and 1,25 dihydroxyvitamin D is low. Oncogenic osteomalacia is usually caused by benign mesenchymal tumors, such as hemangiopericytomas, fibromas, or giant cell tumors, often of the skeletal extremities or head. It has also been described in sarcomas and in patients with prostate and lung cancer. Resection of the tumor reverses the disorder, confirming its humoral basis. The circulating phosphaturic factor is called *phosphatonin*—a factor that inhibits renal tubular reabsorption of phosphate and renal conversion of 25-hydroxyvitamin D to 1,25-dihydroxyvitamin D. Phosphatonin has been identified as fibroblast growth factor 23 (FGF23). The disorder exhibits biochemical features similar to those seen with inactivating mutations in the *PHEX* gene, the cause of hereditary X-linked hypophosphatemia. The *PHEX* gene encodes a protease that activates FGF23. Treatment involves removal of the tumor,

if possible, and supplementation with phosphate and vitamin D. Octreotide treatment reduces phosphate wasting in some patients with tumors that express somatostatin receptor subtype 2. Octreotide scans may also be useful to detect these tumors.

HEMATOLOGIC SYNDROMES

The elevation of granulocyte, platelet, and eosinophil counts in most patients with myeloproliferative disorders is caused by the proliferation of the myeloid elements due to the underlying disease rather than a paraneoplastic syndrome. The paraneoplastic hematologic syndromes in patients with solid tumors are less well characterized than the endocrine syndromes because the ectopic hormone(s) or cytokines responsible have not been identified in most of these tumors (Table 86-2). The severity of the paraneoplastic syndromes parallels the course of the cancer.

ERYTHROCYTOSIS Ectopic production of erythropoietin by cancer cells causes most paraneoplastic erythrocytosis. The ectopically produced erythropoietin stimulates the production of red blood cells in the bone marrow and raises the hematocrit. Other lymphokines and hormones produced by cancer cells may stimulate erythropoietin release but have not been proven to cause erythrocytosis.

Most patients with erythrocytosis have an elevated hematocrit (>52% in men; >48% in women) that is detected on a routine blood count. Approximately 3% of patients with renal cell cancer, 10% of patients with hepatoma, and 15% of patients with cerebellar hemangioblastomas have erythrocytosis. In most cases the erythrocytosis is asymptomatic.

Patients with erythrocytosis due to a renal cell cancer, hepatoma, or CNS cancer should have measurement of red cell mass. If the red cell mass is elevated, the serum erythropoietin level should then be measured. Patients with an appropriate cancer, elevated erythropoietin levels, and no other explanation for erythrocytosis (e.g., hemoglobinopathy that causes increased O_2 affinity; see Chap. 91) have the paraneoplastic syndrome.

℞ TREATMENT

Successful resection of the cancer usually resolves the erythrocytosis. If the tumor cannot be resected or treated effectively with radiation

TABLE 86-2 *Paraneoplastic Hematologic Syndromes*

Syndrome	Proteins	Cancers Typically Associated with Syndrome
Erythrocytosis	Erythropoietin	Renal cancers
		Hepatocarcinoma
		Cerebellar hemangioblastomas
Granulocytosis	G-CSF	Lung cancer
	GM-CSF	Gastrointestinal cancer
	IL-6	Ovarian cancer
		Genitourinary cancer
		Hodgkin's disease
Thrombocytosis	IL-6	Lung cancer
		Gastrointestinal cancer
		Breast cancer
		Ovarian cancer
		Lymphoma
Eosinophilia	IL-5	Lymphoma
		Leukemia
		Lung cancer
Thrombophlebitis	Unknown	Lung cancer
		Pancreatic cancer
		Gastrointestinal cancer
		Breast cancer
		Genitourinary cancer
		Ovarian cancer
		Prostate cancer
		Lymphoma

therapy or chemotherapy, phlebotomy may control any symptoms related to erythrocytosis.

GRANULOCYTOSIS Approximately 30% of patients with solid tumors have granulocytosis (granulocyte count >8000/μL). In about half of patients with granulocytosis and cancer, the granulocytosis has an identifiable nonparaneoplastic etiology (infection, tumor necrosis, glucocorticoid administration, etc.). The other patients have proteins in urine and serum that stimulate the growth of bone marrow cells. Tumors and tumor cell lines from patients with lung, ovarian, and bladder cancers have been documented to produce granulocyte colony-stimulating factor (G-CSF), granulocyte-macrophage colony-stimulating factor (GM-CSF), and/or interleukin 6 (IL-6). However, the etiology of granulocytosis has not been characterized in most patients.

Patients with granulocytosis are nearly all asymptomatic, and the differential white blood cell count does not have a shift to immature forms of neutrophils. Granulocytosis occurs in 40% of patients with lung and gastrointestinal cancers, 20% of patients with breast cancer, 30% of patients with brain tumors and ovarian cancers, and 10% of patients with renal cell carcinoma. Patients with advanced-stage disease are more likely to have granulocytosis than those with early-stage disease.

Paraneoplastic granulocytosis does not require treatment. The granulocytosis resolves when the underlying cancer is successfully treated.

THROMBOCYTOSIS Some 35% of patients with thrombocytosis (platelet count >400,000/μL) have an underlying diagnosis of cancer. IL-6, a candidate molecule for the etiology of paraneoplastic thrombocytosis, stimulates the production of platelets in vitro and in vivo. Some patients with cancer and thrombocytosis have elevated levels of IL-6 in plasma. Another candidate molecule is thrombopoietin, a peptide hormone that stimulates megakaryocyte proliferation and platelet production. The etiology of thrombocytosis has not been established in most cases.

Patients with thrombocytosis are nearly all asymptomatic. Thrombocytosis is not clearly linked to thrombosis in patients with cancer. Thrombocytosis is present in 40% of patients with lung and gastrointestinal cancers, 20% of patients with breast, endometrial, and ovarian cancers, and 10% of patients with lymphoma. Patients with thrombocytosis are more likely to have advanced-stage disease and have a poorer prognosis than patients without thrombocytosis. Paraneoplastic thrombocytosis does not require treatment.

EOSINOPHILIA Eosinophilia is present in ~1% of patients with cancer. Tumors and tumor cell lines from patients with lymphomas or leukemia may produce IL-5, which stimulates eosinophil growth. Activation of IL-5 transcription in lymphomas and leukemias may involve translocation of the long arm of chromosome 5, to which the genes for IL-5 and other cytokines map.

Patients with eosinophilia are typically asymptomatic. Eosinophilia is present in 10% of patients with lymphoma, 3% of patients with lung cancer, and occasional patients with cervical, gastrointestinal, renal, and breast cancer. Patients with markedly elevated eosinophil counts (>5000/μL) can develop shortness of breath and wheezing. A chest radiograph may reveal diffuse pulmonary infiltrates from eosinophil infiltration and activation in the lungs.

℞ TREATMENT

Definitive treatment is directed at the underlying malignancy: tumors should be resected or treated with radiation or chemotherapy. In most patients who develop shortness of breath related to eosinophilia, symptoms resolve with the use of oral or inhaled glucocorticoids.

THROMBOPHLEBITIS Deep venous thrombosis and pulmonary embolism are the most common thrombotic conditions in patients with cancer. Migratory or recurrent thrombophlebitis may be the initial manifestation of cancer. Nearly 15% of patients who develop deep venous thrombosis or pulmonary embolism have a diagnosis of cancer (Chap. 102). The coexistence of peripheral venous thrombosis with visceral carcinoma, particularly pancreatic cancer, is called *Trousseau's syndrome*.

Pathogenesis Patients with cancer are predisposed to thromboembolism because they are often at bedrest or immobilized, and tumors may obstruct or slow blood flow. Chronic intravenous catheters also predispose to clotting. In addition, clotting may be promoted by release of procoagulants or cytokines from tumor cells or associated inflammatory cells, or by platelet adhesion or aggregation. The specific molecules that mediate the increased risk of thromboembolism have not been identified.

Clinical Manifestations Patients with cancer who develop deep venous thrombosis usually develop swelling or pain in the leg, and physical examination reveals tenderness, warmth, and redness. Patients who present with pulmonary embolism develop dyspnea, chest pain, and syncope, and physical examination shows tachycardia, cyanosis, and hypotension. Some 5% of patients with no history of cancer who have a diagnosis of deep venous thrombosis or pulmonary embolism will have a diagnosis of cancer within 1 year. The most common cancers associated with thromboembolic episodes include lung, pancreatic, gastrointestinal, breast, ovarian, and genitourinary cancers, lymphomas, and brain tumors. Patients with cancer who undergo surgical procedures requiring general anesthesia have a 20 to 30% risk of deep venous thrombosis.

Diagnosis The diagnosis of deep venous thrombosis in patients with cancer is made by impedance plethysmography or bilateral compression ultrasonography of the leg veins. Patients with a noncompressible venous segment have deep venous thrombosis. If compression ultrasonography is normal and a high clinical suspicion exists for deep venous thrombosis, venography should be done to look for a luminal filling defect. Elevation of D-dimer is not as predictive of deep venous thrombosis in patients with cancer as it is in patients without cancer.

Patients with symptoms and signs suggesting a pulmonary embolism should be evaluated with a chest radiograph, electrocardiogram, arterial blood gas analysis, and ventilation–perfusion scan. Patients with mismatched segmental perfusion defects have a pulmonary embolus. Patients with equivocal ventilation–perfusion findings should be evaluated as described above for deep venous thrombosis in their legs. If deep venous thrombosis is detected, they should be anticoagulated. If deep venous thrombosis is not detected, they should be considered for a pulmonary angiogram.

Patients without a diagnosis of cancer who present with an initial episode of thrombophlebitis or pulmonary embolus need no additional tests for cancer other than a careful history and physical exam. In light of the many possible primary sites, diagnostic testing in asymptomatic patients is wasteful. However, if the clot is refractory to standard treatment or is in an unusual site, or if the thrombophlebitis is migratory or recurrent, efforts to find an underlying cancer are indicated.

℞ TREATMENT

Patients with cancer and a diagnosis of deep venous thrombosis or pulmonary embolism should be treated initially with intravenous unfractionated heparin or low-molecular-weight heparin for at least 5 days and warfarin started within 1 or 2 days. The warfarin dose should be adjusted so the international normalized ratio (INR) is 2 to 3. Patients with proximal deep venous thrombosis and a relative contraindication to heparin anticoagulation (hemorrhagic brain metastases or pericardial effusion) should be considered for placement of a filter in the inferior vena cava (Greenfield filter) to prevent pulmonary embolism. Warfarin should be administered for 3 to 6 months. An alternative approach is to use low-molecular-weight heparin for 6 months. Patients with cancer who undergo a major surgical procedure should be considered for heparin prophylaxis or pneumatic boots. Breast cancer patients undergoing chemotherapy and patients with implanted catheters should be considered for prophylaxis (1 mg warfarin per day).

→*Cutaneous paraneoplastic syndromes are discussed in Chap. 48. Neurologic paraneoplastic syndromes are discussed in Chap. 87. More extensive discussion of functional endocrine tumors is given in Chap. 329.*

FURTHER READING

JONES PA, BAYLIN SB: The fundamental role of epigenetic events in cancer. Nat Rev Genet 3:415, 2002

LEE AY et al: Clinical utility of a rapid whole-blood D-dimer assay in patients with cancer who present with suspected acute deep venous thrombosis. Ann Intern Med 131:417, 1999

LEVINE MN: Can we optimise treatment of thrombosis? Cancer Treat Rev 29(Suppl 2):19, 2003

RHEE I et al: DNMT1 and DNMT3b cooperate to silence genes in human cancer cells. Nature 416:552, 2002

SEUFERT J et al: Octreotide therapy for tumor-induced osteomalacia. N Engl J Med 345:1883, 2001

STREWLER GJ: The parathyroid hormone-related protein. Endocrinol Metab Clin North Am 29:629, 2000

87 PARANEOPLASTIC NEUROLOGIC SYNDROMES
Josep Dalmau, Myrna R. Rosenfeld

Paraneoplastic neurologic disorders (PNDs) are cancer-related syndromes that can affect any part of the nervous system (Table 87-1). They are remote effects of cancer, caused by mechanisms other than metastasis or by any of the complications of cancer such as coagulopathy, stroke, metabolic and nutritional conditions, infections, and side effects of cancer therapy. In 60% of patients the neurologic symptoms precede the cancer diagnosis. Overall, clinically disabling PNDs occur in 0.5 to 1% of all cancer patients, but they occur in 2 to 3% of patients with neuroblastoma or small-cell lung cancer (SCLC), and in 30 to 50% of patients with thymoma or sclerotic myeloma.

PATHOGENESIS Most PNDs are mediated by immune responses triggered by the tumor expression of neuronal proteins (onconeuronal antigens). In PNDs of the central nervous system (CNS), many antibody-associated immune responses have been identified (Table 87-2). These antibodies usually react with the patient's tumor, and their detection in serum or cerebrospinal fluid (CSF) strongly predicts the presence of cancer. The target antigens are usually intracellular proteins with roles in neuronal development and function. Some of the antibodies react with epitopes located in critical protein domains, disrupting protein function leading to neuronal apoptosis. In addition to onconeuronal antibodies, most PNDs of the CNS are associated with infiltrates of CD4+ and CD8+ T cells, microglial activation, gliosis, and variable neuronal loss. The infiltrating T cells are often in close contact with neurons undergoing degeneration, suggesting a primary pathogenic role. T cell–mediated cytotoxicity may contribute directly to cell death in these PNDs. Thus both humoral and cellular immune mechanisms participate in the pathogenesis of many PNDs. This complex immunopathogenesis may underlie the resistance of many of these conditions to therapy.

Only three of the antibodies listed in Table 87-2 have been shown to play a direct pathogenic role in PNDs; all produce distinctive disorders of the peripheral nervous system. These are: antibodies to P/Q-type voltage-gated calcium channels (VGCC) in patients with the Lambert-Eaton myasthenic syndrome (LEMS); antibodies to acetylcholine receptors in patients with myasthenia gravis; and antibodies to voltage-gated potassium channels (VGKC) in some patients with peripheral nerve hyperexcitability (neuromyotonia). Common features of these three antibodies are that they target cell-surface molecules and that their passive transfer to animals reproduces the disorders. Plasma exchange or immunomodulation with intravenous immunoglobulin (IVIg) usually produces neurologic improvement. Each of these disorders can occur without cancer, and therefore detection of these antibodies does not predict the presence of cancer.

Other PNDs are likely immune-mediated although their antigens are unknown. These include several syndromes of inflammatory neuropathies and myopathies. In addition, many patients with typical PND syndromes are antibody-negative.

For still other PNDs, the cause remains quite obscure. These include, among others, several neuropathies that occur in the terminal stages of cancer and a number of neuropathies associated with plasma cell dyscrasias or lymphoma without evidence of inflammatory infiltrates or deposits of immunoglobulin, cryoglobulin, or amyloid.

TABLE 87-1 Paraneoplastic Syndromes of the Nervous System

Syndromes of the brain, brainstem, and cerebellum
  Focal encephalitis
    Cortical encephalitis
    Limbic encephalitis
    Brainstem encephalitis
    Cerebellar dysfunction
    Autonomic dysfunction
  Paraneoplastic cerebellar degeneration
  Opsoclonus-myoclonus
Syndromes of the spinal cord
  Subacute necrotizing myelopathy
  Motor neuron dysfunction
  Myelitis
  Stiff-person syndrome
Syndromes of dorsal root ganglia
  Sensory neuronopathy
Multiple levels of involvement
  Encephalomyelitis[a], sensory neuronopathy, autonomic dysfunction
Syndromes of peripheral nerve
  Chronic and subacute sensorimotor peripheral neuropathy
  Vasculitis of nerve and muscle
  Neuropathy associated with malignant monoclonal gammopathies
  Peripheral nerve hyperexcitability
  Autonomic neuropathy
Syndromes of the neuromuscular junction
  Lambert-Eaton myasthenic syndrome
  Myasthenia gravis
Syndromes of the muscle
  Polymyositis/dermatomyositis
  Acute necrotizing myopathy
Syndromes affecting the visual system
  Cancer-associated retinopathy (CAR)
  Melanoma-associated retinopathy (MAR)
  Uveitis (usually in association with encephalomyelitis)

[a] Includes cortical, limbic, or brainstem encephalitis, cerebellar dysfunction, myelitis.

APPROACH TO THE PATIENT

The diagnosis and management of PNDs may be difficult for several reasons. First, it is common for symptoms to appear before the presence of a tumor is known. Second, the neurologic syndrome can evolve in a rapidly progressive fashion, producing a severe and usually irreversible neurologic deficit in a short period of time. There is evidence that prompt tumor control improves the course of PNDs. Therefore, the major concern of the physician is to recognize a disorder promptly as paraneoplastic in order to identify and treat the tumor.

PND of the Central Nervous System and Dorsal Root Ganglia When symptoms involve brain, spinal cord, or dorsal root ganglia, the

Antibody	Syndrome	Associated Cancers
Anti-Hu (ANNA-1)	PEM (including cortical, limbic, brainstem encephalitis, cerebellar dysfunction, myelitis), PSN, autonomic dysfunction	SCLC, other neuroendocrine tumors
Anti-Yo (PCA-1)	PCD	Ovary and other gynecologic cancers, breast
Anti-Ri (ANNA-2)	PCD, brainstem encephalitis, opsoclonus-myoclonus	Breast, gynecological, SCLC
Anti-Tr	PCD	Hodgkin's lymphoma
Anti-Zic	PCD, encephalomyelitis	SCLC and other neuroendocrine tumors
Anti-CV$_2$/CRMP5	PEM, PCD, chorea, peripheral neuropathy, uveitis	SCLC, thymoma, other
Anti-Ma proteins[a]	Limbic, hypothalamic, brainstem encephalitis (infrequently PCD)	Germ-cell tumors of testis, lung cancer, other solid tumors
Anti-amphiphysin	Stiff-person syndrome, PEM	Breast, SCLC
Anti-VGCC[b]	LEMS, PCD	SCLC, lymphoma
Anti-AChR[b]	MG	Thymoma
Anti-VGKC[b]	Peripheral nerve hyperexcitability (neuromyotonia)	Thymoma, SCLC, others
Anti-recoverin	Cancer-associated retinopathy (CAR)	SCLC and other
Anti-bipolar cells of the retina	Melanoma-associated retinopathy (MAR)	Melanoma

[a] Patients with antibodies to Ma2 are usually men with testicular cancer. Patients with additional antibodies to other Ma proteins are men or women with a variety of solid tumors.

[b] These antibodies can occur with or without a cancer association.

Note: PEM: paraneoplastic encephalomyelitis; PCD, paraneoplastic cerebellar degeneration; PSN, paraneoplastic sensory neuronopathy; LEMS, Lambert-Eaton myasthenic syndrome; MG, myasthenia gravis; VGCC, voltage-gated calcium channel; AChR, acetylcholine receptor; VGKC, voltage-gated potassium channel; SCLC, small-cell lung cancer.

suspicion of PND is usually based on a combination of clinical, radiologic, and CSF findings. In these cases, a biopsy of the affected tissue is often difficult to obtain, and although useful to rule out other disorders (e.g., metastasis, infection), neuropathologic findings are not specific for PND. Furthermore, there are no specific radiologic or electrophysiologic tests that are diagnostic of PND. The presence of antineuronal antibodies (Table 87-2) may help in the diagnosis with the following caveats: (1) antibodies are detected in only 40 to 50% of PNDs of the CNS; (2) antibodies may be present in both the serum and CSF, but in some patients only the CSF is positive (especially with antibodies to Tr and Ma proteins); (3) antibodies (usually at low titer) are present in a variable proportion of cancer patients without PND; (4) there is an imperfect correlation between antibody titers and the course of the neurologic disorder; (5) several antibodies may associate with a similar syndrome, with the antibody specificity often correlating with the tumor type (e.g., cerebellar degeneration is associated with anti-Tr antibodies if the tumor is Hodgkin's disease but with anti-Yo antibodies if the tumor is ovarian or breast cancer); and (6) several antibodies may be present in the serum or CSF of the same patient (e.g., anti-Hu and anti-CV$_2$/CRMP5, or less frequently anti-Ri).

Magnetic resonance imaging (MRI) and CSF studies are important to rule out neurologic complications due to the direct spread of cancer, particularly metastatic and leptomeningeal disease. In most PNDs the MRI findings are nonspecific. Paraneoplastic limbic encephalitis is usually associated with characteristic MRI abnormalities in the mesial temporal lobes (see below), but similar findings can occur with other disorders [e.g., systemic lupus erythematosus, human herpesvirus (HHV) 6 encephalitis]. The CSF profile of patients with PND of the CNS or dorsal root ganglia typically consists of mild to moderate pleocytosis (<200 mononuclear cells, predominantly lymphocytes), an increase in the protein concentration, intrathecal synthesis of IgG, and a variable presence of oligoclonal bands.

PND of Nerve and Muscle If symptoms involve peripheral nerve, neuromuscular junction, or muscle, the diagnosis of a specific PND is usually established on clinical, electrophysiologic, and pathologic grounds. The clinical history, accompanying symptoms (e.g., anorexia, weight loss), and type of syndrome dictate the studies

and degree of effort needed to demonstrate a neoplasm. For example, the frequent association of LEMS with SCLC should lead to a chest and abdomen computed tomography or body positron emission tomography (PET) scan and, if negative, periodic tumor screening for at least 3 years after the neurologic diagnosis. In contrast, the weak association of polymyositis with cancer calls into question the need for repeated cancer screenings in this situation. Serum and urine immunofixation studies should be considered in patients with peripheral neuropathy of unknown cause; detection of a monoclonal gammopathy suggests the need for additional studies to uncover a B cell or plasma cell malignancy. In paraneoplastic neuropathies, diagnostically useful antineuronal antibodies are limited to anti-CV$_2$/CRMP5 and anti-Hu.

For any type of PND, if antineuronal antibodies are negative, the diagnosis relies on the demonstration of cancer and the exclusion of other cancer-related or independent neurologic disorders. Body PET scans often uncover tumors undetected by other tests.

SPECIFIC PARANEOPLASTIC NEUROLOGIC SYNDROMES (Table 87-3)

PARANEOPLASTIC ENCEPHALOMYELITIS AND FOCAL ENCEPHALITIS The term *encephalomyelitis* describes an inflammatory process with multifocal involvement of the nervous system, including brain, brainstem, cerebellum, and spinal cord. It is often associated with dorsal root ganglia and autonomic dysfunction. For any given patient, the clinical manifestations are determined by the area or areas predominantly involved, but pathology almost always reveals abnormalities (inflammatory infiltrates, neuronal loss, gliosis) beyond the symptomatic regions. Several clinicopathologic syndromes may occur alone or in combination: (1) *cortical encephalitis*, which may present as "epilepsia partialis continua"; (2) *limbic encephalitis*, characterized by confusion, depression, agitation, anxiety, severe short-term memory deficits, partial complex seizures, and dementia; the MRI usually shows unilateral or bilateral medial temporal lobe abnormalities, best seen with T2 and fluid-attenuated inversion recovery sequences, and occasionally enhancing with gadolinium; (3) *brainstem encephalitis,* resulting in eye movement disorders (nystagmus, opsoclonus, supranuclear or nuclear paresis), cranial nerve paresis, dysarthria, dysphagia, and central autonomic dysfunction; (4) *cerebellar gait and limb ataxia*; (5) *myelitis*, which may cause lower or upper motor neuron symptoms, myoclonus, muscle rigidity, and spasms; and (6) *autonomic dysfunction* as a result of involvement of the neuraxis at multiple levels, including hypothalamus, brainstem, and autonomic nerves (see autonomic neuropathy). Cardiac arrhythmias, postural hypotension, or central hypoventilation are frequent causes of death in patients with encephalomyelitis.

Paraneoplastic encephalomyelitis and focal encephalitis are usually associated with SCLC, but many other cancers have also been reported. Patients with SCLC and these syndromes usually have anti-Hu antibodies in serum and CSF. Anti-CV$_2$/CRMP5 antibodies occur less frequently; some of these patients may develop chorea or uveitis. Antibodies to Ma proteins are associated with limbic and brainstem encephalitis and occasionally with cerebellar symptoms; prominent hypothalamic dysfunction, hypersomnia, and cataplexy can also occur. MRI abnormalities are frequent, including those described with limbic

TABLE 87-3 *A Guide to Antibody-Associated Paraneoplastic and Non-Paraneoplastic Syndromes*[a]

| | Antibodies | | |
| | Paraneoplastic | | |
Syndrome	Frequent	Infrequent	Non-Paraneoplastic
Limbic encephalitis	Ma2, Hu, CV$_2$/CRMP5	Tr, VGKC	VGKC
Cerebellar degeneration	Yo, Tr, P/Q VGCC, Hu, Zic, Ri, CV$_2$/CRMP5, Ma1-2	*mGluR1*; *MAZ*	Gliadin GAD
Hypothalamic, brainstem encephalitis	Ma2, Hu	CV$_2$/CRMP5	
Encephalomyelitis	Hu, Zic	CV$_2$/CRMP5, Ri, amphiphysin	
Chorea	CV$_2$/CRMP5		
Opsoclonus-myoclonus	Ri	Hu, Ma2, Yo,	*APC*
Stiff-person syndrome	Amphiphysin	*Gephyrin*, Ri	GAD
PNH (neuromyotonia)	VGKC		VGKC
Myasthenia gravis	AChR		AChR, MuSK
LEMS	P/Q-type VGCC	*MysB*	P/Q-type VGCC
Sensory neuronopathy	Hu		
Axonal sensorimotor neuropathy	Hu, CV$_2$/CRMP5		Monoclonal gammopathy (M protein)[b]
Autonomic neuropathy	Hu	CV$_2$/CRMP5, ganglionic AChR	Ganglionic AChR
Predominant sensory demyelinating neuropathy		MAG, ganglioside antibodies: often present with Waldenström's macroglobulinemia	MAG, ganglioside antibodies, often present with MGUS
Paraneoplastic retinopathy	Recoverin (CAR), anti-bipolar cell antibodies (*MAR*)	*Tubby-like protein 1, PNR*	

[a] Antibodies have been validated by more than one laboratory and/or the protein sequence of the target antigen is known.

[b] The M protein usually does not have specific antibody activity.

Note: Italics indicate that commercial testing for these antibodies is not available. PNH, peripheral nerve hyperexcitability; CAR, cancer-associated retinopathy; MAR, melanoma-associated retinopathy; PNR, photoreceptor-specific nuclear receptor; MGUS, monoclonal gammopathy of uncertain significance; VGKC, voltage-gated potassium channel; GAD, glutamic acid decarboxylase; AChR, acetylcholine receptor; LEMS, Lambert-Eaton myasthenic syndrome; VGCC, voltage-gated calcium channel; MAG, myelin-associated glycoprotein.

encephalitis and variable involvement of the hypothalamus, basal ganglia, or brainstem. The oncologic associations of these antibodies are shown in Table 87-2.

All types of paraneoplastic encephalitis and encephalomyelitis, except limbic encephalitis, respond poorly to treatment. Stabilization of symptoms or partial neurologic improvement may occasionally occur, particularly if there is a satisfactory response of the tumor to treatment. The roles of plasma exchange, IVIg, and immunosuppression have not been established. Rare patients with limbic encephalitis have shown dramatic improvement after treatment, but it is not known whether remission of the cancer, glucocorticoids, or IVIg was responsible.

PARANEOPLASTIC CEREBELLAR DEGENERATION This disorder is often preceded by a prodrome that may include dizziness, oscillopsia, blurry or double vision, nausea, and vomiting. A few days or weeks later, dysarthria, gait and limb ataxia, and variable dysphagia can appear. The examination usually shows downbeating nystagmus and, rarely, opsoclonus. Brainstem dysfunction, upgoing toes, or a mild neuropathy may occur, but more often the symptoms and signs are restricted to the cerebellum. Early in the course, MRI studies are usually normal; in some patients a transient enhancement of the cerebellar cortex has been noted. Later, the MRI typically reveals cerebellar atrophy. The disorder results from extensive degeneration of Purkinje cells, with variable involvement of other cerebellar cortical neurons, deep cerebellar nuclei, and spinocerebellar tracts. An immune-mediated pathogenesis is supported by CSF findings and biopsy studies obtained during the early stage of the disorder. The tumors more frequently involved are SCLC, cancer of the breast and ovary, and Hodgkin's lymphoma.

Anti-Yo antibodies in patients with breast and gynecologic cancers and anti-Tr antibodies in patients with Hodgkin's lymphoma are the two paraneoplastic antibodies typically associated with prominent or pure cerebellar degeneration. Antibodies to P/Q-type VGCC occur in some patients with SCLC and cerebellar dysfunction; only some of these patients develop LEMS. A subacute cerebellar ataxia can also be the presenting symptom of paraneoplastic encephalomyelitis; in this syndrome, symptoms of widespread CNS involvement eventually occur. Of note, a variable degree of cerebellar dysfunction can be associated with virtually any type of antibody-related PND of the CNS

(Table 87-2). A number of single case reports have described neurologic improvement after tumor removal, plasma exchange, IVIg, cyclophosphamide, or glucocorticoids. However, large series of patients with well-defined antibody-positive paraneoplastic cerebellar degeneration show that these disorders rarely improve with any treatment.

PARANEOPLASTIC OPSOCLONUS-MYOCLONUS SYNDROME *Opsoclonus* is a disorder of eye movement characterized by involuntary, chaotic saccades that occur in all directions of gaze; it is frequently associated with myoclonus and ataxia. Opsoclonus-myoclonus may be cancer-related or idiopathic. When the cause is paraneoplastic, the tumors involved are usually cancer of the lung and breast in adults and neuroblastoma in children. The pathologic substrate of opsoclonus-myoclonus is unclear. The majority of SCLC patients do not harbor antineuronal antibodies. A small subset of patients with ataxia, opsoclonus, and other eye movement disorders develop anti-Ri antibodies; in rare instances muscle rigidity, autonomic dysfunction, and dementia also occur. The tumor most frequently involved in anti-Ri-associated syndromes is breast cancer; however, only 50% of patients with anti-Ri antibodies develop opsoclonus.

If the tumor is not successfully treated, the paraneoplastic opsoclonus-myoclonus syndrome in adults often progresses to encephalopathy, coma, and death. In addition to treating the tumor, symptoms may respond to immunotherapy (glucocorticoids and/or IVIg).

At least 50% of children with opsoclonus-myoclonus have an underlying neuroblastoma. Hypotonia, ataxia, behavioral changes, and irritability are frequent accompanying symptoms. Although some patients harbor anti-Hu antibodies, most are antibody-negative. Neurologic symptoms often improve with treatment of the tumor (including chemotherapy) and with glucocorticoids, adrenocorticotropic hormone (ACTH), plasma exchange, and IVIg. The response to treatment varies; patients who do not improve with glucocorticoids may respond to ACTH. Neurologic relapses are frequent, and many patients are left with psychomotor retardation and behavioral and sleep problems.

PARANEOPLASTIC SYNDROMES OF THE SPINAL CORD The number of reports of paraneoplastic spinal cord syndromes, such as *subacute motor neuronopathy* and *acute necrotizing myelopathy*, has decreased in recent years. This may represent a true decrease in incidence, due to improved and prompt oncologic interventions, or may be because of the identification of nonparaneoplastic etiologies; e.g., subacute necrotizing myelopathy may occur with HSV infection, usually HSV-2.

Some patients with cancer develop *upper* or *lower motor neuron dysfunction* or both, resembling amyotrophic lateral sclerosis. Because paraneoplastic antibody markers are lacking, it is unclear whether these disorders have a paraneoplastic etiology or simply coincide with the presence of cancer. There are isolated case reports of cancer patients with motor neuron dysfunction who had neurologic improvement after tumor treatment. A more than coincidental association occurs between lymphoma and motor neuron dysfunction. A search for lymphoma should be undertaken in patients with a motor neuron syndrome who are found to have a monoclonal protein in serum or CSF or an increased protein concentration in the CSF.

Paraneoplastic myelitis may present with upper or lower motor neuron symptoms, segmental myoclonus, and rigidity. This syndrome can appear as the presenting manifestation of encephalomyelitis and may be associated with SCLC and serum anti-Hu, anti-CV$_2$/CRMP5, or anti-amphiphysin antibodies.

Paraneoplastic myelopathy can also produce several syndromes characterized by prominent muscle stiffness and rigidity. The spectrum ranges from focal symptoms in one or several extremities (*stiff-limb syndrome* or *stiff-person syndrome*) to a disorder that also affects the brainstem (known as *encephalomyelitis with rigidity*) and likely has a different pathogenesis.

PARANEOPLASTIC STIFF-PERSON SYNDROME

This disorder is characterized by progressive muscle rigidity, stiffness, and painful spasms triggered by auditory, sensory, or emotional stimuli. Rigidity mainly involves the lower trunk and legs, but it can affect the upper extremities and neck. Symptoms improve with sleep and general anesthetics. Electrophysiologic studies demonstrate continuous motor unit activity. Antibodies associated with the stiff-person syndrome target proteins [glutamic acid decarboxylase (GAD), amphiphysin] involved in the function of inhibitory synapses utilizing γ-aminobutyric acid (GABA) or glycine as neurotransmitters. Paraneoplastic stiff-person syndrome and amphiphysin antibodies are often related to breast cancer. By contrast, antibodies to GAD may occur in some cancer patients but are much more frequently present in the non-paraneoplastic disorder. Optimal treatment of stiff-person syndrome requires therapy of the underlying tumor, glucocorticoids, and symptomatic use of drugs that enhance GABA-ergic transmission (diazepam, baclofen, sodium valproate, vigabatrin). A benefit of IVIg has been demonstrated for the non-paraneoplastic disorder but remains to be established for the paraneoplastic syndrome.

PARANEOPLASTIC SENSORY NEURONOPATHY OR DORSAL ROOT GANGLIONOPATHY

This syndrome is characterized by sensory deficits that may be symmetric or asymmetric, painful dysesthesias, radicular pain, and decreased or absent reflexes. All modalities of sensation and any part of the body including face and trunk can be involved. Specialized sensations such as taste and hearing can also be affected. Electrophysiologic studies show decreased or absent sensory nerve potentials with normal or near-normal motor conduction velocities. Symptoms result from an inflammatory, likely immune-mediated, process that targets the dorsal root ganglia, causing neuronal loss, proliferation of satellite cells, and secondary degeneration of the posterior columns of the spinal cord. The dorsal nerve roots, and less frequently the anterior nerve roots and peripheral nerves, may also be involved.

This disorder often precedes or is associated with encephalomyelitis and autonomic dysfunction and has the same immunologic and oncologic associations, i.e., anti-Hu antibodies and SCLC. As with anti-Hu-associated encephalomyelitis, the therapeutic approach focuses on prompt treatment of the tumor. Glucocorticoids occasionally produce clinical stabilization or improvement. The benefit of IVIg and plasma exchange is not proved.

PARANEOPLASTIC PERIPHERAL NEUROPATHIES

These disorders may develop any time during the course of the neoplastic disease. Neuropathies occurring at late stages of cancer or lymphoma usually cause mild to moderate sensorimotor deficits due to axonal degeneration of unclear etiology. These neuropathies are often masked by concurrent neurotoxicity from chemotherapy and other cancer therapies. In contrast, the neuropathies that develop in the early stages of cancer often show a rapid progression, sometimes with a relapsing and remitting course, and evidence of inflammatory infiltrates and axonal loss or demyelination in biopsy studies. If demyelinating features predominate (Chap. 363), IVIg or glucocorticoids may improve symptoms. These neuropathies are not usually associated with antineuronal antibodies. Occasionally anti-CV$_2$/CRMP5 antibodies are present; detection of anti-Hu suggests concurrent dorsal root ganglionitis.

Guillain-Barré syndrome and *brachial plexitis* have occasionally been reported in patients with lymphoma, but there is no clear evidence of a paraneoplastic association.

Malignant monoclonal gammopathies include: (1) multiple myeloma and sclerotic myeloma associated with IgG or IgA monoclonal proteins; and (2) Waldenström's macroglobulinemia, B cell lymphoma, and chronic B cell lymphocytic leukemia associated with IgM monoclonal proteins. These disorders may cause neuropathy by a variety of mechanisms, including compression of roots and plexuses by metastasis to vertebral bodies and pelvis, deposits of amyloid in peripheral nerves, and paraneoplastic mechanisms. The paraneoplastic variety has several distinctive features. Approximately half of patients with sclerotic myeloma develop a sensorimotor neuropathy with predominantly motor deficits, resembling a chronic inflammatory demyelinating neuropathy (Chap. 365); some patients develop elements of the POEMS syndrome (*p*olyneuropathy, *o*rganomegaly, *e*ndocrinopathy, *M* protein, *s*kin changes). Treatment of the plasmacytoma or sclerotic lesions usually improves the neuropathy. In contrast, the sensorimotor or sensory neuropathy associated with multiple myeloma rarely responds to treatment. Between 5 and 10% of patients with Waldenström's macroglobulinemia develop a distal symmetric sensorimotor neuropathy with predominant involvement of large sensory fibers. These patients may have IgM antibodies in their serum against myelin-associated glycoprotein (Chap. 365). In addition to treating the Waldenström's macroglobulinemia, other therapies may improve the neuropathy, including plasma exchange, IVIg, chlorambucil, cyclophosphamide, fludarabine, or rituximab.

Vasculitis of the nerve and muscle causes a painful symmetric or asymmetric distal sensorimotor neuropathy with variable proximal weakness. It predominantly affects elderly men and is associated with an elevated erythrocyte sedimentation rate and increased CSF protein concentration. SCLC and lymphoma are the primary tumors involved. Pathology demonstrates axonal degeneration and T cell infiltrates involving the small vessels of the nerve and muscle. Immunosuppressants (glucocorticoids and cyclophosphamide) often result in neurologic improvement.

Peripheral nerve hyperexcitability (*neuromyotonia* or *Isaacs' syndrome*) is characterized by spontaneous and continuous muscle fiber activity of peripheral nerve origin. Clinical features include cramps, muscle twitching (fasciculations or myokymia), stiffness, delayed muscle relaxation (pseudomyotonia), and spontaneous or evoked carpal or pedal spasms. The involved muscles may be hypertrophic, and some patients develop paresthesias and hyperhydrosis. CNS dysfunction, including mood changes, sleep disorder, or hallucinations, may occur. The electromyogram (EMG) shows fibrillations; fasciculations; and doublet, triplet, or multiplet single unit (myokymic) discharges that have a high intraburst frequency. An immune pathogenesis is suggested by the frequent presence of serum antibodies to VGKC. The disorder often occurs without cancer; if paraneoplastic, benign and malignant thymomas and SCLC are the usual tumors. Some patients with thymoma develop acetylcholine receptor antibodies with or without myasthenia gravis. Diphenylhydantoin, carbamazepine, and plasma exchange improve symptoms.

The *cramps-fasciculation syndrome* resembes neuromyotonia, but the EMG does not show myokymic discharges. It may also occur with thymoma, lung cancer, and antibodies to VGKC.

Paraneoplastic autonomic neuropathy usually develops as a component of other disorders, such as LEMS and encephalomyelitis. It may rarely occur as a pure or predominantly autonomic neuropathy with adrenergic or cholinergic dysfunction at the pre- or postganglionic levels. Patients can develop several life-threatening complications, such as gastrointestinal paresis with pseudoobstruction, cardiac dysrhythmias, and postural hypotension. Other symptoms include dry mouth, erectile dysfunction, anhidrosis, and sphincter dysfunction. The disorder has been reported to occur in association with several tumors, including SCLC, cancer of the pancreas or testis, carcinoid tumors, and lymphoma. Because autonomic symptoms can also be the presenting feature of encephalomyelitis, serum anti-Hu and anti-CV$_2$/CRMP5 antibodies should also be sought. Serum antibodies to ganglionic acetylcholine receptors have been reported in this syndrome, but they also occur without a cancer association. (See also Table 354-6).

LAMBERT-EATON MYASTHENIC SYNDROME →*LEMS is discussed in Chap. 366.*

MYASTHENIA GRAVIS →*For discussion of myasthenia gravis, see Chap. 366.*

POLYMYOSITIS-DERMATOMYOSITIS →*Polymyositis and dermatomyositis are discussed in detail in Chap. 369.*

ACUTE NECROTIZING MYOPATHY Patients with this syndrome develop myalgias and rapid progression of weakness involving the extremities and the pharyngeal and respiratory muscles, often resulting in death. Serum muscle enzymes are elevated, and muscle biopsy shows extensive necrosis with minimal or absent inflammation and sometimes deposits of complement. The disorder occurs as a paraneoplastic manifestation of a variety of cancers including SCLC and cancer of the gastrointestinal tract, breast, kidney, and prostate, among others. Glucocorticoids or treatment of the underlying tumor rarely control the disorder.

PARANEOPLASTIC VISUAL SYNDROMES This group of disorders involves the retina and, less frequently, the uvea and optic nerves. The term *cancer-associated retinopathy* is used to describe paraneoplastic cone and rod dysfunction characterized by photosensitivity, progressive loss of vision and color perception, central or ring scotomas, night blindness, and attenuation of photopic and scotopic responses in the electroretinogram (ERG). The most commonly associated tumor is SCLC. Melanoma-associated retinopathy affects patients with metastatic cutaneous melanoma. Patients develop the acute onset of night blindness and shimmering, flickering, or pulsating photopsias that often progress to visual loss. The ERG demonstrates reduction in the b-wave amplitude. Paraneoplastic optic neuritis and uveitis are very uncommon and can develop in association with encephalomyelitis. Some patients with paraneoplastic uveitis harbor anti-CV$_2$/CRMP5 antibodies.

Some paraneoplastic retinopathies are associated with serum antibodies that specifically react with the subset of retinal cells undergoing degeneration, supporting an immune-mediated pathogenesis (Tables 87-2 and 87-3). Paraneoplastic retinopathies usually fail to improve with treatment, although rare responses to glucocorticoids, plasma exchange, and IVIg have been reported.

FURTHER READING

CHAN JW: Paraneoplastic retinopathies and optic neuropathies. Surv Ophthalmol 48:12, 2003

DROPCHO EJ: Remote neurologic manifestations of cancer. Neurol Clin 20: 85, 2002

ROSENFELD MR, DALMAU J: Current therapy of paraneoplastic syndromes. Curr Treat Opt Neurol 5:69, 2003

88 ONCOLOGIC EMERGENCIES
Rasim Gucalp, Janice Dutcher

Emergencies in patients with cancer may be classified into three groups: pressure or obstruction caused by a space-occupying lesion, metabolic or hormonal problems (paraneoplastic syndromes, Chap. 86), and complications arising from the effects of treatment.

STRUCTURAL-OBSTRUCTIVE ONCOLOGIC EMERGENCIES

SUPERIOR VENA CAVA SYNDROME Superior vena cava syndrome (SVCS) is the clinical manifestation of superior vena cava (SVC) obstruction, with severe reduction in venous return from the head, neck, and upper extremities. Malignant tumors, such as lung cancer, lymphoma, and metastatic tumors, are responsible for more than 90% of all SVCS cases. Lung cancer, particularly of small-cell and squamous-cell histologies, accounts for approximately 85% of all cases of malignant origin. In young adults, malignant lymphoma is a leading cause of SVCS. Hodgkin's lymphoma involves the mediastinum more commonly than other lymphomas but rarely causes SVCS. When SVCS is noted in a young man with a mediastinal mass, the differential diagnosis is lymphoma vs primary mediastinal germ cell tumor. Metastatic cancers to the mediastinum, such as testicular and breast carcinomas, account for a small proportion of cases. Other causes include benign tumors, aortic aneurysm, thyroid enlargement, thrombosis, and fibrosing mediastinitis caused by prior irradiation or histoplasmosis.

Patients with SVCS usually present with neck and facial swelling (especially around the eyes), dyspnea, and cough. Other symptoms include hoarseness, tongue swelling, headaches, nasal congestion, epistaxis, hemoptysis, dysphagia, pain, dizziness, syncope, and lethargy. Bending forward or lying down may aggravate the symptoms. The characteristic physical findings are dilated neck veins, an increased number of collateral veins covering the anterior chest wall, cyanosis, and edema of the face, arms, and chest. More severe cases include proptosis, glossal and laryngeal edema, and obtundation. The clinical picture is milder if the obstruction is located above the azygos vein.

Signs and symptoms of cerebral and/or laryngeal edema, though rare, are associated with a poorer prognosis and require urgent evaluation. Seizures may be related to brain metastases rather than cerebral edema from venous occlusion. Patients with small cell lung cancer and SVCS have a higher incidence of brain metastases than those without SVCS.

Cardiorespiratory symptoms at rest, particularly with positional changes, suggest significant airway and vascular obstruction and limited physiologic reserve. Cardiac arrest or respiratory failure can occur, particularly in patients receiving sedatives or undergoing general anesthesia.

The diagnosis of SVCS is a clinical one. The most significant chest radiographic finding is widening of the superior mediastinum, most commonly on the right side. Pleural effusion occurs in only 25% of patients, often on the right side. However, a normal chest radiograph is still compatible with the diagnosis if other characteristic findings are present. Computed tomography (CT) provides the most reliable view of the mediastinal anatomy. The diagnosis of SVCS requires diminished or absent opacification of central venous structures with prominent collateral venous circulation. Magnetic resonance imaging (MRI) has no advantages over CT. Invasive procedures, including bronchoscopy, percutaneous needle biopsy, mediastinoscopy, and even thoracotomy, can be performed by a skilled clinician without any major risk of bleeding. For patients with a known cancer, a detailed workup usually is not necessary, and appropriate treatment may be started after obtaining a CT scan of the thorax. For those with no

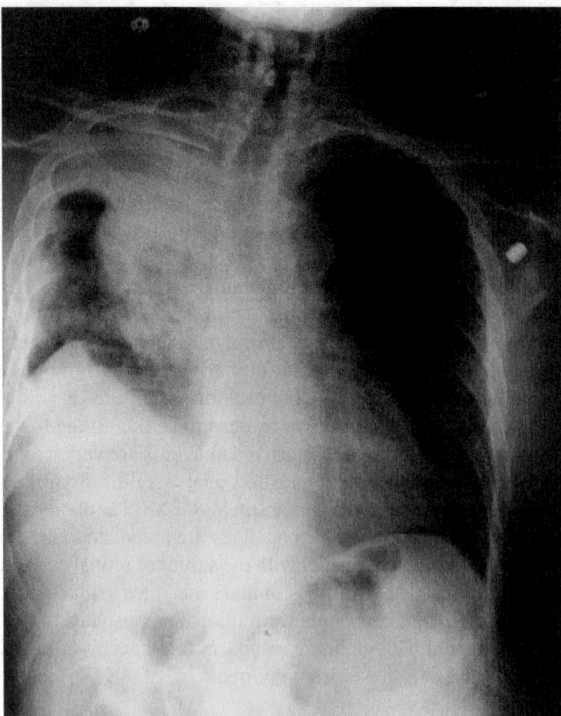

A

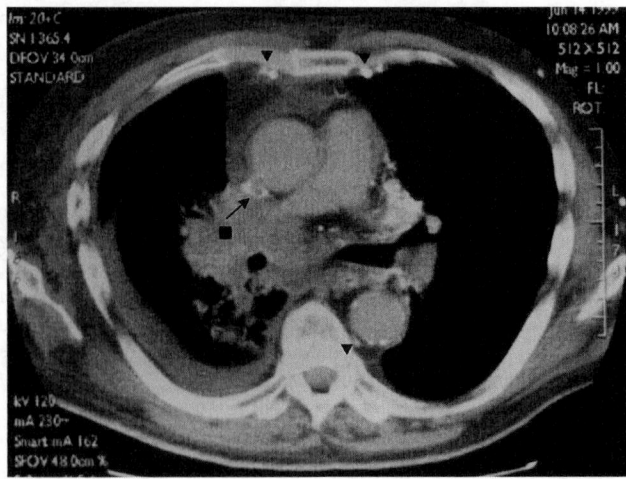

B

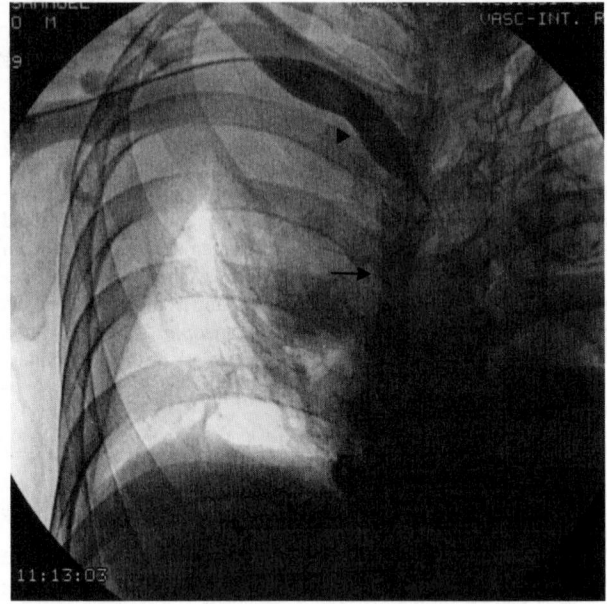

C

FIGURE 88-1 *A.* Chest radiographs of a 59-year-old man with recurrent SVCS caused by non-small cell lung cancer showing right paratracheal mass with right pleural effusion. *B.* Computed tomography of same patient demonstrating obstruction of SVC with thrombosis (arrow) by the lung cancer (square) and collaterals (arrowheads). *C.* Balloon angioplasty (arrowhead) with walstent (arrow) in same patient.

history of malignancy, a detailed evaluation is essential to rule out benign causes and determine a specific diagnosis to direct the appropriate therapy.

℞ TREATMENT

The one potentially life-threatening complication of a superior mediastinal mass is tracheal obstruction. Upper airway obstruction demands emergent therapy. Diuretics with a low salt diet, head elevation, and oxygen may produce temporary symptomatic relief. Glucocorticoids may be useful at shrinking lymphoma masses; they are of no benefit in patients with lung cancer.

Radiation therapy is the primary treatment for SVCS caused by non-small cell lung cancer and other metastatic solid tumors. Chemotherapy is effective when the underlying cancer is small cell carcinoma of the lung or lymphoma. Recurrent SVCS occurs in 10 to 30% of patients after initial therapy; it may be palliated with the use of intravascular self-expanding stents (Fig. 88-1). Early stenting may be necessary in patients with severe symptoms; however, the prompt increase in venous return after stenting may precipitate heart failure and pulmonary edema. Surgery may provide immediate relief for patients in whom a benign process is the cause.

Clinical improvement occurs in most patients, although this improvement may be due to the development of adequate collateral circulation. The mortality associated with SVCS does not relate to caval obstruction, but rather to the underlying cause.

SVCS and Central Venous Catheters in Adults The use of long-term central venous catheters has become common practice in patients with cancer. Major vessel thrombosis may occur. In these cases, catheter removal should be combined with anticoagulation to prevent embolization. SVCS in this setting, if detected early, can be treated by fibrinolytic therapy without sacrificing the catheter. Warfarin (1 mg/d) reduces the incidence of thrombosis without altering coagulation tests.

PERICARDIAL EFFUSION/TAMPONADE Malignant pericardial disease is found at autopsy in 5–10% of patients with cancer, most frequently with lung cancer, breast cancer, leukemias, and lymphomas. Cardiac tamponade as the initial presentation of extrathoracic malignancy is rare. The origin is not malignancy in about 50% of cancer patients with symptomatic pericardial disease, but can be related to irradiation, drug-induced pericarditis, hypothyroidism, idiopathic pericarditis, infection, or autoimmune diseases. Two types of radiation pericarditis occur: an acute inflammatory, effusive pericarditis occurring within months of irradiation, which usually resolves spontaneously, and a chronic effusive pericarditis that may appear up to 20 years after radiation therapy and is accompanied by a thickened pericardium.

Most patients with pericardial metastasis are asymptomatic. However, the common symptoms are dyspnea, cough, chest pain, orthopnea, and weakness. Pleural effusion, sinus tachycardia, jugular venous distension, hepatomegaly, peripheral edema, and cyanosis are the most frequent physical findings. Relatively specific diagnostic findings, such as paradoxical pulse, diminished heart sounds, pulsus alternans (pulse waves alternating between those of greater and lesser amplitude with successive beats), and friction rub are less common than with nonmalignant pericardial disease. Chest radiographs and ECG reveal abnormalities in 90% of patients, but half of these abnormalities are nonspecific. Echocardiography is the most helpful diagnostic test. Pericardial fluid may be serous, serosanguineous, or hemorrhagic, and cytologic examination of pericardial fluid is diagnostic in most patients. False negative cytology may occur in patients with lymphoma and mesothelioma.

℞ TREATMENT

Pericardiocentesis with or without the introduction of sclerosing agents, the creation of a pericardial window, complete pericardial stripping, cardiac irradiation, or systemic chemotherapy are effective treatments. Acute pericardial tamponade with life-threatening hemodynamic instability requires immediate drainage of fluid. This can be quickly achieved by pericardiocentesis. Alternatively, subxiphoid pericardiotomy can be performed in 45 min under local anesthesia. Thoracoscopic pericardial fenestration can be employed for benign causes; however, 60% of malignant pericardial effusions recur after this procedure.

INTESTINAL OBSTRUCTION Intestinal obstruction and reobstruction are common problems in patients with advanced cancer, particularly colorectal or ovarian carcinoma. However, other cancers, such as lung or breast cancer and melanoma, can metastasize within the abdomen, leading to intestinal obstruction. Typically, obstruction occurs at multiple sites. Melanoma has a predilection to involve the small bowel; this involvement may be isolated and resection may result in prolonged survival. Intestinal pseudoobstruction is caused by infiltration of the mesentery or bowel muscle by tumor, involvement of the celiac plexus, or paraneoplastic neuropathy in patients with small cell lung cancer. Paraneoplastic neuropathy is associated with IgG antibodies reactive to neurons of the myenteric and submucosal plexuses of the jejunum and stomach. Ovarian cancer can lead either to authentic luminal obstruction or to pseudoobstruction that results when circumferential invasion of a bowel segment arrests the forward progression of peristaltic contractions.

The onset of obstruction is usually insidious. Pain is the most common symptom and is usually colicky in nature. Pain can also be due to abdominal distention, tumor masses, or hepatomegaly. Vomiting can be intermittent or continuous. Patients with complete obstruction usually have constipation. Physical examination may reveal abdominal distention with tympany, ascites, visible peristalsis, high-pitched bowel sounds, and tumor masses. Erect plain abdominal films may reveal multiple air-fluid levels and dilation of the small or large bowel. Acute cecal dilation to more than 12 to 14 cm is considered a surgical emergency because of the high likelihood of rupture. CT is useful in differentiating benign from malignant causes of obstruction in patients who have undergone surgery for malignancy. Malignant obstruction is suggested by a mass at the site of obstruction or prior surgery, adenopathy, or an abrupt transition zone and irregular bowel thickening at the obstruction site. Benign obstruction is more likely when CT shows mesenteric vascular changes, a large volume of ascites, or a smooth transition zone and smooth bowel thickening at the obstruction site. The prognosis for the patient with cancer who develops intestinal obstruction is poor; median survival is 3 to 4 months. About 25–30% are found to have intestinal obstruction due to causes other than cancer. Adhesions from previous operations are a common benign cause. Ileus induced by vincristine is another reversible cause.

℞ TREATMENT

The management of intestinal obstruction in patients with advanced malignancy depends on the extent of the underlying malignancy and the functional status of the major organs. The initial management should include surgical evaluation. Operation is not always successful and may lead to further complications with a substantial mortality rate (10 to 20%). Self-expanding metal stents placed in the gastric outlet, duodenum, proximal jejunum, colon, or rectum may palliate obstructive symptoms at those sites without major surgery. Patients known to have advanced intraabdominal malignancy should receive a prolonged course of conservative management, including nasogastric decom-

pression. Treatment with antiemetics, antispasmodics, and analgesics may allow patients to remain outside the hospital. The somatostatin analogue octreotide may relieve obstructive symptoms through its inhibitory effect on gastrointestinal secretion.

URINARY OBSTRUCTION Urinary obstruction may occur in patients with prostatic or gynecologic malignancies, particularly cervical carcinoma, or metastatic disease from other primary sites such as carcinomas of the breast, stomach, lung, colon, and pancreas, and lymphomas. Radiation therapy to pelvic tumors may cause fibrosis and subsequent ureteral obstruction. Bladder outlet obstruction is usually due to prostate and cervical cancers and may lead to bilateral hydronephrosis and renal failure.

Flank pain is the most common symptom. Persistent urinary tract infection, persistent proteinuria, or hematuria in patients with cancer should raise suspicion of ureteral obstruction. Total anuria and/or anuria alternating with polyuria may occur. A slow, continuous rise in the serum creatinine level necessitates immediate evaluation. Renal ultrasound is the safest and cheapest way to identify hydronephrosis. The function of an obstructed kidney can be evaluated by a nuclear scan. CT can reveal the point of obstruction and identify a retroperitoneal mass or adenopathy.

℞ TREATMENT

Obstruction associated with flank pain, sepsis, or fistula formation is an indication for immediate palliative urinary diversion. Internal ureteral stents can be placed under local anesthesia. Percutaneous nephrostomy offers an alternative approach for drainage. In the case of bladder outlet obstruction due to malignancy, a suprapubic cystostomy can be used for urinary drainage.

MALIGNANT BILIARY OBSTRUCTION This common clinical problem can be caused by a primary carcinoma arising in the pancreas, ampulla of Vater, bile duct, or liver or by metastatic disease to the periductal lymph nodes or liver parenchyma. The most common metastatic tumors causing biliary obstruction are gastric, colon, breast, and lung cancers. Jaundice, light-colored stools, dark urine, pruritus, and weight loss due to malabsorption are usual symptoms. Pain and secondary infection are uncommon in malignant biliary obstruction. Ultrasound, CT, or percutaneous transhepatic or endoscopic retrograde cholangiography will identify the site and nature of the biliary obstruction.

℞ TREATMENT

Palliative intervention is indicated only in patients with disabling pruritus resistant to medical treatment, severe malabsorption, or infection. Stenting under radiographic control, surgical bypass, or radiation therapy with or without chemotherapy may alleviate the obstruction. The choice of modality should be based on the site of obstruction (proximal versus distal), the type of tumor (sensitive to radiotherapy, chemotherapy, or neither), and the general condition of the patient. In the absence of pruritus, biliary obstruction may be a largely asymptomatic cause of death.

SPINAL CORD COMPRESSION Spinal cord compression occurs in 5–10% of patients with cancer. Epidural tumor is the first manifestation of malignancy in about 10% of patients. The underlying cancer is usually identified during the initial evaluation; lung cancer is most commonly the primary malignancy.

Metastatic tumor involves the vertebral column more often than any other part of the bony skeleton. Lung, breast, and prostate cancer are the most frequent offenders. Multiple myeloma also has a high incidence of spine involvement. Lymphomas, melanoma, renal cell cancer, and genitourinary cancers also cause cord compression. The thoracic spine is the most common site (70%), followed by the lumbosacral spine (20%) and the cervical spine (10%). Involvement of multiple sites is most frequent in patients with breast and prostatic carcinoma. Cord injury develops when metastases to the vertebral body or pedicle enlarge and compress the underlying dura. Another cause of cord compression is direct extension of a paravertebral lesion through the intervertebral foramen. These cases usually involve a lymphoma, myeloma, or pediatric neoplasm. Parenchymal spinal cord metastasis due to hematogenous spread is rare.

Expanding extradural tumors induce injury through several mechanisms. Obstruction of the epidural venous plexus leads to edema. Local production of inflammatory cytokines enhances blood flow and edema formation. Compression compromises blood flow leading to ischemia.

The most common initial symptom in patients with spinal cord compression is localized back pain and tenderness due to involvement of vertebrae by tumor. Pain is usually present for days or months before other neurologic findings appear. It is exacerbated by movement and by coughing or sneezing. It can be differentiated from the pain of disk disease by the fact that it worsens when the patient is supine. Radicular pain is less common than localized back pain and usually develops later. Radicular pain in the cervical or lumbosacral areas may be unilateral or bilateral. Radicular pain from the thoracic roots is often bilateral and is described by patients as a feeling of tight, band-like constriction around the thorax and abdomen. Typical cervical radicular pain radiates down the arm; in the lumbar region, the radiation is down the legs. Lhermitte's sign, a tingling or electric sensation down the back, upper and lower limbs upon flexing or extending the neck, may be an early sign of cord compression. Loss of bowel or bladder control may be the presenting symptom, but usually occurs late in the course.

On physical examination, pain induced by straight leg raising, neck flexion, or vertebral percussion may help to determine the level of cord compression. Patients develop numbness and paresthesias in the extremities or trunk. Loss of sensibility to pinprick is as common as loss of sensibility to vibration or position. The upper limit of the zone of sensory loss is often one or two vertebrae below the site of compression. Motor findings include weakness, spasticity, and abnormal muscle stretching. An extensor plantar reflex reflects significant compression. Deep tendon reflexes may be brisk. Motor and sensory loss usually precede sphincter disturbance. Patients with autonomic dysfunction may present with decreased anal tonus, decreased perineal sensibility, and a distended bladder. The absence of the anal wink reflex or the bulbocavernosus reflex confirms cord (conus or cauda equina) involvement. In doubtful cases, evaluation of post-voiding urinary residual volume can be helpful. A residual volume of more than 150 mL suggests bladder dysfunction. Autonomic dysfunction is an unfavorable prognostic factor. Patients with progressive neurologic symptoms should have frequent neurologic examinations and rapid therapeutic intervention. Other illnesses that may mimic cord compression include osteoporotic vertebral collapse, disc disease, pyogenic abscess or vertebral tuberculosis, radiation myelopathy, neoplastic leptomeningitis, benign tumors, epidural hematoma, and spinal lipomatosis.

Patients with cancer who develop back pain should be evaluated for spinal cord compression as quickly as possible (Fig. 88-2). Treatment is more often successful in patients who are ambulatory and still have sphincter control at the time treatment is initiated. Patients should have a neurologic examination and plain films of the spine. Those whose physical examination suggests cord compression should receive dexamethasone (24 mg intravenously every 6 h), starting immediately.

Erosion of the pedicles (the "winking owl" sign) is the earliest radiologic finding of vertebral tumor. Other radiographic changes include increased intrapedicular distance, vertebral destruction, lytic or sclerotic lesions, scalloped vertebral bodies, and vertebral body collapse. Vertebral collapse is not a reliable indicator of the presence of tumor; about 20% of cases of vertebral collapse, particularly those in older patients and postmenopausal women, are due not to cancer but to osteoporosis. Also, a normal appearance on plain films of the spine does not exclude the diagnosis of cancer. The role of bone scans in

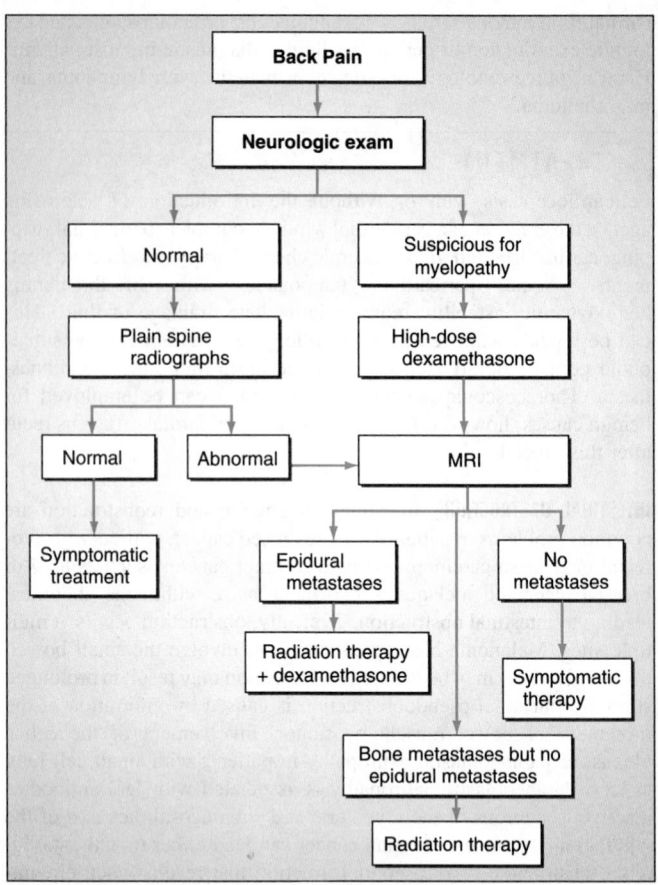

FIGURE 88-2   Management of cancer patients with back pain.

the detection of cord compression is not clear; this method is sensitive but less specific than spinal radiography.

The full-length image of the cord provided by MRI is useful. Multiple epidural metastases are noted in 25% of patients with cord compression and their presence influences treatment plans. On T1-weighted images, good contrast is noted between the cord, cerebrospinal fluid, and extradural lesions. Owing to its sensitivity in demonstrating the replacement of bone marrow by tumor, MRI can show which parts of a vertebra are involved by tumor (the body, pedicle, lamina, spinous process). MRI also visualizes intraspinal extradural masses compressing the cord. T2-weighted images are most useful for the demonstration of intramedullary pathology. Gadolinium-enhanced MRI can help to delineate intramedullary disease. MRI is as good as or better than myelography plus postmyelogram CT in detecting metastatic epidural disease with cord compression. Myelography should be reserved for patients who have poor MR images or who cannot undergo MRI promptly. CT in conjunction with myelography enhances the detection of small areas of spinal destruction.

In patients with cord compression and an unknown primary tumor, a simple workup including chest radiography, mammography, measurement of prostate-specific antigen, and abdominal CT usually reveals the underlying malignancy.

℞ TREATMENT

The treatment of patients with spinal cord compression is aimed at relief of pain and restoration of neurologic function (Fig. 88-2).

Radiation therapy plus glucocorticoids is generally the initial treatment of choice for spinal cord compression. Up to 75% of patients treated when still ambulatory remain ambulatory, but only 10% of patients with paraplegia recover walking capacity. Indications for surgical intervention include unknown etiology, failure of radiation therapy, a radioresistant tumor type (e.g., melanoma or renal cell cancer), pathologic fracture dislocation, and rapidly evolving neurologic symptoms. Until recently, laminectomy was the standard operation for metastatic spinal cord compression, although results were poor. At present, laminectomy should be used only for tissue diagnosis and for the removal of posteriorly localized epidural deposits in the absence of vertebral disease. Because most cases of epidural spinal cord compression are due to anterior or anterolateral extradural disease, resection of the anterior vertebral body along with the tumor, followed by spinal stabilization, has achieved good results and low mortality rate. Chemotherapy may have a role in patients with chemosensitive tumors who have had prior radiation therapy to the same region and who are not candidates for surgery. Most patients with prostate cancer who develop cord compression have already had hormonal therapy; however, for those who have not, androgen deprivation is combined with surgery and radiation therapy.

Patients with metastatic vertebral tumors may benefit from percutaneous vertebroplasty, the injection of acrylic cement into a collapsed vertebra to stabilize the fracture. Pain palliation is common and local antitumor effects have been noted. Cement leakage may cause symptoms in about 10% of patients.

The histology of the tumor is an important determinant of both recovery and survival. Rapid onset and quick progression are poor prognostic features.

INCREASED INTRACRANIAL PRESSURE About 25% of patients with cancer die with intracranial metastases. The cancers that most often metastasize to the brain are lung and breast cancers and melanoma. Brain metastases often occur in the presence of systemic disease, and they frequently cause major symptoms, disability, and early death.

The signs and symptoms of a metastatic brain tumor are similar to those of other intracranial expanding lesions: headache, nausea, vomiting, behavioral changes, seizures, and focal, progressive neurologic changes. Occasionally the onset is abrupt, resembling a stroke, with the sudden appearance of headache, nausea, vomiting, and neurologic deficits. This picture is usually due to hemorrhage into the metastasis. Melanoma, germ cell tumors, and renal cell cancers have a particularly high incidence of intracranial bleeding. The tumor mass and surrounding edema may cause obstruction of the circulation of cerebrospinal fluid, with resulting hydrocephalus. Patients with increased intracranial pressure may have papilledema with visual disturbances and neck stiffness. As the mass enlarges, brain tissue may be displaced through the fixed cranial openings, producing various herniation syndromes.

CT and MRI are equally effective in the diagnosis of brain metastases. CT with contrast should be used as a screening procedure. The CT scan shows brain metastases as multiple enhancing lesions of various sizes with surrounding areas of low-density edema. If a single lesion or no metastases are visualized by contrast-enhanced CT, MRI of the brain should be performed. Gadolinium-enhanced MRI is more sensitive than CT at revealing meningeal involvement and small lesions, particularly in the brainstem or cerebellum.

℞ TREATMENT

If signs and symptoms of brain herniation (particularly headache, drowsiness, and papilledema) are present, the patient should be intubated and hyperventilated to maintain P_{CO_2} between 25 and 30 mmHg and should receive infusions of mannitol (1 to 1.5 g/kg) every 6 h. Dexamethasone is the best initial treatment for all symptomatic patients with brain metastases (see above). Patients with multiple lesions should receive whole-brain radiation therapy. Patients with a single brain metastasis and with controlled extracranial disease may be treated with surgical excision followed by whole-brain radiation therapy, especially if they are younger than 60 years. Radioresistant tumors should be resected if possible. Stereotactic radiosurgery is an effective treatment for inaccessible or recurrent lesions. With a gamma knife or linear accelerator, multiple small, well-collimated beams of ionizing radiation destroy lesions seen on MRI. Some patients with increased intracranial pressure associated with hydrocephalus may benefit from shunt placement. If neurological deterioration is not reversed with

medical therapy, ventriculotomy to remove cerebrospinal fluid (CSF) or craniotomy to remove tumors or hematomas may be necessary.

NEOPLASTIC MENINGITIS Tumor involving the leptomeninges is a complication of both primary tumors of the central nervous system (CNS) and tumors that metastasize to the CNS. The incidence is estimated at 3 to 8% of patients with cancer. Melanoma, breast and lung cancer, lymphoma (including AIDS-associated), and acute leukemia are the most common causes.

Patients typically present with multifocal neurologic signs and symptoms including headache, gait abnormality, mental changes, nausea, vomiting, seizures, back or radicular pain, and limb weakness. Signs include cranial nerve palsies, extremity weakness, paresthesia, and decreased deep tendon reflexes.

Diagnosis is made by demonstrating malignant cells in the cerebrospinal fluid (CSF); however, up to 40% of patients may have false negative CSF cytology. An elevated CSF protein level is nearly always present (except in HTLV-1-associated adult T cell leukemia). Patients with neurologic signs and symptoms consistent with neoplastic meningitis who have a negative CSF cytology but an elevated CSF protein level should have the spinal tap repeated at least three times for repeated cytologic examination before the diagnosis is rejected. MRI findings suggestive of neoplastic meningitis include leptomeningeal, subependymal, dural or cranial nerve enhancement, superficial cerebral lesions, and communicating hydrocephalus. Spinal cord imaging by MRI is a necessary component of the evaluation of non-leukemia neoplastic meningitis as ~20% of patients have cord abnormalities including intradural enhancing nodules that are diagnostic for leptomeningeal involvement. Cauda equina lesions are common but lesions may be seen anywhere in the spinal canal. Radiolabeled CSF flow studies are abnormal in up to 70% of patients with neoplastic meningitis; ventricular outlet obstruction, abnormal flow in the spinal canal, or impaired flow over the cerebral convexities may affect distribution of intrathecal chemotherapy resulting in decreased efficacy or increased toxicity. Radiation therapy may correct CSF flow abnormalities before use of intrathecal chemotherapy.

The development of neoplastic meningitis usually occurs in the setting of uncontrolled cancer outside the CNS; thus, prognosis is poor (median survival 10 to 12 weeks). However, treatment of the neoplastic meningitis may successfully alleviate symptoms and control the CNS spread.

℞ TREATMENT

Intrathecal chemotherapy, usually methotrexate, cytarabine, or thiotepa, is delivered by lumbar puncture or by an intraventricular reservoir (Ommaya) three times a week until the CSF is free of malignant cells. Then injections are given twice a week for a month and then weekly for a month. An extended release preparation of cytarabine (Depocyte) has a longer half-life and is more effective than regular formulations. Among solid tumors, breast cancer responds best to therapy. Patients with neoplastic meningitis from either acute leukemia or lymphoma may be cured of their CNS disease if the systemic disease can be eliminated.

SEIZURES Seizures occurring in a patient with cancer can be caused by the tumor itself, by metabolic disturbances, by radiation injury, by cerebral infarctions, by chemotherapy-related encephalopathies, or by CNS infections. Metastatic disease to the CNS is the most common cause of seizures in patients with cancer. However, seizures occur more frequently in primary brain tumors than in metastatic brain lesions. Seizures are a presenting symptom of CNS metastasis in 6 to 29% of cases. Approximately 10% of patients with CNS metastasis eventually develop seizures. The presence of frontal lesions correlates with early seizures, and the presence of hemispheric symptoms increases the risk for late seizures. Both early and late seizures are uncommon in patients with posterior fossa lesions. Seizures are also common in patients with CNS metastases from melanoma. Very rarely, cytotoxic drugs such as etoposide, busulfan, and chlorambucil cause seizures.

℞ TREATMENT

Patients in whom seizures due to CNS metastases have been demonstrated should receive anticonvulsive treatment with diphenylhydantoin. Prophylactic anticonvulsant therapy is not recommended unless the patient is at a high risk for late seizures (melanoma primary, hemorrhagic metastases, treatment with radiosurgery). In those patients, serum diphenylhydantoin levels should be monitored closely and the dosage adjusted according to serum levels. Phenytoin induces the hepatic metabolism of dexamethasone, reducing its half-life, while dexamethasone may decrease phenytoin levels. Most anti-seizure medications alter the metabolism of antitumor agents.

PULMONARY AND INTRACEREBRAL LEUKOCYTOSTASIS Hyperleukocytosis and the leukostasis syndrome associated with it is a potentially fatal complication of acute leukemia (particularly myeloid leukemia) that can occur when the peripheral blast cell count is greater than 100,000/mL. The frequency of hyperleukocytosis is 5–13% in AML and 10–30% in acute lymphoid leukemia; however, leukostasis is rare in lymphoid leukemia. At such high blast cell counts, blood viscosity is increased, blood flow is slowed by aggregates of tumor cells, and the primitive myeloid leukemic cells are capable of invading through endothelium and causing hemorrhage. Brain and lung are most commonly affected. Patients with brain leukostasis may experience stupor, headache, dizziness, tinnitus, visual disturbances, ataxia, confusion, coma, or sudden death. Administration of 600 cGy of whole-brain irradiation can protect against this complication and can be followed by rapid institution of antileukemic therapy. Pulmonary leukostasis may present as respiratory distress, hypoxemia, and progress to respiratory failure. Chest radiographs may be normal but usually show interstitial or alveolar infiltrates. Leukapheresis may be helpful in decreasing circulating blast counts. Treatment of the leukemia can result in pulmonary hemorrhage from lysis of blasts in the lung, called "leukemic cell lysis pneumopathy." Intravascular volume depletion and unnecessary blood transfusions may increase blood viscosity and worsen leukostasis syndrome. Leukostasis is not a feature of the high white cell counts associated with chronic lymphoid or chronic myeloid leukemia.

When acute promyelocytic leukemia is treated with differentiating agents like tretinoin and arsenic trioxide, cerebral or pulmonary leukostasis may occur. This complication can be largely avoided by using cytotoxic chemotherapy together with the differentiating agents.

HEMOPTYSIS Hemoptysis may be caused by nonmalignant conditions, but lung cancer accounts for a large proportion of cases. Up to 20% of patients with lung cancer have hemoptysis some time in their course. Endobronchial metastases from carcinoid tumors, breast, colon, kidney cancer, and melanoma may also cause hemoptysis. The volume of bleeding is often difficult to gauge. Massive hemoptysis is defined as more than 600 mL of blood produced in 48 h. When respiratory difficulty occurs, hemoptysis should be treated emergently. Often patients can tell where the bleeding is occurring. They should be placed bleeding side down, given supplemental oxygen, and subjected to emergency bronchoscopy. If the site of the lesion is detected, either the patient undergoes a definitive surgical procedure or the lesion is treated with a neodymium:yttrium-aluminum-garnet (Nd:YAG) laser. The surgical option is preferred. Bronchial artery embolization may control brisk bleeding in 75 to 90% of patients, permitting the definitive surgical procedure to be done more safely. Embolization without definitive surgery is associated with rebleeding in 20 to 50% of patients. Recurrent hemoptysis usually responds to a second embolization procedure. A post-embolization syndrome characterized by pleuritic pain, fever, dysphagia, and leukocytosis may occur; it lasts 5–7 days and resolves with symptomatic treatment. Bronchial or

esophageal wall necrosis, myocardial infarction, and spinal cord infarction are rare complications.

Pulmonary hemorrhage with or without hemoptysis in hematologic malignancies is often associated with fungal infections, particularly *Aspergillus* sp. After granulocytopenia resolves, the lung infiltrates in aspergillosis may cavitate and cause massive hemoptysis. Thrombocytopenia and coagulation defects should be corrected, if possible. Surgical evaluation is recommended in patients with aspergillosis-related cavitary lesions.

AIRWAY OBSTRUCTION Generally, airway obstruction refers to a blockage at the level of the mainstem bronchi or above. It may result either from intraluminal tumor growth or from extrinsic compression of the airway. The most common cause of malignant upper airway obstruction is invasion from an adjacent primary tumor, most commonly lung cancer, followed by esophageal, thyroid, and mediastinal malignancies.Extrathoracic primary tumors such as renal cell, colon, or breast cancer can cause airway obtruction through endobronchial and/or mediastinal lymph node metastases. Patients may present with dyspnea, hemoptysis, stridor, wheezing, intractable cough, post-obstructive pneumonia, or hoarseness. Chest radiographs usually demonstrate obstructing lesions. CT scans provide more detailed information about the extent of tumor. Cool humidified oxygen, glucocorticoids, and ventilation with a mixture of helium and oxygen (Heliox) may provide temporary relief. If the obstruction is proximal to the larynx, a tracheostomy may be life-saving. For more distal obstructions, particularly intrinsic lesions incompletely obstucting the airway, bronchoscopy with laser treatment, photodynamic therapy, or stenting can produce immediate relief in most patients. However, radiation therapy (either external-beam irradiation or brachytherapy) given together with glucocorticoids may also open the airway. Symptomatic extrinsic compression may be palliated by stenting. Patients with primary airway tumors such as squamous cell carcinoma, carcinoid tumor, adenocystic carcinoma, or non-small cell lung cancer should have surgery.

METABOLIC EMERGENCIES

HYPERCALCEMIA Hypercalcemia is the most common paraneoplastic syndrome. →*Its pathogenesis and management are fully discussed in Chaps. 86 and 332.*

SYNDROME OF INAPPROPRIATE SECRETION OF ANTIDIURETIC HORMONE (SIADH) Hyponatremia is a common electrolyte abnormality in cancer patients, and SIADH is the most common cause of hyponatremia among patients with cancer. →*SIADH is discussed fully in Chaps. 86 and 319.*

LACTIC ACIDOSIS Lactic acidosis is a rare and potentially fatal metabolic complication of cancer. Lactic acidosis associated with sepsis and circulatory failure is a common preterminal event in many malignancies. Lactic acidosis in the absence of hypoxemia may occur in patients with leukemia, lymphoma, or solid tumors. Extensive involvement of the liver by tumor is present in most cases. Alteration of liver function may be responsible for the lactate accumulation. HIV-infected patients have an increased risk of aggressive lymphoma; lactic acidosis may occur in such patients either related to the rapid growth of the tumor or from toxicity of nucleoside reverse transcriptase inhibitors (components of HAART). Severe liver toxicity manifesting as acute lactic acidosis may be seen from nucleosides. Symptoms of lactic acidosis include tachypnea, tachycardia, change of mental status, and hepatomegaly. The serum level of lactic acid may reach 10 to 20 meq/L (90 to 180 mg/dL). Treatment is aimed at the underlying disease. The danger from lactic acidosis is from the acidosis, not the lactate. Sodium bicarbonate should be added if acidosis is very severe or if hydrogen ion production is very rapid and uncontrolled. The prognosis is poor.

HYPOGLYCEMIA Persistent hypoglycemia occasionally is associated with tumors other than pancreatic islet cell tumors. Usually these tumors are large, and often they are of mesenchymal origin or are hepatomas or adrenocortical tumors. Mesenchymal tumors are usually located in the retroperitoneum or thorax. In these patients, obtundation, confusion, and behavioral aberrations occur in the postabsorptive period and may precede the diagnosis of the tumor. These tumors often secrete incompletely processed insulin-like growth factor II (IGF-II), a hormone capable of activating insulin receptors and causing hypoglycemia. Rarely, hypoglycemia is due to insulin secretion by a non-islet cell carcinoma. Also, the development of hepatic dysfunction from liver metastases and increased glucose consumption by the tumor can contribute to hypoglycemia. If the tumor cannot be resected, hypoglycemia symptoms may be relieved by the administration of glucose, glucocorticoids, or glucagon.

Hypoglycemia can be artifactual; hyperleukocytosis from leukemia, myeloproliferative diseases, leukemoid reactions, or colony stimulating factor treatment can increase glucose consumption in the test tube after blood is drawn, leading to pseudohypoglycemia.

ADRENAL INSUFFICIENCY In patients with cancer, adrenal insufficiency may go unrecognized because the symptoms, such as nausea, vomiting, anorexia, and orthostatic hypotension, are nonspecific and may be mistakenly attributed to progressive cancer or to cancer therapy. Primary adrenal insufficiency may develop owing to replacement of both glands by metastases (lung, breast, colon, or kidney cancer, lymphoma), to removal of both glands, or to hemorrhagic necrosis in association with sepsis or anticoagulation. Impaired adrenal steroid synthesis occurs in patients being treated for cancer with mitotane, ketoconazole, aminoglutethimide, or the investigational agent suramin or in those undergoing rapid reduction in glucocorticoid therapy. Rarely, metastatic replacement causes primary adrenal insufficiency as the first manifestation of an occult malignancy. Metastasis to the pituitary or hypothalamus is found at autopsy in up to 5% of patients with cancer, but associated secondary adrenal insufficiency is rare. Megesterol acetate, used to manage cancer and HIV-related cachexia, may suppress plasma levels of cortisol and adrenocorticotropic hormone (ACTH). Patients taking megesterol may develop adrenal insufficiency, and even those whose adrenal dysfunction is not symptomatic may have inadequate adrenal reserve if they become seriously ill.

Acute adrenal insufficiency is potentially lethal. Treatment of suspected adrenal crisis is initiated after the sampling of serum cortisol and ACTH levels (Chap. 321).

TREATMENT-RELATED EMERGENCIES

TUMOR LYSIS SYNDROME Tumor lysis syndrome is a well-recognized clinical entity that is characterized by various combinations of hyperuricemia, hyperkalemia, hyperphosphatemia, lactic acidosis, and hypocalcemia and is caused by the destruction of a large number of rapidly proliferating neoplastic cells. Frequently, acute renal failure develops as a result of the syndrome.

Tumor lysis syndrome is most frequently associated with the treatment of Burkitt's lymphoma, acute lymphoblastic leukemia, and other high-grade lymphomas, but it also may be seen with chronic leukemias and, rarely, with solid tumors. This syndrome has been seen in patients with chronic lymphocytic leukemia after treatment with fludarabine and cladribine. Tumor lysis syndrome usually occurs during or shortly (1 to 5 days) after chemotherapy. Rarely, spontaneous necrosis of malignancies causes tumor lysis syndrome.

Hyperuricemia may be present at the time of chemotherapy. Effective treatment kills malignant cells and leads to increased serum uric acid levels from the turnover of nucleic acids. Owing to the acidic local environment, uric acid can precipitate in the tubules, medulla, and collecting ducts of the kidney, leading to renal failure. Lactic acidosis and dehydration may contribute to the precipitation of uric acid in the renal tubules. The finding of uric acid crystals in the urine is strong evidence for uric acid nephropathy. The ratio of urinary uric acid to urinary creatinine is >1 in patients with acute hyperuricemic nephropathy and <1 in patients with renal failure due to other causes.

Hyperphosphatemia, which can be caused by the release of intracellular phosphate pools by tumor cell lysis, produces a reciprocal depression in serum calcium, which causes severe neuromuscular irritability and tetany. Deposition of calcium phosphate in the kidney

and hyperphosphatemia may cause renal failure. Potassium is the principal intracellular cation, and massive destruction of malignant cells may lead to hyperkalemia. Hyperkalemia in patients with renal failure may rapidly become life-threatening. Hyperkalemia can cause ventricular arrhythmias and sudden death.

The likelihood that the tumor lysis syndrome will occur in patients with Burkitt's lymphoma is related to the tumor burden and renal function. Hyperuricemia and high serum levels of lactate dehydrogenase (LDH >1500 U/L), both of which correlate with total tumor burden, also correlate with the risk of tumor lysis syndrome. In patients at risk for tumor lysis, pretreatment evaluations should include a complete blood count, serum chemistry evaluation, and urine analysis. High leukocyte and platelet counts may artificially elevate potassium levels ("pseudohyperkalemia") due to lysis of these cells after the blood is drawn. In these cases, plasma potassium instead of serum potassium should be followed. In pseudohyperkalemia, no electrocardiographic abnormalities are present. In patients with abnormal baseline renal function, the kidneys and retroperitoneal area should be evaluated by sonography and/or CT to rule out obstructive uropathy. Urine output should be watched closely.

Rx TREATMENT

Recognition of risk and prevention are the most important steps in the management of this syndrome (Fig. 88-3). The standard preventive approach consists of allopurinol, urinary alkalinization, and aggressive hydration. Intravenous allopurinol may be given in patients who cannot tolerate oral therapy. In some cases, uric acid levels cannot be lowered sufficiently with the standard preventive approach. Rasburicase (recombinant urate oxidase) can be effective in these instances.

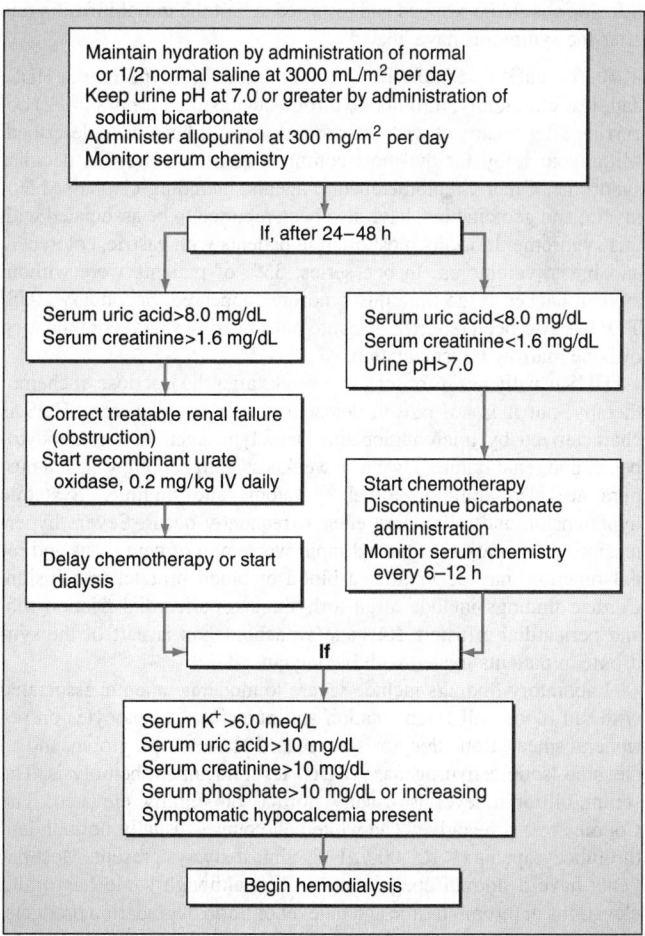

FIGURE 88-3 Management of patients at high risk for the tumor lysis syndrome.

Urate oxidase is missing from primates and catalyzes the conversion of poorly soluble uric acid to readily soluble allantoin. Rasburicase acts rapidly decreasing uric acid levels within hours; however, it may cause hypersensitivity reactions such as bronchospasm, hypoxemia, and hypotension. Rasburicase is contraindicated in patients with glucose-6-phosphate dehydrogenase deficiency who are unable to breakdown hydrogen peroxide, an end product of the urate oxidase reaction. Despite aggressive prophylaxis, tumor lysis syndrome and/or oliguric or anuric renal failure may occur. Care should be taken to prevent worsening of symptomatic hypocalcemia by induction of alkalosis during bicarbonate infusion. Administration of sodium bicarbonate may also lead to urinary precipitation of calcium phosphate, which is less soluble at alkaline pH. Dialysis is often necessary and should be considered early in the course. Hemodialysis is preferred. Hemofiltration offers a gradual, continuous method of removing cellular byproducts and fluid. The prognosis is excellent, and renal function recovers after the uric acid level is lowered to ≤10 mg/dL.

HUMAN ANTIBODY INFUSION REACTIONS   The initial infusion of human or humanized antibodies (e.g., rituximab, gemtuzumab, trastuzumab) is associated with fever, chills, nausea, asthenia, and headache in up to half of treated patients. Bronchospasm and hypotension occur in 1% of patients. The pathogenesis is thought to be activation of immune effector processes (cells and complement). In the presence of high levels of circulating lymphoid tumor cells, thrombocytopenia, a rapid fall in circulating tumor cells, and mild electrolyte evidence of tumor lysis syndrome may also occur. In addition, increase of liver enzymes, D-dimer, LDH, and prolongation of the prothrombin time may occur. This syndrome is related to release of inflammatory cytokines, such as tumor necrosis factor-α and IL-6. Diphenhydramine and acetaminophen can often prevent or suppress the symptoms. If they occur, the infusion should be stopped and restarted at half the initial infusion rate after the symptoms have abated.

HEMOLYTIC-UREMIC SYNDROME   Hemolytic-uremic syndrome (HUS) and, less commonly, thrombotic thrombocytopenic purpura (TTP) occurring after treatment with antineoplastic drugs have been described. Mitomycin is by far the most common agent causing this peculiar syndrome. Other chemotherapeutic agents, including cisplatin, bleomycin, and gemcitabine, have also been reported to be associated with this syndrome. It occurs most often in patients with gastric, colorectal, and breast carcinoma. In one series, 35% of patients were without evident cancer at the time this syndrome appeared. Secondary HUS/TTP has also been reported as a rare but sometimes fatal complication of bone marrow transplantation.

HUS usually has its onset 4 to 8 weeks after the last dose of chemotherapy, but it is not rare to detect it several months later. HUS is characterized by microangiopathic hemolytic anemia, thrombocytopenia, and renal failure. Dyspnea, weakness, fatigue, oliguria, and purpura are also common initial symptoms and findings. Systemic hypertension and pulmonary edema frequently occur. Severe hypertension, pulmonary edema, and rapid worsening of hemolysis and renal function may occur after a blood or blood product transfusion. Cardiac findings include atrial arrhythmias, pericardial friction rub, and pericardial effusion. Raynaud's phenomenon is part of the syndrome in patients treated with bleomycin.

Laboratory findings include severe to moderate anemia associated with red blood cell fragmentation and numerous schistocytes on peripheral smear. Reticulocytosis, decreased plasma haptoglobin, and an elevated lactic dehydrogenase (LDH) level document hemolysis. The serum bilirubin level is usually normal or slightly elevated. The Coombs test is negative. The white cell count is usually normal, and thrombocytopenia ($<100,000/\mu L$) is almost always present. Most patients have a normal coagulation profile, although some have mild elevations in thrombin time and in level of fibrin degradation products. The serum creatinine level is elevated at presentation and shows a pattern of subacute worsening within weeks of the initial azotemia.

The urinalysis reveals hematuria, proteinuria, and granular or hyaline casts; and circulating immune complexes may be present.

The basic pathologic lesion appears to be deposition of fibrin in the walls of capillaries and arterioles, and these deposits are similar to those seen in HUS due to other causes. These microvascular abnormalities involve mainly the kidneys and rarely occur in other organs. The pathogenesis of chemotherapy-related HUS is unknown. Immune complexes have been proposed but not confirmed to be etiologic.

The case fatality rate is high; most patients die within a few months. Plasmapheresis and plasma exchange may normalize the hematologic abnormalities, but renal failure is not reversed in most patients. Immunoperfusion over a staphylococcal protein A column is the most successful treatment. About half of the patients treated with immunoperfusion respond with resolution of thrombocytopenia, improvement in anemia, and stabilization of renal failure. Treatment is well tolerated. It is not clear how the treatment works.

NEUTROPENIA AND INFECTION   These remain the most common serious complications of cancer therapy. →*They are covered in detail in Chap. 72.*

PULMONARY INFILTRATES   Patients with cancer may present with dyspnea associated with diffuse interstitial infiltrates on chest radiographs. Such infiltrates may be due to progression of the underlying malignancy, treatment-related toxicities, infection, and/or unrelated diseases. The cause may be multifactorial; however, most commonly they occur as a consequence of treatment. Infiltration of the lung by malignancy has been described in patients with leukemia, lymphoma, and breast and other solid cancers. Pulmonary lymphatics may be involved diffusely by neoplasm (pulmonary lymphangitic carcinomatosis), resulting in a diffuse increase in interstitial markings on chest radiographs. The patient is often mildly dyspneic at the onset, but pulmonary failure develops over a period of weeks. In some patients, dyspnea precedes changes on the chest radiographs and is accompanied by a nonproductive cough. This syndrome is characteristic of solid tumors. In patients with leukemia, diffuse microscopic neoplastic peribronchial and peribronchiolar infiltration is frequent but may be asymptomatic. However, some patients present with diffuse interstitial infiltrates, an alveolar capillary block syndrome, and respiratory distress. In these situations, glucocorticoids can provide symptomatic relief, but specific chemotherapy should always be started promptly.

Several cytotoxic agents, such as bleomycin, methotrexate, busulfan, and the nitrosoureas, may cause pulmonary damage. The most frequent presentations are interstitial pneumonitis, alveolitis, and pulmonary fibrosis. Some cytotoxic agents, including methotrexate and procarbazine, may cause an acute hypersensitivity reaction. Cytosine arabinoside has been associated with noncardiogenic pulmonary edema. Administration of multiple cytotoxic drugs, as well as radiation therapy and preexisting lung disease, may potentiate the pulmonary toxicity. Supplemental oxygen may potentiate the effects of drugs and radiation injury. Patients should always be managed with the lowest FI_{O_2} that is sufficient to maintain hemoglobin saturation.

The onset of symptoms may be insidious, with symptoms including dyspnea, nonproductive cough, and tachycardia. Patients may have bibasilar crepitant rales, end-inspiratory crackles, fever, and cyanosis. The chest radiograph generally shows an interstitial and sometimes an intraalveolar pattern that is strongest at the lung bases and may be symmetric. A small effusion may occur. Hypoxemia with decreased carbon monoxide diffusing capacity is always present. Glucocorticoids may be helpful in patients in whom pulmonary toxicity is related to radiation therapy or to chemotherapy. Treatment is otherwise supportive.

Radiation pneumonitis and/or fibrosis is a relatively frequent side effect of thoracic radiation therapy when the dosage exceeds 40 Gy; it may be acute or chronic. It has its onset usually from 2 to 6 months after completion of radiation therapy. The clinical syndrome, which varies in severity, consists of dyspnea, cough with scanty sputum, low-grade fever, and an initial hazy infiltrate on chest radiographs. The infiltrate and tissue damage usually are confined to the radiation field.

The patients subsequently may develop a patchy alveolar infiltrate and air bronchograms, which may progress to acute respiratory failure that is sometimes fatal. A lung biopsy may be necessary to make the diagnosis. Asymptomatic infiltrates found incidentally after radiation therapy need not be treated. However, prednisone should be administered to patients with fever or other symptoms. The dosage should be tapered slowly after the resolution of radiation pneumonitis, as abrupt withdrawal of glucocorticoids may cause an exacerbation of pneumonia. Delayed radiation fibrosis may occur years after radiation therapy and is signaled by dyspnea on exertion. Often it is mild, but it can progress to chronic respiratory failure. Therapy is supportive.

Classical radiation pneumonitis that leads to pulmonary fibrosis is due to radiation-induced production of local cytokines such as platelet-derived growth factor β, tumor necrosis factor, and transforming growth factor β in the radiation field. An immunologically mediated sporadic radiation pneumonitis occurs in about 10% of patients; bilateral alveolitis mediated by T cells results in infiltrates outside the radiation field. This form of radiation pneumonitis usually resolves without sequelae.

Pneumonia is a common problem in patients undergoing treatment for cancer. Bacterial pneumonia typically causes a localized infiltrate on chest radiographs. Therapy is tailored to the causative organism. When diffuse interstitial infiltrates appear in a febrile patient, the differential diagnosis is extensive and includes pneumonia due to infection with *Pneumocystis carinii*, cytomegalovirus, or intracellular pathogens such as *mycoplasma* and *Legionella*; effects of drugs or radiation; tumor progression; nonspecific pneumonitis; and fungal disease. Patients with cancer who are neutropenic and have fever and local infiltrates on chest radiograph should be treated with a third generation cephalosporin perhaps together with an aminoglycoside or imipenem. A new or persistent focal infiltrate not responding to broad spectrum antibiotics argues for initiation of empiric antifungal therapy. When diffuse bilateral infiltrates develop in patients with febrile neutropenia, broad spectrum antibiotics plus trimethoprim-sulfamethoxazole with or without erythromycin should be initiated. The empiric administration of trimethoprim-sulfamethoxazole plus erythromycin to patients without neutropenia and these antibiotics plus ceftazidime to patients with neutropenia covers nearly every treatable diagnosis (except tumor progression) and gives as good overall survival as a strategy based on early invasive intervention with bronchoalveolar lavage or open lung biopsy. If the patient does not improve in 4 days, open lung biopsy is the procedure of choice. Bronchoscopy with bronchoalveolar lavage may be used in patients who are poor candidates for surgery.

In patients with pulmonary infiltrates who are afebrile, heart failure and multiple pulmonary emboli form part of the differential diagnosis.

TYPHLITIS Neutropenic enterocolitis (typhlitis) is an inflammation and necrosis of the cecum and surrounding tissues that may complicate the treatment of acute leukemia. This complication has also been seen in patients with other forms of cancer treated with taxanes and in patients receiving high-dose chemotherapy. The patient develops right lower quadrant abdominal pain, often with rebound tenderness and a tense, distended abdomen, in a setting of fever and neutropenia. Watery diarrhea (often containing sloughed mucosa) and bacteremia are com-

mon, and bleeding may occur. Plain abdominal films are generally of little value in the diagnosis; CT scan may show marked bowel wall thickening, particularly in the cecum, with bowel wall edema. Patients with bowel wall thickness >10 mm on ultrasonogram have higher mortality rates. Rapid institution of broad-spectrum antibiotic coverage and nasogastric suction may reverse the disease. Surgical intervention should be considered if there is no improvement by 24 h after the start of antibiotic treatment. If the localized abdominal findings become diffuse, the prognosis is poor.

HEMORRHAGIC CYSTITIS Hemorrhagic cystitis can develop in patients receiving cyclophosphamide or ifosfamide. Both drugs are metabolized to acrolein, which is a strong chemical irritant that is excreted in the urine. Prolonged contact or high concentrations may lead to bladder irritation and hemorrhage. Symptoms include gross hematuria, frequency, dysuria, burning, urgency, incontinence, and nocturia. The best management is prevention. Maintaining a high rate of urine flow minimizes exposure. In addition, 2-mercaptoethanesulfonate (mesna) detoxifies the metabolites and can be coadministered with the instigating drugs. Mesna usually is given three times on the day of ifosfamide administration in doses that are each 20% of the total ifosfamide dose. If hemorrhagic cystitis develops, the maintenance of a high urine flow may be sufficient supportive care. If conservative management is not effective, irrigation of the bladder with an 0.37 to 0.74% formalin solution for 10 min stops the bleeding in most cases. *N*-acetylcysteine may also be an effective irrigant. Prostaglandins (carboprost tromethamine) can inhibit the progress. In extreme cases, ligation of the hypogastric arteries, urinary diversion, or cystectomy may be necessary.

Hemorrhagic cystitis also occurs in patients who undergo bone marrow transplantation (BMT). In the BMT setting, early onset hemorrhagic cystitis is related to drugs in the treatment regimen (e.g. cyclophosphamide) and late onset hemorrhagic cystitis is usually due to the polyoma virus BKV or adenovirus type 11. Viral causes are usually detected by PCR-based diagnostic tests. Treatment of viral hemorrhagic cystitis is largely supportive with reduction in doses of immunosuppressive agents, if possible. No antiviral therapy is in use, though cidofovir is being tested.

FURTHER READING

ALBANELL J, BASELGA J: Systemic therapy emergencies. Semin Oncol 27: 347, 2000

APARICIO A et al: Neoplastic meningitis. Curr Neurol Neurosci Rep 2:225, 2002

DAVIS MP et al: Modern management of cancer-related intestinal obstruction. Curr Oncol Rep 2:343, 2000

JAECKLE KA et al: An open label trial of sustained release cytarabine (DepoCyte) for intrathecal treatment of solid tumor neoplastic meningitis. J Neuro Oncol 57:231, 2002

RIPAMONTI C et al: Respiratory problems in advanced cancer. Support Care Cancer 10:204, 2002

VAITKUS PT et al: Treatment of malignant pericardial effusion. JAMA 272: 59, 1994

YIM BT et al: Rasburicase for the treatment and prevention of hyperuricemia. Ann Pharmacother 37:1047, 2003

89 LATE CONSEQUENCES OF CANCER AND ITS TREATMENT
Michael C. Perry, Dan L. Longo

Over 9 million Americans alive today have had cancer. Virtually all of these survivors will bear some mark of their diagnosis and its therapy, and many will experience long-term complications, including medical problems, psychosocial disturbances, sexual dysfunction, and inability to find employment or insurance.

Problems may be related to the cancer itself (e.g., patients with primary cancers of the head and neck are at increased risk for subsequent lung cancer), or to the normal aging process (surviving one cancer does not necessarily alter the risk of other common tumors that increase in frequency with age). However, many of the problems affecting cured patients are related to the treatments. Individuals carefully followed for periods up to 30 years have taught us the spectrum

TABLE 89-1 *Late Effects of Cancer Therapy*

Surgical Procedure	Effect
Amputation	Functional loss
Lymph node dissection	Risk of lymphedema
Ostomy	Psychosocial impact
Splenectomy	Risk of sepsis
Adhesions	Risk of obstruction
Bowel anastomoses	Malabsorption syndromes

Radiation Therapy		Effect
Organ		
Bone		Premature termination of growth, osteonecrosis
Soft tissues		Atrophy, fibrosis
Brain		Neuropsychiatric deficits, cognitive dysfunction
Thyroid		Hypothyroidism, Graves' disease, cancer
Salivary glands		Dry mouth, caries, dysgeusia
Eyes		Cataracts
Heart		Pericarditis, myocarditis, coronary artery disease
Lung		Pulmonary fibrosis
Kidney		Decreased function, hypertension
Liver		Decreased function
Intestine		Malabsorption, stricture
Gonads		Infertility, premature menopause
Any		Secondary neoplasia

Chemotherapy		Effect
Organ	Drug	
Bone	Glucocorticoids	Osteoporosis, avascular necrosis
Brain	Methotrexate, ara-C, others	Neuropsychiatric deficits, cognitive decline?
Peripheral nerves	Vincristine, platinum	Neuropathy, hearing loss
Eyes	Glucocorticoids	Cataracts
Heart	Anthracyclines, herceptin	Cardiomyopathy
Lung	Bleomycin	Pulmonary fibrosis
	Methotrexate	Pulmonary hypersensitivity
Kidney	Platinum, others	Decreased function, hypomagnesemia
Liver	Various	Altered function
Gonads	Alkylating agents, others	Infertility, premature menopause
Bone marrow	Various	Aplasia, myelodysplasia, secondary leukemia

of problems that can be encountered. Because of heterogeneity in treatment details and in completeness of follow-up, some treatment-related problems went undetected for many years. However, studies of long-term survivors of childhood cancers, acute leukemia, Hodgkin's disease, lymphomas, testicular cancer, and localized solid tumors have identified the features of cancer treatment that are associated with later morbidity and mortality. We have been somewhat slow to act in changing those aspects of primary treatment that contribute to these late problems. This reticence is due to the uncertainty associated with changing a treatment that is known to work before having a replacement that works as well.

The first task is always to eradicate the diagnosed malignancy. Late problems occurring in cured patients reflect the success of treatment. Such problems never develop in those who do not survive the cancer. Morbidity and mortality from iatrogenic disease should be avoided, if possible. However, the risk of late complications should not lead to the failure to apply potentially curative treatment. The challenge is to preserve or augment the cure rate while decreasing the risk of serious treatment-related illness.

The mechanisms of damage vary. Surgical procedures can create abnormal physiology (such as blind loops leading to malabsorption) or interfere with normal organ function (splenectomy leading to impaired immune response). Radiation therapy can damage organ function directly (salivary gland toxicity leading to dry mouth and dental caries), act as a carcinogen (second solid tumors in radiation ports), or promote accelerated aging-associated changes (atherosclerosis). Cancer chemotherapy can produce damage to the bone marrow and immune system and induce a spectrum of organ dysfunctions. Therapy may produce subclinical damage that may only become recognized in

the presence of a second inciting factor (such as the increased incidence of melanoma in patients with dysplastic nevus syndrome treated for Hodgkin's disease with radiation therapy). Finally, although the mechanisms are not elucidated, cancer and its treatment are associated with psychosocial problems that can impair the survivor's ability to adapt to life after cancer.

Late effects by treatment modality are shown in Table 89-1. →*Drug toxicities are discussed in Chap. 70; radiation toxicity is discussed in Chap. 71.*

CONSEQUENCES BY ORGAN SYSTEM ■ **Cardiovascular Dysfunction** Most anthracyclines damage the heart muscle. A dose-dependent dropout of myocardial cells is seen on endomyocardial biopsy, and eventually ventricular failure ensues. About 5% of patients who receive >550 mg/m² of doxorubicin will develop congestive heart failure (CHF). Coexisting cardiac disease, hypertension, advanced age, and concomitant therapy with thoracic radiation therapy or mitomycin may hasten the onset of CHF. Anthracycline-induced CHF is not readily reversible; mortality is as high as 50%, thus, prevention is the best approach. Mitoxantrone is a related drug that has less cardiac toxicity. Administration of doxorubicin by continuous infusion or encapsulated in liposomes appears to decrease the risk of heart damage. Dexrazoxane, an intracellular iron chelator, may protect the heart against anthracycline toxicity by preventing iron-dependent free-radical generation.

Mediastinal radiation therapy that includes the heart can induce acute pericarditis, chronic constrictive pericarditis, myocardial fibrosis, or accelerated premature coronary atherosclerosis. The incidence of acute pericarditis is 5 to 13%; patients may be asymptomatic or have dyspnea on exertion, fever, and chest pain. Onset is insidious, with a peak about 9 months after treatment. Pericardial effusion may be present. Chronic constrictive pericarditis can develop 5 to 10 years after treatment and usually presents with dyspnea on exertion. Myocardial fibrosis may present as unexplained CHF with diagnostic evaluation showing restrictive cardiomyopathy. Patients may have aortic insufficiency from valvular thickening or mitral regurgitation from papillary muscle dysfunction. Patients who receive mantle field radiation therapy have a threefold increased risk of *fatal* myocardial infarction. Similarly, radiation of the carotids is associated with premature atherosclerosis of the carotids and can produce central nervous system embolic disease. At very high doses, cyclosphosphamide can produce a hemorrhagic myocarditis. Herceptin has been associated with heart failure.

Pulmonary Dysfunction Pulmonary fibrosis from bleomycin is dose-related, with potential exacerbation by age, preexisting lung disease, thoracic radiation, high concentrations of inhaled oxygen, and the concomitant use of other chemotherapeutic agents. Several other chemotherapy agents and radiation therapy can cause pulmonary fibrosis, and at least five can cause pulmonary venoocclusive disease, especially following high-dose therapy such as that involved in stem cell/bone marrow transplantation.

Liver Dysfunction Clinically significant long-term damage to the liver from standard-dose chemotherapy is relatively infrequent and mostly confined to patients who have received chronic methotrexate for maintenance therapy of acute lymphoblastic leukemia. Radiation doses to the liver >1500 cGy can produce liver dysfunction. Although rarely seen with standard-dose chemotherapy, hepatic venoocclusive disease is more common with high-dose therapy, such as that given to prepare patients for autologous or allogeneic stem cell transplantation. Endothelial damage is probably the inciting event.

Renal/Bladder Dysfunction   Reduced renal function may be produced by cisplatin; it is usually asymptomatic but may render the patient more susceptible to other renal insults. Cyclophosphamide cystitis may eventually lead to the development of bladder cancer. Ifosfamide produces cystitis and a proximal tubular defect, a Fanconi-like syndrome that is usually, but not always, reversible.

Endocrine Dysfunction   Long-term survivors of childhood cancer who received cranial irradiation are shorter, more likely to be obese, and have reductions in strength, exercise tolerance, and bone mineral density. The obesity may be related to alterations in leptin biology. Growth hormone deficiency is the most common hormone deficiency.

Thyroid disease is common in patients who have received radiation therapy to the neck, such as patients with Hodgkin's disease, with an incidence of up to 62% at 26 years post-therapy. Hypothyroidism is the most common abnormality, followed by Graves' disease, thyroiditis, and cancer. Such patients should have frequent thyroid-stimulating hormone (TSH) levels to detect hypothyroidism early and suppress the TSH drive, which may contribute to thyroid cancer.

Nervous System Dysfunction   Although many patients experience peripheral neuropathy during chemotherapy, only a few have chronic problems, perhaps because they have other coexisting diseases such as diabetes mellitus. High doses of cisplatin can produce severe sensorimotor neuropathy. Vincristine may produce permanent numbness and tingling in the fingers and toes.

Neurocognitive sequelae from intrathecal chemotherapy, with or without radiation therapy, are recognized complications of the successful therapy of childhood acute lymphoblastic leukemia. Cognitive decline has been attributed to radiating the brain in the treatment of a variety of tumor types. In addition, cognitive decline can follow the use of adjuvant chemotherapy in women being treated for breast cancer. Because the agents are given at modest doses and are not thought to cross the blood-brain barrier, the mechanism of the cognitive decline is not defined.

Many patients suffer intrusive thoughts about cancer recurrence for many years after successful treatment. Adjustment to normal expectations can be difficult. Cancer survivors may often have more problems holding a job, staying in a stable relationship, and coping with the usual stresses of daily life.

A dose-related hearing loss can occur with the use of cisplatin, usually with doses >400 mg/m². This is irreversible, and patients should be screened with audiometric examinations periodically during such therapy.

Eyes   Cataracts may be caused by chronic glucocorticoid use, radiation therapy to the head, and, rarely, by tamoxifen.

Sexual and Reproductive Dysfunction   Reversible azoospermia can be caused by many chemotherapy agents. The gonads may also be permanently damaged by radiation therapy or by chemotherapeutic agents, particularly the alkylating agents. The extent of the damage depends upon the patient's age and the total dose administered. As a woman nears menopause, smaller amounts of chemotherapy will produce ovarian failure. In men, chemotherapy may produce infertility, but hormone production is not usually affected. Women, however, commonly lose both fertility and hormone production. The premature induction of menopause in a young woman can have serious medical and psychological consequences. Hormone therapy is controversial. Paroxetine may be useful in controlling hot flashes.

Musculoskeletal Dysfunction   Late consequences of radiation therapy on the musculoskeletal system occur mostly in children and are related to the radiation dose, volume of tissue irradiated, and the age of the child at the time of therapy. Damage to the microvasculature of the epiphyseal growth zone may result in leg length discrepancy, scoliosis, and short stature.

Raynaud's Phenomenon   Up to 40% of patients with testicular cancer treated with bleomycin may experience Raynaud's phenomenon varying in severity from mild and transient to severe. The mechanism is unknown.

Oral Complications   Radiation therapy can damage the salivary glands, producing dry mouth. Without saliva, dental caries develop, and many patients have poor dentition. In rare patients, taste can be adversely affected and appetite can be suppressed.

SECOND MALIGNANCIES   Second malignancies are a major cause of death for those cured of cancer. Second malignancies can be grouped into three categories: those associated with the primary cancer, those caused by radiation therapy, and those caused by chemotherapy.

Primary cancers increase the risk of secondary cancers in a number of settings. Patients with head and neck cancers are at increased risk of developing a lung cancer, and vice versa, probably because of shared risk factors, especially tobacco abuse. Patients with breast cancer are at increased risk of a second breast cancer in the contralateral breast. Patients with Hodgkin's disease are at increased risk of non-Hodgkin's lymphoma. Patients with genetic syndromes, such as multiple endocrine neoplasia type 1 or Lynch syndrome, are at increased risk of second cancers of specific types. In none of these examples does it appear that treatment of the primary cancer is the cause of the secondary cancer, but a role for treatment is difficult to exclude. These predispositions should result in heightened surveillance in persons at risk. Patients with head and neck cancer may have a reduced risk of developing lung cancer with retinoic acid treatment. Other cancer preventions have not been proved effective.

Patients treated with radiation therapy have an increasing and apparently life-long risk of developing second solid tumors, usually in or adjacent to the radiation field. The risk is modest in the first decade after treatment but reaches 1% per year in the second decade, such that populations followed for 25 years or more have a ≥25% chance of developing a second treatment-related tumor. Some organs differ in their susceptibility to radiation carcinogenesis with age; women receiving chest radiation therapy after age 30 have a small increased risk of breast cancer, but those <30 have a 19-fold increased risk. The chances of curing the second malignancies hinge on early diagnosis. Patients who were treated with radiation therapy should be carefully examined on an annual basis and evaluated for any abnormalities in organs and tissues that were in the radiation field. Symptoms in a patient cured of cancer should not be dismissed as they may be an early sign of second cancers.

Chemotherapy produces two clinical syndromes that can be fatal: myelodysplasia and acute myeloid leukemia. Two types of acute leukemia have been described. The first occurs in patients treated with alkylating agents, especially over a protracted period. The malignant cells frequently carry genetic deletions in chromosomes 5 or 7. The lifetime risk is about 2%; the risk is increased by the addition of radiation therapy and is about three times higher in people treated over age 40. It peaks in incidence 4 to 6 years after treatment; the risk returns to baseline if no disease has developed within 10 years of treatment. The second type of acute leukemia occurs after exposure to topoisomerase II inhibitors such as doxorubicin or etoposide. It is morphologically indistinguishable from the first but contains a characteristic chromosome translocation involving 10q23. The incidence is <1%, and it usually occurs 1.5 to 3 years after treatment. Both forms of acute leukemia are highly refractory to treatment, and no preventive strategy has been developed.

Hormonal manipulations can also cause second tumors. Tamoxifen induces endometrial cancer in about 1 to 2% of women taking it for 5 years or longer. Usually these tumors are found at an early stage; mortality from endometrial cancer is very low compared to the benefit from tamoxifen use as adjuvant therapy in women with breast cancer.

CONSEQUENCES BY CANCER TYPE ■ **Pediatric Cancers**   Quality of life is often excellent, although the majority have at least one late effect. About one-third of long-term survivors have moderate to severe problems. Cognitive function may be impaired. Late effects are worse for those with poor socioeconomic status. Functional impairments in the cardiovascular system due to radiation therapy and anthracyclines, and in the lungs due to radiation therapy, are rare. Scoliosis and/or delayed growth due to radiation of the skeleton is more common. Many survivors have psychosocial and sexual problems. Second malignant neoplasms are a significant cause of death.

Hodgkin's Disease   The patient cured of Hodgkin's disease remains subject to long-term medical problems such as thyroid dysfunction, premature coronary artery disease, gonadal dysfunction, postsplenectomy sepsis, and second malignancies. The second malignancies encountered include myelodysplasia and acute myeloid leukemia, non-Hodgkin's lymphomas, breast cancer, lung cancer, and melanoma. The major risk factor for hematologic malignancies is treatment with alkylating agents plus radiation therapy, while solid tumors are more likely to be seen with the use of radiation therapy. Patients cured of Hodgkin's disease seem to have greater fatigue, more psychosocial and sexual problems, and report a poorer quality of life than patients cured of acute leukemia.

Non-Hodgkin's Lymphomas   The patient cured of a non-Hodgkin's lymphoma may be at increased risk of myelodysplasia and acute leukemia if high doses or prolonged courses of alkylating agents were used. Chronic exposure to cyclophosphamide increases the risk of bladder cancer. Patients cured of lymphoma report a very good quality of life.

Acute Leukemia   The late effects of anti-leukemic therapy include second malignancies (hematologic and solid tumors), neuropsychiatric difficulties, subnormal growth, thyroid abnormalities, and infertility.

Head and Neck Cancer   Patients frequently have poor dentition, dry mouth, trismus, difficulty in eating, and poor nutrition. Those with nasopharyngeal cancer report the poorest long-term quality of life, possibly related to the volume of disease that is radiated.

Stem Cell Transplantation   Cured patients are at risk of second cancers, especially if radiation therapy was part of the treatment. They are also subject to gonadal damage and infertility. Graft-versus-host disease is the leading factor contributing to the morbidity and mortality from allogeneic bone marrow transplantation, with an immune-mediated attack against the skin, liver, and gut epithelium. About half of patients report psychosexual problems.

Breast Cancer   Patients treated with adjuvant chemotherapy and/or hormonal therapy for breast cancer are at risk for endometrial cancer from the use of tamoxifen. Those patients who have received chemotherapy may be at risk from doxorubicin- or radiation-induced cardiomyopathy and acute leukemia. Herceptin may contribute to heart failure. The development of premature ovarian failure from chemotherapy may cause hormone-deficient symptoms (hot flashes, decreased vaginal secretions, dyspareunia) and places women at risk for osteoporosis and cardiovascular death. Patients commonly report intrusive thoughts of cancer and psychological distress.

Testicular Cancer   Depending on the modalities used for therapy, patients cured of testicular cancer can anticipate Raynaud's phenomenon, renal and/or pulmonary damage from chemotherapy, and retrograde ejaculation from retroperitoneal lymph node dissection. Sexual dysfunction is reported by 15% of patients cured of testicular cancer.

Colon Cancer   To date the major threat to patients with colorectal cancer treated with chemotherapy and/or radiation therapy remains the risk of a second colorectal cancer. Quality of life is reported as high in long-term survivors.

Prostate Cancer   Radical surgical treatment is often accompanied by impotence, and about 10 to 15% develop some urine incontinence. Use of radiation therapy increases the risk of second cancers.

OUTLOOK   The challenge for the future is to integrate new chemotherapy and biologic agents and newer techniques of delivering radiation therapy in a fashion that increases cure rates and lowers the late effects of treatment. Additional populations at risk for late effects include those with cancers where therapy is becoming more effective, such as ovarian cancer, and cancers where chemotherapy and radiation therapy are used together in an organ-sparing approach, such as bladder, anal, and laryngeal cancers. Patients who have been cured of a cancer represent an important resource for cancer prevention studies.

FURTHER READING

AHLES T et al: Neuropsychiatric impact of standard-dose chemotherapy in long-term survivors of breast cancer and lymphoma. J Clin Oncol 20:485, 2002

BOOKMAN MA et al: Late complications of curative treatment in Hodgkin's disease. JAMA 260:680, 1988

MACKIE E et al: Adult psychosocial outcomes in long-term survivors of acute lymphoblastic leukemia and Wilms' tumor: A controlled study. Lancet 355:1310, 2000

TRAVIS LB: Therapy-associated solid tumors. Acta Oncol 41:323, 2002

Section 2   Hematopoietic Disorders

90 | IRON DEFICIENCY AND OTHER HYPOPROLIFERATIVE ANEMIAS
John W. Adamson

Anemias associated with normocytic and normochromic red cells and an inappropriately low reticulocyte response (reticulocyte index <2.5) are *hypoproliferative anemias*. This category includes early iron deficiency (before hypochromic microcytic red cells develop), acute and chronic inflammation (including many malignancies), renal disease, hypometabolic states such as protein malnutrition and endocrine deficiencies, and anemias from marrow damage. Marrow damage states are discussed in Chap. 94. Hypoproliferative anemias are the most common anemias and anemia associated with acute and chronic inflammation is the most common of these. The anemia of acute and chronic inflammation, like iron deficiency, is related in part to abnormal iron metabolism. The anemias associated with renal disease, inflammation, cancer, and hypometabolic states are characterized by an abnormal erythropoietin response to anemia.

IRON METABOLISM

Iron is a critical element in the function of all cells, although the amount of iron required by individual tissues varies during development. At the same time, the body must protect itself from free iron, which is highly toxic in that it participates in chemical reactions that generate free radicals such as singlet O_2 or OH^-. Consequently, elaborate mechanisms have evolved that allow iron to be made available for critical physiologic functions while at the same time conserving this element and handling it in such a way that toxicity is avoided.

The major role of iron in mammals is to carry O_2 as part of the heme protein that, in turn, is part of hemoglobin. O_2 is also bound by a heme protein in muscle, myoglobin. Iron is a critical element in iron-containing enzymes, including the cytochrome system in mitochondria; iron distribution in the body is shown in Table 90-1. Without

TABLE 90-1 *Body Iron Distribution*

	Iron Content, mg	
	Adult Male, 80 kg	Adult Female, 60 kg
Hemoglobin	2500	1700
Myoglobin/enzymes	500	300
Transferrin iron	3	3
Iron stores	600–1000	0–300

iron, cells lose their capacity for electron transport and energy metabolism; in erythroid cells hemoglobin synthesis is impaired, resulting in anemia and reduced O_2 delivery to tissue.

THE IRON CYCLE IN HUMANS Figure 90-1 outlines the major pathways of internal iron exchange in humans. Iron absorbed from the diet or released from stores circulates in the plasma bound to *transferrin*, the iron transport protein. Transferrin is a bilobed glycoprotein with two iron binding sites. Transferrin that carries iron exists in two forms—*monoferric* (one iron atom) or *diferric* (two iron atoms). The turnover (half-clearance time) of transferrin-bound iron is very rapid—typically 60 to 90 min. Because the overwhelming majority of iron transported by transferrin is delivered to the erythroid marrow, the clearance time of transferrin-bound iron from the circulation is affected most by the plasma iron level and the activity of the erythroid marrow. When erythropoiesis is markedly stimulated, the pool of erythroid cells requiring iron increases and the clearance time of iron from the circulation decreases. The half-clearance time of iron in the presence of iron deficiency is as short as 10 to 15 min; this value reflects the limits of iron delivery as a function of the cardiac output going to the bone marrow. With suppression of the erythroid marrow, the plasma iron level typically is increased and the half-clearance time is prolonged to as much as several hours. Normally, the iron bound to transferrin turns over 10 to 20 times per day. Assuming a normal plasma iron level of 80 to 100 μg/dL, the amount of iron passing through the transferrin pool is 20 to 24 mg/d.

The iron-transferrin complex circulates in the plasma until the iron-carrying transferrin interacts with specific *transferrin receptors* on the surface of marrow erythroid cells. Diferric transferrin has the highest affinity for transferrin receptors; apotransferrin (transferrin not carrying iron) has very little affinity. While transferrin receptors are found on cells in many tissues within the body—and all cells at some time

during development will display transferrin receptors—the cell having the greatest number of receptors (300,000 to 400,000/cell) is the developing erythroblast.

Once the iron-bearing transferrin interacts with its receptor, the iron-transferrin-receptor complex is internalized via clathrin-coated pits and transported to an acidic endosome, where the iron is released at the low pH. The iron is then made available for heme synthesis while the transferrin-receptor complex is recycled to the surface of the cell, where the bulk of the transferrin is released back into the circulation and the transferrin receptor reanchors into the cell membrane. At this point a certain amount of the transferrin receptor protein may be released into circulation. Within the erythroid cell, iron that is in excess of the amount needed for hemoglobin synthesis binds to a storage protein, *apoferritin*, forming *ferritin*. This mechanism of iron exchange also takes place in other cells of the body expressing transferrin receptors, especially liver parenchymal cells where the iron can be incorporated into heme-containing enzymes or stored. The iron incorporated into hemoglobin subsequently enters the circulation as new red cells are released from the bone marrow. The iron is then part of the red cell mass and will not become available for reutilization until the red cell dies.

In a normal individual, the average red cell life span is 120 days. Thus, 0.8 to 1.0% of red cells turn over each day. At the end of its life span, the red cell is recognized as senescent by the cells of the *reticuloendothelial (RE) system*, and the cell undergoes phagocytosis. Once within the RE cell, the hemoglobin from the ingested red cell is broken down, the globin and other proteins are returned to the amino acid pool, and the iron is shuttled back to the surface of the RE cell, where it is presented to circulating transferrin. The "harvesting" of iron from senescent red cells is both efficient and rapid, with newly recycled iron appearing in the circulation within 10 min of ingestion of the red cell. It is the efficient and highly conserved recycling of iron from senescent red cells that supports steady state (and even mildly accelerated) erythropoiesis.

Since each milliliter of red cells contains 1 mg of elemental iron, the amount of iron needed to replace those red cells lost through senescence amounts to 16 to 20 mg/d (assuming an adult with a red cell mass of 2 L). Any additional iron required for daily red cell production comes from the diet. Normally, an adult male will need to absorb at least 1 mg of elemental iron daily to meet needs, while females in the childbearing years will need to absorb an average of 1.4 mg/d. However, to achieve a maximum proliferative erythroid marrow response to anemia, additional iron must be available. With markedly stimulated erythropoiesis, demands for iron are increased by as much as six- to eightfold. With hemolytic anemias, the rate of red cell destruction is increased, but the iron recovered from the red cells is efficiently reutilized for hemoglobin synthesis. In contrast, with blood loss anemia the rate of red cell production is limited by the amount of iron that can be mobilized from ferritin and hemosiderin stores. Typically, the rate of mobilization under these circumstances will not support red cell production more than 2.5 to 3 times normal. If the delivery of iron to the stimulated marrow is suboptimal, the marrow's proliferative response is blunted and normal hemoglobin synthesis is impaired. The result is a hypoproliferative marrow accompanied by microcytic, hypochromic anemia.

While blood loss or hemolysis places a demand for iron to be supplied to the erythroid marrow, other conditions such as inflammation interfere with iron release from stores and can result in a rapid decrease in the serum iron (see below).

NUTRITIONAL IRON BALANCE The balance of iron metabolism in the organism is tightly controlled and designed to conserve iron for reutilization. There is no excretory pathway for iron, and the only mechanisms by which iron is lost from the body are blood loss (via gastrointestinal bleeding, menses, or other forms of bleeding) and the loss of epidermal cells from the skin and gut. Normally, the only route

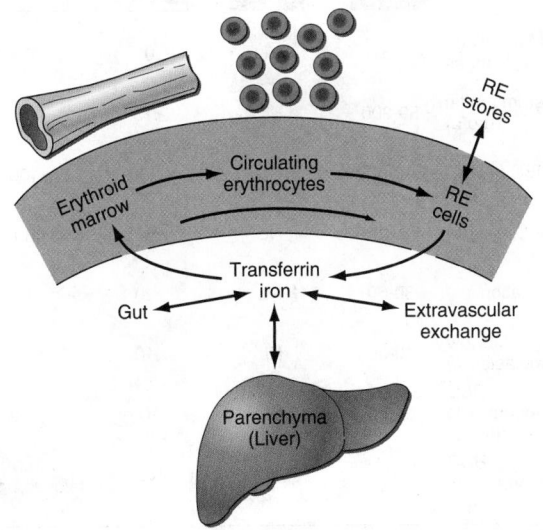

FIGURE 90-1 Internal iron exchange. Normally about 80% of iron passing through the plasma transferrin pool is recycled from broken-down red cells. Absorption of about 1 mg/d is required from the diet in men, 1.4 mg/d in women to maintain homeostasis. As long as transferrin saturation is maintained between 20 to 60% and erythropoiesis is not increased, iron stores are not required. However, in the event of blood loss, dietary iron deficiency, or inadequate iron absorption, up to 40 mg/d of iron can be mobilized from stores. RE, reticuloendothelial.

by which iron comes into the body is via absorption from food (dietary iron intake) or from medicinal iron taken orally. Iron may also enter the body through red cell transfusions or injection of iron complexes. The margin between the amount of iron available for absorption and the requirement for iron in growing infants and the adult female is narrow. The narrowness of this margin accounts for the great prevalence of iron deficiency worldwide—currently estimated at one-half billion people.

External iron exchange—the amount of iron required from the diet to replace losses—averages about 10% of body iron content a year in men and 15% in women of childbearing age, equivalent to 1.0 and 1.4 mg of elemental iron daily, respectively. Dietary iron content is closely related to total caloric intake (approximately 6 mg of elemental iron per 1000 calories). Iron bioavailability is affected by the nature of the foodstuff, with heme iron (e.g., red meat) being most readily absorbed. In the United States, the average iron intake in an adult male is 15 mg/d with 6% absorption; for the average female, the daily intake is 11 mg/d with 12% absorption. An individual with iron deficiency can increase iron absorption to about 20% of the iron present in a meat-containing diet but only 5 to 10% of the iron in a vegetarian diet. As a result, nearly one-third of the female population in the United States has virtually no iron stores. Vegetarians are at an additional disadvantage because certain foodstuffs that include phytates and phosphates reduce iron absorption by about 50%. When ionizable iron salts are given together with food, the amount of iron absorbed is reduced. This is particularly true with iron in the ferric state. When the percentage of iron absorbed from individual food items is compared with the percentage for an equivalent amount of ferrous salt, iron in vegetables is only about one-twentieth as available, egg iron one-eighth, liver iron one-half, and heme iron one-half to two-thirds. Therefore, liver and heme iron are absorbed nearly as well as iron salt added to food, while the iron in vegetables and eggs is much less available.

Infants, children, and adolescents may be unable to maintain normal iron balance because of the demands of body growth and lower dietary intake of iron. In pregnancy during the last two trimesters, daily iron requirements increase to 5 to 6 mg. That is the reason why iron supplements are strongly recommended for pregnant women in developed countries. Enthusiasm for supplementing foods such as bread and cereals with iron has waned in the face of concerns that the very prevalent hemochromatosis gene would result in an unacceptable risk of iron overload.

Iron absorption takes place largely in the proximal small intestine and is a carefully regulated process. For absorption, iron must be taken up by the luminal cell. That process is facilitated by the acidic contents of the stomach, which maintains the iron in solution. At the brush border of the absorptive cell, the ferric iron is converted to the ferrous form by a ferrireductase. Transport across the membrane is accomplished by divalent metal transporter 1 (DMT 1, also known as Nramp 2 or DCT 1). DMT 1 is a general cation transporter. Once iron is inside the gut cell, the iron may be stored as ferritin or transported through the cell to be released at the basolateral surface to plasma transferrin. It is likely that another transporter acts here in concert with hephaestin, another ferroxidase. Hephaestin is similar to ceruloplasmin, the copper-carrying protein.

Iron absorption is influenced by a number of physiologic states. Erythroid hyperplasia, for example, stimulates iron absorption, even in the face of normal or increased iron stores. Patients with anemias associated with high levels of ineffective erythropoiesis absorb excess amounts of dietary iron. Over time, this may lead to iron overload and tissue damage. In iron deficiency, iron is much more efficiently absorbed from a given diet; the contrary is true in the presence of iron overload. This is possibly mediated through signals that become fixed before the jejunal crypt cell migrates up the villus to become an absorptive cell. The normal individual can reduce iron absorption in situations of excessive intake or medicinal iron intake; however, while the percentage of iron absorbed goes down, the absolute amount goes

up. This accounts for the acute iron toxicity occasionally seen when children ingest large numbers of iron tablets. Under these circumstances, the amount of iron absorbed exceeds the transferrin binding capacity of the plasma, resulting in free iron that affects critical organs such as cardiac muscle cells.

IRON DEFICIENCY ANEMIA

STAGES OF IRON DEFICIENCY Iron deficiency anemia is the condition in which there is anemia and clear evidence of iron deficiency. However, iron deficiency occurs in steps (Fig. 90-2). These can be divided into three stages. The first stage is *negative iron balance*, in which the demands for (or losses of) iron exceed the body's ability to absorb iron from the diet. This stage can result from a number of physiologic mechanisms including blood loss, pregnancy (in which the demands for red cell production by the fetus outstrip the mother's ability to provide iron), rapid growth spurts in the adolescent, or inadequate dietary iron intake. Most commonly, the growth needs of the fetus or rapidly growing child exceed the individual's ability to absorb the iron necessary for hemoglobin synthesis from the diet. Blood loss in excess of 10 to 20 mL of red cells per day is greater than the amount of iron that the gut can absorb from a normal diet. Under these circumstances, the iron deficit must be made up by mobilization of iron from RE storage sites. During this period measurements of iron stores—such as the serum ferritin level or the appearance of stainable iron on bone marrow aspirations—will decrease. As long as iron stores are present and can be mobilized, the serum iron, total iron-binding capacity (TIBC), and red cell protoporphyrin levels remain within normal limits. At this stage, red cell morphology and indices are normal.

When iron stores become depleted, the serum iron begins to fall. Gradually, the TIBC increases, as do red cell protoporphyrin levels. By definition, marrow iron stores are absent when the serum ferritin level is <15 μg/L. As long as the serum iron remains within the normal range, hemoglobin synthesis is unaffected despite the dwindling iron stores. Once the transferrin saturation falls to 15 to 20%, hemoglobin synthesis becomes impaired. This is a period of *iron-*

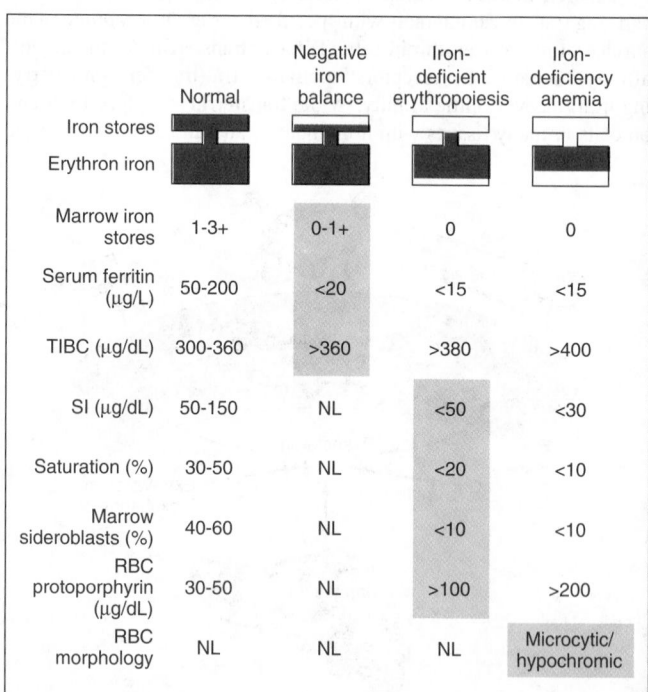

	Normal	Negative iron balance	Iron-deficient erythropoiesis	Iron-deficiency anemia
Iron stores				
Erythron iron				
Marrow iron stores	1-3+	0-1+	0	0
Serum ferritin (μg/L)	50-200	<20	<15	<15
TIBC (μg/dL)	300-360	>360	>380	>400
SI (μg/dL)	50-150	NL	<50	<30
Saturation (%)	30-50	NL	<20	<10
Marrow sideroblasts (%)	40-60	NL	<10	<10
RBC protoporphyrin (μg/dL)	30-50	NL	>100	>200
RBC morphology	NL	NL	NL	Microcytic/hypochromic

FIGURE 90-2 Laboratory studies in the evolution of iron deficiency. Measurements of marrow iron stores, serum ferritin, and total iron-binding capacity (TIBC) are sensitive to early iron-store depletion. Iron-deficient erythropoiesis is recognized from additional abnormalities in the serum iron (SI), percent transferrin saturation, the pattern of marrow sideroblasts, and the red cell protoporphyrin level. Patients with iron deficiency anemia demonstrate all the same abnormalities plus hypochromic microcytic anemia. (*From Hillman and Finch, with permission.*)

deficient erythropoiesis. Careful evaluation of the peripheral blood smear reveals the first appearance of microcytic cells, and if the laboratory technology is available, one finds hypochromic reticulocytes in circulation. Gradually, the hemoglobin and hematocrit begin to fall, reflecting *iron deficiency anemia.* The transferrin saturation at this point is 10 to 15%.

When moderate anemia is present (hemoglobin 10–13 g/dL), the bone marrow remains hypoproliferative. With more severe anemia (hemoglobin 7–8 g/dL), hypochromia and microcytosis become more prominent, misshapen red cells (poikilocytes) appear on the blood smear as cigar- or pencil-shaped forms and target cells, and the erythroid marrow becomes increasingly ineffective. Consequently, with severe prolonged iron deficiency anemia, erythroid hyperplasia of the marrow develops rather than hypoproliferation.

CAUSES OF IRON DEFICIENCY Conditions that increase demand for iron, increase iron loss, or decrease iron intake or absorption can produce iron deficiency (Table 90-2).

CLINICAL PRESENTATION OF IRON DEFICIENCY Certain clinical conditions carry an increased likelihood of iron deficiency. Pregnancy, adolescence, periods of rapid growth, and an intermittent history of blood loss of any kind should alert the clinician to possible iron deficiency. A cardinal rule is that the appearance of iron deficiency in an adult male means gastrointestinal blood loss until proven otherwise. Signs related to iron deficiency depend on the severity and chronicity of the anemia in addition to the usual signs of anemia—fatigue, pallor, and reduced exercise capacity. *Cheilosis* (fissures at the corners of the mouth) and *koilonychia* (spooning of the fingernails) are signs of advanced tissue iron deficiency. The diagnosis of iron deficiency is typically based on laboratory results.

LABORATORY IRON STUDIES ■ Serum Iron and Total Iron-Binding Capacity The serum iron level represents the amount of circulating iron bound to transferrin. The TIBC is an indirect measure of the circulating transferrin. The normal range for the serum iron is 50 to 150 μg/dL; the normal range for TIBC is 300 to 360 μg/dL. Transferrin saturation, which is normally 25 to 50%, is obtained by the following formula: serum iron $\times$ 100 $\div$ TIBC. Iron deficiency states are associated with saturation levels below 18%. In evaluating the serum iron, the clinician should be aware that there is a diurnal variation in the value. A transferrin saturation of >50% indicates that a disproportionate amount of the iron bound to transferrin is being delivered to nonerythroid tissues. If this condition persists for an extended time, tissue iron overload may occur.

Serum Ferritin Free iron is toxic to cells, and the body has established an elaborate set of protective mechanisms to bind iron in various tissue compartments. Within cells, iron is stored complexed to protein as ferritin or hemosiderin. Apoferritin binds to free ferrous iron and stores it in the ferric state. As ferritin accumulates within cells of the RE system, protein aggregates are formed as hemosiderin. Iron in ferritin or hemosiderin can be extracted for release by the RE cells although hemosiderin is less readily available. Under steady state conditions,

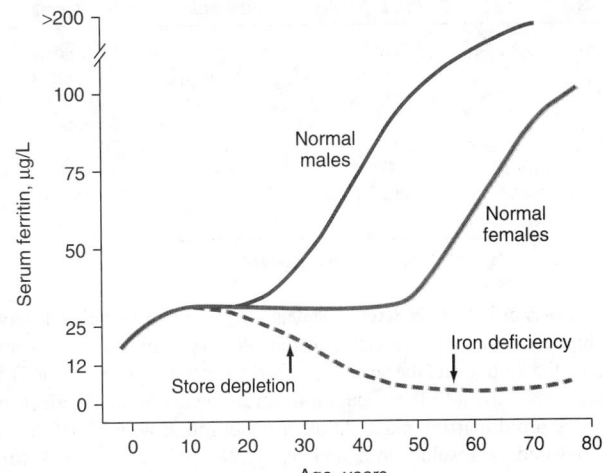

FIGURE 90-3 Serum ferritin levels as a function of sex and age. Iron store depletion and iron deficiency are accompanied by a fall in serum ferritin level below 20 μg/L. *(From Hillman and Ault, with permission.)*

the serum ferritin level correlates with total body iron stores; thus, the serum ferritin level is the most convenient laboratory test to estimate iron stores. The normal value for ferritin varies according to the age and gender of the individual (Fig. 90-3). Adult males have serum ferritin values averaging about 100 μg/L, while adult females have levels averaging 30 μg/L. As iron stores are depleted, the serum ferritin falls to <15 μg/L. Such levels are virtually always diagnostic of absent body iron stores.

Evaluation of Bone Marrow Iron Stores Although RE cell iron stores can also be estimated from the iron stain of a bone marrow aspirate or biopsy, the measurement of serum ferritin has largely supplanted bone marrow aspirates for determination of storage iron (Table 90-3). The serum ferritin level is a better indicator of iron overload than the marrow iron stain. However, in addition to storage iron the marrow iron stain provides information about the effective delivery of iron to developing erythroblasts. Normally, 20 to 40% of developing erythroblasts—called *sideroblasts*—will have visible ferritin granules in their cytoplasm. This represents iron in excess of that needed for hemoglobin synthesis. In states in which release of iron from storage sites is blocked, RE iron will be detectable, and there will be few or no sideroblasts. In the myelodysplastic syndromes, mitochondrial dysfunction occurs, and accumulation of iron in mitochondria appears in a necklace fashion around the nucleus of the erythroblast. Such cells are referred to as *ringed sideroblasts.*

Red Cell Protoporphyrin Levels Protoporphyrin is an intermediate in the pathway to heme synthesis. Under conditions in which heme synthesis is impaired, protoporphyrin accumulates within the red cell. This can reflect an inadequate iron supply to erythroid precursors to support hemoglobin synthesis. Normal values are less than 30 μg/dL of red cells. In iron deficiency, values in excess of 100 μg/dL are seen. The most common causes of increased red cell protoporphyrin levels are absolute or relative iron deficiency and lead poisoning.

TABLE 90-2   Causes of Iron Deficiency

Increased demand for iron and/or hematopoiesis
   rapid growth in infancy or adolescence
   pregnancy
   erythropoietin therapy
Increased iron loss
   chronic blood loss
   menses
   acute blood loss
   blood donation
   phlebotomy as treatment for polycythemia vera
Decreased iron intake or absorption
   inadequate diet
   malabsorption from disease (sprue, Crohn's disease)
   malabsorption from surgery (post-gastrectomy)
   acute or chronic inflammation

TABLE 90-3   Iron Store Measurements

Iron Stores	Marrow Iron Stain, 0–4+	Serum Ferritin, μg/L
0	0	<15
1–300 mg	Trace to 1+	15–30
300–800 mg	2+	30–60
800–1000 mg	3+	60–150
1–2 g	4+	>150
Iron overload	—	>500–1000

TABLE 90-4 *Diagnosis of Microcytic Anemia*

Tests	Iron Deficiency	Inflammation	Thalassemia	Sideroblastic Anemia
Smear	Micro/hypo	Normal micro/hypo	Micro/hypo with targeting	Variable
SI	<30	<50	Normal to high	Normal to high
TIBC	>360	<300	Normal	Normal
Percent saturation	<10	10–20	30–80	30–80
Ferritin (μg/L)	<15	30–200	50–300	50–300
Hemoglobin pattern	Normal	Normal	Abnormal	Normal

Note: SI, serum iron; TIBC, total iron-binding capacity.

Serum Levels of Transferrin Receptor Protein Because erythroid cells have the highest numbers of transferrin receptors on their surface of any cell in the body, and because transferrin receptor protein (TRP) is released by cells into the circulation, serum levels of TRP reflect the total erythroid marrow mass. Another condition in which TRP levels are elevated is absolute iron deficiency. Normal values are 4 to 9 μg/L determined by immunoassay. This laboratory test is becoming increasingly available and has been proposed to measure the serial expansion of the erythroid marrow in response to recombinant erythropoietin therapy.

DIFFERENTIAL DIAGNOSIS Other than iron deficiency, only three conditions need to be considered in the differential diagnosis of a hypochromic microcytic anemia (Table 90-4). The first is inherited defects in globin chain synthesis: the thalassemias. These are differentiated from iron deficiency most readily by serum iron values, since it is characteristic to have normal or increased serum iron levels and transferrin saturation with the thalassemias.

The second condition is chronic inflammatory disease with inadequate iron supply to the erythroid marrow. The distinction between true iron deficiency anemia and the anemia associated with chronic inflammatory states is among the most common diagnostic problems encountered by clinicians (see below). Usually the anemia of chronic disease is normocytic and normochromic. Again, the iron values usually make the differential diagnosis clear, as the ferritin level is normal or increased and the TIBC is typically below normal.

Finally, the myelodysplastic syndromes represent the third and most rare condition. Occasionally, patients with myelodysplasia have impaired hemoglobin synthesis with mitochondrial dysfunction resulting in impaired iron incorporation into heme. The iron values again reveal normal stores and more than an adequate supply to the marrow, despite the microcytosis and hypochromia.

Rx TREATMENT

The severity and cause of iron deficiency anemia will determine the appropriate approach to treatment. As an example, symptomatic elderly patients with severe iron deficiency anemia and cardiovascular instability may require red cell transfusions. Younger individuals who have compensated for their anemia can be treated more conservatively with iron replacement. The foremost issue for the latter patient is the precise identification of the cause of the iron deficiency.

For the majority of cases of iron deficiency (pregnant women, growing children and adolescents, patients with infrequent episodes of bleeding, and those with inadequate dietary intake of iron), oral iron therapy will suffice. For patients with unusual blood loss or malabsorption, specific diagnostic tests and appropriate therapy take priority. Once the diagnosis of iron deficiency anemia and its cause is made, and a therapeutic approach is charted, there are three major approaches.

Red Cell Transfusion Transfusion therapy is reserved for those individuals who have symptoms of anemia, cardiovascular instability, and continued and excessive blood loss from whatever source, and those who require immediate intervention. The management of these patients is less related to the iron deficiency than it is to the consequences of the severe anemia. Not only do transfusions correct the anemia acutely, but the transfused red cells provide a source of iron for reutilization, assuming they are not lost through continued bleeding. Transfusion therapy will stabilize the patient while other options are reviewed.

Oral Iron Therapy In the patient with established iron deficiency anemia who is asymptomatic, treatment with oral iron is usually adequate. Multiple preparations are available ranging from simple iron salts to complex iron compounds designed for sustained release throughout the small intestine (Table 90-5). While the various preparations contain different amounts of iron, they are generally all absorbed well and are effective in treatment. Some come with other compounds designed to enhance iron absorption, such as ascorbic acid. It is not clear whether the benefits of such compounds justify their costs. Typically, for iron replacement therapy up to 300 mg of elemental iron per day is given, usually as three or four iron tablets (each containing 50 to 65 mg elemental iron) given over the course of the day. Ideally, oral iron preparations should be taken on an empty stomach, since foods may inhibit iron absorption. Some patients with gastric disease or prior gastric surgery require special treatment with iron solutions, since the retention capacity of the stomach may be reduced. The retention capacity is necessary for dissolving the shell of the iron tablet before the release of iron. A dose of 200 to 300 mg of elemental iron per day should result in the absorption of iron up to 50 mg/d. This supports a red cell production level of two to three times normal in an individual with a normally functioning marrow and appropriate erythropoietin stimulus. However, as the hemoglobin level rises, erythropoietin stimulation decreases, and the amount of iron absorbed is reduced. The goal of therapy in individuals with iron deficiency anemia is not only to repair the anemia, but also to provide stores of at least 0.5 to 1.0 g of iron. Sustained treatment for a period of 6 to 12 months after correction of the anemia will be necessary to achieve this.

Of the complications of oral iron therapy, gastrointestinal distress is the most prominent and is seen in 15 to 20% of patients. For these patients, abdominal pain, nausea, vomiting, or constipation often lead to noncompliance. Although small doses of iron or iron preparations with delayed release may help somewhat, the gastrointestinal side effects are a major impediment to the effective treatment of a number of patients.

The response to iron therapy varies, depending on the erythropoietin stimulus and the rate of absorption. Typically, the reticulocyte count should begin to increase within 4 to 7 days after initiation of therapy and peak at 1½ weeks. The absence of a response may be due to poor adsorption, noncompliance (which is common), or a confounding diagnosis. If iron deficiency persists, it may be necessary to switch to parenteral iron therapy.

Parenteral Iron Therapy Intravenous iron can be given to patients who are unable to tolerate oral iron, whose needs are relatively acute, or who need iron on an ongoing basis, usually due to persistent gastrointestinal blood loss. Parenteral iron use has been rising rapidly in the last several years with the recognition that recombinant erythropoietin therapy induces a large demand for iron—a demand that frequently

TABLE 90-5 *Oral Iron Preparations*

Generic Name	Tablet (Iron Content), mg	Elixir (Iron Content), mg in 5 mL
Ferrous sulfate	325 (65)	300 (60)
	195 (39)	90 (18)
Extended release	525 (105)	
Ferrous fumarate	325 (107)	
	195 (64)	100 (33)
Ferrous gluconate	325 (39)	300 (35)
Polysaccharide iron	150 (150)	100 (100)
	50 (50)	

cannot be met through the physiologic release of iron from RE sources. Concern has been raised about the safety of parenteral iron—particularly iron dextran. The serious adverse reaction rate to intravenous iron dextran is 0.7%. Fortunately, newer iron complexes are available in the United States that have a much lower rate of adverse effects. The most recently approved preparations are intravenous sodium ferric gluconate (Ferrlecit) and iron sucrose (Venofer).

Parenteral iron is used in two ways: one is to administer the total dose of iron required to correct the hemoglobin deficit and provide the patient with at least 500 mg of iron stores; the second is to give repeated small doses of parenteral iron over a protracted period. The latter approach is common in dialysis centers, where it is not unusual for 100 mg of elemental iron to be given weekly for 10 weeks to augment the response to recombinant erythropoietin therapy. The amount of iron needed by an individual patient is calculated by the following formula:

Body weight (kg) $\times$ 2.3 $\times$ (15 $-$ patient's hemoglobin, g/dL)
$$+ \text{ 500 or 1000 mg (for stores)}.$$

In administering intravenous iron dextran, anaphylaxis is a concern. Anaphylaxis is almost never seen with the newer preparations. The factors that have correlated with a serious anaphylactic-like reaction include a history of multiple allergies or a prior allergic reaction to dextran (in the case of iron dextran). Generalized symptoms appearing several days after the infusion of a large dose of iron can include arthralgias, skin rash, and low-grade fever. This may be dose-related, but it does not preclude the further use of parenteral iron in the patient. To date, patients with sensitivity to iron dextran have been safely treated with iron gluconate. If a large dose of iron dextran is to be given (>100 mg) the iron preparation should be diluted in 5% dextrose in water or 0.9% NaCl solution. The iron solution can then be infused over a 60- to 90-min period (for larger doses) or at a rate convenient for the attending nurse or physician. While a test dose (25 mg) of parenteral iron is recommended, in reality a slow infusion of a larger dose of parenteral iron solution will afford the same kind of early warning as a separately injected test dose. Early in the infusion of iron, if chest pain, wheezing, a fall in blood pressure, or other systemic manifestations occur, the infusion of iron—whether as a large solution or a test dose—should be interrupted immediately.

OTHER HYPOPROLIFERATIVE ANEMIAS

In addition to mild to moderate iron deficiency anemia, the hypoproliferative anemias can be divided into four categories: (1) chronic inflammation/infection; (2) renal disease; (3) endocrine and nutritional deficiencies (hypometabolic states); and (4) marrow damage (Chap. 94). With chronic inflammation, renal disease, or hypometabolism, endogenous erythropoietin production is inadequate for the degree of anemia observed. For the anemia of chronic inflammation (anemia of chronic disease), the erythroid marrow also responds inadequately to stimulation, due in part to defects in *iron reutilization*. As a result of the lack of adequate erythropoietin stimulation, an examination of the peripheral blood smear will disclose only an occasional polychromatophilic ("shift") reticulocyte. In the cases of iron deficiency or marrow damage, appropriate elevations in endogenous erythropoietin levels are typically found, and shift reticulocytes will be present on the blood smear.

ANEMIA OF ACUTE AND CHRONIC INFLAMMATION/INFECTION (THE ANEMIA OF CHRONIC DISEASE) The anemia of chronic disease—which encompasses inflammation, infection, tissue injury, and conditions associated with the release of proinflammatory cytokines (such as cancer)—is one of the most common forms of anemia seen clinically and is probably the most important in the differential diagnosis of iron deficiency, since many of the features of the anemia are brought about by inadequate iron delivery to the marrow, despite the presence of normal or increased iron stores. This is reflected by a low serum iron, increased red cell protoporphyrin, a hypoproliferative marrow, transferrin saturation in the range of 15 to 20%, and a normal or increased serum ferritin. The serum ferritin values are often the most distinguishing

feature between true iron deficiency anemia and the iron-deficient erythropoiesis associated with inflammation. Typically, serum ferritin values increase threefold over basal levels in the face of inflammation. All of these changes are due to the effects of inflammatory cytokines and hepcidin, the storage iron regulator, acting at several levels of erythropoiesis (Fig. 90-4). Interleukin 1 (IL-1) directly decreases erythropoietin production in response to anemia. IL-1, acting through accessory cell release of interferon γ (IFN-γ), suppresses the response of the erythroid marrow to erythropoietin—an effect that can be overcome by increased erythropoietin administration in vitro and in vivo. In addition, tumor necrosis factor (TNF), acting through the release of IFN-γ by marrow stromal cells, also suppresses the response to erythropoietin. Hepcidin, made by the liver, is increased in inflammation and acts to suppress iron absorption and iron release from storage sites. The overall result is a chronic hypoproliferative anemia with classic changes in iron metabolism. The anemia is further compounded by a mild to moderate shortening in red cell survival.

With chronic inflammation/infection, the primary disease will determine the severity and characteristics of the anemia. For instance, many patients with cancer also have anemia that is typically normocytic and normochromic. In contrast, patients with long-standing active rheumatoid arthritis or chronic infections such as tuberculosis will have a microcytic, hypochromic anemia. In both cases, the bone marrow is hypoproliferative, but the differences in red cell indices reflect differences in the availability of iron for hemoglobin synthesis. Occasionally, conditions associated with chronic inflammation are also associated with chronic blood loss. Under these circumstances, a bone marrow aspirate stained for iron may be necessary to rule out absolute iron deficiency. However, the administration of iron in this case will correct the iron deficiency component of the anemia and leave the inflammatory component unaffected.

The anemia associated with acute infection or inflammation is typically mild but becomes more pronounced over time. Acute infection can produce a fall in hemoglobin levels of 2 to 3 g/dL within 1 or 2 days; this is largely related to the hemolysis of red cells near the end of their natural life span. The fever and cytokines released exert a selective pressure against cells with more limited capacity to maintain the red cell membrane. In most individuals the mild anemia is reasonably well tolerated, and symptoms, if present, are associated with the underlying disease. Occasionally, in patients with preexisting cardiac disease, moderate anemia (hemoglobin 10–11 g/dL) may be associated with angina, exercise intolerance, and shortness of breath. The red cell indices vary from normocytic, normochromic to microcytic, hypochromic. The serum iron values tend to correlate with the red cell indices. The erythropoietic profile that distinguishes the anemia of

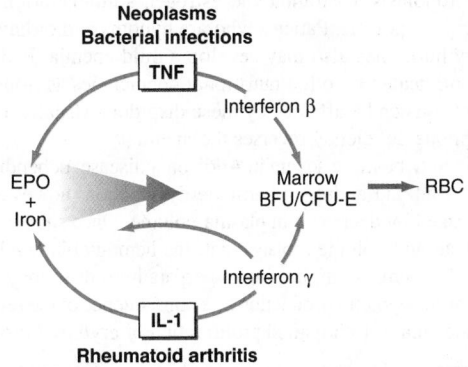

FIGURE 90-4 Suppression of erythropoiesis by inflammatory cytokines. Through the release of tumor necrosis factor (TNF) and interferon γ (IFN-γ) neoplasms and bacterial infections suppress erythropoietin (EPO) production, the release of iron from reticuloendothelial stores, and the proliferation of erythroid progenitors [erythroid burst-forming units and erythroid colony-forming units (BFU/CFU-E)]. The mediators in patients with vasculitis and rheumatoid arthritis include interleukin 1 (IL-1) and IFN-γ. The red arrows indicate sites of inflammatory cytokine inhibitory effects.

TABLE 90-6 *Diagnosis of Hypoproliferative Anemias*

Tests	Iron Deficiency	Inflammation	Renal Disease	Hypometabolic States
Anemia	Mild to severe	Mild	Mild to severe	Mild
MCV (fL)	60–90	80–90	90	90
Morphology	Normo-microcytic	Normocytic	Normocytic	Normocytic
SI	<30	<50	Normal	Normal
TIBC	>360	<300	Normal	Normal
Saturation (%)	<10	10–20	Normal	Normal
Serum ferritin (μg/L)	<15	30–200	115–150	Normal
Iron stores	0	2–4+	1–4+	Normal

Note: MCV, mean corpuscular volume; SI, serum iron; TIBC, total iron-binding capacity.

inflammation from the other causes of hypoproliferative anemias is shown in Table 90-6.

ANEMIA OF RENAL DISEASE Chronic renal failure is usually associated with a moderate to severe hypoproliferative anemia; the level of the anemia correlates with the severity of the renal failure. Red cells are typically normocytic and normochromic. Reticulocytes are decreased. The anemia is due to a failure to produce adequate amounts of erythropoietin and a reduction in red cell survival. In certain forms of acute renal failure, the correlation between the anemia and renal function is weaker. Patients with the hemolytic-uremic syndrome increase erythropoiesis in response to the hemolysis, despite renal failure requiring dialysis. Polycystic renal disease also shows a smaller degree of erythropoietin deficiency for a given level of renal failure. By contrast, patients with diabetes have more severe erythropoietin deficiency for a given level of renal failure.

Assessment of iron status provides information to distinguish the anemia of renal disease from the other forms of hypoproliferative anemia (Table 90-6) and to guide management. Patients with the anemia of renal disease usually present with normal serum iron, TIBC, and ferritin levels. However, those maintained on chronic hemodialysis may develop iron deficiency from blood loss through the dialysis procedure. Iron must be replenished in these patients to ensure an adequate response to erythropoietin therapy (see below).

ANEMIA IN HYPOMETABOLIC STATES Patients who are starving, particularly for protein, and those with a variety of endocrine disorders that produce lower metabolic rates may develop a mild to moderate hypoproliferative anemia. The release of erythropoietin from the kidney is sensitive to the need for O_2, not just O_2 levels. Thus, erythropoietin production is triggered at lower levels of O_2 tension in disease states (such as hypothyroidism and starvation) where metabolic activity, and thus O_2 demand, is decreased.

Endocrine Deficiency States The difference in the levels of hemoglobin between men and women is related to the effects of androgen and estrogen on erythropoiesis. Testosterone and anabolic steroids augment erythropoiesis; castration and estrogen administration to males decrease erythropoiesis. Patients who are hypothyroid or have deficits in pituitary hormones also may develop a mild anemia. Pathogenesis may be complicated by other nutritional deficiencies as iron and folic acid absorption can be affected by these disorders. Usually, correction of the hormone deficiency reverses the anemia.

Anemia may be more severe in Addison's disease, depending on the level of thyroid and androgen hormone dysfunction; however, anemia may be masked by decreases in plasma volume. Once such patients are given cortisol and volume replacement, the hemoglobin level may fall rapidly. Mild anemia complicating hyperparathyroidism may be due to decreased erythropoietin production as a consequence of the renal effects of hypercalcemia or to impaired proliferation of erythroid progenitors.

Protein Starvation Decreased dietary intake of protein may lead to mild to moderate hypoproliferative anemia; this form of anemia may be prevalent in the elderly. The anemia can be more severe in patients with a greater degree of starvation. In marasmus, where patients are both protein- and calorie-deficient, the release of erythropoietin is impaired in proportion to the reduction in metabolic rate; however, the degree of anemia may be masked by volume depletion and becomes apparent after refeeding. Deficiencies in other nutrients (iron, folate) may also complicate the clinical picture but may not be apparent at diagnosis. Changes in the erythrocyte indices on refeeding should prompt evaluation of iron, folate, and B_{12} status.

Anemia in Liver Disease A mild hypoproliferative anemia may develop in patients with chronic liver disease from nearly any cause. The peripheral blood smear may show spur cells and stomatocytes from the accumulation of excess cholesterol in the membrane from a deficiency of lecithin cholesterol acyltransferase. Red cell survival is shortened, and the production of erythropoietin is inadequate to compensate. In alcoholic liver disease, nutritional deficiencies can add complexity to the management. Folate deficiency from inadequate intake, as well as iron deficiency from blood loss and inadequate intake, can alter the red cell indices.

℞ TREATMENT

Many patients with hypoproliferative anemias experience recovery of normal hemoglobin levels when the underlying disease is appropriately treated. For those in whom such reversals are not possible—such as patients with end-stage renal failure, cancer, and chronic inflammatory diseases—symptomatic anemia requires treatment. The two major forms of treatment are transfusions and erythropoietin.

Transfusions Thresholds for transfusion should be altered based on the patient's symptoms. In general, patients without serious underlying cardiovascular or pulmonary disease can tolerate hemoglobin levels above 8 g/dL and do not require intervention until the hemoglobin falls below that level. Patients with more physiologic compromise may need to have their hemoglobin levels kept above 11 g/dL. A typical unit of packed red cells increases the hemoglobin level by 1 g/dL. Transfusions are associated with certain infectious risks (Chap. 99), and chronic transfusions can produce iron overload.

Erythropoietin Erythropoietin is particularly useful in anemias in which endogenous erythropoietin levels are inappropriately low, such as the hypoproliferative anemias. Iron status must be evaluated and iron repleted to obtain optimal effects from erythropoietin. In patients with chronic renal failure, the usual dose of erythropoietin is 50 to 150 U/kg three times a week subcutaneously. Hemoglobin levels of 10 to 12 g/dL are usually reached within 4 to 6 weeks if iron levels are adequate; 90% of these patients respond. Once a target hemoglobin level is reached, the erythropoietin dose can be decreased. A fall in hemoglobin level occurring in the face of erythropoietin therapy usually signifies the development of an infection or iron depletion. Aluminum toxicity and hyperparathyroidism can also compromise the erythropoietin response. When an infection intervenes, it is best to interrupt the erythropoietin therapy and rely on transfusion to correct the anemia until the infection is adequately treated. The dose needed to correct the anemia in patients with cancer is higher, up to 300 U/kg three times a week, and only about 60% of patients respond.

ACKNOWLEDGMENT
Dr. Robert S. Hillman was the author of this chapter in the 14th edition, and material from his chapter has been retained.

FURTHER READING

BAILIE GR et al: Parenteral iron use in the management of anemia in end-stage renal disease patients. Am J Kidney Dis 35:1, 2000

BRUGNARA C: Iron deficiency and erythropoiesis: New diagnostic approaches. Clin Chem 49:1573, 2003

HILLMAN RS, AULT KA: *Hematology in Clinical Practice*, 3d ed. New York, McGraw-Hill, 2002

HILLMAN RS, FINCH CA: *Red Cell Manual*, 7th ed. Philadelphia, Davis, 1996

TSAKIRIS D: Morbidity and mortality reduction associated with the use of erythropoietin. Nephron 85(Suppl S1):2, 2000

WEINSTEIN DA et al: Inappropriate expression of hepcidin is associated with iron refractory anemia: Implications for the anemia of chronic disease. Blood 100:3776, 2002

91 HEMOGLOBINOPATHIES
Edward J. Benz

Hemoglobin is critical for normal oxygen delivery to tissues; it is also present in erythrocytes in such high concentrations that it can alter red cell shape, deformability, and viscosity. Hemoglobinopathies are disorders affecting the structure, function, or production of hemoglobin. These conditions are usually inherited and range in severity from asymptomatic laboratory abnormalities to death in utero. Different forms may present as hemolytic anemia, erythrocytosis, cyanosis, or vasoocclusive stigmata.

PROPERTIES OF THE HUMAN HEMOGLOBINS

HEMOGLOBIN STRUCTURE Different hemoglobins are produced during embryonic, fetal, and adult life (Fig. 91-1). Each consists of a tetramer of globin polypeptide chains: a pair of α-like chains 141 amino acids long and a pair of β-like chains 146 amino acids long. The major adult hemoglobin, HbA, has the structure $\alpha_2\beta_2$. HbF ($\alpha_2\gamma_2$) predominates during most of gestation, and HbA$_2$ ($\alpha_2\delta_2$) is a minor adult hemoglobin. Embryonic hemoglobins need not be considered here.

Each globin chain enfolds a single heme moiety, consisting of a protoporphyrin IX ring complexed with a single iron atom in the ferrous state (Fe^{2+}), positioned in a manner optimal for reversible binding of oxygen. Each heme moiety can bind a single oxygen molecule; every molecule of hemoglobin can thus transport up to four oxygen molecules.

The amino acid sequences of the various globins are highly homologous to one another. Each has a highly helical *secondary structure*. Their globular *tertiary structures* can cause the exterior surfaces to be rich in polar (hydrophilic) amino acids that enhance solubility and the interior to be lined with nonpolar groups, forming a hydrophobic pocket into which heme is inserted. The tetrameric *quaternary structure* of HbA contains two $\alpha\beta$ dimers. Numerous tight interactions (i.e., $\alpha_1\beta_1$ contacts) hold the α and β chains together. The complete tetramer is held together by interfaces (i.e., $\alpha_1\beta_2$ contacts) between the α-like chain of one dimer and the non-α chain of the other dimer.

The hemoglobin tetramer is highly soluble but individual globin chains are insoluble. Unpaired globin precipitates, forming inclusions that damage the cell. Normal globin chain synthesis is balanced so that each newly synthesized α or non-α globin chain will have an available partner with which to pair to form hemoglobin.

Solubility and reversible oxygen binding are the key properties deranged in hemoglobinopathies. Both depend most on the hydrophilic surface amino acids, the hydrophobic amino acids lining the heme pocket, a key histidine in the F helix, and the amino acids forming the $\alpha_1\beta_1$ and $\alpha_1\beta_2$ contact points. Mutations in these strategic regions tend to be the ones that alter clinical behavior.

FUNCTION OF HEMOGLOBIN To support oxygen transport, hemoglobin must bind O$_2$ efficiently at the partial pressure of oxygen (P$_{O_2}$) of the alveolus, retain it, and release it to tissues at the P$_{O_2}$ of tissue capillary beds. Oxygen acquisition and delivery over a relatively narrow range of oxygen tensions depend on a property inherent in the tetrameric arrangement of heme and globin subunits within the hemoglobin molecule called *cooperativity* or *heme-heme interaction*.

At low oxygen tensions, the hemoglobin tetramer is fully deoxygenated (Fig.

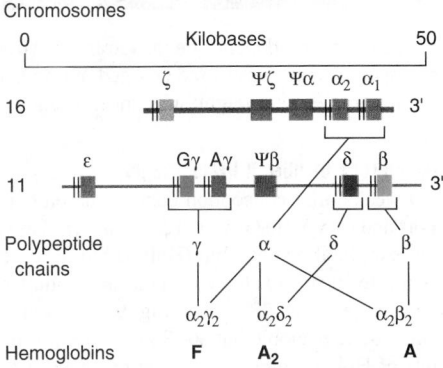

FIGURE 91-1 The globin genes. The α-like genes (α,ζ) are encoded on chromosome 16; the β-like genes ($\beta,\gamma,\delta,\varepsilon$) are encoded on chromosome 11. The ζ and ε genes encode embryonic globins.

91-2). Oxygen binding begins slowly as O$_2$ tension rises. However, as soon as some oxygen has been bound by the tetramer, an abrupt increase occurs in the slope of the curve. Thus, hemoglobin molecules that have bound some oxygen develop a higher oxygen affinity, greatly accelerating their ability to combine with more oxygen. This S-shaped oxygen equilibrium curve (Fig. 91-2), along which substantial amounts of oxygen loading *and unloading* can occur over a narrow range of oxygen tensions, is physiologically more useful than the high-affinity hyperbolic curve of individual monomers.

Oxygen affinity is modulated by several factors. The Bohr effect arises from the stabilizing action of protons on deoxyhemoglobin, which binds protons more readily than oxyhemoglobin because it is a weaker acid (Fig. 91-2). Thus, hemoglobin has a lower oxygen affinity at low pH, facilitating delivery to tissues. The major small molecule that alters oxygen affinity in humans is 2,3-bisphosphoglycerate (2,3-BPG, formerly 2,3-DPG), which lowers oxygen affinity when bound to hemoglobin. HbA has a reasonably high affinity for 2,3-BPG. HbF does not bind 2,3-BPG, so it tends to have a higher oxygen affinity in vivo. Hemoglobin also binds nitric oxide reversibly; this interaction may influence vascular tone, but its physiologic relevance remains unclear.

To understand hemoglobinopathies, it is important to understand

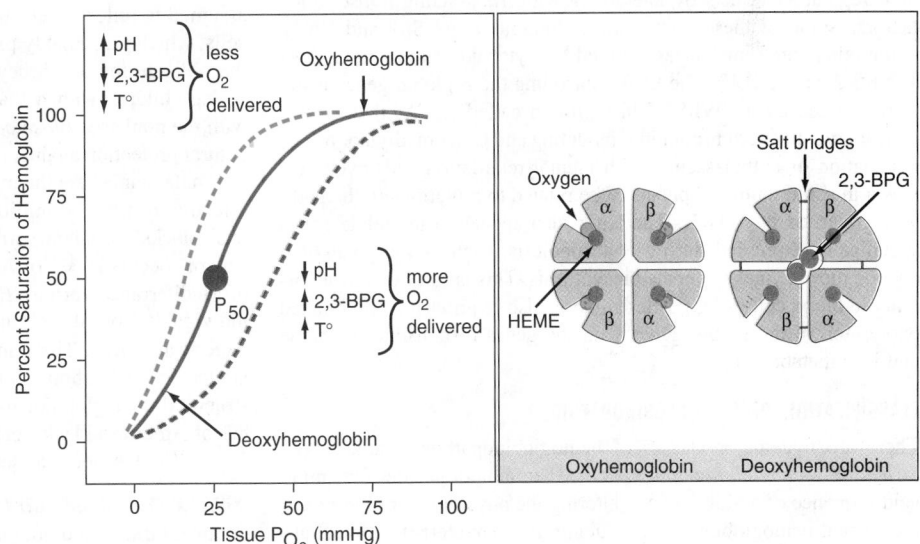

FIGURE 91-2 Hemoglobin-oxygen dissociation curve. The hemoglobin tetramer can bind up to four molecules of oxygen in the iron-containing sites of the heme molecules. As oxygen is bound, 2,3-BPG and CO$_2$ are expelled. Salt bridges are broken, and each of the globin molecules changes its conformation to facilitate oxygen binding. Oxygen release to the tissues is the reverse process, salt bridges being formed and 2,3-BPG and CO$_2$ bound. Deoxyhemoglobin does not bind oxygen efficiently until the cell returns to conditions of higher pH, the most important modulator of O$_2$ affinity (Bohr effect). When acid is produced in the tissues, the dissociation curve shifts to the right, facilitating oxygen release and CO$_2$ binding. Alkalosis has the opposite effect, reducing oxygen delivery.

that proper oxygen transport depends on the tetrameric structure of the proteins, the proper arrangement of the charged amino acids, and interaction with low-molecular-weight substances such as protons or 2,3-BPG.

DEVELOPMENTAL BIOLOGY OF HUMAN HEMOGLOBINS

Red cells first appearing at about 6 weeks after conception contain the embryonic hemoglobins Hb Portland ($\zeta_2\gamma_2$), Hb Gower I ($\zeta_2\varepsilon_2$), and Hb Gower II ($\alpha_2\varepsilon_2$). At 10 to 11 weeks, fetal hemoglobin (HbF; $\alpha_2\gamma_2$) becomes predominant. The switch to nearly exclusive synthesis of adult hemoglobin (HbA; $\alpha_2\beta_2$) occurs at about 38 weeks (Fig. 91-1). Fetuses and newborns therefore require α-globin but not β-globin for normal gestation. Small amounts of HbF are produced during postnatal life. A few red cell clones called *F cells* are progeny of a small pool of immature committed erythroid precursors (BFU-e) that retain the ability to produce HbF. Profound erythroid stress, such as that seen in severe hemolytic anemias, after bone marrow transplant, or during chemotherapy, causes more of the F-potent BFU-e to be recruited. HbF levels thus tend to rise in some patients with sickle cell anemia or thalassemia. This phenomenon is also important because it probably explains the ability of hydroxyurea to increase levels of HbF in adults. Fetal globin genes can also be activated partially after birth by agents such as butyrate that inhibit histone deacetylase and modify the structure of chromatin.

GENETICS AND BIOSYNTHESIS OF HUMAN HEMOGLOBIN

The human hemoglobins are encoded in two tightly linked gene clusters; the α-like globin genes are clustered on chromosome 16, and the β-like genes on chromosome 11 (Fig. 91-1). The α-like cluster consists of two α-globin genes and a single copy of the ζ gene. The non-α gene cluster consists of a single ε gene, the Gγ and Aγ fetal globin genes, and the adult δ and β genes.

Important regulatory sequences flank each gene. Immediately upstream are typical promoter elements needed for the assembly of the transcription initiation complex. Sequences in the 5' flanking region of the γ and the β genes appear to be crucial for the correct developmental regulation of these genes, while elements that function like classic enhancers and silencers are in the 3' flanking regions. The locus control region (LCR) elements located far upstream appear to control the overall level of expression of each cluster. These elements achieve their regulatory effects by interacting with *trans*-acting transcription factors. Some of these factors are ubiquitous (e.g., Sp1 and YY1), while others are more or less limited to erythroid cells (e.g., GATA-1, NFE-2, and EKLF). The LCR controlling the α globin gene cluster is modulated by a SWI/SNF-like protein called *ATRX*; this protein appears to influence chromatin remodeling and DNA methylation. The association of α thalassemia with mental retardation and myelodysplasia in some families appears to be related to mutations in the pathway governed by ATRX. The latter also appear to modulate genes specifically expressed during erythropoiesis, such as the genes that encode the enzymes for heme biosynthesis. This is relevant since normal red blood cell (RBC) differentiation also requires the coordinated expression of the globin genes with the genes responsible for heme and iron metabolism.

CLASSIFICATION OF HEMOGLOBINOPATHIES

There are five major classes of hemoglobinopathies (Table 91-1). *Structural hemoglobinopathies* occur when mutations alter the amino acid sequence of a globin chain, altering the physiologic properties of the variant hemoglobins and producing the characteristic clinical abnormalities. The variant hemoglobins relevant to this chapter polymerize abnormally, as in sickle cell anemia, or exhibit altered solubility or oxygen-binding affinity. *Thalassemia syndromes* arise from mutations that impair production or translation of globin mRNA, leading to deficient globin chain biosynthesis. Clinical abnormalities are attributable to the inadequate supply of hemoglobin and the imbalances in the production of individual globin chains, leading to premature

TABLE 91-1   Classification of Hemoglobinopathies

I. Structural hemoglobinopathies—hemoglobins with altered amino acid sequences that result in deranged function or altered physical or chemical properties
   A. Abnormal hemoglobin polymerization—HbS, hemoglobin sickling
   B. Altered O_2 affinity
      1. High affinity—polycythemia
      2. Low affinity—cyanosis, pseudoanemia
   C. Hemoglobins that oxidize readily
      1. Unstable hemoglobins—hemolytic anemia, jaundice
      2. M hemoglobins—methemoglobinemia, cyanosis
II. Thalassemias—defective biosynthesis of globin chains
   A. α Thalassemias
   B. β Thalassemias
   C. $\delta\beta$, $\gamma\delta\beta$, $\alpha\beta$ Thalassemias
III. Thalassemic hemoglobin variants—structurally abnormal Hb associated with coinherited thalassemic phenotype
   A. HbE
   B. Hb Constant Spring
   C. Hb Lepore
IV. Hereditary persistence of fetal hemoglobin—persistence of high levels of HbF into adult life
V. Acquired hemoglobinopathies
   A. Methemoglobin due to toxic exposures
   B. Sulfhemoglobin due to toxic exposures
   C. Carboxyhemoglobin
   D. HbH in erythroleukemia
   E. Elevated HbF in states of erythroid stress and bone marrow dysplasia

destruction of erythroblasts and red cells. *Thalassemic hemoglobin variants* combine features of thalassemia (e.g., abnormal globin biosynthesis) and of structural hemoglobinopathies (e.g., an abnormal amino acid sequence). *Hereditary persistence of fetal hemoglobin* (HPFH) is characterized by synthesis of high levels of fetal hemoglobin in adult life. *Acquired hemoglobinopathies* include modifications of the hemoglobin molecule by toxins (e.g., acquired methemoglobinemia) and abnormal hemoglobin synthesis (e.g., high levels of HbF production in preleukemia and α thalassemia in myeloproliferative disorders).

EPIDEMIOLOGY   Hemoglobinopathies are especially common in areas in which malaria is endemic. This clustering of hemoglobinopathies is assumed to reflect a selective survival advantage for the abnormal red cells, which presumably provide a less hospitable environment during the obligate intraerythrocytic stages of the parasitic life cycle. Very young children with α thalassemia are *more* susceptible to infection with the nonlethal *Plasmodium vivax*. Thalassemia might then favor a natural protection against infection with the more lethal *P. falciparum*.

Thalassemias are the most common genetic disorders in the world, affecting nearly 200 million people worldwide. About 15% of American blacks are silent carriers for α thalassemia; α-thalassemia trait (minor) occurs in 3% of American blacks and in 1 to 15% of persons of Mediterranean origin. β Thalassemia has a 10 to 15% incidence in individuals from the Mediterranean and Southeast Asia and 0.8% in American blacks. The number of severe cases of thalassemia in the United States is about 1000. Sickle cell disease is the most common structural hemoglobinopathy occurring in heterozygous form in about 8% of American blacks and in homozygous form in 1 in 400. Between 2 and 3% of American blacks carry a hemoglobin C allele.

INHERITANCE AND ONTOGENY   Hemoglobinopathies are autosomal codominant traits—compound heterozygotes who inherit a different abnormal mutant allele from each parent exhibit composite features of each. For example, patients inheriting sickle β thalassemia exhibit features of β thalassemia and sickle cell anemia. The α chain is present in HbA, HbA$_2$, and HbF; α-chain mutations thus cause abnormalities in all three. The α-globin hemoglobinopathies are symptomatic in utero and after birth because normal function of the α-globin gene is required throughout gestation and adult life. In contrast, infants with β-globin hemoglobinopathies tend to be asymptomatic until 3 to 9 months of age, when HbA has largely replaced HbF.

DETECTION AND CHARACTERIZATION OF HEMOGLOBINOPATHIES— GENERAL METHODS

Of the many methods available for hemoglobin analysis, electrophoretic techniques are used for routine clinical purposes. Electrophoresis at pH 8.6 on cellulose acetate membranes is especially simple, inexpensive, and reliable for initial screening. Agar gel electrophoresis at pH 6.1 in citrate buffer is often used as a complementary method because each method detects different variants. Comparison of results obtained in each system usually allows unambiguous diagnosis, but some important variants are electrophoretically silent. These mutant hemoglobins can usually be characterized by more specialized techniques such as isoelectric focusing and/or high pressure liquid chromatography (HPLC).

Quantitation of the hemoglobin profile is often desirable. HbA_2 is frequently elevated in β-thalassemia trait and depressed in iron deficiency. HbF is elevated in HPFH, some β-thalassemia syndromes, and occasional periods of erythroid stress or marrow dysplasia. For characterization of sickle cell trait, sickle thalassemia syndromes, or HbSC disease, and for monitoring the progress of exchange transfusion therapy to lower the percentage of circulating HbS, quantitation of individual hemoglobins is also required. In most laboratories, quantitation is performed only if the test is specifically ordered.

Because some variants can comigrate with HbA or HbS (sickle hemoglobin), electrophoretic assessment should always be regarded as incomplete unless functional assays for hemoglobin sickling, solubility, or oxygen affinity are also performed, as dictated by the clinical presentation. The best sickling assays involve measurement of the degree to which the hemoglobin sample becomes insoluble, or gelated, as it is deoxygenated (i.e., sickle solubility test). Unstable hemoglobins are detected by their precipitation in isopropanol or after heating to 50°C. High-O_2 affinity and low-O_2 affinity variants are detected by quantitating the P_{50}, the partial pressure of oxygen at which the hemoglobin sample becomes 50% saturated with oxygen. Direct tests for the percent carboxyhemoglobin and methemoglobin, employing spectrophotometric techniques, can readily be obtained from most clinical laboratories on an urgent basis.

Complete characterization, including amino acid sequencing or gene cloning and sequencing, is available from several investigational laboratories around the world. The advent of the polymerase chain reaction (PCR), allele-specific oligonucleotide hybridization, and automated DNA sequencing has made it possible to identify globin gene mutations in a few days.

Laboratory evaluation remains an adjunct, rather than the primary diagnostic aid. Diagnosis is best established by recognition of a characteristic history, physical findings, peripheral blood smear morphology, and abnormalities of the complete blood cell count (e.g., profound microcytosis with minimal anemia in thalassemia trait).

STRUCTURALLY ABNORMAL HEMOGLOBINS

SICKLE CELL SYNDROMES The sickle cell syndromes are caused by a mutation in the β-globin gene that changes the sixth amino acid from glutamic acid to valine. HbS ($\alpha_2\beta_2^{6\ Glu\rightarrow Val}$) polymerizes reversibly when deoxygenated to form a gelatinous network of fibrous polymers that stiffen the erythrocyte membrane, increase viscosity, and cause dehydration due to potassium leakage and calcium influx (Fig. 91-3). These changes also produce the char-

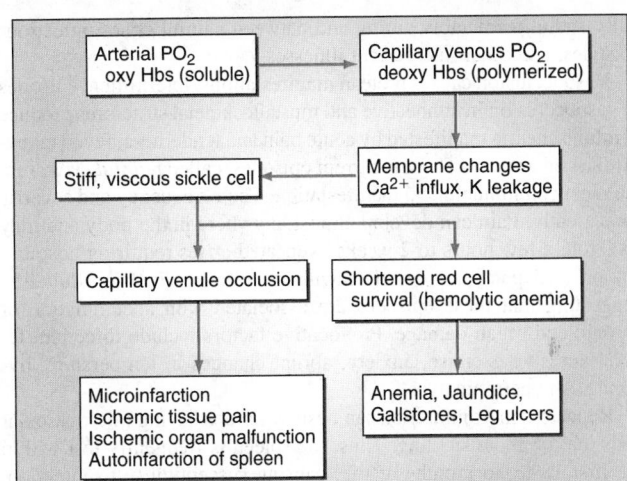

FIGURE 91-3 Pathophysiology of sickle cell crisis.

acteristic sickle shape. Sickled cells lose the pliability needed to traverse small capillaries. They possess altered sticky membranes (especially reticulocytes) that are abnormally adherent to the endothelium of small venules. These abnormalities provoke unpredictable episodes of microvascular vasoocclusion and premature RBC destruction (hemolytic anemia). Hemolysis occurs because the abnormal erythrocytes are destroyed by the spleen. The rigid adherent cells also clog small capillaries and venules, causing tissue ischemia, acute pain, and gradual end-organ damage. This venoocclusive component usually dominates the clinical course. Prominent manifestations include episodes of ischemic pain (i.e., painful crises) and ischemic malfunction or frank infarction in the spleen, central nervous system, bones, liver, kidneys, and lungs (Fig. 91-3).

Several sickle syndromes occur as the result of inheritance of HbS from one parent and another hemoglobinopathy, such as β thalassemia or HbC ($\alpha_2\beta_2^{6\ Glu\rightarrow Lys}$), from the other parent. The prototype disease, sickle cell anemia, is the homozygous state for HbS (Table 91-2).

Clinical Manifestations of Sickle Cell Anemia Most patients with sickling syndromes suffer from hemolytic anemia, with hematocrits from 15 to 30%, and significant reticulocytosis. Anemia was once thought to exert protective effects against vasoocclusion by reducing blood viscosity. However, natural history and drug therapy trials suggest that an *increase* in the hematocrit and feedback inhibition of reticulocytosis might be beneficial, even at the expense of increased blood viscosity. The role of adhesive reticulocytes in vasoocclusion might account for these paradoxical effects.

Granulocytosis is common. The white count can fluctuate substan-

TABLE 91-2 Clinical Features of Sickle Hemoglobinopathies

Condition	Clinical Abnormalities	Hemoglobin Level g/L (g/dL)	MCV, fL	Hemoglobin Electrophoresis
Sickle cell trait	None; rare painless hematuria	Normal	Normal	Hb S/A:40/60
Sickle cell anemia	Vasoocclusive crises with infarction of spleen, brain, marrow, kidney, lung; aseptic necrosis of bone; gallstones; priapism; ankle ulcers	70–100 (7–10)	80–100	Hb S/A:100/0 Hb F:2–25%
S/β° thalassemia	Vasoocclusive crises; aseptic necrosis of bone	70–100 (7–10)	60–80	Hb S/A:100/0 Hb F:1–10%
S/β⁺ thalassemia	Rare crises and aseptic necrosis	100–140 (10–14)	70–80	Hb S/A:60/40
Hemoglobin SC	Rare crises and aseptic necrosis; painless hematuria	100–140 (10–14)	80–100	Hb S/A:50/0 Hb C:50%

tially and unpredictably during and between painful crises, infectious episodes, and other intercurrent illnesses.

Vasoocclusion causes protean manifestations. Intermittent episodes of vasoocclusion in connective and musculoskeletal structures produce painful ischemia manifested by acute pain and tenderness, fever, tachycardia, and anxiety. These recurrent episodes, called *painful crises*, are the most common clinical manifestation. Their frequency and severity vary greatly. Pain can develop almost anywhere in the body and may last from a few hours to 2 weeks. Repeated crises requiring hospitalization (>3 per year) correlate with reduced survival in adult life, suggesting that these episodes are associated with accumulation of chronic end-organ damage. Provocative factors include infection, fever, excessive exercise, anxiety, abrupt changes in temperature, hypoxia, or hypertonic dyes.

Repeated microinfarction can destroy tissues having microvascular beds that promote sickling. Thus, the spleen is frequently lost within the first 18 to 36 months of life, causing susceptibility to infection, particularly by pneumococci. Acute venous obstruction of the spleen (*splenic sequestration crisis*), a rare occurrence in early childhood, may require emergency transfusion and/or splenectomy to prevent trapping of the entire arterial output in the obstructed spleen. Occlusion of retinal vessels can produce hemorrhage, neovascularization, and eventual detachments. Renal papillary necrosis invariably produces isosthenuria. More widespread renal necrosis leads to renal failure in adults, a common late cause of death. Bone and joint ischemia can lead to aseptic necrosis, especially of the femoral or humeral heads; chronic arthropathy; and unusual susceptibility to osteomyelitis, which may be caused by organisms, such as *Salmonella*, rarely encountered in other settings. The *hand-foot syndrome* is caused by painful infarcts of the digits and dactylitis. Stroke is especially common in children, a small subset of whom tend to suffer repeated episodes; stroke is less common in adults and is often hemorrhagic. A particularly painful complication in males is priapism, due to infarction of the penile venous outflow tracts; permanent impotence is a frequent consequence. Chronic lower leg ulcers probably arise from ischemia and superinfection in the distal circulation.

Acute chest syndrome is a distinctive manifestation characterized by chest pain, tachypnea, fever, cough, and arterial oxygen desaturation. It can mimic pneumonia, pulmonary emboli, bone marrow infarction and embolism, myocardial ischemia, or in situ lung infarction. Acute chest syndrome is thought to reflect in situ sickling within the lung producing pain and temporary pulmonary dysfunction. It is frequently difficult or impossible to distinguish among other possibilities. Pulmonary infarction and pneumonia are the most frequent underlying or concomitant conditions in patients with this syndrome. Repeated episodes of acute chest pain correlate with reduced survival. Acutely, reduction in arterial oxygen saturation is especially ominous because it promotes sickling on a massive scale. Chronic acute or subacute pulmonary crises lead to pulmonary hypertension and cor pulmonale, an increasingly common cause of death as patients survive further into adult life.

Sickle cell syndromes are remarkable for their clinical heterogeneity. Some patients remain virtually asymptomatic into or even through adult life, while others suffer repeated crises requiring hospitalization from early childhood. Patients with sickle thalassemia and sickle-HbE tend to have similar, slightly milder, symptoms, perhaps because of the ameliorating effects of production of other hemoglobins within the RBC. Hemoglobin SC disease, one of the more common variants of sickle cell anemia, is frequently marked by lesser degrees of hemolytic anemia and a greater propensity for the development of retinopathy and aseptic necrosis of bones. In most respects, however, the clinical manifestations resemble sickle cell anemia. Some rare hemoglobin variants actually aggravate the sickling phenomenon.

Clinical Manifestations of Sickle Cell Trait Sickle cell trait is usually asymptomatic. Anemia and painful crises are exceedingly rare. An

uncommon, but highly distinctive, symptom is painless hematuria often occurring in adolescent males, probably due to papillary necrosis. Isosthenuria is a more common manifestation of the same process. Sloughing of papillae with ureteral obstruction has been reported, as have isolated cases of massive sickling or sudden death due to exposure to high altitudes or extraordinary extremes of exercise and dehydration.

Diagnosis Sickle cell syndromes are readily suspected on the basis of characteristic hemolytic anemia, red cell morphology (Fig. 91-4), and intermittent episodes of ischemic pain. Diagnosis is confirmed by hemoglobin electrophoresis and the sickling tests already discussed. Thorough characterization of the exact hemoglobin profile of the patient is important, because sickle thalassemia and hemoglobin SC disease are correlated with alterations in prognosis or clinical features. Diagnosis is usually established in childhood, but occasional patients, often with compound heterozygous states, do not develop symptoms until the onset of puberty, pregnancy, or early adult life. Genotyping of family members and potential parental partners is critical for genetic counseling. Details of the childhood history establish prognosis and eligibility for aggressive or experimental therapies. Factors associated with increased morbidity and reduced survival are more than three crises requiring hospitalization per year, a chronic neutrophilia, a history of splenic sequestration or hand-foot syndrome, and second episodes of acute chest syndrome. Patients with a history of cerebrovascular accidents are at higher risk for repeated episodes and require especially close monitoring.

℞ TREATMENT

Patients with sickle cell syndromes require ongoing continuity of care. Familiarity with the pattern of symptoms provides the best safeguard against excessive use of the emergency room, hospitalization, and habituation to addictive narcotics. Additional preventive measures include regular slit-lamp examinations to monitor development of retinopathy; antibiotic prophylaxis appropriate for splenectomized patients during dental or other invasive procedures; and vigorous oral hydration during or in anticipation of periods of extreme exercise, exposure to heat or cold, emotional stress, or infection. Pneumococcal and *Haemophilus influenzae* vaccines are less effective in splenectomized individuals. Thus, patients with sickle cell anemia should be vaccinated early in life.

The management of acute painful crisis includes vigorous hydration, thorough evaluation for underlying causes (such as infection), and aggressive analgesia administered by a standing order and/or patient-controlled analgesia (PCA) pump. Morphine (0.1 to 0.15 mg/kg every 3 to 4 h) or meperidine (0.75 to 1.5 mg/kg every 2 to 4 h) should control severe pain. Meperidine should be used only for acute short-term pain control; as a chronic analgesic, it is unsuitable. Bone pain may respond as well to ketorolac (30 to 60 mg initial dose, then 15 to 30 mg every 6 to 8 h). Inhalation of nitrous oxide can provide short-term pain relief, but great care must be exercised to avoid hypoxia and respiratory depression. Nitrous oxide also elevates O_2 affinity, reducing O_2 delivery to tissues. Its use should be restricted to experts. Many crises can be managed at home with oral hydration and oral analgesia. Use of the emergency room should be reserved for especially severe symptoms or circumstances in which other processes, e.g., infection, are strongly suspected. Nasal oxygen should be employed as appropriate to protect arterial saturation. Most crises resolve in 1 to 7 days.

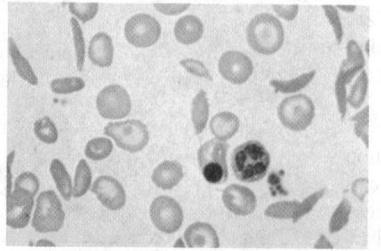

FIGURE 91-4 Sickle cell anemia. The elongated and crescent-shaped red blood cells seen on this smear represent circulating irreversibly sickled cells. Target cells and a nucleated red blood cell are also seen.

Use of blood transfusion should be reserved for extreme cases: no evidence exists for a beneficial effect in shortening the duration of the crisis.

No tests are definitive to diagnose acute painful crisis. Critical to good management is an approach that recognizes that most patients reporting crisis symptoms do indeed have crisis or another significant medical problem. Diligent diagnostic evaluation for underlying causes is imperative, even though these are found infrequently. In adults, the possibility of aseptic necrosis or sickle arthropathy must be considered, especially if pain and immobility become repeated or chronic at a single site. Nonsteroidal anti-inflammatory agents are often effective for sickle cell arthropathy.

Acute chest syndrome is a medical emergency that may require management in an intensive care unit. Hydration should be monitored carefully to avoid the development of pulmonary edema, and oxygen therapy should be especially vigorous for protection of arterial saturation. Diagnostic evaluation for pneumonia and pulmonary embolism should be especially thorough, since these may occur with atypical symptoms. Critical interventions are transfusion to maintain a hematocrit >30, and emergency exchange transfusion if arterial saturation drops to <90%. As patients with sickle cell syndrome increasingly survive into their fifth and sixth decades, end-stage renal failure and pulmonary hypertension are becoming increasingly prominent causes of end-stage morbidity. Anecdotal evidence suggests that a sickle cell cardiomyopathy and/or premature coronary artery disease may compromise cardiac function in later years. Sickle cell patients have received kidney transplants, but they often experience an increase in the frequency and severity of crises, possibly due to increased infection as a consequence of immunosuppression.

The most significant advance in the therapy of sickle cell anemia has been the introduction of hydroxyurea as a mainstay of therapy for patients with severe symptoms. Hydroxyurea (10 to 30 mg/kg per day) increases fetal hemoglobin and may also exert beneficial affects on red cell hydration, vascular wall adherence, and suppression of the granulocyte and reticulocyte counts; indeed, dosage is titrated to maintain a white count between 5000 and 8000 cells/μL. White cells and reticulocytes may play a major role in the pathogenesis of sickle cell crisis, and their suppression may be an important benefit of hydroxyurea therapy.

Hydroxyurea should be considered in patients experiencing repeated episodes of acute chest syndrome or with more than three crises per year requiring hospitalization. The utility of this agent for reducing the incidence of other complications (priapism, retinopathy) is under evaluation, as are the long-term side effects. The preponderance of evidence, however, is that hydroxyurea offers broad benefits to most patients whose disease is severe enough to impair their functional status. One long-term study suggests that hydroxyurea may improve survival. A number of experts are advocating more widespread use of this agent. HbF levels increase in most patients within a few months.

The antitumor drug, 5-azacytidine, was the first agent found to elevate HbF. It never achieved widespread use because of concerns about acute toxicity and carcinogenesis. However, low doses of the related agent, 5-deoxyazacytidine (decitabine) can elevate HbF with acceptable toxicity.

Bone marrow transplantation can provide definitive cures but is known to be effective and safe only in children. Prognostic features justifying bone marrow transplant are the presence of repeated crises early in life, a high neutrophil count, or the development of hand-foot syndrome. Children at risk for stroke can now be identified through the use of Doppler ultrasound techniques. Prophylactic exchange transfusion appears to substantially reduce the risk of stroke in this population. Children who do suffer a cerebrovascular accident should be maintained for at least 3 to 5 years on a program of vigorous exchange transfusion, since the risk of second strokes is extremely high in this population.

Gene therapy for sickle cell anemia is being intensively pursued, but no safe measures are currently available. Agents blocking RBC dehydration or vascular adhesion, such as clotrimazole or magnesium, may have value as an adjunct to hydroxyurea therapy, pending the completion of ongoing trials. Combinations of clotrimazole and magnesium are being evaluated in clinical trials.

UNSTABLE HEMOGLOBINS Amino acid substitutions that reduce solubility or increase susceptibility to oxidation produce unstable hemoglobins that precipitate, forming inclusion bodies injurious to the red cell membrane. Representative mutations are those that interfere with contact points between the α and β subunits [e.g., Hb Philly ($\beta^{35Tyr \rightarrow Phe}$)], alter the helical segments [e.g., Hb Genova ($\beta^{28Leu \rightarrow Pro}$)], or disrupt interactions of the hydrophobic pockets of the globin subunits with heme [e.g., Hb Koln ($\beta^{98Val \rightarrow Met}$)] (Table 91-3). The inclusions, called *Heinz bodies*, are clinically detectable by staining with supravital dyes such as crystal violet (Heinz body test). Removal of these inclusions by the spleen generates pitted, rigid cells that have shortened life spans, producing hemolytic anemia of variable severity, sometimes requiring chronic transfusion support. Splenectomy may be needed to correct the anemia. Leg ulcers and premature gallbladder disease due to bilirubin turnover are frequent stigmata.

Unstable hemoglobins occur sporadically, often by spontaneous new mutations. Heterozygotes are often symptomatic because a significant Heinz body burden can develop even when the unstable variant accounts for a portion of the total hemoglobin. Symptomatic unstable hemoglobins tend to be β-globin variants, because sporadic mutations affecting only one of the four α globins would generate only 20 to 30% abnormal hemoglobin.

HEMOGLOBINS WITH ALTERED OXYGEN AFFINITY *High-affinity hemoglobins* [e.g., Hb Yakima ($\beta^{99 Asp \rightarrow His}$)] bind oxygen more readily but deliver less O_2 to tissues at normal capillary P_{O_2} levels (Fig. 91-2). Mild tissue hypoxia ensues, stimulating RBC production and erythrocytosis (Table 91-3). In extreme cases, the hematocrits can rise to 60 to 65%, increasing blood viscosity and producing typical symptoms (headache, somnolence, or dizziness). Phlebotomy may be required. Typical mutations alter interactions within the heme pocket or disrupt the Bohr effect or salt-bond site. Mutations that impair the interaction of HbA with 2,3-BPG can increase O_2 affinity because 2,3-BPG binding lowers O_2 affinity.

Low-affinity hemoglobins [e.g., Hb Kansas ($\beta^{102Asn \rightarrow Lys}$)] bind sufficient oxygen in the lungs, despite their lower oxygen affinity, to achieve nearly full saturation. At capillary oxygen tensions, they lose sufficient amounts of oxygen to maintain homeostasis at a low hematocrit (Fig. 91-2) (*pseudoanemia*). Capillary hemoglobin desaturation can also be sufficient to produce clinically apparent cyanosis. Despite these findings, patients usually require no specific treatment.

METHEMOGLOBINEMIAS Methemoglobin is generated by oxidation of the heme iron moieties to the ferric state, causing a characteristic bluish-brown muddy color resembling cyanosis. Methemoglobin has such

TABLE 91-3 *Representative Abnormal Hemoglobins with Altered Synthesis or Function*

Designation	Mutation	Population	Main Clinical Effects[a]
Sickle or S	$\beta^{6Glu \rightarrow Val}$	African	Anemia, ischemic infarcts
C	$\beta^{6Glu \rightarrow Lys}$	African	Mild anemia; interacts with HbS
E	$\beta^{26Glu \rightarrow Lys}$	Southeast Asian	Microcytic anemia, splenomegaly, thalassemic phenotype
Köln	$\beta^{98Val \rightarrow Met}$	Sporadic	Hemolytic anemia, Heinz bodies when splenectomized
Yakima	$\beta^{99Asp \rightarrow His}$	Sporadic	Polycythemia
Kansas	$\beta^{102Asn \rightarrow Lys}$	Sporadic	Mild anemia
M. Iwata	$\alpha^{87His \rightarrow Tyr}$	Sporadic	Methemoglobinemia

[a] See text for details.

high oxygen affinity that virtually no oxygen is delivered to tissues. Levels >50 to 60% are often fatal.

Congenital methemoglobinemia arises from globin mutations that stabilize iron in the ferric state [e.g., HbM Iwata ($\alpha^{87 \text{ His} \rightarrow \text{Tyr}}$), Table 91-3] or from mutations that impair the enzymes that reduce methemoglobin to hemoglobin (e.g., methemoglobin reductase, NADP diaphorase). Acquired methemoglobinemia is caused by toxins that oxidize heme iron, notably nitrate and nitrite-containing compounds.

DIAGNOSIS AND MANAGEMENT OF PATIENTS WITH UNSTABLE HEMOGLOBINS, HIGH-AFFINITY HEMOGLOBINS, AND METHEMOGLOBINEMIA *Unstable hemoglobin variants* should be suspected in patients with nonimmune hemolytic anemia, jaundice, splenomegaly, or premature biliary tract disease. Severe hemolysis usually presents during infancy as neonatal jaundice or anemia. Milder cases may present in adult life with anemia or only as unexplained reticulocytosis, hepatosplenomegaly, premature biliary tract disease, or leg ulcers. Because spontaneous mutation is common, family history of anemia may be absent. The peripheral blood smear often shows anisocytosis, abundant cells with punctate inclusions, and irregular shapes (i.e., poikilocytosis).

The two best tests for diagnosing unstable hemoglobins are the Heinz body preparation and the isopropanol or heat stability test. Many unstable Hb variants are electrophoretically silent. A normal electrophoresis does not rule out the diagnosis.

Severely affected patients may require transfusion support for the first 3 years of life, because splenectomy before age 3 is associated with a significantly higher immune deficit. Splenectomy is usually effective thereafter, but occasional patients may require lifelong transfusion support. Even after splenectomy, patients can develop cholelithiasis and leg ulcers. Splenectomy can also be considered in patients exhibiting severe secondary complications of chronic hemolysis, even if anemia is absent. Precipitation of unstable hemoglobins is aggravated by oxidative stress, e.g., infection, antimalarial drugs.

High-O$_2$ affinity hemoglobin variants should be suspected in patients with erythrocytosis. The best test for confirmation is measurement of the P$_{50}$. A high-O$_2$ affinity Hb causes a significant left shift (i.e., lower numeric value of the P$_{50}$); confounding conditions, e.g., tobacco smoking or carbon monoxide exposure, can also lower the P$_{50}$.

High-affinity hemoglobins are often asymptomatic; rubor or plethora may be telltale signs. When the hematocrit reaches to 55 to 60%, symptoms of high blood viscosity and sluggish flow (headache, lethargy, dizziness, etc.) may be present. These persons may benefit from judicious phlebotomy. Erythrocytosis represents an appropriate attempt to compensate for the impaired oxygen delivery by the abnormal variant. Overzealous phlebotomy may stimulate increased erythropoiesis or aggravate symptoms by thwarting this compensatory mechanism. The guiding principle of phlebotomy should be to improve oxygen delivery by reducing blood viscosity and increasing blood flow rather than restoration of a normal hematocrit. Modest iron deficiency may aid in control.

Low-affinity hemoglobins should be considered in patients with cyanosis or a low hematocrit with no other reason apparent after thorough evaluation. The P$_{50}$ test confirms the diagnosis. Counseling and reassurance are the interventions of choice.

Methemoglobin should be suspected in patients with hypoxic symptoms who appear cyanotic but have a Pa$_{O_2}$ sufficiently high that hemoglobin should be fully saturated with oxygen. A history of nitrite or other oxidant ingestions may not always be available; some exposures may be unapparent to the patient, and others may result from suicide attempts. The characteristic muddy appearance of freshly drawn blood can be a critical clue. The diagnostic test of choice is measurement of the methemoglobin content, which is usually available on an emergency basis.

Methemoglobinemia often causes symptoms of cerebral ischemia at levels >15%; levels >60% are usually lethal. Intravenous injection of 1 mg/kg of methylene blue is effective emergency therapy. Milder cases and follow-up of severe cases can be treated orally with methylene blue (60 mg three to four times each day) or ascorbic acid (300 to 600 mg/d).

THALASSEMIA SYNDROMES

The thalassemia syndromes are inherited disorders of α- or β-globin biosynthesis. The reduced supply of globin diminishes production of hemoglobin tetramers, causing hypochromia and microcytosis. Unbalanced accumulation of α and β subunits occurs because the synthesis of the unaffected globins proceeds at a normal rate. Unbalanced chain accumulation dominates the clinical phenotype. Clinical severity varies widely, depending on the degree to which the synthesis of the affected globin is impaired, altered synthesis of other globin chains, and coinheritance of other abnormal globin alleles.

CLINICAL MANIFESTATIONS OF β-THALASSEMIA SYNDROMES Mutations causing thalassemia can affect any step in the pathway of globin gene expression: transcription, processing of the mRNA precursor, translation, and posttranslational metabolism of the β-globin polypeptide chain. The most common forms arise from mutations that derange splicing of the mRNA precursor or prematurely terminate translation of the mRNA.

Hypochromia and microcytosis characterize all forms of β thalassemia because of the reduced amounts of hemoglobin tetramers (Fig. 91-5). In heterozygotes (β-thalassemia trait), this is the only abnormality seen. Anemia is minimal. In more severe homozygous states, unbalanced α- and β-globin accumulation causes accumulation of highly insoluble unpaired α chains. They form toxic inclusion bodies that kill developing erythroblasts in the marrow. Few of the proerythroblasts beginning erythroid maturation survive. The few RBCs surviving bear a burden of inclusion bodies that are detected in the spleen, shortening the RBC life span and producing severe hemolytic anemia. The resulting profound anemia stimulates erythropoietin release and compensatory erythroid hyperplasia, but the marrow response is sabotaged by ineffective erythropoiesis. Anemia persists. Erythroid hyperplasia can become exuberant and produce masses of extramedullary erythropoietic tissue in the liver and spleen.

Massive bone marrow expansion deranges growth and development. Children develop characteristic chipmunk facies due to maxillary marrow hyperplasia and frontal bossing, thinning and pathologic fracture of long bones and vertebrae due to cortical invasion by erythroid elements, and profound growth retardation. Hemolytic anemia causes hepatosplenomegaly, leg ulcers, gallstones, and high-output congestive heart failure. The conscription of caloric resources to support erythropoiesis leads to inanition, susceptibility to infection, endocrine dysfunction, and in the most severe cases, death during the first decade of life. Chronic transfusions with RBCs improves oxygen delivery, suppresses the excessive ineffective erythropoiesis, and prolongs life, but the inevitable side effects, notably iron overload, usually prove fatal by age 30.

Severity is highly variable. Known modulating factors are those that ameliorate the burden of unpaired α-globin inclusions. Alleles associated with milder synthetic defects and coinheritance of α-thalassemia trait reduce clinical severity by reducing accumulation of excess α globin. HbF persists to various degrees in β thalassemias. γ-Globin gene chains can substitute for β chains, simultaneously generating more hemoglobin and reducing the burden of α-globin inclu-

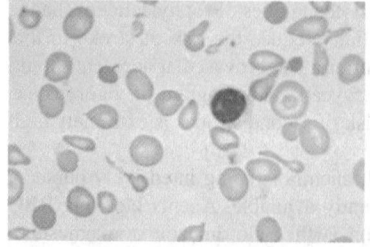

FIGURE 91-5 β-Thalassemia intermedia. Microcytic and hypochromic red blood cells are seen that resemble the red blood cells of severe iron deficiency anemia. Many elliptical and teardrop-shaped red blood cells are noted.

sions. The terms *β-thalassemia major* and *β-thalassemia intermedia* are used to reflect the clinical heterogeneity. Patients with β-thalassemia major require intensive transfusion support to survive. Patients with β-thalassemia intermedia have a somewhat milder phenotype and can survive without transfusion. The terms *β-thalassemia minor* and *β-thalassemia trait* describe asymptomatic heterozygotes for β-thalassemia.

α-THALASSEMIA SYNDROMES The four classic α-thalassemias, most common in Asians, are α-thalassemia-2 trait, in which one of the four α-globin loci is deleted; α-thalassemia-1 trait, with two

TABLE 91-4 The α Thalassemias

Condition	Hemoglobin A, %	Hemoglobin H (β⁴), %	Hemoglobin level, g/L (g/dL)	MCV, fL
Normal	97	0	150 (15)	90
Silent thalassemia: −α/αα	98–100	0	150 (15)	90
Thalassemia trait: −α/−α homozygous α-thal-2[a] or −−/αα heterozygous α-thal-1[a]	85–95	Rare red blood cell inclusions	120–130 (12–13)	70–80
Hemoglobin H disease: −−/−α heterozygous α-thal-1/α-thal-2	70–95	5–30	60–100 (6–10)	60–70
Hydrops fetalis: −−/−− homozygous α-thal-1	0	5–10[b]	Fatal in utero or at birth	

[a] When both α alleles on one chromosome are deleted, the locus is called α-thal-1; when only a single α allele on one chromosome is deleted, the locus is called α-thal-2.

[b] 90–95% of the hemoglobin is hemoglobin Barts (tetramers of γ chains).

deleted loci; HbH disease, with three loci deleted; and hydrops fetalis with Hb Bart's, with all four loci deleted (Table 91-4). Nondeletion forms of α-thalassemia also exist.

α-Thalassemia-2 trait is an asymptomatic, silent carrier state. *α-Thalassemia-1 trait* resembles β-thalassemia minor. Offspring doubly heterozygous for α-thalassemia-2 and α-thalassemia-1 exhibit a more severe phenotype called HbH disease. Heterozygosity for a deletion that removes both genes from the same chromosome (*cis* deletion) is common in Asians and Mediterranean individuals, as is homozygosity for α-thalassemia-2 (*trans* deletion). Both produce asymptomatic hypochromia and microcytosis.

In *HbH disease*, HbA production is only 25 to 30% of normal. Fetuses accumulate some unpaired β chains. In adults, unpaired β chains accumulate and are soluble enough to form $β_4$ tetramers called HbH. HbH forms few inclusions in erythroblasts but does not precipitate in circulating red cells. Patients with HbH disease have thalassemia intermedia characterized by moderately severe hemolytic anemia but milder ineffective erythropoiesis. Survival into mid-adult life without transfusions is common.

The homozygous state for the α-thalassemia-1 *cis* deletion (hydrops fetalis) causes total absence of α-globin synthesis. No physiologically useful hemoglobin is produced beyond the embryonic stage. Excess γ globin forms tetramers called *Hb Barts* ($γ_4$), which has an extraordinarily high oxygen affinity. It delivers almost no O_2 to fetal tissues, causing tissue asphyxia, edema (hydrops fetalis), congestive heart failure, and death in utero. *α-Thalassemia-2 trait* is common (15 to 20%) among people of African descent. The *cis* α-thalassemia-1 deletion is almost never seen, however. Thus, α-thalassemia-2 and the *trans* form of α-thalassemia-1 are very common, but HbH disease and hydrops fetalis are almost never encountered.

It has been known for some time that some patients with myelodysplasia or erythroleukemia produce red cell clones containing HbH. It now appears that this phenomenon is due to mutations in the ATRX pathway that affect the LCR of the α-globin gene cluster.

DIAGNOSIS AND MANAGEMENT OF THALASSEMIAS The diagnosis of β-thalassemia major is readily made during childhood on the basis of severe anemia accompanied by the characteristic signs of massive ineffective erythropoiesis: hepatosplenomegaly, profound microcytosis, a characteristic blood smear (Fig. 91-5), and elevated levels of HbF, HbA₂, or both. Many patients require chronic hypertransfusion therapy designed to maintain a hematocrit of at least 27 to 30% so that erythropoiesis is suppressed. Splenectomy is required if the annual transfusion requirement (volume of RBCs per kilogram of body weight per year) increases by >50%. Folic acid supplements may be useful. Vaccination with Pneumovax in anticipation of eventual splenectomy is advised, as is close monitoring for infection, leg ulcers, and biliary tract disease. Early endocrine evaluation is required for glucose intolerance, thyroid dysfunction, and delayed onset of puberty or secondary sexual characteristics. Many patients develop endocrine deficiencies as a result of iron overload.

Patients with β-thalassemia intermedia exhibit similar stigmata but can survive without chronic hypertransfusion. Management is particularly challenging because a number of factors can aggravate the anemia, including infection, onset of puberty, and development of splenomegaly and hypersplenism. Some patients may eventually benefit from splenectomy. The expanded erythron can cause absorption of excessive dietary iron and hemosiderosis, even without transfusion.

β-Thalassemia minor (i.e., thalassemia trait) usually presents as profound microcytosis and hypochromia with target cells, but only minimal or mild anemia. The mean corpuscular volume is rarely >75 fL; the hematocrit is rarely <30 to 33%. Hemoglobin electrophoresis classically reveals an elevated HbA₂ (3.5 to 7.5%), but some forms are associated with normal HbA₂ and/or elevated HbF. Genetic counseling and patient education are essential. Patients with β-thalassemia trait should be warned that their blood picture resembles iron deficiency and can be misdiagnosed. They should eschew routine use of iron but know that iron deficiency requiring supplementation can develop, as in other persons, during pregnancy or from chronic bleeding.

Persons with α-thalassemia trait may exhibit mild hypochromia and microcytosis usually without anemia. HbA₂ and HbF levels are normal. Affected individuals usually require only genetic counseling. HbH disease resembles β-thalassemia intermedia, with the added complication that the HbH molecule behaves like a moderately unstable hemoglobin. Patients with HbH disease should undergo splenectomy if excessive anemia or a transfusion requirement develops. Oxidative drugs should be avoided. Iron overload leading to death can occur in more severely affected patients.

PREVENTION Antenatal diagnosis of thalassemia syndromes is now widely available. DNA diagnosis is based on PCR amplification of fetal DNA, obtained by amniocentesis or chorionic villus biopsy followed by hybridization to allele-specific oligonucleotides probes. The probes can be designed to detect simultaneously the subset of mutations that account for 95 to 99% of the α- or β-thalassemias that occur in a particular ethnic group.

THALASSEMIC STRUCTURAL VARIANTS

Thalassemic structural variants are characterized by both defective synthesis and abnormal structure.

HEMOGLOBIN LEPORE Hb Lepore [$α_2(δβ)_2$] arises by an unequal crossover and recombination event that fuses the proximal end of the δ-gene with the distal end of the closely linked β-gene. The resulting chromosome contains only the fused δβ gene. The Lepore (δβ) globin is synthesized poorly because the fused gene is under the control of the weak δ-globin promoter. Hb Lepore alleles have a phenotype like β-thalassemia, except for the added presence of 2 to 20% Hb Lepore. Compound heterozygotes for Hb Lepore and a classic β-thalassemia allele may also have severe thalassemia.

HEMOGLOBIN E HbE (i.e., $α_2β_2^{26Glu→Lys}$) is extremely common in Cambodia, Thailand, and Vietnam. The gene has become far more prevalent in the United States as a result of immigration of Asian persons, especially in California, where HbE is the most common variant detected. HbE is mildly unstable but not enough to affect RBC life span significantly. The high frequency of the HbE gene may be a result of the thalassemia phenotype associated with its inheritance. Heterozygotes resemble individuals with mild β-thalassemia trait. Homozygotes have somewhat more marked abnormalities but are asymptomatic. Compound heterozygotes for HbE and a β-thalassemia gene can have β-thalassemia intermedia or β-thalassemia major, depending on the severity of the coinherited thalassemic gene.

The β^E allele contains only a single base change, in codon 26, that causes the amino acid substitution. However, this mutation activates a cryptic RNA splice site generating a structurally abnormal globin mRNA that cannot be translated from about 50% of the initial pre-mRNA molecules. The remaining 40 to 50% that are normally spliced generate functional mRNA that is translated into β^E-globin because the mature mRNA carries the base change that alters codon 26.

Genetic counseling of the persons at risk for HbE should be concerned with the interaction of HbE with β thalassemia rather than HbE homozygosity, a condition associated with asymptomatic microcytosis, hypochromia, and hemoglobin levels rarely <10 g/dL.

HEREDITARY PERSISTENCE OF FETAL HEMOGLOBIN HPFH is characterized by continued synthesis of high levels of HbF in adult life. No deleterious effects are apparent, even when all of the hemoglobin produced is HbF. These rare patients demonstrate convincingly that prevention or reversal of the fetal to adult hemoglobin switch would provide efficacious therapy for sickle cell anemia and β thalassemia.

ACQUIRED HEMOGLOBINOPATHIES The two most important acquired hemoglobinopathies are carbon monoxide poisoning and methemoglobinemia, which is covered elsewhere in this chapter. Carbon monoxide has a higher affinity for hemoglobin than does oxygen; it can replace oxygen and diminish O_2 delivery. Chronic elevation of carboxyhemoglobin levels to 10 or 15%, as occurs in smokers, can lead to secondary polycythemia. Carboxyhemoglobin is cherry red in color and masks the development of cyanosis usually associated with poor O_2 delivery to tissues.

Abnormalities of hemoglobin biosynthesis have also been described in blood dyscrasias. In some patients with myelodysplasia, erythroleukemia, or myeloproliferative disorders, a mild form of HbH disease may also be seen. The abnormalities are not severe enough to alter the course of the underlying disease.

MANAGEMENT OF TRANSFUSIONAL HEMOSIDEROSIS

Chronic blood transfusion can lead to bloodborne infection, alloimmunization, febrile reactions, and lethal iron overload. A unit of packed RBCs contains 250 to 300 mg iron (1 mg/mL). The iron assimilated by single transfusion of two units of packed RBCs is thus equal to a 1- to 2-year intake of iron. Iron accumulates in chronically transfused patients because no mechanisms exist for increasing iron excretion: an expanded erythron causes especially rapid development of iron overload because accelerated erythropoiesis promotes excessive absorption of dietary iron. Vitamin C should not be supplemented because it generates free radicals in iron excess states.

Patients who receive >100 units of packed RBCs usually develop hemosiderosis. The ferritin level rises, followed by early endocrine dysfunction (glucose intolerance and delayed puberty), cirrhosis, and cardiomyopathy. Liver biopsy shows both parenchymal and reticuloendothelial iron. The superconducting quantum-interference device (SQUID) is accurate at measuring hepatic iron but not widely available. Cardiac toxicity is often insidious. Early development of pericarditis is followed by dysrhythmia and pump failure. The onset of heart failure is ominous, often presaging death within a year (Chap. 336).

The decision to start long-term transfusion support should also prompt one to institute therapy with iron-chelating agents. The only approved and available iron chelator, desferoxamine (Desferal), is expensive and poorly absorbed from the gastrointestinal tract. Its iron-binding kinetics require chronic slow infusion via a metering pump.

The constant presence of the drug improves the efficiency of chelation and protects tissues from occasional releases of the most toxic fraction of iron—low-molecular-weight iron—which may not be sequestered by protective proteins. Oral iron-chelating agents such as deferiprone showed initial promise, but long-term trials have raised serious doubts about their efficacy and safety. Newer oral agents are in clinical trials.

Desferoxamine is relatively nontoxic. Occasional cataracts, deafness, and local skin reactions, including urticaria, occur. Skin reactions can usually be managed with antihistamines. Negative iron balance can be achieved, even in the face of a high transfusion requirement, but this alone does not prevent long-term morbidity and mortality in chronically transfused patients. Irreversible end-organ deterioration develops at relatively modest levels of iron overload, even if symptoms do not appear for many years thereafter. To enjoy a significant survival advantage, chelation must begin before 5 to 8 years of age in β thalassemia major.

EXPERIMENTAL THERAPIES

BONE MARROW TRANSPLANTATION, GENE THERAPY, AND MANIPULATION OF HbF
Bone marrow transplantation provides stem cells able to express normal hemoglobin; it has been used in a large number of patients with β thalassemia and a smaller number of patients with sickle cell anemia. Early in the course of disease, before end-organ damage occurs, transplantation is curative in 80 to 90% of patients. In highly experienced centers, the treatment-related mortality is <10%. Since survival into adult life is possible with conventional therapy, the decision to transplant is best made in consultation with specialized centers.

Gene therapy of thalassemia and sickle cell disease has proved to be an exceptionally elusive goal. Uptake of gene vectors into the nondividing hematopoietic stem cells has been disappointingly inefficient. Lentiviral-type vectors that can transduce nondividing cells may solve this problem.

Reestablishing high levels of fetal hemoglobin synthesis should ameliorate the symptoms of β thalassemia. Cytotoxic agents such as hydroxyurea and cytarabine promote high levels of HbF synthesis, probably by stimulating proliferation of the primitive HbF-producing progenitor cell population (i.e., F cell progenitors). Unfortunately, no regimen has yet been identified that ameliorates the clinical manifestations of β thalassemia. Butyrates stimulate HbF production, but only transiently. Pulsed or intermittent administration has recently been found to sustain HbF induction in the majority of patients with sickle cell disease. It is unclear whether butyrates will have similar activity in patients with β thalassemia.

APLASTIC AND HYPOPLASTIC CRISIS IN PATIENTS WITH HEMOGLOBINOPATHIES

Patients with hemolytic anemias sometimes exhibit an alarming decline in hematocrit during and immediately after acute illnesses. Bone marrow suppression occurs in almost everyone during acute inflammatory illnesses. In patients with short RBC life spans, suppression can affect RBC counts more dramatically. These hypoplastic crises are usually transient and self-correcting before intervention is required.

Aplastic crisis refers to a profound cessation of erythroid activity in patients with chronic hemolytic anemias. It is associated with a rapidly falling hematocrit. Episodes are usually self-limited. Aplastic crises are caused by infection with a particular strain of parvovirus, B19A. Children infected with this virus usually develop permanent immunity. Aplastic crises do not often recur and are rarely seen in adults. Management requires close monitoring of the hematocrit and reticulocyte count. If anemia becomes symptomatic, transfusion support is indicated. Most crises resolve spontaneously within 1 to 2 weeks.

FURTHER READING

ATAGA KI, ORRINGA EP: Hypercoagulability in sickle cell disease: a curious paradox. Am J. Med 115:721, 2003

BRUGNARA C et al: Therapy with oral clotrimazole induces inhibition of the Gardos channel and reduction of erythrocyte dehydration in patients with sickle cell disease. J Clin Invest 97:1227, 1996

CLASTA S, VICHINSKY EP: Managing sickle cell disease. BMJ 327:1151, 2003

DESIMONE J et al: Maintenance of elevated fetal hemoglobin levels by decitabine during dose interval treatment of sickle cell anemia. Blood 99:3905, 2002

OLIVIERI NF: The beta-thalassemias. N Engl J Med 341:99, 1999

VICHINSKY E: New therapies in sickle cell disease. Lancet 360:629, 2002

WARE RE et al: Predictors of fetal hemoglobin response in children with sickle cell anemia receiving hydroxyurea therapy. Blood 99:10, 2002

92 | MEGALOBLASTIC ANEMIAS
Bernard M. Babior, H. Franklin Bunn

The megaloblastic anemias are disorders caused by impaired DNA synthesis. Cells primarily affected are those having relatively rapid turnover, especially hematopoietic precursors and gastrointestinal epithelial cells. Cell division is sluggish, but cytoplasmic development progresses normally, so megaloblastic cells tend to be large, with an increased ratio of RNA to DNA. Megaloblastic erythroid progenitors tend to be destroyed in the marrow. Thus, marrow cellularity is often increased but production of red blood cells (RBC) is decreased, an abnormality termed *ineffective erythropoiesis* (Chap. 52).

Most megaloblastic anemias are due to a deficiency of cobalamin (vitamin B_{12}) and/or folic acid. The various clinical entities associated with megaloblastic anemia are listed in Table 92-1.

PHYSIOLOGIC AND BIOCHEMICAL CONSIDERATIONS

FOLIC ACID Folic acid is the common name for pteroylmonoglutamic acid. It is synthesized by many different plants and bacteria. Fruits and vegetables constitute the primary dietary source of the vitamin. Some forms of dietary folic acid are labile and may be destroyed by cooking. The minimum daily requirement is normally about 50 μg, but this may be increased severalfold during periods of enhanced metabolic demand such as pregnancy.

The assimilation of adequate amounts of folic acid depends on the nature of the diet and its means of preparation. Folates in various foodstuffs are largely conjugated to a chain of glutamic acid residues. This highly polar side chain impairs the intestinal absorption of the vitamin. However, conjugases (γ-glutamyl carboxypeptidases) in the lumen of the gut convert polyglutamates to mono- and diglutamates, which are readily absorbed in the proximal jejunum.

Plasma folate is primarily in the form of N^5-methyltetrahydrofolate, a monoglutamate, which is transported into cells by a carrier that is specific for the tetrahydro forms of the vitamin. Once in the cell, the N^5-methyl group is removed in a cobalamin-requiring reaction (see below), and the folate is then reconverted to the polyglutamate form. Conjugation to polyglutamate may be useful for retention of folate within the cell.

A folate-binding protein occurs in plasma, milk, and other body fluids. The function of this folate binder and its membrane-bound precursor is unknown. Neither the binder nor its precursor is related to the tetrahydrofolate carrier.

Normal individuals have about 5 to 20 mg folic acid in various body stores, half in the liver. In light of the minimum daily requirement, it is not surprising that a deficiency will occur within months if dietary intake or intestinal absorption is curtailed.

The prime function of folate compounds is to transfer 1-carbon moieties such as methyl and formyl groups to various organic compounds (Fig. 92-1). The sources of these 1-carbon moieties is usually serine, which reacts with tetrahydrofolate to produce glycine and $N^{5,10}$-methylenetetrahydrofolate. An alternative source is formiminoglutamic acid, an intermediate in histidine catabolism, which gives up its formimino group to tetrahydrofolate to yield N^5-formiminotetrahydrofolate and glutamic acid. These derivatives provide entry into an interconvertible donor pool consisting of tetrahydrofolate derivatives carrying various 1-carbon moieties. The constituents of this pool can donate their 1-carbon moieties to appropriate acceptor compounds to form metabolic intermediates, which are ultimately converted to build-

TABLE 92-1 *Classification of the Megaloblastic Anemias*

COBALAMIN DEFICIENCY

I. Inadequate intake: vegans (rare)
II. Malabsorption
    A. Defective release of cobalamin from food
        1. Gastric achlorhydria
        2. Partial gastrectomy
        3. Drugs that block acid secretion
    B. Inadequate production of intrinsic factor (IF)
        1. Pernicious anemia
        2. Total gastrectomy
        3. Congenital absence or functional abnormality of IF (rare)
    C. Disorders of terminal ileum
        1. Tropical sprue
        2. Nontropical sprue
        3. Regional enteritis
        4. Intestinal resection
        5. Neoplasms and granulomatous disorders (rare)
        6. Selective cobalamin malabsorption (Imerslund's syndrome) (rare)
    D. Competition for cobalamin
        1. Fish tapeworm (*Diphyllobothrium latum*)
        2. Bacteria: "blind loop" syndrome
    E. Drugs: *p*-aminosalicylic acid, colchicine, neomycin
III. Other
    A. Nitrous oxide
    B. Transcobalamin II deficiency (rare)
    C. Congenital enzyme defects (rare)

FOLIC ACID DEFICIENCY

I. Inadequate intake: unbalanced diet (common in alcoholics, teenagers, some infants)
II. Increased requirements
    A. Pregnancy
    B. Infancy
    C. Malignancy
    D. Increased hematopoiesis (chronic hemolytic anemias)
    E. Chronic exfoliative skin disorders
    F. Hemodialysis
III. Malabsorption
    A. Tropical sprue
    B. Nontropical sprue
    C. Drugs: Phenytoin, barbiturates, (?) ethanol
IV. Impaired metabolism
    A. Inhibitors of dihydrofolate reductase: methotrexate, pyrimethamine, triamterene, pentamidine, trimethoprim
    B. Alcohol
    C. Rare enzyme deficiencies: dihydrofolate reductase, others

OTHER CAUSES

I. Drugs that impair DNA metabolism
    A. Purine antagonists: 6-mercaptopurine, azathioprine, etc.
    B. Pyrimidine antagonists: 5-fluorouracil, cytosine arabinoside, etc.
    C. Others: procarbazine, hydroxyurea, acyclovir, zidovudine
II. Metabolic disorders (rare)
    A. Hereditary orotic aciduria
    B. Lesch-Nyhan syndrome
    C. Others
III. Megaloblastic anemia of unknown etiology
    A. Refractory megaloblastic anemia
    B. Di Guglielmo's syndrome[a]
    C. Congenital dyserythropoietic anemia

[a] A form of acute myeloid leukemia with atypical, dysplastic changes in erythroid series.

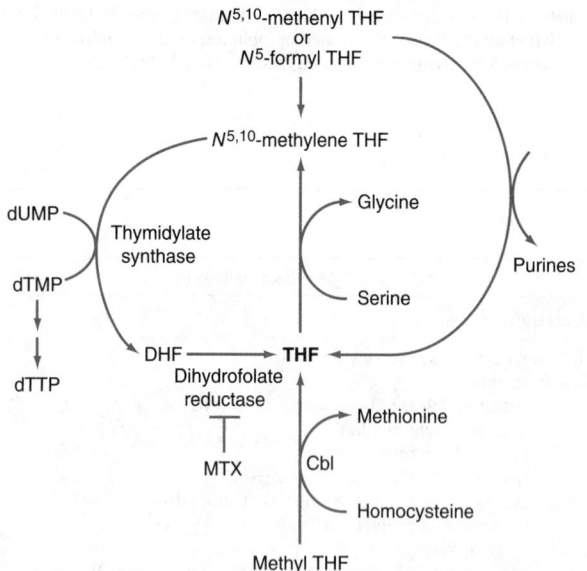

FIGURE 92-1 Folate metabolism. Folate is essential for the de novo synthesis of purines, deoxythymidylate monophosphate (dTMP), and methionine, serving as an intermediate carrier of 1-carbon fragments used in the biosynthesis of these compounds. Its active form is tetrahydrofolate (THF). THF acquires the 1-carbon fragment principally from serine, which is converted to glycine in the course of the reaction. For purine synthesis, the 1-carbon fragment is first oxidized to the level of formic acid, then transferred to substrate. For methionine synthesis, a cobalamin-requiring reaction, the 1-carbon fragment is first reduced to the level of a methyl group, then transferred to homocysteine. In these reactions the cofactor is released as THF, which can immediately participate in another 1-carbon transfer cycle. During the production of dTMP from dUMP, however, the 1-carbon fragment is reduced from formaldehyde to a methyl group in the course of the transfer reaction. The hydrogen atoms used for this reduction come from the cofactor, which is therefore released, not as THF, but as dihydrofolate (DHF). To participate further in the 1-carbon transfer cycle, the DHF has to be re-reduced to THF, a reaction catalyzed by dihydrofolate reductase.

ing blocks used in the synthesis of macromolecules. The most important building blocks are (1) purines, in which the C-2 and C-8 atoms are introduced in folate-dependent reactions; (2) deoxythymidylate monophosphate (dTMP), synthesized from $N^{5,10}$-methylenetetrahydrofolate and deoxyuridylate monophosphate (dUMP); and (3) methionine, formed by the transfer of a methyl group from N^5-methyltetrahydrofolate to homocysteine (two of these three reactions are shown in Fig. 92-1).

In all but one of the 1-carbon transfer reactions, tetrahydrofolate is produced. It can immediately accept a 1-carbon moiety and reenter the donor pool. The single exception is the thymidylate synthase reaction (dUMP → dTMP), in which dihydrofolate is the product (Fig. 92-1). This must be reduced to tetrahydrofolate by the enzyme dihydrofolate reductase before it can reenter the donor pool. A number of drugs are able to inhibit dihydrofolate reductase (Table 92-1), thereby diverting folate from the donor pool and producing what amounts to a state of folate deficiency in the face of normal tissue folate concentrations.

COBALAMIN This vitamin is a complex organometallic compound in which a cobalt atom is situated within a corrin ring, a structure similar to the porphyrin from which heme is formed. Unlike heme, however, cobalamin cannot be synthesized in the human body and must be supplied in the diet. The only dietary source of cobalamin is animal products: meat and dairy foods. The minimum daily requirement for cobalamin is about 2.5 μg.

During gastric digestion, cobalamin in food is released and forms a stable complex with gastric R binder, one of a closely related group of glycoproteins of unknown function that are found in secretions (e.g., saliva, milk, gastric juice, bile), phagocytes, and plasma. On entering the duodenum, the cobalamin–R binder complex is digested, releasing the cobalamin, which then binds to intrinsic factor (IF), a 50-kDa gly-

coprotein produced by the parietal cells of the stomach. The secretion of IF generally parallels that of hydrochloric acid. The cobalamin-IF complex is resistant to proteolytic digestion and travels to the distal ileum, where specific receptors on the mucosal brush border bind and absorb the cobalamin-IF complex. Thus, IF, like iron-binding transferrin, is a cell-directed carrier protein. The receptor-bound cobalamin-IF complex is taken into the ileal mucosal cell, where the IF is destroyed and the cobalamin is transferred to another transport protein, transcobalamin (TC) II. The cobalamin–TC II complex is then secreted into the circulation, from which it is rapidly taken up by the liver, bone marrow, and other cells. The pathway of cobalamin absorption is shown in Fig. 92-2. Normally, about 2 mg cobalamin is stored in the liver, and another 2 mg is stored elsewhere in the body. In view of the minimum daily requirement, about 3 to 6 years would be required for a normal individual to become deficient in cobalamin if absorption were to cease abruptly.

Although TC II is the acceptor for newly absorbed cobalamin, most circulating cobalamin is bound to TC I, a glycoprotein closely related to gastric R binder. TC I appears to be derived in part from leukocytes. The paradox that most circulating cobalamin is bound to TC I rather than TC II, even though TC II initially carries all the cobalamin that is absorbed by the intestine, is explained by the fact that cobalamin bound to TC II is rapidly cleared from the blood ($t_{1/2}$ about 1 h), while clearance of cobalamin bound to TC I requires many days. The function of TC I is unknown.

Cobalamin is an essential cofactor for two enzymes in human cells: methionine synthase and methylmalonyl–coenzyme A (CoA) synthase. Cobalamin exists in two metabolically active forms, identified by the alkyl group attached to the sixth coordination position of the cobalt atom: methylcobalamin and adenosylcobalamin. The vitamin preparation that is used therapeutically is cyanocobalamin (also called vitamin B_{12}). Cyanocobalamin has no known physiologic role and must be converted to a biologically active form before it can be used by tissues.

Methylcobalamin is the form required for methionine synthase,

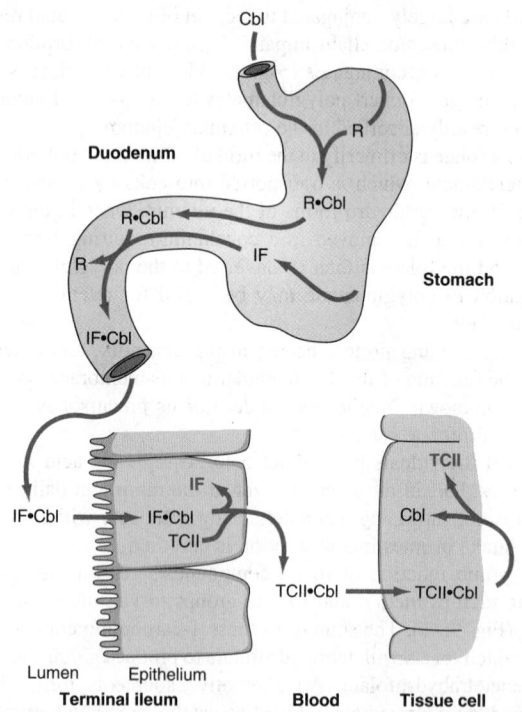

FIGURE 92-2 The assimilation of cobalamin. On entering the stomach, dietary cobalamin (Cbl) forms a complex with R binding protein. As this protein is digested in the small intestine, cobalamin is transferred to intrinsic factor (IF). This complex passes through the intestine until it reaches specific receptors on the mucosa of the distal ileum. The internalized Cbl is then transferred to transcobalamin II (TC II), which circulates in the plasma until it binds to receptors on cells throughout the body and is internalized.

which catalyzes the conversion of homocysteine to methionine (Fig. 92-1). When this reaction is impaired, folate metabolism is deranged; it is this derangement that underlies the defect in DNA synthesis and the megaloblastic maturation pattern in patients who are deficient in cobalamin. In cobalamin deficiency, the unconjugated N^5-methyltetrahydrofolate newly taken from the bloodstream cannot be converted to other forms of tetrahydrofolate by methyl transfer. This is the so-called folate trap hypothesis. Because N^5-methyltetrahydrofolate is a poor substrate for the conjugating enzyme, it largely remains in the unconjugated form and slowly leaks from the cell. Tissue folate deficiency therefore develops, and this results in megaloblastic hematopoiesis. This hypothesis explains why tissue folate stores in cobalamin deficiency are substantially reduced, with a disproportionate reduction in conjugated, as compared with unconjugated, folates, despite normal or supranormal serum folate levels. It also explains why large doses of folate can produce a partial hematologic remission in patients with cobalamin deficiency.

Megaloblastic changes in both cobalamin and folate deficiency as well as in methotrexate treatment are related to a deficiency in production of dTMP. In addition, the excess deoxyuridylate that accumulates can be phosphorylated and mistakenly incorporated into DNA in place of thymidylate; base pairing can be affected by this U-for-T substitution.

Plasma homocysteine levels are elevated in both folate and cobalamin deficiency, and high levels of plasma homocysteine appear to be a risk factor for venous and arterial thrombosis. It is not yet known if hyperhomocysteinemia due to folate or cobalamin deficiency predisposes to thrombosis or alters its response to treatment.

Impairment in the conversion of homocysteine to methionine may also contribute to the neurologic complications of cobalamin deficiency (see below). The methionine formed in this reaction is needed for the production of choline and choline-containing phospholipids. Nervous system damage is postulated to result at least in part from interference with these processes due to decreased methionine production in cobalamin deficiency.

Adenosylcobalamin is required for the conversion of methylmalonyl CoA to succinyl CoA. Lack of this cofactor leads to large increases in the tissue levels of methylmalonyl CoA and its precursor, propionyl CoA. As a consequence, nonphysiologic fatty acids containing an odd number of carbon atoms are synthesized and incorporated into neuronal lipids. This biochemical abnormality may also contribute to the neurologic complications of cobalamin deficiency (see below).

CLINICAL DISORDERS

CLASSIFICATION OF MEGALOBLASTIC ANEMIAS (Table 92-1) The cause of megaloblastic anemia varies in different parts of the world. In temperate zones, folate deficiency in alcoholics and cobalamin deficiency due to pernicious anemia or achlorhydria are the common types of megaloblastic anemias. In certain areas close to the equator, tropical sprue is endemic and an important cause of megaloblastic anemia, while in Scandinavia, infestations by the fish tapeworm, *Diphyllobothrium latum*, may be a cause.

The dietary intake of cobalamin is more than adequate for the body's requirements, except in complete vegetarians (vegans) and their breast-fed infants. Thus deficiency of cobalamin is almost always due to malabsorption. Malabsorption can occur at several levels. In contrast, the dietary intake of folic acid is marginal in many parts of the world. Furthermore, because the body's stores of folate are relatively low, folic acid deficiency can arise rather suddenly during periods of decreased dietary intake or increased metabolic demand. Finally, folic acid deficiency may be due to malabsorption. Often two or more of these factors coexist in a given patient.

Combined deficiencies of cobalamin and folic acid are not uncommon. Patients with tropical sprue are often deficient in both vitamins. The biochemical lesion that results in megaloblastic maturation of bone marrow cells also causes structural and functional abnormalities of the rapidly proliferating epithelial cells of the intestinal mucosa.

Thus severe deficiency of one vitamin can lead to malabsorption of the other. Furthermore, as discussed above, a deficiency of cobalamin causes a secondary reduction in cellular folic acid.

Finally, megaloblastic anemias may occasionally be induced by factors unrelated to a vitamin deficiency. Most such cases are caused by drugs that interfere with DNA synthesis. Less commonly, megaloblastic maturation is a feature of certain acquired hematopoietic stem cell defects. Rarest of all are specific congenital enzyme deficiencies.

COBALAMIN DEFICIENCY The clinical features of cobalamin deficiency involve the blood, the gastrointestinal tract, and the nervous system.

The hematologic manifestations are almost entirely the result of anemia, although very rarely purpura may appear, due to thrombocytopenia. Symptoms of anemia may include weakness, light-headedness, vertigo, and tinnitus, as well as palpitations, angina, and the symptoms of congestive failure. On physical examination, the patient with florid cobalamin deficiency is pale, with slightly icteric skin and eyes. Elevated bilirubin levels are related to high erythroid cell turnover in the marrow. The pulse is rapid, and the heart may be enlarged; auscultation will usually reveal a systolic flow murmur.

The gastrointestinal manifestations reflect the effect of cobalamin deficiency on the rapidly proliferating gastrointestinal epithelium. The patient sometimes complains of a sore tongue, which on inspection will be smooth and beefy red. Anorexia with moderate weight loss may also be evident, possibly accompanied by diarrhea and other gastrointestinal symptoms. These latter manifestations may be caused in part by megaloblastosis of the small intestinal epithelium, which results in malabsorption.

The neurologic manifestations often fail to remit fully on treatment. The initial pathology is demyelination, followed by axonal degeneration and eventual neuronal death; the final stage, of course, is irreversible. Sites of involvement include peripheral nerves; the spinal cord, where the posterior and lateral columns undergo demyelination; and the cerebrum itself. Signs and symptoms include numbness and paresthesia in the extremities (the earliest neurologic manifestations), weakness, and ataxia. There may be sphincter disturbances. Reflexes may be diminished or increased. The Romberg and Babinski's signs may be positive, and position and vibration senses are usually diminished. Disturbances of mentation will vary from mild irritability and forgetfulness to severe dementia or frank psychosis. It should be emphasized that *neurologic disease may occur in a patient with a normal hematocrit* and normal RBC indices. Although it has many benefits, folate supplementation of food may increase the likelihood of neurologic presentations of cobalamin deficiency.

In the classic patient, in whom hematologic problems predominate, the blood and bone marrow show characteristic megaloblastic changes (described under "Diagnosis," below). The anemia may be very severe—hematocrits of 15 to 20 are not infrequent—but is surprisingly well tolerated by the patient because it develops slowly.

Defective Release of Cobalamin from Food Cobalamin in food is tightly bound to enzymes in meat and is split from these enzymes by hydrochloric acid and pepsin in the stomach. People >70 years commonly have achlorhydria. Therefore, they are unable to release cobalamin from food sources but retain the ability to absorb crystalline B_{12}, the form most commonly found in multivitamins. The exact incidence of the defect in cobalamin release from food has not been well defined; estimates vary from 10 to >50% of those over age 70 years. Only a minority of these persons go on to develop frank cobalamin deficiency, but many have biochemical changes, including low levels of cobalamin bound to TC II and elevated homocysteine levels, that augur cobalamin deficiency (see below).

Similarly, patients on drugs that suppress gastric acid production, such as omeprazole, may also fail to release cobalamin from food. However, the proton pump inhibitors do not inhibit IF secretion by parietal cells.

Pernicious Anemia Pernicious anemia, considered the most common cause of cobalamin deficiency, is caused by the absence of IF, due to either atrophy of the mucosa or autoimmune destruction of parietal cells. It is most frequently seen in individuals of northern European descent and African Americans and is much less common in southern Europeans and Asians. Men and women are equally affected. It is a disease of the elderly, the average patient presenting near age 60; it is rare under age 30, although typical pernicious anemia can be seen in children under age 10 (juvenile pernicious anemia). Inherited conditions in which a histologically normal stomach secretes either an abnormal IF or none at all will induce cobalamin deficiency in infancy or early childhood.

The incidence of pernicious anemia is substantially increased in patients with other diseases thought to be of immunologic origin, including Graves' disease, myxedema, thyroiditis, idiopathic adrenocortical insufficiency, vitiligo, and hypoparathyroidism. Patients with pernicious anemia also have abnormal circulating antibodies related to their disease: 90% have antiparietal cell antibody, which is directed against the H^+,K^+-ATPase, while 60% have anti-IF antibody. Antiparietal cell antibody is also found in 50% of patients with gastric atrophy without pernicious anemia, as well as in 10 to 15% of an unselected patient population, but anti-IF antibody is usually absent from these patients. Relatives of patients with pernicious anemia have an increased incidence of the disease, and even clinically unaffected relatives may have anti-IF antibody in their serum. Finally, treatment with glucocorticoids may reverse the disease.

Cytotoxic T cells may also contribute to the destruction of parietal cells in pernicious anemia. Pernicious anemia is unusually common in patients with agammaglobulinemia, supporting a role for the cellular immune system in its pathogenesis. In contrast, *Helicobacter pylori* does not cause parietal cell destruction in pernicious anemia.

The most characteristic finding in pernicious anemia is gastric atrophy affecting the acid- and pepsin-secreting portion of the stomach; the antrum is spared. Other pathologic changes are secondary to the deficiency of cobalamin; these include megaloblastic alterations in the gastric and intestinal epithelium and the neurologic changes described above. The abnormalities in the gastric epithelium appear as cellular atypia in gastric cytology specimens, a finding that must be carefully distinguished from the cytologic abnormalities seen in gastric malignancy.

The *clinical manifestations* are primarily those of cobalamin deficiency, as described above. The disease is of insidious onset and progresses slowly. Laboratory examination will reveal hypergastrinemia and pentagastrin-fast achlorhydria as well as the hematologic and other laboratory abnormalities discussed under "Diagnosis."

Through appropriate replacement therapy, patients with pernicious anemia should experience complete and lifelong correction of all abnormalities that are due to cobalamin deficiency, except to the extent that irreversible changes in the nervous system may have occurred before treatment. These patients, however, are unusually subject to gastric polyps and have about twice the normal incidence of cancer of the stomach. Thus, patients should be followed with frequent stool guaiac examinations and endoscopy when indicated.

Postgastrectomy Following total gastrectomy or extensive damage to gastric mucosa as, for example, by ingestion of corrosive agents, megaloblastic anemia will develop because the source of IF has been removed. In all such patients, the absorption of orally administered cobalamin is impaired. Megaloblastic anemia may also follow partial gastrectomy, but the incidence is lower than after total gastrectomy. The cause of cobalamin deficiency after partial gastrectomy is not clear; defective release of cobalamin from food and intestinal overgrowth of bacteria have been suggested, but response to antibiotics is not common.

Intestinal Organisms Megaloblastic anemia may occur with intestinal stasis due to anatomic lesions (strictures, diverticula, anastomoses,

"blind loops") or pseudoobstruction (diabetes mellitus, scleroderma, amyloid). This anemia is caused by colonization of the small intestine by large masses of bacteria that consume intestinal cobalamin before absorption. Steatorrhea may also be seen under these circumstances because bile salt metabolism is disturbed when the intestine is heavily colonized with bacteria. Hematologic responses have been observed after administration of oral antibiotics such as tetracycline and ampicillin. Megaloblastic anemia is seen in persons harboring the fish tapeworm, *D. latum*, due to competition by the worm for cobalamin. Destruction of the worm eliminates the problem.

Ileal Abnormalities Cobalamin deficiency is common in tropical sprue, while it is an unusual complication of nontropical sprue (gluten-sensitive enteropathy; Chap. 275). Virtually any disorder that compromises the absorptive capacity of the distal ileum can result in cobalamin deficiency. Specific entities include regional enteritis, Whipple's disease, and tuberculosis. Segmental involvement of the distal ileum by disease can cause megaloblastic anemia without any other manifestations of intestinal malabsorption such as steatorrhea. Cobalamin malabsorption is also seen after ileal resection. The Zollinger-Ellison syndrome (intense gastric hyperacidity due to a gastrin-secreting tumor) may cause cobalamin malabsorption by acidifying the small intestine, retarding the transfer of the vitamin from R binder to IF and impairing the binding of the cobalamin-IF complex to the ileal receptors. Chronic pancreatitis may also cause cobalamin malabsorption by impairing the transfer of the vitamin from R binder to IF. This abnormality can be detected by tests of cobalamin absorption (see below, Schilling test), but it is invariably mild and never causes clinical cobalamin deficiency. Finally, a rare congenital disorder, Imerslund-Gräsbeck disease, involves a selective defect in cobalamin absorption accompanied by proteinuria. Affected individuals have a mutation in cubulin, a receptor that mediates intestinal absorption of the cobalamin-IF complex.

Nitrous Oxide Inhalation of nitrous oxide as an anesthetic destroys endogenous cobalamin. As ordinarily used, the magnitude of the effects are not sufficient to cause clinical cobalamin deficiency, but repeated or protracted exposure (>6 h), particularly in older patients with borderline cobalamin stores, can lead to severe megaloblastic anemia and/or acute neurologic deficits.

FOLIC ACID DEFICIENCY Since January 1998, folic acid has been added to all enriched grain products by order of the U.S. Food and Drug Administration; accordingly, the incidence of folic acid deficiency has fallen markedly. Patients with folic acid deficiency are more often malnourished than those with cobalamin deficiency. The gastrointestinal manifestations are similar to but may be more widespread and more severe than those of pernicious anemia. Diarrhea is often present, and cheilosis and glossitis are also encountered. However, in contrast to cobalamin deficiency, neurologic abnormalities do not occur.

The hematologic manifestations of folic acid deficiency are the same as those of cobalamin deficiency. Folic acid deficiency can generally be attributed to one or more of the following factors: inadequate intake, increased demand, or malabsorption.

Inadequate Intake Alcoholics may become folate deficient because their main source of caloric intake is alcoholic beverages. Distilled spirits are virtually devoid of folic acid, while beer and wine do not contain enough of the vitamin to satisfy the daily requirement. In addition, alcohol may interfere with folate metabolism. Narcotic addicts are also prone to become folate deficient because of malnutrition. Many indigent and elderly individuals who subsist primarily on canned foods or "tea and toast" and occasional teenagers whose diet consists of "junk food" develop folate deficiency.

Increased Demand Tissues with a relatively high rate of cell division such as the bone marrow or gut mucosa have a large requirement for folate. Therefore, patients with chronic hemolytic anemias or other causes of very active erythropoiesis may become deficient. Pregnant women formerly were at risk to become deficient in folic acid because of the high demand of the developing fetus. Deficiency in the first weeks of pregnancy can cause neural tube defects in newborns. Often the pregnancy was not detected until the defect had developed; thus, provision of folate supplementation to women after they learned they were pregnant was ineffective. However, folate food supplementation has decreased neural tube defects by >50%. Folate deficiency may also occur during the growth spurts of infancy and adolescence. Patients on chronic hemodialysis may require supplementary folate to replace that lost in the dialysate.

Malabsorption Folic acid deficiency is a common accompaniment of tropical sprue. Both the gastrointestinal symptoms and malabsorption are improved by the administration of either folic acid or antibiotics by mouth. Patients with nontropical sprue (gluten-sensitive enteropathy) may also develop significant folic acid deficiency that parallels other parameters of malabsorption. Similarly, folate deficiency in alcoholics may be due in part to malabsorption. In addition, other primary small-bowel disorders are sometimes associated with folate deficiency (Chap. 275).

DRUGS Next to deficiency of folate or cobalamin, the most common cause of megaloblastic anemia is drugs. Agents that cause megaloblastic anemia do so by interfering with DNA synthesis, either directly or by antagonizing the action of folate. They can be classified as follows:

1. *Direct inhibitors of DNA synthesis.* They include purine analogues (6-thioguanine, azathioprine, 6-mercaptopurine), pyrimidine analogues (5-fluorouracil, cytosine arabinoside), and other drugs that interfere with DNA synthesis by a variety of mechanisms (hydroxyurea, procarbazine). The antiviral agent zidovudine (AZT), used for treating HIV, often causes severe megaloblastic anemia.

2. *Folate antagonists.* The most toxic of these is methotrexate, a powerful inhibitor of dihydrofolate reductase, which is used in the treatment of certain malignancies and rheumatologic disorders. Much less toxic but still capable of inducing a megaloblastic anemia are several weak dihydrofolate reductase inhibitors used to treat a variety of nonmalignant conditions. These drugs include pentamidine, trimethoprim, triamterene, and pyrimethamine.

3. *Others.* A number of drugs antagonize folate by mechanisms that are poorly understood but are thought to involve an effect on absorption of the vitamin by the intestine. In this category are the anticonvulsants phenytoin, primidone, and phenobarbital. Megaloblastic anemia induced by these agents is mild.

OTHER MECHANISMS ■ Hereditary Megaloblastic anemia may be seen in several hereditary disorders. Orotic aciduria is a deficiency of orotidylic decarboxylase and phosphorylase, leading to a defect in pyrimidine metabolism and characterized by retarded growth and development as well as by the excretion of large amounts of orotic acid. Congenital folate malabsorption causes megaloblastic anemia, accompanied by ataxia and mental retardation. A thiamine-responsive megaloblastic anemia accompanied by nerve deafness and diabetes mellitus has been reported in several children. Megaloblastic changes as well as multinuclearity of RBC precursors are seen in the marrow of certain patients with congenital dyserythropoietic anemia, a group of inherited disorders characterized by mild to moderate anemia and a benign course.

TC II deficiency, like the congenital abnormalities in cobalamin absorption, causes pronounced deficiency in cobalamin in infancy or early childhood. Megaloblastic anemia is not seen in hereditary TC I deficiency.

Refractory Megaloblastic Anemia Megaloblastic erythropoiesis may sometimes be seen in myelodysplasia. Megaloblastic changes are restricted to the RBC series (see below). Myelodysplasia often produces a distinct morphologic picture most apparent in orthochromatic normoblasts in which a megaloblastic nucleus is associated with severely hypochromic cytoplasm. This variant has been called "megaloblastoid" and refers to the presence of both nuclear and cytoplasmic maturation defects. "Megaloblastoid" does not mean "mildly megaloblas-

tic." As with other forms of myelodysplasia, refractory megaloblastic anemia is associated with an increased incidence of acute leukemia.

Megaloblastic changes are seen in erythremic myelosis and acute erythroleukemia, where RBC precursors are prominently involved. Here, the marrow is characterized by bizarre erythroid maturation, with multinuclearity and multipolar mitotic figures in the RBC precursors (Chap. 96).

MEGALOBLASTIC DISEASE WITHOUT ANEMIA Megaloblastic disease is easily overlooked in nonanemic patients. It can present in one of two ways.

Acute Megaloblastic Disease Occasionally, a full-blown megaloblastic state can develop over the course of just a few days. This is usually seen following nitrous oxide anesthesia but may occur in any patient with a serious illness requiring intensive care, especially a patient receiving multiple transfusions, dialysis, or total parenteral nutrition. An acute megaloblastic state can also be precipitated by the administration of a weak antifolate (e.g., trimethoprim) to a patient with marginal tissue folate stores.

The condition resembles an immune cytopenia, with a rapidly developing thrombocytopenia and/or leukopenia in the absence of anemia. The blood smear may be completely normal, but the marrow is floridly megaloblastic. Acute megaloblastic anemia responds rapidly to treatment with folate plus cobalamin in the usual therapeutic doses.

Cobalamin Deficiency without Anemia Cobalamin deficiency without hematologic abnormalities is surprisingly common, especially in the elderly. The risk of a nonhematologic presentation for cobalamin deficiency is increased by the folate food fortification because folate can mask the hematologic effects of cobalamin deficiency. Between 10 and 30% of persons over age 70 years have metabolic evidence of cobalamin deficiency, either elevated homocysteine levels, low cobalamin-TC II levels, or both. Only 10% of these patients have defective production of IF, and the remainder often have atrophic gastritis and cannot release cobalamin from their food (see above). Serum cobalamin levels may be normal or low, but serum levels of methylmalonic acid are almost invariably increased due to a deficiency of cobalamin at the tissue level. The neuropsychiatric abnormalities tend to improve, and serum methylmalonic acid levels generally return to normal after treatment with cobalamin. Neurologic defects do not always reverse with cobalamin supplementation.

DIAGNOSIS The finding of significant macrocytosis [mean corpuscular volume (MCV) > 100 fL] suggests the presence of a megaloblastic anemia. Other causes of macrocytosis include hemolysis, liver disease, alcoholism, hypothyroidism, and aplastic anemia. If the macrocytosis is marked (MCV > 110 fL), the patient is much more likely to have a megaloblastic anemia. Macrocytosis is less marked with concurrent iron deficiency or thalassemia. The reticulocyte index is low, and the leukocyte and platelet count may also be decreased, particularly in severely anemic patients. The blood smear (Fig. 92-3) demonstrates marked anisocytosis and poikilocytosis, together with macroovalocytes, which are large, oval, fully hemoglobinized erythrocytes typical of megaloblastic anemias. There is some basophilic stippling, and an occasional nucleated RBC may be seen. In the white blood cell series, the neutrophils show hypersegmentation of the nucleus (Fig. 92-4). This is such a characteristic finding that a single cell with a nucleus of six lobes or more should raise the immediate suspicion of a meg-

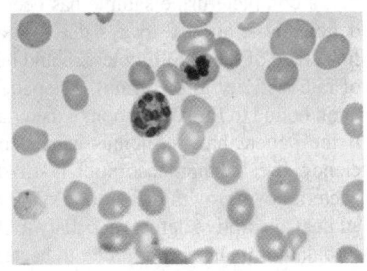

FIGURE 92-3 Megaloblastic anemia. Oval macrocytes, well filled with hemoglobin, are admixed with lesser numbers of large red blood cells, some of which are teardrop-shaped. Note also hypersegmented granulocyte.

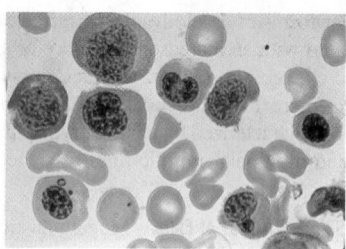

FIGURE 92-4 This marrow section demonstrates nuclear-cytoplasmic dissociation. Nuclei of late stage (orthochromatic) erythroblasts have loose chromatin more characteristic of more immature cells while their cytoplasms are nearly filled with hemoglobin. Slow nuclear maturation is related to a decrese in DNA synthesis related to an insufficient supply of thymidylate. An inadequate supply of reduced folate (usually folate or B12 deficiency) or drugs that inhibit DNA synthesis can produce this picture. (*From RS Hillman, MD, and KA Ault, MD, courtesy of the American Society of Hematology Slide Bank.*)

aloblastic anemia. A rare myelocyte may also be seen. Bizarre, misshapen platelets are also observed. The bone marrow is hypercellular with a decreased myeloid/erythroid ratio and abundant stainable iron. RBC precursors are abnormally large and have nuclei that appear much less mature than would be expected from the development of the cytoplasm (nuclear-cytoplasmic asynchrony). The nuclear chromatin is more dispersed than expected, and it condenses in a peculiar fenestrated pattern that is very characteristic of megaloblastic erythropoiesis. Abnormal mitoses may be seen. Granulocyte precursors are also affected, many being larger than normal, including giant bands and metamyelocytes. Megakaryocytes are decreased and show abnormal morphology.

Megaloblastic anemias are characterized by ineffective erythropoiesis (Chap. 52). In a severely megaloblastic patient, as many as 90% of the RBC precursors may be destroyed before they are released into the bloodstream, compared with 10 to 15% in normal individuals. Enhanced intramedullary destruction of erythroblasts results in an increase in unconjugated bilirubin and lactic acid dehydrogenase (isoenzyme 1) in plasma.

In evaluating a patient with megaloblastic anemia, it is important to determine whether there is a specific vitamin deficiency by measuring serum cobalamin and folate levels. The normal range of cobalamin in serum is 300 to 900 pg/mL; values <200 pg/mL indicate clinically significant deficiency. Measurements of cobalamin bound to TC II would be a more physiologic measure of cobalamin status, but such assays are not yet routinely available. The normal serum concentration of folic acid ranges from 6 to 20 ng/mL; values ≤4 ng/mL are generally considered to be diagnostic of folate deficiency. Unlike serum cobalamin, serum folate levels may reflect recent alterations in dietary intake. Measurement of RBC folate level provides useful information because it is not subject to short-term fluctuations in folate intake and is better than serum folate as an index of folate stores.

Once cobalamin deficiency has been established, its pathogenesis can be delineated by means of a Schilling test. A patient is given radioactive cobalamin by mouth, followed shortly thereafter by an intramuscular injection of unlabeled cobalamin. The proportion of the administered radioactivity excreted in the urine during the next 24 h provides an accurate measure of absorption of cobalamin, assuming that a complete urine sample has been collected. Because cobalamin deficiency is almost always due to malabsorption (Table 92-1), this first stage of the Schilling test should be abnormal (i.e., small amounts of radioactivity in the urine). The patient is then given labeled cobalamin bound to IF. Absorption of the vitamin will now approach normal if the patient has pernicious anemia or some other type of IF deficiency. If cobalamin absorption is still decreased, the patient may have bacterial overgrowth (blind loop syndrome) or ileal disease (including an ileal absorptive defect secondary to the cobalamin deficiency itself). Cobalamin malabsorption due to bacterial overgrowth can frequently

be corrected by the administration of antibiotics. The Schilling test can provide equally reliable information after the patient has had adequate therapy with parenteral cobalamin.

A normal Schilling test in a patient with documented cobalamin deficiency may indicate poor absorption of the vitamin when mixed with food. This can be established by repeating the Schilling test with radioactive cobalamin scrambled with an egg.

Serum methylmalonic acid and homocysteine levels are also useful in the diagnosis of megaloblastic anemias. Both are elevated in cobalamin deficiency, while elevated levels of homocysteine but not methylmalonic acid are seen in folate deficiency. These tests measure tissue vitamin stores and may demonstrate a deficiency even when the more traditional but less reliable folate and cobalamin levels are borderline or even normal. Patients (particularly older patients) without anemia and with normal serum cobalamin levels but elevated levels of serum methylmalonic acid may develop neuropsychiatric abnormalities. Treatment of patients with this "subtle" cobalamin deficiency will usually prevent further deterioration and may result in improvement.

℞ TREATMENT

Cobalamin Deficiency   Apart from specific therapy related to the underlying disorder (e.g., antibiotics for intestinal overgrowth with bacteria), the mainstay of treatment for cobalamin deficiency is replacement therapy. Because the defect is nearly always malabsorption, patients are generally given parenteral treatment, specifically in the form of intramuscular cyanocobalamin. Parenteral treatment begins with 1000 μg cobalamin per week for 8 weeks, followed by 1000 μg cyanocobalamin intramuscularly every month for the rest of the patient's life. Cobalamin deficiency can also be managed very effectively by oral replacement therapy with 2 mg crystalline B_{12} per day; however, compliance is a greater concern with oral than intramuscular treatment.

The response to treatment is gratifying. Shortly after treatment is begun, and several days before a hematologic response is evident in the peripheral blood, the patient will experience an increase in strength and an improved sense of well-being. Marrow morphology begins to revert toward normal within a few hours after treatment is initiated. Reticulocytosis begins 4 to 5 days after therapy is started and peaks at about day 7 (Fig. 92-5), with subsequent remission of the anemia over the next several weeks. If a reticulocytosis does not occur, or if it is less brisk than expected from the level of the hematocrit, a search should be made for other factors contributing to the anemia (e.g., infection, coexisting iron and/or folate deficiency, or hypothyroidism). Hypokalemia and salt retention may occur early in the course of therapy. Thrombocytosis may also be seen.

In most cases, replacement therapy is all that is needed for the treatment of cobalamin deficiency. Occasionally, however, a patient with a severe anemia will have such a precarious cardiovascular status that emergency transfusion is necessary. This must be done with great

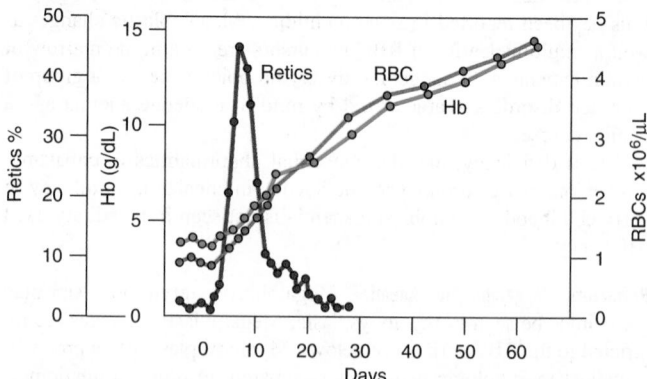

FIGURE 92-5 Hematologic response of a patient with pernicious anemia to an intramuscular injection of 100 μg cobalamin on day 0. Retics, reticulocytes; RBC, red blood cell; Hb, hemoglobin. (*From A Erslev, TG Gabuzda, Pathophysiology of Blood, Philadelphia, Saunders, 1975, with permission.*)

care, because such patients may develop heart failure from fluid over-load. Blood must be administered slowly in the form of packed RBCs, with very close observation. A small volume of packed RBCs will frequently be enough to ameliorate the acute cardiovascular problems. If necessary, blood may be administered by exchanging patient blood (mostly plasma) for packed cells.

With lifelong treatment, patients should experience no further man-ifestations of cobalamin deficiency, although neurologic symptoms may not be fully corrected even by optimal therapy. The potential for late development of gastric carcinoma in pernicious anemia necessi-tates careful follow-up of the patient.

Folate, particularly in large doses, can correct the megaloblastic anemia of cobalamin deficiency without altering the neurologic ab-normalities. The neurologic manifestations may even be aggravated by folate therapy. Cobalamin deficiency can thus be masked in patients who are taking large doses of folate. For this reason, a hematologic response to folate must never be used to rule out cobalamin deficiency in a given patient; cobalamin deficiency can be excluded only by ap-propriate laboratory evaluation.

In light of the high frequency of defective cobalamin absorption in older people and the possible increased risk that overt cobalamin de-ficiency will present with neurologic rather than hematologic symp-toms (because of folate food fortification), some experts have recom-mended the use of 0.1 mg oral crystalline cobalamin prophylaxis daily in people over age 65 years.

Folate Deficiency Like cobalamin deficiency, folate deficiency is treated by replacement therapy. The usual dose of folic acid is 1 mg/d, by mouth, but higher doses (up to 5 mg/d) may be required for folate deficiency due to malabsorption. Parenteral folate is rarely nec-essary. The hematologic response is similar to that seen after replace-ment therapy for cobalamin deficiency, i.e., a brisk reticulocytosis after about 4 days, followed by correction of the anemia over the next 1 to 2 months. The duration of therapy depends on the basis of the defi-

ciency state. Patients with a continuously increased requirement (such as patients with hemolytic anemia) or those with malabsorption or chronic malnutrition should continue to receive oral folic acid indefi-nitely. In addition, the patient should be encouraged to maintain an optimal diet containing adequate amounts of folate.

Other Causes of Megaloblastic Anemia Megaloblastic anemia due to drugs can be treated, if necessary, by reducing the dose of the drug or elim-inating it altogether. The effects of folate antagonists that inhibit di-hydrofolate reductase can be counteracted by folinic acid [5-formyl tetrahydrofolate (THF)] in a dose of 100 to 200 mg/d (Fig. 92-1), which circumvents the block in folate metabolism by providing a form of folate that can be converted to 5,10-methylene THF. For the meg-aloblastic forms of sideroblastic anemia, pyridoxine in pharmacologic doses (as high as 300 mg/d) should be tried. Simple supportive mea-sures are all that appear to be in order for treatment of refractory megaloblastic anemia. Acute erythroleukemia is treated like other types of acute myeloid leukemia (Chap. 96).

FURTHER READING

CARMEL R: Current concepts in cobalamin deficiency. Annu Rev Med 51:357, 2000
D'ANGELO A, SELHUB J: Homocysteine and thrombotic disease. Blood 90:1, 1997
DHAMARAJAN TS et al: Vitamin B12 deficiency: Recognizing subtle symp-toms in older adults. Geriatrics 58:30, 2003
JACQUES PF et al: The effect of folic acid fortification on plasma folate and total homocysteine concentrations. N Engl J Med 340:1449, 1999
KUZMINSKI AM et al: Effective treatment of cobalamin deficiency with oral cobalamin. Blood 92:1191, 1998
TOH BH et al: Pernicious anemia. N Engl J Med 337:1441, 1997
WICKRAMASINGHE SN: The wide spectrum and unresolved issues of mega-loblastic anemia. Semin Hematol 36:3, 1999

93 HEMOLYTIC ANEMIAS AND ACUTE BLOOD LOSS
H. Franklin Bunn, Wendell Rosse

The loss of red cells either through hemorrhage or, less commonly, through premature destruction of the red cells (hemolysis) may cause anemia. Hemolysis or blood loss normally leads to an increase in red cell production, detected by an increase in reticulocyte index.

HEMOLYTIC ANEMIAS

Red blood cells (RBC) normally survive 90 to 120 days in the circu-lation. The life span of RBC may be shortened in a number of disor-ders, often resulting in anemia if the bone marrow is not able to replenish adequately the prematurely destroyed RBC.

In all patients with hemolytic anemia, a careful history and physical examination provide important clues to the diagnosis. The patient may complain of fatigue and other symptoms of anemia (Chap. 52). Less commonly, jaundice and even red-brown urine (hemoglobinuria) are reported. A complete drug and toxin exposure history and the family history often provide crucial information. The physical examination may show jaundice of skin and mucosae. Splenomegaly is encountered in a variety of hemolytic anemias. Other historic and physical findings are associated with specific hemolytic anemias (see below).

Laboratory tests may be used initially to demonstrate the presence of hemolysis (Table 93-1) and define its cause. An elevated reticulo-cyte count in the patient with anemia is the most useful indicator of hemolysis, reflecting erythroid hyperplasia of the bone marrow; biopsy of the bone marrow is often unnecessary. Reticulocytes are also ele-vated in patients with active blood loss, those with myelophthisis, and those who are recovering from suppression of erythropoiesis (Chap. 52). The morphology of the RBC may provide evidence both of he-molysis and of its cause; the characteristic abnormalities and their

associated causes and syndromes are listed in Table 93-2. While the findings on the peripheral blood smear alone are rarely pathogno-monic, they may provide important clues to the presence of hemolysis and to diagnosis.

Hemolysis results in increased heme catabolism and enhanced for-mation of unconjugated bilirubin. The plasma level of unconjugated bilirubin may be high enough to produce readily apparent jaundice (detectable usually when serum bilirubin is >34 μmol/L or 2 mg/dL).

TABLE 93-1 *Laboratory Evaluation of Hemolysis*

	Extravascular	Intravascular
HEMATOLOGIC		
Routine blood film	Polychromatophilia	Polychromatophilia
Reticulocyte count	↑	↑
Bone marrow examination	Erythroid hyperplasia	Erythroid hyperplasia
PLASMA OR SERUM		
Bilirubin	↑ Unconjugated	↑ Unconjugated
Haptoglobin	↓, Absent	Absent
Plasma hemoglobin	N–↑	↑↑
Lactate dehydrogenase	↑ (Variable)	↑↑ (Variable)
URINE		
Bilirubin	0	0
Hemosiderin	0	+
Hemoglobin	0	+ in severe cases

Note: N, normal.

TABLE 93-2 *Red Blood Cell Morphology in the Diagnosis of Hemolytic Anemia*

Morphology	Cause	Syndromes
Spherocytes	Loss of membrane	Hereditary spherocytosis, immunohemolytic anemia
Target cells	Increased ratio of RBC surface area to volume	Hemoglobin disorders: thalassemias, hemoglobin S, C, etc.; liver disease
Schistocytes	Traumatic disruption of membrane	Microangiopathy, intravascular prostheses
Sickled cells	Polymerization of hemoglobin S	Sickle cell syndromes
Acanthocytes	?Abnormal membrane lipids	Severe liver disease (spur cell anemia)
Agglutinated cells	Presence of IgM antibody	Cold agglutinin disease
Heinz bodies	Precipitated hemoglobin	Unstable hemoglobin, oxidant stress

TABLE 93-3 *Classification of Hemolytic Anemias*

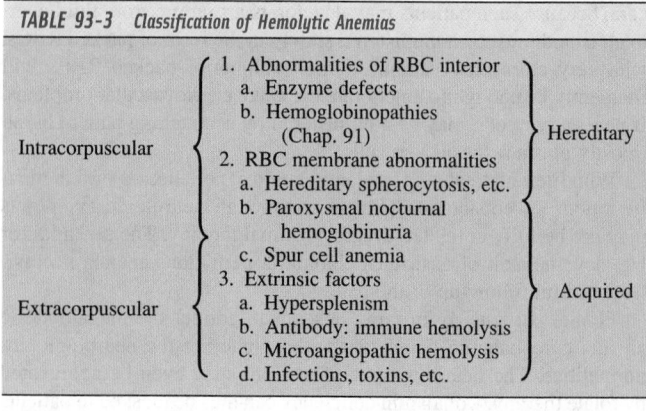

Intracorpuscular	1. Abnormalities of RBC interior a. Enzyme defects b. Hemoglobinopathies (Chap. 91) 2. RBC membrane abnormalities a. Hereditary spherocytosis, etc. b. Paroxysmal nocturnal hemoglobinuria c. Spur cell anemia	Hereditary
Extracorpuscular	3. Extrinsic factors a. Hypersplenism b. Antibody: immune hemolysis c. Microangiopathic hemolysis d. Infections, toxins, etc.	Acquired

The unconjugated (indirect) bilirubin level can be further elevated by a commonly encountered defect in conjugation of bilirubin (Gilbert's syndrome) (Chap. 284). In patients with hemolysis, the level of unconjugated bilirubin never exceeds 70 to 85 μmol/L (4 to 5 mg/dL) unless liver function is impaired.

In the absence of tissue damage in other organs, serum enzyme levels can be useful in the diagnosis and monitoring of patients with hemolysis. Lactate dehydrogenase (LDH), particularly LDH-2, is elevated by accelerated RBC destruction. Serum AST (SGOT) may be somewhat elevated, whereas ALT (SGPT) is not.

Haptoglobin is an α globulin that is present in high concentration (~1.0 g/L) in the serum. It binds specifically to the globin in hemoglobin. The hemoglobin-haptoglobin complex is cleared rapidly by the mononuclear phagocyte system. Thus patients with significant hemolysis, either intravascular or extravascular, have low or absent levels of serum haptoglobin. The fact that haptoglobin synthesis is decreased in patients with hepatocellular disease and increased in inflammatory states must be considered in the interpretation of serum haptoglobin.

Intravascular hemolysis (which is uncommon) results in the release of hemoglobin into the plasma. In these cases, plasma hemoglobin is increased in proportion to the degree of hemolysis (plasma hemoglobin may be falsely elevated due to lysis of RBC in vitro). If the haptoglobin-binding capacity of the plasma is exceeded, free hemoglobin tetramer dissociates into dimers that pass through renal glomeruli. This filtered hemoglobin is reabsorbed by the proximal tubule, where it is catabolized in situ, and the heme iron is incorporated into storage proteins (ferritin and hemosiderin). The presence of hemosiderin in the urine, detected by staining the sediment with Prussian blue, indicates that a significant amount of circulating free hemoglobin has been filtered by the kidneys. When the absorptive capacity of the tubular cells is exceeded, hemoglobinuria ensues and indicates severe intravascular hemolysis. Hemoglobinuria must be distinguished from hematuria (in which case RBC are seen on urine examination) and from myoglobinuria due to rhabdomyolysis; in all three cases, the urine is positive with the benzidine reaction, commonly used in analysis of urine. After centrifugation of an anticoagulated blood specimen, the plasma of patients with hemoglobinuria has a reddish-brown color, whereas that of patients with myoglobinuria is normal in color. Because of its higher molecular weight, hemoglobin has lower glomerular permeability than myoglobin and is less rapidly cleared by the kidneys.

CLASSIFICATION The hemolytic anemias can be grouped into three categories (Table 93-3). Accelerated RBC destruction can be caused by (1) a molecular defect (hemoglobinopathy or enzymopathy) inside the red cell, (2) an abnormality in membrane structure and function, or (3)

an environmental factor such as mechanical trauma or an autoantibody. In *intracorpuscular types* of hemolysis, the patient's RBC have an abnormally short life span in a normal recipient (with a compatible blood type), while compatible normal RBC survive normally in the patient. The opposite is true in *extracorpuscular* types of hemolysis. Finally, hemolytic disorders can be either inherited or acquired.

INHERITED HEMOLYTIC ANEMIAS The inherited hemolytic anemias are due to inborn defects in one of three main components of red cells: the membrane, enzymes, or hemoglobin. These defects are often known at the genomic level, but their identification still largely depends on their clinical and laboratory manifestations.

Red Cell Membrane Disorders These are usually readily detected by morphologic abnormalities of the RBC on the blood film. The three inherited RBC membrane abnormalities are hereditary spherocytosis, hereditary elliptocytosis (including hereditary pyropoikilocytosis), and hereditary stomatocytosis.

HEREDITARY SPHEROCYTOSIS Hereditary spherocytosis is characterized by spherical RBC due to a molecular defect in one of the proteins in the cytoskeleton of the RBC membrane; this leads to a loss of membrane and hence decreased ratio of surface area to volume and consequently spherocytosis. Usually an autosomal dominant trait, this disorder has an incidence of 1:1000 to 1:4500. In ~20% of patients, the absence of hematologic abnormalities in family members suggests either autosomal recessive inheritance or a spontaneous mutation. The disorder is sometimes clinically apparent in early infancy but often escapes detection until adult life.

Clinical Manifestations The major clinical features of hereditary spherocytosis are anemia, splenomegaly, and jaundice. Jaundice may be intermittent and tends to be less pronounced in early childhood. Because of the increased bile pigment production, pigmented gallstones are common, even in childhood. Compensatory erythroid hyperplasia of the bone marrow occurs, with the extension of red marrow into the midshafts of long bones and occasionally with extramedullary erythropoiesis, at times leading to the formation of paravertebral masses visible on chest x-ray. Because the bone marrow's capacity to increase erythropoiesis nearly matches the rate of hemolysis, anemia is usually mild or moderate and may even be absent in an otherwise healthy individual. Compensation may be temporarily interrupted by episodes of relative erythroid hypoplasia precipitated by infections, particularly parvovirus. Splenomegaly is very common. The hemolytic rate may increase transiently during systemic infections, which induce further splenic enlargement. Chronic leg ulcers, similar to those observed in sickle cell anemia, occur occasionally.

The characteristic erythrocyte abnormality is the spherocyte (Fig. 93-1). The mean corpuscular volume (MCV) is usually normal or slightly decreased, and the mean corpuscular hemoglobin concentration (MCHC) is increased to 350 to 400 g/L. Spheroidicity may be quantitatively assessed by measurement of the osmotic fragility of the RBC on exposure to hyposmotic solutions causing a net influx of water (Fig. 93-2). On microscopic examination, spherocytes are usually detected as small cells without central pallor.

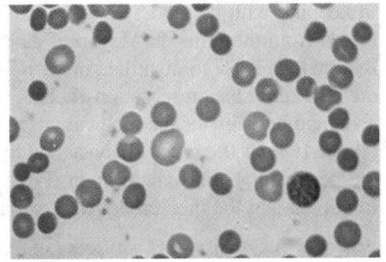

FIGURE 93-1 *Hereditary spherocytosis* Small, densely staining red blood cells are seen that have lost their central area of pallor (microspherocytes). Microspherocytes may also be found in other hemolytic disorders (Fig. 93-5).

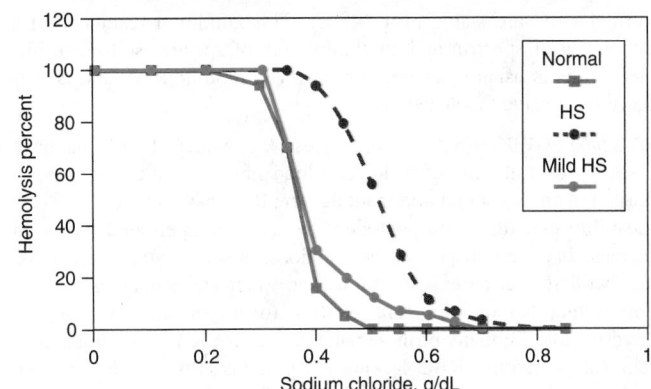

FIGURE 93-2 Osmotic fragility of RBC in hereditary spherocytosis (HS). The results from two patients are compared to those from a normal individual.

Pathogenesis The molecular abnormality in hereditary spherocytosis primarily involves the proteins responsible for tethering the lipid bilayer to the underlying cytoskeletal network. About 50% of patients have a defect in ankyrin, the protein that forms a bridge between protein 3 and spectrin (Fig. 93-3). Homozygotes who have a recessive inheritance pattern for ankyrin deficiency have more severe anemia than heterozygotes with the more common dominant form. About 25% of patients have a mutation of protein 3, resulting in a deficiency of that protein and mild anemia with dominant inheritance. Most of the remaining 25% have mutations of spectrin, leading to impaired synthesis or self-association. β-spectrin mutants are generally mild, with dominant inheritance, while α-spectrin deficiency is severe, with a recessive inheritance pattern. Less often, deficiency of palladin (protein 4.2) is a cause of hereditary spherocytosis. Because the lipid bilayer is not well anchored when these proteins are defective, part of it is lost by vesiculation, resulting in a more spherical and less deformable cell. Because of their shape and rigidity, spherocytes are trapped in the spleen where their increased metabolic rate cannot be sustained, causing a further loss of surface membrane. This "conditioning" produces a subpopulation of hyperspheroidal RBC in the peripheral blood.

Diagnosis Hereditary spherocytosis must be distinguished primarily from the spherocytic hemolytic anemias associated with RBC antibodies. The family history of anemia and/or splenectomy is helpful, when present. The diagnosis of immune spherocytosis is usually readily established by a positive direct Coombs test (see below). Spherocytes are also seen in association with hemolysis induced by splenomegaly in patients with cirrhosis, in clostridial infections, and in certain snake envenomations (due to the action of phospholipases on the membrane). A few spherocytes are seen in the course of a wide variety of hemolytic disorders, particularly glucose-6-phosphate dehydrogenase (G6PD) deficiency.

HEREDITARY ELLIPTOCYTOSIS AND HEREDITARY PYROPOIKILOCYTOSIS *Hereditary elliptocytosis* is an autosomal dominant trait and affects 1 per 4000 to 5000 people, a frequency similar to that of hereditary spherocytosis (rarely, patients with myelodysplastic disorders of the bone marrow may have acquired elliptocytosis). In most affected individuals, a structural abnormality of erythrocyte spectrin leads to impaired assembly of the cytoskeleton. In some families, affected individuals have a deficiency of erythrocyte membrane protein 4.1, which stabilizes the interaction of spectrin and actin in the cytoskeleton (Fig. 93-3). In Southeast Asia, the incidence of hereditary ovalocytosis is high; a small internal deletion of protein 3 makes the membrane rigid and confers resistance against malaria.

The great majority of patients manifest only mild hemolysis, with little or no anemia. RBC destruction occurs predominantly in an enlarged spleen. Hemolysis is corrected by splenectomy.

The blood smear reveals elongated or oval red cells (elliptocytes). Patients with marked hemolysis have microovalocytes, bizarre-shaped RBC, and RBC fragments, all of which increase in number after splenectomy. The degree of hemolysis does not correlate with the percentage of elliptocytes.

Hereditary pyropoikilocytosis is a rare disorder related to hereditary elliptocytosis and is characterized by bizarre-shaped, microcytic RBC that undergo disruption at temperatures of 44 to 45°C (in contrast,

℞ TREATMENT

Splenectomy is recommended in patients with moderate or severe hemolysis. Although the RBC defect and its consequent morphology persist, anemia is ameliorated. The operative risk is low, particularly if performed by laparoscopy. RBC survival after splenectomy is normal or nearly so; if it is not, an accessory spleen or another diagnosis should be sought. Because of the potential for gallstones and for episodes of bone marrow hypoplasia or hemolytic crises, splenectomy should be performed in symptomatic individuals; cholecystectomy should not be performed without splenectomy, as intrahepatic gallstones may result. Splenectomy in children should be postponed until age 4, if possible, to minimize the risk of severe infections with gram-positive encapsulated organisms. Pneumococcal, meningococcal, and *Haemophilus influenzae* vaccines should be administered at least 2 weeks before splenectomy. In patients with severe hemolysis, folic acid (1 mg/d) should be administered prophylactically.

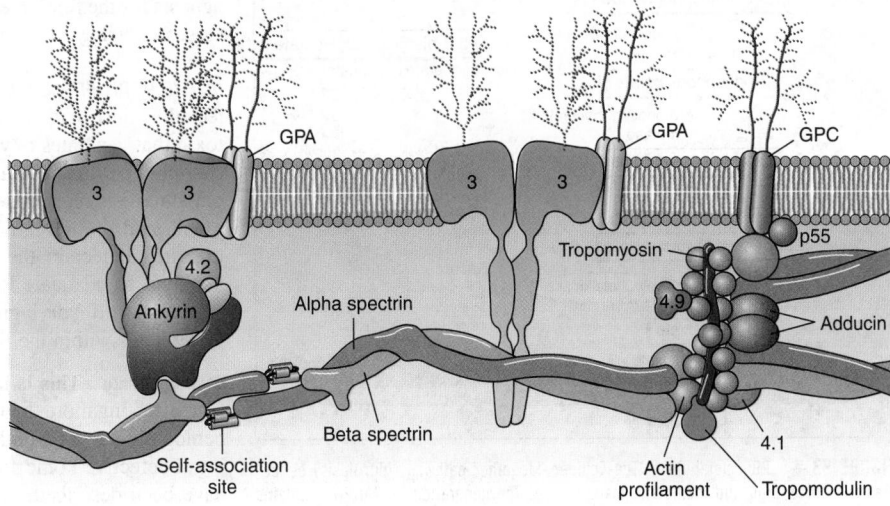

FIGURE 93-3 Diagram of a cross-section of the RBC membrane. Spectrin, actin, tropomyosin, adducin, and protein 4.1 form a meshwork that laminates the inner surface of the membrane. In contrast, other proteins such as the glycophorins (GPA and GPC) and protein 3 (anion transport channel) traverse the lipid bilayer. Long polysaccharide chains are covalently attached to these proteins on the outer surface of the cell and also to glycolipid. Ankyrin and protein 4.2 form a bridge between spectrin and a fraction of the anion transport proteins. Protein 4.1 binds to GPC. [*From Lux SE, Palek J, in Blood: Principles and Practice of Hematology, RI Handin et al (eds). Philadelphia, Lippincott, 1995.*]

normal RBC are stable up to 49°C). This condition results from a deficiency of spectrin and an abnormality of spectrin self-assembly. Hemolysis is usually severe, is recognized in childhood, and is partially responsive to splenectomy.

HEREDITARY STOMATOCYTOSIS   Stomatocytes are cup-shaped RBC that have a slitlike central zone of pallor on blood smears. The disorder is inherited in an autosomal dominant pattern. RBC have an increased permeability to sodium and potassium, which is compensated for by an increased active transport of these cations. In some patients, the RBC are swollen with an excess of ions and water and a decreased mean corpuscular hemoglobin concentration (overhydrated stomatocytes, "hydrocytosis"); many of these patients lack the RBC membrane protein 7.2 (stomatin). RBC lacking Rh proteins (Rh$_{null}$ cells) are also stomatocytic and have a shortened life span. In other patients, the RBC are shrunken, with a decreased ion and water content, appearing as target cells on blood smears. Most patients have splenomegaly and mild anemia. Splenectomy decreases but does not totally correct the hemolytic process.

Red Cell Enzyme Defects   During its maturation, the RBC loses its nucleus, ribosomes, and mitochondria and thus its capability for protein synthesis and oxidative phosphorylation. The mature circulating RBC has a relatively simple pattern of intermediary metabolism (Fig. 93-4)

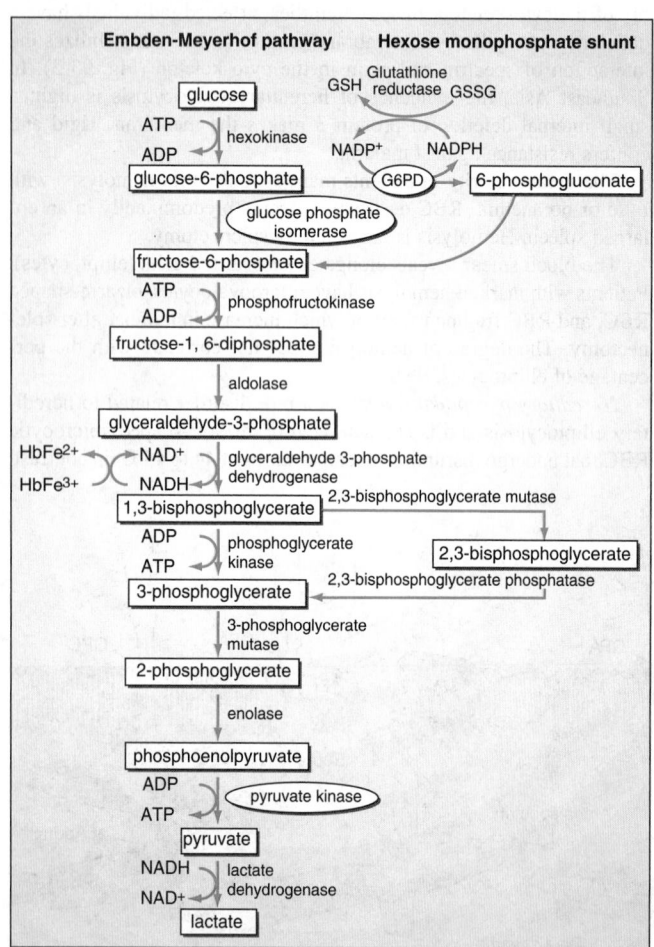

FIGURE 93-4   RBC metabolism. The Embden-Meyerhof pathway (glycolysis) generates ATP for energy and membrane maintenance. The generation of NADPH maintains hemoglobin in a reduced state. The hexose monophosphate shunt generates NADPH that is used to reduce glutathione, which protects the red cell against oxidant stress. Regulation of 2,3-bisphosphoglycerate levels is a critical determinant of oxygen affinity of hemoglobin. Enzyme deficiency states in order of prevalence: glucose-6-phosphate dehydrogenase (G6PD) ≫ pyruvate kinase > glucose-6-phosphate isomerase > rare deficiencies of other enzymes in the pathway. The more common enzyme deficiencies are encircled.

in keeping with its modest metabolic obligations. ATP must be generated from the Embden-Meyerhof pathway to drive the cation pump that maintains the ionic milieu in the RBC. Smaller amounts of energy are needed for the preservation of hemoglobin iron in the ferrous (Fe^{2+}) state and perhaps for the renewal of the lipids in the RBC membrane. About 10% of the glucose consumed by the RBC is metabolized via the hexose-monophosphate shunt (Fig. 93-4), which protects both hemoglobin and the membrane from oxidants, including certain drugs.

DEFECTS IN THE EMBDEN-MEYERHOF PATHWAY   Most of the glycolytic enzyme defects are inherited in an autosomal recessive pattern. Since the gene frequency for this group of defects is low, true heterozygotes are often the offspring of a consanguineous mating. More often, affected individuals are compound homozygotes. Patients with severe hemolysis usually present during early childhood with anemia, jaundice, and splenomegaly. The RBC are often relatively deficient in ATP, resulting in a leak of potassium ion out of these cells. These RBC are rigid and thus more readily sequestered by the mononuclear phagocyte system.

Some of these glycolytic enzyme deficiencies such as pyruvate kinase (PK) deficiency and hexokinase deficiency are localized to the RBC, with no apparent metabolic abnormality in other cells. In other disorders, the enzyme deficiency is more widespread.

About 95% of the clinically significant defects in the glycolytic pathway are due to PK deficiency, and about 4% are due to glucose phosphate isomerase deficiency. The remainder, shown in Fig. 93-4, are extremely rare. Most have been encountered in isolated families; clinical manifestations are variable.

Laboratory Findings   Patients have a normocytic (or slightly macrocytic), normochromic anemia with reticulocytosis. In those with PK deficiency, bizarre erythrocytes, including spiculated cells, are noted on the peripheral smear, especially after splenectomy. Spherocytes are usually absent; the term *congenital nonspherocytic hemolytic anemia* has been applied to these disorders. The diagnosis of this group of anemias depends on specific enzymatic assays. Abnormalities in enzymatic properties may be useful in distinguishing among enzyme mutants. DNA sequencing is the only definitive way to identify a mutant.

℞ TREATMENT

Most patients do not require therapy. Those with severe hemolysis should be given folic acid (1 mg/d). Blood transfusions may be necessary during a hypoplastic crisis. Women with PK deficiency may become very anemic during pregnancy, sometimes leading to the diagnosis for the first time. Patients with PK or glucose phosphate isomerase deficiency may benefit from splenectomy.

DEFECTS IN THE HEXOSE-MONOPHOSPHATE SHUNT   Normal RBC are well protected against oxidant stress. When the cells are exposed to a drug or toxin that generates oxygen radicals, glucose metabolism via the hexose-monophosphate shunt is normally increased severalfold. Reduced glutathione is regenerated, protecting the sulfhydryl groups of hemoglobin and the RBC membrane from oxidation. Individuals with an inherited defect in the hexose-monophosphate shunt are unable to maintain an adequate level of reduced glutathione in their RBC, hemoglobin sulfhydryl groups become oxidized, and the hemoglobin precipitates within the RBC, forming Heinz bodies.

G6PD Deficiency   This is by far the most common congenital shunt defect, affecting more than 200 million people throughout the world; like hemoglobin S, it partially protects the patient from malaria by providing a defective home for the merozoite. Over 400 variants of G6PD have been described, resulting in considerable clinical heterogeneity among affected individuals. Most are missense mutations resulting in altered enzymatic properties.

The normal G6PD is designated as type B. About 20% of individuals of African descent have a G6PD (designated A+) that differs by a single amino acid and is electrophoretically distinguishable but functionally normal. Among the clinically significant G6PD variants, the most common, the so-called A− type, is due to two base substitutions and is encountered primarily in individuals of central African descent. The A− G6PD has the same electrophoretic mobility as the A+ type, but it is unstable and has abnormal kinetic properties. This variant is found in about 11% of African-American males. A second relatively common G6PD variant is encountered among groups of Mediterranean origin, particularly Sardinians and Sephardic Jews; this variant is more severe than the A− variant and may result in nonspherocytic hemolytic anemia in the absence of known oxidative stress. A third relatively common and slightly less severe variant occurs in southern Chinese populations.

The G6PD gene is located on the X chromosome; thus the deficiency state is a sex-linked trait. Affected males (hemizygotes) inherit the abnormal gene from their mothers who are usually carriers (heterozygotes). Because of inactivation of one of the two X chromosomes (Lyon hypothesis: Chap. 56), the heterozygote has two populations of RBC: normal and deficient in G6PD. Most female carriers have no problems. Those who happen to have a high proportion of deficient cells resemble the male hemizygotes. G6PD activity normally declines ∼50% during the 120-day life span of the RBC. This decay is moderately accelerated in A− RBC and markedly so in RBC containing the Mediterranean variant. Individuals with the A− variant normally have a slightly shortened RBC survival time, but they are not anemic. Clinical problems arise only when the affected individual is subjected to some type of environmental stress. Most often, hemolytic episodes are triggered by viral and bacterial infections. The mechanism is unknown. In addition, drugs or toxins that pose an oxidant threat to the RBC (most commonly sulfa drugs, antimalarials, and nitrofurantoin) cause hemolysis in individuals deficient in G6PD (Table 93-4). Although aspirin is frequently mentioned as a likely offender, it has no deleterious effect in A− individuals. Accidental ingestion of toxic compounds such as naphthalene (moth balls) may cause severe hemolysis. Metabolic acidosis can precipitate an episode of hemolysis in individuals deficient in G6PD.

Clinical and Laboratory Features   The patient may experience an acute hemolytic crisis within hours of exposure to the oxidant stress, leading to hemoglobinuria and peripheral vascular collapse in severe cases. Since only the older population of RBC is rapidly destroyed, the hemolytic crisis is usually self-limited, even if the exposure to the oxidant continues. Among black males with the A− variant, the RBC mass decreases by a maximum of 25 to 30%. The oxidation of hemoglobin leads to the formation of Heinz bodies, visualized by means of a supravital stain such as crystal violet. However, Heinz bodies are usually not seen after the first day or so, since these inclusions are readily removed by the spleen. Their removal leads to the formation of "bite cells" (RBC that have lost a peripheral portion of the cell). Multiple bites cause the formation of fragments. A few spherocytes also may be present. Individuals with the Mediterranean type G6PD have much lower overall enzyme activity than those with the A− variant and, therefore, have more severe clinical manifestations. A minority of patients are exquisitely sensitive to fava beans and develop a fulminant hemolytic crisis after exposure. The oxidants in *Vicia fava* are two β-glycosides whose aglycones, when autoxidized, produce oxygen free radicals. The incidence of favism is highly variable due to variations in concentration, in absorption, or in metabolism of the aglycones. Favism is seldom encountered in individuals with the A− variant.

The *diagnosis* of G6PD deficiency should be considered in any individual, particularly a male of African or Mediterranean descent,

TABLE 93-4   *Drugs Causing Hemolysis in Subjects Deficient in G6PD*

Antimalarials: Primaquine, pamaquine, dapsone
Sulfonamides: Sulfamethoxazole
Nitrofurantoin
Analgesics: Acetanilid
Miscellaneous: Vitamin K (water-soluble form), doxorubicin, methylene
    blue, nalidixic acid, furazolidone, niridazole, phenazopyridine

who experiences an acute hemolytic episode. The patient should be questioned about possible exposure to oxidant agents. The diagnosis can be established by a number of tests that assess either the enzyme activity or the effects of its deficiency. However, the test may yield a false-negative result during a hemolytic episode when the old RBC deficient in the enzyme have already lysed.

R_x TREATMENT

Since hemolysis in patients deficient in A− G6PD is usually self-limited, no specific treatment is necessary. Splenectomy does not benefit Mediterranean patients with chronic hemolysis. Blood transfusions are rarely indicated. Adequate urine flow should be maintained if hemoglobinuria develops during an acute hemolytic episode.

Hemolytic episodes can be prevented by warning patients about risks posed by oxidant drugs and fava beans and by prompt treatment of infections.

Other Defects of the Hexose-Monophosphate Shunt   A few kindreds have been found to have congenital deficiency in RBC glutathione due to a defect in either of the two enzymes responsible for the synthesis of this tripeptide. Affected individuals have a hemolytic anemia with Heinz bodies that is aggravated by oxidant drugs.

OTHER ENZYME DEFECTS   Hemolytic anemia may sometimes be caused by abnormalities in enzymes of nucleotide metabolism. Individuals with pyrimidine 5′-nucleotidase deficiency have marked coarse basophilic stippling in their RBC because the mRNA of the cell is not properly metabolized. Hemolytic anemia also has been noted in individuals whose RBC have supranormal levels of adenosine deaminase and relatively low levels of ATP.

Hemoglobinopathies   Hemolysis is a component of anemias related to some hemoglobinopathies (Chap. 91).

ACQUIRED HEMOLYTIC ANEMIAS   In most patients with acquired hemolytic anemia, RBC are made normally but are prematurely destroyed because of damage acquired in the circulation. (The exceptions are rare disorders characterized by acquired dysplasia of the cells of the bone marrow and the production of structurally and functionally abnormal RBC.) The damage that occurs may be mediated by antibodies or toxins or may be due to abnormalities in the circulation, including an overactive mononuclear phagocyte system or traumatic lysis by natural or artificial impediments to circulation. The acquired hemolytic anemias are classified into five categories (Table 93-5).

TABLE 93-5   *Causes of Acquired Hemolytic Anemia*

   I. Entrapment
  II. Immune
     A. Warm-reactive (IgG) antibody
     B. Cold-reactive IgM antibody (cold agglutinin disease)
     C. Cold-reactive IgG antibody (paroxysmal cold hemoglobinuria)
     D. Drug-dependent antibody
       1. Autoimmune
       2. Haptene
  III. Traumatic hemolytic anemia
     A. Impact hemolysis
     B. Macrovascular defects—prostheses
     C. Microvascular causes
       1. Thrombotic thrombocytopenic purpura/hemolytic-uremic
         syndrome
       2. Other causes of microvascular abnormalities
       3. Disseminated intravascular hemolysis
  IV. Hemolytic anemia due to toxic effects on the membrane
     A. Spur cell anemia
     B. External toxins
       1. Animal or spider bites
       2. Metals (e.g., copper)
       3. Organic compounds
   V. Paroxysmal nocturnal hemoglobinuria

Hypersplenism   The spleen is particularly efficient in trapping and destroying RBC that have minimal defects. This unique ability of the spleen to filter mildly damaged RBC results from its unusual vascular anatomy (Chap. 54). Almost all the blood circulating through the spleen flows rapidly from arterioles in the white pulp to sinuses in the spleen's red pulp and then into the venous system. In contrast, a small portion of splenic blood flow (normally 1 to 2%) passes into the "marginal zone" of the lymphatic white pulp. Although the cells that occupy this zone are not phagocytic, they serve as a mechanical filter that hinders the progress of severely damaged blood cells. As RBC leave this zone and enter the red pulp, they flow into narrow cords, rich in macrophages, that end blindly but communicate with sinuses through small openings between the lining cells of the sinuses. These openings, averaging 3 μm in diameter, test the ability of RBC (4.5 μm in diameter) to undergo deformation. RBC that cannot re-enter the vascular sinuses are engulfed by phagocytic cells and destroyed (see Fig. 54-1).

The normal spleen retains reticulocytes for 1 to 2 days but otherwise poses no threat to normal RBC until they become senescent. However, in the face of splenomegaly, increased destruction of the cells of the blood, including the RBC, may take place due to pooling of the blood in a relatively nutrient-poor environment full of phagocytic cells. Splenic sequestration that causes cytopenia is called hypersplenism. In infiltrative diseases of the spleen, substantial splenomegaly may exist with no apparent hemolysis; inflammatory and congestive splenomegaly is commonly associated with modest shortening of RBC survival time, along with more marked granulocytopenia and thrombocytopenia. Patients with cytopenia(s) sufficient to produce symptoms generally benefit from splenectomy.

Immunologic Causes of Hemolysis   Immune hemolysis in the adult is usually induced by IgG or IgM antibodies reacting specifically with antigens associated with the patient's RBC (often called "autoantibodies") or with alloantigens on transfused RBC (alloantibodies) (Chap. 99).

The Coombs antiglobulin test is the major tool for diagnosing autoimmune hemolysis. This test relies on the ability of antibodies specific for immunoglobulins (especially IgG) or complement components (especially C3) to agglutinate RBC coated with these proteins. With specific anti-IgG and anti-C3, the *direct Coombs test* detects IgG or C3 on the patient's RBC, which indicates the presence of immune hemolysis and may help define its cause (Table 93-6). Rarely, neither IgG nor complement may be found on the RBC of the patient (Coombs-negative immune hemolytic anemia).

Antibodies in the serum of the patient that recognize RBC antigens can be detected by reacting the serum with normal RBC bearing the antigen. With the exception of cold-reacting antibodies and some drug-related antibodies (see below), this is of value primarily in compatibility testing for transfusion.

"WARM" ANTIBODIES   Antibodies that react at body temperature (warm antibodies) are nearly always IgG, rarely IgM or IgA. Autologous warm antibodies cause *autoimmune hemolytic (or immunohemolytic) anemia, warm antibody type*.

Clinical Manifestations   Immunohemolytic anemia of the warm antibody type occurs at all ages, but it is more common in adults, particularly women. In approximately one-fourth of patients this disorder occurs as a complication of an underlying disease affecting the immune system, especially lymphoid neoplasms (Chap. 97); collagen vascular diseases, especially systemic lupus erythematosus (SLE); and congenital immunodeficiency diseases (Table 93-7). A wide variety of drugs may stimulate antibody formation, resulting in a similar syndrome (see below).

The presentation and course of IgG immunohemolytic anemia are quite variable. In its mildest form, the only manifestation is a positive direct Coombs test. In this instance, insufficient antibody is present on the RBC surface to permit the reticuloendothelial system to recognize

TABLE 93-6 *Use of the Direct Coombs Test in Diagnosing the Cause of Autoimmune Hemolytic Anemia*

Reaction with		
Anti-IgG	Anti-C3	Causes
Yes	No	Antibodies to Rh proteins, hemolysis caused by α-methyldopa or penicillin
Yes	Yes	Antibodies to glycoprotein antigens, SLE
No	Yes	Cold-reacting antibodies (agglutinins or Donath-Landsteiner antibody), most drug-related antibodies, IgM antibodies, IgG antibodies of low affinity, activation of complement by immune complexes

the cell as abnormal. Most symptomatic patients have a moderate to severe anemia [hemoglobin levels 60 to 100 g/L and reticulocyte counts 10 to 30% (200 to 600 × 10³/μL)], spherocytosis (Fig. 93-5), and splenomegaly. Occasionally, venous thrombosis occurs.

Severe immunohemolytic anemia presents with fulminant hemolysis associated with hemoglobinemia, hemoglobinuria, and shock; this syndrome may be rapidly fatal unless aggressively treated.

The direct Coombs test is positive in 98% of patients; usually IgG is detected with or without C3. The pattern of IgG and C3 fixation on the patient's RBC may indicate the origin of the disorder.

Immune thrombocytopenia also may be present (*Evans syndrome*), a disorder in which separate antibodies are directed against platelets and RBC.

Pathogenesis   IgG antibodies lyse RBC by two mechanisms: (1) immune adherence of RBC to phagocytes mediated by the antibody and by complement components that become fixed to the membrane (by far the more important mechanism of destruction), and (2) complement activation. IgG antibodies bind to Fc receptors on macrophages, activating those cells to engulf the coated RBC. If internalization is only partial, a portion of the RBC membrane is removed, resulting in the formation of spherocytes, which are destroyed in the spleen. Complement-mediated immune adherence involves the interaction of C3b and C4b with receptors on the macrophage; while much less likely to lead to RBC lysis, this mechanism markedly increases the immune adherence due to IgG. Immune adherence, particularly that due to the IgG antibody, is also enhanced by the transit of RBC into splenic cords and sinuses, which brings cells into direct contact with phagocytic cells.

Ⓡ TREATMENT

Patients having a mild degree of hemolysis usually do not require therapy. In those with clinically significant hemolysis, initial therapy consists of glucocorticoids (e.g., prednisone, 1.0 mg/kg per day). A rise in hemoglobin is frequently noted within 3 or 4 days and occurs

TABLE 93-7 *Hemolysis due to Antibodies*

WARM-ANTIBODY IMMUNOHEMOLYTIC ANEMIA

1. Idiopathic
2. Lymphomas: Chronic lymphocytic leukemia, non-Hodgkin's lymphomas, Hodgkin's disease (infrequent)
3. SLE and other collagen-vascular diseases
4. Drugs
   a. α-Methyldopa type (autoantibody to Rh antigens)
   b. Penicillin type (stable hapten)
   c. Quinidine type (unstable hapten)
5. Postviral infections
6. Other tumors (rare)

COLD-ANTIBODY IMMUNOHEMOLYTIC ANEMIA

1. Cold agglutinin disease
   a. Acute: *Mycoplasma* infection, infectious mononucleosis
   b. Chronic: Idiopathic, lymphoma
2. Paroxysmal cold hemoglobinuria

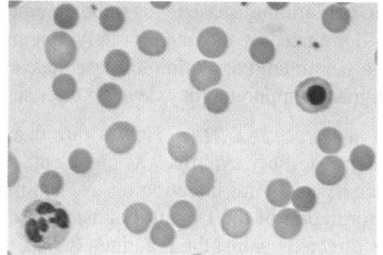

FIGURE 93-5 *Immunohemolytic anemia* Microspherocytes are seen on this blood smear along with several macrocytes with a slight purple tinge (polychromasia). The latter represent new red blood cells released early from the bone marrow. The microspherocytes seen in immunohemolytic anemia may be indistinguishable from the microspherocytes seen in hereditary spherocytosis (Fig. 93-1).

in most patients within 1 to 2 weeks. Prednisone is continued until the hemoglobin level has risen to normal values, and thereafter it is tapered rapidly to about 20 mg/d, then slowly over the course of several months. An algorithm for this tapering process is given in Fig. 93-6. For chronic therapy with prednisone, alternate-day administration is preferred. More than 75% of patients achieve an initial significant and sustained reduction in hemolysis; however, in half these patients the disease recurs, either during glucocorticoid tapering or after its cessation. Glucocorticoids have two modes of action: an immediate effect due to inhibiting clearance of IgG-coated RBC by the mononuclear phagocyte system and a later effect due to inhibiting antibody synthesis. Splenectomy is recommended for patients who cannot tolerate or fail to respond to glucocorticoid therapy.

Patients who have been refractory to glucocorticoid therapy and to splenectomy are treated with immunosuppressive drugs. A success rate of ~50% has been reported. Intravenous gamma globulin may cause rapid cessation of hemolysis; however, it is not nearly as effective in this disorder as in immune thrombocytopenia.

Patients with severe anemia may require blood transfusions. Because the antibody in this disease is usually a "panagglutinin," reacting with nearly all normal donor cells, compatible cross-matching is impossible. The goal in selecting blood for transfusion is to avoid administering RBC with antigens to which the patient may have alloantibodies. A common procedure is to adsorb the panagglutinin

present in the patient's serum with the patient's own RBC from which antibody has been previously eluted. Serum cleared of autoantibody can then be tested for the presence of alloantibody to donor blood groups. ABO-compatible RBC matched in this fashion are administered slowly, with watchfulness for signs of an immediate-type hemolytic transfusion reaction.

Prognosis Immune hemolytic anemia is often transient in children, particularly when it follows a viral infection, but is usually chronic in adults, lasting many years with exacerbations and remissions. In most patients, hemolysis is controlled by glucocorticoid therapy alone, by splenectomy, or by a combination. Fatalities occur among three rare subsets of patients: (1) those with overwhelming hemolysis who die from anemia; (2) those whose host defenses are impaired by glucocorticoids, splenectomy, and/or immunosuppressive agents; and (3) those with major thrombotic events coincident with active hemolysis.

When immunohemolysis develops as a complication of an underlying disorder, the prognosis is often determined by the primary disease.

IMMUNOHEMOLYTIC ANEMIA SECONDARY TO DRUGS Drugs cause immunohemolytic anemia by two mechanisms of action: (1) they induce a disorder identical in almost every respect to warm-antibody immunohemolytic anemia [e.g., α-methyldopa (an antihypertensive; Chap. 230)], or (2) they become associated as haptens with the RBC surface and induce the formation of an antibody directed against the RBC-drug complex (e.g., penicillin, quinidine).

A positive direct Coombs test is observed in up to 10% of patients receiving α-methyldopa therapy in doses of 2 g/d or higher. A small minority of these patients develop spherocytosis and hemolysis, which may be severe. The autoantibodies cross-react with the normal Rh protein.

In most other cases of drug-induced hemolysis, the antibody is directed against the combination of the drug and the membrane glycoprotein to which it is attached. The hemolytic reaction in vivo is dependent on the presence of the drug and usually ceases shortly after the drug has been discontinued. Penicillin and its congeners may cause this type of reaction if the drug is given in very high doses (10 million units per day or more). The direct Coombs test is positive only with anti-IgG; the indirect Coombs test is positive only when the normal cells have been coated with penicillin. Complement is not usually fixed, and the hemolysis in vivo is usually not severe. Since the antibody is usually IgG, spherocytosis and splenic destruction may occur.

Most other drugs (such as quinine, quinidine, sulfonamides, sulfonureas, phenacetin, stibophen, and dipyrone) do not adhere as tightly to their glycoproteins, and the drug-antibody complexes are removed during the washing steps of the direct and indirect Coombs reactions. These antibodies (particularly IgM) are usually able to fix complement, and C3d and C4d remain on the RBC surface; thus the direct Coombs test is positive with anti-C3 but not anti-IgG. The antibody is detected in the *indirect* Coombs test only when the drug is added to the incubation mixture. Hemolysis may be quite severe, sometimes resulting in signs of intravascular hemolysis; resolution is usually prompt after the drug is discontinued.

IMMUNE HEMOLYSIS DUE TO COLD-REACTIVE ANTIBODIES Antibodies that react with polysaccharide antigens are usually IgM and bind antigen better at temperatures lower than 37°C, hence the name *cold-reactive antibodies*. Uncommonly, the antibody is IgG (the Donath-Landsteiner antibody of paroxysmal cold hemoglobinuria).

IgM cold-reacting antibodies readily agglutinate RBC and are called *cold agglutinins*. They arise in two clinical settings: (1) monoclonal antibodies, the product of lymphocytic neoplasia or paraneoplasia; and (2) polyclonal antibodies in response to infection. In many elderly patients, the "neoplasm" is benign monoclonal gammopathy that does not progress, and the paraprotein remains its only manifes-

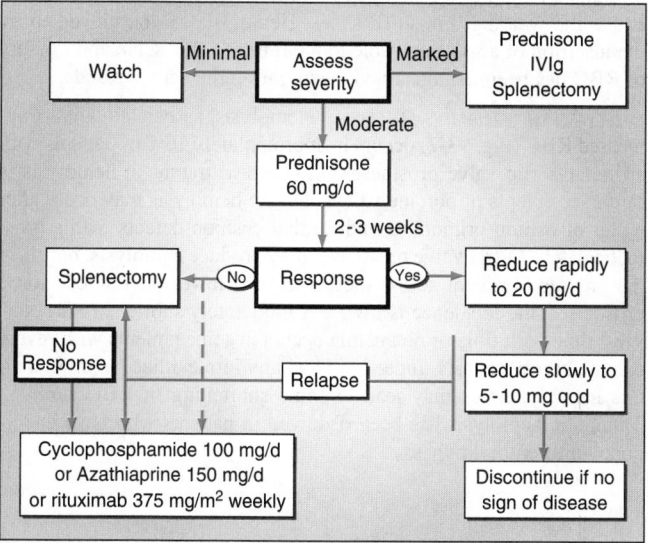

FIGURE 93-6 Algorithm for the treatment of patients with IgG-mediated immune hemolytic anemia. The patient with minimal disease may be watched carefully. The patient with very severe disease may need all modalities of treatment applied at once. The more common patient with moderate disease may be treated with prednisone at a high dose; if no response is seen, then either splenectomy is performed or an immunosuppressive agent is given. If a response is seen, the dose of prednisone is reduced over time. If relapse occurs during this process, splenectomy or chemotherapy may be needed.

tation. Occasionally, cold agglutinins are found in patients with non-lymphoid neoplasms.

Transient cold agglutinins occur commonly in two infections: *Mycoplasma pneumoniae* infection and infectious mononucleosis. In both, the titer of antibody is usually too low to cause clinical symptoms, but its presence is of diagnostic value; only occasionally is hemolysis present. Cold agglutinins are less frequently encountered in a number of other viral infections. Their manifestations are usually benign.

The specificity of the antibody may be of diagnostic value. Cold agglutinins reacting more strongly with adult RBC than fetal (cord) RBC are called *anti-I*; these antibodies are seen in benign lymphoproliferation (chronic cold agglutinin monoclonal gammopathy) and in Mycoplasma infections. Those reacting more strongly with cord RBC cells are called *anti-i*; these antibodies are seen in aggressive lymphomas and in infectious mononucleosis. Rarely, the antibody may react with other antigens that are equally expressed on adult and cord RBC. The clinical manifestations elicited by the antibody on exposure to cold are of two sorts: intravascular agglutination (acrocyanosis) and hemolysis. Acrocyanosis is the marked purpling of the extremities, ears, and nose when the blood becomes cold enough to agglutinate in the veins; it clears on warming and does not have the vasospastic characteristics of Raynaud's phenomenon (Chap. 232). Patients may also have symptoms when swallowing cold food or drinks.

The hemolysis is usually not severe and is manifested by a mild reticulocytosis, agglutination on the blood film, and agglutination during analysis of the blood by particle analysis (giving rise to a falsely high mean corpuscular volume). The degree of hemolysis depends on several variables.

1. *Antibody titer.* The titer in symptomatic patients is usually above 1:2000 dilution of serum and may range to as high as 1:50,000. When collecting samples, great care must be taken to keep the serum separated from the cells while the sample is maintained at 37°C so that the antibody will not adsorb onto the patient's own cells.
2. *Thermal amplitude of the antibody* (the highest temperature at which the antibody will react with the RBC). For most antibodies, this is 23 to 30°C. Those with a higher thermal amplitude (up to 37°C) are more hemolytic, since it is more likely that these temperatures will be encountered during RBC circulation.
3. *Environmental temperature.* Since the reaction can occur only at temperatures below body temperature, frequency and degree of exposure to cold are major determinants of the rate of hemolysis.

The hemolysis that occurs is due primarily to the hemolytic action of complement, since there are no functional Fc receptors for the IgM antibody on phagocytes. Complement is readily fixed; a single molecule of IgM is enough to effect binding of C1 and initiate the cascade. However, normal human RBC are remarkably resistant to the hemolytic action of complement because of several defense mechanisms. Therefore, severe hemolysis with hemoglobinuria occurs only with massive activation of the antibody, such as by sudden cooling. The activation of complement is always marked by the accumulation of a degradation product of C3, C3dg, on the surface; this product is what is detected with appropriate antisera in the direct Coombs test in all patients with significant cold agglutinin disease.

The cutaneous manifestations are best treated by maintaining the patient in a warm environment. Splenectomy is usually not of value in this disorder. Glucocorticoids are of limited value, although patients with the panthermal variety of cold agglutinin disease may respond. Chlorambucil and cyclophosphamide are commonly used to treat patients who have hemolysis associated with monoclonal gammopathy, but their efficacy is usually marginal. Rituximab (anti-CD20) has been effective in some cases. Successful treatment of the neoplasm responsible for the cold agglutinin often lowers the antibody titer and the severity of hemolysis.

Chronic cold agglutinin disease tends to be unremitting. The overall prognosis is dominated by the underlying lymphoma, if present. In those patients in whom cold agglutinin disease appears to arise spontaneously, malignant lymphoma may develop after several years.

PAROXYSMAL COLD HEMOGLOBINURIA (PCH)   Now a rare disorder, PCH was more frequent when tertiary syphilis was prevalent; now, most cases are either secondary to a viral infection or are autoimmune. PCH results from the formation of the Donath-Landsteiner antibody, an IgG antibody that is directed against the P antigen (Chap. 99) and that can induce complement-mediated lysis. Attacks are precipitated by exposure to cold and are associated with hemoglobinemia and hemoglobinuria; chills and fever; back, leg, and abdominal pain; headache; and malaise. Recovery from the acute episode is prompt, and between episodes patients are usually asymptomatic. When this syndrome accompanies acute viral infections (e.g., measles and mumps in children), it is self-limited but may be severe. Although the direct Coombs test may show complement to be present (seldom IgG), this test may be negative. The diagnosis is made by demonstrating cold-reacting IgG antibodies either by lytic tests (when the titer is very high) or by special antiglobulin tests. When PCH is secondary to syphilis, it responds to therapy for syphilis. Chronic autoimmune PCH may respond to prednisone or cytotoxic therapy (azathioprine or cyclophosphamide) but does not respond to splenectomy. The natural history of this disease often extends over many years.

Hemolysis Due to Trauma in the Circulation   RBC may be fragmented by mechanical trauma as they circulate; this circumstance leads to intravascular hemolysis and in most cases to RBC fragments called *schistocytes*. Schistocytes are identified by the sharp points that result from the faulty resealing of the fractured membrane (Fig. 93-7). Mechanical trauma leading to hemolysis occurs in three clinical settings: (1) when RBC flow through small vessels over the surface of bony prominences and are subject to external impact during various physical activities, (2) when RBC flow across a pressure gradient created by an abnormal heart valve or valve prosthesis (macrovascular), and (3) when the deposition of fibrin or small platelet thrombi in the microvasculature exposes RBC to a physical impediment that fragments them (microvascular) (Table 93-8).

EXTERNAL IMPACT   Hemoglobinemia and hemoglobinuria have been observed in a small proportion of individuals who have undergone a prolonged march or a prolonged run, most typically on a hard surface and while wearing thin-soled shoes. Hemolysis can be prevented by the insertion of a soft inner sole in the runner's shoes. No abnormality of RBC has been demonstrated, even during the acute episode.

MACROVASCULAR TRAUMATIC HEMOLYSIS   Hemolysis associated with fragmented RBC (Fig. 93-7) occurs in approximately 10% of patients with artificial aortic valve prostheses. In contrast, traumatic hemolysis is rare in recipients of porcine valves. Severe hemolysis may occur after repair of ostium primum or endocardial cushion defects with a prosthetic patch. Mitral valve prostheses may produce hemolysis, but since the pressure gradient across these valves is lower than across aortic prostheses, the incidence is lower. A moderately shortened RBC survival time with little or no anemia occurs in some patients with severe calcific aortic stenosis. Indeed, almost any intracardiac lesion that alters hemodynamics may lead to some shortening of RBC survival. Traumatic hemolysis has been observed in patients who have undergone aortofemoral bypass.

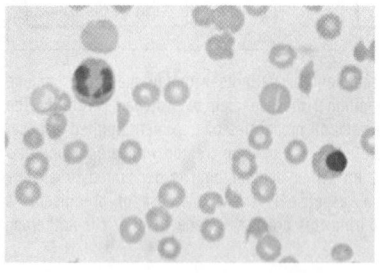

FIGURE 93-7 The helmet-shaped red blood cell and the small triangular-shaped red blood cells seen on this smear represent morphologic evidence of mechanical damage to red blood cells within the blood vessels.

TABLE 93-8 *Changes in RBC and Platelets Induced by Intravascular Trauma*

Etiology	Fragments	Hemolysis	Thrombocytopenia
Impact: march hemoglobinuria, etc.	0	+	0
Cardiac (turbulence):			
Aortic valve prosthesis	++++	++++	0
Mitral valve prosthesis	++	++	0
Calcific aortic stenoses	+	±	0
Vessel disease[a]	+++	+	+
Thrombotic thrombocytopenic purpura	++++	++++	++++
Hemolytic-uremic syndrome	++++	++++	++++
Adenocarcinoma	++++	++++	++++
Disseminated intravascular coagulation	++	±	++++

[a] Malignant hypertension, eclampsia, renal graft rejection, hemangiomas, immune disease (scleroderma).

Clinical Manifestations In severe cases, hemoglobin levels fall to 50 to 70 g/L with reticulocytosis, fragmented RBC in the peripheral blood, depressed haptoglobin, elevated serum LDH, and hemoglobinemia and hemoglobinuria. Iron loss (as hemoglobin or hemosiderin) in the urine may lead to iron deficiency. The direct Coombs test may rarely become positive.

℞ TREATMENT

Iron deficiency should be corrected by the administration of oral iron. The elevated hemoglobin that results may permit a decrease in the cardiac output and a slowing of the hemolytic rate. Limitation in physical activity also lessens the hemolytic rate. When these measures fail, any paravalvular leak must be repaired or the prosthetic valve replaced.

MICROVASCULAR TRAUMATIC HEMOLYSIS If fibrin or platelet microthrombi are deposited in arteriolar sites, RBC may be trapped on the meshwork and fragmented by high shear forces.

Abnormalities of the Vessel Wall Disorders such as malignant hypertension, eclampsia [hemolysis, elevated liver enzymes, low platelets (HELLP) syndrome], renal allograft rejection, disseminated cancer, hemangiomas, or disseminated intravascular coagulation (DIC) may cause traumatic hemolysis (Chaps. 101, 102). The degree of hemolysis induced by this family of disorders is usually quite mild, but a large number of fragments may be seen in the peripheral blood. In some patients, thrombocytopenia may be severe. Therapy is best directed at the primary disease. Thus, reversal of renal graft rejection, treatment of malignant hypertension and eclampsia, control of cancer, and the like lead to a cessation of hemolysis. The relative importance of the primary vascular abnormality versus fibrin deposition is unclear.

THROMBOTIC THROMBOCYTOPENIA PURPURA (TTP) This disorder is characterized by arteriolar lesions in various organs that contain platelet thrombi and produce thrombocytopenia and hemolytic anemia due to fragmentation of RBC (see Chap. 101).

HEMOLYTIC-UREMIC SYNDROME This disorder is similar to TTP and is characterized by the same arteriolar lesions, which may be confined to the kidney, and by similar laboratory findings (see Chap. 101).

DISSEMINATED INTRAVASCULAR COAGULATION Inappropriate activation of the clotting system with deposition of fibrin in small vessels may lead to RBC fragmentation in the microvasculature. RBC fragmentation occurs in about one-fourth of patients with DIC (Chap. 102). The degree of hemolysis is much less in DIC than in either TTP or the hemolytic-uremic syndrome, and anemia with reticulocytosis is rare.

Environmental Alteration of the Red Cell Membrane by "Toxic" Effects A variety of infections may be associated with severe hemolysis. The microbes that cause bartonellosis (Chap. 144), as well as malaria and babesiosis (Chap. 195), directly parasitize RBC. *Clostridium welchii* (Chap. 126) produces a phospholipase that can cleave the phosphoryl bond of lecithin, thereby lysing human RBC. A mild, transient hemolysis frequently accompanies bacteremia with diverse organisms such as pneumococci, staphylococci, and *Escherichia coli*.

Hemolysis may result from the direct action of snake and spider venoms on the RBC. Although cobra venom is directly lytic in vitro, the clinical disease induced by the bite of the cobra is one of moderate hemolysis associated with spherocytosis. Spider bites, particularly the bite of the brown recluse spider, induce acute intravascular hemolysis associated with spherocytosis and fragments of complement components on the RBC. The hemolysis continues for several days up to 1 week.

Copper has a direct hemolytic effect on RBC. Hemolysis has been observed after exposure of individuals to copper salts (such as during hemodialysis). Transient episodes of hemolysis occur in patients with Wilson's disease (Chap. 339).

The RBC membrane is unstable at temperatures above 49°C due to denaturation of the cytoskeletal protein spectrin. The RBC undergoes a process of budding, cleavage, and resealing above this temperature. Patients with extensive burns have prominent spherocytosis, hemoglobinemia, and sometimes hemoglobinuria.

Spur Cell Anemia Hemolytic anemia with bizarre-shaped RBC occurs in about 5% of patients with severe hepatocellular disease, particularly advanced Laennec's cirrhosis.

Clinical Manifestations Anemia is more severe than that observed in otherwise uncomplicated cirrhosis. Splenomegaly is always present and is greater than in patients who have cirrhosis without spur cell anemia. The RBC are irregularly shaped with multiple spicules, and a small number of bizarre-shaped fragments are commonly seen on peripheral blood smears (see Fig. 98-3).

Pathogenesis The surface membrane of a spur cell contains 50 to 70% excess cholesterol, but its total phospholipid content is normal. Cholesterol out of proportion to phospholipid decreases the membrane fluidity and cell deformability. These rigid, cholesterol-laden RBC cannot pass through the filtering system of the spleen, further impeded by congestive splenomegaly in cirrhosis. In contrast, the target-shaped RBC is more common in liver disease and has an excess of both cholesterol and phospholipid.

Diagnosis Patients with spur cell anemia have severe hemolysis and characteristic RBC morphology. Spur cells or acanthocytes have irregular spikes (irregular in length of projections and their spacing) and must be distinguished from regularly spaced, crenated RBC (echinocytes). Echinocytes are a frequent artifact on portions of some blood smears, and they are uniformly present in some patients with uremia ("burr cells") (Fig. 93-8). Small, dense, crenated spheres (spheroechinocytes) are sometimes seen in congenital nonspherocytic hemolytic anemia due to enzyme deficiencies in the Embden-Meyerhof pathway (see above). RBC of similar morphology are seen in patients with abetalipoproteinemia. However, hemolysis is minimal.

℞ TREATMENT

Transfusion therapy is of limited benefit. Lipid-lowering agents have been unsuccessful. Splenectomy has been reported to prevent both the

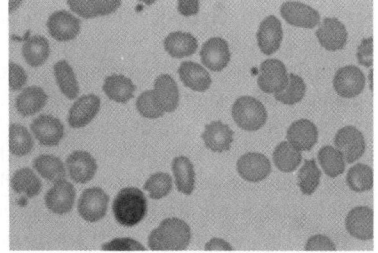

FIGURE 93-8 The red blood cells in uremia may acquire numerous, regularly spaced, small spiny projections. Such cells, called burr cells or echinocytes, are readily distinguishable from irregularly spiculated acanthocytes or spur cells.

conditioning of RBC in the spleen and their premature destruction. However, splenectomy carries a high risk in patients with severe liver disease complicated by portal hypertension and coagulation defects. It must be reserved for patients in whom hemolysis is a major problem and who are relatively good surgical risks.

Prognosis Spur cell anemia occurs during the late stages of cirrhosis, and >90% of patients succumb to their underlying liver disease within 1 year of the diagnosis of spur cell anemia.

Paroxysmal Nocturnal Hemoglobinuria (PNH) This hemolytic disorder is distinctive because it is an intracorpuscular defect acquired at the stem cell level.

Clinical Manifestations The three common manifestations of PNH are hemolytic anemia, venous thrombosis, and deficient hematopoiesis. Anemia is highly variable, with hematocrit values ranging from ≤20% to normal. RBC are normochromic and normocytic unless iron deficiency has occurred from chronic iron loss in the urine.

Clinical hemoglobinuria is intermittent in most patients and never occurs in some, but hemosiderinuria is usually present. Since hemolysis is due to abnormalities of the RBC leading to sensitivity to the hemolytic action of complement, it is manifest when complement is activated, for example, by infection.

Granulocytopenia and thrombocytopenia are common and reflect impaired hematopoiesis. The life span of the platelet is normal. However, the activation of complement indirectly stimulates platelet aggregation and hypercoagulability; this probably accounts for the tendency toward thrombosis seen in PNH.

Venous thrombosis is a common complication of patients of European origin, affecting ~40% at one time or another; it is less common in Asian patients. It occurs primarily in intra-abdominal veins (hepatic, portal, mesenteric) and results in Budd-Chiari syndrome, congestive splenomegaly, and abdominal pain. It may occur in cerebral venous sinuses and is a common cause of death in patients with PNH.

The bone marrow may appear normocellular, but in vitro marrow progenitor assays are abnormal. In about 15 to 30% of long-term survivors of aplastic anemia, PNH cells appear in the circulation; in some patients, the manifestations of PNH become dominant. Patients with PNH may have aplastic periods lasting from weeks to years. PNH may be seen in association with other stem cell disorders, including myelofibrosis and (rarely) other myelodysplastic or myeloproliferative disorders.

Pathogenesis PNH is an acquired clonal disease, arising from an inactivating somatic mutation in a single hematopoietic stem cell of a gene on the X-chromosome (*pig-A*) necessary for the biosynthesis of the glycosylphosphatidylinositol (GPI) anchor. This anchor attaches a number of proteins to the external membrane surface, and its partial or complete absence results in the absence of those proteins; to date, about 20 proteins have been found to be missing on the blood cells of patients with PNH. Two of these are the complement defense proteins CD55 [PNH decay accelerating factor (DAF)] and CD59, which block complement activation on the cell surface. Their absence accounts for the sensitivity of RBC to complement lysis and for the tendency of platelets to abnormally initiate clotting. The normal clones of stem cells do not completely disappear, and the proportion of cells that are abnormal varies among patients and over time in a single patient.

Diagnosis PNH should be suspected in anyone with otherwise unexplained hemolytic anemia, especially with leukopenia and/or thrombocytopenia and with evidence of intravascular hemolysis (hemoglobinemia, hemoglobinuria, hemosiderinuria, elevated LDH). Anyone recovering from aplastic anemia should be examined at intervals for the appearance of the diagnostic cells. The diagnosis is often delayed because (1) it is not considered, (2) hemoglobinuria is confused with hematuria, (3) elevation of the LDH is attributed to liver disease, and (4) the diagnostic tests [the acidified serum lysis test (Ham test) and the sucrose lysis test] are not reliable.

For many years, the diagnosis of PNH depended on the demonstration of the lysis of RBC after complement activation either by acid (Ham test) or by reduction in ionic strength (sucrose lysis test). These tests are inferior to the analysis of GPI-linked proteins (e.g., CD59, DAF) on RBC and granulocytes by flow cytometry.

℞ TREATMENT

Transfusion therapy is useful in PNH not only for raising the hemoglobin level but also for suppressing the marrow production of RBC during episodes of sustained hemoglobinuria. Washed RBC are the preferred source to prevent exacerbation of hemolysis. Therapy with androgens sometimes results in a rise in hemoglobin level. Glucocorticoids reduce the rate of hemolysis in moderate doses (15 to 30 mg prednisone) on alternate days.

Iron deficiency is common. Iron replacement may exacerbate hemolysis because of the formation of many new RBC, which may be sensitive to complement. This occurrence may be minimized by giving prednisone (60 mg/d) or by suppressing the bone marrow with transfusions.

Acute thrombosis in PNH, particularly Budd-Chiari syndrome and cerebral thrombosis, should be treated with thrombolytic agents. Heparin therapy should be instituted rapidly and maintained using low-molecular-weight heparin, at least for several weeks to months and perhaps indefinitely in severe cases. Anyone who has had a major thrombosis should chronically receive at least warfarin therapy. Antithymocyte globulin (total dose, 150 mg/kg over 4 to 10 days) is often of use in treating marrow hypoplasia; prednisone counteracts the immune-complex disease that results from the administration of this foreign protein.

In patients with either hypoplasia or thrombosis who have an appropriate sibling donor, marrow transplantation should be considered early in the course of the disease. The usual conditioning programs are sufficient to eradicate the aberrant clone.

ANEMIA OF ACUTE BLOOD LOSS

The normal capacity to compensate for acute blood loss involves cardiovascular mechanisms, an adjustment in the oxygen affinity of hemoglobin, and an increase in erythropoiesis in the marrow. The signs and symptoms of blood loss relate to the volume of the blood loss and the time frame over which the hemorrhage occurs (Table 93-9). Losses of up to 20% of the blood volume are normally tolerated by redistribution of blood flow mediated by reflex venospasm, but the presence of fever or pain may interfere with this compensation. With larger losses, blood volume redistribution is not adequate to maintain normal blood pressure: initially, hypotension is only seen on standing, but with greater losses the patient has hypotension in sitting or supine positions. If the blood loss is more gradual, plasma volume increases, but albumin production usually lags behind the fluid shifts. It may take 2 to 3 days for the liver to generate the albumin lost in a 1500-mL bleed.

TABLE 93-9 *Signs and Symptoms of Acute Blood Loss*

Blood Loss			
%,[a]	Volume, mL	Symptoms	Signs
<20	<1000	Restlessness	+/− Vasovagal reaction
20–30	1000–1500	Anxiety, DOE	Orthostatic hypotension, tachycardia on exertion
30–40	1500–2000	Syncope on sitting or standing	Orthostatic hypotension, tachycardia at rest
>40	>2000	Confusion, shortness of breath	Shock, poor perfusion

[a] Based on an estimated total blood volume of 5000 mL (70-kg adult).

The most rapid hematologic adjustment to acute blood loss is an increase in oxygen delivery to the tissues. This is first mediated by the Bohr effect, in which the more acidic milieu of the hypoperfused hypoxic tissues shifts the hemoglobin-oxygen dissociation curve to the right. Over several hours the RBC increase their production of 2,3-bisphosphoglycerate, which also enhances the unloading of oxygen to tissues. These two mechanisms can substantially increase the capacity of RBC to deliver oxygen to the tissues.

The marrow response to hemorrhage is related to the erythropoietin response to decreased oxygen tension. A normal response depends on the production of erythropoietin, the presence of normal erythroid progenitors in the marrow, and an adequate supply of iron. If these three elements are normal, reticulocytes begin to increase in the first 2 days based on early release of reticulocytes from the marrow. However, it takes 3 to 6 days for erythroid hyperplasia to appear and 7 to 10 days before the erythropoietic response is maximal, producing reticulocyte counts up to 20 to 30%, a reticulocyte index of ≥ 3, and a marked increase in the marrow erythroid/granulocytic ratio.

DIAGNOSIS Usually it is clear that a patient is bleeding; however, in some cases, large volumes of blood loss can occur internally from the gastrointestinal tract (esophageal varices, cancer in the stomach or colon), a ruptured spleen, fractures and other trauma, or other lesions that can cause massive hemorrhage into the peritoneal cavity, the pleural cavity, or the retroperitoneal space. Patients who have bled sufficiently to develop hypotension generally develop anemia, which is apparent only after volume replacement. The granulocyte count may increase to $\geq 20,000$ cells/μL and include immature cell types such as

metamyelocytes and myelocytes. Epinephrine-induced demargination of peripheral granulocytes and release of cells from the marrow may account for this change. Nucleated RBC may appear in the circulation, and platelet counts may exceed $1 \times 10^6/\mu$L. The basis for the increased platelet count is unclear. Hemorrhage in an internal cavity is accompanied by a rise in unconjugated bilirubin and a fall in serum haptoglobin.

R̲x̲ TREATMENT

Treatment of the underlying cause of the hemorrhage is of paramount importance. If the patient is severely anemic or sufficiently hypovolemic, packed RBC should be transfused. In less severe cases, if the patient has normal kidneys (and presumably a normal erythropoietin response to anemia), normal bone marrow function, and an adequate supply of iron, no specific therapy for the anemia is required.

FURTHER READING

AMIDON TM et al: Mitral and aortic paravalvular leaks with hemolytic anemia. Am Heart J 125:266, 1993

GARRATY G, PETZ LD: Approaches to selecting blood for transfusion to patients with autoimmune hemolytic anemia. Transfusion 42:1390, 2002

MAURO FR et al: Autoimmune hemolytic anemia in chronic lymphocytic leukemia: Clinical, therapeutic, and prognostic features. Blood 95:2786, 2000

PRUSS A et al: Immune hemolysis-serological and clinical aspects. Clin Exp Med 3:55, 2003

ROSSE WF: Paroxysmal nocturnal hemoglobinuria as a molecular disease. Medicine 76:63, 1997

94 | APLASTIC ANEMIA, MYELODYSPLASIA, AND RELATED BONE MARROW FAILURE SYNDROMES
Neal S. Young

The hypoproliferative anemias associated with marrow damage include aplastic anemia, myelodysplasia (MDS), pure red cell aplasia (PRCA), and myelophthisis. Anemia in these disorders, which is normochromic, normocytic or macrocytic, and characterized by low reticulocyte count, is not a solitary or even the major finding in these diseases, which are better described as marrow failure states. In bone marrow failure, pancytopenia—anemia, leukopenia, and thrombocytopenia (sometimes in various combinations)—results from deficient hematopoiesis, as distinguished from blood count depression due to peripheral destruction of red cells (hemolytic anemias), platelets (idiopathic thrombocytopenic purpura or due to splenomegaly), and granulocytes (as in the immune leukopenias).

Hematopoietic failure syndromes are classified by dominant morphologic features of the bone marrow (Table 94-1). While practical distinction among these syndromes usually is clear, they can occur secondary to other diseases, and some processes are so closely related that the differential diagnosis may be arbitrary. Patients may seem to suffer from two or three related diseases simultaneously, or one diagnosis may appear to evolve into another. Finally, many of these syndromes share an immune-mediated pathophysiologic mechanism of marrow destruction and some element of genomic instability resulting in a higher rate of malignant transformation.

APLASTIC ANEMIA

DEFINITION Aplastic anemia is pancytopenia with bone marrow hypocellularity. Acquired aplastic anemia is distinguished from iatrogenic marrow aplasia, the common occurrence of marrow hypocellularity after intensive cytotoxic chemotherapy for cancer. Aplastic anemia can also be constitutional: the genetic diseases Fanconi's anemia and dyskeratosis congenita, while frequently associated with typical physical anomalies and the development of pancytopenia

early in life, can also present as marrow failure in normal-appearing adults. Acquired aplastic anemia is often stereotypical in its manifestations, with the abrupt onset of low blood counts in a previously well young adult; seronegative hepatitis or a course of an incriminated medical drug may precede the onset. The diagnosis in these instances is

TABLE 94-1 Differential Diagnosis of Pancytopenia

PANCYTOPENIA WITH HYPOCELLULAR BONE MARROW

Acquired aplastic anemia
Constitutional aplastic anemia (Fanconi's anemia, dyskeratosis congenita)
Some myelodysplasia syndromes
Rare aleukemic leukemia (AML)
Some acute lymphoid leukemia
Some lymphomas of bone marrow

PANCYTOPENIA WITH CELLULAR BONE MARROW

Primary bone marrow diseases	Secondary to systemic diseases
Myelodysplasia syndromes	Systemic lupus erythematosus
Paroxysmal nocturnal hemoglobinuria	Hypersplenism
	B_{12}, folate deficiency
Myelofibrosis	Overwhelming infection
Some aleukemic leukemia	Alcohol
Myelophthisis	Brucellosis
Bone marrow lymphoma	Sarcoidosis
Hairy cell leukemia	Tuberculosis
	Leishmaniasis

HYPOCELLULAR BONE MARROW ± CYTOPENIA

Q fever
Legionnaires' disease
Anorexia nervosa, starvation
Mycobacteria

uncomplicated. Sometimes blood count depression is moderate or incomplete, resulting in anemia, leukopenia, and thrombocytopenia in some combination. Aplastic anemia is related to both paroxysmal nocturnal hemoglobinuria (PNH; Chap. 93) and to MDS, and in some cases a clear distinction among these disorders may not be possible.

EPIDEMIOLOGY The incidence of acquired aplastic anemia in Europe and Israel is 2 cases per million persons annually. In Thailand and China, rates of 5 to 7 per million have been established. In general, men and women are affected with equal frequency, but there is a biphasic age distribution, with the major peak in the teens and twenties and a second rise in the elderly.

ETIOLOGY The origins of aplastic anemia have been inferred from several recurring clinical associations (Table 94-2); unfortunately, these relationships are neither a reliable guide in an individual patient nor necessarily etiologic. In addition, while most cases of aplastic anemia are idiopathic, little other than history separates these cases from those with a presumed etiology such as a drug exposure.

Radiation Marrow aplasia is a major acute sequela of radiation. Radiation damages DNA; tissues dependent on active mitosis are particularly susceptible. Nuclear accidents can involve not only power plant workers but also employees of hospitals, laboratories, and industry (food sterilization, metal radiography, etc.), as well as innocents exposed to stolen, misplaced, or misused sources. While the radiation dose can be approximated from the rate and degree of decline in blood counts, dosimetry by reconstruction of the exposure can help to estimate the patient's prognosis and also to protect medical personnel from contact with radioactive tissue and excreta. MDS and leukemia, but probably not aplastic anemia, are late effects of irradiation.

Chemicals Benzene is a notorious cause of bone marrow failure. Vast quantities of epidemiologic, clinical, and laboratory data link benzene to aplastic anemia, acute leukemia, and blood and marrow abnormalities. The occurrence of leukemia is roughly correlated with cumulative exposure, but susceptibility must also be important, as only a minority of even heavily exposed workers develop benzene myelotoxicity. The employment history is important, especially in industries where benzene is used for a secondary purpose, usually as a solvent. Benzene-related blood diseases have declined with regulation of industrial exposure. Although benzene is no longer generally available as a household solvent, exposure to its metabolites occurs in the normal diet and in the use of lead-free gasoline. The association between marrow failure and other chemicals is much less well substantiated.

Drugs (See Table 94-3) Many chemotherapeutic drugs have marrow suppression as a major toxicity; effects are dose-dependent and will occur in all recipients. In contrast, idiosyncratic reactions to a large and diverse group of drugs may lead to aplastic anemia without a clear dose-response relationship. These associations rested largely on accumulated case reports until a large international study in Europe in the 1980s quantitated drug relationships, especially for nonsteroidal analgesics, sulfonamides, thyrostatic drugs, some psychotropics, penicillamine, allopurinol, and gold. Not all associations necessarily reflect causation: a drug may have been used to treat the first symptoms of bone marrow failure (antibiotics for fever or the preceding viral illness) or provoked the first symptom of a preexisting disease (petechiae by nonsteroidal anti-inflammatory agents administered to the thrombocytopenic patient). In the context of total drug use, idiosyncratic reactions, while individually devastating, are rare events. Chlor-

TABLE 94-2 *Classification of Aplastic Anemia and Single Cytopenias*

Acquired	Inherited
APLASTIC ANEMIA	
Secondary	Fanconi's anemia
Radiation	Dyskeratosis congenita
Drugs and chemicals	Shwachman-Diamond syndrome
Regular effects	Reticular dysgenesis
Idiosyncratic reactions	Amegakaryocytic
	thrombocytopenia
Viruses	Familial aplastic anemias
Epstein-Barr virus (infectious	Preleukemia (monosomy 7, etc.)
mononucleosis)	Nonhematologic syndrome
Hepatitis (non-A, non-B, non-	(Down's, Dubowitz, Seckel)
C hepatitis)	
Parvovirus B19 (transient	
aplastic crisis, PRCA)	
HIV-1 (AIDS)	
Immune diseases	
Eosinophilic fasciitis	
Hypoimmunoglobulinemia	
Thymoma/thymic carcinoma	
Graft-versus-host disease in	
immunodeficiency	
Paroxysmal nocturnal	
hemoglobinuria	
Pregnancy	
Idiopathic	
CYTOPENIAS	
PRCA (see Table 94-4)	Congenital PRCA (Diamond-
	Blackfan anemia)
Neutropenia/Agranulocytosis	
Idiopathic	Kostmann's Syndrome
Drugs, toxins	Shwachman-Diamond syndrome
Pure white cell aplasia	Reticular dysgenesis
Thrombocytopenia	
Drugs, toxins	Amegakaryocytic
	thrombocytopenia
Idiopathic amegakaryocytic	Thrombocytopenia with absent
	radii

Note: PRCA, pure red cell aplasia.

TABLE 94-3 *Some Drugs and Chemicals Associated with Aplastic Anemia*

Agents that regularly produce marrow depression as major toxicity in commonly employed doses or normal exposures:
  Cytotoxic drugs used in cancer chemotherapy: *alkylating agents*, antimetabolites, antimitotics, some antibiotics

Agents that frequently but not inevitably produce marrow aplasia:
  Benzene

Agents associated with aplastic anemia but with a relatively low probability:
  Chloramphenicol
  Insecticides
  Antiprotozoals: *quinacrine* and chloroquine, mepacrine
  Nonsteroidal anti-inflammatory drugs (including *phenylbutazone*, indomethacin, ibuprofen, sulindac, aspirin)
  Anticonvulsants (*hydantoins*, *carbamazapine*, phenacemide, felbamate)
  Heavy metals (*gold*, arsenic, bismuth, mercury)
  Sulfonamides: some antibiotics, antithyroid drugs (methimazole, methylthiouracil, propylthiouracil), antidiabetes drugs (tolbutamide, chlorpropamide), carbonic anhydrase inhibitors (acetazolamide and methazolamide)
  Antihistamines (*cimetidine*, chlorpheniramine)
  D-Penicillamine
  Estrogens (in pregnancy and in high doses in animals)

Agents whose association with aplastic anemia is more tenuous:
  Other antibiotics (streptomycin, tetracycline, methicillin, mebendazole, trimethoprim/sulfamethoxazole, flucytosine)
  Sedatives and tranquilizers (chlorpromazine, prochlorperazine, piperacetazine, chlordiazepoxide, meprobamate, methyprylon)
  Allopurinol
  Methyldopa
  Quinidine
  Lithium
  Guanidine
  Potassium perchlorate
  Thiocyanate
  Carbimazole

Note: Terms set in italic show the most consistent association with aplastic anemia.

amphenicol, the most infamous culprit, reportedly produced aplasia in only about 1/60,000 therapy courses, and even this number is almost certainly an overestimate (risks are almost invariably exaggerated when based on collections of cases; although the introduction of chloramphenicol was perceived to have created an epidemic of aplastic anemia, its diminished use was not followed by a changed frequency of marrow failure). Risk estimates are usually lower when determined in population-based studies; furthermore, the low absolute risk is also made more obvious: even a 10- or 20-fold increase in risk translates, in a rare disease, to but a handful of drug-induced aplastic anemia cases among hundreds of thousands of exposed patients.

Infections Hepatitis is the most common preceding infection, and posthepatitis marrow failure accounts for about 5% of etiologies in most series. Patients are usually young men who have recovered from a bout of liver inflammation 1 to 2 months earlier; the subsequent pancytopenia is very severe. The hepatitis is seronegative (non-A, non-B, non-C, non-G) and presumably due to a novel, as yet undiscovered, virus. Fulminant liver failure in childhood also follows seronegative hepatitis, and marrow failure occurs at a high rate in these patients. Marrow failure can rarely follow infectious mononucleosis, and Epstein-Barr virus has been found in the marrow of a few aplastic anemia patients, some without a suggestive preceding history. Parvovirus B19, the cause of transient aplastic crisis in hemolytic anemias and of some pure red cell aplasia (see below), does not usually cause generalized bone marrow failure. Blood count depression is frequent in the course of many viral and bacterial infections but is moderate and resolves with the infection.

Immunologic Diseases Aplasia is a major consequence and the cause of death in *transfusion-associated graft-versus-host disease*, which can occur after infusion of unirradiated blood products to an immunodeficient recipient. Aplastic anemia is strongly associated with the rare collagen vascular syndrome called *eosinophilic fasciitis*, which is characterized by painful induration of subcutaneous tissues (Chap. 303). Pancytopenia with marrow hypoplasia can also occur in systemic lupus erythematosus.

Pregnancy Aplastic anemia very rarely may occur and recur during pregnancy and resolve with delivery or with spontaneous or induced abortion.

Paroxysmal Nocturnal Hemoglobinuria An acquired mutation in the *PIG-A* gene in a hematopoietic stem cell is required for the development of PNH, but *PIG-A* mutations probably occur commonly in normal individuals. If the PIG-A mutant stem cell proliferates, the result is a clone of progeny deficient in glycosylphosphatidylinositol-linked cell surface membrane proteins (Chap. 93). Such PNH cells are now most accurately enumerated using fluorescence-activated flow cytometry of CD55 or CD59 expression on granulocytes rather than Ham or sucrose lysis tests on red cells. Small clones of deficient cells can be detected in about half of patients with aplastic anemia at the time of presentation [and PNH cells are also seen in MDS (see below)]; frank hemolysis and thrombotic episodes occur in patients with PNH clones. Functional studies of bone marrow from PNH patients, even those with mainly hemolytic manifestations, show evidence of defective hematopoiesis. Patients with an initial clinical diagnosis of PNH, especially younger individuals, may later develop frank marrow aplasia and pancytopenia; patients with an initial diagnosis of aplastic anemia may suffer from hemolytic PNH years after recovery of blood counts. One explanation for the aplastic anemia/PNH syndrome is selection of the deficient clones, because they are favored for proliferation in the peculiar environment of immune-mediated marrow destruction.

Congenital Disorders Fanconi's anemia, an autosomal recessive disorder, manifests as congenital developmental anomalies, progressive pancytopenia, and an increased risk of malignancy. Chromosomes in Fanconi's anemia are peculiarly susceptible to DNA cross-linking agents, the basis for a diagnostic assay. Patients with Fanconi's anemia typically have short stature, café au lait spots, and anomalies involving the thumb, radius, and genitourinary tract. At least eight different genetic defects have been defined by complementation analysis. The most common, type A Fanconi's anemia, is due to a mutation in *FANCA*. The Fanconi's anemia genes play a role in the cellular response to DNA damage, a response that includes BRCA1, ATM, and NBS1.

Dyskeratosis congenita is characterized by mucous membrane leukoplakia, dystrophic nails, reticular hyperpigmentation, and the development of aplastic anemia during childhood. The common X-linked variety is due to mutations in the *DKC1* (*dyskerin*) gene; the more unusual autosomal dominant type has been linked to *hTERC*, the RNA component of the telomerase complex. These two gene products cooperate in maintaining telomere length. In Shwachman-Diamond syndrome, marrow failure is seen with pancreatic insufficiency and malabsorption.

PATHOPHYSIOLOGY Bone marrow failure results from severe damage to the hematopoietic cell compartment. In aplastic anemia, replacement of the bone marrow by fat is apparent in the morphology of the biopsy specimen (Fig. 94-1) and magnetic resonance imaging (MRI) of the spine; cells bearing the CD34 antigen, a marker of early hematopoietic cells, are greatly diminished; and in functional studies, committed and primitive progenitor cells are virtually absent—in vitro assays have suggested that the stem cell pool is reduced to ≤1% of normal in severe disease at the time of presentation. Qualitative abnormalities, such as limited number of operating stem cell clones or shortened telomere length, may follow from the quantitative deficiency, reflecting the shrunken and stressed state of hematopoiesis. An intrinsic stem cell defect exists for constitutional aplastic anemia, as cells from patients with Fanconi's anemia exhibit chromosome damage and death on exposure to certain chemical agents. Aplastic anemia does not appear to result from defective stroma or growth factor production.

Drug Injury Extrinsic damage to the marrow follows massive physical or chemical insults such as high doses of radiation and toxic chemicals. For the more common idiosyncratic reaction to modest doses of medical drugs, altered drug metabolism has been invoked as a likely mechanism. The metabolic pathways of many drugs and chemicals, especially if they are polar and have limited water solubility, involve enzymatic degradation to highly reactive electrophilic compounds; these intermediates are toxic because of their propensity to bind to cellular macromolecules. For example, derivative hydroquinones and quinolones are responsible for benzene-induced tissue injury. Excessive generation of toxic intermediates or failure to detoxify the intermediates may be genetically determined and apparent only on specific drug challenge; the complexity and specificity of the pathways imply multiple susceptibility loci and would provide an explanation for the rarity of idiosyncratic drug reactions.

Immune-Mediated Injury The recovery of marrow function in some patients prepared for bone marrow transplantation with antilymphocyte globulin (ALG) first suggested that aplastic anemia might be immune-mediated. Consistent with this hypothesis was the frequent failure of simple bone marrow transplantation from a syngeneic twin, without conditioning cytotoxic chemotherapy, which also argued both *against* simple stem cell absence as the cause and *for* the presence of a host factor producing marrow failure. Laboratory data support an important role for the immune system in aplastic anemia. Blood and bone marrow cells of patients can suppress normal hematopoietic progenitor cell growth, and removal of T cells from aplastic anemia bone marrow improves colony formation in vitro. Increased numbers of activated cytotoxic T cells are observed in aplastic anemia patients and usually decline with successful immunosuppressive therapy; cytokine measurements show a T_H1 immune response (interferon γ, interleukin 2, and tumor necrosis factor). Interferon and tumor necrosis factor induce Fas expression on CD34 cells, leading to apoptotic cell death; localization of activated T cells to bone marrow and local production of their soluble factors are probably important in stem cell destruction.

Early immune system events in aplastic anemia are not well understood. Analysis of T cell receptor expression suggests an oligoclonal, antigen-driven cytotoxic T cell response. Many different exogenous antigens appear capable of initiating a pathologic immune response, but at least some of the T cells may recognize true self-antigens. The rarity of aplastic anemia despite common exposures (medicines, hepatitis virus) suggests that genetically determined features of the immune response can convert a normal physiologic response into a sustained abnormal autoimmune process.

CLINICAL FEATURES ■ History Aplastic anemia can appear with seeming abruptness or have a more insidious onset. Bleeding is the most common early symptom; a complaint of days to weeks of easy bruising, oozing from the gums, nose bleeds, heavy menstrual flow, and sometimes petechiae will have been noticed. With thrombocytopenia, massive hemorrhage is unusual, but small amounts of bleeding in the central nervous system can result in catastrophic intracranial or retinal hemorrhage. Symptoms of anemia are also frequent, including lassitude, weakness, shortness of breath, and a pounding sensation in the ears. Infection is an unusual first symptom in aplastic anemia (unlike in agranulocytosis, where pharyngitis, anorectal infection, or frank sepsis occur early). A striking feature of aplastic anemia is the restriction of symptoms to the hematologic system, and patients often feel and look remarkably well despite drastically reduced blood counts. Systemic complaints and weight loss should point to other etiologies of pancytopenia. Prior drug use, chemical exposure, and preceding viral illnesses must often be elicited with repeated questioning. A family history of hematologic diseases or blood abnormalities may indicate a constitutional etiology of marrow failure.

Physical Examination Petechiae and ecchymoses are typical, and retinal hemorrhages may be present. Pelvic and rectal examinations should be performed with great gentleness to avoid trauma; these will often show bleeding from the cervical os and blood in the stool. Pallor of the skin and mucous membranes is common except in the most acute cases or those already transfused. Infection on presentation is unusual but may occur if the patient has been symptomatic for a few weeks. Lymphadenopathy and splenomegaly are highly atypical of aplastic anemia. Café au lait spots and short stature suggest Fanconi's anemia; peculiar nails and leukoplakia suggest dyskeratosis congenita.

LABORATORY STUDIES ■ Blood The smear shows large erythrocytes and a paucity of platelets and granulocytes. Mean corpuscular volume (MCV) is commonly increased. Reticulocytes are absent or few, and lymphocyte numbers may be normal or reduced. The presence of immature myeloid forms suggests leukemia or MDS; nucleated red blood cells suggest marrow fibrosis or tumor invasion; abnormal platelets suggest either peripheral destruction or MDS.

Bone Marrow The bone marrow is usually readily aspirated but appears dilute on smear, and the fatty biopsy specimen may be grossly pale on withdrawal; a "dry tap" suggests fibrosis or myelophthisis. In severe aplasia the smear of the aspirated specimen shows only red cells, residual lymphocytes, and stromal cells; the biopsy, which should be >1 cm in length, is superior for determination of cellularity and shows mainly fat under the microscope, with hematopoietic cells occupying <25% of the marrow space. In the most serious cases the biopsy is virtually 100% fat. The correlation between marrow cellularity and disease severity is imperfect. Some patients with moderate disease by blood counts will have empty iliac crest biopsies, while "hot spots" of hematopoiesis may be seen in severe cases. If an iliac crest specimen is inadequate, cells may also be obtained by aspiration from the sternum. Residual hematopoietic cells should have normal morphology, except for mildly megaloblastic erythropoiesis; megakaryocytes are invariably greatly reduced and usually absent. Areas adjacent to the spicule should be searched for myeloblasts. Granulomas (in cellular specimens) may indicate an infectious etiology of the marrow failure.

Ancillary Studies Chromosome breakage studies of peripheral blood using diepoxybutane (DEB) or mito-

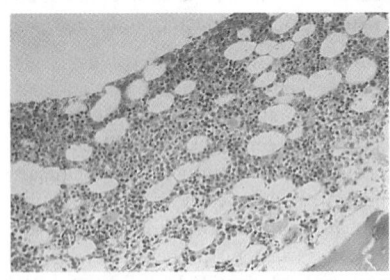

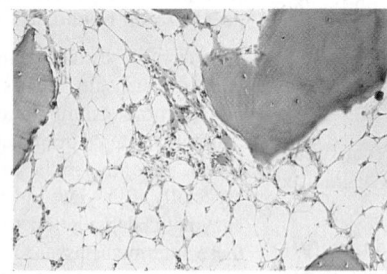

A *C*

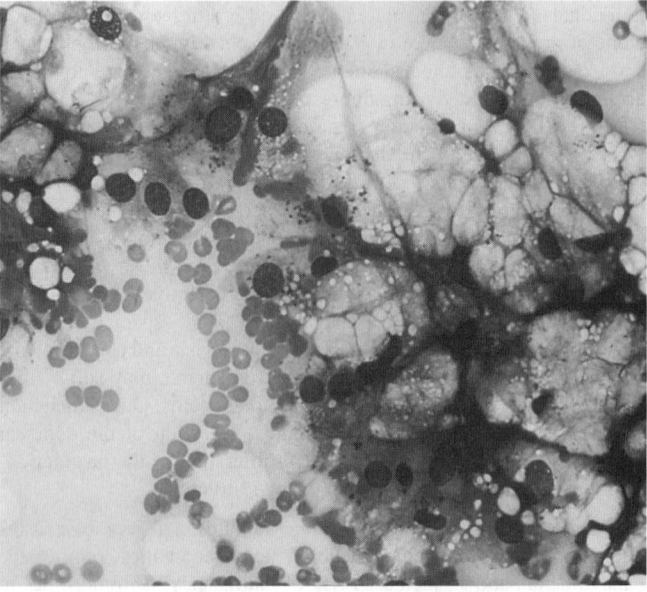

B *D*

FIGURE 94-1 *A.* Normal bone marrow biopsy. *B.* Normal bone marrow aspirate smear. The marrow is normally 30 to 70% cellular, and there is a heterogeneous mix of myeloid, erythroid, and lymphoid cells. *C.* Aplastic anemia biopsy. *D.* Marrow smear in aplastic anemia. The marrow shows replacement of hematopoietic tissue by fat and only residual stromal and lymphoid cells.

mycin C should be performed on children and younger adults to exclude Fanconi's anemia. Chromosome studies of bone marrow cells are often revealing in MDS and should be negative in typical aplastic anemia. Flow cytometric assays have replaced the Ham test for the diagnosis of PNH. Serologic studies may show evidence of viral infection, especially Epstein-Barr virus and HIV. Posthepatitis aplastic anemia is typically seronegative. The spleen size should be determined by scanning if the physical examination of the abdomen is unsatisfactory. MRI may be helpful to assess the fat content on a few vertebrae in order to distinguish aplasia from MDS.

DIAGNOSIS The diagnosis of aplastic anemia is usually straightforward, based on the combination of pancytopenia with a fatty, empty bone marrow. Aplastic anemia is a disease of the young and should be a leading diagnosis in the pancytopenic adolescent or young adult. When pancytopenia is secondary, the primary diagnosis is usually obvious from either history or physical examination: the massive spleen of alcoholic cirrhosis, the history of metastatic cancer or systemic lupus erythematosus, or obvious miliary tuberculosis on chest radiograph (Table 94-1).

Diagnostic problems can occur with atypical presentations and among related hematologic diseases. While pancytopenia is most common, some patients with bone marrow hypocellularity have depression of only one or two of three blood lines, sometimes showing later progression to more recognizable aplastic anemia. The bone marrow in constitutional aplastic anemia is indistinguishable morphologically from the aspirate in acquired disease. The diagnosis can be suggested by family history, abnormal blood counts since childhood, or the presence of associated physical anomalies. Aplastic anemia may be difficult to distinguish from the hypocellular variety of MDS: MDS is favored by finding morphologic abnormalities, particularly of megakaryocytes and myeloid precursor cells, and typical cytogenetic abnormalities (see below).

PROGNOSIS The natural history of severe aplastic anemia is rapid deterioration and death. Provision first of red blood cell and later platelet transfusions and effective antibiotics were of some benefit, but few patients showed spontaneous recovery. The major prognostic determinant is the blood count; severe disease is defined by the presence of two of three parameters: absolute neutrophil count $<500/\mu$L, platelet count $<20,000/\mu$L, and corrected reticulocyte count $<1\%$ (or absolute reticulocyte count $<60,000/\mu$L). Survival of patients who fulfill these criteria is about 20% at 1 year after diagnosis with only supportive care; patients with very severe disease, defined by an absolute neutrophil count $<200/\mu$L, fare even more poorly. Treatment has markedly improved survival in this disease.

Rx TREATMENT

Severe acquired aplastic anemia can be cured by replacement of the absent hematopoietic cells (and the immune system) by stem cell transplant, or it can be ameliorated by suppression of the immune system to allow recovery of the patient's residual bone marrow function. Hematopoietic growth factors have limited usefulness and glucocorticoids are of no value. Suspect exposures to drugs or chemicals should be discontinued; however, spontaneous recovery of severe blood count depression is rare, and a waiting period before beginning treatment may not be advisable unless the blood counts are only modestly depressed.

Bone Marrow Transplantation This is the best therapy for the young patient with a fully histocompatible sibling donor (Chap. 100). Human leukocyte antigen (HLA) typing should be ordered as soon as the diagnosis of aplastic anemia is established in a child or younger adult. In transplant candidates, transfusion of blood from family members should be avoided so as to prevent sensitization to histocompatibility antigens; while transfusions in general should be minimized, limited numbers of blood products probably do not seriously affect outcome.

For allogeneic transplant from fully matched siblings, long-term survival rates for children are 80% or better. Transplant morbidity and

mortality are increased among adults, due mainly to the higher risk of chronic graft-versus-host disease and serious infections. Graft rejection was historically a major determinant of outcome in bone marrow transplant for aplastic anemia; high rates of primary or secondary graft failure may be related to the pathophysiology of marrow failure as well as to alloimmunization from transfusions.

Most patients do not have a suitable sibling donor. Occasionally, a full phenotypic match can be found within the family and serve as well. Far more available are other alternative donors, either unrelated but histocompatible volunteers, or closely but not perfectly matched family members. Survival using alternative donors is about half that of conventional sibling transplants. These patients will be at risk for late complications, especially a higher rate of cancer, if radiation is used as a component of conditioning. Most older adults who undergo alternative donor transplants succumb to transplant-related complications.

Immunosuppression Used alone, ALG or antithymocyte globulin (ATG) induces hematologic recovery (independence from transfusion and a leukocyte count adequate to prevent infection) in about 50% of patients. The addition of cyclosporine to either ALG or ATG has further increased response rates to about 70% and especially improved outcomes for children and for severely neutropenic patients. Combined treatment is now standard for patients with severe disease. Hematologic response strongly correlates with survival. Improvement in granulocyte number is generally apparent within 2 months of treatment. Most recovered patients continue to have some degree of blood count depression, the MCV remains elevated, and the bone marrow cellularity returns toward normal only very slowly, if at all. Relapse (recurrent pancytopenia) is frequent, often occurring as cyclosporine is discontinued; most, but not all, patients respond to reinstitution of immunosuppression, but some responders become dependent on continued cyclosporine administration. Development of MDS, with typical marrow morphologic or cytogenetic abnormalities, occurs in about 15% of treated patients, usually but not invariably associated with a return of pancytopenia, and some patients develop leukemia. Although the laboratory diagnosis of PNH can generally be made at the time of presentation of aplastic anemia by flow cytometry, recovered patients showing frank hemolysis should be retested for PNH. Bone marrow examinations should be performed if there is an unfavorable change in blood counts.

Horse ATG is given at 40 mg/kg per day for 4 days; rabbit ALG is administered at 3.5 mg/kg per day for 5 days. For ATG, anaphylaxis is a rare but occasionally fatal complication; allergy should be tested by a skin-prick test with an undiluted solution and immediate observation; desensitization is feasible. ATG binds to peripheral blood cells; therefore, platelet and granulocyte numbers may fall further during active treatment. Serum sickness, a flulike illness with a characteristic cutaneous eruption and arthralgia, often develops about 10 days after initiating treatment. Most patients are given methylprednisolone, 1 mg/kg per day for 2 weeks, to ameliorate the immune consequences of heterologous protein infusion. Excessive or extended glucocorticoid therapy is associated with avascular joint necrosis. Cyclosporine is administered orally at an initial dose of 12 mg/kg per day in adults (15 mg/kg per day in children), with subsequent adjustment according to blood levels obtained every 2 weeks. Trough levels should be between 150 and 200 ng/mL. The most important side effects of chronic cyclosporine treatment are nephrotoxicity, hypertension, seizures, and opportunistic infections, especially *Pneumocystis carinii* (prophylactic treatment with monthly inhaled pentamidine is recommended).

Most patients with aplastic anemia lack a suitable marrow donor and immunosuppression is the treatment of choice. Long-term survival is equivalent with transplantation and immunosuppression. However, successful transplant cures marrow failure, while patients who recover adequate blood counts after immunosuppression remain at risk of relapse and malignant evolution. Because of the excellent results in children, allogeneic transplant should be performed in the pediatric population if a suitable sibling donor is available. Increasing age and the severity of neutropenia are the most important factors weighing in the decision between transplant and immunosuppression in adults who have a matched family donor: older patients do better with ATG and cyclosporine, whereas transplant is preferred if granulocytopenia is profound. Some reluctant patients may be treated by immunosuppression; transplant is used for failure to recover blood counts or occurrence of late complications.

Outcomes following both transplant and immunosuppression have improved with time. High doses of cyclophosphamide, without stem cell rescue, have been reported to produce durable hematologic recovery, without relapse or evolution to MDS, but this treatment can produce sustained severe fatal neutropenia and response is often delayed. Several new immunosuppressive drugs in clinical trial may further improve outcome.

Other Therapies The effectiveness of androgens has not been verified in controlled trials, but occasional patients will respond or even demonstrate blood count dependence on continued therapy. For patients with moderate disease or those with severe pancytopenia in whom immunosuppression has failed, a 3- to 4-month trial is appropriate. Hematopoietic growth factors, granulocyte colony-stimulating factor (G-CSF), granulocyte-macrophage CSF (GM-CSF), and interleukin 3 are not recommended as initial therapy for severe aplastic anemia, and even their role as adjuncts to immunosuppression is not well defined. Some patients may respond to combinations of growth factors after immunosuppression has failed. Splenectomy may occasionally increase blood counts in relapsed or refractory cases.

Supportive Care Meticulous medical attention is required so that the patient may survive to benefit from definitive therapy or, having failed treatment, to maintain a reasonable existence in the face of pancytopenia. First and most important, infection in the presence of severe neutropenia must be aggressively treated by prompt institution of parenteral, broad-spectrum antibiotics, usually ceftazidime or a combination of an aminoglycoside, cephalosporin, and semisynthetic penicillin. Therapy is empirical and must not await results of culture, although specific foci of infection such as oropharyngeal or anorectal abscesses, pneumonia, sinusitis, and typhlitis (necrotizing colitis) should be sought on physical examination and with radiographic studies. When indwelling plastic catheters become contaminated, vancomycin should be added. Persistent or recrudescent fever implies fungal disease: *Candida* or *Aspergillus* are common, especially after several courses of antibacterial antibiotics, and a progressive course may be averted by timely initiation of antifungal therapy. Granulocyte transfusions using G-CSF–mobilized peripheral blood have been effective in the treatment of overwhelming or refractory infections in a few patients. Hand washing, the single best method of preventing the spread of infection, remains a neglected practice. Nonabsorbed antibiotics for gut decontamination are poorly tolerated and not of proven value. Total reverse isolation does not reduce mortality from infections.

Both platelet and erythrocyte numbers can be maintained by transfusion. Alloimmunization limits the usefulness of platelet transfusions and can be avoided or minimized by several strategies, including use of single donors to reduce exposure and physical or chemical methods to diminish leukocytes in the product; HLA-matched platelets are often effective in patients refractory to random donor products. Inhibitors of fibrinolysis such as aminocaproic acid have not been shown to relieve mucosal oozing; the use of low-dose glucocorticoids to induce "vascular stability" is unproven. Whether platelet transfusions are better used prophylactically or only as needed remains unclear. Any rational regimen of prophylaxis requires transfusions once or twice weekly in order to maintain the platelet count $>10,000/\mu L$ (oozing from the gut, and presumably also from other vascular beds, increases precipitously at counts $<5000/\mu L$). Menstruation should be suppressed either by oral estrogens or nasal follicle-stimulating hormone/luteinizing hormone (FSH/LH) antagonists. Aspirin and other nonsteroidal anti-inflammatory agents inhibit platelet function and must be avoided.

Red blood cells should be transfused to maintain a normal level of activity, usually at a hemoglobin value of 70 g/L (90 g/L if there is underlying cardiac or pulmonary disease); a regimen of 2 units every 2 weeks will replace normal losses in a patient without a functioning bone marrow. In chronic anemia, the iron chelator deferoxamine should be added at around the fiftieth transfusion in order to avoid secondary hemochromatosis.

PURE RED CELL APLASIA

Other, more restricted forms of marrow failure occur, in which only a single circulating cell type is affected and the aregenerative marrow shows corresponding absence or decreased numbers of specific precursor cells: aregenerative anemia as in PRCA (see below), thrombocytopenia with amegakaryocytosis (Chap. 101), and neutropenia without marrow myeloid cells in agranulocytosis (Chap. 55). In general, and in contrast to aplastic anemia and MDS, the unaffected lineages appear quantitatively and qualitatively normal. Agranulocytosis, the most frequent of these syndromes, is usually a complication of medical drug use (with agents similar to those related to aplastic anemia), either by a mechanism of direct chemical toxicity or by immune destruction. Agranulocytosis has an incidence similar to aplastic anemia but is especially frequent among the elderly and in women. The syndrome should resolve with discontinuation of exposure, but significant mortality is attached to neutropenia in the older and often previously unwell patient. Both pure white cell aplasia (agranulocytosis without incriminating drug exposure) and amegakaryocytic thrombocytopenia are exceedingly rare and, like PRCA, appear to be due to destructive antibodies or lymphocytes and can respond to immunosuppressive therapies. In all the single lineage failure syndromes, progression to pancytopenia or leukemia is unusual.

DEFINITION AND DIFFERENTIAL DIAGNOSIS PRCA is characterized by anemia, reticulocytopenia, and absent or rare erythroid precursor cells in the bone marrow. The classification of PRCA is shown in Table 94-4. In adults, PRCA is acquired. An identical syndrome can occur constitutionally: Diamond-Blackfan anemia, or congenital PRCA, is diagnosed at birth or in early childhood and often responds to glucocorticoid treatment. Temporary red cell failure occurs in transient aplastic crisis of hemolytic anemias, due to acute parvovirus infection

TABLE 94-4 *Classification of Pure Red Cell Aplasia*

Self-limited
  Transient erythroblastopenia of childhood
  Transient aplastic crisis of hemolysis (acute B19 parvovirus infection)
Fetal red blood cell aplasia
  Nonimmune hydrops fetalis (in utero B19 parvovirus infection)
Hereditary pure red cell aplasia
  Congenital pure red cell aplasia (Diamond-Blackfan syndrome)
Acquired pure red cell aplasia
  Thymoma and malignancy
    Thymoma
    Lymphoid malignancies (and more rarely other hematologic diseases)
    Paraneoplastic to solid tumors
  Connective tissue disorders with immunologic abnormalities
    Systemic lupus erythematosus, juvenile rheumatoid arthritis, rheumatoid arthritis
    Multiple endocrine gland insufficiency
  Virus
    Persistent B19 parvovirus, hepatitis, adult T cell leukemia virus, Epstein-Barr virus
  Pregnancy
  Drugs
    Especially phenytoin, azathioprine, chloramphenicol, procaineamide, isoniazid
  Idiopathic

(Chap. 168), and in transient erythroblastopenia of childhood, which affects normal children.

CLINICAL ASSOCIATIONS AND ETIOLOGY PRCA has important associations with immune system diseases. A small minority of cases occur with a thymoma. More frequently, red cell aplasia can be the major manifestation of large granular lymphocytosis or may occur in chronic lymphocytic leukemia. Some patients may be hypogammaglobulinemic. As with agranulocytosis, PRCA can be due to an idiosyncratic reaction to a drug.

Like aplastic anemia, PRCA results from diverse mechanisms. Antibodies to red blood cell precursors are frequently present in the blood, but T cell inhibition is probably the more common immune mechanism. Cytotoxic lymphocyte activity restricted by histocompatibility locus or specific for human T cell leukemia/lymphoma virus I–infected cells, as well as natural killer cell activity inhibitory of erythropoiesis, have been demonstrated in particularly well-studied individual cases.

Persistent Parvovirus B19 Infection Chronic parvovirus infection is an important, treatable cause of PRCA. This common virus causes a benign exanthem of childhood (fifth disease) and a polyarthralgia syndrome in adults. In patients with underlying hemolysis (or any condition that increases demand for red blood cell production), parvovirus infection can cause a transient aplastic crisis and an abrupt but temporary worsening of the anemia due to failed erythropoiesis. In normal individuals, acute infection is resolved by production of neutralizing antibodies to the virus, but in the setting of congenital, acquired, or iatrogenic immunodeficiency, persistent viral infection may occur. The bone marrow shows red cell aplasia and the presence of giant pronormoblasts (Fig. 94-2), which is the cytopathic sign of B19 parvovirus infection. Viral tropism for human erythroid progenitor cells is due to its use of erythrocyte P antigen as a cellular receptor for entry. Direct cytotoxicity of virus causes anemia if demands on

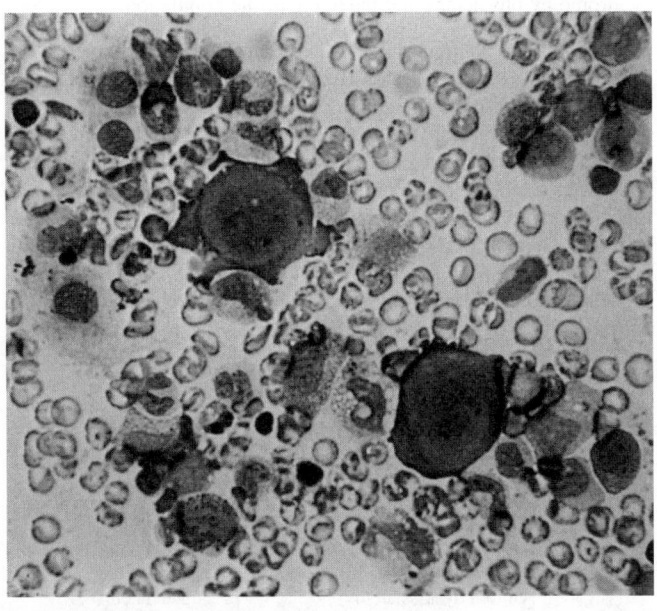

A

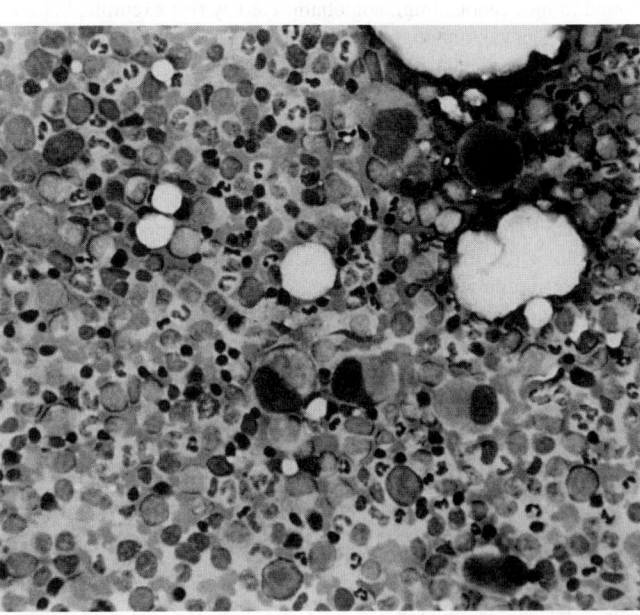

B

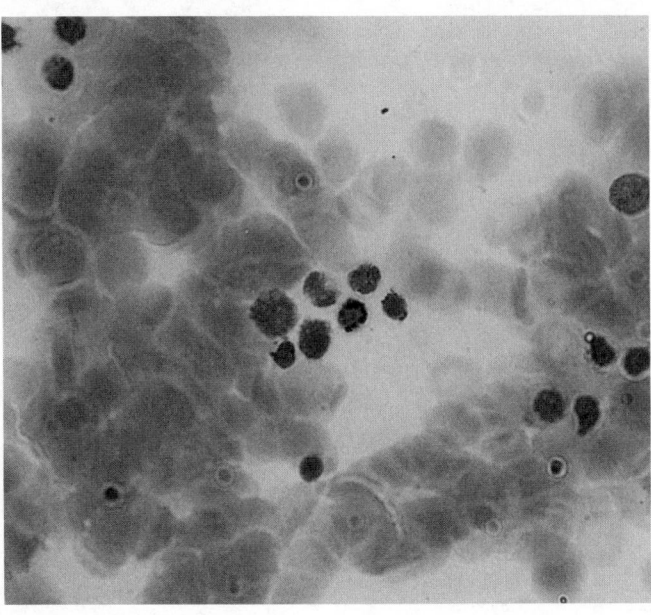

C

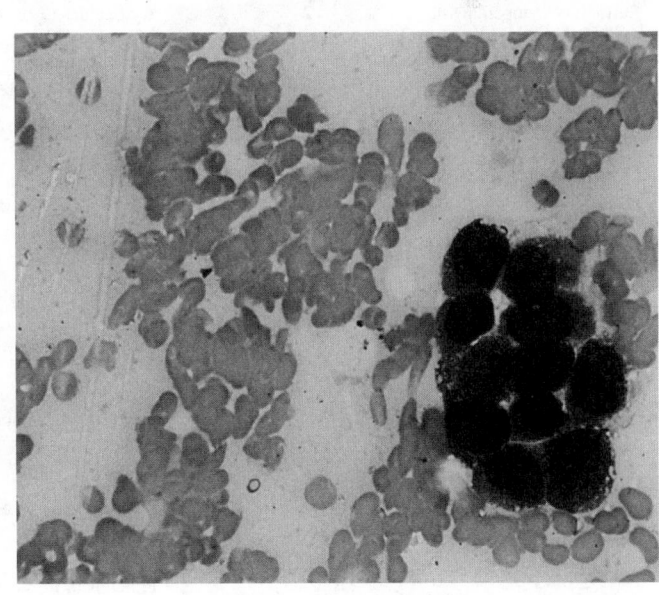

D

FIGURE 94-2 Pathognomonic cells in marrow failure syndromes. *A.* Giant pronormoblast, the cytopathic effect of B19 parvovirus infection of the erythroid progenitor cell. *B.* Uninuclear megakaryocyte and microblastic erythroid precursors typical of the 5q– myelodysplasia syndrome. *C.* Ringed sideroblast showing perinuclear iron granules. *D.* Tumor cells present on a touch preparation made from the marrow biopsy of a patient with metastatic carcinoma.

erythrocyte production are high; in normal individuals, the temporary cessation of red cell production is not clinically apparent, and skin and joint symptoms are mediated by immune complex deposition.

℞ TREATMENT

History, physical examination, and routine laboratory studies may disclose an underlying disease or a suspect drug exposure. Thymoma should be sought by radiographic procedures. Tumor excision is indicated, but anemia does not necessarily improve with surgery. The diagnosis of parvovirus infection requires detection of viral DNA sequences in the blood (IgG and IgM antibodies are commonly absent). The presence of erythroid colonies has been considered predictive of response to immunosuppressive therapy in idiopathic PRCA.

Red cell aplasia is compatible with long survival with supportive care alone: a combination of erythrocyte transfusions and iron chelation. For persistent B19 parvovirus infection, almost all patients respond to intravenous immunoglobulin therapy (for example, 0.4 g/kg daily for 5 days), although relapse and retreatment may be expected, especially in patients with AIDS. The majority of patients with idiopathic PRCA respond favorably to immunosuppression. Most first receive a course of glucocorticoids, followed in the absence of a response by cyclosporine, ATG, azathioprine, or cyclophosphamide.

MYELODYSPLASIA

DEFINITION The myelodysplasias (MDS) are a heterogeneous group of hematologic disorders broadly characterized by cytopenias associated with a dysmorphic (or abnormal appearing) and usually cellular bone marrow, and consequent ineffective blood cell production. A clinically useful nosology of these entities was first developed by the French-American-British Cooperative Group in 1983. Five entities were defined: refractory anemia (RA), refractory anemia with ringed

sideroblasts (RARS), refractory anemia with excess blasts (RAEB), refractory anemia with excess blasts in transformation (RAEB-t), and chronic myelomonocytic leukemia (CMML). The World Health Organization classification (2002) recognizes that the distinction between RAEB-t and acute myeloid leukemia is arbitrary and groups them together as acute leukemia, notes that CMML behaves as a myeloproliferative disease, and separates refractory anemias with dysmorphic change restricted to erythroid lineage from those with multilineage changes (Table 94-5).

EPIDEMIOLOGY Idiopathic MDS is a disease of the elderly; the mean age at onset is 68 years. There is a slight male preponderance. MDS is a relatively common form of bone marrow failure, with reported incidence rates of 35 to >100 per million persons in the general population and 120 to >500 per million in the elderly. MDS is rare in children, but monocytic leukemia can be seen. Therapy-related MDS is not age-related and may occur in as many as 15% of patients within a decade following intensive combined modality treatment for cancer. Rates of MDS have increased over time, due to the recognition of the syndrome by physicians and the aging of the population.

ETIOLOGY AND PATHOPHYSIOLOGY MDS is caused by environmental exposures such as radiation and benzene; other risk factors have been reported inconsistently. Secondary MDS occurs as a late toxicity of cancer treatment, usually with a combination of radiation and the radiomimetic alkylating agents such as busulfan, nitrosourea, or procarbazine (with a latent period of 5 to 7 years) or the DNA topoisomerase inhibitors (2 years). Both acquired aplastic anemia following immunosuppressive treatment and Fanconi's anemia can evolve into MDS.

MDS is a clonal hematopoietic stem cell disorder leading to impaired cell proliferation and differentiation. Cytogenetic abnormalities are found in about half of patients, and some of the same specific lesions are also seen in frank leukemia; aneuploidy is more frequent

TABLE 94-5 *World Health Organization Classification of Myelodysplastic Syndromes*

Disease	Frequency	Blood Findings	Bone Marrow Findings	Prognosis
Refractory anemia (RA)	5–10%	Anemia No or rare blasts	Erythroid dysplasia only <5% blasts <15% ringed sideroblasts	Protracted course Leukemic transformation in ~6%
Refractory anemia with ringed sideroblasts (RARS)	10–12%	Anemia No blasts	Erythroid dysplasia only ≥15% ringed sideroblasts <5% blasts	Protracted course Leukemia in ~1–2%
Refractory cytopenia with multilineage dysplasia (RCMD)	24%	Cytopenias (2 or 3 lineages) No or rare blasts No Auer rods <1 × 10⁹/L monocytes	Dysplasia in ≥10% of cells in ≥2 lineages <5% blasts No Auer rods <15% ringed sideroblasts	Variable clinical course Leukemia in ~11%
RCMD with ringed sideroblasts (RCMD-RS)	15%	Cytopenias (2 or 3 lineages) No or rare blasts No Auer rods <1 × 10⁹/L monocytes	Dysplasia in ≥10% of cells in ≥2 lineages ≥15% ringed sideroblasts <5% blasts No Auer rods	
Refractory anemia with excess blasts-1 (RAEB-1)	40% (RAEB-1 +2)	Cytopenias <5% blasts No Auer rods <1 × 10⁹/L monocytes	Unilineage or multilineage dysplasia 5–9% blasts No Auer rods	Progressive BM failure Leukemia in ~25%
Refractory anemia with excess blasts-2 (RAEB-2)		Cytopenias 5–19% blasts ±Auer rods <1 × 10⁹/L monocytes	Unilineage or multilineage dysplasia 10–19% blasts ±Auer rods	Progressive BM failure Leukemia in ~33%
Myelodysplastic syndrome, unclassified (MDS-U)	Unknown	Cytopenias No or rare blasts No Auer rods	Dysplasia in myeloid or platelet lineage <5% blasts No Auer rods	Unknown
MDS with isolated del(5q)	Unknown	Anemia <5% blasts Platelets nl or increased	Nl or increased megakaryocytes with hypolobated nuclei <5% blasts No Auer rods Isolated del(5q)	Long survival

Note: BM, bone marrow.
Source: Extracted from Jaffe ES et al (eds): *Pathology and Genetics of Tumors of Haematopoietic and Lymphoid Tissues.* Lyon, IARC Press, 2001

than translocations. Both presenting and evolving hematologic manifestations result from the accumulation of multiple genetic lesions, loss of tumor suppressor genes, activating oncogene mutations, or other harmful alterations. Cytogenetic abnormalities are not random (loss of all or part of 5, 7, and 20, trisomy of 8) and may be related to etiology (11q23 following topoisomerase II inhibitors); chronic myelomonocytic leukemia is often associated with t(5;12) that creates a chimeric *tel-PDGFβ* gene. The type and number of cytogenetic abnormalities strongly correlate with the probability of leukemic transformation and survival. Mutations of N-*ras* (an oncogene), *p53* and *IRF-1* (tumor suppressor genes), *Bcl-2* (an antiapoptotic gene), and others have been reported in some patients but may occur relatively late in the sequence leading to leukemic transformation. Apoptosis of marrow cells is increased in MDS, presumably due to these acquired genetic alterations or possibly to an overlaid immune response. Sideroblastic anemia may be related to mutations in mitochondrial genes. Ineffective erythropoiesis and disordered iron metabolism are the functional consequences of the genetic alterations.

CLINICAL FEATURES
Anemia dominates the early course. Most symptomatic patients complain of the gradual onset of fatigue and weakness, dyspnea, and pallor, but at least half the patients are asymptomatic and their MDS is discovered only incidentally on routine blood counts. Previous chemotherapy or radiation exposure is an important historic fact. Fever and weight loss should point to a myeloproliferative rather than myelodysplastic process. Children with Down syndrome are susceptible to MDS, and a family history may indicate a hereditary form of sideroblastic anemia or Fanconi's anemia.

The physical examination is remarkable for signs of anemia; about 20% of patients have splenomegaly. Some unusual skin lesions, including Sweet's syndrome (febrile neutrophilic dermatosis), occur with MDS. Autoimmune syndromes are not infrequent.

LABORATORY STUDIES ■ Blood
Anemia is present in the majority of cases, either alone or as part of bi- or pancytopenia; isolated neutropenia or thrombocytopenia is more unusual. Macrocytosis is common, and the smear may be dimorphic with a distinctive population of large red blood cells. Platelets are also large and lack granules. In functional studies, they may show marked abnormalities, and patients may have bleeding symptoms despite seemingly adequate numbers. Neutrophils are hypogranulated; have hyposegmented, ringed, or abnormally segmented nuclei; contain Dohle bodies; and may be functionally deficient. Circulating myeloblasts usually correlate with marrow blast numbers, and their quantitation is important for classification and prognosis. The total white blood cell count is usually normal or low, except in chronic myelomonocytic leukemia. As in aplastic anemia, MDS also can be associated with a clonal population of PNH cells.

Bone Marrow
The bone marrow is usually normal or hypercellular but in 20% of cases is sufficiently hypocellular to be confused with aplasia. No single characteristic feature of marrow morphology distinguishes MDS, but the following are commonly observed: dyserythropoietic changes (especially nuclear abnormalities) and ringed sideroblasts in the erythroid lineage; hypogranulation and hyposegmentation in granulocytic precursors, with an increase in myeloblasts; and megakaryocytes showing reduced numbers of disorganized nuclei. Megaloblastic nuclei associated with defective hemoglobinization in the erythroid lineage are common. Prognosis strongly correlates with the proportion of marrow blasts. Cytogenetic analysis and fluorescent in situ hybridization can identify genetic lesions.

DIFFERENTIAL DIAGNOSIS
Deficiencies of vitamin B_{12} or folate should be excluded by appropriate blood tests; vitamin B_6 deficiency can be assessed by a therapeutic trial of pyridoxine if the bone marrow shows ringed sideroblasts. Marrow dysplasia can be observed in acute viral infections, drug reactions, or chemical toxicity but should be transient. More difficult are the distinctions between hypocellular MDS and aplasia or between refractory anemia with excess blasts and early acute leukemia. The World Health Organization considers the presence of 20% blasts in the marrow as the criterion that separates acute myeloid leukemia from MDS.

PROGNOSIS
The median survival varies greatly from years for patients with 5q– or sideroblastic anemia to a few months in refractory anemia with excess blasts or severe pancytopenia associated with monosomy 7; an International Prognostic Scoring System (Table 94-6) assists in making predictions. Most patients die as a result of complications of pancytopenia and not due to leukemic transformation; perhaps one-third will succumb to other diseases unrelated to their MDS. Precipitous worsening of pancytopenia, acquisition of new chromosomal abnormalities on serial cytogenetic determination, and increase in the number of blasts are all poor prognostic indicators. The outlook in therapy-related MDS, regardless of type, is poor, and most patients will progress within a few months to refractory acute myeloid leukemia.

Rx TREATMENT

The therapy of MDS is generally unsatisfactory. Only stem cell transplantation offers cure: survival rates of 50% at 3 years have been reported, but older patients are particularly prone to develop treatment-related mortality and morbidity. Results of transplant using matched unrelated donors are comparable, although most series contain younger and more highly selected cases. MDS associated with trisomy 8 may respond to cyclosporine.

MDS has been regarded as particularly refractory to cytotoxic chemotherapy regimens but is probably no more resistant to effective treatment than acute myeloid leukemia in the elderly, in whom drug toxicity is often fatal and remissions, if achieved, are brief. Low doses of cytotoxic drugs have been administered for their "differentiating" potential. 5-azacytidine inhibits DNA methylation and may induce the expression of genes; its use in MDS can improve blood counts and modestly improves survival compared to best supportive care. Amifostine, an organic thiophosphonate that blocks apoptosis, can improve blood counts but has significant toxicities. Both azacytidine and amifostine are approved by the U.S. Food and Drug Administration for use in MDS. ATG may improve blood counts in one-third of MDS patients; those who are young, HLA-D2 positive, and have a PNH clone are more likely to respond.

Hematopoietic growth factors can improve blood counts but, as in most other marrow failure states, have been most beneficial to patients with the least severe pancytopenia. G-CSF treatment alone failed to improve survival in a controlled trial. Erythropoietin alone or in combination with G-CSF can improve hemoglobin levels, especially in those with low serum erythropoietin levels who have no or only a modest need for transfusions.

The same principles of supportive care described for aplastic anemia apply to MDS. Because many patients will be anemic for years,

TABLE 94-6 *International Prognostic Scoring System*

	Score Value				
Prognostic Variable	0	0.5	1.0	1.5	2.0
Bone marrow blasts (%)	<5%	5–10%		11–20%	21–30%
Karyotype[a]	Good	Intermediate	Poor		
Cytopenia[b] (lineages affected)	0 or 1	2 or 3			
Risk Group Scores	**Score**				
Low	0				
Intermediate-1	0.5–1.0				
Intermediate-2	1.5–2.0				
High	≥2.5				

[a] Good, normal, -Y, del(5q), del (20q); intermediate, all other abnormalities; poor, complex (≥3 abnormalities) or chromosome 7 abnormalities.
[b] Cytopenias defined as Hb <100 g/L, platelet count < 100,000/μL, absolute neutrophil count <1500/μL.

erythrocyte transfusion support should be accompanied by iron chelation in order to prevent secondary hemochromatosis.

MYELOPHTHISIC ANEMIAS

Fibrosis of the bone marrow (see Fig. 95-2), usually accompanied by a characteristic blood smear picture called *leukoerythroblastosis*, can occur as a primary hematologic disease, called *myelofibrosis* or *myeloid metaplasia* (Chap. 95), and as a secondary process, called *myelophthisis*. Myelophthisis, or secondary myelofibrosis, is reactive. Fibrosis can be a response to invading tumor cells, usually of an epithelial cancer of breast, lung, and prostate or neuroblastoma. Marrow fibrosis may occur with infection of mycobacteria (both *Mycobacterium tuberculosis* and *M. avium*), fungi, or HIV, and in sarcoidosis. Intracellular lipid deposition in Gaucher disease and obliteration of the marrow space related to absence of osteoclast remodeling in congenital osteopetrosis also can produce fibrosis. Secondary myelofibrosis is a late consequence of radiation therapy or treatment with radiomimetic drugs. Usually, the infectious or malignant underlying processes are obvious. Marrow fibrosis can also be a feature of a variety of hematologic syndromes, especially chronic myeloid leukemia, multiple myeloma, lymphomas, myeloma, and hairy cell leukemia.

The pathophysiology has three distinct features: proliferation of fibroblasts in the marrow space (myelofibrosis); the extension of hematopoiesis into the long bones and, most particularly, into extramedullary sites usually the spleen, liver, and lymph nodes (myeloid metaplasia); and ineffective erythropoiesis. The etiology of fibrosis is unknown but most likely involves dysregulated production of growth factors: platelet-derived growth factor and transforming growth factor β have been implicated. Abnormal regulation of other hematopoietins

would lead to localization of blood-producing cells in nonhematopoietic tissues and uncoupling of the usually balanced processes of stem cell proliferation and differentiation. Myelofibrosis is remarkable for pancytopenia despite extraordinarily large numbers of circulating hematopoietic progenitor cells.

Anemia is dominant in secondary myelofibrosis, usually normocytic and normochromic. The diagnosis is suggested by the characteristic leukoerythroblastic smear (see Fig. 95-1). Erythrocyte morphology is highly abnormal, with circulating nucleated red blood cells, teardrops, and shape distortions. White blood cell numbers are often elevated, sometimes mimicking a leukemoid reaction, with circulating myelocytes, promyelocytes, and myeloblasts. Platelets may be abundant and are often giant size. Inability to aspirate the bone marrow, the characteristic "dry tap," can allow a presumptive diagnosis in the appropriate setting before the biopsy is decalcified.

The course of secondary myelofibrosis is determined by its cause, usually a metastatic tumor or an advanced hematologic malignancy. Treatable causes must be excluded, especially tuberculosis and fungus. Transfusion support can relieve symptoms.

FURTHER READING

D'ANDREA AD, GROMPE M: The Fanconi anaemia/BRCA pathway. Nat Rev Cancer 3:23, 2003

FISCH P et al: Pure red cell aplasia. Br J Haematol 111:1010, 2000

MOLLDREM JJ et al: Antithymocyte globulin for treatment of the bone marrow failure associated with myelodysplastic syndromes. Ann Intern Med 137: 156, 2002

SILVERMAN JR et al: Randomized controlled trial of azacitidine in patients with the myelodysplastic syndrome: A study of the Cancer and Leukemia Group B. J Clin Oncol 20:2429, 2002

YOUNG NS: Acquired aplastic anemia. Ann Intern Med 136:534, 2002

YOUNG NS, BROWN KE: Parvovirus B19. N Engl J Med 350:586, 2004

95 | POLYCYTHEMIA VERA AND OTHER MYELOPROLIFERATIVE DISEASES
Jerry L. Spivak

Polycythemia vera, chronic idiopathic myelofibrosis, essential thrombocytosis, and chronic myeloid leukemia (CML) are commonly classified together under the rubric *the chronic myeloproliferative disorders*, because their pathophysiology involves the clonal expansion of a multipotent hematopoietic progenitor cell with the overproduction of one or more of the formed elements of the blood. These entities may transform into acute leukemia naturally or as a consequence of mutagenic treatment. However, while polycythemia vera, idiopathic myelofibrosis, essential thrombocytosis, and CML share similar phenotypic characteristics, CML is genotypically distinct from the other three disorders because it alone is associated with translocation of genetic material between the long arms of chromosomes 9 and 22, resulting in the production of the unique fusion protein, bcr-abl.

The new World Health Organization classification of myeloid neoplasms has expanded the list of chronic myeloproliferative disorders to include the exceedingly rare entities chronic neutrophilic leukemia, chronic eosinophilic leukemia, and the hypereosinophilic syndrome. In addition, a category of myelodysplastic/myeloproliferative diseases was created to encompass juvenile myelomonocytic leukemia, atypical chronic myeloid leukemia [lacking t(9;22)], and chronic myelomonocytic leukemia. The word "chronic" was also added to idiopathic myelofibrosis to distinguish this disorder from the rarer syndrome of acute panmyelosis with myelofibrosis, a rare form of acute leukemia.

These classification changes were made in recognition of the considerable overlap in clinical presentation and hematopathology that characterizes the chronic myeloproliferative disorders. Systemic mastocytosis, while having phenotypic overlap with the chronic myeloproliferative diseases, was given its own category in recognition of the many distinct clinical syndromes that characterize mast cell proliferation. In this chapter, only polycythemia vera, chronic idiopathic mye-

lofibrosis, and essential thrombocytosis will be discussed as their clinical overlap is substantial and their clinical course distinct from the other myeloproliferative disorders. ➙*CML is discussed in Chap. 96.*

POLYCYTHEMIA VERA

Polycythemia vera is a clonal disorder involving a multipotent hematopoietic progenitor cell in which there is accumulation of phenotypically normal red cells, granulocytes, and platelets in the absence of a recognizable physiologic stimulus. The most common of the chronic myeloproliferative disorders, polycythemia vera occurs in about 2 per 100,000 persons, sparing no adult age group. Vertical transmission has been documented, establishing a genetic basis for the disorder. A slight overall male predominance has been observed, but females predominate within the reproductive age range.

ETIOLOGY The etiology of polycythemia vera is unknown. Although nonrandom chromosome abnormalities such as 20q−, trisomy 8 or 9 have been documented in a small percentage of untreated polycythemia vera patients, no consistent cytogenetic abnormality has been associated with the disorder and no specific genetic defect has yet been identified. Impaired posttranslational processing of the thrombopoietin receptor, Mpl, has been noted in polycythemia vera patients; the extent of the defect correlated with disease duration and splenomegaly. While this defect is specific for polycythemia vera and is not found in secondary erythrocytosis, its role in the pathophysiology of the disorder is still undefined. Polycythemia vera leukocytes also overexpress mRNA for *PRV-1*. In contrast to normal erythroid progenitor cells, polycythemia vera erythroid progenitor cells can grow in vitro in the absence of erythropoietin due to hypersensitivity to insulin-like growth factor I. However, this phenotypic abnormality is not specific for polycythemia vera and has been documented in essential thrombocytosis and secondary erythrocytosis. Polycythemia vera erythroid progenitor cells are more resistant to apoptosis induced by erythropoietin deprivation, due to upregulation of bcl-X_L, an antiapoptotic protein. Polycythemia vera erythroid progenitors do not divide more rapidly than their normal counterparts, but they accumulate because they do not die normally. Additionally, the transformed hematopoietic progenitor cells in polycythemia vera, as in other neoplastic disorders, exhibit clonal dominance and suppress the proliferation of normal hematopoietic progenitor cells by an unknown mechanism. Consequently, the circulating formed elements of the blood represent only progeny of the transformed clone.

CLINICAL FEATURES Although massive splenomegaly may be the initial presenting sign in polycythemia vera, most often the disorder is first recognized by the discovery of a high hemoglobin or hematocrit, but with the exception of aquagenic pruritus, no symptoms distinguish polycythemia vera from other causes of erythrocytosis.

Uncontrolled erythrocytosis can lead to neurologic symptoms such as vertigo, tinnitus, headache, and visual disturbances. Systolic hypertension also accompanies the elevated red cell mass. In some patients, venous or arterial thrombosis may be the presenting manifestation of polycythemia vera. Intraabdominal venous thrombosis is particularly common and may be catastrophic when there is sudden compromise of the hepatic vein. Polycythemia vera should be suspected in any patient who develops the Budd-Chiari syndrome. Digital ischemia may also occur. Easy bruising, epistaxis, or gastrointestinal hemorrhage may be observed, and polycythemia vera patients are frequently hypermetabolic. Hyperuricemia with secondary gout, uric acid stones, and acid-peptic disease also complicate the disorder. Because isolated erythrocytosis is a common initial presentation for polycythemia vera but no clonal marker is available for the disease, the first task of the physician is to distinguish this autonomous clonal form of erythrocytosis from the many other types of erythrocytosis, most of which are correctable (Table 95-1).

Erythropoiesis is normally regulated by the glycoprotein hormone erythropoietin. Erythropoietin, which in adults is produced primarily in the kidneys and to a small extent in the liver, promotes the proliferation of erythroid progenitor cells, maintains their survival, and facilitates their differentiation. Because erythropoietin acts as a survival factor, it is constitutively produced and, like the red cell mass, its level is constant as long as tissue oxygenation is adequate. The plasma erythropoietin level, like the red cell mass, differs among individuals but in adults is not affected by either age or gender. Erythropoietin production is regulated at the level of gene transcription. Hypoxia is the only physiologic stimulus that increases the number of cells producing erythropoietin, and thus the production of erythropoietin is independent of its plasma level. In the absence of renal or hepatic disease, plasma erythropoietin levels reflect erythropoietin production, and therefore the assay for plasma erythropoietin is a surrogate assay for tissue hypoxia. Erythropoietin is active at the picomolar level, and its production is tightly regulated. Thus, the plasma erythropoietin level does not rise outside the normal range until the hemoglobin level falls below 105 g/L. This is not meant to imply that an increase in erythropoietin production does not occur as the hemoglobin level falls below normal, but because the normal range for plasma erythropoietin is wide (4 to 26 mU/mL), unless the patient's baseline level is known, any increase will not be recognized until the hemoglobin falls below 105 g/L. Thereafter, there is a log-linear inverse correlation between the plasma erythropoietin and hemoglobin levels. With erythrocytosis, erythropoietin production is suppressed; this suppression reflects not only the increase in tissue oxygen transport associated with the increase in red cell number but also additional negative-feedback mechanisms unrelated to oxygen transport but related to the increase in blood viscosity and an increase in red cell precursors capable of metabolizing erythropoietin. The summation of these mechanisms accounts for the paradoxical observation that many patients with hypoxic erythrocytosis due to cyanotic congenital heart disease or obstructive lung disease have a "normal" plasma erythropoietin level. The plasma erythropoietin level is a useful diagnostic test in patients with isolated erythrocytosis, because an elevated level excludes polycythemia vera as the cause for the erythrocytosis.

DIAGNOSIS When confronted with an elevated hemoglobin or hematocrit level, it is important to obtain previous values to determine the duration of this abnormality. Because the hemoglobin or hematocrit level is affected by the plasma volume, and hematocrit and red cell mass are not linearly related, a red cell mass determination must also be performed to distinguish absolute erythrocytosis from relative erythrocytosis due to a reduction in plasma volume alone (also known as *stress* or *spurious erythrocytosis* or *Geisböck's syndrome*). Red cell mass determination is important because in polycythemia vera, in contrast to erythropoietin-driven erythrocytosis, the plasma volume is frequently elevated, masking not only the true extent of red cell mass expansion but often its presence. Indeed, a significant proportion of patients with polycythemia vera have a hematocrit within the normal range, particularly patients with a substantial splenomegaly. Failure to recognize this phenomenon is undoubtedly the basis for many of the reported instances of hepatic or portal vein thrombosis in patients with an "undefined" myeloproliferative disorder.

Red cell mass is reliably determined by isotope dilution using the patient's ^{51}Cr-tagged red cells; extrapolations made after determining only the plasma volume are unacceptable. Furthermore, to allow ample time for equilibration of the labeled red cells, measurements should be made over a period of ≥90 min.

Once the presence of absolute erythrocytosis has been established, its cause must be determined. An elevated plasma erythropoietin level suggests either an hypoxic cause for erythrocytosis or autonomous erythropoietin production, in which case assessment of pulmonary function and an abdominal computed tomography scan to evaluate renal and hepatic anatomy are appropriate. A normal erythropoietin level does not exclude an hypoxic cause for erythrocytosis. In polycythemia vera, in contrast to hypoxic erythrocytosis, the arterial oxygen saturation is normal. However, a normal oxygen saturation does not exclude a high-affinity hemoglobin as a cause for erythrocytosis, and it is here that documentation of previous hemoglobin levels and a family study become important. Because there is no clonal marker for polycythemia vera, clinical guidelines have been proposed to define the disease. A modified version is provided in Table 95-2. However, these guidelines do not establish clonality, and in some patients the underlying disorder only becomes apparent over time. Diagnostic ambiguity does not preclude the initiation of therapy.

Other laboratory studies that may aid in diagnosis include the red cell count, mean corpuscular volume, and red cell distribution width (RDW). Only three situations cause microcytic erythrocytosis: β-thalassemia trait, hypoxic erythrocytosis, and polycythemia vera. However, with β-thalassemia trait the RDW is normal, whereas with hy-

---

TABLE 95-1 *Causes of Absolute Erythrocytosis*

Hypoxia	Tumors
Carbon monoxide intoxication	Hypernephroma
High altitude	Hepatoma
Pulmonary disease	Cerebellar hemangioblastoma
High-affinity hemoglobin	Adrenal adenoma
Sleep-apnea syndrome	Pheochromocytoma
Respiratory center	Meningioma
dysfunction	Uterine fibromyoma
Supine hypoventilation	Familial (with normal hemoglobin
Right-to-left cardiac shunts	function)
Renal disease	VHL mutations
Renal cysts	Erythropoietin receptor mutations
Hydronephrosis	BPG mutase deficiency
Renal artery stenosis	Bartter's syndrome
Focal glomerulonephritis	Androgen therapy
Renal transplantation	Recombinant erythropoietin therapy
	Polycythemia vera

Note: BPG, bisphosphoglycerate; VHL, von Hippel–Lindau.

TABLE 95-2 *Suggested Criteria for the Clinical Diagnosis of Polycythemia Vera*[a]

Elevated red cell mass
Normal arterial oxygen saturation
Splenomegaly
In the absence of splenomegaly:
   Leukocytosis and thrombocytosis

[a] It must be emphasized that these criteria do not establish clonality.

poxic erythrocytosis and polycythemia vera, the RDW is usually elevated. A properly made blood smear from a patient with erythrocytosis will be virtually unreadable due to the marked elevation in red cell count, but no specific morphologic abnormalities are seen in the leukocytes or platelets in polycythemia vera. However, when these are also elevated the diagnosis is assured. In many patients, the leukocyte alkaline phosphatase level is also increased, as is the uric acid level. Elevated serum vitamin B_{12} or B_{12}-binding capacity may be present. In patients with associated acid-peptic disease, occult gastrointestinal bleeding may lead to presentation with hypochromic, microcytic anemia.

A bone marrow aspirate and biopsy will provide no specific diagnostic information, and unless there is a need to establish the presence of myelofibrosis or exclude some other disorder, these procedures need not be done. Although the presence of a cytogenetic abnormality such as trisomy 8 or 9 or 20q− in the setting of an expanded red cell mass supports a clonal etiology, no specific cytogenetic abnormality is associated with polycythemia vera, and the absence of a cytogenetic marker does not exclude the diagnosis.

COMPLICATIONS The major clinical complications of polycythemia vera relate directly to the increase in blood viscosity associated with elevation of the red cell mass and indirectly to the increased turnover of red cells, leukocytes, and platelets and the attendant increase in uric acid and cytokine production. The latter appears to be responsible for the increase in peptic ulcer disease and for the pruritus associated with this disorder, although little formal proof for this has been obtained. A sudden massive increase in spleen size is another problem and can be associated with splenic infarction or progressive cachexia. Myelofibrosis and myeloid metaplasia can also develop with transfusion-dependent anemia, but the frequency is low in those not receiving chemotherapy or irradiation. Although acute nonlymphocytic leukemia is reported to be increased in polycythemia vera, the incidence of acute leukemia in patients not exposed to chemotherapy or radiation is low and the development of leukemia is not related to disease duration, suggesting that the treatment exposure may be a more important risk factor than the disease itself.

Erythromelalgia is a curious syndrome of unknown etiology primarily involving the lower extremities and manifested usually by erythema, warmth, and pain of the affected appendage and occasionally digital infarction. It occurs with a variable frequency in patients with a myeloproliferative disorder and is usually responsive to salicylates. Some of the central nervous system symptoms observed in patients with polycythemia vera may represent a variant of erythromelalgia.

If left uncontrolled, erythrocytosis can lead to intravascular thrombosis involving vital organs such as the liver, heart, brain, or lungs. Patients with massive splenomegaly are particularly prone to thrombotic events because the associated increase in plasma volume masks the true extent of the red cell mass elevation as measured by the hematocrit or hemoglobin level. A "normal" hematocrit or hemoglobin level in a polycythemia vera patient with massive splenomegaly should be considered as indicative of an elevated red cell mass until proven otherwise.

℞ **TREATMENT**

Polycythemia vera is generally an indolent disorder whose clinical course can run many decades, and its medical management should

reflect the tempo of the disorder. Maintenance of the hemoglobin level at ≤140 g/L in men and ≤120 g/L in women is mandatory to avoid the thrombotic complications. Thrombosis due to erythrocytosis is the most significant complication of this disorder. Phlebotomy serves initially to reduce hyperviscosity by bringing the red cell mass into the normal range. Periodic phlebotomies thereafter serve to maintain the red cell mass within the range of normal and to induce a state of iron deficiency, which prevents an accelerated reexpansion of the red cell mass. In most polycythemia vera patients, once an iron-deficient state is achieved, phlebotomy is usually required only at 3-month intervals. Although both phlebotomy and iron deficiency, in addition to the disease itself, tend to increase the platelet count, thrombocytosis is not correlated with thrombosis in polycythemia vera, in contrast to the strong correlation between erythrocytosis and thrombosis in this disease. The use of salicylates as a tonic against thrombosis in polycythemia vera patients is potentially harmful, and salicylates should be employed only to treat erythromelalgia. Anticoagulants are not routinely indicated and are difficult to monitor owing to the artifactual imbalance between the test tube anticoagulant and plasma that occurs when blood from these patients is assayed for prothrombin or partial thromboplastin activity. Asymptomatic hyperuricemia requires no therapy, but allopurinol should be administered to avoid further elevation of the uric acid when chemotherapy is employed to reduce splenomegaly, leukocytosis, or pruritus. Generalized pruritus intractable to antihistamines can be a major problem in polycythemia vera, and hydroxyurea, interferon (IFN)-α, and psoralens with ultraviolet light in the A range (PUVA) therapy are methods of palliation. Asymptomatic thrombocytosis requires no therapy. Symptomatic splenomegaly can be treated with hydroxyurea or IFN-α, although each can be associated with significant side effects. Anagrelide, a quinazolin derivative and platelet antiaggregant that also lowers the platelet count, can control thrombocytosis and is preferable to hydroxyrurea or IFN-α. A reduction in platelet number may be necessary in the treatment of erythromelalgia if salicylates are not effective or if the thrombocytosis is associated with migraine-like symptoms. Alkylating agents and sodium phosphate P32 (^{32}P) are leukemogenic in polycythemia vera, and their use should be avoided. If a cytotoxic agent must be used, hydroxyurea is preferred, but it also may be leukemogenic. Chemotherapy should be used for as short a time as possible. In some patients, massive splenomegaly unresponsive to reduction by hydroxyurea or IFN-α therapy and associated with intractable weight loss will require splenectomy. Allogeneic bone marrow transplantation may be curative in young patients.

Patients with polycythemia vera can be expected to live long and useful lives when their red cell mass is effectively managed with phlebotomy. Chemotherapy is never indicated to control the red cell mass unless venous access is impossible.

CHRONIC IDIOPATHIC MYELOFIBROSIS

Chronic idiopathic myelofibrosis (other designations include *agnogenic myeloid metaplasia* or *myelofibrosis with myeloid metaplasia*) is a clonal disorder of a multipotent hematopoietic progenitor cell of unknown etiology characterized by marrow fibrosis, myeloid metaplasia with extramedullary hematopoiesis, and splenomegaly. Chronic idiopathic myelofibrosis is uncommon; in the absence of a specific clonal marker, establishing this diagnosis is difficult because myelofibrosis and myeloid metaplasia with splenomegaly are also features of both polycythemia vera and CML. Furthermore, myelofibrosis and splenomegaly occur in a variety of benign and malignant disorders (Table 95-3), many of which are amenable to specific therapies not effective in chronic idiopathic myelofibrosis. In contrast to the other chronic myeloproliferative disorders and so-called acute or malignant myelofibrosis, which can occur at any age, chronic idiopathic myelofibrosis primarily afflicts individuals in their sixth decade or later.

ETIOLOGY The etiology of chronic idiopathic myelofibrosis is unknown. Although nonrandom chromosome abnormalities such as 20q−, 13q−, and trisomy 1q are not uncommon, no specific cytoge-

TABLE 95-3 *Causes of Myelofibrosis*

Carcinoma metastatic to the marrow	Polycythemia vera
Infection	Chronic idiopathic myelofibrosis
Lymphoma	Systemic mastocytosis
Hodgkin's disease	Thorium dioxide (Thorotrast) exposure
Acute leukemia (lymphoid or myeloid)	Systemic lupus erythematosus
Hairy cell leukemia	Renal osteodystrophy
	HIV infection
Multiple myeloma	Hyperparathyroidism
Chronic myeloid leukemia	Gray-platelet syndrome

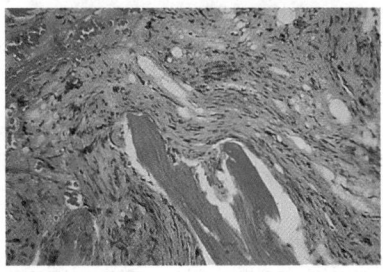

FIGURE 95-2 This marrow section shows the marrow cavity replaced by fibrous tissue composed of reticulin fibers and collagen. When this fibrosis is due to a primary hematologic process, it is called *myelofibrosis*. When the fibrosis is secondary to a tumor or a granulomatous process, it is called *myelophthisis*.

netic abnormality has been identified. The degree of myelofibrosis and the extent of extramedullary hematopoiesis are not related. Fibrosis in this disorder is associated with overproduction of transforming growth factor β and thrombopoietin. Importantly, fibroblasts in chronic idiopathic myelofibrosis are not part of the neoplastic clone.

CLINICAL FEATURES   No specific signs or symptoms are associated with chronic idiopathic myelofibrosis. Most patients are asymptomatic at presentation and usually detected by the discovery of splenic enlargement and/or abnormal blood counts during a routine examination. A blood smear reveals the characteristic features of extramedullary hematopoiesis: teardrop-shaped red cells, nucleated red cells, myelocytes, and promyelocytes; myeloblasts may also be present but have no prognostic significance (Fig. 95-1). Anemia, usually mild initially, is the rule, while the leukocyte and platelet counts are either normal or increased but either can be depressed. Mild hepatomegaly may accompany the splenomegaly, and both the lactate dehydrogenase and serum alkaline phosphatase levels can be elevated. The level of leukocyte alkaline phosphatase can be low, normal, or elevated. Marrow may be unaspirable due to the myelofibrosis (Fig. 95-2), and bone x-rays may reveal osteosclerosis. Exuberant extramedullary hematopoiesis can cause ascites, pulmonary hypertension, intestinal or ureteral obstruction, intracranial hypertension, pericardial tamponade, spinal cord compression, or skin nodules. Splenic enlargement can be sufficiently rapid to cause splenic infarctions with fever and pleuritic chest pain. Hyperuricemia and secondary gout may ensue.

DIAGNOSIS   While the clinical picture described above is characteristic of chronic idiopathic myelofibrosis, all of the clinical features described can be observed in polycythemia vera or CML. Massive splenomegaly commonly masks erythrocytosis in polycythemia vera, and reports of intraabdominal thromboses in chronic idiopathic myelofibrosis likely represent instances of unrecognized polycythemia vera. Furthermore, many other disorders have features that overlap with chronic idiopathic myelofibrosis but respond to distinctly different therapies. Therefore, the diagnosis of chronic idiopathic myelofibrosis is one of exclusion, which requires that the disorders listed in Table 95-3 be ruled out.

The presence of teardrop-shaped red cells, nucleated red cells, myelocytes, and promyelocytes establishes the presence of extramedullary hematopoiesis; the presence of leukocytosis, thrombocytosis with large and bizarre platelets, as well as circulating myeloblasts suggests

the presence of a myeloproliferative disorder as opposed to a secondary form of myelofibrosis (Table 95-3). Marrow is usually not aspirable due to increased marrow reticulin, but marrow biopsy will reveal a hypercellular marrow with trilineage hyperplasia and, in particular, increased megakaryocytes, but there are no characteristic morphologic abnormalities that distinguish idiopathic myelofibrosis from the other chronic myeloproliferative disorders. Splenomegaly due to extramedullary hematopoiesis may be sufficiently massive to cause portal hypertension and variceal formation. In some patients, exuberant extramedullary hematopoiesis can dominate the clinical picture. An intriguing feature of chronic idiopathic myelofibrosis is the occurrence of autoimmune abnormalities such as immune complexes, antinuclear antibodies, rheumatoid factor, or a positive Coombs' test. Whether these represent a host reaction to the disorder or are involved in its pathogenesis is unknown. Cytogenetic analysis of blood or marrow is useful both to exclude CML and for prognostic purposes, because complex karyotype abnormalities portend a poor prognosis in chronic idiopathic myelofibrosis.For unknown reasons, the number of circulating CD34+ cells is markedly increased in chronic idiopathic myelofibrosis.

COMPLICATIONS   Chronic idiopathic myelofibrosis has a median survival of only 5 years (range 1 to 15 years), a duration much shorter than for polycythemia vera or essential thrombocytosis. The natural history of chronic idiopathic myelofibrosis is one of inexorable marrow failure with transfusion-dependent anemia and increasing organomegaly. Patients are prone to deep-seated tissue infections, particularly of the lungs. As with CML, chronic idiopathic myelofibrosis can evolve from a chronic phase to an accelerated phase with constitutional symptoms and increasing marrow failure. About 10% of patients develop an aggressive form of acute leukemia for which therapy is usually ineffective. Important prognostic factors for disease acceleration include anemia; thrombocytopenia; age; the presence of complex cytogenetic abnormalities; and constitutional symptoms such as unexplained fever, night sweats, or weight loss. Any nonrandom cytogenetic abnormality is associated with a shortened life span, and the presence or development of multiple cytogenetic abnormalities is highly indicative of disease acceleration.

℞ TREATMENT

No specific therapy exists for chronic idiopathic myelofibrosis. Anemia may be exacerbated by deficiency of folic acid or iron, and in rare instances, pyridoxine therapy has been effective. However, anemia is more often due to ineffective erythropoiesis not compensated for by the extramedullary hematopoiesis in the spleen and liver; neither androgens nor erythropoietin has been consistently effective therapy. Erythropoietin may worsen splenomegaly. A red cell splenic sequestration study can establish the presence of hypersplenism, for which splenectomy is indicated. Splenectomy may also be necessary if splenomegaly impairs alimentation and should be performed before cachexia sets in. In this situation, splenectomy should not be avoided because of concern over rebound thrombocytosis, loss of hematopoietic capacity, or compensatory hepatomegaly. However, for unexplained reasons, splenectomy increases the risk of blastic transformation. Allopurinol can control significant hyperuricemia, and

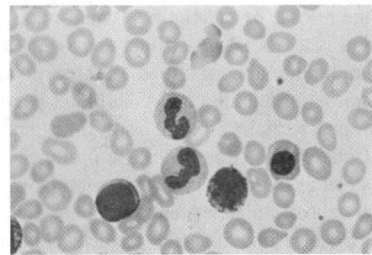

FIGURE 95-1   Teardrop-shaped red blood cells indicative of membrane damage from collagen fibers, a nucleated red blood cell indicative of premature release of erythroid precursors, and immature myeloid cells indicative of extramedullary hematopoiesis are noted. This peripheral blood smear is related to marrow fibrosis, either primary myelofibrosis or secondary myelophthisis.

hydroxyurea has proved useful for controlling organomegaly. The role of IFN-α is undefined, and its side effects are more pronounced in the older individuals who are affected with this disorder, but reversal of myelofibrosis has been observed. Glucocorticoids are used to control autoimmune complications and may ameliorate anemia alone or in combination with thalidomide. Allogeneic bone marrow transplantation should be considered in younger patients.

ESSENTIAL THROMBOCYTOSIS

Essential thrombocytosis (other designations include *essential thrombocythemia, idiopathic thrombocytosis, primary thrombocytosis, hemorrhagic thrombocythemia*) is a clonal disorder of unknown etiology involving a multipotent hematopoietic progenitor cell and is manifested clinically by the overproduction of platelets without a definable cause. Essential thrombocytosis is an uncommon disorder, but its exact frequency is unknown. No clonal marker distinguishes it from the more common nonclonal, reactive forms of thrombocytosis (Table 95-4). Clinical recognition of thrombocytosis is unlikely in the largely asymptomatic persons affected by this disorder. As a consequence, essential thrombocytosis was formerly considered to be a disease of the elderly and to be responsible for significant morbidity due to hemorrhage or thrombosis. However, with the widespread application of platelet counting, it is now clear that essential thrombocytosis can occur at any age in adults and often occurs without symptoms or disturbances of hemostasis. There is an unexplained female predominance, in contrast to the reactive forms of thrombocytosis where no sex bias exists. Because no clonal marker is available for the disorder, clinical criteria have been proposed to distinguish it from the other chronic myeloproliferative disorders, which may also present with thrombocytosis but have differing prognoses and treatment (Table 95-5). These criteria do not establish clonality; therefore, they are truly useful only in identifying disorders such as CML, polycythemia vera, or myelodysplasia, which can masquerade as essential thrombocytosis, as opposed to establishing the presence of essential thrombocytosis. Furthermore, as with "primary" erythrocytosis, nonclonal, benign forms of thrombocytosis exist (such as hereditary overproduction of thrombopoietin) that are not widely recognized because we currently lack the diagnostic tools to do so.

ETIOLOGY Megakaryocytopoiesis and platelet production depend upon thrombopoietin and its receptor, Mpl. As in the case of early erythroid and myeloid progenitor cells, early megakaryocytic progenitors require the presence of interleukin (IL) 3 and stem cell factor for optimal proliferation, and their subsequent development is enhanced by IL-6 and -11. However, megakaryocyte maturation and differentiation require thrombopoietin.

Megakaryocytes are unique among hematopoietic progenitor cells because they undergo endomitotic as opposed to mitotic reduplication of their genome. In the absence of thrombopoietin, endomitotic megakaryocytic reduplication and, by extension, the cytoplasmic development necessary for platelet production are impaired. Like erythropoietin, thrombopoietin is produced in both the liver and the kidneys,

TABLE 95-4 Causes of Thrombocytosis

Iron-deficiency anemia	Idiopathic myelofibrosis
Hyposplenism	Essential thrombocytosis
Postsplenectomy[a]	Chronic myeloid leukemia
Malignancy	Idiopathic sideroblastic anemia
Collagen vascular disease	Myelodysplasia (5q− syndrome)
Inflammatory bowel disease	Postsurgery
Infection	Rebound (cessation of ethanol intake,
Hemolysis	correction of vitamin B_{12} or folate
Hemorrhage	deficiency)
Polycythemia vera	

[a] If the platelet count is greater than $2 \times 10^6/\mu L$, the etiology is most likely a myeloproliferative disorder.

TABLE 95-5 Suggested Criteria for the Clinical Diagnosis of Essential Thrombocytosis[a]

Platelet count $\geq 500,000/\mu L$
Absence of a known cause of reactive thrombocytosis (see Table 95-4)
Absence of the Ph chromosome and the bcr-abl gene rearrangement
Normal red cell mass
Presence of marrow iron
Absence of myelofibrosis
Absence of myelodysplasia clinically and by cytogenetic analysis
Splenomegaly

[a] The concept that a platelet count greater than $1 \times 10^6/\mu L$ distinguishes essential thrombocytosis from other causes of thrombocytosis has no clinical validity.

and an inverse correlation exists between the platelet count and plasma thrombopoietic activity. Like erythropoietin, plasma levels of thrombopoietin are controlled in part by the size of its progenitor cell pool. In contrast to erythropoietin, but like its myeloid counterparts granulocyte and granulocyte-macrophage colony-stimulating factors, thrombopoietin not only enhances the proliferation of its target cells but also enhances the reactivity of their end-stage product, the platelet. In addition to its role in thrombopoiesis, thrombopoietin enhances the survival of multipotent hematopoietic stem cells.

The clonality of essential thrombocytosis was established by the use of the isoenzymes of glucose-6-phosphate dehydrogenase in patients who are hemizygous for this gene, by the use of X-linked DNA polymorphisms, and by the identification of nonrandom, although variable, cytogenetic abnormalities. The multipotent hematopoietic progenitor cell involved in this disorder can vary; in some patients lymphocytes contained the same clonal marker as the megakaryocytes, erythrocytes, and myeloid cells, whereas in others the lymphocytes were not involved. Similar observations have been made in polycythemia vera. Furthermore, a number of families have been described in which essential thrombocytosis was inherited, in one instance as an autosomal dominant trait. In one kindred, in addition to essential thrombocytosis, idiopathic myelofibrosis and polycythemia vera were also individually documented.

CLINICAL FEATURES Clinically, essential thrombocytosis is most often identified incidentally when a platelet count is obtained during the course of a routine evaluation. Occasionally, review of previous platelet counts will reveal that an elevation was present but overlooked. No symptoms or signs are specific for essential thrombocytosis, but patients do have hemorrhagic and thrombotic tendencies expressed as easy bruising for the former or microvascular occlusions for the latter, which may be manifested by erythromelalgia, migraine, or transient ischemic attacks. Physical examination is generally unremarkable except occasionally for mild splenomegaly. Massive splenomegaly is more characteristic of the other myeloproliferative disorders, particularly polycythemia vera or idiopathic myelofibrosis.

Anemia is unusual, but a mild neutrophilic leukocytosis is not. The blood smear, however, is most remarkable for the number of platelets present, some of which may be very large. The leukocyte alkaline phosphatase score is either normal or elevated. The large mass of circulating platelets may prevent the accurate measurement of serum potassium due to the release of platelet potassium upon blood clotting. This hyperkalemia is a laboratory artifact and is not associated with any electrocardiographic abnormalities. Similarly, arterial oxygen measurements can be inaccurate unless the blood is collected on ice. The prothrombin and partial thromboplastin times are normal, while abnormalities of platelet function such as a prolonged bleeding time and impaired platelet aggregation can be present. However, in spite of much study, characteristic platelet function abnormalities are not yet defined, and no platelet function test predicts clinically significant bleeding or thrombosis.

The elevated platelet count may hinder the collection of a marrow aspirate, but marrow biopsy usually reveals both megakaryocyte hyperplasia and hypertrophy, as well as an overall increase in marrow cellularity. A slight increase in marrow reticulin may be present, but if extensive, another diagnosis should be considered. The absence of stainable iron demands an explanation, because iron deficiency alone can cause thrombocytosis and absent marrow iron is a feature of polycythemia vera.

While nonrandom cytogenetic abnormalities have been identified in essential thrombocytosis, no consistently identifiable abnormality is notable, even involving chromosomes 3 and 1 where the genes for thrombopoietin and its receptor Mpl, respectively, are located.

DIAGNOSIS Thrombocytosis is encountered in a variety of clinical disorders (Table 95-4) in which production of cytokines is increased. Thus, the first obligation when confronted with a high platelet count is to determine if it is a consequence of another disorder. Cytogenetic evaluation is mandatory to determine if the thrombocytosis is due to CML or a myelodysplastic disorder such as the 5q− syndrome. Because the bcr-abl translocation can be present in the absence of the Ph chromosome, fluorescence in situ hybridization (FISH) analysis for bcr-abl expression should be performed in all patients with thrombocytosis rather than a cytogenetic study. Anemia and ringed sideroblasts are not features of essential thrombocytosis, but they are features of idiopathic refractory sideroblastic anemia, in which thrombocytosis can also occur. The presence of massive splenomegaly should suggest the possibility of another myeloproliferative disorder, and in this setting a red cell mass determination is mandatory because substantial splenomegaly can mask the presence of erythrocytosis. What appears to be essential thrombocytosis can evolve into polycythemia vera, revealing the true nature of the underlying myeloproliferative disorder.

COMPLICATIONS Perhaps no other condition in clinical medicine has caused otherwise astute physicians to intervene inappropriately more often than thrombocytosis, particularly if the platelet count is $>1 \times 10^6/\mu L$. It is commonly believed that a high platelet count must cause intravascular stasis and thrombosis; however, no controlled clinical study has ever established this association.

To the contrary, very high platelet counts are associated primarily with hemorrhage due to acquired von Willebrand disease, while platelet counts of $<1 \times 10^6/\mu L$ are more often associated with thrombosis. This is not meant to imply that an elevated platelet count cannot cause symptoms in a patient with essential thrombocytosis, but rather that the focus should be on the patient, not the platelet count. For example, some of the most dramatic neurologic problems in essential thrombocytosis are migraine-related and may respond only to lowering of the platelet count; other symptoms may be a manifestation of erythromelalgia and respond simply to platelet cyclooxygenase inhibitors such as aspirin, without a reduction in platelet number. Still others may represent an interaction between an atherosclerotic vascular system and a high platelet count, and others may have no relationship to the platelet count whatsoever. Progress in distinguishing essential thrombocytosis from polycythemia vera and in defining new causes of hypercoagulability (such as factor V Leiden) make the older literature on thrombocytosis less reliable.

℞ TREATMENT

An elevated platelet count in an asymptomatic patient requires no therapy, and before any therapy is initiated in a patient with thrombocytosis, the cause of symptoms must be clearly identified to be a consequence of the elevated platelet count. Platelet pheresis has not been proven efficacious and cannot be recommended. Furthermore, patients with essential thrombocytosis treated with ^{32}P, hydroxyurea, or alkylating agents are placed at risk of developing acute leukemia without any proof of benefit from such therapy. If platelet reduction is deemed necessary on the basis of neurologic symptoms refractory to salicylates, IFN-α or anagrelide, a quinazolin derivative, can reduce the platelet count, but neither is uniformly effective nor without significant side effects. Hydroxyurea should be considered only if these agents are not effective or tolerable. Bleeding associated with thrombocytosis usually responds to ϵ-aminocaproic acid, which can be given prophylactically before and after elective surgery. As more clinical experience is acquired, it appears that essential thrombocytosis is more benign than previously thought, and that evolution to acute leukemia is more likely to be a consequence of prior therapy than of the disease itself. In managing patients with thrombocytosis, the physician's first obligation is to do no harm.

FURTHER READING

BAROSI G: Myelofibrosis with myeloid metaplasia: Diagnostic definition and prognostic classification for clinical studies and treatment guidelines. J Clin Oncol 17:2954, 1999

BUSS DH et al: The incidence of thrombotic and hemorrhagic disorders in association with extreme thrombocytosis: An analysis of 129 cases. Am J Hematol 20:365, 1985

SPIVAK JL: Polycythemia vera: Myths, mechanisms, and management. Blood 100:4272, 2002

SPIVAK JL et al: Chronic myeloproliferative disorders. Hematology (Am Soc Hematol Educ Program):200, 2003

TEFFERI A: The forgotten myeloproliferative disorder: Myeloid metaplasia. Oncologist 8:255, 2003

VARDIMAN JW et al: The World Health Organization (WHO) classification of the myeloid neoplasms. Blood 100:2292, 2002

96 ACUTE AND CHRONIC MYELOID LEUKEMIA
Meir Wetzler, John C. Byrd, Clara D. Bloomfield

The myeloid leukemias are a heterogeneous group of diseases characterized by infiltration of the blood, bone marrow, and other tissues by neoplastic cells of the hematopoietic system. In 2004, the estimated number of new myeloid leukemia cases in the United States was 16,520. These leukemias comprise a spectrum of malignancies that, untreated, range from rapidly fatal to slowly growing. Based on their untreated course, the myeloid leukemias have traditionally been designated acute or chronic.

ACUTE MYELOID LEUKEMIA

INCIDENCE The incidence of acute myeloid leukemia (AML) is ~3.6 per 100,000 people per year, and the age-adjusted incidence is higher in men than in women (4.4 versus 3.0). AML incidence increases with age; it is 1.7 in individuals <65 years and 16.2 in those >65. A significant increase in AML incidence has occurred over the past 10 years.

ETIOLOGY Heredity, radiation, chemical and other occupational exposures, and drugs have been implicated in the development of AML. No direct evidence suggests a viral etiology.

Heredity Certain syndromes with somatic cell chromosome aneuploidy, e.g., Down (chromosome 21 trisomy), Klinefelter (XXY and variants), and Patau (chromosome 13 trisomy), are associated with an increased incidence of AML. Inherited diseases with excessive chromatin fragility, e.g., Fanconi anemia, Bloom syndrome, ataxia telangiectasia, and Kostmann syndrome, are also associated with AML.

Radiation Survivors of the atomic bomb explosions in Japan had an increased incidence of myeloid leukemias that peaked 5 to 7 years after exposure. Therapeutic radiation alone seems to add little risk of AML but can increase the risk in people exposed to alkylating agents.

Chemical and Other Exposures Exposure to benzene, which is used as a solvent in the chemical, plastic, rubber, and pharmaceutical industries, is associated with an increased incidence of AML. Smoking and exposure to petroleum products, paint, embalming fluids, ethylene oxide, herbicides, and pesticides, have also been associated with an increased risk of AML.

Drugs Anticancer drugs are the leading cause of treatment-associated AML. Alkylating agent–associated leukemias occur on average 4 to 6 years after exposure, and affected individuals have aberrations in chromosomes 5 and 7. Topoisomerase II inhibitor–associated leukemias occur 1 to 3 years after exposure, and affected individuals often have aberrations involving chromosome 11q23. Chloramphenicol, phenylbutazone, and, less commonly, chloroquine and methoxypsoralen can result in bone marrow failure that may evolve into AML.

CLASSIFICATION The categorization of acute leukemia into biologically distinct groups is based on morphology, cytochemistry, and immunophenotype as well as cytogenetic and molecular techniques.

Morphologic and Cytochemical Classification The diagnosis of AML is established by the presence of $\geq 20\%$ myeloblasts in blood and/or bone marrow according to the World Health Organization (WHO) classification. Myeloblasts have nuclear chromatin that is uniformly fine or lacelike in appearance and large nucleoli (2 to 5 per cell). If specific cytoplasmic granules, Auer rods, or the nuclear folding and clefting characteristic of monocytoid cells are not present, the morphologic features observed under light microscopy may not be sufficient to clarify the diagnosis. A positive myeloperoxidase reaction in $>3\%$ of the blasts may be the only feature distinguishing AML from acute lymphoblastic leukemia (ALL).

Until 2000, the diagnosis of AML was established by the presence of $\geq 30\%$ myeloblasts in the marrow and further classified based on morphology and cytochemistry according to the French, American, and British (FAB) schema, which includes eight major subtypes, M0 to M7 (Table 96-1). The WHO classification modified the FAB schema by reducing the number of blasts required for a diagnosis and incorporating molecular (including cytogenetic), morphologic (multilineage dysplasia), and clinical features (such as prior hematologic disorder) in defining disease entities (Table 96-1).

Immunophenotypic Classification The phenotype of human myeloid leukemia cells can be studied by multiparameter flow cytometry after the cells are labeled with monoclonal antibodies to cell-surface antigens. For example, M0, which is characterized by immature morphology and no lineage-specific cytochemical reactions, is diagnosed by flow cytometric demonstration of the myeloid-specific antigens cluster designation (CD) 13 or 33. Similarly, M7 can often be diagnosed only by expression of the platelet-specific antigens CD41 and/or CD61 or by electron microscopic demonstration of myeloperoxidase.

Chromosomal Classification Chromosomal analysis of the leukemic cell provides the most important pretreatment prognostic information in AML. Two cytogenetic abnormalities have been invariably associated with a specific FAB group: t(15;17)(q22;q12) with M3 and inv(16)(p13q22) with M4Eo, and many chromosomal abnormalities have been associated primarily with one FAB group, including t(8;21)(q22;q22) with M2, and t(9;11)(p22;q23), and other translocations involving 11q23, with M5. As a result of their prognostic significance and association with specific morphologic features, the WHO classification incorporates cytogenetics (Table 96-1). Many of the recurring chromosomal abnormalities in AML have been associated with specific clinical characteristics. More commonly associated with younger age are t(8;21) and t(15;17), and with older age, del(5q) and del(7q). Myeloid sarcomas (see below) are associated with t(8;21) and disseminated intravascular coagulation (DIC) with t(15;17).

Molecular Classification Molecular study of many recurring cytogenetic abnormalities has revealed genes that may be involved in leukemo-

---

TABLE 96-1   *Acute Myeloid Leukemia (AML) Classification Systems*

French-American-British (FAB) Classification[a]
M0: Minimally differentiated leukemia
M1: Myeloblastic leukemia without maturation
M2: Myeloblastic leukemia with maturation
M3: Hypergranular promyelocytic leukemia
M4: Myelomonocytic leukemia
M4Eo: Variant: Increase in abnormal marrow eosinophils
M5: Monocytic leukemia
M6: Erythroleukemia (DiGuglielmo's disease)
M7: Megakaryoblastic leukemia

World Health Organization Classification[b]
I. AML with recurrent genetic abnormalities
   AML with t(8;21)(q22;q22);*AML1(CBFα)/ETO*
   AML with abnormal bone marrow eosinophils [inv(16)(p13q22) or t(16;16)(p13;q22);*CBFβ/MYH11*]
   Acute promyelocytic leukemia [AML with t(15;17)(q22;q12) (*PML/RARα* and variants]
   AML with 11q23 (*MLL*) abnormalities
II. AML with multilineage dysplasia
   Following a myelodysplastic syndrome or myelodysplastic syndrome/myeloproliferative disorder
   Without antecedent myelodysplastic syndrome
III. AML and myelodysplastic syndromes, therapy-related
   Alkylating agent–related
   Topoisomerase type II inhibitor–related
   Other types
IV. AML not otherwise categorized
   AML minimally differentiated
   AML without maturation
   AML with maturation
   Acute myelomonocytic leukemia
   Acute monoblastic and monocytic leukemia
   Acute erythroid leukemia
   Acute megakaryoblastic leukemia
   Acute basophilic leukemia
   Acute panmyelosis with myelofibrosis
   Myeloid sarcoma

[a] JM Bennett et al: Ann Intern Med 103:620, 1985
[b] ES Jaffe et al: *World Health Organization Classification of Tumours. Pathology and Genetics of Tumours of Haematopoietic and Lymphoid Tissues.* Lyon, IARC Press, 2001.

---

genesis. The 15;17 translocation encodes a chimeric protein, Pml/Rarα, which is formed by the fusion of the retinoic acid receptor-α (*RARα*) gene from chromosome 17 and the promyelocytic leukemia (*PML*) gene from chromosome 15. The *RARα* gene encodes a member of the nuclear hormone receptor family of transcription factors. After binding retinoic acid, *RARα* can promote expression of a variety of genes. The 15;17 translocation juxtaposes *PML* with *RARα* in a head-to-tail configuration that is under the transcriptional control of *PML*. Three different breakpoints in the *PML* gene lead to various fusion proteins. The Pml-Rarα fusion protein tends to suppress gene transcription and blocks differentiation of the cells. Pharmacologic doses of the Rarα ligand, all-*trans*-retinoic acid (tretinoin), relieve the block and promote differentiation (see below).

The inv(16), characteristic of M4Eo or AML with abnormal bone marrow eosinophils, and the t(8;21) both involve subunits of the transcription factor complex core-binding factor (Cbf), also known as polyomavirus enhancer binding protein 2 (Pebp2). This transcription factor contains two subunits, an α subunit, the Am11 protein, and a β subunit, the Pebp2 protein, and is involved in the expression of a number of differentiation-dependent genes in myeloid cells. The inv(16) results in a fusion of the core-binding factor β (*CBFB*) gene on the q arm (encodes Pebp2 protein) and the myosin heavy chain (*MYH11*) gene on the p arm. The 8;21 translocation involves the core binding factor α (*CBFA*) gene on chromosome 21, called the *AML1* (also *RUNX1*) gene, joining the *ETO* gene on chromosome 8. Similar to the t(15;17) gene product, the Am11/Eto protein acts to block transcription of *CBFA-CBFB*-controlled genes.

Most translocations that involve 11q23 rearrange the myeloid-lymphoid [or mixed-lineage leukemia (*MLL*)] gene. The *MLL* gene has two regions that encompass multiple zinc fingers and has at least two additional potential DNA-binding motifs. Abnormalities in the *MLL* gene are relatively common in patients with AML who do not have 11q23 rearrangements cytogenetically.

The above molecular aberrations are increasingly being used for diagnosis and detection of residual disease after treatment. Molecular aberrations are also being identified that are useful for classifying risk of relapse in patients without cytogenetic abnormalities. A partial tandem duplication (PTD) of the *MLL* gene is found in 5 to 10% of patients with normal cytogenetics and results in short remission duration. Flt3 (FMS-like tyrosine kinase 3) is a tyrosine kinase receptor important in the development of myeloid and lymphoid lineages. Activating mutations of *FLT3* are present in ~30% of adult AML patients due to internal tandem duplications (ITD) in the juxtamembrane domain or mutations of the activating loop of the kinase. Continuous activation of Flt3 and downstream target kinases, including signal transducer and activator of transcription protein 5, Ras/mitogen-activated protein kinase, and phosphatidylinositol 3-kinase/Akt, provides increased proliferation and antiapoptotic signals to the myeloid progenitor cell. Several clinical studies have demonstrated that presence of *FLT3* ITD in patients with normal cytogenetics predicts for short remission duration and inferior survival.

CLINICAL PRESENTATION ■ Symptoms

Patients with AML most often present with nonspecific symptoms that begin gradually or abruptly and are the consequence of anemia, leukocytosis, leukopenia or leukocyte dysfunction, or thrombocytopenia. Nearly half have had symptoms for ≥3 months before the leukemia was diagnosed.

Half mention fatigue as the first symptom, but most complain of fatigue or weakness at the time of diagnosis. Anorexia and weight loss are common. Fever with or without an identifiable infection is the initial symptom in ~10% of patients. Signs of abnormal hemostasis (bleeding, easy bruising) are noted first in 5% of patients. On occasion, bone pain, lymphadenopathy, nonspecific cough, headache, or diaphoresis is the presenting symptom.

Rarely patients may present with symptoms from a mass lesion located in the soft tissues, breast, uterus, ovary, cranial or spinal dura, gastrointestinal tract, lung, mediastinum, prostate, bone, or other organs. The mass lesion represents a tumor of leukemic cells and is called a *granulocytic sarcoma*, or *chloroma*. Typical AML may occur simultaneously, later, or not at all in these patients. This rare presentation is more common in patients with 8;21 translocations.

Physical Findings

Fever, splenomegaly, hepatomegaly, lymphadenopathy, sternal tenderness, and evidence of infection and hemorrhage are often found at diagnosis. Significant gastrointestinal bleeding, intrapulmonary hemorrhage, or intracranial hemorrhage occur most often in acute promyelocytic leukemia (APL). Bleeding associated with coagulopathy may also occur in monocytic AML and with extreme degrees of leukocytosis or thrombocytopenia in other morphologic subtypes. Retinal hemorrhages are detected in 15% of patients. Infiltration of the gingivae, skin, soft tissues, or the meninges with leukemic blasts at diagnosis is characteristic of the monocytic subtypes (FAB M4 and M5).

Hematologic Findings

Anemia is usually present at diagnosis and can be severe. The degree varies considerably irrespective of other hematologic findings, splenomegaly, or the duration of symptoms. The anemia is usually normochromic normocytic. Decreased erythropoiesis often results in a reduced reticulocyte count, and erythrocyte survival is decreased by accelerated destruction. Active blood loss also contributes to the anemia.

The median presenting leukocyte count is about 15,000/μl. Between 25 and 40% of patients have counts <5000/μl, and 20% have counts >100,000/μl. Fewer than 5% have no detectable leukemic cells in the blood. Poor neutrophil function may be noted functionally by impaired phagocytosis and migration and morphologically by abnormal lobulation and deficient granulation.

Platelet counts <100,000/μl are found at diagnosis in ~75% of patients, and about 25% have counts <25,000/μl. Both morphologic

and functional platelet abnormalities can be observed, including large and bizarre shapes with abnormal granulation and inability of platelets to aggregate or adhere normally to one another.

Pretreatment Evaluation

Once the diagnosis of AML is suspected, a rapid evaluation and initiation of appropriate therapy should follow (Table 96-2). In addition to clarifying the subtype of leukemia, initial studies should evaluate the overall functional integrity of the major organ systems, including the cardiovascular, pulmonary, hepatic, and renal systems. Factors that have prognostic significance, either for achieving complete remission (CR) or for predicting the duration of CR, should also be assessed before initiating treatment. Leukemic cells

---

TABLE 96-2 *Initial Diagnostic Evaluation and Management of Adult Patients with AML*

History
  Increasing fatigue or decreased exercise tolerance (anemia)
  Excess bleeding or bleeding from unusual sites (DIC, thrombocytopenia)
  Fevers or recurrent infections (granulocytopenia)
  Headache, vision changes, nonfocal neurologic abnormalities (CNS leukemia or bleed)
  Early satiety (splenomegaly)
  Family history of AML (Fanconi, Bloom, or Kostmann syndromes or ataxia telangiectasia)
  History of cancer (exposure to alkylating agents, radiation, topoisomerase II inhibitors)
  Occupational exposures (radiation, benzene, petroleum products, paint, smoking, pesticides)
Physical Examination
  Performance status (prognostic factor)
  Ecchymosis and oozing from IV sites (DIC, possible acute promyelocytic leukemia)
  Fever and tachycardia (signs of infection)
  Papilledema, retinal infiltrates, cranial nerve abnormalities (CNS leukemia)
  Poor dentition, dental abscesses
  Gum hypertrophy (leukemic infiltration, most common in monocytic leukemia)
  Skin infiltration or nodules (leukemia infiltration, most common in monocytic leukemia)
  Lymphadenopathy, splenomegaly, hepatomegaly
  Back pain, lower extremity weakness [spinal granulocytic sarcoma, most likely in t(8;21) patients]
Laboratory and radiologic studies
  CBC with manual differential cell count
  Chemistry tests (electrolytes, creatinine, BUN, calcium, phosphorus, uric acid, hepatic enzymes, bilirubin, LDH, amylase, lipase)
  Clotting studies (prothrombin time, partial thromboplastin time, fibrinogen, D-dimer)
  Viral serologies (CMV, HSV-1, varicella zoster)
  RBC type and screen
  HLA-typing of patient, siblings, and parents for potential allogeneic SCT
  Bone marrow aspirate and biopsy (morphology, cytochemistry, cytogenetics, flow cytometry, molecular studies)
  Cryopreservation of viable leukemia cells
  Echocardiogram
  PA and lateral chest radiograph
  Placement of central venous access device
Interventions for specific patients
  Dental evaluation (for those with poor dentition)
  Lumbar puncture (for those with symptoms of CNS involvement)
  Screening spine MRI (for patients with back pain, lower extremity weakness, paresthesias)
  Social work referral for patient and family psychosocial support
Counseling for all patients
  Provide patient with information regarding their disease, financial counseling, and support group contacts

Abbreviations: BUN, blood urea nitrogen; CBC, complete blood count; CMV, cytomegalovirus; CNS, central nervous system; DIC, disseminated intravascular coagulation; HSV, herpes simplex virus; LDH, lactate dehydrogenase; MRI, magnetic resonance imaging; PA, posteroanterior; RBC, red blood (cell) count; SCT, stem cell transplant.

should be obtained from all patients and cryopreserved for future use as new tests and therapeutics become available. All patients should be evaluated for infection.

Most patients are anemic and thrombocytopenic at presentation. Replacement of the appropriate blood components, if necessary, should begin promptly. Because qualitative platelet dysfunction or the presence of an infection may increase the likelihood of bleeding, evidence of hemorrhage justifies the immediate use of platelet transfusion, even if the platelet count is only moderately decreased.

About 50% of patients have a mild to moderate elevation of serum uric acid at presentation. Only 10% have marked elevations, but renal precipitation of uric acid and the nephropathy that may result is a serious but uncommon complication. The initiation of chemotherapy may aggravate hyperuricemia, and patients are usually started immediately on allopurinol or rasburicase (recombinant uric oxidase) and hydration at diagnosis. Finally, the presence in high concentrations of lysozyme, a marker for monocytic differentiation, may be etiologic in renal tubular dysfunction, which could worsen other renal problems that arise during the initial phases of therapy.

PROGNOSTIC FACTORS   Many factors influence the likelihood of entering CR, the length of CR, and the curability of AML. CR is defined after examination of both blood and bone marrow. The blood neutrophil count must be ≥1500/μl and the platelet count ≥100,000/μl. Hemoglobin concentration or hematocrit are not considered in determining CR. Circulating blasts should be absent. While rare blasts may be detected in the blood during marrow regeneration, they should disappear on successive studies. Bone marrow cellularity should be >20% with trilineage maturation. The bone marrow should contain <5% blasts, and Auer rods should be absent. Extramedullary leukemia should not be present. For patients in CR, reverse transcriptase polymerase chain reaction (RT-PCR) to detect AML-associated molecular abnormalities and fluorescence in situ hybridization (FISH) to detect AML-associated cytogenetic aberrations are currently used to detect residual disease. Such detection of minimal residual disease may become a reliable discriminator between patients in CR who do or do not require additional and/or alternative therapies. Prognostic factors are influenced by the treatment used.

Age at diagnosis remains among the most important pretreatment risk factors, with advancing age being associated with a poorer prognosis primarily because of its influence on the patient's ability to survive induction therapy and thus achieve CR. Age may also influence outcome because AML in older patients differs biologically. The leukemic cells in elderly patients more commonly express CD34 and the multidrug resistance 1 (Mdr1) efflux pump that conveys resistance to natural product–derived agents such as the anthracyclines (see below). With each successive decade of age, a greater proportion of patients have more resistant disease. Chronic and intercurrent diseases impair tolerance to rigorous therapy; acute medical problems at diagnosis reduce the likelihood of survival. Performance status, independent of age, also influences ability to survive induction therapy and thus respond to treatment.

Chromosome findings at diagnosis are an independent prognostic factor. Patients with t(8;21), inv(16), or t(15;17) have good prognoses, while those with no cytogenetic abnormality have a moderately favorable outcome when treated with high-dose cytarabine. Patients with a complex karyotype, inv(3), or −7 have a very poor prognosis. Molecular markers such as the presence of a PTD of *MLL* or the ITD of *FLT3* may also predict poor outcome of AML patients who otherwise have an intermediate prognosis.

A prolonged symptomatic interval with cytopenias preceding diagnosis or a history of an antecedent hematologic disorder are other pretreatment clinical features that are associated with a lower CR rate and shorter survival time. The CR rate is lower in patients who have had anemia, leukopenia, and/or thrombocytopenia for >1 month before the diagnosis of AML when compared to those without such a

history. Responsiveness to chemotherapy declines as the duration of the antecedent disorder(s) increases. Secondary AML developing after treatment with cytotoxic agents for other malignancies is extremely difficult to treat successfully.

A high presenting leukocyte count is an independent prognostic factor; duration of CR is inversely related to the presenting leukocyte count or absolute circulating myeloblast count. Among patients with hyperleukocytosis (>100,000/μl), early central nervous system bleeding and pulmonary leukostasis and relapse contribute to poor outcome.

The FAB classification diagnosis has been found to be an independent prognostic factor in some series. Other characteristics of leukemic cells have been reported to have prognostic significance, including Auer rods, ultrastructural features, in vitro and in vivo growth characteristics and chemotherapeutic sensitivity, and immunophenotype. Expression of the *MDR1* gene adversely influences outcome.

In addition to pretreatment variables, several treatment factors correlate with prognosis in AML, including, most importantly, achievement of CR. Another is the rapidity with which the blast cells disappear from the blood after the institution of therapy. In addition, patients who achieve CR after one induction cycle have longer CR durations than those requiring multiple cycles.

℞ TREATMENT

Treatment of the newly diagnosed patient with AML is usually divided into two phases, induction and postremission management (Fig. 96-1). The initial goal is to quickly induce CR. Once CR is obtained, further therapy must be used to prolong survival and achieve cure. The initial induction treatment and subsequent consolidation therapy are often chosen based upon the patient's age. The influence of intensifying therapy with traditional chemotherapy agents such as cytarabine and

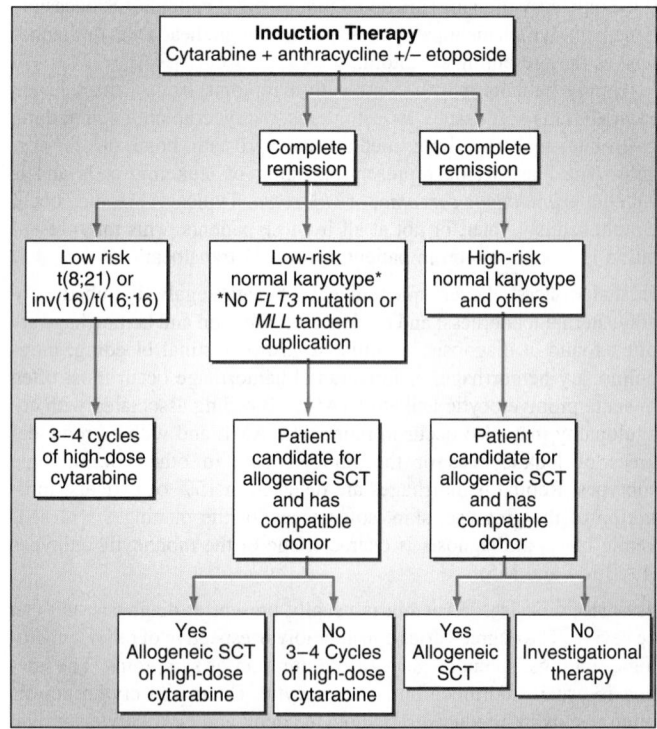

FIGURE 96-1   Flow chart for the therapy of newly diagnosed AML. For all forms of AML except APL, standard therapy includes a 7-day continuous infusion of cytarabine (100–200 mg/m² per day) and a 3-day course of daunorubicin (45–60 mg/m² per day) or idarubicin (12–13 mg/m² per day) with or without 3 days of etoposide. Patients who achieve complete remission undergo some form of consolidation therapy, including sequential courses of high-dose cytarabine, high-dose combination chemotherapy with allogeneic stem cell transplant (SCT), or novel therapies, based on their predicted risk of relapse (i.e., risk-stratified therapy). Patients with APL usually receive tretinoin together with anthracycline chemotherapy for remission induction and then receive consolidation chemotherapy (daunorubicin and cytarabine) followed by maintenance tretinoin, with or without chemotherapy.

anthracyclines in younger patients (<60 years) appears to increase the cure rate of AML. In older patients, the benefit of intensive therapy has been more difficult to document and therefore pursuit of novel therapies as consolidation for these patients has recently been actively pursued.

Induction Chemotherapy The most commonly used CR induction regimens (for patients other than those with APL) consist of combination chemotherapy with cytarabine (cytosine arabinoside) and an anthracycline. Cytarabine is a cell cycle S-phase-specific antimetabolite that becomes phosphorylated intracellularly to an active triphosphate form that interferes with DNA synthesis. Anthracyclines are DNA intercalaters. Their primary mode of action is thought to be inhibition of topoisomerase II, leading to DNA breaks. Cytarabine is usually administered as a continuous intravenous infusion at 100 to 200 mg/m^2 per day for 7 days. Anthracycline therapy generally consists of daunorubicin, 45 to 60 mg/m^2, intravenously on days 1, 2, and 3 (the 7 and 3 regimen). Treatment with idarubicin at 12 or 13 mg/m^2 per day for 3 days in conjunction with cytarabine by 7-day continuous infusion is at least as effective and may be superior to daunorubicin in younger patients. The addition of etoposide does not increase the CR rate but may improve the CR duration.

After induction chemotherapy, the bone marrow is examined to determine if the leukemia has been eliminated. If >5% blasts exist with ≥20% cellularity, the patient has traditionally been retreated with cytarabine and an anthracycline in doses similar to those given initially, but for 5 and 2 days, respectively. Our recommendation, however, is to change therapy in this setting. Patients who fail to attain CR after two induction courses should immediately proceed to an allogeneic stem cell transplant (SCT) if an appropriate donor exists. This approach is only applied to patients under the age of 65 to 70 with acceptable end-organ function.

With the 7 and 3 cytarabine/daunorubicin regimen outlined above, 65 to 75% of adults with de novo AML achieve CR. Two-thirds achieve CR after a single course of therapy, and one-third require two courses. About 50% of patients who do not achieve CR have a drug-resistant leukemia, and 50% do not achieve CR because of fatal complications of bone marrow aplasia or impaired recovery of normal stem cells. A higher induction treatment–related mortality and frequency of resistant disease has been observed as age increases in virtually all studies.

High-dose cytarabine-based regimens have very high CR rates after a single cycle of therapy. When given in high doses, more cytarabine may enter the cells, saturate the cytarabine-inactivating enzymes, and increase the intracellular levels of 1-β-D-arabinofuranylcytosine-triphosphate, the active metabolite incorporated into DNA. Thus, higher doses of cytarabine may increase the inhibition of DNA synthesis and thereby overcome resistance to standard-dose cytarabine. In two randomized studies, high-dose cytarabine with an anthracycline produced CR rates similar to those achieved with standard 7 and 3 regimens. However, the CR duration was longer after high-dose cytarabine than after standard-dose cytarabine.

The hematologic toxicity of high-dose cytarabine-based induction regimens has typically been greater than that associated with 7 and 3 regimens. Toxicity with high-dose cytarabine includes myelosuppression, pulmonary toxicity, and significant and occasionally irreversible cerebellar toxicity. All patients treated with high-dose cytarabine must be closely monitored for cerebellar toxicity. Full cerebellar testing should be performed before each dose, and further high-dose cytarabine should be withheld if evidence of cerebellar toxicity develops. This toxicity occurs more commonly in patients with renal impairment and in those over the age of 60. Indeed, it is the increased toxicity observed with high-dose cytarabine, as opposed to the lack of benefit of this therapy, that has limited the use of this more intensive therapy in elderly AML patients. Clinical trials in the elderly patients have therefore focused upon new agents and attenuated doses of high-dose cytarabine therapy.

Supportive Care Measures geared to supporting patients through several weeks of granulocytopenia and thrombocytopenia are critical to the success of AML therapy. Patients with AML should be treated in centers expert in providing supportive measures for their management.

Recombinant hematopoietic growth factors have been incorporated into clinical trials in AML. These trials have been designed to lower the infection rate after chemotherapy. Both granulocyte colony-stimulating factor (G-CSF) and granulocyte-macrophage colony-stimulating factor (GM-CSF) have reduced the median time to neutrophil recovery by an average of 5 to 7 days. This accelerated rate of neutrophil recovery, however, has not always translated into significant reductions in infection rates. In most randomized studies, both G-CSF and GM-CSF have failed to improve the CR rate, disease-free survival, or overall survival. Although receptors for both G-CSF and GM-CSF are present on AML blasts, therapeutic efficacy is neither enhanced nor inhibited by these agents. The use of growth factors as supportive care for AML patients is controversial. We favor their use in elderly patients, those receiving intensive regimens, patients with uncontrolled infections, or those participating in clinical trials.

Multilumen right atrial catheters should be inserted through a subcutaneous tunnel as soon as patients with newly diagnosed AML have been stabilized. They should be used thereafter for administration of intravenous medications and transfusions, as well as for blood drawing. Antibiotic-impregnated catheters should be considered if the risk or subsequent consequence of line-related infection is high. The separation between the vascular access site and the exit site and the presence of a Dacron cuff in the subcutaneous channel reduce the risk of infection. With meticulous attention to sterile technique in catheter placement and maintenance, catheters may often be left in place for months.

Adequate and prompt blood bank support is critical to therapy of AML. Platelet transfusions should be given as needed to maintain a platelet count >10,000 to 20,000/μl. We believe that the platelet count should be kept at higher levels in febrile patients and during episodes of active bleeding or DIC. Patients with poor posttransfusion platelet count increments may benefit from administration of platelets from human leukocyte antigen (HLA)-matched donors. Red blood cell transfusions should be administered to keep the hemoglobin level >80 g/L (8 g/dL) in the absence of active bleeding, DIC, or congestive heart failure. Blood products leukodepleted by filtration should be used to avert or delay alloimmunization as well as febrile reactions. Blood products should also be irradiated to prevent graft-versus-host disease (GVHD). Cytomegalovirus (CMV)-negative blood products should be used for CMV-seronegative patients who are potential candidates for allogeneic SCT. Leukodepleted products are also effective for these patients if CMV-negative products are not available.

Infectious complications remain the major cause of morbidity and death during induction and postremission chemotherapy for AML. Prophylactic administration of antibiotics in the absence of fever is controversial. Oral nystatin or clotrimazole is recommended to prevent localized candidiasis. For patients who are herpes simplex virus antibody titer–positive, acyclovir prophylaxis is effective in preventing reactivation of latent oral herpes infections.

Fever develops in most patients with AML, but infections are documented in only half of febrile patients. Early initiation of empirical broad-spectrum antibacterial and antifungal antibiotics has significantly reduced the number of patients dying of infectious complications (Chap. 72). An antibiotic regimen adequate to treat gram-negative and gram-positive organisms should be instituted at the onset of fever in a granulocytopenic patient after clinical evaluation, including a detailed physical examination with inspection of the indwelling catheter exit site and a perirectal examination, as well as procurement of cultures and radiographs aimed at documenting the source of fever. Specific antibiotic regimens should be based on antibiotic sensitivity data obtained from the institution at which the patient is being treated. Acceptable regimens include imipenem-cilastin; an antipseudomonal semisynthetic penicillin (e.g., piperacillin) combined with an aminoglycoside; a third-generation cephalosporin with antipseudomonal activity (i.e., ceftazidime or cefepime); or double β-lactam combinations (ceftazidime and piperacillin). Aminoglycosides should be avoided if possible in patients with renal insufficiency. For patients with known immediate-type hypersensitivity reactions to penicillin, aztreonam may be substituted for β-lactams. Aztreonam should be combined with an aminoglycoside or a quinolone antibiotic rather than used alone.

Empirical vancomycin is not given initially in the absence of suspected gram-positive infection or mucositis but should be initiated in neutropenic patients who remain febrile for 3 days; empirical systemic antifungal therapy is added at 7 days if fever persists. While amphotericin B has been used in the past for this, itraconazole and voriconazole have been shown to be equivalent in efficacy and less toxic. Our approach is therefore to use either itraconazole or voriconazole. Liposomal amphotericin, which has also been demonstrated to be equivalent to regular amphotericin and to have less renal toxicity, is utilized when this treatment approach fails. Antibacterial and antifungal antibiotics should be continued until patients are no longer neutropenic, regardless of whether a specific source has been found for the fever.

Treatment of Promyelocytic Leukemia   Tretinoin is an oral drug that induces the differentiation of leukemic cells bearing the t(15;17); it is not effective in other forms of AML. APL is responsive to cytarabine and daunorubicin, but about 10% of patients treated with these drugs die from DIC induced by the release of granule components by dying tumor cells. Tretinoin does not produce DIC but produces another complication called the *retinoic acid syndrome*. Occurring within the first 3 weeks of treatment, it is characterized by fever, dyspnea, chest pain, pulmonary infiltrates, pleural and pericardial effusions, and hypoxia. The syndrome is related to adhesion of differentiated neoplastic cells to the pulmonary vasculature endothelium. Glucocorticoids, chemotherapy, and/or supportive measures can be effective. The mortality of this syndrome is about 10%.

Tretinoin (45 mg/m^2 per day orally until remission is documented) plus concurrent anthracycline chemotherapy appears to be the safest and most effective treatment for APL. Unlike patients with other types of AML, patients with this subtype benefit from maintenance therapy with either tretinoin or chemotherapy. The optimal regimen is being sought in clinical studies.

Arsenic trioxide produces meaningful responses in up to 85% of patients refractory to tretinoin. The use of arsenic trioxide is being explored as part of initial treatment in clinical trials of APL.

The detection of minimal residual disease by RT-PCR amplification of the t(15;17) chimeric gene product appears to predict relapse. Disappearance of the signal is associated with long-term disease-free survival; its persistence predicts relapse. With increases in the sensitivity of the assay, some patients with persistent abnormal gene product have been found who do not suffer a relapse. Studies are underway to determine whether there is a critical threshold level of transcripts that predicts for leukemia relapse.

Postremission Therapy   Induction of a durable first CR is critical to long-term disease-free survival in AML. However, without further therapy virtually all patients experience relapse. Once relapse has occurred, AML is generally curable only by SCT.

Postremission therapy is designed to eradicate any residual leukemic cells; therefore, it should prevent relapse and prolong survival. Approaches to postremission therapy in AML are often based upon age (<55 to 65 and >55 to 65). For younger patients, most studies include intensive chemotherapy and allogeneic or autologous SCT. High-dose cytarabine is more effective than standard-dose cytarabine. The Cancer and Leukemia Group B (CALGB), for example, compared the duration of CR in patients randomly assigned postremission to four cycles of high (3 g/m^2, every 12 h on days 1, 3, and 5), intermediate (400 mg/m^2 for 5 days by continuous infusion), or standard (100 mg/m^2 per day for 5 days by continuous infusion) doses of cytarabine. A

dose-response effect for cytarabine in patients with AML who were ≤60 years was demonstrated. High-dose cytarabine significantly prolonged CR and increased the fraction cured in patients with favorable [t(8;21) and inv(16)] and normal cytogenetics, but it had no significant effect on patients with other abnormal karyotypes. For older patients, exploration of attenuated intensive therapy that includes either chemotherapy or nonmyeloablative allogeneic SCT has been pursued. In addition, early introduction of new agents (Table 96-3) is often pursued.

Allogeneic and autologous SCT in first CR have been studied extensively in younger patients with no major organ dysfunction. Allogeneic SCT is used in patients <65 to 70 years with an HLA-compatible donor. Relapse with this therapy occurs in only a small fraction of patients, but toxicity is relatively high from treatment; complications include venoocclusive disease, GVHD, and infections. Autologous transplantation can be administered in young and older patients and uses the same preparative regimens. Patients subsequently receive their own stem cells collected while in remission. The toxicity is lower with autologous SCT (5% mortality rate), but the relapse rate is higher than with allogeneic SCT. The increased relapse rate is due to the absence of the graft-vs-leukemia (GVL) effect seen with allogeneic SCT and possible contamination of the autologous stem cells with tumor cells. Purging the autologous stem cells does not lower the relapse rate with autologous SCT.

Randomized trials comparing intensive therapy and autologous and allogeneic SCT have shown improved duration of remission with allogeneic SCT compared to autologous SCT or chemotherapy alone. However, overall survival is generally not different; the improved disease control with allogeneic SCT is erased by the increase in fatal toxicity. While stem cells were previously harvested from the bone marrow, virtually all efforts currently collect these from the peripheral blood following mobilization regimens including growth factors with or without chemotherapy. Prognostic factors may help select patients in first CR for whom transplant is most effective.

Our approach includes strong consideration for allogeneic SCT in first CR for patients with high-risk karyotypes. Patients with normal karyotypes who have other poor risk factors (antecedent hematologic disorder, failure to attain remission with a single induction course, hyperleukocytosis, PTD of the *MLL* gene, and *FLT3* abnormalities) are also potential candidates. If a suitable HLA donor does not exist, autologous SCT or novel therapeutic approaches are considered. Other novel transplant strategies including nonmyeloblative SCT are being actively explored for consolidation of high-risk AML patients. Patients with t(8;21) and inv(16) are treated with repetitive doses of high-dose

TABLE 96-3   *Selected New Agents Under Study for Treatment of Adults with AML*

Class of Drugs	Example Agent(s)
MDR1 modulator	Cyclosporine analogues, PSC-833
Demethylating agent	Decitabine, 5-azacytidine
Histone deacetylase inhibitor	Depsipeptide, suberoylanilide hydroxamic acid (SAHA), MS275, Valproic Acid
Heavy metals	Arsenic trioxide, antimony
Farnesyl transferase inhibitors	R115777, SCH66336
FLT3 inhibitors	SU11248, PKC412, MLN518
HSP-90 antagonists	17-Allylaminogeldanamycin (17-AAG)
BCR/ABL PDGFR/c-*kit* inhibitor	Imatinib (ST1571, Gleevec)
Protein kinase C inhibitor	Bryostatin, UCN-01, CGP41251
Cell cycle inhibitor	Flavopiridol
Humanized antibodies	Anti-CD33 (HuM195), Hu1D10 (β-chain, HLA-DR)
Toxin-conjugated antibodies	Gemtuzumab ozogamicin (Mylotarg)
Radiolabeled antibodies	Yttrium-90-labeled human M195
Cytokines	Recombinant human interleukin (IL) 2 and IL-12
Anticytokines	Antivascular endothelial growth factor (Avastin)

cytarabine, which offers a high frequency of cure without the morbidity of transplant.

Relapse   Once relapse occurs after the standard induction and postremission chemotherapy approach described above and outlined in Fig. 96-1, patients are rarely cured with further standard-dose chemotherapy. Patients eligible for allogeneic SCT should receive transplants expeditiously at the first sign of relapse. Long-term disease-free survival is approximately the same (30 to 50%) with allogeneic SCT in first relapse or in second remission. Chemotherapy is administered prior to allogeneic transplant if the AML is rapidly progressing. Autologous SCT rescues about 20% of relapsed patients with AML who have chemosensitive disease. The most important factors predicting response at relapse are the length of the previous CR, whether initial CR was achieved with one or two courses of chemotherapy, and the type of postremission therapy. Because of the poor outcome of patients in early (<12 months) first relapse, it is justified (for patients without HLA-compatible donors) to explore innovative approaches, such as new drugs or immunotherapies (Table 96-3). Patients with longer (>12 months) first CR generally relapse with drug-sensitive disease and have a higher chance of attaining a CR. However, cure for these patients is uncommon, and treatment with novel approaches should be considered if SCT is not possible. New agents (Table 96-3) that may have clinical activity in AML are needed.

For elderly patients (age >60) for whom clinical trials are not available, gemtuzumab ozogamicin (Mylotarg) is another alternative. This therapy is an antibody-targeted chemotherapy consisting of the humanized anti-CD33 antibody linked to calicheamicin, a potent antitumor antibiotic. The CR rate in response to this therapy is ~30%. The effectiveness of this agent in early relapsing (<6 months) or refractory AML patients is limited, possibly due to calicheamicin being a potent Mdr1 substrate. Toxicity, including myelosuppression, infusion toxicity, and venoocclusive disease, can be observed with gemtuzumab ozogamicin. Currently, studies are examining the efficacy of this treatment in combination with chemotherapy for both young and older patients with previously untreated AML.

CHRONIC MYELOGENOUS LEUKEMIA

INCIDENCE   The incidence of chronic myelogenous leukemia (CML) is 1.5 per 100,000 people per year, and the age-adjusted incidence is higher in men than in women (2.0 versus 1.2). The incidence of CML increases slowly with age until the middle forties, when it starts to rise rapidly. CML incidence decreased slightly between 1973 and 1999 (1.9 versus 1.5).

DEFINITION   The diagnosis of CML is established by identifying a clonal expansion of a hematopoietic stem cell possessing a reciprocal translocation between chromosomes 9 and 22. This translocation results in the head-to-tail fusion of the breakpoint cluster region (*BCR*) gene on chromosome 22q11 with the *ABL* (named after the abelson murine leukemia virus) gene located on chromosome 9q34. Untreated, the disease is characterized by the inevitable transition from a chronic phase to an accelerated phase and on to blast crisis.

ETIOLOGY   No clear correlation with exposure to cytotoxic drugs, such as alkylating agents, has been found, and there is no direct evidence of a viral etiology. Cigarette smoking has been shown to accelerate the progression to blast crisis and therefore has an adverse effect on survival in CML. The effect of radiation was demonstrated in a study of the atomic bomb survivors, where it has been estimated that the development of a CML cell mass of $10,000/\mu l$ takes 6.3 years. No increase in CML incidence was found in the survivors of the Chernobyl accident, suggesting that only large doses of radiation can induce CML.

PATHOPHYSIOLOGY   The product of the fusion gene resulting from the t(9;22) plays a central role in the development of CML. This chimeric gene is transcribed into a hybrid *BCR/ABL* mRNA in which exon 1 of *ABL* is replaced by variable numbers of 5′ *BCR* exons. Bcr/Abl fusion proteins, p210$^{BCR/ABL}$, are produced that contain NH$_2$-terminal domains

of Bcr and the COOH-terminal domains of Abl. A rare breakpoint, occurring within the 3′ region of the *BCR* gene, yields a fusion protein of 230 kDa, p230$^{BCR/ABL}$. Bcr/Abl fusion proteins can transform hematopoietic progenitor cells *in vitro*. Furthermore, reconstituting lethally irradiated mice with bone marrow cells infected with retrovirus carrying the gene encoding the p210$^{BCR/ABL}$ leads to the development of a myeloproliferative syndrome resembling CML in 50% of the mice. Specific antisense oligomers to the *BCR/ABL* junction inhibit the growth of t(9;22)-positive leukemic cells without affecting normal colony formation.

The mechanism(s) by which p210$^{BCR/ABL}$ promotes the transition from the benign state to the fully malignant one is still unclear. Messenger RNA for *BCR/ABL* can occasionally be detected in normal individuals. However, attachment of the *BCR* sequences to *ABL* results in three critical functional changes: (1) the Abl protein becomes constitutively active as a tyrosine kinase enzyme, subsequently activating downstream kinases that prevent apoptosis; (2) the DNA-protein-binding activity of Abl is attenuated; and (3) the binding of Abl to cytoskeletal actin microfilaments is enhanced.

Disease Progression   The events associated with transition to the acute phase are poorly understood. Chromosomal instability of the malignant clone, resulting, for example, in the acquisition of an additional t(9;22), trisomy 8, or 17p- (p53 loss), is a fundamental characteristic of CML. Acquisition of these additional genetic and/or molecular abnormalities is critical to the phenotypic transformation. Large deletions adjacent to the translocation breakpoint on the derivative 9 chromosome, detected by microsatellite polymerase chain reaction (PCR) or FISH, are associated with shorter survival time. Heterogeneous structural alterations of the p53 gene, as well as structural alterations and lack of protein production of the retinoblastoma gene, have been associated with disease progression in a subset of patients. Rare patients show alterations in *RAS*. Sporadic reports also document the presence of an altered *MYC* (named after the myelocytomatosis virus) gene. Progressive de novo DNA methylation at the *BCR/ABL* locus has also been shown to herald blastic transformation. Finally, interleukin (IL)-1β may be involved in the progression of CML to the blastic phase. Multiple pathways to disease transformation exist, but the exact timing and relevance of each remain unclear.

CLINICAL PRESENTATION ■ **Symptoms**   The clinical onset of the chronic phase is generally insidious. Accordingly, some patients are diagnosed while still asymptomatic, during health screening tests; other patients present with fatigue, malaise, and weight loss or have symptoms resulting from splenic enlargement, such as early satiety and left upper quadrant pain or mass. Less common are features related to granulocyte or platelet dysfunction, such as infections, thrombosis, or bleeding. Occasionally, patients present with leukostatic manifestations due to severe leukocytosis or thrombosis such as vasoocclusive disease, cerebrovascular accidents, myocardial infarction, venous thrombosis, priapism, visual disturbances, and pulmonary insufficiency. Patients with p230$^{BCR/ABL}$-positive CML have a more indolent course.

Progression of CML is associated with worsening symptoms. Unexplained fever, significant weight loss, increasing dose requirement of the drugs controlling the disease, bone and joint pain, bleeding, thrombosis, and infections suggest transformation into accelerated or blastic phases. Fewer than 10 to 15% of newly diagnosed patients present with accelerated disease or with de novo blastic phase CML.

Physical Findings   In most patients the abnormal finding on physical examination at diagnosis is minimal to moderate splenomegaly; mild hepatomegaly is found occasionally. Persistent splenomegaly despite continued therapy is a sign of disease acceleration. Lymphadenopathy and myeloid sarcomas are unusual except late in the course of the disease; when they are present, the prognosis is poor.

Hematologic Findings   Elevated white blood cell counts, with various degrees of immaturity of the granulocytic series, are present at diagnosis. Usually <5% circulating blasts and <10% blasts and promyelocytes are noted. Cycling of the counts may be observed in patients followed without treatment. Platelet counts are almost always elevated at diagnosis, and a mild degree of normochromic normocytic anemia is present. Leukocyte alkaline phosphatase is characteristically low in CML cells. Serum levels of vitamin B_{12} and vitamin B_{12}–binding proteins are generally elevated. Phagocytic functions are usually normal at diagnosis and remain normal during the chronic phase. Histamine production secondary to basophilia is increased in later stages, causing pruritus, diarrhea, and flushing.

At diagnosis, bone marrow cellularity, primarily of the myeloid and megakaryocytic lineages, with a greatly altered myeloid to erythroid ratio, is increased in almost all patients with CML. The marrow blast percentage is generally normal or slightly elevated. Marrow or blood basophilia, eosinophilia, and monocytosis may be present. While collagen fibrosis in the marrow is unusual at presentation, significant degrees of reticulin stain–measured fibrosis are noted in about half of the patients.

Disease acceleration is defined by the development of increasing degrees of anemia unaccounted for by bleeding or chemotherapy; cytogenetic clonal evolution; or blood or marrow blasts between 10 and 20%, blood or marrow basophils ≥20%, or platelet count <100,000/μl. *Blast crisis* is defined as acute leukemia, with blood or marrow blasts ≥ 20%. Hyposegmented neutrophils may appear (Pelger-Huet anomaly). Blast cells can be classified as myeloid, lymphoid, erythroid, or undifferentiated, based on morphologic, cytochemical, and immunologic features. About half the cases are myeloid, one-third lymphoid, 10% erythroid, and the rest are undifferentiated.

Chromosomal Findings The cytogenetic hallmark of CML, found in 90 to 95% of patients, is the t(9;22)(q34;q11.2). Originally, this was recognized by the presence of a shortened chromosome 22 (22q-), designated as the *Philadelphia chromosome*, that arises from the reciprocal 9;22 translocation. Some patients may have complex translocations (designated as *variant translocations*) involving three, four, or five chromosomes (usually including chromosomes 9 and 22). However, the molecular consequences of these changes appear similar to those resulting from the typical t(9;22). All patients should have evidence of the translocation either by cytogenetics, FISH, or molecularly to make a diagnosis of CML.

PROGNOSTIC FACTORS The clinical outcome of patients with CML is variable. Before imatinib mesylate, death was expected in 10% of patients within 2 years and in about 20% yearly thereafter and the median survival time was ~4 years. Therefore, several prognostic models that identify different risk groups in CML have been developed. The most commonly used staging systems have been derived from multivariate analyses of prognostic factors. The *Sokal index* identified percentage of circulating blasts, spleen size, platelet count, cytogenetic clonal evolution, and age as the most important prognostic indicators. This system was based on chemotherapy-treated patients. The *Hasford system* was developed on interferon α-treated patients. It identified age, spleen size, percentage of circulating blasts, platelet count, and percentage of eosinophils and basophils as the most important prognostic indicators. This system differs from the Sokal index by ignoring clonal evolution and incorporating percentage of eosinophils and basophils. When applied to a data set of 272 patients treated with interferon α (IFN-α), the Hasford system was more potent than the Sokal score for predicting survival time; it identified more low-risk patients but left only a small number of cases in the high-risk group. The Hasford system has not yet been validated in patients undergoing transplantation. However, preliminary results suggest that it is applicable to imatinib-treated patients.

℞ TREATMENT

The therapy of CML is rapidly undergoing evolution because we have a curative treatment (allogeneic transplantation) that has significant

TABLE 96-4 *Response Criteria in CML*

Hematologic	
Complete response[a]	White blood cell count <10,000/μl, normal morphology
	Normal hemoglobin and platelet counts
Incomplete response	White blood cell count ≥ 10,000/μl
Cytogenetic	Percentage of bone marrow metaphases with t(9;22)
Complete response	0
Partial response	≤35
Minor response	36–85[b]
No response	85–100
Molecular	Presence of *BCR/ABL* transcript by RT-PCR
Complete response	None
Incomplete response	Any

[a] Complete hematologic response requires the disappearance of splenomegaly.
[b] Up to 15% normal metaphases are occasionally seen at diagnosis (when 30 metaphases are analyzed).
Note: RT-PCR, reverse transcriptase polymerase chain reaction.

toxicity and a new targeted treatment (imatinib) without long-term follow-up data. Therefore, physician experience and patient preference must be factored into the treatment selection process. Discussion of both treatment options with a patient is indicated. The decision should focus on the outcomes, risks, and toxicities of the various approaches. Some centers would employ allogeneic SCT in patients <30 years, as the risk of transplant-related toxicity is minimal in that population.

At present, the goal of therapy in CML is to achieve prolonged, durable, nonneoplastic, nonclonal hematopoiesis, which entails the eradication of any residual cells containing the *BCR/ABL* transcript. Hence the goal is complete molecular remission and cure (Table 96-4). A proposed treatment plan for the newly diagnosed patient with CML is presented in Fig. 96-2.

Allogeneic SCT Allogeneic SCT is currently the only curative therapy for CML and, when feasible, is the treatment of choice. However, it is complicated by a high early-mortality rate owing to the transplant procedure. Outcome of SCT depends on multiple factors including: (1) the patient (e.g., age and phase of disease); (2) the type of donor [e.g., syngeneic (monozygotic twins) or HLA-compatible allogeneic, related or unrelated]; (3) the preparative regimen; (4) GVHD; and (5) posttransplantation treatment.

THE PATIENT As experience has been gained and safety and efficacy have been established, it has become clear that patients should have acceptable end-organ function, be <65 to 70 years, and have a healthy

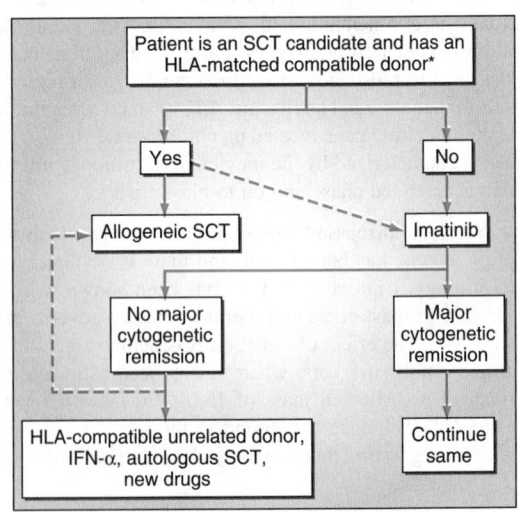

FIGURE 96-2 Flow chart for the therapy of newly diagnosed CML. Patients with an HLA-compatible donor have the possibility to undergo allogeneic stem cell transplant (SCT) as initial therapy or treatment with imatinib. The asterisk denotes that some centers employ allogeneic SCT only if imatinib fails to induce a response. Broken lines denote lack of long-term survival data. IFN, interferon.

and histocompatible donor. Furthermore, survival after SCT in the accelerated and blastic phases of the disease is significantly diminished and is associated with a very high rate of relapse. The Seattle pre-imatinib data demonstrate that bone marrow transplantation (BMT) early in the chronic phase (1 to 2 years from diagnosis) is superior to later BMT.

THE DONOR Transplantation from a family donor, who is either fully matched or mismatched at only one HLA locus, should be considered the only curative therapy for any patient with CML who is a candidate for an HLA-related sibling transplant. Syngeneic BMT in patients with chronic phase CML has been reported from the Seattle group to result in 7-year disease-free survival in 55% of the patients, with a 30% relapse rate. With HLA-identical sibling BMT in the chronic phase, many groups have reported 5-year disease-free survival in 40 to 70% of patients, with a 25% relapse rate. BMT from an HLA-matched unrelated donor in chronic phase <1 year from diagnosis and <30 years resulted in similar 5-year disease-free survival as matched sibling donor transplantation. For all other groups, patients receiving transplants from unrelated individuals have higher rates of graft failure and acute and chronic GVHD and prolonged convalescence after treatment, compared to those who receive allogeneic transplants from related individuals. Peripheral blood is now being studied as a source of hematopoietic progenitor cells; it may offer rapid engraftment and less risk for the donor. With unrelated donors, some studies demonstrated no difference in GVHD and improved disease-free survival when comparing peripheral blood to bone marrow stem cells. No such data are available using matched sibling donors to date. At the current time, some centers collect bone marrow and some peripheral blood from sibling donors for newly diagnosed CML patients. Umbilical-cord blood may permit mismatched SCT with notably less GVHD; GVL effects do not appear to be impaired. A problem with cord blood is obtaining a sufficient number of progenitor cells to reconstitute hematopoiesis in an adult.

PREPARATIVE REGIMENS These regimens have been studied by several groups. A randomized study by the Seattle group compared cyclophosphamide and total-body irradiation with busulphan and cyclophosphamide. They found no significant differences in the 3-year probabilities of survival, relapse, event-free survival, speed of engraftment, or incidence of venoocclusive disease of the liver. Significantly more patients in the total-body irradiation arm experienced major elevations of creatinine, acute GVHD, longer periods of fever, positive blood cultures, hospital admissions, and longer inpatient hospital stays. However, increased chronic GVHD, obstructive bronchiolitis, and alopecia were noted with busulphan. Measurement of busulphan levels revealed no significant association between busulphan levels and regimen-related toxicity, but low levels were associated with an increased risk of relapse. Intravenous busulphan allows better control of serum levels. We tend to favor the use of busulphan and cyclophosphamide. Nonmyeloblative transplants in which the preparative regimen is aimed at eliminating host lymphocytes rather than bone marrow are being tested. Reduced toxicity with preserved antitumor efficacy is the goal.

DEVELOPMENT AND TYPE OF GVHD Development of grade I GVHD, as compared to no GVHD, decreases the risk of relapse. A lower relapse rate was observed also in patients with grade II GVHD but was accompanied by a substantially higher transplant-related mortality rate. The decreased relapse rate may be caused by a GVL effect. Depletion of T lymphocytes from donor marrow can prevent GVHD but results in an increased risk of relapse, which exceeds the relapse rate after syngeneic SCT. Thus, T lymphocytes from the donor marrow mediate a significant antileukemic, or GVL, effect, and even syngeneic marrow may exhibit limited GVL activity in CML.

POSTTRANSPLANTATION TREATMENT Further support for the existence of an immunologically mediated GVL effect came from the observation that donor leukocyte infusions (without any preparative chemotherapy or

GVHD prophylaxis) can induce hematologic and cytogenetic remissions in patients with CML who have relapsed after allogeneic SCT.

Imatinib's effect in the chronic phase of the disease prompted its study in patients who relapse after allogeneic SCT. Studies with small numbers of patients have proved that imatinib can control CML that has recurred after allogeneic SCT but is associated with myelosuppression and recurrence of severe GVHD. Imatinib studies after allogeneic SCT to prevent relapse in patients with advanced disease at the time of transplantation (patients at high risk for relapse) or patients undergoing non-myeloblative transplants are under way.

The activity of IFN-α in patients with early chronic-phase CML was the basis for the use of IFN-α after SCT, either to induce cytogenetic remissions in relapsed patients or to prevent relapse after SCT for high-risk patients. The main concern about IFN-α use after allogeneic SCT has been the development or worsening of GVHD, because IFN-α acts as an immunomodulator. IFN-α has also been combined with mononuclear cells obtained from donor blood to induce cytogenetic remissions in relapsed patients. Cytogenetic remissions have been achieved, but the exact role of IFN-α as opposed to the mononuclear cells is unclear.

Imatinib Mesylate Imatinib mesylate (Gleevec, STI571) functions through competitive inhibition at the adenosine triphosphate (ATP) binding site of the Abl kinase, which leads to inhibition of tyrosine phosphorylation of proteins involved in Bcr/Abl signal transduction. It shows a high degree of specificity for Bcr/Abl, the receptor for platelet-derived growth factor, and c-*kit* tyrosine kinases. Imatinib induces apoptosis in cells expressing Bcr/Abl. Based on its antileukemic activity in vitro it was tested in clinical trials.

Most patients with CML in chronic phase have a rapid hematologic response to imatinib therapy. In the initial studies with imatinib in patients with chronic-phase CML who were intolerant to IFN-α, 95% of patients achieved complete hematologic remission, and 60% achieved major cytogenetic remission, with a complete cytogenetic remission rate of 41%. Those who did not achieve at least a major cytogenetic remission following 3 months of therapy had a higher risk of disease progression to the accelerated/blastic phases of the disease. Patients in the accelerated/blastic phases of the disease are less sensitive to imatinib, and the treatment outcome is less favorable. In newly diagnosed CML, a recent randomized phase III study of imatinib (400 mg/d) versus IFN-α and cytarabine revealed the complete hematologic remission rate, at 18 months, of patients treated with imatinib to be 97% as compared to 69% in patients treated with IFN-α and cytarabine. Similarly, the complete cytogenetic remission rate was 76% in patients treated with imatinib as compared to 14% in patients treated with IFN-α and cytarabine. Progression to accelerated/blastic phases of the disease was noted in 3% of patients treated with imatinib as compared to 8.5% of patients treated with IFN-α and cytarabine. These results led to rapid Food and Drug Administration approval of imatinib for all stages of CML.

Imatinib is administered orally and has an acceptable toxicity profile. The main side effects are fluid retention, nausea, muscle cramps, diarrhea, and skin rashes. The management of these side effects is usually supportive. Myelosuppression is the most common hematologic side effect, and patients who received busulphan are at a greater risk than patients who were treated with IFN-α. It seems to result from the eradication of the malignant clone and delayed recovery of the normal nonclonal progenitor cells. Blood and platelet support should be provided, and therefore dose reduction is rarely recommended in the absence of infection. Doses <300 mg/d seem ineffective and may lead to development of resistance.

Four mechanisms of resistance to imatinib have been described to date. These are (1) gene amplification, (2) mutations at the kinase site, (3) enhanced expression of multidrug exporter proteins, and (4) alternative signaling pathways functionally compensating for the imatinib-sensitive mechanisms. The unfavorable prognosis associated with imatinib-resistance was shown in the accelerated and blast crisis phases of the disease. Specifically, patients who do not achieve major cytogenetic remission within 3 months of initiation of imatinib have shorter survival than patients who achieve that level of remission. Therefore, all four mechanisms are being targeted in clinical trials.

The encouraging results with imatinib have led many clinicians to offer it as a first-line therapy for newly diagnosed CML patients, including those who otherwise would have benefited from transplant (e.g., young patients with a sibling matched donor). This may be unwise since the clinical studies so far have very short follow-up, thus limiting knowledge regarding the curative potential of imatinib. Delaying transplantation until after development of imatinib resistance may worsen outcome.

Interferons When allogeneic SCT is not feasible, IFN-α therapy used to be the treatment of choice before imatinib became available. Only longer follow-up of patients treated with imatinib will prove whether IFN-α will still have a role in the treatment of CML. The interferons are a complex group of naturally occurring proteins produced by eukaryotic cells in response to viruses, antigens, and mitogens. Three distinct groups of IFN species have been identified: IFN-α, -β and -γ. Although various interferons have become available for clinical investigation, most data have been generated with IFN-α preparations.

Interferons have potent, pleiotropic biologic effects, spanning a spectrum of antiviral, microbicidal, immunomodulatory, and antiproliferative properties. While interferons downregulate the expression of several oncogenes and cytokines, they also upregulate the expression of IFN regulatory factor-1 (a transcriptional activator with antioncogenic activity), adhesion molecules, and the histocompatibility genes. Interferons also inhibit angiogenesis and induce a cellular immune response. However, the mode(s) of action in CML is still unknown.

In randomized studies comparing IFN-α and chemotherapy, patients treated with IFN-α survived longer than patients treated with hydroxyurea or busulphan. The 5-year survival rate was 51% with IFN-α and 42% with chemotherapy. Of note, achieving complete cytogenetic or molecular response after IFN-α therapy is associated with a 10-year survival rate as high as 78%.

Patients develop both acute and chronic side effects from IFN-α therapy. Acute side effects (flulike symptoms) appear early in the course of the treatment. Most flulike symptoms respond to acetaminophen, and tachyphylaxis develops within 1 to 2 weeks. Chronic reactions, such as fatigue and lethargy, depression, weight loss, myalgias, and arthralgias, occur in about half of the patients and often require dose reduction. Patients also report cough, postnasal drip, and dryness of the skin. Infrequently, immune-mediated thrombocytopenia and anemia develop. In addition, long-term therapy has been associated with late autoimmune side effects, such as hypothyroidism and occasionally generalized autoimmune phenomena.

The most important persistent side effects in patients with CML who are treated with IFN-α are neurologic. All patients treated with IFN-α are subject to some neurologic toxicity, the most common symptom being lethargy. Up to 20% of patients have neurologic side effects that are associated with compromised quality of life and reduced ability to carry out their regular activity, such as full-time work. In addition, at the required doses, impotence in men is not infrequent. The combination of IFN-α with cytarabine has produced better results in one study but not in another.

Chemotherapy Innovative approaches are still important in CML; the exact role of imatinib in the armamentarium of CML remains undefined. Initial management of patients with chemotherapy is currently reserved for rapid lowering of white blood cell counts, reduction of symptoms, and reversal of symptomatic splenomegaly. Hydroxyurea, a ribonucleotide reductase inhibitor, induces rapid disease control. The initial dose is 1 to 4 g/d; the dose should be halved with each 50% reduction of the leukocyte count. Unfortunately, cytogenetic remissions with hydroxyurea are uncommon. Busulphan, an alkylating

agent that acts on early progenitor cells, has a more prolonged effect. However, we do not recommend its use because of its serious side effects, which include unexpected, and occasionally fatal, myelosuppression in 5 to 10% of patients; pulmonary, endocardial, and marrow fibrosis; and an Addison-like wasting syndrome.

Homoharringtonine (HHT) is a plant alkaloid derived from a tree, *Cephalotaxus fortuneii* sp. *harringtonii*. HHT blocks peptide bond formation after binding of the aminoacyl-transfer RNA to the ribosome. In patients whose disease progressed during treatment with IFN-α or who were in later chronic phase (>1 year from diagnosis), HHT induced 72% complete hematologic responses and 15% major cytogenetic responses. The use of HHT before IFN-α in early chronic phase resulted in a 92% complete hematologic response rate and a 27% major cytogenetic response rate. Toxicity is mainly related to myelosuppression. In vitro synergism between HHT and imatinib have led to the development of combination trials.

Arsenic trioxide gained recognition as a therapeutic agent following reports from China of a high incidence of favorable hematologic responses in patients with APL. The mechanism(s) of action of arsenic trioxide in non-APL leukemias is unknown. Initial studies of arsenic trioxide in Bcr/Abl-expressing cell lines demonstrated downregulation of Bcr/Abl expression as well as activation of apoptosis. More recent studies have demonstrated an initial effect of arsenic trioxide on Bcr/Abl expression prior to activation of the apoptotic pathway. In vitro synergism between arsenic trioxide and imatinib have led to the clinical investigation of this combination.

Intensive combination chemotherapy has also been used in chronic-phase CML, with 30 to 50% of patients achieving complete cytogenetic responses. However, these cytogenetic remissions have been short-lived. Consequently, intensive combination chemotherapy regimens are being used today only to mobilize normal progenitors in the blood in order to collect circulating stem cells for autologous transplantation.

Autologous SCT Autologous SCT could potentially cure CML if a means to select the residual normal progenitors, which coexist with their malignant counterparts, could be developed. As a source of autologous hematopoietic stem cells for transplantation, blood offers certain advantages over marrow (e.g., faster engraftment for the patient and no general anesthesia for the donor). Normal hematopoietic stem cells appear with increased frequency in the blood of patients with CML during the recovery phase after chemotherapy and G-CSF. A role for imatinib before stem cell collection to achieve minimal residual disease and following transplantation to maintain this status is currently being investigated. However, only a few cases have been reported to successfully engraft following imatinib therapy. Therefore such approaches should be performed only in clinical trials.

Leukapheresis and Splenectomy Intensive leukapheresis may control the blood counts in chronic-phase CML; however, it is expensive and cumbersome. It is useful in emergencies where leukostasis-related complications such as pulmonary failure or cerebrovascular accidents are likely. It may also have a role in the treatment of pregnant women in whom it is important to avoid potentially teratogenic drugs.

Splenectomy was used in CML in the past because of the suggestion that evolution to the acute phase might occur in the spleen. However, this does not appear to be the case, and splenectomy is now reserved for symptomatic relief of painful splenomegaly unresponsive to chemotherapy or for significant anemia or thrombocytopenia associated with hypersplenism. Splenic radiation is used rarely to reduce the size of the spleen.

Minimal Residual Disease After allogeneic SCT, RT-PCR analysis may be positive for residual disease during the first 6 months in patients who subsequently achieve a long-lasting remission. However, late persistence of RT-PCR positivity appears to indicate a reduced probability of cure. RT-PCR positivity at any single time point is not predictive of imminent relapse. After allogeneic SCT, patients are often divided according to RT-PCR results into one of three groups: (1) persistently positive, (2) intermittently negative, and (3) persistently negative.

These three groups have low, intermediate, and high probability of maintaining remission and disease free-survival, respectively. Although these data suggest that patients who are persistently RT-PCR positive >6 months after allogeneic SCT need additional therapeutic interventions, this conclusion has not been rigorously established. The studies have used an assortment of techniques for measuring minimal residual disease, the level of sensitivity has been variable, and the follow-up durations of patients are short. Quantitative PCR may provide a more sensitive tool to predict relapse in CML. In patients who do not have any evidence for GVHD and are intermittently RT-PCR negative, GVL may be induced by alloreactive donor cells (without the side effects of GVHD) to suppress the proliferation of the leukemic cells. Another approach may be the use of imatinib to eradicate minimal residual disease.

Following imatinib therapy, only a minority (5 to 10%) of the patients develop molecular remission. Extrapolating from the SCT data, most patients without molecular remission are at risk of relapse. However, patients with AML with t(8;21) who are in long-term remission have persistent multipotent progenitor cells expressing *AML1/ETO* transcripts. Therefore it is unclear whether indeed achieving durable molecular remission should still be the goal of treatment in this disease. Until this issue is sorted out, approaches have been developed to try and improve the current results. Based on improved outcome with higher doses of imatinib in patients with the advanced stages of the disease, trials have been initiated that compare 400 mg to 800 mg of imatinib in newly diagnosed patients. Similarly, combination regimens have been developed; based on the effect of IFN-α in the chronic phase of the disease, imatinib with IFN-α or with its long-acting (pegylated) member are being studied. Likewise, based on the combined effect of cytarabine and IFN-α, a regimen of imatinib and cytarabine is being evaluated. The results from these trials are premature at this point. However, they will most probably lead to a randomized trial of imatinib versus imatinib with IFN-α versus imatinib with cytarabine.

After IFN-α therapy, residual disease was found in all samples tested from patients with complete cytogenetic remissions. More recent studies have demonstrated the eventual elimination of the *BCR/ABL* mRNA transcript after more prolonged IFN-α treatment in some cases.

Future Directions   Abrogation of DNA methylation with 5-aza-2′deoxycytidine (decitabine) has shown clinical activity in the advanced stages of the disease. Inhibition of *Ras* with a farnesyl transferase inhibitor that blocks its insertion into the membrane may have antitumor activity in CML on the basis of early clinical trials. Preclinical efforts to use Bcr/Abl peptides as a tumor vaccine appear promising. The use of *BCR/ABL* antisense oligonucleotides to purge residual leukemic cells from autologous hematopoietic progenitors before reinfusion, as well as new approaches to induce GVL in the setting of minimal residual disease without inducing GVHD, are under way. All these agents and others are being or will be studied in combination with imatinib. Further, treatment with the histone deacetylase inhibitor suberoylanilide hydroxamic acid (SAHA) was shown to enhance imatinib-induced apoptosis of Bcr/Abl-positive cell lines, and the heat-shock protein 90 antagonist 17-allylaminogeldanamycin (17-AAG) inhibited cell growth of cell lines containing mutations at the kinase site.

Treatment of Blast Crisis   The treatment for all forms of blast crisis is generally ineffective, including imatinib. Only 52% of patients treated with imatinib achieved hematologic remission (21% complete hematologic remission), and the median overall survival was 6.6 months. Patients who achieve complete hematologic remission or whose disease returns to a second chronic phase should be considered for allogeneic SCT. Other approaches include induction chemotherapy tailored to the phenotype of the blast cell followed by imatinib, with or without additional chemotherapy and SCT. Blast crisis following initial therapy with imatinib carries a dismal prognosis.

FURTHER READING

AML

KELLY LM, GILLILAND DG: Genetics of myeloid leukemias. Annu Rev Genomics Hum Genet 3:179, 2002

LOWENBERG B et al: Acute myeloid leukemia and acute promyelocytic leukemia. Hematology (Am Soc Hematol Educ Program):82, 2003

STONE RM: The difficult problem of acute myeloid leukemia in the older adult. CA Cancer J Clin 52:363, 2002

TALLMAN MS, NABHAN G: Management of acute promyelocytic leukemia. Curr Oncol Rep 4:381, 2002

CML

CORTES J, KANTARJIAN H: Advanced-phase chronic myeloid leukemia. Semin Hematol 40:79, 2003

DEININGER MW, DRUKER BJ: Specific targeted therapy of chronic myelogenous leukemia with imatinib. Pharmacol Rev 55:401, 2003

GOLDMAN JM, MELO JV: Chronic myeloid leukemia—advances in biology and new approaches to treatment. N Engl J Med 349:1451, 2003

97 | MALIGNANCIES OF LYMPHOID CELLS
James O. Armitage, Dan L. Longo

Malignancies of lymphoid cells range from the most indolent to the most aggressive human malignancies. These cancers arise from cells of the immune system at different stages of differentiation, resulting in a wide range of morphologic, immunologic, and clinical findings. Insights on the normal immune system have allowed a better understanding of these sometimes confusing disorders.

Some malignancies of lymphoid cells almost always present as leukemia (i.e., primary involvement of bone marrow and blood), while others almost always present as lymphomas (i.e., solid tumors of the immune system). However, other malignancies of lymphoid cells can present as either leukemia or lymphoma. In addition, the clinical pattern can change over the course of the illness. This change is more often seen in a patient who seems to have a lymphoma and then develops the manifestations of leukemia over the course of the illness.

BIOLOGY OF LYMPHOID MALIGNANCIES: CONCEPTS OF THE WHO CLASSIFICATION OF LYMPHOID MALIGNANCIES

The classification of lymphoid cancers evolved steadily throughout the twentieth century. The distinction between leukemia and lymphoma was made early, and separate classification systems were developed for each. Leukemias were first divided into acute and chronic subtypes based on average survival. Chronic leukemias were easily subdivided into those of lymphoid or myeloid origin based on morphologic characteristics. However, in recent years, a spectrum of diseases that were formerly all called chronic lymphoid leukemia has become apparent (Table 97-1). The acute leukemias were usually malignancies of blast cells with few identifying characteristics. When cytochemical stains became available, it was possible to divide these objectively into myeloid malignancies and acute leukemias of lymphoid cells. Acute leu-

TABLE 97-1 *Lymphoid Disorders That Can Present as "Chronic Leukemia" and Be Confused with Typical B Cell Chronic Lymphoid Leukemia*

Follicular lymphoma	Prolymphocytic leukemia (B cell or
Splenic marginal zone lymphoma	T cell)
Nodal marginal zone lymphoma	Lymphoplasmacytic lymphoma
Mantle cell lymphoma	Sézary syndrome
Hairy cell leukemia	Smoldering adult T cell leukemia/
	lymphoma

TABLE 97-2 *Classification of Acute Lymphoid Leukemia (ALL)*

Immunologic Subtype	% of Cases	FAB Subtype	Cytogenetic Abnormalities
Pre-B ALL	75	L1, L2	t(9;22), t(4;11), t(1;19)
T cell ALL	20	L1, L2	14q11 or 7q34
B cell ALL	5	L3	t(8;14), t(8;22), t(2;8)

Note: FAB, French-American-British classification.

kemias of lymphoid cells have been subdivided based on morphologic characteristics by the French-American-British (FAB) group (Table 97-2). Using this system, lymphoid malignancies of small uniform blasts (e.g., typical childhood acute lymphoblastic leukemia) were called L1, lymphoid malignancies with larger and more variable size cells were called L2, and lymphoid malignancies of uniform cells with basophilic and sometimes vacuolated cytoplasm were called L3 (e.g., typical Burkitt's lymphoma cells). Acute leukemias of lymphoid cells have also been subdivided based on immunologic (i.e., T cell vs. B cell) and cytogenetic abnormalities (Table 97-2). Major cytogenetic subgroups include the t(9;22) (e.g., Philadelphia chromosome–positive acute lymphoblastic leukemia) and the t(8;14) found in the L3 or Burkitt's leukemia.

Non-Hodgkin's lymphomas were separated from Hodgkin's disease by recognition of the Sternberg-Reed cells early in the twentieth century. The histologic classification for non-Hodgkin's lymphomas was has been one of the most contentious issues in oncology. Imperfect morphologic systems were supplanted by imperfect immunologic systems, and poor reproducibility of diagnosis has hampered progress. In 1999, the World Health Organization (WHO) classification of lymphoid malignancies was devised through a process of consensus development among international leaders in hematopathology and clinical oncology. The WHO classification takes into account morphologic, clinical, immunologic, and genetic information and attempts to divide non-Hodgkin's lymphomas and other lymphoid malignancies into clinical/pathologic entities that have clinical and therapeutic relevance. This system is presented in Table 97-3. Clinical studies have shown that this new system is clinically relevant and has a higher degree of diagnostic accuracy than those used previously. The possibilities for subdividing lymphoid malignancies are extensive. However, Table 97-3 presents in bold those malignancies that occur in at least 1% of patients. Specific lymphoma subtypes will be dealt with in more detail below.

GENERAL ASPECTS OF LYMPHOID MALIGNANCIES

ETIOLOGY AND EPIDEMIOLOGY Chronic lymphoid leukemia (CLL) is the most prevalent form of leukemia in western countries. It occurs most frequently in older adults and is exceedingly rare in children. In 2004, 8190 new cases were diagnosed in the United States, but because of the prolonged survival associated with this disorder, the total prevalence is many times higher. CLL is more common in men than in women and more common in whites than in blacks. This is an uncommon malignancy in Asia. The etiologic factors for typical CLL are unknown.

In contrast to CLL, acute lymphoid leukemias (ALLs) are predominantly cancers of children and young adults. The L3 or Burkitt's leukemia occurring in children in developing countries seems to be associated with infection by the Epstein-Barr virus (EBV) in infancy. However, the explanation for the etiology of more common subtypes of ALL is much less certain. Childhood ALL occurs more often in higher socioeconomic subgroups. Children with trisomy 21 (Down's syndrome) have an increased risk for childhood acute lymphoblastic leukemia as well as acute myeloid leukemia. Exposure to high-energy radiation in early childhood increases the risk of developing T cell acute lymphoblastic leukemia.

The etiology of ALL in adults is also uncertain. ALL is unusual in middle-aged adults but increases in incidence in the elderly. However, acute myeloid leukemia is still much more common in older patients. Environmental exposures including certain industrial exposures, exposure to agricultural chemicals, and smoking might increase the risk of developing ALL as an adult.

The preponderance of evidence suggests that Hodgkin's disease is of B cell origin. The incidence of Hodgkin's disease appears fairly stable, with ~7800 new cases diagnosed in 2004 in the United States. Hodgkin's disease is more common in whites than in blacks and more common in males than in females. A bimodal distribution of age at diagnosis has been observed, with one peak incidence occurring in patients in their 20s and the other in those in their 80s.

TABLE 97-3 *WHO Classification of Lymphoid Malignancies*

B Cell	T Cell	Hodgkin's Disease
Precursor B cell neoplasm	Precursor T cell neoplasm	Nodular lymphocyte-predominant Hodgkin's disease
Precursor B lymphoblastic leukemia/lymphoma (precursor B cell acute lymphoblastic leukemia)	**Precursor T lymphoblastic lymphoma/leukemia (precursor T cell acute lymphoblastic leukemia)**	
Mature (peripheral) B cell neoplasms	Mature (peripheral) T cell neoplasms	Classic Hodgkin's disease
B cell chronic lymphocytic leukemia/small lymphocytic lymphoma	T cell prolymphocytic leukemia	Nodular sclerosis Hodgkin's disease
B cell prolymphocytic leukemia	T cell granular lymphocytic leukemia	Lymphocyte-rich classic Hodgkin's disease
Lymphoplasmacytic lymphoma	Aggressive NK cell leukemia	Mixed-cellularity Hodgkin's disease
Splenic marginal zone B cell lymphoma (± villous lymphocytes)	Adult T cell lymphoma/leukemia (HTLV-I+)	Lymphocyte-depletion Hodgkin's disease
Hairy cell leukemia	Extranodal NK/T cell lymphoma, nasal type	
Plasma cell myeloma/plasmacytoma	Enteropathy-type T cell lymphoma	
Extranodal marginal zone B cell lymphoma of MALT type	Hepatosplenic $\gamma\delta$ T cell lymphoma	
Mantle cell lymphoma	Subcutaneous panniculitis-like T cell lymphoma	
Follicular lymphoma	**Mycosis fungoides/Sézary syndrome**	
Nodal marginal zone B cell lymphoma (± monocytoid B cells)	Anaplastic large cell lymphoma, primary cutaneous type	
Diffuse large B cell lymphoma	**Peripheral T cell lymphoma, not otherwise specified (NOS)**	
Burkitt's lymphoma/Burkitt cell leukemia	**Angioimmunoblastic T cell lymphoma**	
	Anaplastic large cell lymphoma, primary systemic type	

Note: HTLV, human T cell lymphotropic virus; MALT, mucosa-associated lymphoid tissue; NK, natural killer; WHO, World Health Organization.
Source: Adapted from Harris et al.

Some of the late age peak may be attributed to confusion among entities with similar appearance such as anaplastic large cell lymphoma and T cell–rich B cell lymphoma. Patients in the younger age groups diagnosed in the United States largely have the nodular sclerosing subtype of Hodgkin's disease. Elderly patients, patients infected with HIV, and patients in third world countries more commonly have mixed-cellularity Hodgkin's disease or lymphocyte-depleted Hodgkin's disease. Infection by HIV is a risk factor for developing Hodgkin's disease. In addition, an association between infection by EBV and Hodgkin's disease has been demonstrated. A monoclonal or oligoclonal proliferation of EBV-infected cells in 20 to 40% of the patients with Hodgkin's disease has led to proposals for this virus having an etiologic role in Hodgkin's disease. However, the matter is not settled definitively.

For unknown reasons, non-Hodgkin's lymphomas increased in frequency in the United States at the rate of 4% per year between 1950 and the late 1990s. For uncertain reasons, the rate of increase in the past few years seems to be decreasing. About 54,000 new cases of non-Hodgkin's lymphoma were diagnosed in the United States in the year 2004. Non-Hodgkin's lymphomas are more frequent in the elderly and more frequent in men. Patients with both primary and secondary immunodeficiency states are predisposed to developing non-Hodgkin's lymphomas. These include patients with HIV infection; patients who have undergone organ transplantation; and patients with inherited immune deficiencies, the sicca syndrome, and rheumatoid arthritis.

The incidence of non-Hodgkin's lymphomas and the patterns of expression of the various subtypes differ geographically. T cell lymphomas are more common in Asia than in western countries, while certain subtypes of B cell lymphomas such as follicular lymphoma are more common in western countries. A specific subtype of non-Hodgkin's lymphoma known as the angiocentric nasal T/natural killer (NK) cell lymphoma has a striking geographic occurrence, being most frequent in Southern Asia and parts of Latin America. Another subtype of non-Hodgkin's lymphoma associated with infection by human T cell lymphotropic virus (HTLV) I is seen particularly in southern Japan and the Caribbean (Chap. 172).

A number of environmental factors have been implicated in the occurrence of non-Hodgkin's lymphoma, including infectious agents, chemical exposures, and medical treatments. Several studies have demonstrated an association between exposure to agricultural chemicals and an increased incidence in non-Hodgkin's lymphoma. Patients treated for Hodgkin's disease can develop non-Hodgkin's lymphoma; it is unclear whether this is a consequence of the Hodgkin's disease or its treatment. However, the infectious etiology of non-Hodgkin's lymphoma is the area where evidence has been expanding most rapidly in recent years. Table 97-4 illustrates those infectious agents associated with the development of non-Hodgkin's lymphoma. HTLV-I infects T cells and leads directly to the development of adult T cell lymphoma (ATL) in a small percentage of infected patients. The cumulative lifetime risk of developing lymphoma in an infected patient is 2.5%. The virus is transmitted by infected lymphocytes ingested by nursing babies of infected mothers, blood-borne transmission, or sexually. The median age of patients with ATL is about 56 years, emphasizing the long latency. HTLV-I is also the cause of tropical spastic paraparasis—a neurologic disorder that occurs somewhat more frequently than lymphoma and with shorter latency.

EBV is associated with the development of Burkitt's lymphoma in Central Africa and the occurrence of aggressive non-Hodgkin's lymphomas in immunosuppressed patients in western countries. The majority of primary central nervous system (CNS) lymphomas are associated with EBV. EBV infection is strongly associated with the occurrence of extranodal nasal T/NK cell lymphomas in Asia and South America. Infection with HIV predisposes to the development of aggressive, B cell non-Hodgkin's lymphoma. This may be through overexpression of interleukin 6 by infected macrophages. Infection of the stomach by the bacterium *Helicobacter pylori* induces the development of gastric MALT (mucosa-associated lymphoid tissue) lymphomas. This association is supported by evidence that patients treated with antibiotics to eradicate *H. pylori* have regression of their MALT lymphoma. The bacterium does not transform lymphocytes to produce the lymphoma; instead, a vigorous immune response is made to the bacterium and the chronic antigenic stimulation leads to the neoplasia. MALT lymphomas of the skin may be related to *Borrelia* sp. infections.

Chronic hepatitis C virus infection has been associated with the development of lymphoplasmacytic lymphoma. Human herpesvirus 8 is associated with primary effusion lymphoma in HIV-infected persons and multicentric Castleman's disease, a diffuse lymphadenopathy associated with systemic symptoms of fever, malaise, and weight loss.

In addition to infectious agents, a number of other diseases or exposures may predispose to developing lymphoma (Table 97-5).

IMMUNOLOGY All lymphoid cells are derived from a common hematopoietic progenitor that gives rise to lymphoid, myeloid, erythroid, monocyte, and megakaryocyte lineages. Through the ordered and sequential activation of a series of transcription factors, the cell first becomes committed to the lymphoid lineage and then gives rise to B and T cells. About 75% of all lymphoid leukemias and 90% of all lymphomas are of B cell origin. A cell becomes committed to B cell development when it begins to rearrange its immunoglobulin genes. The sequence of cellular changes, including changes in cell-surface phenotype, that characterizes normal B cell development is shown in Fig. 97-1. A cell becomes committed to T cell differentiation upon migration to the thymus and rearrangement of T cell antigen receptor genes. The sequence of the events that characterize T cell development is depicted in Fig. 97-2.

Although lymphoid malignancies often retain the cell-surface phenotype of lymphoid cells at particular stages of differentiation, this information is of little consequence. The so-called stage of differentiation of a malignant lymphoma does not predict its natural history. For example, the clinically most aggressive lymphoid leukemia is

---

TABLE 97-4 *Infectious Agents Associated with the Development of Lymphoid Malignancies*

Infectious Agent	Lymphoid Malignancy
Epstein-Barr virus	Burkitt's lymphoma
	Post–organ transplant lymphoma
	Primary CNS diffuse large B cell lymphoma
	Hodgkin's disease
	Extranodal NK/T cell lymphoma, nasal type
HTLV-I	Adult T cell leukemia/lymphoma
HIV	Diffuse large B cell lymphoma
	Burkitt's lymphoma
Hepatitis C virus	Lymphoplasmacytic lymphoma
Helicobacter pylori	Gastric MALT lymphoma
Human herpesvirus 8	Primary effusion lymphoma
	Multicentric Castleman's disease

Note: CNS, central nervous system; HTLV, human T cell lymphotropic virus; MALT, mucosa-associated lymphoid tissue; NK, natural killer.

TABLE 97-5 *Diseases or Exposures Associated with Increased Risk of Development of Malignant Lymphoma*

Inherited immunodeficiency disease	Autoimmune disease
Klinefelter's syndrome	Sjögren's syndrome
Chédiak-Higashi syndrome	Celiac sprue
Ataxia telangiectasia syndrome	Rheumatoid arthritis and systemic
Wiscott-Aldrich syndrome	lupus erythematosus
Common variable	Chemical or drug exposures
immunodeficiency disease	Phenytoin
Acquired immunodeficiency	Dioxin, phenoxyherbicides
diseases	Radiation
Iatrogenic immunosuppression	Prior chemotherapy and radiation
HIV-1 infection	therapy
Acquired	
hypogammaglobulinemia	

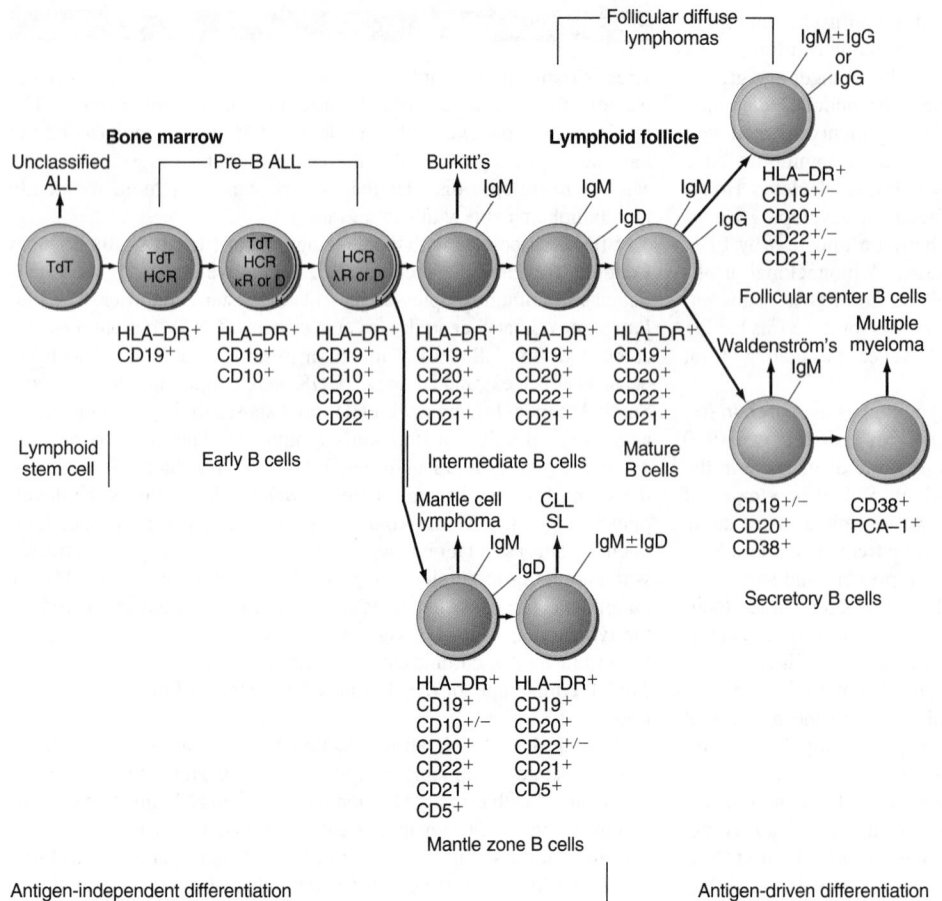

FIGURE 97-1 Pathway of normal B cell differentiation and relationship to B cell lymphomas. HLA-DR, CD10, CD19, CD20, CD21, CD22, CD5, and CD38 are cell markers used to distinguish stages of development. Terminal transferase (TdT) is a cellular enzyme. Immunoglobulin heavy chain gene rearrangement (HCR) and light chain gene rearrangement or deletion (κ R or D, λ R or D) occur early in B cell development. The approximate normal stage of differentiation associated with particular lymphomas is shown. ALL, acute lymphoid leukemia; CLL, chronic lymphoid leukemia; SL, small lymphocytic lymphoma.

Burkitt's leukemia, which has the phenotype of a mature follicle center IgM-bearing B cell. Leukemias bearing the immunologic cell-surface phenotype of more primitive cells (e.g., pre-B ALL, CD10+) are less aggressive and more amenable to curative therapy than the "more mature" appearing Burkitt's leukemia cells. Furthermore, the apparent stage of differentiation of the malignant cell does not reflect the stage at which the genetic lesions that gave rise to the malignancy developed. For example, follicular lymphoma has the cell-surface phenotype of a follicle center cell, but its characteristic chromosomal translocation, the t(14;18), which involves juxtaposition of the anti-apoptotic *bcl-2* gene next to the immunoglobulin heavy chain gene (see below), had to develop early in ontogeny as an error in the process of immunoglobulin gene rearrangement. Why the subsequent steps that led to transformation became manifest in a cell of follicle center differentiation is not clear.

The major value of cell-surface phenotyping is to aid in the differential diagnosis of lymphoid tumors that appear similar by light microscopy. For example, benign follicular hyperplasia may resemble follicular lymphoma; however, the demonstration that all the cells bear the same immunoglobulin light chain isotype strongly suggests the mass is a clonal proliferation rather than a polyclonal response to an exogenous stimulus.

GENETIC CONSIDERATIONS Malignancies of lymphoid cells are associated with recurring genetic abnormalities. While specific genetic abnormalities have not been identified for all subtypes of lymphoid malignancies, it is presumed that they exist. Genetic abnormalities can be identified at a variety of levels including gross chromosomal changes (i.e., translocations, additions, or deletions); re-

arrangement of specific genes that may or may not be apparent from cytogenetic studies; and overexpression, underexpression, or mutation of specific oncogenes. Altered expression or mutation of specific proteins is particularly important. Many lymphomas contain balanced chromosomal translocations involving the antigen receptor genes; immunoglobulin genes on chromosomes 2, 14, and 22 in B cells; and T cell antigen receptor genes on chromosomes 7 and 14 in T cells. The rearrangement of chromosome segments to generate mature antigen receptors must create a site of vulnerability to aberrant recombination. B cells are even more susceptible to acquiring mutations during their maturation in germinal centers; the generation of antibody of higher affinity requires the introduction of mutations into the variable region genes in the germinal centers. Other nonimmunoglobulin genes, for example *bcl-6*, may acquire mutations as well.

In the case of diffuse large B cell lymphoma, the translocation t(14;18) occurs in ~30% of patients and leads to overexpression of the *bcl-2* gene found on chromosome 18. Some other patients without the translocation also overexpress the BCL-2 protein. This protein is involved in suppressing apoptosis—i.e., the mechanism of cell death most often induced by cytotoxic chemotherapeutic agents. A higher relapse rate has been observed in patients whose tumors overexpress the BCL-2 protein, but not in those patients whose lymphoma cells show only the translocation. Thus, particular genetic mechanisms have clinical ramifications.

Table 97-6 presents the best documented translocations and associated oncogenes for various subtypes of lymphoid malignancies. In some cases, such as the association of the t(14;18) in follicular lymphoma, the t(2;5) in anaplastic large T/null-cell lymphoma, the t(8;14) in Burkitt's lymphoma, and the t(11;14) in mantle cell lymphoma, the great majority of tumors in patients with these diagnoses display these abnormalities. In other types of lymphoma where a minority of the patients have tumors expressing specific genetic abnormalities, the defects may have prognostic significance. No specific genetic abnormalities have been identified in Hodgkin's disease other than aneuploidy.

In typical B cell CLL, trisomy 12 conveys a poorer prognosis. In ALL in both adults and children, genetic abnormalities have important prognostic significance. Patients whose tumor cells display the t(9;22) have a much poorer outlook than patients who do not have this translocation. Other genetic abnormalities that occur frequently in adults with ALL include the t(4;11) and the t(8;14). The t(4;11) is associated with younger age, female predominance, high white cell counts, and L1 morphology. The t(8;14) is associated with older age, male predominance, frequent CNS involvement, and L3 morphology. Both are associated with a poor prognosis. In childhood ALL, hyperdiploidy has been shown to have a favorable prognosis.

Gene profiling using array technology allows the simultaneous assessment of the expression of thousands of genes. This technology provides the possibility to identify new genes with pathologic importance in lymphomas, the identification of patterns of gene expression with diagnostic and/or prognostic significance, and the identification

T CELL DIFFERENTIATION	THYMUS	T CELL MALIGNANCIES
Stage I Prothymocyte	CD: 2, 7, 38, 71	Majority of T cell ALL
Stage II Thymocyte	CD: 1, 2, 4, 7, 8, 38	Minority of T-ALL Majority of T-LL
Stage III Thymocyte	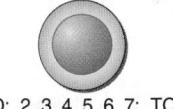 CD: 2, 3, 4/8, 5, 6, 7; TCR	Minority of T-LL Rare T-ALL

PERIPHERAL BLOOD AND NODES

Mature T Helper Cell	CD: 2, 3, 4, 5, 6, 7; TCR	Majority of T-CLL, CTCL, Sezary Cell, NHL
Mature T Cytotoxic/ Suppressor Cell	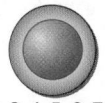 CD: 2, 3, 4, 5, 6, 7; TCR	Minority of T-CLL, NHL

FIGURE 97-2 Pathway of normal T cell differentiation and relationship to T cell lymphomas. CD1, CD2, CD3, CD4, CD5, CD6, CD7, CD8, CD38, and CD71 are cell markers used to distinguish stages of development. T cell antigen receptors (TCR) rearrange in the thymus, and mature T cells emigrate to nodes and peripheral blood. ALL, acute lymphoid leukemia; T-ALL, T cell ALL; T-LL, T cell lymphoblastic lymphoma; T-CLL, T cell chronic lymphoid leukemia; CTCL, cutaneous T cell lymphoma; NHL, non-Hodgkin's lymphoma.

of new therapeutic targets. Recognition of patterns of gene expression is complicated and requires sophisticated mathematical techniques. Early successes using this technology in lymphoma include the identification of previously unrecognized subtypes of diffuse large B cell lymphoma whose gene expression patterns resemble either those of follicular center B cells or activated peripheral blood B cells (Fig. 97-3). Patients whose lymphomas have a germinal center B cell pattern of gene expression have a considerably better prognosis than those whose lymphomas have a pattern resembling that seen in activated

TABLE 97-6 *Cytogenetic Translocation and Associated Oncogenes Often Seen in Lymphoid Malignancies*

Disease	Cytogenetic Abnormality	Oncogene
CLL/small lymphocytic lymphoma	t(14;15)(q32;q13)	—
MALT lymphoma	t(11;18)(q21;q21)	—
Precursor B cell acute lymphoid leukemia	t(9;22)(q34;q11) or variant	BCR/ABL
	t(4;11)(q21;q23)	AF4, ALLI
Precursor acute lymphoid leukemia	t(9;22)	BCR, ABL
	t(1;19)	E2A, PBX
	t(17;19)	HLF, E2A
	t(5;14)	IL3, IGμ
Mantle cell lymphoma	t(11;14)(q13;q32)	BCL-1, IgH
Follicular lymphoma	t(14;18)(q32;q21)	BCL-2, IgH
Diffuse large-cell lymphoma	t(3;-)(q27;-)[a]	BCL-6
	t(17;-)(p13;-)	p53
Burkitt's lymphoma, Burkitt's leukemia	t(8;-)(q24;-)[a]	C-MYC
CD30+ Anaplastic large cell lymphoma	t(2;5)(p23;q35)	ALK
Lymphoplasmacytoid lymphoma	t(9;14)(p13;q32)	—

[a] Numerous sites of translocation may be involved with these genes.
Note: CLL, chronic lymphoid leukemia; MALT, mucosa-associated lymphoid tissue; IgH, immunoglobulin heavy chain.

peripheral blood B cells. This improved prognosis is independent of other known prognostic factors and provides the opportunity to identify better treatments for these subgroups of patients. Similar information is being generated in follicular lymphoma and mantle cell lymphoma. The challenge remains to provide information from such techniques in a clinically useful time frame.

APPROACH TO THE PATIENT

Regardless of the type of lymphoid malignancy, the initial evaluation of the patient should include performance of a careful history and physical examination. These will help confirm the diagnosis, identify those manifestations of the disease that might require prompt attention, and aid in the selection of further studies to optimally characterize the patient's status to allow the best choice of therapy. It is difficult to overemphasize the importance of a carefully done history and physical examination. They might provide observations that lead to reconsidering the diagnosis, provide hints at etiology, clarify the stage, and allow the physician to establish rapport with the patient that will make it possible to develop and carry out a therapeutic plan.

For patients with ALL, evaluation is usually completed after a complete blood count, chemistry studies reflecting major organ function, a bone marrow biopsy with genetic and immunologic studies, and a lumbar puncture. The latter is necessary to rule out occult CNS involvement. At this point, most patients would be ready to begin therapy. In ALL, prognosis is dependent upon the genetic characteristics of the tumor, the patient's age, the white cell count, and the patient's overall clinical status and major organ function.

In CLL, the patient evaluation should include a complete blood count, chemistry tests to measure major organ function, serum protein electrophoresis, and a bone marrow biopsy. However, some physicians believe that the diagnosis would not always require a bone marrow biopsy. Patients often have imaging studies of the chest and abdomen looking for pathologic lymphadenopathy. Patients with typical B cell CLL can be subdivided into three major prognostic groups. Those patients with only blood and bone marrow involvement by leukemia but no lymphadenopathy, organomegaly, or signs of bone marrow failure have the best prognosis. Those with lymphadenopathy and organomegaly have an intermediate prognosis, and patients with bone marrow failure, defined as hemoglobin <100 g/L (10 g/dL) or platelet count <100,000/μL, have the worst prognosis. The pathogenesis of the anemia or thrombocytopenia is important to discern. The prognosis is adversely affected when either or both of these abnormalities are due to progressive marrow infiltration and loss of productive marrow. However, either or both may be due to autoimmune phenomena or to hypersplenism that can develop during the course of the disease. These destructive mechanisms are usually completely reversible (glucocorticoids for autoimmune disease; splenectomy for hypersplenism) and do not influence disease prognosis.

Two popular staging systems have been developed to reflect these prognostic groupings (Table 97-7). Patients with typical B cell CLL can have their course complicated by immunologic abnormalities including autoimmune hemolytic anemia, autoimmune thrombocytopenia, and hypogammaglobulinemia. Patients with hypogammaglobulinemia benefit from regular (monthly) γ globulin administration. Because of expense, γ globulin is often withheld until the patient experiences a significant infection. These abnormalities do not have a clear prognostic significance and should not be used to assign a higher stage.

The initial evaluation of a patient with Hodgkin's disease or non-Hodgkin's lymphoma is similar. In both situations, the determination of an accurate anatomic stage is an important part of the evaluation. The staging system is the Ann Arbor staging system originally developed for Hodgkin's disease (Table 97-8).

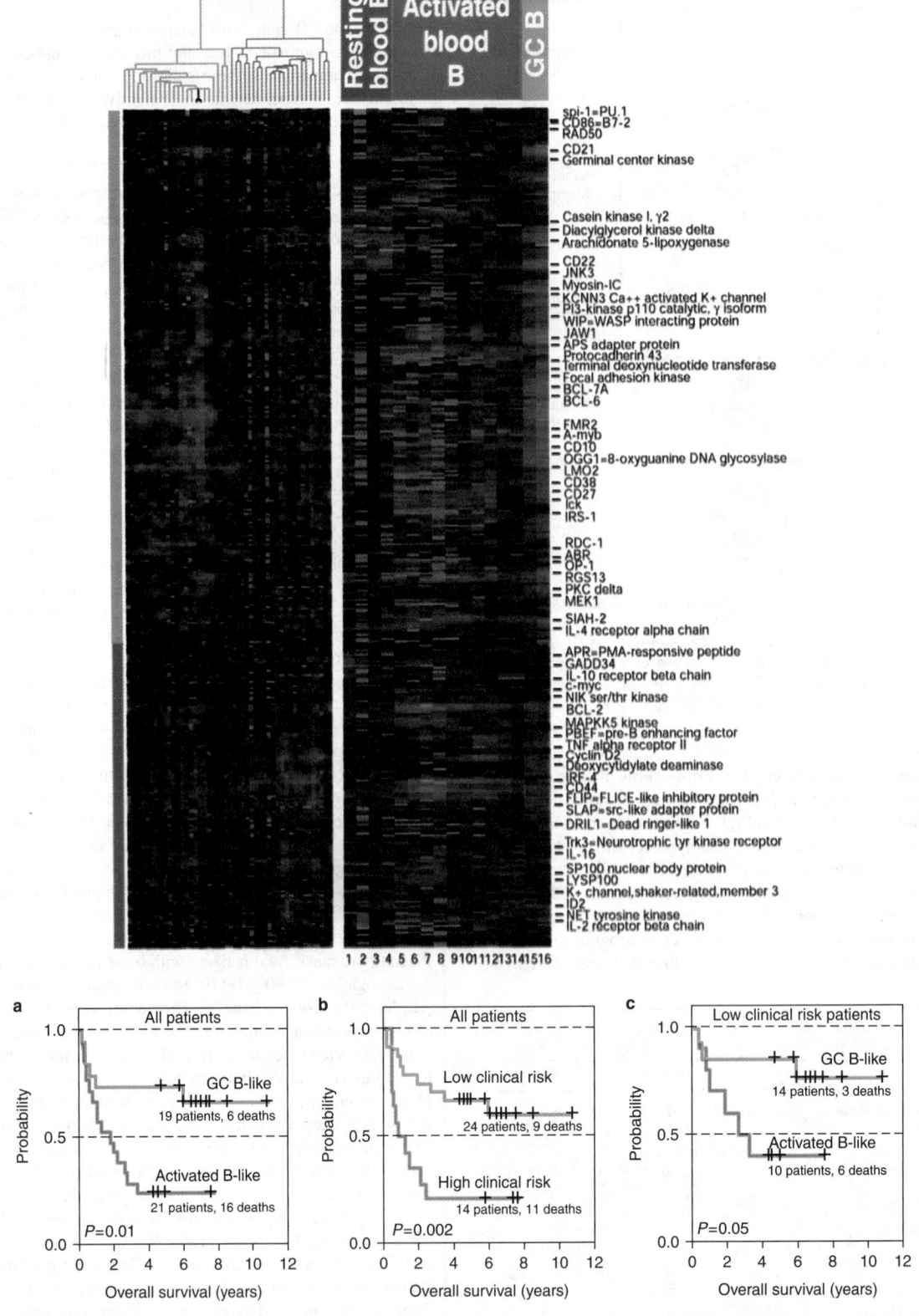

FIGURE 97-3 Relationship of different gene expression patterns to outcome of treatment for diffuse large B cell lymphoma. The top panel reveals the pattern of expression of a large number of lymphocyte-expressed genes in tumors from patients with diffuse large B cell lymphoma, a lymphoma recognized as morphologically heterogeneous but before now not classifiable reproducibly. Two dominant patterns are seen, one mimicking germinal center B cells and one mimicking activated peripheral blood B cells. The bottom panels show the relationship between gene expression pattern and clinical outcome. *A.* Kaplan-Meier survival plots of all patients according to gene profile showing significant differences between follicular center and activated B cell types. *B.* Kaplan-Meier survival of patients based upon the IPI scores. *C.* Kaplan-Meier survival plots showing that among patients with IPI low risk, the gene expression profile has prognostic significance. (IPI, International Prognostic Index.)

TABLE 97-7   *Staging of Typical B Cell Lymphoid Leukemia*

Stage	Clinical Features	Median Survival, Years
RAI SYSTEM		
0: Low risk	Lymphocytosis only in blood and marrow	>10
I: Intermediate risk	Lymphocytosis + lymphadenopathy + splenomegaly ± hepatomegaly	7
II		
III: High risk	Lymphocytosis + anemia	1.5
IV	Lymphocytosis + thrombocytopenia	
BINET SYSTEM		
A	Fewer than three areas of clinical lymphadenopathy; no anemia or thrombocytopenia	>10
B	Three or more involved node areas; no anemia or thrombocytopenia	7
C	Hemoglobin ≤10 g/dL and/or platelets <100,000/μl	2

Evaluation of patients with Hodgkin's disease will typically include a complete blood count; erythrocyte sedimentation rate; chemistry studies reflecting major organ function; computed tomography (CT) scans of the chest, abdomen, and pelvis; and a bone marrow biopsy. Neither a positron emission tomography (PET) scan nor a gallium scan is absolutely necessary for primary staging, but one performed at the completion of therapy allows evaluation of persisting radiographic abnormalities, particularly the mediastinum. Knowing that the PET scan or gallium scan is abnormal before treatment is initiated can help in this assessment. In most cases, these studies will allow assignment of anatomic stage and the development of a therapeutic plan.

In patients with non-Hodgkin's lymphoma, the same evaluation described for patients with Hodgkin's disease is usually carried out. In addition, serum levels of lactate dehydrogenase (LDH) and β_2-

TABLE 97-8   *The Ann Arbor Staging System for Hodgkin's Disease*

Stage	Definition
I	Involvement of a single lymph node region or lymphoid structure (e.g., spleen, thymus, Waldeyer's ring)
II	Involvement of two or more lymph node regions on the same side of the diaphragm (the mediastinum is a single site; hilar lymph nodes should be considered "lateralized" and, when involved on both sides, constitute stage II disease)
III	Involvement of lymph node regions or lymphoid structures on both sides of the diaphragm
III$_1$	Subdiaphragmatic involvement limited to spleen, splenic hilar nodes, celiac nodes, or portal nodes
III$_2$	Subdiaphragmatic involvement includes paraaortic, iliac, or mesenteric nodes plus structures in III$_1$
IV	Involvement of extranodal site(s) beyond that designated as "E"
	More than one extranodal deposit at any location
	Any involvement of liver or bone marrow
A	No symptoms
B	Unexplained weight loss of >10% of the body weight during the 6 months before staging investigation
	Unexplained, persistent, or recurrent fever with temperatures >38°C during the previous month
	Recurrent drenching night sweats during the previous month
E	Localized, solitary involvement of extralymphatic tissue, excluding liver and bone marrow

TABLE 97-9   *International Prognostic Index for NHL*

Five clinical risk factors:
   Age ≥ 60 years
   Serum lactate dehydrogenase levels elevated
   Performance status ≥ 2 (ECOG) or ≤ 70 (Karnofsky)
   Ann Arbor stage III or IV
   >1 site of extranodal involvement
Patients are assigned a number for each risk factor they have
Patients are grouped differently based upon the type of lymphoma
For diffuse large B cell lymphoma:

0,1 factor = low risk	35% of cases; 5-year survival, 73%
2 factors = low-intermediate risk	27% of cases; 5-year survival, 51%
3 factors = high-intermediate risk	22% of cases; 5-year survival, 43%
4,5 factors = high risk	16% of cases; 5-year survival, 26%

microglobulin and serum protein electrophoresis are often included in the evaluation. Anatomic stage is assigned in the same manner as used for Hodgkin's disease. However, the prognosis of patients with non-Hodgkin's lymphoma is best assigned using the International Prognostic Index (IPI) (Table 97-9). This is a powerful predictor of outcome in all subtypes of non-Hodgkin's lymphoma. Patients are assigned an IPI score based on the presence or absence of five adverse prognostic factors and may have none or all five of these adverse prognostic factors. Figure 97-4 shows the prognostic significance of this score in 1300 patients with all types of non-Hodgkin's lymphoma. CT scans are routinely used in the evaluation of patients with all subtypes of non-Hodgkin's lymphoma but PET and gallium scans are much more useful in aggressive subtypes such as diffuse large B cell lymphoma than in more indolent subtypes such a follicular lymphoma or small lymphocytic lymphoma.

CLINICAL FEATURES, TREATMENT, AND PROGNOSIS OF SPECIFIC LYMPHOID MALIGNANCIES

PRECURSOR CELL B CELL NEOPLASMS ▪ Precursor B Cell Lymphoblastic Leukemia/Lymphoma   The most common cancer in childhood is B cell ALL. Although this disorder can also present as a lymphoma in either adults or children, presentation as lymphoma is quite rare.

The malignant cells in patients with precursor B cell lymphoblastic leukemia are most commonly of pre-B cell origin. Patients typically present with signs of bone marrow failure such as pallor, fatigue, bleeding, fever, and infection related to peripheral blood cytopenias. Peripheral blood counts regularly show anemia and thrombocytopenia but might show leukopenia, a normal leukocyte count, or leukocytosis based largely on the number of circulating malignant cells (Fig. 97-5). Extranodal sites of disease are frequently involved in patients who

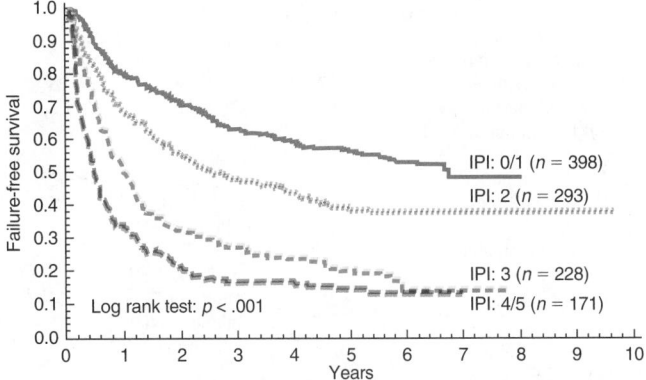

FIGURE 97-4   Relationship of International Prognostic Index (IPI) to survival. Kaplan-Meier survival curves for 1300 patients with various kinds of lymphoma stratified according to the IPI.

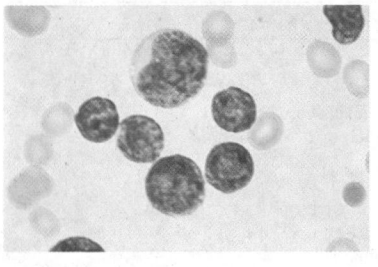

FIGURE 97-5 Acute lymphoblastic leukemia. The cells are heterogeneous in size, have round or convoluted nuclei, high nuclear/cytoplasmic ratio, and absence of cytoplasmic granules.

present with leukemia, which might be manifested by lymphadenopathy, hepato- or splenomegaly, CNS disease, testicular enlargement, and/or cutaneous infiltration.

The diagnosis is usually made by bone marrow biopsy, which shows infiltration by malignant lymphoblasts. Demonstration of a pre-B cell immunophenotype (Fig. 97-1) and, often, characteristic cytogenetic abnormalities (Table 97-6) confirm the diagnosis. An adverse prognosis in patients with precursor B cell ALL is predicted by a very high white cell count, the presence of symptomatic CNS disease, and unfavorable cytogenetic abnormalities. For example, t(9;22) is frequently found in adults with B cell lymphoblastic leukemia and is associated with a very poor outlook.

℞ TREATMENT

The treatment of patients with precursor B cell lymphoblastic leukemia involves remission induction with combination chemotherapy, a consolidation phase that includes administration of high-dose systemic therapy and treatment to eliminate disease in the CNS, and a period of continuing therapy to prevent relapse and effect cure. The overall cure rate in children is 85%, while about 50% of adults are long-term disease-free survivors. This reflects the high proportion of adverse cytogenetic abnormalities seen in adults with precursor B cell lymphoblastic leukemia.

Precursor B cell lymphoblastic lymphoma is a rare presentation of precursor B cell lymphoblastic malignancy. These patients often have a rapid transformation to leukemia, and similar treatment approaches as are used in patients presenting with leukemia are appropriate. In the few patients who present with the disease confined to lymph nodes, a high cure rate has been reported.

MATURE (PERIPHERAL) B CELL NEOPLASMS ■ B Cell Chronic Lymphoid Leukemia/Small Lymphocytic Lymphoma
B cell CLL/small lymphocytic lymphoma represents by far the most common lymphoid leukemia, and

when presenting as a lymphoma, it accounts for ~7% of non-Hodgkin's lymphomas. As the name implies, presentation can be as either leukemia or lymphoma. The major clinical characteristics of B cell CLL/small lymphocytic lymphoma are presented in Table 97-10.

The diagnosis of typical B cell CLL is made when an increased number of circulating lymphocytes (i.e., $>4 \times 10^9$/L and usually $>10 \times 10^9$/L) is found (Fig. 97-6) that are monoclonal B cells and display the CD5 antigen. Finding bone marrow infiltration by the same cells confirms the diagnosis. The peripheral blood smear in such patients typically shows many "smudge" or "basket" cells, nuclear remnants of cells damaged by the physical shear stress of making the blood smear. If cytogenetic studies are performed, trisomy 12 is found in ~25 to 30% of patients. Abnormalities in chromosome 13 are also seen.

If the primary presentation is lymphadenopathy and a lymph node biopsy is performed, pathologists usually have little difficulty in making the diagnosis of small lymphocytic lymphoma based on morphologic findings and immunophenotype. However, even in these patients, ~70 to 75% will be found to have bone marrow involvement and the search for circulating monoclonal B lymphocytes is often positive.

The differential diagnosis of typical B cell CLL is extensive and presented in Table 97-1. Immunophenotyping will eliminate the T cell disorders and can often help sort out other B cell malignancies. For example, only mantle cell lymphoma and typical B cell CLL are usually CD5 positive. Typical B cell small lymphocytic lymphoma can be confused with other B cell disorders including lymphoplasmacytic lymphoma (i.e., the tissue manifestation of Waldenström's macroglobulinemia), nodal marginal zone B cell lymphoma, and mantle cell lymphoma. In addition, some small lymphocytic lymphomas have areas of large cells that can lead to confusion with diffuse large B cell lymphoma. An expert hematopathologist is vital for making this distinction.

Typical B cell CLL is often found incidentally when a complete blood count is done for another reason. However, complaints that might lead to the diagnosis include fatigue, frequent infections, and new lymphadenopathy. The diagnosis of typical B cell CLL should be considered in a patient presenting with an autoimmune hemolytic anemia or autoimmune thrombocytopenia. B cell CLL has also been associated with red cell aplasia. When this disorder presents as lymphoma, the most common abnormality is asymptomatic new lymphadenopathy, with or without splenomegaly. The staging systems used to predict prognosis in patients with typical B cell CLL are presented in Table 97-7. The IPI for non-Hodgkin's lymphomas, which also predicts prognosis in these patients, is presented in Table 97-9. The evaluation of a new patient with typical B cell CLL/small lym-

TABLE 97-10 *Clinical Characteristics of Patients with Common Types of Non-Hodgkin's Lymphomas (NHL)*

Disease	Median Age, years	Frequency in Children	% Male	Stage I/II vs III/IV, %	B Symptoms, %	Bone Marrow Involvement, %	Gastrointestinal Tract Involvement, %	% Surviving 5 years
B cell chronic lymphocytic leukemia/small lymphocytic lymphoma	65	Rare	53	9 vs 91	33	72	3	51
Mantle cell lymphoma	63	Rare	74	20 vs 80	28	64	9	27
Extranodal marginal zone B cell lymphoma of MALT type	60	Rare	48	67 vs 33	19	14	50	74
Follicular lymphoma	59	Rare	42	33 vs 67	28	42	4	72
Diffuse large B cell lymphoma	64	~25% of childhood NHL	55	54 vs 46	33	16	18	46
Burkitt's lymphoma	31	~30% of childhood NHL	89	62 vs 38	22	33	11	45
Precursor T cell lymphoblastic lymphoma	28	~40% of childhood NHL	64	11 vs 89	21	50	4	26
Anaplastic large T/null cell lymphoma	34	Common	69	51 vs 49	53	13	9	77
Peripheral T cell non-Hodgkin's lymphoma	61	~5% of childhood NHL	55	20 vs 80	50	36	15	25

Note: MALT, mucosa-associated lymphoid tissue.

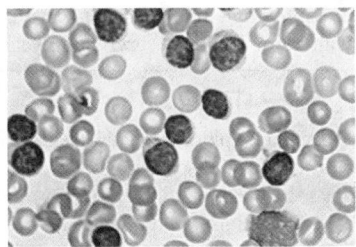

FIGURE 97-6 Chronic lymphocytic leukemia. The peripheral white blood cell count is high due to increased numbers of small, well-differentiated, normal-appearing lymphocytes. The leukemia lymphocytes are fragile, and substantial numbers of broken, smudged cells are usually also present on the blood smear.

phocytic lymphoma will include many of the studies included in Table 97-11, which describes the initial evaluation of a new patient with non-Hodgkin's lymphoma. In addition, particular attention needs to be given to detecting immune abnormalities such as autoimmune hemolytic anemia, autoimmune thrombocytopenia, hypogammaglobulinemia, and red cell aplasia. Molecular analysis of immunoglobulin gene sequences in CLL has demonstrated that about half the patients have tumors expressing mutated immunoglobulin genes and half have tumors expressing unmutated or germ-line immunoglobulin sequences. Patients with unmutated immunoglobulins tend to have a more aggressive clinical course and are less responsive to therapy. Unfortunately, immunoglobulin gene sequencing is not routinely available. CD38 expression is said to be low in the better-prognosis patients expressing mutated immunoglobulin and high in poorer-prognosis patients expressing unmutated immunoglobulin, but this test has not been confirmed as a reliable means of distinguishing the two groups.

℞ TREATMENT

Patients whose presentation is typical B cell CLL with no manifestations of the disease other than bone marrow involvement and lymphocytosis (i.e., Rai stage O and Binet stage A; Table 97-7) can be followed without specific therapy for their malignancy. These patients have a median survival >10 years, and some will never require therapy for this disorder. If the patient has an adequate number of circulating normal blood cells and is asymptomatic, many physicians would not initiate therapy for patients in the intermediate stage of the disease manifested by lymphadenopathy and/or hepatosplenomegaly. However, the median survival for these patients is ~7 years, and most will require treatment in the first few years of follow-up. Patients who present with bone marrow failure (i.e., Rai stage III or IV or Binet stage C) will require initial therapy in almost all cases. These patients have a serious disorder with a median survival of only 1.5 years. It must be remembered that immune manifestations of typical B cell CLL should be managed independently of specific antileukemia therapy. For example, glucocorticoid therapy for autoimmune cytopenias and γ globulin replacement for patients with hypogammaglobulinanemia should be used whether or not antileukemia therapy is given.

Patients who present primarily with lymphoma and have a low IPI score have a 5-year survival of ~75%, but those with a high IPI score

---

TABLE 97-11 *Staging Evaluation for Non-Hodgkin's Lymphoma*

Physical examination
Documentation of B symptoms
Laboratory evaluation
  Complete blood counts
  Liver function tests
  Uric acid
  Calcium
  Serum protein electrophoresis
  Serum β_2-microglobulin
Chest radiograph
CT scan of abdomen, pelvis, and usually chest
Bone marrow biopsy
Lumbar puncture in lymphoblastic, Burkitt's, and diffuse large B cell
  lymphoma with positive marrow biopsy
Gallium scan (SPECT) or PET scan in large-cell lymphoma

Note: CT, computed tomography; SPECT, single photon emission CT; PET, position emission tomography.

---

have a 5-year survival of <40% and are more likely to require early therapy.

The most common treatments for patients with typical B cell CLL/small lymphocytic lymphoma have been single-agent chlorambucil or fludarabine alone or in combination. Chlorambucil can be administered orally with few immediate side effects, while fludarabine is administered intravenously and is associated with significant immune suppression. However, fludarabine is by far the more active agent and is the only drug associated with a significant incidence of complete remission. The combination of rituximab (375 to 500 mg/m² day 1), fludarabine (25 mg/m² days 2 to 4 on cycle 1 and 1 to 3 in subsequent cycles), and cyclophosphamide (250 mg/m² with fludarabine) achieves complete responses in 69% of patients and those responses are associated with molecular remissions in half of the cases. Half the patients experience grade III or IV neutropenia. For young patients presenting with leukemia requiring therapy, regimens containing fludarabine are today the treatment of choice. Because fludarabine is an effective second-line agent in patients with tumors unresponsive to chlorambucil, the latter agent is often chosen in elderly patients who require therapy. Many patients who present with lymphoma will receive a combination chemotherapy regimen used in other lymphomas such as CVP (cyclophosphamide, vincristine, and prednisone), or CHOP (cyclophosphamide, doxorubicin, vincristine, and prednisone) although fludarabine-containing regimens may be preferrable. Alemtuzimab (anti-CD52) is another antibody with activity in the disease, but it kills both B and T cells and is associated with more immune compromise that rituximab. Young patients with this disease can be candidates for bone marrow transplantation. Allogeneic bone marrow transplantation can be curative but is associated with a significant treatment-related mortality. The use of autologous transplantation in patients with this disorder has been discouraging.

Extranodal Marginal Zone B Cell Lymphoma of MALT Type Extranodal marginal zone B cell lymphoma of MALT type makes up ~8% of non-Hodgkin's lymphomas. This small-cell lymphoma presents in extranodal sites. It was previously considered a small lymphocytic lymphoma or sometimes a pseudolymphoma. The recognition that the gastric presentation of this lymphoma was associated with *H. pylori* infection was an important step in recognizing it as a separate entity. The clinical characteristics of extranodal marginal zone B cell lymphoma of MALT type are presented in Table 97-10.

The diagnosis of extranodal marginal zone B cell lymphoma of MALT type can be made accurately by an expert hematopathologist based on a characteristic pattern of infiltration of small lymphocytes that are monoclonal B cells and CD5 negative. In some cases, transformation to diffuse large B cell lymphoma occurs, and both diagnoses may be made in the same biopsy. The differential diagnosis includes benign lymphocytic infiltration of extranodal organs and other small-cell B cell lymphomas.

Extranodal marginal zone B cell lymphoma of MALT type may occur in the stomach, orbit, intestine, lung, thyroid, salivary gland, skin, soft tissues, bladder, kidney, and CNS. It may present as a new mass, be found on routine imaging studies, or be associated with local symptoms such as upper abdominal discomfort in gastric lymphoma. Most MALT lymphomas are gastric in origin. At least two genetic forms of gastric MALT exist: one (accounting for ~50% of cases) characterized by t(11;18)(q21;q21) that juxtaposes the amino terminal of the *API2* gene with the carboxy terminal of the *MALT1* gene creating an API2/MALT1 fusion product, and the other characterized by multiple sites of genetic instability including trisomies of chromosomes 3, 7, 12, and 18. Ninety-five percent of gastric MALT lymphomas are associated with *H. pylori* infection, and those that are not usually express t(11;18). The t(11;18) usually results in activation of NF-κB, which acts a survival factor for the cells. Lymphomas with t(11;18) translocations are genetically stable and do not evolve to diffuse large B cell lymphoma. By contrast, t(11;18)-negative MALT lymphomas often acquire *BCL6* mutations and progress to aggressive histology lymphoma. MALT lymphomas are localized to the organ of origin in ~40% of cases and to the organ and regional lymph nodes in ~30% of patients. However, distant metastasis can occur—particularly with transformation to diffuse large B cell lymphoma. Many patients who develop this lymphoma will have an autoimmune or inflammatory process such as Sjögren's syndrome (salivary gland MALT), Hashimoto's thyroiditis (thyroid MALT), or *Helicobacter* gastritis (gastric MALT).

Evaluation of patients with extranodal marginal zone B cell lymphoma of MALT type follows the pattern set forth in Table 97-11 for staging a patient with non-Hodgkin's lymphoma. In particular, patients with gastric lymphoma need to have studies performed to document the presence or absence of *H. pylori* infection. Endoscopic studies including ultrasound can help define the extent of gastric involvement. Most patients with extranodal marginal zone B cell lymphoma of MALT type have a good prognosis, with a 5-year survival of ~75%. In patients with a low IPI score, the 5-year survival is ~90%, while it drops to ~40% in patients with a high IPI score.

℞ TREATMENT

Extranodal marginal zone B cell lymphoma of MALT type is curable when localized. Local therapy such as radiation or surgery can effect cure, and this is one of the few times where surgery might be a reasonable primary therapy for a patient with non-Hodgkin's lymphoma. Patients with gastric MALT lymphomas who are infected with *H. pylori* can achieve remission in the majority of cases with eradication of the infection. These remissions can be durable, but molecular evidence of persisting neoplasia is frequent and the long-term outcome is uncertain. Patients who present with more extensive disease are most often treated with single-agent chemotherapy such as chlorambucil. Coexistent diffuse large B cell lymphoma must be treated with combination chemotherapy. The additional acquired mutations that mediate the histologic progression also convey *Helicobacter* independence to the growth.

Mantle Cell Lymphoma Mantle cell lymphoma makes up ~6% of all non-Hodgkin's lymphomas. Recognized as a separate entity only in the past decade, this lymphoma was previously placed in a number of other subtypes. Its existence was confirmed by the recognition that these lymphomas have a characteristic chromosomal translocation, t(11;14), between the immunoglobulin heavy chain gene on chromosome 14 and the *bcl-1* gene on chromosome 11, and regularly overexpress the BCL-1 protein. The clinical characteristics of mantle cell lymphoma are presented in Table 97-10.

The diagnosis of mantle cell lymphoma can be made accurately by an expert hematopathologist based on morphologic findings and proof that the tumor is a B cell lymphoma. As with all subtypes of lymphoma, an adequate biopsy is important. The differential diagnosis of mantle cell lymphoma includes other small-cell B cell lymphomas. In particular, mantle cell lymphoma and small lymphocytic lymphoma share a characteristic expression of CD5. Mantle cell lymphoma usually has a slightly indented nucleus.

The most common presentation of mantle cell lymphoma is with palpable lymphadenopathy, frequently accompanied by systemic symptoms. Approximately 70% of patients will be stage IV at the time of diagnosis, with frequent bone marrow and peripheral blood involvement. Of the extranodal organs that can be involved, gastrointestinal involvement is particularly important to recognize. Patients who present with lymphomatosis polyposis in the large intestine usually have mantle cell lymphoma. The evaluation of patients with mantle cell lymphoma involves the studies presented in Table 97-11 for staging of patients with non-Hodgkin's lymphoma. Patients who present with gastrointestinal tract involvement often have Waldeyer's ring involvement, and vice versa. The 5-year survival for all patients with mantle cell lymphoma is ~25%, with only occasional patients who present with a high IPI score surviving 5 years and ~50% of patients with a low IPI score surviving 5 years.

℞ TREATMENT

Current therapies for mantle cell lymphoma are unsatisfactory. Patients with localized disease might be treated with combination chemotherapy followed by radiotherapy; however, these patients are exceedingly rare. For the usual presentation with disseminated disease, treatments have been unsatisfactory, with the minority of patients achieving complete remission. Aggressive combination chemotherapy regimens followed by autologous or allogeneic bone marrow transplantation are frequently offered to younger patients. For the occasional elderly, asymptomatic patient, observation followed by single-agent chemotherapy might be the most practical approach. An intensive combination chemotherapy regimen originally used in the treatment of acute leukemia, HyperC-VAD (cyclophosphamide, vincristine, doxorubicin, dexamethasone, cytarabine, and methotrexate) in combination with rituximab seems to be associated with better response rates—particularly in younger patients. CHOP plus rituximab has shown better response rates than CHOP alone, but long-term follow-up is lacking.

Follicular Lymphoma Follicular lymphomas make up 22% of non-Hodgkin's lymphomas worldwide and at least 30% of non-Hodgkin's lymphomas diagnosed in the United States. This type of lymphoma can be diagnosed accurately on morphologic findings alone and has been the diagnosis in the majority of patients in therapeutic trials for "low-grade" lymphoma in the past. The clinical characteristics of follicular lymphoma are presented in Table 97-10.

Evaluation of an adequate biopsy by an expert hematopathologist is sufficient to make a diagnosis of follicular lymphoma. The tumor is composed of small cleaved and large cells in varying proportions organized in a follicular pattern of growth (Fig. 97-7). Confirmation of B cell immunophenotype and the existence of the t(14;18) and abnormal expression of BCL-2 protein are confirmatory. The major differential diagnosis is between lymphoma and reactive follicular hyperplasia. The coexistence of diffuse large B cell lymphoma must be considered. Patients with follicular lymphoma are often subclassified into those with predominantly small cells, those with a mixture of small and large cells, and those with predominantly large cells. While this distinction cannot be made simply or very accurately, these subdivisions do have prognostic significance. Patients with follicular lymphoma with predominantly large cells have a higher proliferative fraction, progress more rapidly, and have a shorter overall survival with simple chemotherapy regimens.

The most common presentation for follicular lymphoma is with new, painless lymphadenopathy. Multiple sites of lymphoid involvement are typical, and unusual sites such as epitrochlear nodes are sometimes seen. However, essentially any organ can be involved, and extranodal presentations do occur. Most patients do not have fevers, sweats, or weight loss, and an IPI score of 0 or 1 is found in ~50% of patients. Fewer than 10% of patients have a high (i.e., 4 or 5) IPI score. The staging evaluation for patients with follicular lymphoma should include the studies included in Table 97-11 for the staging of patients with non-Hodgkin's lymphoma.

℞ TREATMENT

Follicular lymphoma is one of the malignancies most responsive to chemotherapy and radiotherapy. In addition, as many as 25% of the patients undergo spontaneous regression—usually transient—when followed without therapy. In an asymptomatic patient, no initial treatment and watchful waiting can be an appropriate management strategy and is particularly likely to be adopted for older patients. For patients who do require treatment, single-agent chlorambucil or cyclophosphamide or combination chemotherapy with CVP or CHOP are most frequently used. With adequate treatment, 50 to 75% of patients will achieve a complete remission. While most patients relapse (median response duration is ~2 years), at least 20% of complete responders

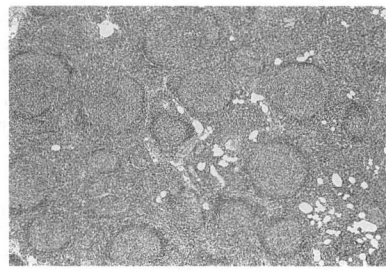

FIGURE 97-7 Follicular lymphoma. The normal nodal architecture is effaced by nodular expansions of tumor cells. Nodules vary in size and contain predominantly small lymphocytes with cleaved nuclei along with variable numbers of larger cells with vesicular chromatin and prominent nucleoli.

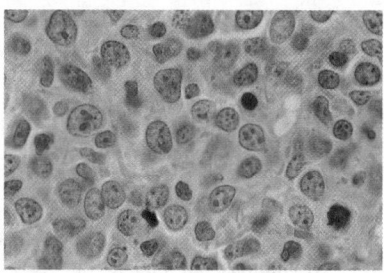

FIGURE 97-8 Diffuse large B cell lymphoma. The neoplastic cells are heterogeneous but predominantly large cells with vesicular chromatin and prominent nucleoli.

will remain in remission for >10 years. For the rare patient with localized follicular lymphoma, involved field radiotherapy produces an excellent treatment result.

A number of new therapies have been shown to be active in the treatment of patients with follicular lymphoma. These include new cytotoxic agents such as fludarabine, and biologic agents such as interferon α, monoclonal antibodies with or without radionuclides, and lymphoma vaccines. In patients treated with a doxorubicin-containing combination chemotherapy regimen, interferon α given to patients in complete remission seems to prolong survival. The monoclonal antibody rituximab can cause objective responses in 35 to 50% of patients with relapsed follicular lymphoma, and radiolabeled antibodies appear to have response rates well in excess of 50%. Trials with tumor vaccines have been encouraging. Both autologous and allogeneic hematopoietic stem cell transplantation yield high complete response rates in patients with relapsed follicular lymphoma, and long-term remissions can occur.

Patients with follicular lymphoma with a predominance of large cells have a shorter survival when treated with single-agent chemotherapy but seem to benefit from receiving an anthracycline-containing combination chemotherapy regimen. When their disease is treated aggressively, the overall survival for such patients is no lower than for patients with other follicular lymphomas, and the failure-free survival is superior.

Patients with follicular lymphoma have a high rate of histologic transformation to diffuse large B cell lymphoma (~7% per year). This is recognized ~40% of the time during the course of the illness by repeat biopsy and is present in almost all patients at autopsy. This transformation is usually heralded by rapid growth of lymph nodes—often localized—and the development of systemic symptoms such as fevers, sweats, and weight loss. Although these patients have a poor prognosis, aggressive combination chemotherapy regimens can sometimes cause a complete remission in the diffuse large B cell lymphoma, often leaving the patient with persisting follicular lymphoma.

Diffuse Large B Cell Lymphoma Diffuse large B cell lymphoma is the most common type of non-Hodgkin's lymphoma, representing approximately one-third of all cases. This lymphoma makes up the majority of cases in previous clinical trials of "aggressive" or "intermediate-grade" lymphoma. The clinical characteristics of diffuse large B cell lymphoma are presented in Table 97-10.

The diagnosis of diffuse large B cell lymphoma can be made accurately by an expert hematopathologist when review of an adequate biopsy and proof of B cell immunophenotype are available (Fig. 97-8). Cytogenetic and molecular genetic studies are not necessary for diagnosis, but some evidence has accumulated that patients who overexpress the BCL-2 protein might be more likely to relapse than others. Patients with prominent mediastinal involvement are sometimes diagnosed as a separate subgroup having primary mediastinal diffuse large B cell lymphoma. This latter group of patients has a younger median age (i.e., 37 years) and a female predominance (66%). Subtypes of diffuse large B cell lymphoma, including those with an immunoblastic subtype and tumors with extensive fibrosis, are recognized by pathologists but do not appear to have important, independent prognostic significance.

Diffuse large B cell lymphoma can present as either primary lymph node disease or at extranodal sites. More than 50% of patients will have some site of extranodal involvement at diagnosis, with the most common sites being the gastrointestinal tract and bone marrow, each being involved in 15 to 20% of patients. Essentially any organ can be involved, making a diagnostic biopsy imperative. For example, diffuse large B cell lymphoma of the pancreas has a much better prognosis than pancreatic carcinoma but would be missed without biopsy. Primary diffuse large B cell lymphoma of the brain is being diagnosed with increasing frequency. Other unusual subtypes of diffuse large B cell lymphoma such as pleural effusion lymphoma and intravascular lymphoma have been difficult to diagnose and associated with a very poor prognosis.

The initial evaluation of patients with diffuse large B cell lymphoma involves the studies presented in Table 97-11 for staging of patients with non-Hodgkin's lymphoma. After a careful staging evaluation, ~50% of patients will be found to have stage I or II disease and ~50% will have widely disseminated lymphoma. Bone marrow biopsy shows involvement by lymphoma in about 15% of cases, with marrow involvement by small cells more frequent than with large cells.

℞ TREATMENT

The initial treatment of all patients with diffuse large B cell lymphoma should be with a combination chemotherapy regimen. The most popular regimen in the United States is CHOP, sometimes in combination with rituximab, although a variety of other anthracycline-containing combination chemotherapy regimens appear to be equally efficacious. Patients with stage I or nonbulky stage II can be effectively treated with three to four cycles of combination chemotherapy followed by involved field radiotherapy. The results are at least equal and probably superior to six to eight cycles of combination therapy, and cure rates of 60 to 70% in stage II disease and 80 to 90% in stage I disease can be expected.

For patients with bulky stage II, stage III, or stage IV, six to eight cycles of a combination chemotherapy regimen such as CHOP, often in combination with rituximab, are usually administered. A large randomized trial showed the superiority of CHOP combined with rituximab over CHOP alone in elderly patients. A frequent approach would be to administer four cycles of therapy and then reevaluate. If the patient has achieved a complete remission after four cycles, two more cycles of treatment might be given and then therapy discontinued. Using this approach, 70% of patients can be expected to achieve a complete remission, and 50 to 70% of complete responders will be cured. The chances for a favorable response to treatment are predicted by the IPI. In fact, the IPI was developed specifically to predict outcome in patients with diffuse large B cell lymphoma. For the 35% of patients with a low IPI score of 0 to 1, the 5-year survival is >70%, while for the 20% of patients with a high IPI score of 4 to 5, the 5-year survival is ~20%. A number of other factors, including molecular features of the tumor, levels of circulating cytokines and soluble receptors, and other surrogate markers, have been shown to influence prognosis. However, they have not been validated as rigorously as the IPI and have not been uniformly applied clinically.

Because a large number of patients with diffuse large B cell lymphoma are either initially refractory to therapy or relapse after apparently effective chemotherapy, nearly half of patients will be candidates for salvage treatment at some point. Alternative combination chemotherapy regimens can induce complete remission in as many as 50% of these patients, but long-term disease-free survival is seen in ≤10%. Autologous bone marrow transplantation has been shown to be superior to salvage chemotherapy at usual doses and leads to long-term disease-free survival in ~40% of patients whose lymphomas remain chemotherapy-sensitive after relapse.

Burkitt's Lymphoma/Leukemia Burkitt's lymphoma/leukemia is a rare disease in adults in the United States, making up <1% of non-Hodgkin's lymphomas, but it makes up ~30% of childhood non-Hodgkin's lymphoma. Burkitt's leukemia, or L3 ALL, makes up a small proportion of childhood and adult acute leukemias. The clinical features of Burkitt's lymphoma occurring in adults are presented in Table 97-10.

Burkitt's lymphoma can be diagnosed morphologically by an expert hematopathologist with a high degree of accuracy. The cells are homogeneous in size and shape (Fig. 97-9). Demonstration of a very high proliferative fraction and the presence of the t(8;14) or one of its variants, t(2;8) (*c-myc* and the λ light chain gene) or t(8;22) (*c-myc* and the κ light chain gene), can be confirmatory. Burkitt's cell leukemia is recognized by the typical monotonous mass of medium-sized cells with round nuclei, multiple nucleoli, and basophilic cytoplasm with cytoplasmic vacuoles. Demonstration of a B cell immunophenotype and one of the above-noted cytogenetic abnormalities is confirmatory.

The three distinct clinical forms of Burkitt's lymphoma that are recognized are endemic, sporadic, and immunodeficiency-associated. Endemic and sporadic Burkitt's lymphomas occur frequently in children in Africa, and the sporadic form in western countries. Immuno-deficiency-associated Burkitt's lymphoma is seen in patients with HIV infection.

Pathologists sometimes have difficulty distinguishing between Burkitt's lymphoma and diffuse large B cell lymphoma. In the past, a separate subgroup of non-Hodgkin's lymphoma intermediate between the two was recognized. When tested, this subgroup could not be diagnosed accurately. Distinction between the two major types of B cell aggressive non-Hodgkin's lymphoma can sometimes be made based on the extremely high proliferative fraction seen in patients with Burkitt's lymphoma (i.e., essentially 100% of tumor cells are in cycle) caused by *c-myc* deregulation.

Most patients in the United States with Burkitt's lymphoma present with peripheral lymphadenopathy or an intraabdominal mass. The disease is typically rapidly progressive and has a propensity to metastasize to the CNS. Initial evaluation should always include an examination of cerebral spinal fluid to rule out metastasis in addition to the other staging evaluations noted in Table 97-11. Once the diagnosis of Burkitt's lymphoma is suspected, a diagnosis must be made promptly and staging evaluation must be accomplished expeditiously. This is the most rapidly progressive human tumor, and any delay in initiating therapy can adversely affect the patient's prognosis.

℞ TREATMENT

Treatment of Burkitt's lymphoma in both children and adults should begin within 48 h of diagnosis and involves the use of intensive combination chemotherapy regimens incorporating high doses of cyclophosphamide. Prophylactic therapy to the CNS is mandatory. Burkitt's

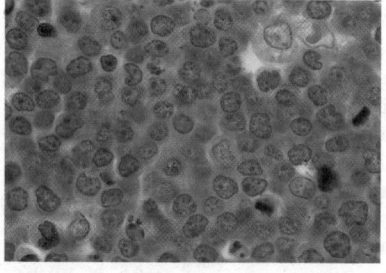

FIGURE 97-9 Burkitt's lymphoma. The neoplastic cells are homogenous, medium-sized B cells with frequent mitotic figures, a morphologic correlate of high growth fraction. Reactive macrophages are scattered through the tumor and their pale cytoplasm in a background of blue-staining tumor cells give the tumor a so-called starry sky appearance.

lymphoma was one of the first cancers shown to be curable by chemotherapy. Today, cure can be expected in 70 to 80% of both children and young adults when effective therapy is administered precisely. Salvage therapy has been generally ineffective in patients failing the initial treatment, emphasizing the importance of the initial treatment approach.

Other B Cell Lymphoid Malignancies *B-cell prolymphocytic leukemia* involves blood and marrow infiltration by large lymphocytes with prominent nucleoli. Patients typically have a high white cell count, splenomegaly, and minimal lymphadenopathy. The chances for a complete response to therapy are poor.

Hairy cell leukemia is a rare disease that presents predominantly in older males. Typical presentation involves pancytopenia, although occasional patients will have a leukemic presentation. Splenomegaly is usual. The malignant cells appear to have "hairy" projections on light and electron microscopy and show a characteristic staining pattern with tartrate-resistant acid phosphatase. Bone marrow is typically not able to be aspirated, and biopsy shows a pattern of fibrosis with diffuse infiltration by the malignant cells. Patients with this disorder are prone to unusual infections including infection by *Mycobacterium avium intracellulare*, and vasculitic syndromes have been described. Hairy cell leukemia is responsive to chemotherapy with interferon α, pentostatin, or cladribine, with the latter being the usually preferred treatment. Clinical complete remissions with cladribine occur in the majority of patients, and long-term disease-free survival is frequent.

Splenic marginal zone lymphoma involves infiltration of the splenic white pulp by small, monoclonal B cells. This is a rare disorder that can present as leukemia as well as lymphoma. Definitive diagnosis is often made at splenectomy, which is also an effective therapy. This is an extremely indolent disorder, but when chemotherapy is required, the most usual treatment has been chlorambucil.

Lymphoplasmacytic lymphoma is the tissue manifestation of Waldenström's macroglobulinemia (Chap. 98). This type of lymphoma has been associated with chronic hepatitis C virus infection, and an etiologic association has been proposed. Patients typically present with lymphadenopathy, splenomegaly, bone marrow involvement, and occasionally peripheral blood involvement. The tumor cells do not express CD5. Patients often have a monoclonal IgM protein, high levels of which can dominate the clinical picture with the symptoms of hyperviscosity. Treatment of lymphoplasmacytic lymphoma can be aimed primarily at reducing the abnormal protein, if present, but will usually also involve chemotherapy. Chlorambucil, fludarabine, and cladribine have been utilized. The median 5-year survival for patients with this disorder is ~60%.

Nodal marginal zone lymphoma, also known as *monocytoid B cell lymphoma*, represents ~1% of non-Hodgkin's lymphomas. This lymphoma has a slight female predominance and presents with disseminated disease (i.e., stage III or IV) in 75% of patients. Approximately one-third of patients have bone marrow involvement, and a leukemic presentation occasionally occurs. The staging evaluation and therapy should use the same approach as used for patients with follicular lymphoma. Approximately 60% of the patients with nodal marginal zone lymphoma will survive 5 years after diagnosis.

PRECURSOR CELL T CELL MALIGNANCIES ■ Precursor T Cell Lymphoblastic Leukemia/Lymphoma Precursor T cell malignancies can present either as ALL or as an aggressive lymphoma. These malignancies are more common in children and young adults, with males more frequently affected than females.

Precursor T cell ALL can present with bone marrow failure, although the severity of anemia, neutropenia, and thrombocytopenia is often less than in precursor B cell ALL. These patients sometimes have very high white cell counts, a mediastinal mass, lymphadenopathy, and hepatosplenomegaly. Precursor T cell lymphoblastic lymphoma is most often found in young men presenting with a large mediastinal mass and pleural effusions. Both presentations have a propensity to metastasize to the CNS, and CNS involvement is often present at diagnosis.

Children with precursor T cell ALL seem to benefit from very intensive remission induction and consolidation regimens. The majority of patients treated in this manner can be cured. Older children and young adults with precursor T cell lymphoblastic lymphoma are also often treated with "leukemia-like" regimens. Patients who present with localized disease have an excellent prognosis. However, advanced age is an adverse prognostic factor. Adults with precursor T cell lymphoblastic lymphoma who present with high LDH levels or bone marrow or CNS involvement are often offered bone marrow transplantation as part of their primary therapy.

MATURE (PERIPHERAL) T CELL DISORDERS ■ Mycosis Fungoides Mycosis fungoides is also known as *cutaneous T cell lymphoma*. This lymphoma is more often seen by dermatologists than internists. The median age of onset is in the mid-fifties, and the disease is more common in males and in blacks.

Mycosis fungoides is an indolent lymphoma with patients often having several years of eczematous or dermatitic skin lesions before the diagnosis is finally established. The skin lesions progress from patch stage to plaque stage to cutaneous tumors. Early in the disease, biopsies are often difficult to interpret, and the diagnosis may only become apparent by observing the patient over time. In advanced stages, the lymphoma can metastasize to lymph nodes and visceral organs. A particular syndrome in patients with this lymphoma involves erythroderma and circulating tumor cells. This is known as *Sézary's syndrome*.

Rare patients with localized early stage mycosis fungoides can be cured with radiotherapy, often total-skin electron beam irradiation. More advanced disease has been treated with topical glucocorticoids, topical nitrogen mustard, phototherapy, psoralen with ultraviolet A (PUVA), electron beam radiation, interferon, antibodies, fusion toxins, and systemic cytotoxic therapy. Unfortunately, these treatments are palliative.

Adult T Cell Lymphoma/Leukemia Adult T cell lymphoma/leukemia is one manifestation of infection by the HTLV-I retrovirus. Patients can be infected through transplacental transmission, blood transfusion, and by sexual transmission of the virus. Patients who acquire the virus from their mother through breast milk are most likely to develop lymphoma, but the risk is still only 2.5% and the latency averages 55 years. Nationwide testing for HTLV-I antibodies and the aggressive implementation of public health measures could theoretically lead to the disappearance of adult T cell lymphoma/leukemia. Tropical spastic paraparesis, another manifestation of HTLV-I infection (Chap. 172), occurs after a shorter latency (1 to 3 years) and is most common in people who acquire the virus during adulthood from transfusion or sex.

The diagnosis of adult T cell lymphoma/leukemia is made when an expert hematopathologist recognizes the typical morphologic picture, a T cell immunophenotype (i.e., CD4 positive) of malignant cells has been demonstrated, and the existence of antibodies to HTLV-I is proven. Examination of the peripheral blood will usually reveal characteristic, pleomorphic abnormal CD4-positive cells with indented nuclei, which have been called "flower" cells (Fig. 97-10).

A subset of patients have a smoldering clinical course and long survival, but most patients present with an aggressive disease mani-

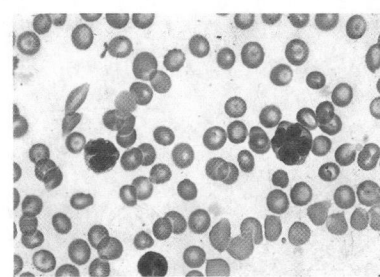

FIGURE 97-10 Adult T cell leukemia/lymphoma. Peripheral blood smear showing leukemia cells with typical "flower-shaped" nucleus.

fested by lymphadenopathy, hepatosplenomegaly, skin infiltration, hypercalcemia, lytic bone lesions, and elevated LDH levels. The skin lesions can be papules, plaques, tumors, and ulcerations. Bone marrow involvement is not usually extensive, and anemia and thrombocytopenia are not usually prominent. Although treatment by combination chemotherapy regimens can result in objective responses, true complete remissions are unusual, and the median survival of patients is about 7 months.

Anaplastic Large T/Null Cell Lymphoma Anaplastic large T/null cell lymphoma was previously usually diagnosed as undifferentiated carcinoma or malignant histiocytosis. Discovery of the CD30, or Ki-1, antigen and the recognition that some patients with previously unclassified malignancies displayed this antigen led to the identification of a new type of lymphoma. Subsequently, discovery of the t(2;5) and the resultant frequent overexpression of the anaplastic lymphoma kinase (ALK) protein confirmed the existence of this entity. This lymphoma accounts for ~2% of all non-Hodgkin's lymphomas. The clinical characteristics of patients with anaplastic large T/null cell lymphoma are presented in Table 97-10.

The diagnosis of anaplastic large T/null cell lymphoma is made when an expert hematopathologist recognizes the typical morphologic picture and a T cell or null cell immunophenotype is demonstrated along with CD30 positivity. Documentation of the t(2;5) and/or overexpression of ALK protein confirm the diagnosis. Some diffuse large B cell lymphomas can also have an anaplastic appearance but have the same clinical course or response to therapy as other diffuse large B cell lymphomas.

Patients with anaplastic large T/cell null cell lymphoma are typically young (median age, 33 years) and male (~70%). Some 50% of patients present in stage I/II, and the remainder with more extensive disease. Systemic symptoms and elevated LDH levels are seen in about one-half of patients. Bone marrow and the gastrointestinal tract are rarely involved, but skin involvement is frequent. Some patients with disease confined to the skin have a different and more indolent disorder that has been termed *cutaneous anaplastic large T/null cell lymphoma* and might be related to lymphomatoid papulosis.

R̶x̶ TREATMENT

Treatment regimens appropriate for other aggressive lymphomas, such as diffuse large B cell lymphoma, should be utilized in patients with anaplastic large T/null cell lymphoma. Surprisingly, given the anaplastic appearance, this disorder has the best survival rate of any aggressive lymphoma. The 5-year survival is >75%. While traditional prognostic factors such as the IPI predict treatment outcome, overexpression of the ALK protein is an important prognostic factor, with patients overexpressing this protein having a superior treatment outcome.

Peripheral T Cell Lymphoma The peripheral T cell lymphomas make up a heterogenous morphologic group of aggressive neoplasms that share a mature T cell immunophenotype. They represent ~7% of all cases of non-Hodgkin's lymphoma. A number of distinct clinical syndromes are included in this group of disorders. The clinical characteristics of patients with peripheral T cell lymphoma are presented in Table 97-10.

The diagnosis of peripheral T cell lymphoma, or any of its specific subtypes, requires an expert hematopathologist, an adequate biopsy, and immunophenotyping. Most peripheral T cell lymphomas are CD4+, but a few will be CD8+, both CD4+ and CD8+, or have an NK cell immunophenotype. No characteristic genetic abnormalities have yet been identified, but translocations involving the T cell antigen receptor genes on chromosomes 7 or 14 may be detected. The differential diagnosis of patients suspected of having peripheral T cell lymphoma includes reactive T cell infiltrative processes. In some cases, demonstration of a monoclonal T cell population using T cell receptor gene rearrangement studies will be required to make a diagnosis.

The initial evaluation of a patient with a peripheral T cell lymphoma should include the studies in Table 97-11 for staging patients with non-Hodgkin's lymphoma. Unfortunately, patients with peripheral T cell lymphoma usually present with adverse prognostic factors, with >80% of patients having an IPI score ≥2 and >30% having an IPI score ≥4. As this would predict, peripheral T cell lymphomas are associated with a poor outcome, and only 25% of the patients survive 5 years after diagnosis. Treatment regimens are the same as those used for diffuse large B cell lymphoma, but patients with peripheral T cell lymphoma have a poorer response to treatment. Because of this poor treatment outcome, hematopoietic stem cell transplantation is often considered early in the care of young patients.

A number of specific clinical syndromes are seen in the peripheral T cell lymphomas. *Angioimmunoblastic T cell lymphoma* is one of the more common subtypes, making up ~20% of T cell lymphomas. These patients typically present with generalized lymphadenopathy, fever, weight loss, skin rash, and polyclonal hypergammaglobulinemia. In some cases, it is difficult to separate patients with a reactive disorder from those with true lymphoma.

Extranodal T/NK cell lymphoma of nasal type has also been called *angiocentric lymphoma* and was previously termed *lethal midline granuloma*. This disorder is more frequent in Asia and South America than in the United States and Europe. Although most frequent in the upper airway, it can involve other organs. The course is aggressive, and patients frequently have the hemophagocytic syndrome. When marrow and blood involvement occur, distinction between this disease and leukemia might be difficult. Some patients will respond to aggressive combination chemotherapy regimens, but the overall outlook is poor.

Enteropathy-type intestinal T cell lymphoma is a rare disorder that occurs in patients with untreated gluten-sensitive enteropathy. Patients are frequently wasted and sometimes present with intestinal perforation. The prognosis is poor. *Hepatosplenic γδ T cell lymphoma* is a systemic illness that presents with sinusoidal infiltration of the liver, spleen, and bone marrow by malignant T cells. Tumor masses generally do not occur. The disease is associated with systemic symptoms and is often difficult to diagnosis. Treatment outcome is poor. *Subcutaneous panniculitis-like T cell lymphoma* is a rare disorder that is often confused with panniculitis. Patients present with multiple subcutaneous nodules, which progress and can ulcerate. Hemophagocytic syndrome is common. Response to therapy is poor. The development of the hemophagocytic syndrome (profound anemia, ingestion of erythrocytes by monocytes and macrophages) in the course of any peripheral T cell lymphoma is generally associated with a fatal outcome.

HODGKIN'S DISEASE ■ **Classic Hodgkin's Disease**   Hodgkin's disease occurs in 7600 patients in the United States each year, and the disease does not appear to be increasing in frequency. Most patients present with palpable lymphadenopathy that is nontender; in most patients, these lymph nodes are in the neck, supraclavicular area, and axilla. More than half the patients will have mediastinal adenopathy at diagnosis, and this is sometimes the initial manifestation. Subdiaphragmatic presentation of Hodgkin's disease is unusual and more common in older males. Approximately one-third of patients present with fevers, night sweats, and/or weight loss—B symptoms in the Ann Arbor staging classification (Table 97-8). Occasionally, Hodgkin's disease can present as a fever of unknown origin. This is more common in older patients who are found to have mixed-cellularity Hodgkin's disease in an abdominal site. Rarely, the fevers persist for days to weeks, followed by afebrile intervals and then recurrence of the fever. This pattern is known as *Pel-Epstein fever*. Hodgkin's disease can occasionally present with unusual manifestations. These include severe and unexplained itching, cutaneous disorders such as erythema nodosum

and ichthyosiform atrophy, paraneoplastic cerebellar degeneration and other distant effects on the CNS, nephrotic syndrome, immune hemolytic anemia and thrombocytopenia, hypercalcemia, and pain in lymph nodes on alcohol ingestion.

The diagnosis of Hodgkin's disease is established by review of an adequate biopsy specimen by an expert hematopathologist. In the United States, most patients would be classified as having nodular sclerosing Hodgkin's disease, with a minority of patients having mixed-cellularity Hodgkin's disease. Lymphocyte-predominant and lymphocyte-depleted Hodgkin's disease are rare. Mixed-cellularity Hodgkin's disease or lymphocyte-depletion Hodgkin's disease are seen more frequently in patients infected by HIV (Fig. 97-11). The differential diagnosis of a lymph node biopsy suspicious for Hodgkin's disease includes inflammatory processes, mononucleosis, non-Hodgkin's lymphoma, phenytoin-induced lymphadenopathy, and nonlymphomatous malignancies.

The staging evaluation for a patient with Hodgkin's disease would typically include a careful history and physical examination; complete blood count; erythrocyte sedimentation rate; serum chemistry studies including LDH; chest radiograph; CT scan of the chest, abdomen, and pelvis; and bone marrow biopsy. Many patients would also have a PET scan or a gallium scan. Although rarely utilized, a bipedal lymphangiogram can be helpful. PET and gallium scans are most useful at the completion of therapy to document remission. Staging laparotomies were once popular for most patients with Hodgkin's disease but are now done rarely because of an increased reliance on systemic rather than local therapy.

℞ TREATMENT

Patients with localized Hodgkin's disease are cured >90% of the time. In patients with good prognostic factors, extended field radiotherapy has a high cure rate. Increasingly, patients with all stages of Hodgkin's disease are treated initially with chemotherapy. Patients with localized or good-prognosis disease receive a brief course of chemotherapy followed by radiotherapy to sites of node involvement. Patients with more extensive disease or those with B symptoms receive a complete course of chemotherapy. The most popular chemotherapy regimens used in the treatment of Hodgkin's disease include doxorubicin, bleomycin, vinblastine, and dacarbazine (ABVD) and mechlorethamine, vincristine, procarbazine, and prednisone (MOPP), or combinations of the drugs in these two regimens. Today, most patients in the United States receive ABVD, but a weekly chemotherapy regimen administered for 12 weeks called *Stanford V* is becoming increasingly popular, but includes radiation therapy, which has been associated with life-threatening late toxicities such as premature coronary artery disease and second solid tumors. In Europe a high-dose regimen called *BEACOPP* incorporating alkylating agents has become popular and might have a better response rate in very high risk patients. Long-term disease-free survival in patients with advanced disease can be achieved in >75% of patients who lack systemic symptoms and in 50 to 70% of patients with systemic symptoms.

Patients who relapse after primary therapy of Hodgkin's disease can frequently still be cured. Patients who relapse after initial treatment only with radiotherapy have an excellent outcome when treated with chemotherapy. Patients who relapse after an effective chemotherapy regimen are usually not curable with subsequent chemotherapy administered at standard doses. However, patients with a long initial

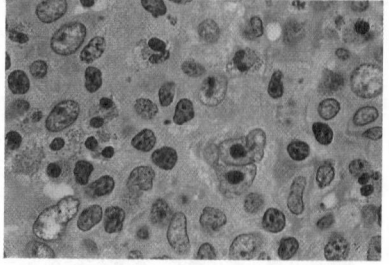

FIGURE 97-11   Mixed cellularity Hodgkin's disease. A Reed-Sternberg cell is present near the center of the field; a large cell with a bilobed nucleus and prominent nucleoli giving an "owl's eyes" appearance. The majority of the cells are normal lymphocytes, neutrophils, and eosinophils that form a pleiomorphic cellular infiltrate.

remission can be an exception to this rule. Autologous bone marrow transplantation can cure half of patients who fail effective chemotherapy regimens.

Because of the very high cure rate in patients with Hodgkin's disease, long-term complications have become a major focus for clinical research. In fact, in some series of patients with early-stage disease, more patients died from late complications of therapy than from Hodgkin's disease itself. This is particularly true in patients with localized disease. The most serious late side effects include second malignancies and cardiac injury. Patients are at risk for the development of acute leukemia in the first 10 years after treatment with combination chemotherapy regimens that contain alkylating agents plus radiation therapy. The risk for development of acute leukemia appears to be greater after MOPP-like regimens than with ABVD. The risk of development of acute leukemia after treatment for Hodgkin's disease is also related to the number of exposures to potentially leukemogenic agents (i.e., multiple treatments after relapse) and the age of the patient being treated, with those >60 years at particularly high risk. The development of carcinomas as a complication of treatment for Hodgkin's disease has become a major problem. These tumors usually occur ≥10 years after treatment and are associated with use of radiotherapy. For this reason, young women treated with thoracic radiotherapy for Hodgkin's disease should institute screening mammograms 5 to 10 years after treatment, and all patients who receive thoracic radiotherapy for Hodgkin's disease should be discouraged from smoking. Thoracic radiation also accelerates coronary artery disease, and patients should be encouraged to minimize risk factors for coronary artery disease such as smoking and elevated cholesterol levels.

A number of other late side effects from the treatment of Hodgkin's disease are well known. Patients who receive thoracic radiotherapy are at very high risk for the eventual development of hypothyroidism and should be observed for this complication; intermittent measurement of thyrotropin should be made to identify the condition before it becomes symptomatic. Lhermitte's syndrome occurs in ~15% of patients who receive thoracic radiotherapy. This syndrome is manifested by an "electric shock" sensation into the lower extremities on flexion of the neck. Infertility is a concern for all patients undergoing treatment for Hodgkin's disease. In both women and men, the risk of permanent infertility is age-related, with younger patients more likely to recover fertility. In addition, treatment with ABVD rather than MOPP increases the chances to retain fertility.

Nodular Lymphocyte-Predominant Hodgkin's Disease Nodular lymphocyte-predominant Hodgkin's disease is now recognized as an entity distinct from classic Hodgkin's disease. Previous classification systems recognized that biopsies from a subset of patients diagnosed as having Hodgkin's disease contained a predominance of small lymphocytes and rare Reed-Sternberg cells. A subset of these patients have tumors with nodular growth pattern and a clinical course that varied from that of patients with classic Hodgkin's disease. This is an unusual clinical entity and represents <5% of cases of Hodgkin's disease.

Nodular lymphocyte-predominant Hodgkin's disease has a number of characteristics that suggest its relationship to non-Hodgkin's lymphoma. These include a clonal proliferation of B cells and a distinctive immunophenotype; tumor cells express J chain and display CD45 and epithelial membrane antigen (ema) and do not express two markers normally found on Sternberg-Reed cells, CD30 and CD15. This lymphoma tends to have a chronic, relapsing course and sometimes transforms to diffuse large B cell lymphoma.

The treatment of patients with nodular lymphocyte-predominant Hodgkin's disease is controversial. Some clinicians favor no treatment and merely close follow-up. In the United States, most physicians will treat localized disease with radiotherapy and disseminated disease with regimens utilized for patients with classic Hodgkin's disease. Regardless of the therapy utilized, most series report a long-term survival of >80%.

LYMPHOMA-LIKE DISORDERS

The most common condition that pathologists and clinicians might confuse with lymphoma is reactive, atypical lymphoid hyperplasia. Patients might have localized or disseminated lymphadenopathy and might have the systemic symptoms characteristic of lymphoma. Underlying causes include a drug reaction to phenytoin or carbamezepine. Immune disorders such as rheumatoid arthritis and lupus erythematosus, viral infections such as cytomegalovirus and EBV, and bacterial infections such as cat-scratch disease may cause adenopathy (Chap. 54). In the absence of a definitive diagnosis after initial biopsy, continued follow-up, further testing, and repeated biopsies, if necessary, are the appropriate approach rather than instituting therapy.

Specific conditions that can be confused with lymphoma include *Castleman's disease*, which can present with localized or disseminated lymphadenopathy; some patients have systemic symptoms. The disseminated form is often accompanied by anemia and polyclonal hypergammaglobulinemia, and the condition has been associated with overproduction of interleukin 6, possibly produced by human herpesvirus 8. Patients with localized disease can be treated effectively with local therapy, while the initial treatment for patients with disseminated disease is usually with systemic glucocorticoids.

Sinus histiocytosis with massive lymphadenopathy (Rosai-Dorfman's disease) usually presents with bulky lymphadenopathy in children or young adults. The disease is usually nonprogressive and self-limited, but patients can manifest autoimmune hemolytic anemia.

Lymphomatoid papulosis is a cutaneous lymphoproliferative disorder that is often confused with anaplastic large-cell lymphoma involving the skin. The cells of lymphomatoid papulosis are similar to those seen in lymphoma and stain for CD30, and T cell receptor gene rearrangements are sometimes seen. However, the condition is characterized by waxing and waning skin lesions that usually heal, leaving small scars. In the absence of effective communication between the clinician and the pathologist regarding the clinical course in the patient, this disease will be misdiagnosed. Since the clinical picture is usually benign, misdiagnosis is a serious mistake.

FURTHER READING

ARMITAGE JO et al: *Text Atlas of Lymphomas*. London, Martin Dunitz, 2002

DIEHL V et al: Hodgkin's lymphoma—diagnosis and treatment. Lancet Oncol 5:19, 2004

HARRIS NL et al: World Health Organization classification of neoplastic diseases of the hematopoietic and lymphoid tissues: Report of the Clinical Advisory Committee Meeting, Airlie House, Virginia, November, 1997. J Clin Oncol 17:3835, 1999

HAUKE RJ, ARMITAGE JO: A new approach to non-Hodgkin's lymphoma. Intern Med 39:197, 2000

ROSENWALD A et al: The use of molecular profiling to predict survival after chemotherapy for diffuse large B cell lymphoma. N Engl J Med 346:1937, 2002

URBA WJ, LONGO DL: Hodgkin's disease. N Engl J Med 326:678, 1992

YUNG L, LINCH D: Hodgkin's lymphoma. Lancet 361:943, 2003

98 | PLASMA CELL DISORDERS
Dan L. Longo, Kenneth C. Anderson

GENERAL PRINCIPLES The *plasma cell disorders* are monoclonal neoplasms related to each other by virtue of their development from common progenitors in the B lymphocyte lineage. Multiple myeloma, Waldenström's macroglobulinemia, primary amyloidosis (Chap. 310), and the heavy chain diseases comprise this group and may be designated by a variety of synonyms such as *monoclonal gammopathies, paraproteinemias, plasma cell dyscrasias*, and *dysproteinemias*. Mature B lymphocytes destined to produce IgG bear surface immunoglobulin molecules of both M and G heavy chain isotypes with both isotypes having identical idiotypes (variable regions). Under normal circumstances, maturation to antibody-secreting plasma cells is stimulated by exposure to the antigen for which the surface immunoglobulin is specific; however, in the plasma cell disorders the control over this process is lost. The clinical manifestations of all the plasma cell disorders relate to the expansion of the neoplastic cells, to the secretion of cell products (immunoglobulin molecules or subunits, lymphokines), and to some extent to the host's response to the tumor. →*Normal development of B lymphocytes is discussed in Chap. 295.*

There are three categories of structural variation among immunoglobulin molecules that form antigenic determinants, and these are used to classify immunoglobulins (Chap. 295). *Isotypes* are those determinants that distinguish among the main classes of antibodies of a given species and are the same in all normal individuals of that species. Therefore, isotypic determinants are, by definition, recognized by antibodies from a distinct species (heterologous sera) but not by antibodies from the same species (homologous sera). There are five heavy chain isotypes (M, G, A, D, E) and two light chain isotypes (κ, λ). *Allotypes* are distinct determinants that reflect regular small differences between individuals of the same species in the amino acid sequences of otherwise similar immunoglobulins. These differences are determined by allelic genes; by definition, they are detected by antibodies made in the same species. *Idiotypes* are the third category of antigenic determinants. They are unique to the molecules produced by a given clone of antibody-producing cells. Idiotypes are formed by the unique structure of the antigen-binding portion of the molecule.

Antibody molecules (Fig. 295-9) are composed of two heavy chains (mol wt ~50,000) and two light chains (mol wt ~25,000). Each chain has a constant portion (limited amino acid sequence variability) and a variable region (extensive sequence variability). The light and heavy chains are linked by disulfide bonds and are aligned so that their variable regions are adjacent to one another. This variable region forms the antigen recognition site of the antibody molecule; its unique structural features form a particular set of determinants, or idiotypes, that are reliable markers for a particular clone of cells because each antibody is formed and secreted by a single clone. Each chain is specified by distinct genes, synthesized separately, and assembled into an intact antibody molecule after translation (Fig. 98-1). Because of the mechanics of the gene rearrangements necessary to specify the immunoglobulin variable regions (VDJ joining for the heavy chain, VJ joining for the light chain), a particular clone rearranges only one of the two chromosomes to produce an immunoglobulin molecule of only one light chain isotype and only one allotype (allelic exclusion). After exposure to antigen, the variable region may become associated with a new heavy chain isotype (class switch). Each clone of cells performs these sequential gene arrangements in a unique way. This results in each clone producing a unique immunoglobulin molecule. In most cells, light chains are synthesized in slight excess, are secreted as free light chains by plasma cells, and are cleared by the kidney, but <10 mg of such light chains is excreted per day.

Electrophoretic analysis of components of the serum proteins permits determination of the amount of immunoglobulin in the serum (Fig. 98-2). The variety of immunoglobulins move heterogeneously in an electric field and form a broad peak in the gamma region. The γ globulin region of the electrophoretic pattern is usually increased in the sera of patients and animals with plasma cell tumors. There is a sharp spike in this region called an *M component* (M for monoclonal). Less commonly, the M component may appear in the β_2 or α_2 globulin region. The antibody must be present at a concentration of at least 5 g/L (0.5 g/dL) to be detectable by this method. This corresponds to approximately 10^9 cells producing the antibody. Confirmation that such an M component is truly monoclonal relies on the use of immunoelectrophoresis that shows a single light and heavy chain type. Hence immunoelectrophoresis and electrophoresis provide qualitative and quantitative assessment of the M component, respectively. Once the presence of an M component has been confirmed, electrophoresis provides the more practical information for managing patients with monoclonal gammopathies. In a given patient, the amount of M component in the serum is a reliable measure of the tumor burden. This makes the M component an excellent tumor marker, yet it is not specific enough to be used to screen asymptomatic patients. In addition

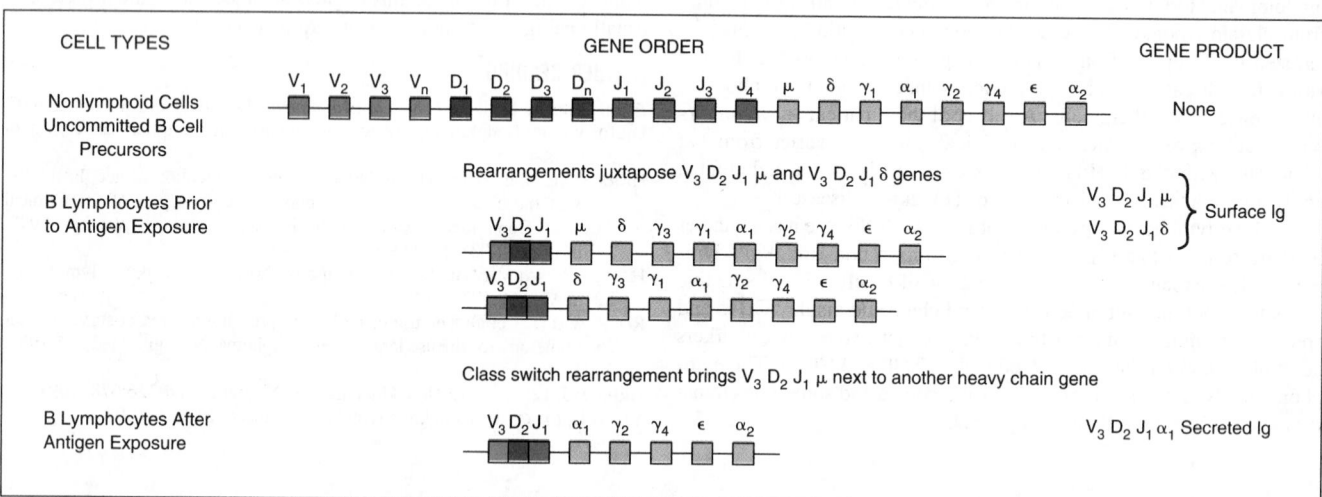

FIGURE 98-1 Immunoglobulin heavy chains are encoded by four distinct genetic elements: variable (Igh-V), diversity (Igh-D), joining (Igh-J), and constant (Igh-C) genes. The variable region of the immunoglobulin heavy chain is encoded by the V, D, and J genes. The same variable region may be associated with any of the 10 heavy chain constant region genes. In the germ-line genome (all cells except B cells) the V, D, and J genes are widely separated and exist in numerous forms. Once a cell becomes committed to B cell differentiation, a single V gene and a single D gene translocate to a single J gene, and the intervening genetic material is excised (VDJ joining). The newly formed VDJ gene is transcribed into a single message along with either an M or D isotype C gene. Upon exposure to antigen, another rearrangement may occur so that the VDJ gene may be associated with a G, A, or E isotype C gene. In light chain genes there appear to be no D genes, and thus light chain variable regions are formed by VJ joining.

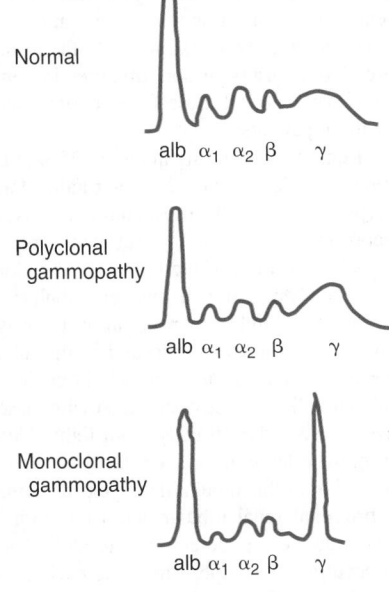

FIGURE 98-2 Representative patterns of serum electrophoresis. The upper panel illustrates the normal pattern of serum protein on electrophoresis. Since there are many different immunoglobulins in the serum, their differing mobilities in an electric field produce a broad peak. In conditions associated with increases in polyclonal immunoglobulin, the broad peak is more prominent (middle panel). In monoclonal gammopathies, the predominance of a product of a single cell produces a "church spire" sharp peak, usually in the γ globulin region (bottom panel).

to the plasma cell disorders, M components may be detected in other lymphoid neoplasms such as chronic lymphocytic leukemia and lymphomas of B or T cell origin; nonlymphoid neoplasms such as chronic myeloid leukemia, breast cancer, and colon cancer; a variety of nonneoplastic conditions such as cirrhosis, sarcoidosis, parasitic diseases, Gaucher disease, and pyoderma gangrenosum; and a number of autoimmune conditions, including rheumatoid arthritis, myasthenia gravis, and cold agglutinin disease. A very rare skin disease known as lichen myxedematosus or papular mucinosis is associated with a monoclonal gammopathy. Highly cationic IgG is deposited in the dermis of patients with this disease. This organ specificity may reflect the specificity of the antibody for some antigenic component of the dermis.

The nature of the M component is variable in plasma cell disorders. It may be an intact antibody molecule of any heavy chain subclass, or it may be an altered antibody or fragment. Isolated light or heavy chains may be produced. In some plasma cell tumors such as extramedullary or solitary bone plasmacytomas, <1/3 of patients will have an M component. In about 20% of myelomas, only light chains are produced and in most cases are secreted in the urine as Bence Jones proteins. The frequency of myelomas of a particular heavy chain class is roughly proportional to the serum concentration, and therefore IgG myelomas are more common than IgA and IgD myelomas.

MULTIPLE MYELOMA ■ Definition Multiple myeloma represents a malignant proliferation of plasma cells derived from a single clone. The terms *multiple myeloma* and *myeloma* may be used interchangeably. The tumor, its products, and the host response to it result in a number of organ dysfunctions and symptoms of bone pain or fracture, renal failure, susceptibility to infection, anemia, hypercalcemia, and occasionally clotting abnormalities, neurologic symptoms, and vascular manifestations of hyperviscosity.

Etiology The cause of myeloma is not known. Myeloma occurred with increased frequency in those exposed to the radiation of nuclear warheads in World War II after a 20-year latency. A variety of chromosomal alterations have been found in patients with myeloma; 13q14 deletions, 17p13 deletions, and 11q abnormalities predominate. The most common translocation is t(11;14)(q13;q32), and evidence is strong that errors in switch recombination—the genetic mechanism to change antibody heavy chain isotype—participate in the transformation pathway. Overexpression of *myc* or *ras* genes has been noted in some cases. Mutations in p53 and Rb-1 have also been described, but no common molecular pathogenesis has yet emerged.

Myeloma has been seen more commonly than expected among farmers, wood workers, leather workers, and those exposed to petroleum products. The neoplastic event in myeloma may involve cells

earlier in B cell differentiation than the plasma cell. Circulating B cells bearing surface immunoglobulin that share the idiotype of the M component are present in myeloma patients. Interleukin (IL) 6 may play a role in driving myeloma cell proliferation; a large fraction of myeloma cells exposed to IL-6 in vitro respond by proliferating. The IL-6 dependency of myeloma is controversial. It remains difficult to distinguish benign from malignant plasma cells on the basis of morphologic criteria in all but a few cases (Fig. 98-3).

Incidence and Prevalence About 15,270 cases of myeloma were diagnosed in 2004, and 11,070 people died from the disease. Myeloma increases in incidence with age. The median age at diagnosis is 68 years; it is rare under age 40. The yearly incidence is around 4 per 100,000 and remarkably similar throughout the world. Males are slightly more commonly affected than females, and blacks have nearly twice the incidence of whites. In the age group over 25 the incidence is 30 per 100,000. Myeloma accounts for about 1% of all malignancies in whites and 2% in blacks; 13% of all hematologic cancers in whites and 33% in blacks.

Pathogenesis and Clinical Manifestations (Table 98-1) Bone pain is the most common symptom in myeloma, affecting nearly 70% of patients. The pain usually involves the back and ribs, and unlike the pain of metastatic carcinoma, which often is worse at night, the pain of myeloma is precipitated by movement. Persistent localized pain in a patient with myeloma usually signifies a pathologic fracture. The bone lesions of myeloma are caused by the proliferation of tumor cells and the activation of osteoclasts that destroy the bone. The osteoclasts respond to osteoclast activating factors (OAF) made by the myeloma cells [OAF activity can be mediated by several cytokines, including IL-1, lymphotoxin, vascular endothelial growth factor (VEGF), receptor activator of NF-κB (RANK) ligand, macrophage inhibitory factor (MIP)-1α, and tumor necrosis factor (TNF)]. However, production of these factors decreases following administration of glucocorticoids or interferon (IFN)-α. The bone lesions are lytic in nature and are rarely associated with osteoblastic new bone formation. Therefore, radioisotopic bone scanning is less useful in diagnosis than is plain radiography. The bony lysis results in substantial mobilization of calcium from bone, and serious acute and chronic complications of hypercalcemia may dominate the clinical picture (see below). Localized bone lesions may expand to the point that mass lesions may be palpated, especially on the skull (Fig. 98-4), clavicles, and sternum, and the collapse of vertebrae may lead to spinal cord compression.

The next most common clinical problem in patients with myeloma is susceptibility to bacterial infections. The most common infections are pneumonias and pyelonephritis, and the most frequent pathogens are *Streptococcus pneumoniae*, *Staphylococcus aureus*, and *Klebsiella pneumoniae* in the lungs and *Escherichia coli* and other gram-negative organisms in the urinary tract. In about 25% of patients, recurrent infections are the presenting features, and over 75% of patients will have a serious infection at some time in their course. The susceptibility to infection has several contributing causes. First, patients with myeloma have diffuse hypogammaglobulinemia if the M component is excluded. The hypogammaglobulinemia is related to both decreased production and increased destruction of normal antibodies. Moreover, some patients generate a population of circulating regulatory cells in response to their myeloma that can suppress normal antibody synthe-

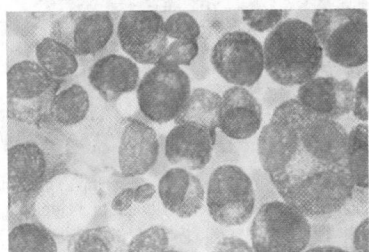

FIGURE 98-3 Multiple myeloma (marrow). The cells bear characteristic morphologic features of plasma cells, round or oval cells with an eccentric nucleus composed of coarsely clumped chromatin, a densely basophilic cytoplasm, and a perinuclear clear zone (hof) containing the Golgi apparatus. Binucleate and multinucleate malignant plasma cells can be seen.

TABLE 98-1 Pathogenesis and Clinical Manifestations of Multiple Myeloma

Clinical Finding	Underlying Cause	Pathogenic Mechanism
Hypercalcemia, pathologic fractures, cord compression, lytic bone lesions, osteoporosis, bone pain	Skeletal destruction	Tumor expansion; production of osteoclast activating factors (OAF) by tumor cells
Renal failure	Light chain proteinuria, hypercalcemia, urate nephropathy, amyloid glomerulopathy (rare) Pyelonephritis	Toxic effects of tumor products, light chains, OAF, DNA breakdown products Hypogammaglobulinemia
Anemia	Myelophthisis, decreased production, increased destruction	Tumor expansion; production of inhibitory factors and autoantibodies by tumor cells
Infection	Hypogammaglobulinemia, decreased neutrophil migration	Decreased production due to tumor-induced suppression; increased IgG catabolism
Neurologic symptoms	Hyperviscosity, cryoglobulins, amyloid deposits Hypercalcemia, cord compression	Products of tumor; properties of M component; light chains OAF
Bleeding	Interference with clotting factors, amyloid damage of endothelium, platelet dysfunction	Products of tumor; antibodies to clotting factors; light chains; antibody coating of platelets
Mass lesions		Tumor expansion

sis. In the case of IgG myeloma, normal IgG antibodies are broken down more rapidly than normal because the catabolic rate for IgG antibodies varies directly with the serum concentration. The large M component results in fractional catabolic rates of 8 to 16% instead of the normal 2%. These patients have very poor antibody responses, especially to polysaccharide antigens such as those on bacterial cell walls. Most measures of T cell function in myeloma are normal, but

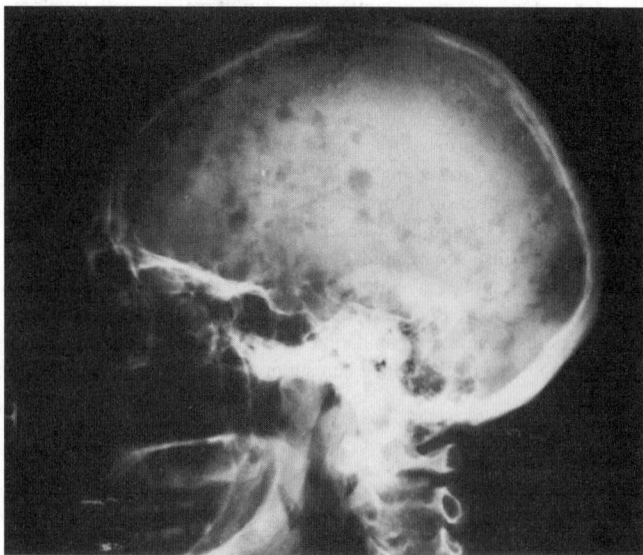

FIGURE 98-4 Bony lesions in multiple myeloma. The skull demonstrates the typical "punched out" lesions characteristic of multiple myeloma. The lesion represents a purely osteolytic lesion with little or no osteoblastic activity. (Courtesy of Dr. Geraldine Schechter.)

a subset of CD4+ cells may be decreased. Granulocyte lysozyme content is low, and granulocyte migration is not as rapid as normal in patients with myeloma, probably the result of a tumor product. There are also a variety of abnormalities in complement functions in myeloma patients. All these factors contribute to the immune deficiency of these patients.

Renal failure occurs in nearly 25% of myeloma patients, and some renal pathology is noted in over half. Many factors contribute to this. Hypercalcemia is the most common cause of renal failure. Glomerular deposits of amyloid, hyperuricemia, recurrent infections, and occasional infiltration of the kidney by myeloma cells all may contribute to renal dysfunction. However, tubular damage associated with the excretion of light chains is almost always present. Normally, light chains are filtered, reabsorbed in the tubules, and catabolized. With the increase in the amount of light chains presented to the tubule, the tubular cells become overloaded with these proteins, and tubular damage results either directly from light chain toxic effects or indirectly from the release of intracellular lysosomal enzymes. The earliest manifestation of this tubular damage is the adult Fanconi syndrome (a type 2 proximal renal tubular acidosis), with loss of glucose and amino acids, as well as defects in the ability of the kidney to acidify and concentrate the urine. The proteinuria is not accompanied by hypertension, and the protein is nearly all light chains. Generally, very little albumin is in the urine because glomerular function is usually normal. When the glomeruli are involved, the proteinuria is nonselective. Patients with myeloma also have a decreased anion gap [i.e., $Na^+ - (Cl^- + HCO_3^-)$] because the M component is cationic, resulting in retention of chloride. This is often accompanied by hyponatremia that is felt to be artificial (pseudohyponatremia) because each volume of serum has less water as a result of the increased protein. Myeloma patients are susceptible to developing acute renal failure if they become dehydrated.

Anemia occurs in about 80% of myeloma patients. It is usually normocytic and normochromic and related both to the replacement of normal marrow by expanding tumor cells and to the inhibition of hematopoiesis by factors made by the tumor. In addition, mild hemolysis may contribute to the anemia. A larger than expected fraction of patients may have megaloblastic anemia due to either folate or vitamin B_{12} deficiency. Granulocytopenia and thrombocytopenia are very rare. Clotting abnormalities may be seen due to the failure of antibody-coated platelets to function properly or to the interaction of the M component with clotting factors I, II, V, VII, or VIII. Raynaud's phenomenon and impaired circulation may result if the M component forms cryoglobulins, and hyperviscosity syndromes may develop depending on the physical properties of the M component (most common with IgM, IgG3, and IgA paraproteins). Hyperviscosity is defined on the basis of the relative viscosity of serum as compared with water. Normal relative serum viscosity is 1.8 (i.e., serum is normally almost twice as viscous as water). Symptoms of hyperviscosity occur at a level of 5 to 6, a level usually reached at paraprotein concentrations of around 40 g/L (4 g/dL) for IgM, 50 g/L (5 g/dL) for IgG3, and 70 g/L (7 g/dL) for IgA.

Although neurologic symptoms occur in a minority of patients, they may have many causes. Hypercalcemia may produce lethargy, weakness, depression, and confusion. Hyperviscosity may lead to headache, fatigue, visual disturbances, and retinopathy. Bony damage and collapse may lead to cord compression, radicular pain, and loss of bowel and bladder control. Infiltration of peripheral nerves by amyloid can be a cause of carpal tunnel syndrome and other sensorimotor mono- and polyneuropathies.

Many of the clinical features of myeloma, e.g., cord compression, pathologic fractures, hyperviscosity, sepsis, and hypercalcemia, can present as medical emergencies. Despite the widespread distribution of plasma cells in the body, tumor expansion is dominantly within bone and bone marrow and, for reasons unknown, rarely causes enlargement of spleen, lymph nodes, or gut-associated lymphatic tissue.

Diagnosis and Staging The classic triad of myeloma is marrow plasmacytosis (>10%), lytic bone lesions, and a serum and/or urine M component. The diagnosis may be made in the absence of bone lesions if the plasmacytosis is associated with a progressive increase in the M component over time or if extramedullary mass lesions develop. There are two important variants of myeloma, solitary bone plasmacytoma and extramedullary plasmacytoma. These lesions are associated with an M component in fewer than 30% of the cases, they may affect younger individuals, and both are associated with median survivals of 10 or more years. Solitary bone plasmacytoma is a single lytic bone lesion without marrow plasmacytosis. Extramedullary plasmacytomas usually involve the submucosal lymphoid tissue of the nasopharynx or paranasal sinuses without marrow plasmacytosis. Both tumors are highly responsive to local radiation therapy. If an M component is present, it should disappear after treatment. Solitary bone plasmacytomas may recur in other bony sites or evolve into myeloma. Extramedullary plasmacytomas rarely recur or progress.

The most difficult differential diagnosis in patients with myeloma involves their separation from individuals with benign monoclonal gammopathies or monoclonal gammopathies of uncertain significance (MGUS). MGUS are vastly more common than myeloma, occurring in 1% of the population over age 50 and in up to 10% over age 75. Patients with MGUS usually have <10% bone marrow plasma cells; <30 g/L (3 g/dL) of M components; no urinary Bence Jones protein; and no anemia, renal failure, lytic bone lesions, or hypercalcemia. When bone marrow cells are exposed to radioactive thymidine in order to quantitate dividing cells, patients with MGUS always have a labeling index <1%; patients with myeloma always have a labeling index >1%. With long-term follow-up, about 1% per year of patients with MGUS go on to develop myeloma. Typically, patients with MGUS require no therapy. Their survival is about 2 years shorter than age-matched controls without MGUS.

The clinical evaluation of patients with myeloma includes a careful physical examination searching for tender bones and masses. Only a small minority of patients has an enlargement of the spleen and lymph nodes, the physiologic sites of antibody production. Chest and bone radiographs may reveal lytic lesions or diffuse osteopenia. MRI offers a sensitive means to document cord or root compression in patients with pain syndromes. A complete blood count with differential may reveal anemia. Erythrocyte sedimentation rate is elevated. Rare patients (~2%) may have plasma cell leukemia with more than 2000 plasma cells/μL. This may be seen in disproportionate frequency in IgD (12%) and IgE (25%) myelomas. Serum calcium, urea nitrogen, creatinine, and uric acid levels may be elevated. Protein electrophoresis and measurement of serum immunoglobulins are useful for detecting and characterizing M spikes, supplemented by immunoelectrophoresis, which is especially sensitive for identifying low concentrations of M components not detectable by protein electrophoresis. A 24-h urine specimen is necessary to quantitate protein excretion, and a concentrated aliquot is used for electrophoresis and immunologic typing of any M component. Serum alkaline phosphatase is usually normal even with extensive bone involvement because of the absence of osteoblastic activity. It is also important to quantitate serum β_2-microglobulin (see below). Serum soluble IL-6 receptor levels and C-reactive protein may reflect physiologic IL-6 levels in the patient.

The serum M component will be IgG in 53% of patients, IgA in 25%, and IgD in 1%; 20% of patients will have only light chains in serum and urine. Dipsticks for detecting proteinuria are not reliable at identifying light chains, and the heat test for detecting Bence Jones protein is falsely negative in about 50% of patients with light chain myeloma. Fewer than 1% of patients have no identifiable M component; these patients usually have light chain myelomas in which renal catabolism has made the light chains undetectable in the urine. IgD myeloma may also present as light chain myeloma. About two-thirds of patients with serum M components also have urinary light chains. The light chain isotype may have an impact on survival. Patients secreting lambda light chains have a significantly shorter overall survival than those secreting kappa light chains. It is not clear whether this is due to some genetically important determinant of cell proliferation or

because lambda light chains are more likely to cause renal damage and form amyloid than are kappa light chains. The heavy chain isotype may have an impact on patient management as well. About half of patients with IgM paraproteins develop hyperviscosity compared with only 2 to 4% of patients with IgA and IgG M components. Among IgG myelomas, it is the IgG3 subclass that has the highest tendency to form both concentration- and temperature-dependent aggregates, leading to hyperviscosity and cold agglutination at lower serum concentrations.

The staging system for patients with myeloma is a functional system for predicting survival and is based on a variety of clinical and laboratory tests, unlike the anatomic staging systems for solid tumors. Details of the staging system are given in Table 98-2. Based on the hemoglobin, calcium, M component, and degree of skeletal involvement, the total-body tumor burden is estimated to be low (stage I, $<0.6 \times 10^{12}$ cells/m^2), intermediate (stage II, 0.6 to 1.2×10^{12} cells/ m^2), or high (stage III, $>1.2 \times 10^{12}$ cells/m^2), and the stages are further subdivided on the basis of renal function [A if serum creatinine <177 mol/L (<2 mg/dL), B if >177 (>2). Patients in stage IA have a median survival of more than 5 years and those in stage IIIB about 15 months. β_2-Microglobulin is a protein of 11,000 mol wt with homologies with the constant region of immunoglobulins that is the light chain of the class I major histocompatibility antigens (HLA-A, -B, -C) on the surface of every cell. Serum β_2-microglobulin is the single most powerful predictor of survival and can substitute for staging. Patients with β_2-microglobulin levels <0.004 g/L have a median survival of 43 months and those with levels >0.004 g/L only 12 months. It is also felt that once the diagnosis of myeloma is firm, histologic features of atypia may also exert an influence on prognosis. IL-6 may be an autocrine and/or paracrine growth factor for myeloma cells; el-

TABLE 98-2 *Myeloma Staging System*

Stage	Criteria	Estimated Tumor Burden, $\times 10^{12}$ cells/m^2

I	All of the following:
	1. Hemoglobin >100 g/L (>10 g/dL)
	2. Serum calcium <3 mmol/L (<12 mg/dL)
	3. Normal bone x-ray or solitary lesion
	4. Low M-component production
	   a. IgG level <50 g/L (<5 g/dL)
	   b. IgA level <30 g/L (<3 g/dL)
	   c. Urine light chain <4 g/24 h
		<0.6 (low)

II	Fitting neither I nor III	0.6–1.20 (intermediate)

III	One or more of the following:
	1. Hemoglobin <85 g/L (<8.5 g/dL)
	2. Serum calcium >3 mmol/L (>12 mg/dL)
	3. Advanced lytic bone lesions
	4. High M-component production
	   a. IgG level >70 g/L (>7 g/dL)
	   b. IgA level >50 g/L (>5 g/dL)
	   c. Urine light chains >12 g/24 h
		>1.20 (high)

Level	Stage	Median Survival, Months
SUBCLASSIFICATION BASED ON SERUM CREATININE LEVELS		
A < 177 μmol/L (<2 mg/dL)	IA	61
B > 177 μmol/L (>2 mg/dL)	IIA,B	55
	IIIA	30
	IIIB	15
STAGING BASED ON SERUM β_2-MICROGLOBULIN LEVELS		
<0.004 g/L (<4 μg/mL)	I	43
>0.004 g/L (>4 μg/mL)	II	12

evated levels are associated with more aggressive disease. High labeling index and high levels of lactate dehydrogenase and thymidine kinase are also associated with poor prognosis.

Other factors that may influence prognosis are the number of cytogenetic abnormalities, chromosome 13q deletion, % plasma cells in the marrow, circulating plasma cells, performance status, and serum levels of IL-6, soluble IL-6 receptors, C-reactive protein, hepatocyte growth factor, C-terminal cross-linked telopeptide of collagen I, TGF-β, and syndecan-1.

℞ TREATMENT

About 10% of patients with myeloma will have an indolent course demonstrating only very slow progression of disease over many years. Such patients only require antitumor therapy when the serum myeloma protein level rises above 50 g/L (5 g/dL) or progressive bone lesions develop. Patients with solitary bone plasmacytomas and extramedullary plasmacytomas may be expected to enjoy prolonged disease-free survival after local radiation therapy to a dose of around 40 Gy. There is a low incidence of occult marrow involvement in patients with solitary bone plasmacytoma. Such patients are usually detected because their serum M component falls slowly or disappears initially only to return after a few months. These patients respond well to systemic chemotherapy.

The vast majority of patients with myeloma require therapeutic intervention. In general such therapy is of two sorts: systemic chemotherapy to control the progression of myeloma, and symptomatic supportive care to prevent serious morbidity from the complications of the disease. All patients with stage II or III disease and stage I patients exhibiting Bence Jones proteinuria, progressive lytic bone lesions, vertebral compression fractures, recurrent infections, or rising serum M component should be treated with systemic combination chemotherapy. Therapy can prolong and improve the quality of life for myeloma patients.

The standard treatment has consisted of intermittent pulses of an alkylating agent [L-phenylalanine mustard (L-PAM, melphalan), cyclophosphamide, or chlorambucil] and prednisone administered for 4 to 7 days every 4 to 6 weeks. The alkylating agents appear to be roughly equally active, but resistance to one agent is often accompanied by resistance to the others. The usual doses are as follows: melphalan, 8 mg/m^2 per day; cyclophosphamide, 200 mg/m^2 per day; chlorambucil, 8 mg/m^2 per day; prednisone, 25 to 60 mg/m^2 per day. Melphalan is used most commonly, but because of their near equivalence in antitumor efficacy, we favor cyclophosphamide as the alkylating agent because it is less toxic to the marrow stem cell compartment and results in a lower incidence of myelodysplastic syndromes than do the other alkylating agents. Doses may need adjustment based on marrow tolerance. However, there are few constraints on the dose of the steroid pulse, and it appears that more is better. Patients responding to therapy generally have a prompt and gratifying reduction in bone pain, hypercalcemia, and anemia, and often have fewer infections. The serum M component lags substantially behind the symptomatic improvement, often taking 4 to 6 weeks to fall. This fall depends on the rate of tumor kill and the fractional catabolic rate of immunoglobulin, which in turn depends on the serum concentration (for IgG). Light chain excretion, with a functional half-life of approximately 6 h, may fall within the first week of treatment. However, since urine light chain levels may relate to renal tubular function, they are not a reliable measure of tumor cell kill. Calculations of tumor cell kill are made by extrapolation of the serum M component level and rely heavily on the assumption that every tumor cell produces immunoglobulin at a constant rate. About 60% of patients will achieve at least a 75% reduction in serum M component level and tumor cell mass in response to an alkylating agent and prednisone. Although this is a tumor reduction of less than 1 log, clinical responses may last many months. The important feature of the level of the M protein is

not how far or how fast it falls, but the rate of its increase after therapy. Efforts to improve the fraction of patients responding and the degree of response have involved adding other active chemotherapeutic agents to the treatment program. Patients with more advanced disease may benefit most from such an approach. High-dose therapy with hematopoietic stem cell support can modestly extend progression-free and overall survival but few, if any, patients are cured. Sequential treatment with combination chemotherapy regimens followed by two successive high-dose melphalan treatments, each supported with peripheral blood stem cell transplants, have achieved complete responses in 50% of patients treated within a year of diagnosis. Complete responses are rare (<10%) with standard therapy. Long-term follow-up is not yet available. Allogeneic transplants may also produce high response rates, but treatment-related mortality may be as high as 40%. Nonmyeloablative allogeneic transplantation is now under evaluation to reduce toxicity while permitting an immune graft-vs-tumor effect.

The ideal duration of therapy has not been determined. Most physicians treat every 4 to 6 weeks for 1 or 2 years. Cessation of therapy is followed by relapse, usually within a year. Retreatment may be associated with a second response in up to 80% of patients. Maintenance therapy (e.g., with IFN-α) may prolong the duration of response, but this therapy is toxic and has generally not prolonged survival. Oral prednisone maintenance therapy appears to improve response duration and survival. The regrowth rate of the tumor during relapse accelerates with each relapse. This observation suggests that kinetic resistance to therapy (i.e., increase in cycling cells) is perhaps more important than drug resistance controlled by mdr-1 expression. Patients often respond to treatment, but the length of the response progressively shortens. Patients primarily resistant to initial therapy have a median survival of less than a year. High-dose pulsed glucocorticoids used alone (200 mg prednisone every other day or 1 g/m^2 per day methylprednisolone for 5 days) or VAD combination chemotherapy (vincristine, 0.4 mg/d in a 4-day continuous infusion; doxorubicin, 9 mg/m^2 per day in a 4-day continuous infusion; dexamethasone, 40 mg/d for 4 days per week for 3 weeks) may offer useful palliation in patients resistant to primary therapy. High-dose melphalan has activity in patients with refractory disease. Thalidomide, which inhibits angiogenesis, also produces responses in refractory cases, but at doses that may cause somnolence. Novel agents, including immunomodulatory derivatives of thalidomide (IMIDs) and the proteasome inhibitor, PS-341, target not only the tumor cell but also the tumor cell-bone marrow interaction and production of myeloma growth, survival, drug resistance, and migration factors. These agents can achieve responses in relapsed refractory disease and are under evaluation for efficacy earlier in the disease course.

About 15% of patients die within the first 3 months after diagnosis; subsequently, the death rate is about 15% per year. The disease usually follows a chronic course for 2 to 5 years before developing an acute terminal phase, usually marked by the development of pancytopenia with a cellular marrow that is refractory to treatment. Widespread organ infiltration by myeloma cells occurs, and survival is less than 6 months. About 46% of patients die in the chronic phase of disease from progressive myeloma (16%) and renal failure (10%), sepsis (14%), or both (6%). Death in the acute terminal phase (26%) is chiefly from progressive myeloma (13%) and sepsis (9%). Five percent of patients die of acute leukemia, myeloblastic or monocytic. Although it has been debated that this is related to the primary disease, it appears more likely to be the result of chronic therapy with alkylating agents. Nearly 23% of patients die of myocardial infarction, chronic lung disease, diabetes, or stroke, all intercurrent illnesses related more to the age of the patient group than to the tumor.

Supportive care directed at the anticipated complications of the disease may be as important as primary antitumor therapy. The hypercalcemia generally responds well to bisphosphonates, glucocorticoid therapy, hydration, and natriuresis. Calcitonin may add to the inhibitory effects of steroids on bone resorption. Bisphosphonates (e.g., pamidronate 90 mg or zoledronate 4 mg once a month) reduce osteoclastic bone resorption and preserve performance status and quality of life; antitumor effects are also possible. Treatments aimed at strengthening the skeleton, such as fluorides, calcium, and vitamin D, with or without androgens, have been suggested but are not of proven efficacy. Iatrogenic worsening of renal function may be prevented by the use of allopurinol during chemotherapy to avoid urate nephropathy and by maintaining a high fluid intake to prevent dehydration and to help excrete light chains and calcium. In the event of acute renal failure, plasmapheresis is approximately 10 times more effective at clearing light chains than peritoneal dialysis, and acutely reducing the protein load may result in functional improvement. Urinary tract infections should be watched for and treated early. Chronic dialysis probably should not be initiated in patients who have failed to respond to antitumor therapy. Plasmapheresis may be the treatment of choice for hyperviscosity syndromes. Although the pneumococcus is a dreaded pathogen in myeloma patients, pneumococcal polysaccharide vaccines may not elicit an antibody response. Prophylactic administration of intravenous γ globulin preparations is used in the setting of recurrent serious infections. Chronic oral antibiotic prophylaxis is probably not warranted. Patients developing neurologic symptoms in the lower extremities, severe localized back pain, or problems with bowel and bladder control may need emergency myelography and radiation therapy for palliation. Most bone lesions respond to analgesics and chemotherapy, but certain painful lesions may respond most promptly to localized radiation. The chronic anemia may respond to hematinics (iron, folate, cobalamin), and some have responded to androgens. The pathogenesis of the anemia should be established and specific therapy instituted, where possible. In the setting of renal disease and low serum erythropoietin levels, erythropoietin is useful to increase red cell mass.

WALDENSTRÖM'S MACROGLOBULINEMIA In 1948, Waldenström described a malignancy of lymphoplasmacytoid cells that secreted IgM. In contrast to myeloma, the disease was associated with lymphadenopathy and hepatosplenomegaly, but the major clinical manifestation was the hyperviscosity syndrome. The disease resembles the related diseases chronic lymphocytic leukemia, myeloma, and lymphocytic lymphoma. Waldenström's macroglobulinemia and IgM myeloma both follow a similar clinical course. The diagnosis of IgM myeloma is usually reserved for patients with lytic bone lesions and is important only because of the hazard of pathologic fractures.

The cause of macroglobulinemia is unknown. The disease is similar to myeloma in being slightly more common in men and occurring with increased incidence with age (median 64 years). There have been reports that the IgM in some patients with macroglobulinemia may have specificity for myelin-associated glycoprotein (MAG), a protein that has been associated with demyelinating disease of the peripheral nervous system and may be lost earlier and to a greater extent than the better known myelin basic protein in patients with multiple sclerosis. Sometimes patients with macroglobulinemia develop a peripheral neuropathy before the appearance of the neoplasm. There is speculation that the whole process begins with a viral infection that may elicit an antibody response that cross-reacts with a normal tissue component.

Like myeloma, the disease involves the bone marrow, but unlike myeloma, it does not cause bone lesions or hypercalcemia. Like myeloma, a serum M component is present in the serum in excess of 30 g/L (3 g/dL), but unlike myeloma, the size of the IgM paraprotein results in little renal excretion and only around 20% of patients excrete light chains. Therefore, renal disease is not common. The light chain isotype is kappa in 80% of the cases. Patients present with weakness, fatigue, and recurrent infections, similar to myeloma patients, but epistaxis, visual disturbances, and neurologic symptoms such as peripheral neuropathy, dizziness, headache, and transient paresis are much more common in macroglobulinemia. Physical examination reveals adenopathy and hepatosplenomegaly, and ophthalmoscopic examination may reveal vascular segmentation and dilatation of the retinal veins characteristic of hyperviscosity states. Patients may have a normocytic, normochromic anemia, but rouleaux formation and a positive Coombs' test are much more common than in myeloma. Malignant

lymphocytes are usually present in the peripheral blood. About 10% of macroglobulins are cryoglobulins. These are pure M components and are not the mixed cryoglobulins seen in rheumatoid arthritis and other autoimmune diseases. Mixed cryoglobulins are composed of IgM or IgA complexed with IgG, for which they are specific. In both cases, Raynaud's phenomenon and serious vascular symptoms precipitated by the cold may occur, but mixed cryoglobulins are not commonly associated with malignancy. Patients suspected of having a cryoglobulin based on history and physical examination should have their blood drawn into a warm syringe and delivered to the laboratory in a container of warm water to avoid errors in quantitating the cryoglobulin.

℞ TREATMENT

Control of serious hyperviscosity symptoms such as an altered state of consciousness or paresis can be achieved acutely by plasmapheresis because 80% of the IgM paraprotein is intravascular. Fludarabine (25 mg/m^2 per day for 5 days every 4 weeks) or cladribine (0.1 mg/kg per day for 7 days every 4 weeks) are highly effective single agents. About 80% of patients respond to chemotherapy, and their median survival is over 3 years. Rituximab (anti-CD20) can produce responses alone or combined with chemotherapy. The absence of other serious organ toxicities results in a longer life span of patients with macroglobulinemia compared with those with myeloma.

POEMS SYNDROME The features of this syndrome are *p*olyneuropathy, *o*rganomegaly, *e*ndocrinopathy, *m*ultiple myeloma, and *s*kin changes (POEMS). Patients usually have a severe, progressive sensorimotor polyneuropathy associated with sclerotic bone lesions from myeloma. Polyneuropathy occurs in about 1.4% of myelomas, but the POEMS syndrome is only a rare subset of that group. Unlike typical myeloma, hepatomegaly and lymphadenopathy occur in about two-thirds of patients, and splenomegaly is seen in one-third. The lymphadenopathy frequently resembles Castleman's disease histologically, a condition that has been linked to IL-6 overproduction. The endocrine manifestations include amenorrhea in women and impotence and gynecomastia in men. Hyperprolactinemia due to loss of normal inhibitory control by the hypothalamus may be associated with other central nervous system manifestations such as papilledema and elevated cerebrospinal fluid pressure and protein. Type 2 diabetes mellitus occurs in about one-third of patients. Hypothyroidism and adrenal insufficiency are occasionally noted. Skin changes are diverse: hyperpigmentation, hypertrichosis, skin thickening, and digital clubbing. Other manifestations include peripheral edema, ascites, pleural effusions, fever, and thrombocytosis.

The pathogenesis of the disease is unclear, but high circulating levels of the proinflammatory cytokines IL-1, IL-6, VEGF, and TNF have been documented and levels of the inhibitory cytokine transforming growth factor (TGF-β) are lower than expected. Treatment of the myeloma may result in an improvement in the other disease manifestations.

HEAVY CHAIN DISEASES The heavy chain diseases are rare lymphoplasmacytic malignancies. Their clinical manifestations vary with the heavy chain isotype. Patients secrete a defective heavy chain that usually has an intact Fc fragment and a deletion in the Fd region. Gamma, alpha, and mu heavy chain diseases have been described, but no reports of delta or epsilon heavy chain diseases have appeared. Molecular biologic analysis of these tumors has revealed structural genetic defects that may account for the aberrant chain secreted.

Gamma Heavy Chain Disease (Franklin's Disease) This disease affects people of widely different age groups and countries of origin. It is characterized by lymphadenopathy, fever, anemia, malaise, hepatosplenomegaly, and weakness. Its most distinctive symptom is palatal edema, resulting from node involvement of Waldeyer's ring, and this may progress to produce respiratory compromise. The diagnosis depends on the demonstration of an anomalous serum M component [often <20 g/L (<2 g/dL) that reacts with anti-IgG but not anti-light chain reagents. *The M component is typically present in both serum and urine.* Most of the paraproteins have been of the gamma$_1$ subclass, but other subclasses have been seen. The patients may have thrombocytopenia, eosinophilia, and nondiagnostic bone marrow. Patients usually have a rapid downhill course and die of infection; however, some patients have survived 5 years with chemotherapy.

Alpha Heavy Chain Disease (Seligmann's Disease)

This is the most common of the heavy chain diseases. It is closely related to a malignancy known as *Mediterranean lymphoma*, a disease that affects young people in parts of the world where intestinal parasites are common, such as the Mediterranean, Asia, and South America. The disease is characterized by an infiltration of the lamina propria of the small intestine with lymphoplasmacytoid cells that secrete truncated alpha chains. Demonstrating alpha heavy chains is difficult because the alpha chains tend to polymerize and appear as a smear instead of a sharp peak on electrophoretic profiles. Despite the polymerization, hyperviscosity is not a common problem in alpha heavy chain disease. Without J chain–facilitated dimerization, viscosity does not increase dramatically. Light chains are absent from serum and urine. The patients present with chronic diarrhea, weight loss, and malabsorption and have extensive mesenteric and para-aortic adenopathy. Respiratory tract involvement occurs rarely. Patients may vary widely in their clinical course. Some may develop diffuse aggressive histologies of malignant lymphoma. Chemotherapy may produce long-term remissions. Rare patients appear to have responded to antibiotic therapy, raising the question of the etiologic role of antigenic stimulation, perhaps by some chronic intestinal infection. Chemotherapy plus antibiotics may be more effective than chemotherapy alone.

Mu Heavy Chain Disease

The secretion of isolated mu heavy chains into the serum appears to occur in a very rare subset of patients with chronic lymphocytic leukemia. The only features that may distinguish patients with mu heavy chain disease are the presence of vacuoles in the malignant lymphocytes and the excretion of kappa light chains in the urine. The diagnosis requires ultracentrifugation or gel filtration to confirm the nonreactivity of the paraprotein with the light chain reagents, because some intact macroglobulins fail to interact with these serums. The tumor cells seem to have a defect in the assembly of light and heavy chains, because they appear to contain both in their cytoplasm. There is no evidence that such patients should be treated differently from other patients with chronic lymphocytic leukemia (Chap. 97).

FURTHER READING

BARLOGIE B et al: Treatment of myeloma. Blood 103:20, 2004

BERENSON JR et al: Maintenance therapy with alternate-day prednisone improves survival in multiple myeloma patients. Blood 99:3163, 2002

BERENSON JR et al: American Society of Clinical Oncology clinical practice guidelines: The role of bisphosphonates in multiple myeloma. J Clin Oncol 20:3719, 2002

GHOBRIAL IM et al: Waldenstrom macroglobulinaemia. Lancet Oncol 4:679, 2003

HIDESHIMA T, ANDERSON KC: Novel therapeutic approaches for multiple myeloma. Nature Rev Cancer 2:927, 2002

KUEHL WM, BERGSAGEL PL: Multiple myeloma: Evolving genetic events and host interactions. Nature Rev Cancer 2:175, 2002

KYLE RA et al: A long-term study of prognosis in monoclonal gammopathy of undetermined significance. N Engl J Med 346:564, 2002

KYLE RA et al: Review of 1027 patients with newly diagnosed multiple myeloma. Mayo Clin Proc 78:21, 2003

WAHNER-ROEDLER DL et al: Gamma-heavy chain disease: review of 23 cases. Medicine 82:236, 2003

---

99 TRANSFUSION BIOLOGY AND THERAPY
Jeffery S. Dzieczkowski, Kenneth C. Anderson

BLOOD GROUP ANTIGENS AND ANTIBODIES

The study of red blood cell (RBC) antigens and antibodies forms the foundation of transfusion medicine. Serologic studies initially characterized these antigens, but now the molecular composition and structure of many are known. Antigens, either carbohydrate or protein, are assigned to a blood group system based upon the structure and similarity of the determinant epitopes. Other cellular blood elements and plasma proteins are also antigenic and can result in *alloimmunization*, the production of antibodies directed against the blood group antigens of another individual. These antibodies are called *alloantibodies*.

Antibodies directed against RBC antigens may result from "natural" exposure, particularly to carbohydrates that mimic some blood group antigens. Those antibodies that occur via natural stimuli are usually produced by a T cell–independent response (thus, generating no memory) and are IgM isotype. *Autoantibodies* (antibodies against autologous blood group antigens) arise spontaneously or as the result of infectious sequelae (e.g., from *Mycoplasma pneumoniae*) and are also often IgM. These antibodies are often clinically insignificant due to their low affinity for antigen at body temperature. However, IgM antibodies can activate the complement cascade and result in hemolysis. Antibodies that result from allogeneic exposure, such as transfusion or pregnancy, are usually IgG. IgG antibodies commonly bind to antigen at warmer temperatures and may hemolyze RBCs. Unlike IgM antibodies, IgG antibodies can cross the placenta and bind fetal erythrocytes bearing the corresponding antigen, resulting in hemolytic disease of the newborn, or *hydrops fetalis*.

Alloimmunization to leukocytes, platelets, and plasma proteins may also result in transfusion complications such as fevers and urticaria but generally does not cause hemolysis. Assay for these other alloantibodies is not routinely performed; however, they may be detected using special assays.

ABO ANTIGENS AND ANTIBODIES The first blood group antigen system, recognized in 1900, was ABO, the most important in transfusion medicine. The major blood groups of this system are A, B, AB, and O. O type RBCs lack A or B antigens. These antigens are carbohydrates attached to a precursor backbone, may be found on the cellular membrane either as glycosphingolipids or glycoproteins, and are secreted into plasma and body fluids as glycoproteins. H substance is the immediate precursor upon which the A and B antigens are added. This H substance is formed by the addition of fucose to the glycolipid or glycoprotein backbone. The subsequent addition of *N*-acetylgalactosamine creates the A antigen, while the addition of galactose produces the B antigen.

The genes that determine the A and B phenotypes are found on chromosome 9p and are expressed in a Mendelian codominant manner. The gene products are glycosyl transferases, which confer the enzymatic capability of attaching the specific antigenic carbohydrate. Individuals who lack the "A" and "B" transferases are phenotypically type "O," while those who inherit both transferases are type "AB." Rare individuals lack the H gene, which codes for fucose transferase, and cannot form H substance. These individuals are homozygous for the silent h allele (hh) and have Bombay phenotype (O_h).

The ABO blood group system is important because essentially all individuals produce antibodies to the ABH carbohydrate antigen that they lack. The naturally occurring anti-A and anti-B antibodies are termed *isoagglutinins*. Thus, type A individuals produce anti-B, while type B individuals make anti-A. Neither isoagglutinin is found in type AB individuals, while type O individuals produce both anti-A and anti-B. Thus, persons with type AB are "universal recipients" because they do not have antibodies against any ABO phenotype, while persons with type O blood can donate to essentially all recipients because their cells are not recognized by any ABO isoagglutinins. The rare individuals with Bombay phenotype produce antibodies to H substance (which is present on all red cells except those of hh phenotype) as well as to both A and B antigens and are therefore compatible only with other hh donors.

In most people, A and B antigens are secreted by the cells and are present in the circulation. Nonsecretors are susceptible to a variety of infections (e.g., *Candida albicans, Neisseria meningitidis, Streptococcus pneumoniae, Haemophilus influenzae*) as many organisms may bind to polysaccharides on cells. Soluble blood group antigens may block this binding.

Rh SYSTEM The Rh system is the second most important blood group system in pretransfusion testing. The Rh antigens are found on a 30- to 32-kDa RBC membrane protein that has no defined function. Although >40 different antigens in the Rh system have been described, five determinants account for the vast majority of phenotypes. The presence of the D antigen confers Rh "positivity," while persons who lack the D antigen are Rh negative. Two allelic antigen pairs, E/e and C/c, are also found on the Rh protein. The three Rh genes, E/e, D, and C/c, are arranged in tandem on chromosome 1 and inherited as a haplotype, i.e., cDE or Cde. Two haplotypes can result in the phenotypic expression of two to five Rh antigens.

The D antigen is a potent alloantigen. About 15% of individuals lack this antigen. Exposure of these Rh-negative people to even small amounts of Rh-positive cells, by either transfusion or pregnancy, can result in the production of anti-D alloantibody.

OTHER BLOOD GROUP SYSTEMS AND ALLOANTIBODIES More than 100 blood group systems are recognized, composed of more than 500 antigens. The presence or absence of certain antigens has been associated with various diseases and anomalies; antigens also act as receptors for infectious agents. Alloantibodies of importance in routine clinical practice are listed in Table 99-1.

Antibodies to *Lewis system* carbohydrate antigens are the most common cause of incompatibility during pretransfusion screening. The Lewis gene product is a fucosyl transferase and maps to chromosome 19. The antigen is not an integral membrane structure but is adsorbed to the RBC membrane from the plasma. Antibodies to Lewis antigens are usually IgM and cannot cross the placenta. Lewis antigens may be adsorbed onto tumor cells and may be targets of therapy.

I system antigens are also oligosaccharides related to H, A, B, and Le. I and i are not allelic pairs but are carbohydrate antigens that differ only in the extent of branching. The i antigen is an unbranched chain that is converted by the I gene product, a glycosyltransferase, into a branched chain. The branching process affects all the ABH antigens, which become progressively more branched in the first 2 years of life. Some patients with cold agglutinin disease or lymphomas can produce anti-I autoantibodies that cause RBC destruction. Occasional patients with mononucleosis or *Mycoplasma* pneumonia may develop cold agglutinins of either anti-I or anti-i specificity. Most adults lack i expression; thus, finding a donor for patients with anti-i is not difficult.

Even though most adults express I antigen, binding is generally low at body temperature. Thus, administration of warm blood prevents isoagglutination.

The *P system* is another group of carbohydrate antigens controlled by specific glycosyltransferases. Its clinical significance is in rare cases of syphilis and viral infection that lead to paroxysmal cold hemoglobinuria. In these cases, an unusual autoantibody to P is produced that binds to RBCs in the cold and fixes complement upon warming. Antibodies with these biphasic properties are called *Donath-Landsteiner antibodies*. The P antigen is the cellular receptor of parvovirus B19 and also may be a receptor for *Escherichia coli* binding to urothelial cells.

The *MNSsU system* is regulated by genes on chromosome 4. M and N are determinants on glycophorin A, an RBC membrane protein, and S and s are determinants on glycophorin B. Anti-S and anti-s IgG antibodies may develop after pregnancy or transfusion and lead to hemolysis. Anti-U antibodies are rare but problematic; virtually every donor is incompatible because nearly all persons express U.

The *Kell* protein is very large (720 amino acids) and its secondary structure contains many different antigenic epitopes. The immunogenicity of Kell is third behind the ABO and Rh systems. The absence of the Kell precursor protein (controlled by a gene on X) is associated with acanthocytosis, shortened RBC survival, and a progressive form of muscular dystrophy that includes cardiac defects. This rare condition is called the *McLeod phenotype*. The K$_x$ gene is linked to the 91-kDa component of the NADPH-oxidase on the X chromosome, deletion or mutation of which accounts for about 60% of cases of chronic granulomatous disease.

The *Duffy* antigens are codominant alleles, Fy^a and Fy^b, that also serve as receptors for *Plasmodium vivax*. More than 70% of persons in malaria-endemic areas lack these antigens, probably from selective influences of the infection on the population.

The *Kidd* antigens, Jk^a and Jk^b, may elicit antibodies transiently. A delayed hemolytic transfusion reaction that occurs with blood tested as compatible is often related to delayed appearance of anti-Jk^a.

PRETRANSFUSION TESTING

Pretransfusion testing of a potential recipient consists of the "type and screen." The "forward type" determines the ABO and Rh phenotype of the recipient's RBC by using antisera directed against the A, B, and D antigens. The "reverse type" detects isoagglutinins in the patient's serum and should correlate with the ABO phenotype, or forward type.

The alloantibody screen identifies antibodies directed against other RBC antigens. The alloantibody screen is performed by mixing patient serum with type O RBCs that contain the major antigens of most blood group systems and whose extended phenotype is known. The specificity of the alloantibody is identified by correlating the presence or absence of antigen with the results of the agglutination.

Cross-matching is ordered when there is a high probability that the patient will require a packed RBC (PRBC) transfusion. Blood selected for cross-matching must be ABO compatible and lack antigens for which the patient has alloantibodies. Nonreactive cross-matching confirms the absence of any major incompatibility and reserves that unit for the patient.

In the case of Rh-negative patients, every attempt must be made to provide Rh-negative blood components to prevent alloimmunization to the D antigen. In an emergency, Rh-positive blood can be safely transfused to a Rh-negative patient who lacks anti-D; however, the recipient is likely to become alloimmunized and produce anti-D. Rh-negative women of childbearing age who are transfused with products containing Rh-positive RBCs should receive passive immunization with anti-D (RhoGam or WinRho) to reduce or prevent sensitization.

BLOOD COMPONENTS

Blood products intended for transfusion are routinely collected as whole blood (450 mL) in various anticoagulants. Most donated blood is processed into components: PRBCs, platelets, and fresh-frozen

TABLE 99-1 *RBC Blood Group Systems and Alloantigens*

Blood Group System	Antigen	Alloantibody	Clinical Significance
Rh (D, C/c, E/e)	RBC protein	IgG	HTR, HDN
Lewis (Le^a, Le^b)	Oligosaccharide	IgM/IgG	Rare HTR
Kell (K/k)	RBC protein	IgG	HTR, HDN
Duffy (Fy^a/Fy^b)	RBC protein	IgG	HTR, HDN
Kidd (Jk^a/Jk^b)	RBC protein	IgG	HTR (often delayed), HDN (mild)
I/i	Carbohydrate	IgM	None
MNSsU	RBC protein	IgM/IgG	Anti-M rare HDN, anti-S, -s, and -U HDN, HTR

Note: RBC, red blood cell; HDN, hemolytic disease of the newborn; HTR, hemolytic transfusion reaction.

TABLE 99-2 *Characteristics of Selected Blood Components*

Component	Volume, mL	Content	Clinical Response
PRBC	180–200	RBCs with variable leukocyte content and small amount of plasma	Increase hemoglobin 10 g/L and hematocrit 3%
Platelets	50–70	5.5×10^{10}/RD unit	Increase platelet count 5000–10,000/μL
	200–400	$\geq 3.0 \times 10^{11}$/SDAP product	CCI $\geq 10 \times 10^9$/L within 1 h and $\geq 7.5 \times 10^9$/L within 24 h posttransfusion
FFP	200–250	Plasma proteins—coagulation factors, proteins C and S, antithrombin	Increases coagulation factors about 2%
Cryoprecipitate	10–15	Cold-insoluble plasma proteins, fibrinogen, factor VIII, vWF	Topical fibrin glue, also 80 IU factor VIII

Note: PRBC, packed red blood cells; RBC, red blood cell; RD, random donor; SDAP, single-donor apheresis platelets; CCI, corrected count increment; FFP, fresh frozen plasma; vWF, von Willebrand factor.

plasma (FFP) or cryoprecipitate (Table 99-2). Whole blood is first separated into PRBCs and platelet-rich plasma by slow centrifugation. The platelet-rich plasma is then centrifuged at high speed to yield one unit of random donor (RD) platelets and one unit of FFP. Cryoprecipitate is produced by thawing FFP to precipitate the plasma proteins, then separated by centrifugation.

Apheresis technology is used for the collection of multiple units of platelets from a single donor. These single-donor apheresis platelets (SDAP) contain the equivalent of at least six units of RD platelets and have fewer contaminating leukocytes than pooled RD platelets.

Plasma may also be collected by apheresis. Plasma derivatives such as albumin, intravenous immunoglobulin, antithrombin, and coagulation factor concentrates are prepared from pooled plasma from many donors and are treated to eliminate infectious agents.

WHOLE BLOOD Whole blood provides both oxygen-carrying capacity and volume expansion. It is the ideal component for patients who have sustained acute hemorrhage of ≥25% total blood volume loss. Whole blood is stored at 4°C to maintain erythrocyte viability, but platelet dysfunction and degradation of some coagulation factors occurs. In addition, 2,3-bisphosphoglycerate levels fall over time, leading to an increase in the oxygen affinity of the hemoglobin and a decreased capacity to deliver oxygen to the tissues, a problem with all red cell storage. Whole blood is not readily available since it is routinely processed into components.

PACKED RED BLOOD CELLS This product increases oxygen-carrying capacity in the anemic patient. Adequate oxygenation can be maintained with a hemoglobin content of 70 g/L in the normovolemic patient without cardiac disease; however, comorbid factors often necessitate transfusion at a higher threshold. The decision to transfuse should be guided by the clinical situation and not by an arbitrary laboratory value. In the critical care setting, liberal use of transfusions to maintain near normal levels of hemoglobin may have unexpected negative effects on survival. In most patients requiring transfusion, levels of hemoglobin of 100 g/L are sufficient to keep oxygen supply from being critically low.

PRBCs may be modified to prevent certain adverse reactions. Leukocyte reduction of cellular blood products is increasingly common, and universal prestorage leukocyte reduction has been recommended. Prestorage filtration appears superior to bedside filtration as smaller amounts of cytokines are generated in the stored product. These PRBC units contain $<5 \times 10^6$ donor white blood cells (WBCs), and their use lowers the incidence of posttransfusion fever, cytomegalovirus (CMV) infections, and alloimmunization. Other theoretical benefits include less immunosuppression in the recipient and lower risk of infections. Plasma, which may cause allergic reactions, can be removed from cellular blood components by washing.

PLATELETS Thrombocytopenia is a risk factor for hemorrhage, and platelet transfusion reduces the incidence of bleeding. The threshold

for prophylactic platelet transfusion is 10,000/μL. In patients without fever or infections, a threshold of 5000/μL may be sufficient to prevent spontaneous hemorrhage. For invasive procedures, 50,000/μL platelets is the usual target level.

Platelets are given either as pools prepared from five to eight RDs or as SDAPs from a single donor. In an unsensitized patient without increased platelet consumption [splenomegaly, fever, disseminated intravascular coagulation (DIC)], six to eight units of RD platelets (about 1 unit per 10 kg body weight) are transfused, and each unit is anticipated to increase the platelet count 5000 to 10,000/μL. Patients who have received multiple transfusions may be alloimmunized to many HLA- and platelet-specific antigens and have little or no increase in their posttransfusion platelet counts. Patients who may require multiple transfusions are best served by receiving SDAP and leukocyte-reduced components to lower the risk of alloimmunization.

Refractoriness to platelet transfusion may be evaluated using the corrected count increment (CCI):

$$CCI = \frac{\text{posttransfusion count} - \text{pretransfusion count}}{\text{number of platelets transfused} \times 10^{11}} \times BSA$$

where BSA is body surface area measured in square meters. The platelet count performed 1 h after the transfusion is acceptable if the CCI is 10×10^9/mL, and after 18 to 24 h an increment of 7.5×10^9/mL is expected. Patients who have suboptimal responses are likely to have received multiple transfusions and have antibodies directed against class I HLA antigens. Refractoriness can be investigated by detecting anti-HLA antibodies in the recipient's serum. Patients who are sensitized will often react with 100% of the lymphocytes used for the HLA-antibody screen, and HLA-matched SDAPs should be considered for those patients who require transfusion. Although ABO-identical HLA-matched SDAPs provide the best chance for increasing the platelet count, locating these products is difficult. Platelet cross-matching is available in some centers. Additional clinical causes for a low platelet CCI include fever, bleeding, splenomegaly, DIC, or medications in the recipient.

FRESH-FROZEN PLASMA FFP contains stable coagulation factors and plasma proteins: fibrinogen, antithrombin, albumin, as well as proteins C and S. Indications for FFP include correction of coagulopathies, including the rapid reversal of warfarin; supplying deficient plasma proteins; and treatment of thrombotic thrombocytopenic purpura. FFP should not be routinely used to expand blood volume. FFP is an acellular component and does not transmit intracellular infections, e.g., CMV. Patients who are IgA-deficient and require plasma support should receive FFP from IgA-deficient donors to prevent anaphylaxis (see below).

CRYOPRECIPITATE Cryoprecipitate is a source of fibrinogen, factor VIII, and von Willebrand factor (vWF). It is ideal for supplying fibrinogen to the volume-sensitive patient. When factor VIII concentrates are not available, cyroprecipitate may be used since each unit contains approximately 80 units of factor VIII. Cryoprecipitate may also supply vWF to patients with dysfunctional (type II) or absent (type III) von Willebrand disease.

PLASMA DERIVATIVES Plasma from thousands of donors may be pooled to derive specific protein concentrates, including albumin, intravenous immunoglobulin, antithrombin, and coagulation factors. In addition, donors who have high-titer antibodies to specific agents or antigens provide hyperimmune globulins, such as anti-D (RhoGam, WinRho), and antisera to hepatitis B virus (HBV), varicella-zoster virus, CMV, and other infectious agents.

ADVERSE REACTIONS TO BLOOD TRANSFUSION

Adverse reactions to transfused blood components occur despite multiple tests, inspections, and checks. Fortunately, the most common reactions are not life-threatening, although serious reactions can present with mild symptoms and signs. Some reactions can be reduced or prevented by modified (filtered, washed, or irradiated) blood components. When an adverse reaction is suspected, the transfusion should be stopped and reported to the blood bank for investigation.

Transfusion reactions may result from immune and nonimmune mechanisms. Immune-mediated reactions are often due to preformed donor or recipient antibody; however, cellular elements may also cause adverse effects. Nonimmune causes of reactions are due to the chemical and physical properties of the stored blood component and its additives.

Transfusion-transmitted viral infections are increasingly rare due to improved screening and testing. As the risk of viral infection is reduced, the relative risk of other reactions increases, such as hemolytic transfusion reactions and sepsis from bacterially contaminated components. More effort is being directed at improving pretransfusion quality assurance to further increase the safety of transfusion therapy. Infections, like any adverse transfusion reaction, must be brought to the attention of the blood bank for appropriate studies (Table 99-3).

IMMUNE-MEDIATED REACTIONS ■ Acute Hemolytic Transfusion Reactions

Immune-mediated hemolysis occurs when the recipient has preformed antibodies that lyse donor erythrocytes. The ABO isoagglutinins are responsible for the majority of these reactions, although alloantibodies directed against other RBC antigens, i.e., Rh, Kell, and Duffy, may result in hemolysis.

Acute hemolytic reactions may present with hypotension, tachypnea, tachycardia, fever, chills, hemoglobinemia, hemoglobinuria, chest and/or flank pain, and discomfort at the infusion site. Monitoring the patient's vital signs before and during the transfusion is important to identify reactions promptly. When acute hemolysis is suspected, the transfusion must be stopped immediately, intravenous access maintained, and the reaction reported to the blood bank. A correctly labeled posttransfusion blood sample and any untransfused blood should be sent to the blood bank for analysis. The laboratory evaluation for hemolysis includes the measurement of serum haptoglobin, lactate dehydrogenase (LDH), and indirect bilirubin levels.

TABLE 99-3 *Risks of Transfusion Complications*

	Frequency, Episodes:Unit
Reactions	
Febrile (FNHTR)	1–4:100
Allergic	1–4:100
Delayed hemolytic	1:1,000
TRALI	1:5,000
Acute hemolytic	1:12,000
Fatal hemolytic	1:100,000
Anaphylactic	1:150,000
Infections[a]	
Hepatitis B	1:63,000
Hepatitis C	1:1,600,000
HIV-1	1:1,960,000
HIV-2	None reported
HTLV-I and -II	1:641,000
Malaria	1:4,000,000
Other complications	
RBC allosensitization	1:100
HLA allosensitization	1:10
Graft-versus-host disease	Rare

[a] Infectious agents rarely associated with transfusion, theoretically possible or of unknown risk include: Hepatitis A virus, parvovirus B-19, *Babesia microti* (babesiosis), *Borrelia burgdorferi* (Lyme disease), *Trypanosoma cruzi* (Chagas disease), and *Treponema pallidum*, human herpesvirus-8 and hepatitis G virus.
Note: FNHTR, febrile nonhemolytic transfusion reaction; TRALI, transfusion-related acute lung injury; HTLV, human T lymphotropic virus; RBC, red blood cell

The immune complexes that result in RBC lysis can cause renal dysfunction and failure. Diuresis should be induced with intravenous fluids and furosemide or mannitol. Tissue factor released from the lysed erythrocytes may initiate DIC. Coagulation studies including prothrombin time (PT), activated partial thromboplastin time (aPTT), fibrinogen, and platelet count should be monitored in patients with hemolytic reactions.

Errors at the patient's bedside, such as mislabeling the sample or transfusing the wrong patient, are responsible for the majority of these reactions. The blood bank investigation of these reactions includes examination of the pre- and posttransfusion samples for hemolysis and repeat typing of the patient samples; direct antiglobulin test (DAT), sometimes called the direct Coombs test, of the posttransfusion sample; repeating the cross-matching of the blood component; and checking all clerical records for errors. DAT detects the presence of antibody or complement bound to RBCs in vivo.

Delayed Hemolytic and Serologic Transfusion Reactions Delayed hemolytic transfusion reactions (DHTRs) are not completely preventable. These reactions occur in patients previously sensitized to RBC alloantigens who have a negative alloantibody screen due to low antibody levels. When the patient is transfused with antigen-positive blood, an anamnestic response results in the early production of alloantibody that binds donor RBCs. The alloantibody is detectable 1 to 2 weeks following the transfusion, and the posttransfusion DAT may become positive due to circulating donor RBCs coated with antibody or complement. The transfused, alloantibody-coated erythrocytes are cleared by the reticuloendothelial system. These reactions are detected most commonly in the blood bank when a subsequent patient sample reveals a positive alloantibody screen or a new alloantibody in a recently transfused recipient.

No specific therapy is usually required, although additional RBC transfusions may be necessary. Delayed serologic transfusion reactions are similar to DHTR, as the DAT is positive and alloantibody is detected; however, RBC clearance is not increased.

Febrile Nonhemolytic Transfusion Reaction The most frequent reaction associated with the transfusion of cellular blood components is a febrile nonhemolytic transfusion reaction (FNHTR). These reactions are characterized by chills and rigors and a $\geq 1°C$ rise in temperature. FNHTR is diagnosed when other causes of fever in the transfused patient are ruled out. Antibodies directed against donor leukocyte and HLA antigens may mediate these reactions; thus, multiply transfused patients and multiparous women are felt to be at increased risk. Although antibodies may be demonstrated in the recipient's serum, investigation is not routinely done because of the mild nature of most FNHTR. The use of leukocyte-reduced blood products may prevent or delay sensitization to leukocyte antigens and thereby reduce the incidence of these febrile episodes. Cytokines released from cells within stored blood components may mediate FNHTR; thus, leukoreduction before storage may prevent these reactions. The incidence and severity of these reactions can be decreased in patients with recurrent reactions by premedicating with acetaminophen or other antipyretic agents.

Allergic Reactions Urticarial reactions are related to plasma proteins found in transfused components. Mild reactions may be treated symptomatically by temporarily stopping the transfusion and administering antihistamines (diphenhydramine, 50 mg orally or intramuscularly). The transfusion may be completed after the signs and/or symptoms resolve. Patients with a history of allergic transfusion reaction should be premedicated with an antihistamine. Cellular components can be washed to remove residual plasma for the extremely sensitized patient.

Anaphylactic Reaction This severe reaction presents after transfusion of only a few milliliters of the blood component. Symptoms and signs include difficulty breathing, coughing, nausea and vomiting, hypotension, bronchospasm, loss of consciousness, respiratory arrest, and shock. Treatment includes stopping the transfusion, maintaining vascular access, and administering epinephrine (0.5 to 1.0 mL of 1:1000 dilution subcutaneously). Glucocorticoids may be required in severe cases.

Patients who are IgA-deficient may be sensitized to this Ig class and are at risk for anaphylactic reactions associated with plasma transfusion. Individuals with severe IgA deficiency should therefore receive only IgA-deficient plasma and washed cellular blood components. Patients who have anaphylactic or repeated allergic reactions to blood components should be tested for IgA deficiency.

Graft-versus-Host Disease Graft-versus-host disease (GVHD) is a frequent complication of allogeneic stem cell transplantation, in which lymphocytes from the donor attack and cannot be eliminated by an immunodeficient host. Transfusion-related GVHD is mediated by donor T lymphocytes that recognize host HLA antigens as foreign and mount an immune response, which is manifested clinically by the development of fever, a characteristic cutaneous eruption, diarrhea, and liver function abnormalities. GVHD can also occur when blood components that contain viable T lymphocytes are transfused to immunodeficient recipients or to immunocompetent recipients who share HLA antigens with the donor (e.g., a family donor). In addition to the aforementioned clinical features of GVHD, transfusion-associated GVHD (TA-GVHD) is characterized by marrow aplasia and pancytopenia. TA-GVHD is highly resistant to treatment with immunosuppressive therapies, including glucocorticoids, cyclosporine, antithymocyte globulin, and ablative therapy followed by allogeneic bone marrow transplantation. Clinical manifestations appear at 8 to 10 days, and death occurs at 3 to 4 weeks posttransfusion.

TA-GVHD can be prevented by irradiation of cellular components (minimum of 2500 cGy) before transfusion to patients at risk. Patients at risk for TA-GVHD include fetuses receiving intrauterine transfusions, selected immunocompetent (e.g., lymphoma patients) or immunocompromised recipients, recipients of donor units known to be from a blood relative, and recipients who have undergone marrow transplantation. Directed donations by family members should be discouraged (they are not less likely to transmit infection); lacking other options, the blood products from family members should always be irradiated.

Transfusion-Related Acute Lung Injury This uncommon reaction results from the transfusion of donor plasma that contains high-titer anti-HLA antibodies that bind recipient leukocytes. The leukocytes aggregate in the pulmonary vasculature and release mediators that increase capillary permeability. The recipient develops symptoms of respiratory compromise and signs of noncardiogenic pulmonary edema, including bilateral interstitial infiltrates on chest x-ray. Treatment is supportive, and patients usually recover without sequelae. Testing the donor's plasma for anti-HLA antibodies can support this diagnosis. The implicated donors are frequently multiparous women, and transfusion of their plasma component should be avoided.

Posttransfusion Purpura This reaction presents as thrombocytopenia 7 to 10 days after platelet transfusion and occurs predominantly in women. Platelet-specific antibodies are found in the recipient's serum, and the most frequently recognized antigen is HPA-1a found on the platelet glycoprotein IIIa receptor. The delayed thrombocytopenia is due to the production of antibodies that react to both donor and recipient platelets. Additional platelet transfusions can worsen the thrombocytopenia and should be avoided. Treatment with intravenous immunoglobulin may neutralize the effector antibodies, or plasmapheresis can be used to remove the antibodies.

Alloimmunization A recipient may become alloimmunized to a number of antigens on cellular blood elements and plasma proteins. Alloantibodies to RBC antigens are detected during pretransfusion testing, and their presence may delay finding antigen-negative cross-match-compatible products for transfusion. Women of childbearing age who are sensitized to certain RBC antigens (i.e., D, c, E, Kell, or Duffy) are at

risk for bearing a fetus with hemolytic disease of the newborn. Matching for D antigen is the only pretransfusion selection test to prevent RBC alloimmunization.

Alloimmunization to antigens on leukocytes and platelets can result in refractoriness to platelet transfusions. Once alloimmunization has developed, HLA-compatible platelets from donors who share similar antigens with the recipient may be difficult to find. Hence, prudent transfusion practice is directed at preventing sensitization through the use of leukocyte-reduced cellular components, as well as limiting antigenic exposure by the judicious use of transfusions and use of SDAPs.

NONIMMUNOLOGIC REACTIONS ■ **Fluid Overload** Blood components are excellent volume expanders, and transfusion may quickly lead to volume overload. Monitoring the rate and volume of the transfusion, along with the use of a diuretic, can minimize this problem.

Hypothermia Refrigerated (4°C) or frozen (−18°C or below) blood components can result in hypothermia when rapidly infused. Cardiac dysrhythmias can result from exposing the sinoatrial node to cold fluid. Use of an in-line warmer will prevent this complication.

Electrolyte Toxicity RBC leakage during storage increases the concentration of potassium in the unit. Neonates and patients in renal failure are at risk for hyperkalemia. Preventive measures, such as using fresh or washed RBCs, are warranted for neonatal transfusions because this complication can be fatal.

Citrate, commonly used to anticoagulate blood components, chelates calcium and thereby inhibits the coagulation cascade. Hypocalcemia, manifested by circumoral numbness and/or tingling sensation of the fingers and toes, may result from multiple rapid transfusions. Because citrate is quickly metabolized to bicarbonate, calcium infusion is seldom required in this setting. If calcium or any other intravenous infusion is necessary, it must be given through a separate intravenous line.

Iron Overload Each unit of RBCs contains 200 to 250 mg of iron. Symptoms and signs of iron overload affecting endocrine, hepatic, and cardiac function are common after 100 units of RBCs have been transfused (total body iron load of 20 g). Preventing this complication by using alternative therapies (e.g., erythropoietin) and judicious transfusion is preferable and cost effective. Deferoxamine and other chelating agents are available, but the response is often suboptimal.

Hypotensive Reactions Transient hypotension may be noted among transfused patients who take angiotensin-converting enzyme (ACE) inhibitors. Since blood products contain bradykinin that is normally degraded by ACE, patients on ACE inhibitors may have increased bradykinin levels that cause hypotension. The blood pressure typically returns to normal without intervention.

Immunomodulation Transfusion of allogeneic blood is immunosuppressive. Multiply transfused renal transplant recipients are less likely to reject the graft, and transfusion may result in poorer outcomes in cancer patients and increase the risk of infections. Transfused leukocytes are thought to mediate the immunosuppression. Leukocyte-depleted cellular products may cause less immunosuppression, though controlled data have not been obtained and are unlikely to be obtained as the blood supply becomes universally leukocyte-depleted.

INFECTIOUS COMPLICATIONS Nucleic acid amplification testing (NAT) has been used since 1999 to screen donated blood for the presence of HIV and hepatitis C virus RNA.

Viral Infections ■ *HEPATITIS C VIRUS (HCV)* Fewer than 150 donors have been found to be HCV RNA positive in the absence of HCV antibodies, and the risk of acquiring HCV through transfusion is now 1 in 1,600,000 units. Infection with HCV may be asymptomatic or lead to chronic active hepatitis, cirrhosis, and liver failure.

HUMAN IMMUNODEFICIENCY VIRUS TYPE 1 Improved donor screening and testing (NAT) have dramatically reduced the risk of HIV-1 infection by blood transfusion. Donated blood is tested for HIV-1 p24 antigen.

Only eight seronegative donors have been shown to harbor HIV RNA. The risk of HIV-1 infection per transfusion episode is 1 in 1.9 million. Antibodies to HIV-2 are also measured in donated blood. No cases of HIV-2 infection have been reported in the United States since 1992.

HEPATITIS B VIRUS Donated blood is screened for HBV using assays for hepatitis B surface antigen (HbsAg). NAT testing is not practical because of slow viral replication and lower levels of viremia. The risk of transfusion-associated HBV infection is 1 in 63,000 units, twentyfold greater than for HCV. Vaccination of individuals who require long-term transfusion therapy can prevent this complication.

OTHER HEPATITIS VIRUSES Hepatitis A virus is rarely transmitted by transfusion, and the disease is typically asymptomatic and does not lead to chronic infection. Hepatitis G virus, now called GBV-C, along with two other transfusion-transmitted viruses, TTV and SEN-V, do not cause chronic hepatitis or other disease states. Routine testing does not appear to be warranted.

CYTOMEGALOVIRUS This ubiquitous virus infects ≥50% of the general population and is transmitted by the infected "passenger" WBCs found in transfused PRBCs or platelet components. Cellular components that are leukocyte-reduced have a decreased risk of transmitting CMV, regardless of the serologic status of the donor. Groups at risk for CMV infections include immunosuppressed patients, CMV-seronegative transplant recipients, and neonates; these patients should receive leukocyte-depleted components or CMV seronegative products.

HUMAN T LYMPHOTROPIC VIRUS (HTLV) TYPE I Assays to detect HTLV-I and -II are used to screen all donated blood. HTLV-1 is associated with adult T cell leukemia/lymphoma and tropical spastic paraparesis in a small percentage of infected persons (Chap. 172). The risk of HTLV-I infection via transfusion is 1 in 641,000 transfusion episodes. HTLV-II is not clearly associated with any disease.

PARVOVIRUS B-19 Blood components and products derived from pooled plasma can transmit this virus, the etiologic agent of erythema infectiosum, or fifth disease, in children. Parvovirus B-19 shows tropism for erythroid precursors and inhibits both erythrocyte production and maturation. Pure red cell aplasia, presenting either as acute aplastic crisis or chronic anemia with shortened RBC survival, may occur in individuals with an underlying hematologic disease, such as sickle cell disease or thalassemia (Chap. 94). The fetus of a seronegative woman is at risk for developing hydrops from this virus. NAT testing has reduced the risk of transfusion transmission.

Bacterial Contamination Most bacteria do not grow well at cold temperatures; thus, PRBCs and FFP are not common sources of bacterial contamination. However, some gram-negative bacteria, notably *Yersinia* and *Pseudomonas* species, can grow at 1° to 6°C. Platelet concentrates, which are stored at room temperature, are more likely to contain skin contaminants such as gram-positive organisms, including coagulase-negative staphylococci.

Recipients of transfusions contaminated with bacteria may develop fever and chills, which can progress to septic shock and DIC. These reactions may occur abruptly, within minutes of initiating the transfusion, or after several hours. The onset of symptoms and signs is often sudden and fulminant, which distinguishes bacterial contamination from a FNHTR. The reactions, particularly those related to gram-negative contaminants, are the result of infused endotoxins formed within the contaminated stored component.

When contaminated transfusions are suspected (i.e., when there is sudden development of shock), the transfusion must be stopped immediately. Therapy is directed at supporting the recipient's blood pressure, cardiac output, oxygenation, and renal function. The laboratory investigation should include cultures of any untransfused component, along with the routine blood bank clerical checks and serologic studies. Broad-spectrum antibiotic coverage should be started immediately and may be adjusted based on culture and sensitivity.

Other Infectious Agents Various parasites including those causing malaria, babesiosis, and Chagas disease can be transmitted by blood transfusion rarely. Geographic migration and travel of donors can shift the incidence of these rare infections. West Nile virus may be transmitted by transfusion. Other agents implicated in transfusion transmission include Lyme disease and varian Creutzfeld-Jakob disease. Because these infections can prove fatal, they should be considered in the transfused patient in the appropriate clinical setting.

ALTERNATIVES TO TRANSFUSION

Alternatives to allogeneic blood transfusions that avoid homologous donor exposures with attendant immunologic and infectious risks remain attractive. Autologous blood is the best option when transfusion is anticipated. However, the cost:benefit ratio of autologous transfusion remains high. No transfusion is a zero-risk event; clerical errors and bacterial contamination remain potential complications even with autologous transfusions. Additional methods of autologous transfusion in the surgical patient include preoperative hemodilution, recovery of shed blood from sterile surgical sites, and postoperative drainage collection. Directed or designated donation from friends and family of the potential recipient has not been safer than volunteer donor component transfusions. Such directed donations may in fact place the recipient at higher risk for complications such as GVHD and alloimmunization.

Oxygen-carrying blood substitutes, such as perfluorocarbons and aggregated hemoglobin solution, are presently in various stages of clinical trials. Granulocyte and granulocyte-macrophage colony-stimulating factor are clinically useful to hasten leukocyte recovery in patients with leukopenia related to high-dose chemotherapy. Erythropoietin stimulates erythrocyte production in patients with anemia of chronic renal failure and other conditions, thus avoiding or reducing the need for transfusion. This hormone can also stimulate erythropoiesis in the autologous donor to enable additional donation. Thrombopoietin, a cytokine that promotes megakaryocyte proliferation and maturation, is being tested for its ability to reduce the need for platelet transfusion.

FURTHER READING

BARON JF et al: The effect of universal leukodepletion of packed red blood cells on postoperative infections in high-risk patients undergoing abdominal aortic surgery. Anesth Analg 94:529, 2002

BRECHER ME et al: *The Technical Manual*, 14th ed. Arlington, VA, American Association of Blood Banks, 2002

DODD RY et al: Current prevalence and incidence of infectious disease markers and estimated window-period risk in the American Red Cross blood donor population. Transfusion 42:975, 2002

DZIK WH et al: Patient safety and blood tranfusion: New solutions. Transfus Med Rev 17:169, 2003

GOODNOUGH LT: Risks of blood transfusion. Crit Care Med 31(12 Suppl): 5678, 2003

RUBELLA P et al: A multicenter randomized study of the threshold for prophylactic platelet transfusions in adults with acute myeloid leukemia. N Engl J Med 337:1870, 1997

TABOR E et al: NAT screening of blood and plasma donations: Evolution of technology and regulatory policy. Transfusion 42:1230, 2002

Bone marrow transplantation was the original term used to describe the collection and transplantation of hematopoietic stem cells, but with the recent demonstration that the peripheral blood and umbilical cord blood are also useful sources of stem cells, *hematopoietic cell transplantation* has become the preferred generic term for this process. The procedure is usually carried out for one of two purposes: (1) to replace an abnormal but nonmalignant lymphohematopoietic system with one from a normal donor, or (2) to treat malignancy by allowing the administration of higher doses of myelosuppressive therapy than would otherwise be possible. The use of bone marrow transplantation has been steadily increasing, both because of its demonstrated effectiveness in selected diseases and because of increasing availability of donors. The International Bone Marrow Transplant Registry (*http://www.ibmtr.org*) estimates that about 50,000 transplants are performed each year.

THE HEMATOPOIETIC STEM CELL

Several features of the hematopoietic stem cell make transplantation clinically feasible, including its remarkable regenerative capacity, its ability to home to the marrow space following intravenous injection, and the ability of the stem cell to be cryopreserved. Transplantation of a single stem cell can replace the entire lymphohematopoietic system of an adult mouse. In humans, transplantation of a few percent of a donor's bone marrow volume regularly results in complete and sustained replacement of the recipient's entire lymphohematopoietic system, including all red cells, granulocytes, B and T lymphocytes, and platelets, as well as cells comprising the fixed macrophage population, including Kupffer cells of the liver, pulmonary alveolar macrophages, osteoclasts, Langerhans cells of the skin, and brain microglial cells. The ability of the hematopoietic stem cell to home to the marrow following intravenous injection is mediated, at least in part, by the interaction of specific cell molecules, termed *selectins*, on bone marrow endothelial cells with their unique ligands, termed *integrins*, on early hematopoietic cells. Human hematopoietic stem cells can survive freezing and thawing with little, if any, damage, making it possible to remove and store a portion of the patient's own bone marrow for later reinfusion following treatment of the patient with high-dose myelotoxic therapy.

CATEGORIES OF HEMATOPOIETIC CELL TRANSPLANTATION

Hematopoietic cell transplantation can be described according to the relationship between the patient and the donor and by the anatomic source of stem cells. In ~1% of cases, patients have identical twins who can serve as donors. Syngeneic donors represent the best source of stem cells; unlike the use of allogeneic donors, there is no risk of graft-versus-host disease (GVHD) and, unlike the use of autologous marrow, there is no risk that the stem cells are contaminated with tumor cells.

Allogeneic transplantation involves a donor and recipient who are not immunologically identical. Following allogeneic transplantation immune cells transplanted with the marrow or developing from it can react against the patient, causing GVHD. Alternatively, if the immunosuppressive preparative regimen used to treat the patient before transplant is inadequate, immunocompetent cells of the patient can cause graft rejection. The risks of these complications are greatly influenced by the degree of matching between donor and recipient for antigens encoded by genes of the major histocompatibility complex.

The human leukocyte antigen (HLA) molecules are responsible for binding antigenic proteins and presenting them to T cells. The antigens presented by HLA molecules may derive from exogenous sources (e.g., during active infections) or may be endogenous proteins produced by the cell. If individuals are not matched for HLA, T cells from one individual will react strongly to the mismatched HLA, or "major

antigens," of the second. Even if the individuals are HLA-matched, the T cells of the donor may react to differing endogenous, or "minor antigens," presented by the HLA of the recipient. Reactions to minor antigens tend to be less vigorous. The genes of major relevance to transplantation include HLA-A, -B, -C, and -D; they are closely linked and therefore tend to be inherited as haplotypes, with only rare crossovers between them. Thus, the odds that any one full sibling will match a patient are one in four, and the probability that the patient has an HLA-identical sibling is $1 - (0.75)^n$, where n equals the number of siblings.

With current techniques, the risk of graft rejection is 1 to 3%, and the risk of severe, life-threatening acute GVHD is ~15% following transplantation between HLA-identical siblings. The incidence of graft rejection and GVHD increases progressively with the use of family member donors mismatched for one, two, or three antigens. While survival following a one-antigen mismatched transplant is not markedly altered, survival following two- or three-antigen mismatched transplants is significantly impaired, and such transplants should be performed only as part of clinical trials.

The formation of the National Marrow Donor Program has allowed for the identification of HLA-matched unrelated donors for many patients. The genes encoding HLA antigens are highly polymorphic, and thus the odds of any two unrelated individuals being HLA-identical are extremely low, somewhat less than 1 in 10,000. However, by identifying and typing >7 million volunteer donors, HLA-matched donors can now be found for ~50% of patients for whom a search is initiated. It takes, on average, 3 to 4 months to complete a search and schedule and initiate an unrelated donor transplant. Results so far suggest that GVHD is somewhat increased and survival somewhat poorer with such donors than with HLA-matched siblings.

Autologous transplantation involves the removal and storage of the patient's own stem cells with subsequent reinfusion after the patient receives high-dose myeloablative therapy. Unlike allogeneic transplantation, there is no risk of GVHD or graft rejection with autologous transplantation. On the other hand, autologous transplantation lacks a graft-versus-tumor (GVT) effect, and the autologous stem cell product can be contaminated with tumor cells that could lead to relapse. A variety of techniques have been developed to "purge" autologous products of tumor cells. Some use antibodies directed at tumor-associated antigens plus complement, antibodies linked to toxins, or antibodies conjugated to immunomagnetic beads. In vitro incubation with certain chemotherapeutic agents such as 4-hydroperoxycyclophosphamide and long-term culture of bone marrow have also been shown to diminish tumor cell numbers in stem cell products. Another technique is positive selection of stem cells using antibodies to CD34, with subsequent column adherence or flow techniques to select normal stem cells while leaving tumor cells behind. All these approaches can reduce the number of tumor cells from 1000- to 10,000-fold and are clinically feasible; however, no prospective randomized trials have yet shown that any of these approaches results in a decrease in relapse rates or improvements in disease-free or overall survival.

Bone marrow aspirated from the posterior and anterior iliac crests has traditionally been the source of hematopoietic stem cells for transplantation. Typically, anywhere from 1.5 to 5×10^8 nucleated marrow cells per kilogram are collected for allogeneic transplantation. Several recent studies have found improved survival in the settings of both matched sibling and unrelated transplantation by transplanting higher numbers of bone marrow cells.

Hematopoietic stem cells circulate in the peripheral blood but in very low concentrations. Following the administration of certain hematopoietic growth factors, including granulocyte colony-stimulating factor (G-CSF) or granulocyte-macrophage colony-stimulating factor (GM-CSF), and during recovery from intensive chemotherapy, the concentration of hematopoietic progenitor cells in blood, as measured either by colony-forming units or expression of the CD34 antigen, increases markedly. This has made it possible to harvest adequate numbers of stem cells from the peripheral blood for transplantation. Donors are typically treated with 4 or 5 days of hematopoietic growth factor, following which stem cells are collected in one or two 4-h pheresis sessions. In the autologous setting, transplantation of $>2.5 \times 10^6$ CD34 cells per kilogram, a number easily collected in most circumstances, leads to rapid and sustained engraftment in virtually all cases. Compared to the use of autologous marrow, use of peripheral blood stem cells results in more rapid hematopoietic recovery, with granulocytes recovering to $500/\mu L$ by day 12 and platelets recovering to $20,000/\mu L$ by day 14. While this more rapid recovery diminishes the morbidity of transplantation, no studies show an improvement in survival.

Hesitation in studying the use of peripheral blood stem cells for allogeneic transplantation was because peripheral blood stem cell products contain as much as one log more T cells than are contained in the typical marrow harvest; in animal models, the incidence of GVHD is related to the number of T cells transplanted. Nonetheless, phase II and randomized phase III trials have shown that the use of growth factor–mobilized peripheral blood stem cells from HLA-matched family members leads to faster engraftment without an increase in acute GVHD. Chronic GVHD may be increased with peripheral blood stem cells, but in trials conducted so far, this has been more than balanced by reductions in relapse rates and nonrelapse mortality, with the use of peripheral blood stem cells resulting in improved overall survival.

Umbilical cord blood contains a high concentration of hematopoietic progenitor cells, allowing for its use as a source of stem cells for transplantation. Cord blood transplantation from family members has been explored in the setting where the immediate need for transplantation precludes waiting the 9 or so months generally required for the baby to mature to the point of donating marrow. Use of cord blood in such settings results in somewhat slower engraftment than seen with marrow but a low incidence of GVHD, perhaps reflecting the low number of T cells in cord blood. Several banks have been developed to harvest and store cord blood for possible transplantation to unrelated patients from material that would otherwise be discarded. A summary of the first 562 unrelated cord blood transplants, facilitated by the New York Blood Center, reported engraftment in ~85% of patients but at a slower pace than seen with marrow. Severe GVHD was seen in 23% of patients. The risk of graft failure was related to the dose of cord blood cells per kilogram infused. The low cell content of most cord blood collections has limited the use of this approach as a source of stem cells for adult patients.

THE TRANSPLANT PREPARATIVE REGIMEN

The treatment regimen administered to patients immediately preceding transplantation is designed to eradicate the patient's underlying disease and, in the setting of allogeneic transplantation, immunosuppress the patient adequately to prevent rejection of the transplanted marrow. The appropriate regimen, therefore, depends on the disease setting and source of marrow. For example, when transplantation is performed to treat severe combined immunodeficiency and the donor is a histocompatible sibling, no treatment is required because no host cells require eradication and the patient is already too immunoincompetent to reject the transplanted marrow. For aplastic anemia, there is no large population of cells to eradicate and high-dose cyclophosphamide plus antithymocyte globulin are sufficient to immunosuppress the patient adequately to accept the marrow graft. In the setting of thalassemia and sickle cell anemia, high-dose busulfan is frequently added to cyclophosphamide in order to eradicate the hyperplastic host hematopoiesis. A variety of different regimens have been developed to treat malignant diseases. Most of these regimens include agents that have high activity against the tumor in question at conventional doses and have myelosuppression as their predominant dose-limiting toxicity. Therefore, these regimens commonly include busulfan, cyclophospha-

mide, melphalan, thiotepa, carmustine, etoposide, and total-body irradiation in various combinations.

Although high-dose treatment regimens have typically been used in transplantation, the understanding that much of the antitumor effect of transplantation derives from an immunologically mediated GVT response has led investigators to ask if less intensive "nonmyeloablative" regimens might be effective and more tolerable. Evidence for a GVT effect comes from studies showing posttransplant relapse rates are lowest in patients who develop acute and chronic GVHD, higher in those without GVHD, and higher still in recipients of T cell–depleted allogeneic or syngeneic marrow. The demonstration that complete remissions can be obtained in many patients who have relapsed posttransplant by simply administering viable lymphocytes from the original donor further strengthens the argument for a potent GVT effect. Accordingly, a variety of less intensive nonmyeloablative regimens have been studied, ranging in intensity from the very minimum required to achieve engraftment (e.g., fludarabine plus 200 cGy total-body irradiation) to regimens of more immediate intensity (e.g., fludarabine plus melphalan). Studies to date document that engraftment can be readily achieved with less toxicity than seen with conventional transplantation. Complete sustained responses have been documented in many patients, particularly those with more indolent hematologic malignancies. The precise role of nonmyeloablative transplants in any one disease category, however, has not yet been fully defined.

THE TRANSPLANT PROCEDURE

Marrow is usually collected from the donor's posterior and sometimes anterior iliac crests with the donor under general or spinal anesthesia. Typically, 10 to 15 mL/kg of marrow is aspirated, placed in heparinized media, and filtered through 0.3- and 0.2-mm screens to remove fat and bony spicules. The collected marrow may undergo further processing depending on the clinical situation, such as the removal of red cells to prevent hemolysis in ABO-incompatible transplants, the removal of donor T cells to prevent GVHD, or attempts to remove possible contaminating tumor cells in autologous transplantation. Marrow donation is safe, with only very rare complications reported.

Peripheral blood stem cells are collected by leukopheresis after the donor has been treated with hematopoietic growth factors or, in the setting of autologous transplantation, sometimes after treatment with a combination of chemotherapy and growth factors. Stem cells for transplantation are generally infused through a large-bore central venous catheter. Such infusions are usually well tolerated, although occasionally patients develop fever, cough, or shortness of breath. These symptoms usually resolve with slowing of the infusion. When the stem cell product has been cryopreserved using dimethyl sulfoxide, patients more often experience short-lived nausea or vomiting due to the odor and taste of the cryoprotectant.

ENGRAFTMENT

Peripheral blood counts usually reach their nadir several days to a week posttransplant as a consequence of the preparative regimen, then cells produced by the transplanted stem cells begin to appear in the peripheral blood. The rate of recovery depends on the source of stem cells, the use of posttransplant growth factors, and the form of GVHD prophylaxis employed. If marrow is the source of stem cells, recovery to 100 granulocytes/μL occurs by day 16 and $500/\mu L$ by day 22. Use of G-CSF-mobilized peripheral blood stem cells speeds the rate of recovery by ~1 week when compared to marrow. Use of myeloid growth factor (G-CSF or GM-CSF) posttransplant can further accelerate recovery by 3 to 5 days, while use of methotrexate to prevent GVHD delays engraftment by a similar period. Following allogeneic transplantation, engraftment can be documented using fluorescence in situ hybridization of sex chromosomes if donor and recipient are sex-mismatched, HLA-typing if HLA-mismatched, or restriction fragment length polymorphism analysis if sex- and HLA-matched.

COMPLICATIONS FOLLOWING HEMATOPOIETIC CELL TRANSPLANT

EARLY DIRECT CHEMORADIOTOXICITIES The transplant preparative regimens commonly used cause a spectrum of acute toxicities that vary according to the specific regimen but frequently result in nausea, vomiting, and mild skin erythema (Fig. 100-1). Regimens that include high-dose cyclophosphamide can result in hemorrhagic cystitis, which can usually be prevented by bladder irrigation or with the sulfhydryl compound, mercaptoethanesulfonate (MESNA); rarely, acute hemorrhagic carditis is seen. Most preparative regimens will result in oral mucositis, which typically develops 5 to 7 days posttransplant and often requires narcotic analgesia. Use of a patient-controlled analgesic pump provides the greatest patient satisfaction and results in a lower cumulative dose of narcotic. Patients begin losing their hair 5 to 6 days posttransplant and by 1 week are usually profoundly pancytopenic.

Approximately 10% of patients will develop venoocclusive disease of the liver, a syndrome resulting from direct cytotoxic injury to hepatic-venular and sinusoidal endothelium, with subsequent deposition of fibrin and the development of a local hypercoagulable state. This chain of events results in the clinical symptoms of tender hepatomegaly, ascites, jaundice, and fluid retention. These symptoms can develop any time during the first month posttransplant, with the peak incidence at day 16. The mortality of venoocclusive disease is ~30%, with progressive hepatic failure culminating in a terminal hepatorenal syndrome. Both thrombolytic and antithrombotic agents, such as tissue plasminogen activator, heparin, and prostaglandin E, have been studied as therapy, but none has proven of consistent major benefit in controlled trials and all have significant toxicity. Early studies with defibrotide, a polydeoxyribonucleotide, seem encouraging.

Although most pneumonias developing posttransplant are caused by infectious agents, in ~5% of patients a diffuse interstitial pneumonia will develop that is thought to be the result of direct toxicity of the preparative regimen. Bronchoalveolar lavage typically shows alveolar hemorrhage, and biopsies are typically characterized by diffuse alveolar damage, although some cases may have a more clearly interstitial pattern. High-dose glucocorticoids are often used as treatment, although randomized trials testing their utility have not been reported.

LATE DIRECT CHEMORADIOTOXICITIES Late complications of the preparative regimen include decreased growth velocity in children and delayed development of secondary sex characteristics. These complications can be partly ameliorated with the use of appropriate growth and sex hormone replacement. Most men become azoospermic, and most postpubertal women will develop ovarian failure, which

should be treated. Thyroid dysfunction, usually well compensated, is sometimes seen. Cataracts develop in 10 to 20% of patients and are most common in patients treated with total-body irradiation and those who receive glucocorticoid therapy posttransplant for treatment of GVHD. Aseptic necrosis of the femoral head is seen in 10% of patients and is particularly frequent in those receiving chronic glucocorticoid therapy.

GRAFT-VERSUS-HOST DISEASE GVHD is the result of allogeneic T cells that were either transferred with the donor's stem cell inoculum or develop from it, reacting with antigenic targets on host cells. GVHD developing within the first 3 months posttransplant is termed *acute GVHD*, while GVHD developing or persisting beyond 3 months posttransplant is termed *chronic GVHD*. Acute GVHD most often first becomes apparent 2 to 4 weeks posttransplant and is characterized by an erythematous maculopapular rash; persistent anorexia or diarrhea, or both; and by liver disease with increased serum levels of bilirubin, alanine and aspartate aminotransferase, and alkaline phosphatase. Since many conditions can mimic acute GVHD, diagnosis usually requires skin, liver, or endoscopic biopsy for confirmation. In all these organs, endothelial damage and lymphocytic infiltrates are seen. In skin, the epidermis and hair follicles are damaged; in liver, the small bile ducts show segmental disruption; and in intestines, destruction of the crypts and mucosal ulceration may be noted. A commonly used rating system for acute GVHD is shown in Table 100-1. Grade I acute GVHD is of little clinical significance, does not affect the likelihood of survival, and does not require treatment. In contrast, grades II to IV GVHD are associated with significant symptoms and a poorer probability of survival and require aggressive therapy. The incidence of acute GVHD is higher in recipients of stem cells from mismatched or unrelated donors, in older patients, and in patients unable to receive full doses of drugs used to prevent the disease.

One general approach to the prevention of GVHD is the administration of immunosuppressive drugs early after transplant. Combinations of methotrexate and either cyclosporine or tacrolimus are among the most effective and widely used regimens. Prednisone, anti–T cell antibodies, mycophenolate mofetil, and other immunosuppressive agents have also been or are being studied in various combinations. A second general approach to GVHD prevention is removal of T cells from the stem cell inoculum. While effective in preventing GVHD, T cell depletion is associated with an increased incidence of graft failure and of tumor recurrence posttransplant; as yet, little evidence suggests that this approach improves cure rates in any specific setting.

Despite prophylaxis, significant acute GVHD will develop in ~30% of recipients of stem cells from matched siblings and in as many as 60% of those receiving stem cells from unrelated donors. The disease is usually treated with glucocorticoids, antithymocyte globulin, or monoclonal antibodies targeted against T cells or T cell subsets.

Between 20 and 50% of patients surviving >6 months after allogeneic transplantation will develop chronic GVHD. The disease is more common in older patients, in recipients of mismatched or unrelated stem cells, and in those with a preceding episode of acute GVHD. The disease resembles an autoimmune disorder with malar rash, sicca syndrome, arthritis, obliterative bronchiolitis, and bile duct degeneration and cholestasis. Single-agent prednisone or cyclosporine is standard treatment at present, although trials of other agents, including thalidomide, are under way. In most patients, chronic GVHD resolves, but it may require 1 to 3 years of immunosuppressive treatment before these agents can be withdrawn without the disease recurring. Because patients with chronic GVHD are susceptible to significant infection, they should receive prophylactic trimethoprim-sulfamethoxazole, and all suspected infections should be investigated and treated aggressively.

GRAFT FAILURE While complete and sustained engraftment are usually seen posttransplant, occasionally marrow function either does not return or, after a brief period of engraftment, is lost. Graft failure after autologous transplantation can be the result of inadequate numbers of stem cells being transplanted, damage during ex vivo treatment or

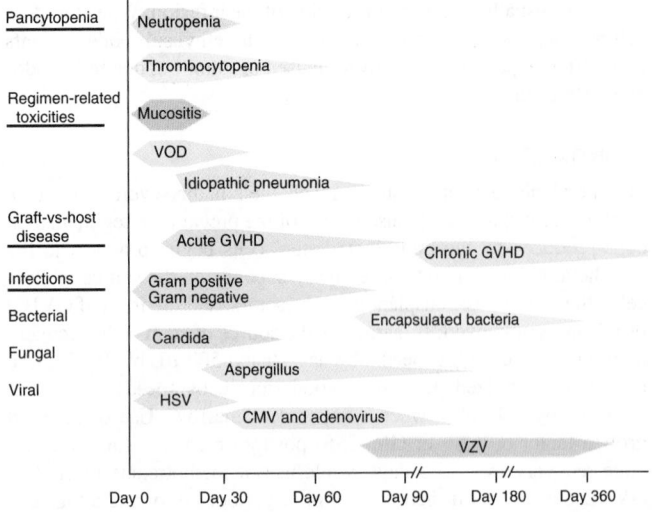

FIGURE 100-1 Major syndromes complicating marrow transplantation. VOD, venoocclusive disease; GVHD, graft-versus-host disease; HSV, herpes simplex virus; CMV, cytomegalovirus; VZV, varicella-zoster virus. The size of the shaded area roughly reflects the risk of the complication.

storage, or exposure of the patient to myelotoxic agents posttransplant. Infections with cytomegalovirus (CMV) or human herpes virus type 6 have also been associated with loss of marrow function. Graft failure after allogeneic transplantation can also be due to immunologic rejection of the graft by immunocompetent host cells. Immunologically based graft rejection is more common following use of less immunosuppressive preparative regimens, in recipients of T cell–depleted stem cell products, and in patients receiving grafts from HLA-mismatched donors.

Treatment of graft failure usually involves removing all potentially myelotoxic agents from the patient's regimen and attempting a short trial of myeloid growth factor. Persistence of lymphocytes of host origin in allogeneic transplant recipients with graft failure indicates immunologic rejection. Reinfusion of donor stem cells in such patients is usually unsuccessful unless preceded by a second immunosuppressive preparative regimen. Standard preparative regimens are generally tolerated poorly if administered within 100 days of a first transplant because of cumulative toxicities. However, use of regimens combining, for example, anti-CD3 antibodies with high-dose glucocorticoids have been successful in achieving engraftment in >50% of patients.

INFECTION Posttransplant patients, particularly recipients of allogeneic transplantation, require unique approaches to the problem of infection. Early after transplantation, patients are profoundly neutropenic, and because the risk of bacterial infection is so great, most centers initiate antibiotic treatment once the granulocyte count falls to <500/μL. Fluconazole prophylaxis at a dose of 200 to 400 mg/kg per day reduces the risk of candidal infections. Patients seropositive for herpes simplex should receive acyclovir prophylaxis. One approach to infection prophylaxis is shown in Table 100-2. Despite these prophylactic measures, most patients will develop fever and signs of infection posttransplant. The management of patients who become febrile despite bacterial and fungal prophylaxis is a difficult challenge and is guided by individual aspects of the patient and by the institution's experience. →*The general problem of infection in the immunocompromised host is discussed in Chap. 117.*

Once patients engraft, the incidence of bacterial infection diminishes; however, patients, particularly allogeneic transplant recipients, remain at significant risk of infection. During the period from engraftment until about 3 months posttransplant, the most common causes of infection are gram-positive bacteria, fungi (particularly *Aspergillus*) and viruses including CMV. CMV infection, which in the past was frequently seen and often fatal, can be prevented in seronegative patients by the use of seronegative blood products. The use of ganciclovir, either as prophylaxis beginning at the time of engraftment or initiated when CMV first reactivates as evidenced by development of antigenemia, can significantly reduce the risk of CMV disease in seropositive patients. Foscarnet is effective for some patients who develop CMV antigenemia or infection despite the use of ganciclovir or who cannot tolerate the drug.

Pneumocystis carinii pneumonia, once seen in 5 to 10% of patients, can be prevented by treating patients with oral trimethoprim-sulfamethoxazole for 1 week pretransplant and resuming the treatment once patients have engrafted.

The risk of infection diminishes considerably beyond 3 months after transplant unless chronic GVHD develops, requiring continuous immunosuppression. Most transplant centers recommend continuing trimethoprim-sulfamethoxazole prophylaxis while patients are receiving any immunosuppressive drugs and also recommend careful monitoring for late CMV reactivation. In addition, many centers recommend prophylaxis against varicella zoster, using acyclovir for 1 year posttransplant.

TABLE 100-1 *Clinical Staging and Grading of Acute Graft-versus-Host Disease*

Clinical Stage	Skin	Liver— Bilirubin, μmol/L (mg/dL)	Gut
1	Rash <25% body surface	34–51 (2–3)	Diarrhea 500–1000 mL/d
2	Rash 25–50% body surface	51–103 (3–6)	Diarrhea 1000–1500 mL/d
3	Generalized erythroderma	103–257 (6–15)	Diarrhea >1500 mL/d
4	Desquamation and bullae	>257 (> 15)	Ileus

Overall Clinical Grade	Skin Stage	Liver Stage	Gut Stage
I	1–2	0	0
II	1–3	1	1
III	1–3	2–3	2–3
IV	2–4	2–4	2–4

TREATMENT OF SPECIFIC DISEASES USING HEMATOPOIETIC CELL TRANSPLANTATION

NONMALIGNANT DISEASES ■ **Immunodeficiency Disorders** By replacing abnormal stem cells with cells from a normal donor, hematopoietic cell transplantation can cure patients of a variety of immunodeficiency disorders including severe combined immunodeficiency, Wiskott-Aldrich syndrome, and Chédiak-Higashi syndrome. The widest experience has been with severe combined immunodeficiency disease, where cure rates of 90% can be expected with HLA-identical donors and success rates of 50 to 70% have been reported using haplotype-mismatched parents as donors (Table 100-3).

Aplastic Anemia Transplantation from matched siblings after a preparative regimen of high-dose cyclophosphamide and antithymocyte globulin can cure up to 90% of patients <40 years with severe aplastic anemia. Results in older patients and in recipients of mismatched family member or unrelated marrow are less favorable; therefore, a trial of immunosuppressive therapy is generally recommended for such patients before considering transplantation. Transplantation is effective in all forms of aplastic anemia including, for example, the syndromes associated with paroxysmal nocturnal hemoglobinuria and Fanconi's anemia. Patients with Fanconi's anemia are abnormally sensitive to the toxic effects of alkylating agents and so less intensive preparative regimens must be used in their treatment (Chap. 94).

Hemoglobinopathies Marrow transplantation from an HLA-identical sibling following a preparative regimen of busulfan and cyclophosphamide can cure 70 to 90% of patients with thalassemia major. The best outcomes can be expected if patients are transplanted before they develop hepatomegaly or portal fibrosis and if they have been given adequate iron chelation therapy. Among such patients, the probabilities of 5-year survival and disease-free survival are 95 and 90%, respectively. Although prolonged survival can be achieved with aggressive chelation therapy, transplantation is the only curative treatment for

TABLE 100-2 *Approach to Infection Prophylaxis in Allogeneic Transplant Recipients*

Organism		Approach
Bacterial	Ceftazidime	2 g IV q8h while neutropenic
Fungal	Fluconazole	400 mg PO qd to day 75 posttransplant
Pneumocystis carinii	Trimethoprim-sulfamethoxazole	1 double-strength tablet PO bid 2 days/week until day 180 or off immunosuppression
Viral		
Herpes simplex	Acyclovir	800 mg PO bid to day 30
Varicella zoster	Acyclovir	800 mg PO bid to day 365
Cytomegalovirus	Ganciclovir	5 mg/kg IV bid for 7 days, then 5 (mg/kg)/d 5 days/week to day 100

TABLE 100-3 *Estimated 5-Year Survival Rates following Transplantation[a]*

Disease	Allogeneic, %	Autologous, %
Severe combined immunodeficiency	90	N/A
Aplastic anemia	90	N/A
Thalassemia	90	N/A
Acute myeloid leukemia		
First remission	55–60	50
Second remission	40	30
Acute lymphocytic leukemia		
First remission	50	40
Second remission	40	30
Chronic myeloid leukemia		
Chronic phase	70	ID
Accelerated phase	40	ID
Blast crisis	15	ID
Chronic lymphocytic leukemia	50	ID
Myelodysplasia	45	ID
Multiple myeloma	30	35
Non-Hodgkin's lymphoma		
First relapse/second remission	40	40
Hodgkin's disease		
First relapse/second remission	40	50
Breast cancer		
High-risk stage II	N/A	70
Stage IV	N/A	15

[a] These estimates are generally based on data reported by the International Bone Marrow Transplant Registry. The analysis has not been reviewed by their Advisory Committee.
Note: N/A, not applicable; ID, insufficient data.

thalassemia. Transplantation is being studied as a curative approach to patients with sickle cell anemia. Two-year survival and disease-free survival rates of 90 and 80%, respectively, have been reported following matched sibling transplantation. Decisions about patient selection and the timing of transplantation remain difficult, but transplantation seems to represent a reasonable option for younger patients who suffer repeated crises or other significant complications and who have not responded to other interventions (Chap. 91).

Other Nonmalignant Diseases Theoretically, hematopoietic cell transplantation should be able to cure any disease that results from an inborn error of the lymphohematopoietic system. Transplantation has been used successfully to treat congenital disorders of white blood cells such as Kostmann's syndrome, chronic granulomatous disease, and leukocyte adhesion deficiency. Congenital anemias such as Blackfan-Diamond anemia can also be cured with transplantation. Infantile malignant osteopetrosis is due to an inability of the osteoclast to resorb bone, and since osteoclasts derive from the marrow, transplantation can cure this rare inherited disorder.

Hematopoietic cell transplantation has been used as treatment for a number of storage diseases caused by enzymatic deficiencies, such as Gaucher's disease, Hurler's syndrome, Hunter's syndrome, and infantile metachromatic leukodystrophy. Transplantation for these diseases has not been uniformly successful, but treatment early in the course of these diseases, before irreversible damage to extramedullary organs has occurred, increases the chance for success.

Transplantation is being explored as a treatment for severe acquired autoimmune disorders. These trials are based on studies demonstrating that transplantation can reverse autoimmune disorders in animal models and on the observation that occasional patients with coexisting autoimmune disorders and hematologic malignancies have been cured of both with transplantation.

MALIGNANT DISEASES ■ Acute Leukemia Allogeneic hematopoietic cell transplantation cures 15 to 20% of patients who do not achieve complete response from induction chemotherapy for acute myeloid leukemia (AML) and is the only form of therapy that can cure such patients. Cure rates of 30 to 35% are seen when patients are transplanted in second remission or in first relapse. The best results with allogeneic transplantation are achieved when applied during first re-

mission, with disease-free survival rates averaging 55 to 60%. Chemotherapy alone can cure a portion of AML patients, and so the relative merits of transplanting all patients during first remission versus only transplanting very high risk patients and those who relapse continue to be discussed. Autologous transplantation is also able to cure a portion of patients with AML. The rates of disease recurrence with autologous transplantation are higher than seen after allogeneic transplantation, and cure rates are generally somewhat less.

Similar to patients with AML, adults with acute lymphocytic leukemia who do not achieve a complete response to induction chemotherapy can be cured in 15 to 20% of cases with immediate transplantation. Cure rates improve to 30 to 50% in second remission, and therefore transplantation can be recommended for adults who have persistent disease after induction chemotherapy or who have subsequently relapsed. Transplantation in first remission results in cure rates around 55%. While transplantation appears to offer a clear advantage over chemotherapy for patients with high-risk disease, such as those with Philadelphia chromosome–positive disease, debate continues about whether adults with standard-risk disease should be transplanted in first remission or whether transplantation should be reserved until relapse. Autologous transplantation is associated with a higher relapse rate but a somewhat lower risk of nonrelapse mortality when compared to allogeneic transplantation. On balance, most experts recommend use of allogeneic stem cells if an appropriate donor is available.

Chronic Leukemia Allogeneic hematopoietic cell transplantation is the only therapy shown to cure a substantial portion of patients with chronic myeloid leukemia (CML). Five-year disease-free survival rates are 15 to 20% for patients transplanted for blast crisis, 25 to 50% for accelerated-phase patients, and 60 to 70% for chronic phase patients, with cure rates as high as 80% at selected centers. Time from diagnosis to transplantation influences outcome, with best results obtained among patients transplanted within 1 year of diagnosis. Use of unrelated donors results in more GVHD and slightly worse survival than seen with matched siblings, although, at some large centers, 3-year disease-free survival rates of 70% have been reported. Autologous transplantation is being studied; however, few data suggest that this approach has curative potential in this disease. The timing of transplantation in CML has become more complicated with the introduction of imatinib mesylate, a remarkably effective, relatively nontoxic oral agent. Because imatinib does not generally result in complete molecular remissions, many would argue that allogeneic transplantation remains the treatment of choice for younger patients with matched donors. For older patients and those without matched donors, an initial trial of imatinib is appropriate (Chap. 96).

Allogeneic transplantation has been used to only a limited extent for chronic lymphocytic leukemia, in large part because of the chronic nature of the disease and because of the age profile of patients. With allogeneic transplantation, complete remissions have been achieved in the majority of patients so far reported, with disease-free survival rates of ~50% at 3 years. However, treatment-related mortality has been substantial, and further follow-up is needed. There is even less experience with autologous transplantation in this disorder.

Myelodysplasia Between 40 and 50% of patients with myelodysplasia appear to be cured with allogeneic transplantation. Results are better among younger patients and those with less advanced disease. However, some patients with myelodysplasia can live for extended periods without intervention, and so transplantation is generally recommended only for patients with disease categorized as intermediate risk I or greater according to the International Prognostic Scoring System (Chap. 94).

Lymphoma Patients with disseminated intermediate- or high-grade non-Hodgkin's lymphoma who have not been cured by first-line chemotherapy and are transplanted in first relapse or second remission can still be cured in 40 to 50% of cases. This represents a clear advantage over results obtained with salvage chemotherapy. It is unsettled whether patients with high-risk disease benefit from transplantation in first remission. Most experts favor the use of autologous rather than allogeneic transplantation for patients with non-Hodgkin's lymphoma, because fewer complications occur with this approach and survival appears equivalent. The role of transplantation in patients with indolent non-Hodgkin's lymphoma is less well defined. Long-term remissions can be obtained in many patients with acceptable toxicity and results with transplantation in patients with recurrent disease generally appear better than one would expect with conventional-dose chemotherapy. However, late relapses are seen after transplantation, and no randomized study has confirmed its superiority.

The role of transplantation in Hodgkin's disease is similar to that in non-Hodgkin's lymphoma. With transplantation, 5-year disease-free survival is 20 to 30% in patients who never achieve a first remission with standard chemotherapy and up to 60% for those transplanted in second remission. Transplantation has no defined role in first remission in Hodgkin's disease.

Myeloma Patients with myeloma who have progressed on first-line therapy can sometimes benefit from allogeneic or autologous transplantation. Autologous transplantation has been studied as part of the initial therapy of patients, and in randomized trials, both disease-free survival as well as overall survival were improved with this approach. A strategy of autologous transplantation followed by nonmyeloablative allogeneic transplantation has shown encouraging results.

Solid Tumors Among women with metastatic breast cancer, 15 to 20% disease-free survival rates at 3 years have been reported, with better results seen in younger patients who have responded completely to standard-dose therapy before undergoing transplantation. Randomized trials have not shown superior survival for patients treated for metastatic disease with high-dose chemotherapy plus stem cell support. Randomized trials evaluating transplantation as treatment for primary breast cancer are being conducted, but final results are not yet available.

Patients with testicular cancer who have failed first-line chemotherapy have been treated with autologous transplantation; ~10 to 20% of such patients apparently have been cured with this approach.

The use of high-dose chemotherapy with autologous stem cell support is being studied for several other solid tumors, including ovarian cancer, small cell lung cancer, neuroblastoma, and pediatric sarcomas. As in most other settings, the best results have been obtained in patients with limited amounts of disease and where the remaining tumor retains sensitivity to conventional-dose chemotherapy. Few randomized trials of transplantation in these diseases have been completed.

Partial and complete responses have been reported following non-myeloablative allogeneic transplantation for several solid tumors, most notably renal cell carcinomas. These results suggest that the GVT effect, well documented in the treatment of hematologic malignancies, may under certain circumstances apply to selected solid tumors.

Posttransplant Relapse Patients who relapse following autologous transplantation sometimes respond to further chemotherapy, particularly if the remission following transplantation was long. More options are available for patients who relapse following allogeneic transplantation. Of particular interest are the response rates seen with infusion of unirradiated donor lymphocytes. Complete responses in as many as 75% of patients with chronic myeloid leukemia, 40% in myelodysplasia, 25% in AML, and 15% in myeloma have been reported. Major complications of donor lymphocyte infusions include transient myelosuppression and the development of GVHD. These complications appear to be dependent on the number of donor lymphocytes given and the schedule of infusions, with less GVHD seen with lower dose, fractionated schedules.

FURTHER READING

APPELBAUM FR: Haematopoietic cell transplantation as immunotherapy. Nature 411:385, 2001

BENSINGER WI et al: Transplantation of bone marrow as compared with peripheral-blood cells from HLA-identical relatives in patients with hematologic cancers. N Engl J Med 344:175, 2001

HANSEN JA et al: Bone marrow transplants from unrelated donors for patients with chronic myeloid leukemia. N Engl J Med 338:962, 1998

PHILIP T et al: Autologous bone marrow transplantation as compared with salvage chemotherapy in relapses of chemotherapy-sensitive non-Hodgkin's lymphoma. N Engl J Med 333:1540, 1995

RUBINSTEIN P et al: Outcomes among 562 recipients of placental-blood transplants from unrelated donors. N Engl J Med 339:1565, 1998

Section 3 Disorders of Hemostasis

101 | DISORDERS OF THE PLATELET AND VESSEL WALL
Robert I. Handin

Patients with platelet or vessel wall disorders usually bleed into superficial sites such as the skin, mucous membranes, or genitourinary or gastrointestinal tract. Bleeding begins immediately after trauma and either responds to simple measures, such as pressure and packing, or requires systemic therapy with glucocorticoids, desmopressin, plasma fractions, or platelet concentrates. The most common platelet/vessel wall disorders are (1) various forms of thrombocytopenia, (2) von Willebrand's disease (vWD), and (3) drug-induced platelet dysfunction. This chapter reviews the diagnosis and treatment of quantitative and qualitative platelet disorders as well as vessel wall defects that cause bleeding. →*For further discussion of the physiology of normal hemostasis and the cardinal manifestations of bleeding arising from hemostatic disorders, see Chap. 53.*

PLATELET DISORDERS

Platelets arise from the fragmentation of megakaryocytes, which are very large, polyploid bone marrow cells produced by the process of endomitosis. They undergo from three to five cycles of chromosomal duplication without cytoplasmic division. After leaving the marrow space, about one-third of the platelets are sequestered in the spleen, while the other two-thirds circulate for 7 to 10 days. Normally, only a small fraction of the platelet mass is consumed in the process of hemostasis, so most platelets circulate until they become senescent and are removed by phagocytic cells. The normal blood platelet count is 150,000 to 450,000/μL. A decrease in platelet count stimulates an increase in the number, size, and ploidy of megakaryocytes, releasing additional platelets into the circulation. This process is regulated by thrombopoietin (TPO) binding to its megakaryocyte receptor, a proto-oncogene c-mpl. TPO (c-mpl ligand) is secreted continuously at a low level and binds tightly to circulating platelets. A reduction in platelet count increases the level of free TPO and thereby stimulates megakaryocyte and platelet production.

The platelet count varies during the menstrual cycle, rising following ovulation and falling at the onset of menses. It is also influenced by the patient's nutritional state and can be decreased in severe iron, folic acid, or vitamin B_{12} deficiency. Platelets are acute-phase reac-

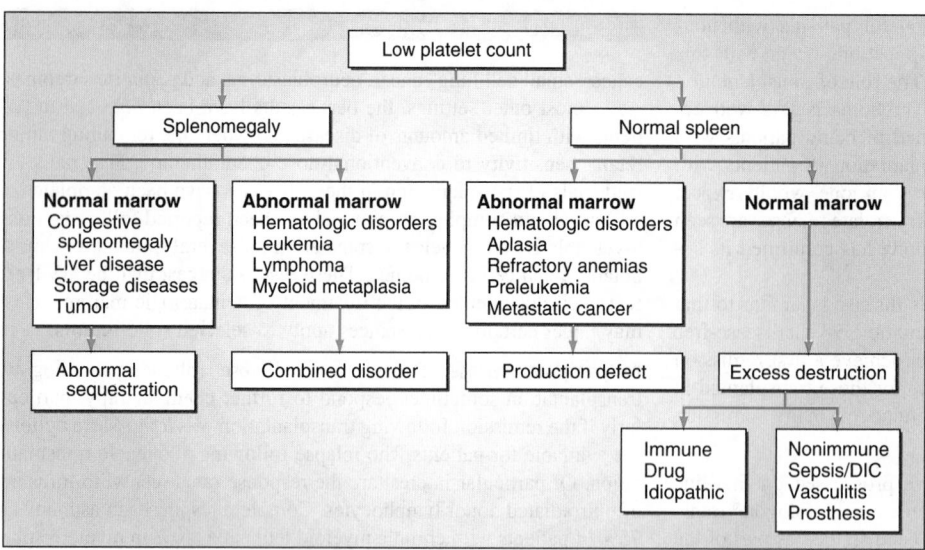

FIGURE 101-1 Clinical evaluation of patients with thrombocytopenia. [*Modified from RI Handin, in W Beck (ed), Hematology, 4th ed. Cambridge, MA, MIT Press, 1985.*]

tants, and patients with systemic inflammation, tumors, bleeding, and mild iron deficiency may have an increased platelet count, a benign condition called *secondary, or reactive, thrombocytosis*. The cytokines interleukin (IL) 3, IL-6, and IL-11 may stimulate platelet production in acute inflammation. In these conditions, the platelet count is usually < 1 million/μL. In contrast, the increase in platelet count that is characteristic of the myeloproliferative disorders such as polycythemia vera, chronic myeloid leukemia, myeloid metaplasia, and essential thrombocytosis can be much higher and cause either severe bleeding or thrombosis. In these patients, unregulated platelet production is secondary to a clonal stem cell abnormality affecting all bone marrow progenitors.

THROMBOCYTOPENIA Thrombocytopenia is caused by one of three mechanisms—decreased bone marrow production, increased splenic sequestration, or accelerated destruction of platelets. In order to determine the etiology of thrombocytopenia, each patient should have a careful examination of the peripheral blood film, an assessment of marrow morphology by examination of an aspirate or biopsy, and an estimate of splenic size by bedside palpation supplemented, if necessary, by ultrasonography or computed tomography (CT). Occasional patients have "pseudothrombocytopenia," a benign condition in which platelets agglutinate or adhere to leukocytes when blood is collected with EDTA as anticoagulant. This is a laboratory artifact, and the actual platelet count in vivo is normal. A scheme for classifying patients with thrombocytopenia based on these clinical observations and laboratory tests is outlined in Fig. 101-1.

Impaired Production Disorders that injure stem cells or prevent their proliferation frequently cause thrombocytopenia. They usually affect multiple hematopoietic cell lines so that thrombocytopenia is accompanied by varying degrees of anemia and leukopenia. Diagnosis of a platelet production defect is readily established by examination of a bone marrow aspirate or biopsy, which should show a reduced number of megakaryocytes. The most common causes of decreased platelet production are marrow aplasia, fibrosis, or infiltration with malignant cells, all of which produce highly characteristic marrow abnormalities. Occasionally, thrombocytopenia is the presenting laboratory abnormality in these disorders. Cytotoxic drugs impair megakaryocyte proliferation and maturation and frequently cause thrombocytopenia. Rare marrow disorders, such as congenital amegakaryocytic hypoplasia and thrombocytopenia with absent radii (TAR syndrome), produce a selective decrease in megakaryocyte production.

Splenic Sequestration Since one-third of the platelet mass is normally sequestered in the spleen, splenectomy will increase the platelet count by 30%. Postsplenectomy thrombocytosis is a benign self-limited con-

dition that does not require specific therapy. In contrast, when the spleen enlarges, the fraction of sequestered platelets increases, lowering the platelet count. The most common causes of splenomegaly are portal hypertension secondary to liver disease and splenic infiltration with tumor cells in myeloproliferative or lymphoproliferative disorders (Chap. 54). Isolated splenomegaly is rare, and in most patients it is accompanied by other clinical manifestations of an underlying disease. Many patients with leukemia, lymphoma, or a myeloproliferative syndrome have both marrow infiltration and splenomegaly and develop thrombocytopenia from a combination of impaired marrow production and splenic sequestration of platelets.

Accelerated Destruction Abnormal vessels, fibrin thrombi, and intravascular prostheses can all shorten platelet survival and cause nonimmunologic thrombocytopenia. Thrombocytopenia is common in patients with vasculitis, the hemolytic uremic syndrome (HUS), thrombotic thrombocytopenic purpura (TTP), or as a manifestation of disseminated intravascular coagulation (DIC). In addition, platelets coated with antibody, immune complexes, or complement are rapidly cleared by mononuclear phagocytes in the spleen or other tissues, inducing immunologic thrombocytopenia. The most common causes of immunologic thrombocytopenia are viral or bacterial infections, drugs (often heparin), and a chronic autoimmune disorder referred to as *idiopathic thrombocytopenic purpura* (ITP). Patients with immunologic thrombocytopenia do not usually have splenomegaly and have an increased number of bone marrow megakaryocytes.

DRUG-INDUCED THROMBOCYTOPENIA Many common drugs can cause thrombocytopenia (Table 101-1). Cancer chemotherapeutic agents may depress megakaryocyte production. Ingestion of large quantities of alcohol has a marrow-depressing effect leading to transient thrombocytopenia, particularly in binge drinkers. Thiazide diuretics, used to treat hypertension or congestive heart failure, impair megakaryocyte production and can produce mild thrombocytopenia (50,000 to 100,000/μL), which may persist for several months after the drug is discontinued.

Most drugs induce thrombocytopenia by eliciting an immune response in which the platelet is an innocent bystander. The platelet is damaged by complement activation following the formation of drug-antibody complexes. Current laboratory tests can identify the causative agent in 10% of patients with clinical evidence of drug-induced thrombocytopenia. The best proof of a drug-induced etiology is a prompt rise in the platelet count when the suspected drug is discontinued. Patients with drug-induced platelet destruction may also have a secondary increase in megakaryocyte number without other marrow abnormalities.

Although most patients recover within 7 to 10 days and do not require therapy, occasional patients with platelet counts <10,000 to 20,000/μL have severe hemorrhage and may require temporary support with glucocorticoids, plasmapheresis, or platelet transfusions

TABLE 101-1 *Drugs That May Cause Thrombocytopenia*

1. Chemotherapeutic agents—especially carboplatin, alkylating agents, anthracyclines, antimetabolites
2. Antibiotics—sulfonamides, penicillins, cephalosporins
3. Heparins—highest incidence is with unfractionated products
4. Cardiovascular agents—thiazide diuretics, rarely angiotensin converting enzyme inhibitors

while waiting for the platelet count to rise. A patient who has recovered from drug-induced immunologic thrombocytopenia should be instructed to avoid the offending drug in the future, since only minute amounts of drug are needed to set up subsequent immune reactions. Certain drugs that are cleared from body storage depots quite slowly, such as phenytoin, may induce prolonged thrombocytopenia.

Heparin is a common cause of thrombocytopenia in hospitalized patients. Between 10 and 15% of patients receiving therapeutic doses of unfractionated heparin develop thrombocytopenia (heparin-induced thrombocytopenia, HIT) and, occasionally, may have severe bleeding or intravascular platelet aggregation and paradoxical thrombosis. Heparin-induced thrombosis, sometimes called the "white clot syndrome," can be fatal unless recognized promptly. Heparin can cause mild thrombocytopenia by directly agglutinating platelets (type I HIT). The more serious form (type II HIT) results from an immune reaction. The offending antigen is a complex formed between heparin and the platelet-derived heparin-neutralizing protein, platelet factor 4. Type II HIT is particularly severe because the heparin–PF-4 antibody complexes bind the platelet Fc receptor and induce platelet activation and secretion. Prompt cessation of heparin will reverse the thrombocytopenia and lepirudin can reduce the risk of thrombosis. Low-molecular-weight heparin products have reduced the incidence of HIT. They are effective antithrombotic agents (Chap. 103) and are less immunogenic. Unfortunately, 80 to 90% of the antibodies generated against conventional heparins cross-react with low-molecular-weight heparins, so only a minority of patients with preformed antibody can be treated with these products. Several potent thrombin inhibitors with different structures from heparin can be used to treat patients with HIT (Chap. 103). Argatroban is the current drug of choice, but pentasaccharides that mimic heparin's active site are in development.

IDIOPATHIC THROMBOCYTOPENIC PURPURA The immunologic thrombocytopenias can be classified on the basis of the pathologic mechanism, the inciting agent, or the duration of the illness. The explosive onset of severe thrombocytopenia following recovery from a viral exanthem or upper respiratory illness (*acute ITP*) is common in children and accounts for 90% of the pediatric cases of immunologic thrombocytopenia. Of these patients, 60% recover in 4 to 6 weeks and >90% recover within 3 to 6 months. Transient immunologic thrombocytopenia also complicates some cases of infectious mononucleosis, acute toxoplasmosis, or cytomegalovirus infection and can be part of the prodromal phase of viral hepatitis and initial infection with HIV. Acute ITP is rare in adults and accounts for <10% of postpubertal patients with immune thrombocytopenia. Acute ITP is caused by immune complexes containing viral antigens that bind to platelet Fc receptors or by antibodies produced against viral antigens that cross-react with the platelet. In addition to these viral disorders, the differential diagnosis includes atypical presentations of aplastic anemia, acute leukemias, or metastatic tumor. A bone marrow examination is essential to exclude these disorders, which can occasionally mimic acute ITP.

Most adults present with a more indolent form of thrombocytopenia that may persist for many years and is referred to as *chronic ITP*. Women age 20 to 40 are afflicted most commonly and outnumber men by a ratio of 3:1. They may present with an abrupt fall in platelet count and bleeding similar to patients with acute ITP. More often they have a prior history of easy bruising or menometrorrhagia. These patients have an autoimmune disorder with antibodies directed against target antigens on the glycoprotein (Gp) IIb/IIIa or, less frequently, the Gp Ib/IX complex (Fig. 53-2). Although most antibodies function as opsonins and accelerate platelet clearance by phagocytic cells, occasional antibodies bind to epitopes on critical regions of these glycoproteins and impair platelet function. Platelet-associated IgG can be measured, but specificity is a problem. High "background" level of IgG on normal platelets and elevations in plasma immunoglobulin levels or in circulating immune complexes will nonspecifically increase platelet-associated IgG. Few clinical situations require platelet-associated IgG testing.

A low platelet count may be the initial manifestation of systemic lupus erythematosus (SLE) or the first sign of a primary hematologic disorder. Thus, patients with chronic ITP should have a bone marrow examination and an antinuclear antibody determination. In addition, patients with hepatic or splenic enlargement, lymphadenopathy, or atypical lymphocytes should have serologic studies for hepatitis viruses, cytomegalovirus, Epstein-Barr virus, *Toxoplasma*, and HIV. HIV infection is a common cause of immunologic thrombocytopenia. Thrombocytopenia can be the initial symptom of HIV infection or a complication of fully developed clinical AIDS.

Rx TREATMENT

Treatment of patients with ITP must take into account the age of the patient, the severity of the illness, and the anticipated natural history. Although adults have a higher incidence of intracranial bleeding than children, specific therapy may not be necessary unless the platelet count is $<20,000/\mu L$ or there is extensive bleeding. Hemorrhage in patients with either acute or chronic ITP can usually be controlled with glucocorticoids but, in rare cases, may require temporary phagocytic blockade with intravenous immunoglobulin (IVIg) or anti-RhD (WinRho). Although antibody preparations are effective, they are expensive and should be reserved for patients with severe thrombocytopenia and clinical bleeding who are refractory to other measures. Emergency splenectomy is usually reserved for patients with acute or chronic ITP who are desperately ill and have not responded to any medical measures. The treatment of symptomatic thrombocytopenia in patients with HIV infection is more complex because the administration of glucocorticoids or splenectomy may increase susceptibility to opportunistic infections. Splenectomy has been effective in the course of HIV before the onset of symptomatic AIDS. Treatment with zidovudine (AZT) and other antiviral agents that reduce viral load can improve the platelet count in patients with HIV-induced thrombocytopenia.

Symptomatic patients with chronic ITP are usually placed on prednisone, 60 mg/d for 4 to 6 weeks. The drug is then decreased slowly over another few weeks. About 50% of patients with chronic ITP will normalize their platelet count on high doses of prednisone. However, the majority will have a fall in platelet count following steroid withdrawal. Patients with chronic ITP who fail to maintain a normal platelet count after a course of prednisone are eligible for elective splenectomy. These glucocorticoid-responsive but glucocorticoid-dependent patients are very likely to respond to splenectomy, and 70% will have a normal platelet count within 1 week after surgery. Splenectomy can now often be performed by minimally invasive laparoscopic techniques that reduce morbidity and shorten hospital stay. Some patients who do not respond to glucocorticoids may still respond to splenectomy. Occasionally, patients may fail to respond to splenectomy because of the failure to remove an accessory spleen. In other patients, a small, inactive accessory spleen may grow or new splenic foci may develop from splenic cells shed at the time of surgery and cause the late onset of thrombocytopenia. In either case, the presence of splenic tissue can be diagnosed by examination of the blood smear for Howell-Jolly bodies that appear in the red cells of asplenic individuals. Persistent splenic tissue can be confirmed by a radionuclide scan.

Patients still thrombocytopenic after splenectomy or who relapse months to years after initial therapy have received a variety of immunosuppressive drugs including azathioprine, cyclophosphamide, vincristine, vinblastine, and cyclosporine. Danazol has also been used with some success. Although each of these drugs may be beneficial, they have serious side effects and should be used judiciously. IVIg and anti-RhD are only transiently effective and expensive. IVIg can cause meningismus and headache, and some lots have carried hepatitis C virus. Anti-RhD can cause hemolysis. These drugs should be used to raise the platelet count temporarily and to support patients before surgery or labor and delivery; they are not substitutes for splenectomy. If a patient is not bleeding and maintains a platelet count >20,000/

μL, consideration should be given to withholding therapy. Patients with severe chronic thrombocytopenia may live with their disease for two or three decades.

Rituximab, an anti-CD20 monoclonal antibody used to treat lymphoma, has also proven an effective approach to ITP and is probably preferable to long-term glucocorticoid therapy. Rituximab eliminates normal B cells, including those producing the antiplatelet antibody. This B cell depletion is transient (lasting 12 to 18 months, normally) and has surprisingly few side effects or toxicities.

FUNCTIONAL PLATELET DISORDERS   As described in Chap. 53, normal hemostasis requires three critical platelet reactions—adhesion, aggregation, and granule release. Clinical bleeding can result from a failure of any of these important functions. Table 101-2 lists the major functional platelet disorders. Table 101-3 lists methods to assess platelet function.

von Willebrand's Disease   vWD is the most common inherited bleeding disorder, occurring in 1 in 100 to 500 individuals. The von Willebrand factor (vWF) is a heterogeneous multimeric plasma glycoprotein with two major functions: (1) It facilitates platelet adhesion under conditions of high shear stress by linking platelet membrane receptors to vascular subendothelium; and (2) it serves as the plasma carrier for factor VIII, the antihemophilic factor, a critical blood coagulation protein. Discrete domains in each vWF subunit mediate each of these important functions. The normal plasma vWF level is 10 mg/L. The vWF activity is distributed among a series of plasma multimers with estimated molecular weights ranging from 400,000 to >20 million. A single large vWF precursor subunit is synthesized in endothelial cells and megakaryocytes, where it is cleaved and assembled into the disulfide-linked multimers present in plasma, platelets, and vascular subendothelium. A modest reduction in plasma vWF concentration or a selective loss in the high-molecular-weight multimers decreases platelet adhesion and causes clinical bleeding.

Although vWD is heterogeneous, certain clinical features are common to all the syndromes. With one exception (type III disease), all forms are inherited as autosomal dominant traits, and affected patients are heterozygous with one normal and one abnormal vWF allele. In mild cases, bleeding occurs only after surgery or trauma. More severely affected patients have spontaneous epistaxis or oral mucosal, gastrointestinal, or genitourinary bleeding. The laboratory findings are variable. The most diagnostic pattern is the combination of (1) a pro-

---

TABLE 101-2   Classification of Functional Platelet Disorders

I. Disorders of adhesion
  A. Inherited
    1. Bernard-Soulier syndrome
    2. von Willebrand's disease (vWD)
  B. Acquired
    1. Uremia
    2. Acquired vWD
II. Disorders of aggregation
  A. Inherited
    1. Glanzmann's thrombasthenia
    2. Afibrinogenemia
  B. Acquired
    1. Fibrin degradation product inhibition
    2. Dysproteinemias
    3. Drugs—e.g., ticlopidine, Gp IIb/IIIa inhibitors
III. Disorders of granule release
  A. Inherited
    1. Oculocutaneous albinism (Hermansky-Pudlak syndrome)
    2. Chédiak-Higashi syndrome
    3. Isolated dense (δ) granule deficiency
    4. Gray-platelet syndrome—combined α and β granule deficiency
  B. Acquired
    1. Cardiopulmonary bypass
    2. Myeloproliferative disorders
    3. Drugs—aspirin and other nonsteroidal anti-inflammatory agents

---

TABLE 101-3   Evaluation of Platelet Function

Bleeding time
  Modified Ivy method
  Skin incision—time to stop bleeding
  Global screen of platelet role in hemostasis
von Willebrand factor assays
  vWF Ag—immunoassay of total vWF protein
  vWF: RCof—bioassay of vWF that measures ability of patient plasma to support agglutination of normal platelets in the presence of ristocetin
  Factor VIII—coagulation assay of factor VIII bound and carried by plasma vWF
Platelet aggregometry
  Measures platelet aggregation in response to a panel of agonists, usually ADP, collagen, arachidonic acid, and epinephrine
Membrane glycoproteins
  Presence of glycoproteins Ib/IX and IIb/IIIa can be measured using monoclonal antibodies and flow cytometry
Platelet granule content
  Dense granules—electron microscopy or uptake and retention of radiolabeled serotonin
  Alpha granules—electron microscopy and/or immunoassays for platelet-associated proteins—vWF, fibrinogen, platelet factor 4

Note: vWF, von Willebrand factor; ADP, adenosine diphosphate; Ag, antigen, R:Cof, ristocetin cofactor.

---

longed bleeding time, (2) a reduction in plasma vWF concentration, (3) a parallel reduction in biologic activity as measured with the ristocetin cofactor assay, and (4) reduced factor VIII activity. The variability in laboratory tests is related to both the heterogeneous nature of the defects in vWD and the fact that plasma levels are influenced by ABO blood group type, central nervous system disorders, systemic inflammation, and pregnancy. Since vWD is an autosomal dominant disorder, some vWF is produced by the remaining normal allele. Thus patients with mild defects may have laboratory values that fluctuate over time and may occasionally be within the normal range.

There are three major types of vWD. Their mode of inheritance and laboratory findings are shown in Fig. 101-2. Patients with type I disease, the most common abnormality, have a mild to moderate decrease in plasma vWF. In the milder cases, although hemostasis is impaired, the vWF level is just below normal (50% activity, or 5 mg/L). In type I disease, vWF antigen, factor VIII activity, and ristocetin cofactor activity are decreased with a normal spectrum of multimers detected by sodium dodecyl sulfate (SDS)–agarose gel electrophoresis.

The variant forms of vWD (type II disease) are much less common and characterized by normal or near-normal levels of a dysfunctional protein. Patients with the type IIa variant of vWD have a deficiency in the high- and medium-molecular-weight forms of vWF multimer detected by SDS-agarose electrophoresis. This is due either to an inability to secrete the high-molecular-weight vWF multimers or to proteolysis of the multimers soon after they leave the endothelial cell and enter the circulation. Mutations in a localized region of the vWF A-2 domain have been identified in families with type IIa vWD (Fig. 101-3). The quantity of vWF antigen and the amount of associated factor VIII are usually normal. In the type IIb variant, high-molecular-weight multimers are also decreased; however, the decrease is due to the inappropriate binding of vWF to platelets. Intravascular platelet aggregates form that are rapidly cleared from the circulation, causing mild, variable thrombocytopenia. Mutations in a disulfide-bonded loop in the A-1 domain that binds to Gp Ib/IX are the cause of the type IIb defect (Fig. 101-3). A few patients have a platelet membrane disorder that mimics type IIb vWD—*platelet-type vWD*. It is due to mutations in the portion of Gp Ib/IX that interacts with vWF. Levels of total vWF antigen and factor VIII are normal.

Approximately 1 in 1 million individuals has a very severe form of vWD that is phenotypically recessive (type III disease). Type III patients are usually the offspring of two parents (usually asymptomatic) with mild type I disease. Type III patients may inherit a different abnormality from each parent (a doubly heterozygous or compound

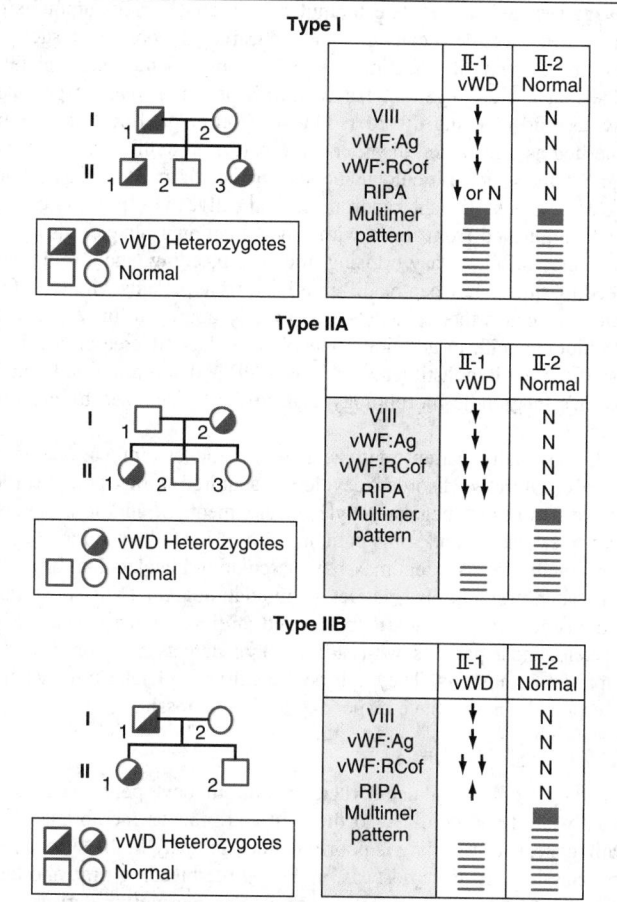

FIGURE 101-2 Pattern of inheritance and laboratory findings in von Willebrand's disease. The assays of platelet function include a coagulation assay of factor VIII bound and carried by von Willebrand factor (vWF), abbreviated as VIII; immunoassay of total vWF protein, abbreviated vWF:Ag; bioassay of the ability of patient plasma to support ristocetin-induced agglutination of normal platelets, abbreviated vWF:RCoF; and ristocetin-induced aggregation of patient platelets, abbreviated RIPA. The multimer pattern illustrates the protein bonds present when plasma is electrophoresed in a polyacrylamide gel. The II-1 and II-2 columns refer to the phenotypes of the second-generation offspring.

heterozygous state) or be homozygous for a single defect. Type III patients have severe mucosal bleeding and no detectable vWF antigen or activity and, like patients with mild hemophilia, may have sufficiently low factor VIII that they have occasional hemarthroses. Major deletions in the vWF gene have been found in some type III families. Families with nonsense mutations and the combination of a deleted and nonsense mutant allele have also been described.

Type IIn disease is due to a defect in the factor VIII binding site of vWF. Patients resemble those with mild hemophilia and have low levels of factor VIII. The presence of disease in both males and females in a family is a clue to the role of vWF in this disease.

℞ TREATMENT

There are two therapeutic options. Factor VIII concentrates retain high-molecular-weight vWF multimers (Humate-P, Alfanate), are highly purified and heat-treated to destroy HIV, and are appropriate treatments for all the inherited forms of vWD. During surgery or after major trauma, patients should receive factor VIII concentrates twice daily for 2 to 3 days to assure optimal hemostasis. Minor bleeding episodes such as prolonged epistaxis or severe menorrhagia may respond to a single infusion. Recurrent menorrhagia, a major

problem for women with severe vWD, can be treated effectively with oral contraceptive agents that suppress menses.

A second therapeutic option, which avoids the use of plasma, is the use of desmopressin, a vasopressin analogue that has minimal blood pressure–elevating and fluid-retaining properties and raises the plasma vWF level in both normal individuals and patients with mild vWD. Patients with type I disease are the best candidates for desmopressin therapy. However, they must be tested for an adequate response before anticipated surgery, and vWF levels must be monitored closely during therapy, since the patient may develop tachyphylaxis when therapy is continued for >48 h. Desmopressin should not be given to patients with variant forms of vWD without prior testing, since it may not improve multimer pattern or hemostasis in type IIa patients and may actually worsen the defect by depleting high-molecular-weight multimers, inducing intravascular platelet aggregation, and lowering the platelet count in type IIb patients. It is ineffective therapy for the severe (type III) form of vWD.

ACQUIRED vWD Although most cases of vWD are inherited, acquired vWD may be caused by antibodies that inhibit vWF function or by lymphoid or other tumors that selectively adsorb vWF multimers onto their surfaces. Anti-vWF antibodies have developed in patients with severe vWD following multiple transfusions, as well as in patients with autoimmune and lymphoproliferative disorders. Adsorption of vWF to tumor surfaces has been documented in patients with Waldenström's macroglobulinemia and Wilms' tumor and inferred in other patients with lymphoma. Treatment of acquired vWD should focus on the underlying disease, since plasma derivatives and desmopressin are often not effective and the disorder can be fatal.

Platelet Membrane Defects Receptors that modulate platelet adhesion and aggregation are located on the two major platelet surface glycoproteins. vWF facilitates platelet adhesion by binding to Gp Ib/IX, while fibrinogen links platelets into aggregates via sites on the Gp IIb/IIIa complex. Two rare platelet defects are characterized by a loss of or a defect in these Gp receptors. Patients with the *Bernard-Soulier syndrome* have markedly reduced platelet adhesion and cannot bind vWF to their platelets due to deficiency or dysfunction of the Gp Ib/IX complex. They also have reduced levels of another membrane protein (GpV that associates with Gp Ib/II), mild thrombocytopenia, and extremely large, lymphocytoid platelets. Platelets from patients with *Glanzmann's disease*, or *thrombasthenia*, are deficient or defective in the Gp IIb/IIIa complex. Their platelets do not bind fibrinogen and cannot form aggregates, although the platelets undergo shape change and secretion and are of normal size.

Both these disorders are autosomal recessive traits and markedly

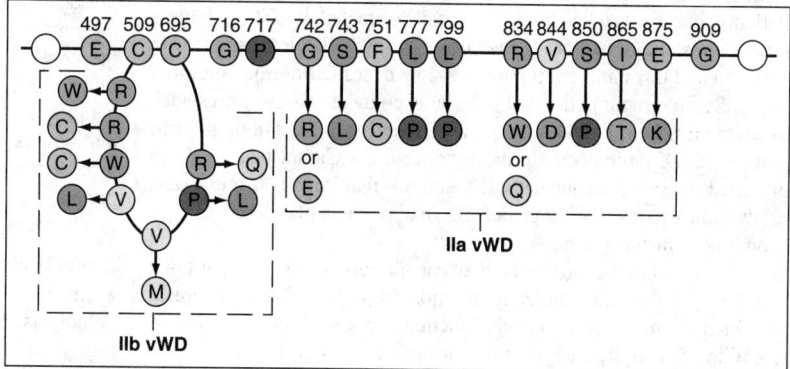

FIGURE 101-3 Location of mutations in types IIa and IIb von Willebrand's disease. Mutations in the region of the protein between amino acids 742 and 875 have been identified in patients with type IIa disease. These result in a deficiency in high- and medium-molecular-weight multimers due either to failure to secrete high-molecular-weight forms of von Willebrand factor (vWF) or to their proteolytic degradation in the circulation. In type IIb disease, there is also a decrease in high-molecular-weight vWF, but the defect is due to the failure of vWF with mutations in the A-1 domain of the protein (amino acids 509–695) to bind properly to platelet glycoprotein Ib/IX.

impair hemostasis, leading to recurrent episodes of severe mucosal hemorrhage. Bernard-Soulier platelets react normally to all stimuli except ristocetin. In contrast, thrombasthenic platelets adhere normally and will agglutinate with ristocetin but will not aggregate with any of the agonists that require fibrinogen binding, such as adenosine diphosphate (ADP), thrombin, or epinephrine.

The only effective therapy for hemorrhagic episodes in these two disorders is transfusion with normal platelets. Alloimmunization will eventually limit the life span of infused platelets. In addition, a few patients have developed inhibitor antibodies with specificity for the missing protein. These antibodies bind to the protein that is expressed on the transfused normal platelets and impair their function.

Platelet Release Defects   The most common mild bleeding disorders arise from the ingestion of aspirin and other nonsteroidal anti-inflammatory drugs (NSAIDs) that inhibit platelet production of thromboxane A_2, an important mediator of platelet secretion and aggregation (Figs. 53-3 and 53-4). These drugs inhibit cyclooxygenase (COX), which converts arachidonic acid to a labile endoperoxide intermediate that is critical for thromboxane formation. Aspirin is the most potent of these agents; it irreversibly acetylates the platelet enzyme so that a single dose impairs hemostasis for 5 to 7 days. The other agents are competitive and reversible inhibitors with more transient effects. Blocking thromboxane A_2 synthesis partially inhibits platelet release and aggregation with weak agonists, such as ADP and epinephrine, and produces a mild hemostatic defect. Cyclooxygenase exists in two isoforms, COX-1, which is constitutively expressed and active in the normal platelet, and COX-2, which is induced, especially in inflamed tissue. The selective COX-2 inhibitors, such as celecoxib, are increasingly being used to control arthritis pain and in other settings where NSAIDs are clinically useful. The COX-2 inhibitors are long-acting reversible inhibitors that have no adverse effects on platelet function. Their chronic use may be associated with high blood pressure and risk of thrombosis. The administration of high doses of certain antibiotics, particularly penicillin, can coat the platelet surface, block platelet release, and impair hemostasis.

Patients with release defects generally have minimal symptoms such as easy bruising, and bleeding is usually confined to the skin. Occasional patients will have prolonged oozing after surgery, particularly with procedures involving mucous membranes such as periodontal, oral, or reconstructive plastic surgery. The antiplatelet effect of drugs such as aspirin is more dramatic when they are administered to patients with underlying defects such as vWD or hemophilia. Patients with drug-induced COX deficiency often have a mildly prolonged bleeding time, and their platelets fail to aggregate when incubated with arachidonic acid, epinephrine, or low doses of ADP. Patients who have taken aspirin should be treated as if they have a mild hemostatic defect for the next 5 to 7 days. Platelet responses to collagen and thrombin are impaired at low doses but normal at higher doses. Symptomatic patients should be encouraged to use drugs such as acetaminophen that do not impair platelet function. Although most cases of COX deficiency are drug-induced, occasional patients have inherited disorders in platelet COX activity that impair thromboxane production or receptor level defects that prevent platelets from responding to thromboxane A_2.

Of the metabolic disorders that can perturb hemostasis, uremic platelet dysfunction is clinically the most important. The mechanism by which uremia impairs platelet function is not well understood, and retention of phenolic and guanidinosuccinic acids, excess prostacyclin production, or impaired vWF-platelet interactions have all been implicated. The degree of uremia correlates with bleeding symptoms and anemia. Bleeding can usually be reversed by dialysis and often improves after red cell transfusion or treatment with erythropoietin. In addition, factor VIII concentrate or desmopressin, both of which raise plasma vWF levels, can also improve hemostasis. Conjugated estrogens improve hemostasis and can be used as long-term therapy.

Storage Pool Defects   Platelet granules have considerable amounts of adenine nucleotides, calcium, and adhesive glycoproteins such as thrombospondin, fibronectin, and vWF, all of which promote platelet adhesion and aggregation. Patients with defective platelet granules have a mild bleeding disorder. Platelet storage pool defects may be inherited as an isolated disorder or be part of systemic granule packaging defects such as oculocutaneous albinism or the Hermansky-Pudlak or Chédiak-Higashi syndromes. Clinically, these patients cannot be distinguished from those with other functional platelet disorders, since they all have easy bruising, mucosal bleeding, and a prolonged bleeding time. They can be differentiated from patients with the COX defects because their platelets will usually aggregate in response to arachidonic acid. In addition, their platelets have decreased levels of specific granule constituents such as ADP and serotonin and abnormalities in granule morphology that are best visualized by electron microscopy.

Occasionally, patients with acute or chronic leukemia or one of the myeloproliferative disorders develop an acquired storage pool disorder due to dysplastic megakaryocyte development. In addition, patients with liver disease and some patients with SLE or other immune complex–mediated disorders may have circulating platelets that have degranulated prematurely. Platelet degranulation and a transient storage pool disorder may occur after prolonged cardiopulmonary bypass. Fortunately, most patients with storage pool defects have only mildly impaired hemostasis. They can be treated with platelet transfusions. Occasional patients have responded to desmopressin.

VESSEL WALL DISORDERS

Bleeding from vascular disorders (nonthrombocytopenic purpura) is usually mild and confined to the skin and mucous membranes. The pathogenesis of bleeding is poorly defined in many of the syndromes, and classic tests of hemostasis, including the bleeding time and tests of platelet function, are usually normal. Vascular purpura arises from damage to capillary endothelium, abnormalities in the vascular subendothelial matrix or extravascular connective tissues that support blood vessels, or from the formation of abnormal blood vessels. Several idiopathic disorders involve the vessel wall and can cause more severe bleeding and organ dysfunction.

THROMBOTIC THROMBOCYTOPENIC PURPURA   TTP is a fulminant, often lethal disorder that may be initiated by endothelial injury and subsequent release of vWF and other procoagulant materials from the endothelial cell. Causes include pregnancy, metastatic cancer, mitomycin C, high-dose chemotherapy, HIV infection, and certain drugs, such as the antiplatelet agent ticlopidine. Characteristic findings include the microvascular deposition of hyaline fibrin thrombi, thrombocytopenia, microangiopathic hemolytic anemia, fever, renal failure, fluctuating levels of consciousness, and evanescent focal neurologic deficits. The presence of hyaline thrombi in arterioles, capillaries, and venules without any inflammatory changes in the vessel wall is diagnostic. The presence of a severe Coombs-negative hemolytic anemia with schistocytes or fragmented red blood cells in the peripheral blood smear, coupled with thrombocytopenia, and minimal activation of the coagulation system help to confirm the clinical suspicion of TTP. This disorder should be distinguished from vasculitis and SLE, which can predispose patients to TTP. Platelet-associated IgG and complement levels are usually normal in TTP.

Clinical Manifestations   The classic pentad of TTP consists of hemolytic anemia with fragmentation of erythrocytes and signs of intravascular hemolysis, thrombocytopenia, diffuse and nonfocal neurologic findings, decreased renal function, and fever. These signs and symptoms occur variably, depending on the number and sites of the arteriolar lesions. The anemia may be very mild to very severe, and the thrombocytopenia often parallels it. The neurologic and renal symptoms are usually seen only when the platelet count is markedly diminished (<20 to $30 \times 10^3/\mu L$). Fever is not reliably present. TTP may be acute in onset, but its course spans days to weeks in most patients and occasionally continues for months. Proteinuria and a moderate elevation of blood urea nitrogen may be found on initial presentation; the latter continues to rise while urine output falls if the patient develops renal failure. Neurologic symptoms develop in >90% of patients whose disease terminates in death. Initially, changes in mental status such as confusion, delirium, or altered states of consciousness may occur. Focal findings include seizures, hemiparesis, aphasia, and visual field defects. These neurologic symptoms may fluctuate and terminate in coma. Involvement of myocardial blood vessels may be a cause of sudden death. The severity of the disorder can be estimated from the degree of anemia and thrombocytopenia and the serum lactic dehydrogenase level. Prothrombin time, partial thromboplastin time, fibrinogen concentration, and the level of fibrin split products are usually normal or only mildly abnormal. If the coagulation tests indicate a major consumption of clotting factors, the diagnosis of TTP is doubtful. A positive antinuclear antibody (ANA) determination is obtained in ~20% of patients.

Pathogenesis TTP is due to a deficiency in the activity of a specific metalloproteinase called *ADAMTS 13*, a normal plasma constituent that cleaves the ultra-high-molecular-weight (UHMW) forms of vWF secreted by endothelial cells to yield the heterogeneous set of multimers normally present in plasma (Fig. 101-4). A small number of patients have recurrent episodes of a TTP-like illness (*Upshaw-Schulman syndrome*) and are deficient in ADAMTS 13; the syndrome is inherited as an autosomal recessive trait. The more common acquired form of TTP is due to an inhibitory antibody that blocks ADAMTS 13 activity. These findings have led to more reliable diagnostic tests based on ADAMTS 13 enzyme activity and may have implications beyond TTP. Studies are underway to see if asymptomatic carriers with 50% levels of ADAMTS 13 are at increased risk of thromboembolism.

℞ TREATMENT

The treatment of acute TTP has focused on the use of exchange transfusion or intensive plasmapheresis coupled with infusion of fresh-frozen plasma. Therapy may remove abnormal forms of vWF, lower the concentration of ADAMTS 13 inhibitor, and replenish the deficient enzyme. Overall mortality has been markedly reduced, and the majority of patients with TTP recover from this formerly fatal disorder. Most patients surviving the acute illness recover completely, with no residual renal or neurologic disease. Occasional patients with a chronic, relapsing form of TTP require maintenance plasmapheresis and plasma infusion, and a few patients are controlled only with glucocorticoids. They presumably have persistence of the ADAMTS 13 inhibitor. In the future, TTP patients may be treated with some combination of enzyme replacement and immunosuppression to block inhibitor production.

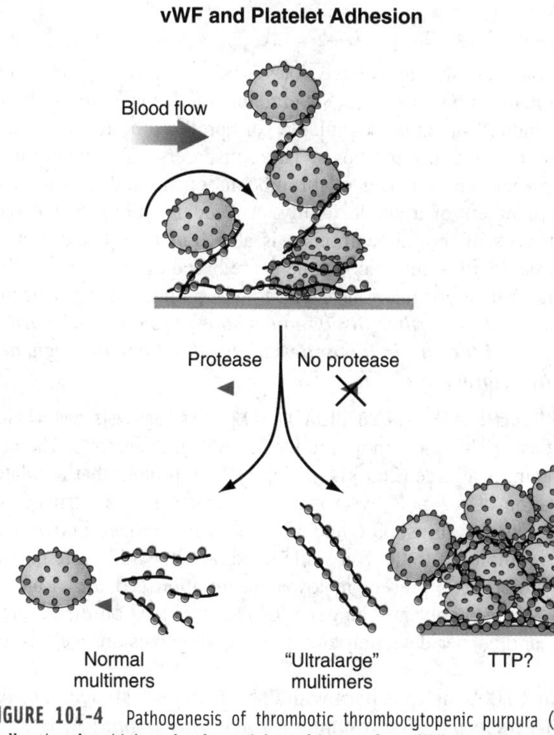

HEMOLYTIC-UREMIC SYNDROME HUS is a disease of infancy and early childhood that closely resembles TTP. Patients present with fever, thrombocytopenia, microangiopathic hemolytic anemia, hypertension, and varying degrees of acute renal failure. In many cases, onset is preceded by a minor febrile or viral illness, and an infectious or immune complex–mediated cause has been proposed. Epidemics related to infection with a specific strain of *Escherichia coli* (O157:H7) have been documented. The bacteria contain a *Shigella*-like toxin that damages endothelial cells. As in TTP, DIC is not found. In contrast to TTP, the disorder remains localized to the kidney, where hyaline thrombi are seen in the afferent arterioles and glomerular capillaries. Thrombi are not present in other vessels, and neurologic symptoms, other than those associated with uremia, are uncommon. No therapy is proven effective; however, with dialysis for acute renal failure, the initial mortality is only 5% in children but may be higher in adults. Between 10 and 50% of patients have some chronic renal impairment. ADAMTS 13 levels are normal, and no inhibitors of the enzyme are present in this disorder.

HENOCH-SCHÖNLEIN PURPURA Henoch-Schönlein, or anaphylactoid, purpura is a distinct, self-limited type of vasculitis that occurs in children and young adults. Patients have an acute inflammatory reaction in capillaries, mesangial tissues, and small arterioles that leads to increased vascular permeability, exudation, and hemorrhage. Vessel lesions contain IgA and complement components. The syndrome may be preceded by an upper respiratory infection or streptococcal pharyngitis or be associated with food or drug allergies. Patients develop a purpuric or urticarial rash on the extensor surfaces of the arms and legs and on the buttocks as well as polyarthralgias or arthritis, colicky abdominal pain, and hematuria from focal glomerulonephritis. Despite the hemorrhagic features, all coagulation tests are normal. A small number of patients may develop fatal acute renal failure, and 5 to 10% develop chronic nephritis. Glucocorticoids provide symptomatic relief of the joint and abdominal pains but do not alter the course of the illness.

METABOLIC AND INFLAMMATORY DISORDERS Acute febrile illnesses may cause capillary fragility and skin bleeding. Immune complexes containing viral antigens or the viruses themselves may damage endothelial cells. In addition, certain pathogens such as the rickettsiae that cause Rocky Mountain spotted fever replicate in endothelial cells and damage them. Thrombocytopenia is also a frequent finding in acute infectious disorders and may contribute to skin bleeding. In addition, whenever the platelet count is <10,000/μL, gaps develop between endothelial cells, which allow the diapedesis of red cells into the dermis, forming petechiae. Drugs such as the sulfonamides, penicillin, and allopurinol may cause vascular inflammation, resulting in maculopapular or urticarial rashes. Some of these mechanisms are additive, and drug reactions in thrombocytopenic individuals cause an intensely hemorrhagic rash.

Occasionally, patients with diffuse polyclonal hyperglobulinemia will develop purpuric lesions on the lower limbs—a benign condition referred to as *hyperglobulinemic purpura*. Vascular purpura may occur in patients with various monoclonal gammopathies, including Waldenström's macroglobulinemia, multiple myeloma, and cryoglobuli-

vWF and Platelet Adhesion

FIGURE 101-4 Pathogenesis of thrombotic thrombocytopenic purpura (TTP). Normally, the ultra-high-molecular-weight multimers of von Willebrand factor (vWF) produced by the endothelial cells are processed into smaller multimers by a plasma metalloproteinase called ADAMTS 13. In TTP, the activity of the protease is inhibited, and the ultra-high-molecular-weight multimers of vWF initiate platelet aggregation and thrombosis. (*From Vesely et al., Copyright American Society of Hematology.*)

nemia. These proteins markedly increase serum viscosity and may impair blood flow through capillaries and lead to retinal hemorrhage, central nervous system dysfunction, and skin necrosis. In addition, the globulins may impair platelet aggregation and adhesion and interfere with fibrin polymerization. Patients with mixed cryoglobulinemia develop a more extensive maculopapular lesion due to immune complex–mediated damage to the vessel wall. The mixed cryoglobulinemia (usually IgG and anti-IgG) may be associated with arthralgias, diffuse weakness, and unexplained nephritis. Plasmapheresis will temporarily lower the level of globulins, remove immune complexes, and improve symptoms in these patients. However, long-term management must include control of the underlying disease that produces the abnormal globulins or immune complexes.

Patients with *scurvy* (vitamin C deficiency) develop painful episodes of perifollicular skin bleeding as well as bleeding into muscles and, occasionally, into the gastrointestinal and genitourinary tracts. The diagnosis is confirmed by the presence of hyperkeratosis of skin, gum swelling, and low levels of the vitamin in leukocytes. Vitamin C is needed to synthesize hydroxyproline, an essential constituent of collagen. Thus, collagen synthesis is impaired by scurvy. Patients with *Cushing's syndrome*, an excess production of glucocorticoids, or patients on large doses of glucocorticoids develop generalized protein wasting and may show skin bleeding or easy bruising due to atrophy of the supporting connective tissue around blood vessels. Aging causes a similar atrophy of perivascular connective tissue on the extensor surfaces of the hands and arms, leading to *senile purpura*—dark purple, irregularly shaped hemorrhagic areas due to abnormal skin mobility that tears small blood vessels.

Patients with inherited disorders of the connective tissue matrix such as *Marfan's syndrome*, *Ehlers-Danlos syndrome*, and *pseudoxanthoma elasticum* also have easy bruising. In addition to having fragile skin vessels and easy bruising, patients with Ehlers-Danlos syndrome may develop aneurysms in intraabdominal vessels and apoplectic rupture and hemorrhage due to defects in the vascular collagen network. Primary vascular abnormalities can also lead to bleeding. Patients with *Osler-Rendu-Weber disease* [hereditary hemorrhagic telangiectasia (HHT)], an inherited autosomal dominant disorder, have frequent episodes of nasal and gastrointestinal bleeding from abnormal telangiectatic capillaries. They may develop pulmonary arteriovenous fistulas. Two genetic defects have been identified in these patients, both involving proteins that bind to transforming growth factor β (TGF-β); HHT-1 has mutations in endoglin, and HHT-2 has mutations in ALK-1. Patients with *angiodysplasia of the colon* have increased incidence of gastrointestinal bleeding. In the *Kasabach-Merritt syndrome*, patients may have very extensive and progressively enlarging vascular malformation that may involve large portions of their extremities. Bleeding is secondary to DIC triggered by stagnant blood flow through the tortuous vessels.

FURTHER READING

ALVING BM: How I treat heparin-induced thrombocytopenia and thrombosis. Blood 101:31, 2003

Guidelines for the investigation and management of idiopathic thrombocytopenic purpura in adults, children, and pregnancy. Br J Haematol 120:574, 2003

HANDIN RI, EWENSTEIN BM: von Willebrand's disease, in *Blood: Principles and Practice of Hematology*, 2d ed, RI Handin et al (eds). Philadelphia, Lippincott Williams & Wilkins, 2003, pp 1103–1130

VESELY SK et al: ADAMTS 13 activity in thrombotic thrombocytopenic purpura—hemolytic uremic syndrome: Relation to presenting features and clinical outcomes in a prospective cohort of 142 patients. Blood 102:60, 2003

———: Management of adult patients with persistent idiopathic thrombocytopenic purpura following splenectomy: A systematic review. Ann Intern Med 140:112, 2004

102   DISORDERS OF COAGULATION AND THROMBOSIS
Robert I. Handin

Patients with congenital plasma coagulation defects characteristically bleed into muscles, joints, and body cavities hours or days after an injury. Most of the *inherited* plasma coagulation disorders are due to defects in single coagulation proteins, with the two X-linked disorders, factors VIII and IX deficiency, accounting for the majority. These patients may have severe bleeding and chronic disability and require specialized medical therapy. With rare exceptions, the known disorders prolong either the prothrombin time (PT), partial thromboplastin time (PTT), or both. If they are abnormal, quantitative assays of specific coagulation proteins are then carried out using the PT or PTT tests with plasma from congenitally deficient individuals as substrate. The corrective effect of varying concentrations of patient plasma is measured and expressed as a percentage of a normal pooled plasma standard. The interval range for most coagulation factors is 50 to 150% of this average value, and the minimal level of most individual factors needed for adequate hemostasis is 25%.

Acquired coagulation disorders are both more frequent and more complex, arising from deficiencies of multiple coagulation proteins and simultaneously affecting both primary and secondary hemostasis. The most common acquired hemorrhagic disorders are (1) disseminated intravascular coagulation (DIC), (2) the hemorrhagic diathesis of liver disease, and (3) vitamin K deficiency and complications of anticoagulant therapy.

Although congenital and acquired bleeding disorders are relatively rare, venous and arterial thrombosis and embolism are common medical disorders that have been recognized for >100 years. Although risk factors such as atherosclerotic vascular disease, congestive heart failure, malignancy, and immobility predispose patients to thrombosis, specific coagulation defects have not yet been identified in most patients with thromboembolism. Several inherited coagulation abnormalities induce a hypercoagulable or prethrombotic state and predispose patients to thrombosis. These disorders affect young people, cause recurrent episodes of thromboembolism, and may involve multiple members of a single family. An understanding of the biochemical basis of thromboembolism is also important because anticoagulant and antithrombotic regimens are based on the premise that modifying critical coagulation reactions will reduce the incidence of thrombosis. →*For further discussion of the physiology of normal hemostasis and the cardinal manifestations of the hemorrhagic and thrombotic disorders, see Chap. 53.*

FACTOR VIII DEFICIENCY—HEMOPHILIA A ■ **Pathogenesis and Clinical Manifestations**   The antihemophilic factor (AHF), or factor VIII coagulant protein, is a large (265-kDa), single-chain protein that regulates the activation of factor X by proteases generated in the intrinsic coagulation pathway (Figs. 53-6 and 53-7). It is synthesized in liver and circulates complexed to the von Willebrand factor (vWF) protein. Factor VIII molecule is present in low concentration (10 μg/L) and is susceptible to proteolysis. The gene for factor VIII is on the X chromosome, and carrier detection and prenatal diagnosis are well established.

One in 10,000 males is born with deficiency or dysfunction of the factor VIII molecule. The resulting disorder, *hemophilia A*, is characterized by bleeding into soft tissues, muscles, and weight-bearing joints. Symptomatic patients usually have factor VIII levels <5%, with a close correlation between the clinical severity of hemophilia and plasma AHF level. Patients with <1% factor VIII activity have *severe* disease; they bleed frequently even without discernible trauma. Patients with levels of 1 to 5% have *moderate* disease with less frequent bleeding episodes. Those with levels >5% have *mild* disease with infrequent bleeding that is usually secondary to trauma. Occasional patients with factor VIII levels as high as 25% are discovered when they bleed after major trauma or surgery. The majority of patients with hemophilia A have factor VIII levels <5%.

Hemophilic bleeding occurs hours or days after injury, can involve any organ, and, if untreated, may continue for days or weeks. This can result in large collections of partially clotted blood putting pressure on adjacent normal tissues and can cause necrosis of muscle (compartment syndromes), venous congestion (pseudophlebitis), or ischemic damage to nerves. Patients with hemophilia often develop femoral neuropathy due to pressure from an unsuspected retroperitoneal hematoma. They can also develop large calcified masses of blood and inflammatory tissue that are mistaken for cancers (pseudotumor syndrome).

Patients with severe hemophilia are usually diagnosed shortly after birth because of an extensive cephalhematoma or profuse bleeding at circumcision. However, young children with moderate disease may not bleed until they begin to walk or crawl, and individuals with mild hemophilia may not be diagnosed until they are adolescents or young adults. Typically, a hemophilia patient presents with pain followed by swelling in a weight-bearing joint, such as the hip, knee, or ankle. The presence of blood in the joint (*hemarthrosis*) causes synovial inflammation, and repetitive bleeding erodes articular cartilage and causes osteoarthritis, articular fibrosis, joint ankylosis, and eventually muscle atrophy. Bleeding may occur into any joint, but after a joint has been damaged, it may become a site for subsequent bleeding episodes.

Hematuria, without any genitourinary pathology, is also common. It is usually self-limited and may not require specific therapy. The most feared complications of hemophilia are oropharyngeal and central nervous system bleeding. Patients with oropharyngeal bleeding may require emergency intubation to maintain an adequate airway. Central nervous system bleeding can occur without antecedent trauma or without evidence of a specific lesion.

Patients suspected of having hemophilia should have a platelet count, bleeding time, PT, and PTT determination. Typically, the patient will have a prolonged PTT with all other tests normal. Because of the clinical similarity of factor VIII deficiency and factor IX deficiency, any male with an appropriate bleeding history and a prolonged PTT should have specific assays for factor VIII and factor IX.

Rx TREATMENT

Tenets regarding the treatment of bleeding in hemophilia patients include the following: (1) Symptoms often precede objective evidence of bleeding. (2) Signs of bleeding may not appear until several days after well-documented trauma. The patients can generally be relied upon to identify early symptoms, usually pain. Early treatment is more effective, less costly, and can be lifesaving. (3) Avoid the use of aspirin or aspirin-containing drugs, which impair platelet function and may cause severe hemorrhage. Cyclooxygenase inhibitors can be used, as they do not impair platelet function.

Plasma products enriched in factor VIII reduce the degree of orthopedic deformity and permit virtually any form of elective and emergency surgery. The widespread use of factor VIII concentrates has also produced serious complications, including viral hepatitis, chronic liver disease, and AIDS. *Cryoprecipitate*, which contains about half the factor VIII activity of fresh-frozen plasma in one-tenth the original volume, is simple to prepare and is produced in hospital or regional blood banks.

Three developments have increased the safety of factor VIII therapy and have changed medical practice. First, heating of lyophilized factor VIII concentrates under carefully controlled conditions can inactivate HIV without destroying factor VIII activity. Second, highly purified factor VIII can be produced by adsorbing and eluting factor VIII from monoclonal antibody columns. Third, recombinant factor

VIII is now available. Patients with hemophilia should receive either monoclonal purified or recombinant factor VIII to minimize viral infections and exposure to irrelevant proteins.

Each unit of factor VIII infused, defined as the amount present in 1 mL normal plasma, will raise the plasma level of the recipient by 2%/kg of body weight. Factor VIII has a half-life of 8 to 12 h, making it necessary to infuse it continuously or at least twice daily to sustain a chosen factor VIII level. In patients with mild hemophilia, an alternative treatment is desmopressin (DDAVP), which transiently increases the factor VIII level. Desmopressin will increase the factor level two- to threefold. Although generally safe, it occasionally causes hyponatremia or may precipitate thrombosis in elderly patients.

An uncomplicated episode of soft tissue bleeding or an early hemarthrosis can be treated with one infusion of sufficient factor VIII concentrate to raise the factor VIII level to 15 or 20%. A more extensive hemarthrosis or retroperitoneal bleeding requires twice-daily or continuous infusions in order to keep the factor VIII level at 25 to 50% for at least 72 h. Life-threatening bleeding into the central nervous system or major surgery may require therapy for 2 weeks with levels kept at a minimum of 50% normal. Patients also need skilled orthopedic care, with immobilization of inflamed joints to promote healing and to prevent contractures, and physical therapy to strengthen muscles and maintain joint mobility.

Before surgery, every hemophilia patient should be screened for the presence of an inhibitor to factor VIII. Patients with hemophilia who do not have an inhibitor should receive factor VIII infusions just before surgery and will require daily monitoring so that the factor VIII level is maintained >50% for 10 to 14 days after surgery. When patients undergo joint replacement or other major orthopedic surgery, therapy should be continued for 3 weeks to permit wound healing and the institution of physical therapy.

Hemophilia patients also require treatment before dental procedures. Filling of a carious tooth can be managed by a single infusion of factor VIII concentrate coupled with the administration of 4 to 6 g of ε-aminocaproic acid (EACA) four times daily for 3 to 4 days after the dental procedure. EACA is a potent antifibrinolytic agent that inhibits plasminogen activators present in oral secretions and stabilizes clot formation in oral tissue. Alternatives include tranexamic acid, a longer-acting antifibrinolytic. EACA is also effective when used as a mouthwash. For major oral and periodontal surgery and extractions of permanent teeth, patients should probably be hospitalized briefly and also treated with factor VIII concentrates. Therapy should begin just before surgery and continue for at least 2 to 3 days.

Many centers have organized home-care programs so that patients can administer their own factor VIII infusions with the onset of symptoms. Occasional patients with very frequent bleeding receive regularly scheduled infusions. Despite the expense and inconvenience of "prophylactic" infusions, their use in early childhood has reduced or eliminated hemarthroses. Concern about transmission of AIDS has made some patients reluctant to treat themselves, despite the fact that current blood products carry a very low or no risk of transmitting HIV.

The prospects for correcting factor VIII deficiency by gene therapy are promising; some success has been achieved in dogs. Clinical studies in humans are underway. Concerns about the side effects of current viral vectors used to deliver the factor VIII cDNA are slowing clinical trials.

Complications Most hemophilia patients have had multiple episodes of hepatitis, and a majority have elevated hepatocellular enzyme levels and abnormalities on liver biopsy. Donated blood is now being screened for various types of hepatitis, so the risk of this disease is diminishing. Between 10 and 20% of patients also have hepatosplenomegaly, and a small number develop chronic active or persistent hepatitis or cirrhosis. A few patients with hemophilia and end-stage liver disease have received liver transplants with cure of both diseases. Along with homosexuals and intravenous drug abusers, long-time hemophilia patients are at high risk for AIDS because they frequently received blood products before the era of testing them for HIV; they can also present with the full range of AIDS-related syndromes, including diffuse lymphadenopathy and immune thrombocytopenia. Although up to 50% of current multiply transfused hemophiliacs are HIV-positive and many have clinical AIDS, the advances in factor VIII concentrate production should prevent future HIV infection.

Despite frequent bleeding, severe iron-deficiency anemia is uncommon because most of the bleeding is internal and iron is effectively recycled. Mild iron deficiency from chronic epistaxis or gastrointestinal bleeding occurs in some patients. In addition, some patients have developed a mild Coombs-positive hemolytic anemia due to small amounts of anti-A and anti-B antibody that are present in intermediate purity factor VIII concentrates.

Following multiple transfusions, 10 to 20% of patients with severe hemophilia develop inhibitors to factor VIII. Inhibitors are usually IgG antibodies that rapidly neutralize factor VIII activity. Two types of inhibitors are found with different biologic characteristics and different clinical presentations. Patients with type I inhibitors have a typical anamnestic response and raise their antibody titer following exposure to factor VIII. Patients with a type II inhibitor have a low antibody titer that is not stimulated by factor VIII infusion. Patients with the type I inhibitor should not receive factor VIII. Control of bleeding may require the infusion of either porcine factor VIII concentrates, which may not be affected by inhibitors, or prothrombin complex concentrates, which contain trace quantities of activated coagulation factors and can bypass the block in coagulation produced by the inhibitor. Patients with low-titer type II antibodies may respond to higher doses of factor VIII. Another alternative is the infusion of recombinant factor VIIa; it activates factor X directly and bypasses the inhibitor-induced block.

Protocols to induce tolerance to human factor VIII use massive doses of the factor coupled with immunosuppression. Tolerance induction is expensive and not always effective; it should be reserved for severely affected patients.

Genetic Counseling and Carrier Detection   It is possible to trace the defective allele in some families by examining the inheritance of restriction fragment length polymorphisms (RFLP) linked to the factor VIII gene. In addition, in families in which a specific mutation has been defined in the factor VIII gene, it can be readily detected by gene amplification and allele-specific oligonucleotide hybridization. For example, 45% of patients with severe hemophilia A have a chromosomal inversion arising from homologous recombination between sequences in intron 22 and an upstream gene. The inversion is readily detected by polymerase chain reaction (PCR) or Southern blotting. Precise diagnosis is possible early in pregnancy from either chorionic villus biopsy or amniocentesis.

Female carriers of hemophilia, who are heterozygotes, usually produce sufficient factor VIII from the factor VIII allele on their normal X chromosome for normal hemostasis. However, occasional hemophilia carriers will have factor VIII levels far below 50% due to random inactivation of normal X chromosomes in tissue producing factor VIII. These symptomatic carriers may bleed with major surgery or bleed occasionally with menses. Rarely, true female hemophiliacs arise from consanguinity within families with hemophilia or from concomitant Turner's syndrome or XO mosaicism in a carrier female.

FACTOR IX DEFICIENCY—HEMOPHILIA B   Factor IX is a single-chain, 55-kDa proenzyme that is converted to an active protease (IXa) by factor XIa or by the tissue factor–VIIa complex. Factor IXa then activates factor X in conjunction with activated factor VIII. Factor IX is one of six proteins synthesized in the liver that require vitamin K for biologic activity. Vitamin K is a cofactor for a unique posttranslational modification that inserts a second carboxyl group onto certain glutamic acid residues on factor IX (Chap. 53). This modification permits calcium binding and adsorption onto phospholipid surfaces. Factor IX gene is on the X chromosome.

Factor IX deficiency or dysfunction (hemophilia B, Christmas disease) occurs in 1 in 100,000 male births. Accurate laboratory diagnosis is critical, since it is indistinguishable clinically from factor VIII deficiency (hemophilia A) but requires different treatment. Either fresh-frozen plasma or a plasma fraction enriched in the prothrombin complex proteins is used. Monoclonally purified or recombinant factor IX preparations are now available. In addition to the expected complications of hepatitis, chronic liver disease, and AIDS, the therapy of factor IX deficiency has a special hazard. Trace quantities of activated coagulation factors in prothrombin complex concentrates may activate the coagulation system and cause thrombosis and embolism. This is particularly common in immobilized surgical patients and patients with liver disease. As a result, some centers have returned to fresh-frozen plasma for factor IX–deficient surgical patients, while others have recommended the addition of small doses of heparin to the concentrate to activate antithrombin III during the infusion and reduce hypercoagulability. The recombinant or monoclonally purified products are less likely to be thrombogenic.

FACTOR XI DEFICIENCY   Factor XI is a 160-kDa dimeric protein activated to an active protease (XIa) by factor XIIa, in conjunction with high-molecular-weight kininogen and kallikrein (Figs. 53-6 and 53-7). Factor XI deficiency is inherited as an autosomal recessive trait and is especially common in Ashkenazi Jews. In contrast to deficiency in factors VIII and IX, the correlation between factor level and propensity to bleed is not as precise, spontaneous bleeding is less, and hemarthroses are rare. Many patients with factor XI deficiency present with posttraumatic bleeding or with bleeding in the perioperative period, and occasional factor XI–deficient women have menorrhagia. Daily infusions of fresh-frozen plasma are sufficient, since the half-life of factor XI is approximately 24 h. The majority of defective factor XI alleles were accounted for by a limited number of mutations.

OTHER FACTOR DEFICIENCIES   Deficiencies in factors V, VII, X, and prothrombin (factor II) are exceedingly rare autosomal recessive disorders. Spontaneous or posttraumatic musculoskeletal bleeding or menorrhagia can occur with these deficiencies, but hemarthroses are uncommon. Fresh-frozen plasma is the appropriate therapy, although prothrombin concentrates may be employed for patients with severe prothrombin deficiency or decreases in factors VII and X as long as the risks of hepatitis and thrombosis are recognized.

Defects in the contact activation pathway involving Hageman factor (factor XII), high-molecular-weight kininogen, and prekallikrein cause laboratory abnormalities but no clinical bleeding. Despite dramatic prolongation of the PTT, often to greater than 100 s, deficient individuals have normal hemostasis and can undergo major surgery without plasma replacement therapy. Direct activation of factor IX by the tissue factor–VIIa complex may bypass this defective step in coagulation (Fig. 53-8). Patients with these disorders should neither be treated inappropriately with plasma nor denied indicated surgery on the basis of these laboratory abnormalities.

AFIBRINOGENEMIA AND DYSFIBRINOGENEMIA   Fibrinogen is a 340-kDa dimeric molecule made up of two sets of three covalently linked polypeptide chains. Thrombin sequentially cleaves fibrinopeptides A and B from the $A\alpha$ and $B\beta$ chains of fibrinogen to produce fibrin monomer, which then polymerizes to form a fibrin clot. Although fibrinogen is needed for platelet aggregation and fibrin formation, severe fibrinogen deficiency does not usually cause serious bleeding except after surgery. Patients with afibrinogenemia, who have no detectable fibrinogen in plasma or platelets, may have infrequent, mild bleeding episodes. Genetic analyses do not show any gross deletion or structural changes in the genes encoding the α, β, and γ chains of fibrinogen despite the total absence of plasma fibrinogen.

Fibrinogen is an abundant plasma protein (2.5 g/L). Mutations have been identified that alter the release of fibrinopeptides from the $A\alpha$ and $B\beta$ chains of fibrinogen, the rate of polymerization of fibrin monomers, and the sites for fibrin cross-linking. These dysfibrinogenemias are almost always inherited as autosomal dominant traits, so patients have nearly equal concentrations of normal and mutant fibrinogen in their plasma. Patients with dysfibrinogenemia have a slightly prolonged PT and PTT, a prolonged thrombin time, and a disparity in levels of fibrinogen measured with functional and immunologic assays. Despite these abnormalities, most patients have no symptoms or only moderate bleeding. A few dysfibrinogenemias induce a hypercoagulable state and increase the risk of thrombosis, and others have been associated with an increased incidence of abortion (Chap. 103). Some patients with liver disease, hepatomas, AIDS, and lymphoproliferative disorders develop an acquired form of dysfibrinogenemia.

FACTOR XIII DEFICIENCY AND DEFECTIVE FIBRIN CROSS-LINKING Factor XIII is a transglutaminase that stabilizes fibrin clots by forming ε-amino–γ-glutamyl cross-links between adjacent α and γ chains of fibrin. Factor XIII deficiency is an extremely rare inherited syndrome. Patients usually bleed in the neonatal period from their umbilical stump or circumcision. In addition to hemorrhage, these patients may have poor wound healing, a high incidence of infertility among males and abortion among affected females, and a high incidence of intracerebral hemorrhage. These observations suggest that the enzyme may be important in other physiologic processes beyond hemostasis, including placental implantation, spermatogenesis, and wound healing. Several drugs, including isoniazid, may bind to cross-linking sites on fibrinogen and mimic factor XIII deficiency by blocking enzyme activity. Normal hemostasis requires only 1% of normal enzyme activity; a single infusion of fresh-frozen plasma or a purified factor XIII–rich product derived from human placenta called Fibrogammin is effective. Factor XIII has a 14-day half-life.

VITAMIN K DEFICIENCY Vitamin K is a fat-soluble vitamin that plays a critical role in hemostasis. Dietary vitamin K is absorbed in the small intestine and stored in the liver. The vitamin is also synthesized by endogenous bacterial flora in the small intestine and colon; however, the quantity of endogenous vitamin K absorbed from the large intestine is debated. Following absorption, vitamin K is converted to an active epoxide in liver microsomes and serves as a cofactor in the enzymatic carboxylation of glutamic acid residues on prothrombin complex proteins (Fig. 102-1).

The three major causes of vitamin K deficiency are inadequate dietary intake, intestinal malabsorption, and loss of storage sites due to hepatocellular disease. Neonatal vitamin K deficiency, which causes hemorrhagic disease of the newborn, has disappeared from western countries with the routine administration of vitamin K to all newborn infants. Although a 30-day supply of vitamin K is stored in the normal liver, acutely ill patients can become deficient within 7 to 10 days. Acute vitamin K deficiency is particularly common in patients recovering from biliary tract surgery who have no dietary intake of vitamin K, have T-tube drainage of bile, and are on broad-spectrum antibiotics. Vitamin K deficiency is also seen in chronic liver disease, particularly primary biliary cirrhosis, and in some malabsorption states (Chaps. 275 and 286). The cephalosporins inhibit the reduction and recycling of vitamin K, much like warfarin.

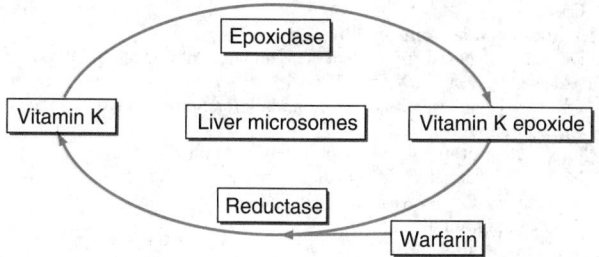

FIGURE 102-1 The mechanism of action of vitamin K, a cofactor in the formation of di-γ-carboxyglutamic acid residues on coagulation proteins, is depicted. Vitamin K is converted to an epoxide in liver microsomes. The epoxide is the active form and is reduced back to vitamin K by a liver membrane reductase. Warfarin blocks the action of the reductase and competitively inhibits the effects of vitamin K.

With vitamin K deficiency, plasma levels of all the prothrombin complex proteins (factors II, VII, IX, X; proteins C and S) decrease. Those with the shortest half-lives, factor VII and protein C, decrease first. Because of the rapid fall in factor VII, patients with mild vitamin K deficiency may have a prolonged PT and a normal PTT. Later, as the levels of the other factors fall, the PTT will also become prolonged. Parenteral administration of 10 mg vitamin K rapidly restores vitamin K levels in the liver and permits normal production of prothrombin complex proteins within 8 to 10 h. Severe hemorrhage can be treated with fresh-frozen plasma, which immediately corrects the hemostatic defect. If the cause of vitamin K deficiency cannot be eliminated, patients may need monthly injections. Purified prothrombin complex concentrates should be avoided because they contain trace quantities of activated forms of the prothrombin complex proteins and can cause thrombosis in patients with liver disease. They also carry an increased risk of hepatitis.

DISSEMINATED INTRAVASCULAR COAGULATION DIC can be either an explosive and life-threatening bleeding disorder or a relatively mild or subclinical disorder. Although a long list of diseases can be complicated by DIC, it is most frequently associated with obstetric catastrophes, metastatic malignancy, massive trauma, and bacterial sepsis (Table 102-1). Tentative triggering mechanisms have been identified. Tumors and traumatized or necrotic tissue release tissue factor into the circulation. Endotoxin from gram-negative bacteria activates several steps in the coagulation cascade. In addition to a direct effect on the activation of Hageman factor (factor XII), endotoxin induces the expression of tissue factor on the surface of monocytes and endothelial cells. These activated cell surfaces then accelerate coagulation reactions. These potent thrombogenic stimuli cause the deposition of small thrombi and emboli throughout the microvasculature. This early thrombotic phase of DIC is then followed by a phase of procoagulant consumption and secondary fibrinolysis. Continued fibrin formation and fibrinolysis lead to hemorrhage from the coagulation factor and platelet depletion and the antihemostatic effects of fibrin degradation products (Fig. 102-2).

The clinical presentation varies with the stage and severity of the

TABLE 102-1 *Etiologic Factors and Disorders Causing Disseminated Intravascular Coagulation*

Liberation of tissue factors	Obstetric syndromes—abruptio placentae, amniotic fluid embolism, retained dead fetus, second trimester abortion
	Hemolysis
	Neoplasms, particularly mucinous adenocarcinomas, acute promyelocytic leukemia
	Intravascular hemolysis
	Fat embolism
	Tissue damage—burns, frostbite, head injury, gunshot wounds
Endothelial damage	Aortic aneurysm
	Hemolytic uremic syndrome
	Acute glomerulonephritis
	Rocky Mountain spotted fever
Vascular malformation, decreased blood flow	Kasabach-Merritt syndrome
Infections	Bacterial: staphylococci, streptococci, pneumococci, meningococci, gram-negative bacilli
	Viral: arboviruses, varicella, variola, rubella
	Parasitic: malaria, kala-azar
	Rickettsial: Rocky Mountain spotted fever
	Mycotic: acute histoplasmosis

Source: Modified from RI Handin, RD Rosenberg, in *Hematology*, 4th ed, WS Beck (ed), Cambridge, MA, MIT Press, 1985.

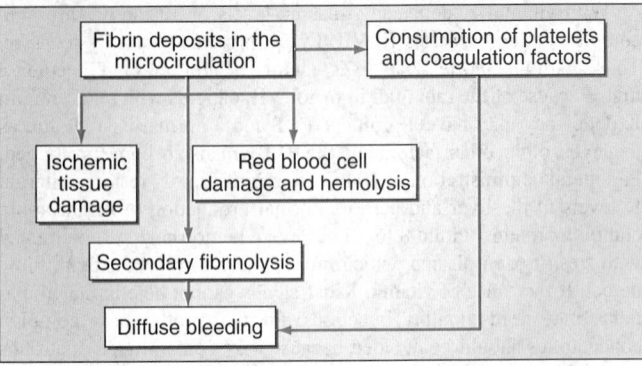

FIGURE 102-2 The pathophysiology of disseminated intravascular coagulation (DIC). Shown are the interactions between coagulation and fibrinolytic pathways that result in bleeding in patients with DIC.

syndrome. Most patients have extensive skin and mucous membrane bleeding and hemorrhage from surgical incisions or venipuncture or catheter sites. Less often, patients present with peripheral acrocyanosis, thrombosis, and pregangrenous changes in digits, genitalia, and nose—areas where blood flow is markedly reduced by vasospasm or microthrombi. Some patients, particularly those with chronic DIC and malignancy, have laboratory abnormalities without any evidence of thrombosis or hemorrhage.

The laboratory manifestations include thrombocytopenia and the presence of schistocytes or fragmented red blood cells that arise from cell trapping and damage within fibrin thrombi; prolonged PT and PTT and thrombin time and a reduced fibrinogen level from depletion of coagulation proteins; and elevated fibrin degradation products (FDP) from intense secondary fibrinolysis. The D dimer immunoassay, which measures cross-linked fibrin derivatives (i.e., those that have been in blood clots), is a more specific FDP assay. Low fibrinogen levels in DIC predict more bleeding.

℞ TREATMENT

DIC, although sometimes indolent, can cause life-threatening hemorrhage and may require emergency treatment including (1) an attempt to correct any reversible cause of DIC; (2) measures to control the major symptom, either bleeding or thrombosis; and (3) a prophylactic regimen to prevent recurrence in cases of chronic DIC. Treatment will vary with the clinical presentation. In patients with an obstetric complication such as abruptio placentae or acute bacterial sepsis, prompt delivery of the fetus and placenta or treatment with appropriate antibiotics will reverse the DIC syndrome. In patients with metastatic tumor causing DIC, control of the primary disease may not be possible, and long-term prophylaxis may be necessary.

Patients with bleeding as a major symptom should receive fresh-frozen plasma to replace depleted clotting factors and platelet concentrates to correct thrombocytopenia. Those with acrocyanosis and incipient gangrene or other thrombotic problems need immediate anticoagulation with intravenous heparin. The use of heparin in the treatment of bleeding is still controversial. Although it is a logical way to reduce thrombin generation and prevent further consumption of clotting proteins, it should be reserved for patients with thrombosis or who continue to bleed despite vigorous treatment with plasma and platelets.

Patients who initially have mild asymptomatic DIC may begin to bleed following surgery or chemotherapy. For example, mild DIC, without clinical bleeding, has been documented during saline- or prostaglandin-induced midtrimester abortions. Prophylactic treatment of patients with heparin may prevent progression of a mild DIC syndrome and has been used in the treatment of patients with acute promyelocytic leukemia and in some patients with a retained dead fetus who require surgical extraction. However, most patients with low-grade DIC can be managed with plasma and platelet replacement and do not require

heparin. Chronic DIC does not respond to oral warfarin anticoagulants, but it can be controlled with long-term heparin infusion. Occasional patients with indolent tumors and severe DIC have been maintained on heparin administered by intermittent subcutaneous injection or continuous infusion with portable pumps.

Despite our detailed understanding of the pathophysiology of DIC and a vigorous approach to therapy, treatment does not usually change the natural history of the underlying disorder. Therapy will only stabilize the patient, prevent exsanguination or massive thrombosis, and permit institution of definitive therapy.

COAGULATION DISORDERS IN LIVER DISEASE   Liver dysfunction is frequently accompanied by a hemostatic defect. The major causes of hemorrhage in patients with liver disease are shown in Table 102-2. Bleeding is usually due to an anatomic lesion that is exacerbated by a hemostatic defect. Most patients bleed from complications of portal hypertension, esophageal varices, or gastritis and peptic ulcer disease. Portal hypertension also causes splenomegaly, with splenic sequestration of platelets and thrombocytopenia, which contributes to the hemostatic defect.

Patients with hepatocellular liver disease cannot store vitamin K optimally and may have some degree of vitamin K deficiency. Cholestasis, a frequent feature of liver disease, impairs vitamin K absorption and further decreases liver vitamin K stores. Abnormalities in the γ-carboxylation of prothrombin complex proteins independent of vitamin K and the production of abnormal proteins have also been described. Patients may also have decreased production of other coagulation proteins, including fibrinogen and factor V. The liver also produces inhibitors of coagulation such as antithrombin III and proteins C and S and is the clearance site for activated coagulation factors and fibrinolytic enzymes. Thus patients with liver disease are also "hypercoagulable" and predisposed to developing DIC or systemic fibrinolysis. Coagulation defects in advanced liver failure are often difficult to distinguish from those of DIC.

Each patient with hemorrhage and liver disease should have a PT, PTT, platelet count, and fibrinogen determination, although it is not always possible to determine the major hemostatic abnormality from a single set of laboratory values. It is helpful to have previous laboratory data available for patients with chronic liver disease who develop an acute complication. The degree of prolongation of the PT predicts the risk of bleeding. Most patients present with moderate prolongation of the PT and PTT, mild thrombocytopenia, and a normal fibrinogen level. However, they may also present with a more complex defect combining defective synthesis, abnormal clearance, and active consumption of coagulation proteins. Since vitamin K deficiency is so common, a single parenteral dose of vitamin K is given after initial

TABLE 102-2   *Causes of Bleeding in Liver Disease*

Anatomic Factors
  Portal hypertension
    Varices
    Splenomegaly and secondary thrombocytopenia
  Peptic ulceration
  Gastritis
Hepatic Function Abnormalities
  Decreased synthesis of procoagulant proteins: fibrinogen, prothrombin, factors V, VII, IX, X, XI
  Decreased synthesis of coagulation inhibitors: protein C, protein S, antithrombin III
  Impaired absorption and metabolism of vitamin K
  Failure to clear activated coagulation proteins leading to:
    Disseminated intravascular coagulation
    Systemic fibrinolysis
Complications of Therapy
  Dilution of platelets and coagulation proteins from massive transfusions
  Infusion of activated coagulation proteins in prothrombin complex concentrates
  Bleeding from heparin; thrombosis from ε-aminocaproic acid (EACA)

laboratory studies have been obtained, even though this may only partially correct the laboratory abnormalities. The presence of severe thrombocytopenia or a low fibrinogen level suggests the additional complication of DIC and may require further studies and therapy.

The safest replacement therapy for a patient with liver disease is fresh-frozen plasma, since it supplies all known coagulation factors. However, even this form of therapy has drawbacks, since large quantities of plasma may precipitate hepatic encephalopathy and cause fluid and sodium overload. Prothrombin complex concentrates should be avoided because they replace only the vitamin K–dependent factors, may be contaminated with hepatitis and AIDS virus, and contain trace quantities of activated coagulation proteins. Similarly, fibrinogen concentrates (or cryoprecipitate), rich in factor VIII and fibrinogen, should not be used without additional fresh-frozen plasma. Anticoagulation with heparin has been advocated to control DIC, but this is particularly hazardous and not recommended in cirrhosis because heparin is metabolized erratically and may lead to severe bleeding.

FIBRINOLYTIC DEFECTS Bleeding can also occur from defects in the fibrinolytic system. Patients with α_2 plasmin inhibitor deficiency or plasminogen activator inhibitor (PAI) 1 have rapid fibrinolysis following fibrin deposition after trauma or surgery and may experience recurrent hemorrhage. Similarly, patients with cirrhosis have an impaired clearance of tissue plasminogen activator (tPA) and systemic fibrinolysis that may contribute to their hemorrhagic defect. Rarely, patients with tumors such as metastatic prostatic cancer may develop diffuse bleeding from primary fibrinolysis rather than DIC. Clues to the diagnosis include a disproportionately low fibrinogen level with a relatively normal PT and PTT and the presence of a normal or nearly normal platelet count. With rare exceptions, patients with primary fibrinolysis should have an elevated titer of FDP but a normal D dimer level. However, it is sometimes difficult or impossible to differentiate primary fibrinolysis from the secondary fibrinolysis in DIC. Patients with clearly established primary fibrinolysis should not receive heparin; they require plasma therapy and, occasionally, fibrinolytic inhibitors such as EACA. However, EACA should not be given to patients suspected of having DIC unless they are also receiving heparin, since EACA can cause massive, often fatal, thrombosis in a patient with DIC.

CIRCULATING ANTICOAGULANTS Circulating anticoagulants, or inhibitors, are usually IgG antibodies that interfere with coagulation reactions. Specific inhibitors inactivate individual coagulation proteins and may cause severe hemorrhage. They arise in 15 to 20% of patients with factor VIII or factor IX deficiency who have received plasma infusions. Specific inhibitors also occur in previously normal individuals. Although the most common target protein is factor VIII, inhibitors with specificity for each of the coagulation proteins occur. In addition to hemophiliacs, anti-factor VIII antibodies are seen in postpartum females, in patients on various drugs, as part of the spectrum of autoantibodies in systemic lupus erythematosus (SLE) patients, and in normal elderly individuals. Circulating anticoagulants also occur in patients with AIDS.

Nonspecific (lupus-like) inhibitors prolong coagulation tests by binding to phospholipids. They are assayed by their anticoagulant effect [lupus anticoagulant (LA) activity] or their ability to bind to the complex phospholipid cardiolipin [anticardiolipin antibody (ACLA) activity]. While most often encountered in patients with SLE, these nonspecific inhibitors may develop in patients with many other disorders and also in otherwise normal individuals.

The critical laboratory feature that identifies the presence of either type of inhibitor is the failure of normal plasma to correct a prolonged PT, PTT, or both. Plasma from patients with a specific inhibitor will progressively inactivate a coagulation protein and thus prolong whichever of these screening tests requires the participation of that clotting factor. This effect persists after dilution. Nonspecific inhibitors immediately prolong the PT and PTT and, at low dilution, block multiple coagulation reactions. However, these effects can be overcome by altering the quantity or type of phospholipid or by diluting the plasma.

Hemorrhage in patients with specific inhibitors may require treatment with massive plasma or concentrate infusion, the use of activated prothrombin complex concentrates to bypass the antibodies against factors VIII or IX, and plasmapheresis or exchange transfusion to lower antibody titer. Chronic immunosuppressive regimens have been particularly useful in otherwise normal individuals with an acquired factor VIII antibody. Many patients lose their antibody and recover within 6 to 12 months, although the acute mortality rate from bleeding may approach 10%.

Patients with LA activity have normal hemostasis and will not bleed unless they have concomitant thrombocytopenia or prothrombin deficiency. Both thrombocytopenia and hypoprothrombinemia are secondary to autoantibodies that bind either to platelets or the prothrombin molecule. While these antibodies have no effect on function, they accelerate clearance of the coated platelets or the antibody-prothrombin complexes.

The presence of LA activity may predispose patients to venous and arterial thromboembolism and may cause midtrimester abortions. However, the risk of thrombosis is difficult to estimate, and the appropriate therapy for individual patients difficult to choose. Tests for either LA or ACLA activity are not well standardized, and results vary among and within patients. The best predictor is a consistent prolongation of more than one coagulation test coupled with a high titer of ACLA activity. Second, the risk of thrombosis is increased in patients who have SLE compared with those with idiopathic LA or ACLA activity. Prophylactic therapy is not clearly beneficial, and treatments aimed at reducing the titer of antibody are not superior to conventional antithrombotic therapy.

Therapy should be individualized. Patients with SLE and either LA or ACLA activity who have had a thrombotic episode are at high risk for a recurrence and should receive long-term anticoagulant therapy. Women who have had more than one midtrimester abortion, especially those with SLE, should have a trial of anticoagulant therapy. Patients with a single thrombotic episode (stroke or pulmonary embolus) and no other risk factor except LA or ACLA activity should be treated. No consensus has been reached about treatment after an initial minor event [deep venous thrombosis (DVT)]. Asymptomatic patients with only laboratory abnormalities should not be treated. Glucocorticoids should be administered only in conjunction with antithrombotic agents and are not of proven efficacy.

INHERITED PROTHROMBOTIC DISORDERS Coagulation is carefully regulated by a series of inhibitors that limit thrombin generation and fibrin formation and by the fibrinolytic system, which effectively removes fibrin thrombi (Figs. 53-6 and 53-7). Inherited defects in the natural coagulation inhibitors (i.e., antithrombin, proteins C and S), abnormalities in the fibrinolytic system, and certain dysfibrinogenemias predispose patients to thrombosis (Table 53-5). A single point mutation in the factor V gene (factor V Leiden), which converts arginine 506 to glutamine and makes the molecule resistant to degradation by activated protein C, may account for 25% of inherited prethrombotic states. Antithrombin, protein C, and protein S defects are all autosomal dominant traits, so heterozygous individuals, who have a 50% reduction in protein concentration or a mixture of mutant and normal molecules, will have an increased risk of thrombosis. The patients have similar clinical presentations with a strong family history of thrombosis, episodes of recurrent venous thromboembolism, and symptoms by their early twenties. Any patient with this distinctive history should be tested for specific abnormalities.

ANTITHROMBIN DEFICIENCY Antithrombin complexes with activated coagulation proteins and blocks their biologic activity (Fig. 53-6). The rate of this reaction is enhanced by heparin-like molecules within the vessel wall or on endothelial cells. Plasma antithrombin III content is 5 to 15 mg/L (50 to 150%), with values only slightly below normal increasing the risk of thrombosis. For optimal screening, the antithrombin III concentration is measured by immunoassay and the plasma antithrombin and heparin cofactor activity assessed with functional assays. The most common defect (1 in 2000 indidivuals) is mild (heterozygous) antithrombin deficiency. Dysfunctional antithrombin molecules with mutations affecting either the serine protease or heparin-binding site or activation of inhibitor by heparin have also been described.

Patients with antithrombin deficiency who develop acute thrombosis or embolism can be treated with intravenous heparin, since there is usually sufficient normal antithrombin to act as a heparin cofactor. Following their first episode of thromboembolism, patients should be placed on oral anticoagulants for life to prevent recurrent thrombosis. Family studies should be conducted when an antithrombin-deficient individual is discovered, since up to half the members of a kindred may be affected. Asymptomatic individuals with antithrombin deficiency should receive prophylactic anticoagulation with heparin or plasma infusions to raise their antithrombin level before medical or surgical procedures that may increase their risk of thrombosis. Chronic oral anticoagulation is not recommended until individuals at risk have a thrombotic episode.

DEFICIENCIES OF PROTEINS C AND S   Protein C is a vitamin K–dependent hepatic protein that binds to the endothelial cell surface protein thrombomodulin and is converted to an active protease by thrombin (Fig. 53-6). Activated protein C, in conjunction with protein S, proteolyzes factors Va and VIIIa, which shuts off fibrin formation. Activated protein C may also stimulate fibrinolysis and accelerate clot lysis. Deficiencies of proteins C and S are usually autosomal dominant disorders, and deficiencies in the two proteins cause an identical syndrome of recurrent venous thrombosis and pulmonary embolism. Dysfunctional molecules have also been identified in some patients with thrombosis. Rare patients with homozygous protein C deficiency have fulminant neonatal intravascular coagulation and require prompt diagnosis and treatment.

The correlation between levels of proteins C and S and the risk of thrombosis is not as precise as for antithrombin III deficiency. In fact, some asymptomatic individuals with protein C "deficiency" have been discovered. In some well-studied protein C–deficient kindreds, asymptomatic individuals may have protein C levels as low as or lower than relatives with recurrent thrombosis. It is possible that an undiscovered cofactor is present in symptomatic patients. Finally, since a fraction of the available protein S is bound to C4b-binding protein and is unavailable for coagulation reactions, both free and total protein S levels or C4b-binding protein levels should be assessed for maximum accuracy.

Heterozygous patients with protein C or S deficiencies who develop acute thrombosis should be heparinized and then placed on oral anticoagulants. There are, however, two potential problems with the use of warfarin anticoagulants in these patients. First, these vitamin K antagonists (Fig. 102-1), which lower the level of the procoagulant factors II, VII, IX, and X, may also reduce the concentration of proteins C and S sufficiently to nullify the desired antithrombotic effect. In addition, patients who are protein C–deficient may develop warfarin-induced skin necrosis; this defect may predispose patients to a rare but serious complication. Patients with homozygous protein C deficiency require periodic plasma infusions rather than oral anticoagulants to prevent recurrent intravascular coagulation and thrombosis.

RESISTANCE TO ACTIVATED PROTEIN C AND THE FACTOR V LEIDEN MUTATION
Some patients with familial or recurrent venous thromboembolism were found not to prolong their PTT when activated protein C was added to their plasma. These patients were found to have an identical mutation in which arginine 506 in factor V is converted to glutamine. This amino acid substitution abolishes a protein C cleavage site in factor V and thus prolongs the thrombogenic effect of factor V activation. About 3% of the population worldwide is heterozygous for this mutation. The mutation is absent in certain populations, e.g., Asians,

TABLE 102-3   *Relationship between Coagulation Defect and Site of Thrombosis*

Abnormality	Arterial	Venous
Factor V Leiden R506 Q	–	+
Prothrombin G20210A	–	+
Antithrombin III	–	+
Protein C	–	+
Protein S	–	+
Homocysteinemia	+	+
Antiphospholipid antibody[a]	+	+

[a] Anticardiolipin antibody—lupus anticoagulant.

African Americans, and Native Americans. It may account for 25% of patients with recurrent DVT or pulmonary embolism.

Heterozygosity at this allele increases an individual's lifetime risk of venous thromboembolism sevenfold. The risk rises steadily with age. A homozygote has a twentyfold increased risk of thrombosis. Heterozygosity coupled with ingestion of oral contraceptives or pregnancy increases the risk at least fifteenfold. Coinheritance of factor V Leiden and another low-penetrance defect such as protein C or S deficiency is also additive. Many previous studies of risk factors predisposing patients to venous thromboembolism are being reevaluated to take into account this common mutation.

PROTHROMBIN GENE MUTATION   A specific point mutation in the prothrombin gene [conversion of G to A at position 20210 (G20210A)] also predisposes to venous thrombosis and embolism. This mutation is in the 3'-untranslated region of the gene and results in a 30% increase in plasma prothrombin levels, either through more efficient translation or greater stability of the message. Heterozygotes account for ~18% of cases with family histories of venous thrombosis and 6% of patients with first episodes of DVT.

The inheritance of multiple mutations increases the risk of thrombosis. The relationship between known mutations and the type of thrombosis is shown in Table 102-3. The fraction of patients with DVT with known mutations is shown in Table 102-4.

℞ TREATMENT

Patients who develop venous thromboembolism without a clear predisposing factor, have a strong family history, present under age 30, or have more than one episode should have assays for antithrombin III, proteins C and S, and factor V Leiden. Patients who present with DVT or pulmonary embolism during pregnancy or while using oral contraceptives have a 30% chance of having factor V Leiden.

Treatment recommendations for patients with the inherited prethrombotic disorders are still evolving. All patients should receive standard initial therapy with heparin, either conventional or low dose (Chap. 103), followed by 3 months of oral warfarin. This regimen should allow for maximal healing and reendothelialization of the thrombosed vessels and minimize recurrence in the damaged vascular beds. It is not clear which patients should go on to receive long-term (perhaps lifelong) anticoagulation, a judgment that depends on assessing the risk/benefit ratio.

Patients with antithrombin III deficiency who become symptomatic have a high likelihood of recurrent events and should be placed on lifelong anticoagulation. Patients with protein C or S deficiency or heterozygous factor V Leiden and prothrombin G20210A patients have a lower likelihood of recurrent disease. Long-term anticoagula-

TABLE 102-4   *Prevalence of Coagulation Defects in Patients with Venous Thrombosis*

Defect	Prevalence, %
Factor V Leiden (Arg506Gln) R506 Q	12–40
Hyperhomocysteinemia	10–20
Prothrombin G20210A	6–18
Deficiencies of antithrombin III, proteins C and S	5–15
Antiphospholipid antibody syndrome	10–20

tion should be reserved until their second or subsequent episode of thromboembolism. Homozygous factor V Leiden patients should be placed on long-term anticoagulation after their initial episode, and all patients should receive replacement therapy or receive heparin prophylaxis during surgery or after trauma; women with these defects should avoid the use of oral contraceptives. The asymptomatic relatives of patients shown to have these disorders should be screened to determine if they have inherited the defective gene. If so, they should receive appropriate prophylaxis but not start anticoagulation until they are symptomatic. In the absence of a congenital defect predisposing a patient to thrombosis, recurring or migratory thrombophlebitis may indicate an underlying malignancy.

DYSFIBRINOGENEMIAS AND FIBRINOLYTIC DEFECTS Recurrent venous thrombosis and embolism may be due to familial defects in fibrinogen or plasminogen or decreased synthesis or release of tPA. While most dysfibrinogenemias cause bleeding, several variants have excessively rapid release of fibrinopeptides and recurrent thromboembolism. Patients with this disorder and those with an abnormal plasminogen that resists activation by streptokinase and urokinase have been treated successfully with heparin and oral anticoagulants. Defects in tPA content or release have not been completely characterized. One group of patients with recurrent venous thrombosis and embolism failed to increase venous blood fibrinolytic activity when challenged with local ischemia or physical exercise. The other group had impaired fibrinolytic activity in extracts prepared from biopsied veins. Young patients with acute myocardial infarction may have impaired fibrinolysis due to increased plasma levels of PAI, a serine protease inhibitor that binds to tPA and is derived from endothelial cells.

Many common illnesses are associated with an increased risk of thrombosis (Table 53-5). These patients are said to have a "hypercoagulable" or "prethrombotic" state. This increased risk is seen in patients with chronic congestive heart failure and metastatic cancer and in patients undergoing major surgery. The generation of tissue factor activity in damaged or ischemic tissue or metastatic tumor, coupled with venous stasis and endothelial injury, induces the formation of venous and, more rarely, arterial thrombi. Several hematologic disorders, paroxysmal nocturnal hemoglobinuria, essential thrombocythemia, and polycythemia vera predispose patients to venous and arterial thrombosis through diverse mechanisms related to increased blood viscosity and abnormal blood cells. Diseases that affect the endothelial cell, such as Behçet's syndrome, Kawasaki's disease, and homocystinuria, or the administration of drugs such as oral contraceptives, which lower antithrombin III levels, or L-asparaginase, which inhibits production of multiple coagulation factors, may also predispose patients to thrombosis. Infusion of granulocyte-macrophage colony-stimulating factor (GM-CSF) has been associated with thrombosis. Tamoxifen, an estrogen receptor antagonist, can cause venous thrombosis. The mechanism is unclear.

Plasma homocysteine levels influence the risk of both venous and arterial thromboembolism. Individuals with the congenital homocystinuria syndrome have, in addition to their Marfanoid habitus, an increased incidence of strokes and coronary artery disease. These patients have well-recognized enzyme defects (Chap. 343), excrete homocysteine in their urine, and have very high plasma levels of the amino acid. Some patients with early-onset cerebral vascular events have mild homocystinuria that can be brought out by a methionine loading test. Epidemiologic studies show a relationship between homocysteine levels that are nearer to the normal range and coronary artery disease. Vitamin B_{12} deficiency occurs in about 30% of people over age 70, produces elevated homocysteine levels, and may be a reversible cause of thrombotic disease.

FURTHER READING

ARNOUT J, VERYLEN J: Current status and implications of autoimmune antiphospholipid antibodies in relation to thrombotic disease. J Thromb Haemost 1:931, 2003

CROWTHER MA, KELTON JG: Congenital thrombophilic states associated with venous thrombosis: A qualitative overview and proposed classification system. Ann Intern Med 138:128, 2003

HEDNER U: Recombinant factor VIIa (NovoSeven) as a hemostatic agent. Dis Mon 49:39, 2003

HIGH KA: Gene transfer as an approach to treating hemophilia. Semin Thromb Hemost 1:107, 2003

LEE C: Recombinant clotting factors in the treatment of hemophilia. Thromb Haemost 82:516, 1999

LEVI M, TEN CATE H: Current concepts: Disseminated intravascular coagulation. N Engl J Med 341:586, 1999

MANNUCCI PM: Hemophilia: Treatment options in the twenty-first century. J Thromb Haemost 1:1349, 2003

103   ANTIPLATELET, ANTICOAGULANT, AND FIBRINOLYTIC THERAPY
Steven R. Deitcher

Arterial and venous thrombosis together with complicating embolic phenomena are major causes of mortality in the developed countries of the world. In the United States alone, myocardial infarction (MI) and thromboembolic stroke account for >800,000 deaths annually, and from one-half to 2 million venous thromboembolic events (VTE) including deep venous thrombosis (DVT) and pulmonary embolism (PE) occur annually. A common feature of the management of *all* thromboembolic vascular diseases is the use of antithrombotic agents. Antithrombotic agents, including antiplatelet drugs, anticoagulants, and fibrinolytic agents, are used to prevent thrombotic events, prevent or mitigate the complications of thrombotic events, and restore vascular patency in order to prevent loss of tissue, limb, and organ function as well as life. The pathologic basis of thrombosis in different vascular beds dictates the choice of agents: drugs that inhibit platelet activation and aggregation play a primary role in arterial disease management; drugs that inhibit thrombin and fibrin generation play a primary role in venous disease.

ANTIPLATELET DRUGS

Antiplatelet treatment reduces overall mortality from vascular disease by 15% and nonfatal vascular events by 30%. Multiple targets exist for antiplatelet therapy (Fig. 103-1), including cyclooxygenase (COX), adenosine diphosphate (ADP) receptors, the platelet adhesion glycoprotein (Gp) Ib, and the platelet agonist thrombin. Prostaglandin E_1 and stable analogues of prostacyclin inhibit platelet activation by increasing platelet cyclic AMP levels. Dipyridamole inhibits platelet activation by inhibiting phosphodiesterase to increase cyclic AMP. Because expression of functionally active GpIIb/IIIa on platelet surfaces is the final common pathway of platelet activation regardless of initial stimulus, it is a logical therapeutic target.

ASPIRIN   Aspirin (acetylsalicylic acid) irreversibly inactivates by acetylation the activity of platelet prostaglandin H synthase-1 and -2 (COX-1 and -2). COX inhibition leads to the prevention of thromboxane A_2 synthesis and impairment of platelet secretion and aggregation. Non-enteric-coated aspirin is rapidly absorbed from the upper gastrointestinal tract; plasma salicylate concentrations peak within 1 h of ingestion. The effects of aspirin on platelet function occur within 1 h and last for the duration of the affected platelets' life span (1 week). Toxicities including gastrointestinal discomfort, blood loss, and systemic bleeding are dose-related. Aspirin doses as low as 30 mg/d are antithrombotic. Aspirin has been convincingly shown to be effective in treatment of stable and unstable angina, acute MI, transient ischemic

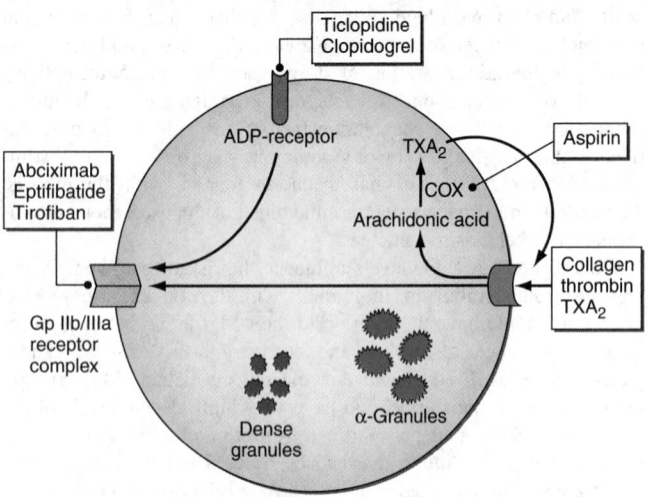

FIGURE 103-1 Antiplatelet drugs and targets for platelet function inhibition. The thienopyridines, ticlopidine and clopidogrel, inhibit the ADP-receptor of platelets. Aspirin targets platelet cyclooxygenase (COX). The disintegrins bind to and inhibit the final common pathway of platelet activation, namely the glycoprotein (Gp) IIb/IIIa complex. (TXA$_2$, thromboxane A$_2$.)

attack and incomplete stroke, stroke following carotid artery surgery, and atrial fibrillation. The minimum effective aspirin dose for these indications is 75 to 325 mg/d. Aspirin reduces mortality after coronary artery bypass surgery. In patients with acute MI or stroke, aspirin prevents 35 to 40 cardiovascular events per 1000 patients treated (secondary prevention). For primary prevention in persons >50 years of age with at least one major risk factor for coronary artery disease, aspirin prevents 4 events per 1000 patients treated. Aspirin is advisable following peripheral arterial bypass surgery and carotid endarterectomy and in patients with intermittent claudication. Though beneficial when compared to placebo, aspirin cannot be recommended as first-line VTE prophylaxis in hip fracture patients because the benefit of aspirin is less than with anticoagulants.

THIENOPYRIDINES   Ticlopidine and clopidogrel are structurally related compounds that selectively inhibit ADP-induced platelet aggregation and likely ADP-mediated amplification of the platelet response to other agonists. Though more effective than aspirin in reducing vascular events in many settings, enthusiasm for ticlopidine is dampened by hematologic toxicities, including thrombotic thrombocytopenic purpura (TTP). Clopidogrel is rapidly absorbed, extensively metabolized, and inhibits ADP-induced platelet aggregation in a dose-dependent fashion with inhibition detectable 2 h after an oral dose of 400 mg. The plasma half-life of the main metabolite, SR 26334, is ~8 h. On repeated daily dosing of 50 to 100 mg, 25 to 30% inhibition of ADP-induced platelet aggregation is noted on the second day of therapy, with 50 to 60% steady-state inhibition noted after 4 to 7 days. Platelet function returns to normal about 7 days after the last dose of clopidogrel. The CAPRIE trial demonstrated a modest reduction in ischemic events in patients with recent stroke or MI and in those with symptomatic peripheral arterial disease randomly assigned to clopidogrel, 75 mg/d, compared to aspirin (5.32% vs. 5.83%). The majority of the difference in efficacy occurred in the patients who entered because of symptomatic peripheral arterial disease, with a 23.8% relative risk reduction. Another trial (PCI-CURE) demonstrated an advantage of pretreatment clopidogrel plus aspirin followed by long-term therapy over aspirin alone in patients with acute coronary syndromes. Clopidogrel rarely precipitates TTP.

GpIIb/IIIa (αIIbβ3) ANTAGONISTS   GpIIb/IIIa is a member of the integrin family of receptors. These receptors recognize the amino acid sequence arginine-glycine-aspartate (Arg-Gly-Asp; RGD), which represents the cell attachment recognition sequence present in adhesive proteins such

as fibrinogen. Three potent parenteral GpIIb/IIIa inhibitors (disintegrins) have been extensively studied, primarily in the settings of percutaneous coronary intervention (PCI), unstable angina, and non-Q-wave MI. Abciximab (c7E3 Fab) is a chimeric monoclonal Fab fragment of human and murine protein that binds to GpIIb/IIIa. Eptifibatide is a synthetic cyclic heptapeptide with a KGD sequence more specific for GpIIb/IIIa than RGD. Tirofiban is a synthetic peptidomimetic based on the RGD sequence. Oral, in contrast to intravenous, GpIIb/IIIa inhibitors have been generally disappointing.

ANTICOAGULANT DRUGS

Anticoagulant drugs are used to prevent and treat thrombosis in medical and surgical patients. Narrow-spectrum (single-protein target) anticoagulants (e.g., fondaparinux and ximelagatran) are being developed to supplant more broad-spectrum anticoagulants (e.g., heparin and warfarin). The molecular targets of selected agents are shown in Fig. 103-2. Oral delivery and lack of obligatory therapeutic monitoring are desired anticoagulant characteristics.

HEPARIN   Commercial unfractionated heparin (UFH), obtained from bovine lung or porcine intestinal mucosa, consists of a heterogeneous mixture of highly sulfated polysaccharides (glycosaminoglycans) with molecular masses ranging from 4 to 30 kDa, with a mean molecular mass of ~15 kDa ($\approx$45 saccharide units). UFH molecules contain a randomly distributed unique pentasaccharide sequence that binds to antithrombin. Once bound to UFH, the natural anticoagulant effect of antithrombin is potentiated, resulting in accelerated binding and inactivation of serine proteases such as the common pathway coagulation factors, factor Xa and thrombin. Heparin is active when given intravenously or subcutaneously. Delivery systems utilizing synthetic amino acids such as sodium N-[8(2-hydroxybenzoyl)amino] caprylate (SNAC) facilitate oral heparin gut absorption. The half-life of heparin increases with increasing dosage. A 100-U/kg intravenous dose is cleared with a half-life of ~1 h. Heparin is cleared by the reticuloendothelial system and metabolized by the liver, and metabolic products are excreted in the urine. "True" heparin resistance, manifesting as inadequate anticoagulant [activated partial thromboplastin time (aPTT) prolongation] and antithrombotic (anti-factor Xa activity) responses from what would otherwise be perceived as an adequate heparin dose, likely results from the nonspecific heparin binding to white blood cells, vascular endothelial cells, and acute-phase proteins. In "apparent" heparin resistance, usually as a result of elevated factor VIII levels, the aPTT may be normal or near normal while the anti-factor Xa activity assay reveals a therapeutic heparin activity level. Simply escalating the dose of heparin to achieve the desired aPTT without checking a heparin assay may result in a pronounced bleeding

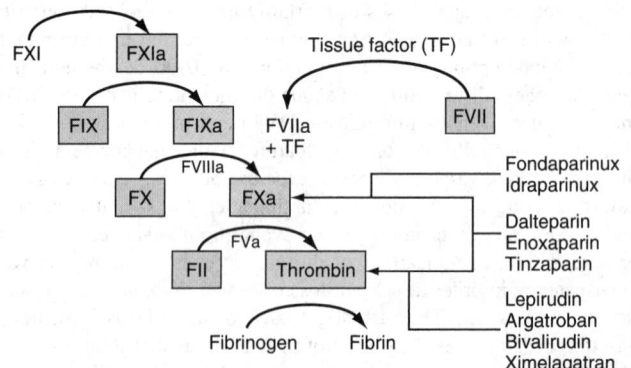

FIGURE 103-2 Anticoagulant drugs and molecular targets of anticoagulation. Unfractionated heparin targets the serine protease coagulation factors (highlighted in pale red); warfarin affects the vitamin K–dependent factors (highlighted in pale gray); pentasaccharide-based agents such as fondaparinux and idraparinux are select factor Xa inhibitors; the low-molecular-weight heparins target both factor Xa and thrombin with preference for factor Xa; and the direct thrombin inhibitors selectively target thrombin.

risk. These variables warrant close laboratory monitoring of heparin therapy.

LOW-MOLECULAR-WEIGHT HEPARINS (LMWHS)
LMWHs are derived from the enzymatic or chemical cleavage of UFH into a mixture of glycosaminoglycans with a mean molecular mass of ~5 kDa (≈15 saccharide units). LMWHs bind antithrombin via the same pentasaccharide sequence as UFH. Due to the predominance of molecules <18 saccharide units in length, LMWHs have limited antithrombin activity compared to anti-factor Xa activity, and LMWH therapy is unable to be monitored by aPTT. Whereas UFH has an anti-factor Xa:antithrombin activity ratio of 1:1, LMWHs have reported ratios of 1.9:1 to 4.1:1. LMWHs differ in their degree of tissue factor pathway inhibitor release, degree of sulfation, and degree of stimulated von Willebrand factor (vWF) release. Superior bioavailability, limited nonspecific binding, and non-dose-dependent half-lives facilitate once- or twice-daily subcutaneous dosing based solely on weight and without laboratory monitoring. LMWH is cleared by renal mechanisms; therefore, multiday use in patients with severe renal insufficiency (creatinine clearance <30 mL/min) should be avoided. Reversible elevations of liver transaminases may occur during the administration of LMWH and UFH. LMWHs are associated with less heparin-induced thrombocytopenia (HIT) (Chap. 101) and osteopenia than UFH but are only partially (≈60%) neutralized by protamine sulfate.

HEPARINOIDS
The heparinoid dermatan sulfate acts as an anticoagulant by activating heparin cofactor II. Danaparoid is a glycosaminoglycan mixture derived from porcine intestinal mucosa composed of heparan sulfate (84%), dermatan sulfate (12%), and chondroitin sulfate (4%). Danaparoid has an anti-factor Xa:antithrombin activity ratio of >22:1. Danaparoid's potential for heparin cross-reactivity and longer half-life (24 h) make it less desirable than a direct thrombin inhibitor for the treatment of patients with HIT, the main indication for heparinoid use.

PENTASACCHARIDES
Fondaparinux is a synthetic pentasaccharide that causes selective indirect inhibition of factor Xa. Fondaparinux is administered subcutaneously and does not require therapeutic monitoring. Fondaparinux elimination is prolonged in patients with renal impairment, in those >75 years, and in those weighing <50 kg. Fondaparinux is primarily used for thromboprophylaxis in patients with hip fracture undergoing surgery and in those undergoing elective knee and hip joint replacement. Fondaparinux does not bind platelet factor 4 and may result in less HIT than UFH and LMWH. A long-acting pentasaccharide, idraparinux, has a half-life of 130 h, which may facilitate once-weekly dosing for primary and/or secondary prevention of thromboembolic events.

DIRECT THROMBIN INHIBITORS (DTI)
Despite elimination of all heparin exposure and platelet count recovery, patients with isolated, serologically confirmed HIT have up to a 50% risk of developing a confirmed thrombotic event during the 30-day period following HIT diagnosis. The persistent prothrombotic tendency associated with HIT, the presence of thrombus in HIT with thrombosis, and a patient's original indication for heparin therapy all warrant use of an alternative anticoagulant agent such as DTI following heparin cessation.

Lepirudin Lepirudin is a recombinant hirudin that, unlike native hirudin in medicinal leech saliva, lacks sulfation on tyrosine 63 and has a leucine at position 1. Lepirudin is a potent, irreversible DTI that lacks any structural homology with heparin, does not cross-react with heparin, has a short half-life (1.5 h), inactivates clot-bound thrombin, and can be monitored by the aPTT assay or ecarin clotting time. The rate of death, amputation, and new thromboembolic events is reduced by >50% in HIT patients treated with lepirudin, compared with historic controls. Current lepirudin dosing recommendations for acute HIT management are 0.4 mg/kg as a bolus followed by 0.15 mg/kg per hour (up to 110 kg). The target aPTT is 1.5 to 2.5 times the median value for the normal range. The target plasma lepirudin concentration during heart bypass is 2.0 μg/mL. Outpatient subcutaneous lepirudin has been used to treat patients with HIT and patients refractory to other

anticoagulant therapy. The major challenges of lepirudin treatment are the lack of an antidote, the extreme care needed when treating patients with even mild renal insufficiency, and immunogenicity. Marked bolus and infusion rate reductions are necessary in patients with a creatinine clearance of <60 mL/min. Lepirudin should be avoided completely or administered with extreme care in the settings of hemodialysis and acute renal failure. Approximately 40% of HIT patients treated with lepirudin develop IgG anti-hirudin antibodies that decrease renal elimination of the drug rather than exerting any in vivo neutralizing effect. This enhancement of anticoagulant effect often warrants a major reduction of the infusion rate.

Argatroban Argatroban is a synthetic, small-molecule, L-arginine derivative, rapid, and reversible DTI capable of inhibiting both free and fibrin-bound thrombin. Argatroban exerts its antithrombotic effects by inhibiting thrombin-mediated fibrin formation; coagulation factor V, VII, and XIII activation; and platelet activation. Argatroban does not cross-react with heparin. Argatroban is hepatically metabolized with biliary excretion and has a half-life of 40 min. Dose reduction is required in patients with significant hepatic disease. In HIT, the combined incidence of death, amputation, and new thromboembolic events is significantly lower in argatroban recipients compared with controls. The recommended starting intravenous infusion rate is 2 μg/kg per min with a target aPTT of 1.5 to 3 times the baseline value. Prothrombin time (PT) prolongation makes an accurate International Normalized Ratio (INR) determination during conversion to oral warfarin a challenge. Argatroban [350-μg/kg bolus followed by 25 μg/kg per min titrated to achieve an activated clotting time (ACT) of 300 to 450 s] provides adequate anticoagulation with minimal bleeding risk while enabling procedural success in HIT patients undergoing a PCI.

Bivalirudin Bivalirudin is a semisynthetic, bivalent DTI consisting of a dodecapeptide analogue of the carboxyterminus of hirudin. Bivalirudin has four glycine residues that connect the thrombin exocite 1 and thrombin active-site binding moieties. Bivalirudin has a very short half-life (25 min) and is a reversible DTI. Bivalirudin is primarily used during PCI, where it is at least as effective as heparin with an improved safety profile.

Ximelagatran Ximelagatran is an oral prodrug of the DTI melagatran. Ximelagatran is administered in a fixed-dose fashion, does not require therapeutic monitoring, and has no apparent major food or drug interactions. Ximelagatran is rapidly absorbed (peak levels in 15 to 30 min) and rapidly converted to melagatran (peak levels in 1 to 2 h). Melagatran is renally eliminated. Melagatran binds to the thrombin active site resulting in inhibition of thrombin-mediated activation of coagulation factors and platelets. It is active against free and clot-bound thrombin. Ximelagatran is promising as a treatment of acute VTE, chronic management of atrial fibrillation, and prevention of VTE in high-risk settings such as following surgery and HIT. Reversible liver function abnormalities have been reported.

WARFARIN
Warfarin inhibits vitamin K epoxide reductase and vitamin K reductase, thus inhibiting γ-carboxylation of select glutamic acid residues in the N-terminus of prothrombin; factors VII, IX, and X; and protein C and protein S. Inhibition of γ-carboxylation leads to synthesis of hypofunctional coagulation proteins that are unable to bind to cellular surfaces to mediate coagulation reactions. Commercially available warfarin is a racemic mixture of levo- and dextrorotatory forms of the drug. The half-life of warfarin in plasma is ~36 h. Because factor X and prothrombin have half-lives >2 days, reduction of all vitamin K–dependent coagulation proteins into the therapeutic range (~20% of normal) requires 4 to 5 days of therapy. Warfarin dosage is influenced by dietary stores of vitamin K, liver function, coexisting medical disorders, concurrent medications, and presence or absence of a common cytochrome P450 2C9 gene mutation. Warfarin metabolism is affected by other drugs metabolized by the cytochrome P450, by drugs that displace albumin-bound warfarin and impair gas-

trointestinal absorption, and by antibiotics that alter the natural flora of the colon (an endogenous source of vitamin K). The PT assay is useful to monitor warfarin therapy because this assay measures three vitamin K–dependent coagulation proteins—factors VII, X, and prothrombin. The PT is particularly sensitive to factor VII deficiency; with a half-life of 4 to 6 h, the factor VII level may drop rapidly after only 1 day of warfarin therapy and prolong the PT value. Large loading doses of warfarin result in a more rapid drop in factor VII levels, delay in attainment of a stable PT, a precipitous fall in protein C levels, and predisposition to warfarin-induced skin necrosis. The INR is a method that standardizes PT assays. Each new PT reagent (thromboplastin) is calibrated against the World Health Organization reference thromboplastin. A relative sensitivity of the unknown preparation compared with the reference called the International Sensitivity Index (ISI) is derived. By adjusting for the ISI of a particular thromboplastin, an INR, defined as the PT ratio (patient PT divided by the mean normal PT) that would have been obtained if the reference thromboplastin had been used, can be determined. The INR is calculated using the following formula: $INR = (PT ratio)^{ISI}$. An INR of 2.0 to 3.0 is recommended for all indications except prosthetic mechanical heart valves and prophylaxis of recurrent MI, for which higher-intensity warfarin therapy (INR 2.5 to 3.5) is suggested, and primary prophylaxis where an INR <2.0 is usually desired. In part because many patients with lupus anticoagulants have elevated baseline PTs, the INR may not be an accurate means of monitoring warfarin therapy in this setting. Factors contributing to warfarin-associated bleeding include an INR > 3.0, structural gastrointestinal lesions, concomitant antiplatelet therapy, hypertension, renal disease, and cerebrovascular disease. Visceral bleeding while on warfarin therapy often results in identification of structural lesions. In pregnant women, warfarin can cause an embryopathy consisting of nasal hypoplasia and epiphyseal stippling. The risk may be greatest between weeks 6 and 12 of gestation and may reflect the effect of warfarin on a vitamin K–dependent bone matrix protein, osteocalcin. Most practitioners avoid warfarin during pregnancy. Warfarin-induced skin necrosis is a devastating complication of warfarin therapy, occurring within the first week of therapy and associated in some with protein C deficiency. The skin lesions often begin on fatty body parts (breasts, abdomen, thighs) as erythematous patches and progress to blebs followed by demarcated skin necrosis. Skin biopsy reveals generalized thrombosis of skin vessels. The "purple-toe syndrome" is an uncommon syndrome described in patients with underlying atherosclerotic vascular disease receiving warfarin. These patients present with atheroembolic symptoms including ischemic (purple) toes, livedo reticularis, gangrene, abdominal pain, or symptoms of renal infarction. Skin biopsy reveals cholesterol emboli in the purple-toe syndrome.

FIBRINOLYTIC DRUGS

Most thrombolytic agents are recombinant forms of physiologic plasminogen activators (PAs) that differ in plasma half-life, fibrin specificity, primary clinical usage, primary infusion strategy, and immunogenicity. Therapeutic PAs are fashioned after endogenous tissue-type plasminogen activator (t-PA) or urokinase that converts plasminogen into the active enzyme plasmin. Plasmin degrades fibrinogen and fibrin into fibrin(ogen) degradation products. Major goals of new thrombolytic agent development include increasing fibrin specificity to theoretically reduce bleeding complications, prolonging initial plasma half-life to facilitate bolus administration, and reducing sensitivity to inactivation by plasminogen activator inhibitor (PAI) 1.

STREPTOKINASE Streptokinase is obtained from cultures of β-hemolytic streptococci. By itself, streptokinase has no PA activity, but when complexed with plasminogen, it can convert other plasminogen molecules to plasmin. It is not fibrin-selective in that the so-called lytic state resulting from its therapeutic use is due to lysis of fibrinogen as well as fibrin. Platelet function may be perturbed because plasmin can

proteolyze key platelet membrane receptors. The half-life of streptokinase is ~20 min. Because streptokinase is a bacterial protein, it is antigenic; allergic reactions occur in up to 6% of patients, and anaphylaxis occurs in ~0.1% of patients. Patients previously exposed to streptokinase or with previous streptococcal infections may acquire antistreptococcal antibody levels sufficient to neutralize its activity. Streptokinase has been primarily used to treat VTE and MI as well as to treat central venous line–associated thrombosis.

UROKINASE-TYPE PLASMINOGEN ACTIVATOR Native urokinase is obtained from human fetal kidney cell cultures. Recombinant high-molecular-weight urokinase is produced using nonhuman, mammalian tissue cultures. Urokinase is not fibrin-selective and thus produces a lytic state. Its half-life is ~20 min, and it is used to treat DVT, PE, MI, peripheral arterial thrombosis, and occluded catheters.

TISSUE-TYPE PLASMINOGEN ACTIVATOR Recombinant tissue-type plasminogen activator (rt-PA) produced by recombinant technology demonstrates high in vitro affinity for fibrin with which it forms a ternary complex with plasminogen. Despite reported fibrin-specificity, the lytic state is produced with dosages currently used. Bleeding complications with t-PA are similar to those of streptokinase or urokinase. The half-life of t-PA is ~5 min. t-PA is used to treat DVT, PE, acute MI, acute thrombotic stroke, and dysfunctional central venous lines.

TISSUE-TYPE PLASMINOGEN ACTIVATOR VARIANTS Recombinant PA (r-PA; reteplase) is a nonglycosylated deletion mutant of wild-type human t-PA composed of only the kringle 2 and the protease domains of the parent molecule. Lack of the finger domain imparts lower fibrin-binding affinity. Lack of glycosylation, a finger domain, and epidermal growth factor domain imparts an extended half-life (15 min versus 5 min). TNK-t-PA differs from t-PA by three sets of mutations. The $Asn^{117} \rightarrow Gln$ and $Thr^{103} \rightarrow Asn$ mutations promote a lower plasma clearance rate and greater fibrin specificity. The Lys^{296}-His^{297}-Arg^{298}-$Arg^{299} \rightarrow$ Ala-Ala-Ala-Ala mutation imparts an 80-fold increased resistance to PAI-1. The longer half-lives of r-PA and TNK-rt-PA compared with rt-PA facilitate bolus administration primarily for acute coronary thrombosis.

NEWER NON-t-PA FIBRINOLYTICS Recombinant glycosylated pro-urokinase is a rapid acting and safe fibrin-specific PA. Staphylokinase produced by *Staphylococcus aureus* possesses substantial thrombolytic activity but may be immunogenic. Vampire bat (*Desmodus rotundus*) salivary PA, possessing 85% primary structure homology to human t-PA but lacking a kringle 2 domain, holds promise as a potent thrombolytic. Alfimiprase is a novel thrombolytic based on the snake venom–derived protein fibrolase. Alfimiprase is a direct fibrinolytic (not a PA) neutralized by α_2-macroglobulin that holds promise as a rapid and safe catheter-delivered thrombolytic.

THROMBOLYTIC THERAPY–ASSOCIATED BLEEDING Bleeding associated with all PAs stems from plasmin's inability to differentiate between hemostatic and pathologic thrombi. Bleeding complications range from minor bleeding to life-threatening hemorrhage including intracranial hemorrhage. Older age, female sex, black ethnicity, systolic blood pressure ≥ 140 mmHg, diastolic blood pressure ≥ 100 mmHg, history of stroke, t-PA dose > 1.5 mg/kg, and lower body weight are all associated with increased intracranial hemorrhage risk. The ability of a thrombolytic agent (PA) to distinguish between plasminogen in the general circulation and plasminogen bound to fibrin surfaces dictates its fibrin specificity. Activation of fibrin-bound plasminogen results in the generation of fibrin-bound plasmin that is protected from inactivation by α_2-antiplasmin. Bound plasmin generates soluble fibrin degradation products, whereas circulating plasmin degrades fibrinogen into fibrinogen degradation products. High fibrin specificity is thought to be associated with lower risk for hemorrhagic complications because of the belief that plasmin born on the fibrin surface of a thrombus will restrict its activity only to that surface. This view is not supported by available data from large-scale clinical trials. Unlike in acute MI where intravenous bolus PA dosing is necessary to facilitate rapid lysis of a relatively small thrombus, lysis of larger diameter and longer peripheral thromboses is best achieved with catheter-directed infusions of PA over several hours to days. Drugs designed for bolus infusion to treat acute coronary thrombosis (e.g., r-PA and TNK-t-PA) may be associated with loss of fibrin specificity, accumulation of fragment X, and increased bleeding rates when given by extended continuous infusion.

MANAGEMENT OF VENOUS THROMBOEMBOLIC DISEASE (Fig. 103-3)

The major clinical consequences of extremity DVT include the post-thrombotic syndrome (swelling, stasis dermatitis, ulceration, and venous claudication all due to venous insufficiency), PE, and paradoxical embolism resulting in stroke. The major clinical consequences of PE include chronic dyspnea, pulmonary hypertension, pulmonary infarction, and death. Inadequately treated DVT involving the popliteal or more proximal leg veins is associated with a 20 to 50% risk of clinically relevant recurrence and is strongly associated with both symptomatic and fatal pulmonary embolism. Death from PE occurs most frequently within 2 days of presentation in untreated patients. All-cause mortality rates in treated patients with PE run as high as 11% at 2 weeks and 17% at 3 months.

CALF DEEP VENOUS THROMBOSIS While calf DVT and proximal DVT may be considered separate diseases at their outset, 15 to 25% of calf DVTs propagate and convert into proximal DVT. Symptomatic and asymptomatic calf DVT appear to propagate with equal frequency. Such "proximal conversion" renders what was initially a calf DVT just as dangerous as any proximal DVT. Proximal conversion has been shown to occur within the initial 2 weeks after diagnosis in the majority of cases and warrants treatment accordingly. The most essential goal of calf DVT treatment should be to prevent early proximal conversion. Treatment approaches for isolated calf DVT range from identical therapy as is used for proximal DVT to a complete lack of any pharmacologic therapy. Appropriate management, which falls between these extremes, includes serial duplex ultrasound surveillance (twice-weekly for 2 to 3 weeks) with therapy begun only in the event of proximal conversion and abbreviated courses of standard anticoagulation. Serial surveillance seems especially prudent in situations such as recent gastrointestinal bleeding where the risk of anticoagulation likely exceeds the benefit. Situational calf DVT (DVT with a clear precipitant) can be safely treated with anticoagulation for only 6 weeks, assuming the precipitating illness or event has resolved. Infe-

rior vena cava (IVC) filter placement is not recommended for calf DVT in most circumstances.

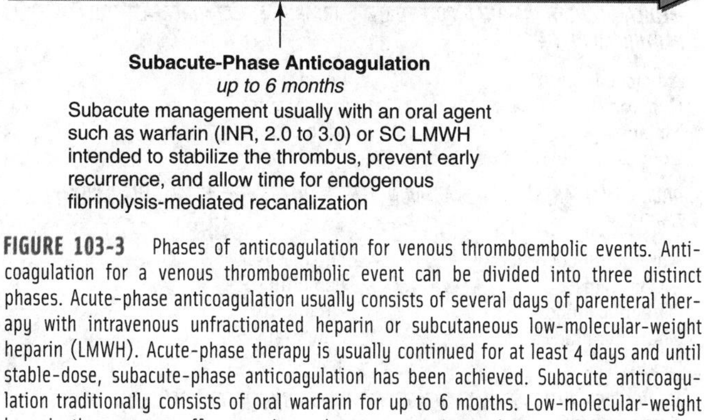

PROXIMAL DEEP VENOUS THROMBOSIS The goals of proximal DVT therapy include restoration of venous patency and prevention of embolization, thrombus extension, early and late recurrence, and postthrombotic syndrome. Studies done before the routine use of anticoagulant therapy demonstrated that 20% of patients with untreated DVT died of PE. Intravenous, aPTT-adjusted UFH and weight-based LMWH effectively prevent embolization, extension, and recurrence. LMWHs appear to be slightly but significantly better than standard heparin at restoring venous patency and may reduce the incidence of early postthrombotic syndrome. Placement of an IVC filter prevents PE in the short run but probably at the expense of a greater long-term DVT recurrence rate.

PULMONARY EMBOLISM In general, acute PE should be treated in the same fashion as acute proximal DVT. It is advisable to start anticoagulation at the time of suspected PE even before diagnostic testing has been performed. LMWHs have been shown to be safe and effective in patients with acute PE treated in hospital. Outpatient treatment of PE is investigational. Placement of an IVC filter at the time of PE diagnosis is usually reserved for those with an absolute contraindication to anticoagulation. Filters may be reasonable in select patients with underlying cardiac or pulmonary disease perceived as being at high risk for death in the event of even a small PE. Placement of a filter because of a "free-floating" DVT is probably not indicated.

INITIAL VTE ANTICOAGULATION Initial anticoagulation refers to the therapy begun at the time of VTE diagnosis and continued only until stable, usually oral, more long-term therapy has been achieved. Treatment with heparin or LMWH should be begun as soon as possible unless an absolute contraindication exists. A delay in achieving a therapeutic intensity of initial parenteral therapy may increase a patient's long-term VTE recurrence rate. Weight-based initial dosing of heparin (80 U/kg bolus followed by 18 U/kg per hour) with subsequent dose adjustments based on any published standardized nomogram facilitates achieving a target aPTT. An aPTT that correlates with an anti-FXa activity level of 0.3 to 0.7 IU/mL is considered therapeutic. The aPTT should be checked every 4 to 6 h until the aPTT surpasses the minimum of the target range. Fixed-dose boluses and initial infusions are preferred by some and are not necessarily inferior to weight-based dosing. Active bleeding, HIT or a history of HIT, and known sensitivity to UFH or pork products are absolute contraindications to heparin therapy. Patients with acute DVT and active bleeding require placement of an IVC filter. In patients with filters placed because of bleeding, appropriate anticoagulation should be begun as soon as the bleeding source has been properly and completely treated. Because of the risk of re-bleeding, such a patient may benefit from inpatient anticoagulation initiation. Placement and subsequent removal of a temporary (or retrievable) IVC filter once the contraindication to anticoagulation has passed seems ideal. Patients who are excessively anticoagulated with heparin without serious bleeding can be treated simply by stopping the drug; the short half-life (1 to 2 h) of heparin ensures rapid return of the aPTT to the therapeutic range. In occasional patients with thrombosis, such as those with lupus anticoagulants, the aPTT assay may not be reliable in monitoring heparin therapy. For these patients, one can follow heparin levels determined using the anti-factor Xa method or give a LMWH, with the dosage determined solely by body weight. Excessively anticoagulated and actively bleeding patients should be considered for reversal of anticoagulation with protamine sulfate. Protamine is given by slow IV infusion, with 1 mg of protamine neutralizing ~100 U of heparin. Protamine infusion may be associated with anaphylaxis, and excess protamine may lead to a paradoxical bleeding disorder. Weight-based subcutaneous LMWH is an established standard of care. Whether to use LMWH or UFH for acute anticoagulation should be determined for each patient taking into account the individual patient medical history, bleeding risk, ambu-

Initial-Phase Anticoagulation
4 to 14 days
Acute management usually with a parenteral agent (heparin or LMWH) intended to rapidly abrogate thrombin generation, prevent thrombus extension, and serve as a "bridge" to subacute anticoagulation

Chronic-Phase Anticoagulation
Long term
Chronic management usually with subacute-phase intensity or reduced-intensity (INR, 1.5 to 2.0) oral warfarin and perhaps in the future with oral ximelagatran or once-weekly SC idraparinux

Subacute-Phase Anticoagulation
up to 6 months
Subacute management usually with an oral agent such as warfarin (INR, 2.0 to 3.0) or SC LMWH intended to stabilize the thrombus, prevent early recurrence, and allow time for endogenous fibrinolysis-mediated recanalization

FIGURE 103-3 Phases of anticoagulation for venous thromboembolic events. Anticoagulation for a venous thromboembolic event can be divided into three distinct phases. Acute-phase anticoagulation usually consists of several days of parenteral therapy with intravenous unfractionated heparin or subcutaneous low-molecular-weight heparin (LMWH). Acute-phase therapy is usually continued for at least 4 days and until stable-dose, subacute-phase anticoagulation has been achieved. Subacute anticoagulation traditionally consists of oral warfarin for up to 6 months. Low-molecular-weight heparin therapy may offer superior and more convenient subacute anticoagulation in select populations. Long-term, chronic-phase anticoagulation consists of identical intensity therapy as is employed during subacute-phase therapy in high-risk patients and attenuated-intensity warfarin in others.

latory status, and insurance coverage. LMWHs are at least as safe and effective as UFH for the initial treatment of DVT. The major advantage of subcutaneous LMWH is its ability to be self-administered at home without the need for therapeutic monitoring. This translates into a significant reduction in mean hospital length of stay (6.5 days for UFH versus 1.1 days for LMWH in one study). Patients may be started on LMWH in the hospital and then discharged in an "accelerated" fashion to continue their conversion to oral warfarin or treated exclusively in the outpatient setting. Meta-analyses have shown a survival advantage in patients with acute DVT treated initially with LMWH versus those treated initially with UFH. This survival advantage seems primarily derived from a survival advantage in cancer patients with DVT. Enoxaparin is dosed at 1 mg/kg body weight every 12 h or 1.5 mg/kg once daily. Dalteparin is dosed at 200 IU/kg (up to 18,000 IU) once-daily. Tinzaparin is dosed at 175 IU/kg once daily. Patients at increased risk for bleeding should probably be treated initially in an inpatient setting. Such patients include those with active bleeding (including occult stool blood), a history of recent surgery, past gastrointestinal tract or neuraxial bleeding, recent trauma or stroke, concomitant regular use of nonsteroidal anti-inflammatory drugs (NSAIDs), thrombocytopenia, and renal insufficiency. Severe renal dysfunction (creatinine clearance < 30 mL/min) results in a ≥25% reduction in LMWH clearance and thus results in drug accumulation. LMWH therapy may not be suitable for the morbidly obese. Monitored heparin therapy is always a choice for the obese patient with acute DVT or PE. Therapeutic monitoring of LMWH therapy using the anti-factor Xa activity assay is not indicated in most patients. An exact therapeutic range has not been carefully determined, and adjusting the dose of LMWH based on such testing has not been shown to be superior to weight-based dosing. Fondaparinux has been shown to be equivalent to enoxaparin for the initial management of DVT and equivalent to intravenous UFH for the initial management of PE. Ximelagatran holds promise as an oral acute VTE treatment. Warfarin therapy *alone* is contraindicated as initial therapy of acute thrombosis because of the inherent delay in achieving therapeutic anticoagulation and the theoretical transient exacerbation of hypercoagulability caused by a rapid reduction in protein C functional activity. This warfarin-induced paradoxical hypercoagulability may explain warfarin-induced skin necrosis and warfarin-induced limb gangrene in patients with HIT.

SUBACUTE VTE ANTICOAGULATION *Subacute anticoagulation* refers to treatment (usually oral warfarin) that follows acute-phase therapy and continues for up to 6 months (Table 103-1). Warfarin therapy (oral or intravenous) can be started as soon as an aPTT > 1.5 times control has been achieved with heparin or an initial weight-based dose of LMWH has been given. Bolus dosing of warfarin does not help achieve a stable, target INR faster and may actually delay achievement of a stable INR and prolong hospitalization. Initial dosing with 2.5 to 7.5 mg/d (based on patient weight and nutritional status) seems prudent. Heparin and LMWH therapy must overlap oral warfarin therapy for a minimum of 4 days and ideally until a stable, target range (2.0 to 3.0) INR has been achieved. Starting warfarin therapy early after heparin therapy (day 1 or 2) facilitates earlier hospital discharge and potential reduction in the incidence of HIT. Patients with massive DVT

or PE may benefit from 7 to 10 days of initial heparin or LMWH therapy. Because of its teratogenic effects, warfarin therapy is contraindicated in pregnancy, so continued heparin or LMWH is prudent. Patients should be encouraged to consume a constant intake of dietary vitamin K and avoid large variations or fluctuations in their diet. Because of the number of pharmacologic interactions that exist between warfarin and other drugs, patients should be instructed to inform their physician of the addition or withdrawal of any medication, vitamin, and herbal preparation (Table 103-2). Recently completed studies (LITE, ONCENOX, and CLOT) provide strong evidence to support the use of LMWH as acute *plus* subacute VTE treatment. Once-daily tinzaparin (175 IU/kg) was as effective and safer than INR-adjusted oral warfarin in a mixed population of acute DVT patients. Once-daily tinzaparin, enoxaparin, and dalteparin were shown to be more effective than oral warfarin at preventing recurrent VTE in cancer patients with thrombosis. Patients with DVT secondary to a transient risk such as surgery, trauma, or pregnancy may be anticoagulated for a duration of 6 weeks to 3 months, as long as the risk factor has passed. Patients with a first idiopathic VTE should be anticoagulated for a minimum of 3 to 6 months.

CHRONIC ANTICOAGULATION FOR VTE Patients with persistent risk factors for thrombosis such as an anti-phospholipid antibody, hyperhomocysteinemia, active malignancy, or a deficiency of a natural anticoagulant (protein C, protein S, and antithrombin), homozygous factor V Leiden, and those with recurrent idiopathic VTE may benefit from long-term therapy (Table 103-1). The risk of VTE recurrence is very low as long as therapeutic anticoagulation is continued. It is the up to 3 to 4% annual risk of major hemorrhage secondary to warfarin (INR 2.0 to 3.0) that prevents physicians from prescribing long-term anticoagulation with abandon. The long-term risks and inconvenience of chronic (>6 months) therapeutic-intensity warfarin anticoagulation have led to the study of alternative approaches to chronic-phase anticoagulation following VTE. Extended secondary prevention with the oral DTI ximelagatran (24 mg bid) for 18 months after 6 months of standard anticoagulation in patients with VTE (THRIVE III) revealed recurrence rates of 2.0% and 11.6% ($p < .0001$) in the ximelagatran and placebo groups, respectively. Reported major and minor bleeding rates on therapy were not different between groups. Another successful approach

---

TABLE 103-1 Duration of Anticoagulation for Venous Thromboembolic Events (VTE)

Event	Duration of Anticoagulation
Situational DVT	6 weeks to 3 months
Idiopathic DVT	3 to 6 months (minimum)
Recurrent idiopathic DVT	12 months (minimum)
VTE with ongoing risk factors[a]	Long-term/indefinite
Pulmonary embolism	6 months (minimum)
Massive pulmonary embolism	Long-term/indefinite

[a] Malignancy, anti-phospholipid antibodies, homozygous factor V Leiden, natural anticoagulant deficiency, etc.
Note: DVT, deep venous thrombosis.

TABLE 103-2 Effect of Select Drugs and Medical Conditions on Oral Warfarin Anticoagulation

DRUGS THAT POTENTIATE WARFARIN EFFECT (INCREASE THE PROTHROMBIN TIME)

Acetaminophen	Phenylbutazone
Anabolic steroids	Phenytoin
Broad-spectrum antibiotics	Propranolol
Cimetidine	Protease inhibitors (except retinovir)
Fluconazole	Quinidine
Lovastatin	Salicylate
Metronidazole	Tamoxifen
Omeprazole	Trimethoprim-sulfamethoxazole

MEDICAL CONDITIONS THAT POTENTIATE WARFARIN EFFECT (INCREASE THE PROTHROMBIN TIME)

Advanced age	Fever
Hepatobiliary disease	Hyperthyroidism
Malabsorption	Malnutrition
Congestive heart failure	Cancer

DRUGS THAT ANTAGONIZE WARFARIN EFFECT (DECREASE THE PROTHROMBIN TIME)

Adrenal glucocorticoids	Griseofulvin
Barbiturates	Penicillin
Carbamazepine	Rifampin
Cholestyramine	Sulcrafate
Efavirenz	Trazadone

MEDICAL CONDITIONS THAT ANTAGONIZE WARFARIN EFFECT (DECREASE THE PROTHROMBIN TIME)

Excess dietary vitamin K	Hypothyroidism
Inherited warfarin resistence	Nephrotic syndrome

to chronic-phase anticoagulation involves long-term, low-intensity oral warfarin therapy with infrequent (every 8 weeks) INR monitoring (PREVENT). In this landmark study, patients with idiopathic VTE who had received standard acute- and subacute-phase anticoagulant therapy were randomly assigned to placebo or low-intensity warfarin (target INR 1.5 to 2.0). Recurrent VTE rates were 7.2 per 100 person-years and 2.6 per 100 person-years in the placebo and warfarin groups, respectively. This 64% risk reduction was accomplished in both those with and without inherited thrombophilia without any increase in major hemorrhage rates. Such safe and effective regimens have the potential to redefine the standard of care for VTE.

THROMBOLYSIS FOR VTE Benefits of DVT thrombolysis include the ability to subsequently diagnosis and treat underlying venous stenosis, venous compression (as in May-Thurner syndrome) or venous webs. Thrombolysis results in improved venous patency and symptom resolution and in a decrease in postthrombolic syndrome symptoms, and it may improve health-related quality of life. Because of the bleeding risk, thrombolysis is best reserved to treat iliofemoral DVT in the young and those with extensive thrombosis resulting in venous limb gangrene (*phlegmasia cerulea dolens*). Intravenous thrombolysis has been demonstrated to improve survival in patients with massive PE plus shock and is probably indicated in these patients. When compared to anticoagulation alone, thrombolytic therapy results in more rapid thrombus lysis, an early improvement in pulmonary blood flow, and improvement of right ventricular function. However, these improvements in cardiopulmonary function alone have not resulted in decreased mortality in stable patients without significant hemodynamic compromise. It remains unclear whether patients with PE and evidence of right ventricular dysfunction and/or elevated cardiac troponin levels are subgroups that benefit more from thrombolysis. Major hemorrhage rates have varied between 4 and 22% when thrombolytic agents are used in studies at the currently recommended doses.

VENOUS THROMBOEMBOLIC DISEASE PREVENTION If physicians focused more on VTE prophylaxis, much less time would need to be dedicated to emphasizing methods for VTE treatment. Fatal PE is the most common preventable cause of hospital death. A key to proper prophylaxis is the recognition of risk factors for thrombosis. Established clinical risk factors include: advanced age; prolonged immobility, stroke, or paralysis; prior VTE; active malignancy and its treatment; major surgery especially involving the abdomen, pelvis, and lower extremities; trauma, especially involving fracture of the pelvis, hip, or leg; obesity; varicose veins; depressed left ventricular ejection fraction; central venous access devices; inflammatory bowel disease; lobar pneumonia; nephrotic syndrome; pregnancy; estrogen use; and inherited and acquired hypercoagulable states. The number of risk factors, risk of DVT, risk of clinical PE, risk of fatal PE, and the required intensity of prophylactic therapy necessary to mitigate the risk all seem to increase in parallel. Medically ill patients (predominantly those immobilized with severe cardiopulmonary disease) have a 14.9% risk of developing DVT within 14 days of admission in the absence of active prophylaxis (MEDENOX). The DVT rate is reduced to 5.5% by the addition of a once-daily dose of LMWH (enoxaparin, 40 mg) without a significant increase in bleeding risk. Other studies have demonstrated equivalency between LMWH and heparin (5000 U tid) in medical patients with acute cardiac or pulmonary disease. Not all patients at risk will develop a thrombosis, and not all thromboses will result in symptoms, morbidity, or death. The benefit of pharmacologic thromboprophylaxis must always be weighed against the bleeding risk. Patients at high risk for bleeding should still receive prophylaxis in the form of intermittent pneumatic compression and/or thromboembolism-deterrence stockings.

FURTHER READING

DEITCHER SR, CARMAN TL: Heparin-induced thrombocytopenia: Natural history, diagnosis, and management. Vasc Med 6:113, 2001

——, ——: Deep venous thrombosis and pulmonary embolism. Curr Treat Options Cardiovasc Med 4:223, 2002

——: Cancer and thrombosis: Mechanisms and treatment. J Thromb Thrombolysis 16:21, 2003

GOLDHABER SZ: Thrombolysis in pulmonary embolism: A debatable indication. Thromb Haemost 86:444, 2001

HAYDEN M et al: Aspirin for the primary prevention of cardiovascular events: A summary of the evidence for the U.S. Preventive Services Task Force. Ann Intern Med 136:161, 2002

VERSTRAETE M: Third-generation thrombolytic drugs. Am J Med 109:52, 2001

104 | INTRODUCTION TO INFECTIOUS DISEASES: HOST–PATHOGEN INTERACTIONS
Lawrence C. Madoff, Dennis L. Kasper

Despite decades of dramatic progress in their treatment and prevention, infectious diseases remain a major cause of death and debility and are responsible for worsening the living conditions of many millions of people around the world. Infections frequently challenge the physician's diagnostic skill and must be considered in the differential diagnoses of syndromes affecting every organ system.

CHANGING EPIDEMIOLOGY OF INFECTIOUS DISEASES With the advent of antimicrobial agents, some medical leaders believed that infectious diseases would soon be eliminated and become of historic interest only. Indeed, the hundreds of chemotherapeutic agents developed since World War II, most of which are potent and safe, include drugs effective not only against bacteria but also against viruses, fungi, and parasites. Nevertheless, we now realize that as we developed antimicrobial agents, microbes developed the ability to elude our best weapons and to counterattack with new survival strategies. Antibiotic resistance occurs at an alarming rate among all classes of mammalian pathogens. Pneumococci resistant to penicillin and enterococci resistant to vancomycin have become commonplace. Even *Staphylococcus aureus* that is resistant to vancomycin has appeared. Such pathogens present real clinical problems in managing infections that were easily treatable just a few years ago. Diseases once thought to have been nearly eradicated from the developed world—tuberculosis, cholera, and rheumatic fever, for example—have rebounded with renewed ferocity. Newly discovered and emerging infectious agents appear to have been brought into contact with humans by changes in the environment and by movements of human and animal populations. An example of the propensity for pathogens to escape from their usual niche is the alarming 1999 outbreak in New York of encephalitis due to West Nile virus, which had never previously been isolated in the Americas. In 2003, severe acute respiratory syndrome (SARS) was first recognized. This emerging clinical entity is caused by a novel coronavirus that may have jumped from an animal niche to become a significant human pathogen. In early 2004, avian influenza spread rapidly through poultry farms in Asia and caused deaths in exposed humans, raising the specter of a new influenza pandemic.

Many infectious agents have been discovered only in recent decades (Fig. 104-1). Ebola virus, human metapneumovirus, *Anaplasma phagocytophila* (the agent of human granulocytotropic ehrlichiosis), and retroviruses such as HIV humble us despite our deepening understanding of pathogenesis at the most basic molecular level. Even in developed countries, infectious diseases have made a resurgence. Between 1980 and 1996, mortality from infectious diseases in the United States increased by 64% to levels not seen since the 1940s.

The role of infectious agents in the etiology of diseases once believed to be noninfectious is being increasingly recognized. For example, it is now widely accepted that *Helicobacter pylori* is the causative agent of peptic ulcer disease and perhaps of gastric malignancy. Human papillomavirus is likely to be the most important cause of invasive cervical cancer. Human herpesvirus type 8 is believed to be the cause of most cases of Kaposi's sarcoma. Epstein-Barr virus is a cause of certain lymphomas and may play a role in the genesis of Hodgkin's disease. The possibility certainly exists that other diseases of unknown cause, such as rheumatoid arthritis, sarcoidosis, or inflammatory bowel disease, have infectious etiologies. There is even evidence that atherosclerosis may have an infectious component. In contrast, there are data to suggest that decreased exposures to pathogens in childhood may be contributing to an increase in the observed rate of allergic diseases.

Medical advances over infectious diseases have been hindered by changes in the patient population. Immunocompromised hosts now constitute a significant proportion of the seriously infected population. Physicians immunosuppress their patients to prevent the rejection of

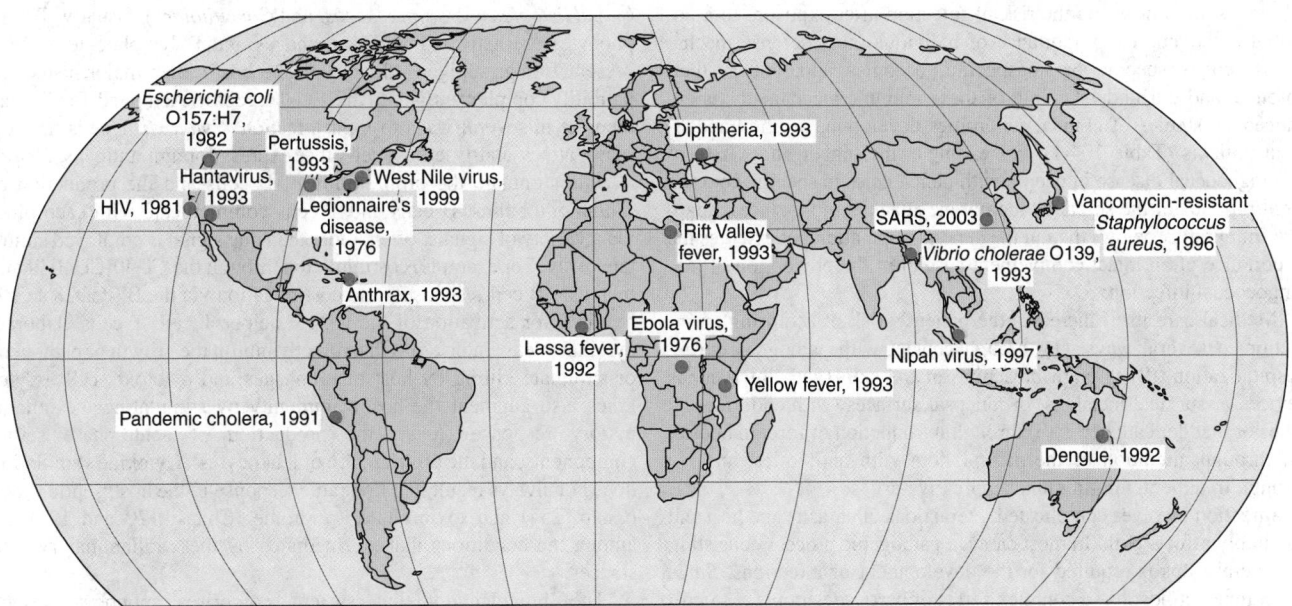

FIGURE 104-1 Map of the world showing examples of geographic locales where infectious diseases were noted to have emerged or resurged. (Adapted from *Addressing Emerging Infectious Disease Threats: A Prevention Strategy for the United States,* Department of Health and Human Services, Centers for Disease Control and Prevention, 1994.)

transplants and to treat neoplastic and inflammatory diseases. Some infections, most notably that caused by HIV, immunocompromise the host in and of themselves. Lesser degrees of immunosuppression are associated with other infections, such as influenza and syphilis. Infectious agents that coexist peacefully with immunocompetent hosts wreak havoc in those who lack a complete immune system. AIDS has brought to prominence once-obscure organisms such as *Pneumocystis*, *Cryptosporidium parvum*, and *Mycobacterium avium*.

HOST FACTORS IN INFECTION For any infectious process to occur, the pathogen and the host must first encounter each other. Factors such as geography, environment, and behavior thus influence the likelihood of infection. Although the initial encounter between a susceptible host and a virulent organism frequently results in disease, some organisms can be harbored in the host for years before disease becomes clinically evident. For a complete view, individual patients must be considered in the context of the population to which they belong. Infectious diseases do not often occur in isolation; rather, they spread through a group exposed from a point source (e.g., a contaminated water supply) or from individual to individual (e.g., via respiratory droplets). Thus, the clinician must be alert to infections prevalent in the community as a whole. A detailed history, including information on travel, behavioral factors, exposures to animals or potentially contaminated environments, and living and occupational conditions, must be elicited. For example, the likelihood of infection by *Plasmodium falciparum* can be significantly affected by altitude, climate, terrain, season, and even time of day. Antibiotic-resistant strains are localized to specific geographic regions, and a seemingly minor alteration in a travel itinerary can dramatically influence the likelihood of acquiring chloroquine-resistant malaria. If such important details in the history are overlooked, inappropriate treatment may result in the death of the patient. Likewise, the chance of acquiring a sexually transmitted disease can be greatly affected by a relatively minor variation in sexual practices, such as the method used for birth control. Knowledge of the relationship between specific risk factors and disease allows the physician to influence a patient's health even before the development of infection by modification of these risk factors and—when a vaccine is available—by immunization.

Many specific host factors influence the likelihood of acquiring an infectious disease. Age, immunization history, prior illnesses, level of nutrition, pregnancy, coexisting illness, and perhaps emotional state all have some impact on the risk of infection after exposure to a potential pathogen. The importance of individual host defense mechanisms, either specific or nonspecific, becomes apparent in their absence, and our understanding of these immune mechanisms is enhanced by studies of clinical syndromes developing in immunodeficient patients (Table 104-1). For example, the higher attack rate of meningococcal disease in people with deficiencies in specific complement proteins of the so-called membrane attack complex (see "Adaptive Immunity," below) than in the general population underscores the importance of an intact complement system in the prevention of meningococcal infection.

Medical care itself increases the patient's risk of acquiring an infection in several ways: (1) through contact with pathogens during hospitalization, (2) through breaching of the skin (with intravenous devices or surgical incisions) or mucosal surfaces (with endotracheal tubes or bladder catheters), (3) through introduction of foreign bodies, (4) through alteration of the natural flora with antibiotics, and (5) through treatment with immunosuppressive drugs.

Infection involves complicated interactions of parasite and host and inevitably affects both. In most cases, a pathogenic process consisting of several steps is required for the development of infections. Since the competent host has a complex series of barricades in place to prevent infection, the successful parasite must use specific strategies at each of these steps. The specific strategies used by bacteria, viruses, and parasites (Chap. 105) have some remarkable conceptual similari-

ties, but the strategic details are unique not only for each class of organism but also for individual species within a class.

THE IMMUNE RESPONSE ■ Innate Immunity As they have co-evolved with microbes, higher organisms have developed mechanisms for recognizing and responding to microorganisms. Many of these mechanisms, referred to together as *innate immunity*, are evolutionarily ancient, having been conserved from insects to humans (Fig. 104-2). In general, innate immune mechanisms exploit molecular patterns found specifically in pathogenic microorganisms. These "pathogen signatures" are recognized by host molecules that either directly interfere with the pathogen or initiate a response that does so. Innate immunity serves to protect the host without prior exposure to an infectious agent—i.e., before specific or adaptive immunity has had a chance to develop. Innate immunity also functions as a warning system that activates components of adaptive immunity early in the course of infection.

Examples of innate immune effectors include defensins, simple peptides found on the skin and mucosal surfaces with activity against bacteria, fungi, and viruses. Macrophages that engulf and kill microbes (and other cells with similar function) are found even in invertebrates, such as *Drosophila*. The complement system (described below and discussed in more detail in Chap. 295) can respond to microbes without prior exposure.

The response to lipopolysaccharide (LPS), a molecule found uniquely in gram-negative bacteria, is instructive in understanding innate immunity. Even minuscule amounts of LPS are detected by LPS-binding protein, CD14, and Toll-like receptor 4 (Fig. 104-2). The interaction of LPS with these components of the innate immune system prompts macrophages, via the transcriptional activator NFκB, to produce cytokines that lead to inflammation and enzymes that enhance the clearance of microbes. These initial responses serve not only to limit infection but also to initiate specific or adaptive immune responses.

Adaptive Immunity Once in the bloodstream or a normally sterile body site, the microorganism faces the host's tightly integrated cellular and humoral immune systems. Cellular immunity (Chap. 295), comprising T lymphocytes, macrophages, and natural killer cells, primarily recognizes and combats pathogens that proliferate intracellularly. Cellular immune mechanisms are important in immunity to all classes of infectious agents, including most viruses and many bacteria (e.g., *Mycoplasma*, *Chlamydia*, *Listeria*, *Salmonella*, and *Mycobacterium*), parasites (e.g., *Trypanosoma*, *Toxoplasma*, and *Leishmania*), and fungi (e.g., *Histoplasma*, *Cryptococcus*, and *Coccidioides*). Usually, T lymphocytes are activated by macrophages and B lymphocytes, which present foreign antigens along with the host's own major histocompatibility complex antigen to the T cell receptor. Activated T cells may then act in several ways to fight infection. *Cytotoxic* T cells may directly attack and lyse host cells that express foreign antigens. *Helper* T cells stimulate the proliferation of B cells and the production of immunoglobulins. B cells and T cells communicate with each other via a variety of signals; often, more than one signal is employed simultaneously. For example, costimulation through the CD40-CD40 ligand increases B cell responses, and costimulation via the B7-CD28 axis is required for activation of the CD4+ helper T cell. T cells elaborate cytokines (e.g., interferon) that directly inhibit the growth of pathogens or stimulate killing by host macrophages and cytotoxic cells. Cytokines also augment the host's immunity by stimulating the inflammatory response (fever, the production of acute-phase serum components, and the proliferation of leukocytes). Cytokine stimulation does not always result in a favorable response in the host; septic shock (Chap. 254) and toxic shock syndrome (Chaps. 120 and 121) are among the conditions that are mediated by these inflammatory substances.

The reticuloendothelial system comprises monocyte-derived phagocytic cells that are located in the liver (Kupffer cells), lung (alveolar macrophages), spleen, kidney (mesangial cells), brain (microglia), and lymph nodes and that clear circulating microorganisms.

TABLE 104-1 Infections Associated with Selected Defects in Immunity

Host Defect	Disease or Therapy Associated with Defect	Common Etiologic Agent of Infection
NONSPECIFIC IMMUNITY		
Impaired cough	Rib fracture, neuromuscular dysfunction	Bacteria causing pneumonia, aerobic and anaerobic oral flora
Loss of gastric acidity	Achlorhydria, histamine blockade	*Salmonella* spp., enteric pathogens
Loss of cutaneous integrity	Penetrating trauma, athlete's foot	*Staphylococcus* spp., *Streptococcus* spp.
	Burn	*Pseudomonas aeruginosa*
	Intravenous catheter	*Staphylococcus* spp., *Streptococcus* spp., gram-negative rods, coagulase-negative staphylococci
Implantable device	Heart valve	*Streptococcus* spp., coagulase-negative staphylococci, *Staphylococcus aureus*
	Artificial joint	*Staphylococcus* spp., *Streptococcus* spp., gram-negative rods
Loss of normal bacterial flora	Antibiotic use	*Clostridium difficile*, *Candida* spp.
Impaired clearance		
Poor drainage	Urinary tract infection	*Escherichia coli*
Abnormal secretions	Cystic fibrosis	Chronic pulmonary infection with *P. aeruginosa*
INFLAMMATORY RESPONSE		
Neutropenia	Hematologic malignancy, cytotoxic chemotherapy, aplastic anemia, HIV infection	Gram-negative enteric bacilli, *Pseudomonas* spp., *Staphylococcus* spp., *Candida* spp.
Chemotaxis	Chédiak-Higashi syndrome, Job's syndrome, protein-calorie malnutrition	*S. aureus*, *Streptococcus pyogenes*, *Haemophilus influenzae*, gram-negative bacilli
	Leukocyte adhesion defects 1 and 2	Bacteria causing skin and systemic infections, gingivitis
Phagocytosis (cellular)	Systemic lupus erythematosus (SLE), chronic myelogenous leukemia, megaloblastic anemia	*Streptococcus pneumoniae*, *H. influenzae*
Splenectomy	—	*H. influenzae*, *S. pneumoniae*, other streptococci, *Capnocytophaga* spp., *Babesia microti*, *Salmonella* spp.
Microbicidal defect	Chronic granulomatous disease	Catalase-positive bacteria and fungi: staphylococci, *E. coli*, *Klebsiella* spp., *P. aeruginosa*, *Aspergillus* spp., *Nocardia* spp.
	Chédiak-Higashi syndrome	*S. aureus*, *S. pyogenes*
	Interferon γ receptor defect, interleukin 12 deficiency, interleukin 12 receptor defect	*Mycobacterium* spp., *Salmonella* spp.
INNATE IMMUNITY		
Complement system		
C3	Congenital liver disease, SLE, nephrotic syndrome	*S. aureus*, *S. pneumoniae*, *Pseudomonas* spp., *Proteus* spp.
C5	Congenital	*Neisseria* spp., gram-negative rods
C6, C7, C8	Congenital, SLE	*Neisseria meningitidis*, *N. gonorrhoeae*
Alternative pathway	Sickle cell disease	*S. pneumoniae*, *Salmonella* spp.
Toll-like receptor 4	Congenital	Gram-negative bacilli
Interleukin 1 receptor–associated kinase (IRAK) 4	Congenital	*S. pneumoniae*, *S. aureus*, other bacteria
Mannan-binding lectin	Congenital	*N. meningitidis*, other bacteria
ADAPTIVE IMMUNITY		
T lymphocyte deficiency/dysfunction	Thymic aplasia, thymic hypoplasia, Hodgkin's disease, sarcoidosis, lepromatous leprosy	*Listeria monocytogenes*, *Mycobacterium* spp., *Candida* spp., *Aspergillus* spp., *Cryptococcus neoformans*, herpes simplex virus, varicella-zoster virus
	AIDS	*Pneumocystis*, cytomegalovirus, herpes simplex virus, *Mycobacterium avium-intracellulare*, *C. neoformans*, *Candida* spp.
	Mucocutaneous candidiasis	*Candida* spp.
	Purine nucleoside phosphorylase deficiency	Fungi, viruses
B cell deficiency/dysfunction	Bruton's X-linked agammaglobulinemia	*S. pneumoniae*, other streptococci
	Agammaglobulinemia, chronic lymphocytic leukemia, multiple myeloma, dysglobulinemia	*H. influenzae*, *N. meningitidis*, *S. aureus*, *Klebsiella pneumoniae*, *E. coli*, *Giardia lamblia*, *Pneumocystis*, enteroviruses
	Selective IgM deficiency	*S. pneumoniae*, *H. influenzae*, *E. coli*
	Selective IgA deficiency	*G. lamblia*, hepatitis virus, *S. pneumoniae*, *H. influenzae*
Mixed T and B cell deficiency/dysfunction	Common variable hypogammaglobulinemia	*Pneumocystis*, cytomegalovirus, *S. pneumoniae*, *H. influenzae*, various other bacteria
	Ataxia-telangiectasia	*S. pneumoniae*, *H. influenzae*, *S. aureus*, rubella virus, *G. lamblia*
	Severe combined immunodeficiency	*S. aureus*, *S. pneumoniae*, *H. influenzae*, *Candida albicans*, *Pneumocystis*, varicella-zoster virus, rubella virus, cytomegalovirus
	Wiskott-Aldrich syndrome	Agents of infections associated with T and B cell abnormalities
	X-linked hyper-IgM syndrome	*Pneumocystis*, cytomegalovirus, *Cryptosporidium parvum*

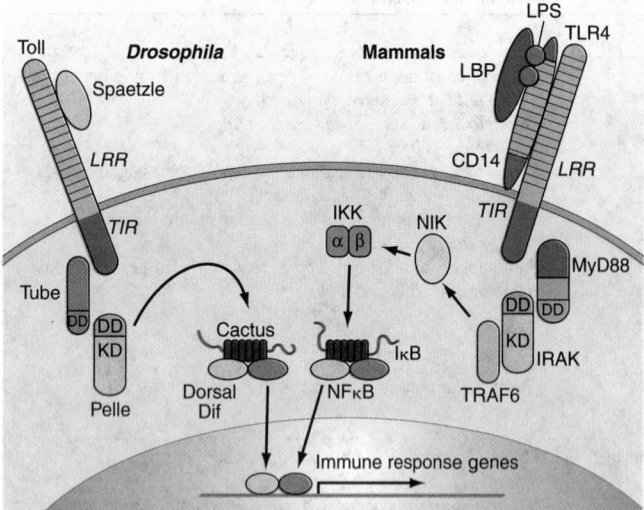

FIGURE 104-2 Conserved pathways in innate immunity in *Drosophila* and mammals. Examples chosen are, left, the induction of the antifungal gene drosomycin by binding of processed Spaetzle protein to the transmembrane receptor Toll and, right, activation of costimulatory protein genes by binding of an LPS-LBP-CD14 complex to a human Toll homologue, TLR4. DD, death domain; IκB, inhibitor of κB; IKK, IκB kinase; IRAK, interleukin 1 receptor–associated kinase; KD, kinase domain; LBP, LPS-binding protein; LPS, lipopolysaccharide; LRR, leucine-rich domain; NFκB, nuclear factor κB; NIK, NFκB-inducing kinase; TIR, Toll/IL-1 receptor homology domain; TRAF6, tumor necrosis factor receptor–associated factor 6. (*Reprinted with permission from JA Hoffman et al: Science 284:1315, 1999. Copyright 1999 American Association for the Advancement of Science.*)

Although these tissue macrophages and polymorphonuclear leukocytes (PMNs) are capable of killing microorganisms without help, they function much more efficiently when pathogens are first *opsonized* (Greek, "to prepare for eating") by components of the complement system such as C3b and/or by antibodies.

Extracellular pathogens, including most encapsulated bacteria (those surrounded by a complex polysaccharide coat), are attacked by the humoral immune system, which includes antibodies, the complement cascade, and phagocytic cells. Antibodies are complex glycoproteins (also called immunoglobulins) that are produced by mature B lymphocytes, circulate in body fluids, and are secreted on mucosal surfaces. Antibodies specifically recognize and bind to foreign antigens. One of the most impressive features of the immune system is the ability to generate an incredible diversity of antibodies capable of recognizing virtually every foreign antigen yet not reacting with self. In addition to being exquisitely specific for antigens, antibodies come in different structural and functional classes: IgG predominates in the circulation and persists for many years after exposure; IgM is the earliest specific antibody to appear in response to infection; secretory IgA is important in immunity at mucosal surfaces, while monomeric IgA appears in the serum; and IgE is important in allergic and parasitic diseases. Antibodies may directly impede the function of an invading organism, neutralize secreted toxins and enzymes, or facilitate the removal of the antigen (invading organism) by phagocytic cells. Immunoglobulins participate in cell-mediated immunity by promoting the antibody-dependent cellular cytotoxicity functions of certain T lymphocytes. Antibodies also promote the deposition of complement components on the surface of the invader.

The complement system (Chap. 295) consists of a group of serum proteins functioning as a cooperative, self-regulating cascade of enzymes that adhere to—and in some cases disrupt—the surface of invading organisms. Some of these surface-adherent proteins (e.g., C3b) can then act as opsonins for destruction of microbes by phagocytes. The later, "terminal" components (C7, C8, and C9) can directly kill some bacterial invaders (notably, many of the neisseriae) by forming a membrane attack complex and disrupting the integrity of the bacterial

membrane, thus causing bacteriolysis. Other complement components, such as C5a, act as chemoattractants for PMNs. Complement activation and deposition occur by either or both of two pathways: the classic pathway is activated primarily by immune complexes (i.e., antibody bound to antigen), and the alternative pathway is activated by microbial components, frequently in the absence of antibody. PMNs have receptors for both antibody and C3b, and antibody and complement function together to aid in the clearance of infectious agents.

PMNs, short-lived white blood cells that engulf and kill invading microbes, are first attracted to inflammatory sites by chemoattractants such as C5a, which is a product of complement activation at the site of infection. PMNs localize to the site of infection by adhering to cellular adhesion molecules expressed by endothelial cells. Endothelial cells express these receptors, called *selectins* (CD-62, ELAM-1), in response to inflammatory cytokines such as tumor necrosis factor (TNF) α and interleukin 1. The binding of these selectin molecules to specific receptors on PMNs results in the adherence of the PMNs to the endothelium. Cytokine-mediated upregulation and expression of intercellular adhesion molecule 1 (ICAM 1) on endothelial cells then take place, and this latter receptor binds to β_2 integrins on PMNs, thereby facilitating diapedesis into the extravascular compartment. Once the PMNs are in the extravascular compartment, various molecules such as arachidonic acids further enhance the inflammatory process.

APPROACH TO THE PATIENT

The clinical manifestations of infectious diseases at presentation are myriad, varying from fulminant life-threatening processes to brief and self-limited conditions to indolent chronic maladies. The clinician must use all the skills of medicine to diagnose the infection and prescribe appropriate treatment. First, a careful history is essential and must include details on underlying chronic diseases; medications; occupation; travel; and risk factors for exposure to certain types of pathogens, such as those associated with sexual contacts, family illnesses, illicit drug use, particular animals, blood transfusions, ingestion of contaminated liquids or foods, or bites of insect vectors. Since infectious diseases may involve many organ systems, a careful review of systems may elicit important clues as to the disease process. The physical examination must be thorough, and attention must be paid to seemingly minor details: a soft heart murmur that might indicate bacterial endocarditis; an evanescent skin rash that suggests rheumatic fever; or a retinal lesion that suggests disseminated candidiasis or cytomegalovirus (CMV) infection.

LABORATORY INVESTIGATIONS Laboratory studies must be carefully considered and directed toward establishing an etiologic diagnosis in the shortest possible time, at the lowest possible cost, and with the least possible discomfort to the patient. Cultures must be performed in a manner that minimizes the likelihood of contamination with normal flora while maximizing the yield. A sputum sample is far more likely to be valuable when elicited with careful coaching by the clinician than when collected in a container simply left at the bedside with cursory instructions. Gram's stains of specimens should be interpreted carefully and the quality of the specimen assessed. The findings on Gram's staining should correspond to the results of culture; a discrepancy may suggest diagnostic possibilities such as infection due to fastidious or anaerobic bacteria.

The microbiology laboratory must be an ally in the diagnostic endeavor. Astute laboratory personnel will suggest optimal culture and transport conditions or alternative tests to facilitate diagnosis. If informed about specific potential pathogens, an alert laboratory staff will allow sufficient time for these organisms to become evident in culture, even when present in small numbers or when slow-growing. The parasitology technician who is attuned to the specific diagnostic considerations relevant to a particular case may be able to detect the rare, otherwise-elusive egg or cyst in a stool specimen. In cases where a diagnosis appears difficult, serum should be stored during the early acute phase of the illness so that a diagnostic rise in titer of antibody to a specific pathogen can be detected later. Bacterial and fungal antigens can sometimes be detected in body fluids, even when cultures are negative or are rendered sterile by antibiotic therapy. Techniques such as the polymerase chain reaction allow the amplification of specific DNA sequences so that minute quantities of foreign nucleic acids can be recognized in host specimens.

℞ TREATMENT

Optimal therapy for infectious diseases requires a broad knowledge of medicine and careful clinical judgment. Life-threatening infections such as bacterial meningitis or sepsis, viral encephalitis, or falciparum malaria must be treated immediately, often before a specific causative organism is identified. Antimicrobial agents must be chosen empirically and must be active against the range of potential infectious agents consistent with the clinical scenario. In contrast, good clinical judgment sometimes dictates withholding of antimicrobials in a self-limited process or until a specific diagnosis is made. The dictum *primum non nocere* should be adhered to, and it should be remembered that all antimicrobials carry a risk (and a cost) to the patient. Direct toxicity may be encountered—e.g., ototoxicity due to aminoglycosides, lipodystrophy due to antiretroviral agents, and hepatotoxicity due to antituberculous agents such as isoniazid and rifampin. Allergic reactions are common and can be serious. Since superinfection sometimes follows the eradication of the normal flora and colonization by a resistant organism, one invariable principle is that infectious disease therapy should be directed toward as narrow a spectrum of infectious agents as possible. Treatment specific for the pathogen should result in as little perturbation as possible of the host's microflora. With few exceptions, abscesses require surgical or percutaneous drainage for cure. Foreign bodies, including medical devices, must generally be removed in order to eliminate an infection of the device or of the adjacent tissue. Other infections, such as necrotizing fasciitis, peritonitis due to a perforated organ, gas gangrene, and chronic osteomyelitis, require surgery as the primary means of cure; in these conditions, antibiotics play only an adjunctive role.

The role of immunomodulators in the management of infectious diseases has received increasing attention. Glucocorticoids have been shown to be of benefit in the treatment of *Haemophilus influenzae* meningitis in children and in therapy for *Pneumocystis* pneumonia in patients with AIDS. The use of these agents in other infectious processes remains less clear and in some cases (in cerebral malaria and septic shock, for example) is detrimental. Activated protein C is the first immunomodulatory agent widely available for the treatment of severe sepsis. Its usefulness demonstrates the interrelatedness of the clotting cascade and systemic immunity. Other agents that modulate the immune response include prostaglandin inhibitors, specific lymphokines, and TNF inhibitors. Specific antibody therapy plays a role in the treatment and prevention of many diseases. Specific immunoglobulins have long been known to prevent the development of symptomatic rabies and tetanus. More recently, CMV immune globulin has been recognized as important not only in preventing the transmission of the virus during organ transplantation but also in treating CMV pneumonia in bone marrow transplant recipients. There is a strong need for well-designed clinical trials to evaluate each new interventional modality.

PERSPECTIVE The genetic simplicity of many infectious agents allows them to undergo rapid evolution and to develop selective advantages that result in constant variation in the clinical manifestations of infection. Moreover, changes in the environment and the host can predispose new populations to a particular infection. The dramatic march of West Nile virus from a single focus in New York City in 1999 to locations across the North American continent by the summer of 2002

caused widespread alarm, illustrating the fear that new plagues induce in the human psyche. The intentional release of deadly spores of *Bacillus anthracis* awakened many from a sense of complacency regarding biological weapons.

"The terror of the unknown is seldom better displayed than by the response of a population to the appearance of an epidemic, particularly when the epidemic strikes without apparent cause." Edward Kass made this statement in 1977 in reference to the newly discovered Legionnaire's disease, but it could apply equally to SARS or to any other new and mysterious disease. The potential for infectious agents to emerge in novel and unexpected ways requires that physicians and public health officials be knowledgeable, vigilant, and open-minded in their approach to unexplained illness. The emergence of antimicrobial-resistant pathogens (e.g., enterococci that are resistant to all known antimicrobial agents and cause infections that are essentially untreatable) has led some to conclude that we are entering the "post-antibiotic era." Others have held to the perception that infectious diseases no longer represent as serious a concern to world health as they once did. The progress that science, medicine, and society as a whole have made in combating these maladies is impressive, and it is ironic that, as we stand on the threshold of an understanding of the most basic biology of the microbe, infectious diseases are posing renewed problems. We are threatened by the appearance of new diseases such as AIDS, SARS, hepatitis C, and Ebola virus infection and by the reemergence of old foes such as tuberculosis, cholera, plague, and *Streptococcus pyogenes* infection. True students of infectious diseases were perhaps less surprised than anyone else by these developments. Those who know pathogens are aware of their incredible adaptability and diversity. As ingenious and successful as therapeutic approaches may be, our ability to develop methods to counter infectious agents so far has not matched the myriad strategies employed by the sea of microbes that surrounds us. Their sheer numbers and the rate at which they can evolve are daunting. Moreover, environmental changes, rapid global travel, population movements, and medicine itself—through its use of antibiotics and immunosuppressive agents—all increase the impact of infectious diseases. Although new vaccines, new antibiotics, improved global communication, and new modalities for treating and preventing infection will be developed, pathogenic microbes will continue to develop new strategies of their own, presenting us with an unending and dynamic challenge.

FURTHER READING

ARMSTRONG G et al: Trends in infectious disease mortality in the United States during the 20th century. JAMA 281:61, 1999

BARTLETT JG: Update in infectious diseases. Ann Intern Med 133:285, 2000

BERKELMAN RL, HUGHES JM: The conquest of infectious diseases: Who are we kidding? Ann Intern Med 119:426, 1993

BUCKLEY RH: Immunodeficiency diseases. JAMA 268:2797, 1992

DE JONG R et al: Severe mycobacterial and *Salmonella* infections in interleukin-12 receptor–deficient patients. Science 280:1435, 1998

GOLD HS, EISENSTEIN BI: Introduction to bacterial diseases, in *Principles and Practice of Infectious Diseases*, 5th ed, GL Mandell et al (eds). New York, Churchill Livingstone, 2000, p 2065

HENDERSON DA: Bioterrorism as a public health threat. Emerg Infect Dis 4: 488, 1998

HOFFMAN J et al: Phylogenetic perspectives in innate immunity. Science 284: 1313, 1999

PROMED-MAIL: The Program for Monitoring Emerging Diseases. http://www.promedmail.org

PUCK JM: Primary immunodeficiency diseases. JAMA 278:1835, 1997

TYLER KL, NATHANSON N: Pathogenesis of viral infections, in *Fields Virology*, DM Knipe, PM Howley (eds). Philadelphia, Lippincott Williams & Wilkins, 2001, pp 199–244

WEISS ST: Eat dirt—the hygiene hypothesis and allergic diseases. N Engl J Med 347:930, 2002

Over the past three decades, molecular studies of the pathogenesis of microorganisms have yielded an explosion of information about the various microbial and host molecules that contribute to the processes of infection and disease. These processes can be classified into several stages: microbial encounter with and entry into the host; microbial growth after entry; avoidance of innate host defenses; tissue invasion and tropism; tissue damage; and transmission to new hosts. *Virulence* is the measure of an organism's capacity to cause disease and is a function of the pathogenic factors elaborated by microbes. These factors promote *colonization* (the simple presence of potentially pathogenic microbes in or on a host), *infection* (attachment and growth of pathogens and avoidance of host defenses), and *disease* (often, but not always, the result of activities of secreted toxins or toxic metabolites). In addition, the host's inflammatory response to infection greatly contributes to disease and its attendant clinical signs and symptoms.

MICROBIAL ENTRY AND ADHERENCE

ENTRY SITES A microbial pathogen can potentially enter any part of a host organism. In general, the type of disease produced by a particular microbe is often a direct consequence of its route of entry into the body. The most common sites of entry are mucosal surfaces (the respiratory, alimentary, and urogenital tracts) and the skin. Ingestion, inhalation, and sexual contact are typical routes of microbial entry. Other portals of entry include sites of skin injury (cuts, bites, burns, trauma) along with injection via natural (i.e., vector-borne) or artificial (i.e., needle-stick injury) routes. A few pathogens, such as *Schistosoma* spp., can penetrate unbroken skin. The conjunctiva can serve as an entry point for pathogens of the eye.

Microbial entry usually relies on the presence of specific microbial factors needed for persistence and growth in a tissue. Fecal-oral spread via the alimentary tract requires a biology consistent with survival in the varied environments of the gastrointestinal tract (including the low pH of the stomach and the high bile content of the intestine) as well as in contaminated food or water outside the host. Organisms that gain entry via the respiratory tract survive well in small moist droplets produced during sneezing and coughing. Pathogens that enter by venereal routes often survive best on the warm moist environment of the urogenital mucosa and have restricted host ranges (e.g., *Neisseria gonorrhoeae*, *Treponema pallidum*, and HIV).

The biology of microbes entering through the skin is highly varied. Some of these organisms can survive in a broad range of environments, such as the salivary glands or alimentary tracts of arthropod vectors, the mouths of larger animals, soil, and water. A complex biology allows protozoan parasites such as *Plasmodium*, *Leishmania*, and *Trypanosoma* spp. to undergo morphogenic changes that permit transmission of the organism to mammalian hosts during insect feeding for blood meals. Plasmodia are injected as infective sporozoites from the salivary glands during mosquito feeding. *Leishmania* parasites are regurgitated as promastigotes from the alimentary tract of sandflies and injected by bite into a susceptible host. Trypanosomes are first ingested from infected hosts by reduviid bugs; the pathogens then multiply in the gastrointestinal tract of the insects and are released in feces onto the host's skin during subsequent feedings. Most microbes that land directly on intact skin are destined to die, as survival on the skin or in hair follicles requires resistance to fatty acids, low pH, and other antimicrobial factors on skin. Once it is damaged (and particularly if it becomes necrotic), the skin can be a major portal of entry and growth for pathogens or their toxic products. Tetanus and burn wound infections are clear examples. After animal bites, pathogens resident in the animal's saliva gain access to the victim's tissues through the skin. Rabies is the paradigm for this pathogenic process; rabies virus grows in striated muscle cells at the site of inoculation.

MICROBIAL ADHERENCE Once in or on a host, most microbes must anchor themselves to a tissue or tissue factor; the possible exceptions are organisms that directly enter the bloodstream and multiply there. Specific ligands or adhesins for host receptors constitute a major area of study in the field of microbial pathogenesis. Adhesins comprise a wide range of surface structures, not only anchoring the microbe to a tissue and promoting cellular entry where appropriate but also eliciting host responses critical to the pathogenic process (Table 105-1). Most microbes produce multiple adhesins specific for multiple host receptors. These adhesins are often redundant, are serologically variable, and act additively or synergistically with other microbial factors to promote microbial sticking to host tissues. In addition, some microbes adsorb host proteins onto their surface and utilize the natural host protein receptor for microbial binding and entry into target cells.

TABLE 105-1 *Examples of Microbial Ligand-Receptor Interactions*

Microorganism	Type of Microbial Ligand	Host Receptor
VIRAL PATHOGENS		
Influenza virus	Hemagglutinin	Sialic acid
Measles virus		
Vaccine strain	Hemagglutinin	CD46/moesin
Wild-type strains	Hemagglutinin	Signaling lymphocytic activation molecule (SLAM)
Human herpesvirus type 6	?	CD46
Herpes simplex virus	Glycoprotein C	Heparin sulfate
HIV	Surface glycoprotein	CD4 and chemokine receptors (CCR5 and CXCR4)
Epstein-Barr virus	Envelope protein	CD21 (=CR2)
Adenovirus	Fiber protein	Coxsackie-adenovirus receptor (CAR)
Coxsackievirus	Fiber protein	CAR and major histocompatibility class I antigens
BACTERIAL PATHOGENS		
Neisseria species	Pili	Membrane cofactor protein (CD46)
Pseudomonas aeruginosa	Pili and flagella	Asialo-GM1
	Lipopolysaccharide	Cystic fibrosis transmembrane conductance regulator (CFTR)
Escherichia coli	Pili	Ceramides/mannose and digalactosyl residues
Yersinia spp.	Invasin/accessory invasin locus	β_1 Integrins
Bordetella pertussis	Filamentous hemagglutinin	CR3
Legionella pneumophila	Adsorbed C3bi	CR3
Mycobacterium tuberculosis	Adsorbed C3bi	CR3
FUNGAL PATHOGENS		
Blastomyces dermatitidis	WI-1	Possibly matrix proteins and integrins
Candida albicans	Int1p	Extracellular matrix proteins
PROTOZOAL PATHOGENS		
Plasmodium vivax	Merozoite form	Duffy Fy antigen
Plasmodium falciparum	EBA-175	Glycophorin A
Entamoeba histolytica	Surface lectin	*N*-Acetylglucosamine

Viral Adhesins All viral pathogens must bind to host cells, enter them, and replicate within them. Viral coat proteins serve as the ligands for cellular entry, and more than one ligand-receptor interaction may be needed; for example, HIV utilizes its envelope glycoprotein (gp) 120 to enter host cells by binding to both CD4 and one of two receptors for chemokines (designated CCR5 and CXCR4). Similarly, the measles virus H glycoprotein binds to both CD46 and the membrane-organizing protein moesin on host cells. The gC protein on herpes simplex virus binds to heparin sulfate; this step is followed by attachment to mammalian cells mediated by the viral gD (and possibly gH) protein. CD46 has now been shown to be the cellular receptor for human herpesvirus type 6.

Bacterial Adhesins Among the microbial adhesins studied in greatest detail are bacterial pili and flagella (Fig. 105-1). *Pili* or *fimbriae* are commonly used by gram-negative bacteria for attachment to host cells and tissues. In electron micrographs, these hairlike projections (up to several hundred per cell) may be confined to one end of the organism (polar pili) or distributed more evenly over the surface. An individual cell may have pili with a variety of functions. Most pili are made up of a major pilin protein subunit (molecular weight, 17,000 to 30,000) that polymerizes to form the pilus. Many strains of *Escherichia coli* express mannose-binding type 1 pili, whose binding to host tissues is inhibited by D-mannose. Other strains produce the Pap (pyelonephritis-associated) or P pilus adhesin that mediates binding to digalactose (gal-gal) residues on globosides of the human P blood groups. These pili have proteins located at the tips of the main pilus unit that are critical to the binding specificity of the whole pilus unit. Immunization with the mannose-binding FimH tip protein of type 1 pili prevents experimental *E. coli* bladder infections in mice and monkeys. *E. coli* cells causing diarrheal disease express pilus-like receptors for enterocytes on the small bowel, along with other receptors termed *colonization factors*.

A common type of pilus found in *Neisseria* spp., *Moraxella* spp., *Vibrio cholerae*, and *Pseudomonas aeruginosa* mediates adherence of these organisms to target surfaces. These pili tend to have a relatively conserved amino-terminal region and a more variable carboxyl-terminal region. For some species such as *N. gonorrhoeae* and *Neisseria meningitidis*, the pili are critical for attachment to mucosal epithelial cells. For others, such as *P. aeruginosa*, the pili only partially mediate the cells' adherence to host tissues. *V. cholerae* cells appear to use two different types of pili for intestinal colonization. Whereas interference with this stage of colonization would appear to be an effective antibacterial strategy, attempts to develop pilus-based vaccines for human diseases have not been highly successful to date.

Flagella are long appendages attached at either one or both ends of the bacterial cell (polar flagella) or distributed over the entire cell surface (peritrichous flagella). Flagella, like pili, are composed of a polymerized or aggregated basic protein. In flagella, the protein subunits form a tight helical structure and vary serologically with the species. Spirochetes such as *T. pallidum* and *Borrelia burgdorferi* have axial filaments similar to flagella running down the long axis of the center of the cell, and they "swim" by rotation around these filaments. Some bacteria can glide over a surface in the absence of obvious motility structures.

Other bacterial structures involved in adherence to host tissues include specific staphylococcal and streptococcal proteins that bind to human extracellular matrix proteins such as fibrin, fibronectin, laminin, and collagen. Fibronectin appears to be a commonly used receptor for various pathogens; a particular amino acid sequence in fibronectin, Arg-Gly-Asp or RGD, is critical for bacterial binding. The surface lipopolysaccharide (LPS) of *P. aeruginosa* mediates binding to the cystic fibrosis transmembrane conductance regulator (CFTR) on airway epithelial cells. Coagulase-negative staphylococci and *Staphylococcus aureus* readily colonize prosthetic devices and catheters commonly used in medical care; a surface polysaccharide composed of poly-N-acetyl glucosamine elaborated by these organisms promotes binding to the prosthetic material. High-powered imaging techniques such as atomic force microscopy have revealed that bacterial cells have a nonhomogeneous surface that is likely attributable to different concentrations of cell surface molecules, including microbial adhesins, at specific places on the cell surface (Fig. 105-1D).

Fungal Adhesins Several fungal adhesins have been described that mediate colonization of epithelial surfaces, particularly adherence to structures like fibronectin, laminin, and collagen. The product of the *Candida albicans INT1* gene, Int1p, bears similarity to mammalian integrins that bind to extracellular matrix proteins. Transformation of normally nonadherent *Saccharomyces cerevisiae* with this gene allows these yeast cells to adhere to human epithelial cells. Disruption of *INT1* in *C. albicans* diminishes but does not eliminate epithelial cell adhesion; this result indicates that other adhesins participate in binding of *C. albicans* to epithelial cells. Moreover, Int1p is needed for filamentous growth of *C. albicans*—a phenotype linked to virulence, and particularly to the ability to penetrate keratinized epithelium. *INT1*-deficient *C. albicans* exhibits markedly reduced virulence in a mouse model of infection.

For several fungal pathogens that initiate infections after inhalation of infectious material, the inoculum is ingested by alveolar macrophages, in which the fungal cells transform to pathogenic phenotypes. Like *C. albicans*, *Blastomyces dermatitidis* binds to CD11b/CD18 integrins as well as to CD14 on macrophages. *B. dermatitidis* produces a 120-kDa surface protein, designated WI-1, that mediates this adherence. The binding domain of WI-1 is homologous to the invasin protein of *Yersinia* that binds to the same type of host cell receptor. An unidentified factor on *Histoplasma capsulatum* also mediates binding of this fungal pathogen to the integrin surface proteins.

Eukaryotic Pathogen Adhesins Eukaryotic parasites use complicated surface glycoproteins as adhesins, some of which are lectins (proteins that

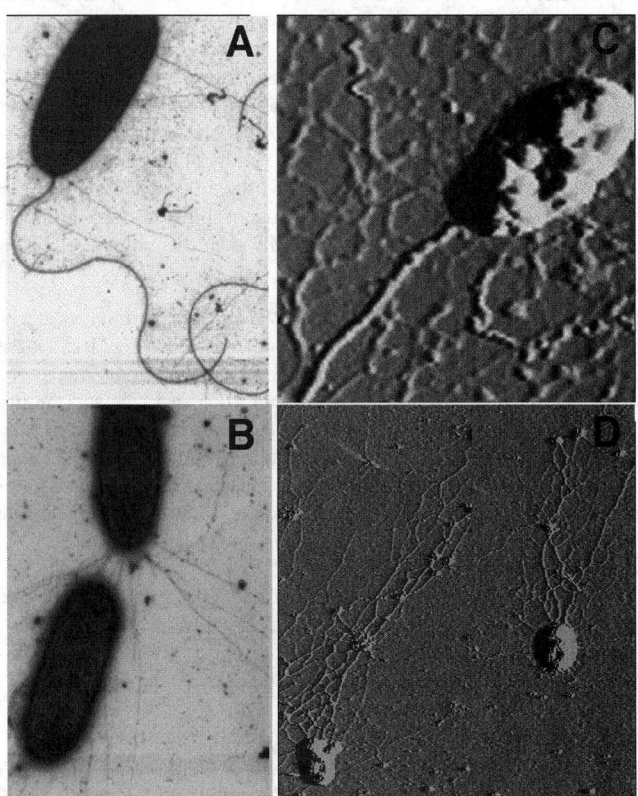

FIGURE 105-1 Bacterial surface structures. *A and B.* Traditional electron micrographic images of fixed cells of *Pseudomonas aeruginosa*. Flagella (*A*) and pili (*B*) projecting out from the bacterial poles can be seen. *C and D.* Atomic force microscopic image of live *P. aeruginosa* freshly planted onto a smooth mica surface. This new technology reveals the fine, three-dimensional detail of the bacterial surface structures. *(Images courtesy of Dr. Martin Lee and Mr. Milan Bajmociz, Harvard Medical School.)*

bind to specific carbohydrates on host cells). For example, *Plasmodium vivax*, one of four *Plasmodium* species causing malaria, binds (via Duffy-binding protein) to the Duffy blood group carbohydrate antigen Fy on erythrocytes. *Entamoeba histolytica*, the third leading cause of death from parasitic diseases, expresses two proteins that bind to the disaccharide galactose/N-acetyl galactosamine. Reports indicate that children with mucosal IgA antibody to one of these lectins are resistant to reinfection with virulent *E. histolytica*. A major surface glycoprotein (gp63) of *Leishmania* promastigotes is needed for these parasites to enter human macrophages—the principal target cell of infection. This glycoprotein promotes complement binding but inhibits complement lytic activity, allowing the parasite to use complement receptors for entry into macrophages; gp63 also binds to fibronectin receptors on macrophages. In addition, the pathogen can express a carbohydrate that mediates binding to host cells. Evidence suggests that, as part of hepatic granuloma formation, *Schistosoma mansoni* expresses a carbohydrate epitope related to the Lewis X blood group antigen that promotes adherence of helminthic eggs to vascular endothelial cells under inflammatory conditions.

HOST RECEPTORS   Host receptors are found both on target cells (such as epithelial cells lining mucosal surfaces) and within the mucus layer covering these cells. Microbial pathogens bind to a wide range of host receptors to establish infection (Table 105-1). Selective loss of host receptors for a pathogen may confer natural resistance to an otherwise susceptible population. For example, 70% of individuals in West Africa lack Fy antigens and are resistant to *P. vivax* infection. *Salmonella typhi*, the etiologic agent of typhoid fever, uses CFTR to enter the gastrointestinal submucosa after being ingested. As homozygous mutations in *CFTR* are the cause of the life-shortening disease cystic fibrosis, heterozygote carriers (e.g., 4 to 5% of individuals of European ancestry) may have had a selective advantage due to decreased susceptibility to *S. typhi* infection.

Numerous virus–target cell interactions have been described, and it is now clear that different viruses can use similar host cell receptors for entry. The list of certain and likely host receptors for viral pathogens is long. Among the host membrane components that can serve as receptors for viruses are sialic acids, gangliosides, glycosaminoglycans, integrins and other members of the immunoglobulin superfamily, histocompatibility antigens, and regulators and receptors for complement components.

MICROBIAL GROWTH AFTER ENTRY

Once established on a mucosal or skin site, pathogenic microbes must replicate before causing full-blown infection and disease. Within cells, viral particles release their nucleic acids, which may be directly translated into viral proteins (positive-strand RNA viruses), transcribed from a negative strand of RNA into a complementary mRNA (negative-strand RNA viruses), or transcribed into a complementary strand of DNA (retroviruses); for DNA viruses, mRNA may be transcribed directly from viral DNA, either in the cell nucleus or in the cytoplasm. To grow, bacteria must acquire specific nutrients or synthesize them from precursors in host tissues. Many infectious processes are usually confined to specific epithelial surfaces—influenza to the respiratory mucosa, gonorrhea to the urogenital epithelium, shigellosis to the gastrointestinal epithelium. While there are multiple reasons for this specificity, one important consideration is the ability of these pathogens to obtain from these specific environments the nutrients needed for growth and survival.

Temperature restrictions also play a role in limiting certain pathogens to specific tissues. Rhinoviruses, a cause of the common cold, grow best at 33°C and replicate in cooler nasal tissues but not in the lung. Leprosy lesions due to *Mycobacterium leprae* are found in and on relatively cool body sites. Fungal pathogens that infect the skin, hair follicles, and nails (dermatophyte infections) remain confined to the cooler, exterior, keratinous layer of the epithelium.

A topic of major interest is the ability of many bacterial, fungal, and protozoal species to grow in multicellular masses referred to as *biofilms*. These masses are biochemically and morphologically quite distinct from the free-living individual cells referred to as *planktonic cells*. Growth in biofilms leads to altered microbial metabolism, production of extracellular virulence factors, and decreased susceptibility to biocides, antimicrobial agents, and host defense molecules and cells. *P. aeruginosa* growing on the bronchial mucosa during chronic infection, staphylococci and other pathogens growing on implanted medical devices, and dental pathogens growing on tooth surfaces to form plaques represent several examples of microbial biofilm growth associated with human disease. Many other pathogens can form biofilms during in vitro growth, but the data are insufficient to determine whether this property is related to microbial virulence and induction of disease.

AVOIDANCE OF INNATE HOST DEFENSES

As microbes have probably interacted with mucosal/epithelial surfaces since the emergence of multicellular organisms, it is not surprising that multicellular hosts have a variety of innate surface defense mechanisms that can sense when pathogens are present and contribute to their elimination. The skin is acidic and is bathed with fatty acids toxic to many microbes. Successful skin pathogens such as staphylococci must tolerate these adverse conditions. Mucosal surfaces are covered by a barrier composed of a thick mucus layer that entraps microbes and facilitates their transport out of the body by such processes as mucociliary clearance, coughing, and urination. Mucous secretions, saliva, and tears contain antibacterial factors such as lysozyme and antimicrobial peptides as well as antiviral factors such as interferons. Gastric acidity is inimical to the survival of many ingested pathogens, and many mucosal surfaces—particularly the nasopharynx, the vaginal tract, and the gastrointestinal tract—contain a resident flora of commensal microbes that interfere with the ability of pathogens to colonize and infect a host.

Pathogens that survive these factors must still contend with host endocytic, phagocytic, and inflammatory responses as well as with host genetic factors that determine the degree to which a pathogen can survive and grow. The growth of viral pathogens entering skin or mucosal epithelial cells can be limited by a variety of host genetic factors, including production of interferons, modulation of receptors for viral entry, and age- and hormone-related susceptibility factors; by nutritional status; and even by personal habits such as smoking and exercise.

ENCOUNTERS WITH EPITHELIAL CELLS   Over the past decade, many bacterial pathogens have been shown to enter epithelial cells (Fig. 105-2); the bacteria often use specialized surface structures that bind to receptors, with consequent internalization. However, the exact role and the importance of this process in infection and disease are not well defined for most of these pathogens. Bacterial entry into host epithelial cells is seen as a means for dissemination to adjacent or deeper tissues or as a route to sanctuary to avoid ingestion and killing by professional phagocytes. Epithelial cell entry appears, for instance, to be a critical aspect of dysentery induction by *Shigella*.

Curiously, the less virulent strains of many bacterial pathogens are more adept at entering epithelial cells than are more virulent strains; examples include pathogens that lack the surface polysaccharide capsule needed to cause serious disease. Thus, for *Haemophilus influenzae*, *Streptococcus pneumoniae*, *Streptococcus agalactiae* (group B *Streptococcus*), and *Streptococcus pyogenes*, isogenic mutants or variants lacking capsules enter epithelial cells better than the wild-type, encapsulated parental forms that cause disseminated disease. These observations have led to the proposal that epithelial cell entry may be a manifestation of host defense, resulting in bacterial clearance by both shedding of epithelial cells containing internalized bacteria and initiation of a subclinical inflammatory response. However, a consequence of this process would be the opening of a hole in the epithelium, potentially allowing uningested organisms to enter the submucosa.

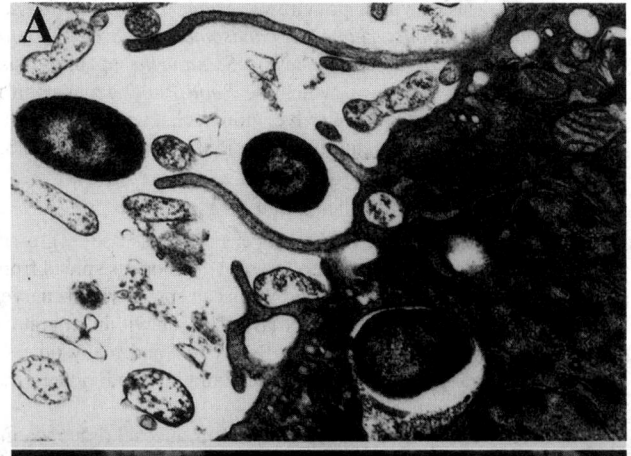

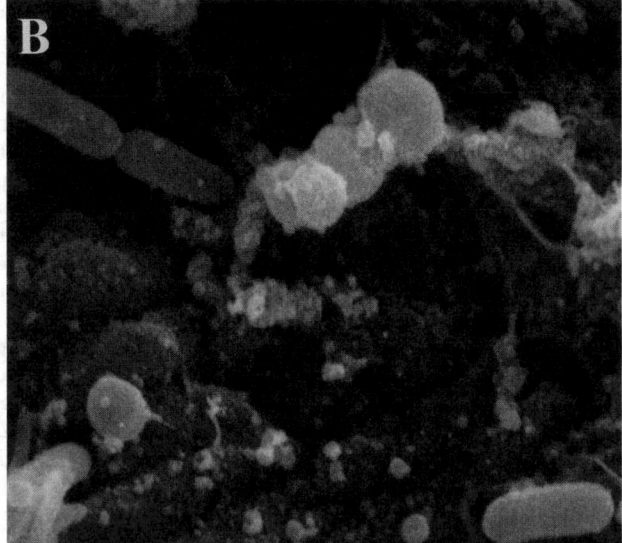

FIGURE 105-2   Entry of bacteria into epithelial cells. *A.* Internalization of *P. aeruginosa* by cultured airway epithelial cells expressing wild-type cystic fibrosis transmembrane conductance regulator (CFTR), the cell receptor for bacterial ingestion. *B.* Entry of *P. aeruginosa* into murine tracheal epithelial cells after murine infection by the intranasal route.

This scenario has been documented in murine *Salmonella typhimurium* infections and in experimental bladder infections with uropathogenic *E. coli*. In the latter system, bacterial pili mediate cell attachment to integral membrane glycoproteins called *uroplakins* that coat the host cells, resulting in exfoliation of the cells with attached bacteria. Subsequently, infection is produced by residual bacterial cells that invade the denuded epithelium. Perhaps at low bacterial inocula epithelial cell ingestion and subclinical inflammation are efficient means to eliminate pathogens, while at higher inocula a proportion of surviving bacterial cells enter the host tissue through the damaged mucosal surface and multiply, producing disease. Alternatively, failure of the appropriate epithelial cell response to a pathogen may allow the organism to survive on a mucosal surface where, if it avoids other host defenses, it can grow and cause a local infection. Along these lines, as noted above, *P. aeruginosa* is taken into epithelial cells by CFTR, a protein missing or nonfunctional in most severe cases of cystic fibrosis. The major clinical consequence of this disease is chronic airway-surface infection with *P. aeruginosa* in 80 to 90% of patients with cystic fibrosis. The failure of airway epithelial cells to ingest and promote the removal of *P. aeruginosa* has been proposed as a key component of the hypersusceptibility of these patients to chronic airway infection.

ENCOUNTERS WITH PHAGOCYTES ■ Phagocytosis and Inflammation   Phagocytosis of microbes is a major innate host defense that limits the growth and spread of pathogens. Phagocytes appear rapidly at sites of infection in conjunction with the initiation of inflammation. Ingestion

of microbes by both tissue-fixed macrophages and migrating phagocytes probably accounts for the limited ability of most microbial agents to cause disease. A family of related molecules called *collectins, soluble defense collagens,* or *pattern-recognition molecules* are found in blood (mannose-binding lectins), in lung (surfactant proteins A and D), and most likely in other tissues as well and bind to carbohydrates on microbial surfaces to promote phagocyte clearance. Bacterial pathogens seem to be ingested principally by polymorphonuclear neutrophils (PMNs), while eosinophils are frequently found at sites of infection by protozoan or multicellular parasites. Successful pathogens, by definition, must avoid being cleared by professional phagocytes. One of several antiphagocytic strategies employed by bacteria and by the fungal pathogen *Cryptococcus neoformans* is to elaborate large-molecular-weight surface polysaccharide antigens, often in the form of a capsule that coats the cell surface. Most pathogenic bacteria produce such antiphagocytic capsules.

As activation of local phagocytes in tissues is a key step in initiating inflammation and migration of additional phagocytes into infected sites, much attention has been paid to microbial factors that initiate inflammation. Encounters with phagocytes are governed largely by the structure of the microbial constituents that elicit inflammation, and detailed knowledge of these structures for bacterial pathogens has contributed greatly to our understanding of molecular mechanisms of microbial pathogenesis (Fig. 105-3). One of the best-studied systems involves the interaction of LPS from gram-negative bacteria and the glycosylphosphatidylinositol (GPI)-anchored membrane protein CD14 found on the surface of professional phagocytes, including migrating and tissue-fixed macrophages and PMNs. A soluble form of CD14 is also found in plasma and on mucosal surfaces. A plasma protein, LPS-binding protein (LBP), transfers LPS to membrane-bound CD14 on myeloid cells and promotes binding of LPS to soluble CD14. Soluble CD14/LPS/LBP complexes bind to many cell types and may be internalized to initiate cellular responses to microbial pathogens. It has been shown that peptidoglycan and lipoteichoic acid from gram-positive bacteria and cell-surface products of mycobacteria and spirochetes can interact with CD14 (Fig. 105-3).

GPI-anchored receptors do not have intracellular signaling domains, and mammalian Toll-like receptors (TLRs) transduce signals for cellular activation due to LPS binding. TLRs initiate cellular activation through a series of signal-transducing molecules (Fig. 105-3) that lead to nuclear translocation of the transcription factor NF-κB, a master-switch for production of important inflammatory cytokines such as tumor necrosis factor α (TNF-α) and interleukin (IL) 1.

The initiation of inflammation can occur not only with LPS and peptidoglycan but also with viral particles and other microbial products such as polysaccharides, enzymes, and toxins. Bacterial flagella activate inflammation by binding to TLR5. Bacteria also produce a high proportion of DNA molecules with unmethylated CpG residues that activate inflammation through TLR9. TLR3 recognizes double-stranded RNA, a pattern-recognition molecule produced by many viruses during their replicative cycle. TLR1 and TLR6 associate with TLR2 to promote recognition of acylated microbial proteins and peptides.

The myeloid differentiation factor 88 (MyD88) molecule is a generalized adaptor protein that binds to the cytoplasmic domains of all known TLRs and also to receptors that are part of the IL-1 receptor (IL-1Rc) family. Numerous studies have shown that MyD88-mediated transduction of signals from TLRs and IL-1Rc is critical for innate resistance to infection. Mice lacking MyD88 are more susceptible than normal mice to infection with group B *Streptococcus, Listeria monocytogenes,* and *Mycobacterium tuberculosis.*

Additional Interactions of Microbial Pathogens and Phagocytes   Other ways that microbial pathogens avoid destruction by phagocytes include production of factors that are toxic to the phagocytes or that interfere with the chemotactic and ingestion function of phagocytes. Hemolysins,

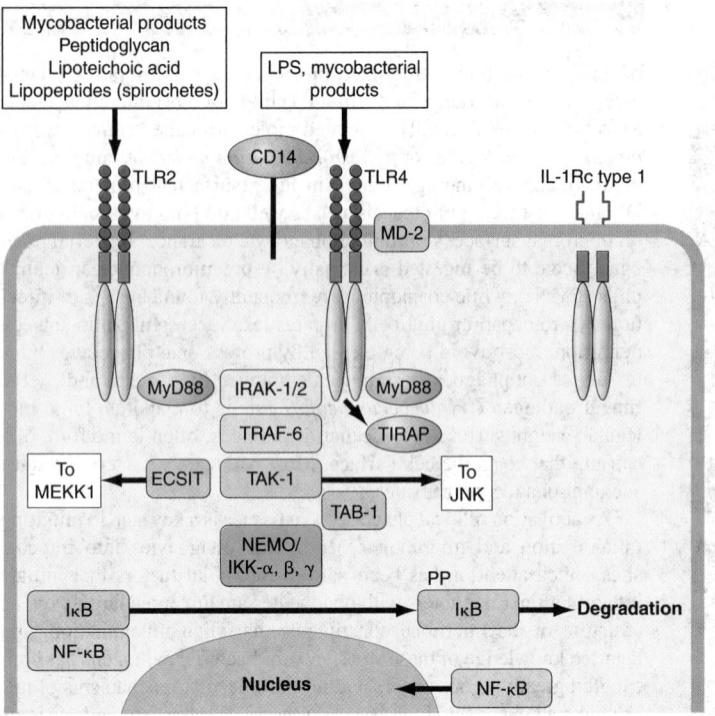

FIGURE 105-3 Cellular signaling pathways for production of inflammatory cytokines in response to microbial products. Various microbial cell-surface constituents interact with CD14, which in turn interacts in a currently unknown fashion with Toll-like receptors (TLRs). Some microbial factors do not need CD14 to interact with TLRs. Associating with TLR4 (and to some extent with TLR2) is MD-2, a cofactor that facilitates the response to lipopolysaccharide (LPS). Both CD14 and TLRs contain extracellular leucine-rich domains. The cytoplasmic domains of TLRs are oligomerized for binding to the general adaptor protein MyD88, which also binds to members of the interleukin-1 receptor (IL-1Rc) transmembrane proteins because of homology in the intracellular domain. TIRAP (TIR domain-containing adaptor protein) participates in the transduction of signals from TLR4. The receptor complex clusters or oligomerizes; oligomerization is followed by activation of signal-transducing molecules such as IRAK-1/2 (IL-1Rc-associated kinase 1 or 2), TRAF-6 (tumor necrosis factor receptor–associated factor 6), TAK-1 (transforming growth factor β–activating kinase 1), and TAB1 (TAK1-binding protein 1)/NIK (Nck-interacting kinase). In addition to activating other signaling pathways leading to cytokine production and stress responses, such as the c-Jun N-terminal kinase (JNK) pathway and MAP kinase kinase kinase (MEKK1) pathway [via evolutionarily conserved signaling intermediate in Toll pathways (ECSIT)], TLR-mediated signaling leads to activation of the inducible kinase complex, IKK-α, -β, and -γ. IKK-γ is also called NEMO [nuclear factor κB (NF-κB) essential modulator]. These are part of a larger complex that phosphorylates the inhibitory portion (I) of NF-κB, resulting in release of IκB from NF-κB. Phosphorylated (PP) IκB is then degraded, and NF-κB translocates to the nucleus, where it binds to transcriptional sites on target genes, many of which encode inflammatory proteins. *(Figure courtesy of Dr. Terry Means and Dr. Douglas Golenbock.)*

leukocidins, and the like are microbial proteins that can kill phagocytes that are attempting to ingest organisms elaborating these substances. For example, staphylococcal hemolysins inhibit macrophage chemotaxis and kill these phagocytes. Streptolysin O made by *S. pyogenes* binds to cholesterol in phagocyte membranes and initiates a process of internal degranulation, with the release of normally granule-sequestered toxic components into the phagocyte's cytoplasm. *Entamoeba histolytica*, an intestinal protozoan that causes amebic dysentery, can disrupt phagocyte membranes after direct contact via the release of protozoal phospholipase A and pore-forming peptides.

Microbial Survival Inside Phagocytes Many important microbial pathogens use a variety of strategies to survive inside phagocytes (particularly macrophages) after ingestion. Inhibition of fusion of the phagocytic vacuole (the phagosome) containing the ingested microbe with the lysosomal granules containing antimicrobial substances (the lysosome) allows *M. tuberculosis*, *S. typhi*, and *Toxoplasma gondii* to survive inside macrophages. Some organisms, such as *L. monocytogenes*, escape into the phagocyte's cytoplasm to grow and eventually spread to other cells. Resistance to killing within the macrophage and subsequent growth are critical to successful infection by herpes-type

viruses, measles virus, poxviruses, *Salmonella*, *Yersinia*, *Legionella*, *Mycobacterium*, *Trypanosoma*, *Nocardia*, *Histoplasma*, *Toxoplasma*, and *Rickettsia*. *Salmonella* spp. use a master regulatory system, in which the *PhoP/PhoQ* genes control other genes, to enter and survive within cells, with intracellular survival entailing structural changes in the cell envelope LPS.

TISSUE INVASION AND TISSUE TROPISM

TISSUE INVASION Most viral pathogens cause disease by growth at skin or mucosal entry sites, but some pathogens spread from the initial site to deeper tissues. Virus can spread via the nerves (rabies virus) or plasma (picornaviruses) or within migratory blood cells (poliovirus, Epstein-Barr virus, and many others). Specific viral genes determine where and how individual viral strains can spread.

Bacteria may invade deeper layers of mucosal tissue via intracellular uptake by epithelial cells, traversal of epithelial cell junctions, or penetration through denuded epithelial surfaces. Among virulent *Shigella* strains and invasive *E. coli*, outer-membrane proteins are critical to epithelial cell invasion and bacterial multiplication. *Neisseria* and *Haemophilus* spp. penetrate mucosal cells by poorly understood mechanisms before dissemination into the bloodstream. Staphylococci and streptococci elaborate a variety of extracellular enzymes, such as hyaluronidase, lipases, nucleases, and hemolysins, that are probably important in breaking down cellular and matrix structures and allowing the bacteria access to deeper tissues and blood. Organisms that colonize the gastrointestinal tract can often translocate through the mucosa into the blood and, under circumstances in which host defenses are inadequate, cause bacteremia. *Yersinia enterocolitica* can invade the mucosa through the activity of the invasin protein. Some bacteria (e.g., *Brucella*) can be carried from a mucosal site to a distant site by phagocytic cells (e.g., PMNs) that ingest but fail to kill the bacteria.

Fungal pathogens almost always take advantage of host immunocompromise to spread hematogenously to deeper tissues. The AIDS epidemic has resoundingly illustrated this principle: the immunodeficiency of many HIV-infected patients permits the development of life-threatening fungal infections of the lung, blood, and brain. Other than the capsule of *C. neoformans*, specific fungal antigens involved in tissue invasion are not well characterized. Both fungal pathogens and protozoal pathogens (e.g., *Plasmodium* spp. and *E. histolytica*) undergo morphologic changes to spread within a host. Malarial parasites grow in liver cells as merozoites and are released into the blood to invade erythrocytes and become trophozoites. *E. histolytica* is found as both a cyst and a trophozoite in the intestinal lumen, through which this pathogen enters the host, but only the trophozoite form can spread systemically to cause amebic liver abscesses. Other protozoal pathogens, such as *T. gondii*, *Giardia lamblia*, and *Cryptosporidium*, also undergo extensive morphologic changes after initial infection to spread to other tissues.

TISSUE TROPISM The propensity of certain microbes to cause disease by infecting specific tissues has been known since the early days of bacteriology, yet the molecular basis for this propensity is understood somewhat better for viral pathogens than for other agents of infectious disease. Specific receptor-ligand interactions clearly underlie the ability of certain viruses to enter cells within tissues and disrupt normal tissue function, but the mere presence of a receptor for a virus on a target tissue is not sufficient for tissue tropism. Factors in the cell, route of viral entry, viral capacity to penetrate into cells, viral genetic elements that regulate gene expression, and pathways of viral spread in a tissue all affect tissue tropism. Some viral genes are best transcribed in specific target cells, such as hepatitis B genes in liver cells and Epstein-Barr virus genes in B lymphocytes. The route of inoculation of poliovirus determines its neurotropism, although the molecular basis for this circumstance is not understood.

The lesser understanding of the tissue tropism of bacterial and parasitic infections is exemplified by *Neisseria* spp. There is no well-accepted explanation of why *N. gonorrhoeae* colonizes and infects the human genital tract while the closely related species *N. meningitidis* principally colonizes the human oropharynx. *N. meningitidis* expresses a capsular polysaccharide, while *N. gonorrhoeae* does not; however, there is no indication that this property plays a role in the different tissue tropisms displayed by these two bacterial species. *N. gonorrhoeae* can use cytidine monophosphate *N*-acetylneuraminic acid from host tissues to add *N*-acetylneuraminic acid (sialic acid) to its lipooligosaccharide (LOS) O side chain, and this alteration appears to make the organism resistant to host defenses. Lactate, present at high levels on genital mucosal surfaces, stimulates sialylation of gonococcal LOS. Bacteria with sialic acid sugars in their capsules, such as *N. meningitidis*, *E. coli* K1, and group B streptococci, have a propensity to cause meningitis, but this generalization has many exceptions. For example, all recognized serotypes of group B streptococci contain sialic acid in their capsules, but only one serotype (III) is responsible for most cases of group B streptococcal meningitis. Moreover, both *H. influenzae* and *S. pneumoniae* can readily cause meningitis, but these organisms do not have sialic acid in their capsules.

TISSUE DAMAGE AND DISEASE

Disease is a complex phenomenon resulting from tissue invasion and destruction, toxin elaboration, and host response. Viruses cause much of their damage by exerting a cytopathic effect on host cells and inhibiting host defenses. The growth of bacterial, fungal, and protozoal parasites in tissue, which may or may not be accompanied by toxin elaboration, can also compromise tissue function and lead to disease. For some bacterial and possibly some fungal pathogens, toxin production is one of the best-characterized molecular mechanisms of pathogenesis, while host factors such as IL-1, TNF-α, kinins, inflammatory proteins, products of complement activation, and mediators derived from arachidonic acid metabolites (leukotrienes) and cellular degranulation (histamines) readily contribute to the severity of disease.

VIRAL DISEASE Viral pathogens are well known to inhibit host immune responses by a variety of mechanisms. Immune responses can be affected by downregulating production of most major histocompatibility complex (MHC) molecules (adenovirus E3 protein), by diminishing cytotoxic T-cell recognition of virus-infected cells (Epstein-Barr virus EBNA1 antigen and cytomegalovirus IE protein), by producing virus-encoded complement receptor proteins that protect infected cells from complement-mediated lysis (herpesvirus and vaccinia virus), by making proteins that interfere with the action of interferon (influenza virus and poxvirus), and by elaborating superantigen-like proteins (mouse mammary tumor virus and related retroviruses, rabies nucleocapsid, and possibly the Nef protein of HIV). Superantigens activate large populations of T cells that express particular subsets of the T cell receptor β protein, causing massive cytokine release and subsequent host reactions. Another molecular mechanism of viral virulence involves the production of peptide growth factors for host cells, which disrupt normal cellular growth, proliferation, and differentiation. In addition, viral factors can bind to and interfere with the function of host receptors for signaling molecules. Modulation of cytokine production during viral infection can stimulate viral growth inside cells with receptors for the cytokine, and virus-encoded cytokine homologues (e.g., the Epstein-Barr virus BCRF1 protein, which is highly homologous to the immunoinhibitory IL-10 molecule) can potentially prevent immune-mediated clearance of viral particles. Viruses can cause disease in neural cells by interfering with levels of neurotransmitters without necessarily destroying the cells, or they may induce either programmed cell death (apoptosis) to destroy tissues or inhibitors of apoptosis to allow for prolonged viral infection of cells. Overall, any disruption of normal cellular and tissue function due to viral infection can underlie the resultant clinical disease.

BACTERIAL TOXINS Among the first infectious diseases to be understood were those due to toxin-elaborating bacteria. Diphtheria, botulism, and tetanus toxins are responsible for the diseases associated with local infections due to *Corynebacterium diphtheriae*, *Clostridium botulinum*, and *Clostridium tetani*, respectively. Enterotoxins produced by *E. coli*, *Salmonella*, *Shigella*, *Staphylococcus*, and *V. cholerae* contribute to diarrheal disease caused by these organisms. Staphylococci, streptococci, *P. aeruginosa*, and *Bordetella* elaborate various toxins that cause or contribute to disease, including toxic shock syndrome toxin 1 (TSST-1); erythrogenic toxin; exotoxins A, S, and U; and pertussis toxin. A number of these toxins (e.g., cholera toxin, diphtheria toxin, pertussis toxin, *E. coli* heat-labile toxin, and *P. aeruginosa* exotoxin) have adenosine diphosphate (ADP)-ribosyltransferase activity; i.e., the toxins enzymatically catalyze the transfer of the ADP-ribosyl portion of nicotinamide adenine dinucleotide to target proteins and inactivate them. The staphylococcal enterotoxins, TSST-1, and the streptococcal pyogenic exotoxins behave as superantigens, stimulating certain T cells to proliferate without processing of the protein toxin by antigen-presenting cells. Part of this process involves stimulation of the antigen-presenting cells to produce IL-1 and TNF-α, which have been implicated in many of the clinical features of diseases like toxic shock syndrome and scarlet fever. A number of gram-negative pathogens (*Salmonella*, *Yersinia*, and *P. aeruginosa*) can inject toxins directly into host target cells by means of a complex set of proteins referred to as the type III secretion system. Loss or inactivation of this virulence system usually greatly reduces the capacity of a bacterial pathogen to cause disease.

ENDOTOXIN The lipid A portion of gram-negative LPS has potent biologic activities that cause many of the clinical manifestations of gram-negative bacterial sepsis, including fever, muscle proteolysis, uncontrolled intravascular coagulation, and shock. The effects of lipid A appear to be mediated by the production of potent cytokines due to LPS binding to CD14 and signal transduction via TLRs, particularly TLR4. Cytokines exhibit potent hypothermic activity through effects on the hypothalamus; they also increase vascular permeability, alter the activity of endothelial cells, and induce endothelial-cell procoagulant activity. Numerous therapeutic strategies aimed at neutralizing the effects of endotoxin are under investigation, but so far the results have been disappointing.

INVASION Many diseases are caused primarily by pathogens growing in tissue sites that are normally sterile. Pneumococcal pneumonia is mostly attributable to the growth of *S. pneumoniae* in the lung and the attendant host inflammatory response, although specific factors that enhance this process (e.g., pneumolysin) may be responsible for some of the pathogenic potential of the pneumococcus. Disease that follows bacteremia and invasion of the meninges by meningitis-producing bacteria such as *N. meningitidis*, *H. influenzae*, *E. coli* K1, and group B streptococci appears to be due solely to the ability of these organisms to gain access to these tissues, multiply in them, and provoke cytokine production leading to tissue-damaging host inflammation.

Specific molecular mechanisms accounting for tissue invasion by fungal and protozoal pathogens are less well described. Except for studies pointing to factors like capsule and melanin production by *C. neoformans* and possibly levels of cell wall glucans in some pathogenic fungi, the molecular basis for fungal invasiveness is not well defined. Melanism has been shown to protect the fungal cell against death caused by phagocyte factors such as nitric oxide, superoxide, and hypochlorite. Morphogenic variation and production of proteases (e.g., the *Candida* aspartyl proteinase) have been implicated in fungal invasion of host tissues.

If pathogens are effectively to invade host tissues (particularly the blood), they must avoid the major host defenses represented by complement and phagocytic cells. Bacteria most often avoid these defenses through their cell surface polysaccharides—either capsular polysaccharides or long O-side-chain antigens characteristic of the smooth LPS of gram-negative bacteria. These molecules can prevent the activation and/or deposition of complement opsonins or limit the access of phagocytic cells with receptors for complement opsonins to these molecules when they are deposited on the bacterial surface below the capsular layer. Another potential mechanism of microbial virulence is the ability of some organisms to present the capsule as an apparent self antigen through molecular mimicry. For example, the polysialic acid capsule of group B *N. meningitidis* is chemically identical to an oligosaccharide found on human brain cells.

Immunochemical studies of capsular polysaccharides have led to an appreciation of the tremendous chemical diversity that can result from the linking of a few monosaccharides. For example, three hexoses can link up in more than 300 different, potentially serologically distinct ways, while three amino acids have only six possible peptide combinations. Capsular polysaccharides have been used as effective vaccines against meningococcal meningitis as well as against pneumococcal and *H. influenzae* infections and may prove to be of value as vaccines against any organisms that express a nontoxic, immunogenic capsular polysaccharide. In addition, most encapsulated pathogens become virtually avirulent when capsule production is interrupted by genetic manipulation; this observation emphasizes the importance of this structure in pathogenesis.

HOST RESPONSE   The inflammatory response of the host is critical for interruption and resolution of the infectious process but also is often responsible for the signs and symptoms of disease. Infection promotes a complex series of host responses involving the complement, kinin, and coagulation pathways. The production of cytokines such as IL-1, TNF-α, and other factors regulated in part by the NF-κB transcription factor leads to fever, muscle proteolysis, and other effects, as noted above. An inability to kill or contain the microbe usually results in further damage due to the progression of inflammation and infection. For example, in many chronic infections, degranulation of host inflammatory cells can lead to release of host proteases, elastases, histamines, and other toxic substances that can degrade host tissues. Chronic inflammation in any tissue can lead to the destruction of that tissue and to clinical disease associated with loss of organ function, such as sterility from pelvic inflammatory disease caused by chronic infection with *N. gonorrhoeae*.

The nature of the host response elicited by the pathogen often determines the pathology of a particular infection. Local inflammation produces local tissue damage, while systemic inflammation, such as that seen during sepsis, can result in the signs and symptoms of septic shock. The severity of septic shock is associated with the degree of production of host effectors. Disease due to intracellular parasitism results from the formation of granulomas, wherein the host attempts to wall off the parasite inside a fibrotic lesion surrounded by fused epithelial cells that make up so-called multinucleated giant cells. A number of pathogens, particularly anaerobic bacteria, staphylococci, and streptococci, provoke the formation of an abscess, probably because of the presence of zwitterionic surface polysaccharides such as the capsular polysaccharide of *Bacteroides fragilis*. The outcome of an infection depends on the balance between an effective host response that eliminates a pathogen and an excessive inflammatory response that is associated with an inability to eliminate a pathogen and with the resultant tissue damage that leads to disease.

TRANSMISSION TO NEW HOSTS

As part of the pathogenic process, most microbes are shed from the host, often in a form infectious for susceptible individuals. However, the rate of transmissibility may not necessarily be high, even if the disease is severe in the infected individual, as these traits are not linked. Most pathogens exit via the same route by which they entered: respiratory pathogens by aerosols from sneezing or coughing or through salivary spread, gastrointestinal pathogens by fecal-oral spread, sexually transmitted diseases by venereal spread, and vector-borne organisms by either direct contact with the vector through a blood meal or indirect contact with organisms shed into environmental sources such as water. Microbial factors that specifically promote transmission are not well characterized. Respiratory shedding is facilitated by overproduction of mucous secretions, with consequently enhanced sneezing and coughing. Diarrheal toxins such as cholera toxin, *E. coli* heat-labile toxins, and *Shigella* toxins probably facilitate fecal-oral spread of microbial cells in the high volumes of diarrheal fluid produced during infection. The ability to produce phenotypic variants that resist hostile environmental factors (e.g., the highly resistant cysts of *E. histolytica* shed in feces) represents another mechanism of pathogenesis relevant to transmission. Blood parasites such as *Plasmodium* spp. change phenotype after ingestion by a mosquito—a prerequisite for the continued transmission of this pathogen. Venereally transmitted pathogens may undergo phenotypic variation due to the production of specific factors to facilitate transmission, but shedding of these pathogens into the environment does not result in the formation of infectious foci.

In summary, the molecular mechanisms used by pathogens to colonize, invade, infect, and disrupt the host are numerous and diverse. Each phase of the infectious process involves a variety of microbial and host factors interacting in a manner that can result in disease. Recognition of the coordinated genetic regulation of virulence factor elaboration when organisms move from their natural environment into the mammalian host emphasizes the complex nature of the host-parasite interaction. Fortunately, the need for diverse factors in successful infection and disease implies that a variety of therapeutic strategies may be developed to interrupt this process and thereby prevent and treat microbial infections.

FURTHER READING

BASSLER BL: Small talk. Cell-to-cell communication in bacteria. Cell 17:421, 2002

CAROFF M et al: Structural and functional analyses of bacterial lipopolysaccharides. Microbes Infect 4:915, 2002

CLAPHAM PR, MCKNIGHT A: Cell surface receptors, virus entry and tropism of primate lentiviruses. J Gen Virol 83:1809, 2002

DOBROVOLSKAIA MA, VOGEL SN: Toll receptors, CD14, and macrophage activation and deactivation by LPS. Microbes Infect 4:903, 2002

MODLIN RL: Mammalian Toll-like receptors. Ann Allergy Asthma Immunol 88:543, 2002

PORTNOY DA: The cell biology of *Listeria monocytogenes* infection: The intersection of bacterial pathogenesis and cell-mediated immunity. J Cell Biol 5:409, 2002

SOLL DR: *Candida* commensalism and virulence: The evolution of phenotypic plasticity. Acta Trop 81:101, 2002

WEISS RA: Virulence and pathogenesis. Trends Microbiol 10:314, 2002

106   APPROACH TO THE ACUTELY ILL INFECTED FEBRILE PATIENT
Tamar F. Barlam, Dennis L. Kasper

The physician treating the acutely ill febrile patient must be able to recognize infections that require emergent attention. If such infections are not adequately evaluated and treated at initial presentation, the opportunity to alter an adverse outcome may be lost. In this chapter, the clinical presentations of and approach to patients with relatively common infectious disease emergencies are discussed. These infectious processes are discussed in detail in other chapters. →*Noninfectious causes of fever are not covered in this chapter; information on the approach to fever of unknown origin, including that eventually shown to be of noninfectious etiology, is presented in Chap. 18.*

APPEARANCE A physician must have a consistent approach to acutely ill patients. Even before the history is elicited and a physical examination performed, an immediate assessment of the patient's general appearance yields valuable information. The perceptive physician's subjective sense that a patient is septic or toxic often proves accurate. Visible agitation or anxiety in a febrile patient can be a harbinger of critical illness.

HISTORY Presenting symptoms are frequently nonspecific. In addition to a general description of symptoms, it is important to obtain a sense of disease progression. Detailed questions should be asked about the onset and duration of symptoms and about changes in severity or rate of progression over time. Host factors and comorbid conditions may enhance the risk of infection with certain organisms or of a more fulminant course than is usually seen. Lack of splenic function, alcoholism with significant liver disease, intravenous drug use, HIV infection, diabetes, malignancy, and chemotherapy all predispose to specific infections and frequently to increased severity. The patient should be questioned about factors that might help identify a nidus for invasive infection, such as recent upper respiratory tract infections, influenza, or varicella; prior trauma; disruption of cutaneous barriers due to lacerations, burns, surgery, or decubiti; and the presence of foreign bodies, such as nasal packing after rhinoplasty, barrier contraceptives, tampons, arteriovenous fistulas, or prosthetic joints. Travel, contact with pets or other animals, or activities that might result in tick exposure can lead to diagnoses that would not otherwise be considered. Recent dietary intake, medication use, social or occupational contact with ill individuals, vaccination history, recent sexual contacts, and menstrual history may be relevant. A review of systems should focus on any neurologic signs or sensorium alterations, rashes or skin lesions, and focal pain or tenderness and should also include a general review of respiratory, gastrointestinal, or genitourinary symptoms. It is especially important to determine the duration and progression of these symptoms in order to gain an appreciation of the pace and urgency of the process.

PHYSICAL EXAMINATION A complete physical examination should be performed, with special attention to some areas that are sometimes given short shrift in routine examinations. Assessment of the patient's general appearance and vital signs, skin and soft tissue examination, and the neurologic evaluation are of particular importance.

The patient may appear either anxious and agitated or lethargic and apathetic. Fever is usually present, although elderly patients and compromised hosts (e.g., patients who are uremic or cirrhotic and those who are taking glucocorticoids or nonsteroidal anti-inflammatory agents) may be afebrile despite serious underlying infection. Measurement of blood pressure, heart rate, and respiratory rate helps determine the degree of hemodynamic and metabolic compromise. The patient's airway must be evaluated to rule out the risk of obstruction from an invasive oropharyngeal infection.

The etiologic diagnosis may become evident in the context of a thorough skin examination (see also Chap. 17). Petechial rashes are typically seen with meningococcemia or Rocky Mountain spotted fever (RMSF); erythroderma is usual with toxic shock syndrome (TSS) and drug fever. The soft tissue and muscle examination is critical. Areas of erythema or duskiness, edema, and tenderness may indicate underlying necrotizing fasciitis, myositis, or myonecrosis. The neurologic examination must include a careful assessment of mental status for signs of early encephalopathy. Evidence of nuchal rigidity or focal neurologic findings should be sought. Focal findings, depressed mental status, or papilledema should be evaluated by brain imaging prior to lumbar puncture, which, in this setting, could initiate herniation.

DIAGNOSTIC WORKUP After a quick clinical assessment, diagnostic material should be obtained rapidly and antibiotic and supportive treatment begun. Blood (for cultures; baseline complete blood count with differential; measurement of serum electrolytes, blood urea nitrogen, serum creatinine, and serum glucose; and liver function tests) can be obtained at the time an intravenous line is placed and before antibiotics are administered. For patients with possible acute endocarditis, three sets of blood cultures should be performed. Asplenic patients should have a blood smear examined to confirm the presence of Howell-Jolly bodies (indicating the absence of splenic function) and a buffy coat examined for bacteria; these patients can have $>10^6$ organisms per milliliter of blood (compared with 10^4/mL in patients with an intact spleen). Blood smears from patients at risk for severe parasitic disease, such as malaria or babesiosis, must be examined for the diagnosis and quantitation of parasitemia. Blood smears may also be diagnostic in ehrlichiosis.

Patients with possible meningitis should have cerebrospinal fluid (CSF) obtained before the initiation of antibiotic therapy. *If focal neurologic signs, abnormal mental status, or papilledema mandates brain imaging before a lumbar puncture, antibiotics should be administered prior to imaging but after blood for cultures has been drawn.* If CSF cultures are negative, laboratory examination of CSF by latex agglutination or immunoprecipitation can be attempted to make an etiologic diagnosis. However, blood cultures will provide the diagnosis in 50 to 70% of cases.

Focal abscesses necessitate immediate computed tomography or magnetic resonance imaging (MRI) as part of an evaluation for surgical intervention. Other diagnostic procedures, such as cultures of wounds or scraping of skin lesions, should not delay the initiation of treatment for more than minutes. Once emergent evaluation, diagnostic procedures, and (if appropriate) surgical consultation (see below) have been completed, other laboratory tests can be conducted. Appropriate radiography, computed axial tomography, MRI, urinalysis, erythrocyte sedimentation rate (ESR) determination, and transthoracic or transesophageal echocardiography may all prove important.

℞ TREATMENT

In the acutely ill patient, empirical antibiotic therapy is critical and should be administered without undue delay. Table 106-1 lists first-line treatments for the infections considered in this chapter. (For a more detailed discussion of treatment, see specific chapters.) In addition to the initiation of parenteral antibiotic therapy, several of these infections require urgent surgical attention. General surgery for possible necrotizing fasciitis or myonecrosis, neurosurgical evaluation for subdural empyema or spinal epidural abscess, otolaryngologic surgery for possible mucormycosis, and cardiothoracic surgery for critically ill patients with acute endocarditis are as important as the rapid commencement of antibiotic therapy. For infections such as necrotizing fasciitis and clostridial myonecrosis, rapid surgical intervention supersedes other diagnostic or therapeutic maneuvers.

Adjunctive treatments, such as intravenous immunoglobulin administration for TSS, can be considered after initial stabilization. Some adjunctive treatments, such as dexamethasone for bacterial meningitis or protein C replacement for meningococcemia, must be considered in conjunction with the initiation of antibiotic treatment.

SPECIFIC PRESENTATIONS

For most infections, there is time for careful evaluation, diagnostic testing, and consultation with other physicians before therapy commences. However, the infections considered below according to common clinical presentation can have rapidly catastrophic outcomes, and their immediate recognition and treatment can be life-saving. Recommended empirical therapeutic regimens are presented in Table 106-1.

SEPSIS WITHOUT AN OBVIOUS FOCUS OF PRIMARY INFECTION These patients initially have a brief prodrome of nonspecific symptoms and signs that progresses quickly to hemodynamic instability with hypotension, tachycardia, tachypnea, or respiratory distress. A patient may display altered mental status. Disseminated intravascular coagulation (DIC)

TABLE 106-1   *Common Infectious Disease Emergencies*

Clinical Syndrome	Possible Etiologies	Treatment	Comments	Reference(s)
SEPSIS WITHOUT A CLEAR FOCUS				
Gram-negative sepsis	*Pseudomonas* spp., gram-negative enteric bacilli	Piperacillin/tazobactam (3.75 g q4h) *or* Ceftazidime (2 g q8h) *plus* Tobramycin (5 mg/kg per day)	See Chap. 254.	136, 254
Gram-positive sepsis	*Staphylococcus* spp., *Streptococcus* spp.	Vancomycin (1 g q12h) *plus* Gentamicin (5 mg/kg per day)	If a β-lactam-sensitive strain is identified, antibiotics should be altered.	120, 121, 254
Overwhelming post-splenectomy sepsis	*Streptococcus pneumoniae, Haemophilus influenzae, Neisseria meningitidis*	Ceftriaxone (2 g q12h)[a]	If the isolate is penicillin-sensitive, penicillin is the drug of choice.	254
Babesiosis	*Babesia microti* (U.S.), *B. divergens* (Europe)	**Either:** Clindamycin (600 mg tid) *plus* Quinine (650 mg tid) *or* Atovaquone (750 mg q12h) *plus* Azithromycin (500-mg loading dose, then 250 mg/d)	Atovaquone and azithromycin have been shown to be as effective as clindamycin and quinine and are associated with fewer side effects. Treatment with doxycycline (100 mg bid) for potential coinfection with *Borrelia burgdorferi* or *Ehrlichia* spp. may be prudent.	193, 195
SEPSIS WITH SKIN FINDINGS				
Petechiae: Meningococcemia	*N. meningitidis*	Penicillin (4 mU q4h) *or* Ceftriaxone (2 g q12h)	Consider protein C replacement in fulminant meningococcemia.	127, 158
Rocky Mountain spotted fever	*Rickettsia rickettsii*	Doxycycline (100 mg bid)	If both meningococcemia and Rocky Mountain spotted fever are being considered, use chloramphenicol (50–75 mg/kg per day in four divided doses). *Do not add doxycycline to a regimen including a β-lactam agent.* If Rocky Mountain spotted fever is diagnosed, doxycycline is the proven superior agent.	
Purpura fulminans	*S. pneumoniae, H. influenzae, N. meningitidis*	Ceftriaxone (2 g q12h)[a]	If the isolate is penicillin-sensitive, penicillin is the drug of choice.	127, 254
Erythroderma: toxic shock syndrome	Group A *Streptococcus, Staphylococcus aureus*	Penicillin (2 mU q4h) *or* Oxacillin (2 g q4h) *plus* Clindamycin (600 mg q8h)	Site of toxigenic bacteria should be debrided; if necessary, intravenous immunoglobulin can be used in severe cases. The optimal dose of IVIG has not been determined, but the median dose in observational studies is 2 g/kg (total dose administered over 1–5 days).	120, 121
SEPSIS WITH SOFT TISSUE FINDINGS				
Necrotizing fasciitis	Group A *Streptococcus*, mixed aerobic/anaerobic flora	Penicillin (2 mU q4h) *plus* Clindamycin (600 mg q8h) *plus* Gentamicin (5 mg/kg per day)	Urgent surgical evaluation is critical.	110, 121
Clostridial myonecrosis	*Clostridium perfringens*	Penicillin (2 mU q4h) *plus* Clindamycin (600 mg q8h)	Urgent surgical evaluation is critical.	126
NEUROLOGIC INFECTIONS				
Bacterial meningitis	*S. pneumoniae, N. meningitidis*	Ceftriaxone (2 g q12h)[a]	If the isolate is penicillin-sensitive, penicillin is the drug of choice. If the patient is >50 years old, add ampicillin for *Listeria* coverage. Dexamethasone (10 mg q6h × 4 days) improves outcome in adult patients with meningitis (especially that due to *S. pneumoniae*) and cloudy CSF, positive CSF Gram's stain, or CSF leukocyte count >1000/μL.	360
Suppurative intracranial infections	*Staphylococcus* spp., *Streptococcus* spp., anaerobes, gram-negative bacilli	Oxacillin (2 g q4h)[b] *plus* Metronidazole (500 mg tid) *plus* Ceftriaxone (2 g q12h)	Urgent surgical evaluation is critical.	360
Brain abscess	*Streptococcus* spp., anaerobes, *Staphylococcus* spp.	Penicillin (4 mU q4h) *or* Oxacillin (2 g q4h)[b] *plus* Metronidazole (500 mg tid)	Surgical evaluation is essential.	360

(continued)

TABLE 106-1—(Continued)

Clinical Syndrome	Possible Etiologies	Treatment	Comments	Reference(s)
Cerebral malaria	*Plasmodium falciparum*	Quinine (650 mg tid for 3 days) **plus** Tetracycline (250 mg tid for 7 days)	Do not use glucocorticoids.	193, 195
Spinal epidural abscess	*Staphylococcus* spp.	Oxacillin (2 g q4h)[c]	Surgical evaluation is essential.	356
FOCAL INFECTIONS				
Acute bacterial endocarditis	*S. aureus*, β-hemolytic streptococci, HACEK group,[d] *Neisseria* spp., *S. pneumoniae*	Ceftriaxone (2 g q12h) **plus** Vancomycin (1 g q12h)	Adjust treatment when culture data become available. Surgical evaluation is essential.	109

[a] If resistant pneumococci are prevalent, add vancomycin (1 g q12h).

[b] Vancomycin (1 g q12h) should replace oxacillin if methicillin-resistant strains are highly prevalent.

[c] In HIV-infected intravenous drug users with suspected spinal epidural abscess, empirical therapy must cover gram-negative rods and methicillin-resistant *S. aureus*.

[d] *Haemophilus aphrophilus, H. paraphrophilus, H. parainfluenzae, Actinobacillus actinomycetemcomitans, Cardiobacterium hominis, Eikenella corrodens,* and *Kingella kingae.*

Note: References refer to chapters.

with clinical evidence of a hemorrhagic diathesis is a poor prognostic sign.

Septic Shock (See also Chap. 254)   Patients with bacteremia leading to septic shock may have a primary site of infection (e.g., pneumonia, pyelonephritis, or cholangitis) that is not evident initially. Elderly patients with comorbid conditions, hosts compromised by malignancy and neutropenia, or patients who have recently undergone a surgical procedure or hospitalization are at increased risk for an adverse outcome. Gram-negative bacteremia with organisms such as *Pseudomonas aeruginosa, Aeromonas hydrophila,* or *Escherichia coli* and gram-positive infection with organisms such as *Staphylococcus aureus* or group A streptococci can present as intractable hypotension and multiorgan failure. Treatment can usually be initiated empirically on the basis of the presentation (Table 254-4).

Overwhelming Infection in Asplenic Patients (See also Chap. 254)   Patients without splenic function are at risk for overwhelming bacterial sepsis. Asplenic adult patients succumb to sepsis at 58 times the rate of the general population; 50 to 70% of cases occur within the first 2 years after splenectomy, with a mortality rate of up to 80%. However, in the asplenic individual, an increased risk of overwhelming sepsis continues throughout life. In asplenia, encapsulated bacteria cause the majority of infections, and adults are at lower risk than children because they are more likely to have antibody to these organisms. *Streptococcus pneumoniae* infection is most common, causing 50 to 70% of cases, but the risk of infection with *Haemophilus influenzae* or *Neisseria meningitidis* is also high. Severe clinical manifestations of infections due to *E. coli, S. aureus,* group B streptococci, *P. aeruginosa, Capnocytophaga, Babesia,* and *Plasmodium* have been described.

Babesiosis (See also Chap. 195)   A history of recent travel to endemic areas should raise the possibility of infection with *Babesia.* Between 1 and 4 weeks after a tick bite, the patient experiences chills, fatigue, anorexia, myalgia, arthralgia, shortness of breath, nausea, and headache; ecchymosis and/or petechiae are occasionally seen. The tick that most commonly transmits *Babesia, Ixodes scapularis,* also transmits *Borrelia burgdorferi* (the agent of Lyme disease) and *Ehrlichia,* and co-infection can occur, resulting in more severe disease. Infection with the European species *Babesia divergens* is more frequently fulminant than that due to the U.S. species *Babesia microti,* causing a febrile syndrome with hemolysis, jaundice, hemoglobinemia, and renal failure and a mortality rate of >50%. Severe babesiosis is especially common in asplenic hosts but does occur in hosts with normal splenic function, particularly those >60 years of age. Complications include renal failure, acute respiratory failure, and DIC.

Other Sepsis Syndromes   Tularemia (Chap. 142) is seen throughout the United States but occurs primarily in Arkansas, Oklahoma, and Missouri. This disease is associated with wild rabbit, tick, and tabanid fly contact. The uncommon typhoidal form can be associated with gram-negative septic shock and a mortality rate of >30%. In the United States, plague (Chap. 143) occurs primarily in New Mexico, Arizona, and Colorado after contact with ground squirrels, prairie dogs, or chipmunks. The septic form is particularly rare and is associated with shock, multiorgan failure, and a 30% mortality rate. These rare infections should be considered in the appropriate epidemiologic setting. Tularemia and plague, along with anthrax, are listed by the Centers for Disease Control and Prevention as important biological agents that might be intentionally used for bioterrorism (Table 106-2 and Chap. 205).

SEPSIS WITH SKIN MANIFESTATIONS (See also Chap. 17)   Maculopapular rashes may reflect early meningococcal or rickettsial disease but are usually associated with nonemergent infections. Exanthems are usually viral. It is noteworthy that primary HIV infection commonly presents with rash. Untreated, symptomatic HIV-seroconversion illness is associated with rapid progression to late-stage disease. The rash is typically maculopapular and involves the upper part of the body but can spread to the palms and soles. In addition, the patient is febrile and can have lymphadenopathy, severe headache, dysphagia, diarrhea, myalgias, and arthralgias. Recognition of this syndrome not only can prevent the spread of HIV to other individuals but also provides an opportunity for early treatment and improved prognosis.

Petechiae   Petechial rashes caused by viruses are seldom associated with hypotension or a toxic appearance, although severe measles can be an exception. In other settings, petechial rashes require more urgent attention.

MENINGOCOCCEMIA (See also Chap. 127)   Almost three-quarters of patients with bacteremic *N. meningitidis* infection have a rash. Meningococcemia most often affects young children (i.e., those 6 months to 5 years old, often in day care). However, sporadic cases and outbreaks occur in schools (grade school through college) and army barracks. Between 10 and 20% of all cases have a fulminant course, with shock, DIC, and multiorgan failure. Of these patients, 50 to 60% die, and survivors often require extensive debridement or amputation of gangrenous extremities. Patients may exhibit fever, headache, nausea, vomiting, myalgias, change in mental status, and meningismus. However, the rapidly progressive form of disease is not usually associated with meningitis. The rash is initially pink, blanching, and maculopapular, appearing on the trunk and extremities, but then becomes hemorrhagic, forming petechiae. Petechiae are first seen at the ankles, wrists, axillae, mucosal surfaces, and palpebral and bulbar conjunctiva, with subsequent spread to the lower extremities and trunk. A cluster of petechiae may be seen at pressure points—e.g., where a blood pressure cuff has been inflated. In rapidly progressive meningococcemia, the petechial rash quickly becomes purpuric (see Fig. 46-5) and patients develop DIC. Hypotension with petechiae for <12 h is associated with significant mortality. The mortality rate can exceed 90% among patients without meningitis who have rash, hypotension, and a normal or low white blood cell count and ESR. Cyanosis, coma, oliguria, metabolic acidosis, and elevated partial thromboplastin time are also associated with a fatal outcome. A better prognosis has been re-

Clinical Presentation	Agent	Signs and Symptoms	First-Line Treatment[b]	Comments	Reference Chapters
Sepsis without an obvious focus	Plague[c] Tularemia[d]	Fever, fatigue, headache, dyspnea, chest pain progressing to fulminant course of sepsis, shock, multiorgan failure, DIC	Streptomycin (1 g IM q12h) *or* Gentamicin (5 mg/kg per day) *plus* Ciprofloxacin (400 mg IV q12h)	Alternatives: Doxycycline (100 mg IV q12h) *or* Chloramphenicol (15 mg/ kg IV q6h) *or* A different fluoroquinolone	142, 143, 180, 181, 205
	Smallpox[e] and hemorrhagic fevers[f]	Patients can present before rash develops with severe nonspecific febrile illness.			
Sepsis with skin manifestations	Hemorrhagic fevers	Viral prodrome, high fevers, myalgias, encephalitis, bleeding diatheses with progression to petechial rash and mucous membrane hemorrhages	Provide supportive care and begin ribavirin. Continue if an arenavirus or bunyavirus is identified.	Person-to-person transmission with arenaviruses, Ebola virus, and Marburg virus	180, 181, 205
	Smallpox	Fever, myalgias, toxicity. Rash begins on face, extremities—vesicular lesions in one crop progressing to deep pustules	Supportive care	Person-to-person transmission Petechial or hemorrhagic forms described	
Neurologic infections with/without septic shock	Botulism[g]	No fever, sensation intact, mental status normal, symmetric cranial-nerve palsies, symmetric descending flaccid paralysis starting in bulbar region	Supportive care and antitoxin	Distinguish from Guillain-Barré and poliomyelitis—no antecedent infection, normal CSF, no sensory signs	125, 205
	Anthrax	Hemorrhagic meningitis can be associated with presentation.	Include rifampin, penicillin, or chloramphenicol along with primary treatment below.		
Focal infection with fulminant course	Anthrax[h] (inhalational)	Fever, cough, sweats, chest pain, abnormal chest x-rays—mediastinal widening, effusions	Ciprofloxacin (400 mg IV q12h) *or* Doxycycline (100 mg q12h) *plus* 1–2 additional agents	Consider clindamycin (600 mg q8h) for possible inhibition of toxin production.	142, 143, 205
	Plague	Fever, cough, cyanosis; bloody, watery sputum	See above.		
	Tularemia	Fulminant pneumonia	See above.		

[a] For details, see Chap. 205. The Centers for Disease Control and Prevention has defined three categories of biological agents that can be used as weapons of terror on the basis of their ease of dissemination or transmission, potential for public health impact, potential for public panic, and requirements for preparedness. Category A agents are those of greatest concern.

[b] Recommendations for mass casualty situations and special populations differ. Consult appropriate consensus statements.

[c] Inglesby TV et al: Plague as a biological weapon. JAMA 283:2281, 2000.
[d] Dennis DT et al: Tularemia as a biological weapon. JAMA 285:2763, 2001.
[e] Henderson DA et al: Smallpox as a biological weapon. JAMA 281:2127, 1999.
[f] Borio L et al: Hemorrhagic fever viruses as biological weapons. JAMA 287:2391, 2002.
[g] Arnon SS et al: Botulinum toxin as a biological weapon. JAMA 285:1059, 2001.
[h] Inglesby TV et al: Anthrax as a biological weapon. JAMA 287:2236, 2002.

ported in cases where antibiotics are given before admission by the primary care provider. This observation suggests that early initiation of treatment may be life-saving. In addition, several small experimental and clinical studies have suggested that correction of the protein C deficiency that is evident in meningococcal purpura fulminans can improve outcome.

ROCKY MOUNTAIN SPOTTED FEVER (See also Chap. 158) RMSF occurs throughout the United States. A history of known tick bite is common; however, if such a history is lacking, a history of travel or outdoor activity (e.g., camping in tick-infested areas) can be ascertained. RMSF is caused by *Rickettsia rickettsii*. For the first 3 days, headache, fever, malaise, myalgias, nausea, vomiting, and anorexia are present. By day 3, half of patients have skin findings. Blanching macules develop initially on the wrists and ankles and then spread over the legs and trunk. The lesions become hemorrhagic and are frequently petechial. The rash spreads to palms and soles later in the course. The centripetal spread is a classic feature of RMSF. However, 10 to 15% of patients with RMSF never develop a rash. The patient can be hypotensive and develop noncardiogenic pulmonary edema, confusion, lethargy, and encephalitis progressing to coma. The CSF contains 10 to 100 cells/μL, usually with a predominance of mononuclear cells. The CSF glucose level is often normal; the protein concentration may be slightly elevated. Renal and hepatic injury and bleeding secondary to vascular damage are noted. Untreated infection has a mortality rate of 30%.

Purpura Fulminans (See also Chaps. 127 and 254) Purpura fulminans is the cutaneous manifestation of DIC and presents as large ecchymotic areas and hemorrhagic bullae. Progression of petechiae to purpura and ecchymoses is associated with congestive heart failure, septic shock, acute renal failure, acidosis, hypoxia, hypotension, and death. Purpura fulminans has been associated primarily with *N. meningitidis* but, in splenectomized patients, may be associated with *S. pneumoniae* and *H. influenzae*.

Ecthyma Gangrenosum Septic shock caused by *P. aeruginosa* and *A. hydrophila* can be associated with ecthyma gangrenosum (see Fig. 136-1): hemorrhagic vesicles surrounded by a rim of erythema with central necrosis and ulceration. These gram-negative bacteremias are most common among patients with neutropenia, extensive burns, and hypogammaglobulinemia.

Other Emergent Infections Associated with Rash *Vibrio vulnificus* and other noncholera *Vibrio* bacteremic infections (Chap. 140) can cause focal skin lesions and overwhelming sepsis in the host with liver disease. After ingestion of contaminated shellfish, there is a sudden onset of malaise, chills, fever, and hypotension. The patient develops bullous or hemorrhagic skin lesions, usually on the lower extremities, and 75% of patients have leg pain. The mortality rate can be as high as 50%. *Capnocytophaga canimorsus* can cause septic shock in asplenic patients. Infection with this fastidious gram-negative rod typically presents after a dog bite as fever, chills, myalgia, vomiting, diarrhea, dyspnea, confusion, and headache. Findings can include an exanthem or erythema multiforme (see Fig. 46-9), cyanotic mottling or peripheral cyanosis, petechiae, and ecchymosis. About 30% of patients with this fulminant form die of overwhelming sepsis and DIC, and survivors may require amputation because of gangrene.

Erythroderma TSS (Chaps. 120 and 121) is usually associated with erythroderma. The patient presents with fever, malaise, myalgias, nausea, vomiting, diarrhea, and confusion. There is a sunburn-type rash that may be subtle and patchy but is usually diffuse and is found on the face, trunk, and extremities. Erythroderma, which desquamates after 1 to 2 weeks, is more common in *Staphylococcus*-associated than in *Streptococcus*-associated TSS. Hypotension develops rapidly—often within hours—after the onset of symptoms. Multiorgan failure is seen. Commonly there is no indication of a primary focal infection, although possible cutaneous or mucosal portals of entry for the organism can be ascertained when a careful history is taken. Colonization rather than overt infection of the vagina or a postoperative wound, for example, is typical with staphylococcal TSS, and the mucosal areas appear hyperemic but not infected. Early renal failure may precede hypotension and distinguishes this syndrome from other septic shock syndromes. Clinical evaluation constitutes the diagnosis because TSS is defined by the clinical criteria of fever, rash, hypotension, and multiorgan involvement. The mortality rate is 5% for menstruation-associated TSS, 10 to 15% for nonmenstrual TSS, and 30 to 70% for streptococcal TSS.

SEPSIS WITH A SOFT TISSUE/MUSCLE PRIMARY FOCUS (See also Chap. 110)

■ Necrotizing Fasciitis This infection may arise at a site of minimal trauma or postoperative incision and may also be associated with recent varicella, childbirth, or muscle strain. The most common causes of necrotizing fasciitis are group A streptococci alone (Chap. 121) and a mixed facultative and anaerobic flora (Chap. 110). Diabetes mellitus, peripheral vascular disease, and intravenous drug use are associated risk factors. Use of nonsteroidal anti-inflammatory agents adversely affects granulocyte chemotaxis, phagocytosis, and bacterial killing, allowing progression of skin or soft tissue infections. The patient may have bacteremia and hypotension without other organ-system failure. Physical findings are minimal compared with the severity of pain and the degree of fever. The examination is often unremarkable except for soft tissue edema and erythema. The infected area is red, hot, shiny, swollen, and exquisitely tender. In untreated infection, the overlying skin develops blue-gray patches after 36 h, and cutaneous bullae and necrosis develop after 3 to 5 days. Necrotizing fasciitis due to a mixed flora, but not that due to group A streptococci, can be associated with gas production. Without treatment, pain decreases because of thrombosis of the small blood vessels and destruction of the peripheral nerves—an ominous sign. The mortality rate is >30% overall, >70% in association with TSS, and nearly 100% without surgical intervention. Life-threatening necrotizing fasciitis may also be due to *Clostridium perfringens* (Chap. 126); in this condition, the patient is extremely toxic and the mortality rate is high. Within 48 h, rapid tissue invasion and systemic toxicity associated with hemolysis and death ensue. The distinction between this entity and clostridial myonecrosis is made by muscle biopsy.

Clostridial Myonecrosis (See also Chap. 126) Myonecrosis is often associated with trauma or surgery but can be spontaneous. The incubation period is usually 12 to 24 h long, and massive necrotizing gangrene develops within hours of onset. Systemic toxicity, shock, and death can occur within 12 h. The patient's pain and toxic appearance are out of proportion to physical findings. On examination, the patient is febrile, apathetic, tachycardic, and tachypneic and may express a feeling of impending doom. Hypotension and renal failure

develop later, and hyperalertness is evident preterminally. The skin over the affected area is bronze-brown, mottled, and edematous. Bullous lesions with serosanguineous drainage and a mousy or sweet odor can be present. Crepitus can occur secondary to gas production in muscle tissue. The mortality rate is >65% with spontaneous myonecrosis, which is often associated with *Clostridium septicum* and underlying malignancy. The mortality rates associated with trunk and limb infection are 63 and 12%, respectively, and any delay in surgical treatment increases the risk of death.

NEUROLOGIC INFECTIONS WITH OR WITHOUT SEPTIC SHOCK ■ Bacterial Meningitis (See also Chap. 360) Bacterial meningitis is one of the most common infectious emergencies involving the central nervous system. Although hosts with cell-mediated immune deficiency (including transplant recipients, diabetic patients, elderly patients, and cancer patients treated with certain chemotherapeutic agents) are at particular risk for *Listeria monocytogenes* meningitis, most cases in adults are due to *S. pneumoniae* (30 to 50%) and *N. meningitidis* (10 to 35%). An early presentation of headache, meningismus, and fever is classic but is seen in only one-half to two-thirds of patients. The elderly can present without fever or meningeal signs despite lethargy and confusion. Cerebral dysfunction is evidenced by confusion, delirium, and lethargy that can progress to coma. The presentation is fulminant, with sepsis and brain edema, in some cases; papilledema at presentation is unusual and suggests another diagnosis (e.g., an intracranial lesion). Focal signs, including cranial nerve palsies (IV, VI, VII), can be seen in 10 to 20% of cases; 50 to 60% of patients have bacteremia. A poor outcome is associated with coma at any time during the course, hypotension, meningitis due to *S. pneumoniae*, or a CSF glucose level of <0.6 mmol/L (<10 mg/dL). Mortality is associated with coma, respiratory distress, shock, a CSF protein level of >2.5 g/L, a peripheral white blood cell count of <5000/μL, and a serum sodium level of <135 mmol/L.

Suppurative Intracranial Infections (See also Chap. 360) Other rare intracranial lesions that present with sepsis and hemodynamic instability are subdural empyema, septic cavernous sinus thrombosis, and septic superior sagittal sinus thrombosis. Rapid recognition of the toxic patient with central neurologic signs is crucial to improvement of the dismal prognosis of these entities.

SUBDURAL EMPYEMA This infection arises from the paranasal sinus in 60 to 70% of cases. Microaerophilic streptococci and staphylococci are the predominant etiologic organisms. The patient is toxic, with fever, headache, and nuchal rigidity. Of all patients, 75% have focal signs and 6 to 20% die. Despite improved survival rates, 15 to 44% of patients are left with permanent neurologic deficits.

SEPTIC CAVERNOUS SINUS THROMBOSIS This condition follows a facial or sphenoid sinus infection; 70% of cases are due to staphylococci and the remainder are due primarily to aerobic or anaerobic streptococci. A unilateral or retroorbital headache progresses to a toxic appearance and fever within days. Three-quarters of patients have unilateral periorbital edema that becomes bilateral and then progresses to ptosis, proptosis, ophthalmoplegia, and papilledema. The mortality rate is as high as 30%.

SEPTIC THROMBOSIS OF THE SUPERIOR SAGITTAL SINUS This infection spreads from the ethmoid or maxillary sinuses. Its bacterial causes include *S. pneumoniae*, other streptococci, and staphylococci. The fulminant course is characterized by headache, nausea, vomiting, rapid progression to confusion and coma, nuchal rigidity, and brainstem signs. If the sinus is totally thrombosed, the mortality rate exceeds 80%.

Brain Abscess (See also Chap. 360) Brain abscess often occurs without systemic signs. Almost half of patients are afebrile, and presentations are more consistent with a space-occupying lesion in the brain; 70% of patients have headache, 50% have focal neurologic signs, and 25% have papilledema. Abscesses can present as single or multiple lesions resulting from contiguous foci or hematogenous infection, such as unrecognized endocarditis. The infection progresses over several days from cerebritis to an abscess with a mature capsule. More than half of infections are polymicrobial, with an etiology consisting of aerobic bacteria (primarily streptococcal species) and anaerobes. Abscesses arising hematogenously are especially apt to rupture into the ventricular space, causing a sudden and severe deterioration in clinical status and high mortality. Otherwise, mortality is low but morbidity is high (30 to 55%). Patients presenting with stroke and a parameningeal infectious focus, such as sinusitis or otitis, may have a brain abscess, and physicians must maintain a high level of suspicion. Prognosis worsens in patients with a fulminant course, delayed diagnosis, abscess rupture into the ventricles, multiple abscesses, or abnormal neurologic status at presentation.

Cerebral Malaria (See also Chap. 195)   This entity should be urgently considered if patients who have recently traveled to areas endemic for malaria present with a febrile illness and lethargy or other neurologic signs. Fulminant malaria is caused by *Plasmodium falciparum* and is associated with temperatures of >40°C (>104°F), hypotension, jaundice, adult respiratory distress syndrome, and bleeding. By definition, any patient with a change in mental status or repeated seizure in the setting of fulminant malaria has cerebral malaria. In adults, this nonspecific febrile illness progresses to coma over several days; occasionally, coma occurs within hours and death within 24 h. Nuchal rigidity and photophobia are rare. On physical examination, symmetric encephalopathy is typical, and upper motor neuron dysfunction with decorticate and decerebrate posturing can be seen in advanced disease. Unrecognized infection results in a 20 to 30% mortality rate.

SPINAL EPIDURAL ABSCESSES (See also Chap. 356)   Patients with spinal epidural abscesses often present with back pain and develop neurologic deficits late in their course. At-risk patients include those with diabetes mellitus; intravenous drug use; chronic alcohol abuse; recent spinal trauma, surgery, or epidural anesthesia; and other comorbid conditions, such as HIV infection. The thoracic or lumbar spine is the most common location, and staphylococci are the most common etiologic agents; in HIV-infected intravenous drug users, therapy must cover gram-negative rods and methicillin-resistant *S. aureus*. If a patient gives a history of antecedent back pain and has new neurologic symptoms, this diagnosis must immediately be considered. Almost 60% of patients have fever and almost 90% have back pain. Paresthesia, bowel and bladder dysfunction, radicular pain, and weakness are frequent neurologic complaints, and examination of the patient may reveal abnormal reflexes and motor and sensory deficits. The ESR and leukocyte counts are usually elevated. Rapid recognition and treatment, including immediate drainage, can prevent or minimize permanent neurologic sequelae.

FOCAL SYNDROMES WITH A FULMINANT COURSE   Infection at virtually any primary focus (e.g., osteomyelitis, pneumonia, pyelonephritis, or cholangitis) can result in bacteremia and sepsis. TSS has been associated with focal infections such as septic arthritis, peritonitis, sinusitis, and wound infection. Death occurs secondary to septic shock or toxin production with hemodynamic instability and multiorgan failure. Rapid clinical deterioration and death can be associated with destruction of the primary site of infection, as is seen in endocarditis and in necrotizing infections of the oropharynx (in which edema suddenly compromises the airway).

Rhinocerebral Mucormycosis (See also Chap. 189)   Patients with diabetes or malignancy are at risk for invasive rhinocerebral mucormycosis. Patients present with low-grade fever, dull sinus pain, diplopia, decreased mental status, decreased ocular motion, chemosis, proptosis, dusky or necrotic nasal turbinates, and necrotic hard-palate lesions that respect the midline. Without rapid recognition and intervention, the process continues an inexorable invasive course with high mortality.

Acute Bacterial Endocarditis (See also Chap. 109)   This entity presents with a much more aggressive course than subacute endocarditis. Bacteria such as *S. aureus*, *S. pneumoniae*, *L. monocytogenes*, *Haemophilus* spp., and streptococci of groups A, B, and G attack native valves. Mortality rates range from 10 to 40%. The host may have comorbid conditions such as underlying malignancy, diabetes mellitus, intravenous drug use, or alcoholism. The patient presents with fever, fatigue, and malaise <2 weeks after onset of infection. On physical examination, a changing murmur and congestive heart failure may be noted. Hemorrhagic macules on palms or soles (*Janeway lesions*) sometimes develop. Petechiae, Roth's spots, splinter hemorrhages, and splenomegaly are unusual. Rapid valvular destruction, particularly of the aortic valve, results in pulmonary edema and hypotension. Myocardial abscesses can form, eroding through the septum or into the conduction system and causing life-threatening arrhythmias or highdegree conduction block. Large friable vegetations can result in major arterial emboli, metastatic infection, or tissue infarction. Emboli can lead to stroke, change in mental status, visual disturbances, aphasia, ataxia, headache, meningismus, brain abscess, cerebritis, spinal cord infarct with paraplegia, arthralgia, osteomyelitis, splenic abscess, septic arthritis, and hematuria. Older patients with *S. aureus* endocarditis are especially likely to present with nonspecific symptoms—a circumstance that delays diagnosis and worsens prognosis. Rapid intervention is crucial for a successful outcome.

Inhalational Anthrax (See also Chap. 205)   Inhalational anthrax, the most severe form of disease caused by *Bacillus anthracis*, had not been reported in the United States for more than 25 years until the recent use of this organism as an agent of bioterrorism (Table 106-2 and Chap. 205). Patients presented with malaise, fever, cough, nausea, drenching sweats, shortness of breath, and headache. Rhinorrhea was unusual. All patients had abnormal chest roentgenograms at presentation. Mediastinal widening, pulmonary infiltrates, and pleural effusions were the most common findings. All patients who developed fulminant disease before receiving antibiotics died. Hemorrhagic meningitis has been seen in up to 50% of patients in other large outbreaks. Without urgent intervention with antimicrobial agents and supportive care, inhalational anthrax progresses rapidly to hypotension, cyanosis, and death.

CONCLUSION

Acutely ill febrile patients, with the syndromes discussed in this chapter, require close observation, aggressive supportive measures, and—in most cases—admission to intensive care units. The most important task of the physician is to distinguish these patients from other infected febrile patients who will not progress to fulminant disease. The alert physician must recognize the acute infectious emergency and then proceed with appropriate urgency.

FURTHER READING

ALBERIO L et al: Protein C replacement in severe meningococcemia: Rationale and clinical experience. Clin Infect Dis 32:1338, 2001

ASTIZ ME et al: Septic shock. Lancet 351:1501, 1998

DE GANS J et al: Dexamethasone in adults with bacterial meningitis. N Engl J Med 347:1549, 2002

HENRETIG FM et al: Medical management of the suspected victim of bioterrorism: An algorithmic approach to the undifferentiated patient. Emerg Med Clin North Am 20:351, 2002

KRAUSE PJ: Babesiosis. Med Clin North Am 86:361, 2002

NEWTON CRJC et al: Cerebral malaria. J Neurol Neurosurg Psychiatry 69:433, 2000

SEXTON DJ et al: Rocky Mountain spotted fever. Med Clin North Am 86:351, 2002

STEVENS DL: Streptococcal toxic shock syndrome associated with necrotizing fasciitis. Annu Rev Med 51:271, 2000

SUMARAJU V et al: Infectious complications in asplenic hosts. Infect Dis Clin North Am 15:551, 2001

Most humans live their lives ignoring the certainty of their own mortality. Perhaps this fact explains why the adage "an ounce of prevention is worth a pound of cure" has so little effect on their everyday behavior. Even when it comes to acting to protect their young, parents are capable of ignoring the potential for the death of their children in the developed world and of accepting the certainty of childhood deaths in the developing world. In both settings, parents all too often fail to seek out and demand the best preventive measures available. Unless mandated by the law in wealthy societies or provided by benevolent organizations or governments in poor nations, universal immunization has invariably remained an unattained goal.

Vaccination is ranked as one of the greatest public health achievements of the twentieth century and is the principal factor contributing to the reduction of morbidity and mortality among children around the world. The integration of immunization practices (a major component of primary disease prevention) into routine health care services has provided caregivers with control over a substantial proportion of the disease and mortality that plagued the United States during the first half of the twentieth century (Table 107-1). For society today, immunization is one of the few cost-saving interventions to prevent infectious disease. At present, >50 biologic products are licensed in the United States. A total of 21 antigens, many in the form of combined vaccines, are used for routine immunization during the first 18 months of life, including diphtheria/tetanus/acellular pertussis (DTaP) vaccine, trivalent inactivated poliovirus vaccine (IPV), measles/mumps/rubella (MMR) vaccine, *Haemophilus influenzae* type b (Hib) vaccine, hepatitis B (HepB) and hepatitis A (HepA) vaccines, and varicella vaccine. Recently, a heptavalent pneumococcal vaccine has been recommended for routine use in children, as has influenza vaccine (given annually). Five vaccines are designed for routine use in adults: tetanus/diphtheria (Td) toxoids formulated for adult use; HepB vaccine; influenza virus vaccine; polyvalent pneumococcal polysaccharide vaccine; and varicella vaccine. Some preparations are designated as special-use vaccines for outbreak response, prophylaxis in travelers, or regional use (e.g., vaccines against *Neisseria meningitidis*, Japanese B encephalitis virus, yellow fever virus, and *Salmonella typhi* and HepA vaccine). Unfortunately, vaccines for eukaryotic pathogens (protozoa and helminths), which affect a large proportion of the world's population, have been difficult to develop and remain only a hope for the future.

Healthy People 2010 Objectives for the Nation includes a set of immunization indicators. By 2010, 80% of children should have received DTaP, poliovirus, MMR, Hib, and HepB vaccines, while 90% of adults are expected to have received influenza and pneumococcal vaccines.

IMPACT OF IMMUNIZATION
The epidemiologically appropriate use of vaccines has resulted in the global eradication of smallpox and, until recently, the cessation of smallpox vaccination. Immunization has eliminated naturally transmitted poliomyelitis from the Western Hemisphere, Europe, and the Western Pacific. Similarly, measles, which had a nearly 100% infectivity rate in the prevaccination era, has been effectively eliminated from most of the Western Hemisphere by widespread immunization. Current debate centers around whether it is possible to eradicate an organism from the world and cease immunization or whether the best that can be hoped for is the elimination of clinical disease worldwide, with continued routine immunization. Already achieved in the United States are the virtual elimination of congenital rubella syndrome, tetanus, and diphthe-

ria as well as a dramatic reduction in pertussis, rubella, measles, and mumps. The introduction of Hib conjugate vaccines for immunization of infants has all but eliminated invasive *Haemophilus* infections (including meningitis and pneumonia) because this vaccine both elicits durable immunity by the time maternal-derived antibodies have dissipated and reduces nasopharyngeal carriage of Hib, thereby reducing the risk of transmission. Polyvalent pneumococcal polysaccharide conjugate vaccine is having a significant impact on invasive pneumococcal disease, including otitis media.

DEFINITIONS
Vaccination and *immunization* are often used as interchangeable terms. However, the former denotes only the administration of a vaccine, whereas the latter describes the process of inducing or providing immunity by any means, whether active or passive. Thus, vaccination does not guarantee immunization. Active immunization refers to the induction of immune defenses by the administration of antigens in appropriate forms, whereas passive immunization involves the provision of temporary protection by the administration of exogenously produced immune substances (Table 107-2).

PRINCIPLES OF IMMUNIZATION
Artificial induction of immunity closely follows two well-tested principles of nature. The first, active immunization, can be traced at least as far back as Thucydides, who noted that people surviving epidemics of plague in Athens were spared during later outbreaks of the same disease. The second, passive immunization, is a natural process as well and is exemplified by the transplacental transmission of maternal antibodies to the fetus to provide protection against several diseases during the first months of life. Use of the two measures together may produce a complementary effect (as with HepB vaccine plus hepatitis B immune globulin) or may actually interfere with the development of immunity (as when measles vaccine is administered within 6 weeks of measles immunoglobulin). Depending on whether there are multiple species or serotypes of an organism and—if so—whether there are common, cross-reactive, protective antigens, a specific vaccine may induce protection against all representative forms of an infectious agent or against the immunizing strain only. One of the intrinsic virtues of whole-organism vaccines is that they potentially contain all protective antigens of the organism. However, this virtue is counterbalanced by an inherent problem with such vaccines: the possibility of adverse responses to reactive but nonprotective antigens present in the mix. Because the immune response to specific antigens is controlled genetically, all individuals cannot be expected to respond identically to the same vaccine.

APPROACHES TO ACTIVE IMMUNIZATION
The two standard approaches to active immunization are (1) the use of live, generally attenuated, in-

TABLE 107-1 *Reduction in Morbidity due to Vaccine-Preventable Diseases in the United States, 1900–2002*

Disease	Reporting Period	Annual Morbidity Prior to Vaccine	2001 Morbidity	2002 Morbidity[a]	Decrease, %[b]
Smallpox	1900–1904	48,164	0	0	100
Diphtheria	1920–1922	175,885	2	1	100
Pertussis	1922–1925	147,271	7580	8296	94.6
Tetanus	1922–1926	1314	27	23	98.1
Neonatal tetanus	1972–1985	785	29	1	98.1
Poliomyelitis (paralytic)	1951–1954	16,316	0	0	100
Measles	1958–1962	503,282	116	37	99.9
Mumps	1968	152,209	266	238	99.8
Rubella	1966–1968	47,745	23	14	99.9
Congenital rubella syndrome	1969	823	3	3	99.6
Haemophilus influenzae type b	Before 1985	20,000	27	27	99.9

[a] Provisional data.
[b] Average of figures for 2001 and 2002 compared with peak incidence.

TABLE 107-2 *Definitions of Immunizing Agents*

Term	Definition
Vaccine	A preparation of attenuated live or killed microorganisms or antigenic portions of these agents presented to a potential host to induce immunity and prevent disease
Toxoid	A modified bacterial toxin that has been made nontoxic but retains the capacity to stimulate the formation of antitoxin
Immune globulin	An antibody-containing protein fraction derived from human plasma and used primarily for maintenance of the immunity of persons with immunodeficiency disorders or for passive immunization when there is no opportunity for active immunization[a]
Antitoxin	An antibody derived from the serum of animals after stimulation with specific antigens and used to provide passive immunity to the toxin protein to which it is directed

[a] Both intramuscular and intravenous preparations are available.

fectious agents (e.g., measles virus); and (2) the use of inactivated agents or their constituents or products obtained by genetic recombination (e.g., acellular pertussis vaccines). For many diseases (e.g., poliomyelitis), both approaches have been employed.

Live attenuated vaccines consisting of selected or genetically altered organisms that are avirulent or dramatically attenuated, yet remain immunogenic, generally produce long-lasting immunity. These agents are expected to cause a subclinical illness and immunologic response mimicking natural infection (except for the lack of clinically significant disease). They offer the advantage of replication in vivo, which increases the antigenic load presented to the host's immune system; they may confer lifelong protection with one dose; they present all expressed antigens, thus overcoming immunogenetic restrictions in some hosts; they may reach the local sites most relevant to the induction of protective immunity; and they may produce important protective antigens in vivo that are not efficiently expressed in vitro.

Inactivated vaccines typically require multiple doses and periodic boosters thereafter for the maintenance of immunity. The exception to this rule is pure polysaccharide vaccine, whose effects cannot be boosted by additional exposures. Nonviable vaccines administered parenterally fail to elicit mucosal IgA-mediated immunity, as they lack a delivery system that can effectively transport them to local antigen-processing cells. However, killed vaccines can be extremely successful. For example, the nonviable HepA vaccine formulation appears to be close to 100% effective in inducing protective immunity. Currently available nonviable vaccines consist of inactivated whole organisms (e.g., plague vaccine); detoxified protein exotoxins (e.g., tetanus toxoid); recombinant protein antigens (e.g., HepB vaccine); or carbohydrate antigens, either present as soluble purified capsular material (e.g., *Streptococcus pneumoniae* polysaccharides) or conjugated to a protein carrier (e.g., Hib polysaccharide conjugated to diphtheria or tetanus toxoids).

Despite their advantages, live vaccines are not always preferable. For example, live oral poliovirus vaccine (OPV) is contraindicated for use in children with immune deficiency diseases or their adult contacts. In addition, even though killed poliovirus vaccine does not completely immunize the gut or immunize contacts of vaccine recipients, the United States has now switched to a four-dose schedule of this vaccine because of the rare but real risk of vaccine-associated polio posed by live OPV.

APPROACHES TO PASSIVE IMMUNIZATION   Passive immunization is generally used to provide temporary immunity in an unimmunized subject exposed to an infectious disease when active immunization either is unavailable (e.g., for respiratory syncytial virus) or has not been implemented before exposure (e.g., for rabies). Passive immunization is used in the treatment of certain disorders associated with toxins (e.g., diphtheria), in certain bites (those of snakes and spiders), and as a specific or nonspecific immunosuppressant [Rho(D) immune globulin and antilymphocyte globulin, respectively]. Three types of preparations are used in passive immunization: (1) standard human immune serum globulin for general use (e.g., γ globulin), administered intramuscularly or intravenously; (2) special immune serum globulins with a known content of antibody to specific agents [e.g., hepatitis B virus (HBV) or varicella-zoster immune globulin]; and (3) animal sera and antitoxins.

ROUTE OF ADMINISTRATION   The route of administration in part determines the rapidity and nature of the immune responses to vaccines. Vaccines can be administered orally, intranasally, intradermally, subcutaneously, or intramuscularly. Parenterally administered vaccine may not induce mucosal secretory IgA, and mucosal immunization may not induce good systemic responses. Vaccines must be administered by the licensed route to ensure immunogenicity and safety. For example, administration of HepB vaccine into the gluteal rather than the deltoid muscle often fails to induce an adequate immune response, while subcutaneous rather than intramuscular administration of diphtheria/tetanus/pertussis vaccine (DTP) increases the risk of reactions.

AGE   Because age influences the response to vaccines, schedules for immunization are based on age-dependent responses determined empirically from clinical trials. The presence of high levels of maternal antibody and/or the immaturity of the immune system in the early months of life impairs the initial immune response to some vaccines (e.g., measles or Hib polysaccharide) but not to others (e.g., HepB). In the elderly, vaccine responses may be diminished because of natural waning of the immune system. Hence, larger amounts of an antigen may be required to produce the desired response (e.g., in vaccination against influenza).

ADJUVANT POTENTIATION   The immune response to some antigens is potentiated by the addition of adjuvants such as aluminum salts or, in the case of polysaccharides (e.g., the polyribose phosphate oligosaccharide of Hib), by conjugation to a carrier protein. Adjuvants—nonspecific boosters of immune responses—are used with inactivated products such as diphtheria and tetanus toxoids, acellular pertussis vaccine, and HepB vaccine. The mechanism for adjuvant enhancement of immunogenicity is not well defined but relates in part to the rendering of soluble antigens into a particulate form; the mobilization of phagocytes to the site of antigen deposition; and the slowing down of the release of antigens, which prolongs stimulation of the immune response.

THE IMMUNE RESPONSE   While many constituents of infectious microorganisms and their products, such as exotoxins, are or can be made to be immunogenic, only a limited number stimulate a protective immune response. The immune system is complex, and antigen composition and presentation are critical for stimulation of the desired immune responses.

The Primary Response   In the primary response to a vaccine antigen, an apparent latent period of several days precedes the detection of humoral and cell-mediated immunity. Although the immune response begins with initial recognition of the antigen by the immune system, measurable circulating antibodies do not appear for 7 to 10 days. The immunoglobulin class of the response also changes over time. The primary response is characterized by early-appearing IgM antibodies. These generally exhibit only low affinity for the antigen, whereas later-appearing IgG antibodies display high affinity. For "thymus-dependent" antigens, CD4+ T-helper lymphocytes control the switch from IgM to IgG. Some individuals do not respond, even when presented repeatedly with a vaccine antigen, often because they lack the major histocompatibility complex determinants required to recognize the antigen. This situation is known as *primary vaccine failure*.

The Secondary Response   Heightened humoral or cell-mediated responses are elicited by a second exposure to the same antigen and occur rapidly, usually within 4 or 5 days. The secondary response depends on immunologic memory after the first exposure and is characterized by a marked proliferation of IgG antibody–producing B lymphocytes and/or effector T cells. Whereas polysaccharide vaccines, such as that for *S. pneumoniae*, evoke immune responses that are independent of T cells and are not enhanced by repeated administration, conjugation to proteins converts the polysaccharides to T cell–dependent antigens that induce immunologic memory and secondary responses to revaccination. Although levels of vaccine-induced antibodies may decline over time (*secondary vaccine failure*), revaccination or exposure to the organism generally elicits a rapid protective secondary response consisting of IgG antibodies with little or no detectable IgM. This anamnestic response indicates that immunity has persisted. Thus, lack of measurable antibody does not necessarily mean that the individual is unprotected. Furthermore, the mere presence of detectable antibodies after the administration of some vaccines and toxoids does not ensure clinical protection. A minimal circulating level of antibody is known to be required for protection from some diseases (e.g., 0.01 IU/mL for tetanus antitoxin).

Hypersensitivity Reactions   Independent of antibody production, the stimulation of the immune system by vaccination may elicit unanticipated responses, especially hypersensitivity reactions. In the past, killed measles vaccine induced incomplete humoral immunity and cell-mediated hypersensitivity, resulting in the development of a syndrome of atypical measles in some children after subsequent exposure; thus this type of vaccine is no longer in use.

Mucosal Immunity   Some pathogens are confined to and replicate only at mucosal surfaces (e.g., *Vibrio cholerae*), while others are able to penetrate the mucosa and replicate (e.g., poliovirus, rubella virus, and influenza virus). At the mucosal site, these organisms induce secretory IgA. The induction of secretory IgA by vaccines may be an efficient way to block the essential first steps in pathogenesis, whether the organism is restricted to mucosal surfaces or invades the host across mucosal surfaces.

Measurement of the Immune Response   Immune responses to vaccines are often gauged by the concentration of specific antibody in serum. While seroconversion serves as a dependable indicator of an immune response, it measures only one immunologic parameter and does not necessarily indicate protection. The development of circulating antibodies after immunization often correlates directly with clinical protection (e.g., against measles or rubella). Some responses may not in themselves confer immunity but may be sufficiently associated with protection that they remain useful proxy measures of protective immunity (e.g., vibriocidal serum antibodies in cholera).

HERD IMMUNITY   Vaccination provides direct protection against infection of individuals, thereby decreasing the percentage of susceptible persons within a population. At a definable prevalence of immunity in the population (*herd immunity*), an organism can no longer circulate freely among the susceptibles. This indirect protection of unvaccinated (nonimmune) persons is called the *herd immunity effect*. The level of vaccination coverage needed to elicit a herd immunity effect is dependent on the mixing patterns of the population and the biology of the specific infectious agents. For example, measles and varicella viruses have high transmission rates and therefore require a higher level of vaccine coverage to elicit herd immunity than do organisms with lower transmission rates, such as *S. pneumoniae*. Wherever herd immunity for poliomyelitis and measles has been induced with vaccines, transmission of infection has ceased. It is not surprising that herd immunity may wane if immunization programs are interrupted (as was the case for diphtheria in the former Soviet Union) or if a sufficient percentage of individuals refuse to be immunized (as occurred for pertussis in the United Kingdom and Japan because concern about infrequent—albeit severe—vaccine reactions came to exceed the fear of the disease itself). In each setting, loss of herd immunity led to renewed circulation of the organism and subsequent large outbreaks.

TARGET POPULATIONS AND TIMING OF IMMUNIZATION   Different age groups have different disease attack rates, and the effectiveness of vaccines depends on a variety of factors, including the individual's responsiveness to vaccines, the demographic features of the populations at risk, and the duration and character of the immunologic response. In vaccination programs, which are as much community as individual endeavors, schedules for immunization are based on careful consideration of the variables affecting age-dependent responses and population interactions (e.g., school entry, college enrollment, military induction) as well as the feasibility of implementation.

For common and highly communicable childhood diseases like measles, the target population is the universe of susceptible individuals, and the time to immunize is as early in life as is feasible. Yet epidemiologic differences in measles transmission in different settings dictate different strategies for immunization. In the industrialized world, immunization with live-virus vaccine at 12 to 15 months of age has been the norm because the vaccine protects >95% of those immunized at this age and there is little measles morbidity or mortality among very young infants. In contrast, in the developing world, measles is a significant cause of death in young infants. Thus, it is desirable to immunize children earlier to narrow the window of vulnerability between the rapid decline of maternal antibody after 4 to 6 months and the development of vaccine-induced active immunity.

Hib causes meningitis, epiglottitis, and pneumonia in early childhood, with rates rising sharply after the disappearance of maternally derived antibody. The first Hib polysaccharide vaccines often failed when administered during infancy, mainly because of an age-related inability to respond to polysaccharide antigens. To overcome this problem, the protective polysaccharide was converted to a T cell–dependent antigen by conjugation to proteins to which infants could respond.

In contrast, rubella is primarily a threat to the fetus; young infants and children are not at risk of serious illness. An ideal strategy would be to immunize all women of reproductive age before pregnancy. Because it is difficult to systematically vaccinate adolescent and young-adult females and to assure the protection of as many women as possible, rubella is included in a combination vaccine (MMR vaccine) that is administered during infancy. Screening for rubella antibodies during pregnancy should be followed up with postpartum vaccination of seronegative individuals.

Some vaccines were originally formulated primarily for adults. For example, influenza virus and polyvalent pneumococcal polysaccharide vaccines are used to prevent pneumonia, hospitalizations, and deaths among the elderly. Unfortunately, these vaccines are underutilized, in part because physicians and otherwise-healthy individuals in the target group ignore the indications and in part because there is still a tendency to think about disease prevention with vaccines as a strategy for children. With the advent of pneumococcal conjugate vaccines and the cold-adapted influenza strain as well as of administration by nasal spray, infants can also be targeted to receive these vaccines.

THE DEVELOPMENT OF VACCINES

BIOLOGIC IMPEDIMENTS   There are often major technical problems to overcome in vaccine development. Although just one major antigenic type of influenza virus is typically in circulation at any one time, the virus is characterized biologically by its antigenic drift. Thus, a new antigenic version capable of causing a global pandemic emerges regularly, and a new vaccine must be rapidly devised, produced, distributed, and administered. In contrast, many prevalent pneumococcal polysaccharide serotypes circulate at all times. Because immunity to the pneumococcus is serotype specific, an individual is susceptible to all serotypes against which he or she lacks antibody. Serotype-specific protection has made it more difficult to develop an effective pneumococcal vaccine than it was to develop a vaccine against *H. influenzae*, of which one capsular serotype (type b) is associated with nearly all cases of severe disease. To overcome this problem, pneumococcal vaccine currently includes 23 polysaccharides that represent ~80% of the virulent serotypes commonly encountered in the United States. Unfortunately, some serotypes are poorly immunogenic, and immunized individuals remain susceptible to the serotypes not included in the vaccine.

STRATEGY FOR VACCINE DEVELOPMENT   Vaccine development depends on the systematic application of a four-phase strategy: (1) studies in animals to identify protective antigens, (2) determination of how to present this antigen effectively to the immune system, (3) assessment of the safety and immunogenicity of the preparation in small and then in large human populations at various ages, and (4) evaluation of safety and efficacy in the target population. Each of these steps is simple in concept but difficult in execution; failure at any level stops the process. Progress in immunology has taught us much about the organization and function of the immune system (Chap. 295); it has also taught us that the immune system is complex and that details of antigen composition and presentation are critical for stimulating desired immune responses.

Ultimately, vaccines for humans must be tested in humans. After initial animal studies and small phase 1 and 2 human studies to assess immune responses, optimal dosage, and safety, clinical trials of vaccine efficacy are performed with informed volunteers who are challenged with a virulent strain. Larger clinical effectiveness trials in the community, typically involving 1000 to 10,000 vaccinees, may lead to application for licensure. Because of their limited size, however, these trials cannot be expected to detect rare adverse effects. Thus, licensing does not guarantee that a new vaccine is completely safe, and postlicensing monitoring is needed to ensure effectiveness and to document the occurrence of adverse events of low frequency. In 1999, the recently licensed rhesus rotavirus vaccine was withdrawn because postmarketing surveillance suggested an association with a rare event in infants: intussusception of the bowel.

The development of vaccines goes beyond technology and proof of principle to issues such as development costs, manufacturers' liability and indemnity, perceived public health needs, and the likelihood that a product will be used or sold. Given the complex science required, the costs of vaccine development are high and success is uncertain, adding risk to the development decision. It is unfortunate that the one sure implication of uncertainty in vaccine development is increased cost. In addition, a rational assignment of costs for development between the public and private sectors in the United States has never been achieved.

VACCINE FORMULATIONS   Studies of clinical immunology have shown that living and dead antigens do not induce the same immune responses and that the requirements for the development of protective immunity may differ with the organism. These insights, together with the refinement of epidemiologic concepts surrounding immunization, have changed the strategy of vaccine development. The goal is not only to select the correct antigens but also to ensure that the vaccines will result in the type of immune response needed for protection, whether T cell–mediated activation of macrophages or the generation of cytotoxic T cells, B cell–mediated secretory IgA, or a particular IgG subtype response to a specific polysaccharide epitope. To create a deliverable vaccine, constituents other than antigens are also required (Table 107-3). These constituents can affect the immunogenicity, efficacy, and safety of a vaccine and can render one formulation superior to another.

PRODUCTION OF VACCINES   As products to be given to healthy individuals to prevent disease, vaccines must not only be efficacious but also cause no harm. In the United States, quality assurance is the responsibility of vaccine manufacturers. Standards of manufacture of biologics (known as good manufacturing practices, or GMPs) are regulated and supervised by the U.S. Food and Drug Administration (FDA). Proof of the safety, efficacy, sterility, and purity of products is required before licensure, and sterility and purity are continually monitored for

TABLE 107-3   *Constituents of Vaccines*

Constituent(s)	Examples/Purpose
Preservatives, stabilizers, antibiotics	These components are used to prevent deterioration of the vaccine before use, to inhibit or prevent bacterial growth, or to stabilize the vaccine. Any of these additions can cause allergic responses.
Adjuvants	This type of additive (e.g., aluminum salts, or alum) is intended to enhance the immune response (e.g., to toxoids, hepatitis B vaccine).
Suspending fluid	The suspending fluid can be sterile water, saline, buffer, or more complex fluids derived from the growth medium or biologic system in which the agent is produced (e.g., egg antigens, cell culture ingredients, serum proteins).

all lots of vaccine after licensure. Postmarketing studies of safety (phase 4 studies) are part of routine regulatory control. On rare occasions, either GMP or quality assurance breaks down; for example, the release of incompletely killed Salk polio vaccine in 1955 caused an outbreak of poliomyelitis in nearly 200 vaccine recipients and their contacts. Unregulated and/or uncontrolled manufacture of vaccines in developing countries has sometimes led to immunization with inactive products that fail to provide the expected protective immunity (e.g., tetanus toxoid produced in Bangladesh).

There is a serious new problem affecting the production of vaccines. For various reasons, including the high costs of vaccine development and the prospect of much higher profitability from investments in other products, the number of vaccine manufacturers in the United States has declined and the cost of some basic childhood vaccines has increased. These changes raise concerns about the future availability of these essential biologics for national use. Furthermore, pricing decisions made within the private-sector pharmaceutical industry can have a major impact on vaccine use. This situation has stimulated an initiative toward increased public involvement in supplying vaccine to individuals for whom price is an issue as well as in oversight of the vaccine supply and of price negotiations with industry.

ADMINISTRATION OF VACCINES   Health care workers administering vaccines must take the precautions necessary to minimize the risk of spreading disease—for example, hand washing between immunizations. Different vaccines should not be mixed in the same syringe unless such a practice is specifically endorsed by licensure. Disposable needles and syringes must be safely discarded to prevent inadvertent needlestick injury or, in resource-poor settings, the reuse of these items.

The addition of new, individually injectable vaccines to the childhood immunization schedule has heightened parental concerns about multiple injections being administered at a single clinic visit. The development and use of combinations of vaccines are intended to mitigate these concerns. Even when multiple injections are required, providers must make every effort to administer all indicated vaccines at each visit.

Wherever effective primary health care systems ensure access to medical services for the majority and the population is educated about the need for and efficacy of vaccines, coverage rates for basic immunization are usually high, regardless of the route of vaccine administration or the number of doses necessary. However, without systematic attention to the completion of multiple-dose vaccine schedules, coverage rates for second, third, and booster doses may drop off significantly.

USE OF VACCINES

Several professional groups develop recommendations for vaccine use in the United States: the Advisory Committee on Immunization Practices, the American Academy of Pediatrics (AAP), the American Academy of Family Practice, the American College of Obstetricians and Gynecologists, the American College of Physicians, and the Infectious Diseases Society of America. These recommendations are the

Vaccine	Year Licensed	Type of Immunizing Agent	Protective Antibody	Route of Administration	Efficacy, %	Adverse Events
DT, Td (adult)	1949	Toxoid	Diphtheria and tetanus neutralizing antitoxins, 0.1 IU/mL each	IM	D: 95 T: 95	Local reactions; hypersensitivity to tetanus toxoid
aP	1991	Inactivated bacterial antigen	Not established	IM	80–90	Reduced local reactions compared with whole-cell pertussis vaccines;
DTaP	1996	Acellular	Not established	IM	80–90	no serious reactions reported
Hib	1987	Bacterial polysaccharide–protein conjugate	Antibody to capsular polysaccharide, 0.15 μg/mL	IM	90	Few local, no serious reactions reported
HepB	1981 1987	Inactivated serum-derived antigen Recombinant antigen	Antibody to surface antigen, 10 mIU/mL	IM	80–95	Few (? Guillain-Barré syndrome)
Influenza	1945	Inactivated virus or viral components	Neutralizing antibody	IM	40–60	? Guillain-Barré syndrome with swine influenza vaccine
MMR	1971	Live viruses	Neutralizing measles antibody, 200 mIU/mL; not known for mumps or rubella	SC	M: 95 Mu: 90 R: 95	Acute encephalopathy (measles) Rare parotitis or orchitis (mumps) Arthralgia and rare arthropathy (rubella)
Pneumococcal polysaccharide	1983	Capsular polysaccharide (23 types)	Antibody to polysaccharides	IM or SC	60–80	Local reactions; rare anaphylaxis
Pneumococcal conjugate	2000	Polysaccharide-protein conjugates (7–11 types)	Antibody to polysaccharides	IM	73–94	None thus far
IPV	1967	Inactivated virus of 3 types, enhanced immunogenicity	Neutralizing antibody	SC	95	No significant reactions
Varicella	1995	Live virus	Neutralizing antibody	SC	86–100	Local reaction; varicella-like rash

Abbreviations: DT, diphtheria and tetanus toxoids, adsorbed; Td, tetanus and diphtheria toxoids, adsorbed, for adult use; aP, acellular pertussis; DTaP, diphtheria/tetanus/acellular pertussis vaccine; Hib, *Haemophilus influenzae* type b; HepB, hepatitis B virus vaccine; MMR, measles/mumps/rubella; IPV, inactivated poliovirus vaccine.
Source: Recommendations of the Advisory Committee on Immunization Practices, the American Academy of Pediatrics, and the American College of Physicans.

result of a collaborative process among the recommending groups, the pharmaceutical industry, and the FDA.

Vaccines recommended in 2003 for routine administration to infants, children, and adults are shown in Table 107-4; vaccines recommended for special use are shown in Table 107-5; and schedules for immunization of children and adolescents and of adults are shown in Fig. 107-1 and Fig. 107-2, respectively. The recommendations on route, site, and dosages for vaccination have been derived from theoretical considerations, experimental trials, and clinical experience; deviation from these recommendations can result in inadequate protection. The administration of doses at intervals longer than those recommended does not diminish the ultimate protective response but merely delays it. In contrast, giving vaccines at shorter-than-recommended intervals may result in poor responses. When a scheduled dose is missed, it is not necessary to restart from the beginning or to add an extra dose (www.cdc.gov/nip/recs/child-catchup.pdf).

RECORDING AND REPORTING REQUIREMENTS Certain aspects of vaccine use are regulated by the National Childhood Vaccine Injury Act (NCVIA) of 1986 (modified in 1995 and 2002). The act requires that all mandated childhood vaccinations be recorded by health care providers in the child's permanent medical record, including date of administration, manufacturer and lot number, and name of the provider administering the vaccine. State-based immunization information systems and electronic registries have been developed to help public and private providers manage their immunization activities and particularly to address the problem of assessing immunization coverage when an individual's records are divided among multiple medical facilities. By permitting active and targeted recall of children who are overdue for immunization and by providing data on immunization status at the time of an office visit, these systems improve vaccination rates and offer important public health benefits.

Parents must be informed about the benefits and risks of immunization and should maintain an up-to-date immunization record on their children. Educational materials providing the required information (Vaccine Information Statements) are available from the AAP or the Centers for Disease Control and Prevention (CDC; www.cdc.gov/nip/publications/vis/). The National Network for Immunization Informa-

tion website (www.immunizationinfo.org) is an excellent source of authoritative information for parents.

VACCINES FOR ROUTINE USE ■ Infants and Children (See Fig. 107-1 and www.cdc.gov/nip/recs/child-catchup.pdf) It is current practice for all children in the United States to receive DTaP, poliovirus, MMR, Hib, HepB, varicella, and pneumococcal conjugate vaccines unless there are specific contraindications. The administration of HepA vaccine is currently recommended when there is a special risk of exposure to infection due to residence in communities with elevated rates of hepatitis A or travel to highly endemic countries. Influenza vaccine is recommended for children 6 to 24 months of age, especially those who have certain risk factors or who reside with persons with certain chronic disorders. In several European countries, meningococcal C conjugate vaccine is routinely recommended.

Adults (See Fig. 107-2) Immunization recommendations for adults (>18 years old) fall into four categories: (1) routine vaccines for all adults; (2) vaccines for high-risk exposure groups (health care and other institutional workers, prisoners, students, military personnel, travelers to endemic areas, injection drug users, men who have sex with men); (3) vaccines for persons at high risk for severe outcomes of infection (pregnant women; the elderly; persons with chronic medical conditions, including diabetes, alcoholism, immunodeficiency, and renal, hepatic, respiratory, or cardiac disease); and (4) vaccines for household contacts of persons in group 3. A substantial proportion of adults in the United States no longer have protective levels of antibodies against tetanus or diphtheria. All adults who completed the pediatric series should be boosted with Td (adult formulation) every 10 years (once after age 50). If not previously immunized, however, adults require a primary immunizing course of Td. Young adults without laboratory evidence or a reliable history of past vaccination or disease should be immunized against measles, mumps, rubella, and varicella. A second dose of MMR vaccine is recommended for groups with a higher risk of exposure and for health care workers with certain other indications. Unless they have documented proof of immunity, rubella vaccine should be given to all nonpregnant women of childbearing age. Rubella-susceptible pregnant women should be vacci-

TABLE 107-5 Special Vaccines for Infants, Children, and Adults

Vaccine	Year Licensed	Type of Immunizing Agent	Route of Administration	Indications	Efficacy	Adverse Events
Anthrax	1970	Inactivated avirulent bacteria	SC (6 doses primary; annual booster)	For high risk of exposure (e.g., persons in contact with or involved in manufacture of animal hides, furs, bone meal, wool, goat hair) and military risk of biowarfare exposure	90% antibody response; efficacy uncertain	No serious adverse effects known
Tuberculosis (BCG)	1950	Living bacteria (attenuated *Mycobacterium bovis*)	ID	PPD-negative individuals in prolonged contact with active TB patients	Controversial, maximal for children <15 years	Regional adenitis, disseminated BCG in immunocompromised hosts
HepA	1995	Killed virus antigen	IM	Travelers or persons living in high-risk areas	94%	Local reactions, mild
Cholera	1914	Inactivated whole bacteria	SC or IM	Not recommended for public health use because of limited efficacy; two new vaccines licensed in Europe	?50% (short duration)	Frequent fever and local reactions, pain, swelling
Meningococcus A, C, Y, W-135	1981	Bacterial polysaccharides from 4 serotypes, not type B	SC	Military personnel; travelers to endemic areas; college students in dormitories	90% for 2- to 3-year olds	Rare
Plague	1994	Inactivated bacteria	IM	Laboratory workers; foresters in endemic areas; ? travelers	90% antibody response; efficacy uncertain	10% local reactions; rare sterile abscesses and hypersensitivity
Rabies (human diploid)	1980	Inactivated virus grown in cell culture	IM or ID	Travelers; laboratory workers; veterinarians	Virtually 100%	25% local reactions; 6% arthropathy, arthritis, angioedema
Yellow fever	1978	Live attenuated virus	SC	Laboratory workers	High	Encephalitis, encephalopathy, death
Japanese B encephalitis	1992	Inactivated virus	SC	Travelers to endemic areas	80–90%	Anaphylactic/severe delayed allergic reactions common; recipient should be observed for 10 days
Typhoid	1952	Heat- or phenol-killed bacteria	IM	Not routinely recommended in U.S.; used for travelers, contacts of carriers	50–70% (short duration)	Frequent fever, local swelling, pain
		Purified Vi polysaccharide	IM	Travelers	70–75%	Local reactions, mild
Lyme disease	1998	Recombinant outer-membrane protein	IM	For high risk of exposure to infected ticks	76% (3 doses)	Local reactions

Abbreviations: SC, subcutaneous; BCG, bacille Calmette-Guérin; PPD, purified protein derivative; TB, tuberculosis.

Source: Recommendations of the Advisory Committee on Immunization Practices, the American Academy of Pediatrics, and the American College of Physicians.

nated as early as possible in the postpartum period. Live-virus vaccines, such as MMR and varicella vaccines, are contraindicated in pregnant women and immunosuppressed individuals. Routine immunization against polio is not recommended for adults unless they are at particular risk of exposure because of travel to the remaining endemic areas. College students, particularly freshmen living at close quarters, are at increased risk of meningococcal meningitis and should be offered the meningococcal polysaccharide vaccine for serogroups A, C, Y, and W-135.

Current recommendations also include influenza vaccine for routine annual administration to individuals with chronic illness at any age, to persons living in the same household as chronically ill individuals, and to all adults >50 years of age. Polyvalent pneumococcal polysaccharide vaccine is similarly recommended for adults ≥65 years of age and for all chronically ill persons. HepB vaccine is recommended for individuals at high risk from clinical, occupational, behavioral, and travel exposures, including patients undergoing hemodialysis, routine recipients of clotting factors, health care workers exposed to potentially infected blood or blood products, individuals living and working in institutions for the mentally handicapped, travelers to highly endemic countries, persons at elevated risk for sexually transmitted diseases, injection drug users, and household contacts of known carriers of hepatitis B surface antigen. HepA vaccine is recommended for these same groups and for persons with clotting dis-

orders or chronic liver disease. There are a number of other special-use vaccines whose administration is related to travel and occupational exposures (e.g., Japanese B encephalitis, typhoid, yellow fever, rabies); specific recommendations for the use of these vaccines in the United States can be found at www.cdc.gov/nip.

Adverse Events Given the success of vaccination programs and the virtual disappearance of many vaccine-preventable diseases in the United States, concerns about vaccine safety have sometimes become inflated in conjunction with complacency about the consequences of infection. An *adverse reaction* or *vaccine side effect* is an untoward effect caused by a vaccine that is extraneous to its primary purpose (to produce immunity). In contrast, an *adverse event* can be either a true vaccine reaction or a coincidental event. A small number of highly publicized claims unsubstantiated by valid data have heightened the suspicion that some or all vaccines routinely cause unacceptable adverse events. Antivaccine advocacy groups actively encourage avoidance of immunization because of the unproven belief that vaccines can cause certain disorders (e.g., autism). Websites maintained by such groups commonly appear in the first 10 listings identified by search engines. This situation presents a challenge to physicians and public health officials who must educate parents about vaccine benefits and risks.

In fact, modern vaccines, while safe and effective, are associated with adverse events that range from infrequent and mild to rare and life-threatening. The decision to recommend the use of a vaccine involves an assessment of the risks of disease and the benefits and risks of vaccination. Because these factors may change over time, continual assessment of the balance between societal benefits and individual risks is essential. Valid and invalid contraindications to childhood immunization and appropriate precautions in the use of specific vaccines can be found at www.cdc.gov/nip/recs/contraindications.pdf.

Ironically, ongoing efforts to enhance vaccine safety through quality improvement and changes in vaccine policy (e.g., the decision to eliminate the mercury-based preservative thimerosol from vaccines) have actually led to an even greater awareness of the possible adverse events associated with routine vaccine administration. It has been claimed that increased rates of diabetes mellitus in the general pediatric population are due to an increase in exposure to vaccine antigens in childhood, although rigorous studies have refuted this hypothesis. A putative link of measles immunization to autism has been the subject of intense international controversy. The Institute of Medicine issued four recent reports whose findings (1) fail to support hypotheses that vaccines are associated with multiple sclerosis, neurodevelopmental disorders, or immune dysfunction; (2) provide no evidence for a temporal association of these conditions with vaccination; and (3) elucidate no biologically plausible basis for the purported relationships.

Within 9 months of the introduction of routine administration of the rhesus reassortant rotavirus vaccine (Rotashield) in the United States, cases of intussusception were reported by the CDC to be temporally associated with administration of the initial dose. This report led first to the cessation of the vaccine's use and subsequently to the withdrawal of the vaccine from the market and the discontinuation of its production. Although other analyses have failed to support the association, rotavirus vaccine has not been introduced into developing countries, where the risk of any real increase in intussusception would be dramatically outweighed by the benefit of decreased rotavirus mortality.

The ramifications of these events for future vaccine development and introduction have yet to be assessed. Vaccine components, including protective antigens, animal proteins introduced during vaccine production, and antibiotics or other preservatives or stabilizers, can certainly cause allergic reactions in some recipients. These reactions may be local or systemic and include urticaria and serious anaphylaxis. The most common extraneous allergen is egg protein introduced when vaccines such as those for measles, mumps, influenza, and yellow fever are prepared in embryonated eggs. Gelatin, which is used as a heat stabilizer, has been implicated in rare but severe allergic reactions. Local or systemic reactions (probably due to antigen-antibody complexes) can result from too-frequent administration of vaccines such as Td, diphtheria/tetanus vaccine, or rabies vaccine. Because live-virus vaccines can interfere with tuberculin test responses, necessary tuberculin testing should be done either on the day of immunization or at

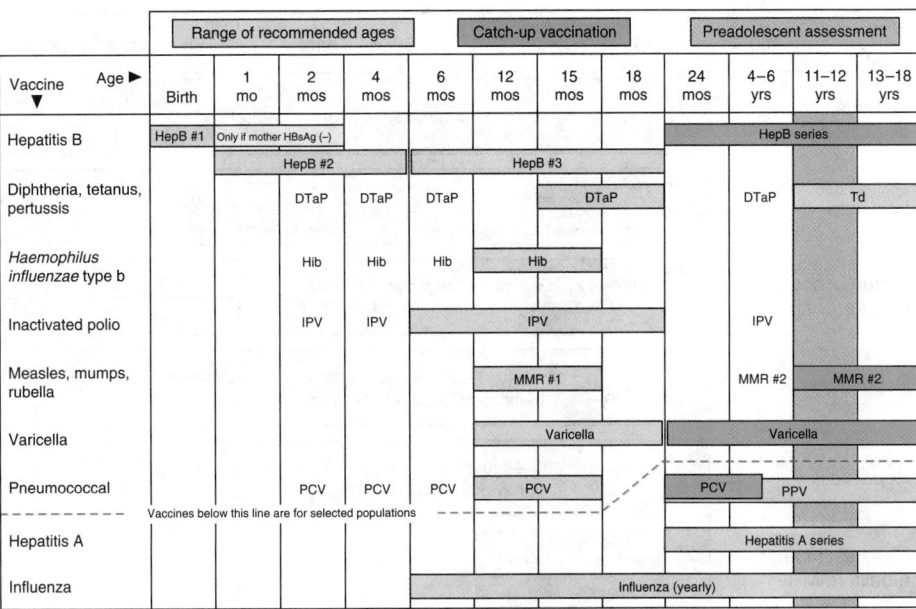

FIGURE 107-1 Recommended childhood and adolescent immunization schedule—United States, 2003. Any dose not given at the recommended age should be given at any subsequent time when indicated and feasible. Green bars indicate age groups that warrant special efforts to administer those vaccines not previously given. Infants born to mothers positive for hepatitis B surface antigen (HBsAg) should receive hepatitis B vaccine (HepB) and 0.5 mL of hepatitis B immune globulin (HBIG) at separate sites within 12 h of birth. The second dose of HepB is recommended at age 1 to 2 months. The last dose in the series should not be administered before age 6 months. Infants born to mothers whose HBsAg status is unknown should receive the first dose of the HepB series within 12 h of birth. The mother's HBsAg status should be tested as soon as possible; if positive, the infant should receive HBIG as soon as possible. The number of *Haemophilus influenzae* type b (Hib) conjugate vaccine doses depends on the vaccine used. PRP-OMP (PedvaxHIB or ComVax) is administered just twice: at ages 2 and 4 months. Diphtheria/tetanus/acellular pertussis (DtaP)/Hib combination products should not be used for primary immunization but can be used as boosters following a primary series with any Hib vaccine. Influenza vaccine is now recommended annually for children age ≥6 months with certain risk factors (including but not limited to asthma, cardiac disease, sickle cell disease, HIV infection, and diabetes mellitus) and household members of persons in groups at high risk; it can be administered to all others wishing to obtain immunity. If feasible, influenza vaccination of healthy children age 6 to 23 months is encouraged because of a substantially increased risk for influenza-related hospitalizations in this group. Children ≥12 years old should receive influenza vaccine in a dosage appropriate for their age. Children ≤8 years old who are receiving influenza vaccine for the first time should receive two doses separated by at least 4 weeks. Hepatitis A vaccine is recommended for children and adolescents in selected states and regions and for certain high-risk groups; hepatitis A immunization can begin during any visit, and the two doses should be administered at least 6 months apart. The heptavalent pneumococcal conjugate vaccine (PCV) is recommended for all children age 2 to 23 months. It is also recommended for certain children age 24 to 59 months. Pneumococcal polysaccharide vaccine (PPV) is recommended in addition to the conjugate vaccine for certain high-risk groups. Further information can be obtained via the National Immunization Program website (www.cdc.gov/nip) or at the National Immunization Information Hotline (800-232-2522 for English and 800-232-0233 for Spanish). MMR, measles/mumps/rubella vaccine; IPV, inactivated poliovirus vaccine; Td, tetanus and diphtheria toxoids, adsorbed, for adult use. (*Adapted from recommendations approved by the Advisory Committee on Immunization Practices, the American Academy of Pediatrics, and the American College of Family Physicians.*)

least 6 weeks later. When influenza vaccine is given to children <13 years old, only "split-virus" preparations should be used since whole-virus vaccines are associated with higher rates of adverse reactions in this age group.

The U.S. government conducts vaccine safety surveillance through a network of active and passive reporting. All detected adverse events whose occurrence is temporally related to vaccination must be reported to both the local health department and the vaccine manufacturer. For the purpose of postlicensure passive surveillance of vaccines, health care providers are required to report certain suspected adverse events following the administration of a mandated vaccine to the FDA's Vaccine Adverse Events Reporting System. The NCVIA has established criteria for reimbursable vaccine-related adverse events (www.hrsa.gov/osp/vicp/table.htm). Although a temporal relationship does not establish cause and effect, this surveillance system remains the only mechanism for collecting the data needed for analysis, conclusions, and decision-making. The CDC has established an active-surveillance system for ongoing evaluation of vaccine safety in large populations of vaccinated individuals. The Vaccine Safety Datalink is a population-based network in which four large health maintenance organizations (HMOs) continuously monitor immunization records linked to the medical records of 600,000 children <7 years of age. A

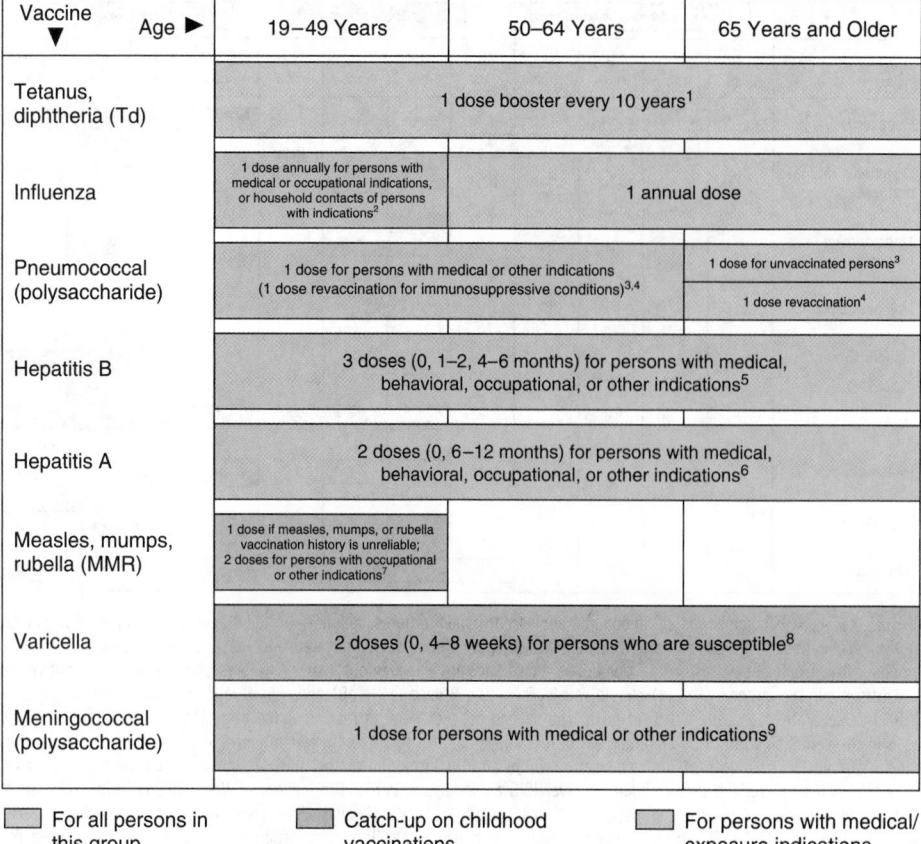

Vaccine ▼ / Age ▶	19–49 Years	50–64 Years	65 Years and Older
Tetanus, diphtheria (Td)	1 dose booster every 10 years[1]		
Influenza	1 dose annually for persons with medical or occupational indications, or household contacts of persons with indications[2]	1 annual dose	
Pneumococcal (polysaccharide)	1 dose for persons with medical or other indications (1 dose revaccination for immunosuppressive conditions)[3,4]		1 dose for unvaccinated persons[3]
			1 dose revaccination[4]
Hepatitis B	3 doses (0, 1–2, 4–6 months) for persons with medical, behavioral, occupational, or other indications[5]		
Hepatitis A	2 doses (0, 6–12 months) for persons with medical, behavioral, occupational, or other indications[6]		
Measles, mumps, rubella (MMR)	1 dose if measles, mumps, or rubella vaccination history is unreliable; 2 doses for persons with occupational or other indications[7]		
Varicella	2 doses (0, 4–8 weeks) for persons who are susceptible[8]		
Meningococcal (polysaccharide)	1 dose for persons with medical or other indications[9]		

☐ For all persons in this group   ▨ Catch-up on childhood vaccinations   ☐ For persons with medical/ exposure indications

FIGURE 107-2   Recommended adult immunization schedule—United States, 2002–2003. (1) *Tetanus and diphtheria (Td)*: A primary series for adults is 3 doses, with the first 2 doses at least 4 weeks apart and the third dose 6 to 12 months after the second. One dose suffices if a primary series was completed >10 years before. In addition to a teenage/young adult booster, adults >50 years of age who have completed the full series plus booster should receive one more dose. (2) *Influenza vaccination*: Indications include chronic cardiovascular or pulmonary disease, asthma, diabetes, renal disease, hemoglobinopathy, immunosuppression (due to medications or HIV infection), pregnancy (second or third trimester during the influenza season), health care employment, residence in a nursing home or another long-term-care facility, and high likelihood of transmitting influenza to those at high risk. (3) *Pneumococcal polysaccharide vaccination*: Indications include chronic cardiovascular or pulmonary disease (except asthma), diabetes, chronic liver disease, chronic renal failure or nephrotic syndrome, asplenia, immunosuppression, certain cancer chemotherapy, and long-term systemic glucocorticoid therapy. Vaccination is also indicated in Alaskan natives, certain Native American populations, and residents of nursing homes and other long-term-care facilities. (4) *Revaccination with pneumococcal polysaccharide vaccine*: One-time revaccination after age 5 is indicated for persons with chronic renal failure or nephrotic syndrome, asplenia, immunosuppression, certain cancer chemotherapy, or long-term systemic glucocorticoid therapy. Persons >65 years old should undergo one-time revaccination if their prior vaccination was at least 5 years before and was given before age 65. (5) *Hepatitis B vaccination*: Vaccination is indicated for hemodialysis patients, patients receiving clotting factor concentrates, health care workers and public safety workers exposed to blood, students in the health professions, injection drug users, persons with multiple sex partners within 6 months, patients with recent sexually transmitted disease (STD), clients of STD clinics, men who have sex with men, household contacts and sex partners of persons with chronic hepatitis B virus infection, clients and staff of institutions for the mentally disabled, inmates of correctional institutions, and international travelers to countries with high prevalence. (6) *Hepatitis A vaccination*: For the combined HepA/HepB vaccine, use 3 doses at 0, 1, and 6 months. Hepatitis A vaccination is indicated in persons with clotting factor disorders or chronic liver disease, men who have sex with men, users of injection and noninjection illegal drugs, persons working with hepatitis A virus–infected primates or working with the virus in a laboratory, and persons traveling to or working in countries with high prevalence. (7) *Measles/mumps/rubella vaccination (MMR)*: Measles component: Adults born before 1957 are considered immune to measles. Adults born after 1957 should have at least 1 dose of MMR vaccine barring a medical contraindication or documentation of prior immunization. A second dose is recommended for adults who have recently been exposed to measles in an outbreak setting, who have previously received killed measles vaccine, who were vaccinated with an unknown measles vaccine between 1963 and 1967, who are students at a college or university, who work in health care facilities, or who plan to travel internationally. *Mumps component*: 1 dose of MMR vaccine is adequate. *Rubella component*: 1 dose of MMR vaccine should be given to women whose history is unreliable, with counseling to avoid becoming pregnant for 4 weeks. The rubella immune status of women of childbearing age should be ascertained and counseling provided regarding congenital rubella. (8) *Varicella vaccination*: Vaccination is recommended for all persons without a reliable clinical history of varicella or serologic evidence of immunity, health care workers, family contacts of immunosuppressed persons, those who live or work in high-risk settings (teachers of young children, daycare workers, residents and staff members working in institutional settings), adolescents and adults living in households with children, and women who are not pregnant but intend to become pregnant in the future. (9) *Meningococcal vaccine, quadrivalent*: Vaccination should be considered for adults with terminal complement component deficiencies, those with anatomical or functional asplenia, college freshmen (especially those living in dormitories), and travelers to the "meningitis belt" in sub-Saharan Africa or to Mecca for the Hajj. High-risk persons can be revaccinated in 5 years. (*Adapted from recommendations approved by the Advisory Committee on Immunization Practices and accepted by the American College of Obstetricians and Gynecologists and the American Academy of Family Physicians.*)

similar system is in place for immunized adult members of four HMOs.

USE OF VACCINES IN SPECIAL CIRCUMSTANCES

■ **Influenza Pandemic Preparedness**   Influenza pandemics occur at irregular intervals and are characterized by excess deaths, hospitalizations, public concern, and social and economic disruption. A National Preparedness Plan has been developed to assess the incidence of disease and the antigenic characteristics of the prevalent strain and to promote flexibility in vaccine manufacture and vaccination. This plan is based on enhancement of current capacities for virologic surveillance, disease surveillance, and emergency medical responses.

Pregnancy   Because of the theoretical risk to the fetus and the real risk of litigation to the practitioner, routine immunization of pregnant women is best avoided. However, wherever hygienic conditions during delivery cannot be guaranteed, it is essential to ensure that pregnant women are immune to tetanus because the transfer of maternal antitoxin is an important means of preventing neonatal tetanus. Pregnant women can safely receive tetanus as well as diphtheria toxoids. Live-virus vaccines, such as rubella, measles, mumps, and varicella, should be withheld during pregnancy. However, if the risk of exposure is great, polio and yellow fever vaccines may be safely administered. If indicated, some inactivated vaccines (e.g., HepB, influenza, and pneumococcal vaccines) may be given during the second and third trimesters of pregnancy (Fig. 107-3).

Breast Feeding   Neither killed nor live vaccine affects the safety of breast feeding for either mother or infant. Breastfed infants can be immunized on a normal schedule.

Occupational Exposure   Immunization recommendations for most occupational groups remain to be developed. Specific practices are now mandated by the Occupational Safety and Health Administration for the immunization of health care workers against hepatitis B in the United States. Rubella is transmitted to and from health care workers in medical facilities, particularly in pediatric practice. Health care workers who might transmit rubella to pregnant patients should be immune to rubella; it is prudent to screen these employees for antibodies to rubella virus and to immunize susceptible individuals. Persons providing health care are also at greater risk from measles and varicella than the general public, and those who are likely to come into contact with measles- and varicella-infected patients should be immune. Persons employed in caring for patients with chronic diseases can transmit influenza; such workers should be vaccinated annually.

HIV Infection and Other Immunocompromised States
Limited studies in HIV-infected individuals have found no increase in the risk of adverse events from live or inactivated vaccines. However, immune responses may not be as vigorous in immunocompromised individuals as in those with a normal immune system. Persons known to be infected with HIV should be immunized with recommended vaccines in the same manner as individuals with a normal immune system and as early in the course of their disease as possible, before immune function becomes significantly impaired (Fig. 107-3). Live attenuated MMR vaccine can be administered to this group. When vaccination against polio is indicated, IPV should be administered to immunocompromised HIV-infected individuals and to their household contacts. Albeit prudent, it is not necessary in practice to test for HIV before making decisions about the immunization of asymptomatic individuals from known HIV risk groups.

Live attenuated vaccines are also contraindicated in other immunocompromised patients, including those with congenital immunodeficiency syndromes and those receiving immunosuppressive therapy. Passive immunization with immunoglobulin preparations or antitoxins can be considered in individual cases, either as postexposure prophylaxis or as part of the treatment of established infection.

Postexposure Immunization
For certain infections, active or passive immunization soon after exposure prevents or attenuates disease expression. Recommended postexposure immunization regimens are compiled in Table 107-6. Measles immune globulin given within 6 days of exposure may prevent or modify infection, and measles vaccine given within the first few days after exposure may prevent symptomatic infection. Although clinical manifestations of rubella in pregnant women are minimized by postexposure passive immunization, this approach may not prevent maternal viremia, fetal infection, and congenital rubella syndrome. Therefore, the administration of immune globulin is recommended only for women developing rubella during pregnancy who will not consider abortion under any circumstances. Proper immunization for tetanus plays an important role in wound management. The need for active immunization—with or without passive immunization—depends on the condition of the wound and the patient's immunization history (Table 107-7). Rarely have cases of tetanus occurred in persons with a documented primary series of tetanus toxoid. Tetanus immune globulin is useful in patients with tetanus. Survivors with no history of tetanus immunization should receive a primary series of toxoid since disease does not produce protective levels of antitoxin. Administration of rabies immune globulin plus rabies vaccine in the immediate postexposure period is highly effective in preventing disease. Similarly, for persons who have not been actively immunized, the use of hepatitis A immune globulin within 2 weeks of exposure to hepatitis A is likely to prevent clinical illness. Sound data indicate the efficacy of human hepatitis B immune globulin in preventing disease after exposure. While no high-titer preparation is available for postexposure protection against non-A, non-B hepatitis, standard human immune serum globulin is efficacious.

Simultaneous Administration of Multiple Vaccines
There are no contraindications to the simultaneous administration of several vaccines. The use of combination vaccines can potentially reduce the required number of injections from 9 to 3 during a child's first 6 months of life and from 21 to 13 during the first 2 years. Simultaneous administration of the most widely used live and inactivated vaccines has not resulted in impaired antibody responses or in increased rates of adverse reactions. Moreover, this approach increases the probability that a child will ultimately be fully immunized. Simultaneous administration is useful in any age group when the potential exists for exposure to multiple infectious diseases during travel to endemic countries. Combination DTaP/Hib vaccines should not be used for primary immunization of infants because the result is a blunted, suboptimal response to Hib; however, the combination may be used for booster immunizations.

Medical conditions ▼ / Vaccine ▶	Tetanus-Diphtheria (Td)	Influenza	Pneumococcal (Polysaccharide)	Hepatitis B	Hepatitis A	Measles, Mumps, Rubella (MMR)	Varicella
Pregnancy		A					
Diabetes, heart disease, chronic pulmonary disease, chronic liver disease, including chronic alcoholism		B	C		D		
Congenital immunodeficiency, leukemia, lymphoma, generalized malignancy, therapy with alkylating agents, antimetabolites, radiation or large amounts of glucocorticoids			E				F
Renal failure/end stage renal disease, recipients of hemodialysis or clotting factor concentrates			E	G			
Asplenia (including elective splenectomy) and terminal complement component deficiencies			E, H, I				
HIV infection			E, J			K	

Legend: □ For all persons in this group □ Catch-up on childhood vaccinations ▨ For persons with medical/exposure indications ▧ Contraindicated

FIGURE 107-3 Recommended immunizations for adults with medical conditions—United States, 2002–2003. **A.** Vaccine may be given if pregnancy is at second or third trimester during influenza season. **B.** Although chronic liver disease and alcoholism are not indicator conditions for influenza vaccination, give 1 dose annually if the patient is ≥50 years old, has other indications for influenza vaccine, or requests vaccination. **C.** Asthma is an indicator condition for influenza vaccination but not for pneumococcal vaccination. **D.** Vaccinate all persons with chronic liver disease. **E.** Revaccinate once after ≥5 years have elapsed since initial vaccination. **F.** Persons with impaired humoral (but not cellular) immunity may be vaccinated [*MMWR* 1999; 48 (RR-06), 1–5]. **G.** *Hemodialysis patients:* Use special formulation of vaccine (40 μg/mL) or two 1.0-mL, 20-μg doses given at one site. Vaccinate early in the course of renal disease. Assess antibody titers to hepatitis B surface antigen annually; administer additional doses if titers decline to <10 mIU/mL. **H.** Also administer meningococcal vaccine. **I.** In persons undergoing elective splenectomy, vaccinate at least 2 weeks before surgery. **J.** Vaccinate as close to diagnosis as possible, when CD4+ cell counts are highest. **K.** Withhold MMR or other measles-containing vaccines from HIV-infected persons with evidence of severe immunosuppression [*MMWR* 1996; 45, 603–606; *MMWR* 1992; 41 (RR-17), 1–19]. (Approved by the Advisory Committee on Immunization Practices and accepted by the American College of Obstetricians and Gynecologists and the American Academy of Family Physicians.)

Disease	Indicated	Comments
Measles	Yes	Standard human immune globulin is recommended for exposed infants and adults with normal immunocompetence (but with a contraindication to measles vaccine) and for immunocompromised patients exposed to measles (regardless of immunization status). Patients should be actively immunized 3 to 6 months after immunoglobulin administration. Recommended dose: 0.25–0.50 mL/kg (40–80 mg of IgG/kg) IM; 80 mg of IgG/kg for immunocompromised contact; maximum, 15 mL.
Rubella	No	Efficacy is unreliable; therefore, standard human immune globulin is recommended for administration only to antibody-negative pregnant women in the first trimester who have a documented rubella exposure and will not consider terminating the pregnancy. Recommended dose is 0.55 mL/kg (90 mg of IgG/kg) IM.
Tetanus	Yes	Human tetanus immune globulin (TIG) has replaced equine tetanus antitoxin because of the risk of serum sickness with equine serum. Recommended dose for postexposure prophylaxis is 250–500 units of TIG (10–20 mg of IgG/kg) IM. Recommended dose for treatment of tetanus is 3000–6000 units of TIG IM.
Rabies	Yes	Human rabies immune globulin (RIG) is preferred over equine rabies antiserum because of the risk of serum sickness with equine serum. RIG or antiserum is recommended for nonimmunized individuals with animal bites in whom rabies cannot be ruled out and with other exposures to known rabid animals. Recommended dose of RIG is 20 IU/kg (22 mg of IgG/kg). Recommended dose of antiserum is 40 IU/kg. Rabies vaccine is given as well at 0, 3, 7, 14, and 28 days.
Hepatitis A	Yes	Standard immune serum globulin is given in a single dose of 0.02–0.04 mL/kg or (for continuous exposure) in a dose up to 0.06 mL/kg every 5 months. Postexposure treatment with hepatitis A immune globulin has not been studied.

When live-virus vaccines are not given together on the same day, an interval of at least 30 days should be allowed.

Because high doses of immune globulin may inhibit the efficacy of measles and rubella vaccines, an interval of at least 3 months is recommended between the administration of immune globulin and that of MMR vaccine or its components. Postpartum vaccination of rubella-susceptible women should not be delayed because of the administration of anti-Rho(D) immune globulin or any other blood product during the last trimester or at delivery. Should administration of an immune globulin preparation become necessary after vaccination, it should be postponed, if possible, for at least 14 days to allow time for vaccine-virus replication and development of immunity. In general, there is little interaction of immune globulin with inactivated vaccines, and postexposure passive prophylaxis can be given together with HepB vaccine or tetanus toxoid, resulting in both immediate and long-lasting protection.

Travel (See also Chap. 108) The International Sanitary Regulations allow countries to impose requirements for yellow fever and killed cholera vaccines as a condition for admission, even though the latter is not an effective public health tool. Travelers should know whether these vaccines are required for entry into the countries on their itinerary to avoid being turned back or immunized on the spot, with the inherent danger of unsafe injections. Infants, children, and adults should have all routine immunizations updated before traveling, with particular attention to polio, measles, and DTP/DTaP or Td vaccines. The use of HepA vaccine may be advisable for travelers to some locales. Special-use vaccines (Table 107-5), including rabies, meningococcal polysaccharide, typhoid, Japanese B encephalitis, and plague vaccines, should be considered for those individuals who expect to go beyond the usual tourist routes or to spend extended periods in rural areas in disease-endemic regions. Most U.S. cities have travel clinics that maintain up-to-date epidemiologic information and can provide the appropriate vaccines. The CDC also maintains a website for travelers (www.cdc.gov/travel).

DELIVERY OF VACCINES Over the past 25 years, considerable progress has been made to ensure that every child in the United States is fully immunized by the time of school entry. All 50 states now require immunization for school entry, and most have laws addressing attendance at preschools and day-care centers. Despite the dramatic impact of immunization and of other improvements in the health care provided to the American population on the incidence of vaccine-preventable illness (Table 107-1), many children are not fully immunized—both in poor communities (as a result of inadequate health services) and in affluent communities (where parental concern about potential adverse events may exceed concern about now-uncommon diseases). The failure to vaccinate preschool children was largely responsible for the resurgence of measles in the United States between 1989 and 1991, with >55,000 cases and >130 measles-related deaths. Outbreaks of pertussis, mumps, and congenital rubella syndrome have occurred wherever immunization rates among preschool children are low. While measles (36 cases in 2002) and rubella (14 cases in 2002) have reached historic lows, the risk of imported infection and spread to susceptibles persists.

ACCESS TO IMMUNIZATION Four major barriers to infant and childhood immunization have been identified within the health care system: (1) low public awareness and lack of public demand for immunization, (2) inadequate access to immunization services, (3) missed opportunities to administer vaccines, and (4) inadequate resources for public health and preventive programs. These problems are sources of public concern, and their solution must be a priority for national health policy in the United States. At the national level, outreach and educational campaigns promote parental awareness of the value of vaccination and encourage health care providers to use every opportunity to vaccinate the children in their care. At the state and local levels, community and business groups, religious and service groups, schools, and the media have joined together in community-based networks. Those who remain unvaccinated do so largely because health care practices and providers do not always perform optimally in delivering vaccines. The AFIX Program (*A*ssessment of coverage, *F*eedback of diagnostic information, *I*ncentives or recognition, and e*X*change of information among providers) is one effort by the CDC to change the attitude of health care personnel who lack an appreciation of low immunization rates in their practices to one of awareness, concern, and knowledge. The CDC has also developed two approaches to immunization assessment: CASA (Clinic Assessment Software Application) and LQA (Lot Quality Assessment). CASA requires review of up to 200 immunization records to assess whether record keeping and documentation are adequate, whether children start their vaccine series on time, whether and when patients drop out of the system, whether recall is used effectively, and whether vaccines are given simultaneously. LQA requires the review of only 30 records and does not yield a precise immunization rate or a diagnosis of the problem. A National Immunization Week each April has been established to focus attention on the vac-

TABLE 107-7 *Tetanus Wound Management*

Vaccination History	Clean, Minor Wounds		All Other Wounds	
	Td	TIG	Td	TIG
Unknown or <3 doses	Yes	No	Yes	Yes
3 doses	No[a]	No	No[b]	No

[a] Yes, if >10 years since last dose.
[b] Yes, if >5 years since last dose.

Pediatric Practice
1. Immunization services are readily available.
2. There are no barriers to or unnecessary prerequisites for the receipt of vaccines.
3. Immunization services are available free or for a minimal fee.
4. Providers use all clinical encounters to screen and, when indicated, immunize children.
5. Providers educate parents and guardians about immunization in general terms.
6. Providers question parents or guardians about contraindications and, before immunizing a child, inform them in specific terms about the risks and benefits of the immunizations their child is to receive.
7. Providers follow only true contraindications.
8. Providers administer simultaneously all vaccine doses for which a child is eligible at the time of each visit.
9. Providers use accurate and complete recording procedures.
10. Providers coschedule immunization appointments in conjunction with appointments for other child health services.
11. Providers report adverse events following immunization promptly, accurately, and completely.
12. Providers operate a tracking system.
13. Providers adhere to appropriate procedures for vaccine management.
14. Providers conduct semiannual audits to assess immunization coverage levels and to review immunization records for the patient populations they serve.
15. Providers maintain up-to-date, easily retrievable medical protocols at all locations where vaccines are administered.
16. Providers operate with patient-oriented and community-based approaches.
17. Vaccines are administered by properly trained individuals.
18. Providers receive ongoing education and training on current immunization recommendations.

Adult Practice
1. Appropriate vaccine use is promoted through information campaigns for health care practitioners and trainees, employers, and the public about the benefits of immunizations.
2. Providers are completely immunized to protect themselves and prevent transmission to patients.
3. Providers routinely determine the immunization status of their adult patients, offer vaccines to those for whom they are indicated, and maintain complete immunization records.
4. Providers identify high-risk patients in need of influenza vaccine and develop a system to recall them for annual immunization.
5. Providers and institutions identify high-risk adult patients in hospitals and other treatment centers and ensure that appropriate vaccination is considered either before discharge or as part of discharge planning.
6. Licensing/accreditation agencies support the development by health care institutions of comprehensive immunization programs for staff, trainees, volunteer workers, inpatients, and outpatients.
7. States establish preenrollment immunization requirements for colleges and other institutions of higher learning.
8. Institutions that train health care professionals, deliver health care, or provide laboratory or other medical support services require appropriate immunizations for persons at risk of contracting or transmitting vaccine-preventable diseases.
9. Health care benefit programs, third-party payers, and government health care programs provide coverage for adult immunization services.
10. A standard personal and institutional immunization record is adopted as a means of verifying the immunization status of patients and staff.

cination needs of infants and children. To improve the quality and quantity of vaccination services, expanded immunization-clinic hours and computerization of immunization records have been implemented as well. State-mandated school-entry immunity requirements have also helped to raise population immunity.

Although special vaccination target groups (e.g., college students, military personnel, and health care workers) have been successfully immunized, there has been only modest progress toward immunization goals for older adults in the United States. As many as 60,000 adults

die each year of vaccine-preventable diseases for which effective vaccines are not being optimally used. More than 30% of persons >65 years of age do not receive influenza vaccine each year, and even fewer have ever received pneumococcal vaccine. Health care providers more often miss vaccination opportunities with adults than with infants and children. From 60 to 90% of adults hospitalized for or dying of influenza-associated respiratory disease have received medical care during the previous year and could have been immunized at that time. Medicare reimbursement for excess hospitalization during influenza epidemics ranges from $750 million to $1 billion. Additional efforts are required to ensure that adults receive Td and HepB vaccines as well.

A special setting for adult immunization is the administration of certain vaccines (e.g., tetanus toxoid) to pregnant women to enhance passive immunity in their offspring. In most cases, the mother herself derives important benefits as well. Immunization of the mother should be undertaken at least 6 weeks before delivery to allow for efficient transplacental transfer of antibody to the fetus.

Recent childhood vaccine shortages in the United States have prompted federal authorities to recommend deferring some vaccinations and have caused states to reduce vaccination requirements. Efforts to resolve supply-and-demand issues have yielded plans to increase national stockpiles of vaccines.

HANDLING OF VACCINES Vaccines must be handled and stored with care. Vaccines should be kept at 2° to 8°C and, with the exception of varicella vaccine, should not be frozen. Varicella should be kept frozen at −15°C. Measles vaccine must be protected from light, which inactivates the virus.

STANDARDS FOR IMMUNIZATION PRACTICE National standards of immunization for adult and pediatric practice have been established to define common policies and practices for public health clinics and physicians' private offices (Table 107-8). These standards highlight the need to distinguish between valid contraindications and conditions that are often considered to be but are not in fact contraindications (www.cdc.gov/nip/recs/contraindications.pdf). Among the valid contraindications applicable to all vaccines are a history of anaphylaxis or other serious allergic reactions to a vaccine or vaccine component and the presence of a moderate or severe illness, with or without fever. Infants who develop encephalopathy within 72 h of a dose of DTP or DTaP should not receive further doses; those who develop a "precaution" should not normally receive further doses. Because of theoretical risks to the fetus, pregnant women should not receive MMR or varicella vaccine. Diarrhea, minor respiratory illness (with or without fever), mild to moderate local reactions to a previous dose of vaccine, the concurrent or recent use of antimicrobial agents, mild to moderate malnutrition, and the convalescent phase of an acute illness are not valid contraindications to routine immunization. Failure to vaccinate children because of these conditions is increasingly viewed as a missed opportunity for immunization.

THE NATIONAL VACCINE INJURY COMPENSATION PROGRAM The use of mandated vaccines benefits society as a whole by reducing morbidity and the cost of care for preventable diseases and by reducing childhood mortality. Thus, in the United States, society has assumed the obligation to care for those injured by the administration of mandated vaccines. The NCVIA of 1986 (modified in 1995 and 2002) is the instrument in use to ensure both fairness to injured persons and protection for federal, state, and local immunization programs; private immunization providers; and vaccine manufacturers. The act was designed to implement two vital public policies: (1) to provide prompt and fair compensation to the families of children who have died or have been injured as a result of routine mandated immunization; and (2) to reduce the adverse impact of the tort system on vaccine supply, cost, and innovation/development. The success of immunization programs in the United States depends upon the continued viability of the National Vaccine Injury Compensation Program.

CONTROL OF VACCINE-PREVENTABLE DISEASE

A continuing task of public health practice is to maintain individual and herd immunity. The job is not over once a population is fully vaccinated; rather, it is imperative to immunize each subsequent generation as long as the threat of the reintroduction of the disease from anywhere in the world persists. Ongoing surveillance and prompt reporting of disease to local or state health departments are essential to this goal, ensuring a continuing awareness of the possibility of vaccine-preventable illness. Nearly all vaccine-preventable diseases are notifiable, and individual case data are routinely forwarded to the CDC. These data are used to detect outbreaks or other unusual events that require investigation and to evaluate prevention and control policies, practices, and strategies.

RESEARCH ON VACCINES AND IMMUNIZATION

The potential to eliminate selected diseases and to build sustainable immunization programs that reach every child is not being fulfilled with existing vaccines and delivery technology. New vaccines or new formulations that will not only improve protective responses but also simplify the immunization schedule are needed. The ideal would be vaccines that can be administered orally early in life, that provide lifelong protection against multiple infections, that can be given as one or only a few doses, and that are less reactive and more heat stable than current vaccines. Diseases for which safe and effective vaccines have not been achieved represent the more difficult immunologic challenges and mark the frontiers of vaccine development. To attain these ambitious goals may take decades. However, progress is already being made in combining current vaccines to facilitate complete immunization, and prototypes of new vaccines are being assessed in early clinical trials. The results will be applicable to immunization programs in both developed and developing countries.

REEMERGENCE OF CONTROLLED DISEASE AND EMERGENCE OF NEW DISEASE

The emergence of new pathogens is fostered by the genetic potential of microbes to evolve and exchange genetic material as well as by rapid changes in human demographics and behavior and in global ecology that create new or more favorable niches and hosts. Proof of the need for continuing vaccine research is provided by the emergence of new infectious diseases, including HIV infection, Lyme borreliosis, hantavirus pulmonary syndrome, hepatitis C, and—most recently—the severe acute respiratory syndrome (SARS) caused by a coronavirus; the sudden outbreak of epidemic cholera due to a previously unknown serotype (O139 Bengal); and the increase in global incidence and drug resistance of familiar diseases that were once considered under control (e.g., tuberculosis and malaria). In addition, some common illnesses without a previously known etiology, such as peptic ulcer disease and cervical and nasopharyngeal cancer, have now been epidemiologically linked to specific infectious agents and thus, by definition, are vaccine-preventable conditions.

NEW VACCINE APPROACHES   The first generation of vaccines included whole killed bacteria, partially purified microbial products that induced protective antibodies (e.g., tetanus and diphtheria toxoids), or live attenuated microorganisms. The second generation of vaccines has taken advantage of molecular genetics and protein chemistry: purified proteins or subunits of organisms have been isolated and manipulated, and genetically engineered and attenuated live native organisms have been generated, as have cloned antigens expressed by harmless vector organisms. One conceptual leap is the production of edible transgenic plants (e.g., potatoes, bananas) that express protective vaccine antigens (as a result of insertion of the relevant microbial genes) and that, when eaten, induce mucosal and systemic immune responses to homologous infectious challenges. While the practical use of this technique awaits further refinement, the concept that protective immunity can be induced in this manner has been proved in both animals and humans. Ease of production, stability, ease of administration without equipment, and low cost are the obvious advantages.

TABLE 107-9 *Advantages and Disadvantages of DNA Vaccines*

Advantages	Disadvantages
Safe; cannot cause infection; stable and heat resistant	Potential risk of integration of viral genes from the vector
No need to express or purify antigens in vitro; no need for adjuvants; can be genetically engineered	Tumor promotion from integration near proto-oncogenes or tumor suppressor genes
Normal processing of gene product closely resembling native conformation	Possible induction of tolerance or autoimmunity by vaccine persistence
Persistence for prolonged periods; induction of durable immune response	Possible influence of strong promoters on expression of host genes, with adverse consequences
Induction of both humoral and cell-mediated immunity, including cytotoxic T cells	
Likely to be safe in pregnant women, immunosuppressed patients, or (in the presence of maternal antibody) infants	

Another conceptual leap has led to a third generation of vaccines, in which nucleic acids (either DNA or RNA) are used to induce immunity. The principle is simple and offers many advantages (Table 107-9). First, a DNA plasmid containing the gene sequence for the immunogenic protein or fragment of interest is assembled and placed under the control of a strong promoter and an appropriate transcription termination sequence. A single immunization with the plasmid by a number of possible routes results in DNA uptake into cells, where the gene is expressed and processed normally. The resulting protein product of the vaccine DNA induces an immune response. It should be possible to manipulate the DNA construct, its mode of administration, or the coadministration of cytokine genes to drive a T_H1, T_H2, or cytotoxic T cell response that optimizes the protective immune response. Recently, a technique known as *prime-boost* has been used to convert antibody responses to an antigen into cell-mediated responses. In prime-boost, a priming dose—most often naked DNA encoding the antigen of interest—is followed at the optimal interval by the same DNA inserted into a viral vector (e.g., the modified vaccinia virus vector MVA). DNA vaccines may be particularly useful for the induction of tumor immunity, for the treatment of allergy by suppression of IgE production, or for gene therapy. Because RNA is less stable and does not persist or integrate into the chromosome or result in insertional mutagenesis, the value of RNA vaccines would be to diminish concerns about adverse events associated with the effects of DNA integration into the chromosome (Table 107-9). These virtues of RNA paradoxically represent the hurdles to overcome in producing stable, inexpensive, and effective RNA vaccines.

INTERNATIONAL CONSIDERATIONS

Since the establishment of the Expanded Programme on Immunization (EPI) by the World Health Organization (WHO) in 1981 and the involvement of UNICEF in the program's implementation, levels of coverage for the recommended basic children's vaccines (bacille Calmette-Guérin, poliomyelitis, DTP/DTaP, and measles) have risen from 5 to ~80% worldwide, although coverage does not necessarily translate into protective immunity. Each year, at least 2.7 million deaths from measles, neonatal tetanus, and pertussis and 200,000 cases of paralysis due to polio are prevented by immunization. Despite the successes of this program, many vaccine-preventable diseases remain prevalent in the developing world. Measles, for example, continues to kill an estimated 800,000 children each year, and diphtheria, whooping cough, polio, and neonatal tetanus still occur at unacceptably high rates. An estimated 20 to 35% of all deaths of children <5 years old are still associated with vaccine-preventable diseases.

In addition to the antigens included in the EPI for routine use in the developing world, others (hepatitis B, Hib, Japanese B encephalitis, yellow fever, meningococcus, mumps, and rubella) are used regionally, depending on disease epidemiology and resources. The rationale for inclusion of HepB vaccine in Africa and Asia is to prevent the subsequent development of hepatocellular carcinoma, which is strongly linked with the persistence of HBV from early childhood. The delivery of vaccines in mass campaigns on national immunization days, superseding even civil wars and insurgencies, has resulted in the cessation of transmission of poliomyelitis and the virtual elimination of clinical measles from the Western Hemisphere. Periodic vaccination campaigns complement routine infant and childhood vaccination services under the rubric "catch up, follow up, and keep up." Despite these successes, ongoing concerns remain about inadequate long-term strategies to ensure continuity, the impact of vaccine campaigns on the provision of routine services, and unsafe injection practices.

Because infectious diseases know no geographic or political boundaries, uncontrolled disease anywhere in the world poses a threat to the United States, even without the threat of bioterrorism (Chap. 205). Although the expectation of eradicating infectious agents and ceasing immunization altogether no longer seems realistic, vaccines offer the opportunity to effectively control and even eliminate some diseases through individual and herd protection. Vaccines also represent the best societal hope for stopping the pandemic of HIV infection throughout the world and efficiently controlling malaria and tuberculosis. Issues of cost, liability, risk, and profitability limit the interest of the pharmaceutical industry in the development of vaccines (e.g., for malaria) that will be used primarily in poor developing countries. Global recognition of the powerful effect that vaccines have on reduction of the disease burden has led to the creation of the Global Alliance for Vaccines and Immunization, which coordinates partnerships in public research and privately funded vaccine development. WHO, UNICEF, and other organizations (such as the International AIDS Vaccine Initiative, Rotary International, the Bill and Melinda Gates Foundation, and the Rockefeller Foundation) have helped to move the process forward with new strategies, investment in development, and implementation or with new funding for basic research. New international collaborations are being considered by wealthy industrial nations to attract increasing interest from the private sector—for example, advance-purchase schemes in which the purchase of effective vaccines is guaranteed, ensuring the profitability that the marketplace has provided for industry in wealthy countries. The effectiveness of such approaches remains to be seen, but they offer much-needed hope for at-risk populations around the world.

SOURCES OF INFORMATION ON IMMUNIZATION

- Official vaccine package circulars and Vaccine Administration Statements from the CDC
- Report of the Committee on Infectious Diseases of the American Academy of Pediatrics ("Red Book")
- Recommendations of the Advisory Committee on Immunization Practices, CDC
- Guide for Adult Immunization, American College of Physicians
- Health Information for International Travel (published yearly) and Advisory Memoranda on Travel (published periodically), CDC
- Control of Communicable Diseases in Man, American Public Health Association
- Technical Bulletin of the College of Obstetrics and Gynecology
- National Network for Immunization Information, Infectious Diseases Society of America/Pediatric Infectious Diseases Society/American Academy of Pediatrics/American Nurses Association

FURTHER READING

AVERY RK: Immunizations in adult immunocompromised patients: Which to use and which to avoid. Cleve Clin J Med 68:337, 2001

DENNEHY PH: Active immunization in the United States: Developments over the past decade. Clin Microbiol Rev 14:872, 2001

HINMAN A: Eradication of vaccine-preventable diseases. Annu Rev Public Health 20:211, 1999

KELLER MA, STIEHM ER: Passive immunity in prevention and treatment of infectious diseases. Microbiol Rev 13:602, 2000

MAHONEY RT, MAYNARD JE: The introduction of new vaccines into developing countries. Vaccine 17:646, 1999

MUNOZ FM, ENGLUND JA: Vaccines in pregnancy. Infect Dis Clin North Am 15:253, 2001

PETER G, GARDNER P: Standards for immunization practice for vaccines in children and adults. Infect Dis Clin North Am 15:9, 2001

WILSON ME: Travel-related vaccines. Infect Dis Clin North Am 15:231, 2001

WEBSITES OF INTEREST: www.cdc.gov/nip; www.idsociety.org/vaccine/resources; www.immunizationinfo.org; www.genweb.com/Dnavax/dnavax

ZIMMERMAN RK, BALL JA: Adult vaccinations. Prim Care 28:763, 2001

108 | HEALTH ADVICE FOR INTERNATIONAL TRAVEL
J.S. Keystone, P.E. Kozarsky

According to the World Tourism Organization, the number of international tourist arrivals in 2001 amounted to 693 million—the highest figure ever documented. Not only are more people traveling; travelers are seeking more exotic and remote destinations. In 1999, more than 75 million people traveled from industrialized to developing countries; this figure represents a 50% increase from 1993. Studies show that between 50 and 75% of short-term travelers to the tropics or subtropics report some health impairment. Most of these health problems are minor, with only 5% requiring medical attention and fewer than 1% requiring hospitalization. Although infectious agents contribute substantially to morbidity among travelers, these pathogens account for only ~1% of deaths in this population. Cardiovascular disease and injuries are the most frequent causes of death among travelers from the United States, accounting for 49 and 22% of deaths, respectively. Age-specific rates of death due to cardiovascular disease are similar among travelers and nontravelers. In contrast, rates of death due to injury (the majority from motor vehicle, drowning, or aircraft accidents) are several times higher among travelers. Figure 108-1 summarizes the monthly incidence of health problems during travel in developing countries.

GENERAL ADVICE

Staying healthy during travel requires familiarity with the various health risks that may be encountered at a given destination. However, health maintenance recommendations are based not only on the traveler's destination but also on risk assessment, which is determined by health status, specific itinerary, and lifestyle during travel. Detailed information regarding country-specific risks and recommendations may be obtained from the Centers for Disease Control and Prevention (CDC) publication *Health Information for International Travel* (www.cdc.gov/travel).

Fitness for travel is an issue of growing concern in view of the increased numbers of elderly and chronically ill individuals journeying to exotic destinations (see "Travel and Special Hosts," below). Since most commercial aircraft are pressurized to 2500 m (8000 ft) above sea level (corresponding to a Pa_{O_2} of ~55 mmHg), individuals with serious cardiopulmonary problems should be evaluated before travel. In addition, those who have recently had surgery, a myocardial infarction, a cerebrovascular accident, or a deep-vein thrombosis (among other events) may be at high risk for adverse events in flight. A summary of current recommendations regarding fitness to fly has been

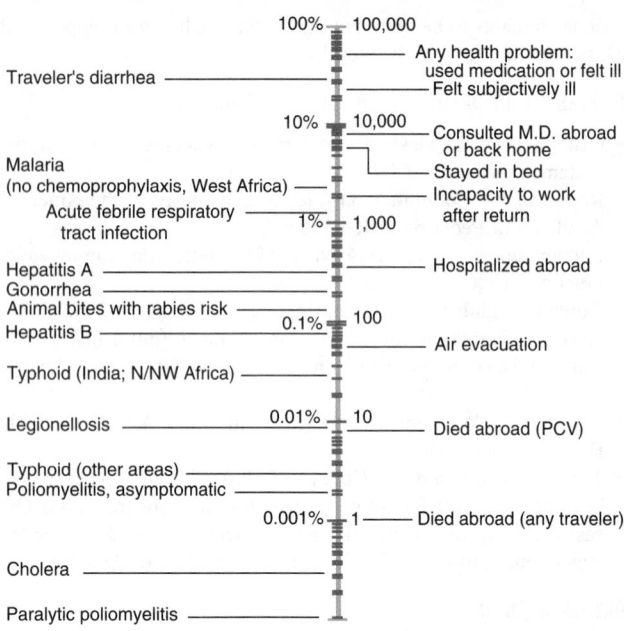

FIGURE 108-1   Incidence rate, per month, of health problems during a stay in developing countries. PCV, Peace Corps volunteer. (*From Steffen R, Lobel HO: Epidemiologic basis for the practice of travel medicine. J Wilderness Med 5:56, 1994. Reprinted with permission from Chapman and Hall, New York.*)

published by the Aerospace Medical Association Air Transport Medical Committee. A pretravel health assessment may also be advisable for individuals considering particularly adventurous recreational activities, such as mountain climbing and scuba diving.

TABLE 108-1   *Vaccines Commonly Used for Travel*

Vaccine	Primary Series	Booster Interval
Cholera, live oral (CVD 103 - HgR)	1 dose	6 months
Hepatitis A (Havrix), 1440 enzyme immunoassay U/mL	2 doses, 6–12 months apart, IM	None required
Hepatitis A (VAQTA, AVAXIM, EPAXAL)	2 doses, 6–12 months apart, IM	None required
Hepatitis A/B combined (Twinrix)	3 doses at 0, 1, and 6–12 months *or* 0, 7, and 21 days plus booster of B at 1 year, IM	None required *except* 12 months (once only, for accelerated schedule)
Hepatitis B (Engerix B): accelerated schedule	3 doses at 0, 1, and 2 months *or* 0, 7, and 21 days plus booster at 1 year, IM	12 months, once only
Hepatitis B (Engerix B or Recombivax): standard schedule	3 doses at 0, 1, and 6 months, IM	None required
Immune globulin (hepatitis A prevention)	1 dose IM	Intervals of 3–5 months, depending on initial dose
Japanese encephalitis (JEV, Biken)	3 doses, 1 week apart, SC	12–18 months (first booster), then 4 years
Meningococcus, quadrivalent	1 dose SC	>3 years (optimum booster schedule not yet determined)
Rabies (HDCV), rabies vaccine absorbed (RVA), or purified chick embryo cell vaccine (PCEC)	3 doses at 0, 7, and 21 or 28 days, IM	None required except with exposure
Typhoid Ty21a, oral live attenuated (Vivotif)	1 capsule every other day × 4 doses	5 years
Typhoid Vi capsular polysaccharide, injectable (Typhim Vi)	1 dose IM	2 years
Yellow fever	1 dose SC	10 years

IMMUNIZATIONS FOR TRAVEL   Immunizations for travel fall into three broad categories: routine (childhood/adult boosters that are necessary regardless of travel), required (immunizations that are mandated by international regulations for entry into certain areas or for border crossings), and recommended (immunizations that are desirable because they confer protection against a variety of illnesses for which travel increases the risk). Vaccines commonly given to travelers are listed in Table 108-1.

Routine Immunizations ■ *Diphtheria, Tetanus, and Polio*   Diphtheria continues to be a problem worldwide; large outbreaks have occurred over the past decade in the independent states formerly encompassed by the Soviet Union. Serosurveys show that tetanus antitoxin is lacking in many North Americans, especially in women over the age of 50. The risk of polio to the international traveler is extremely low, and wild poliovirus has been eradicated from the western hemisphere and Europe. However, studies in the United States have found varying levels of immunity in the general population, and data suggest that 12% of adult travelers from the United States are unprotected against at least one poliovirus serogroup. Foreign travel offers an ideal opportunity to have these immunizations updated.

Measles   Measles (rubeola) continues to be a major cause of morbidity and mortality in the developing world (Chap. 176). Several outbreaks of measles in the United States have been linked to imported cases. The group at highest risk consists of persons born after 1956 and vaccinated before 1980, in many of whom primary vaccination failed. Travelers in this group should be reimmunized.

Influenza   Influenza occurs year-round in the tropics and during the summer months in the southern hemisphere (coinciding with the winter months in the northern hemisphere). Vaccination should be considered for all travelers to these regions, particularly those who are elderly or chronically ill. The largest outbreak of travel-related influenza occurred in the summer of 1998 in Alaska and the Northwest Territories of Canada among cruise ship passengers and staff. Such outbreaks continue to occur; unfortunately, however, influenza vaccine is generally not available during the summer months in the United States (Chap. 171).

Pneumococcal Infection   Pneumococcal vaccine should be administered routinely to persons at high risk of serious infection, such as individuals with chronic heart, lung, or renal disease and those who have been splenectomized or have sickle cell disease.

Required Immunizations ■ *Yellow Fever*   Documentation of yellow fever vaccination may be required as a condition of entry into or passage through countries of sub-Saharan Africa and equatorial South America, where the disease is endemic or epidemic, or into countries that are at risk of having the infection introduced. This vaccine is given only by state-authorized yellow fever centers, and its administration must be documented on an official International Certificate of Vaccination. In Africa, the risk of yellow fever has been estimated to be as high as 1 case per 267 travelers per 2-week stay during epidemics and as low as 1 case per 2000 travelers per 2-week stay where the disease is endemic. The incidence of yellow fever among travelers is extremely low, probably because the vaccine is highly efficacious. However, recent data suggest that fewer than 50% of travelers entering areas endemic for yellow fever are immunized, and both American and European travelers have died of this very serious illness on their return home. It is also of concern that yellow fever–endemic areas may be expanding. Education about the importance of preventing this illness is crucial.

Cholera   According to the World Health Organization, cholera vaccination should no longer be required for entry into any country. The inactivated injectable vaccine is no longer available in the United States.

Meningococcal Meningitis Protection against meningitis (using the quadrivalent polysaccharide vaccine) is required for entry into Saudi Arabia during the Hajj.

Recommended Immunizations ■ *Hepatitis A and B* Hepatitis A is the most frequent vaccine-preventable infection of travelers; Swiss data show that the incidence of symptomatic infection during a 1-month stay in a developing country ranges from 3 to 6 cases per 1000. The risk is six times greater for travelers who stray from the usual tourist routes. The results of a recent Canadian study showed that rates of hepatitis A among short-term vacationers to Mexico and the Caribbean were considerably lower (1 case per 10,000 to 20,000 travelers per month of stay). The mortality rate for hepatitis A increases with age, reaching almost 3% among symptomatic individuals over age 50. Of the four hepatitis A vaccines currently available in North America (two in the United States), all are interchangeable and have an efficacy rate of >95%. The monthly incidence of hepatitis B infection, both symptomatic and asymptomatic, is 80 to 240 cases per 100,000. For reasons that are not entirely clear, long-stay overseas workers are at considerable risk for hepatitis B infection. A combined hepatitis A and B vaccine is now available and has been approved for administration on a 3-week accelerated schedule in Canada and Europe.

Typhoid Fever The attack rate for typhoid fever is 1 case per 30,000 per month of travel to the developing world (Chap. 137). However, the attack rates in India, Senegal, and North Africa are tenfold higher; in these areas, rates are especially high among travelers to relatively remote destinations and among persons who are returning to their homelands to stay with relatives or friends. Between 1994 and 1999 in the United States, 77% of imported cases involved the latter group. The two available vaccines—one oral and the other injectable—have an efficacy rate of ~70%.

Meningococcal Meningitis Although the risk of meningococcal disease among travelers has not been quantified, it is likely to be higher among travelers who live with poor indigenous populations in overcrowded conditions. Meningococcal polysaccharide vaccine is recommended for persons traveling to sub-Saharan Africa during the dry season or to areas of the world where there are epidemics. The vaccine, which protects against serogroups A, C, Y, and W-135, has an efficacy rate of >90%.

Japanese Encephalitis The risk of Japanese encephalitis, an infection transmitted by mosquitoes in rural Asia and Southeast Asia, is ~1 case per 5000 travelers per month of stay in an endemic area. Most symptomatic infections among U.S. residents have involved military personnel or their families. The vaccine efficacy rate is >90%; serious allergic reactions sometimes occur. The vaccine is recommended for persons staying >1 month in rural endemic areas.

Cholera The risk of cholera is extremely low, with ~1 case per 500,000 journeys to endemic areas. Cholera vaccine, no longer available in the United States, was rarely recommended but was considered for aid and health care workers in refugee camps or in disaster/war-torn areas. A more effective oral cholera vaccine is available in other countries.

Rabies Many cases of rabies have been reported in travelers, but there are no data on the risk of infection. Domestic animals, primarily dogs, are the major transmitters of rabies in developing countries (Chap. 179). Several studies have shown that the risk of rabies posed by a dog bite in an endemic area ranges from 1 to 3.6 cases per 1000 travelers per month of stay. Countries where canine rabies is highly endemic include Mexico, the Philippines, Sri Lanka, India, Thailand, and Vietnam. The three vaccines available in the United States provide >90% protection. Rabies vaccine is recommended for long-stay travelers, particularly children, and persons who may be occupationally exposed to rabies in endemic areas.

PREVENTION OF MALARIA AND OTHER INSECT-BORNE DISEASES It is estimated that more than 30,000 American and European travelers develop malaria each year (Chap. 195). The risk of malaria is highest in Oceania and sub-Saharan Africa (estimated at 1:5 and 1:50 per month of stay, respectively, among persons not using chemoprophylaxis) and during the past decade has increased by more than fivefold for travelers to Kenya. The risk is intermediate (1:250 to 1:1000 per month) for travelers to malarious areas on the Indian subcontinent and in Southeast Asia and is low (1:2500 to 1:10,000 per month) for travelers to South and Central America. Of the more than 1000 cases of malaria reported annually in the United States, 90% of those due to *Plasmodium falciparum* occur in travelers returning or immigrating from Africa and Oceania. With the worldwide increase in chloroquine- and multidrug-resistant falciparum malaria, decisions about chemoprophylaxis have become more difficult. In addition, the spread of malaria due to primaquine- and chloroquine-resistant strains of *Plasmodium vivax* has added to the complexity of treatment. The case-fatality rate of falciparum malaria in the United States is 4%; however, in only one-third of patients who die is the diagnosis of malaria considered before death.

Several recent studies indicate that fewer than 50% of travelers adhere to basic recommendations for malaria prevention. Keys to the prevention of malaria include both personal protection measures against mosquito bites, especially between dusk and dawn, and malaria chemoprophylaxis. The former measures include the use of DEET-containing insect repellents, permethrin-impregnated bed-nets and clothing, screened sleeping accommodations, and protective clothing. These practices also help prevent other insect-transmitted illnesses, such as dengue fever. Over the past decade, the incidence of dengue has increased, particularly in the Caribbean region, Latin America, and Southeast Asia. Dengue virus is transmitted by an urban-dwelling mosquito that bites at dawn and dusk.

The decision about whether to use malaria prophylaxis is based on the traveler's destination; the particular medication is determined by the destination as well as the traveler's preference and medical history. Table 108-2 lists the currently recommended drugs of choice for prophylaxis of malaria, by destination. Primaquine is an alternative medication used for prophylaxis by some physicians; although popular in parts of Europe, the chloroquine/proguanil combination is not recommended because of its low efficacy.

PREVENTION OF GASTROINTESTINAL ILLNESS Diarrhea, the leading cause of illness in travelers (Chap. 113), is usually a short-lived, self-limited condition; however, 40% of affected individuals need to alter their scheduled activities, and another 20% are confined to bed. The most important determinant of risk is the destination. Incidence rates per 2-week stay have been reported to be as low as 8% in industrialized countries and as high as 55% in parts of Africa, Central and South America, and Southeast Asia. Infants and young adults are at particularly high risk. The incidence of diarrhea is proportional to the num-

TABLE 108-2 *Malaria Chemosuppressive Regimens According to Geographic Area*[a]

Geographic Area	Drug of Choice	Alternatives
Central America (north of Panama), Haiti, Dominican Republic, Iraq, Egypt, Turkey, northern Argentina, and Paraguay	Chloroquine	Mefloquine Doxycycline Atovaquone/proguanil
South America including Panama (except northern Argentina and Paraguay); Asia (including Southeast Asia); Africa; and Oceania	Mefloquine Doxycycline Atovaquone-proguanil (Malarone)	Primaquine
Thai, Myanmar, and Cambodian borders	Doxycycline Atovaquone-proguanil (Malarone)	

[a] See CDC's *Health Information for International Travel 2003–2004*.
Note: See also Chap. 195.

ber of dietary indiscretions. Studies of U.S. students in Mexico showed that eating meals in restaurants and cafeterias or consuming food from street vendors was associated with increased risk.

Etiology (See also Table 113-2)   The most frequently identified pathogen causing traveler's diarrhea is toxigenic *Escherichia coli*, although in some parts of the world (notably northern Africa and Southeast Asia) *Campylobacter* infections appear to predominate. Other common causative organisms include *Salmonella*, *Shigella*, rotavirus, and the Norwalk agent. Except for giardiasis, parasitic infections are uncommon causes of traveler's diarrhea. A growing problem for travelers is the development of antibiotic resistance by many bacterial pathogens, including strains of *Campylobacter* resistant to quinolones and strains of *E. coli*, *Shigella*, and *Salmonella* resistant to trimethoprim-sulfamethoxazole.

Precautions   Although the mainstay of prevention of traveler's diarrhea involves food and water precautions, the literature has repeatedly documented dietary indiscretions in 98% of travelers within the first 48 h after arrival at their destination. The maxim "Boil it, cook it, peel it, or forget it!" is easy to remember but apparently difficult to follow. General food and water precautions include eating foods piping hot; avoiding foods that are raw, poorly cooked, or sold by street vendors; and drinking only boiled or commercially bottled beverages, particularly those that are carbonated. Heating kills diarrhea-causing organisms, whereas freezing does not; therefore, ice cubes made from unpurified water should be avoided.

Self-Treatment (See also Table 113-4)   As traveler's diarrhea often occurs despite rigorous food and water precautions, travelers should carry medications for self-treatment. For mild to moderate diarrhea, loperamide and fluid replacement may be sufficient. An antibiotic is useful in reducing the frequency of bowel movements and duration of illness in moderate to severe diarrhea. The standard regimen is a 3-day course of a quinolone taken twice daily (or, in the case of some newer formulations, once daily). However, studies have shown that a single double dose of a quinolone may be equally effective, particularly if infection with a multidrug-resistant organism is not suspected. For diarrhea acquired in areas such as Thailand, where >90% of *Campylobacter* infections are quinolone resistant, azithromycin may be a better alternative.

Prophylaxis   Prophylaxis of traveler's diarrhea with bismuth subsalicylate is widely used but only ~60% effective. For certain individuals (e.g., athletes, persons with a repeated history of traveler's diarrhea, and persons with chronic diseases), a single daily dose of a quinolone during travel of <1 month's duration is highly effective.

Illness after Return   Although extremely common, acute traveler's diarrhea is usually self-limited or amenable to antibiotic therapy. Persistent bowel problems after the traveler returns home have a less well-defined etiology and may require medical attention from a specialist. Infectious agents appear to be responsible for only a small proportion of cases with persistent bowel symptoms. Of the pathogens detected in these instances, *Giardia lamblia* (Chap. 199) is by far the most common; *Cyclospora cayetanensis*, *Cryptosporidium* species, and *Entamoeba histolytica* are rarely isolated. Studies suggest that enteroadherent *E. coli* may be important. By far the most frequent causes of persistent diarrhea after travel are postinfectious sequelae, such as lactose intolerance or an irritable bowel syndrome. In the latter, intermittent diarrhea often alternates with constipation. When no infectious etiology can be identified, a trial of metronidazole therapy for presumed giardiasis, a strict lactose-free diet for 1 week, or a several-week trial of high-dose hydrophilic mucilloid (plus lactulose for persons with constipation) relieves the symptoms of many patients.

PREVENTION OF OTHER TRAVEL-RELATED PROBLEMS   Travelers are at high risk for *sexually transmitted diseases*. Surveys have shown that large numbers engage in casual sex, and there is a reluctance to use condoms

consistently. An increasing number of travelers are being diagnosed with *schistosomiasis*. Travelers should be cautioned to avoid bathing, swimming, or wading in freshwater lakes, streams, or rivers in parts of tropical South America, the Caribbean, Africa, and Southeast Asia where this infection can be acquired. Prevention of *travel-associated injury* depends mostly on common-sense precautions. Riding on motorcycles and in overcrowded public vehicles is not recommended; in particular, individuals should not travel by road after dark in rural areas. In addition to its association with motor vehicle accidents, excessive alcohol use has been a significant factor in drownings, assaults, and injuries. Travelers are cautioned to avoid walking barefoot because of the risk of hookworm and *Strongyloides* infections (Chap. 201) and snakebites (Chap. 378).

THE TRAVELER'S MEDICAL KIT   A traveler's medical kit is strongly advisable, particularly for long-stay travelers. The contents may vary widely, depending on the itinerary, duration of stay, style of travel, and local medical facilities. While many medications are available abroad, often over the counter, directions for their use may be nonexistent or in a foreign language, or a product may be outdated or counterfeit. Therefore, if possible, a complete supply of medications should accompany the traveler. In the kit, the short-term traveler should consider carrying an analgesic, an antidiarrheal agent, antihistamines, a laxative, oral rehydration salts, a sunscreen with a skin-protection factor of at least 30, a DEET-containing insect repellent for the skin, an insecticide for clothing (permethrin), and (if necessary) an antimalarial drug. To these medications the long-stay traveler might add a broad-spectrum general-purpose antibiotic (levofloxacin or azithromycin), an antibacterial eye and skin ointment, and a topical antifungal cream. Regardless of the duration of travel, a first-aid kit containing such items as scissors, tweezers, and bandages should be considered.

TRAVEL AND SPECIAL HOSTS

PREGNANCY AND TRAVEL   A woman's medical history and itinerary, the quality of medical care at her destinations, and her degree of flexibility determine whether travel is wise during pregnancy. According to the American College of Obstetrics and Gynecology, the safest part of pregnancy in which to travel is between 18 and 24 weeks, when there is the least danger of spontaneous abortion or premature labor. Some obstetricians prefer that women stay within a few hundred miles of home after the 28th week of pregnancy in case problems arise; in general, however, healthy women may be advised that it is acceptable to travel.

Despite this general recommendation, there are some relative contraindications to international travel during pregnancy, including certain obstetric risk factors: a history of miscarriage, premature labor, incompetent cervix, or toxemia. General medical problems such as diabetes, heart failure, severe anemia, or a history of thromboembolic disease should also prompt the pregnant woman to postpone her travels. Finally, regions in which the pregnant woman and her fetus may be at excessive risk (e.g., those at high altitudes and those where live-virus vaccines are required or where multidrug-resistant malaria is endemic) are not ideal destinations during any trimester.

Malaria   Malaria during pregnancy carries a significant risk of morbidity and death. Levels of parasitemia are highest and failure to clear the parasites after treatment is most frequent among primigravidae. Severe disease, with complications such as cerebral malaria, massive hemolysis, and renal failure, is especially likely in pregnancy. Fetal sequelae include spontaneous abortion, stillbirth, preterm delivery, and congenital infection.

Traveler's Diarrhea   Because dehydration due to traveler's diarrhea can lead to inadequate placental blood flow, pregnant travelers must be extremely cautious regarding their food and beverage intake. The exclusive consumption of bottled (carbonated) or boiled drinks without ice, the eating of well-cooked meats and pasteurized dairy products, and the avoidance of pre-prepared salad items should help protect against traveler's diarrhea due to the usual causes as well as against infections such as toxoplasmosis, hepatitis E, and listeriosis, which can have serious sequelae in pregnancy.

The mainstay of therapy for traveler's diarrhea is rehydration. Loperamide may be used if necessary, but many of the usual antibiotics are contraindicated during pregnancy. Ampicillin alone or with clavulanic acid may be used, but many strains of *E. coli* and other organisms implicated in traveler's diarrhea are resistant. Azithromycin may be the best option.

Because of the major problems encountered when infants are given local foods and beverages, women are strongly encouraged to breast-feed when traveling with a neonate. A nursing mother with traveler's diarrhea should not stop breast-feeding but should increase her fluid intake.

Air Travel and High-Altitude Destinations Commercial air travel is not a risk to the healthy pregnant woman or to the fetus. Fetal oxygenation is not adversely affected by decreased cabin pressures because of the fetal hemoglobin dissociation curve; the higher radiation levels reported at altitudes of >10,500 m (>35,000 ft) should pose no problem to the healthy pregnant traveler. Since each airline has a policy regarding pregnancy and flying, it is best to check with the specific carrier when booking reservations. Domestic air travel is usually permitted until the 36th week, whereas international air travel is generally curtailed after the 32nd week.

There are no known risks for pregnant women who travel to high-altitude destinations and stay for short periods. However, there are likewise no data on the safety of pregnant women at altitudes of >4500 m (15,000 ft). Because of the harsh conditions usually associated with such trips, they are generally contraindicated for other reasons.

THE HIV-INFECTED TRAVELER The traveler infected with HIV is at special risk of serious infections due to a number of pathogens that may be more prevalent at travel destinations than at home. However, the degree of risk depends primarily on the state of the immune system at the time of travel. For persons whose CD4+ cell counts are normal or >500/μL, no data suggest a greater risk during travel than for persons without HIV infection. Individuals with AIDS (CD4+ cell counts of <200/μL) and others who are symptomatic need special counseling and should visit a travel medicine practitioner before departure, especially when traveling to the developing world.

Several countries now routinely deny entry to HIV-positive individuals, even though no data show that these restrictions decrease rates of transmission of the virus. In general, HIV testing is required of those individuals who wish to stay abroad >3 months or who intend to work or study abroad. Some countries will accept an HIV serologic test done within 6 months of departure, whereas others will not accept a blood test done at any time in the traveler's home country. In addition, border officials often have the authority to make inquiries of individuals entering a country and to check the medications they are carrying. If a drug such as zidovudine is identified, the person may be barred from entering the country. Information on testing requirements for specific countries is available from consular offices but is subject to frequent change.

Health insurance policies should be checked to make sure they are valid for care in other countries. The HIV-positive traveler should strongly consider obtaining trip cancellation insurance and evacuation insurance in case of illness. It is ideal to have the name of a physician at the travel destination who is familiar with the treatment of patients with AIDS, as the clinical findings associated with infection may be atypical in a patient with AIDS, and several infections may exist simultaneously. The traveler should be encouraged to visit the physician promptly if problems arise.

Immunizations All of the HIV-infected traveler's routine immunizations should be up to date (Chap. 107). The response to immunization may be impaired at CD4+ cell counts of <200/μL (and in some cases at even higher counts). Thus HIV-infected persons should be vaccinated as early as possible to ensure adequate immune response to all

vaccines. In patients receiving highly active antiretroviral therapy, at least 3 months must elapse before regenerated CD4+ cells can be considered fully functional; therefore, in these patients, vaccinations should be delayed, if possible, until the CD4+ cell count has been stable for this length of time. However, when the risk of illness is high or the sequelae of illness are serious, immunization is recommended. In certain circumstances, it may be prudent to check the adequacy of the serum antibody response before departure (e.g., yellow fever neutralization inhibition if exposure is unavoidable).

Because of the increased risk of infections due to *Streptococcus pneumoniae* and other bacterial pathogens that cause pneumonia following influenza, pneumococcal polysaccharide and influenza vaccines should be administered. The estimated rates of response to influenza vaccine are >80% among persons with asymptomatic HIV infection and <50% among those with AIDS.

In general, live attenuated vaccines are contraindicated for persons with immune dysfunction. Because measles (rubeola) can be a severe and lethal infection in HIV-positive patients, these patients should receive the measles vaccine (or the combination measles-mumps-rubella vaccine) unless they are severely immunocompromised (CD4+ cell count, <200/μL). Between 18 and 58% of symptomatic HIV-infected vaccinees develop adequate antibody titers, and between 50 and 100% of asymptomatic persons infected with HIV seroconvert. Immune globulin should be considered for measles-susceptible, severely immunosuppressed HIV-infected persons who are planning to travel to measles-endemic countries.

The decision of whether to administer any of the special vaccines to an HIV-infected traveler should be based on the individual's risk. Inactivated vaccines can be administered without concern for safety but with concern about adequate protection. For example, data suggest that HIV-infected persons do not have as strong an antibody response to the meningococcal meningitis vaccine as do uninfected persons. Moreover, few data are available on the efficacy of many of the other vaccines (e.g., those for hepatitis A and typhoid).

It is recommended that the live yellow fever vaccine not be given to HIV-infected travelers. Although the potential adverse affects of a live vaccine in an HIV-infected individual are always a consideration, there appear to have been no reported cases of illness in those who have inadvertently received this vaccine. Nonetheless, if the CD4+ count is <200/μL, an alternative itinerary that poses no risk of exposure to yellow fever is recommended. If the traveler is passing through or traveling to an area where the vaccine is required but the disease risk is low, a physician's waiver should be issued. Bacille Calmette-Guérin vaccine should not be given because of reports of disseminated infection in HIV-infected persons.

A transient increase in viremia (lasting days to weeks) has been demonstrated in HIV-infected individuals following immunization with vaccines for such diseases as influenza, pneumococcal infection, and tetanus (Chap. 173). However, at this point, there is no evidence that this transient increase in HIV levels in the bloodstream is detrimental over time. Furthermore, it is likely that immune activation associated with infection with the live organisms in question would result in increases in viremia of greater magnitude and duration than those associated with vaccination. Therefore, the vaccination recommendations discussed above need not be modified at this time.

Gastrointestinal Illness Decreased levels of gastric acid, abnormal gastrointestinal mucosal immunity, other complications of HIV infection, and medications taken by HIV-infected patients make traveler's diarrhea especially problematic in these individuals. Traveler's diarrhea is likely to occur more frequently, be more severe, and be more difficult to treat in association with HIV infection. *Salmonella*, *Shigella*, and *Campylobacter* infections are also more protracted and more often accompanied by bacteremia in HIV-infected persons.

Cryptosporidium (Chap. 199), a common cause of diarrhea in tropical countries, produces severe chronic diarrhea and cholecystitis with increased mortality among patients with AIDS. *Isospora belli* causes infections at high rates among AIDS patients in the developing world; this infection is associated with malabsorption, weight loss, and relapses after treatment. Persistent diarrhea due to microsporidiosis has been reported.

Because of these potential problems, the HIV-infected traveler must be careful to consume only appropriately prepared foods and beverages. In addition, this group of individuals may benefit from prophylaxis for traveler's diarrhea, using bismuth subsalicylate or a daily antibiotic (ideally a quinolone derivative) for short-term travel to the developing world. If the traveler is already taking a sulfonamide preparation for prophylaxis of *Pneumocystis* pneumonia, a regimen of self-treatment with a quinolone would be appropriate.

Other Travel-Related Infections   Data are lacking on the severity of many vector-borne diseases in HIV-infected individuals. Malaria is especially severe in asplenic and certain immunocompromised hosts, including those with AIDS. *Babesia* infection is known to cause serious illness and to recur in HIV-infected patients; this tick-transmitted illness occurs in parts of the United States but is not known to be a widespread problem.

Visceral leishmaniasis (Chap. 196) has been reported in numerous HIV-infected travelers. The diagnosis may be difficult to make, given that splenomegaly and hyperglobulinemia are often lacking and serologic results are frequently negative. This infection is difficult to treat, and its associated mortality is high. Even short-term travelers to southern Europe have developed the illness; thus the avoidance of sandfly bites is critical.

Certain respiratory illnesses, such as histoplasmosis and coccidioidomycosis, cause greater morbidity and mortality among patients with AIDS than in the general population. Although tuberculosis is common among HIV-infected persons (especially in developing countries), the acquisition of this infection by the short-term traveler is not a major concern. The possibility of acquiring *Legionella* infections from spas should be considered, although no data confirm an increase in the severity of such infections in AIDS.

Finally, the HIV-infected traveler should always be cautioned about safe sexual practices, which may help prevent both the transmission of HIV to others and the acquisition by the traveler of other sexually transmitted diseases that may be drug resistant or may result in serious sequelae (e.g., syphilis).

Medications   Adverse events due to medications and drug interactions are common and raise complex issues for HIV-infected persons. Rates of cutaneous reaction (e.g., increased cutaneous sensitivity to sulfonamides) are unusually high among patients with AIDS. Physicians advising HIV-infected travelers need to consider the problems that may arise from the use of agents such as antimalarial drugs, medications for altitude acclimation, or antidiarrheal compounds. Since zidovudine is metabolized by hepatic glucuronidation, inhibitors of this process may elevate serum levels of the drug. Concomitant administration of mefloquine and ritonavir may result in decreased plasma levels of ritonavir. In contrast, no significant influence of concomitant mefloquine administration on plasma levels of indinavir or nelfinavir was detected in two HIV-infected travelers.

CHRONIC ILLNESS, DISABILITY, AND TRAVEL   Chronic health problems should not prevent travel, but special measures can make the journey safer and more comfortable.

Heart Disease   Cardiovascular events are the main cause of deaths among travelers and of in-flight emergencies on commercial aircraft. Persons with underlying heart disease should review their itineraries with a physician prior to departure; travel in harsh environments or to remote destinations is not wise. Extra supplies of all medications should be kept in carry-on luggage, along with a copy of a recent electrocardiogram and the name and telephone number of the traveler's physician at home. Pacemakers are not affected by airport security

devices, but electronic telephone checks of pacemaker function cannot be transmitted by international satellites. The traveler may benefit from supplemental oxygen, which should be ordered by a physician (since oxygen delivery systems are not standard) 48 to 72 h before flight time. Personal oxygen tanks are not permitted aboard aircraft. Travelers should request aisle seating and should walk, perform stretching and flexing exercises, and remain hydrated during the flight to prevent venous thrombosis and pulmonary embolism.

Chronic Lung Disease   Chronic obstructive pulmonary disease is one of the most common diagnoses in patients who require emergency-room evaluation for symptoms occurring during airline flights. Patients with such disease experience dyspnea, edema, wheezing, cyanosis, and chest pain. The best predictor of the development of these symptoms is the sea level Pa_{O_2}. A Pa_{O_2} of at least 72 mmHg corresponds to an in-flight arterial Pa_{O_2} of $\sim$55 mmHg when the cabin is pressurized to 2500 m (8000 ft). Therefore, if the traveler's baseline Pa_{O_2} is <72 mmHg, the provision of supplemental oxygen during the flight should be considered. Pulmonary function is also maximized by continuing bronchodilator treatment and the use of glucocorticoids as prescribed. Contraindications to flight include active bronchospasm, lower respiratory infection, lower-limb deep-vein phlebitis, pulmonary hypertension, and recent thoracic surgery (within the preceding 3 weeks) or pneumothorax. Consideration should be given to decreasing the amount of outdoor activity at the destination if there is excessive air pollution.

Diabetes Mellitus   Alterations in glucose control and changes in insulin requirements are common problems among patients with diabetes who travel. Changes in time zone, in the amount and timing of food intake, and in physical activity demand more vigilant assessment of metabolic control. The traveler with diabetes should pack medication (including a bottle of regular insulin for emergencies), insulin syringes and needles, equipment and supplies for glucose monitoring, and snacks in carry-on luggage. Insulin is stable for $\sim$3 months at room temperature but should be kept as cool as possible. The name and telephone number of the home physician and a card and necklace listing the patient's medical problems and the type and dose of insulin used should accompany the traveler. When six or more time zones are crossed, insulin requirements may be temporarily altered, depending on food intake and physical activity. In traveling eastward (e.g., from the United States to Europe), the morning insulin dose on arrival may need to be decreased. The blood glucose can then be checked during the day to determine whether additional insulin is required. For flights westward, with lengthening of the day, an additional dose of regular insulin may be required. Comfortable footwear is essential for the traveler with diabetes.

Other Special Groups   Other groups for whom special travel measures are encouraged include patients undergoing dialysis, those with transplants, and those with other disabilities. Up to 13% of travelers have some disability, but few advocacy groups and tour companies dedicate themselves to this growing population. The key to safe travel in each case is adequate research ahead of time. Patients undergoing chronic ambulatory peritoneal dialysis may ship their dialysis solutions to their destinations before traveling. They should carry essential medical records as well as antibiotics for self-treatment of presumed peritonitis. Hemodialysis patients need to reserve appointments at dialysis centers prior to their departure from home. Travel by transplant recipients to distant destinations should ideally be scheduled at least 1 year after surgery, as most rejection episodes occur early. Medication interactions are a source of serious concern for these travelers, and appropriate medical information should be carried, along with the home physician's name and telephone number. Some travelers taking glucocorticoids carry stress doses in case they become ill. Immunization of these immunocompromised travelers may result in less than adequate protection against certain diseases. Thus the traveler and physician must carefully consider which destinations are appropriate.

The most common medical problems encountered by travelers after their return home are diarrhea, fever, respiratory illnesses, and skin diseases. Frequently ignored problems are fatigue and emotional stress, especially in long-stay travelers. The approach to diagnosis requires some knowledge of geographic medicine, in particular the epidemiology and clinical presentation of infectious disorders. A geographic history should focus on the traveler's exact itinerary, including dates of arrival and departure; exposure history (food indiscretions, drinking-water sources, freshwater contact, sexual activity, animal contact, insect bites); location and style of travel (urban vs. rural, first-class hotel accommodation vs. camping); immunization history; and use of antimalarial chemosuppression.

DIARRHEA See "Prevention of Gastrointestinal Illness," above.

FEVER Fever in a traveler who has returned from a malarious area should be considered a medical emergency because death from *P. falciparum* malaria can follow an illness of only several days' duration. Although "fever from the tropics" does not always have a tropical cause, malaria should be the first diagnosis considered. The risk of *P. falciparum* malaria is highest among travelers returning from Africa or Oceania and among those who become symptomatic within the first 2 months after return. Other important causes of fever after travel include viral hepatitis (hepatitis A and E), typhoid fever, bacterial enteritis, arbovirus infections (e.g., dengue fever), rickettsial infections (including tick and scrub typhus and Q fever), and—in rare instances—leptospirosis, acute HIV infection, and amebic liver abscess. In at least 25% of cases, no etiology can be found, and the illness resolves spontaneously. Clinicians should keep in mind that no present-day antimalarial agent guarantees protection from malaria and that some immunizations (notably, that against typhoid fever) are only partially protective.

As noted above, the approach to the febrile returned traveler begins with a detailed medical and geographic history. Knowing exact dates of arrival and departure from tropical areas enables the physician to ascertain the shortest and longest possible incubation periods for illnesses in the differential diagnosis. For example, a traveler who develops fever <1 week after arrival in a malarious area cannot have malaria because the incubation period is too short, whereas a fever whose onset comes >2 weeks after departure from an endemic area cannot be dengue fever because the incubation period is too long. In the physical examination, particular attention should be given to the skin so as not to miss a subtle rash or eschar.

When no specific diagnosis is forthcoming, the following investigations, where applicable, are suggested: complete blood count, liver function tests, thick/thin blood films for malaria (repeated twice if necessary), urinalysis, urine and blood cultures (repeated once), chest x-ray, and collection of an acute-phase serum sample to be held for subsequent examination along with a paired convalescent-phase serum sample.

SKIN DISEASES Pyodermas, sunburn, insect bites, skin ulcers, and cutaneous larva migrans are the most common skin conditions encountered in travelers after their return home. In those with persistent skin ulcers, a diagnosis of cutaneous leishmaniasis, mycobacterial infec-

tion, or fungal infection should be considered. Careful, complete inspection of the skin is important in detecting the rickettsial eschar in a febrile patient or the central breathing hole in a "boil" due to myiasis.

EMERGING INFECTIOUS DISEASES In recent years, travel and commerce have fostered the worldwide spread of HIV infection, led to the reemergence of cholera as a global health threat, and created considerable fear about the possible spread of Ebola virus infection and severe acute respiratory syndrome (SARS). For travelers, there are more realistic concerns. One of the largest outbreaks of dengue fever ever documented is now raging in Latin America; schistosomiasis is being described in previously unaffected lakes in Africa; and antibiotic-resistant strains of sexually transmitted and enteric pathogens are emerging at an alarming rate in the developing world. In addition, concerns have been raised regarding the potential for bioterrorism involving not only standard strains of unusual agents but mutant strains as well. Time will tell whether travelers (as well as persons at home) will routinely be vaccinated against diseases such as anthrax and smallpox. As Nobel Laureate Dr. Joshua Lederberg pointed out, "The microbe that felled one child in a distant continent yesterday can reach yours today and seed a global pandemic tomorrow." The vigilant clinician understands that the importance of a thorough travel history cannot be overemphasized.

FURTHER READING

AEROSPACE MEDICAL ASSOCIATION AIR TRANSPORT MEDICINE COMMITTEE: Medical guidelines for air travel. Aviat Space Environ Med 67(Suppl 10):b1, 1996

CAUMES E et al: Dermatoses associated with travel to tropical countries: A prospective study of the diagnosis and management of 269 patients presenting to a tropical disease unit. Clin Infect Dis 20:542, 1995

CENTERS FOR DISEASE CONTROL AND PREVENTION: *Health Information for International Travel 2003-2004.* HHS publication no (CDC) 92-8280. Washington, DC, Government Printing Office, 2003 (www.cdc.gov/travel/yb/index.htm)

ERICSSON CD: Travelers' diarrhea: Epidemiology, prevention and self-treatment. Infect Dis Clin North Am 12:285, 1998

FRADIN MS: Mosquitoes and mosquito repellents: A clinician's guide. Ann Intern Med 128:931, 1998

KAIN KC et al: Malaria chemoprophylaxis in the age of drug resistance. I. Currently recommended drug regimens. Clin Infect Dis 33:226, 2001

KEYSTONE JS et al: *Travel Medicine.* Mosby, Philadelphia, 2004

—— et al: Internet and computer-based resources for travel medicine practitioners. Clin Infect Dis 32:757, 2001

——: GIDEON computer program for diagnosing and teaching geographic medicine. J Travel Med 6:152, 1999

MILENO MD, BIA FJ: The compromised traveler. Infect Dis Clin North Am 12:369, 1998

RYAN ET et al: Illness after international travel. N Engl J Med 347:505, 2002

——, KAIN KC: Health advice and immunizations for travelers. N Engl J Med 342:1716, 2000

SAMUEL B, BARRY M: The pregnant traveler. Infect Dis Clin North Am 12: 323, 1998

SPIRA A: Assessment of travellers who return. Lancet 361:1459, 2003

——: Preparing the traveller. Lancet 361:1368, 2003

WEBSITES OF INTEREST: Chronic renal failure: www.kidney.org. Diabetes: www.diabetesmonitor.com/other-14.htm. Dialysis: www.dialysisfinder.com. Disability: www.access-able.com. HIV: www.aegis.com

Section 2   Clinical Syndromes: Community-Acquired Infections

109 INFECTIVE ENDOCARDITIS
Adolf W. Karchmer

The proliferation of microorganisms on the endothelium of the heart results in infective endocarditis. The prototypic lesion at the site of infection, the *vegetation* (Fig. 109-1), is a mass of platelets, fibrin, microcolonies of microorganisms, and scant inflammatory cells. In-

fection most commonly involves heart valves (either native or prosthetic) but may also occur on the low-pressure side of the ventricular septum at the site of a defect, on the mural endocardium where it is damaged by aberrant jets of blood or foreign bodies, or on intracardiac devices themselves. The analogous process involving arteriovenous shunts, arterioarterial shunts (patent ductus arteriosus), or a coarctation of the aorta is called *infective endarteritis*.

Endocarditis may be classified according to the temporal evolution

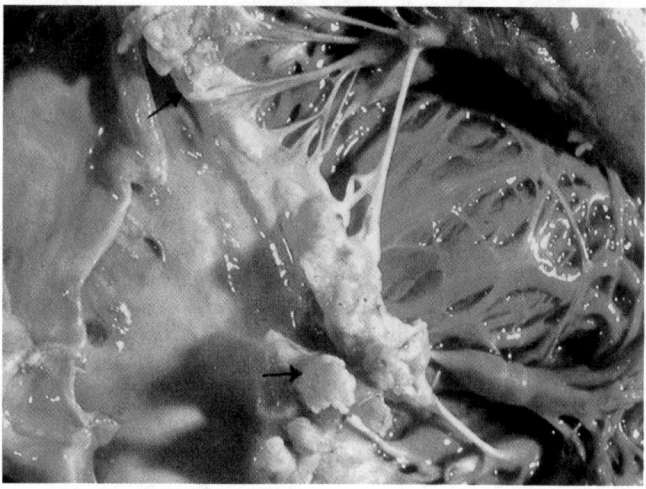

FIGURE 109-1 Vegetations (*arrows*) due to viridans streptococcal endocarditis involving the mitral valve.

of disease, the site of infection, the cause of infection, or a predisposing risk factor such as injection drug use. While each classification criterion provides therapeutic and prognostic insight, none is sufficient alone. The classification of endocarditis as acute and subacute was initially used to describe the illness and the time elapsed until death; presently it is applied to the features and progression of infection until diagnosis. *Acute endocarditis* is a hectically febrile illness, rapidly damages cardiac structures, hematogenously seeds extracardiac sites, and, if untreated, progresses to death within weeks. *Subacute endocarditis* follows an indolent course; causes structural cardiac damage only slowly, if at all; rarely causes metastatic infection; and is gradually progressive unless complicated by a major embolic event or ruptured mycotic aneurysm.

In developed countries, the incidence of endocarditis ranges from 1.5 to 6.2 cases per 100,000 population per year. In the late 1980s in a metropolitan area of the United States (Philadelphia), endocarditis occurred in 9.3 persons per 100,000 population per year. However, half of these cases arose as a consequence of injection drug use. The incidence of endocarditis is notably increased among the elderly. The cumulative rate of prosthetic valve endocarditis is 1.5 to 3.0% at 1 year after valve replacement and 3 to 6% at 5 years; the risk is greatest during the first 6 months after valve replacement.

ETIOLOGY   Many species of bacteria and fungi have been reported to cause sporadic episodes of endocarditis; nevertheless, a small number of bacterial species cause the majority of cases (Table 109-1). The causative microorganisms vary somewhat among the major clinical types of endocarditis, in part because of the different portals of entry. The oral cavity, skin, and upper respiratory tract are the respective primary portals for the viridans streptococci, staphylococci, and HACEK organisms (*Haemophilus, Actinobacillus, Cardiobacterium, Eikenella,* and *Kingella*) causing community-acquired native valve endocarditis. *Streptococcus bovis* originates from the gastrointestinal tract, where it is associated with polyps and colonic tumors, and enterococci enter the bloodstream from the genitourinary tract. Nosocomial native valve endocarditis is largely the consequence of bacteremia arising from intravascular catheters and less commonly from nosocomial wound and urinary tract infection. Endocarditis complicates 6 to 25% of episodes of catheter-associated *Staphylococcus aureus* bacteremia; the higher rates are detected by careful transesophageal echocardiography (TEE) screening (see "Echocardiography," below).

Prosthetic valve endocarditis arising within 2 months of valve surgery is generally the result of intraoperative contamination of the prosthesis or a bacteremic postoperative complication. The nosocomial nature of these infections is reflected in their primary microbial causes: coagulase-negative staphylococci, *S. aureus,* facultative gram-negative bacilli, diphtheroids, and fungi. The portals of entry and organisms causing cases beginning >12 months after surgery are similar to those in community-acquired native valve endocarditis. Epidemiologic evidence suggests that prosthetic valve endocarditis due to coagulase-negative staphylococci that presents between 2 and 12 months after surgery is often nosocomial in origin but with a delayed onset. At least 85% of coagulase-negative staphylococci that cause prosthetic valve endocarditis within 12 months of surgery are methicillin-resistant; the rate of methicillin resistance decreases to 25% among coagulase-negative staphylococci causing prosthetic endocarditis that presents >1 year after valve surgery.

Transvenous pacemaker lead– and/or implanted defibrillator–associated endocarditis is usually a nosocomial infection. The majority of episodes occur within weeks of implantation or generator change and are caused by *S. aureus* or coagulase-negative staphylococci.

Endocarditis occurring among injection drug users, especially when infection involves the tricuspid valve, is commonly caused by *S. aureus* strains, many of which are methicillin-resistant. Left-sided valve infections in addicts have a more varied etiology and involve abnormal valves, often ones damaged by prior episodes of endocarditis. A number of these cases are caused by *Pseudomonas aeruginosa*

TABLE 109-1   *Organisms Causing Major Clinical Forms of Endocarditis*

	Percent of Cases							
	Native Valve Endocarditis		Prosthetic Valve Endocarditis at Indicated Time of Onset (Months) after Valve Surgery			Endocarditis in Injection Drug Users		
Organism	Community-Acquired (n = 683)	Nosocomial (n = 82)	< 2 (n = 144)	2–12 (n = 31)	> 12 (n = 194)	Right-Sided (n = 346)	Left-Sided (n = 204)	Total (n = 675)
Streptococci[a]	32	7	1	9	31	5	15	12
Pneumococci	1	—	—	—	—	—	—	—
Enterococci	8	16	8	12	11	2	24	9
Staphylococcus aureus	35	55	22	12	18	77	23	57
Coagulase-negative staphylococci	4	10	33	32	11	—	—	—
Fastidious gram-negative coccobacilli (HACEK group)[b]	3	—	—	—	6	—	—	—
Gram-negative bacilli	3	5	13	3	6	5	13	7
Candida spp.	1	4	8	12	1	—	12	4
Polymicrobial/miscellaneous	6	1	3	6	5	8	10	7
Diphtheroids	—	—	6	—	3	—	—	0.1
Culture-negative	5	2	5	6	8	3	3	3

[a] Includes viridans streptococci; *Streptococcus bovis;* other non–group A, groupable streptococci; and *Abiotrophia* spp. (nutritionally variant, pyridoxal-requiring streptococci).

[b] Includes *Haemophilus* spp., *Actinobacillus actinomycetemcomitans, Cardiobacterium hominis, Eikenella* spp., and *Kingella kingae.*

Note: Data are compiled from multiple studies.

and *Candida* species, and sporadic cases are due to unusual organisms such as *Bacillus*, *Lactobacillus*, and *Corynebacterium* species. Polymicrobial endocarditis occurs more frequently in injection drug users than in patients who do not inject drugs. The presence of HIV in this population does not significantly impact the causes of endocarditis.

From 5 to 15% of patients with endocarditis have negative blood cultures; in one-third to one-half of these cases, cultures are negative because of prior antibiotic exposure. The remainder of these patients are infected by fastidious organisms, such as pyridoxal-requiring streptococci (now designated *Abiotrophia* species), the gram-negative coccobacillary HACEK organisms, *Bartonella henselae*, or *Bartonella quintana*. Some fastidious organisms that cause endocarditis have characteristic epidemiologic settings (e.g., *Coxiella burnetii* in Europe, *Brucella* species in the Middle East). *Tropheryma whipplei* causes an indolent, culture-negative, afebrile form of endocarditis.

PATHOGENESIS Unless it is injured, the normal endothelium is resistant to infection by most bacteria and to thrombus formation. Endothelial injury (e.g., at the site of impact of high-velocity jets or on the low-pressure side of a cardiac structural lesion) causes aberrant flow and allows either direct infection by virulent organisms or the development of an uninfected platelet-fibrin thrombus—a condition called *nonbacterial thrombotic endocarditis* (NBTE). The thrombus subsequently serves as a site of bacterial attachment during transient bacteremia. The cardiac lesions most commonly resulting in NBTE are mitral regurgitation, aortic stenosis, aortic regurgitation, ventricular septal defects, and complex congenital heart disease. These lesions result from rheumatic heart disease (particularly in the developing world, where rheumatic fever remains prevalent), mitral valve prolapse, degenerative heart disease, and congenital malformations. NBTE also arises as a result of a hypercoagulable state; this phenomenon gives rise to the clinical entity of *marantic endocarditis* (uninfected vegetations seen in patients with malignancy and chronic diseases) and to bland vegetations complicating systemic lupus erythematosus and the antiphospholipid antibody syndrome.

Organisms that cause endocarditis generally enter the bloodstream from mucosal surfaces, the skin, or sites of focal infection. Except for more virulent bacteria (e.g., *S. aureus*) that can adhere directly to intact endothelium or exposed subendothelial tissue, microorganisms in the blood adhere to thrombi. If resistant to the bactericidal activity of serum and the microbicidal peptides released by platelets, the organisms proliferate and induce a procoagulant state at the site by eliciting tissue factor from adherent monocytes or, in the case of *S. aureus*, from monocytes and from intact endothelium. Fibrin deposition, resulting from tissue factor initiation of the coagulation cascade, combines with platelet aggregation, stimulated by tissue factor and independently by proliferating microorganisms, to generate an infected vegetation. The organisms that commonly cause endocarditis bear surface components that facilitate adherence to injured endothelium and host proteins or, in the case of *S. aureus*, to intact endothelial cells or to thrombi. Fibronectin-binding proteins present on many gram-positive bacteria, clumping factor (a fibrinogen- and fibrin-binding surface protein) on *S. aureus*, and glucans on streptococci facilitate adherence. Fibronectin-binding proteins are required for *S. aureus* invasion of intact endothelium; thus these surface proteins may facilitate infection of previously normal valves. In the absence of host defenses, organisms enmeshed in the growing platelet-fibrin vegetation proliferate to form dense microcolonies. Organisms deep in vegetations are metabolically inactive (nongrowing) and relatively resistant to killing by antimicrobial agents. Proliferating surface organisms are shed into the bloodstream continuously, whereupon some are cleared by the reticuloendothelial system and others are redeposited on the vegetation and stimulate further vegetation growth.

The pathophysiologic consequences and clinical manifestations of endocarditis—other than constitutional symptoms, which are probably a result of cytokine production—arise from damage to intracardiac structures; embolization of vegetation fragments, leading to infection or infarction of remote tissues; hematogenous infection of sites during

bacteremia; and tissue injury due to the deposition of circulating immune complexes or immune responses to deposited bacterial antigens.

CLINICAL MANIFESTATIONS The clinical syndrome of infective endocarditis is highly variable and spans a continuum between acute and subacute presentations. Native valve endocarditis (whether acquired in the community or nosocomially), prosthetic valve endocarditis, and endocarditis due to injection drug use share clinical and laboratory manifestations (Table 109-2). Although the relationship is not absolute, the causative microorganism is primarily responsible for the temporal course of endocarditis. β-Hemolytic streptococci, *S. aureus*, and pneumococci typically result in an acute course, although *S. aureus* occasionally causes subacute disease. Endocarditis caused by *Staphylococcus lugdunensis* (a coagulase-negative species) or by enterococci may present acutely. Subacute endocarditis is typically caused by viridans streptococci, enterococci, coagulase-negative staphylococci, and the HACEK group. Endocarditis caused by *Bartonella* species and the agent of Q fever, *C. burnetii*, is exceptionally indolent.

The clinical features of endocarditis are nonspecific. However, these symptoms in a febrile patient with valvular abnormalities or a behavior pattern (injection drug use) that predisposes to endocarditis suggest the diagnosis, as do bacteremia with organisms that frequently cause endocarditis, otherwise-unexplained arterial emboli, and progressive cardiac valvular incompetence. In patients with subacute presentations, fever is typically low-grade and rarely exceeds 39.4°C (103°F); in contrast, temperatures between 39.4 and 40°C (103 and 104°F) are often noted in acute endocarditis. Fever may be blunted or absent in patients who are elderly or severely debilitated or who have marked cardiac or renal failure.

Cardiac Manifestations Although heart murmurs are usually indicative of the predisposing cardiac pathology rather than of endocarditis, valvular damage and ruptured chordae may result in new regurgitant murmurs. In acute endocarditis involving a normal valve, murmurs are heard on presentation in only 30 to 45% of patients but ultimately are detected in 85%. Congestive heart failure develops in 30 to 40% of patients; it is usually a consequence of valvular dysfunction but occasionally is due to endocarditis-associated myocarditis or an intracardiac fistula. The temporal progression of heart failure is variable; failure due to aortic valve dysfunction progresses more rapidly than that due to mitral valve dysfunction. Extension of infection beyond valve leaflets into adjacent annular or myocardial tissue results in perivalvular abscesses, which in turn may cause fistulae (from the root of

TABLE 109-2 *Clinical and Laboratory Features of Infective Endocarditis*

Feature	Frequency, %
Fever	80–90
Chills and sweats	40–75
Anorexia, weight loss, malaise	25–50
Myalgias, arthralgias	15–30
Back pain	7–15
Heart murmur	80–85
New/worsened regurgitant murmur	10–40
Arterial emboli	20–50
Splenomegaly	15–50
Clubbing	10–20
Neurologic manifestations	20–40
Peripheral manifestations (Osler's nodes, subungual hemorrhages, Janeway lesions, Roth's spots)	2–15
Petechiae	10–40
Laboratory manifestations	
Anemia	70–90
Leukocytosis	20–30
Microscopic hematuria	30–50
Elevated erythrocyte sedimentation rate	>90
Rheumatoid factor	50
Circulating immune complexes	65–100
Decreased serum complement	5–40

the aorta into cardiac chambers or between cardiac chambers) with new murmurs. Abscesses may burrow from the aortic valve annulus through the epicardium, causing pericarditis. Extension of infection into paravalvular tissue adjacent to either the right or the noncoronary cusp of the aortic valve may interrupt the conduction system in the upper interventricular septum, leading to varying degrees of heart block. Although perivalvular abscesses arising from the mitral valve may potentially interrupt conduction pathways near the atrioventricular node or in the proximal bundle of His, such interruption occurs infrequently. Emboli to a coronary artery may result in myocardial infarction; nevertheless, embolic transmural infarcts are rare.

Noncardiac Manifestations   The classic nonsuppurative peripheral manifestations of subacute endocarditis are related to the duration of infection and, with early diagnosis and treatment, have become infrequent. In contrast, septic embolization mimicking some of these lesions (subungual hemorrhage, Osler's nodes) is common in patients with acute *S. aureus* endocarditis (Fig. 109-2). Musculoskeletal symptoms, including nonspecific inflammatory arthritis and back pain, usually remit promptly with treatment but must be distinguished from focal metastatic infection. Hematogenously seeded focal infection may involve any organ but most often is clinically evident in the skin, spleen, kidneys, skeletal system, and meninges. Arterial emboli are clinically apparent in up to 50% of patients. Vegetations >10 mm in diameter (as measured by echocardiography) and those located on the mitral valve are more likely to embolize than are smaller or nonmitral vegetations. Embolic events—often with infarction—involving the extremities, spleen, kidneys (Fig. 109-3), bowel, or brain are often noted at presentation. With antibiotic treatment, the frequency of embolic events decreases from 13 per 1000 patient-days during the initial week to 1.2 per 1000 patient-days after the third week. Emboli occurring late during or after effective therapy do not in themselves constitute evidence of failed antimicrobial treatment. Neurologic symptoms, most often resulting from embolic strokes, occur in up to 40% of patients. Other neurologic complications include aseptic or purulent meningitis, intracranial hemorrhage due to hemorrhagic infarcts or ruptured mycotic aneurysms, seizures, and encephalopathy. (*Mycotic aneurysms* are focal dilations of arteries occurring at points in the artery wall that have been weakened by infection in the vasa vasorum or where septic emboli have lodged.) Microabscesses in brain and meninges occur commonly in *S. aureus* endocarditis; surgically drainable abscesses are infrequent.

Immune complex deposition on the glomerular basement membrane causes diffuse hypocomplementemic glomerulonephritis and renal dysfunction, which typically improve with effective antimicrobial

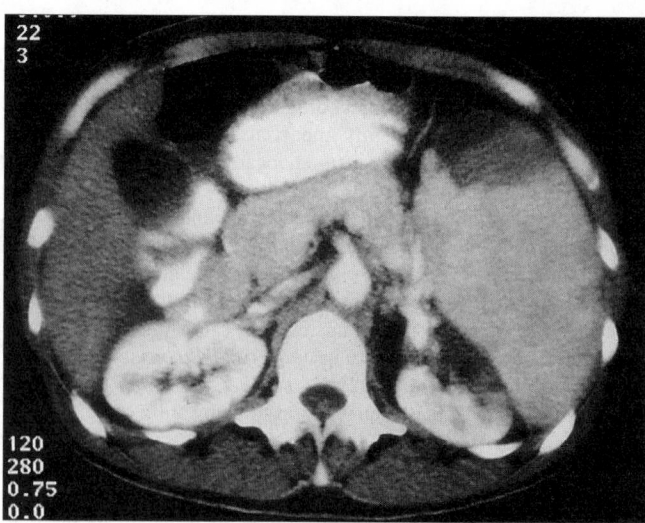

FIGURE 109-3   Computed tomography of the abdomen showing large embolic infarcts in the spleen and left kidney of a patient with *Bartonella* endocarditis.

therapy. Embolic renal infarcts cause flank pain and hematuria but rarely cause renal dysfunction.

Manifestations of Specific Predisposing Conditions   In almost 50% of patients who have endocarditis associated with injection drug use, infection is limited to the tricuspid valve. These patients present with fever, faint or no murmur, and (in 75% of cases) prominent pulmonary findings, including cough, pleuritic chest pain, nodular pulmonary infiltrates, and occasionally pyopneumothorax. Infection involving valves on the left side of the heart presents with the typical clinical features of endocarditis.

Nosocomial endocarditis (defined as that which results from hospital care within the prior month and most commonly presenting as intravascular catheter–associated bacteremia), if not associated with a retained intracardiac device, has typical manifestations. Endocarditis associated with flow-directed pulmonary artery catheters is often cryptic, with symptoms masked by comorbid critical illness, and is commonly diagnosed at autopsy. Transvenous pacemaker lead– and/or implanted defibrillator–associated endocarditis commonly follows initial implantation or a generator unit change; may be associated with obvious or cryptic generator pocket infection; and results in fever, minimal murmur, and pulmonary symptoms similar to those encountered in addicts with tricuspid endocarditis.

Prosthetic valve endocarditis presents with typical clinical features. Cases arising within 60 days of valve surgery (early onset) lack peripheral vascular manifestations and may be obscured by comorbidity associated with recent surgery. In both early-onset and more delayed presentations, paravalvular infection is common and often results in partial valve dehiscence, regurgitant murmurs, congestive heart failure, or disruption of the conduction system.

DIAGNOSIS ■ The Duke Criteria   The diagnosis of infective endocarditis is established with certainty only when vegetations obtained at cardiac surgery, at autopsy, or from an artery (an embolus) are examined histologically and microbiologically. Nevertheless, a highly sensitive and specific diagnostic schema—known as the *Duke criteria*—has been developed on the basis of clinical, laboratory, and echocardiographic findings (Table 109-3). Documentation of two major criteria, of one major and three minor criteria, or of five minor criteria allows a clinical diagnosis of definite endocarditis. The diagnosis of endocarditis is rejected if an alternative diagnosis is established, if symptoms resolve and do not recur with ≤4 days of antibiotic therapy, or if surgery or autopsy after ≤4 days of antimicrobial therapy yields no histologic evidence of endocarditis. Illnesses not classified as definite endocarditis or rejected are considered cases of possible infective endocarditis when either one major and one minor criteria or three minor criteria are identified. Requiring the identification of clinical features of en-

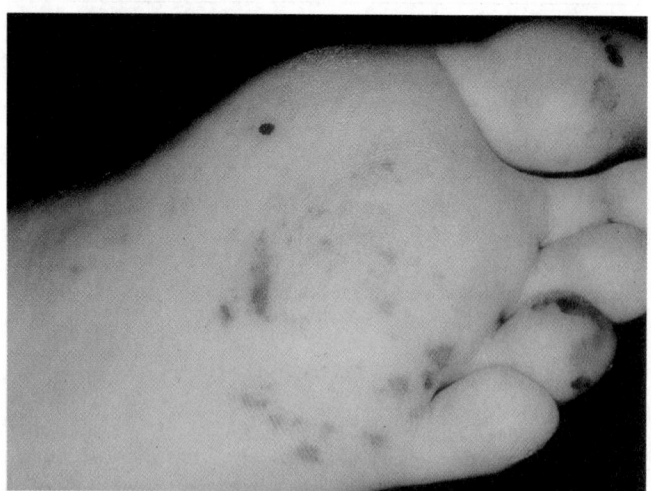

FIGURE 109-2   Septic emboli with hemorrhage and infarction due to acute *Staphylococcus aureus* endocarditis. (*Courtesy of L. Baden.*)

docarditis for classification as possible infective endocarditis increases the specificity of the schema without significantly reducing its sensitivity.

The roles of bacteremia and echocardiographic findings in the diagnosis of endocarditis are appropriately emphasized in the Duke criteria. That multiple blood cultures obtained over time are positive is consistent with the known continuous low-density nature of bacteremia characteristic of patients with endocarditis ($\leq$100 organisms per milliliter). Among untreated endocarditis patients who ultimately have a positive blood culture, 95% of all blood cultures are positive, and in 98% of cases one of the initial two sets of cultures yields the microorganism. The diagnostic criteria attach significance to the species of organism isolated from blood cultures. To fulfill a major criterion, the isolation of an organism that causes both endocarditis and bacteremia in the absence of endocarditis (e.g., *S. aureus*, enterococci) must take place repeatedly (i.e., persistent bacteremia) and in the absence of a primary focus of infection. Organisms that rarely cause endocarditis but commonly contaminate blood cultures (e.g., diphtheroids, coagulase-negative species) must be isolated repeatedly if their isolation is to serve as a major criterion.

Blood Cultures Isolation of the causative microorganism from blood cultures is critical not only for diagnosis but also for determination of antimicrobial susceptibility and planning of treatment. In the absence of prior antibiotic therapy, a total of three blood culture sets, ideally with the first separated from the last by at least 1 h, should be obtained from different venipuncture sites over 24 h. If the cultures remain negative after 48 to 72 h, two or three additional blood cultures, including a lysis-centrifugation culture, should be obtained, and the laboratory should be asked to pursue fastidious microorganisms by prolonging incubation time and performing special subcultures. Empirical antimicrobial therapy should not be administered initially to hemodynamically stable patients with subacute endocarditis, especially those who have received antibiotics within the preceding 2 weeks; thus, if necessary, additional blood cultures can be obtained without the confounding effect of empirical treatment. Patients with acute endocarditis or with deteriorating hemodynamics that may require urgent surgery should be treated empirically immediately after the initial three sets of blood cultures are obtained.

Non-Blood-Culture Tests for the Etiologic Agent Serologic tests can be used to identify some organisms causing endocarditis that are difficult to recover by blood culture: *Brucella, Bartonella, Legionella,* and *C. burnetii.* Pathogens can also be identified in vegetations by culture, by microscopic examination with special stains (i.e., the periodic acid–Schiff stain for *T. whipplei*), and by use of polymerase chain reaction to recover unique microbial DNA or 16S rRNA.

Echocardiography Cardiac imaging with echocardiography allows anatomic confirmation of infective endocarditis, sizing of vegetations, detection of intracardiac complications, and assessment of cardiac function. A two-dimensional study with color flow and continuous as well as pulsed Doppler is optimal. Transthoracic echocardiography (TTE) is noninvasive and exceptionally specific; however, it cannot image vegetations <2 mm in diameter, and in 20% of patients it is technically inadequate because of emphysema or body habitus. Thus, TTE detects vegetations in only 65% of patients with definite clinical

TABLE 109-3 The Duke Criteria for the Clinical Diagnosis of Infective Endocarditis
MAJOR CRITERIA
1. Positive blood culture
Typical microorganism for infective endocarditis from two separate blood cultures
Viridans streptococci, *Streptococcus bovis*, HACEK group, *Staphylococcus aureus*, or
Community-acquired enterococci in the absence of a primary focus, *or*
Persistently positive blood culture, defined as recovery of a microorganism consistent with infective endocarditis from:
Blood cultures drawn >12 h apart; *or*
All of three or a majority of four or more separate blood cultures, with first and last drawn at least 1 h apart
Single positive blood culture for *Coxiella burnetii* or phase I IgG antibody titer of >1:800
2. Evidence of endocardial involvement
Positive echocardiogram
Oscillating intracardiac mass on valve or supporting structures or in the path of regurgitant jets or in implanted material, in the absence of an alternative anatomic explanation, *or*
Abscess, *or*
New partial dehiscence of prosthetic valve, *or*
New valvular regurgitation (increase or change in preexisting murmur not sufficient)
MINOR CRITERIA
1. Predisposition: predisposing heart condition or injection drug use
2. Fever $\geq$38.0°C ($\geq$100.4°F)
3. Vascular phenomena: major arterial emboli, septic pulmonary infarcts, mycotic aneurysm, intracranial hemorrhage, conjunctival hemorrhages, Janeway lesions
4. Immunologic phenomena: glomerulonephritis, Osler's nodes, Roth's spots, rheumatoid factor
5. Microbiologic evidence: positive blood culture but not meeting major criterion as noted previously[a] or serologic evidence of active infection with organism consistent with infective endocarditis

[a] Excluding single positive cultures for coagulase-negative staphylococci and diphtheroids, which are common culture contaminants, and organisms that do not cause endocarditis frequently, such as gram-negative bacilli.
Note: HACEK, *Haemophilus* spp., *Actinobacillus actinomycetemcomitans, Cardiobacterium hominis, Eikenella corrodens, Kingella kingae.*
Source: Adapted from Li et al., with permission from the University of Chicago Press.

endocarditis (i.e., it has a sensitivity of 65%). Moreover, TTE is not adequate for evaluating prosthetic valves or detecting intracardiac complications. TEE is safe and significantly more sensitive than TTE. It detects vegetations in >90% of patients with definite endocarditis; nevertheless, false-negative studies are noted in 6 to 18% of endocarditis patients. TEE is the optimal method for the diagnosis of prosthetic endocarditis or the detection of myocardial abscess, valve perforation, or intracardiac fistulae.

Experts favor echocardiographic evaluation of all patients with a clinical diagnosis of endocarditis; however, the test should not be used to screen patients with otherwise-explained positive blood cultures or patients with unexplained fever. In patients with a low pretest likelihood of endocarditis (<5%), a high-quality TTE that is negative is sufficient to exclude endocarditis. For patients whose habitus makes them difficult to study with TTE and for those who may have prosthetic valve endocarditis or who are at high risk of intracardiac complications, TEE is the preferred imaging modality. For patients with a pretest probability of endocarditis ranging from 5 to 50%, initial evaluation by TEE—in lieu of a sequential strategy of TTE, which, if negative, will be followed by TEE—is cost-effective. A negative TEE when endocarditis is likely does not exclude the diagnosis but rather warrants repetition of the study in 7 to 10 days with optimal multiplanar technique.

Other Studies Many laboratory studies that do not aid in diagnostic evaluation are nevertheless important in the management of patients with endocarditis; these studies include complete blood counts, creatinine measurement, chest radiography, and electrocardiography. The erythrocyte sedimentation rate, C-reactive protein level, circulating immune complex titer, and rheumatoid factor concentration are commonly increased in endocarditis (Table 109-2). Cardiac catheterization is useful primarily to assess coronary artery patency in older individuals who are to undergo surgery for endocarditis.

℞ TREATMENT

ANTIMICROBIAL THERAPY It is difficult to eradicate bacteria from the avascular vegetation in infective endocarditis because this site is relatively inaccessible to host defenses and because the bacteria are non-growing and metabolically inactive. Since all bacteria in the vegetation must be killed, therapy for endocarditis must be bactericidal and must be given for prolonged periods. Antibiotics are generally given parenterally and must reach high serum concentrations that will, through passive diffusion, lead to effective concentrations in the depths of the vegetation. The choice of effective therapy requires precise knowledge of the susceptibility of the causative microorganisms. The initiation of treatment before a cause is defined must balance the need to establish a microbiologic diagnosis against the potential progression of disease or the need for urgent surgery (see "Blood Cultures," above). The individual vulnerabilities of the patient should be weighed in the selection of therapy—e.g., simultaneous infection at other sites (such as meningitis), allergies, end-organ dysfunction, interactions with concomitant medications, and risks of adverse events.

Although given for several weeks longer, the regimens recommended for the treatment of endocarditis involving prosthetic valves (except for staphylococcal infections) are similar to those used to treat native valve infection (Table 109-4). Recommended doses and duration of therapy should be adhered to unless alterations are required by adverse events.

Organism-Specific Therapies ■ *STREPTOCOCCI* Although most strains of viridans streptococci and *S. bovis* that cause endocarditis are susceptible to penicillin [minimum inhibitory concentration (MIC) ≤0.1 μg/mL], recent reports indicate increasing penicillin resistance among viridans streptococci recovered from blood cultures. In the selection of optimal therapy, the penicillin MIC must be determined (Table 109-4). The 2-

TABLE 109-4 *Antibiotic Treatment for Infective Endocarditis Caused by Common Organisms*[a]

Organism	Drug, Dose, Duration	Comments
Streptococci		
Penicillin-susceptible[b] streptococci, *S. bovis*	Penicillin G 2–3 million units IV q4h for 4 weeks	—
	Penicillin G 2–3 million units IV q4h *plus* gentamicin[c] 1 mg/kg IM or IV q8h, both for 2 weeks	Avoid penicillin plus gentamicin if risks of aminoglycoside toxicity are increased or case is complicated
	Ceftriaxone 2 g/d IV as single dose for 4 weeks	Can use ceftriaxone in patients with nonimmediate penicillin allergy
	Vancomycin[d] 15 mg/kg IV q12h for 4 weeks	Use vancomycin in patients with severe or immediate β-lactam allergy
Relatively penicillin-resistant[e] streptococci	Penicillin G 3 million units IV q4h for 4–6 weeks *plus* gentamicin[c] 1 mg/kg IV q8h for 2 weeks	Preferred for treatment of prosthetic valve endocarditis caused by penicillin-susceptible streptococci; continue penicillin for 6 weeks in this setting
Moderately penicillin-resistant[f] streptococci, pyridoxal-requiring streptococci (*Abiotrophia* spp.)	Penicillin G 3–4 million units IV q4h *plus* gentamicin[c] 1 mg/kg IV q8h, both for 4–6 weeks	—
Enterococci[g]	Penicillin G 3–4 million units IV q4h *plus* gentamicin[c] 1 mg/kg IV q8h, both for 4–6 weeks	Can use streptomycin 7.5 mg/kg q12h in lieu of gentamicin if there is not high-level resistance to streptomycin
	Ampicillin 2 g IV q4h *plus* gentamicin[c] 1 mg/kg IV q8h, both for 4–6 weeks	Do not use cephalosporins or carbapenems for treatment of enterococcal endocarditis
	Vancomycin[d] 15 mg/kg IV q12h *plus* gentamicin[c] 1 mg/kg IV q8h, both for 4–6 weeks	Use vancomycin plus gentamicin for penicillin-allergic patients or desensitize to penicillin
Staphylococci		
Methicillin-susceptible, infecting native valves (no foreign devices)	Nafcillin or oxacillin 2 g IV q4h for 4–6 weeks *plus* (optional) gentamicin[c] 1 mg/kg IM or IV q8h for 3–5 days	May use penicillin 3–4 million units q6h if isolate is penicillin-susceptible (does not produce β-lactamase)
	Cefazolin 2 g IV q8h for 4–6 weeks *plus* (optional) gentamicin[c] 1 mg/kg IM or IV q8h for 3–5 days	Can use cefazolin regimen for patients with nonimmediate penicillin allergy
	Vancomycin[d] 15 mg/kg IV q12h for 4–6 weeks	Use vancomycin for patients with immediate (urticarial) or severe penicillin allergy
Methicillin-resistant, infecting native valves (no foreign devices)	Vancomycin[d] 15 mg/kg IV q12h for 4–6 weeks	No role for routine use of rifampin
Methicillin-susceptible, infecting prosthetic valves	Nafcillin or oxacillin 2 g IV q4h for 6–8 weeks *plus* gentamicin[c] 1 mg/kg IM or IV q8h for 2 weeks *plus* rifampin[h] 300 mg PO q8h for 6–8 weeks	Use gentamicin during initial 2 weeks; determine susceptibility to gentamicin before initiating rifampin (see text); if patient is highly allergic to penicillin, use regimen for methicillin-resistant staphylococci; if β-lactam allergy is of the minor, nonimmediate type, can substitute cefazolin for oxacillin/nafcillin
Methicillin-resistant, infecting prosthetic valves	Vancomycin[d] 15 mg/kg IV q12h for 6–8 weeks *plus* gentamicin[c] 1 mg/kg IM or IV q8h for 2 weeks *plus* rifampin[h] 300 mg PO q8h for 6–8 weeks	Use gentamicin during initial 2 weeks; determine gentamicin susceptibility before initiating rifampin (see text)
HACEK organisms	Ceftriaxone 2 g/d IV as single dose for 4 weeks	May use another third-generation cephalosporin at comparable dosage
	Ampicillin 2 g IV q4h *plus* gentamicin[c] 1 mg/kg IM or IV q8h, both for 4 weeks	Determine ampicillin susceptibility; do not use ampicillin if β-lactamase is produced

[a] Doses are for adults with normal renal function. Doses of gentamicin, streptomycin, and vancomycin must be adjusted for reduced renal function. Ideal body weight is used to calculate doses per kilogram (men = 50 kg + 2.3 kg per inch over 5 feet; women = 45.5 kg + 2.3 kg per inch over 5 feet).
[b] MIC ≤ 0.1 μg/mL.
[c] Aminoglycosides should not be administered as single daily doses and should be introduced as part of the initial treatment. Target peak and trough serum concentrations of gentamicin 1 h after a 20- to 30-min infusion or IM injection are 3–5 μg/mL and ≤1 μg/mL, respectively; the target peak serum concentration of streptomycin (timing as with gentamicin) is 20–25 μg/mL.
[d] Desirable peak vancomycin level 1 h after completion of a 1-h infusion is 30–45 μg/mL.
[e] MIC > 0.1 μg/mL and <0.5 μg/mL.
[f] MIC ≥ 0.5 μg/mL and <8.0 μg/mL.
[g] Antimicrobial susceptibility must be evaluated; see text.
[h] Rifampin increases warfarin and dicumarol requirements for anticoagulation.

week penicillin/gentamicin regimen should not be used to treat complicated native valve infection or prosthetic valve endocarditis. Although small studies have suggested that a 2-week regimen of single daily doses of ceftriaxone (2 g IV) plus gentamicin (3 mg/kg) or netilmicin (4 mg/kg) is effective for penicillin-susceptible streptococcal endocarditis, the data are not sufficient to support routine use of this regimen. Penicillin/gentamicin is recommended for the treatment of endocarditis caused by group B streptococci.

ENTEROCOCCI Enterococci are resistant to oxacillin, nafcillin, and the cephalosporins and are inhibited only by penicillin, ampicillin, teicoplanin (not available in the United States), and vancomycin. To kill enterococci requires the synergistic interaction of a cell wall–active antibiotic (penicillin, ampicillin, vancomycin, or teicoplanin) that is effective at achievable serum concentrations and an aminoglycoside (gentamicin or streptomycin) to which the isolate does not exhibit high-level resistance. An isolate's resistance to cell wall–active agents or ability to replicate in the presence of gentamicin at ≥ 500 μg/mL or streptomycin at 2000 μg/mL—a phenomenon called *high-level aminoglycoside resistance*—indicates that the ineffective antimicrobial cannot participate in the interaction to produce killing. High-level resistance to gentamicin predicts that tobramycin, netilmicin, amikacin, and kanamycin will also be ineffective. In fact, even when enterococci are not highly resistant to gentamicin, it is difficult to predict the ability of these other aminoglycosides to participate in synergistic killing; consequently, they should not in general be used to treat enterococcal endocarditis.

Clearly, enterococci causing endocarditis must be tested for high-level resistance to streptomycin and gentamicin, β-lactamase production, and susceptibility to penicillin and ampicillin (MIC ≤ 16 μg/mL) and to vancomycin (MIC ≤ 8 μg/mL). If the isolate produces β-lactamase, ampicillin/sulbactam or vancomycin can be used as the cell wall–active component; if the penicillin/ampicillin MIC is >16 μg/mL, vancomycin can be considered; and if the vancomycin MIC is >8 μg/mL, penicillin or ampicillin may be considered. Based on the absence of high-level resistance, gentamicin or streptomycin should be used as the aminoglycoside. If there is high-level resistance to both these drugs, no aminoglycoside should be given; instead, an 8- to 12-week course of a single cell wall–active agent is suggested. If single-drug therapy fails or the isolate is resistant to all of the commonly used agents, surgical treatment is advised. The role of newer agents potentially active against multidrug-resistant enterococci (quinupristin/dalfopristin, linezolid, and daptomycin) in the treatment of endocarditis has not been established. Although the dose of gentamicin used to achieve bactericidal synergy in treating enterococcal endocarditis is smaller than that used in standard therapy, nephrotoxicity is not uncommon during treatment with recommended regimens for 4 to 6 weeks. Regimens wherein gentamicin treatment has been truncated at 2 to 3 weeks because of nephrotoxicity have been curative. Thus, discontinuation of gentamicin is recommended when progressive nephrotoxicity develops in patients with enterococcal endocarditis who have responded satisfactorily to therapy.

STAPHYLOCOCCI The regimens used to treat staphylococcal endocarditis are not based upon coagulase production but rather upon the presence or absence of a prosthetic valve or foreign device, the native valve(s) involved, and the resistance of the isolate to penicillin and methicillin. Penicillinase is produced by 95% of staphylococci; thus, all isolates should be considered penicillin-resistant until shown not to produce this enzyme. The addition of gentamicin (if the isolate is susceptible) to a β-lactam antibiotic to enhance therapy for native mitral or aortic valve endocarditis is optional. Its addition hastens eradication of bacteremia but does not improve survival rates. If added, gentamicin should be limited to the initial 3 to 5 days of therapy to avoid nephrotoxicity. Gentamicin generally is not added to the vancomycin regimen in this setting.

Methicillin-susceptible *S. aureus* endocarditis that is uncomplicated and limited to the tricuspid or pulmonic valve—a condition occurring almost exclusively in injection drug users—can often be treated with a 2-week course that combines oxacillin or nafcillin (but not vancomycin) with gentamicin. Prolonged fevers (≥ 5 days) during therapy suggest that these patients should receive standard therapy.

Staphylococcal prosthetic valve endocarditis is treated for 6 to 8 weeks with a multidrug regimen. Rifampin is an essential component because it kills staphylococci that are adherent to foreign material. Two other agents (selected on the basis of susceptibility testing) are combined with rifampin to prevent in vivo emergence of resistance. Because many staphylococci, particularly methicillin-resistant *S. aureus* and *S. epidermidis*, are resistant to gentamicin, the utility of gentamicin should be established before rifampin treatment is begun. If the isolate is resistant to gentamicin, another aminoglycoside or a fluoroquinolone (chosen in light of susceptibility results) should be substituted.

OTHER ORGANISMS Endocarditis caused by *Streptococcus pneumoniae*, with a penicillin MIC ≤ 1.0 can be treated with intravenous penicillin (4 million units every 4 h), ceftriaxone (2 g/d as a single dose), or cefotaxime (at a comparable dosage). Infection caused by strains with a penicillin MIC ≥ 2.0 should be treated with vancomycin. Until the strain's susceptibility to penicillin is established, therapy should consist of vancomycin plus ceftriaxone, especially if concurrent meningitis is suspected. *P. aeruginosa* endocarditis is treated with an antipseudomonal penicillin (ticarcillin or piperacillin) and high doses of tobramycin (8 mg/kg per day in three divided doses). Endocarditis caused by Enterobacteriaceae is treated with a potent β-lactam antibiotic plus an aminoglycoside. Corynebacterial endocarditis is treated with penicillin plus an aminoglycoside (if the organism is susceptible to the aminoglycoside) or with vancomycin, which is highly bactericidal for most strains. Therapy for *Candida* endocarditis consists of amphotericin B plus flucytosine and early surgery; long-term (if not indefinite) suppression with fluconazole is used increasingly.

Empirical Therapy In designing and executing therapy without culture data (i.e., before culture results are known or when cultures are negative), clinical and epidemiologic clues to etiology must be weighed, and both the pathogens associated with the specific endocarditis syndrome and the hazards of suboptimal therapy must be considered. Thus, empirical therapy for acute endocarditis in an injection drug user should cover methicillin-resistant *S. aureus* and gram-negative bacilli. The initiation of treatment with vancomycin plus gentamicin immediately after blood is obtained for cultures covers these as well as many other potential causes. In treating culture-negative episodes, marantic endocarditis must be excluded and fastidious organisms sought serologically. In the absence of confounding prior antibiotic therapy, it is unlikely that *S. aureus*, coagulase-negative staphylococcal, or enterococcal infection will present with negative blood cultures. Thus, in this situation, these organisms are not the determinants of therapy for subacute endocarditis. Blood culture–negative subacute native valve endocarditis is treated with ceftriaxone plus gentamicin; these two antimicrobials plus vancomycin should be used if prosthetic valves are involved.

Outpatient Antimicrobial Therapy Fully compliant patients who have sterile blood cultures, are afebrile during therapy, and have no clinical or echocardiographic findings that suggest an impending complication may complete therapy as outpatients. Careful follow-up and a stable home setting are necessary, as are predictable intravenous access and selection of antimicrobials that are stable in solution.

Monitoring Antimicrobial Therapy The serum bactericidal titer—the highest dilution of the patient's serum during therapy that kills 99.9% of the standard inoculum of the infecting organism—is no longer recommended for assessment of patients receiving standard regimens. However, in the treatment of endocarditis caused by unusual organisms, this measurement, although not standardized and difficult to interpret, may provide a patient-specific assessment of in vivo antibiotic effect. Serum concentrations of aminoglycosides and vancomycin should be monitored.

TABLE 109-5 *Indications for Cardiac Surgical Intervention in Patients with Endocarditis*

Surgery required for optimal outcome
  Moderate to severe congestive heart failure due to valve dysfunction
  Partially dehisced unstable prosthetic valve
  Persistent bacteremia despite optimal antimicrobial therapy
  Lack of effective microbicidal therapy (e.g., fungal or *Brucella* endocarditis)
  S. aureus prosthetic valve endocarditis with an intracardiac complication
  Relapse of prosthetic valve endocarditis after optimal antimicrobial therapy
Surgery to be strongly considered for improved outcome[a]
  Perivalvular extension of infection
  Poorly responsive *S. aureus* endocarditis involving the aortic or mitral valve
  Large (>10-mm diameter) hypermobile vegetations with increased risk of embolism
  Persistent unexplained fever (≥10 days) in culture-negative native valve endocarditis
  Poorly responsive or relapsed endocarditis due to highly antibiotic-resistant enterococci or gram-negative bacilli

[a] Surgery must be carefully considered; findings are often combined with other indications to prompt surgery.

Antibiotic toxicities, including allergic reactions, occur in 25 to 40% of patients and commonly arise during the third week of therapy. Blood tests to detect antibiotic-specific potential end-organ toxicity should be performed periodically.

In most patients, effective antibiotic therapy results in subjective improvement and resolution of fever within 5 to 7 days. Blood cultures should be repeated daily until sterile, rechecked if there is recrudescent fever, and performed again 4 to 6 weeks after therapy to document cure. Blood cultures become sterile within 2 days after the start of appropriate therapy when infection is caused by viridans streptococci, enterococci, or HACEK organisms. In *S. aureus* endocarditis, β-lactam therapy results in sterile cultures in 3 to 5 days, whereas positive cultures may persist for 7 to 9 days with vancomycin treatment. When fever persists for 7 days in spite of appropriate antibiotic therapy, patients should be evaluated for paravalvular abscess and for extracardiac abscesses (spleen, kidney) or complications (embolic events). Recrudescent fever raises the question of these complications but also of drug reactions or complications of hospitalization. Serologic abnormalities (e.g., erythrocyte sedimentation rate, rheumatoid factor) resolve slowly and do not reflect response to treatment. Vegetations

become smaller with effective therapy, but at 3 months after cure half are unchanged and 25% are slightly larger.

SURGICAL TREATMENT Intracardiac and central nervous system complications of endocarditis are important causes of the morbidity and mortality associated with this infection. In some cases, effective treatment for these complications requires surgery. Most of the clinical indications for surgical treatment of endocarditis are not absolute (Table 109-5). The risks and benefits as well as the timing of surgical treatment must therefore be individualized (Table 109-6).

Intracardiac Surgical Indications Most surgical interventions are warranted by intracardiac findings, often detected by echocardiography. Because of the highly invasive nature of prosthetic valve endocarditis, as many as 40% of affected patients merit surgical treatment. In many patients, coincident rather than single intracardiac events necessitate surgery.

CONGESTIVE HEART FAILURE Moderate to severe refractory congestive heart failure caused by new or worsening valve dysfunction is the major indication for cardiac surgical treatment of endocarditis. Of patients with moderate to severe heart failure due to valve dysfunction who are treated medically, 60 to 90% die within 6 months. In the setting of similar hemodynamic dysfunction, surgical treatment is associated with mortality rates of 20 to 40% with native valve endocarditis and 35 to 55% with prosthetic valve infection. Surgery may be required to relieve functional stenosis due to large vegetations or to restore competence to damaged regurgitant valves.

PERIVALVULAR INFECTION This complication, which occurs in 10 to 15% of native valve and 45 to 60% of prosthetic valve infections, is suggested by persistent unexplained fever during appropriate therapy, new electrocardiographic conduction disturbances, and pericarditis. Extension can occur from any valve but is most common with aortic valve infection. TEE with color Doppler is the test of choice to detect perivalvular abscesses (sensitivity ≥ 85%). Although occasional perivalvular infections are cured medically, surgery is warranted when fever persists, fistulae develop, prostheses are dehisced and unstable, and invasive infection relapses after appropriate treatment. Cardiac rhythm must be monitored since high-grade heart block may require insertion of a pacemaker.

UNCONTROLLED INFECTION Continued positive blood cultures or otherwise-unexplained persistent fevers (in patients with either blood culture–positive or –negative endocarditis) despite optimal antibiotic therapy may reflect uncontrolled infection and warrant surgery. Surgical treatment is also advised for endocarditis caused by those organisms against which clinical experience indicates that effective antimicrobial

TABLE 109-6 *Timing of Cardiac Surgical Intervention in Patients with Endocarditis*

| | Indication for Surgical Intervention | |
Timing	Strong Supporting Evidence	Conflicting Evidence, but Majority of Opinions Favor Surgery
Emergent (same day)	Acute aortic regurgitation plus preclosure of mitral valve	
	Sinus of Valsalva abscess ruptured into right heart	
	Rupture into pericardial sac	
Urgent (within 1–2 days)	Valve obstruction by vegetation	Major embolus plus persisting large vegetation (>10 mm in diameter)
	Unstable (dehisced) prosthesis	
	Acute aortic or mitral regurgitation with heart failure (New York Heart Association class III or IV)	
	Septal perforation	
	Perivalvular extension of infection with/without new electrocardiographic conduction system changes	
	Lack of effective antibiotic therapy	
Elective (earlier usually preferred)	Progressive paravalvular prosthetic regurgitation	Staphylococcal PVE
	Valve dysfunction plus persisting infection after ≥7–10 days of antimicrobial therapy	Early PVE (≤2 months after valve surgery)
		Fungal endocarditis (*Candida* spp.)
	Fungal (mold) endocarditis	Antibiotic-resistant organisms

Abbreviation: PVE, prosthetic valve endocarditis.
Source: Adapted from I Olaison, G Pettersson: Infect Dis Clin North Am 16:453, 2002.

TABLE 109-7 *Procedures for which Endocarditis Prophylaxis Is Advised in Patients at High or Moderate Risk for Endocarditis[a]*

Dental procedures
  Extractions
  Periodontal procedures, cleaning causing gingival bleeding
  Implant placement, reimplantation of avulsed teeth
  Endodontic instrumentation (root canal) or surgery beyond the apex
  Subgingival placement of antibiotic fibers or strips
  Placement of orthodontic bands but not brackets
  Intraligamentary injections (anesthetic)
Respiratory procedures
  Operations involving the mucosa
  Bronchoscopy with rigid bronchoscope
Gastrointestinal procedures[b]
  Esophageal: Sclerotherapy of varices, stricture dilation
  Biliary tract: Endoscopic retrograde cholangiography with biliary
    obstruction, biliary tract surgery
  Intestinal tract: Surgery involving the mucosa
Genitourinary procedures
  Urethral dilation, prostate or urethral surgery
  Cystoscopy

[a] Prophylaxis is optional for high-risk patients undergoing bronchoscopy or gastrointestinal endoscopy with/without biopsy, vaginal delivery, vaginal hysterectomy, or transesophageal echocardiography.
[b] Prophylaxis is recommended for high-risk patients and optional for moderate-risk group (see Table 109-8).
Source: Adapted from AS Dajani et al: JAMA 277:1794, 1997; with permission.

therapy is lacking. This category includes infections caused by yeasts, fungi, *P. aeruginosa*, other highly resistant gram-negative bacilli, *Brucella* species, and probably *C. burnetii*.

S. AUREUS ENDOCARDITIS Mortality rates for *S. aureus* prosthetic valve endocarditis exceed 70% with medical treatment but are reduced to 25% with surgical treatment. In patients with intracardiac complications associated with *S. aureus* prosthetic valve infection, surgical treatment reduces mortality by twentyfold. Surgical treatment should be considered for patients with *S. aureus* native aortic or mitral valve infection who have TTE-demonstrable vegetations and remain septic during the initial week of therapy. Isolated tricuspid valve endocarditis, even with persistent fever, rarely requires surgery.

PREVENTION OF SYSTEMIC EMBOLI Mortality and persisting morbidity due to emboli are largely limited to patients suffering occlusion of cerebral or coronary arteries. Echocardiographic determination of vegetation size and anatomy, although predictive of patients at high risk of systemic emboli, does not identify those patients in whom the benefits of surgery to prevent emboli clearly exceed the risks of the surgical procedure and an implanted prosthetic valve. Net benefits favoring surgery are most likely when the risk of embolism is high and other surgical benefits can be achieved simultaneously—e.g., repair of a moderately dysfunctional valve or debridement of a paravalvular abscess. Reduced overall risks of surgical intervention (e.g., use of vegetation resection and valve repair to avoid insertion of a prosthesis) make the benefit-to-risk ratio more favorable and this intervention more attractive.

TABLE 109-8 *Cardiac Lesions for which Endocarditis Prophylaxis Is Advised*

High Risk	Moderate Risk
Prosthetic heart valves	Congenital cardiac malformations
Prior bacterial endocarditis	(other than high-/low-risk
Complex cyanotic congenital heart	lesions), ventricular septal defect,
disease; other complex congenital	bicuspid aortic valve
lesions after correction (see text)	Acquired aortic and mitral valve
Patent ductus arteriosus	dysfunction
Coarctation of the aorta	Hypertrophic cardiomyopathy
Surgically constructed systemic-	(asymmetric septal hypertrophy)
pulmonary shunts	Mitral valve prolapse with valvular
	regurgitation and/or thickened
	leaflets

TABLE 109-9 *Cardiac Conditions That Are Considered to Pose a Low Risk of Endocarditis and for which Antibiotic Prophylaxis Is Not Recommended*

Isolated secundum ASD
Surgically repaired ASD, VSD, PDA (without residual defect, >6 months after repair)
Prior coronary artery bypass graft
Mitral valve prolapse without regurgitation or thickened leaflets
Physiologic or functional murmur
Prior Kawasaki disease or acute rheumatic fever without valve dysfunction
Cardiac pacemakers or implanted defibrillators

Abbreviations: ASD, atrial septal defect; VSD, ventricular septal defect; PDA, patent ductus arteriosus.
Source: Adapted from AS Dajani et al: JAMA 277:1794, 1997; with permission.

Timing of Cardiac Surgery In general, when indications for surgical treatment of infective endocarditis are identified, surgery should not be delayed simply to permit additional antibiotic therapy, since this course of action increases the risk of death (Table 109-6). Delay is justified only when infection is controlled and congestive heart failure is fully compensated with medical therapy. Recrudescent endocarditis involving a prosthetic valve follows surgery in 2% of patients with culture-positive native valve endocarditis and in 6 to 15% of patients with active prosthetic valve endocarditis. These risks are more acceptable than the high mortality rates that result when surgery is inappropriately delayed or not performed.

Among patients who have experienced a neurologic complication of endocarditis, further neurologic deterioration can occur as a consequence of cardiac surgery. The risk of significant neurologic exacerbation is related to the interval between the complication and surgery. Where feasible, cardiac surgery should be delayed for 2 to 3 weeks after a nonhemorrhagic embolic stroke and for 4 weeks after a

TABLE 109-10 *Antibiotic Regimens for Prophylaxis of Endocarditis in Adults at Moderate or High Risk[a]*

I. Oral cavity, respiratory tract, or esophageal procedures[b]
  A. Standard regimen
    1. Amoxicillin 2.0 g PO 1 h before procedure
  B. Inability to take oral medication
    1. Ampicillin 2.0 g IV or IM within 30 min of procedure
  C. Penicillin allergy
    1. Clarithromycin 500 mg PO 1 h before procedure
    2. Cephalexin[c] or cefadroxil[c] 2.0 g PO 1 h before procedure
    3. Clindamycin 600 mg PO 1 h before procedure or IV 30 min before procedure
  D. Penicillin allergy, inability to take oral medication
    1. Cefazolin[c] 1.0 g IV or IM 30 min before procedure
II. Genitourinary and gastrointestinal tract[d] procedures
  A. High-risk patients
    1. Ampicillin 2.0 g IV or IM *plus* gentamicin 1.5 mg/kg (not to exceed 120 mg) IV or IM within 30 min of procedure; repeat ampicillin 1.0 g IV or IM or amoxicillin 1.0 g PO 6 h later
  B. High-risk, penicillin-allergic patients
    1. Vancomycin 1.0 g IV over 1–2 h *plus* gentamicin 1.5 mg/kg (not to exceed 120 mg) IV or IM within 30 min before procedure; no second dose recommended
  C. Moderate-risk patients
    1. Amoxicillin 2.0 g PO 1 h before procedure or ampicillin 2.0 g IV or IM within 30 min before procedure
  D. Moderate-risk, penicillin-allergic patients
    1. Vancomycin 1.0 g IV infused over 1–2 h and completed within 30 min of procedure

[a] Dosing for children: for amoxicillin, ampicillin, cephalexin, or cefadroxil, use 50 mg/kg PO; cefazolin, 25 mg/kg IV; clindamycin, 20 mg/kg PO, 25 mg/kg IV; clarithromycin, 15 mg/kg PO; gentamicin, 1.5 mg/kg IV or IM; and vancomycin, 20 mg/kg IV.
[b] For patients at high risk (Table 109-8), administer a half-dose 6 h after the initial dose.
[c] Do not use cephalosporins in patients with immediate hypersensitivity (urticaria, angioedema, anaphylaxis) to penicillin.
[d] Excludes esophageal procedures.
Source: Adapted from AS Dajani et al: JAMA 277:1794, 1997; with permission.

hemorrhagic embolic stroke. A ruptured mycotic aneurysm should be clipped and cerebral edema allowed to resolve prior to cardiac surgery.

Extracardiac Complications Splenic abscess develops in 3 to 5% of patients with endocarditis. Effective therapy requires either computed tomography–guided percutaneous drainage or splenectomy. Mycotic aneurysms occur in 2 to 15% of endocarditis patients; half of these cases involve the cerebral arteries and present as headaches, focal neurologic symptoms, or hemorrhage. Cerebral aneurysms should be monitored by angiography. Some will resolve with effective antimicrobial therapy, but those that persist, enlarge, or leak should be treated surgically if possible. Extracerebral aneurysms present as local pain, a mass, local ischemia, or bleeding; generally these aneurysms are treated by resection.

OUTCOME The outcome of infective endocarditis is affected by a variety of factors, some of which are interrelated. Factors with an adverse impact include older age, severe comorbid conditions, delayed diagnosis, involvement of prosthetic valves or the aortic valve, an invasive (*S. aureus*) or antibiotic-resistant (*P. aeruginosa*, yeast) pathogen, intracardiac complications, and major neurologic complications. Death and poor outcome often are related not to failure of antibiotic therapy but rather to the interactions of comorbidities and endocarditis-related end-organ complications. The overall survival rate for patients with native valve endocarditis caused by viridans streptococci, HACEK organisms, or enterococci (susceptible to synergistic therapy) ranges from 85 to 90%. For *S. aureus* native valve endocarditis in patients who do not inject drugs, survival rates are 55 to 70%, whereas 85 to 90% of injection drug users survive this infection. Prosthetic valve endocarditis beginning within 2 months of valve replacement results in mortality rates of 40 to 50%, whereas rates are only 10 to 20% in later-onset cases.

PREVENTION Antibiotics have been administered in conjunction with selected procedures considered to entail a risk for bacteremia and endocarditis. The benefits of antibiotic prophylaxis are not established and in fact may be modest: only 50% of patients with native valve endocarditis know that they have a valve lesion predisposing to infection, most endocarditis cases do not follow a procedure, and 35% of cases are caused by organisms not targeted by prophylaxis. Dental treatments, the procedures most widely accepted as predisposing to endocarditis, are no more frequent during the 3 months preceding this diagnosis than in uninfected matched controls. Nevertheless, an expert committee of the American Heart Association, along with similar advisory groups in other developed countries, has identified procedures that may precipitate bacteremia with organisms that cause endocarditis (Table 109-7), patients who should receive prophylaxis based on the relative risk for developing endocarditis and the severity of subsequent infection (Table 109-8), patients who are at low risk and do not require prophylaxis (Table 109-9), and regimens that may be used for prophylaxis (Table 109-10). Except for an isolated secundum atrial septal defect and a totally corrected patent ductus arteriosus, ventricular septal defect, or pulmonary stenosis, patients with congenital heart defects continue to experience high rates of endocarditis despite total surgical correction of the defect. In vulnerable patients, maintaining good dental hygiene and aggressively treating local infections may reduce the risk of endocarditis.

FURTHER READING

ANDREWS MM, VON REYN CF: Patient selection criteria and management guidelines for outpatient parenteral antibiotic therapy for native valve infective endocarditis. Clin Infect Dis 33:203, 2001

BAYER AS et al: Diagnosis and management of infective endocarditis and its complications. Circulation 98:2936, 1998

DURACK DT (ed): Infective endocarditis. Infect Dis Clin North Am 16:255, 2002

KARCHMER AW: Infections of prosthetic valves and intravascular devices, in *Mandell, Douglas, and Bennett's Principles and Practice of Infectious Diseases*, 5th ed, GL Mandell et al (eds). New York, Churchill Livingstone, 2000, pp 903–917

————: Infective endocarditis, in *Heart Disease*, 6th ed, E Braunwald et al (eds). Philadelphia, Saunders, 2000

LI JS et al: Proposed modifications to the Duke criteria for the diagnosis of infective endocarditis. Clin Infect Dis 30:633, 2000

MYLONAKIS E, CALDERWOOD SB: Infective endocarditis in adults. N Engl J Med 345:1318, 2001

110 INFECTIONS OF THE SKIN, MUSCLE, AND SOFT TISSUES
Dennis L. Stevens

ANATOMICAL RELATIONSHIPS: CLUES TO THE DIAGNOSIS OF SOFT TISSUE INFECTIONS Protection against infection of the epidermis is dependent on the mechanical barrier afforded by the stratum corneum, since the epidermis itself is devoid of blood vessels (Fig. 110-1). Disruption of this layer by burns or bites, abrasions, foreign bodies, primary dermatologic disorders (e.g., herpes simplex, varicella, and ecthyma gangrenosum), surgery, or vascular or pressure ulcer allows penetration of bacteria to the deeper structures. Similarly, the hair follicle can serve as a portal either for components of the normal flora (e.g., *Staphylococcus*) or for extrinsic bacteria (e.g., *Pseudomonas* in hot-tub folliculitis). Intracellular infection of the squamous epithelium with vesicle formation may arise from cutaneous inoculation, as in infection with herpes simplex virus (HSV) type 1; from the dermal capillary plexus, as in varicella and infections due to other viruses associated with viremia; or from cutaneous nerve roots, as in herpes zoster. Bacteria infecting the epidermis, such as *Streptococcus pyogenes*, may be translocated laterally to deeper structures via lymphatics, an event that results in the rapid superficial spread of erysipelas. Later, engorgement or obstruction of lymphatics causes flaccid edema of the epidermis, another characteristic of erysipelas.

The rich plexus of capillaries beneath the dermal papillae provides nutrition to the stratum germinativum, and physiologic responses of this plexus produce important clinical signs and symptoms. For ex-

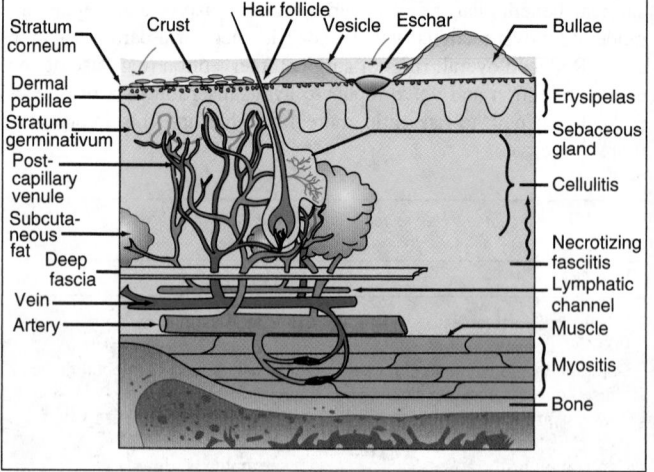

FIGURE 110-1 Structural components of the skin and soft tissue, superficial infections, and infections of the deeper structures. The rich capillary network beneath the dermal papillae plays a key role in the localization of infection and in the development of the acute inflammatory reaction.

ample, infective vasculitis of the plexus results in petechiae, Osler's nodes, Janeway lesions, and palpable purpura, which, if present, are important clues to the existence of endocarditis (Chap. 109). In addition, metastatic infection within this plexus can result in cutaneous manifestations of disseminated fungal infection (Chap. 187), gonococcal infection (Chap. 128), *Salmonella* infection (Chap. 137), *Pseudomonas* infection (i.e., ecthyma gangrenosum; Chap. 136), meningococcemia (Chap. 127), and staphylococcal infection (Chap. 120). The plexus also provides access for bacteria to the circulation, thereby facilitating local spread or bacteremia. The postcapillary venules of this plexus are a major site of polymorphonuclear leukocyte sequestration, diapedesis, and chemotaxis to the site of cutaneous infection.

Exaggeration of these physiologic mechanisms by excessive levels of cytokines or bacterial toxins causes leukostasis, venous occlusion, and pitting edema. Edema with purple bullae, ecchymosis, and cutaneous anesthesia suggests loss of vascular integrity and necessitates exploration of the deeper structures for evidence of necrotizing fasciitis or myonecrosis. An early diagnosis requires a high level of suspicion in instances of unexplained fever and of pain and tenderness in the soft tissue, even in the absence of acute cutaneous inflammation.

INFECTIONS ASSOCIATED WITH VESICLES (Table 110-1) Vesicle formation due to infection is caused by viral proliferation within the epidermis. In varicella and variola, viremia precedes the onset of a diffuse centripetal rash that progresses from macules to vesicles, then to pustules, and finally to scabs over the course of 1 to 2 weeks. Vesicles of varicella have a "dewdrop" appearance and develop in crops randomly about the trunk, extremities, and face over 3 to 4 days (see Fig. 164-1). Herpes zoster occurs in a single dermatome; the appearance of vesicles is preceded by pain for several days (see Figs. 164-2 and 164-3). Zoster may occur in persons of any age but is most common among immunosuppressed individuals and elderly patients, whereas most cases of varicella occur in young children. Vesicles due to HSV are found on or around the lips (HSV-1) or genitals (HSV-2) but may appear on the head and neck of young wrestlers (herpes gladiatorum) or on the digits of health care workers (herpetic whitlow). Recurrent herpes labialis (HSV-1) and herpes genitalis are common following primary infection. Coxsackievirus A16 characteristically causes vesicles on the hands, feet, and mouth of children. Orf is caused by a DNA virus related to smallpox virus and infects the fingers of individuals who work around goats and sheep. Molluscum contagiosum virus induces flaccid vesicles on the skin of healthy and immunocompromised individuals. Although variola (smallpox) in nature was eradicated as of 1977, recent terrorist events have renewed interest in this devastat-

TABLE 110-1 *Skin and Soft Tissue Infections*

Lesion, Clinical Syndrome	Infectious Agent	Chapter(s)
Vesicles		
Smallpox	Variola virus	205
Chickenpox	Varicella-zoster virus	164
Shingles (herpes zoster)	Varicella-zoster virus	164
Cold sores, herpetic whitlow, herpes gladiatorum	Herpes simplex virus	163
Hand-foot-and-mouth disease	Coxsackievirus A16	175
Orf	Parapoxvirus	167
Molluscum contagiosum	Pox-like virus	167
Rickettsialpox	*Rickettsia akari*	158
Blistering distal dactylitis	*Staphylococcus aureus* or *Streptococcus pyogenes*	120, 121
Bullae		
Staphylococcal scalded-skin syndrome	*S. aureus*	120
Necrotizing fasciitis	*S. pyogenes, Clostridium* spp., mixed aerobes and anaerobes	148
Gas gangrene	*Clostridium* spp.	126
Halophilic vibrio	*Vibrio vulnificus*	140
Crusted lesions		
Bullous impetigo/ecthyma	*S. aureus*	120
Impetigo contagiosa	*S. pyogenes*	121
Ringworm	Superficial dermatophyte fungi	190
Sporotrichosis	*Sporothrix schenckii*	190
Histoplasmosis	*Histoplasma capsulatum*	183
Coccidioidomycosis	*Coccidioides immitis*	184
Blastomycosis	*Blastomyces dermatitidis*	185
Cutaneous leishmaniasis	*Leishmania* spp.	196
Cutaneous tuberculosis	*Mycobacterium tuberculosis*	150
Nocardiosis	*Nocardia asteroides*	146
Folliculitis		
Furunculosis	*S. aureus*	120
Hot-tub folliculitis	*Pseudomonas aeruginosa*	136
Swimmer's itch	*Schistosoma* spp.	203
Acne vulgaris	*Propionibacterium acnes*	47
Papular and nodular lesions		
Fish-tank or swimming-pool granuloma	*Mycobacterium marinum*	152
Creeping eruption (cutaneous larva migrans)	*Ancylostoma braziliense*	200
Dracunculiasis	*Dracunculus medinensis*	202
Cercarial dermatitis	*Schistosoma mansoni*	203
Verruca vulgaris	Human papillomaviruses 1, 2, 4	169
Condylomata acuminata (anogenital warts)	Human papillomaviruses 6, 11, 16, 18	169
Onchocerciasis nodule	*Onchocerca volvulus*	202
Cutaneous myiasis	*Dermatobia hominis*	379
Verruca peruana	*Bartonella bacilliformis*	144
Cat-scratch disease	*Bartonella henselae*	144
Lepromatous leprosy	*Mycobacterium leprae*	151
Secondary syphilis (papulosquamous, nodular, and condylomata lata lesions)	*Treponema pallidum*	153
Tertiary syphilis (nodular gummatous lesions)	*T. pallidum*	153
Ulcers with or without eschars		
Anthrax	*Bacillus anthracis*	205
Ulceroglandular tularemia	*Francisella tularensis*	142, 205
Bubonic plague	*Yersinia pestis*	143, 205
Buruli ulcer	*Mycobacterium ulcerans*	152
Leprosy	*M. leprae*	151
Cutaneous tuberculosis	*M. tuberculosis*	150
Chancroid	*Haemophilus ducreyi*	130
Primary syphilis	*T. pallidum*	153
Erysipelas	*S. pyogenes*	121
Cellulitis	*Staphylococcus* spp., *Streptococcus* spp., various other bacteria	Various
Necrotizing fasciitis		
Streptococcal gangrene	*S. pyogenes*	121
Fournier's gangrene	Mixed aerobic and anaerobic bacteria	148
Myositis and myonecrosis		
Pyomyositis	*S. aureus*	120
Streptococcal necrotizing myositis	*S. pyogenes*	121
Gas gangrene	*Clostridium* spp.	126
Nonclostridial (crepitant) myositis	Mixed aerobic and anaerobic bacteria	148
Synergistic nonclostridial anaerobic myonecrosis	Mixed aerobic and anaerobic bacteria	148

ing infection (see Chap. 205). Viremia beginning after an incubation period of 12 days is followed by a diffuse maculopapular rash, with rapid evolution to vesicles, pustules, and then scabs. Secondary cases can occur among close contacts.

Rickettsialpox begins after mite-bite inoculation of *Rickettsia akari* into the skin. A papule with a central vesicle evolves to form a 1- to 2.5-cm painless crusted black eschar with an erythematous halo and proximal adenopathy. While more common in the northeastern United States and the Ukraine in 1940–1950, rickettsialpox has recently been described in Ohio, Arizona, and Utah. Blistering dactylitis is a painful, vesicular, localized *Staphylococcus aureus* or group A streptococcal infection of the pulps of the distal digits of the hands.

INFECTIONS ASSOCIATED WITH BULLAE (Table 110-1) Staphylococcal scalded-skin syndrome (SSSS) in neonates is caused by a toxin (exfoliatin) from phage group II *S. aureus*. SSSS must be distinguished from toxic epidermal necrolysis (TEN), which occurs primarily in adults, is drug-induced, and has a higher mortality. Punch biopsy with frozen section is useful in making this distinction since the cleavage plane is the stratum corneum in SSSS (Fig. 110-1) and the stratum germinativum in TEN. Intravenous γ-globulin is a promising treatment for TEN. Necrotizing fasciitis and gas gangrene also induce bulla formation (see "Necrotizing Fasciitis," below). Halophilic vibrio infection can be as aggressive and fulminant as necrotizing fasciitis; a helpful clue in its diagnosis is a history of exposure to waters of the Gulf of Mexico or the Atlantic seaboard or (in a patient with cirrhosis) the ingestion of raw seafood. The etiologic organism (*Vibrio vulnificus*) is highly susceptible to tetracycline.

INFECTIONS ASSOCIATED WITH CRUSTED LESIONS (Table 110-1) Impetigo contagiosa is caused by *S. pyogenes*, and bullous impetigo is due to *S. aureus* (see Fig. 121-2). Both skin lesions may have an early bullous stage but then appear as thick crusts with a golden-brown color. Streptococcal lesions are most common among children 2 to 5 years of age, and epidemics may occur in settings of poor hygiene, particularly among children of lower socioeconomic status in tropical climates. It is important to recognize impetigo contagiosa because of its relationship to poststreptococcal glomerulonephritis. Rheumatic fever is not a complication of skin infection caused by *S. pyogenes*. Superficial dermatophyte infection (ringworm) can occur on any skin surface, and skin scrapings with KOH staining are diagnostic. Primary infections with dimorphic fungi such as *Blastomyces dermatitidis* and *Sporothrix schenckii* can initially present as crusted skin lesions resembling ringworm. Disseminated infection with *Coccidioides immitis* can also involve the skin, and biopsy and culture should be performed on crusted lesions in patients from endemic areas. Crusted nodular lesions caused by *Mycobacterium chelonei* have been described in HIV-seropositive patients. Treatment with clarithromycin looks promising.

FOLLICULITIS (Table 110-1) Hair follicles serve as portals for a number of bacteria, although *S. aureus* is the most common cause of localized folliculitis. Sebaceous glands empty into hair follicles and ducts and, if blocked, form sebaceous cysts, which may resemble staphylococcal abscesses or may become secondarily infected. Infection of sweat glands (hidradenitis suppurativa) can also mimic infection of hair follicles, particularly in the axillae. Chronic folliculitis is uncommon except in acne vulgaris, where constituents of the normal flora (e.g., *Propionibacterium acnes*) may play a role.

Diffuse folliculitis occurs in two settings. "Hot-tub folliculitis" is caused by *Pseudomonas aeruginosa* in waters that are insufficiently chlorinated and maintained at temperatures between 37 and 40°C. Infection is usually self-limited, though bacteremia and shock have been reported. Swimmer's itch occurs when a skin surface is exposed to water infested with freshwater avian schistosomes. Warm water temperatures and alkaline pH are suitable for mollusks that serve as intermediate hosts between birds and humans. Free-swimming schistosomal cercariae readily penetrate human hair follicles or pores but

quickly die and elicit a brisk allergic reaction, causing intense itching and erythema.

PAPULAR AND NODULAR LESIONS (Table 110-1) Raised lesions of the skin occur in many different forms. *Mycobacterium marinum* infections of the skin may present as cellulitis or as raised erythematous nodules. Erythematous papules are early manifestations of cat-scratch disease (primary site of inoculation) and bacillary angiomatosis (*Bartonella henselae*). Raised serpiginous or linear eruptions are characteristic of cutaneous larva migrans, which is caused by burrowing larvae of dog or cat hookworms (*Ancylostoma braziliense*) and which humans acquire through contact with soil that has been contaminated with dog or cat feces. Similar burrowing raised lesions are present in dracunculiasis caused by migration of the adult female nematode *Dracunculus medinensis*. Nodules caused by *Onchocerca volvulus* may range from 1 to 10 cm in diameter and occur largely in persons bitten by *Simulium* flies in Africa. The nodules contain the adult worm encased in fibrous tissue. Migration of microfilariae into the eyes may result in blindness. Verruca peruana is caused by *Bartonella bacilliformis*, which is transmitted to humans by the sandfly *Phlebotomus*. This condition can take the form of single gigantic lesions (several centimeters in diameter) or multiple small lesions (several millimeters in diameter). Numerous subcutaneous nodules may also be present in cysticercosis caused by larvae of *Taenia solium*. Multiple erythematous papules develop in schistosomiasis; each represents a cercarial invasion site. Skin nodules as well as thickened subcutaneous tissue are prominent features of lepromatous leprosy. Large nodules or gummas are features of tertiary syphilis, whereas flat papulosquamous lesions are characteristic of secondary syphilis. Human papillomavirus may cause singular warts (verruca vulgaris) or multiple warts in the anogenital area (condylomata acuminata). The latter are major problems in HIV-infected individuals.

ULCERS WITH OR WITHOUT ESCHARS (Table 110-1) Cutaneous anthrax begins as a pruritic papule, which develops within days into an ulcer with surrounding vesicles and edema and then into an enlarging ulcer with a black eschar. Cutaneous anthrax may cause chronic nonhealing ulcers with an overlying dirty-gray membrane, although lesions may also mimic psoriasis, eczema, or impetigo. Ulceroglandular tularemia may have associated ulcerated skin lesions with painful regional adenopathy. Although buboes are the major cutaneous manifestation of plague, ulcers with eschars, papules, or pustules are also present in 25% of cases.

Mycobacterium ulcerans typically causes chronic skin ulcers on the extremities of individuals living in the tropics. *Mycobacterium leprae* may be associated with cutaneous ulcerations in patients with lepromatous leprosy related to Lucio's phenomenon, in which immune-mediated destruction of tissue bearing high concentrations of *M. leprae* bacilli occurs, usually several months after initiation of effective therapy. *Mycobacterium tuberculosis* may also cause ulcerations, papules, or erythematous macular lesions of the skin in both normal and immunocompromised patients.

Decubitus ulcers are due to tissue hypoxia secondary to pressure-induced vascular insufficiency and may become secondarily infected with components of the skin and gastrointestinal flora, including anaerobes. Ulcerative lesions on the anterior shins may be due to pyoderma gangrenosum, which must be distinguished from similar lesions of infectious etiology by histologic evaluation of biopsy sites. Ulcerated lesions on the genitals may be either painful (chancroid) or painless (primary syphilis).

ERYSIPELAS (Table 110-1) Erysipelas is due to *S. pyogenes* and is characterized by an abrupt onset of fiery-red swelling of the face or extremities. The distinctive features of erysipelas are well-defined indurated margins, particularly along the nasolabial fold; rapid progression; and intense pain (see Fig. 121-3). Flaccid bullae may develop during the second or third day of illness, but extension to deeper soft tissues is rare. Treatment with penicillin is effective; swelling may progress despite appropriate treatment, although fever, pain, and the intense red color diminish. Desquamation of the involved skin occurs 5 to 10 days into the illness. Infants and elderly adults are most commonly afflicted, and the severity of systemic toxicity varies.

CELLULITIS (Table 110-1)   Cellulitis is an acute inflammatory condition of the skin that is characterized by localized pain, erythema, swelling, and heat. Cellulitis may be caused by indigenous flora colonizing the skin and appendages (e.g., *S. aureus* and *S. pyogenes*) or by a wide variety of exogenous bacteria. Because the exogenous bacteria involved in cellulitis occupy unique niches in nature, a thorough history (including epidemiologic data) provides important clues to etiology. When there is drainage, an open wound, or an obvious portal of entry, Gram's stain and culture provide a definitive diagnosis. In the absence of these findings, the bacterial etiology of cellulitis is difficult to establish, and in some cases staphylococcal and streptococcal cellulitis may have similar features. Even with needle aspiration of the leading edge or a punch biopsy of the cellulitis tissue itself, cultures are positive in only 20% of cases. This observation suggests that relatively low numbers of bacteria may cause cellulitis and that the expanding area of erythema within the skin may be a direct effect of extracellular toxins or of the soluble mediators of inflammation elicited by the host.

Bacteria may gain access to the epidermis through cracks in the skin, abrasions, cuts, burns, insect bites, surgical incisions, and intravenous catheters. Cellulitis caused by *S. aureus* spreads from a central localized infection, such as an abscess, folliculitis, or an infected foreign body (e.g., a splinter, a prosthetic device, or an intravenous catheter). In contrast, cellulitis due to *S. pyogenes* is a more rapidly spreading, diffuse process frequently associated with lymphangitis and fever. Recurrent streptococcal cellulitis of the lower extremities may be caused by organisms of group A, C, or G in association with chronic venous stasis or with saphenous venectomy for coronary artery bypass surgery. Streptococci also cause recurrent cellulitis among patients with chronic lymphedema resulting from elephantiasis, lymph node dissection, or Milroy's disease. Recurrent staphylococcal cutaneous infections are more common among individuals who have eosinophilia and elevated serum levels of IgE (Job's syndrome) and among nasal carriers of staphylococci. Cellulitis caused by *Streptococcus agalactiae* (group B *Streptococcus*) occurs primarily in elderly patients and those with diabetes mellitus or peripheral vascular disease. *Haemophilus influenzae* typically causes periorbital cellulitis in children in association with sinusitis, otitis media, or epiglottitis. It is unclear whether this form of cellulitis will (like meningitis) become less common as a result of the impressive efficacy of the *H. influenzae* type b vaccine.

Many other bacteria also cause cellulitis. Fortunately, these organisms occur in such characteristic settings that a good history provides useful clues to the diagnosis. Cellulitis associated with cat bites and, to a lesser degree, with dog bites is commonly caused by *Pasteurella multocida*, although in the latter case *Staphylococcus intermedius* and *Capnocytophaga canimorsus* (formerly DF-2) must also be considered. Sites of cellulitis and abscesses associated with dog bites and human bites also contain a variety of anaerobic organisms, including *Fusobacterium*, *Bacteroides*, aerobic and anaerobic streptococci, and *Eikenella corrodens*. *Pasteurella* is notoriously resistant to dicloxacillin and nafcillin but is sensitive to all other β-lactam antimicrobials as well as to quinolones, tetracycline, and erythromycin. Ampicillin/clavulanate, ampicillin/sulbactam, and cefoxitin are good choices for the treatment of animal or human bite infections. *Aeromonas hydrophila* causes aggressive cellulitis in tissues surrounding lacerations sustained in fresh water (lakes, rivers, and streams). This organism remains sensitive to aminoglycosides, fluoroquinolones, chloramphenicol, trimethoprim-sulfamethoxazole, and third-generation cephalosporins; it is resistant to ampicillin, however.

P. aeruginosa causes three types of soft tissue infection: ecthyma gangrenosum in neutropenic patients, hot-tub folliculitis, and cellulitis following penetrating injury. Most commonly, *P. aeruginosa* is introduced into the deep tissues when a person steps on a nail. Treatment includes surgical inspection and drainage, particularly if the injury also involves bone or joint capsule. Choices for empirical treatment while

antimicrobial susceptibility data are awaited include an aminoglycoside, a third-generation cephalosporin (ceftazidime, cefoperazone, or cefotaxime), a semisynthetic penicillin (ticarcillin, mezlocillin, or piperacillin), or a fluoroquinolone (although drugs of the last class are not indicated for the treatment of children <13 years old).

Gram-negative bacillary cellulitis, including that due to *P. aeruginosa*, is most common among hospitalized, immunocompromised hosts. Cultures and sensitivity tests are critically important in this setting because of multidrug resistance (Chap. 136).

The gram-positive aerobic rod *Erysipelothrix rhusiopathiae* is most often associated with fish and domestic swine and causes cellulitis primarily in bone renderers and fishmongers. *E. rhusiopathiae* remains susceptible to most β-lactam antibiotics (including penicillin), erythromycin, clindamycin, tetracycline, and cephalosporins but is resistant to sulfonamides, chloramphenicol, and vancomycin. Its resistance to vancomycin, which is unusual among gram-positive bacteria, is of potential clinical significance since this agent is sometimes used in empirical therapy for skin infection. Fish food containing the water flea *Daphnia* is sometimes contaminated with *M. marinum*, which can cause cellulitis or granulomas on skin surfaces exposed to the water in aquariums or injured in swimming pools. Rifampin plus ethambutol has been an effective therapeutic combination in some cases, although no comprehensive studies have been undertaken. In addition, some strains of *M. marinum* are susceptible to tetracycline or to trimethoprim-sulfamethoxazole.

NECROTIZING FASCIITIS (Table 110-1)   Necrotizing fasciitis, formerly called streptococcal gangrene, may be associated with group A *Streptococcus* or mixed aerobic-anaerobic bacteria or may occur as part of gas gangrene caused by *Clostridium perfringens*. Early diagnosis may be difficult when pain or unexplained fever is the only presenting manifestation. Swelling then develops and is followed by brawny edema and tenderness. With progression, dark red induration of the epidermis appears, along with bullae filled with blue or purple fluid. Later the skin becomes friable and takes on a bluish, maroon, or black color. By this stage, thrombosis of blood vessels in the dermal papillae (Fig. 110-1) is extensive. Extension of infection to the level of the deep fascia causes this tissue to take on a brownish-gray appearance. Rapid spread occurs along fascial planes, through venous channels and lymphatics. Patients in the later stages are toxic and frequently manifest shock and multiorgan failure.

Necrotizing fasciitis caused by mixed aerobic-anaerobic bacteria begins with a breach in the integrity of a mucous membrane barrier, such as the mucosa of the gastrointestinal or genitourinary tract. The portal can be a malignancy, diverticulum, hemorrhoid, anal fissure, or urethral tear. Other predisposing factors include peripheral vascular disease, diabetes mellitus, surgery, and penetrating injury to the abdomen. Leakage into the perineal area results in a syndrome called *Fournier's gangrene*, characterized by massive swelling of the scrotum and penis with extension into the perineum or the abdominal wall and legs.

Necrotizing fasciitis caused by *S. pyogenes* has increased in frequency and severity since 1985. It frequently begins deep at the site of a nonpenetrating minor trauma, such as a bruise or a muscle strain. Seeding of the site via transient bacteremia is likely, although most patients deny antecedent streptococcal infection. Alternatively, *S. pyogenes* may reach the deep fascia from a site of cutaneous infection or penetrating trauma. Toxicity is severe, and renal impairment may precede the development of shock. In 20 to 40% of cases, myositis occurs concomitantly, and, as in gas gangrene (see below), serum creatine phosphokinase values may be markedly elevated. Necrotizing fasciitis due to mixed aerobic-anaerobic bacteria may be associated with gas in the deep tissue, but gas is not usually present when the cause is *S. pyogenes*. Prompt surgical exploration down to the deep fascia and muscle is essential. Necrotic tissue must be surgically removed, and Gram's staining and culture of excised tissue are useful in establishing whether group A streptococci, mixed aerobic-anaerobic bacteria, or *Clostridium* species are present (see "Treatment," below).

MYOSITIS/MYONECROSIS (Table 110-1)   Muscle involvement can occur with viral infection (e.g., influenza, dengue, or coxsackievirus B infection) or parasitic invasion (e.g., trichinellosis, cysticercosis, or toxoplasmosis). Although myalgia can occur in most of these infections, severe muscle pain is the hallmark of pleurodynia (coxsackievirus B), trichinellosis, and bacterial infection. Acute rhabdomyolysis predictably occurs with clostridial and streptococcal myositis but may also be associated with influenza virus, echovirus, coxsackievirus, Epstein-Barr virus, and *Legionella* infection.

Pyomyositis is usually due to *S. aureus*, is common in tropical areas, and generally has no known portal of entry. Infection remains localized, and shock does not develop unless organisms produce toxic shock syndrome toxin 1 or certain enterotoxins and the patient lacks antibodies to the toxin produced by the infecting organisms. In contrast, *S. pyogenes* may induce primary myositis (referred to as *streptococcal necrotizing myositis*) in association with severe systemic toxicity. Myonecrosis occurs concomitantly with necrotizing fasciitis in ~50% of cases. Both are part of the streptococcal toxic shock syndrome.

Gas gangrene usually follows severe penetrating injuries that result in interruption of the blood supply and introduction of soil into wounds. Such cases of traumatic gangrene are usually caused by the clostridial species *C. perfringens*, *C. septicum*, or *C. histolyticum*. Rarely, latent or recurrent gangrene can occur years after penetrating trauma; dormant spores that reside at the site of previous injury are most likely responsible. Spontaneous nontraumatic gangrene among patients with neutropenia, gastrointestinal malignancy, diverticulosis, or recent radiation therapy to the abdomen is caused by several clostridial species, of which *C. septicum* is the most commonly involved. The tolerance of this anaerobe to oxygen probably explains why it can initiate infection spontaneously in normal tissue anywhere in the body.

Synergistic nonclostridial anaerobic myonecrosis, also known as necrotizing cutaneous myositis and synergistic necrotizing cellulitis, is a variant of necrotizing fasciitis caused by mixed aerobic and anaerobic bacteria with the exclusion of clostridial organisms (see "Necrotizing Fasciitis," above).

DIAGNOSIS   This chapter has emphasized the physical appearance and location of lesions within the soft tissues as important diagnostic clues. The temporal progression of the lesions as well as the patient's travel history, animal exposure or bite history, age, underlying disease status, and lifestyle are also crucial considerations in the formulation of a narrowed differential diagnosis. However, even the astute clinician may find it challenging to diagnose all infections of the soft tissues by history and inspection alone. Soft tissue radiography, computed tomography, and magnetic resonance imaging may be useful in determining the depth of infection and should be performed in patients with rapidly progressing lesions or in those with evidence of systemic inflammatory response syndrome. These tests are particularly valuable

---

TABLE 110-2 *Treatment of Common Infections of the Skin*

Diagnosis/Condition	Primary Treatment	Alternative Treatment	See Also Chap(s).
Animal bite (prophylaxis or early infection)[a]	Amoxicillin/clavulanate, 875/125 mg PO bid	Doxycycline, 100 mg PO bid	. . .
Animal bite[a] (established infection)	Ampicillin/sulbactam, 1.5–3.0 g IV q6h	Clindamycin, 600–900 mg IV q8h *plus* Ciprofloxacin, 400 mg IV q12h *or* Cefoxitin, 2 g IV q6h	. . .
Bacillary angiomatosis	Erythromycin, 500 mg PO qid	Doxycycline, 100 mg PO bid	144
Herpes simplex (primary genital)	Acyclovir, 400 mg PO tid for 10 days	Famciclovir, 250 mg PO tid for 5–10 days *or* Valacyclovir, 1000 mg PO bid for 10 days	163
Herpes zoster (immunocompetent host >50 years of age)	Acyclovir, 800 mg PO 5 times daily for 7–10 days	Famciclovir, 500 mg PO tid for 7–10 days *or* Valacyclovir, 1000 mg PO tid for 7 days	164
Cellulitis (staphylococcal or streptococcal[b,c])	Nafcillin or oxacillin, 2 g IV q4–6h	Cefazolin, 1–2 g q8h *or* Ampicillin/sulbactam, 1.5–3.0 g IV q6h *or* Erythromycin, 0.5–1.0 g IV q6h *or* Clindamycin, 600–900 mg IV q8h	120, 121
Necrotizing fasciitis (group A streptococcal[b])	Clindamycin, 600–900 mg IV q6–8h *plus* Penicillin G, 4 million units IV q4h	Clindamycin, 600–900 mg IV q6–8h *plus* Cephalosporin (first- or second-generation)	121
Necrotizing fasciitis (mixed aerobes and anaerobes)	Ampicillin, 2 g IV q4h *plus* Clindamycin, 600–900 mg IV q6–8h *plus* Ciprofloxacin, 400 mg IV q6–8h	Vancomycin, 1 g IV q6h *plus* Metronidazole, 500 mg IV q6h *plus* Ciprofloxacin, 400 mg IV q6–8h	148
Gas gangrene	Clindamycin, 600–900 mg IV q6–8h *plus* Penicillin G, 4 million units IV q4–6h	Clindamycin, 600–900 mg IV q6–8h *plus* Cefoxitin, 2 g IV q6h	126

[a] *Pasteurella multocida*, a species commonly associated with both dog and cat bites, is resistant to cephalexin, dicloxacillin, clindamycin, and erythromycin. *Eikenella corrodens*, a bacterium commonly associated with human bites, is resistant to clindamycin, penicillinase-resistant penicillins, and metronidazole but is sensitive to trimethoprim-sulfamethoxazole and fluoroquinolones.

[b] The frequency of erythromycin resistance in group A *Streptococcus* is currently ~5% in the United States but has reached 70 to 100% in some other countries. Most, but not all, erythromycin-resistant group A streptococci are susceptible to clindamycin. Approximately 90 to 95% of *Staphylococcus aureus* strains are sensitive to clindamycin.

[c] Severe hospital-acquired *S. aureus* infections or community-acquired *S. aureus* infections that are not responding to the β-lactam antibotics recommended in this table may be caused by methicillin-resistant strains, requiring a switch to vancomycin or linezolid.

for defining a localized abscess or detecting gas in tissue. Unfortunately, they may reveal only soft tissue swelling and thus are not specific for fulminant infections such as necrotizing fasciitis or myonecrosis caused by group A *Streptococcus*, where gas is not found in lesions.

Aspiration of the leading edge or punch biopsy with frozen section may be helpful if the results are positive, but false-negative results occur in ~80% of cases. There is some evidence that aspiration alone may be superior to injection and aspiration using normal saline. Frozen sections are especially useful in distinguishing SSSS from TEN and are quite valuable in cases of necrotizing fasciitis. Open surgical inspection with debridement as indicated is clearly the best way to determine the extent and severity of infection and to obtain material for Gram's staining and culture. Such an aggressive approach is important and may be lifesaving if undertaken early in the course of fulminant infections where there is evidence of systemic toxicity.

℞ TREATMENT

A full description of the treatment of all the clinical entities described herein is beyond the scope of this chapter. As a guide to the clinician in selecting appropriate treatment, the antimicrobial agents useful in the most common and the most fulminant cutaneous infections are listed in Table 110-2.

Early and aggressive surgical exploration is essential in patients with suspected necrotizing fasciitis, myositis, or gangrene in order to (1) visualize the deep structures, (2) remove necrotic tissue, (3) reduce compartment pressure, and (4) obtain suitable material for Gram's staining and for aerobic and anaerobic cultures. Appropriate empirical antibiotic treatment for mixed aerobic-anaerobic infections could consist of ampicillin/sulbactam, cefoxitin, or the following combination: (1) clindamycin (600 to 900 mg intravenously every 8 h) or metronidazole (750 mg every 6 h) plus (2) ampicillin or ampicillin/sulbactam (2 to 3 g intravenously every 6 h) plus (3) gentamicin (1.0 to 1.5 mg/

kg every 8 h). Group A streptococcal and clostridial infection of the fascia and/or muscle carries a mortality rate of 20 to 50% with penicillin treatment. In experimental models of streptococcal and clostridial necrotizing fasciitis/myositis, clindamycin has exhibited markedly superior efficacy, but no comparative trials have been performed in humans. Hyperbaric oxygen treatment may also be useful in gas gangrene due to clostridial species. Antibiotic treatment should be continued until all signs of systemic toxicity have resolved, all devitalized tissue has been removed, and granulation tissue has developed (Chaps. 121, 126, and 148).

In summary, infections of the skin and soft tissues are diverse in presentation and severity and offer a great challenge to the clinician. This chapter provides an approach to diagnosis and understanding of the pathophysiologic mechanisms involved in these infections. More in-depth information is found in chapters on specific infections.

FURTHER READING

BISNO AI, STEVENS DL: Streptococcal infections in skin and soft tissues. N Engl J Med 334:240, 1996

BREMAN JG, HENDERSON DA: Diagnosis and management of smallpox. N Engl J Med 346:1300, 2002

NORRBY-TEGLUND A, STEVENS DL: Novel therapies in streptococcal toxic shock syndrome: Attenuation of virulence factor expression and modulation of host response. Curr Opin Infect Dis 11:285, 1998

STEVENS DL: Streptococcal toxic shock syndrome associated with necrotizing fasciitis. Annu Rev Med 51:271, 2000

———: Necrotizing soft tissue infections. Curr Treat Opt Infect Dis 2:359, 2000

TALAN DA et al: Bacteriologic analysis of infected dog and cat bites. Emergency Medicine Animal Bite Infection Study Group. N Engl J Med 340: 85, 1999

TRAYLOR KK, TODD JK: Needle aspirate culture method in soft tissue infections: Injection of saline vs. direct aspiration. Pediatr Infect Dis J 17:840, 1998

111 | OSTEOMYELITIS
Jeffrey Parsonnet, James H. Maguire

Osteomyelitis, an infection of bone, is caused most commonly by pyogenic bacteria and mycobacteria. As a useful framework for evaluating the patient and planning treatment, cases are classified on the basis of the causative agent; the route, duration, and anatomical location of infection; and local and systemic host factors.

PATHOGENESIS AND PATHOLOGY Microorganisms enter bone by the hematogenous route, by direct introduction from a contiguous focus of infection, or by a penetrating wound. Trauma, ischemia, and foreign bodies enhance the susceptibility of bone to microbial invasion by exposing sites to which bacteria can bind. Phagocytes attempt to contain the infection and, in the process, release enzymes that lyse bone. Bacteria escape host defenses by adhering tightly to damaged bone, by entering and persisting within osteoblasts, and by coating themselves and underlying surfaces with a protective polysaccharide-rich biofilm. Pus spreads into vascular channels, raising intraosseous pressure and impairing the flow of blood; as the untreated infection becomes chronic, ischemic necrosis of bone results in the separation of large devascularized fragments (*sequestra*). When pus breaks through the cortex, subperiosteal or soft tissue abscesses form, and the elevated periosteum deposits new bone (an *involucrum*) around the sequestrum.

Microorganisms, infiltrates of neutrophils, and congested or thrombosed blood vessels are the principal histologic findings of acute osteomyelitis. The distinguishing feature of chronic osteomyelitis is necrotic bone, which is characterized by the absence of living osteocytes. Mononuclear cells predominate in chronic infections, and granulation and fibrous tissues replace bone that has been resorbed by osteoclasts. In the chronic stage, organisms may be too few to be seen on staining.

HEMATOGENOUS OSTEOMYELITIS Hematogenous infection accounts for ~20% of cases of osteomyelitis and primarily affects children, in whom the long bones are infected, and older adults and intravenous drug users, in whom the spine is the most common site of infection.

Acute Hematogenous Osteomyelitis Infection usually involves a single bone, most commonly the tibia, femur, or humerus in children and vertebral bodies in older adults and injection drug users. Bacteria settle in the well-perfused metaphysis of growing bones where functioning phagocytes are scarce, a network of venous sinusoids slows the flow of blood, and fenestrations in capillaries allow organisms to escape into the extravascular space. Because vascular anatomy changes with age, hematogenous infection of long bones is uncommon during adulthood and, when it occurs, usually involves the diaphysis.

On presentation, the child with osteomyelitis usually appears acutely ill, with high fever, chills, and localized pain and tenderness and often with restriction of movement or difficulty bearing weight. Cutaneous erythema and swelling indicate extension of pus through the cortex. During infancy and after puberty, infection may spread through the epiphysis into the joint space. In children of other ages, extension of infection through the cortex results in involvement of joints if the metaphysis is intracapsular. Thus, septic arthritis of the elbow, shoulder, and hip may complicate osteomyelitis of the proximal radius, humerus, and femur, respectively. In children, the source of bacteremia is usually inapparent. A history is often obtained of recent blunt trauma to the area involved; presumably, this event results in a small intraosseous hematoma or vascular obstruction. Adults with osteomyelitis may present in the context of an apparent infection elsewhere, such as the lung, sinuses, or urinary tract, or without an obvious source of bacteremia.

Plain radiographs obtained early in the course of infection may show soft tissue swelling, but the first change in bone—a periosteal reaction—is not evident until at least 10 days after the onset of infection. Lytic changes can be detected after 2 to 6 weeks, when 50 to 75% of bone density has been lost. Rarely, a well-circumscribed lytic lesion, or *Brodie's abscess*, is seen in a child who has been in pain for several months but has had no fever.

Vertebral Osteomyelitis   The vertebral bodies are the most common sites of acute hematogenous osteomyelitis in adults. Organisms reach the well-perfused vertebral body via spinal arteries and quickly spread from the end plate into the disk space and then to the adjacent vertebral body. The infection may originate in the urinary tract, and it does so particularly often among men over age 50. Other sources of bacteremia include endocarditis, dental abscess, soft tissue infection, and a contaminated intravenous line; these sources may or may not be obvious. Diabetes mellitus, hemodialysis, and injection drug use carry an increased risk of spinal infection. Many patients have a history of degenerative joint disease involving the spine, and some report an episode of trauma preceding the onset of infection. Penetrating injuries and surgical procedures to the spine may cause nonhematogenous vertebral osteomyelitis or infection localized to the disk.

Most patients with vertebral osteomyelitis report neck or back pain; patients may describe atypical pain in the chest, the abdomen, or an extremity that is due to irritation of nerve roots. Symptoms are localized to the lumbar spine more often than to the thoracic spine (>50% vs. 35% of cases) or the cervical spine in pyogenic infections, but the thoracic spine is involved most commonly in tuberculous spondylitis (Pott's disease). More than 50% of patients experience a subacute illness in which a vague, dull pain gradually intensifies over 2 to 3 months. Fever is usually low grade or absent, but some patients recall having had an episode of fever and chills prior to or at the onset of pain. An acute presentation with high fever and toxicity is less common and suggests ongoing bacteremia. Percussion over the involved vertebra elicits tenderness, and physical examination may reveal spasm of the paraspinal muscles and limitation of motion.

Laboratory findings at the time of presentation include a normal or modestly elevated white blood cell count and, almost invariably, an increased erythrocyte sedimentation rate (ESR) and C-reactive protein (CRP) level. Blood cultures are positive only 20 to 50% of the time.

Usually, by the time the patient seeks medical attention, plain radiographs show irregular erosions in the end plates of adjacent vertebral bodies and narrowing of the intervening disk space. This radiographic pattern is virtually diagnostic of bacterial infection because tumors and other diseases of the spine rarely cross the disk space. Computed tomography (CT) or magnetic resonance imaging (MRI) may demonstrate epidural, paraspinal, retropharyngeal, mediastinal, retroperitoneal, or psoas abscesses that originate in the spine.

A spinal epidural abscess may evolve suddenly or over several weeks; the classic clinical presentation is spinal pain progressing to radicular pain and/or weakness. Irreversible paralysis may result from failure to recognize epidural abscess before the development of neurologic deficits. MRI is the best procedure for detection of epidural abscess and should be performed in all cases of vertebral osteomyelitis accompanied by subjective weakness or objective neurologic abnormalities.

Microbiology   More than 95% of cases of hematogenous osteomyelitis are caused by a single organism. *Staphylococcus aureus* accounts for 50% of isolates. Other common pathogens include group B streptococci and *Escherichia coli* during the newborn period and group A streptococci in early childhood. Vertebral osteomyelitis is due to *E. coli* and other enteric bacilli in ~25% of cases. *S. aureus, Pseudomonas aeruginosa,* and *Serratia* infections are associated with intravenous drug use in some parts of the United States and may involve the sacroiliac, sternoclavicular, or pubic joints as well as the spine. *Salmonella* spp. and *S. aureus* are the major causes of long-bone osteomyelitis complicating sickle cell anemia and other hemoglobinopathies. Tuberculosis and brucellosis affect the spine more often than

other bones. Other common sites of tuberculous osteomyelitis include the small bones of the hands and feet, the metaphyses of long bones, the ribs, and the sternum.

Unusual causes of hematogenous osteomyelitis include disseminated histoplasmosis, coccidioidomycosis, and blastomycosis in endemic areas. Immunocompromised persons on rare occasions develop osteomyelitis due to atypical mycobacteria, *Bartonella henselae,* or *Pneumocystis* or to species of *Candida, Cryptococcus,* or *Aspergillus.* Hematogenous osteomyelitis with *Mycobacterium bovis* has been reported following intravesicular instillation of bacille Calmette-Guérin (BCG) for cancer of the bladder. The etiology of chronic relapsing multifocal osteomyelitis, an inflammatory condition of children that is characterized by recurrent episodes of painful lytic lesions in multiple bones, has not been identified.

OSTEOMYELITIS SECONDARY TO A CONTIGUOUS FOCUS OF INFECTION ■ Clinical Features   This broad category of osteomyelitis accounts for ~80% of all cases and occurs most commonly in adults. It includes infections introduced by penetrating injuries, such as bites, puncture wounds, and open fractures; by surgical procedures; and by direct extension of infection from adjacent soft tissues. Generalized vascular insufficiency and the presence of a foreign body are important predisposing factors and make infection more difficult to cure.

Frequently, the diagnosis of this type of osteomyelitis is not made until the infection has already become chronic. The pain, fever, and inflammatory signs due to acute infection may be attributed to the original injury or to overlying soft tissue infection. An indolent infection may become apparent only weeks or months later, when a sinus tract develops, a surgical wound breaks down, or a fracture fails to heal. It may be impossible to distinguish radiographic abnormalities due to osteomyelitis from those due to the precipitating condition.

A special type of contiguous-focus osteomyelitis occurs in the setting of peripheral vascular disease and nearly always involves the small bones of the feet of adult diabetic patients. This type of infection is a major cause of morbidity and hospitalization for patients with diabetes and results in many thousands of amputations per year. Diabetic neuropathy exposes the foot to frequent trauma and pressure sores, and the patient may be unaware of infection as it spreads into bone. Poor tissue perfusion impairs normal inflammatory responses and wound healing and creates a milieu that is conducive to anaerobic infections. It is often during the evaluation of a nonhealing ulcer, a swollen toe, or acute cellulitis that a radiograph provides the first evidence of osteomyelitis. If bone is palpable during examination of the base of an ulcer with a blunt surgical probe, osteomyelitis is likely.

Microbiology   *S. aureus* is a pathogen in more than half of cases of contiguous-focus osteomyelitis. However, in contrast to hematogenous osteomyelitis, these infections are often polymicrobial and are more likely to involve gram-negative and anaerobic bacteria. Hence a mixture of staphylococci, streptococci, enteric organisms, and anaerobic bacteria may be isolated from a diabetic foot infection or pelvic osteomyelitis underlying a decubitus ulcer. Aerobic and anaerobic bacteria cause osteomyelitis following surgery or soft tissue infection of the oropharynx, paranasal sinuses, gastrointestinal tract, or female genital tract. A human bite may result in mixed infection of the hand, with anaerobes included among the etiologic agents. *S. aureus* is the principal cause of postoperative infections; coagulase-negative staphylococci are common pathogens after implantation of orthopedic appliances; and these organisms as well as gram-negative enteric bacilli, atypical mycobacteria, and *Mycoplasma* may cause sternal osteomyelitis after cardiac surgery. Infection with *P. aeruginosa* is frequently associated with puncture wounds of the foot (especially by a nail through a sneaker) or with thermal burns, and *Pasteurella multocida* infection commonly follows cat bites.

CHRONIC OSTEOMYELITIS   With prompt treatment, fewer than 5% of cases of acute hematogenous osteomyelitis progress to chronic osteomyelitis. Chronic osteomyelitis is more likely to develop in contiguous-focus than in hematogenous osteomyelitis. The presence of a foreign body makes establishment of chronic infection especially likely.

A protracted clinical course, long periods of quiescence, and recurrent exacerbations are characteristic of chronic osteomyelitis. Sinus tracts between bone and skin may drain purulent material and occasionally pieces of necrotic bone. An increase in drainage, pain, or ESR signals an exacerbation. Fever is unusual except when obstruction of a sinus tract leads to soft tissue infection. Rare late complications include pathologic fractures, squamous cell carcinoma of the sinus tract, and amyloidosis.

DIAGNOSIS Early diagnosis of acute osteomyelitis is critical because prompt antibiotic therapy may prevent the necrosis of bone. The ESR and CRP levels are elevated in most cases of active osteomyelitis, including those in which constitutional symptoms and leukocytosis are lacking. These findings are not specific to osteomyelitis, however, and the ESR is occasionally normal in early infections. Baseline values are often useful in monitoring the efficacy of treatment. A variety of radiologic tests are available for evaluation of osteomyelitis (Table 111-1). Evaluation usually begins with plain radiographs because of their ready availability, although they frequently show no abnormalities during early infection. Three-phase bone scans (^{99}Tc-monodiphosphonate) offer high sensitivity but often have low specificity, especially in the presence of underlying bony abnormalities. There is a lack of consensus over the optimal use of other radionuclide studies, and there is considerable variation between institutions in their use. Although the use of MRI (Fig. 111-1) is expanding because of high sensitivity and specificity, this modality is not available at all institutions.

The role of diagnostic imaging in chronic osteomyelitis is to detect active infection and delineate the extent of debridement necessary to

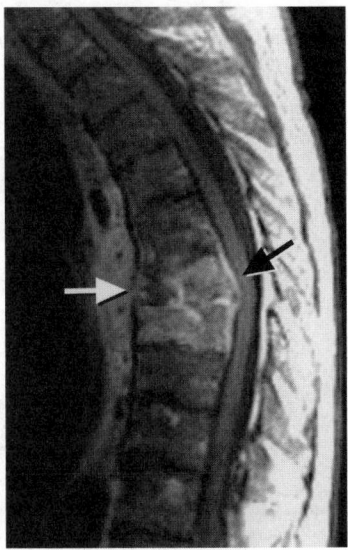

FIGURE 111-1 Osteomyelitis of the thoracic spine demonstrated on a sagittal, fat-suppressed T1-weighted magnetic resonance image after the administration of intravenous gadolinium. At T8–T9, there is involvement of the adjacent vertebral bodies and intervening disk. Abnormally enhancing inflammatory tissue extends from the disk space anteriorly (*white arrow*) as well as posteriorly into the epidural space, compressing the thecal sac (*black arrow*).

remove necrotic bone and abnormal soft tissues. Although plain films accurately reflect chronic changes, CT is more sensitive for the detection of sequestra, sinus tracts, and soft tissue abscesses. Both CT and ultrasound are useful for guiding percutaneous aspiration of subperiosteal and soft tissue fluid collections. Sequential technetium and gallium or indium scans may help determine whether infection is active and may distinguish infection from noninflammatory bone changes. MRI provides superior information about the anatomical extent of infection but does not always distinguish osteomyelitis from healing fractures and tumors. MRI is particularly useful in distinguishing cellulitis from osteomyelitis in the diabetic foot; however, no imaging modality consistently distinguishes infection from neuropathic osteopathy.

Appropriate samples for microbiologic studies should be obtained in all cases of suspected osteomyelitis before the initiation of antimicrobial therapy. Blood cultures are indicated in acute cases and are positive in more than one-third of cases of hematogenous osteomyelitis in children and in 25% of cases of vertebral osteomyelitis in adults. The presence of sepsis occasionally requires initiation of empirical therapy after blood samples alone have been obtained for culture. If blood cultures are negative, samples from needle aspiration of pus in bone or soft tissues or from a bone biopsy should be obtained for culture; in the case of vertebral osteomyelitis, these samples can usually be obtained with the guidance of fluoroscopy or CT scan.

The results of culture of specimens obtained by swabbing of a sinus tract or the base of an ulcer correlate poorly with the organisms infecting the bone. For this reason, in cases of chronic osteomyelitis and contiguous-focus osteomyelitis, samples for aerobic and anaerobic culture should be obtained from several sites by percutaneous needle aspiration, percutaneous biopsy, or intraoperative biopsy at the time of debridement. Isolates of coagulase-negative staphylococci and other organisms of low virulence should not automatically be disregarded as contaminants, especially in the presence of prosthetic materials. Special culture media may be necessary for the isolation of mycobacteria, fungi, and less common pathogens. In some cases, histopathologic examination of biopsy specimens may be the only way to make a diagnosis.

TABLE 111-1	Diagnostic Imaging Studies for Osteomyelitis
Type of Study	**Comments**
Plain radiographs	Insensitive, especially in early osteomyelitis. May show periosteal elevation after 10 days, lytic changes after 2–6 weeks. Useful to look for anatomical abnormalities (e.g., fractures, bony variants, or deformities), foreign bodies, and soft tissue gas.
Three-phase bone scan (^{99m}Tc-MDP)	Characteristic finding in osteomyelitis: increased uptake in all three phases of scan. Highly sensitive (~95%) in acute infection; somewhat less sensitive if blood flow to bone is poor. Specificity moderate if plain films are normal, but poor in presence of neuropathic arthropathy, fractures, tumor, infarction.
Other radionuclide scans	Examples: ^{67}Ga-citrate, ^{111}In-labeled WBCs. ^{111}In-WBCs more specific than gallium but not always available. Often used in conjunction with bone scan because its greater specificity for inflammation than ^{99m}Tc-MDP helps to distinguish infectious from noninfectious processes. Lack of consensus over role in routine evaluation.
Ultrasound	May detect subperiosteal fluid collection or soft tissue abscess adjacent to bone, but largely supplanted by CT and MRI.
CT	Limited role in acute osteomyelitis. In chronic osteomyelitis, excellent for detection of sequestra, cortical destruction, soft tissue abscesses, and sinus tracts. Use may be limited by metallic foreign body.
MRI	As sensitive as ^{99m}Tc-MDP bone scan for acute osteomyelitis (~95%); detects changes in water content of marrow before disruption of cortical bone. High specificity (~87%), with better anatomical detail than nuclear studies. Procedure of choice for vertebral osteomyelitis because of high sensitivity for epidural abscess. Use may be limited by metallic foreign body.

Abbreviations: CT, computed tomography; MDP, monodiphosphonate; MRI, magnetic resonance imaging; WBCs, white blood cells.

℞ TREATMENT

Antibiotic Therapy (Table 111-2) Antibiotics are administered only after appropriate specimens have been obtained for culture. The antibiotics selected should be bactericidal, should be given at a high dose, and—at least initially—should be given intravenously. When necessary, empirical therapy is guided by findings on Gram's staining of a specimen from the bone or abscess or is chosen to cover the most

Organism	Suggested Regimen[a]	
	Primary	Alternative[b]
Staphylococcus aureus		
Penicillin-resistant, methicillin-sensitive (MSSA)	Nafcillin or oxacillin, 2 g IV q4h	Cefazolin, 1 g IV q8h; ceftriaxone, 1 g IV q24h; clindamycin, 900 mg IV q8h[c]
Penicillin-sensitive	Penicillin 3–4 million U IV q4h	Cefazolin, ceftriaxone, clindamycin (as above)
Methicillin-resistant (MRSA)	Vancomycin, 15 mg/kg (up to 1 g) IV q12h	Clindamycin[c] (as above); linezolid, 600 mg IV or PO q12h[d]; daptomycin, 4–6 mg/kg per day IV[d]
Streptococci (including *S. milleri*, β-hemolytic streptococci)	Penicillin (as above)	Cefazolin, ceftriaxone, clindamycin (as above)
Gram-negative aerobic bacilli		
Escherichia coli, other "sensitive" species	Ampicillin, 2 g IV q4h; cefazolin, 1 g IV q8h	Ceftriaxone, 1 g IV q24h; parenteral or oral fluoroquinolone (e.g., ciprofloxacin, 400 mg IV or 750 mg PO q12h)[e]
Pseudomonas aeruginosa	Extended-spectrum β-lactam agent (e.g., piperacillin, 3–4 g IV q4–6h or ceftazidime, 2 g IV q12h) *plus* tobramycin, 5–7 mg/kg q24h[f]	May substitute parenteral or oral fluoroquinolone for β-lactam agent
Enterobacter spp., other "resistant" species	Extended-spectrum β-lactam agent IV or fluoroquinolone IV or PO[e] (as above)	
Mixed infections possibly involving anaerobic bacteria	Ampicillin/sulbactam, 1.5–3 g IV q6h; piperacillin/tazobactam 3.375 g IV q6h	Cefotetan, 1–2 g IV q12h; combination of fluoroquinolone plus clindamycin (as above)

[a] Duration of treatment is discussed in the text.
[b] Cephalosporins may be used for the treatment of patients allergic to penicillin whose reaction did not consist of anaphylaxis or urticaria (immediate-type hypersensitivity).
[c] Because of the possibility of inducible resistance, clindamycin must be used with caution for the treatment of strains resistant to erythromycin. Consult clinical microbiology laboratory.
[d] Experience is limited; there are anecdotal reports of efficacy.
[e] Oral fluoroquinolones must not be coadministered with divalent cations (calcium, magnesium, iron, aluminum), which block the drugs' absorption.
[f] Tobramycin levels and renal function must be monitored closely to minimize the risks of nephro- and ototoxicity.

likely pathogens. Empirical therapy in most cases should include high doses of an agent active against *S. aureus* (such as oxacillin, nafcillin, cefazolin, or vancomycin) and—if gram-negative organisms are likely to be involved—a third-generation cephalosporin, an aminoglycoside, or a fluoroquinolone.

Specific intravenous therapy is based on the in vitro susceptibility of the organism(s) isolated from bone or blood. At-home intravenous administration of antibiotics or oral therapy is appropriate for motivated and medically stable patients and represents a significant advance in management. Antibiotics that require infrequent dosing, such as ceftriaxone, may facilitate home therapy. Many antibiotics can be given automatically by portable infusion pump, which decreases the disruption otherwise caused by the frequent administration of drug. Use of a peripherally inserted central catheter (PICC line) also facilitates outpatient administration of antibiotics. Outpatient therapy requires close coordination of nursing, pharmacy, and physician care, with clear delineations of responsibility for monitoring safety and efficacy.

Children with acute hematogenous osteomyelitis routinely receive oral antibiotics after 5 to 10 days of parenteral therapy if signs of active infection have resolved; such treatment has been as successful as standard parenteral therapy. The doses of oral penicillins or cephalosporins required for the treatment of osteomyelitis are several times higher than the doses of these drugs given for common infections. Adults may not tolerate these high doses as well as children, and, except in the case of the fluoroquinolones and rifampin, few data support the use of oral antibiotics by adults. For treatment of osteomyelitis due to Enterobacteriaceae, oral administration of a fluoroquinolone has been as successful as intravenous administration of β-lactam antibiotics.

Caution should be exercised in the use of fluoroquinolones as the sole agents for treatment of infection due to *S. aureus* or *P. aeruginosa* because resistance may develop during therapy. Addition of rifampin to a fluoroquinolone or a β-lactam agent has yielded encouraging results in infections due to *S. aureus*, but potential drug toxicity and drug interactions make this option desirable only for selected patients, such as those with necrotic bone that cannot be adequately debrided. Oral administration of clindamycin (300 to 450 mg every 6 h) or metronidazole (500 mg every 8 h) results in high drug levels in serum and can take the place of intravenous regimens for the treatment of *Bacteroides* infections. Oral clindamycin has produced good results for continuation treatment of osteomyelitis due to *S. aureus*, but consultation with the microbiology laboratory is advised because of inducible resistance exhibited by some strains. The bacteriostatic drug linezolid (600 mg by mouth every 12 h) and the bactericidal drug daptomycin (4 to 6 mg/kg per day intravenously) have been used successfully in a small number of patients with infection caused by methicillin-resistant *S. aureus* and vancomycin-resistant *Enterococcus*, but data are currently insufficient to recommend their routine use. Data do not support the routine use of the serum minimal bactericidal concentration in guiding therapy.

Acute Hematogenous Osteomyelitis Early treatment of acute hematogenous osteomyelitis of childhood with 4 to 6 weeks of an appropriate antibiotic is usually successful; treatment for <3 weeks has resulted in a 10-fold greater rate of failure. Surgical intervention in childhood cases is indicated for intraosseous or subperiosteal abscesses, concomitant septic arthritis, and failure of the acute signs of infection to improve in 24 to 48 h. Acute hematogenous osteomyelitis of bones other than the spine in adults often requires surgical debridement.

Vertebral Osteomyelitis A 4- to 6-week course of treatment with an appropriate antibiotic is usually sufficient to cure vertebral osteomyelitis. Failure of the ESR to drop by two-thirds or more of its pretreatment level or of CRP to normalize is an indication for reevaluation and (possibly) longer treatment. Surgery is seldom necessary, even in cases of many months' duration, except in instances of spinal instability, new or progressive neurologic deficits, or large soft-tissue abscesses that cannot be drained percutaneously. All but small and asymptomatic epidural abscesses should be surgically drained. Patients should maintain bed rest until back pain has declined to the point at which ambulation is possible. Body casts are no longer used except for comfort.

Contiguous-Focus Osteomyelitis Even when diagnosed early, contiguous-focus osteomyelitis usually requires surgery in addition to 4 to 6 weeks of appropriate antibiotic therapy because of underlying soft tissue infection or damage to bone from an injury or surgery. A 2-week course of antibiotics following thorough debridement and soft tissue coverage has yielded excellent results in the treatment of superficial osteomyelitis involving only the outer cortex of bone.

Chronic Osteomyelitis The risks and benefits of aggressive therapy for chronic osteomyelitis should be weighed before any attempt is made to eradicate the infection. Some patients with extensive disease prefer to live with their infections rather than undergo multiple surgical procedures, take prolonged courses of antimicrobial therapy, and face the risk of loss of an extremity. Such persons often benefit from intermittent courses of oral antibiotics to suppress acute exacerbations.

Once the decision has been made to treat chronic osteomyelitis aggressively, the patient's nutritional and metabolic status should be optimized to expedite healing of soft tissues and bone. Antibiotic administration should be started several days before surgery to reduce inflammation if the etiology of the infection is known; if not, antibiotic therapy should be withheld until debridement. A 4- to 6-week course of appropriate antibiotic therapy is given postoperatively on the basis of the susceptibility pattern of organisms isolated from bone. The benefit of prolonged oral antibiotic therapy after 4 to 6 weeks of parenteral therapy remains unproven. There is insufficient information to recommend either the routine use of hyperbaric oxygen or the use of antibiotic-impregnated methacrylate beads or other depots to deliver high levels of antibiotics to the bone. The success of therapy for chronic osteomyelitis still rests largely on the complete surgical removal of necrotic bone and abnormal soft tissues. In the past, the inability to repair large defects in bone and soft tissue limited the extent of debridement. Muscle flaps and skin grafts are now used routinely to cover large soft-tissue defects and to fill dead space, and bone grafts and vascularized bone transfer may restore a seriously compromised bone to a functional state.

In infections of recent fractures, internal fixators are often left in place, and the infection is controlled by limited debridement and suppressive antibiotic therapy. Definitive surgical/antimicrobial therapy is delayed until after bony union of the fracture is achieved. If there is nonunion of the fracture or loosening of the fixator, the appliance must be removed, the bone debrided, and an external fixator or a new internal fixator applied.

Osteomyelitis of the small bones of the feet in persons with vascular disease usually requires surgical treatment. The effectiveness of the surgery is limited by the blood supply to the site and the body's ability to heal the wound. Revascularization of the extremity is indicated if the vascular disease involves large arteries. In cases of decreased perfusion due to small-vessel disease, foot-sparing surgery may fail, and the best option is often suppressive therapy or amputation. The duration of antibiotic therapy depends on the surgical procedure performed. When the infected bone is removed entirely but residual infection of soft tissues remains, antibiotic therapy should be given for 2 weeks; if amputation eliminates infected bone and soft tissue, standard surgical prophylaxis is given; otherwise, postoperative antibiotics must be given for 4 to 6 weeks.

FURTHER READING

KAIM AH et al: Imaging of chronic posttraumatic osteomyelitis. Eur Radiol 12:1193, 2002

KHATRI G et al: Effect of bone biopsy in guiding antimicrobial therapy for osteomyelitis complicating open wounds. Am J Med Sci 321:367, 2001

LEW DP, WALDVOGEL FA: Osteomyelitis. N Engl J Med 336:999, 1997

LIPSKY BA: Osteomyelitis of the foot in diabetic patients. Clin Infect Dis 25:1318, 1997

MADER JT et al: Staging and staging application in osteomyelitis. Clin Infect Dis 25:1303, 1997

MCHENRY MC et al: Vertebral osteomyelitis: Long-term outcome for 253 patients from 7 Cleveland-area hospitals. Clin Infect Dis 34:1342, 2002

REZAI AR et al: Contemporary management of spinal osteomyelitis. Neurosurgery 44:1018, 1999

RISSING JP: Antimicrobial therapy for chronic osteomyelitis in adults: Role of the quinolones. Clin Infect Dis 25:1327, 1997

TICE AD et al: Outcomes of osteomyelitis among patients treated with outpatient parenteral antimicrobial therapy. Am J Med 114:723, 2003

TSUKAYAMA DT: Pathophysiology of posttraumatic osteomyelitis. Clin Orthop 360:22, 1999

112 INTRAABDOMINAL INFECTIONS AND ABSCESSES
Dennis L. Kasper, Dori F. Zaleznik

Intraperitoneal infections generally arise because a normal anatomical barrier is disrupted. This disruption may occur when the appendix, a diverticulum, or an ulcer ruptures; when the bowel wall is weakened by ischemia, tumor, or inflammation (e.g., in inflammatory bowel disease); or with adjacent inflammatory processes, such as pancreatitis or pelvic inflammatory disease, in which enzymes (in the former case) or organisms (in the latter) may leak into the peritoneal cavity. Whatever the inciting event, once inflammation develops and organisms usually contained within the bowel or another organ enter the normally sterile peritoneal space, a predictable series of events takes place. Intraabdominal infections occur in two stages: peritonitis and—if the patient survives this stage and goes untreated—abscess formation. The types of microorganisms predominating in each stage of infection are responsible for the pathogenesis of disease.

PERITONITIS

Peritonitis is a life-threatening event that is often accompanied by bacteremia and sepsis syndrome (Chap. 254). The peritoneal cavity is large but is divided into compartments. The upper and lower peritoneal cavities are divided by the transverse mesocolon; the greater omentum extends from the transverse mesocolon and from the lower pole of the stomach to line the lower peritoneal cavity. The pancreas, duodenum, and ascending and descending colon are located in the anterior retroperitoneal space; the kidneys, ureters, and adrenals are found in the posterior retroperitoneal space. The other organs, including liver, stomach, gallbladder, spleen, jejunum, ileum, transverse and sigmoid colon, cecum, and appendix, are found within the peritoneal cavity itself. Normally the cavity is lined with a serous membrane that can serve as a conduit for fluids—a property utilized in peritoneal dialysis.

A small amount of fluid, sufficient to allow movement of organs, is normally present in the peritoneal space. This fluid is serous, with a protein content (consisting mainly of albumin) of <30 g/L and <300 white blood cells (WBCs, generally mononuclear cells) per microliter. In the presence of infection, some compartments collect fluid or pus more often than others. These compartments include the pelvis (the lowest portion), the subphrenic spaces on the right and left sides, and Morrison's pouch, which is a posterosuperior extension of the subhepatic spaces and is the lowest part of the paravertebral groove when a patient is recumbent. The falciform ligament separating the right and left subphrenic spaces appears to act as a barrier to the spread of infection; consequently, it is unusual to find bilateral subphrenic collections. In bacterial infections, leukocyte recruitment into the infected peritoneal cavity consists of an early influx of polymorphonuclear leukocytes (PMNs) and a prolonged subsequent phase of mononuclear cell migration. The phenotype of the infiltrating leukocytes during the course of inflammation is regulated primarily by resident-cell chemokine synthesis.

PRIMARY (SPONTANEOUS) BACTERIAL PERITONITIS Peritonitis is either primary (without an apparent source of contamination) or secondary. The types of organisms found and the clinical presentations of these two processes are different. In adults, primary bacterial peritonitis (PBP) occurs most commonly in conjunction with cirrhosis of the liver (frequently the result of alcoholism). However, the disease has been reported in adults with metastatic malignant disease, postnecrotic cirrhosis, chronic active hepatitis, acute viral hepatitis, congestive heart failure, systemic lupus erythematosus, and lymphedema as well as in patients with no underlying disease. PBP virtually always develops in patients with ascites. Nevertheless, it is not a common event, occurring in ≤10% of cirrhotic patients. The cause of PBP has not been established definitively but is believed to involve hematogenous spread of organisms in a patient in whom a diseased liver and altered portal circulation result in a defect in the usual filtration function. Organisms are able to multiply in ascites, a good medium for growth. The proteins of the complement cascade have been found in peritoneal fluid, with lower levels in cirrhotic patients than in patients with ascites of other etiologies. The opsonic and phagocytic properties of neutrophils are diminished in patients with advanced liver disease.

The presentation of PBP differs from that of secondary peritonitis. The most common manifestation is fever, which is reported in as many as 80% of patients. Ascites is found but virtually always predates infection. Abdominal pain, an acute onset of symptoms, and peritoneal irritation detected during physical examination can be helpful diagnostically, but the absence of any of these findings does not exclude this often-subtle diagnosis. It is vital to sample the peritoneal fluid of any cirrhotic patient with ascites and fever. The finding of >300 PMNs per microliter is diagnostic for PBP, according to Conn. This criterion does not apply to secondary peritonitis (see below). The microbiology of PBP is also distinctive. While enteric gram-negative bacilli such as *Escherichia coli* are most commonly encountered, gram-positive organisms such as streptococci, enterococci, or even pneumococci are sometimes found. In PBP, a single organism is typically isolated; anaerobes are found less frequently in PBP than in secondary peritonitis, in which a mixed flora including anaerobes is the rule. In fact, if PBP is suspected and multiple organisms including anaerobes are recovered from the peritoneal fluid, the diagnosis must be reconsidered and a source of secondary peritonitis sought.

The diagnosis of PBP is not easy. It depends on the exclusion of a primary intraabdominal source of infection. Contrast-enhanced computed tomography (CT) is very useful in identifying an intraabdominal source for infection. It may be difficult to recover organisms from cultures of peritoneal fluid, presumably because the burden of organisms is low. However, the yield can be improved if 10 mL of peritoneal fluid is placed directly into a blood culture bottle. Since bacteremia frequently accompanies PBP, blood should be cultured simultaneously. No specific radiographic studies are helpful in the diagnosis of PBP. A plain film of the abdomen would be expected to show ascites. Chest and abdominal radiography should be performed in patients with abdominal pain to exclude free air, which signals a perforation.

℞ TREATMENT

Treatment for PBP is directed at the isolate from blood or peritoneal fluid. Gram's staining of peritoneal fluid often gives negative results in PBP. Therefore, until culture results become available, empirical therapy should cover gram-negative aerobic bacilli and gram-positive cocci. Third-generation cephalosporins such as cefotaxime [2 g q8h, administered intravenously (IV)] provide reasonable initial coverage in moderately ill patients. Broad-spectrum antibiotics, such as penicillin/β-lactamase inhibitor combinations (e.g., piperacillin/tazobactam, 3.375 g q6h IV) or ceftriaxone (2 g q24h IV), are also options. Empirical coverage for anaerobes is not necessary. After the infecting organism is identified, therapy should be narrowed to target the specific pathogen. Patients with PBP usually respond within 72 h to appropriate antibiotic therapy. Antimicrobial therapy can be administered for as little as 5 days if rapid improvement occurs and blood cultures are negative, but a course of up to 2 weeks may be required for patients with bacteremia and for those whose improvement is slow. Persistence of leukocytes in the ascitic fluid after therapy should initiate a search for additional diagnoses.

Prevention PBP has a high rate of recurrence. Up to 70% of patients reportedly experience a recurrence within 1 year. Antibiotic prophy-

laxis reduces the rate of recurrence to <20%. Recommended prophylactic regimens include fluoroquinolones (ciprofloxacin, 750 mg weekly; norfloxacin, 400 mg/d) or trimethoprim-sulfamethoxazole (one double-strength tablet per day). However, long-term administration of broad-spectrum antibiotics in this setting has been shown to increase the risk of severe hospital-acquired staphylococcal infections and of high-level resistance to antibiotics.

SECONDARY PERITONITIS Secondary peritonitis develops when bacteria contaminate the peritoneum as a result of spillage from an intraabdominal viscus. The organisms found almost always constitute a mixed flora in which facultative gram-negative bacilli and anaerobes predominate, especially when the contaminating source is colonic. Early in the course of infection, when the host response is directed toward containment of the infection, exudate containing fibrin and PMNs is found. Early death in this setting is attributable to gram-negative bacillary sepsis and to potent endotoxins circulating in the bloodstream (Chap. 254). Gram-negative bacilli, particularly *E. coli*, are common bloodstream isolates, but *Bacteroides fragilis* bacteremia occurs as well. The severity of abdominal pain and the clinical course depend on the inciting process. The species of organisms isolated from the peritoneum also vary with the source of the initial process and the normal flora present at that site. Secondary peritonitis can result primarily from chemical irritation or bacterial contamination. For example, as long as the patient is not achlorhydric, a ruptured gastric ulcer will release low-pH gastric contents that will serve as a chemical irritant. The normal flora of the stomach comprises the same organisms found in the oropharynx (Chap. 148) but in lower numbers. The surfaces of teeth contain ~10^7 aerobic and 10^7 anaerobic organisms per milliliter of saliva; the normally acidic stomach contains an equal ratio of aerobic and anaerobic species, but in concentrations more in the range of 10^5/mL. After meals, when gastric acidity is highest, this number may fall to 10^3/mL. Thus, the bacterial burden in a ruptured gastric ulcer—or even a duodenal ulcer—is negligible compared with that in a ruptured appendix. The normal flora of the colon below the ligament of Treitz contains ~10^{11} anaerobic organisms per gram of feces but only 10^8 aerobes per gram; therefore, anaerobic species account for 99% of the bacteria. Leakage of colonic contents (pH 7 to 8) does not cause significant chemical peritonitis, but infection is intense because of the heavy bacterial load.

Depending on the inciting event, local symptoms may initially be found in secondary peritonitis—for example, epigastric pain from a ruptured gastric ulcer. In appendicitis (Chap. 281), the initial presenting symptoms are often vague, with periumbilical discomfort and nausea followed in a number of hours by pain more localized to the right lower quadrant. Unusual locations of the appendix (including a retrocecal position) can complicate this presentation further. Once infection has spread to the peritoneal cavity, however, pain increases, particularly with infection involving the parietal peritoneum, which is innervated extensively. Patients usually lie motionless, often with knees drawn up to avoid stretching the nerve fibers of the peritoneal cavity. Coughing and sneezing, which increase pressure within the peritoneal cavity, are associated with sharp pain. There may or may not be pain localized to the infected or diseased organ from which secondary peritonitis has arisen. Patients with secondary peritonitis generally have abnormal findings on abdominal examination, with marked voluntary and involuntary guarding of the anterior abdominal musculature. Later findings include tenderness, especially rebound tenderness. In addition, there may be localized findings in the area of the inciting event. In general, patients are febrile, with marked leukocytosis and a left shift of the WBCs to earlier granulocyte forms.

While recovery of organisms from peritoneal fluid is easier in secondary than in primary peritonitis, a tap of the abdomen is rarely the procedure of choice in secondary peritonitis. An exception is in cases involving trauma, where the possibility of a hemoperitoneum may need to be excluded early. Etiologic studies to find the source of peritoneal contamination should be undertaken.

Rx TREATMENT

Treatment for secondary peritonitis includes early administration of antibiotics aimed particularly at aerobic gram-negative bacilli and anaerobes (see below). Mild to moderate disease can be treated with many drugs covering these organisms, including broad-spectrum penicillin/β-lactamase inhibitor combinations (e.g., ticarcillin/clavulanate, 3.1 g q6h IV) or cefoxitin (2 g q24h IV). Patients requiring hospitalization in intensive care should receive imipenem (500 mg q6h IV), meropenem (1 g q8h IV), or combinations of drugs, such as ampicillin plus metronidizole plus ciprofloxacin. Secondary peritonitis usually requires both surgical intervention to address the inciting process and antibiotic administration to treat early bacteremia, to decrease the incidence of abscess formation and wound infection, and to prevent more distant spread of infection. Whereas surgery is rarely indicated in PBP in adults, it may be life-saving in secondary peritonitis.

PERITONITIS IN PATIENTS UNDERGOING CAPD A third type of peritonitis arises in patients who are undergoing continuous ambulatory peritoneal dialysis (CAPD). Unlike primary and secondary peritonitis, which are caused by endogenous bacteria, peritonitis in CAPD patients usually involves skin organisms. The pathogenesis of infection is similar to that of intravascular-device infection, in which skin organisms migrate along the catheter, which both serves as an entry point and exerts the effects of a foreign body. Exit-site or tunnel infection may or may not accompany CAPD peritonitis. Like PBP, CAPD peritonitis is usually caused by a single organism. Peritonitis is, in fact, the most common reason for discontinuation of CAPD. Improvements in equipment design, especially that of the Y-set connector, have resulted in a decrease from one case of peritonitis per 9 months of CAPD to one case per 15 months.

The clinical presentation of CAPD peritonitis resembles that of secondary peritonitis in that diffuse pain and peritoneal signs are common. The dialysate is usually cloudy and contains >100 WBCs per microliter, >50% of which are neutrophils. The most common etiologic organism is coagulase-negative *Staphylococcus*, which accounts for ~30% of cases. *Staphylococcus aureus* causes ~10% of cases, is more commonly identified among patients who are nasal carriers of the organism, and is the most frequent pathogen in those with an overt exit-site infection. Gram-negative bacilli and fungi such as *Candida* species are also found. Vancomycin-resistant enterococci (VRE) and vancomycin-intermediate *S. aureus* (VISA) have been reported to produce peritonitis in CAPD patients. The finding of more than one organism in dialysate culture should prompt a search for a cause of secondary peritonitis. As with primary peritonitis, culture of dialysate fluid in blood culture bottles improves the yield. To facilitate diagnosis, several hundred milliliters of removed dialysis fluid should be concentrated by centrifugation before culture.

Rx TREATMENT

Empirical therapy for CAPD peritonitis should be directed at *S. aureus*, coagulase-negative *Staphylococcus*, and gram-negative bacilli until the results of cultures are available. Since the advent of VRE and VISA, a first-generation cephalosporin such as cefazolin and a third-generation cephalosporin such as ceftazidime constitute the treatment of choice. A loading dose of cefazolin is administered intraperitoneally along with ceftazidime; doses depend on the dialysis method and the patient's renal function. If methicillin-resistant *S. aureus* is a relatively common isolate in a community, vancomycin may be a reasonable first choice for empirical therapy, especially in a toxic-appearing patient or a patient with an overt exit-site infection. The dose (2 g) is allowed to remain in the peritoneal cavity for 6 h. If the patient is severely ill, intravenous antibiotics similar to those in the dialysis bag should be added to the regimen at doses appropriate for the patient's degree of renal failure. The clinical response to an empirical treatment regimen should be rapid; if the patient has not responded after 48 h of treatment, catheter removal should be considered.

TUBERCULOUS PERITONITIS See Chap. 150.

FAMILIAL MEDITERRANEAN FEVER (See Chap. 279) Familial Mediterranean fever is an autosomal recessive disorder usually presenting with episodic bouts of peritonitis without an infectious etiology.

INTRAPERITONEAL ABSCESSES

Abscess formation is common in untreated peritonitis if overt gram-negative sepsis either does not develop or develops but is not fatal. In experimental models of abscess formation, mixed aerobic and anaerobic organisms have been implanted intraperitoneally. Without therapy directed at anaerobes, animals develop intraabdominal abscesses. As in humans, these experimental abscesses may stud the peritoneal cavity, lie within the omentum or mesentery, or even develop on the surface of or within viscera such as the liver.

PATHOGENESIS AND IMMUNITY There is often disagreement about whether an abscess represents a disease state or a host response. In a sense, it represents both: While an abscess is an infection in which viable infecting organisms and PMNs are contained in a fibrous capsule, it is also a process by which the host confines microbes to a limited space, thereby preventing further spread of infection. In any event, abscesses do cause significant symptoms, and patients with abscesses can be quite ill. Experimental work has helped to define both the host cells and the bacterial virulence factors responsible—most notably, in the case of *B. fragilis*. This organism, although accounting for only 0.5% of the normal colonic flora, is the anaerobe most frequently isolated from intraabdominal infections, is especially prominent in abscesses, and is the most common anaerobic bloodstream isolate. On clinical grounds, therefore, *B. fragilis* appears to be uniquely virulent. Moreover, *B. fragilis* acts alone to cause abscesses in animal models of intraabdominal infection, whereas most other *Bacteroides* species must act synergistically with a facultative organism to induce abscess formation.

Of the several virulence factors identified in *B. fragilis*, one is critical: the capsular polysaccharide complex (CPC) found on the bacterial surface. The CPC comprises at least eight distinct surface polysaccharides. Structural analysis of some of the polysaccharides in the CPC has shown an unusual motif of oppositely charged sugars. Polysaccharides having these *zwitterionic* characteristics, such as polysaccharide A (PS A), evoke a host response in the peritoneal cavity that localizes bacteria into abscesses. *B. fragilis* and PS A have been found to adhere to primary mesothelial cells in vitro; this adherence, in turn, stimulates the production of tumor necrosis factor α (TNF-α) and intercellular adhesion molecule 1 (ICAM-1) by peritoneal macrophages. Although abscesses characteristically contain PMNs, the process of abscess induction depends on the stimulation of T lymphocytes by these unique zwitterionic polysaccharides. The stimulated CD4+ lymphocytes secrete leukoattractant cytokines and chemokines. The alternative pathways of complement and fibrinogen also participate in abscess formation.

While antibodies to the CPC enhance bloodstream clearance of *B. fragilis*, CD4+ T cells are critical in immunity to abscesses. When administered subcutaneously, *B. fragilis* PS A has immunomodulatory characteristics and stimulates CD4+ T regulatory (Treg) cells via an interleukin (IL) 2–dependent mechanism to produce IL-10. IL-10 downregulates the inflammatory response, thereby preventing abscess formation.

CLINICAL PRESENTATION Most intraperitoneal abscesses result from fecal spillage from a colonic source, such as an inflamed appendix. Of all intraabdominal abscesses, 74% are intraperitoneal or retroperitoneal and are not visceral. Abscesses can also arise from a number of other processes. They usually form within weeks of the development of peritonitis and may be found in a variety of locations—from omentum to mesentery, pelvis to psoas muscles, and subphrenic space to a visceral organ such as the liver, where they may develop either on the surface of the organ or within it. Periappendiceal and diverticular abscesses occur commonly. Diverticular abscesses are least likely to rupture. Infections of the female genital tract and pancreatitis are also among the more common causative events. When abscesses occur in the female genital tract—either as a primary infection (e.g., tubo-ovarian abscess) or as an infection extending into the pelvic cavity or peritoneum—*B. fragilis* figures prominently among the organisms isolated. *B. fragilis* is not found in large numbers in the normal vaginal flora. It is encountered less commonly in pelvic inflammatory disease and endometritis, for example, without an associated abscess. In pancreatitis with leakage of damaging pancreatic enzymes, inflammation is prominent. Therefore, clinical findings such as fever, leukocytosis, and even abdominal pain do not distinguish pancreatitis itself from complications such as pancreatic pseudocyst, pancreatic abscess (Chap. 294), or intraabdominal collections of pus. Especially in cases of necrotizing pancreatitis, in which the incidence of local pancreatic infection may be as high as 30%, needle aspiration under CT guidance is performed as often as once a week to sample fluid for culture. Many centers prescribe prophylactic antibiotics to prevent infection in patients with necrotizing pancreatitis. Imipenem is the drug most frequently used for this purpose since it reaches high tissue levels in the pancreas (although it is not unique in this regard). If needle aspiration yields infected fluid, most experts agree that surgery is superior to percutaneous drainage.

DIAGNOSIS   A variety of scanning procedures have considerably facilitated the diagnosis of intraabdominal abscesses. Abdominal CT probably has the highest yield, although ultrasonography is particularly useful for the right upper quadrant, kidneys, and pelvis. Both indium-labeled WBCs and gallium tend to localize in abscesses and may be useful in finding a collection. Since gallium is taken up in the bowel, indium-labeled WBCs may have a slightly greater yield for abscesses near the bowel. Neither indium-labeled WBC nor gallium scans serve as a basis for a definitive diagnosis, however; both need to be followed by other, more specific studies, such as CT, if an area of possible abnormality is identified. Abscesses contiguous with or contained within outpouchings of bowel are particularly difficult to diagnose with scanning procedures. Occasionally, a barium enema may detect a diverticular abscess not diagnosed by other procedures, although barium should not be injected if a free perforation is suspected. If one study is negative, a second study sometimes reveals a collection. Although exploratory laparotomy has been less commonly used since the advent of CT, this procedure still must be undertaken on occasion if an abscess is strongly suspected on clinical grounds.

℞ TREATMENT

An algorithm for the management of patients with intraabdominal abscesses is presented in Fig. 112-1. The treatment of intraabdominal infections involves the determination of the initial focus of infection, the administration of broad-spectrum antibiotics targeted at organisms involved in the associated infection, and the performance of a drainage procedure if one or more definitive abscesses have already formed. Antimicrobial therapy, in general, is adjunctive to drainage and/or surgical correction of an underlying lesion or process in intraabdominal abscesses. Unlike the intraabdominal abscesses precipitated by most infections, for which drainage of some kind is generally required, abscesses associated with diverticulitis usually wall off locally after rupture of a diverticulum, so that surgical intervention is not routinely required.

A number of antimicrobial agents exhibit excellent activity against aerobic gram-negative bacilli. Since mortality in intraabdominal sepsis is linked to gram-negative bacteremia, empirical therapy for intraabdominal infection always needs to include adequate coverage of gram-negative aerobic, facultative, and anaerobic organisms. Even if anaerobes are not cultured from clinical specimens, they still must be

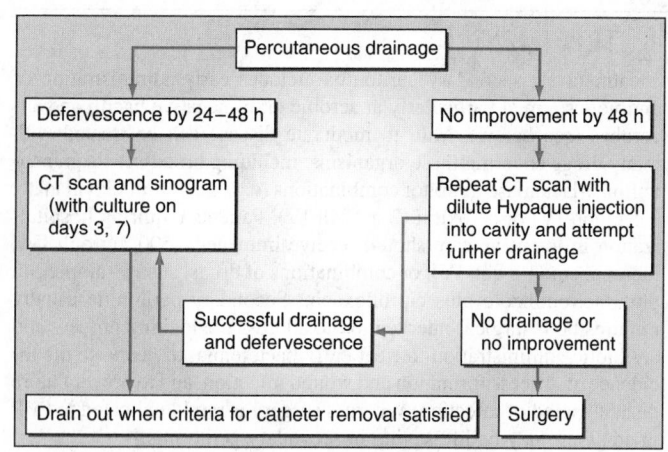

FIGURE 112-1   Algorithm for the management of patients with intraabdominal abscesses using percutaneous drainage. Antimicrobial therapy should be administered concomitantly. CT, computed tomography. [*Reprinted with permission from B Lorber (ed): Atlas of Infectious Diseases, vol VII: Intra-abdominal Infections, Hepatitis, and Gastroenteritis. Philadelphia, Current Medicine, 1995, pp 1–101, as adapted from OD Rotstein, RL Simmons, in SL Gorbach et al (eds): Infectious Diseases, Philadelphia, Saunders, 1992, p. 668.*]

covered by the therapeutic regimen. Broad-spectrum empirical antibiotic therapy should be the same as that discussed above for secondary peritonitis.

VISCERAL ABSCESSES ■ **Liver Abscesses**   The liver is the organ most subject to the development of abscesses. In one study of 540 intraabdominal abscesses over a 12-year period, 26% of these abscesses were visceral. Liver abscesses made up 13% of the total number of abscesses, or 48% of all visceral abscesses. Liver abscesses may be solitary or multiple; they may arise from hematogenous spread of bacteria or from local spread from contiguous sites of infection within the peritoneal cavity. In the past, appendicitis with rupture and subsequent spread of infection was the most common route for the development of a liver abscess. Currently, associated disease of the biliary tract is most often the etiology. Suppurative pylephlebitis (suppurative thrombosis of the portal vein), usually arising from infection in the pelvis but sometimes from infection elsewhere in the peritoneal cavity, is another common source for bacterial seeding of the liver.

Fever is the most common presenting sign of liver abscess. Some patients, particularly those with active associated disease of the biliary tract, have symptoms and signs localized to the right upper quadrant, including pain, guarding, punch tenderness, and even rebound tenderness. Nonspecific symptoms, such as chills, anorexia, weight loss, nausea, and vomiting, may also develop. Only 50% of patients with liver abscesses, however, have hepatomegaly, right-upper-quadrant tenderness, or jaundice; thus, half of patients have no symptoms or signs that would direct attention to the liver. Fever of unknown origin (FUO) may be the only presenting manifestation of liver abscess, especially in the elderly. Diagnostic studies of the abdomen, especially the right upper quadrant, should be a part of any FUO workup. The single most reliable laboratory finding is an elevated serum concentration of alkaline phosphatase, which is documented in 70% of patients with liver abscesses. Other tests of liver function may yield normal results, but 50% of patients have elevated serum levels of bilirubin, and 48% have elevated concentrations of aspartate aminotransferase. Other associated laboratory findings include leukocytosis in 77% of patients, anemia (usually normochromic, normocytic) in 50%, and hypoalbuminemia in 33%. Concomitant bacteremia is found in one-third of patients. A liver abscess is sometimes suggested by chest radiography, especially if a new elevation of the right hemidiaphragm is seen; other suggestive findings include a right basilar infiltrate and a right pleural effusion.

Imaging studies are the most reliable methods for diagnosing liver abscesses. These studies include ultrasonography, CT (Fig. 112-2), indium-labeled WBC or gallium scans, and magnetic resonance im-

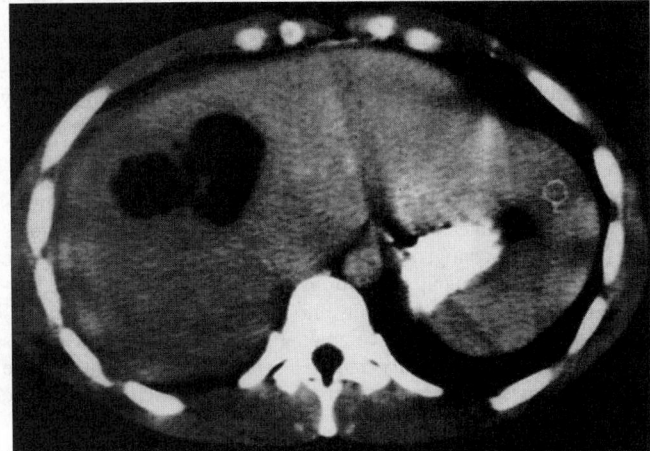

FIGURE 112-2 Multilocular liver abscess on computed tomography scan. Multiple or multilocular abscesses are more common than solitary abscesses. [*Reprinted with permission from B Lorber (ed): Atlas of Infectious Diseases, Vol VII: Intra-abdominal Infection, Hepatitis, and Gastroenteritis. Philadelphia, Current Medicine, 1996, Fig. 1-70.*]

aging. In an occasional case, more than one such study may be required. Organisms recovered from liver abscesses vary with the etiology. In liver infection arising from the biliary tree, enteric gram-negative aerobic bacilli and enterococci are common isolates. Unless previous surgery has been performed, anaerobes are not generally involved in liver abscesses arising from biliary infections. In contrast, in liver abscesses arising from pelvic and other intraperitoneal sources, a mixed flora including both aerobic and anaerobic species is common; *B. fragilis* is the species most frequently isolated. With hematogenous spread of infection, usually only a single organism is encountered; this species may be *S. aureus* or a streptococcal species such as *S. milleri*. Results of cultures obtained from drain sites are not reliable for defining the etiology of infections. Liver abscesses may also be caused by *Candida* species; such abscesses usually follow fungemia in patients receiving chemotherapy for cancer and often present when neutrophils return after a period of neutropenia. However, the recovery of *Candida* from a drain site does not necessarily implicate this organism as a cause of infection. Amebic liver abscesses are not an uncommon problem (Chap. 194). Amebic serologic testing gives positive results in >95% of cases; thus, a negative result helps to exclude this diagnosis.

Rx TREATMENT

While drainage—either percutaneous (with a pigtail catheter kept in place) or surgical—remains the mainstay of therapy for intraabdominal abscesses (including liver abscesses), there is growing interest in medical management alone for pyogenic liver abscesses. The drugs used for empirical broad-spectrum antibiotic therapy include the same ones used in intraabdominal sepsis and secondary bacterial peritonitis. Usually, a diagnostic aspirate of abscess contents should be obtained before the initiation of empirical therapy, with antibiotic choices adjusted when the results of Gram's staining and culture become available. Cases treated without definitive drainage generally require longer courses of antibiotic therapy. When percutaneous drainage was compared with open surgical drainage, the average length of hospital stay for the former was almost twice that for the latter, although both the time required for fever to resolve and the mortality rate were the same for the two procedures. Mortality was appreciable despite treatment, averaging 15%. Several factors may predict the failure of percutaneous drainage and therefore may favor primary surgical intervention. These factors include the presence of multiple, sizable abscesses; viscous abscess contents that tend to plug the catheter; associated disease (e.g., disease of the biliary tract) that requires surgery; or the lack of a clinical response to percutaneous drainage in 4 to 7 days.

Treatment of candidal liver abscesses usually entails lengthy ad-

ministration of amphotericin B, although reports have described successful maintenance therapy with fluconazole after an initial course of amphotericin (Chap. 187).

Splenic Abscesses Splenic abscesses are much less common than liver abscesses. The incidence of splenic abscesses has ranged from 0.14 to 0.7% in various autopsy series. The clinical setting and the organisms isolated usually differ from those for liver abscesses. The degree of clinical suspicion for splenic abscess needs to be high, as this condition is frequently fatal if left untreated. Even in the most recently published series, diagnosis was made only at autopsy in 37% of cases. While splenic abscesses may arise occasionally from contiguous spread of infection or from direct trauma to the spleen, hematogenous spread of infection is the usual mode of development. Bacterial endocarditis is the most common associated infection (Chap. 109). Splenic abscesses can develop in patients who have received extensive immunosuppressive therapy (particularly those with malignancy involving the spleen) and in patients with hemoglobinopathies or other hematologic disorders (especially sickle cell anemia).

While ~50% of patients with splenic abscesses have abdominal pain, the pain is localized to the left upper quadrant in only half of these cases. Splenomegaly is found in ~50% of cases. Fever and leukocytosis are generally present; the development of fever preceded diagnosis by an average of 20 days in one series. Left-sided chest findings may include abnormalities to auscultation, and chest radiographic findings may include an infiltrate or a left-sided pleural effusion. When splenic abscesses are being considered in a differential diagnosis, CT scan of the abdomen has been the most sensitive diagnostic tool. Ultrasonography can yield the diagnosis, but cases have been missed with this modality. Liver-spleen scan or gallium scan may also be useful. Streptococcal species are the most common bacterial isolates from splenic abscesses, and *S. aureus* is the next most common; presumably these prevalences reflect the bacterial cause of the associated endocarditis. An increase in the frequency of isolation of gram-negative aerobic organisms from splenic abscesses has been reported; these organisms often derive from a urinary tract focus, with associated bacteremia, or from another intraabdominal source. *Salmonella* species are seen fairly commonly, especially in patients with sickle cell hemoglobinopathy. Anaerobic species accounted for only 5% of isolates in the largest collected series, but the reporting of a number of "sterile abscesses" may indicate that optimal techniques for the isolation of anaerobes were not employed.

Rx TREATMENT

Because of the high mortality figures reported for splenic abscesses, the treatment of choice is splenectomy with adjunctive antibiotics. However, percutaneous drainage has been successful. The most important factor in successful treatment of splenic abscesses is early consideration of the diagnosis.

Perinephric and Renal Abscesses Perinephric and renal abscesses are not common: The former accounted for only ~0.02% of hospital admissions and the latter for ~0.2% in Altemeier's series of 540 intraabdominal abscesses. While liver abscesses generally arise from contiguous foci of infection or track from other intraabdominal sources and splenic abscesses usually arise from hematogenous spread (e.g., spread from bacterial endocarditis), perinephric and renal abscesses have a different pathogenesis. Before antibiotics became available, most renal and perinephric abscesses were hematogenous in origin, with *S. aureus* most commonly recovered. Now, in contrast, >75% of perinephric and renal abscesses arise from an initial urinary tract infection. Infection ascends from the bladder to the kidney, with pyelonephritis occurring first. Bacteria may directly invade the renal parenchyma from medulla to cortex. Local vascular channels within the kidney may also facilitate the transport of organisms. Areas of abscess developing within the parenchyma may rupture into the perinephric space. The kidneys and adrenal glands are surrounded by a layer of perirenal fat that, in turn, is surrounded by Gerota's fascia, which extends superiorly to the diaphragm and inferiorly to the pelvic fat. When abscesses extend into the perinephric space, tracking may occur through Gerota's fascia into the psoas or transversalis muscles, into the anterior peritoneal cavity, superiorly to the subdiaphragmatic space, or inferiorly to the pelvis. Of the several risk factors that have been associated with the development of perinephric abscesses, the most important is the presence of concomitant nephrolithiasis producing local obstruction to urinary flow. Of patients with perinephric abscess, 20 to 60% have renal stones. In addition, other structural abnormalities of the urinary tract, a history of urologic surgery, trauma, and diabetes mellitus have all been identified as risk factors.

The organisms most frequently encountered in perinephric and renal abscesses are *E. coli*, *Proteus* species, and *Klebsiella* species. *E. coli*, the aerobic species most commonly found in the colonic flora, seems to have unique virulence properties in the urinary tract, including factors promoting adherence to uroepithelial cells. The urease of *Proteus* species splits urea, thereby creating a more alkaline and more hospitable environment for bacterial proliferation. *Proteus* species are frequently found in association with large struvite stones caused by the precipitation of magnesium ammonium sulfate in an alkaline environment. These stones serve as a nidus for recurrent urinary tract infection. While a single bacterial species is usually recovered from a perinephric or renal abscess, multiple species may also be found. If a urine culture is not contaminated with periurethral flora and is found to contain more than one organism, a perinephric abscess or renal abscess should be considered in the differential diagnosis. Urine cultures may also be polymicrobial in cases of bladder diverticulum.

Candida species should be considered in the etiology of renal abscesses. This fungus may spread to the kidney via the hematogenous route or by ascension from the bladder. The hallmark of the latter route of infection is ureteral obstruction with large fungal balls.

The presentation of perinephric and renal abscesses is quite nonspecific. Flank pain and abdominal pain are common. At least 50% of patients are febrile. Pain may be referred to the groin or leg, particularly with extension of infection. The diagnosis of perinephric abscess, like that of splenic abscess, is frequently delayed, and the mortality rate in some series is appreciable, although lower than in the past. Perinephric or renal abscess should be most seriously considered when a patient presents with symptoms and signs of pyelonephritis and remains febrile after 4 or 5 days, by which time the fever should have resolved. Moreover, when a urine culture yields a polymicrobial flora, when a patient is known to have renal stone disease, or when fever and pyuria coexist with a sterile urine culture, the diagnosis of perinephric or renal abscess should be entertained.

Renal ultrasonography and abdominal CT are the most useful diagnostic modalities. If a renal abscess or perinephric abscess is diagnosed, nephrolithiasis should be excluded, especially when a high urinary pH suggests the presence of a urea-splitting organism.

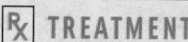

TREATMENT

Treatment for perinephric or renal abscesses, like that for other intraabdominal abscesses, includes drainage of pus and antibiotic therapy directed at the organism(s) recovered. For perinephric abscesses, percutaneous drainage is usually successful.

Psoas Abscesses The psoas muscle is another location in which abscesses are encountered. Psoas abscesses may arise from a hematogenous source, by contiguous spread from an intraabdominal or pelvic process, or by contiguous spread from nearby bony structures (e.g., vertebral bodies). Associated osteomyelitis due to spread from bone to muscle or from muscle to bone is common in psoas abscesses. When Pott's disease was common, *Mycobacterium tuberculosis* was a frequent cause of psoas abscess. Currently, either *S. aureus* or a mixture of enteric organisms including aerobic and anaerobic gram-negative bacilli is usually isolated from psoas abscesses in the United States. *S. aureus* is most likely to be isolated when a psoas abscess arises from hematogenous spread or a contiguous focus of osteomyelitis; a mixed enteric flora is the most likely etiology when the abscess has an intraabdominal or pelvic source. Patients with psoas abscesses frequently present with fever, lower abdominal or back pain, or pain referred to the hip or knee. CT is the most useful diagnostic technique.

TREATMENT

Treatment includes surgical drainage and the administration of an antibiotic regimen directed at the inciting organism(s).

Pancreatic Abscesses See Chap. 294.

FURTHER READING

Bassi C et al: Controlled clinical trial of pefloxacin versus imipenem in severe acute pancreatitis. Gastroenterology 115:1513, 1998

Campillo B et al: Epidemiology of severe hospital-acquired infections in patients with liver cirrhosis: Effect of long-term administration of norfloxacin. Clin Infect Dis 26:1066, 1998

Finegold SM: Anaerobic bacteria: General concepts, in *Principles and Practice of Infectious Diseases*, 5th ed, GL Mandell et al (eds). New York, Churchill Livingstone, 2000, pp 2519–2537

Gibson FC III et al: Cellular mechanism of intraabdominal abscess formation by *Bacteroides fragilis*. J Immunol 160:5000, 1998

Levison ME, Bush LM: Peritonitis and other intra-abdominal infections, in *Principles and Practice of Infectious Diseases*, 5th ed, GL Mandell et al (eds). New York, Churchill Livingstone, 2000, pp 821–856

Robson RI et al: Differential regulation of chemokine production in human peritoneal mesothelial cells: IFN-gamma controls neutrophil migration across the mesothelium in vitro and in vivo. J Immunol 167:1028, 2001

Solomkin JS et al: Guidelines for the selection of anti-infective agents for complicated intra-abdominal infections. Clin Infect Dis 37:997, 2003

———— et al: Results of a randomized trial comparing sequential intravenous/oral treatment with ciprofloxacin plus metronidazole to imipenem/cilastatin for intra-abdominal infections. Ann Surg 223:303, 1996

Tzianabos AO et al: T cells activated by zwitterionic molecules prevent abscesses induced by pathogenic bacteria. J Biol Chem 275:6733, 2000

113 ACUTE INFECTIOUS DIARRHEAL DISEASES AND BACTERIAL FOOD POISONING
Joan R. Butterton, Stephen B. Calderwood

Ranging from mild annoyances during vacations to devastating dehydrating illnesses that can kill within hours, acute gastrointestinal illnesses rank second only to acute upper respiratory illnesses as the most common diseases worldwide. In children <5 years old, attack rates range from 2 to 3 illnesses per child per year in developed countries to as high as 10 to 18 illnesses per child per year in developing countries. In Asia, Africa, and Latin America, acute diarrheal illnesses are not only a leading cause of morbidity in children—with an estimated 1 billion cases per year—but also a major cause of mortality,

being responsible for 4 to 6 million deaths per year, or a sobering total of 12,600 deaths per day. In some areas, >50% of childhood deaths are directly attributable to acute diarrheal illnesses. In addition, by contributing to malnutrition and thereby reducing resistance to other infectious agents, gastrointestinal illnesses may be indirect factors in a far greater burden of disease.

The wide range of clinical manifestations of acute gastrointestinal illnesses is matched by the wide variety of infectious agents involved, including viruses, bacteria, and parasitic pathogens (Table 113-1). This chapter will discuss factors that enable gastrointestinal pathogens to cause disease, will review host defense mechanisms, and will delineate an approach to the evaluation and treatment of patients presenting with acute diarrhea. Individual organisms causing acute gastrointestinal illnesses are discussed in detail in subsequent chapters.

PATHOGENIC MECHANISMS Enteric pathogens have developed a variety of tactics to overcome host defenses. Understanding the virulence factors employed by these organisms is important in the diagnosis and treatment of clinical disease.

Inoculum Size The number of microorganisms that must be ingested to cause disease varies considerably from species to species. For *Shigella*, enterohemorrhagic *Escherichia coli*, *Giardia lamblia*, or *Entamoeba*, as few as 10 to 100 bacteria or cysts can produce infection, while 10^5 to 10^8 *Vibrio cholerae* organisms must be ingested orally to cause disease. The infective dose of *Salmonella* varies widely, depending on the species, host, and food vehicle. The ability of organisms to overcome host defenses has important implications for transmission; *Shigella*, enterohemorrhagic *E. coli*, *Entamoeba*, and *Giardia* can spread by person-to-person contact, whereas under some circumstances *Salmonella* may have to grow in food for several hours before reaching an effective infectious dose.

Adherence Many organisms must adhere to the gastrointestinal mucosa as an initial step in the pathogenic process; thus, organisms that can compete with the normal bowel flora and colonize the mucosa have an important advantage in causing disease. Specific cell-surface proteins involved in attachment of bacteria to intestinal cells are important virulence determinants. *V. cholerae*, for example, adheres to the brush border of small-intestinal enterocytes via specific surface adhesins, including the toxin-coregulated pilus and other accessory colonization factors. Different pathogenic varieties of *E. coli* have different adherence mechanisms. Enterotoxigenic *E. coli*, which causes watery diarrhea, produces an adherence protein called *colonization factor antigen* that is necessary for colonization of the upper small intestine by the organism prior to the production of enterotoxin. Enteropathogenic *E. coli*, an agent of diarrhea in young children, and enterohemorrhagic *E. coli*, which causes hemorrhagic colitis and the hemolytic-uremic syndrome, produce virulence determinants that allow these organisms to attach to and efface the brush border of the intestinal epithelium.

Toxin Production The production of one or more exotoxins is important in the pathogenesis of numerous enteric organisms. Such toxins include *enterotoxins*, which cause watery diarrhea by acting directly on secretory mechanisms in the intestinal mucosa; *cytotoxins*, which cause destruction of mucosal cells and associated inflammatory diarrhea; and *neurotoxins*, which act directly on the central or peripheral nervous system. Some exotoxins act by more than one mechanism; *Shigella dysenteriae* type 1, for example, produces an exotoxin that has both enterotoxic and cytotoxic activities.

The prototypical enterotoxin is cholera toxin, a heterodimeric protein composed of one A and five B subunits. The A subunit contains the enzymatic activity of the toxin, while the B subunit pentamer binds holotoxin to the enterocyte surface receptor, the ganglioside G_{M1}. After the binding of holotoxin, a fragment of the A subunit is translocated across the eukaryotic cell membrane into the cytoplasm, where it catalyzes the ADP-ribosylation of a GTP-binding protein and causes persistent activation of adenylate cyclase. The end result is an increase of cyclic AMP in the intestinal mucosa, which increases Cl^- secretion and decreases Na^+ absorption, leading to loss of fluid and the production of diarrhea.

Enterotoxigenic strains of *E. coli* may produce a protein called *heat-labile enterotoxin* (LT) that is similar to cholera toxin and causes secretory diarrhea by the same mechanism. Alternatively, enterotoxigenic strains of *E. coli* may produce *heat-stable enterotoxin* (ST), one form of which causes diarrhea by activation of guanylate cyclase and elevation of intracellular cyclic GMP. Some enterotoxigenic strains of *E. coli* produce both LT and ST.

Bacterial cytotoxins, in contrast, destroy intestinal mucosal cells and produce the syndrome of dysentery, with bloody stools containing inflammatory cells. Enteric pathogens that produce such cytotoxins include *S. dysenteriae* type 1, *Vibrio parahaemolyticus*, and *Clostridium difficile*. Shiga toxin–producing strains of *E. coli* (a group that includes enterohemorrhagic strains and whose most common serotype in the United States is O157:H7) produce potent cytotoxins that are highly related to the Shiga toxin of *S. dysenteriae* type 1. Such strains of *E. coli* have been associated with outbreaks of hemorrhagic colitis and hemolytic-uremic syndrome.

Neurotoxins are usually produced by the responsible organism outside the host and therefore cause symptoms soon after ingestion. Included are the staphylococcal and *Bacillus cereus* toxins, which act on the central nervous system to produce vomiting.

Invasion Dysentery may result not only from the production of cytotoxins but also from bacterial invasion and destruction of intestinal mucosal cells. Infections due to *Shigella* and enteroinvasive *E. coli*, for example, are characterized by the organisms' invasion of mucosal epithelial cells, intraepithelial multiplication, and subsequent spread to adjacent cells. *Salmonella*, on the other hand, causes inflammatory diarrhea by invasion of the bowel mucosa but generally is not associated with the destruction of enterocytes or the full clinical syndrome of dysentery. *Salmonella typhi* and *Yersinia enterocolitica* can penetrate intact intestinal mucosa, multiply intracellularly in Peyer's patches and intestinal lymph nodes, and then disseminate through the

TABLE 113-1 *Gastrointestinal Pathogens Causing Acute Diarrhea*

Mechanism	Location	Illness	Stool Findings	Examples of Pathogens Involved
Noninflammatory (enterotoxin)	Proximal small bowel	Watery diarrhea	No fecal leukocytes; mild or no increase in fecal lactoferrin	*Vibrio cholerae*, enterotoxigenic *Escherichia coli* (LT and/or ST), *Clostridium perfringens*, *Bacillus cereus*, *Staphylococcus aureus*, *Aeromonas hydrophila*, *Plesiomonas shigelloides*, rotavirus, Norwalk-like viruses, enteric adenoviruses, *Giardia lamblia*, *Cryptosporidium* spp., *Cyclospora* spp., microsporidia
Inflammatory (invasion or cytotoxin)	Colon or distal small bowel	Dysentery or inflammatory diarrhea	Fecal polymorphonuclear leukocytes; substantial increase in fecal lactoferrin	*Shigella* spp., *Salmonella* spp., *Campylobacter jejuni*, enterohemorrhagic *E. coli*, enteroinvasive *E. coli*, *Yersinia enterocolitica*, *Vibrio parahaemolyticus*, *Clostridium difficile*, ?*A. hydrophila*, ?*P. shigelloides*, *Entamoeba histolytica*
Penetrating	Distal small bowel	Enteric fever	Fecal mononuclear leukocytes	*Salmonella typhi*, *Y. enterocolitica*, ?*Campylobacter fetus*

Abbreviations: LT, heat-labile enterotoxin; ST, heat-stable enterotoxin.
Source: After Guerrant and Steiner.

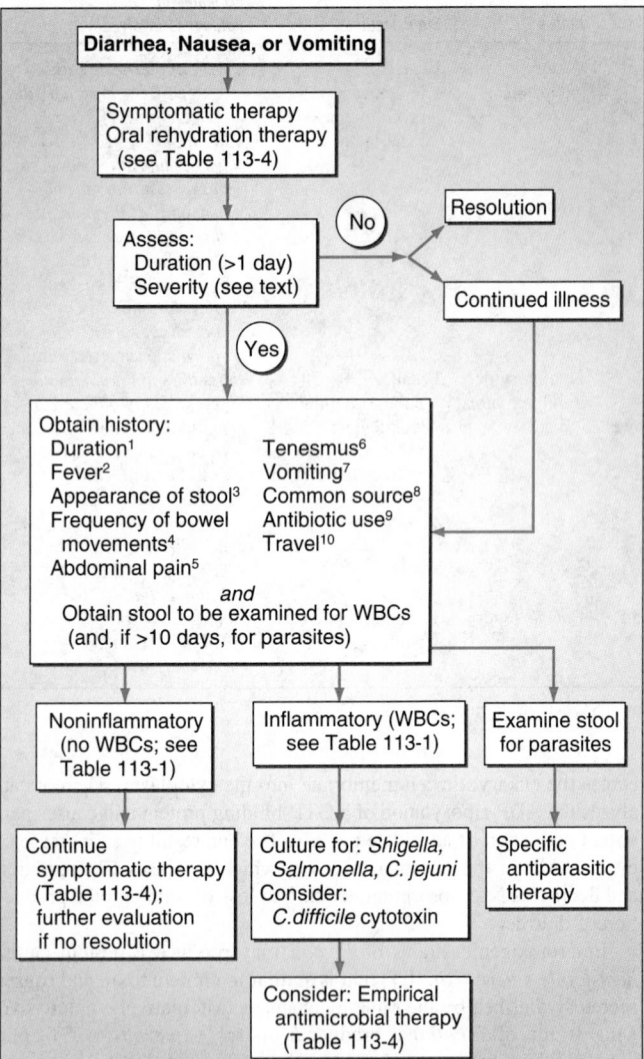

Diarrhea, Nausea, or Vomiting

Symptomatic therapy
Oral rehydration therapy
(see Table 113-4)

Assess:
Duration (>1 day)
Severity (see text)

No → Resolution

Continued illness

Yes

Obtain history:
Duration[1]   Tenesmus[6]
Fever[2]   Vomiting[7]
Appearance of stool[3]   Common source[8]
Frequency of bowel   Antibiotic use[9]
  movements[4]   Travel[10]
Abdominal pain[5]
            and
Obtain stool to be examined for WBCs
(and, if >10 days, for parasites)

Noninflammatory
(no WBCs; see
Table 113-1)

Inflammatory (WBCs;
see Table 113-1)

Examine stool
for parasites

Continue
symptomatic therapy
(Table 113-4);
further evaluation
if no resolution

Culture for: *Shigella,
Salmonella, C. jejuni*
Consider:
C.difficile cytotoxin

Specific
antiparasitic
therapy

Consider: Empirical
antimicrobial therapy
(Table 113-4)

FIGURE 113-1   Clinical algorithm for the approach to patients with community-acquired infectious diarrhea or bacterial food poisoning. Key to superscripts: 1. Diarrhea lasting >2 weeks is generally defined as chronic; in such cases, many of the causes of acute diarrhea are much less likely, and a new spectrum of causes needs to be considered. 2. Fever often implies invasive disease, although fever and diarrhea may also result from infection outside the gastrointestinal tract, as in malaria. 3. Stools that contain blood or mucus indicate ulceration of the large bowel. Bloody stools without fecal leukocytes should alert the laboratory to the possibility of infection with Shiga toxin–producing enterohemorrhagic *Escherichia coli*. Bulky white stools suggest a small-intestinal process that is causing malabsorption. Profuse "rice-water" stools suggest cholera or a similar toxigenic process. 4. Frequent stools over a given period can provide the first warning of impending dehydration. 5. Abdominal pain may be most severe in inflammatory processes like those due to *Shigella, Campylobacter,* and necrotizing toxins. Painful abdominal muscle cramps, caused by electrolyte loss, can develop in severe cases of cholera. Bloating is common in giardiasis. An appendicitis-like syndrome should prompt a culture for *Yersinia enterocolitica* with cold enrichment. 6. Tenesmus (painful rectal spasms with a strong urge to defecate but little passage of stool) may be a feature of cases with proctitis, as in shigellosis or amebiasis. 7. Vomiting implies an acute infection (e.g., a toxin-mediated illness or food poisoning) but can also be prominent in a variety of systemic illnesses (e.g., malaria) and in intestinal obstruction. 8. Asking patients whether anyone else they know is sick is a more efficient means of identifying a common source than is constructing a list of recently eaten foods. If a common source seems likely, specific foods can be investigated. See text for a discussion of bacterial food poisoning. 9. Current antibiotic therapy or a recent history of treatment suggests *Clostridium difficile* diarrhea (Chap. 114). Stop antibiotic treatment if possible and consider tests for *C. difficile* toxins. Antibiotic use may increase the risk of other infections, such as salmonellosis. 10. See text (and Chap. 108) for a discussion of traveler's diarrhea. (*After Guerrant and Steiner; RL Guerrant, DA Bobak: N Engl J Med 325:327, 1991; with permission.*)

bloodstream to cause enteric fever, a syndrome characterized by fever, headache, relative bradycardia, abdominal pain, splenomegaly, and leukopenia.

HOST DEFENSES   Given the enormous number of microorganisms ingested with every meal, the normal host must possess effective defense mechanisms to combat a constant influx of potential enteric pathogens. Studies of infections in patients with alterations in these defenses have led to a greater understanding of the variety of ways in which the normal host can protect itself against disease.

Normal Flora   The large numbers of bacteria that normally inhabit the intestine act as an important host defense by preventing colonization by potential enteric pathogens. Persons with fewer intestinal bacteria, such as infants who have not yet developed normal enteric colonization or patients receiving antibiotics, are at significantly greater risk of developing infections with enteric pathogens. The composition of the intestinal flora is as important as the number of organisms present. More than 99% of the normal colonic flora is made up of anaerobic bacteria, and the acidic pH and volatile fatty acids produced by these organisms appear to be critical elements in resistance to colonization.

Gastric Acid   The acidic pH of the stomach is an important barrier to enteric pathogens, and an increased frequency of infections due to *Salmonella, G. lamblia,* and a variety of helminths has been reported among patients who have undergone gastric surgery or are achlorhydric for some other reason. Neutralization of gastric acid with antacids or H_2 blockers—common among hospitalized patients—similarly increases the risk of enteric colonization. Some microorganisms, however, can survive the extreme acidity of the gastric environment; rotavirus, for example, is highly stable to acidity.

Intestinal Motility   Normal peristalsis is the major mechanism for clearance of bacteria from the proximal small intestine, although gastric acidity and secreted immunoglobulins also play a role in limiting the number of organisms present. When intestinal motility is impaired—for example, by treatment with opiates or other antimotility drugs, anatomic abnormalities (diverticula, fistulas, or afferent-loop stasis following surgery), or hypomotility states (as in diabetes mellitus or scleroderma)—the frequency of bacterial overgrowth and infection of the small bowel with enteric pathogens is much increased. Some patients in whom *Shigella* infection is treated with diphenoxylate hydrochloride with atropine (Lomotil) experience prolonged fever and shedding of organisms, while patients treated with opiates for mild *Salmonella* gastroenteritis have a higher frequency of bacteremia than those not treated with opiates.

Immunity   Both cellular immune responses and antibody production play important roles in protecting susceptible hosts from enteric infections. The wide spectrum of viral, bacterial, parasitic, and fungal gastrointestinal infections in patients with AIDS highlights the significance of cell-mediated immunity in protecting the normal host from these pathogens. Humoral immunity is also important and consists of systemic IgG and IgM as well as secretory IgA. Growing evidence supports the concept of a mucosal immune system for secretory IgA in which binding of bacterial antigens to the luminal surface of M cells in the distal small bowel and subsequent presentation of antigens to subepithelial lymphoid tissue lead to the proliferation of sensitized lymphocytes. These lymphocytes circulate and populate all of the mucosal tissues of the body as IgA-secreting plasma cells.

APPROACH TO THE PATIENT

The approach to the patient with possible infectious diarrhea or bacterial food poisoning is shown in Fig. 113-1.

History   The answers to questions with high discriminating value can quickly narrow the range of potential causes of diarrhea and help determine whether treatment is needed. Important elements of the narrative history are detailed in Fig. 113-1.

Physical Examination The examination of patients for signs of dehydration provides essential information about the severity of the diarrheal illness and the need for rapid therapy. Mild dehydration is indicated by thirst, dry mouth, decreased axillary sweat, decreased urine output, and slight weight loss. Signs of moderate dehydration include an orthostatic fall in blood pressure, skin tenting, and sunken eyes (or, in infants, a sunken fontanelle). Signs of severe dehydration range from hypotension and tachycardia to confusion and frank shock.

Diagnostic Approach After the severity of illness is assessed, the most important distinction that the clinician must make is between *inflammatory* and *noninflammatory* disease. Using the history and epidemiologic features of the case as guides in making this distinction, the clinician can rapidly evaluate the need for further efforts to define a specific etiology and for therapeutic intervention. Examination of a stool sample is an important supplement to the narrative history. Grossly bloody or mucoid stool suggests an inflammatory process. A test for fecal leukocytes (preparation of a thin smear of stool on a glass slide, addition of a drop of methylene blue, and examination of the wet mount) can suggest inflammatory disease in patients presenting with diarrhea, although the predictive value of this test is still debated. A test for fecal lactoferrin, which is a marker of fecal leukocytes, is more sensitive and is available in latex agglutination and enzyme-linked immunosorbent assay formats. Causes of acute infectious diarrhea, categorized as inflammatory and noninflammatory, are listed in Table 113-1.

TABLE 113-2 *Epidemiology of Traveler's Diarrhea*

Etiologic Agent	Approximate Percentage of Cases	Comments
Enterotoxigenic *Escherichia coli*	15–50	Single most important agent, particularly in summertime in semitropical areas; percentage of cases ranges from 15% in Asia to 50% in Latin America
Enteroaggregative *E. coli*	10–20	May cause one-third of culture-negative cases
Shigella and enteroinvasive *E. coli*	10–25	Major causes of fever and dysentery
Salmonella	5–10	Causes fever and dysentery
Campylobacter jejuni	3–15	More common in winter in semitropical areas; more common in Asia
Aeromonas	5	Important in Thailand
Plesiomonas	5	Related to tropical travel and seafood consumption
Vibrio cholerae	0–10	Most common in India and Asia; also common in Central and South America
Rotavirus and Norwalk-like virus	10–40	Latin America, Asia, and Africa; Norwalk-like virus associated with seafood ingestion on cruise ships
Entamoeba histolytica	5	Particularly important in Mexico and Thailand
Giardia lamblia	<2	Zoonotic reservoirs in northern United States; affects hikers and campers who drink from freshwater streams; contaminates water supplies in Russia
Cryptosporidium	2	Affects travelers to Russia, Mexico, and Africa; causes large-scale urban outbreaks in United States
Cyclospora	<1	Affects travelers to Nepal, Haiti, and Peru; contaminates water or food
Unknown	20	Illness improves with antibacterial therapy, implicating bacterial diarrhea

Source: After Dupont.

EPIDEMIOLOGY

Travel History Of the several million people who travel from temperate industrialized countries to tropical regions of Asia, Africa, and Central and South America each year, 20 to 50% experience a sudden onset of abdominal cramps, anorexia, and watery diarrhea; thus *traveler's diarrhea* is the most common travel-related illness (Chap. 108). The time of onset is usually 3 days to 2 weeks after the traveler's arrival in a tropical area; most cases begin within the first 3 to 5 days. The illness is generally self-limited, lasting 1 to 5 days. The high rate of diarrhea among travelers to underdeveloped areas is related to the ingestion of contaminated food or water.

The organisms that cause traveler's diarrhea vary considerably with location (Table 113-2). In all areas, enterotoxigenic *E. coli* is the most common isolate from persons with the classic secretory traveler's diarrhea syndrome.

Location Day-care centers have particularly high attack rates of enteric infections. Rotavirus is most common among children <2 years old, with attack rates of 75 to 100% among those exposed. *G. lamblia* is more common among older children, with somewhat lower attack rates. Other common organisms, often spread by fecal-oral contact, are *Shigella*, *Campylobacter jejuni*, and *Cryptosporidium*. A characteristic feature of infection among children attending day-care centers is the high rate of secondary cases among family members.

Similarly, hospitals are sites in which enteric infections are concentrated. In medical intensive-care units and pediatric wards, diarrhea is among the most common nosocomial infections. *C. difficile* is the predominant cause of nosocomial diarrhea among adults in the United States; viral pathogens, especially rotavirus, can spread rapidly in pediatric wards. Enteropathogenic *E. coli* has been associated with outbreaks of diarrhea in nurseries for newborns. One-third of elderly patients in chronic-care institutions develop a significant diarrheal illness each year. Surveillance stool cultures suggest that 25% of the residents of these institutions harbor cytotoxin-producing *C. difficile*, which causes more than half of all cases of diarrhea in this population. Antimicrobial therapy can predispose to pseudomembranous colitis by altering the normal colonic flora and allowing the multiplication of *C. difficile* (Chap. 114).

Age Most of the morbidity and mortality from enteric pathogens involves children <5 years of age. Breast-fed infants are protected from contaminated food and water and derive some protection from maternal antibodies, but their risk of infection rises dramatically when they begin to eat solid foods. Infants and younger children are more likely than adults to develop rotavirus disease, while older children and adults are more commonly infected with Norwalk-like viruses. Other organisms with higher attack rates among children than among adults include enterotoxigenic, enteropathogenic, and enterohemorrhagic *E. coli*; *C. jejuni*; and *G. lamblia*. In children, the incidence of *Salmonella* infections is highest among those <1 year of age, while the attack rate for *Shigella* infections is greatest among those 6 months to 4 years of age.

Bacterial Food Poisoning If the history and the stool examination indicate a noninflammatory etiology of diarrhea and there is evidence of a common-source outbreak, questions concerning the ingestion of specific foods and the time of onset of the diarrhea after a meal can provide clues to the bacterial cause of the illness. Potential causes of bacterial food poisoning are shown in Table 113-3.

Bacterial disease caused by an enterotoxin elaborated outside the host, such as that due to *Staphylococcus aureus* or *B. cereus*, has the shortest incubation period (1 to 6 h) and generally lasts <12 h. Most cases of staphylococcal food poisoning are caused by contamination from infected human carriers. Staphylococci can multiply at a wide range of temperatures; thus, if food is left to cool slowly and remains at room temperature after cooking, the organisms will have the opportunity to form enterotoxin. Outbreaks following picnics where potato salad, mayonnaise, and cream pastries have been served offer classic examples of staphylococcal food poisoning. Diarrhea,

TABLE 113-3 *Bacterial Food Poisoning*

Incubation Period, Organisms	Symptoms	Common Food Sources
1 TO 6 H		
Staphylococcus aureus	Nausea, vomiting, diarrhea	Ham, poultry, potato or egg salad, mayonnaise, cream pastries
Bacillus cereus	Nausea, vomiting, diarrhea	Fried rice
8 TO 16 H		
Clostridium perfringens	Abdominal cramps, diarrhea (vomiting rare)	Beef, poultry, legumes, gravies
B. cereus	Abdominal cramps, diarrhea (vomiting rare)	Meats, vegetables, dried beans, cereals
>16 H		
Vibrio cholerae	Watery diarrhea	Shellfish
Enterotoxigenic *Escherichia coli*	Watery diarrhea	Salads, cheese, meats, water
Enterohemorrhagic *E. coli*	Bloody diarrhea	Ground beef, roast beef, salami, raw milk, raw vegetables, apple juice
Salmonella spp.	Inflammatory diarrhea	Beef, poultry, eggs, dairy products
Campylobacter jejuni	Inflammatory diarrhea	Poultry, raw milk
Shigella spp.	Dysentery	Potato or egg salad, lettuce, raw vegetables
Vibrio parahaemolyticus	Dysentery	Mollusks, crustaceans

nausea, vomiting, and abdominal cramping are common, while fever is less so.

B. cereus can produce either a syndrome with a short incubation period—the *emetic* form, mediated by a staphylococcal type of enterotoxin—or one with a longer incubation period (8 to 16 h)—the *diarrheal* form, caused by an enterotoxin resembling *E. coli* LT, in which diarrhea and abdominal cramps are characteristic but vomiting is uncommon. The emetic form of *B. cereus* food poisoning is associated with contaminated fried rice; the organism is common in uncooked rice, and its heat-resistant spores survive boiling. If cooked rice is not refrigerated, the spores can germinate and produce toxin. Frying before serving may not destroy the preformed, heat-stable toxin.

Food poisoning due to *Clostridium perfringens* also has a slightly longer incubation period (8 to 14 h) and results from the survival of heat-resistant spores in inadequately cooked meat, poultry, or legumes. After ingestion, toxin is produced in the intestinal tract, causing moderately severe abdominal cramps and diarrhea; vomiting is rare, as is fever. The illness is self-limited, rarely lasting for more than 24 h.

Not all food poisoning has a bacterial cause. Diagnostic confusion can result from diarrhea caused by nonbacterial agents of short-incubation food poisoning, including capsaicin, which is found in hot peppers, and a variety of toxins found in fish and shellfish (Chap. 378).

LABORATORY EVALUATION Many cases of noninflammatory diarrhea are self-limited or can be treated empirically, and in these instances the clinician may not need to determine a specific etiology. Potentially pathogenic *E. coli* cannot be distinguished from normal fecal flora by routine culture. Special tests to detect LT and ST are not available in most clinical laboratories. In situations in which cholera is a concern, stool should be cultured on thiosulfate–citrate–bile salts–sucrose (TCBS) agar. A latex agglutination test has made the rapid detection of rotavirus in stool practical for many laboratories, while reverse-transcriptase polymerase chain reaction and specific antigen enzyme immunoassays have been developed for the identification of Norwalk-like viruses. At least three stool specimens should be examined for *Giardia* cysts or stained for *Cryptosporidium* if the level of clinical suspicion regarding the involvement of these organisms is high.

All patients with fever and evidence of inflammatory disease acquired outside the hospital should have stool cultured for *Salmonella*, *Shigella*, and *Campylobacter*. *Salmonella* and *Shigella* can be selected on MacConkey's agar as non-lactose-fermenting (colorless) colonies or can be grown on *Salmonella-Shigella* agar or in selenite enrichment broth, both of which inhibit most organisms except these pathogens. Evaluation of nosocomial diarrhea should initially focus on *C. difficile*; stool culture for other pathogens in this setting has an extremely low yield and is not cost-effective. Pathogenic strains of *C. difficile* generally produce two toxins, A and B. Toxin B can be detected with a cytotoxin assay; if the toxin is present, a monolayer culture of fibroblasts will show cytopathic effects within 6 to 24 h. Rapid enzyme immunoassays and latex agglutination tests for both toxin A and toxin B have been developed (Chap. 114). Isolation of *C. jejuni* requires inoculation of fresh stool onto selective growth medium and incubation at 42°C in a microaerophilic atmosphere. In many laboratories in the United States, *E. coli* O157:H7 is among the most common pathogens isolated from visibly bloody stools. Strains of this enterohemorrhagic serotype can be identified in specialized laboratories by serotyping but also can be identified presumptively in hospital laboratories as lactose-fermenting, indole-positive colonies of sorbitol nonfermenters (white colonies) on sorbitol MacConkey plates. Fresh stools should be examined for amebic cysts and trophozoites.

R_x TREATMENT

In many cases, a specific diagnosis is not necessary or not available to guide treatment. The clinician can proceed with the information obtained from the history, stool examination, and evaluation of the severity of dehydration. Empirical regimens for the treatment of traveler's diarrhea are listed in Table 113-4.

The mainstay of treatment is adequate rehydration. The treatment of cholera and other dehydrating diarrheal diseases was revolutionized by the promotion of oral rehydration solutions, the efficacy of which depends on the fact that glucose-facilitated absorption of sodium and water in the small intestine remains intact in the presence of cholera toxin. The use of oral rehydration solutions has reduced mortality due to cholera from >50% (in untreated cases) to <1%. The World Health Organization recommends a solution containing 3.5 g sodium chloride, 2.5 g sodium bicarbonate, 1.5 g potassium chloride, and 20 g glucose (or 40 g sucrose) per liter of water. Oral rehydration solutions containing rice or cereal as the carbohydrate source may be even more effective than glucose-based solutions. Patients who are severely dehydrated or in whom vomiting precludes the use of oral therapy should receive intravenous solutions such as Ringer's lactate.

Although most secretory forms of traveler's diarrhea—usually due to enterotoxigenic *E. coli*—can be treated effectively with rehydration, bismuth subsalicylate, or antiperistaltic agents, antimicrobial agents can shorten the duration of illness from between 3 and 4 days to between 24 and 36 h.

The antibiotic treatment of children who present with bloody diarrhea raises special concerns. Laboratory studies of enterohemorrhagic *E. coli* strains have demonstrated that a number of antibiotics induce replication of Shiga toxin–producing lambdoid bacteriophages, significantly increasing toxin production by these strains. Clinical studies have supported these laboratory results, and antibiotics are not recommended for the treatment of enterohemorrhagic *E. coli* infections in children.

PROPHYLAXIS Improvements in hygiene to limit fecal-oral spread of enteric pathogens will be necessary if the prevalence of diarrheal diseases is to be significantly reduced in developing countries. Travelers

TABLE 113-4 *Treatment of Traveler's Diarrhea on the Basis of Clinical Features*

Clinical Syndrome	Suggested Therapy
Watery diarrhea (no blood in stool, no fever), 1 or 2 unformed stools per day without distressing enteric symptoms	Oral fluids (Pedialyte, Lytren, or flavored mineral water) and saltine crackers
Watery diarrhea (no blood in stool, no fever), 1 or 2 unformed stools per day with distressing enteric symptoms	Bismuth subsalicylate (for adults): 30 mL or 2 tablets (262 mg/tablet) every 30 min for 8 doses; or loperamide[a]: 4 mg initially followed by 2 mg after passage of each unformed stool, not to exceed 8 tablets (16 mg) per day (prescription dose) or 4 caplets (8 mg) per day (over-the-counter dose); drugs can be taken for 2 days
Watery diarrhea (no blood in stool, no distressing abdominal pain, no fever), >2 unformed stools per day	Antibacterial drug[b] plus (for adults) loperamide[a] (see dose above)
Dysentery (passage of bloody stools) or fever (>37.8°C)	Antibacterial drug[b]
Vomiting, minimal diarrhea	Bismuth subsalicylate (for adults; see dose above)
Diarrhea in infants (<2 y old)	Fluids and electrolytes (Pedialyte, Lytren); continue feeding, especially with breast milk; seek medical attention for moderate dehydration, fever lasting >24 h, bloody stools, or diarrhea lasting more than several days
Diarrhea in pregnant women	Fluids and electrolytes; can consider attapulgite, 3 g initially, with dose repeated after passage of each unformed stool or every 2 h (whichever is earlier), for a total dosage of 9 g/d; seek medical attention for persistent or severe symptoms
Diarrhea despite trimethoprim-sulfamethoxazole prophylaxis	Fluoroquinolone—with loperamide[a] (see dose above) if no fever and no blood in stool, alone in cases of fever/dysentery
Diarrhea despite fluoroquinolone prophylaxis	Bismuth subsalicylate (see dose above) for mild to moderate disease; consult physician for moderate to severe disease or if disease persists

[a] Loperamide should not be used by patients with fever or dysentery; its use may prolong diarrhea in patients with infection due to *Shigella* or other invasive organisms.

[b] The recommended antibacterial drugs are as follows:

Travel to high-risk country other than Thailand:

Adults: A fluoroquinolone, such as ciprofloxacin, 500 mg bid; levofloxacin, 500 mg/d; norfloxacin, 400 mg bid; or ofloxacin, 400 mg bid on day 1; repeat on days 2 and 3 if diarrhea persists. Alternative agent: azithromycin, 500 mg on day 1, 250 mg on days 2 and 3 if diarrhea persists.

Children: Azithromycin, 10 mg/kg on day 1, 5 mg/kg on days 2 and 3 if diarrhea persists. Alternative agent: furazolidone, 7.5 mg/kg per day in four divided doses for 5 days.

Travel to Thailand (with risk of fluoroquinolone-resistant *Campylobacter*):

Adults: Azithromycin (at above dose for adults). Alternative agent: a fluoroquinolone (at above doses for adults).

Children: Same as for children traveling to other areas (see above).

All patients should take oral fluids (Pedialyte, Lytren, or flavored mineral water) plus saltine crackers. If diarrhea becomes moderate or severe, if fever persists, or if bloody stools or dehydration develops, the patient should seek medical attention.

Source: After Dupont.

can reduce their risk of diarrhea by eating only hot, freshly cooked food; by avoiding raw vegetables, salads, and unpeeled fruit; and by drinking only boiled or treated water and avoiding ice. In one cross-sectional epidemiologic survey, fewer than 3% of all European and North American travelers to Jamaica adhered to prescribed dietary restrictions, and travel health advice had no impact on the incidence of traveler's diarrhea; overall, the diarrhea attack rate among these travelers was 23.6%, with classic traveler's diarrhea in 11.7%.

Bismuth subsalicylate is an inexpensive agent for the prophylaxis of traveler's diarrhea; it is taken at a dosage of 2 tablets (525 mg) four times a day. Treatment appears to be effective and safe for up to 3 weeks. Prophylactic antimicrobial agents, although effective, are not generally recommended for the prevention of traveler's diarrhea, except when travelers are immunosuppressed or have other underlying illnesses that place them at high risk for morbidity from gastrointestinal infection. The risk of side effects and the possibility of developing an infection with a drug-resistant organism or with more harmful, invasive bacteria make it more reasonable to institute an empirical short course of treatment if symptoms develop.

The possibility of exerting a major impact on the worldwide morbidity and mortality associated with diarrheal diseases has led to intense efforts to develop effective vaccines against the common bacterial and viral enteric pathogens. Recent research has shown promising advances in the development of vaccines against rotavirus, *Shigella*, *V. cholerae*, *S. typhi*, and enterotoxigenic *E. coli*.

FURTHER READING

ANSDELL VE, ERICSSON CD: Prevention and empiric treatment of traveler's diarrhea. Med Clin North Am 83:945, 1999

BARTLETT JG: Clinical practice. Antibiotic-associated diarrhea. N Engl J Med 346:334, 2002

DUPONT HL: Travelers' diarrhea, in *Infections of the Gastrointestinal Tract*, 2d ed, MJ Blaser et al (eds). Philadelphia, Lippincott Williams & Wilkins, 2002, Chap 19

GUERRANT RL, STEINER TS: Principles and syndromes of enteric infection, in *Mandell, Douglas and Bennett's Principles and Practice of Infectious Diseases*, 5th ed, GL Mandell et al (eds). Philadelphia, Churchill Livingstone, 2000, Chap 81

RYAN ET et al: Illness after international travel. N Engl J Med 347:505, 2002

TALAN D et al: Etiology of bloody diarrhea among patients presenting to United States emergency departments: Prevalence of *Escherichia coli* O157:H7 and other enteropathogens. Clin Infect Dis 32:573, 2001

TAUXE RV et al: Foodborne disease, in *Mandell, Douglas and Bennett's Principles and Practice of Infectious Diseases*, 5th ed, GL Mandell et al (eds). Philadelphia, Churchill Livingstone, 2000, Chap 87

WONG CS et al: The risk of the hemolytic-uremic syndrome after antibiotic treatment of *Escherichia coli* O157:H7 infections. N Engl J Med 342:1930, 2000

DEFINITION *Clostridium difficile*–associated disease (CDAD) is a unique colon infection that is acquired almost exclusively in association with antimicrobial use and the consequent disruption of the normal colonic flora. The most commonly diagnosed diarrheal illness acquired in the hospital, CDAD results from the ingestion of spores of *C. difficile* that vegetate, multiply, and secrete toxins, causing diarrhea and pseudomembranous colitis (PMC).

ETIOLOGY AND EPIDEMIOLOGY *C. difficile* is an obligately anaerobic, gram-positive, spore-forming bacillus whose spores are found widely in nature, particularly in the environment of hospitals and chronic care facilities. CDAD occurs most frequently in hospitals and nursing homes where the level of antimicrobial use is high and the environment is contaminated by *C. difficile* spores.

Clindamycin, ampicillin, and cephalosporins were the first antibiotics associated with CDAD; the second- and third-generation cephalosporins, particularly cefotaxime, ceftriaxone, cefuroxime, and ceftazidime, are now the agents most frequently responsible for this condition. Penicillin/β-lactamase-inhibitor combinations such as ticarcillin/clavulanate and piperacillin/tazobactam pose significantly less risk. However, all antibiotics, including vancomycin and metronidazole (the agents most commonly used to treat CDAD), have been found to carry a risk of subsequent CDAD.

C. difficile is acquired exogenously, most frequently in the hospital, and is carried in the stool of symptomatic and asymptomatic patients. The rate of fecal colonization is often ≥20% among adult patients hospitalized for >1 week; in contrast, the rate is 1 to 3% among community residents. The risk of *C. difficile* acquisition increases in proportion to length of hospital stay. Asymptomatic fecal carriage of *C. difficile* in healthy neonates is very common, often exceeding 50% during the first 6 months of life. Spores of *C. difficile* are found on environmental surfaces (where the organism can persist for months) and on the hands of hospital personnel who fail to practice good hand hygiene. Hospital epidemics of CDAD have been attributed to a single *C. difficile* strain and to multiple strains present simultaneously. Other identified risk factors for CDAD include older age, greater severity of illness, use of electronic rectal thermometers, enteral tube feeding, antacid treatment, and gastrointestinal surgery.

PATHOLOGY AND PATHOGENESIS Spores of toxigenic *C. difficile* are ingested, survive gastric acidity, germinate in the small bowel, and colonize the lower intestinal tract, where they elaborate two large toxins: toxin A, an enterotoxin, and toxin B, a cytotoxin. These toxins initiate processes resulting in the disruption of epithelial-cell barrier function, diarrhea, and pseudomembrane formation. Toxin A is a potent neutrophil chemoattractant, and both toxins glucosylate the GTP-binding proteins of the Rho subfamily that regulate the actin cell cytoskeleton. Disruption of the cell cytoskeleton results in loss of cell shape, adherence, and tight junctions, with resultant fluid leakage. The pseudomembranes of PMC are confined to the colonic mucosa and initially appear as 1- to 2-mm whitish-yellow plaques. The intervening mucosa appears unremarkable, but, as the disease progresses, the pseudomembranes coalesce to form larger plaques and become confluent over the entire colon wall (Fig. 114-1). The whole colon is usually involved, but 10% of patients have rectal sparing. Viewed microscopically, the pseudomembranes have a mucosal attachment point and contain necrotic leukocytes, fibrin, mucus, and cellular debris. The epithelium is eroded and necrotic in focal areas, with neutrophil infiltration of the mucosa.

Patients colonized with *C. difficile* were initially thought to be at high risk for CDAD. However, four prospective studies have shown that colonized patients actually have a decreased risk of subsequent CDAD. At least three events are proposed as essential for the devel-

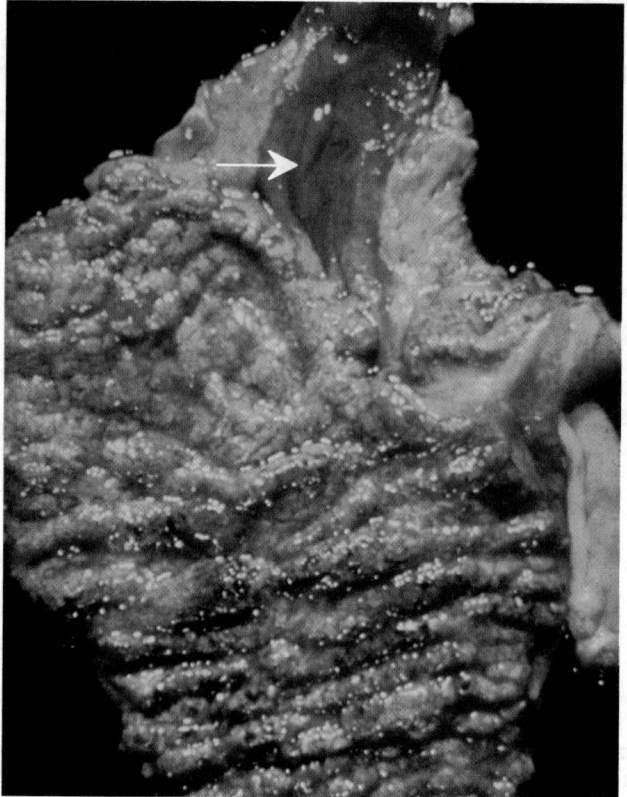

FIGURE 114-1 Autopsy specimen showing confluent pseudomembranes covering the cecum of a patient with pseudomembranous colitis. Note the sparing of the terminal ileum (*arrow*).

opment of CDAD (Fig. 114-2). Exposure to antimicrobial agents is the first event and establishes susceptibility to *C. difficile* infection. The second event is exposure to toxigenic *C. difficile*. Given that the majority of patients do not develop CDAD after the first two events, a third event is clearly essential for its occurrence. Candidate third

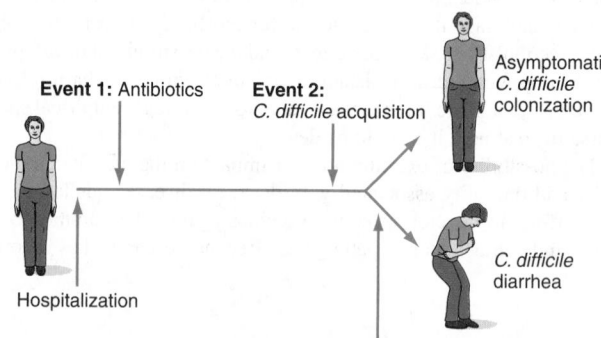

Event 1: Antibiotics

Event 2: *C. difficile* acquisition

Asymptomatic *C. difficile* colonization

C. difficile diarrhea

Hospitalization

Event 3: Inadequate anamnestic IgG host response to toxin A of toxigenic *C. difficile*

FIGURE 114-2 Pathogenesis model for hospital-acquired *Clostridium difficile*–associated diarrhea (CDAD). At least three events are integral to *C. difficile* pathogenesis. Exposure to antibiotics establishes susceptibility to infection. Once susceptible, the patient may acquire nontoxigenic (nonpathogenic) or toxigenic strains of *C. difficile* as a second event. Acquisition of toxigenic *C. difficile* may be followed by asymptomatic colonization or CDAD, depending on one or more additional events, including an inadequate host anamnestic IgG response to *C. difficile* toxin A.

events include exposure to a *C. difficile* strain of particular virulence, exposure to antimicrobial agents especially likely to cause CDAD, and an inadequate host immune response. The host anamnestic serum IgG antibody response to toxin A of *C. difficile* is the most likely third event that determines which patients will develop diarrhea and which patients will remain asymptomatic. The majority of humans first develop antibody to *C. difficile* toxins when colonized asymptomatically during the first year of life. Infants are thought not to develop symptomatic CDAD because they lack suitable mucosal toxin receptors that develop later in life. In adulthood, levels of antitoxin A IgG in serum increase more in response to infection in individuals who become asymptomatic carriers than in those who develop CDAD. For persons who develop CDAD, higher levels of antitoxin A correlate with a lower risk of recurrence of CDAD.

TABLE 114-1 *Relative Sensitivity and Specificity of Diagnostic Tests for Clostridium difficile–Associated Disease (CDAD)*

Type of Test	Relative Sensitivity[a]	Relative Specificity[a]	Comment
Stool culture for *C. difficile*	++++	+++	Most sensitive test; specificity is ++++ if the *C. difficile* isolate tests positive for toxin; with clinical data, is diagnostic of CDAD
Cell culture cytotoxin test on stool	+++	++++	With clinical data, is diagnostic of CDAD; highly specific but not as sensitive as stool culture
Enzyme immunoassay for toxin A or toxins A and B in stool	++ to +++	+++	With clinical data, is diagnostic of CDAD; rapid but not as sensitive as stool culture or cell culture cytotoxin test; rapid results
Latex test for *C. difficile* antigen in stool	++	+++	Detects glutamate dehydrogenase found in toxigenic and nontoxigenic strains of *C. difficile* and other stool organisms; less sensitive and specific than other tests; rapid results
Colonoscopy or sigmoidoscopy	+	++++	Highly specific if pseudomembranes are seen; insensitive compared with other tests

[a] According to both clinical and test-based criteria.
Note: ++++, >90%; +++, 71–90%; ++, 51–70%; +, ~50%.

CLINICAL MANIFESTATIONS Diarrhea is the most common symptom caused by *C. difficile*. Stools are almost never grossly bloody and range from soft and unformed to watery or mucoid in consistency, with a characteristic odor. Patients may have as many as 20 bowel movements per day. Clinical and laboratory findings include fever in 28% of cases, abdominal pain in 22%, and leukocytosis in 50%. When adynamic ileus (which is seen on x-ray in ~20% of cases) results in cessation of stool passage, the diagnosis of CDAD is frequently overlooked. A clue to the presence of unsuspected CDAD in these patients is unexplained leukocytosis with ≥15,000 cells/mm³. Such patients are at high risk for complications of *C. difficile* infection, particularly toxic megacolon and sepsis.

C. difficile diarrhea recurs after treatment in ~20% of cases. Recurrences may represent either relapses due to the same strain or reinfections with a new strain. Recurrence of clinical CDAD is likely to be a result of continued disruption of the normal fecal flora by the antibiotic used to treat CDAD.

DIAGNOSIS The diagnosis of CDAD is based on a combination of clinical criteria: (1) diarrhea (≥3 unformed stools per 24 h for ≥2 days), with no other recognized cause; plus (2) toxin A or B detected in the stool, toxin-producing *C. difficile* detected by stool culture, or pseudomembranes seen in the colon. PMC is a more advanced form of CDAD and is visualized at endoscopy in only ~50% of patients with diarrhea who have a positive stool culture and toxin assay for *C. difficile* (Table 114-1). Endoscopy is a rapid diagnostic tool in seriously ill patients with suspected PMC and an acute abdomen, but a negative result in this examination does not rule out CDAD.

Despite the array of tests available for *C. difficile* and its toxins (Table 114-1), no single test has high sensitivity, high specificity, and rapid turnaround. The turnaround time for reporting of a positive result in the cell cytotoxicity test can be shortened to <24 h if cell cultures are examined at intervals as short as 4 h. However, this approach is labor intensive, and observation for 48 h is required for a conclusive test result. Most laboratory tests for toxins lack sensitivity; thus, if the first specimen is negative and diarrhea persists, testing of additional stool specimens increases the likelihood of diagnosis. Empirical treatment is appropriate if CDAD is strongly suspected on clinical grounds. Testing of asymptomatic patients is not recommended except for epidemiologic study purposes. In particular, so-called "tests of cure" of asymptomatic treated patients are not recommended because many patients continue to harbor the organism and toxin after diarrhea has ceased and test results do not correlate with recurrence of CDAD. These test results should not be used to restrict placement of patients in long-term-care or nursing home facilities.

℞ **TREATMENT**

PRIMARY CDAD CDAD resolves in 15 to 23% of patients within 2 to 3 days after administration of the precipitating antimicrobial agent is discontinued, but most patients require specific treatment. General treatment guidelines include hydration and the avoidance of antiperistaltic agents and opiates, which may mask symptoms and possibly worsen disease. However, antiperistaltic agents have been used safely with vancomycin or metronidazole for mild to moderate CDAD. As mentioned above, test-of-cure cultures or toxin assays after treatment are not recommended; their results are not predictive of recurrence, and treatment of asymptomatic patients does not eradicate *C. difficile* from the stool.

Prospective randomized clinical trials show no statistical differences among the major therapeutic agents for the primary outcome end point of CDAD treatment: cessation of diarrhea (Table 114-2). The clinical response rate for bacitracin is 10 to 20% lower than that for vancomycin; therefore, bacitracin use for first-line therapy is discouraged. All drugs, particularly vancomycin, should be given orally if possible. When metronidazole is given intravenously, fecal bactericidal drug concentrations are achieved during acute diarrhea, and CDAD treatment has been successful; however, in the presence of adynamic ileus, intravenous metronidazole treatment of PMC has

TABLE 114-2 *Expected Treatment Outcomes Based on Randomized Comparative Trials of Oral Therapy for Initial Episodes of Clostridium difficile–Associated Diarrhea (CDAD)*

Treatment or Medication	Dose and Duration	Expected Resolution of Diarrhea, %	Expected Recurrence, %
Placebo or discontinuation of offending antibiotics	None	21	Unknown
Metronidazole	250 mg qid × 10 d	95	5
	500 mg tid × 10 d	94	17
Vancomycin[a]	500 mg tid × 10 d	94	17
	500 mg qid × 10 d	100	15
	125 mg qid × 7 d	86	33
	125 mg qid × 5 d	75	Unknown
Teicoplanin	400 mg bid × 10 d	96	7
	100 mg bid × 10 d	96	8
Fusidic acid	500 mg tid × 10 d	93	28
Bacitracin	25,000 U qid × 10 d	80	42

[a] Vancomycin treatment for first episodes of CDAD is discouraged because of possible development of vancomycin resistance in other nosocomial bacteria, such as enterococci.

failed. Diarrhea response rates to oral therapy with vancomycin or metronidazole are ≥94%. The mean interval to resolution of diarrhea is 2 to 4 days. Treatment should not be deemed a failure until a drug has been given for at least 6 days. On the basis of data for shorter courses of vancomycin (Table 114-2), it is recommended that treatment be given for 10 days, although no controlled comparisons are available. Metronidazole, although not approved by the U.S. Food and Drug Administration (FDA) for the treatment of CDAD, is the drug of first choice and the least expensive agent. Metronidazole-resistant isolates have been reported rarely, but treatment failure has not been attributed to resistance. Vancomycin as first-line treatment is discouraged because it may increase the incidence of vancomycin-resistant enterococci in hospitals.

Recurrent CDAD   In all, 15 to 25% of patients experience recurrences of CDAD, either as relapses caused by the original organism or as reinfections following treatment (Table 114-2). Re-treatment with metronidazole is recommended for first recurrences of CDAD. There is no standard treatment for multiple recurrences. Approaches include the administration of vancomycin, metronidazole, or bacitracin followed by the yeast *Saccharomyces boulardii* or *Lactobacillus* GG; the administration of vancomycin followed by synthetic fecal bacterial enema; and the intentional colonization of the patient with a nontoxigenic strain of *C. difficile*. None of these biotherapeutic agents is available in the United States as an FDA-approved pharmaceutical for treating CDAD. Other approaches include the use of vancomycin in tapering doses over 21 days, with subsequent pulse-dosing every several days for 21 days; the administration of vancomycin followed by that of the anion-exchange binding resin cholestyramine; and combined treatment with vancomycin and rifampin—the approach the authors favor (vancomycin, 125 mg four times daily, and rifampin, 300 mg twice daily, for 10 days). In antibody-deficient children, intravenous immunoglobulin has been used successfully to treat CDAD.

Fulminant CDAD   Fulminant CDAD is the most difficult treatment challenge in the rare patients who present with or develop toxic megacolon or ileus. These patients often do not have diarrhea, and their illness mimics an acute surgical abdomen. Sepsis (hypotension, fever, tachycardia, leukocytosis) may result from severe CDAD. An acute abdomen (with or without toxic megacolon) may include signs of obstruction, ileus, bowel-wall thickening, and ascites on abdominal computed tomography (CT), often with peripheral-blood leukocytosis (≥25,000 cells/mm³). Whether or not the patient has diarrhea, the differential diagnosis of an acute abdomen, sepsis, or toxic megacolon should include CDAD if the patient has received antibiotics in the past

2 months. Cautious sigmoidoscopy or colonoscopy to visualize PMC and an abdominal CT examination are the best diagnostic tests in patients without diarrhea.

Medical management of fulminant CDAD is suboptimal because of the difficulty of delivering metronidazole or vancomycin to the colon by the oral route in the presence of ileus. Six patients with severe ileus have been successfully treated by the authors with vancomycin—given via nasogastric tube and by retention enema—plus intravenous metronidazole. Surgical intervention is indicated for patients with suspected perforation of the colon or fulminant CDAD that does not respond to medical management. The incidence of fulminant CDAD requiring colectomy may be increasing, and surgical mortality may be >50% in this setting.

PROGNOSIS   The mortality rate attributed to CDAD is 0.6 to 3.5%, with the highest figures among the elderly. Most patients recover, but some have recurrences over months or years.

PREVENTION AND CONTROL   Strategies for the prevention of CDAD are of two types: those aimed at preventing transmission of the organism to the patient and those aimed at reducing the risk of CDAD if the organism is transmitted. Transmission of *C. difficile* in clinical practice has been prevented by gloving of personnel and elimination of the use of contaminated electronic thermometers. CDAD outbreaks have been most successfully controlled by restricting use of specific antibiotics, such as clindamycin and second- and third-generation cephalosporins. Outbreaks of CDAD due to clindamycin-resistant strains have resolved promptly when clindamycin use was restricted.

FURTHER READING

BIGNARDI GE: Risk factors for *Clostridium difficile* infection. J Hosp Infect 40:1, 1998

DALLAL RM et al: Fulminant *Clostridium difficile*: An underappreciated and increasing cause of death and complications. Ann Surg 235:363, 2002

FEKETY R: Guidelines for the diagnosis and management of *Clostridium difficile*–associated diarrhea and colitis. Am J Gastroenterol 92:739, 1997

GERDING DN et al: Society for Healthcare Epidemiology of America position paper on *Clostridium difficile*–associated diarrhea and colitis. Infect Control Hosp Epidemiol 16:459, 1995

JOHNSON S, GERDING DN: *Clostridium difficile* infection. Clin Infect Dis 26:1027, 1998

KYNE L et al: Association between antibody response to toxin A and protection against recurrent *Clostridium difficile* diarrhea. Lancet 357:189, 2001

WANAHITA A et al: Conditions associated with leukocytosis in a tertiary care hospital, with particular attention to the role of infection caused by *Clostridium difficile*. Clin Infect Dis 34:1585, 2002

WENISCH C et al: Comparison of vancomycin, teicoplanin, metronidazole, and fusidic acid for the treatment of *Clostridium difficile*–associated diarrhea. Clin Infect Dis 22:813, 1996

115   SEXUALLY TRANSMITTED DISEASES: OVERVIEW AND CLINICAL APPROACH
King K. Holmes

CLASSIFICATION AND EPIDEMIOLOGY

Certain sexually transmitted diseases (STDs), such as syphilis, gonorrhea, HIV infection, hepatitis B, and chancroid, are most concentrated within "core populations" having high rates of partner change, concurrent partners, or "dense" sexual networks—for example, prostitutes and their clients, some homosexual men, and persons involved in the use of illicit drugs, particularly crack cocaine and methamphetamine. Other STDs are distributed more evenly throughout society. For example, chlamydial infections, genital infections with human papillomavirus (HPV), and genital herpes can spread efficiently in relatively low-risk populations.

In general, the product of three factors determines the initial rate of spread of any sexually transmitted infection (STI) within a population: rate of exposure of susceptible to infectious people, efficiency of transmission per exposure, and duration of infectivity of those in-

fected. Efforts to prevent and control STIs attempt to decrease the duration of infectivity (through early diagnosis and curative or suppressive treatment), to decrease the efficiency of transmission (e.g., through promotion of condom use and safer sexual practices), and to decrease the rate of exposure of susceptibles to infected persons (e.g., through individual counseling and efforts to change the norms of sexual behavior).

In all societies, STDs rank among the most common of all infectious diseases, with >30 infections now classified as predominantly sexually transmitted or as frequently sexually transmissible (Table 115-1). In developing countries, with three-quarters of the world's population and 90% of the world's STDs, such factors as population growth (especially in adolescent and young-adult age groups), rural-to-urban migration, wars, and poverty create exceptional vulnerability to disease resulting from risky sexual behaviors. During the 1990s, in

China, Russia, the other states of the former Soviet Union, and South Africa, internal social structures changed rapidly as borders opened to the West, unleashing enormous new epidemics of HIV infection and other STDs. HIV has become the leading cause of death in some developing countries, and HPV and hepatitis B virus (HBV) remain important causes of cervical and hepatocellular carcinoma, respectively—two of the most common malignancies in the developing world. Sexually transmitted herpes simplex virus (HSV) infections now cause most genital ulcer disease throughout the world and an increasing proportion of cases of genital herpes in developing countries with generalized HIV epidemics, where the positive feedback loop between HSV and HIV transmission is a growing, intractable problem. Globally, five curable STDs—gonorrhea, chlamydial infections, syphilis, chancroid, and trichomoniasis—caused ~350 million new infections annually in the mid-1990s. Up to 50% of women of reproductive age in developing countries have bacterial vaginosis (arguably acquired sexually). All six of these curable infections have been associated with increased risk of HIV transmission or acquisition.

In the industrialized countries, fear of HIV infection since the mid-1980s, coupled with widespread behavioral interventions and better-organized systems of care for the curable STDs, have helped curb the transmission of the latter diseases. Nonetheless, foci of hyperendemic transmission persist in the southeastern United States and in most large U.S. cities. Rates of gonorrhea and syphilis remain higher in the United States than in any other Western industrialized country. The remarkable resurgence of gonorrhea and syphilis among homosexual and bisexual men in many parts of the United States and Europe since the 1990s reflects increased risk-taking since the advent of potent antiretroviral therapy and has been accompanied by increasing HIV transmission in this group. The prevalence of antibody to HSV-2 has begun to fall only recently (since the mid-1990s), and genital HPV remains the most common sexually transmitted pathogen, infecting one-third of a cohort of U.S. college women within 2 years in a study conducted during the 1990s.

MANAGEMENT OF COMMON STD SYNDROMES

Although other chapters discuss management of specific STIs, delineating treatment based on diagnosis of a specific infection, most patients are actually managed (at least initially) on the basis of presenting symptoms and signs and associated risk factors, even in industrialized countries. Table 115-2 lists some of the most common clinical STD syndromes and their microbial etiologies. Strategies for their management are outlined below. →*Chapters 172 and 173 address the management of infections with human retroviruses.*

STD care and management begin with risk assessment and proceed to clinical assessment, diagnostic testing or screening, treatment, and prevention. Indeed, the routine care of any patient begins with risk assessment (e.g., for risk of heart disease, cancer). STD/HIV risk assessment is important in primary care, urgent care, and emergency care settings as well as in specialty clinics providing adolescent, prenatal, and family planning services. STD/HIV risk assessment guides interpretation of symptoms that could reflect an STD; decisions on screening or prophylactic/preventive treatment; risk reduction counseling and intervention (e.g., hepatitis B vaccination); and notification of partners of patients with known infections. Consideration of routine demographic data (e.g., gender, age, marital status, area of residence) is a simple first step in STD/HIV risk assessment. For example, national guidelines now recommend routine screening of sexually active fe-

males ≤25 years of age for *Chlamydia trachomatis* infection. Table 115-3 provides a set of 10 STD/HIV risk-assessment questions that clinicians can pose verbally or that health care systems can adapt (with yes/no responses) into a routine self-administered questionnaire for use in clinics. The initial framing statement gives permission to discuss taboo topics.

Risk assessment is followed by clinical assessment (elicitation of information on specific current symptoms and signs of STDs). Confirmatory diagnostic tests (for persons with symptoms or signs) or screening tests (for those without symptoms or signs) may involve microscopic examination, culture, antigen detection tests, genetic probe or amplification tests, or serology. Initial syndrome-based treatment should cover the most likely causes. For certain syndromes, results of rapid tests can narrow the spectrum of this initial therapy (e.g., wet mount of vaginal fluid for women with vaginal discharge, Gram's stain of urethral discharge for men with urethral discharge, rapid plasma reagin test for genital ulcer). After the institution of treatment, STD management proceeds to the "4 C's" of prevention and control: contact tracing (see "Prevention and Control of STDs," below), ensuring compliance with therapy, and counseling on risk reduction, including condom promotion and provision.

URETHRITIS IN MEN During the 1990s, the incidence of reported gonorrhea among men in the United States fell to 126 cases per 100,000 population; the incidence figures then leveled off through 2002. The incidence of reported *C. trachomatis* infections among men has been increasing steadily (with increased testing), reaching 130 cases per 100,000 in 2002. Until recently, *C. trachomatis* caused ~30 to 40% of cases of nongonococcal urethritis (NGU); however, the proportion of cases due to this organism may have declined in some populations served by effective chlamydial-control programs. HSV and *Trichomonas vaginalis* each cause a small proportion of NGU cases in the United States. Recently, multiple studies have consistently implicated *Mycoplasma genitalium* as a probable cause of many *Chlamydia*-negative cases, while fewer studies than in the past have implicated *Ureaplasma urealyticum*. Coliform bacteria can cause urethritis in men who practice insertive anal intercourse. The initial diagnosis of urethritis in men currently includes specific tests only for *Neisseria gonorrhoeae*

TABLE 115-1 *Sexually Transmitted and Sexually Transmissible Microorganisms*

Bacteria	Viruses	Other[a]
TRANSMITTED IN ADULTS PREDOMINANTLY BY SEXUAL INTERCOURSE		
Neisseria gonorrhoeae	HIV (types 1 and 2)	*Trichomonas vaginalis*
Chlamydia trachomatis	Human T-cell lymphotropic virus type I	*Phthirus pubis*
Treponema pallidum	Herpes simplex virus type 2	
Haemophilus ducreyi	Human papillomavirus (multiple genotypes)	
Calymmatobacterium granulomatis	Hepatitis B virus[b]	
Ureaplasma urealyticum	Molluscum contagiosum virus	
SEXUAL TRANSMISSION REPEATEDLY DESCRIBED BUT NOT WELL DEFINED OR NOT THE PREDOMINANT MODE		
Mycoplasma hominis	Cytomegalovirus	*Candida albicans*
Mycoplasma genitalium	Human T-cell lymphotropic virus type II	*Sarcoptes scabiei*
Gardnerella vaginalis and other vaginal bacteria	(?) Hepatitis C, D viruses	
Group B *Streptococcus*	Herpes simplex virus type 1	
Mobiluncus spp.	(?) Epstein-Barr virus	
Helicobacter cinaedi	Kaposi's sarcoma–associated herpesvirus[c]	
Sporothrix fennelliae	Transfusion-transmitted virus	
TRANSMITTED BY SEXUAL CONTACT INVOLVING ORAL-FECAL EXPOSURE; OF DECLINING IMPORTANCE IN HOMOSEXUAL MEN		
Shigella spp.	Hepatitis A virus	*Giardia lamblia*
Campylobacter spp.		*Entamoeba histolytica*

[a] Includes protozoa, ectoparasites, and fungi.
[b] Among U.S. patients for whom a risk factor can be ascertained, most hepatitis B virus infections are transmitted sexually or by injection drug use.
[c] Human herpesvirus type 8.

TABLE 115-2 *Major STD Syndromes and Sexually Transmitted Microbial Etiologies*

Syndrome	ST Microbial Etiologies
AIDS	HIV types 1 and 2
Urethritis: males	*Neisseria gonorrhoeae, Chlamydia trachomatis, Mycoplasma genitalium, Ureaplasma urealyticum, Trichomonas vaginalis,* HSV
Epididymitis	*C. trachomatis, N. gonorrhoeae*
Lower genital tract infections: females	
Cystitis/urethritis	*C. trachomatis, N. gonorrhoeae,* HSV
Mucopurulent cervicitis	*C. trachomatis, N. gonorrhoeae, M. genitalium*
Vulvitis	*Candida albicans,* HSV
Vulvovaginitis	*C. albicans, T. vaginalis*
Bacterial vaginosis (BV)	BV-associated bacteria (see text)
Acute pelvic inflammatory disease	*N. gonorrhoeae, C. trachomatis,* BV-associated bacteria, group B streptococci, *M. genitalium*
Infertility	*N. gonorrhoeae, C. trachomatis,* BV-associated bacteria
Ulcerative lesions of the genitalia	HSV-1, HSV-2, *Treponema pallidum, Haemophilus ducreyi, C. trachomatis* (LGV strains), *Calymmatobacterium granulomatis*
Complications of pregnancy/puerperium	Several agents implicated
Intestinal infections	
Proctitis	*C. trachomatis, N. gonorrhoeae,* HSV, *T. pallidum*
Proctocolitis or enterocolitis	*Campylobacter* spp., *Shigella* spp., *Entamoeba histolytica,* other enteric pathogens
Enteritis	*Giardia lamblia*
Acute arthritis with urogenital infection or viremia	*N. gonorrhoeae* (e.g., DGI), *C. trachomatis* (e.g., Reiter's syndrome), HBV
Genital and anal warts	HPV (30 genital types)
Mononucleosis syndrome	CMV, HIV, EBV
Hepatitis	Hepatitis viruses, *T. pallidum,* CMV, EBV
Neoplasias	
Squamous cell dysplasias and cancers of the cervix, anus, vulva, vagina, or penis	HPV (especially types 16, 18, 31, 45)
Kaposi's sarcoma, body-cavity lymphomas	HHV-8
T cell leukemia	HTLV-I
Hepatocellular carcinoma	HBV
Tropical spastic paraparesis	HTLV-I
Scabies	*Sarcoptes scabiei*
Pubic lice	*Phthirus pubis*

Note: HSV, herpes simplex virus; LGV, lymphogranuloma venereum; DGI, disseminated gonococcal infection; HPV, human papillomavirus; CMV, cytomegalovirus; EBV, Epstein-Barr virus; HBV, hepatitis B virus; HTLV, human T-cell lymphotropic virus; HHV-8, human herpesvirus type 8.

and *C. trachomatis.* The following summarizes the approach to the patient with suspected urethritis:

1. *Establish the presence of urethritis.* If proximal-to-distal "milking" of the urethra does not express a purulent or mucopurulent discharge, even after the patient has not voided for several hours or preferably overnight, a Gram's-stained smear of overt discharge or of an anterior urethral specimen obtained by passage of a small urethrogenital swab 2 to 3 cm into the urethra usually reveals ≥5 neutrophils per $1000\times$ field in areas containing cells; in gonococcal infection, such a smear usually reveals gram-negative intracellular diplococci as well. Alternatively, the centrifuged sediment

of the first 20 to 30 mL of voided urine can be examined for inflammatory cells, either by microscopy showing ≥10 leukocytes per high-power field or by the leukocyte esterase test. Patients with symptoms who lack objective evidence of urethritis may have functional rather than organic problems and generally do not benefit from repeated courses of antibiotics.

2. *Evaluate for complications or alternative diagnoses.* A brief history and examination will exclude epididymitis and systemic complications, such as disseminated gonococcal infection (DGI) and Reiter's syndrome. Although digital examination of the prostate gland seldom contributes to the evaluation of sexually active young men with urethritis, men with dysuria who lack evidence of urethritis as well as sexually inactive men with urethritis should undergo prostate palpation, urinalysis, and urine culture to exclude bacterial prostatitis and cystitis.

3. *Evaluate for gonococcal and chlamydial infection.* An absence of typical gram-negative diplococci on Gram's-stained smear of urethral exudate containing inflammatory cells warrants a preliminary diagnosis of NGU and should lead to testing of the urethral specimen for *C. trachomatis.* Culture or DNA detection tests for *N. gonorrhoeae* may be positive when Gram's staining is negative; certain strains of *N. gonorrhoeae* can result in negative urethral Gram's stains in up to 30% of cases of urethritis. Results of tests for gonococcal and chlamydial infection predict the patient's prognosis (with greater risk for recurrent NGU if neither chlamydiae nor gonococci are found than if either is detected) and can

TABLE 115-3 *Ten-Question STD/HIV Risk Assessment*

Framing Statement:
In order to provide the best care for you today and to understand your risk for certain infections, it is necessary for us to talk about your sexual behavior.
Screening Questions:
(1) Do you have any reason to think you might have a sexually transmitted disease? If so, what reason?
(2) For all adolescents <18 years old: Have you begun having any kind of sex yet?
STD History:
(3) Have you ever had any sexually transmitted diseases or any genital infections? If so, which ones?
Sexual Preference:
(4) Have you had sex with men, women, or both?
Injection Drug Use:
(5) Have you ever injected yourself ("shot up") with drugs? (If yes, have you ever shared needles or injection equipment?)
(6) Have you ever had sex with a gay or bisexual man or with anyone who had ever injected drugs?
Characteristics of Partner(s):
(7) Has your sex partner(s) had any sexually transmitted infections? If so, which ones?
STD Symptoms Checklist:
(8) Have you recently developed any of these symptoms?

For Men	**For Women**
(a) Discharge of pus (drip) from the penis	(a) Abnormal vaginal discharge (increased amount, abnormal odor, abnormal yellow color)
(b) Genital sores (ulcers) or rash	(b) Genital sores (ulcers), rash, or itching

Sexual Practices, Past 2 Months (for patients answering yes to any of the above questions, to guide examination and testing):
(9) Now I'd like to ask what parts of your body may have been sexually exposed to an STD (e.g., your penis, mouth, vagina, anus)?
Query about Interest in STD Screening Tests (for patients answering no to all of the above questions):
(10) Would you like to be tested for HIV or any other STDs today? (If yes, clinician can explore which STD and why.)

Source: Adapted from JR Curtis, KK Holmes, in KK Holmes et al (eds): *Sexually Transmitted Diseases*, 3d ed. New York, McGraw-Hill, 1999.

TABLE 115-4 *Management of Urethral Discharge in Men*

Usual causes	Usual initial evaluation
Chlamydia trachomatis	Demonstration of urethral discharge or
Neisseria gonorrhoeae	pyuria
Ureaplasma urealyticum	Exclusion of local or systemic
Trichomonas vaginalis	complications
Herpes simplex virus	Urethral Gram's stain to confirm
Mycoplasma genitalium	urethritis, detect gram-negative
	diplococci
	Test for *N. gonorrhoeae, C. trachomatis*

INITIAL TREATMENT FOR PATIENT AND PARTNERS

Treat gonorrhea (unless excluded):	plus	Treat chlamydial infection:
Cefpodoxime, 400 mg PO; *or*		Azithromycin, 1 g PO;
Ceftriaxone, 125 mg IM; *or*		*or*
Fluoroquinolone (e.g., cipro-floxacin, 500 mg PO)		Doxycycline, 100 mg bid for 7 days

MANAGEMENT OF RECURRENCE

Confirm objective evidence of urethritis. If patient was reexposed to untreated or new partner, repeat treatment of patient and partner.
If patient was not reexposed, consider infection with *T. vaginalis*[a] or doxycycline-resistant *Ureaplasma*, and consider treatment with metronidazole or azithromycin.

[a] In men, the diagnosis of *T. vaginalis* infection requires culture (or nucleic acid amplification test, where available) of early-morning first-voided urine sediment or of a urethral swab specimen obtained before voiding.

guide both the counseling given to the patient and the management of the patient's sexual partner(s).

4. *Treat urethritis.*

Table 115-4 summarizes the steps in management of sexually active men with symptoms of urethral discharge and/or dysuria.

℞ TREATMENT

In practice, if Gram's stain does not reveal gonococci, urethritis is treated with a regimen effective for NGU, such as azithromycin (1.0 g orally in a single dose) or doxycycline (100 mg orally bid for 7 days). If gonococci are demonstrated by Gram's stain or if no diagnostic tests are performed to definitively exclude gonorrhea, treatment should include a single-dose regimen for gonorrhea (Chap. 128) plus azithromycin or doxycycline treatment for *C. trachomatis.* Sexual partners should be tested for gonorrhea and chlamydial infection and should receive the same regimen given to the male index case. Patients with confirmed persistence or recurrence of urethritis after treatment should be re-treated with the initial regimen if they did not comply with the original treatment or were reexposed to an untreated partner. Otherwise, an intraurethral swab specimen and a first-voided urine sample should be cultured for *T. vaginalis.* If compliance with initial treatment is confirmed and reexposure excluded, treatment with metronidazole (2 g orally in a single dose) plus erythromycin base (500 mg orally qid for 7 days) is recommended.

EPIDIDYMITIS Acute epididymitis, almost always unilateral, must be differentiated from testicular torsion, tumor, and trauma. Torsion, a surgical emergency, usually occurs in the second or third decade of life and produces a sudden onset of pain, elevation of the testicle within the scrotal sac, rotation of the epididymis from a posterior to an anterior position, and absence of blood flow on Doppler examination or ^{99m}Tc scan. Persistence of symptoms after a course of therapy for epididymitis suggests the possibility of testicular tumor. In sexually active men under age 35, acute epididymitis is caused most frequently by *C. trachomatis* and less commonly by *N. gonorrhoeae* and is usually associated with overt or subclinical urethritis. Acute epididymitis occurring in older men or following urinary tract instrumentation is usually caused by urinary pathogens. Similarly, epididymitis in men who have practiced insertive rectal intercourse is often caused by Enterobacteriaceae. These men usually have no urethritis but do have bacteriuria.

℞ TREATMENT

Ceftriaxone (250 mg as a single dose IM) followed by doxycycline (100 mg orally bid for 10 days) is effective for epididymitis caused by *N. gonorrhoeae* or *C. trachomatis.* Alternatively, ofloxacin (300 mg orally bid for 10 days) or levofloxacin (500 mg orally once daily for 10 days) is also effective for syndrome-based treatment of epididymitis because of effectiveness against Enterobacteriaceae as well as *N. gonorrhoeae* and *C. trachomatis;* however, emerging gonococcal resistance to fluoroquinolones now limits the use of these drugs in some areas.

URETHRITIS AND THE URETHRAL SYNDROME IN WOMEN *C. trachomatis, N. gonorrhoeae,* and occasionally HSV cause symptomatic urethritis—known as the urethral syndrome in women—characterized by "internal" dysuria (usually without urinary urgency or frequency) and pyuria, with *Escherichia coli* or other uropathogens not present in urine at counts of $\geq 10^2$/mL. In contrast, the dysuria associated with vulvar herpes or vulvovaginal candidiasis (and perhaps with trichomoniasis) is often described as "external," being caused by painful contact of urine with the inflamed or ulcerated labia or introitus. Acute onset, association with urinary urgency or frequency, hematuria, or suprapubic bladder tenderness suggests bacterial cystitis. Among women with symptoms of acute bacterial cystitis, costovertebral pain and tenderness or fever suggests acute pyelonephritis. →*The management of bacterial urinary tract infection (UTI) is discussed in Chap. 269.*

Signs of vulvovaginitis, coupled with symptoms of external dysuria, suggest vulvar infection (e.g., with HSV or *Candida albicans*). Among dysuric women without signs of vulvovaginitis, bacterial UTI must be differentiated from the urethral syndrome by assessment of risk, evaluation of the pattern of symptoms and signs, and specific microbiologic testing. An STD etiology of the urethral syndrome is suggested by young age, more than one current sexual partner, a new partner within the past month, a partner with urethritis, or coexisting mucopurulent cervicitis (see below). The finding of a single urinary pathogen, such as *E. coli* or *Staphylococcus saprophyticus,* at a concentration of $\geq 10^2$/mL in a properly collected specimen of midstream urine from a dysuric woman with pyuria indicates probable bacterial UTI, whereas pyuria with $<10^2$ conventional uropathogens per milliliter of urine ("sterile" pyuria) suggests acute urethral syndrome due to *C. trachomatis* or *N. gonorrhoeae.* Gonorrhea and chlamydial infection should be sought by specific tests (e.g., nucleic acid amplification tests on the first 10 mL of voided urine). Among dysuric women with sterile pyuria caused by infection with *N. gonorrhoeae* or *C. trachomatis,* appropriate treatment alleviates dysuria.

VULVOVAGINAL INFECTIONS ■ **Abnormal Vaginal Discharge** If directly questioned about vaginal discharge during routine health checkups, many women acknowledge having nonspecific symptoms of vaginal discharge that do not correlate with objective signs of inflammation or with actual infection. However, unsolicited reporting of abnormal vaginal discharge does suggest bacterial vaginosis or trichomoniasis. Specifically, an abnormally increased amount or an abnormal odor of the discharge is associated with one or both of these conditions. Cervical infection with *N. gonorrhoeae* or *C. trachomatis* does not appear to cause an increased amount or abnormal odor of discharge, but cervicitis, like trichomoniasis, can include the production of an increased number of neutrophils in vaginal fluid, resulting in a yellow color. Vulvar conditions such as genital herpes or vulvovaginal candidiasis can cause vulvar pruritus, burning, irritation, or lesions as well as external dysuria (as urine passes over the inflamed vulva) or vulvar dyspareunia.

Certain vulvovaginal infections may have serious sequelae. Trichomoniasis, bacterial vaginosis, and vulvovaginal candidiasis have all been associated with increased risk of acquisition of HIV infection. Vaginal trichomoniasis and bacterial vaginosis early in pregnancy independently predict premature onset of labor. Bacterial vaginosis can also lead to anaerobic bacterial infection of the endometrium and salpinges. Vaginitis may be an early and prominent feature of toxic shock syndrome, and recurrent or chronic vulvovaginal candidiasis develops with increased frequency among women with systemic illnesses, such as diabetes mellitus or HIV-related immunosuppression (although only a very small proportion of women with recurrent vulvovaginal candidiasis in the United States actually have a serious predisposing illness).

Thus vulvovaginal symptoms or signs warrant careful evaluation, including pelvic examination, simple rapid diagnostic tests, and appropriate therapy specific for the anatomical site and type of infection. Unfortunately, a recent survey in the United States indicated that clinicians seldom perform the tests required to establish the cause of such symptoms. Further, comparison of telephone and office management of vulvovaginal complaints has documented the inaccuracy of the former, and comparison of evaluations by nurse-midwives with those by physician-practitioners showed that the practitioners' clinical evaluations correlated poorly both with the nurses' evaluations and with diagnostic tests. The diagnosis and treatment of the three most common types of vaginal infection are summarized in Table 115-5.

Inspection of the vulva and perineum may reveal tender genital ulcerations (typically due to HSV infection, occasionally due to chancroid) or fissures (typically due to vulvovaginal candidiasis) or discharge visible at the introitus before insertion of a speculum (suggestive of bacterial vaginosis or trichomoniasis). Speculum examination permits the clinician to discern whether the discharge in fact looks abnormal and whether any abnormal discharge in the vagina emanates from the cervical os (mucoid and, if abnormal, yellow) or from the vagina (not mucoid, since the vaginal epithelium does not produce mucus). Symptoms or signs of abnormal vaginal discharge should prompt testing of vaginal fluid for pH, fishy odor when mixed with 10% KOH, and microscopic features when mixed with saline and with 10% KOH. Additional objective laboratory tests useful for establishing the cause of abnormal vaginal discharge include Gram's staining to

TABLE 115-5 *Diagnostic Features and Management of Vaginal Infection*

Feature	Normal Vaginal Examination	Vulvovaginal Candidiasis	Trichomonal Vaginitis	Bacterial Vaginosis
Etiology	Uninfected; lactobacilli predominant	*Candida albicans*	*Trichomonas vaginalis*	Associated with *Gardnerella vaginalis*, various anaerobic bacteria, and mycoplasmas
Typical symptoms	None	Vulvar itching and/or irritation	Profuse purulent discharge; vulvar itching	Malodorous, slightly increased discharge
Discharge				
Amount	Variable; usually scant	Scant	Often profuse	Moderate
Color[a]	Clear or white	White	White or yellow	White or gray
Consistency	Nonhomogeneous, floccular	Clumped; adherent plaques	Homogeneous	Homogeneous, low viscosity; uniformly coats vaginal walls
Inflammation of vulvar or vaginal epithelium	None	Erythema of vaginal epithelium, introitus; vulvar dermatitis common	Erythema of vaginal and vulvar epithelium; colpitis macularis	None
pH of vaginal fluid[b]	Usually ≤4.5	Usually ≤4.5	Usually ≥5.0	Usually >4.5
Amine ("fishy") odor with 10% KOH	None	None	May be present	Present
Microscopy[c]	Normal epithelial cells; lactobacilli predominant	Leukocytes, epithelial cells; mycelia or pseudomycelia in up to 80% of *C. albicans* culture-positive persons with typical symptoms	Leukocytes; motile trichomonads seen in 80 to 90% of symptomatic patients, less often in the absence of symptoms	Clue cells; few leukocytes; no lactobacilli or only a few outnumbered by profuse mixed flora, nearly always including *G. vaginalis* plus anaerobic species on Gram's stain
Usual treatment	None	Azole cream, tablet, or suppository—e.g., miconazole 100-mg vaginal suppository or clotrimazole 100-mg vaginal tablet, once daily for 7 days Fluconazole, 150 mg orally (single dose)	Metronidazole, 2 g orally (single dose) Metronidazole, 500 mg PO bid for 7 days	Metronidazole, 500 mg PO bid for 7 days Clindamycin, 2% cream, one full applicator vaginally each night for 7 days Metronidazole gel, 0.75%, one full applicator vaginally twice daily for 5 days Metronidazole, 2 g PO (single dose)[d]
Usual management of sexual partner	None	None; topical treatment if candidal dermatitis of penis is detected	Examination for STD; treatment with metronidazole, 2 g PO (single dose)	Examination for STD; no treatment if normal

[a] Color of discharge is best determined by examination against the white background of a swab.

[b] pH determination is not useful if blood is present.

[c] To detect fungal elements, vaginal fluid is digested with 10% KOH prior to microscopic examination; to examine for other features, fluid is mixed (1:1) with physiologic saline.

Gram's stain is also excellent for detecting yeasts and pseudomycelia and for distinguishing normal flora from the mixed flora seen in bacterial vaginosis, but it is less sensitive than the saline preparation for detection of *T. vaginalis*.

[d] Single-dose regimen is less effective than 7-day metronidazole regimen.

detect alterations in the vaginal flora; card tests for bacterial vaginosis, as described below; and a new DNA probe test (the Affirm test) to detect *T. vaginalis* and *C. albicans* as well as the increased concentrations of *Gardnerella vaginalis* associated with bacterial vaginosis.

℞ TREATMENT

Patterns of treatment for vaginal discharge vary widely. In developing countries, where clinics or pharmacies often dispense treatment based on symptoms alone without examination or testing, oral treatment with metronidazole—either as a 2-g single dose or as a 7-day regimen—provides reasonable coverage against both trichomoniasis and bacterial vaginosis, the usual causes of symptoms of vaginal discharge; metronidazole treatment of sex partners prevents reinfection of women with trichomoniasis, even though it does not help prevent the recurrence of bacterial vaginosis. Guidelines promulgated during the 1990s by the World Health Organization suggested treatment for cervical infection and for vulvovaginal candidiasis in women with symptoms of abnormal vaginal discharge; in retrospect, these recommendations were faulty, since these conditions seldom produce such symptoms.

In industrialized countries, clinicians treating symptoms and signs of abnormal vaginal discharge should at least differentiate between bacterial vaginosis and trichomoniasis, because optimal management of patients and partners differs for these two conditions (as discussed briefly below).

Vaginal Trichomoniasis (See also Chap. 199) Symptomatic trichomoniasis characteristically produces a profuse, yellow, purulent, homogeneous vaginal discharge and vulvar irritation, often with visible inflammation of the vaginal and vulvar epithelium and petechial lesions on the cervix (the so-called strawberry cervix, usually evident only by colposcopy). The pH of vaginal fluid usually rises to ≥5.0. In women with typical symptoms and signs of trichomoniasis, microscopic examination of vaginal discharge mixed with saline reveals motile trichomonads in most culture-positive cases. However, in the absence of symptoms or signs, culture is often required for detection of the organism. Polymerase chain reaction (PCR) tests for *T. vaginalis* compare favorably with culture, and PCR testing of urine is now disclosing surprisingly high prevalences of this pathogen among men at several STD clinics in the United States. Treatment of asymptomatic as well as symptomatic cases reduces rates of transmission and prevents later development of symptoms.

℞ TREATMENT

Only nitroimidazoles consistently cure trichomoniasis. Tinidazole and ornidazole have longer half-lives than metronidazole but do not give better results than a single 2-g oral dose of metronidazole, which is much less expensive. Treatment of male sexual partners—often facilitated by dispensing metronidazole to the female patient to give to her partner(s), with a warning about avoiding the concurrent use of alcohol—significantly reduces both the risk of reinfection and the reservoir of infection. Treatment with 0.75% metronidazole gel intravaginally, although moderately effective for bacterial vaginosis, is not reliable for vaginal trichomoniasis. Systemic use of metronidazole is not recommended during the first trimester of pregnancy but is considered safe thereafter. In a large randomized trial, metronidazole treatment of trichomoniasis during pregnancy did not reduce the frequency of perinatal morbidity.

Bacterial Vaginosis This syndrome (formerly termed *nonspecific vaginitis, Haemophilus vaginitis, anaerobic vaginitis,* or *Gardnerella-associated vaginal discharge*) is characterized by symptoms of vaginal malodor and a slightly to moderately increased white discharge, which appears homogeneous, is low in viscosity, and smoothly coats the vaginal mucosa. An interesting observation is that new genital HPV infection in young women is associated with increased subsequent risk of developing bacterial vaginosis. Other risk factors include multiple sexual partners and recent intercourse with a new partner, but metro-

nidazole treatment of male partners has not reduced the rate of recurrence among affected women.

The vaginal fluid of women with bacterial vaginosis is characterized by markedly increased prevalences and concentrations of *G. vaginalis, Mycoplasma hominis,* and several anaerobic bacteria [e.g., *Mobiluncus* spp., *Prevotella* spp. (formerly *Bacteroides* spp.), and some *Peptostreptococcus* spp.]. The vaginal fluid usually lacks hydrogen peroxide–producing *Lactobacillus* spp., which constitute most of the normal vaginal flora and perhaps help protect against certain cervical and vaginal infections. Vaginal douching, use of intravaginal nonoxynol-9 spermicide, and new sexual partners can all result in loss of vaginal colonization by hydrogen peroxide–producing lactobacilli.

Bacterial vaginosis is conventionally diagnosed clinically with the Amsel criteria, which include any three of the following four clinical abnormalities: (1) objective signs of increased white homogeneous vaginal discharge; (2) a vaginal discharge pH of >4.5; (3) liberation of a distinct fishy odor (attributable to volatile amines such as trimethylamine) immediately after vaginal secretions are mixed with a 10% solution of KOH; and (4) microscopic demonstration of "clue cells" (vaginal epithelial cells coated with coccobacillary organisms giving them a granular appearance and indistinct borders; Fig. 115-1) on a wet mount prepared by mixing vaginal secretions with normal saline in a ratio of ~1:1. A diagnostic card test facilitates screening of vaginal fluid for pH > 4.5 and amines, and a dipstick test detects proline aminopeptidase, an enzyme associated with this syndrome.

℞ TREATMENT

The standard dosage of metronidazole for the treatment of bacterial vaginosis is 500 mg orally bid for 7 days. The single 2-g oral dose of metronidazole recommended for trichomoniasis produces somewhat

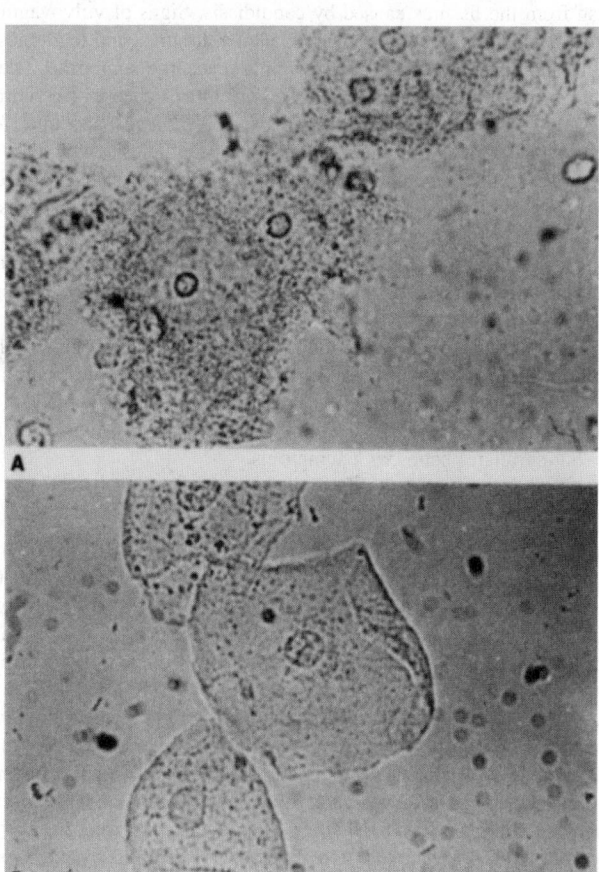

FIGURE 115-1 *A.* Vaginal epithelial "clue cells." Note granular appearance due to adherent *Gardnerella vaginalis* and indistinct cell margins (400×). *B.* Normal vaginal epithelial cells. The cell margins are distinct and lack granularity.

lower short-term cure rates. Intravaginal treatment with 2% clindamycin cream [one full applicator (5 g containing 100 mg of clindamycin phosphate) each night for 7 nights] or with 0.75% metronidazole gel [one full applicator (5 g containing 37.5 mg of metronidazole) twice daily for 5 days] is also approved for use in the United States and does not elicit systemic adverse reactions. Oral clindamycin (300 mg bid for 7 days) and clindamycin ovules (100 g intravaginally once at bedtime for 3 days) have also been approved. Unfortunately, long-term recurrence (i.e., several months later) is distressingly common after either oral or intravaginal treatment. Treatment of male partners with metronidazole does not prevent recurrence of bacterial vaginosis.

No controlled data support the use of currently available vaginal or oral preparations of lactobacilli for the treatment or prevention of recurrence of bacterial vaginosis. In a randomized trial, repeated intravaginal inoculation of a vaginal peroxide-producing *Lactobacillus* species following treatment of bacterial vaginosis with metronidazole did not reduce the frequency of recurrence. A meta-analysis of 18 studies concluded that bacterial vaginosis during pregnancy substantially increased the risk of preterm delivery and of spontaneous abortion. Although intravaginal treatment of bacterial vaginosis during pregnancy has not reduced perinatal morbidity, oral clindamycin treatment of this syndrome early in pregnancy significantly reduced the risk of late miscarriage and of preterm delivery. Oral antimicrobial treatment of bacterial vaginosis for ≥7 days early in pregnancy may reduce the risk of preterm delivery for women with a history of this pregnancy outcome.

Vulvovaginal Pruritus, Burning, or Irritation   Vulvovaginal candidiasis produces vulvar pruritus, burning, or irritation, generally without symptoms of increased vaginal discharge or malodor. Genital herpes can produce similar symptoms, with lesions sometimes difficult to distinguish from the fissures caused by candidiasis. Signs of vulvovaginal candidiasis include vulvar erythema, edema, fissures, and tenderness. With candidiasis, a white scanty vaginal discharge sometimes takes the form of white thrush-like plaques or cottage cheese–like curds adhering loosely to the vaginal mucosa. *C. albicans* accounts for nearly all cases of symptomatic vulvovaginal candidiasis, which probably arise from endogenous strains of *C. albicans* that have colonized the vagina or the intestinal tract. Complicated vulvovaginal candidiasis includes cases that recur four or more times per year; are unusually severe; are caused by non-*albicans Candida* spp.; or occur in women with uncontrolled diabetes, debilitation, immunosuppression, or pregnancy.

The diagnosis of vulvovaginal candidiasis usually involves the demonstration of pseudohyphae or hyphae by microscopic examination of vaginal fluid mixed with saline or 10% KOH or subjected to Gram's staining. Microscopic examination is less sensitive than culture but correlates better with symptoms.

R̥ TREATMENT

Symptoms and signs of vulvovaginal candidiasis warrant treatment, usually intravaginal administration of any of several imidazole antibiotics (e.g., miconazole or clotrimazole) for 3 to 7 days. Over-the-counter marketing of such preparations has reduced the cost of care and made treatment more convenient for many women with recurrent yeast vulvovaginitis. However, most women who purchase these preparations do not have vulvovaginal candidiasis, while many do have other vaginal infections that require different treatment. Therefore, only women with classic symptoms of vulvar pruritus and a history of previous episodes of yeast vulvovaginitis documented by an experienced clinician should self-treat. Single-dose oral treatment with fluconazole (150 mg) is also effective and is preferred by many patients. Management of complicated cases (see above) and those that do not respond to the usual intravaginal or single-dose oral therapy often involves prolonged or periodic oral therapy; this situation is discussed extensively in the *2002 STD Treatment Guidelines* published

by the Centers for Disease Control and Prevention (CDC). Treatment of sexual partners is not routinely indicated.

Other Causes of Vaginal Discharge or Vaginitis   In the ulcerative vaginitis associated with staphylococcal toxic shock syndrome, *Staphylococcus aureus* should be promptly identified in vaginal fluid by Gram's stain and by culture. In desquamative inflammatory vaginitis, smears of vaginal fluid reveal neutrophils, massive vaginal epithelial-cell exfoliation with increased numbers of parabasal cells, and gram-positive cocci; this syndrome may respond to treatment with 2% clindamycin cream. Additional causes of vaginitis and vulvovaginal symptoms include retained foreign bodies (e.g., tampons), cervical caps, vaginal spermicides, vaginal antiseptic preparations or douches, vaginal epithelial atrophy (in postmenopausal women or during prolonged breast-feeding in the postpartum period), allergic reactions to latex condoms, vaginal aphthae associated with HIV infection or Behçet's syndrome, and vestibulitis (a poorly understood syndrome).

MUCOPURULENT CERVICITIS   Mucopurulent cervicitis (MPC) refers to inflammation of the columnar epithelium and subepithelium of the endocervix and of any contiguous columnar epithelium that lies exposed in an ectopic position on the exocervix. MPC in women represents the "silent partner" of urethritis in men, being equally common and often caused by the same agents (*N. gonorrhoeae, C. trachomatis,* or—in a significant association shown by two recent case-control studies—*M. genitalium*); however, MPC is more difficult to recognize. As the most common manifestation of these serious bacterial infections in women, MPC can be a harbinger or sign of upper genital tract infection, also known as pelvic inflammatory disease (PID; see below). In pregnant women, MPC can lead to obstetric complications. More than half of all cases of MPC in the United States today remain idiopathic.

The diagnosis of MPC rests on the detection of yellow mucopurulent discharge from the cervical os or of increased numbers of polymorphonuclear leukocytes (PMNs) in Gram's-stained or Papanicolaou-stained smears of endocervical mucus. MPC due to *C. trachomatis* can also produce edematous cervical ectopy (see below) and endocervical bleeding upon gentle swabbing. Unlike the endocervicitis produced by gonococcal or chlamydial infection, cervicitis caused by HSV produces ulcerative lesions on the stratified squamous epithelium of the exocervix as well as on the columnar epithelium. Yellow cervical mucus on a white swab removed from the endocervix indicates the presence of PMNs. The mucus should be rolled thinly on a slide for Gram's staining. The presence of ≥20 polymorphonuclear cells per 1000× microscopic field within strands of cervical mucus not contaminated by vaginal squamous epithelial cells or vaginal bacteria indicates endocervicitis (Fig. 115-2). Detection of intracellular gram-negative diplococci in carefully collected endocervical mucus is quite specific but ≤50% sensitive for gonorrhea. Therefore, specific and sensitive tests for *N. gonorrhoeae* as well as *C. trachomatis* are also indicated in the evaluation of MPC.

R̥ TREATMENT

Although the above criteria for MPC are neither highly specific nor highly predictive of gonococcal or chlamydial infection in many settings, current CDC guidelines call for consideration of empirical treatment for MPC, pending test results, "for a patient who has suspected gonorrhea or chlamydial infection, if (a) the prevalences of these infections are high in the patient population, and (b) the patient might be difficult to locate after treatment." In this situation, therapy should include a single-dose regimen effective for gonorrhea plus treatment for chlamydial infection, as outlined in Table 115-4 for the treatment of urethritis. In settings where gonorrhea is much less common than chlamydial infection, initial therapy for chlamydial infection alone suffices, pending test results for gonorrhea. The etiology and potential benefit of treatment of endocervicitis not associated with gonorrhea or chlamydial infection remain undefined. Although the antimicrobial susceptibility of *M. genitalium* is not yet well defined, it currently seems reasonable to use azithromycin to treat possible *M. genitalium*

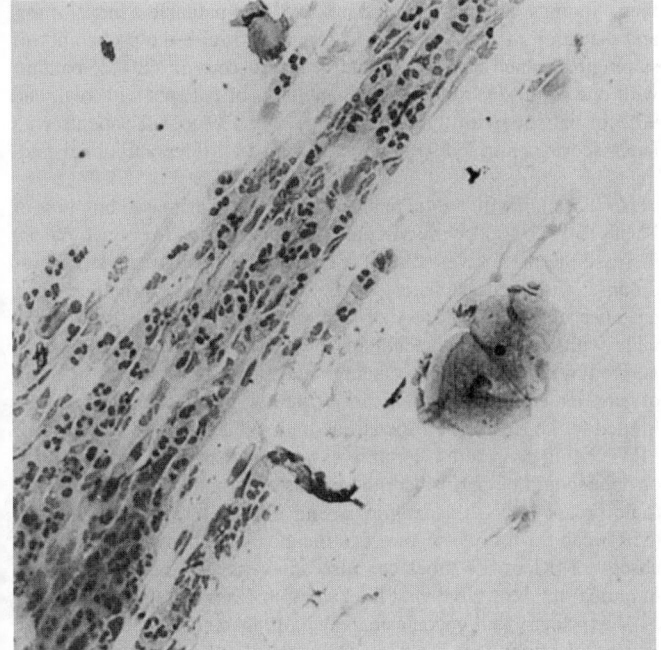

FIGURE 115-2 Gram's stain of cervical mucus, showing a strand of cervical mucus containing many polymorphonuclear leukocytes. This picture is typical of mucopurulent cervicitis. Note that leukocytes are not seen in areas of the slide containing vaginal epithelial cells, adjacent to the mucus strands.

infection in such cases. Sexual partner(s) of a woman with MPC should be examined and given a regimen similar to that chosen for the woman unless results of tests for gonorrhea or chlamydial infection in either partner warrant different therapy or no therapy.

CERVICAL ECTOPY Cervical ectopy, often mislabeled "cervical erosion," is easily confused with infectious endocervicitis. Ectopy represents the presence of the one-cell-thick columnar epithelium extending from the endocervix out onto the visible ectocervix. In ectopy, the cervical os may contain clear or slightly cloudy mucus but usually not yellow mucopus. Colposcopy shows intact epithelium. Normally found during adolescence and early adulthood, ectopy gradually recedes through the second and third decades of life, as squamous metaplasia replaces the ectopic columnar epithelium. Oral contraceptive use favors the persistence or reappearance of ectopy, while smoking apparently accelerates squamous metaplasia. Cauterization of ectopy is not warranted. Ectopy may render the cervix more susceptible to infection with *N. gonorrhoeae*, *C. trachomatis*, or HIV.

PELVIC INFLAMMATORY DISEASE The term *pelvic inflammatory disease* usually refers to infection that ascends from the cervix or vagina to involve the endometrium and/or fallopian tubes. Infection can extend beyond the reproductive tract to cause pelvic peritonitis, generalized peritonitis, perihepatitis, or pelvic abscess. In rare instances, infection extends secondarily to the pelvic organs from adjacent foci of inflammation (e.g., appendicitis, regional ileitis, or diverticulitis), as a result of hematogenous dissemination (e.g., of tuberculosis), or as a rare complication of certain tropical diseases (e.g., schistosomiasis). Intrauterine infection can be primary (spontaneously occurring and usually sexually transmitted) or secondary to invasive intrauterine surgical procedures [e.g., dilatation and curettage, termination of pregnancy, insertion of an intrauterine device (IUD), or hysterosalpingography] or to parturition.

Etiology The agents most often implicated in acute PID include those that are primary causes of endocervicitis (*N. gonorrhoeae* and *C. trachomatis*) and those that can be regarded as components of an altered vaginal flora. In general, PID is most often associated with gonorrhea where there is a high incidence of gonorrhea—e.g., in developing countries and in indigent, inner-city populations in the United States.

In recent case-control studies, detection of *M. genitalium* by PCR in endometrial specimens has also been significantly associated with histopathologic diagnoses of endometritis.

Anaerobic and facultative organisms (especially *Prevotella* species, peptostreptococci, *E. coli*, *Haemophilus influenzae*, and group B streptococci) as well as genital mycoplasmas have been isolated from specimens obtained at laparoscopy from the peritoneal fluid or fallopian tubes in a varying proportion (typically one-fourth to one-third) of women with PID studied in the United States. The difficulty of determining the exact microbial etiology of an individual case of PID has implications for the approach to empirical antimicrobial treatment of this infection.

Epidemiology In the United States in 2002, women 15 to 44 years of age made ~200,000 initial visits to physician's offices for PID, and an estimated 66,000 women were hospitalized for acute PID. Important risk factors for acute PID include the presence of endocervical infection or bacterial vaginosis, a history of salpingitis or of recent vaginal douching, and the use of an IUD (especially among nulliparous women, during the first few months after IUD insertion, and among women with multiple sex partners). Certain other iatrogenic factors, such as dilatation and curettage or cesarean section, can increase the risk of PID, especially among women with endocervical gonococcal or chlamydial infection or bacterial vaginosis. The onset of symptoms of *N. gonorrhoeae*–associated and *C. trachomatis*–associated PID often occurs during or soon after the menstrual period; this timing suggests that menstruation is a risk factor in women with endocervical infection. Experimental inoculation of the fallopian tubes of lower primates has shown that repeated exposure to *C. trachomatis* leads to the greatest degree of tissue inflammation and damage; thus, immunopathology probably contributes to the pathogenesis of chlamydial salpingitis. Women using oral contraceptives appear to be at decreased risk of symptomatic PID, and tubal sterilization reduces the risk of salpingitis by preventing intraluminal spread of infection into the tubes.

Clinical Manifestations ■ *ENDOMETRITIS: A CLINICAL PATHOLOGIC SYNDROME* A study of women with clinically suspected PID who were undergoing both endometrial biopsy and laparoscopy showed that those with endometritis alone differed from those who also had salpingitis in that they significantly less often had lower quadrant, adnexal, or cervical motion or abdominal rebound tenderness; fever; or elevated C-reactive protein levels. In addition, women with endometritis alone differed from those with neither endometritis nor salpingitis in that they more often had gonorrhea, chlamydial infection, and risk factors such as douching or IUD use. Thus, women with endometritis alone were intermediate between those with neither endometritis nor salpingitis and those with salpingitis with respect to risk factors, clinical manifestations, cervical infection prevalence, and elevated C-reactive protein.

SALPINGITIS Symptoms of nontuberculous salpingitis classically evolve from a yellow or malodorous vaginal discharge caused by MPC and/or bacterial vaginosis to midline abdominal pain and abnormal vaginal bleeding caused by endometritis and then to bilateral lower abdominal and pelvic pain caused by salpingitis, with nausea, vomiting, and increased abdominal tenderness caused by peritonitis.

The abdominal pain in nontuberculous salpingitis is usually described as dull or aching. In some cases, pain is lacking or is atypical, but active inflammatory changes are found in the course of an unrelated evaluation or procedure, such as a laparoscopic evaluation for infertility. Abnormal uterine bleeding precedes or coincides with the onset of pain in ~40% of women with PID, symptoms of urethritis (dysuria) occur in 20%, and symptoms of proctitis (anorectal pain, tenesmus, and rectal discharge or bleeding) are occasionally seen in women with gonococcal or chlamydial infection.

Speculum examination shows evidence of MPC (yellow endocervical discharge, easily induced endocervical bleeding) in the majority of women with gonococcal or chlamydial PID. Cervical motion tenderness is produced by stretching of the adnexal attachments on the side toward which the cervix is pushed. Bimanual examination reveals uterine fundal tenderness due to endometritis and abnormal adnexal tenderness due to salpingitis that is usually, but not necessarily, bilateral. Adnexal swelling is palpable in about one-half of women with acute salpingitis, but evaluation of the adnexae in a patient with marked tenderness is not reliable. The initial temperature is >38°C in only about one-third of patients with acute salpingitis. Laboratory findings include elevation of the erythrocyte sedimentation rate (ESR) in 75% of patients with acute salpingitis and elevation of the peripheral white blood cell count in up to 60%.

Unlike nontuberculous salpingitis, genital tuberculosis often occurs in older women, many of whom are postmenopausal. Presenting symptoms include abnormal vaginal bleeding, pain (including dysmenorrhea), and infertility. About one-quarter of these women have had adnexal masses. Endometrial biopsy shows tuberculous granulomas and provides optimal specimens for culture.

PERIHEPATITIS AND PERIAPPENDICITIS   Pleuritic upper abdominal pain and tenderness (usually localized to the right upper quadrant) develop in 3 to 10% of women with acute PID. Symptoms of perihepatitis arise during or after the onset of symptoms of PID and may overshadow lower abdominal symptoms, thereby leading to a mistaken diagnosis of cholecystitis. In perhaps 5% of cases of acute salpingitis, early laparoscopy reveals perihepatic inflammation ranging from edema and erythema of the liver capsule to exudate with fibrinous adhesions between the visceral and parietal peritoneum. When treatment is delayed and laparoscopy is performed late, dense "violin-string" adhesions can be seen over the liver; chronic exertional or positional right upper quadrant pain ensues when traction is placed on the adhesions. Although perihepatitis, also known as the *Fitz-Hugh–Curtis syndrome*, was for many years specifically attributed to gonococcal salpingitis, most cases are now attributed to chlamydial salpingitis. In patients with chlamydial salpingitis, serum titers of microimmunofluorescent antibody to *C. trachomatis* are typically much higher when perihepatitis is present than when it is absent.

Physical findings include right upper quadrant tenderness and usually include adnexal tenderness and cervicitis, even in patients whose symptoms do not suggest salpingitis. Results of liver function tests and right upper quadrant ultrasonography are nearly always normal. The presence of MPC and pelvic tenderness in a young woman with subacute pleuritic right upper quadrant pain and normal ultrasonography of the gallbladder points to a diagnosis of perihepatitis.

Periappendicitis (appendiceal serositis without involvement of the intestinal mucosa) has been found in ~5% of patients undergoing appendectomy for suspected appendicitis and can occur as a complication of gonococcal or chlamydial salpingitis.

Among women with salpingitis, HIV infection is associated with increased severity of salpingitis and with tuboovarian abscess requiring hospitalization and surgical drainage. Nonetheless, among women with HIV infection and salpingitis, the clinical reponse to conventional antimicrobial therapy (coupled with drainage of tuboovarian abscess, when found) has been satisfactory.

Diagnosis   Treatment appropriate for PID must not be withheld from patients who have an equivocal diagnosis; it is better to err on the side of overdiagnosis and overtreatment. On the other hand, it is essential to differentiate between salpingitis and other pelvic pathology, particularly surgical emergencies such as appendicitis and ectopic pregnancy.

Nothing short of laparoscopy definitively identifies salpingitis, but routine laparoscopy to confirm suspected salpingitis is generally impractical. Most patients with acute PID have lower abdominal pain of <3 weeks' duration, pelvic tenderness on bimanual pelvic examination, and evidence of lower genital tract infection (e.g., MPC). Approximately 60% of such patients have salpingitis at laparoscopy, and perhaps 10 to 20% have endometritis alone. Among the patients with

these findings, a rectal temperature >38°C, a palpable adnexal mass, and elevation of the ESR to >15 mm/h also raise the probability of salpingitis, which has been found at laparoscopy in 68% of patients with one of these additional findings, 90% of patients with two, and 96% of patients with three. However, only 17% of all patients with laparoscopy-confirmed salpingitis have had all three additional findings.

In a woman with pelvic pain and tenderness, increased numbers of PMNs (30 per 1000× microscopic field in strands of cervical mucus) increase the predictive value of a clinical diagnosis of acute PID, as do onset with menses, history of recent abnormal menstrual bleeding, presence of an IUD, history of salpingitis, and sexual exposure to a male with urethritis. Appendicitis or another disorder of the gut is favored by the early onset of anorexia, nausea, or vomiting; the onset of pain later than day 14 of the menstrual cycle; or unilateral pain limited to the right or left lower quadrant. Whenever the diagnosis of PID is being considered, serum assays for human β-chorionic gonadotropin should be performed; these tests are usually positive with ectopic pregnancy. Ultrasonography and magnetic resonance imaging (MRI) can be useful for the identification of tuboovarian or pelvic abscess. MRI of the tubes can also show increased tubal diameter, intratubal fluid, or tubal wall thickening in cases of salpingitis.

The primary and uncontested value of laparoscopy in women with lower abdominal pain is for the exclusion of other surgical problems. Some of the most common or serious problems that may be confused with salpingitis (e.g., acute appendicitis, ectopic pregnancy, corpus luteum bleeding, ovarian tumor) are unilateral. Unilateral pain or pelvic mass, although not incompatible with PID, is a strong indication for laparoscopy unless the clinical picture warrants laparotomy instead. Atypical clinical findings, such as the absence of lower genital tract infection, a missed menstrual period, a positive pregnancy test, or failure to respond to appropriate therapy, are other common indications for laparoscopy. Endometrial biopsy is relatively sensitive and specific for the diagnosis of endometritis, which correlates well with the presence of salpingitis.

Endocervical swab specimens should be examined by Gram's staining for PMNs and gram-negative diplococci and by nucleic acid amplification tests for *N. gonorrhoeae* and *C. trachomatis*. The clinical diagnosis of PID made by expert gynecologists is confirmed by laparoscopy or endometrial biopsy in ~90% of women who also have cultures positive for *N. gonorrhoeae* or *C. trachomatis*. Even among women with no symptoms suggestive of acute PID who were attending an STD clinic or gynecology clinic in Pittsburgh, endometritis was significantly associated with endocervical gonorrhea or chlamydial infection or bacterial vaginosis, being detected in 26, 27, and 15% of women with these conditions, respectively.

℞ TREATMENT

Women with PID can be treated as either outpatients or inpatients. In the multicenter Pelvic Inflammatory Disease Evaluation and Clinical Health (PEACH) trial, 831 women with mild to moderately severe symptoms and signs of PID were randomized to receive either inpatient treatment with intravenous (IV) cefoxitin and doxycycline or outpatient treatment with a single intramuscular (IM) dose of cefoxitin plus oral doxycycline. Short-term clinical and microbiologic outcomes and long-term outcomes were equivalent in the two groups. Nonetheless, hospitalization should be considered when (1) the diagnosis is uncertain and surgical emergencies such as appendicitis and ectopic pregnancy cannot be excluded, (2) pelvic abscess is suspected, (3) severe illness or nausea and vomiting preclude outpatient management, (4) the patient has HIV infection, (5) the patient is assessed as unable to follow or tolerate an outpatient regimen, or (6) the patient has failed to respond to outpatient therapy. Some experts also prefer to hospitalize adolescents with PID for initial therapy.

Recommended combination regimens for ambulatory or parenteral management of PID are presented in Table 115-6. Women managed as outpatients should receive a combined regimen with broad activity,

TABLE 115-6 *Combination Antimicrobial Regimens Recommended for Outpatient Treatment or for Parenteral Treatment of PID*

Outpatient Regimens	Parenteral Regimens
Regimen A Ofloxacin 400 mg PO bid for 14 days *or* Levofloxacin 500 mg PO once daily for 14 days *plus*[a] Metronidazole 500 mg PO bid for 14 days **Regimen B** Ceftriaxone 250 mg IM once *plus* Doxycycline 100 mg PO bid for 14 days *plus*[a] Metronidazole 500 mg PO bid for 14 days	Initiate parenteral therapy with either of the following regimens; continue parenteral therapy until 48 h after clinical improvement; then change to outpatient therapy, as described in text. **Regimen A** Cefotetan 2 g IV q12h *or* Cefoxitin 2 g IV q6h *plus* Doxycycline 100 mg IV or PO q12h **Regimen B** Clindamycin 900 mg IV q8h *plus* Gentamicin, loading dose of 2 mg/kg IV or IM, then maintenance dose of 1.5 mg/kg q8h

[a] The addition of metronidazole is recommended by some experts.
Source: Adapted from Centers for Disease Control and Prevention: MMWR 51(RR-6):1, 2002.

such as ceftriaxone followed by doxycycline. Metronidazole can be added, if tolerated, to enhance activity against anaerobes. Alternatively, oral ofloxacin or levofloxacin, each continued for 14 days and given with or without metronidazole, provides good coverage of the major pathogens. Although few methodologically sound clinical trials (especially with prolonged follow-up) have been conducted, one meta-analysis suggested a benefit of providing good coverage against anaerobes.

The following two parenteral regimens have given nearly identical results in a multicenter randomized trial:

1. Doxycycline (100 mg bid, given IV or by mouth) plus cefotetan (2.0 g IV every 12 h) or cefoxitin (2.0 g IV every 6 h). Administration of these drugs should be continued by the IV route for at least 48 h after the patient's condition improves and then followed with doxycycline (100 mg bid by mouth) to complete 14 days of therapy.

2. Clindamycin (900 mg IV every 8 h) plus gentamicin (2.0 mg/kg IV or IM, followed by 1.5 mg/kg every 8 h) in patients with normal renal function. Once-daily dosing of gentamicin (with combination of the total daily dose into a single daily dose) has not been evaluated in PID but has been efficacious in other serious infections and could be substituted.

Treatment with these drugs should be continued for at least 48 h after the patient's condition improves and then followed with oral doxycycline (100 mg bid by mouth) or clindamycin (450 mg qid by mouth) to complete 14 days of therapy. In cases with tuboovarian abscess, clindamycin rather than doxycycline for continued therapy may provide better coverage for anaerobic infection.

FOLLOW-UP Hospitalized patients should show substantial clinical improvement within 3 to 5 days. Women treated as outpatients should be clinically reevaluated within 72 h. A follow-up telephone survey of women seen in an emergency room and given a prescription for 10 days of oral doxycycline for PID found that 28% never filled the prescription and 41% stopped taking medication early (after an average of 4.1 days), often because of persistent symptoms, lack of symptoms, or side effects. Women not responding favorably to ambulatory therapy should be hospitalized. After completion of treatment, tests for persistent or recurrent infection with *N. gonorrhoeae* or *C. trachomatis* should be performed if symptoms persist or recur or if the patient has not complied with therapy or has been reexposed to an untreated sex partner.

SURGERY Surgery is necessary for the treatment of salpingitis only in the face of life-threatening infection (such as rupture or threatened rupture of a tuboovarian abscess) or for drainage of an abscess. Conservative surgical procedures are usually sufficient. Pelvic abscesses can often be drained by posterior colpotomy, and peritoneal lavage can be used if there is generalized peritonitis.

Prognosis Among 900 women in Sweden who underwent long-term follow-up for a mean period of 8 years after successful treatment of an acute episode of PID with various regimens (that today would often not be considered to provide optimal broad antimicrobial activity), late sequelae included infertility due to bilateral tubal occlusion, ectopic pregnancy due to tubal scarring without occlusion, chronic pelvic pain, and recurrent salpingitis. The postsalpingitis risk of infertility due to tubal occlusion among sexually active women not using contraceptives was 14% at 15 to 24 years of age and 26% at 25 to 34 years of age; the risk for women of all ages combined was 11% after one episode of salpingitis, 23% after two episodes, and 54% after three or more episodes. A study at the University of Washington found a sevenfold increase in the risk of ectopic pregnancy and an eightfold increase in the rate of hysterectomy after PID.

Prevention A randomized controlled trial designed to determine whether selective screening for chlamydial infection reduced the risk of subsequent PID showed that women randomized to undergo screening had a 56% lower rate of PID over the following year than did women receiving the usual care without screening. This report helped to prompt the establishment of U.S. national guidelines for risk-based chlamydial screening of young women as a highly effective way to reduce the incidence of PID and the prevalence of post-PID sequelae, while also reducing sexual transmission of *C. trachomatis*.

ULCERATIVE GENITAL LESIONS Genital ulceration reflects a set of important STIs, most of which sharply increase the risk of sexual acquisition and shedding of HIV. In a 1996 study of genital ulcers in 10 of the U.S. cities with the highest rates of primary syphilis, PCR testing of ulcer specimens demonstrated HSV in 62% of patients, *Treponema pallidum* in 13%, and *Haemophilus ducreyi* in 12 to 20%.

In Asia and Africa, chancroid (Fig. 115-3) was once considered the most common type of genital ulcer, followed in frequency by primary

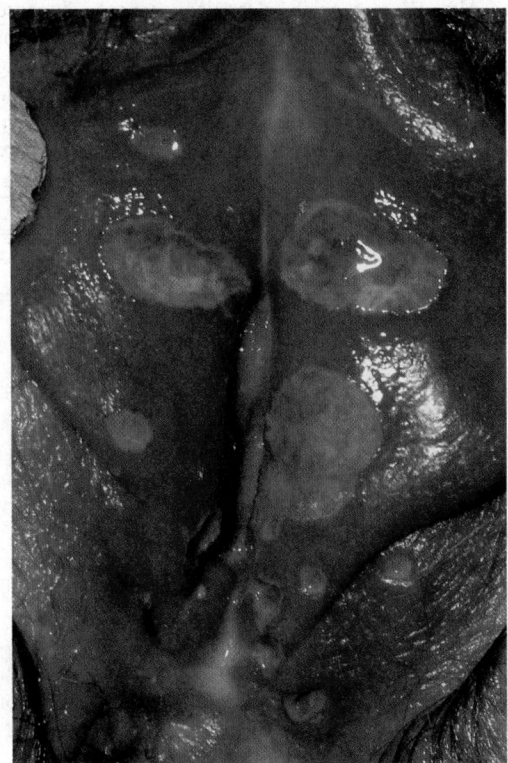

FIGURE 115-3 Chancroid: multiple, painful, punched-out ulcers with undermined borders on the labia occurring after autoinoculation.

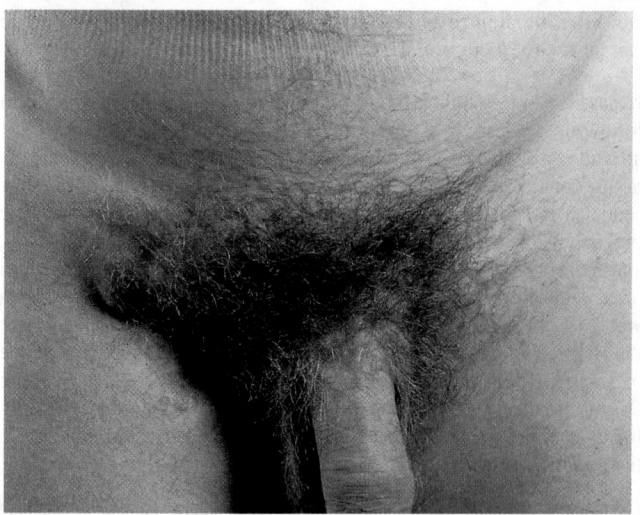

FIGURE 115-4 Lymphogranuloma venereum: striking tender lymphadenopathy occurring at the femoral and inguinal lymph nodes, separated by a groove made by Poupart's ligament.

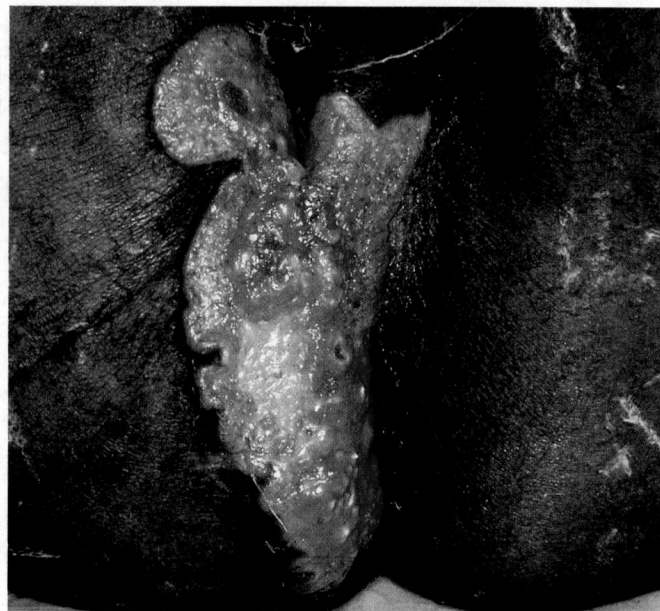

FIGURE 115-5 Donovanosis, ulcerovegetative type: extensive granulation-tissue formation, ulceration, and scarring of the perineum, scrotum, and penis.

syphilis and then genital herpes. With increased efforts to control chancroid and syphilis, together with more frequent recurrences or persistence of genital herpes attributable to HIV infection, PCR testing of genital ulcers now clearly implicates genital herpes as the most common cause of genital ulceration in many developing countries. Lymphogranuloma venereum (LGV; Fig. 115-4) and donovanosis (granuloma inguinale; Fig. 115-5) continue to cause genital ulceration in developing countries but rarely occur today in North America or Europe. Other causes of genital ulcer include (1) candidiasis and traumatized genital warts—both readily recognized; (2) lesions due to genital involvement of more widespread dermatoses; and (3) cutaneous manifestations of systemic diseases, such as genital mucosal ulceration in Stevens-Johnson syndrome or Behçet's disease.

Diagnosis   Although most genital ulcerations cannot be diagnosed confidently on clinical grounds alone, clinical findings plus epidemiologic considerations (Table 115-7) can usually guide initial management (Table 115-8) pending results of further tests. Clinicians should order a rapid serologic test for syphilis in all cases of genital ulcer and a dark-field or direct immunofluorescence test (or PCR test, where avail-

able) for *T. pallidum* in all lesions except those highly characteristic of infection with HSV (i.e., those with herpetic vesicles). All patients presenting with genital ulceration should be asked to undergo serologic testing for HIV infection.

Typical vesicles or pustules or a cluster of painful ulcers preceded by vesiculopustular lesions suggests genital herpes. These typical clinical presentations make detection of the virus optional; however, many patients want confirmation of the diagnosis, and differentiation of HSV-1 from HSV-2 has prognostic implications, since the latter causes more frequent genital recurrences.

Painless, nontender, indurated ulcers with firm, nontender inguinal adenopathy suggest primary syphilis. If dark-field examination and a rapid serologic test for syphilis are initially negative and the patient will comply with follow-up and sexual abstinence, the performance of two more dark-field examinations on successive days before treatment is begun will improve the sensitivity of the diagnosis of syphilis. Repeated serologic testing for syphilis 1 or 2 weeks after treatment of seronegative primary syphilis usually demonstrates seroconversion.

TABLE 115-7   *Clinical Features of Genital Ulcers*

Feature	Syphilis	Herpes	Chancroid	Lymphogranuloma Venereum	Donovanosis
Incubation period	9–90 days	2–7 days	1–14 days	3 days–6 weeks	1–4 weeks (up to 6 months)
Early primary lesions	Papule	Vesicle	Pustule	Papule, pustule, or vesicle	Papule
No. of lesions	Usually one	Multiple, may coalesce	Usually multiple, may coalesce	Usually one	Variable
Diameter	5–15 mm	1–2 mm	Variable	2–10 mm	Variable
Edges	Sharply demarcated, elevated, round, or oval	Erythematous	Undermined, ragged, irregular	Elevated, round, or oval	Elevated, irregular
Depth	Superficial or deep	Superficial	Excavated	Superficial or deep	Elevated
Base	Smooth, nonpurulent, relatively nonvascular	Serous, erythematous, nonvascular	Purulent, bleeds easily	Variable, nonvascular	Red and velvety, bleeds readily
Induration	Firm	None	Soft	Occasionally firm	Firm
Pain	Uncommon	Frequently tender	Usually very tender	Variable	Uncommon
Lymphadenopathy	Firm, nontender, bilateral	Firm, tender, often bilateral with initial episode	Tender, may suppurate, loculated, usually unilateral	Tender, may suppurate, loculated, usually unilateral	None; pseudobuboes

Source: From RM Ballard, in KK Holmes et al (eds): *Sexually Transmitted Diseases*, 3d ed. New York, McGraw-Hill, 1999.

| TABLE 115-8 | Initial Management of Genital Ulcer |

Usual causes
  Herpes simplex virus (HSV)
  Treponema pallidum (primary syphilis)
  Haemophilus ducreyi (chancroid)
Usual initial laboratory evaluation
  Dark-field exam, direct FA, or PCR for *T. pallidum*; RPR test (if
    negative but primary syphilis suspected, repeat RPR in 1 week);
    culture, direct FA, ELISA, or PCR for HSV. In chancroid-endemic
    area: PCR or culture for *H. ducreyi*

INITIAL TREATMENT

Herpes confirmed or suspected (history or sign of vesicles):
  Treat for genital herpes with acyclovir, valacyclovir, or famciclovir
Syphilis confirmed (dark-field, FA, or PCR showing *T. pallidum*, or
  RPR reactive):
  Benzathine penicillin 2.4 million units IM once to patient, recent (e.g.,
    within 3 months) seronegative partner(s), and every seropositive
    partner
Chancroid confirmed or suspected (diagnostic test positive, or HSV
  and syphilis excluded, and lesion persists):
  Ciprofloxacin 500 mg PO as single dose *or*
  Ceftriaxone 250 mg IM as single dose *or*
  Azithromycin 1 g PO as single dose

Note: FA, fluorescent antibody; PCR, polymerase chain reaction; RPR, rapid plasma reagin; ELISA, enzyme-linked immunosorbent assay; HSV, herpes simplex virus.

"Atypical" or clinically trivial ulcers may be more common manifestations of genital herpes than classic vesiculopustular lesions. Specific tests for HSV in such lesions are therefore indicated (Chap. 163). Type-specific serologic tests for serum antibody to HSV-2, now commercially available, may give negative results, especially when patients present early with the initial episode of genital herpes or when HSV-1 is the cause of genital herpes (as is often the case today). Furthermore, a positive test for HSV-2 antibody does not prove that the current lesions are herpetic, since nearly one-fourth of the general population of the United States becomes seropositive for HSV-2 during early adulthood. Nonetheless, a positive HSV-2 serology does enable the clinician to tell the patient that he or she has had genital herpes, should learn to recognize symptoms, should avoid sex during recurrences, and should consider use of condoms or suppressive antiviral therapy, both of which can reduce transmission to a sexual partner.

Demonstration of *H. ducreyi* by culture (or by PCR test, when available) is most useful when ulcers are painful and purulent, especially if inguinal lymphadenopathy with fluctuance or overlying erythema is noted; if chancroid is prevalent in the community; or if the patient has recently had a sexual exposure elsewhere in a chancroid-endemic area (e.g., a developing country). Enlarged, fluctuant lymph nodes should be aspirated for culture or PCR tests to detect *H. ducreyi* as well as for Gram's staining and culture to rule out the presence of other pyogenic bacteria.

When genital ulcers persist beyond the natural history of initial episodes of herpes (2 to 3 weeks) or of chancroid or syphilis (up to 6 weeks) and do not resolve with syndrome-based antimicrobial therapy, then—in addition to the usual tests for herpes, syphilis, and chancroid—biopsy is indicated to exclude donovanosis, carcinoma, and other nonvenereal dermatoses. HIV serology should also be undertaken, since chronic, persistent genital herpes is common in AIDS.

R̽ **TREATMENT**

Immediate syndrome-based treatment for acute genital ulcerations (after collection of all necessary diagnostic specimens) is often appropriate before all test results become available, because patients with typical initial or recurrent episodes of genital or anorectal herpes can benefit from prompt oral antiviral therapy (Chap. 163); because early treatment of sexually transmitted causes of genital ulcers decreases further transmission; and because some patients do not return for test results and treatment. The patient with nonvesicular ulcerative lesions

who may not return for follow-up or may continue sexual activity should receive initial treatment for syphilis, together with empirical therapy for chancroid if there has been an exposure in an area where chancroid occurs or if regional lymph node suppuration is evident. In resource-poor settings lacking ready access to diagnostic tests, this approach to syndromic treatment for syphilis and chancroid has helped bring these two diseases under control. Finally, empirical antimicrobial therapy may be indicated if ulcers persist and the diagnosis remains unclear after a week of observation despite attempts to diagnose herpes, syphilis, and chancroid.

PROCTITIS, PROCTOCOLITIS, ENTEROCOLITIS, AND ENTERITIS Sexually acquired *proctitis*, with inflammation limited to the rectal mucosa (the distal 10 to 12 cm), results from direct rectal inoculation of typical STD pathogens. In contrast, inflammation extending from the rectum to the colon (*proctocolitis*), involving both the small and the large bowel (*enterocolitis*), or involving the small bowel alone (*enteritis*) can result from ingestion of typical intestinal pathogens through oral-anal exposure during sexual contact. Anorectal pain and mucopurulent, bloody rectal discharge suggest proctitis or protocolitis. Proctitis commonly produces tenesmus (causing frequent attempts to defecate, but not true diarrhea) and constipation, whereas proctocolitis and enterocolitis more often cause true diarrhea. In all three conditions, anoscopy usually shows mucosal exudate and easily induced mucosal bleeding (i.e., a positive "wipe test"), sometimes with petechiae or mucosal ulcers. Exudate should be sampled for Gram's staining and other microbiologic studies. Sigmoidoscopy or colonoscopy shows inflammation limited to the rectum in proctitis or disease extending at least up into the sigmoid colon in proctocolitis.

The AIDS era brought an extraordinary shift in the clinical and etiologic spectrum of intestinal infections among homosexual men. The number of cases of the acute intestinal STIs described above fell as high-risk sexual behaviors became less common in this group. At the same time, the number of AIDS-related opportunistic intestinal infections increased rapidly, many associated with chronic or recurrent symptoms. The incidence of these infections has since fallen with increasingly effective antiretroviral therapy.

Acquisition of *N. gonorrhoeae*, HSV, or *C. trachomatis* during receptive anorectal intercourse causes most cases of infectious proctitis in women or homosexual men. Primary and secondary syphilis can also produce anal or anorectal lesions, with or without symptoms. Gonococcal or chlamydial proctitis typically involves the most distal rectal mucosa and the anal crypts and is clinically mild, without systemic manifestations. In contrast, primary proctitis due to HSV and proctocolitis due to the strains of *C. trachomatis* that cause LGV usually produce severe anorectal pain and often cause fever. Perianal ulcers and inguinal lymphadenopathy, most commonly due to HSV, can also occur in LGV or syphilis. Sacral nerve root radiculopathies, usually presenting as urinary retention, laxity of the anal sphincter, or constipation, may complicate primary herpetic proctitis. In LGV, rectal biopsy typically shows crypt abscesses, granulomas, and giant cells—findings resembling those in Crohn's disease; such findings should always prompt rectal culture and serology for LGV, which is a curable infection. Syphilis can also produce rectal granulomas, usually in association with infiltration by plasma cells or other mononuclear cells. Syphilis, LGV, and HSV infection involving the rectum can produce perirectal adenopathy that is sometimes mistaken for malignancy; syphilis, LGV, HSV infection, and chancroid involving the anus can produce inguinal adenopathy, because anal lymphatics drain to inguinal lymph nodes.

Diarrhea and abdominal bloating or cramping pain without anorectal symptoms and with normal findings on anoscopy and sigmoidoscopy occur with inflammation of the small intestine (enteritis) or with proximal colitis. In homosexual men without HIV infection, enteritis is often attributable to *Giardia lamblia*. Sexually acquired proctocolitis is most often due to *Campylobacter* or *Shigella* spp.

℞ TREATMENT

Acute proctitis in persons who have practiced receptive intercourse is usually sexually acquired. Such patients should undergo anoscopy to detect rectal ulcers or vesicles and petechiae after swabbing of the rectal mucosa; to examine rectal exudates for PMNs and gram-negative diplococci; and to obtain rectal swab specimens for testing for rectal gonorrhea, chlamydial infection, herpes, and syphilis. Pending test results, patients with proctitis should receive empirical syndromic treatment—e.g., with ceftriaxone (a single IM dose of 125 mg for gonorrhea) plus doxycycline (100 mg bid by mouth for 7 days for possible chlamydial infection) plus treatment for herpes or syphilis if indicated.

PREVENTION AND CONTROL OF STDS

Prevention and control of STDs require (1) reduction of the average rate of sexual exposure through alteration of behaviors and behavioral norms among both susceptible and infected persons in all population groups; (2) reduction of the efficiency of transmission through the promotion of safer sexual practices, the use of condoms during casual or commercial sex, hepatitis B immunization, and many other approaches (e.g., early detection and treatment of other STIs to reduce the efficiency of sexual transmission of HIV); and (3) shortening of the duration of infectivity of STDs through early detection and curative or suppressive treatment of patients and their sexual partners.

Financial and time constraints imposed by managed-care practice patterns often curtail screening and prevention services. As outlined in Fig. 115-6, the success of clinicians' efforts to detect and treat STDs depends in part on societal efforts to teach young people how to recognize symptoms of STDs; to motivate those with symptoms to seek care promptly; and to make such care accessible, affordable, and acceptable, especially to the young indigent patients most likely to acquire an STD.

Since many infected individuals develop no symptoms or fail to recognize and report symptoms, clinicians should routinely perform an STI risk assessment for teenagers and young adults as a guide to selective screening. U.S. Preventive Services Task Force Guidelines recommend screening sexually active female patients ≤25 years of age for *C. trachomatis* whenever they present for health care (at least once a year); older women should be tested if they have more than one sexual partner, have begun a new sexual relationship since the previous test, or have another STD diagnosed. In the United States, widespread selective screening of young women for cervical *C. trachomatis* infection in some regions has been associated with a 50 to 60% drop in prevalence, and such screening also protects the individual woman from PID. Sensitive urine-based genetic amplification tests permit expansion of screening to men, teenage boys, and girls in settings where examination is not planned or is impractical (e.g., during pre-participation sports examinations).

Although gonorrhea is now substantially less common than chlamydial infection in industrialized countries, screening tests for *N. gonorrhoeae* are still appropriate for women and teenage girls attending STD clinics and for sexually active teens and young women from areas of high gonorrhea prevalence. However, multiplex nucleic acid amplification tests that combine screening for *N. gonorrhoeae* and *C. trachomatis* in a single low-cost assay may facilitate the prevention and control of both infections in populations at high risk.

All patients with newly detected STIs or at high risk for STIs according to routine risk assessment as well as all pregnant women should be encouraged to undergo serologic testing for syphilis and HIV infection, with appropriate HIV counseling before and after testing. Randomized trials have shown that risk-reduction counseling of patients with STDs significantly lowers subsequent risk of acquiring an STD; such counseling should now be considered a standard component of STD management. Preimmunization serologic testing for antibody to HBV is indicated for unvaccinated persons who are known to be at high risk, such as homosexually active men and injection drug users. In most young persons, however, it is more cost-effective to vaccinate against HBV without serologic screening.

Partner notification is the process of identifying and informing partners of infected patients of possible exposure to an STI and of examining, testing, and treating partners as appropriate. In a series of 22 reports concerning partner notification during the 1990s, index patients with gonorrhea or chlamydial infection named a mean of 0.75 to 1.6 partners, of whom one-fourth to one-third were infected; those with syphilis named 1.8 to 6.3 partners, with one-third to one-half infected; and those with HIV infection named 0.76 to 5.31 partners, with up to one-fourth infected. Persons who transmit infection or who have recently been infected and are still in the incubation period usually have no symptoms or only mild symptoms and seek medical attention only when notified of their exposure. Therefore, the clinician must encourage patients to participate in partner notification, must ensure that exposed persons are notified, and must guarantee confidentiality to all involved. In the United States, local health departments often offer assistance in partner notification, treatment, and/or counseling. It seems both feasible and most useful to notify those partners exposed within the patient's likely period of infectiousness, which is often considered the preceding 1 month for gonorrhea, 1 to 2 months for chlamydial infection, and up to 3 months for early syphilis.

Persons with a new-onset STD always have a *source* contact who gave them the infection; in addition, they may have a *secondary* (*spread* or *exposed*) contact with whom they had sex after becoming infected. The identification and treatment of these two types of contacts have different objectives. Treatment of the source contact (often a casual contact) benefits the community by preventing further transmission; treatment of the recently exposed secondary contact (typically a spouse or another steady sexual partner) prevents both the development of serious complications (such as PID) in the partner and reinfection of the index patient. A recent survey of a random sample of U.S. physicians found that most instructed patients to abstain from sex during treatment, to use condoms, and to inform their sex partners after being diagnosed with gonorrhea, chlamydial infection, or syphilis; physicians sometimes gave the patients drugs for their partners. However, follow-up of the partners by physicians was infrequent. A recent randomized trial compared patients' delivery of therapy to partners exposed to gonorrhea or chlamydial infection with conventional notification and advice to partners to seek evaluation for STD; patients' delivery of therapy to their partners significantly reduced rates of re-

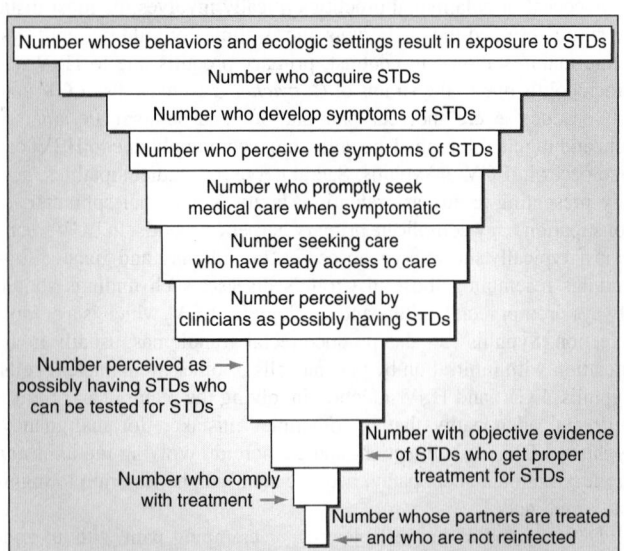

FIGURE 115-6 Critical control points for preventive and clinical interventions against sexually transmitted diseases (STDs). [*Adapted from HT Waller and MA Piot: Bull World Health Organ 41:75, 1969 and 43:1, 1970; and from "Resource allocation model for public health planning—a case study of tuberculosis control," Bull World Health Organ 84(Suppl) 1973.*]

infection of the index patient. State-by-state variations in regulations on this approach have not been well defined.

In summary, clinicians and public health agencies share responsibility for the prevention and control of STDs. In the managed-care era, the role of primary care clinicians has become increasingly important in prevention as well as in diagnosis and treatment.

FURTHER READING

ALLEN-DAVIS JT et al: Assessment of vulvovaginal complaints: Accuracy of telephone triage and in-office diagnosis. Obstet Gynecol 99:18, 2002

CENTERS FOR DISEASE CONTROL AND PREVENTION: Sexually transmitted diseases treatment guidelines 2002. MMWR 51(RR-6):1, 2002

———: Incorporating HIV prevention into the medical care of persons living with HIV. MMWR 52(RR-12):1, 2003

DALABETTA G et al (eds): Syndromic management of sexually transmitted diseases. Sex Transm Dis 74(Suppl 1):S1, 1998

ECKERT LO et al: Endometritis: The clinical-pathologic syndrome. Am J Obstet Gynecol 186:690, 2002

GROSSKURTH H et al: Impact of improved treatment of sexually transmitted diseases on HIV infection in rural Tanzania: Randomized controlled trial. Lancet 346:530, 1995

KAMB ML et al: Efficacy of risk-reduction counseling to prevent human immunodeficiency virus and sexually transmitted diseases: A randomized controlled trial. Project RESPECT Study Group. JAMA 280:1161, 1998

MCCREE DH et al: National survey of doctors' actions following the diagnosis of a bacterial STD. Sex Transm Infect 79:254, 2003

NESS RB et al: Effectiveness of inpatient and outpatient treatment strategies for women with pelvic inflammatory disease: Results from the Pelvic Inflammatory Disease Evaluation and Clinical Health (PEACH) Randomized Trial. Am J Obstet Gynecol 186:929, 2002

TAO G et al: Missed opportunities to assess sexually transmitted diseases in U.S. adults during routine medical checkups. Am J Prev Med 18:109, 2000

Section 3   Clinical Syndromes: Nosocomial Infections

116   HOSPITAL-ACQUIRED INFECTIONS
Robert A. Weinstein

The costs of nosocomial (hospital-acquired) infections are great. It is estimated that nosocomial infections affect more than 2 million patients, cost $4.5 billion, and contribute to 88,000 deaths in U.S. hospitals annually. Efforts to lower infection risks have been challenged by the growing numbers of immunocompromised patients, antibiotic-resistant bacteria, fungal and viral superinfections, and invasive devices and procedures. Nevertheless, evidence-based guidelines for prevention and control are now available (Table 116-1); according to some estimates, the consistent application of these guidelines may reduce the risk of nosocomial infection by more than one-third. This chapter reviews hospital-acquired and device-related infections and the basic surveillance, prevention, and control and treatment activities that have been developed to deal with these problems.

ORGANIZATION AND RESPONSIBILITIES OF INFECTION-CONTROL PROGRAMS   The standards of the Joint Commission on Accreditation of Healthcare Organizations require all accredited hospitals to have an active program for surveillance, prevention, and control of nosocomial infections. A multidisciplinary infection-control committee usually oversees the program. The agents of the committee are the chairperson, who is preferably an infectious disease physician, and the infection-control

practitioners, who are usually trained in nursing or medical technology and in epidemiology and public health. Education of physicians in infection control and hospital epidemiology is required in infectious disease fellowship programs and is available in courses provided by professional societies, primarily the Society for Healthcare Epidemiology of America.

Diagnosis-related reimbursement has led hospital administrators to place increased emphasis on cost containment and on documentation of the cost-effectiveness of infection control. The quality-improvement movements and the Joint Commission have redirected infection-control attention, in part, beyond the mere writing of policies and procedures to improvement of the actual processes and optimization of outcomes. In many hospitals, epidemiology programs have taken on additional pharmacoepidemiologic and antibiotic-use review responsibilities as well as broader quality-assurance activities under the rubic "patient safety." All programs must respond to governmental regulation of hospital waste and to standards mandated by the Occupational Safety & Health Administration for protecting health care workers from occupational exposure to bloodborne pathogens and tuberculosis.

SURVEILLANCE   Traditionally, infection-control practitioners have surveyed inpatients for infections acquired in hospitals (defined as those neither present nor incubating at the time of admission). Surveillance involves a review of microbiology laboratory results, "shoe-leather" epidemiology on the nursing wards, application of standardized defi-

TABLE 116-1   Sources of Infection-Control Guidance and Oversight

Organization	Role	Major Constituents	Web Site
JCAHO	Regulatory	Hospitals, long-term-care facilities, laboratories	www.jcaho.org
CAP	Regulatory	Laboratories	www.cap.org
OSHA	Regulatory	Workers	www.osha.gov
CMS (formerly HCFA)	Regulatory	Medicare/Medicaid providers	www.cms.hhs.gov
CDC			
DHQP	Advisory	Health care facilities and personnel	www.cdc.gov/ncidod/hip/default.htm
HICPAC	Advisory	Health care facilities and personnel	www.cdc.gov/ncidod/hip/HICPAC/hicpac.htm
NIOSH	Advisory	Workers	www.cdc.gov/niosh/homepage.htm
AHRQ	Advisory	Broad (e.g., health care personnel)	www.ahrq.org
NQF	Advisory	Broad (e.g., health care personnel)	www.qualityforum.org
IOM	Advisory	Broad (e.g., health care personnel)	www.iom.edu
IDSA	Professional society	Infectious disease physicians/researchers	www.idsociety.org
SHEA	Professional society	Hospital epidemiologists	www.shea-online.org
APIC	Professional society	Infection-control practitioners	www.apic.org

Abbreviations: JCAHO, Joint Commission on Accreditation of Healthcare Organizations; CAP, College of American Pathologists; OSHA, Occupational Safety & Health Administration; CMS, Centers for Medicare & Medicaid Services; HCFA, Health Care Financing Administration; CDC, Centers for Disease Control and Prevention; DHQP, Division of Healthcare Quality Promotion; HICPAC, Healthcare Infection Control Practices Advisory Committee; NIOSH, National Institute for Occupational Safety and Health; AHRQ, Agency for Healthcare Research and Quality; NQF, National Quality Forum; IOM, Institute of Medicine; IDSA, Infectious Diseases Society of America; SHEA, Society for Healthcare Epidemiology of America, Inc.; APIC, Association for Professionals in Infection Control and Epidemiology, Inc.

nitions of infection, ongoing dialogue with hospital workers, and common sense. Some innovative infection-control programs have taken advantage of the increased use of computerized pharmacy, microbiology, and other databases in hospitals to create algorithm-driven surveillance.

Most hospitals aim surveillance at infections that (1) are associated with a high level of morbidity [e.g., intensive care unit (ICU)–related infections and nosocomial pneumonia]; (2) are costly (e.g., cardiac surgical wound infections); (3) are difficult to treat (e.g., infections due to antibiotic-resistant bacteria); (4) pose recurrent epidemic problems (e.g., *Clostridium difficile*–related diarrhea); and (5) are potentially preventable (e.g., vascular access–related infections). Quality-assurance activities in infection control have led to increased surveillance of the compliance of personnel with infection-control policies (e.g., monitoring of actual adherence to hand hygiene recommendations).

The results of surveillance are expressed as rates; in general, 5 to 10% of patients develop nosocomial infections. Such overall statistics have little value unless qualified by duration of risk, by site of infection, by patient population, and by exposure to risk factors. Meaningful denominators for infection rates include the number of patients exposed to a specific risk (e.g., rates of pneumonia among patients using mechanical ventilators) and the number of intervention days (e.g., rates of pneumonia per 1000 patient-days on a ventilator).

Temporal trends in rates should be reviewed, and rates should be compared with regional and national norms. However, even comparison rates generated by the ongoing National Nosocomial Infections Surveillance System [a program of the Centers for Disease Control and Prevention (CDC)], which collects data from more than 350 hospitals that use standardized definitions of nosocomial infections, have not been validated independently and represent a nonrandom sample of hospitals. Interhospital comparisons are easily confounded by the wide range in risk factors and in severity of underlying illnesses; unless rates are adjusted for these factors, comparisons may be misleading. Unfortunately, systems for making such adjustments either are rudimentary or have not been well validated.

The ongoing analysis of an individual hospital's infection rates helps to determine whether control efforts are succeeding and where increased education and control measures should be focused. Knowledge of infection rates is also useful in discussions with the hospital administration regarding areas to which additional resources should be directed.

EPIDEMIOLOGIC BASIS AND GENERAL MEASURES FOR PREVENTION AND CONTROL

Nosocomial infections follow basic epidemiologic patterns that can help to direct prevention and control measures. Nosocomial pathogens have reservoirs, are transmitted by predictable routes, and require susceptible hosts. Reservoirs and sources exist in the inanimate environment (e.g., tap water contaminated with *Legionella*) and in the animate environment (e.g., infected or colonized health care workers, patients, and hospital visitors). The mode of transmission most often is either cross-infection (e.g., indirect spread of pathogens from one patient to another on the inadequately cleaned hands of hospital personnel) or autoinoculation (e.g., aspiration of oropharyngeal flora into the lung along an endotracheal tube). Occasionally, pathogens (e.g., group A streptococci and many respiratory viruses) are spread indirectly from person to person via infectious droplets released by coughing or sneezing. Much less common—but often devastating in terms of epidemic risk—is true airborne spread of droplet nuclei (as in nosocomial chickenpox) or common-source spread by contaminated materials (e.g., iodophors contaminated with *Pseudomonas*). Factors that increase host susceptibility include underlying conditions and the many medical-surgical interventions and procedures that bypass or compromise normal host defenses.

Through its program, the hospital's infection-control committee must determine the general and specific measures used to control infections

and must review and recommend specific antiseptics and disinfectants for hospital use. Given the prominence of cross-infection, hand hygiene is the single most important preventive measure in hospitals (Table 116-2). Health care workers' rates of adherence to hand-hygiene recommendations are abysmally low (<50%). Reasons cited include inconvenience, time pressures, and skin damage from frequent washing. Sinkless alcohol rubs are quick and highly effective and actually improve hand condition since they contain emollients and allow the retention of natural protective oils that are removed with repeated rinsing. Use of alcohol hand rubs between patient contacts is now recommended for all health care workers except when the hands are visibly soiled, in which case washing with soap and water is still required.

NOSOCOMIAL AND DEVICE-RELATED INFECTIONS   The fact that 25 to 50% of nosocomial infections are due to the combined effect of the patient's own flora and invasive devices highlights the importance of improvements in the use and design of such devices. Intensive educational programs can be associated with at least a temporary reduction in infection rates through improved asepsis in handling and earlier removal of invasive devices, but the maintenance of such gains is often difficult. Of particular note, shortages of trained personnel jeopardize safe and effective patient care and have been associated with increased rates of infection and death among patients.

Urinary Tract Infections   Urinary tract infections (UTIs) account for as many as 40 to 45% of nosocomial infections; up to 3% of bacteriuric patients develop bacteremia. Although UTIs contribute only 10 to 15% to prolongation of hospital stay and to extra costs, these infections are important reservoirs and sources for spread of antibiotic-resistant bacteria in hospitals. Almost all nosocomial UTIs are associated with preceding instrumentation or indwelling bladder catheters, which create a 3 to 10% risk of infection each day. UTIs generally are caused by pathogens that spread up the periurethral space from the patient's perineum or gastrointestinal tract—the most common pathogenesis in women—or via intraluminal contamination of urinary catheters, usually due to cross-infection by caregivers who are irrigating catheters or emptying drainage bags. Pathogens occasionally come from inadequately disinfected urologic equipment and rarely come from contaminated supplies (e.g., dilute aqueous benzalkonium chloride, an ineffective disinfectant).

The most important measures for preventing nosocomial UTIs are (1) the placement of catheters only when absolutely necessary and not solely for the convenience of caregivers, (2) the use of aseptic technique for catheter insertion and for urinary tract instrumentation, (3) the manipulation and opening of drainage systems as infrequently as possible, and (4) the removal of catheters as soon as feasible. Hospitals

---

TABLE 116-2 *Examples of Ways in which Physicians Can Contribute to Infection-Control Efforts*

- Act as role models for other personnel by paying careful attention to hand-hygiene recommendations and barrier precautions during contact with patients and by observing posted isolation precautions.
- Give corrective feedback to caregivers who do not adhere to hand-hygiene recommendations or isolation precautions.
- Place invasive devices based on clinical need (not just on convenience).
- Remove invasive devices promptly when they are no longer needed clinically.
- Limit surgical antimicrobial prophylaxis to the perioperative period.
- Exercise care in initial empirical antibiotic selection (avoid "shotgun" approaches).
- Narrow the spectrum of antibiotic therapy once a pathogen is recovered.
- Discontinue antibiotic therapy in a timely fashion.
- Become familiar with the hospital's bloodborne pathogen and tuberculosis control plans.
- Order appropriate isolation precautions promptly for infected patients.
- During patient rounds, alert nursing staff to lapses in asepsis (e.g., soiled dressings at sites of intravascular catheters) and to infection-predisposing situations (e.g., aspiration-prone positioning of patients).
- Notify infection-control practitioners of potential infection-control problems (e.g., surgical wound infections that manifest after a patient's discharge).

should develop criteria for and closely monitor these four performance measures.

Sealed catheter–drainage tube junctions can help to prevent breaks in the system. Approaches to the prevention of UTIs also have included the use of topical meatal antimicrobials, drainage bag disinfectants, and anti-infective catheters. A meta-analysis and more recent studies suggest that silver alloy–coated catheters may reduce the incidence of bacteriuria, at least during short-term catheterization. However, because of conflicting study results, none of the latter three measures is considered routine.

Systemic antimicrobials given for other purposes decrease the risk of UTI during the first 4 days of catheterization, after which resistant bacteria or yeasts emerge as pathogens. Selective decontamination of the gut is also associated with a reduced risk. Again, however, neither approach is routine.

Irrigation of catheters, with or without antimicrobials, may actually increase the risk of infection. A condom catheter for men without bladder obstruction may be more acceptable than an indwelling catheter, but the infection risks with the two types are similar unless the condom catheter is carefully maintained. The role of suprapubic catheters in preventing infection is not well defined.

Treatment of UTIs is based on the results of quantitative cultures of urine (see Chap. 269); the most common pathogens are *Escherichia coli*, nosocomial gram-negative bacilli, enterococci, and *Candida*. Several caveats apply in the treatment of institutionally acquired infection. First, in patients with chronic indwelling bladder catheters, especially those in long-term-care facilities, the "catheter flora"—microorganisms living in the biofilm or on encrustations within the catheter lumen—may differ from the actual urinary tract pathogens. Therefore, for suspected infection in the setting of chronic catheterization (especially in women), it is useful to replace the bladder catheter and to obtain a freshly voided urine specimen. Second, as in all nosocomial infections, at the time treatment is initiated on the basis of a positive culture, it is useful to repeat the culture to verify the persistence of infection. Third, the frequency with which UTIs occur may lead to the erroneous assumption that this site alone is the source of infection in a febrile hospitalized patient. Thus, in the treatment of nosocomial UTIs, it is important to assess the patient for symptoms, especially of upper-pole infection (e.g., flank pain in conscious patients), and for signs of abnormal urinary sediment. Since nosocomial UTIs usually occur in the setting of catheterization or recent instrumentation, lower-tract symptoms (e.g., dysuria) may not be reliable. Fourth, recovery of *Staphylococcus aureus* from urine cultures may result from hematogenous seeding and may indicate an occult systemic infection. Finally, although *Candida* is now the most common pathogen in nosocomial UTIs in ICU patients, it is not clear that candiduria in the absence of upper-pole invasion, obstruction, neutropenia, or immunosuppression warrants treatment.

Pneumonia Pneumonia accounts for 15 to 20% of nosocomial infections but has been responsible for 24% of extra hospital days and 39% of extra costs—i.e., 6 days and $6000 (based on 1992 dollars) per episode. Almost all cases of bacterial nosocomial pneumonia are caused by aspiration of endogenous or hospital-acquired oropharyngeal (and occasionally gastric) flora. Nosocomial pneumonias are associated with more deaths than are infections at any other body site. However, attributable mortality for ventilator-associated pneumonia—the most common and lethal form of nosocomial pneumonia—is in the 6 to 14% range; this figure suggests that the risk of dying from nosocomial pneumonia is affected greatly by other factors, including comorbidities, inadequate antibiotic treatment, and the involvement of specific pathogens (particularly *Pseudomonas aeruginosa* and *Acinetobacter*). Surveillance and accurate diagnosis of pneumonia are often problematic in hospitals because many patients, especially those in the ICU, have abnormal chest roentgenographs, fever, and leukocytosis potentially attributable to multiple causes. →*Viral pneumonias, which are particularly important in pediatric and immunocompromised patients, are discussed in the virology section and in Chap. 239.*

Risk factors for nosocomial pneumonia, particularly ventilator-associated pneumonia, include those events that increase the risk of colonization by potential pathogens (e.g., prior antimicrobial therapy, contaminated ventilator circuits or equipment, or decreased gastric acidity); those that heighten the possibility of aspiration of oropharyngeal contents into the lower respiratory tract (e.g., intubation, decreased levels of consciousness, or presence of a nasogastric tube); and those that reduce host defense mechanisms in the lung and permit overgrowth of aspirated pathogens (e.g., chronic obstructive pulmonary disease, old age, or upper abdominal surgery).

Control measures for pneumonia are aimed at the remediation of risk factors in general patient care (e.g., minimizing aspiration-prone supine positioning) and at meticulous aseptic care of respirator equipment (e.g., disinfecting or sterilizing all inline reusable components such as nebulizers, replacing tubing circuits at intervals of >48 h—rather than more frequently—to lessen the number of breaks in the system, and teaching aseptic technique for suctioning). In a large multicenter trial, sucralfate, which provides stress-ulcer prophylaxis without altering gastric pH, did not reduce the risk of ventilator-associated pneumonia, despite the theoretical advantage of lessened risk for gastric colonization by gram-negative bacilli. The benefits of selective decontamination of the oropharynx and gut with nonabsorbable antimicrobials and/or use of short-course postintubation systemic antibiotics have been controversial. Among the logical preventive measures that require further investigation are the use of endotracheal tubes that provide channels for subglottic drainage of secretions and the use of noninvasive mechanical ventilation whenever feasible. Of note, even interventions that have reduced the rate of ventilator-associated pneumonia most often have not reduced overall ICU mortality; this fact suggests that this infection is a marker for patients with an otherwise-heightened risk of death.

The most likely pathogens for nosocomial pneumonia and treatment options are discussed in Chap. 239. Several considerations regarding diagnosis and treatment are worth emphasizing. Clinical criteria for diagnosis (e.g., fever, leukocytosis, development of purulent secretions, new or changing radiographic infiltrates, change in oxygen requirement or ventilator settings) have high sensitivity but relatively low specificity. These criteria are most useful for selecting patients for bronchoscopic or nonbronchoscopic procedures that yield lower respiratory tract samples protected from upper-tract contamination; quantitative cultures of such specimens have diagnostic sensitivities in the range of 80%. Early-onset nosocomial pneumonia, which manifests within the first 4 days of hospitalization, is most often caused by community-acquired pathogens, such as *Streptococcus pneumoniae* and *Haemophilus* species. Late-onset pneumonias most commonly are due to *S. aureus*, *P. aeruginosa*, *Enterobacter* species, *Klebsiella pneumoniae*, or *Acinetobacter*—a pathogen of increasing concern in many ICUs. When invasive techniques are used to diagnose ventilator-associated pneumonia, the proportion of isolates accounted for by gram-negative bacilli decreases from 50–70% to 35–45%. Infection is polymicrobial in as many as 20 to 40% of cases. The role of anaerobic bacteria in ventilator-associated pneumonia is not well defined. The appropriate duration of therapy for nosocomial pneumonia, although generally stated to be in the 10- to 21-day range, is not well studied. Finally, in febrile patients (particularly those who have endotracheal and/or nasogastric tubes), more occult sources of respiratory tract infection, especially bacterial sinusitis and otitis media, should be considered.

Surgical Wound Infections Wound infections account for up to 20 to 30% of nosocomial infections but contribute up to 57% of extra hospital days and 42% of extra costs. Because the average wound infection has an incubation period of 5 to 7 days, which is longer than many postoperative stays, and because many procedures now are performed on an outpatient basis, the incidence of wound infections has become difficult to assess. These infections usually are caused by the patient's endogenous or hospital-acquired skin and mucosal flora and occasionally are due to airborne spread of skin squames that may be shed into the wound from members of the operating-room team. True airborne spread of infection through droplet nuclei is rare in operating rooms unless there is a "disseminator" (e.g., of group A streptococci or staphylococci) among the staff. In general, the most common risks for postoperative wound infection are deficits in the surgeon's technical skill, the patient's underlying diseases (e.g., diabetes mellitus, obesity), and inappropriate timing of antibiotic prophylaxis. Additional risk factors include the presence of drains, prolonged preoperative hospital stays, shaving of the operative site the day before surgery, a long duration of surgery, and infection at remote sites (e.g., untreated UTI).

The substantial literature related to risk factors for surgical-site infections and the recognized morbidity and cost of these infections have led to careful evaluation of a number of interventions. The most important control measures include the use of antimicrobial prophylaxis at the start of high-risk procedures (see Chap. 118), attention to technical surgical issues and operating-room asepsis (e.g., not shaving the operative site until surgery and avoiding open or prophylactic drains), and preoperative therapy for active infection. Reporting of surveillance results to surgeons has been associated with reductions in infection rates. Measures that improve patients' resistance to infection are rare; thus the reductions in postoperative wound-infection rates associated with use of supplemental oxygen, maintenance of normothermia, or improved perioperative glucose control in recent studies are particularly exciting. The increasingly extensive review of infection rates by regulatory agencies and third-party payers emphasizes the importance of stratifying rates by patient-related risk factors and of developing meaningful systems for interhospital comparisons and for wound surveillance after the patient's discharge from the hospital or clinic (when more than 50% of infections first become apparent). The epidemic of mad cow disease, centered in the United Kingdom, and associated cases of variant Creutzfeldt-Jakob disease in humans (Chap. 362) caused by disinfection-resistant prion agents are leading to new recommendations for decontamination of surgical instruments, especially those used for operations on the central nervous system or in patients with a dementing illness of unknown etiology.

The process of diagnosing and treating wound infections begins with a careful assessment of the surgical site in the febrile postoperative patient. Clinical findings range from obvious cellulitis or abscess formation to subtle clues such as a sternal "click" following open heart surgery. Diagnosis of deeper organ-space infections or subphrenic abscesses requires a high index of suspicion and the use of computed tomography or magnetic resonance imaging. Diagnosis of infections of prosthetic devices, such as orthopedic implants, may be particularly difficult and often requires the use of interventional radiographic techniques to obtain periprosthetic specimens for culture. The most common pathogens in postoperative wound infections are *S. aureus*, coagulase-negative staphylococci, and enteric and anaerobic bacteria. In rapidly progressing postoperative infections, which manifest within 24 to 48 h of a surgical procedure, the level of suspicion regarding group A streptococcal or clostridial infection (Chaps. 121 and 126) should be high. Treatment of postoperative wound infections requires drainage or surgical excision of infected or necrotic material and antibiotic therapy aimed at the most likely or laboratory-confirmed pathogens.

Infections Related to Vascular Access and Monitoring   Intravascular devices are common causes of local site infection and cause up to 50% of nosocomial bacteremias; central vascular catheters account for 80 to 90% of these infections. National estimates indicate that as many as 250,000 bloodstream infections associated with central vascular catheters occur each year in the United States, with an attributable mortality of 12 to 25% and an estimated cost of $25,000 per episode; one-third to one-half of these episodes occur in ICUs. With increasing care of seriously ill patients in the community, vascular catheter–associated bloodstream infections acquired by outpatients are receiving more at-

tention than in the past. A recent study of bacteremia patients at three hospitals showed that the numbers of patients being treated for device-associated bacteremia acquired in the hospital or in the community setting (e.g., home or clinic intravascular therapy) were similar. This finding emphasizes the need to broaden surveillance activities.

Catheter-related bloodstream infections derive largely from the cutaneous microflora of the insertion site, with pathogens migrating extraluminally to the catheter tip, usually during the first week after insertion. In addition, contamination of hubs of central vascular catheters may lead to intraluminal infection over longer periods, particularly with surgically implanted or cuffed catheters. Intrinsic contamination of infusate, although rare, is the most common cause of epidemic device-related bloodstream infection; extrinsic contamination may cause up to half of endemic bacteremias related to arterial infusions used for hemodynamic monitoring. The most common pathogens isolated from vascular device–associated bacteremias include coagulase-negative staphylococci, *S. aureus* (with up to 50% of isolates potentially resistant to methicillin), enterococci, nosocomial gram-negative bacilli, and *Candida*.

Infections related to vascular catheters and monitoring devices may be the most preventable of nosocomial infections. Evidence-based control measures include implementing educational programs with didactic and interactive components for persons who insert and maintain catheters, using maximal sterile barrier precautions (e.g., gowns, gloves, masks, and large drapes) during catheter placement, using chlorhexidine for skin antisepsis prior to catheter placement, and ensuring that "idle catheters" are removed. Hospitals should periodically monitor adherence to these performance indicators. Use of antimicrobial- or antiseptic-impregnated central venous catheters is a reasonable control measure for adults whose catheters are expected to remain in place for >5 days if, after implementation of the performance measures just listed, the rates of catheter-related bloodstream infection remain above the goals set by individual institutions based on benchmark national rates and local factors. Additional control measures for infections associated with vascular access include avoiding the femoral site for catheterization because of an unusually high risk of infection (most likely related to the density of the skin flora); moving peripheral catheters to a new site at specified intervals (e.g., every 72 to 96 h), which may be facilitated by use of an intravenous therapy team; and applying disposable transducers for pressure monitoring and aseptic technique for accessing transducers or other vascular ports. Improvements in composition of semitransparent access-site dressings and potential nursing benefits (ease of bathing and site inspection, protection of site from secretions) favor the use of such coverings. Unresolved issues include the best frequency for rotation of central vascular catheter sites (given that guidewire-assisted catheter changes at the same site do not lessen infection risk); the appropriate role of mupirocin ointment, a topical antibiotic with excellent antistaphylococcal activity, in site care; the relative degrees of risk posed by peripherally inserted central catheters (PICC lines); and the risk-benefit of prophylactic use of heparin to avoid catheter thrombi, which may be associated with increased risk of infection.

Vascular device–related infection is suspected on the basis of the appearance of the catheter site or the presence of fever or bacteremia without another source in patients with vascular catheters. The diagnosis is confirmed by the recovery of the same species of microorganism from peripheral-blood cultures (preferably two cultures drawn from peripheral veins by separate venipunctures) and from semiquantitative or quantitative cultures of the vascular catheter tip. Less commonly used diagnostic measures include differential time to positivity (>2 h) for blood drawn through the vascular access device compared with a sample from a peripheral vein or differences in quantitative cultures (a 5- to 10-fold or greater "step-up") for blood samples drawn simultaneously from a peripheral vein and from a central vascular catheter. When infusion-related sepsis is considered (e.g., because of the abrupt onset of fever or shock temporally related to infusion therapy), a sample of the infusate or blood product should be retained for culture.

Therapy for vascular access–related infection is directed at the pathogen recovered from the blood and/or infected site. Important considerations in treatment are the need for an echocardiogram (to evaluate the patient for bacterial endocarditis), the duration of therapy, and the need to remove potentially infected catheters. In one report, approximately one-fourth of patients with intravascular catheter–associated *S. aureus* bacteremia studied by transesophageal echocardiography had evidence of endocarditis; the implication is that this test may be useful in determining the appropriate duration of treatment. Detailed consensus guidelines for the management of intravascular catheter–related infections have been published and recommend catheter removal in most cases of bacteremia or fungemia due to nontunneled central venous catheters. When attempting to salvage a potentially infected catheter, some clinicians use the "antibiotic lock" technique (instillation of concentrated antibiotic solution into the catheter lumen) in addition to systemic antimicrobial therapy. In one study of hemodialysis catheters, only about one-third of salvage attempts were successful, although delayed removal did not appear to increase the risk of complications. When feasible, a potentially infected central vascular catheter may be exchanged over a guidewire. If cultures of the removed catheter tip are positive, the replacement catheter will be moved to a new site; if the tip cultures are negative, the replacement catheter can remain in the original site. For patients with track-site infection, successful therapy without catheter removal is unusual. For patients with suppurative venous thrombophlebitis, excision of the affected vein is required. The authors of the consensus guidelines advise that the decision to remove a tunneled catheter or implanted device suspected to be the source of bacteremia or fungemia should be based on the severity of the patient's illness, the strength of the evidence that the device is infected, an assessment of the specific pathogens, and the presence of local or systemic complications.

ISOLATION TECHNIQUES Written policies for the isolation of infectious patients are a standard component of infection-control programs. In 1996, the CDC revised its isolation guidelines to make them simpler; to recognize the importance of all body fluids, secretions, and excretions in the transmission of nosocomial pathogens; and to focus precautions on the major routes of infection transmission.

The revised guidelines contain two tiers of precautions. *Standard precautions* are designed for the care of all patients in hospitals to reduce the risk of transmission of microorganisms from both recognized and unrecognized sources of infection. These precautions include gloving as well as hand cleansing for potential contact with (1) blood; (2) all other body fluids, secretions, and excretions, whether or not they contain visible blood; (3) nonintact skin; and (4) mucous membranes. Depending on exposure risks, standard precautions also include use of masks, eye protection, and gowns.

In the second tier are precautions for the care of patients with suspected or diagnosed colonization or infection with transmissible pathogens. These transmission-based guidelines collapse the older category- and disease-specific isolation guidelines into three sets of precautions based on probable routes of transmission: *airborne precautions*, *droplet precautions*, and *contact precautions*. Sets of precautions may be combined for diseases that have more than one route of transmission (e.g., varicella). Potentially contagious clinical syndromes, such as acute diarrhea, are included in the revised guidelines.

Because some prevalent antibiotic-resistant pathogens, particularly vancomycin-resistant enterococci (VRE), may be present on *intact* skin of patients in hospitals, some experts recommend gloving for all contact with patients who are acutely ill and/or from high-risk units, such as ICUs. In recent trials, wearing gloves did not replace the need for hand hygiene because hands occasionally became contaminated during wearing or removal of gloves. Some studies have suggested that use of gowns and gloves compared with routine care of patients (i.e., using neither of these barriers) decreases the risk of nosocomial infection; however, more recent evaluation suggests that gowning by personnel does not add benefit beyond that conferred by gloving and hand hygiene. Nevertheless, requiring increased precaution levels can

improve the compliance of health care workers with isolation recommendations by 30%.

EPIDEMIC AND EMERGING PROBLEMS Outbreaks and emerging pathogens are always big news but probably account for fewer than 5% of nosocomial infections. Concern about emerging pathogens often prompts authorities to require hospitals to develop contingency and response plans. The investigation and control of nosocomial epidemics require that infection-control personnel develop a case definition, confirm that an outbreak really exists (since many apparent epidemics are actually pseudo-outbreaks due to surveillance or laboratory artifacts), review aseptic practices and disinfectant use, determine the extent of the outbreak, perform an epidemiologic investigation to determine modes of transmission, work closely with microbiology personnel to culture for common sources or personnel carriers as appropriate and to type epidemiologically important isolates, and heighten surveillance to judge the effect of control measures. Control measures generally include the early reinforcement of routine aseptic practices and hand hygiene during a search for compliance problems that may have fostered the outbreak, the ensuring of the appropriate isolation of cases (and the institution of cohort isolation and nursing if needed), and the implementation of further controls on the basis of the investigation's findings. Examples of some emerging and potential epidemic problems follow.

Chickenpox When health care workers are exposed to chickenpox in the community or through patients with initially unrecognized infections, or when these employees work during the 24 h before developing chickenpox, infection-control practitioners institute a varicella exposure investigation and control plan. The names of exposed workers and patients are obtained; medical histories are reviewed, and (if necessary) serologic tests for immunity are conducted; physicians are notified of susceptible exposed patients; postexposure prophylaxis with varicella-zoster immune globulin (VZIG) is considered for immunocompromised or pregnant contacts (see Table 164-1); preemptive use of acyclovir is considered as an alternative strategy in some susceptible persons; and susceptible exposed employees are furloughed during the at-risk period for disease (8 to 21 days, or 28 days if VZIG has been administered). Routine varicella vaccination of children and susceptible employees can markedly decrease risk and frequency of exposures.

Tuberculosis The resurgence of pulmonary tuberculosis in the United States since 1987 and a series of nosocomial outbreaks of infection with multidrug-resistant strains—primarily involving patients with AIDS and their caregivers—led to a successful revamping of tuberculosis control. Important control measures include prompt recognition, isolation, and treatment of cases; recognition of atypical presentations (e.g., lower-lobe infiltrates without cavitation); use of negative-pressure, 100% exhaust, private isolation rooms with closed doors and 6 to 12 or more air changes per hour; use of face masks ("respirators" approved by the National Institute for Occupational Safety and Health) by caregivers entering isolation rooms; possible use of high-efficiency particulate air filter units and/or ultraviolet lights for disinfecting air when other engineering controls are not feasible or reliable; and follow-up skin-testing of susceptible personnel who have been exposed to infectious patients before isolation.

Group A Streptococci The potential for a group A streptococcal outbreak should be considered when even a single nosocomial case occurs. Most outbreaks involve surgical wounds and are due to the presence of an asymptomatic carrier in the operating room. Investigation can be confounded by carriage at extrapharyngeal sites such as the rectum and vagina. Health care workers in whom carriage has been linked to nosocomial transmission of group A streptococci are removed from the patient-care setting and are not permitted to return until carriage has been eliminated by antimicrobial therapy.

Aspergillus Fungal spores are common in the environment, particularly on dusty surfaces. When hospital ceiling tiles are removed to provide access for repairs or when dusty areas are disturbed during hospital renovation, the spores become airborne. Inhalation of spores by immunosuppressed (especially neutropenic) patients creates a risk of pulmonary and/or paranasal sinus infection and disseminated aspergillosis. Routine surveillance among neutropenic patients for infections with filamentous fungi, such as *Aspergillus* and *Fusarium*, helps hospitals to determine whether they have unduly large environmental risks. As a matter of routine, hospitals should inspect and clean air-handling equipment, review all planned renovations with infection-control personnel and subsequently construct appropriate barriers, remove immunosuppressed patients from renovation sites, and consider the use of high-efficiency particulate air intake filters for rooms housing immunosuppressed patients.

Legionella Sporadic and epidemic cases of nosocomial *Legionella* pneumonia are most often due to the contamination of potable water and predominantly affect immunosuppressed patients, particularly those receiving glucocorticoid medication. The risk varies greatly within and among geographic regions, depending on the extent of hospital hot-water contamination, on the presence or absence of high-risk patient populations, and on specific hospital practices (e.g., inappropriate use of nonsterile water in respiratory therapy equipment). Laboratory-based surveillance for nosocomial *Legionella* should be performed, and a diagnosis of legionellosis should probably be considered more often than it is. If cases are detected, environmental samples (e.g., tap water) should be cultured. If cultures yield *Legionella* and if typing of clinical and environmental isolates reveals a correlation, eradication measures should be pursued (Chap. 132). An alternative approach is to periodically culture tap water in wards housing high-risk patients. If *Legionella* is found, a concerted effort should be made to culture samples from all patients with nosocomial pneumonia for *Legionella*.

Antibiotic-Resistant Bacteria Outbreaks of antibiotic resistance can depend on any of the following events: Darwinian selection of bacterial chromosomal mutations, spread of plasmid- and/or transposon-borne resistance among bacterial species, and (re)admission to the hospital of patients chronically infected with resistant bacteria. After the introduction of resistant strains, dissemination occurs by cross-infection on contaminated hands of caregivers or, occasionally, via personnel carriage and/or environmental contamination. Outbreak control (Table 116-3) depends on close laboratory surveillance, with early detection of problems; on the reinforcement of routine asepsis (e.g., hand hygiene); on the implementation of barrier precautions for all colonized and/or infected patients; on the use of patient-surveillance cultures to more fully ascertain the extent of patient colonization; and on the timely initiation of an epidemiologic investigation when rates increase. Colonized personnel who are implicated in nosocomial transmission and patients who pose a threat may be decontaminated; for example, colonization with methicillin-resistant *S. aureus* may be controlled

with oral antibiotics, including trimethoprim-sulfamethoxazole and rifampin, and with topical agents, including hexachlorophene or chlorhexidine and mupirocin. In a few ICUs, selective decontamination has been used successfully as a temporary emergency control measure for outbreaks of infection due to gram-negative bacilli.

An emerging bacterial-resistance problem to plague hospitals is the presence of VRE. Initially an ICU problem, VRE have now spread onto general wards in many hospitals. VRE are particularly problematic because of a substantial "iceberg" effect (i.e., the fact that, for each individual with a clinical infection, many other patients are colonized); the occurrence of both gastrointestinal and skin colonization (reflecting fecal contamination on the skin of ill, hospitalized patients); and the propensity for these organisms to contaminate the patient's environment, which may increase the risk of cross-infection. Control of VRE requires strict attention to hand hygiene by personnel, concerted use of barrier precautions or cohort nursing for patients known to be colonized or infected, and emphasis on thorough cleaning of the rooms of these patients.

Spread of vancomycin resistance to *S. aureus* is a major concern. Clinical infections with methicillin-resistant *S. aureus* strains that exhibit high-level vancomycin resistance due to VRE-derived plasmids have now been reported in the setting of prolonged or repeated treatment with vancomycin and/or VRE colonization. The detection of these strains appears to be readily accomplished in clinical microbiology laboratories and should trigger an aggressive epidemiologic investigation and infection-control measures.

Because the excessive use of broad-spectrum antibiotics underlies many resistance problems, aggressive antibiotic-control policies must be considered a cornerstone of resistance-control efforts. Although the efficacy of antibiotic-control measures in reducing rates of antimicrobial resistance has not been proved in prospective controlled trials, it seems worthwhile to restrict the use of particular agents to narrowly defined indications or possibly to cycle the use of antibiotic classes to limit selective pressure on the nosocomial flora.

Bioterrorism Preparedness The terrorist attack on the World Trade Center in New York City; other horrific events of September 11, 2001; and the subsequent mailings of anthrax spores in the United States have made bioterrorism a prominent source of concern to hospital

---

TABLE 116-3 *Controlling Antibiotic Resistance: Approaches to Consider*

- Conduct surveillance for antibiotic resistance.
- Perform molecular typing (e.g., pulsed-field gel electrophoresis) when rates increase.
- For clonal expansion (e.g., single-strain outbreaks): Stress hand hygiene (alcohol hand rub and universal gloving); monitor adherence and give feedback.
- For polyclonal expansion (e.g., multistrain outbreaks): Stress antibiotic prudence (consider antibiotic rotation for ICUs); monitor adherence and give feedback.
- For continued problems: Obtain patient-surveillance cultures and isolate or provide cohort nursing for colonized/infected patients.
- Control device-related infections.
- Enlist administrative support proactively.

Source: Adapted from: RA Weinstein, *Emerg Infect Dis* 7:188, 2001.

TABLE 116-4 *Highlights of Hospital Preparedness for Bioterrorism*

Emergency Department: Educate staff regarding bioterrorism diagnoses, case definitions, and appropriate syndrome-based isolation precautions.

Laboratory: Identify protocols and laboratory safety procedures for agents of bioterrorism.

Pharmacy: Develop medication and vaccine par stock, allocation, and delivery plans.

Nursing: Assess bed and isolation surge capacity; help develop contingency plans to free bed space by early discharges and deferred admissions.

Hospital Police: Plan for responsibilities as first responders and providers of risk assessment.

Mailroom: Plan for risk assessment and need/indications-for-use of personal protective equipment as appropriate.

Engineering/Buildings and Grounds: Evaluate air-handling systems and ensure familiarity with shutoffs and controls; educate staff about environmental decontamination.

Outpatient Areas: Develop plans for family and community evaluation and staging for delivery of prophylactic medications and/or vaccines.

Public Health: Ascertain local public health resources and open lines of communication, education, and surveillance.

The Community: Plan for infection-control practitioners to serve as liaisons/links/facilitators for emergency departments, laboratories, and community providers.

Administration: Perform resource assessment for medical supplies, transportation capabilities, potable water, sanitation facilities, provider backup, bed-space backup, etc. Oversee development of an incident command system.

"Morale Officer": Establish this position to help survey and keep staff functioning.

infection-control programs. The essentials for hospital preparedness (Table 116-4) entail education, internal and external communication, and risk assessment. Among the category A agents of bioterrorism (Chap. 205), smallpox is of major concern to the U.S. intelligence community. Consequently, in December 2002, the President of the United States recommended smallpox vaccination of a core group of military and hospital personnel; up-to-date information on a variety of vaccination-related and other bioterrorism-associated issues is available from the CDC (see www.bt.cdc.gov).

EMPLOYEE HEALTH SERVICE ISSUES An institution's employee health service is a critical component of its infection-control efforts. New employees should be processed through the service, where a contagious-disease history can be taken; evidence of immunity to a variety of diseases, such as hepatitis B, chickenpox, measles, and rubella, can be sought; immunizations for hepatitis B, measles, rubella, and varicella can be given as needed and a reminder about the need for yearly influenza immunization can be imparted; baseline and "booster" purified protein derivative of tuberculin skin-testing can be performed; and education about personal responsibility for infection control can be initiated. Evaluations of employees should be codified to meet the requirements of accrediting and regulatory agencies.

The employee health service must have protocols for dealing with workers who have been exposed to contagious diseases, such as those percutaneously or mucosally exposed to the blood of patients infected with HIV or hepatitis B or C virus. For example, postexposure HIV prophylaxis with a combination of two or three antiretroviral agents is recommended; free consultation is available from the CDC PEPLine (1-888-HIV-4911). Protocols are also needed for dealing with caregivers who have common contagious diseases, such as chickenpox,

group A streptococcal infections, respiratory infections, and infectious diarrhea, and for those who have less common but high-visibility public health problems, such as chronic hepatitis B or C or HIV infection, for which exposure-control guidelines have been published by the CDC and by the Society for Healthcare Epidemiology of America.

FURTHER READING

CENTERS FOR DISEASE CONTROL AND PREVENTION: Guideline for hand hygiene in health-care settings: Recommendations of the Healthcare Infection Control Practices Advisory Committee and the HICPAC/SHEA/APIC/IDSA Hand Hygiene Task Force. MMWR 51(RR-16):1, 2002

———: Guidelines for preventing opportunistic infections among hematopoietic stem cell transplant recipients: Recommendations of CDC, the Infectious Diseases Society of America, and the American Society of Blood and Marrow Transplantation. MMWR 49(RR-10):1, 2000

HUBMAYR RD: Statement of the 4th International Consensus Conference in Critical Care on ICU-Acquired Pneumonia. Intensive Care Med 28:1521, 2002

MAKI DG, WEINSTEIN RA: Nosocomial infection in the intensive care unit, in *Critical Care Medicine—Principles of Diagnosis and Management in the Adult*, 2d ed, JE Parillo, RP Dellinger (eds). Saunders, Philadelphia, 2001, pp 981–1046

MERMEL LA et al: Guidelines for the management of intravascular catheter–related infections. Clin Infect Dis 32:1249, 2001

O'GRADY NP et al: Guidelines for the prevention of intravascular catheter–related infections. Clin Infect Dis 35:1281, 2002

SCHWARTZ DS, WEINSTEIN RA: Fever in hospitalized patients, in *Clinical Infectious Diseases: A Practical Approach*, R Root et al (eds). Oxford, New York, 1999, pp 449–458

WEINSTEIN RA, BONTEN M (eds): *Infection Control in the ICU Environment*. Boston, Kluwer, 2002

117 INFECTIONS IN TRANSPLANT RECIPIENTS
Robert Finberg, Joyce Fingeroth

The evaluation of infections in transplant recipients involves consideration of both the donor and the recipient of the transplanted organ. Infections following transplantation are complicated by the use of drugs that are necessary to enhance the likelihood of survival of the transplanted organ but that also cause the host to be immunocompromised. Thus what might have been a latent or asymptomatic infection in an immunocompetent donor or in the recipient prior to therapy becomes a life-threatening problem when the recipient becomes immunosuppressed.

A variety of organisms have been transmitted by organ transplantation (Table 117-1). Careful attention to the sterility of the medium used to process the organ combined with meticulous microbiologic evaluation reduces rates of transmission of bacteria that may be present or grow in the organ culture medium. From 2% to >20% of donor kidneys are estimated to be contaminated with bacteria—in most cases, with the organisms that colonize the skin or grow in the tissue culture medium used to bathe the donor kidney while it awaits implantation. The reported rate of bacterial contamination of transplanted bone marrow is as high as 17% but is most commonly ~1%. The use of enrichment columns and monoclonal-antibody depletion procedures results in a higher incidence of contamination. Approximately 2% of cryopreserved marrow and peripheral-blood stem cells transfused as part of treatment for cancer are contaminated. In one series of patients receiving contaminated products, 14% had fever or bacteremia, but none died. Results of cultures performed at the time of cryopreservation and at the time of thawing were helpful in guiding therapy for the recipient.

In many transplantation centers, transmission of infections that may be latent or clinically inapparent in the donor organ has resulted in the development of specific donor-screening protocols. In addition to ordering serologic studies focusing on viruses such as herpes-group viruses [herpes simplex virus (HSV) 1, HSV-2], varicella-zoster virus (VZV), cytomegalovirus (CMV), human herpesvirus (HHV) type 6, Epstein-Barr virus (EBV), HHV-8, hepatitis B and C viruses, HIV, and human T-cell lymphotropic virus (HTLV) type I and on parasites such as *Toxoplasma gondii*, clinicians caring for organ donors should consider assessing stool (for parasites) and should perform skin testing for *Mycobacterium tuberculosis*. An investigation of the patient's dietary habits (e.g., consumption of raw meat or fish or of unpasteurized dairy products), occupations or avocations (e.g., gardening or spelunking), and travel history (e.g., travel to areas with endemic fungi) is mandatory. It is expected that the recipient will have been likewise assessed. This chapter considers aspects of infection unique to various transplantation settings.

INFECTIONS IN BONE MARROW AND HEMATOPOIETIC STEM CELL TRANSPLANT RECIPIENTS

Bone marrow or hematopoietic stem cell transplantation for either immunodeficiency or cancer results in a transient state of complete immune incompetence. Immediately after transplantation, both phagocytes and immune cells (T and B cells) are absent, and the host is extremely susceptible to infection. The reconstitution that follows transplantation has been likened to maturation of the immune system in neonates. The analogy does not entirely predict infections seen in bone marrow transplant (BMT) and hematopoietic stem cell transplant (HSCT) recipients because the new marrow matures in an old host who has several latent infections already. Nevertheless, infections occur in a predictable time frame after transplantation (Table 117-2).

BACTERIAL INFECTIONS In the first month after bone marrow or hematopoietic stem cell transplantation, infectious complications are similar to those in granulocytopenic patients receiving chemotherapy for acute leukemia (Chap. 72). Because of the anticipated 1- to 4-week duration

TABLE 117-1　*Organisms Transmitted by Organ Transplantation and Sites of Reactivation Disease*[a]

	Blood	Lungs	Heart	Brain	Liver	Skin
Viruses						
Cytomegalovirus[b]	+	+	+/–	+	+	+
Epstein-Barr virus[c]	+	+	+	+	+	+
Herpes simplex virus		+			+	+
Human herpesvirus type 6	+	+		+		+
Human herpesvirus type 8[b]	+	+/–			+/–	+
Hepatitis B and C viruses					+	
Bovine spongiform encephalopathy (prion)[d]				+		
Rabies virus[e]				+		
West Nile virus				+		
Fungi						
Candida albicans	+	+			+	+
Histoplasma capsulatum	+	+			+	
Cryptococcus neoformans	+	+		+		+
Parasites						
Toxoplasma gondii[f]		+	+	+		
Strongyloides stercoralis[g,h]		+				
Trypanosoma cruzi[h]			+			
Plasmodium falciparum[h]	+					

[a] +, well documented; ±, probably occurs.
[b] Cytomegalovirus reactivation is prone to occur in the transplanted organ. The same may be true for human herpesvirus type 8 (Kaposi's sarcoma–associated herpesvirus).
[c] Epstein-Barr virus reactivation usually presents as an extranodal proliferation of transformed B cells and can be present either as a diffuse disease or as a mass lesion in a single organ.
[d] Bovine spongiform encephalopathy, a prion-mediated disease, can be transmitted with organs.
[e] Rabies has been transmitted through corneal transplants.
[f] T. gondii usually causes disease in the brain. In bone marrow transplant recipients, acute pulmonary disease may also occur. Heart transplant recipients develop disease in the allograft.
[g] Strongyloides "hyperinfection" may present with pulmonary disease—often associated with gram-negative bacterial pneumonia.
[h] While transmission with organs has been described, it is unusual.

of neutropenia and the high rate of bacterial infection in this population, many centers give prophylactic antibiotics to patients upon initiation of chemotherapy. Levofloxacin decreases the incidence of gram-negative bacteremia among these patients. Bacterial infections are common in the first few days after bone marrow transplantation.

The organisms involved are predominantly aerobic bacteria found in the bowels (*Escherichia coli*, *Klebsiella*, *Pseudomonas*) and those found on the skin or in intravenous catheters (*Staphylococcus aureus*, coagulase-negative staphylococci). Beyond the first few days of neutropenia, infections with filamentous bacteria (*Nocardia* and the organisms that cause actinomycosis) become more common. Episodes of bacteremia due to encapsulated organisms mark the late posttransplantation period (>6 months after bone marrow reconstitution).

FUNGAL INFECTIONS　Beyond the first week after transplantation, fungal infections become increasingly common. As in most granulocytopenic patients, *Candida* infections are most commonly seen in this setting. With increased use of prophylactic fluconazole, infections with resistant fungi, such as *Candida glabrata* and *Aspergillus*, have become more common. In patients with graft-versus-host disease (GVHD) who require prolonged or indefinite courses of glucocorticoids and other immunosuppressive agents [e.g., cyclosporine, tacrolimus, mycophenolate mofetil, rapamycin, alemtuzumab (an antilymphocyte and antimonocyte antibody)], there is a high risk of fungal infection (usually with *Candida* or *Aspergillus*), even after engraftment and resolution of neutropenia. These patients are also at high risk of reactivation of fungal infection (histoplasmosis, coccidioidomycosis, blastomycosis) in areas where endemic fungi reside and if they are involved in activities such as spelunking or gardening. Because of the high and prolonged risk of *Pneumocystis* pneumonia (especially among patients being treated for hematologic malignancies), most patients should receive maintenance prophylaxis with trimethoprim-sulfamethoxazole (TMP-SMX) starting 1 month after engraftment and continuing for at least 1 year.

PARASITIC INFECTIONS　The regimen just described for *Pneumocystis* pneumonia may also protect patients seropositive for *T. gondii*, which may cause pneumonia as well as central nervous system (CNS) lesions. The advantages of maintaining patients on daily TMP-SMX for 1 year after transplantation include protection against *Listeria monocytogenes* and nocardial disease as well as late infections with *Streptococcus pneumoniae* and *Haemophilus influenzae*, which are a consequence of the inability of the immature bone marrow to respond to polysaccharide antigens.

VIRAL INFECTIONS　BMT/HSCT recipients are susceptible to infection with a variety of viruses, including reactivation syndromes caused by most HHVs (Table 117-3) and infections caused by viruses that circulate in the community.

Herpes Simplex Virus　Within the first 2 weeks after transplantation, most patients who are seropositive for HSV-1 excrete the virus from the oropharynx. The ability to isolate HSV declines with time. Administration of prophylactic acyclovir (or valacyclovir) to seropositive BMT/HSCT recipients has been shown to reduce mucositis and prevent HSV pneumonia (a rare condition reported almost exclusively in BMT recipients). Both esophagitis (usually due to HSV-1) and anogenital disease (commonly induced by HSV-2) may be prevented with acyclovir prophylaxis. →*For further discussion, see Chap. 163.*

Varicella-Zoster Virus　Reactivation of herpes zoster may occur within the first month but more commonly occurs several months after transplantation. Reactivation rates are ~40% for allogeneic recipients and 25% for autologous recipients. Localized zoster can spread locally in an immunosuppressed patient. Fortunately, disseminated disease can usually be controlled with high doses of acyclovir. Because of the high incidence of dissem-

TABLE 117-2　*Infections After Bone Marrow Transplantation*

| Infection Site | Period after Transplantation | | |
	Early (<1 Month)	Middle (1–4 Months)	Late (>6 Months)
Disseminated	Bacteria (aerobic gram-negative, gram-positive)	Bacteria (*Nocardia*, agents of actinomycosis) Fungi (*Candida*, *Aspergillus*)	Encapsulated bacteria (*Streptococcus pneumoniae*, *Haemophilus influenzae*, *Neisseria meningitidis*)
Skin and mucous membranes	Herpes simplex virus	Human herpesvirus type 6	Varicella-zoster virus
Lungs	Herpes simplex virus	Viruses (cytomegalovirus, human herpesvirus type 6) Parasites (*Toxoplasma gondii*) Fungi (*Pneumocystis*)	
Kidneys			Viruses (BK)
Brain			Parasites (*T. gondii*) Viruses (JC)

TABLE 117-3 *Herpes-Group Virus Syndromes in Transplant Recipients*

Virus	Reactivation Disease
Herpes simplex virus type 1	Oral lesions, may be associated with pneumonia, described only in BMT recipients Hepatitis
Herpes simplex virus type 2	Severe and/or persistent anogenital lesions Hepatitis
Varicella-zoster virus	Zoster (potentially disseminated)
Cytomegalovirus	Associated with graft rejection, fever, bone marrow failure, pneumonitis, gastrointestinal disease, other
Epstein-Barr virus	B cell lymphoproliferative disease Oral hairy leukoplakia (rare)
Human herpesvirus type 6	Fever, rash,[a] pneumonitis, bone marrow suppression, encephalitis (manifestations controversial)
Human herpesvirus type 7	Undefined
Kaposi's sarcoma–associated herpesvirus/human herpesvirus type 8	Kaposi's sarcoma Primary effusion lymphoma (rare) Multicentric Castleman's disease (rare)

[a] A rash may be seen with primary infections, but it is difficult to distinguish from other rashes seen in these patients.

Note: BMT, bone marrow transplant.

ination of herpes zoster among patients with skin lesions, acyclovir is given prophylactically in some centers to prevent severe disease. Low doses of acyclovir (400 mg orally, three times daily) appear to be effective in preventing reactivation of VZV. However, acyclovir also inhibits the development of VZV-specific immunity. Thus, its administration for only 6 months after transplantation does not prevent zoster from occurring when treatment is stopped. Some data suggest that administration of low doses of acyclovir for an entire year after transplantation is effective and may eliminate most cases of posttransplantation zoster. →*For further discussion, see Chap. 164.*

Cytomegalovirus The onset of CMV disease (interstitial pneumonia, bone marrow suppression, or graft failure) usually comes between 30 and 90 days after transplantation, when the granulocyte count is adequate but immunologic reconstitution has not occurred. CMV disease rarely develops earlier than 14 days after transplantation and may become evident as late as 4 months after the procedure. It is of great concern in the second month after transplantation, particularly in allogeneic BMT/HSCT recipients. In cases in which the donor marrow is depleted of T cells (to prevent GVHD or eliminate a T cell tumor), the disease may be manifested earlier. The use of αCD52 antibody (alemtuzumab) to prevent GVHD in nonmyeloablative transplantation has been associated with an increase in CMV disease. Patients who receive ganciclovir (for prophylaxis, preemptive treatment, or treatment; see below) may develop CMV infection even later than 4 months after transplantation; treatment appears to delay the development of the normal immune response to CMV infection. Although CMV disease may present as isolated fever, granulocytopenia, or gastrointestinal disease, the foremost cause of death from CMV infection in this setting is pneumonia.

With the standard use of CMV-negative or filtered blood products, primary CMV infection should be a risk in allogeneic transplantation only when the donor is CMV-seropositive and the recipient is CMV-seronegative. Reactivation disease or superinfection with another strain from the donor is also common in CMV-positive recipients, and most seropositive patients who undergo bone marrow transplantation excrete CMV, with or without clinical findings. Serious CMV disease is much more common among allogeneic than autologous recipients and is often associated with GVHD. In addition to pneumonia and marrow suppression (and, less often, graft failure), manifestations of CMV disease in BMT/HSCT recipients include fever with or without arthralgias, myalgias, and esophagitis. CMV ulcerations occur in both the lower and the upper gastrointestinal tract, and it may be difficult to distinguish diarrhea due to GVHD from that due to CMV infection.

The finding of CMV in the liver of a patient with GVHD does not necessarily mean that CMV is responsible for hepatic enzyme abnormalities.

Management of CMV disease in BMT/HSCT recipients includes strategies directed at prophylaxis, suppression, preemptive therapy, or treatment. Prophylaxis results in a lower incidence of disease at the cost of treating many patients who otherwise would not require therapy. Because of the high fatality rate associated with CMV pneumonia in these patients and the difficulty of early diagnosis of CMV infection, prophylactic intravenous ganciclovir (or oral valganciclovir) has been used in some centers and has been shown to abort CMV disease during the period of maximal vulnerability (from engraftment to day 120 after transplantation). The foremost problem with the administration of ganciclovir relates to adverse effects, which include dose-related bone marrow suppression (thrombocytopenia, leukopenia, anemia, and pancytopenia). Because the frequency of CMV pneumonia is lower among autologous BMT recipients (2 to 7%) than among allogeneic BMT recipients (10 to 40%), prophylaxis in the former group will not become the rule until a less toxic antiviral agent becomes available.

Like prophylaxis, suppressive treatment, which targets patients with polymerase chain reaction evidence of CMV or urine cultures positive for CMV, entails the unnecessary treatment of many individuals (on the basis of a laboratory test that is not highly predictive of disease) with drugs that have adverse effects. Currently, because of the neutropenia associated with ganciclovir in BMT/HSCT recipients, a preemptive approach—treatment of those patients in whose blood CMV is detected by an antigen or DNA test—is used at most centers. This approach is almost as effective as prophylaxis or suppression and causes less toxicity. Quantitative viral load assays, which are not dependent on circulating polymorphonuclear leukocytes, have supplanted antigen-based assays and are used by most centers. A positive test (or increase in titer) prompts the initiation of preemptive therapy.

Treatment of CMV pneumonia in BMT/HSCT recipients requires both intravenous immune globulin (IVIg) and ganciclovir. In patients who cannot tolerate ganciclovir, foscarnet is a useful alternative, although it may produce nephrotoxicity and electrolyte imbalance. Transfusion of CMV-specific T cells from the donor decreased viral load in a small series of patients; this result suggests that immunotherapy may play a role in the treatment of this disease in the future. →*For further discussion, see Chap. 166.*

Human Herpesviruses 6 and 7 HHV-6, the cause of roseola in children, is a ubiquitous herpesvirus that reactivates (as determined by culture of the virus from the blood) in ~50% of transplant recipients between 2 and 4 weeks after surgery. In some cases, reactivation of HHV-6 appears to be associated with neutropenia; since, like CMV, this virus can be found in marrow cells, it is possible that HHV-6 reactivation is responsible for some of the neutropenia that follows bone marrow transplantation. Although encephalitis developing after transplantation has been associated with HHV-6 in cerebrospinal fluid (CSF), the causality of the association is not well defined. HHV-6 DNA is sometimes found in lung samples after transplantation. However, its role in pneumonitis is unclear. While HHV-6 has been shown to be susceptible to foscarnet (and possibly to ganciclovir) in vitro, the efficacy of antiviral treatment has not been well studied. Little is known about the related herpesvirus HHV-7 or its role in posttransplantation infection. →*For further discussion, see Chap. 166.*

Epstein-Barr Virus Primary EBV infection can be fatal to transplant recipients; EBV reactivation can cause EBV–B cell lymphoproliferative disease (LPD), which may also be fatal to patients taking immunosuppressive drugs. The localization of EBV to B cells leads to several interesting phenomena in BMT/HSCT recipients. The marrow ablation that occurs as part of the BMT/HSCT procedure may eliminate latent EBV from the host. Infection can then be reacquired immediately after transplantation by transfer of infected donor B cells.

Rarely, transplantation from a seronegative donor may result in cure. The recipient is then at risk for a second primary infection.

EBV-LPD can develop in the recipient's B cells (if any should survive marrow ablation) but is more likely to be a consequence of outgrowth of infected donor cells. Both lytic and latent EBV replication are more likely during immunosuppression (e.g., they are associated with GVHD and the use of antibodies to T cells). Although less likely in autologous transplantation, reactivation can occur in T cell–depleted autologous recipients (e.g., patients being given antibodies to T cells for the treatment of a T cell lymphoma with marrow depletion). EBV-LPD, which can become apparent as soon as 1 to 3 months after engraftment, causes high fevers and cervical adenopathy resembling the symptoms of infectious mononucleosis but more commonly presents as an extranodal mass. The incidence of 0.6% among allogeneic BMT/HSCT recipients contrasts with figures of ~5% for renal transplant recipients and up to 20% for cardiac transplant patients. In all cases, EBV-LPD is more likely to occur with continued immunosuppression (especially that caused by the use of antibodies to T cells and cyclosporine or other T cell–suppressive agents).

EBV-specific T cells generated from the donor have been used experimentally to prevent and to treat EBV-LPD in the allogeneic recipient. Administration of a monoclonal antibody to CD20 (rituximab) for the treatment of B cell lymphomas that express this surface protein has elicited dramatic responses and currently constitutes first-line therapy for EBV-LPD, although long-term suppression of new antibody responses accompanies therapy. The role of antivirals is uncertain because no available agents have been documented to have activity against latent EBV infection. Ganciclovir has been postulated to have activity on the basis of its ability to inhibit proliferation of B cells, but this activity is associated with toxicity. High-dose zidovudine shows promise for the treatment of EBV-positive CNS lymphomas—another EBV-associated complication of transplantation. Both interferon α and retinoic acid have been used in the treatment of EBV-LPD, as has IVIg, but no large studies have assessed the efficacy of these agents. Chemotherapeutic regimens have been used as a last resort, even though patients' tolerance and long-term results have been disappointing in this setting. *→For further discussion, see Chap. 165.*

Human Herpesvirus 8   The EBV-related gamma herpesvirus HHV-8, which is causally associated with Kaposi's sarcoma, with primary effusion lymphoma, and sometimes with multicentric Castleman's disease, has rarely resulted in disease in BMT/HSCT recipients. The reasons may be a relatively low seroprevalence in the population and the limited duration of profound T cell suppression after bone marrow/hematopoietic stem cell transplantation. *→For further discussion, see Chap. 166.*

Other (Nonherpes) Viruses   The diagnosis of pneumonia in BMT/HSCT recipients poses some special problems. Because patients have undergone treatment with multiple chemotherapeutic agents and sometimes radiation, their differential diagnosis should include—in addition to bacterial pneumonia—CMV pneumonitis, pneumonia of other viral or fungal etiology, parasitic pneumonia, diffuse alveolar hemorrhage, and chemical- or radiation-associated pneumonitis. Since fungal disease and viruses such as respiratory syncytial virus (RSV), parainfluenza virus (types 1, 2, and 3), influenza A and B viruses, and adenovirus are also causes of pneumonia in this setting, it is important to diagnose CMV specifically (see above). *M. tuberculosis* has been an uncommon cause of pneumonia among BMT/HSCT recipients in Western countries (<0.1 to 0.2%) but is common in Hong Kong (5.5%) and in countries where the prevalence of tuberculosis is high. The exposure history of the recipient is clearly critical in an assessment of posttransplantation infections.

Both RSV and parainfluenza viruses, particularly type 3, can cause severe or even fatal pneumonia in BMT recipients. Infections with both of these agents sometimes occur as disastrous nosocomial epidemics. Therapy with aerosolized ribavirin as well as RSV immuno-

globulin or monoclonal antibody to RSV (palivizumab) has been reported to lessen the severity of RSV disease, but there are no large studies to prove efficacy. Influenza also occurs in BMT recipients and generally mirrors the presence of infection in the community. Several drugs are available for the treatment of influenza (amantadine/rimantadine, ribavirin?) but have limited effects, primarily reducing symptoms and shortening the duration of illness. The neuraminidase inhibitors (oseltamivir and zanamivir) are active against both influenza A virus and influenza B virus and are a reasonable treatment option. Adenovirus can be isolated from BMT recipients at rates varying from 5 to 18%. Although hemorrhagic cystitis, pneumonia, and fatal disseminated infection have been reported, adenovirus infection, which (like CMV infection) usually occurs in the first or second month after transplantation, is often asymptomatic. Cidofovir has proved effective in animal models and in case reports. Infections with parvovirus B19 (presenting as anemia or occasionally as pancytopenia) and enteroviruses (sometimes fatal) can occur. Parvovirus infection can be treated with IVIg (Chap. 168). Pleconaril, a capsid-binding agent, is being studied for the treatment of enterovirus infection. Rotaviruses are a common cause of gastroenteritis in BMT/HSCT recipients. Polyomavirus BK is found at high titers in the urine of patients who are highly immunosuppressed. BK viruria may be associated with hemorrhagic cystitis. Progressive multifocal leukoencephalopathy caused by JC virus is rare among BMT/HSCT recipients compared with the rate among patients with impaired T cell function due to HIV infection. There is no known treatment for this disease. When transmitted by mosquitoes or by blood transfusion, West Nile virus can cause encephalitis and death after bone marrow transplantation.

INFECTIONS IN SOLID ORGAN TRANSPLANT RECIPIENTS

Morbidity and mortality among solid organ transplant recipients have been reduced by the use of more effective antibiotics. The organisms that cause infections in recipients of solid organ transplants are different from those that infect BMT/HSCT recipients because solid organ recipients do not go through a period of neutropenia. As the transplantation procedure involves surgery, however, solid organ recipients are subject to infections at anastomotic sites and to wound infections. Compared with BMT/HSCT recipients, organ transplant patients are immunosuppressed for longer periods (often permanently). Thus they are susceptible to the same organisms as patients with chronically impaired T cell immunity (Chap. 72, especially Table 72-1).

During the early period (<1 month after transplantation), infections are most commonly caused by extracellular bacteria (staphylococci, streptococci, *E. coli*, other gram-negative organisms), which often originate in surgical wound or anastomotic sites. The spectrum of infection is largely determined by the type of transplant.

In subsequent weeks, the consequences of the administration of agents that suppress cell-mediated immunity and of the acquisition or reactivation (from the transplanted organ) of viruses and parasites become apparent. CMV infection is often a problem in the first 6 months after transplantation and may present as severe systemic disease or as infection of the transplanted organ. HHV-6 reactivation (assessed by blood culture) occurs within the first 2 to 4 weeks after transplantation and may be associated with fever and granulocytopenia. Data suggest that HHV-6 and HHV-7 may exacerbate CMV-induced disease. CMV is associated not only with generalized immunosuppression but also with organ-specific, rejection-related syndromes: glomerulopathy in kidney transplant recipients, bronchiolitis obliterans in lung transplant recipients, vasculopathy in heart transplant recipients, and the vanishing bile duct syndrome in liver transplant recipients. A complex interplay between increased CMV replication and enhanced graft rejection is well established: Increasing immunosuppression leads to increased CMV replication, which is associated with graft rejection. For this reason, considerable attention has been focused on the diagnosis, treatment, and prophylaxis of CMV infection in organ transplant recipients. Early transmission of West Nile virus to transplant recipients from an organ donor has been reported.

Beyond 6 months after transplantation, infections characteristic of patients with defects in cell-mediated immunity—e.g., infections with *Listeria*, *Nocardia*, various fungi, and other intracellular pathogens—may be a problem. Elimination of these late infections will not be possible until specific tolerance to the transplanted organ can be achieved without the administration of drugs that lead to generalized immunosuppression. Meanwhile, vigilance, prophylaxis/preemptive therapy (when indicated), and rapid diagnosis and treatment of infections can be lifesaving in solid organ transplant recipients, who, unlike most BMT recipients, continue to be immunosuppressed.

Solid organ transplant recipients are susceptible to EBV-LPD from as early as 2 months to many years after transplantation. The prevalence of this complication is increased by potent and prolonged use of T cell–suppressive drugs. The condition may be reversed (in some cases) by decreasing the degree of immunosuppression. Among organ transplant patients, those with heart and lung transplants—who receive the most intensive immunosuppressive regimens—are most likely to develop EBV-LPD, particularly in the lungs. Although the disease usually originates in recipient B cells, several cases of donor origin have been reported. There is a notable tendency for EBV-LPD to develop in the transplanted organ. High organ-specific content of B lymphoid tissues (i.e., bronchial-associated lymphoid tissue in the lung), anatomical factors (i.e., lack of access of host T cells to the transplanted organ because of disturbed lymphatics), and differences in major histocompatibility loci between the host T cells and the organ (i.e., lack of cell migration or lack of effective T cell/macrophage cooperation) may result in defective elimination of EBV-infected B cells. Solid organ transplant recipients are also highly susceptible to the development of Kaposi's sarcoma and to B cell proliferative disorders associated with Kaposi's sarcoma–associated herpesvirus (KSHV) (primary effusion lymphoma, multicentric Castleman's disease). Kaposi's sarcoma can develop very rapidly after transplantation and can occur in the allograft. However, because the seroprevalence of KSHV is very low in Western countries, Kaposi's sarcoma is infrequent in these areas.

KIDNEY TRANSPLANTATION (See Table 117-4) ■ **Early Infections** Infections developing soon after kidney transplantation are often caused by bacteria associated with skin or wound infections. There is a role for perioperative antibiotic prophylaxis, and many centers give cephalosporins to decrease the risk of postoperative complications. Urinary tract infections developing soon after transplantation are usually related to anatomical alterations resulting from surgery. Such early infections may require prolonged treatment (e.g., 6 weeks of antibiotic administration for pyelonephritis). Urinary tract infections that occur >6 months after transplantation do not seem to be associated with the high rate of pyelonephritis or relapse seen with infections that occur in the first 3 months and may be treated for shorter periods.

Prophylaxis with TMP-SMX [1 double-strength tablet (800 mg of sulfamethoxazole, 160 mg of trimethoprim) per day] for the first 4 months after transplantation decreases the incidence of early and middle-period infections (see below and Tables 117-4 and 117-5).

Middle-Period Infections Because of continuing immunosuppression, kidney transplant recipients are predisposed to lung infections characteristic of those in patients with T cell deficiency (i.e., infections with intracellular bacteria, mycobacteria, nocardiae, fungi, viruses, and parasites). The high mortality associated with *Legionella pneumophila* infection (Chap. 132) led to the closing of renal transplant units in hospitals with endemic legionellosis.

About 50% of all renal transplant recipients presenting with fever 1 to 4 months after transplantation have evidence of CMV disease; CMV itself accounts for the fever in more than two-thirds of cases and thus is the predominant pathogen during this period. CMV infection (Chap. 166) may also present as arthralgias or myalgias. During this period, this infection may represent primary disease (in the case of a seronegative recipient of a kidney from a seropositive donor) or may present as reactivation disease or superinfection. Patients may have atypical lymphocytosis. Unlike immunocompetent patients, however, they often do not have lymphadenopathy or splenomegaly. Therefore, clinical suspicion and laboratory confirmation are necessary for diagnosis. The clinical syndrome may be accompanied by bone marrow suppression (particularly leukopenia). CMV also causes glomerulopathy and is associated with an increased incidence of other opportunistic infections. Because of the frequency and severity of CMV disease, a considerable effort has been made to prevent and treat it in renal transplant recipients. Administration of an immune globulin preparation enriched with antibodies to CMV decreases the incidence in the group at highest risk for severe infections (seronegative recipients of

TABLE 117-4 *Infections After Kidney Transplantation*

Infection Site	Period after Transplantation		
	Early (<1 Month)	Middle (1–4 Months)	Late (>6 Months)
Urinary tract	Bacteria (*Escherichia coli*, *Klebsiella*, Enterobacteriaceae, *Pseudomonas*, *Enterococcus*) associated with bacteremia and pyelonephritis, *Candida*	Cytomegalovirus (CMV; fever alone is common)	Bacteria; late infections usually not associated with bacteremia
Lungs	Bacteria (*Legionella* in endemic settings)	CMV diffuse interstitial pneumonitis, *Pneumocystis*, *Aspergillus*, *Legionella*	*Nocardia*, *Aspergillus*, *Mucor*
Central nervous system		*Listeria* meningitis, CMV encephalitis, *Toxoplasma gondii*	CMV retinitis, *Listeria* meningitis, cryptococcal meningitis, *Aspergillus*, *Nocardia*

TABLE 117-5 *Prophylaxis of Infections in Transplant Recipients*

Risk Factor	Organism	Prophylactic Antibiotics	Examinations
Travel to or residence in area with known risk of fungal infection	Coccidioidomycosis, histoplasmosis, blastomycosis	Imidazoles (fluconazole, itraconazole, voriconazole)	Chest radiography
Latent viruses	HSV, VZV, EBV, CMV	Acyclovir after bone marrow transplantation for HSV and VZV; ganciclovir in some settings	Serologic test for HSV, VZV, CMV, HHV-6, EBV, HHV-8
Latent parasites	*Pneumocystis*, *Toxoplasma gondii*	Trimethoprim-sulfamethoxazole or dapsone plus pyrimethamine	Serologic test for *Toxoplasma*
History of exposure to tuberculosis or latent tuberculosis	*Mycobacterium tuberculosis*	Isoniazid if recent conversion for positive chest x-ray and no previous treatment	PPD skin test and chest radiography

Note: CMV, cytomegalovirus; EBV, Epstein-Barr virus; HHV, human herpesvirus; HSV, herpes simplex virus; PPD, purified protein derivative; VZV, varicella-zoster virus.

seropositive kidneys). Ganciclovir is useful for prophylaxis and the treatment of serious CMV disease. One study showed a significant (50%) reduction in CMV disease and rejection at 6 months in patients who received prophylactic valacyclovir (an acyclovir congener) for the first 90 days after renal transplantation. The availability of valganciclovir and valacyclovir has allowed most centers to move to oral prophylaxis for transplant recipients.

Infection with the other herpes-group viruses may become evident within 6 months after transplantation or later. Early after transplantation, HSV may cause either oral or anogenital lesions that are usually responsive to acyclovir. Large ulcerating lesions in the anogenital area may lead to bladder and rectal dysfunction as well as predisposing to bacterial infection. VZV may cause fatal disseminated infection in nonimmune kidney transplant recipients, but in immune patients reactivation zoster usually does not disseminate outside the dermatome; thus disseminated VZV infection is a less fearsome complication in kidney transplantation than in bone marrow transplantation. HHV-6 may reactivate and (although usually asymptomatic) may be associated with fever, rash, marrow suppression, or encephalitis.

EBV reactivation disease is more serious; it may present as an extranodal proliferation of B cells that invade the CNS, nasopharynx, liver, small bowel, heart, and transplanted kidney. The disease is diagnosed by the finding of a proliferation of EBV-positive B cells. The incidence of EBV-LPD is higher among patients given high doses of cyclosporine, tacrolimus, or other immunosuppressive agents (including anti–T cell antibodies). Disease may regress once immunocompetence is restored. HHV-8 infection can be transmitted with the donor kidney and is associated with the development of Kaposi's sarcoma in the recipient. Kaposi's sarcoma (primary vs. reactivation of HHV-8) often appears within 1 year after transplantation, although the range of onset times is wide (1 month to ~20 years).

The papovaviruses BK and JC (polyomavirus hominis types 1 and 2) have been cultured from the urine of kidney transplant recipients (as they have from that of BMT recipients). The excretion of BK virus is associated with ureteral strictures, BK nephropathy, and—in rare instances—vasculopathy. JC virus is associated with progressive multifocal leukoencephalopathy (rare). Adenoviruses may persist with continued immunosuppression in these patients.

Kidney transplant recipients are also subject to infections with other intracellular organisms. These patients may develop pulmonary infections with Nocardia, Aspergillus, and Mucor as well as infections with other pathogens in which the T cell/macrophage axis plays an important role. In patients without intravenous catheters, L. monocytogenes is a common cause of bacteremia ≥1 month after renal transplantation and should be seriously considered in renal transplant recipients presenting with fever and headache. Kidney transplant recipients may develop Salmonella bacteremia, which can lead to endovascular infections and require prolonged therapy. Pulmonary infections with Pneumocystis are common unless the patient is maintained on TMP-SMX prophylaxis. Nocardia infection (Chap. 146) may present in the skin, bones, and lungs or in the CNS, where it usually takes the form of single or multiple brain abscesses. Nocardia infection generally occurs ≥1 month after transplantation and may follow immunosuppressive treatment for an episode of rejection. Pulmonary findings are nonspecific: localized disease with or without cavities is most common, but the disease may disseminate. The diagnosis is made by culture of the organism from sputum or from the involved nodule. As with Pneumocystis, prophylaxis with TMP-SMX is often efficacious in the prevention of disease. The occurrence of Nocardia infections >2 years after transplantation suggests that a long-term prophylactic regimen may be justified.

Toxoplasmosis can occur in seropositive patients but is less common than in other transplant settings, usually developing in the first few months after kidney transplantation. Again, TMP-SMX is helpful in prevention. In endemic areas, histoplasmosis, coccidioidomycosis, and blastomycosis may cause pulmonary infiltrates or disseminated disease.

Late Infections Late infections (>6 months after kidney transplantation) include CMV retinitis and a variety of CNS complications. Patients (particularly those whose immunosuppression has been increased) are at risk for subacute meningitis due to *Cryptococcus neoformans*. Cryptococcal disease may present in an insidious manner (sometimes as a skin infection before the development of clear CNS findings). *Listeria* meningitis may have an acute presentation and requires prompt therapy to avoid a fatal outcome.

Patients who continue to take glucocorticoids are predisposed to infection. "Transplant elbow" is a recurrent bacterial infection in and around the elbow that is thought to result from a combination of poor tensile strength of the skin of steroid-treated patients and steroid-induced proximal myopathy that requires patients to push themselves up with their elbows to get out of chairs. Bouts of cellulitis (usually caused by S. aureus) recur until patients are provided with elbow protection.

Kidney transplant recipients are susceptible to invasive fungal infections—such as those due to *Aspergillus* and *Rhizopus*, which may present as superficial lesions before dissemination. Mycobacterial infection (particularly that with *Mycobacterium marinum*) can be diagnosed by skin examination. Infection with *Prototheca wickerhamii* (an achlorophyllic alga) has been diagnosed by skin biopsy. Warts caused by human papillomaviruses (HPVs) are a late consequence of persistent immunosuppression; imiquimod or other forms of local therapy are usually satisfactory.

HEART TRANSPLANTATION ■ Early Infections Sternal wound infection and mediastinitis are early complications of heart transplantation. An indolent course is common, with fever or a mildly elevated white blood cell count preceding the development of site tenderness or drainage. Clinical suspicion based on evidence of sternal instability and failure to heal may lead to the diagnosis. Although common microbial residents of the skin (e.g., S. aureus and Staphylococcus epidermidis) as well as gram-negative organisms (e.g., Pseudomonas aeruginosa) and fungi (e.g., Candida) are often involved, mediastinitis in heart transplant recipients (in rare cases) can also be due to Mycoplasma hominis (Chap. 159). Since this organism requires an anaerobic environment for growth and may be difficult to see on conventional medium, the laboratory should be alerted that M. hominis infection is suspected. M. hominis mediastinitis has been cured with a combination of surgical debridement (sometimes requiring muscle-flap placement) plus clindamycin and tetracycline. Organisms associated with mediastinitis may be cultured from accompanying pericardial fluid.

Middle-Period Infections T. gondii (Chap. 198) resident in the heart of a seropositive donor may be transmitted to a seronegative recipient. Thus serologic screening for T. gondii infection is important before and in the months after cardiac transplantation. Rarely, active disease can be introduced at the time of transplantation. The overall incidence of toxoplasmosis is so high in this setting that some prophylaxis is always warranted. Although alternatives are available, the most frequently used agent is TMP-SMX, which prevents infection with Pneumocystis as well as with Nocardia and other bacterial pathogens. CMV has also been transmitted by heart transplantation. CNS infections can be caused by Toxoplasma, Nocardia, and Aspergillus. L. monocytogenes meningitis should be considered in heart transplant recipients with fever and headache.

CMV infection is associated with poor outcomes after heart transplantation. The virus is usually cultivable 1 to 2 months after transplantation, causes early signs and laboratory abnormalities (usually fever and atypical lymphocytosis or leukopenia and thrombocytopenia) at 2 to 3 months, and produces severe disease (e.g., pneumonia) at 3 to 4 months. Seropositive recipients usually develop cultivable virus faster than patients whose primary CMV infection is a consequence of transplantation. Between 40 and 70% of patients develop symptomatic CMV disease in the form of (1) CMV pneumonia, the most likely form of CMV disease to be fatal; (2) CMV esophagitis and gastritis, sometimes accompanied by abdominal pain with or without ulcerations and bleeding; and (3) the CMV syndrome, consisting of CMV in the blood along with fever, leukopenia, thrombocytopenia, and hepatic enzyme abnormalities. Ganciclovir is efficacious in the treatment of CMV infection; prophylaxis with ganciclovir or possibly with other antivirals, as described for renal transplantation, may reduce the incidence of CMV-related disease.

Late Infections EBV infection usually presents as a lymphoma-like proliferation of B cells late after heart transplantation, particularly in patients maintained on heavy immunosuppression. A subset of heart and heart-lung transplant recipients may develop early (within 2 months) fulminant EBV-LPD. Treatment includes the reduction of immunosuppression if possible and the consideration of B cell antibodies (rituximab), immunomodulatory agents, or chemotherapy, as discussed earlier under bone marrow/hematopoietic stem cell transplantation. HHV-8-associated disease, including primary effusion lymphoma, has been reported in heart transplant recipients. Prophylaxis for *Pneumocystis* infection is required for these patients (see below).

LUNG TRANSPLANTATION ■ **Early Infections** It is not surprising that lung transplant recipients are predisposed to the development of pneumonia. The combination of ischemia and the resulting mucosal damage together with accompanying denervation and lack of lymph drainage probably contributes to the high rate of pneumonia (66% in one series). The prophylactic use of high doses of broad-spectrum antibiotics for the first 3 or 4 days after surgery decreases the incidence of pneumonia. Gram-negative pathogens (Enterobacteriaceae and *Pseudomonas* species) are troublesome in the first 2 weeks after surgery (the period of maximal vulnerability). Pneumonia can also be caused by *Candida* (possibly as a result of colonization of the donor lung), *Aspergillus*, and *Cryptococcus*.

Mediastinitis may occur at an even higher rate among lung transplant recipients than among heart transplant recipients and most commonly develops within 2 weeks of surgery. Pneumonitis due to CMV (which may be transmitted as a consequence of transplantation) usually presents between 2 weeks and 3 months after surgery, with primary disease occurring later than reactivation disease.

Middle-Period Infections The incidence of CMV infection, either reactivated or primary, is between 75 and 100% if either the donor or the recipient is seropositive for CMV. CMV-induced disease appears to be most severe in recipients of lung and heart-lung transplants. Whether this severity relates to the mismatch in lung antigen-presenting and host immune cells or is attributable to other (nonimmune) factors is not known. More than half of lung transplant recipients with symptomatic CMV disease have pneumonia. Difficulty in distinguishing the radiographic picture of CMV infection from organ rejection further complicates therapy. CMV can also cause bronchiolitis obliterans in lung transplants. The development of pneumonitis related to HSV has led to the prophylactic use of acyclovir. Such prophylaxis may also decrease rates of CMV disease, but ganciclovir is more active against CMV and is also active against HSV. Prophylaxis of CMV infection with intravenous ganciclovir (or with valganciclovir, the oral alternative) is recommended for lung transplant recipients.

Late Infections The incidence of *Pneumocystis* infection (which may present with a paucity of findings) is high among lung and heart-lung transplant recipients. Some form of prophylaxis for *Pneumocystis* pneumonia is indicated in all organ transplant situations (Table 117-5). TMP-SMX prophylaxis for 12 months after transplantation may be sufficient to prevent *Pneumocystis* disease in patients whose degree of immunosuppression is not increased.

As in other transplant recipients, infection with EBV may cause either a mononucleosis-like syndrome or LPD. The tendency of the B cell blasts to present in the lung appears to be greater after lung transplantation than after the transplantation of other organs. Reduction of immunosuppression causes remission in some cases, but airway compression can be fatal and more rapid intervention may therefore become necessary. The approach to EBV-LPD is similar to that described in other sections.

LIVER TRANSPLANTATION ■ **Early Infections** As in other types of transplantation, early bacterial infections are a major problem after liver transplantation. Many centers administer systemic broad-spectrum antibiotics for the first 5 days after surgery, even in the absence of documented infection. However, despite prophylaxis, infectious complications are common and are correlated with the duration of the surgical procedure and the type of biliary drainage. An operation lasting >12 h is associated with an increased likelihood of infection. Patients who have a choledochojejunostomy with drainage of the biliary duct to a Roux-en-Y jejunal bowel loop have more fungal infections than those whose bile is drained via a choledochocholedochostomy with anastomosis of the donor common bile duct to the recipient common bile duct.

Peritonitis and intraabdominal abscesses are common complications of liver transplantation. Bacterial peritonitis may result from biliary leaks and primary or secondary infection after leakage of bile. Peritonitis in liver transplant recipients is often polymicrobial, commonly involving enterococci, aerobic gram-negative bacteria, staphylococci, anaerobes, or *Candida*. Only one-third of patients with intraabdominal abscesses have bacteremia. Abscesses within the first month after surgery may occur not only over the liver but also in the spleen, pericolic area, and pelvis. Treatment includes antibiotic administration and drainage as necessary.

Liver transplant patients have a high incidence of fungal infections, and the occurrence of fungal infection (often candidiasis) correlates with preoperative use of glucocorticoids, a long duration of treatment with antibacterial agents, and posttransplantation use of immunosuppressive agents.

Middle-Period Infections The development of postsurgical biliary stricture predisposes patients to cholangitis. These patients may lack the characteristic signs and symptoms of cholangitis: fever, abdominal pain, and jaundice. Alternatively, these findings may be present but may suggest graft rejection. The diagnosis of cholangitis in liver transplant recipients therefore requires documentation of bacteremia or demonstration of aggregated neutrophils in bile duct biopsy specimens. Unfortunately, invasive studies of the biliary tract (either T-tube cholangiography or endoscopic retrograde cholangiopancreatography) may themselves lead to cholangitis. For this reason, many clinicians recommend prophylaxis with antibiotics covering gram-negative organisms and anaerobes when these procedures are performed in liver transplant recipients.

Viral hepatitis is a common complication of liver transplantation (Chap. 285). Reactivation of hepatitis B and C infections, for which transplantation may be performed, is problematic. To prevent hepatitis B infection, high-dose intravenous hepatitis B immune globulin is administered. The long-term efficacy of lamivudine (3TC) and adefovir in inhibiting hepatitis B viral replication after transplantation is being studied. A combination of interferon α and ribavirin is being tested for treatment/prophylaxis of hepatitis C infection.

As in other transplantation settings, reactivation disease with herpes-group viruses is common (Table 117-3). Herpesviruses can be transmitted in donor organs. Although CMV hepatitis occurs in ~4% of liver transplant recipients, it is usually not so severe as to require retransplantation. CMV disease develops in the majority of seronegative recipients of organs from CMV-positive donors, but fatality rates are lower among liver transplant recipients than among lung or heart-lung transplant recipients. Disease due to CMV is associated with the vanishing bile duct syndrome after liver transplantation. Patients respond to treatment with ganciclovir; prophylaxis with CMV immune globulin and acyclovir or oral ganciclovir may modify disease. A role for HHV-6 in posttransplantation fever and leukopenia has been proposed. HHV-6 and HHV-7 appear to exacerbate CMV disease in this setting. EBV-LPD after liver transplantation shows a propensity for involvement of the liver, and such disease may be of donor origin.

PANCREAS TRANSPLANTATION Transplantation of the pancreas can be complicated by early abdominal infection. To prevent contamination of the allograft with enteric bacteria and yeasts, some surgeons, instead of draining the pancreas through the bowel, drain secretions into the urinary tract or bladder. A cuff of duodenum is used in the anastomosis between the pancreatic graft and either the bladder or the gut. In addition to bicarbonate loss, bladder drainage causes a high rate of urinary tract infection and sterile cystitis. Prophylactic antimicrobials are commonly used at the time of surgery. An alternative method—the transplantation of islet cells only—may eliminate the problems characteristically posed by wound and urinary tract sepsis in pancreas transplant recipients.

Issues related to the development of CMV infection, EBV-LPD, and infections with opportunistic pathogens in patients receiving a pancreas are similar to those in other solid organ transplant recipients.

MISCELLANEOUS INFECTIONS IN SOLID ORGAN TRANSPLANTATION ■ **Indwelling Intravenous Catheter Infections** The prolonged use of indwelling intravenous catheters for administration of medications, blood products, and nutrition is common in diverse transplantation settings and poses a risk of local and bloodstream infection. Significant insertion-site infection is most commonly caused by *S. aureus*. Bloodstream infection most frequently develops within a week of catheter placement or in patients who become neutropenic. Coagulase-negative staphylococci are the most common isolates from the blood. →*For further discussion of differential diagnosis and therapeutic options, see Chap. 72.*

Tuberculosis The incidence of tuberculosis occurring within 12 months after solid organ transplantation ranges broadly worldwide (0.35 to 15%), reflecting prevalences in local populations. Nonrenal transplantation, GVHD within 6 months, and intensity of immunosuppression are predictive of tuberculosis reactivation and development of disseminated disease in a host with latent disease. The use of antibodies to tumor necrosis factor is associated with the development of active tuberculosis. Tuberculosis has rarely been transmitted from the donor organ. In contrast to the low mortality in BMT/HSCT recipients, mortality in solid organ transplant patients is reported to be 29%. Isoniazid toxicity has not been a significant problem except in the liver transplantation setting.

Virus-Associated Malignancies In addition to malignancy associated with gammaherpesvirus infection (EBV, HHV-8) and simple warts (HPV), other tumors that are virus-associated or suspected of being virus-associated are more likely to develop in transplant recipients, particularly those who require long-term immunosuppression, than in the general population. The interval to tumor development is usually >1 year. Transplant recipients develop nonmelanoma skin or lip cancers that, in contrast to de novo skin cancers, have a high ratio of squamous cells to basal cells. HPV appears to play a major role in these lesions. Cervical and vulvar carcinomas, quite clearly associated with HPV, develop with increased frequency in female transplant recipients. Among renal transplant recipients, rates of melanoma are modestly increased and rates of cancers of the kidney and bladder are increased.

VACCINATION OF TRANSPLANT RECIPIENTS

In addition to receiving antibiotic prophylaxis, transplant recipients should be vaccinated against likely pathogens (Table 117-6). In the case of BMT recipients, optimal responses cannot be achieved until after immune reconstitution, despite previous immunization of both donor and recipient. Recipients of allogeneic BMTs must be reimmunized if they are to be protected against pathogens. The situation is less clear-cut in the case of autologous transplantation. T and B cells in the peripheral blood may reconstitute the immune response if they

TABLE 117-6 *Vaccination for Bone Marrow or Solid Organ Transplant Recipients*

Vaccine	Type of Transplantation	
	Bone Marrow	Solid Organ
Streptococcus pneumoniae, Haemophilus influenzae, Neisseria meningitidis	Immunize after transplantation (optimal timing not established); preimmunize graft[a]	Immunize before transplantation and every 5 years for Pneumovax (others not established)
Seasonal influenza	Vaccinate in the fall; vaccinate close contacts	Vaccinate in the fall
Poliomyelitis	Administer inactivated vaccine	Administer inactivated vaccine
Measles/mumps/ rubella	Immunize 24 months after transplantation if patient does not have graft-versus-host disease	Immunize before transplantation
Tetanus, diphtheria	Reimmunize after transplantation	Immunize before transplantation; give boosters at 10 years or as required; a new primary series is not required

[a] Studies indicate that it is possible to "immunize the graft" before transplantation.

are transferred in adequate numbers. However, cancer patients (particularly those with Hodgkin's disease, in whom vaccination has been extensively studied) who are undergoing chemotherapy do not respond normally to immunization, and titers of antibodies to infectious agents fall more rapidly than in healthy individuals. Therefore, even immunosuppressed patients who have not had marrow transplants may need booster vaccine injections. If memory cells are specifically eliminated as part of a marrow "cleanup" procedure, it will be necessary to reimmunize the recipient with a new primary series. Optimal times for immunizations of different transplant populations are being evaluated. Immunization of household and other contacts (including health care personnel) against influenza every season is likely to benefit the patient by preventing local spread.

In the absence of compelling data as to optimal timing, it is reasonable to administer the pneumococcal and *H. influenzae* type b conjugate vaccines to both autologous and allogeneic BMT recipients 12 months after transplantation and again 12 months later (since the response to the initial vaccine dose is weak in the early posttransplantation period). Recent studies indicate that the use of the pneumococcal conjugate vaccines will be more effective than previous products. The pneumococcal and *H. influenzae* type b vaccines are particularly important for patients who have undergone splenectomy. In addition, *Neisseria meningitidis* polysaccharide vaccine, diphtheria vaccine, tetanus vaccine, and inactivated polio vaccine can all be given at these same intervals (12 and 24 months after transplantation). Some authorities recommend a new primary series for tetanus/diphtheria and inactivated polio vaccine (vaccination 12, 14, and 16 months after transplantation). Because of the risk of spread, household contacts of BMT recipients (or of patients immunosuppressed as a result of chemotherapy) should receive only inactivated polio vaccine. Live-virus measles/mumps/rubella (MMR) vaccine can be given to autologous BMT recipients 24 months after transplantation and to most allogeneic BMT recipients at the same point if they are not receiving maintenance therapy with immunosuppressive drugs and do not have ongoing GVHD. The risk of spread from a household contact is lower for MMR vaccine than for polio vaccine. Neither patients nor household contacts of patients should be vaccinated with vaccinia unless they have been exposed to the smallpox virus. In patients who have active GVHD and/or are taking high maintenance doses of glucocorticoids, it may be prudent to avoid all live-virus vaccines. In the absence of detectable antibody titers, vaccination to prevent hepatitis B and hepatitis A also seems advisable.

In the case of solid organ transplant recipients, administration of all the usual vaccines and of the indicated booster doses should be completed before immunosuppression, if possible, to maximize responses. For patients taking immunosuppressive agents, the administration of pneumococcal vaccine should be repeated every 5 years. No data are available for meningococcal polysaccharide vaccine, but it is probably reasonable to administer it along with the pneumococcal vaccine or more frequently (every 3 years for persons with significant exposure risk). *H. influenzae* conjugate vaccine is safe and should be efficacious in this population; therefore, its administration before transplantation is recommended. Booster doses of this vaccine are not recommended for adults. Solid organ transplant recipients who continue to receive immunosuppressive drugs (glucocorticoids, cyclosporine) should not receive live-virus vaccines. A person in this group exposed to measles should be given immune globulin. Similarly, an immunocompromised patient who is seronegative for varicella and who comes into contact with a person who has chickenpox should be given varicella-zoster immune globulin as soon as possible (and certainly within 96 h) or, if this is not possible, should be started immediately on a 10- to 14-day course of acyclovir therapy. Susceptible household contacts of transplant recipients should receive live attenuated VZV vaccine, but vaccinees should avoid direct contact with the patient if a rash develops.

Immunocompromised patients who travel may benefit from some but not all vaccines. In general, they should receive any killed or inactivated vaccine preparation appropriate to the area they are visiting; this recommendation includes the vaccines for Japanese encephalitis, hepatitis A and B, poliomyelitis, meningococcal infection, and typhoid. The live typhoid vaccines are not recommended for use in most immunocompromised patients, but inactivated typhoid or the purified polysaccharide vaccine can be used. Live yellow fever vaccine should not be administered. Phenol-inactivated cholera vaccine is probably of little use in this setting. On the other hand, immunization with the purified-protein hepatitis B vaccine is indicated if patients are likely to be exposed. Patients who will reside for >6 months in areas where hepatitis B is common (Africa, Southeast Asia, the Middle East, Eastern Europe, parts of South America, and the Caribbean) should receive hepatitis B vaccine. Inactivated hepatitis A vaccine should be used in the appropriate setting (Chap. 107). If hepatitis A vaccine is not administered, travelers should consider receiving passive protection with immune globulin (the dose depending on the duration of travel in the high-risk area).

FURTHER READING

CONE RW et al: Human herpesvirus 6 infections after bone marrow transplantation: Clinical and virologic manifestations. J Infect Dis 179:311, 1999

EUVRARD S et al: Skin cancers after organ transplantation. N Engl J Med 348: 1681, 2003

FEHR T et al: Disseminated varicella infection in adult renal allograft recipients: Four cases and a review of the literature. Transplantation 73:608, 2002

HIRSCH HH et al: Prospective study of polyomavirus type BK replication and nephropathy in renal transplant recipients. N Engl J Med 347:488, 2002

LO C-M et al: Prophylaxis and treatment of recurrent hepatitis B after liver transplantation. Transplantation 75:S41, 2003

MOLRINE DC et al: Donor immunization with pneumococcal conjugate vaccine and early protective antibody responses following allogeneic hematopoietic cell transplantation. Blood 101:831, 2003

MYLONAKIS E et al: Combination antiviral therapy for ganciclovir-resistant cytomegalovirus infection in solid-organ transplant recipients. Clin Infect Dis 34:1337, 2002

SINGH N et al: Safety and efficacy of isoniazid chemoprophylaxis administered during liver transplant candidacy for the prevention of posttransplant tuberculosis. Transplantation 74:892, 2002

Section 4 Approach to Therapy for Bacterial Diseases

118 TREATMENT AND PROPHYLAXIS OF BACTERIAL INFECTIONS
Gordon L. Archer, Ronald E. Polk

The development of vaccines and drugs that prevent and cure bacterial infections was one of the twentieth century's major contributions to human longevity and quality of life. Antibacterial agents are among the most commonly prescribed drugs of any kind worldwide. Used appropriately, these drugs are lifesaving. However, their indiscriminate use drives up the cost of health care, leads to a plethora of side effects and drug interactions, and fosters the emergence of bacterial resistance, rendering previously valuable drugs useless. The rational use of antibacterial agents depends on an understanding of their mechanisms of action, pharmacokinetics, pharmacodynamics, toxicities, and interactions; bacterial strategies for resistance; and bacterial susceptibility in vitro. In addition, patient-associated parameters, such as the site of infection and the immune and excretory status of the host, are critically important to appropriate therapeutic decisions. This chapter provides specific data required for making an informed choice of antibacterial agent.

MECHANISMS OF ACTION

Antibacterial agents, like all antimicrobial drugs, are directed against unique targets not present in mammalian cells. The goal is to limit toxicity to the host and maximize chemotherapeutic activity affecting invading microbes only. *Bactericidal drugs* kill the bacteria that are within their spectrum of activity; *bacteriostatic drugs* only inhibit bacterial growth. While bacteriostatic activity is adequate for the treatment of most infections, bactericidal activity may be necessary for cure in patients with altered immune systems (e.g., neutropenia), protected infectious foci (e.g., endocarditis or meningitis), or specific infections (e.g., complicated *Staphylococcus aureus* bacteremia). The mechanisms of action of the antibacterial agents to be discussed in this section are summarized in Table 118-1 and are depicted in Fig. 118-1.

INHIBITION OF CELL-WALL SYNTHESIS One major difference between bacterial and mammalian cells is the presence in bacteria of a rigid wall external to the cell membrane. The wall protects bacterial cells from osmotic rupture, which would result from the cell's usual marked hyperosmolarity (by up to 20 atm) relative to the host environment. The structure conferring cell-wall rigidity and resistance to osmotic lysis in both gram-positive and gram-negative bacteria is peptidoglycan, a large, covalently linked sacculus that surrounds the bacterium. In gram-positive bacteria, peptidoglycan is the only layered structure external to the cell membrane and is thick (20 to 80 nm); in gram-negative bacteria, there is an outer membrane external to a very thin (1-nm) peptidoglycan layer.

Chemotherapeutic agents directed at any stage of the synthesis, export, assembly, or cross-linking of peptidoglycan lead to inhibition of bacterial cell growth and, in most cases, to cell death. Peptidoglycan is composed of (1) a backbone of two alternating sugars, *N*-acetylglucosamine and *N*-acetylmuramic acid; (2) a chain of four amino acids that extends down from the backbone (stem peptides); and (3) a peptide bridge that cross-links the peptide chains. Peptidoglycan is formed by the addition of subunits (a sugar with its five attached amino acids) that are assembled in the cytoplasm and transported through the cytoplasmic membrane to the cell surface. Subsequent cross-linking is

Letter for Fig. 118-1	Antibacterial Agent[a]	Major Cellular Target	Mechanism of Action	Major Mechanisms of Resistance
A	β-Lactams (penicillins and cephalosporins)	Cell wall	Inhibit cell-wall cross-linking	1. Drug inactivation (β-lactamase) 2. Insensitivity of target (altered penicillin-binding proteins) 3. Decreased permeability (altered gram-negative outer-membrane porins) 4. Active efflux
B	Vancomycin	Cell wall	Interferes with addition of new cell-wall subunits (muramyl pentapeptides)	Alteration of target (substitution of terminal amino acid of peptidoglycan subunit)
	Bacitracin	Cell wall	Prevents addition of cell-wall subunits by inhibiting recycling of membrane lipid carrier	Not defined
C	Macrolides (erythromycin)	Protein synthesis	Bind to 50S ribosomal subunit	1. Alteration of target (ribosomal methylation and mutation of 23S rRNA) 2. Active efflux
	Lincosamides (clindamycin)	Protein synthesis	Bind to 50S ribosomal subunit	Alteration of target (ribosomal methylation)
D	Chloramphenicol	Protein synthesis	Binds to 50S ribosomal subunit	1. Drug inactivation (chloramphenicol acetyltransferase) 2. Active efflux
E	Tetracycline	Protein synthesis	Binds to 30S ribosomal subunit	1. Decreased intracellular drug accumulation (active efflux) 2. Insensitivity of target
F	Aminoglycosides (gentamicin)	Protein synthesis	Bind to 30S ribosomal subunit	1. Drug inactivation (aminoglycoside-modifying enzyme) 2. Decreased permeability through gram-negative outer membrane 3. Active efflux
G	Mupirocin	Protein synthesis	Inhibits isoleucine tRNA synthetase	Mutation of gene for target protein or acquisition of new gene for drug-insensitive target
H	Quinupristin/ dalfopristin (Synercid)	Protein synthesis	Bind to 50S ribosomal subunit	1. Alteration of target (ribosomal methylation: dalfopristin) 2. Active efflux (quinupristin) 3. Drug inactivation (quinupristin and dalfopristin)
I	Linezolid	Protein synthesis	Bind to 50S ribosomal subunit	Alteration of target (mutation of 23S rRNA)
J	Sulfonamides and trimethoprim	Cell metabolism	Competitively inhibit enzymes involved in two steps of folic acid biosynthesis	Production of insensitive targets [dihydropteroate synthetase (sulfonamides) and dihydrofolate reductase (trimethoprim)] that bypass metabolic block
K	Rifampin	Nucleic acid synthesis	Inhibits DNA-dependent RNA polymerase	Insensitivity of target (mutation of polymerase gene)
L	Metronidazole	Nucleic acid synthesis	Intracellularly generates short-lived reactive intermediates that damage DNA by electron transfer system	Not defined
M	Quinolones (ciprofloxacin)	DNA synthesis	Inhibit DNA gyrase (A subunit) and topoisomerase IV	1. Insensitivity of target (mutation of gyrase genes) 2. Decreased intracellular drug accumulation (active efflux)
	Novobiocin	DNA synthesis	Inhibits DNA gyrase (B subunit)	Not defined
N	Polymyxins (polymyxin B)	Cell membrane	Disrupt membrane permeability by charge alteration	Not defined
	Gramicidin	Cell membrane	Forms pores	Not defined

[a] Compounds in parentheses are major representatives for the class.

driven by cleavage of the terminal stem-peptide amino acid. Antibacterial agents act to inhibit cell-wall synthesis in several ways, as described below.

Bacitracin Bacitracin, a cyclic peptide antibiotic, inhibits the conversion to its active form of the lipid carrier that moves the water-soluble cytoplasmic peptidoglycan subunits through the cell membrane to the cell exterior. Cell-wall subunits accumulate in the cytoplasm and cannot be added to the growing peptidoglycan chain.

Glycopeptides Glycopeptides (vancomycin and teicoplanin) are high-molecular-weight antibiotics that bind to the terminal D-alanine–D-alanine component of the stem peptide while the subunits are external to the cell membrane but still linked to the lipid carrier. This binding sterically inhibits the addition of subunits to the peptidoglycan backbone.

β-Lactam Antibiotics β-Lactam antibiotics (penicillins, cephalosporins, carbapenems, and monobactams; Table 118-2) are characterized by a four-membered β-lactam ring and prevent the cross-linking reaction called *transpeptidation*. The energy for attaching a peptide cross-bridge from the stem peptide of one peptidoglycan subunit to another is derived from the cleavage of a terminal D-alanine residue from the subunit stem peptide. The cross-bridge amino acid is then attached to the penultimate D-alanine by transpeptidase enzymes. The β-lactam ring of the antibiotic forms an irreversible covalent acyl bond with the transpeptidase enzyme (probably because of the antibiotic's steric similarity to the enzyme's D-alanine–D-alanine target), preventing the cross-linking reaction. Transpeptidases and similar enzymes involved in cross-linking are called *penicillin-binding proteins* (PBPs) because they all have active sites that bind β-lactam antibiotics.

Virtually all the antibiotics that inhibit bacterial cell-wall synthesis are bactericidal. That is, they eventually result in the cell's death due to osmotic lysis. However, much of the loss of cell-wall integrity following treatment with cell wall–active agents is due to the bacteria's own cell-wall remodeling enzymes (autolysins) that cleave peptido-

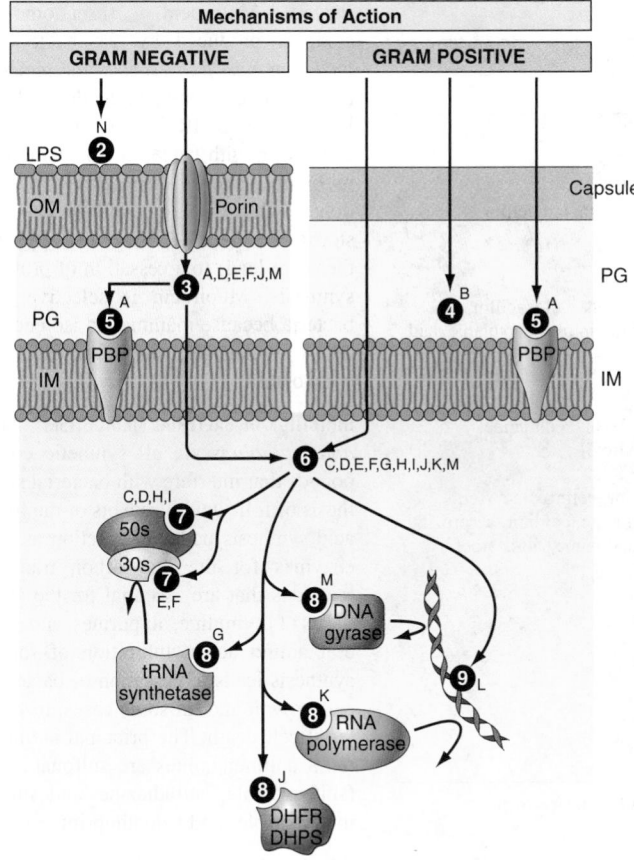
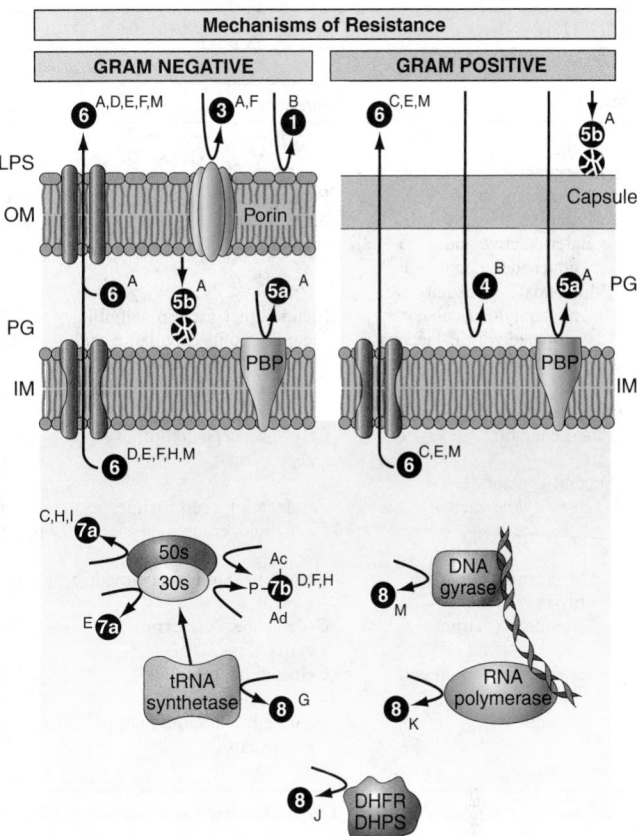

2 Detergent action on lipid gram ⊖ outer membrane.

3 Penetration of hydrophilic drugs through porin channels in gram ⊖ outer membrane.

4 Free diffusion through gram ⊕ cell envelope with binding to cell wall PG **or**

5 Binding to cell membrane PBP. Drug confined to space external to IM.

6 Diffusion or transport of drugs with intracellular target through IM.

7 Binding to ribosomal target for protein synthesis inhibition.

8 Antibiotic interaction with target protein leading to metabolic (DHFR, DHPS), protein synthetic (tRNA synthetase), or nucleic acid (DNA gyrase, RNA polymerase) abnormalities.

9 Direct interaction of reactive intermediates with nucleic acid.

1 **Intrinsic resistance:** Inability of antibiotic to penetrate gram ⊖ envelope (e.g., vancomycin).

3 Mutant porin channels **decrease** antimicrobial **penetration**.

4 **Production of insensitive target** by acquired gene mediating production of altered peptidoglycan.

5a **Production of β-lactam-insensitive PBP target** by mutation of gene or acquisition of new gene.

5b **Inactivation** of β-lactam antibiotic by β-lactamases in periplasm (gram ⊖) or surrounding medium (gram ⊕).

6 **Active efflux** of drugs from cytoplasm or from gram ⊖ periplasm.

7a Decreased ribosomal binding due to **target site alteration**.

7b **Inactivation** of drug by chemical modification leading to decreased ribosomal interaction.

8 Mutation of target gene or acquisition of new gene producing a **drug-insensitive target** protein.

FIGURE 118-1 Mechanisms of action of and resistance to antibacterial agents. Black lines trace the routes of drug interaction with bacterial cells, from entry to target site. The letters in each figure indicate specific antibacterial agents or classes of agents, as shown in Table 118-1. The numbers correspond to mechanisms listed beneath each panel. Abbreviations: LPS, lipopolysaccharide; OM, outer membrane; PG, peptidoglycan; PBP, penicillin-binding protein; IM, inner (cytoplasmic) membrane; 50s and 30s, large and small ribosome subunits; DHFR, dihydrofolate reductase; DHPS, dihydropteroate synthetase; Ac, acetylation; Ad, adenylation; P, phosphorylation.

glycan bonds in the normal course of cell growth. In the presence of antibacterial agents that inhibit cell-wall growth, autolysis proceeds without normal cell-wall repair; weakness and eventual cellular lysis occur.

INHIBITION OF PROTEIN SYNTHESIS Most of the antibacterial agents that inhibit protein synthesis interact with the bacterial ribosome. The difference between the composition of bacterial and mammalian ribosomes gives these compounds their selectivity.

Aminoglycosides Aminoglycosides (gentamicin, kanamycin, tobramycin, streptomycin, netilmicin, neomycin, and amikacin) are a group of structurally related compounds containing three linked hexose sugars. They exert a bactericidal effect by binding irreversibly to the 30S subunit of the bacterial ribosome and blocking initiation of protein synthesis. The reason for the lethal effect of aminoglycosides, as opposed to the largely bacteriostatic effect of other protein synthesis–

inhibiting antibacterial drugs, is not completely understood. Uptake of aminoglycosides and their penetration through the cell membrane constitute an aerobic, energy-dependent process. Thus, aminoglycoside activity is markedly reduced in an anaerobic environment. *Spectinomycin*, an aminocyclitol antibiotic, also acts on the 30S ribosomal subunit but has a different mechanism of action from the aminoglycosides and is bacteriostatic rather than bactericidal.

Macrolide Antibiotics Macrolide antibiotics (erythromycin, clarithromycin, and azithromycin) consist of a large lactone ring to which sugars are attached. *Ketolide antibiotics*, including telithromycin, replace the cladinose sugar on the macrolactone ring with a ketone group. These drugs bind specifically to the 50S portion of the bacterial ribosome. After attachment of mRNA to the initiation site of the 30S ribosomal subunit (the process blocked by aminoglycosides), the 50S subunit becomes bound to the 30S component to form the 70S ribosomal com-

TABLE 118-2 Classification of β-Lactam Antibiotics

Class	Route of Administration	
	Parenteral	Oral
Penicillins		
β-Lactamase–susceptible		
Narrow-spectrum	Penicillin G	Penicillin V
Enteric-active	Ampicillin	Amoxicillin, ampicillin
Enteric-active and antipseudomonal	Ticarcillin	None
β-Lactamase–resistant		
Antistaphylococcal	Methicillin, oxacillin, nafcillin	Cloxacillin, dicloxacillin
Combined with β-lactamase inhibitors	Ticarcillin plus clavulanic acid, ampicillin plus sulbactam, piperacillin plus tazobactam	Amoxicillin plus clavulanic acid
Cephalosporins		
First-generation	Cefazolin, cephalothin, cephapirin	Cephalexin, cephradine, cefadroxil
Second-generation		
Haemophilus-active	Cefamandole, cefuroxime, cefonicid, ceforanide	Cefaclor, cefuroxime axetil, ceftibuten, cefdinir, cefprozil, cefpodoxime,[a] loracarbef
Bacteroides-active	Cefoxitin, cefotetan, cefmetazole	None
Third-generation		
Extended-spectrum	Ceftriaxone, cefotaxime, ceftizoxime	None
Extended-spectrum and antipseudomonal	Ceftazidime, cefepime	None
Carbapenems	Imipenem-cilastatin, meropenem, ertapenem	None
Monobactams	Aztreonam	None

[a] Some sources classify cefpodoxime as a third-generation oral agent because of a marginally broader spectrum.

plex, and protein chain elongation proceeds. When these drugs bind to the 50S ribosomal subunit, protein chain elongation is inhibited.

Although structurally unrelated to the macrolides, *lincosamides* (clindamycin and lincomycin) bind to a site on the 50S ribosome nearly identical to the binding site for macrolides. Although the mechanism and site of action of macrolides and lincosamides are similar, the number and types of bacteria against which these two groups of agents are active differ.

Streptogramins Streptogramins [quinupristin (streptogramin B) and dalfopristin (streptogramin A)], which are supplied as a combination in Synercid, are peptide macrolactones that also bind to the 50S ribosomal subunit and block protein synthesis. Streptogramin B binds to a ribosomal site similar to the binding site for macrolides and lincosamides, whereas streptogramin A binds to a different ribosomal site, blocking the late phase of protein synthesis. The two streptogramins act synergistically to kill bacteria if the strain is susceptible to both components.

Chloramphenicol Chloramphenicol consists of a single aromatic ring and a short side chain. This antibiotic binds reversibly to the 50S portion of the bacterial ribosome at a site close to but not identical with the binding sites for the macrolides and lincosamides. The ribosomal binding of chloramphenicol inhibits peptide bond formation.

Linezolid Linezolid is the first drug in a new, completely synthetic class of antimicrobial agents, the oxazolidinones. Linezolid binds to the 50S ribosomal subunit and blocks the initiation of protein synthesis.

Tetracyclines Tetracyclines (tetracycline, doxycycline, and minocycline) consist of four aromatic rings with various substituent groups. They interact reversibly with the bacterial 30S ribosomal subunit, blocking the binding of aminoacyl tRNA to the mRNA-ribosome complex. This mechanism is markedly different from that of the aminoglycosides, which also bind to the 30S subunit. The specificity of tetracyclines for bacteria depends both on their selectivity for bacterial ribosomes and on their requirement for active, energy-dependent transport into the bacterial cell by a system not found in mammalian cell membranes.

Mupirocin Mupirocin (pseudomonic acid) is produced by the bacterium *Pseudomonas fluorescens*. Its mechanism of action is unique: the drug inhibits isoleucine tRNA synthetase by competing with bacterial isoleucine for its binding site on the enzyme. Inhibition of this enzyme depletes cellular stores of isoleucine-charged tRNA and therefore leads to a cessation of protein synthesis. Mupirocin is selective for bacteria because mammalian isoleucine tRNA synthetase lacks affinity for the compound.

INHIBITION OF BACTERIAL METABOLISM The *antimetabolites* are all synthetic compounds that interfere with bacterial synthesis of folic acid. Products of the folic acid synthesis pathway function as coenzymes for the one-carbon transfer reactions that are essential for the synthesis of thymidine, all purines, and several amino acids. Inhibition of folate synthesis leads to cessation of bacterial cell growth and, in some cases, to bacterial cell death. The principal antibacterial antimetabolites are sulfonamides (sulfisoxazole, sulfadiazine, and sulfamethoxazole) and trimethoprim.

Sulfonamides Sulfonamides are structural analogues of *p*-aminobenzoic acid (PABA), one of the three structural components of folic acid (the other two being pteridine and glutamate). The first step in the synthesis of folic acid is the addition of PABA to pteridine by the enzyme dihydropteroic acid synthetase. Sulfonamides compete with PABA as substrates for the enzyme. The selective effect of sulfonamides is due to the fact that bacteria synthesize folic acid, while mammalian cells cannot synthesize the cofactor and must have exogenous supplies. However, the activity of sulfonamides can be greatly reduced by the presence of excess PABA or by the exogenous addition of end products of one-carbon transfer reactions (e.g., thymidine and purines). High concentrations of the latter substances may be present in some infections as a result of tissue and white cell breakdown, compromising sulfonamide activity.

Trimethoprim Trimethoprim is a diaminopyrimidine, a structural analogue of the pteridine moiety of folic acid. Trimethoprim is a competitive inhibitor of dihydrofolate reductase; this enzyme is responsible for reduction of dihydrofolic acid to tetrahydrofolic acid—the essential final component in the folic acid synthesis pathway that is necessary for all one-carbon transfer reactions. Like the sulfonamides, trimethoprim is bactericidal in the absence of thymine but is only bacteriostatic when this pyrimidine is present in high concentration. The selective antibacterial activity of trimethoprim is based on the much (~50,000-fold) greater sensitivity of bacterial dihydrofolate reductase than of the mammalian enzyme to inhibition by this drug.

INHIBITION OF NUCLEIC ACID SYNTHESIS OR ACTIVITY Numerous antibacterial compounds have disparate effects on nucleic acids. The *quinolones*, including nalidixic acid and its fluorinated derivatives (ciprofloxacin, levofloxacin, gatifloxacin, and moxifloxacin), are synthetic compounds that inhibit the activity of the A subunit of the bacterial enzyme DNA gyrase as well as topoisomerase IV. DNA gyrase and topoisomerases are responsible for negative supercoiling of DNA—an essential conformation for DNA replication in the intact cell. Inhibition of the activity of DNA gyrase and topoisomerase IV is lethal to bacterial cells. The antibiotic *novobiocin* also interferes with the activity of DNA gyrase, but it interferes with the B subunit.

Rifampin Rifampin, used primarily against *Mycobacterium tuberculosis*, is also active against a variety of other bacteria. Rifampin binds tightly to the B subunit of bacterial DNA-dependent RNA polymerase, thus inhibiting transcription of DNA into RNA. Mammalian-cell RNA polymerase is not sensitive to this compound.

Nitrofurantoin Nitrofurantoin, a synthetic compound, causes DNA damage. The nitrofurans, compounds containing a single five-membered ring, are reduced by a bacterial enzyme to highly reactive, short-lived intermediates that are thought to cause DNA strand breakage, either directly or indirectly.

Metronidazole Metronidazole, a synthetic imidazole, is active against a wide range of anaerobic bacteria and protozoa. Its activity is totally dependent on its anaerobic electron-transport system for energy production. In the presence of this system, the nitro group of metronidazole is reduced to a series of transiently produced, reactive intermediates that are thought to cause DNA damage. The unique redox system of anaerobes accounts for the selective antibacterial activity of metronidazole. This compound is also a mutagen and a radiosensitizer of hypoxic mammalian cells.

ALTERATION OF CELL-MEMBRANE PERMEABILITY The *polymyxins* (polymyxin B and colistin, or polymyxin E) are cyclic, basic polypeptides. They behave as cationic, surface-active compounds that disrupt the permeability of both the outer and the cytoplasmic membranes of gram-negative bacteria.

Gramicidin A is a polypeptide of 15 amino acids that acts as an ionophore, forming pores or channels in lipid bilayers.

MECHANISMS OF RESISTANCE

Some bacteria exhibit *intrinsic resistance* to certain classes of antibacterial agents (e.g., obligate anaerobic bacteria to aminoglycosides and gram-negative bacteria to vancomycin). In addition, bacteria that are ordinarily susceptible to antibacterial agents can acquire resistance. *Acquired resistance* is one of the major limitations to effective antibacterial chemotherapy. Resistance can develop by mutation of resident genes or by acquisition of new genes. New genes mediating resistance are usually spread from cell to cell by way of mobile genetic elements such as plasmids, transposons, and bacteriophages. The resistant bacterial populations flourish in areas of high antimicrobial use, where they enjoy a selective advantage over susceptible populations.

The major mechanisms used by bacteria to resist the action of antimicrobial agents are inactivation of the compound, alteration or overproduction of the antibacterial target through mutation of the target protein's gene, acquisition of a new gene that encodes a drug-insensitive target, decreased permeability of the cell envelope to the agent, and active efflux of the compound from the periplasm or interior of the cell. Specific mechanisms of bacterial resistance to the major antibacterial agents are outlined below, summarized in Table 118-1, and depicted in Fig. 118-1.

β-LACTAMS Bacteria develop resistance to β-lactam antibiotics by a variety of mechanisms. Most common is the destruction of the drug by β-lactamases. The β-lactamases of gram-negative bacteria are confined to the periplasm, between the inner and outer membranes, while gram-positive bacteria secrete their β-lactamases into the surrounding medium. These enzymes have a higher affinity for the antibiotic than the antibiotic has for its target. Binding results in hydrolysis of the β-lactam ring. Genes encoding β-lactamases have been found in both chromosomal and extrachromosomal locations and in both gram-positive and gram-negative bacteria; these genes are often on mobile genetic elements. Many "advanced-generation" β-lactam antibiotics, such as ceftriaxone and ceftazidime, are stable in the presence of plasmid-mediated β-lactamases and are active against bacteria resistant to earlier-generation β-lactam antibiotics. However, some β-lactamases either acquired by gram-negative bacteria (e.g., *Klebsiella pneumoniae* and *Escherichia coli*) on mobile genetic elements or present as stable chromosomal genes in other gram-negative species (e.g., *Enterobacter*

spp.) have a broad substrate specificity, hydrolyzing virtually all penicillins and cephalosporins. One strategy that has been devised for circumventing resistance mediated by β-lactamases is to combine the β-lactam agent with an inhibitor that avidly binds the inactivating enzyme, preventing its attack on the antibiotic. Unfortunately, the inhibitors (e.g., clavulanic acid, sulbactam, and tazobactam) do not bind all chromosomal β-lactamases (e.g., *Enterobacter* chromosomal β-lactamase) and thus cannot be depended on to prevent the inactivation of β-lactam antibiotics by such enzymes. No β-lactam antibiotic or inhibitor has been produced that can resist all of the many β-lactamases that have been identified.

A second mechanism of bacterial resistance to β-lactam antibiotics is an alteration in PBP targets so that the PBPs have a markedly reduced affinity for the drug. While this alteration may occur by mutation of existing genes, the acquisition of new PBP genes (as in staphylococcal resistance to methicillin) or of new pieces of PBP genes (as in streptococcal, gonococcal, and meningococcal resistance to penicillin) is more important.

A final resistance mechanism is the coupling, in gram-negative bacteria, of a decrease in outer-membrane permeability with rapid efflux of the antibiotic from the periplasm to the cell exterior. Mutations of genes encoding outer-membrane protein channels called *porins* decrease the entry of β-lactam antibiotics into the cell, while additional proteins form channels that actively pump β-lactams out of the cell. Resistance of Enterobacteriaceae to some cephalosporins and resistance of *Pseudomonas* spp. to cephalosporins and ureidopenicillins are the best examples of this mechanism.

VANCOMYCIN Clinically important resistance to vancomycin was first described among enterococci in France in 1988. Vancomycin-resistant enterococci have subsequently become disseminated worldwide. The genes encoding resistance are carried on plasmids that can transfer themselves from cell to cell and on transposons that can jump from plasmids to chromosomes. Resistance is mediated by enzymes that substitute D-lactate for D-alanine on the peptidoglycan stem peptide so that there is no longer an appropriate target for vancomycin binding. This alteration does not appear to affect cell-wall integrity, however. This type of acquired vancomycin resistance was confined for 14 years to enterococci—more specifically, to *Enterococcus faecium* rather than the more common pathogen *E. faecalis*. However, in 2002, *S. aureus* isolates that were highly resistant to vancomycin were recovered from two patients in the United States. Both isolates contained the gene that mediated vancomycin resistance in enterococci. In addition, since 1996, a few isolates of both *S. aureus* and *S. epidermidis* that display a four- to eightfold reduction in susceptibility to vancomycin have been found worldwide, and many more isolates may contain subpopulations with reduced vancomycin susceptibility. These isolates have not acquired the genes that mediate vancomycin resistance in enterococci but are mutant bacteria with markedly thickened cell walls. These mutants were apparently selected in patients who were undergoing prolonged vancomycin therapy. The failure of vancomycin therapy in some patients infected with *S. aureus* or *S. epidermidis* strains exhibiting only intermediate susceptibility to this drug is thought to have been a result of this resistance.

AMINOGLYCOSIDES The most common aminoglycoside resistance mechanism is inactivation of the antibiotic. Aminoglycoside-modifying enzymes, usually encoded on plasmids, transfer phosphate, adenyl, or acetyl residues from intracellular molecules to hydroxyl or amino side groups on the antibiotic. The modified antibiotic is less active because of diminished binding to its ribosomal target. Modifying enzymes that can inactivate any of the available aminoglycosides have been found in both gram-positive and gram-negative bacteria.

A second aminoglycoside resistance mechanism, which has been identified predominantly in clinical isolates of *Pseudomonas aeruginosa*, is decreased antibiotic uptake, presumably due to alterations in the bacterial outer membrane.

MACROLIDES, KETOLIDES, LINCOSAMIDES, AND STREPTOGRAMINS Resistance in gram-positive bacteria, which are the usual target organisms for macrolides, lincosamides, and streptogramins, can be due to the production of an enzyme—most commonly plasmid-encoded—that methylates ribosomal RNA, interfering with binding of the antibiotics to their target. Methylation mediates resistance to erythromycin, clarithromycin, azithromycin, clindamycin, and streptogramin B. Resistance to streptogramin B converts quinupristin/dalfopristin from a bactericidal to a bacteriostatic antibiotic. Streptococci can also actively cause the efflux of macrolides, and staphylococci can cause the efflux of clindamycin and streptogramin A. In addition, staphylococci can inactivate streptogramin A by acetylation and streptogramin B by either acetylation or hydrolysis. Finally, mutations in 23S ribosomal RNA that alter macrolide binding to their targets have been found in both staphylococci and streptococci. Ketolides retain activity against most isolates of *Streptococcus pneumoniae* resistant to macrolides.

CHLORAMPHENICOL Most bacteria resistant to chloramphenicol produce a plasmid-encoded enzyme, chloramphenicol acetyltransferase, that inactivates the compound by acetylation.

TETRACYCLINES The most common mechanism of tetracycline resistance in gram-negative bacteria is a plasmid-encoded active-efflux pump that is inserted into the cytoplasmic membrane and extrudes antibiotic from the cell. Resistance in gram-positive bacteria is due either to active efflux or to ribosomal alterations that diminish binding of the antibiotic to its target. Genes involved in ribosomal protection are found on mobile genetic elements.

MUPIROCIN Although the topical compound mupirocin was introduced into clinical use relatively recently, resistance is already becoming widespread in some areas. The mechanism appears to be either mutation of the target isoleucine tRNA synthetase so that it is no longer inhibited by the antibiotic or plasmid-encoded production of a form of the target enzyme that binds mupirocin poorly.

TRIMETHOPRIM AND SULFONAMIDES The most prevalent mechanism of resistance to trimethoprim and the sulfonamides in both gram-positive and gram-negative bacteria is the acquisition of plasmid-encoded genes that produce a new, drug-insensitive target—specifically, an insensitive dihydrofolate reductase for trimethoprim and an altered dihydropteroate synthetase for sulfonamides.

QUINOLONES Resistance to the newer fluoroquinolones emerged rapidly among *Staphylococcus* and *Pseudomonas* spp. after the introduction of these agents. Widespread use of fluoroquinolones in the community has resulted in increasing rates of resistance in *S. pneumoniae*. The most common mechanism is the development of one or more mutations in target DNA gyrases and topoisomerase IV that prevent the antibacterial agent from interfering with the activity of the enzyme. Some gram-negative bacteria develop mutations that both decrease outer-membrane porin permeability and cause active drug efflux from the cytoplasm. Mutations that result in active quinolone efflux are also found in gram-positive bacteria.

RIFAMPIN Bacteria rapidly become resistant to rifampin by developing mutations in the B subunit of RNA polymerase that render the enzyme unable to bind the antibiotic. The rapid selection of resistant mutants is the major limitation to the use of this antibiotic against otherwise-susceptible staphylococci and requires that the drug be used in combination with another antistaphylococcal agent.

LINEZOLID Enterococci, streptococci, and staphylococci become resistant to linezolid in vitro by mutation of the 23S rRNA binding site. Clinical isolates of *E. faecium* and *E. faecalis* acquire resistance to linezolid readily by this mechanism, often during therapy, but linezolid-resistant staphylococcal and streptococcal isolates are rare.

MULTIPLE ANTIBIOTIC RESISTANCE The acquisition by one bacterium of resistance to multiple antibacterial agents is becoming increasingly common. The two major mechanisms are the acquisition of multiple unrelated resistance genes and the development of mutations in a single gene or gene complex that mediate resistance to a series of unrelated compounds. The construction of multiresistant strains by acquisition of multiple genes occurs by sequential steps of gene transfer and environmental selection in areas of high-level antimicrobial use. In contrast, mutations in a single gene can conceivably be selected in a single step. Bacteria that are multiresistant by virtue of the acquisition of new genes include hospital-associated gram-negative bacteria, enterococci, and staphylococci and community-acquired strains of salmonellae, gonococci, and pneumococci. Mutations that confer resistance to multiple unrelated antimicrobial agents occur in the genes encoding outer-membrane porins and efflux proteins of gram-negative bacteria. These mutations decrease bacterial intracellular and periplasmic accumulation of β-lactams, quinolones, tetracyclines, chloramphenicol, and aminoglycosides. Multiresistant bacterial isolates pose increasing problems in U.S. hospitals; strains resistant to all available antibacterial chemotherapy have already been identified.

PHARMACOKINETICS OF ANTIBIOTICS

The *pharmacokinetic profile* of an antibacterial agent refers to concentrations in serum and tissue versus time and reflects the processes of absorption, distribution, metabolism, and excretion. Important characteristics include peak and trough serum concentrations and mathematically derived parameters such as half-life, clearance, and distribution volume. Pharmacokinetic information is useful for estimating the appropriate antibacterial dose and frequency of administration, for adjusting dosages in patients with impaired excretory capacity, and for comparing one drug with another. In contrast, the *pharmacodynamic profile* of an antibiotic refers to the relationship between serum and tissue concentrations of the antibiotic and its minimal inhibitory concentrations (MICs) for bacteria. →*For further discussion of basic pharmacokinetic principles, see Chap. 3.*

ABSORPTION Antibiotic *absorption* refers to the rate and extent of a drug's systemic bioavailability after oral, intramuscular, or intravenous administration.

Oral Administration Most patients with infection are treated with oral antibacterial agents in the outpatient setting. Advantages of oral therapy over parenteral therapy include lower cost, generally fewer adverse effects (including complications of indwelling lines), and greater acceptance by patients. The percentage of an orally administered antibacterial agent that is absorbed (i.e., its *bioavailability*) ranges from as little as 10 to 20% (erythromycin and penicillin G) to nearly 100% [amoxicillin, clindamycin, metronidazole, doxycycline, trimethoprim-sulfamethoxazole (TMP-SMX), linezolid, and most fluoroquinolones]. These differences in bioavailability are not clinically important as long as drug concentrations at the site of infection are sufficient to inhibit or kill the pathogen. However, therapeutic efficacy may be compromised when absorption is reduced as a result of physiologic or pathologic conditions (such as the presence of food for some drugs or the shunting of blood away from the gastrointestinal tract in patients with hypotension), drug interactions (such as that of quinolones and metal cations), or noncompliance. The oral route is usually used for patients with relatively mild infections in whom absorption is not thought to be compromised by the preceding conditions. In addition, the oral route can often be used in more severely ill patients after they have responded to parenteral therapy ("switch" therapy).

Intramuscular Administration Although the intramuscular route of administration usually results in 100% bioavailability, it is not as widely used in the United States as the oral and intravenous routes, in part because of the pain often associated with intramuscular injections and the relative ease of intravenous access in the hospitalized patient. Intramuscular injection may be suitable for specific indications requiring an "immediate" and reliable effect (e.g., with long-acting forms of penicillin, including benzathine and procaine, and with single doses of ceftriaxone for acute otitis media or uncomplicated gonococcal infection).

Intravenous Administration The intravenous route is appropriate when oral antibacterial agents are not effective against a particular pathogen, when bioavailability is uncertain, or when larger doses are required than are feasible with the oral route. After intravenous administration, bioavailability is 100%; serum concentrations are maximal at the end of the infusion. For many patients in whom long-term antimicrobial therapy is required and oral therapy is not feasible, outpatient parenteral antibiotic therapy, including the use of convenient portable pumps, may be cost-effective and safe. Alternatively, some oral antibacterial drugs (e.g., fluoroquinolones) are sufficiently active against Enterobacteriaceae to provide potency equal to that of parenteral therapy; their use may allow the patient to return home from the hospital earlier or to avoid hospitalization entirely.

DISTRIBUTION To be effective, an antibacterial agent must exceed the pathogen's MIC. Serum concentrations usually exceed the MIC for susceptible bacteria, but since most infections are extravascular, the antibiotic must also distribute to the site of the infection. Concentrations of most antibacterial agents in interstitial fluid are similar to free-drug concentrations in serum. However, when the infection is located in a "protected" site where penetration is poor, such as cerebrospinal fluid (CSF), the eye, the prostate, or infected cardiac vegetations, high parenteral doses or local administration for prolonged periods may be required for cure. In addition, even though an antibacterial agent may penetrate to the site of infection, its activity may be antagonized by factors in the local environment, such as an unfavorable pH or inactivation by cellular degradation products. For example, since the activity of aminoglycosides is reduced at acidic pH, the acidic environment in many infected tissues may be partly responsible for the relatively poor efficacy of aminoglycoside monotherapy. In addition, the abscess milieu reduces the penetration and local activity of many antibacterial compounds, so that surgical drainage may be required for cure.

Most bacteria that cause human infections are located extracellularly. Intracellular pathogens such as *Legionella*, *Chlamydia*, *Brucella*, and *Salmonella* may persist or cause relapse if the antibacterial agent does not enter the cell. In general, β-lactams, vancomycin, and aminoglycosides penetrate cells poorly, whereas macrolides, ketolides, tetracyclines, metronidazole, chloramphenicol, rifampin, TMP-SMX, and quinolones penetrate cells well.

METABOLISM AND ELIMINATION Like other drugs, antibacterial agents are disposed of by hepatic elimination (metabolism or biliary elimination), by renal excretion of the unchanged or metabolized form, or by a combination of the two processes. For most antibacterial drugs, metabolism leads to loss of in vitro activity, although some agents, such as cefotaxime, rifampin, rifabutin, and clarithromycin, have bioactive metabolites that may contribute to their overall efficacy.

The most practical application of knowing the mode of excretion of an antibacterial agent is adjustment of the dosage when elimination capability is impaired (Table 118-3). Direct, nonidiosyncratic toxicity from antibacterial drugs may result from failure to reduce the dosage in a patient with impaired elimination. For agents that are primarily cleared intact by glomerular filtration, drug clearance is linearly correlated with creatinine clearance. Unfortunately, for drugs whose elimination is primarily hepatic, no simple marker (such as serum creatinine) is useful for dosage adjustment in patients with liver disease. Even in patients with severe hepatic disease, residual metabolic capability is usually sufficient to preclude accumulation and toxic effects.

PRINCIPLES OF ANTIBACTERIAL CHEMOTHERAPY

The choice of an antibacterial compound for a particular patient and a specific infection involves more than just a knowledge of the agent's pharmacokinetic profile and in vitro activity. The basic tenets of chemotherapy, to be elaborated below, include the following: When appropriate, material containing the infecting organism(s) should be obtained before the start of treatment so that presumptive identification can be made by microscopic examination of stained specimens and

TABLE 118-3 *Antibacterial Drug Dose Adjustments in Patients with Renal Impairment*

Antibiotic	Major Route of Excretion	Dosage Adjustment with Renal Impairment
Aminoglycosides	Renal	Yes
Azithromycin	Biliary	No
Cefazolin	Renal	Yes
Cefepime	Renal	Yes
Ceftazidime	Renal	Yes
Ceftriaxone	Renal/biliary	Modest reduction in severe renal impairment
Ciprofloxacin	Renal/biliary	Only in severe renal insufficiency
Clarithromycin	Renal/biliary	Only in severe renal insufficiency
Erythromycin	Biliary	Only when given in high IV doses
Levofloxacin	Renal	Yes
Linezolid	Metabolism	No
Metronidazole	Biliary	No
Nafcillin	Biliary	No
Penicillin G	Renal	Yes (when given in high IV doses)
Piperacillin	Renal	Only with Cl_{cr} of <40 mL/min
Quinupristin/ dalfopristin	Metabolism	No
Ticarcillin	Renal	Yes
TMP-SMX	Renal/biliary	Only in severe renal insufficiency
Vancomycin	Renal	Yes

Abbreviations: Cl_{cr}, creatinine clearance rate; TMP-SMX, trimethoprim-sulfamethoxazole.

the organism can be grown for definitive identification and susceptibility testing. Awareness of local susceptibility patterns is useful when the patient is treated empirically. Once the organism is identified and its susceptibility to antibacterial agents is determined, the regimen with the narrowest effective spectrum should be chosen. The choice of antibacterial agent is guided by the pharmacokinetic and adverse-reaction profile of active compounds, the site of infection, the immune status of the host, and evidence of efficacy from well-performed clinical trials. If all other factors are equal, the least expensive antibacterial regimen should be chosen.

SUSCEPTIBILITY OF BACTERIA TO ANTIBACTERIAL DRUGS IN VITRO Determination of the susceptibility of the patient's infecting organism to a panel of appropriate antibacterial agents is an essential first step in devising a chemotherapeutic regimen. Standard susceptibility testing is designed to estimate the susceptibility of a bacterial isolate to an antibacterial drug under standardized conditions. These conditions favor rapidly growing aerobic or facultative organisms and assess bacteriostasis only. Specialized testing is required for the assessment of bactericidal antimicrobial activity; for the detection of resistance among such fastidious organisms as obligate anaerobes, *Haemophilus* spp., and pneumococci; and for the determination of resistance phenotypes with variable expression, such as resistance to methicillin or oxacillin among staphylococci. Antimicrobial susceptibility testing is important when susceptibility is unpredictable, most often as a result of increasing acquired resistance among hospitalized patients.

PHARMACODYNAMICS: RELATIONSHIP OF PHARMACOKINETICS AND IN VITRO SUSCEPTIBILITY TO CLINICAL RESPONSE Bacteria are often considered to be *susceptible* to a drug if the achievable peak serum concentration exceeds the MIC by approximately fourfold. The *breakpoint* is the concentration of the antibiotic that separates susceptible from resistant bacteria (Fig. 118-2). When a majority of the isolates of a given bacterial species are inhibited at concentrations below the breakpoint, the species is considered to be within the spectrum of the antibiotic (see "Choice of Antibacterial Therapy," below).

The pharmacodynamic profile of an antibiotic refers to the quantitative relationships between the time course of antibiotic concentrations in serum and tissue, in vitro susceptibility, and microbial response (inhibition of growth or rate of killing). Three pharmacodynamic parameters quantify these relationships: the ratio of the area

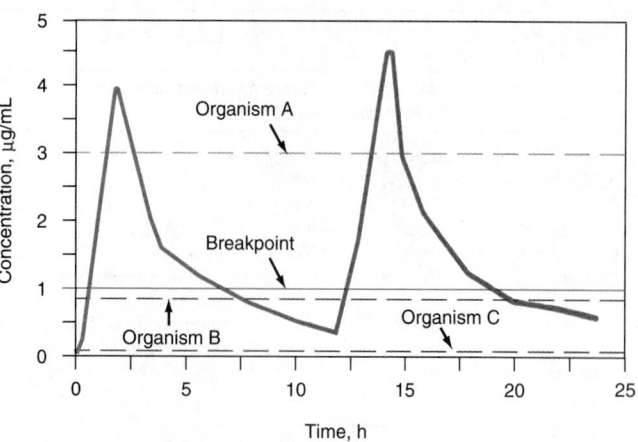

FIGURE 118-2 Relationship between pharmacokinetics of an antibiotic and susceptibility. Organism A is resistant, organism B is moderately susceptible, and organism C is very susceptible.

under the curve for the plasma concentration vs. time curve to MIC (AUC/MIC), the ratio of the maximal serum concentration to the MIC (C_{max}/MIC), and the time during a dosing interval that plasma concentrations exceed the MIC ($t >$ MIC). The pharmacodynamic profile of an antibiotic class is characterized as either *concentration dependent* (fluoroquinolones, aminoglycosides), such that the increase in antibiotic concentration leads to a more rapid rate of bacterial death, or *time dependent* (β-lactams), such that the reduction in bacterial density is proportional to the time that concentrations exceed the MIC. For concentration-dependent antibiotics, the C_{max}/MIC or AUC/MIC ratio correlates best with the reduction in microbial density in vitro and in animal investigations. Dosing strategies attempt to maximize these ratios by the administration of a large dose relative to the MIC for anticipated pathogens, often at long intervals (relative to the serum half-life). Once-daily dosing of aminoglycoside antibiotics is the most practical consequence of these relationships. In contrast, dosage strategies for time-dependent antibiotics emphasize the administration of doses sufficient to maintain serum concentrations above the MIC for a critical portion of the dose interval. Response to β-lactam antibiotics, measured as the decline in bacterial density at the site of infection, appears to be maximal when serum and tissue concentrations are maintained above the MIC for 30 to 50% of the dose interval. For example, the use of high-dose amoxicillin (90 to 100 mg/kg per day) in the treatment of acute otitis media increases not only the penetration of amoxicillin into the inner ear but also the duration of time that concentrations exceed the MIC for pneumococci. This approach provides effective therapy in most patients, including those whose pneumococcal isolates are penicillin resistant. The clinical implications of these pharmacodynamic relationships are in the early stages of investigation; their elucidation should eventually result in more rational antibacterial dosage regimens. Table 118-4 summarizes the pharmacodynamic properties of the major antibiotic classes.

STATUS OF THE HOST Various host factors must be considered in the devising of antibacterial chemotherapy. The host's antibacterial *immune function* is of importance, particularly as it relates to opsonophagocytic function. Since the major host defense against acute, overwhelming bacterial infection is the polymorphonuclear leukocyte, patients with neutropenia must be treated aggressively and empirically with bactericidal drugs for suspected infection (Chap. 72). Likewise, patients who have deficient humoral immunity (e.g., those with chronic lymphocytic leukemia and multiple myeloma) and individuals with surgical or functional asplenia (e.g., those with sickle cell disease) should be treated empirically for infections with encapsulated organisms, especially the pneumococcus.

Pregnancy increases the risk of toxicity of certain antibacterial drugs for the mother (e.g., hepatic toxicity of tetracycline), affects drug

disposition and pharmacokinetics, and—because of the risk of fetal toxicity—severely limits the choice of agents for treating infections. Certain antibacterial agents are contraindicated in pregnancy either because their safety has not been established or because they are known to be toxic. These agents include all fluoroquinolones, clarithromycin, erythromycin estolate (but not erythromycin base), and tetracyclines (Table 118-5). Data on the safety of many other antibacterial drugs are limited, but these drugs may be used cautiously when there is no suitable alternative and the perceived benefit outweighs the risk. These agents include the aminoglycosides, azithromycin, clindamycin, imipenem, metronidazole, trimethoprim, and vancomycin. Nitrofurantoin and the sulfonamides are contraindicated in the third trimester but can be used cautiously in the first two trimesters.

In patients with *concomitant viral infections*, the incidence of adverse reactions to antibacterial drugs may be unusually high. For example, persons with infectious mononucleosis and those infected with HIV react more often to ampicillin and folic acid synthesis inhibitors, respectively.

In addition, the patient's age, sex, racial heritage, genetic background, and excretory status all determine the incidence and type of side effects that can be expected with certain antibacterial agents.

SITE OF INFECTION The location of the infected site may play a major role in the choice and dose of antimicrobial drug. Patients with suspected *meningitis* should receive drugs that can cross the blood-CSF barrier; in addition, because of the relative paucity of phagocytes and opsonins at the site of infection, the agents should be bactericidal. Chloramphenicol, an older drug but occasionally useful in the treatment of meningitis, is bactericidal for common organisms causing meningitis (i.e., meningococci, pneumococci, and *Haemophilus influenzae*, but *not* enteric gram-negative bacilli), is highly lipid-soluble, and enters the CSF well. However, β-lactam drugs, the mainstay of therapy for most of these infections, do not normally reach high levels in CSF. Their efficacy is based on the increased permeability of the blood-brain and blood-CSF barriers to hydrophilic molecules during inflammation and the extreme susceptibility of most infectious organisms to even small amounts of β-lactam drug.

The vegetation, which is the major site of infection in *bacterial endocarditis*, is also a focus that is protected from normal host-defense mechanisms. Antibacterial therapy needs to be bactericidal, with the selected agent administered parenterally over a long period and at a dose that produces serum levels at least eight times higher than the minimal bactericidal concentration (MBC) for the infecting organism. Likewise, *osteomyelitis* involves a site that is somewhat resistant to opsonophagocytic removal of infecting bacteria; furthermore, avascular bone (sequestrum) represents a foreign body that thwarts normal host-defense mechanisms. *Chronic prostatitis* is exceedingly difficult to cure because most antibiotics do not penetrate through the capillaries serving the prostate, especially when acute inflammation is absent. *Intraocular infections*, especially endophthalmitis, are difficult to treat because retinal capillaries lacking fenestration hinder drug penetration into the vitreous from blood. Inflammation does little to disrupt this barrier. Thus, direct injection into the vitreous is necessary in many cases. Antibiotic penetration into *abscesses* is usually poor, and local conditions (e.g., low pH or the presence of enzymes that hydrolyze the drug) may further antagonize antibacterial activity.

TABLE 118-4 *Pharmacodynamic Parameters of Major Antimicrobial Classes*

Parameter Predicting Response	Drug or Drug Class
Time above the MIC	Penicillins, cephalosporins, carbapenems, aztreonam
24-h AUC/MIC	Aminoglycosides, fluoroquinolones, tetracyclines, vancomycin, macrolides, clindamycin, quinupristin/dalfopristin
Peak to MIC	Aminoglycosides, fluoroquinolones

Abbreviations: MIC, minimal inhibitory concentration: AUC, area under the concentration curve.

In contrast, *urinary tract infections*, when confined to the bladder, are relatively easy to cure, in part because of the higher concentration of most antibiotics in urine than in blood. Since blood is the usual reference fluid in defining susceptibility (Fig. 118-2), even organisms found to be resistant to achievable serum concentrations may be susceptible to achievable urine concentrations. For drugs that are used only for the treatment of urinary tract infections, such as nitrofurantoin and methenamine salts, achievable urine concentrations are used to determine susceptibility.

TABLE 118-5 *Antibacterial Drugs in Pregnancy*

Antibacterial Drug	Toxicity in Pregnancy	Recommendation
Aminoglycosides	Possible 8th nerve toxicity	Caution[a]
Chloramphenicol	Gray syndrome in newborn	Caution at term
Fluoroquinolones	Arthropathy in immature animals	Caution
Clarithromycin	Teratogenicity in animals	Contraindicated
Ertapenem	Decreased weight in animals	Caution
Erythromycin estolate	Cholestatic hepatitis	Contraindicated
Imipenem/cilastatin	Toxicity in some pregnant animals	Caution
Linezolid	Embryonic and fetal toxicity in rats	Caution
Meropenem	Unknown	Caution
Metronidazole	None known, but carcinogenic in rats	Caution
Nitrofurantoin	Hemolytic anemia in newborns	Caution; contraindicated at term
Quinupristin/dalfopristin	Unknown	Caution
Sulfonamides	Hemolysis in newborn with G6PD[b] deficiency; kernicterus in newborn	Caution; contraindicated at term
Tetracyclines	Tooth discoloration, inhibition of bone growth in fetus; hepatotoxicity	Contraindicated
Vancomycin	Unknown	Caution

[a] Use only for strong clinical indication in the absence of a suitable alternative.
[b] G6PD, glucose-6-phosphate dehydrogenase.
Source: *Medical Letter Handbook of Antimicrobial Therapy*, 16th ed, 2002.

COMBINATION CHEMOTHERAPY One of the tenets of antibacterial chemotherapy is that if the infecting bacterium has been identified, the most specific chemotherapy possible should be used. The use of a single agent with a narrow spectrum of activity against the pathogen diminishes the alteration of normal flora and thus limits the overgrowth of resistant nosocomial organisms (e.g., *Candida albicans*, enterococci, *Clostridium difficile*, or methicillin-resistant staphylococci), avoids the potential toxicity of multiple-drug regimens, and reduces cost. However, certain circumstances call for the use of more than one antibacterial agent. These are summarized below.

1. *Prevention of the emergence of resistant mutants.* Spontaneous mutations occur at a detectable frequency in certain genes encoding the target proteins for some antibacterial agents. The use of these agents can eliminate the susceptible population, select out resistant mutants at the site of infection, and result in the failure of chemotherapy. Resistant mutants are usually selected when the MIC of the antibacterial agent for the infecting bacterium is close to achievable levels in serum or tissues and/or when the site of infection limits the access or activity of the agent. Among the most common examples are rifampin for staphylococci, imipenem for *Pseudomonas*, and fluoroquinolones for staphylococci and *Pseudomonas*. Small-colony variants of staphylococci resistant to aminoglycosides also emerge during monotherapy with these antibiotics. A second antibacterial agent with a mechanism of action different from that of the first is added to prevent the emergence of these resistant mutants (e.g., imipenem plus an aminoglycoside for systemic *Pseudomonas* infections). However, since resistant mutants have emerged following combination chemotherapy, this approach clearly is not uniformly successful.

2. *Synergistic or additive activity.* Synergistic or additive activity involves a lowering of the MIC or MBC of each or all of the drugs tested in combination against a specific bacterium. In *synergy*, each agent is more active when combined with a second drug than it would be alone, and the drugs' combined activity is therefore greater than the sum of the individual activities of each drug. In an *additive relationship*, the combined activity of the drugs is equal to the sum of their individual activities. Among the best examples of a synergistic or additive effect, confirmed both in vitro and by animal studies, are the enhanced bactericidal activities of certain β-lactam/aminoglycoside combinations against enterococci, viridans streptococci, and *P. aeruginosa*. The synergistic or additive activity of these combinations has also been demonstrated against selected isolates of enteric gram-negative bacteria and staphylococci. The combination of trimethoprim and sulfamethoxazole has synergistic or additive activity against many enteric gram-negative bacteria. Most other antimicrobial combinations display indifferent activity (i.e., the combination is *no better* than the more active of the two agents alone), and some combinations (e.g.,

penicillin plus tetracycline against pneumococci) may be antagonistic (i.e., the combination is *worse* than either drug alone).

3. *Therapy directed against multiple potential pathogens.* For certain infections, either a mixture of pathogens is suspected or the patient is desperately ill with an as-yet-unidentified infection (see "Empirical Therapy," below). In these situations, the most important of the likely infecting bacteria must be covered by therapy until culture and susceptibility results become available. Examples of the former infections are intraabdominal or brain abscesses and infections of limbs in diabetic patients with microvascular disease. The latter situations include fevers in neutropenic patients, acute pneumonia from aspiration of oral flora by hospitalized patients, and septic shock or sepsis syndrome.

EMPIRICAL THERAPY In many situations, antibacterial therapy is begun before a specific bacterial pathogen has been identified. The choice of agent is guided by the results of studies identifying the usual pathogens at that site or in that clinical setting, by pharmacodynamic considerations, and by the resistance profile of the expected pathogens in a particular hospital or geographic area. Situations in which empirical therapy is appropriate include the following:

1. *Life-threatening infection.* Any suspected bacterial infection in a patient with a life-threatening illness should be treated presumptively. Therapy is usually begun with more than one agent and is later tailored to a specific pathogen if one is eventually identified.

2. *Treatment of community-acquired infections.* In many situations, it is appropriate to treat non-life-threatening infections without obtaining cultures. These situations include outpatient infections such as community-acquired upper and lower respiratory tract infections, cystitis, cellulitis or local wound infection, urethritis, and prostatitis. However, if any of these infections recurs or fails to respond to initial therapy, every effort should be made to obtain cultures to guide retreatment.

CHOICE OF ANTIBACTERIAL THERAPY

The antibacterial spectrum of specific agents and the infections for which they represent the treatment of choice are detailed below. No attempt has been made to include all the potential situations in which antibacterial agents may be used. A more detailed discussion of specific bacteria and infections that they cause can be found elsewhere in this volume.

β-LACTAMS (Table 118-2) All *penicillins* (except for the semisynthetic, penicillinase-resistant antistaphylococcal agents) are hydrolyzed by β-lactamases and are ineffective against isolates that produce these enzymes. Penicillin G has a spectrum that includes spirochetes

(*Treponema pallidum*, *Borrelia*, and *Leptospira*), streptococci (groups A and B, viridans, and many strains of *S. pneumoniae*), *E. faecalis*, most *Neisseria* spp., a few staphylococci, many fastidious oral bacteria (including many *Porphyromonas* and *Prevotella* spp., streptococci, *Actinomyces*, and *Fusobacterium*), *Clostridium* spp. (except *C. difficile*), *Pasteurella multocida*, *Erysipelothrix rhusiopathiae*, and *Streptobacillus moniliformis*. However, penicillin G resistance is widespread among staphylococci; is increasing rapidly among gonococci and pneumococci; and is emerging among meningococci, viridans streptococci, and oral anaerobes such as *Porphyromonas* and *Prevotella*. Penicillin G is the *drug of choice* for syphilis, yaws, leptospirosis, group A and B streptococcal infections, actinomycosis, oral and periodontal infections, meningococcal meningitis and meningococcemia, viridans streptococcal endocarditis, clostridial myonecrosis, tetanus, anthrax, rat-bite fever, *P. multocida* infections, and erysipeloid (*E. rhusiopathiae*).

Ampicillin extends the spectrum of penicillin G to some gram-negative rods. It is active against some isolates of *Escherichia coli*, *Proteus mirabilis*, *Salmonella*, *Shigella*, and *H. influenzae* and is one of the *drugs of choice* for susceptible organisms causing salmonellosis, acute otitis media, *H. influenzae* meningitis and epiglottitis, and *Listeria monocytogenes* meningitis. *E. faecalis* is usually susceptible, and amoxicillin is the *drug of choice* for urinary tract infections caused by this organism. High rates of resistance have lessened the value of ampicillin and amoxicillin as empirical therapy in some situations. For example, >80% of isolates of *E. coli* and *P. mirabilis* are resistant in many hospitals, as are ~30% of isolates of *H. influenzae*; moreover, in some outbreaks of infection due to salmonellae, all isolates are resistant to ampicillin.

The *penicillinase-resistant penicillins* are used solely for the treatment of staphylococcal infections and are the *drugs of choice* for systemic or deep staphylococcal infections caused by susceptible organisms. Unfortunately, on average, ~40% of *S. aureus* isolates and >70% of coagulase-negative staphylococcal isolates acquired in U.S. hospitals are resistant to these agents (i.e., methicillin-resistant). The spectrum of these agents also includes most of the same gram-positive bacteria that are susceptible to penicillin G.

The spectrum of the *antipseudomonal penicillins* includes the bacteria covered by ampicillin as well as some nonpseudomonal enteric gram-negative bacilli. For example, piperacillin is active against many indole-positive *Proteus*, *Enterobacter*, *Klebsiella*, *Providencia*, and *Serratia* spp. However, the susceptibility of these penicillins to β-lactamase markedly limits their utility as empirical therapy when infections caused by gram-negative enteric organisms are suspected. The "antipseudomonal penicillins" are no longer commercially available or have been formulated in combination with β-*lactamase inhibitors*. The addition of a β-lactamase inhibitor (clavulanic acid, sulbactam, or tazobactam) to ampicillin, amoxicillin, ticarcillin, or piperacillin extends the spectrum of the β-lactam agent to include many organisms that are resistant by virtue of β-lactamase production. These organisms include many strains of *E. coli*, *Klebsiella* spp., all *Proteus* spp., *H. influenzae*, *Moraxella catarrhalis*, *Providencia* spp., and anaerobes (including *Bacteroides* spp.). Such combinations are also active against staphylococci that produce β-lactamase but are not resistant to methicillin. However, the efficacy of these combinations in serious staphylococcal infections has not been adequately proven. Furthermore, *Serratia*, indole-positive *Proteus*, *Citrobacter*, *Enterobacter*, *Pseudomonas*, *Acinetobacter*, and various enteric gram-negative isolates either produce chromosomal β-lactamases that are not inhibited by these compounds or develop resistance attributable to non-β-lactamase-mediated mechanisms.

The *first-generation cephalosporins* have a spectrum that includes penicillinase-producing, methicillin-susceptible staphylococci and penicillin-susceptible streptococci. While these drugs may be used when infections with gram-positive bacteria are suspected, they are *not* the drugs of choice for such infections. They have excellent activity against many isolates of *E. coli*, *Klebsiella pneumoniae*, and *P. mirabilis* and are among the *drugs of choice* in presumptive therapy for community-acquired urinary tract infections. They have no activity against *Bacteroides fragilis*, enterococci, methicillin-resistant staphylococci, *Pseudomonas*, *Acinetobacter*, *Enterobacter*, indole-positive *Proteus*, and *Serratia* and only poor activity against *H. influenzae*.

The *parenteral second-generation cephalosporins* extend the gram-negative spectrum of first-generation compounds. The various second-generation agents have differing activities. Cefuroxime retains activity against gram-positive cocci and is also active against *H. influenzae*, *Neisseria*, and indole-positive *Proteus* but exhibits poor activity against *B. fragilis*. Cefoxitin and cefotetan have reasonably good activity against *B. fragilis*, but cefotetan is less effective against some other *Bacteroides* spp. (Chaps. 112 and 148). Both of the latter drugs display poor activity against gram-positive cocci and *Enterobacter*. No second-generation cephalosporin is active against *Pseudomonas* or *Acinetobacter*.

Oral second- and third-generation cephalosporins have fair activity against gram-positive cocci and *H. influenzae* and are widely used in outpatient therapy for otitis media, sinusitis, and lower respiratory tract infections, although cheaper agents that are equally effective are preferable. Cefditoren, cefdinir, and cefpodoxime have good activity against most respiratory pathogens and methicillin-susceptible *S. aureus*.

Third-generation parenteral cephalosporins all have a broad spectrum of activity against enteric gram-negative rods and are especially useful for treating hospital-acquired infections caused by multiresistant organisms. In addition, ceftazidime and cefepime have good antipseudomonal activity; the other drugs have poor activity. Since resistance to third-generation cephalosporins is increasing among all nosocomial gram-negative rods, the use of these agents should be guided by susceptibility testing. The gram-positive spectrum of the third-generation cephalosporins is variable. All are less active than first-generation cephalosporins against methicillin-susceptible staphylococci; ceftazidime has the least antistaphylococcal activity of this group. However, ceftriaxone and cefotaxime have excellent activity against streptococci, especially *S. pneumoniae*. Ceftazidime is not recommended for treatment of streptococcal infections.

Ceftriaxone has an excellent gram-negative spectrum; is active against *Haemophilus*, most *S. pneumoniae* strains, and penicillin-resistant *Neisseria*; has a long serum half-life; and reaches high serum and CSF levels (with inflammation). Thus it has become one of the *drugs of choice* for empirical therapy for bacterial meningitis (except that caused by *Listeria* and by highly penicillin-resistant pneumococcal strains), all gonococcal infections, salmonellosis, and typhoid fever. The third-generation cephalosporins are among the *drugs of choice* for nonpseudomonal hospital-acquired pneumonia. Cefepime is more resistant to chromosomal β-lactamase produced by *Enterobacter* spp. than are other third-generation cephalosporins and is more active against methicillin-susceptible *S. aureus*. Third-generation cephalosporins have poor activity against *Bacteroides* and no activity against methicillin-resistant staphylococci, *Enterococcus*, *Acinetobacter*, or *Stenotrophomonas*.

The *carbapenems* currently available in the United States are imipenem, meropenem, and ertapenem. Imipenem is marketed in combination with the renal dipeptidase inhibitor cilastatin, which enables imipenem to escape renal inactivation and thus to reach higher urinary levels. Imipenem and meropenem have excellent activity in vitro against virtually all bacterial pathogens except *Stenotrophomonas*, methicillin-resistant staphylococci, and *E. faecium*. Imipenem has dose-related central nervous system side effects that are less frequent with meropenem. Resistance to imipenem and meropenem is a problem among nosocomial isolates of *P. aeruginosa*, ~20% of which are resistant. Ertapenem has poor activity against enterococci, *P. aeruginosa*, and *Acinetobacter* but exhibits activity similar to that of meropenem against Enterobacteriaceae. Because of their broad spectrum, imipenem and meropenem can be used as empirical therapy for serious nosocomial infections thought to be caused by multiple bacterial species or multiresistant organisms. Imipenem and meropenem are often used to treat hospital-acquired infections caused by *Enterobacter* spp. because these organisms produce inducible β-lactamases that inactivate third-generation cephalosporins but not the carbapenems. The latter antibiotics are often held in reserve as therapy for nosocomial infections due to gram-negative pathogens that are resistant to third-generation cephalosporins.

The only *monobactam* currently available is aztreonam. This antibiotic has a spectrum limited to gram-negative enteric bacilli. It has no activity against any gram-positive or anaerobic bacterium. Its gram-negative spectrum is similar to that of ceftazidime, with equally good activity against *Pseudomonas*. Aztreonam's primary advantages are its theoretical ability to preserve the normal gram-positive and anaerobic flora and the lack of cross-reactive immediate hypersensitivity in patients who have had this type of reaction to other β-lactam antibiotics.

VANCOMYCIN The spectrum of vancomycin is limited to gram-positive cocci, especially enterococci, streptococci, and staphylococci. Vancomycin serves as second-line therapy for most gram-positive bacterial infections but is the *drug of choice* for infections caused by methicillin-resistant staphylococci or *Corynebacterium jeikeium* and for serious infections in penicillin-allergic patients. Given orally (a route by which it is not absorbed), vancomycin can be used to treat antibiotic-associated pseudomembranous colitis caused by *C. difficile* in patients who have failed to respond to metronidazole—the *drug of choice*. Vancomycin has also been recommended as initial empirical therapy for presumed pneumococcal meningitis because of increasing pneumococcal resistance to penicillins and cephalosporins. Resistance to vancomycin is increasing rapidly among isolates of *E. faecium* in large hospitals, particularly in areas of high vancomycin use. In addition, *S. aureus* isolates with both high-level resistance and reduced susceptibility to vancomycin have now been detected. Because of the growing threat of vancomycin-resistant enterococci and the potential for increasing resistance among staphylococci, a national advisory committee has established guidelines for appropriate and limited use of this antibiotic (Table 118-6).

AMINOGLYCOSIDES The aminoglycosides are rapidly bactericidal in vitro at low concentrations, with activity limited to gram-negative bacteria and staphylococci. They have no activity against anaerobic bacteria and are not effective in environments that are acidic or have a low oxygen tension. However, their spectrum includes virtually all gram-negative bacteria that are not strict anaerobes, and they are among the *drugs of choice* for any suspected gram-negative bacteremic infection, particularly in neutropenic patients. Aminoglycosides are synergistically bactericidal in combination with a penicillin for the treatment of staphylococcal, enterococcal, or viridans streptococcal endocarditis and are usually combined with a β-lactam antibiotic for the treatment of gram-negative bacteremia. Aminoglycosides are also among the *drugs of choice* for severe infections of the upper urinary tract. The major limitations to use of aminoglycosides are their renal and otic toxicity, their diminished activity at certain sites of infection (e.g., abscesses and the central nervous system), and the resistance of target bacteria. Among the available agents, gentamicin and tobramycin are generally preferred because of their low cost. Tobramycin has slightly greater activity against *P. aeruginosa*, and amikacin retains activity against many tobramycin- and gentamicin-resistant gram-negative bacteria because it is inactivated by fewer aminoglycoside-modifying enzymes. Streptomycin is still one of the *drugs of choice* in initial therapy for tularemia, plague, glanders, and brucellosis and is a second-line agent for the treatment of *tuberculosis*.

MACROLIDES AND KETOLIDES Erythromycin has broad-spectrum activity against gram-positive bacteria, with additional activity against *Legionella*, *Mycoplasma*, *Campylobacter*, *Bordetella pertussis*, and some *Chlamydia* isolates. It is the *drug of choice* for infections due to *Legionella*, *Campylobacter*, and *Mycoplasma* and is among the *drugs of choice* for community-acquired pneumococcal pneumonia and group A streptococcal pharyngitis in penicillin-allergic patients. However, resistance to erythromycin among group A streptococci and especially pneumococci is increasing dramatically in some areas. Erythromycin also appears to be one of the *drugs of choice* for infections caused by the agent of bacillary angiomatosis (*Bartonella henselae*) in immunocompromised patients. Clarithromycin and azithromycin have an antibacterial spectrum similar to that of erythromycin in vitro. However, azithromycin has greater activity against *Chlamydia*. Clarithromycin, in combination with a proton pump inhibitor, has been designated a *drug of choice* for the treatment of gastric infections due to *Helicobacter pylori* (gastritis, gastric and duodenal ulcers). Both azithromycin and clarithromycin are active against nontuberculous mycobacteria, and both appear to have fewer gastrointestinal side effects than does erythromycin. Bacteria that are resistant to erythromycin are also resistant to clarithromycin and azithromycin. Telithromycin is a ketolide antibiotic that is similar to erythromycin in structure, spectrum of activity, and mechanism of action. However, telithromycin is active against most macrolide-resistant strains of *S. pneumoniae*.

LINCOSAMIDES The only lincosamide used in the United States is clindamycin. It shares the gram-positive coccal spectrum of erythromycin but is more active (in some cases showing bactericidal activity) against susceptible staphylococci. However, resistance among staphylococci and some streptococci, mediated by the same genes responsible for macrolide resistance, limits clindamycin's usefulness against gram-positive cocci. In general, all staphylococci resistant to erythromycin should be considered resistant to clindamycin regardless of the results of in vitro susceptibility testing. However, at least half of the streptococci resistant to erythromycin are truly susceptible to clindamycin. In these bacteria, resistance is mediated by a drug-efflux pump that removes macrolides but not lincosamides. Despite increasing resistance, clindamycin remains useful for most anaerobic infections because of its broad spectrum of activity against most gram-positive and gram-negative strict anaerobes. It is also a *drug of choice* for the treatment of severe, invasive group A streptococcal infections. In contrast, clindamycin, like erythromycin, has no clinically significant activity against facultative gram-negative enteric bacilli. The appropriate use of clindamycin is limited only by resistance or the development of pseudomembranous colitis, the major serious side effect of this drug.

CHLORAMPHENICOL Chloramphenicol has a broad spectrum of activity against gram-positive and gram-negative bacteria, although plasmid-mediated resistance has diminished its effective spectrum. This antibiotic is rarely used in adult infections because of the rare idiosyncratic side effect of irreversible bone-marrow aplasia and the availability of other agents with similar activity. It remains one of the *drugs of choice* for the treatment of typhoid fever and plague and is still useful for the treatment of brucellosis and both pneumococcal and meningococcal meningitis in patients with severe penicillin allergy.

TABLE 118-6   *Guidelines for Appropriate and Limited Use of Vancomycin*

Acceptable Use	Discourage Use
Infection with methicillin-resistant *Staphylococcus aureus*	When culture reveals a β-lactam-susceptible organism
Infection with gram-positive bacteria in penicillin-allergic patient (where vancomycin is one of the drugs of choice)	Continued empirical use without indication (e.g., no evidence of infection)
Antibiotic-associated colitis unresponsive to metronidazole	Coagulase-negative staphylococcal bacteremia, single positive culture
Endocarditis prophylaxis during dental procedures for patients allergic to β-lactam antibiotics	Routine empirical therapy
Cardiovascular surgical prophylaxis (with unusually high rates of postoperative infection with β-lactam-resistant organisms)	Routine surgical prophylaxis or prophylaxis in the dialysis patient

TETRACYCLINES Tetracyclines have a broad spectrum of bacteriostatic activity against gram-positive and gram-negative bacteria and are widely used in a variety of community-acquired infections. These agents are among the *drugs of choice* for acute bacterial exacerbations of chronic bronchitis, granuloma inguinale, brucellosis (with streptomycin), tularemia, glanders, melioidosis, spirochetal infections caused by *Borrelia* (Lyme disease and relapsing fever; doxycycline), infections caused by *Vibrio vulnificus*, some *Aeromonas* infections, infections due to *Stenotrophomonas* (minocycline), plague, ehrlichiosis, chlamydial infections (doxycycline), and granulomatous skin infections due to *Mycobacterium marinum* (minocycline). The tetracyclines are also used in penicillin-allergic patients for the treatment of leptospirosis, syphilis, actinomycosis, and skin and soft tissue infections caused by gram-positive cocci. Doxycycline is also among the drugs recommended for the treatment of community-acquired pneumonia, although clinical data are few and resistance in *S. pneumoniae* is increasing.

SULFONAMIDES AND TRIMETHOPRIM The folic acid synthesis inhibitors have a broad spectrum of bacteriostatic activity individually; in combination, they can be bactericidal against facultative gram-negative bacteria and staphylococci. The fixed combination of sulfamethoxazole and trimethoprim, the major folic acid synthesis inhibitors used in therapy for bacterial infections, has modest activity against some streptococci and no activity against strict anaerobes. However, resistance to TMP-SMX is common among methicillin-resistant staphylococci and penicillin-resistant pneumococci and is increasing among *E. coli* strains that cause urinary tract infections. The individual sulfonamides are rarely used in the treatment of bacterial infections but are among the *drugs of choice* for the treatment of nocardial infections, leprosy (dapsone, a sulfone), and toxoplasmosis (sulfadiazine). Although increasing resistance has been reported among gram-negative organisms, TMP-SMX remains one of the *drugs of choice* for the treatment of uncomplicated urinary tract infections (except for those caused by enterococci) and had been used in the treatment of otitis media. It can be used in therapy for upper respiratory tract infections in which *S. pneumoniae*, *H. influenzae*, or *M. catarrhalis* is suspected (although resistance in *S. pneumoniae* is now common in some areas); for gonococcal and meningococcal infections; for chancroid; and for infections thought to be caused by *Aeromonas*, *Stenotrophomonas*, *Burkholderia cepacia*, *Acinetobacter*, and *Yersinia enterocolitica*. For nosocomial infections due to *Stenotrophomonas*, TMP-SMX is the *drug of choice*.

FLUOROQUINOLONES The fluoroquinolones have excellent activity against most facultative gram-negative rods and variable activity against gram-positive cocci. The quinolones are the oral agents with greatest activity against *P. aeruginosa*; ciprofloxacin is the most active against this species, although a high rate of acquired resistance limits its utility in many hospitals. All the quinolones except norfloxacin are well absorbed orally; ciprofloxacin, levofloxacin, moxifloxacin, and gatifloxacin are also administered as intravenous formulations. The quinolones are among the *drugs of choice* for urinary tract infections, bacterial gastroenteritis, community-acquired pneumonia, and enteric fever and are useful for serious hospital-acquired infections caused by gram-negative organisms. While older quinolones (such as ciprofloxacin) have limited activity against gram-positive bacteria, the newer quinolones have an expanded spectrum of activity against gram-positive cocci, including staphylococci (methicillin-susceptible) and streptococci (especially *S. pneumoniae*). Quinolones can also be used as prophylaxis for persons at risk for meningococcal meningitis. However, use of quinolones should be coupled with the realization that, in conjunction with rapidly expanding usage, resistance is being reported increasingly among all bacteria targeted by these drugs, including *S. pneumoniae*, *Neisseria gonorrhoeae*, *E. coli*, and *P. aeruginosa*.

RIFAMPIN Rifampin has been used in combinations for the treatment of serious infections due to methicillin-resistant staphylococci (e.g.,

coagulase-negative staphylococcal foreign-body infections). Because the spontaneous selection of rifampin-resistant mutants occurs rapidly, rifampin should never be used alone in the treatment of staphylococcal infections. Rifampin is also used for chemoprophylaxis in persons at risk of meningococcal meningitis and for the treatment of *Legionella* pneumonia.

METRONIDAZOLE Metronidazole has a spectrum limited to anaerobic bacteria, especially gram-negative species (e.g., *Bacteroides* spp.). It is less active against anaerobic gram-positive cocci (e.g., *Peptostreptococcus* and *Peptococcus* spp.). Because of its spectrum and its ability to penetrate into the area of infection, metronidazole is one of the *drugs of choice* for the treatment of any abscess in which the involvement of obligate anaerobes is suspected (e.g., lung, brain, or intraabdominal abscesses). Other antibacterial agents should be used in combination with metronidazole if facultative and aerobic pathogens are also thought to be involved. Metronidazole is the *drug of choice* for the treatment of bacterial vaginosis and antibiotic-associated pseudomembranous colitis.

LINEZOLID This antibacterial agent has a spectrum limited to gram-positive bacteria and is indicated for the treatment of infections caused by streptococci, staphylococci, and enterococci. Because there is very little preexisting resistance to linezolid, the drug is active against gram-positive bacteria that are resistant to other antibacterial agents. In particular, it is active against vancomycin-resistant enterococci (both *E. faecium* and *E. faecalis*) and is one of the *drugs of choice* for treating infections due to these organisms. However, since this drug has only bacteriostatic activity, it has limited utility in treating complicated *S. aureus* infections.

POLYMYXINS Polymyxins B and E have a broad spectrum of activity that includes virtually all gram-negative bacteria. However, while polymyxin B is still used as a component of topical preparations (see "Topical Antibacterial Agents," below), polymyxin E (colistin) has been used little since the early 1980s because of the high incidence of severe renal toxicity associated with its systemic use. The occurrence in recent years of nosocomial infections caused by strains of bacteria such as *P. aeruginosa*, *Acinetobacter baumanii*, and *Stenotrophomonas maltophilia* that are resistant to all available therapy but susceptible to colistin has prompted a reexamination of its use in certain patients for whom there are no other options. Recent data suggest that colistin is reasonably safe and effective when used with caution.

STREPTOGRAMINS The combination of streptogramin B (quinupristin) and streptogramin A (dalfopristin) has a spectrum that is limited to gram-positive bacteria and is indicated for the treatment of infections caused by staphylococci, streptococci, and *E. faecium*. It is not active against *E. faecalis*. Quinupristin/dalfopristin is used primarily as therapy for infections caused by vancomycin-resistant *E. faecium*. The agent has bactericidal activity against isolates of *S. aureus* and *S. epidermidis* that are susceptible to both components. However, since ~80% of oxacillin (methicillin)-resistant *S. aureus* and *S. epidermidis* and 20 to 40% of oxacillin-susceptible staphylococci are resistant to streptogramin A (dalfopristin) as a result of ribosomal methylation, quinupristin/dalfopristin has only bacteriostatic activity against most hospital-acquired staphylococci. It is *not*, therefore, a drug of choice for serious nosocomial staphylococcal infections and should be used for complicated *S. aureus* infections only when complete susceptibility to both components can be demonstrated.

URINARY TRACT ANTISEPTICS Urinary tract antiseptics are active only in the lower urinary tract and cannot be used for the treatment of upper urinary tract or systemic infections. The available agents in this category include nitrofurantoin and methenamine salts, which are most active against susceptible gram-negative enteric bacteria. Nitrofurantoin is often active against vancomycin-resistant enterococci and is a less expensive alternative to linezolid for the treatment of lower urinary tract infections.

TOPICAL ANTIBACTERIAL AGENTS Mupirocin is available only as a topical preparation for use against staphylococci and streptococci. Its major applications are for impetigo and eradication of the staphylococcal carrier state. It is the *drug of choice* for the elimination of nasal carriage of both methicillin-susceptible and methicillin-resistant staphylococci. Unfortunately, the emergence of resistance is limiting its usefulness in some hospitals.

Although their efficacy has never been well documented, topical preparations that include sulfonamides, polymyxin B, neomycin, bacitracin, gramicidin, and novobiocin in a variety of combinations are widely used as eyedrops, irrigation solutions, and ointments for superficial skin infections.

ADVERSE REACTIONS

Adverse drug reactions are frequently classified by mechanism as either dose-related ("toxic") effects or unpredictable reactions. Unpredictable reactions are either idiosyncratic or allergic. Dose-related reactions include aminoglycoside-induced nephrotoxicity, linezolid-induced thrombocytopenia, penicillin-induced seizures, and vancomycin-induced anaphylactoid reactions. Many of these reactions can be avoided by reducing dosage, limiting the duration of therapy, or reducing the frequency or rate of administration. Adverse reactions to antibacterial agents are a common cause of morbidity, requiring alteration in therapy and additional expense, and they occasionally result in death. The elderly, often those with the more severe infections, may be especially prone to certain adverse reactions. →*For further discussion of adverse drug reactions, see Chap. 3.*

β-LACTAMS The therapeutic index for β-lactam antibiotics is broad, and dose-related adverse reactions are uncommon and largely preventable. The greatest concern is allergic reactions. All types can occur, including anaphylaxis (type 1, immediate-hypersensitivity reactions), nephritis and Coombs-positive hemolytic anemia (type 2, cytotoxic reactions), drug fever and serum sickness (type 3, immune-complex formation), contact dermatitis (type 4, cell-mediated effects), and maculopapular eruption (type 5, idiopathic reactions). Approximately 1 to 4% of treatment courses result in an allergic reaction, and ~0.004 to 0.015% of treatment courses result in anaphylaxis. Only 10 to 20% of the patients who claim an allergy to penicillin react to skin testing with the major and minor determinants (penicilloyl-polylysine and benzylpenicillin degradation products, respectively); those with negative skin tests only rarely react adversely to subsequent therapeutic doses. Generally, a suitable alternative to β-lactams is available for patients who have a severe allergy, and penicillin desensitization can be carefully undertaken if there is no suitable alternative. A small proportion (<2%) of persons who are allergic to penicillin react similarly when a cephalosporin is administered; thus, cephalosporins are contraindicated in patients with a history of an immediate reaction to penicillin, although they are often used in patients with a history of mild reactions. The same precaution applies to carbapenems, but aztreonam is antigenically distinct and can be administered safely to the penicillin-allergic patient.

Other reactions thought to have an allergic basis include nephritis (associated with methicillin and occasionally nafcillin), hepatitis (related to oxacillin), leukopenia (following high doses of most β-lactams administered for prolonged periods), and severe skin rashes (toxic epidermal necrolysis and Stevens-Johnson syndrome). These reactions are not IgE-mediated, and skin testing is not predictive of their occurrence. For unclear reasons, most patients who have infectious mononucleosis or cytomegalovirus infection develop a rash when given ampicillin or amoxicillin.

Miscellaneous reactions to β-lactams include gastrointestinal side effects ranging in severity from mild diarrhea (5 to 10%) to pseudomembranous colitis (<1%). Although the probability of antibiotic-associated colitis is low, a large number of cases occur because β-lactams are so commonly prescribed. Drugs excreted to a large extent through the bile, such as ampicillin and ceftriaxone, may be especially prone to cause diarrhea. The addition of clavulanic acid to amoxicillin further increases the frequency of diarrhea. Ceftriaxone, because of extremely high concentrations in bile, can cause "sludging"

in the gallbladder and occasionally produces symptoms compatible with acute cholecystitis.

In high doses—and most often in patients with renal impairment who receive an excessive dose—penicillins (especially ticarcillin and penicillin G) can cause bleeding from impaired platelet aggregation. Seizures are occasionally observed with β-lactams, especially penicillin G and imipenem. This reaction is most common when excessive doses relative to renal function are administered or when the patient has a history of seizures.

VANCOMYCIN When vancomycin was first used clinically in 1956, local intolerance at the infusion site was common, as were systemic reactions, including ototoxicity and nephrotoxicity. Current formulations are of higher purity and, when proper dosage guidelines are followed, are very safe, although phlebitis can still be troublesome. The most common adverse reaction is called *red man syndrome* and is characterized by pruritus, flushing, and erythema of the head and upper torso. This anaphylactoid reaction usually follows the first dose, is dependent on dose size and infusion time, and results from vancomycin-induced release of histamine. The reaction is usually mild in adult patients who receive 1 g over 60 min and diminishes with repeated doses. If vancomycin is mistakenly given as a bolus, severe hypotension may result. In unusually sensitive patients, extending the infusion time or administering H$_1$ receptor antagonists is usually effective in preventing this reaction or reducing its severity. Patients with this reaction must not be mislabeled as having an allergy to vancomycin, since vancomycin may be the only effective treatment for certain infections (e.g., those due to methicillin-resistant staphylococci).

Nephrotoxicity from vancomycin is mild and uncommon. Although some data suggest that aminoglycosides and vancomycin are synergistically nephrotoxic, this point is difficult to prove, and the simultaneous use of these agents should not be avoided if clinically indicated, as in the treatment of enterococcal endocarditis in penicillin-allergic patients.

Ototoxicity from vancomycin is rare as long as doses are appropriately reduced in patients with renal insufficiency. Other uncommon adverse reactions include leukopenia, skin rashes, and true allergy. Serum concentrations of vancomycin are of little use in predicting toxicity but may be of value in selecting dosages for patients with unstable renal function.

AMINOGLYCOSIDES Aminoglycoside antibiotics have a narrow therapeutic index. The two most common adverse reactions are nephrotoxicity and ototoxicity. Rarely, respiratory depression is observed. Nephrotoxicity results from accumulation of the aminoglycoside in the peritubular space, with damage to the proximal tubule and a corresponding reduction in the glomerular filtration rate. The incidence of nephrotoxicity, defined as an increase of >0.5 mg/dL over baseline in the serum creatinine level, is ~5 to 10% among adult patients who receive therapy for 10 to 14 days. However, many cofactors also influence the frequency of toxicity, such as extremes of age (toxicity is uncommon among children, more common among the elderly), concomitant drug therapy, and hydration status. Nephrotoxicity is manifested clinically by a gradual rise in serum creatinine levels after a few days of therapy and is reversible if the dosage is reduced or treatment is discontinued. Serum creatinine levels should be monitored every 3 to 5 days or more often if changes are seen. There is not an important difference among the most useful agents (gentamicin, tobramycin, and amikacin) in terms of the frequency of nephrotoxicity; streptomycin is a rare cause of nephrotoxicity. Some data suggest that once-daily administration of aminoglycosides may cause less nephrotoxicity than more frequent administration.

Ototoxicity from aminoglycoside therapy presents as either auditory or vestibular damage. Since the aminoglycosides can destroy hair cells in the inner ear, ototoxicity may be permanent. The risk of ototoxicity increases with prolonged therapy, higher serum concentrations (especially in patients with renal impairment), hypovolemia, and concurrent treatment with other ototoxins, especially ethacrynic acid. There is evidence of a genetic predisposition to ototoxicity in some persons. Clinically apparent ototoxicity, manifested by diminished acuity or vestibular imbalance, is uncommon (probably occurring in <1% of cases) when the duration of therapy is kept to a minimum. With more sensitive monitoring (e.g., audiograms), asymptomatic high-tone hearing loss is more commonly noted. There are no clinically important differences among the aminoglycosides in the overall frequency of ototoxicity.

Neuromuscular depression from aminoglycosides is caused by reduced acetylcholine activity at postsynaptic membranes and can result in rare but severe respiratory depression. Risk factors include hypocalcemia, peritoneal administration, use of neuromuscular blockers, and preexisting respiratory depression. This complication can be largely avoided if the aminoglycoside is administered intravenously over 30 min or by intramuscular injection; if respiratory depression occurs, it is reversed by the administration of calcium.

Fear of toxicity should not prevent the use of aminoglycosides for a legitimate indication, since toxicity is usually mild and reversible. The value of measuring serum concentrations is controversial; these measurements are usually unnecessary when the patient is receiving once-daily therapy, especially when the duration is <7 to 10 days.

MACROLIDES Serious adverse reactions to the macrolide antibiotics are very rare. Gastrointestinal effects, such as burning, nausea, and vomiting, are the most common adverse reactions to the macrolides; depending on dosage, these reactions may occur in up to 50% of patients, occasionally requiring early discontinuation of therapy. The mechanism is thought to be the binding of erythromycin to motilin receptors, with a consequent increase in gastrointestinal motility. Gastrointestinal side effects appear equally common for all the oral formulations and also occur with intravenous administration. Clarithromycin and azithromycin are better tolerated than erythromycin, although gastrointestinal distress is still their most common adverse effect.

Less common reactions include hepatotoxicity and ototoxicity. Hepatotoxicity is a rare, nonfatal complication that is usually associated with erythromycin estolate and presents as an allergic cholestatic jaundice. Ototoxicity is rare after oral administration but may occur in a dose-dependent pattern in up to 20% of adults who receive intravenous erythromycin (4 g/d) and have audiograms performed. Ototoxicity is usually reversible and mild. Allergic cutaneous reactions are observed in rare cases. Macrolides are among the many drugs that can prolong the QT_c interval in some patients. The clinical significance of this effect continues to be investigated. The limited data suggest that the ketolide telithromycin has adverse effects similar to those of erythromycin.

LINCOSAMIDES The most common adverse effect of clindamycin is gastrointestinal distress. Diarrhea has been reported in up to 20% of patients and pseudomembranous colitis in 0.01 to 10%. The mechanism of pseudomembranous colitis is production of a toxin by *C. difficile* (Chap. 114). *C. difficile* colonizes the gastrointestinal tract and may produce a toxin when the normal flora is suppressed by clindamycin and other antibiotics, especially β-lactams. This toxin causes mucosal damage that results in cramps, pain, and diarrhea that may be bloody. Pseudomembranous colitis may follow both intravenous and oral administration and may not become manifest until after completion of therapy. Oral metronidazole or oral vancomycin is effective in treating symptomatic patients with toxin-positive stools, but some spores may survive, and relapse is frequent. Metronidazole is the *drug of choice* since oral treatment with vancomycin can select for vancomycin-resistant enterococci. Although diarrhea and pseudomembranous colitis can be caused by most antibacterial agents, the incidence in relation to the amount used may be highest for clindamycin. Allergic reactions (such as rashes and fever), hepatotoxicity, and neutropenia are observed only rarely.

CHLORAMPHENICOL Chloramphenicol causes two types of bone marrow suppression: a dose-related, reversible suppression of all elements, which occurs commonly during therapy at the maximal recommended doses (4 g/d in adults), and an idiosyncratic, irreversible aplastic anemia, which occurs in ~1 of every 25,000 to 40,000 exposures. The irreversible form has been reported to follow all types of chloramphenicol treatment, including ocular administration, and often develops months after therapy is discontinued.

In premature neonates and infants, chloramphenicol can cause a dose-related "gray syndrome" that is characterized by cyanosis, hypotension, and death and that results from an inability of the newborn to metabolize the drug. These potentially serious toxicities and the availability of newer drugs have substantially reduced the indications for chloramphenicol use.

TETRACYCLINES Gastrointestinal effects are the most common adverse reactions to the tetracyclines. These problems may be related to a direct irritant effect, since tetracyclines can also cause esophageal ulceration when they dissolve before reaching the stomach. It is important that nighttime doses be taken with sufficient fluid. Concurrent food intake may improve tolerance, but absorption of tetracycline HCl is impaired when the drug is taken with food.

Hepatotoxicity has been reported after administration of >2 g of tetracycline intravenously and at lower doses during pregnancy. There are currently no indications for intravenous tetracycline treatment in pregnancy. All tetracyclines can cause phototoxic skin reactions; these reactions are most common with doxycycline. Other dermal reactions, including rash, are uncommon. Tetracyclines are contraindicated in children <8 years of age because of mottling of the permanent teeth; doxycycline may be less likely than the other tetracyclines to cause this problem. Worsening of renal function in patients with preexisting renal dysfunction has been reported with use of tetracycline. Doxycycline and perhaps minocycline appear to be free from these renal side effects. Alternative effective agents are nearly always available for use in patients with renal dysfunction. Minocycline can cause vertigo in up to 70% of women receiving therapeutic doses and in a lower percentage of men.

SULFONAMIDES AND TRIMETHOPRIM The sulfonamides are generally safe, but the list of possible adverse reactions is very long. These compounds occasionally cause a number of allergic reactions, from relatively minor skin rashes (including maculopapular rashes and urticarial reactions typically appearing after a week of therapy) to severe or even life-threatening reactions such as erythema multiforme, Stevens-Johnson syndrome, and toxic epidermal necrolysis. The severe hypersensitivity reactions have occurred most commonly after treatment with the long-acting sulfonamides, such as sulfamethoxypyridazine, which are no longer used. Pyrimethamine plus sulfadoxine (Fansidar), used for malaria prophylaxis, may cause severe allergic reactions, including hepatic and hematologic toxicities, in addition to dermatologic toxicity. Photosensitivity reactions are also relatively common with sulfonamides.

Many patients infected with HIV who receive TMP-SMX have adverse dermatologic reactions. These reactions are usually not life-threatening and appear to regress in many cases despite continuation of therapy. In high doses, trimethoprim interferes with the renal secretion of potassium. Hyperkalemia is relatively common among HIV-positive patients and is most often found after 7 days of TMP-SMX therapy for pneumonia caused by *Pneumocystis*.

Sulfonamides and trimethoprim may also cause severe hematologic complications, including agranulocytosis, hemolytic and megaloblastic anemia, and thrombocytopenia. These dose-related side effects may be more frequent and more severe in patients with renal insufficiency. Hemolytic anemia is most common in patients with glucose-6-phosphate dehydrogenase deficiency who take long-acting compounds; TMP-SMX rarely causes hemolysis in such subjects. Granulocytopenia from TMP-SMX is especially common among HIV-infected patients, occurring in 10 to 50% of this group.

Renal insufficiency, caused by crystals of the relatively insoluble acetyl metabolite, is observed primarily with the long-acting sulfonamides. Many cases of crystalluria in HIV-infected patients taking sulfadiazine for toxoplasmosis have been reported. A high level of fluid intake may prevent this complication.

It is recommended that sulfonamides not be administered to newborns because of concerns that bilirubin may be displaced from protein-binding sites, with subsequent jaundice and kernicterus.

In addition to the preceding problems, sulfonamides may occasionally cause drug fever with serum sickness, hepatic toxicity (including necrosis), and systemic lupus erythematosus.

FLUOROQUINOLONES Fluoroquinolones are relatively safe; adverse reactions rarely require discontinuation of therapy. The most common reactions include gastrointestinal distress, such as nausea or diarrhea (<5%), and central nervous system effects, including insomnia and dizziness (<5%). Phototoxicity is occasionally severe. Rarely, hepatic and renal dysfunction and anaphylactoid and allergic reactions are observed. Quinolones can cause tendon rupture in rare instances. The use of these drugs is currently contraindicated in patients <18 years of age because of evidence in animals of cartilage damage in developing joints. In carefully selected situations in which the perceived benefits outweigh the risks (e.g., in adolescent patients with cystic fibrosis who have pulmonary exacerbations), fluoroquinolones may be useful for short-term therapy. They are contraindicated in pregnancy because of concern for the developing fetus. Quinolones can also increase the QT_c interval; it is unclear whether the currently available quinolones differ in a clinically important way in this respect. Hypo- and hyperglycemia have been reported and may be more common with gatifloxacin. As of 2003, a number of fluoroquinolones—including temafloxacin, sparfloxacin, grepafloxacin, and trovafloxacin—have been removed from the U.S. market because of rare but severe adverse effects. It may be prudent to limit the use of the newest drugs in this class until their safety has been fully established.

RIFAMPIN Rifampin is generally well tolerated but has several important side effects. Some patients have transient rises in hepatic aminotransferases, but these levels usually return to normal without discontinuation of the drug. Although hepatitis from rifampin itself develops only rarely, the drug is thought by some investigators to potentiate the hepatic toxicity of concomitantly administered isoniazid. Intermittent administration of rifampin (usually fewer than three times per week) has been associated with signs and symptoms that seem to have an immunologic basis. These include flulike symptoms and (rarely) hemolysis, thrombocytopenia, shock, and renal failure. Minor gastrointestinal side effects, skin rashes, and interstitial nephritis have also been reported. Patients should be warned that rifampin and its metabolites cause secretions such as urine, tears, sweat, and saliva to turn orange and that contact lenses may be stained.

METRONIDAZOLE Serious adverse reactions to metronidazole are uncommon. Gastrointestinal side effects such as nausea are most frequent but rarely necessitate discontinuation of therapy. Pseudomembranous colitis in association with metronidazole has been reported but is very rare. A metallic taste is relatively common, and stomatitis and glossitis are occasionally reported. Peripheral neuropathy develops in some patients, and seizures and encephalopathy have been reported after high doses and in patients with hepatic failure.

Concerns about mutagenicity and carcinogenicity from metronidazole have led to recommendations that it not be used in pregnancy (especially during the first trimester) when alternative agents are available. Although retrospective studies have found no association between metronidazole and carcinogenesis, long-term administration of high doses should be avoided when therapeutic alternatives exist.

LINEZOLID The most common adverse events accompanying linezolid therapy include gastrointestinal upset (nausea, vomiting, and diarrhea) and headache. Of most concern is a reversible myelosuppression that is directly related to the duration of therapy. Thrombocytopenia is the most likely hematologic abnormality, although anemia and leukopenia are also observed. If the duration of therapy is expected to exceed 1 week, then weekly complete blood counts are recommended.

QUINUPRISTIN/DALFOPRISTIN Quinupristin/dalfopristin is not well tolerated. In particular, venous irritation is a frequent and potentially serious adverse effect when the drug is given by peripheral intravenous infusion. Administration via a central line is often required to complete a course of therapy. In addition, arthralgia and myalgia are substan-

TABLE 118-7 Interactions of Antibacterial Agents with Other Drugs

Antibiotic	Interacts with	Potential Consequence (Clinical Significance[a])
Erythromycin/clarithromycin/ telithromycin	Theophylline	Theophylline toxicity (1)
	Carbamazepine	CNS depression (1)
	Digoxin	Digoxin toxicity (2)
	Triazolam/midazolam	CNS depression (2)
	Ergotamine	Ergotism (1)
	Warfarin	Bleeding (2)
	Cyclosporine/tacrolimus	Nephrotoxicity (1)
	Cisapride	Cardiac arrhythmias (1)
	Statins[b]	Rhabdomyolysis (2)
	Valproate	Valproate toxicity (2)
	Vincristine/vinblastine	Excess neurotoxicity (2)
Quinupristin/dalfopristin	Similar to erythromycin[c]	
Fluoroquinolones[d]	Theophylline	Theophylline toxicity (2)
	Antacids/sucralfate/iron	Subtherapeutic antibiotic levels (1)
Tetracycline	Antacids/sucralfate/iron	Subtherapeutic antibiotic levels (1)
Trimethoprim- sulfamethoxazole	Phenytoin	Phenytoin toxicity (2)
	Oral hypoglycemics	Hypoglycemia (2)
	Warfarin	Bleeding (1)
	Digoxin	Digoxin toxicity (2)
Metronidazole	Ethanol	Disulfiram-like reactions (2)
	Fluorouracil	Bone marrow suppression (1)
	Warfarin	Bleeding (2)
Rifampin	Warfarin	Clot formation (1)
	Oral contraceptives	Pregnancy (1)
	Cyclosporine/tacrolimus	Rejection (1)
	HIV-1 protease inhibitors	Increased viral load, resistance (1)
	Nonnucleoside reverse- transcriptase inhibitors	Increased viral load, resistance (1)
	Glucocorticoids	Loss of steroid effect (1)
	Methadone	Narcotic withdrawal symptoms (1)
	Digoxin	Subtherapeutic digoxin levels (1)
	Itraconazole	Subtherapeutic itraconazole levels (1)
	Phenytoin	Loss of seizure control (1)
	Statins	Hypercholesterolemia (1)
	Diltiazem	Subtherapeutic diltiazem levels (1)
	Verapamil	Subtherapeutic verapamil levels (1)

[a] 1 = a well-documented interaction with clinically important consequences; 2 = an interaction of uncertain frequency but of potential clinical importance.
[b] Lovastatin and simvastatin are most affected; pravastatin and atorvastatin are less prone to clinically important effects.
[c] The macrolide antibiotics and quinupristin/dalfopristin inhibit the same human metabolic enzyme, CYP3A4, and similar interactions are anticipated.
[d] Ciprofloxacin only. Levofloxacin, moxifloxacin, and gatifloxacin do not inhibit theophylline metabolism.
Note: New interactions are commonly reported after marketing. Consult the most recent prescribing information for updates.
Abbreviation: CNS, central nervous system.

TABLE 118-8 *Prophylaxis of Bacterial Infections in Adults*

Condition	Antibacterial Agent	Timing or Duration of Prophylaxis
Nonsurgical		
Cardiac lesions susceptible to bacterial endocarditis	Amoxicillin[a]	Before and after procedures causing bacteremia
Recurrent *S. aureus* infections	Mupirocin	5 days (intranasal)
Contact with patient with meningococcal meningitis	Rifampin Fluoroquinolone	2 days Single dose
Bite wounds[b]	Penicillin V or amoxicillin/ clavulanic acid	3–5 days
Recurrent cystitis	Trimethoprim-sulfamethoxazole or a fluoroquinolone or nitrofurantoin	3 times per week for up to 1 year or after sexual intercourse
Surgical		
Clean (cardiac, vascular, neurologic, or orthopedic surgery)	Cefazolin (vancomycin)[c]	Before and during procedure
Ocular	Topical combinations and subconjunctival cefazolin	During and at end of procedure
Clean-contaminated (head and neck, high-risk gastroduodenal or biliary tract surgery; high-risk cesarean section; hysterectomy)	Cefazolin (or clindamycin for head and neck)	Before and during procedure
Clean-contaminated (vaginal or abdominal hysterectomy)	Cefazolin or cefoxitin or cefotetan	Before and during procedure
Clean-contaminated (high-risk genitourinary surgery)	Fluoroquinolone	Before and during procedure
Clean-contaminated (colorectal surgery or appendectomy)	Cefoxitin or cefotetan (add oral neomycin + erythromycin for colorectal)	Before and during procedure
Dirty[b] (ruptured viscus)	Cefoxitin or cefotetan ± gentamicin (clindamycin + gentamicin) or another appropriate regimen directed at anaerobes and gram-negative aerobes	Before and for 3–5 days after procedure
Dirty[b] (traumatic wound)	Cefazolin	Before and for 3–5 days after trauma

[a] Gentamicin should be added to the amoxicillin regimen for high-risk gastrointestinal and genitourinary procedures; vancomycin should be used in penicillin-allergic patients.
[b] In these cases, use of antibacterial agents actually constitutes treatment of infection rather than prophylaxis.
[c] Vancomycin is recommended only in institutions that have a high incidence of infection with methicillin-resistant staphylococci.

tially more common among patients treated with quinupristin/dalfopristin than among those receiving other antimicrobial agents. Other side effects include rash, elevated serum bilirubin levels, and gastrointestinal distress.

DRUG INTERACTIONS

Antimicrobial drugs are a common cause of drug-drug interactions. Table 118-7 lists the most common and best-documented interactions of antibacterial agents with other drugs and characterizes the clinical relevance of these interactions. Coadministration of drugs paired in the tables does not necessarily result in clinically important adverse consequences. Recognition of the potential for an interaction before the administration of an antibacterial agent is crucial to the rational use of these drugs, since adverse consequences can often be prevented if the interaction is anticipated. Table 118-7 is intended only to heighten awareness of the potential for an interaction. Additional sources should be consulted to identify appropriate options. →*For further discussion of drug interactions, see Chap. 3.*

MACROLIDES AND KETOLIDES Erythromycin, clarithromycin, and telithromycin inhibit the P450 enzyme CYP3A4 and thus the metabolism of many other drugs, including cyclosporine, certain statins (lovastatin, simvastatin), theophylline, carbamazepine, warfarin, certain antineoplastic agents (e.g., vincristine, irinotecan), and ergot alkaloids. When erythromycin and other inhibitors of CYP3A4 are given to patients receiving terfenadine, astemizole, cisapride, and pimozide, cardiac arrhythmias (including torsades de pointes) can occur; the availability

of the latter drugs has been severely restricted or they have been removed from the U.S. market. Azithromycin has little effect on the metabolism of other drugs. In ~10% of patients receiving digoxin, concentrations increase when these drugs are given.

QUINUPRISTIN/DALFOPRISTIN Quinupristin/ dalfopristin is an inhibitor of CYP3A4. Its interactions with other drugs should be similar to those of erythromycin.

LINEZOLID Linezolid is a monoamine oxidase inhibitor. Its concomitant administration with sympathomimetics such as phenylpropanolamine, with selective serotonin reuptake inhibitors, and with foods with high concentrations of tyramine should be avoided.

TETRACYCLINES The most important interaction involving tetracyclines is the reduction in absorption when these drugs are coadministered with divalent and trivalent cations, such as antacids, iron compounds, or dairy products. Food also adversely affects absorption of most tetracyclines. Inducers of hepatic isoenzymes, such as phenytoin and rifampin, increase the clearance of doxycycline; although the clinical significance of this effect is unknown, use of an alternative antibiotic may be appropriate.

SULFONAMIDES Sulfonamides, including sulfamethoxazole, increase the hypoprothrombinemic effect of warfarin by inhibition of its metabolism and possibly by protein-binding displacement. Sulfonamides may also potentiate the effects of oral hypoglycemic agents and phenytoin through reduction in metabolism or displacement from serum protein.

FLUOROQUINOLONES There are two clinically important drug interactions involving fluoroquinolones. First, like tetracyclines, all fluoroquinolones are chelated by divalent and trivalent cations, which prevent most of the dose from being absorbed. Second, certain fluoroquinolones, including ciprofloxacin, inhibit hepatic enzymes that metabolize theophylline, with consequent theophylline toxicity. The same mechanism accounts for increases in serum caffeine concentrations, but the clinical significance of this interaction is unknown. Scattered case reports suggest that quinolones can also potentiate the effects of warfarin, but this effect has not been observed in most controlled trials.

RIFAMPIN Rifampin is an excellent inducer of many cytochrome P450 enzymes and increases the hepatic clearance of a number of drugs, including the following (with the indicated predictable outcomes): HIV-1 protease inhibitors (loss of viral suppression), oral contraceptives (pregnancy), warfarin (decreased prothrombin times), cyclosporine and prednisone (organ rejection or exacerbations of any underlying inflammatory condition), and verapamil and diltiazem (increased dosage requirements). Before rifampin is prescribed for any patient, a review of concomitant drug therapy is essential.

METRONIDAZOLE Metronidazole can cause a disulfiram-like syndrome when alcohol is ingested; thus, patients taking metronidazole should be instructed to avoid alcohol. Inhibition of the metabolism of warfarin by metronidazole leads to significant rises in prothrombin times.

PROPHYLAXIS OF BACTERIAL INFECTIONS

Antibacterial agents are occasionally indicated for use in patients who have no evidence of infection but who have been or are expected to be exposed to bacterial pathogens under circumstances that constitute a major risk of infection. The basic tenets of antimicrobial prophylaxis are as follows: (1) the risk or potential severity of infection should be greater than the risk of side effects from the antibacterial agent, (2) the antibacterial agent should be given for the shortest period necessary to prevent target infections, and (3) the antibacterial agent should be given before the expected period of risk (e.g., surgical prophylaxis) or as soon as possible after contact with an infected individual (e.g., prophylaxis for meningococcal meningitis).

Table 118-8 lists the major indications for antibacterial prophylaxis in adults. (The use of antibacterial agents in children to prevent rheumatic fever and otitis media under certain circumstances is also common practice.) The table includes only those indications that are widely accepted, supported by well-designed studies, or recommended by expert panels. Prophylaxis is also used but is less widely accepted for recurrent cellulitis in conjunction with lymphedema, recurrent pneumococcal meningitis in conjunction with deficiencies in humoral immunity or CSF leaks, traveler's diarrhea, gram-negative sepsis in conjunction with neutropenia, and spontaneous bacterial peritonitis in conjunction with ascites.

The major use of antibacterial prophylaxis in the United States is for infections following surgical procedures. Antibacterial agents are administered just before the surgical procedure—and, for long operations, during the procedure as well—to ensure high levels in serum and tissues during surgery. The objective is to eradicate bacteria originating from the air of the operating suite, the skin of the surgical team, or the patient's own flora that may contaminate the wound. In all but colorectal surgical procedures, prophylaxis is predominantly directed against staphylococci. Prophylaxis is intended to prevent wound infection or infection of implanted devices, not all infections that may occur during the postoperative period (e.g., urinary tract infections or pneumonia). Prolonged prophylaxis merely alters the normal flora and favors infections with organisms resistant to the antibacterial agents used.

DURATION OF THERAPY AND TREATMENT FAILURE

It is often difficult to determine the proper duration of therapy for bacterial infections. There are few infections for which trials have established the appropriate treatment duration. Table 118-9 lists those common bacterial infections for which guidelines have been established or for which there is sufficient clinical experience to establish treatment durations. The ultimate test of cure for a bacterial infection is the absence of relapse when therapy is discontinued. *Relapse* is defined as a recurrence of infection with the identical organism that caused the first infection. In general, therefore, the duration of therapy should be long enough to prevent relapse yet not excessive. Therapy extended beyond the limit of effectiveness will increase side effects of medication and encourage the selection of resistant bacteria. The art of treating bacterial infections lies in the ability to determine the appropriate duration of therapy for infections that are not covered by established guidelines. Re-treatment of infections for which therapy has failed usually requires a prolonged course (>4 weeks) with combinations of antibacterial agents.

ANTIBACTERIAL COSTS AND INAPPROPRIATE USE

Use of antibacterial agents in U.S. hospitals can represent the largest expenditure for any single pharmacologic class. It is not unusual for the purchase cost of a newer parenteral antibiotic (in 2003 dollars) to be $1000 to $2000 for a 10- to 14-day course of treatment. Therapy for 5 to 10 days with a new oral antibiotic can easily cost $60 to $100, compared with a few dollars for older drugs such as doxycycline and amoxicillin. Administration costs, monitoring costs, and pharmacy charges must be added to these figures. While some newer antibacterial agents undeniably represent important advances in therapy, many newer drugs offer no advantage over older, less expensive agents. With

TABLE 118-9 *Duration of Therapy for Bacterial Infections*

Duration of Therapy	Infections
Single dose	Gonococcal urethritis, streptococcal pharyngitis (penicillin G benzathine), primary and secondary syphilis (penicillin G benzathine)
3 days	Cystitis in young women, community- or travel-acquired diarrhea
7–10 days	Community-acquired pneumonia, community-acquired meningitis (pneumococcal or meningococcal), antibiotic-associated diarrhea (10 days), *Giardia* enteritis, cellulitis, epididymitis
2 weeks	*Helicobacter pylori*–associated peptic ulcer, neurosyphilis (penicillin IV), penicillin-susceptible viridans streptococcal endocarditis (penicillin plus aminoglycoside), disseminated gonococcal infection with arthritis, acute pyelonephritis, uncomplicated *S. aureus* catheter-associated bacteremia
3 weeks	Lyme disease, septic arthritis (nongonococcal)
4 weeks	Acute and chronic prostatitis, infective endocarditis (penicillin-resistant streptococcal)
>4 weeks	Acute and chronic osteomyelitis, *S. aureus* endocarditis, foreign-body infections (prosthetic-valve and joint infections), relapsing pseudomembranous colitis

rare exceptions, newer drugs are usually found to be no more effective than the comparison antibiotic in controlled trials, despite the "high prevalence of resistance" often touted to market the advantage of the new antibiotic over older therapies.

Clinicians are understandably confused by the bewildering array of available drugs and their competing claims of superiority. Numerous surveys have reported that ~50% of antibiotic use is in some way "inappropriate." Aside from the monetary cost of unnecessary antibiotics, there are the costs of excess morbidity from adverse effects and drug interactions and the eventual costs of treating more resistant organisms. The following suggestions are intended to provide guidance through the antibiotic maze.

First, objective evidence regarding the merits of newer drugs is available through publications such as *The Medical Letter* (including periodic updates of the *Drugs of Choice*) and through online references such as those on the Johns Hopkins website (http://hopkins-abxguide.org), which offers much current information. Second, clinicians should become comfortable using a few drugs recommended by independent experts and professional organizations and should resist the temptation to use a new drug unless the merits are clear. A new antibacterial agent with a "broader spectrum and greater potency," a "longer half-life and higher tissue levels," or a "higher serum concentration-to-MIC ratio" does not necessarily translate into greater clinical efficacy. Third, clinicians should become familiar with local bacterial susceptibility profiles. It may not be necessary to use a new drug with "improved activity against *P. aeruginosa*" if that pathogen is rarely encountered or if it retains full susceptibility to older drugs. Finally, with regard to inpatient use of antibacterial drugs, appropriate empirical treatment with one or more broad-spectrum agents may often be simplified, with use of a narrower-spectrum agent or even an oral drug, once the results of cultures and susceptibility tests become available. While there is an understandable temptation not to alter effective therapy, switching to a more specific agent once the patient has improved clinically does not compromise outcome. A promising and active area of research includes shorter durations of antimicrobial therapy. Many antibiotics that once were given for 7 to 14 days can probably be given for 3 to 7 days. As these clinical trials of shorter duration and equal efficacy are published, prompt adoption of the shorter courses by the clinical community may be an effective counter to the problems of increasing resistance. Adoption of these guidelines will not undermine the care of patients, many unnecessary complications and expenses will be avoided, and the useful life of valuable drugs will be extended.

FURTHER READING

ANTIMICROBIAL PROPHYLAXIS IN SURGERY. Med Lett Drugs Ther 43:92, 2001

AVORN J, SOLOMON DH: Cultural and economic factors that (mis)shape antibiotic use: The nonpharmacologic basis of therapeutics. Ann Intern Med 133:128, 2000

CRAIG WA: Does the dose matter? Clin Infect Dis 33(Suppl 3):S233, 2001

HOSPITAL INFECTION CONTROL PRACTICES ADVISORY COMMITTEE: Recommendations for preventing the spread of vancomycin resistance. Infect Control Hosp Epidemiol 16:105, 1995

LEVIN AS et al: Intravenous colistin as therapy for nosocomial infections caused by multidrug-resistant *Pseudomonas aeruginosa* and *Acinetobacter baumanii*. Clin Infect Dis 28:1008, 1999

THE CHOICE OF ANTIBACTERIAL DRUGS. Med Lett Drugs Ther 43:69, 2001

Section 5   Diseases Caused by Gram-Positive Bacteria

119 PNEUMOCOCCAL INFECTIONS
Daniel M. Musher

Streptococcus pneumoniae (the pneumococcus) was recognized as the major cause of pneumonia in the 1880s and has been a central focus of study leading to the modern understanding of humoral immunity. The name *Diplococcus pneumoniae* was assigned to the organism in 1926 because of its appearance in Gram-stained sputum. In 1974, the organism was renamed *Streptococcus pneumoniae* because it grows in chains in liquid medium. Around 1900, pneumococcal serotypes were recognized when the injection of killed organisms into a rabbit stimulated the production of serum antibody that agglutinated the immunizing strain and protected rabbits against challenge with that strain and with some but not all other pneumococcal isolates. Ninety serotypes have now been identified, each possessing a unique polysaccharide capsule.

MICROBIOLOGY Pneumococci are identified in the clinical laboratory as gram-positive cocci that grow in chains and are catalase-negative. They produce pneumolysin, a toxin that breaks down hemoglobin into a greenish degradation product, thereby causing α-hemolysis on blood agar. More than 98% of pneumococcal isolates are susceptible to ethylhydrocupreine (optochin), and virtually all pneumococcal colonies are dissolved by bile salts; these reactions are the basis for laboratory identification.

Peptidoglycan and teichoic acid are the principal constituents of the pneumococcal cell wall. The cell wall's integrity depends on the presence of numerous peptide side chains cross-linked by the activity of enzymes such as trans- and carboxypeptidases. β-Lactam antibiotics inactivate these enzymes by covalently binding their active site. Unique to *S. pneumoniae* and present in all strains is C (for "cell-wall") substance, a polysaccharide consisting of teichoic acid with a phosphorylcholine residue. Surface-exposed choline residues serve as a site of attachment for potential virulence factors, such as pneumococcal surface protein A (PspA), which may prevent phagocytosis. Except for strains that cause conjunctivitis, nearly every clinical isolate of *S. pneumoniae* has a polysaccharide capsule.

There are two systems for numbering the 90 known distinct capsules of *S. pneumoniae*. In the American system, serotypes are numbered in the order in which they were identified. The strains that most frequently cause human disease were generally the earliest to be identified and thus tend to have lower numbers. The more widely accepted Danish system places serotypes into groups based on antigenic similarities; for example, Danish group 19 includes types 19F ("first recognized"), 19A, 19B, and 19C, which in the American system would be types 19, 57, 58, and 59, respectively. Serotyping was clinically relevant in the 1930s, when type-specific antisera were administered as therapy, and again in the 1990s, when it was used to track the spread of antibiotic-resistant isolates (although this method has largely been replaced by molecular biologic techniques such as pulsed-field gel electrophoresis and multilocus sequence typing). Capsule switching has been documented and further limits the epidemiologic reliability of serotyping.

EPIDEMIOLOGY *S. pneumoniae* colonizes the nasopharynx and, on any single occasion, can be isolated from 5 to 10% of healthy adults and from 20 to 40% of healthy children. Once the organisms have colonized an adult, they are likely to persist for 4 to 6 weeks but may persist for as long as 6 months. Pneumococci spread from one individual to another by direct or droplet transmission as a result of close contact; transmission may be enhanced by crowding or poor ventilation. Day-care centers have been a site of spread, especially of penicillin-resistant strains of serotypes 6B, 14, 19F, and 23F. Outbreaks occur among adults in crowded living conditions—e.g., in military barracks, prisons, and shelters for the homeless—as well as among susceptible populations in settings such as nursing homes. The risk of pneumococcal pneumonia is not increased by contact in schools or workplaces (including hospitals).

The incidence of bacteremic pneumococcal infection is relatively high among infants up to 2 years of age and low among teenagers and young adults; rates increase with increasing age beginning at around age 55. A surveillance study in South Carolina showed the incidences of pneumococcal bacteremia among infants, young adults, and persons $\geq$70 years of age to be 160, 5, and 70 cases per 100,000 population, respectively. (These results antecede implementation of vaccination for infants and young children.) Most cases of pneumococcal bacteremia in adults are due to pneumonia, and there are three to four cases of nonbacteremic pneumonia for every bacteremic case. Thus an estimated 20 cases of pneumococcal pneumonia per 100,000 young adults and 280 cases per 100,000 persons over the age of 70 occur annually. The incidence of pneumococcal bacteremia among adults exhibits a distinct midwinter peak and a striking dip in summer. In children, the incidence of bacteremia is relatively constant throughout the year except for a marked dip in midsummer. For reasons that are unclear but probably are multifactorial, Native Americans, Native Alaskans, and African Americans are unusually susceptible to invasive pneumococcal disease. This enhanced susceptibility is thought to have a genetic basis that thus far remains unelucidated.

PATHOGENETIC MECHANISMS *S. pneumoniae* attaches to human nasopharyngeal cells through the specific interaction of bacterial surface adhesins, such as pneumococcal surface antigen A or choline-binding proteins (including PspA), with epithelial cell receptors. Epithelial cell glycoconjugates containing the disaccharide GlcNAcβ1-4Gal or asialo-GM1 glycolipid are possible binding sites. Pneumococcal phase variation, in which organisms may form transparent or opaque colonies, may also play a role in adherence. Organisms from opaque colonies have relatively little peptidoglycan and large capsules; those from transparent colonies have much more phosphorylcholine (which contributes to their capacity to adhere to mammalian cells) and less capsular polysaccharide. When pneumococci are inoculated intranasally into an experimental animal, organisms that form transparent colonies persist; in contrast, after intraperitoneal inoculation, organisms that yield transparent colonies are rapidly cleared from the blood, whereas those that make opaque colonies resist clearance.

Once the nasopharynx has been colonized, infection results if the organisms are carried into anatomically contiguous areas such as the eustachian tubes or the nasal sinuses and if their clearance is hindered, for example, by mucosal edema due to allergy or viral infection. Similarly, pneumonia ensues if organisms are inhaled or aspirated into the bronchioles or alveoli and then are not cleared—especially, for example, if viral infection or cigarette smoke or other toxic substances have increased mucus production and/or damaged ciliary action. A mechanism by which pneumococci may bind to pneumocytes after viral infection has been suggested. Pneumocytes activated by cytokines express the receptor for platelet-activating factor, which binds the phosphorylcholine residue of pneumococcal C substance, enhancing the adherence of pneumococci. Pneumococci may invade tissues by penetrating mucosal layers; the clinical significance of this finding remains to be determined.

Once pneumococci reach an area where they do not naturally belong, they activate complement by classic and alternative pathways and stimulate cytokine production, which leads to the attraction of polymorphonuclear leukocytes (PMNs). The polysaccharide capsule, however, renders the organisms resistant to phagocytosis. In the absence of anticapsular antibody, phagocytic cells such as alveolar macrophages have a limited capacity to ingest and kill pneumococci; a large bacterial inoculum and/or a compromise of phagocytic function allows the initiation of lung infection. Infection of the meninges, joints, bones, and peritoneal cavity may result from the spread of pneumococci through the bloodstream, usually but not always from a respiratory tract focus of infection.

The capacity to cause disease reflects the capacities of pneumococci to escape ingestion and killing by host phagocytic cells, on the one hand, and to stimulate an inflammatory response and damage tissues, on the other. Encapsulated pneumococci are poorly ingested and killed in vivo in the immunologically naïve host or in vitro by mammalian phagocytic cells in the absence of anticapsular antibody and complement. Unencapsulated pneumococci virtually never cause invasive disease (although they can cause conjunctivitis), and mutants lacking a capsule are essentially avirulent in mice. Symptoms of disease are largely attributable to the generation of an inflammatory response that may cause pain by increasing pressure (as in sinusitis or otitis media) or may interfere with vital bodily functions by preventing oxygenation of blood (as in pneumonia) or by inhibiting blood flow (as in vasculitis due to meningitis). Cell-wall constituents of *S. pneumoniae*, including teichoic acid, C substance, and (in particular) peptidoglycan, activate complement by the alternative pathway; the reaction between cell-wall structures and antibody that is present in all humans also activates the classic complement pathway. The result is the release of C5a, a potent attractant for PMNs, into the surrounding medium. Peptidoglycan can also directly stimulate the release of proinflammatory cytokines such as interleukin (IL) 1β, tumor necrosis factor (TNF) α, and IL-6 that activate a cascade of inflammation mediators. These cytokines increase expression of selectins on endothelial cells and integrins on leukocytes, thereby enhancing PMN migration. Pneumolysin, a thiol-activated toxin, exerts a variety of effects on ciliary cells and PMNs and also activates the classic complement pathway by direct binding of Clq. Injection of pneumolysin into the lungs of experimental animals produces the histologic features of pneumonia; in mice, immunization with this substance or challenge with genetically engineered mutants that do not produce it is associated with a significant reduction in virulence. Autolysin may contribute to the pathogenesis of pneumococcal disease by lysing bacteria, thereby releasing their constituents and heightening the reaction with human tissues. Inflammation in the central nervous system (CNS) during meningitis is a major contributor to neuronal cell injury. The release of matrix metalloproteinases, reactive oxygen species, and reactive nitrogen intermediates in neuronal tissue also contributes to damage caused by meningitis.

HOST DEFENSE MECHANISMS Mechanisms of host defense may be immunologically nonspecific or specific. Nonspecific mechanisms that protect against pneumonia include laminar airflow across mucous layers that filter inspired air, the glottal reflex, laryngeal closure, the cough reflex, clearance of organisms from the lower airways by ciliated cells, and ingestion by pulmonary macrophages and PMNs of small bacterial inocula that manage to reach alveolar spaces. Respiratory virus infection, chronic pulmonary disease, or heart failure compromises these mechanisms, predisposing to the development of pneumococcal pneumonia.

Anticapsular antibody provides the best specific protection against pneumococcal infection. Most healthy adults lack IgG antibody to the majority of pneumococcal capsular polysaccharides. Antibody appears after colonization, infection, or vaccination. In the first few weeks after colonization, nonspecific mechanisms probably protect the host from infection. Thereafter, newly developed anticapsular antibody provides a high degree of specific protection. Adults who are at risk of aspirating pharyngeal contents and/or who have diminished mechanisms of lower airway clearance are at risk of developing pneumonia before antibody is produced. Similarly, children whose nasal mucosal membranes become acutely congested around the time of colonization are at risk of developing otitis media. Persons with a diminished capacity to form antibody remain susceptible for as long as they are colonized. Antibody to PspA and other pneumococcal constituents, such as pneumolysin, is prevalent in the population and may contribute to immunity that is immunologically specific but not type specific.

The risk of serious pneumococcal infection is greatly increased in persons with conditions that compromise IgG synthesis and/or the phagocytic function of PMNs and macrophages; this risk is also elevated in the presence of conditions associated with debilitation or malnutrition. Nearly all adults who are hospitalized for pneumococcal pneumonia have at least one predisposing condition and/or fall into a group known to be at high risk epidemiologically (Table 119-1). Prior hospitalization either predisposes to or serves as a strong marker for subsequent pneumococcal infection. The susceptibility of elderly individuals to pneumococcal pneumonia is multifactorial, reflecting diminished clearance mechanisms as well as debilitation, malnutrition, and the presence of comorbid diseases. Although IgG responses to

---

TABLE 119-1 *Conditions That Commonly Predispose to Pneumococcal Infection*

Increased risk of exposure	Defective complement function
Day-care centers	Defective clearance of
Military training camps	pneumococcal bacteremia[a]
Prisons	Congenital asplenia,
Shelters for the homeless	hyposplenia
Respiratory infection,	Splenectomy
inflammation	Sickle cell disease
Influenza, other viral	Multifactorial conditions
respiratory infections	Infancy and aging
Air pollution	Chronic disease, hospitalization
Allergies	Alcoholism
Cigarette smoking	Malnutrition
Chronic obstructive pulmonary	HIV infection
disease	Chronic lung disease
Other causes of chronic	Glucocorticoid treatment
pulmonary inflammation or	Cirrhosis of the liver
obstruction	Renal insufficiency
Anatomical disruption of	Diabetes mellitus
meninges (dural tear)	Anemia
Defective antibody formation	Coronary artery disease
Common variable	Fatigue, stress, and/or exposure
hypogammaglobulinemia	to cold
Selective IgG subclass	
deficiency	
Multiple myeloma	
Chronic lymphocytic leukemia	
Lymphoma	

[a] The absence of a spleen predisposes to more fulminant infection (see text).

some capsular polysaccharides, as measured by enzyme-linked immunosorbent assay (ELISA), are more or less normal in elderly persons, postvaccination levels of antibody to others are reduced, and the functional capacity of the antibody appears to be decreased. A remarkably high incidence of pneumococcal infection—perhaps 100-fold above baseline—among persons with AIDS is largely related to poor formation of antibody to capsular polysaccharides.

Once a pneumococcal infection has been initiated, the absence of a spleen predisposes to fulminant disease. The liver is able to remove opsonized (antibody-coated) pneumococci from the circulation; in the absence of antibody, however, only the slow passage of blood through the splenic sinuses and prolonged contact with reticuloendothelial cells in the cords of Billroth allow time for bacterial clearance. Patients without spleens may die of pneumococcal pneumonia and sepsis at such an early stage of the illness that pulmonary consolidation is not evident on x-ray but rather is found only at autopsy.

SPECIFIC INFECTIONS CAUSED BY *S. PNEUMONIAE* *S. pneumoniae* causes infections of the middle ear, sinuses, trachea, bronchi, and lungs (Table 119-2) by direct spread from the nasopharyngeal site of colonization. Infections of the CNS, heart valves, bones, joints, and peritoneal cavity usually arise by hematogenous spread; peritoneal infection also results from ascent via the fallopian tubes. The CNS may also be infected by contiguous spread of organisms, as in patients who have a tear in the dura. Primary pneumococcal bacteremia—i.e., the presence of pneumococci in the blood with no apparent source—occurs commonly in children <2 years of age and as a small percentage of all pneumococcal bacteremias in adults; if no therapy is given, a source and/or a secondary site of infection may become apparent. Pleural infection results either from direct extension of pneumonia to the visceral pleura or from hematogenous spread of bacteria from a pulmonary or extrapulmonary focus to the pleural space; the route cannot be determined in any individual case. Infections listed after meningitis in Table 119-2 are uncommon or rare.

Otitis Media and Sinusitis When fluid from the middle ear is cultured during acute otitis media or fluid from a paranasal sinus is cultured during acute sinusitis, *S. pneumoniae* is the most common isolate or is second only to nontypable *Haemophilus influenzae*. Whether in adults or in children, pneumococci are identified in ~40 to 50% of cases of otitis in which an etiologic agent is isolated. Prior infection by a respiratory virus or allergy is thought to contribute significantly to these pneumococcal infections by causing congestion of the openings to the eustachian tubes or the paranasal sinuses. Prospective studies of young children have shown that colonization precedes infection in most cases. For reasons that are unclear, serotypes 6B, 14, 19F, and 23F predominate both as colonizing and as infecting organisms of children.

Pneumonia The distinctive symptoms and signs of pneumonia, whether due to the pneumococcus or to other bacteria, are (1) cough and sputum production, which reflect the proliferation of bacteria and the resulting inflammatory response in the alveoli; (2) fever; and (3) radiographic detection of an infiltrate.

TABLE 119-2 *Most Common Infections Caused by Streptococcus pneumoniae in Adults*

Acute sinusitis	Septic arthritis
Pneumonia	Peritonitis
Acute purulent tracheobronchitis	Endocarditis
Otitis media	Pericarditis
Empyema	Endometritis
Meningitis	Cellulitis
Primary bacteremia	Brain abscess
Osteomyelitis	

Note: The order of the list very roughly approximates the order of frequency among adults, from most to least common.

PREDISPOSING CONDITIONS Pneumococcal pneumonia is most common at the extremes of age. Despite the undisputed role of *S. pneumoniae* as a major pathogenic bacterium for humans, the great majority of adults with pneumococcal pneumonia have underlying diseases that predispose them to infection. Otherwise-healthy military recruits involved in outbreaks of infection may be an exception to this rule; however, many of those affected have an exposure to stress and/or an antecedent viral-type illness that may reduce normal host resistance. In addition to prior viral respiratory illness, the most common predisposing conditions are alcoholism, malnutrition, chronic pulmonary disease of any kind, cigarette smoking, infection with HIV, diabetes mellitus, cirrhosis of the liver, anemia, prior hospitalization for any reason, renal insufficiency, and coronary artery disease (with or without recognized congestive heart failure). HIV infection is such an important predisposing factor that some authorities recommend that any young adult with pneumococcal pneumonia be tested for antibody to HIV.

PRESENTING SYMPTOMS Patients often present with a preexisting respiratory condition that has distinctly deteriorated. If a viral respiratory illness is the predisposing factor, the patient may have felt unwell for several days, with coryza or a nonproductive cough and low-grade fever. At the time of onset of pneumonia, the patient feels distinctly worse. The temperature may rise to 38.9 to 39.4°C (102 to 103°F); however, one series of cases documented temperatures from 33.3 to 40.5°C (92 to 104.9°F), with only one-third of bacteremic patients having a temperature of ≥37.5°C (≥99.5°F) at admission. Sputum production may become prominent; in a patient who has chronic bronchitis, the sputum may increase in volume and may become yellow or green and thicker than usual. In a small proportion of cases, the onset of disease follows a hyperacute pattern in which the patient suddenly has a single episode of shaking chills followed by sustained fever and a cough productive of blood-tinged sputum. This clinical picture is unfortunately called "classic," a vague term that is best avoided because many physicians believe that it means "most common," which is clearly not the case. In elderly subjects, the onset of disease may be especially insidious and may not suggest pneumonia at all. Elderly patients may have minimal cough, no sputum production, and no fever, instead appearing tired or confused. Nausea and vomiting or diarrhea, sometimes quite prominent, occur in up to 20% of cases of pneumococcal pneumonia. Symptoms of myocardial ischemia or an actual infarction may be present in 5% of cases. The most abrupt progression of pneumococcal disease is seen in patients who have undergone splenectomy; given their defective clearance of pneumococci from the bloodstream, these individuals may go from apparent good health to death in as little as 24 h. An inapparent pulmonary focus is often responsible. In pneumonia, pleuritic chest pain may result from extension of the inflammatory process to the visceral pleura; persistence of this pain, especially after the first day or two of treatment, raises concern about empyema (see "Complications," below). Clearly, the range of symptoms is sufficiently broad that no characteristic presentation distinguishes pneumococcal from other types of bacterial pneumonia (or from some types of nonbacterial pneumonia).

PHYSICAL FINDINGS Patients with pneumococcal pneumonia usually appear ill and have a grayish, anxious appearance that differs from that of persons with viral or mycoplasmal pneumonia. Temperature, pulse, and respiratory rate are typically elevated. Elderly patients may have only a slight temperature elevation or may be afebrile. Hypothermia is associated with increased morbidity and mortality. Herpes labialis appears in a small percentage of cases. Pain may cause diminished respiratory excursion (splinting) on the affected side. Dullness to percussion is noted in about half of cases, and vocal fremitus is increased. Breath sounds may be bronchial or tubular, and crackles are heard in most cases if enough air is being moved to generate them. Flatness to percussion at the lung base, absent fremitus, and lack of the expected degree of diaphragmatic motion suggest the presence of pleural fluid, which raises the possibility that empyema is present. The finding of a heart murmur, certainly if new, raises concern about endocarditis, a rare but serious complication. Hypoxia or the generalized response to pneumonia may cause the patient to be confused, but the appearance of confusion should also raise concern about meningitis. Obtundation or neck stiffness should lead to an immediate consideration of this complication.

RADIOGRAPHIC FINDINGS Pneumococcal pneumonia involves only one lung segment or a portion thereof in one-fourth of cases; it involves more than one segment but only one lobe or a portion thereof in another one-fourth of instances. Thus multilobar disease is seen in half of cases. Air-space consolidation is the predominant finding and is detected in 80% of cases (Fig. 119-1). Air bronchogram (visualization of the air-filled bronchus against a background of consolidation in the alveoli) is evident in fewer than half of cases and is more common in bacteremic than in nonbacteremic disease. In rare instances, pneu-

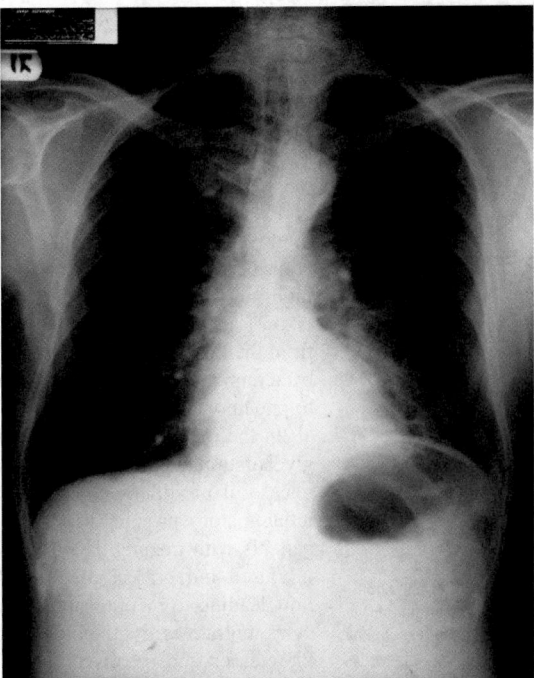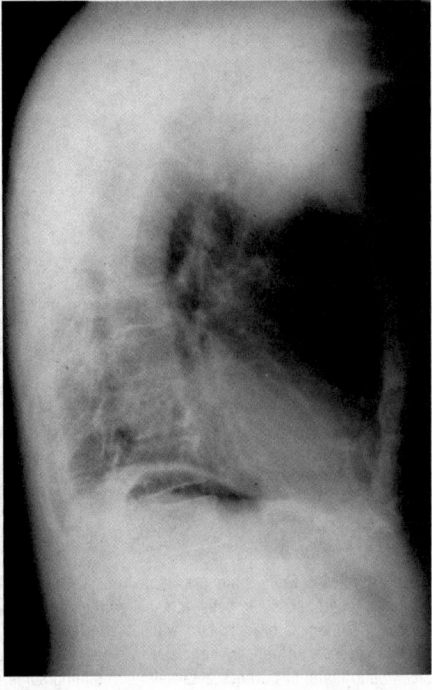

FIGURE 119-1 A retrocardiac infiltrate in a patient with pneumococcal pneumonia. Consolidation is apparent on posterior-anterior view (left) but is better visualized on lateral view of the chest (right).

mococcal pneumonia leads to a lung abscess; an underlying malignancy may be present, and co-infection with a mixture of anaerobic and microaerophilic organisms may be documented as well. Although some pleural fluid may actually be present in half of cases, no more than 20% of patients have a sufficient volume of fluid to allow aspiration, and in only a minority of these patients is empyema documented.

GENERAL LABORATORY FINDINGS Anemia (a hemoglobin level of <10 g/dL) is present in 25% of cases. The peripheral-blood white blood cell (WBC) count exceeds 12,000/μL in the great majority of patients with pneumococcal pneumonia. However, the count is <6000/μL in 5 to 10% of persons hospitalized for pneumococcal pneumonia. Such a low count is strongly associated with lethal disease and is often but not always associated with bone marrow suppression due to alcohol ingestion. The serum bilirubin level is modestly elevated in one-third of cases; hypoxia, inflammatory changes in the liver, and breakdown of red blood cells in the lung are all thought to contribute to this increase. A serum albumin level of <2.5 g/dL in 30% of cases may indicate predisposing malnutrition or may be secondary to sepsis. About 20% of patients have serum sodium concentrations of ≤130 meq/L, and another 20% have serum creatinine concentrations of ≥2 mg/dL. →*Abnormalities of pleural fluid in empyema are reviewed in Chap. 239.*

DIFFERENTIAL DIAGNOSIS Patients who present with community-acquired pneumonia may actually have infection due to one of many organisms. The extensive list includes the following: *H. influenzae* or *Moraxella catarrhalis* in persons with little to predispose them other than chronic or acute inflammation of the airways; *Staphylococcus aureus* in persons who take glucocorticoids or who have major anatomical disruption of the airways; *Streptococcus pyogenes*; *Neisseria meningitidis*; anaerobic species in persons who have seizures or who may have aspirated oropharyngeal contents for some other reason; *Legionella*; *Pasteurella multocida* in dog or cat owners; gram-negative bacilli, especially in persons with severely damaged lungs who are taking glucocorticoids; viruses, especially influenza virus (in season), adenovirus, or respiratory syncytial virus; *Mycobacterium tuberculosis*; fungi, including *Pneumocystis* (depending on epidemiologic factors and the possible presence of HIV infection); *Mycoplasma*; *Chlamydia pneumoniae*, especially in older adults; and *Chlamydia psittaci* in bird owners. Many older men with lung cancer present with pneumonia, as

do persons who have acute-onset inflammatory pulmonary conditions of uncertain etiology or those with pulmonary embolus and infarction. The breadth of this list vividly illustrates the deficiency of empirical therapy for community-acquired pneumonia (Table 119-3). Many of these diseases require evaluation, and specific therapy is available for an increasing number. Moreover, pneumococci—perhaps the most common cause of community-acquired pneumonia—are increasingly resistant to available antibiotics. Taken together, these factors favor precise determination of the etiology of a pneumonia syndrome whenever possible.

DIAGNOSTIC MICROBIOLOGY An etiologic role for the pneumococcus in pneumonia is strongly suggested by the microscopic demonstration of large numbers of PMNs and slightly elongated gram-positive cocci in pairs and chains in the sputum (Fig. 119-2). Capsules may be seen surrounding the bacterial forms. Examined areas of the slide must be free of buccal epithelial cells, which indicate the admixture of saliva with sputum; saliva may contain viridans streptococci at counts of >10^7/mL. When characteristic microscopic findings are noted, the identification of *S. pneumoniae* in sputum culture strongly indicates pneumococcal infection of the lower respiratory tract. In the absence of such microscopic findings, the identification of pneumococci by culture may be nonspecific, reflecting colonization of the upper airways. Culture is, however, more sensitive than microscopic exami-

TABLE 119-3 Causes of a Pneumonia Syndrome Leading to Hospitalization of Adults in Houston, Texas[a]

Common	Less Common
Streptococcus pneumoniae	*Moraxella catarrhalis*
Haemophilus influenzae	*Staphylococcus aureus*
Lung cancer	*Legionella* species
Mycobacterium tuberculosis	Pulmonary infarction
Pneumocystis	*Klebsiella pneumoniae*
Influenza (seasonal)	Respiratory syncytial virus
	Microaerophilic and anaerobic mouth flora
	Pseudomonas aeruginosa
	Chlamydia pneumoniae
	Cryptococcus, Histoplasma
	Hamman-Rich syndrome, others

[a] Pneumonia was defined as a syndrome consisting of fever, increased cough, sputum production, and an abnormal pulmonary shadow on chest x-ray.

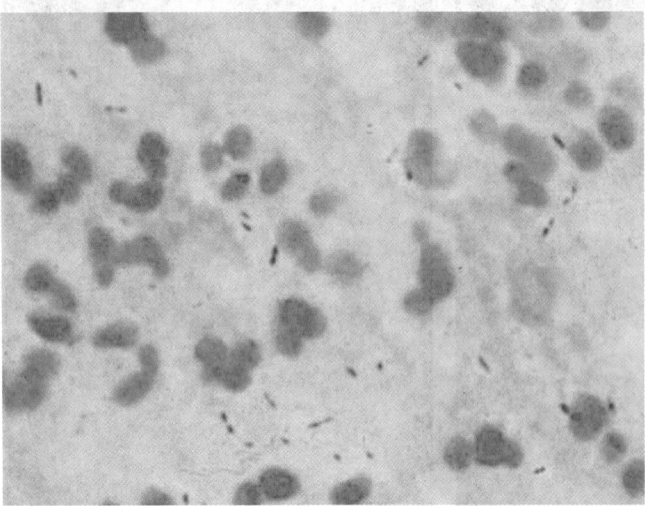

FIGURE 119-2 Gram-stained sputum from a patient with pneumococcal pneumonia shows polymorphonuclear cells with no epithelial cells, indicating the origin of the sample in inflammatory exudate without contamination. Slightly pleomorphic gram-positive coccobacilli appear, generally in pairs. Displacement of stained proteinaceous background material outlines a capsule surrounding some of the organisms. When obtained from a patient with pneumonia, a sample like this one is highly specific in identifying the pneumococcus as the etiologic agent.

nation for identifying pneumococci. Since most pneumococci do not produce distinctively mucoid colonies, their identification in the laboratory depends on the ability to select putative pneumococcal colonies for further study from among α-hemolytic streptococci of the mouth. In short, laboratory diagnosis by sputum culture depends on the quality of the specimen provided, the care with which the relevant purulent component is separated for study, and the assiduity with which α-hemolytic colonies are studied. Prior treatment with antibiotics can also rapidly clear pneumococci from sputum. These factors need to be considered when sputum cultures from patients who appear to have pneumococcal pneumonia are said to yield only "normal mouth flora" and when the medical literature describes what appear to be poor results of sputum culture. Because of the central role of microscopic examination in diagnosis, physicians may wish to view the slides with the microbiologist. Blood cultures yield *S. pneumoniae* in ~25% of cases of pneumococcal pneumonia, often within 12 h after the sample is obtained.

COMPLICATIONS Empyema is the most common complication of pneumococcal pneumonia, occurring in ~2% of cases. Some fluid appears in the pleural space in a substantial proportion of cases of pneumococcal pneumonia, but this parapneumonic effusion usually reflects an inflammatory response to infection that has been contained within the lung, and its presence is self-limited. When bacteria reach the pleural space—either hematogenously or as a result of contiguous spread, possibly across lymphatics of the visceral pleura—empyema results. The finding of frank pus, a positive result on Gram's staining, or the presence of fluid with a pH of ≤7.1 indicates the need for aggressive and complete drainage, preferably by prompt insertion of a chest tube, with verification by computed tomography (CT) that fluid has been removed. Failure to drain most or all of the fluid usually indicates the need for thoracotomy. Persistence of fever (even if low-grade) and leukocytosis after 4 or 5 days of appropriate antibiotic treatment for pneumococcal pneumonia suggests empyema. In this setting, the diagnosis is exceedingly likely if the x-ray shows pleural fluid; at this stage, thoracotomy is often needed for cure. Aggressive drainage is likely to reduce morbidity and mortality from empyema (Chap. 245).

Meningitis Except during outbreaks of meningococcal infection, *S. pneumoniae* is the most common cause of bacterial meningitis in adults. Because of the remarkable success of *H. influenzae* type b vac-

cine, *S. pneumoniae* now predominates among cases in infants and toddlers as well (but not among those in newborns). Meningitis develops either by the direct extension of infection from the sinuses or the middle ear or as a result of seeding of meningeal endothelial cells or the choroid plexus during bacteremia. Favoring the former pathogenesis are the association between acute otitis media or sinusitis and meningitis and the role of *S. pneumoniae* as the most common cause of recurrent meningitis associated with head trauma, cerebrospinal fluid (CSF) leak, and/or dural tear. Favoring the latter are the association between pneumococcal bacteremia from any source and meningitis as well as an autopsy study of temporal bone from children who died of bacterial meningitis, which yielded no evidence of extension from the middle ear. In adults, meningitis is usually a complication of bacteremia, which in turn is attributable, in the great majority of cases, to pneumonia.

In the meninges and subarachnoid space, pneumococcal peptidoglycan stimulates an intense inflammatory response mediated by the release of proinflammatory cytokines such as IL-8 and macrophage inflammatory protein (MIP)-1, which are detectable in the CSF of patients with meningitis. The ensuing inflammatory response results in raised intracranial pressure, brain edema, and decreased blood flow leading to meningismus, drowsiness, or coma. Activated leukocytes migrate across the blood-brain barrier and release matrix metalloproteases and reactive oxygen and nitrogen species that damage neurons. Focal neurologic signs may result from vasculitis with venous or arterial thrombosis, cranial neuropathy due to entrapment or infarction, local cerebritis, subdural effusion, or brain herniation (Chap. 360).

No distinctive clinical or laboratory feature differentiates meningitis due to *S. pneumoniae* from that due to other bacteria. Patients note the sudden onset of fever, headache, and stiffness or pain in the neck. Without treatment, there is a progression over 24 to 48 h to confusion and then obtundation. On physical examination, the patient looks acutely ill and has a rigid neck. In such cases lumbar puncture should not be delayed for CT of the head unless papilledema or focal neurologic signs are evident. Typical CSF findings consist of pleocytosis (500 to 10,000 cells/μL) with ≥85% PMNs, an elevated protein level (100 to 500 mg/dL), and a decrease in glucose content (<30 mg/dL). If antibiotics have not been given, large numbers of pneumococci can be seen in a Gram-stained specimen of CSF in all cases, and specific therapy can be administered, although, because of its similar appearance, *Listeria* may be misidentified as the pneumococcus. If an effective antibiotic has already been given, the number of bacteria may be greatly decreased and microscopic examination of a Gram-stained specimen may yield negative results. In this situation, immunologic methods for the detection of pneumococcal capsule in the CSF may be positive in up to two-thirds of cases, although these methods have fallen out of favor.

OTHER SYNDROMES The appearance of pneumococcal infection at other, ordinarily sterile body sites indicates hematogenous spread, usually during frank pneumonia or, in a small proportion of cases, from an inapparent focus of infection. A case of pneumococcal endocarditis is seen every few years at large tertiary-care hospitals. Purulent pericarditis, occurring as a separate entity or together with endocarditis, is even rarer. Septic arthritis can arise spontaneously in a natural or prosthetic joint or as a complication of rheumatoid arthritis. Osteomyelitis in adults tends to involve vertebral bones. Pneumococcal peritonitis occurs by one of three pathogenetic pathways: (1) hematogenous spread when ascites or other preexisting peritoneal disease is present; (2) local spread from a perforated viscus (usually appendicitis or perforated ulcer); or (3) transit via the fallopian tubes. Salpingitis may be recognized with or without accompanying peritonitis. Epidural and brain abscesses arise as a complication of sinusitis or mastoiditis. Cellulitis develops most often in persons who have connective tissue diseases or HIV infection. The appearance of any of these unusual pneumococcal infections may suggest that tests for HIV infection should be undertaken. Finally, for reasons that are unclear, unencapsulated (but not encapsulated) pneumococci cause sporadic or epidemic conjunctivitis.

Antibiotic Susceptibility β-Lactam antibiotics, the cornerstone of therapy for serious pneumococcal infection, bind covalently to the active site and thereby block the action of enzymes (endo-, trans-, and carboxypeptidases) needed for cell-wall synthesis. Because these enzymes were identified by their reaction with radiolabeled penicillin, they are called *penicillin-binding proteins*. In the 1960s, virtually all clinical isolates of *S. pneumoniae* were susceptible to penicillin (i.e., were inhibited in vitro by concentrations of <0.06 μg/mL). During the past two decades, an increasing number of isolates have shown some degree of resistance to penicillin. Resistance results when spontaneous mutation or acquisition of new genetic material alters penicillin-binding proteins in a manner that reduces their affinity for penicillin, thereby necessitating a higher concentration of penicillin for their saturation. The genetic

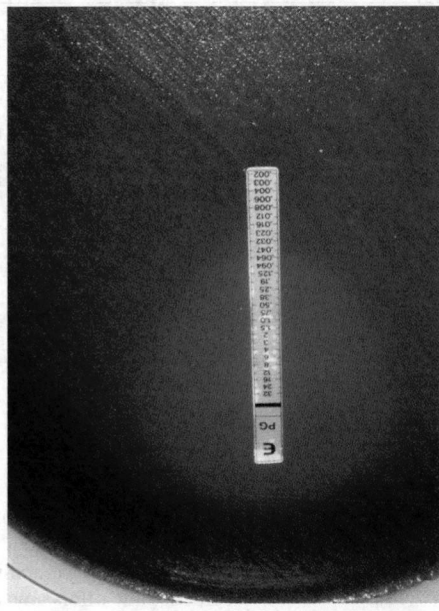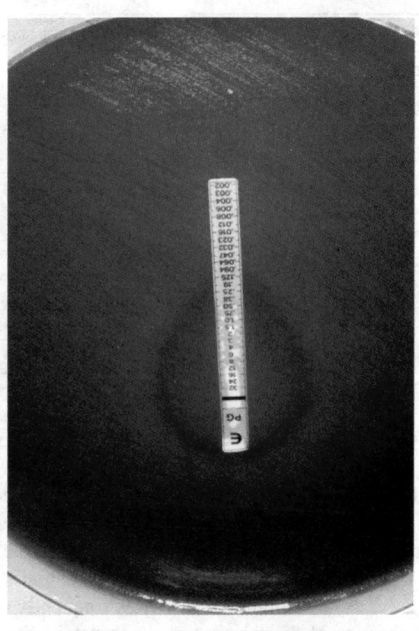

FIGURE 119-3 The e-strip method currently used by most laboratories to determine the susceptibility of *S. pneumoniae* to antibiotics. After the plate is streaked with a suspension of pneumococci, a strip that has been impregnated with graded concentrations of the antibiotic under study (penicillin in the example shown) is placed on the surface, and the plate is incubated overnight at 37°C. The organism on the left is inhibited by a penicillin concentration of 0.016 μg/mL and is fully susceptible to this drug. The organism on the right is inhibited only by a penicillin concentration of 0.25 μg/mL and is intermediately resistant to this agent.

information that renders pneumococci resistant to penicillin is generally acquired from oral streptococci and conveys resistance to other antibiotics as well. Selection of antibiotic-resistant strains in the United States—especially in areas of high antibiotic use, such as day-care centers—and importation of strains from other countries where antibiotics are available without prescription have contributed to the prevalence of multidrug resistance.

At present, ~20% of pneumococcal isolates in the United States are intermediately susceptible to penicillin [minimal inhibitory concentration (MIC) 0.1 to 1.0 μg/mL], and 15% are resistant (MIC ≥2.0 μg/mL; Fig. 119-3). These definitions were based on drug levels achievable in CSF during treatment of meningitis, whereas levels reached in the bloodstream, lungs, and sinuses are actually much higher. Thus the MIC needs to be interpreted in light of the infection being treated. Pneumonia caused by a penicillin-resistant strain is likely to respond to 24 million units of penicillin daily, whereas meningitis will not. The recently revised definition of amoxicillin resistance (susceptible, MIC ≤2 μg/mL; intermediately resistant, MIC = 4 μg/mL; resistant, MIC ≥8 μg/mL) is based on serum levels, assuming that no physician would knowingly treat meningitis with this oral medication. Pneumonia due to an intermediately amoxicillin-resistant strain may not respond to treatment with this drug, and that due to a resistant strain is likely not to respond. On the assumption that antibiotic concentrations in middle-ear fluid or sinus cavities approach those in serum, similar inferences can be made about the treatment of otitis or sinusitis.

Penicillin-susceptible pneumococci are susceptible to all commonly used cephalosporins. Penicillin-intermediate strains tend to be resistant to all first- and many second-generation cephalosporins (of which cefuroxime retains the best efficacy), but most are susceptible to certain third-generation cephalosporins, including cefotaxime, ceftriaxone, cefepime, and cefpodoxime. One-half of highly penicillin-resistant pneumococci are also resistant to cefotaxime, ceftriaxone, and cefepime, and nearly all are resistant to cefpodoxime. Just as in the case of penicillin, susceptibility to cefotaxime and ceftriaxone is defined on the basis of achievable CSF levels. Thus pneumonia caused by intermediately resistant strains (MIC = 2 μg/mL) will respond well to usual doses of these drugs, and pneumonia due to a resistant organism (MIC ≥ 4 μg/mL) is likely to respond. Meningitis due to inter-

mediately resistant strains may not respond, and meningitis due to a resistant strain is likely not to respond to treatment with cefotaxime or ceftriaxone.

About one-quarter of all pneumococcal isolates in the United States are resistant to erythromycin and the newer macrolides, including azithromycin and clarithromycin, with much higher rates of resistance in penicillin-resistant strains. This resistance will certainly affect empirical therapy for bronchitis, sinusitis, and pneumonia. In the United States, the majority of macrolide-resistant pneumococci bear the so-called M phenotype (erythromycin MIC = 1 to 8 μg/mL) and are susceptible to clindamycin. In this case, resistance is mediated by an efflux pump mechanism; to some extent, M-type resistance can be overcome by clinically achievable levels of macrolides. In Europe, most macrolide resistance is due to a mutation in *ermB*, which confers high-level resistance not only to macrolides but also to clindamycin; more than 90% of pneumococcal isolates in the United States are susceptible to clindamycin. Rates of doxycycline resistance among pneumococci of varying susceptibility to penicillin are similar to those observed for macrolides. One-third of pneumococcal isolates exhibit reduced susceptibility to trimethoprim-sulfamethoxazole. The newer fluoroquinolones remain highly effective against pneumococci, with equal efficacy against penicillin-susceptible and -resistant strains; the rate of resistance is generally <1% but approaches 2 to 3% in areas where quinolones are widely used and is increasing. Ketolides appear to be uniformly effective against pneumococci, as does vancomycin, although it is feared that the acquisition of vancomycin resistance by enterococci and other gram-positive bacteria may eventually lead to pneumococcal transformation to resistance. Oxazolidinones and glycopeptides also appear to be effective in vitro, with MICs no higher for drug-resistant *S. pneumoniae* strains than for penicillin-susceptible strains. Resistance to streptogramins parallels that to macrolides, limiting the usefulness of these drugs for the treatment of pneumonia.

Pneumococcal susceptibility patterns vary greatly between and even within individual communities, and the data are in a state of flux. It does appear, however, that the constant trend is toward more widespread antibiotic resistance.

Otitis Media and Acute Sinusitis (Table 119-4) Current treatment recommendations for otitis media and acute sinusitis—conditions whose pathogenesis and microbial etiology are similar—are based on the

TABLE 119-4 Regimens for the Treatment of Pneumococcal Otitis Media or Sinusitis in Adults[a]

Regimen	Drug, Dose	Duration	Comments
First-line	Amoxicillin, 1 g q8h	Otitis: 3–5 days after clinical response, not to exceed 7 days total; sinusitis: 7–10 days after clinical response, not to exceed 2 weeks total	If this regimen fails, try second-line regimen.
Second-line	Amoxicillin, 1 g q8h, plus clavulanic acid[b]	Same as above	If this regimen fails, try third-line regimen.
Third-line	Ceftriaxone, 1 g qd	3–5 days for otitis; longer for sinusitis	If this regimen fails, consider complications; consult otolaryngologist and/or infectious disease specialist.

[a] Treatment for otitis media or sinusitis is empirical, since aspiration of the involved area to establish an etiologic diagnosis is rarely undertaken, except under the conditions of a research protocol.
[b] Give half as amoxicillin alone and half as amoxicillin with clavulanic acid.

following points: (1) Acute otitis media is the most common infection for which antibiotics are prescribed in the United States. (2) As noted above, *S. pneumoniae* is the most likely treatable cause; taken together, *H. influenzae* and *M. catarrhalis*, many strains of which produce β-lactamases, are implicated nearly as frequently as pneumococci. (3) In the absence of diagnostic tympanocentesis, the etiologic diagnosis is nearly always presumptive. (4) Because penetration into a closed space is required, high serum levels of an effective antibiotic are required to treat otitis caused by intermediately or fully resistant pneumococci. (5) *S. pneumoniae* is more likely than *Haemophilus* to cause progression to serious complications without specific therapy. (6) Antibiotics that are effective against pneumococci and yet resist β-lactamases tend to be very expensive compared with amoxicillin.

As a result of these considerations, the Otitis Media Working Group of the Centers for Disease Control and Prevention (CDC) recommended that initial therapy be amoxicillin in a high dosage—e.g., 80 to 90 mg/kg per day in two or three divided doses for infants and toddlers or 1 g three times daily for adults. If this regimen fails, highly penicillin-resistant pneumococci or β-lactamase-producing bacteria may be responsible, and amoxicillin may be given at the same total dosage but with one-half of the dose in the form of amoxicillin/clavulanic acid. If this regimen fails, three doses of ceftriaxone at daily intervals are likely to be curative. A quinolone or ketolide may also be tried in adults. Patients must be monitored closely for a response. Despite the detection (by molecular analysis) of pneumococcal DNA in middle-ear fluid, chronic serous otitis ("glue ear") is probably not due to active infection and does not require antibiotic therapy. Treatment for otitis is recommended for a total of 5 to 7 days; treatment for acute sinusitis is given for 10 to 14 days.

Pneumonia (Table 119-5) This section will deal primarily with the treatment of pneumonia that is known to be due to *S. pneumoniae*. The broader issue of empirical therapy for community-acquired pneumonia is covered in detail elsewhere (Chap. 239). However, a few general comments on empirical therapy apply. Without a good sputum sample that can be Gram-stained and examined microscopically, the etiologic agent is not known at the time when treatment needs to be initiated and is not likely to become known later. Empirical therapy in such cases must be effective against *S. pneumoniae*, which remains the most likely causative agent of community-acquired pneumonia, unless epidemiologic, clinical, and radiologic findings strongly favor another etiologic entity. In the past, when pneumococci were uniformly susceptible to nearly all antibiotics, it did not matter which drug was selected. Now that pneumococci are resistant, it clearly makes a difference. If a good sputum sample reveals only organisms consistent with *S. pneumoniae*, therapy can be focused on this organism, although additional treatment may be added for organisms that are not visualized microscopically—e.g., influenza virus in a patient hospitalized during an influenza outbreak. Even if the pneumococcus is suspected, a certain degree of empiricism is required, because the antibiotic susceptibility of the strain involved will not be known for 1 or 2 days.

There has been increased emphasis on outpatient therapy in patients who are at low risk (as determined by PORT score according to criteria described by the Pneumonia Outcomes Research Team; Chap. 239). This approach appears to be safe. However, if the physician is in doubt about the severity of illness, the social circumstances, or the likelihood of compliance with the prescribed antibiotic regimen, it may be best to hospitalize the patient, at least briefly. Predictions based on PORT score have been validated for pneumococcal pneumonia.

OUTPATIENT THERAPY Amoxicillin (1 g three times daily) effectively treats all cases of pneumococcal pneumonia except those caused by the most highly penicillin-resistant isolates. Neither cefuroxime nor cefpodoxime offers any advantages over amoxicillin since these drugs are less likely, even at high dosages, to be active against highly resistant pneumococcal strains. One of the newer fluoroquinolones or a ketolide in an accepted dosage for pneumonia is highly likely to be effective. Clindamycin will be effective in 90% and doxycycline, azithromycin, or clarithromycin in 75% of cases—levels of resistance that make their use questionable unless the organism is known to be susceptible. Because one-third of all isolates are now resistant to trimethoprim-sulfamethoxazole, this agent can no longer be recommended. Since none of these therapies ensures the kind of antibiotic coverage that it would have had in the past, patients should be instructed to remain in close contact with the prescribing physician, especially if there is any deterioration in their condition.

INPATIENT THERAPY Pneumonia caused by penicillin-susceptible or intermediately penicillin-resistant pneumococcal isolates is readily treatable with β-lactam antibiotics. The dosages that follow are acceptable against intermediately resistant strains and against many or most fully resistant isolates, although they are excessive for use against susceptible isolates. Lower doses, however, cannot be recommended initially because susceptibility is usually not known until 48 to 72 h after treatment is begun. Patients who are sick enough to be hospitalized should

TABLE 119-5 Regimens for the Treatment of Pneumococcal Pneumonia in Adults[a]

Route, Drug	Dose, Schedule[b]
ORAL THERAPY	
Amoxicillin	1 g q8h
Quinolone, e.g., gatifloxacin	400 mg q24h
PARENTERAL THERAPY	
Penicillin[c]	3–4 mU q4h
Ampicillin[d]	1–2 g q6h
Ceftriaxone	1 g q12–24h
Cefotaxime	1–2 g q6–8h
Quinolone, e.g., gatifloxacin	400 mg q24h
Imipenem	500 mg q6h
Vancomycin[e]	500 mg q6h

[a] These regimens are recommended for treatment after a presumptive diagnosis is made on the basis of examination of a Gram-stained sputum sample or as a replacement for more broad-spectrum empirical therapy after a diagnosis of pneumococcal pneumonia is proven by culture. When a valid sputum specimen cannot be obtained, concern for other likely pathogens should prompt the selection of more all-inclusive therapeutic regimens.
[b] Therapy should continue for 5 days after defervescence, not to exceed 7–10 days total. A switch from parenteral to oral drug administration may be made as soon as the patient can tolerate oral medications.
[c] This regimen is listed more for historic than for practical reasons. The spectrum is overly narrow, although perfectly acceptable if a Gram-stained sputum specimen shows only pneumococci. However, the need for frequent administration, mandated by the short half-life of penicillin, renders this regimen impractical.
[d] Usually given in the form of ampicillin/sulbactam.
[e] Not proven to be effective by the extensive clinical experience that applies to the other regimens.

be treated promptly. Most physicians favor parenteral antibiotics, although oral administration of well-absorbed drugs may be acceptable if the patient is not vomiting or hypotensive. Recommended regimens include ceftriaxone (1 g every 12 to 24 h) or cefotaxime (1 to 2 g every 6 to 8 h); the lower doses should suffice except against highly resistant strains. Ampicillin (1 to 2 g every 6 h) is also widely used, usually in the form of ampicillin/sulbactam. Quinolones are effective against all but a small percentage of pneumococcal strains and can be given parenterally or orally. Clindamycin is effective against ~90% of isolates. On the basis of in vitro considerations, vancomycin (500 mg every 6 h) is likely to be uniformly effective against pneumococci, and this drug or a quinolone should be used together with a third-generation cephalosporin for initial therapy in a patient who is likely to be infected with a highly antibiotic-resistant strain or in one who has had a severe allergic reaction to penicillins and cephalosporins. As noted above, there have always been treatment failures unrelated to the antimicrobial susceptibility of the organism; nevertheless, the failure of a patient to respond promptly should raise the question of resistance, and another drug should be given until the susceptibility of the infecting strain has been documented. Of course, evidence for loculated infections (such as empyema) and/or other causes of fever should be sought and addressed appropriately.

DURATION OF THERAPY The optimal duration of treatment for pneumococcal pneumonia is uncertain. Penicillin-susceptible strains begin to disappear from the sputum within several hours of the first dose of penicillin, and a single dose of procaine penicillin, which results in the maintenance of an effective antimicrobial level for 24 h, was said to cure pneumococcal pneumonia in otherwise-healthy young adults at the time when all isolates were susceptible. Most older physicians treated pneumococcal pneumonia for 5 to 7 days. In the absence of reports of therapy failure, younger physicians have tended to treat the infection for 10 to 14 days. Prolongation of therapy is a two-edged sword, especially in debilitated patients, because the risk of complications increases with each day of antibiotic treatment, particularly in the hospital setting. A few days of close observation and parenteral therapy followed by an oral antibiotic—with the entire course of treatment continuing for no more than 5 days after the patient becomes afebrile—may be the best approach.

Meningitis (Table 119-6) Pneumococcal meningitis should be treated initially with ceftriaxone (1 to 2 g every 12 h) plus vancomycin (500 mg every 6 h or 1 g every 12 h). At this time, studies in experimental animals suggest benefits of the addition of rifampin, but in vitro studies indicate antagonism between this drug and ceftriaxone or vancomycin. This author does not recommend that rifampin be added. Two drugs are given initially because the cephalosporin is likely to be effective against most isolates and readily penetrates the blood-brain barrier, whereas, although all isolates are susceptible to vancomycin, this drug has a somewhat unpredictable capacity to cross the blood-brain barrier. If the isolate is shown to be susceptible or intermediately resistant, treatment can be continued with ceftriaxone, and vancomycin may be discontinued. If the organism is resistant, continued treatment with two drugs is indicated. Cefotaxime (2 g every 6 h) may be used instead of ceftriaxone. Imipenem (500 mg every 6 h) may be used in patients who have had life-threatening reactions to β-lactam antibiotics. As noted above, the author of this chapter does not recommend the addition of rifampin. The total duration of therapy for pneumococcal meningitis is 10 days. Consistent with the central pathogenic role of inflammation in meningitis, a recent study demonstrates clear benefit from the addition of glucocorticoids; heretofore, relevant data were conflicting (Chap. 360). Meningitis should be treated in an intensive care unit and with the participation of appropriate consultants, generally including a neurologist and a specialist in infectious diseases.

Endocarditis Pneumococcal endocarditis is associated with rapid destruction of heart valves. Pending results of susceptibility studies, treatment should be initiated with ceftriaxone or cefotaxime; as the prevalence of highly resistant strains increases, it might be prudent to add vancomycin until results of susceptibility studies are available.

TABLE 119-6 *Treatment of Pneumococcal Meningitis*

Circumstance	Appropriate Course[a]
Diagnosis of pneumococcal meningitis; antibiotic susceptibility unknown	Treat with ceftriaxone, 1–2 g q12h, plus vancomycin, 500 mg q6h, until antibiotic susceptibility of organism is known.
Susceptibility results available	Continue treatment with ceftriaxone alone if organism is susceptible or intermediate; continue both ceftriaxone and vancomycin if organism is resistant.
Life-threatening penicillin allergy	Treat with imipenem, 500 mg q6h, rather than a β-lactam antibiotic.

[a] Treatment should be administered for 5–7 days after defervescence or for a total of 10 days.

There is no clear evidence that adding another antibiotic to the regimen is beneficial; aminoglycosides are somewhat synergistic and rifampin or quinolones are antagonistic with β-lactams. Patients with endocarditis should probably be treated in an intensive care unit in collaboration with an infectious disease consultant, a cardiologist, and a cardiovascular surgeon.

Other Therapeutic Modalities A variety of agents that block the action of TNF-α, IL-1, or platelet-activating factor have conferred no benefit and may even have had a detrimental effect on pneumococcal sepsis. Similar results have been obtained with glucocorticoids except in cases of meningitis.

PREVENTION Pneumococcal polysaccharide vaccine contains 25 μg of capsular polysaccharide from the 23 most prevalent serotypes of *S. pneumoniae*; vaccination stimulates antibody to most serotypes in most recipients. In adults <55 years old, protection rates are at least 85% even 5 years or longer after vaccination (Table 119-7). The level and duration of protection decrease with advancing age, perhaps because of a diminished avidity of the antibody for the capsular polysaccharide. As a result, 50% of persons in their eighties are protected for up to 3 years, with very little or no protection thereafter. In subgroups of the population at high risk (e.g., debilitated elderly persons and individuals with severe chronic lung disease), vaccine has not been shown conclusively to be effective. Persons who most need the vaccine because of poor IgG responses are not likely to respond to immunization with significant increases in antibody level. Nevertheless, in light of the safety and low cost of the vaccine, some experts believe that the poor average rate of response should not deter physicians from administering vaccine to individual patients who are at increased risk of pneumococcal infection.

The CDC's Immunization Practices Advisory Committee has broadened its recommendations for pneumococcal vaccination to include all persons over the age of 2 years who are at substantially increased risk of developing pneumococcal infection and/or of having

TABLE 119-7 *Protective Efficacy of Polyvalent Pneumococcal Polysaccharide Vaccine[a]*

Age, Years	No. of Subject Pairs	Years since Last Vaccination		
		<3	3–5	>5
<55	125	93	89	85
55–64	149	88	82	75
65–74	213	80	71	58
75–84	188	67	53	32
≥85	133	46	22	−13

[a] Results of a case-control study involving all cases of invasive pneumococcal disease in Connecticut during 7 years (1984–1990). Vaccinated subjects were matched with controls, and the rate of invasive pneumococcal disease was related to age and time since vaccination. The data, showing protective efficacy, suggest that, within 5 years of vaccination, protection rates decline with age—i.e., from ~90% in persons <65 years of age to <50% in persons ≥85 years old. Protection also declines with increasing time from vaccination to infection, and this decline is more prominent in older patients.

Source: Data adapted Ed Shapiro et al: N Engl J Med 325:1453, 1991; with permission.

a serious complication of such an infection. Perhaps most important are those with anatomical or functional asplenia who are at risk for overwhelming, life-threatening infections. Others who might fall within these recommendations are persons (1) over the age of 65; (2) with CSF leak, diabetes mellitus, alcoholism, cirrhosis, chronic renal insufficiency, chronic pulmonary disease, or advanced cardiovascular disease; (3) who have an immunocompromising condition associated with increased risk of pneumococcal disease, such as multiple myeloma, lymphoma, Hodgkin's disease, HIV infection, organ transplantation, or chronic use of glucocorticoids; (4) who are genetically at increased risk, such as Native Americans and Alaskans; or (5) who live in environments where outbreaks are particularly likely to occur, such as nursing homes.

Recommendations regarding revaccination seem to be somewhat inconsistent. A single revaccination is advocated for persons over the age of 65 if more than 5 years have transpired since the first vaccination. Since antibody levels decline and there is no anamnestic response, it seems more reasonable simply to recommend revaccination at 5-year intervals, especially in persons over the age of 65, who tend to have almost no adverse reaction to vaccination, and in splenectomized patients, who are most in need.

Pneumococcal polysaccharide vaccine is not useful in children <2 years of age, whose immune system does not respond well to polysaccharide antigens. Conjugating the polysaccharide to a protein alters the form in which the antigen is presented to immune-processing cells, yielding an effective immunogen. A heptavalent protein-conjugate pneumococcal polysaccharide vaccine, approved for use in 2000, protects infants and young children against pneumococcal otitis media, pneumonia, bacteremia, and meningitis; efficacy for serotypes contained in the vaccine, which are responsible for about two-thirds of all cases of pneumococcal disease in young children, is 67% for otitis and 97% for bacteremia and meningitis. The rate of nasopharyngeal carriage of vaccine serotypes is also reduced. By its "herd effect" (i.e., the effect on nonvaccinated members of the population), widespread

use of this vaccine appears to have decreased the overall incidence of invasive pneumococcal disease in the population. Protein conjugate vaccines that contain antigen from the 11 most common infecting serotypes are being studied. The usefulness of these products may ultimately be limited because they may lead to replacement of serotypes contained in the vaccine with nonvaccine serotypes. Vaccines that contain surface-expressed proteins present in all pneumococci, such as pneumococcal surface protein A (PspA) and surface adhesin A (PsaA), are in the early phases of investigation. Conjugate vaccines do not appear to offer any advantage over polysaccharide vaccine in healthy or diseased adults, although a subpopulation of persons who, on a genetic basis, fail to respond to pneumococcal polysaccharide vaccine may respond to a conjugate vaccine.

FURTHER READING

BARTLETT JG et al: Practice guidelines for the management of community-acquired pneumonia in adults. Clin Infect Dis 31:347, 2000

FEDSON DS, MUSHER DM: Pneumococcal vaccine, in *Vaccines,* 4th ed, SA Plotkin, EA Mortimer Jr (eds). Philadelphia, Saunders, 2003

HAUSDORFF WP et al: The contribution of specific pneumococcal serogroups to different disease manifestations: Implications for conjugate vaccine formulation and use, part II. Clin Infect Dis 30:122, 2000

MUSHER DM et al: A fresh look at the definition of susceptibility of *Streptococcus pneumoniae* to beta-lactam antibiotics. Arch Intern Med 161:2538, 2001

───── et al: Bacteremic and nonbacteremic pneumococcal pneumonia: A prospective study. Medicine 79:210, 2000

─────: *Streptococcus pneumoniae,* in *Principles and Practice of Infectious Diseases,* 6th ed, GL Mandell et al (eds). New York, Churchill Livingstone, 2004 (in press)

THORNSBERRY C et al: Regional trends in antimicrobial resistance among clinical isolates of *Streptococcus pneumoniae, Haemophilus influenzae,* and *Moraxella catarrhalis* in the United States: Results from the TRUST Surveillance Program, 1999–2000. Clin Infect Dis 34(Suppl 1):S4, 2002

TUOMANEN EI et al: Pathogenesis of pneumococcal infection. N Engl J Med 332:1280, 1995

WATANAKUNAKORN C et al: Adult bacteremic pneumococcal pneumonia in a community teaching hospital, 1992–1996. A detailed analysis of 108 cases. Arch Intern Med 157:1965, 1997

120 STAPHYLOCOCCAL INFECTIONS
Franklin D. Lowy

Staphylococcus aureus, the most virulent of the many staphylococcal species, has demonstrated its versatility by remaining a major cause of morbidity and mortality despite the availability of numerous effective antistaphylococcal antibiotics. *S. aureus* is a pluripotent pathogen, causing disease through both toxin-mediated and non-toxin-mediated mechanisms. This organism is responsible for both nosocomial and community-based infections that range from relatively minor skin and soft tissue infections to life-threatening systemic infections.

The "other" staphylococci, collectively designated *coagulase-negative staphylococci* (CoNS), are considerably less virulent than *S. aureus* but remain important pathogens in selected clinical settings. These include but are not limited to infections associated with prosthetic devices.

MICROBIOLOGY AND TAXONOMY

The 33 staphylococcal species (with additional staphylococcal species under review) are pathogenic members of the family Micrococcaceae. A simple strategy for identification of the more clinically important species is outlined in Fig. 120-1. Automated diagnostic systems as well as kits are available for biochemical characterization of all the staphylococcal species. 16S ribosomal RNA analysis has proved a reliable method for distinguishing among species. With few exceptions, *S. aureus* is distinguished from other staphylococcal species by its production of coagulase, a surface enzyme that converts fibrinogen to fibrin. Most other clinically relevant staphylococci are coagulase-

negative. *S. aureus* also ferments mannitol, is positive for protein A, and produces DNase. On blood agar plates, *S. aureus* tends to form golden β-hemolytic colonies; in contrast, CoNS produce white non-hemolytic colonies.

Staphylococci are gram-positive cocci that form grapelike clusters on Gram's stain (Fig. 120-2). They are catalase-positive (unlike streptococcal species), nonmotile, aerobic, and facultatively anaerobic. These hardy organisms are capable of prolonged survival on environmental surfaces in varying conditions.

Determining whether multiple isolates (especially of CoNS) from a particular patient are the same or different is often an important factor in distinguishing contaminants from genuine pathogens. Determining whether multiple isolates from different patients are the same or different is relevant when there is concern that a nosocomial outbreak may have been due to a common point source (e.g., a contaminated medical instrument). Biochemical tests, often performed in conjunction with antimicrobial susceptibility testing, have been used as a relatively simple means of distinguishing among staphylococcal species or strains. More discriminating molecular typing techniques, such as pulsed-field gel electrophoresis, have also been used for this purpose.

S. AUREUS INFECTIONS

EPIDEMIOLOGY *S. aureus* is a part of the normal human flora. The anterior nares is the most frequent site of human colonization, although the skin (especially when damaged), vagina, axilla, perineum, and oropharynx may also be colonized. Approximately 25 to 50% of healthy persons may be persistently or transiently colonized with *S. aureus*. The rate of colonization is higher among insulin-dependent diabetics, HIV-infected patients, injection drug users, patients under-

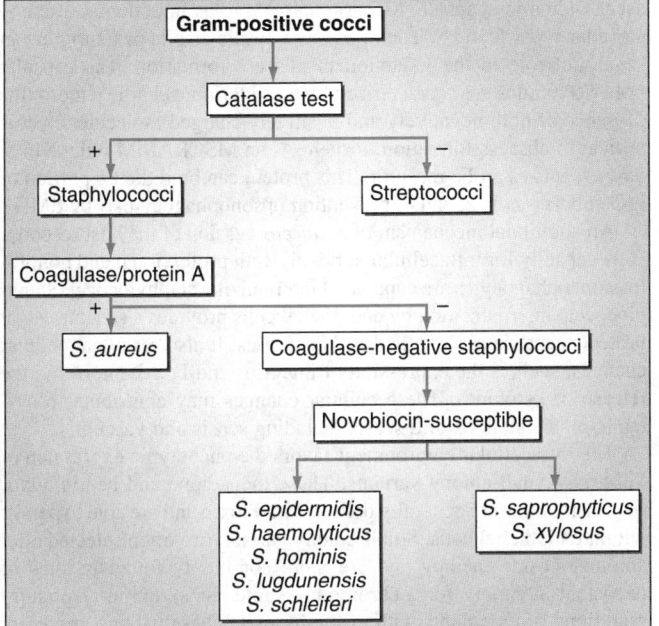

FIGURE 120-1 Biochemical characterization of staphylococci: algorithm of biochemical tests used to discriminate among the clinically important staphylococci. Additional tests are necessary to identify all of the different species.

going hemodialysis, and individuals with skin damage. Sites of colonization serve as a reservoir of strains for future *S. aureus* infections, and persons colonized with *S. aureus* are at greater risk of subsequent infection (with their colonizing strain) than are uncolonized individuals.

Overall, *S. aureus* is a leading cause of nosocomial infections. It is the most common cause of surgical wound infections and is second only to CoNS as a cause of primary bacteremia. Increasingly, nosocomial isolates are resistant to multiple drugs. In the community, *S. aureus* remains an important cause of skin and soft tissue infections, respiratory infections, and (among injection drug users) infective endocarditis. As the number of patients receiving home infusion therapy increases, so does the number of community-acquired staphylococcal infections.

Several reports have described community-acquired infections (in

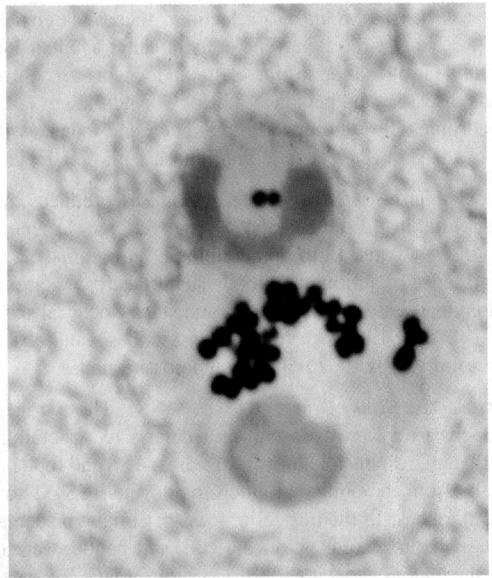

FIGURE 120-2 Gram's stain of *S. aureus* in a sputum sample with polymorphonuclear leukocytes. (*From Lowy, 1998; with permission of the New England Journal of Medicine. Copyright 1998 Massachusetts Medical Society. All rights reserved.*)

both rural and urban settings) caused by methicillin-resistant *S. aureus* (MRSA) in individuals with no prior medical exposure. In contrast to hospital-acquired MRSA strains, these community isolates have remained susceptible to many non-β-lactam antibiotics. Of concern has been the apparent capacity of community-acquired MRSA strains to cause serious disease in immunocompetent individuals. This ability may be due to the presence of different toxin-producing genes in these strains as well as the use of β-lactam agents for empirical treatment of patients infected with these strains.

Most individuals who develop *S. aureus* infections do so with their own colonizing strains. However, *S. aureus* may also be acquired from other people or from environmental exposures. Transmission most frequently results from transient colonization of the hands of hospital personnel, who then transfer strains from one patient to another. Spread of staphylococci in aerosols of respiratory or nasal secretions from heavily colonized individuals has also been reported.

PATHOGENESIS ■ General Concepts *S. aureus* is a pyogenic pathogen known for its capacity to induce abscess formation at sites of both local and metastatic infections. This classic pathologic response to *S. aureus* defines the framework within which the infection will progress. The bacteria elicit an inflammatory response characterized by an initial intense polymorphonuclear leukocyte (PMN) response and the subsequent infiltration of macrophages and fibroblasts. Either the host cellular response (including the deposition of fibrin and collagen) contains the infection, or infection spreads to the adjoining tissue or the bloodstream.

In toxin-mediated staphylococcal disease, the clinical infection is not invariably present. For example, once toxin has been elaborated into food, staphylococcal food poisoning can develop in the absence of viable bacteria. In the staphylococcal toxic shock syndrome (TSS), conditions that allow elaboration of toxin at sites of colonization (e.g., the presence of a superabsorbent tampon) are sufficient for initiation of clinical illness.

The *S. aureus* Genome The entire genome has been sequenced for several strains of *S. aureus*. Among the interesting revelations are the following: (1) There is a high degree of nucleotide sequence similarity among the different strains. (2) A relatively large amount of genetic information is acquired by horizontal transfer from other bacterial species. (3) *S. aureus* contains a number of unique "pathogenicity" or "genomic" islands. These islands are mobile genetic elements that contain clusters of enterotoxin and exotoxin genes or antimicrobial resistance determinants. (4) Among the genes contained in these islands are those carrying *mecA*, the gene responsible for methicillin resistance. These methicillin resistance–containing islands have been designated *staphylococcal cassette chromosomes* (SCC*mec*) and range in size from ~20 to 60 kb. To date, four SCC*mecs* have been identified. The type 4 SCC*mec* has been associated with the community-acquired MRSA strains that have been responsible for numerous outbreaks.

Regulation of Virulence Gene Expression In both toxin-mediated and non-toxin-mediated diseases due to *S. aureus*, the expression of virulence determinants associated with infection is dependent on a series of regulatory genes [e.g., accessory gene regulator (*agr*) and staphylococcal accessory regulator (*sar*)] that coordinately control the expression of the virulence genes. The regulatory gene *agr* is part of a quorum-sensing signal transduction pathway that senses and responds to bacterial density. Staphylococcal surface proteins are synthesized during the bacterial exponential growth phase in vitro. In contrast, secreted proteins, such as α toxin, the enterotoxins, and assorted enzymes, are released during the postexponential growth phase.

It has been hypothesized that these regulatory genes serve a similar function in vivo. Successful invasion requires the sequential expression of these different bacterial elements. Bacterial adhesins are needed to initiate colonization of host tissue surfaces. The subsequent release of various enzymes enables the colony to obtain nutritional support and permits bacteria to spread to adjacent tissues. Studies using mutant strains with these regulatory genes inactivated show reduced virulence in several animal models of *S. aureus* infection.

Pathogenesis of Invasive *S. aureus* Infection   Staphylococci are opportunists. For these organisms to invade the host and cause infection, some or all of the following steps are necessary: inoculation and local colonization of tissue surfaces, invasion, evasion of the host response, and metastatic spread. The initiation of staphylococcal infection requires a breach in cutaneous or mucosal barriers. Colonizing strains or strains transferred from other individuals are inoculated into damaged skin, a wound, or the bloodstream. Except under these circumstances, staphylococci generally persist as harmless commensals.

In *S. aureus* infections, recurrences develop relatively frequently, apparently because of the capacity of these pathogens to survive, to persist in a quiescent state in various tissues, and then to cause recrudescent infections when suitable conditions arise.

Nasal Colonization   The anterior nares are the principal site of staphylococcal colonization in humans. Surprisingly little is known about the biology of this colonization process. It appears to involve the attachment of *S. aureus* to both nasal mucin and keratinized epithelial cells of the anterior nares. Other factors that may contribute to colonization include the influence of other resident nasal flora and their bacterial density, nasal mucosal damage (e.g., that resulting from inhalational drug use), the antimicrobial properties of nasal secretions, and host genetic factors [e.g., human leukocyte antigen (HLA) type].

Inoculation and Colonization of Tissue Surfaces   Staphylococci may be introduced into tissue as a result of minor abrasions, administration of medications such as insulin, or establishment of intravenous access with catheters. After their introduction into a tissue site, bacteria replicate and colonize the host tissue surface. A family of structurally related *S. aureus* surface proteins referred to as MSCRAMMs (microbial surface components recognizing adhesive matrix molecules) plays an important role as a mediator of adherence to these sites. MSCRAMMs such as fibronectin-binding protein, clumping factor, and collagen-binding protein enable the bacteria to colonize different tissue surfaces; these proteins contribute to the pathogenesis of invasive infections such as endocarditis and arthritis by facilitating the adherence of *S. aureus* to surfaces with exposed fibronectin, fibrinogen, or collagen.

Although CoNS are classically known for their ability to elaborate a biofilm and colonize prosthetic devices, *S. aureus* also possesses the genes responsible for biofilm formation—the intercellular adhesion (*ica*) locus. Binding to these devices often involves staphylococcal adherence to serum constituents that have coated the device surface. As a result, *S. aureus* is frequently isolated from biomedical-device infections.

Invasion   After colonization, staphylococci replicate at the initial site of infection, elaborating enzymes that include serine proteases, hyaluronidases, thermonucleases, and lipases. These enzymes facilitate bacterial survival and local spread across tissue surfaces, although their precise role in infections is still not well defined. The lipases may also facilitate survival in lipid-rich areas such as the hair follicles, where *S. aureus* infections are often initiated. The *S. aureus* toxin Panton-Valentine leukocidin is cytolytic to PMNs, macrophages, and monocytes. Strains elaborating this toxin have been epidemiologically linked with cutaneous infections such as furuncles and carbuncles as well as with serious pulmonary infections in adolescents.

Constitutional findings may result from either localized or systemic infections. The cell wall—consisting of alternating N-acetyl muramic acid and N-acetyl glucosamine units in combination with an additional cell wall component, lipoteichoic acid—can initiate an inflammatory response that includes the sepsis syndrome. Staphylococcal α toxin, which causes pore formation in various eukaryotic cells, can also initiate an inflammatory response with findings suggestive of sepsis.

Evasion of Host Defense Mechanisms   Evasion of host defense mechanisms is critical to invasion. Staphylococci possess an antiphagocytic polysaccharide microcapsule. Most human *S. aureus* infections are due to capsular types 5 and 8. The *S. aureus* capsule also appears to play an important role in the induction of abscess formation. The capsular polysaccharides are characterized by a zwitterionic charge pattern (the presence of both negatively and positively charged molecules) that is critical to abscess formation. Protein A, an MSCRAMM unique to *S. aureus*, acts as an Fc receptor. This protein can bind the Fc portion of IgG subclasses 1, 2, and 4, preventing opsonophagocytosis by PMNs.

An additional mechanism of *S. aureus* evasion of the host response is its capacity for intracellular survival. Both professional and nonprofessional phagocytes are capable of internalizing staphylococci. Staphylococcal internalization by endothelial cells provides a sanctuary that protects bacteria against the host's defenses. It also results in cellular changes, such as the expression of integrins and Fc receptors and the release of cytokines. These cellular changes may contribute to systemic manifestations of disease, including sepsis and vasculitis.

The intracellular environment favors the phenotypic expression of *S. aureus* small-colony variants. These menadione and hemin auxotrophic mutants are generally deficient in α toxin and are able to persist within endothelial cells. Small-colony variants are often selected after aminoglycoside therapy and are more commonly found in sites of persistent infections (e.g., chronic bone infections) and in respiratory secretions from patients with cystic fibrosis. These variants represent another mechanism for prolonged staphylococcal survival that may enhance the likelihood of recurrences. Finally, *S. aureus* can survive within PMNs and may use these cells to spread and to seed other tissue sites.

Host Response to *S. aureus* Infection   The primary host response to *S. aureus* infection is the PMN. PMNs are attracted to sites of infection by bacterial components such as formylated peptides or peptidoglycan. These cells are also attracted by the cytokines tumor necrosis factor (TNF) and interleukins (ILs) 1 and 6, which are released by activated macrophages and endothelial cells.

Although most individuals have antistaphylococcal antibodies, it is not clear that the antibody levels are qualitatively or quantitatively sufficient to protect against infection. Anticapsular and anti-MSCRAMM antibodies facilitate opsonization in vitro and have been protective against infection in several animal models.

Groups at Increased Risk of Infection   Some diseases appear to entail multiple risk factors for *S. aureus* infection; diabetes, for example, entails an increased rate of colonization with *S. aureus*, the use of injectable insulin, and the possibility of impaired leukocyte function. Individuals with congenital or acquired qualitative or quantitative defects in PMNs are at increased risk of *S. aureus* infections; these include neutropenic patients (e.g., those receiving chemotherapeutic agents), individuals with defective intracellular killing of staphylococci (e.g., chronic granulomatous disease), and persons with Job's syndrome or Chédiak-Higashi syndrome. Other groups at risk include individuals with abnormalities of the skin (e.g., eczema) and those with prosthetic devices.

Pathogenesis of Toxin-Mediated Disease   *S. aureus* produces three types of toxin: cytotoxins (discussed above), pyrogenic-toxin superantigens, and exfoliative toxins. Both epidemiologic and animal data suggest that the presence of antitoxin antibodies is protective against illness in TSS, staphylococcal food poisoning, and staphylococcal scalded-skin syndrome (SSSS). Illness develops after synthesis and absorption of the toxin followed by the toxin-initiated host response.

Enterotoxin and Toxic Shock Syndrome Toxin 1 (TSST-1)   The pyrogenic toxin superantigens are a family of small-molecular-size, structurally similar proteins that are responsible for two diseases: TSS and food poisoning. TSS results from the ability of enterotoxins and TSST-1 to function as T cell mitogens. In the normal process of antigen presentation, the antigen is first processed within the cell, and peptides are then presented in the major histocompatibility complex (MHC) class II groove, initiating a measured T cell response. In contrast, enterotoxins bind directly to the invariant region of MHC—outside the MHC class II groove. The enterotoxins can then bind T cell receptors via the $v\beta$

chain, resulting in a dramatic overexpansion of T cell clones (up to 20% of the total T cell population).

As a result of this T cell expansion, there is the equivalent of a "cytokine storm," with the release of inflammatory mediators that include interferon (IFN) γ, IL-1, IL-6, TNF-α, and TNF-β. The result is a multisystem disease that produces a constellation of findings, including myalgias, fever, rash, and hypotension. These findings mimic those found in endotoxin shock; however, the pathogenic mechanisms differ. It has been hypothesized that a contributing factor to TSS is the release of endotoxin from the gastrointestinal tract, which may synergistically enhance the effects of the toxin.

A different region of the enterotoxin molecule is responsible for the symptoms of food poisoning. The enterotoxins are heat stable and can survive conditions that kill the bacteria. Illness results from the ingestion of preformed toxin. As a result, the incubation period is short (1 to 6 h). The toxin stimulates the vagus nerve and the vomiting center of the brain. It also appears to stimulate intestinal peristaltic activity.

Exfoliative Toxins and the Staphylococcal Scalded-Skin Syndrome   The exfoliative toxins are responsible for SSSS. The toxins that produce disease in humans have been divided into two serotypes: ETA and ETB. These toxins disrupt the desmosomes that link adjoining cells. Although the mechanism of this disruption remains uncertain, studies suggest that the toxins possess serine protease activity, which—through as-yet-undefined mechanisms—triggers exfoliation. The result is a split in the epidermis at the granular level, and this event is responsible for the superficial desquamation of the skin that typifies this illness.

DIAGNOSIS   *S. aureus* infections are readily diagnosed by Gram's stain (Fig. 120-2) and microscopic examination of abscess contents or of infected tissue. Staphylococci appear as large gram-positive cocci that are present singly, in pairs, or in clusters. Routine culture of infected material usually yields positive results, and blood cultures are sometimes positive even when infections are localized to extravascular sites. Polymerase chain reaction (PCR)–based assays have been applied to the rapid diagnosis of *S. aureus* infection and are increasingly being used in clinical microbiology laboratories. To date, serologic assays have not proved useful for the diagnosis of staphylococcal infections. Determining whether patients with documented *S. aureus* bacteremia also have infective endocarditis or a metastatic focus of infection remains a diagnostic challenge (see "Bacteremia, Sepsis, and Infective Endocarditis," below).

CLINICAL SYNDROMES (Table 120-1) ■ **Skin and Soft Tissue Infections**   *S. aureus* causes a variety of cutaneous infections. Common predisposing factors include skin diseases, damage to the skin (e.g., insect bites, minor trauma), injections (e.g., in diabetes, injection drug use), and poor personal hygiene. These infections are characterized by the formation of pus-containing blisters, which often begin in hair follicles and spread to adjoining tissues. *Folliculitis* is a superficial infection that involves the hair follicle, with a central area of purulence (pus) surrounded by induration and erythema. *Furuncles* (boils) are more extensive, painful lesions that tend to occur in hairy, moist regions of the body and extend from the hair follicle to become a true abscess with an area of central purulence. *Carbuncles* are most often located in the lower neck and are even more severe and painful, resulting from the coalescence of other lesions that extend to a deeper layer of the subcutaneous tissue. In general, furuncles and carbuncles are readily apparent, with pus often expressible or discharging from the abscess.

Mastitis develops in 1 to 3% of nursing mothers. The infection, which generally presents within 2 to 3 weeks after delivery, is characterized by findings that range from cellulitis to abscess formation. Systemic signs, such as fever and chills, are often present in more severe cases.

Other cutaneous *S. aureus* infections include impetigo, cellulitis, and hidradenitis suppurativa (recurrent follicular infections in regions such as the axilla). *S. aureus* is also one of the most common causes of surgical wound infection.

TABLE 120-1   Common Illnesses Caused by Staphylococcus aureus

Skin and Soft Tissue Infections
  Folliculitis
  Furuncle, carbuncle
  Cellulitis
  Impetigo
  Mastitis
  Surgical wound infections
  Hidradenitis suppurativa
Musculoskeletal Infections
  Septic arthritis
  Osteomyelitis
  Pyomyositis
  Psoas abscess
Respiratory Tract Infections
  Ventilator-associated or nosocomial pneumonia
  Septic pulmonary emboli
  Postviral pneumonia (e.g., influenza)
  Empyema
Bacteremia and Its Complications
  Sepsis, septic shock
  Metastatic foci of infection (kidney, joints, bone, lung)
  Infective endocarditis
Infective Endocarditis
  Injection drug use–associated
  Native-valve
  Prosthetic-valve
  Nosocomial
Device-Related Infections (e.g., intravascular catheters, prosthetic joints)
Toxin-Mediated Illnesses
  Toxic shock syndrome
  Food poisoning
  Staphylococcal scalded-skin syndrome

Musculoskeletal Infections   *S. aureus* is among the most common causes of bone infections—both those resulting from hematogenous dissemination and those arising from contiguous spread from a soft tissue site.

Hematogenous osteomyelitis in children most often involves the long bones. Infections present with fever and bone pain or with a child's reluctance to bear weight. The white blood cell count and erythrocyte sedimentation rate are often elevated. Blood cultures are positive in ~50% of cases. When necessary, bone biopsies for culture and histopathologic examination are usually diagnostic. Routine x-rays may be normal for up to 14 days after the onset of symptoms. ^{99m}Tc-phosphonate scanning often detects early evidence of infection. Magnetic resonance imaging (MRI) is more sensitive than other techniques in establishing a radiologic diagnosis.

In adults, hematogenous osteomyelitis involving the long bones is less common. However, *vertebral osteomyelitis* is among the more common clinical presentations. These infections are most often seen in patients with endocarditis, those undergoing hemodialysis, diabetics, and injection drug users. Vertebral bone infections may present with intense back pain and fever but may also be clinically occult, presenting with chronic back pain and low-grade fever. *S. aureus* is the most common cause of epidural abscess, a complication that can result in neurologic compromise. Patients complain of difficulty voiding or walking and of radicular pain in addition to the symptoms associated with their osteomyelitis. Surgical intervention in this setting often constitutes a medical emergency. MRI most reliably establishes the diagnosis (Fig. 120-3).

Bone infections that result from contiguous spread tend to develop from soft tissue infections, such as those associated with diabetic or vascular ulcers, surgery, or trauma. Exposure of bone, a draining fistulous tract, failure to heal, or continued drainage suggests involvement of underlying bone. Bone involvement is established by bone culture and histopathologic examination. Contamination of culture material from adjacent tissue can make the diagnosis of osteomyelitis difficult in the absence of pathologic confirmation. In addition, it is

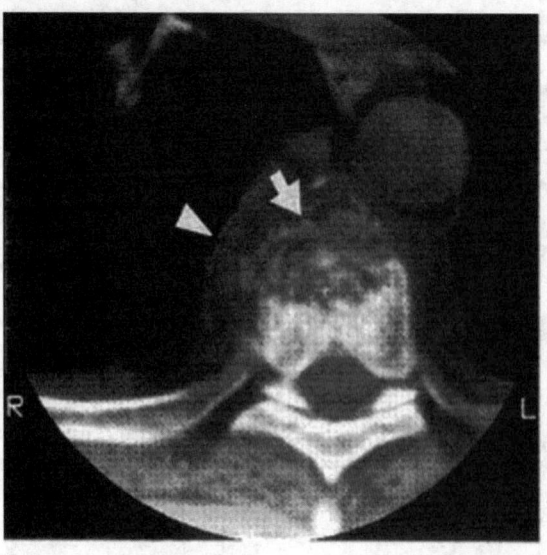
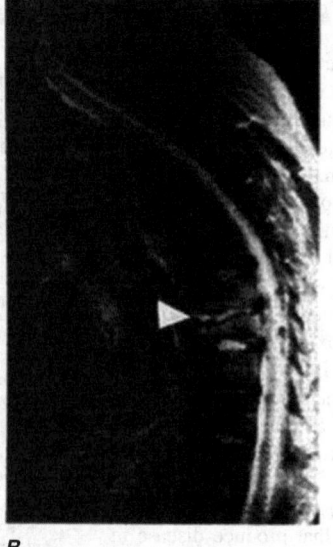

A   **B**

FIGURE 120-3   *S. aureus* vertebral osteomyelitis involving the thoracic disk between T8 and T9 in a 63-year-old man. *A.* The lower end plate is damaged (*arrow*), and there is an adjacent paraspinal mass (*arrowhead*). *B.* Sagittal T2-weighted magnetic resonance image of the spine, illustrating anterior wedging of the body of T8. (*From MA Artinian et al: Images in clinical medicine. Vertebral osteomyelitis.* N Engl J Med *329:399, 1993. Copyright 1993 Massachusetts Medical Society. All rights reserved. Reprinted with permission.*)

sometimes difficult to distinguish radiologically between osteomyelitis and overlying soft tissue infection with underlying osteitis.

S. aureus is the most common cause of *septic arthritis* in children. This infection is rapidly progressive and may be associated with extensive joint destruction if left untreated. It presents with intense pain on motion of the affected joint, swelling, and fever. Aspiration of the joint reveals turbid fluid, with >50,000 PMNs/μL and gram-positive cocci in clusters on Gram's stain. In adults, arthritis may result from trauma, surgery, or hematogenous dissemination. The most commonly involved joints include the knees, shoulders, hips, and phalanges. Infection frequently develops in joints previously damaged by osteoarthritis or rheumatoid arthritis. Iatrogenic infections resulting from aspiration or injection of agents into the joint also occur. In these settings, the patient experiences increased pain and swelling in the involved joint in association with fever.

Pyomyositis is an unusual infection of skeletal muscles that is seen primarily in tropical climates. In addition to occurring in seriously immunocompromised patients, it has recently been reported in HIV-infected individuals. Pyomyositis presents with fever, swelling, and pain overlying the involved muscle. Aspiration of fluid from the involved tissue reveals pus containing numerous white blood cells and gram-positive bacteria in clusters. Although a history of trauma may be associated with the infection, its pathogenesis is poorly understood.

Respiratory Tract Infections   Respiratory tract infections caused by *S. aureus* occur in selected clinical settings. *S. aureus* is a cause of serious infections in newborns and infants; these infections present with shortness of breath, fever, and respiratory failure. Chest x-ray may reveal pneumatoceles (shaggy, thin-walled cavities). Pneumothorax and empyema are recognized complications of this type of infection.

In adults, nosocomial *S. aureus* pulmonary infections are commonly seen in intubated patients on intensive care units. The clinical presentation is no different from that encountered in pulmonary infections of other bacterial etiologies. Patients produce increased volumes of purulent sputum and develop respiratory distress, fever, and new pulmonary infiltrates. Distinguishing bacterial pneumonia from other causes of respiratory failure or new pulmonary infiltrates in critically ill patients is often difficult and relies on a constellation of clinical, radiologic, and laboratory findings.

Community-acquired respiratory tract infections due to *S. aureus* are most commonly seen as postviral infections or as a result of septic pulmonary emboli (e.g., in injection drug users). Influenza is the most

common cause of the former type of presentation. Patients may present with fever, bloody sputum production, and midlung field pneumatoceles or multiple, patchy pulmonary infiltrates. Diagnosis is made by sputum Gram's stain and culture. Blood cultures, although useful, are usually negative.

Bacteremia, Sepsis, and Infective Endocarditis   *S. aureus* bacteremia may be complicated by sepsis, endocarditis, vasculitis, or metastatic seeding (establishment of suppurative collections at other tissue sites). The frequency of metastatic seeding during bacteremia has been estimated to be as high as 31%. Among the more commonly seeded tissue sites are bones, joints, kidneys, and lungs.

Recognition that these complications have developed is often difficult if clinical and laboratory diagnostic methods alone are used. Comorbid conditions that are frequently seen in association with *S. aureus* bacteremia and that increase the risk of complications include diabetes, HIV infection, and renal insufficiency. Other host factors associated with an increased risk of complications include presentation with community-acquired *S. aureus* bacteremia (except in injection drug users), lack of an identifiable primary focus, and presence of prosthetic devices.

Clinically, *S. aureus* sepsis presents in a manner similar to that documented for sepsis due to other bacteria. The well-described progression of hemodynamic changes—beginning with respiratory alkalosis and clinical findings of hypotension and fever—is commonly seen. The microbiologic diagnosis is established by positive blood cultures.

The overall incidence of *S. aureus* endocarditis has increased over the past 20 years. Depending on the series, *S. aureus* now accounts for 25 to 35% of all cases of bacterial endocarditis. This increase is due, at least in part, to the increased use of intravascular devices; the incidence of infective endocarditis among patients with *S. aureus* bacteremia and intravascular catheters was 25% when studied with transesophageal echocardiography. Other factors associated with an increased risk of endocarditis are injection drug use, hemodialysis, the presence of intravascular prosthetic devices, and immunosuppression. Despite the availability of effective antibiotics, mortality from these infections continues to range from 20 to 40%, depending on both the host and the nature of the infection. Complications of *S. aureus* endocarditis include cardiac valvular insufficiency, peripheral emboli, metastatic seeding, and central nervous system involvement. *S. aureus* brain abscess is a recognized complication of left-sided endocarditis.

S. aureus endocarditis is encountered in four clinical settings: (1) right-sided endocarditis in association with injection drug use, (2) left-sided native-valve endocarditis, (3) prosthetic-valve endocarditis, and (4) nosocomial endocarditis. In each of these settings, the diagnosis is established by recognition of clinical stigmata suggestive of endocarditis. These findings include cardiac manifestations such as new or changing cardiac valvular murmurs; cutaneous evidence of endocarditis such as vasculitic lesions, Osler's nodes, or Janeway lesions; evidence of embolic disease; and a history suggesting a risk for *S. aureus* bacteremia. In the absence of antecedent antibiotic therapy, blood cultures are almost uniformly positive. Transthoracic echocardiography, while less sensitive than transesophageal echocardiography, is less invasive and often establishes the presence of valvular vegetations.

Acute right-sided tricuspid valvular *S. aureus* endocarditis is most often seen in injection drug users. The classic presentation includes a high fever, a toxic clinical appearance, pleuritic chest pain, and the production of purulent (sometimes bloody) sputum. Chest x-rays reveal evidence of septic pulmonary emboli (small, periph[eral] lesions that may cavitate with time). A high percentage of the[se] patients have no history of antecedent valvular damage. At t[he onset] of their illness, patients may present with fever alone, withou[t heart murmur] or other localizing findings. As a result, a high index of clin[ical sus]picion is essential to the diagnosis.

Individuals with antecedent cardiac valvular damage mor[e com]monly present with left-sided native-valve endocarditis involvi[ng the] previously affected valve. These patients tend to be older than [those] with right-sided endocarditis, their prognosis is worse, and their [inci]dence of complications (including peripheral emboli, cardiac de[com]pensation, and metastatic seeding) is higher.

S. aureus is one of the more common causes of prosthetic-v[alve] endocarditis. This infection is especially fulminant in the early post-operative period and is associated with a high mortality rate. In most instances, medical therapy alone is not sufficient and urgent valve replacement is necessary. Patients are prone to develop valvular in-sufficiency or myocardial abscesses originating from the region of valve implantation.

The increased frequency of nosocomial endocarditis (15 to 30% of cases, depending on the study) reflects in part the increased use of intravascular devices. This form of endocarditis is most commonly caused by *S. aureus*; because patients often are critically ill, are re-ceiving antibiotics for various other indications, and have comorbid conditions, the diagnosis is not easily recognized.

Urinary Tract Infections   Urinary tract infections are infrequently caused by *S. aureus*. In contrast with that of most other urinary pathogens, the presence of *S. aureus* in the urine is suggestive of hematogenous dissemination. Ascending *S. aureus* infections occasionally result from instrumentation of the genitourinary tract.

Prosthetic Device–Related Infections   *S. aureus* accounts for a large pro-portion of prosthetic device–related infections. These infections often involve intravascular catheters, prosthetic valves, orthopedic devices, peritoneal or intraventricular catheters, and vascular grafts. Recently, *S. aureus* isolates have also been responsible for a sizable proportion of infections of left-ventricular-assist devices. In contrast with the more indolent presentation of CoNS infections, *S. aureus* device-re-lated infections often present more acutely, with both localized and systemic manifestations. The latter infections also tend to be more rapidly progressive. It is relatively common for a pyogenic collection to be present at the device site. Aspiration of these collections and performance of blood cultures are important components in establish-ing a diagnosis. *S. aureus* infections tend to occur more commonly in the early postimplantation period unless the device is used for access (e.g., intravascular or hemodialysis catheters). In the latter instance, infections can occur as long as the device is used. As in most pros-thetic-device infections, successful therapy usually involves removal of the device. Left in place, the device is a potential nidus for either persistent or recurrent infections.

Toxin-Mediated Diseases ■ *Toxic Shock Syndrome*   TSS was first recognized as a disease in children in 1978. The disease gained national attention in the early 1980s, when a nationwide outbreak occurred among young, otherwise healthy, menstruating women. Epidemiologic inves-tigation demonstrated that these cases were strongly associated with menstruation and the use of a highly absorbent tampon that had re-cently been introduced to the market. Subsequent studies established the role of TSST-1 in these illnesses. Withdrawal of the tampon from the market resulted in a rapid decline in the incidence of this disease. However, menstrual and nonmenstrual cases continue to be reported.

The clinical presentation is similar in menstrual and nonmenstrual TSS, although the nature of the risk clearly differs. Evidence of a clinical *S. aureus* infection is not a prerequisite for the development of the illness. TSS results from the elaboration of an enterotoxin or the structurally related enterotoxin-like TSST-1. More than 90% of menstrual cases are caused by TSST-1, whereas a high percentage of nonmenstrual cases are caused by enterotoxins.

TSS begins with relatively nonspecific flulike symptoms. In men-strual cases, the onset usually comes 2 or 3 days after the start of menstruation. Patients present with fever, hypotension, and erythro-[d]erma of variable intensity. Mucosal involvement is common (e.g., [co]njunctival hyperemia). The illness can rapidly progress to symptoms [th]at include vomiting, diarrhea, confusion, myalgias, and abdominal [pa]in. These symptoms reflect the multisystemic nature of the disease, [wit]h involvement of the liver, kidneys, gastrointestinal tract, and/or [cen]tral nervous system. Desquamation of the skin occurs during con-[vale]scence, usually 1 or 2 weeks after the onset of illness. Laboratory [find]ings may include azotemia, leukocytosis, hypoalbuminemia, [throm]bocytopenia, and liver function abnormalities.

Diagnosis of TSS still depends on the presence of a constellation of findings rather than on one specific finding (Table 120-2). Part of the case definition is the absence of laboratory evidence of other ill-nesses that are often included in the differential (e.g., Rocky Mountain spotted fever, rubeola, leptospirosis). Other diagnoses to be considered are drug toxicities, viral exanthems, sepsis, and Kawasaki disease. Ill-ness occurs only in persons who lack antibody to TSST-1. Recurrences are possible if antibody fails to develop after the illness.

Food Poisoning   *S. aureus* is among the most common causes of food-borne outbreaks of infection in the United States. *S. aureus* food poi-soning results from the inoculation of toxin-producing *S. aureus* into food by colonized food handlers. Toxin is then elaborated in such growth-promoting food as custards, potato salad, or processed meats. Even if the bacteria are killed by warming, the heat-stable toxin is not destroyed. The onset of illness is rapid and explosive, occurring within 1 to 6 h of ingestion. The illness is characterized by nausea and vom-iting, although diarrhea, hypotension, and dehydration may also occur. The differential diagnosis includes diarrhea of other etiologies, espe-cially that caused by similar toxins (e.g., the toxins elaborated by *Ba-cillus cereus*). The rapidity of onset, the absence of fever, and the epidemic nature of the presentation arouse suspicion regarding this diagnosis. Symptoms generally resolve within 8 to 10 h. The diagnosis can be established by the demonstration of bacteria or the documen-tation of enterotoxin in the implicated food. Treatment is entirely sup-portive.

Staphylococcal Scalded-Skin Syndrome   SSSS most often affects newborns and children. The illness may vary from localized blister formation to exfoliation of much of the skin surface. The skin is usually fragile and often tender, with thin-walled, fluid-filled bullae. Gentle pressure re-sults in rupture of the lesions, leaving denuded underlying skin (Ni-

---

TABLE 120-2   *Case Definition of S. aureus Toxic Shock Syndrome*

1. Fever: temperature of ≥38.9°C (≥102°F)
2. Hypotension: systolic blood pressure of ≤90 mmHg, or orthostatic hy-potension (orthostatic drop in diastolic blood pressure by ≥15 mmHg, orthostatic syncope, or orthostatic dizziness)
3. Diffuse macular rash with subsequent desquamation in 1 to 2 weeks after onset (including the palms and soles)
4. Multisystem involvement
   a. Hepatic: bilirubin or aminotransferase levels ≥2 times normal
   b. Hematologic: platelet count ≤100,000/μL)
   c. Renal: blood urea nitrogen or serum creatinine level ≥2 times the normal upper limit
   d. Mucous membranes: vaginal, oropharyngeal, or conjunctival hyper-emia
   e. Gastrointestinal: vomiting or diarrhea at onset of illness
   f. Muscular: severe myalgias or serum creatine phosphokinase level ≥2 times the upper limit
   g. Central nervous system: disorientation or alteration in consciousness without focal neurologic signs and in the absence of fever and hy-potension
5. Negative serologic or other tests for measles, leptospirosis, and Rocky Mountain spotted fever as well as negative blood or cerebrospinal fluid cultures for organisms other than *S. aureus*

Source: M Wharton et al: Case definitions for public health surveillance. MMWR 39:1, 1990; with permission.

kolsky's sign; Fig. 120-4). The mucous membranes are usually spared. In more generalized infection, there are often constitutional symptoms, including fever, lethargy, and irritability with poor feeding. Significant amounts of fluid can be lost in more extensive cases. Illness usually follows localized infection at one of a number of possible sites. SSSS is much less common among adults but can follow infections caused by exfoliative toxin–producing strains.

PREVENTION Prevention of the spread of *S. aureus* infections in the hospital setting involves hand washing and careful attention to appropriate isolation procedures. Through strict isolation practices, some Scandinavian countries have been remarkably successful at preventing the introduction and dissemination of MRSA in hospitals. Other countries, such as the United States and Great Britain, have been less successful.

The use of topical antimicrobial agents (e.g., mupirocin) to eliminate nasal colonization with *S. aureus* and to prevent subsequent infection has been investigated in a number of clinical settings. Elimination of nasal carriage of *S. aureus* has reduced the incidence of infections among patients undergoing hemodialysis and peritoneal dialysis. A randomized, placebo-controlled study attempted to reduce rates of wound infection among patients undergoing surgery with the prophylactic application of topical mupirocin to the nares. The results failed to demonstrate an overall benefit from the use of mupirocin but did suggest that the incidence of infections might be reduced if the use of mupirocin were limited to patients nasally colonized with *S. aureus*.

The ability of a capsular polysaccharide–protein conjugate vaccine to prevent staphylococcal infections in hemodialysis patients was studied. The results, while inconclusive, did show promise. Other potential vaccine candidates, including those incorporating the ligand-binding domains of several MSCRAMMs, are also under investigation.

COAGULASE-NEGATIVE STAPHYLOCOCCAL INFECTIONS

CoNS, although considerably less virulent than *S. aureus*, are among the most common causes of prosthetic-device infections. Approximately half of the 32 identified CoNS species have been associated with human infections. Of these species, *S. epidermidis* is the most common human pathogen overall; this component of the normal human flora is found on the skin (where it is the most abundant bacterial species) as well as in the oropharynx and vagina. *S. saprophyticus*, a novobiocin-resistant species, is a pathogen in urinary tract infections.

PATHOGENESIS Among CoNS, *S. epidermidis* is the species most commonly associated with prosthetic-device infections. Infection is a two-

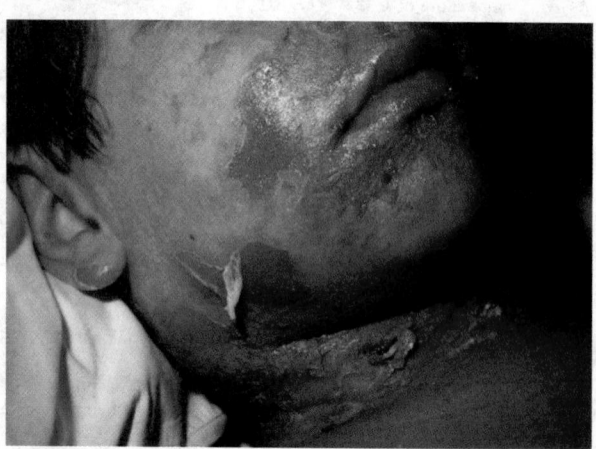

FIGURE 120-4 Evidence of staphylococcal scalded-skin syndrome in a 6-year-old boy. Nikolsky's sign, with separation of the superficial layer of the outer epidermal layer, is visible. (*From LA Schenfeld et al: Images in clinical medicine. Staphylococcal scalded skin syndrome. N Engl J Med 42:1178, 2000. Copyright 2000 Massachusetts Medical Society. All rights reserved. Reprinted with permission.*)

step process, with initial adhesion to the device followed by colonization. *S. epidermidis* is uniquely adapted to colonize these devices by its capacity to elaborate the extracellular polysaccharide (slime) that facilitates formation of a protective biofilm on the device surface.

Implanted prosthetic material is often coated with host serum or tissue constituents such as fibrinogen or fibronectin. These molecules serve as potential bridging ligands, facilitating bacterial attachment to the device surface. The surface-associated staphylococcal enzyme autolysin (AtlE) may play a role in attachment to either modified or unmodified prosthetic surfaces. In addition to AtlE, other surface molecules, such as fibrinogen-binding protein and cell wall teichoic acid, appear to mediate adherence to fibrinogen and fibronectin, respectively. The polysaccharide intercellular adhesin facilitates subsequent staphylococcal colonization and accumulation on the device surface. The genes responsible for synthesis of this polysaccharide (the *ica* genes) are also present in *S. aureus*, although their role in the two species may differ. In *S. epidermidis*, the *ica* genes are more commonly found in strains associated with device infections than in strains associated with colonization of mucosal surfaces. Biofilm appears to act as a barrier protecting bacteria from host defense mechanisms as well as from antibiotics, while providing a suitable environment for bacterial survival.

Two additional staphylococcal species, *S. lugdunensis* and *S. schleiferi*, produce more serious infections (native-valve endocarditis and osteomyelitis) than do other CoNS. The basis for this enhanced virulence is not known, although both species appear to share more virulence determinants with *S. aureus* (e.g., clumping factor and lipase) than do other CoNS.

The capacity of *S. saprophyticus* to cause urinary tract infections in young women appears to be related to its enhanced capacity to adhere to uroepithelial cells. A 160-kDa hemagglutinin/adhesin may contribute to this affinity.

DIAGNOSIS While the detection of CoNS at sites of infection or in the bloodstream is not difficult by standard microbiologic culture methods, interpretation of these results is frequently problematic. Since these organisms are present in large numbers on the skin, they often contaminate cultures. It has been estimated that only 10 to 25% of blood cultures positive for CoNS reflect true bacteremia. Similar problems arise with cultures of other sites. Among the clinical findings suggestive of true bacteremia are fever, evidence of local infection (e.g., erythema or purulent drainage at the intravenous catheter site), leukocytosis, and systemic signs of sepsis. Laboratory findings suggestive of true bacteremia include multiple positive cultures of the same strain (i.e., the same species with the same antibiogram or a closely related DNA fingerprint) from separate cultures, growth of the strain within 48 h, and bacterial growth in both aerobic and anaerobic bottles.

CLINICAL SYNDROMES CoNS cause diverse prosthetic device–related infections, including those that involve prosthetic cardiac valves and joints, vascular grafts, intravascular devices, and central nervous system shunts. In all of these settings, the clinical presentation is similar. The signs of localized infection are often subtle, the rate of disease progression is slow, and the systemic findings are often limited. Signs of infection such as purulent drainage, pain at the site, or loosening of prosthetic implants are sometimes evident. Fever is frequently but not always present, and there may be mild leukocytosis.

Infections that are not associated with prosthetic devices are infrequent, although native-valve endocarditis due to CoNS has accounted for ~5% of cases in some reviews. *S. lugdunensis* appears to be a more aggressive pathogen in this setting, causing greater mortality and rapid valvular destruction with abscess formation.

℞ TREATMENT

General Principles of Therapy In addition to the selection of appropriate antimicrobial therapy for staphylococcal infections, surgical incision and drainage of all suppurative collections are necessary. Prosthetic-device infections are unlikely to be successfully managed unless the device is removed. In the limited number of situations in which removal is not possible or the infection is due to CoNS, an initial attempt at medical therapy without device removal may be warranted. Because of the well-recognized risk of complications associated with *S. aureus* bacteremia, therapy is generally prolonged (4 to 8 weeks) unless the patient is identified as being one of the small percentage of individuals who are at low risk for complications—e.g., immunocompetent patients and patients whose *S. aureus* infection is associated with a removable focus (such as an intravenous catheter) and whose device is promptly removed.

Duration of Antimicrobial Therapy Debate continues regarding the duration of therapy for bacteremic *S. aureus* infections. No carefully controlled, prospective study has addressed this question. A meta-analysis reviewing studies relevant to this issue concluded that insufficient information was currently available to determine which patients were candidates for short-course therapy (2 weeks rather than 4 to 8 weeks).

Among the findings associated with an increased risk of complicated bacteremia are persistently positive blood cultures 48 to 96 h after institution of therapy, acquisition of the infection in the community, a removable focus of infection (i.e., intravascular catheters) that is not removed, and cutaneous or embolic manifestations of infection. In those immunocompetent patients for whom short-course therapy is planned, a transesophageal echocardiogram to rule out endocarditis is warranted since neither clinical nor laboratory findings are adequate to detect cardiac involvement. In addition, an aggressive radiologic investigation to identify potential metastatic collections is indicated. All symptomatic sites need to be carefully evaluated.

Choice of Antimicrobial Agents The choice of antimicrobial agents to treat both coagulase-positive staphylococcal and CoNS infections has become increasingly problematic because of the prevalence of multidrug-resistant strains. Data collected by the Centers for Disease Control and Prevention from intensive care units in the United States (1988 to 1998) show a dramatic increase in the number of isolates that are now susceptible only to vancomycin. This trend is even more apparent with CoNS: more than 80% of nosocomial isolates are resistant to methicillin, and these MRSA strains are usually resistant to most other antibiotics as well. Because the selection of antimicrobial agents for the treatment of *S. aureus* infections is similar to that for CoNS infections, treatment options for these pathogens are discussed together and are summarized in Table 120-3.

As a result of the widespread dissemination of plasmids containing the enzyme penicillinase, few strains of staphylococci (<5%) remain susceptible to penicillin. However, against susceptible strains, penicillin remains the drug of choice. Penicillin-resistant isolates are treated with semisynthetic penicillinase-resistant penicillins (SPRPs) such as oxacillin or nafcillin. Methicillin, the first of the SPRPs, is now used infrequently. Cephalosporins are alternative therapeutic agents for these infections. Second- and third-generation cephalosporins do not have a therapeutic advantage over first-generation cephalosporins for the treatment of staphylococcal infections. The carbapenem imipenem has excellent activity against methicillin-sensitive *S. aureus* (MSSA) but not MRSA.

The isolation of MRSA was reported within 1 year of the introduction of methicillin. The prevalence of MRSA has since increased steadily. In many hospitals, 40 to 50% of *S. aureus* isolates are now resistant to methicillin. Resistance to methicillin indicates resistance to all SPRPs as well as all cephalosporins. Many MRSA isolates are also resistant to other antimicrobial families, including aminoglycosides, quinolones, and macrolides.

Production of a novel penicillin-binding protein (PBP 2a or 2′) is responsible for methicillin resistance. This protein is synthesized by the *mecA* gene, which (as stated above) is part of a large mobile genetic element—a pathogenicity or genomic island—called the staphylococcal cassette chromosome (SCC*mec*). It is hypothesized that acquisition of this genetic material resulted from horizontal transfer from a related staphylococcal species, such as *S. sciuri*. Phenotypic expression of methicillin resistance may be constitutive (i.e., expressed in all organisms in a population) or heterogeneous (i.e., displayed by only

a proportion of the total organism population). Detection of methicillin resistance in the clinical microbiology laboratory can be difficult if the strain expresses heterogeneous resistance. Therefore, susceptibility studies are routinely performed at reduced temperatures (30° to 35°C for 24 h), with increased concentrations of salt in the medium to enhance the expression of resistance. In addition to PCR-based techniques, a number of rapid methods for the detection of methicillin resistance have recently been developed.

Vancomycin is the drug of choice for the treatment of methicillin-resistant staphylococcal infections. Because it is less bactericidal than the β-lactams, it should be used only after careful consideration in patients with a history of β-lactam allergies. In 1997, an *S. aureus* strain with reduced susceptibility to vancomycin (VISA) was reported from Japan. Subsequently, additional clinical isolates of VISA were reported from geographically disparate locations. These strains were all resistant to methicillin and many other antimicrobial agents. The VISA strains appear to evolve (under vancomycin selective pressure) from strains that are susceptible to vancomycin but are heterogeneous, with a small proportion of the bacterial population expressing the resistance phenotype. The mechanism of VISA resistance is uncertain but appears to be an abnormal cell wall, which was first noted by electron microscopy. Vancomycin is trapped by the abnormal peptidoglycan cross-linking and is unable to gain access to its target site.

In 2002, the first clinical isolate of fully vancomycin-resistant *S. aureus* was reported. Resistance in this and one subsequently reported clinical isolate was due to the presence of *vanA*, the gene responsible for expression of vancomycin resistance in enterococci. This observation suggested that resistance was acquired as a result of horizontal conjugal transfer from a vancomycin-resistant strain of *Enterococcus faecalis*. The patients had both MRSA and vancomycin-resistant enterococci cultured from sites of infection. The isolates remained susceptible to chloramphenicol, linezolid, minocycline, quinupristin/dalfopristin, and trimethoprim-sulfamethoxazole (TMP-SMX). The *vanA* gene is responsible for the synthesis of the dipeptide D-Ala-D-Lac in place of D-Ala-D-Ala. Vancomycin is not able to bind to the altered peptide.

Alternatives to the β-lactams and vancomycin have less antistaphylococcal activity. Although the quinolones have reasonable in vitro activity against staphylococci, the frequency of fluoroquinolone resistance has increased progressively, especially among methicillin-resistant isolates. Methicillin-susceptible staphylococci have remained more susceptible to the fluoroquinolones than have methicillin-resistant strains. Of particular concern in methicillin-resistant strains is the possible emergence of quinolone resistance during therapy. Resistance to the quinolones is most commonly chromosomal and results from mutations of the topoisomerase IV or DNA gyrase genes, although multidrug efflux pumps may also contribute. While the newer quinolones exhibit increased in vitro activity against staphylococci, it is uncertain whether this increase translates into enhanced in vivo activity. Other antibiotics such as minocycline and TMP-SMX have been successfully used to treat methicillin-resistant staphylococcal infections in the face of vancomycin toxicity or intolerance.

Among the newer antistaphylococcal agents, the parenteral streptogramin quinupristin/dalfopristin displays bactericidal activity against all staphylococci, including VISA strains. This drug has been used successfully to treat serious MRSA infections. In cases of erythromycin or clindamycin resistance, it is bacteriostatic against staphylococci.

Linezolid—the first member of a new drug family, the oxazolidinones—is bacteriostatic against staphylococci, has been well tolerated, and offers the advantage of comparable bioavailability after oral or parenteral administration. Cross-resistance with other inhibitors of protein synthesis has not been reported. Resistance to linezolid has been limited, although at least one resistant clinical isolate has been reported. The efficacy of linezolid in the treatment of deep-seated infections such as osteomyelitis has not yet been established. There are currently insufficient data on the efficacy of either quinupristin/dalfopristin or linezolid for the treatment of infective endocarditis. Dap-

TABLE 120-3 Antimicrobial Therapy for Serious S. aureus Infections[a]

Sensitivity/Resistance of Isolate	Drug of Choice	Alternative(s)	Comments
Sensitive to penicillin	Penicillin G (4 mU q4h)	Nafcillin (2 g q4h) or oxacillin (2 g q4h), cefazolin (2 g q8h), vancomycin (1 g q12h[b])	Fewer than 5% of isolates are sensitive to penicillin.
Sensitive to methicillin	Nafcillin or oxacillin (2 g q4h)	Cefazolin (2 g q8h[b]), vancomycin (1 g q12h[b])	Patients with penicillin allergy can be treated with a cephalosporin if the allergy does not involve an anaphylactic or accelerated reaction; vancomycin is the alternative. Desensitization to β-lactams may be indicated in selected cases of serious infection where maximal bactericidal activity is needed (e.g., prosthetic-valve endocarditis[c]). Type A β-lactamase may rapidly hydrolyze cefazolin and reduce its efficacy in endocarditis.
Resistant to methicillin	Vancomycin (1 g q12h[b])	TMP-SMX (TMP, 5 mg/kg q12h[b]), minocycline (100 mg PO q12h[b]), ciprofloxacin (400 mg q12h[b]), levofloxacin (500 mg q24h[b]), quinupristin/dalfopristin (7.5 mg/kg q8h), linezolid (600 mg q12h *except*: 400 mg q12h for uncomplicated skin infections); daptomycin (4 mg/kg q24h[b]) for complicated skin infections; investigational drugs: oritavancin, tigecycline	Sensitivity testing is necessary before an alternative drug is used. Adjunctive drugs (those that should be used only in combination with other antimicrobial agents) include gentamicin (1 mg/kg q8h[b]), rifampin (300 mg PO q8h), and fusidic acid (500 mg q8h; not readily available in the United States). Quinupristin/dalfopristin is bactericidal against methicillin-resistant isolates unless the strain is resistant to erythromycin or clindamycin. The newer quinolones may retain in vitro activity against ciprofloxacin-resistant isolates; resistance may develop during therapy. The efficacy of adjunctive therapy is not well established in many settings. Both linezolid and quinupristin/dalfopristin have had in vitro activity against most VISA and VRSA strains. See footnote for treatment of prosthetic-valve endocarditis.[c]
Resistant to methicillin with intermediate or complete resistance to vancomycin[d]	Uncertain	Same as for methicillin-resistant strains; check antibiotic susceptibilities	Same as for methicillin-resistant strains; check antibiotic susceptibilities
Not yet known (i.e., empirical therapy)	Vancomycin (1 g q12h)	—	Empirical therapy is given when the susceptibility of the isolate is not known. Vancomycin with or without an aminoglycoside is recommended for suspected community- or hospital-acquired S. aureus infections because of the increased frequency of methicillin-resistant strains in the community.

[a] Recommended dosages are for adults with normal renal and hepatic function. The route of administration is intravenous unless otherwise indicated.

[b] The dosage must be adjusted in patients with reduced creatinine clearance.

[c] For the treatment of prosthetic-valve endocarditis, the addition of gentamicin (1 mg/kg q8h) and rifampin (300 mg PO q8h) is recommended, with adjustment of the gentamicin dosage if the creatinine clearance rate is reduced.

[d] Vancomycin-resistant S. aureus isolates from clinical infections have recently been reported.

Source: Modified with permission of the *New England Journal of Medicine* (Lowy, 1998). Copyright 1998 Massachusetts Medical Society. All rights reserved.

Note: TMP-SMX, trimethoprim-sulfamethoxazole; VISA, vancomycin-intermediate *S. aureus*; VRSA, vancomycin-resistant *S. aureus*.

tomycin, a new parenteral bactericidal agent with antistaphylococcal activity, was recently approved for the treatment of complicated skin infections. This drug disrupts the cytoplasmic membrane. Oritavancin, a new glycopeptide, is undergoing clinical trials.

Combinations of antistaphylococcal agents are sometimes used to enhance bactericidal activity in the treatment of serious infections such as endocarditis or osteomyelitis. In selected instances (e.g., right-sided endocarditis), drug combinations are also used to shorten the duration of therapy. Among the antimicrobial agents used in combinations are rifampin, aminoglycosides (e.g., gentamicin), and fusidic acid (which is not readily available in the United States). While these agents are not effective singly because of the frequent emergence of resistance, they have proved useful in combination with other agents because of their bactericidal activity against staphylococci.

In vitro studies have demonstrated synergy against staphylococci with the following combinations: (1) β-lactams and aminoglycosides; (2) vancomycin and gentamicin; (3) vancomycin, gentamicin, and rifampin (against CoNS); and (4) vancomycin and rifampin. In several instances, these in vitro observations have been supported by studies using the experimental animal model of endocarditis.

Antimicrobial Therapy for Selected Settings For uncomplicated skin and soft tissue infections, the use of oral antistaphylococcal agents is usually successful. For other infections, parenteral therapy is indicated.

S. aureus endocarditis is usually an acute, life-threatening infection. Thus blood cultures need to be obtained promptly and followed by the immediate institution of empirical antimicrobial therapy. For *S. aureus* native-valve endocarditis, a combination of antimicrobial agents is often used. In a large prospective study, an SPRP combined with an aminoglycoside did not alter the clinical outcome but did reduce the duration of *S. aureus* bacteremia. As a result, many clinicians begin therapy for life-threatening infections with a 3- to 5-day course of a β-lactam and an aminoglycoside (gentamicin, 1 mg/kg intravenously every 8 h). If a MRSA strain is isolated, vancomycin (30 mg/kg every 24 h, given in two equal doses up to a total of 2 g) is recommended. Patients are treated for 4 to 6 weeks, depending on the clinical response.

In prosthetic-valve endocarditis, surgery in addition to antibiotic therapy is often necessary. The combination of a β-lactam agent—or, if the isolate is β-lactam resistant, vancomycin (30 mg/kg every 24 h, given in two equal doses up to a total of 2 g)—with an aminoglycoside (gentamicin, 1 mg/kg intravenously every 8 h) and rifampin (300 mg orally every 8 h) is recommended. This combination is used to avoid the possible emergence of rifampin resistance during therapy if only two drugs are used.

For hematogenous osteomyelitis or septic arthritis in children, a 4-week course of therapy is usually adequate. In adults, treatment is often more prolonged. For chronic forms of osteomyelitis, surgical debridement is necessary in combination with antimicrobial therapy. For joint infections, a critical component of therapy is the repeated aspiration or arthroscopy of the affected joint to prevent damage from leukocytes.

The combination of rifampin with ciprofloxacin has been used successfully to treat prosthetic-joint infections, especially when the device cannot be removed. The efficacy of this combination may reflect the enhanced activity against staphylococci in biofilms as well as the attainment of effective intracellular concentrations.

The choice of empirical therapy for staphylococcal infections depends in part on susceptibility data for the local geographic area. Increasingly, vancomycin (in combination with an aminoglycoside or rifampin for serious infections) is the drug of choice for both community- and hospital-acquired infections.

Therapy for Toxic Shock Syndrome   Supportive therapy with reversal of hypotension is the mainstay of therapy for TSS. Both fluids and pressors may be necessary. Tampons or other packing material should be promptly removed. The role of antibiotics is less clear. Some investigators recommend a combination of clindamycin and a semisynthetic penicillin. Clindamycin is advocated because, as a protein synthesis inhibitor, it reduces toxin synthesis in vitro. A semisynthetic penicillin is suggested to eliminate any potential focus of infection as well as to eradicate persistent carriage that might increase the likelihood of recurrent illness. Anecdotal reports document the successful use of intravenous immunoglobulin to treat TSS. The role of glucocorticoids in the treatment of this disease is uncertain at present.

Therapy for Other Toxin-Mediated Diseases   Therapy for staphylococcal food poisoning is entirely supportive. For SSSS, antistaphylococcal therapy targets the primary site of infection.

FURTHER READING

BABA T et al: Genome and virulence determinants of high virulence community-acquired MRSA. Lancet 359:1819, 2002

CHAMBERS HF: Methicillin resistance in staphylococci: Molecular and biochemical basis and clinical implications. Clin Microbiol Rev 10:781, 1997

FOWLER VG JR et al: Role of echocardiography in evaluation of patients with Staphylococcus aureus bacteremia: Experience in 103 patients. J Am Coll Cardiol 30:1072, 1997

HIRAMATSU K et al: The emergence and evolution of methicillin-resistant Staphylococcus aureus. Trends Microbiol 9:486, 2001

ING MB et al: Bacteremia and infective endocarditis: Pathogenesis, diagnosis, and complications, in The Staphylococci in Human Disease, KB Crossley, GL Archer (eds). New York, Churchill Livingstone, 1997, pp 331–354

LOWY FD:Antimicrobial resistance: The example of Staphylococcus aureus. J Clin Invest 111:1265, 2003

————: Staphylococcus aureus infections. N Engl J Med 339:520, 1998

MCCORMICK JK et al: Toxic shock syndrome and bacterial superantigens: An update. Annu Rev Microbiol 55:77, 2001

MYLOTTE JM, TAYARA A: Staphylococcus aureus bacteremia: Predictors of 30-day mortality in a large cohort. Clin Infect Dis 31:1170, 2000

VON EIFF C et al: Pathogenesis of infections due to coagulase-negative staphylococci. Lancet Infect Dis 2:677, 2002

121   STREPTOCOCCAL AND ENTEROCOCCAL INFECTIONS
Michael R. Wessels

Many varieties of streptococci are found as part of the normal human flora colonizing the respiratory, gastrointestinal, and genitourinary tracts. Several species are important causes of human disease. Group A *Streptococcus*, or *S. pyogenes*, is responsible for streptococcal pharyngitis, one of the most common bacterial infections of school-age children, and for the postinfectious syndromes of acute rheumatic fever and poststreptococcal glomerulonephritis. Group B *Streptococcus*, or *S. agalactiae*, is the leading cause of bacterial sepsis and meningitis in newborns and a major cause of endometritis and fever in parturient women. Enterococci are important causes of urinary tract infection, nosocomial bacteremia, and endocarditis. Viridans streptococci are the most common cause of bacterial endocarditis.

Streptococci are gram-positive bacteria of spherical to ovoid shape that characteristically form chains when grown in liquid media. Most streptococci that cause human infections are facultative anaerobes, although some are strict anaerobes. Streptococci are relatively fastidious organisms, requiring enriched media for growth in the laboratory. No single scheme for classification of streptococci is entirely satisfactory. Consequently, clinicians and clinical microbiologists often identify streptococci by any of several classification systems, including hemolytic pattern, Lancefield group, species name, and common or trivial name. Many of the streptococci associated with human infection produce a zone of complete hemolysis around the bacterial colony when cultured on blood agar, a pattern known as β hemolysis. The β-hemolytic streptococci can be classified by the Lancefield system, a serologic grouping based on the reaction of specific antisera with cell-wall carbohydrate antigens of the bacteria. With rare exceptions, organisms belonging to Lancefield groups A, B, C, and G are all β-hemolytic streptococci, and each is associated with characteristic patterns of human infection. Other streptococci produce a zone of partial (α) hemolysis, often imparting a greenish appearance to the agar. These α-hemolytic streptococci are further identified by biochemical testing and include *S. pneumoniae*, an important cause of pneumonia, meningitis, and other infections, and several species of streptococci referred to collectively as the *viridans streptococci*, which are part of

the normal oral flora and are important as agents of subacute bacterial endocarditis. Finally, some streptococci are nonhemolytic, a pattern sometimes called γ hemolysis. The classification of the major groups of streptococci responsible for human infections is outlined in Table 121-1. Among the organisms classified serologically as group D streptococci, the enterococci are now considered to constitute a separate genus on the basis of DNA homology studies. Thus species previously designated as *S. faecalis* and *S. faecium* have been renamed *Enterococcus faecalis* and *E. faecium*, respectively. →*For further discussion of pneumococcal infections, see Chap. 119.*

GROUP A STREPTOCOCCI

Lancefield's group A consists of a single species, *S. pyogenes*. As its species name implies, this organism is associated with a variety of suppurative infections. In addition, group A streptococci can trigger the postinfectious syndromes of acute rheumatic fever (which is uniquely associated with *S. pyogenes* infection; Chap. 302) and poststreptococcal glomerulonephritis (Chap. 264).

PATHOGENESIS   Group A streptococci elaborate a number of cell-surface components and extracellular products important both in the pathogenesis of infection and in the immune response of the human host. The cell wall contains a carbohydrate antigen that may be released by treatment with acid. The reaction of such acid extracts with group A–specific antiserum is the basis for the definitive identification of a streptococcal strain as *S. pyogenes*. The major surface protein of group A streptococci is M protein, which occurs in more than 100 antigenically distinct types and is the basis for the serotyping of strains with specific antisera. The M protein molecules are fibrillar structures anchored in the cell wall of the organism that extend as hairlike projections away from the cell surface. The amino acid sequence of the distal or amino-terminal portion of the M protein molecule is quite variable, accounting for the antigenic variation of the different M types, while more proximal regions of the protein are relatively conserved. A newer technique for assignment of M type to group A streptococcal isolates uses the polymerase chain reaction to amplify the

TABLE 121-1 Classification of Streptococci

Lancefield Group	Representative Species	Hemolytic Pattern	Typical Infections
A	S. pyogenes	β	Pharyngitis, impetigo, cellulitis, scarlet fever
B	S. agalactiae	β	Neonatal sepsis and meningitis, puerperal infection, urinary tract infection, diabetic ulcer infection, endocarditis
C	S. equisimilis	β	Cellulitis, bacteremia, endocarditis
D	Enterococci: E. faecalis; E. faecium	Usually nonhemolytic	Urinary tract infection, nosocomial bacteremia, endocarditis
	Nonenterococci: S. bovis	Usually nonhemolytic	Bacteremia, endocarditis
G	S. canis	β	Cellulitis, bacteremia, endocarditis, septic arthritis
Variable or nongroupable	Viridans streptococci: S. sanguis; S. mitis	α	Endocarditis, dental abscess, brain abscess
	Intermedius, milleri, or anginosus group: S. intermedius, S. anginosus, S. constellatus	Variable	Brain abscess, visceral abscess
	Anaerobic streptococci: Peptostreptococcus magnus	Usually nonhemolytic	Sinusitis, pneumonia, empyema, brain abscess, liver abscess

variable region of the M protein gene. DNA sequence analysis of the amplified gene segment can be compared with an extensive database [developed at the Centers for Disease Control and Prevention (CDC)] for assignment of M type. This method eliminates the need for typing sera, which are available in only a few reference laboratories. The presence of M protein on a group A streptococcal isolate correlates with its capacity to resist phagocytic killing in fresh human blood; this phenomenon appears to be due, at least in part, to the binding of plasma fibrinogen to M protein molecules on the streptococcal surface, which interferes with complement activation and deposition of opsonic complement fragments on the bacterial cell. This resistance to phagocytosis may be overcome by M protein–specific antibodies; thus individuals with antibodies to a given M type acquired as a result of prior infection are protected against subsequent infection with organisms of the same M type but not against that with different M types.

Group A streptococci also elaborate, to varying degrees, a polysaccharide capsule composed of hyaluronic acid. The production of large amounts of hyaluronic acid capsule by certain strains lends a characteristic mucoid appearance to the bacterial colonies. The capsular polysaccharide also plays an important role in protecting the organisms from ingestion and killing by phagocytes. In contrast to M protein, the hyaluronic acid capsule is a weak immunogen, and antibodies to hyaluronate have not been shown to be important in protective immunity; the presumed explanation is the apparent structural identity between streptococcal hyaluronic acid and the hyaluronic acid of mammalian connective tissues. The capsular polysaccharide may also play a role in group A streptococcal colonization of the pharynx by binding to CD44, a hyaluronic acid–binding protein expressed on human pharyngeal epithelial cells.

Group A streptococci produce a large number of extracellular products that may be important in local and systemic toxicity and in the spread of infection through tissues. These products include streptolysins S and O, toxins that damage cell membranes and account for the hemolysis produced by the organisms; streptokinase; DNases; protease; and pyrogenic exotoxins A, B, and C. The pyrogenic exotoxins, previously known as erythrogenic toxins, cause the rash of scarlet fever. Since the mid-1980s, pyrogenic exotoxin–producing strains of group A Streptococcus have been linked to unusually severe invasive infections, including necrotizing fasciitis and a systemic syndrome termed the streptococcal toxic shock syndrome. Several extracellular products stimulate specific antibody responses useful in the serodiagnosis of recent streptococcal infection. Tests for these antibodies are

used primarily for the detection of preceding streptococcal infection in cases of suspected acute rheumatic fever or poststreptococcal glomerulonephritis.

CLINICAL MANIFESTATIONS ■ Pharyngitis

Although seen in patients of all ages, group A streptococcal pharyngitis is one of the most common bacterial infections of childhood, accounting for 20 to 40% of all cases of exudative pharyngitis in children; it is rare among those under the age of 3. Younger children may manifest streptococcal infection with a syndrome of fever, malaise, and lymphadenopathy without exudative pharyngitis. Infection is acquired through contact with another individual carrying the organism. Respiratory droplets are the usual mechanism of spread, although other routes, including food-borne outbreaks, have been well described.

The incubation period is 1 to 4 days. Symptoms include sore throat, fever and chills, malaise, and sometimes abdominal complaints and vomiting, particularly in children. Both symptoms and signs are quite variable, ranging from mild throat discomfort with minimal physical findings to high fever and severe sore throat associated with intense erythema and swelling of the pharyngeal mucosa and the presence of purulent exudate over the posterior pharyngeal wall and tonsillar pillars. Enlarged, tender anterior cervical lymph nodes commonly accompany exudative pharyngitis.

The differential diagnosis of streptococcal pharyngitis includes the many other bacterial and viral causes of pharyngitis (Table 121-2). Streptococcal infection is unlikely to be the cause of pharyngitis when symptoms and signs suggestive of viral infection are prominent (conjunctivitis, coryza, cough, hoarseness, or discrete ulcerative lesions of

TABLE 121-2 Infectious Etiologies of Acute Pharyngitis

Organism	Associated Clinical Syndrome(s)
VIRUSES	
Rhinovirus	Common cold
Coronavirus	Common cold
Adenovirus	Pharyngoconjunctival fever
Influenza virus	Influenza
Parainfluenza virus	Cold, croup
Coxsackievirus	Herpangina, hand-foot-and-mouth disease
Herpes simplex virus	Gingivostomatitis (primary infection)
Epstein-Barr virus	Infectious mononucleosis
Cytomegalovirus	Mononucleosis-like syndrome
HIV	Acute (primary) infection syndrome
BACTERIA	
Group A streptococci	Pharyngitis, scarlet fever
Group C or G streptococci	Pharyngitis
Mixed anaerobes	Vincent's angina
Arcanobacterium haemolyticum	Pharyngitis, scarlatiniform rash
Neisseria gonorrhoeae	Pharyngitis
Treponema pallidum	Secondary syphilis
Francisella tularensis	Pharyngeal tularemia
Corynebacterium diphtheriae	Diphtheria
Yersinia enterocolitica	Pharyngitis, enterocolitis
Yersinia pestis	Plague
Chlamydiae	
Chlamydia pneumoniae	Bronchitis, pneumonia
Chlamydia psittaci	Psittacosis
Mycoplasmas	
Mycoplasma pneumoniae	Bronchitis, pneumonia

the buccal or pharyngeal mucosa). Other infections commonly producing exudative pharyngitis include infectious mononucleosis and adenovirus infection. Now rare in the United States, the pseudomembrane of diphtheria may give a similar appearance. The coryneform organism *Arcanobacterium haemolyticum* may cause pharyngitis, often in association with a scarlet fever–like rash (Chap. 122). Other causes of pharyngitis, usually without a purulent exudate, include coxsackievirus, influenza virus, mycoplasmas, and *Neisseria gonorrhoeae* and acute infection with HIV. Because of the range of clinical presentations of streptococcal pharyngitis and the large number of other agents that can produce the same clinical picture, diagnosis of streptococcal pharyngitis on clinical grounds alone is not reliable.

The throat culture remains the diagnostic "gold standard." Culture of a throat specimen that is properly collected (i.e., by vigorous rubbing of a sterile swab over both tonsillar pillars) and properly processed is the most sensitive and specific means available to make a definitive diagnosis. A rapid diagnostic kit for latex agglutination or enzyme immunoassay of swab specimens can serve as a useful adjunct to the throat culture. While precise figures on sensitivity and specificity vary among studies, the rapid diagnostic kits generally are >95% specific. Thus a positive result can be relied upon for definitive diagnosis and eliminates the need for a throat culture. However, because the rapid diagnostic tests are less sensitive than throat culture (with a relative sensitivity ranging from 55 to 90% in comparative studies), a negative result should be confirmed with a throat culture.

℞ TREATMENT

In the usual course of uncomplicated streptococcal pharyngitis, symptoms resolve after 3 to 5 days. The course is shortened little by treatment, which is given primarily to prevent suppurative complications and rheumatic fever. Prevention of rheumatic fever depends on eradication of the organism from the pharynx, not simply on resolution of symptoms, and requires 10 days of penicillin treatment—either a single intramuscular dose of benzathine penicillin G or a 10-day course of oral penicillin (Table 121-3). Erythromycin may be substituted for penicillin in the treatment of individuals allergic to penicillin. Once-daily azithromycin is a more convenient but expensive alternative. Although azithromycin is approved for a 5-day course of treatment, only limited data support equivalent efficacy to a standard 10-day treatment course. Resistance to erythromycin and other macrolides is common in isolates from several countries, including Spain, Italy, Finland, Japan, and Korea. Macrolide resistance may be becoming more prevalent elsewhere with the increasing use of this class of antibiotics. In areas in which resistance rates exceed 5 to 10%, macrolides should be

TABLE 121-3 *Treatment of Group A Streptococcal Infections*

Infection	Treatment[a]
Pharyngitis	Benzathine penicillin G, 1.2 mU IM; *or* penicillin V, 250 mg PO tid or 500 mg PO bid × 10 days (Children <27 kg: Benzathine penicillin G, 600,000 units IM; *or* penicillin V, 250 mg PO bid or tid × 10 days)
Impetigo	Same as pharyngitis
Erysipelas/cellulitis	Severe: Penicillin G, 1–2 mU IV q4h Mild to moderate: Procaine penicillin, 1.2 mU IM bid
Necrotizing fasciitis/myositis	Surgical debridement; *plus* penicillin G, 2–4 mU IV q4h; *plus* clindamycin,[b] 600–900 mg q8h
Pneumonia/empyema	Penicillin G, 2–4 mU IV q4h; *plus* drainage of empyema
Streptococcal toxic shock syndrome	Penicillin G, 2–4 mU IV q4h; *plus* clindamycin,[b] 600–900 mg q8h; *plus* intravenous immunoglobulin,[b] 2 g/kg as a single dose

[a] Penicillin allergy: Erythromycin (10 mg/kg PO qid up to a maximum of 250 mg per dose) may be substituted for oral penicillin. Alternative agents for parenteral therapy include first-generation cephalosporins—if the nature of the allergy is not an immediate hypersensitivity reaction (anaphylaxis or urticaria) or another potentially life-threatening manifestation (e.g., severe rash and fever)—or vancomycin.
[b] Efficacy unproven, but recommended by several experts. See text for discussion.

avoided unless results of susceptibility testing are known. Follow-up culture after treatment is no longer routinely recommended but may be warranted in selected cases, such as those involving patients or families with frequent streptococcal infections or those occurring in situations in which the risk of rheumatic fever is thought to be high (e.g., when cases of rheumatic fever have recently been reported in the community).

COMPLICATIONS Suppurative complications of streptococcal pharyngitis have become uncommon with the widespread use of antibiotics for most cases of symptomatic streptococcal infection. The complications result from the spread of infection from the pharyngeal mucosa to deeper tissues by direct extension or by the hematogenous or lymphatic route and may include cervical lymphadenitis, peritonsillar or retropharyngeal abscess, sinusitis, otitis media, meningitis, bacteremia, endocarditis, and pneumonia. Local complications, such as abscess formation in the peritonsillar or parapharyngeal space, should be considered in a patient with unusually severe or prolonged symptoms or localized pain associated with high fever and a toxic appearance. Nonsuppurative complications include acute rheumatic fever (Chap. 302) and poststreptococcal glomerulonephritis (Chap. 264), both of which are thought to result from immune responses to streptococcal infection. Penicillin treatment of streptococcal pharyngitis has been shown to reduce the likelihood of acute rheumatic fever but not that of poststreptococcal glomerulonephritis.

Bacteriologic Treatment Failure and the Asymptomatic Carrier State Surveillance cultures have shown that up to 20% of individuals in certain populations may have asymptomatic pharyngeal colonization with group A streptococci. There are no definitive guidelines for management of these asymptomatic carriers or of asymptomatic individuals who still have a positive throat culture after a full course of treatment for symptomatic pharyngitis. A reasonable course of action is to give a single 10-day course of penicillin for symptomatic pharyngitis and, if positive cultures persist, not to re-treat unless symptoms recur. Studies of the natural history of streptococcal carriage and infection have shown that the risk both of developing rheumatic fever and of transmitting infection to others is substantially lower among asymptomatic carriers than among individuals with symptomatic pharyngitis. Therefore, overly aggressive attempts to eradicate carriage are probably not justified under most circumstances. An exception is the situation in which an asymptomatic carrier is a potential source of infection to others. Outbreaks of food-borne infection and nosocomial puerperal infection have been traced to asymptomatic carriers who may harbor the organisms in the throat, on the skin, or in the vagina or anus.

℞ TREATMENT

In cases in which a carrier is transmitting infection to others, attempts to eradicate carriage are warranted, although data are limited on the best regimen to use to clear the organism after penicillin alone has failed. The combination of penicillin V (500 mg four times daily for 10 days) and rifampin (600 mg twice daily for the last 4 days) has been used to eliminate pharyngeal carriage. A 10-day course of oral vancomycin (250 mg four times daily) and rifampin (600 mg twice daily) has eradicated rectal colonization. However, experience is not extensive with any regimen.

Scarlet Fever Scarlet fever consists of streptococcal infection, usually pharyngitis, accompanied by a characteristic rash (Fig. 121-1). The rash arises from the effects of one of three toxins, currently designated streptococcal pyrogenic exotoxins A, B, and C, and previously known as erythrogenic or scarlet fever toxins. In the past, scarlet fever was thought to reflect infection of an individual lacking toxin-specific immunity with a toxin-producing strain of group A *Streptococcus*. Susceptibility to scarlet fever was correlated with results of the Dick test, in which a small amount of erythrogenic toxin injected intradermally produced local erythema in susceptible individuals but elicited no re-

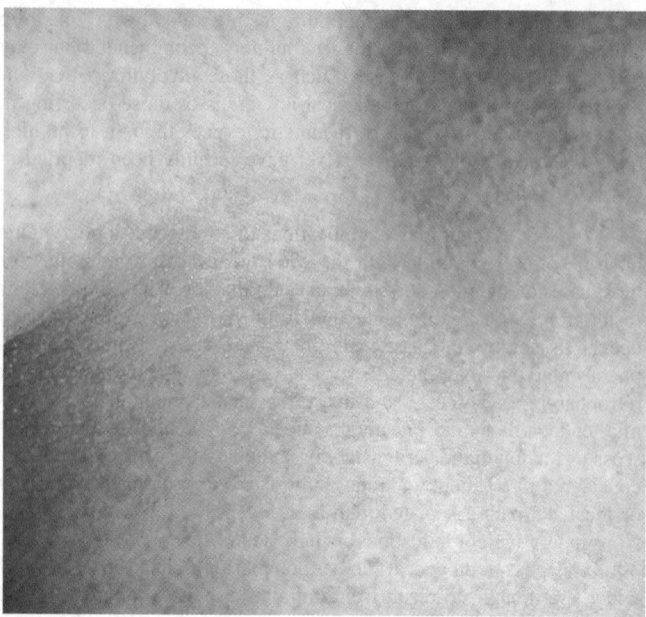

FIGURE 121-1   Scarlet fever exanthem. Finely punctated erythema has become confluent (scarlatiniform); petechiae can occur and have a linear configuration within the exanthem in body folds (Pastia's lines). *(From Fitzpatrick, Johnson, Wolff: Color Atlas and Synopsis of Clinical Dermatology, 4th ed., New York, McGraw-Hill, 2001, with permission.)*

action in those with specific immunity. Subsequent studies have suggested that development of the scarlet fever rash may reflect a hypersensitivity reaction requiring prior exposure to the toxin. For reasons that are not clear, scarlet fever has become less common in recent years, although strains of group A streptococci that produce pyrogenic exotoxins continue to be prevalent in the population.

The symptoms of scarlet fever are the same as those of pharyngitis alone. The rash typically begins on the first or second day of illness over the upper trunk, spreading to involve the extremities but sparing the palms and soles. The rash is made up of minute papules, giving a characteristic "sandpaper" feel to the skin. Associated findings include circumoral pallor, "strawberry tongue" (enlarged papillae on a coated tongue, which later may become denuded), and accentuation of the rash in the skin folds (Pastia's lines). Subsidence of the rash in 6 to 9 days is followed after several days by desquamation of the palms and soles. The differential diagnosis of scarlet fever includes other causes of fever and generalized rash, such as measles and other viral exanthems, Kawasaki disease, toxic shock syndrome, and systemic allergic reactions (e.g., drug eruptions).

Skin and Soft Tissue Infections   Group A streptococci—and occasionally other streptococcal species—cause a variety of infections involving the skin, subcutaneous tissues, muscles, and fascia. While several clinical syndromes, recognized according to the tissues involved, offer a useful means for classification of skin and soft tissue infections, not all cases fit exactly into a single category. The classic syndromes should be considered as general guides to predicting the level of tissue involvement in a particular patient, the probable clinical course, and the likelihood that surgical intervention or aggressive life-support will be required.

IMPETIGO (PYODERMA)   Impetigo is a superficial infection of the skin caused primarily by group A streptococci and occasionally by other streptococci or by *Staphylococcus aureus*. Impetigo is seen most often in young children, tends to occur during the warmer months, and is more common in semitropical or tropical climates than in cooler regions. Infection is more common among children living under conditions of poor hygiene. Prospective studies have shown that colonization of unbroken skin with group A streptococci precedes the de-

velopment of clinical infection. Minor trauma, such as a scratch or an insect bite, may then serve to inoculate organisms into the skin. Impetigo is best prevented, therefore, by attention to adequate hygiene. The usual sites of involvement are the face (particularly around the nose and mouth) and the legs, although lesions may occur at other locations. Individual lesions begin as red papules, which evolve quickly into vesicular and then pustular lesions that break down and coalesce to form characteristic honeycomb-like crusts (Fig. 121-2). Lesions are generally not painful, and patients do not appear ill. Fever is not a feature of impetigo and, if present, suggests either infection extending to deeper tissues or another diagnosis.

The classic presentation of impetigo usually poses little diagnostic difficulty. Cultures of impetiginous lesions often yield *S. aureus* as well as group A streptococci, but longitudinal studies have shown that, in almost all cases, streptococci can be isolated initially, with staphylococci appearing later, presumably as secondary colonizing flora. In the past, penicillin was nearly always effective against these infections; in recent years, however, penicillin treatment failures have become more common, an observation suggesting that *S. aureus* infection may have become more prominent as a cause of impetigo. *Bullous impetigo* due to *S. aureus* is distinguished from typical streptococcal infection by the presence of more extensive, bullous lesions that break down and leave thin paper-like crusts instead of the thick amber crusts of streptococcal impetigo. Other skin lesions that may be confused with impetigo include herpetic lesions—either those of orolabial herpes simplex or those of chickenpox or zoster. Herpetic lesions can generally be distinguished by their appearance as more discrete, grouped vesicles and by a positive Tzanck test. In difficult cases, cultures of vesicular fluid should yield group A streptococci in impetigo and the responsible virus in *Herpesvirus* infections.

℞ TREATMENT

Treatment of streptococcal impetigo is the same as that for streptococcal pharyngitis. In view of evidence that *S. aureus* has become a relatively frequent cause of impetigo, empirical regimens should cover both streptococci and *S. aureus*. For example, either dicloxacillin or cephalexin can be given at a dose of 250 mg four times daily for 10 days. Topical mupirocin ointment is also effective. Rheumatic fever is not a sequela to streptococcal skin infections, although poststreptococcal glomerulonephritis may follow either skin or throat infection. The reason for this difference is not known. One hypothesis is that the immune response necessary for development of rheumatic fever occurs only after infection of the pharyngeal mucosa. In addition, the strains of group A streptococci that cause pharyngitis are generally of different M protein types than those associated with skin infections; thus the strains that cause pharyngitis may have rheumatogenic potential, while the skin-infecting strains may not.

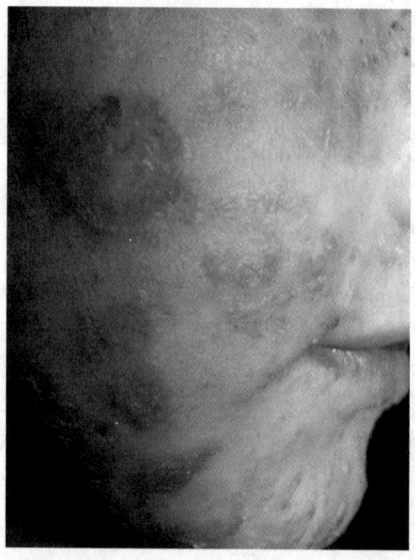

FIGURE 121-2 Impetigo contagiosa is a superficial streptococcal or *Staphylococcus aureus* infection consisting of honey-colored crusts and erythematous weeping erosions. Occasionally, bullous lesions may be seen. *(Courtesy of Mary Spraker, MD.)*

CELLULITIS   Inoculation of organisms into the skin may lead to infection involving the skin and subcutaneous tissues, or *cellulitis*. The portal of entry may be a traumatic or surgical wound, an insect bite, or any other break in skin integrity. Often, no entry site is apparent.

One form of streptococcal cellulitis, *erysipelas*, is characterized by a bright red appearance of the involved skin, which forms a plateau sharply demarcated from surrounding normal skin (Fig. 121-3). The lesion is warm to the touch, may be tender, and appears shiny and swollen. The skin often has a *peau d'orange* texture, which is thought to reflect involvement of superficial lymphatics; superficial blebs or bullae may form, usually 2 or 3 days after onset. The lesion typically develops over a few hours and is associated with fever and chills. Erysipelas tends to occur in certain characteristic locations: the malar area of the face (often with extension over the bridge of the nose to the contralateral malar region) and the lower extremities. After one episode, recurrence at the same site—sometimes years later—is not uncommon.

Classic cases of erysipelas, with the typical features described above, are almost always due to β-hemolytic streptococci, usually those of group A and occasionally those of group C or G. Often, however, the appearance of streptococcal cellulitis is not sufficiently distinctive to permit a specific diagnosis on clinical grounds. The area of involvement may not be one of the typical sites for erysipelas, the lesion may be less intensely red than usual and may fade into surrounding skin, and/or the patient may appear only mildly ill. In such cases, it is prudent to broaden the spectrum of empiric antimicrobial therapy to include other pathogens, particularly *S. aureus*, that can produce cellulitis with the same appearance. Staphylococcal infection should be suspected if cellulitis develops around a wound or an ulcer.

Streptococcal cellulitis tends to develop at anatomic sites in which normal lymphatic drainage has been disrupted, such as sites of prior episodes of cellulitis, the arm ipsilateral to a mastectomy and axillary lymph node dissection, a lower extremity previously involved in deep venous thrombosis or chronic lymphedema, or the leg from which a saphenous vein has been harvested for coronary artery bypass grafting. The organism may enter via a breach in the dermal barrier at a location some distance from the eventual site of clinical cellulitis. For example, some patients with recurrent episodes of leg cellulitis following saphenous vein removal stop having recurrent episodes only after treatment of tinea pedis on the affected extremity. Fissures in the skin presumably serve as a portal of entry for streptococci, which then produce infection more proximally in the leg at the site of previous injury. Streptococcal cellulitis may also involve recent surgical wounds. Group A streptococci are among the few bacterial pathogens that typically produce signs of wound infection and surrounding cellulitis within the first 24 h after surgery. These wound infections are usually associated with a thin exudate and may spread rapidly, either as cellulitis in the skin and subcutaneous tissue or as a deeper tissue infection (see below). Streptococcal wound infection or localized cellulitis may also be associated with *lymphangitis*, manifested by red streaks extending proximally along superficial lymphatics from the site of infection.

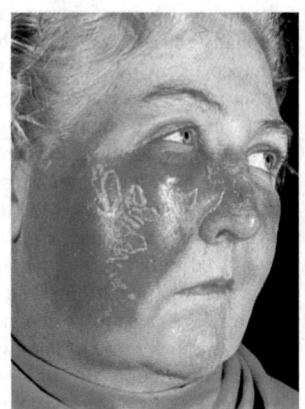

FIGURE 121-3   Erysipelas is a streptococcal infection of the superficial dermis and consists of well-demarcated, erythematous, edematous, warm plaques.

℞ TREATMENT

See Table 121-3 and Chap. 110.

Deep Soft-Tissue Infections   *Necrotizing fasciitis*, also referred to as *hemolytic streptococcal gangrene*, is an infection involving the superficial and/or deep fascia investing the muscles of an extremity or the trunk. The source of the infection is either the skin, with organisms introduced into the tissue as a result of trauma (sometimes trivial), or the bowel flora, with organisms released during abdominal surgery or from an occult enteric source, such as a diverticular or appendiceal abscess. The site of inoculation in both forms of necrotizing fasciitis may be inapparent and is often some distance from the site of clinical involvement; e.g., the introduction of organisms via minor trauma to the hand may be associated with clinical infection of the tissues overlying the shoulder or chest. In cases associated with the bowel flora, the infection is usually polymicrobial, involving a mixture of anaerobic bacteria (such as *Bacteroides fragilis* or anaerobic streptococci) and facultative organisms (usually gram-negative bacilli). Cases unrelated to contamination from bowel organisms are most commonly caused by group A streptococci, either alone or in combination with other organisms (most often *S. aureus*). Overall, group A streptococci are implicated in about 60% of cases of necrotizing fasciitis. The onset of symptoms is usually quite acute and is marked by severe pain at the site of involvement, malaise, fever, chills, and a toxic appearance. The physical findings, particularly early in the illness, may not be striking, with only minimal erythema of the overlying skin. Pain and tenderness are usually severe; in contrast, in more superficial cellulitis, the skin appearance is more abnormal, but pain and tenderness are only mild or moderate. As the infection progresses (often in a matter of several hours), the severity and extent of symptoms worsen, and skin changes become more evident, with the appearance of dusky or mottled erythema and edema. The marked tenderness of the involved area may evolve into anesthesia as the spreading inflammatory process produces infarction of cutaneous nerves.

Although myositis is more commonly due to *S. aureus* infection, group A streptococci occasionally produce abscesses in skeletal muscles (*streptococcal myositis*), with little or no involvement of the surrounding fascia or overlying skin. The presentation is usually subacute, but a fulminant form has been described in association with severe systemic toxicity, bacteremia, and a high mortality rate. The fulminant form may reflect the same basic disease process as that seen in necrotizing fasciitis, but with the necrotizing inflammatory process extending into the muscles themselves rather than remaining limited to the fascial layers.

℞ TREATMENT

Once necrotizing fasciitis is suspected, early surgical exploration is both diagnostically and therapeutically indicated. Surgery reveals necrosis and inflammatory fluid tracking along the fascial planes above and between muscle groups, without involvement of the muscles themselves. The process usually extends beyond the area of clinical involvement, and extensive debridement is required. Drainage and debridement are central to the management of necrotizing fasciitis; antibiotic treatment is a useful adjunct (Table 121-3), but surgery is life-saving.

Treatment for streptococcal myositis consists of surgical drainage—usually by an open procedure that permits evaluation of the extent of the infection and ensures adequate debridement of involved tissues—and high-dose penicillin (Table 121-3).

Pneumonia and Empyema   Group A streptococci are an occasional cause of pneumonia, generally in previously healthy individuals. The onset of symptoms may be abrupt or gradual. Pleuritic chest pain, fever, chills, and dyspnea are the characteristic symptoms. Cough is usually present but may not be prominent. Approximately one-half of patients with group A streptococcal pneumonia have an accompanying pleural effusion. In contrast to the sterile parapneumonic effusions typical of pneumococcal pneumonia, those complicating streptococcal pneumonia are almost always infected. The empyema fluid is usually visible by chest radiography on initial presentation and may enlarge rapidly. These pleural collections should be drained early, as they tend to become loculated rapidly, resulting in a chronic fibrotic reaction that may require thoracotomy for removal.

Bacteremia, Puerperal Sepsis, and Streptococcal Toxic Shock Syndrome

Group A streptococcal bacteremia is usually associated with an identifiable local infection. Bacteremia occurs rarely with otherwise uncomplicated pharyngitis, occasionally with cellulitis or pneumonia, and relatively frequently with necrotizing fasciitis. Bacteremia without an identified source raises the possibility of endocarditis, an occult abscess, or osteomyelitis. A variety of focal infections may arise secondarily from streptococcal bacteremia, including endocarditis, meningitis, septic arthritis, osteomyelitis, peritonitis, and visceral abscesses.

Group A streptococci are occasionally implicated in infectious complications of childbirth, usually endometritis and associated bacteremia. In the preantibiotic era, puerperal sepsis was commonly caused by group A streptococci, but currently it is more often caused by group B streptococci. Several nosocomial outbreaks of puerperal infection due to group A streptococci have been traced to an asymptomatic carrier, usually an individual present at the delivery of the infant. The site of carriage may be the skin, throat, anus, or vagina.

Beginning in the late 1980s, several reports described patients who had group A streptococcal infections associated with shock and multisystem organ failure. This syndrome has been called the streptococcal toxic shock syndrome (TSS) because it shares certain features with staphylococcal TSS. In 1993, a case definition for group A streptococcal TSS was formulated by a group of clinicians, microbiologists, and epidemiologists in conjunction with the CDC (Table 121-4). The general features of the illness include fever, hypotension, renal impairment, and respiratory distress syndrome. Various types of rash have been described, but rash usually does not develop. Laboratory abnormalities include a marked shift to the left in the white blood cell differential, with many immature granulocytes; hypocalcemia; hypoalbuminemia; and thrombocytopenia, which usually becomes more pronounced on the second or third day of illness. In contrast to those with staphylococcal TSS, the majority of patients with streptococcal TSS are bacteremic. The most common associated infection is a soft tissue infection—necrotizing fasciitis, myositis, or cellulitis—although a variety of other associated local infections have been described, including pneumonia, peritonitis, osteomyelitis, and myometritis. Streptococcal TSS is associated with a mortality rate of 30%, with most deaths secondary to shock and respiratory failure. Because of its rapidly progressive and lethal course, early recognition of the syndrome is essential. Patients should be given aggressive supportive care in the form of fluid resuscitation, pressors, and mechanical ventilation in addition to antimicrobial therapy and, in cases associated with necrotizing fasciitis, surgical debridement. Exactly why certain patients develop this fulminant syndrome is not known. Early studies of the streptococcal strains isolated from these patients demonstrated a strong association with the production of pyrogenic exotoxin A. This association has been inconsistent in subsequent cases series. Pyrogenic exotoxin A and several other streptococcal exotoxins act as superantigens to trigger release of inflammatory cytokines from T lymphocytes. Fever, shock, and organ dysfunction in streptococcal TSS may reflect, in part, the systemic effects of superantigen-mediated cytokine release.

℞ TREATMENT

In light of the possible role of pyrogenic exotoxins or other streptococcal toxins in streptococcal TSS, treatment of the affected patients with clindamycin has been advocated by some authorities, who argue that, through its direct action on protein synthesis, clindamycin is more effective in rapidly terminating toxin production than penicillin—a cell-wall agent (Table 121-3). Support for this view comes from studies of an experimental model of streptococcal myositis, in which mice treated with clindamycin had a higher rate of survival than those given penicillin. Comparable data on the treatment of human infections are not available. Although clindamycin resistance in group A streptococci is uncommon (<2% among U.S. isolates), it has been documented. Thus, if clindamycin is used for initial treatment of a critically ill patient, penicillin should be given as well until the antibiotic susceptibility of the streptococcal isolate is known.

Intravenous immunoglobulin has been used as adjunctive therapy for streptococcal TSS; pooled immunoglobulin preparations contain antibodies capable of neutralizing the effects of streptococcal toxins (Table 121-3). Anecdotal reports and case series have suggested favorable clinical responses to intravenous immunoglobulin, but no prospective controlled trials of this modality of therapy have yet been reported.

STREPTOCOCCI OF GROUPS C AND G

Group C and group G streptococci are β-hemolytic bacteria that occasionally cause human infections similar to those caused by group A streptococci, including pharyngitis, cellulitis and soft-tissue infections, pneumonia, bacteremia, endocarditis, and septic arthritis. Puerperal sepsis, meningitis, epidural abscess, intraabdominal abscess, urinary tract infection, and neonatal sepsis have also been reported. Group C streptococci are a common cause of infection in domesticated animals, especially horses and cattle, and some human infections have been acquired through contact with animals or through consumption of unpasteurized milk. Bacteremia and septic arthritis more frequently involve group G than group C streptococci. Group C or G streptococcal bacteremia occurs most often in patients who are elderly or chronically ill and, in the absence of an obvious local infection, is likely to reflect endocarditis. Septic arthritis, sometimes involving multiple joints, may complicate endocarditis or develop in its absence.

TABLE 121-4 *Proposed Case Definition for the Streptococcal Toxic Shock Syndrome[a]*

I. Isolation of group A streptococci (*Streptococcus pyogenes*)
  A. From a normally sterile site (e.g., blood, cerebrospinal fluid, pleural or peritoneal fluid, tissue biopsy, surgical wound)
  B. From a nonsterile site (e.g., throat, sputum, vagina, superficial skin lesion)

II. Clinical signs of severity
  A. Hypotension: Systolic blood pressure of ≤90 mmHg in adults or in the 5th percentile for age in children *and*
  B. Two or more of the following signs:
    1. Renal impairment: Serum creatinine level of ≥177 μmol/L (≥2 mg/dL) for adults or at least twice the upper limit of normal for age; in patients with preexisting renal disease, elevation over baseline by a factor of at least 2
    2. Coagulopathy: Platelet count of ≤100 × 10⁹/L (100,000/μL) *or* disseminated intravascular coagulation, defined by prolonged clotting times, low fibrinogen level, and the presence of fibrin degradation products
    3. Liver involvement: Alanine aminotransferase (SGOT), aspartate aminotransferase (SGPT), or total bilirubin level at least twice the upper limit of normal for age; in patients with preexisting liver disease, elevation over baseline by a factor of at least 2
    4. Adult respiratory distress syndrome, defined by acute onset of diffuse pulmonary infiltrates and hypoxemia in the absence of cardiac failure; *or* evidence of diffuse capillary leak manifested by acute onset of generalized edema; *or* pleural or peritoneal effusions with hypoalbuminemia
    5. Generalized erythematous macular rash that may desquamate
    6. Soft tissue necrosis, including necrotizing fasciitis or myositis; *or* gangrene

[a] An illness fulfilling criteria IA, IIA, and IIB is defined as a *definite* case. An illness fulfilling criteria IB, IIA, and IIB is defined as a *probable* case if no other etiology for the illness is identified.

Source: Working Group on Severe Streptococcal Infections, 1993.

℞ TREATMENT

Penicillin is the drug of choice for treatment of infections due to group C or G streptococci. Antibiotic treatment is the same as for patients with similar syndromes due to group A *Streptococcus* (Table 121-3). Patients with bacteremia or septic arthritis should receive intravenous penicillin (2 to 4 mU every 4 h). All group C and G streptococci are sensitive to penicillin; nearly all are inhibited in vitro by concentrations of ≤ 0.03 $\mu g/mL$. Occasional isolates exhibit tolerance: although inhibited by low concentrations of penicillin, they are killed only by significantly higher concentrations. The clinical significance of tolerance is unknown. Because of the poor clinical response of some patients to penicillin alone, the addition of gentamicin (1 mg/kg every 8 h for patients with normal renal function) is recommended by some authorities for treatment of endocarditis or septic arthritis due to group C or G streptococci; however, combination therapy has not been shown to be superior to treatment with penicillin alone. Patients with joint infections often require repeated aspiration or open drainage and debridement for cure; the response to treatment may be slow, particularly in debilitated patients and those with involvement of more than one joint. Infection of prosthetic joints almost always requires removal of the prosthesis in addition to antibiotic therapy.

GROUP B STREPTOCOCCI

Identified first as a cause of mastitis in cows, streptococci belonging to Lancefield's group B have since been recognized as a major cause of sepsis and meningitis in human neonates. Group B streptococci are also a frequent cause of peripartum fever in women and an occasional cause of serious infection in nonpregnant adults. Lancefield group B consists of a single species, *S. agalactiae*, which is definitively identified with specific antiserum to the group B cell wall–associated carbohydrate antigen. A streptococcal isolate can be classified presumptively as belonging to group B on the basis of biochemical tests, including hydrolysis of sodium hippurate (in which 99% of isolates are positive), hydrolysis of bile esculin agar (in which 99 to 100% are negative), bacitracin susceptibility (in which 92% are resistant), and production of CAMP factor (in which 98 to 100% are positive). CAMP factor is a phospholipase produced by group B streptococci that results in synergistic hemolysis with β lysin produced by certain strains of *S. aureus*. Its presence can be demonstrated by cross-streaking of the test isolate and an appropriate staphylococcal strain on a blood agar plate. Group B streptococci causing human infections are encapsulated by one of nine antigenically distinct polysaccharides. The capsular polysaccharide has been shown experimentally to be important in the virulence of the organism. Antibodies to the capsular polysaccharide afford protection against group B streptococci of the same (but not of a different) capsular type.

INFECTION IN NEONATES Two general types of group B streptococcal infection in infants are defined by the age of the patient at presentation. *Early-onset infections* occur within the first week of life, with a median age of 20 h at the onset of illness. Approximately half of these infants have signs of group B streptococcal disease at birth. The infection is acquired during or shortly before birth from organisms colonizing the maternal genital tract. Surveillance studies have shown that 5 to 40% of women are vaginal or rectal carriers of group B streptococci. Approximately 50% of infants delivered vaginally by carrier mothers become colonized, although only 1 to 2% of those colonized develop clinically evident infection. Prematurity and maternal risk factors (prolonged labor, obstetric complications, and maternal fever) are often involved. The presentation of early-onset infection is the same as that of other forms of neonatal sepsis. Typical findings include respiratory distress, lethargy, and hypotension. Essentially all infants with early-onset disease are bacteremic, one-third to one-half have pneumonia and/or respiratory distress syndrome, and one-third have meningitis.

Late-onset infections occur in infants between 1 week and 3 months of age, with a mean age at onset of 3 to 4 weeks. The infecting organism may be acquired during delivery (as in early-onset cases) or during later contact with a colonized mother, nursery personnel, or another source. Meningitis is the most common manifestation of late-onset infection and in most cases is associated with a strain of capsular type III of the organism. Infants present with fever, lethargy or irritability, poor feeding, and seizures. The various other types of late-onset infection include bacteremia without an identified source, osteomyelitis, septic arthritis, and facial cellulitis associated with submandibular or preauricular adenitis.

℞ TREATMENT

Penicillin is the treatment of choice for all group B streptococcal infections. Empiric broad-spectrum therapy for suspected bacterial sepsis, consisting of ampicillin and gentamicin, is generally administered until culture results become available. If cultures yield group B streptococci, many pediatricians continue to administer gentamicin, along with ampicillin or penicillin, for a few days until clinical improvement becomes evident. Infants with bacteremia or soft-tissue infection should receive penicillin at a dosage of 200,000 units/kg per day in divided doses; those with meningitis should receive 400,000 units/kg per day. Meningitis should be treated for at least 14 days because of the risk of relapse with shorter courses.

Prevention The incidence of group B streptococcal infection is unusually high among infants of women with risk factors: preterm delivery, early rupture of membranes (>24 h before delivery), prolonged labor, fever, or chorioamnionitis. Because the usual source of the organisms infecting a neonate is the mother's birth canal, efforts have been made to prevent group B streptococcal infections by the identification of high-risk carrier mothers and their treatment with various forms of antibiotic or immunoprophylaxis. Prophylactic administration of ampicillin or penicillin to such patients during delivery has been shown to reduce the risk of infection in the newborn. This approach has been hampered by the logistical difficulties of identifying colonized women before delivery, since the results of vaginal cultures early in pregnancy are poor predictors of carrier status at delivery. The CDC has recommended that women be screened for anogenital colonization at 35 to 37 weeks of pregnancy by means of a swab culture of the lower vagina and anorectum; intrapartum chemoprophylaxis is recommended for women who are culture-positive and to all women, regardless of culture status, who have previously given birth to an infant with group B streptococcal infection or who have a history of group B streptococcal bacteriuria during pregnancy. Women whose culture status is unknown and who develop premature labor (<37 weeks), prolonged rupture of membranes (>18 h), or intrapartum fever should also receive intrapartum chemoprophylaxis. The recommended regimen for chemoprophylaxis is 5 million units of penicillin G followed by 2.5 million units every 4 h until delivery. Cefazolin is an alternative for women with a history of penicillin allergy who are thought not to be at high risk for anaphylaxis. For women with a history of an immediate hypersensitivity reaction, clindamycin or erythromycin may be substituted, but only if the colonizing isolate has been demonstrated to be susceptible. If susceptibility testing results are not available or indicate resistance, vancomycin should be used in this situation.

Treatment of all pregnant women who are colonized or who have risk factors for neonatal infection will result in exposure of 15 to 25% of pregnant women and newborns to antibiotics, with the attendant risks of allergic reactions and selection for resistant organisms. Although still in the developmental stages, a group B streptococcal vaccine may ultimately offer a better solution to prevention. Because transplacental passage of maternal antibodies produces protective antibody levels in the newborn, efforts are under way to develop a vaccine against group B streptococci that can be given to childbearing women before or during pregnancy. Results of phase 1 clinical trials of group B streptococcal capsular polysaccharide–protein conjugate vaccines suggest that a multivalent conjugate vaccine would be safe and highly immunogenic.

INFECTION IN ADULTS   The majority of group B streptococcal infections in adults are related to pregnancy and parturition. Peripartum fever, the most common manifestation, is sometimes accompanied by symptoms and signs of endometritis or chorioamnionitis (abdominal distention and uterine or adnexal tenderness). Blood cultures are often positive, as are cultures of vaginal swabs. Bacteremia is usually transitory but occasionally results in meningitis or endocarditis. Infections in adults that are not associated with the peripartum period generally involve individuals who are elderly or have some underlying chronic illness, such as diabetes mellitus or a malignancy. Among the infections that develop with some frequency in adults are cellulitis and soft tissue infection (including infected diabetic skin ulcers), urinary tract infection, pneumonia, endocarditis, and septic arthritis. Other reported infections include meningitis, osteomyelitis, and intraabdominal or pelvic abscesses.

℞ TREATMENT

Group B streptococci are less sensitive to penicillin than group A organisms, requiring somewhat higher doses. Adults with serious localized infections (pneumonia, pyelonephritis, abscess) should receive doses in the range of 12 million units of penicillin G daily, while patients with endocarditis or meningitis should receive 18 to 24 million units per day in divided doses. Vancomycin is an acceptable alternative for patients allergic to penicillin.

ENTEROCOCCI AND NONENTEROCOCCAL GROUP D STREPTOCOCCI

ENTEROCOCCI   Lancefield group D includes the enterococci, organisms now classified in a separate genus from other streptococci, and nonenterococcal group D streptococci. Enterococci are distinguished from nonenterococcal group D streptococci by their ability to grow in the presence of 6.5% sodium chloride and by the results of other biochemical tests. The enterococcal species that are significant pathogens for humans are *E. faecalis* and *E. faecium*. These organisms tend to produce infection in patients who are elderly or debilitated or in whom mucosal or epithelial barriers have been disrupted or the balance of the normal flora altered by antibiotic treatment. Urinary tract infections due to enterococci are quite common, particularly among patients who have received antibiotic treatment or undergone instrumentation of the urinary tract. Enterococci are a frequent cause of nosocomial bacteremia in patients with intravascular catheters. These organisms account for 10 to 20% of cases of bacterial endocarditis on both native and prosthetic valves. The presentation of enterococcal endocarditis is usually subacute but may be acute, with rapidly progressive valve destruction. Enterococci are frequently cultured from bile and are involved in infectious complications of biliary surgery and in liver abscesses. Moreover, enterococci are often isolated from polymicrobial infections arising from the bowel flora (e.g., intraabdominal abscesses), from abdominal surgical wounds, and from diabetic foot ulcers. While such mixed infections are frequently cured by antimicrobials not active against enterococci, specific therapy directed against enterococci is warranted when these organisms are the predominant species or are isolated from blood cultures.

℞ TREATMENT

Unlike streptococci, enterococci are not reliably killed by penicillin or ampicillin alone at concentrations achieved clinically in the blood or tissues. Ampicillin reaches sufficiently high urinary concentrations to constitute adequate monotherapy for uncomplicated urinary tract infections. Because in vitro testing has shown evidence of synergistic killing of most enterococcal strains by the combination of penicillin or ampicillin with an aminoglycoside, combined therapy is recommended for enterococcal endocarditis and meningitis; the regimen is penicillin (3 to 4 million units every 4 h) or ampicillin (2 g every 4 h) plus moderate-dose gentamicin (1 mg/kg every 8 h for patients with normal renal function). Enterococcal endocarditis should be treated for

a minimum of 4 weeks and for 6 weeks if symptoms have been present for ≥3 months or if the infection involves a prosthetic heart valve. For nonendocarditis bacteremia and other serious enterococcal infections, it is not known whether the efficacy of single-agent β-lactam therapy is improved by the addition of gentamicin, but many infectious disease specialists use combination therapy for such infections, especially in critically ill patients. Vancomycin, in combination with gentamicin, may be substituted for penicillin in allergic patients. Enterococci are resistant to all cephalosporins; therefore, this class of antibiotics should not be used for treatment of enterococcal infections.

Antimicrobial susceptibility testing should be performed routinely on enterococcal isolates from patients with serious infections, and therapy should be adjusted according to the results (Table 121-5). Most enterococci are resistant to streptomycin, and this drug should not be used for treatment of enterococcal infection unless in vitro testing of the strain indicates susceptibility. Though less widespread than streptomycin resistance, high-level resistance to gentamicin—with a minimum inhibitory concentration (MIC) of >2000 μg/mL—has become common. Gentamicin-resistant enterococci should be tested for susceptibility to streptomycin; occasional gentamicin-resistant enterococci are sensitive to streptomycin. If the isolate is resistant to all aminoglycosides, treatment with penicillin or ampicillin alone may be successful. The prolonged administration (i.e., for at least 6 weeks) of high-dose ampicillin (e.g., 12 g/d) is recommended for endocarditis due to these highly resistant enterococci.

Enterococci may be resistant to penicillins via two distinct mechanisms. The first is the production of β-lactamase (mediating resistance to penicillin and ampicillin), which has been reported for *E. faecalis* isolates from several locations in the United States and other countries. Because the amount of β-lactamase produced by enterococci may be insufficient for detection by routine antibiotic susceptibility testing, isolates from serious infections should be screened specifically for β-lactamase production with use of a chromogenic cephalosporin or by another method. For the treatment of β-lactamase-producing strains, vancomycin, ampicillin/sulbactam, amoxicillin/clavulanate, or imipenem may be used in combination with gentamicin.

The second mechanism of penicillin resistance is not mediated by β-lactamase and may be due to altered penicillin-binding proteins. This intrinsic penicillin resistance is common among *E. faecium* isolates, which routinely are more resistant to β-lactam antibiotics than are isolates of *E. faecalis*. Moderately resistant enterococci (MICs of penicillin and ampicillin, 16 to 64 μg/mL) may be susceptible to high-dose penicillin or ampicillin plus gentamicin, but strains with MICs of ≥200 μg/mL must be considered resistant to clinically achievable levels of β-lactam antibiotics, including imipenem. Vancomycin plus gentamicin is the recommended regimen for infections due to enterococci with high-level intrinsic resistance to β-lactams.

Vancomycin-resistant enterococci, first reported from clinical sources in the late 1980s, have become common in many hospitals.

TABLE 121-5   *Treatment Options for Antibiotic-Resistant Enterococcal Infections*

Resistance Pattern	Recommended Therapy
β-Lactamase production	Gentamicin plus ampicillin/sulbactam, amoxicillin/clavulanate, imipenem, or vancomycin
β-Lactam resistance, but no β-lactamase production	Gentamicin plus vancomycin
High-level gentamicin resistance	Streptomycin-sensitive isolate: Streptomycin plus ampicillin or vancomycin Streptomycin-resistant isolate: No proven therapy (continuous-infusion ampicillin, prolonged treatment)
Vancomycin resistance	Ampicillin plus gentamicin
Vancomycin and β-lactam resistance	No uniformly bactericidal drugs; linezolid (all enterococci) or quinupristin/dalfopristin (*E. faecium* only)

Three major vancomycin resistance phenotypes have been described: VanA, VanB, and VanC. The VanA phenotype is associated with high-level resistance to vancomycin and to teicoplanin, a related glycopeptide antibiotic not currently available in the United States. VanB and VanC strains are resistant to vancomycin but susceptible to teicoplanin, although teicoplanin resistance may develop during treatment in VanB strains. For enterococci resistant to both vancomycin and β-lactams, there are no established therapies that provide uniformly bactericidal activity. Regimens that have been tried with some success in individual cases or experimentally include ciprofloxacin plus rifampin plus gentamicin; ampicillin plus vancomycin (particularly if in vitro testing shows synergistic bacteriostatic activity); and chloramphenicol or tetracycline (if the strain is susceptible in vitro). Two newer agents with activity against vancomycin-resistant enterococci are quinupristin/dalfopristin and linezolid, which were approved for use in the United States in 1999 and 2000, respectively. Quinupristin/dalfopristin is a streptogramin combination with in vitro bacteriostatic activity against *E. faecium*, including vancomycin-resistant isolates, but not against *E. faecalis* or other enterococcal species. Favorable clinical responses have been obtained in approximately three-quarters of patients treated with this agent. Linezolid is an oxazolidinone antibiotic with good bacteriostatic activity against nearly all enterococci, including vancomycin-resistant enterococci. Limited clinical experience suggests that linezolid is at least as efficacious as quinupristin/dalfopristin.

OTHER GROUP D STREPTOCOCCI The main nonenterococcal group D streptococcal species that causes human infections is *S. bovis*. *S. bovis* endocarditis is often associated with neoplasms of the gastrointestinal tract—most frequently a colon carcinoma or polyp—but is also reported in association with other bowel lesions. When occult gastrointestinal lesions are carefully sought, abnormalities are found in ≥60% of patients with *S. bovis* endocarditis. In contrast to the enterococci, nonenterococcal group D streptococci like *S. bovis* are reliably killed by penicillin as a single agent, and penicillin is the treatment of choice for *S. bovis* infections.

VIRIDANS AND OTHER STREPTOCOCCI

VIRIDANS STREPTOCOCCI Consisting of multiple species of α-hemolytic streptococci, the viridans streptococci are a heterogeneous group of organisms that are important as agents of bacterial endocarditis (Chap. 109). Several species of viridans streptococci, including *S. salivarius*, *S. mitis*, *S. sanguis*, and *S. mutans*, are part of the normal flora of the mouth, where they live in close association with the teeth and gingiva. Some species contribute to the development of dental caries. The transient viridans streptococcal bacteremia induced by eating, tooth-brushing, flossing, and other sources of minor trauma, together with adherence to biologic surfaces, is thought to account for the predilection of these organisms to cause endocarditis (see Fig. 109-1). Viridans streptococci are also isolated, often as part of a mixed flora, from sites of sinusitis, brain abscess, and liver abscess.

Viridans streptococcal bacteremia occurs relatively frequently in neutropenic patients, particularly after bone marrow transplantation or high-dose chemotherapy for cancer. Some of these patients develop a sepsis syndrome with high fever and shock. Risk factors for viridans streptococcal bacteremia include chemotherapy with high-dose cytosine arabinoside, prior treatment with trimethoprim-sulfamethoxazole or a fluoroquinolone, treatment with antacids or histamine antagonists, mucositis, and profound neutropenia.

The *S. milleri* group (also referred to as the *S. intermedius* or *S. anginosus* group) includes three species that cause human disease: *S. intermedius*, *S. anginosus*, and *S. constellatus*. These organisms are often considered viridans streptococci, although they differ somewhat from other viridans streptococci in both their hemolytic pattern (they may be α-, β-, or nonhemolytic) and the disease syndromes they cause. This group commonly produces suppurative infections, particularly abscesses of brain and abdominal viscera, and infections related to the oral cavity or respiratory tract, such as peritonsillar abscess, lung abscess, and empyema.

Rx TREATMENT

Isolates from neutropenic patients with bacteremia are often resistant to penicillin; thus these patients should be treated presumptively with vancomycin until the results of susceptibility testing become available. Viridans streptococci isolated in other clinical settings usually are sensitive to penicillin.

ABIOTROPHIA SPECIES (NUTRITIONALLY VARIANT STREPTOCOCCI)

Occasional isolates cultured from the blood of patients with endocarditis fail to grow when subcultured on solid media. These *nutritionally variant streptococci* require supplemental thiol compounds or active forms of vitamin B$_6$ (pyridoxal or pyridoxamine) for growth in the laboratory. The nutritionally variant streptococci are generally grouped with the viridans streptococci because they cause similar types of infections. However, they have been reclassified on the basis of 16S ribosomal RNA sequence comparisons into a separate genus, *Abiotrophia*, with two species: *A. defectivus* and *A. adjacens*.

Rx TREATMENT

Treatment failure and relapse appear to be more common in cases of endocarditis due to nutritionally variant streptococci than in those due to the usual viridans streptococci. Thus the addition of gentamicin (1 mg/kg every 8 h for patients with normal renal function) to the penicillin regimen is recommended in therapy for endocarditis due to the nutritionally variant organisms.

OTHER STREPTOCOCCI

S. suis is an important pathogen in swine and has been reported to cause meningitis in humans, usually in individuals with occupational exposure to pigs. Strains of *S. suis* associated with human infections have generally reacted with Lancefield group R typing serum and sometimes with group D typing serum as well. Isolates may be α- or β-hemolytic and are sensitive to penicillin. *S. iniae*, a pathogen of fish, has been associated with infections in humans who have handled live or freshly killed fish. Cellulitis of the hand is the most common form of human infection, although bacteremia and endocarditis have been reported. *Anaerobic streptococci*, or *peptostreptococci*, are part of the normal flora of the oral cavity, bowel, and vagina. Infections caused by the anaerobic streptococci are discussed in Chap. 148.

FURTHER READING

BISNO AL, STEVENS DL: Streptococcal infections of skin and soft tissues. N Engl J Med 334:240, 1996

——— et al: Practice guidelines for the diagnosis and management of group A streptococcal pharyngitis. Clin Infect Dis 35:113, 2002

BRUCKNER LB et al: High incidence of penicillin resistance among α-hemolytic streptococci isolated from the blood of children with cancer. J Pediatr 140:20, 2002

CENTERS FOR DISEASE CONTROL AND PREVENTION: Prevention of perinatal group B streptococcal disease. MMWR 51(RR-11):1, 2002

EDWARDS MS, BAKER CJ: *Streptococcus agalactiae* (group B *Streptococcus*), in *Principles and Practice of Infectious Diseases*, 5th ed, GL Mandell et al (eds). New York, Churchill Livingstone, 2000

GOLD HS: Vancomycin-resistant enterococci: Mechanism and clinical observations. Clin Infect Dis 33:210, 2001

JACKSON LA et al: Risk factors for group B streptococcal disease in adults. Ann Intern Med 123:415, 1995

KAUL R et al: Intravenous immunoglobulin therapy for streptococcal toxic shock syndrome—a comparative observational study. The Canadian Streptococcal Study Group. Clin Infect Dis 28:800, 1999

ZURAWSKI CA et al: Invasive group A streptococcal disease in metropolitan Atlanta: A population-based assessment. Clin Infect Dis 27:150, 1998

DIPHTHERIA

DEFINITION Diphtheria is a localized infection of mucous membranes or skin that is caused by *Corynebacterium diphtheriae* and may be associated with a characteristic pseudomembrane at the site of infection (Fig. 122-1). Some strains of *C. diphtheriae* produce diphtheria toxin, a protein that can cause myocarditis, polyneuropathy, and other systemic toxic effects. Respiratory diphtheria is usually caused by toxinogenic (tox⁺) *C. diphtheriae*, but infections of the skin (cutaneous diphtheria) and other anatomical sites are often caused by nontoxinogenic (tox⁻) *C. diphtheriae*. Respiratory diphtheria caused by either tox⁺ or tox⁻ isolates of *C. diphtheriae*—but not cutaneous diphtheria—is a nationally notifiable infectious disease in the United States.

ETIOLOGY *C. diphtheriae* is an aerobic, nonmotile, nonsporulating, irregularly staining, gram-positive rod. The bacteria are club-shaped and are often arranged in clusters (*Chinese letters*) or parallel arrays (*palisades*). Selective media containing either tellurite or colisitin plus nalidixic acid are recommended for cultivation of *C. diphtheriae*. The gravis, mitis, and intermedius biotypes are distinguished by colonial morphology and laboratory tests. Both tox⁺ and tox⁻ strains are infectious, but tox⁺ strains can produce toxemic diphtheria and are more likely to cause pseudomembranes. Diphtheria toxin is encoded by specific corynephages, and tox⁻ *C. diphtheriae* (or other *Corynebacterium* species, such as *C. ulcerans* and *C. pseudotuberculosis*) can acquire the ability to produce diphtheria toxin by infection with tox⁺ phages (*phage conversion*). Growth of *C. diphtheriae* under low-iron conditions that mimic the environment of host tissues induces production of diphtheria toxin and expression of systems for siderophore-dependent iron uptake, utilization of iron from heme, and several other iron-regulated functions.

IMMUNOLOGY Treatment of diphtheria toxin with formaldehyde converts it to a nontoxic but immunogenic product (*diphtheria toxoid*). Immunization with toxoid elicits antibody (*antitoxin*) that neutralizes the toxin and prevents diphtheria. The attack rate and mortality rate

for diphtheria are low in immune individuals with antitoxin titers of >0.01 unit per milliliter. Antitoxin neither prevents colonization by *C. diphtheriae* nor eradicates the *carrier state*. When most individuals in a population have protective levels of antitoxin (*herd immunity*), the carrier rate for tox⁺ strains of *C. diphtheriae* falls to a low level, and the risk that susceptible individuals will be exposed to tox⁺ *C. diphtheriae* decreases dramatically. Susceptible individuals may contract diphtheria if they travel to regions where the disease is present or if tox⁺ strains of *C. diphtheriae* are introduced into their community.

EPIDEMIOLOGY AND IMMUNITY Humans are the principal reservoir for *C. diphtheriae*. Transmission occurs primarily by close personal contact. The risk that *C. diphtheriae* will be transmitted to susceptible individuals from patients with diphtheria is greater than the risk that it will be transmitted to them from carriers. The incubation period for respiratory diphtheria is typically 2 to 5 days (range, 1 to 10 days). Cutaneous diphtheria is usually a secondary infection whose signs develop an average of 7 days (range, 1 to >21 days) after the appearance of other primary dermatologic lesions.

In temperate climates, diphtheria primarily involves the respiratory tract. It occurs throughout the year, with a peak incidence in colder months, and it is usually caused by tox⁺ *C. diphtheriae*. Before immunization was introduced, diphtheria was primarily a disease of children; it affected up to 10% of individuals in this group and sometimes caused devastating epidemics. Most young infants were immune because of transplacental transfer of maternal IgG antitoxin, but children became susceptible by 6 to 12 months of age. Approximately 75% of individuals became immune by 10 years of age as a result of contact with *C. diphtheriae*. Mortality rates of 30 to 40% were common in untreated disease and were sometimes >50% in epidemics. Treatment with antitoxin reduced the case-fatality rate to 5 to 10%.

Routine immunization of children in the United States resulted in a progressive decrease of diphtheria from the peak of 206,939 cases (incidence rate, 191 cases per 100,000 population) in 1921 to ≤5 cases per year since 1980. Circulation of tox⁺ strains of *C. diphtheriae* among the population decreased dramatically throughout this period, but endemic foci of clonally related tox⁺ and tox⁻ strains, belonging predominantly to the ET215 complex, have persisted for the past 25 years in South Dakota and Ontario. As the incidence of diphtheria decreased, a higher proportion of cases occurred in older persons (who were never immunized or whose immunity waned because they did not receive booster doses of vaccine or did not have contact with *C. diphtheriae*), but the case-fatality ratio remained unchanged at 5 to 10%. High rates of immunization are achieved by school entry (>96%), but immunization rates for younger children are substantially lower. Immunity to diphtheria among adults declines gradually with increasing age, and only 30% of men in the 60- to 69-year-old age group have protective levels of diphtheria antitoxin. Among adults immunity to diphtheria is typically lower among women than among men; likewise, it is lower among Mexican-Americans than among other racial or ethnic groups. The most recent large diphtheria outbreak in the United States (about 1100 cases) occurred in Seattle, Washington, between 1972 and 1982. Alcoholism, low socioeconomic status, crowded living conditions, and Native-American ethnic background were significant risk factors in this outbreak.

A massive diphtheria epidemic (>157,000 cases and >5000 deaths) occurred during the 1990s in Russia and the newly independent states of the former Soviet Union and accounted for >80% of diphtheria cases reported worldwide during that decade. The epidemic began in 1990 with 1436 cases (0.49 per 100,000 population) and peaked in 1995 with 50,425 cases (17.29 per 100,000 population). Clonally related tox⁺ *C. diphtheriae* stains of the ET8 complex, which constituted only a small percentage of archival *C. diphtheriae* isolates from Russia before that epidemic, increased dramatically in prevalence, ac-

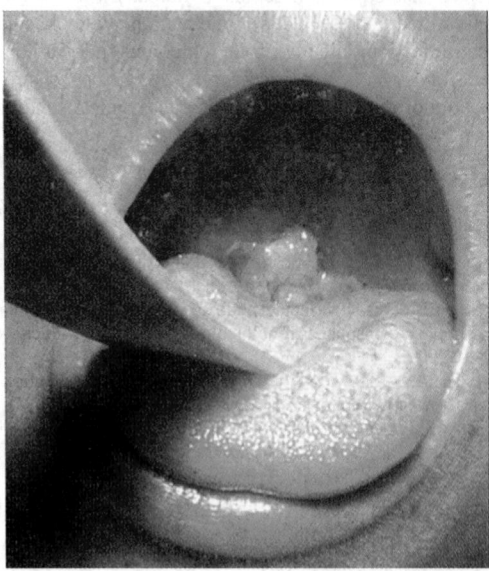

FIGURE 122-1 Pseudomembrane of diphtheria. Diphtheria is now a rare cause of exudative pharyngitis in the United States, but outbreaks continue to occur in under-immunized countries and regions. The pharyngitis has an acute onset, is characterized by severe dysphagia, and is accompanied by a thick, tenacious, gray-white exudate on the tonsils, uvula, and pharynx. As the exudate coagulates, it forms a so-called pseudomembrane, which may result in respiratory obstruction. [*From Upper Respiratory and Head and Neck Infections, Vol. IV, I. Brook (ed), in Atlas of Infectious Diseases, GL Mandell (ed). Philadelphia, Current Medicine, Inc., with permission.*]

counting for >80% of isolates by 1994. Molecular analysis of *tox* gene alleles from isolates of the ET8 complex demonstrated that the existing diphtheria toxoid vaccine remained appropriate for ongoing use as a protective immunogen, and a mass vaccination program succeeded in reducing the number of cases to 2720 in 1998 (0.93 per 100,000 population). A majority of cases throughout this epidemic occurred in persons ≥15 years old, and adults from 40 to 49 years old had very high incidence and death rates. In 1994, case-fatality rates varied from 2.8% in the Russian Federation to 23% in Lithuania and Turkmenistan. Factors that facilitated the spread of this epidemic included large-scale population movements, socioeconomic instability, deteriorating health infrastructure, delayed implementation of aggressive control measures in response to the epidemic, inadequate information for physicians and the public, and frequent shortages of supplies for prevention and treatment of the disease. The most important risk factor for diphtheria in the Republic of Georgia was lack of vaccination (matched odds ratio, 19.2), but household diphtheria exposure, exposure to skin lesions, the presence of tonsils, a history of eczema, preceding fever with myalgia, sharing a bed, sharing glasses and cups, and taking a bath less often than weekly were also significant risk factors. Although small numbers of imported cases from this epidemic occurred in western European countries, none resulted in secondary transmission of diphtheria, notwithstanding a high proportion of susceptible adults in countries with imported cases. Inadequate primary immunization of children in the states of the former Soviet Union in the years preceding the epidemic, along with failure to maintain adequate immunity in adults by booster immunization, appear to have been primary factors in the development of the massive diphtheria epidemic in this region.

In the tropics, cutaneous diphtheria is more common than respiratory diphtheria, occurs throughout the year, and often develops as a secondary infection complicating other dermatoses. Isolates of *C. diphtheriae* from skin lesions are more often tox⁻ than tox⁺. Cutaneous diphtheria is increasingly recognized in temperate climates and accounted for 86% of the 1100 cases in the Seattle epidemic of 1972 to 1982. Since 1980, cutaneous diphtheria has not been a reportable disease in the United States, and recent health statistics include only respiratory diphtheria.

During the 1990s, tox⁻ strains of *C. diphtheriae* were associated with new types of infections. In the United Kingdom, these strains caused symptomatic pharyngitis, predominantly among homosexual men, that was sometimes accompanied by tonsillar exudate. In Switzerland, strains with a high potential for invasiveness were isolated from 38 intravenous drug users and shown by ribotyping to be clonally related. The latter strains caused infections of the skin (15 cases), respiratory tract (10 cases), and blood (13 cases). Among the patients with bloodstream infections, 9 had endocarditis, and 4 of these 9 patients died.

PATHOLOGY AND PATHOGENESIS *C. diphtheriae* infects mucous membranes, most commonly in the respiratory tract, and also invades open skin lesions resulting from insect bites or trauma. In infections caused by tox⁺ *C. diphtheriae*, initial edema and hyperemia are often followed by epithelial necrosis and acute inflammation. Coagulation of the dense fibrinopurulent exudate produces a pseudomembrane (Fig. 122-1), and the inflammatory reaction accompanied by vascular congestion extends into the underlying tissues. The pseudomembrane contains large numbers of *C. diphtheriae* organisms, but the bacteria are rarely isolated from the blood or internal organs.

Diphtheria toxin acts both locally and systemically, and the lethal dose for humans is ~0.1 μg/kg. Toxin contributes locally to pseudomembrane formation; systemically, it can cause myocarditis, polyneuropathy, and focal necrosis in various organs, including the kidneys, liver, and adrenal glands. Changes in the myocardium include cloudy swelling of muscle fibers and interstitial edema. These changes are followed within weeks by hyaline and granular degeneration (sometimes with fatty degeneration), progressing to myolysis and finally to the replacement of lost muscle by fibrosis. Thus, diphtheria can cause permanent cardiac damage. In diphtheritic polyneuropathy, pathologic changes include patchy breakdown of myelin sheaths in peripheral and autonomic nerves, but recovery of nerve damage is the rule if the patient survives.

Diphtheria toxin is produced by *C. diphtheriae* as an extracellular polypeptide. Proteolytic cleavage of the intact toxin forms nicked toxin consisting of fragments A and B. Fragment B binds to a plasma-membrane receptor (a precursor of a heparin-binding growth factor resembling epidermal growth factor), and the bound toxin is internalized by receptor-mediated endocytosis. Fragment A is translocated across the membrane of acidified endosomes and released into the cytoplasm, where it catalyzes the transfer of the adenosine diphosphate ribose moiety from nicotinamide adenine dinucleotide (NAD) to a modified histidine residue (diphthamide) on elongation factor 2 (EF-2), thereby inactivating EF-2 and inhibiting protein synthesis. One molecule of fragment A in the cytoplasm can kill a cell. Other metabolic alterations are secondary to inhibition of protein synthesis.

CLINICAL MANIFESTATIONS ■ Respiratory Diphtheria The current epidemiologic case definition of diphtheria used by the Centers for Disease Control and Prevention (CDC) is based on both a clinical syndrome [upper respiratory tract illness with sore throat, low-grade fever, and an adherent membrane of the tonsil(s), pharynx, and/or nose] and laboratory criteria (isolation of *C. diphtheriae* from a clinical specimen or a histopathologic diagnosis of diphtheria). Clinically compatible cases are classified as *confirmed* if they are either confirmed by the laboratory or epidemiologically linked to a laboratory-confirmed case and as *probable* if they are neither confirmed by the laboratory nor linked to a laboratory-confirmed case. By these criteria, both asymptomatic individuals and patients with respiratory findings but no pseudomembrane are classified as *carriers* if *C. diphtheriae* is isolated from the respiratory tract. On clinical grounds, diphtheria is graded as *tonsillar* if pseudomembranes are localized to the tonsils, as *combined types* or *delayed diagnosis* if more extensive pseudomembranes are present, and as *severe* if cervical adenopathy or cervical edema is also present. Onset is often gradual, but most patients seek medical care within a few days of becoming ill. Fever [a temperature of 37.8° to 38.9°C (100° to 102°F)], sore throat, and weakness are the most common symptoms, while dysphagia, headache, and change of voice occur in fewer than half of patients. Neck edema and difficulty breathing are noted in ≤10% of patients and are associated with an increased risk of death. Systemic manifestations are due primarily to toxic effects of diphtheria toxin. Patients without toxicity exhibit discomfort and malaise associated with local infection, whereas severely toxic patients may develop listlessness, pallor, and tachycardia that can progress rapidly to vascular collapse.

Primary infection in the respiratory tract is most often tonsillopharyngeal but may also be (in decreasing order of frequency) laryngeal, nasal, and tracheobronchial. Multiple sites are frequently involved, and secondary spread of pharyngeal infection upward to the nasal mucosa or downward to the larynx and tracheobronchial tree is much more common than primary infection at those sites. Systemic toxicity is usually most severe when extensive pseudomembrane extends from the tonsils and pharynx into contiguous regions. A small percentage of patients present with malignant or "bull-neck" diphtheria, with extensive pseudomembrane formation, foul breath, massive swelling of the tonsils and uvula, thick speech, cervical lymphadenopathy, striking edematous swelling of the submandibular region and anterior neck, and severe toxicity.

In tonsillopharyngeal diphtheria, isolated spots of gray or white exudate may appear first. These spots often extend and coalesce within a day to form a confluent, sharply demarcated pseudomembrane (Fig. 122-1) that becomes progressively thicker, more tightly adherent to the underlying tissue, and darker gray in color. Unlike the exudate in streptococcal pharyngitis, the diphtheritic pseudomembrane often extends beyond the margin of the tonsils onto the tonsillar pillars, palate, or uvula. Dislodging the membrane is likely to cause bleeding. Laryngeal diphtheria often presents as hoarseness and cough. Demonstration of laryngeal pseudomembrane by laryngoscopy helps distinguish diphtheria from other infectious forms of laryngitis. Patients with nasal diphtheria may present with unilateral or bilateral serosanguineous nasal discharge associated with irritation of the nares or lip. Primary or secondary diphtheritic infection occasionally involves other mucous membranes, including the conjunctiva and the membranes of the genitourinary and gastrointestinal tracts.

Cutaneous Diphtheria Cutaneous diphtheria usually presents as an infection by *C. diphtheriae* of preexisting dermatoses involving the lower extremities, upper extremities, head, or trunk. The clinical features are similar to those of other secondary cutaneous bacterial infections. In the tropics, cutaneous diphtheria may present as a primary cutaneous lesion, typically with morphologically distinct "punched-out" ulcers that are covered by necrotic slough or membrane and have well-demarcated edges.

Other Clinical Presentations *C. diphtheriae* is an occasional cause of invasive infections, including endocarditis and septic arthritis. Risk factors for such infections include preexisting cardiac abnormalities, abuse of intravenous drugs, and alcoholic cirrhosis.

COMPLICATIONS Obstruction of the respiratory tract can be caused by extensive pseudomembrane formation and swelling early in the disease or by sloughed pseudomembrane that becomes lodged in the airways later in the disease. The risk is greater when infection involves the larynx or the tracheobronchial tree and in children because of the small size of the airways.

Myocarditis and polyneuropathy are the prominent toxic manifestations of diphtheria. The risk of each is proportional to the severity of local disease. Myocarditis occurred in 22% and neuropathy in 5% of 656 hospitalized patients (54% female, 70% ≥15 years old) with diphtheria in the Kyrgyz Republic in 1995; 7% of patients with myocarditis and 2% of patients without myocarditis died. The median interval from hospitalization to death was 4.5 days (range, 0 to 13 days). Manifestations of diphtheritic myocarditis include various dysrhythmias, conduction disturbances, and dilated cardiomyopathy. Although complete heart block from diphtheritic myocarditis was almost always fatal before temporary cardiac pacemakers were developed, approximately one-fourth of patients with this complication have recently been treated successfully.

Polyneuropathy typically begins 3 to 5 weeks after onset of diphtheria and has a slow course. It appears earliest in patients who experience the most severe and prolonged neurologic abnormalities. The initial presentation commonly involves gingival, lingual, or facial numbness as well as dysphonia, dysphagia, and paresthesias of the extremities. These findings may be followed by cranial motor nerve pareses, respiratory and abdominal muscle weakness that may require artificial ventilation, quadriparesis or quadriplegia, peripheral sensory disturbances, sensory ataxia, pain in the extremities, and a variety of autonomic disturbances. Cranial nerve dysfunction typically appears earlier than motor disturbances of the trunk and extremities. In severely affected patients, paresis or paralysis of the trunk and extremities may become worse during the second month, as cranial nerve dysfunction is improving, and peak at 7 to 9 weeks after the onset of polyneuropathy. Severe arterial hypotension attributable to autonomic dysfunction may occur from 4 to 7 weeks after the onset of polyneuropathy and last from 3 to 10 days. Polyneuropathy usually resolves completely in patients who survive.

Pneumonia occurs in more than one-half of fatal cases of diphtheria. Less common complications include renal failure, encephalitis, cerebral infarction, pulmonary embolism, and bacteremia or endocarditis due to invasive infection by *C. diphtheriae*. Serum sickness may result from antitoxin therapy.

COURSE AND PROGNOSIS Most cases of diphtheria develop in nonimmunized patients. The attack rate, severity of disease, and risk of

complications are much lower in immunized patients. The pseudomembrane may continue to increase in size during the first day after administration of antitoxin. During the next several days to a week, it becomes softer, less adherent, and nonconfluent and eventually disappears. In the preantibiotic era, *C. diphtheriae* persisted in the throat for ~2 weeks in one-half of patients and for ≥1 month in about one-fifth. Mortality increases with the severity of local disease, the extent of pseudomembrane formation, and the delay between onset of local disease and administration of antitoxin. The death rate is highest during the first week of illness; among patients with bull-neck diphtheria; among patients with myocarditis who develop ventricular tachycardia, atrial fibrillation, or complete heart block; among patients with laryngeal or tracheobronchial involvement; among infants and patients >60 years of age; and among alcoholics. Both the mortality rate and the risk of myocarditis or peripheral neuropathy are significantly lower in cutaneous diphtheria than in respiratory diphtheria.

DIAGNOSIS A characteristic pseudomembrane (Fig. 122-1) on the mucosa of the tonsils, palate, oropharynx, nasopharynx, nose, or larynx suggests diphtheria but is not uniformly present. Diphtheritic pseudomembrane must be distinguished from other pharyngeal exudates, including those of group A β-hemolytic streptococcal infections, infectious mononucleosis, viral pharyngitis, fusospirochetal infection, and candidiasis. Diphtheria should be considered in patients with sore throat, cervical adenopathy or swelling, and low-grade fever, especially when these manifestations are accompanied by systemic toxicity, hoarseness, stridor, palatal paralysis, or serosanguineous nasal discharge with or without demonstrable pseudomembrane. Treatment with diphtheria antitoxin should begin as soon as the clinical diagnosis of diphtheria is made.

Definitive diagnosis of respiratory diphtheria is based on compatible clinical findings supported by the isolation of *C. diphtheriae* from local lesions or by histopathology. Rarely, respiratory diphtheria may be caused by infection with tox+ *C. ulcerans*, and such cases should be managed like cases caused by *C. diphtheriae*. *C. pseudodiphtheriticum*, a tox− organism that is often part of the normal throat flora, can be associated with pseudomembranous pharyngitis or lower respiratory tract infection; however, unlike *C. diphtheriae*, it does not pose a significant risk to contacts of infected patients. Specimens from the nose, throat, and membrane (and, when possible, from beneath the membrane) should be submitted for culture. The laboratory should be notified that diphtheria is suspected to ensure that one appropriate selective medium, such as cysteine-tellurite blood agar or Tinsdale medium, is used in addition to a nonselective medium (e.g., sheep blood agar) for primary plating of the specimens. Biochemical tests needed to differentiate *C. diphtheriae* from corynebacteria of the normal flora (diphtheroids) require several days. Group A β-hemolytic streptococci and *Staphylococcus aureus* are also isolated frequently from patients with diphtheria. All laboratory isolates of *C. diphtheriae*, whether or not they are associated with disease, should be submitted to the Diphtheria Laboratory, National Center for Infectious Diseases, CDC, for confirmation of biotype and toxinogenicity and for other specialized tests.

Cutaneous diphtheria may present as a characteristic "punched-out" ulcer with a membrane, but it is more often indistinguishable from other inflammatory dermatoses. Diagnosis depends on a high degree of suspicion and on culture of cutaneous lesions on laboratory media appropriate for isolation of *C. diphtheriae*. Throat samples from all patients with cutaneous diphtheria should be cultured for *C. diphtheriae*.

℞ TREATMENT

Administration of diphtheria antitoxin is the most import element in the treatment of respiratory diphtheria. The decision to administer diphtheria antitoxin must be based on the clinical diagnosis of respiratory diphtheria, without waiting for definitive laboratory confirmation. Since antitoxin cannot neutralize toxin that is already bound to tissues, each day of delay in initiating treatment with antitoxin is associated with a significant increase in mortality risk. Because diphtheria antitoxin is produced in horses, it is necessary to question patients about possible allergy to horse serum and to perform a conjunctival or intracutaneous test with diluted antitoxin for immediate hypersensitivity. Epinephrine must be available for immediate administration to patients with severe allergic reactions. Patients with immediate hypersensitivity should be desensitized before a full therapeutic dose of antitoxin is given. The risk of serum sickness associated with administration of equine antitoxin is acceptable because of the established therapeutic value of antitoxin in decreasing mortality from respiratory diphtheria. Since 1997, diphtheria antitoxin has been available in the United States only from the CDC and is distributed under an Investigational New Drug (IND) protocol. Physicians should promptly notify their state health departments of suspected diphtheria cases. To obtain diphtheria antitoxin and consultation on its use, physicians should promptly contact staff at the National Immunization Program at (404) 639-8255 during office hours from 8:00 A.M. to 4:30 P.M. eastern standard time or through the CDC operator at (404) 639-2889 or (404) 639-2888 at any time.

Antibiotics have little demonstrated effect on the healing of local infection in diphtheria patients treated with antitoxin. The primary goal of antibiotic therapy for patients or carriers is therefore to eradicate *C. diphtheriae* and prevent its transmission from the patient to susceptible contacts. Regimens currently recommended by the CDC for the treatment of patients with respiratory diphtheria are erythromycin given orally or by injection for 14 days (40 mg/kg per day; maximum, 2 g/d) or procaine penicillin G given intramuscularly for 14 days (300,000 U/d for patients weighing ≤10 kg and 600,000 U/d for those weighing >10 kg). Rifampin or clindamycin has also been used successfully and is an acceptable alternative for treating patients who cannot take penicillin G or erythromycin. Eradication of *C. diphtheriae* should be documented by negative cultures of samples taken on two or three successive days at least 24 h after the completion of antibiotic therapy. Some authorities also recommend a repeat throat culture 2 weeks later. The small percentage of patients who continue to be infected with *C. diphtheriae* after treatment with penicillin or erythromcyin should receive an additional 10-day course of oral erythromycin followed by a repeat culture for *C. diphtheriae*. Plasmid-mediated resistance to erythromycin emerged transiently in *C. diphtheriae* during the Seattle epidemic, but its frequency declined dramatically after the routine use of erythromycin was discontinued.

Patients with respiratory or cutaneous diphtheria caused by tox⁺ *C. diphtheriae* or by *C. diphtheriae* strains of unknown toxinogenicity should be hospitalized, kept in bed initially, handled with isolation procedures appropriate for the site of infection, and given supportive care as needed. Respiratory and cardiac function must be monitored closely. Early intubation or tracheostomy is recommended when the larynx is involved or signs of impending airway obstruction are detected. Tracheobronchial membrane can sometimes be removed mechanically via the endotracheal tube or tracheostomy. Primary or secondary pneumonia should be diagnosed and treated promptly. Sedative or hypnotic drugs that may mask respiratory symptoms are contraindicated. Close electrocardiographic monitoring, treatment of arrhythmias, and electrical pacing for heart block are essential. Congestive heart failure should be treated as described in Chap. 216. Glucocorticoids do not reduce the risk of diphtheritic myocarditis or polyneuropathy. Ulcerative or ecthymatous cutaneous lesions should be treated with Burow's solution applied on wet compresses after debridement of necrotic areas, and treatment for associated conditions such as pediculosis, scabies, or underlying dermatoses should be instituted. Recovery from diphtheria does not always confer active immunity, and initiation of an immunization regimen for diphtheria that is appropriate for the patient's age should be an integral part of the treatment plan.

PREVENTION DTaP (diphtheria and tetanus toxoids and acellular pertussis vaccine adsorbed) is currently recommended for all doses in the primary immunization schedule for children up to age 7 years who do not have contraindications. Td (tetanus and diphtheria toxoids adsorbed; for adult use) is currently recommended for routine booster immunizations at 10-year intervals in adults who do not have contraindications. Td is also recommended for adults who require prophylactic booster immunizations for tetanus-prone wounds. Currently recommended schedules for primary immunization of children and adults against diphtheria and for maintenance of immunity by periodic booster doses of appropriate vaccines throughout life are summarized in Chap. 107.

Close contacts of patients with respiratory diphtheria, especially household contacts, should have throat and nasal specimens collected and cultured for *C. diphtheriae*, should receive a 7- to 10-day course of either benzathine penicillin G (600,000 U for persons <6 years old or 1,200,000 U for persons ≥6 years old) or oral erythromycin (40 mg/kg per day for children and 1 g/d for adults), and should promptly receive diphtheria antitoxin if they become ill. Contacts whose immunization status is inadequate should receive a booster dose of diphtheria toxoid appropriate for their age. In situations where surveillance of contacts cannot be maintained, the benzathine penicillin G regimen should be used for treatment to ensure compliance. Contacts of patients with cutaneous diphtheria should be treated similarly, except that ongoing investigation of contacts can be discontinued if the strain of *C. diphtheriae* from the patient is found to be nontoxinogenic. Identified carriers of *C. diphtheriae* in the community should also be treated with the recommended regimen for contacts.

OTHER CORYNEBACTERIAL INFECTIONS

DEFINITION Medically important coryneform bacteria include 36 of 59 currently recognized species in the genus *Corynebacterium* plus numerous other taxonomically related organisms that share specific 16S rDNA signature nucleotides and belong to the high-guanosine-plus-cytosine lineage of gram-positive bacteria. They include environmental organisms and members of the normal flora that cause opportunistic infections, human pathogens of relatively low virulence, and animal pathogens that cause zoonotic infections. Reported infections caused by coryneform bacteria have increased substantially in number over the past several decades. Isolates of *C. jeikeium* and *C. urealyticum* are often resistant to multiple antibiotics.

ETIOLOGY AND LABORATORY DIAGNOSIS Because coryneform bacteria are potential pathogens, it is important not to dismiss them arbitrarily as components of the normal flora or as contaminants when they are found in clinical specimens. Coryneform bacteria should be identified to the species level when they are isolated from normally sterile body sites (unless only one of several specimens is positive for growth), when they represent the predominant organisms in appropriately collected clinical specimens, and when they are present as the only organism in urine at a count of >10⁴/mL or as the predominant organisms in urine with a total bacterial count of >10⁵/mL.

The coryneform bacteria are a large, heterogeneous group of gram-positive, pleomorphic, irregularly staining bacilli or coccobacilli that superficially resemble *C. diphtheriae*, have widely varying guanosine-plus-cytosine contents (from 46 to 74% guanosine plus cytosine) for members of the genus *Corynebacterium*, and are often difficult to identify and classify. Club-shaped rod forms are observed only for true *Corynebacterium* species. The genus *Corynebacterium* is currently divided into three groups: the nonlipophilic, fermentative corynebacteria (including *C. diphtheriae*, *C. ulcerans*, *C. pseudotuberculosis*, *C. xerosis*, *C. striatum*, *C. minutissimum*, and others); the nonlipophilic, nonfermentative corynebacteria (including *C. pseudodiphtheriticum* and others); and the lipophilic corynebacteria (including *C. jeikeium*, *C. urealyticum*, and others). The coryneform group includes additional genera, such as *Arcanobacterium* and *Rhodococcus*. Classification of coryneform bacteria is based on routine and molecular genetics–based diagnostic methods; these methods are often supplemented by chemotaxonomic methods that include identification of the short-chain mycolic acids present in most *Corynebacterium* species but absent in other coryneform bacteria, determination of the specific diamino acid present in peptidoglycan, and characterization of the major cellular fatty acids. The classification system for coryneform bacteria is evolving rapidly, with 14 new species defined in the past 5 years. All coryneform bacteria that are clinically significant but cannot be readily identified in routine diagnostic laboratories should be submitted to an appropriate reference laboratory experienced in this area.

ECOLOGY AND EPIDEMIOLOGY   Humans are the probable natural reservoir for *C. xerosis*, *C. pseudodiphtheriticum*, *C. striatum*, *C. minutissimum*, *C. jeikeium*, *C. urealyticum*, and *Arcanobacterium haemolyticum*. Animals are the probable natural reservoir for *Arcanobacterium pyogenes* (cows, sheep, pigs), *C. ulcerans* (cows, horses), and *C. pseudotuberculosis* (sheep, horses, goats, cattle). The natural reservoir for *Rhodococcus equi* is soil. The ecologic niches for many other coryneform bacteria of medical importance are not well defined.

Corynebacterial species that are found frequently as components of the normal human flora include *C. pseudodiphtheriticum* (pharynx, skin), *C. xerosis* (conjunctival sac, nasopharynx, skin), *C. auris* (external auditory canal), and *C. striatum* (anterior nares, skin). Corynebacterial species that commonly colonize the skin of hospitalized patients include *C. jeikeium* (axilla, groin, perineum) and *C. urealyticum*. *C. jeikeium* most often colonizes patients with malignancies or severe immunodeficiency; it is also isolated from environmental sources (surfaces, air) in hospitals and from the hands of ward staff. *C. ulcerans* infections are acquired by consumption of raw milk. *C. pseudotuberculosis* infections are acquired by contact with animals or animal products or by consumption of raw milk.

PATHOGENESIS AND CLINICAL MANIFESTATIONS   *C. ulcerans* infections of humans usually present as pharyngitis and can mimic respiratory diphtheria, whereas infections caused by *C. pseudotuberculosis* typically present as suppurative granulomatous lymphadenitis. Some strains of *C. ulcerans* and *C. pseudotuberculosis* can produce diphtheria toxin, but infections of humans with tox⁻ strains have been reported only for *C. ulcerans*. *C. ulcerans* infections that are presumed on clinical grounds to be caused by tox⁺ strains should be managed like diphtheria, and diphtheria antitoxin should be administered. *C. pseudodiphtheriticum*, a tox⁻ commensal of low virulence, is an uncommon cause of pneumonia in men with AIDS and of pharyngitis. It has also been associated with necrotizing tracheitis, tracheobronchitis, endocarditis, and urinary tract infection in patients without known immune deficiencies. Pharyngeal infections associated with *C. pseudodiphtheriticum* can be confused with diphtheria until the bacteriologic diagnosis is established; however, unlike diphtheria, these infections do not pose a danger to contacts. *C. xerosis* and *C. striatum* are constituents of the normal human flora that are of low virulence and rarely cause human infections.

C. jeikeium causes severe infections primarily in patients with hematologic malignancies and neutropenia. Skin colonization precedes clinical infection. Risk factors for nosocomial *C. jeikeium* sepsis include prolonged hospitalization, breaks in the integument, chronic intravascular catheterization, and prior treatment with broad-spectrum antibiotics. Other presentations of *C. jeikeium* infection include endocarditis, device-related infections, pulmonary infiltrates, cutaneous septic emboli, soft tissue infections, and rashes. Endocarditis due to *C. jeikeium* occurs primarily in patients with prosthetic heart valves. *C. jeikeium* is a rare cause of central nervous system infections in patients with ventricular shunts.

C. urealyticum is a significant cause of nosocomial urinary tract infections, including acute and chronic cystitis and pyelonephritis. The organism closely resembles *C. jeikeium* but differs from the latter by producing urease and failing to convert glucose to acidic metabolites. Hydrolysis of urea by urease causes alkalinization of the urine and formation of ammonium magnesium phosphate (struvite) stones. *C. urealyticum* is a cause of alkaline-encrusted cystitis in patients with preexisting bladder lesions that serve as foci for precipitation of struvite crystals. Risk factors associated with symptomatic urinary tract infections include preexisting immunosuppression, recent urologic

procedures (including renal transplantation), underlying disorders of the genitourinary tract, and a history of urinary tract infections.

C. minutissimum is frequently isolated from the lesions of erythrasma, a common superficial skin infection characterized by the presence in intertriginous areas of reddish-brown, scaly, pruritic, macular patches that exhibit coral-red fluorescence under a Wood's light. The etiology of erythrasma appears to be polymicrobial; infection of the skin by *C. minutissimum* follows the onset of maceration and scaling. Deep infections caused by *C. minutissimum*, which are rare, include abscesses, bacteremia, endocarditis, peritonitis, pyelonephritis, and infection of central venous catheters.

A. haemolyticum causes pharyngitis and chronic skin ulcers. Less frequently, it causes a variety of deep tissue infections, septicemia, and endocarditis. Some 90% of *A. haemolyticum* infections occur in patients between 10 and 30 years old. *A. haemolyticum* pharyngitis in this age group is 5 to 13% as frequent as *Streptococcus pyogenes* pharyngitis. An erythematous rash is present in 30 to 67% of cases. The rash is usually scarlatiniform and most pronounced on the trunk and proximal extremities, but it sometimes resembles urticaria or erythema multiforme. Because rash is more frequent in *A. haemolyticum* infections than in *S. pyogenes* infections, *A. haemolyticum* should be considered as a possible etiology in older children and adults who present with the scarlet fever syndrome. Infection due to *A. haemolyticum* can also present as extensive pharyngeal exudate and can mimic diphtheria. *A. haemolyticum* occasionally causes peritonsillar abscess, sepsis, endocarditis, or meningitis.

A. pyogenes causes bovine mastitis, a disease transmitted by flies. Yearly epidemics of leg ulcers infected with *A. pyogenes* among schoolchildren in Thailand occurred between 1979 and 1984 and were postulated to have resulted from introduction of the organism into traumatic skin lesions by flies. Reported *A. pyogenes* infections in adults in Denmark have included abscesses, cystitis, intraabdominal infections, and mastoiditis with bacteremia.

R. equi, which causes bronchopneumonia in horses and occasional infections in other animals, has emerged as an important intracellular opportunistic pathogen in immunocompromised patients. Most reported cases are necrotizing pulmonary infections that resemble tuberculosis or nocardiosis in patients with severely defective cell-mediated immunity, including those with AIDS.

DIAGNOSIS   Pharyngitis caused by tox⁺ strains of *C. ulcerans* may be clinically indistinguishable from diphtheria. The presentations of infections caused by other coryneform bacteria are not pathognomonic, and diagnosis of these infections is based on a high index of suspicion, identification of the organism by culture in appropriate clinical specimens, and exclusion of other likely causes of infection. Sheep blood agar containing fosfomycin (100 μg/mL) or colistin–nalidixic acid blood agar is useful as a selective medium for most coryneform bacteria, and medium containing 0.1 to 1% Tween 80 is useful for isolation of lipophilic coryneform bacteria.

Since *C. urealyticum* is often undetected by routine urine cultures; it is necessary to incubate cultures for 24 to 48 h on blood agar or on special media for selected patients (especially elderly men with preexisting genitourinary abnormalities) with alkaline urine, ammonium magnesium phosphate stones, gram-positive bacilli in the urine, or negative standard urine cultures despite clinical evidence of bacteriuria. Other microbes that can cause urinary tract infections with alkaline urine include *Proteus*, *Ureaplasma*, and some staphylococci and streptococci. Alkaline-encrusted cystitis is an anatomic diagnosis made by cystoscopy.

The differential diagnosis of *A. haemolyticum* pharyngitis with rash includes scarlet fever; rubella; staphylococcal and streptococcal toxic shock syndromes; infections caused by Epstein-Barr virus, cytomegalovirus, and enteroviruses (especially coxsackieviruses); disseminated gonococcal infection; secondary syphilis; and drug allergy. Routine diagnostic methods for throat cultures are not ideal for the detection of *A. haemolyticum*, nor is this organism detected by the rapid tests for *S. pyogenes* that are sometimes substituted for throat cultures. Pharyngitis caused by *A. haemolyticum* in adolescents and adults is likely to remain underdiagnosed until improved tests for the organism are developed and used by diagnostic laboratories.

Erythrasma is diagnosed clinically. Because of uncertainty about the etiologic role of *C. minutissimum*, culture of erythrasma lesions is not currently recommended.

℞ TREATMENT

Since prediction of susceptibility patterns on the basis of isolate identification to the species level is not necessarily reliable, antimicrobial susceptibility testing should be performed on all isolates of clinically significant coryneform bacteria. In light of the emergence and spread of vancomycin resistance in several gram-positive bacterial species as well as the observation of intrinsic vancomycin resistance in some species of coryneform bacteria (e.g., *Microbacterium resistens*), some authorities have recently recommended that glycopeptide antibiotics not be used as first-line agents to treat infections caused by coryneform bacteria. Physicians treating infections caused by coryneform bacteria that are likely to exhibit resistance to multiple antibiotics should obtain expert consultation concerning current treatment recommendations.

Strains of *C. jeikeium* are typically resistant to most antibiotics. Vancomycin has been recommended most often as the drug of choice for empirical treatment of infections caused by this organism, although antimicrobial susceptibility testing may reveal other antibiotic options for some isolates. For device-related *C. jeikeium* infections, removal of the infected device is usually required in addition to appropriate antibiotic therapy.

C. urealyticum is often resistant to the antibiotics used commonly for the treatment of urinary tract infections. Empirical treatment with vancomycin has often been recommended pending the results of antimicrobial susceptibility testing. Several courses of antibiotic therapy may be necessary for bacteriologic cure. Patients with alkaline-encrusted cystitis require resection of the encrusted lesions in addition to antibiotic therapy.

No controlled trials of treatment for *A. haemolyticum* infections have been performed. In vitro tests usually demonstrate susceptibility to penicillins, erythromycin, azithromycin, clindamycin, doxycycline, ciprofloxacin, and vancomycin, but treatment failures have been reported with appropriate doses of penicillins. Limited data suggest that the clinical course of *A. haemolyticum* pharyngitis may be shortened by treatment with erythromycin.

Infections with *C. ulcerans* that present like diphtheria or are known to be caused by tox+ strains should be treated like diphtheria. Oral erythromycin is usually effective for treatment of erythrasma. For infections caused by *R. equi*, vancomycin has often been recommended as the drug of choice. Possible alternatives include erythromycin, rifampin, aminoglycosides, and chloramphenicol; the combination of erythromycin and rifampin is attractive because of possible synergy. Penicillins should not be used, because *R. equi* rapidly develops resistance. Many weeks of antibiotic treatment, sometimes supplemented by surgical intervention, are often needed for infections caused by *R. equi*. Suppressive therapy with antibiotics should be continued indefinitely in patients with AIDS after initial treatment of infections caused by *R. equi*. Initial treatment of infections caused by other coryneform bacteria should be based on the identity of the organism and published data regarding antibiotic susceptibility. Therapy should be modified, when necessary, in light of the results of antibiotic susceptibility tests.

FURTHER READING

Brown AE: Other corynebacteria and *Rhodococcus*, in *Mandell, Douglas, and Bennett's Principles and Practice of Infectious Diseases*, vol 2, 5th ed, GL Mandell et al (eds). Philadelphia, Churchill Livingstone, 2000, pp 2198–2208

Funke G, Bernard KA: Coryneform gram-positive rods, in *Manual of Clinical Microbiology*, 8th ed, PR Murray et al (eds). Washington, DC, ASM Press, 2003, pp 472–501

Hadfield TL: The pathology of diphtheria. J Infect Dis 181(Suppl 1):S116, 2000

Holmes RK: Biology and molecular epidemiology of diphtheria toxin and the *tox* gene. J Infect Dis 181(Suppl 1):S156, 2000

Kadirova R et al: Clinical characteristics and management of 676 hospitalized diphtheria cases, Kyrgyz Republic, 1995. J Infect Dis 181(Suppl 1): S110, 2000

McQuillan GM et al: Serologic immunity to diphtheria and tetanus in the United States. Ann Intern Med 136:660, 2002

Ohuabunowo CJ et al: Diphtheria, in *Centers for Disease Control and Prevention. Manual for the Surveillance of Vaccine-Preventable Diseases*, 3d ed, M Wharton et al (eds). 2002, pp 1-1–1-8 [http://www.cdc.gov/nip/publications/surv-manual/default.htm]

123 INFECTIONS CAUSED BY *LISTERIA MONOCYTOGENES*
Anne Schuchat, Claire V. Broome

Listeria monocytogenes is a gram-positive rod that can be isolated from soil, vegetation, and many animal reservoirs. Human disease due to *L. monocytogenes* generally occurs in the setting of pregnancy or of immunosuppression caused by illness or medication. Increasing evidence suggests that a substantial portion of cases of human listeriosis are attributable to the food-borne transmission of *L. monocytogenes*. Unlike most food-borne pathogens, which cause primarily gastrointestinal illness, *L. monocytogenes* causes invasive syndromes, such as meningitis, sepsis, chorioamnionitis, and stillbirth.

ETIOLOGY Listeriae are aerobic or facultatively anaerobic, nonsporulating gram-positive bacilli that grow at 1 to 45°C and typically have tumbling motility when cultured at 20 to 25°C. Characteristics that help distinguish *L. monocytogenes* from other *Listeria* spp. include the formation of a narrow zone of β hemolysis on sheep blood agar and the production of acid from glucose, maltose, L-rhamnose, and α-methyl-D-mannoside but not from D-xylose. Determination of the serotype of *L. monocytogenes* is based on somatic (O) and flagellar (H) antigens. Most cases of human disease are caused by serotypes 1/2a, 1/2b, and 4b. Subtyping, especially by pulsed-field gel electrophoresis, has made it easier to discriminate among strains of *Listeria* and thus to link environmental or food isolates with clinical infections.

PATHOGENESIS *L. monocytogenes* is an intracellular pathogen—characteristic consistent with its predilection for causing illness in persons with deficient cell-mediated immunity. The organism can be found as part of the gastrointestinal flora in healthy individuals. Lack of gastric acidity and abnormal gastrointestinal functioning may increase the risk of invasive disease following exposure to the organism in the gastrointestinal tract. The increased risk of *L. monocytogenes* infection in pregnant women may be due to both systemic and local immunologic changes associated with pregnancy. For example, local immunosuppression at the maternal-fetal interface of the placenta may facilitate intrauterine infection following transient maternal bacteremia.

The molecular pathogenesis of *L. monocytogenes* has been elucidated. The cell-surface protein internalin interacts with specific receptors to induce phagocytosis. Both listeriolysin O and phospholipases permit the organism to escape from the phagosome into the cytosol while avoiding intracellular killing. Through the surface protein Act A, *L. monocytogenes* uses actin-based motility to move to the cell membrane. Efficient cell-to-cell spread is accomplished by both actin filament formation and phospholipase production. Genetic determinants of these proteins have been characterized. Because the organism is adapted for both intracellular survival and direct cell-to-cell spread, it is not eliminated by antibodies.

EPIDEMIOLOGY Long recognized as a veterinary pathogen, *L. mono-cytogenes* causes basilar meningitis ("circling disease") and stillbirth in sheep and cattle. The occurrence of listeriosis among humans has received increasing attention as the role of contaminated foods in the pathogenesis of epidemic listeriosis has been recognized and reports of disease associated with the expanding immunosuppressed population have accumulated.

Invasive listeriosis—confirmed by culture of blood or cerebrospinal fluid (CSF)—occurs in approximately 3 to 5 individuals per million population annually in the United States. Perinatal listeriosis complicates 9 births per 100,000. A 40% decline in incidence since the period from 1986 through 1990 may be attributable to aggressive food regulation and industrial clean-up efforts. Incidence further declined by 35% from 1996 through 2001. Multistate surveillance for sporadic listeriosis suggests that 20% of infections are fatal or result in stillbirth, although higher case-fatality rates have been reported during listeriosis epidemics and were described in early series. Most cases of disease due to *L. monocytogenes* are sporadic; however, investigation of several outbreaks of listeriosis since 1980 has demonstrated common-source food-borne transmission as a cause of human illness and has shown that the incubation period for disease following consumption of contaminated food can be 2 to 6 weeks. The largest North American outbreak, which took place in Los Angeles in 1985, involved more than 100 cases and 48 deaths or stillbirths. A nationwide outbreak in France in 1992 involved 279 cases and 63 deaths. Foods implicated in outbreaks of listeriosis include contaminated coleslaw, pasteurized milk, soft cheeses, pâté, ready-to-eat turkey and pork products, hot dogs, butter, and prepared salads; epidemiologic studies have implicated undercooked chicken, uncooked hot dogs, soft cheeses, and food from store delicatessen counters in sporadic disease. Listerial contamination of foods is relatively common. Among foods contaminated with the organism, those that are purchased ready to eat, are contaminated with serotype 4b, and are contaminated at a relatively high level may be the most likely to cause illness. The long incubation period associated with listeriosis contributes to the difficulty of implicating specific foods as the cause of either common-source outbreaks or sporadic cases.

Although food-borne transmission appears to be the foremost cause of epidemic and sporadic disease, several clusters of late-onset neonatal infection suggest nosocomial transmission of *L. monocytogenes*. Contaminated multiuse materials and equipment have been suggested as causes of some nosocomial clusters. Listeriosis has been reported in veterinarians and other persons in close contact with infected animals.

CLINICAL PRESENTATION *Pregnancy-associated listeriosis* may occur during any stage of pregnancy, although most infections are detected during the third trimester, possibly because of failure to obtain specimens for bacterial culture earlier during gestation in instances of abortion and stillbirth. One-half to two-thirds of pregnant women with perinatal listeriosis experience a mild illness characterized by fever, myalgias, malaise, and backache, which sometimes are accompanied by diarrhea, abdominal pain, nausea, and/or vomiting during the bacteremic phase. Blood cultures should be used for diagnosis. Transplacental spread of the organism results in intrauterine infection, which can lead to chorioamnionitis, premature labor, intrauterine fetal demise, or early-onset disease of the newborn. Women with listeriosis diagnosed during pregnancy have a favorable clinical outcome after antibiotic therapy or delivery. Although often included in the differential diagnosis of recurrent spontaneous abortion, infection with *L. monocytogenes* appears to cause fewer than 2% of stillbirths.

Neonatal listeriosis can be classified under the same categories used for group B streptococcal infection (Chap. 121), with early-onset disease evident during the first week of life and late-onset disease developing thereafter. Infants may be symptomatic at birth; most infants with early-onset disease are symptomatic by the second day of life. Aspiration of infected amniotic fluid contributes to pathogenesis. Early-onset disease may include sepsis, respiratory distress, skin le-

sions, and the syndrome called *granulomatosis infantisepticum*, which is characterized by disseminated abscesses involving the liver, spleen, adrenal glands, lungs, and other sites. Infants with late-onset neonatal disease are more likely than those with early-onset disease to develop meningitis. While early-onset disease is often associated with obstetric complications such as premature delivery and chorioamnionitis, late-onset disease typically affects infants born at term by uncomplicated deliveries. Infants may acquire *L. monocytogenes* during passage through the birth canal; except in several clusters of late-onset neonatal infections linked to nosocomial transmission, the pathogenesis of late-onset disease is not well understood.

Listeriosis not associated with pregnancy usually affects persons with immunosuppressive conditions, although invasive disease can also affect immunocompetent adults, particularly elderly persons. The most common underlying conditions in nonpregnant adults with listeriosis are chronic glucocorticoid therapy, solid or hematologic malignancies (particularly in fludarabine-treated patients), diabetes mellitus, renal disease, liver disease, and AIDS. Although the prevalence of listeriosis among persons infected with HIV is much higher than that in the general population, listeriosis is a relatively uncommon opportunistic infection in AIDS.

Sepsis Clinical studies have shown that bacteremic infection without an evident focus is the most common clinical manifestation of listeriosis among immunocompromised hosts, while infection of the central nervous system (CNS) ranks second in frequency. Listerial sepsis cannot be distinguished clinically from bacteremia involving other organisms. Patients are usually febrile, often appear extremely ill, and may have prodromal symptoms including myalgia, nausea, vomiting, and diarrhea. Immunocompromised patients with listeriosis are less likely than other *Listeria*-infected adults to present with CNS infection, possibly because they are more likely to have blood cultured during febrile episodes and thus to have transient listerial bacteremia recognized.

CNS Infection The most common presentation of CNS infection due to *L. monocytogenes* is meningitis, which can present as either an acute or (less often) a subacute illness. Presenting symptoms include fever, headache, and an altered level of consciousness. Examination of CSF usually reveals pleocytosis, increased protein concentrations, and normal glucose levels, although other patterns are sometimes found. Gram's stain is positive in only 25% of cases. The diagnosis is made when *L. monocytogenes* is identified on culture. Despite its name, *L. monocytogenes* is rarely associated with monocytosis of either CSF or blood. Other syndromes seen in CNS infection include meningoencephalitis; cerebritis; and brainstem, spinal cord, or intracranial abscesses. The unusual syndrome of rhombencephalitis includes asymmetric cranial-nerve palsies, altered consciousness, cerebellar signs, and motor or sensory loss. Symptoms of other nonmeningitic CNS infections include fever, ataxia, seizures, personality changes, and coma. Nuchal rigidity is rare in nonmeningitic infections. CSF cultures may be sterile; blood cultures are usually diagnostic.

Endocarditis Like most forms of bacterial endocarditis, listerial endocarditis typically occurs in patients with prosthetic or previously damaged valves. The organism has a predilection for the left side of the heart. Endocarditis due to *L. monocytogenes* is often associated with systemic embolization.

Focal Infections Other focal infections that can follow unrecognized bacteremia include endophthalmitis, peritonitis, osteomyelitis, visceral abscess, pleuropulmonary infection, and cholecystitis. Cutaneous lesions may develop without systemic involvement and have been reported in veterinarians and poultry workers.

Gastrointestinal Illness Several common-source outbreaks of acute febrile gastroenteritis suggest that *L. monocytogenes* can cause an acute diarrheal syndrome in persons without immunocompromising conditions. The importance of *L. monocytogenes* in sporadic diarrheal illness is unclear. Although the organism is not identified by the culture methods routinely used for stool specimens, studies using selective enrichment media for evaluation of consecutive specimens from patients hospitalized with acute diarrhea have suggested that *L. monocytogenes* is not a major cause of sporadic diarrhea.

Recurrences Recurrent infection with *L. monocytogenes* has been reported but is rare. Many recurrences are due to the subtype responsible for the initial infection. The implication is that such recurrences result either from insufficient treatment of a focus of primary infection or from repeated exposure to a persistently contaminated source.

DIAGNOSIS Invasive listeriosis is diagnosed when the organism is cultured from a site that is usually sterile, such as blood, CSF, or amniotic fluid. The organism grows readily within 36 h on routine culture media, but morphologic similarities between *Listeria* and diphtheroids make it necessary to use biochemical tests to identify the species. Serologic assays with whole-cell antigens have not been useful for the diagnosis of listeriosis, both because exposure to the organism (and thus the presence of antibody) may be common and because infected individuals may not produce antibody. Assays for antibody to listeriolysin O have been applied in epidemiologic investigations and, retrospectively, in the diagnosis of culture-negative CNS infection. Culture of the organism from nonsterile sites such as the vagina and rectum is not useful for clinical diagnosis, as the organism may be carried at these sites by ~5% of healthy individuals.

Differential diagnosis of prematurity, spontaneous abortion, or stillbirth includes infectious diseases such as group B streptococcal infection, congenital syphilis, and toxoplasmosis; pathogens such as group B streptococci and *Escherichia coli* are more common than *L. monocytogenes* as causes of meningitis and sepsis in the newborn period. Listerial infection should always be considered in the differential diagnosis of meningitis in immunosuppressed persons, particularly transplant recipients and others undergoing glucocorticoid treatment, patients with hematologic malignancy, and HIV-infected patients. Among healthy adults, meningitis is much more likely to be caused by *Neisseria meningitidis*, *Streptococcus pneumoniae*, or viral pathogens than by *L. monocytogenes*.

℞ TREATMENT

The treatment of choice for listeriosis is intravenous administration of either ampicillin or penicillin, often in combination with an aminoglycoside for synergy. Trimethoprim-sulfamethoxazole is bactericidal against *L. monocytogenes* and has been used successfully in the treatment of patients with penicillin allergy. *L. monocytogenes* is susceptible in vitro to penicillin G, ampicillin, erythromycin, trimethoprim-sulfamethoxazole, chloramphenicol, rifampin, tetracyclines, aminoglycosides, and imipenem. However, chloramphenicol and rifampin may antagonize the bactericidal effect of penicillins. Because *L. monocytogenes* is not sensitive to cephalosporins, these agents should not be used for single-agent empirical treatment of neonatal sepsis or of meningitis in newborns or immunocompromised hosts.

Dosages and durations of therapy have not been subjected to controlled trials. For nonpregnant adults with listeriosis, the regimen of choice is either ampicillin (12 g intravenously per day in six divided doses) or penicillin G (15 to 20 million units intravenously per day in six divided doses); for immunosuppressed patients with meningitis, some experts add gentamicin (1.3 mg/kg intravenously every 8 h) for synergy. Penicillin-allergic patients may be treated with trimethoprim-sulfamethoxazole (15/75 mg/kg intravenously per day in three equal portions every 8 h). Meningitis in an immunocompetent patient may require 2 to 3 weeks of antibiotic therapy after defervescence. Meningitis, bacteremia, endocarditis, and nonmeningitic listeriosis in immunosuppressed patients should be treated longer, probably for 4 to 6 weeks. Neonatal listeriosis can be treated with a 2-week course of ampicillin. Infants weighing <2000 g should receive 100 mg/kg per day in two equal doses during the first week of life and 150 mg/kg per day during the second week. Infants weighing ≥2000 g should receive 150 mg/kg per day in three equal doses during the first week of life and 200 mg/kg per day during the second week. The addition of an aminoglycoside should be considered for neonatal infection (genta-

TABLE 123-1 *Dietary Recommendations for the Prevention of Food-Borne Listeriosis*

Recommendations to all individuals
1. Thoroughly cook raw food from animal sources, such as beef, pork, and poultry.
2. Wash raw vegetables thoroughly before eating them.
3. Keep uncooked meats separate from vegetables and from cooked and ready-to-eat foods.
4. Avoid raw (unpasteurized) milk or foods made from raw milk.
5. Wash hands, knives, and cutting boards after handling uncooked foods.

Additional recommendations to high-risk individuals[a]
6. Avoid soft cheeses such as Mexican-style, feta, Brie, Camembert, and blue-veined cheese. There is no need to avoid hard cheeses, cream cheese, cottage cheese, or yogurt.
7. Leftover foods or ready-to-eat foods, such as hot dogs, should be reheated until steaming hot before being eaten.
8. Although the risk of listeriosis associated with foods from delicatessen counters is relatively low and poorly characterized, pregnant women and immunosuppressed persons may choose to avoid these foods or to thoroughly reheat cold cuts before eating them.

[a] Persons immunocompromised by illness or medications; pregnant women.

micin, 5 mg/kg per day in two divided doses during the first week of life; 7.5 mg/kg per day in three equal doses during the second week). For listeriosis in pregnant women, a 2-week course of ampicillin (4 to 6 g per day in four equal doses) is recommended. During the last month of pregnancy, infected women with serious penicillin allergies may be treated with erythromycin.

PROGNOSIS Treatment of maternal bacteremia during pregnancy can prevent neonatal infection. Antibiotic therapy for the newborn can limit sequelae, although the widely disseminated disease characteristic of granulomatosis infantisepticum is frequently fatal regardless of treatment. Early-onset disease carries a higher mortality risk than late-onset infection, and immunocompromised hosts have a worse prognosis than do otherwise-healthy adults with listeriosis.

PREVENTION *L. monocytogenes* is frequently isolated from food; the Food and Drug Administration, the U.S. Department of Agriculture, and manufacturers are pursuing further measures to reduce *L. monocytogenes* contamination of foods that have been subjected to listericidal processing. Prevention of listeriosis requires dietary counseling of persons at increased risk of disease (Table 123-1). There is no role for the administration of prophylaxis to contacts of patients with listeriosis. Clinicians are encouraged to report cases of listeriosis to local or state health departments. Case reporting and subtyping of clinical isolates can facilitate early recognition of outbreaks and prevention of subsequent cases.

FURTHER READING

AURELI P et al: An outbreak of febrile gastroenteritis associated with corn contaminated by *Listeria monocytogenes*. N Engl J Med 342:1236, 2000
PINNER RW et al: Role of foods in sporadic listeriosis: II. Microbiologic and epidemiologic investigation. JAMA 267:2046, 1992
RYSER ET, MARTH EH (eds): *Listeria, Listeriosis, and Food Safety*, 2d ed. New York, Marcel Dekker, 1999
SCHLECH WF III: Foodborne listeriosis. Clin Infect Dis 31:770, 2000
SCHUCHAT A et al: Role of foods in sporadic listeriosis: I. Case-control study of dietary risk factors. JAMA 267:2041, 1992
SLUTSKER L et al: Listeriosis, in *Emerging Infections 4*, W Scheld et al (eds). Washington, DC, ASM Press, 2000, pp 83–106
SOUTHWICK FS, PURICH DL: Intracellular pathogenesis of listeriosis. N Engl J Med 334:770, 1996
TAPPERO JW et al: Reduction in the incidence of human listeriosis in the United States—effectiveness of prevention efforts? JAMA 273:1118, 1995

124 | TETANUS
Elias Abrutyn

DEFINITION Tetanus is a neurologic disorder, characterized by increased muscle tone and spasms, that is caused by tetanospasmin, a powerful protein toxin elaborated by *Clostridium tetani*. Tetanus occurs in several clinical forms, including generalized, neonatal, and localized disease.

ETIOLOGIC AGENT *C. tetani* is an anaerobic, motile gram-positive rod that forms an oval, colorless, terminal spore and thus assumes a shape resembling a tennis racket or drumstick. The organism is found worldwide in soil, in the inanimate environment, in animal feces, and occasionally in human feces. Spores may survive for years in some environments and are resistant to various disinfectants and to boiling for 20 min. Vegetative cells, however, are easily inactivated and are susceptible to several antibiotics (metronidazole, penicillin, and others).

Tetanospasmin is formed in vegetative cells under plasmid control. It is a single polypeptide chain. With autolysis, the single-chain toxin is released and cleaved to form a heterodimer consisting of a heavy chain (100 kDa), which mediates binding to nerve-cell receptors and entry into these cells, and a light chain (50 kDa), which acts to block neurotransmitter release. The genome sequence of *C. tetani* has been reported. The amino acid structures of the two most powerful toxins known, botulinum toxin and tetanus toxin, are partially homologous.

EPIDEMIOLOGY Tetanus occurs sporadically and almost always affects nonimmunized persons, partially immunized persons, or fully immunized individuals who fail to maintain adequate immunity with booster doses of vaccine. Although tetanus is entirely preventable by immunization, the burden of disease is large worldwide. The disease is common in areas where soil is cultivated, in rural areas, in warm climates, during summer months, and among males. In countries without a comprehensive immunization program, tetanus occurs predominantly in neonates and other young children. It is noteworthy that international programs to eliminate neonatal tetanus have been in place for some time. In the United States and other nations with successful immunization programs, neonatal tetanus is rare (only one case was reported in the United States during the period 1998–2000), and the disease affects other age groups and groups inadequately covered by immunization (such as nonwhites). The success of immunization in the United States is depicted in Fig. 124-1. Since 1976, fewer than 100 cases have been reported yearly; this figure contrasts remarkably with that of 500 to 600 cases reported annually in the late 1940s, when vaccine administration became routine and tetanus became notifiable. In 1947, the incidence of tetanus was 3.9 cases per 1 million population. In contrast, the average annual incidence rate for 1998–2000 was

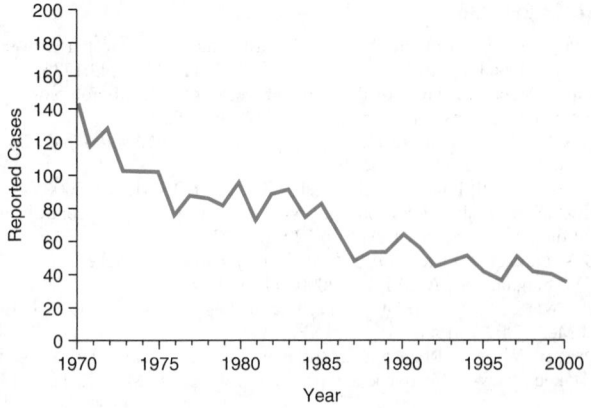

FIGURE 124-1 Tetanus: Reported cases by year—United States, 1970–2000. *[From Centers for Disease Control and Prevention: Summary of notifiable diseases, United States, 2000. MMWR 49(53):74, 2000.]*

0.16 per 1 million population. The risk for the development of tetanus is highest among the elderly. A large-scale national serologic survey for tetanus and diphtheria antibody performed in 1988–1994 showed that, overall, 72% of Americans over the age of 6 years were protected against tetanus. Whereas 91% of children 6 to 11 years old were protected, the percentage protected fell with age: only 30% of persons >70 years old (men, 45%; women, 21%) had adequate antibody levels. Notably, individuals 20 to 49 years old now account for a large proportion of cases, because fewer cases occurred in the elderly without a similar reduction among young and middle-aged adults.

In the United States, most cases of tetanus follow an acute injury, such as a puncture wound, laceration, or abrasion. Tetanus is acquired indoors or during farming, gardening, and other outdoor activities. The injury may be major but often is trivial, so that medical attention is not sought; in some instances no injury can be identified. The disease may complicate chronic conditions such as skin ulcers, abscesses, and gangrene. Tetanus is also associated with burns, frostbite, middle-ear infection, surgery, abortion, childbirth, body piercing, and drug abuse, notably "skin popping." In some patients no portal of entry for the organism can be identified.

PATHOGENESIS Contamination of wounds with spores of *C. tetani* is probably a frequent occurrence. Germination and toxin production, however, take place only in wounds with low oxidation-reduction potential, such as those with devitalized tissue, foreign bodies, or active infection. *C. tetani* does not itself evoke inflammation, and the portal of entry retains a benign appearance unless infection with other organisms is present.

Toxin released in the wound binds to peripheral motor neuron terminals, enters the axon, and is transported to the nerve-cell body in the brainstem and spinal cord by retrograde intraneuronal transport. The toxin then migrates across the synapse to presynaptic terminals, where it blocks release of the inhibitory neurotransmitters glycine and γ-aminobutyric acid (GABA). The blocking of neurotransmitter release by tetanospasmin, a zinc metalloprotease, involves the cleavage of protein(s) critical to proper function of the synaptic vesicle release apparatus. With diminished inhibition, the resting firing rate of the α motor neuron increases, producing rigidity. With lessened activity of reflexes that limit polysynaptic spread of impulses (a glycinergic activity), agonists and antagonists may be recruited rather than inhibited, with the consequent production of spasms. Loss of inhibition may also affect preganglionic sympathetic neurons in the lateral gray matter of the spinal cord and produce sympathetic hyperactivity and high circulating catecholamine levels. Tetanospasmin, like botulinum toxin, may block neurotransmitter release at the neuromuscular junction and produce weakness or paralysis; recovery requires sprouting of new nerve terminals.

In local tetanus, only the nerves supplying the affected muscles are involved. Generalized tetanus occurs when toxin released in the wound enters the lymphatics and bloodstream and is spread widely to distant nerve terminals; the blood-brain barrier blocks direct entry into the central nervous system. If it is assumed that intraneuronal transport times are equal for all nerves, short nerves are affected before long nerves: this fact explains the sequential involvement of nerves of the head, trunk, and extremities in generalized tetanus.

CLINICAL MANIFESTATIONS *Generalized tetanus,* the most common form of the disease, is characterized by increased muscle tone and generalized spasms. The median time of onset after injury is 7 days; 15% of cases occur within 3 days and 10% after 14 days.

Typically, the patient first notices increased tone in the masseter muscles (trismus, or lockjaw). Dysphagia or stiffness or pain in the neck, shoulder, and back muscles appears concurrently or soon thereafter. The subsequent involvement of other muscles produces a rigid abdomen and stiff proximal limb muscles; the hands and feet are relatively spared. Sustained contraction of the facial muscles results in a grimace or sneer (risus sardonicus), and contraction of the back muscles produces an arched back (opisthotonos). Some patients develop paroxysmal, violent, painful, generalized muscle spasms that may cause cyanosis and threaten ventilation. These spasms occur repetitively and may be spontaneous or provoked by even the slightest stimulation. A constant threat during generalized spasms is reduced ventilation or apnea or laryngospasm. The severity of illness may be mild (muscle rigidity and few or no spasms), moderate (trismus, dysphagia, rigidity, and spasms), or severe (frequent explosive paroxysms). The patient may be febrile, although many have no fever; mentation is unimpaired. Deep tendon reflexes may be increased. Dysphagia or ileus may preclude oral feeding.

Autonomic dysfunction commonly complicates severe cases and is characterized by labile or sustained hypertension, tachycardia, dysrhythmia, hyperpyrexia, profuse sweating, peripheral vasoconstriction, and increased plasma and urinary catecholamine levels. Periods of bradycardia and hypotension may also be documented. Sudden cardiac arrest sometimes occurs, but its basis is unknown. Other complications include aspiration pneumonia, fractures, muscle rupture, deep-vein thrombophlebitis, pulmonary emboli, decubitus ulcer, and rhabdomyolysis.

Neonatal tetanus usually occurs as the generalized form and is usually fatal if left untreated. It develops in children born to inadequately immunized mothers, frequently after unsterile treatment of the umbilical cord stump. Its onset generally comes during the first 2 weeks of life. Poor feeding, rigidity, and spasms are typical features of neonatal tetanus. *Local tetanus* is an uncommon form in which manifestations are restricted to muscles near the wound. The prognosis is excellent. *Cephalic tetanus*, a rare form of local tetanus, follows head injury or ear infection. Trismus and dysfunction of one or more cranial nerves, often the seventh nerve, are found. The incubation period is a few days and the mortality is high.

DIAGNOSIS The diagnosis of tetanus is based entirely on clinical findings. Tetanus is unlikely if a reliable history indicates the completion of a primary vaccination series and the receipt of appropriate booster doses. Wounds should be cultured in suspected cases. However, *C. tetani* can be isolated from wounds of patients without tetanus and frequently cannot be recovered from wounds of those with tetanus. The leukocyte count may be elevated. Cerebrospinal fluid examination yields normal results. Electromyograms may show continuous discharge of motor units and shortening or absence of the silent interval normally seen after an action potential. Nonspecific changes may be evident on the electrocardiogram. Muscle enzyme levels may be raised. Serum antitoxin levels of ≥0.15 U/mL are considered protective and make tetanus unlikely, although cases developing despite protective antitoxin levels have been reported.

The differential diagnosis includes local conditions also producing trismus, such as alveolar abscess, strychnine poisoning, dystonic drug reactions (e.g., to phenothiazines and metoclopramide), and hypocalcemic tetany. Other conditions sometimes confused with tetanus include meningitis/encephalitis, rabies, and an acute intraabdominal process (because of the rigid abdomen). Markedly increased tone in central muscles (face, neck, chest, back, and abdomen) with superimposed generalized spasms and relative sparing of the hands and feet strongly suggests tetanus.

Rx TREATMENT

General Measures The goals of therapy are to eliminate the source of toxin, neutralize unbound toxin, and prevent muscle spasms, monitoring the patient's condition and providing support—especially respiratory support—until recovery. Patients should be admitted to a quiet room in an intensive care unit, where observation and cardiopulmonary monitoring can be maintained continuously but stimulation can be minimized. Protection of the airway is vital. Wounds should be explored, carefully cleansed, and thoroughly debrided.

Antibiotic Therapy Although of unproven value, antibiotic therapy is administered to eradicate vegetative cells—the source of toxin. The

use of penicillin (10 to 12 million units intravenously, given daily for 10 days) has been recommended, but metronidazole (500 mg every 6 h or 1 g every 12 h) is preferred by some experts on the basis of this drug's excellent antimicrobial activity, a survival rate higher than that obtained with penicillin in one nonrandomized trial, and the absence of activity antagonistic to GABA, as seen with penicillin. Clindamycin and erythromycin are also alternatives for the treatment of penicillin-allergic patients. Additional specific antimicrobial therapy should be given for active infection with other organisms.

Antitoxin Given to neutralize circulating toxin and unbound toxin in the wound, antitoxin effectively lowers mortality; toxin already bound to neural tissue is unaffected. Human tetanus immune globulin (TIG) is the preparation of choice and should be given promptly. The dose is 3000 to 6000 units intramuscularly, usually in divided doses because the volume is large. The optimal dose is not known, however, and results from one study indicated that a 500-unit dose was as effective as higher doses. Pooled intravenous immunoglobulin may be an alternative to TIG, but the specific antitoxin concentration in this formulation is not standardized. It may be best to administer antitoxin before manipulating the wound; the value of injecting a dose proximal to the wound or infiltrating the wound is unclear. Additional doses are unnecessary because the half-life of antitoxin is long. Antibody does not penetrate the blood-brain barrier. Intrathecal administration should be considered experimental. Equine tetanus antitoxin (TAT) is not available in the United States but is used elsewhere. It is cheaper than human antitoxin, but its half-life is shorter and its administration commonly elicits hypersensitivity and serum sickness.

Control of Muscle Spasms Many agents, alone and in combination, have been used to treat the muscle spasms of tetanus, which are painful and can threaten ventilation by causing laryngospasm or sustained contraction of ventilatory muscles. The ideal therapeutic regimen would abolish spasmodic activity without causing oversedation and hypoventilation. Diazepam, a benzodiazepine and GABA agonist, is in wide use. The dose is titrated, and large doses (≥250 mg/d) may be required. Lorazepam, with a longer duration of action, and midazolam, with a short half-life, are other options. Barbiturates and chlorpromazine are considered second-line agents. Therapeutic paralysis with a nondepolarizing neuromuscular blocking agent and mechanical ventilation may be required for the treatment of spasms unresponsive to medication or spasms that threaten ventilation. However, prolonged paralysis after the discontinuation of therapy with such agents has been described, and both the need for continued paralysis and the occurrence of complications should be assessed daily. Alternative agents include propofol, which is expensive; dantrolene and intrathecal baclofen, which are being investigated in the hope of shortening the period of therapeutic paralysis; succinylcholine, which has been associated with hyperkalemia; and magnesium sulfate, which requires monitoring of neurologic (patellar reflex) and respiratory function as well as daily measurement of serum magnesium levels.

Respiratory Care Intubation or tracheostomy, with or without mechanical ventilation, may be required for hypoventilation due to oversedation or laryngospasm or for the avoidance of aspiration by patients with trismus, disordered swallowing, or dysphagia. The need for these procedures should be anticipated, and they should be undertaken electively and early.

Autonomic Dysfunction The optimal therapy for sympathetic overactivity has not been defined. Agents that have been considered include labetalol (an α- and β-adrenergic blocking agent that is recommended by some experts but that reportedly has caused sudden death), esmolol administered by continuous infusion (a beta blocker whose short half-life may be advantageous in the event of severe hypertension from unopposed α-adrenergic activity), clonidine (a central-acting antiadrenergic drug), and morphine sulfate. Parenteral magnesium sulfate and continuous spinal or epidural anesthesia have been used but may be more difficult to administer and monitor. The relative efficacy of these modalities has yet to be determined. Hypotension or bradycardia may require volume expansion, use of vasopressors or chronotropic agents, or pacemaker insertion.

Vaccine Patients recovering from tetanus should be actively immunized (see below) because immunity is not induced by the small amount of toxin that produces disease.

Additional Measures Additional therapeutic measures include hydration to control insensible and other fluid losses, which may be significant; the meeting of the patient's increased nutritional requirements by enteral or parenteral means; physiotherapy to prevent contractures; and administration of heparin or another anticoagulant to prevent pulmonary emboli. Bowel, bladder, and renal function must be monitored. Gastrointestinal bleeding and decubitus ulcers must be prevented, and intercurrent infection should be treated.

PREVENTION ■ Active Immunization All partially immunized and unimmunized adults should receive vaccine, as should those recovering from tetanus. The primary series for adults consists of three doses: the first and second doses are given 4 to 8 weeks apart, and the third dose is given 6 to 12 months after the second. A booster dose is required every 10 years and may be given at mid-decade ages—35, 45, and so on. Combined tetanus and diphtheria toxoid, adsorbed (Td, for adult use)—rather than single-antigen tetanus toxoid—is preferred for persons >7 years of age. Adsorbed vaccine is preferred because it produces more persistent antibody titers than fluid vaccine. In response to a vaccine shortage in 2001, the Centers for Disease Control and Prevention recommended that routine booster doses of Td for adolescents and adults be deferred until 2002, pending a better supply, but that all other existing recommendations for vaccine use be followed.

Wound Management Proper wound management requires consideration of the need for (1) passive immunization with TIG and (2) active immunization with vaccine, preferably Td in persons over age 7 (Table 124-1). The dose of TIG for passive immunization of persons with wounds of average severity is 250 units intramuscularly, which produces a protective antibody level in the serum for at least 4 to 6 weeks; the appropriate dose of TAT, an equine-derived product, is 3000 to 6000 units. Vaccine and TAT should be administered at separate sites with separate syringes.

Neonatal Tetanus Measures aimed at preventing neonatal tetanus include maternal vaccination, even during pregnancy; efforts to increase the proportion of births that take place in the hospital; and the provision of training for nonmedical birth attendants.

PROGNOSIS The application of methods to monitor and support oxygenation has markedly improved the prognosis in tetanus; mortality rates as low as 10% have been reported from units accustomed to handling such cases. In the United States during the periods 1995–

TABLE 124-1 *Wound Care: Administration of Tetanus Toxoid and Tetanus Immune Globulin*

History of Adsorbed Tetanus Toxoid	Clean Minor Wound		All Other Wounds[a]	
	Td[b]	TIG	Td[b]	TIG
Unknown or <3 doses	Yes	No	Yes	Yes
3 doses[c]	No, unless >10 years since last dose	No	No, unless >5 years since last dose	No

[a] Such as, but not limited to, wounds contaminated with dirt, feces, soil, and saliva; puncture wounds; avulsions; and wounds resulting from missile or crushing injuries, burns, and frostbite.

[b] For children <7 years old, DTP (or DT, if pertussis vaccine is contraindicated) is preferred to tetanus toxoid alone. Td is preferred to tetanus toxoid alone in adults.

[c] If only three doses of fluid toxoid have been received, then a fourth dose of toxoid—preferably an adsorbed toxoid—should be given.

Note: DT, diphtheria and tetanus vaccine; DTP, diphtheria, tetanus, and pertussis vaccine; Td, tetanus-diphtheria toxoid, adsorbed; TIG, tetanus immune globulin.

Source: Modified from Centers for Disease Control and Prevention: Diphtheria, tetanus, and pertussis: Recommendations for vaccine use and other preventive measures: Recommendations of the Immunization Practices Advisory Committee (ACIP). MMWR 40(RR-10):1, 1991.

1997 and 1998–2000, the case-fatality rates were 11% and 16%, respectively. In the latter period, there were 20 deaths among the 113 cases with known outcome (total, 130 cases). The outcome is poor in neonates and the elderly and in patients with a short incubation period, a short interval from the onset of symptoms to admission, or a short period from the onset of symptoms to the first spasm (period of onset). Outcome is also related to the extent of prior vaccination.

The course of tetanus extends over 4 to 6 weeks, and patients may require prolonged ventilator support. Increased tone and minor spasms can last for months, but recovery is usually complete.

FURTHER READING

ABRUTYN E, BERLIN JA: Intrathecal therapy of tetanus: A meta-analysis. JAMA 266:2262, 1991

AHMADSYAH I, SALIM A: Treatment of tetanus: An open study to compare the efficacy of procaine penicillin and metronidazole. BMJ 291:648, 1985

BLECK TP: *Clostridium tetani* (tetanus), in *Principles and Practice of Infectious Diseases*, 5th ed, GL Mandell et al (eds). New York, Churchill Livingstone, 2000, pp 2537–2543

BRUGGEMANN H et al: The genome sequence of *Clostridium tetani,* the causative agent of tetanus disease. Proc Natl Acad Sci USA 100:1316, 2003

CENTERS FOR DISEASE CONTROL AND PREVENTION: Tetanus—Puerto Rico, 2002. MMWR 51:613, 2002

———: Tetanus surveillance—United States, 1998–2000. Surveillance summaries, June 20, 2003. MMWR 52(SS-3):1, 2003

COOK TM et al: Tetanus: A review of the literature. Br J Anaesth 87:477, 2001

HSU SS et al: Tetanus in the emergency department: A current review. J Emerg Med 20:357, 2001

MCQUILLAN CM et al: Serologic immunity to diphtheria and tetanus in the United States. Ann Intern Med 136:660, 2002

TURTON K et al: Botulinum and tetanus neurotoxins: Structure, function and therapeutic utility. Trends Biochem Sci 27:552, 2002

125   BOTULISM
Elias Abrutyn

DEFINITION Botulism is a paralytic disease caused by potent protein neurotoxins elaborated by *Clostridium botulinum*. Illness begins with cranial nerve involvement, and progression proceeds caudally to involve the extremities. Cases may be classified as (1) *food-borne botulism*, from ingestion of preformed toxin in food contaminated with *C. botulinum*; (2) *wound botulism*, from toxin produced in wounds contaminated with the organism; and (3) *intestinal botulism*, from in-

gestion of spores and production of toxin in the intestine of infants (infant botulism) or adults. Botulinum toxin, because of its extraordinary potency, has long been considered a threat as an agent of bioterrorism or biological warfare (see Chap. 205).

ETIOLOGIC AGENT *C. botulinum*, a species encompassing a heterogeneous group of anaerobic gram-positive organisms that form subterminal spores, is found in soil and marine environments throughout the world and elaborates the most potent bacterial toxin known. Organisms of types A through G have been distinguished by the antigenic specificities of their toxins; a classification system based on physiologic characteristics has also been described. Rare strains of other clostridial species—*C. butyricum* and *C. baratii*—have also been found to produce toxin. *C. botulinum* strains with proteolytic activity can digest food and produce a spoiled appearance; nonproteolytic types leave the appearance of food unchanged.

Of the eight distinct toxin types described (A, B, C_1, C_2, D, E, F, and G), all except C_2 are neurotoxins; C_2 is a cytotoxin of unknown clinical significance. Botulinum neurotoxin, whether ingested, inhaled, or produced in the intestine or a wound, enters the vascular system and is transported to peripheral cholinergic nerve terminals, including neuromuscular junctions, postganglionic parasympathetic nerve endings, and peripheral ganglia. The central nervous system is not involved. Active neurotoxin (150 kDa) is composed of a heavy chain (a 100-kDa fragment responsible for neurospecific binding and translocation in the nerve cell) and a light chain (a 50-kDa fragment responsible for intracellular catalytic activity). The steps involved in neurotoxin activity include (1) specific binding to presynaptic nerve cells at the myoneural junction, (2) internalization of the toxin inside the nerve cell in endocytic vesicles, (3) translocation of the toxin into the cytosol, and (4) proteolysis by toxin (a zinc endopeptidase) of components of the neuroexocytosis apparatus curtailing release of the neurotransmitter acetylcholine. Cure follows sprouting of new nerve terminals.

Toxin is heat-labile, but spores are highly heat-resistant; both can be inactivated under appropriate conditions (see "Prevention," below). In the gastrointestinal tract, toxin is complexed with nontoxin proteins and resists degradation. Toxin types A, B, E, and (rarely) F cause human disease; type G (from *C. argentinense*) has been associated with sudden death, but not with neuroparalytic illness, in a few patients in Switzerland; and types C and D cause animal disease.

EPIDEMIOLOGY Human botulism occurs worldwide. In the United States, the geographic distribution of cases by toxin type parallels the distribution of organism types found in the environment. Type A predominates west of the Rocky Mountains; type B is generally distributed but is more common in the East; and type E is found in the Pacific Northwest, Alaska, and the Great Lakes area. In the United States, food-borne botulism has been associated primarily with home-canned food, particularly vegetables, fruit, and condiments, and less commonly with meat and fish. Type E outbreaks are frequently associated with fish products. Commercial products occasionally cause outbreaks, but some of these outbreaks have resulted from improper handling after purchase. Outbreaks in restaurants, schools, and private homes have been traced to uncommon sources (commercial potpies, beef stew, turkey loaf, sautéed onions, baked potatoes, and chopped garlic in oil). Food-borne botulism can occur when (1) a food to be preserved is contaminated with spores, (2) preservation does not inactivate the spores but kills other putrefactive bacteria that might inhibit growth of *C. botulinum* and provides anaerobic conditions at a pH and temperature that allow germination and toxin production, and (3) food is not heated to a temperature that destroys toxin before being eaten.

CLINICAL MANIFESTATIONS ■ **Food-Borne Botulism** After ingestion of food containing toxin, illness varies from a mild condition for which no medical advice is sought to very severe disease that can result in death within 24 h. The incubation period is usually 18 to 36 h but, depending on toxin dose, can extend from a few hours to several days. Symmetric descending paralysis is characteristic and can lead to respiratory failure and death. Cranial nerve involvement, which almost always marks the onset of symptoms, usually produces diplopia, dysarthria, dysphonia, and/or dysphagia. Weakness progresses, often rapidly, from the head to involve the neck, arms, thorax, and legs; occasionally, weakness is asymmetric. Nausea, vomiting, and abdominal pain may precede or follow the onset of paralysis. Dizziness, blurred vision, dry mouth, and very dry, occasionally sore throat are common. Patients are generally alert and oriented, but they may be drowsy, agitated, and anxious. Typically, they have no fever. Ptosis is frequent; the pupillary reflexes may be depressed, and fixed or dilated pupils are noted in half of patients. The gag reflex may be suppressed, and deep tendon reflexes may be normal or decreased. Sensory findings are usually absent. Paralytic ileus, severe constipation, and urinary retention are common.

Wound Botulism Wound botulism occurs when the spores contaminating a wound germinate and form vegetative organisms that produce toxin. This rare condition resembles food-borne illness except that the incubation period is longer, averaging about 10 days, and gastrointestinal symptoms are lacking. Wound botulism has been documented after traumatic injury involving contamination with soil; in injection drug users, for whom black-tar heroin use has been identified as a risk factor; and after cesarean delivery. The illness has occurred even after antibiotics have been given to prevent wound infection. When present, fever is probably attributable to concurrent infection with other bacteria. The wound may appear benign.

Intestinal Botulism In intestinal botulism, toxin is produced in and absorbed from the intestine after the germination of ingested spores. Infant botulism is the most common form of botulism. The severity ranges from mild illness with failure to thrive to fulminant severe paralysis with respiratory failure. Infant botulism may be one cause of sudden infant death. The identification of contaminated honey as one source of spores has led to the recommendation that honey not be fed to children <12 months of age. Most cases cannot be attributed to a particular food source. The factors permitting intestinal colonization with *C. botulinum* are not fully defined, but cases usually involve infants <6 months of age; susceptibility may decrease as the normal intestinal flora develops. Intestinal botulism involving adults is uncommon. The patient may have a history of gastrointestinal disease, gastrointestinal surgery, or recent antibiotic therapy. Toxin and organisms may be identified in the stool.

Bioterrorism and Biological Warfare (See also Chap. 205) Botulinum toxin could be dispersed as an aerosol (producing inhalational botulism) or as a contaminant in material to be ingested (producing food-borne botulism). Inhalational botulism resembles food-borne illness, but gastrointestinal symptoms are absent. Botulism follows adsorption of toxin from mucosal surfaces (gut, lung) and wounds, but the toxin does not penetrate intact skin. As a toxin-mediated illness, botulism is noncommunicable, and standard isolation precautions are sufficient unless bacterial meningitis is being considered. Features suggestive of an outbreak due to deliberate release of botulinum toxin are shown in Table 125-1.

DIAGNOSIS A diagnosis of botulism must be considered in patients with symmetric descending paralysis who are afebrile and mentally intact. The bulbar musculature is involved initially, but sensory findings are absent and, early on, deep tendon reflexes remain intact. The differential diagnosis of botulism and differentiating features are listed in Table 125-2.

The demonstration of toxin in serum by bioassay in mice is definitive, but this test may be negative, particularly in wound and infant botulism. It is performed only by specific laboratories, which can be identified through regional public health authorities. Other assays are

---

TABLE 125-1 *Features of Outbreaks Suggesting Deliberate Release of Botulinum Toxin*[a]

- Outbreak of large number of cases of acute flaccid paralysis with prominent bulbar palsies
- Outbreak with an unusual botulinum toxin type (i.e., type C, D, F, or G or type E toxin not associated with food of aquatic origin)
- Outbreak with a common geographic factor among cases (e.g., airport, work location) but without a common dietary exposure (i.e., features suggesting an aerosol attack)
- Multiple simultaneous outbreaks with no common source

[a] A careful travel and activity history, as well as a dietary history, should be taken in any suspected botulism outbreak. Patients should also be asked whether they know of other persons with similar symptoms.
Source: Reproduced with permission of the publisher from Arnon et al, 2002

TABLE 125-2 *Selected Mimics That May Lead to Misdiagnosis of Botulism*

Condition	Features Distinguishing Condition from Botulism
COMMON MISDIAGNOSES	
Guillain-Barré syndrome[a] and its variants, especially Miller-Fisher variant	History of antecedent infection; paresthesias; often ascending paralysis; early areflexia; eventual CSF protein increase; EMG findings
Myasthenia gravis[a]	Recurrent paralysis; EMG findings; sustained response to anticholinesterase
Stroke[a]	Paralysis often asymmetric; abnormal CNS image
Intoxication with depressants (e.g., acute alcohol intoxication), organophosphates, carbon monoxide, or nerve gas	History of exposure; excessive drug levels detected in body fluids
Lambert-Eaton syndrome	Increased strength with sustained contraction; evidence of lung carcinoma; EMG findings similar to botulism
Tick paralysis	Paresthesias; ascending paralysis; tick attached to skin
OTHER MISDIAGNOSES	
Poliomyelitis	Antecedent febrile illness; asymmetric paralysis; CSF pleocytosis
CNS infections, especially of the brainstem	Mental status changes; CSF and EEG abnormalities
CNS tumor	Paralysis often asymmetric; abnormal CNS image
Streptococcal pharyngitis[b]	Absence of bulbar palsies; positive rapid antigen test result or throat culture
Psychiatric illness[a]	Normal EMG in conversion paralysis
Viral syndrome[a]	Absence of bulbar palsies and flaccid paralysis
Inflammatory myopathy[a]	Elevated creatine kinase level
Diabetic complications[a]	Sensory neuropathy; few cranial nerve palsies
Hyperemesis gravidarum[a]	Absence of bulbar palsies and acute flaccid paralysis
Hypothyroidism[a]	Abnormal thyroid function tests
Laryngeal trauma[a]	Absence of flaccid paralysis; dysphonia without flaccid paralysis
Overexertion[a]	Absence of bulbar palsies and acute flaccid paralysis

[a] Misdiagnoses made in a large outbreak of botulism (St. Louis ME et al: Botulism from chopped garlic: Delayed recognition of a major outbreak. Ann Intern Med 108:363, 1988).
[b] Pharyngeal erythema can occur in botulism.
Note: CNS, central nervous system; CSF, cerebrospinal fluid; EEG, electroencephalogram; EMG, electromyogram.
Source: Reproduced with the permission of the publisher from Arnon et al, 2002.

being developed and remain experimental. The demonstration of the organism or its toxin in vomitus, gastric fluid, or stool is strongly suggestive of the diagnosis, because intestinal carriage is rare. Isolation of the organism from food without toxin is insufficient grounds for the diagnosis. Wound cultures yielding the organism are suggestive of botulism. The edrophonium chloride (Tensilon) test for myasthenia gravis may be falsely positive in botulism but is usually less dramatically positive than in the former condition. Nerve conduction velocity is normal, but compound muscle action potentials on routine nerve stimulation studies are decreased with a supramaximal stimulus, and facilitation is evident after repetitive stimulation at high frequency. Single-fiber electromyography may be helpful. The white blood cell count and erythrocyte sedimentation rate are normal.

℞ TREATMENT

Patients should be hospitalized and monitored closely, both clinically and by spirometry, pulse oximetry, and measurement of arterial blood gases for incipient respiratory failure. Intubation and mechanical ventilation should be strongly considered when the vital capacity is <30% of predicted, especially when paralysis is progressing rapidly and hypoxemia with absolute or relative hypercarbia is documented (Chap. 252). Serial measurements of the maximal static inspiratory pressure may be useful in predicting respiratory failure.

In food-borne illness, equine antitoxin should be administered as soon as possible after specimens are obtained for laboratory analysis. Treatment should not await laboratory analyses, which may take days. The previous trivalent antitoxin (types A, B, and E) preparation is no longer available. Instead, a bivalent preparation containing toxin types A and B and an investigational monovalent type E preparation can be obtained. The bivalent preparation is given routinely; monovalent type E antitoxin is given in addition when exposure to type E toxin is suspected (after seafood ingestion, for example). In the United States, antitoxin as well as help in clinical management and laboratory confirmation are available at *any* time from state health departments or from the Centers for Disease Control and Prevention (CDC: 404-639-2206; emergency number, 404-639-2888). A limited supply of an investigational heptavalent antitoxin (types A through G) is maintained by the U.S. military for emergency use.

After testing for hypersensitivity to horse serum, antitoxin is given as recommended by the CDC; repeated doses are not considered necessary. Anaphylaxis and serum sickness are risks inherent in use of the equine product, and desensitization of allergic patients may be required. If there is no ileus, cathartics and enemas may be given to purge the gut of toxin; emetics or gastric lavage can also be used if the time since ingestion is brief (only a few hours). Neither the use of antibiotics to eliminate an intestinal source for possible continued toxin production nor the administration of guanidine hydrochloride and other drugs to reverse paralysis is of proven value.

Treatment of infant botulism requires supportive care and administration of human botulism immune globulin (obtainable at all times from the California Department of Health Services at 510-540-2646). Neither equine antitoxin nor antibiotics have been shown to be beneficial. In wound botulism, equine antitoxin is administered. The wound should be thoroughly explored and debrided, and an antibiotic such as penicillin should be given to eradicate *C. botulinum* from the site, even though the benefit of this therapy is unproven. Results of wound cultures should guide the use of other antibiotics.

Botulinum toxins have been approved for therapeutic use. Botulinum toxin type A has been approved for the treatment of strabismus, blepharospasm, cervical dystonia, and glabellar lines; therapy appears safe and effective. Botulinum toxin type B has been approved for the treatment of cervical dystonia. The value of these preparations in many other conditions is being evaluated. Generalized botulism-like weakness complicating therapy has been reported but is rare.

PROGNOSIS Type A disease is generally more severe than type B, and mortality from botulism is higher among patients above age 60 than among younger patients. With improved respiratory and intensive care, the case-fatality rate in food-borne illness has been reduced to ~7.5% and is low in infant botulism as well. Artificial respiratory support may be required for months in severe cases. Some patients experience residual weakness and autonomic dysfunction for as long as a year after disease onset.

PREVENTION A pentavalent vaccine (A–E) is available for use in highly exposed individuals. Spores can be inactivated by exposure to high temperature (116° to 121°C) and pressure, as in steam sterilizers or pressure cookers used in accordance with the manufacturer's instructions. Toxin can be inactivated by exposure to a temperature of 100°C for 10 min. Newly identified cases should be reported immediately to public health authorities.

FURTHER READING

ANGULO FJ et al: Large outbreak of botulism: The hazardous baked potato. Clin Infect Dis 178:172, 1998

ARNON SS et al: Botulinum toxin as a biological weapon, in *Bioterrorism: Guidelines for Medical and Public Health Management*, DA Henderson et al (eds). Chicago, AMA Press, 2002, pp 141–165

CHERINGTON M: Clinical spectrum of botulism. Muscle Nerve 21:701, 1998

HATHEWAY CL: Botulism: The present status of disease. Curr Top Microbiol Immunol 195:55, 1995

LONG SS: Infant botulism. Pediatr Infect Dis J 20:707, 2001

MEUNIER FA et al: Botulinum neurotoxins: From paralysis to recovery of functional neuromuscular transmission. J Physiol Paris, 96:105, 2002

SHAPIRO RL: Botulism in the United States: A clinical and epidemiologic review. Ann Intern Med 129:221, 1998

WERNER SB et al: Wound botulism in California, 1951–1998: Recent epidemic in heroin injectors. Clin Infect Dis 31:1018, 2000

126 GAS GANGRENE AND OTHER CLOSTRIDIAL INFECTIONS
Dennis L. Kasper, Lawrence C. Madoff

DEFINITION Bacteria of the genus *Clostridium* are gram-positive, spore-forming, obligate anaerobes that are ubiquitous in nature. There are >60 recognized species of clostridia, many of which are generally considered saprophytic. Some of these species are pathogenic for humans and animals, particularly under conditions of lowered oxidation-reduction potential. Infections associated with these organisms range from localized wound contamination to overwhelming systemic disease. The four major disease categories for which clostridia are responsible are intestinal disorders, suppurative deep-tissue infections, skin and soft tissue infections, and bacteremia. Toxins play a major role in some of these syndromes. →*Colitis caused by C. difficile is discussed in Chap. 114.*

ETIOLOGY In humans, clostridia normally reside in the gastrointestinal tract and in the female genital tract, although they occasionally are isolated from the skin or the mouth. Of the known species of the genus *Clostridium*, at least 30 have been isolated from human infections. Like several other pathogenic anaerobic bacterial species, clostridia are quite aerotolerant, but they do not grow on artificial media in the presence of oxygen. Clostridia characteristically produce abundant gas in artificial media and form subterminal endospores. *C. perfringens*, one of the most important species, is encapsulated and nonmotile and rarely sporulates in artificial media; the spores can usually be destroyed by boiling. →*C. tetani and C. botulinum are discussed in detail in Chaps. 124 and 125, respectively.*

Clostridia are present in the normal colonic flora at concentrations of 10^9 to 10^{10}/g. Of the ≥30 species that normally colonize humans, *C. ramosum* is the most abundant and is followed in frequency by *C. perfringens*. These organisms are universally present in soil at concentrations of up to 10^4/g. *C. perfringens* strains are classified (on the basis of their production of several lethal toxins) into five types, designated A through E. Type A predominates in fecal flora of humans as well as in soil, whereas the habitats of types B through E are thought to be the intestinal tracts of other animals. Although clostridia are gram-positive organisms, many species may appear to be gram-negative in clinical specimens or stationary-phase cultures. Therefore, the results of Gram's staining of cultures or clinical material should be interpreted with great care.

C. perfringens is the most common of the clostridial species isolated from tissue infections and bacteremias; next in frequency are *C. novyi* and *C. septicum*. In the category of enteric infections, *C. difficile* is an important cause of antibiotic-associated colitis, and *C. perfringens* is associated with food poisoning (type A) and enteritis necroticans (type C).

PATHOGENESIS Despite the isolation of clostridial species from many serious traumatic wounds, the prevalence of severe infections due to these organisms is low. Two factors that appear to be essential to the development of severe disease are tissue necrosis and a low oxidation-reduction potential. *C. perfringens* requires about 14 amino acids and at least 6 additional growth factors for optimal growth. These nutrients are not found in appreciable concentrations in normal body fluids but are present in necrotic tissue. When *C. perfringens* grows in necrotic tissue, a zone of tissue damage due to the toxins elaborated by the organism allows progressive growth. In contrast, when only a few bacteria leak into the bloodstream from a small defect in the intestinal wall, the organisms do not have the opportunity to multiply rapidly because blood as a medium for growth is relatively deficient in certain amino acids and growth factors. Therefore, in a patient without tissue necrosis, bacteremia is usually benign.

C. perfringens possesses at least 17 possible virulence factors, including 12 active tissue toxins and enterotoxins. The enterotoxins include four major lethal toxins: α, β, ϵ, and ι. The α toxin is a phospholipase C (lecithinase) that splits lecithin into phosphorylcholine and diglyceride. It has been associated with gas gangrene and is known to be hemolytic, to destroy platelets and polymorphonuclear leukocytes (PMNs), and to cause widespread capillary damage. When injected intravenously, it causes massive intravascular hemolysis and damages liver mitochondria. The α toxin may be important in the initiation of muscle infections that may progress to gas gangrene. Experimentally, the higher the concentration of α toxin in the culture fluid, the smaller the dose of *C. perfringens* required to produce infection. The protective effect of antiserum is directly proportional to its content of α antitoxin. Studies suggest that θ *toxin*, a thiol-activated cytolysin that is also called *perfringolysin O*, may also play an important role in pathogenesis by promoting vascular leukostasis, endothelial cell injury, and regional tissue hypoxia. The resulting perfusion defects extend the anaerobic environment and contribute to rapidly advancing tissue destruction. A characteristic pathologic finding in gas gangrene is the near absence of PMNs despite extensive tissue destruction. Experimental data indicate that both α and θ toxins are essential in the leukocyte aggregation that occurs at the margins of tissue injury instead of the expected infiltration of these cells into the area of damage. Genetically altered strains induce less leukocyte aggregation when α toxin is absent and none when θ toxin is missing. The other major toxins, β, ϵ, and ι, are known to increase capillary permeability.

CLINICAL MANIFESTATIONS ■ **Intestinal Disorders** ■ *FOOD POISONING* *C. perfringens*, primarily type A, is the second or third most common cause of food poisoning in the United States (Chap. 113). The responsible toxin is thought to be a cytotoxin produced by >75% of strains isolated from cases of foodborne disease. The cytotoxin binds to a receptor on the small-bowel brush border and induces a calcium ion–dependent alteration in permeability. The associated loss of ions alters intracellular metabolism, resulting in cell death. Outbreaks generally have resulted from problems in the cooling and storage of food cooked in bulk. The food sources primarily involved are meat, meat products, and poultry. Generally, the implicated meats have been cooked, allowed to cool, and then recooked the following day, often in a stew or hash. Strains of *C. perfringens* that contaminate meat manage to survive initial cooking. During reheating, the organisms sporulate and germinate. The disease is associated with an attack rate that is often as high as 70%. Symptoms of food poisoning from type A strains develop 8 to 24 h after ingestion of foods heavily contaminated with the organism. The primary symptoms include epigastric pain, nausea, and watery diarrhea usually lasting 12 to 24 h. Fever and vomiting are uncommon. Molecular methods including ribotyping and pulsed-field gel electrophoresis have been used to detect fecal cytotoxin in outbreaks of food poisoning caused by *C. perfringens*.

C. perfringens has also been implicated in a more severe form of diarrhea than that of classic food poisoning. This more severe disease tends to occur in the elderly and has been associated with antibiotic use in hospitalized populations. In this form of disease, diarrhea is generally more profuse, of longer duration, and accompanied by abdominal pain. Blood and mucus have been detected in the feces of the affected patients. In one hospital-based study of a cluster of cases, widespread environmental contamination with *C. perfringens* spores was documented.

ENTERITIS NECROTICANS Necrotizing enteritis (enteritis necroticans, or *pigbel*) is caused by β toxin produced by type C strains of *C. perfringens* following ingestion of a high-protein meal in conjunction with trypsin inhibitors (e.g., in sweet potatoes) by a susceptible host who has limited intestinal proteolytic activity. This disease has been reported among children and adults in New Guinea. A similar disease, *darmbrand*, was epidemic in Germany after World War II. Clinical features of pigbel include acute abdominal pain, bloody diarrhea, vomiting, shock, and peritonitis; 40% of patients die. Pathologic studies reveal an acute ulcerative process of the bowel restricted to the small intestine. The mucosa is lifted off the submucosa, with the formation of large denuded areas. Pseudomembranes composed of sloughed epithelium are common, and gas may dissect into the submucosa. The source of the organisms may be the patient's own intestinal flora; cultures of ingested pork have failed to yield the organism. Antibodies to the β toxin of *C. perfringens* have been of considerable benefit in changing the course of established disease. In a large-scale trial, children immunized with *C. perfringens* β toxoid were protected.

NEUTROPENIC ENTEROCOLITIS (TYPHLITIS) See Chaps. 72 and 148.

Suppurative Deep Tissue Infections Clostridia are frequently recovered from various suppurative conditions in conjunction with other anaerobic and aerobic bacteria but can also be the only organisms isolated. These suppurative conditions, which exist with severe local inflammation but usually without the characteristic systemic signs induced by clostridial toxins, include intraabdominal sepsis, empyema, pelvic abscess, subcutaneous abscess, frostbite with gas gangrene, infection of a stump in an amputee, brain abscess, prostatic abscess, perianal abscess, conjunctivitis, infection of a renal cell carcinoma, and infection of an aortic graft.

Clostridia are isolated from approximately two-thirds of patients with intraabdominal infections resulting from intestinal perforation. *C. ramosum*, *C. perfringens*, and *C. bifermentans* are the most commonly isolated species. The presence of clostridial species does not affect the clinical presentation or outcome of these infections (Chap. 148).

An association has been made between malignancy and the isolation of *C. septicum* in the absence of grossly contaminated deep traumatic wounds. A major site for such a malignancy is the gastrointestinal tract, particularly the colon. An association with leukemia or with other solid tumors has also been noted, and one case of fatal myonecrosis has been reported in a patient with ovarian cancer. Some of these patients present with *C. septicum* bacteremia; these cases have a fulminant clinical course (discussed below). Others develop localized suppurative infection in the abdomen or the abdominal wall without bacteremia. Presumably, this infection arises from a silent perforation that leads to intraabdominal abscess formation.

Clostridia have been isolated from suppurative infections of the female genital tract, particularly tuboovarian and pelvic abscesses. The major species involved has been *C. perfringens*. Most of these are mild suppurative infections without evidence of uterine gangrene. *C. perfringens* has been isolated from as many as 20% of diseased gallbladders at surgery. One clinical syndrome, *emphysematous cholecystitis*, is caused by clostridial species at least 50% of the time. In this syndrome, gas forms in the biliary radicles and the wall of the gallbladder.

Emphysematous cholecystitis is seen most often in diabetic patients. Although the mortality rate in this entity is higher than in more common forms of cholecystitis, there is no evidence of myonecrosis.

Clostridia are among the many organisms found in empyema fluid or isolated by transtracheal aspiration from patients with lung abscesses. There is no unique clinical clue to the presence of clostridia (as opposed to other organisms) in these infections. *C. perfringens* has been reported as a cause of empyema arising from aspiration pneumonia, pulmonary emboli, and infarction. However, the majority of cases of clostridial empyema are secondary to trauma.

Skin and Soft Tissue Infections Various categories of traumatic wound infections due to clostridia have been described: simple contamination, anaerobic cellulitis, fasciitis with or without systemic manifestations, and anaerobic myonecrosis.

SIMPLE CONTAMINATION Clostridia are cultured most often from wounds in the absence of clinical signs of sepsis. As many as 30% of battle wounds are contaminated by clostridia without signs of suppuration, and 16% of penetrating abdominal wounds yield clostridia on culture despite treatment with cephalothin and kanamycin. In cases of trauma, clostridia are isolated with equal frequency from suppurative and well-healing wounds. Thus the diagnosis of clostridial infection should be based on clinical rather than bacteriologic criteria.

LOCALIZED INFECTION OF THE SKIN AND SOFT TISSUE WITHOUT SYSTEMIC SIGNS This condition, originally referred to as *anaerobic cellulitis*, is a localized infection involving the skin and soft tissue and is due to clostridia alone or with other bacteria. There are no systemic signs of toxicity, although the infection may invade locally, producing necrosis. These infections tend to be relatively indolent, spreading slowly to contiguous areas. Localized infections are relatively free of pain and edema. Perhaps because of the lack of edema, gas that is limited to the wound and the immediately surrounding tissue may be more evident than in gas gangrene. In these localized infections, gas is never found intramuscularly. Cellulitis, perirectal abscesses, and diabetic foot ulcers are typical infections from which clostridial species can be isolated. If inadequately treated, these localized infections advance by extension through subcutaneous tissue and fascial planes into muscle and may produce severe systemic disease with signs of toxemia.

A localized form of suppurative myositis has been described in heroin addicts. These patients develop local pain and tenderness in discrete areas (particularly the thigh and forearm), with the subsequent appearance of fluctuance and crepitance that require surgical drainage. The unusual aspect of these infections is that they remain localized without systemic signs of toxicity. Moreover, the affected local areas are not necessarily sites of trauma or heroin injection. Pathologic examination reveals subcutaneous abscesses, purulent myositis, and fasciitis from which clostridia are recovered in pure culture; on occasion, mixed infections involving aerobes and anaerobes are found. Wound botulism has been reported in association with the injection of black tar heroin.

SPREADING CELLULITIS AND FASCIITIS WITH SYSTEMIC TOXICITY This condition involves diffuse spreading cellulitis and fasciitis, without myonecrosis and with only mild inflammation in muscle. Patients present with the abrupt onset of a syndrome that progresses rapidly (within hours) through the fascial planes. In cases with suppuration and gas in soft tissues as well as overwhelming toxemia, the infection is rapidly fatal. On physical examination there is subcutaneous crepitation but little localized pain. Surgery is of no proven value because there are no discretely involved tissues amenable to resection, as may be the case in myonecrosis. However, in rapidly advancing fasciitis, incision of the affected area is still the cornerstone of therapy. The initial local lesion may be quite innocuous and arises from an area involved by tumor or other infection and not by injury. The systemic toxic effects include hemolysis and injury of capillary membranes. Usually, this infection is fatal within 48 h, despite intensive therapy involving antitoxin and exchange transfusion. This syndrome is seen most commonly in patients with carcinoma, especially of the sigmoid or the cecum. Presumably, the tumor invades the fascia, and colonic contents leak into the abdominal wall. Patients present with extreme toxicity and occasionally with total-body crepitation. The syndrome differs from necrotizing fasciitis caused by other organisms in three respects: (1) rapid mortality, (2) rapid tissue invasion, and (3) the systemic effects of the toxin, typified by massive hemolysis.

GAS GANGRENE (CLOSTRIDIAL MYONECROSIS) Gas gangrene is characterized by rapid and extensive necrosis of muscle accompanied by gas formation and systemic toxicity and occurs when bacteria invade healthy muscle from adjacent traumatized muscle or soft tissue. The infection originates in a wound contaminated with clostridia. Although >30% of deep wounds are infected with clostridia, the incidence of clostridial myonecrosis is quite low. These infections occur in both military and civilian settings. An essential factor in the genesis of gas gangrene appears to be trauma, particularly involving deep muscle laceration. The entity of clostridial myonecrosis is relatively uncommon after simple, through-and-through bullet wounds without shattering of bone and is relatively common following shrapnel fragmentation wounds, particularly when deep muscle is involved. In civilian cases, gas gangrene can follow trauma, surgery, or intramuscular injection. The trauma need not be severe; however, the wound must be deep, necrotic, and without communication to the surface.

The incubation period of gas gangrene is usually short: almost always <3 days and frequently <24 h. Some 80% of cases are caused by *C. perfringens*, while *C. novyi*, *C. septicum*, and *C. histolyticum* cause most of the remaining cases. Typically, gas gangrene begins with the sudden onset of pain in the region of the wound, which helps to differentiate it from spreading cellulitis. Once established, the pain increases steadily in severity but remains localized to the infected area and spreads only if the infection spreads. Soon after pain develops, local swelling and edema—accompanied by a thin, often hemorrhagic exudate—appear. Patients frequently develop marked tachycardia, but elevation in temperature may be only minimal. Gas is usually not obvious at this early stage and may be completely absent. Frothiness of the wound exudate may be noted. The skin is tense, white, often marbled with blue, and cooler than normal. The symptoms progress rapidly; swelling, edema, and toxemia increase, and a profuse serous discharge, which may have a peculiar sweetish smell, appears. Gram's staining of the wound exudate shows many gram-positive rods with relatively few inflammatory cells.

At surgery, muscle may appear pale because of the intensity of edema, but it does not contract when probed with a scalpel. When dissected, the muscle is beefy red and nonviable and can progress to become black, friable, and gangrenous. It is important to establish a diagnosis early, preferably by frozen-section biopsy of muscle.

Despite hypotension, renal failure, and (often) body crepitation, patients with myonecrosis frequently have a heightened awareness of their surroundings until just before death, when they lapse into toxic delirium and coma. In untreated cases, as the local wounds progress, the skin becomes bronzed; bullae appear, become filled with dark red fluid, and are accompanied by dark patches of cutaneous gangrene. Gas appears in later phases (Fig. 126-1) but may not be as obvious as in anaerobic cellulitis. Jaundice is rare in wound gas gangrene (in contrast to uterine infections) and, when it does appear, is almost invariably associated with hemoglobinuria, hemoglobinemia, and septicemia. Cases of clostridial myonecrosis without a history of trauma have been reported. These patients have bullous lesions and crepitation of the skin; they present with a rapidly worsening course that includes myonecrosis, especially of the extremities.

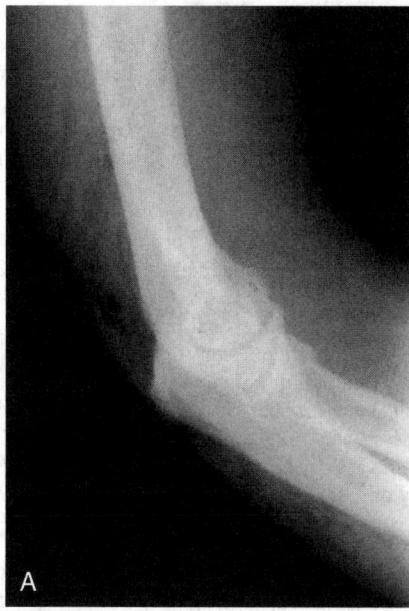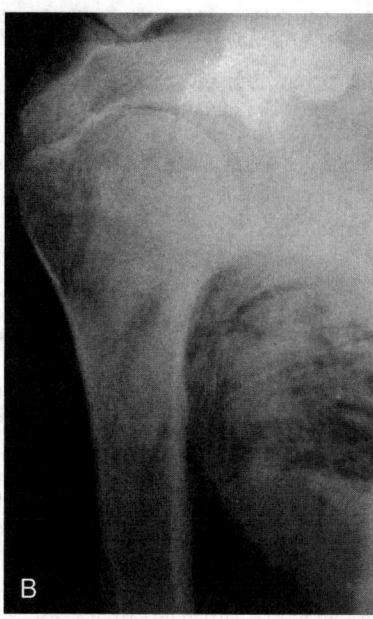

FIGURE 126-1 Spontaneous gas gangrene. Radiographs of the elbow (*A*) and shoulder (*B*) show gas in tissue. The patient developed spontaneous gas gangrene of the hand, which spread rapidly up the arm and onto the thorax. *C. septicum* was grown from blood and necrotic tissue of the arm. [*Reprinted with permission from DL Stevens (ed): Atlas of Infectious Diseases, vol II: Skin, Soft Tissue, Bone and Joint Infections. Philadelphia, Current Medicine, 1995.*]

Bacteremia and Clostridial Sepsis The relatively common entity of transient clostridial bacteremia can arise in any hospitalized patient but is most common with a predisposing focus in the gastrointestinal tract, biliary tract, or uterus. Fever frequently resolves within 24 to 48 h without therapy. Despite the finding of clostridial bacteremia following septic abortions and the frequent isolation of clostridia from the lochia, most of the patients involved do not have evidence of sepsis. In one series of 60 patients with clostridial bacteremia, half had an infected site that could be associated with the bacteremia, while the other half had a totally unrelated illness, such as tuberculous pneumonia, meningitis, or benign gastroenteritis. By the time blood culture reports are returned, patients frequently are completely well and sometimes have been discharged. Therefore, when a blood culture is positive for clostridia, the patient must be assessed clinically rather than simply treated on the basis of the culture result.

Clostridial sepsis is an uncommon but almost invariably fatal illness following clostridial infection—primarily that of the uterus, colon, or biliary tract. This entity must be differentiated from transient clostridial bacteremia, which is much more common. *C. perfringens* causes the majority of cases of both sepsis and transient bacteremia. *C. septicum*, *C. sordellii*, and *C. novyi* account for most of the remainder of cases. Clostridia account for 1 to 2.5% of all positive blood cultures in major hospital centers.

The majority of cases of clostridial sepsis originate from the female genital tract and follow septic abortion. Introduction of a foreign body is a common antecedent event. In the uterus, residual necrotic fetal and placental tissues and traumatized endometrium may allow the growth of clostridia. Only a small fraction of cases of septic abortion (1%) are followed by serious sepsis. In these patients, sepsis, fever, and chills begin from 1 to 3 days after the attempted abortion. The initial signs are malaise, headache, severe myalgias, abdominal pain, nausea, vomiting, and occasionally diarrhea. Frequently, a bloody or brown vaginal discharge is noted. Patients may rapidly develop oliguria, hypotension, jaundice, and hemoglobinuria. The hemolysis, which is secondary to *C. perfringens* α toxin, causes a characteristic bronzing of the skin. As in myonecrosis, the mental status of severely ill patients is characterized by increased alertness and apprehension. Local examination of the pelvis reveals foul cervical discharge, occasionally with gas. Frequently, laceration marks around the cervix or perforation of the cervical segment is evident. If the infection involves the myometrium or has spread to the adnexa, extreme tenderness, guarding, and an adnexal mass may be found.

Laboratory studies in patients with sepsis reveal an elevated white blood cell count and may show pink, hemoglobin-tinged plasma. Anemia is proportional to the degree of hemolysis, and the hematocrit may be extremely low. Platelet counts may be reduced, and there is often evidence of disseminated intravascular coagulation (DIC). Oliguria or anuria, increasingly refractory hypotension, and hemorrhage and bruising may develop.

Clostridia may enter the bloodstream from the gastrointestinal or biliary tract. This occurrence is associated with ulcerative lesions or obstruction of the small or large intestine, necrotic or infiltrating malignancy, bowel surgery, or various abdominal catastrophes. The patient may present with an acute febrile illness, with chills and fever but no other signs of localized infection. Intravascular hemolysis occurs in as many as half of such cases. Biliary or gastrointestinal symptoms, if present, may be the only clue to the etiology. Positive blood cultures provide the definitive clue to the diagnosis.

Patients with malignant disease can also develop rapidly fatal clostridial sepsis, particularly from a gastrointestinal focus. The most common species in this setting is *C. septicum*. Characteristic signs and symptoms include fever, tachycardia, hypotension, abdominal pain or tenderness, nausea, vomiting, and (preterminally) coma. The tachycardia may be out of proportion to the fever. Only ~20 to 30% of patients develop hemolysis. A striking feature of this syndrome is the rapidity of death, which frequently occurs in <12 h.

DIAGNOSIS The diagnosis of clostridial disease, in association with positive cultures, must be based primarily on clinical findings. Because of the presence of clostridia in many wounds, their mere isolation from any site, including the blood, does not necessarily indicate severe disease. Smears of wound exudates, uterine scrapings, or cervical discharge may show abundant large gram-positive rods as well as other organisms. Cultures should be placed in selective media and incubated anaerobically for identification of clostridia. The diagnosis of clostridial myonecrosis can be established by frozen-section biopsy of muscle.

The urine of patients with severe clostridial sepsis may contain protein and casts, and some patients may develop severe uremia. Profound alterations of circulating erythrocytes are seen in severely toxemic patients. Patients have hemolytic anemia, which develops extremely rapidly, along with hemoglobinemia, hemoglobinuria, and elevated levels of serum bilirubin. Spherocytosis, increased osmotic and mechanical red blood cell fragility, erythrophagocytosis, and methemoglobinemia have been described. DIC may develop in patients with severe infection. In patients with severe sepsis, Wright's or Gram's staining of a smear of peripheral blood or buffy coat may demonstrate clostridia.

X-ray examination sometimes provides an important clue to the diagnosis by revealing gas in muscles, subcutaneous tissue, or the uterus. However, the finding of gas is not pathognomonic for clostridial infection. Other anaerobic bacteria, frequently mixed with aerobic organisms, may produce gas.

℞ TREATMENT (Table 126-1)

Traumatic wounds should be thoroughly cleansed and debrided. Traditionally, the antibiotic treatment of choice for severe clostridial infection has been penicillin G (20 million units per day in adults). Penicillin G treatment of gas gangrene has become more controversial because of increasing resistance to this drug and data obtained from animal models of infection. In a mouse model of gas gangrene, antibiotics inhibiting toxin synthesis appeared to be preferable to cell wall–active drugs; clindamycin treatment enhanced survival more than therapy with penicillin; and the combination of clindamycin and penicillin was superior to penicillin alone. For severe clostridial sepsis, clindamycin may be used at a dose of 600 mg every 6 h in combination with high-dose penicillin (3 to 4 million units every 4 h). Although no clinical trials validate this choice, it is gaining acceptance in the infectious disease community.

In cases of penicillin sensitivity or allergy, other antibiotics should be considered, but all should be tested for in vitro activity because of the occasional isolation of resistant strains. Clostridia are frequently, but not universally, susceptible in vitro to cefoxitin, carbenicillin, chloramphenicol, clindamycin, metronidazole, doxycycline, imipenem, minocycline, tetracycline, third-generation cephalosporins, and vancomycin. For severe clostridial infections, sensitivity testing should be done before an antimicrobial agent with unpredictable activity is used. Simple contamination of a wound with clostridia should not be treated with antibiotics. Localized skin and soft tissue infection can be managed by debridement rather than with systemic antibiotics. Drugs are required when the process extends into adjacent tissue or when fever and systemic signs of sepsis are present. Surgery is a mainstay of therapy for gas gangrene. Amputation is often required for rapidly spreading infection involving a limb, as the process frequently fails to respond to antibiotics. Hysterectomy is required for uterine myonecrosis. Abdominal wall myonecrosis usually continues despite initial aggressive surgery and antibiotic therapy and requires repeated surgical debridement of all involved muscle.

Suppurative infections should be treated with antibiotics. Frequently, broad-spectrum antibiotics must be used because of the mixed flora involved in these infections. Aminoglycosides can be used for the aerobic gram-negative bacteria involved in mixed infections.

The use of a polyvalent gas gangrene antitoxin is still recommended by some authorities. At present, no such antitoxin is produced in the United States, and most centers have discontinued its use in the management of patients with suspected gas gangrene or clostridial postabortion sepsis because of questionable efficacy and the substantial risk of hypersensitivity to horse serum, from which the antitoxin is derived.

The use of hyperbaric oxygen in the treatment of gas gangrene is also controversial. Studies in humans are not well designed to an-

TABLE 126-1 *Treatment of Clostridial Infections*[a]

Condition	Antibiotic Treatment	Penicillin Allergy	Adjunctive Treatment/Note
Contamination	None	—	
Gas gangrene	Penicillin, 3 to 4 million units IV q4h, *plus* Clindamycin, 600 mg IV q6h	Chloramphenicol, metronidazole, imipenem, doxycycline (see text)[b]	Surgical debridement with wide excision is essential; consider hyperbaric oxygen
Clostridial sepsis	Penicillin, 3 to 4 million units IV q4h, *plus* Clindamycin, 600 mg IV q6h	Chloramphenicol, metronidazole, imipenem, doxycycline (see text)[b]	Transient bacteremia may be clinically insignificant
Suppurative deep-tissue infections (e.g., abdominal wall, gynecologic)	Penicillin, 3 to 4 million units IV q4h, *plus* Gentamicin, 5 mg/kg IV q24h, *or* A third-generation cephalosporin (e.g., ceftriaxone, 2 g IV q12h)	As above, plus gentamicin or a quinolone	Empirical therapy should be given; therapy should be based on Gram's stain and culture results when available

[a] Treatment recommendations for *C. difficile* colitis, tetanus, and botulism are found in Chaps. 114, 124, and 125, respectively.
[b] Perform sensitivity testing; consider desensitization.

swer questions on efficacy, but several knowledgeable authors believe that hyperbaric oxygen therapy has contributed to dramatic clinical improvement. Such therapy may, however, be associated with untoward effects due to oxygen toxicity and high atmospheric pressure. Some centers without hyperbaric chambers have reported acceptable mortality rates; thus expert surgical and medical management and control of complications are probably the most important factors in the treatment of gas gangrene. Fasciotomy should not be delayed for hyperbaric oxygen therapy.

ACKNOWLEDGMENT
The authors acknowledge the contributions of Dori F. Zaleznik, MD, to this chapter in earlier editions.

FURTHER READING

BORRIELLO SP: Clostridial disease of the gut. Clin Infect Dis 20:S242, 1995

LORBER B: Gas gangrene and other *Clostridium*-associated diseases, in *Principles and Practice of Infectious Diseases*, 5th ed, GL Mandell et al (eds). New York, Churchill Livingstone, 2000, pp 2549–2560

PRINSSEN HM et al: *Clostridium septicum* myonecrosis and ovarian cancer: A case report and review of literature. Gynecol Oncol 72:116, 1999

ROOD JI: Virulence genes of *Clostridium perfringens*. Annu Rev Microbiol 52:333, 1998

STEVENS DL, BRYANT AE: The role of clostridial toxins in the pathogenesis of gas gangrene. Clin Infect Dis 35:S93, 2002

WANG C et al: Hyperbaric oxygen for treating wounds: A systematic review of the literature. Arch Surg 138:272, 2003

Section 6   Diseases Caused by Gram-Negative Bacteria

127 MENINGOCOCCAL INFECTIONS
David S. Stephens, Robert S. Munford, Lee M. Wetzler

DEFINITION *Neisseria meningitidis* is the etiologic agent of two life-threatening diseases: meningococcal meningitis and fulminant meningococcemia. Meningococci also cause pneumonia, septic arthritis, pericarditis, urethritis, and conjunctivitis. Most cases are potentially preventable by vaccination.

ETIOLOGIC AGENT Meningococci are gram-negative aerobic diplococci. Unlike the other neisseriae, they have a polysaccharide capsule. They are transmitted among humans—their only known habitat—via respiratory secretions. Colonization of the nasopharynx or pharynx is much more common than invasive disease.

MICROBIOLOGY AND CLASSIFICATION On the basis of genome sequencing, *N. meningitidis* is categorized as a β-proteobacterium related to *Bordetella*, *Burkholderia*, *Kingella*, and *Methylomonas* and—more distantly—to *Vibrio*, *Haemophilus*, and *Escherichia coli*. Meningococci are traditionally classified by serologic typing systems based on structural differences in capsule (serogroup), major outer-membrane protein (OMP) porins (serotype), other OMPs (serosubtype), and lipooligosaccharide (LOS; immunotype). Thus, the meningococcal strain designation B:2b:P1.5:L3,7,9 reflects the serogroup (B), serotype (2b), serosubtype (P1.5), and immunotype (L3,7,9).

Meningococci are classified into serogroups according to the antigenicity of their capsular polysaccharides, which reflects structural differences in these carbohydrates. Five serogroups (A, B, C, Y, and W-135) are responsible for >90% of cases of meningococcal disease worldwide. Serogroup A strains, which caused most of the large epidemics of meningococcal disease during the first half of the twentieth century, are now associated with recurring epidemics in sub-Saharan Africa and other locales in the developing world. Serogroups B and C cause most cases of sporadic and epidemic meningococcal disease in industrialized countries. In the United States and Canada during the 1990s, serogroup B was the most common cause of sporadic disease, while serogroup C was a more frequent cause of outbreaks. Serogroup Y has recently been isolated from almost one-third of cases of meningococcal disease in the United States. In general, patients with serogroup Y disease are older and more likely to be African American or to have a chronic underlying illness than are patients with disease caused by other serogroups. Serogroups Y and W-135 are isolated more often than the other serogroups from patients with pneumonia.

One limitation of the serogroup classification is that the genes for capsule biosynthesis can be transferred from one strain to another, with consequent changes in the capsule structure of the recipient strain and

therefore in its serogroup. Other methods for tracking meningococcal strains have thus become increasingly useful. Meningococcal serotypes and subtypes are defined by antigenic differences in specific OMPs, whereas multilocus enzyme electrophoresis classifies bacteria into electrophoretic types (ETs). Other techniques for establishing strain identity or nonidentity are pulsed-field gel electrophoresis and amplification of bacterial genomic sequences by polymerase chain reaction (PCR). These techniques are used for the identification of the strains associated with outbreaks of disease. For example, the virulent III-1 clonal complex of serogroup A was first recognized in Nepal in 1983 to 1984; it spread to Mecca, then to sub-Saharan Africa, and subsequently to temperate Africa. The serogroup B ET-5 complex was first identified in Norway in the 1970s and later caused outbreaks in Europe, Cuba, and South and North America (most recently, in the Pacific Northwest). Serogroup C ET-24 (the ET-37 complex) has caused sporadic cases and outbreaks in Canada and the United States; in some analyses, it has been associated with high rates of mortality and morbidity.

EPIDEMIOLOGY Meningococcal disease occurs worldwide as isolated (sporadic) cases, institution- or community-based outbreaks, and large epidemics. Despite effective antibiotics and partially effective vaccines, *N. meningitidis* is still a leading global cause of meningitis and rapidly fatal sepsis, often in otherwise-healthy individuals.

N. meningitidis is unique among the major bacterial agents of meningitis in that it causes epidemic as well as endemic (sporadic) disease. In all, 300,000 to 500,000 cases of meningococcal disease occur worldwide each year—numbers that frequently are increased by large epidemics. The annual incidence of meningococcal disease is 1 to 2 cases per 100,000 population for sporadic disease, 5 to 10 per 100,000 for hypersporadic disease (localized outbreaks and case clusters), and 10 to >1000 per 100,000 for pandemic and epidemic disease (e.g., serogroup A epidemics). The African meningitis belt (i.e., sub-Saharan Africa) continues to have high levels of sporadic disease and major outbreaks. In the largest meningococcal epidemic outbreak recorded, >300,000 cases and 30,000 deaths occurred in sub-Saharan Africa in 1996 to 1997 due to serogroup A *N. meningitidis*. Large serogroup B epidemics and/or outbreaks of serogroup A or C meningococcal disease have also occurred in Europe, the United States, Canada, China, Nepal, Mongolia, New Zealand, Cuba, Brazil, Chile, Saudi Arabia, and South Africa since 1980. In 2000, 2001, and 2002, worldwide epidemics of serogroup W-135 meningococcal disease occurred in association with the Muslim pilgrimage to Mecca (the Hajj) and in the meningitis belt of sub-Saharan Africa.

In the United States, the attack rate for sporadic meningococcal disease is ~1 case per 100,000 persons per year. Disease attack rates are highest among infants 3 to 9 months of age (10 to 15 cases per

100,000 infants per year). Attack rates are higher among children than among adults, and there is a second peak of incidence among teenagers, in whom outbreaks have often been tied to residence in barracks, dormitories, or other crowded conditions. Although the age-specific incidence is much lower among adults (<1 case per 100,000 persons per year), one-third to one-half of all cases of sporadic meningococcal disease occur in individuals ≥18 years of age. Peak disease incidence coincides with the winter peak of respiratory viral illnesses. During epidemics, disease incidence increases disproportionately among teenagers and young adults. In sub-Saharan Africa, epidemic outbreaks occur with the dry season and the coming of the dry dusty winds of the harmattan.

Meningococcal disease occurs more commonly among the household contacts of primary cases than in the general population. The secondary attack rate is 400 to 1000 per 100,000 household members. School-based clusters of cases have also been described; the attack rate among school contacts of cases has been estimated at 2 to 4 cases per 100,000 exposed individuals. In outbreaks on college campuses, attack rates have been highest among students living in dormitories. Most secondary cases occur within 2 weeks of the primary case, although some cases may develop as long as several months later. Secondary cases account for <2% of all cases reported each year in the United States.

Meningococcal colonization of the nasopharynx (asymptomatic carriage) can persist for months. In nonepidemic periods, ~10% of healthy individuals are colonized. Factors that predispose individuals to colonization with *N. meningitidis* include residence in the same household with a person who has meningococcal disease or is a carrier, household or institutional crowding, active or passive exposure to tobacco smoke, and a recent history of a viral upper respiratory infection. These factors have also been associated with an increased risk of meningococcal disease.

PATHOGENESIS (Fig. 127-1)   Meningococci that colonize the upper respiratory tract are internalized by nonciliated mucosal cells and may traverse them to enter the submucosa, from which they can make their way into the bloodstream. While meningococcal colonization occurs often in healthy humans, bloodstream infection is an infrequent event that is not essential for the organisms' survival and spread. The pro-

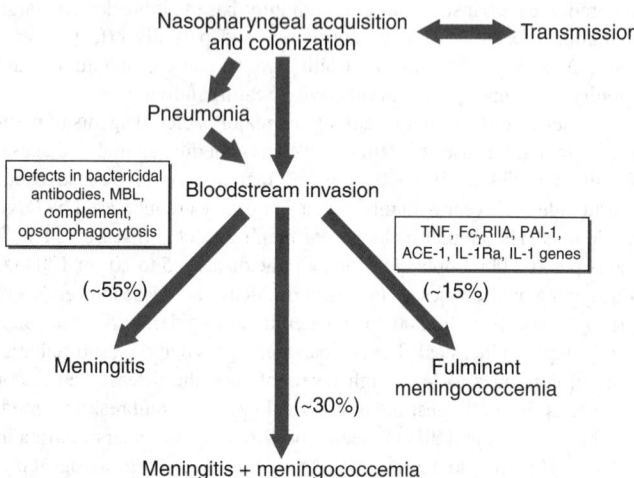

FIGURE 127-1   Meningococcal disease pathogenesis, susceptibility, and severity. After human-to-human transmission, environmental factors (smoking, coinfections), polymorphisms in innate immunity or other genes, and absence of mucosal antibodies may confer susceptibility to meningococcal invasion from the nasopharynx into the bloodstream. In individuals who lack bactericidal antibodies, terminal or alternative pathway complement-deficiency states and other genetic polymorphisms may influence the severity of the ensuing host response and the clinical presentation. Although each of these gene associations has been reported, most of them require confirmation in different ethnic groups. MBL, mannose-binding lectin; TNF, tumor necrosis factor; FcγRIIA, FCγRIIA R131 allele; PAI-1, plasminogen activator inhibitor 1; ACE-1, angiotensin-converting enzyme 1; IL, interleukin.

duction of human disease has no obvious evolutionary advantage for either pathogen or host. Although some strains of *N. meningitidis* are thought to cause more severe disease in humans than do other strains, the basis for this difference is not understood. Meningococci may undergo important phenotypic changes when they adapt to growth in vivo; presumed virulence traits include the antiphagocytic capsular polysaccharide, an ability to sialylate LOS so that it mimics host-cell carbohydrate moieties, the secretion of IgA protease, and mechanisms for iron acquisition. The ET-5 strain of serogroup B *N. meningitidis* has been associated with high case-fatality rates in some populations but not in others; this discrepancy suggests that host factors also contribute importantly to disease pathogenesis.

A meningococcus that enters the bloodstream from the nasopharynx and survives host defenses generally has one of two fates. If multiplication occurs slowly, the bacteria eventually may seed local sites, such as the meninges and/or (less commonly) the joints or the pericardium. More rapid multiplication in the bloodstream is associated with the clinical features of meningococcemia, with petechiae, purpura, disseminated intravascular coagulation (DIC), and shock, which usually causes symptoms before local sites become infected. Thus compartmentalization of bacterial growth and host inflammation either in the blood or at a local site (usually the meninges) can occur.

Outer-Membrane Components Associated with Virulence   Invasive meningococcal strains are characterized by the expression of capsular polysaccharide and other outer-membrane structures, including LOS (endotoxin). Outer-membrane blebbing, meningococcal autolysis, molecular mimicry, genome plasticity, horizontal DNA exchange, and phase and/or antigenic variation are all important in meningococcal virulence.

CAPSULE   The polysaccharide capsule is a major—if not the major—virulence factor of *N. meningitidis*. As stated above, meningococci isolated from the blood or cerebrospinal fluid (CSF) of patients with invasive meningococcal disease most often express capsules of serogroups A, B, C, Y, and W-135. Isolates from asymptomatic nasopharyngeal carriers are nongroupable or express B, Y, X, Z, or 29E capsular serogroups. Capsules impart antiphagocytic and antibactericidal properties to the meningococcus and thus enhance meningococcal survival during invasion of the bloodstream or CSF. Capsules also provide protective properties (e.g., preventing desiccation and phagocytic killing) and antiadherent properties; these properties promote meningococcal transmission, spread, and survival externally and within intracellular compartments such as phagocytic vacuoles.

Except in serogroup A, the major meningococcal capsular polysaccharides associated with invasive disease are composed of sialic acid (*N*-acetyl neuraminic acid, NANA) derivatives. The serogroup B capsule is composed of ($\alpha2\rightarrow8$)-linked NANA, the serogroup C capsule of ($\alpha2\rightarrow9$)-linked NANA, the serogroup Y capsule of alternating D-glucose and NANA, and the serogroup W-135 capsule of D-galactose and NANA. The differences in sialic acid capsule composition are derived from the distinct polysialyltransferases encoded by the fourth gene of the capsule biosynthesis operon, which is also used as a basis for capsule-specific PCR diagnosis. A four-gene operon encoding the capsule transport apparatus (ctr) is conserved among different serogroups and is also used in PCR diagnosis. The serogroup A capsule is composed of repeating units of (α)-linked *N*-acetyl-mannosamine-1-phosphate and is encoded by a four-gene biosynthesis cassette unique for this serogroup.

OUTER-MEMBRANE PROTEINS   Meningococci isolated from sites of colonization or invasive disease are piliated. Pili are complex outer-membrane, protein-based organelles that facilitate adhesion—the first step in meningococcal host-cell interactions. Meningococci express two major OMP porins, PorA and PorB. Human opsonins and bactericidal antibodies induced during meningococcal disease have been shown to recognize PorA and PorB. Vaccines based on PorA-containing outer-membrane vesicles are under development. Another OMP, Opc, is involved in cell attachment and is also a target of bactericidal antibodies. Meningococci encounter iron-restricted environments during infection. The majority of host iron is presented intracellularly as hemoglobin and extracellularly as human transferrin and lactoferrin. Meningococci have evolved systems for acquisition of these iron-carrying molecules.

LIPOOLIGOSACCHARIDE Meningococcal LOS is structurally related to the lipopolysaccharide (LPS) expressed by many gram-negative bacilli. However, LOS does not have repeating O-antigen subunits of sugars. The lipid A moiety of LOS, which has been classically termed *endotoxin* (as opposed to the bacterial exotoxins), is the portion that mediates the induction of inflammatory cytokines often seen in disease. The effect of lipid A is due to an interaction with the innate immune receptor Toll-like receptor 4 (TLR4) in association with the membrane protein MD2. TLR4 and MD2 are found mainly on macrophages/monocytes, dendritic cells, and other phagocytes. The morbidity and mortality of meningococcal bacteremia and meningitis have been directly correlated with the amount of circulating meningococcal endotoxin.

Other Virulence Mechanisms The outer-membrane components of *N. meningitidis* (e.g., pili, LOS, Opa proteins, Opc, capsule) vary in expression or structure at high frequencies (10^{-2} to 10^{-4} per cell per generation). Variation is the result of genetic switches that turn expression of a component on or off, regulate the amount of a component, or alter the structure of a component. Genetic events leading to phase and structural variation allow immune escape and create variability in the structures that are important in pathogenesis (on and off expression of attachment ligands, protection against serum killing, invasion determinants). The serogroup B capsule provides an example of how meningococci downregulate the human immune response through the expression of host-like antigens. The ($\alpha2{\rightarrow}8$)-linked polysialic acid capsule of serogroup B meningococci is identical to structures on the human neural cell adhesion molecule N-CAM. Meningococci are also characterized by frequent vesiculation (blebbing) of the outer membrane, and the amount of blebbing may vary between strains. Blebs may contribute to the rapid initiation of the inflammatory and clotting cascades. They may also be related to the natural autolysis of meningococci that results in DNA release and facilitates genetic transformation.

Specific disease manifestations of meningococcal infections have specific virulence and pathogenic mechanisms as described below for fulminant meningococcemia and meningitis.

Fulminant Meningococcemia (Purpura Fulminans) Fulminant meningococcemia is perhaps the most rapidly lethal form of septic shock experienced by humans. It differs from most other forms of septic shock by the prominence of hemorrhagic skin lesions (petechiae, purpura; see Fig. 46-5) and the consistent development of DIC.

The dominant proinflammatory molecule in the meningococcal cell wall is the endotoxin or LOS, and the outer membrane that contains it is poorly tethered to the underlying peptidoglycan. This structural peculiarity seems to account for the fact that meningococci shed LOS-containing membrane blebs as they grow. The bacteria can multiply to very high concentrations in the blood. The concentrations of endotoxin detected in the blood of patients with fulminant meningococcemia are 10- to 1000-fold higher than those found in the blood of patients with bacteremia due to other gram-negative bacteria. The bacteria and endotoxin-containing blebs stimulate monocytes, neutrophils, and endothelial cells, which then release cytokines and other mediators that can activate many distant targets, including other leukocytes, platelets, and endothelial cells. In addition, meningococci can invade the vascular endothelium. When activated, the endothelium produces molecules that can be procoagulant as well as adhesive for leukocytes.

Patients with fulminant meningococcemia usually have extremely high blood levels of both proinflammatory mediators—i.e., tumor necrosis factor (TNF), interleukin (IL) 1, interferon γ, and IL-8—and anti-inflammatory mediators—i.e., IL-1 receptor antagonist (IL-1Ra), soluble IL-1 receptors, soluble TNF receptors, and IL-10. The plasma of patients with meningococcal shock can decrease the responses of normal leukocytes to stimuli such as LOS; the implication is that anti-inflammatory mediators predominate in the blood late in infection.

Procoagulant, antifibrinolytic forces are also active in the blood of patients with fulminant meningococcemia (Fig. 127-2). Monocytes express large amounts of tissue factor. Fibrinopeptide A and thrombin-antithrombin levels are high, reflecting active clotting, while antithrombin and fibrinogen levels are low. Although the tissue factor–regulated ("extrinsic") arm of coagulation predominates, the contact system (factors XII and XI, prekallikrein, high-molecular-weight kininogen) is also activated. Striking deficiencies of antithrombin and proteins C and S can occur; studies have found a strong negative correlation between protein C activity and both the size of purpuric skin lesions and the mortality rate. Plasminogen levels are decreased, while plasmin-antiplasmin complexes and plasminogen activator inhibitor 1 (PAI-1) levels in the blood are very high. PAI-1 levels have been correlated with mortality risk.

Fibrin deposition is therefore favored both by the procoagulant tendency (promoted through activation of tissue factor and deficiencies of proteins C and S and antithrombin) and by an antifibrinolytic tendency (favored by excessive PAI-1). Both platelets and leukocytes doubtless contribute to the formation of microthrombi and to the vascular injury that ensues. Thrombosis of small to mid-sized arteries can produce peripheral necrosis and gangrene necessitating limb or digit amputation.

Meningitis Meningococcal bacteremia can result in the seeding of the meninges, pericardium, and large joints. Up to one-third of patients with meningococcal disease present with meningitis or other closed-space infections without signs of sepsis. How meningococci traverse the blood-brain barrier and enter the CSF or reach other closed sites is unclear. Meningococci have been shown to invade endothelial cells both experimentally and in vivo. The choroid plexus is also a potential site of meningococcal entry into the CSF. Meningococcal pili may bind CD46, a complement-regulatory protein that is expressed by the choroid plexus and meningeal epithelia. Upon meningococcal entry into the CSF, a vigorous local inflammatory response ensues, probably triggered by endotoxin-containing meningococcal membranes. Both bacterial growth and the inflammatory response occur within the CSF, where levels of endotoxin, IL-6, TNF, IL-1β, IL-1Ra, and IL-10 exceed the concentrations found in plasma by 100- to 1000-fold. The inflammatory response is largely confined to the subarachnoid space and contiguous structures. The inflammatory cytokines TNF and IL-1 released in meningococcal bacteremia may also enhance the permeability of the blood-brain barrier. Meningitis and other closed-space infections (e.g., arthritis, pericarditis) are the result of bacterial survival and multiplication at these sites. For example, meningitis and its sequelae are due to the induction of local inflammatory cytokines and other mediators (e.g., nitric oxide), leukocyte infiltration across the blood-brain barrier, breakdown of the blood-brain barrier with edema,

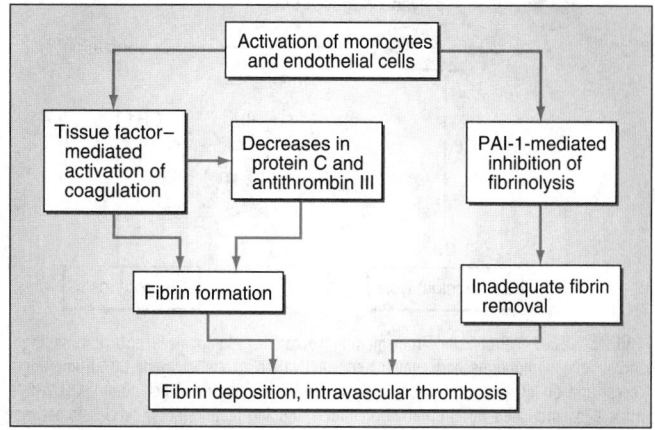

FIGURE 127-2 The pathogenesis of fibrin deposition in patients with fulminant meningococcemia. PAI-1, plasminogen activator inhibitor 1. (*Adapted from M Levi et al: Eur J Clin Invest 27:3, 1997.*)

release of metalloproteases, induction of cellular apoptosis, coagulation of vessels, and ischemia.

Patients who develop meningitis without meningococcemia may be individuals in whom meningococci do not grow rapidly in or have been cleared from the blood; may have antibodies or phagocytes that slow meningococcal growth; or may lack the (unknown) factors that allow *N. meningitidis* to multiply rapidly in vivo. If disease is recognized early, the prognosis of patients with meningococcal meningitis is substantially better than that of patients with fulminant meningococcemia.

HOST DEFENSE MECHANISMS Preventing meningococcal growth in blood requires bactericidal and opsonic antibodies, complement, and phagocytes (Fig. 127-3). The major bactericidal antibodies are IgM and IgG, which (except for serogroup B) bind to the capsular polysaccharide. Immunity to meningococci is therefore serogroup specific. Antibodies to other surface (subcapsular) antigens may confer cross-serogroup protection. PorA, PorB, Opc, and LOS appear to be major targets of cross-reactivity and of serogroup B bactericidal antibodies. Infants are protected from meningococcal disease during the first months of life by passively transferred maternal IgG antibodies. As maternal antibody levels wane, the attack rate increases, peaking from 3 to 9 months of age. Disease incidence declines as protective antibodies are induced by colonization with nonpathogenic bacteria that have cross-reactive antigens. In addition to *Neisseria lactamica*, which frequently colonizes young children, some enteric bacteria have antigens that cross-react with those of meningococci. One theory relates the occurrence of some cases of meningococcal disease to the presence of high levels of IgA antibodies to meningococci, since these antibodies can block the bactericidal activity of IgM.

Complement is required for bactericidal activity and for efficient opsonophagocytosis. Individuals deficient in any of the late complement components (C5 to C9) cannot assemble the membrane-attack complex (MAC) needed to kill *Neisseria*. These persons typically develop less severe meningococcal disease than complement-sufficient individuals, do so at an older age, and tend to have disease due to uncommon serogroups (W-135, X, Y, Z, and 29E). Although only one-half of individuals with known late-complement-component deficiency ever experience meningococcal disease, some affected persons have several episodes. Deficiency of each of the terminal complement components is inherited in an autosomal recessive fashion. Properdin deficiency, in contrast, is X-linked; some affected males develop overwhelming meningococcal disease, an observation indicating that the alternative complement pathway is also needed for antimeningococcal host defense. Disease onset in properdin-deficient individuals typically occurs in the teens or twenties. There is also recent evidence that inherited differences in the mannose-binding lectin (MBL) pathway of complement activation may influence the risk of acquiring meningococcal disease in childhood. Alleles that decrease MBL synthesis have been associated with increased risk in the few studies reported to date.

Activation of the classic pathway of complement by antigen-antibody complexes or of the alternative pathway by LOS or capsular polysaccharide is important for producing and maintaining C3b (Fig. 127-3). Without C3b, neither bactericidal lysis nor phagocytosis can proceed effectively. When C3b is generated, meningococcal growth is probably checked by the MAC, which produces bacterial lysis, and by robust phagocytosis. Most IgG antibodies to the meningococcal polysaccharide are of the IgG_2 isotype; a phagocytic cell defect (the FcγRIIA R131 allele) that impairs the phagocytosis of IgG_2-coated particles has been associated with more severe meningococcal disease. This allele has also been associated with a more severe clinical course in patients with late-complement-component deficiency; thus effective phagocytosis may contribute to the relatively mild meningococcal disease usually observed in these individuals.

The available studies of gene polymorphism–disease associations are summarized in Figs. 127-1 and 127-3. In individuals who lack bactericidal antibodies, protection from acquiring meningococcal bacteremia may be provided, at least in part, by innate immune mechanisms such as the MBL pathway for activating complement, complement factor C4b, and the TLR4 pathway for LOS recognition. Other genes may influence meningococcal survival in vivo [FcγIIA (CD32)], while still others seem to regulate the host inflammatory (IL-1β, IL-1Ra, TNF, angiotensin-converting enzyme) and clotting (PAI-1) responses to invading meningococci. Although many of these associations await confirmation in other populations of patients, in sum they point to important genetic influences on the acquisition and severity of meningococcal disease. This conclusion is supported by the overrepresentation of ABO blood group nonsecretors among patients with meningococcal disease and by the striking variability in meningococcal disease incidence among different racial groups.

CLINICAL MANIFESTATIONS ■ **Upper Respiratory Tract Infections** Although many patients who develop meningococcal meningitis or meningococcemia report having had throat soreness or other upper respiratory symptoms during the preceding week, it is uncertain whether these symptoms are due to infection with meningococci. Meningococcal pharyngitis is rarely diagnosed. Adult patients with *N. meningitidis* bacteremia more often have clinically apparent disease of the respiratory tract (pneumonia, sinusitis, tracheobronchitis, conjunctivitis) than do younger patients.

Meningococcemia Patients with meningococcal disease may have both meningococcemia and meningitis. These conditions have a wide clinical spectrum, with many overlapping features.

Approximately 10 to 30% of patients with meningococcal disease have meningococcemia without clinically apparent meningitis. Although meningococcal bacteremia may occasionally be transient and asymptomatic, in most individuals it is associated with fever, chills, nausea, vomiting, and myalgias. Prostration is common. The most distinctive feature is rash. Erythematous macules rapidly become petechial and, in severe cases, purpuric (see Fig. 46-5). Although the lesions are typically found on the trunk and lower extremities, they may also occur on the face, arms, and mucous membranes. The petechiae may coalesce into hemorrhagic bullae or may undergo necrosis and ulcerate. Patients with severe coagulopathy may develop ischemic extremities or digits, often with a sharp line of demarcation between normal and ischemic tissue.

In many patients with fulminant meningococcemia, the CSF may be normal and the CSF culture negative. Indeed, the absence of meningitis in a patient with meningococcemia is a poor prognostic sign; it suggests that the bacteria have multiplied so rapidly in the blood that meningeal seeding has not yet occurred or had time to elicit in-

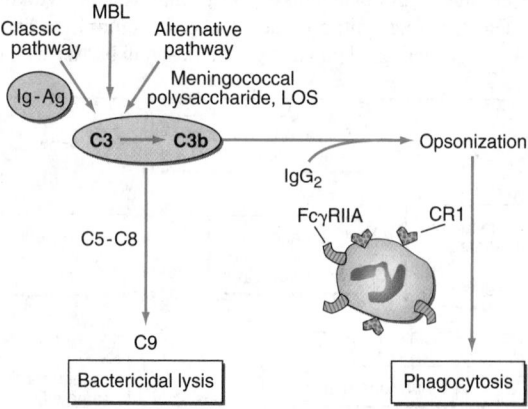

FIGURE 127-3 Protection from meningococcal disease involves both antimeningococcal immunoglobulins and complement. Activation of complement by antimeningococcal IgM or IgG promotes bacterial lysis via the membrane attack complex (C5–C9), while C3b [produced by alternative, mannose-binding lectin (MBL), or classic pathway activation] and antimeningococcal IgG_2 cooperate to produce effective opsonophagocytosis. A neutrophil defect in binding IgG_2 (the FcγRIIA R131 allele) has been associated with more severe meningococcal disease. CR1, complement receptor 1; LOS, lipooligosaccharide.

flammation in the CSF. Most of these patients also lack evidence of an acute-phase response; i.e., the erythrocyte sedimentation rate is normal, and the C-reactive protein concentration in blood is low.

The *Waterhouse-Friderichsen syndrome* is a dramatic example of DIC-induced microthrombosis, hemorrhage, and tissue injury. Although overt adrenal failure is infrequently documented in patients with fulminant meningococcemia, patients may have partial adrenal insufficiency and be unable to mount the normal hypercortisolemic response to severe stress or cosyntropin stimulation. Almost all patients who die from fulminant meningococcemia have adrenal hemorrhages at autopsy.

Chronic meningococcemia (Fig. 127-4) is a rare syndrome of episodic fever, rash, and arthralgias that can last for weeks to months. The rash may be maculopapular; it is occasionally petechial. Splenomegaly may develop. If untreated or if treated with glucocorticoids, chronic meningococcemia may evolve into meningitis, fulminant meningococcemia, or (rarely) endocarditis.

Meningitis (See also Chap. 360) Patients with meningococcal meningitis have usually been sick for ≥24 h before they seek medical attention. Common presenting symptoms include nausea and vomiting, headache, neck stiffness, lethargy, and confusion. The symptoms and signs of meningococcal meningitis cannot be distinguished from those elicited by other meningeal pathogens. Many patients with meningococcal meningitis have concurrent meningococcemia, however, and petechial or purpuric skin lesions (Fig. 46-5) may suggest the correct diagnosis. CSF findings are consistent with those of purulent meningitis: hypoglycorrhachia, an elevated protein concentration, and a neutrophilic leukocytosis. A Gram's stain of CSF is usually positive (see "Diagnosis," below); when this finding is unaccompanied by CSF leukocytosis, the prognosis for normal recovery is often poor.

Other Manifestations Arthritis occurs in ~10% of patients with meningococcal disease. When arthritis develops during the first few days of the patient's illness, it usually reflects direct meningococcal invasion of the joint. Arthritis that begins later in the course is thought to be due to immune complex deposition. Primary meningococcal pneumonia occurs principally in adults, often in military populations, and is often due to serogroup Y. While meningococcal pericarditis is occasionally seen, endocarditis due to *N. meningitidis* is now exceedingly rare. Primary meningococcal conjunctivitis can be complicated by meningococcemia; systemic therapy is therefore warranted when this condition is diagnosed. Meningococcal urethritis has been reported in individuals who practice oral sex.

Complications Patients with meningococcal meningitis may develop cranial nerve palsies, cortical venous thrombophlebitis, and cerebral edema. Children may develop subdural effusions. Permanent sequelae

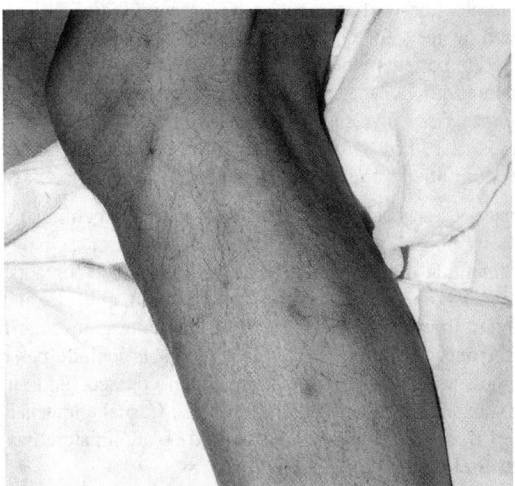

FIGURE 127-4 Erythematous papular lesions are seen on the leg of this patient with chronic meningococcemia. (*Courtesy of Kenneth M. Kaye, M.D., and Elaine T. Kaye, M.D.*)

can include mental retardation, deafness, and hemiparesis. The major long-term morbidity of fulminant meningococcemia is the loss of skin, limbs, or digits that results from ischemic necrosis and infarction.

DIAGNOSIS Few clinical clues help the physician distinguish the patient with early meningococcal disease from patients with other acute systemic infections. The most useful clinical finding is the petechial or purpuric rash (see Fig. 46-5), but it must be differentiated from the petechial lesions seen with gonococcemia (see Fig. 128-1), Rocky Mountain spotted fever (see Fig. 158-1), hypersensitivity vasculitis (see Fig. 46-4), endemic typhus, and some viral infections. In one case series, one-half of the adults with meningococcal bacteremia had neither meningitis nor a rash.

The definitive diagnosis is established by recovering *N. meningitidis*, its antigens, or its DNA from normally sterile body fluids, such as blood, CSF, or synovial fluid, or from skin lesions. Meningococci grow best on Mueller-Hinton or chocolate blood agar at 35°C in an atmosphere that contains 5 to 10% CO_2. Specimens should be plated without delay. *N. meningitidis* bacteria are oxidase-positive, gram-negative diplococci that typically utilize maltose and glucose.

A Gram's stain of CSF reveals intra- or extracellular organisms in ~85% of patients with meningococcal meningitis. The latex agglutination test for meningococcal polysaccharides is less sensitive. PCR amplification of DNA in buffy coat or CSF samples is more sensitive than either of these tests; like the latex agglutination test, this method is unaffected by prior antibiotic therapy.

Throat or nasopharyngeal specimens should be cultured on Thayer-Martin medium, which suppresses the competing oral flora. Throat or nasopharyngeal cultures are recommended only for research or epidemiologic purposes, since a positive result merely confirms the carrier state and does not establish the existence of systemic disease.

℞ TREATMENT (Table 127-1)

A third-generation cephalosporin, such as cefotaxime (2 g intravenously every 4 h) or ceftriaxone (2 g intravenously every 12 h), is preferred for initial therapy. One of these cephalosporins in combination with other agents may cover other bacteria (such as *Streptococcus pneumoniae* and *Haemophilus influenzae*) that can cause the same syndromes (Chap. 360). Penicillin G (18 to 24 million units intravenously per day) remains an acceptable alternative for confirmed invasive meningococcal disease in most countries. However, the prevalence of meningococci with reduced susceptibility to penicillin has been increasing, and high-level penicillin resistance has been reported. Other options include meropenem (1 g intravenously every 8 h). In the patient who is allergic to β-lactam drugs, chloramphenicol (75 to 100 mg/kg per day) is a suitable alternative; chloramphenicol-resistant meningococci have been reported from Vietnam and France. The newer fluoroquinolones gatifloxacin, moxifloxacin, and gemifloxacin have excellent in vitro activity against *N. meningitidis*, with measurable CNS penetration, and appear promising in animal models. Patients with meningococcal meningitis should be given antimicrobial therapy for at least 5 days. While glucocorticoid therapy for meningitis in adults is controversial, many experts administer dexamethasone, beginning if possible before antibiotic therapy is initiated; the schedule is 10 mg intravenously 15 to 20 min before the first antibiotic dose and then every 6 h for 4 days.

Patients with fulminant meningococcemia often experience diffuse leakage of fluid into extravascular spaces, shock, and multiple-organ dysfunction (Chaps. 253 and 254). Myocardial depression may be prominent. Supportive therapy, although never studied in randomized, placebo-controlled trials, is recommended. Standard measures include vigorous fluid resuscitation (often requiring several liters over the first 24 h), elective ventilation, and pressors. Some authorities recommend early hemodialysis or hemofiltration. Fresh-frozen plasma is often given to patients who are bleeding extensively or who have severely deranged clotting parameters. Many European experts have adminis-

ANTIBIOTIC TREATMENT[a]

1. Ceftriaxone 2 g IV q12h (100 mg/kg per day) or cefotaxime 2 g IV q4h
2. For penicillin-sensitive *N. meningitidis*: Penicillin G 18–24 million units per day in divided doses q4h (250,000 units/kg per day)
3. Chloramphenicol 75–100 mg/kg per day in divided doses q6h
4. Meropenem 1.0 g (children, 40 mg) IV q8h
5. In an outbreak setting in developing countries: Long-acting chloramphenicol in oil suspension (Tifomycin), single dose
   Adults: 3.0 g (6 mL)
   Children 1–15 years old: 100 mg/kg
   Children <1 year old: 50 mg/kg

CHEMOPROPHYLAXIS[b]

Rifampin (oral)
   Adults: 600 mg bid for 2 days
   Children ≥1 month old: 10 mg/kg bid for 2 days
   Children <1 month old: 5 mg/kg bid for 2 days
Ciprofloxacin (oral)
   Adults: 500 mg, 1 dose
Ofloxacin (oral)
   Adults: 400 mg, 1 dose
Ceftriaxone (IM)
   Adults: 250 mg, 1 dose
   Children <15 years old: 125 mg, 1 dose
Azithromycin (oral)
   500 mg, 1 dose

VACCINATION[c]

A, C, Y, W-135 vaccine (Memomune, Aventis Pasteur) or A, C vaccine
   Single 0.5-mL subcutaneous injection
New C; A, C; and A, C, Y, W-135 meningococcal conjugate vaccines[d]

[a] Patients with meningococcal meningitis should receive antimicrobial therapy for at least 5 days.
[b] Use is recommended for close contacts of cases.
[c] At present, use is generally limited to the control of epidemics and to individuals with increased risk of meningococcal disease. Vaccine efficacy wanes after 3–5 years, and vaccine is not effective in recipients <2 years of age.
[d] These vaccines appear to provide immunity in young children, a prolonged immune response, and herd immunity (decreased transmission and colonization).

tered antithrombin III to such patients. Patients with fulminant meningococcemia in whom shock persists despite vigorous fluid resuscitation should receive supplemental glucocorticoid treatment (hydrocortisone, 1 mg/kg every 6 h) pending tests of adrenal reserve.

Although it has not been formally tested in patients with fulminant meningococcemia, activated protein C (drotrecogin alfa, Xigris) is approved for use in patients with severe sepsis and dysfunction of more than one organ (APACHE II score, >25). Because of the pathophysiology, patients with meningococcemia may represent a group most likely to benefit from administration of activated protein C. The recommended dose is 24 μg/kg per hour, given as a continuous intravenous infusion for 96 h. Drotrecogin alfa is contraindicated when the peripheral-blood platelet count is <50,000/μL, however, and when there is active bleeding or a high risk of bleeding. Clotting parameters should be monitored closely while the drug is being infused; its administration should be discontinued 4 to 6 h before the performance of an invasive procedure. Drotrecogin alfa should not be used in patients with meningitis pending further evidence that it does not induce intracranial bleeding when the meninges are inflamed.

PROGNOSIS When patients are first evaluated, the clinical features most strongly associated with a fatal outcome are shock, a purpuric or ecchymotic rash, a low or normal blood leukocyte count, an age of ≥60 years, and coma. The absence of meningitis, the presence of thrombocytopenia, low blood concentrations of antithrombin or proteins S and C, high blood levels of PAI-1, and a low erythrocyte sedimentation rate (or C-reactive protein level) have also been associated with increased mortality from meningococcal disease. In contrast, the receipt of antibiotics before hospital admission has been associated with lower mortality rates in some studies.

PREVENTION ■ **Meningococcal Polysaccharide Vaccines** A single injection of quadrivalent meningococcal polysaccharide vaccine (serogroups A, C, W-135, and Y) immunizes ~80 to 95% of immunocompetent adults (Table 127-1). Children ≥3 months of age can be vaccinated to prevent serogroup A disease, but multiple doses are required; the vaccine is otherwise ineffective in children <2 years old. The duration of vaccine-induced immunity in adults is probably <5 years. There is currently no vaccine for serogroup B; its polysaccharide is a sialic acid homopolymer that is poorly immunogenic in humans. In addition to individuals with late-complement-component or properdin deficiency, persons with sickle cell anemia, asplenia, or splenectomy should receive the quadrivalent vaccine. Vaccination is also recommended for military recruits, pilgrims on the Hajj, and individuals traveling to sub-Saharan Africa during the dry months (June to December) or to other areas with epidemic meningococcal disease. The Advisory Committee on Immunization Practices (ACIP) of the Centers for Disease Control and Prevention (CDC) recommends vaccination of incoming college freshmen who will live in dormitories. In general, the vaccine should be given only to persons >2 years of age.

New meningococcal capsular oligosaccharide and polysaccharide conjugate vaccines (C; A and C; A, C, Y, and W-135) are being developed; some are currently undergoing clinical trials, and some are now in use in Europe and Canada. These vaccines are based on the approach used for the highly successful *H. influenzae* type b conjugate vaccines. Covalent linkage of the polysaccharide to a carrier protein converts the polysaccharide to a thymus-dependent antigen enhancing IgG anticapsular antibodies and memory B cells. Because levels of antibody in mucosal secretions are much higher after the administration of a conjugate vaccine than after vaccination with an unconjugated preparation, a major benefit of these vaccines may be the introduction of herd immunity. Memory response to meningococcal polysaccharide also appears to be an important effect of the conjugate vaccines. Meningococcal conjugate vaccines are not yet licensed in the United States. However, in the United Kingdom, serogroup C conjugate vaccines introduced in 2000 have had a marked impact on the incidence of serogroup C disease in the population vaccinated. If conjugate meningococcal vaccines prove to be capable of providing durable antibody or memory responses (particularly in infants and young children), their integration into the routine childhood immunization schedule would appear warranted. Vaccines for serogroup B meningococcal disease remain elusive; none of the group B vaccines studied in clinical trials has proven to be broadly effective, but these products have a role in the control of serogroup B epidemics. The identification of new meningococcal protective antigens and the development of better meningococcal vaccines are areas of continued research and hold promise for the prevention of diseases due to *N. meningitidis*.

Screening tests for complement-component deficiency should be conducted in patients who have a family history of meningococcal or disseminated gonococcal disease; in patients who have a recurrence; in patients whose first case occurs at ≥15 years of age; in patients with cases caused by serogroups other than A, B, or C; and in family members of patients found to have a complement deficiency.

Antimicrobial Chemoprophylaxis The attack rate for meningococcal disease among household or other close contacts of cases is >400-fold greater than that in the population as a whole. Close contacts of cases should receive chemoprophylaxis with rifampin, ciprofloxacin, ofloxacin, or azithromycin (Table 127-1). A single intramuscular injection of ceftriaxone is also effective. Close contacts include persons who live in the same household, day-care center contacts, and anyone directly exposed to a patient's oral secretions. Casual contacts are not at increased risk. Chemoprophylaxis should be administered as soon as possible after the case is identified.

Isolation Precautions The CDC recommends that patients with meningococcal disease who are hospitalized be placed in respiratory isolation for the first 24 h.

Outbreak Control An organization- or community-based outbreak of meningococcal disease is defined as the occurrence of three or more cases within ≤3 months in persons who have a common affiliation or reside in the same area but who are not close contacts of one another; in addition, the primary disease attack rate must exceed 10 cases per 100,000 persons, and the case strains of *N. meningitidis* must be of the same molecular type. Mass vaccination should be considered when such outbreaks occur, and mass chemoprophylaxis may be used to control school- or other institution-based outbreaks. Consultation with public health authorities is recommended when such campaigns are contemplated.

FURTHER READING

BRANDTZAEG P et al: Net inflammatory capacity of human septic shock plasma evaluated by a monocyte-based target cell assay: Identification of interleukin-10 as a major functional deactivator of human monocytes. J Exp Med 184:51, 1996

CENTERS FOR DISEASE CONTROL AND PREVENTION: Prevention and control of meningococcal disease: Recommendations of the Advisory Committee on Immunization Practices (ACIP). MMWR 49(RR-7):1, 2000

FIJEN CA et al: Assessment of complement deficiency in patients with meningococcal disease in the Netherlands. Clin Infect Dis 28:98, 1999

HIBBERD ML et al: Association of variants of the gene for mannose-binding lectin with susceptibility to meningococcal disease. Lancet 353:1049, 1999

JOHANSSON L et al: CD46 in meningococcal disease. Science 301:373, 2003

MACDONALD NE et al: Induction of immunologic memory by conjugated vs plain meningococcal C polysaccharide vaccine in toddlers—a randomized controlled trial. JAMA 280:1685, 1998

PLATONOV AE et al: Meningococcal disease and polymorphism of FcγRIIA (CD32) in late complement component–deficient individuals. Clin Exp Immunol 111:97, 1998

ROSENSTEIN NE et al: Meningococcal disease. N Engl J Med 344:1378, 2001

SMIRNOVA I et al: Assay of locus-specific genetic load implicates rare Toll-like receptor 4 mutations in meningococcal susceptibility. Proc Natl Acad Sci USA 100:6075, 2003

128 GONOCOCCAL INFECTIONS
Sanjay Ram, Peter A. Rice

DEFINITION Gonorrhea is a sexually transmitted infection of epithelium and commonly manifests as cervicitis, urethritis, proctitis, and conjunctivitis. If untreated, infections at these sites can lead to local complications such as endometritis, salpingitis, tuboovarian abscess, bartholinitis, peritonitis, and perihepatitis in the female; periurethritis and epididymitis in the male; and ophthalmia neonatorum in the newborn. Disseminated gonococcemia is an uncommon event whose manifestations include skin lesions, tenosynovitis, arthritis, and (in rare cases) endocarditis or meningitis.

Neisseria gonorrhoeae is a gram-negative, nonmotile, non-spore-forming organism that grows in pairs (diplococci). Each individual organism is shaped like a coffee bean, with adjacent concave sides seen on Gram's stain. Gonococci, like all other *Neisseria* spp., are oxidase positive. They are distinguished from other neisseriae by their ability to grow on selective media and to utilize glucose but not maltose, sucrose, or lactose.

EPIDEMIOLOGY The incidence of gonorrhea has declined significantly in the United States, but there were still ~362,000 newly reported cases in 2002. Gonorrhea remains a major public health problem worldwide, is a significant cause of morbidity in developing countries, and may play a role in enhancing transmission of HIV.

Gonorrhea predominantly affects young, nonwhite, unmarried, less educated members of urban populations. The number of reported cases probably represents half of the true number of cases—a discrepancy resulting from underreporting, self-treatment, and nonspecific treatment without a culture-proven diagnosis. The number of reported cases of gonorrhea in the United States rose from ~250,000 in the early 1960s to a high of 1.01 million in 1978. The peak recorded incidence of gonorrhea in modern times was reported in 1975, with 468 cases per 100,000 population in the United States. This peak was attributable to the interaction of several variables, including improved accuracy of diagnosis, changes in patterns of contraceptive use, and changes in sexual behavior. The incidence of the disease has since gradually declined and is currently estimated at 120 cases per 100,000, a figure that is still the highest among industrialized countries. A further decline in the overall incidence of gonorrhea in the United States over the past decade may reflect increased condom use resulting from public health efforts to curtail HIV transmission. Presently, the attack rate in the United States is highest in the 20- to 24-year age group, in which 75% of all cases occur. With adjustment for sexual experience, the risk is highest among sexually active 15- to 19-year-old women. In terms of ethnicity, rates are highest among African Americans and lowest among persons of Asian or Pacific Island descent.

The incidence of gonorrhea is highest in developing countries. The exact incidence of any of the sexually transmitted diseases (STDs) is difficult to ascertain in developing countries because of limited surveillance and variable diagnostic criteria. For example, in Kenya, it was estimated in 1987 that 10% of all live births were adversely affected by STDs, and gonococcal ophthalmia neonatorum reportedly affected 4% of all live-born infants. The median prevalence of gonorrhea in unselected populations of pregnant women has been estimated at 10% in Africa, 5% in Latin America, and 4% in Asia. Studies in Africa have clearly demonstrated that nonulcerative STDs such as gonorrhea are an independent risk factor for the transmission of HIV (Chap. 173).

Gonorrhea is transmitted from males to females more efficiently than in the opposite direction. The rate of transmission to a woman following a single unprotected sexual encounter with an infected man is on the order of 40 to 60%. Oropharyngeal gonorrhea occurs in ~20% of women who practice fellatio with infected partners. Transmission in either direction by cunnilingus is rare.

There exists in any population a small minority of individuals who have high rates of new-partner acquisition. These "core-group members" or "high-frequency transmitters" are vital in sustaining STD transmission at the population level. Another instrumental factor in sustaining gonorrhea in the population is the large number of infected individuals who are asymptomatic or have minor symptoms that are ignored. These persons, unlike symptomatic individuals, do not cease sexual activity and therefore continue to transmit the disease. This situation underscores the importance of contact tracing and empirical treatment of sex partners of index cases.

PATHOGENESIS, IMMUNOLOGY, AND ANTIMICROBIAL RESISTANCE ■ **Outer-Membrane Proteins** ■ *PILI* Fresh clinical isolates of *N. gonorrhoeae* initially form piliated (fimbriated) colonies distinguishable on translucent agar. Pilus expression is rapidly switched off with unselected subculture because of rearrangements in pilus genes. This change is a basis for phase variation of gonococci. Piliated strains adhere better to cells derived from human mucosal surfaces and are more virulent in organ culture models and human inoculation experiments than nonpiliated variants. In a fallopian tube explant model, pili mediate gonococcal attachment to nonciliated columnar epithelial cells. This event initiates gonococcal phagocytosis and transport through these cells to intercellular spaces near the basement membrane or directly into the subepithelial tissue. Damage to nearby ciliated columnar epithelial cells, which is caused by the release of cytokines, results in loss of cilia and sloughing of ciliated cells and diminishes the integrity of the fallopian tube. Nonpiliated gonococci cause epithelial damage at a much slower rate. CD46 (membrane cofactor protein) is present on urogenital epithelial cells in both men and women and has been determined to be a receptor for PilC; this subunit is located at the tip of the pilus molecule and is critical in mediating adherence. Pili are also essential for genetic competence and transformation of *N. gonorrhoeae*, which permit horizontal transfer of genetic material between different gonococcal lineages in vivo.

OPACITY-ASSOCIATED PROTEIN Another gonococcal surface protein that is important in adherence to epithelial cells is opacity-associated protein (Opa, formerly called protein II). Opa contributes to intergonococcal adhesion, which is responsible for the opaque nature of gonococcal colonies on translucent agar and the organism's adherence to a variety of eukaryotic cells, including polymorphonuclear leukocytes (PMNs). Certain Opa variants promote invasion of epithelial cells, and this effect has been linked with the ability of Opa to bind vitronectin, glycosaminoglycans, and several members of the carcinoembryonic antigen–related cell adhesion molecule (CEACAM, previously known as CD66) receptor family. Each strain of *N. gonorrhoeae* possesses as many as 11 different *opa* genes, but usually no more than three types are expressed at any given time. Isolates from normally sterile sites such as the fallopian tube and synovial fluid usually fail to express Opa, while isolates from mucosal sites usually form opaque colonies. Female commercial sex workers with antibodies to Opa may be less likely to develop pelvic inflammatory disease (PID) than women without such antibodies. *N. gonorrhoeae* Opa proteins that bind CEACAM 1, which is expressed by primary CD4+ T lymphocytes, suppress the activation and proliferation of these lymphocytes. This phenomenon may serve to explain the transient decrease in CD4+ T-lymphocyte counts associated with gonococcal infection.

PORIN Porin (previously designated protein I) is the most abundant gonococcal surface protein, accounting for >50% of the organism's total outer-membrane protein. Porin molecules exist as trimers that provide anion aqueous channels through the otherwise-hydrophobic outer membrane. Porin shows stable interstrain antigenic variation and forms the basis for gonococcal serotyping. Two main serotypes have been identified: Por1A strains are often associated with disseminated gonococcal infection (DGI), while Por1B strains usually cause local genital infections only. DGI strains are generally resistant to the killing action of normal human serum, do not incite a significant local inflammatory response, and therefore may not cause symptoms at genital sites. These characteristics may be related to the ability of Por1A strains to bind to complement-downregulatory molecules, resulting in a diminished inflammatory response. Porin can translocate to the cytoplasmic membrane of host cells—a process that could initiate gonococcal endocytosis and invasion. In addition, porin is an immunologic target of bactericidal and opsonophagocytic antibodies that may arise in response to immune stimulation resulting from infection or immunization with porin-containing vaccine candidates.

OTHER OUTER-MEMBRANE PROTEINS Other notable outer-membrane proteins include H.8, a lipoprotein that is present in high concentration on the surface of all gonococcal strains and is an excellent target for antibody-based diagnostic testing. Transferrin-binding proteins (Tbp1 and Tbp2) and lactoferrin-binding protein are required for scavenging iron from transferrin and lactoferrin in vivo. Transferrin and iron have been shown to increase attachment of iron-deprived *N. gonorrhoeae* to human endometrial cells. Studies with volunteers have demonstrated that gonococci deficient in transferrin- and lactoferrin-binding proteins cannot establish infection in men. IgA1 protease is produced by *N. gonorrhoeae* and may protect the organism from the action of mucosal IgA.

Lipooligosaccharide Gonococcal lipooligosaccharide (LOS) consists of a lipid A and a core oligosaccharide that lacks the repeating O-carbohydrate antigenic side chain seen in other gram-negative bacteria (Chap. 105). Gonococcal LOS possesses marked endotoxic activity and contributes to the local cytotoxic effect in the fallopian tube model. LOS core sugars undergo a high degree of antigenic variation under different conditions of growth; this variation reflects genetic regulation

and expression of glycotransferase genes that dictate the carbohydrate structure of LOS. These phenotypic changes may affect interactions of *N. gonorrhoeae* with elements of the humoral immune system (antibodies and complement) and may also influence direct binding of organisms to both professional phagocytes and nonprofessional phagocytes (epithelial cells). For example, gonococci that are sialylated at their LOS sites bind complement factor H and downregulate the alternative pathway of complement. LOS sialylation may also mask bactericidal antibody–binding epitopes on LOS and porin and may decrease opsonophagocytosis and inhibit the oxidative burst in PMNs. While sialylation of LOS confers on the bacteria the ability to attenuate the inflammatory response and evade the innate immune system, experiments in male volunteers suggest that sialylated gonococci may be less capable of establishing infection than their unsialylated counterparts. This difference could be explained by the observation that the unsialylated terminal lactosamine residue of LOS binds to an asialoglycoprotein receptor on male epithelial cells that would otherwise facilitate binding and subsequent gonococcal invasion of these cells.

Host Factors In addition to gonococcal structures that interact with epithelial cells, host factors seem to be important in mediating entry of gonococci into nonphagocytic cells. Activation of phosphatidylcholine-specific phospholipase C and acidic sphingomyelinase by *N. gonorrhoeae*, which results in the release of diacylglycerol and ceramide, is a requirement for the entry of *N. gonorrhoeae* into epithelial cells. Ceramide accumulation within cells leads to apoptosis, which may disrupt epithelial integrity and facilitate entry of gonococci into subepithelial tissue. Release of chemotactic factors as a result of complement activation contributes to inflammation, as does the toxic effect of LOS in provoking the release of inflammatory cytokines.

The importance of humoral immunity in host defenses against neisserial infections is best illustrated by the predisposition of persons deficient in terminal complement components (C5 through C9) to recurrent bacteremic gonococcal infections and to recurrent meningococcal meningitis or meningococcemia. Gonococcal porin induces T cell–proliferative responses in persons with urogenital gonococcal disease. A significant increase in porin-specific interleukin (IL) 4–producing CD4+ as well as CD8+ lymphocytes is seen in individuals with mucosal gonococcal disease. A portion of these lymphocytes that show a porin-specific T_H2-type response could traffic to mucosal surfaces and play a role in immune protection against the disease. Few data clearly indicate that protective immunity is acquired from a previous gonococcal infection, although bactericidal and opsonophagocytic antibodies to porin and LOS may offer partial protection. On the other hand, women who are infected and acquire high levels of antibody to another outer-membrane protein, Rmp (reduction modifiable protein, formerly called protein III), may be especially likely to become reinfected with *N. gonorrhoeae* because Rmp antibodies block the effect of bactericidal antibodies to porin and LOS. Rmp shows little, if any, interstrain antigenic variation; therefore, Rmp antibodies potentially may block antibody-mediated killing of all gonococci. The mechanism of blocking has not been fully characterized, but Rmp antibodies noncompetitively inhibit binding of porin and LOS antibodies because of the proximity of these structures in the gonococcal outer membrane. Less well understood is how blocking antibody may divert complement binding to the gonococcal surface or otherwise hasten inactivation of complement. In male volunteers who have no history of gonorrhea, the net effect of these events may influence the outcome of experimental challenge with *N. gonorrhoeae*. Because Rmp bears extensive homology to enterobacterial OmpA and meningococcal class 4 proteins, it is possible that these blocking antibodies result from prior exposure to cross-reacting proteins from these species and also play a role in first-time infection with *N. gonorrhoeae*.

Gonococcal Resistance to Antimicrobial Agents It is no surprise that *N. gonorrhoeae*, with its remarkable capacity to alter its antigenic structure and adapt to changes in the microenvironment, has become resistant to numerous antibiotics. The first effective agents against gonorrhea were the sulfonamides, which were introduced in the 1930s. Within a decade, antibiotic resistance emerged, resulting in treatment failures in one-third of patients. Penicillin was then employed as the drug of choice for the treatment of gonorrhea. By 1965, 42% of gonococcal isolates had developed low-level resistance to penicillin G. To prevent treatment failures, the Centers for Disease Control and Prevention (CDC) at that time recommended doubling the dose of penicillin for the treatment of gonorrhea. Resistance due to the production of penicillinase arose later.

Gonococci become fully resistant to antibiotics either by chromosomal mutations or by acquisition of R factors (plasmids). Two types of chromosomal mutations have been described. The first type, which is drug specific, is a single-step mutation leading to high-level resistance. The second type involves mutations at several chromosomal loci that combine to determine the level as well as the pattern of resistance. Strains with mutations in chromosomal genes were first observed in the late 1950s. As recently as 1997, strains with chromosomal resistance (CMRNG) accounted for resistance to penicillin, tetracycline, or both in ~20% of strains surveyed in the United States.

β-Lactamase (penicillinase)–producing strains of *N. gonorrhoeae* (PPNG) carrying plasmids with the Pc^r determinant were seen almost simultaneously in the United States, England, western Africa, and the Philippines in the late 1970s. PPNG strains have since spread worldwide and by the early 1980s accounted for >50% of all gonococcal isolates in some parts of the developing world. The average prevalence of PPNG in the United States dropped by two-thirds after most penicillin use was discontinued and is now on the order of 4%, with higher rates reported from certain areas. *N. gonorrhoeae* strains with plasmid-borne tetracycline resistance (TRNG) can mobilize some β-lactamase plasmids, and PPNG and TRNG occur together, sometimes along with CMRNG. Penicillin, ampicillin, and tetracycline are no longer reliable agents for the treatment of gonorrhea and should not be used. Third-generation cephalosporins have remained highly effective as single-dose therapy for gonorrhea. Even though the minimal inhibitory concentrations (MICs) of ceftriaxone for certain strains may reach 0.015 to 0.125 mg/L (higher than MICs of 0.0001 to 0.008 mg/L for fully susceptible strains), these levels are greatly exceeded in blood, the urethra, and the cervix when the routinely recommended ceftriaxone and cefixime regimens are administered (see below). These regimens almost always result in an effective cure.

Quinolone-containing regimens are also recommended for treatment of gonococcal infections; the fluoroquinolones offer the advantage of antichlamydial activity when administered for 7 days. Serum concentrations following therapeutic dosages of the quinolones exceed the MIC for *N. gonorrhoeae* by ~100-fold. However, quinolone-resistant *N. gonorrhoeae* (QRNG) appeared soon after these agents were first used to treat gonorrhea, particularly in Southeast Asia. QRNG strains have been reported recently in the United States, mostly in the far western states. Alterations in DNA gyrase and topoisomerase IV have been implicated as mechanisms of fluoroquinolone resistance.

Resistance to spectinomycin, which is used as an alternative agent, has been reported, but resistance to this agent is usually not associated with resistance to other antibiotics. Therefore, spectinomycin can be reserved for use against multiresistant strains of *N. gonorrhoeae*. Nevertheless, outbreaks caused by strains resistant to spectinomycin have been documented in Korea and England when the drug was used as a primary agent to treat gonorrhea.

CLINICAL MANIFESTATIONS ■ Gonococcal Infection in Males
Acute urethritis is the most common clinical manifestation of gonorrhea in males. The usual incubation period following exposure is 2 to 7 days, although the interval can be longer and some men remain asymptomatic. Strains of the Por1A serotype, with nutritional requirements for arginine, hypoxanthine, and uracil (i.e., the AHU auxotype), tend to cause a greater proportion of cases of mild and asymptomatic urethritis than Por1B strains. Urethral discharge and dysuria, usually without urinary frequency or urgency, are the major symptoms. The discharge initially is scant and mucoid but becomes profuse and purulent within a day

or two. The clinical manifestations of gonococcal urethritis are usually more severe and overt than those of nongonococcal urethritis, including urethritis caused by *Chlamydia trachomatis* (Chap. 160); however, exceptions are common, and it is often impossible to differentiate the causes of urethritis on clinical grounds alone. The majority of cases of urethritis seen in the United States today are not caused by *N. gonorrhoeae* and/or *C. trachomatis*. Although a number of other organisms may be responsible, most cases do not have a specific etiologic agent identified. Most symptomatic males with gonorrhea seek treatment and cease to be infectious. The remaining men, who are largely asymptomatic, accumulate in number over time and constitute about two-thirds of all infected men at any point in time. Together with men incubating the organism (who shed the organism but are asymptomatic), they serve as the source of spread of infection. Prior to the antibiotic era, symptoms of urethritis persisted for about 8 weeks. Epididymitis is now an uncommon complication, and gonococcal prostatitis occurs rarely, if at all. Other unusual local complications of gonococcal urethritis include edema of the penis due to dorsal lymphangitis or thrombophlebitis, submucous inflammatory "soft" infiltration of the urethral wall, periurethral abscess or fistulae, inflammation or abscess of Cowper's gland, and seminal vesiculitis. Balanitis may develop in uncircumcised men. After a decline in gonococcal infections among homosexual men early in the era of AIDS, a disturbing increase in gonorrhea was observed among young homosexual men in the 1990s, probably related to decreased condom use. The clinical features of anorectal and pharyngeal gonorrhea are discussed below.

Gonococcal Infections in Females ■ GONOCOCCAL CERVICITIS Mucopurulent cervicitis is the most common STD diagnosis in American women and may be caused by *N. gonorrhoeae*, *C. trachomatis*, and other organisms. Cervicitis may coexist with candidal or trichomonal vaginitis. *N. gonorrhoeae* primarily infects the cervical os but can also infect more peripheral areas of the cervix where columnar epithelium meets stratified squamous epithelium. Except in rare instances, the vaginal mucosa, which is lined by stratified squamous epithelium, does not become infected. Bartholin's glands occasionally become infected.

Women infected with *N. gonorrhoeae* usually develop symptoms. However, the women who either remain asymptomatic or have only minor symptoms may delay in seeking medical attention. These symptoms may include scant discharge from the vagina that may issue forth from the inflamed cervix (not vaginitis or vaginosis per se) and dysuria (often without urgency or frequency) that may be associated with gonococcal urethritis. Although the incubation period of gonorrhea is less well defined in women than in men, symptoms usually develop within 10 days of infection and are more acute and intense than those of chlamydial cervicitis.

The physical examination may reveal a mucopurulent discharge (mucopus) issuing from the cervical os. The examiner may check for mucopurulent discharge by swabbing a sample of mucus from the endocervix and observing its color against the white background of the swab; yellow or green mucus suggests mucopus. However, only 35% of women with gonococcal cervicitis actually have a mucopurulent discharge defined by these criteria. Because Gram's stain is not sensitive for the diagnosis of gonorrhea in women, specimens should be submitted for culture or a nonculture assay (see below). Edematous and friable cervical ectopy as well as endocervical bleeding induced by gentle swabbing are more often seen in chlamydial infection.

N. gonorrhoeae may be recovered from the urethra and rectum of women with cervicitis, but these are rarely the sole infected sites. Urethritis in women may produce symptoms of internal dysuria, which is often attributed to "cystitis." Pyuria in the absence of bacteriuria seen on Gram's stain of unspun urine, accompanied by urine cultures that fail to yield >10^5 colonies of bacteria usually associated with urinary tract infection, signifies the possibility of urethritis due to *C. trachomatis*. Urethral infection with *N. gonorrhoeae* may also occur in this context, but in this instance urethral cultures will usually be positive. Compression of the urethra through the anterior vaginal wall against the symphysis pubis may express urethral exudate.

COMPLICATIONS OF GONOCOCCAL CERVICITIS　　Gonococcal infection may extend deep enough to produce dyspareunia and lower abdominal or back pain. In such cases, it is imperative to consider a diagnosis of PID and to administer treatment for that disease (Chap. 115). Ascending infection of the genital tract follows ~20% of cases of gonococcal cervicitis and may result in acute endometritis accompanied by abnormal menstrual bleeding, midline lower abdominal pain and tenderness, and dyspareunia. Spread to the fallopian tubes results in acute salpingitis, whose symptoms may be accompanied by signs of cervical motion tenderness and abnormal adnexal mass on pelvic examination. Patients may be febrile, and leukocytosis and an elevated erythrocyte sedimentation rate or C-reactive protein level may be detected. Co-infection with *C. trachomatis* may increase the risk of PID, which is the clinical counterpart of endometritis and salpingitis. Tubal scarring leading to infertility is the most devastating sequela of salpingitis; the increased risk of ectopic pregnancy is also significant. Prompt and appropriate antibiotic therapy for gonococcal salpingitis (prior to the development of an adnexal mass) can prevent tubal infertility in nearly all cases. Bilateral tubal damage occurs in ~20% of women with an adnexal mass. More than half of women with tubal infertility give no history of PID. These women with "silent salpingitis" may report abdominal or pelvic discomfort (such as dysmenorrhea or dyspareunia) that may be attributed to other diagnoses (such as endometriosis). Spread of infection to the pelvis may result in pelvic peritonitis characterized by nausea and vomiting. Spread of gonococci—or, more commonly, of chlamydiae—via the peritoneal cavity to the upper abdomen may cause perihepatitis (Fitz-Hugh–Curtis syndrome; Chap. 115).

GONOCOCCAL VAGINITIS　　The vaginal mucosa of healthy women is lined by stratified squamous epithelium and is usually not infected by *N. gonorrhoeae*. However, gonococcal vaginitis can occur in anestrogenic women (e.g., prepubertal girls and postmenopausal women), in whom the vaginal stratified squamous epithelial layers are often thinned down to the basilar layer, which can be infected by *N. gonorrhoeae*. The intense inflammation of the vagina makes the physical (speculum and bimanual) examination extremely painful. The vaginal mucosa is red and edematous, and an abundant purulent discharge is present. Infection in the urethra and in Skene's and Bartholin's glands often accompanies gonococcal vaginitis. Inflamed cervical erosion or abscesses in nabothian cysts may also occur. Coexisting cervicitis may result in pus in the cervical os.

Differential Diagnosis of Genital Gonococcal Infections　　The clinical features of uncomplicated gonococcal infections closely resemble those of genital infections caused by *C. trachomatis*. Although the symptoms produced by chlamydial infections tend to be milder, the two infections are often indistinguishable on clinical grounds alone. Co-infection with *N. gonorrhoeae* and *C. trachomatis* is seen in up to 40% of cases. →*The differential diagnosis of urethritis, epididymitis, and proctitis in men; of cervicitis and PID in women; and of vaginitis in prepubertal girls is discussed in Chap. 115.*

Anorectal Gonorrhea　　Because the female anatomy permits the spread of cervical exudate to the rectum, *N. gonorrhoeae* is sometimes recovered from the rectum of women with uncomplicated gonococcal cervicitis. The rectum is the sole site of infection in only 5% of women with gonorrhea. Such women are usually asymptomatic but occasionally have acute proctitis manifested by anorectal pain or pruritus, tenesmus, purulent rectal discharge, and rectal bleeding. Among homosexual men, the frequency of gonococcal infection, including rectal infection, fell by ≥90% throughout the United States in the early 1980s, but a resurgence of gonorrhea among homosexual men was documented in several cities during the 1990s. Gonococcal isolates from the rectum of homosexual men tend to be more resistant than other gonococcal

isolates to antimicrobials. Gonococcal isolates with a mutation in mtrR (multiple transferable resistance repressor) or in the promoter region of the gene that encodes for this transcriptional repressor develop increased resistance to antimicrobial hydrophobic agents such as bile acids and fatty acids in feces and thus are found with increased frequency in homosexual men. The mutation, which curtails the production of a DNA-binding protein called MtrR, results in derepression of the expression of other *mtr* genes that encode the production of an energy-dependent efflux pump, thereby resulting in increased resistance to hydrophobic agents. This situation may have been responsible for higher rates of failure of treatment for rectal gonorrhea with older regimens consisting of penicillin or tetracyclines.

Pharyngeal Gonorrhea　　Pharyngeal gonorrhea is usually mild or asymptomatic, although symptomatic pharyngitis does occasionally occur with cervical lymphadenitis. The mode of acquisition is oral-genital sexual exposure, with fellatio being a more efficient means of transmission than cunnilingus. It is important to solicit a sexual history as part of the evaluation of pharyngitis so that appropriate cultures for *N. gonorrhoeae* can be performed. Acute HIV infection should also be considered in the differential diagnosis of pharyngitis in persons with appropriate risk factors. Most cases resolve spontaneously, and transmission from the pharynx to sexual contacts is rare. Pharyngeal infection almost always coexists with genital infection. Swabs from the pharynx should be plated directly onto gonococcal selective media. Because pharyngeal colonization with *N. meningitidis* needs to be differentiated from that with other *Neisseria* species, the diagnosis of pharyngeal gonorrhea is more expensive and difficult than that of anogenital gonorrhea.

Ocular Gonorrhea in Adults　　Ocular gonorrhea in an adult usually results from autoinoculation from an infected genital site. As in genital infection, the manifestations range from severe to occasionally mild or asymptomatic disease. The variability in clinical manifestations may result from differences in the ability of the infecting strain to elicit an inflammatory response.

Infection may result in a markedly swollen eyelid, severe hyperemia and chemosis, and a profuse purulent discharge. The massively inflamed conjunctiva may be draped over the cornea and limbus. Lytic enzymes from the infiltrating PMNs occasionally cause corneal ulceration and rarely cause perforation.

Prompt recognition and treatment of this condition are of paramount importance. Gram's stain and culture of the purulent discharge establish the diagnosis. Genital cultures should also be performed.

Gonorrhea in Pregnant Women, Neonates, and Children　　Gonorrhea in pregnancy can have serious consequences for both the mother and the infant. Therefore, early detection and eradication of the disease in the mother are extremely important. Recognition of gonorrhea early in pregnancy also identifies a population at risk for other STDs, particularly chlamydial infection and syphilis. These women should be monitored closely for these infections throughout pregnancy. The incidence of gonorrhea in pregnancy ranges from rare to ~10%, depending upon the population surveyed. Salpingitis and PID can occur during the first trimester and are associated with a high rate of fetal loss. In the second and third trimesters, the relative impermeability of the cervical mucus (under the influence of progesterone) and the obliteration of the intrauterine cavity (resulting from the attachment of the chorion to the endometrial decidua by around the twelfth week of gestation) pose physical barriers that usually prevent ascending infection. Pharyngeal infection, most often asymptomatic, may be more common during pregnancy because of altered sexual practices. Acquisition of gonococcal infection late in pregnancy can adversely affect labor and delivery as well as the well-being of the fetus. Prolonged rupture of the membranes, premature delivery, chorioamnionitis, funisitis (infection of the umbilical cord stump), and sepsis in the infant (with *N. gonorrhoeae* detected in the gastric aspirate of the newborn during delivery) are common complications of maternal gonococcal infection at term. Hazards to the fetus include spontaneous abortion, perinatal death, premature delivery, perinatal distress, and premature rupture of membranes. Other microorganisms and conditions, including *Mycoplasma hominis, Ureaplasma urealyticum, C. trachomatis,* and bacterial vaginosis, have been associated with similar complications.

The most common form of gonorrhea in neonates is ophthalmia neonatorum, which results from exposure to infected cervical secretions during parturition. Ocular neonatal instillation of a prophylactic agent (e.g., 1% silver nitrate eyedrops or ophthalmic preparations containing erythromycin or tetracycline) is a cost-effective measure for the prevention of ophthalmia neonatorum but is not effective for its treatment, which requires systemic antibiotics. The clinical manifestations are acute and begin 2 to 5 days after birth. A small inoculum of organisms, low virulence of the infecting strain, or partial suppression by ophthalmic prophylaxis can result in a more indolent course. Therefore, gonococcal infection must be ruled out by culture in every case of conjunctivitis in infants. An initial nonspecific conjunctivitis with a serosanguineous discharge is followed by tense edema of both eyelids, chemosis, and a profuse, thick, purulent discharge. Corneal ulcerations that result in nebulae or perforation may lead to anterior synechiae, anterior staphyloma, panophthalmitis, and blindness. Infections described at other mucosal sites in infants, including vaginitis, rhinitis, and anorectal infection, are likely to be asymptomatic. Pharyngeal colonization has been demonstrated in 35% of infants with gonococcal ophthalmia, and coughing is the most prominent symptom in these cases. Septic arthritis (see below) is the most common manifestation of systemic infection or DGI in the newborn. The primary focus of DGI in most of these cases is uncertain. The onset usually comes at 3 to 21 days of age, and polyarticular involvement is common. Sepsis, meningitis, and pneumonia are seen in rare instances.

Any STD in children beyond the neonatal period raises the possibility of sexual abuse. In most cases of abuse, the perpetrator is a male assailant known to the child. Gonococcal vulvovaginitis is the most common manifestation of gonococcal infection in children beyond infancy. Anorectal and pharyngeal infections are common in these children and are frequently asymptomatic. The urethra, Bartholin's and Skene's glands, and the upper genital tract are rarely involved. All children with gonococcal infection should also be evaluated for chlamydial infection, syphilis, and possibly HIV infection. All cases of suspected and confirmed child abuse should be reported to the appropriate social service agency in the county where the child resides.

Gonococcal Arthritis (DGI) DGI or gonococcal arthritis results from gonococcal bacteremia. In the 1970s, DGI occurred in ~0.5 to 3% of persons with untreated gonococcal mucosal infection. The lower incidence at present is probably attributable to a decline in the prevalence of particular strains that are likely to disseminate and has resulted in fewer cases that present in the bacteremic stage of the disease (see below). DGI strains resist the bactericidal action of human serum and generally do not incite inflammation at genital sites, probably because of limited generation of chemotactic factors. These strains are often of the Por1A serotype, are highly susceptible to penicillin, and have special growth requirements (i.e., the AHU auxotype) that makes the organism more fastidious and more difficult to isolate. Menstruation is a risk factor for dissemination, and approximately two-thirds of cases of DGI are in women. In about half of affected women, symptoms of DGI begin within 7 days of onset of menses. Complement deficiencies, especially of the components involved in the assembly of the membrane attack complex (C5 through C9), predispose to neisserial bacteremia. Up to 13% of patients with DGI have complement deficiencies, and persons with more than one episode of DGI should be screened with an assay for total hemolytic complement activity.

The clinical manifestations of DGI have sometimes been classified into two stages: a bacteremic stage, which is less common today, and a joint-localized stage with suppurative arthritis. A clear-cut progression usually is not evident. Patients in the bacteremic stage have higher temperatures, and their fever is more frequently accompanied by chills. Painful joints are common and often occur in conjunction with tenosynovitis and skin lesions. Polyarthralgias usually include the knees,

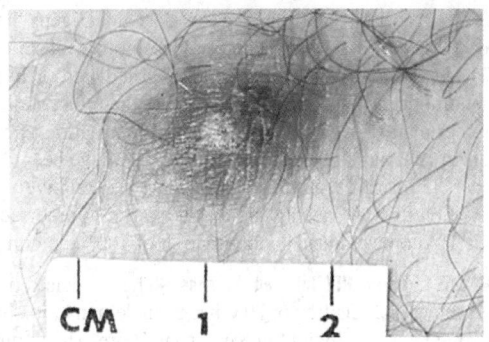

FIGURE 128-1 Disseminated gonococcemia in the skin is seen as hemorrhagic papules and pustules with purpuric centers in a centrifugal distribution.

elbows, and more distal joints; the axial skeleton is generally spared. Skin lesions are seen in ~75% of patients and include papules and pustules, often with a hemorrhagic component (Fig. 128-1). These lesions are usually on the extremities and number between 5 and 40. The differential diagnosis of the bacteremic stage of DGI includes Reiter's syndrome, acute rheumatoid arthritis, sarcoidosis, erythema nodosum, drug-induced arthritis, and viral infections (e.g., hepatitis B and acute HIV infection). The distribution of joint symptoms in Reiter's syndrome differs from DGI (Fig. 128-2), as do the skin and genital manifestations (Chap. 305).

Suppurative arthritis involves one or two joints, most often (in decreasing order of frequency) the knees, wrists, ankles, and elbows. The occurrence of arthritis in the absence of signs and symptoms of the bacteremic stage has led to the suggestion that these are separate syndromes. Other joints, such as the small joints of the hands and feet and the sternoclavicular and temporomandibular joints, are occasionally involved. Most patients who develop gonococcal septic arthritis do so without prior polyarthralgias or skin lesions; in the absence of symptomatic genital infection, this disease cannot be distinguished from septic arthritis caused by other pathogens. The differential diagnosis of acute arthritis in young adults is discussed in Chap. 314. Rarely, osteomyelitis complicates septic arthritis involving small joints of the hand.

Although it has been postulated that the initial arthritis and skin lesions are due to direct tissue invasion by *N. gonorrhoeae*, the organism has been recovered from <5% of skin lesions cultured. This low isolation rate has been attributed to either a small inoculum of infecting organisms or the fastidious growth requirements of *N. gon-*

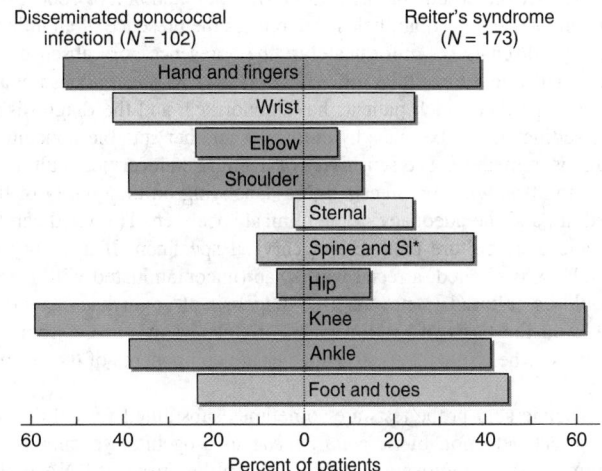

FIGURE 128-2 Distributions of joints with arthritis in 102 patients with disseminated gonococcal infection and 173 patients with Reiter's syndrome. "Sternal" includes the sternoclavicular joints. *SI denotes the sacroiliac joint. (*Reprinted with permission from M Kousa et al: Sex Transm Dis 5:57, 1978; with permission.*)

orrhoeae strains that disseminate. Gonococcal antigens have been identified in "sterile" skin lesions by immunofluorescent staining techniques. There is also evidence that immune-mediated or hypersensitivity phenomena caused by gonococcal antigens account for skin lesions. Other manifestations of noninfectious dermatitis, such as nodular lesions, urticaria, and erythema multiforme, have been described. Gonococcal endocarditis, although rare today, was relatively common in the preantibiotic era, causing about one-quarter of reported cases of endocarditis. Another unusual complication of DGI is meningitis.

Gonococcal Infection in HIV-Infected Persons The association between gonorrhea and the acquisition of HIV has been demonstrated in several well-controlled studies, mainly in Kenya and Zaire. The nonulcerative STDs enhance the transmission of HIV by three- to fivefold, possibly because of increased viral shedding in persons with urethritis or cervicitis (Chap. 173). HIV has been detected by polymerase chain reaction (PCR) more commonly in ejaculates from HIV-positive men with gonococcal urethritis than in those from HIV-positive men with nongonococcal urethritis. PCR positivity diminishes by twofold following appropriate therapy for urethritis. Not only does gonorrhea enhance the transmission of HIV, it may also increase the individual's risk for acquisition of HIV. A proposed mechanism is the significantly greater number of CD4+ lymphocytes and dendritic cells that can be infected by HIV in endocervical secretions of women with nonulcerative STDs than in those of women with ulcerative STDs.

LABORATORY DIAGNOSIS A rapid diagnosis of gonococcal infection in men may be obtained by Gram's staining of urethral exudates. The detection of gram-negative intracellular diplococci is usually highly specific and sensitive in diagnosing gonococcal urethritis in symptomatic males but is only ~50% sensitive in diagnosing gonococcal cervicitis. Samples should be collected with Dacron or rayon swabs. Part of the sample should be inoculated onto a plate of modified Thayer-Martin or other gonococcal selective medium for culture. It is important to process all samples immediately because gonococci do not tolerate drying. If plates cannot be incubated immediately, they can be held safely for several hours at room temperature in candle extinction jars prior to incubation. If processing is to occur within 6 h, transport of specimens may be facilitated by the use of nonnutritive swab transport systems such as Stuart or Amies medium. For longer holding periods (e.g., when specimens for culture are to be mailed), culture media with self-contained CO_2-generating systems (such as the JEMBEC or Gono-Pak systems) may be used. Specimens should also be obtained for the diagnosis of chlamydial infection.

PMNs are often seen in the endocervix on a Gram's stain, and an abnormally increased number [≥30 PMNs per field in five 1000X oil-immersion (microscopic) fields] establishes the presence of an inflammatory discharge. Unfortunately, the presence or absence of gram-negative intracellular diplococci in cervical smears does not accurately predict which patients have gonorrhea, and the diagnosis in this setting should be made by culture or another suitable nonculture diagnostic method. The sensitivity of a single endocervical culture is ~80 to 90%, with the precise figure depending on the quality of the medium and the adequacy of the clinical specimen. The yield can be enhanced by culture of a second cervical specimen. If a history of rectal sex is elicited, a rectal wall swab (uncontaminated with feces) should be cultured. A presumptive diagnosis of gonorrhea cannot be made on the basis of gram-negative diplococci in smears from the pharynx, where other *Neisseria* species are components of the normal flora.

Nucleic acid probe tests are sometimes substituted for culture for the direct detection of *N. gonorrhoeae* in urogenital specimens. A common assay employs a nonisotopic chemiluminescent DNA probe that hybridizes specifically with gonococcal 16S ribosomal RNA. Studies assessing the utility of the nucleic acid probe system in high-risk outpatients undergoing screening for STDs have revealed that it is at least as sensitive as conventional culture techniques and may be

a cost-effective alternative to culture, especially in high-risk males. A disadvantage of non-culture-based assays in general is that specimens submitted in probe-transport systems cannot be cultured subsequently. Therefore, a culture-confirmatory test is not possible, and formal antimicrobial susceptibility testing, if needed, cannot be performed. Low-cost point-of-care tests are under development for use in resource-poor settings, where specific diagnosis often gives way to syndromic management. Nucleic acid amplification tests (NAATs, including Roche Amplicor, Gen-Probe APTIMA, and BDProbeTec) have been cleared by the U.S. Food and Drug Administration (FDA) and offer the advantage of testing urine samples with a sensitivity similar to that of culture and other non-NAATs on urethral or cervical swab samples.

Because of the legal implications, the preferred method for the diagnosis of gonococcal infection in children is a standardized culture. Two positive NAATs, each targeting a different nucleic acid sequence, may be substituted for culture of the cervix or the urethra as legal evidence of infection; however, cervical specimens are not recommended for prepubertal girls. Nonculture tests for gonococcal infection have not been approved by the FDA for use with specimens obtained from the pharynx and rectum of infected children. Cultures should be obtained from the pharynx and anus of both girls and boys, the vagina of girls, and the urethra of boys. For boys with a urethral discharge, a meatal specimen of the discharge is adequate for culture. Presumptive colonies of *N. gonorrhoeae* should be identified definitively by at least two independent methods (e.g., biochemical, enzyme substrate, or serologic).

Blood should be cultured in suspected cases of DGI. The use of Isolator blood culture tubes may enhance the yield. The probability of positive blood cultures decreases after 48 h of illness. Synovial fluid should be inoculated into blood culture broth medium and plated onto chocolate agar rather than selective medium because this fluid is not likely to be contaminated with commensal bacteria. Gonococci are infrequently recovered from early joint effusions containing <20,000 leukocytes/μL but may be recovered from effusions containing >80,000 leukocytes/μL. The organisms are seldom recovered from blood and synovial fluid of the same patient.

R̲x̲ TREATMENT

Although clinical isolates of *N. gonorrhoeae* vary in their antimicrobial susceptibility patterns in different parts of the world, they remain susceptible to a wide variety of agents. Because failure of treatment can lead to continued transmission and the emergence of antibiotic resistance, the importance of adequate treatment with a regimen that the patient will adhere to cannot be overemphasized. Thus highly effective single-dose regimens have been developed for the treatment of uncomplicated gonococcal infections. The 2002 CDC treatment guidelines for gonococcal infections are summarized in Table 128-1; the recommendations for uncomplicated gonorrhea apply to HIV-infected as well as HIV-uninfected patients.

The third-generation cephalosporins cefixime (given orally) and ceftriaxone (given intramuscularly), both as a single dose, have been the mainstay of therapy with this class of antibiotics for uncomplicated gonococcal infection of the urethra, cervix, rectum, or pharynx. The recent discontinuation of cefixime production in the United States has prompted further examination of alternative oral options for urogenital and pharyngeal gonococcal infections. To be considered as a recommended treatment for uncomplicated gonorrhea, an antimicrobial regimen should cure >95% of urogenital infections. (The therapeutic efficacy for anorectal infection is typically comparable to that for urogenital infection.) Studies documenting efficacy should have sufficient sample size so that the lower limit of the confidence interval (CI) of the cure rate is also >95%. The available data do not demonstrate that any single-dose oral antimicrobial regimen other than cefixime or a fluoroquinolone (see below) meets these efficacy criteria for urogenital gonococcal infection; published data on the efficacy of alternative oral regimens in treating pharyngeal gonococcal infection are even more limited. Single doses of ciprofloxacin, ofloxacin, or levofloxacin are effective first-line regimens. Other quinolones, such as gatifloxacin, norfloxacin, and lomefloxacin, are probably efficacious for treating uncomplicated gonorrhea, but data regarding their use are also limited, and they offer no advantage over the other recommended quinolones. Because of resistance to fluoroquinolones in several parts of Asia and the Pacific (including Hawaii), these agents should not be used to treat gonorrhea acquired in these regions. Several states, including California, are now recommending the curtailment of quinolone treatment for gonorrhea infection altogether, and in these regions ceftriaxone should be used.

Because co-infection with *C. trachomatis* occurs frequently, initial treatment regimens must incorporate an agent (e.g., azithromycin or doxycycline) effective against chlamydial infection. Routine dual therapy without testing for *Chlamydia* can be cost-effective for populations where chlamydial infection accompanies 10 to 30% of gonococcal infections. Pregnant women with gonorrhea should receive concurrent treatment with a macrolide antibiotic for possible chlamydial infection; doxycycline should not be used during pregnancy. A single 1-g dose of azithromycin, which is effective therapy for uncomplicated chlamydial infections, results in an unacceptably low cure rate (93%) for gonococcal infections and should not be used alone.

Uncomplicated gonococcal infections in penicillin-allergic persons who cannot tolerate quinolones may be treated with a single dose of spectinomycin.

Persons with uncomplicated infections who receive a recommended regimen need not return for a test of cure. Cultures for *N. gonorrhoeae* should be performed if symptoms persist after therapy with an established regimen, and any gonococci isolated should be tested for antimicrobial susceptibility.

Symptomatic gonococcal pharyngitis is more difficult to eradicate than genital infection. Few regimens result in cure rates of >90%. Persons who cannot tolerate cephalosporins or quinolones can be treated with spectinomycin, but this agent results in a cure rate of ≤52%. Therefore, persons given spectinomycin should have a pharyngeal culture performed 3 to 5 days after treatment as a test of cure.

Treatments for gonococcal epididymitis and PID are discussed in Chap. 115. Ocular gonococcal infections in older children and adults should be managed with a single dose of ceftriaxone combined with saline irrigation of the conjunctivae (both undertaken expeditiously), and patients should undergo a careful ophthalmologic evaluation that includes a slit-lamp examination.

DGI may require higher dosages and longer durations of therapy (Table 128-1). Hospitalization is indicated if the diagnosis is uncertain, if the patient has localized joint disease that requires aspiration, or if the patient cannot be relied on to comply with treatment. Open drainage is necessary only occasionally—e.g., for management of hip infections that may be difficult to drain percutaneously. Nonsteroidal anti-inflammatory agents may be indicated to alleviate pain and hasten improvement of affected joints. Gonococcal meningitis and endocarditis should be treated in the hospital with high-dose intravenous ceftriaxone (1 to 2 g every 12 h); therapy should continue for 10 to 14 days for meningitis and for at least 4 weeks for endocarditis. All persons who experience more than one episode of DGI should be evaluated for complement deficiency.

PREVENTION AND CONTROL Condoms, if properly used, provide effective protection against the transmission and acquisition of gonorrhea as well as other infections that are transmitted to and from genital mucosal surfaces. Spermicidal preparations used with a diaphragm or cervical sponges impregnated with nonoxynol 9 offer some protection against gonorrhea and chlamydial infection. However, the frequent use of preparations that contain nonoxynol 9 is associated with mucosal disruption that paradoxically may enhance the risk of HIV infection

---

TABLE 128-1 *Recommended Treatment for Gonococcal Infections: 2002 Guidelines of the Centers for Disease Control and Prevention*

Diagnosis	Treatment of Choice
Uncomplicated gonococcal infection of the cervix, urethra, pharynx, or rectum[a]	
First-line regimens	Ceftriaxone (125 mg IM, single dose) *or* Ciprofloxacin (500 mg PO, single dose)[b] *or* Ofloxacin (400 mg PO, single dose)[b] *or* Levofloxacin (250 mg PO, single dose)[b] *or* Cefixime (400 mg PO, single dose)[c] *plus* If chlamydial infection is not ruled out: Azithromycin (1 g PO, single dose) *or* Doxycycline (100 mg PO bid for 7 days)
Alternative regimens	Spectinomycin (2 g IM, single dose) *or* Ceftizoxime (500 mg IM, single dose) *or* Cefotaxime (500 mg IM, single dose) *or* Cefotetan (1 g IM, single dose) plus probenecid (1 g PO, single dose) *or* Cefoxitin (2 g IM, single dose) plus probenecid (1 g PO, single dose)
Epididymitis	See Chap. 115
Pelvic inflammatory disease	See Chap. 115
Gonococcal conjunctivitis in an adult	Ceftriaxone (1 g IM, single dose)[d]
Ophthalmia neonatorum[e]	Ceftriaxone (25–50 mg/kg IV, single dose, not to exceed 125 mg)
Disseminated gonococcal infection[f]	
Initial therapy[g]	
Patient tolerant of β-lactam drugs	Ceftriaxone (1 g IM or IV q24h; recommended) *or* Cefotaxime (1 g IV q8h) *or* Ceftizoxime (1 g IV q8h)
Patients allergic to β-lactam drugs	Ciprofloxacin (500 mg IV q12h)[b] *or* Ofloxacin (400 mg IV q12h)[b] *or* Levofloxacin (500 mg IV q24h)[b] *or* Spectinomycin (2 g IM q12h)
Continuation therapy	Ciprofloxacin (500 mg PO bid)[b] *or* Ofloxacin (400 mg PO bid)[b] *or* Levofloxacin (500 mg PO qd)[b] *or* Cefixime (400 mg PO bid)[c]
Meningitis or endocarditis	See text[h]

[a] True failure of treatment with a recommended regimen is rare and should prompt an evaluation for reinfection or consideration of an alternative diagnosis. In cases of quinolone failure, the isolate should be tested for drug resistance if possible.

[b] Quinolones should not be used for infections acquired in Asia or the Pacific, including Hawaii and California. The use of quinolones is also inadvisable for treating infections acquired in other areas where the prevalence of quinolone-resistant *N. gonorrhoeae* (QRNG) is >1%, or in areas that are reporting increasing numbers of QRNG strains.

[c] Cefixime, a first-line recommendation for treatment of uncomplicated gonococcal infection (or continuation therapy for DGI), is currently unavailable in the United States.

[d] Plus lavage of the infected eye with saline solution (once).

[e] Prophylactic regimens are discussed in the text.

[f] Hospitalization is indicated if the diagnosis is uncertain, if the patient has frank arthritis with an effusion, or if the patient cannot be relied on to adhere to treatment.

[g] All initial regimens should be continued for 24 to 48 h after clinical improvement begins, at which time therapy may be switched to one of the continuation regimens to complete a full week of antimicrobial treatment.

[h] Hospitalization is indicated to exclude suspected meningitis or endocarditis.

in the event of exposure. All patients should be instructed to refer sex partners for evaluation and treatment. All sex partners of persons with gonorrhea should be evaluated and treated for *N. gonorrhoeae* and *C. trachomatis* infections if their last contact with the patient took place within 60 days before the onset of symptoms or the diagnosis of infection in the patient. If the patient's last sexual encounter was >60 days before onset of symptoms or diagnosis, the patient's most recent sex partner should be treated. Patients should be instructed to abstain from sexual intercourse until therapy is completed and until they and their sex partners no longer have symptoms. Greater emphasis must be placed on prevention by public health education, individual patient counseling, and behavior modification. Sexually active persons, especially adolescents, should be offered screening for STDs. For males, a NAAT on urine or a urethral swab may be used for screening. Preventing the spread of gonorrhea may help reduce the transmission of HIV. No effective vaccine for gonorrhea is yet available, but efforts to test a porin vaccine candidate are under way.

ACKNOWLEDGMENT

The authors acknowledge the contributions of Dr. King K. Holmes and Dr. Stephen A. Morse to the chapter on this subject in earlier editions of Harrison's.

FURTHER READING

CENTERS FOR DISEASE CONTROL AND PREVENTION: Annual Report; Gonococcal Isolate Surveillance Project (GISP); *www.cdc.gov/ncidod/dastlr/gcdir/Resist/gisp.html*

————: 2002 Sexually transmitted diseases treatment guidelines. MMWR 51(RR-6):1, 2002

————: Screening tests to detect *Chlamydia trachomatis* and *Neisseria gonorrhoeae* infections—2002. MMWR 51 (RR-15):1, 2002

HOOK EW III, HOLMES KK: Gonococcal infections. Ann Intern Med 102:229, 1985

LAGA M et al: Non-ulcerative sexually transmitted diseases as risk factors for HIV-1 transmission in women: Results from a cohort study. AIDS 7:95, 1993

O'BRIEN JP et al: Disseminated gonococcal infection: A prospective analysis of 49 patients and a review of pathophysiology and immune mechanisms. Medicine (Baltimore) 62:395, 1983

129 | *MORAXELLA CATARRHALIS* AND OTHER *MORAXELLA* SPECIES
Daniel M. Musher

MORAXELLA CATARRHALIS

The gram-negative coccus *Moraxella catarrhalis* is a component of the normal bacterial flora of the upper airways and has been increasingly recognized as a cause of otitis media, sinusitis, and bronchopulmonary infection. Over the past several decades, this organism has been variously designated as *Micrococcus catarrhalis*, *Neisseria catarrhalis*, and *Branhamella catarrhalis*.

BACTERIOLOGY AND IMMUNITY   On Gram's staining, *M. catarrhalis* organisms appear as gram-negative cocci, sometimes occurring in pairs and retaining the side-by-side kidney-bean configuration of *Neisseria* (Fig. 129-1). These cocci tend to retain crystal violet during the decolorizing step and may be confused with *Staphylococcus aureus*. *Moraxella* colonies grow well on blood or chocolate agar but may be overlooked because of their resemblance to *Neisseria* spp. (a major component of the normal pharyngeal flora). *Moraxella* is readily distinguishable from *Neisseria* spp. by biochemical tests.

Strains of *M. catarrhalis* show a surprising degree of homogeneity in terms of their outer-membrane proteins. Antibody to some of these proteins is generally present in serum of children >4 years old; however, colonizing or disease-causing isolates may survive in serum despite this naturally present antibody and complement. Bactericidal antibody emerges after natural infection and may be directed against one or more conserved outer-membrane proteins—a property of potential value in vaccine development. The presence of certain outer-membrane proteins is associated with virulence in mice, and antibody may be protective. Antibody to lipooligosaccharide may also provide some degree of protection. These and other bacterial constituents are under investigation for use as vaccines.

EPIDEMIOLOGY   With repeated cultures and the use of selective media, *M. catarrhalis* can be isolated from the upper respiratory tract or saliva of 50% of healthy schoolchildren and of up to 7% of healthy adults. When conventional microbiologic techniques are used, *Moraxella* can be isolated from sputum of about 10% of persons who have chronic bronchitis and 25% of those who have bronchiectasis in the absence of acute infection. Investigators in both the northern and southern hemispheres have reported a striking seasonal variation in the isolation of this organism from clinical specimens, with a peak in late winter/early spring and a nadir in late summer/early fall. Direct contact has not been shown to contribute to community-acquired infection, but nosocomial spread of infection has been documented occasionally.

CLINICAL MANIFESTATIONS ■ **Otitis Media and Sinusitis**   *M. catarrhalis* has repeatedly been shown to be the third most common bacterial isolate from middle-ear fluid of children who have otitis media, being surpassed only by *Streptococcus pneumoniae* and nontypable *Haemophilus influenzae*. Recent studies have shown that this organism is also a prominent isolate from sinus cavities in acute and chronic sinusitis.

Purulent Tracheobronchitis and Pneumonia   *M. catarrhalis* causes acute exacerbations of chronic bronchitis (increased production and/or purulence of sputum), purulent tracheobronchitis (the latter also involving fever and leukocytosis), and pneumonia; acquisition of a new bacterial strain is often responsible. The great majority of infected persons are >50 years old and have a long history of cigarette smoking and underlying chronic obstructive pulmonary disease (COPD); many have lung cancer as well. In one study, 76% of affected persons had COPD (severe in many cases), and one-third of those with COPD had lung cancer; most patients also had clinical evidence of malnutrition. In one extensive series of cases, *M. catarrhalis* pneumonia did not occur in otherwise-healthy hosts.

Symptoms of *M. catarrhalis* infection have been regarded as modest in severity. Both cough and the amount and purulence of sputum are usually increased above baseline. Chills are reported in one-quarter

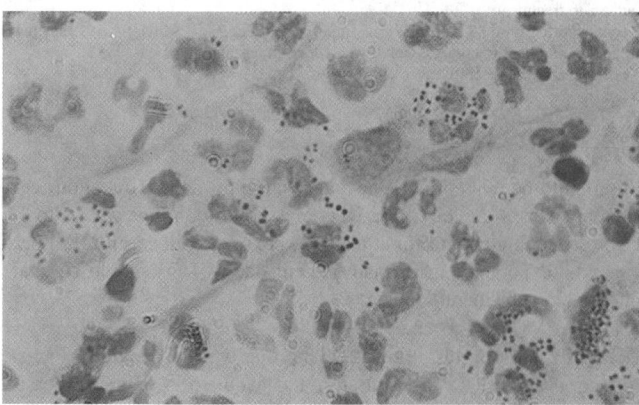

FIGURE 129-1   Gram-stained sputum from a patient with acute purulent tracheobronchitis. Many polymorphonuclear neutrophils and a few macrophages are seen along with many gram-negative cocci (*Moraxella catarrhalis*), a few of which appear as pairs. Nearly all organisms are cell associated and probably have been taken up by phagocytes, consistent with the notion that *Moraxella* is a lower-grade pathogen than organisms such as *Streptococcus pneumoniae*.

of patients, pleuritic pain in one-third, and malaise in 40%. Most patients have peak temperatures of <38.3°C (<101°F), and peripheral white blood cell counts are <10,000/μL in nearly one-quarter of cases. Microscopic examination of a good sputum specimen following Gram's staining regularly reveals profuse organisms, and quantitative culture yields ∼ 2 × 10⁸ colony-forming units per milliliter. The radiologic appearance is variable; in one study, 43% of subjects had segmental or lobar infiltrates, and the remainder had a mixed pattern of subsegmental, segmental, interstitial, and diffuse involvement. These clinical, laboratory, and radiographic findings do not differ from those of pneumococcal or *Haemophilus* pneumonia in an older patient population. However, a far lesser degree of bloodstream invasion occurs in *M. catarrhalis* infection; in one series, none of 25 patients with *M. catarrhalis* pneumonia had bacteremia. Nevertheless, pneumonia due to *M. catarrhalis* is a marker for severe underlying disease: nearly half of patients die within 3 months of onset.

Other Syndromes Local extension causing empyema is very uncommon, and, as might be inferred from the low rate of bacteremia, metastatic complications of *M. catarrhalis* pneumonia, such as septic arthritis, are exceedingly rare. As of 1995, 58 cases of bacteremic infection due to *M. catarrhalis* had been reported, mainly in children <10 years old or adults >60 years old; most of these patients had severe underlying lung disease and/or were immunocompromised. The syndromes reported have included bacteremia with no apparent focus, pneumonia, endocarditis, and meningitis. A petechial or purpuric rash, reminiscent of that observed in meningococcal sepsis and associated with disseminated intravascular coagulation, has been described in a few cases.

DIAGNOSIS Microscopic examination of Gram-stained sputum yields characteristic findings (Fig. 129-1). The presence of many polymorphonuclear leukocytes without epithelial cells indicates that the sputum sample is of good quality; since most patients with *Moraxella* infection have chronic lung disease, it is usually not difficult to obtain a good specimen. Large numbers of *Moraxella* organisms are seen as gram-negative cocci, often lining up side by side and thus resembling pairs of kidneys.

℞ TREATMENT

Treatment of *M. catarrhalis* infection with a penicillin/clavulanic acid combination seems highly appropriate. Penicillin resistance first appeared in isolates in the mid-1970s and is now found in 94% of clinical isolates. Resistance is mediated by two closely related β-lactamases, BRO-1 and BRO-2, which are present in 90% and 10% of resistant isolates, respectively. These enzymes are active against penicillin, ampicillin, and amoxicillin but less so against cephalosporins, especially third-generation cephalosporins, and they bind avidly to clavulanic acid and sulbactam. Thus a β-lactam/β-lactamase inhibitor combination offers an effective mode of treatment. Cephalosporins, especially those of the second and third generations, are effective alternatives. Isolates in the United States are also nearly uniformly susceptible to tetracycline, newer macrolides, ketolides, trimethoprim-sulfamethoxazole (TMP-SMX), quinolones, and chloramphenicol. A 5-day course of therapy has been shown to cure respiratory infection, although a longer course is required in sinusitis.

Treatment of sinusitis or otitis media is empirical, as appropriate specimens are usually obtained only in research studies. In the treatment of pneumonia during the period between the identification of gram-negative cocci in a Gram-stained specimen and the final identification of the organisms by culture, the severity of the condition and the potential presence of other infecting organisms should guide antibiotic selection. For example, an exacerbation of bronchitis caused by *M. catarrhalis* might be treated with tetracycline or TMP-SMX; however, in a patient with pneumonia, the possibility that pneumo-

TABLE 129-1 *Moraxella* Species

Moraxella Species	Number of Isolates	Common Sites/Clinical Association	Number (Percent) for Each Site
M. osloensis[a]	199	Blood	44 (22)
		CSF	18 (9)
		Urine	17 (9)
		Respiratory tract	24 (12)
M. nonliquefaciens	356	Blood	27 (8)
		CSF	6 (2)
		Respiratory tract	196 (55)
M. canis	74	Dog-bite wound	53 (72)
M-6	47	Blood, bone	15 (32)
M. lacunata	33	Conjunctivitis, keratitis	23 (70)
M. urethralis	28	Urine	16 (57)
		Genital tract	3 (11)
M. phenylpyruvica	73	Blood	19 (26)
		CSF	8 (11)
		Urine	12 (16)
M. atlantae	44	Blood	20 (45)
		CSF	5 (11)

[a] Some of these isolates would now be distinguished as a new species, *Moraxella lincolnii*.
Note: CSF, cerebrospinal fluid.
Source: Adapted from a summary of CDC experience (Graham et al).

cocci resistant to these agents also might be present dictates the choice of ampicillin/sulbactam, a third-generation cephalosporin, or a quinolone, at least until culture results become available.

OTHER *MORAXELLA* SPECIES

Other *Moraxella* species cause a wide range of infections, including bronchitis, pneumonia, empyema, endocarditis, meningitis, conjunctivitis, endophthalmitis, urinary tract infection, septic arthritis, and wound infection. In a report on all *Moraxella* isolates submitted to the Centers for Disease Control and Prevention (CDC) between 1953 and 1980, certain clinical associations were apparent (Table 129-1). *M. osloensis* and *M. nonliquefaciens*, the most commonly isolated species, were cultured from a wide range of normally sterile body sites, including blood, cerebrospinal fluid, and joints. *M. osloensis* was the *Moraxella* species most frequently isolated from blood; *M. nonliquefaciens* tended to be isolated from the ears, nose, or throat (47%) or the sputum (8%) and has since been implicated as a cause of conjunctivitis and keratitis. *M. urethralis* was isolated most often from urine and the genital tract and probably represents the *Moraxella* species implicated previously in urethritis. More than half of isolates of *M. phenylpyruvica* and *M. atlantae* were obtained from normally sterile sites. A recent study found *Moraxella* spp., including *M. catarrhalis*, in 35% of infected wounds following cat bites and in 10% of those following dog bites. The clinical features of infections due to *Moraxella* spp. other than *M. catarrhalis* and the nature of the hosts in which they occur have not been fully characterized.

FURTHER READING

GRAHAM D et al: Infections caused by *Moraxella, Moraxella urethralis, Moraxella*-like groups M-5 and M-6, and *Kingella kingae* in the United States, 1953–1980. Rev Infect Dis 12:423, 1990

IOANNIDIS JPA et al: Spectrum and significance of bacteremia due to *Moraxella catarrhalis*. Clin Infect Dis 21:390, 1995

SETHI S et al: New strains of bacteria and exacerbations of chronic obstructive pulmonary disease. N Engl J Med 347:465, 2002

TALAN DA et al: Bacteriologic analysis of infected dog and cat bites. N Engl J Med 340:85, 1999

VERDUIN CM et al: *Moraxella catarrhalis*: From emerging to established pathogen. Clin Microbiol Rev 15:125, 2002

WRIGHT PW et al: A descriptive study of 42 cases of *Branhamella catarrhalis* pneumonia. Am J Med 88(Suppl 5A):2S, 1990

HAEMOPHILUS INFLUENZAE

MICROBIOLOGY *Haemophilus influenzae* was first recognized in 1892 by Pfeiffer, who erroneously concluded that the bacterium was the cause of influenza. The bacterium is a small (1- by 0.3-μm) gram-negative organism of variable shape; hence, it is often described as a pleomorphic coccobacillus. In clinical specimens such as cerebrospinal fluid (CSF) and sputum, it frequently stains only faintly with phenosafranin and therefore can easily be overlooked.

H. influenzae grows both aerobically and anaerobically. Its aerobic growth requires two factors: hemin (X factor) and nicotinamide adenine dinucleotide (V factor). These requirements are used in the clinical laboratory to identify the bacterium. Six major serotypes of *H. influenzae* have been identified; designated *a* through *f*, they are based on antigenically distinct polysaccharide capsules. In addition, some strains lack a polysaccharide capsule and are referred to as *nontypable* strains. Type b and nontypable strains are the most relevant strains clinically (Table 130-1), although encapsulated strains other than type b can cause disease. *H. influenzae* was the first free-living organism to have its entire genome sequenced.

The antigenically distinct type b capsule is a linear polymer composed of ribosyl-ribitol phosphate. Strains of *H. influenzae* type b (Hib) cause disease primarily in infants and children under the age of 6 years. Nontypable strains are primarily mucosal pathogens, although these strains occasionally cause invasive disease.

EPIDEMIOLOGY AND TRANSMISSION *H. influenzae* is an exclusively human pathogen. The organism is spread by airborne droplets or by direct contact with secretions or fomites. Nontypable strains colonize the upper respiratory tract of up to three-fourths of healthy adults. Colonization with nontypable *H. influenzae* is a dynamic process; new strains are acquired and other strains are replaced periodically.

The widespread use of Hib conjugate vaccines has resulted in striking decreases in the rate of nasopharyngeal colonization by Hib and the incidence of Hib infection (Fig. 130-1). Invasive Hib disease now occurs predominantly in underimmunized children and in infants who have not completed the primary immunization series.

Certain population groups have a higher incidence of invasive Hib disease than the general population. The incidence of meningitis due to Hib has been three to four times higher among black children than among white children in several studies. In some Native American groups, the incidence of invasive Hib disease is 10 times higher than that in the general population. Although this increased incidence has not yet been accounted for, several factors may be relevant, including age at exposure to the bacterium, socioeconomic conditions, and genetic differences in the ability to mount an immune response.

PATHOGENESIS Hib strains cause systemic disease by invasion and hematogenous spread to distant sites such as the meninges, bones, and

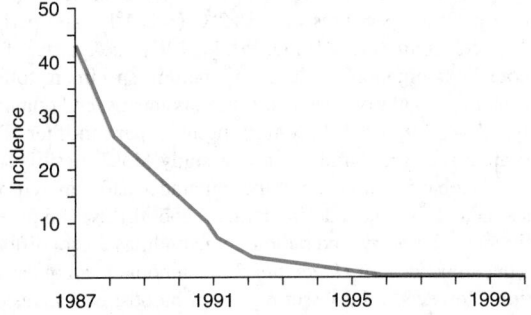

FIGURE 130-1 Estimated incidence (rate per 100,000) of invasive disease due to *Haemophilus influenzae* type b among children <5 years of age: 1987–2000. (*Data from the Centers for Disease Control and Prevention.*)

joints. The type b polysaccharide capsule is an important virulence factor affecting the bacterium's ability to avoid opsonization and cause systemic disease.

Nontypable strains cause disease by local invasion of mucosal surfaces. Otitis media results when bacteria reach the middle ear by way of the eustachian tube. Adults with chronic bronchitis experience recurrent lower respiratory tract infection due to nontypable strains. The incidence of invasive disease caused by nontypable strains is low.

IMMUNE RESPONSE Antibody to capsule is important in protection from infection by Hib strains. The level of (maternally acquired) serum antibody to the capsular polysaccharide, which is a polymer of polyribitol ribose phosphate (PRP), declines from birth to 6 months of age and, in the absence of vaccination, remains low until around 2 or 3 years of age. The age at the antibody nadir correlates with that of the peak incidence of type b disease. Antibody to PRP then appears partly as a result of exposure to Hib or cross-reacting antigens. Systemic Hib disease is unusual after the age of 6 years because of the presence of protective antibody. Vaccines in which PRP is conjugated to protein carrier molecules have been developed and are now used widely. These vaccines generate an antibody response to PRP in infants and are effective in preventing invasive infections in infants and children.

Since nontypable strains lack a capsule, the immune response to infection is directed at noncapsular antigens. These noncapsular antigens of *H. influenzae* have generated considerable interest as targets of the human immune response and as potential vaccine components. The human immune response to nontypable strains appears to be strain-specific, accounting in part for the propensity of these strains to cause recurrent otitis media and recurrent exacerbations of chronic bronchitis in immunocompetent hosts.

CLINICAL MANIFESTATIONS ■ **Hib** The most serious manifestation of infection with Hib is meningitis. The age of peak incidence varies somewhat among populations, depending in part on the use of vaccine, but this infection primarily affects infants <2 years of age. The clinical manifestations of meningitis caused by Hib are similar to those of meningitis caused by other bacterial pathogens. Fever and altered central nervous system function are the most common features at presentation. Nuchal rigidity may or may not be evident. Subdural effusion, the most common complication, is suspected when, despite 2 or 3 days of appropriate antibiotic therapy, the infant has seizures, hemiparesis, or continued obtundation. The overall mortality from meningitis caused by Hib is ~5%, and the rate of morbidity is high. Of survivors, 6% have permanent sensorineural hearing loss, and about one-fourth have a significant handicap of some type. If more subtle handicaps are sought, up to half of survivors are found to have some neurologic sequelae, such as partial hearing loss and delay in language development.

Epiglottitis is a life-threatening infection involving cellulitis of the epiglottis and supraglottic tissues. It can lead to acute upper airway obstruction. Its unique epidemiologic features are its occurrence in an older age group (2 to 7 years old) than other Hib infections and its absence among Navajo Indians and Alaskan Eskimos. Sore throat and

TABLE 130-1 *Characteristics of Type b and Nontypable Strains of Haemophilus influenzae*

Feature	Type b Strains	Nontypable Strains
Capsule	Ribosyl-ribitol phosphate	Unencapsulated
Pathogenesis	Invasive infections due to hematogenous spread	Mucosal infections due to contiguous spread
Clinical manifestations	Meningitis and invasive infections in incompletely immunized infants and children	Otitis media in infants and children; lower respiratory tract infections in adults with chronic bronchitis
Evolutionary history	Basically clonal	Genetically diverse
Vaccine	Highly effective conjugate vaccines	None available; under development

fever rapidly progress to dysphagia, drooling, and airway obstruction. Epiglottitis also occurs in adults.

Cellulitis due to Hib occurs in young children. The most common location is on the head or neck, and the involved area sometimes takes on a characteristic bluish-red color. Most patients have bacteremia, and 10% have an additional focus of infection.

Hib causes *pneumonia* in infants. The infection is clinically indistinguishable from other types of bacterial pneumonia (e.g., pneumococcal pneumonia) except that Hib is more likely to involve the pleura.

Several less common invasive conditions can be important clinical manifestations of Hib infection in children. These include osteomyelitis, septic arthritis, pericarditis, orbital cellulitis, endophthalmitis, urinary tract infection, abscesses, and bacteremia without an identifiable focus. As has already been mentioned, infections due to Hib are unusual among patients older than 6 years.

Nontypable *H. influenzae*   Nontypable *H. influenzae* is a common cause of community-acquired bacterial pneumonia in adults. Nontypable *H. influenzae* pneumonia is especially common among patients with chronic obstructive pulmonary disease (COPD) or AIDS. The clinical features of pneumonia due to *H. influenzae* are similar to those of other types of bacterial pneumonia (including pneumococcal pneumonia). Patients present with fever, cough, and purulent sputum, usually of several days' duration. Chest radiography reveals alveolar infiltrates in a patchy or lobar distribution. Gram-stained sputum contains a predominance of small, pleomorphic, coccobacillary gram-negative bacteria.

Exacerbations of COPD caused by nontypable *H. influenzae* are characterized by increased cough, sputum production, and shortness of breath. Fever is low-grade, and no infiltrates are evident on chest x-ray.

Nontypable *H. influenzae* is one of the three most common causes of childhood otitis media (the other two being *Streptococcus pneumoniae* and *Moraxella catarrhalis*). Infants are febrile and irritable, while older children report ear pain. Symptoms of viral upper respiratory infection often precede otitis media. The diagnosis is made by pneumatic otoscopy. An etiologic diagnosis, although not routinely sought, can be established by tympanocentesis and culture of middle-ear fluid.

Nontypable *H. influenzae* also causes puerperal sepsis and is an important cause of neonatal bacteremia. These nontypable strains tend to be of biotype IV and cause invasive disease after colonizing the female genital tract.

Nontypable *H. influenzae* causes sinusitis in adults and children. In addition, the bacterium is a less common cause of various invasive infections that are reported primarily as small-series descriptions and case reports. These infections include empyema, adult epiglottitis, pericarditis, cellulitis, septic arthritis, osteomyelitis, endocarditis, cholecystitis, intraabdominal infections, urinary tract infections, mastoiditis, aortic graft infection, and bacteremia without a detectable focus.

DIAGNOSIS   The most reliable method for establishing a diagnosis of Hib infection is recovery of the organism in culture. The CSF of a patient in whom meningitis is suspected should be subjected to Gram's staining and culture. The presence of gram-negative coccobacilli in Gram-stained CSF is strong evidence for Hib meningitis. Recovery of the organism from CSF confirms the diagnosis. Cultures of other normally sterile body fluids, such as blood, joint fluid, pleural fluid, pericardial fluid, and subdural effusion, are confirmatory in other infections.

Detection of PRP is an important adjunct to culture in rapid diagnosis. Immunoelectrophoresis, latex agglutination, coagglutination, and enzyme-linked immunosorbent assay are effective in detecting PRP. These assays are particularly helpful when patients have received prior antimicrobial therapy and thus are especially likely to have negative cultures.

Before the early 1980s, nontypable strains of *H. influenzae* were frequently misidentified as Hib because of their autoagglutination when serotypes were determined in agglutination assays. Since non-typable *H. influenzae* is primarily a mucosal pathogen, it is a component of a mixed flora; this situation makes etiologic diagnosis challenging. Nontypable *H. influenzae* infection is strongly suggested by the predominance of gram-negative coccobacilli among abundant polymorphonuclear leukocytes in a Gram-stained sputum specimen from a patient in whom pneumonia or tracheobronchitis is suspected. A sputum culture is helpful when interpreted along with the results of Gram's staining. Although bacteremia is detectable in a small proportion of patients with pneumonia due to nontypable *H. influenzae*, most such patients have negative blood cultures.

A diagnosis of otitis media is based on the detection by pneumatic otoscopy of fluid in the middle ear. An etiologic diagnosis requires tympanocentesis but is not routinely sought. An invasive procedure is also required to determine the etiology of sinusitis; thus, treatment is often empirical once the diagnosis is suspected in light of clinical symptoms and sinus radiographs.

℞ TREATMENT

Initial therapy for meningitis due to Hib should consist of a cephalosporin such as ceftriaxone or cefotaxime. For children, the dosage of ceftriaxone is 75 to 100 mg/kg daily given in two doses 12 h apart. The pediatric dosage of cefotaxime is 200 mg/kg daily given in four doses 6 h apart. Adult dosages are 2 g every 12 h for ceftriaxone and 2 g every 4 to 6 h for cefotaxime. An alternative regimen for initial therapy is ampicillin (200 to 300 mg/kg daily in four divided doses) plus chloramphenicol (75 to 100 mg/kg daily in four divided doses). Therapy should continue for a total of 1 to 2 weeks.

Administration of glucocorticoids to patients with Hib meningitis reduces the incidence of neurologic sequelae. The presumed mechanism is reduction of the inflammation induced by bacterial cell-wall mediators of inflammation when cells are killed by antimicrobial agents. Dexamethasone (0.6 mg/kg per day intravenously in four divided doses for 2 days) is recommended for the treatment of Hib meningitis in children >2 months of age.

Invasive infections other than meningitis are treated with the same antimicrobial agents. For epiglottitis, the dosage of ceftriaxone is 50 mg/kg daily, and the dosage of cefotaxime is 150 mg/kg daily, given in three divided doses 8 h apart. Epiglottitis constitutes a medical emergency, and maintenance of an airway is critical. The duration of therapy is determined by the clinical response. A course of 1 to 2 weeks is usually appropriate.

Many infections caused by nontypable strains of *H. influenzae*, such as otitis media, sinusitis, and exacerbations of COPD, can be treated with oral antimicrobial agents. Approximately 25% of nontypable strains produce β-lactamase and are resistant to ampicillin. Infections caused by ampicillin-resistant strains can be treated with a variety of agents, including trimethoprim-sulfamethoxazole, amoxicillin/clavulanic acid, various extended-spectrum cephalosporins, and newer macrolides (azithromycin and clarithromycin). Fluoroquinolones are highly active against *H. influenzae* but are not currently recommended for the treatment of children or pregnant women because of possible effects on articular cartilage.

PREVENTION ■ Vaccination (See also Chap. 107)   The development of conjugate vaccines that prevent invasive infections with Hib in infants and children has been a dramatic success. Three such vaccines are licensed in the United States. In addition to eliciting protective antibody, these vaccines prevent disease by reducing pharyngeal colonization with Hib.

All children should be immunized with an Hib conjugate vaccine, receiving the first dose at ~2 months of age, the rest of the primary series between 2 and 6 months of age, and a booster dose at 12 to 15 months of age. Specific recommendations vary for the different conjugate vaccines. The reader is referred to the recommendations of the American Academy of Pediatrics. Currently, no vaccines are available for the prevention of disease caused by nontypable *H. influenzae*.

Chemoprophylaxis The risk of secondary disease is greater than normal among household contacts of patients with Hib disease. The attack rate is as high as 4% among susceptible infants. Therefore, all children and adults (except pregnant women) in households with at least one contact <4 years of age who is incompletely immunized should receive prophylaxis with oral rifampin. (This rule does not apply when all household contacts under the age of 4 years have been completely immunized with conjugate vaccine.) Children <12 years old should receive rifampin at a dose of 20 mg/kg once daily for 4 days, and adults should receive 600 mg daily for 4 days. The index case should receive rifampin before or at the time of discharge from the hospital because antimicrobial agents used for the treatment of meningitis do not reliably eradicate Hib from the nasopharynx.

When two or more cases of invasive Hib disease have occurred within 60 days at a child-care facility attended by incompletely vaccinated children, administration of rifampin to all attendees and personnel is indicated, as is recommended for household contacts. Chemoprophylaxis is not indicated in nursery and child-care contacts of a single index case. The reader is referred to the recommendations of the American Academy of Pediatrics.

HAEMOPHILUS INFLUENZAE BIOGROUP AEGYPTIUS

H. influenzae biogroup aegyptius was formerly called *Haemophilus aegyptius* because of phenotypic characteristics distinct from those of *H. influenzae*. However, later studies involving DNA hybridization and DNA transformation demonstrated that *H. aegyptius* and *H. influenzae* are members of the same species.

H. influenzae biogroup aegyptius has long been associated with conjunctivitis. Moreover, this strain is now known to be the cause of Brazilian purpuric fever (BPF), which was first recognized in 1984 in the rural Brazilian town of Promissao. The sharing of many phenotypic and genotypic characteristics by the various strains of *H. influenzae* biogroup aegyptius that cause BPF indicates that these strains represent a clone of *H. influenzae*. The age of peak incidence of BPF is 1 to 4 years, with a range of 3 months to 8 years. The illness can occur sporadically or in outbreaks. Typically, after an episode of purulent conjunctivitis, high fever occurs in association with vomiting and abdominal pain. Within 12 to 48 h after onset, the patient develops petechiae, purpura, and peripheral necrosis and experiences vascular collapse. The characteristic laboratory features are thrombocytopenia, prolonged prothrombin time, uniformly unrevealing CSF findings, and blood cultures positive for *H. influenzae* biogroup aegyptius. Initial reports cited high mortality (70%), but subsequent studies have indicated that milder forms of the illness exist. Most patients have resolved or resolving purulent conjunctivitis, and culture of the conjunctiva is positive in approximately one-third of cases. BPF has been seen in several towns in Brazil and on two occasions in Australia.

HAEMOPHILUS DUCREYI

Haemophilus ducreyi is the etiologic agent of chancroid (Chap. 115), a sexually transmitted disease characterized by genital ulceration and inguinal adenitis. *H. ducreyi* poses a significant health problem in developing countries. Although this infection is less common in the United States, its incidence has increased dramatically in the past several years. In addition to being a cause of morbidity in itself, chancroid is associated with infection with HIV because of the role of genital ulceration in the transmission of HIV.

MICROBIOLOGY *H. ducreyi* is a highly fastidious coccobacillary gram-negative bacterium whose growth requires X factor (hemin). Although, in light of this requirement, the bacterium has been classified in the genus *Haemophilus*, DNA homology and chemotaxonomic studies have established substantial differences between *H. ducreyi* and other *Haemophilus* species. Taxonomic reclassification of the organism is likely in the future but awaits further study.

The histology of the genital ulcer of chancroid is characterized by perivascular and interstitial infiltrates of macrophages and of CD4+ and CD8+ lymphocytes. The appearance is consistent with a delayed-type hypersensitivity, cell-mediated immune response. The presence of CD4+ cells and macrophages in the ulcer may explain, in part, the facilitation of transmission of HIV in patients with chancroid.

EPIDEMIOLOGY AND PREVALENCE Chancroid is a common cause of genital ulcers in developing countries. In the United States, chancroid is now endemic in some regions, and several large outbreaks have occurred since 1981. Recurring epidemiologic themes have been apparent in these outbreaks: (1) transmission has been predominantly heterosexual; (2) males have outnumbered females by ratios of 3:1 to 25:1; (3) prostitutes have been important in transmission of the infection; and (4) chancroid has been strongly associated with illicit drug use. The incidence of chancroid in the United States will likely increase in the coming years, and the genital ulcers associated with this infection will continue to play a role in the transmission of HIV.

CLINICAL MANIFESTATIONS Infection is acquired as the result of a break in the epithelium during sexual contact with an infected individual. After an incubation period of 4 to 7 days, the initial lesion—a papule with surrounding erythema—appears. In 2 to 3 days, the papule evolves into a pustule, which spontaneously ruptures and forms a sharply circumscribed ulcer that is generally not indurated (Fig. 130-2). The ulcers are painful and bleed easily; little or no inflammation of the surrounding skin is evident. Approximately half of patients develop enlarged, tender inguinal lymph nodes, which frequently become fluctuant and spontaneously rupture. Patients usually seek medical care after 1 to 3 weeks of painful symptoms.

The presentation of chancroid does not usually include all of the typical clinical features and is sometimes atypical. Multiple ulcers can coalesce to form giant ulcers. Ulcers can appear and then resolve, with inguinal adenitis (Fig. 130-2) and suppuration following 1 to 3 weeks later; this clinical picture can be confused with that of lymphogranuloma venereum. Multiple small ulcers can resemble folliculitis. Other differential diagnostic considerations include the various infections causing genital ulceration, such as primary syphilis, condyloma latum of secondary syphilis, genital herpes, and donovanosis. In rare cases chancroid lesions become secondarily infected with bacteria; the result is extensive inflammation.

DIAGNOSIS Clinical diagnosis of chancroid is often inaccurate, and laboratory confirmation should be attempted in suspected cases. Gram's staining of a swab of the lesion may reveal a predominance of characteristic gram-negative coccobacilli, but the presence of other bacteria often makes it difficult to interpret this result. An accurate diagnosis of chancroid relies on cultures of *H. ducreyi* from the lesion. In addition, aspiration and culture of suppurative lymph nodes should be considered. Since the organism can be difficult to grow, the use of selective and supplemented media is necessary. A new multiplex

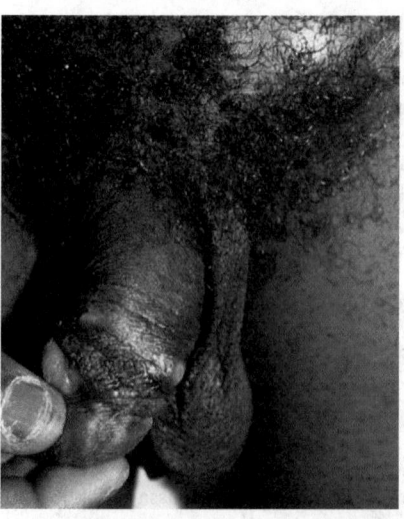

FIGURE 130-2 Chancroid with characteristic penile ulcers and associated left inguinal adenitis (bubo).

polymerase chain reaction (PCR) assay has been developed to amplify simultaneously DNA targets from *H. ducreyi*, *Treponema pallidum*, and herpes simplex virus types 1 and 2. When this assay becomes commercially available, it will be a useful diagnostic method with which to identify the etiology of genital ulcers.

℞ TREATMENT

The treatment regimen recommended by the Centers for Disease Control and Prevention is a single 1-g oral dose of azithromycin. Alternative regimens include ceftriaxone (250 mg intramuscularly in a single dose), ciprofloxacin (500 mg orally twice a day for 3 days), or erythromycin base (500 mg orally three times a day for 7 days). Isolates from patients who do not respond promptly to treatment should be tested for antimicrobial susceptibility. In patients with HIV infection, healing may be slow and longer courses of treatment may be necessary. Clinical treatment failure in HIV-seropositive patients may reflect co-infection, especially with herpes simplex virus. Contacts of patients with chancroid should be identified and treated whether or not symptoms are present if they had sexual contact with the patient during the 10 days preceding the patient's onset of symptoms.

OTHER *HAEMOPHILUS* SPECIES

Haemophilus species are often recovered as components of the flora of the normal human upper respiratory tract. However, these bacteria are infrequent causes of infection because of their low pathogenic potential. *Haemophilus* species have fastidious growth requirements and are generally rather slow-growing. The species implicated in human infections include *H. parainfluenzae*, *H. aphrophilus*, and *H. paraphrophilus* (Chap. 131); *H. parahaemolyticus*; *H. haemolyticus*; and *H. segnis*. *Haemophilus* species are differentiated from one another by several characteristics, primarily their requirements for X and V factors. Species designated *para-* require V factor but not X factor for growth, whereas the others require either X and V or X only.

Haemophilus species, particularly *H. parainfluenzae*, are an increasingly recognized cause of endocarditis and should be considered as such, especially when initial blood cultures are negative but clinical suspicion of endocarditis is high. Blood cultures should be incubated for 2 weeks to increase the likelihood of isolating slow-growing *Hae-*

mophilus species. Endocarditis due to *Haemophilus* species usually presents with a subacute course, but the presentation varies.

A variety of other infections involving almost all organ systems can be caused by *Haemophilus* species. Most of these unusual manifestations have been reported as single cases and small series.

℞ TREATMENT

The antimicrobial susceptibility characteristics of other *Haemophilus* species are similar to those of *H. influenzae*. Some strains produce β-lactamase and are thereby resistant to ampicillin. Other strains are sensitive to ampicillin, and this agent has been used successfully to treat many infections. Alternative agents with good activity against most *Haemophilus* species include trimethoprim-sulfamethoxazole, third-generation cephalosporins, tetracycline, chloramphenicol, and aminoglycosides. Endocarditis caused by ampicillin-sensitive strains should be treated with ampicillin plus an aminoglycoside.

FURTHER READING

BONG CT et al: *Haemophilus ducreyi*: Clinical features, epidemiology, and prospects for disease control. Microbes Infect 4:1141, 2002

COMMITTEE ON INFECTIOUS DISEASES: *Haemophilus influenzae* infections, in *2000 Red Book, Report of the Committee on Infectious Diseases*, LK Pickering et al (eds). Elk Grove Village, IL, American Academy of Pediatrics, 2000

FOXWELL AR et al: Nontypeable *Haemophilus influenzae*: Pathogenesis and prevention. Microbiol Mol Biol Rev 62:294, 1998

HOBAN DJ et al: Worldwide prevalence of antimicrobial resistance in *Streptococcus pneumoniae*, *Haemophilus influenzae*, and *Moraxella catarrhalis* in the SENTRY antimicrobial surveillance program, 1997–1999. Clin Infect Dis 32(Suppl):S81, 2001

PELTOLA H: Worldwide *Haemophilus influenzae* type b disease at the beginning of the 21st century: Global analysis of the disease burden 25 years after the use of the polysaccharide vaccine and a decade after the advent of conjugates. Clin Microbiol Rev 13:302, 2000

SARANGI J et al: Invasive *Haemophilus influenzae* disease in adults. Epidemiol Infect 124:441, 2000

SETHI S et al: New strains of bacteria and exacerbations of chronic obstructive pulmonary disease. N Engl J Med 347:465, 2002

131 INFECTIONS DUE TO HACEK GROUP AND MISCELLANEOUS GRAM-NEGATIVE BACTERIA
Dennis L. Kasper, Tamar F. Barlam

HACEK GROUP ORGANISMS

HACEK organisms are a group of fastidious, slow-growing, gram-negative bacteria whose growth requires an atmosphere of carbon dioxide. Species belonging to this group include several *Haemophilus* species, *Actinobacillus actinomycetemcomitans*, *Cardiobacterium hominis*, *Eikenella corrodens*, and *Kingella kingae*. HACEK bacteria normally reside in the oral cavity and have been associated with local infections in the mouth. They are also known to cause severe systemic infections, most often bacterial endocarditis (Chap. 109).

Of the HACEK group, the *Haemophilus* species, *A. actinomyce-temcomitans*, and *C. hominis* are most frequently associated with endocarditis, which can develop on either native or prosthetic valves. In large series, up to 3% of cases of infective endocarditis are attributable to HACEK organisms. The clinical course of HACEK endocarditis tends to be subacute; however, embolization is common. The overall prevalence of major emboli associated with HACEK endocarditis ranges from 28 to 71% in different series. On echocardiography, valvular vegetations are seen in up to 85% of patients. The vegetations are frequently large, although vegetation size has not been directly correlated with risk of embolization. Cultures of blood from patients with suspected HACEK endocarditis may require up to 30 days to

become positive, and the microbiology laboratory should be alerted if a HACEK organism is being considered. However, most cultures that ultimately yield a HACEK organism become positive within the first week, especially with improved culture systems such as BACTEC. In addition, polymerase chain reaction techniques are facilitating the diagnosis of HACEK infections. Because of the organisms' slow growth, antimicrobial testing may be difficult, and strains producing β-lactamase may not be identified accurately. This factor should be considered in the selection of a therapeutic regimen. E-test methodology may improve the accuracy of susceptibility testing.

Native-valve endocarditis should be treated for 4 weeks with antibiotics, whereas prosthetic-valve endocarditis requires 6 weeks of therapy. The cure rates for HACEK prosthetic-valve endocarditis appear to be high. Unlike prosthetic-valve endocarditis caused by other gram-negative organisms, HACEK endocarditis is often cured with antibiotic treatment alone—i.e., without surgical intervention. Recommendations for the treatment of HACEK endocarditis are presented in Table 131-1.

***HAEMOPHILUS* SPECIES** *Haemophilus* species cause more than half of all cases of HACEK endocarditis. *H. aphrophilus* and *H. parainfluenzae* are most common; *H. paraphrophilus* is less common. Up to 50%

TABLE 131-1 *Treatment of Endocarditis Caused by HACEK Group Organisms*[a]

Organism	Initial Therapy	Alternative Agents	Comments
Haemophilus species	Ceftriaxone (2 g/d)	Fluoroquinolones,[b] ampicillin/sulbactam	Ampicillin ± aminoglycoside can be used if organism does not produce β-lactamase.
Actinobacillus actinomycetemcomitans	Ceftriaxone (2 g/d)	Semisynthetic penicillins (e.g., mezlocillin), TMP-SMX, fluoroquinolones,[b] azithromycin	Limited data exist on efficacy of regimens other than semisynthetic penicillins or third-generation cephalosporins.
Cardiobacterium hominis	Penicillin (16–18 mU/d in 6 divided doses) ± gentamicin (5–6 mg/kg/d in 3 divided doses)	Ceftriaxone, ampicillin/sulbactam	Value of aminoglycoside has not been proven. Organism is usually pan-sensitive, but high-level resistance to penicillin has been reported.
Eikenella corrodens	Ampicillin (2 g q4h)	Ceftriaxone, fluoroquinolones[b]	Organism is resistant to clindamycin and metronidazole.
Kingella kingae	Ceftriaxone (2 g/d) or ampicillin/sulbactam (3 g of ampicillin q6h)	Fluoroquinolones,[b] vancomycin, clindamycin, macrolides, TMP-SMX	Prevalence of β-lactamase-producing strains is increasing. Efficacy for invasive infections is best demonstrated for first-line treatments.

[a] Susceptibility testing should be performed to guide therapy.
[b] Fluoroquinolones are not recommended for treatment of children <17 years of age.

Note: TMP-SMX, trimethoprim-sulfamethoxazole.

of patients with native-valve endocarditis due to *Haemophilus* species report a history of cardiac valvular disease, 60% have been ill for <2 months before presentation, and 50% are anemic at presentation. Some 19% to 50% of these patients develop congestive heart failure. Mortality rates as high as 30% to 50% have been reported in older series, with most deaths attributed to cerebral embolism; however, recent studies have documented mortality rates of <5%. In rare cases, *H. parainfluenzae* has been isolated from other infections, such as meningitis; brain, dental, and liver abscess; pneumonia; and septicemia.

 TREATMENT

See Table 131-1.

ACTINOBACILLUS ACTINOMYCETEMCOMITANS *A. actinomycetemcomitans*, another slow-growing inhabitant of the oral cavity, can be isolated from soft tissue infections and abscesses in association with *Actinomyces israelii*. About 30% of actinomycotic lesions also yield *A. actinomycetemcomitans* on culture. *A. actinomycetemcomitans* has been associated with severe destructive periodontal disease, characterized by loss of alveolar bone of the molars and incisors, in both children and adults. Patients who develop endocarditis with this organism typically have severe periodontal disease and underlying cardiac valvular damage as well as high rates of embolic phenomena. *A. actinomycetemcomitans* has been isolated from patients with brain abscess, meningitis, parotitis, osteomyelitis, urinary tract infection, pneumonia, and empyema, among other infections.

 TREATMENT

See Table 131-1.

CARDIOBACTERIUM HOMINIS *C. hominis* primarily causes endocarditis in patients with underlying valvular heart disease or with prosthetic valves. Unlike other HACEK bacteria, *C. hominis* most frequently affects the aortic valve. Many patients have signs and symptoms of long-standing infection before diagnosis and have evidence of arterial embolization, vasculitis, cerebrovascular accidents, immune complex glomerulonephritis, or arthritis at presentation. As in endocarditis due to other HACEK organisms, embolization, mycotic aneurysms, and congestive heart failure are frequent.

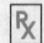 **TREATMENT**

See Table 131-1.

EIKENELLA CORRODENS *E. corrodens*, a fastidious, facultative gram-negative organism, is part of the endogenous flora of the mouth and nasopharynx. It is most frequently recovered from sites of infection in

conjunction with other bacterial species. Clinical sources of *E. corrodens* include sites of human bite wounds (clenched-fist injuries), endocarditis, soft tissue infections of the head and neck, soft tissue infections in injection drug users, osteomyelitis, respiratory infections, chorioamnionitis, gynecologic infections associated with intrauterine devices, meningitis and brain abscesses, and visceral abscesses.

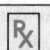 **TREATMENT**

See Table 131-1.

KINGELLA KINGAE *K. kingae* is a β-hemolytic, fastidious, nonmotile gram-negative rod. Because of improved microbiologic methodology, isolation of this organism is increasingly common. In recent series, *K. kingae* was the cause of up to half of all cases of previously undiagnosed osteomyelitis and septic arthritis in children <2 years old. *K. kingae* has been the third most common cause of septic arthritis in children <24 months of age; staphylococcal and streptococcal species remain most prevalent. In children <4 years of age, there is evidence for prolonged nasopharyngeal colonization, with carriage rates of 10%. Invasive *K. kingae* infections with bacteremia are associated with stomatitis. Both *K. kingae* colonization and primary herpes—a major cause of stomatitis—peak in children 6 to 48 months of age. *K. kingae* bacteremia can present with a petechial rash similar to that seen with *Neisseria meningitidis* sepsis.

Infective endocarditis, unlike other infections with *K. kingae*, occurs in older children and adults. The majority of patients have pre-existing valvular disease. As in endocarditis caused by the other HACEK organisms, there is a high incidence of complications, including arterial emboli, cerebrovascular accidents, tricuspid insufficiency, and congestive heart failure with cardiovascular collapse.

 TREATMENT

See Table 131-1.

OTHER GRAM-NEGATIVE BACTERIA
ACINETOBACTER SPECIES See Chap. 134.

ACHROMOBACTER XYLOSOXIDANS Previously known as *Alcaligenes xylosoxidans*, this gram-negative bacillus is probably part of the endogenous intestinal flora and has been isolated from water sources. Immunocompromised hosts appear to be at increased risk for infection with this organism. Nosocomial sources to which outbreaks of infection with *A. xylosoxidans* have been attributed include contaminated intravenous fluids, pressure transducers, and disinfectants. Clinical illness has been associated with isolates from many sites, including blood (often in the setting of infected intravascular devices), urine, respiratory secretions, cerebrospinal fluid, peritoneal and pleural fluids, and endocarditic prosthetic valves. Community-acquired bacteremia with *A. xylosoxidans* usually occurs in the setting of pneumonia. Metastatic skin lesions are present in one-fifth of cases. The reported mortality rate is 67%, similar to rates for other bacteremic gram-negative pneumonias.

℞ TREATMENT

In vitro susceptibility testing of all clinically relevant isolates is essential to the selection of appropriate therapy.

AGROBACTERIUM RADIOBACTER (TUMEFACIENS) This organism has been associated with intravascular catheter–related infections in immunocompromised hosts, especially individuals infected with HIV. Clinically important infections associated with *A. radiobacter* include prosthetic-joint and prosthetic-valve infections, bacteremia, peritonitis, and urinary tract infections.

℞ TREATMENT

Antibiotic sensitivity testing is essential in the choice of therapy.

CAPNOCYTOPHAGA SPECIES This genus of fusiform, long, thin, gram-negative coccobacilli is facultatively anaerobic and requires an atmosphere enriched in carbon dioxide for optimal growth. *C. ochracea*, *C. gingivalis*, and *C. sputigena* are inhabitants of the healthy human oral cavity and have been isolated from the female genital tract. Their isolation has also been reported from blood, cerebrospinal fluid, and respiratory fluids (including pleural collections). These organisms have been associated with sepsis in immunocompromised hosts; particularly at risk are neutropenic patients with acute myelogenous leukemia or acute lymphocytic leukemia. In the immunocompetent host, these three species probably play a role in localized juvenile periodontitis; however, they have been isolated from many other sites as well, usually as part of a polymicrobial infection. In vitro sensitivity testing of these organisms is difficult because they are slow-growing and fastidious.

C. canimorsus and *C. cynodegmi* are endogenous to the canine mouth. Patients infected with these species frequently have a history of dog bites or of exposure to dogs without scratches or bites. Asplenia, glucocorticoid therapy, and alcohol abuse are predisposing conditions and are associated with relatively fulminant infections. The interval from dog bite to presentation averages 5 days but ranges from 1 day to 1 month. *C. canimorsus* causes a wide range of infections, including severe sepsis with shock and disseminated intravascular coagulation, meningitis, endocarditis, cellulitis, and septic arthritis. In the asplenic individual who has recently sustained a dog bite, infection with this organism must be considered early because of a potentially rapid progression to death.

℞ TREATMENT

Although penicillin has been considered first-line therapy for infections due to *C. ochracea*, *C. gingivalis*, and *C. sputigena*, an increasing number of isolates reportedly produce β-lactamase. Fluoroquinolone resistance is also increasing. Clindamycin (600 to 900 mg every 6 to 8 h) or drug combinations including a penicillin derivative plus a β-lactamase inhibitor—such as ampicillin/sulbactam (1.5 to 3.0 g of ampicillin every 6 h)—are currently recommended for empirical therapy. Penicillin (12 to 18 million units daily in 6 divided doses) is the drug of choice for documented infections with *C. canimorsus*. This regimen or ampicillin/sulbactam should also be given prophylactically to asplenic patients sustaining dog-bite injuries. Patients with suspected infection due to *C. canimorsus* should be treated empirically, because identification of this organism and determination of its antibiotic sensitivity can take many days. Other drugs to which *C. canimorsus* is reportedly susceptible include clindamycin, imipenem, quinolones, and third-generation cephalosporins.

CHROMOBACTERIUM VIOLACEUM This organism is rarely a human pathogen but reportedly has been responsible for life-threatening infections

with severe sepsis and metastatic abscesses, particularly in children. A slender, slightly curved, gram-negative rod that is facultatively anaerobic, *C. violaceum* inhabits tropical water and soil and causes infection after contamination of skin wounds. Patients with defective neutrophil function (e.g., those with chronic granulomatous disease) are infected by this organism with unusual frequency. The mortality rate in the United States from infection with *C. violaceum* has been reported at >60%.

℞ TREATMENT

C. violaceum is generally susceptible to ciprofloxacin (500 mg every 12 h orally or 400 mg every 12 h intravenously), trimethoprim-sulfamethoxazole (TMP-SMX), gentamicin, and chloramphenicol.

CHRYSEOBACTERIUM SPECIES *C. meningosepticum* and *C. indologenes* were previously classified as *Flavobacterium* species. *C. meningosepticum* is a ubiquitous organism and an important cause of nosocomial infections. It has been associated with outbreaks due to contaminated fluids, such as disinfectants, arterial catheter flush solutions, and aerosolized antibiotics, and with sporadic infections due to indwelling devices, vials, sink traps, feeding tubes, and other fluid-associated apparatus. Patients with nosocomial *C. meningosepticum* infection usually have underlying immunosuppression (e.g., related to malignancy). *C. meningosepticum* has been reported to cause meningitis (primarily in neonates), sepsis, endocarditis, bacteremia, soft tissue infections, and pneumonia. *C. indologenes* has caused bacteremia, sepsis, and pneumonia, typically in immunocompromised patients with indwelling devices.

℞ TREATMENT

Antibiotic treatment should be based on susceptibility results because of the high likelihood that a *C. meningosepticum* isolate will produce β-lactamase. Early reports suggested that vancomycin might be efficacious, but more recent data refute this conclusion.

PLESIOMONAS SHIGELLOIDES This freshwater organism is a cause of acute diarrhea (Chap. 113) and occasionally of serious extraintestinal disease. *P. shigelloides* is transmitted to humans via contaminated water or food. This motile, facultatively anaerobic gram-negative rod most often produces mild, watery diarrhea. Severe extraintestinal infections have been reported, most commonly in immunocompromised hosts, and include bacteremia, cellulitis, neonatal sepsis and meningitis, and septic arthritis.

℞ TREATMENT

There is great variability among strains in terms of antibiotic sensitivity patterns, and isolates must be tested before appropriate therapy can be selected.

AEROMONAS SPECIES Five species of *Aeromonas* are known to be associated with disease in humans, but more than 85% of these *Aeromonas* infections are caused by *A. hydrophila*, *A. caviae*, and *A. veronii* biovar *sobria*. *Aeromonas* proliferates in potable and fresh water and in soil. It remains controversial whether *Aeromonas* is a cause of bacterial gastroenteritis. Although many case reports have associated *Aeromonas* with gastroenteritis, no clear outbreaks with a single isolate have been documented, no conclusive animal model exists, and asymptomatic colonization of the intestinal tract with *Aeromonas* occurs frequently. However, rare cases of hemolytic-uremic syndrome following bloody diarrhea have been shown to be secondary to the presence of *Aeromonas*. In addition, identification of an enterotoxin (different from the Shiga-like toxin produced by *Escherichia coli* O157:H7) in these cases supports the hypothesis that *Aeromonas* causes gastroenteritis.

Aeromonas causes sepsis and bacteremia in infants with multiple medical problems and in immunocompromised hosts, particularly those with cancer or hepatobiliary disease. *Aeromonas* infection and sepsis can occur in trauma patients with myonecrosis or in burn patients exposed to *Aeromonas* by environmental contamination of their wounds from fresh water or soil sources. Mortality ranges from 25% among immunocompromised adults with sepsis to >90% among patients with myonecrosis. *Aeromonas* can produce skin lesions resembling the ecthyma gangrenosum lesions seen in *Pseudomonas aeruginosa* infection. These lesions are hemorrhagic vesicles surrounded by a rim of erythema with central necrosis and ulceration.

Aeromonas wound infections can occur in healthy adults who sustain minor trauma with environmental contamination, usually water-related; after severe trauma and crush injuries with sepsis and environmental exposure, usually to soil; and in nosocomial infections related to catheters, surgical incisions, or use of leeches. Other clinical manifestations include meningitis, peritonitis, pneumonia, and ocular infections.

℞ TREATMENT

Treatment should be guided by antimicrobial susceptibility testing. *Aeromonas* species are generally susceptible to fluoroquinolones (e.g., ciprofloxacin at a dosage of 500 mg every 12 h orally or 400 mg every 12 h intravenously), TMP-SMX (at a trimethoprim dosage of 10 mg/kg per day in 3 or 4 divided doses), third-generation cephalosporins, and aminoglycosides. However, resistance is increasing.

MISCELLANEOUS ORGANISMS Many other gram-negative rods have been reported to cause occasional infections in hosts who are immunologically unprepared to deal with relatively avirulent organisms or who are unfortunate enough to encounter an exceptionally large inoculum. Such organisms include *Weeksella* species; various CDC groups, such as EF-4, Ve-2 (*Flavimonas* species), IVc-2, NO-1, WO-1, and Gilardi Group WO-1; *Sphingobacterium* species; *Protomonas* species; *Ochrobactrum anthropi*; *Oligella urethralis*; and *Shewanella putrefaciens*. The reader is advised to consult subspecialty texts and references for further guidance on these organisms.

FURTHER READING

BROUQUI P, RAOULT D: Endocarditis due to rare and fastidious bacteria. Clin Microbiol Rev 14:177, 2001

DARRAS-JOLY C et al: *Haemophilus* endocarditis: Report of 42 cases in adults and review. Clin Infect Dis 24:1087, 1997

DAS M et al: Infective endocarditis caused by HACEK microorganisms. Annu Rev Med 48:25, 1997

JANDA JM et al: Evolving concepts regarding the genus *Aeromonas*: An expanding panorama of species, disease presentations, and unanswered questions. Clin Infect Dis 27:332, 1998

MARTINO R et al: Bacteremia caused by *Capnocytophaga* species in patients with neutropenia and cancer: Results of a multicenter study. Clin Infect Dis 33:E20, 2001

PAUL K, PATEL SS: *Eikenella corrodens* infections in children and adolescents: Case report and review of the literature. Clin Infect Dis 33:54, 2001

SHIGEMATSU M et al: An epidemiological study of *Plesiomonas shigelloides* diarrhoea among Japanese travelers. Epidemiol Infect 125:523, 2000

YAGUPSKY P, DAGAN R: Population-based study of invasive *Kingella kingae* infections. Emerg Infect Dis 6:85, 2000

132 LEGIONELLA INFECTION
Feng-Yee Chang, Victor L. Yu

DEFINITION *Legionellosis* refers to the two clinical syndromes caused by bacteria of the genus *Legionella*. *Pontiac fever* is an acute, febrile, self-limited illness that has been serologically linked to *Legionella* species, whereas *Legionnaires' disease* is the designation for pneumonia caused by these species.

HISTORY Legionnaires' disease was first recognized in 1976, when an outbreak of pneumonia took place at a hotel in Philadelphia during the American Legion Convention. The causative agent proved to be a newly discovered bacterium, *Legionella pneumophila*, that was isolated from lung specimens obtained from the victims at autopsy.

MICROBIOLOGY The family Legionellaceae comprises 41 species with 64 serogroups. The species *L. pneumophila* causes 80 to 90% of human infections and includes at least 14 serogroups; serogroups 1, 4, and 6 are most commonly implicated in human infections. To date, 17 species other than *L. pneumophila* have been associated with human infections, among which *L. micdadei* (Pittsburgh pneumonia agent), *L. bozemanii*, *L. dumoffii*, and *L. longbeachae* are the most common.

Members of the Legionellaceae are aerobic gram-negative bacilli that do not grow on routine microbiologic media. Buffered charcoal yeast extract (BCYE) agar is the medium used to grow *Legionella*. Antibiotics added to the medium suppress the growth of competing flora from nonsterile sites, and dyes color the colonies and assist in identification.

The direct fluorescent antibody (DFA) test can definitively identify a number of individual species. In *L. pneumophila*, lipopolysaccharide is a prominent constituent of the outer membrane, and the serogroup-specific antigen and antibodies detected by immunofluorescence are directed primarily at the lipopolysaccharide. Both polyclonal and monoclonal DFA reagents are commercially available. The monoclonal antibody reagent is less cross-reactive but is specific for *L. pneumophila*.

ECOLOGY AND TRANSMISSION The natural habitats for *L. pneumophila* are aquatic bodies, including lakes and streams. *L. longbeachae* has been isolated from soil. *Legionella* can survive under a wide range of environmental conditions; for example, the organisms can live for years in refrigerated water samples. Natural bodies of water contain only small numbers of *Legionella*. However, once the organisms enter human-constructed aquatic reservoirs (such as water-distribution systems), they can grow and proliferate. Factors known to enhance colonization by and amplification of legionellae include warm temperatures (25° to 42°C), stagnation, and scale and sediment. *L. pneumophila* can form microcolonies within biofilms; its eradication from water-distribution systems requires disinfectants that can penetrate the biofilm. The presence of symbiotic microorganisms, including algae, amebas, ciliated protozoa, and other water-dwelling bacteria, promotes the growth of *L. pneumophila*. *Legionella* can invade and multiply within free-living protozoa.

Hot-water tanks colonized with *L. pneumophila* are significantly more likely than uncolonized tanks to be cooler, to have a vertical configuration, to be older, and to have higher concentrations of calcium and magnesium. Vertical tanks, especially those that are electric coil-heated rather than gas-heated, have a pronounced temperature stratification and thick sediment accumulation at the bottom.

The source of *Legionella* is water. Early investigations that implicated cooling towers antedated the discovery that the organism could also exist in potable-water distribution systems. It is now known that, in most previously reported outbreaks, cases of Legionnaires' disease continued to occur despite disinfection of cooling towers and the potable water supply was the actual source. Koch's postulates have been fulfilled in epidemiologic studies using molecular fingerprinting methods to link potable water sources (rather than cooling towers) to *Legionella* infection in humans. Community-acquired Legionnaires' disease has also been linked to colonization of residential and industrial water supplies.

Multiple modes of transmission of *Legionella* to humans exist, including aerosolization, aspiration, and direct instillation into the lung during respiratory tract manipulations. Aspiration is the predominant mode of transmission, but it is unclear whether *Legionella* enters the lung via oropharyngeal colonization or directly via the drinking of contaminated water. Nasogastric tubes have been linked to nosocomial Legionnaires' disease in several reports; microaspiration of contaminated water was the hypothesized mode of transmission. Surgery with general anesthesia is a known risk factor that is consistent with aspiration. Especially compelling is the reported 30% incidence of postoperative *Legionella* pneumonia among patients undergoing head and neck surgery at a hospital with a contaminated water supply; aspiration is a recognized sequela in such cases. Studies of patients with hospital-acquired Legionnaires' disease have shown that these individuals underwent endotracheal intubation significantly more often and for a significantly longer duration than patients with nosocomial pneumonia of other etiologies.

Aerosolization of *Legionella* by devices filled with tap water, including nebulizers and humidifiers, has been implicated in disease causation. An ultrasonic mist machine in the produce section of a grocery store was implicated in a community outbreak. Pontiac fever has been linked to *Legionella*-containing aerosols from water-using machinery, a cooling tower, air-conditioners, and whirlpools.

EPIDEMIOLOGY   The incidence of Legionnaires' disease depends on the degree of contamination of the aquatic reservoir, the immune status of the persons exposed to water from that reservoir, the intensity of exposure, and the availability of specialized laboratory tests on which the correct diagnosis can be based.

Numerous prospective studies have ranked *Legionella* among the top four microbial causes of community-acquired pneumonia (with *Streptococcus pneumoniae*, *Haemophilus influenzae*, and *Chlamydia pneumoniae* usually ranked first, second, and third, respectively), accounting for 3 to 15% of cases. On the basis of a multihospital study of community-acquired pneumonia in Ohio, it is estimated that only 3% of sporadic cases of Legionnaires' disease are correctly diagnosed. *Legionella* is responsible for 10 to 50% of nosocomial pneumonias when a hospital's water system is colonized with the organisms. One situation in which the diagnosis of Legionnaires' disease should be considered is that in which the presenting patient has been hospitalized within 10 days before the onset of symptoms.

The most common risk factors for Legionnaires' disease are cigarette smoking, chronic lung disease, advanced age, and immunosuppression (including receipt of glucocorticoids). However, in a large prospective study of community-acquired pneumonia, 28% of patients with Legionnaires' disease did not have these classic risk factors. Surgery is a prominent predisposing factor in hospital-acquired infection, with transplant recipients at highest risk. Hospital-acquired cases are now being recognized among neonates and children with immunosuppression or underlying pulmonary disease.

Pontiac fever occurs in epidemics. The high attack rate (>90%) reflects airborne transmission.

PATHOGENESIS AND IMMUNITY   *Legionella* enters the lungs through aspiration or direct inhalation. Attachment of the bacteria to host cells is mediated by type IV pili, heat-shock protein Hsp60, and the major outer-membrane protein. *Legionella* binds to complement CR1 and CR3 integrin receptors on the surface of the host cell. Because the organisms possess pili that may mediate adherence to respiratory tract epithelial cells, conditions that impair mucociliary clearance, including cigarette smoking, lung disease, or alcoholism, predispose to Legionnaires' disease.

Cell-mediated immunity is the primary mechanism of host defense against *Legionella*, as it is against other intracellular pathogens, including *Mycobacterium tuberculosis*, *Listeria*, and *Toxoplasma*. Alveolar macrophages readily phagocytose *Legionella*. The attachment of the bacteria to phagocytes is mediated via Fc receptors and complement receptors, which attach to the bacterial major outer-membrane protein. Binding to these receptors promotes phagocytosis but fails to trigger an oxidative burst. The *L. pneumophila* phagosome resists acidification and evades fusion with late endocytic compartments and lysosomes. Although many *Legionella* organisms are killed, some proliferate intracellularly until the cells rupture; the bacteria are then phagocytosed again by newly recruited phagocytes, and the cycle begins anew.

Two general types of bacterial virulence genes required for intracellular growth have been identified: those that affect trafficking of the bacterial phagosome (establishment factors) and those that affect replication after trafficking (maintenance factors). Establishment factor mutants exhibit severe intracellular-growth defects because they cannot alter phagosome trafficking to inhibit fusion with lysosomes. Genes of the *L. pneumophila* chromosome that harbor this phenotype, referred to as *dot* (defective organelle trafficking) or *icm* (intracellular multiplication) genes, play an essential role in redirecting phagosome trafficking and establishing an intracellular site for bacterial growth. The Dot/Icm apparatus is hypothesized to be a translocase that exports effector molecules into host cells. *Legionella* does not require this transporter for growth once a replicative niche has been established. Among the *L. pneumophila* maintenance factors is the macrophage infectivity potentiator protein (Mip), which is exported to the bacterial surface and is involved in establishing intracellular infection. *L. pneumophila* Mip mutants have macrophage uptake and replicative phagosome formation kinetics that are similar to those of wild-type bacteria. However, these activities are delayed once the replicative phagosome is established.

Legionnaires' disease is more common and its manifestations are more severe among patients with depressed cell-mediated immunity, including transplant recipients, patients infected with HIV, and patients receiving glucocorticoids. The disease also occurs with unusual frequency among patients with hairy cell leukemia (which is characterized by monocyte deficiency and dysfunction) but not among patients with other types of leukemia.

The role of neutrophils in immunity appears to be minimal: neutropenic patients are not predisposed to Legionnaires' disease. Although *L. pneumophila* is susceptible to oxygen-dependent microbiologic systems in vitro, it resists killing by neutrophils.

The humoral immune system is active against *Legionella*. Type-specific IgM and IgG antibodies are measurable within weeks of infection. In vitro, antibodies promote killing of *Legionella* by phagocytes (neutrophils, monocytes, and alveolar macrophages). Immunized animals develop a specific antibody response, with subsequent resistance to *Legionella* challenge. However, antibodies neither enhance lysis by complement nor inhibit intracellular multiplication within phagocytes.

Some *L. pneumophila* strains are clearly more virulent than others, although the precise factors mediating virulence remain uncertain. For example, although multiple strains may colonize water-distribution systems, only a few cause disease in patients exposed to water from these systems. At least one surface epitope of *L. pneumophila* serogroup 1 is associated with virulence. *L. pneumophila* serogroup 6 is more commonly involved in hospital-acquired Legionnaires' disease and is more likely to be associated with a poor outcome.

PATHOLOGY   The consistent pathologic features of Legionnaires' disease are confined to the lungs. Multifocal pneumonia with patchy lobular inflammation and extensive multilobar consolidation has been observed. Visible abscesses with central necrosis were seen in 20% of autopsied cases in one study. On histologic examination, fibrinopurulent pneumonia with intensive alveolitis and bronchiolitis is evident. Lesions of longer standing can have a nodular appearance with a central area of necrosis surrounded by macrophages and other cells. The alveoli are filled with fibrin, neutrophils, and alveolar macrophages. The direct fluorescent stain is not only specific but also the most sensitive option for visualization of the organism in tissues. Polyvalent DFA stains but not monoclonal DFA stain can be used for formalinized specimens. Culture is the preferred method for diagnosis based on clinical specimens.

CLINICAL AND LABORATORY FEATURES ■ **Pontiac Fever** Pontiac fever is an acute, self-limiting, flulike illness with a 24- to 48-h incubation period. Pneumonia does not develop. Malaise, fatigue, and myalgias are the most frequent symptoms, occurring in 97% of cases. Fever (usually with chills) develops in 80 to 90% of cases and headache in 80%. Other symptoms (seen in fewer than 50% of cases) include arthralgias, nausea, cough, abdominal pain, and diarrhea. Modest leukocytosis with a neutrophilic predominance is sometimes detected. Complete recovery takes place within only a few days without antibiotic therapy; a few patients may experience lassitude for many weeks thereafter. The diagnosis is established by antibody seroconversion.

Legionnaires' Disease (Pneumonia) Legionnaires' disease is often included in the differential diagnosis of "atypical pneumonia," along with infection due to *C. pneumoniae*, *Chlamydia psittaci*, *Mycoplasma pneumoniae*, *Coxiella burnetii*, and some viruses. The clinical similarities among these types of pneumonia include a relatively nonproductive cough and a low incidence of grossly purulent sputum. However, the clinical manifestations of Legionnaires' disease are usually more severe than those of most "atypical" pneumonias, and the course and prognosis of *Legionella* pneumonia more closely resemble those of bacteremic pneumococcal pneumonia than those of pneumonia due to other "atypical" pathogens. Patients with community-acquired Legionnaires' disease are significantly more likely than patients with pneumonia of other etiologies to be admitted to an intensive care unit on presentation.

The incubation period for Legionnaires' disease is 2 to 10 days. The symptoms and signs may range from a mild cough and a slight fever to stupor with widespread pulmonary infiltrates and multisystem failure. Nonspecific symptoms—malaise, fatigue, anorexia, and headache—are seen early in the illness. Myalgias and arthralgias are uncommon but are prominent in a few patients. Upper respiratory symptoms, including coryza, are rare.

The mild cough of Legionnaires' disease is only slightly productive. Sometimes the sputum is streaked with blood. Chest pain—either pleuritic or nonpleuritic—can be a prominent feature and, when coupled with hemoptysis, can lead to an incorrect diagnosis of pulmonary embolism. Shortness of breath is reported by one-third to one-half of patients.

Gastrointestinal difficulties are often pronounced; abdominal pain, nausea, and vomiting affect 10 to 20% of patients. Diarrhea (watery rather than bloody) is reported in 25 to 50% of cases. The most common neurologic abnormalities are confusion or changes in mental status; however, the multitudinous neurologic symptoms reported range from headache and lethargy to encephalopathy.

Patients with Legionnaires' disease virtually always have fever. Temperatures in excess of 40.5°C (104.9°F) were recorded in 20% of the cases in one series. Relative bradycardia has been overemphasized as a useful diagnostic finding; it occurs primarily in older patients with severe pneumonia. Chest examination reveals rales early in the course and evidence of consolidations as the disease progresses. Abdominal examination may reveal generalized or local tenderness.

Although the clinical manifestations often considered classic for Legionnaires' disease (Table 132-1) may suggest the diagnosis, prospective comparative studies have shown that clinical manifestations are generally nonspecific and that Legionnaires' disease is not readily distinguishable from pneumonia of other etiologies. In a review of 13 studies of community-acquired pneumonia, clinical manifestations that occurred significantly more often in Legionnaires' disease included diarrhea, neurologic findings (including confusion), and a temperature of >39°C. Hyponatremia, elevated values in liver function tests, and hematuria also occurred more frequently in Legionnaires' disease. Other laboratory abnormalities include creatine phosphokinase elevation, hypophosphatemia, serum creatinine elevation, and proteinuria.

Extrapulmonary Legionellosis Since the portal of entry for *Legionella* is the lung in virtually all cases, extrapulmonary manifestations usually result from bloodborne dissemination from the lung. In a prospective survey of patients with Legionnaires' disease diagnosed by isolation of the organism from sputum, *Legionella* was isolated from the blood by a special culture method in 38% of cases.

Legionella has been identified in lymph nodes, spleen, liver, or kidneys in autopsied cases of Legionnaires' disease. The most common extrapulmonary site of legionellosis is the heart; numerous reports have described myocarditis, pericarditis, postcardiotomy syndrome, and prosthetic-valve endocarditis. Most cases have been hospital-acquired. In some patients who have not had overt evidence of pneumonia, the organisms may have gained entry through a postoperative sternal wound exposed to contaminated tap water or through a mediastinal-tube insertion site. Sinusitis, peritonitis, pyelonephritis, skin and soft tissue infection, septic arthritis, and pancreatitis have been seen predominantly in immunosuppressed patients.

Chest Radiographic Abnormalities Virtually all patients with Legionnaires' disease have abnormal chest radiographs showing pulmonary infiltrates at the time of clinical presentation. In a few cases of hospital-acquired disease, fever and respiratory tract symptoms have preceded the appearance of the infiltrate on chest radiography. Findings on chest radiography are useful for assessing the severity of illness in that they identify multilobar involvement and permit monitoring of disease progression. However, these findings are nonspecific and do not serve to distinguish Legionnaires' disease from pneumonias of other etiologies. Pleural effusion is evident in 28 to 63% of cases on hospital admission. In immunosuppressed patients, especially those receiving glucocorticoids, distinctive rounded nodular opacities may be seen; these lesions may expand and cavitate (Fig. 132-1). Likewise, pulmonary abscesses can occur in immunosuppressed hosts. The progression of infiltrates and pleural effusion on chest radiography despite appropriate antibiotic therapy within the first week is common, and radiographic improvement lags behind clinical improvement by several days. Complete clearing of infiltrates requires 1 to 4 months.

DIAGNOSIS The diagnosis of Legionnaires' disease requires special microbiologic tests (Table 132-2). The sensitivity of bronchoscopy specimens is approximately the same as that of sputum samples for culture on selective media; if sputum is not available, bronchoscopy specimens may yield the organism. Bronchoalveolar lavage fluid gives higher yields than bronchial wash specimens. Thoracentesis should be performed if pleural effusion is found, and the fluid should be evaluated by DFA staining, culture, and the antigen assay designed for use with urine.

Staining Gram's staining of material from normally sterile sites, such as pleural fluid or lung tissue, occasionally suggests the diagnosis; efforts to detect *Legionella* in sputum by Gram's staining typically reveal numerous leukocytes but no organisms. When they are visualized, the organisms appear as small, pleomorphic, faint, gram-negative bacilli. *L. micdadei* organisms can be detected as weakly or partially acid-fast bacilli in clinical specimens. Modified acid-fast staining substitutes 1% sulfuric acid for the traditional 3% hydrochloric acid; the less aggressive decolorizer increases the yield of *L. micdadei*. *Legionella*-infected patients have occasionally been treated empirically with

---

TABLE 132-1 *Clinical Clues Suggestive of Legionnaires' Disease*

Diarrhea
High fever (>40°C or >104°F))
Numerous neutrophils but no organisms revealed by Gram's staining of respiratory secretions
Hyponatremia (serum sodium level of <131 meq/L)
Failure to respond to β-lactam drugs (penicillins or cephalosporins) and aminoglycoside antibiotics
Occurrence of illness in an environment in which the potable water supply is known to be contaminated with *Legionella*
Onset of symptoms within 10 days after discharge from the hospital

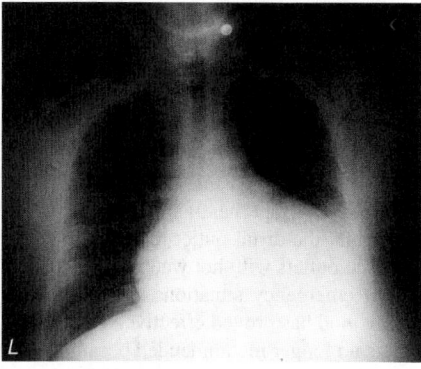
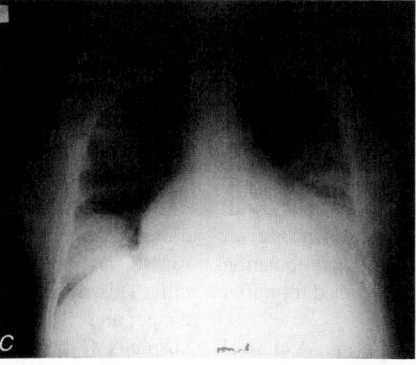
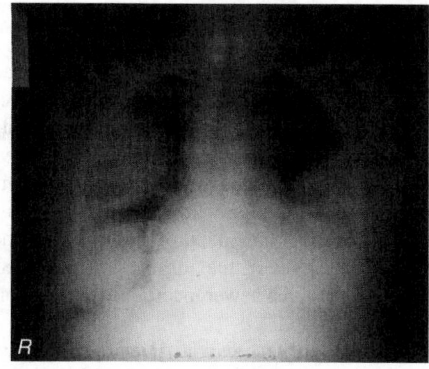

FIGURE 132-1 Chest radiographic findings in a 52-year-old man who presented with pneumonia subsequently diagnosed as Legionnaires' disease. The patient was a cigarette smoker with chronic obstructive pulmonary disease and alcoholic cardiomyopathy; he had received glucocorticoids. *L. pneumophila* was identified by DFA staining and culture of sputum. *Left:* Baseline chest radiograph showing long-standing cardiomegaly. *Center:* Admission chest radiograph showing new rounded opacities. *Right:* Chest radiograph taken 3 days after admission, during treatment with erythromycin.

antituberculosis medications because of false-positive acid-fast smears.

The DFA test is rapid and highly specific but is less sensitive than culture because large numbers of organisms are required for microscopic visualization. This test is more likely to be positive in advanced than in early disease.

Culture The definitive method for diagnosis of *Legionella* infection is isolation of the organism from respiratory secretions or other specimens. Multiple selective BCYE media are required for maximal sensitivity. Colonies grow slowly, requiring 3 to 5 days to become grossly visible. When culture plates are overgrown with other microflora, pretreatment of the specimen with acid or heat can markedly improve the yield. *L. pneumophila* is often isolated from sputum that is not grossly or microscopically purulent; sputum containing more than 25 epithelial cells per high-power field (a finding that classically suggests contamination) may still yield *L. pneumophila*.

Antibody Detection Antibody testing of both acute- and convalescent-phase sera is necessary. A fourfold rise in titer is diagnostic; 12 weeks are often required for the detection of an antibody response. A single titer of 1:128 in a patient with pneumonia constitutes presumptive (but not definitive) evidence for Legionnaires' disease. Serology is of use primarily in epidemiologic studies. The specificity of serology for *Legionella* species other than *L. pneumophila* is uncertain; there is cross-reactivity with *Legionella* spp. and some gram-negative bacilli.

Urinary Antigen The assay for *Legionella* soluble antigen in urine (Binax, Portland, ME) is rapid, relatively inexpensive, easy to perform, second only to culture in terms of sensitivity, and highly specific. Its use in every clinical laboratory is recommended. The test is available only for *L. pneumophila* serogroup 1, which, as has been mentioned, causes about 80% of *Legionella* infections. Cross-reactivity with other *L. pneumophila* serogroups and other *Legionella* species has been detected in up to 22% of urine samples from patients with culture-proven cases. Antigen in urine is detectable 3 days after the onset of clinical disease, and urinary antigen positivity persists for several weeks. The test is not affected by antibiotic administration.

Molecular Methods Polymerase chain reaction (PCR) with DNA probes is theoretically more sensitive and specific than other methods, but the results have been disappointing to date. PCR has proved useful in the identification of *Legionella* from environmental water specimens.

℞ TREATMENT

Since *Legionella* is an intracellular pathogen, antibiotics that can reach intracellular concentrations exceeding the minimal inhibitory concentration are most likely to be efficacious in the clinical setting. The dosages for various drugs used in the treatment of *Legionella* infection are listed in Table 132-3.

The newer macrolides (especially azithromycin) and respiratory tract quinolones (levofloxacin, gemifloxacin, moxifloxacin) are now the antibiotics of choice and are effective as monotherapy. Compared with erythromycin, the newer macrolides have superior in vitro activity, display greater intracellular activity, and reach higher concentrations in respiratory secretions and in lung tissue. The pharmacokinetics of the newer macrolides and quinolones also allow once- or twice-daily dosing. Finally, the large fluid volume required for intravenous administration, symptomatic ototoxicity, and gastrointestinal side effects have rendered erythromycin obsolete for the treatment of *Legionella* infection. Quinolones are the preferred antibiotics for transplant recipients because both macrolides and rifampin interact

TABLE 132-2 *Utility of Special Laboratory Tests for the Diagnosis of Legionnaires' Disease*

Test	Sensitivity, %	Specificity, %
Culture		
Sputum[a]	80	100
Transtracheal aspirate	90	100
DFA staining of sputum	50–70	96–99
Urinary antigen testing[b]	70	100
Antibody serology[c]	40–60	96–99

[a] Use of multiple selective media with dyes.
[b] Serogroup 1 only.
[c] IgG and IgM testing of both acute- and convalescent-phase sera. A single titer of ≥1:256 is considered presumptive, while fourfold seroconversion is considered definitive.

TABLE 132-3 *Antibiotic Therapy for Legionella Infection*

Antimicrobial Agent	Dosage[a]
Macrolides	
Azithromycin	500 mg[b] PO or IV[c] q24h
Clarithromycin	500 mg PO or IV[c] q12h
Quinolones	
Levofloxacin	750 mg IV q24h
	500 mg[b] PO q24h
Ciprofloxacin	400 mg IV q8h
	750 mg PO q12h
Ofloxacin	400 mg PO or IV q12h
Moxifloxacin	400 mg[b] PO q24h
Tetracyclines	
Doxycycline	100 mg[b] PO or IV q12h
Minocycline	100 mg[b] PO or IV q12h
Tetracycline	500 mg PO or IV q6h
Others	
Trimethoprim-sulfamethoxazole	160/800 mg IV q8h
	160/800 mg PO q12h
Rifampin[d]	300–600 mg PO or IV q12h

[a] Dosages are derived from clinical experience.
[b] We recommend doubling the first dose.
[c] Intravenous formulation is not available in some countries.
[d] Rifampin should be used only in combination with a macrolide or a quinolone.

pharmacologically with cyclosporine and tacrolimus. One uncontrolled retrospective study has suggested that complications are fewer and clinical response is more rapid in patients receiving quinolones than in those receiving macrolides. Alternative agents include tetracycline and its analogues doxycycline and minocycline. Anecdotal reports have described both successes and failures with trimethoprim-sulfamethoxazole, imipenem, and clindamycin. For severely ill patients with extensive pulmonary infiltrates, a combination of rifampin with a newer macrolide or quinolone can be used for initial treatment.

Initial therapy should be given by the intravenous route. A clinical response usually occurs within 3 to 5 days, after which oral therapy can be substituted. The total duration of therapy in the immunocompetent host is 10 to 14 days; a longer course (3 weeks) may be appropriate for immunosuppressed patients and those with advanced disease. For azithromycin, with its long half-life, a 5- to 10-day course is sufficient.

Pontiac fever requires only symptom-based treatment, not antimicrobial therapy.

PROGNOSIS Mortality rates for Legionnaires' disease vary, depending on the patient's underlying disease and its severity, the patient's immune status, the severity of pneumonia, and the timing of administration of appropriate antimicrobial therapy. Mortality rates are highest (80%) among immunosuppressed patients who do not receive appropriate antimicrobial therapy early in the course of illness. With appropriate and timely antibiotic treatment, mortality from community-acquired Legionnaires' disease among immunocompetent patients ranges from 0 to 11%; without treatment, the figure may be as high as 31%. In an observational study of survivors of an outbreak of community-acquired Legionnaires' disease, sequelae of fatigue, neurologic symptoms, and weakness were found in 63% to 75% of patients 17 months after receipt of antibiotics.

PREVENTION Routine environmental culture of the hospital water supply is recommended as an approach to the prevention of hospital-acquired Legionnaires' disease. Positive cultures from the water supply mandate the use of specialized laboratory tests (especially culture on selective media and urinary antigen assay) for patients with hospital-acquired pneumonia. Studies have shown that neither a high degree of outward cleanliness nor routine application of maintenance measures decreases the frequency or intensity of *Legionella* colonization. Thus, engineering guidelines and building codes, although routinely advocated as preventive measures, have little impact on *Legionella* colonization.

Disinfection of the water supply is now feasible. Two methods have proven reliable and cost-effective. The superheat-and-flush method requires heating of the water so that the distal-outlet temperature is 70 to 80°C and flushing of the distal outlets with hot water for at least 30 min. This method is ideal for emergency situations. A commercial copper and silver ionization method has proved effective in numerous hospitals. Hyperchlorination is no longer recommended because of its expense, carcinogenicity, corrosive effects on piping, and unreliable efficacy.

FURTHER READING

FIORE AE et al: A survey of methods used to detect nosocomial legionellosis among participants in the NNIS system. Infect Control Hosp Epidemiol 20: 412, 1999

FORMICA N et al: The impact of diagnosis by *Legionella* urinary antigen test on the epidemiology and outcomes of Legionnaires' disease. Epidemiol Infect 127:275, 2001

MARRE R et al: *Legionella*. Washington, DC, ASM Press, 2002

MUDER R, YU VL: Infection due to *Legionella* species other than *L. pneumophila*. Clin Infect Dis 35:990, 2002

MULAZIMOGLU L, YU VL: Can Legionnaires' disease be diagnosed by clinical criteria? A critical review. Chest 120:1049, 2001

PEDRO-BOTET ML et al: Legionnaires' disease contracted from patient homes: The coming of the third plague? Eur J Clin Microbiol Infect Dis 21:699, 2002

SABRIA M, YU VL: Hospital-acquired legionellosis: Solutions for preventable infection. Lancet Infect Dis 2:368, 2002

STOUT JE, YU VL: Experience of the first 16 hospitals using copper-silver ionization for *Legionella* control: Implications for the evaluation of other disinfection modalities. Infect Control Hosp Epidemiol 24:563, 2003

———: Current concepts: Legionellosis. N Engl J Med 337:682, 1997

SWANSON MS, HAMMER BK: *Legionella pneumophila* pathogenesis: A fateful journey from amoebae to macrophages. Annu Rev Microbiol 54:567, 2000

TAN MJ et al: The radiologic manifestations of Legionnaire's disease. Chest 116:398, 2000

YU VL: Resolving the controversy on environmental cultures for *Legionella*. Infect Control Hosp Epidemiol 19:893, 1998

133 PERTUSSIS AND OTHER *BORDETELLA* INFECTIONS
Scott A. Halperin

Pertussis is an acute infection of the respiratory tract caused by *Bordetella pertussis*. The name *pertussis* means "violent cough," which aptly describes the most consistent and prominent feature of the illness. The inspiratory sound made at the end of an episode of paroxysmal coughing gives rise to the common name for the illness, "whooping cough"; however, this feature is variable, being uncommon in infants ≤6 months of age and frequently absent in older children and adults. The Chinese name for pertussis is "the 100-day cough," which accurately describes the clinical course of the illness. The identification of *B. pertussis* was first reported by Bordet and Gengou in 1906, and vaccines were produced over the following two decades.

MICROBIOLOGY Six species have been identified in the genus *Bordetella*: *B. pertussis*, *B. parapertussis*, *B. bronchiseptica*, *B. avium*, *B. holmesii*, and *B. hinzii*. *B. pertussis* infects only humans and is the most important *Bordetella* species causing human disease. *B. parapertussis* causes an illness in humans that is similar to pertussis but is typically milder; coinfections with *B. parapertussis* and *B. pertussis* have been documented. *B. bronchiseptica* is an important pathogen of domestic animals that causes kennel cough in dogs, atrophic rhinitis and pneumonia in pigs, and pneumonia in cats. Both respiratory infection and opportunistic infection are occasionally reported in humans. *B. avium* is an important cause of respiratory illness in turkeys. The remaining two species, *B. hinzii* and *B. holmesii*, have been recognized as unusual causes of bacteremia. Both of these species have been isolated from patients with sepsis, most often from those who are immunocompromised.

Bordetella species are gram-negative pleomorphic aerobic bacilli that share common genotypic characteristics. *B. pertussis* and *B. parapertussis* are the most similar of the species but differ in that *B. parapertussis* does not express the gene coding for pertussis toxin. *B. pertussis* is a slow-growing fastidious organism that requires selective medium and forms small glistening bifurcated colonies. Suspicious colonies are presumptively identified as *B. pertussis* by direct fluorescent antibody testing or by agglutination with species-specific antiserum. *B. pertussis* is further differentiated from other *Bordetella* species by biochemical and motility characteristics.

B. pertussis produces a wide array of toxins and biologically active products that are important in its pathogenesis and in immunity. Most of these virulence factors are under the control of a single genetic locus that regulates their production, resulting in antigenic modulation and phase variation. Although these processes occur both in vitro and in vivo, their importance in the pathobiology of the organism is unknown; they may play a role in intracellular persistence and person-to-person spread. The organism's most important virulence factor is *pertussis toxin*, which is composed of a B oligomer–binding subunit and an enzymatically active A protomer that ADP-ribosylates a guanine nucleotide-binding regulatory protein (G protein) in target cells, producing a variety of biologic effects. Pertussis toxin has important mitogenic activity, affects the circulation of lymphocytes, and serves as an adhesin for bacterial binding to respiratory ciliated cells. In animal models, the toxin's effects include histamine sensitization, lymphocytosis promotion, and insulin secretion. Another virulence factor is *filamentous hemagglutinin*, a component of the cell wall and a bacterial adhesin. *Pertactin* is an outer-membrane protein and another important adhesin. *Fimbriae* are bacterial appendages that also play a role in bacterial attachment; they are the major antigens against which agglutinating antibodies are directed. These agglutinating antibodies have historically been the primary means of serotyping *B. pertussis* strains. Other virulence factors include tracheal cytotoxin, which causes respiratory epithelial damage; adenylate cyclase toxin, which impairs host immune-cell function; dermonecrotic toxin, which may contribute to respiratory mucosal damage; and lipooligosaccharide, which has properties similar to those of other gram-negative bacterial endotoxins.

PATHOGENESIS Infection with *B. pertussis* is initiated by attachment of the organism to the ciliated epithelial cells of the nasopharynx. Attachment is mediated by surface adhesins (e.g., pertactin and filamentous hemagglutinin), which bind to the integrin family of cell-surface proteins, probably in conjunction with pertussis toxin. The role of fimbriae in adhesion or maintenance of infection has not been fully delineated. At the site of attachment, the organism multiplies, producing a variety of other toxins that cause local mucosal damage (tracheal cytotoxin, dermatonecrotic toxin). Impairment of host defense by *B. pertussis* is mediated by pertussis toxin and adenylate cyclase toxin. There is local cellular invasion, with intracellular bacterial persistence; however, systemic dissemination does not occur. Systemic manifestations (lymphocytosis) result from the effects of the toxins.

The pathogenesis of the clinical manifestations of pertussis is poorly understood. It is not known what causes the paroxysmal cough that is the hallmark of pertussis. A pivotal role for pertussis toxin has been proposed. Proponents of this position point to the efficacy of preventing clinical symptoms with a vaccine containing only pertussis toxoid. Detractors counter that pertussis toxin is not the critical factor because paroxysmal cough also occurs in patients infected with *B. parapertussis*, which does not produce pertussis toxin. It is thought that the neurologic events observed in pertussis, such as seizures and encephalopathy, are due to hypoxia from coughing paroxysms or apnea rather than to the effects of specific bacterial products. *B. pertussis* pneumonia, which occurs in up to 10% of infants with pertussis, is usually a diffuse bilateral primary infection. In older children and adults with pertussis, pneumonia is often due to secondary bacterial infection with streptococci or staphylococci.

IMMUNITY Both humoral and cell-mediated immunity are thought to be important in pertussis. Antibodies to pertussis toxin, filamentous hemagglutinin, pertactin, and fimbriae are all protective in animal models. Pertussis agglutinins were correlated with protection in early studies of whole-cell pertussis vaccines. Serologic correlates of protection conferred by acellular pertussis vaccines have not been established, although antibody to pertactin, fimbriae, and (to a lesser degree) pertussis toxin correlated best with protection in two acellular pertussis vaccine efficacy trials. The duration of immunity after whole-cell pertussis vaccination is short-lived, with little protection remaining after 10 to 12 years. Data on the duration of protection after acellular pertussis vaccination are still being collected. Although immunity after natural infection has been said to be lifelong, seroepidemiologic evidence suggests that it may not be and that subsequent episodes of clinical pertussis are prevented by intermittent subclinical infection.

EPIDEMIOLOGY Pertussis is a highly communicable disease, with attack rates of 80 to 100% among unimmunized household contacts and 20% within households in well-immunized populations. The infection has a worldwide distribution, with cyclical outbreaks every 3 to 5 years (a pattern that has persisted despite widespread immunization). Pertussis occurs in all months; however, in North America, pertussis activity peaks in the summer and autumn.

Before the institution of widespread immunization programs, pertussis was one of the most common infectious causes of morbidity and death. In the United States prior to the 1940s, between 115,000 and 270,000 cases of pertussis were reported annually, with an average yearly rate of 150 cases per 100,000 population. With universal childhood immunization, the number of reported cases fell by >95%, with even more dramatic decreases in mortality. Only 1010 cases of pertussis were reported in 1976. Since that time, however, rates have slowly increased. In 2000, more than 7800 cases of pertussis were reported in the United States.

Although thought of as a disease of childhood, pertussis can affect people of all ages and is increasingly being identified as a cause of prolonged coughing illness in adolescents and adults. In unimmunized populations, pertussis incidence peaks in the preschool years, and well over half of children have the disease before reaching adulthood. In highly immunized populations such as those in North America, the peak incidence is among infants <1 year of age who have not completed the three-dose primary immunization series. Recent trends, however, show an increasing incidence of pertussis among adolescents and adults. In the United States in 2000, 24% of patients were <7 months of age, 36% were adolescents, and 20% were adults. The figures for adolescents and adults are probably underestimates because of a greater degree of underrecognition and underreporting in these age groups. A number of studies of prolonged coughing illness suggest that pertussis may be the etiologic agent in 12 to 30% of adults with cough that does not improve within 2 weeks. In a recent study of the efficacy of an acellular pertussis vaccine in adolescents and adults, the incidence of pertussis in the placebo group was 3.7 to 4.5 cases per 1000 person-years. Although this prospective cohort study yielded a lower estimate than the studies of cough illness, its results still translate to between 600,000 and 800,000 cases of pertussis in adults annually in the United States. Severe morbidity and mortality, however, are virtually restricted to infants. In Canada, there were 10 deaths from pertussis between 1991 and 1998; all those who died were infants ≤6 months of age. Although school-age children are the source of infection for most households, adults are the likely source for high-risk infants and may serve as the reservoir of infection between epidemic years. In developing countries, pertussis remains an important cause of infant morbidity and mortality. The World Health Organization estimated that in 1995 over 40 million people worldwide were infected by *B. pertussis* and that 355,000 children died of pertussis.

CLINICAL MANIFESTATIONS Pertussis is a prolonged coughing illness with clinical manifestations that vary by age (Table 133-1). Classic pertussis is most often seen in preschool and school-age children, although it is not uncommon among adolescents and adults. After an incubation

TABLE 133-1 *Clinical Features of Pertussis, by Age Group and Diagnostic Status*

	Percentage of Patients		
	Adolescents and Adults		
Feature	Laboratory Confirmation	No Laboratory Confirmation	Children
Cough	95–100	95–100	95–100
Prolonged	60–80	60–80	60–95
Paroxysmal	60–90	50–90	80–95
Sleep-disturbing	50–80	50–80	90–100
Whoop	10–40	5–30	40–80
Posttussive vomiting	20–50	5–30	80–90

period averaging 7 to 10 days, an illness develops that is indistinguishable from the common cold and is characterized by coryza, lacrimation, mild cough, low-grade fever, and malaise. After 1 to 2 weeks, this *catarrhal phase* evolves into the *paroxysmal phase*: the cough becomes more frequent and spasmodic with repetitive bursts of 5 to 10 coughs, often within a single expiration. Posttussive vomiting is frequent, with a mucous plug occasionally expelled at the end of an episode. The episode may be terminated by an audible whoop, which occurs upon rapid inspiration against a closed glottis at the end of a paroxysm. During a spasm, there may be impressive neck-vein distension, bulging eyes, tongue protrusion, and cyanosis. Paroxysms may be precipitated by noise, eating, or physical contact. Between attacks, the patient's appearance is normal but increasing fatigue is evident. The frequency of paroxysmal episodes varies widely, from several per hour to 5 to 10 per day. Episodes are often worse at night and interfere with sleep. Weight loss is not uncommon as a result of the illness's interference with eating. Most complications occur during the paroxysmal stage. Fever is uncommon and suggests bacterial superinfection.

After 2 to 4 weeks, the coughing episodes become less frequent and less severe—changes heralding the onset of the *convalescent phase*. This phase can last from 1 to 3 months and is characterized by a gradual resolution of the coughing episodes. For 6 months to a year, intercurrent viral infections may be associated with a recrudescence of paroxysmal cough.

Not all individuals who develop pertussis have classic disease. The clinical manifestations in adolescents and adults are more often atypical. In a German study of pertussis in adults, more than two-thirds had paroxysmal cough and more than one-third had whoop. Adult illness in North America differs from this experience: the cough may be severe and prolonged but is less frequently paroxysmal, and a whoop is uncommon. Vomiting with cough is the best predictor of a diagnosis of pertussis as the cause of a prolonged cough in adults. Other features predictive of this diagnosis are a cough at night and exposure to other individuals with a prolonged coughing illness.

COMPLICATIONS Complications are frequently associated with pertussis and are more common among infants than among older children or adults. Subconjunctival hemorrhages, abdominal and inguinal hernias, pneumothoraces, and facial and truncal petechiae can result from increased intrathoracic pressure generated by severe fits of coughing. Weight loss can follow decreased caloric intake. In a series of more than 1100 children <2 years of age who were hospitalized with pertussis, 27.1% had apnea, 9.4% had pneumonia, 2.6% had seizures, and 0.4% had encephalopathy; 10 children (0.9%) died. Pneumonia is reported in <5% of adolescents and adults and increases in frequency after 50 years of age. In contrast to the primary *B. pertussis* pneumonia that develops in infants, pneumonia in adolescents and adults with pertussis is usually caused by a secondary infection with encapsulated organisms such as *Streptococcus pneumoniae* or *Haemophilus influenzae*. Pneumothorax, severe weight loss, inguinal hernia, rib fracture, carotid artery aneurysm, and cough syncope have all been reported in adolescents and adults with pertussis.

DIAGNOSIS If the classic symptoms of pertussis are present, clinical diagnosis is not difficult. However, particularly in older children and adults, it is difficult to differentiate infections caused by *B. pertussis* and *B. parapertussis* from other respiratory tract infections on clinical grounds. Therefore, laboratory confirmation should be attempted in all cases. Lymphocytosis (absolute lymphocyte count, $>10 \times 10^9$/L) is common among young children (in whom it is unusual with other infections) but not among adolescents and adults. Culture of nasopharyngeal secretions remains the "gold standard" of diagnosis; the best specimen is collected by nasopharyngeal aspiration, in which a fine flexible plastic catheter attached to a 10-mL syringe is passed into the nasopharynx and withdrawn while gentle suction is applied. Since *B. pertussis* is highly sensitive to drying, secretions should be inoculated without delay onto appropriate media (Bordet-Gengou or Regan-

Lowe) or the catheter should be flushed with a phosphate-buffered saline solution. An alternative is a nasopharyngeal culture with a calcium alginate swab; again, inoculation of culture plates should be immediate or an appropriate transport medium (such as Regan-Lowe charcoal medium) should be used. Cultures become positive by day 5 of incubation, and *B. pertussis* and *B. parapertussis* can be differentiated by agglutination with specific antisera or by direct immunofluorescence.

Nasopharyngeal cultures in untreated pertussis remain positive for a mean of 3 weeks after the onset of illness; these cultures become negative within 5 days of the institution of appropriate antimicrobial therapy. Since much of the period during which the organism can be recovered from the nasopharynx falls into the catarrhal phase, when the etiology of the infection is not suspected, there is only a small window of opportunity for culture-proven diagnosis. Cultures from infants and young children are more frequently positive than those from older children and adults; this difference may reflect earlier presentation of the former age group for medical care. The increasing availability of the polymerase chain reaction for pertussis in diagnostic laboratories is enhancing the sensitivity of the organism's detection. This method may further laboratory confirmation but does not solve problems related to the long delays in specimen procurement that often are encountered in pertussis cases. Direct fluorescent antibody tests of nasopharyngeal secretions for direct diagnosis may still be available in some laboratories but should not be used because of poor sensitivity and specificity.

As a result of the difficulties with laboratory diagnosis of pertussis in adolescents, adults, and any patient who has been symptomatic for >4 weeks, increasing attention is being given to serologic diagnosis. Enzyme immunoassays detecting IgA and IgG antibodies to pertussis toxin, filamentous hemagglutinin, pertactin, and fimbriae have been developed and assessed for reproducibility. Two- or fourfold increases in antibody titer are suggestive of pertussis, although cross-reactivity of some antigens (such as filamentous hemagglutinin and pertactin) among *Bordetella* species makes it difficult to depend diagnostically on seroconversion involving a single type of antibody. Late presentation for medical care and prior immunization also complicate serologic diagnosis because the first sample obtained may in fact be a convalescent-phase specimen. Proposed criteria for serologic diagnosis based on a single serum specimen call for comparison of the patient's antibody levels with established population values; for example, a patient with serologically confirmed pertussis might be required to have a titer greater than two or three standard deviations above the mean titer for a normal population. However, at present, no antibody test is widely or commercially available, and no specific serologic criteria are universally accepted.

DIFFERENTIAL DIAGNOSIS A child presenting with paroxysmal cough, posttussive vomiting, and whoop is likely to have an infection caused by *B. pertussis* or *B. parapertussis*; lymphocytosis increases the likelihood of a *B. pertussis* etiology. Viruses such as respiratory syncytial virus and adenovirus have been isolated from patients with clinical pertussis but probably represent coinfection. In adolescents and adults, among whom paroxysmal cough and whoop are frequently absent, the differential diagnosis of a prolonged coughing illness is more extensive. Pertussis should be suspected in anyone with a cough that does not improve within 14 days, a paroxysmal cough of any duration, or any respiratory symptoms after contact with a laboratory-confirmed case of pertussis. Other etiologies to consider include infections caused by *Mycoplasma pneumoniae*, *Chlamydia pneumoniae*, adenovirus, influenza virus, and other respiratory viruses. Use of angiotensin-converting enzyme (ACE) inhibitors, reactive airway disease, and gastroesophageal reflux disease are well-described noninfectious causes of prolonged cough in adults.

℞ TREATMENT

Antibiotics The purpose of antibiotic therapy for pertussis is to eradicate the infecting bacteria from the nasopharynx; therapy does not substantially alter the clinical course unless given early in the catarrhal phase. Macrolide antibiotics are the drugs of choice for treatment of pertussis (Table 133-2); a macrolide-resistant *B. pertussis* strain has been reported from a single case in an outbreak in Arizona. Trimethoprim-sulfamethoxazole is recommended as an alternative for individuals allergic to macrolides.

Supportive Care Young infants have the highest rates of complication and death from pertussis; therefore, most infants and older children with severe disease should be hospitalized. A quiet environment may decrease the stimulation that can trigger paroxysmal episodes. Use of β-adrenergic agonists and/or glucocorticoids has been advocated by some authorities but has not been proved to be effective. Cough suppressants are not effective and play no role in the management of pertussis.

Infection Control Measures Hospitalized patients with pertussis should be placed in respiratory isolation, with the use of precautions appropriate for pathogens spread by large respiratory droplets. Isolation should continue for 5 days after initiation of erythromycin therapy or for 3 weeks (i.e., until nasopharyngeal cultures are consistently negative) in those individuals unable to tolerate antimicrobial therapy.

PREVENTION ■ Chemoprophylaxis Because the risk of transmission of *B. pertussis* within households is high, chemoprophylaxis is widely recommended for household contacts of pertussis cases. The effectiveness of chemoprophylaxis, although unproven, is supported by several epidemiologic studies of institutional and community outbreaks of pertussis. In the only randomized placebo-controlled study, erythromycin estolate (50 mg/kg per day in three divided doses; maximum dose, 1 g/d) was effective in reducing the incidence of bacteriologically confirmed pertussis by 67%; however, there was no decrease in the incidence of clinical disease. Despite these disappointing results, many authorities continue to recommend chemoprophylaxis, particularly in households with members at high risk of severe disease (children <1 year of age). Data are not yet available on use of the newer macrolides for chemoprophylaxis.

Immunization (See also Chap. 107) The mainstay of pertussis prevention is active immunization. Pertussis vaccine has been available for over 70 years and became widely used in North America after 1940; reported cases of pertussis have since fallen by >90%. Whole-cell pertussis vaccines are prepared through the heating, chemical inactivation, and purification of whole *B. pertussis* organisms. Although effective (average efficacy estimate, 85%, with results in various studies of different products ranging from 30 to 100%), whole-cell pertussis vaccines are associated with adverse events—both common (fever; injection-site pain, erythema, and swelling; irritability) and uncommon (febrile seizures, hypotonic hyporesponsive episodes). Alleged associations of whole-cell pertussis vaccine with encephalopathy, sudden infant death syndrome, and autism, although not substantiated, have spawned an active anti-immunization lobby. The development of acellular pertussis vaccines, which are effective but less reactogenic, has greatly alleviated concerns about the inclusion of pertussis vaccine in the combined infant immunization series. Although whole-cell vaccines are still extensively used worldwide, acellular pertussis vaccines are used exclusively for childhood immunization in the United States and elsewhere (Canada, Sweden, Germany, Japan). In North America, acellular pertussis vaccines are given as a three-dose primary series at 2, 4, and 6 months of age, with a reinforcing dose between 15 and 18 months of age and a booster dose at 4 to 6 years of age.

A wide variety of acellular pertussis vaccines have been developed, although not all are available in every country. All acellular pertussis vaccines currently available contain pertussis toxoid. Only one monovalent pertussis toxoid vaccine has been licensed in the United States; the remainder of the fully developed vaccines contain filamentous hemagglutinin as well as toxoid. At least four acellular pertussis vaccines also contain pertactin, and two products also contain one or more types of fimbriae. All of the licensed acellular pertussis vaccines have undergone phase 3 efficacy testing. Although differences in study design make direct comparisons difficult, an effort to standardize case definitions and the similarity of some of the studies, which used common vaccine arms to allow "bridging" of the data between studies, have permitted some general conclusions. Even though some would still disagree, most experts have concluded that two-component acellular pertussis vaccines are more effective than monocomponent vaccines and that the addition of pertactin further increases efficacy. The further addition of fimbriae appears to provide some additional protective efficacy against milder disease. In two studies, protection against pertussis by vaccines correlated best with the production of antibody to pertactin, fimbriae, and pertussis toxin.

The development of acellular pertussis vaccines has sparked interest in the potential for control of pertussis in adolescents and adults and in the possibility that pertussis control in those groups will enhance the protection of infants too young to be immunized. Whole-cell pertussis vaccine is contraindicated in individuals ≥7 years of age because of their poor toleration of possible adverse events. However, adult formulations of acellular pertussis vaccines, both alone and in combination with adult-formulation diphtheria-tetanus toxoid, have been demonstrated to be safe, immunogenic, and efficacious in clinical trials in adolescents and adults and are now recommended for routine immunization of adolescents in several countries. Further epidemiologic studies will help public health authorities and advisory committees determine the role of pertussis immunization in the control of pertussis in adults.

FURTHER READING

DE SERRES G et al: Morbidity of pertussis in adolescents and adults. J Infect Dis 182:174, 2000

HALPERIN SA et al: A randomized, placebo-controlled trial of erythromycin estolate chemoprophylaxis for household contacts of children with culture-positive *Bordetella pertussis* infection. Pediatrics 104:e42, 1999

——— et al: Epidemiological features of pertussis in hospitalized patients in Canada, 1991–1997: Report of the Immunization Monitoring Program—Active (IMPACT). Clin Infect Dis 28:1238, 1999

SENZILET LD et al: Pertussis is a frequent cause of prolonged cough illness in adults and adolescents. Clin Infect Dis 32:1691, 2001

SKOWRONSKI DM et al: The changing age and seasonal profile of pertussis in Canada. J Infect Dis 185:1448, 2002

WIRSING VON KÖNIG CH et al: Pertussis in adults: Frequency of transmission after household exposure. Lancet 346:1326, 1995

YIH WK et al: The increasing incidence of pertussis in Massachusetts adolescents and adults, 1989–1998. J Infect Dis 182:1409, 2000

TABLE 133-2 Antimicrobial Therapy for Pertussis

Drug	Adult Daily Dose	Frequency	Duration (Days)	Comments
Erythromycin estolate	1–2 g	3 divided doses	7–14	Frequent gastrointestinal side effects
Clarithromycin	500 mg	2 divided doses	7	
Azithromycin	500 mg on day 1, 250 mg subsequently	1 daily dose	5	
Trimethoprim-sulfamethoxazole	160 mg of trimethoprim, 800 mg of sulfamethoxazole	2 divided doses	14	For patients allergic to macrolides; data on effectiveness limited

Extraintestinal infections are the predominant presentation of disease caused by gram-negative bacilli (GNB) belonging to medically important genera of the family Enterobacteriaceae (*Escherichia, Klebsiella, Proteus, Enterobacter, Serratia, Citrobacter, Morganella, Providencia,* and *Edwardsiella*) and by the genus *Acinetobacter* from the family Neisseriaceae. However, certain strains of *Escherichia coli* have evolved to be strictly intestinal pathogens, causing gastroenteritis by a variety of unique pathogenic mechanisms. The virulence traits of intestinal pathogenic *E. coli* are for the most part distinct from those of extraintestinal pathogenic *E. coli* and other GNB that cause disease outside the bowel. This difference reflects site-dependent differences in host environments and defense mechanisms.

E. COLI AS AN INTESTINAL PATHOGEN

Certain strains of *E. coli* are capable of causing intestinal infection. Other important intestinal pathogens are discussed in Chaps. 113, 126, and 137–140.

ETIOLOGY, EPIDEMIOLOGY, AND MANIFESTATIONS Intestinal pathogenic strains of *E. coli* are rarely encountered in the fecal flora of healthy hosts and instead appear to be essentially obligate pathogens. These strains have evolved a special ability to cause enteritis, enterocolitis, and colitis whenever ingested in sufficient quantities by a naive host. At least six distinct "pathotypes" of intestinal pathogenic *E. coli* exist: (1) Shiga toxin–producing *E. coli* (STEC)/enterohemorrhagic *E. coli* (EHEC), (2) enterotoxigenic *E. coli* (ETEC), (3) enteropathogenic *E. coli* (EPEC), (4) enteroinvasive *E. coli* (EIEC), (5) enteroaggregative *E. coli* (EAEC), and (6) diffusely adherent *E. coli* (DAEC). Organisms of these pathotypes are acquired via the fecal-oral route. Transmission occurs predominantly via contaminated food and water for ETEC, STEC, EIEC, EAEC, and DAEC and by person-to-person spread for EPEC (and occasionally STEC). Humans appear to be the major reservoir (except for STEC), since the host range appears to be dictated by species-specific attachment factors. Although there is some overlap, each pathotype possesses a unique combination of virulence traits that results in a distinctive intestinal pathogenic mechanism (Table 134-1); however, these strains are largely incapable of causing disease outside the intestinal tract. Except in the case of STEC, disease due to this group of pathogens occurs primarily in developing countries.

Shiga Toxin–Producing E. coli STEC strains constitute an emerging group of pathogens that can cause hemorrhagic colitis and the hemolytic-uremic syndrome (HUS). Several large outbreaks resulting from the consumption of undercooked ground beef and other foods have received significant attention from the media. O157:H7 is the most prominent serotype, but O6, O26, O55, O91, O103, O111, O113, and OX3 have also been associated with these syndromes. The ability to produce Shiga toxins (Stx2 and/or Stx1) or related toxins is the critical factor dictating whether a bacterium can cause the STEC syndrome. *Shigella dysenteriae* strains that produce the closely related Shiga toxin Stx can cause the same syndrome. Stx2 appears to be more important than Stx1 in the development of HUS and other severe disease. All Shiga toxins studied to date consist of an enzymatically active A subunit and five identical B subunits that mediate binding to globoceramides. The A subunit cleaves an adenine from the 28S rRNA, which irreversibly inhibits ribosomal function. Therefore, Shiga toxins belong to the class of toxins known as *ribosome-inactivating proteins* (RIPs).

Additional factors, such as acid tolerance and adherence, are necessary for maximal pathogenicity of STEC. The genomes of the majority of isolates responsible for disease possess the locus for enterocyte effacement (LEE). This pathogenicity island was first described in EPEC strains and contains genes that mediate adherence to intestinal epithelial cells. It has been proposed that the subgroup of STEC strains that possess stx_1 and/or stx_2 as well as LEE be termed *enterohemorrhagic E. coli* (EHEC).

Domesticated ruminant animals, particularly cattle and young calves, serve as the major reservoir for STEC. Ground beef—the most common food source of STEC strains—is often contaminated during processing. Furthermore, manure from cattle or other animals that is used as fertilizer can contaminate produce (potatoes, lettuce, sprouts, fallen apples) and water (fecal runoff). It is estimated that $<10^3$ CFU (colony-forming units) of STEC can cause disease. Therefore, not only can low levels of food or environmental contamination (e.g., in water swallowed while swimming) result in disease, but person-to-person transmission (e.g., at day-care centers and in institutions) becomes an important vehicle for secondary spread. Laboratory-associated infections also take place. Both outbreaks and sporadic cases are attributable to this group of pathogens, with a seasonal peak in the summer months.

In contrast to the other pathotypes, STEC causes infections more frequently in developed countries, where the consumption of processed foods is more common than in developing regions. O157 strains are the fourth most commonly reported cause of bacterial diarrhea in the United States (after *Campylobacter, Salmonella,* and *Shigella*). Colonization of the colon and perhaps the ileum results in symptoms after an incubation period of 3 or 4 days. Colonic edema and an initial secretory diarrhea may develop into the STEC syndrome's hallmark trait of grossly bloody diarrhea (detected by history or examination) in >90% of cases. Significant abdominal pain and fecal leukocytes are commonly present (70% of cases), but fever is usually absent. Occasionally, *Clostridium difficile, Campylobacter,* and *Salmonella* infection present in a similar fashion, as do noninfectious diseases (e.g., inflammatory bowel disease). STEC disease is usually self-limited, lasting 5 to 10 days. This infection can be complicated by HUS, which occurs 2 to 14 days after diarrhea in 2 to 8% of cases, most often affecting the very young and the elderly. It is estimated that >50% of all cases of HUS in the United States are caused by STEC. This complication is probably mediated by the systemic translocation of Shiga toxins. Erythrocytes may serve as carriers of Stx to small-vessel renal and cerebral endothelial cells. The subsequent development of thrombotic microangiopathy (perhaps with direct toxin-mediated effects on various cells) most commonly results in some combination of fever, thrombocytopenia, renal failure, and encephalopathy. Although the mortality rate with dialysis support is <10%, residual renal dysfunction and neurologic sequelae may persist.

Enterotoxigenic E. coli In tropical or developing countries, ETEC is a major cause of endemic diarrhea. After weaning, children experience several episodes of ETEC infection during the first 3 years of life. The incidence of disease diminishes with age, a pattern that correlates with the development of mucosal immunity to colonization factors. In industrialized countries, infection usually follows travel to endemic areas. ETEC is the most common agent of traveler's diarrhea, causing 25 to 75% of cases. The incidence of infection is decreased by the prudent avoidance of potentially contaminated fluids and foods (Chap. 108). ETEC infection is uncommon in the United States, but outbreaks secondary to consumption of food products imported from endemic areas have occurred. A large inoculum (10^6 to 10^{10} CFU) is needed to produce disease. After ingestion of contaminated water or food (particularly items poorly cooked, unpeeled, or unrefrigerated), colonization factor–mediated intestinal adherence occurs over 12 to 72 h.

Disease is mediated primarily by heat-labile toxin (LT-1) and/or a heat-stable toxin (STa) that causes net fluid secretion via activation of adenylate cyclase (LT-1) and/or guanylate cyclase (STa) in the jejunum and ileum; the result is watery diarrhea accompanied by cramps. LT-1 consists of an A and a B subunit and is structurally and functionally similar to cholera toxin. Strong binding of the B subunit to the GM_1 ganglioside leads to the intracellular translocation of the A subunit, which functions as an ADP-ribosyltransferase. The mature STa toxin is an 18- or 19-amino-acid secreted peptide whose biologic activity is mediated by binding to the guanylate cyclase C found in the brush-border membrane of intestinal epithelial cells; this binding results in increased intracellular concentrations of cyclic GMP. Characteristically absent are histopathologic changes of the small bowel; mucus, blood, and inflammatory cells in stool; and fever. The disease spectrum ranges from a mild illness to a life-threatening cholera-like illness. Although symptoms are usually self-limited (typically lasting for 3 days), infection may result in significant morbidity and mortality when health care is poor and when small and/or undernourished children are affected.

Enteropathogenic *E. coli*

EPEC causes disease primarily in young children, including neonates. The first *E. coli* pathotype recognized as an agent of diarrheal disease, EPEC was responsible for outbreaks of infantile diarrhea (including some outbreaks in hospital nurseries) in industrialized countries in the 1940s and 1950s. At present, however, infection due to EPEC is uncommon in developed countries. In contrast, EPEC is an important cause of infant diarrhea (both sporadic and epidemic) in developing countries. Breast-feeding diminishes the incidence of EPEC infection. Rapid person-to-person spread may occur. Upon colonization of the small bowel, symptoms develop after a brief incubation period (1 or 2 days). Initial localized adherence leads to a characteristic effacement of microvilli, with the formation of cuplike, actin-rich pedestals. Diarrheal stool often contains mucus but not blood. Although usually self-limited (lasting for 5 to 15 days), EPEC diarrhea may persist for weeks.

Enteroinvasive *E. coli*

EIEC, a relatively uncommon cause of diarrhea, is rarely identified in the United States, although a few food-related outbreaks have been described. In developing countries, sporadic disease is infrequently recognized in children and travelers. EIEC shares many genetic and clinical features with *Shigella*; however, unlike *Shigella*, EIEC produces disease only at a large inoculum (10^8 to 10^{10} CFU), with onset generally occurring after an incubation period of 1 to 3 days. Initially, enterotoxins are believed to induce secretory small-bowel diarrhea. Subsequently, colonization and invasion of the colonic mucosa, followed by replication therein and cell-to-cell spread, result in the development of inflammatory colitis characterized by fever, abdominal pain, tenesmus, and scant stool containing mucus, blood, and inflammatory cells. Symptoms are usually self-limited (7 to 10 days).

Enteroaggregative and Diffusely Adherent *E. coli*

EAEC and DAEC have been described primarily in developing countries and in young children. These strains can cause traveler's diarrhea. A large inoculum is required for infection. In vitro, the organisms exhibit a diffuse or "stacked-brick" adherence pattern. Clinical disease has been associated with prolonged watery diarrhea.

DIAGNOSIS A practical approach to the evaluation of diarrhea is to distinguish noninflammatory from inflammatory cases (Chap. 113). ETEC, EPEC, EAEC, and DAEC are uncommon causes of noninflammatory diarrhea in the United States. Their diagnosis requires specialized assays that are not routinely available and whose use is rarely indicated since these diseases are self-limited. ETEC causes the majority of cases of noninflammatory traveler's diarrhea; EAEC and DAEC cause a minority of these cases. Definitive diagnosis generally is not necessary, and empirical antimicrobial treatment is a reasonable approach. If diarrhea persists despite treatment, *Giardia* or *Cryptosporidium* should be sought. The diagnosis of infection with EIEC, a rare

cause of inflammatory diarrhea in the United States, also requires specialized assays. However, evaluation for STEC infection, particularly when bloody diarrhea is reported or observed, is appropriate. Although screening for *E. coli* strains that do not ferment sorbitol and subsequent serotyping for O157 constitute the most common method presently used to detect STEC, testing for Shiga toxins or toxin genes is more sensitive, specific, and rapid. The latter approach offers another advantage as well: it detects both non-O157 strains and sorbitol-fermenting strains of O157, which otherwise are difficult to identify. DNA-based, enzyme-linked immunosorbent, and cytotoxicity assays are in various stages of development and are likely to emerge as the diagnostic standards in time.

TREATMENT

The mainstay of treatment for all diarrheal syndromes is the appropriate replacement of water and electrolytes (Chap. 113). The use of prophylactic antibiotics to prevent traveler's diarrhea should be discouraged, especially in light of high rates of antibiotic resistance. When stools are free of mucus and blood, early patient-initiated treatment of traveler's diarrhea with a quinolone decreases the duration of illness, and the use of loperamide may halt symptoms within a few hours (Chap. 113). Although dysentery caused by EIEC is self-limited, treatment hastens the resolution of symptoms, particularly in severe cases. Treatment of STEC infection should be avoided since antibiotics may increase the incidence of HUS (possible via increased release of Stx).

EXTRAINTESTINAL PATHOGENS

GENERAL FEATURES AND PRINCIPLES ■ Epidemiology Extraintestinal pathogenic *E. coli*, *Klebsiella*, *Proteus*, *Enterobacter*, *Serratia*, *Citrobacter*, *Morganella*, *Providencia*, *Edwardsiella*, and *Acinetobacter* are components of the normal animal and human colonic flora and/or of the flora of a variety of environmental habitats (including long-term-care facilities and hospitals). In healthy humans, *E. coli* is the predominant gram-negative bacillus in the colonic flora. GNB (primarily *E. coli*, *Klebsiella*, and *Proteus*) only transiently colonize the oropharynx and skin of healthy individuals. In contrast, in long-term-care and hospital settings, a variety of GNB emerge as the dominant colonizing flora of both mucosal and skin surfaces, particularly with antimicrobial use, severe illness, and extended length of stay. Acquisition of the GNB (from various reservoirs) leads to infection.

Pathogenesis Multiple bacterial traits are required for various aspects of the pathogenesis of GNB. The possession of specialized virulence genes is what defines pathogens and enables them to infect the host efficiently. As more is learned about these genes, it is becoming clear

TABLE 134-1	Intestinal Pathogenic E. coli		
Pathotype[a]	Clinical Syndrome(s)[b]	Defining Molecular Trait	Responsible Genetic Element[c]
STEC	Hemorrhagic colitis, hemolytic-uremic syndrome	Shiga toxin	Lambda-like Stx1 or Stx2 encoding bacteriophage
ETEC	Traveler's diarrhea	Heat-stable and -labile enterotoxins, colonization factors	Virulence plasmid(s)
EPEC	Watery diarrhea in young children	Localized adherence, attaching and effacing lesion on intestinal epithelium	EPEC adherence factor plasmid pathogenicity island (locus for enterocyte effacement)
EIEC	Dysentery	Invasion of colonic epithelial cells, intracellular multiplication, cell-to-cell spread	Multiple genes contained primarily in large virulence plasmid
EAEC/DAEC	Traveler's diarrhea, persistent diarrhea	Aggregative/diffuse adherence	Chromosomal or plasmid-associated adherence genes

[a] STEC, Shiga toxin–producing *E. coli*; ETEC, enterotoxigenic *E. coli*; EPEC, enteropathogenic *E. coli*; EIEC, enteroinvasive *E. coli*; EAEC, enteroaggregative *E. coli*; DAEC, diffusely adherent *E. coli*.
[b] Classic syndromes; see text for details on spectrum of disease.
[c] Pathogenesis is multigenic and requires genes in addition to those listed.

TABLE 134-2 *Interactions of Extraintestinal Pathogenic E. coli with the Human Host: A Paradigm for Extracellular, Extraintestinal Gram-Negative Bacterial Pathogens*

Bacterial Goal	Host Obstacle	Bacterial Solution
Extraintestinal attachment	Flow of urine, mucociliary blanket	Multiple adhesins (e.g., type 1 fimbriae, Sfa/Foc, P pili)
Nutrient acquisition for growth	Nutrient sequestration (e.g., iron via intracellular storage and extracellular scavenging via lactoferrin and transferrin)	Cellular lysis (e.g., hemolysin); multiple mechanisms for competing for extracellular iron (e.g., siderophores) and other nutrients
Initial avoidance of host bactericidal activity	Complement, phagocytic cells, antimicrobial peptides	Capsular polysaccharide, lipopolysaccharide
Transmission	?	Irritant tissue damage resulting in increased excretion (e.g., toxins such as hemolysin)
Late avoidance of host bactericidal activity	Acquired immunity (e.g., specific antibodies), treatment with antibiotics	? Cell entry, acquisition of antimicrobial resistance

that hosts and their cognate pathogens have been coadapting throughout evolutionary history. In fact, it has been speculated that infection is just a point on the spectrum of evolutionary development between microbes and hosts. At one end of this spectrum is a commensal/symbiotic interaction (e.g., mitochondria—formerly bacteria—within eukaryotic cells); at the other end is a lethal outcome that results in a "dead-end relationship" (e.g., Ebola virus). During this host-pathogen "chess match" over time, various and redundant solutions have emerged both in pathogens and in their hosts that enable these partners to maintain their coexistence (Table 134-2).

Extraintestinal pathogenic strains of *E. coli* (ExPEC) and the other genera discussed in this chapter cause infection outside the bowel. All are extracellular pathogens and therefore share certain pathogenic features. Innate defense systems (complement, antimicrobial peptides, professional phagocytes) and humoral immunity are the most critical host-defense components. As a result, both susceptibility to and severity of infection are increased with dysfunction or deficiencies of these components (e.g., neutrophils) (Chap. 104).

A given pathogen usually possesses multiple adhesins for binding to a variety of host cells (e.g., in *E. coli*: type 1 fimbriae, Sfa/Foc, P pili). Nutrient acquisition (e.g., iron via siderophores) requires many genes that are necessary but not sufficient for pathogenesis. The ability to resist the bactericidal activity of complement and professional phagocytes in the absence of antibody [e.g., conferred by capsule or O antigen of lipopolysaccharide (LPS)] is one of the defining traits of an extracellular pathogen. Tissue damage (e.g., hemolysis in the case of *E. coli*) may facilitate spread. Many important virulence genes await identification, and our understanding of many aspects of the pathogenesis of GNB is in its infancy (Chap. 105).

The ability to induce septic shock is another defining feature of these genera. GNB are the most common cause of this dangerous complication. The lipid A moiety of LPS (via interaction with host Toll-like receptors) and probably other bacterial factors as well (including capsule) stimulate a proinflammatory host response, which, if over-exuberant, results in shock (Chap. 254).

Lastly, many serotypes exist in most genera of GNB; for example, there are >100 O-specific antigens and >80 capsular antigens in *E. coli*. This antigenic variability, which permits immune evasion and successful recurrent infection by strains of the same species, has also impeded vaccine development (Chap. 107).

Infectious Syndromes Depending on both the host and the pathogen, nearly every organ or body cavity can be infected with GNB. *E. coli* and, to a lesser degree, *Klebsiella* and *Proteus* account for the majority of infections and are the most virulent pathogens of this group. However, the other genera are becoming increasingly important, particularly among persons in long-term care and hospitalized patients. This expanding role is in large part due to the innate or acquired resistance of these organisms to antimicrobial agents and to the increasing number of immunocompromised hosts. The mortality rate is significant in many GNB infections and correlates with the severity of illness. Especially problematic are pneumonia and bacteremia from any source complicated by severe sepsis (with or without shock); these conditions have associated mortality rates of 20 to 50%.

Diagnosis Isolation of GNB from ordinarily sterile sites almost always implies infection. Their isolation from nonsterile sites, particularly from soft-tissue and respiratory cultures, requires clinical correlation to differentiate colonization from infection. Results of an assessment of lactose fermentation (described for each genus below) are usually available before final identification of the organism and its antimicrobial susceptibilities and may assist in guiding empirical therapy.

℞ TREATMENT

The antimicrobial resistance of GNB is variable and is influenced by both geographic location and regional antibiotic use. Empirical antimicrobial choices should be based on local susceptibility patterns. Extended-spectrum β-lactamases (ESBLs, class A) and AmpC β-lactamases (class C) are responsible for the majority of multidrug resistance in GNB. The acquisition of ESBLs via transferable plasmids is increasing. To date, ESBLs are most prevalent in *Klebsiella* and *E. coli*, but they have also been described (and are probably underrecognized) in *Enterobacter* and other enteric GNB. Plasmids encoding for ESBLs confer resistance to third-generation cephalosporins and aztreonam and frequently contain linked resistance determinants for aminoglycosides, tetracyclines, and trimethoprim-sulfamethoxazole (TMP-SMX). Up to 50% of strains expressing ESBLs have associated fluoroquinolone resistance. Outbreaks due to strains possessing ESBLs have been associated with extensive institutional use of third-generation cephalosporins, particularly ceftazidime. The carbapenems (e.g., imipenem) are the only β-lactam agents that are reliably efficacious against strains expressing an ESBL.

Derepression of inducible chromosomal AmpC β-lactamases, another important resistance mechanism, may be preexisting or may develop during therapy. This determinant confers resistance to second- and third-generation cephalosporins, to aztreonam, and often to β-lactam/β-lactamase inhibitor combinations. Chromosomal AmpC β-lactamases occur in *Enterobacter*, *Serratia*, *Citrobacter*, *Proteus vulgaris*, *Proteus penneri*, *Providencia*, *Morganella*, and *Acinetobacter*. In addition, some strains of *E. coli*, *Klebsiella pneumoniae*, and other Enterobacteriaceae that carry chromosomal AmpC β-lactamases have acquired plasmids that contain AmpC β-lactamases.

Although relevant data are suboptimal or conflicting, combination therapy may increase antibiotic efficacy (particularly for serious infections, such as pneumonia) and diminish the emergence of resistance. Furthermore, drainage of abscesses and removal of infected foreign bodies are often needed for cure.

GNB are commonly involved in polymicrobial infections, in which it is difficult to determine the role of each specific pathogen (Chap. 148). Although some GNB are more pathogenic than others, it is usually prudent, if possible, to design an antimicrobial regimen that includes activity against all of the GNB identified, since each is capable of pathogenicity in its own right.

Prevention Diligent hand hygiene by health care personnel and avoidance of inappropriate antimicrobial use are key in preventing infection and the further development of antimicrobial resistance.

ESCHERICHIA COLI INFECTIONS ■ **Commensal Strains** Commensal *E. coli* variants, which constitute the major portion of the normal facultative intestinal flora in most humans, for the most part confer benefits (such as resistance to colonization) to their hosts. These strains generally lack the specialized virulence traits that enable intestinal and extra-intestinal pathogenic *E. coli* strains to cause disease within and outside the gastrointestinal tract, respectively. However, commensal *E. coli* are sometimes involved in extraintestinal infections when an aggravating factor is present, such as a foreign body (e.g., a urinary catheter), host compromise (e.g., local anatomical or functional abnormalities such as urinary or biliary tract obstruction or immunocompromise), or an inoculum that is large or contains a mixture of bacterial species (e.g., fecal contamination of the peritoneal cavity).

Extraintestinal Pathogenic Strains (ExPEC) The majority of *E. coli* isolates from symptomatic infections of the urinary tract, bloodstream, cerebrospinal fluid, respiratory tract, and peritoneum (spontaneous bacterial peritonitis) are distinct from commensal and intestinal pathogenic strains of *E. coli* by virtue of their functionally similar virulence factor profiles (Table 134-2) and clonal background. It has recently been proposed that these extraintestinal strains of *E. coli* be termed *ExPEC*. Evaluation of a limited number of strains has established that ExPEC can also cause surgical wound infection, osteomyelitis, and myositis, but the number of cases evaluated to date is too small for a reliable assessment of proportions. Studies on the nature of *E. coli* strains responsible for other extraintestinal infections are in progress.

Like commensal *E. coli* (but in contrast to intestinal pathogenic *E. coli*), ExPEC strains are often found in the normal intestinal flora and do not cause gastroenteritis in humans. Although acquisition of an ExPEC strain by the host is a prerequisite for ExPEC infection, it is not the rate-limiting step, which instead is entry of a colonizing ExPEC strain from its site of colonization (e.g., the colon, vagina, or oropharynx) into a normally sterile extraintestinal site (e.g., the urinary tract, peritoneal cavity, or lungs). ExPEC strains have acquired genes encoding diverse extraintestinal virulence factors that enable the bacteria to cause infections outside the gastrointestinal tract in both normal and compromised hosts (Table 134-2). These virulence genes are, for the most part, distinct from those that enable intestinal pathogenic strains to cause intestinal disease. All age groups, all types of hosts, and nearly all organs and sites are susceptible to infection by ExPEC. Previously healthy hosts infected with ExPEC can become severely ill and even die; however, adverse outcomes are more prevalent in the presence of coincidental disease and abnormalities in host defenses. *E. coli* is the most common enteric gram-negative species to cause extraintestinal infection in ambulatory, long-term-care, and hospital settings. The diversity and the medical and economic impact of ExPEC infections are evident from a review of the following specific syndromes.

Infectious Syndromes ■ *URINARY TRACT INFECTION (UTI)* The urinary tract is the site most frequently infected by ExPEC. A common infection among ambulatory patients, UTI accounts for 1% of ambulatory care visits in the United States and is second only to lower respiratory tract infection among infections responsible for hospitalization. UTIs are best considered by clinical syndrome (e.g., uncomplicated cystitis, catheter-associated) within the context of specific hosts (e.g., premenopausal women, compromised host; Chap. 269). *E. coli* is the single most prevalent pathogen for all UTI syndrome/host group combinations. Each year in the United States, for example, *E. coli* causes 85 to 95% of an estimated 6 to 8 million episodes of uncomplicated cystitis in premenopausal women, with an estimated $1 billion in direct health care costs. Furthermore, 20% of women with an initial infection develop frequent recurrences (0.3 to >20 per year). Except in the first year of life, acceptance of the diagnosis of UTI in males requires clear documentation since such infection is unusual in the absence of a history of instrumentation or anal intercourse.

Uncomplicated urethritis or cystitis occurs most commonly and is characterized by symptoms of dysuria, frequency, and suprapubic pain. Fever and/or back pain suggests progression to pyelonephritis. Pregnant women are at unusually high risk for this complication, which can adversely affect the outcome of pregnancy. As a result, prenatal screening for bacteriuria, with treatment when the results are positive, is the standard of care. Fever may take 5 to 7 days to resolve completely in appropriately treated patients with pyelonephritis but should fall over time. Persistently elevated or increasing fever and neutrophil counts should prompt evaluation for intrarenal or perinephric abscess and/or obstruction. Renal parenchymal damage and loss of renal function occur primarily in the setting of obstruction. Prostatic infection is generally a complication of UTI in men with a history of instrumentation and/or prostatic hypertrophy. The diagnosis and treatment of UTI are detailed in Chap. 269 and are tailored according to the individual host, the nature and site of infection, and the local pattern of antimicrobial susceptibility.

ABDOMINAL AND PELVIC INFECTION The abdomen/pelvis is the second most frequent site of extraintestinal infection due to *E. coli*. A wide variety of clinical syndromes occur in this location, including acute peritonitis secondary to fecal contamination, spontaneous bacterial peritonitis, peritoneal dialysis–associated peritonitis, diverticulitis, appendicitis, intraperitoneal or visceral abscesses (hepatic, pancreatic, splenic), infected pancreatic pseudocysts, and septic cholangitis and/or cholecystitis. In intraabdominal infections, *E. coli* can be isolated either alone or (as is often the case) along with other facultative and/or anaerobic members of the intestinal flora (Chap. 112).

PNEUMONIA *E. coli* is not usually considered a cause of pneumonia (Chap. 239). Indeed, enteric GNB account for only 2 to 5% of cases of community-acquired pneumonia (CAP), in part because these organisms only transiently colonize the oropharynx of a minority of healthy individuals. In contrast, rates of oral colonization with *E. coli* and other GNB increase with the severity of illness and with antibiotic use. Thus, GNB are a common cause of pneumonia among residents of long-term-care institutions and are the most frequent cause (60 to 70% of cases) of hospital-acquired pneumonia (Chap. 116), particularly among postoperative and intensive care patients. Infection is usually acquired by small-volume aspiration but occasionally occurs via hematogenous spread, in which case multifocal nodular infiltrates can be seen. Tissue necrosis, probably due to cytotoxins produced by GNB, is common. Despite significant institutional variation, *E. coli* is generally the third or fourth most commonly isolated gram-negative bacillus in these settings, accounting for 5 to 8% of episodes in both U.S.- and European-based studies. Regardless of the host, pneumonia due to enteric GNB is a serious disease, with high crude and attributable mortality rates (20 to 60% and 10 to 20%, respectively).

MENINGITIS (See also Chap. 360) *E. coli* is one of the two leading causes of neonatal meningitis (the other being group B *Streptococcus*). The majority of responsible strains possess the K1 capsular serotype. Outside this setting, meningitis due to *E. coli* is uncommon, occurring predominantly in the setting of disruption of the meninges due to craniotomy or trauma or in the presence of cirrhosis. In these instances, the meninges are presumably seeded from poorly cleared portal-source episodes of bacteremia or via direct extension from an otogenic or sinus source.

CELLULITIS/MUSCULOSKELETAL INFECTION Infections of decubitus ulcers and the lower extremities in diabetic patients (or other hosts with neurovascular compromise) are usually polymicrobial. *E. coli* contributes frequently to decubitus infections and occasionally to lower-extremity infections in these patients. In addition, *E. coli* may occasionally cause cellulitis or burn-site or surgical-wound infection, particularly when the infection originates close to the perineum. Osteomyelitis secondary to contiguous spread can occur in these settings. Hematogenously acquired osteomyelitis, particularly of vertebral bodies, is more commonly caused by *E. coli* than is generally appreciated; this organism accounts for 10% of cases in some series (Chap. 111). *E. coli* occasionally causes orthopedic device–associated infection or septic arthritis and is a rare cause of hematogenously acquired myositis. Myositis or fasciitis of the upper leg should prompt an evaluation for an abdominal source with contiguous spread.

ENDOVASCULAR INFECTION Despite being one of the most common causes of bacteremia, *E. coli* rarely seeds native heart valves and is an uncommon cause of prosthetic-valve endocarditis. Likewise, *E. coli* infections of aneurysms and vascular grafts are uncommon.

MISCELLANEOUS INFECTIONS *E. coli* can cause infection in nearly every organ and site. It is responsible for 8% of surgical site infections (superficial, deep tissue, or organ/space—e.g., mediastinitis), occasional cases of complicated sinusitis, and uncommon cases of endophthalmitis or brain abscess.

BACTEREMIA *E. coli* bacteremia can arise from primary infection at any extraintestinal site. In addition, primary *E. coli* bacteremia can arise from percutaneous intravascular devices or can result from the increased intestinal mucosal permeability seen in neonates and in the settings of neutropenia and chemotherapy-induced mucositis, trauma, and burns. Roughly equal proportions of bacteremia cases originate in the community and in the hospital. *E. coli* and *Staphylococcus aureus* are the most common clinically significant blood isolates; *E. coli*, which is isolated in 17 to 37% of cases, is the gram-negative bacillus most often isolated from the blood in the ambulatory setting as well as in most long-term-care and hospital settings. Isolation of *E. coli* from the blood is almost always clinically significant and typically is accompanied by the sepsis syndrome, severe sepsis (sepsis-induced dysfunction of at least one organ or system), or septic shock (Chap. 254). Calculations based on a conservative estimate for severe *E. coli* sepsis (i.e., 17% of all cases of severe sepsis) translate into an estimated 40,000 deaths among the affected patients in the United States in 2001.

The urinary tract is the most common source of *E. coli* bacteremia, accounting for two-thirds of episodes. Bacteremia from a urinary tract source is particularly common with pyelonephritis, urinary tract obstruction, or instrumentation in the presence of infected urine. The abdomen is the second most common source, accounting for 25% of episodes. Although obstructive biliary tract disease (stones, tumor) and overt disruption of bowel are responsible for many of these cases, some abdominal sources (e.g., abscesses) are remarkably silent clinically and require identification via imaging studies (e.g., computed tomography). Therefore, the physician should be cautious in designating the urinary tract as the source of *E. coli* bacteremia in the absence of appropriate signs and symptoms. Soft tissue, bone, and pulmonary infections are the next most common sources for bacteremia.

Diagnosis Strains of *E. coli* that cause extraintestinal infections usually grow both aerobically and anaerobically within 24 h on standard diagnostic media and are easily identified by the clinical microbiology laboratory according to standard biochemical criteria. More than 90% of ExPEC strains are rapid lactose fermenters.

℞ TREATMENT

In the past, *E. coli* has typically been highly susceptible to antibiotics and readily eradicated with antibiotic therapy. Unfortunately, this situation has changed. In general, the frequency of ampicillin resistance precludes its empirical use, even in community-acquired infections. Rates of resistance to first-generation cephalosporins and TMP-SMX are increasing among community-acquired strains in the United States (with current rates of 10 to 40%) and are even higher in Europe and developing countries. Until recently, TMP-SMX was the drug of choice for the treatment of uncomplicated cystitis in many locales. Although continued empirical use of TMP-SMX will predictably result in ever-diminishing cure rates, a wholesale switch to alternative agents (e.g., fluoroquinolones) will just as predictably accelerate the widespread emergence of resistance to these antimicrobial classes, as has already occurred in some areas. It is not surprising that rates of resistance among isolates from long-term-care facilities and hospitals are particularly high. Significant resistance (30 to 40%) to amoxicillin/clavulanic acid and piperacillin has been increasingly reported. For-

tunately, rates of resistance to cephalosporins (second-, third-, and fourth-generation), quinolones, monobactams (e.g., aztreonam), carbapenems (e.g., imipenem), and aminoglycosides are generally <10%. [The mean rate of resistance to third-generation cephalosporins was 3.2% among isolates reported to the National Nosocomial Infections Surveillance (NNIS) system in 1998.] An exception involves settings where extensive use of quinolone prophylaxis has led to the emergence of significant quinolone resistance (e.g., in patients with leukemia, transplant recipients, and patients with cirrhosis). Whatever the current rates, the frequency of acquisition of plasmids containing ESBLs and other resistance determinants is likely to increase.

KLEBSIELLA INFECTIONS *K. pneumoniae* is the most important *Klebsiella* species from a medical standpoint, causing community-acquired, long-term-care, and nosocomial infections. *K. oxytoca* is primarily a pathogen in long-term-care and hospital settings. *K. rhinoscleromatis* and *K. ozaenae* are usually isolated from patients in tropical climates. *Klebsiella* species are broadly prevalent in the environment and colonize mucosal surfaces of mammals. In healthy humans, *K. pneumoniae* colonization rates range from 5 to 35% in the colon and from 1 to 5% in the oropharynx; the skin is usually colonized only transiently. In long-term-care facilities and hospitals, colonization occurs with *K. oxytoca* as well, and carriage rates are significant among both workers and patients. Person-to-person spread is thought to be the predominant mode of acquisition. Classically, *Klebsiella* is associated with CAP, primarily in alcoholics. However, the majority of *Klebsiella* infections now occur in long-term-care facilities and hospitals. *Klebsiella* causes a spectrum of extraintestinal infections similar to that caused by *E. coli*. However, extraintestinal infections due to *Klebsiella* occur at a lower incidence in all sites except the respiratory tract. These variances in infection rates are probably due to differences in colonization and site-specific virulence traits. Antibiotic-resistant strains have been responsible for a number of nosocomial outbreaks of infection in intensive care units (ICUs) and neonatal nurseries. The most common clinical syndromes are pneumonia, UTI, abdominal infection, surgical site infection, soft tissue infection, and subsequent bacteremia. *K. rhinoscleromatis* is the causative agent of rhinoscleroma, a slowly progressive (months to years) mucosal upper respiratory infection that causes necrosis and occasional obstruction of the nasal passages. *K. ozaenae* has been implicated as a cause of chronic atrophic rhinitis.

Infectious Syndromes ■ *PNEUMONIA* *K. pneumoniae* causes only a small proportion of cases of CAP (Chap. 239). This infection occurs primarily in hosts with underlying disease, such as alcoholics, diabetics, and individuals with chronic lung disease. As in all pneumonias due to enteric GNB, purulent sputum production and "airspace" disease on x-ray are typical. Presentation with earlier, less extensive infection is more common than that with the classic lobar infiltrate with a bulging fissure. Pulmonary necrosis, pleural effusion, and empyema occur with progression. Pulmonary infection in residents of long-term-care facilities and in hospitalized patients is especially frequent because of increased oropharyngeal colonization rates. Mechanical ventilation is an important risk factor.

UTI The incidence of *K. pneumoniae* UTI among healthy adults is only 1 to 2%. However, in complicated UTIs (including those associated with indwelling bladder catheters), the incidence of *Klebsiella* infection increases to 5 to 17%.

ABDOMINAL INFECTION *Klebsiella* causes a spectrum of abdominal infections similar to that caused by *E. coli* but is less frequently isolated from these infections.

OTHER INFECTIONS *Klebsiella* cellulitis or soft tissue infection occurs most frequently in devitalized tissue (e.g., decubitus ulcers, diabetes, burn sites) or in immunocompromised hosts. *Klebsiella* causes a significant minority of surgical site infections, hematogenously derived endophthalmitis cases, and nosocomial sinusitis cases as well as occasional cases of osteomyelitis contiguous to soft tissue infection, temperate myositis, and neonatal meningitis or meningitis associated with neurosurgery.

BACTEREMIA *Klebsiella* infection at any site can result in bacteremia. Infections of the urinary tract, respiratory tract, and abdomen each account for 15 to 30% of *Klebsiella* bacteremias. Intravascular device–related infection is another important source (5 to 15%). Surgical site infection and other miscellaneous infections account for the rest. *Klebsiella* is one of the agents that causes sepsis neonatorum and bacteremia with fever and neutropenia. Like enteric GNB in general, *Klebsiella* rarely causes endocarditis or endovascular infection.

Diagnosis Except for *K. rhinoscleromatis* and *K. ozaenae*, klebsiellae are readily isolated and identified by the laboratory and usually ferment lactose.

℞ TREATMENT

K. pneumoniae and *K. oxytoca* have similar antibiotic resistance profiles. They are intrinsically resistant to ampicillin and ticarcillin. NNIS data from 1998 indicated that 10.7% of ICU patients were infected with strains resistant to third-generation cephalosporins. This increasing degree of resistance is primarily mediated by plasmids containing genes that encode ESBLs. In addition, these plasmids usually possess linked resistance determinants for aminoglycosides, tetracyclines, and TMP-SMX. In specific hospitals or geographic locales (e.g., Brooklyn, NY), the prevalence of ESBL-containing isolates is significantly higher. Resistance to β-lactam/β-lactamase inhibitor combinations and second-generation cephalosporins independent of ESBL-containing plasmids has also been increasingly described. Up to 50% of ESBL-containing strains have displayed associated fluoroquinolone resistance. At this time, rates of resistance to quinolones, cephamycins (e.g., cefoxitin), fourth-generation cephalosporins (e.g., cefepime), and amikacin are generally <10%, but these rates will probably increase. Carbapenems (e.g., imipenem) remain the most active antibiotic class against *Klebsiella*.

***PROTEUS* INFECTIONS** *P. mirabilis* causes 90% of *Proteus* infections. These infections occur in the community, in long-term-care facilities, and in hospitals. *P. vulgaris* and *P. penneri* are isolated primarily from infections contracted in long-term-care facilities or hospitals. *Proteus* species are part of the colonic flora of a wide variety of mammals, birds, fish, and reptiles. Their ability to generate histamine from contaminated fish has implicated these GNB in the pathogenesis of scombroid (fish) poisoning (Chap. 378). *P. mirabilis* colonizes healthy humans (prevalence, 50%), but *P. vulgaris* and *P. penneri* are isolated primarily from individuals with underlying disease. The urinary tract is overwhelmingly the favored site of *Proteus* infection, with adhesins, flagella, IgA protease, and urease as the important virulence factors. However, *Proteus* less commonly causes infection in a variety of extraintestinal sites.

Infectious Syndromes ■ *UTI* *P. mirabilis* causes only 1 to 2% of cases of UTI in healthy women, and *Proteus* species cause only 5% of cases of hospital-acquired UTI. However, *Proteus* is responsible for 10 to 15% of cases of complicated UTI, primarily those associated with catheterization; in the setting of long-term catheterization, their prevalence rate ranges from 20 to 45%. This high prevalence is due in part to the ability of *Proteus* to produce high levels of urease, which hydrolyzes urea to ammonia and results in alkalization of the urine. This situation, in turn, leads to precipitation of organic and inorganic compounds, with the formation of struvite and carbonate-apatite crystals, biofilm formation on catheters, and/or the development of calculi. *Proteus* becomes associated with the stones and can usually be eradicated only by complete stone removal. Over time, staghorn calculi may form and lead to obstruction and renal failure. Therefore, an unexplained alkaline urine should be cultured for *Proteus*, and identification of a *Proteus* species should prompt an evaluation for calculi.

OTHER INFECTIONS Although the majority of *Proteus* infections arise from the urinary tract, these bacteria occasionally cause pneumonia (primarily in long-term-care or hospitalized patients), nosocomial si-

nusitis, intraabdominal abscesses, biliary tract infection, surgical site infection, soft tissue infection (especially decubitus and diabetic ulcers), and osteomyelitis (primarily contiguous); they rarely cause temperate myositis. In addition, *Proteus* occasionally causes neonatal meningitis (with the umbilicus often implicated as the source), which is often complicated by the development of a cerebral abscess. Otogenic brain abscess is also seen.

BACTEREMIA The majority of *Proteus* bacteremias originate from the urinary tract; however, any of the less common sites of infection are also potential sources. Infection of intravascular devices should also be considered. Endovascular infection is rare. *Proteus* species are occasional agents of sepsis neonatorum and bacteremia with fever and neutropenia.

Diagnosis *Proteus* is readily isolated and identified by the laboratory. The majority of strains are lactose negative, and most demonstrate characteristic "swarming" motility on agar plates.

℞ TREATMENT

P. mirabilis remains susceptible to most antimicrobial agents except tetracycline. Resistance to ampicillin and first-generation cephalosporins has been acquired by 10 to 50% of strains. Overall, 5% of *P. mirabilis* isolates in the United States now possess an ESBL. *P. vulgaris* and *P. penneri* are more resistant than *P. mirabilis*. Resistance to ampicillin and first-generation cephalosporins is the rule for these species. Derepression of an inducible chromosomal AmpC β-lactamase (not present in *P. mirabilis*) occurs in up to 30% of strains. Imipenem, fourth-generation cephalosporins (e.g., cefepime), aminoglycosides, TMP-SMX, and quinolones have excellent activity (90 to 100%).

***ENTEROBACTER* INFECTIONS** *E. cloacae* and *E. aerogenes* are responsible for most *Enterobacter* infections (65 to 75% and 15 to 25%, respectively); *E. agglomerans*, *E. sakazakii*, and *E. gergoviae* are less commonly isolated (5%, 1%, and <1%, respectively). These organisms cause primarily health care–related or hospital-related infections. They are widely prevalent in foods, environmental sources (including health care facility equipment), and a wide variety of animals. Only a minority of healthy humans are colonized, but the percentage increases significantly in the setting of long-term care or hospitalization. Although colonization is an important prelude to infection, direct introduction via intravenous lines (e.g., contaminated intravenous fluids, pressure monitors) also occurs. Significant antibiotic resistance has developed in *Enterobacter* species and has contributed to their emergence as prominent nosocomial pathogens. Individuals who have received prior antibiotic treatment, who have comorbid disease, and who are patients in ICUs are at greatest risk for infection. *Enterobacter* causes a spectrum of extraintestinal infections similar to that described for other GNB in this chapter.

Infectious Syndromes Pneumonia, UTI (particularly catheter-related), intravascular device–related infection, surgical site infection, and abdominal infection (primarily postoperative or device-related—e.g., biliary stents) are the most common syndromes encountered. Nosocomial sinusitis, meningitis related to neurosurgical procedures (including use of pressure monitors), osteomyelitis, and endophthalmitis after eye surgery are less frequent. *E. sakazakii* is commonly responsible for neonatal meningitis/sepsis (particularly in premature infants); contaminated formula has been implicated as a source of this infection, which is often complicated by brain abscess or ventriculitis. Bacteremia can result from infection at any of these sites. In the setting of *Enterobacter* bacteremia, contamination of intravenous fluids or medications, blood components or plasma derivatives, catheter-flushing fluids, pressure monitors, and dialysis equipment should always be considered, particularly with epidemic infection. *Enterobacter* can also cause bacteremia in patients with fever and neutropenia. *Enterobacter* endocarditis is rare, occurring primarily in association with intravenous drug abuse or prosthetic valves.

Diagnosis *Enterobacter* is readily isolated and identified by the laboratory. Most strains are lactose positive.

℞ TREATMENT

Significant antimicrobial resistance exists among *Enterobacter* strains. Ampicillin and the first- and second-generation cephalosporins have little or no activity. The extensive use of third-generation cephalosporins has resulted in the selection of strains that produce high levels of AmpC β-lactamase, which confers resistance to second- and third-generation cephalosporins, monobactams (e.g., aztreonam), and (frequently) β-lactam/β-lactamase inhibitor combinations. Resistant isolates may emerge during therapy; their presence should be considered a possibility when clinical deterioration follows several days of improvement. A 34% resistance rate to third-generation cephalosporins was reported in ICU isolates in 1998 (NNIS data). Imipenem, fourth-generation cephalosporins (e.g., cefepime), aminoglycosides (amikacin > gentamicin), TMP-SMX, and quinolones have retained excellent activity (90 to 99%). However, increasing resistance to quinolones, in conjunction with the increased use of these agents, is a concern.

ACINETOBACTER INFECTIONS *A. baumannii* is responsible for the majority of *Acinetobacter* infections; a minority are due to *A. calcoaceticus*, *A. junii*, and *Acinetobacter* genospecies 3 and 13TU. *Acinetobacter* is highly prevalent in the environment. It is found in most water and soil samples and has a wide habitat. *Acinetobacter* has been cultured from the moist skin of healthy humans; increased colonization of the skin and the respiratory and gastrointestinal tracts occurs in individuals in long-term-care facilities and hospitals. Reservoirs for acquisition in these settings include health care personnel, medical equipment, food, and the surrounding environment. The overwhelming majority of infections are acquired in the hospital or in long-term-care facilities. The spectrum of extraintestinal infections caused by *Acinetobacter* is similar to that caused by other GNB. *Acinetobacter* species account for 1 to 3% of hospital-acquired infections and primarily affect immunocompromised hosts and patients with comorbid disease. ICUs are a prominent site of *Acinetobacter* infection. In some centers, the incidence of *Acinetobacter* infections, particularly those due to antibiotic-resistant strains, is increasing. Both sporadic and epidemic infections occur, usually after the first week of hospitalization.

Infectious Syndromes The respiratory tract (particularly in ventilated patients) and intravascular devices (particularly for non–*A. baumannii* species) are the favored sites of infection. *A. baumannii* uncommonly causes severe CAP, usually in compromised hosts (e.g., alcoholics), with the preponderance of cases reported from warm, humid geographic locales. Infections of a catheterized urinary tract, postoperative sites, burn sites, biliary stents, and sinuses (with tube-related ostial obstruction) are less common, as are neurosurgical infections (site- or device-associated—e.g., pressure monitors). Uncommon infections include contiguous osteomyelitis, peritonitis associated with continuous ambulatory peritoneal dialysis, and ophthalmic infection. The respiratory tract and intravascular devices are the most common sources for bacteremia.

Diagnosis On Gram's stain, *Acinetobacter* organisms usually appear as short GNB or coccobacilli. They are strictly aerobic, nonfermenting, and readily isolated and identified.

℞ TREATMENT

Many strains of *Acinetobacter* are highly resistant to antimicrobial agents. Empirical combination therapy is prudent pending susceptibility studies. Ampicillin, aztreonam, and the first- and second-generation cephalosporins possess little or no activity against these species. Resistance rates are 20 to 50% for mezlocillin, piperacillin,

quinolones, third-generation cephalosporins, and gentamicin. Imipenem is presently the most active antimicrobial (>95% sensitivity); β-lactam/β-lactamase inhibitor combinations, cefepime, and amikacin are often active.

SERRATIA INFECTIONS *S. marcescens* causes the majority of *Serratia* infections (>90%), and *S. liquefaciens* is occasionally isolated. Serratiae are found primarily in the environment (including health care institutions) and particularly in moist foci. Although strains have been isolated from a variety of animals, healthy humans are rarely colonized. In long-term-care facilities or hospitals, diverse reservoirs for the organisms include health care personnel, food, milk in neonatal units, sinks, respiratory and other hospital equipment, pressure monitors, intravenous solutions, multiply accessed medication vials, blood products (e.g., platelets), lotions, irrigation solutions, and even disinfectants. Infection results from either direct inoculation (e.g., via intravenous fluid) or colonization (primarily of the respiratory tract) and subsequent infection. Sporadic infection is most common, but occasional epidemics and common-source outbreaks occur. The spectrum of extraintestinal infections caused by *Serratia* is similar to that for other GNB. *Serratia* species account for 1 to 3% of hospital-acquired infections.

Infectious Syndromes The respiratory tract, the genitourinary tract, intravascular devices, and surgical wounds are the most common sites of *Serratia* infection and sources of *Serratia* bacteremia. Soft tissue infections, including myositis, osteomyelitis, abdominal and biliary tract infection (postprocedural), contact lens–associated keratitis, endophthalmitis, septic arthritis (primarily with intraarticular injections), and infusion-related bacteremias occur less commonly. Serratiae are uncommon causes of neonatal or postsurgical meningitis and bacteremia associated with fever and neutropenia. Endocarditis is rare.

Diagnosis Serratiae are readily cultured and identified by the laboratory and are usually lactose negative. A minority of *S. marcescens* strains are red-pigmented.

℞ TREATMENT

A high proportion of *Serratia* strains (>80%) are resistant to ampicillin and the first-generation cephalosporins. Although derepression of inducible chromosomal AmpC β-lactamases may be preexistent or may develop during therapy, >90% of isolates are susceptible to other GNB-appropriate antibiotics.

CITROBACTER INFECTIONS *C. freundii* and *C. koseri* (formerly *C. diversus*) cause the majority of human *Citrobacter* infections, which are similar epidemiologically and clinically to *Enterobacter* and *Acinetobacter* infections. *Citrobacter* organisms are commonly present in water, food, soil, and the intestinal tracts of animals. *Citrobacter* is part of the normal fecal flora in a minority of healthy humans, but colonization rates increase in long-term-care facilities and hospitals—the settings in which nearly all infections occur. *Citrobacter* species account for 1 to 2% of nosocomial infections. The affected hosts are usually immunocompromised or have comorbid disease. *Citrobacter* causes extraintestinal infections whose spectrum is similar to that described for other GNB.

Infectious Syndromes The urinary tract is the site of 40 to 50% of infections due to *Citrobacter*. Less commonly infected sites include the biliary tree (particularly with stones or obstruction), the respiratory tract, surgical sites, soft tissue (e.g., decubitus ulcers), the peritoneum, and intravascular devices. Osteomyelitis (usually contiguous), neurosurgery-related infection, and myositis occur rarely. *Citrobacter* is also an uncommon cause of neonatal meningitis; *C. koseri* accounts for 90% of cases due to this genus. A frequent and devastating complication of this infection (occurring in 50 to 80% of cases) is the development of brain abscesses. Bacteremia is most commonly due to UTI, biliary or abdominal infection, or intravascular devices. *Citrobacter* is an uncommon cause of bacteremia in the setting of fever and neutropenia. Endocarditis or endovascular infection is rare.

Diagnosis *Citrobacter* species are readily isolated and identified, often as part of a polymicrobial culture; 35 to 50% of isolates are lactose positive.

℞ TREATMENT

C. freundii is generally more resistant to antibiotics than *C. koseri*. Ampicillin and the first- and second-generation cephalosporins display poor activity against *Citrobacter*. Resistance is variable but increasing to ticarcillin, mezlocillin, piperacillin, aztreonam, quinolones, gentamicin, and third-generation cephalosporins; such resistance may evolve during therapy. The β-lactamase inhibitors usually do not improve susceptibility to β-lactam agents. Imipenem, amikacin, and the fourth-generation cephalosporins are most active, with >90% of strains sensitive.

MORGANELLA AND PROVIDENCIA INFECTIONS *M. morganii* (formerly *Proteus morganii*), *P. stuartii*, and (less frequently) *P. rettgeri* (formerly *Proteus rettgeri*) are the members of these genera that are responsible for human infections. The epidemiologic, pathogenic, and clinical manifestations of these organisms are similar to those of *Proteus* species; however, *Morganella* and *Providencia* are almost exclusively pathogens of persons in long-term-care facilities and, to a lesser degree, hospitalized patients.

Infectious Syndromes These species are primarily urinary tract pathogens, most often associated with long-term (>30-day) catheterization. UTI in uncatheterized or short-term-catheterized individuals is uncommon. Biofilm formation or encrustation of the catheter usually develops and may lead to catheter obstruction. Likewise, infection may result in the development of struvite bladder or renal stones, which, in turn, may lead to renal obstruction and serve as foci for relapse. Other infectious syndromes occur less commonly but include surgical site infection, soft tissue infection (primarily decubitus and diabetic ulcers), burn site infection, pneumonia (particularly ventilator-associated), intravascular device infection, and intraabdominal infection. Rarely, the other extraintestinal infections described for GNB also occur. Bacteremia is uncommon; although any infected site can serve as the source, the urinary tract accounts for the majority of cases, with surgical site and soft tissue infections less frequently responsible.

Diagnosis *M. morganii* and *Providencia* are readily isolated and identified. Nearly all isolates are unable to ferment lactose.

℞ TREATMENT

Morganella and *Providencia* may be highly resistant to antimicrobial agents. Ampicillin and the first-generation cephalosporins exhibit poor activity against these organisms. Of *Providencia* isolates, 40% are resistant to fluoroquinolones. Variable resistance is emerging (and may evolve during therapy) against ticarcillin, mezlocillin, piperacillin, aztreonam, gentamicin, TMP-SMX, and the second- and third-generation cephalosporins. The β-lactamase inhibitor tazobactam (but not sulbactam or clavulanic acid) somewhat improves susceptibility to β-lactam agents. Imipenem, amikacin, and the fourth-generation cephalosporins are most active, with >90% of strains susceptible. Removal of an infected catheter or stones is critical for eradication of the organisms from the urinary tract.

EDWARDSIELLA INFECTION *E. tarda* is the only member of this genus associated with human disease. This organism is found predominantly

in both freshwater and marine environments and in the animals that live in these environments. Human acquisition occurs primarily during interaction with these reservoirs. *E. tarda* infection is rare in the United States; most recently reported cases are from Southeast Asia. This pathogen shares some of the clinical features of both *Salmonella* species and *Vibrio vulnificus*.

Infectious Syndromes Gastroenteritis is the predominant infectious syndrome reported (50 to 80% of infections). Self-limiting watery diarrhea is most frequent; however, cases of severe colitis responding to therapy have also been described. The most common extraintestinal infection is wound infection due to direct inoculation, which is often associated with freshwater, marine, or snake-related injuries. Other infectious syndromes appear to be due to invasion of the gastrointestinal tract and subsequent bacteremia. The majority of afflicted hosts have either liver disease or an iron-overload state (e.g., sickle cell disease). A primary bacteremic syndrome, sometimes complicated by meningitis, has been described and has a 40% case-fatality rate. Visceral (primarily hepatic) or intraperitoneal abscesses have also been reported.

Diagnosis Although *E. tarda* can readily be isolated and identified, most laboratories do not routinely identify it from stool.

℞ TREATMENT

E. tarda is sensitive to most GNB-appropriate antimicrobial agents. Gastroenteritis is generally self-limiting, but treatment with TMP-SMX or a quinolone may expedite its resolution. In the setting of overwhelming sepsis, quinolones, third- or fourth-generation cephalosporins, imipenem, and aminoglycosides—alone or in combination—are the safest choices pending susceptibility information.

INFECTIONS CAUSED BY MISCELLANEOUS GENERA Species from genera of GNB such as *Hafnia*, *Kluyvera*, *Cedecea*, *Pantoea*, and *Ewingella* are occasionally isolated from a variety of clinical specimens, including blood, sputum, cerebrospinal fluid, joint fluid, biliary drainage, and wounds. Although their role in disease has not always been defined, these strains appear to be rare and usually opportunistic human pathogens. The primary medical literature should be consulted for details on their potential role as infectious agents.

FURTHER READING

DONNENBERG M (ed): *Escherichia coli: Virulence Mechanisms of a Versatile Pathogen.* San Diego, Academic Press, 2002

GRANSDEN WR et al: Bacteremia due to *Escherichia coli*: A study of 861 episodes. Rev Infect Dis 12:1008, 1990

HEJAZI A, FALKINER FR: *Serratia marcescens.* J Med Microbiol 46:903, 1997

LEVISON ME: Plasmid-mediated extended-spectrum β-lactamases in organisms other than *Klebsiella pneumoniae* and *Escherichia coli*: A hidden reservoir of transferable resistance genes. Curr Infect Dis Rep 4:181, 2002

PODSCHUN R, ULLMANN U: *Klebsiella* spp. as nosocomial pathogens: Epidemiology, taxonomy, typing methods, and pathogenicity factors. Clin Microbiol Rev 11:589, 1998

SANDERS WE JR, SANDERS CC: *Enterobacter* spp.: Pathogens poised to flourish at the turn of the century. Clin Microbiol Rev 10:220, 1997

SHIH CC et al: Bacteremia due to *Citrobacter* species: Significance of primary intraabdominal infection. Clin Infect Dis 23:543, 1996

SLAVEN EM et al: Myonecrosis caused by *Edwardsiella tarda*: A case report and case series of extraintestinal *E. tarda* infections. Clin Infect Dis 32:1430, 2001

WATANAKUNAKORN C, PERNI SC: *Proteus mirabilis* bacteremia: A review of 176 cases during 1980–1992. Scand J Infect Dis 26:361, 1994

DEFINITION *Helicobacter pylori* persistently colonizes the human stomach and is of etiologic importance in peptic ulcer disease (Chap. 274) and gastric malignancy (Chap. 77). Other gastric *Helicobacter* species colonize animals, some with a narrow range and others with a broad range of host species specificity. Those with broad specificity are occasionally found in humans, probably as zoonoses. The two most common of these species among isolates from humans are *Helicobacter bizzozeronii* (formerly known as *Helicobacter heilmannii* or *Gastrospirillum hominis*) and *Helicobacter felis*. It is unclear whether these helicobacters cause human disease. Numerous species of nongastric helicobacters are found in humans and animals and have been increasingly recognized as causes of human disease, especially in immunocompromised hosts.

ETIOLOGIC AGENT *H. pylori* is a gram-negative, spiral, flagellated bacillus that has naturally colonized humans for at least tens of thousands of years. It is noninvasive, living in gastric mucus; a small proportion of the bacterial cells are adherent to the mucosa. Its spiral shape and flagella render *H. pylori* motile in the mucus environment. This organism has several acid-resistance mechanisms, most notably a highly expressed urease that catalyzes urea hydrolysis to produce buffering ammonia. In vitro, *H. pylori* is microaerophilic and slow-growing and requires complex growth media. Publication of the complete genomic sequence of *H. pylori* in 1997 led to significant advances in the understanding of the organism's biology.

EPIDEMIOLOGY The prevalence of *H. pylori* is ~30% in the United States and other developed countries as opposed to >80% in most developing countries. In the United States, prevalence varies with age: ~50% of 60-year-old persons and 20% of 30-year-old persons are colonized. *H. pylori* is usually acquired in childhood. The age association is due mostly to a birth-cohort effect whereby current 60-year-olds were more commonly colonized as children than current 30-year-olds. Spontaneous acquisition or loss of the bacterium in adulthood is uncommon. Other than age, the main risk factor for *H. pylori* positivity is low socioeconomic status; crowding and markers of poor hygiene in childhood are particularly strong risk factors. Thus, the falling incidence among children is likely due, at least in part, to improvements in living standards and increased use of antibiotics.

Humans are the only important reservoir of *H. pylori*. Members of a family may carry the same strain, and colonization is particularly common in childhood institutions. These findings imply direct person-to-person spread, but whether transmission takes place by the fecal-oral or the oral-oral route is unknown. *H. pylori* is easily cultured from vomitus and gastroesophageal refluxate and is less easily cultured from stool.

PATHOLOGY AND PATHOGENESIS *H. pylori* colonization induces chronic superficial gastritis, which includes both mononuclear and polymorphonuclear cell infiltration of the mucosa. (The term *gastritis* should be used specifically to describe histologic features; it also has been used to describe endoscopic appearances and even symptoms, which do not correlate closely with microscopic findings or with the presence of *H. pylori*.) The immune response to *H. pylori* includes both the production of antibody (local and systemic) and a cell-mediated response but is ineffective in clearing the bacterium. The pattern of gastric inflammation is associated with disease risk: antral-predominant gastritis is most closely linked with duodenal ulceration, whereas pangastritis is linked with gastric ulceration and adenocarcinoma. This probably explains why patients with duodenal ulceration rarely develop gastric adenocarcinoma later, despite being colonized by *H. pylori*. Longitudinal analyses of gastric biopsy specimens taken years apart from the same patient show that inflammation may progress stepwise through atrophy, intestinal metaplasia, and dysplasia to carcinoma. Continuous proton pump inhibitor (PPI) therapy—for example,

for gastroesophageal reflux disease (GERD)—may speed progression to atrophy when *H. pylori* is present, but it remains unclear whether this situation increases cancer risk.

Most *H. pylori*–colonized persons do not develop clinical sequelae. That some persons develop overt disease whereas others do not is probably due to a combination of bacterial strain differences, host susceptibility to disease, and environmental factors. Several *H. pylori* virulence factors are more common in disease-associated strains. The *cag* PaI is a group of genes including those that encode a secretion system through which a specific protein, CagA, is translocated into epithelial cells. CagA interferes with host cell signaling, causing proliferation and cytoskeletal changes. The secretion system also induces a proinflammatory cytokine response, which results in enhanced inflammation. The CagA protein is highly immunogenic, and patients with peptic ulcer disease or gastric adenocarcinoma are more likely than persons without these conditions to have antibodies to CagA. However, patients with severe reflux esophagitis, the premalignant condition Barrett's esophagus, or esophageal adenocarcinoma are less likely to harbor *cag*$^+$ strains than are persons with a normal esophagus. The *H. pylori* vacuolating cytotoxin VacA occurs in several forms that exhibit different levels of toxicity. Strains with the more toxic forms are more commonly isolated from patients with peptic ulcer disease or gastric carcinoma than from persons without these conditions. BabA, an adhesin expressed by only some strains, is associated with increased gastric inflammation and with increased risk of peptic ulceration and gastric adenocarcinoma.

The best-characterized host determinant of disease is the possession of genetic polymorphisms leading to enhanced *H. pylori*–stimulated secretion of the proinflammatory cytokine interleukin 1β. If they are *H. pylori*–positive, individuals with these polymorphisms are at increased risk of hypochlorhydria and gastric adenocarcinoma. Environmental cofactors are also important in pathogenesis. Smoking increases ulcer and cancer risk in *H. pylori*–positive individuals. Diets high in salt and preserved foods increase cancer risk, whereas diets high in antioxidants and vitamin C are protective.

The pathogenesis of duodenal ulceration is becoming clearer. Antral *H. pylori* colonization diminishes the number of somatostatin-producing cells. Since somatostatin inhibits gastrin release, gastrin levels are higher than normal in *H. pylori*–positive persons. Individuals with antral-predominant gastritis (and thus a normally functioning acid-producing gastric corpus) develop increased acid secretion, which induces protective gastric metaplasia in the duodenum; the duodenum becomes colonized by *H. pylori*, inflamed, and then ulcerated. The pathogenesis of gastric ulceration is less well understood. These ulcers usually occur at the junction of antral and corpus-type mucosa, and this region is particularly inflamed. Gastric cancer probably stems from progressive DNA damage and the survival of abnormal epithelial cell clones. The DNA damage is thought to be due principally to reactive oxygen and nitrogen species arising from inflammatory cells and perhaps from other bacteria that survive in the achlorhydric stomachs in which gastric malignancies occur.

CLINICAL MANIFESTATIONS Essentially all *H. pylori*–colonized persons have gastric inflammation, but fewer than 10% of these individuals develop associated illnesses such as peptic ulceration, gastric adenocarcinoma, or gastric lymphoma (Fig. 135-1).

More than 80% of duodenal ulcers and 60% of gastric ulcers are related to *H. pylori* colonization (Chap. 274), most of the remainder being due to aspirin or nonsteroidal anti-inflammatory drugs (NSAIDs). The main lines of evidence for an ulcer-promoting role of *H. pylori* are (1) that the presence of the organism is a risk factor for the development of ulcers, (2) that (non-NSAID-induced) ulcers rarely develop in the absence of *H. pylori*, (3) that eradication of *H. pylori* markedly reduces rates of ulcer relapse, and (4) that experimental *H. pylori* infection of gerbils causes gastric ulceration.

Prospective nested case-control studies have shown that *H. pylori* colonization is a risk factor for adenocarcinomas of the distal stomach (Chap. 77). Long-term experimental infection of gerbils also may result in gastric adenocarcinoma. The presence of *H. pylori* is strongly associated with gastric lymphoma, although this is a rarer condition. Many low-grade gastric B cell lymphomas arising from mucosa-associated lymphoid tissue (MALT) are driven by T cell stimulation, which in turn is driven by *H. pylori* antigen stimulation; *H. pylori* antigen–driven tumors may regress either fully or partially after *H. pylori* eradication.

Many patients have upper gastrointestinal symptoms but normal results in upper gastrointestinal endoscopy (so-called functional or nonulcer dyspepsia; Chap. 274). Because *H. pylori* is common, some of these patients will be positive for the organism. *H. pylori* eradication leads to symptom resolution more commonly than does placebo treatment, but only by a little (<10%). Whether such patients have peptic ulcers in remission at the time of endoscopy or whether a subgroup of patients with true functional dyspepsia respond to *H. pylori* treatment is unclear.

Much interest has focused on a possible protective role for *H. pylori* against GERD (Chap. 273) and adenocarcinoma of the esophagus and gastric cardia (Chap. 77). The main lines of evidence for this role are (1) that there is a temporal relationship between a falling prevalence of *H. pylori* colonization and a rising incidence of these conditions; (2) that in most studies, the prevalence of *H. pylori* colonization (especially with proinflammatory *cagA+* strains) is significantly lower among patients with these esophageal diseases than among control subjects; and (3) that in some studies, eradication of *H. pylori* leads to the development or worsening of GERD. The mechanism underlying this protective effect appears to be *H. pylori*–induced hypochlorhydria. Since—at the individual level—GERD symptoms may decrease, worsen, or remain unchanged after *H. pylori* treatment, concerns about GERD should not affect treatment decisions where a definite indication exists.

H. pylori has a less-well-established role in other gastric pathologies. *H. pylori* may be one initial precipitant of autoimmune gastritis and pernicious anemia and also may predispose to iron deficiency in some patients through hypochlorhydria and reduced iron absorption. In addition, several extragastrointestinal pathologies have been linked epidemiologically with *H. pylori* colonization, the most notable being ischemic heart disease and cerebrovascular disease. However, the strength of these associations is reduced if confounding factors are considered, and most authorities consider them to be noncausal.

DIAGNOSIS   Tests for *H. pylori* can be divided into two groups: invasive tests, which require upper gastrointestinal endoscopy and are based on the analysis of gastric biopsy specimens, and noninvasive tests (Table 135-1). Endoscopy often is not performed in the initial management of young dyspeptic patients without worrying symptoms but is commonly used in older people to exclude malignancy. If endoscopy is performed, the most convenient biopsy-based test is the biopsy urease test, in which one large or two small antral biopsy specimens are placed into a gel containing urea and an indicator. The presence of *H. pylori* urease elicits a color change, which often occurs within minutes but can require up to 24 h. Histologic examination of biopsy specimens is accurate, provided that a special stain (e.g., a modified Giemsa or silver stain) permitting optimal visualization of *H. pylori* is used. If biopsies from both antrum and corpus are obtained, histologic study yields additional information, including the degree and pattern of inflammation, atrophy, metaplasia, and dysplasia. Microbiologic culture is most specific but may be insensitive because of difficulty with *H. pylori* isolation. Once cultured, the identity of *H. pylori* can be confirmed by its typical appearance on Gram's stain and its positive reactions in oxidase, catalase, and urease tests. Moreover, the organism's antibiotic sensitivities can be determined. The occasional biopsy specimens containing the less common non-*pylori* helicobacters give only weakly positive results in the biopsy urease test.

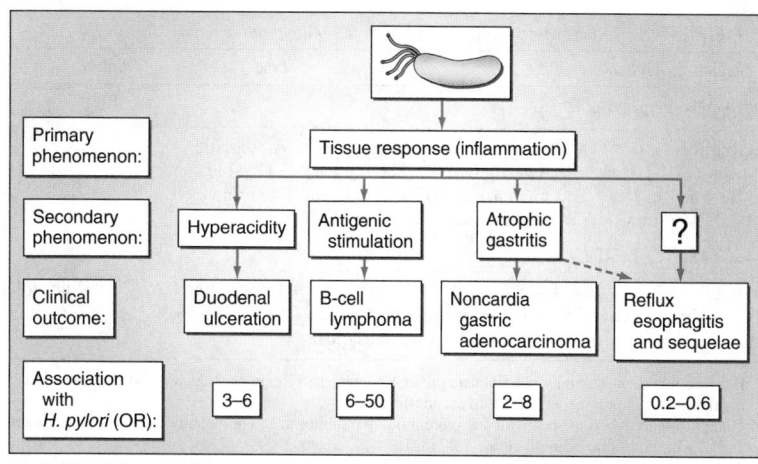

FIGURE 135-1   Schematic of the relationships between colonization with *Helicobacter pylori* and diseases of the upper gastrointestinal tract among persons in developed countries. Essentially all persons colonized with *H. pylori* develop a host response, which is generally termed *chronic gastritis*. The nature of the interaction of the host with the particular bacterial population determines the clinical outcome. *H. pylori* colonization increases the lifetime risk of peptic ulcer disease, noncardia gastric cancer, and B cell non-Hodgkin's gastric lymphoma [odds ratios (ORs) for all, >3]. In contrast, a growing body of evidence indicates that *H. pylori* colonization (especially with *cag+* strains) protects against adenocarcinoma of the esophagus (and the related gastric cardia) and premalignant lesions such as Barrett's esophagus (OR, <1). While the incidences of peptic ulcer disease (cases not due to nonsteroidal anti-inflammatory drugs) and noncardia gastric cancer are declining in developed countries, the incidence of adenocarcinoma of the esophagus is rapidly increasing. (*Adapted from Blaser 1999, with permission.*)

Positive identification of these bacteria requires visualization of the characteristic long, tight spiral bacteria in histologic sections.

Noninvasive *H. pylori* testing is now the norm if gastric cancer does not need to be excluded. The most consistently accurate test is the urea breath test. In this simple test, the patient drinks a labeled urea solution and then blows into a tube. The urea is labeled with either the nonradioactive isotope ^{13}C or a minute dose of the radioactive isotope ^{14}C. If *H. pylori* urease is present, the urea is hydrolyzed and labeled carbon dioxide is detected in breath samples. The stool antigen test is another simple assay that is dependent on the detection of *H. pylori* antigens in stool. It is more convenient and less expensive than the urea breath test but has been slightly less accurate in some

TABLE 135-1   *Tests Commonly Used to Detect Helicobacter pylori*

Test	Advantages	Disadvantages
INVASIVE (BASED ON ENDOSCOPIC BIOPSY)		
Biopsy urease test	Quick, simple	Some commercial tests not fully sensitive before 24 h
Histology	May give additional histologic information	Sensitivity dependent on experience and use of special stains
Culture	Permits determination of antibiotic susceptibility	Sensitivity dependent on experience
NONINVASIVE		
Serology	Inexpensive and convenient	Cannot be used for early follow-up; some commercial kits inaccurate
^{13}C or ^{14}C urea breath test	Inexpensive and simpler than endoscopy; useful for follow-up after treatment	Low-dose irradiation in ^{14}C test
Stool antigen test	Inexpensive and convenient; useful for follow-up after treatment; may be useful in children	New test; role not fully established; appears less accurate than urea breath test

TABLE 135-2 *Recommended Treatment Regimens for Helicobacter pylori*

Regimen, Duration	Drug 1	Drug 2	Drug 3	Drug 4
FIRST-LINE TREATMENT				
Regimen 1: OCA (7 days)[a]	Omeprazole[b] (20 mg bid)	Clarithromycin (500 mg bid)	Amoxicillin (1 g bid)	—
Regimen 2: OCM (7 days)	Omeprazole[b] (20 mg bid)	Clarithromycin (500 mg bid)	Metronidazole (500 mg bid)	—
SECOND-LINE TREATMENT[c]				
Regimen 3: OBTM (14 days)[d]	Omeprazole[b] (20 mg bid)	Bismuth subsalicylate (2 tabs qid)	Tetracycline HCl (500 mg qid)	Metronidazole (500 mg tid)

[a] For first-line therapy, many practitioners prefer Regimen 1 to Regimen 2, as it avoids the use of metronidazole—an important constituent of second-line therapy.

[b] Omeprazole may be replaced with any protein pump inhibitor at an equivalent dosage or, in Regimens 1 and 2, with ranitidine bismuth citrate (400 mg).

[c] An alternative to this second-line therapy is to culture *H. pylori* and to be guided by antibiotic susceptibility data. Patients in whom second-line therapy fails should undergo endoscopy for *H. pylori* culture and antibiotic susceptibility testing.

[d] Data supporting this regimen come mainly from Europe and are based on the use of bismuth subcitrate and metronidazole (400 mg tid).

comparative studies. The urea breath test, the stool antigen test, and biopsy-based tests can all be used to assess the success of treatment. However, because these tests are dependent on *H. pylori* load, their use <4 weeks after treatment may lead to false-negative results. These tests are also unreliable if performed within 4 weeks of intercurrent treatment with antibiotics or bismuth compounds or within 2 weeks of the discontinuation of PPI treatment. In the assessment of treatment success, noninvasive tests are normally preferred; however, after gastric ulceration, endoscopy should be repeated to ensure healing and to exclude gastric carcinoma by further histologic sampling.

The simplest tests for ascertaining *H. pylori* status are serologic assays measuring specific IgG levels in serum by enzyme-linked immunosorbent assay (ELISA) or immunoblot. The best of these tests are as accurate as other diagnostic methods, but many commercial tests, especially rapid office tests, perform poorly. In quantitative tests, a defined drop in antibody titer between matched serum samples taken before and 6 months after treatment (no sooner because of the slow decline in titer) accurately indicates that *H. pylori* has been eradicated. However, serologic tests are not commonly used in this context because of the inconvenient wait and the logistics. Although serology can distinguish between *cag⁺* and *cag⁻* strains, this technique is not yet commercially available in the United States.

℞ TREATMENT

The most clear-cut indications for treatment are *H. pylori*–related duodenal or gastric ulceration and low-grade gastric B cell lymphoma. *H. pylori* should be eradicated in patients with documented ulcer disease, whether or not the ulcers are currently active, to reduce the likelihood of relapse. Many guidelines now recommend *H. pylori* treatment in uninvestigated simple dyspepsia following noninvasive diagnosis; others also recommend treatment in functional dyspepsia, in case the patient is one of the perhaps 5 to 10% to benefit (beyond placebo effects) from such treatment. People with a strong family history of gastric cancer should be treated for *H. pylori* in the hope that this therapy will reduce their risk. For many reasons, widespread community screening for and treatment of *H. pylori* as primary prophylaxis for gastric cancer and peptic ulcers are not currently recommended. It is unclear whether treatment of *H. pylori* (as opposed to never having acquired the organism) reduces cancer risk, except in certain high-risk populations. Treatment has side effects, which are severe in rare cases. Antibiotic resistance may arise in *H. pylori* or other incidentally carried bacteria. Otherwise healthy people may become anxious, especially if treatment is unsuccessful. Finally, there is a possible risk of provoking or worsening GERD.

Although *H. pylori* is susceptible to a wide range of antibiotics in vitro, monotherapy has been disappointing in vivo, probably because

of inadequate antibiotic delivery to the full locus of colonization. Failure of monotherapy has led to the development of multidrug regimens, the most successful of which are triple and quadruple combinations that produce *H. pylori* eradication rates of >90% in many trials and >75% in clinical practice. Current regimens consist of a PPI or ranitidine bismuth citrate and two or three antimicrobial agents given for 7 to 14 days (Table 135-2).

The two most important goals in *H. pylori* eradication are to obtain the patient's close compliance with the dosing regimen and to use drugs to which *H. pylori* has not acquired resistance. Treatment failure following minor lapses in compliance is common and often leads to acquired resistance to metronidazole or clarithromycin. To stress the importance of compliance, written instructions should be given to the patient, and minor side effects of the regimen should be explained. Resistance to metronidazole and clarithromycin is of growing concern. Clarithromycin resistance is less prevalent but, if present, usually results in treatment failure. Metronidazole-resistant strains of *H. pylori* are more common, but infections with these strains may still respond to metronidazole-containing regimens. Assessment of antibiotic susceptibilities before treatment would be optimal but is not usually undertaken. In the absence of susceptibility information, a history of antibiotic use should be obtained, and, even if only distant exposure is identified (e.g., previous metronidazole consumption for giardiasis or trichomoniasis), use of the agent should be avoided if possible. If initial *H. pylori* treatment fails, two strategies are commonly used. One is re-treatment with a quadruple drug regimen (Table 135-2). The second is endoscopy and biopsy culture plus treatment based on documented antibiotic sensitivities. If re-treatment fails, susceptibility testing should always be performed.

Clearance of non-*pylori* gastric helicobacters following the use of bismuth compounds alone or triple-therapy regimens has been described. However, in the absence of trials, it is unclear whether this result represents successful treatment or natural clearance of the bacterium.

PREVENTION Carriage of *H. pylori* has considerable public health significance in developed countries, where it is associated with peptic ulcer disease and gastric adenocarcinoma, and in developing countries, where gastric adenocarcinoma is an even more common cause of cancer death late in life. However, given that *H. pylori* has co-evolved with its human host over millennia, preventing or eliminating colonization on a population basis may have distinct disadvantages. For example, absence of *H. pylori* has been reported to increase the risk of diarrheal diseases and, as has been mentioned, appears to increase the risk of GERD and esophageal adenocarcinoma. If mass prevention were contemplated, vaccination would be the most obvious method, and experimental immunization of animals has given promising results. However, in the United States and other developed countries, rates of *H. pylori* carriage, peptic ulceration, and gastric adenocarcinoma are falling. Thus, prevention of colonization in these countries may be unnecessary or even unwise.

FURTHER READING

Blaser MJ: Hypothesis: The changing relationships of *Helicobacter pylori* and humans: Implications for health and disease. J Infect Dis 179:1523, 1999

Ghose C et al: East Asian genotypes of *Helicobacter pylori* strains in Amerindians provide evidence for its ancient human carriage. Proc Natl Acad Sci USA 99:15107, 2002

Hansson LE et al: The risk of stomach cancer in patients with gastric or duodenal ulcer disease. N Engl J Med 335:242, 1996

Kuipers E et al: Atrophic gastritis and *Helicobacter pylori* infection in patients with reflux esophagitis treated with omeprazole or fundoplication. N Engl J Med 334:1018, 1996

Parsonnet J et al: *Helicobacter pylori* infection and gastric lymphoma. N Engl J Med 330:1267, 1994

PEEK RM JR, BLASER MJ: *Helicobacter pylori* and gastrointestinal tract adenocarcinomas. Nat Rev Cancer 2:28, 2002

UEMURA N et al: *Helicobacter pylori* infection and the development of gastric cancer. N Engl J Med 345:784, 2001

ZUCCA E et al: Molecular analysis of the progression from *Helicobacter py-lori*–associated chronic gastritis to mucosa-associated lymphoid-tissue lymphoma of the stomach. N Engl J Med 338:804, 1998

136 INFECTIONS DUE TO *PSEUDOMONAS* SPECIES AND RELATED ORGANISMS

Christopher A. Ohl, Matthew Pollack

Pseudomonas species and phylogenetically related bacteria are ubiquitous, free-living, opportunistic gram-negative pathogens. *Pseudomonas aeruginosa*, the most common human pathogen in this group, is the primary subject of this chapter. Also discussed are *Burkholderia cepacia* (formerly *Pseudomonas cepacia*), *Stenotrophomonas maltophilia* (formerly *Xanthomonas maltophilia*), and *Burkholderia pseudomallei* and *Burkholderia mallei* (the causative agents of melioidosis and glanders, respectively).

INFECTIONS DUE TO *P. AERUGINOSA*

MICROBIOLOGY *P. aeruginosa* is a small, nonsporulating, aerobic gram-negative rod belonging to the family Pseudomonadaceae. It is motile by virtue of its single polar flagellum. More than half of all clinical isolates produce the blue-green pigment pyocyanin; this pigment is helpful in the identification of the organism and accounts for the species name *aeruginosa*, which refers to the distinctive color of copper oxide. The organism, which can easily be identified in culture by the clinical laboratory, is differentiated from enteric gram-negative bacilli by its ability to oxidize indophenol and its inability to ferment lactose.

EPIDEMIOLOGY *P. aeruginosa* is widespread in nature, inhabiting soil, water, plants, and animals (including humans). It has a predilection for moist environments. This organism occasionally colonizes the skin, external ear, upper respiratory tract, or large bowel of healthy humans. Rates of carriage are relatively low, however, except among patients who have serious underlying disease, whose host defenses have been naturally or iatrogenically compromised, who have previously received antibiotic therapy, and/or who have been exposed to the hospital environment. Under these circumstances, colonization with *P. aeruginosa* frequently precedes infection, and factors that predispose to the former also increase the likelihood of the latter.

Most *P. aeruginosa* infections are acquired in the hospital, where intensive care units (ICUs) account for higher rates of infection than other hospital units. According to the National Nosocomial Infections Surveillance (NNIS) System, between 1992 and 1999, *P. aeruginosa* was the second most common cause of pneumonia, the fourth most common cause of urinary tract infection, and the sixth most common bloodstream isolate in ICUs. Many potential reservoirs of infection have been identified in the hospital environment, including respiratory equipment, cleaning solutions, disinfectants, sinks, vegetables, flowers, endoscopes, and physiotherapy pools. Most reservoirs are associated with moisture. While some infecting strains of *P. aeruginosa* appear to be endemic within the hospital, others are traced to a common source associated with a specific outbreak or epidemic. Nosocomial outbreaks of *Pseudomonas* infection have been specifically traced to the hands and fingernails of health care workers, and the majority of instances of patient-to-patient transmission in the hospital are thought to occur via this route. Epidemiologic investigation of health care–associated outbreaks is facilitated by the use of molecular techniques such as pulsed-field gel electrophoresis.

PATHOGENESIS The pathogenesis of *Pseudomonas* disease is complex, as is suggested by the clinical diversity of the infections related to this organism and by the multiplicity of putative virulence factors it produces. *P. aeruginosa* rarely causes disease in the healthy host but is highly virulent for persons in whom the normal cutaneous or mucosal barriers have been breached or bypassed, the immunologic defense mechanisms have been compromised, or the protective function of the normal bacterial flora has been disrupted (Table 136-1). The organism's ubiquity, flexible nutritional and metabolic requirements, invasive capacity, toxinogenicity, and innate antibiotic resistance help account for the frequency and success with which it acts as an opportunistic pathogen.

Infections caused by *P. aeruginosa* usually begin with bacterial attachment and superficial colonization of cutaneous or mucosal surfaces and progress to localized bacterial invasion and damage to underlying tissues. The infection may remain anatomically localized or may spread by direct extension to contiguous structures. This process may continue with bloodstream invasion, dissemination, the systemic inflammatory response syndrome (SIRS), multiple-organ dysfunction, and ultimately death. Not only is local infection more likely to occur in immunocompromised hosts (e.g., those with profound neutropenia), it is also more likely to culminate in bloodstream invasion and dissemination in these patients. Both intrinsic and extrinsic virulence factors appear to play roles in the pathogenicity of *P. aeruginosa* (Table 136-2). The organism's 6.3-million base-pair genome has been sequenced in its entirety, and a number of genes with specific regulatory, catabolic, and transport functions have been identified. These findings will undoubtedly increase our understanding of the pathogenicity and virulence of *P. aeruginosa*.

The production and secretion of many of the extracellular virulence factors of *P. aeruginosa* as well as the assembly and maturation of its biofilm are under the regulatory control of a complex cell-to-cell signaling system termed *quorum sensing*. Through lactones and other signal molecules secreted by each individual bacterium, the entire population of *P. aeruginosa* in a biofilm, colonized mucosa, or infected tissue senses its environment, communicates, and discerns its own cell density. This regulatory system may conceivably allow the bacteria to produce extracellular virulence factors in a coordinated manner that depends on cell density and thus may give the pathogen an appreciable advantage over host defense mechanisms.

Some of the exotoxins produced by *P. aeruginosa* (ExoS, ExoT, ExoU, and ExoY) are introduced directly from the bacterial cytosol into the host cell cytoplasm via a complex array of transmembrane proteins that together make up the *type III secretion apparatus*. This

TABLE 136-1 *Factors Predisposing to Pseudomonas aeruginosa Infections*

DISRUPTION OF CUTANEOUS OR MUCOSAL BARRIERS	
Burn injury	Endotracheal intubation
Cystic fibrosis	Indwelling central venous
Dermatitis	catheterization
Penetrating trauma	Urinary bladder catheterization
Surgery	Injection drug use

IMMUNOSUPPRESSION	
Neutropenia	Extremes of age
Qualitative white blood cell defects	Diabetes mellitus
	Steroid therapy
Hypogammaglobulinemia	Cancer
Defective cell-mediated immunity	AIDS

DISRUPTION OF NORMAL BACTERIAL FLORA
Broad-spectrum antibiotic therapy
Exposure to the hospital environment

TABLE 136-2 *Putative Virulence Factors of Pseudomonas aeruginosa*

Virulence Factor	Function(s)
Pili or fimbriae	Attachment to epithelial cells
Mucoid exopolysaccharide (alginate)	Attachment to epithelial cells, inhibition of mucociliary and opsonophagocytic clearance, biofilm formation
Alkaline protease	Tissue breakdown, proteolysis of immunoglobulin and complement
Elastase	Destruction of elastic tissues, including lamina of blood vessels
Phospholipase C (a hemolysin)	Breakdown of lipids and lecithin, tissue necrosis
Lipopolysaccharide (LPS or endotoxin)	Fever, leukocytosis or leukopenia, hypotension, shock; disseminated intravascular coagulation; adult respiratory distress syndrome; systemic inflammatory response syndrome
Exotoxins	
ExoA	Inhibition of protein synthesis through interference with adenosine diphosphate ribosylation of elongation factor-2
ExoS	Ribosylation of guanosine triphosphate binding proteins; disruption of cellular actin cytoskeleton
ExoT	Disruption of cellular actin cytoskeleton
ExoU	Acute cytotoxicity
ExoY	Increase in intracellular cyclic adenosine monophosphate

system requires direct cell contact and allows the injection of virulence factors from the bacterium into host cells without interference from humoral immune defenses.

CLINICAL MANIFESTATIONS AND DIAGNOSIS ■ Respiratory Tract Infections
Primary pneumonia or *nonbacteremic pneumonia* results from the aspiration of upper respiratory tract secretions and often develops in patients with previous antibiotic use who are exposed to the hospital environment, particularly the ICU. It is a common cause of ventilator-associated pneumonia and is noted especially often in patients with chronic lung disease, congestive heart failure, or AIDS. Community-aquired pneumonia due to *P. aeruginosa* is uncommon among normal hosts. Fever, chills, severe dyspnea, cyanosis, productive cough, apprehension, confusion, and other signs of severe systemic toxicity characterize this acute, often life-threatening infection. Chest roentgenograms typically show bilateral bronchopneumonia with nodular infiltrates and small areas of radiolucency; pleural effusions are common; empyema is relatively uncommon; and lobar consolidation is occasionally seen. Cavitary lesions are unusually common among AIDS patients with *P. aeruginosa* pneumonia. Pathologic lesions include alveolar necrosis, focal hemorrhages, and microabscesses.

Bacteremic pneumonia due to *P. aeruginosa* begins as a respiratory infection. However, unlike primary pneumonia, it is typically associated with neutropenia, subsequent bloodstream invasion, and metastatic spread that produces characteristic lesions in the lungs and other viscera. Alveolar hemorrhage and necrosis are common. The signs and symptoms of this fulminant disease include those described for nonbacteremic pneumonia caused by this organism as well as those associated with gram-negative sepsis. Chest roentgenograms characteristically demonstrate a rapid progression from pulmonary vascular congestion to interstitial edema, then to alveolar edema, and finally to diffuse necrotizing bronchopneumonia with cavity formation. The patient typically dies 3 or 4 days after initial presentation.

Chronic infection of the lower respiratory tract with *P. aeruginosa* is caused almost exclusively by mucoid strains that produce alginate and is prevalent among older children and young adults with cystic fibrosis as well as in some patients with bronchiectasis or AIDS. In patients with cystic fibrosis, mucoid strains invariably colonize and infect patients with increasing prevalence over time and contribute to the acute exacerbations and chronic progression that characterize pulmonary disease in these individuals. Airway obstruction appears to begin with bronchiolitis, which causes mucus plugging and predisposes to *P. aeruginosa* infection. The latter produces more mucus plugging, chronic suppuration, bronchiectasis, atelectasis, and ultimately fibrosis. This process progresses to pulmonary insufficiency, hypoxemia, and alterations in cardiopulmonary dynamics resulting in pulmonary hypertension and cor pulmonale.

Clinical manifestations of lower respiratory tract infections due to *P. aeruginosa* in patients with cystic fibrosis vary with the severity and duration of underlying lung disease, the frequency and intensity of acute episodes, and the presence of co-infecting pathogens such as *B. cepacia* (Chap. 241). Early in the disease, patients may experience recurrent upper respiratory symptoms followed by a lingering cough. Episodes of pneumonia develop later, with persistent cough between acute episodes. Eventually, patients exhibit a chronic productive cough, wheezing, diminished appetite, weight loss, growth retardation, and decreased activity. Acute exacerbations are typically accompanied by low-grade fever and heightened respiratory symptoms. Physical signs include evidence of malnutrition, an increase in anteroposterior diameter, intercostal retractions, cyanosis, inspiratory and expiratory wheezing, rhonchi, moist rales, abdominal distention, and clubbing of the fingers and toes. Laboratory abnormalities include leukocytosis with a left shift and hypoxemia with or without hypercarbia. Tests of pulmonary function demonstrate obstructive and restrictive defects. Chest roentgenograms reveal overaeration, patchy atelectasis, peribronchial fibrosis, and patchy infiltrates associated with pneumonia. In more advanced disease, there may be evidence of severe overaeration, depressed diaphragm, further increased anteroposterior diameter, extensive peribronchial infiltration, generalized bronchiectasis, and cyst formation.

Bacteremia *P. aeruginosa* remains an important cause of life-threatening bloodstream infection in immunocompromised patients, particularly those with hematologic malignancies complicated by neutropenia. Bacteremia is frequently iatrogenic and is usually seen in hospitalized patients with various comorbid conditions (Table 136-1). Bloodstream infection may be primary (with no identifiable source) or secondary to a discrete focus of infection. Common primary sites of infection include the urinary and gastrointestinal tracts, lungs, skin and soft tissues, and intravascular foci, including indwelling central venous catheters.

The clinical features of *P. aeruginosa* bacteremia are similar to those of other forms of bacteremia. Fever, tachypnea, tachycardia, and prostration are common. Disorientation, confusion, or obtundation may be evident. Hypotension can progress to refractory shock. Renal failure, adult respiratory distress syndrome, disseminated intravascular coagulation, and other manifestations of SIRS occur as complications.

Pathognomonic skin lesions termed *ecthyma gangrenosum* (Fig. 136-1) develop in a relatively small minority of patients with *P. aeruginosa* bacteremia. The lesions begin as small hemorrhagic vesicles

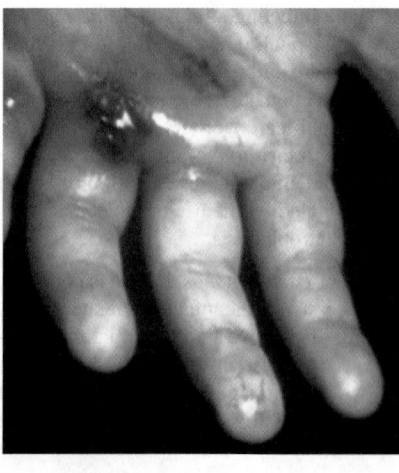

FIGURE 136-1 Ecthyma gangrenosum in a neutropenic patient with *Pseudomonas aeruginosa* bacteremia.

surrounded by a rim of erythema and undergo central necrosis with subsequent ulceration. They occur singly or in small numbers on the perineum, buttocks, and extremities; in the axillae; and elsewhere. Bacterial invasion of blood vessels, documented histologically, is the sine qua non of ecthyma lesions. Bacteria are visible on Gram's staining or are recoverable by culture of aspirated material from lesions.

Endocarditis (See also Chap. 109)　*P. aeruginosa* infects the native heart valves of intravenous drug users as well as prosthetic heart valves. The source of *P. aeruginosa* strains infecting drug users appears to be standing water contaminating drug paraphernalia. Foreign materials mixed with heroin may cause injury to valve leaflets or mural endocardium, with resulting fibrosis and an increased risk for valve infection. Exposure of the tricuspid valve to both trauma and bacteria apparently accounts for the high incidence of tricuspid involvement in association with intravenous drug use.

The tricuspid, pulmonic, mitral, or aortic valve and the mural endocardium of either atrium may be affected in *P. aeruginosa* endocarditis. Multiple-valve infections are common. Tricuspid or right-sided involvement is often associated with septic pulmonary emboli. Right-sided *P. aeruginosa* endocarditis usually presents subacutely, while the appearance of left-sided disease is likely to be more acute or even fulminant. Fever is virtually invariable, and murmurs are usually detectable at initial presentation or shortly thereafter. Septic pulmonary emboli associated with right-sided disease result in cough, pleuritic chest pain, sputum production, pulmonary infiltration (with or without abscess formation), and pleural effusion. Left-sided infections may present as intractable heart failure or large systemic emboli. Mycotic aneurysms, cerebritis, or brain abscess may occur; septic infarcts are occasionally found in the spleen. Skin and soft tissue manifestations, including Janeway lesions, Osler's nodes, and ecthyma gangrenosum, are relatively uncommon.

The diagnosis of *P. aeruginosa* endocarditis is based on positive blood culture in the absence of an extracardiac source; an indication of valvular dysfunction or vegetation on an echocardiogram; evidence of septic pulmonary lesions on a chest roentgenogram (in right-sided disease); and the actual demonstration of infected heart valves at the time of surgery.

Central Nervous System Infections　*P. aeruginosa* infections of the central nervous system include meningitis and brain abscess. These infections follow extension from a contiguous parameningeal structure such as the ear, mastoid, or paranasal sinus; direct inoculation into the subarachnoid space or brain through head trauma, surgery, or diagnostic procedures; or bacteremic spread from infection at a distant site. Like *P. aeruginosa* infections at other anatomical sites, central nervous system infections are documented almost exclusively in patients with compromised local or systemic immune-defense mechanisms. Mortality rates from these infections are high.

The clinical signs of *P. aeruginosa* meningitis, like those of other forms of acute bacterial meningitis, include fever, headache, stiff neck, confusion, and obtundation. The onset of illness may be acute or even fulminant, particularly in bacteremic patients, with a precipitous downhill course, shock, coma, and early death. In nonbacteremic patients, *P. aeruginosa* meningitis or brain abscess may present more insidiously, with a paucity of systemic symptoms. This presentation is especially common in infections resulting from recent neurosurgery, cancer of the head and neck, or direct extension from a parameningeal focus of chronic infection. Occasionally, *P. aeruginosa* meningitis runs a subacute or relapsing course that is thought to be related to the intermittent release of bacteria from a loculated site of infection.

Ear Infections　*P. aeruginosa* is often found in the external auditory canal, particularly under moist conditions and in the presence of inflammation or maceration (as in "swimmer's ear"). Moreover, this organism is the predominant pathogen associated with external otitis, a usually benign inflammatory process affecting the external auditory canal. The ear is painful or merely itchy, there is a purulent discharge, and pain is elicited by pulling on the pinna. The external canal appears edematous and is filled with detritus that often prevents visualization of the tympanic membrane.

P. aeruginosa occasionally penetrates the epithelium overlying the floor of the external auditory canal at the junction between bone and cartilage and invades underlying soft tissue. The ensuing invasive process, which involves soft tissue, cartilage, and cortical bone, is typically slow but destructive. Termed *malignant external otitis*, this condition occurs predominantly in elderly diabetic patients but is reported occasionally in infants with other underlying diseases and rarely in elderly nondiabetic patients. Virtually all cases of malignant external otitis are caused by *P. aeruginosa*. From the external ear, the infection advances to the retromandibular area or parotid space and enters the mastoid air cells and temporal bone. Advancing osteomyelitis at the base of the skull often involves the seventh, ninth, tenth, and eleventh cranial nerves. The cavernous sinus can become involved, as can the contralateral petrous apex. The middle ear is commonly spared; meningitis and brain abscess are relatively rare complications.

Otorrhea and severe otalgia are common presenting symptoms of malignant external otitis. Facial-nerve paralysis tends to occur early, while other cranial-nerve palsies appear later. There may be a loss of hearing. Constitutional symptoms such as fever and weight loss are relatively uncommon. Physical examination almost always reveals remarkable tenderness of the pinna and abnormalities of the external auditory canal, including swelling, erythema, purulent discharge, debris, and granulation tissue in the canal wall. The tympanic membrane is often hidden from view and is sometimes perforated. Inflammation may involve the pinna as well as the periauricular, retromandibular, and mastoid areas.

Peripheral leukocytosis is relatively infrequent in malignant external otitis, while the erythrocyte sedimentation rate (ESR) is usually markedly elevated. Cerebrospinal fluid occasionally exhibits pleocytosis and an elevation in the protein level. Computed tomography (CT) or magnetic resonance imaging (MRI) of the mastoid or temporal bone typically reveals bony erosions and new bone formation, while the floor of the skull may have soft tissue densities associated with areas of cellulitis. In addition, technetium 99m bone scans and gallium 67 scans frequently give positive results. Cultures of samples from the external auditory canal and of surgical specimens are almost always positive for *P. aeruginosa*.

Eye Infections (See also Chap. 25)　*P. aeruginosa* causes bacterial keratitis or corneal ulcer and endophthalmitis in the human eye. Keratitis due to *P. aeruginosa* may result from even minor corneal injury, which interrupts the integrity of the superficial epithelial surface and permits bacterial access to the underlying stroma. Corneal ulcer may complicate contact lens use, particularly when extended-wear soft contact lenses are involved. Contact lens solutions or the lenses themselves may be the source of the organism, which is probably inoculated into the eye at sites of minor lens-induced corneal damage. Patients who have sustained serious burns, have undergone ocular irradiation or tracheostomy, have been exposed to the intensive care environment, and/or are in a coma are also susceptible to *P. aeruginosa*–associated corneal ulcers. Contaminated eye medications are occasionally implicated in these infections. *P. aeruginosa* keratitis usually starts as a small central ulcer; spreads concentrically to involve a large portion of the cornea, sclera, and underlying stroma; and in some cases progresses to posterior corneal perforation.

The clinical manifestations of *P. aeruginosa* keratitis include a rapidly expanding, necrotic stromal infiltrate in the bed of an epithelial injury; surrounding epithelial edema; an anterior chamber reaction; and mucopurulent discharge adherent to the ulcer's surface. Corneal ulcer due to *P. aeruginosa* may advance rapidly to involve the entire cornea in ≤2 days or may evolve subacutely over several days. Systemic symptoms are uncommon. Complications include corneal perforation, anterior chamber involvement, and endophthalmitis.

P. aeruginosa endophthalmitis is typically a rapidly progressive, sight-threatening condition that demands immediate therapeutic intervention. It may complicate penetrating injuries of the eye, intraocular surgery, hematogenous spread from other sites of *Pseudomonas* infection, or posterior perforation of corneal ulcers. Clinical manifestations may include eye pain, conjunctival hyperemia, chemosis, lid edema, decreased visual acuity, hypopyon, severe anterior uveitis, and signs of possible vitreous involvement. Panophthalmitis may result from this intraocular infection.

Bone and Joint Infections   Sternoclavicular pyarthrosis caused by *P. aeruginosa* is often a complication of injection drug use and is rarely associated with *P. aeruginosa* endocarditis. Joint involvement is usually monarticular, with the sternoclavicular joint more often affected than sternochondral joints. Patients present with acute or chronic pain in the anterior chest wall, often associated with fever and restricted movement of the homolateral shoulder. Physical examination reveals tenderness, erythema, and swelling over the affected joint. Leukocytosis is common, and the ESR is almost invariably elevated. Roentgenograms show soft tissue edema, bone demineralization, lytic lesions, and periosteal elevation of the clavicular head, rib, or sternum. Material obtained by arthrocentesis or synovial biopsy yields *P. aeruginosa* in culture.

P. aeruginosa infections of the symphysis pubis are associated with pelvic surgery and injection drug use. The symphysis pubis, like other fibrocartilaginous joints, exhibits a peculiar susceptibility to bloodborne infection with *P. aeruginosa*. Affected patients report pain in the groin, hip, thigh, and/or lower abdomen that is made worse by walking. Fever is variable, and the duration of symptoms before diagnosis ranges from days to months. The ESR is markedly elevated. Roentgenograms or CT scans show irregularities of the pubic margins, separation of the symphysis pubis, and osteomyelitic abnormalities of the pubic rami that may be extensive. Bone scans are usually positive. Needle aspiration or biopsy is necessary to obtain material for culture. A positive culture is particularly important for the discrimination of *P. aeruginosa* infections and other pyogenic infections from osteitis pubis, which is thought to be a noninfectious condition complicating pelvic surgery, childbirth, or trauma.

P. aeruginosa is the most common cause of osteochondritis of the foot following plantar puncture wounds. This infection is seen primarily in children and is usually acquired via the direct inoculation of *P. aeruginosa* that inhabits the moist environment found in the soles of shoes. The organism infects the small joints and bones, including the proximal phalanges, metatarsals, metatarsophalangeal joints, tarsal bones, and calcaneus. On average, local pain and swelling last for several weeks, and systemic symptoms are usually lacking. There may be plantar cellulitis over the involved area or tenderness upon deep palpation. Results of roentgenograms and bone scans are generally positive. Aspiration of the affected joint frequently yields purulent material in which *P. aeruginosa* can be demonstrated by Gram's staining and by culture.

Vertebral osteomyelitis due to *P. aeruginosa* is associated with complicated urinary tract infection, genitourinary instrumentation or surgery, and injection drug use. Vertebral infections that are associated with a urinary tract source most often develop in the elderly and usually affect the lumbosacral spine. Presumably the route of infection in these patients is a shared venous plexus between the pelvis and spine. Drug use–related infections typically occur in younger patients and may affect the cervical or lumbosacral spine. *P. aeruginosa* vertebral osteomyelitis is usually an indolent disease. Accordingly, symptoms may develop weeks or even months before diagnosis. Back or neck pain is generally reported, while fever and systemic symptoms are relatively uncommon. Local tenderness and decreased range of motion of the affected spine are typical. Leukocytosis may be noted, the ESR is almost always markedly elevated, and blood cultures are sometimes positive. Roentgenograms reveal loss of bone density, narrowed intervertebral space, destruction of vertebral end plates, lytic lesions of

vertebral bodies, sclerosis, and possible osteophyte formation. MRI or CT is the most sensitive and specific means of defining lesions. Technetium bone scans and gallium scans usually yield positive results but have lower specificity. An etiologic diagnosis requires the culture of material obtained by needle aspiration or biopsy of the affected spine under fluoroscopic guidance; open biopsy is occasionally needed.

P. aeruginosa is one of the most common causative agents in a variety of other, less specific syndromes involving nonhematogenous infections of bones and joints and collectively referred to as *chronic contiguous osteomyelitis*. These infections may result, for example, from compound fractures, contamination associated with open reduction and fixation of closed fractures, sternotomy performed in conjunction with cardiac surgery, contiguous spread from infected ischemic ulcers related to peripheral vascular disease or diabetes mellitus, and cellulitis in general. The chronicity, indolence, and heterogeneity of these infections explain their varied clinical manifestations and the frequent need for complicated long-term management.

Urinary Tract Infections   *P. aeruginosa* is one of the most common causes of complicated and nosocomial infections of the urinary tract. These infections may result from urinary tract catheterization, instrumentation, surgery (including renal transplantation), or obstruction; they may arise from persistent foci (e.g., the prostate or stones) and may be chronic or recurrent. The urinary tract may be a target for bloodborne infection in patients with *P. aeruginosa* bacteremia but more often is the source of bacteremia. Chronic *P. aeruginosa* infections of the urinary tract are relatively common among patients with indwelling bladder catheters, altered urinary tract anatomy secondary to diversionary procedures, and paraplegia. Chronic or recurrent urinary tract infection caused by *Pseudomonas* often involves multidrug-resistant (MDR) strains.

The clinical features of urinary tract infections due to *P. aeruginosa* are usually indistinguishable from those of other bacterial infections. However, *P. aeruginosa* infections exhibit a propensity for persistence, chronicity, and recurrence. More unusual forms of urinary tract involvement peculiar to *P. aeruginosa* include (1) ulcerative lesions of the renal pelvis, ureters, and bladder that cause sloughing of vesical membranes in the urine; and (2) ecthyma-like lesions of the renal cortex that are seen in association with *Pseudomonas* sepsis.

Skin and Soft Tissue Infections (See also Chap. 110)   As indicated above, *P. aeruginosa* bacteremia may be associated with the disseminated skin lesions of ecthyma gangrenosum (Fig. 136-1). Less common skin manifestations of *P. aeruginosa* sepsis include vesicular or pustular lesions, bullae, subcutaneous nodules, deep abscesses, and cellulitis. Metastatic lesions of the skin or mucous membranes complicate *Pseudomonas* sepsis and occasionally produce massive necrosis or gangrene of the extremities, perineum, face, or oropharynx.

Primary *P. aeruginosa* pyoderma occurs when the skin breaks down secondary to surgery, trauma, burn injury, dermatitis, or ulcers related to peripheral vascular disease or pressure sores. Moist conditions and neutropenia may predispose to this condition. The clinical appearance of primary *P. aeruginosa* pyoderma, which frequently includes hemorrhage and necrosis, resembles that of metastatic *P. aeruginosa* skin lesions. Histologic studies document vascular invasion by bacteria in both diseases. A rare distinguishing feature of *P. aeruginosa* pyoderma is its association with a characteristic fruity odor and an exudate of blue-green hue (due to pyocyanin) that is occasionally noted on dressings or bandages rather than on the wound itself.

P. aeruginosa wound infection complicating extensive third-degree burn injuries typically occurs at least 1 to 2 weeks after the injury and results from colonization of the burn site or burn eschar. Invasion of the subeschar space and underlying dermis, vascular invasion, and systemic spread may occur and are associated with an elevated mortality rate. The development and progression of *P. aeruginosa* burn wound sepsis are facilitated by the injury-associated breakdown of normal skin, selection of antibiotics with inadequate coverage for this pathogen, and burn-related immune defects. Local manifestations include black, dark brown, or violaceous discoloration of the burn eschar; degeneration of underlying granulation tissue, hemorrhage, and premature eschar separation; edema, hemorrhage, and necrosis of skin adjacent to the burn site; and erythematous nodular lesions in unburned skin. Systemic manifestations include fever or hypothermia and other signs of sepsis, SIRS, or multiple-organ system failure. The diagnosis of *P. aeruginosa* burn sepsis is based on these local and systemic clinical manifestations and on a burn wound biopsy that reveals both >10^5 colony-forming units of *P. aeruginosa* per gram of tissue and histologic evidence of bacterial invasion of unburned tissue, vasculitis, or intense inflammation at the burn margin.

P. aeruginosa causes diffuse, pruritic, maculopapular, and vesiculopustular rashes associated with exposure to contaminated hot tubs, spas, whirlpools, and swimming pools. Most cases of *P. aeruginosa* dermatitis have occurred as part of a common-source outbreak. At least two nosocomial common-source outbreaks—one related to a physiotherapy pool—have been reported. Skin rashes may be limited to areas covered by swimsuits or may be more diffuse, sparing only the head and neck. Low-grade fever or other associated symptoms are uncommon. The illness is usually self-limited, and the rash resolves without specific therapy after cessation of exposure. A related benign condition has been reported in children exposed to *P. aeruginosa*–contaminated wading pools. Termed *pseudomonas hot-foot syndrome*, this infection presents with painful nodules on the plantar aspect of the foot.

P. aeruginosa Infections in Patients with AIDS

During the 1980s and 1990s, *P. aeruginosa* infections were increasingly associated with AIDS. The vast majority of these infections are currently seen in patients with advanced AIDS, previous opportunistic infections, and CD4+ lymphocyte counts <100/μL (often <50/μL). The specific immunologic factors that lead to *P. aeruginosa* infections in patients with AIDS are not well understood but are thought to result from a loss of mucosal integrity, defects in cellular and humoral immunity, and qualitative leukocyte abnormalities. Notably, the majority of *P. aeruginosa* infections in this population are community-acquired, in contrast to the nosocomial transmission observed for most infections in non-AIDS patients.

Pneumonia accounts for a substantial proportion of *P. aeruginosa* infections in patients with AIDS. In most instances, pneumonia presents as a necrotizing infection of the pulmonary parenchyma, frequently with cavitary lesions, or as a chronic relapsing bronchopulmonary infection reminiscent of the bronchopulmonary disease seen in patients with cystic fibrosis. Also observed are bloodstream infections, including those associated with indwelling central venous catheters, and infections of the paranasal sinuses, skin and soft tissue, and urinary tract. Bacteremia, either primary or secondary to infection at a remote site, is often recurrent, associated with high mortality, and occasionally accompanied by skin manifestations similar to those seen in non-AIDS patients.

Because *P. aeruginosa* infections occur in patients with advanced AIDS, survival after recovery from the initial infection may be limited to a few months. However, with the widespread use of highly active antiretroviral therapy and the resultant increase in CD4+ cell count, the incidence of *P. aeruginosa* infection among patients with AIDS appears to have declined and the natural history of infection to have been modified. For example, a small number of patients with recalcitrant, relapsing *P. aeruginosa* bronchopulmonary infections have reportedly experienced the resolution of infection soon after initiation of intensive antiretroviral therapy. For those patients infected with HIV that has developed antiretroviral resistance, the risk of *Pseudomonas* infection remains elevated.

Rx TREATMENT

Approach to Therapy Table 136-3 lists antimicrobial agents available in the United States that are generally active against *P. aeruginosa*. Table 136-4 outlines suggested antibiotic choices and an approach to therapy for infections at selected sites. The initial antibiotic selection should take into account the local patterns of antimicrobial susceptibility, and the susceptibilities of the isolate from a particular case should guide definitive antibiotic therapy (see below).

In most severe or life-threatening infections due to *P. aeruginosa*, two antipseudomonal antibiotics to which the infecting strain is (or is likely to be) sensitive should be administered together. The putative benefits of this combined therapy, as determined by in vitro studies, are to increase efficacy, to achieve additive or synergistic killing, and to prevent the emergence of antibiotic resistance. Despite widespread acceptance of combination therapy for *P. aeruginosa* infections, there are few clinical data collected since the advent of newer β-lactam antibiotics to document that combination therapy is in fact more efficacious than monotherapy or that it actually forestalls the acquisition of antimicrobial resistance. Nevertheless, combination therapy continues to be recommended—at least as initial treatment—for most fulminant infections, as outlined in Table 136-4.

The appropriate duration of antibiotic therapy for disease caused by *P. aeruginosa* depends on the type, location, and severity of infection. In general, chronic infections associated with extensive tissue injury, disruption of normal anatomy, foreign or prosthetic material, or suboptimal antibiotic accessibility require therapy for weeks or even months rather than days. More acute infections may be treated aggressively but for shorter periods.

P. aeruginosa infections of the lower respiratory tract in cystic fibrosis pose a special challenge because of their long-standing nature (Chap. 241). In general, antibiotic therapy for acute exacerbations results in short-term clinical improvement, while periodic expectant courses of antimicrobial therapy may limit disease progression. The clinical response to antimicrobial therapy may have little relation to the identity and antimicrobial susceptibility of cultured sputum isolates. A more novel approach to antimicrobial treatment—the use of intermittent, cyclical inhaled tobramycin—has been shown to improve pulmonary function, decrease the risk of hospitalization, and reduce the density of *P. aeruginosa* in sputum of older patients with cystic fibrosis. In addition, lung transplantation has been employed with good results in selected cystic fibrosis patients with severe, progressive lower respiratory tract infections due to *P. aeruginosa*.

Antimicrobial Resistance Antibiotic resistance in *P. aeruginosa* is both intrinsic (as reflected by the relative paucity of antibiotics with inherent activity against wild-type strains) and acquired (as defined by high-level resistance to agents that normally would be expected to exhibit antimicrobial activity). Acquired resistance is rapidly increasing among isolates of *P. aeruginosa*, particularly those associated with cystic fibrosis and with ICUs. Escalating resistance among ICU isolates is especially alarming. Data from NNIS and the Intensive Care Antimicrobial Resistance Epidemiology (ICARE) project on the resistance of *P. aeruginosa* between 1998 and 2002 show that the pooled mean figures for resistance to piperacillin, ceftazidime, imipenem, and ciprofloxacin increased from previous years and represented 14.3, 10.5, 13.7, and 28.9% of ICU-associated isolates, respectively. Factors responsible for this increase may include the expanding use of immunosuppressive therapies, the increased severity of illness in hospitalized patients, inadequate infection-control procedures, and growing antibiotic use. Resistant organisms can be transmitted directly to patients from the hospital staff, other patients, or the environment, or they may arise de novo during therapy with any given agent. The emergence of MDR strains has been associated with increases in secondary bacteremia and mortality and has led in some cases to longer hospital stays and increased hospitalization costs. Therapy for resistant *P. aeruginosa* infections should consist of antimicrobial agents selected on the basis of extended susceptibility testing and may involve increased treatment duration as well as surgical drainage or removal of infected tissues. Infections due to strains resistant to all commonly available antimicrobial agents may respond to parenteral or inhaled therapy with the relatively toxic antibiotics polymyxin B and colistin.

TABLE 136-3 *Antimicrobial Agents Active Against Pseudomonas aeruginosa and Available in the United States*

Agent	Dose,[a] Route	Comments
ANTIPSEUDOMONAL PENICILLINS		
Piperacillin	3–4 g q4–6h IV	Drugs in class are listed in order of decreasing in
Piperacillin/tazobactam	3.375 g q4h IV	vitro activity. Piperacillin/tazobactam or ticarcil-
Mezlocillin	3 g q4h IV	lin/clavulanate has little more activity against *P.*
Ticarcillin	3 g q3–6h IV	*aeruginosa* than piperacillin or ticarcillin alone.
Ticarcillin/clavulanate	3.1 g q4–6h IV	Monotherapy should not be used for serious infections.
ANTIPSEUDOMONAL CEPHALOSPORINS		
Ceftazidime[b]	2 g q8–12h IV	Use more frequent indicated doses for CNS infec-
Cefoperazone[b]	2 g q6h IV	tions or infections in neutropenic or severely im-
Cefepime	2 g q8–12h IV	munocompromised patients. The antipseudomonal activity of cefepime is equivalent to that of cefta-zidime, with less potential for β-lactamase induction in gram-negative enteric bacteria.
CARBAPENEMS[b,c]		
Imipenem/cilastatin	0.5 g q6h IV	Class is active against strains producing β-lacta-
Meropenem	1 g q8h IV	mases. Imipenem may cause seizures in patients with renal failure (avoid by reducing dose) or CNS infections or lesions. Meropenem is slightly more active in vitro against *P. aeruginosa* than imipenem.
MONOBACTAMS		
Aztreonam	2 g q6–8h IV	Drug can usually be administered to patients with β-lactam hypersensitivity.
AMINOGLYCOSIDES[b]		
Tobramycin	MD: 2 mg/kg load, then 1.7 mg/kg q8h IV ODD: 5–7 mg/kg q24h IV	Tobramycin has greater in vitro activity against *P. aeruginosa* than gentamicin, but the drugs' clini-
Gentamicin	MD: Same as tobramycin ODD: Same as tobramycin	cal efficacies are probably equivalent. Some *P. aeruginosa* isolates that are resistant to tobramy-cin or gentamicin may be susceptible to amikacin.
Amikacin	MD: 7.5 mg/kg load, then 7.5 mg/kg q12h IV ODD: 15 mg/kg q24h IV	Except in urinary tract infection, this class should not be used for monotherapy. ODD may reduce adverse effects. Serum levels must be monitored.
FLUOROQUINOLONES[b,d]		
Ciprofloxacin	0.4 g q12h IV or 0.5–0.75 g bid PO	Ciprofloxacin is the most active of the available quinolones against *P. aeruginosa*. Serum levels
Levofloxacin	0.75 g q24h IV or PO	attained with oral therapy approximate those after IV therapy; thus oral formulations are useful for long-duration therapy in selected patients.
OTHER AGENTS		
Polymyxin B	0.75–1.25 mg/kg q12h IV	These drugs are reserved for use in multidrug-resis-
Colistin	1.5 mg/kg q8h IV	tant infections. Nephrotoxicity and neurotoxicity occur. Colistin inhalational therapy consists of 75 mg in 3 mL of normal saline via nebulizer, given twice daily.

[a] Indicated dosages are for the treatment of infections due to *P. aeruginosa* in adults. Doses should be adjusted in renal insufficiency. Higher doses may be required in patients with cystic fibrosis, and lower doses may be adequate for the treatment of uncomplicated urinary tract infections.

[b] Some strains of *P. aeruginosa* may rapidly develop resistance to these agents during therapy.

[c] Ertapenem, an additional drug in this class, has less in vitro activity and should not be used for the treatment of *Pseudomonas* infections.

[d] Trovafloxacin, an additional fluoroquinolone with antipseudomonal activity, has limited usefulness because of its hepatotoxicity. Gatifloxacin and moxifloxacin have in vitro activity against *P. aeruginosa* (albeit less than ciprofloxacin and levofloxacin), but there are no clinical studies to support their use in *Pseudomonas* or nosocomial infections.

Abbreviations: MD, multidose; ODD, once-daily dosing; CNS, central nervous system.

INFECTIONS CAUSED BY OTHER *PSEUDOMONAS* SPECIES AND RELATED BACTERIA

Burkholderia cepacia Like *P. aeruginosa*, *B. cepacia* is primarily an opportunistic pathogen that is implicated in both sporadic endemic infections and occasional nosocomial outbreaks. *B. cepacia* is actually a complex of closely related bacteria, and the species is now divided into nine distinct genomovars based on molecular sequencing and biochemical analysis. Hospital epidemics are most frequently associated with a liquid reservoir or a moist environmental surface. Colonization by this organism precedes infection, and distinction between the two is often difficult. *B. cepacia* has been reported to cause pneumonia, urinary tract infections, meningitis, peritonitis, surgical and burn wound infections, bacteremia, and endocarditis related to injection drug use. In addition, *B. cepacia* has been implicated as a cause of chronic lower respiratory tract infections in patients with chronic granulomatous disease, in patients with sickle cell hemoglobinopathies, and—together with *P. aeruginosa*—in patients with cystic fibrosis. For cystic fibrosis patients, chronic *B. cepacia* respiratory infection (especially that involving genomovar III) is of special concern, as it portends an unusually rapid decline in pulmonary function and a poor clinical prognosis. Moreover, in some patients with cystic fibrosis, *B. cepacia* has been associated with fulminant necrotizing pneumonia, bacteremia, and a rapid downhill course.

Rx TREATMENT

The treatment of *B. cepacia* infections typically is complicated by intrinsic resistance of the organism to several antimicrobial drugs, including many β-lactam agents, the aminoglycosides, colistin, and polymyxin B. Trimethoprim-sulfamethoxazole (TMP-SMX; 15 to 20 mg/kg per day for patients with normal renal function) is preferred for the treatment of *B. cepacia* infections, although acquired resistance to this agent has been reported. Carbapenems, third-generation cephalosporins, fluoroquinolones, minocycline, and chloramphenicol may offer activity against sensitive strains. For infections with MDR strains or those not responding to a single antibiotic, combinations of agents may display in vitro synergy and clinical efficacy. Some cystic fibrosis centers segregate patients infected with *B. cepacia* in an attempt to reduce horizontal transmission to uninfected patients. In addition, many centers consider lung transplantation contraindicated in patients with chronic infection due to genomovar III because of an unacceptably high mortality rate following surgery.

Stenotrophomonas maltophilia A ubiquitous free-living opportunistic bacterium, *S. maltophilia* has emerged as an important pathogen among hospitalized patients, particularly at cancer centers and in ICUs. Most infections are sporadic; however, nosocomial outbreaks of *S. maltophilia* infection have been linked to contaminated respiratory and inhalational equipment and water faucets. As with *P. aeruginosa* and *B. cepacia*, infection can be difficult to discriminate from colonization. Risk factors for either include prolonged hospitalization, malignancy, chemotherapy-induced mucositis and neutropenia, instrumentation (e.g., urinary, peritoneal, and central venous catheterization), and prior administration of broad-spectrum antibiotics. Intrinsic antibiotic resistance of *S. maltophilia*, based on both low outer-membrane permeability and inducible β-lactamases, is at least partly responsible for the emergence of this organism as a nosocomial pathogen under the selective pressure of antibiotic treatment.

Anatomical Site or Diagnosis	Preferred Therapy[a,b]	Alternative Therapy[a,b]	Comments
Bacteremia, endocarditis, wound infections, or pneumonia	Antipseudomonal penicillin *plus* aminoglycoside	Antipseudomonal penicillin *plus* ciprofloxacin (IV) *or* Antipseudomonal cephalosporin, aztreonam, or carbapenem *plus* aminoglycoside *or* ciprofloxacin (IV)	Bacteremia due to infection of an indwelling central venous catheter usually necessitates catheter removal. Monotherapy with an antipseudomonal penicillin, cephalosporin, carbapenem, or fluoroquinolone may be acceptable for patients without neutropenia, concomitant *Pseudomonas* pneumonia, septic shock, or life-threatening co-morbidity. Endocarditis: Use highest indicated doses from Table 136-3. MD is preferable to ODD for aminoglycosides. Serum aminoglycoside levels should be 10 times the MBC for the isolate. Valve replacement is often required. Wounds: Debridement is required. Pneumonia: Combination therapy should initially be employed for severe pneumonia if *P. aeruginosa* is highly suspected or confirmed by culture. Repeated or prolonged therapy may be required in patients with AIDS. Inhalational therapy for cystic fibrosis: Give 300 mg of tobramycin inhalation solution (TOBI) q12h via jet nebulizer.
Central nervous system	Ceftazidime *plus or minus* aminoglycoside	Cefepime[c] or ciprofloxacin (IV)[c] or aztreonam[c] or meropenem[c]	Aminoglycosides should be administered intrathecally for central nervous system infections not responding to initial IV therapy. Brain abscesses >2 cm in diameter require drainage.
Bone and joint	Antipseudomonal penicillin *plus* either aminoglycoside or ciprofloxacin	Antipseudomonal cephalosporin *or* aztreonam *or* fluoroquinolone *or* carbapenem	A 4- to 6-week course of therapy is often suggested. Limited data suggest that prolonged therapy with an oral fluoroquinolone may be equivalent to IV administration. Surgical debridement is often required for osteomyelitis that is chronic or associated with trauma, direct inoculation of bone, or extension from adjacent tissues.
Malignant external otitis	Antipseudomonal cephalosporin *or* carbapenem *or* ciprofloxacin (IV or PO)	Antipseudomonal penicillin or cephalosporin *plus* aminoglycoside	Surgical debridement is usually required. At least 4–6 weeks of therapy is suggested. Oral ciprofloxacin can be used with close follow-up for limited disease or after initial IV therapy.
Eye			
Keratitis and corneal ulcer	Tobramycin (14 mg/mL, topical solution[d]) *plus or minus* piperacillin or ticarcillin (6–12 mg/mL topical solution[d])	Ciprofloxacin *or* ofloxacin (0.3% topical solution[d])	Fortified aminoglycoside eyedrops require pharmacy preparation. Systemic antibiotics are reserved for severe infections with impending perforation or extension beyond the cornea (see endophthalmitis). If combination therapy is used, the second agent should be administered at least 5 min after the first.
Endophthalmitis	Same as for corneal ulcer above *plus* intravitreal amikacin (0.4 mg in 0.1 mL) *or* ceftazidime (2.25 mg in 0.1 mL)	Same as for corneal ulcer above *plus* intravitreal amikacin (0.4 mg in 0.1 mL) *or* ceftazidime (2.25 mg in 0.1 mL)	Surgical vitrectomy is usually indicated. Addition of systemic therapy with ceftazidime or an antipseudomonal penicillin plus ciprofloxacin or an aminoglycoside and subconjunctival injection of an intravitreal agent may be beneficial.
Urinary tract	Ciprofloxacin (PO or IV)	Aminoglycoside, *or* antipseudomonal penicillin or cephalosporin, *or* carbapenem	Relieve obstructions and remove foreign bodies (e.g., chronic urinary catheters and stones). Monotherapy is usually sufficient.
Dermatitis or folliculitis	None	None	Diffuse folliculitis related to spas, whirlpools, or hot tubs does not require therapy in normal hosts.

[a] Susceptibility testing should be performed on all significant *Pseudomonas* isolates in order to direct definitive therapy. Empirical antibiotic therapy for suspected *Pseudomonas* infections should take into account the institution's antimicrobial susceptibility patterns.

[b] Dosages for individual agents from each antimicrobial class are listed in Table 136-3.

[c] Clinical experience is limited for treatment of this infection with this agent. Addition of a second antipseudomonal agent is advised.

[d] 1 drop q5min X 1 h, then q15–30min for 24–48 h; frequency can then be gradually decreased.

Abbreviations: MD, multidose; ODD, once-daily dosing; MBC, minimal bactericidal concentration.

S. maltophilia has most commonly been associated with pneumonia but also causes bacteremia, urinary tract infection, wound infection, peritonitis, cholangitis, meningitis, and (rarely) endocarditis. Acute *S. maltophilia* pneumonia, an uncommon but devastating disease associated with bacteremia, is usually seen in debilitated patients in ICUs. Bacteremia is most often related to central venous catheter infection, although it may arise secondary to any focal *S. maltophilia* infection.

℞ TREATMENT

TMP-SMX is the drug of choice for the treatment of most *S. maltophilia* infections. Other agents include ticarcillin/clavulanate, minocycline, or doxycycline, either alone or in combination with TMP-SMX. The third-generation cephalosporins cefoperazone and ceftazidime and the fluoroquinolones are occasionally active against *S. maltophilia*, but in vitro susceptibility data may not reflect the clin-

ical efficacy of these agents. The aminoglycosides and carbapenems are almost always inactive. Indwelling catheters or appliances that are associated with infection should be removed.

Melioidosis ■ *ETIOLOGY AND EPIDEMIOLOGY* Infections caused by *B. pseudomallei* (formerly *P. pseudomallei*) constitute a broad spectrum of acute and chronic, local and systemic, clinical and subclinical disease processes collectively called *melioidosis*. *B. pseudomallei* and the infections it causes are found mainly in the tropics and are endemic in Southeast Asia, northern Australia, and—to a lesser extent—southern Asia and southern China. Melioidosis is sometimes seen outside of these regions, however, in immigrants or travelers arriving from endemic areas.

B. pseudomallei is a free-living, small, motile, aerobic gram-negative bacillary saprophyte normally found in soil, ponds, and rice paddies and on produce from endemic areas. It is occasionally a pathogen for animals, but zoonotic transmission to humans is rare. Humans contract the disease during contact with *B. pseudomallei*–contaminated soil or water through exposure of abraded skin, percutaneous inoculation, nasal instillation, inhalation, or possibly ingestion. Unlike *B. cepacia*, *B. pseudomallei* does not cause colonization without infection and is only rarely transmitted from person to person. *B. pseudomallei* is listed as a category B biological agent by the Centers for Disease Control and Prevention (CDC) because of its potential to cause considerable morbidity and mortality if deliberately disseminated as a weapon of mass destruction.

MANIFESTATIONS Melioidosis presents in different forms. The infection may be acute, subacute, or chronic. High rates of seropositivity in endemic areas such as Vietnam, Thailand, and Malaysia suggest that many infections are clinically inapparent. The occasional diagnosis based solely on abnormal routine chest roentgenography represents asymptomatic pneumonitis. Acute pulmonary infections are the most common manifestation of melioidosis and may result from hematogenous spread or originate in the respiratory tract; these infections vary from mild bronchitis to extensive necrotizing pneumonia. Their onset may be sudden or gradual. Fever, rigors, productive cough, and marked tachypnea are common. More chronic pulmonary infections may present as productive cough, hemoptysis, and indolent fever with night sweats mimicking tuberculosis. Chest roentgenograms typically reveal upper-lobe infiltrates, occasionally with thin-walled cavities. Another common manifestation of melioidosis is an acute, localized skin infection with ulceration or abscess that is associated with nodular lymphangitis and regional lymphadenitis. Melioidosis may also present as suppurative parotitis, particularly in children. More rarely, *B. pseudomallei* may cause liver or splenic abscesses, septic arthritis, osteomyelitis, or genitourinary or central nervous system infection. Recrudescent disease arising from inactive sites of infection and perhaps triggered by intercurrent illness or other events may present in an acute or chronic form.

Either acute suppurative infections or pulmonary disease may give rise to hematogenous dissemination and the acute septicemic form of melioidosis. This progression is more likely in chronically debilitated patients, such as those with diabetes mellitus, chronic renal disease, or alcoholism. Septicemic patients may present with severe tachypnea, confusion, headache, pharyngitis, diarrhea, and pustular lesions of the head, trunk, and extremities. The skin may be flushed or cyanotic, signs of meningitis or arthritis may be apparent, the liver and spleen may be enlarged, and muscle tenderness may be striking. Chest roentgenograms show diffuse nodular densities that may expand, coalesce, and finally cavitate. The acute septicemic form of melioidosis usually follows a rapid downhill course, ending in early death. Mortality rates remain high despite optimal therapy.

DIAGNOSIS The diagnosis of melioidosis should be entertained when a febrile patient who has been in an endemic area presents with an acute lower respiratory tract illness, parotitis, lymphadenitis, or unusual skin or subcutaneous lesions or has a chest roentgenogram suggesting tuberculosis in the absence of sputum-associated tubercle bacilli. An etiologic diagnosis is suggested by the microscopic demonstration in exudate material of small, bipolar, irregularly staining, gram-negative rods with a characteristic "safety-pin" appearance and is confirmed by a culture positive for *B. pseudomallei* and/or a fourfold or greater rise in the titer of serum antibody to the organism.

℞ TREATMENT

The mainstay of treatment for melioidosis is antibiotic administration combined with appropriate surgical drainage of abscesses and aggressive support for patients with septicemic forms of the disease. The guidelines for antibiotic therapy are somewhat imprecise. Ceftazidime or carbapenems such as imipenem or meropenem appear to be the agents of choice for clinical disease, including severe infections. TMP-SMX, cefotaxime, and amoxicillin/clavulanate are possible alternatives. Fluoroquinolones are not active against *B. pseudomallei* and

have no role in the treatment of melioidosis. Combination therapy with ceftazidime or imipenem plus TMP-SMX may be indicated in severe forms of melioidosis, including septicemia. Unfortunately, the increasing resistance of many strains of *B. pseudomallei* to TMP-SMX, particularly in Southeast Asia, is of concern. Patients with acute pulmonary infections who are treated with either ceftazidime or carbapenems should receive antibiotics until they show definite evidence of clinical improvement (often in 10 to 30 days), at which time they can be switched to oral maintenance or eradication therapy with a combination of chloramphenicol, TMP-SMX, and doxycycline or with the single agent amoxicillin/clavulanate for 12 to 20 weeks. Chronic disease associated with persistently positive sputum cultures and extrapulmonary suppurative disease may require treatment for up to 1 year.

Glanders ■ *ETIOLOGY AND EPIDEMIOLOGY* Glanders is primarily a systemic equine disease that is caused by *B. mallei*. Once widespread, glanders was eradicated from North America in 1938 through the extensive culling of infected or exposed horses. The disease still occurs sporadically, however, in Africa, Asia, and South America. Historically, glanders was occasionally transmitted to humans during close contact with infected horses, mules, or donkeys. *B. mallei* is believed to have been used deliberately as an agent of biological warfare during World War I, an effort resulting in the infection of large numbers of Russian horses and mules. Research on *B. mallei* as an agent of biological warfare may have continued into more recent times, including work to develop an antibiotic-resistant aerosolized form of the bacterium. The first human case of glanders since 1949 was reported in the United States in 2001 and was acquired through laboratory exposure to *B. mallei* during the course of research on defense against agents of biological warfare and terrorism. Like *B. pseudomallei*, *B. mallei* has been classified by the CDC as a category B biological agent.

MANIFESTATIONS Glanders can assume the following forms in humans: acute localized suppurative infection, acute pulmonary infection, acute septicemic infection, and chronic suppurative infection. Disease develops several days or weeks after the inoculation of *B. mallei* into the skin, usually of the hand or arm. A localized skin nodule or suppurative focus is associated with regional lymphadenitis, fever, malaise, and prostration. Mucous membrane infection results in the production of a mucopurulent discharge from the eye, nose, or lips, with the subsequent development of granulomatous ulcers. Inhalation of the organism is accompanied by the typical symptoms and signs of pneumonia. The acute septicemic form of the infection may follow local infection and is characterized by signs of sepsis frequently associated with shock and multiorgan system failure. Evidence of acute *B. mallei* dissemination may include lymphadenopathy, splenomegaly, lung abscesses, lobar consolidation, liver and splenic abscesses, and a diffuse papular or pustular eruption resembling smallpox. Mortality rates from septicemic and acute disseminated disease are high. Chronic suppurative glanders presents as multiple subcutaneous, intramuscular, and visceral abscesses. Any form of glanders could follow aerosolized dissemination of the organism—e.g., in a bioterrorist event.

DIAGNOSIS The diagnosis of glanders may be suggested by the epidemiology and clinical setting of the infection together with evidence of irregularly staining, small, bipolar, gram-negative rods in suppurative exudates. *B. mallei* can be cultured and identified with standard bacteriologic media but may be misidentified as *Pseudomonas fluorescens* or *P. putida* by automated identification systems. Molecular methods, such as 16S rRNA gene sequencing, can be used for rapid identification of *B. mallei* from culture and can discriminate this organism from closely related organisms, including *B. pseudomallei*. A single high titer of serum antibody or a fourfold increase in titer suggests recent infection. A diagnosis of glanders in the absence of close contact with an infected equine should raise suspicion regarding the deliberate, bioterrorism-related dissemination of *B. mallei*.

Rx TREATMENT

Treatment of glanders includes appropriate supportive measures for sepsis and the surgical drainage of abscesses. Optimal antimicrobial therapy for glanders has not been adequately defined because of a lack of human infections in the antibiotic era. Ceftazidime, gentamicin, imipenem, doxycycline, and ciprofloxacin all have in vitro activity against *B. mallei*. A recent laboratory-acquired case of human glanders responded to a combination of imipenem and doxycycline, and experimental glanders in primates responds to a combination of sulfamonomethoxine (not available in the United States) and trimethoprim. It has been suggested that rational therapy for glanders should consist of the same antibiotics recommended for the treatment of melioidosis, with the specific agent chosen on the basis of in vitro susceptibility testing. As in melioidosis, long-term antimicrobial therapy is probably necessary. The antimicrobial susceptibilities of *B. mallei* organisms disseminated in the context of bioterrorism or biowarfare may not be predictable, given the possibility of bioengineered antimicrobial resistance.

Other Species *P. fluorescens* occasionally causes human disease; it is implicated particularly often in infections related to the administration of contaminated (stored) blood products and in pseudoinfections. Additional bacterial species that are associated only rarely with human infections include *P. putida*, *Pseudomonas luteola*, *Pseudomonas stutzeri*, *Pseudomonas alcaligenes*, *Pseudomonas pseudoalcaligenes*, and (all formerly *Pseudomonas* species) *Burkholderia gladioli*, *Burkholderia pickettii*, *Comamonas acidovorans*, *Comamonas testosteroni*, *Brevundimonas diminuta*, and *Brevundimonas vesicularis*.

FURTHER READING

ACHARYA A, PATERSON DL: *Pseudomonas aeruginosa*, in *Antimicrobial Therapy and Vaccines*, 2d ed, VL Yu et al (eds). New York, Apple Trees Productions, 2002, pp 549–562

BALTCH AL, SMITH RP (eds): *Pseudomonas aeruginosa Infections and Treatment*. New York, Marcel Dekker, 1994

MORRISON AF, WENZEL RP: Epidemiology of infections due to *Pseudomonas aeruginosa*. Rev Infect Dis 6(Suppl):S267, 1984

NEUHAUSER MM et al: Antibiotic resistance among gram-negative bacilli in US intensive care units: Implications for fluoroquinolone use. JAMA 289: 885, 2003

OHL CA, POLLACK M: *Pseudomonas aeruginosa* and related bacteria, in *Infectious Diseases*, 3d ed, SL Gorbach et al (eds). New York, Lippincott Williams & Wilkins, 2004, pp 1703–1717

SHEPP DH et al: Serious *Pseudomonas aeruginosa* infection in AIDS. J Acquir Immun Defic Syndr 7:823, 1994

SIMPSON AJ et al: Comparison of imipenem and ceftazidime as therapy for severe melioidosis. Clin Infect Dis 29:381, 1999

SMITH RS, IGLEWSKI BH: *P. aeruginosa* quorum-sensing systems and virulence. Curr Opin Microbiol 6:56, 2003

VARTIVARIAN S, ANAISSIE E: *Stenotrophomonas maltophilia* and *Burkholderia cepacia*, in *Principles and Practice of Infectious Diseases*, 5th ed, GL Mandell et al (eds). New York, Churchill Livingstone, 2000, pp 2335–2339

WHITE NJ: Melioidosis. Lancet 361:1715, 2003

137 SALMONELLOSIS
Cammie F. Lesser, Samuel I. Miller

Salmonellae constitute a genus of more than 2300 serotypes that are highly adapted for growth in both humans and animals and that cause a wide spectrum of disease. The growth of *S. typhi* and *S. paratyphi* is restricted to human hosts, in whom these organisms cause enteric (typhoid) fever. The remainder of *Salmonella* serotypes, referred to as nontyphoidal *Salmonella*, can colonize the gastrointestinal tracts of a broad range of animals, including mammals, reptiles, birds, and insects. More than 200 of these serotypes are pathogenic to humans, in whom they often cause gastroenteritis and can also be associated with localized infections and/or bacteremia.

ETIOLOGY Salmonellae make up a large genus of gram-negative bacilli within the family Enterobacteriaceae. In 1983, more than 2000 bacterial strains exhibiting a high degree of DNA similarity among their genomes were grouped into one species, *S. choleraesuis*. This species was further divided into seven subgroups based on host range specificity and additional DNA similarity. Almost all the strains pathogenic for humans are in subgroup 1 (*enterica* or *choleraesuis*) except for those causing rare infections [subgroups 3a (*S. arizonae*) and 3b]. The nomenclature of this large species is quite complex. For example, the correct taxonomic name for the organism that causes enteric fever is *Salmonella choleraesuis* ssp. *choleraesuis* (or subgroup 1), serovar *typhi*. A simplified system is commonly used in which the species name that predated the reclassification is accepted. For example, *S. choleraesuis* ssp. *choleraesuis*, serovar *typhi*, is referred to by its common name, *S. typhi*.

The initial identification of *Salmonella* in the clinical microbiology laboratory is based on growth characteristics. Salmonellae, like other Enterobacteriaceae, produce acid on glucose fermentation, reduce nitrates, and do not produce cytochrome oxidase. They are facultatively anaerobic and do not form spores. In addition, all salmonellae except *S. gallinarum-pullorum* are motile by means of peritrichous flagella, and all but *S. typhi* produce gas (H_2S) on sugar fermentation. Notably, only 1% of clinical isolates ferment lactose; a high level of suspicion must be maintained to detect these rare clinical lactose-fermenting isolates.

The genus *Salmonella* can be further divided into serovars based on the detection of three major antigenic determinants: the somatic O antigen [lipopolysaccharide (LPS) cell-wall components], the surface Vi antigen (restricted to *S. typhi* and *S. paratyphi* C), and the flagellar H antigen. In general, clinical laboratories initially divide *Salmonella* into serogroups (A, B, C_1, C_2, D, and E) based on reactivity to somatic O-antigen antisera. These initial groupings provide only limited clinical information since there is a high degree of cross-reactivity. Additional biochemical and serologic tests are needed to identify specific serotypes. Bacteriophage typing, plasmid profile determination, and pulsed-field gel electrophoresis analyses are used to determine whether a specific *Salmonella* strain within a serovar is responsible for an outbreak.

PATHOGENESIS All *Salmonella* infections begin with ingestion of organisms in contaminated food or water. The infectious dose of *Salmonella* varies from 10^3 to 10^6 colony-forming units. This variability probably reflects the ability of salmonellae to resist the low pH of the stomach—a powerful component of host defense. Conditions that decrease stomach acidity (an age of <1 year, antacid ingestion, or achlorhydric disease) or conditions that decrease intestinal integrity (inflammatory bowel disease, history of gastrointestinal surgery, or alteration of the intestinal flora by antibiotic administration) increase susceptibility to *Salmonella* infection.

Once salmonellae reach the small intestines, the bacteria again encounter numerous host defenses, including bile salts, lysozyme, complement, and cationic antimicrobial peptides—all components of the host's innate immune response. The salmonellae next penetrate the mucous layer of the gut and subsequently traverse the intestinal layer through phagocytic microfold (M) cells that reside within Peyer's patches. Salmonellae can also trigger the formation of membrane ruffles in normally nonphagocytic epithelial cells. These ruffles reach out and enclose adherent bacteria within large vesicles by a process referred to as *bacteria-mediated endocytosis* (BME). BME is dependent on the direct delivery of *Salmonella* proteins into the cytoplasm of epithelial cells by a specialized bacterial secretion system (*type III secretion*). These bacterial proteins mediate alterations in the actin cytoskeleton that are required for *Salmonella* uptake.

After crossing the epithelial layer of the small intestine, *S. typhi* and *S. paratyphi*, which cause enteric (typhoid) fever, are phagocytosed by macrophages. Once internalized, the salmonellae are protected from polymorphonuclear leukocytes (PMNs), the complement system, and the acquired immune response (antibodies). However, these bacteria must survive the antimicrobial environment of the macrophage, which includes the production of reactive oxygen and nitrogen species, antimicrobial peptides, and hydrolytic enzymes. Environmental signals within the macrophage trigger alterations in regulatory systems of the phagocytosed bacteria. The best-characterized regulatory system is PhoP/PhoQ, a two-component regulon that senses changes in bacterial location and alters bacterial protein expression. For example, PhoP/PhoQ triggers the expression of outer-membrane proteins and mediates modifications in LPS so that the bacteria's outer surface can resist microbicidal activities and potentially alter host cell signaling. In addition, salmonellae encode a second type III secretion system that directly delivers bacterial proteins from the phagosome into the macrophage cytoplasm. This secretion system is essential for survival within macrophages.

Once phagocytosed, salmonellae disseminate throughout the body in macrophages via the lymphatics and colonize reticuloendothelial tissues (liver, spleen, lymph nodes, and bone marrow). Patients have relatively few or no signs and symptoms during this initial incubation stage. Signs and symptoms, including fever and abdominal pain, probably result from secretion of cytokines by macrophages when a critical number of organisms have replicated. For example, the development of hepatosplenomegaly is likely to be related to the recruitment of mononuclear cells and the development of a cell-mediated immune response to *S. typhi* colonization. The recruitment of additional mononuclear cells and lymphocytes to Peyer's patches during the several weeks after initial colonization/infection can result in marked enlargement and necrosis of the Peyer's patches.

In contrast to enteric fever, which is characterized by an infiltration of mononuclear cells into the small-bowel mucosa, nontyphoidal *Salmonella* gastroenteritis is characterized by massive PMN infiltration into both the large- and the small-bowel mucosa. This response appears to depend on the induction of interleukin (IL) 8, a strong neutrophil chemotactic factor, which is secreted by intestinal cells. The degranulation and release of toxic substances by neutrophils may result in damage to the intestinal mucosa, causing the inflammatory diarrhea observed with nontyphoidal gastroenteritis.

It is not yet known why *S. typhi* and *S. paratyphi* cause systemic disease and are host restricted, whereas the vast majority of pathogenic *Salmonella* strains cause gastroenteritis in a broad range of hosts. Recently generated genome sequences show that *S. typhi* contains more than 200 pseudogenes, which appear to be functional genes in *S. typhimurium*. These pseudogenes may have been dispensable for *S. typhi* growth in humans.

ENTERIC (TYPHOID) FEVER

Typhoid fever is a systemic disease characterized by fever and abdominal pain caused by dissemination of *S. typhi* or *S. paratyphi*. The disease was initially called *typhoid fever* because of its clinical similarity to typhus. However, in the early 1800s, typhoid fever was clearly defined pathologically as a unique illness on the basis of its association with enlarged Peyer's patches and mesenteric lymph nodes. In 1869, given the anatomical site of infection, the term *enteric fever* was proposed as an alternative designation to distinguish typhoid fever from typhus. However, to this day, the two designations are used interchangeably.

EPIDEMIOLOGY   In contrast to other *Salmonella* serotypes, the etiologic agents of enteric fever—*S. typhi* and *S. paratyphi*—have no known hosts other than humans. Thus, enteric fever is transmitted only

through close contact with acutely infected individuals or chronic carriers. While direct person-to-person transmission through the fecal-oral route has been documented, it is quite rare. Rather, most cases of disease result from ingestion of contaminated food or water. Health care workers occasionally acquire enteric fever after exposure to infected patients, while laboratory workers can acquire the disease after laboratory accidents.

Over the past four decades, with the advent of improvements in food handling and water/sewage treatment, enteric fever has become a rare occurrence in developed nations. Over the past 10 years, ~400 cases of typhoid fever and even fewer cases of paratyphoid fever have been reported annually in the United States. In contrast, enteric fever continues to be a global health problem, with an estimated 13 to 17 million cases worldwide resulting in ~600,000 deaths per year. Children <1 year of age appear to be most susceptible to initial infection and to the development of severe disease.

Enteric fever is endemic in most developing regions, especially the Indian subcontinent, South and Central America, and Asia, and is related to rapid population growth, increased urbanization, inadequate human waste treatment, limited water supply, and overburdened health care systems. These conditions most likely account for the recent epidemics of typhoid fever in Eastern Europe. Antibiotic resistance among salmonellae is also a rising concern and has been linked to antibiotic use in livestock. Many *S. typhi* strains contain plasmids encoding resistance to chloramphenicol, ampicillin, and trimethoprim—antibiotics that have long been used to treat enteric fever. In addition, resistance to ciprofloxacin, either chromosomally or plasmid encoded, has been observed in Asia (India and Vietnam). Morbidity and mortality are increased in outbreaks associated with antibiotic-resistant strains, presumably because of inadequate or delayed treatment.

The high worldwide prevalence of enteric fever serves as a reservoir for cases in the United States. More than 70% of U.S. cases are related to international travel within 30 days before onset. Only 3% of travelers diagnosed with enteric fever give a history of vaccination against *S. typhi* within the previous 2 years. Of U.S. cases of internationally acquired enteric fever, 80% can be linked to travel in six countries: Mexico (28%), India (25%), the Philippines (10%), Pakistan (8%), El Salvador (5%), and Haiti (4%). While the percentage of cases associated with travel to Mexico is declining, travel to the Indian subcontinent is becoming much riskier, with an incidence 18 times higher than for any other area. The trend toward an increased incidence of multidrug-resistant (MDR) *Salmonella* (see "Treatment," below) in developing countries is reflected by the increase in the proportion of U.S. cases caused by MDR strains from 0.6% in 1985–1989 to 12% in 1990–1994.

Almost 30% of the reported cases of enteric fever in the United States are domestically acquired. Although the majority of these cases (80%) are sporadic, large outbreaks do occur. In 1993, 47 culture-proven and 24 potential cases were linked to contaminated orange juice at a resort in New York. Evaluation of this outbreak led to the identification of a previously unknown chronic carrier. Similarly, evaluation of 25% of the 571 cases of domestically acquired enteric fever reported between 1985 and 1994 led to the identification of previously unknown chronic carriers.

CLINICAL COURSE   Enteric fever is a misnomer, in that the hallmark features of this disease—fever and abdominal pain—are variable. While fever is documented at presentation in more than 75% of cases, abdominal pain is reported in only 20 to 40%. Thus, a high index of suspicion for this potentially lethal systemic illness is necessary when a person presents with fever and a history of recent travel to a developing country.

The incubation period for *S. typhi* ranges from 3 to 21 days. This variability is most likely related to the size of the initial inoculum and the health and immune status of the host. The most prominent symptom of this systemic infection is prolonged fever (38.8° to 40.5°C, or 101.8° to 104.9°F). A prodrome of nonspecific symptoms often precedes fever and includes chills, headache, anorexia, cough, weakness, sore throat, dizziness, and muscle pains. Gastrointestinal symptoms are quite variable. Patients can present with either diarrhea or constipation; diarrhea is more common among patients with AIDS and among children <1 year of age. As stated above, only 20 to 40% of patients present with abdominal pain, although the majority have abdominal tenderness over the course of the disease. In general, the symptoms associated with *S. typhi* are more severe than those associated with *S. paratyphi*.

Early physical findings of enteric fever include rash ("rose spots"), hepatosplenomegaly, epistaxis, and relative bradycardia. Rose spots (Fig. 137-1) make up a faint, salmon-colored, blanching, maculopapular rash located primarily on the trunk and chest. The rash is evident in ~30% of patients at the end of the first week and resolves after 2 to 5 days without leaving a trace. Patients can have two or three crops of lesions, and *Salmonella* can be cultured from punch biopsies of these lesions. The faintness of the rash makes it difficult to detect in dark-skinned patients. On occasion, patients who remain toxic manifest neuropsychiatric symptoms described as a "muttering delirium" or "coma vigil," with picking at bedclothes or imaginary objects.

Late complications, occurring in the third and fourth weeks of infection, are most common in untreated adults and include intestinal perforation and/or gastrointestinal hemorrhage. These complications can develop despite clinical improvement and presumably result from necrosis at the initial site of *Salmonella* infiltration at the Peyer's patches of the small intestine. Both complications are life-threatening and require immediate medical and surgical interventions, with broadened antibiotic coverage for polymicrobial peritonitis (Chap. 112) and treatment of gastrointestinal hemorrhages, including bowel resection.

Rare complications whose incidences are reduced by prompt antibiotic treatment include pancreatitis, hepatic and splenic abscesses, endocarditis, pericarditis, orchitis, hepatitis, meningitis, nephritis, myocarditis, pneumonia, arthritis, osteomyelitis, and parotitis. Despite prompt antibiotic treatment, relapse rates remain at ~10% in immunocompetent hosts.

Approximately 1 to 5% of patients with enteric fever become long-term, asymptomatic, chronic carriers who shed *S. typhi* in either urine or stool for >1 year. The incidence of chronic carriage is higher among women and among persons with biliary abnormalities (e.g., gallstones, carcinoma of the gallbladder) and gastrointestinal malignancies. The anatomical abnormalities associated with these conditions presumably allow prolonged colonization.

DIAGNOSIS   Since the clinical presentation of typhoid fever is relatively nondescript, the diagnosis needs to be considered in any febrile traveler returning from a developing country, especially the Indian subcontinent, the Philippines, or Latin America. Other diagnoses that should be considered in this patient population include malaria, hepatitis, bacterial enteritis, dengue fever, rickettsial infections, leptospirosis, amebic liver abscesses, and acute HIV infection (Chap. 108). Other than a positive culture, no specific laboratory test is diagnostic for enteric fever. In 15 to 25% of cases, leukopenia and neutropenia are detectable. In the majority of cases, the white blood cell count is normal despite high fever. However, leukocytosis can develop in typhoid fever (especially in children) during the first 10 days of the illness, or later if the disease course is complicated by intestinal perforation or secondary infection. Other nonspecific laboratory results include moderately elevated values in liver function tests (aminotransferases, alkaline phosphatase, and lactate dehydrogenase). In addition, nonspecific ST and T wave abnormalities can be seen on electrocardiograms.

The diagnostic "gold standard" is a culture positive for *S. typhi* or *S. paratyphi*. The yield of blood cultures is quite variable: it can be as high as 90% during the first week of infection and decrease to 50% by the third week. A low yield is related to low numbers of *Salmonella* (<15 organisms per milliliter) in infected patients and/or to recent antibiotic treatment. Centrifugation to isolate and culture the buffy coat, which contains abundant blood mononuclear cells associated with the bacteria, decreases time to isolation but does not affect culture sensitivity.

A diagnosis can also be based on positive cultures of stool, urine, rose spots, bone marrow, and gastric or intestinal secretions. Unlike blood cultures, bone marrow cultures remain highly (90%) sensitive despite ≤5 days of antibiotic therapy. Culture of intestinal secretions (best obtained by a noninvasive duodenal string test) can be positive despite a negative bone marrow culture. If blood, bone marrow, and intestinal secretions are all cultured, the yield of a positive culture is >90%. Stool cultures, while negative in 60 to 70% of cases during the first week, can become positive during the third week of infection in untreated patients. Although the majority of patients (90%) clear bacteria from the stool by the eighth week, a small percentage become chronic carriers and continue to have positive stool cultures for at least 1 year.

Several serologic tests, including the classic Widal test for "febrile agglutinins," are available; however, given high rates of false-positivity and false-negativity, these tests are not clinically useful. Polymerase chain reaction and DNA probe assays are being developed.

℞ TREATMENT

In the preantibiotic era, the mortality rate from typhoid fever was as high as 15%. The introduction of treatment with chloramphenicol in 1948 greatly altered the disease course, decreasing mortality to <1% and the duration of fever from 14–28 days to 3–5 days. Chloramphenicol remained the standard treatment for enteric fever until the emergence of plasmid-mediated resistance to this drug in the 1970s. Given the increased mortality associated with resistance to chloramphenicol and the rare chloramphenicol-induced bone marrow toxicity, ampicillin (1 g orally every 6 h) and trimethoprim-sulfamethoxazole (TMP-SMX; one double-strength tablet twice daily) became the mainstays of treatment.

In 1989, MDR *S. typhi* emerged. These bacteria are resistant to chloramphenicol, ampicillin, trimethoprim, streptomycin, sulfonamides, and tetracycline. Like chloramphenicol resistance, resistance to ampicillin and trimethoprim is plasmid-encoded. In 1994, 12% of *S. typhi* isolates in the United States were MDR. Thus either quinolones or third-generation cephalosporins are currently recommended for empirical antibiotic treatment (Table 137-1). Despite efficient in vitro killing of *Salmonella*, first- and second-generation cephalosporins as well as aminoglycosides are ineffective in treating clinical infections.

Quinolones are the only available oral antibiotics for the treatment of MDR *S. typhi* infections. The greatest experience has been gained for ciprofloxacin (500 mg orally twice a day for 10 days). Shorter courses of ofloxacin (10 to 15 mg/kg in divided doses twice daily for 2 to 3 days) have also been successful. Limited data suggest that treatment with fluoroquinolones is associated with fewer treatment failures

FIGURE 137-1   "Rose spots," the rash of enteric fever due to *S. typhi* or *S. paratyphi*.

TABLE 137-1 *Antibiotic Therapy Options for Typhoid Fever*

Antibiotic	Dosage
First-line	
Ciprofloxacin	500 mg PO bid for 10 days
Ceftriaxone	1–2 g IV or IM for 10–14 days
Alternative (NARST[a])	
Azithromycin	1 g PO daily for 5 days
Ciprofloxacin	10 mg/kg PO bid for 10 days

[a] Nalidixic acid—resistant *S. typhi*.

and more rapid resolution of symptoms than treatment with β-lactam agents. However, quinolone resistance is emerging. In 1993, an outbreak of nalidixic acid–resistant *S. typhi* (NARST) infections in Vietnam was linked to chromosomal mutations in the gene encoding DNA gyrase (the target of the quinolones). NARST strains have also been isolated in India. Thus, all strains of *S. typhi* must be screened for resistance to nalidixic acid and tested for sensitivity to a clinically appropriate quinolone. Patients infected with NARST strains need to be treated with higher doses of ciprofloxacin (10 mg/kg twice a day for 10 days) or longer courses of ofloxacin (10 to 15 mg/kg in divided doses twice daily for 7 to 10 days) or with other antibiotics to which the strains are sensitive.

Ceftriaxone (1 to 2 g intravenously or intramuscularly) for 10 to 14 days is equivalent to oral or intravenous chloramphenicol in the treatment of susceptible strains. An alternative agent shown to be effective in an open-label study for the treatment of NARST strains is azithromycin (1 g orally once a day for 5 days or 1 g orally on day 1 followed by 500 mg orally for 6 days).

In cases of severe typhoid fever (fever; an abnormal state of consciousness—i.e., delirium, obtundation, stupor, or coma—or septic shock; and a positive culture for *S. typhi* or *S. paratyphi* A), dexamethasone treatment should be considered. In a single trial in Jakarta in the early 1980s in chloramphenicol-treated patients, treatment with dexamethasone (a single dose of 3 mg/kg followed by eight doses of 1 mg/kg, given every 6 h) decreased the mortality rate from 56% to 10%.

The 1 to 4% of patients who develop chronic carriage of *Salmonella* can be treated for 6 weeks with an appropriate antibiotic. Treatment with oral amoxicillin, TMP-SMX, ciprofloxacin, or norfloxacin has been shown to be ~80% effective in eradicating chronic carriage of susceptible organisms. However, in cases of anatomical abnormality (e.g., biliary or kidney stones), eradication of the infection often cannot be achieved by antibiotic therapy alone and requires surgical correction of the abnormalities.

PREVENTION AND CONTROL Theoretically, it is possible to eliminate salmonellae that cause enteric fever since the bacteria survive only in human hosts and are spread by contaminated food and water. However, given the high prevalence of the disease in developing countries that lack good facilities for sewage disposal and water treatment, this goal is currently unrealistic. Thus, travelers to developing countries should be advised to monitor their food and water intake carefully and to consider vaccination.

Three vaccine alternatives are currently available: (1) a heat-killed, phenol-extracted, whole-cell vaccine (two parenteral doses); (2) Ty21a, an attenuated *S. typhi* vaccine (four oral doses); and (3) ViCPS, consisting of purified Vi polysaccharide from the bacterial capsule (one parenteral dose). In addition, an acetone-killed whole-cell vaccine is available only for use by the U.S. military. The minimal ages for vaccination with the Ty21a, ViCPS, and Vi-rEPA (see below) vaccines are 6 years, 2 years, and 6 months, respectively. A large-scale meta-analysis of vaccine trials comparing the whole-cell vaccine, Ty21a, and ViCPS in populations of endemic areas indicates that, while all three vaccines have similar efficacy for the first year, the 3-year cumulative efficacy of the whole-cell vaccine (73%) exceeds that of both Ty21a (51%) and purified Vi (55%). In addition, the heat-killed whole-cell vaccine maintains its efficacy for 5 years, while Ty21a and ViCPS most likely maintain their efficacy for 4 and 2 years, respectively. However, the whole-cell vaccine is associated with a much higher incidence of side effects than the other two vaccines: 16% of whole-cell vaccine recipients develop fever and 10% miss a day of work or school, while only 1 to 2% of persons receiving the alternative vaccines have any fever. A fourth vaccine, Vi-rEPA, has been developed. This vaccine consists of Vi polysaccharide bound to a nontoxic recombinant protein that is identical to *Pseudomonas aeruginosa* exotoxin A; two parenteral doses are given. Coupling of the Vi polysaccharide to exotoxin A results in impressive T cell responses. In a trial in 2- to 5-year-old children, the vaccine provided 90% efficacy and was very well tolerated, with no serious adverse reactions. Trials of this vaccine in adults and infants are under way.

Although data on typhoid vaccines in travelers are limited, some evidence suggests that efficacy may be substantially lower than that for populations in endemic areas. The Centers for Disease Control and Prevention (CDC) currently recommends vaccination for persons traveling to developing countries who will have prolonged exposure to contaminated food and water or close contact with indigenous populations in rural areas. The only recommendations for domestic vaccination include people who have intimate or household contact with a chronic carrier or laboratory workers who frequently work with *S. typhi*. Given their decreased incidence of side effects and their similar short-term efficacy, the current bias is toward the use of Ty21a or ViCPS for vaccination of travelers.

Enteric fever is a reportable disease in the United States. Individual health departments have their own guidelines for allowing food handlers or health care workers to return to work. The reporting system enables public health departments to track down potential source patients and thus to identify and treat chronic carriers in order to prevent further outbreaks. In addition, since 1 to 4% of patients with *S. typhi* infection become chronic carriers, it is important to monitor patients (especially those employed in child care or food handling) for chronic carriage and to treat this condition if indicated.

NONTYPHOIDAL SALMONELLOSIS

EPIDEMIOLOGY The incidence of nontyphoidal salmonellosis has doubled in the United States over the past two decades. Currently, the CDC estimates that there are 2 million cases annually, with 500 to 2000 deaths. Although more than 200 serovars of *Salmonella* are considered to be human pathogens, the majority of the reported cases in the United States are caused by *S. typhimurium* or *S. enteritidis*. The incidence of salmonellosis is highest during the rainy season in tropical climates and during the warmer months in temperate climates, coinciding with the peak in food-borne outbreaks. Morbidity and mortality associated with salmonellosis are highest among the elderly, infants, and immunocompromised individuals, including those with hemoglobinopathies and those infected with HIV or with pathogens that cause blockade of the reticuloendothelial system (e.g., patients with bartonellosis, malaria, schistosomiasis, or histoplasmosis).

Unlike *S. typhi* and *S. paratyphi*, whose only reservoir is humans, nontyphoidal salmonellosis is acquired from multiple animal reservoirs. The main mode of transmission is from food products contaminated with animal products or waste—most commonly eggs and poultry but also undercooked meat, unpasteurized dairy products, seafood, and fresh produce.

S. enteritidis associated with chicken eggs is emerging as a major cause of food-borne disease. *S. enteritidis* causes infection of the ovaries and upper oviduct tissue of hens, resulting in contamination of the contents of eggs prior to shell deposition. Approximately 1 in 20,000 eggs is thought to be infected with *S. enteritidis*. Between 1974 and 1994, there was a fivefold increase (from 5% to 25%) in the isolation of *S. enteritidis* from eggs in the United States; in 1998, the U.S. Department of Agriculture estimated that 80% of all salmonellosis cases were caused by infected eggs. Eradication of *S. enteritidis* from hens has proved difficult, given that infection is spread to egg-laying hens both vertically from breeding flocks and horizontally through contact with rodents and manure. Transmission via contaminated eggs can be prevented by cooking of eggs such that the liquid yolk is solidified or through pasteurization of egg products.

Another factor in the increasing incidence of nontyphoidal salmonellosis in developed countries, including the United States, is related to the centralization of food processing and widespread distribution. For example, a 1994 outbreak of ~250,000 cases was linked to a pasteurized ice-cream premix most likely contaminated in tanker trucks that had previously carried unpasteurized eggs. Similar outbreaks have been traced to manufactured foods including pasteurized milk, infant formula, powdered-milk products, paprika-powdered potato chips, and a ready-to-eat savory snack. In addition, large outbreaks have been linked to fresh produce, including alfalfa sprouts, cantaloupe, fresh-squeezed orange juice, and sliced tomatoes, contaminated by manure or water at a single site and then broadly distributed.

A less common source of nontyphoidal *Salmonella* infections is exposure to pets, especially reptiles. Fecal carriage rates in reptiles can be >90%. In the 1970s, 14% of cases of salmonellosis were attributed to small turtles; the U.S. Food and Drug Administration subsequently prohibited the distribution of these pets, with a resultant decline in rates of reptile-associated salmonellosis. However, since 1986, an increase in the popularity of nonbanned reptiles, including iguanas, has been followed by increases in rates of *Salmonella* infections. Other pets, including African hedgehogs, snakes, birds, rodents, baby chicks, ducklings, dogs, and cats, can also serve as potential vectors.

Antibiotic resistance is an increasing phenomenon among nontyphoidal *Salmonella* serovars. In particular, *S. typhimurium* of definitive phage type 104 (DT104)—a serotype resistant to ampicillin, chloramphenicol, streptomycin, sulfonamides, and tetracyclines—has become prominent in the United Kingdom. This serotype is associated with greater mortality and morbidity than other nontyphoidal *Salmonella* serotypes. Its acquisition is associated with exposure to ill farm animals and to a variety of meat products. The prevalence of *S. typhimurium* DT104 in the United States increased from 0.6% in 1979–1980 to 34% in 1996. Of concern is the isolation in the United Kingdom in 1996 of *S. typhimurium* DT104 strains resistant to ciprofloxacin (14%) or trimethoprim (24%).

Also of concern is the recent increase in ceftriaxone- and fluoroquinolone-resistant nontyphoidal *Salmonella* strains in the United States. The CDC reported that the prevalence of ceftriaxone-resistant strains increased from 0 to 0.5% from 1995 to 1998. Each resistant strain appears to be an independent isolate. The majority of resistant strains have been isolated from children, where the clinical use of fluoroquinolones is limited. The likely source of resistant strains appears to be cattle and chickens treated with ceftiofur, since 2% of *S. typhimurium* strains isolated from these livestock in the United States are also resistant to ceftriaxone. In addition, at least two outbreaks of fluoroquinolone-resistant *S. typhimurium* have been reported in this country. In each instance, the index case presumably originated in the Philippines. Fluoroquinolone-resistant *S. choleraesuis* has also been documented in Taiwan. One outbreak was associated with fluoroquinolone-treated swine; thus the source of these resistant strains also appears to be livestock treated with antibiotics.

CLINICAL MANIFESTATIONS ■ Gastroenteritis

Infection with nontyphoidal *Salmonella* most often results in gastroenteritis indistinguishable from that caused by other bacterial and viral pathogens. Nausea, vomiting, and diarrhea occur 6 to 48 h after the ingestion of contaminated food or water. Patients often experience abdominal cramping and fever (38° to 39°C, or 100.5° to 102.2°F). The diarrhea is usually characterized as loose, nonbloody stools of moderate volume. However, large-volume watery stools, bloody stools, or symptoms of dysentery do not rule out the diagnosis. Rarely, *Salmonella* causes a syndrome of pseudoappendicitis or an illness that mimics inflammatory bowel disease.

Gastroenteritis caused by nontyphoidal *Salmonella* is usually self-limited. Diarrhea resolves within 3 to 7 days and fever within 72 h. Stool cultures remain positive for 4 to 5 weeks after infection and—

in rare cases of chronic carriage (<1%)—remain positive for >1 year. Antibiotic treatment usually is not recommended and in some studies has prolonged carriage of *Salmonella*. Neonates, the elderly, and the immunosuppressed (e.g., HIV-infected patients) with nontyphoidal *Salmonella* gastroenteritis are especially susceptible to dehydration and dissemination and may require hospitalization and antibiotic therapy.

Bacteremia and Endovascular Infections Up to 5% of patients with nontyphoidal *Salmonella* gastroenteritis have positive blood cultures, and 5 to 10% of these bacteremic persons develop localized infections. Bacteremia is particularly common and persistent among infants, the elderly, and patients with severe underlying infection or immunosuppression (e.g., transplant recipients, HIV-infected patients). Salmonellae have a propensity for infection of vascular sites; if >50% of three or more blood cultures are positive, an endovascular infection should be suspected. Preexisting valvular heart disease is a strong risk factor for the development of endocarditis, while atherosclerotic plaque, prosthetic grafts, and aortic aneurysms are associated with arteritis. Arteritis should be suspected in elderly patients who have a history of prolonged fever with associated back, chest, or abdominal pain preceded by gastroenteritis. Endocarditis and arteritis are rare (<1% of cases) but are associated with potentially morbid complications. Endocarditis can be complicated by cardiac valve perforation or by ring or septal abscesses, while arteritis can be associated with mycotic aneurysms, ruptured aneurysms, or vertebral osteomyelitis.

Unlike most nontyphoidal *Salmonella* serotypes, *S. choleraesuis* and *S. dublin* are frequently associated with sustained bacteremia and fever, often in the absence of a history of gastroenteritis. Similarly, these serotypes appear to be especially invasive and are often associated with metastatic infection.

Localized Infections ■ *INTRAABDOMINAL INFECTIONS* Intraabdominal infections due to nontyphoidal *Salmonella* are rare and usually manifest as hepatic or splenic abscesses or as cholecystitis. Involvement of the pancreas and adrenals and even an infected pheochromocytoma have been reported. Risk factors include anatomical abnormalities of the hepatobiliary system, including gallstones; abdominal malignancy; and sickle cell disease (especially with splenic abscesses). Eradication of the infection often requires surgical correction of anatomical abnormalities and drainage of abscesses.

CENTRAL NERVOUS SYSTEM INFECTIONS *Salmonella* infections of the central nervous system usually manifest as meningitis, although cerebral abscesses have been found. Meningitis is usually seen in neonates (<4 months old) and is associated with severe sequelae, including residual seizures, hydrocephalus, ventriculitis, abscess formation, subdural empyema, and permanent disability (e.g., mental retardation and paralysis).

PULMONARY INFECTIONS Nontyphoidal *Salmonella* pulmonary infections usually present as lobar pneumonia, sometimes complicated by lung abscesses, empyemas, pleural effusions, and bronchopleural fistulas. The majority of cases occur in patients with a preexisting abnormality of lung or pleura, including malignancy. Additional risk factors include sickle cell disease and glucocorticoid use. It is important to determine whether the pulmonary infection is in fact due to *Salmonella* or whether it is a secondary infection.

URINARY AND GENITAL TRACT INFECTIONS Urinary tract infections caused by nontyphoidal salmonellae present as either cystitis or pyelonephritis, usually in association with malignancy, urolithiasis, structural abnormalities, or immunosuppression (HIV infection, renal transplantation). Genital infections due to these bacteria are rare and present as ovarian and testicular abscesses, prostatitis, or epididymitis. Like other focal infections, both genital and urinary tract infections can be complicated by abscess formation.

BONE, JOINT, AND SOFT TISSUE INFECTIONS *Salmonella* osteomyelitis most commonly affects the femur, tibia, humerus, or lumbar vertebrae and is most often seen in association with sickle cell disease, hemoglobinopathies, or preexisting bone disease (e.g., fractures). Prolonged antibiotic treatment is recommended to decrease the incidence of relapse and chronic osteomyelitis. Septic arthritis occurs in the same patient population as osteomyelitis and usually presents in the knee, hip, or shoulder joints. Reactive arthritis (Reiter's syndrome) can follow *Salmonella* gastroenteritis and is seen most frequently in persons with the HLA-B27 histocompatibility antigen. *Salmonella* can cause rare soft tissue infections, usually at sites of local trauma in immunosuppressed patients.

DIAGNOSIS Nontyphoidal *Salmonella* gastroenteritis is diagnosed when *Salmonella* is cultured from stool. All salmonellae isolated in clinical laboratories should be sent to local public health departments. In cases where there is concern about bacteremia (i.e., those including prolonged or recurrent fever), blood cultures are indicated. Once bacteremia is documented, it is important to determine whether it is high-grade (>50% of three or more blood cultures positive); if so, endovascular infection is possible and further evaluation to identify the source is indicated. In addition, depending on clinical symptoms and on whether metastatic disease is suspected, other body fluids, such as joint fluid or cerebrospinal fluid, should be cultured.

℞ TREATMENT

Antibiotic treatment is not generally recommended for *Salmonella* gastroenteritis. The symptoms are usually self-limited and have not been demonstrated to be altered by short courses of antibiotics. In addition, in case-control and double-blind placebo-controlled trials, antibiotic treatment has been associated with increased rates of relapse and prolonged gastrointestinal carriage. Dehydration secondary to diarrhea should be treated with fluid and electrolyte replacement.

However, preemptive antibiotic treatment should be considered in patients at increased risk for metastatic infection. These patients include neonates (probably up to 3 months of age); persons >50 years old (because of the high risk of atherosclerotic plaque or aneurysm); transplant recipients; and patients with lymphoproliferative disease, HIV infection, prosthetic joints, vascular grafts, significant joint disease, or underlying sickle cell disease. This group should receive a course of oral or intravenous antibiotics lasting for 2 or 3 days or until defervescence in immunologically normal patients. Limited data exist regarding the treatment of highly immunocompromised individuals; however, these individuals may require a longer course of therapy—perhaps 7 to 14 days, depending on the clinical scenario. Rare cases of chronic nontyphoidal *Salmonella* carriage should be treated with a prolonged antibiotic course, as described above for chronic carriage of *S. typhi*.

Focal infections or life-threatening bacteremia with nontyphoidal *Salmonella* should be treated with antibiotics (at the same doses used for enteric fever). Given the increasing prevalence of antibiotic resistance, empirical therapy should include a third-generation cephalosporin or a quinolone. If the bacteremia is low-grade (<50% of blood cultures positive), the patient should be treated for 7 to 14 days. Pa-

tients with AIDS and *Salmonella* bacteremia should receive 1 to 2 weeks of intravenous antibiotic therapy followed by 4 weeks of oral therapy with quinolones. Patients who relapse after this regimen should receive long-term suppressive therapy with a quinolone or TMP-SMX, as indicated by bacterial sensitivities.

If the patient has an endovascular infection or endocarditis, treatment for 6 weeks with intravenous β-lactam antibiotics is indicated. Chloramphenicol treatment has been associated with high failure rates and is not recommended. Limited case reports have described the successful treatment of *Salmonella* endovascular infections with quinolones, which may prove an alternative approach in cases caused by sensitive strains. However, concern remains about the development of quinolone resistance during prolonged therapy. Surgical resection of infected aneurysms or other infected endovascular sites is often required. If surgical resection is not possible, lifelong suppressive antibiotic therapy may be indicated. For extraintestinal nonvascular infections, 2 to 4 weeks of antibiotic therapy (depending on the site) are usually recommended. In cases of chronic osteomyelitis, abscesses, and urinary or biliary tract abnormality, surgical interventions may be required in addition to prolonged antibiotic therapy to eradicate infection.

PREVENTION AND CONTROL The incidence of nontyphoidal salmonellosis continues to rise along with rates of emergence of antibiotic-resistant strains. The increased centralization of food production plays a prominent role in the growing incidence, as one oversight can result in rapid, widespread distribution of contaminated food. Thus, it is important to monitor every step of food production, from handling of raw products to preparation of finished foods. In particular, with the increasing prevalence of *S. enteritidis* in egg-laying hens, it is recommended that pasteurized eggs be substituted for bulk-pooled eggs at all nursing homes, hospitals, and commercial food-service establishments. All cases of nontyphoidal salmonellosis should be reported to public health departments, since tracking and monitoring of these cases result in the identification of the sources of local outbreaks and help authorities anticipate large-scale international outbreaks. Lastly, the prudent use of antimicrobial agents in both humans and animals is necessary to minimize the further emergence of antibiotic-resistant strains.

FURTHER READING

COHEN JI et al: Extra-manifestations of *Salmonella* infections. Medicine 66: 349, 1987

GLYNN MK et al: Emergence of multidrug-resistant *Salmonella enterica* serotype *typhimurium* DT104 infections in the United States. N Engl J Med 338:1333, 1998

LIN FY et al: The efficacy of a *Salmonella typhi* Vi conjugate vaccine in two-to-five-year-old children. N Engl J Med 344:1263, 2001

MERMIN JH et al: Typhoid fever in the United States, 1985–1994: Changing risks of international travel and increasing antimicrobial resistance. Arch Intern Med 158:633, 1998

OHL ME, MILLER, SI: *Salmonella*: A model for bacterial pathogenesis. Annu Rev Med 52:259, 2001

TAUXE RV: Emerging foodborne diseases: An evolving public health challenge. Emerg Infect Dis 3:425, 1997

138 SHIGELLOSIS
Gerald T. Keusch, Dennis J. Kopecko

DEFINITION *Shigellosis* is an acute infectious inflammatory colitis due to one of the members of the genus *Shigella*. Although the disease is often referred to as "bacillary dysentery," many patients have only mild watery diarrhea and never develop dysenteric symptoms. Less severe illness predominates in industrialized countries such as the United States, whereas more severe, often fatal dysentery occurs commonly in patients in developing countries.

ETIOLOGIC AGENT Shigellae are small, gram-negative, nonmotile bacilli and are members of the family Enterobacteriaceae and the tribe Escherichieae. They are so closely related to *Escherichia coli* that the two genera cannot be distinguished by DNA hybridization methods. In fact, shigellae are now thought to be differentiated pathogenic *E. coli*. The four *Shigella* species (*S. dysenteriae*, *S. flexneri*, *S. boydii*, and *S. sonnei*) are defined on the basis of somatic O antigens and carbohydrate fermentation patterns. Overall, there are 43 O serotypes of *Shigella*; *S. sonnei* is the only species that exists as a single serotype. Because acquired immunity is serotype-specific, an individual can be infected multiple times by different serotypes. Shigellae are classically lactose-negative; the exception is *S. sonnei*, which is a late, weak lactose fermenter. All shigellae produce acid but not gas from glucose; the result is a typical acid butt and alkaline slant in triple sugar iron agar without H_2S production. The genus is characterized by its ability to invade intestinal epithelial cells and to cause infection and illness in humans with a very small number of ingested bacteria, from a few hundred to a few thousand organisms.

EPIDEMIOLOGY Worldwide, it is estimated that at least 200 million clinical cases and more than 650,000 deaths due to shigellosis occur annually, primarily in developing countries and especially among children <5 years old. Shigellae are ubiquitous but have no known animal hosts other than higher primates. Poor environmental sanitation and crowding facilitate transmission from person to person. For example, a major outbreak took place in the makeshift camps for refugees fleeing the Rwandan civil war in 1994, with thousands of cases and high mortality.

The Centers for Disease Control and Prevention (CDC) maintain a national *Shigella* surveillance system based on data collected by state public health laboratories. In 2001, 10,598 isolates (primarily *S. sonnei*) were reported to the CDC, representing an apparent 45% decrease from 1991; this figure translates to an isolation rate in 2001 of 3.8/100,000 population—down from 6/100,000 a decade earlier. As in the past, the young were most susceptible, with one-fourth of isolates obtained from children <5 years old and another one-fourth from persons 5 to 19 years old. However, the reporting system seriously underestimates the number of infections occurring in the United States, both because some individuals are not sick enough to seek care and because no culture is performed in some instances when care is sought. Thus, the CDC-estimated number of *Shigella* infections in the United States approaches half a million per year. Rates are similar among males and females except among women aged 20 to 39; in this group, the rate is almost twice that among males, presumably because of greater contact with young children, especially those in day care. Cases are detected most commonly in counties with a relatively high proportion of low-income minority-group residents, including African Americans, Hispanics, and Native Americans; rates are especially high in poor urban communities, in day-care centers, and among retarded children in custodial care. Incidence rates in communities bordering Mexico are 228% higher than those in nonborder states; even so, they are several hundred times lower than those recorded among young children in many developing countries.

Since the discovery of the genus *Shigella* in 1896, major unexplained global shifts in the prevalence of its four species have been noted. Until World War I, *S. dysenteriae* type 1 was the predominant isolate, frequently causing devastating epidemics with high mortality until it was replaced by *S. flexneri*. Since World War II, *S. flexneri* has been steadily replaced by *S. sonnei* in industrialized countries. Since 1969, epidemic *S. dysenteriae* type 1 has reappeared in Latin America, in the Indian subcontinent and elsewhere in Asia, and in sub-Saharan Africa and has been associated with relatively high mortality rates due to multidrug resistance and inadequate diagnosis and case management. In contrast, *S. boydii*, the fourth species, has remained largely confined to the Indian subcontinent. The reasons for these epidemiologic trends are not clear. *Shigella* is highly host-adapted and is a natural pathogen only of humans and higher primates. It is transmitted from feces to the mouth, generally via direct person-to-person contact, although intermediate vectors such as food, water, flies, and fomites can be involved. In the United States, imported herbs and salads have recently caused multistate outbreaks. *Shigella* infection can also be transmitted during participation in recreational water sports in poorly chlorinated pools or lakes fecally contaminated by infected infants and young children and can spread rapidly among confined populations in close contact—for example, in day-care centers, in institutions for the mentally retarded, on cruise ships, or on military bases. Moreover, *Shigella* is transmitted by anal-oral sexual practices among gay men; although these infections were previously caused primarily by *S. flexneri*, *S. sonnei* now accounts for two-thirds of isolates. Similar trends are reported from Canada, Australia, and New Zealand. Rates of *Shi-*

gella infection and recurrent disease among HIV-infected individuals greatly exceed those in the HIV-uninfected population (Chap. 173).

Shigellosis is associated with a high rate of secondary household transmission. As many as 40% of children and 20% of adults who are household contacts of a case (generally a preschool child) develop *Shigella* infection. The infection is often symptomatic in children but asymptomatic in adults, presumably because of acquired immunity in adults. In contrast, epidemic disease due to newly introduced strains affects all ages, with severe and fatal cases occurring primarily in the very young and the very old. Prolonged asymptomatic carriage of *Shigella* in humans is uncommon; unless there is underlying malnutrition, the organisms are generally cleared rapidly. However, veterinary reports suggest that long-term asymptomatic carriage of *Shigella* by non-human primates is not uncommon.

PATHOGENESIS AND PATHOLOGY Shigellae enter the host via the mouth. Because they are genetically equipped to survive low pH, they readily pass the gastric acid barrier. An essential step in pathogenesis is invasion of the colonic mucosa and cell-to-cell spread of infection. It was originally thought that shigellae invade the host across the absorptive epithelial cells. However, the luminal surface of colonic cells appears to be resistant to invasion. More recent experimental studies show that *Shigella* uptake occurs primarily through the antigen-sampling M cells, resulting in initial limited penetration of the lamina propria, where the organisms encounter and are ingested by resident macrophages. Shigellae multiply within and trigger apoptosis of the infected macrophage, but not before initiating the production of the proinflammatory cytokine interleukin (IL) 1β. Viable shigellae released from dead macrophages then invade the basolateral surface of the colonic epithelium, spread from cell to cell via a novel host actin-based propulsion mechanism, and provoke the synthesis of IL-8 from the epithelium. IL-8 is a chemokine that induces the migration of polymorphonuclear neutrophils (PMNs) through the epithelial cell layer into the intestinal lumen; the tight junctions are damaged as the PMNs traverse the mucosa, and this damage allows further *Shigella* invasion and exacerbates inflammation. The consequences are mucosal ulcerations and characteristic dysenteric small-volume stools consisting of mucus, cellular debris, neutrophil exudates, and blood. The host inflammatory response is essential to disease pathogenesis, and its blockade by any number of interventions interrupts the cascade from invasion to illness.

After attaching to the colonic epithelium, shigellae induce their own uptake via a host endocytic mechanism (i.e., a phagocytosis-like process) in which the bacteria are initially engulfed within plasma membrane–enclosed endosomes. Subsequently, the bacteria dissolve the endosomal vacuole and are released into the nutrient-rich cytoplasm—a step that is essential for their intracellular replication. This intracellular existence also provides the organism with a means to evade extracellular host defenses, to move within the cell to the plasma membrane, and to spread directly from cell to cell via protrusions it creates at the interface between adjacent cells.

Many of the microbial virulence features as well as the host cell biologic responses occurring during pathogenesis have been defined during the past decade, and this information has led to the following understanding of this complex process: Virulence requires the function of multiple genes and regulatory elements encoded both on the chromosome and on a large (180- to 210-kilobase pair) plasmid present in all virulent shigellae as well as in enteroinvasive *E. coli* (EIEC, which causes a *Shigella*-like disease). Some of these gene products convey acid resistance, some mediate the endocytic cell invasion process, others underlie the subsequent escape from the endosomal vacuole, and still others underlie the movement of the organism to the plasma membrane, leading to cell-to-cell transfer. The plasmid-borne invasion genes encode a type III bacterial secretion system that, upon contact with the host cell, injects invasion effectors into that cell via needle-like microbial structures. These effectors cause an actin-dependent rearrangement of the local plasma membrane, which engulfs the attached bacterium into a plasma membrane–bound endosome.

Shigellae lack flagella and are nonmotile. To move within the cell, they have evolved a novel mechanism involving the formation of a growing tail of polymerized host actin created by the microbial protein IcsA (an ATPase) localized to one pole of the bacterium. Actin polymerization and cross-linking at one end of the bacterium propel it randomly through the cytosol. Some organisms reach the plasma membrane, where they form protrusions into the adjacent cell. When these protrusions are pinched off and the resulting double host-cell membrane surrounding the organism is lysed, the bacterium lies within the cytoplasm of the newly invaded cell, and the process is repeated. Inactivation of IcsA by host phosphorylases may serve as a molecular host-defense mechanism to modulate virulence by limiting microbial spread. Another important host protein essential for cell-to-cell spread is the cadherin L-CAM. Mutations in L-CAM alter the long finger-like protrusions induced by shigellae at the plasma membrane and impair their subsequent fusion with the adjacent cell. Once a single *Shigella* organism has invaded a host epithelial cell, the entire process of bacterial escape from the endosome into the host cell's cytoplasm, multiplication, and cell-to-cell spread can take place without exposure of the bacterium to the extracellular milieu and host immune defenses. Invaded host epithelial cells ultimately die.

Another property of apparent importance in the virulence of *S. dysenteriae* type 1 (which causes the most clinically severe form of shigellosis) is the ability to produce Shiga toxin, a protein encoded by the iron-regulated chromosomal gene *stx*. Related members of this toxin family are produced by some strains of *E. coli*, including serotype O157: H7. Such strains, designated Shiga toxin–producing *E. coli* (STEC), cause hemorrhagic colitis and hemolytic-uremic syndrome (HUS). Shiga toxins are composed of two distinct peptide subunits, each with highly conserved active regions. The first, located on the larger A subunit, is an *N*-glycosidase that hydrolyzes adenine from specific sites of ribosomal RNA of the mammalian 60S ribosomal subunit, irreversibly inhibiting protein synthesis. The second conserved region is a binding site on the B subunit that recognizes the receptor glycolipid Gb3 on host cells. Receptor specificity is determined by a terminal galactose $\alpha1\rightarrow4$-galactose disaccharide. Wild-type toxigenic *S. dysenteriae* causes more severe illness than does an isogenic toxin-negative mutant in an experimental monkey model. The related Shiga toxins all target endothelial cells and appear to play a role in the pathogenesis of the microangiopathic complications associated with toxin-producing shigellae and *E. coli*: HUS and thrombotic thrombocytopenic purpura (TTP). Two other *Shigella* enterotoxins, ShET-1 and -2, have been described; the former is restricted almost exclusively to *S. flexneri* 2a, whereas the latter is distributed more widely (e.g., in the physiologically similar EIEC). These two enterotoxins, encoded by chromosomal and plasmid-encoded genes, respectively, alter electrolyte transport by gut segments in vitro and cause net fluid secretion in ligated rabbit ileal loops in vivo. Although both toxins induce antibody in infected humans, their role (if any) in the pathogenesis of the watery-diarrhea phase of shigellosis remains uncertain.

The characteristic pathology of human bacillary dysentery is extensive ulceration of the epithelial surface of the colonic mucosa, with an exudate consisting of desquamated colonic cells, PMNs, and erythrocytes that may resemble a pseudomembrane in severely affected areas. Marked mucus depletion and increased mitotic activity are evident in the crypt regions and presumably reflect a response to the loss of surface colonic cells. The lamina propria is edematous and hemorrhagic and is infiltrated by neutrophils and plasma cells. There is also swelling of capillary and venular endothelial cells, with margination of neutrophils. At the ultrastructural level, intraepithelial-cell bacteria can be seen within endosomes as well as free in the cytoplasm. Histologic examination of colon from dysenteric humans shows an alteration of mucosal endothelial cells similar to that induced by endotoxin (lipopolysaccharide, LPS). Shiga toxin also targets endothelial cells, especially when toxin receptor expression is upregulated by exposure to LPS or proinflammatory cytokines. Circulating LPS is de-

tectable in human shigellosis and is present in blood at especially high levels in *S. dysenteriae* type 1 infection, even without detectable bacteremia. Variation in the lipid A component of LPS is related to virulence—an observation that further suggests the importance of LPS in pathogenesis. One likely mechanism involves the ability of LPS to induce cytokine gene transcription and the strong association of cytokine secretion and inflammation. However, bacterial invasion of the colonic mucosa itself activates the transcription factor NF-κB, which is involved in regulation of cytokine synthesis. Cytokine-producing cells are present in the colonic mucosa of patients infected with *S. dysenteriae* or *S. flexneri* and in their stools as well. In fact, the number of cells producing IL-1, IL-6, interferon γ, and transforming growth factor β is directly related to the severity of inflammation. These inflammatory processes persist longer in children than in adults; this difference may reflect the lesser efficacy of the immune responses of the young in clearing the offending pathogen. Resolution of disease symptoms probably involves clearance of the organisms by both nonspecific immune defenses (i.e., PMNs and accelerated intestinal cell turnover) and specific immune defenses, with down-modulation of inflammation and repair of damaged mucosa.

Epidemiologic evidence indicates that protective immunity develops and is serotype-specific (i.e., LPS-related). Despite much effort, the precise nature of this immunity has not been elucidated. Common surface outer-membrane proteins involved in invasion elicit serum antibodies that, although cross-reactive among *Shigella* species and serotypes, do not seem to be protective. The serotype-specific determinants are likely to be the somatic antigens, as serum antibody to LPS predicts resistance to infection and evidence exists for IgA-mediated mucosal responses to LPS during convalescence from shigellosis.

CLINICAL MANIFESTATIONS Shigellosis in the United States, due primarily to *S. sonnei*, is typically a pediatric ambulatory disease, presenting as a self-limited nonbloody but inflammatory watery diarrhea containing many neutrophils. The clinical spectrum of shigellosis was clearly shown in an experiment in which adult volunteers ingested 10,000 virulent *S. flexneri* type 2a organisms. Approximately one-fourth of the volunteers never became ill. However, over the first 24 to 48 h, one-fourth developed transient fever, another one-fourth had fever and self-limited watery diarrhea, and the remaining one-fourth had fever and watery diarrhea that progressed to bloody diarrhea and dysentery. In young children in particular, body temperature can rise rapidly to 40° to 41°C, sometimes resulting in generalized seizures; however, they rarely recur or result in serious sequelae. Fever is part of a cytokine-mediated response to infection that includes anorexia and muscle catabolism initiating negative nitrogen balance; additional energy is consumed in raising body temperature. This response is of significance in patients who are already poorly nourished, sometimes precipitating severe protein-energy malnutrition that can lead to later death. Dysentery is a syndrome characterized by frequent passage (usually 10 to 30 times per day) of small-volume stools consisting of blood, mucus, and pus; this diarrhea is accompanied by severe abdominal cramps and tenesmus—the painful straining with stooling that may lead to rectal prolapse (especially in young children, in whom the ligamentous support of the rectum is still poorly developed). Severe dysentery most likely involves infection due to *S. dysenteriae* type 1, occurs less commonly with *S. flexneri*, and is least likely with *S. sonnei* or *S. boydii*. Patients with mild disease generally recover without specific therapy in a few days to a week. Severe shigellosis can progress to toxic dilatation and colonic perforation, either of which may be fatal. In developing countries, shigellosis almost doubles the risk of persistent diarrhea; the mortality rate increases by tenfold when persistent *Shigella* diarrhea develops.

Endoscopy shows the mucosa to be hemorrhagic, with mucous discharge and focal ulcerations and sometimes an overlying exudate resembling a pseudomembrane. The majority of lesions are in the distal colon, with progressively fewer in the more proximal segments of large bowel. Mild dehydration is common among patients with watery diarrhea; severe dehydration is very rare. With extensive colonic involvement, protein-losing enteropathy can occur and can have important adverse nutritional consequences, especially for already poorly nourished children. The majority of extraintestinal complications of shigellosis arise in patients in developing countries and are related both to the prevalence of infections caused by *S. dysenteriae* type 1 and *S. flexneri* and to the poor nutritional state of the hosts. For example, bacteremia, thought to occur relatively infrequently among patients with shigellosis in the United States, develops in up to 8% of patients hospitalized for shigellosis in Dacca, Bangladesh. The causative *Shigella* species is isolated from half of these patients, while other Enterobacteriaceae are found in the remainder. Bacteremia is associated with higher-than-usual mortality and is more common among infants (<1 year old) and among persons with protein-energy malnutrition. Persistent and clinically severe *Shigella* bacteremia has been encountered in the United States only in patients with AIDS (Chap. 173).

HUS may occur with *S. dysenteriae* type 1 infection. In the United States, STEC strains (such as *E. coli* O157:H7) producing high levels of Shiga-family toxins are the most likely causes of HUS. Manifestations of HUS usually develop toward the end of the first week of shigellosis, when dysentery is already resolving. Oliguria and a marked drop in hematocrit (by as much as 10% within 24 h) are the first signs and may progress to anuria with renal failure and to severe anemia with congestive heart failure, respectively. Even with advanced therapy, 5 to 10% of patients with HUS die of the acute illness. In addition, renal damage progresses slowly over several decades in survivors, some of whom will develop significant renal failure and require long-term dialysis or renal transplantation for survival. Leukemoid reactions, with leukocyte counts of <50,000/μL, usually accompany HUS; thrombocytopenia, with 30,000 to 100,000 platelets/μL, is common and in adults can lead to TTP, which is part of the spectrum of the toxin-mediated microangiopathy. Profound hyponatremia and severe hypoglycemia are also encountered, especially in developing countries, and may underlie central nervous system abnormalities such as seizures and altered consciousness. *S. flexneri* is associated with a rare toxic encephalopathy that is manifested by bizarre posturing and lethal cerebral edema.

Reactive arthritis is a less common extraintestinal manifestation that is usually associated with *S. flexneri* strains. In patients expressing histocompatibility antigen HLA-B27, the full triad of Reiter's syndrome sometimes develops weeks to months after diarrheal illness (Chap. 305). Pneumonia, meningitis, vaginitis (in prepubertal girls), keratoconjunctivitis, and "rose spot" rashes are rare events.

DIAGNOSIS AND LABORATORY FINDINGS Shigellosis is the principal bacterial cause of dysentery and should be considered whenever a patient presents with bloody diarrhea. However, in the United States, because *S. sonnei* is the most common infecting *Shigella* species, most patients present with fever and nonbloody watery diarrhea that are indistinguishable from the signs caused by other bacterial or viral agents of mild to moderate diarrhea. In this country, many patients with bloody diarrhea have STEC or *Campylobacter jejuni* identified as the cause. The specific diagnosis is based on culture of *Shigella* from the stool; sensitive and specific diagnostic methods based on the polymerase chain reaction have been developed but are not yet widely available. A commercial enzyme immunoassay to detect Shiga-family toxins in stool can identify most patients infected with *S. dysenteriae* type 1 (rare in the United States) or STEC within 3 h. The yield of *Shigella* in culture is increased if the patient has fecal leukocytes or bloody diarrhea. The organism is very labile and must be transferred quickly to plates or holding media (such as buffered glycerol saline) if it is to be isolated. Stool samples are preferable to swabs; when the latter are used, a rectal sample should be obtained. More than one differential selective medium should be used for culture—i.e., MacConkey and one other medium, such as Hektoen enteric or xylose-lysine-deoxycholate. Stool cultures to diagnose nonbloody watery diarrhea have a very low yield of positives and are not considered to be cost-effective in the United States.

Serologic tests can be performed, since antibodies to somatic antigens develop early in the acute phase of disease. However, the reagents for such tests generally are not available, even in the United

States, and serologic assessments are usually used only for epidemiologic studies.

The differential diagnosis includes inflammatory colitis due to other microbial agents: STEC, EIEC, *C. jejuni*, *Salmonella enteritidis*, *Yersinia enterocolitica*, *Clostridium difficile*, and the protozoan *Entamoeba histolytica*. Ulcerative colitis and Crohn's colitis are among the "noninfectious" conditions that should be considered (Chap. 276). All these infections except that due to *E. histolytica* are associated with the presence of large numbers of fecal leukocytes. Amebiasis can be diagnosed by the detection of erythrophagocytic trophozoites in the stool or by immunoassay (Chap. 194).

Other laboratory studies are nonspecific and may disclose neutrophilic leukocytosis, anemia due to blood loss with hemorrhagic diarrhea, prerenal azotemia, or (if watery diarrhea has been pronounced) hyperchloremic acidosis. Laboratory findings in shigellosis complicated by HUS are discussed above.

℞ TREATMENT

The mild to moderate dehydration in shigellosis is readily corrected with oral rehydration solutions (Chap. 140). The role of antibiotic therapy depends on the bacterial species involved and the severity of disease. Since *S. sonnei* infection is usually self-limited, culture results generally do not become available until the patient is better and there is little clinical need for further therapy. The use of antibiotics in severe cases with bloody diarrhea or dysentery reduces the duration of illness and can shorten the carriage state. Resistance to sulfonamides, streptomycin, chloramphenicol, and tetracyclines is almost universal, and many shigellae are now resistant to ampicillin and trimethoprim-sulfamethoxazole (TMP-SMX) as well. Knowledge of the pattern of resistance in a given population, which can change with time, is essential. In the United States, multiresistant strains are most likely to be acquired during travel abroad; therefore, for domestically acquired infection, either ampicillin or TMP-SMX remains the drug of choice unless resistance is known to be prevalent in particular communities (Table 138-1). Amoxicillin should not be substituted for ampicillin; it is ineffective because it is too well absorbed proximally and does not reach bacteria in the colonic lumen. Similarly, nonabsorbable antibiotics are ineffective because they do not reach the mucosal bacterial population. Short courses of treatment (1 or 3 days) or even single doses of a fluoroquinolone such as ciprofloxacin or the macrolide azithromycin have been employed with success. In developing countries, where resistance to ampicillin and TMP-SMX is commonplace, the drug of choice for the treatment of multiresistant *S. dysenteriae* type 1 infections is nalidixic acid; however, resistance to the latter agent is increasing in prevalence with its increasing use. The fluoroquinolones (e.g., ciprofloxacin, ofloxacin) are highly effective against all strains (Chap. 118) but are currently too costly for use in the developing world and are not yet approved for use in children <17 years old in the United States; these drugs have caused cartilage damage in young rodents during toxicity tests, although there is no evidence for a similar effect at therapeutic doses in humans. Alternative drugs shown to be effective include oral pivamdinocillin (amdinocillin, pivoxil, pivmecillinam; still not available in the United States), azithromycin, and intravenous ceftriaxone (50 mg/kg per day for 5 days). In small-scale clinical trials, 2 to 5 days of cefixime treatment resulted in the resolution of clinical symptoms due to *S. sonnei*, but the relapse rate was 20 to 24%. (Cefixime is not currently available in the United States.) Single doses of ceftriaxone may be effective, but more clinical data are needed. No antibiotic treatment is recommended for the convalescent carrier state, which usually lasts no more than a few weeks—i.e., for a much shorter period than is seen with nontyphoidal *Salmonella* or *Salmonella typhi*. Patients with AIDS can develop chronic carriage of *Shigella* and may be subject to relapsing infection with bacteremia (Chap. 173). This cycle can be interrupted by several weeks of treatment with a quinolone.

The role of antimotility agents such as atropine sulfate and di-

TABLE 138-1 *Options for Oral Antibiotic Treatment of Shigellosis*

| Drug | Dose/Duration | | Daily Cost ($US)[a] | Comments |
	Children	Adults		
UNITED STATES				
Ampicillin	100 mg/kg q6h × 5 d	500 mg q6h × 5 d	$0.12/kg, liquid form $0.88, capsule form	Resistance varies with locale and is very common when infection is acquired abroad. Diarrhea is a frequent side effect.
Trimethoprim-sulfamethoxazole	10/50 mg/kg bid × 3–5 d	160/800 mg (1 DS tablet) bid × 3–5 d	$0.26/kg, liquid form $0.64, tablet form	Resistance varies with locale and is very common when infection is acquired abroad.
Ciprofloxacin	15 mg/kg q12h × 3–5 d; 500 mg max/dose	500 mg bid × 3 d	$0.17/kg, liquid form $10.80, tablet form	Resistance rates are low. Regimen is not licensed for use in children <17 years old, but there is no evidence of toxicity.
Azithromycin	12 mg/kg on day 1 (max, 500 mg), 6 mg/kg on days 2–5 (max, 250 mg/d)	1 g (single dose)	$0.37/kg day 1 (liquid) $27.00, adult tablet form	Single-dose regimen for adults is attractive but has not been tested in children.
Cefixime[b]	8 mg/kg (max, 400 mg) once daily × 5 d	400 mg/d × 5 d	$0.30/kg, liquid form $8.80, adult tablet form	Efficacy differs in different studies. Some studies show bacteriologic relapse rates of 20–24%.
DEVELOPING COUNTRIES				
Naladixic acid	55 mg/kg, divided into daily dose × 5 d	1 g qid × 5 d	$0.20/kg, children $16.00/d, adults	This is not an FDA-approved indication for either children or adults. Prices are likely to be lower in developing countries.

[a] Redbook 2003 average wholesale prices; for comparison only, as actual cost to pharmacies and charges to patients vary greatly.

[b] Cefixime is not currently available in the United States.

Note: DS, double strength; FDA; U.S. Food and Drug Adminstration.

phenoxylate (Lomotil) and loperamide (Imodium) in the early phases of shigellosis is controversial. Loperamide, in particular, may reduce diarrhea volume and in one study was highly effective in combination with antimicrobial therapy. However, antimotility drugs are suspected of enhancing the severity of disease by delaying excretion of organisms and facilitating further invasion of the mucosa, potentially increasing the likelihood of complicating toxic megacolon. Therefore, they are contraindicated in infants and young children. In adults, these agents are contraindicated for use in the dysenteric phase of disease.

Unique therapies are also being tested. Hyperimmune bovine colostrum containing high titers of antibody to *S. dysenteriae* type 1 LPS did not alter the clinical course of disease when coadministered with an effective antibiotic. An energy-dense diet did not improve the outcome of acute shigellosis in malnourished children but appeared to hasten the resolution of rectal prolapse. An interesting experimental approach is the use of engineered avirulent bacteria hyperexpressing Shiga toxin receptors to bind and prevent the biologic effects of the toxin.

Treatment of complications of shigellosis often differs in developed and developing countries. For example, antibiotic-unresponsive toxic megacolon, with or without perforation, is often managed by colectomy and ileostomy in the United States. Surgery is less often employed in developing countries because of a lack of surgical services or difficulties in ileostomy management; instead, management concentrates on antibiotic administration and conservative fluid and electrolyte support. HUS often requires dialysis; however, in developing countries, the threshold for dialysis may be higher than in the United States because azotemia is slow to develop and the risk of significant hyperkalemia is often diminished by a preexisting deficiency in total-body potassium due to malnutrition and wasting of lean body mass. The management of hyponatremia, usually caused by inappropriate secretion of antidiuretic hormone (vasopressin), is governed by the severity of the condition and the symptomatic state of the patient, as outlined in Chap. 41. Infusion of glucose can reverse clinical manifestations caused by hypoglycemia, and responses can be monitored by finger-stick blood glucose tests if no biochemistry laboratory is available. In developing countries, optimal nutritional management is needed to correct deficiencies due to underlying malnutrition as well as the superimposed catabolic stress and protein-losing enteropathy of shigellosis. Nutritional support should begin during the acute illness and is required for months thereafter (Chap. 63).

PREVENTION There are no licensed vaccines against *Shigella*, although considerable effort is being directed toward the development of a safe and effective vaccine. Direct-contact transmission of shigellosis can be prevented by appropriate environmental and personal hygiene. Hand washing with soap and water when caring for infected infants, handling diapers, or preparing food is effective, and efficacy can be enhanced by the use of a triclosan antibacterial soap. Safe water supplies and sanitary latrines or toilets significantly reduce the primary and secondary transmission of *Shigella* infection. In highly endemic developing countries, infants are protected during the period of exclusive breast-feeding, which should be encouraged wherever HIV transmission via breast-feeding is not a consideration. Any measures that reduce the burden of malnutrition also reduce the burden of shigellosis in the population. Stool precautions should be instituted for hospitalized infected patients to ensure safe disposal of infected excreta and linens, and hospital personnel must wash and disinfect their hands and medical instruments (such as stethoscopes) after each contact with an infected patient. In the United States, cohorting of asymptomatic infected children, use of antibiotics to reduce infectiousness, and scrupulous attention to hygiene are usually successful in nosocomial outbreaks. Children in day care must be kept at home while clinically ill and ideally should have one negative stool culture before returning to the day-care facility. Likewise, food handlers who develop shigellosis should be culture-negative before returning to work. Antibiotic treatment is not indicated for the asymptomatic carrier state.

FURTHER READING

AHMED F et al: Epidemiology of postshigellosis persistent diarrhea in young children. Pediatr Infect Dis J 20:525, 2001

D'HAUTEVILLE H et al: Two msbB genes encoding maximal acylation of lipid A are required for invasive *Shigella flexneri* to mediate inflammatory rupture and destruction of the intestinal epithelium. J Immunol 168:5240, 2002

KOTLOFF KL et al: Global burden of *Shigella* infection: Implications for vaccine development and implementation of control strategies. Bull World Health Organ 77:651, 1999

LOPEZ EL et al: *Shigella* and Shiga toxin–producing *Escherichia coli* causing bloody diarrhea in Latin America. Infect Dis Clin North Am 14:41, 2000

MEAD PS et al: Food-related illness and death in the United States. Emerg Infect Dis 5:607, 1999

SHANE AL et al: Sharing *Shigella*: Risk factors for a multicommunity outbreak of shigellosis. Arch Pediatr Adolesc Med 157:601, 2003

ZIMBABWE, BANGLADESH, SOUTH AFRICA DYSENTERY STUDY GROUP: Multicenter, randomized, double blind clinical trial of short course versus standard course oral ciprofloxacin for *Shigella dysenteriae* type 1 dysentery in children. Pediatr Infect Dis J 21:1136, 2002

DEFINITION Bacteria of the genus *Campylobacter* and of the related genera *Arcobacter* and *Helicobacter* (Chap. 135) cause a variety of inflammatory conditions. Although acute diarrheal illnesses are most common, these organisms may cause infections in virtually all parts of the body, especially in compromised hosts, and these infections may have late nonsuppurative sequelae. The designation *Campylobacter* comes from the Greek for "curved rod" and refers to the organism's vibrio-like morphology.

ETIOLOGY Campylobacters are motile, non-spore-forming, curved gram-negative rods. Originally known as *Vibrio fetus*, these bacilli were reclassified as a new genus in 1973, after it was recognized that they were quite dissimilar to other vibrios. Since then, >15 species have been identified. These species are currently divided into three genera: *Campylobacter*, *Arcobacter*, and *Helicobacter*. Not all of the species are pathogens of humans. The human pathogens can be divided into two major groups: those that primarily cause diarrheal disease and those that cause extraintestinal infection. The principal diarrheal pathogen is *C. jejuni*, which accounts for 80 to 90% of all cases of recognized illness due to campylobacters. Other organisms that cause diarrheal disease include *C. coli*, *C. upsaliensis*, *C. lari*, and *C. fetus*. The major species causing extraintestinal illnesses is *C. fetus*; however, any of the diarrheal agents may cause systemic or localized infection as well. Neither aerobes nor strict anaerobes, these microaerophilic organisms are adapted for survival in the gastrointestinal mucous layer. This chapter will focus on *C. jejuni* and *C. fetus* as the major pathogens and prototypes for their groups; the key features of infection are listed by species (excluding *C. jejuni*, described in detail in the text below) in Table 139-1.

EPIDEMIOLOGY Campylobacters are found in the gastrointestinal tract of many animals used for food (including poultry, cattle, sheep, and swine) and of many household pets (including birds, dogs, and cats). These microorganisms usually do not cause illness in their animal hosts. In most cases, campylobacters are transmitted to humans in raw or undercooked food products or through direct contact with infected animals. In the United States and other developed countries, ingestion of contaminated poultry that has not been sufficiently cooked is the most common means of acquiring infection (50 to 70% of cases). Other modes of transmission include ingestion of raw (unpasteurized) milk or untreated water, contact with infected household pets, travel to developing countries (campylobacters being among the causes of traveler's diarrhea; Chap. 113), oral-anal sexual contact, and (occasionally) contact with an index case who is incontinent of stool.

Campylobacter infections are common. Several studies indicate that, in the United States, diarrheal disease due to campylobacters is more common than that due to *Salmonella* and *Shigella* combined. Infections occur throughout the year, but their incidence peaks during summer and early autumn. Persons of all ages are affected; however, attack rates for *C. jejuni* are highest among young children and young adults, while those for *C. fetus* are highest at the extremes of age. Systemic infections due to *C. fetus* (and to other *Campylobacter* and related species) are most common in compromised hosts. Persons at increased risk include those with AIDS, hypogammaglobulinemia, neoplasia, liver disease, diabetes mellitus, and generalized atherosclerosis as well as neonates and pregnant women. However, apparently healthy nonpregnant persons occasionally develop transient *Campylobacter* bacteremia as part of a gastrointestinal illness.

In developing countries, *C. jejuni* infections are hyperendemic, with the highest rates among children <2 years old. Infection rates fall with age, as does the illness-to-infection ratio; these observations suggest that frequent exposure to *C. jejuni* leads to the acquisition of immunity.

PATHOLOGY AND PATHOGENESIS Many *C. jejuni* infections are subclinical, especially in hosts in developing countries who have had multiple prior infections and thus are partially immune. Most illnesses occur within 2 to 4 days (range, 1 to 7 days) of exposure to the organism in food or water. The sites of tissue injury include the jejunum, ileum, and colon. Biopsies show an acute nonspecific inflammatory reaction, with neutrophils, monocytes, and eosinophils in the lamina propria, as

TABLE 139-1 *Clinical Features Associated with Infection Due to "Atypical" Campylobacter and Related Species Implicated as Causes of Human Illness*

Species	Common Clinical Features	Less Common Clinical Features	Additional Information
Campylobacter coli	Fever, diarrhea, abdominal pain	Bacteremia[a]	Clinically indistinguishable from *C. jejuni*
Campylobacter fetus	Bacteremia,[a] sepsis, meningitis, vascular infections	Diarrhea, relapsing fevers	Not usually isolated from media containing cephalothin or incubated at 42°C
Campylobacter upsaliensis	Watery diarrhea, low-grade fever, abdominal pain	Bacteremia, abscesses	Difficult to isolate because of cephalothin susceptibility
Campylobacter lari	Abdominal pain, diarrhea	Colitis, appendicitis	Seagulls frequently colonized; organism often transmitted to humans via contaminated water
Campylobacter hyointestinalis	Watery or bloody diarrhea, vomiting, abdominal pain	Bacteremia	Causes proliferative enteritis in swine
Helicobacter fennelliae	Chronic mild diarrhea, abdominal cramps, proctitis	Bacteremia[a]	Best treated with fluoroquinolones
Helicobacter cinaedi	Chronic mild diarrhea, abdominal cramps, proctitis	Bacteremia[a]	Best treated with fluoroquinolones; identified in healthy hamsters
Campylobacter jejuni subspecies *doylei*	Diarrhea	Chronic gastritis, bacteremia[b]	Uncertain role as human pathogen
Arcobacter cryaerophila	Diarrhea	Bacteremia	Cultured under aerobic conditions
Arcobacter butzleri	Fever, diarrhea, abdominal pain, nausea	Bacteremia, appendicitis	Cultured under aerobic conditions; enzootic in nonhuman primates
Campylobacter sputorum	Pulmonary, perianal, groin, and axillary abscesses	Bacteremia	Three clinically relevant biovars: *C. sputorum* subspecies *sputorum*, *C. sputorum* subspecies *bubulus*, and *Campylobacter mucosalis*

[a] In immunocompromised hosts, especially HIV-infected persons.
[b] In children.

Source: Adapted from Allos and Blaser.

well as damage to the epithelium, including loss of mucus, glandular degeneration, and crypt abscesses. Biopsy findings may be consistent with Crohn's disease or ulcerative colitis, but these "idiopathic" chronic inflammatory diseases should not be diagnosed unless infectious colitis, *specifically including* that due to infection with *Campylobacter* species and related organisms, has been ruled out.

The high frequency of *C. jejuni* infections and their severity and recurrence among hypogammaglobulinemic patients suggest that antibodies are important in protective immunity. The pathogenesis of infection is uncertain. Both the motility of the strain and its capacity to adhere to host tissues appear to favor disease, but classic enterotoxins and cytotoxins (although described and including cytolethal distending toxin, or CLDT) appear not to play any substantial role in tissue injury or disease production. The organisms have been visualized in the epithelium, albeit in low numbers. The documentation of a significant tissue response and occasionally of *C. jejuni* bacteremia further suggests that tissue invasion is clinically significant.

The pathogenesis of *C. fetus* infections is better defined. Virtually all clinical isolates of *C. fetus* possess a proteinaceous capsule-like structure (an S-layer) that renders the organism resistant to complement-mediated killing and opsonization. As a result, *C. fetus* can cause bacteremia and can seed sites beyond the intestinal tract. The ability of the organism to switch the S-layer proteins expressed, a phenomenon that results in antigenic variability, may contribute to the chronicity and high rate of recurrence of these infections in compromised hosts.

CLINICAL MANIFESTATIONS OF *C. JEJUNI* AND *C. FETUS* INFECTIONS

The clinical features of infections due to all of the *Campylobacter* and related species causing enteric disease appear to be highly similar. There is often a prodrome, with fever, headache, myalgia, and/or malaise, 12 to 48 h before the onset of diarrheal symptoms. The most common signs and symptoms of the intestinal phase are diarrhea, abdominal pain, and fever. The degree of diarrhea varies from several loose stools to grossly bloody stools; most patients presenting for medical attention have 10 or more bowel movements on the worst day of illness. Abdominal pain usually consists of cramping and may be the most prominent symptom. Pain is usually generalized but may become localized; *C. jejuni* infection may cause pseudoappendicitis. Fever may be the only initial manifestation of *C. jejuni* infection, a situation mimicking the early stages of typhoid fever. Febrile young children may develop convulsions. *Campylobacter* enteritis is generally self-limited; however, symptoms persist for >1 week in 10 to 20% of patients seeking medical attention, and relapses occur in 5 to 10% of untreated patients.

C. fetus may cause a diarrheal illness similar to that due to *C. jejuni*, especially in normal hosts, or may cause either intermittent diarrhea or nonspecific abdominal pain without localizing signs. Sequelae are uncommon, and outcome is benign. *C. fetus* may also cause a prolonged relapsing systemic illness (with fever, chills, and myalgias) that has no obvious primary source; this manifestation is especially common in compromised hosts. Secondary seeding of an organ (e.g., meninges, brain, bone, urinary tract, or soft tissue) complicates the course, which may be fulminant. *C. fetus* infections have a tropism for vascular sites: endocarditis, mycotic aneurysm, and septic thrombophlebitis may all occur. Infection during pregnancy often leads to fetal death. *H. cinaedi* causes recurrent cellulitis with fever and bacteremia in immunocompromised hosts.

COMPLICATIONS

Except in the case of infection with *C. fetus*, bacteremia is uncommon, developing most often in immunocompromised hosts and at the extremes of age. Three patterns of extraintestinal infection have been noted: (1) transient bacteremia in a normal host with enteritis (benign course, no specific treatment needed); (2) sustained bacteremia or focal infection in a normal host (bacteremia originating from enteritis, with patients responding well to antimicrobial therapy); and (3) sustained bacteremia or focal infection in a compromised host. Enteritis may not be clinically apparent. Antimicrobial therapy, possibly prolonged, is necessary for suppression or cure of the infection.

Campylobacter infections in patients with AIDS or hypogammaglobulinemia may be severe, persistent, and extraintestinal; relapse after cessation of therapy is common. Hypogammaglobulinemic patients may also develop osteomyelitis and an erysipelas-like rash.

Local suppurative complications of infection include cholecystitis, pancreatitis, and cystitis; distant complications include meningitis, endocarditis, arthritis, peritonitis, cellulitis, and septic abortion. All are rare. Hepatitis, interstitial nephritis, and the hemolytic-uremic syndrome occasionally complicate acute infection. Reactive arthritis and other rheumatologic complaints may develop several weeks after infection, especially in persons with the HLA-B27 phenotype. Guillain-Barré syndrome follows *Campylobacter* infections uncommonly (i.e., in 1 of every 1000 to 2000 cases). For certain *C. jejuni* serotypes, such as O19, Guillain-Barré syndrome may occur once following 100 or 200 cases. Because of their high incidence, it is now estimated that *Campylobacter* infections may trigger 20 to 40% of all cases of Guillain-Barré syndrome.

DIAGNOSIS

In patients with *Campylobacter* enteritis, peripheral leukocyte counts reflect the severity of the inflammatory process. However, stools from nearly all *Campylobacter*-infected patients presenting for medical attention in the United States contain leukocytes or erythrocytes. Fecal smears should be treated with Gram's or Wright's stain and examined in all suspected cases. When the diagnosis of *Campylobacter* enteritis is suspected on the basis of findings indicating inflammatory diarrhea (fever, fecal leukocytes), clinicians can ask the laboratory to attempt the visualization of organisms with characteristic vibrioid morphology by direct microscopic examination of stools with Gram's staining or to use phase-contrast or dark-field microscopy to identify the organisms' characteristic "darting" motility. Confirmation of the diagnosis of *Campylobacter* infection is based on identification of an isolate from cultures of stool, blood, or another site. *Campylobacter*-specific media should be used to culture stools from all patients with inflammatory or bloody diarrhea. Since all *Campylobacter* species are fastidious, they will not be isolated unless selective media or other selective techniques are used. Not all media are equally useful for isolation of the broad array of campylobacters; therefore, failure to isolate campylobacters from stool does not entirely rule out their presence. The detection of the organisms in stool almost always implies infection; there is a brief period of postconvalescent fecal carriage and no commensalism in humans. In contrast, *C. sputorum* and related organisms found in the oral cavity are commensals with rare pathogenic significance.

DIFFERENTIAL DIAGNOSIS

The symptoms of *Campylobacter* enteritis are not sufficiently unusual to distinguish this illness from that due to *Salmonella*, *Shigella*, or *Yersinia*, among other pathogens. The combination of fever and fecal leukocytes or erythrocytes is indicative of inflammatory diarrhea, and definitive diagnosis is based on culture or demonstration of the characteristic organisms on stained fecal smears. Similarly, extraintestinal *Campylobacter* illness is diagnosed by culture. Infection due to *Campylobacter* should be suspected in the setting of septic abortion and that due to *C. fetus* specifically in the setting of septic thrombophlebitis. It is important to reiterate that the presentation of *Campylobacter* enteritis may mimic that of ulcerative colitis or Crohn's disease, that *Campylobacter* enteritis is much more common than either of the latter (especially among young adults), and that biopsy may not be able to distinguish among these entities. Thus a diagnosis of inflammatory bowel disease should not be made until *Campylobacter* infection has been ruled out, especially in persons with a history of foreign travel, significant animal contact, immunodeficiency, or exposure incurring a high risk of transmission.

℞ TREATMENT

Fluid and electrolyte replacement is central to the treatment of diarrheal illnesses (Chap. 113). Even among patients presenting for medical attention with *Campylobacter* enteritis, fewer than half will clearly benefit from specific antimicrobial therapy. Indications for such therapy include high fever, bloody diarrhea, severe diarrhea, persistence for >1 week, and worsening of symptoms. A 5- to 7-day course of erythromycin (250 mg orally four times daily or—for children—30 to 50 mg/kg per day, in divided doses) is the regimen of choice. Although no relevant clinical trials have been conducted, the in vitro susceptibility of *Campylobacter* species to macrolides such as clarithromycin and azithromycin suggests that these antibiotics would also be useful therapeutic agents. An alternative regimen for adults is ciprofloxacin (500 mg orally twice daily) or another fluoroquinolone for 5 to 7 days, but resistance to this class of agents is increasing. Other alternatives include tetracycline and furazolidone. Use of antimotility agents, which may prolong the duration of symptoms and has been associated with toxic megacolon and with death, is not recommended.

For systemic infections, treatment with gentamicin (1.7 mg/kg intravenously every 8 h after a loading dose of 2 mg/kg), imipenem (500 mg intravenously every 6 h), or chloramphenicol (50 mg/kg intravenously each day in three or four divided doses) should be started empirically, but susceptibility testing should then be performed. Ciprofloxacin and amoxicillin/clavulanate are alternative agents for susceptible strains. In the absence of immunocompromise or endovascular infections, therapy should be administered for 14 days. For immunocompromised patients with systemic infections due to *C. fetus* and for patients with endovascular infections, prolonged therapy (for up to 4 weeks) is usually necessary.

PROGNOSIS Nearly all patients recover fully from *Campylobacter* enteritis, either spontaneously or after antimicrobial therapy. Volume depletion likely contributes to the few deaths that are reported. As stated above, occasional patients develop reactive arthritis or Guillain-Barré syndrome. Systemic infection with *C. fetus* is much more often fatal than that due to related species; this higher mortality reflects in part the population affected. Prognosis is dependent on the rapidity with which appropriate therapy is begun. Otherwise healthy hosts usually survive *C. fetus* infections without sequelae. Compromised hosts often have recurrent infections.

FURTHER READING

ALLOS BM, BLASER MJ: *Campylobacter jejuni* and the expanding spectrum of related infections. Clin Infect Dis 20:1092, 1995

LANG DR et al (eds): Development of Guillain-Barré syndrome following *Campylobacter* infection. J Infect Dis 176(Suppl 2):S91, 1997

MEAD PS et al: Food-related illness and death in the United States. Emerg Infect Dis 5:607, 1999

NACHAMKIN I, BLASER MJ (eds): *Campylobacter jejuni*, 2d ed. Washington, American Society for Microbiology, 2000

SMITH KE et al: Quinolone-resistant *Campylobacter jejuni* infections in Minnesota, 1992–1998. Investigation Team. N Engl J Med 340:1525, 1999

140 CHOLERA AND OTHER VIBRIOSES
Matthew K. Waldor, Gerald T. Keusch

Members of the genus *Vibrio* cause a number of important infectious syndromes. Classic among them is cholera, a devastating diarrheal disease caused by *V. cholerae* that has been responsible for seven global pandemics and much suffering over the past two centuries. Epidemic cholera remains a significant public health concern in the developing world today. Other vibrioses have also been described, including syndromes of diarrhea, soft tissue infection, or primary sepsis caused by additional named species in the genus *Vibrio*.

All members of the genus are highly motile, facultatively anaerobic, curved gram-negative rods with one or more flagella. Except for *V. cholerae* and *V. mimicus*, all vibrios are halophilic (i.e., require salt for growth). In nature, vibrios most commonly reside in tidal rivers and bays under conditions of moderate salinity. They proliferate in the summer months when water temperatures exceed 20°C. As might be expected, the illnesses they cause also increase in frequency during the warm months.

CHOLERA

DEFINITION Cholera is an acute diarrheal disease that can, in a matter of hours, result in profound, rapidly progressive dehydration and death. Accordingly, cholera gravis (the severe form of cholera) is a much-feared disease, particularly in its epidemic presentation. Fortunately, prompt aggressive fluid repletion and supportive care can obviate the high mortality that cholera has historically wrought. While the term *cholera* has occasionally been applied to any severely dehydrating secretory diarrheal illness, whether infectious in etiology or not, it has generally referred to disease caused by *V. cholerae* serogroup O1. In 1992, however, a new serogroup (O139) that causes epidemic cholera emerged on the Indian subcontinent and has since killed thousands of people.

MICROBIOLOGY AND EPIDEMIOLOGY The species *V. cholerae* comprises a host of organisms classified on the basis of the carbohydrate determinants of their lipopolysaccharide (LPS) O antigens. Some 200 serogroups have now been recognized. They are divided into those that agglutinate in antisera to the O1 group antigen (*V. cholerae* O1) and those that do not (non-O1 *V. cholerae*). Although some non-O1 *V. cholerae* serogroups have occasionally caused sporadic outbreaks of diarrhea, serogroup O1 was, until the emergence of serogroup O139, the exclusive cause of epidemic cholera.

Two biotypes of *V. cholerae* O1, *classical* and *El Tor*, are distinguished. Each biotype is further subdivided into two serotypes, termed *Inaba* and *Ogawa*.

The natural habitat of *V. cholerae* is coastal salt water and brackish estuaries, where the organism lives in close relation to plankton and where it may survive in a viable but nonculturable form. Humans become infected incidentally but, once infected, can act as vehicles for spread. Ingestion of water contaminated by human feces is the most common means of acquisition of *V. cholerae*. Consumption of contaminated food can also contribute to spread. There is no known animal reservoir. While the infectious dose is relatively high, it is markedly reduced in hypochlorhydric persons, in those using antacids, and when gastric acidity is buffered by a meal. Cholera is predominantly a pediatric disease in endemic areas, but it affects adults and children equally when newly introduced into a population. In endemic areas, the disease is more common in the summer and fall months. While this seasonality has not been explained fully, it may be due to environmental conditions that affect the multiplication of vibrios or to seasonal alterations in human behavior that affect contact with water. In endemic areas, children <2 years of age are less likely to develop severe cholera than are older children, perhaps because of passive immunity acquired from breast milk. For unexplained reasons, susceptibility to cholera is significantly influenced by ABO blood group status; those with type O blood are at greatest risk, while those with type AB are at least risk.

Cholera is native to the Ganges delta in the Indian subcontinent. Since 1817, seven global pandemics have occurred. The current (seventh) pandemic—the first due to the El Tor biotype—began in Indonesia in 1961 and spread throughout Asia as *V. cholerae* El Tor displaced the endemic classical strain in many areas. In the early 1970s, El Tor cholera exploded in Africa, causing major epidemics before becoming a persistent endemic problem. Its recent history in Africa has been punctuated by severe outbreaks, often fed by the chaos of war and genocide. Such was the case in the camps for Rwandan refugees set up in 1994 around Goma, Zaire. Tens of thousands of cases occurred and mortality was high. In 1995, the occurrence of hundreds of cases in Romania and the Black Sea states of the former Soviet Union demonstrated the potential of this organism to cause epidemics whenever public health measures break down.

Since 1973, sporadic endemic infections due to vibrios related to the seventh-pandemic strain have been recognized along the U.S. Gulf Coast of Louisiana and Texas. These infections are typically associated with the consumption of contaminated, locally harvested shellfish. Occasionally, cases in U.S. locations remote from the Gulf Coast have been linked to shipped-in Gulf Coast seafood.

It was not until 1991 that the current cholera pandemic reached Latin America. Beginning along the Peruvian coast in January 1991, the disease spread in an explosive epidemic to virtually all of South and Central America and to Mexico (Fig. 140-1). About 400,000 cases were reported in the first year of the outbreak, and >1 million had been reported by the end of 1994. While the cumulative mortality rate has been <1%, the mortality rate approached 30% in the communities first affected, where a lack of familiarity with the disease led initially to the deployment of ineffective treatment. Intensive education of health care providers and of the community at large has enhanced awareness of the disease and its appropriate management and has greatly diminished mortality. As it did in Africa two decades earlier, the epidemic El Tor strain proved capable of establishing itself in inland waters rather than in its classic niche of coastal salt waters; the organism has already become endemic in many of the Latin American countries into which it was recently introduced. Cases linked to the Latin American epidemic have occurred (via importation of contaminated seafood) in the United States. Although secondary spread of this strain has not taken place in the United States, these events underscore the need for vigilance among health care professionals, even in locations remote from an epidemic.

In October 1992, a large-scale outbreak of clinical cholera occurred in southeastern India. The etiologic agent proved to be a novel strain of *V. cholerae* belonging neither to the O1 serogroup that typically causes epidemic cholera nor to any of the 137 other serogroups known at the time. This strain spread rapidly up and down the coast of the Bay of Bengal, reaching Bangladesh in December 1992. There alone, it caused more than 100,000 cases of cholera in the first 3 months of 1993. It subsequently spread across the Indian subcontinent and to neighboring countries, affecting Pakistan, Nepal, western China, Thailand, and Malaysia by the end of 1994 (Fig. 140-2). The organism has since been designated *V. cholerae* O139 Bengal in recognition of its novel O antigen and its geographic origin. The clinical manifestations and epidemiologic features of the disease caused by *V. cholerae* O139

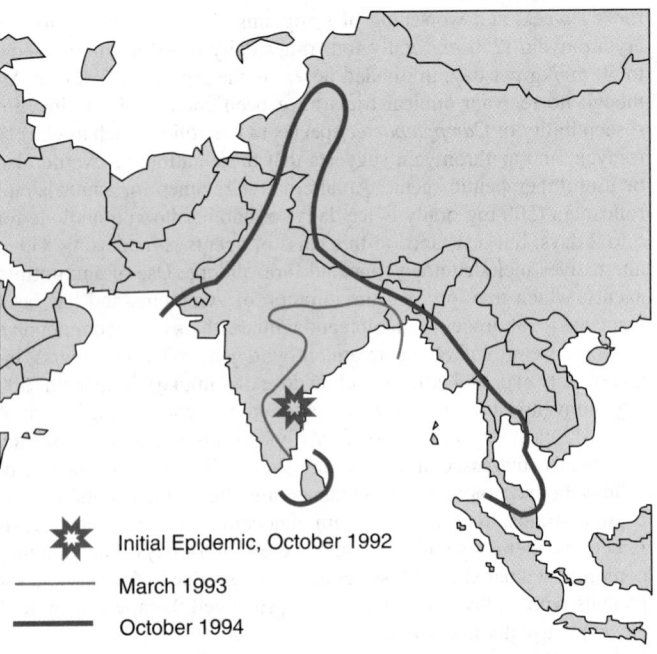

✳ Initial Epidemic, October 1992

─── March 1993

━━━ October 1994

FIGURE 140-2 Spread of *Vibrio cholerae* O139 in the Indian subcontinent and elsewhere in Asia, 1992–1994. *(Courtesy of Dr. Robert V. Tauxe, Centers for Disease Control and Prevention, Atlanta.)*

Bengal are indistinguishable from those of O1 cholera. Immunity to the latter, however, is not protective against the former. Because naturally acquired immunity to *V. cholerae* O1 does not cross-protect against *V. cholerae* O139 Bengal, vaccines being developed against the former are unlikely to be effective against the latter.

Some authorities believed that the emergence of *V. cholerae* O139 signaled the beginning of the eighth global cholera pandemic. Indeed, just as O1 El Tor replaced the classical biotype that preceded it, O139 Bengal in 1993 rapidly replaced O1 El Tor as the most common environmental isolate and the predominant cause of clinical cholera in the areas in which it had appeared. However, by the beginning of 1994, O1 El Tor resumed its dominance in Bangladesh. Currently, in most regions of Southest Asia, O1 *V. cholerae* remains dominant; in others, O139 periodically reemerges.

PATHOGENESIS In the final analysis, cholera is a toxin-mediated disease. Its characteristic watery diarrhea is due to the action of cholera toxin (CT), a potent protein enterotoxin elaborated by the organism following its colonization of the small intestine. For *V. cholerae* to colonize the small intestine and produce CT, it must first recognize, contend with, and traverse several hostile environments. The first of these is the acidic milieu of the stomach. To elude the bactericidal effects of gastric acidity, *V. cholerae* relies, at least in part, on a relatively large inoculum size (compared to that needed for colonization by *Shigella*, for instance). The organism must next traverse the mucous layer lining the small bowel. *V. cholerae* chemotaxis and motility and a variety of proteases may allow the organism to traverse this gel covering the intestinal epithelium. Adherence to the intestinal epithelium is believed to be mediated by the toxin-coregulated pilus (TCP), so named because its synthesis is regulated in parallel with that of CT. CT, TCP, and several other virulence factors are coordinately regulated by the *toxR* gene product. The ToxR protein modulates the expression of virulence genes in response to environmental signals via a cascade of regulatory proteins. Additional regulatory processes, including the density of the bacterial population (in a phenomenon known as *quorum sensing*), control the virulence of *V. cholerae*.

Once established in the human small bowel, the organism produces CT, which consists of a monomeric enzymatic moiety (the A subunit) and a pentameric binding moiety (the B subunit). The B pentamer binds to G_{M1} ganglioside, a glycolipid on the surface of epithelial cells that serves as the toxin receptor and makes possible the delivery of

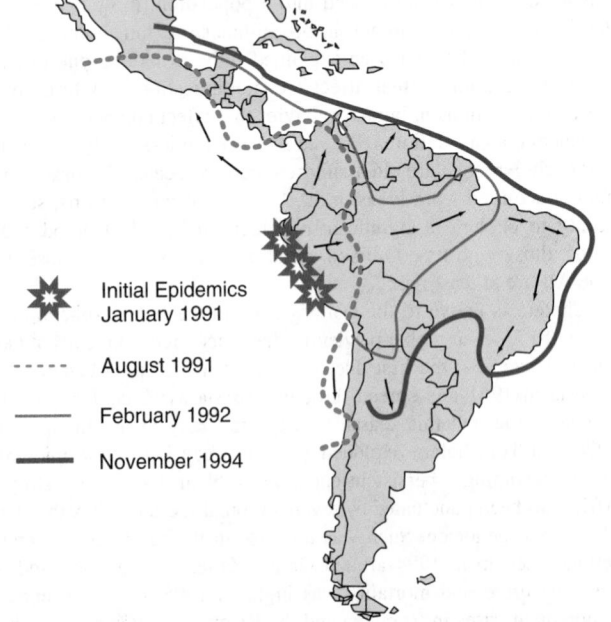

✳ Initial Epidemics
    January 1991

----- August 1991

─── February 1992

━━━ November 1994

FIGURE 140-1 Spread of *Vibrio cholerae* O1 in the Americas, 1991–1994. *(Courtesy of Dr. Robert V. Tauxe, Centers for Disease Control and Prevention, Atlanta.)*

the A subunit to its cytosolic target. The activated A subunit (A_1) irreversibly transfers ADP-ribose from nicotinamide adenine dinucleotide to its specific target protein, the GTP-binding regulatory component of adenylate cyclase in intestinal epithelial cells. The ADP-ribosylated G protein upregulates the activity of adenylate cyclase; the result is the intracellular accumulation of high levels of cyclic AMP. In intestinal epithelial cells, cyclic AMP inhibits the absorptive sodium transport system in villus cells and activates the secretory chloride transport system in crypt cells, and these events lead to the accumulation of sodium chloride in the intestinal lumen. Since water moves passively to maintain osmolality, isotonic fluid accumulates in the lumen. When the volume of that fluid exceeds the capacity of the rest of the gut to resorb it, watery diarrhea results. Unless the wasted fluid and electrolytes are adequately replaced, shock (due to profound dehydration) and acidosis (due to loss of bicarbonate) follow. Although perturbation of the adenylate cyclase pathway is the primary mechanism by which CT causes excess fluid secretion, it is not the only one. Increasing evidence indicates that CT also enhances intestinal secretion via prostaglandins and/or neural histamine receptors.

The genes encoding CT (*ctxAB*) are part of the genome of a bacteriophage designated CTXΦ. The receptor for this phage on the *V. cholerae* surface is the essential *V. cholerae* intestinal colonization factor TCP. After the infection of TCP+ *ctxAB− V. cholerae* cells, the CTXΦ genome stably integrates at a specific site on the *V. cholerae* chromosome. Since *ctxAB* is part of a mobile genetic element (CTXΦ), horizontal transfer of this bacteriophage may account for the emergence of new toxigenic *V. cholerae* serogroups. Many of the other genes important for *V. cholerae* pathogenicity, including the genes encoding the biosynthesis of TCP, those encoding accessory colonization factors, and those regulating virulence gene expression, are clustered together in the *V. cholerae* pathogenicity island. Similar clustering of virulence genes is found in other bacterial pathogens. It is believed that pathogenicity islands are acquired by horizontal gene transfer.

V. cholerae O139 Bengal is closely related to the O1 El Tor strains of the seventh pandemic and seems to have arisen from them by horizontal gene transfer. It shares the virulence attributes and general pathogenic mechanisms of O1 vibrios. *V. cholerae* O139 Bengal is in fact virtually identical to the seventh-pandemic strains of *V. cholerae* O1 El Tor except for two important differences: production of the novel O139 LPS and of an immunologically related O-antigen polysaccharide capsule. The ability to produce the O139 LPS is due to a replacement of a 22-kb DNA segment encoding O1 antigen biosynthesis with a 35-kb segment containing the genes encoding O139 LPS and capsule biosynthesis. Encapsulation is not a feature of O1 strains and may explain the resistance of O139 strains to human serum in vitro as well as the occasional development of O139 bacteremia.

CLINICAL MANIFESTATIONS After a 24- to 48-h incubation period, cholera begins with the sudden onset of painless watery diarrhea that may quickly become voluminous and is often followed shortly by vomiting. In severe cases, stool volume can exceed 250 mL/kg in the first 24 h. If fluids and electrolytes are not replaced, hypovolemic shock and death ensue. Fever is usually absent. Muscle cramps due to electrolyte disturbances are common. The stool has a characteristic appearance: a nonbilious, gray, slightly cloudy fluid with flecks of mucus, no blood, and a somewhat sweet, inoffensive odor. It has been called "rice-water" stool because of its resemblance to the water in which rice has been washed. Clinical symptoms parallel volume contraction: At losses of 3 to 5% of normal body weight, thirst develops; at 5 to 8%, postural hypotension, weakness, tachycardia, and decreased skin turgor are documented; and at >10%, oliguria, weak or absent pulses, sunken eyes (and, in infants, sunken fontanelles), wrinkled ("washerwoman") skin, somnolence, and coma are characteristic. Complications derive exclusively from the effects of volume and electrolyte depletion and include renal failure due to acute tubular necrosis. Thus, if the patient is adequately treated with fluid and electrolytes, complications are averted and the process is self-limited, resolving in a few days.

Laboratory data usually reveal an elevated hematocrit (due to hemoconcentration) in nonanemic patients; mild neutrophilic leukocytosis; elevated levels of blood urea nitrogen and creatinine consistent with prerenal azotemia; normal sodium, potassium, and chloride levels; a markedly reduced bicarbonate level (<15 mmol/L); and an elevated anion gap (due to increases in serum lactate, protein, and phosphate). Arterial pH is usually low (about 7.2).

DIAGNOSIS The clinical suspicion of cholera can be confirmed by the identification of *V. cholerae* in stool; however, the organism must be specifically sought. With experience, it can be detected directly by dark-field microscopy on a wet mount of fresh stool, and its serotype can be discerned by immobilization with Inaba- or Ogawa-specific antiserum. Laboratory isolation of the organism requires the use of a selective medium. The best of these is thiosulfate–citrate–bile salts–sucrose (TCBS) agar, on which the organism grows as a flat yellow colony. If a delay in sample processing is expected, Carey-Blair transport medium and/or alkaline-peptone water-enrichment medium should be inoculated as well. In endemic areas there is little need for biochemical confirmation and characterization, although these tasks may be worthwhile in places where *V. cholerae* is an uncommon isolate. Standard microbiologic biochemical testing for Enterobacteriaceae will suffice for identification of *V. cholerae*. All vibrios are oxidase-positive.

The yield of stool cultures for the diagnosis of *V. cholerae* infection declines late in the course of the illness or when effective antibacterial therapy is initiated. Although not generally performed in clinical laboratories, measurement of serum vibriocidal antibody titers can be used to confirm the diagnosis in non-cholera-endemic regions of the world. Monoclonal antibody–based diagnostic kits and methods based on the polymerase chain reaction and on DNA probes have also been developed for detection of *V. cholerae* O1 and O139.

Rx TREATMENT

Cholera is simple to treat; only the rapid and adequate replacement of fluids, electrolytes, and base is required. The mortality rate for appropriately treated disease is usually <1%. However, analysis of a large outbreak of cholera among airline travelers from an endemic country to the United States revealed frequent misdiagnoses by U.S. health professionals and poor appreciation on their part of the principles of management. It has been proved conclusively that fluid may be given orally. This approach takes advantage of the hexose-Na^+ cotransport mechanism to move Na^+ across the gut mucosa together with an actively transported molecule such as glucose. Since Na^+ losses in the stool are high, a fluid containing Na^+ at 90 mmol/L has been recommended by the World Health Organization (WHO) (Table 140-1). This amount of Na^+ is higher than that needed to treat diarrhea due to most other causes. The solution is safe, even for infants, if its intake is alternated with the consumption of sodium-free fluids such as breast milk or water. For the sake of simplicity, WHO advises routine use of

TABLE 140-1 *Composition of World Health Organization Oral Rehydration Solution (ORS)[a,b]*

Constituent	Concentration, mmol/L
Na^+	90
K^+	20
Cl^-	80
Citrate[c]	10
Glucose	110

[a] Contains (per package, to be added to 1 L of drinking water): NaCl, 3.5 g; $Na_3C_6H_5O_7 \cdot 2H_2O$, 2.9 g; KCl, 1.5 g; and glucose, 20 g.
[b] If prepackaged ORS is unavailable, a simple homemade alternative can be prepared by combining 5 g NaCl (about 1 level teaspoon) with either 50 g precooked rice cereal or 40 g sucrose in 1 L of drinking water. In that case, potassium must be supplied separately (e.g., in orange juice or coconut water).
[c] 10 mmol citrate per liter, which supplies 30 mmol HCO_3/L.

this single solution for diarrheal disease rather than attempts to choose among multiple formulations according to etiology.

Cereal-based formulations are receiving increased attention as alternative oral rehydration solutions. Because of their lower osmolarity, they may reduce stool output. A mixture with a lower sugar and salt content has also been evaluated in cholera patients, with favorable results. However, concerns have been raised over the safety of its use—in particular, whether it could cause significant hyponatremia in patients with moderate or severe diarrhea. Because commercial oral rehydration solutions also contain concentrations of glucose and sodium lower than those of the WHO formulation, they should not yet be used routinely to treat cholera.

For initial management of severely dehydrated patients, intravenous fluid replacement is preferable, if available. Because profound acidosis (pH < 7.2) is common in this group, Ringer's lactate is the best choice among commercial products (Table 140-2). It must be used with additional potassium supplements, preferably given by mouth. The total fluid deficit in severely dehydrated patients ($\geq$10% of body weight) can be replaced safely within the first 4 h of therapy, half within the first hour. Thereafter, oral therapy can usually be initiated, with the goal of maintaining fluid intake equal to fluid output. However, patients with continued large-volume diarrhea may require prolonged intravenous treatment to keep up with gastrointestinal fluid losses. Severe hypokalemia can develop but will respond to potassium given either intravenously or orally. In the absence of adequate staff to monitor the patient's progress, the oral route of rehydration and potassium replacement is safer than the intravenous route.

Although not necessary for cure, the use of an antibiotic to which the organism is susceptible will diminish the duration and volume of fluid loss and will hasten clearance of the organism from the stool. Single-dose tetracycline (2 g) or doxycycline (300 mg) is effective in adults but is not recommended for children <8 years of age because of possible deposition in bone and developing teeth. Emerging drug resistance is an ever-present concern. For adults with cholera in areas where tetracycline resistance is prevalent, ciprofloxacin—either in a single dose (30 mg/kg, not to exceed a total dose of 1 g) or in a short course (15 mg/kg twice daily for 3 days, not to exceed a total daily dose of 1 g)—or erythromycin (a total of 40 mg/kg daily in three divided doses for 3 days) is a clinically effective substitute. Both drugs are highly effective in reducing total stool output, and each is significantly better than trimethoprim-sulfamethoxazole. Because of the high cost of quinolones, WHO recommends erythromycin as the first alternative to tetracycline. For children, furazolidone has been the recommended agent and trimethoprim-sulfamethoxazole the second choice. Because of cost and/or toxicity issues related to the other drugs, erythromycin is a good choice for pediatric cholera.

CONTROL In outbreaks, efforts should first be made to identify case contacts and to treat incubating carriers. Next, epidemiologic studies should be undertaken to establish the modes of transmission in order to define the best strategy to interrupt them. Both the establishment of rehydration centers and instruction in rehydration techniques are essential to the reduction of mortality.

PREVENTION Provision of safe water and facilities for sanitary disposal of feces, improved nutrition, and attention to food preparation and storage in the household could significantly reduce the incidence of cholera. Much effort has been devoted to the development of an effective cholera vaccine over the past two decades, with a particular focus on oral vaccine strains. Traditional killed cholera vaccine given intramuscularly provides little protection to nonimmune subjects and predictably causes adverse effects, including pain at the injection site, malaise, and fever. The vaccine's limited efficacy is at least partially due to its failure to induce a local immune response at the intestinal mucosal surface.

Two types of oral cholera vaccines are under development. The first is a killed whole-cell (WC) vaccine. Two formulations of the killed WC vaccine have been prepared: one that also contains the nontoxic B subunit of CT (WC/BS) and one composed solely of killed bacteria. In field trials in Bangladesh, both of the killed vaccines were compared with placebo and conferred ~50% protection over a 3-year evaluation period. The protective efficacy of WC/BS was superior to that of WC during the initial 8 months of follow-up (69 versus 41%) but equivalent or inferior thereafter. Immunity was relatively sustained in persons vaccinated at an age of >5 years but was not well sustained in younger vaccinees. The WC/BS vaccine is now available in Europe but not in the United States.

The second approach is that of a live attenuated vaccine strain developed, for example, by the isolation or creation of mutants lacking the genes encoding CT. Strain CVD 103-HgR, an oral live cholera vaccine licensed for immunization of travelers in Europe, is derived from a classical biotype strain of *V. cholerae* and contains a deletion of the CT A subunit gene. This strain has been extensively tested in volunteers; although it is poorly excreted in the stool of human vaccinees, a single dose produces a significant increase in the titer of vibriocidal antibody in ~75% of recipients, including children between the ages of 2 and 4 years, with almost no side effects. Unfortunately, in a large field trial in Indonesian children, this vaccine failed to induce protection against clinical cholera. Other live attenuated vaccine candidate strains have been prepared from El Tor and O139 *V. cholerae* and are now undergoing clinical trials. Because of the minimal efficacy of existing parenteral vaccines, cholera immunization is recommended for U.S. travelers only if it is mandated by the countries they plan to visit.

OTHER *VIBRIO* SPECIES

The genus *Vibrio* includes several human pathogens that do not cause clinical cholera. Abundant in coastal waters throughout the world, noncholera vibrios can reach high concentrations in the tissues of filter-feeding mollusks. As a result, human infection commonly follows the ingestion of seawater or of raw or undercooked shellfish (Table 140-3). Most noncholera vibrios can be cultured on blood or MacConkey agar, which contains enough salt to support the growth of these halophilic species. In the microbiology laboratory, the species of noncholera vibrios are distinguished by standard biochemical tests. The most important of these organisms are *V. parahaemolyticus* and *V. vulnificus*.

The two major types of syndromes for which these species are responsible are gastrointestinal illness (due to *V. parahaemolyticus*, non-O1 *V. cholerae*, *V. mimicus*, *V. fluvialis*, *V. hollisae*, and *V. furnissii*) and soft tissue infections (due to *V. vulnificus*, *V. alginolyticus*, and *V. damsela*). *V. vulnificus* is also a cause of primary sepsis in some compromised individuals. *V. parahaemolyticus* causes rare cases of wound infection and otitis and very rare cases of sepsis.

SPECIES ASSOCIATED PRIMARILY WITH GASTROINTESTINAL ILLNESS ■ *V. parahaemolyticus* Widespread in marine environments, *V. parahaemolyticus* grows in saline concentrations up to 8 to 10%. This species was originally implicated in enteritis in Japan in 1953, accounting for 24% of reported cases in one study—a rate that presumably was due to the common practice of eating raw seafood in that country. *V. parahaemolyticus* has since been identified as a significant intestinal path-

TABLE 140-2 *Electrolyte Composition of Cholera Stool and of Intravenous Rehydration Solution*

Substance	Concentration, mmol/L			
	Na+	K+	Cl−	Base
Stool				
Adult	135	15	90	30
Child	100	25	90	30
Ringer's lactate	130	4[a]	109	28

[a] Potassium supplements, preferably administered by mouth, are required to replace the usual potassium losses from stool.

ogen in many regions of the world. In the United States, common-source outbreaks of diarrhea caused by this organism have been linked to the consumption of undercooked or improperly handled seafood or of other foods contaminated by seawater. Since the mid-1990s, the incidence of *V. parahaemolyticus* infections has increased in several countries, including the United States. Serotypes O3:K6, O4:K68, and O1:K-untypable, which are genetically related to one another, account for this increase. The enteropathogenicity of *V. parahaemolyticus* is closely linked to its ability to cause hemolysis on Wagatsuma agar (i.e., the *Kanagawa phenomenon*). The genome sequence of *V. parahaemolyticus* contains a pathogenicity island—a cluster of likely virulence-associated genes. Although the mechanism by which the organism causes diarrhea remains unclear, it should be considered a possible etiologic agent in all cases of diarrhea that can be linked epidemiologically to seafood consumption or to the sea itself.

Infections with *V. parahaemolyticus* can result in two distinct gastrointestinal presentations. The more common of the two presentations (including nearly all cases in North America) is characterized by watery diarrhea, usually occurring in conjunction with abdominal cramps, nausea, and vomiting and accompanied in ~25% of cases by fever and chills. After an incubation period of 4 h to 4 days, symptoms develop and persist for a median of 3 days. Dysentery, the less common presentation, is characterized by severe abdominal cramps, nausea, vomiting, and bloody or mucoid stools. This syndrome is reported from India and Bangladesh.

Most cases of *V. parahaemolyticus*–associated gastrointestinal illness, regardless of the presentation, are self-limited and require neither antimicrobial treatment nor hospitalization. Deaths are extremely rare. Severe infections are associated with underlying diseases, including diabetes, preexisting liver disease, iron-overload states, or immunosuppression. The occasional severe case should be treated with fluid replacement and antibiotics, as described above for cholera.

Non-O1 *V. cholerae* The heterogeneous non-O1 *V. cholerae* organisms cannot be distinguished from *V. cholerae* O1 by routine biochemical tests but do not agglutinate in O1 antiserum. Non-O1 strains have caused several well-studied food-borne outbreaks of gastroenteritis and have also been responsible for sporadic cases of otitis media, wound infection, and bacteremia. Like other vibrios, non-O1 *V. cholerae* organisms are widely distributed in marine environments. In most instances, recognized cases in the United States have been associated with the consumption of raw oysters or with recent travel, typically to Mexico. The broad clinical spectrum of diarrheal illness caused by these organisms is probably due to the group's heterogeneous virulence attributes. *V. cholerae* O139 Bengal, although technically a non-O1 vibrio, is not grouped with these pathogens because it can cause epidemic cholera.

In the United States, about half of all non-O1 *V. cholerae* isolates are from stool samples. The typical incubation period for gastroenteritis due to these organisms is <2 days, and the illness lasts for ~2 to 7 days. Patients' stools may be copious and watery or may be partly formed, less voluminous, and bloody or mucoid. Diarrhea can result in severe dehydration. Many cases include abdominal cramps, nausea, vomiting, and fever. Like those with cholera, patients who are seriously dehydrated should receive oral or intravenous fluids; the value of antibiotics is not clear.

Extraintestinal infections due to non-O1 *V. cholerae* commonly follow occupational or recreational exposure to seawater. Around 10% of non-O1 *V. cholerae* isolates come from cases of wound infection, 10% from cases of otitis media, and 20% from cases of bacteremia (which is particularly likely to develop in patients with liver disease). Extraintestinal infections should be treated with antibiotics. Information to guide agent selection and dosing is limited, but most strains are sensitive in vitro to tetracycline, ciprofloxacin, and third-generation cephalosporins.

SPECIES ASSOCIATED PRIMARILY WITH SOFT TISSUE INFECTION OR BACTEREMIA (See also Chap. 110) ■ *V. vulnificus* *V. vulnificus* is the most common cause of severe *Vibrio* infections in the United States. Like most vibrios, this organism proliferates in the warm summer months and requires a saline environment for growth. In this country, infections in humans typically occur in coastal states between May and October and most commonly affect men >40 years of age. *V. vulnificus* has been linked unequivocally to two distinct syndromes: primary sepsis, which usually occurs in patients with underlying liver disease, and primary wound infection, which generally affects people without underlying disease. Some authors have suggested that *V. vulnificus* also causes gastroenteritis independent of other clinical manifestations. *V. vulnificus* is endowed with a number of virulence attributes, including a capsule that confers resistance to phagocytosis and to the bactericidal activity of human serum as well as a cytolysin. Measured as the 50% lethal dose in mice, the organism's virulence is considerably increased under conditions of iron overload; this observation is consistent with the propensity of *V. vulnificus* to infect patients who have hemochromatosis.

Primary sepsis most often develops in patients who have cirrhosis or hemochromatosis. However, *V. vulnificus* bacteremia can also affect individuals who have hematopoietic disorders or chronic renal insufficiency, those who are using immunosuppressive medications or alcohol, or (in rare instances) those who have no known underlying disease. After a median incubation period of 16 h, the patient develops malaise, chills, fever (mean temperature, 39.8°C), and prostration. One-third of patients develop hypotension, which is often apparent at admission. Cutaneous manifestations develop in most cases (usually within 36 h of onset) and characteristically involve the extremities (the lower more often than the upper). In a common sequence, erythematous patches are followed by ecchymoses, vesicles, and bullae. In fact, sepsis and bullous skin lesions suggest the diagnosis in appropriate settings. Necrosis and sloughing may also be evident. Laboratory studies reveal leukopenia more often than leukocytosis, thrombocytopenia, or elevated levels of fibrin split products. *V. vulnificus* can be cultured from blood or cutaneous lesions. The mortality rate approaches 50%, with most deaths due to uncontrolled sepsis. Accordingly, prompt treatment is critical and should include empirical antibiotic administration, aggressive debridement, and general supportive care. *V. vulnificus* is sensitive in vitro to a number of antibiotics, including tetracycline, fluoroquinolones, and third-generation cephalosporins. Data from animal models suggest that either a fluoroquinolone or the combination of minocycline and cefotaxime should be used in the treatment of *V. vulnificus* septicemia.

V. vulnificus can infect either a fresh or an old wound that comes into contact with seawater; the patient may or may not have underlying disease. After a short incubation period (4 h to 4 days; mean, 12 h), the disease begins with swelling, erythema, and (in many cases) intense pain around the wound. These signs and symptoms are followed by cellulitis, which spreads rapidly and is sometimes accompanied by vesicular, bullous, or necrotic lesions. Metastatic events are uncommon. Most patients have a fever (median temperature, 38.9°C) and leukocytosis. *V. vulnificus* can be cultured from skin lesions and occasionally from the blood. Prompt antibiotic therapy and debridement are usually curative.

V. alginolyticus   First identified as a pathogen of humans in 1973, *V. alginolyticus* occasionally causes eye, ear, and wound infections. This species is the most salt-tolerant of the vibrios and can grow in salt concentrations of >10%. Most clinical isolates come from superinfected wounds that presumably become contaminated at the beach. Although severity varies, *V. alginolyticus* infection tends not to be serious and generally responds well to antibiotic therapy and drainage. A few cases of otitis externa, otitis media, and conjunctivitis due to this pathogen have been described. Tetracycline treatment usually results in cure. *V. alginolyticus* is a rare cause of bacteremia in immunocompromised hosts.

ACKNOWLEDGMENT
The authors gratefully acknowledge the valuable contributions of Dr. Robert Deresiewicz, a coauthor of this chapter for the 14th edition of Harrison's.

FURTHER READING

COLWELL RR: Global climate and infectious disease: The cholera paradigm. Science 274:2025, 1996

DANIELS NA et al: *Vibrio parahaemolyticus* infections in the United States, 1973–1998. J Infect Dis 181:1661, 2000

MAKINO K et al: Genome sequence of *Vibrio parahaemolyticus*: A pathogenic mechanism distinct from that of *V. cholerae*. Lancet 361:743, 2003

MILLER MB et al: Parallel quorum sensing systems converge to regulate virulence in *Vibrio cholerae*. Cell 110:303, 2002

RAMAKRISHNA BS et al: Amylase-resistant starch plus oral rehydration solution for cholera. N Engl J Med 342:308, 2000

RAUFMAN JP: Cholera. Am J Med 104:386, 1998

RYAN ET, CALDERWOOD SB: Cholera vaccines. Clin Infect Dis 31:561, 2000

TANG HJ et al: In vitro and in vivo activities of newer fluoroquinolones against *Vibrio vulnificus*. Antimicrob Agents Chemother 46:3580, 2002

141 | BRUCELLOSIS
Michael J. Corbel, Nicholas J. Beeching

DEFINITION   Brucellosis is a bacterial zoonosis transmitted directly or indirectly to humans from infected animals, predominantly domesticated ruminants and swine. The disease is known colloquially as *undulant fever* because of its remittent character. Its distribution is worldwide apart from the few countries where it has been eradicated from the animal reservoir (see "Epidemiology," below). Although brucellosis commonly presents as an acute febrile illness, its clinical manifestations can be quite varied, and definitive signs to indicate the diagnosis can be lacking. Thus the clinical diagnosis must usually be supported by the results of bacteriologic and/or serologic tests.

ETIOLOGIC AGENT   Human brucellosis is caused by strains of *Brucella*, a bacterial genus considered on genetic grounds to comprise a single species, *Brucella melitensis*, with a number of biologic variants that exhibit particular host preferences. For the sake of convenience, the traditional classification into nomen species is still in general use; this scheme, which closely follows the epidemiologic patterns of the infection, recognizes *B. melitensis*, which is the commonest cause of symptomatic disease in humans and for which the main sources are sheep, goats, and camels; *B. abortus*, which is usually acquired from cattle or buffalo: *B. suis*, which is generally acquired from swine except for one variant enzootic in reindeer and caribou and another enzootic in rodents; and *B. canis*, which is most often acquired from dogs. *B. ovis*, which causes reproductive disease in sheep, and *B. neotomae*, which is specific for desert rodents, have not been clearly implicated in human disease. Other brucellae have been isolated from marine mammals and probably correspond to at least three distinctive nomen species. At least one case of laboratory-acquired human disease due to these marine types has been described, and apparent cases of natural infection have been reported.

All brucellae are small, gram-negative, unencapsulated, nonsporulating rods or coccobacilli. They grow aerobically on peptone-based media incubated at 37°C; the growth of some types is enhanced by supplementary CO_2. In vivo, brucellae behave as facultative intracellular parasites. The organisms are sensitive to sunlight, ionizing radiation, and moderate heat; they are killed by boiling and pasteurization but are resistant to freezing and drying. Their resistance to drying renders brucellae stable in aerosol form and facilitates airborne transmission. Brucellae can survive for up to 2 months in soft cheeses made from goat or sheep milk; for at least 6 weeks in dry soil contaminated with infected urine, vaginal discharge, or placental or fetal tissues; and for at least 6 months in damp soil or liquid manure kept under cool, dark conditions. The bacteria are easily killed by a wide range of common disinfectants used under optimal conditions but are likely to be much more resistant at low temperatures or in the presence of heavy organic contamination.

EPIDEMIOLOGY   Brucellosis is a zoonosis whose occurrence is closely related to its prevalence in domesticated animals. The true global prevalence of human brucellosis is unknown because of the imprecision of diagnosis and the inadequacy of reporting and surveillance systems in many countries. Even in developed countries, the true incidence may be 10 to 20 times higher than the reported figures. Bovine brucellosis has been the subject of control programs in many parts of the world and has been eradicated from the cattle populations of Australia, New Zealand, Bulgaria, Canada, Cyprus, Great Britain (including the Channel Islands), Japan, Luxembourg, Romania, the Scandinavian countries, Switzerland, and the Czech and Slovak Republics. Its incidence in cattle has been reduced to a low level in the United States and most Western European countries, with a varied picture in other parts of the world. There is evidence of some resurgence of brucellosis in cattle in Eastern Europe following economic changes in recent years. Efforts to eradicate *B. melitensis* infection from sheep and goat populations have been much less successful. These efforts have relied heavily on vaccination programs, which have tended to fluctuate with changing economic and political conditions. In some countries, such as Israel, *B. melitensis* has caused serious outbreaks in cattle. Brucellosis still represents a major public health problem in Mediterranean countries; in western, central, and southern Asia; and in parts of Africa and South and Central America.

Human brucellosis is usually associated with occupational or domestic exposure to infected animals or their products. Farmers, shepherds, goatherds, veterinarians, and workers in slaughterhouses and meat-processing plants in endemic areas are occupationally exposed to infection. Family members (including children) of individuals involved in animal husbandry may also be at risk, although it is often difficult to differentiate food-borne infection from environmental contamination under these circumstances. Laboratory workers involved in handling cultures or infected samples are also at risk. Travelers and urban dwellers usually acquire the infection through consumption of contaminated foods. In countries that have eradicated the disease, new cases are most often acquired abroad. Dairy products, especially soft cheeses, unpasteurized milk, and ice cream, are the most frequently implicated sources; raw meat and bone marrow may be sources of infection under exceptional circumstances. Infection resulting from contact with cosmetic products containing infected fetal materials has been recorded. Person-to-person transmission is extremely rare, as is transfer of infection by blood or tissue donation. Although brucellosis is a chronic intracellular infection, there is no evidence for increased prevalence or severity among individuals with HIV infection or other forms of immune deficiency or immune suppression.

Brucellosis may be acquired by ingestion or inhalation or through mucosal or percutaneous exposure. *B. melitensis* and *B. suis* are known to have been developed as biological weapons by several countries and could be exploited as weapons of bioterrorism (Chap. 205). This possibility should be borne in mind in the event of sudden unexplained outbreaks.

IMMUNITY AND PATHOGENESIS The mechanisms of protective immunity against human brucellosis are presumed to be similar to those documented in laboratory animals. Exposure to infection generates both humoral and cell-mediated immune responses. Although antibodies promote clearance of extracellular brucellae by bactericidal action and through the facilitation of phagocytosis by polymorphonuclear phagocytes, the antibody response cannot eradicate the infection. Organisms taken up by macrophages and other cell types can establish persistent intracellular infections. Early in the course of infection, cytokines such as interleukin (IL) 12 promote production of interferon γ, which drives T_H1-type responses and stimulates macrophage activation. Activated macrophages can kill intracellular brucellae (probably mainly through the production of reactive oxygen intermediates) and can clear the infection. Tumor necrosis factor α (TNF-α) is produced early in the immune response and stimulates cytotoxic lymphocytes, which can achieve partial clearance; however, the ability of virulent *Brucella* cells to suppress the TNF-α response may explain its limited role in protection. Inflammatory cytokines, including IL-6 and IL-10, down-regulate the protective response. As in other types of intracellular infection, it is assumed that initial replication of brucellae takes place within cells of the lymph nodes draining the point of entry. Subsequent hematogenous spread may result in chronic localizing infection at almost any site, although the reticuloendothelial system, musculoskeletal tissues, and the genitourinary system are most frequently involved. Both acute and chronic inflammatory responses develop in brucellosis, and the local tissue response may include granuloma formation, with or without necrosis and caseation. Abscesses may also develop, especially in chronic localized infection.

The determinants of pathogenicity of *Brucella* have not been fully characterized, and the mechanisms underlying the manifestations of brucellosis are incompletely understood. The survival strategy of the organism is centered on processes that enable it to persist within monocytic cells. The smooth *Brucella* lipopolysaccharide, which has an unusual O-chain composition, possesses endotoxin activity and plays a key role in pyrogenicity and in resistance to phagocytosis and serum killing in the nonimmune host. Specific exotoxins have not been isolated, but a type IV secretion system responsible for secreting proteins that regulate intracellular survival and trafficking has been identified. This system is activated by low pH, and brucellae produce acid-stable proteins that facilitate survival in phagosomes and depress activation of the oxidative burst. Macrophage apoptosis and phagosome-lysosome fusion are also suppressed. Virulent brucellae are resistant to defensins and produce a Cu-Zn superoxide dismutase that enhances resistance to reactive oxygen intermediates.

CLINICAL FEATURES Brucellosis almost invariably causes fever, which may be associated with profuse sweats, especially at night. In endemic areas, brucellosis may be difficult to distinguish from the many other causes of fever. However, two features were recognized in the nineteenth century to distinguish brucellosis from other tropical fevers, such as typhoid and malaria: (1) Left untreated, the fever of brucellosis shows an undulating pattern that persists for weeks before the commencement of an afebrile period that may be followed by relapse, and (2) the fever of brucellosis is associated with musculoskeletal symptoms and signs in about one-half of all patients.

The clinical syndromes caused by the different nomen species are similar, although *B. melitensis* tends to be associated with a more acute and aggressive presentation and *B. suis* with focal abscess induction. *B. abortus* infections may be more insidious in onset and more likely to become chronic.

The incubation period varies from 1 week to several months, and the onset of fever and other symptoms may be abrupt or insidious. In

addition to fever and sweats, patients become increasingly apathetic and fatigued; lose appetite and weight; and have nonspecific myalgia, headache, and chills. Overall, the presentations of brucellosis often fit into one of three patterns: febrile illness that resembles typhoid but is less severe; fever and acute monarthritis, typically of hip or knee, in a young child; or long-lasting fever, misery, and low-back pain or hip pain in an older man. In an endemic area (e.g., much of the Middle East), a patient with fever and difficulty walking into the clinic would be regarded as having brucellosis until it was proved otherwise.

Diagnostic clues in the patient's history include travel to an endemic area, employment in a diagnostic microbiology laboratory, consumption of unpasteurized milk products (including soft cheeses), contact with animals, and—in an endemic setting—a history of similar illness in the family (documented in almost 50% of cases).

Focal features are present in the majority of patients. The most common is musculoskeletal pain and physical findings in the peripheral and axial skeleton ($\sim$40% of cases). Osteomyelitis more commonly involves the lumbar and lower thoracic vertebrae than the cervical and high thoracic spine. Individual joints that are most commonly affected by septic arthritis are the knee, hip, sacroiliac, shoulder, and sternoclavicular joints, and the pattern may be one of either monarthritis or polyarthritis. Osteomyelitis may also accompany septic arthritis.

In addition to the usual causes of vertebral osteomyelitis or septic arthritis, the most important differential diagnosis is tuberculosis. This point has an impact on the therapeutic approach as well as on the prognosis, given that several antimicrobial agents used to treat brucellosis are also used to treat tuberculosis. Septic arthritis in brucellosis progresses slowly, starting with small pericapsular erosions. In the vertebrae, anterior erosions of the superior end plate are typically the first features to become evident, with eventual involvement and sclerosis of the whole vertebra. Anterior osteophytes eventually develop, but vertebral destruction or impingement on the spinal cord is rare and usually suggests tuberculosis (Table 141-1).

Other systems may be involved in a manner that resembles typhoid. About one-quarter of patients have a dry cough, usually with few changes visible on the chest x-ray, although pneumonia, empyema, intrathoracic adenopathy, or lung abscess can occur. One-quarter of patients have hepatosplenomegaly, and 10 to 20% have significant lymphadenopathy; the differential diagnosis includes glandular fever–like illness such as that caused by Epstein-Barr virus, *Toxoplasma*, and cytomegalovirus; HIV infection; or tuberculosis. Up to 10% of men have acute epididymoorchitis, which must be distinguished from that due to mumps or surgical problems such as torsion. Prostatitis, inflammation of the seminal vesicles, salpingitis, and pyelonephritis all occur. There is an increased incidence of fetal loss among infected pregnant women, although teratogenicity has not been described and

TABLE 141-1 *Radiology of the Spine: Differentiation of Brucellosis from Tuberculosis*

	Brucellosis	Tuberculosis
Site	Lumbar and others	Dorsolumbar
Vertebrae	Multiple or contiguous	Contiguous
Diskitis	Late	Early
Body	Intact until late	Morphology lost early
Canal compression	Rare	Common
Epiphysitis	Anterosuperior	General: upper, lower disk region, central, subperiosteal
Osteophyte	Anterolateral	Unusual
Deformity	Wedging uncommon	Anterior wedge, gibbus
Recovery	Sclerosis, whole body	Variable
Paravertebral abscess	Small, well-localized	Common and discrete loss, transverse process
Psoas abscess	Rare	More likely

the tendency to cause abortions is much less pronounced in humans than in farm animals.

Neurologic involvement is common, with depression and lethargy whose severity may not be fully appreciated by either the patient or the physician until after treatment. A small proportion of patients develop lymphocytic meningoencephalitis that mimics neurotuberculosis or noninfectious conditions and that may be complicated by intracerebral abscess, a variety of cranial nerve deficits, and ruptured mycotic aneurysms.

Endocarditis occurs in ~1% of cases, most often affecting the aortic valve (natural or prosthetic). Any site in the body may be involved in metastatic abscess formation or inflammation; the female breast and the thyroid gland are affected particularly often. Nonspecific maculopapular rashes and other skin manifestations are uncommon and are rarely noticed by the patient even if they are present.

DIAGNOSIS Because the clinical picture of brucellosis is not distinctive, the diagnosis must be based on a history of potential exposure, a presentation consistent with the disease, and supporting laboratory findings. Routine biochemical assays are usually within normal limits, although serum levels of hepatic enzymes and bilirubin may be elevated. Peripheral leukocyte counts are usually normal or low, with relative lymphocytosis. Mild anemia may be documented. Thrombocytopenia and disseminated intravascular coagulation with raised levels of fibrinogen degradation products can develop. The erythrocyte sedimentation rate and C-reactive protein levels are often normal but may be raised.

In body fluids such as cerebrospinal fluid (CSF) or joint fluid, lymphocytosis and low glucose levels are the norm. Elevated CSF levels of adenosine deaminase cannot be used to distinguish tubercular meningitis, as they may also be found in brucellosis. Biopsied samples of tissues such as lymph node or liver may show noncaseating granulomas (Fig. 141-1) without acid/alcohol-fast bacilli. The radiologic features of bony disease develop late in brucellosis and are much more subtle than those of tuberculosis or septic arthritis of other etiologies, with less bone and joint destruction. Isotope scanning is more sensitive than plain x-ray and continues to give positive results long after successful treatment.

Isolation of brucellae from blood, CSF, bone marrow, or joint fluid or from a tissue aspirate or biopsy sample is definitive, and attempts at isolation are usually successful in 50 to 70% of cases. Duplicate cultures (in air and 10% CO_2, respectively) should be incubated for up to 6 weeks. Concentration and lysis of buffy coat cells before culture may increase the isolation rate. Cultures in modern nonradiometric or similar signaling systems (e.g., BACTEC) usually become positive within 7 to 10 days but should be maintained for at least 3 weeks before the results are declared negative.

Nucleic acid amplification techniques are not yet widely available for the diagnosis of human brucellosis, and no single standardized procedure has been adopted. The peripheral blood–based polymerase chain reaction (PCR) has enormous potential to detect bacteremia, to predict relapse, and to exclude "chronic brucellosis" (see "Prognosis and Follow-Up," below); PCR is probably more sensitive and is certainly quicker than blood culture, and it does not carry the attendant biohazard risk posed by culture. Primers for the spacer region between the genes encoding the 16S and 23S ribosomal RNAs (*rrs–rrl*), outermembrane protein Omp2, insertion sequence IS711, or protein BCSP31 are sensitive and specific. Blood or other tissues are the most suitable samples for PCR testing.

Serologic examination often provides the only positive laboratory findings in brucellosis. In acute infection, IgM antibodies appear early and are followed by IgG and IgA antibodies. All these antibodies are active in agglutination tests, whether performed by tube, plate, or microagglutination methods. The majority of patients have detectable agglutinins at this stage. As the disease progresses, IgM levels decline, and the avidity and subclass distribution of IgG and IgA change. The result is reduced or undetectable agglutinin titers. However, the antibodies are detectable by alternative tests, including the complement fixation test, Coombs' antiglobulin test, and enzyme-linked immunosorbent assay. There is no clear cutoff value for a diagnostic titer. Rather, serologic results must be interpreted in the context of exposure history and clinical presentation. In endemic areas or in settings of potential occupational exposure, agglutinin titers of ≥1:320 to 1:640 are considered diagnostic; in nonendemic areas, a titer of ≥1:160 is considered significant. Repetition of tests after 2 to 4 weeks may demonstrate a rising titer.

In most centers, the standard agglutination test (SAT) is still the mainstay of serologic diagnosis, although some investigators rely on the rose bengal test, which has not been fully validated for human diagnostic use. Dipstick assays for anti-*Brucella* IgM are useful for the diagnosis of acute infection but are less sensitive for infection with symptoms of several months' duration. In an endemic setting, >90% of patients with acute bacteremia have SAT titers of at least 1:320.

Antibody to the *Brucella* lipopolysaccharide O chain—the dominant antigen—is detected by all the conventional tests that employ smooth *B. abortus* cells as antigen. Since *B. abortus* cross-reacts with *B. melitensis* and *B. suis*, there is no advantage in replicating the tests with these antigens. Cross-reactions also occur with the O chains of some other gram-negative bacteria, including *Escherichia coli* O157, *Francisella tularensis*, *Salmonella enterica* group N, *Stenotrophomonas maltophilia*, and *Vibrio cholerae*. Cross-reactions do not occur with the cell-surface antigens of rough *Brucella* strains such as *B. canis* or *B. ovis*; serologic tests for these nomen species must employ an antigen prepared from either one. Most protein antigens are shared by all *Brucella* strains, and some are also common to *Ochrobactrum* species.

℞ TREATMENT

The broad aims of antimicrobial therapy for brucellosis are to treat current infection and relieve its symptoms and to prevent relapse. Focal disease presentations may require surgical intervention (e.g., cardiac valve replacement, abscess drainage, joint replacement) in addition to more prolonged and tailored antibiotic therapy. In addition, tuberculosis must always be excluded, or—to prevent the emergence of resistance—the regimen must be tailored to specifically exclude monotherapy with agents active against tuberculosis (e.g., rifampin) or to include a full antituberculous regimen.

Early experience with streptomycin monotherapy for brucellosis showed that relapse was common; thus dual therapy with streptomycin and tetracyclines became the norm. This is still the most effective combination, but alternatives may be used, with the options depending on local or national policy about the use of rifampin for the treatment of nonmycobacterial infection. Antimicrobial efficacy can usually be predicted by in vitro testing. The efficacy of fluoroquinolone monotherapy has been disappointing, with a high relapse rate, despite the good in vitro activity and white-cell penetration of most agents of this class.

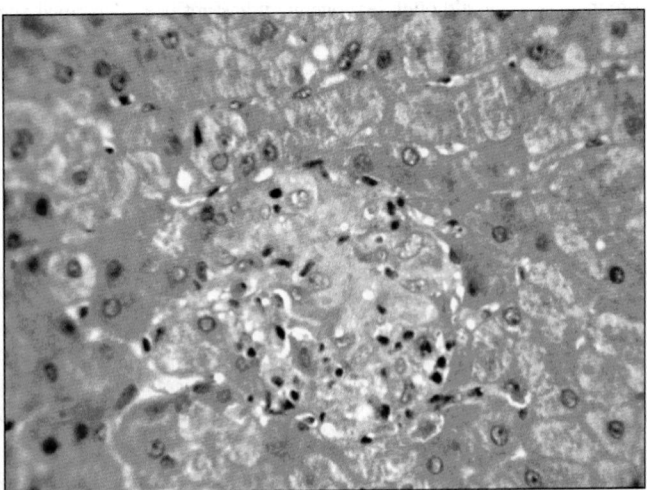

FIGURE 141-1 Liver biopsy specimen from a patient with brucellosis shows a noncaseating granuloma. [*From Mandell's Atlas of Infectious Diseases, Vol II, in DL Stevens (ed): Skin, Soft Tissue, Bone and Joint Infections, Fig. 5-9; with permission.*]

For adults with acute nonfocal brucellosis (duration, <1 month), a 6-week course of therapy incorporating at least two antimicrobial agents is required. Complex or focal disease necessitates ≥3 months of therapy. Adherence to the therapeutic regimen is very important, and poor compliance underlies almost all cases of apparent treatment failure; such failure is rarely due to the emergence of drug resistance, although increasing resistance to trimethoprim-sulfamethoxazole (TMP-SMX) has been reported at one center. There is good retrospective evidence that a 3-week course of two agents is as good as a 6-week course for treatment and prevention of relapse in children, but this point has not yet been proved in prospective studies.

The "gold standard" for the treatment of brucellosis in adults is intramuscular streptomycin (750 mg to 1 g daily for 14 to 21 days) together with doxycycline (100 mg twice daily for 6 weeks). In both clinical trials and observational studies, relapse follows such treatment in 5 to 10% of patients. The usual alternative regimen (and the current World Health Organization recommendation) is rifampin (600 to 900 mg/d) plus doxycycline (100 mg twice daily) for 6 weeks. In trial conditions, the relapse/failure rate is ~10%, but this rate rises to >20% in many nontrial situations, possibly because doxycycline levels are reduced and clearance rates increased by concomitant rifampin administration. Patients who cannot tolerate or receive tetracyclines (children, pregnant women) can be given high-dose TMP-SMX instead (2 or 3 standard-strength tablets twice daily for adults, depending on weight).

Evidence is beginning to accumulate that other aminoglycosides can be substituted for streptomycin—e.g., netilmicin or gentamicin given at a dosage of 5 to 6 mg/kg per day for at least 2 weeks. (Shorter courses have been associated with high failure rates in adults.) A 5- to 7-day course of therapy with gentamicin (and a 3-week course of TMP-SMX) is probably adequate for children with uncomplicated disease. Early experience with fluoroquinolone monotherapy was disappointing, but high-dose ofloxacin (400 mg twice daily) or ciprofloxacin (500 mg twice daily), given for 6 weeks with rifampin, may become accepted as an alternative to the other 6-week regimens for adults.

Significant neurologic disease due to *Brucella* requires prolonged treatment (i.e., for 6 to 12 months), usually with ceftriaxone supplementation of a standard regimen. *Brucella* endocarditis is treated with at least three drugs (an aminoglycoside, a tetracycline, and rifampin), and many experts add ceftriaxone and/or a fluoroquinolone to reduce the need for valve replacement. Treatment is usually given for at least 6 months, and clinical end points for its discontinuation are often difficult to define. Surgery is still required for the majority of cases of infection of prosthetic heart valves and prosthetic joints.

There is no evidence base to guide prophylaxis after exposure to brucellae in the laboratory, inadvertent immunization with live vaccine intended for use in animals, or exposure to deliberately released brucellae. Most authorities recommend the administration of rifampin plus doxycycline for 3 weeks after a low-risk exposure (e.g., a nonspecific laboratory accident) and for 6 weeks after a major exposure to aerosol or injected material.

PROGNOSIS AND FOLLOW-UP Relapse occurs in up to 30% of poorly compliant patients. Thus patients ideally should be followed clinically for up to 2 years to detect relapse, which responds to a prolonged

course of the same therapy that was originally used. The general well-being and body weight of the patient are more useful guides than serology to lack of relapse. IgG antibody levels detected by SAT and variants of this test can remain in the diagnostic range for >2 years after successful treatment. Complement fixation titers usually fall to normal within 1 year of cure. Immunity is not solid; patients can be reinfected after repeated exposures. Fewer than 1% of patients die of brucellosis. When the outcome of this infection is fatal, death is usually a consequence of cardiac involvement; more rarely, it results from severe neurologic disease. Despite the low mortality rate, recovery from brucellosis is slow, and the illness in humans can cause prolonged inactivity, with consequent domestic difficulties and economic losses.

The existence of a prolonged chronic brucellosis state after successful treatment remains controversial. Evaluation of patients in whom this state is considered (often those with work-related exposure to brucellae) includes careful exclusion of malingering, nonspecific chronic fatigue syndromes and other causes of excessive sweating, such as alcohol abuse and obesity. In the future, the availability of more sensitive assays to detect *Brucella* antigen or DNA may help to identify patients with ongoing infection.

PREVENTION Vaccines based on live attenuated *Brucella* strains, such as *B. abortus* strain 19BA or 104M, have been used in some countries to protect high-risk populations but have displayed only short-term efficacy and a high incidence of local and systemic side effects (local inflammation, pain, lymphadenopathy, fever, malaise, nausea). Subunit vaccines have been developed but are of uncertain value and cannot be recommended at present. Interest in biodefense has stimulated research in this area (Chap. 205). The mainstay of veterinary prevention is a national commitment to testing and slaughter of infected herds and flocks (with compensation for owners), control of animal movement, and active immunization of animals. These measures are usually sufficient to control human disease as well. In their absence, pasteurization of all milk products before consumption is sufficient to prevent animal-to-human transmission. All cases of *Brucella* infection in animals and humans should be reported to the appropriate public health authorities.

FURTHER READING

ALMUNEEF M, MEMISH ZA: Prevalence of brucella antibodies after acute brucellosis. J Chemother 15:148, 2003

CORBEL MJ, MACMILLAN AP: Brucellosis, in *Topley and Wilson's Microbiology and Microbial Infections*, vol 3, *Bacterial Infections*, WJ Hausler Jr, M Sussman (eds). London, Arnold, 1999, pp 819–847

———, BANAI M: Genus *Brucella* Meyer and Shaw 1920,173[AL], in *Bergey's Manual of Systematic Bacteriology*, 2d ed, vol 2. Berlin, Springer-Verlag, 2004 (in press)

HALLING SM, BOYLE SM (eds): Brucellosis [special issue]. Vet Microbiol 90: Issues 1–4, 2003

KHAN MY et al: Brucellosis in pregnant women. Clin Infect Dis 32:1172, 2000

MEMISH Z et al: Brucella bacteraemia: Clinical and laboratory observations in 160 patients. J Infect 40:59, 2000

MONTEJO JM et al: Open, randomized therapeutic trial of six antimicrobial regimens in the treatment of human brucellosis. Clin Infect Dis 16:671, 1993

142 TULAREMIA
Richard F. Jacobs

DEFINITION Tularemia is a zoonosis caused by *Francisella tularensis*. Humans of any age, sex, or race are universally susceptible to this systemic infection. Tularemia is primarily a disease of wild animals and persists in contaminated environments, ectoparasites, and animal carriers. Human infection is incidental and usually results from interaction with biting or blood-sucking insects, wild or domestic animals, or the environment. Tularemia is common in Arkansas, Oklahoma,

and Missouri, where more than 50% of the cases in the United States occur. An increasing number of cases of tularemia have been reported from the Scandinavian countries, eastern Europe, and Siberia. The illness is characterized by various clinical syndromes, the most common of which consists of an ulcerative lesion at the site of inoculation, with regional lymphadenopathy and lymphadenitis. Systemic manifestations, including pneumonia, typhoidal tularemia, and fever without localizing findings, pose a greater diagnostic challenge.

ETIOLOGY AND EPIDEMIOLOGY With rare exceptions, tularemia is the only disease produced by *F. tularensis*—a small (0.2 μm by 0.2 to 0.7 μm), gram-negative, pleomorphic, nonmotile, non-spore-forming bacillus. Bipolar staining results in a coccoid appearance. The organism is a thinly encapsulated, nonpiliated strict aerobe that invades host cells. In nature, *F. tularensis* is a hardy organism that persists for weeks or months in mud, water, and decaying animal carcasses. Dozens of biting and blood-sucking insects, especially ticks and tabanid flies, serve as vectors. Ticks and wild rabbits are the source for most of the human cases in the endemic areas of the southeastern and Rocky Mountain states. In Utah, Nevada, and California, tabanid flies are the most common vectors. Animal reservoirs include wild rabbits, squirrels, birds, sheep, beavers, muskrats, and domestic dogs and cats. Humans become infected by various modes, including bites by infected arthropods; handling of infected animal tissues or fluids; direct contact with or ingestion of contaminated water, food, or soil; and inhalation of infected aerosols.

The two main biovars of *F. tularensis*—*tularensis* (type A) and *palearctica* (type B)—are both found in the United States. Type A produces more serious disease in humans; without treatment, the associated fatality rate is ~5%. Type B produces a milder, often subclinical infection that is usually contracted from water or marine mammals. Although all strains appear serologically identical, individual strains may possess varying degrees of virulence. *F. tularensis* does not produce an exotoxin, but an endotoxin similar to that of other gram-negative bacilli has been identified. The progression of illness depends on the organism's virulence, the inoculum size, the portal of entry, and the host's immune status.

Ticks pass the organism to their offspring via a transovarian route. The organism is found in tick feces but not in large quantities in tick salivary glands. In the United States, the disease can be carried by *Dermacentor andersoni* (Rocky Mountain wood tick), *D. variabilis* (American dog tick), *D. occidentalis* (Pacific coast dog tick), and *Amblyomma americanum* (Lone Star tick). *F. tularensis* is transmitted frequently during blood meals taken by embedded ticks following hours of attachment. It is the taking of a blood meal through a fecally contaminated field that transmits the organism. Tularemia is more common among men than among women. Person-to-person transmission is rare or nonexistent. Transmission of the organism by ticks and tabanid flies takes place mainly in the spring and summer. However, continued transmission in the winter months by trapped or hunted animals has been documented. The organism is extremely infectious. Biosafety level 2 is recommended for clinical laboratory work with material whose contamination is suspected, and biosafety level 3 is required for culture of the organism in large quantities. Issues related to the intentional spread of tularemia through ingestion or inhalation are discussed in Chap. 205.

PATHOGENESIS AND PATHOLOGY   The most common portal of entry for human infection is through skin or mucous membranes, either directly—through the bite of ticks, other arthropods, or other animals— or via inapparent abrasions. Inhalation or ingestion of *F. tularensis* can also result in infection. Although more than 10^8 organisms are usually required to produce infection via the oral route (oropharyngeal or gastrointestinal tularemia), fewer than 50 organisms will result in infection when injected into the skin (ulceroglandular/glandular tularemia) or inhaled (pneumonia). After inoculation into the skin, the organism multiplies locally; within 2 to 5 days (range, 1 to 10 days), it produces an erythematous, tender, or pruritic papule. The papule rapidly enlarges and forms an ulcer with a black base (chancriform lesion). The bacteria spread to regional lymph nodes, producing lymphadenopathy (buboes), and, with bacteremia, may spread to distant organs.

Tularemia is characterized by mononuclear cell infiltration with pyogranulomatous pathology. The histopathologic findings can be quite similar to those in tuberculosis, although tularemia develops more rapidly. As a facultatively intracellular bacterium, *F. tularensis* can parasitize both phagocytic and nonphagocytic host cells and sur-

vive intracellularly for prolonged periods. In the acute phase of infection, the primary organs affected (skin, lymph nodes, liver, and spleen) include areas of focal necrosis, initially surrounded by polymorphonuclear leukocytes (PMNs). Subsequently, granulomas form, with epithelioid cells, lymphocytes, and multinucleated giant cells surrounded by areas of necrosis. These areas may resemble caseation necrosis but later coalesce to form abscesses.

Conjunctival inoculation can result in infection of the eye, with regional lymph node enlargement (preauricular lymphadenopathy, Parinaud's complex). Aerosolization and inhalation or hematogenous spread of organisms can result in pneumonia. In the lung, an inflammatory reaction develops, including foci of alveolar necrosis and cell infiltration (initially polymorphonuclear and later mononuclear) with granulomas. Chest roentgenograms usually reveal bilateral patchy infiltrates rather than large areas of consolidation. Pleural effusions are common and may contain blood. Lymphadenopathy occurs in regions draining infected organs. Therefore, in pulmonary infection, mediastinal adenopathy may be evident, whereas patients with oropharyngeal tularemia develop cervical lymphadenopathy. In gastrointestinal or typhoidal tularemia, mesenteric lymphadenopathy may follow the ingestion of large numbers of organisms. The term *typhoidal tularemia* may be used to describe severe bacteremic disease, irrespective of the mode of transmission or portal of entry. Meningitis has been reported as a primary or secondary manifestation of bacteremia. Patients may also present with fever and no localizing signs.

IMMUNOLOGY   Infection with *F. tularensis* stimulates the host to produce antibodies. However, this antibody response probably plays only a minor role in the containment of infection. In contrast, cell-mediated immunity, which develops over 2 to 4 weeks, plays a major role in containment and eradication. Macrophages, once activated, can kill *F. tularensis*. Recovery from infection generally renders the patient resistant to reinfection; this point is not completely understood.

Immunospecific protection against tularemia can be afforded either by natural infection or by vaccination with live attenuated strains of *F. tularensis*. Killed vaccines, on the other hand, induce no protection against virulent *F. tularensis*. After natural infection or vaccination, serum antibodies to surface-exposed carbohydrate antigens predominate, whereas T cell determinants are located on membrane proteins beneath the bacterial capsule. T cell responses are thought to be due to priming by the organism. The anamnestic T cell response to *F. tularensis* seems to involve a multitude of microbial proteins, each with a distinct set of T cell determinants. A predominant role for CD4+ T cells is supported by the results of experiments in mice, which indicated that resistance to infection was restricted at the level of the major histocompatibility complex (MHC) class II determinants. Humans primed to *F. tularensis* (like those primed to *Mycobacterium tuberculosis*) show a T_H1-like response. T cell proliferation is associated with the production of interleukin (IL) 2 and interferon γ but with little or no production of IL-4. Recent evidence indicates that the percentage of $\gamma\delta$ T cells expressing tumor necrosis factor α is decreased during the first 7 to 40 days after infection. This decrease may reflect the modulation of an inflammatory response. Investigations of neutrophils in tularemia suggest that PMNs are needed for defense against primary infection. PMNs may restrict the growth of *F. tularensis* before the organism becomes intracellular.

CLINICAL MANIFESTATIONS   Tularemia often starts with a sudden onset of fever, chills, headache, and generalized myalgias and arthralgias (Table 142-1). This onset takes place when the organism penetrates the skin, is ingested, or is inhaled. An incubation period of 2 to 10 days is followed by the formation of an ulcer at the site of penetration, with local inflammation. The ulcer may persist for several months as organisms are transported via the lymphatics to the regional lymph nodes. These nodes enlarge and may become necrotic and suppurative. If the organism enters the bloodstream, widespread dissemination as well as signs and symptoms of endotoxemia may result.

In the United States, most patients with tularemia (75 to 85%) acquire the infection by inoculation of the skin. In adults, the most

TABLE 142-1 *Clinical Presentation of Tularemia*

Sign or Symptom	Rate of Occurrence, %	
	Children	Adults
Lymphadenopathy	96	65
Fever (≥38.3°C or ≥101°F)	87	21
Ulcer/eschar/papule	45	51
Myalgias/arthralgias	39	2
Headache	9	5
Cough	9	5
Pharyngitis	43	—
Diarrhea	43	—

Source: Adapted from Jacobs and Narain (1985).

common localized form is inguinal/femoral lymphadenopathy; in children, it is cervical lymphadenopathy. About 20% of patients develop a generalized maculopapular rash, which occasionally becomes pustular. Erythema nodosum occurs infrequently. The clinical manifestations of tularemia have been divided into various syndromes, which are listed in Table 142-2.

Ulceroglandular/Glandular Tularemia These two forms of tularemia account for ~75 to 85% of cases. The predominant form in children involves cervical or posterior auricular lymphadenopathy and is usually related to tick bites on the head and neck. In adults, the most common form is inguinal/femoral lymphadenopathy resulting from insect and tick exposures on the lower limbs. In cases related to wild game, the usual portal of entry for *F. tularensis* is either an injury sustained while skinning or cleaning an animal carcass or a bite (usually on the hand). Epitrochlear lymphadenopathy/lymphadenitis is common in patients with bite-related injuries.

In ulceroglandular tularemia, the ulcer is erythematous, indurated, and nonhealing, with a punched-out appearance that lasts from 1 to 3 weeks. The papule may begin as an erythematous lesion that is tender or pruritic; it evolves over several days into an ulcer with sharply demarcated edges and a yellow exudate. The ulcer gradually develops a black base, and simultaneously the regional lymph nodes become tender and severely enlarged (Fig. 142-1). The affected lymph nodes may become fluctuant and drain spontaneously, but usually the condition resolves with effective treatment. Late suppuration of lymph nodes has been described in up to 25% of patients with ulceroglandular/glandular tularemia. Examination of material taken from these late fluctuant nodes after successful antimicrobial treatment has revealed sterile necrotic tissue. In 5 to 10% of patients, the skin lesion may be inapparent, with lymphadenopathy plus systemic signs and symptoms the only physical findings (*glandular tularemia*). Conversely, a tick or deerfly bite on the trunk may result in an ulcer without evident lymphadenopathy.

Oculoglandular Tularemia In ~1% of patients, the portal of entry for *F. tularensis* is the conjunctiva. Usually, the organism reaches the conjunctiva through contact with contaminated fingers. The inflamed conjunctiva is painful, with numerous yellowish nodules and pinpoint ulcers. Purulent conjunctivitis with regional lymphadenopathy (preauricular, submandibular, or cervical) is evident. Because of debilitating pain, the patient may seek medical attention before regional

TABLE 142-2 *Clinical Syndromes of Tularemia*

Syndrome	Rate of Occurrence, %	
	Children	Adults
Ulceroglandular	45	51
Glandular	25	12
Pulmonary (pneumonia)	14	18
Oropharyngeal	4	—
Oculoglandular	2	—
Typhoidal	2	12
Unclassified	6	11

Source: Adapted from Jacobs and Narain (1985).

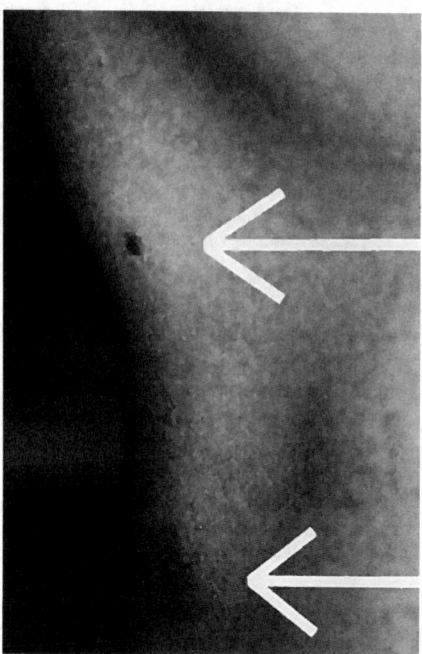

FIGURE 142-1 An ulcerative lesion (*lower arrow*) with adjacent lymphadenitis (*upper arrow*) on the lateral chest wall of a patient with ulceroglandular tularemia.

lymphadenopathy develops. Painful preauricular lymphadenopathy is unique to tularemia and distinguishes it from cat-scratch disease, tuberculosis, sporotrichosis, and syphilis. Corneal perforation may occur.

Oropharyngeal and Gastrointestinal Tularemia Rarely, tularemia follows the ingestion of contaminated undercooked meat, the oral inoculation of *F. tularensis* from the hands in association with the skinning and cleaning of animal carcasses, or the consumption of contaminated food or water. Oral inoculation may result in acute, exudative, or membranous pharyngitis associated with cervical lymphadenopathy or in ulcerative intestinal lesions associated with mesenteric lymphadenopathy, diarrhea, abdominal pain, nausea, vomiting, and gastrointestinal bleeding. Infected tonsils become enlarged and develop a yellowish-white pseudomembrane, which can be confused with that of diphtheria. The clinical severity of gastrointestinal tularemia varies from mild, unexplained, persistent diarrhea with no other symptoms to a fulminant, fatal disease. In fatal cases, the extensive intestinal ulceration found at autopsy suggests an enormous inoculum.

Pulmonary Tularemia Tularemia pneumonia presents as variable parenchymal infiltrates that are unresponsive to treatment with β-lactam antibiotics. Tularemia must be considered in the differential diagnosis of atypical pneumonia in a patient with a history of travel to an endemic area. The disease can result from either inhalation of an infectious aerosol or can spread to the lungs and pleura after bloodstream dissemination. Inhalation-related pneumonia has been described in laboratory workers after exposure to contaminated materials and is associated with a relatively high mortality rate. Exposure to *F. tularensis* in aerosols from live domestic animals or dead wildlife (including birds) has been reported to cause pneumonia. Hematogenous dissemination to the lungs occurs in 10 to 15% of cases of ulceroglandular tularemia and in about half of cases of typhoidal tularemia. Previously, tularemia pneumonia was thought to be a disease of older patients, but as many as 10 to 15% of children with clinical manifestations of tularemia have parenchymal infiltrates detected by chest roentgenography. Patients with pneumonia usually have a nonproductive cough and may have dyspnea or pleuritic chest pain. Roentgenograms of the chest usually reveal bilateral patchy infiltrates (described as ovoid or lobar densities), lobar parenchymal infiltrates, and cavitary lesions. Pleural effusions may have a predominance of mononuclear

TABLE 142-3 *Tularemia: Differential Diagnosis, by Clinical Disease Category*

Glandular	Oropharyngeal	Typhoidal	Pneumonia
Pyogenic bacterial infection[a]	Group A streptococcal pharyngitis	Typhoid fever	*Mycoplasma pneumoniae* pneumonia
Nontuberculous mycobacterial infection	*Arcanobacterium haemolyticum* pharyngitis	Other *Salmonella* bacteremias	*Chlamydia pneumoniae* pneumonia
Sporotrichosis	Diphtheria	Rocky Mountain spotted fever	Psittacosis
Tuberculosis	Infectious mononucleosis	Human monocytotropic ehrlichiosis	*Legionella pneumophila* pneumonia
Syphilis	Various viruses[b]	Human granulocytotropic ehrlichiosis	Q fever
Anthrax		Infectious mononucleosis	Histoplasmosis
Rat-bite fever		Brucellosis	Blastomycosis
Scrub typhus		Toxoplasmosis	Coccidioidomycosis
Plague		Tuberculosis	Various viruses[c]
Lymphogranuloma venereum		Sarcoidosis	
Cat-scratch disease		Malignancy[d]	

[a] *Staphylococcus aureus*, *Streptococcus pyogenes*.
[b] Adenovirus, enteroviruses, parainfluenza virus, influenza virus A and B, respiratory syncytial virus.
[c] Influenza virus A and B, parainfluenza virus, respiratory syncytial virus, adenovirus, enteroviruses, hantavirus.
[d] Hematologic and reticuloendothelial malignancies.

leukocytes or PMNs and sometimes red blood cells. Empyema may develop. Blood cultures may be positive for *F. tularensis*.

Typhoidal Tularemia The typhoidal presentation is now considered rare in the United States. The source of infection in typhoidal tularemia is usually associated with pharyngeal and/or gastrointestinal inoculation or bacteremic disease. Fever usually develops without apparent skin lesions or lymphadenopathy. Some patients have cervical and mesenteric lymphadenopathy. In the absence of a history of possible contact with a vector, diagnosis can be extremely difficult. Blood cultures may be positive and patients may present with classic sepsis or septic shock in this acute systemic form of the infection. Typhoidal tularemia is usually associated with a huge inoculum or with a preexisting compromising condition. High continuous fevers, signs of endotoxemia, and severe headache are common. The patient may be delirious and may develop prostration and shock. If presumptive antibiotic therapy in culture-negative cases does not include an aminoglycoside, the mortality rate can approach 30%.

Other Manifestations *F. tularensis* infection has been associated with meningitis, pericarditis, hepatitis, peritonitis, endocarditis, osteomyelitis, and sepsis and septic shock with rhabdomyolysis and acute renal failure. In the rare cases of tularemia meningitis, a predominantly lymphocytic response is demonstrated in cerebrospinal fluid.

DIFFERENTIAL DIAGNOSIS When patients in endemic areas present with fever, chronic ulcerative skin lesions, and large tender lymph nodes (Fig. 142-1), a diagnosis of tularemia should be made presumptively, and confirmatory diagnostic testing and appropriate therapy should be undertaken. When the possibility of tularemia is considered in a non-endemic area, an attempt should be made to identify contact with a potential animal vector. The level of suspicion should be especially high in hunters, trappers, game wardens, veterinarians, laboratory workers, and individuals exposed to an insect or another animal vector. However, up to 40% of patients with tularemia have no known history of epidemiologic contact with an animal vector.

The characteristic presentation of ulceroglandular tularemia does not pose a diagnostic problem, but a less classic progression of regional lymphadenopathy or glandular tularemia must be differentiated from other diseases (Table 142-3). The skin lesion of tularemia may resemble those seen in various other diseases but is generally accompanied by more impressive regional lymphadenopathy. In children, the differentiation of tularemia from cat-scratch disease is made more difficult by the chronic papulovesicular lesion associated with *Bartonella henselae* infection (Chap. 144). Oropharyngeal tularemia can resemble and must be differentiated from pharyngitis due to other bacteria or viruses. Tularemia pneumonia may resemble any atypical pneumonia. Typhoidal tularemia may resemble a variety of other infections.

LABORATORY DIAGNOSIS Direct microscopic examination of polychromatically stained tissue smears or clinical specimens reveals *F. tularensis* organisms, singly and in groups, both intra- and extracellularly. Gram's staining of clinical or biopsy material is of little value, as the small, weakly staining organisms cannot be readily distinguished from the background. An indirect fluorescent antibody test with commercially available antisera can be useful, although false-positive results due to *Legionella* spp. have been reported.

The diagnosis of tularemia is most frequently confirmed by serologic testing. In the standard tube agglutination test, a single titer of ≥1:160 is interpreted as a presumptive positive result. A fourfold increase in titer between paired serum samples collected 2 to 3 weeks apart is considered diagnostic. False-negative serologic responses are obtained early in infection; up to 30% of patients infected for 3 weeks have sera that test negative. Late in infection, titers into the thousands are common, and titers of 1:20 to 1:80 may persist for years. A microagglutination test that may be as much as 100-fold more sensitive than the standard tube agglutination test has been described and is currently being used in many clinical microbiology laboratories. Enzyme-linked immunosorbent assays have proved useful for the detection of both antibodies and antigens. Analysis of urine for *F. tularensis* antigen has yielded promising results in clinical trials, but facilities for this type of analysis are not widely available. A skin test for delayed hypersensitivity to *F. tularensis* turns positive during the first week of illness and remains positive for years. The skin-test antigen, which is not commercially available, can boost titers of agglutinating antibody.

Culture and isolation of *F. tularensis* are difficult. In one study the organism was isolated in only 10% of more than 1000 human cases, 84% of which were confirmed by serology. The medium of choice is cysteine-glucose-blood agar. *F. tularensis* can be isolated directly from infected ulcer scrapings, lymph-node biopsy specimens, gastric washings, sputum, and blood cultures. Colonies are blue-gray, round, smooth, and slightly mucoid. On media containing blood, a small zone of α hemolysis usually surrounds the colony. Slide agglutination tests or direct fluorescent antibody tests with commercially available antisera can be applied directly to culture suspensions for identification.

The polymerase chain reaction (PCR) has been used to detect *F. tularensis* DNA in multiple clinical specimens. During one outbreak, a multiplex PCR was used to target 16S rRNA and to diagnose ulceroglandular tularemia with DNA extracted from wound swabs; the PCR result was positive in 29 (73%) of 40 serologically confirmed cases. However, this test has not been shown to be more sensitive than direct culture and at present remains a research tool.

℞ TREATMENT

F. tularensis cannot be subjected to standardized antimicrobial susceptibility testing because the organism will not grow on the media used. A wide variety of antibiotics, including all β-lactam antibiotics and the newer cephalosporins, are ineffective for the treatment of this infection. Several studies indicated that third-generation cephalosporins were active against *F. tularensis* in vitro, but clinical case reports suggested a nearly universal failure rate of ceftriaxone in pediatric patients with tularemia. Although in vitro data indicate that imipenem may be active, therapy with imipenem, sulfanilamides, and macrolides is not presently recommended because of the lack of relevant clinical data. Fluoroquinolones have shown promise in terms of their relatively low toxicity and their potential for oral administration. With intracellular activity, fluoroquinolones have been used for successful treatment of tularemia and are candidates for primary or alternative therapy, pending clinical trials. The use of these agents should also be considered when patients are allergic or intolerant to other treatments. When used, ciprofloxacin should be given for a total of 10 days. Chloramphenicol and tetracycline have been used successfully for treatment of the acute stages of tularemia but have been associated with higher relapse rates (up to 20%) than conventionally used agents. Oral chloramphenicol is no longer available in the United States.

Streptomycin, given intramuscularly at a dose of 7.5 to 10 mg/kg every 12 h, is considered the drug of choice for adults. In severe cases, 15 mg/kg every 12 h may be used for the first 48 to 72 h. Streptomycin is also considered the drug of choice for children; the appropriate dose is 30 to 40 mg/kg daily in two divided doses administered intramuscularly. In children, after a clinical response is demonstrated at 3 to 5 days, the dose can be reduced to 10 to 15 mg/kg daily in two divided doses. Therapy is typically continued for 7 to 10 days; however, in mild to moderate cases of tularemia in which the patient becomes afebrile within the first 48 to 72 h of streptomycin treatment, a 5- to 7-day course has been successful.

Gentamicin, at a dose of 1.7 mg/kg given intravenously or intramuscularly every 8 h, is also effective and may be more readily available. The published experience in adults consists of two reports describing, respectively, nine and eight patients who were treated effectively with gentamicin. The eight patients in one of the reports all had fever before treatment, and all eight became afebrile within 24 to 72 h. In a pediatric study, other symptoms, such as tender lymphadenitis and pharyngitis, also responded within 24 to 72 h of the start of gentamicin therapy.

Virtually all strains of *F. tularensis* are susceptible to streptomycin and gentamicin. In successfully treated patients, defervescence usually occurs within 2 days, but skin lesions and lymph nodes may take 1 to 2 weeks to heal. When therapy is not initiated within the first several days of illness, defervescence may be delayed. Relapses are uncommon with streptomycin or gentamicin therapy. Late lymph-node suppuration, however, occurs in ~40% of children, regardless of the treatment received. These nodes have typically been found to contain sterile necrotic tissue without evidence of active infection. Patients with fluctuant nodes should receive several days of antibiotic therapy before drainage to minimize the risk to hospital personnel. Unlike streptomycin and gentamicin, tobramycin is ineffective in the treatment of tularemia and should not be used.

PROGNOSIS   If tularemia goes untreated, symptoms usually last 1 to 4 weeks but may continue for months. The mortality rate from severe untreated infection (including all cases of untreated tularemia pneu-

monia and typhoidal tularemia) can be as high as 30%. However, the overall mortality rate for untreated tularemia is <8%. Mortality is <1% with appropriate treatment. Poor outcomes are often associated with long delays in diagnosis and treatment. Lifelong immunity usually follows tularemia.

PREVENTION   The prevention of tularemia is based on avoidance of exposure to biting and blood-sucking insects, especially ticks and deerflies. An intradermal vaccine made from live attenuated *F. tularensis* is available from the Centers for Disease Control and Prevention. This vaccine is effective in reducing the frequency and severity of infection. Vaccination of high-risk individuals working with large quantities of cultured organisms is recommended. Others who come into contact with the organisms, such as veterinarians, hunters, or game wardens, should consider vaccination, particularly if they live in endemic areas. The avoidance of skinning wild animals, especially rabbits, and the wearing of gloves while handling animal carcasses decrease the risk of transmission. Use of insect repellents and preparations that prevent tick attachment as well as prompt removal of ticks can be helpful. Prophylaxis of tularemia has not proved effective in patients with embedded ticks or insect bites. However, in patients who are known to have been exposed to large quantities of organisms (e.g., in the laboratory) and who have incubating infection with *F. tularensis*, early treatment can prevent the development of significant clinical disease.

FURTHER READING

CENTERS FOR DISEASE CONTROL AND PREVENTION: Tularemia—United States, 1990–2000. MMWR 51:181, 2002

DENNIS DT et al: Tularemia as a biological weapon: Medical and public health management. JAMA 285:2763, 2001

ENDERLIN G et al: Streptomycin and alternative agents for the treatment of tularemia: Review of the literature. Clin Infect Dis 19:42, 1994

FELDMAN KA et al: Outbreak of primary pneumonic tularemia on Martha's Vineyard. N Engl J Med 345:1601, 2001

JACOBS RF, NARAIN JP: Tularemia in adults and children: A changing presentation. Pediatrics 76:818, 1985

PENN RL, KINASEWITZ GT: Factors associated with a poor outcome in tularemia. Arch Intern Med 147:265, 1987

SCHEEL O et al: Treatment of tularemia with ciprofloxacin. Eur J Microbiol Infect Dis 11:447, 1992

TAYLOR JP et al: Epidemiologic characteristics of human tularemia in the southwest-central states, 1981–1987. Am J Epidemiol 133:1032, 1991

143 PLAGUE AND OTHER *YERSINIA* INFECTIONS
David T. Dennis, Grant L. Campbell

PLAGUE

DEFINITION   Plague is an acute, febrile, zoonotic disease caused by infection with *Yersinia pestis*. Although human cases are infrequent and are curable with antibiotics, plague is one of the most virulent and potentially lethal bacterial diseases known. The plague bacterium occurs in widely scattered foci in Asia, Africa, and the Americas, where its usual hosts are various wild rodents and human-associated rats. Infection is transmitted to humans typically by flea bite and less commonly by direct contact with infected animal tissues or by airborne droplet. The principal clinical forms of plague are bubonic, septicemic, and pneumonic. Although most cases are now sporadic, occurring singly or in small clusters, the potential for outbreaks and epidemic spread remains. Because of its virulence and transmissibility, *Y. pestis* is considered an important potential agent of biological terrorism that requires special countermeasures to protect the public's health (Chap. 205).

ETIOLOGIC AGENT   *Y. pestis* is a gram-negative coccobacillus in the family Enterobacteriaceae. Genomic analysis suggests that it has recently

evolved from *Y. pseudotuberculosis*. *Y. pestis* is microaerophilic, nonmotile, nonsporulating, oxidase and urease negative, and biochemically unreactive. The organism is nonfastidious and infective for laboratory rodents. It grows well, if slowly, on routinely used microbiologic media (e.g., sheep blood agar, brain-heart infusion broth, and MacConkey agar). *Y. pestis* can multiply within a wide range of temperatures ($-2°C$ to $45°C$) and pH values (5.0 to 9.6), but optimal growth occurs at $28°C$ and at pH ~7.4. When stained with a polychromatic stain (e.g., Wayson or Giemsa), *Y. pestis* isolated from clinical specimens exhibits a characteristic bipolar appearance, resembling closed safety pins. The bacterium is nonencapsulated but when grown at $\geq30°C$ produces a plasmid-expressed envelope glycoprotein, fraction 1 (F1) antigen—a virulence factor that serves as the principal immunodiagnostic marker of infection.

HISTORIC BACKGROUND   Plague's deadly epidemic potential is notorious and well documented. The Justinian pandemic (542 to 767 A.D.) spread from central Africa to the Mediterranean littoral and thence to Asia Minor, causing an estimated 40 million deaths. The second pandemic began in central Asia, was carried to Sicily by ship from Constantinople in 1347, and within a few years swept through Europe and the British Isles; successive epidemics of lesser magnitude occurred over the next four centuries. At its height, the second plague pandemic killed as many as a quarter of the affected population and became known as the Black Death. In the third (modern) pandemic, plague appeared in Yunnan, China, in the latter half of the nineteenth century; established itself in Hong Kong in 1894; and spread by ship to Bombay in 1896 and subsequently to major port cities throughout the world, including San Francisco and several other West Coast and Gulf Coast ports in the United States. The plague bacillus was first cultured by Alexandre Yersin in Hong Kong in 1894. In 1898, Paul-Louis Simond, a French scientist sent to investigate epidemic bubonic plague in Bombay, identified the bacillus in the tissues of dead rats and proposed transmission by rat fleas. Waldemar Haffkine, also in Bombay at that time, developed a crude vaccine.

By 1910, plague had circled the globe and was established in rodent populations on all inhabited continents other than Australia. After 1920, however, the spread of plague was largely halted by international regulations that mandated control of rats in harbors and inspection and rat-proofing of ships. Before subsiding, the third pandemic had resulted in an estimated 26 million plague cases and >12 million deaths, the vast majority in India. By 1950, plague outbreaks around the world had become isolated, sporadic, and manageable with modern techniques of surveillance, flea and rat control, and antimicrobial treatment of patients. Plague has nearly disappeared from cities and now occurs mostly in rural and semirural areas, where it is maintained in various rodents and their fleas. In the United States, the last outbreak of urban plague occurred in Los Angeles in 1924 and 1925, and human cases since then have, with very few exceptions, resulted from exposures in rural areas of western states.

Plague remains one of three quarantinable diseases subject to international health regulations (the other two being cholera and yellow fever). The alarm that plague is still able to evoke was highlighted by the public panic and exaggerated official responses to reported outbreaks of bubonic and pneumonic plague in India in 1994. The plague bacillus is considered to have a high potential for use in biological terrorism; the agent is available around the world, has been "weaponized" for airborne delivery, and would be expected to cause a high primary fatality rate as well as secondary spread among an affected population (Chap. 205).

EPIDEMIOLOGY *Y. pestis* is maintained in well-established "silent" enzootic cycles involving relatively resistant wild rodents and their fleas in remote, lightly populated areas of Asia, Africa, and the Americas and in limited rural foci in extreme southeastern Europe near the Caspian Sea. Humans and mammals other than rodents are incidental hosts. Outbreaks (epizootics) of plague in susceptible rodent populations may result in widespread die-offs of these animals, an avid search by their fleas for new hosts, and an increased risk of spread of infection to humans. In the United States, the principal epizootic hosts are various ground squirrels, prairie dogs, and chipmunks; a variety of burrowing rodents act as epizootic hosts in rural areas elsewhere in the world. *Y. pestis* occasionally spills over from wild rodents to rat species that inhabit cultivated fields and adjacent homes, villages, and towns. The organism can then be transported from towns to cities by these highly adaptable rats and their fleas.

Plague in populated areas is most likely to develop when sanitation is poor and rats are numerous—especially the common black or roof rat (*Rattus rattus*), its close relatives, and the larger brown sewer or Norway rat (*R. norvegicus*). The cosmopolitan oriental rat flea *Xenopsylla cheopis* and (in southern Africa and Brazil) the related species *X. brasiliensis* are efficient vectors of the plague bacillus from rat to rat and from rats to humans. *Y. pestis* multiplies to enormous numbers in the foregut (proventriculus) of these fleas, resulting in a bolus of organisms and clotted blood that blocks the passage of subsequent

blood meals. This situation occurs only at temperatures of ≤28°C and depends on a single protease expressed by the plasminogen activator (*pla*) gene of a 9.5-kb plasmid of *Y. pestis*. Regurgitation by a "blocked" flea while it feeds facilitates transmission of the plague bacillus to the new host. Except for large outbreaks of pneumonic plague in Manchuria in the early part of the twentieth century, person-to-person respiratory transmission of plague has since occurred only sporadically and has been limited to clusters of close, direct contacts of pneumonic plague patients, such as household members and caregivers.

International health regulations require that national authorities immediately report plague cases to the World Health Organization. From 1987 through 2001, 36,876 human plague cases (mean, 2458 cases per year) and 2847 deaths (mortality, 8%) were reported by 24 countries. In the same 15-year period, the United States reported 125 cases and 12 deaths (mortality, 10%). Cases reported by the United States are confirmed by the plague laboratory of the Centers for Disease Control and Prevention (CDC). Animal plague occurs in 17 contiguous western states, extending from the Great Plains states and eastern Texas to the Pacific Coast; around 80% of human cases in this country now occur in New Mexico, Arizona, and Colorado and around 10% in California. The arid Native American reservations of New Mexico and Arizona are active plague foci, and Native Americans account for a disproportionately high percentage of plague cases in the United States. Although plague is a rural disease in this country, >50% of cases are thought to be caused by peridomestic exposures, especially in the southwestern states, where homes are often situated in natural surroundings that provide a favorable habitat for plague-susceptible animals (such as rock squirrels and wood rats) and their fleas. In the Sierra Nevadas of California and Nevada, epizootic plague in chipmunks and ground squirrels poses a risk to visitors in public parks. Hikers, campers, and hunters in natural areas throughout the western states are at a small but finite risk of exposure to plague, especially in the summer months.

Plague can be transmitted during the skinning and handling of carcasses of wild animals such as rabbits and hares, prairie dogs, wildcats, and coyotes. Such direct inoculation of mammal-adapted organisms expressing the F1 antigen is associated with primary septicemia and high mortality. Pharyngeal plague can result from the ingestion of undercooked contaminated meat, from inhaling respiratory droplets, and perhaps from the manual transfer of infected fluids to the mouth during the handling of infected animal tissues.

Carnivores, including dogs and cats, can become infected with *Y. pestis* by eating infected rodents and possibly by being bitten by infective fleas. Although clinical plague commonly develops in infected cats, it rarely does so in infected dogs. Both dogs and cats may transport infected fleas from rodent-infested areas to the home environment.

From 1947 through 2001, 421 plague cases were reported in the United States. Of the 409 evaluable cases, 349 cases (85%) presented as primary lymphadenitic (bubonic) plague, almost all of them thought to be associated with flea bites; 55 cases (13%) presented as primary septicemic plague, many of them following direct animal exposures; and 8 cases (2%) presented as primary pneumonic plague, 6 resulting from the inhalation of respiratory droplets released by infected cats and 2 from unknown sources. The last case of human-to-human plague transmission in the United States occurred in Los Angeles in 1924.

PATHOGENESIS AND PATHOLOGY *Y. pestis* is highly invasive and pathogenic. The mechanisms by which the organism causes disease are incompletely understood, but both chromosome- and plasmid-encoded gene products as well as altered cell-mediated immune responses are involved. Three plasmids encode for a variety of known or presumed virulence factors; these include the F1 envelope antigen and various *Yersinia* outer-membrane proteins (Yops), which confer bacterial resistance to phagocytosis; the V antigen, which is essential for virulence and immunocompromises the host by suppressing the synthesis of various proinflammatory cytokines (e.g, interferon γ and tumor necrosis factor α); pesticin, which interferes with iron uptake; a protease that

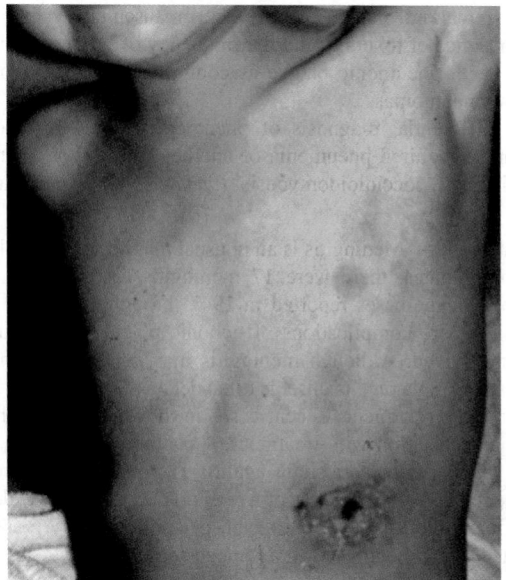

FIGURE 143-1   Plague patient in the southwestern United States with a left axillary bubo and an unusual plague ulcer and eschar at the site of the infective flea bite.

common. Diffuse interstitial myocarditis with cardiac dilatation is sometimes found. If disseminated intravascular coagulation (DIC) ensues, vascular necrosis may lead to widespread cutaneous, mucosal, and serosal ecchymoses and petechiae. Acral ischemia and resulting gangrene sometimes develop.

Primary plague pneumonia generally begins as a lobular process and then extends by confluence, becoming lobar and then multilobar (Fig. 143-2). Plague organisms are typically most numerous in the alveoli. Secondary plague pneumonia begins more diffusely, with organisms at first most numerous in the interstitium. In advanced cases of both primary and secondary plague pneumonia, affected lung tissue is characterized by edema, hemorrhagic necrosis, and infiltration by neutrophilic leukocytes.

MANIFESTATIONS   Plague is characterized by a rapid onset of fever and other systemic manifestations of gram-negative bacterial infection. If it is not quickly and correctly treated, plague can follow a toxic course, resulting in shock, multiple-organ failure, and death. In humans, the three principal forms of plague are bubonic, septicemic, and pneumonic. Bubonic plague, the most common form, is almost always caused by the bite of an infected flea but occasionally results from direct contact with infectious materials. Septicemic and pneumonic plague can be either primary or secondary to metastatic spread. Unusual forms include plague meningitis, endophthalmitis, and lymphadenitis at multiple sites. Primary plague pharyngitis has been documented by culture of organisms from throat swabs and can result from respiratory exposure or ingestion of undercooked flesh of infected animals.

Bubonic Plague   Bubonic plague has a usual incubation period of 2 to 6 days. Patients experience chills; fever, with temperatures that rise within hours to ≥38°C; myalgias; arthralgias; headache; and a feeling of weakness. Soon—usually within 24 h—the patient notices tenderness and pain in one or more regional lymph nodes proximal to the site of inoculation of the plague bacillus (Fig. 143-1). Because fleas most often bite the legs, femoral and inguinal nodes are most commonly involved; axillary and cervical nodes are next most commonly affected. Within hours, the enlarging bubo becomes progressively painful and tender, sometimes exquisitely so. The patient usually guards against palpation and limits movement, pressure, and stretch around the bubo. The surrounding tissue often becomes edematous, sometimes markedly so, and the overlying skin may be erythematous, warm, and tense. Inspection of the skin surrounding or distal to the bubo sometimes reveals the site of a flea bite marked by a papule, pustule, or ulcer. The ulcer may be covered by an eschar (Fig. 143-1). A list of lymphadenitic conditions that could be confused with bubonic plague includes *Staphylococcus aureus* and group A β-hemolytic streptococcal infections, cat-scratch disease, tularemia, and—in filariasis endemic areas—acute filarial lymphadenitis. The bubo of plague

activates plasminogen and degrades serum complement and is thought to enhance dissemination of *Y. pestis* following inoculation of the skin; a coagulase; and a fibrinolysin. A chromosomally encoded lipopolysaccharide endotoxin is important in sepsis, triggering the systemic inflammatory response syndrome and its complications.

Y. pestis organisms inoculated through the skin or mucous membranes are typically carried to regional lymph nodes via lymphatic channels, although direct bloodstream inoculation and dissemination may take place. Mononuclear phagocytes, which can phagocytize *Y. pestis* organisms without destroying them, may play a role in dissemination of the infection to distant sites. Plague can involve almost any organ, and untreated plague generally results in widespread and massive tissue destruction. In the early stages, infected lymph nodes (*buboes*, Fig. 143-1) are characterized by edema and congestion without inflammatory infiltrates or apparent vascular injury. Fully developed buboes contain huge numbers of infectious plague organisms and show distorted or obliterated lymph node architecture with loss of vascular integrity, hemorrhage, necrosis, infiltration of polymorphonuclear neutrophils (PMNs), and extensive serosanguineous effusion. The effusion typically involves perinodal tissues. If several adjacent lymph nodes are involved, a boggy edematous mass can result.

Primary septicemic plague consists of sepsis in the absence of a bubo; secondary septicemic plague is a complication of bubonic or pneumonic plague that occurs when local host defenses are breached. In fatal septicemic plague, multifocal hepatic and splenic necrosis is

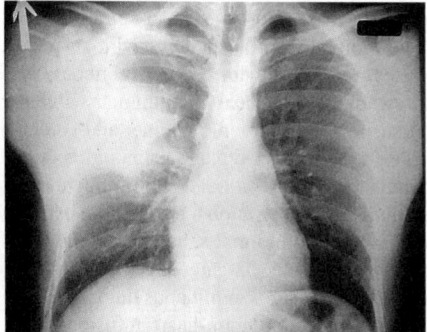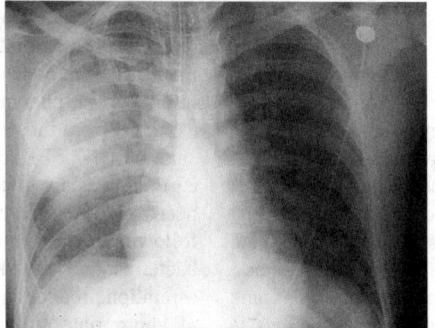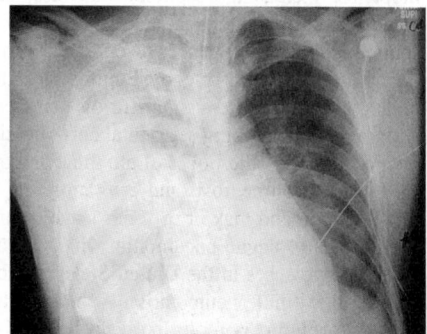

FIGURE 143-2   Sequential chest radiographs of a patient with fatal primary plague pneumonia. *Left*: Upright posteroanterior film taken at admission to hospital emergency department on third day of illness, showing segmental consolidation of right upper lobe. *Center*: Portable anteroposterior film taken 8 h after admission, showing extension of pneumonia to right middle and right lower lobes. *Right*: Portable anteroposterior film taken 13 h after admission (when patient had clinical adult respiratory distress syndrome), showing diffuse infiltration throughout right lung and patchy infiltration of left lower lung. A cavity later developed at the site of initial right-upper-lobe consolidation.

is distinguishable from lymphadenitis of most other causes, however, by its rapid onset, its extreme tenderness, the accompanying signs of toxemia, and the absence of cellulitis or obvious ascending lymphangitis. The pain and swelling of bubonic plague can be confused with a strangulated hernia or trauma.

Treated in the uncomplicated state with an appropriate antibiotic, bubonic plague usually responds quickly, with resolution of fever and alleviation of other systemic manifestations over 2 to 5 days. Buboes often remain enlarged and tender for a week or more after the initiation of treatment and can become fluctuant. Without effective antimicrobial treatment, patients with typical bubonic plague manifest an increasingly toxic state of fever, tachycardia, lethargy leading to prostration, agitation and confusion, and (occasionally) convulsions and delirium. Secondary plague sepsis may result in an alarmingly rapid and refractory cascade of DIC, bleeding, shock, and organ failure. Mild forms of bubonic plague, called *pestis minor*, have been described in South America and other plague endemic areas; in these cases, the patients are ambulatory, are only mildly febrile, and have subacute buboes.

Septicemic Plague Septicemic plague is a progressive, overwhelming gram-negative infection. Primary septicemia develops in the absence of a bubo, and the diagnosis is often not suspected until preliminary blood culture results are reported to be positive by the laboratory. *Y. pestis*, however, can also be cultured from the blood of most bubonic plague patients, and bacteremia should be distinguished from septicemia, in which the patient is desperately ill and requires aggressive care. Septic patients often present with gastrointestinal symptoms of nausea, vomiting, diarrhea, and abdominal pain, which may further confound the correct diagnosis. If not treated early with appropriate antibiotics, septicemic plague can be fulminant and fatal. In the United States in 1947 through 2001, 55 cases of primary septicemic plague with 13 deaths were reported, for a case-fatality rate of 24%. Petechiae, ecchymoses, bleeding from puncture wounds and orifices, and gangrene of acral parts are manifestations of DIC; refractory hypotension, renal shutdown, obtundation, and other signs of shock are preterminal events. Adult respiratory distress syndrome (ARDS), which can occur at any stage of septicemic plague, is sometimes confused with other conditions, such as hantavirus pulmonary syndrome. The differential diagnosis of septicemic plague includes sepsis of other gram-negative bacterial etiology, meningococcemia, and acute severe viral infections such as hantavirus illness.

Pneumonic Plague Of all forms of the disease, pneumonic plague develops most rapidly and is most frequently fatal. The incubation period for primary pneumonic plague is usually 3 to 5 days (range, 1 to 7 days). The onset is most often sudden, with chills, fever, headache, myalgias, weakness, and dizziness. Pulmonary signs, including tachypnea and dyspnea, cough, sputum production, and chest pain, typically arise on the second day of illness and may be accompanied by hemoptysis, increasing respiratory distress, cardiopulmonary insufficiency, and circulatory collapse. In primary plague pneumonia, the sputum is most often watery or mucoid, frothy, and blood-tinged, but it may become frankly bloody. Pulmonary signs in primary pneumonic plague may indicate involvement of a single lobe in the early stage, with rapidly developing segmental consolidation before bronchopneumonic spread to other lobes of the same and opposite lungs (Fig. 143-2). Liquefaction necrosis and cavitation may occur early in areas of consolidation and may or may not leave significant residual scarring.

Secondary plague pneumonia, which occurs in 10 to 15% of bubonic plague cases in the United States, typically manifests first as a diffuse interstitial pneumonitis in which sputum production is scant; since the sputum is more likely to be inspissated and tenacious in character than the sputum found in primary pneumonia, it may be less infectious. In the United States in 1947 through 2001, 46 cases of secondary pneumonic plague and 8 cases of primary pneumonic plague were described, with no known transmission to contacts and an overall case-fatality rate of 41%. Observers in the early twentieth century remarked on the relative lack of auscultatory findings, the usual presence of toxemia, and the frequency of sudden death among patients with pneumonic plague as compared to patients with other bacterial pneumonias.

The differential diagnosis of pneumonic plague includes acute community-acquired pneumonia of another bacterial or a viral etiology, tularemia, coccidioidomycosis, *Pneumocystis* pneumonia, and Q fever.

Plague Meningitis Meningitis is an unusual manifestation of plague. In the United States, there were 17 meningitis cases among the 409 evaluable plague cases reported in 1947 through 2001. All cases of meningitis were complications of bubonic plague, and all but three patients survived. Although meningitis may be a part of the initial presentation of plague, its onset is often delayed and is a manifestation of insufficient treatment. Recent cases in the United States have occurred in association with treatment of bubonic plague with tetracyclines, which are bacteriostatic against *Y. pestis*. Chronic relapsing meningeal plague over periods of weeks or even months was described in the preantibiotic era. The affected patients typically present with fever, headache, meningismus, and neutrophilic pleocytosis.

Plague Pharyngitis Plague pharyngitis presents as fever, sore throat, cervical lymphadenitis, and headache and is often indistinguishable clinically from pharyngitis and tonsillitis of other infectious etiologies, especially streptococcal pharyngitis. Plague pharyngitis can be difficult to distinguish from cervical bubonic plague arising from an infective flea bite on the head and neck region. Caregivers working in endemic areas must be alert to plague in the differential diagnosis of pharyngitis to avoid delayed and/or inappropriate treatment.

LABORATORY FINDINGS AND DIAGNOSIS Since plague is a rare disease in the United States, a high index of clinical suspicion as well as the elicitation of a thorough clinical and epidemiologic history and a careful physical examination are required for timely diagnosis and prompt institution of specific therapy. When the diagnosis of plague is delayed or missed altogether, a high case-fatality rate results; infected travelers who seek medical care after they have left endemic areas (peripatetic plague cases) are at especially high risk. Plague must be considered in the differential diagnosis of acute regional lymphadenitis, sepsis, or acute severe pneumonia in an otherwise-healthy person who has a history of recent travel to or residence in the rural western United States. When the diagnosis of plague is being considered, close communication between clinicians and the diagnostic laboratory and between the diagnostic laboratory and a qualified reference laboratory is essential. Tests for plague are highly reliable when conducted by laboratory personnel experienced with *Y. pestis*, but such expertise is usually limited to selected reference laboratories, including state health department laboratories in some plague-endemic states and the CDC plague laboratory (Fort Collins, Colorado; tel. 970-221-6400).

When plague is suspected, specimens should be collected promptly for laboratory studies, chest roentgenograms should be obtained, and specific antimicrobial therapy should be initiated pending confirmation. Appropriate diagnostic specimens for smear and culture include citrated or heparinized whole blood from all patients with suspected plague; lymph node aspirates from those with suspected buboes; sputum samples, pharyngeal swabs, and tracheal or pulmonary alveolar aspirates from those with suspected pneumonic plague; and cerebrospinal fluid (CSF) from those with suspected plague meningitis. Since early buboes are often exquisitely tender and are seldom fluctuant or necrotic, these lesions usually require aspiration under local anesthesia following the injection of 1 to 2 mL of normal saline (sterile but nonbacteriostatic) into the bubo with a 20- to 22-gauge needle. Typically, aspiration produces a scant amount of serosanguineous fluid. A variety of appropriate culture media (including brain-heart infusion broth, sheep blood agar, and MacConkey agar) should be inoculated with a portion of each specimen. Moreover, for each specimen, at least one smear should be examined immediately with Wayson or Giemsa stain and at least one with Gram's stain; a smear should also be submitted to a reference laboratory for direct fluorescent antibody testing, antigen-capture enzyme-linked immunosorbent assay (ELISA), polymerase chain reaction (PCR) analysis, or testing by another rapid detection method (e.g., immunochromatographic hand-held assay). An acute-phase serum specimen should be tested for antibody to *Y. pestis*; whenever possible, a convalescent-phase serum specimen collected 3 to 4 weeks later should also be tested. When a patient dies and plague is suspected, appropriate autopsy tissues for culture, direct fluorescent antibody testing, and immunohistochemical staining include buboes, all solid organs (especially liver, spleen, and lung), and bone marrow. If culture of such specimens is to be attempted, they should be sent to the laboratory either fresh or frozen on dry ice, not in preservatives or fixatives. If necessary, Cary-Blair or a similar medium can be used to transport *Y. pestis*–infected tissues.

Laboratory confirmation of plague depends on the isolation of *Y. pestis* from cultures of body fluids or tissues. Cultures of three blood samples taken over a 45-min period before treatment will usually result in isolation of the bacterium. *Y. pestis* strains are readily distinguished from those of the closely related species *Y. pseudotuberculosis* by differences in biochemical profile, temperature-dependent susceptibility to lysis by a *Y. pestis*–specific bacteriophage, and motility. Automated bacteriologic test systems can be used to assist in the identification of isolates as *Y. pestis*, but *Y. pestis* can be misidentified (e.g., as *Y. pseudotuberculosis*) or overlooked if these systems are improperly programmed.

In the absence of *Y. pestis* isolation, plague cases can be confirmed either by the demonstration of seroconversion (a fourfold or greater titer rise) to *Y. pestis* F1 antigen in passive hemagglutination tests of acute- and convalescent-phase serum specimens or by detection of an antibody titer of >128 in a single serum sample from a patient with a plague-compatible illness who has not received plague vaccine. The specificity of a positive passive-hemagglutination test requires confirmation with the F1 antigen hemagglutination-inhibition test. A few plague patients seroconvert to F1 antigen as early as 5 days after the onset of illness; most seroconvert between 1 and 2 weeks after onset; a few seroconvert >3 weeks after onset; and a few (<5%) fail to seroconvert at all. Early, specific antibiotic treatment may delay seroconversion by several weeks. After seroconversion, positive serologic titers diminish gradually over months to years. ELISAs for IgM and IgG antibodies to *Y. pestis* are replacing hemagglutination tests in some laboratories. Other new test methods include those mentioned above: antigen-capture ELISAs, PCR, and immunochromatographic hand-held assays for rapid identification of *Y. pestis* in aspirates, sputum, and other infected body fluids or tissues. The hand-held assays can be used at the bedside in the remote rural settings where most plague cases occur and could prove important in responding to bioterrorism (Chap. 205).

Patients with plague typically have white blood cell (WBC) counts of 10,000 to 25,000/μL, with a predominance of PMNs and a left shift. Leukemoid reactions with WBC counts as high as 100,000/μL can occur. Modest thrombocytopenia is usually documented, and fibrin-fibrinogen split products are often detected even in patients without frank DIC. Serum levels of aminotransferases and bilirubin may be elevated. In plague pneumonia, stained respiratory secretions usually contain PMNs and characteristic bipolar-staining bacilli. In *Y. pestis* septicemia, visualization of the characteristic bacilli in a routine blood smear or a buffy-coat smear is an uncommon but grave prognostic sign (Fig. 143-3). In patients with plague meningitis, PMN pleocytosis is typical, and the bacilli are usually visible in stained CSF smears.

℞ TREATMENT

Left untreated, plague is fatal in >50% of cases of bubonic disease and in nearly all cases of septicemic and pneumonic disease. The overall mortality rate for plague cases in the United States since 1950 has been ~14%; deaths are almost always due to delays in seeking treatment, misdiagnosis, delays in the institution of treatment, or incorrect treatment. Rapid diagnosis and appropriate antimicrobial therapy are essential.

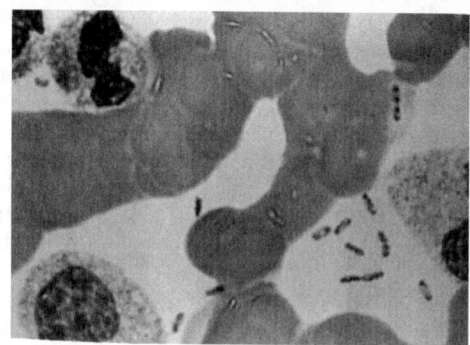

FIGURE 143-3 Peripheral blood smear from a patient with fatal plague septicemia and shock, showing characteristic bipolar-staining *Y. pestis* bacilli (Wright's stain, oil immersion).

Guidelines for the treatment of plague are given in Table 143-1. Although streptomycin is the drug of choice, gentamicin is increasingly used for the treatment of plague in the United States because of its ready availability; it is probably as effective as streptomycin and less toxic, although results of controlled studies in humans have not been published. Alternative antibiotics include the tetracyclines and chloramphenicol; these agents are usually given orally with initial loading doses but may be given intravenously to critically ill patients and to patients unable to tolerate oral medication. Doxycycline is considered the tetracycline of choice. Penicillins, cephalosporins, and macrolides are suboptimal and should not be used. Trimethoprim-sulfamethoxazole (TMP-SMX) has been used successfully to treat bubonic plague but is not considered a first-line agent. Chloramphenicol may be indicated for the treatment of plague meningitis, pleuritis, endophthalmitis, and myocarditis because of its superior tissue penetration; it is used alone or in combination with streptomycin or another first-line agent. In general, antimicrobial treatment should be continued for 7 to 10 days or for at least 3 days after the patient has become afebrile and has made a clinical recovery. Patients initially given intravenous antibiotics may be switched to oral regimens upon clinical improvement. Such improvement is usually evident 2 or 3 days after the start of treatment, even though fever may continue for several days. National bioterrorism-response protocols propose gentamicin, ciprofloxacin, and doxycycline as antimicrobial agents of first choice for treatment and postexposure prophylaxis in the event of an attack using *Y. pestis* (Chap. 205).

Consequences of delayed treatment of plague include DIC, ARDS, and other complications of gram-negative sepsis. Patients with these

TABLE 143-1 *Guidelines for the Treatment of Plague*

Drug	Daily Dosage	Interval, h	Route(s) of Administration
Streptomycin			
Adults	2 g	12	IM
Children	30 mg/kg	12	IM
Gentamicin			
Adults	3–5 mg/kg[a]	8	IM or IV
Children	6.0–7.5 mg/kg	8	IM or IV
Infants/neonates	7.5 mg/kg	8	IM or IV
Tetracycline			
Adults	2 g	6	PO or IV
Children ≥8 y	25–50 mg/kg	6	PO or IV
Doxycycline			
Adults	200 mg	12 or 24	PO or IV
Children ≥8 y	4.4 mg/kg	12 or 24	PO or IV
Chloramphenicol			
Adults	50 mg/kg[b]	6	PO or IV
Children ≥1 y	50 mg/kg[b]	6	PO or IV

[a] Dosage should be reduced to 3 mg/kg daily as soon as clinically indicated.
[b] For meningitis, up to 100 (mg/kg)/d initially.

disorders require intensive monitoring and close physiologic support, as outlined elsewhere (Chaps. 102 and 251). Buboes may require surgical drainage. Abscessed nodes can cause recurrent fever in patients who have apparently recovered; the cause may be occult if intrathoracic or intraabdominal nodes are involved. Although *Y. pestis* is considered to be genetically stable, a multidrug-resistant strain was recently isolated from a plague patient in Madagascar. This strain exhibited resistance (mediated by a transferable plasmid) to principal first-line antibiotics used for treatment and prophylaxis of plague.

PREVENTION AND CONTROL Persons at greatest risk for plague in the United States are individuals who live, work, and participate in outdoor recreational activities in areas of those western states in which plague is enzootic. Surveillance, education, and environmental management are the cornerstones of prevention and control. A network of biologists and public health specialists coordinates these activities through local and state health departments and the CDC. Personal protective measures include the avoidance of areas with known epizootic plague (in which warning signs may be posted) and of sick or dead animals; the use of repellents, insecticides, and protective clothing when at risk of exposure to rodents' fleas; and the wearing of gloves when handling animal carcasses. Short-term antibiotic prophylaxis (Table 143-2) is recommended for persons known to have had close contact with a patient with suspected or confirmed pneumonic plague and occasionally for persons who are unable to avoid an area where a plague outbreak is in progress or who may be caring for patients with plague. Patients in whom respiratory plague is suspected should be managed under isolation, with use of respiratory-droplet precautions until pneumonia has been ruled out or until 48 h of effective antimicrobial therapy has been administered, after which standard infection-control precautions are adequate. Masks are considered to be protective against respiratory transmission of plague and would be expected to be an important tool to prevent secondary plague spread in the event of bioterrorism (Chap. 205).

Rodent food (garbage, pet food) and habitats (brush piles, junk heaps, woodpiles) should be eliminated in domestic, peridomestic, and working environments; buildings and food stores should be rodent-proofed. The control of fleas with insecticides is a key public health measure in situations where epizootic plague activity places humans at high risk; this effort includes dusting and spraying of rodent burrows, rodent runs, and other sites where rodents and their fleas are found. In plague-endemic areas of the western United States, persons should keep their dogs and cats free of fleas and restrained. The decision to control plague by killing rodents should be left to public health authorities, and such a program should be carried out only in conjunction with effective flea control. Killing of rodents has no lasting benefit without environmental sanitation.

TABLE 143-2 *Guidelines for Plague Prophylaxis*

Drug	Daily Dosage	Interval, h	Route of Administration
Tetracycline			
Adults	1–2 g	6 or 12	PO
Children ≥8 y	25–50 mg/kg	6 or 12	PO
Doxycycline			
Adults	100–200 mg	12 or 24	PO
Children ≥8 y	2–4 mg/kg	12 or 24	PO
Trimethoprim-sulfamethoxazole			
Adults	320 mg[a]	12	PO
Children ≥2 mo	8 mg/kg[a]	12	PO
Ciprofloxacin[b]			
Adults	1 g	12	PO
Children	40 mg/kg	12	PO

[a] Trimethoprim component.
[b] Recommended as an alternative to doxycycline in bioterrorism-response plans.

The previously used killed, whole-cell plague vaccine is no longer available in the United States. New and improved vaccines are being evaluated that use recombinant F1 and V antigens to induce protective antibodies. In the United States, the indications for use of these newer vaccines would probably be similar to those for the previously available killed vaccine, which was mostly limited to protecting laboratory personnel who routinely worked with *Y. pestis* and some persons whose vocations brought them into regular contact with wild rodents and their fleas in areas with enzootic or epizootic plague. In addition, a vaccine might be useful in protecting selected persons at risk from biowarfare or bioterrorism.

OTHER *YERSINIA* INFECTIONS

DEFINITION Yersiniosis is an uncommon bacterial zoonosis caused primarily by infection with either of two enteropathogenic *Yersinia* species: *Y. enterocolitica* or *Y. pseudotuberculosis*. Reservoir hosts of these bacteria include swine and other wild and domestic animals, and transmission to humans is predominantly via the oral route. Both sporadic cases and common-source outbreaks occur. The most frequent acute clinical manifestations are (1) enteritis or enterocolitis with self-limited diarrhea (especially with *Y. enterocolitica*) and (2) mesenteric adenitis and terminal ileitis (especially with *Y. pseudotuberculosis*), which can be confused with acute appendicitis. Septicemia and metastatic focal infections are less common. Yersiniosis can be complicated by nonsuppurative, extraintestinal, inflammatory sequelae—e.g., reactive arthritis (Chap. 305) and erythema nodosum (Chap. 17). Other nonplague *Yersinia* species, including *Y. intermedia*, *Y. frederiksenii*, and *Y. kristensenii*, have been associated with enteritis or enterocolitis in humans (particularly immunocompromised adults), but little is known about their pathogenicity, public health importance, or clinical management.

ETIOLOGIC AGENTS *Y. enterocolitica* and *Y. pseudotuberculosis* are pleomorphic gram-negative bacilli in the family Enterobacteriaceae. They can multiply within a wide temperature range ($-1°C$ to $45°C$). Pathogenic *Y. enterocolitica* isolates are most commonly identified by biotyping based on biochemical profiles and serotyping according to somatic O and H antigens. Six biotypes and >60 serotypes of *Y. enterocolitica* are recognized. A separate serotyping system for *Y. pseudotuberculosis* (also based on somatic antigens) has distinguished six major serotypes (I through VI) and their subtypes.

EPIDEMIOLOGY ■ *Yersinia enterocolitica* *Y. enterocolitica* is distributed worldwide and has been isolated from soil, fresh water, contaminated foodstuffs (e.g., meat, milk, and vegetables), and a wide variety of wild and domestic animals. Many serotypes isolated from environmental sources, however, evidently are not human pathogens. Most human infections have been caused by *Y. enterocolitica* serotypes O:3, O:5,27, O:8, and O:9, which are primarily associated with wild and domestic mammals. The recognized incidence of these infections and their sequelae is highest in Scandinavia and some other northern European countries, but reliable population-based estimates of incidence are unavailable.

All age groups are susceptible to *Y. enterocolitica* infections, but the majority of cases of enterocolitis are in children aged 1 to 4. Moreover, these infections show a modest predilection for males. Mesenteric adenitis and terminal ileitis are most common among older children and young adults. Risk factors for *Y. enterocolitica* septicemia and metastatic focal infections include chronic liver disease, malignancy, diabetes mellitus, immunosuppressive therapy, alcoholism, malnutrition, advanced age, iron overload (see below), and hemolytic anemias (including the thalassemias). The nonsuppurative sequelae of yersiniosis are most common among adults. HLA-B27 is expressed in 70 to 80% of patients who develop reactive arthritis associated with yersiniosis. HLA-B27 is not a risk factor for *Yersinia*-induced erythema nodosum; females with this condition outnumber males by 2 to 1.

Among *Y. enterocolitica* strains isolated from patients in recent decades, serotypes O:3 and O:9 have predominated in Europe, while serotype O:3 has predominated in Canada, Japan, and the United States. The apparent incidence of *Yersinia*-induced nonsuppurative sequelae reportedly is 10 to 30% in Scandinavia and much lower in most other countries, including the United States.

Common-source outbreaks of *Y. enterocolitica* enteritis have been traced to such vehicles as raw milk, contaminated pasteurized milk, and foods prepared with contaminated fresh water. Because *Y. enterocolitica* commonly colonizes the gastrointestinal tracts of swine, sporadic human cases and outbreaks of yersiniosis have also been associated with the preparation or ingestion of raw pork products (e.g., chitterlings). In some cases of yersiniosis, circumstantial evidence suggests transmission via contact with dogs and cats or their feces. Several nosocomial outbreaks of *Y. enterocolitica* infection have been described; fecal-oral transmission from person to person was suspected. Fecal-oral transmission among family members may also explain occasional secondary cases in households. In a prospective study of 50 children with *Y. enterocolitica* enteritis, fecal excretion of the organism persisted for an average of 27 days (range, 4 to 79 days) after the cessation of symptoms. A chronic carrier state, however, has not been demonstrated. *Y. enterocolitica* is a rare but often lethal cause of transfusion-associated septicemia. The explanation is that blood donors occasionally have transient, occult *Y. enterocolitica* bacteremia and that this organism can slowly multiply to high concentrations in blood refrigerated for at least 10 days.

Yersinia pseudotuberculosis The ecology of *Y. pseudotuberculosis* seems to parallel that of *Y. enterocolitica* closely. *Y. pseudotuberculosis* is also widespread in wild and domestic animals and is isolated from many environmental sources. Human infections with *Y. pseudotuberculosis*, however, appear to be rare. Swine appear to be an important reservoir for pathogenic strains of *Y. pseudotuberculosis*.

PATHOGENESIS AND PATHOLOGY With rare exceptions (e.g., transmission via contaminated blood products or direct cutaneous inoculation), the enteropathogenic yersiniae are thought to enter the host via the oral route. The incubation period averages 5 days (range, 1 to 11 days). Studies of animals have shown that the organisms initially invade the ileal epithelium, then are translocated via M cells into the lamina propria, and finally enter Peyer's patches, where they are able to replicate. They subsequently drain into the mesenteric lymph nodes, which undergo hyperplasia and from which the bacteria can be disseminated. The mesenteric lymph nodes can become intensely swollen and matted and are occasionally detected on physical examination as a tender right-lower-quadrant mass. Intestinal inflammation (most commonly of the distal ileum and less commonly of the ascending colon) develops and may be accompanied by mucosal ulcerations and by the shedding of PMNs and red blood cells into the intestinal lumen. In relatively severe cases, thrombosis of mesenteric blood vessels, intestinal hemorrhage, and necrosis can occur. In patients with enteropathogenic yersinial infections who undergo exploratory laparotomy, the appendix usually is histologically normal or shows only lymphoid hyperplasia, but frank suppuration is sometimes evident.

A plasmid of ~70 kb is essential for virulence of the enteropathogenic yersiniae because it encodes at least six Yops, which confer a variety of pathogenic properties—e.g., cytotoxicity; resistance to phagocytosis by PMNs; and the ability to cause monocyte apoptosis (programmed cell death), to suppress the host's expression of tumor necrosis factor α, and to interfere with platelet aggregation and host complement activation. A chromosomal gene (*inv*) encodes for the surface protein invasin, which is necessary for yersinial invasion of nonphagocytic host cells (e.g., epithelial cells) in vitro and which facilitates the translocation of bacteria across the intestinal epithelium. Both *Y. enterocolitica* and *Y. pseudotuberculosis* can express at least one protein superantigen that selectively stimulates the proliferation of T cells. Many strains of *Y. enterocolitica* produce a heat-stable enterotoxin that is similar to *Escherichia coli* enterotoxin. The cell walls of *Y. enterocolitica* and *Y. pseudotuberculosis* contain a lipopolysaccharide (endotoxin). Some *Yersinia* strains are unable to synthesize bacterial iron chelators called *siderophores*. However, they can

exploit host-chelated iron stores and the drug deferoxamine (a siderophore produced by *Streptomyces pilosus*). Therefore, iron overload (e.g., caused by hemodialysis or multiple transfusions) and deferoxamine therapy appear to be independent risk factors for *Y. enterocolitica* bacteremia, especially that involving serotypes O:3 and O:9, and to a lesser degree for *Y. pseudotuberculosis* bacteremia.

Immunogenetic factors and cell-mediated immune responses are clearly involved in the pathogenesis of reactive arthritis following infection with the enteropathogenic yersiniae. As noted above, most patients with *Yersinia*-induced reactive arthritis express HLA-B27. In addition, *Y. pseudotuberculosis* shares at least one cross-reactive epitope with HLA-B27, and *Y. enterocolitica* infection alters the expression of serologic HLA-B27 epitopes on lymphocytes and monocytes. In patients with reactive arthritis following *Y. enterocolitica* infection, yersinial antigens are commonly detectable in synovial fluid cells in the apparent absence of whole organisms. Thus, it is unknown whether the arthritis results from occult bacterial persistence through self-tolerance of HLA-B27 with a failure of cross-reactive immune responses to yersiniae, from an immune response to common antigenic determinants shared by the bacteria and host HLA-B27 (i.e., molecular mimicry), or from other mechanisms. The pathogenesis of *Yersinia*-induced erythema nodosum is obscure.

In some assays, patients with Graves' disease have an increased prevalence of serum antibodies to *Y. enterocolitica*, and the immunoglobulins of patients recovering from *Y. enterocolitica* infections react with the human thyroid-stimulating hormone receptor. However, a link between *Y. enterocolitica* infection and the subsequent development of autoimmune thyroiditis has not been convincingly demonstrated.

MANIFESTATIONS ■ ***Yersinia enterocolitica*** The principal clinical manifestations of *Y. enterocolitica* infection are enteritis, enterocolitis, mesenteric adenitis, and terminal ileitis. Less common manifestations include exudative pharyngitis, septicemia, metastatic focal infections, reactive polyarthritis, and erythema nodosum. When age groups are combined, the most common presentation of *Y. enterocolitica* infection is acute diarrhea from enteritis or enterocolitis. Low-grade fever and cramping abdominal pain occur in most cases, nausea and vomiting in 15 to 40%, hematochezia in up to 30%, and a generalized maculopapular skin rash in a few cases. Diarrhea persists for an average of 2 weeks (range, 1 day to many months), during which the frequency of bowel movements diminishes. Uncommonly, enteritis or enterocolitis can be complicated by severe abdominal pain and high fever. Rare (and sometimes fatal) complications include diffuse inflammation, ulceration, hemorrhage, and necrosis of the small bowel and colon; intestinal perforation; peritonitis; ascending cholangitis; mesenteric vein thrombosis; diverticulitis; toxic megacolon; and ileocecal intussusception.

The syndrome of mesenteric adenitis and terminal ileitis without diarrhea is easily confused with appendicitis. Low-grade fever and right-lower-quadrant pain, tenderness, guarding, and rebound tenderness are common. During six recognized common-source outbreaks in the United States, 10% of 444 patients with symptomatic undiagnosed *Y. enterocolitica* infections underwent laparotomy for suspected appendicitis; surgical incisions became infected with *Y. enterocolitica* in a few of these cases.

Acute pharyngitis and pharyngotonsillitis, with or without cervical adenitis or intestinal illness, are less common but potentially lethal manifestations of *Y. enterocolitica* infection, particularly in adults. *Y. enterocolitica* septicemia generally presents as a severe illness with fever and leukocytosis, often with abdominal pain and jaundice and without localized signs of infection. Metastatic focal *Y. enterocolitica* infections can occur with or without clinically apparent bacteremia and can affect almost any organ system. Examples include abscess formation (e.g., in liver, spleen, kidney, lung, skeletal muscle, lymph node, or cutaneous tissue), osteomyelitis, meningitis, peritonitis, urinary tract infection, pneumonia, empyema, endocarditis, pericarditis, mycotic aneurysm, septic arthritis, suppurative conjunctivitis, panophthalmitis, Parinaud's oculoglandular syndrome, and cutaneous pustules or bullae.

In Scandinavia, the incidence of reactive arthritis following *Y. enterocolitica* infection among adults is estimated to be at least 10%. About 80% of these patients have preceding symptoms such as fever, diarrhea, or abdominal pain. Typically, these symptoms precede the arthritis by 1 week and are of short duration. The most commonly affected joints are the knees and ankles, but other joints can be involved. Typically, multiple (two to eight) joints become involved sequentially and asymmetrically over a period of a few days to 2 weeks, after which no additional joints are affected. Monarticular arthritis occurs less commonly. In two-thirds of cases, the acute arthritis remits spontaneously within 1 to 3 months. Chronic joint disease is documented in a minority of cases. A few HLA-B27-positive patients with *Y. enterocolitica*–induced arthritis have subsequent ankylosing spondylitis, but this development is best explained by the fact that HLA-B27 is a major risk factor for each of these diseases. Mild, self-limited myocarditis accompanies ~10% of cases of *Yersinia*-induced arthritis and can occur independently. Typical manifestations include cardiac murmurs and transient electrocardiographic abnormalities, such as prolongation of the PR interval and nonspecific ST-segment and T-wave changes. The syndrome of *Yersinia*-induced arthritis and carditis can be confused with acute rheumatic fever. In Scandinavia, erythema nodosum occurs in 15 to 20% of patients with yersiniosis, usually within a few days to 3 weeks after the onset of intestinal illness. Lesions typically are located on the lower extremities and resolve within 1 month. Less commonly reported nonsuppurative sequelae of *Y. enterocolitica* infections include reactive uveitis, iritis, conjunctivitis, urethritis, and glomerulonephritis. The complete triad of Reiter's syndrome (arthritis, conjunctivitis, and urethritis) is seen in 5 to 10% of patients with *Yersinia*-induced arthritis.

Yersinia pseudotuberculosis   The most common clinical presentation of *Y. pseudotuberculosis* infection is fever and abdominal pain caused by mesenteric adenitis; diarrheal illness is less common than in *Y. enterocolitica* infection. Systemic manifestations, including septicemia, focal infections, reactive arthritis, and erythema nodosum, are generally similar to those associated with *Y. enterocolitica* infection. In addition, *Y. pseudotuberculosis* has been associated with a scarlet fever–like syndrome, acute interstitial nephritis, and hemolytic-uremic syndrome.

LABORATORY FINDINGS AND DIAGNOSIS   Results of routine laboratory tests in most patients with yersiniosis are nonspecific. Leukocyte counts are usually normal or slightly elevated, often with a modest left shift. Standard microbiologic methods are sufficient to isolate *Y. enterocolitica* and *Y. pseudotuberculosis* from otherwise-sterile sites, such as blood, CSF, lymph node tissue, and peritoneal fluid, and from abscesses. Isolation of these organisms from feces is impeded by their slow growth and the overgrowth of normal fecal flora on culture media routinely used to select for enteric bacteria. The yield from feces and other grossly contaminated specimens can be increased by the use of *Yersinia*-selective [e.g., cefsulodin-Irgasan-novobiocin (CIN)] agar and by cold enrichment. Because bacteriologic procedures designed to isolate yersiniae from feces are not considered cost-effective, many laboratories undertake them by special request only.

The results of serologic tests can be used to support a diagnosis of yersiniosis. Agglutination tests or ELISAs are used most commonly; immunoblotting has also been used. The existence of multiple serotypes makes routine serologic tests laborious; thus these tests are generally conducted only in research laboratories or large commercial laboratories. Since these tests are experimental and are neither standardized nor well validated, and since some strains of *Yersinia* cross-react with other bacteria (e.g., *Brucella*, *Salmonella*, and *Vibrio*) and with serum from some patients with thyroiditis, results should be interpreted with caution. In typical uncomplicated cases of yersiniosis,

agglutinin titers begin to rise within the first week of illness, peak in the second week, and then gradually diminish and return to normal within 3 to 6 months, although agglutinating antibody may remain detectable for several years in some cases. Because an initial serum specimen is often collected a week or more after the onset of illness, when agglutinin titers are already high, it is usually impossible to document a fourfold or greater rise in titer between paired specimens (although a fourfold or greater fall in titer may be found). Immunohistochemical techniques and PCR tests to detect yersinial antigens and DNA, respectively, in clinical specimens are experimental at this time.

In patients with *Yersinia*-induced reactive arthritis, synovial fluid is sterile and the leukocyte count ranges from a few hundred to 60,000/μL, with a majority of PMNs. The erythrocyte sedimentation rate is often >100 mm/h. Rheumatoid factor and antinuclear antibodies are usually absent. The diagnosis of *Yersinia*-induced reactive arthritis or other nonsuppurative inflammatory sequelae can be difficult, especially when triggering infections are asymptomatic or clinically mild or occur several weeks before the diagnosis is attempted. Because the isolation of a pathogenic *Yersinia* strain from feces is the most specific diagnostic test in such cases, it should be attempted. Since culture is of limited sensitivity in this clinical setting, a high index of suspicion and positive results of serologic tests for *Y. enterocolitica* or *Y. pseudotuberculosis* are usually required for diagnosis.

℞ TREATMENT

The effectiveness of antimicrobial agents in the treatment of yersinial enteritis, enterocolitis, mesenteric adenitis, or terminal ileitis has not been established. These conditions are usually self-limited, and their treatment is symptom-based and supportive. In uncomplicated cases, diarrhea should be treated with fluid and electrolyte replacement, with the route of delivery dependent on clinical severity. Enteric precautions are advisable for patients hospitalized with yersinial diarrhea. In general, antimicrobial treatment should be reserved for patients with septicemia, metastatic focal infections, or immunosuppression and enterocolitis. Controlled clinical comparisons of antimicrobial agents in the treatment of severe cases of yersiniosis have not yet been conducted. In such cases, drug selection should ultimately be guided by clinical response and bacterial sensitivity patterns. Clinical isolates of *Y. enterocolitica* and *Y. pseudotuberculosis* are usually susceptible in vitro to aminoglycosides, third-generation cephalosporins, chloramphenicol, quinolones, tetracyclines, and TMP-SMX. In laboratory animals infected with enteropathogenic yersiniae, the fluoroquinolones have exerted the strongest bactericidal effects in vivo; clinical experience with these drugs against these pathogens in humans is promising but limited. Because they produce β-lactamases, isolates typically are resistant to penicillin, ampicillin, carbenicillin, and first-generation and most second-generation cephalosporins. Optimal dosages and durations of therapy have not been established. Mortality from *Y. enterocolitica* septicemia is ~10% despite treatment. Focal extraintestinal infections may require at least 3 weeks of therapy. No role for antimicrobial agents in the management of the nonsuppurative inflammatory manifestations of yersiniosis has been established. Patients with reactive arthritis may benefit from treatment with nonsteroidal anti-inflammatory drugs, intraarticular steroid injections, and physical therapy.

PREVENTION AND CONTROL   The importance of safe food-handling and food-preparation practices in the prevention of yersiniosis cannot be overemphasized. Caution is particularly warranted in the case of pork and other animal products. The consumption of raw or undercooked meats, especially pork, should be avoided. Increased efforts to prevent the spread of enteric pathogens in household, pet-care, day-care, and hospital settings and in the food industry would be likely to decrease the incidence of yersiniosis. Current regulations of the U.S. Food and Drug Administration require visual inspection of packed red cell units before transfusion, with the discarding of units in which bacterial contamination is suspected on the basis of darkening (reflecting decreased oxygen saturation and hemolysis). Since the risk is minimal, more specific measures to further decrease the likelihood of transfusion of *Y. enterocolitica*–contaminated blood products (e.g., limiting the period for which red cells can be stored before transfusion) have not been widely implemented.

Yersiniosis is not routinely reportable to public health authorities in most jurisdictions. However, clinicians who suspect a common-source outbreak (e.g., because they have documented a familial case cluster) or some other public health threat (e.g., because they have found *Y. enterocolitica* bacteremia in a recent blood donor) should consult promptly with local public health officials.

FURTHER READING

BOTTONE EJ: *Yersinia enterocolitica*: Overview and epidemiologic correlates. Microbes Infect 1:323, 1999

CENTERS FOR DISEASE CONTROL AND PREVENTION: Imported plague—New York City, 2002. MMWR 52:725, 2003

———: *Yersinia enterocolitica* gastroenteritis among infants exposed to chitterlings—Chicago, Illinois, 2002. MMWR 52:956, 2003

CHANTEAU S et al: Development and testing of a rapid diagnostic test for bubonic and pneumonic plague. Lancet 361:211, 2003

INGLESBY TV et al: Plague as a biological weapon: Medical and public health management. JAMA 283:2281, 2000

LOFTUS CG et al: Clinical features of patients with novel *Yersinia* species. Dig Dis Sci 47:2805, 2002

RATSITORAHINA M et al: Epidemiological and diagnostic aspects of the outbreak of pneumonic plague in Madagascar. Lancet 355:111, 2000

SMEGO RA et al: Yersiniosis I: Microbiological and clinicoepidemiological aspects of plague and non-plague *Yersinia* infections. Eur J Clin Microbiol Infect Dis 18:1, 1999

144 BARTONELLA INFECTIONS, INCLUDING CAT-SCRATCH DISEASE
Lucy Stuart Tompkins

Bartonella species, including *B. bacilliformis*, *B. henselae*, and *B. quintana*, are tiny gram-negative bacilli that can adhere to and invade mammalian cells, including endothelial cells and erythrocytes. Previously classified as *Rochalimaea* species within the rickettsia group, *Bartonella* species have now been removed from the order Rickettsiales on the grounds that they are not obligate intracellular parasites. These agents cause a wide spectrum of clinical illnesses, including trench fever, cat-scratch disease (CSD), bacillary angiomatosis, peliosis hepatis, endocarditis, Oroya fever, and verruga peruana. The pathologic manifestations of *Bartonella* disease vary with the immune status of the host. Key features of major *Bartonella* infections are summarized in Table 144-1.

OROYA FEVER AND VERRUGA PERUANA

DEFINITION AND ETIOLOGY Oroya fever and verruga peruana are caused by *B. bacilliformis*. Oroya fever is characterized by fever, profound anemia, and—unless antibiotic treatment is given—high mortality. The lesions referred to as verruga peruana may develop during the convalescent phase of Oroya fever or during chronic infection with *B. bacilliformis*. In 1885 Daniel Carrion, a Peruvian medical student, inoculated himself with material from a patient with verruga peruana and subsequently died of Oroya fever, thus proving that a single agent causes both diseases.

EPIDEMIOLOGY Infection with *B. bacilliformis* follows the bite of the sandfly vector *Phlebotomus*, an insect found in the river valleys of the Andes Mountains at altitudes of 600 to 2500 m. Oroya fever develops in nonimmune individuals who are not residents of the endemic region, whereas verruga peruana occurs in persons who apparently have been exposed in the past, including those who have recently had Oroya fever. The infection has not been acquired in the United States.

PATHOLOGY During initial infection in the nonimmune host, *B. bacilliformis* cells adhere to erythrocytes and produce indentations in the cell membrane; the bacteria subsequently enter the erythrocytes and cause persistent deformation of the cytoskeleton. The parasitized erythrocytes are ultimately phagocytosed and destroyed. Although the life span of infected erythrocytes is markedly shortened, not all of this

TABLE 144-1 *Bartonella Infections: Clinical Syndromes, Risk Factors, and Therapy*

Bartonella *Species*	Clinical Syndrome	Risk Factors	Therapy[a]
Bartonella henselae	Cat-scratch disease	Cat scratch or bite	Azithromycin for 5 days (500 mg on day 1, 250 mg on days 2–5); or variable duration of rifampin (300 mg daily or bid), doxycycline (100 mg/d), or ciprofloxacin (500 mg/d)
	Bacillary angiomatosis/peliosis	Cat scratch or bite	Erythromycin (500 mg qid) or doxycycline (100 mg/d) for 3–6 weeks
	Endocarditis	Cat exposure	If patient is *Bartonella* culture-positive or seropositive: Give azithromycin (250 mg/d) or doxycycline (100 mg/d) for 4–6 months (surgery may be required)
			If *Bartonella* is suspected but unconfirmed: Treat for culture-negative endocarditis with ceftriaxone (2 g/d IV) plus gentamicin for 6–8 weeks[b]
Bartonella quintana	Trench fever	Homelessness; alcoholism; body lice	Doxycycline (100 mg bid) or azithromycin (500 mg/d) for 4–6 weeks
	Bacillary angiomatosis	Homelessness ± body lice; HIV infection	Same as for bacillary angiomatosis due to *B. henselae*
	Endocarditis	Same as for other *B. quintana* infections	Same as for endocarditis due to *B. henselae*
Bartonella bacilliformis	Oroya fever	Lack of immunity; sandfly bite	Chloramphenicol for 10 days (in South America); ampicillin (1 g q6h IV or PO) or cephalexin (500 mg qid PO) for 10–14 days
	Verruga peruana	Previous exposure to *B. bacilliformis*	Rifampin (300 mg bid) or ciprofloxacin (500 mg/d) for 7–10 days

[a] Azithromycin therapy for cat-scratch disease is based on clinical-trial data; all other recommendations are based on case reports or case series.

[b] If culture results confirm *Bartonella* infection, ceftriaxone may be discontinued and therapy with azithromycin or doxycycline given for a prolonged period.

change can be attributed to the mechanical fragility induced by the internalization of bacteria. Decreased bone marrow erythropoiesis also contributes to anemia.

CLINICAL MANIFESTATIONS   The onset of symptoms in Oroya fever may be either insidious or abrupt, after an incubation period of ~3 weeks. The subacute presentation may include low-grade fever, malaise, headache, and anorexia. Sudden-onset disease commences with high fever, chills, diaphoresis, headaches, and changes in mental status. These manifestations are followed by the sudden development of profound anemia, which is due to a marked decrease in erythrocyte numbers and is associated with macrocytic changes, poikilocytosis, Howell-Jolly bodies, nucleated erythrocytes, and immature myeloid cells. The leukocyte differential usually shifts to the left, although the total leukocyte count may be normal. The erythrocyte count may fall to extremely low levels. In eosin/thiazine-stained peripheral-blood smears, numerous microorganisms can be seen adhering to most erythrocytes.

During the acute phase, muscle and joint pain and headache may be severe; central nervous system changes include insomnia, delirium, and a decreased level of consciousness. Thrombocytopenic purpura may develop. If the patient survives, a convalescent phase ensues, characterized by the sudden disappearance of bacteria from blood smears, declining fever, and an increase in the erythrocyte count. Although much of the mortality associated with Oroya fever is due to profound anemia and toxicity, secondary bacterial infections (including salmonellosis and other enteric infections, malaria, and tuberculosis) are often an important contributing factor.

After convalescence from acute Oroya fever, nodular dermal eruptions known as *verrugas*, *verruga peruana*, or *Peruvian warts* may develop. These red or purple cutaneous lesions may be either tiny and sessile or large, pedunculated, and nodular. They bear a marked resemblance to the lesions of bacillary angiomatosis and to Kaposi's sarcoma.

DIAGNOSIS   During acute infection, bacteria can be cultured from the blood on agar containing rabbit blood, with incubation at 28°C. The hallmark of verruga peruana is the formation of new blood vessels (angiogenesis) at the sites of bacterial replication.

℞ TREATMENT

Oroya fever responds to a variety of antimicrobial agents, including chloramphenicol, tetracyclines, penicillin, and streptomycin. In South America, chloramphenicol is used most often because of its simultaneous efficacy against most *Salmonella* infections (which may develop intercurrently). Ampicillin (1 g every 6 h) has also been used, as has cephalexin (500 mg every 6 h). Verruga peruana may respond similarly; rifampin (300 mg twice a day) and ciprofloxacin (500 mg/d) have also been used. Failure to respond to therapy and relapse are common and require the reinstitution of prolonged therapy.

CAT-SCRATCH DISEASE

DEFINITION AND ETIOLOGY   Typical CSD is manifest by painful regional lymphadenopathy persisting for several weeks or months after a cat scratch. Occasionally, infection may disseminate and produce more generalized lymphadenopathy and systemic manifestations, which may be confused with the manifestations of lymphoma. *B. henselae* is the causative agent of CSD. There is no evidence that other *Bartonella* species cause CSD. The role of *Afipia felis* (originally proposed as the agent of CSD) is unclear inasmuch as only a few cases are associated with its isolation. Several reports suggest that *B. clarridgeiae* may cause feline lymphadenopathy.

EPIDEMIOLOGY   Acquisition of *B. henselae* has been significantly associated with exposure to young cats infested with fleas (*Ctenocephalides felis*). The finding that a high proportion of cats with fleas

have persistent asymptomatic *B. henselae* bacteremia suggests that the domestic cat is the animal reservoir of this microorganism. The flea can serve as a transmitting vector in the cross-infection of cats, but its role in human infection is not clear. Regions of the United States where fleas are endemic have higher rates of CSD. Approximately 60% of cases occur in children.

MICROBIOLOGY   *B. henselae* may be isolated from blood and rarely from lymph nodes or other tissues. Co-cultivation with endothelial cell monolayers has been employed to detect growth. Colonies develop after prolonged incubation (1 to 4 weeks) with 5 to 10% CO_2 at 37°C on blood-containing media (rabbit blood is preferred); the colonies pit the agar. Bacterial cells are gram-negative.

CLINICAL MANIFESTATIONS   A localized papule, progressing to a pustule that often crusts over, develops 3 to 5 days after a cat scratch. Tender regional lymphadenopathy develops within 1 to 2 weeks after inoculation; by this time, the papule may have healed spontaneously. Scratches are most often sustained on the hands or face, producing epitrochlear, axillary, pectoral, or cervical lymph node involvement. The involved nodes occasionally become suppurative; bacterial superinfection with staphylococci or other cutaneous pathogens may develop. Although most patients do not have fever, systemic symptoms are frequent and include malaise, anorexia, and weight loss. Without treatment, lymphadenopathy persists for weeks or even months and may be confused with lymphatic malignancy. Other manifestations in apparently immunocompetent patients include encephalitis, seizures and coma (especially in children), meningitis, transverse myelitis, granulomatous hepatitis and splenitis, osteomyelitis, and disseminated infection. Conjunctival inoculation may cause Parinaud's oculoglandular syndrome, with conjunctivitis and periauricular lymphadenopathy. *B. henselae* is considered the most common cause of acute neuroretinitis. This condition may present as an acute change in vision associated with a stellate macular lesion; other pathologic changes of the retina may also occur.

PATHOLOGY   The histopathologic hallmark of CSD is granulomatous inflammation with stellate necrosis but no evidence of angiogenesis. Infection by *B. henselae* can produce two entirely different pathologic reactions, depending on the immune status of the host: granulomatous inflammation or angiogenesis.

DIAGNOSIS   CSD should be suspected if the patient has a history of exposure to cats and develops lymphadenopathy and a skin lesion. The diagnosis can be confirmed by pathologic examination of the involved nodes. Tiny bacilli in clusters can sometimes be seen in biopsy samples stained with Warthin-Starry silver. The CSD skin test, in which lymph node material obtained from patients with CSD serves as an antigen, is no longer used. Specific serologic tests have been developed and produce positive results in 70 to 90% of patients with intact immunity. These tests are commercially available. The identification of *B. henselae* 16S ribosomal RNA genes in biopsy material by polymerase chain reaction (PCR) amplification with specific oligonucleotide primers can also be diagnostically useful; however, these methods are not commercially available. Cultures of lymph nodes, cerebrospinal fluid, or other tissues are rarely positive.

℞ TREATMENT

Although CSD is generally self-limited, tender regional lymphadenopathy and systemic symptoms may be debilitating. Patients with encephalitis or other serious manifestations should be treated with antibiotics. A randomized, double-blind, placebo-controlled trial demonstrated significant clinical benefit of treatment with oral azithromycin for 5 days in cases of typical CSD (regimen for adults weighing >100 lb: one dose of 500 mg on day 1, 250 mg on days 2 through 5). Several reports suggest that aminoglycoside treatment (e.g., intravenous gentamicin at standard doses calculated to result in therapeutic levels) is effective in patients with encephalitis and other systemic infections. On the basis of case reports and case series, the oral agents that appear to be useful are those that also are most effective for the treatment of bacillary angiomatosis; they include doxycycline (100 mg/d), rifampin (300 mg daily or twice daily), and azithromycin (250 mg/d). Unlike bacillary angiomatosis, CSD may also respond to treatment with ciprofloxacin (500 mg/d). The necessary duration of therapy is variable. Antibiotic treatment of neuroretinitis is followed by partial or complete resolution.

TRENCH FEVER

DEFINITION AND ETIOLOGY Trench fever was first described as a debilitating febrile illness associated with prolonged *B. quintana* bacteremia in soldiers fighting in Europe during World War I. Cases have since occurred throughout the world. In recent years, trench fever has re-emerged in the United States and France among urban homeless patients.

EPIDEMIOLOGY Although trench fever was once thought to have disappeared from the United States, recent cases have been diagnosed in homeless persons with alcohol abuse. Similar epidemiologic features have been noted in Marseilles, France. An outbreak of infection occurred in Seattle, Washington, in 1993, and few cases have been documented subsequently. In World War I, *B. quintana* was transmitted from person to person by the human body louse, and recent cases in Seattle and Marseilles have also been associated with lice.

CLINICAL MANIFESTATIONS Trench fever is characterized by the sudden onset of headache, aseptic meningitis, persistent or relapsing fever (which can be high-grade and is commonly paroxysmal), malaise, weight loss, and other nonspecific symptoms. Some patients may have an indolent course with minimal clinical manifestations. The incubation period is 3 to 38 days. Severe musculoskeletal pain is more common among immunocompetent than among immunocompromised patients. Bacteremia can persist for days or weeks, and relapses have followed short courses of antibiotic therapy. Localized findings are uncommon.

DIAGNOSIS The infection is diagnosed by the finding of sustained bacteremia. *B. quintana* grows slowly, and colonies may develop on rabbit blood agar after 1 to 4 weeks of incubation under conditions of increased CO_2. The infection may also be detected serologically, although these tests are not standardized.

℞ TREATMENT

A prolonged course (4 to 6 weeks) of antimicrobial therapy may be required. Agents that can cross the mammalian cell membrane are most effective, including doxycycline (100 mg by mouth twice daily), erythromycin (2 g/d), or azithromycin (500 mg/d). Data on the efficacy of these agents come from a limited number of case reports.

BACILLARY ANGIOMATOSIS

DEFINITION AND ETIOLOGY Bacillary angiomatosis was initially described as a condition occurring primarily in patients with AIDS and characterized by vascular cutaneous lesions resembling verruga peruana and Kaposi's sarcoma. The disease can disseminate to involve virtually any organ system, including the liver (peliosis hepatis). Immunocompromised individuals, especially those infected with HIV, are at particularly high risk for bacillary angiomatosis, although in rare instances the patient is not obviously immunosuppressed. Both *B. henselae* and *B. quintana* produce bacillary angiomatosis in persons with immunodeficiency.

EPIDEMIOLOGY A case-control study revealed that *B. henselae* and *B. quintana* differ significantly in terms of epidemiologic risk factors. All cases of *B. henselae* infection were associated with exposure to cats and their fleas and occurred sporadically, whereas the cases of *B. quintana* bacillary angiomatosis occurred in clusters and were associated with low socioeconomic status, homelessness, and exposure to body lice. Direct transmission of *B. henselae* from cats to their owners,

presumably through cutaneous trauma, was supported by the matching DNA fingerprint patterns of isolates from the two sources.

PATHOGENESIS AND PATHOLOGY Bacillary angiomatosis is characterized by a lobular proliferation of new blood vessels (angiogenesis) and a neutrophilic inflammatory response to myriad bacilli located within collagen-rich microscopic and macroscopic nodules. The organisms can be visualized with Warthin-Starry silver stain. The endothelial cells lining the vascular spaces have a typical epithelioid appearance, and the lesions may resemble Kaposi's sarcoma histopathologically, although the characteristic spindle cell of the latter disease is usually absent. The bacterial and eukaryotic host factors that elicit the pathologic response are unknown.

CLINICAL MANIFESTATIONS The skin lesions of bacillary angiomatosis (also called *epithelioid angiomatosis*) are vascular nodules, papules, or tumors that range from tiny lesions resembling cherry angiomas or pyogenic granulomas to large, pedunculated, exophytic masses (Fig. 144-1). Characteristically, the lesions are red or purple, resembling Kaposi's sarcoma; they may be surrounded by an epithelial collarette, may be located anywhere on the skin, and may involve mucous membranes. The overlying epidermis may be focally ulcerated, and the underlying bone may be invaded and destroyed.

Dissemination of *B. henselae* infection occurs primarily in patients with cellular immune defects. Clinical manifestations accompanying dissemination are often nonspecific and include persistent fever, abdominal pain, weight loss, and malaise. Although the liver, spleen, bone marrow, and lymph nodes are primarily affected, HIV-infected patients may also develop central nervous system abnormalities (including psychiatric disorders and brain lesions), which are responsive to antibiotic therapy. Skin lesions usually are not evident in disseminated infection. Involvement of the liver or spleen may produce bacillary peliosis hepatis. Patients with the latter condition may report localized pain on palpation of the abdomen. Nodular lesions of variable size can be demonstrated by computed tomography or magnetic resonance imaging, with or without contrast agents. As these lesions are associated with neovascularization, percutaneous biopsy may lead to hemorrhage.

In a case-control study of bacillary angiomatosis (see "Epidemiology" above), only *B. henselae* was associated with hepatosplenic disease (peliosis hepatis) and displayed a predilection for lymph nodes. *B. quintana*, in contrast, was associated with osseous and subcutaneous infection.

DIAGNOSIS The diagnosis of bacillary angiomatosis is based primarily on the typical histopathologic findings of angiomas in association with clumps of tiny bacilli revealed by Warthin-Starry silver stain. Infection can also be established by blood cultures performed with a lysis-centrifugation system or by identification of specific DNA sequences. Bacilli picked from new colonies growing on blood agar but not subcultured may not stain, even with acridine orange; they stain weakly with

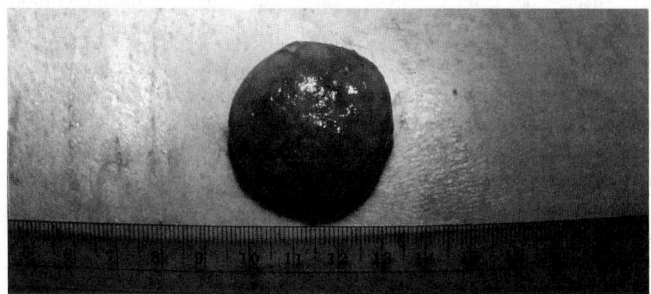

FIGURE 144-1 Characteristic skin lesion of bacillary angiomatosis in an HIV-positive young woman. This large, pedunculated tumor exhibits the typical angiomatous appearance. The patient was treated with oral erythromycin, with nearly complete resolution of the lesion; however, on discontinuation of antibiotic therapy after a 4-week course, the lesion recurred.

safranin. Identification of *B. henselae* and *B. quintana* is based primarily on cellular fatty-acid analysis and PCR-based restriction fragment length polymorphism analysis. Definitive identification of *Bartonella* species depends on DNA sequence analysis of 16S ribosomal RNA genes. The sensitivity and specificity of serologic tests have not been determined.

DIFFERENTIAL DIAGNOSIS   The differential diagnosis of cutaneous bacillary angiomatosis includes Kaposi's sarcoma, angiomas, and pyogenic granulomas. These conditions can be distinguished by histopathologic examination of biopsied material. AIDS patients may have both Kaposi's sarcoma lesions and bacillary angiomatosis lesions simultaneously; thus biopsy is essential to differentiate the two.

℞ TREATMENT

Cutaneous lesions have been treated with a wide variety of antimicrobial drugs, including macrolides, tetracyclines, and antituberculous agents; *B. henselae* is susceptible to most antibiotics in vitro. Erythromycin (2 g/d), given orally for 3 weeks, is usually effective, as are newer macrolides; however, relapse may require prolonged therapy (3 weeks to 2 months) with an antibiotic that reaches an intracellular compartment, such as a macrolide or doxycycline (100 mg/d). Patients with peliosis hepatis should be treated with intravenous antibiotics, and those with disseminated disease or bacteremia should be treated with a prolonged course of a systemic antibiotic. In a case-control study of bacillary angiomatosis, treatment with a macrolide was associated with a therapeutic response and sterile tissue samples and may have been protective, whereas treatment with trimethoprim-sulfamethoxazole, ciprofloxacin, penicillins, or cephalosporins had no protective effect. Cutaneous lesions may or may not regress spontaneously, perhaps depending on the status of the host's immunity. The safety of ciprofloxacin in pregnant or lactating women has not been established. No antimicrobial agent has been studied prospectively, and information on efficacy comes only from case reports.

OTHER *BARTONELLA* INFECTIONS, INCLUDING CULTURE-NEGATIVE ENDOCARDITIS

The application of molecular methods to the detection of microorganisms that are difficult to cultivate in the laboratory has revealed new *Bartonella* species and has established *Bartonella* species as a cause of endocarditis cases previously classified as being of unknown etiology. *B. quintana* is the *Bartonella* species most frequently isolated from patients with endocarditis. Two other species, *B. elizabethae* and *B. clarridgeiae*, as well as *B. henselae* have also been identified as agents of subacute and chronic endocarditis.

The diagnosis of *Bartonella* endocarditis is confirmed by blood cultures. A presumptive diagnosis can be made on the basis of epidemiologic history and by serology. Infection may elicit antibodies that cross-react with *Chlamydia pneumoniae*, and *Coxiella burnetii* infection (Q fever) elicits antibodies that cross-react with *B. quintana*.

In culture-positive or seropositive endocarditis, initial treatment with azithromycin (250 mg/d) or doxycycline (100 mg/d) for 4 to 6 months is recommended. A third-generation cephalosporin or an aminoglycoside may be added for the initial 2 to 3 weeks of therapy. If *Bartonella* infection is suspected but not yet confirmed, therapy for culture-negative endocarditis with ceftriaxone (2 g/d by the intravenous route) plus an aminoglycoside for 6 to 8 weeks is recommended. If culture results prove positive, ceftriaxone administration may be discontinued and treatment with a macrolide (azithromycin) or doxycycline given for a prolonged period.

FURTHER READING

BASS JW et al: Prospective randomized double blind placebo-controlled evaluation of azithromycin for treatment of cat-scratch disease. Pediatr Infect Dis J 17:447, 1998

BROUQUI P et al: Chronic *Bartonella quintana* bacteremia in homeless patients. N Engl J Med 340:184, 1999

CARITHERS HA: Cat scratch disease: An overview based on a study of 1,200 patients. Am J Dis Child 139:1124, 1985

COCKERELL DJ, LEBOIT PE: Bacillary angiomatosis: A newly characterized, pseudoneoplastic, infectious, cutaneous vascular disorder. J Am Acad Dermatol 22:501, 1990

FOURNIER P-E et al: Epidemiologic and clinical characteristics of *B. quintana* and *B. henselae* endocarditis. Medicine 80:245, 2001

MAGUINA C et al: Bartonellosis (Carrion's disease) in the modern era. Clin Infect Dis 33:772, 2001

OHL ME, SPACH DH: *Bartonella quintana* and urban trench fever. Clin Infect Dis 31:131, 2000

SPACH DH et al: *Bartonella (Rochalimaea) quintana* bacteremia in inner-city patients with chronic alcoholism. N Engl J Med 332:425, 1995

---

145 | DONOVANOSIS
Gavin Hart

Donovanosis is a chronic, progressively destructive bacterial infection of the genital region that is generally regarded as sexually transmitted. The disease has been known by many other names, the most common of which are granuloma inguinale and granuloma venereum.

ETIOLOGY   Donovanosis is caused by *Calymmatobacterium granulomatis*, an intracellular, gram-negative, pleomorphic, encapsulated (when mature) bacterium measuring 1.5 by 0.7 μm. *C. granulomatis* shares many morphologic and serologic characteristics and >99% homology at the nucleotide level with *Klebsiella* species that are pathogenic to humans. Polymerase chain reaction (PCR) amplification of the *phoE* gene shows it to be closely related to that in *Klebsiella pneumoniae*, *K. rhinoscleromatis*, and *K. ozaenae*. Electron microscopy shows typical gram-negative morphology and a large capsule but no flagella. Filiform or vesicular protrusions occur on a corrugated cell wall.

EPIDEMIOLOGY   Donovanosis is endemic among Aborigines in central Australia as well as in Papua New Guinea, southeastern India, southern Africa, and the Caribbean and adjacent areas of South America. In the first half of the twentieth century, the disease was endemic in parts of the United States (with an estimated 5000 to 10,000 cases in 1947); small epidemics still occur in this country and in other developed countries. The decline in the United States to fewer than 20 reported cases annually in the past decade has probably resulted from lower transmission rates due to earlier presentation for increasingly effective antibiotic therapy. Over 70% of cases involve persons 20 to 40 years of age. The infection is predominantly sexually transmitted, but extragenital skin lesions can follow transmission from concurrent genital lesions via the fingers or through other nonsexual contact, and autoinoculation may produce new lesions from contact with adjacent skin ("kissing" lesions). Infants born to infected mothers have acquired infection at birth.

The classification of donovanosis as a sexually transmitted disease (STD) has been disputed because of cases in young children and occasionally in sexually inactive individuals, transmission by direct body contact and via inanimate intermediaries, and the low and variable prevalence of donovanosis among sexual partners (0.4 to 52%). The dominance of sexual transmission is suggested by the combined factors of lesions predominantly affecting the genitalia, the highest prevalence among persons in age and socioeconomic groups that are most

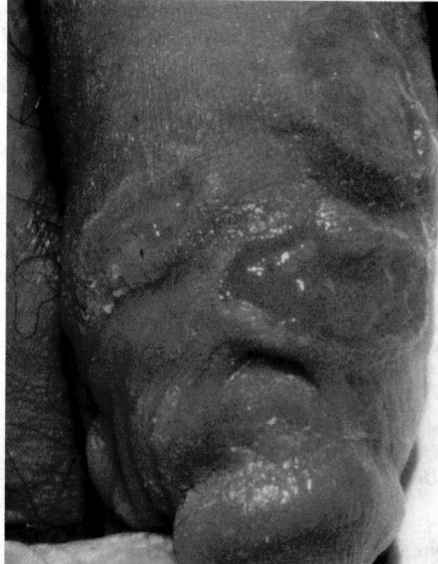

FIGURE 145-1 Multiple granulomatous lesions of the penis in a patient with donovanosis.

TABLE 145-1 *Differential Diagnosis of Donovanosis*

Disease (Chapter)	Distinguishing Features
Secondary syphilis: condylomata lata (153)	White or pale moist plaques in anogenital region (as opposed to bright red donovanosis lesions); lesions subside within 1 week of treatment with benzathine penicillin, 2.4 mU (whereas donovanosis lesions remain unchanged)
Squamous cell carcinoma (73)	Histologic appearance
Penile amebiasis (194)	Microscopic identification of *Entamoeba histolytica*
Chancroid: pseudogranuloma inguinale (130)	Culture of *Haemophilus ducreyi*
Tuberculosis (150)	Histologic features of bony lesions
Actinomycosis (147)	Microscopic identification of sulfur granules
Rhinoscleroma (134)	Histologic features
Leishmaniasis (196)	Histologic features
Histoplasmosis (183)	Histologic features

often affected by STDs, and the predictable occurrence of disease in visitors to areas of endemicity following sexual exposure.

CLINICAL MANIFESTATIONS The incubation period is usually 1 to 4 weeks but may extend to 1 year. Skin lesions have been detected in infants 6 weeks to 6 months after birth. The disease begins as one or more subcutaneous nodules that erode through the skin to produce clean, granulomatous, sharply defined, usually painless lesions (Fig. 145-1). These lesions, which bleed readily on contact, slowly enlarge. The genitalia are involved in 90% of cases, the inguinal region in 10%, and the anal region in 5 to 10%. Genital swelling, particularly of the labia, is a common feature and occasionally progresses to pseudoelephantiasis. Phimosis and paraphimosis are common local complications, and progressive erosion of affected tissues may completely destroy the penis or other organs. Less common clinical variants include a hypertrophic form (cauliflower- or wartlike lesions), a necrotic form (destructive lesions with foul-smelling exudate, often resembling amebiasis), and a sclerotic or cicatricial form, which has a dry base with extensive scar tissue.

Extragenital lesions occur in at least 6% of cases. Oral donovanosis, the most common extragenital manifestation, presents as pain or bleeding in the mouth, lesions on the lips, or extensive swelling of the gums and palate. Donovanosis may affect most bones, and sometimes many bones are affected at the same time; the tibia is involved in over 50% of such cases. Bony lesions are associated with constitutional symptoms (weight loss, fever, night sweats, and malaise) and are usually found in women. More than 50% of women with donovanosis have primary lesions on the cervix. Prompt pelvic examinations and early diagnosis are likely to substantially decrease the morbidity and mortality (likely outcomes in misdiagnosed spinal lesions) associated with extragenital donovanosis in women.

DIAGNOSIS ■ Laboratory Diagnosis The preferred diagnostic method involves demonstration of typical intracellular Donovan bodies within large mononuclear cells visualized in smears prepared from lesions or biopsy specimens. With typical beefy lesions, a small piece of tissue is removed with forceps and scalpel, and a crush impression of the deep surface is made on a glass slide. The smear is air-dried, heat-fixed, and stained with Giemsa, Leishman's, or Wright's stain. For dry, flat, or necrotic lesions, a punch-biopsy specimen should be obtained from the advancing edge. This specimen can be used to prepare a smear or embedded for histologic examination (with a silver stain). Histologic examination shows epithelial proliferation, often simulating

neoplasia, with a heavy inflammatory infiltrate of plasma cells, some neutrophils, and few if any lymphocytes. The large mononuclear cells are 25 to 90 μm in diameter, with a vesicular or pyknotic nucleus. Up to 20 intracytoplasmic vacuoles contain pleomorphic Donovan bodies in either young unencapsulated forms (which often resemble closed safety pins) or mature encapsulated forms. *C. granulomatis* has never been grown on artificial solid media but has been cultured in chicken embryonic yolk sacs, on human monocytes, and on human epithelial (HEp-2) cells. A diagnostic PCR test has been developed and incorporated into a colorimetric detection system for *C. granulomatis*. A serologic test, based on indirect immunofluorescence, is more useful in confirming the diagnosis in cases with long-standing lesions than in early disease.

Differential Diagnosis The differential diagnosis of donovanosis is summarized in Table 145-1. Syphilis and donovanosis frequently coexist because syphilis is usually highly prevalent in areas where donovanosis is endemic; thus positive syphilis serology does not exclude a diagnosis of donovanosis. Genital ulcers are a risk factor for HIV acquisition in developing countries, and patients with donovanosis should be tested for HIV infection.

℞ TREATMENT

Table 145-2 shows the most effective regimens for treating donovanosis. Doxycycline offers the advantage of convenient administration and has been widely used in developed countries, but azithromycin is increasingly being used as first-choice therapy. Extensive lesions have been cured with oral azithromycin at a dosage of 500 mg/d, but the more convenient dose of 1 g weekly is also effective. Although chlor-

TABLE 145-2 *The Most Effective Antibiotic Regimens for Treatment of Donovanosis*[a]

Antibiotic	Oral Dosage
Azithromycin	1 g weekly or 500 mg/d
Erythromycin	500 mg qid
Tetracycline	500 mg qid
Doxycycline	100 mg bid
Trimethoprim-sulfamethoxazole	1 double-strength tablet[b] bid
Chloramphenicol	500 mg tid

[a] Patients should be examined weekly, and therapy should be continued until lesions have healed (3 to 5 weeks, except in severe cases).
[b] 160 mg/800 mg.

amphenicol is the drug of choice in some developing countries, it is unlikely to be acceptable in developed countries because of bone marrow toxicity. Penicillin is not effective for treating donovanosis. Patients should be examined weekly, and therapy should be continued until lesions have healed (3 to 5 weeks, except in severe cases). If antibiotic therapy is stopped earlier, lesions often continue to heal, but the relapse rate is higher. If the lesions are unchanged after 2 weeks of treatment, an alternative antibiotic regimen should be used.

The treatment regimens listed in Table 145-2 are usually adequate in HIV-infected patients without immunosuppression, but an increas-ing failure rate has been reported in immunosuppressed patients, for whom daily administration of azithromycin is recommended if other regimens fail to elicit a response.

FURTHER READING

See www.stdservices.on.net/std/donovanosis/Default.htm for an illustrated lec-ture and a comprehensive bibliography on donovanosis.
CARTER JS, KEMP DJ: A colorimetric detection system for Calymmatobac-terium granulomatis. Sex Trans Infect 76:134, 2000
HART G: Donovanosis (granuloma inguinale), in *Atlas of Infectious Diseases*, vol V: *Sexually Transmitted Diseases*, MF Rein (ed). Philadelphia, Church-ill Livingstone, 1996, pp 17.1–17.10
————: Donovanosis. Clin Infect Dis 25:24, 1997
O'FARRELL N: Donovanosis: An update. Int J STD AIDS 12:423, 2001

Section 7   Miscellaneous Bacterial Infections

146 | NOCARDIOSIS
Gregory A. Filice

Nocardiosis refers to disease associated with members of the genus *Nocardia*. Of several distinctive syndromes associated with these bac-teria, pneumonia and disseminated disease are most common. Others include cellulitis, lymphocutaneous syndrome, actinomycetoma, and keratitis.

MICROBIOLOGY Nocardiae are saprophytic aerobic actinomycetes that are common worldwide in soil, where they contribute to decay of organic matter. Nocardial taxonomy is complex and incompletely un-derstood. Seven species have been clearly associated with human dis-ease: *N. asteroides*, *N. brasiliensis*, *N. otitidis-caviarum* (formerly *N. caviae*), *N. farcinica*, *N. nova*, *N. transvalensis*, and *N. pseudobrasi-liensis*. In addition, two newly described species have been associated with disease in humans: *N. abscessus* from soft-tissue abscesses and *N. africana* from respiratory secretions of patients in the Sudan with pneumonia.

N. asteroides is the species most commonly associated with inva-sive disease. *N. farcinica* disease is less common, but this species is more virulent and prone to dissemination. *N. pseudobrasiliensis* is most often associated with invasive disease, and *N. brasiliensis* is usu-ally associated with disease limited to the skin. *N. transvalensis* is generally associated with pulmonary or systemic disease in immuno-suppressed persons or with *actinomycetoma*, an indolent, slowly pro-gressive disease of skin and underlying tissues with nodular swellings and draining sinuses.

EPIDEMIOLOGY Approximately 1000 cases of nocardial infection are diagnosed annually in the United States, 85% of them pulmonary and/or systemic. The disease is more common among adults than among children and among males than among females. Nearly all cases are sporadic, but outbreaks have been associated with contamination of the hospital environment, solutions, or drug injection equipment. Per-son-to-person spread is not well documented. There is no known sea-sonality.

The risk of pulmonary or disseminated disease is greater than usual among persons with deficient cell-mediated immunity, especially that associated with lymphoma, transplantation, glucocorticoid therapy, or AIDS. In AIDS, nocardiosis usually affects persons with <250 CD4+ lymphocytes/μL. Nocardiosis has also been associated with pulmo-nary alveolar proteinosis, tuberculosis and other mycobacterial dis-eases, chronic granulomatous disease, and interleukin 12 deficiency.

N. brasiliensis, *N. asteroides*, *N. otitidis-caviarum*, and *N. trans-valensis* are associated with actinomycetoma. Cases occur mainly in tropical and subtropical regions, especially those of Mexico, Central and South America, Africa, and India. The most important risk factor is frequent contact with soil or vegetable matter.

PATHOLOGY AND PATHOGENESIS Pneumonia and disseminated disease are both thought to follow inhalation of fragmented bacterial mycelia. The characteristic histologic feature of nocardiosis is an abscess with ex-tensive neutrophil infiltration and prominent necrosis. Granulation tis-sue usually surrounds the lesions, but extensive fibrosis or encapsu-lation is uncommon. Actinomycetoma is characterized by suppurative inflammation with sinus tract formation. Granules—microcolonies composed of dense masses of bacterial filaments extending radially from a central core—are occasionally observed in histologic prepa-rations. They are frequently found in discharges from lesions of acti-nomycetoma but almost never from lesions in other forms of nocar-diosis. Infrequently, nocardiae and other indolent pathogens, including fungi or mycobacteria, are isolated from the same patient.

Nocardiae have evolved a number of properties that enable them to survive within phagocytes, including neutralization of oxidants, pre-vention of phagosome-lysosome fusion, and prevention of phagosome acidification. Neutrophils phagocytose the organisms and limit their growth but do not kill them efficiently. Cell-mediated immunity is important for definitive control and elimination of nocardiae.

CLINICAL MANIFESTATIONS ■ **Respiratory Tract Disease** Pneumonia is by far the most common respiratory tract nocardial disease. Nocardial pneumonia is typically subacute; symptoms have usually been present for days or weeks at presentation. The onset is more acute in some immunosuppressed patients. Cough is prominent and produces small amounts of thick, purulent sputum that is not malodorous. Fever, an-orexia, weight loss, and malaise are common; dyspnea, pleuritic pain, and hemoptysis are less common. Remissions and exacerbations over several weeks are frequent.

Roentgenographic patterns vary, but some are highly suggestive of nocardial pneumonia. Infiltrates vary in size and are typically of at least moderate density. Single or multiple nodules are common, some-times suggesting tumor metastases (Fig. 146-1). Infiltrates and nodules tend to cavitate. Empyema is present in one-third of cases.

Nocardiosis may spread directly from the lungs to adjacent tissues. Pericarditis, mediastinitis, and the superior vena cava syndrome have all been reported. Nocardial laryngitis, tracheitis, and bronchitis are much less common than pneumonia. In the major airways, disease often presents as a nodular or granulomatous mass. A few cases of sinusitis have been reported.

Nocardiae are sometimes isolated from respiratory secretions of patients without apparent nocardial disease. Most of these patients have chronic pulmonary disease with abnormal airways or parenchyma and do not necessarily require treatment for nocardiosis (see "Diag-nosis," below).

Extrapulmonary Disease In half of all cases of pulmonary nocardiosis, disease appears outside the lungs. In one-fifth of cases of disseminated disease, lung disease is not apparent. The most common site of dis-semination is the brain. Other common sites include the skin and sup-

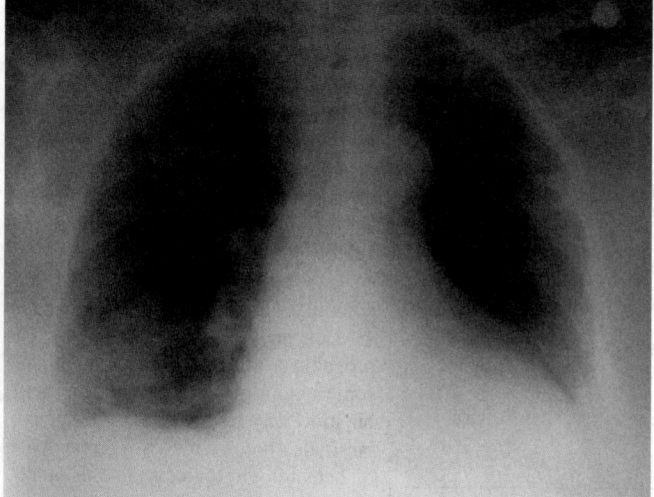

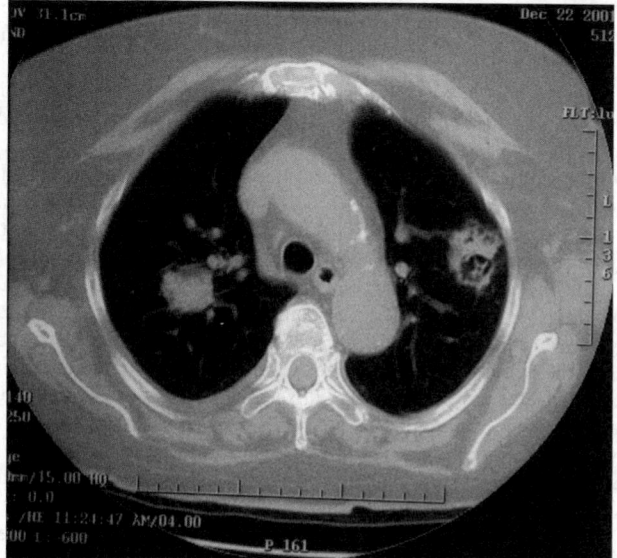

FIGURE 146-1 Nocardial pneumonia. *Top:* Three large nodules with apparent cavitation are apparent on the anterior-posterior chest roentgenograph. *Bottom:* A computed tomographic scan of the same patient confirms the presence of bilateral nodules and cavitation in the nodule in the left midlung field.

porting structures, kidneys, bone, and muscle, but almost any organ can be involved. Peritonitis has been reported. Nocardiae have been recovered from blood in a few cases of pneumonia or disseminated disease. Nocardial endocarditis occurs rarely and can affect either native or prosthetic valves. A few cases of nocardial bacteremia associated with infected central venous catheters have been reported.

The typical manifestation of extrapulmonary dissemination is a subacute abscess. A minority of abscesses outside the lungs or central nervous system (CNS) form fistulae and discharge small amounts of pus.

In CNS infections, brain abscesses are usually supratentorial, are often multiloculated, and may be single or multiple (Fig. 146-2). Brain abscesses tend to burrow into the ventricles or extend out into the subarachnoid space. The symptoms and signs are somewhat more indolent than those of other types of bacterial brain abscess. Meningitis is uncommon and is usually due to spread from a nearby brain abscess. Nocardiae are not easily recovered from cerebrospinal fluid (CSF).

Disease Following Transcutaneous Inoculation Disease following transcutaneous nocardial inoculation usually takes one of three forms: cellulitis, lymphocutaneous syndrome, or actinomycetoma.

Cellulitis generally begins 1 to 3 weeks after a recognized breach of the skin, often with soil contamination. Subacute cellulitis with pain, swelling, erythema, and warmth develops over days to weeks. The

lesions are usually firm and nonfluctuant. Disease may progress to involve underlying muscle, tendon, bones, or joints. Dissemination is rare. *N. asteroides* is common in colder climates, while *N. brasiliensis* predominates in warmer climates.

Lymphocutaneous disease usually begins with a pyodermatous lesion at the site of inoculation, with central ulceration and purulent or honey-colored drainage. Subcutaneous nodules often appear along lymphatics that drain the primary lesion. The lymphangitic form closely resembles lymphocutaneous sporotrichosis (Chap. 190). Most cases of the lymphocutaneous syndrome are associated with *N. brasiliensis*.

Actinomycetoma usually begins with a nodular swelling, sometimes at a site of local trauma. Lesions typically develop on the feet or hands but may involve the posterior part of the neck, the upper back, the head, and other sites. The nodule eventually breaks down and a fistula appears, which is then accompanied by others. The fistulas tend to come and go, with new ones forming as old ones disappear. The discharge is serous or purulent, may be bloody, and often contains 0.1- to 2-mm white granules consisting of masses of mycelia. The lesions spread slowly along fascial planes to involve adjacent areas of skin, subcutaneous tissue, and bone. Over months or years, there may be extensive deformation of the affected part. Lesions involving soft tissues are only mildly painful; those affecting bones or joints are more so. Systemic symptoms are absent or minimal. Infection rarely disseminates from actinomycetoma, and lesions on the hands and feet usually cause only local disability. Lesions on the head, neck, and trunk can invade locally to involve deep organs and result in severe disability or death.

Keratitis *Nocardia* species, usually *N. asteroides*, are uncommon causes of subacute keratitis. The infection usually follows eye trauma. Nocardial infection of lacrimal glands has been reported. Endophthalmitis and other diseases involving deeper eye structures are usually manifestations of dissemination.

DIAGNOSIS The first step in diagnosis is examination of sputum or pus for crooked, branching, beaded, gram-positive filaments 1 μm wide and up to 50 μm long. Most nocardiae are acid-fast in direct smears if a weak acid is used for decolorization (e.g., in the modified Kinyoun, Ziehl-Neelsen, and Fite-Faraco methods). The organisms often take up silver stains. Nocardiae grow relatively slowly; colonies may take

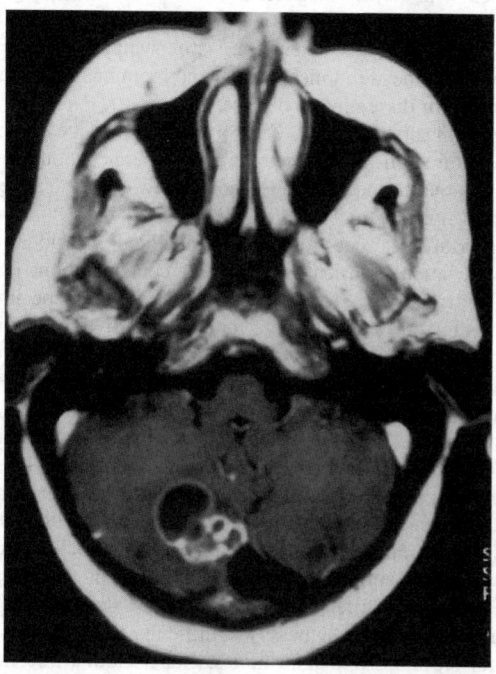

FIGURE 146-2 Nocardial abscesses in the right cerebellum. The appearance suggests one large abscess and multiple daughter abscesses.

TABLE 146-1 *Treatment for Nocardiosis*

Disease	Duration	Drugs (Daily Dose)[a]
Pulmonary or systemic		Systemic therapy
Intact host defenses	6–12 mo	Oral
Deficient host defenses	12 mo[b]	1. Sulfonamides (6–8 g) or combination of
CNS disease	12 mo[c]	trimethoprim (10–20 mg/kg) and
Cellulitis, lympho-		sulfamethoxazole (50–100 mg/kg)
cutaneous syndrome	2 mo	2. Minocycline (200–400 mg)
Osteomyelitis, arthritis,		Parenteral
laryngitis, sinusitis	4 mo	1. Amikacin (10–15 mg/kg)
Actinomycetoma	6–12 mo after	2. Cefotaxime (6 g), ceftizoxime (6 g),
	clinical cure	ceftriaxone (2 g), imipenem (2 g)
Keratitis	Topical: Until apparent cure	1. Sulfonamide drops
		2. Amikacin drops
	Systemic: Until 2–4 mo after apparent cure	Drugs for systemic therapy as listed above

[a] For each category, choices are numbered in order of preference.
[b] In some patients with AIDS or chronic granulomatous disease, therapy for pulmonary or systemic disease must be continued indefinitely.
[c] If all apparent CNS disease has been excised, the duration of therapy may be reduced to 6 months.

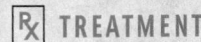

TREATMENT

Sulfonamides are the drugs of choice for nocardiosis (Table 146-1). Initially, 6 to 8 g/d of sulfadiazine or sulfisoxazole in four divided doses should be used. After disease is controlled, 4 g/d can be used to complete therapy. In difficult cases, sulfonamide levels should be measured and dosages adjusted to keep serum levels between 100 and 150 μg/mL. The combination of sulfamethoxazole (SMX) and trimethoprim (TMP) is probably equivalent to sulfonamides; some authorities believe that the combination may in fact be more effective, but it also poses a modestly greater risk of hematologic toxicity. At the outset, 10 to 20 mg of TMP per kg and 50 to 100 mg of SMX per kg should be given each day in two divided doses. Later, the daily doses can be decreased to as little as 5 mg/kg and 25 mg/kg, respectively. In persons with sulfonamide allergies, desensitization usually allows continuation of therapy with these effective and inexpensive drugs.

Minocycline is the best-established alternative oral drug and should be given in doses of 100 to 200 mg twice a day. Other tetracyclines are usually ineffective. *N. nova* infections can be treated with erythromycin (500 to 750 mg four times a day) and/or ampicillin (1 g four times a day), but other *Nocardia* species are often resistant to both drugs. Amoxicillin (500 mg) combined with clavulanic acid (125 mg), given three times a day, has been effective in a few cases but should be avoided in cases due to *N. nova*, in which clavulanate induces β-lactamase production. Ofloxacin (400 mg twice a day) and clarithromycin (500 mg twice a day) have each been successful in a few cases. Linezolid is active in vitro against most *Nocardia* isolates, but there is little clinical experience with this drug as nocardiosis therapy.

Amikacin, the best-established parenteral drug, is given in doses of 5 to 7.5 mg/kg every 12 h. Serum levels should be monitored during prolonged therapy in patients with diminished renal function and in the elderly. Newer β-lactam antibiotics, including cefotaxime, ceftizoxime, ceftriaxone, and imipenem, are usually effective. These agents may be less effective in some cases caused by *N. farcinica*.

In vitro, strains of *N. farcinica* differ from most in that they are usually resistant to cephalosporins and in one-fifth of cases are resistant to imipenem. *N. pseudobrasiliensis* strains often exhibit resistance to minocycline or amoxicillin/clavulanic acid and susceptibility to ciprofloxacin or clarithromycin. *N. transvalensis* displays increased resistance to many antimicrobial agents, including amikacin, tobramycin, cefotaxime, ceftriaxone, and amoxicillin/clavulanic acid. *N. nova* isolates appear to be susceptible to ampicillin and erythromycin in vitro but also produce β-lactamase constitutively or in the presence of a β-lactam.

Use of SMX and TMP in high-risk populations to prevent *Pneumocystis carinii* disease or urinary tract infections appears to reduce the risk of nocardiosis as well. However, the incidence of nocardiosis is infrequent enough that prophylaxis of this disease is not recommended.

In patients with nocardiosis who need immunosuppressive therapy for an underlying disease or prevention of transplant rejection, such therapy should be continued. In many cases, two or more antimicrobial agents have been used to treat nocardiosis, often in combinations including drugs that are usually effective by themselves, like a sulfonamide or minocycline. Whether such combination therapy is better than monotherapy is not known, and it certainly increases the risk of toxicity.

Surgical management of nocardial disease is similar to that of other bacterial diseases. Brain abscesses should be aspirated, drained, or excised if the diagnosis is unclear, if an abscess is large and accessible,

up to 2 weeks to appear and may not develop their characteristic appearance for up to 4 weeks. Several blood culture systems support nocardial growth. Yield is enhanced when blood cultures are incubated aerobically for up to 4 weeks and when blind subcultures are performed. Nocardial growth is so different from that of more common pathogens that the laboratory should be alerted when nocardiosis is suspected to maximize the likelihood of isolation. Since nocardiae are among the few aerobic microorganisms that use paraffin as a carbon source, paraffin baiting can be used to isolate the organisms from mixed cultures.

In cases of pneumonia, sputum smears are often negative. Unless the diagnosis can be made in these cases by sampling lesions in other, more accessible sites, bronchoscopy or lung aspiration is usually necessary. Transtracheal aspiration should be avoided, as it frequently leads to nocardial cellulitis in tissues around the puncture wound.

In patients with nocardial pneumonia, a careful history should be obtained and a thorough physical examination performed to evaluate the possibility of dissemination. Suggestive symptoms or signs should be pursued with further diagnostic tests. Computed tomography or magnetic resonance imaging of the head, with and without contrast material, should be undertaken if signs or symptoms suggest brain involvement. Some authorities recommend brain imaging in all cases of pulmonary or disseminated disease.

When clinically indicated, CSF or urine should be concentrated and then cultured. In actinomycetoma cases, granules should be sought in the discharge. Suspect particles should be washed in saline, examined microscopically, and cultured.

Isolation of nocardiae from sputum or blood occasionally represents colonization, transient infection, or contamination. In typical cases of respiratory tract colonization, Gram-stained specimens are negative and cultures are only intermittently positive. A positive sputum culture in an immunosuppressed patient usually reflects disease. When nocardiae are isolated from an immunocompetent patient without apparent nocardial disease, the patient should be observed carefully without treatment. A patient with a host-defense defect that increases the risk of nocardiosis should usually receive antimicrobial treatment.

Nocardia spp. are difficult to differentiate from one another with standard biochemical tests, and isolates from patients with systemic or severe disease should be sent to a reference laboratory for definitive identification and antimicrobial susceptibility testing. Susceptibility results, which help differentiate species, are of less certain clinical value but sometimes guide therapy in difficult cases.

Several presumptive diagnostic tests for nocardial infection have been studied, including tests for antibodies, nocardial metabolites, and nocardial DNA. None is ready for clinical use at this time.

or if an abscess fails to respond to chemotherapy. Brain abscesses that are small or inaccessible should be treated medically; in these cases, clinical improvement should be noticeable within 1 to 2 weeks. Brain imaging should be repeated to document the resolution of lesions, although abatement on images often lags behind clinical improvement.

Antimicrobial therapy usually suffices for nocardial actinomycetoma. In deep or extensive cases, drainage or excision of heavily involved tissue may facilitate healing, but structure and function should be preserved whenever possible.

Nocardial infections tend to relapse (particularly in patients with chronic granulomatous disease), and long courses of antimicrobial therapy are necessary. If disease is unusually extensive, if the patient is immunosuppressed, or if the response to therapy is slow, the recommendations in Table 146-1 should be exceeded.

The mortality rate for pulmonary or disseminated nocardiosis outside the CNS should be <5%. CNS disease carries a higher mortality rate. Patients should be followed carefully for at least 6 months after therapy has ended. Any child with nocardiosis and no known cause of immunosuppression should undergo tests to determine the adequacy of the phagocytic respiratory burst.

FURTHER READING

CHOUCIÑO C et al: Nocardial infections in bone marrow transplant recipients. Clin Infect Dis 23:1012, 1996

HAMID ME et al: *Nocardia africana* sp. nov., a new pathogen isolated from patients with pulmonary infections. J Clin Microbiol 39:625, 2001

KONTOYIANNIS DP et al: *Nocardia* bacteremia. Report of 4 cases and review of the literature. Medicine 77:255, 1998

MINAMOTO GY, SORDILLO EM: Disseminated nocardiosis in a patient with AIDS: Diagnosis by blood and cerebrospinal fluid cultures. Clin Infect Dis 26:242, 1998

SMEGO RA JR et al: Lymphocutaneous syndrome. A review of non-sporothrix causes. Medicine 78:38, 1999

UTTAMCHANDANI RB et al: Nocardiosis in 30 patients with advanced human immunodeficiency virus infection: Clinical features and outcome. Clin Infect Dis 18:348, 1994

WATSON A et al: *Nocardia asteroides* native valve endocarditis. Clin Infect Dis 32:660, 2001

YASSIN AF et al: *Nocardia abscessus* sp. nov. Int J Syst Evol Microbiol 50:1487, 2000

147 ACTINOMYCOSIS
Thomas A. Russo

Actinomycosis is an indolent, slowly progressive infection caused by anaerobic or microaerophilic bacteria, primarily of the genus *Actinomyces*, that colonize the mouth, colon, and vagina. Mucosal disruption may lead to infection at virtually any site in the body. In vivo growth of actinomycetes usually results in the formation of characteristic clumps called *grains* or *sulfur granules*. The clinical presentations of actinomycosis are myriad. Common in the preantibiotic era, actinomycosis has diminished in incidence, as has its timely recognition. Actinomycosis has been called "the most misdiagnosed disease," and it has been said that "no disease is so often missed by experienced clinicians." Thus this entity remains a diagnostic challenge. Three clinical presentations that should prompt consideration of this unique infection are (1) the combination of chronicity, progression across tissue boundaries, and mass-like features (mimicking malignancy, with which it is often confused); (2) the development of a sinus tract, which may spontaneously resolve and recur; and (3) a refractory or relapsing infection after a short course of therapy, since cure of established actinomycosis requires prolonged treatment. An awareness of the full spectrum of the disease will expedite its diagnosis and treatment and will minimize the unnecessary surgical interventions, morbidity, and mortality that are reported all too often.

ETIOLOGIC AGENTS   Actinomycosis is most commonly caused by *A. israelii*. *A. naeslundii*, *A. odontolyticus*, *A. viscosus*, *A. meyeri*, *A. gerencseriae*, and *Propionibacterium propionicum* are established but less common causes of the disease. Most if not all actinomycotic infections are polymicrobial. *Actinobacillus actinomycetemcomitans*, *Eikenella corrodens*, Enterobacteriaceae, and species of *Fusobacterium*, *Bacteroides*, *Capnocytophaga*, *Staphylococcus*, and *Streptococcus* are commonly isolated with actinomycetes in various combinations, depending on the site of infection. The contribution of these other species to the pathogenesis of actinomycosis is uncertain.

Comparative 16S rRNA gene sequencing has led to the identification of *A. europaeus*, *A. neuii*, *A. radingae*, *A. graevenitzii*, *A. turicensis*, and *A. funkei* in clinical specimens. Increasing data suggest that these species may also cause actinomycosis.

EPIDEMIOLOGY   Actinomycosis occurs throughout life, with a peak incidence in the middle decades. Males have a threefold higher incidence of infection than females, possibly because of poorer dental hygiene and/or more frequent trauma. Likely contributing factors to the decrease in the incidence of actinomycosis since the preantibiotic era include improved dental hygiene and the initiation of antimicrobial treatment early on—before the full development of the disease. Individuals who do not seek or have access to health care are undoubtedly at higher risk.

PATHOGENESIS AND PATHOLOGY   The etiologic agents of actinomycosis are members of the normal oral flora and are often cultured from the bronchi, the gastrointestinal tract, and the female genital tract. The critical step in the development of actinomycosis is disruption of the mucosal barrier. Local infection may consequently ensue. Once established, actinomycosis spreads contiguously in a slow progressive manner, ignoring tissue planes. Although acute inflammation may initially develop at the site of infection, the hallmark of actinomycosis is the characteristic chronic, indolent phase. This stage is manifested by lesions that usually appear as single or multiple indurations. Central necrosis consisting of neutrophils and sulfur granules develops and is virtually diagnostic of this disease. The fibrotic walls of the mass are typically described as "wooden." The responsible bacterial and/or host factors have not yet been identified. Over time, sinus tracts to the skin, adjacent organs, or bone may develop. In rare instances, distant hematogenous seeding may occur. As mentioned above, these unique features of actinomycosis mimic malignancy, with which it is often confused.

Foreign bodies appear to facilitate infection. This association most frequently involves intrauterine contraceptive devices (IUCDs). In addition, an increasing number of reports have described an association of actinomycosis with HIV infection, transplantation, and radio- or chemotherapy. Ulcerative mucosal infections (e.g., by herpes simplex virus or cytomegalovirus) and abnormalities in host defenses may facilitate the development of actinomycosis in the latter settings.

CLINICAL MANIFESTATIONS ■ Oral-Cervicofacial Disease   Actinomycosis occurs most frequently at an oral, cervical, or facial site, usually as a soft tissue swelling, abscess, or mass lesion that is often mistaken for a neoplasm. The angle of the jaw is generally involved, but a diagnosis of actinomycosis should be considered with any mass lesion or relapsing infection in the head and neck (Chap. 27). Otitis, sinusitis, and canaliculitis can also develop. Pain, fever, and leukocytosis are variably reported. Contiguous extension to the cranium, cervical spine, or thorax is a potential sequela.

Thoracic Disease   Thoracic actinomycosis usually follows an indolent progressive course, with involvement of the pulmonary parenchyma and/or the pleural space. Chest pain, fever, and weight loss are common. A cough, when present, is variably productive. The usual radiographic appearance is either a mass lesion or pneumonia. On computed tomography (CT), central areas of low attenuation and ringlike rim

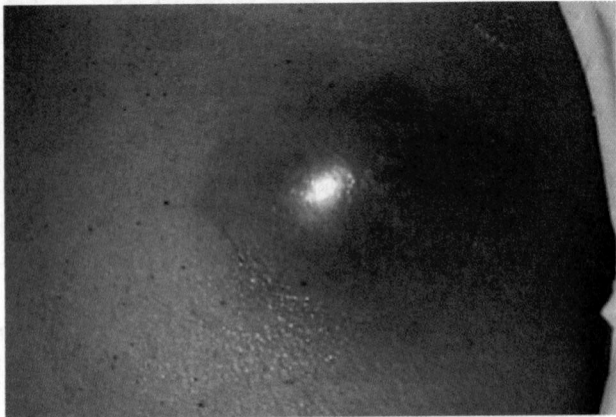

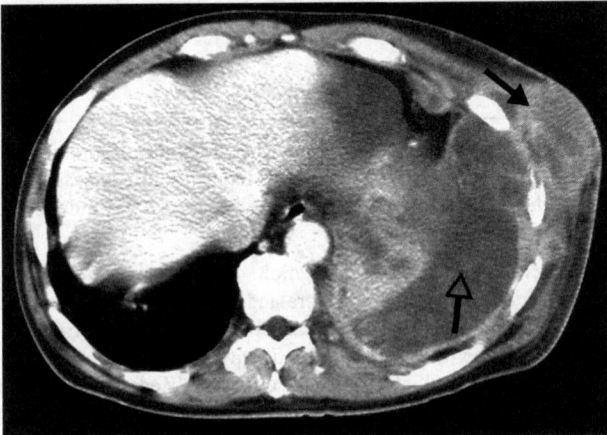

FIGURE 147-1 Thoracic actinomycosis. *Top*: A chest wall mass from extension of pulmonary infection. *Bottom*: Pulmonary infection is complicated by empyema (*open arrow*) and extension to the chest wall (*closed arrow*). (*Courtesy of Dr. C. B. Hsiao, Division of Infectious Diseases, Department of Medicine, State University of New York at Buffalo.*)

enhancement may be seen. Cavitary disease or hilar adenopathy may develop. More than 50% of cases include pleural thickening, effusion, or empyema (Fig. 147-1). Rarely, pulmonary nodules or endobronchial lesions occur. Pulmonary lesions suggestive of actinomycosis may cross fissures or pleura; may involve the mediastinum, contiguous bone, or chest wall; or may be associated with a sinus tract. In the absence of these findings, thoracic actinomycosis is usually mistaken for a neoplasm or for pneumonia due to more usual causes.

Mediastinal infection is uncommon, usually arising from thoracic extension but rarely resulting from perforation of the esophagus, from trauma, or from head and neck or abdominal disease. The structures within the mediastinum and the heart can be involved in various combinations; consequently, the possible presentations are diverse. Primary endocarditis and isolated disease of the breast have been described.

Abdominal Disease Abdominal actinomycosis poses a great diagnostic challenge. Months or years usually pass from the inciting event (e.g., appendicitis, diverticulitis, peptic ulcer disease, foreign-body perforation, bowel surgery, or ascension from IUCD-associated pelvic disease) to clinical recognition. Because of the flow of peritoneal fluid and/or the direct extension of primary disease, virtually any abdominal organ, region, or space can be involved. The disease usually presents as an abscess, a mass, or a mixed lesion that is often fixed to underlying tissue and mistaken for a tumor. On CT, enhancement is most often heterogeneous and adjacent bowel is thickened. Sinus tracts to the abdominal wall, to the perianal region, or between the bowel and other organs may develop and mimic inflammatory bowel disease. Recurrent disease or a wound or fistula that fails to heal suggests actinomycosis.

Hepatic infection usually presents as single or multiple abscesses or masses. Isolated disease presumably develops via hematogenous seeding from cryptic foci. Presently available imaging and percutaneous techniques have resulted in improved diagnosis and treatment.

All levels of the urogenital tract can be infected. Renal disease usually presents as pyelonephritis and/or renal and perinephric abscess. Bladder involvement, usually due to extension of pelvic disease, may result in ureteral obstruction or fistulas to bowel, skin, or uterus. *Actinomyces* can be detected in urine with use of appropriate stains and cultures.

Pelvic Disease Actinomycotic involvement of the pelvis occurs most commonly in association with an IUCD. Pelvic symptoms when an IUCD is in place or has recently been removed should prompt consideration of actinomycosis. Although the risk has not yet been quantified, it appears to be small. The disease rarely develops when the IUCD has been in place for <1 year, but the risk increases with time. Actinomycosis can also present months after the removal of the device. Symptoms are typically indolent; fever, weight loss, abdominal pain, and abnormal vaginal bleeding or discharge are the most common. The earliest stage of disease—often endometritis—commonly progresses to pelvic masses or a tuboovarian abscess (Fig. 147-2). Unfortunately, because the diagnosis is often delayed, a "frozen pelvis" mimicking malignancy or endometriosis can develop by the time of recognition.

An unresolved issue is whether screening of cervical or endometrial specimens for *Actinomyces*-like organisms (ALOs) can predict or prevent IUCD-associated disease. Although the risk appears to be small, the consequences of infection are significant. Therefore, until more quantitative data become available, it would appear prudent to remove the IUCD in the presence of symptoms that cannot be accounted for, regardless of whether ALOs or immunofluorescence-positive organisms are detected, and—if advanced disease is excluded—to initiate a 14-day course of empirical treatment for possible early pelvic actinomycosis. The detection of ALOs or immunofluorescence-positive organisms in the absence of symptoms warrants education of the patient and close follow-up but not removal of the IUCD unless an equally suitable means of contraception can be agreed upon.

Central Nervous System Disease Actinomycosis of the central nervous system is rare. Single or multiple brain abscesses are most common. An abscess usually appears on CT as a ring-enhancing lesion with a thick wall that may be irregular or nodular. Meningitis, epidural or subdural space infection, and cavernous sinus syndrome have also been described.

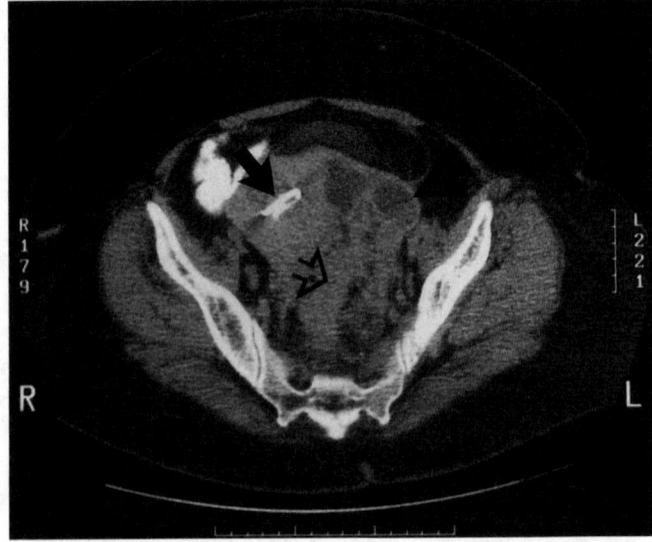

FIGURE 147-2 Computed tomogram showing pelvic actinomycosis associated with an intrauterine contraceptive device. The device is encased by endometrial fibrosis (*solid arrow*); also visible are paraendometrial fibrosis (*open triangular arrowhead*) and an area of suppuration (*open arrow*).

Musculoskeletal and Soft Tissue Infection Actinomycotic infection of the bone is usually due to adjacent soft-tissue infection but may be associated with trauma (e.g., fracture of the mandible) or hematogenous spread. Because of slow disease progression, new bone formation and bone destruction are seen concomitantly. Infection of an extremity is uncommon and is usually a result of trauma. Skin, subcutaneous tissue, muscle, and bone (with periostitis or acute or chronic osteomyelitis) are involved alone or in various combinations. Cutaneous sinus tracts frequently develop.

Disseminated Disease Hematogenous dissemination of disease from any location rarely results in multiple-organ involvement. The lungs and liver are most commonly affected, with the presentation of multiple nodules mimicking disseminated malignancy. The clinical presentation may be surprisingly indolent given the extent of disease.

DIAGNOSIS The diagnosis of actinomycosis is rarely considered. All too often, the first mention of actinomycosis is by the pathologist after extensive surgery has been performed. Since medical therapy alone is often sufficient for cure, the challenge for the clinician is to consider the possibility of actinomycosis in time to diagnose it in the least invasive fashion and to avoid unnecessary surgery. The clinical and radiographic presentations that suggest actinomycosis have been discussed above. Aspirations and biopsies (with or without CT or ultrasound guidance) are being used successfully to obtain clinical material for diagnosis, although surgery may be required. The diagnosis is most commonly made by microscopic identification of sulfur granules (an in vivo matrix of bacteria, calcium phosphate, and host material) in pus or tissues. Occasionally these granules can be grossly identified from draining sinus tracts or pus. Although sulfur granules are a defining characteristic of actinomycosis, granules are also found in mycetoma (Chaps. 146 and 190) and botryomycosis (a chronic suppurative bacterial infection of soft tissue or, in rare cases, visceral tissue that produces clumps of bacteria resembling granules); however, these entities can easily be differentiated from actinomycosis with appropriate histopathologic and microbiologic studies. Microbiologic identification of actinomycetes is often precluded by the administration of prior antimicrobial therapy or the failure to perform appropriate microbiologic cultures. For optimal yield, the avoidance of even a single dose of antibiotics is mandatory. Primary isolation usually requires 5 to 7 days but may take as long as 2 to 4 weeks. Immunofluorescence testing for *A. israelii*, *A. naeslundii*, and *P. propionicum* (available through the Centers for Disease Control and Prevention in Atlanta) is a useful diagnostic alternative. Although 16S rRNA gene amplification and sequencing would be predicted to have increased diagnostic sensitivity, this method apparently has not been used so far. Because these organisms are components of the normal oral and genital-tract flora, their identification in the absence of sulfur granules in sputum, bronchial washings, and cervicovaginal secretions is of little significance.

℞ TREATMENT

Decisions about treatment are based on the collective clinical experience of the past 50 years. Actinomycosis must be treated with high doses of antimicrobials for a prolonged period. The need for this intensive treatment is presumably due to difficulty encountered by antimicrobial agents in penetrating the thick-walled masses that commonly occur in this infection and/or the sulfur granules themselves. Although therapy needs to be individualized, the intravenous administration of 18 to 24 million units of penicillin daily for 2 to 6 weeks, followed by oral therapy with penicillin or amoxicillin for 6 to 12 months, is a reasonable guideline for serious infections. Less extensive disease, particularly that involving the oral-cervicofacial region, may require less intensive therapy. If therapy is extended beyond the point

TABLE 147-1 *Appropriate and Inappropriate Antibiotic Therapy for Actinomycosis*[a]

Category	Agent
Agents for which there is extensive successful clinical experience[b]	Penicillin: 18–24 mU/d IV q4h, 1–2 g/d PO q6h Amoxicillin: 1.5 g/d PO q8h Erythromycin: 2–4 g/d IV q6h, 1–2 g/d PO q6h Tetracycline: 1–2 g/d PO q6h Doxycycline: 200 mg/d IV or PO q12–24 h Minocycline: 200 mg/d IV or PO q12h Clindamycin: 2.7 g/d IV q8h, 1.2–1.8 g/d PO q6–8h
Agents for which there is anecdotal successful clinical experience	Ceftriaxone Ceftizoxime Imipenem Ciprofloxacin
Agents that should be avoided	Metronidazole Aminoglycosides Oxacillin Dicloxacillin Cephalexin

[a] Additional coverage for concomitant "companion" bacteria may be required.
[b] Controlled evaluations have not been performed. Dosing regimens require individualization according to the site and extent of infection. As a general rule, parenteral administration of the maximal antimicrobial dose for 2 to 6 weeks followed by oral therapy, for a total duration of 6 to 12 months, is required for most infections.

of resolution of measurable disease, the risk of relapse—a clinical hallmark of this infection—will be minimized; CT and magnetic resonance imaging (MRI) are generally the most sensitive and objective techniques by which to accomplish this goal. A similar approach is reasonable for immunocompromised patients, although refractory disease has been described in HIV-infected individuals. Suitable alternative antimicrobial agents and those deemed unreliable are listed in Table 147-1. Although the role played by "companion" microbes in actinomycosis is unclear, many isolates are pathogens in their own right, and a regimen covering these organisms during the initial treatment course is reasonable.

Combined medical-surgical therapy is still advocated by some authorities. However, an increasing body of literature now supports an initial attempt at cure with medical therapy alone, even in extensive disease. CT and MRI should be used to monitor the response to therapy. In most cases, either surgery can be avoided or a less extensive procedure can be used. This approach is particularly valuable in sparing critical organs, such as the bladder or the reproductive organs in women of child-bearing age. For a well-defined abscess, percutaneous drainage in combination with medical therapy is a reasonable approach. When a critical location is involved (e.g., the epidural space, the central nervous system) or when suitable medical therapy fails, surgical intervention may be appropriate.

FURTHER READING

DE FEITER PW, SOETERS PB: Gastrointestinal actinomycosis: An unusual presentation with obstructive uropathy: Report of a case and review of the literature. Dis Colon Rectum 44:1521, 2001

LEE YC et al: Computed tomography guided core needle biopsy diagnosis of pelvic actinomycosis. Gynecol Oncol 79:318, 2000

MILLER M, HADDAD AJ: Cervicofacial actinomycosis. Oral Surg Oral Med Oral Pathol Oral Radiol Endod 85:496, 1998

RUSSO TA: Actinomycosis, in *Principles and Practice of Infectious Diseases*, 5th ed, GL Mandell et al (eds). New York, Churchill Livingstone, 2000, pp 2645–2654

SMEGO RA, FOGLIA G: Actinomycosis. Clin Infect Dis 26:1255, 1998

DEFINITIONS *Anaerobic bacteria* are organisms that require reduced oxygen tension for growth, failing to grow on the surface of solid media in 10% CO_2 in air. (In contrast, *microaerophilic bacteria* can grow in an atmosphere of 10% CO_2 in air or under anaerobic or aerobic conditions, although they grow best in the presence of only a small amount of atmospheric oxygen, and *facultative bacteria* can grow in the presence or absence of air.) This chapter describes infections caused by nonsporulating anaerobic bacteria. In general, anaerobes associated with human infections are relatively aerotolerant. They can survive for as long as 72 h in the presence of oxygen, although generally they will not multiply in this environment. A far smaller number of pathogenic anaerobic bacteria (which are also part of the normal flora) die after brief contact with oxygen, even in low concentrations.

The nonsporulating anaerobic bacteria exist as components of the normal flora on the mucosal surfaces of humans and animals. The major reservoirs of these bacteria are the mouth, lower gastrointestinal tract, skin, and female genital tract. Among the constituents of the oral flora, anaerobes are the predominant commensal organisms, ranging in concentration from 10^9/mL in saliva to 10^{12}/mL in gingival scrapings. In the oral cavity, the ratio of anaerobic to aerobic bacteria ranges from 1:1 on the surface of a tooth to 1000:1 in the gingival crevice. Anaerobic bacteria are not found in appreciable numbers in the normal upper intestine until the distal ileum. In the colon, the proportion of anaerobes increases significantly, as does the overall bacterial count. For example, in the colon there are 10^{11} to 10^{12} organisms per gram of stool, with an anaerobe-to-aerobe ratio of $\sim$1000:1. In the female genital tract, there are $\sim$$10^9$ organisms per milliliter of secretions, with an anaerobe-to-aerobe ratio of $\sim$10:1.

It is becoming clear that anaerobes play a key role in maintaining the balance between the host and its colonizing organisms. Hundreds of species of anaerobic bacteria have been identified as part of the normal flora of humans. Identification of as many as 500 different anaerobic species in fecal specimens reflects the diversity of the anaerobic flora. Despite the complex array of bacteria in the normal flora, relatively few species are isolated commonly from human infection. Anaerobic infections occur when the harmonious relationship between the host and the bacteria is disrupted. Any site in the body is susceptible to infection with these indigenous organisms when a mucosal barrier or the skin is compromised by surgery, trauma, tumor, or ischemia or necrosis, all of which can reduce local tissue redox potentials. Because the sites that are colonized by anaerobes contain many species of bacteria, disruption of anatomical barriers allows the penetration of many organisms, resulting in mixed infections involving multiple species of anaerobes combined with facultative or microaerophilic organisms. Such mixed infections are seen in the head and neck (chronic sinusitis, chronic otitis media, Ludwig's angina, and periodontal abscesses). Brain abscesses and subdural empyema are the most common anaerobic infections of the central nervous system. Anaerobes are responsible for pleuropulmonary diseases such as aspiration pneumonia, necrotizing pneumonia, lung abscess, and empyema. These organisms also play an important role in various intraabdominal infections, such as peritonitis and intraabdominal and liver abscesses (Chap. 112). They are isolated frequently in female genital tract infections, such as salpingitis, pelvic peritonitis, tuboovarian abscess, vulvovaginal abscess, septic abortion, and endometritis (Chap. 115). Anaerobic bacteria are also found often in infections of the skin, soft tissues, and bones and in bacteremia.

ETIOLOGY The taxonomic classification of anaerobes is a rapidly evolving field, with frequent changes in nomenclature based on newly discovered relationships among bacterial species. The major anaerobic gram-positive cocci that produce disease are *Peptostreptococcus* spp. The major species of this genus that are involved in infections are *Peptostreptococcus micros*, *P. magnus*, *P. asaccharolyticus*,

P. anaerobius, and *P. prevotii*. Clostridia (Chap. 126) are gram-positive rods that are isolated from wounds, abscesses, sites of abdominal infection, and blood. The principal anaerobic gram-negative bacilli found in human infections are the *Bacteroides fragilis* group as well as *Fusobacterium*, *Prevotella*, and *Porphyromonas* spp. Other members of the Bacteroidaceae family include *Bilophila wadsworthia*, an organism that has been isolated from infected sites and has been reported to cause serious infections, including bacteremia, necrotizing fasciitis, and abscesses; this organism is frequently resistant to several antimicrobial agents, including imipenem, cefoxitin, and other β-lactam drugs. Gram-positive anaerobic non-spore-forming bacilli are uncommon as etiologic agents of human infection. *Propionibacterium acnes*, a rare cause of foreign-body infections, is one of the few nonclostridial gram-positive rods associated with infections.

The *B. fragilis* group contains the anaerobic pathogens most frequently isolated from clinical infections. Members of this group are part of the normal bowel flora; they include several distinct species, such as *B. fragilis*, *B. thetaiotaomicron*, *B. distasonis*, *B. vulgatus*, *B. uniformis*, and *B. ovatus*. Of this group, *B. fragilis* is the most important clinical isolate. However, *B. fragilis* is isolated from the normal fecal flora in lower numbers than some of the other *Bacteroides* spp.

A second major group of phenotypically similar organisms is part of the indigenous oral flora. Thus these organisms are found at infected sites that can be seeded with oral microflora. Many of these species are pigment-producing bacteria previously classified as *Bacteroides melaninogenicus*. The nomenclature of this group has changed so that two distinct genera, *Prevotella* and *Porphyromonas*, are now recognized; these genera comprise several pathogenic species, including *Porphyromonas gingivalis*, *Porphyromonas asaccharolytica*, and *Prevotella oralis*. *Porphyromonas* and *Prevotella* spp. cause localized infections that can spread contiguously.

In female genital tract infections, organisms normally colonizing the vagina, such as *Prevotella bivia* and *Prevotella disiens*, are the most frequent isolates, although *B. fragilis* is not uncommon. The *Fusobacterium* species *Fusobacterium necrophorum*, *F. nucleatum*, and *F. varium*, which reside primarily in the oral cavity and the gastrointestinal tract, are also isolated from clinical infections, including necrotizing pneumonia and abscesses.

Infections caused by anaerobic bacteria most frequently are due to more than one organism. These polymicrobial infections may be caused by one or several anaerobic species or by a combination of anaerobic organisms and microaerophilic or facultative bacteria acting synergistically.

APPROACH TO THE PATIENT

The physician must consider several points when approaching the patient with presumptive infection due to anaerobic bacteria.

1. Most of the organisms colonizing mucosal sites are harmless commensals; very few cause disease.
2. For anaerobes to cause tissue infection, they must spread beyond the normal mucosal barriers.
3. Conditions favoring the propagation of these bacteria, particularly a lowered oxidation-reduction potential, are necessary. These conditions exist at sites of trauma, tissue destruction, compromised vascular supply, and complications of preexisting infection, which produce necrosis.
4. There is a complex array of infecting flora. For example, as many as 12 different types of organisms can be isolated from a suppurative site.
5. Anaerobic organisms tend to be found in abscess cavities or in necrotic tissue. The failure of an abscess to yield organisms on routine culture is a clue that the abscess is likely to contain

anaerobic bacteria. Often smears of this "sterile pus" are found to be teeming with bacteria when Gram's stain is applied. Malodorous pus suggests anaerobic infection. Although some facultative organisms, such as *Staphylococcus aureus*, are also capable of causing abscesses, abscesses in organs or deeper body tissues should call to mind anaerobic infection.

6. Gas is found in many anaerobic infections of deep tissues.
7. Some species (the best example being the *B. fragilis* group) require specific therapy. However, many synergistic infections can be cured with antibiotics directed at some but not all of the organisms involved. Antibiotic therapy, combined with debridement and drainage, disrupts the interdependent relationship among the bacteria, and some species that are resistant to the antibiotic do not survive without the coinfecting organisms.
8. Manifestations of disseminated intravascular coagulation are unusual in patients with purely anaerobic infection.

EPIDEMIOLOGY Difficulties in the performance of appropriate cultures, contamination of cultures by aerobic bacteria or components of the normal flora, and the lack of readily available, reliable culture techniques have made it impossible to obtain accurate incidence or prevalence data. However, anaerobic infections are encountered frequently in hospitals with active surgical, trauma, and obstetric and gynecologic services. In some centers, anaerobic bacteria, particularly *B. fragilis*, account for ~4% of positive blood cultures.

PATHOGENESIS Anaerobic bacterial infections usually occur when an anatomical barrier becomes disrupted and constituents of the local flora enter a site that was previously sterile. Because of the specific growth requirements of anaerobic organisms and their presence as commensals on mucosal surfaces, conditions must arise that allow these organisms to penetrate mucosal barriers and enter tissue with a lowered oxidation-reduction potential. Therefore, tissue ischemia, trauma, surgery, perforated viscus, shock, and aspiration provide environments conducive to the proliferation of anaerobes. In the case of a perforated viscus, hundreds of species of anaerobic bacteria are spilled into the peritoneal cavity, but many of these organisms are unable to survive because the highly vascularized tissue provides a sufficiently high redox potential. The entry of oxygen into the environment results in the selection of the more aerotolerant anaerobic organisms.

The ability of an organism to adhere to host tissues is important to the establishment of infection. Some oral species adhere to crevicular epithelium in the oral cavity. *Prevotella melaninogenica* actually attaches to other microorganisms; *P. gingivalis* is a common isolate in periodontal disease. These organisms have fimbriae that facilitate attachment. Some unencapsulated *Bacteroides* strains appear to be piliated, a characteristic that may account for their ability to adhere.

The most extensively studied virulence factor of the nonsporulating anaerobes is the polysaccharide capsule of *B. fragilis*. This polysaccharide possesses distinct biologic properties, such as the ability (owing to a unique zwitterionic motif of charged sugars) to promote abscess formation. Intraabdominal abscess induction is related to the capacity of the polysaccharide to stimulate the release of cytokines and chemokines—in particular interleukin (IL) 8, IL-17, and tumor necrosis factor (TNF) α—from resident peritoneal cells. The release of cytokines and chemokines results in the chemotaxis of polymorphonuclear neutrophils (PMNs) into the peritoneum, where they adhere to mesothelial cells induced by TNF-α to upregulate their expression of intercellular adhesion molecule 1 (ICAM-1). PMNs adherent to ICAM-1-expressing cells probably represent the nidus for an abscess. Prophylactic or therapeutic administration of the polysaccharide or a zwitterionic mimetic to experimental animals confers protection against abscess induction following challenge with intestinal microorganisms capable of inducing abscesses. This protection is mediated by T cells controlling cytokine release; IL-10 appears to be the cytokine primarily responsible for downregulating the tissue response of abscess formation. Although abscesses constitute a host response

that localizes and contains infecting bacteria, abscess formation in patients with sepsis often results in severe and chronic illness that requires surgical drainage in combination with antimicrobial therapy.

Anaerobic bacteria produce a number of exoproteins that are capable of enhancing the organisms' virulence. The collagenase produced by *P. gingivalis* may enhance tissue destruction. An enterotoxin has been identified in *B. fragilis* strains associated with diarrheal disease in animals and young children. This 20-kDa zinc-dependent metalloprotease reversibly alters the morphology of the tight junctional complexes of intestinal epithelial cells. Both *B. fragilis* and *P. melaninogenica* possess lipopolysaccharides (endotoxins) that are less biologically potent than endotoxins associated with aerobic gram-negative bacteria. This relative biologic inactivity may account for the lower frequency of disseminated intravascular coagulation and purpura in *Bacteroides* bacteremia than in facultative and aerobic gram-negative bacillary bacteremia.

CLINICAL MANIFESTATIONS ■ **Anaerobic Infections of the Mouth, Head, and Neck** (See also Chap. 27) Infections of the mouth can arise from either the supragingival or the subgingival dental plaque. Supragingival plaque formation begins with the adherence of gram-positive bacteria to the tooth surface. This form of plaque is influenced by salivary and dietary components, oral hygiene, and local host factors. Once the supragingival plaque is established, the acquisition of pathogenic bacteria and an increase in the amount of plaque are responsible for the ultimate development of gingivitis. Early bacteriologic changes in the supragingival plaque initiate an inflammatory response in the gingiva, including edema, swelling, and increased gingival fluid, and cause the development of caries and endodontic (pulp) infections. In addition, these changes contribute to the subsequent pathogenic alteration in the subgingival plaque that arises from poor or inadequate oral hygiene.

Subgingival plaque is associated with periodontal disease and disseminated infection arising from the oral cavity. Bacteria that colonize the subgingival area are primarily anaerobic. The black-pigmented gram-negative anaerobic bacilli (principally *P. gingivalis*, *P. asaccharolytica*, and *P. melaninogenica*) are the most important. Infections in this area are frequently mixed and involve both anaerobic and aerobic bacteria. After establishment of local infection either in root canals or in the periodontal area, infection may extend into the mandible, causing osteomyelitis of the maxillary sinuses, or to local tissues in the submandibular or submental spaces, depending on which teeth are involved. Periodontitis may also result in spreading infection that can involve adjacent bone or soft tissues.

NECROTIZING ULCERATIVE GINGIVITIS Gingivitis may become a necrotizing infection (trench mouth, Vincent's stomatitis). The onset of disease is usually sudden and is associated with tender bleeding gums, foul breath, and a bad taste. The gingival mucosa, especially the papillae between the teeth, becomes ulcerated and may be covered by a gray exudate, which is removable with gentle pressure. Patients may become systemically ill, developing fever, cervical lymphadenopathy, and leukocytosis. Occasionally, ulcerative gingivitis can spread to the buccal mucosa, the teeth, and the mandible or maxilla, resulting in widespread destruction of bone and soft tissue. This infection is termed *acute necrotizing ulcerative mucositis* (cancrum oris, noma). It destroys tissue rapidly, causing the teeth to fall out and large areas of bone—or even the whole mandible—to be sloughed. A strong putrid odor is frequently detected, although the lesions are not painful. The gangrenous lesions eventually heal, leaving large disfiguring defects. This infection most commonly follows a debilitating illness or affects severely malnourished children. It has been known to complicate leukemia or to develop in individuals with a genetic deficiency of catalase.

ACUTE NECROTIZING INFECTIONS OF THE PHARYNX These infections usually occur in association with ulcerative gingivitis. Symptoms include an extremely sore throat, foul breath, and a bad taste accompanied by fever and a sensation of choking. Examination of the pharynx demonstrates that the tonsillar pillars are swollen, red, ulcerated, and covered with a grayish membrane that peels easily. Lymphadenopathy and leukocytosis are common. The disease may last for only a few days or, if not treated, may persist for weeks. Lesions begin unilaterally but may spread to the other side of the pharynx or the larynx. Aspiration of the infected material by the patient can result in lung abscesses. Soft tissue infection of the oral-facial area may or may not be odontogenic. Ludwig's angina, a periodontal infection usually arising from the tissues surrounding the third molar, may produce submandibular soft tissue infection that results in marked local swelling of tissues, with pain, trismus, and superior and posterior displacement of the tongue. Submandibular swelling of the neck can impair swallowing and cause respiratory obstruction. In some cases, tracheotomy may be lifesaving.

FASCIAL INFECTIONS   These infections arise from the spread of organisms originating in the upper airways to potential spaces formed by the fascial planes of the head and neck. Perimandibular space infection most commonly involves the submandibular, peritonsillar, and parapharyngeal spaces. Peritonsillar abscesses occur in association with pharyngitis. Complicated dental infections spread to the submandibular and buccal spaces. Entry of organisms by either portal can result in parapharyngeal space infections. Although there are few well-documented reports on the microbiology of these syndromes, anaerobes from the oral flora have been implicated in many cases. Fascial infections associated with *S. aureus* or *Streptococcus pyogenes* may arise from boils or impetigo, whereas anaerobes are associated with space infections either occurring spontaneously or arising from diseases of the mucous membranes or from dental manipulations.

SINUSITIS AND OTITIS   The role of anaerobic bacteria in acute sinusitis may be underestimated because of improper collection of specimens. In a study of chronic sinusitis, anaerobic bacteria were found in 52% of specimens collected during external frontoethmoidotomy or radical antrotomy. However, antibiotic therapy against anaerobes alone is not usually curative. Anaerobic bacteria are much more easily implicated in chronic suppurative otitis media than in acute otitis media. Purulent exudate from chronically draining ears has been found to contain anaerobes, particularly *Bacteroides* spp., in up to 50% of cases. *B. fragilis* has been isolated from up to 28% of patients with chronic otitis media.

COMPLICATIONS OF ANAEROBIC HEAD AND NECK INFECTIONS   Contiguous craniad spread of these infections may result in osteomyelitis of the skull or mandible or in intracranial infections such as brain abscess and subdural empyema. Caudad spread can produce mediastinitis or pleuropulmonary infection. Hematogenous complications may also result from anaerobic infections of the head and neck. Bacteremia, which occasionally is polymicrobial, can lead to endocarditis or other distant infections. Lemierre syndrome, which has been uncommon in the antimicrobial era, is an acute oropharyngeal infection with secondary septic thrombophlebitis of the internal jugular vein and frequent metastatic infections (see also "Bone and Joint Infections," below). *F. necrophorum* is the usual cause. This infection typically begins with pharyngitis, which is followed by local invasion in the lateral pharyngeal space with resultant internal jugular vein thrombophlebitis. The most common site for metastatic infection is the lungs. A typical clinical triad seen in recent series is pharyngitis, a tender/swollen neck, and noncavitating pulmonary infiltrates.

Central Nervous System Infections   Brain abscesses are frequently associated with anaerobic bacteria (Chap. 360). If optimal bacteriologic techniques are employed, as many as 85% of brain abscesses yield anaerobic bacteria—most often anaerobic gram-positive cocci (especially peptostreptococci), which are followed in frequency by *Fusobacterium* and *Bacteroides* spp. Facultative or microaerophilic streptococci and coliforms are often are part of a mixed infecting flora in brain abscesses.

Pleuropulmonary Infections   Anaerobic pleuropulmonary infections result from the aspiration of oropharyngeal contents, often in the context of an altered state of consciousness or an absent gag reflex. Four clinical syndromes are associated with anaerobic pleuropulmonary infection produced by aspiration: simple aspiration pneumonia, necrotizing pneumonia, lung abscess, and empyema.

ASPIRATION PNEUMONITIS   Aspiration pneumonitis must be distinguished from two other clinical syndromes associated with aspiration that are not of bacterial etiology. One syndrome results from aspiration of solids, usually food. Obstruction of major airways typically results in atelectasis and moderate nonspecific inflammation. Therapy consists of removal of the foreign body.

The second aspiration syndrome is more easily confused with bacterial aspiration. *Mendelson's syndrome* results from regurgitation of stomach contents and aspiration of chemical material, usually gastric juices. Pulmonary inflammation—including the destruction of the alveolar lining, with transudation of fluid into the alveolar space—occurs with remarkable rapidity. Typically this syndrome develops within hours, often following anesthesia when the gag reflex is depressed. The patient becomes tachypneic, hypoxic, and febrile. The leukocyte count may rise, and the chest x-ray may evolve suddenly from normal to a complete bilateral "whiteout" within 8 to 24 h. Sputum production is minimal. The pulmonary signs and symptoms can resolve quickly with symptom-based therapy or can culminate in respiratory failure, with the subsequent development of bacterial superinfection over a period of days. Antibiotic therapy is not indicated unless bacterial infection supervenes. The signs of bacterial infection include sputum production, persistent fever, leukocytosis, and clinical evidence of sepsis.

In contrast to these syndromes, bacterial aspiration pneumonia develops more slowly. It is seen in patients who are hospitalized and have a depressed gag reflex, impaired swallowing, or a tracheal or nasogastric tube; elderly patients; or those with transiently impaired consciousness in the wake of seizures, cerebrovascular accidents, or alcoholic blackouts. Patients who enter the hospital with this syndrome typically have been ill for several days and generally report low-grade fever, malaise, and sputum production. Usually the history reveals factors predisposing to aspiration, such as alcohol overdose or residence in a nursing home. Sputum characteristically is not malodorous unless the process has been underway for at least a week. A mixed bacterial flora with many PMNs is evident on Gram's staining of sputum. The most commonly encountered anaerobes in sputum in these infections are pigmented and nonpigmented *Prevotella* spp., *F. nucleatum*, *Peptostreptococcus* spp., and *Bacteroides* spp. Cultures are reliable only if contamination with the normal oral flora is avoided—that is, if specimens are obtained by open lung biopsy. In general, this procedure is not indicated in the evaluation of these patients. Chest x-rays show consolidation in dependent pulmonary segments: in the basilar segments of the lower lobes if the patient has aspirated while upright and in either the posterior segment of the upper lobe (usually on the right side) or the superior segment of the lower lobe if the patient has aspirated while supine. The organisms isolated from the lungs reflect the pharyngeal flora; *P. melaninogenica*, *Fusobacterium* spp., and anaerobic cocci are the most common isolates. The patient who aspirates in the hospital may also have a mixed infection involving enteric gram-negative rods.

NECROTIZING PNEUMONITIS   This form of anaerobic pneumonia is characterized by numerous small abscesses that spread to involve several pulmonary segments. The process can be indolent or fulminating. This syndrome is less common than either aspiration pneumonia or lung abscess and includes features of both types of infection.

ANAEROBIC LUNG ABSCESSES   These abscesses result from subacute anaerobic pulmonary infection. The clinical syndrome typically involves a history of constitutional symptoms, including malaise, weight loss, fever, chills, and foul-smelling sputum, perhaps over a period of weeks (Chap. 239). Patients who develop lung abscesses characteristically have dental infection and periodontitis, but lung abscesses in edentulous patients have been reported. Abscess cavities may be single or multiple and generally occur in dependent pulmonary segments (Fig. 148-1). Anaerobic abscesses must be distinguished from those associated with tuberculosis, neoplasia, and other conditions. Oral anaerobes predominate, although *B. fragilis* is isolated in up to 10% of cases. *S. aureus* may be found as well.

EMPYEMA Empyema is a manifestation of long-standing anaerobic pulmonary infection. The clinical presentation, which includes the presence of foul-smelling sputum, resembles that of other anaerobic pulmonary infections. Patients may report pleuritic chest pain and marked chest-wall tenderness.

Empyema may be masked by overlying pneumonitis and should be considered especially in cases of persistent fever despite antibiotic therapy. Diligent physical examination and the use of ultrasound to localize a loculated empyema are important diagnostic tools. The collection of a foul-smelling exudate by thoracentesis is typical. Cultures of infected pleural fluid yield an average of 3.5 anaerobes and 0.6 facultative or aerobic bacterial species. Drainage is required. Defervescence, a return to a feeling of well-being, and resolution of the process may require several months.

Extension from a subdiaphragmatic infection may also result in anaerobic empyema. Septic pulmonary emboli may originate from intraabdominal or female genital tract infections and can produce anaerobic pneumonia.

Intraabdominal Infections Enterotoxigenic *B. fragilis* has been associated with watery diarrhea in a small number of young children and adults. In case-control studies of children with undiagnosed diarrheal disease, enterotoxigenic *B. fragilis* was isolated from significantly more children with diarrhea than children in the control group. This organism may play a role in a small proportion of childhood diarrhea cases. Neutropenic enterocolitis (typhlitis) has been associated with anaerobic infection of the cecum but—in the setting of neutropenia (Chap. 72)—may involve the entire bowel. Patients usually present with fever; abdominal pain, tenderness, and distention; and watery diarrhea. The bowel wall is edematous with hemorrhage and necrosis. The primary pathogen is thought by some authorities to be *Clostridium septicum*, but other clostridia and mixed anaerobic infections have also been implicated. More than 50% of patients developing early clinical signs can benefit from antibiotic therapy and bowel rest. Surgery is sometimes required to remove gangrenous bowel. →*See Chap. 112 for a complete discussion of intraabdominal infections.*

Pelvic Infections The vagina of a healthy woman is one of the major reservoirs of anaerobic and aerobic bacteria. In the normal flora of the female genital tract, anaerobes outnumber aerobes by a ratio of ~10:1 and include anaerobic gram-positive cocci and *Bacteroides* spp. Anaerobes are isolated from most women with genital tract infections that are not caused by a sexually transmitted pathogen. The major anaerobic pathogens are *B. fragilis, P. bivia, P. disiens, P. melaninogenica*, anaerobic cocci, and *Clostridium* spp. Anaerobes are frequently encountered in tuboovarian abscess, septic abortion, pelvic abscess, endometritis, and postoperative wound infection, particularly following hysterectomy. Although these infections are often of mixed etiology, involving both anaerobes and coliforms, pure anaerobic infections without coliform or other facultative bacterial species occur more often in pelvic than in intraabdominal sites and are characterized by drainage of foul-smelling pus or blood from the uterus, generalized uterine or local pelvic tenderness, and continued fever and chills. Suppurative thrombophlebitis of the pelvic veins may complicate the infections and lead to repeated episodes of septic pulmonary emboli.

Anaerobic bacteria have been thought to be contributing factors in the etiology of bacterial vaginosis. This syndrome of unknown etiology is characterized by a profuse malodorous discharge and an increase in the number of bacteria in the vagina, including *Gardnerella vaginalis, Prevotella* spp., *Mobiluncus* spp., peptostreptococci, and genital mycoplasmas. Anaerobic bacteria are thought to play a role in the etiology of pelvic inflammatory disease (Chap. 115), and several investigations have shown an association between bacterial vaginosis and the development of pelvic inflammatory disease.

Pelvic infections due to *Actinomyces* spp. have been associated with use of intrauterine devices (Chap. 147).

Skin and Soft Tissue Infections Injury to skin, bone, or soft tissue by trauma, ischemia, or surgery creates a suitable environment for anaerobic infections. These infections are most frequently found in sites prone to contamination with feces or with upper airway secretions—for example, wounds associated with intestinal surgery, decubitus ulcers, or human bites. Anaerobic bacteria can be isolated in cases of crepitant cellulitis, synergistic cellulitis, or gangrene and necrotizing fasciitis (Chaps. 110 and 126). Moreover, these organisms have been isolated from cutaneous abscesses, rectal abscesses, and axillary sweat gland infections (hidradenitis suppurativa). Anaerobes are frequently cultured from foot ulcers in diabetic patients.

These soft tissue or skin infections are usually polymicrobial. A mean of 4.8 bacterial species are isolated, with an anaerobe-to-aerobe ratio of ~3:2. The most frequently isolated organisms include *Bacteroides* spp., peptostreptococci, enterococci, clostridia, and *Proteus* spp. The involvement of anaerobes in these types of infections is associated with a higher frequency of fever, foul-smelling lesions, gas in the tissues, and visible foot ulcer.

Anaerobic bacterial *synergistic gangrene (Meleney's gangrene)* is characterized by exquisite pain, redness, and swelling followed by induration. Erythema surrounds a central zone of necrosis. A granulating ulcer forms at the original center as necrosis and erythema extend outward. Symptoms are limited to pain; fever is not typical. These infections usually involve a combination of *Peptostreptococcus* spp. and *S. aureus*; the usual site of infection is an abdominal surgical wound or the area surrounding an ulcer on an extremity. Treatment includes surgical removal of necrotic tissue and antimicrobial administration.

Necrotizing fasciitis, a rapidly spreading destructive disease of the fascia, is usually attributed to group A streptococci (Chap. 121) but can also be a mixed infection involving anaerobes and aerobes. The most frequently isolated anaerobes in these infections are *Peptostreptococcus* and *Bacteroides* spp. Gas may be found in the tissues. Similarly, myonecrosis can be associated with mixed anaerobic infection. *Fournier's gangrene* consists of cellulitis involving the scrotum, perineum, and anterior abdominal wall, with mixed anaerobic organisms spreading along deep external fascial planes and causing extensive loss of skin.

Bone and Joint Infections Although actinomycosis (Chap. 147) accounts on a worldwide basis for most anaerobic infections in bone, organisms including peptostreptococci or microaerophilic cocci, *Bacteroides* spp., *Fusobacterium* spp., and *Clostridium* spp. can also be found. These infections frequently arise adjacent to soft tissue infections. Hematogenous seeding of bone is uncommon. *Prevotella* and *Porphyromonas* spp. are detected in infections involving the maxilla and

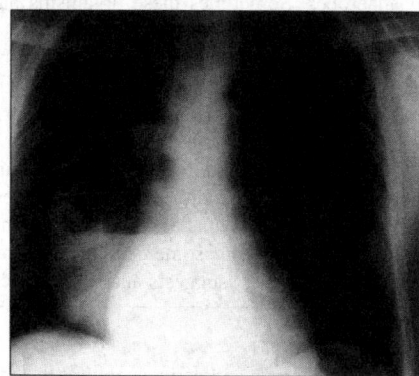

FIGURE 148-1 Chest radiograph of right-lower-lobe lung abscess in a 60-year-old alcoholic. *[From GL Mandell (ed): Atlas of Infectious Diseases, Vol VI. Philadelphia, Current Medicine Inc, Churchill Livingstone, 1996; with permission.]*

mandible, whereas *Clostridium* spp. have been reported as anaerobic pathogens in cases of osteomyelitis of the long bones following fracture or trauma. Fusobacteria have been isolated in pure culture from sites of osteomyelitis adjacent to the perinasal sinuses. Peptostreptococci and microaerophilic cocci have been reported as significant pathogens in infections involving the skull, mastoid, and prosthetic implants placed in bone. In patients with osteomyelitis (Chap. 111), the most reliable culture specimen is a bone biopsy sample free of normal uninfected skin and subcutaneous tissue. In patients with anaerobic osteomyelitis, a mixed flora is frequently isolated from a bone biopsy specimen.

In cases of anaerobic septic arthritis, the most common isolates are *Fusobacterium* spp. Most of the patients involved have uncontrolled peritonsillar infections progressing to septic cervical venous thrombophlebitis (Lemierre syndrome) and resulting in hematogenous dissemination with a predilection for the joints. Unlike anaerobic osteomyelitis, anaerobic pyoarthritis in most cases is not polymicrobial and may be acquired hematogenously. Anaerobes are important pathogens in infections involving prosthetic joints; in these infections, the causative organisms (such as *Peptostreptococcus* spp. and *P. acnes*) are part of the normal skin flora.

Bacteremia   Transient bacteremia is a well-known event in healthy people whose anatomical mucosal barriers have been injured (e.g., during dental extractions or dental scaling). These bacteremic episodes, which are often due to anaerobes, have no pathologic consequences. However, anaerobic bacteria are found in cultures of blood from clinically ill patients when proper culture techniques are used. *B. fragilis* is the single most common anaerobic isolate from the bloodstream.

In recent years, the rate of isolation of anaerobic bacteria from blood cultures has been decreasing. Studies from the 1970s and early 1980s found that 10 to 15% of positive blood cultures yielded anaerobes, while more recent surveys have found rates as low as 4%. The cause of this change is unknown but may be related to the administration of antibiotic prophylaxis before intestinal surgery, the earlier recognition of localized infections, and the empirical use of broad-spectrum antibiotics for presumed infection.

Once the organism has been identified, both the portal of bloodstream entry and the underlying problem that probably led to seeding of the bloodstream can often be deduced from an understanding of the organism's normal site of residence. For example, mixed anaerobic bacteremia including *B. fragilis* usually implies colonic pathology with mucosal disruption from neoplasia, diverticulitis, or some other inflammatory lesion. The initial manifestations are determined by the portal of entry and reflect the localized condition. When bloodstream invasion occurs, patients can become extremely ill, with rigors and hectic fevers ranging up to 40.6°C (105°F). The clinical picture may be quite similar to that seen in sepsis involving aerobic gram-negative bacilli. Although other complications of anaerobic bacteremia, such as septic thrombophlebitis and septic shock, have been reported, the incidence of these complications in association with anaerobic bacteremia is low. Anaerobic bacteremia is potentially fatal and requires rapid diagnosis and appropriate therapy. Mortality appears to increase with the age of the patient (with reported rates of >66% among patients >60 years old), with the isolation of multiple species from the bloodstream, and with the failure to surgically remove a focus of infection.

Endocarditis and Pericarditis (See also Chap. 109)   Endocarditis due to anaerobes is uncommon. However, anaerobic streptococci, which are often classified incorrectly, are responsible for this disease more frequently than is generally appreciated. Gram-negative anaerobes are unusual causes of endocarditis. Signs and symptoms of anaerobic endocarditis are similar to those of endocarditis due to facultative organisms. The mortality rate for anaerobic endocarditis has been reported at 21 to 43%.

Anaerobes, particularly *B. fragilis* and *Peptostreptococcus* spp., are uncommonly found in infected pericardial fluids. Anaerobic pericarditis is associated with a mortality rate of >50%.

DIAGNOSIS   There are three critical steps in the diagnosis of anaerobic infection: (1) proper specimen collection; (2) rapid transport of the specimens to the microbiology laboratory, preferably in anaerobic transport media; and (3) proper handling of the specimens by the laboratory. Specimens must be collected by meticulous sampling of infected sites, with avoidance of contamination by the normal flora. When such contamination is likely, the specimen is unacceptable. Examples of specimens unacceptable for anaerobic culture include sputum collected by expectoration or nasal tracheal suction, bronchoscopy specimens, samples collected directly through the vaginal vault, urine collected by voiding, and feces. Specimens that can be cultured for anaerobes include blood, pleural fluid, transtracheal aspirates, pus obtained by direct aspiration from an abscess cavity, fluid obtained by culdocentesis, suprapubic bladder aspirates, cerebrospinal fluid, and lung puncture specimens.

Because even brief exposure to oxygen may kill some anaerobic organisms and result in failure to isolate them in the laboratory, air must be expelled from the syringe used to aspirate the abscess cavity, and the needle must be capped with a sterile rubber stopper. Proper precautions should be used in the handling of contaminated needles. Specimens can be injected into transport bottles containing a reduced medium or taken immediately in syringes to the laboratory for direct culture on anaerobic media. In general, swabs should not be used. If a swab must be used, it should be placed in a reduced semisolid carrying medium before transport to the laboratory. Delays in transport may lead to a failure to isolate anaerobes due to exposure to oxygen or overgrowth of facultative organisms, which may eliminate or obscure any anaerobes that are present. All clinical specimens from suspected anaerobic infections should be Gram-stained and examined for organisms with characteristic morphology. It is not unusual for organisms to be observed on Gram's staining but not isolated in culture. If purulent materials are found to be sterile or organisms are seen on Gram's staining but do not grow in the culture, the involvement of anaerobes should be suspected.

Because of the time and difficulty involved in the isolation of anaerobic bacteria, diagnosis of anaerobic infections must frequently be based on presumptive evidence. Certain sites (such as avascular necrotic tissues) with lowered oxidation-reduction potential favor the diagnosis of an anaerobic infection. When infections occur in proximity to mucosal surfaces normally harboring an anaerobic flora, such as the gastrointestinal tract, female genital tract, or oropharynx, anaerobes should be considered as potential etiologic agents. A foul odor is often indicative of anaerobes, which produce certain organic acids as they proliferate in necrotic tissue. Although these odors are nearly pathognomonic for anaerobic infection, the absence of odor does not exclude an anaerobic etiology. Because anaerobes often coexist with other bacteria to cause mixed or synergistic infection, Gram's staining of exudate frequently reveals numerous pleomorphic cocci and bacilli suggestive of anaerobes. Sometimes these organisms have morphologic characteristics associated with specific species.

The presence of gas in tissues is highly suggestive, but not diagnostic, of anaerobic infection. When cultures of obviously infected sites yield no growth, streptococci only, or a single aerobic species (such as *Escherichia coli*) and Gram's staining reveals a mixed flora, the implication is that the anaerobic microorganisms failed to grow because of inadequate transport and/or culture techniques. Failure of a patient to respond to antibiotics that are not active against anaerobes (e.g., aminoglycosides and—in some circumstances—penicillin, cephalosporins, or tetracyclines) suggests anaerobic infection.

Rx TREATMENT

Successful therapy for anaerobic infections requires the administration of a combination of appropriate antibiotics, surgical resection, debridement of devitalized tissues, and drainage. Perforations must be closed promptly, closed spaces drained, tissue compartments decompressed, and an adequate blood supply established. Abscess cavities should be drained as soon as fluctuation or localization occurs. Surgery was formerly required to establish drainage; however, computed tomography (CT), magnetic resonance imaging (MRI), and ultrasound now allow diagnostic radiologists to drain many abscess sites percutaneously.

Antibiotic Therapy and Resistance Decisions about the treatment of anaerobic infections with antibiotics are usually based on known resistance patterns in certain species, on the likelihood of encountering a given species in the case at hand, and on Gram's stain findings. Antibiotics active against *Bacteroides* spp., penicillin-resistant *Prevotella* and *Porphyromonas* spp., and *Fusobacterium* spp. can be grouped into four categories on the basis of their predicted activity against anaerobes (Table 148-1). (Nearly all the drugs listed have toxic side effects, which are described in detail in Chap. 118.) In many infections, anaerobes are mixed with coliforms and other facultative organisms. The best therapeutic regimens, therefore, are usually those active against both aerobic and anaerobic bacteria. The choice of empirical antibiotics for the anaerobes in mixed infections can nearly always be made reliably, since patterns of antimicrobial susceptibility are usually predictable (Chap. 118 and Table 148-1).

Antibiotic susceptibility testing of anaerobic bacteria has been difficult and controversial. Owing to the slow growth rate of many anaerobes, the lack of standardized testing methods and of clinically relevant standards for resistance, and the generally good results obtained with empirical therapy, there has been limited interest in testing these organisms for antibiotic susceptibility. However, a recent study found mortality rates of 45 and 16% among antibiotic-treated patients with *Bacteroides* blood isolates deemed resistant and sensitive, respectively, to the agent used. These figures suggest that in vitro susceptibility testing should be performed for *Bacteroides* isolates from hospitalized patients with bacteremia and that the results of this testing should guide treatment.

Clinically important *Bacteroides* spp. are essentially all resistant to penicillin, and penicillin resistance rates among *Porphyromonas*, *Prevotella*, and *Fusobacterium* spp. are increasing rapidly. Failures of therapy are common when documented *Bacteroides* (especially *B. fragilis*) infection is treated with penicillin or first-generation cephalosporins. The number of antimicrobial agents effective against *Bacteroides* spp. has expanded, and there are currently several useful choices (Table 148-1). In general, cure rates of >80% can be attained in patients with *Bacteroides* infection by means of appropriate antimicrobial therapy and drainage.

Resistance to metronidazole has been reported only rarely in *Bacteroides* spp. This well-tolerated drug, which reaches significant levels in serum and can also be found at high concentrations in abscess cavities, should be considered first-line therapy against *Bacteroides* infection. However, if metronidazole is used to treat mixed anaerobic and aerobic infections, it is imperative that other appropriate antibiotics be used in conjunction. Metronidazole is inactive against aerobic and facultative bacteria, *Actinomyces* spp., and *Propionibacterium* spp. The sensitivity of peptostreptococci to metronidazole is unpredictable, and penicillin remains the drug of choice.

If a patient fails to respond to one of the category 1 or category 2 drugs (Table 148-1), consideration should be given to alternative therapy and to determination of the resistance patterns among *Bacteroides* isolates. Although in vitro resistance of *Bacteroides* spp. to chloramphenicol has not been reported, this drug may not be as effective as other category 1 drugs. Ampicillin/sulbactam, ticarcillin/clavulanic acid, piperacillin/tazobactam, imipenem, and meropenem have been effective in the treatment of *B. fragilis* infection. Some newer quinolones, such as moxifloxacin, appear to be highly active in vitro against certain anaerobes, including *B. fragilis*, but not against all members of the *B. fragilis* group; consideration of their use must await appropriate clinical trials.

TABLE 148-1 Antimicrobial Therapy for Infections Involving Commonly Encountered Anaerobic Gram-Negative Rods

Category 1 (<2% Resistance)	Category 2 (<15% Resistance)	Category 3 (Variable Resistance)	Category 4 (Resistance)
Imipenem	Cefoxitin	Penicillin	Aminoglycosides
Meropenem	Clindamycin	Cephalosporins	Quinolones[b]
Metronidazole[a]	High-dose	Tetracycline	Monobactams
Ampicillin/	antipseudomonal	Vancomycin	
sulbactam	penicillins	Erythromycin	
Ticarcillin/			
clavulanic acid			
Piperacillin/			
tazobactam			
Chloramphenicol[c]			

[a] Usually needs to be given in combination with aerobic bacterial coverage. For infections originating below the diaphragm, aerobic gram-negative coverage is essential. For infections from an oral source, aerobic gram-positive coverage is added. Metronidazole also is not active against *Actinomyces*, *Propionibacterium*, or other gram-positive non-spore-forming bacilli (e.g., *Eubacterium*, *Bifidobacterium*) and is unreliable against peptostreptococci.
[b] Moxifloxacin appears to have in vitro activity against many anaerobes.
[c] Chloramphenicol is probably not as effective as other category 1 antimicrobials in treating anaerobic infections.

Treatment of Infections at Specific Sites In clinical situations, specific regimens must be tailored to the initial site of infection. The duration of therapy also depends on the infection site; the reader is referred to specific chapters on sites of infection for recommendations.

β-Lactamase production has been reported in anaerobic strains that are usually isolated from infections originating above the diaphragm. Up to 60% of clinical isolates classified as *Prevotella* or *Porphyromonas* spp., non-*B. fragilis* species of *Bacteroides*, or *Fusobacterium* spp. reportedly produce β-lactamase. The clinical significance of resistance in these organisms has been suggested by studies showing clindamycin to be superior to penicillin (which for many years was considered the therapeutic "gold standard") for the treatment of lung abscesses. Presumably, the success of clindamycin is attributable to a broader spectrum of activity against oral anaerobes; thus, a combination of penicillin and metronidazole or another antibiotic combination that is active against both oral anaerobes and aerobes is likely to be as effective as clindamycin. Bronchoscopy in lung abscess is indicated only to rule out airway obstruction and does not enhance drainage; in any event, it should be delayed until the antimicrobial regimen has begun to affect the disease process so that the procedure does not spread the infection. Surgery is almost never indicated because of the danger of spilling the abscess contents into the lungs.

Although many oral anaerobic infections and most cases of anaerobic pneumonia still respond to penicillin therapy, some infections due to oral organisms fail to respond to this drug, and in these cases the use of a drug that is effective against penicillin-resistant anaerobes is recommended (Table 148-1). Life-threatening infections involving the anaerobic flora of the mouth, such as space infections of the head and neck, should be treated empirically as if penicillin-resistant anaerobes are involved. Less serious infections involving the oral microflora can be treated with penicillin alone; metronidazole can be added (or clindamycin can be substituted) if the patient responds poorly to penicillin therapy. Combinations of antibiotics used to treat mixed infections of oral origin must include drugs active against the gram-positive aerobic flora of the mouth.

Chloramphenicol has been used successfully against anaerobic central nervous system infections at doses of 30 to 60 mg/kg per day, with the exact dose depending on the severity of illness. However, penicillin G and metronidazole also cross the blood-brain barrier and are bactericidal for many anaerobic organisms (Chap. 360).

Anaerobic infections arising below the diaphragm (e.g., colonic and intraabdominal infections) must be treated specifically with agents active against *Bacteroides* spp. (Table 148-1). In intraabdominal sepsis (Chap. 112), the use of antibiotics effective against penicillin-resistant anaerobes has clearly reduced the incidence of postoperative infections and serious infectious complications. Specifically, a drug from cate-

TABLE 148-2 *Doses and Schedules for Treatment of Serious Infections Due to Commonly Encountered Anaerobic Gram-Negative Rods*

First-Line Therapy	Dose	Schedule[a]
Metronidazole[b]	500 mg	q6h
Ticarcillin/clavulanic acid	3.1 g	q4h
Piperacillin/tazobactam	3.375 g	q6h
Imipenem	0.5 g	q6h
Meropenem	1.0 g	q8h

[a] See disease-specific chapters for recommendations on duration of therapy.
[b] Should generally be used in conjunction with drugs active against aerobic or facultative organisms.
Note: All drugs are given by the intravenous route.

gory 1 (Table 148-1) must be included for broad-spectrum coverage. Recommended doses for commonly used category 1 drugs are given in Table 148-2. Therapy for intraabdominal sepsis must also include drugs active against the gram-negative aerobic flora of the bowel. If the involvement of gram-positive bacteria such as enterococci is suspected, either ampicillin or vancomycin should be added.

Cases of anaerobic osteomyelitis in which a mixed flora is isolated from a bone biopsy specimen should be treated with a regimen that covers all the isolates. When an anaerobic organism is recognized as a major or sole pathogen infecting a joint, the duration of treatment should be similar to that used for arthritis caused by aerobic bacteria (Chap. 314). Therapy includes the management of underlying disease states, the administration of appropriate antimicrobial agents, temporary joint immobilization, percutaneous drainage of effusions, and (usually) the removal of infected prostheses or internal fixation devices. Surgical drainage and debridement procedures such as sequestrectomy are essential for the removal of necrotic tissue that can sustain anaerobic infections.

The outcome of anaerobic bacteremia is significantly better in patients either initially given or switched to appropriate therapy based on known antibiotic susceptibilities.

Failure of Therapy   Anaerobic infections that fail to respond to treatment or that relapse should be reassessed. Consideration should be given to additional surgical drainage or debridement. Superinfections with resistant gram-negative facultative or aerobic bacteria should be ruled out. The possibility of drug resistance must be entertained; if resistance is involved, repeated cultures may yield the pathogenic organism.

Supportive Measures   Other supportive measures in the management of anaerobic infections include careful attention to fluid and electrolyte balance (since extensive local edema may lead to hypoalbuminemia), hemodynamic support for septic shock, immobilization of infected extremities, maintenance of adequate nutrition during chronic infections by parenteral hyperalimentation, relief of pain, and anticoagulation with heparin for thrombophlebitis. For patients with severe anaerobic infections of soft tissues, hyperbaric oxygen therapy is advocated by some experts, but its value has not been proven in controlled trials.

FURTHER READING

ALDRIDGE KE et al: Bacteremia due to *Bacteroides fragilis* group: Distribution of species, beta-lactamase production and antimicrobial susceptibility patterns. Antimicrob Agents Chemother 47:148, 2003

CITRON DM et al: 2001: An anaerobe odyssey. Clin Infect Dis 35:S1, 2002

FINEGOLD SM: Anaerobic bacteria: General concepts, in *Principles and Practice of Infectious Diseases*, 5th ed, GL Mandell et al (eds). New York, Churchill Livingstone, 2000, pp 2519–2537

———: Overview of clinically important anaerobes. Clin Infect Dis 20:S205, 1995

NGUYEN MH et al: Antimicrobial resistance and clinical outcome of *Bacteroides* bacteremia: Findings of a multicenter prospective observational trial. Clin Infect Dis 30:870, 2000

SALONEN JH et al: Clinical significance and outcome of anaerobic bacteremia. Clin Infect Dis 26:1413, 1998

SOLOMKIN JS et al: Guidelines for the selection of anti-infective agents for complicated intra-abdominal infections. Clin Infect Dis 37:997, 2003

TZIANABOS AO et al: Role of T cells in abscess formation, in *Current Opinion in Microbiology*, J Davies, P Cossart (eds). London, Elsevier Science, 2002, pp 92–96

Section 8   Mycobacterial Diseases

149 ANTIMYCOBACTERIAL AGENTS
Richard J. Wallace, Jr., David E. Griffith

The physician is greatly challenged to provide optimal therapy for mycobacterial illnesses because of the increase in both drug-susceptible and multidrug-resistant tuberculosis; the increasing number of pathogenic nontuberculous mycobacteria (NTM); drug-related toxicities and drug-drug interactions (especially in patients who have AIDS, with their complex antiretroviral drug regimens); and the plethora of new antibiotics with antimycobacterial potential. This chapter reviews the therapeutic agents used for treatment of tuberculosis, leprosy (Hansen's disease), and diseases caused by NTM, including *Mycobacterium avium-intracellulare* (MAI), *M. kansasii*, the rapidly growing mycobacteria, and *M. marinum*. The use of antimycobacterial agents in patients with renal or hepatic disease and in pregnant women is summarized in Table 149-1. The effects of antimycobacterial agents on the levels, activity, and toxicity of other commonly used drugs are summarized in Table 149-2.

TUBERCULOSIS

Drugs used to treat tuberculosis have been classified into first-line and second-line agents. *First-line essential* antituberculous agents are the most effective and are a necessary component of any short-course therapeutic regimen. The three drugs in this category are rifampin, isoniazid, and pyrazinamide. The *first-line supplemental* agents, which are highly effective and infrequently toxic, include ethambutol and streptomycin. Favorable experience in patients with tuberculosis resistant to first-line essential drugs suggests that rifabutin and the fluoroquinolones ciprofloxacin and levofloxacin are important additions to multidrug antituberculous regimens; thus these agents have now been added to the list of first-line supplemental drugs. *Second-line* antituberculous drugs are clinically much less effective than first-line agents and elicit severe reactions much more frequently. These drugs are rarely used in therapy and then only by caregivers experienced with their use. The older agents include para-aminosalicylic acid (PAS), ethionamide, cycloserine, amikacin, and capreomycin. *Newer* antituberculous drugs, which have not yet been placed in the above categories, include rifapentine and the 8-methoxyfluoroquinolones gatifloxacin and moxifloxacin.

FIRST-LINE ESSENTIAL ANTITUBERCULOUS DRUGS ◼ **Rifampin**   Rifampin, a semisynthetic derivative of *Streptomyces mediterranei*, is considered the most important and potent antituberculous agent. It is also active against a wide spectrum of other organisms, including some gram-positive and gram-negative bacteria, *Legionella* spp., *M. kansasii*, and *M. marinum*.

MECHANISM OF ACTION   Rifampin has both intracellular and extracellular bactericidal activity. It blocks RNA synthesis by specifically binding and inhibiting DNA-dependent RNA polymerase. Susceptible strains

Agent	Severe Hepatic Disease	Use in Indicated Circumstances		Pregnancy[a]
		Renal Disease: Creatinine Clearance Rate		
		>30 mL/min	≤30 mL/min	
Azithromycin	No change	No change	?Decrease dose	No evidence of risk (B)
Clarithromycin	No change	No change	Decrease dose	Risk cannot be ruled out (C)
Ethambutol	No change	No change	No change	Risk cannot be ruled out (C)
Isoniazid	Avoid use or decrease dose	No change	Decrease dose	Risk cannot be ruled out (C)
Pyrazinamide	Avoid use or decrease dose	No change	Decrease dose[b]	Risk cannot be ruled out (C)[c]
Rifabutin	No change	No change	No change	No evidence of risk (B)
Rifampin	Avoid use or decrease dose	No change	No change	Risk cannot be ruled out (C)
Rifapentine	Avoid use or decrease dose	No change	No change	Risk cannot be ruled out (C)
Streptomycin	No change	Decrease dose	Decrease dose and frequency	Definite evidence of risk (D)

[a] Based on Food and Drug Administration pregnancy categories of A–D, X.
[b] Prudent but not absolutely necessary.
[c] Use in pregnancy is recommended by international organizations outside the United States.

of *M. tuberculosis* as well as *M. kansasii* and *M. marinum* are inhibited by ≤1 μg/mL.

PHARMACOLOGY   Rifampin is a fat-soluble complex macrocyclic antibiotic that is absorbed readily after either oral or intravenous administration. Serum levels of 10 to 20 μg/mL follow a standard adult oral dose of 600 mg. Rifampin distributes well throughout most body tissues, including inflamed meninges. The fact that rifampin turns body fluids (urine, saliva, sputum, tears) a red-orange color makes it simple and inexpensive to check on patients' compliance with therapy. Rifampin is excreted primarily through the bile and the enterohepatic circulation, while 30 to 40% of a dose is excreted via the kidneys. The drug is administered either twice weekly or daily at a dose of 600 mg for adults (10 mg/kg) and 10 to 20 mg/kg for children. As mentioned above, rifampin is also available for intravenous administration.

TABLE 149-2   *Effects of Major Antimycobacterial Agents on Levels/Activity/Toxicity of Other Commonly Used Drugs[a]*

Rifampin/rifabutin[b]	Isoniazid
Acetaminophen (↓)	Alcohol (↑ in risk of hepatitis)
Antiarrhythmics (↓)	Carbamazepine (↑)
Anticonvulsants (↓)	Diphenylhydantoin (↑)
Azole antifungals (↓)	Enflurane (↑ in risk of renal failure)
Barbiturates (↓)	Warfarin (↑)
β Blockers (↓)	**Clarithromycin**
Calcium channel blockers (↓)	Astemizole (↑)
Chloramphenicol (↓)	Carbamazepine (↑)
Clarithromycin (↓)	Digoxin (↑)
Cyclosporine (↓)	Rifabutin (↑)
Dapsone (↓)	Ritonavir (↓)
Delavirdine (↓)	Terfenadine (↑)
Diazepam (↓)	Zidovudine (↓)
Digoxin (↓)	
Doxycycline (↓)	
Fluoroquinolones (↓)	
Glucocorticoids (↓)	
Halothane (↓)	
Hormonal contraceptives (↓)	
Narcotics (↓)	
NNRTIs[c] (↓)	
Oral hypoglycemics (↓)	
Probenecid (↓)	
Protease inhibitors (↓)	
Quinidine (↓)	
Theophylline (↓)	
Tricyclic antidepressants (↓)	
Warfarin (↓)	
Zidovudine (↓)	

[a] The following antimycobacterial agents have no or minimal effects on other drugs: amikacin, azithromycin, capreomycin, ethambutol, streptomycin, pyrazinamide.
[b] Rifabutin, which induces the cytochrome P450 system, has the same effects (↓) as rifampin but to a lesser degree. All drugs whose half-life is decreased by rifampin induction of hepatic microsomal enzymes may be subject to the same effect when coadministered with rifabutin; however, this point has not yet been studied.
[c] NNRTIs, nonnucleoside reverse transcriptase inhibitors.

ADVERSE EFFECTS (Table 149-3)   Rifampin is generally well tolerated; the most common adverse event is gastrointestinal upset. Patients with chronic liver disease, especially those with alcoholism and the elderly, appear to be at unusually high risk for the most serious adverse drug reaction: hepatitis. Other adverse effects of rifampin include rash (0.8%), hemolytic anemia (<1%), thrombocytopenia, and immunosuppression of unknown clinical importance. Rifampin is a potent inducer of the hepatic microsomal enzymes and thereby decreases the half-life of a number of drugs, including digoxin, warfarin, prednisone, cyclosporine, methadone, oral contraceptives, clarithromycin, the HIV protease inhibitors, the HIV nonnucleoside reverse transcriptase inhibitors, and quinidine (Table 149-2). The dose of rifampin generally does not require reduction in patients with renal failure, especially those receiving intermittent rifampin administration (Table 149-1).

RESISTANCE   Resistance to rifampin results from spontaneous point mutations that alter the β subunit of the RNA polymerase (*rpoB*) gene. Studies have shown that 96% of rifampin-resistant strains have a missense mutation within a 91-bp central core region of the gene. Rifampin-resistant strains of *M. leprae* have similar mutations that alter a single serine residue (Ser-425) in the same core region of the *rpoB* gene.

Isoniazid

After rifampin, isoniazid is considered the best antituberculous drug currently available. Isoniazid should be included in all tuberculosis treatment regimens unless the organism is resistant. Isoniazid is inexpensive, readily synthesized, available worldwide, highly selective for mycobacteria, and well tolerated, with only 5% of patients exhibiting adverse effects.

MECHANISM OF ACTION   Isoniazid is the hydrazide of isonicotinic acid, a small, water-soluble molecule that easily penetrates the cell. Its mechanism of action involves inhibition of mycolic acid cell-wall synthesis via oxygen-dependent pathways such as the catalase-peroxidase reaction. Isoniazid is bacteriostatic against resting bacilli and bactericidal against rapidly multiplying organisms, both extracellularly and intracellularly. The minimal inhibitory concentrations (MICs) of isoniazid for wild-type (untreated) strains of *M. tuberculosis* are <0.1 μg/mL, while those for *M. kansasii* are usually 0.5 to 2.0 μg/mL. The MICs of this drug for other NTM are often higher.

PHARMACOLOGY   Both oral and intramuscular preparations of isoniazid are readily absorbed. The standard adult daily oral dose of 300 mg produces peak serum levels of 3 to 5 μg/mL. Isoniazid diffuses well throughout the body and reaches therapeutic concentrations in serum, cerebrospinal fluid (CSF), and infected tissue, including caseous granulomas. Isoniazid is metabolized in the liver via acetylation and hydrolysis; its metabolites are excreted into the urine. The rate of acetylation is genetically controlled. The recommended daily dose for the treatment of tuberculosis in the United States is 5 mg/kg for adults and 10 to 20 mg/kg for children, with a maximal daily dose of 300 mg for both groups. (Tuberculosis organizations outside the United States have recommended 5 mg/kg daily for both groups.) For inter-

TABLE 149-3   *Monitoring Side Effects of Common Antituberculous Drugs*

Drug	Side Effect	Management
Rifampin	Rash	Observe patient/stop drug if significant
	Liver dysfunction	Monitor AST/limit alcohol consumption/monitor for hepatitis symptoms
	Flulike syndrome	Administer at least twice weekly/limit dose to 10 mg/kg (adults)
	Red-orange urine	Reassure patient
	Drug interactions	Consider monitoring levels of other drugs affected by rifampin, especially with contraceptives, anticoagulants, and digoxin/avoid use with protease inhibitors
	Fever, chills	Stop drug
Isoniazid	Hepatitis	Monitor AST/limit alcohol consumption/monitor for hepatitis symptoms/educate patient/stop drug at first symptoms of hepatitis (nausea, vomiting, anorexia, flulike syndrome)
	Peripheral neuritis	Administer vitamin B_6
	Optic neuritis	Administer vitamin B_6/stop drug
	Seizures	Administer vitamin B_6
Pyrazinamide	Hepatitis	Monitor AST/limit daily dosage to 15–30 mg/kg/discontinue with signs or symptoms of hepatitis
	Hyperuricemia	Monitor uric acid level only in cases of gout or renal failure
Ethambutol	Optic neuritis	Use 25 mg/kg daily only for first 2 months (except in drug-resistant tuberculosis), then use lower daily dose (15 mg/kg) when possible/monitor visual acuity (eye chart) and red-green color vision (Ishihara Color Book) at baseline and with any visual complaint/educate patient/stop drug at first change in vision, get ophthalmologic evaluation
Streptomycin, amikacin, capreomycin	Ototoxicity, renal toxicity	Limit dose and duration of therapy as much as possible/avoid daily therapy in patients >50 years old/monitor BUN and serum creatinine levels and possibly conduct audiometry before and as needed during therapy/question patient regularly about tinnitus, dizziness, vertigo, and decreased hearing/measure serum drug levels if possible/educate patient/stop drug at first development of adverse effect (usually tinnitus)

Note: AST, aspartate aminotransferase; BUN, blood urea nitrogen.

mittent therapy (usually directly observed), a maximal dose of 900 mg twice or thrice weekly is used. Even in moderate to severe renal failure, the adult dose rarely needs to be reduced below 200 mg/d. Although not approved by the Food and Drug Administration (FDA), intravenous isoniazid can be given in an urgent situation.

ADVERSE EFFECTS (Table 149-3)   The two most important adverse effects of isoniazid therapy are hepatotoxicity and peripheral neuropathy. Other adverse reactions are either rare or less significant and include rash (2%), fever (1.2%), anemia, acne, arthritic symptoms, a systemic lupus erythematosus–like syndrome, optic atrophy, seizures, and psychiatric symptoms. Isoniazid-associated hepatitis is idiosyncratic and increases in incidence with age, daily alcohol consumption, concomitant rifampin administration, and HIV infection as well as in women who are pregnant or in the immediate (3 months) postpartum period. Appropriate clinical monitoring of patients receiving isoniazid includes at least monthly questioning about hepatitis-related symptoms and filling of prescriptions for no more than 1 month's worth of medication. Clinical monitoring is essential for all patients since discontinuation of the drug at the onset of hepatitis symptoms reduces the risk of progression to fatal hepatitis. The Centers for Disease Control and Prevention (CDC) and the American Thoracic Society (ATS) recommend that serum concentrations of aspartate aminotransferase (AST) or alanine aminotransferase (ALT) be determined at baseline in patients with liver disorders or HIV infection, in women who are pregnant or in the immediate postpartum period (3 months), in persons with a history of liver disease (e.g., hepatitis B or C, alcoholic hepatitis, or cirrhosis), in persons who use alcohol regularly, and in other individuals at risk for chronic liver disease who are receiving isoniazid for treatment of latent tuberculosis. Baseline testing is no longer routinely indicated in persons >35 years of age. Routine laboratory monitoring during isoniazid treatment is indicated for patients whose baseline liver function tests yield abnormal results and for persons at risk for hepatic disease, including the groups just mentioned. Measurement of the ALT or AST level is certainly mandatory whenever a patient notices the onset of symptoms suggestive of isoniazid-associated hepatitis (e.g., fever, anorexia, nausea, vomiting, and/or a flulike syndrome including fever and myalgias), and treatment should be discontinued until the relationship between therapy and symptoms is ascertained. Several studies have demonstrated that many patients with isoniazid intolerance can be desensitized. The CDC/ATS recommends that discontin-

uation of isoniazid be strongly considered whenever an asymptomatic elevation of the AST or ALT level exceeds 150 to 200 IU (three to five times the upper limit of normal) in high-risk patients whose baseline values were normal. In one study, only 11 (0.1%) of 11,141 patients had hepatotoxic reactions to isoniazid during preventive treatment.

Peripheral neuritis associated with isoniazid is uncommon and probably relates to interference with pyridoxine (vitamin B_6) metabolism. The risk of isoniazid-related neurotoxicity is greatest for patients with preexisting disorders that also pose a risk of neuropathy, such as diabetes, alcohol abuse, or malnutrition. In these patients, the prophylactic administration of 25 to 50 mg of pyridoxine daily should be considered.

RESISTANCE   Isoniazid-resistant mutants of *M. tuberculosis* occur spontaneously at a rate of 1 in 10^5 to 10^6 organisms. The molecular sites of isoniazid resistance have been detailed. Most isoniazid-resistant strains have amino acid changes in either the catalase-peroxidase gene (*katG*) or the promoter of a two-gene locus known as *inhA*. Missense mutations or deletion of *katG* is also associated with reduced catalase and peroxidase activity. Rates of primary isoniazid resistance in untreated patients are much higher in many foreign-born populations than in populations born in the United States.

Pyrazinamide   A derivative of nicotinic acid, pyrazinamide is an important bactericidal drug used in short-course therapy for tuberculosis.

MECHANISM OF ACTION   Pyrazinamide is similar to isoniazid in its narrow spectrum of antibacterial activity, which essentially includes only *M. tuberculosis*. The drug is bactericidal to slowly metabolizing organisms located within the acidic environment of the phagocyte or caseous granuloma; it is active only at a pH of <6.0. Pyrazinamide is considered a prodrug and is converted by the tubercle bacillus to the active form pyrazinoic acid. The target for this compound is thought to be a fatty acid synthase gene (*fasI*). Susceptible strains of *M. tuberculosis* are inhibited by 20 μg/mL.

PHARMACOLOGY   Pyrazinamide is well absorbed after oral administration, with a plasma concentration range of 20 to 60 μg/mL 1 to 2 h after oral ingestion of the currently recommended adult daily dose of 15 to 30 mg/kg (maximum, 2 g/d). The drug is well distributed throughout the body. Levels in CSF are excellent, reaching 50 to 100% of levels in serum. The serum half-life of the drug is 9 to 11 h. Pyrazinamide is metabolized by at least two major pathways and one minor pathway in the liver; its several metabolites include pyrazinoic acid, 5-hydroxy-pyrazinamide, and 5-hydroxypyrazinoic acid. Pyrazinamide is not available in a parenteral formulation.

ADVERSE EFFECTS (Table 149-3) At the high dosages used in the past, hepatotoxicity was a prominent complication of pyrazinamide therapy. However, at the currently recommended dosages, the frequency of hepatotoxicity is no higher than that for concomitant isoniazid and rifampin therapy. Although pyrazinamide is recommended by international tuberculosis organizations for routine use in pregnancy, it is not recommended in the United States because of inadequate teratogenicity data (Table 149-1). The combination of rifampin/pyrazinamide once recommended for treatment of latent tuberculosis has recently been shown to have an unacceptably high rate of hepatitis. Hyperuricemia is a common adverse effect of pyrazinamide therapy; the incidence is probably reduced by concurrent rifampin therapy. Clinical gout is seen only rarely. Polyarthralgias are encountered fairly commonly but are not related to the hyperuricemia.

RESISTANCE Resistance to pyrazinamide is associated with loss of pyrazinamidase activity such that pyrazinamide is no longer converted to pyrazinoic acid. More than 90% of isolates with MICs of >100 μg/mL have mutations in the *pncA* gene, which encodes for pyrazinamidase. All strains of *M. bovis* are naturally resistant to pyrazinamide and have a point substitution within the *pncA* gene.

FIRST-LINE SUPPLEMENTAL DRUGS ■ Ethambutol A derivative of ethylenediamine, ethambutol is a water-soluble compound that is active only against mycobacteria. Susceptible species include *M. tuberculosis, M. marinum, M. kansasii,* and MAI. Among first-line drugs, ethambutol is the least potent against *M. tuberculosis.* It is used most often with rifampin for treatment of tuberculosis in patients who cannot tolerate isoniazid or who are thought or known to be infected with isoniazid-resistant organisms.

MECHANISM OF ACTION Ethambutol at standard doses is bacteriostatic against *M. tuberculosis.* Its primary mechanism of action appears to be inhibition of an arabinosyltransferase that mediates the polymerization of arabinose into arabinogalactan within the cell wall.

PHARMACOLOGY After oral administration, 75 to 80% of a dose of ethambutol is absorbed from the gastrointestinal tract. Peak serum levels of 2 to 4 μg/mL are achieved 2 to 4 h after the standard adult daily dose of 15 mg/kg. The drug's distribution throughout the body is adequate except in the CSF, where it reaches only low levels. However, ethambutol can reach CSF levels up to 50% as high as peak plasma levels when administered at a daily dosage of 25 mg/kg (which may be given in one daily dose) for the first 2 months, with subsequent reduction to 15 mg/kg. In cases of drug-resistant tuberculosis or where re-treatment is necessary, the higher dose may be given for the duration. For intermittent therapy, the dosage is 50 mg/kg twice weekly or 30 mg/kg thrice weekly. The dosage must be lowered for patients with renal insufficiency (a creatinine clearance rate of <50 mL/min) to prevent drug accumulation and toxicity.

ADVERSE EFFECTS (Table 149-3) Ethambutol is usually well tolerated. Retrobulbar optic neuritis is the most serious adverse effect; axial or central neuritis—the only form reported in patients taking doses of <30 mg/kg—involves the papillomacular bundle of fibers and results in reduced visual acuity, central scotoma, and loss of ability to see green. Symptoms of ocular toxicity typically develop several months after initiation of therapy, but rapid-onset optic neuritis has been reported. The risk of optic neuritis depends on the dose and duration of therapy: this reaction develops in 5% of patients receiving a daily dose of 25 mg/kg but in fewer than 1% of patients given a daily dose of 15 mg/kg. Patients taking the lower dose should be tested at baseline and whenever there is a subjective visual change for visual acuity and red-green color discrimination. Patients taking the higher dose should be tested at baseline, monthly thereafter, and whenever there is subjective

visual change. Intermittent (three times weekly) administration of ethambutol at 25 mg/kg per dose appears to be better tolerated than daily administration of 15 mg/kg, especially in elderly populations being treated for *M. avium* complex infection. Optic neuritis with associated visual loss is usually reversible, but recovery may take >6 months.

Other adverse effects of ethambutol are infrequent. Hyperuricemia occurs but is usually asymptomatic. Peripheral sensory neuropathy occurs in rare instances. Optic neuritis is rare at the low dose in children; however, the use of ethambutol in very young children is problematic because visual complications are difficult to monitor.

RESISTANCE Ethambutol resistance in *M. tuberculosis* most commonly relates to missense mutations in the *embB* gene that encodes for arabinosyltransferase. Such mutations have been found in 70% of resistant strains and involve amino acid replacements at position 306 or 406 in ~90% of cases. Species of NTM that are intrinsically resistant to ethambutol have variant amino acids in this region of the gene, while susceptible species have the same amino acid sequences as *M. tuberculosis.*

Streptomycin An aminoglycoside isolated from *Streptomyces griseus,* streptomycin is available for intramuscular and intravenous administration only. In the United States, it is the least-used first-line supplemental drug for tuberculosis because of its toxicity, the difficulty in obtaining adequate CSF levels, and the inconvenience of parenteral administration. In developing countries, however, streptomycin is frequently used because of its low cost. The drug is active against untreated strains of *M. tuberculosis, M. kansasii,* and *M. marinum* and against some strains of the *M. avium* complex at achievable serum levels.

MECHANISM OF ACTION Streptomycin inhibits protein synthesis by disruption of ribosomal function.

PHARMACOLOGY Serum levels of streptomycin peak at 25 to 40 μg/mL after a 1.0-g dose. Streptomycin is bactericidal for rapidly dividing extracellular mycobacteria but is ineffective in the acidic environment within the macrophage. It diffuses poorly into the meninges and, in patients with meningitis, reaches CSF levels that are only 20% of serum levels.

The usual adult dose of streptomycin for a 70-kg patient is 0.5 to 1.0 g (10 to 15 mg/kg) given intramuscularly daily or five times per week; the pediatric dose is 20 to 40 mg/kg daily, with a maximum of 1 g/d. Because streptomycin is eliminated almost exclusively by the kidneys, the dosage must be lowered and the frequency of administration reduced (to only two or three times per week) in most patients >50 years of age and in any patient with renal impairment (Table 149-1) or reduced body weight. Although this approach is not approved by the FDA, streptomycin can be given intravenously.

ADVERSE EFFECTS (Table 149-3) Adverse reactions to streptomycin therapy occur in 10 to 20% of recipients. Ototoxicity and renal toxicity are the most common and the most serious. Renal toxicity, usually manifested as nonoliguric renal failure, is less common with streptomycin than with other frequently used aminoglycosides, such as gentamicin. Ototoxicity involves both hearing loss and vestibular dysfunction. The latter is more common and includes loss of balance, vertigo, and tinnitus. Patients receiving streptomycin must be monitored carefully for these adverse effects. Less serious reactions include perioral paresthesia, eosinophilia, rash, and drug fever.

RESISTANCE Spontaneous resistance to streptomycin occurs in 1 in 10^5 to 10^7 organisms. In two-thirds of streptomycin-resistant strains of *M. tuberculosis,* mutations have been identified in one of two targets: a 16S rRNA gene (*rrs*) or the gene encoding ribosomal protein S12 (*rpsL*). Both targets are believed to be involved in streptomycin ribosomal binding. No mutational change has been identified in the other one-third of resistant isolates. Strains of *M. tuberculosis* resistant to streptomycin are not cross-resistant to capreomycin or amikacin.

SECOND-LINE ANTITUBERCULOUS DRUGS   Second-line and/or newer anti-tuberculosis agents are used either when tuberculosis is drug resistant or when first-line supplemental drugs are not available. The more important second-line drugs are discussed below in their general (descending) order of usefulness.

Quinolones   A surprisingly large number of fluorinated quinolones are being developed and studied as inhibitors of mycobacteria. Their mode of action presumably is the prevention of DNA synthesis through the inhibition of DNA gyrase. Ofloxacin, levofloxacin, ciprofloxacin, gatifloxacin, and moxifloxacin are active against many mycobacteria, including *M. tuberculosis*, *M. leprae*, *M. marinum*, *M. kansasii*, and *M. fortuitum*. These drugs are well absorbed orally, reach high serum levels, and distribute well to body tissues and fluids. While not approved for antituberculous therapy in the United States, ofloxacin—used in combination with isoniazid and rifampin for the treatment of pulmonary tuberculosis—has been as active and safe as ethambutol in initial trials. Adverse effects are relatively uncommon, occurring in 0.5 to 10% of cases and consisting mostly of benign reactions such as gastrointestinal intolerance, rashes, dizziness, and headache. However, more serious adverse effects are being reported and include confusion, seizures, interstitial nephritis, skin vasculitis, and acute renal failure. The quinolones are rapidly becoming some of the most important and effective drugs for the treatment of tuberculosis resistant to first-line essential drugs. Some experts would classify the quinolones as first-line supplemental agents. The quinolones can also be administered intravenously.

Mycobacterial resistance to the fluoroquinolones develops rapidly. Its molecular basis is complex; only some strains exhibit missense mutations in the A subunit (*gyrA* gene) of DNA gyrase. Fluoroquinolone-resistant tuberculosis is a source of growing concern. Antituberculous therapy with quinolones should be reserved for patients with multidrug resistance and for those who cannot tolerate first-line drugs.

Capreomycin   Capreomycin, a complex cyclic polypeptide antibiotic derived from *Streptomyces capreolus*, is similar to streptomycin in terms of dosing, mechanism of action, pharmacology, and toxicity. It is administered only by the intramuscular route in doses of 10 to 15 mg/kg daily or five times per week (maximal daily dose, 1 g), with peak blood levels of 20 to 40 μg/mL. After 2 to 4 months, the dosage should be reduced to 1 g two or three times a week. Cross-resistance to kanamycin and amikacin—but not to streptomycin—is common. After streptomycin, capreomycin is the injectable drug of choice for tuberculosis.

Rifabutin   Rifabutin, a semisynthetic rifamycin spiropiperidyl derivative, shares many characteristics with rifampin, including its activity against *M. tuberculosis*. Rifabutin is also active against some strains of rifampin-resistant *M. tuberculosis* and is more active than rifampin against the *M. avium* complex and other NTM. To date, rifabutin has been most useful in the prophylaxis of disseminated MAI infection and in the treatment of drug-resistant tuberculosis. Because it seems to exhibit more antituberculous activity than rifampin in vitro and in animals, its possible clinical advantages over rifampin are being evaluated. In a multinational trial in which either rifampin (600 mg/d) or rifabutin (150 mg/d) was administered in combination with isoniazid plus a 2-month regimen of pyrazinamide and ethambutol, the two rifamycins were equally effective and well tolerated in the treatment of newly diagnosed pulmonary tuberculosis. Rifabutin is recommended in place of rifampin for the treatment of HIV-positive individuals who are also taking a protease inhibitor because its effect on these agents is less pronounced (Table 149-2).

MECHANISM OF ACTION   In *Escherichia coli* and *Bacillus subtilis*, rifabutin inhibits DNA-dependent RNA polymerase in the same manner as rifampin. Its mode of action against mycobacteria is believed to be the same.

PHARMACOLOGY   The pharmacology of rifabutin is dramatically different from that of rifampin. Rifabutin is readily absorbed after a single oral dose of 300 mg and reaches peak serum levels (0.35 μg/mL) in 2 to 4 h. This lipophilic drug distributes best to tissues: tissue levels are 5 to 10 times higher than plasma levels. CSF concentrations are 30 to 70% of plasma levels in HIV-infected patients who have meningitis. The drug's slow clearance via hepatic metabolism and renal excretion results in a mean serum half-life of 45 h, which is much longer than the 3- to 5-h half-life of rifampin. Clarithromycin (but not azithromycin) and fluconazole appear to block the hepatic metabolism of rifabutin, with consequent increases in serum levels. When rifabutin is administered orally with food, its rate of absorption is slowed but the extent of absorption is unchanged. Adjustment of dosage is usually unnecessary in elderly patients and in patients with reduced hepatic or renal function (Table 149-1).

ADVERSE EFFECTS   The majority of rifabutin's adverse effects are dose related and occur most frequently in patients receiving >300 mg/d. Discontinuation of therapy because of adverse drug reactions is reported in 16% of patients receiving rifabutin as opposed to 8% of those receiving a placebo. The most common symptoms are gastrointestinal; other reactions include rash, headache, asthenia, chest pain, myalgia, and insomnia. Like those taking rifampin, most patients taking rifabutin have discolored (orange to tan) urine and other body fluids. Less common adverse reactions include fever, chills, a flulike syndrome, hepatitis, *Clostridium difficile*–associated diarrhea, a diffuse polymyalgia syndrome, and a yellow skin discoloration ("pseudojaundice"). After a rifabutin dose of 450 or 600 mg in combination with clarithromycin, anterior uveitis is reported in up to 40% of patients; also common at these high doses are hyperpigmentation and the polymyalgia/arthralgia syndrome. All of these conditions are reversible when treatment is discontinued. Laboratory abnormalities include neutropenia, leukopenia, thrombocytopenia, and increased levels of liver enzymes.

Rifabutin induces the hepatic cytochrome P450 enzymes but does so much less strongly than rifampin. Drugs whose metabolism is enhanced by rifabutin include anticoagulants, quinidine, oral contraceptives, sulfonylureas, analgesics, dapsone, narcotics, glucocorticoids, clarithromycin, zidovudine, protease inhibitors, nonnucleoside reverse transcriptase inhibitors, and cardiac glycosides.

RESISTANCE   Resistance to rifabutin is attributable to the same mechanism as that to rifampin—i.e., mutations involving the *rpoB* gene. However, of the 14 mutant *rpoB* alleles that confer resistance to rifampin, only 9 confer high-level resistance to rifabutin, while the remaining 5 result in only small changes in rifabutin MICs, which remain at ≤0.5 μg/mL. The MIC of rifabutin for susceptible strains of *M. tuberculosis* is low (<0.06 μg/mL), and the drug is considered clinically active against partially resistant strains that are inhibited by plasma levels of ≤0.5 μg/mL. Thus rifabutin inhibits about one-quarter of rifampin-resistant strains of *M. tuberculosis*.

Amikacin   This well-known aminoglycoside is bactericidal to extracellular organisms. Amikacin is active against *M. tuberculosis* and several of the nontuberculous species, including the rapidly growing mycobacteria, *M. kansasii*, *M. leprae*, and the *M. avium* complex. The usual adult dosage is 7 to 10 mg/kg intramuscularly or intravenously three to five times per week (generally no more than 500 to 750 mg/d). Resistance relates to a single A → G base-pair change at position 1408 in the 16S ribosomal RNA gene.

Ethionamide   Like isoniazid and pyrazinamide, ethionamide is a derivative of isonicotinic acid. This agent is bacteriostatic against metabolizing *M. tuberculosis* and some NTM. It is most useful in the treatment of multidrug-resistant tuberculosis. However, its use is severely limited by its toxicity and frequent side effects, which include intense gastrointestinal intolerance (anorexia, vomiting, and dysgeusia), serious neurologic reactions, reversible hepatitis (5% of cases), hypersensitivity reactions, and hypothyroidism. Ethionamide is well absorbed orally and is widely distributed throughout the body at sites including the CSF.

Para-Aminosalicylic Acid PAS as a calcium or sodium salt inhibits the growth of *M. tuberculosis* by impairing folate synthesis. It is rarely indicated for the treatment of tuberculosis because of its low level of antituberculous activity and its high level of gastrointestinal toxicity (manifesting as nausea, vomiting, and diarrhea). Enteric-coated PAS granules (4 g every 8 h) may be better tolerated than other formulations and produce higher therapeutic blood levels. PAS is well absorbed after oral administration but reaches only low concentrations in the CSF. The drug has a short half-life (1 h), and 80% of the dose is excreted in the urine.

Cycloserine Cycloserine (D-4-amino-3-isoxazolidinone) is produced by *Streptomyces orchidaceus* and is active against a broad spectrum of bacteria, including *M. tuberculosis*. Cycloserine is well absorbed after oral administration and is widely distributed throughout body fluids, including the CSF. Serious side effects limit the use of this drug and include psychosis (with suicide in some cases), seizures, peripheral neuropathy, headaches, somnolence, and allergic reactions. Cycloserine should not be given to patients with epilepsy, active alcohol abuse, severe renal insufficiency, or a history of depression or psychosis.

NEWER ANTITUBERCULOUS DRUGS A number of drugs are being evaluated for their antituberculous activity. This group includes rifapentine, the newer 8-methoxyfluoroquinolones gatifloxacin and moxifloxacin, clarithromycin, linezolid and other oxazolidinones, and rifamycins not yet approved by the FDA, such as KRM-1648 (benzoxazinorifamycin).

Rifapentine A semisynthetic cyclopentyl rifamycin antibiotic, rifapentine has received accelerated approval from the FDA for the treatment of tuberculosis. It is the first new drug approved for tuberculosis in the United States in 25 years. While similar to rifampin, rifapentine is lipophilic and longer acting—characteristics that enhance patient compliance; the drug can be administered at a dose of 600 mg once or twice weekly. It is active against *M. tuberculosis* but has undergone only minimal testing against NTM. Rifapentine has not yet been approved for the treatment of patients with HIV disease because rifapentine/rifampin monoresistance frequently develops in HIV-positive patients receiving isoniazid plus once-weekly rifapentine. Like rifampin, rifapentine is active against many nonmycobacterial organisms, including *Haemophilus influenzae*, *Bordetella pertussis*, *Bordetella parapertussis*, *Brucella* spp., *Legionella* spp., *Neisseria* spp., streptococci, and staphylococci.

In a randomized comparative study, 672 Chinese patients received isoniazid plus either rifapentine or rifampin. The isoniazid/rifapentine group had a higher relapse rate than the isoniazid/rifampin group (10% vs 5%). Nevertheless, this disadvantage was considered acceptable in light of the lower rate of adverse effects and the less frequent administration for isoniazid/rifapentine.

MECHANISM OF ACTION Rifapentine exerts its bactericidal effect by inhibiting DNA-dependent RNA polymerase in susceptible bacteria. The MICs of rifapentine for rifampin-susceptible strains of *M. tuberculosis* range from 0.03 to 0.12 μg/mL.

PHARMACOLOGY Food enhances the oral absorption of rifapentine, whereas antacids impair its absorption. After oral administration with food, this drug reaches peak serum concentrations in 5 to 6 h and achieves a steady state in 10 days. The half-life of rifapentine and its active metabolite 25-desacetyl rifapentine is ~13 h. The administered dose is excreted via the liver (70%). Oral clearance is more rapid in males than in females (2.51 vs 1.69 L/h), but the clinical significance of this difference is unknown.

ADVERSE EFFECTS Rifapentine demonstrates an adverse-event pattern similar to that of rifampin. Both drugs are frequently associated with hyperuricemia when administered with pyrazinamide and with elevated hepatocellular enzyme levels in 3 to 4% of patients when ad-

ministered with other antituberculous agents. Liver enzyme levels should be monitored in patients receiving rifapentine who already have elevated liver enzyme concentrations or known liver disease. Like rifampin, rifapentine causes an orange-red discoloration of body fluids, including urine, saliva, and tears, and stains contact lenses.

Rifapentine induces the hepatic cytochrome P450 enzymes CYP3A4 and 2C8/9. Current induction studies suggest that its potential for drug-drug interaction may be less than that of rifampin but greater than that of rifabutin. Other drugs potentially affected by concomitant administration of rifapentine are listed in Table 149-2.

Rifapentine is in category C for use in pregnancy (Table 149-1) because of its teratogenesis in rats and rabbits. There are insufficient data concerning use of this drug in pregnant and breast-feeding patients.

RESISTANCE Strains of *M. tuberculosis* resistant to rifapentine, rifampin, and rifabutin all involve spontaneous point mutations in the *rpoB* gene. All strains resistant to rifampin are also resistant to rifapentine.

LEPROSY (HANSEN'S DISEASE)

Therapy for leprosy remains difficult, especially in developing countries. Obstacles include the long courses of drug therapy required, the high cost and low availability of most drugs, the frequency of adverse drug reactions, the difficulty of determining a treatment endpoint, and (given that *M. leprae* still cannot be grown in vitro) the difficulty of conducting susceptibility testing. While many drugs are active against *M. leprae*, efficacy in the treatment of leprosy has been established only for dapsone, rifampin, clofazimine, and ethionamide. Initiation of multidrug treatment has reduced the problem of acquired drug resistance seen previously with dapsone monotherapy.

Rifampin Rifampin is considered the most active agent for the treatment of leprosy. Its worldwide use is limited only by its cost. This drug is highly bactericidal against *M. leprae* and reduces the number of viable bacilli in patients' tissues faster than any other available agent. Rifampin must be combined with other antileprosy drugs to forestall resistance. For cost reasons, the drug dose of 600 mg is given once a month (supervised) outside the United States, but it is given daily in the United States. For details on pharmacology, adverse events, and resistance, see relevant sections under "Tuberculosis." Allergic interstitial nephritis is a rare but significant complication of rifampin use in Hansen's disease.

Dapsone Dapsone (4,4'-diaminodiphenylsulfone) inhibits bacterial folic acid synthesis. It is now considered the second most active drug (after rifampin) in the treatment of Hansen's disease because of its ready availability, low cost, and low toxicity and the susceptibility of untreated strains of *M. leprae* to low concentrations.

PHARMACOLOGY Dapsone is well absorbed orally and distributes well throughout the body. The usual daily dosage is 100 mg for adults and 0.9 to 1.4 mg/kg for children. Plasma concentrations peak within 1 to 3 h. The median elimination half-life is 22 h. Dapsone is cleared by acetylation in the liver, with genetic variation similar to that documented for the acetylation of isoniazid. The drug is 70% bound to plasma protein. Usual daily doses produce serum concentrations of 10 to 15 μg/mL, which far exceed the MIC for *M. leprae* (0.01 to 0.001 μg/mL).

ADVERSE EFFECTS Hemolysis and methemoglobinemia are common untoward reactions to dapsone. Patients should be screened for glucose-6-phosphate dehydrogenase deficiency to prevent serious drug-induced hemolysis. However, most patients tolerate dapsone therapy well with adequate clinical and laboratory supervision. Other side effects include gastrointestinal intolerance, headache, pruritus, peripheral neuropathies, nephrotic syndrome, fever, and rash. In lepromatous and borderline lepromatous leprosy, erythema nodosum leprosum (ENL) may occur. ENL and other reactions of leprosy may be difficult to distinguish from drug reactions and the infectious mononucleosis–like syndrome due to dapsone.

Clofazimine A phenazine iminoquinone dye, clofazimine is weakly bactericidal against *M. leprae*. It is useful in treating dapsone-resistant leprosy and may lessen the severity of ENL. Clofazimine's mode of action is not well understood, but the drug may inhibit DNA binding. It is absorbed orally and distributed to the fatty tissues and the reticuloendothelial system. Its serum half-life is ~60 to 70 days; only a small proportion of the dose is excreted daily into the urine or bile. Bactericidal activity is very slow and is evident for ~50 days after administration. The usual adult dosage is 50 to 100 mg/d, 100 mg three times a week, or (for treatment of ENL) 300 mg/d. Untoward effects include skin discoloration and, less commonly, gastrointestinal intolerance. Clofazimine was reported to be responsible for a case of cardiotoxicity induced via ventricular arrhythmia. Even though clofazimine-resistant disease has been reported only rarely when this agent is used alone, it should be used with other effective antibiotics. Clofazimine is active in vitro against some NTM species, including MAI, *M. kansasii*, *M. simiae*, and *M. abscessus*.

Ethionamide While ethionamide (250 mg/d) has not been approved by the FDA for the treatment of leprosy, it is sometimes used in the United States in combination with rifampin (600 mg/d) to treat dapsone-resistant leprosy in patients who cannot accept the skin-pigmentation effect of clofazimine. Because resistance to ethionamide develops quickly when the drug is used alone, it must be used with other effective agents. Patients should be monitored closely for hepatotoxicity when taking ethionamide (especially in combination with rifampin), and treatment should be discontinued if the patient's ALT levels exceed 2.5 times the normal value. Prothionamide, a congener of ethionamide that is not available in the United States, has pharmacologic properties similar to those of ethionamide and is widely used throughout the world.

Other Agents A number of other drugs exhibit significant activity against *M. leprae*, but clinical experience with these agents is lacking. Thalidomide is now approved by the FDA for treatment of ENL. This drug is sedating and extremely teratogenic and should *never* be taken by anyone who is or may become pregnant. Physicians wishing to prescribe thalidomide must register with the System for Thalidomide Education and Prescription Safety (S.T.E.P.S) at 1-888-423-5436 (Celgene Corporation); the sole exceptions to this registration requirement are physicians at Hansen's disease clinics that are receiving medication support from the national Hansen's disease program. It is noteworthy that ENL may be a presenting feature of Hansen's disease *before* treatment. It is not considered an adverse drug reaction but may be confused with drug reactional states.

The newer macrolide antibiotics (particularly clarithromycin), minocycline (a long-acting tetracycline), and a number of fluoroquinolones (including ofloxacin, sparfloxacin, and pefloxacin) have shown promising bactericidal activity against *M. leprae*. Ofloxacin and minocycline are being investigated with rifampin in short-course regimens for lepromatous disease. All of these newer leprosy drugs have low toxicity profiles, modes of action different from those of the established agents, and bactericidal activity against *M. leprae*. However, their levels of bactericidal activity are lower than that of rifampin.

NONTUBERCULOUS MYCOBACTERIA

Although less pathogenic than *M. tuberculosis*, NTM can cause pulmonary, skin, bone, joint, lymph node, and soft tissue infection as well as disseminated disease in immunocompromised hosts, including patients with AIDS. MAI and *M. kansasii* are the two most common causes of NTM pulmonary infection. Up to 40% of AIDS patients with CD4+ cell counts of $<50/\mu L$ develop disseminated disease due to *M. avium* unless they are receiving specific *M. avium* prophylaxis.

Clarithromycin Clarithromycin (6-0-methylerythromycin) is a newer macrolide that is similar to erythromycin in its mechanism of action. It is well absorbed with or without meals and elicits little gastrointestinal intolerance at low doses. Clarithromycin distributes well into body tissues and fluids and is highly concentrated in macrophages. The drug is metabolized in the liver, with ~30% of a given dose excreted in the urine. The dosage should be reduced if the creatinine clearance rate is ≤ 30 mL/min. Like erythromycin, clarithromycin binds with plasma proteins (65 to 70%) and can raise the levels of drugs such as theophylline and carbamazepine. Serum levels of clarithromycin are reduced by rifampin and, to a lesser degree, by rifabutin; clarithromycin increases serum levels of rifabutin and some antihistamines (e.g., terfenadine), thus potentially increasing their toxicity. Clarithromycin and (probably) azithromycin are the most active agents for the treatment of MAI infections; one of these drugs is considered an essential component of any regimen for this purpose. However, because of the risk of mutational drug resistance, clarithromycin should be given in combination with other agents, such as ethambutol and rifampin or rifabutin. The drug is also highly active against almost all other NTM, including *M. marinum*, *M. kansasii*, *M. haemophilum*, *M. genavense*, *M. xenopi*, *M. abscessus*, *M. chelonae*, and most isolates of *M. fortuitum*. Standard antimycobacterial doses have been 500 mg twice daily or, in the case of MAI pulmonary disease, three times weekly. The more common side effects of high doses include nausea, vomiting, and (occasionally) abnormal liver function tests. A bitter taste is common even with routine doses. Most gastrointestinal side effects can be minimized by reducing the dose. Clarithromycin is teratogenic in laboratory animals and is in category C for use in pregnancy (Table 149-1). Resistance results from point mutations involving adenine at positions 2058 or 2059 in the 23S ribosomal RNA gene macrolide binding site. Mutational resistance occurs in 1 in 10^8 to 10^9 organisms and develops with monotherapy, especially for all slowly growing species and the rapid growers *M. chelonae* and *M. abscessus*, which have only a single copy of the ribosomal genes.

Azithromycin Azithromycin is a macrolide that belongs to the family of azalides. This drug reaches much lower serum levels than clarithromycin (usually ≤ 0.5 $\mu g/mL$), but its high tissue and macrophage concentrations and longer half-life suggest the feasibility of intermittent therapy. Azithromycin is involved in few drug interactions since it does not affect the cytochrome P450 system. The usual doses are 250 to 500 mg three times weekly (MAI therapy) or 1200 mg once a week (prophylaxis for disseminated *M. avium*). No alteration in dose is required in renal failure. The most common side effects are gastrointestinal symptoms and reversible hearing loss. Azithromycin appears to be less active than clarithromycin for both pulmonary and disseminated MAI disease. Resistance to azithromycin develops by the same mechanism as that to clarithromycin, with cross-resistance between the two macrolides.

Therapy for Specific NTM Infections ■ *MAI*   Therapy for MAI lung disease in the adult usually involves the administration of clarithromycin (500 mg morning and night), ethambutol (25 mg/kg), and rifampin (600 mg) on a Monday-Wednesday-Friday schedule. Therapy is generally continued until cultures have been negative for 12 months.

For disseminated disease in AIDS, daily administration of one of the newer macrolides (clarithromycin or azithromycin) and ethambutol (15 mg/kg) is considered an essential component of any treatment regimen, with rifabutin (300 mg) a commonly used third drug. Other alternative drugs include streptomycin and amikacin. Clofazimine appears to increase mortality and should be avoided. For prophylaxis of disseminated MAI disease, rifabutin (300 mg/d), clarithromycin (500 mg twice daily), and azithromycin (1200 mg once weekly) have all been demonstrated to be effective in controlled or comparative clinical trials. Once-weekly azithromycin is the drug most often used.

MYCOBACTERIUM KANSASII   *M. kansasii* is usually susceptible to most antituberculous drugs except for pyrazinamide. Current ATS recommendations for the treatment of *M. kansasii* pulmonary disease are 18 to 24 months of daily isoniazid (300 mg), rifampin (600 mg), and ethambutol (15 mg/kg). In patients taking protease inhibitors, rifabutin (150 mg/d) or clarithromycin (500 mg twice daily) should be substituted for rifampin. The potential advantages of the highly active rifabutin and the newer macrolides in immunocompetent patients have not been studied.

RAPIDLY GROWING MYCOBACTERIA   The *M. fortuitum* group, *M. abscessus*, and *M. chelonae* account for more than 80% of cases of clinical disease due to rapidly growing mycobacteria. These organisms are resistant to antituberculous agents other than amikacin but are variably susceptible to several traditional antibiotics Clarithromycin has dramatically changed the approach to therapy for infection with these organisms, as it inhibits all rapidly growing mycobacteria (except for 20% of *M. fortuitum* strains and most *M. smegmatis* strains) at concentrations of ≤ 4 μg/mL. Other drugs with good activity include amikacin (which inhibits 80 to 100% of strains), cefoxitin (80% of *M. abscessus* and *M. fortuitum* strains), doxycycline (50% of *M. fortuitum* strains), imipenem (100% of *M. fortuitum* strains, 70% of *M. chelonae* strains, and 70% of *M. abscessus* strains), the fluorinated quinolones (100% of *M. fortuitum* strains), sulfonamides (90% of *M. fortuitum* strains), and linezolid (>90% of isolates of *M. chelonae* and *M. fortuitum*).

MYCOBACTERIUM MARINUM   *M. marinum*, a cause of posttraumatic localized skin infection, is typically susceptible to minocycline, rifampin, ethambutol, clarithromycin, and trimethoprim-sulfamethoxazole and is resistant to isoniazid.

MYCOBACTERIUM HAEMOPHILUM   Infection due to *M. haemophilum* occurs most commonly as disseminated cutaneous disease in immunocompromised patients with or without AIDS. Isolates typically show in vitro resistance to most drugs but may be susceptible to rifampin, rifabutin, quinolones, and clarithromycin.

MYCOBACTERIUM XENOPI   In the United States, *M. xenopi* is best known as a cause of nosocomial pseudoinfections associated with contamination of the hospital's hot-water system. Drug therapy for *M. xenopi* infection is difficult. *M. xenopi* is often resistant to first-line antituberculous agents but susceptible to the newer macrolides, quinolones, streptomycin, and ethionamide. Patients usually respond to multidrug regimens that include clarithromycin, but relapses are common.

MYCOBACTERIUM GENAVENSE   *M. genavense* is a fastidious organism that grows only in liquid media, such as BACTEC 12B or 13A, after prolonged incubation. This organism almost exclusively infects AIDS patients, causing disseminated disease and being isolated from blood, bone marrow, liver, lymph node, spleen, and intestinal cultures. The in vitro susceptibility profile of *M. genavense* has not been well established. Some isolates are susceptible to amikacin, clarithromycin, ofloxacin, rifampin, and rifabutin. Isolates generally respond to macrolide-containing regimens similar to those used for disseminated *M. avium* infection.

MYCOBACTERIUM SIMIAE   *M. simiae* is a cause of chronic lung disease, especially in Texas and other southwestern states. It is highly drug resistant, and no satisfactory treatment regimen has yet been established.

FURTHER READING

ALANGADEN GJ, LERNER SA: The clinical use of fluoroquinolones for the treatment of mycobacterial disease. Clin Infect Dis 25:1213, 1997

AMERICAN THORACIC SOCIETY: Targeted tuberculin testing and treatment of latent tuberculosis infection. Am J Respir Crit Care Med 161:S221, 2000

AMERICAN THORACIC SOCIETY/CENTERS FOR DISEASE CONTROL AND PREVENTION/INFECTIOUS DISEASES SOCIETY OF AMERICA: Treatment of tuberculosis. Am J Respir Crit Care Med 167:603–622, 2003 [special issue]

BOCK NN et al: A prospective, randomized, double-blind study of the tolerability of rifapentine 600, 900, and 1,200 mg plus isoniazid in the continuation phase of tuberculosis treatment. Am J Respir Crit Care Med 165: 1526, 2002

MUSSER JM: Antimicrobial agent resistance in mycobacteria: Molecular genetic insights. Clin Microbiol Rev 8:496, 1995

JASMER RM et al: Short-course rifampin and pyrazinamide compared with isoniazid for latent tuberculosis infection: A multicenter clinical trial. Ann Intern Med 137:640, 2002

WALLACE RJ JR et al: American Thoracic Society Statement: Diagnosis and treatment of disease caused by nontuberculous mycobacteria. Am J Respir Crit Care Med 156:S1, 1997

WHO EXPERT COMMITTEE ON LEPROSY: Seventh Report. Geneva, World Health Organization, 1998, Technical Report Series, No. 874

150   TUBERCULOSIS
Mario C. Raviglione, Richard J. O'Brien

DEFINITION   Tuberculosis, one of the oldest diseases known to affect humans, is caused by bacteria belonging to the *Mycobacterium tuberculosis* complex. The disease usually affects the lungs, although in up to one-third of cases other organs are involved. If properly treated, tuberculosis caused by drug-susceptible strains is curable in virtually all cases. If untreated, the disease may be fatal within 5 years in more than half of cases. Transmission usually takes place through the airborne spread of droplet nuclei produced by patients with infectious pulmonary tuberculosis.

ETIOLOGIC AGENT   Mycobacteria belong to the family Mycobacteriaceae and the order Actinomycetales. Of the pathogenic species belonging to the *M. tuberculosis* complex, the most frequent and important agent of human disease is *M. tuberculosis*. The complex includes *M. bovis* (the bovine tubercle bacillus, once an important cause of tuberculosis transmitted by unpasteurized milk and currently the cause of a small percentage of cases in developing countries), *M. africanum* (isolated from cases in West, Central, and East Africa), *M. microti* (the "vole" bacillus, a less virulent and rarely encountered organism), and *M. canettii* (a very rare isolate in African cases).

M. tuberculosis is a rod-shaped, non-spore-forming, thin aerobic bacterium measuring 0.5 μm by 3 μm. Mycobacteria, including *M. tuberculosis*, are often neutral on Gram's staining. However, once stained, the bacilli cannot be decolorized by acid alcohol, a character-istic justifying their classification as acid-fast bacilli (AFB; Fig. 150-1). Acid fastness is due mainly to the organisms' high content of mycolic acids, long-chain cross-linked fatty acids, and other cell-wall lipids. Microorganisms other than mycobacteria that display some acid fastness include species of *Nocardia* and *Rhodococcus*, *Legionella micdadei*, and the protozoa *Isospora* and *Cryptosporidium*. In the mycobacterial cell wall, lipids (e.g., mycolic acids) are linked to underlying arabinogalactan and peptidoglycan. This structure confers very low permeability of the cell wall, thus reducing effectiveness of most antibiotics. Another molecule in the mycobacterial cell wall, lipoarabinomannan, is involved in the pathogen-host interaction and facilitates the survival of *M. tuberculosis* within macrophages. The several proteins characteristic of *M. tuberculosis* include those in purified protein derivative (PPD) tuberculin, a precipitate of non-species-specific molecules obtained from filtrates of heat-sterilized, concentrated broth cultures. The complete genome sequence of *M. tuberculosis* comprises ~4000 genes and has a high guanine-plus-cytosine content. A large proportion of genes are devoted to the production of enzymes involved in cell wall metabolism.

EPIDEMIOLOGY   More than 3.8 million new cases of tuberculosis—all forms (pulmonary and extrapulmonary), 90% of them from developing countries—were reported to the World Health Organization (WHO) in 2001. However, because of a low level of case detection and incomplete notifications, reported cases represent only a fraction of the total. It is estimated that 8.5 million new cases of tuberculosis occurred worldwide in 2001, 95% of them in developing countries of Asia (5 million), Africa (2 million), the Middle East (0.6 million), and Latin

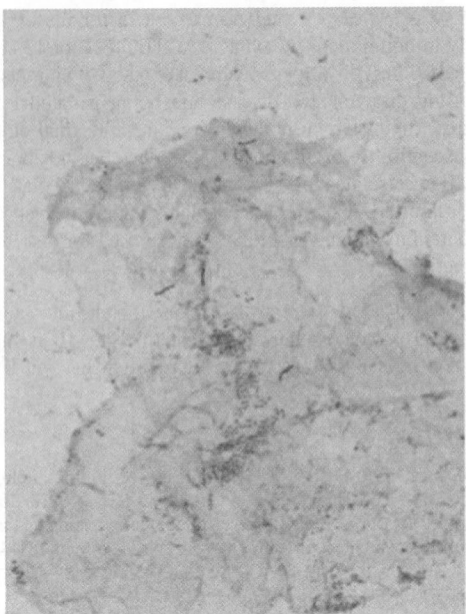

FIGURE 150-1   Acid-fast bacillus (AFB) smear showing *M. tuberculosis* bacilli. (*Courtesy of the CDC, Atlanta.*)

America (0.4 million). It is also estimated that 1.8 million deaths from tuberculosis occurred in 2000, 98% of them in developing countries. Estimates of tuberculosis incidence rates (per 100,000 population) and numbers of tuberculosis-related deaths in 2001 are depicted in Fig. 150-2 and Fig. 150-3, respectively.

After an increase in the late 1980s, numbers of cases have declined during the past few years in several industrialized countries, including the United States. The increases in the 1980s were largely related to immigration from countries with a high prevalence of tuberculosis; infection with HIV; social problems, such as poverty, homelessness, and drug abuse; and dismantling of tuberculosis services. In the United States, with the implementation of stronger control programs, the decrease resumed in 1993. In 2002, 15,075 cases of tuberculosis (5.2 cases per 100,000 population) were reported to the U.S. Centers for Disease Control and Prevention (CDC)—a 43% decrease from the 1992 peak.

In the United States, tuberculosis is uncommon among young adults of European descent, who have only rarely been exposed to *M. tuberculosis* infection during recent decades. In contrast, because of a

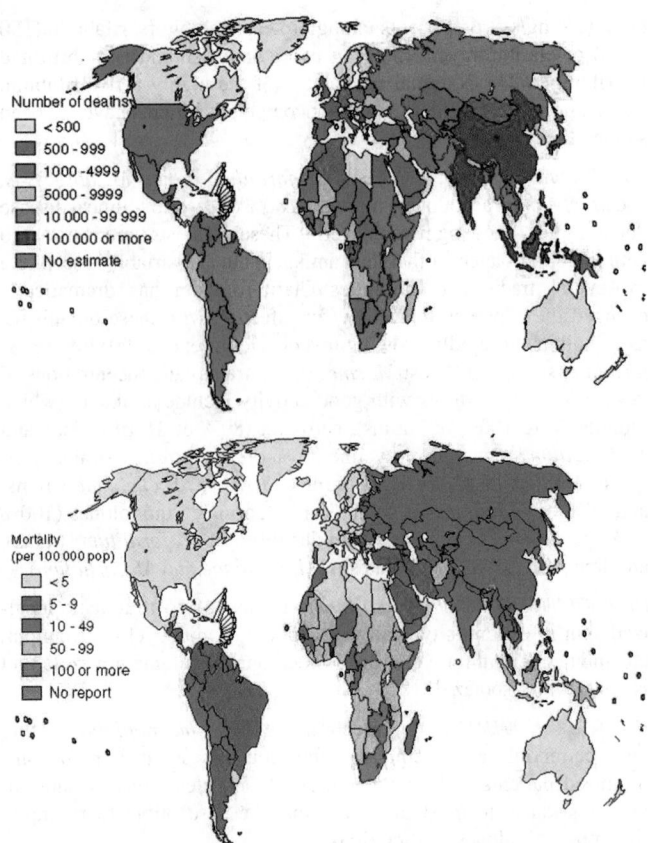

FIGURE 150-3   Maps of the world showing the estimated number of tuberculosis-related deaths and estimated tuberculosis mortality figures in 2001. (*See also disclaimer in Fig. 150-2. Courtesy of the Stop TB Department, WHO.*)

high risk in the past, the prevalence of *M. tuberculosis* infection is relatively high among elderly Caucasians, who remain at increased risk of developing active tuberculosis. Tuberculosis in the United States is also a disease of young adult members of the HIV-infected, immigrant, and disadvantaged/marginalized populations. Similarly, in Europe, tuberculosis has reemerged as an important public health problem, mainly as a result of cases among immigrants from high-prevalence countries.

Recent tuberculosis trends in developing countries indicate a stable situation, with almost no decline. There are two exceptions. First, in sub-Saharan Africa, the spread of the HIV epidemic has resulted in doubling or tripling of the number of reported cases of tuberculosis during the past 15 years. Second, in countries of the former Soviet Union and in Romania, numbers of cases have increased by two- or threefold in the past 10 years, largely as the result of deterioration in socioeconomic conditions and the health care infrastructure.

From Exposure to Infection   *M. tuberculosis* is most commonly transmitted from a patient with infectious pulmonary tuberculosis to other persons by droplet nuclei, which are aerosolized by coughing, sneezing, or speaking. The tiny droplets dry rapidly; the smallest (<10 μm in diameter) may remain suspended in the air for several hours and may gain direct access to the terminal air passages when inhaled. There may be as many as 3000 infectious nuclei per cough. Other routes of transmission of tubercle bacilli, such as through the skin or the placenta, are uncommon and of no epidemiologic significance.

The probability of contact with a case of tuberculosis, the intimacy and duration of that contact, the degree of infectiousness of the case, and the shared environment of the contact are all important determinants of transmission. Several studies of close contacts have clearly demonstrated that tuberculosis patients whose sputum contains AFB visible by microscopy play the greatest role in the spread of infection. These patients often have cavitary pulmonary disease or tuberculosis of the respiratory tract (endobronchial or laryngeal tuberculosis) and

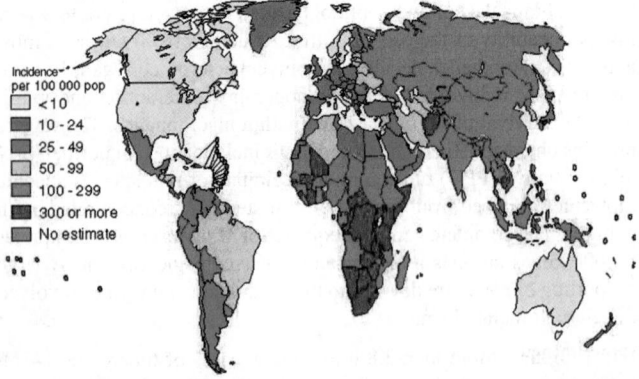

FIGURE 150-2   Map of the world showing the estimated tuberculosis incidence rates (per 100,000 population) in 2001. The designations employed and the presentation of material on this map do not imply the expression of any opinion whatsoever on the part of the WHO concerning the legal status of any country, territory, city or area or of its authorities, or concerning the delimitation of its frontiers or boundaries. White lines on maps represent approximate border lines for which there may not yet be full agreement. (*Courtesy of the Stop TB Department, WHO.*)

produce sputa containing as many as 10^5 AFB/mL. Patients with sputum smear–negative/culture-positive tuberculosis are less infectious, and those with culture-negative pulmonary disease and extrapulmonary tuberculosis are essentially noninfectious. The frequent absence of cavities among HIV-infected patients may reduce their infectiousness. Crowding in poorly ventilated rooms is one of the most important factors in the transmission of tubercle bacilli, since it increases the intensity of contact with a case.

In short, the risk of acquiring *M. tuberculosis* infection is determined mainly by exogenous factors. Because of delays in seeking care and in diagnosis, it is estimated that up to 20 contacts may be infected by each AFB-positive case before detection in high-prevalence settings.

From Infection to Disease   Unlike the risk of acquiring infection with *M. tuberculosis*, the risk of developing disease after being infected depends largely on endogenous factors, such as the individual's innate susceptibility to disease and level of function of cell-mediated immunity. Clinical illness directly following infection is classified as *primary tuberculosis* and is common among children up to 4 years of age. Although this form may be severe and disseminated, it is usually not transmissible. When infection is acquired later in life, the chance is greater that the immune system will contain it, at least temporarily. The majority of infected individuals who ultimately develop tuberculosis do so within the first year or two after infection. Dormant bacilli, however, may persist for years before reactivating to produce *secondary* (or *postprimary*) *tuberculosis*, which is often infectious. Overall, it is estimated that ~10% of persons infected in their youth will eventually develop active tuberculosis. This risk, however, is greatly increased among HIV-infected persons. Reinfection of a previously infected individual, which is common in areas with high rates of tuberculosis transmission, may also favor the development of disease. Molecular typing and comparison of strains of *M. tuberculosis* have suggested that up to one-third of cases of active tuberculosis in U.S. inner-city communities are due to recent transmission rather than to reactivation of latent infection.

Age is an important determinant of the risk of disease after infection. Among infected persons, the incidence of tuberculosis is highest during late adolescence and early adulthood; the reasons are unclear. The incidence among women peaks at 25 to 34 years of age. In this age group rates among women are usually higher than those among men, while at older ages the opposite is true. The risk may increase in the elderly, possibly because of waning immunity and comorbidity.

A variety of diseases and conditions favor the development of active tuberculosis (Table 150-1). The most potent risk factor for tuberculosis among infected individuals is clearly HIV co-infection, which suppresses cellular immunity. The risk that latent *M. tuberculosis* infection will proceed to active disease is directly related to the patient's degree of immunosuppression. In a study of HIV-infected, PPD-positive persons, this risk varied from 2.6 to 13.3 cases per 100 person-years and depended upon the CD4+ cell count.

TABLE 150-1   *Risk Factors for Active Tuberculosis among Persons Who Have Been Infected with Tubercle Bacilli*

Factor	Relative Risk/Odds[a]
Recent infection (<1 year)	12.9
Fibrotic lesions (spontaneously healed)	2–20
Comorbidity	
HIV infection	100
Silicosis	30
Chronic renal failure/hemodialysis	10–25
Diabetes	2–4
Intravenous drug use	10–30
Immunosuppressive treatment	10
Gastrectomy	2–5
Jejunoileal bypass	30–60
Posttransplantation period (renal, cardiac)	20–70
Malnutrition and severe underweight	2

[a] Old infection = 1.

NATURAL HISTORY OF DISEASE   Studies conducted in various countries before the advent of chemotherapy showed that untreated tuberculosis is often fatal. About one-third of patients died within 1 year after diagnosis, and one-half died within 5 years. Five-year mortality among sputum smear–positive cases was 65%. Of the survivors at 5 years, ~60% had undergone spontaneous remission, while the remainder were still excreting tubercle bacilli.

With effective, timely, and proper chemotherapy, patients have a very high chance of being cured. However, improper use of antituberculosis drugs, while reducing mortality, may also result in large numbers of chronic infectious cases, often with drug-resistant bacilli.

PATHOGENESIS AND IMMUNITY   The interaction of *M. tuberculosis* with the human host begins when droplet nuclei containing microorganisms from infectious patients are inhaled. While the majority of inhaled bacilli are trapped in the upper airways and expelled by ciliated mucosal cells, a fraction (usually <10%) reach the alveoli. There, nonspecifically activated alveolar macrophages ingest the bacilli. Invasion of macrophages by mycobacteria may result in part from association of C2a with the bacterial cell wall followed by C3b opsonization of the bacteria and recognition by the macrophages. The balance between the bactericidal activity of the macrophage and the number and virulence of the bacilli (with virulence partially linked to the bacterium's lipid-rich cell wall and to its glycolipid capsule, both of which confer resistance to complement and free radicals of the phagocyte) determines the events following phagocytosis.

Several genes thought to confer virulence to *M. tuberculosis* have been identified; *katG* encodes for catalase, an enzyme protective against oxidative stress; *rpoV* is the main sigma factor initiating transcription of several genes. Defects in these two genes result in loss of virulence. The *erp* gene, encoding a protein required for multiplication, also contributes to virulence. Outbreaks of tuberculosis in Tennessee and Kentucky in 1994 through 1996 exemplify how infection with virulent strains can result in enhanced transmission with high rates of disease. Strains of the Beijing/W genotype family have been identified in outbreak conditions in a variety of settings worldwide and have been associated with high mortality and drug resistance.

Several observations suggest that genetic factors play a key role in innate nonimmune resistance to infection with *M. tuberculosis*. The existence of this resistance is suggested by the differing degrees of susceptibility to tuberculosis in different populations. In mice, a gene called *Nramp1* (natural resistance–associated macrophage protein 1) has a regulatory role in resistance/susceptibility to mycobacteria. The human homologue NRAMP1, cloned to chromosome 2q, may have a role in determining susceptibility to tuberculosis, as is suggested by a study among West Africans.

In the initial stage of host-bacterium interaction, either the host's macrophages contain bacillary multiplication by producing proteolytic enzymes and cytokines or the bacilli begin to multiply. If the bacilli multiply, their growth quickly kills the macrophages, which lyse. Nonactivated monocytes attracted from the bloodstream to the site by various chemotactic factors ingest the bacilli released from the lysed macrophages. These initial stages of infection are usually asymptomatic.

About 2 to 4 weeks after infection, two additional host responses to *M. tuberculosis* develop: a tissue-damaging response and a macrophage-activating response. The *tissue-damaging response* is the result of a delayed-type hypersensitivity (DTH) reaction to various bacillary antigens; it destroys nonactivated macrophages that contain multiplying bacilli. The *macrophage-activating response* is a cell-mediated phenomenon resulting in the activation of macrophages that are capable of killing and digesting tubercle bacilli. Although both of these responses can inhibit mycobacterial growth, it is the balance between the two that determines the form of tuberculosis that will develop subsequently.

With the development of specific immunity and the accumulation of large numbers of activated macrophages at the site of the primary lesion, granulomatous lesions (tubercles) are formed. These lesions consist of lymphocytes and activated macrophages, such as epithelioid cells and giant cells. Initially, the newly developed tissue-damaging response is the only event capable of limiting mycobacterial growth within macrophages. This response, mediated by various bacterial products, not only destroys macrophages but also produces early solid necrosis in the center of the tubercle. Although *M. tuberculosis* can survive, its growth is inhibited within this necrotic environment by low oxygen tension and low pH. At this point, some lesions may heal by fibrosis and calcification, while others undergo further evolution.

Cell-mediated immunity is critical at this early stage. In the majority of infected individuals, local macrophages are activated when bacillary antigens processed by macrophages stimulate T lymphocytes to release a variety of lymphokines. These activated cells aggregate around the lesion's center and effectively neutralize tubercle bacilli without causing further tissue destruction. In the central part of the lesion, the necrotic material resembles soft cheese (*caseous necrosis*)—a phenomenon that may also be observed in other conditions, such as neoplasms. Even when healing takes place, viable bacilli may remain dormant within macrophages or in the necrotic material for years or even throughout the patient's lifetime. These "healed" lesions in the lung parenchyma and hilar lymph nodes may later undergo calcification.

In a minority of cases, the macrophage-activating response is weak, and mycobacterial growth can be inhibited only by intensified DTH reactions, which lead to tissue destruction. The lesion tends to enlarge further, and the surrounding tissue is progressively damaged. At the center of the lesion, the caseous material liquefies. Bronchial walls as well as blood vessels are invaded and destroyed, and cavities are formed. The liquefied caseous material, containing large numbers of bacilli, is drained through bronchi. Within the cavity, tubercle bacilli multiply well and spread into the airways and the environment through expectorated sputum.

In the early stages of infection, bacilli are usually transported by macrophages to regional lymph nodes, from which they disseminate widely to many organs and tissues. The resulting lesions may undergo the same evolution as those in the lungs, although most tend to heal. In young children with poor natural immunity, hematogenous dissemination may result in fatal miliary tuberculosis or tuberculous meningitis.

Cell-mediated immunity confers partial protection against *M. tuberculosis*, while humoral immunity has no defined role in protection. Two types of cells are essential: macrophages, which directly phagocytize tubercle bacilli, and T cells (mainly CD4+ lymphocytes), which induce protection through the production of lymphokines, especially interferon γ (IFN-γ).

After infection with *M. tuberculosis*, alveolar macrophages secrete a number of cytokines: interleukin (IL) 1 contributes to fever; IL-6 contributes to hyperglobulinemia; and tumor necrosis factor α (TNF-α) contributes to the killing of mycobacteria, the formation of granulomas, and a number of systemic effects, such as fever and weight loss. Macrophages are also critical in processing and presenting antigens to T lymphocytes; the result is a proliferation of CD4+ lymphocytes, which are crucial to the host's defense against *M. tuberculosis*. Qualitative and quantitative defects of CD4+ T cells explain the inability of HIV-infected individuals to contain mycobacterial proliferation. Reactive CD4+ lymphocytes produce cytokines of the T_H1 pattern and participate in MHC class II–restricted killing of cells infected with *M. tuberculosis*. T_H1 CD4+ cells produce IFN-γ and IL-2 and promote cell-mediated immunity. T_H2 cells produce IL-4, IL-5, and IL-10 and promote humoral immunity. The interplay of these various cytokines and their cross-regulation determine the host's response. The role of cytokines in promoting intracellular killing of mycobacteria has not been entirely elucidated. IFN-γ may induce release of nitric oxide, and TNF-α also seems to be important. Obser-

vations in transgenic knockout mice suggest that other T cell subsets (especially CD8+ cells) restricted by alternative antigen-presenting molecules containing a $β_2$-microglobulin subunit may play an important role. Lipids have been involved in mycobacterial recognition by the innate immune system, and lipoproteins have been proven to trigger potent signals through Toll-like receptors. Finally, a recently described subset of T cells capable of recognizing lipid elements of the bacillus presented by CD1 molecules may be implicated in protection.

M. tuberculosis possesses various protein antigens. Some are present in the cytoplasm and cell wall; others are secreted. That the latter are more important in eliciting a T lymphocyte response is suggested by experiments documenting the appearance of protective immunity in animals after immunization with live, protein-secreting mycobacteria. Among the antigens with a potential protective role are the 30-kDa (or 85B) and the ESAT-6 antigens. Protective immunity is probably the result of reactivity to a large number of different mycobacterial antigens.

Coincident with the appearance of immunity, DTH to *M. tuberculosis* develops. This reactivity is the basis of the PPD skin test, which is used primarily for the detection of *M. tuberculosis* infection in persons without symptoms. The cellular mechanisms responsible for PPD reactivity are related mainly to previously sensitized CD4+ lymphocytes, which are attracted to the skin-test site. There, they proliferate and produce cytokines.

While DTH is associated with protective immunity (PPD-positive persons being less susceptible to a new *M. tuberculosis* infection than PPD-negative persons), it by no means guarantees protection against reactivation. In fact, severe cases of active tuberculosis are often accompanied by strongly positive skin-test reactions.

CLINICAL MANIFESTATIONS   Tuberculosis is classified as pulmonary or extrapulmonary. Before the recognition of HIV infection, >80% of all cases of tuberculosis were limited to the lungs. However, up to two-thirds of HIV-infected patients with tuberculosis may have both pulmonary and extrapulmonary disease or extrapulmonary disease alone.

Pulmonary Tuberculosis   Pulmonary tuberculosis can be categorized as primary or postprimary (secondary).

PRIMARY DISEASE   Primary pulmonary tuberculosis results from an initial infection with tubercle bacilli. In areas of high tuberculosis prevalence, this form of disease is often seen in children and is frequently localized to the middle and lower lung zones. The lesion forming after infection is usually peripheral and accompanied by hilar or paratracheal lymphadenopathy, which may not be detectable on chest radiography. In the majority of cases, the lesion heals spontaneously and may later be evident as a small calcified nodule (*Ghon lesion*).

In children and in persons with impaired immunity (e.g., those with malnutrition or HIV infection), primary pulmonary tuberculosis may progress rapidly to clinical illness. The initial lesion increases in size and can evolve in different ways. Pleural effusion, a frequent finding, results from the penetration of bacilli into the pleural space from an adjacent subpleural focus. In severe cases, the primary site rapidly enlarges, its central portion undergoes necrosis, and acute cavitation develops (progressive primary tuberculosis). Tuberculosis in young children is almost invariably accompanied by hilar or mediastinal lymphadenopathy due to the spread of bacilli from the lung parenchyma through lymphatic vessels. Enlarged lymph nodes may compress bronchi, causing obstruction and subsequent segmental or lobar collapse. Partial obstruction may cause obstructive emphysema, and bronchiectasis may also develop. Hematogenous dissemination, which is common and is often asymptomatic, may result in the most severe manifestations of primary *M. tuberculosis* infection. Bacilli reach the bloodstream from the pulmonary lesion or the lymph nodes and disseminate into various organs, where they may produce granulomatous lesions. Although healing frequently takes place, immunocompromised persons (e.g., patients with HIV infection) may develop miliary tuberculosis and/or tuberculous meningitis.

POSTPRIMARY DISEASE Also called adult-type, reactivation, or secondary tuberculosis, postprimary disease results from endogenous reactivation of latent infection and is usually localized to the apical and posterior segments of the upper lobes, where the high oxygen concentration favors mycobacterial growth. In addition, the superior segments of the lower lobes are frequently involved. The extent of lung parenchymal involvement varies greatly, from small infiltrates to extensive cavitary disease. With cavity formation, liquefied necrotic contents are ultimately discharged into the airways, resulting in satellite lesions within the lungs that may in turn undergo cavitation (Fig. 150-4). Massive involvement of pulmonary segments or lobes, with coalescence of lesions, produces tuberculous pneumonia. While up to one-third of untreated patients reportedly succumb to severe pulmonary tuberculosis within a few weeks or months after onset, others undergo a process of spontaneous remission or proceed along a chronic, progressively debilitating course ("consumption"). Under these circumstances, some pulmonary lesions become fibrotic and may later calcify, but cavities persist in other parts of the lungs. Individuals with such chronic disease continue to discharge tubercle bacilli into the environment. Most patients respond to treatment, with defervescence, decreasing cough, weight gain, and a general improvement in well-being within several weeks.

Early in the course of disease, symptoms and signs are often nonspecific and insidious, consisting mainly of fever and night sweats, weight loss, anorexia, general malaise, and weakness. However, in the majority of cases, cough eventually develops—often initially nonproductive and subsequently accompanied by the production of purulent sputum. Blood streaking of the sputum is frequently documented. Massive hemoptysis may ensue as a consequence of the erosion of a fully patent vessel located in the wall of a cavity. Hemoptysis, however, may also result from rupture of a dilated vessel in a cavity (*Rasmussen's aneurysm*) or from aspergilloma formation in an old cavity. Pleuritic chest pain sometimes develops in patients with subpleural parenchymal lesions but can also result from muscle strain due to persistent coughing. Extensive disease may produce dyspnea and (occasionally) adult respiratory distress syndrome (ARDS).

Physical findings are of limited use in pulmonary tuberculosis. Many patients have no abnormalities detectable by chest examination, while others have detectable rales in the involved areas during inspiration, especially after coughing. Occasionally, rhonchi due to partial bronchial obstruction and classic amphoric breath sounds in areas with

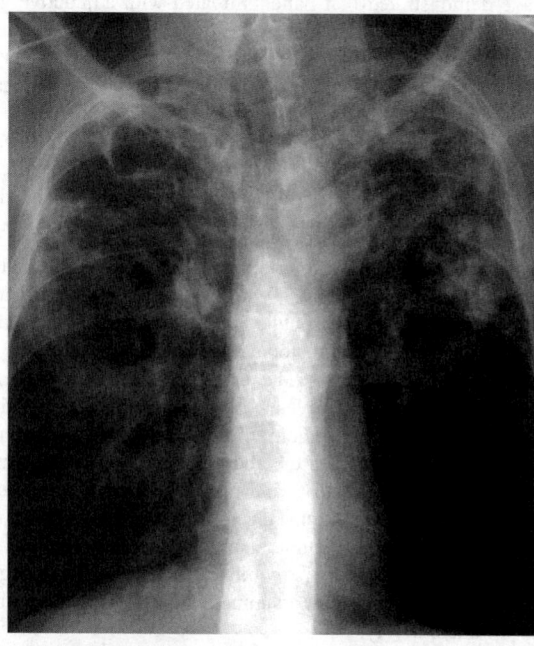

FIGURE 150-4 Chest radiograph showing bilateral upper-lobe infiltrates and cavities in a patient with active tuberculosis. (*Courtesy of L. Richeldi, G. Ferrera, and L. M. Fabbri, University of Modena and Reggio Emilia, Italy.*)

large cavities may be heard. Systemic features include fever (often low-grade and intermittent) and wasting. In some cases, pallor and finger clubbing develop. The most common hematologic findings are mild anemia and leukocytosis. Hyponatremia due to the syndrome of inappropriate secretion of antidiuretic hormone (SIADH) has also been reported.

Extrapulmonary Tuberculosis In order of frequency, the extrapulmonary sites most commonly involved in tuberculosis are the lymph nodes, pleura, genitourinary tract, bones and joints, meninges, peritoneum, and pericardium. However, virtually all organ systems may be affected. As a result of hematogenous dissemination in HIV-infected individuals, extrapulmonary tuberculosis is seen more commonly today than in the past.

LYMPH-NODE TUBERCULOSIS (TUBERCULOUS LYMPHADENITIS) The most common presentation of extrapulmonary tuberculosis (documented in >25% of cases), lymph-node disease is particularly frequent among HIV-infected patients. In the United States, children and women (particularly non-Caucasians) also seem to be especially susceptible. Once caused mainly by *M. bovis*, tuberculous lymphadenitis is today due largely to *M. tuberculosis*. Lymph-node tuberculosis presents as painless swelling of the lymph nodes, most commonly at cervical and supraclavicular sites (a condition often referred to as *scrofula*). Lymph nodes are usually discrete in early disease but may be inflamed and have a fistulous tract draining caseous material. Systemic symptoms are usually limited to HIV-infected patients, and concomitant lung disease may or may not be present. The diagnosis is established by fine-needle aspiration or surgical biopsy. AFB are seen in up to 50% of cases, cultures are positive in 70 to 80%, and histologic examination shows granulomatous lesions. Among HIV-infected patients, granulomas are usually not seen. Differential diagnosis includes a variety of infectious conditions as well as neoplastic diseases such as lymphomas or metastatic carcinomas.

PLEURAL TUBERCULOSIS Involvement of the pleura is common in primary tuberculosis and results from penetration by tubercle bacilli into the pleural space. Depending on the extent of reactivity, the effusion may be small, remain unnoticed, and resolve spontaneously or may be sufficiently large to cause symptoms such as fever, pleuritic chest pain, and dyspnea. Physical findings are those of pleural effusion: dullness to percussion and absence of breath sounds. A chest radiograph reveals the effusion and, in no more than one-third of cases, also shows a parenchymal lesion. Thoracentesis is required to ascertain the nature of the effusion. The fluid is straw colored and at times hemorrhagic; it is an exudate with a protein concentration >50% of that in serum, a normal to low glucose concentration, a pH that is generally <7.2, and detectable white blood cells (usually 500 to 2500/μL). Neutrophils may predominate in the early stage, while mononuclear cells are the typical finding later. Mesothelial cells are generally rare or absent. AFB are very rarely seen on direct smear, but cultures may be positive for *M. tuberculosis* in up to one-third of cases. Needle biopsy of the pleura is often required for diagnosis and reveals granulomas and/or yields a positive culture in up to 70% of cases. This form of pleural tuberculosis responds well to chemotherapy and may resolve spontaneously. The usefulness of glucocorticoids is debatable.

Tuberculous empyema is a less common complication of pulmonary tuberculosis. It is usually the result of the rupture of a cavity, with delivery of a large number of organisms into the pleural space, or of a bronchopleural fistula from a pulmonary lesion. A chest radiograph may show pyopneumothorax with an air-fluid level. The effusion is purulent and thick and contains large numbers of lymphocytes. An acid-fast smear of pleural fluid is often found to be positive when examined by microscopy, as is culture of the pleural fluid. Surgical drainage is usually required as an adjunct to chemotherapy. Tuberculous empyema may result in severe pleural fibrosis and restrictive lung disease.

TUBERCULOSIS OF THE UPPER AIRWAYS   Nearly always a complication of advanced cavitary pulmonary tuberculosis, tuberculosis of the upper airways may involve the larynx, pharynx, and epiglottis. Symptoms include hoarseness and dysphagia in addition to chronic productive cough. Findings depend on the site of involvement, and ulcerations may be seen on laryngoscopy. Acid-fast smear of the sputum is often positive, but biopsy may be necessary in some cases to establish the diagnosis. Cancer may have similar features but is usually painless.

GENITOURINARY TUBERCULOSIS   Genitourinary tuberculosis accounts for ~15% of all extrapulmonary cases, may involve any portion of the genitourinary tract, and is usually due to hematogenous seeding following primary infection. Local symptoms predominate. Urinary frequency, dysuria, hematuria, and flank pain are common presentations. However, patients may be asymptomatic and the disease discovered only after severe destructive lesions of the kidneys have developed. Urinalysis gives abnormal results in 90% of cases, revealing pyuria and hematuria. The documentation of culture-negative pyuria in acidic urine raises the suspicion of tuberculosis. An intravenous pyelogram helps in diagnosis. Calcifications and ureteral strictures are suggestive findings. Culture of three morning urine specimens yields a definitive diagnosis in nearly 90% of cases. Severe ureteral strictures may lead to hydronephrosis and renal damage.

Genital tuberculosis is diagnosed more commonly in female than in male patients. In female patients, it affects the fallopian tubes and the endometrium and may cause infertility, pelvic pain, and menstrual abnormalities. Diagnosis requires biopsy or culture of specimens obtained by dilatation and curettage. In male patients, tuberculosis preferentially affects the epididymis, producing a slightly tender mass that may drain externally through a fistulous tract; orchitis and prostatitis may also develop. In almost half of cases of genitourinary tuberculosis, urinary tract disease is also present. Genitourinary tuberculosis responds well to chemotherapy.

SKELETAL TUBERCULOSIS   In the United States, tuberculosis of the bones and joints is responsible for ~10% of extrapulmonary cases. In bone and joint disease, pathogenesis is related to reactivation of hematogenous foci or to spread from adjacent paravertebral lymph nodes. Weight-bearing joints (spine, hips, and knees—in that order) are affected most commonly. Spinal tuberculosis (Pott's disease or tuberculous spondylitis; Fig. 150-5) often involves two or more adjacent vertebral bodies. While the upper thoracic spine is the most common site of spinal tuberculosis in children, the lower thoracic and upper lumbar vertebrae are usually affected in adults. From the anterior superior or inferior angle of the vertebral body, the lesion reaches the adjacent body, also destroying the intervertebral disk. With advanced disease, collapse of vertebral bodies results in kyphosis (*gibbus*). A paravertebral "cold" abscess may also form. In the upper spine, this abscess may track to the chest wall as a mass; in the lower spine, it

may reach the inguinal ligaments or present as a psoas abscess. Computed tomography (CT) or magnetic resonance imaging (MRI) reveals the characteristic lesion and suggests its etiology, although the differential diagnosis includes other infections and tumors. Aspiration of the abscess or bone biopsy confirms the tuberculous etiology, as cultures are usually positive and histologic findings highly typical. A catastrophic complication of Pott's disease is paraplegia, which is usually due to an abscess or a lesion compressing the spinal cord. Paraparesis due to a large abscess is a medical emergency and requires abscess drainage. Tuberculosis of the hip joints causes pain and limping; tuberculosis of the knee produces pain and swelling and sometimes follows trauma. If the disease goes unrecognized, the joints may be destroyed. Skeletal tuberculosis responds to chemotherapy, but severe cases may require surgery.

TUBERCULOUS MENINGITIS AND TUBERCULOMA   Tuberculosis of the central nervous system accounts for ~5% of extrapulmonary cases. It is seen most often in young children but also develops in adults, especially those who are infected with HIV. Tuberculous meningitis results from the hematogenous spread of primary or postprimary pulmonary disease or from the rupture of a subependymal tubercle into the subarachnoid space. In more than half of cases, evidence of old pulmonary lesions or a miliary pattern is found on chest radiography. The disease may present subtly as headache and mental changes or acutely as confusion, lethargy, altered sensorium, and neck rigidity. Typically, the disease evolves over 1 or 2 weeks, a course longer than that of bacterial meningitis. Paresis of cranial nerves (ocular nerves in particular) is a frequent finding, and the involvement of cerebral arteries may produce focal ischemia. Hydrocephalus is common. Lumbar puncture is the cornerstone of diagnosis. In general, examination of the cerebrospinal fluid (CSF) reveals a high leukocyte count (usually with a predominance of lymphocytes but often with a predominance of neutrophils in the early stage), a protein content of 1 to 8 g/L (100 to 800 mg/dL), and a low glucose concentration; however, any of these three parameters can be within the normal range. AFB are seen on direct smear of CSF sediment in only 20% of cases, but repeated lumbar punctures increase the yield. Culture of CSF is diagnostic in up to 80% of cases. Imaging studies (CT and MRI) may show hydrocephalus and abnormal enhancement of basal cisterns or ependyma. If unrecognized, tuberculous meningitis is uniformly fatal. This disease responds to chemotherapy; however, neurologic sequelae are documented in 25% of treated cases, in most of which the diagnosis has been delayed. Clinical trials have demonstrated that patients treated with adjunctive glucocorticoids experience a significantly faster resolution of CSF abnormalities and elevated CSF pressure. Adjunctive glucocorticoids (e.g., dexamethasone, up to 12 mg/d for 4 to 6 weeks) enhance the chances of survival and reduce the frequency of neurologic sequelae.

Tuberculoma, an uncommon manifestation of tuberculosis, presents as one or more space-occupying lesions and usually causes seizures and focal signs. CT or MRI reveals contrast-enhanced ring lesions, but biopsy is necessary to establish the diagnosis.

GASTROINTESTINAL TUBERCULOSIS   Any portion of the gastrointestinal tract may be affected by tuberculosis. Various pathogenetic mechanisms are involved: swallowing of sputum with direct seeding, hematogenous spread, or (although rare today) ingestion of milk from cows affected by bovine tuberculosis. The terminal ileum and the cecum are the sites most commonly involved. Abdominal pain (at times similar to that associated with appendicitis), diarrhea, obstruction, hematochezia, and a palpable mass in the abdomen are common findings at presentation. Fever, weight loss, and night sweats are also frequent. With intestinal-wall involvement, ulcerations and fistulae may simulate Crohn's disease. Anal fistulae should prompt an evaluation for rectal tuberculosis. As surgery is required in most cases, the diagnosis can be established by histologic examination and culture of specimens obtained intraoperatively.

Tuberculous peritonitis follows either the direct spread of tubercle bacilli from ruptured lymph nodes and intraabdominal organs or hematogenous seeding. Nonspecific abdominal pain, fever, and ascites

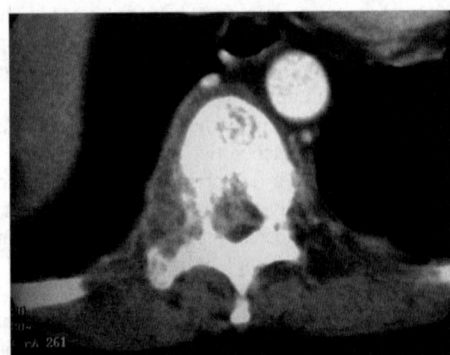

FIGURE 150-5   Computed tomography scan demonstrating destruction of the right pedicle of T10 due to Pott's disease. The patient, a 70-year-old Asian woman, presented with back pain and weight loss and had biopsy-proven tuberculosis. (*Courtesy of Charles L. Daley, M.D., University of California, San Francisco.*)

should raise the suspicion of tuberculous peritonitis. The coexistence of cirrhosis (Chap. 288) in patients with tuberculous peritonitis complicates the diagnosis. In tuberculous peritonitis, paracentesis reveals an exudative fluid with a high protein content and leukocytosis that is usually lymphocytic (although neutrophils occasionally predominate). The yield of direct smear and culture is relatively low; culture of a large volume of ascitic fluid can increase the yield, but peritoneal biopsy is often needed to establish the diagnosis.

PERICARDIAL TUBERCULOSIS (TUBERCULOUS PERICARDITIS) Due to direct progression of a primary focus within the pericardium, to reactivation of a latent focus, or to rupture of an adjacent lymph node, pericardial tuberculosis has often been a disease of the elderly in countries with low tuberculosis prevalence but also develops frequently in HIV-infected patients. Case-fatality rates are as high as 40% in some series. The onset may be subacute, although an acute presentation, with fever, dull retrosternal pain, and a friction rub, is possible. An effusion eventually develops in many cases; cardiovascular symptoms and signs of cardiac tamponade may ultimately appear (Chap. 222). In the presence of effusion detected on chest radiography, tuberculosis must be suspected if the patient belongs to a high-risk population (HIV-infected, originating in a high-prevalence country), if there is evidence of previous tuberculosis or disease in other organs, or if echocardiography shows thick strands crossing the pericardial space. Diagnosis can be facilitated by pericardiocentesis under echocardiographic guidance. The pericardial fluid must be submitted for biochemical, cytologic, and microbiologic study. The effusion is exudative in nature, with a high count of leukocytes (predominantly mononuclear cells). Hemorrhagic effusion is frequent. Culture of the fluid reveals *M. tuberculosis* in ~30% of cases, while biopsy has a higher yield. High levels of adenosine deaminase and IFN-γ may also suggest a tubercular etiology. Without treatment, pericardial tuberculosis is usually fatal. Even with treatment, complications may develop, including chronic constrictive pericarditis with thickening of the pericardium, fibrosis, and sometimes calcification, which may be visible on a chest radiograph. A course of glucocorticoid treatment (e.g., prednisone, 20 to 60 mg/d for up to 6 weeks) is useful in the management of acute disease, reducing effusion, facilitating hemodynamic recovery, and thus decreasing mortality. Progression to chronic constrictive pericarditis, however, seems unaffected by such therapy.

MILIARY OR DISSEMINATED TUBERCULOSIS Miliary tuberculosis is due to hematogenous spread of tubercle bacilli. Although in children it is often the consequence of a recent primary infection, in adults it may be due to either recent infection or reactivation of old disseminated foci. Lesions are usually yellowish granulomas 1 to 2 mm in diameter that resemble millet seeds (thus the term *miliary*, coined by nineteenth-century pathologists).

Clinical manifestations are nonspecific and protean, depending on the predominant site of involvement. Fever, night sweats, anorexia, weakness, and weight loss are presenting symptoms in the majority of cases. At times, patients have a cough and other respiratory symptoms due to pulmonary involvement as well as abdominal symptoms. Physical findings include hepatomegaly, splenomegaly, and lymphadenopathy. Eye examination may reveal choroidal tubercles, which are pathognomonic of miliary tuberculosis, in up to 30% of cases. Meningismus occurs in <10% of cases.

A high index of suspicion is required for the diagnosis of miliary tuberculosis. Frequently, chest radiography reveals a miliary reticulonodular pattern (more easily seen on underpenetrated film), although no radiographic abnormality may be evident early in the course and among HIV-infected patients. Other radiologic findings include large infiltrates, interstitial infiltrates (especially in HIV-infected patients), and pleural effusion. A sputum smear is negative in 80% of cases. Various hematologic abnormalities may be seen, including anemia with leukopenia, neutrophilic leukocytosis and leukemoid reactions, and polycythemia. Disseminated intravascular coagulation has been reported. Elevation of alkaline phosphatase levels and other abnormal values in liver function tests are detected in patients with severe hepatic involvement. The PPD test may be negative in up to half of cases, but reactivity may be restored during chemotherapy. Bronchoalveolar lavage and transbronchial biopsy are more likely to permit bacteriologic confirmation, and granulomas are evident in liver or bone-marrow biopsy specimens from many patients. If it goes unrecognized, miliary tuberculosis is lethal; with proper treatment, however, it is amenable to cure.

A rare presentation seen in the elderly is *cryptic miliary tuberculosis*, which has a chronic course characterized by mild intermittent fever, anemia, and—ultimately—meningeal involvement preceding death. An acute septicemic form, *nonreactive miliary tuberculosis*, occurs very rarely and is due to massive hematogenous dissemination of tubercle bacilli. Pancytopenia is common in this form of disease, which is rapidly fatal. At postmortem examination, multiple necrotic but nongranulomatous ("nonreactive") lesions are detected.

LESS COMMON EXTRAPULMONARY FORMS Tuberculosis may cause chorioretinitis, uveitis, panophthalmitis, and painful hypersensitivity-related phlyctenular conjunctivitis. Tuberculous otitis is rare and presents as hearing loss, otorrhea, and tympanic membrane perforation. In the nasopharynx, tuberculosis may simulate Wegener's granulomatosis. Cutaneous manifestations of tuberculosis include primary infection due to direct inoculation, abscesses and chronic ulcers, scrofuloderma, lupus vulgaris, miliary lesions, and erythema nodosum. Adrenal tuberculosis is a manifestation of advanced disease presenting as signs of adrenal insufficiency. Finally, congenital tuberculosis results from transplacental spread of tubercle bacilli to the fetus or from ingestion of contaminated amniotic fluid. This rare disease affects the liver, spleen, lymph nodes, and various other organs.

HIV-Associated Tuberculosis (See also Chap. 173) Tuberculosis is an important opportunistic disease among HIV-infected persons worldwide. In some African countries, the rate of HIV infection among tuberculosis patients may reach 70 to 80% in certain urban settings. A person with skin test–documented *M. tuberculosis* infection who acquires HIV infection has a 3 to 15% annual risk of developing active tuberculosis.

Tuberculosis can appear at any stage of HIV infection, and its presentation varies with the stage. When cell-mediated immunity is only partially compromised, pulmonary tuberculosis presents as a typical pattern (Fig. 150-4) of upper lobe infiltrates and cavitation, without significant lymphadenopathy or pleural effusion. In late stages of HIV infection, a primary tuberculosis–like pattern, with diffuse interstitial or miliary infiltrates, little or no cavitation, and intrathoracic lymphadenopathy, is more common. Overall, sputum smears may be positive less frequently among tuberculosis patients with HIV infection than among those without; thus the diagnosis of tuberculosis may be unusually difficult, especially in view of the variety of HIV-related pulmonary conditions mimicking tuberculosis.

Extrapulmonary tuberculosis is common among HIV-infected patients. In various series, extrapulmonary tuberculosis—alone or in association with pulmonary disease—has been documented in 40 to 60% of all cases in HIV co-infected individuals. The most common forms are lymphatic, disseminated, pleural, and pericardial. Mycobacteremia and meningitis are also frequent, particularly in advanced HIV disease.

The diagnosis of tuberculosis in HIV-infected patients may be difficult not only because of the increased frequency of sputum-smear negativity (up to 40% in culture-proven pulmonary cases) but also because of atypical radiographic findings, a lack of classic granuloma formation in the late stages, and negative results in PPD skin tests. Delays in treatment may prove fatal.

Recommendations for the prevention and treatment of tuberculosis in HIV-infected individuals are provided below.

DIAGNOSIS The key to the diagnosis of tuberculosis is a high index of suspicion. Diagnosis is not difficult with a high-risk patient—e.g., a homeless alcoholic who presents with typical symptoms and a classic chest radiograph showing upper lobe infiltrates with cavities (Fig.

150-4). On the other hand, the diagnosis can easily be missed in an elderly nursing-home resident or a teenager with a focal infiltrate.

Often, the diagnosis is first entertained when the chest radiograph of a patient being evaluated for respiratory symptoms is abnormal. If the patient has no complicating medical conditions that favor immunosuppression, the chest radiograph may show the typical picture of upper lobe infiltrates with cavitation (Fig. 150-4). The longer the delay between the onset of symptoms and the diagnosis, the more likely is the finding of cavitary disease. In contrast, immunosuppressed patients, including those with HIV infection, may have "atypical" findings on chest radiography—e.g., lower-zone infiltrates without cavity formation.

AFB Microscopy   A presumptive diagnosis is commonly based on the finding of AFB on microscopic examination of a diagnostic specimen such as a smear of expectorated sputum or of tissue (for example, a lymph node biopsy). Most modern laboratories processing large numbers of diagnostic specimens use auramine-rhodamine staining and fluorescence microscopy. The more traditional method—light microscopy of specimens stained with Kinyoun or Ziehl-Neelsen basic fuchsin dyes—is satisfactory, although more time-consuming. For patients with suspected pulmonary tuberculosis, three sputum specimens, preferably collected early in the morning, should be submitted to the laboratory for AFB smear and mycobacteriology culture. If tissue is obtained, it is critical that the portion of the specimen intended for culture not be put in formaldehyde. The use of AFB microscopy on urine or gastric lavage fluid is limited by the presence of mycobacterial commensals, which can cause false-positive results.

Mycobacterial Culture   Definitive diagnosis depends on the isolation and identification of *M. tuberculosis* from a diagnostic specimen—in most cases, a sputum specimen obtained from a patient with a productive cough. Specimens may be inoculated onto egg- or agar-based medium (e.g., Löwenstein-Jensen or Middlebrook 7H10) and incubated at 37°C under 5% CO_2. Because most species of mycobacteria, including *M. tuberculosis*, grow slowly, 4 to 8 weeks may be required before growth is detected. Although *M. tuberculosis* may be presumptively identified on the basis of growth time and colony pigmentation and morphology, a variety of biochemical tests have traditionally been used to speciate mycobacterial isolates. In today's laboratories, the use of liquid media for isolation and speciation by nucleic acid probes or high-pressure liquid chromatography of mycolic acids has replaced the traditional methods of isolation on solid media and identification by biochemical tests. These new methods have decreased the time required for bacteriologic confirmation to 2 to 3 weeks.

Nucleic Acid Amplification   Several test systems based on amplification of mycobacterial nucleic acid are available. These systems permit the diagnosis of tuberculosis in as little as several hours. However, their applicability is limited by low sensitivity (lower than culture, but higher than AFB smear microscopy) and high cost. At present, these tests are most useful for the rapid confirmation of tuberculosis in persons with AFB-positive sputa. However, they may also have utility for the diagnosis of AFB-negative pulmonary and extrapulmonary tuberculosis in selected patients.

Drug Susceptibility Testing   In general, the initial isolate of *M. tuberculosis* should be tested for susceptibility to isoniazid, rifampin, and ethambutol. In addition, expanded susceptibility testing is mandatory when resistance to one or more of these drugs is found or the patient either fails to respond to initial therapy or has a relapse after the completion of treatment (see below). Susceptibility testing may be conducted directly (with the clinical specimen) or indirectly (with mycobacterial cultures) on solid or liquid medium. Results are obtained most rapidly by direct susceptibility testing on liquid medium, with an average reporting time of 3 weeks. With indirect testing on solid medium, results may not be available for ≥8 weeks. Molecular methods for the rapid identification of drug resistance are becoming

available. One of the most promising uses polymerase chain reaction (PCR) to detect mutations in the *rpoB* gene associated with resistance to rifampin.

Radiographic Procedures   As noted above, the initial suspicion of pulmonary tuberculosis is often based on abnormal chest radiographic findings in a patient with respiratory symptoms. Although the "classic" picture is that of upper lobe disease with infiltrates and cavities (Fig. 150-4), virtually any radiographic pattern—from a normal film or a solitary pulmonary nodule to diffuse alveolar infiltrates in a patient with ARDS—may be seen. In the era of AIDS, no radiographic pattern can be considered pathognomonic.

PPD Skin Testing and Diagnosis of Latent Tuberculosis Infection   In 1891, Robert Koch discovered components of *M. tuberculosis* in a concentrated liquid culture medium. Subsequently named "old tuberculin" (OT), this material was initially believed to be useful in the treatment of tuberculosis (although this idea was later disproved). It soon became clear that OT was capable of eliciting a skin reaction when injected subcutaneously into patients with tuberculosis. In 1932, Seibert and Munday purified this product by ammonium sulfate precipitation. The result was an active protein fraction known as *tuberculin PPD*. However, the complexity and diversity of the constituents of PPD rendered its standardization difficult. PPD-S, developed by Seibert and Glenn in 1941, was chosen as the international standard. Later, the WHO and UNICEF sponsored large-scale production of a master batch of PPD, termed *RT23*, and made it available for general use. The greatest limitation of PPD is its lack of mycobacterial species specificity, a property that is due to the large number of proteins in this product that are highly conserved in the various species of mycobacteria.

Skin testing with PPD is most widely used in screening for *M. tuberculosis* infection (see below). The test is of limited value in the diagnosis of active tuberculosis because of its low sensitivity and specificity. False-negative reactions are common in immunosuppressed patients and in those with overwhelming tuberculosis. Positive reactions are obtained when patients have been infected with *M. tuberculosis* but do not have active disease and when persons have been sensitized by nontuberculous mycobacteria (Chap. 152) or bacille Calmette-Guérin (BCG) vaccination. Although BCG vaccine is not used in the United States for tuberculosis prevention, many immigrants will have received it. In the absence of a history of BCG vaccination, a positive skin test may provide additional support for the diagnosis of tuberculosis in culture-negative cases.

Because results of anergy testing in HIV-infected populations do not seem useful to clinicians making decisions about preventive therapy, anergy testing based on other DTH antigens is no longer recommended as a routine component of tuberculosis screening among HIV-infected persons. However, some experts support the use of anergy testing to help guide individual decisions regarding preventive therapy, and some recommend that PPD skin testing be performed for patients previously classified as anergic if evidence indicates that these patients' immune systems have responded to therapy with antiretroviral drugs.

Cytokine Release Assays   A commercially available whole-blood cytokine assay, the QuantiFERON-TB test (Cellestis Ltd), has been approved by the U.S. Food and Drug Administration (FDA) as an aid in the diagnosis of latent tuberculosis infection. The test requires overnight incubation of a peripheral-blood sample with PPD and control antigens followed by measurement of IFN-γ released by sensitized lymphocytes in an enzyme-linked immunosorbent assay (ELISA). A multicenter study conducted by the CDC indicated good agreement between this assay and the PPD skin test, although the assay's ability to predict the development of active tuberculosis is not known. At present, the QuantiFERON-TB test is recommended for screening for latent tuberculosis infection in populations at low to moderate risk of tuberculosis. Studies are under way to assess the performance of this test in contact investigations, persons with suspected tuberculosis disease, HIV-infected persons, and children. The test's performance will probably be enhanced by the use of antigens such as ESAT-6 and CPF-

10 that are present in *M. tuberculosis* but absent from BCG strains and most nontuberculous mycobacteria.

Additional Diagnostic Procedures Other diagnostic tests may be used when pulmonary tuberculosis is suspected. Sputum induction by ultrasonic nebulization of hypertonic saline may be useful for patients unable to produce a sputum specimen spontaneously. Frequently, patients with radiographic abnormalities that are consistent with other diagnoses (e.g., bronchogenic carcinoma) undergo fiberoptic bronchoscopy with bronchial brushings or transbronchial biopsy of the lesion. Bronchoalveolar lavage of a lung segment containing an abnormality may also be performed. In all cases, it is essential that specimens be submitted for AFB smear and mycobacterial culture. For the diagnosis of primary pulmonary tuberculosis in children, who often do not expectorate sputum, specimens from early-morning gastric lavage may yield positive cultures.

Invasive diagnostic procedures are indicated for patients with suspected extrapulmonary tuberculosis. In addition to specimens of involved sites (e.g., CSF for tuberculous meningitis, pleural fluid and biopsy samples for pleural disease), bone marrow and liver biopsy and culture have a good diagnostic yield in disseminated (miliary) tuberculosis, particularly in HIV-infected patients, who also have a high frequency of positive blood cultures.

In some cases, cultures will be negative, but a clinical diagnosis of tuberculosis will be supported by consistent epidemiologic evidence (e.g., a history of close contact with an infectious patient), a positive PPD skin test, and a compatible clinical and radiographic response to treatment. In the United States and other industrialized countries with low rates of tuberculosis, some patients with limited abnormalities on chest radiographs and sputum positive for AFB are infected with organisms of the *M. avium* complex or *M. kansasii* (Chap. 152). Factors favoring the diagnosis of nontuberculous mycobacterial disease over tuberculosis include an absence of risk factors for tuberculosis, a negative PPD skin test, and underlying chronic obstructive pulmonary disease.

Patients with HIV-associated tuberculosis pose several diagnostic problems, as noted above in the description of clinical manifestations. Moreover, HIV-infected patients with sputum culture–positive and AFB-positive tuberculosis may present with a normal chest radiograph. With the advent of highly active antiretroviral therapy (HAART), the occurrence of disseminated *M. avium* complex disease that can be confused with tuberculosis has become much less common.

Adjunctive Diagnostic Tests A number of methods have been evaluated as adjuncts to standard laboratory diagnosis. The most thoroughly investigated is serologic diagnosis based on detection of antibody to a variety of mycobacterial antigens. However, tests with most of the target antigens have a low predictive value when used in a population with a low probability of disease. Tests aimed at detection of mycobacterial antigen by serologic methods have generally been insufficiently sensitive to be useful.

℞ TREATMENT

The two aims of tuberculosis treatment are to interrupt tuberculosis transmission by rendering patients noninfectious and to prevent morbidity and mortality by curing patients with tuberculosis disease. Chemotherapy for tuberculosis became possible with the discovery of streptomycin in the mid-1940s. Randomized clinical trials clearly indicated that the administration of streptomycin to patients with chronic tuberculosis reduced mortality and led to cure in the majority of cases. However, monotherapy with streptomycin was frequently associated with the development of resistance to this drug and the attendant failure of treatment. With the discovery of para-aminosalicylic acid (PAS) and isoniazid, it became axiomatic that cure of tuberculosis required the concomitant administration of at least two agents to which the organism was susceptible. Furthermore, early clinical trials demonstrated that a long period of treatment—i.e., 12 to 24 months—was required to prevent the recurrence of tuberculosis.

The introduction of rifampin in the early 1970s heralded the era of effective short-course chemotherapy, with a treatment duration of <12 months. The discovery that pyrazinamide, which was first used in the 1950s, augmented the potency of isoniazid/rifampin regimens led to the use of a 6-month course of this triple-drug regimen as standard therapy.

DRUGS Four major drugs are considered the first-line agents for the treatment of tuberculosis: isoniazid, rifampin, pyrazinamide, and ethambutol (Table 150-2). These drugs are well absorbed after oral administration, with peak serum levels at 2 to 4 h and nearly complete elimination within 24 h. These agents are recommended on the basis of their bactericidal activity (ability to rapidly reduce the number of viable organisms and render patients noninfectious), their sterilizing activity (ability to kill all bacilli and thus sterilize the affected organ, measured in terms of the ability to prevent relapses), and their low rate of induction of drug resistance. Rifapentine and rifabutin, two drugs related to rifampin, are also available in the United States and are useful for selected patients. →*For a detailed discussion of the drugs used for the treatment of tuberculosis, see Chap. 149.*

Because of a lower degree of efficacy and a higher degree of intolerability and toxicity, a number of second-line drugs are generally used only for the treatment of patients with tuberculosis resistant to first-line drugs. Included in this group are the injectable drugs streptomycin (formerly a first-line agent), kanamycin, amikacin, and capreomycin and the oral agents ethionamide, cycloserine, and PAS. Recently, fluoroquinolone antibiotics have become the most commonly used second-line drugs. Of available agents, ofloxacin is the most widely used, but levofloxacin, gatifloxacin, and moxifloxacin are the most active. Other drugs of doubtful efficacy that have been used in the treatment of patients with resistance to most of the first- and second-line agents include clofazimine, amithiozone (thiacetazone, still used in less wealthy countries but not marketed in North America or Europe), amoxicillin/clavulanic acid, and linezolid.

REGIMENS Short-course regimens are divided into an initial, or bactericidal, phase and a continuation, or sterilizing, phase. During the initial phase, the majority of the tubercle bacilli are killed, symptoms resolve, and the patient becomes noninfectious. The continuation phase is required to eliminate persisting mycobacteria and prevent relapse.

The treatment regimen of choice for virtually all forms of tuberculosis in both adults and children consists of a 2-month initial phase of isoniazid, rifampin, pyrazinamide, and ethambutol followed by a 4-month continuation phase of isoniazid and rifampin (Table 150-3). Treatment may be given daily throughout the course or intermittently (either three times weekly throughout the course or twice weekly following an initial phase of daily therapy). A continuation phase of once-weekly rifapentine and isoniazid is equally effective for HIV-

TABLE 150-2 *Recommended Dosage for Initial Treatment of Tuberculosis in Adults[a]*

Drug	Dosage	
	Daily Dose	Thrice-Weekly Dose[b]
Isoniazid	5 mg/kg, max 300 mg	15 mg/kg, max 900 mg
Rifampin	10 mg/kg, max 600 mg	10 mg/kg, max 600 mg
Pyrazinamide	20–25 mg/kg, max 2 g	30–40 mg/kg, max 3 g
Ethambutol[c]	15–20 mg/kg	25–30 mg/kg

[a] Dosages for children are similar, except that some authorities recommend higher doses of isoniazid (10–15 mg/kg daily; 20–30 mg/kg intermittent) and rifampin (10–20 mg/kg).

[b] Dosages for twice-weekly administration are the same for isoniazid and rifampin but are higher for pyrazinamide (50 mg/kg, with a maximum of 4 g/d) and ethambutol (40–50 mg/d).

[c] In certain settings, streptomycin (15 mg/kg daily, with a maximum dose of 1 g; or 25–30 mg/kg thrice weekly, with a maximum dose of 1.5 g) can replace ethambutol in the initial phase of treatment. However, streptomycin is no longer considered a first-line drug by the ATS, the IDSA, or the CDC.

Source: Based on American Thoracic Society, Infectious Diseases Society of America, and Centers for Disease Control and Prevention.

TABLE 150-3 *Recommended Antituberculosis Treatment Regimens*

Indication	Initial Phase Duration, Months	Initial Phase Drugs	Continuation Phase Duration, Months	Continuation Phase Drugs
New smear- or culture-positive cases	2	HRZE[a,b]	4	HR[a,c,d]
New culture-negative cases	2	HRZE[a]	2	HR[a]
Pregnancy	2	HRE[e]	7	HR
Failure and relapse[f]	—	—	—	—
Resistance (or intolerance) to H	Throughout (6)	RZE[g]		
Resistance to H + R	Throughout (18–24)	ZEQ + S (or another injectable agent[h])		
Resistance to all first-line drugs	Throughout (24)	1 injectable agent[h] + 3 of these 4: ethionamide, cycloserine, Q, PAS		
Standardized re-treatment (susceptibility testing unavailable)	3	HRZES[i]	5	HRE
Drug intolerance to R	Throughout (12)[j]	HZE		
Drug intolerance to Z	2	HRE	7	HR

[a] All drugs can be given daily or intermittently (three times weekly throughout or twice weekly after 2 to 8 weeks of daily therapy during the initial phase).

[b] Streptomycin can be used in place of ethambutol but is no longer considered to be a first-line drug by ATS/IDSA/CDC.

[c] The continuation phase should be extended to 7 months for patients with cavitary pulmonary tuberculosis who remain sputum culture–positive after the initial phase of treatment.

[d] HIV-negative patients with noncavitary pulmonary tuberculosis who have negative sputum AFB smears after the initial phase of treatment can be given once-weekly rifapentine/isoniazid in the continuation phase.

[e] The 6-month regimen with pyrazinamide can probably be used safely during pregnancy and is recommended by the WHO and the International Union Against Tuberculosis and Lung Disease. If pyrazinamide is not included in the initial treatment regimen, the minimum duration of therapy is 9 months.

[f] Regimen is tailored according to the results of drug susceptibility tests.

[g] A fluoroquinolone (Q) may strengthen the regimen for patients with extensive disease.

[h] Amikacin, kanamycin, or capreomycin. All these agents should be discontinued after 2 to 6 months, depending upon tolerance and response.

[i] Streptomycin should be discontinued after 2 months. This regimen is less effective for patients in whom treatment has failed, who have an increased probability of rifampin-resistant disease. In such cases, the re-treatment regimen might include second-line drugs chosen in light of the likely pattern of drug resistance.

[j] Streptomycin for the initial 2 months or a fluoroquinolone might strengthen the regimen for patients with extensive disease.

Note: H, isoniazid; R, rifampin; Z, pyrazinamide; E, ethambutol; S, streptomycin; Q, a quinolone antibiotic; PAS, para-aminosalicylic acid.

seronegative patients with noncavitary pulmonary tuberculosis who have negative sputum cultures at 2 months. Intermittent treatment is especially useful for patients whose therapy is being directly observed (see below). Patients with cavitary pulmonary tuberculosis and delayed sputum-culture conversion (i.e., those who remain culture-positive at 2 months) should have their treatment extended by 3 months, for a total course of 9 months. For patients with sputum culture–negative pulmonary tuberculosis, the duration of treatment may be reduced to a total of 4 months. To prevent isoniazid-related neuropathy, pyridoxine (10 to 25 mg/d) should be added to the regimen given to persons at high risk of vitamin B6 deficiency (e.g., alcoholics; malnourished persons; pregnant and lactating women; and patients with conditions such as chronic renal failure, diabetes, and HIV infection or AIDS, which are also associated with neuropathy). A full course of therapy (completion of treatment) is defined more accurately by the total number of doses taken than by the length of treatment. Specific recommendations on the required numbers of doses for each of the various treatment regimens have been published jointly by the American Thoracic Society (ATS), the Infectious Diseases Society of America (IDSA), and the CDC.

Lack of adherence to treatment is recognized worldwide as the most important impediment to cure. Moreover, the tubercle bacilli infecting patients who do not adhere to the prescribed regimen are likely to become drug resistant. Both patient- and provider-related factors may affect compliance. Patient-related factors include a lack of belief that the illness is significant and/or that treatment will have a beneficial effect; the existence of concomitant medical conditions (notably substance abuse); lack of social support; and poverty, with attendant joblessness and homelessness. Provider-related factors that may promote compliance include the education and encouragement of patients, the offering of convenient clinic hours, and the provision of incentives and enablers such as meals and bus tokens.

In addition to specific measures addressing noncompliance, two other strategic approaches are used: direct observation of treatment and provision of fixed-drug-combination (FDC) products. Because it is difficult to predict which patients will adhere to the recommended treatment, all patients should have their therapy directly supervised, especially during the initial phase. In the United States, personnel to supervise therapy are usually available through tuberculosis control programs of local public health departments. Supervision increases the proportion of patients completing treatment and greatly lessens the chances of relapse and acquired drug resistance. FDC products (e.g., isoniazid/rifampin, isoniazid/rifampin/pyrazinamide, and isoniazid/rifampin/pyrazinamide/ethambutol) are available (except, in the United States, for the four-drug FDC) and strongly recommended as a means of minimizing the likelihood of prescription error and of the development of drug resistance as the result of monotherapy. In some formulations of these combination products, the bioavailability of rifampin has been found to be substandard. In North America and Europe, regulatory authorities ensure that combination products are of good quality; however, this type of quality assurance cannot be assumed to take place in less affluent countries. Alternative regimens for patients who exhibit drug intolerance or adverse reactions are listed in Table 150-3. However, severe side effects prompting discontinuation of any of the first-line drugs and use of these alternative regimens are uncommon.

MONITORING TREATMENT RESPONSE AND DRUG TOXICITY Bacteriologic evaluation is the preferred method of monitoring the response to treatment for tuberculosis. Patients with pulmonary disease should have their sputum examined monthly until cultures become negative. With the recommended regimen, >80% of patients will have negative sputum cultures at the end of the second month of treatment. By the end of the third month, virtually all patients should be culture-negative. In some patients, especially those with extensive cavitary disease and large numbers of organisms, AFB smear conversion may follow culture conversion. This phenomenon is presumably due to the expectoration and microscopic visualization of dead bacilli. As noted above, patients with cavitary disease who do not achieve sputum culture conversion by 2 months require extended treatment. When a patient's sputum cultures remain positive at ≥3 months, treatment failure and drug resistance should be suspected (see below). A sputum specimen should be collected by the end of treatment to document cure. If mycobacterial cultures are not practical, then monitoring by AFB smear examination should be undertaken at 2, 5, and 6 months. Smears positive after 5 months are indicative of treatment failure.

Bacteriologic monitoring of patients with extrapulmonary tuberculosis is more difficult and often is not feasible. In these cases, the response to treatment must be assessed clinically.

Monitoring of the response to treatment during chemotherapy by serial chest radiographs is not recommended, as radiographic changes may lag behind bacteriologic response and are not highly sensitive. After the completion of treatment, neither sputum examination nor chest radiography is recommended for follow-up purposes. However, a chest radiograph may be obtained at the end of treatment and used for comparative purposes should the patient develop symptoms of recurrent tuberculosis months or years later. Patients should be instructed to report promptly for medical assessment should they develop any such symptoms.

During treatment, patients should be monitored for drug toxicity (Table 149-3). The most common adverse reaction of significance is hepatitis. Patients should be carefully educated about the signs and symptoms of drug-induced hepatitis (e.g., dark urine, loss of appetite) and should be instructed to discontinue treatment promptly and see their health care provider should these symptoms occur. Although biochemical monitoring is not routinely recommended, all adult patients should undergo baseline assessment of liver function (e.g., measurement of serum levels of hepatic aminotransferases and serum bilirubin). Older patients, those with concomitant diseases, those with a history of hepatic disease, and those using alcohol daily should be monitored especially closely (i.e., monthly), with repeated measurements of aminotransferases, during the initial phase of treatment. Up to 20% of patients have small increases in aspartate aminotransferase (up to three times the upper limit of normal) that are accompanied by no symptoms and are of no consequence. For patients with symptomatic hepatitis and those with marked (five- to sixfold) elevations in serum levels of aspartate aminotransferase, treatment should be stopped and drugs reintroduced one at a time after liver function has returned to normal.

Hypersensitivity reactions usually require the discontinuation of all drugs and rechallenge to determine which agent is the culprit. Because of the variety of regimens available, it is usually not necessary—although it is possible—to desensitize patients. Hyperuricemia and arthralgia caused by pyrazinamide can usually be managed by the administration of acetylsalicylic acid; however, pyrazinamide treatment should be stopped if the patient develops gouty arthritis. Individuals who develop autoimmune thrombocytopenia secondary to rifampin therapy should not receive the drug thereafter. Similarly, the occurrence of optic neuritis with ethambutol is an indication for permanent discontinuation of this drug. Other common manifestations of drug intolerance, such as pruritus and gastrointestinal upset, can generally be managed without the interruption of therapy.

TREATMENT FAILURE AND RELAPSE As stated above, treatment failure should be suspected when a patient's sputum cultures remain positive after 3 months or when AFB smears remain positive after 5 months. In the management of such patients, it is imperative that the current isolate be tested for susceptibility to first- and second-line agents. When the results of susceptibility testing are expected to become available within a few weeks, changes in the regimen can be postponed until that time. However, if the patient's clinical condition is deteriorating, an earlier change in regimen may be indicated. A cardinal rule in the latter situation is always to add more than one drug at a time to a failing regimen: at least two and preferably three drugs that have never been used and to which the bacilli are likely to be susceptible should be added. The patient may continue to take isoniazid and rifampin along with these new agents pending the results of susceptibility tests.

The mycobacterial strains infecting patients who experience a relapse after apparently successful treatment are less likely to have acquired drug resistance (see below) than are strains from patients in whom treatment has failed. However, if the regimen administered initially does not contain rifampin (and thus is not a short-course regimen), the probability of isoniazid resistance is high. Acquired resistance is uncommon among strains from patients who relapse after completing a short-course regimen. However, it is prudent to begin the treatment of all relapses with all five first-line drugs pending the results of susceptibility testing. In less affluent countries and other settings where facilities for culture and drug susceptibility testing are not available, a standard regimen should be used in all instances of relapse and treatment failure (Table 150-3).

HIV-ASSOCIATED TUBERCULOSIS In general, the standard treatment regimens are equally efficacious in HIV-negative and HIV-positive patients. However, adverse drug effects may be more pronounced in HIV-infected patients. Since these effects may include serious or even fatal skin reactions to amithiozone (thiacetazone), this drug, which has been used in place of ethambutol in developing countries, is no longer recommended by WHO.

There are three important considerations relevant to tuberculosis treatment in HIV-infected patients: an increased frequency of paradoxical reactions, drug interactions between HAART and rifamycins, and development of rifampin monoresistance with widely spaced intermittent treatment. Exacerbations in symptoms, signs, and laboratory or radiographic manifestations of tuberculosis—termed *paradoxical reactions*—have been associated with the administration of HAART regimens. The presumed pathogenesis of paradoxical reactions is an immune response to antigens released as bacilli are killed by effective chemotherapy. In patients in whom HAART has recently been started, paradoxical reactions may be due to improving immune function. The first priority in the management of a possible paradoxical reaction is to ensure that the clinical syndrome does not represent a failure of tuberculosis treatment or the development of another infection. Mild paradoxical reactions can be managed with symptom-based treatment. Glucocorticoids have been used for more severe reactions, although this practice has not been formally evaluated in clinical trials.

Most HIV-infected tuberculosis patients are candidates for HAART, although the optimal timing for antiretroviral treatment is not known. Rifampin, a potent inducer of enzymes of the cytochrome P450 system, lowers serum levels of many HIV protease inhibitors and some nonnucleoside reverse transcriptase inhibitors, essential drugs used in HAART regimens. In such cases, rifabutin, which has much less enzyme-inducing activity, has been recommended in place of rifampin. However, dose adjustments for rifabutin and/or the antiretroviral drugs may be necessary. Because recommendations are frequently updated, consultation of the CDC website is advised (www.cdc.gov/nchstp/tb).

Several clinical trials of HIV-associated tuberculosis have found that patients with advanced immunosuppression (CD4+ cell counts of <100) are prone to treatment failure and relapse with rifampin-resistant organisms when treated with "highly intermittent" (i.e., once- or twice-weekly) rifamycin-containing regimens. Consequently, it is recommended that these patients receive daily or thrice-weekly therapy for the entire course.

DRUG-RESISTANT TUBERCULOSIS Strains of *M. tuberculosis* resistant to individual drugs arise by spontaneous point mutations in the mycobacterial genome, which occur at low but predictable rates. Because there is no cross-resistance among the commonly used drugs, the probability that a strain will be resistant to two drugs is the product of the probabilities of resistance to each drug and thus is low. The development of drug-resistant tuberculosis is invariably the result of monotherapy—i.e., the failure of the health care provider to prescribe at least two drugs to which tubercle bacilli are susceptible or of the patient to take properly prescribed therapy.

Drug-resistant tuberculosis may be either primary or acquired. Primary drug resistance is that in a strain infecting a patient who has not previously been treated. Acquired resistance develops during treatment with an inappropriate regimen. In North America and Europe, rates of primary resistance are generally low, and isoniazid resistance is most common. In the United States, while primary isoniazid resistance was stable at about 7 to 8% between 1993 and 2002, the rate of primary multidrug-resistant (MDR) tuberculosis declined from 2.5% to 1%. Resistance rates are higher among foreign-born and HIV-infected patients. Worldwide, MDR tuberculosis is a serious problem in some regions, especially in the former Soviet Union and parts of Asia. As noted above, drug-resistant tuberculosis can be prevented by adherence to the principles of sound therapy: the inclusion of at least two bactericidal drugs to which the organism is susceptible and the verification that patients complete the prescribed course.

Although the 6-month regimen described in Table 150-3 is generally effective for patients with initial isoniazid-resistant disease, it is prudent to include ethambutol and pyrazinamide for the full 6 months. In such cases, isoniazid probably does not contribute to a successful outcome and should be omitted. MDR tuberculosis is more difficult to manage than is disease caused by a drug-susceptible organism, especially because resistance to other first-line drugs as well as to isoniazid and rifampin is common. For strains resistant to isoniazid and rifampin, combinations of a fluoroquinolone, ethambutol, pyrazinamide, and streptomycin (or, for those resistant to streptomycin as well, another injectable agent such as amikacin), given for 18 to 24 months and for at least 9 months after sputum culture conversion, may be effective. For patients with bacilli resistant to all of the first-line agents, cure may be attained with a combination of four second-line drugs, including one injectable agent (Table 150-3). The optimal duration of treatment in this situation is not known; however, a duration of 24 months is recommended. For patients with localized disease and sufficient pulmonary reserve, lobectomy or pneumonectomy may be helpful. Because the management of patients with MDR tuberculosis is complicated by both social and medical factors, care of these patients should be restricted to specialists and tuberculosis control programs.

SPECIAL CLINICAL SITUATIONS Although comparative clinical trials of treatment for extrapulmonary tuberculosis are limited, the available evidence indicates that most forms of disease can be treated with the 6-month regimen recommended for patients with pulmonary disease. The American Academy of Pediatrics recommends that children with bone and joint tuberculosis, tuberculous meningitis, or miliary tuberculosis receive 9 to 12 months of treatment.

Treatment for tuberculosis may be complicated by underlying medical problems that require special consideration (Table 149-1). As a rule, patients with chronic renal failure should not receive aminoglycosides and should receive ethambutol only if serum levels can be monitored. Isoniazid, rifampin, and pyrazinamide may be given in the usual doses in cases of mild to moderate renal failure, but the dosages of isoniazid and pyrazinamide should be reduced for all patients with severe renal failure except those undergoing hemodialysis. Patients with hepatic disease pose a special problem because of the hepatotoxicity of isoniazid, rifampin, and pyrazinamide. Patients with severe hepatic disease may be treated with ethambutol and streptomycin and, if required, with isoniazid and rifampin under close supervision. The use of pyrazinamide by patients with liver failure should be avoided. Silicotuberculosis necessitates the extension of therapy by at least 2 months. The regimen of choice for pregnant women (Tables 149-1 and 150-3) is 9 months of treatment with isoniazid and rifampin supplemented by ethambutol for the first 2 months. When required, pyrazinamide may be given, although there are no data concerning its safety in pregnancy. Streptomycin is contraindicated because it is known to cause eighth-cranial-nerve damage in the fetus. Treatment for tuberculosis is not a contraindication to breast feeding; most of the drugs administered will be present in small quantities in breast milk, albeit at concentrations far too low to provide any therapeutic or prophylactic benefit to the child.

PREVENTION By far the best way to prevent tuberculosis is to diagnose infectious cases rapidly and administer appropriate treatment until cure. Additional strategies include BCG vaccination and treatment of persons with latent tuberculosis infection who are at high risk of developing active disease.

BCG Vaccination BCG was derived from an attenuated strain of *M. bovis* and was first administered to humans in 1921. Many BCG vaccines are available worldwide; all are derived from the original strain, but the vaccines vary in efficacy. In fact, estimates of efficacy from randomized, placebo-controlled trials have ranged from 80% to nil. A similar range of efficacy was found in recent observational studies (case-control, historic cohort, and cross-sectional) in areas where infants are vaccinated at birth. These studies also found higher rates of efficacy in the protection of infants and young children from relatively

serious forms of tuberculosis, such as tuberculous meningitis and miliary tuberculosis.

BCG vaccine is safe and rarely causes serious complications. The local tissue response begins 2 to 3 weeks after vaccination, with scar formation and healing within 3 months. Side effects—most commonly, ulceration at the vaccination site and regional lymphadenitis—occur in 1 to 10% of vaccinated persons. Some vaccine strains have caused osteomyelitis in ~1 case per million doses administered. Disseminated BCG infection and death have occurred in 1 to 10 cases per 10 million doses administered, although this problem is restricted almost exclusively to persons with impaired immunity, such as children with severe combined immunodeficiency syndrome or adults with HIV infection. BCG vaccination induces PPD reactivity, which tends to wane with time. The presence or size of PPD skin-test reactions after vaccination does not predict the degree of protection afforded.

BCG vaccine is recommended for routine use at birth in countries with high tuberculosis prevalence. However, because of the low risk of transmission of tuberculosis in the United States and the unreliable protection afforded by BCG, the vaccine has never been recommended for general use in the United States. The CDC has recommended that HIV-infected adults and children not receive BCG vaccine, although the WHO has recommended that asymptomatic HIV-infected children residing in tuberculosis-endemic areas receive BCG.

Treatment of Latent Tuberculosis Infection A major component of tuberculosis control in the United States is the treatment of selected persons with latent tuberculosis infection to prevent active disease. This intervention (formerly called preventive chemotherapy or chemoprophylaxis) is based on the results of a large number of randomized, placebo-controlled clinical trials demonstrating that a 6- to 12-month course of isoniazid reduces the risk of active tuberculosis in infected people by ≥90%. Analysis of available data indicates that the optimal duration of treatment is 9 to 10 months. In the absence of reinfection, the protective effect is believed to be lifelong. Clinical trials have also shown that isoniazid reduces rates of tuberculosis among PPD-positive persons with HIV infection. Studies in HIV-infected patients have demonstrated the effectiveness of shorter courses of rifampin-based treatment.

In most cases, candidates for treatment of latent tuberculosis (Table 150-4) are identified by PPD skin testing of persons in defined high-risk groups. For skin testing, 5 tuberculin units of polysorbate-stabilized PPD should be injected intradermally into the volar surface of the forearm (Mantoux method). Multipuncture tests, which may be useful for screening large populations, are not recommended for this purpose; any positive reaction to a multipuncture test must be confirmed by Mantoux testing. Reactions are read at 48 to 72 h as the transverse diameter in millimeters of induration; the diameter of erythema is not considered. In some persons, PPD reactivity wanes with time but can be recalled by a second skin test administered ≥1 week after the first (i.e., two-step testing). For persons undergoing periodic

TABLE 150-4 *Tuberculin Reaction Size, Treatment of Latent Tuberculosis Infection*

Risk Group	Tuberculin Reaction Size, mm
HIV-infected persons or persons receiving immunosuppressive therapy	≥5
Close contacts of tuberculosis patients	≥5[a]
Persons with fibrotic lesions on chest radiography	≥5
Recently infected persons (≤2 years)	≥10
Persons with high-risk medical conditions[b]	≥10
Low-risk persons[c]	≥15

[a] Tuberculin-negative contacts, especially children, should receive prophylaxis for 2 to 3 months after contact ends and should then be retested with PPD. Those whose results remain negative should discontinue prophylaxis. HIV-infected contacts should receive a full course of treatment regardless of PPD results.

[b] Includes diabetes mellitus, some hematologic and reticuloendothelial diseases, injection drug use (with HIV seronegativity), end-stage renal disease, and clinical situations associated with rapid weight loss.

[c] Decision to treat should be based on individual risk/benefit considerations.

PPD skin testing, such as health care workers and individuals admitted to long-term-care institutions, initial two-step testing may preclude subsequent misclassification of persons with boosted reactions as PPD converters.

The cutoff for a positive skin test (and thus for treatment) is related both to the probability that the reaction represents true infection and to the likelihood that the individual, if truly infected, will develop tuberculosis (Table 150-4). Thus positive reactions for close contacts of infectious cases, persons with HIV infection, persons receiving drugs that suppress the immune system, and previously untreated persons whose chest radiograph is consistent with healed tuberculosis are defined as an area of induration ≥5 mm in diameter. A 10-mm cutoff is used to define positive reactions in most other at-risk persons. For persons with a very low risk of developing tuberculosis if infected, a cutoff of 15 mm is used. Treatment should be considered for persons from tuberculosis-endemic countries who have a history of BCG vaccination.

Some PPD-negative individuals are also candidates for treatment. Infants and children who have come into contact with infectious cases should be treated and should have a repeat skin test 2 or 3 months after contact ends. Those whose test results remain negative should discontinue treatment. HIV-infected persons who have been exposed to an infectious tuberculosis patient should receive treatment regardless of the PPD test result.

Isoniazid is administered at a daily dose of 5 mg/kg (up to 300 mg/d) for 9 months (Table 150-5). On the basis of cost-benefit analyses, a 6-month period of treatment has been recommended in the past and may be considered for HIV-negative adults with normal chest radiographs when financial considerations are important. When supervised treatment is desirable and feasible, isoniazid may be given at a dose of 15 mg/kg (up to 900 mg) twice weekly. An alternative regimen for adults is 4 months of daily rifampin. A previously recommended regimen of 2 months of rifampin and pyrazinamide has been associated with serious and fatal hepatotoxicity and is now generally not recommended for use. The rifampin regimen should be considered for persons who are likely to have been infected with an isoniazid-resistant strain.

Isoniazid should not be given to persons with active liver disease. All persons at increased risk of hepatotoxicity (e.g., those abusing alcohol daily and those with a history of liver disease) should undergo baseline and then monthly assessment of liver function. All patients should be carefully educated about hepatitis and instructed to discontinue use of the drug immediately should any symptoms develop. Moreover, patients should be seen and questioned monthly during therapy about adverse reactions and should be given no more than 1 month's supply of drug at each visit.

It may be more difficult to ensure compliance when treating persons with latent infection than when treating those with active tuberculosis. If family members of active cases are being treated, compliance and monitoring may be easier. When feasible, twice-weekly supervised therapy may increase the likelihood of completion. As in active cases, the provision of incentives may also be helpful.

BASICS OF CONTROL The highest priority in any tuberculosis control program is the prompt detection of cases and the provision of short-course chemotherapy to all tuberculosis patients under proper case-management conditions, including directly observed therapy, with emphasis on the cure of sputum smear–positive cases. In addition, in low-prevalence countries with adequate resources, screening of high-risk groups (such as immigrants from high-prevalence countries and HIV-seropositive persons) is recommended. Identification of active cases of tuberculosis should be followed by treatment. PPD-positive high-risk persons should be treated for latent infection. Contact investigation is an important component of efficient tuberculosis control. In the United States, a great deal of attention has been given to the transmission of tuberculosis (particularly in association with HIV infection) in institutional settings such as hospitals, homeless shelters, and prisons. Measures to limit such transmission include respiratory isolation of persons with suspected tuberculosis until they are proven to be noninfectious (i.e., by sputum AFB smear negativity), proper ventilation in rooms of patients with infectious tuberculosis, use of ultraviolet lights in areas of increased risk of tuberculosis transmission, and

TABLE 150-5 Revised Drug Regimens for Treatment of Latent Tuberculosis Infection (LTBI) in Adults

Drug	Interval and Duration	Comments[a]	Rating[b] (Evidence[c]) HIV-Negative	HIV-Infected
Isoniazid	Daily for 9 months[d,e]	In HIV-infected persons, isoniazid may be administered concurrently with nucleoside reverse transcriptase inhibitors, protease inhibitors, or nonnucleoside reverse transcriptase inhibitors (NNRTIs).	A (II)	A (II)
	Twice weekly for 9 months[d,e]	Directly observed therapy (DOT) must be used with twice-weekly dosing.	B (II)	B (II)
	Daily for 6 months[e]	Regimen is not indicated for HIV-infected persons, those with fibrotic lesions on chest radiographs, or children.	B (I)	C (I)
	Twice weekly for 6 months[e]	DOT must be used with twice-weekly dosing.	B (II)	C (I)
Rifampin[f]	Daily for 4 months	Regimen is used for contacts of patients with isoniazid-resistant, rifampin-susceptible tuberculosis. In HIV-infected persons, most protease inhibitors and delavirdine should not be administered concurrently with rifampin. Rifabutin, with appropriate dose adjustments, can be used with protease inhibitors (saquinavir should be augmented with ritonavir) and NNRTIs (except delavirdine). Clinicians should consult web-based updates for the latest specific recommendations.	B (II)	B (III)
Rifampin plus pyrazinamide (RZ)	Daily for 2 months	Regimen generally should not be offered for treatment of LTBI in either HIV-infected or HIV-negative persons.	D (II)	D (II)
	Twice weekly for 2–3 months		D (III)	D (III)

[a] Interactions with HIV-related drugs are updated frequently and are available at http://www.aidsinfo.nih.gov/guidelines.
[b] Strength of the recommendation: A. Both strong evidence of efficacy and substantial clinical benefit support recommendation for use. Should always be offered. B. Moderate evidence for efficacy or strong evidence for efficacy, but only limited clinical benefit, supports recommendation for use. Should generally be offered. C. Evidence for efficacy is insufficient to support a recommendation for or against use, or evidence for efficacy might not outweigh adverse consequences (e.g., drug toxicity, drug interactions) or cost of the treatment or alternative approaches. Optional. D. Moderate evidence for lack of efficacy or for adverse outcome supports a recommendation against use. Should generally not be offered. E. Good evidence for lack of efficacy or for adverse outcome supports a recommendation against use. Should never be offered.
[c] Quality of evidence supporting the recommendation: I. Evidence from at least one properly randomized controlled trial. II. Evidence from at least one well-designed clinical trial without randomization, from cohort or case-controlled analytic studies (preferably from more than one center), from multiple time-series studies, or from dramatic results in uncontrolled experiments. III. Evidence from opinions of respected authorities based on clinical experience, descriptive studies, or reports of expert committees.
[d] Recommended regimen for persons aged <18 years.
[e] Recommended regimen for pregnant women.
[f] The substitution of rifapentine for rifampin is not recommended because rifapentine's safety and effectiveness have not been established for patients with LTBI.
Source: Adapted from CDC: Targeted tuberculin testing and treatment of latent tuberculosis infection. MMWR 49(RR-6), 2000

periodic screening of personnel who may come into contact with known or unsuspected cases of tuberculosis. In the past, radiographic surveys, especially those conducted with portable equipment and miniature films, were advocated for case finding. Today, however, the prevalence of tuberculosis in industrialized countries is sufficiently low that "mass miniature radiography" is not cost-effective.

In high-prevalence countries, tuberculosis control programs should be based on the following key elements defining the DOTS strategy promoted by the WHO: (1) political commitment by the government to sustained tuberculosis control; (2) case detection through microscopic examination of sputum from patients who present to health care facilities with cough of >2 to 3 weeks' duration; (3) administration of standard short-course chemotherapy to all sputum smear–positive patients under proper case-management conditions, including direct observation of drug ingestion; (4) establishment and maintenance of a system of regular drug supply; and (5) establishment and maintenance of an effective surveillance and monitoring system that allows assessment of treatment outcomes (e.g., cure, completion of treatment without bacteriologic proof of cure, death, treatment failure, and default) in all cases registered and notified.

FURTHER READING

AMERICAN THORACIC SOCIETY, CENTERS FOR DISEASE CONTROL AND PREVENTION: Targeted tuberculin testing and treatment of latent tuberculosis infection. Am J Respir Crit Care Med 161:S221, 2000

———, INFECTIOUS DISEASES SOCIETY OF AMERICA, CENTERS FOR DISEASE CONTROL AND PREVENTION: Treatment of tuberculosis. Am J Respir Crit Care Med 167:603, 2003

BURMAN WG, JONES BE: Treatment of HIV associated tuberculosis in the era of effective antiretroviral therapy. Am J Respir Crit Care Med 164:7, 2002

CEGIELSKI JP et al: The global tuberculosis situation: Progress and problems in the 20th century, prospects for the 21st century. Infect Dis Clin North Am 16:1, 2002

CORBETT EL et al: The growing burden of tuberculosis: Global trends and interaction with the HIV epidemic. Arch Intern Med 163:1009, 2003

TUBERCULOSIS TRIALS CONSORTIUM: Rifapentine and isoniazid once a week versus rifampicin and isoniazid twice a week for treatment of drug-susceptible pulmonary tuberculosis in HIV-negative patients: A randomized clinical trial. Lancet 360:528, 2002

WORLD HEALTH ORGANIZATION: *Treatment of Tuberculosis.* Guidelines for National Programmes. Geneva, World Health Organization, 2003

YOUNG DB: Ten years of research progress and what's to come. Tuberculosis 83:77, 2003

151 LEPROSY (HANSEN'S DISEASE)
Robert H. Gelber

Leprosy, first described in ancient Indian texts from the sixth century B.C., is a nonfatal, chronic infectious disease caused by *Mycobacterium leprae*, whose clinical manifestations are largely confined to the skin, peripheral nervous system, upper respiratory tract, eyes, and testes. The unique tropism of *M. leprae* for peripheral nerves (from large nerve trunks to microscopic dermal nerves) and certain immunologically mediated reactional states are the major causes of morbidity in leprosy. The propensity of the disease, when untreated, to result in characteristic deformities and the recognition in most cultures that the disease is communicable from person to person have resulted historically in a profound social stigma. Today, with early diagnosis and the institution of appropriate and effective antimicrobial therapy, patients can lead productive lives in the community, and deformities and other visible manifestations can largely be prevented.

ETIOLOGY *M. leprae* is an obligate intracellular bacillus (0.3 to 1 μm wide and 1 to 8 μm long) that is acid-fast, indistinguishable microscopically from other mycobacteria, and ideally detected in tissue sections by a modified Fite stain. Strain variability was recently discovered in this organism. *M. leprae* produces no known toxins and is well adapted to penetrate and reside within macrophages, yet it may survive outside the body for months. In untreated patients, only ~1% of *M. leprae* organisms are viable. The morphologic index (MI), a measure of the number of acid-fast bacilli (AFB) in skin scrapings that stain uniformly bright, correlates with viability. The bacteriologic index (BI), a logarithmic-scaled measure of the density of *M. leprae* in the dermis, may be as high as 4+ to 6+ in untreated patients, falling by one unit per year during effective therapy; the rate of fall is independent of the relative potency of effective antimicrobial therapy. A rising MI or BI suggests relapse and perhaps—if the patient is being treated—drug resistance; the latter possibility can be confirmed or excluded in the mouse model.

As a result of reductive evolution, almost half of the *M. leprae* genome contains nonfunctional genes; only 1605 genes encode for proteins. In contrast, *M. tuberculosis* uses 91% of its genome to encode for 4000 proteins. Among the lost genes in *M. leprae* are those for catabolic and respiratory pathways; transport systems; purine, methionine, and glutamine synthesis; and nitrogen regulation. The genome of *M. leprae* provides a metabolic rationale for its obligate intracellular existence and reliance on host biochemical support, a template for targets of drug development, and ultimately a pathway to cultivation. The recent finding of strain variability among *M. leprae* isolates provides a powerful tool with which to address anew the organism's epidemiology and pathobiology. The bacterium's complex cell wall has a peptidoglycan backbone, which is linked to arabinogalactan and mycolic acids. Lipoarabinomannan is a key component of the cell membrane, and the outer capsule contains large amounts of an *M. leprae*–specific phenolic glycolipid (PGL-1), which is detected in serologic tests.

Among the mycobacteria, *M. leprae* is unique in exhibiting dopa oxidase activity and an acid-fastness that is pyridine-extractable. Although it was the first bacterium to be etiologically associated with human disease, *M. leprae* remains one of the few bacterial species that still has not been cultivated on artificial medium or tissue culture. The multiplication of *M. leprae* in mouse footpads (albeit limited, with a doubling time of ~2 weeks) has provided a means to evaluate antimicrobial agents, monitor clinical trials, and screen vaccines. *M. leprae* grows best in cooler tissues (the skin, peripheral nerves, anterior chamber of the eye, upper respiratory tract, and testes), sparing warmer areas of the skin (the axilla, groin, scalp, and midline of the back).

EPIDEMIOLOGY ■ **Demographics** Leprosy is almost exclusively a disease of the developing world, affecting areas of Asia, Africa, Latin America, and the Pacific. While Africa has the highest disease prevalence, Asia has the most cases. More than 80% of the world's cases occur in a few countries: India, China, Myanmar, Indonesia, Brazil, Nigeria, Madagascar, and Nepal. Within endemic locales, the distribution of leprosy is quite uneven, with areas of high prevalence bordering on areas with little or no disease. In Brazil the majority of cases occur in the Amazon basin and two western states, while in Mexico leprosy is mostly confined to the Pacific coast. Except as imported cases, leprosy is largely absent from the United States, Canada, and northwestern Europe. In the United States, ~4000 persons have leprosy and 100 to 200 new cases are reported annually, most of them in California, Texas, New York, and Hawaii among immigrants from Mexico, Southeast Asia, the Philippines, and the Caribbean.

The global prevalence of leprosy is difficult to assess, given that many of the locales with high prevalence lack a significant medical or public health infrastructure. Estimates range from 0.6 to 8 million affected individuals. The lower estimate includes only persons who have not completed chemotherapy, excluding those who may be physically or psychologically damaged from leprosy and who may yet relapse or develop immune-mediated reactions; the higher figure includes patients whose infections probably are already cured and many who have no leprosy-related deformity or disability. Although the figures on the worldwide prevalence of leprosy are debatable, it is generally agreed that the annual incidence of new cases is rising (529,000 estimated new cases in 1995 and 719,000 in 2001, with 60% of the latter number from India alone).

Leprosy is associated with poverty and rural residence. It appears not to be associated with AIDS, perhaps because of leprosy's long incubation period. Most people appear to be naturally immune to leprosy and do not develop disease manifestations following exposure. The time of peak onset is in the second and third decades of life. The most severe polar form of leprosy is twice as common among men as among women and is rarely encountered in children. The frequency of the polar forms of leprosy in different countries varies widely and may in part be genetically determined; certain HLA associations are known for both polar forms of leprosy (see below). In India and Africa, 90% of cases are tuberculoid; in Southeast Asia, 50% are tuberculoid and 50% lepromatous; and in Mexico, 90% are lepromatous. (For definitions of disease types, see Table 151-1 and "Clinical, Histologic, and Immunologic Spectrum," below).

Transmission   The route of transmission of leprosy remains uncertain and may be multiple; nasal droplet infection, contact with infected soil, and even insect vectors have been considered the prime candidates. Aerosolized *M. leprae* can cause infection in immunosuppressed mice, and a sneeze from an untreated lepromatous patient may contain >10^{10} AFB. Furthermore, both IgA antibody to *M. leprae* and genes of *M. leprae*—demonstrable by polymerase chain reaction (PCR)—have been found in the nose of individuals without signs of leprosy from endemic areas and in 19% of occupational contacts of lepromatous patients.

Several lines of evidence implicate soil transmission of leprosy: (1) in endemic countries such as India, leprosy is primarily a rural and not an urban disease; (2) *M. leprae* products have been demonstrated to be resident in soil in endemic locales; and (3) direct dermal inoculation (e.g., during tattooing) may transmit *M. leprae*, and common sites of leprosy in children are the buttocks and thighs, suggesting that microinoculation of infected soil may transmit the disease.

Evidence for insect vectors of leprosy includes the demonstration that bedbugs and mosquitoes in the vicinity of leprosaria regularly harbor *M. leprae* and that experimentally infected mosquitoes can transmit infection to mice. Skin-to-skin contact is generally not considered an important route of transmission.

In endemic countries, ~50% of leprosy patients have a history of intimate contact with an infected person (often a household member), while, for unknown reasons, leprosy patients in nonendemic locales can identify such contact only 10% of the time. Moreover, household contact with an infected lepromatous case carries an eventual risk of disease acquisition of ~10% in endemic areas as opposed to only 1% in nonendemic locales. Contact with a tuberculoid case carries a very low risk. Physicians and nurses caring for leprosy patients and the coworkers of these patients are not at risk for leprosy.

M. leprae causes disease primarily in humans. However, in Texas and Louisiana, 15% of nine-banded armadillos are infected, and armadillo contact occasionally results in human disease; armadillos develop a disseminated infection following intravenous inoculation of live *M. leprae*.

CLINICAL, HISTOLOGIC, AND IMMUNOLOGIC SPECTRUM   The incubation period prior to manifestation of clinical disease can vary between 2 and 40 years, although it is generally 5 to 7 years in duration. Leprosy presents as a spectrum of clinical manifestations that have bacteriologic, pathologic, and immunologic counterparts. The spectrum from polar tuberculoid (TT) to borderline tuberculoid (BT) to mid-borderline (BB, which is rarely encountered) to borderline lepromatous (BL) to polar lepromatous (LL) disease is associated with an evolution from asymmetric localized macules and plaques to nodular and indurated symmetric generalized skin manifestations, an increasing bacterial

TABLE 151-1   *Clinical, Bacteriologic, Pathologic, and Immunologic Spectrum of Leprosy*

Clinical and Histologic Features	Tuberculoid (TT) Leprosy	Borderline Tuberculoid (BT) Leprosy	Mid-Borderline (BB) Leprosy	Borderline Lepromatous (BL) Leprosy	Lepromatous (LL) Leprosy
Skin Lesions	Up to 3 in number; sharply defined asymmetric macules or plaques with tendency toward central clearing, elevated borders	Smaller or larger than in TT; potentially more numerous than in TT; usually annular lesions with sharp margination on exterior and interior borders; borders not as elevated as in TT	Dimorphic lesions intermediate between BT and BL	LL-type lesions; ill-defined plaques with an occasional sharp margin; few or many in number, shiny appearance	Symmetric, poorly marginated, multiple infiltrated nodules and plaques or diffuse infiltration; xanthoma-like or dermatofibroma papules; leonine facies and eyebrow alopecia
Nerve lesions	Skin lesions anesthetic early; nerve near lesions sometimes enlarged	Skin lesions anesthetic early; nerve trunk palsies asymmetric; nerve abscesses most common in BT	Anesthetic skin lesions; nerve trunk palsies	Skin lesions usually hypoesthetic, may be anesthetic; nerve trunk palsies common and frequently symmetric	Hypesthesia a late sign; nerve palsies variable; acral, distal, symmetric anesthesia common
Acid-fast bacilli (BI)	3	0–1+	3–4+	4–5+	4–6+
Lymphocytes	3+	2+	1+	1+	0–1+
Macrophage differentiation	Epithelioid	Epithelioid	Epithelioid	Usually undifferentiated; epithelioid foci sometimes present; may show foamy change	Foamy change the rule; may be undifferentiated in early lesions
Langhans' giant cells	1–3+	2+	—	—	—
Lepromin skin test	+++	+++	—	—	—
Lymphocyte transformation test	95%	40%	10%	1–2%	1–2%
CD4+/CD8+ T-cell ratio in lesions	1.35	1.11	NT	0.48	0.50
M. leprae PGL-1 antibodies	1+ (60%+)	2+	2+	3+	3+ (95%+)

Abbreviations: BI, bacteriologic index; PGL-1, phenolic glycolipid 1.

load, and loss of *M. leprae*–specific cellular immunity (Table 151-1). Distinguishing dermatopathologic characteristics include the number of lymphocytes, giant cells, and AFB as well as the nature of epithelioid cell differentiation. Where a patient presents on the clinical spectrum largely determines prognosis, complications, reactional states, and the intensity of antimicrobial therapy required.

Tuberculoid Leprosy   At the less severe end of the spectrum is tuberculoid leprosy, which encompasses TT and BT disease. In general, these forms of leprosy result in symptoms confined to the skin and peripheral nerves. The skin lesions of tuberculoid leprosy consist of one or a few hypopigmented macules or plaques that are sharply demarcated and hypesthetic, often have erythematous or raised borders, and are devoid of the normal skin organs (sweat glands and hair follicles) and thus are dry, scaly, and anhidrotic. AFB are generally absent or few in number. Tuberculoid leprosy patients may have asymmetric enlargement of one or a few peripheral nerves. Indeed, leprosy and certain rare hereditary neuropathies are the only human diseases associated with peripheral-nerve enlargement. Although any peripheral nerve may be enlarged (including small digital and supraclavicular nerves), those most commonly affected are the ulnar, posterior auricular, peroneal, and posterior tibial nerves, with associated hypesthesia and myopathy. TT leprosy is the most common form of the disease encountered in India and Africa but is virtually absent in Southeast Asia, where BT leprosy is frequent.

In tuberculoid leprosy, T cells breach the perineurium, and destruction of Schwann cells and axons may be evident, resulting in fibrosis of the epineurium, replacement of the endoneurium with epithelial granulomas, and occasionally caseous necrosis. Such invasion and destruction of nerves in the dermis by T cells are pathognomonic for leprosy.

Circulating lymphocytes from patients with tuberculoid leprosy readily recognize *M. leprae* and its constituent proteins, and patients have positive lepromin skin tests (see "Diagnosis," below). In tuberculoid leprosy tissue, there is a 2:1 predominance of helper CD4+ over CD8+ T lymphocytes. Tuberculoid tissues are rich in the mRNAs of the proinflammatory T_H1 family of cytokines: interleukin (IL) 2, interferon γ (IFN-γ), and IL-12; in contrast, IL-4, IL-5, and IL-10 mRNAs are scarce.

Lepromatous Leprosy   Lepromatous leprosy patients present with symmetrically distributed skin nodules, raised plaques, or diffuse dermal infiltration, which, when on the face, results in leonine facies. Late manifestations include loss of eyebrows (initially the lateral margins only; Fig. 151-1) and eyelashes, pendulous earlobes, and dry scaling skin, particularly on the feet. In LL leprosy, bacilli are numerous in the skin (as many as 10^9/g), where they are often found in large clumps (*globi*), and in peripheral nerves, where they initially invade Schwann cells, resulting in foamy degenerative myelination and axonal degeneration and later in Wallerian degeneration. In addition, bacilli are plentiful in circulating blood and in all organ systems except the lungs and the central nervous system. Nevertheless, patients are afebrile, and there is no evidence of major organ system dysfunction. Almost exclusively found in western Mexico and the Caribbean is a form of lepromatous leprosy without visible skin lesions but with diffuse dermal infiltration and a demonstrably thickened dermis, termed *diffuse lepromatosis*. In lepromatous leprosy, nerve enlargement and damage tend to be symmetric, result from actual bacillary invasion, and are more insidious but ultimately more extensive than in tuberculoid leprosy. Patients with LL leprosy have acral, distal, symmetric peripheral neuropathy and a tendency toward symmetric nerve-trunk enlargement. They may also have signs and symptoms related to involvement of the upper respiratory tract, the anterior chamber of the eye, and the testes.

In untreated LL patients, lymphocytes regularly fail to recognize either *M. leprae* or its protein constituents, and lepromin skin tests are negative (see "Diagnosis," below). This loss of protective cellular im-

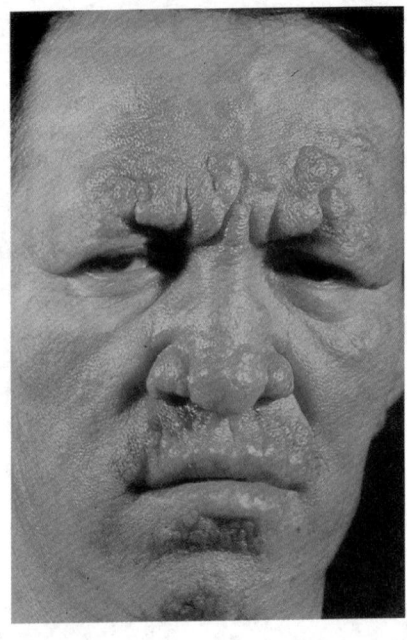

munity appears to be antigen-specific, as patients are not unusually susceptible to opportunistic infections, cancer, or AIDS and maintain delayed-type hypersensitivity to *Candida*, *Trichophyton*, mumps, tetanus toxoid, and even purified protein derivative of tuberculin. At times, *M. leprae*–specific anergy is reversible with effective chemotherapy. In LL tissues, there is a 2:1 ratio of CD8+ to CD4+ T lymphocytes. LL tissues demonstrate a T_H2 cytokine profile, being rich in mRNAs for IL-4, IL-5, and IL-10 and poor in those for IL-2, IFN-γ, and IL-12. It appears that cytokines mediate a protective tissue response in leprosy, as injection of IFN-γ or IL-2 into lepromatous lesions causes a loss of AFB and histopathologic conversion toward a tuberculoid pattern. Macrophages of lepromatous leprosy patients appear to be functionally intact; circulating monocytes exhibit normal microbicidal function and responsiveness to IFN-γ.

Reactional States   Lepra reactions comprise several common immunologically mediated inflammatory states that cause considerable morbidity. Some of these reactions precede diagnosis and the institution of effective antimicrobial therapy. Indeed, these reactions may precipitate presentation for medical attention and diagnosis; others occur after the initiation of appropriate chemotherapy. In the latter circumstances, patients often lose confidence in conventional therapy, perceiving that their leprosy is worsening. Only by warning patients of the potential for these reactions and describing their manifestations can physicians treating leprosy patients ensure continued credibility.

TYPE 1 LEPRA REACTIONS (DOWNGRADING AND REVERSAL REACTIONS)   These reactions occur in almost half of patients with borderline forms of leprosy but not in patients with polar disease. Manifestations include classic signs of inflammation within previously involved macules, papules, and plaques and, on occasion, the appearance of new skin lesions, neuritis, and (less commonly) fever—generally low-grade. The nerve trunk most commonly involved in this process is the ulnar nerve at the elbow, which may be painful and exquisitely tender. If patients with affected nerves are not treated promptly with glucocorticoids (see below), irreversible nerve damage may result in as little as 24 h. The most dramatic manifestation is footdrop, which occurs when the peroneal nerve is involved.

When type 1 lepra reactions precede the initiation of appropriate antimicrobial therapy, they are termed *downgrading reactions*, and the case becomes histologically more lepromatous; when they occur after the initiation of therapy, they are termed *reversal reactions*, and the case becomes more tuberculoid. Reversal reactions often occur in the first months or years after the initiation of therapy but may also develop several years thereafter.

Edema is the most characteristic microscopic feature of type 1 lepra lesions, whose diagnosis is primarily clinical. Reversal reactions are typified by a T_H1 cytokine profile, with an influx of CD4+ helper cells and increased levels of IFN-γ and IL-2. In addition, type 1 reactions are associated with large numbers of T cells bearing γ/∂ receptors—a unique feature of leprosy.

TYPE 2 LEPRA REACTIONS (ERYTHEMA NODOSUM LEPROTICUM, ENL) ENL occurs exclusively in patients near the lepromatous end of the leprosy spectrum (BL-LL), affecting nearly 50% of this group. Although ENL may precede leprosy diagnosis and initiation of therapy—sometimes, in fact, prompting the diagnosis—in 90% of cases it follows the institution of chemotherapy, generally within 2 years. The most common features of ENL are crops of painful erythematous papules that resolve spontaneously in a few days to a week but may recur; malaise; and fever that can be profound. However, patients may also experience symptoms of neuritis, lymphadenitis, uveitis, orchitis, and glomerulonephritis and may develop anemia, leukocytosis, and abnormal liver function tests, particularly increased aminotransferase levels. Individual patients may have either a single bout of ENL or chronic recurrent manifestations. Bouts may be either mild or severe and generalized; in rare instances, ENL results in death.

Skin biopsy of ENL papules reveals vasculitis or panniculitis, sometimes with many lymphocytes but characteristically with polymorphonuclear leukocytes as well.

Elevated levels of circulating tumor necrosis factor (TNF) have been demonstrated in ENL; thus, TNF may play a central role in the pathobiology of this syndrome. ENL is thought to be a consequence of immune complex deposition, given its T_H2 cytokine profile and its high levels of IL-6 and IL-8. However, in ENL tissue, the presence of HLA Dr framework antigen of epidermal cells—considered a marker for a delayed-type hypersensitivity response—and evidence for higher levels of IL-2 and IFN-γ than are usually seen in polar lepromatous disease suggest an alternative mechanism.

LUCIO'S PHENOMENON This unusual reaction is seen exclusively in patients from the Caribbean and Mexico who have the diffuse lepromatosis form of lepromatous leprosy, most often those who are untreated. Patients with this reaction develop recurrent crops of large, sharply marginated, ulcerative lesions—particularly on the lower extremities—that may be generalized and, when so, are frequently fatal as a result of secondary infection and consequent septic bacteremia. Histologically, the lesions are characterized by ischemic necrosis of the epidermis and superficial dermis, heavy parasitism of endothelial cells with AFB, and endothelial proliferation and thrombus formation in the larger vessels of the deeper dermis. Like ENL, the Lucio phenomenon is probably mediated by the immune complex.

Complications ■ *THE EXTREMITIES* Complications of the extremities in leprosy patients are primarily a consequence of neuropathy leading to insensitivity and myopathy. Insensitivity affects fine touch, pain, and heat receptors but generally spares position and vibration appreciation. The most commonly affected nerve trunk is the ulnar nerve at the elbow, whose involvement results in clawing of the fourth and fifth fingers, loss of dorsal interosseous musculature in the affected hand, and loss of sensation in these distributions. Median nerve involvement in leprosy impairs thumb opposition and grasp, while radial nerve dysfunction, though rare in leprosy, leads to wristdrop. Tendon transfers can restore hand function but should not be performed until 6 months after the initiation of antimicrobial therapy and the conclusion of episodes of acute neuritis.

Plantar ulceration, particularly at the metatarsal heads, is probably the most frequent complication of leprous neuropathy. Therapy requires careful debridement; administration of appropriate antibiotics; avoidance of weight-bearing until ulcerations are healed, with slowly progressive ambulation thereafter; and wearing of specialized shoes to prevent recurrence.

Footdrop as a result of peroneal nerve palsy should be treated with a simple nonmetallic brace within the shoe or surgical correction attained by tendon transfers. Although uncommon, Charcot's joints, particularly of the foot and ankle, may result from leprosy.

The loss of distal digits in leprosy is a consequence of insensitivity, trauma, secondary infection, and—in lepromatous patients—a poorly understood and sometimes profound osteolytic process. Conscientious protection of the extremities during cooking and work and the early institution of therapy have substantially reduced the frequency and severity of distal digit loss in recent times.

THE NOSE In lepromatous leprosy, bacillary invasion of the nasal mucosa can result in chronic nasal congestion and epistaxis. Saline nose drops may relieve these symptoms. Long-untreated LL leprosy may further result in destruction of the nasal cartilage, with consequent saddle-nose deformity or anosmia (more common in the preantibiotic era than at present). Nasal reconstructive procedures can ameliorate significant cosmetic defects.

THE EYE Owing to cranial nerve palsies, lagophthalmus and corneal insensitivity may complicate leprosy, resulting in trauma, secondary infection, and (without treatment) corneal ulcerations and opacities. For patients with these conditions, eyedrops during the day and ointments at night provide some protection from such consequences. Furthermore, in LL leprosy, the anterior chamber of the eye is invaded by bacilli, and ENL may result in uveitis, with consequent cataracts and glaucoma. Thus leprosy is a major cause of blindness in the developing world. Slit-lamp evaluation of LL patients often reveals "corneal beading," representing globi of *M. leprae*.

THE TESTES *M. leprae* invades the testes, while ENL may cause orchitis. Thus males with lepromatous leprosy often manifest mild to severe testicular dysfunction, with an elevation of luteinizing and follicle-stimulating hormones, decreased testosterone, and aspermia or hypospermia in 85% of LL patients but in only 25% of BL patients. LL patients may become impotent and infertile. Impotence is sometimes responsive to testosterone replacement.

AMYLOIDOSIS Secondary amyloidosis is a complication of LL leprosy and ENL that is encountered infrequently in the antibiotic era. This complication may result in abnormalities of hepatic and particularly renal function.

NERVE ABSCESSES Patients with various forms of leprosy, but particularly those with the BT form, may develop abscesses of nerves (most commonly the ulnar) with an adjacent cellulitic appearance of the skin. In such conditions, the affected nerve is swollen and exquisitely tender. Although glucocorticoids may reduce signs of inflammation, rapid surgical decompression is necessary to prevent irreversible sequelae.

DIAGNOSIS Leprosy most commonly presents with both characteristic skin lesions and skin histopathology. Thus the disease should be suspected when a patient from an endemic area has suggestive skin lesions or peripheral neuropathy; the diagnosis should be confirmed by histopathology. In tuberculoid leprosy, lesional areas—preferably the advancing edge—must be biopsied because normal-appearing skin does not have pathologic features. In lepromatous leprosy, nodules, plaques, and indurated areas are optimal biopsy sites, but biopsies of normal-appearing skin are also generally diagnostic. Lepromatous leprosy is associated with diffuse hyperglobulinemia, which may result in false-positive serologic tests (e.g., VDRL, RA, ANA) and therefore may cause diagnostic confusion. On occasion, tuberculoid lesions may not (1) appear typical, (2) be hypesthetic, and (3) contain granulomas but only nonspecific lymphocytic infiltrates. In such instances, two of these three characteristics are considered sufficient for a diagnosis. It is preferable to overdiagnose leprosy rather than to allow a patient to remain untreated.

IgM antibodies to PGL-1 are found in 95% of untreated lepromatous leprosy patients; the titer decreases with effective therapy. However, in tuberculoid leprosy—the form of disease most often associated with diagnostic uncertainty owing to the absence or paucity of AFB—patients have significant antibodies to PGL-1 only 60% of the time; moreover, in endemic locales, exposed individuals without clinical leprosy may harbor antibodies to PGL-1. Thus PGL-1 serology is of little diagnostic utility in tuberculoid leprosy. Heat-killed *M. leprae* (lepromin) has been used as a skin test reagent. It generally elicits a reaction in tuberculoid leprosy patients, may do so in individuals without leprosy, and gives negative results in lepromatous leprosy patients; consequently, it is likewise of little diagnostic value. Unfortunately, PCR of the skin for *M. leprae*, although positive in LL and BL leprosy, yields negative results in 50% of tuberculoid leprosy cases, again offering little diagnostic assistance.

Included in the differential diagnosis of lesions that resemble leprosy are sarcoidosis, leishmaniasis, lupus vulgaris, lymphoma, syphilis, yaws, granuloma annulare, and various other disorders causing hypopigmentation. Sarcoidosis may result in perineural inflammation, but actual granuloma formation within dermal nerves is pathognomonic for leprosy. In lepromatous leprosy, sputum specimens may be loaded with AFB—a finding that can be inappropriately interpreted as representing pulmonary tuberculosis.

℞ TREATMENT

Antimicrobial Therapy ■ *ACTIVE AGENTS* Established agents used to treat leprosy include dapsone (50 to 100 mg/d), clofazimine (50 to 100 mg/d, 100 mg three times weekly, or 300 mg monthly), and rifampin (600 mg daily or monthly). Of these drugs, only rifampin is bactericidal. The sulfones (folate antagonists), the foremost of which is dapsone, were the first antimicrobials found to be effective for the treatment of leprosy and are still the mainstay of therapy. With sulfone treatment, skin lesions resolve and numbers of viable bacilli in the skin are reduced. Although primarily bacteriostatic, dapsone monotherapy results in only a 2.5% resistance-related relapse rate; after ≥18 years of therapy and subsequent discontinuation, only another 10% of patients relapse, developing new, usually asymptomatic, shiny, "histoid" nodules. Dapsone is generally safe and inexpensive. Individuals with glucose-6-phosphate dehydrogenase deficiency who are treated with dapsone may develop severe hemolysis; those without this deficiency also have reduced red cell survival and a hemoglobin decrease averaging 1 g/dL. Dapsone's usefulness is limited occasionally by allergic dermatitis and rarely by the sulfone syndrome (including high fever, anemia, exfoliative dermatitis, and a mononucleosis-type picture). It must be remembered that rifampin induces microsomal enzymes, necessitating increased doses of medications such as glucocorticoids and oral birth control regimens. Clofazimine is often cosmetically unacceptable to light-skinned leprosy patients because it causes a red-black skin discoloration that accumulates, particularly in lesional areas, and makes the patient's diagnosis obvious to members of the community.

Other antimicrobial agents active against *M. leprae* in animal models and at the usual daily doses used in clinical trials include ethionamide/prothionamide; the aminoglycosides streptomycin, kanamycin, and amikacin (but not gentamicin or tobramycin); minocycline; clarithromycin; and several fluoroquinolones, particularly ofloxacin. Next to rifampin, minocycline, clarithromycin, and ofloxacin appear to be most bactericidal for *M. leprae*, but these drugs have not been used extensively in leprosy control programs. Most recently, rifapentine and moxifloxacin have been found to be especially potent against *M. leprae*.

CHOICE OF REGIMENS Antimicrobial therapy for leprosy must be individualized, depending on the clinical/pathologic form of the disease encountered. Tuberculoid leprosy, which is associated with a low bacterial burden and a protective cellular immune response, is the easier form to treat and can be reliably cured with a finite course of chemotherapy. In contrast, lepromatous leprosy may have a higher bacillary load than any other human bacterial disease, and the absence of a salutary T cell repertoire requires prolonged or even lifelong chemotherapy. Hence, careful classification of disease prior to therapy is important. In developed countries, clinical experience with leprosy

classification is limited; fortunately, however, the resources needed for skin biopsy are highly accessible and pathologic interpretation is readily available. In developing countries, clinical expertise is greater but is now waning substantially as the care of leprosy patients is integrated into general health services. In addition, access to dermatopathology services is often limited. In such instances, skin smears may prove useful, but in many locales access to the resources needed for their preparation and interpretation may also be unavailable. Use of skin smears is no longer encouraged by the World Health Organization (WHO) and is often replaced by mere counting of lesions, which, together with the lack of histopathology, may negatively affect decisions about chemotherapy, increase the potential for reactions, and worsen the ultimate prognosis.

A reasoned approach to the treatment of leprosy is confounded by these and several other issues:

1. Even without therapy, TT leprosy may heal spontaneously, and prolonged dapsone monotherapy (even for LL leprosy) is generally curative in 80% of cases.
2. In tuberculoid disease, there are often no bacilli found in the skin prior to therapy, and thus there is no objective measure of therapeutic success. Furthermore, despite adequate treatment, TT and particularly BT lesions often resolve little or incompletely, while relapse and late type 1 lepra reactions can be difficult to distinguish.
3. LL leprosy patients commonly harbor viable persistent *M. leprae* organisms after prolonged intensive therapy; the propensity of these organisms to initiate clinical relapse is unclear. Because relapse in LL patients after discontinuation of rifampin-containing regimens usually begins only after 7 to 10 years, follow-up over the very long term is necessary to assess ultimate clinical outcomes.
4. Even though primary dapsone resistance is exceedingly rare and multidrug therapy is generally recommended (at least for lepromatous leprosy), there is a paucity of information from experimental animals and clinical trials on the optimal combination of antimicrobials, dosing schedule, or duration of therapy.

In 1982, the WHO made recommendations for "the chemotherapy of leprosy for control programs." These recommendations came on the heels of the demonstration of the relative success of long-term dapsone monotherapy and in the context of concerns about dapsone resistance. Other complicating considerations included the limited resources available for leprosy care in the very areas where it is most prevalent and the frustration and discouragement of patients and program managers with the previous requirement for lifelong therapy for many leprosy patients. The WHO delineated for the first time a finite duration of therapy for all forms of leprosy and—given the prohibitive cost of daily rifampin treatment in developing countries—encouraged the monthly administration of this agent as part of a multidrug regimen.

Over the ensuing years, these WHO recommendations have been broadly implemented, and the duration of therapy required, particularly for lepromatous leprosy, has been progressively shortened. For treatment purposes, the WHO classifies patients as paucibacillary and multibacillary. Previously, patients without demonstrable AFB in the dermis were classified as paucibacillary and those with AFB as multibacillary. Currently, owing to the perceived unreliability of skin smears in the field, patients are classified as multibacillary if they have six or more skin lesions and as paucibacillary if they have fewer. The WHO recommends that paucibacillary adults be treated with 100 mg of dapsone daily and 600 mg of rifampin monthly (supervised) for 6 months (Table 151-2). For patients with single-lesion paucibacillary leprosy, the WHO recommends as an alternative a single dose of rifampin (600 mg), ofloxacin (400 mg), and minocycline (100 mg). Multibacillary adults should be treated with 100 mg of dapsone plus 50 mg of clofazimine daily (unsupervised) and with 600 mg of rifampin plus 300 mg of clofazimine monthly (supervised). Originally, the WHO recommended that lepromatous patients be treated for 2 years or until smears became negative (generally in ~5 years); subsequently,

TABLE 151-2 *Antimicrobial Regimens Recommended for the Treatment of Leprosy in Adults*

Form of Leprosy	More Intensive Regimen	WHO Recommended Regimen (1982)
Tuberculoid (paucibacillary)	Dapsone (100 mg/d) for 5 years	Dapsone (100 mg/d, unsupervised) *plus* rifampin (600 mg/month, supervised) for 6 months
Lepromatous (multibacillary)	Rifampin (600 mg/d) for 3 years *plus* dapsone (100 mg/d) indefinitely	Dapsone (100 mg/d) *plus* clofazimine (50 mg/d), unsupervised; *and* rifampin (600 mg) *plus* clofazimine (300 mg) monthly (supervised) for 1–2 years

Note: See text for discussion and comparison of WHO recommendations and more intensive approach as well as alternative WHO regimen for single-lesion paucibacillary leprosy.

the acceptable course was reduced to 1 year—a change that remains especially controversial in the absence of supporting clinical trials.

Several factors have caused many authorities to question the WHO recommendations and to favor a more intensive approach. Among these factors are—for multibacillary patients—a high (double-digit) relapse rate in three locales (reaching 20 to 40% in one locale, with the rate directly related to the initial bacterial burden) and—for paucibacillary patients—demonstrable lesional activity for years in fully half of patients after the completion of therapy. The more intensive approach (Table 151-2) calls for tuberculoid leprosy to be treated with dapsone (100 mg/d) for 5 years and for lepromatous leprosy to be treated with rifampin (600 mg/d) for 3 years and with dapsone (100 mg/d) throughout life.

On effective antimicrobial therapy, new skin lesions and signs and symptoms of peripheral neuropathy cease appearing. Nodules and plaques of lepromatous leprosy noticeably flatten in 1 to 2 months and resolve in 1 year or a few years, while tuberculoid skin lesions may disappear, improve, or remain relatively unchanged. Although the peripheral neuropathy of leprosy may improve somewhat in the first few months of therapy, rarely is it significantly ameliorated by treatment.

Therapy for Reactions ■ *TYPE 1* Type 1 lepra reactions are best treated with glucocorticoids (e.g., prednisone, initially at doses of 40 to 60 mg/d). As the inflammation subsides, the glucocorticoid dose can be tapered, but steroid therapy must be continued for at least 3 months lest recurrence supervene. Because of the myriad toxicities of prolonged glucocorticoid therapy, the indications for its initiation are strictly limited to lesions whose intense inflammation poses a threat of ulceration; lesions at cosmetically important sites, such as the face; and cases in which neuritis is present. Mild to moderate lepra reactions that do not meet these criteria should be tolerated and glucocorticoid treatment withheld. Thalidomide is ineffective against type 1 lepra reactions; clofazimine (200 to 300 mg/d) is of questionable benefit but in any event is far less efficacious than glucocorticoids.

TYPE 2 Treatment of ENL must be individualized. If ENL is mild (i.e., without fever or other organ involvement, with occasional crops of only a few skin papules), it may be treated with antipyretics alone. However, in cases with many skin lesions, fever, malaise, and other tissue involvement, brief courses (1 to 2 weeks) of glucocorticoids (initially 40 to 60 mg/d) are often effective. With or without therapy, individual inflamed papules last for >1 week. Successful therapy is defined by the cessation of skin lesion development and the disappearance of other systemic signs and symptoms. If, despite two courses of glucocorticoid therapy, ENL appears to be recurring and persisting, treatment with thalidomide (100 to 300 mg nightly) should be initiated, with the dose depending on the initial severity of the reaction. Because even a single dose of thalidomide administered early in pregnancy may result in severe birth defects, including phocomelia, the use of this drug in the United States for the treatment of fertile female patients is tightly regulated and requires informed consent, prior pregnancy testing, and maintenance of birth control measures. Although the mech-

anism of thalidomide's dramatic action against ENL is not entirely clear, the drug's efficacy is probably attributable to its reduction of TNF levels and IgM synthesis and its slowing of polymorphonuclear leukocyte migration. After the reaction is controlled, lower doses of thalidomide (50 to 200 mg nightly) are effective in preventing relapses of ENL. Clofazimine in high doses (300 mg nightly) has some efficacy against ENL, but its use permits only a modest reduction of the glucocorticoid dose necessary for ENL control.

LUCIO'S PHENOMENON Neither glucocorticoids nor thalidomide is effective against this syndrome. Optimal wound care and therapy for bacteremia are indicated. Ulcers tend to be chronic and heal poorly. In severe cases, exchange transfusion may prove useful.

PREVENTION AND CONTROL Vaccination at birth with bacille Calmette-Guérin (BCG) has proved variably effective in preventing leprosy: the results have ranged from total inefficacy to 80% efficacy. The addition of heat-killed *M. leprae* to BCG does not increase vaccine efficacy. Because whole mycobacteria contain large amounts of lipids and carbohydrates that have proven in vitro to be immunosuppressive for lymphocytes and macrophages, *M. leprae* proteins may prove to be superior vaccines. Data from a mouse model support this possibility.

Chemoprophylaxis with dapsone may reduce the number of cases of tuberculoid leprosy but not of lepromatous leprosy and hence is not recommended, even for household contacts. Because leprosy transmission appears to require close prolonged household contact, hospitalized patients need not be isolated.

In 1992, the WHO—on the basis of that organization's treatment recommendations—launched a landmark campaign to eliminate leprosy as a public health problem by the year 2000 (goal, <1 case per 10,000 population). The campaign mobilized and energized nongovernmental organizations and national health services to treat leprosy with multiple drugs and to clean up outdated registries; in these respects, the effort has proven hugely successful, with >6 million patients completing therapy. However, the target of leprosy elimination has not yet been reached. In fact, the success of the WHO campaign in reducing the number of cases worldwide has been largely attributable to the redefinition of what constitutes a case of leprosy: Formerly calculated by disease prevalence, the case count is now limited to those not yet treated with multiple drugs. In each of the 23 countries with the largest number of leprosy cases, the annual incidence of leprosy is stable or actually rising. Furthermore, after the completion of therapy, when a patient is no longer considered to represent a "case," half of all patients continue to manifest disease activity for years; relapse rates (at least for multibacillary patients) are unacceptably high; disabilities and deformities go unchecked; and the social stigma of the disease persists.

During most of the twentieth century, nongovernmental organizations, particularly Christian missionaries, provided a medical infrastructure devoted to the care and treatment of leprosy patients—the envy of those with other medical priorities in the developing world. With the public perception that leprosy is near eradication, resources for patient care are rapidly being diverted, and the burden of patient care is being transferred to nonexistent or overloaded national health services and to health workers who lack the tools and skills needed for disease diagnosis, classification, and nuanced therapy (particularly in cases of reactional neuritis). Thus the prerequisites for a salutary outcome are increasingly unmet.

FURTHER READING

BAOHONG JI: Does there exist a subgroup of MB patients at greater risk of relapse after MDT? Lepr Rev 72:3, 2001

COLE ST et al: Massive gene decay in the leprosy bacillus. Nature 409:1007, 2001

GELBER RH: Chemotherapy of lepromatous leprosy: Recent developments and prospects for the future. Eur J Clin Microbiol Infect Dis 13:942, 1994

——— et al: Vaccination of mice with a soluble protein fraction of *Mycobac-*

terium leprae provides consistent and long-term protection against *M. leprae* infection. Infect Immun 60:1840, 1992

JAMET P et al: Marchoux Chemotherapy Study Group. Relapse after long-term follow up of multibacillary patients treated by WHO multidrug regimen. Int J Lepr 63:195, 1995

LOCKWOOD D: Leprosy elimination—a virtual phenomenon or a reality? BMJ 324:1516, 2002

MODLIN RL, REA TH: Immunology of leprosy granulomas. Springer Semin Immunopathol 10:359, 1998

RIDLEY DS: Histological classification and the immunological spectrum of leprosy. Bull World Health Organ 51:451, 1974

SHEPARD CC: The experimental disease that follows injection of human leprosy bacilli into foot pads of mice. J Exp Med 112:445, 1960

WHO EXPERT COMMITTEE ON LEPROSY: Seventh Report. WHO Tech Rep Ser No. 874. Geneva, World Health Organization, 1998

152 NONTUBERCULOUS MYCOBACTERIA
C. Fordham von Reyn

The designation *nontuberculous mycobacteria* (NTM) encompasses the mycobacterial species other than organisms of the *Mycobacterium tuberculosis* complex and *M. leprae*. The NTM are distributed widely in the environment, are typically acquired from environmental sources, and therefore are also referred to as *environmental mycobacteria*. Most species are less virulent for humans than is *M. tuberculosis*. Thus symptomatic infections are often associated with local or generalized defects in host defenses. Because isolation of an NTM species from a clinical specimen may represent true infection, colonization, or environmental contamination, strict criteria are required to assess the clinical significance of a positive culture. Although the >90 species of NTM have been associated with a wide variety of infections, most NTM infections are due to a relatively limited number of species that cause characteristic patterns of disease (Table 152-1).

MICROBIOLOGY Similar to *M. tuberculosis*, NTM organisms resist decolorization after staining and are referred to as *acid-fast bacilli* (AFB). NTM have conventionally been characterized by the time required for clinical specimens to yield visible growth on solid media. Rapidly growing NTM species, such as *M. abscessus*, *M. fortuitum*, and *M. chelonae*, appear within 7 days. These organisms grow on standard microbiologic media and thus may be reported even when the clinician has not explicitly requested cultures for mycobacteria. Slow-growing species, in contrast, often take 2 to 3 weeks to grow on solid media and require special mycobacterial media such as Lowenstein-Jensen or Middlebrook. Accordingly, slow-growing NTM species are usually isolated only when the clinician specifically requests cultures for mycobacteria. Representative species include *M. avium*, *M. kansasii*, *M. ulcerans*, and *M. marinum*. Automated broth culture systems are now used in many laboratories and may permit isolation of slow-growing NTM organisms within 10 to 14 days, thus tending to blur species distinctions based on growth rate.

Further classification based on colony pigmentation (Runyon classification) has been replaced by the use of DNA probes for identification of common species such as *M. avium*, *M. intracellulare*, *M. gordonae* (which is rarely pathogenic), and *M. kansasii*. Less common species may be identified rapidly on the basis of fatty acid composition or DNA sequencing. Molecular strain typing ("fingerprinting") based on analysis of polymorphisms among large restriction fragments can be used to determine whether two or more isolates are genotypically—and, by implication, epidemiologically—related. This technique has been useful for identifying common-source outbreaks of infection or contamination.

Antibiotic susceptibility testing should be performed for rapidly growing NTM species. However, susceptibility testing of slow-growing species is of limited value: testing methods are not well standardized, and the relevance of the results to outcome is uncertain since patients are usually treated with multiple-drug regimens. Testing of *M. avium* or *M. kansasii* for susceptibility to specific drugs may be useful in certain situations (see below).

DISTRIBUTION NTM have a waxy, hydrophobic, triple-layered cell wall that renders them unusually resistant to physical conditions and chemical agents (including disinfectants such as chlorine at concentrations used in drinking water). These organisms can make use of a wide variety of carbon and nitrogen sources and can survive in nutrient-poor environments. Thus they are widely distributed in water, biofilms, and soil as well as in numerous animal species. Optimal growth temperatures vary and may influence distribution. For example, *M. avium* and *M. intracellulare* are often isolated from potable hot-water sources, whereas *M. marinum* is found in the cooler water of fish tanks. Most species of NTM are obligate aerobes and grow best at acid pH. Soil and natural water samples from most regions of the world contain numerous species of NTM, which are as common in northern regions (e.g., Finland) as they are in more temperate areas (e.g., the southern United States).

EPIDEMIOLOGY Asymptomatic infections with NTM are common in humans and are probably acquired most often from childhood contact with soil, water, and possibly animals. Studies with skin tests derived from NTM indicate that 30 to 40% of adults in the northern and southern United States have had prior unrecognized or asymptomatic infection with NTM—most often with organisms of the *M. avium* complex (MAC). Since latent infection is not a recognized characteristic of NTM, most symptomatic infections are thought to represent recent exposure. Molecular methods have identified clusters of infections and pseudoinfections associated with potable water as well as with clinical procedures such as endoscopy and surgery. Environmental exposures are assumed to cause most symptomatic infections; however, this point has been difficult to document by molecular methods, presumably because there are many potential exposures (some of which are sporadic) and because a specific NTM species may be present only transiently or in low numbers in any given source.

TABLE 152-1 *Main Species of NTM and Patterns of Disease*

Species	Growth on Solid Media	Environmental Reservoir	Patterns of Disease[a]			
			Cutaneous	Pulmonary	Disseminated	Other
M. avium	Slow	Hot water systems, natural water, soil	−	++	+++	Lymphadenitis
M. intracellulare	Slow	Hot water systems, natural water, soil	−	+++	+	Lymphadenitis
M. kansasii	Slow	Potable and natural water	−	+++	++	
M. abscessus, M. chelonae, M. fortuitum	Rapid	Potable and natural water, soil	++	+	−	Sporotrichoid spread
M. marinum	Slow	Fish tanks, salt water	++	−	−	Sporotrichoid spread
M. ulcerans	Slow	Natural water	++	−	−	"Buruli ulcer," osteomyelitis

[a] Symbols indicate relative prevalence among NTM infections of the indicated species and pattern of disease: +++, most common; ++, common; +, reported but uncommon; −, rare or not reported.

PATHOGENESIS NTM may be acquired through cutaneous, respiratory, gastrointestinal, or (rarely) parenteral exposure. Organisms are ingested by host macrophages and may survive within these cells to replicate and cause symptomatic infection. Disease manifestations in immunocompetent hosts are due to host cellular immune responses and the formation of granulomas. Intracellular killing of mycobacteria, with ultimate control of infection, requires the action of cellular immune mechanisms including proliferation of CD4+ T lymphocytes and elaboration of interferon γ (IFN-γ) and interleukin 12. Deficiencies in CD4+ T cell function due to HIV infection and inherited deficiencies in the production of or response to IFN-γ are associated with disseminated NTM infection (Chap. 173).

There is no convincing evidence that NTM can establish latent infection with subsequent clinical reactivation—a pattern characteristic of *M. tuberculosis*. Asymptomatic infection with NTM in a healthy host may induce beneficial immunity; persons with skin-test reactivity to NTM antigens (e.g., *M. intracellulare*) are at decreased risk for the subsequent development of tuberculosis. Likewise, immunization with bacille Calmette-Guérin (BCG) from *M. bovis* provides protection against childhood cervical adenitis due to NTM.

CLINICAL SYNDROMES ■ Cutaneous Disease NTM can cause a variety of cutaneous disease syndromes when directly inoculated from an environmental source into an area of open or diseased skin or into a surgical wound. *M. abscessus*, *M. fortuitum*, *M. chelonae*, *M. marinum*, and *M. ulcerans* are the most commonly involved species. Cutaneous disease may be nodular or ulcerating, sometimes with reddish-blue discoloration and typically with minimal drainage. Lesions may be single, or the infection may spread proximally up the lymphatics, producing additional nodules (sporotrichoid spread). In compromised hosts, disseminated lesions may appear as a result of bacteremic spread. Clinical suspicion of NTM infection is based on chronicity, the absence of bacterial growth on routine culture, and the failure to respond to standard antibacterial therapy. Biopsies often reveal granuloma formation, and acid-fast stains may be positive.

Pulmonary Disease NTM species cause chronic progressive pulmonary infection both in normal hosts and in those with underlying pulmonary disease. The clinical features may resemble slowly progressive pulmonary tuberculosis, which is often the initial diagnosis in patients with positive AFB smears. Among patients born in the United States, pulmonary disease due to acid-fast organisms is more likely to be due to NTM than to *M. tuberculosis*.

The diagnosis of pulmonary NTM infection is complicated by the variability in clinical and radiologic manifestations, the frequent presence of significant prior pulmonary disease, and the fact that isolation of NTM from the sputum may represent harmless colonization of the lower respiratory tract. The diagnosis should be based on specific, validated criteria that emphasize a compatible clinical syndrome, characteristic findings on computed tomography (CT), and repeated isolation of NTM from the sputum or growth of NTM from a lung biopsy (Table 152-2).

In normal hosts, infection may result in the onset of chronic cough, dyspnea, and fatigue; fever is unusual. Pathologic and radiologic manifestations of NTM pulmonary infection include the formation of solitary or multiple nodules, chronic pneumonitis, bronchiectasis, cavity formation, or a combination of these features. In some patients with NTM pulmonary disease, CT shows the characteristic formation of small cylindrical bronchiectasis and multiple small (<5-mm) nodules and fibrosis. Patients with these findings and negative results of routine sputum cultures for mycobacteria should have bronchoscopy and transbronchial biopsy performed in an attempt to identify granulomas and acid-fast organisms. In patients with chronic pulmonary disease, the superimposition of infection with NTM may not be associated with easily recognizable changes in symptoms or radiologic features.

MAC organisms (especially *M. intracellulare*) are the most common cause of pulmonary disease due to NTM in developed countries; next in frequency are *M. kansasii* (United States, Europe, South Africa), *M. abscessus* (United States), *M. xenopi* (Europe, Canada), and

---

TABLE 152-2 *Criteria for the Diagnosis of Pulmonary Disease Due to NTM[a]*

Category	Requirement
Clinical	Compatible symptoms (e.g., fever, cough), *and* deterioration in clinical status (if underlying lung disease present), *and* reasonable exclusion of other disease
Radiologic	Chest radiograph: Infiltrates with or without nodules, either persistent ($\geq$2 months) or progressive; *or* cavitation; *or* multiple nodules alone
	High-resolution CT: Multiple small nodules; *or* multifocal bronchiectasis, with or without small nodules
Bacteriologic	Sputum/bronchial wash: At least 3 positive cultures in 1 year
	Bronchial wash only: At least 1 positive culture with moderate growth or positive AFB smear
	Lung biopsy: Positive culture

[a] Diagnosis requires clinical criteria plus one radiologic criterion and one bacteriologic criterion.
Abbreviations: AFB, acid-fast bacilli; CT, computed tomography.
Source: Adapted from RJ Wallace et al: Am Rev Respir Crit Care Med 156:S1, 1997.

M. malmoense (United Kingdom, northern Europe). However, isolation of NTM from the sputum must be considered in the context of clinical manifestations. For example, NTM (most prominently MAC organisms, less commonly *M. abscessus*) can be cultured from 13% of cystic fibrosis patients in the United States (Chap. 241); however, not all of these patients appear to have invasive NTM disease. Although invasive disease is particularly strongly suspected when the same NTM species is isolated on multiple occasions from a patient with lung disease, even persistent organisms may represent colonization or slowly progressive disease apparent only on long-term follow-up. Additional laboratory tests (e.g., immunologic assessments) are of no value in the diagnosis.

Although treatment should be considered in patients who meet clinical, radiologic, and microbiologic criteria for disease (Table 152-2), several other factors require consideration. For example, species such as *M. kansasii* are usually pathogenic, and a single isolate may be significant, while species such as *M. gordonae* are rarely pathogenic, even when isolated repeatedly. In addition, in some patients with true invasive disease, infection may progress so slowly that it is unlikely to have much impact on longevity determined by such factors as age or comorbid illness. Since therapy for NTM requires prolonged administration of multiple drugs and is associated with significant side effects, the decision to institute treatment in patients with noncavitary disease who do not have clearly progressive pulmonary disease should be made with careful deliberation after a period of clinical and radiologic follow-up.

Disseminated Disease Patients with impaired cellular immunity—most notably, patients with advanced HIV disease (Chap. 173)—are susceptible to disseminated disease due to NTM. Other conditions that predispose patients to this syndrome include treatment with glucocorticoids or other immunosuppressive agents (e.g., for organ transplantation), lymphoma and leukemia (especially hairy cell leukemia), and heritable disorders of IFN-γ production and function. *M. avium* and *M. kansasii* are the species most commonly isolated in disseminated disease, but numerous other organisms (e.g., *M. genavense*, *M. haemophilum*) have also been recovered.

Patients with disseminated infection present with fever, weight loss, and fatigue and sometimes with hepatosplenomegaly or lymphadenopathy. Chest radiographs are typically normal in infection with *M. avium* (although they may show a miliary pattern) but are usually abnormal in that with *M. kansasii*. Laboratory studies may demonstrate anemia and an elevated level of alkaline phosphatase in serum. Disseminated disease is characterized by the widespread presence of foamy macrophages with AFB, which may be demonstrated in biopsy samples of bone marrow, intestine, or liver. Granulomas are typically absent in patients with impaired cellular immunity. In most cases, the diagnosis can be established by one or two sets of myco-bacterial blood cultures, which will be positive for the etiologic my-cobacteria in 2 to 3 weeks. Treatment requires long-term administra-tion of a multiple-drug antimycobacterial regimen and attempts to ameliorate the defect in cellular immunity (e.g., institution of antiretro-viral therapy, discontinuation of glucocorticoid administration).

Other Disease   NTM species have been associated with disease at nu-merous other anatomical locations, including ocular infections, mas-toiditis, sinusitis, mastitis, catheter site infections, endocarditis, men-ingitis, peritonitis, appendicitis, pericarditis, pyelonephritis, prostatitis, tenosynovitis, bursitis, septic arthritis, osteomyelitis, and lymphade-nitis (especially in children). Accumulating data support an association between infection with *M. avium* subspecies *paratuberculosis* and Crohn's disease.

ORGANISMS

M. AVIUM COMPLEX ■ **Pulmonary Disease**   MAC organisms (*M. avium*, *M. intracellulare*, and genetically related unnamed species) are more common than *M. tuberculosis* as a cause of mycobacterial pulmonary disease among persons born in the United States. Epidemiologic data support a marked increase in the incidence of MAC infection over the past two to three decades. Two patterns of MAC disease are recog-nized: a primary form in apparently healthy nonsmokers and a sec-ondary form in patients with preexisting pulmonary disease (Table 152-3). The description of subtle defects in cellular immune responses and body morphotype in patients with primary disease raises the pos-sibility of an as-yet-undefined immune defect predisposing to MAC infection. Patients with secondary disease include those with chronic obstructive pulmonary disease, prior tuberculosis, cystic fibrosis, or pulmonary alveolar proteinosis. The sources of infection have not been identified.

CLINICAL FEATURES AND DIAGNOSIS   Symptoms and diagnostic studies are described above (see "Clinical Syndromes"). CT identifies character-istic cylindrical bronchiectasis with nodule formation, documents the extent of disease, and establishes a baseline for possible treatment. Standard diagnostic criteria should be applied (Table 152-2), and an-tibiotic susceptibility testing should be reserved for patients with pro-longed prior macrolide exposure and for those in whom treatment fails.

℞ TREATMENT

Treatment should be initiated in most patients with cavitary disease and those with documented progression of a pulmonary process who meet diagnostic criteria for NTM infection. A period of observation prior to consideration of treatment may be useful when there is no evidence of an otherwise-explainable progressive pulmonary process

TABLE 152-3   *Typical Features of Primary and Secondary Pulmonary Disease Due to the M. avium Complex*

Feature	Primary	Secondary
Age	>50 years	30–70 (mean, 60) years
Sex	F > M	M > F
Underlying disease	None definitively identified; subtle defect in cellular immunity postulated	Chronic obstructive pulmonary disease, cystic fibrosis, prior tuberculosis, alveolar proteinosis
Clinical features	Early disease may be limited to cylindrical bronchiectasis, <5-mm nodules, and midzone involvement on chest radiography	Infiltrates, <5-mm nodules, cavities

and when the patient's age or underlying disease is likely to be the critical determinant of survival over the next few years.

Recommended treatment for pulmonary disease includes daily ethambutol and rifabutin plus a macrolide (either daily clarithromycin or thrice-weekly azithromycin; Table 152-4). Concomitant strepto-mycin therapy for the first 2 months should be considered in patients with extensive or cavitary disease. As many as 30% of patients treated with standard drugs and doses are unable to tolerate therapy, generally because of gastrointestinal side effects. Rifabutin appears to have the highest rate of side effects. Thus, doses often need to be reduced or drugs eliminated or replaced with alternatives. A fluoroquinolone may be considered as a substitute drug, although clinical data on this option are limited.

For patients with positive sputum cultures who receive a macrolide-containing regimen, treatment should be continued for at least 12 months after cultures revert to negative—typically for ≥18 months. The duration of therapy with other regimens may need to be extended to 24 months. In some cases, cough and radiographic findings may improve after several months; in others, treatment may serve only to prevent the progression of disease. Approximately 20% of patients experience treatment failure or relapse; some apparent treatment fail-ures may actually represent reinfection. Surgical resection is an option for patients with localized disease who are intolerant or unresponsive to multiple-drug therapy; however, this approach is associated with postoperative complications in as many as 20% of patients and should be undertaken only by surgeons who have considerable experience with this intervention.

Disseminated Disease   Disseminated MAC disease occurs principally among patients with advanced HIV disease who live in developed countries but are not receiving antiretroviral therapy. Almost all cases occur at CD4+ T cell counts of <100/μL, and the risk is ~20% per year for untreated patients with CD4+ T cell counts of <50/μL. The risk of disease is essentially eliminated for patients given highly active antiretroviral therapy (HAART) who have an increase in CD4+ T cell count to >100/μL for 3 months. Most cases are due to *M. avium*, and molecular studies indicate that as many as 25% of disseminated in-fections involve more than one strain. Strains causing bacteremia differ genetically from those typically isolated from respiratory sources or the environment. Molecular techniques have documented nosocomial acquisition from potable hot water and have demonstrated common genotypes among isolates from humans and those from peat used in potting soil. Epidemiologic studies have demonstrated an increased risk associated with consumption of untreated spring water and of raw or partially cooked fish or shellfish and a decreased risk associated with showering. Overall, sources of acquisition appear to be diverse and exposure is probably unavoidable; at this time, no specific behav-ioral changes are recommended for at-risk patients.

CLINICAL FEATURES AND DIAGNOSIS   Disseminated *M. avium* infection in AIDS is associated with fever, weakness, and weight loss and usually presents as a wasting syndrome in patients who are not receiving HAART or chemoprophylaxis for *M. avium* (Chap. 173). Untreated disease shortens the survival period of patients with advanced AIDS by 4 to 5 months. Laboratory findings may include anemia, hypoal-buminemia, and elevated serum levels of alkaline phosphatase and lactate dehydrogenase. HIV-infected patients with prior disseminated MAC infection or unrecognized or subclinical MAC infection may experience an immune reconstitution syndrome when they start to re-ceive HAART (Chap. 173). This syndrome presents 1 to 12 weeks after the institution of HAART and manifests as localized (or gener-alized) culture-positive lymphadenitis with negative blood cultures for *M. avium*.

℞ TREATMENT

Disseminated *M. avium* disease requires treatment with the combina-tion of clarithromycin and ethambutol, with or without rifabutin (Table

152-4), along with HAART for HIV. Antimycobacterial treatment should be continued for at least 12 months and until the CD4+ T cell count has been >100/μL for at least 6 months. The immune reconstitution syndrome should be treated with initiation or continuation of the same antimycobacterial regimen.

PREVENTION Chemoprophylaxis is highly effective for the prevention of disseminated *M. avium* infection in AIDS. Weekly azithromycin administration should be instituted when the CD4+ T cell count is <50/μL or when a patient with HIV infection has had an AIDS-defining opportunistic infection (e.g., *Pneumocystis* infection). Chemoprophylaxis may be discontinued when the CD4+ T cell count has been >100/μL for >6 months.

M. KANSASII ■ Pulmonary Disease Pulmonary disease due to *M. kansasii* has been reported from many areas of the world, including North America, Europe, and South Africa. In the United States, *M. kansasii* is the second most common cause of lung disease due to NTM and is distributed largely in central and southern states and California. The average age of onset is 60 years, and most patients have predisposing factors, such as chronic obstructive pulmonary disease, carcinoma of the lung, silicosis, or prior tuberculosis. However, pulmonary infection sometimes occurs in persons without predisposing disease and has also been associated with poverty. Disease may sometimes wax and wane over many years; this pattern is assumed to represent chronic infection rather than reactivation. Localized pulmonary infection has been described in South African miners with early HIV infection and preserved CD4+ T cell counts. The source of infection has not been identified, although *M. kansasii* has been isolated from both potable and natural water sources.

CLINICAL FEATURES AND DIAGNOSIS *M. kansasii* is the most pathogenic nontuberculous mycobacterial species affecting the lung, and the clinical features of *M. kansasii* disease resemble those of tuberculosis. Most cases include cough and sputum production; 30% include frank hemoptysis. Systemic signs and symptoms, including fever, night sweats, and weight loss, are reported by as many as 50% of patients. However, symptoms may be subtle or absent in patients with underlying malignancy. Chest radiographs show cavitation in 50% of patients, pleural scarring in 40%, and infiltrates in 30%; abnormalities are most prominent in the apices. Clinical and radiographic effects progress in the absence of treatment.

Sputum samples should be obtained for AFB staining and mycobacterial culture. The isolation of *M. kansasii* sometimes represents colonization; the diagnostic criteria in Table 152-2 are useful when multiple sputum samples can be obtained. However, the growth of *M. kansasii* from even a single sputum culture should be considered to have potential clinical significance, especially in HIV-positive patients. Testing of *M. kansasii* isolates for susceptibility to rifampin is recommended.

℞ TREATMENT

For susceptible strains of *M. kansasii*, rifampin is the foundation of a multiple-drug regimen. The recommended regimen consists of daily rifampin (600 mg), isoniazid (300 mg), and ethambutol (25 mg/kg for the initial 2 months, 15 mg/kg subsequently) for at least 18 months. Sputum cultures almost always become negative by 4 months; patients with delayed conversion should be treated for at least 12 months after the last positive culture. Resistance to rifampin may develop, in which case clarithromycin or azithromycin may be substituted.

Disseminated Disease Disseminated *M. kansasii* disease occurs principally among patients with advanced AIDS and CD4+ T cell counts

TABLE 152-4 Regimens for Prevention and Treatment of Disease Due to the *M. avium* Complex

Category	Regimen	Indication and Duration
Pulmonary disease treatment	Clarithromycin 500 mg bid (or azithromycin 600 mg 3 times/week), ethambutol 15 mg/kg/d, and rifabutin 150–300 mg/d; consider adding streptomycin 500–1000 mg 2 or 3 times/week for first 2 months	Treat for 18 months or until 12 months after conversion of sputum culture.
Disseminated disease Treatment	Clarithromycin 500 mg PO bid (or azithromycin 500 mg/d[a]) plus ethambutol 15 mg/kg per day[b]	Treat when MAC blood culture is positive or MAC organism is isolated from ordinarily sterile site. Continue with secondary prevention.
Primary prevention	Azithromycin 1200 mg PO weekly[a] or clarithromycin 500 mg PO bid	Treat when CD4+ T cell count is <50/μL. Discontinue if CD4+ T cell count exceeds 100/μL for >3 months during HAART.
Secondary prevention	Clarithromycin 500 mg PO bid (or azithromycin 500 mg/d[a]) plus ethambutol 15 mg/kg per day[b]	Discontinue if disease resolves with >12 months of MAC therapy and CD4+ T cell count exceeds 100/μL for >6 months during HAART.

[a] Azithromycin is preferred to clarithromycin in pregnancy.
[b] Concomitant rifabutin (150–300 mg/d) may protect against the development of clarithromycin resistance and improve survival but can cause interactions with antiretroviral therapy.
Abbreviations: HAART, highly active antiretroviral therapy.

of <100/μL. It has also been reported in patients with leukemia, lymphoma, or solid-organ transplantation.

CLINICAL FEATURES AND DIAGNOSIS Symptoms are similar to those reported for disseminated MAC infection, although cough is more common with disseminated *M. kansasii* infection and chest radiographs often demonstrate alveolar or interstitial infiltrates or cavities. An immune reconstitution syndrome may occur after the institution of HAART in HIV-infected patients and manifests as cervical or mediastinal lymphadenitis (Chap. 173).

The diagnosis is established by the isolation of *M. kansasii* from a normally sterile parenchymal site or from blood. In one series of cases, concurrent disseminated infection with a second NTM species (most often *M. avium*), was found in one-third of patients. The isolation of *M. kansasii* from sputum from a patient with advanced HIV disease suggests possible disseminated infection and is an indication for mycobacterial blood culture.

℞ TREATMENT

Antimycobacterial treatment of disseminated *M. kansasii* disease is the same as that for pulmonary disease due to this organism. Patients with AIDS who are receiving HAART should have rifabutin (150 mg/d) or clarithromycin (500 mg twice daily) substituted for rifampin because of drug interactions. Untreated disease is associated with shortened survival, and the response to treatment is good in patients who do not have rapidly progressive HIV infection. HIV-positive patients who experience clearing of systemic symptoms and have positive cultures with sustained recovery of the CD4+ T cell count can probably have treatment discontinued (as described above for *M. avium* infection), although there are no clinical data on this point. Azithromycin prophylaxis for disseminated *M. avium* infection may also be effective in preventing disseminated *M. kansasii* infection.

M. ABSCESSUS, M. CHELONAE, AND M. FORTUITUM Three rapidly growing NTM species are prominent in reports of human infection and colonization: *M. abscessus*, *M. chelonae*, and *M. fortuitum*. These organisms are acquired from water, soil, or nosocomial sources. The most common clinical manifestation of infection is disseminated cutaneous disease in patients who have defects in cellular immunity or are receiving glucocorticoid therapy. Normal hosts develop localized cutaneous infection in surgical or traumatic wounds, from contaminated injections, or after body piercing. Cutaneous lesions are cellulitic or nodular; are typically erythematous, indurated, and tender; and may progress to ulceration and purulent drainage. Proximal sporotrichoid spread has also been reported. Pulmonary infections (usually due to *M. abscessus*) are the next most common manifestation and occur principally in patients with underlying lung disease, such as cystic fibrosis.

The rapidly growing NTM species may be isolated from clinical specimens submitted for routine microbiologic testing. However, reliable evaluation requires inoculation onto special mycobacterial media and an extended incubation period. Because rapidly growing NTM species are also common laboratory contaminants, numerous false alarms in the form of pseudoepidemics have been reported.

℞ TREATMENT

Treatment varies with the patient group and with the species of rapidly growing NTM. Susceptibility tests should be performed and used to guide antibiotic selection. All three species are usually susceptible to clarithromycin and amikacin; *M. abscessus* and *M. fortuitum* are also susceptible to cefoxitin. Other agents that may be active include imipenem, doxycycline, and fluoroquinolones. Patients with localized cutaneous disease may respond to a single active agent (e.g., clarithromycin, 500 mg twice daily by mouth for ≥2 weeks). Up to 6 months of therapy may be optimal for bacteremic or disseminated cutaneous disease, and a second agent should be added on the basis of susceptibility tests. Pulmonary disease is especially difficult to treat since prolonged therapy is required and the most active drugs require parenteral administration. Current recommendations are to administer intravenous amikacin (5 to 7.5 mg/kg every 12 h) and cefoxitin (3 g every 6 h) with oral clarithromycin (500 mg twice daily) and to continue treatment for 6 to 12 months. Surgery can be considered for localized disease.

M. MARINUM *M. marinum* is widely distributed in water and causes chronic cutaneous infection when an open cutaneous lesion is exposed to a colonized water source. Most infections are due to hand or upper-extremity exposure to fish tanks, and some are due to shellfish or marine exposures. Swimming pools are no longer a common source of infection because of current chlorination standards. *M. marinum* grows optimally at 30°C—a lower temperature than is optimal for most pathogenic mycobacteria. After a median incubation period of 21 days (≥30 days in 35% of cases), a granulomatous or ulcerating skin lesion develops at the site of entry with subsequent sporotrichoid spread in many cases. In some patients, especially those with serious underlying disease and those receiving immunosuppressive therapy, infection may extend to deeper structures, producing tenosynovitis or osteomyelitis. The diagnosis is established by mycobacterial culture of a biopsied lesion or by demonstration of granulomas or AFB in a biopsy sample from a patient with a compatible exposure history.

℞ TREATMENT

Treatment consists of the combination of clarithromycin and ethambutol, with administration continuing for 1 to 2 months after resolution of lesions—typically 3 to 4 months in total. Surgical debridement may

be necessary in extensive or deep disease; however, in contrast to pyogenic infections, routine incision and drainage are not helpful. Persons with occupational or avocational exposure to fish tanks or salt water should wear waterproof gloves to prevent infection of open cutaneous lesions.

M. ULCERANS *M. ulcerans* causes cutaneous infection ("Buruli ulcer") in endemic regions of Central and West Africa, Central and South America, Malaysia, Indonesia, Papua New Guinea, and Australia. The organism is closely related to *M. marinum*, has a similar temperature for optimal growth, and has been isolated from natural bodies of water. Most cases of human infection occur on the bare arms or legs of children or young adults living near rivers, lakes, or swamps. Transmission is thought to result from minor trauma or the bite of an aquatic insect. The initial lesion is a small painless nodule that progresses to a deep ulcer. The ulcer expands, resulting in sloughing of skin and subcutaneous tissue; osteomyelitis may also occur. Stellate scarring and deforming contractures may result from extensive necrosis.

Biopsy analyses demonstrate extracellular AFB in early lesions, with a limited inflammatory reaction. Tissue destruction extends beyond the area of demonstrable bacterial infection and has been attributed to a unique mycobacterial toxin, mycolactone.

℞ TREATMENT

Antimicrobial therapy has not yet been shown to be beneficial, although rifampin, dapsone, clarithromycin, streptomycin, and amikacin display in vitro activity against *M. ulcerans*. Surgical treatment is primary and may require skin grafting. Immunization with BCG reduces the risk of disease by ~50%.

OTHER NTM SPECIES Numerous other NTM species have been associated with human disease, although they may represent contaminants in clinical specimens. Species and sites of possible infection include *M. celatum* (lung, lymph nodes), *M. genavense* (disseminated), *M. gordonae* (skin, contaminant), *M. haemophilum* (skin, disseminated), *M. malmoense* (lung), *M. simiae* (lung, disseminated), *M. scrofulaceum* (lymphadenitis), *M. szulgai* (skin, lung), and *M. xenopi* (lung, disseminated).

FURTHER READING

CENTERS FOR DISEASE CONTROL AND PREVENTION: Guidelines for preventing opportunistic infections among HIV-infected persons—2002 recommendations of the U.S. Public Health Service and the Infectious Diseases Society of America. MMWR 51(RR-8):10, 2002

FALKINHAM JO: Nontuberculous mycobacteria in the environment. Clin Chest Med 23:529, 2002

HAVLIR DV et al: Prophylaxis against disseminated *Mycobacterium avium* complex with weekly azithromycin, daily rifabutin, or both. N Engl J Med 335:392, 1996

HORSBURGH CR et al: Disseminated *Mycobacterium avium* complex disease among patients infected with human immunodeficiency virus, 1985–2000. Clin Infect Dis 33:1938, 2001

JERNIGAN JA, FARR BM: Incubation period and sources of exposure for cutaneous *Mycobacterium marinum* infection: A case report and review of the literature. Clin Infect Dis 31:439, 2000

VON REYN CF et al: Skin test reactions to *Mycobacterium tuberculosis* purified protein derivative and *Mycobacterium avium* sensitin among health care workers and medical students in the United States. Int J Tuberc Lung Dis 5:1122, 2001

WITZIG RS et al: Clinical manifestations and implications of coinfection with *Mycobacterium kansasii* and human immunodeficiency virus type 1. Clin Infect Dis 21:77, 1995

153 | SYPHILIS
Sheila A. Lukehart

DEFINITION Syphilis, a chronic systemic infection caused by *Treponema pallidum* subspecies *pallidum*, is usually sexually transmitted and is characterized by episodes of active disease interrupted by periods of latency. After an incubation period averaging 2 to 6 weeks, a primary lesion appears, often associated with regional lymphadenopathy. A secondary bacteremic stage, associated with generalized mucocutaneous lesions and generalized lymphadenopathy, is followed by a latent period of subclinical infection lasting many years. In about one-third of untreated cases, the tertiary stage is characterized by progressive destructive mucocutaneous, musculoskeletal, or parenchymal lesions; aortitis; or symptomatic central nervous system (CNS) disease.

ETIOLOGY The Spirochaetales include three genera that are pathogenic for humans and for a variety of other animals: *Leptospira*, which causes human leptospirosis (Chap. 155); *Borrelia*, which causes relapsing fever and Lyme disease (Chaps. 156 and 157); and *Treponema*, which causes the diseases known as treponematoses (see also Chap. 154). The genus *Treponema* includes *T. pallidum* subspecies *pallidum*, which causes venereal syphilis; *T. pallidum* subspecies *pertenue*, which causes yaws; *T. pallidum* subspecies *endemicum*, which causes endemic syphilis or bejel; and *T. carateum*, which causes pinta. Until recently, the subspecies were distinguished primarily by the clinical syndromes they produce. Researchers have now identified molecular signatures that can differentiate *T. pallidum* subspecies *pallidum* from the other pathogenic *T. pallidum* subspecies by culture-independent, polymerase chain reaction (PCR)–based methods. Other *Treponema* species found in the human mouth, genital mucosa, and gastrointestinal tract have no proven pathogenic role in human disease. These spirochetes can be confused with *T. pallidum* on dark-field examination.

T. pallidum subspecies *pallidum* (hereafter referred to in this chapter simply as *T. pallidum*), a thin delicate organism with 6 to 14 spirals and tapered ends, measures 6 to 15 μm in total length and 0.2 μm in width. The cytoplasm is surrounded by a trilaminar cytoplasmic membrane, which in turn is surrounded by a delicate peptidoglycan layer providing some structural rigidity. This layer is surrounded by a lipid-rich outer membrane that contains relatively few integral membrane proteins. Endoflagella wind around the cell body in the periplasmic space and appear to be responsible for motility.

The sequencing of the genome of *T. pallidum* has yielded information about the organism's metabolic capabilities. *T. pallidum* lacks the genes required to synthesize enzyme cofactors, fatty acids, and nucleotides de novo. In addition, it lacks genes encoding the enzymes of the Krebs cycle and oxidative phosphorylation. To compensate, the organism contains numerous genes predicted to code for transporters of amino acids, carbohydrates, and cations. In addition, the genome analyses and other studies have revealed the existence of a 12-member gene family (called *tpr*) that bears similarities to variable outer-membrane antigens of other spirochetes. One member, TprK, has discrete variable (V) regions that are targets of the humoral immune response. Data suggest that sequence variation occurs in TprK during infection and that this variation is a mechanism for immune invasion.

The only known natural host for *T. pallidum* is the human. *T. pallidum* can infect many mammals, but only humans, higher apes, and a few laboratory animals regularly develop syphilitic lesions. Virulent strains of *T. pallidum* are grown and maintained in rabbits, as none of the pathogenic treponemes has been successfully cultured.

EPIDEMIOLOGY Nearly all cases of syphilis are acquired by sexual contact with infectious lesions (i.e., the chancre, mucous patch, skin rash, or condyloma latum). Less common modes of transmission include nonsexual personal contact, infection in utero, and blood transfusion.

The total number of cases of syphilis reported annually in the United States declined from 575,593 in 1943 to a low of 31,575 in 2000—a 95% decrease. This downward trend was interrupted by an epidemic peaking in 1990. Surveillance of the number of new cases of infectious syphilis—a better indicator of disease activity—has revealed four cycles of 7 to 10 years, each with a rapid rise and fall in incidence (with peaks in 1965, 1975, 1982, and 1990). From 1990 to 2000, the number of reported cases of infectious syphilis declined by >88%. In 1997, however, the number of cases of early syphilis began to rise in Seattle, Washington, marking the beginning of a trend that, by 2000, included Los Angeles and San Francisco. Infectious syphilis rates have also begun to rise in the southern region of the United States.

The populations at highest risk for acquiring syphilis have changed. Between 1977 and 1982, approximately half of all patients with early syphilis in the United States were homosexual or bisexual men. The epidemic of syphilis that peaked in 1990 predominantly involved African-American heterosexual men and women and occurred largely in urban areas, where infectious syphilis has been correlated significantly with the exchange of sex for crack cocaine. Since 1996, syphilis rates have declined steadily among African Americans but remain higher than those for other racial/ethnic groups. Foci of syphilis still exist in a small number of counties in the southern United States, and rates are still increasing there. The current outbreak of syphilis in large cities on the West Coast of the United States is focused in men who have sex with men; a high proportion of the individuals in this group who have syphilis are also infected with HIV.

The incidence of congenital syphilis roughly parallels that of infectious syphilis in females. The number of reported cases of congenital syphilis in infants ≤1 year of age was lowest (107 cases) in 1978, when infectious syphilis was most prevalent among homosexual and bisexual men. The dramatic increase in the incidence of primary and secondary syphilis among women from 1986 to 1990 resulted in a proportionate increase in the number of infants born with congenital syphilis—to 4424 infants in 1991. The incidence of early syphilis among women has declined since 1991, as has the number of reported cases of congenital syphilis in infants (with 529 cases in 2000). It is important to note that the case definition for congenital syphilis was broadened in 1989 and now includes all live or stillborn infants delivered to women with untreated or inadequately treated syphilis at delivery.

Approximately one of every two individuals named as sexual contacts of persons with infectious syphilis becomes infected. Many sexual contacts will already have developed manifestations of syphilis when they are first seen, and ~30% of apparently uninfected contacts who are examined within 30 days of exposure actually have incubating infection and will later develop infectious syphilis if not treated. Thus, the identification and "epidemiologic" treatment of all recently exposed sexual contacts constitute an important aspect of syphilis control. Also important is the identification of infected persons by serologic testing of pregnant women, persons admitted to hospitals, military inductees, and persons undergoing examination in physicians' offices. Still controversial are laws and regulations requiring routine premarital serologic testing for syphilis, where—though national data are not available—the yield is undoubtedly lower.

NATURAL COURSE AND PATHOGENESIS OF UNTREATED SYPHILIS *T. pallidum* rapidly penetrates intact mucous membranes or microscopic abrasions in skin and within a few hours enters the lymphatics and blood to produce systemic infection and metastatic foci long before the appearance of a primary lesion. Blood from a patient with incubating or early syphilis is infectious. The generation time of *T. pallidum* during early active disease in vivo is estimated to be 30 to 33 h, and the incubation period of syphilis is inversely proportional to the number of organisms inoculated. The concentration of treponemes generally reaches at least 10^7/g of tissue before the appearance of a clinical lesion. On the basis of intradermal injection of graded doses of *T. pallidum* into eight volunteers, the 50% infectious dose was calculated to be 57 organisms. The median incubation period in humans (~21 days) suggests an average inoculum of 500 to 1000 infectious organisms for naturally acquired disease. The incubation period (from inoculation until the primary lesion becomes discernible) rarely exceeds 6 weeks. Subcurative therapy during the incubation period may delay the onset of the primary lesion, but it is not certain that such treatment reduces the probability that symptomatic disease will ultimately develop.

The primary lesion appears at the site of inoculation, usually persists for 4 to 6 weeks, and then heals spontaneously. Histopathologic examination of primary lesions shows perivascular infiltration, chiefly by lymphocytes (including CD8+ and CD4+ cells), plasma cells, and macrophages, with capillary endothelial proliferation and subsequent obliteration of small blood vessels. The cellular infiltration displays a T_H1-type cytokine profile consistent with the activation of macrophages. At this time *T. pallidum* is demonstrable in the chancre in spaces between epithelial cells; within invaginations or phagosomes of epithelial cells, fibroblasts, plasma cells, and the endothelial cells of small capillaries; within lymphatic channels; and in the regional lymph nodes. Phagocytosis of organisms by activated macrophages ultimately causes their destruction, which results in spontaneous resolution of the chancre.

The generalized parenchymal, constitutional, and mucocutaneous manifestations of secondary syphilis usually appear about 6 to 8 weeks after healing of the chancre, although 15% of patients with secondary syphilis still have persisting or healing chancres. In other patients, secondary lesions may appear several months after the chancre has healed, and some patients may enter the latent stage without ever recognizing secondary lesions. The histopathologic features of secondary maculopapular skin lesions are hyperkeratosis of the epidermis; capillary proliferation with endothelial swelling in the superficial corium; and dermal papillae with transmigration of polymorphonuclear leukocytes and, in the deeper corium, perivascular infiltration by CD8+ lymphocytes, CD4+ lymphocytes and macrophages, and plasma cells. Treponemes are found in many tissues, including the aqueous humor of the eye and the cerebrospinal fluid (CSF). Invasion of the CNS by *T. pallidum* occurs during the first weeks or months of infection, and CSF abnormalities are detected in as many as 40% of patients during the secondary stage. Clinical hepatitis and immune complex–induced membranous glomerulonephritis are relatively rare but recognized manifestations of secondary syphilis; liver function tests may yield abnormal results in up to a quarter of patients with early syphilis. Generalized nontender lymphadenopathy is noted in 85% of patients with secondary syphilis. The paradoxical appearance of secondary manifestations despite high titers of antibody (including immobilizing antibody) to *T. pallidum* is unexplained but may result from changes in expression of surface antigens. Secondary lesions subside within 2 to 6 weeks, and the infection enters the latent stage, which is detectable only by serologic testing. In the preantibiotic era, up to 25% of untreated patients experienced at least one generalized or localized mucocutaneous relapse, usually during the first year; therefore, identification and examination of sexual contacts are most important for patients with syphilis of <1 year's duration. Recurrent generalized rash is now rare.

In the preantibiotic era, about one-third of patients with untreated latent syphilis developed clinically apparent tertiary disease; today, in industrialized countries, specific treatment and coincidental therapy for early and latent syphilis have all but eliminated tertiary disease except for sporadic cases of neurosyphilis in persons infected with HIV. In the past, the most common type of tertiary disease was the gumma, a usually benign granulomatous lesion. Today, gummas are very uncommon. Cardiovascular syphilis, now also rare, is caused by obliterative small-vessel endarteritis, usually involving the vasa vasorum of the ascending aorta and resulting in aneurysm. Asymptomatic CNS involvement is demonstrable in up to 25% of patients with late latent syphilis. The factors that contribute to the development and progression of tertiary disease are unknown.

The course of untreated syphilis was studied retrospectively in a group of nearly 2000 patients with primary or secondary disease diagnosed clinically (the Oslo Study, 1891–1951) and was assessed prospectively in 431 African-American men with seropositive latent syphilis of ≥3 years' duration (the notorious Tuskegee Study, 1932–1972). In the Oslo Study, 24% of patients developed relapsing secondary lesions within 4 years, and 28% eventually developed one or more manifestations of tertiary syphilis. Cardiovascular syphilis, including aortitis, was detected in 10% of patients, none of whom had been infected before age 15; 7% of patients developed symptomatic neurosyphilis, and 16% developed benign tertiary syphilis (gummas of the skin, mucous membranes, and skeleton). Syphilis was the primary cause of death in 15% of men and 8% of women. Cardiovascular syphilis was documented in 35% of men and 22% of women who eventually came to autopsy. In general, serious late complications were nearly twice as common among men as among women.

The Tuskegee Study showed that the death rate among untreated African-American men with syphilis (25 to 50 years old) was 17% higher than that among uninfected subjects and that 30% of all deaths were attributable to cardiovascular or CNS syphilis. By far the most important factor in increased mortality was cardiovascular syphilis. Anatomic evidence of aortitis was found in 40 to 60% of autopsied subjects with syphilis (vs. 15% of control subjects), whereas CNS syphilis was found in only 4%. Rates of hypertension were also higher among the infected subjects. The ethical issues eventually raised by this study, begun in the preantibiotic era but continuing into the early 1970s, had a major influence on the development of current guidelines for human medical experimentation, and the history of the study may still contribute to a reluctance of some African Americans to participate as subjects in clinical research.

These two studies both showed that about one-third of patients with untreated syphilis develop clinical or pathologic evidence of tertiary syphilis, that about one-fourth die as a direct result of tertiary syphilis, and that there is additional excess mortality not directly attributable to tertiary syphilis.

MANIFESTATIONS ■ Primary Syphilis The typical primary chancre usually begins as a single painless papule that rapidly becomes eroded and usually becomes indurated, with a characteristic cartilaginous consistency on palpation of the edge and base of the ulcer. In heterosexual men the chancre is usually located on the penis (Fig. 153-1), whereas in homosexual men it is often found in the anal canal or rectum, in the mouth, or on the external genitalia. In women, common primary

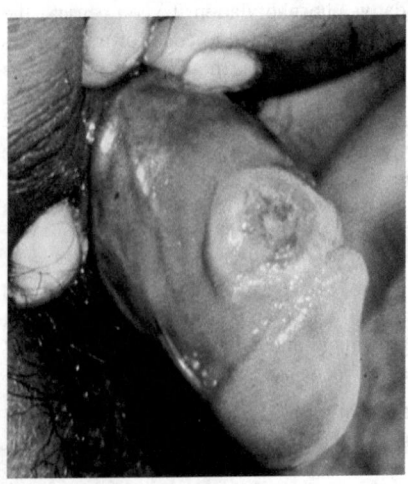

FIGURE   153-1 Primary syphilis with a firm, nontender chancre.

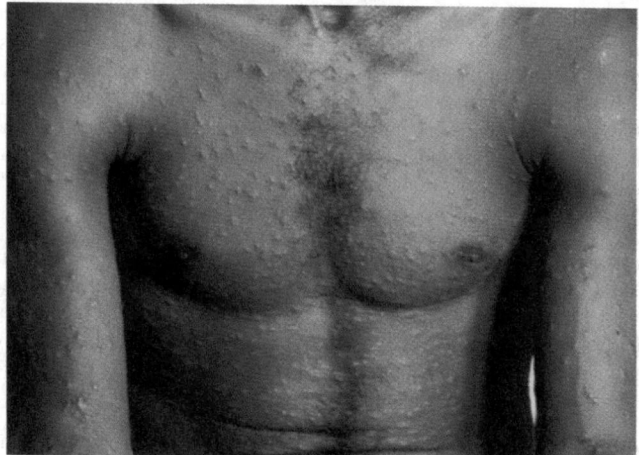

FIGURE 153-2 Secondary syphilis demonstrating the papulosquamous truncal eruption.

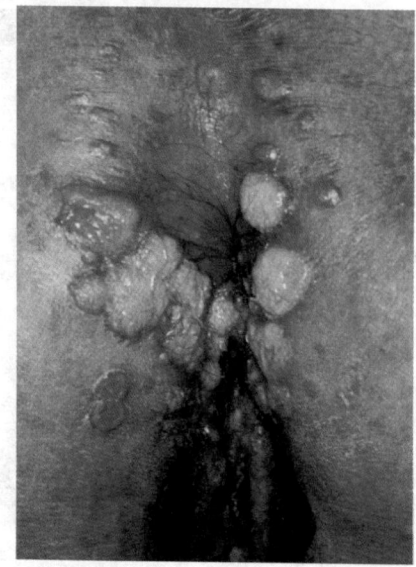

FIGURE 153-4 Condylomata lata are moist, somewhat verrucous intertriginous plaques seen in secondary syphilis.

sites are the cervix and labia. Consequently, primary syphilis goes unrecognized in women and homosexual men more often than in heterosexual men. Multiple primary lesions may be more common among men with concurrent HIV infection.

Atypical primary lesions are common. The clinical appearance depends on the number of treponemes inoculated and on the immunologic status of the patient. A large inoculum produces a dark-field-positive ulcerative lesion in nonimmune volunteers but may produce a small dark-field-negative papule, an asymptomatic but seropositive latent infection, or no response at all in individuals with a history of syphilis. A small inoculum may produce only a papular lesion, even in nonimmune individuals. Therefore, syphilis should be considered even in the evaluation of trivial or atypical dark-field-negative genital lesions. The genital lesions that most commonly must be differentiated from those of primary syphilis include those caused by herpes simplex virus infection (Chap. 163), chancroid (Chap. 130), traumatic injury, and donovanosis (Chap. 145). *Primary genital herpes* may produce inguinal adenopathy, but the nodes are tender and the lesions consist of multiple painful vesicles, which later ulcerate and are often accompanied by systemic symptoms, including fever. *Recurrent genital herpes* typically begins with a unilateral cluster of painful vesicles, usually without associated adenopathy. *Chancroid* produces painful, superficial, exudative, nonindurated ulcers, more often multiple than in syphilis (see Fig. 130-2); adenopathy is common, can be either unilateral or bilateral, is tender, and may be suppurative. Donovanosis, which is rare in the United States and Europe, is usually seen as a granulomatous ulcer that, although painless, is friable.

Regional lymphadenopathy usually accompanies the primary syphilitic lesion, appearing within 1 week of the onset of the lesion. The

nodes are firm, nonsuppurative, and painless. Inguinal lymphadenopathy is bilateral and may occur with anal as well as with external genital chancres. The chancre generally heals within 4 to 6 weeks (range, 2 to 12 weeks), but lymphadenopathy may persist for months.

Secondary Syphilis The protean manifestations of the secondary stage usually include localized or diffuse symmetric mucocutaneous lesions and generalized nontender lymphadenopathy. The healing primary chancre is still present in 15% of cases, and the stages may overlap more frequently in persons with concurrent HIV infection than in those without this co-infection. The skin rash consists of macular, papular, papulosquamous, and occasionally pustular syphilides; often more than one form is present simultaneously. The eruption may be very subtle. Approximately 25% of patients with a discernible rash of secondary syphilis may be unaware that they have dermatologic manifestations. Initial lesions are bilaterally symmetric, pale red or pink, nonpruritic, discrete, round macules that measure 5 to 10 mm in diameter and are distributed on the trunk and proximal extremities. After several days or weeks, red papular lesions 3 to 10 mm in diameter also appear (Fig. 153-2). These lesions, which may progress to necrotic lesions (resembling pustules) in association with increasing endarteritis and perivascular mononuclear infiltration, are distributed widely, frequently involve the palms and soles (Fig. 153-3), and may occur on the face and scalp. Tiny papular *follicular syphilides* involving hair follicles may result in patchy alopecia, with loss of scalp hair, eyebrows, or beard in up to 5% of cases.

In warm, moist, intertriginous body areas, including the perianal area, vulva, scrotum, inner thighs, axillae, and skin under pendulous breasts, papules can enlarge and become eroded to produce broad, moist, pink or gray-white, highly infectious lesions called *condylomata lata* (Fig. 153-4); these lesions develop in 10% of patients with secondary syphilis. Superficial mucosal erosions, called *mucous patches*, occur in 10 to 15% of patients and may involve the lips, oral mucosa, tongue (Fig. 153-5), palate, pharynx, vulva and vagina, glans penis, or inner prepuce. The typical mucous patch is a painless silver-gray erosion surrounded by a red periphery. During relapses of secondary syphilis, condylomata lata are particularly common, and skin lesions tend to be asymmetrically distributed and more infiltrated, resembling skin lesions of late syphilis. These characteristics may reflect increasing cellular immunity.

Constitutional symptoms that may accompany or precede secondary syphilis include sore throat (15 to 30%), fever (5 to 8%), weight loss (2 to 20%), malaise (25%), anorexia (2 to 10%), headache (10%), and meningismus (5%). *Acute meningitis* occurs in only 1 to 2% of cases, but numbers of cells and levels of protein in CSF are increased

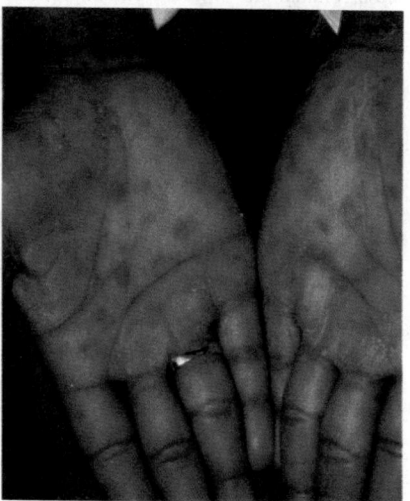

FIGURE 153-3 Secondary syphilis commonly affects the palms and soles with scaling, firm, red-brown papules.

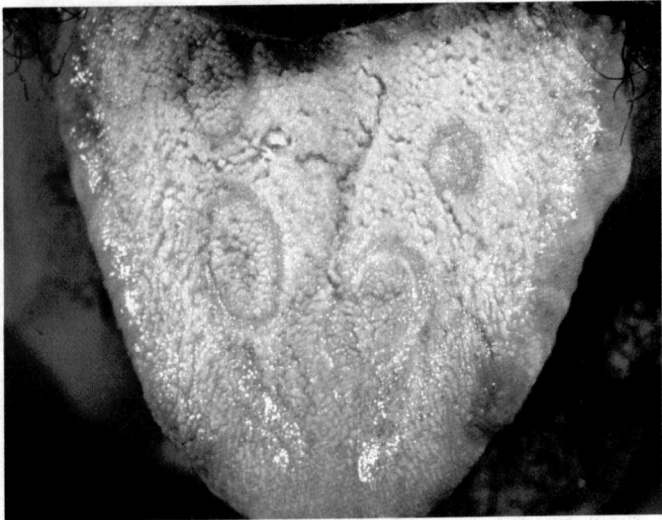

FIGURE 153-5 Mucous patches on the tongue of a patient with secondary syphilis. (*Courtesy of Ron Roddy.*)

in ≥30% of cases. *T. pallidum* has been recovered from CSF during primary and secondary syphilis in 30% of cases; this finding is often but not always associated with other CSF abnormalities.

Less common complications of secondary syphilis include hepatitis, nephropathy, gastrointestinal involvement (hypertrophic gastritis, patchy proctitis, ulcerative colitis, or a rectosigmoid mass), arthritis, and periostitis. Ocular findings that suggest secondary syphilis include otherwise-unexplained pupillary abnormalities, optic neuritis, and a retinitis pigmentosa syndrome as well as the classic iritis (especially granulomatous iritis) or uveitis. The diagnosis of secondary syphilis is often considered in such patients only after they fail to respond to steroid therapy. Anterior uveitis has been reported in 5 to 10% of patients with secondary syphilis, and *T. pallidum* has been demonstrated in the aqueous humor from such patients. Hepatic involvement is common in syphilis; although it is usually asymptomatic, at least 25% of patients may have abnormal liver function tests. Frank *syphilitic hepatitis* is distinguished by an unusually high serum level of alkaline phosphatase and by a nonspecific histologic appearance that is unlike that of viral hepatitis and includes moderate inflammation with polymorphonuclear leukocytes and lymphocytes, some hepatocellular damage, and no cholestasis. *Renal involvement* produces proteinuria associated with an acute nephrotic syndrome (or rarely with hemorrhagic glomerulonephritis) and is characterized by subepithelial electron-dense deposits and glomerular immune complexes—findings suggesting immune-complex glomerulonephritis. Like those of primary syphilis, the manifestations of the secondary stage resolve spontaneously, usually within 1 to 6 months.

Latent Syphilis   Positive serologic tests for syphilis, together with a normal CSF examination and the absence of clinical manifestations of syphilis, indicate a diagnosis of latent syphilis. The diagnosis is often suspected on the basis of a history of primary or secondary lesions, a history of exposure to syphilis, or the delivery of an infant with congenital syphilis. A previous negative serologic test or a history of lesions or exposure may help establish the duration of latent infection, which is an important factor in the selection of appropriate therapy. *Early latent* syphilis encompasses the first year after infection, whereas *late latent* syphilis (beginning ≥1 year after infection in the untreated patient) is associated with relative immunity to infectious relapse. *T. pallidum* may still seed the bloodstream intermittently during the latent stage, and pregnant women with latent syphilis may infect the fetus in utero. Moreover, syphilis has been transmitted through the transfusion of blood from patients with latent syphilis of many years' duration. It was previously thought that untreated late latent syphilis had three

possible outcomes: (1) it could persist throughout the lifetime of the infected individual; (2) it could end in the development of late syphilis; or (3) it could end with the spontaneous cure of infection, with reversion of serologic tests to negative. It is now apparent, however, that the more sensitive treponemal antibody tests rarely, if ever, become negative without treatment. About 70% of untreated patients with latent syphilis never develop clinically evident late syphilis, but the occurrence of spontaneous cure is in doubt.

Involvement of the Central Nervous System   Traditionally, neurosyphilis has been considered to be a late manifestation of syphilis, but this view is inaccurate. CNS syphilis represents a continuum encompassing early invasion (usually within the first weeks or months of infection), months to years of asymptomatic involvement, and, in some cases, development of early or late neurologic manifestations.

ASYMPTOMATIC NEUROSYPHILIS   The diagnosis of asymptomatic neurosyphilis is made in patients who lack neurologic symptoms and signs but who have CSF abnormalities including mononuclear pleocytosis, increased protein concentrations, or a reactive Venereal Disease Research Laboratory (VDRL) slide test. Such abnormalities are found in up to one-quarter of patients with untreated latent syphilis, and these are the patients who are known to be at risk for neurologic complications. In primary and secondary syphilis, such abnormalities may be found in up to 40% of untreated patients, and *T. pallidum* can be isolated from CSF of 30% of patients even in the absence of other CSF abnormalities. Although the therapeutic implications of these findings in early syphilis are uncertain, it seems appropriate to conclude that even patients with early syphilis who have such findings do indeed have asymptomatic neurosyphilis and should be treated for neurosyphilis. In patients with untreated asymptomatic neurosyphilis, the overall cumulative probability of progression to clinical neurosyphilis is about 20% in the first 10 years but increases with time; the likelihood is highest among patients with the greatest degree of pleocytosis or protein elevation. Patients with untreated latent syphilis and normal CSF probably run no risk of subsequent neurosyphilis. In one study, neurosyphilis was associated with a rapid plasma reagin (RPR) titer of ≥1:32, regardless of clinical stage or HIV infection status.

SYMPTOMATIC NEUROSYPHILIS   Although mixed features are common, the major clinical categories of symptomatic neurosyphilis include meningeal, meningovascular, and parenchymatous syphilis. The last category includes general paresis and tabes dorsalis. The onset of symptoms usually comes <1 year after infection for meningeal syphilis, at 5 to 10 years for meningovascular syphilis, at 20 years for general paresis, and at 25 to 30 years for tabes dorsalis. However, symptomatic neurosyphilis, particularly in the antibiotic era, often presents not as a classic picture but rather as mixed and subtle or incomplete syndromes.

Meningeal syphilis may involve either the brain or the spinal cord, and patients may present with headache, nausea, vomiting, neck stiffness, cranial nerve involvement, seizures, and changes in mental status. This condition may be concurrent with or may follow the secondary stage. Patients presenting with uveitis or iritis frequently have meningeal syphilis. *Meningovascular syphilis* reflects diffuse inflammation of the pia and arachnoid together with evidence of focal or widespread arterial involvement of small, medium, or large vessels. The most common presentation is a stroke syndrome involving the middle cerebral artery of a relatively young adult; however, unlike the usual thrombotic or embolic stroke syndrome of sudden onset, meningovascular syphilis often becomes manifest after a subacute encephalitic prodrome (with headaches, vertigo, insomnia, and psychological abnormalities), which is followed by a gradually progressive vascular syndrome.

The manifestations of *general paresis* reflect widespread late parenchymal damage and include abnormalities corresponding to the mnemonic *paresis*: *p*ersonality, *a*ffect, *r*eflexes (hyperactive), *e*ye (e.g., Argyll Robertson pupils), *s*ensorium (illusions, delusions, hallucinations), *i*ntellect (a decrease in recent memory and in the capacity for orientation, calculations, judgment, and insight), and *s*peech. *Tabes* *dorsalis* is also a late manifestation of syphilis that presents as symptoms and signs of demyelination of the posterior columns, dorsal roots, and dorsal root ganglia. Symptoms include ataxic wide-based gait and footslap; paresthesia; bladder disturbances; impotence; areflexia; and loss of position, deep pain, and temperature sensations. Trophic joint degeneration (Charcot's joints) and perforating ulceration of the feet can result from loss of pain sensation. The small, irregular Argyll Robertson pupil, a feature of both tabes dorsalis and paresis, reacts to accommodation but not to light. *Optic atrophy* also occurs frequently in association with tabes.

Other Manifestations of Late Syphilis The slowly progressive inflammatory disease leading to tertiary manifestations begins early during the pathogenesis of syphilis, although these manifestations may not become clinically apparent for years. Early syphilitic aortitis becomes evident soon after secondary lesions subside, and treponemes that trigger the development of gummas may have seeded the tissue years earlier.

CARDIOVASCULAR SYPHILIS Cardiovascular manifestations are attributable to endarteritis obliterans of the vasa vasorum, which provide the blood supply to large vessels. This condition results in uncomplicated aortitis, aortic regurgitation, saccular aneurysm, or coronary ostial stenosis, with symptoms usually appearing 10 to 40 years after infection. In the preantibiotic era, symptomatic cardiovascular complications developed in ~10% of persons with late untreated syphilis, although syphilitic aortitis was demonstrated at autopsy in about one-half of African-American men with untreated syphilis.

Linear calcification of the ascending aorta on chest x-ray films suggests asymptomatic syphilitic aortitis, as arteriosclerosis seldom produces this sign. Syphilitic aneurysms—usually saccular, occasionally fusiform—do not lead to dissection. Only 1 in 10 aortic aneurysms of syphilitic origin involves the abdominal aorta.

LATE BENIGN SYPHILIS (GUMMA) Gummas may be multiple or diffuse but are usually solitary lesions that range from microscopic in size to several centimeters in diameter. Histologic examination shows a granulomatous inflammation with a central area of necrosis. Although rarely demonstrated microscopically, *T. pallidum* has reportedly been recovered from these lesions. The most commonly involved sites include the skin and skeletal system, the mouth and upper respiratory tract, the larynx, the liver, and the stomach; however, any organ may be involved. Gummas of the skin produce painless and indurated nodular, papulosquamous, or ulcerative lesions that are usually indolent. These lesions may resemble those of many other chronic granulomatous conditions, including tuberculosis and sarcoidosis, leprosy, and deep fungal infections. Skeletal gummas most frequently involve the long bones of the legs, although any bone may be affected. Radiographic abnormalities with advanced gummas of bone include periostitis or destructive or sclerosing osteitis. Upper respiratory gummas can lead to perforation of the nasal septum or palate.

Because the histologic changes may be suggestive but are nonspecific, the diagnosis of late benign syphilis is confirmed by serologic testing and by therapeutic trial. Treatment with penicillin results in rapid healing of active gummatous lesions.

Congenital Syphilis Transmission of *T. pallidum* from a syphilitic woman to her fetus across the placenta may occur at any stage of pregnancy, but the lesions of congenital syphilis generally have their onset after the fourth month of gestation, when fetal immunologic competence begins to develop. This timing suggests that the pathogenesis of congenital syphilis depends on the immune response of the host rather than on a direct toxic effect of *T. pallidum*. The risk of infection of the fetus during untreated early maternal syphilis is estimated to be 75 to 95%, decreasing to about 35% for maternal syphilis of >2 years' duration. Adequate treatment of the mother before the 16th week of pregnancy should prevent fetal damage. Untreated maternal infection may result in a rate of fetal loss of up to 40% (with stillbirth more common than abortion because of the late onset of fetal pathology), prematurity, neonatal death, or nonfatal congenital syph-

ilis. Among infants born alive, only fulminant congenital syphilis is clinically apparent at birth, and these babies have a very poor prognosis. The most common clinical problem is the healthy-appearing baby born to a mother with a positive serologic test. Routine serologic testing in early pregnancy is considered cost-effective in virtually all populations, even in areas with a low prenatal prevalence of syphilis. Where the prevalence of syphilis is high or when the patient is at high risk, serologic testing should be repeated in the third trimester and at delivery.

The manifestations of congenital syphilis can be divided into three types according to their timing: (1) early manifestations, which appear within the first 2 years of life (often between 2 and 10 weeks of age), are infectious and resemble the manifestations of severe secondary syphilis in the adult; (2) late manifestations, which appear after 2 years and are noninfectious; and (3) residual stigmata. The earliest sign of congenital syphilis is usually rhinitis, or "snuffles" (23%), which is soon followed by other mucocutaneous lesions (35 to 41%). These may include bullae (syphilitic pemphigus), vesicles, superficial desquamation, petechiae, and (later) papulosquamous lesions, mucous patches, and condylomata lata. The most common early manifestations are bone changes (61%), including osteochondritis, osteitis, and periostitis. Hepatosplenomegaly (50%), lymphadenopathy (32%), anemia (34%), jaundice (30%), thrombocytopenia, and leukocytosis are common. *T. pallidum* can be isolated, by rabbit inoculation, from the CSF of 22% of infected neonates without prior antibiotic exposure.

Neonatal congenital syphilis must be differentiated from other generalized congenital infections, including rubella, cytomegalovirus or herpes simplex virus infection, and toxoplasmosis, as well as from erythroblastosis fetalis. Neonatal death is usually due to pulmonary hemorrhage, secondary bacterial infection, or severe hepatitis.

Late congenital syphilis is that which remains untreated after 2 years of age. In 60% of cases, the infection remains subclinical; the clinical spectrum in the remainder of cases differs in certain respects from that of acquired late syphilis in the adult. For example, cardiovascular syphilis rarely develops in late congenital syphilis, whereas interstitial keratitis is much more common and occurs between the ages of 5 and 25. Other manifestations include eighth-nerve deafness and recurrent arthropathy. Bilateral knee effusions are known as *Clutton's joints*. Asymptomatic neurosyphilis is present in about one-third of untreated patients, and clinical neurosyphilis occurs in one-quarter of untreated individuals >6 years old. Gummatous periostitis occurs between the ages of 5 and 20 and, as in nonvenereal endemic syphilis, tends to cause destructive lesions of the palate and nasal septum.

Characteristic stigmata include *Hutchinson's teeth*—centrally notched, widely spaced, peg-shaped upper central incisors—and "mulberry" molars—sixth-year molars with multiple, poorly developed cusps. The abnormal facies of patients with congenital syphilis include frontal bossing, saddle nose, and poorly developed maxillae. Saber shins, characterized by anterior tibial bowing, are rare. *Rhagades* are linear scars at the angles of the mouth and nose that are caused by secondary bacterial infection of the early facial eruption.

LABORATORY EXAMINATIONS ▪ Demonstration of the Organism *T. pallidum* cannot be detected by culture; therefore, other tests are necessary. Dark-field microscopic examination of lesion exudate is useful in evaluating moist cutaneous lesions, such as the chancre of primary syphilis or the condylomata lata of secondary syphilis. The identification of a single characteristic motile organism by a trained observer is sufficient for diagnosis. Examination of oral lesions and anal ulcers by this method is not recommended, as it is difficult to differentiate *T. pallidum* from other spirochetes that may be present.

Most syphilis is diagnosed in settings where dark-field microscopy is not available. The direct fluorescent antibody *T. pallidum* (DFA-TP) test, an alternative available at central laboratories, uses fluorescein-conjugated polyclonal antitreponemal antibody for the detection of *T. pallidum* in fixed smears prepared from suspect lesions. More sensitive PCR tests have been developed but are available only in research laboratories.

T. pallidum can be found in tissue with appropriate silver stains, although these results should be interpreted with caution because artifacts resembling *T. pallidum* are often seen. Treponemes can be demonstrated more reliably in tissue by immunofluorescence or immunohistochemical methods using specific monoclonal or polyclonal antibodies to *T. pallidum*.

Serologic Tests for Syphilis There are two types of serologic test for syphilis: nontreponemal and treponemal. Both types of test are reactive in persons with any treponemal infection, including yaws, pinta, and endemic syphilis.

The nontreponemal tests measure IgG and IgM directed against a cardiolipin-lecithin-cholesterol antigen complex. The most widely used nontreponemal antibody tests for syphilis are the RPR test, which can be automated (ART), and the VDRL slide test. The RPR test is easier to perform and uses unheated serum; it is the test of choice for rapid serologic diagnosis in a clinic or office setting. The VDRL test, however, remains the standard for use with CSF.

The RPR and VDRL tests are equally sensitive and may be used for initial screening or for quantitation of serum antibody. The titer reflects the activity of the disease. Titers rise during the evolution of early syphilis; VDRL titers usually reach 1:32 or higher in secondary syphilis. A persistent fall by two dilutions (fourfold) or more after treatment of early syphilis provides essential evidence of an adequate response to therapy. VDRL titers do not correspond directly to RPR titers, and sequential quantitative testing (as for response to therapy) must employ a single test.

Two standard treponemal tests are used for confirmation of reactive nontreponemal results: the fluorescent treponemal antibody–absorbed (FTA-ABS) test and the agglutination assays for antibodies to *T. pallidum*. The microhemagglutination assay for *T. pallidum* (MHA-TP) has been replaced by the Serodia TP-PA test (Fujirebio, Tokyo), which is more sensitive for primary syphilis. The *T. pallidum* hemagglutination test (TPHA) is widely used in Europe but is not available in the United States. Both the agglutination assays and the FTA-ABS test are very specific and, when used for confirmation of positive nontreponemal tests, have a very high positive predictive value for the diagnosis of syphilis. However, even these tests give false-positive results at rates as high as 1 to 2% when used for the screening of normal populations. New enzyme-linked immunosorbent assays have also been approved as confirmatory tests.

The relative sensitivities of the VDRL and RPR tests, the FTA-ABS test, and the TP-PA test in the various stages of untreated syphilis are shown in Table 153-1. The nontreponemal tests may be nonreactive in very early primary syphilis, and the detection of antibody can be maximized by the performance of a treponemal test. All treponemal and nontreponemal tests are reactive during secondary syphilis, and a nonreactive result virtually excludes syphilis in a patient with otherwise-compatible mucocutaneous lesions. (Fewer than 1% of patients with secondary syphilis have a VDRL test that is nonreactive or weakly reactive with undiluted serum but is positive at higher serum dilutions—the *prozone phenomenon*.) Although the nontreponemal tests will become nonreactive or will be reactive at lower titers after therapy for early syphilis, the treponemal tests often remain reactive after therapy and therefore are not helpful in determining the infection status of persons with past syphilis. Treatment of early primary syphilis may result in seroreversion in treponemal tests.

For practical purposes, most clinicians need to be familiar with the three uses of serologic tests for syphilis: (1) testing of large numbers of sera for screening or diagnostic purposes (e.g., the RPR or VDRL test), (2) quantitative measurement of antibody titer to assess the clinical activity of syphilis or to monitor the response to therapy (e.g., the RPR or VDRL test), and (3) confirmation of the diagnosis of syphilis in a patient with a positive nontreponemal antibody test or with a

TABLE 153-1 *Sensitivity of Serodiagnostic Tests in Untreated Syphilis*

Test[a]	Mean Percentage Positive (Range) at Indicated Stage of Disease[b]			
	Primary	Secondary	Latent	Tertiary
VDRL, RPR	78 (74–87)	100	95 (88–100)	71 (37–94)
FTA-ABS	84 (70–100)	100	100	96
TP-PA[c]	89	100	100	NA

[a] The specificity for each of these tests is 94 to 99%.
[b] In CDC studies.
[c] Limited numbers of sera have been evaluated by TP-PA.
Source: Modified from SA Larsen et al: Clin Microbiol Rev 8:1, 1995; and V Pope et al: J Clin Microbiol 38:2543, 2000.

suspected clinical diagnosis of syphilis (e.g., the FTA-ABS test or the Serodia TP-PA test).

For measurement of IgM in neonates in whom congenital syphilis is suspected, the syphilis Captia-M test (Trinity Biotech, Jamestown, NY) and the 19S IgM FTA-ABS test are available.

False-Positive Serologic Tests for Syphilis Because the antigen used in nontreponemal tests is found in other tissues, the tests may be reactive in persons without treponemal infection, although rarely do titers exceed 1:8 in such patients. In a population selected for screening because of clinical suspicion, history of exposure, or increased risk for sexually transmitted infections, fewer than 1% of reactive tests are falsely positive. The modern VDRL and RPR tests are 97 to 99% specific, and false-positive reactions are now limited largely to those conditions listed in Table 153-2. False positivity is common among persons with autoimmune disorders. The prevalence of false-positive nontreponemal tests increases with advancing age; 10% of people >70 years of age have false-positive reactions. In the patient with a false-positive nontreponemal test, syphilis is excluded by a nonreactive treponemal test.

Evaluation for Neurosyphilis Involvement of the CNS is detected by examination of CSF for pleocytosis (>5 white blood cells/mm^3), increased protein concentration (>45 mg/dL), or VDRL reactivity. CSF abnormalities can be demonstrated in up to 40% of cases of primary or secondary syphilis and in 25% of cases of latent syphilis. In older asymptomatic seropositive individuals, the yield of lumbar puncture is relatively low. *T. pallidum* has been recovered by CSF inoculation into rabbits from up to 30% of patients with primary or secondary syphilis but rarely from those with latent syphilis. The demonstration of *T. pallidum* in CSF is often associated with other CSF abnormalities; however, organisms can be recovered from patients with otherwise-normal CSF. Before the advent of penicillin, the risk of developing clinical neurosyphilis was roughly proportional to the intensity of CSF changes. CSF examination is recommended by the Centers for Disease Control and Prevention (CDC) in the evaluation of any sero-

TABLE 153-2 *Causes of False-Positive Reactions in Nontreponemal Serologic Tests for Syphilis*

Cause	Rate of False-Positive Reactions, %[a]
ACUTE FALSE-POSITIVE REACTION (<6 MONTHS)	
Recent viral illness or immunization	1–2
Genital herpes	4
Human immunodeficiency virus infection	1–4
Malaria	11
Parenteral drug use	20–25
CHRONIC FALSE-POSITIVE REACTION (≥6 MONTHS)	
Aging	9–11
Autoimmune disorders	1–20
Systemic lupus erythematosus	11–20
Rheumatoid arthritis	5
Parenteral drug use	20–25

[a] Data were collected from a variety of published reports.

positive patient with neurologic signs and symptoms, patients with other late syphilis, cases of suspected treatment failure, and HIV-infected patients with untreated syphilis of unknown duration or of >1 year's duration. The possibility of asymptomatic neurosyphilis in some patients with early disease is not addressed by these recommendations. Because standard therapy with penicillin G benzathine (benzathine benzylpenicillin) for early syphilis fails to result in treponemicidal drug levels in the CSF, some experts also advise lumbar puncture in early syphilis, particularly in patients with HIV infection or with nontreponemal test titers of ≥1:32.

The CSF VDRL test is highly specific but is insensitive and may be nonreactive even in cases of progressive symptomatic neurosyphilis. The degree of sensitivity is highest in meningovascular syphilis and paresis and is lower in asymptomatic neurosyphilis and tabes dorsalis. The unabsorbed FTA test on CSF is reactive far more often than the CSF VDRL test in all stages of syphilis, but FTA reactivity may reflect passive transfer of serum antibody into the CSF. A nonreactive CSF FTA test, however, may be used to rule out neurosyphilis.

TABLE 153-3 *Recommendations for the Treatment of Syphilis[a]*

Stage of Syphilis	Patients without Penicillin Allergy	Patients with Confirmed Penicillin Allergy
Primary, secondary, or early latent	Penicillin G benzathine (single dose of 2.4 mU IM)	Tetracycline hydrochloride (500 mg PO qid) or doxycycline (100 mg PO bid) for 2 weeks
Late latent (or latent of uncertain duration), cardiovascular, or benign tertiary	Lumbar puncture CSF normal: Penicillin G benzathine (2.4 mU IM weekly for 3 weeks) CSF abnormal: Treat as neurosyphilis	Lumbar puncture CSF normal and patient not infected with HIV: Tetracycline hydrochloride (500 mg PO qid) or doxycycline (100 mg PO bid) for 4 weeks CSF normal and patient infected with HIV: Densensitization and treatment with penicillin if compliance cannot be ensured CSF abnormal: Treat as neurosyphilis
Neurosyphilis (asymptomatic or symptomatic)	Aqueous penicillin G (18–24 mU/d IV, given as 3–4 mU q4h or continuous infusion) for 10–14 days *or* Aqueous penicillin G procaine (2.4 mU/d IM) plus oral probenecid (500 mg qid), both for 10–14 days	Desensitization and treatment with penicillin
Syphilis in pregnancy	According to stage	Desensitization and treatment with penicillin

[a] See text for full discussion of syphilis therapy in HIV-infected individuals.
Abbreviation: mU, million units.
Source: These recommendations are based on those issued by the Centers for Disease Control and Prevention in 2002.

Evaluation for Syphilis in Patients Infected with HIV
Because persons at highest risk for syphilis (inner-city populations, homosexually active men, and people in many developing countries) are also at increased risk for HIV infection, these two infections frequently coexist. There is evidence that syphilis and other genital-ulcer diseases may be important risk factors for the acquisition and transmission of HIV infection.

The manifestations of syphilis may be altered in patients with concurrent HIV infection, and multiple cases of neurologic relapse after standard therapy have been reported in HIV-infected patients. *T. pallidum* has been isolated from the CSF of several patients after therapy for early syphilis with penicillin G benzathine. A multicenter U.S. study of early syphilis found similar clinical responses to therapy in persons with and without concurrent HIV infection, although the study lacked sufficient statistical power to exclude an effect of HIV and 41% of subjects were lost to follow-up. Serologically defined treatment failure was more common among HIV-infected patients than among those without this co-infection. This investigation confirmed the high rate of CNS invasion in early syphilis and the persistence of *T. pallidum* after standard therapy: 11 of 43 HIV-infected patients and 21 of 88 HIV-uninfected patients had *T. pallidum* detectable in CSF before therapy; 7 of the 35 patients who underwent lumbar puncture after therapy (some HIV-infected and others uninfected) still had *T. pallidum* detectable in CSF.

There is no clear evidence that the sensitivity of serologic tests for syphilis differs in HIV-infected versus HIV-uninfected patients. Rates of decline of serologic titers appear to be slower in HIV-infected individuals. The clinical significance of this observation is unclear.

Persons with newly diagnosed HIV infection should be tested for syphilis; conversely, all patients with newly diagnosed syphilis should be tested for HIV infection. Some authorities, persuaded by reports of the persistence of *T. pallidum* in the CSF of HIV-infected persons after standard penicillin benzathine therapy for early syphilis, recommend examination of CSF for evidence of neurosyphilis for all co-infected patients, regardless of the clinical stage of syphilis, with treatment for neurosyphilis if CSF abnormalities are found or if CSF examination is not performed. Others do not recommend routine CSF examination for HIV-co-infected patients with early syphilis and believe that standard therapy is sufficient. Serologic testing after treatment is important for all patients with syphilis, particularly those also infected with HIV.

℞ TREATMENT

Treatment of Acquired Syphilis The CDC's 2002 guidelines for the treatment of syphilis are summarized in Table 153-3 and are discussed below. Penicillin G is the drug of choice for all stages of syphilis. *T. pallidum* is killed by very low concentrations of penicillin G, although a long period of exposure to penicillin is required because of the unusually slow rate of multiplication of the organism. The efficacy of penicillin against syphilis remains undiminished after 50 years of use. Other antibiotics effective in syphilis include the tetracyclines, erythromycin, and the cephalosporins. Aminoglycosides and spectinomycin inhibit *T. pallidum* only in very large doses, and the sulfonamides and the quinolones are inactive. Azithromycin shows significant promise as an effective oral agent against *T. pallidum*.

Serum levels of penicillin G of ≥0.03 μg/mL for at least 7 days are considered necessary for the cure of early syphilis. Recurrence rates for a given regimen increase as infection progresses from incubating to seronegative primary to seropositive primary to secondary to late syphilis. Therefore, it is probable, but unproven, that a longer duration of therapy is required to effect cure as the infection progresses.

PATIENTS WITH EARLY SYPHILIS AND THEIR CONTACTS Preventive (abortive, "epidemiologic") treatment is recommended for seronegative individuals without signs of syphilis who have been exposed to infectious syphilis within the previous 3 months. Before treatment is given, every effort should be made to establish a diagnosis by examination and serologic testing. *The regimens recommended for prevention are the same as those recommended for early syphilis.*

Penicillin G benzathine is the most widely used agent for the treatment of early syphilis, although it is more painful on injection than penicillin G procaine. A single dose of 2.4 million units cures more than 95% of cases of primary syphilis. Because the drug's efficacy in secondary syphilis may be slightly lower, some physicians administer a second dose of 2.4 million units 1 week after the initial dose at this stage of disease. Clinical relapse can follow treatment with penicillin G benzathine in patients with both HIV infection and early syphilis. Because the risk of neurorelapse may be higher in HIV-infected patients, examination of CSF from HIV-seropositive individuals with syphilis of any stage is recommended by some experts; therapy appropriate for neurosyphilis should be given if there is any evidence of CNS syphilis.

For penicillin-allergic patients with early syphilis, a 2-week course of therapy with doxycycline or tetracycline is recommended. These regimens appear to be effective, although no well-controlled studies have been performed and poor compliance may be problematic. Limited studies suggest that ceftriaxone (1 g/d, given intramuscularly or intravenously, for 8 to 10 days) and azithromycin (a single oral dose of 2 g) may be effective against early syphilis. These nonpenicillin regimens have not been evaluated in HIV-infected individuals and should be used with caution.

LATE LATENT AND LATE SYPHILIS   If CSF abnormalities are found, the patient should be treated for neurosyphilis. The recommended treatment for late latent syphilis with normal CSF, for cardiovascular syphilis, and for late benign syphilis (gumma) is penicillin G benzathine, 2.4 million units intramuscularly once a week for 3 successive weeks (7.2 million units total). Doxycycline or tetracycline (given for 4 weeks) offers an untested alternative for penicillin-allergic patients with latent or late syphilis and normal CSF. Penicillin-allergic HIV-infected persons with late latent or late syphilis should be desensitized and treated with penicillin if compliance and follow-up cannot be ensured. The clinical response to treatment for benign tertiary syphilis is usually impressive; however, responses to therapy for cardiovascular syphilis are not dramatic because aortic aneurysm and aortic regurgitation cannot be reversed by antibiotic treatment.

NEUROSYPHILIS   Penicillin G benzathine, given in total doses of up to 7.2 million units to adults, or 50,000 units/kg to infants, does not produce detectable concentrations of penicillin G in CSF, and asymptomatic neurosyphilis may relapse in patients treated with 2.4 million units; the risk may be higher in HIV-infected patients. Therefore, the use of penicillin G benzathine alone for the treatment of neurosyphilis is not recommended. On the other hand, administration of intravenous penicillin G in recommended doses is thought to ensure treponemicidal concentrations of penicillin G in CSF. The clinical response to penicillin therapy for meningeal syphilis is dramatic, but the response to treatment for parenchymal neurosyphilis is variable. In general, treatment of neurosyphilis with existing damage may produce no clinical change but may arrest disease progression.

Several recent publications have reported neurologic relapse after high-dose intravenous penicillin therapy for neurosyphilis in HIV-infected patients. No alternative therapies have been explored, but careful follow-up is essential, and re-treatment is warranted in such patients.

No data support the use of antibiotics other than penicillin G for the treatment of neurosyphilis; however, some of the third-generation cephalosporins and azithromycin may deserve further evaluation. In patients with penicillin allergy demonstrated by skin testing, desensitization and treatment with penicillin is the recommended course.

MANAGEMENT OF SYPHILIS IN PREGNANCY   Every pregnant woman should undergo a nontreponemal test at her first prenatal visit, and women at high risk of exposure should have a repeat test in the third trimester and at delivery. In the untreated pregnant patient with presumed syphilis, expeditious evaluation and initiation of treatment appropriate to the stage of the disease are essential. Patients should be warned of the

risk of a Jarisch-Herxheimer reaction, which may be associated with mild premature contractions but rarely results in premature delivery.

Penicillin is the only recommended therapy for syphilis in pregnancy. If the patient has a well-documented penicillin allergy, desensitization and penicillin therapy should be undertaken according to the CDC's 2002 treatment guidelines. After treatment, a quantitative nontreponemal test should be repeated monthly throughout pregnancy. Treated women whose titers rise by fourfold or who do not show a fourfold decrease in titer over a 3-month period should be re-treated.

Evaluation and Management of Congenital Syphilis   Newborn infants of mothers with reactive serologic tests may themselves have reactive tests, whether or not they have become infected, because of transplacental transfer of maternal IgG antibody. Rising or persistent titers indicate infection, and the infant should be treated. Neonatal IgM antibody can be detected in cord or neonatal serum with the syphilis Captia-M or 19S IgM FTA-ABS test; its detection indicates active infection. For asymptomatic infants born to women treated adequately with penicillin during pregnancy, monthly quantitative nontreponemal tests may be performed to monitor for appropriate declines in titer.

An infant should be treated at birth if the seropositive mother has received penicillin therapy in the third trimester, inadequate penicillin treatment, or therapy with a drug other than penicillin; if her treatment status is unknown; or if the infant may be difficult to follow. It is unwise to require proof of diagnosis before treatment in such cases. The CSF should be examined to obtain baseline values before treatment. Penicillin is the only recommended drug for syphilis in infants. The penicillin dosage used for the treatment of the patient with late congenital syphilis is calculated in the same way as for the infant, until dosage based on weight reaches that used for adult neurosyphilis. Specific recommendations for the treatment of infants are included in the CDC's 2002 guidelines.

Jarisch-Herxheimer Reaction   A dramatic though usually mild reaction consisting of fever (average temperature elevation, 1.5°C), chills, myalgias, headache, tachycardia, increased respiratory rate, increased circulating neutrophil count, and vasodilation with mild hypotension may follow the initiation of treatment for syphilis. This reaction occurs in ~50% of patients with primary syphilis, 90% of those with secondary syphilis, and 25% of those with early latent syphilis, and defervescence takes place within 12 to 24 h. The reaction is more delayed in neurosyphilis, with fever peaking after 12 to 14 h. In patients with secondary syphilis, erythema and edema of the mucocutaneous lesions may increase. Patients should be warned to expect such symptoms, which can be managed with symptom-based treatment. Steroid and other anti-inflammatory therapy is not required for this mild transient reaction.

Follow-Up Evaluation of Responses to Therapy   The response of syphilis to treatment should be determined by monitoring of the quantitative VDRL or RPR titer (Table 153-4). More frequent serologic examination is recommended for patients concurrently infected with HIV. Because the FTA-ABS and agglutination tests remain positive in most patients treated for seropositive syphilis, these tests are not useful in following the response to therapy. After successful treatment of seropositive first-episode primary or secondary syphilis, the VDRL titer progressively declines, becoming negative by 12 months in 40 to 75% of seropositive primary cases and in 20 to 40% of secondary cases. Patients with a history of syphilis have less rapid declines in titer and are less likely to become VDRL- or RPR-negative. Re-treatment should be considered if serologic responses are not adequate or if clinical signs persist or recur. Every effort should be made to differentiate treatment failure from reinfection, and the CSF should be examined. Patients in whom treatment failure is suspected, especially those with abnormal CSF, should be treated for neurosyphilis. If the patient remains seropositive but asymptomatic after such re-treatment, no further therapy is necessary. Patients treated for late latent syphilis frequently have low initial VDRL or RPR titers and may not have a fourfold drop after therapy with penicillin; about half of these patients remain seropositive (with low titers) for years after therapy. Re-treat-

Stage of Syphilis	Tests to Perform	When to Perform	Re-Treatment[a] Considered If:
Primary or secondary	Quantitative RPR or VDRL[b]	HIV-uninfected: 6 and 12 months HIV-infected: 3, 6, 9, and 12 months	1. Titer increases by fourfold *or* 2. Titer fails to decline by fourfold or test fails to become nonreactive by 6 months *or* 3. Clinical signs persist or recur
Latent or late	Quantitative RPR or VDRL[b]	6, 12, and 24 months	1. Titer increases by fourfold *or* 2. Initial titer of ≥1:32 fails to decline by fourfold by 6 months *or* 3. New clinical signs develop
Neurosyphilis (asymptomatic or symptomatic)	1. If CSF pleocytosis was documented initially, repeat CSF exam. 2. Monitor decline in CSF protein and CSF-VDRL. (Note: Rate of decline may be slow.) 3. Quantitative RPR or VDRL[b]	1. Every 6 months until CSF cell count is normal 2. Until normal 3. At 6, 12, 18, and 24 months	1. CSF cell count has not decreased at 6 months *or* 2. CSF is not normal after 2 years

[a] Try to distinguish between reinfection and treatment failure. If evidence of treatment failure exists, perform CSF examination. If CSF is normal, treat as for late latent syphilis (Table 153-3). If CSF is abnormal, treat as for neurosyphilis (Table 153-3).

[b] VDRL and RPR titers cannot be compared; use the same test for each follow-up sample.

ment is not warranted unless the titer rises or signs and symptoms of syphilis appear.

The activity of neurosyphilis correlates best with CSF pleocytosis, and this measure provides the most sensitive index of response to treatment. An elevated CSF cell count falls to normal in 3 to 12 months in adequately treated HIV-uninfected patients. The persistence of mild pleocytosis in HIV-infected patients may be due to the presence of HIV in CSF; this scenario may be difficult to distinguish from treatment failure. Elevated levels of CSF protein fall more slowly, and the CSF VDRL titer declines gradually over a period of several years.

IMMUNITY TO AND PREVENTION OF SYPHILIS The rate of development of acquired resistance to *T. pallidum* after natural or experimental infection is related to the size of the antigenic stimulus, which depends on both the size of the infecting inoculum and the duration of infection before treatment. The role of serum antibody in conferring immunity to syphilis remains undefined, although antibodies have been implicated in strain-specific immunity. Cellular immunity is considered to be of major importance in immunity and in the healing of early lesions. The cellular infiltration, predominantly T lymphocytes and macrophages, produces a T_H1 cytokine milieu consistent with the clearance of organisms by activated macrophages. Specific antibody enhances phagocytosis and is required for macrophage-mediated killing of *T. pallidum*. Recent unpublished studies indicate that sequence variation

of TprK occurs during *T. pallidum* infection. This observation suggests a role for antigenic variation in the persistence of infection and in susceptibility to reinfection with another strain.

FURTHER READING

CENTERS FOR DISEASE CONTROL AND PREVENTION: 2002 sexually transmitted diseases treatment guidelines. MMWR 51(RR-6):18, 2002

HOOK EW III et al: A randomized, comparative pilot study of azithromycin versus benzathine penicillin G for treatment of early syphilis. Sex Transm Dis 29:486, 2002

LUKEHART SA et al: Invasion of the central nervous system by *Treponema pallidum*: Implications for diagnosis and treatment. Ann Intern Med 109: 855, 1988

MARRA CM et al: Risk factors for neurosyphilis (late-breaker abstract). 2002 National STD Prevention Conference (http://www.cdc.gov/nchstp/dstd/2002ConfAbstracts/2002ConfAbLatebreaker.htm)

MCBROOM RL et al: Secondary syphilis in persons infected with and not infected with HIV-1: A comparative immunohistologic study. Am J Dermatopathol 21:432, 1999

MICHELOW IC et al: Central nervous system infection in congenital syphilis. N Engl J Med 346:1792, 2002

ROLFS RT et al: A randomized trial of enhanced therapy for early syphilis in patients with and without human immunodeficiency virus infection. N Engl J Med 337:307, 1997

ROMPALO AM et al: Modification of syphilitic genital ulcer manifestations by coexistent HIV infection. Sex Transm Dis 28:448, 2001

154 ENDEMIC TREPONEMATOSES
Sheila A. Lukehart

The endemic, or nonvenereal, treponematoses are bacterial infections that are caused by close relatives of *Treponema pallidum* subspecies *pallidum*, the etiologic agent of venereal syphilis (Chap. 153). Yaws, pinta, and endemic syphilis are distinguished from venereal syphilis by mode of transmission, age of acquisition, geographic distribution, and clinical features. These infections are limited primarily to rural areas of developing nations and are seen in the United States and Europe only in recent immigrants from endemic regions. Much of our "knowledge" about the endemic treponematoses is based upon impressions and observations of health care workers who have visited endemic areas; virtually no well-designed studies of the natural history, diagnosis, or treatment of these infections have been conducted. The treponemal infections are compared and contrasted in Table 154-1.

EPIDEMIOLOGY The endemic treponematoses are chronic diseases acquired during childhood and, like syphilis, can cause severe late manifestations years after initial infection. These infections were very common in Africa, Asia, and South America when the World Health Organization (WHO) and UNICEF embarked on a highly successful mass eradication campaign. From 1952 to 1969, it is estimated that over 160 million people were examined for treponemal infections and over 50 million cases, contacts, and latent infections were treated. This categorical program is one of WHO's outstanding successes in that the prevalence of active yaws was reduced from >20% to <1% in many rural areas and endemic syphilis was eradicated in Bosnia. In the decades since the eradication programs, lack of focused surveillance and diversion of resources to other pressing needs have resulted in a resurgence of these infections in some regions, particularly in Africa. The estimated geographic distribution of the endemic treponematoses in the 1990s is shown in Fig. 154-1. In the early 1980s, WHO sponsored a series of regional meetings on the endemic treponematoses, and areas of resurgent yaws morbidity were identified in West Africa (Ivory Coast, Ghana, Togo, Benin) and extending into the Central African Republic and rural Democratic Republic of Congo (formerly Zaire). The prevalence of endemic syphilis is estimated to be >10% in some regions of Mali, Niger, Burkina Faso, and Senegal. In Asia and the western Pacific, yaws is still prevalent in Indonesia,

TABLE 154-1 *Comparison of the Treponemes and Associated Diseases*

Feature	Venereal Syphilis	Yaws	Endemic Syphilis	Pinta
Organism	*T. pallidum* subspecies *pallidum*	*T. pallidum* subspecies *pertenue*	*T. pallidum* subspecies *endemicum*	*T. carateum*
Mode of transmission	Sexual, transplacental	Skin-to-skin	Household contacts: mouth-to-mouth or via shared drinking/ eating utensils	Skin-to-skin
Usual age of acquisition	Adulthood	Early childhood	Early childhood	Late childhood
Primary lesion	Cutaneous ulcer (chancre)	Papilloma, often ulcerative	Rarely seen	Nonulcerating papule with satellites, pruritic
Location	Genital, oral, anal	Extremities	Oral	Extremities, face
Secondary lesions	Mucocutaneous lesions; condylomata lata	Cutaneous papulo-squamous lesions; osteoperiostitis	Florid mucocutaneous lesions (mucous patch, split papule, condyloma latum); osteoperiostitis	Pintides, pigmented, pruritic
Infectious relapses	~25%	Common	Unknown	None
Late complications	Gummas, cardiovascular and CNS involvement[a]	Destructive gummas of skin, bone, cartilage	Destructive gummas of skin, bone, cartilage	Nondestructive, dyschromic, achromic macules

[a] CNS involvement in the endemic treponematoses has been postulated by some investigators (see text).

Papua New Guinea, and the Solomon Islands; cases have also been identified in Laos and Kampuchea. In the Americas, foci of yaws persist in Haiti and other Caribbean islands, Peru, Colombia, Ecuador, Brazil, Guyana, and Surinam. Pinta is limited to Central America and northern South America, where it is found rarely and only in remote villages. No accurate prevalence data are available for any of the endemic treponematoses because of a lack of active surveillance for these diseases. WHO estimates that there are 2.6 million cases overall, of which 460,000 are infectious.

MICROBIOLOGY The etiologic agents of the endemic treponematoses are *T. pallidum* subspecies *pertenue* (yaws), *T. pallidum* subspecies *endemicum* (endemic syphilis), and *T. carateum* (pinta). These little-studied organisms are morphologically identical to *T. pallidum* subspecies *pallidum*, and no antigenic differences among the pathogenic treponemes have been identified to date. A controversy has existed about whether the treponematoses are caused by different organisms or by the same organism, with clinical manifestations and routes of transmission defined by the climate of the region and the culture of

the population. Three of the four organisms have been placed in the same species because of their genetic similarity; the fourth (*T. carateum*) remains a separate species simply because no organisms have been available for genetic studies. However, a molecular signature has been defined that can be used to differentiate *T. pallidum* subspecies *pallidum* from the nonvenereal subspecies of *T. pallidum*, and unpublished studies have identified a number of distinct differences in the *tpr* gene family between venereal and nonvenereal treponemes. Whether these differences are related to the different clinical courses has not yet been determined.

CLINICAL FEATURES All of the treponemal infections are characterized by defined disease stages, with a localized primary lesion, disseminated secondary lesions, periods of latency, and possible late lesions. Primary and secondary stages are more frequently overlapping in yaws and endemic syphilis, and the late manifestations of pinta are very mild relative to the destructive lesions of the other treponematoses. The current preference is to divide the clinical course of the endemic treponematoses into "early" and "late" stages.

The major clinical features differing between venereal syphilis and the nonvenereal infections are the apparent lack of congenital transmission and the lack of central nervous system (CNS) involvement in the nonvenereal infections. It is not known whether these distinctions are accurate. Because of the high degree of genetic relatedness among the organisms, there is little biologic reason to think that *T. pallidum* subspecies *endemicum* and *T. pallidum* subspecies *pertenue* would be unable to cross the blood-brain barrier or to invade the placenta. These organisms obviously can disseminate from the site of primary infection to other tissues, and they can persist for decades. In this respect, they are like *T. pallidum* subspecies *pallidum*. The lack of recognized congenital infection may be due to the fact that the nonvenereal treponematoses are usually acquired during childhood. By the time an infected girl becomes sexually mature, she would be at low risk for

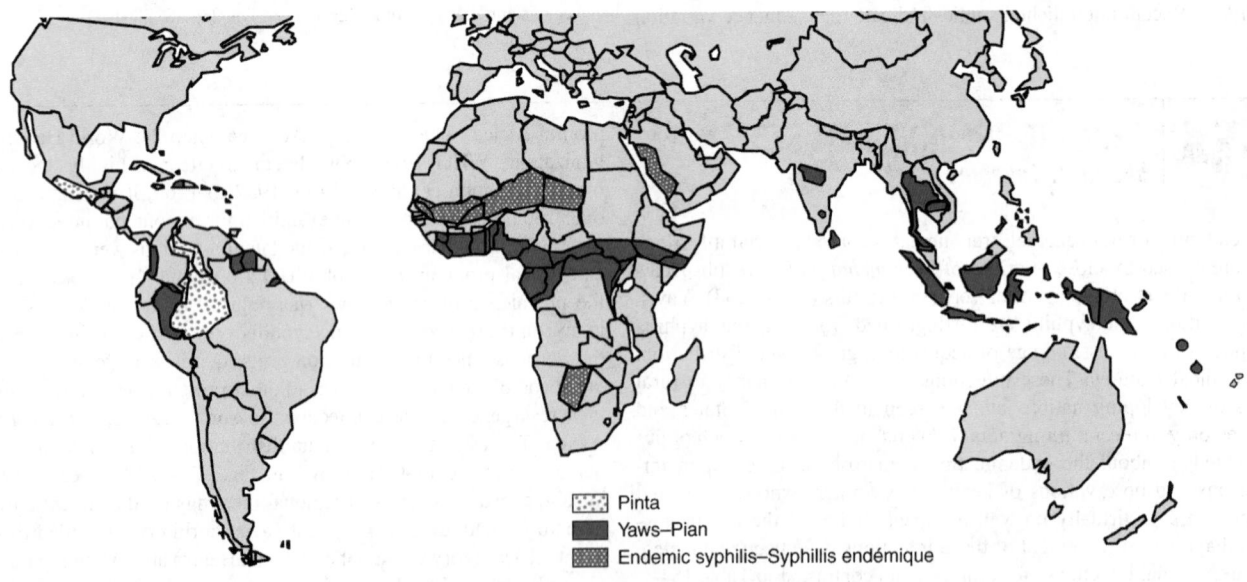

Pinta
Yaws–Pian
Endemic syphilis–Syphillis endémique

WHO 92522

FIGURE 154-1 Geographic distribution of endemic treponematoses in the 1990s. (*Courtesy of the World Health Organization.*)

transplacental transmission. Neurologic involvement may not have been recognized in nonvenereal treponemal infection because of the lack of trained medical personnel in endemic regions, the lag of years to decades between acquisition of infection and possible CNS manifestations, or a low rate of symptomatic CNS disease.

Some published evidence supports congenital transmission as well as cardiovascular, ophthalmologic, and CNS involvement in yaws. Although the case is strong, particularly for CNS involvement, most studies that have shown a relatively high incidence (average, 24.9%) of cerebrospinal fluid (CSF) abnormalities in patients with yaws were not controlled for other possible causes of CSF abnormalities, did not include treponeme-specific tests, or did not follow patients for resolution of abnormalities after antitreponemal therapy. Thus, while no firm conclusions can be drawn about the invasion of the CNS and placenta by the non-*pallidum* treponemes, it may be erroneous to accept unquestioningly the frequently repeated belief that these organisms fail to cause such manifestations.

Yaws Also known as *pian*, *framboesia*, or *bouba*, yaws is a chronic infection that is usually acquired in childhood and is caused by *T. pallidum* subspecies *pertenue*. The disease is characterized by the development of one or several primary lesions (called the "mother yaw"), followed by the appearance of multiple disseminated skin lesions. The early lesions may persist for many months, are infectious, and usually recur several times within the early years of infection. Late manifestations are destructive and can involve skin, bone, and joints.

The infection is transmitted by direct contact with infectious lesions, and transmission may be enhanced by disruption of the skin by insect bites or abrasions. Children with open lesions and without covering clothing are most likely to transmit infection during play or group sleeping. After an average incubation period estimated at 3 to 4 weeks, the first lesion begins as a papule, usually on an extremity, and then enlarges (particularly during moist warm weather) to become papillomatous or "raspberry-like" (thus the name "framboesia") (Fig. 154-2). Regional lymphadenopathy develops, and the lesion usually heals within 6 months; dissemination is thought to occur during the early weeks and months of infection. A generalized secondary eruption, accompanied by generalized lymphadenopathy, appears either concurrent with or following the primary lesion, may take several forms (macular, papular, or papillomatous), and may become secondarily infected with other bacteria. Painful papillomatous lesions on the soles of the feet result in a painful crablike gait ("crab yaws"), and periostitis may result in nocturnal bone pain and polydactylitis. All early skin lesions are infectious, and cutaneous relapses are common during the first 5 years. Late yaws is recognized in ~10% of untreated patients and is manifested by gummas of the skin and long bone, hyperkeratoses of the palms and soles, osteitis and periostitis, and hydrarthrosis. The late gummatous lesions are characteristically very destructive and extensive. Destruction of the nose, maxilla, palate, and pharynx is termed *gangosa* and is similar to the destructive lesions seen in leprosy and leishmaniasis.

Endemic Syphilis Endemic syphilis, also called *bejel, siti, dichuchwa, njovera*, or *skerljevo*, is a chronic infection caused by *T. pallidum* subspecies *endemicum*. Like other endemic treponematoses, endemic syphilis is chronic and is acquired in childhood. The early lesions are primarily localized to the mucocutaneous and mucosal surfaces, and the infection may be transmitted by direct contact, by kissing, or by sharing drinking and eating utensils. A role for insects in transmission has been suggested but is unproved. The initial lesion, usually an intraoral papule (Fig. 154-2), often goes unrecognized and is followed by mucous patches on the oral mucosa and mucocutaneous lesions resembling the condylomata lata of secondary syphilis. This eruption may last for months or even years, and treponemes can readily be demonstrated in early lesions. Periostitis and regional lymphadenopathy are common. After a variable period of latency, late manifestations may appear, including osseous and cutaneous gummas. Destructive gummas, osteitis, and gangosa are more common in endemic syphilis than in late yaws. Gummas of the nipples develop in women who have previously had endemic syphilis and who breast-feed infants with oral lesions. Thus, it appears that the late lesion may result from repeated exposure of a sensitized host.

Pinta Pinta (also called *mal del pinto, carate, azul*, or *purupuru*) is the most benign of the treponemal infections and is caused by *T. carateum*. This disease has three stages that are characterized by marked changes in skin color (Fig. 154-2), but it does not appear to cause destructive lesions or to involve other tissues. Transmission occurs by direct contact, usually during late childhood. The initial papule is most often located on the extremities or face and is pruritic. After one to many months of infection, numerous disseminated secondary lesions (*pintides*) appear. These lesions are initially red but become deeply pigmented, ultimately turning a dark slate blue. The secondary lesions are infectious and highly pruritic and may persist for years. Late pigmented lesions are called *dyschromic macules* and contain treponemes. Over time, most pigmented lesions show varying degrees of depigmentation, becoming brown and eventually white and giving the skin a mottled appearance. White achromic lesions are characteristic of the late stage.

DIAGNOSIS Diagnosis of the endemic treponematoses is based upon clinical manifestations and, when available, dark-field microscopy and serologic testing. The same tests that are used for venereal syphilis (Chap. 153) become reactive during all treponemal infections, and there is no serologic test that can discriminate among the different infections. The nonvenereal treponemal infections should be considered in the evaluation of a reactive syphilis serology in any person who has emigrated from an endemic area.

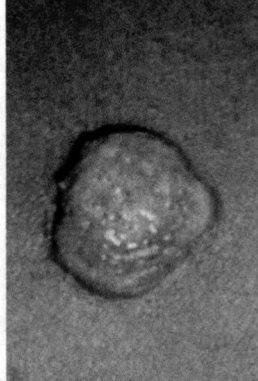
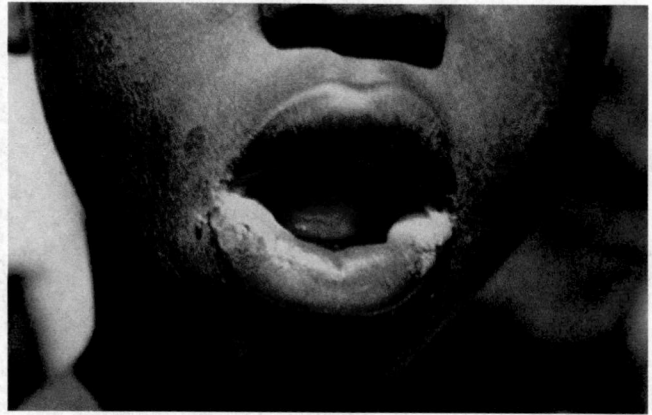
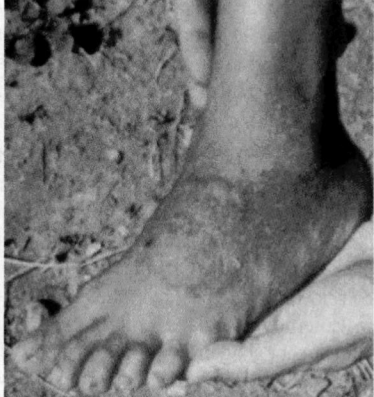

FIGURE 154-2 Clinical manifestations of endemic treponematoses. *Left:* Papillomatous primary lesion of yaws. *Center:* Split papules of early endemic syphilis. *Right:* Pigmented macules of pinta. *(From PL Perine et al.)*

Rx TREATMENT

The recommended therapy for patients and their contacts is benzathine penicillin at a dose of 1.2 million units intramuscularly; the dose for children <10 years of age is 600,000 units. There have been no controlled studies to show that the recommended lower dose (which is half the dose recommended for patients and contacts in early venereal syphilis) is effective in stopping relapse or progression to late disease. Definitive evidence of resistance to penicillin is lacking. However, because failure to heal existing lesions and frequent relapse following treatment for yaws have been described in Papua New Guinea, some health workers have suggested doubling the recommended dose of benzathine penicillin. Limited data suggest the efficacy of tetracycline for the treatment of yaws, but no such data exist for other endemic treponematoses. Solely on the basis of experience with venereal syphilis, it is thought that doxycycline, tetracycline, and erythromycin (at doses appropriate for syphilis; Chap. 153) are therapeutic alternatives for patients allergic to penicillin. A Jarisch-Herxheimer reaction (Chap. 153) may follow treatment of endemic treponematoses. Nontreponemal serologic titers [in the Venereal Disease Research Laboratory (VDRL) slide test or the rapid plasma reagin (RPR) test] usually decline after effective therapy, but patients may not become seronegative.

CONTROL   The endemic treponematoses can be controlled with inexpensive therapy. However, remote locations of affected populations can limit the availability of medical care. Although the mass treatment programs of three decades ago were widely successful, time has shown that sustained control requires vigilance in regular screening and in the investigation of outbreaks—luxuries that are often impossible in countries with more pressing medical needs. There is concern that, as HIV spreads throughout developing countries, it may markedly affect the manifestations and transmission of the endemic treponematoses.

FURTHER READING

ANTAL GM et al: The endemic treponematoses. Microbes Infect 4:83, 2002

BACKHOUSE JL et al: Failure of penicillin treatment of yaws on Karkar Island, Papua New Guinea. Am J Trop Med 59:388, 1998

CENTURION-LARA A et al: The flanking region sequences of the 15 kD lipoprotein gene differentiate pathogenic treponemes. J Infect Dis 177:1036, 1998

——— et al: Multiple alleles of *Treponema pallidum* repeat gene D in *Treponema pallidum* isolates. J Bacteriol 182:2332, 2000

ENGELKENS HJH et al: Nonvenereal treponematoses in tropical countries. Clin Dermatol 17:143, 1999

PARISH JL: Treponemal infections in the pediatric population. Clin Dermatol 18:687, 2000

WALKER SL et al: Yaws—a review of the last 50 years. Int J Dermatol 39:258, 2000

---

155 LEPTOSPIROSIS
Peter Speelman

Leptospirosis is an emerging infectious disease, as illustrated by recent large outbreaks in Asia, Central and South America, and the United States. The disease is caused by pathogenic leptospires and characterized by a broad spectrum of clinical manifestations, varying from inapparent infection to fulminant, fatal disease. In its mild form, leptospirosis may present as an influenza-like illness with headache and myalgias. Severe leptospirosis, characterized by jaundice, renal dysfunction, and hemorrhagic diathesis, is referred to as *Weil's syndrome*.

ETIOLOGIC AGENTS   Leptospires are spirochetes belonging to the order Spirochaetales and the family Leptospiraceae. Traditionally, the genus *Leptospira* comprised two species: the pathogenic *L. interrogans* and the free-living *L. biflexa*. Although 16 genomospecies of pathogenic leptospires are now recognized on the basis of their DNA relatedness, it is more practical clinically and epidemiologically to use a classification based on serologic differences. The pathogenic leptospires are divided into serovars according to their antigenic composition. More than 200 serovars make up the 25 serogroups.

Leptospires are coiled, thin, highly motile organisms with hooked ends and two periplasmic flagella that permit burrowing into tissue (Fig. 155-1). These organisms are 6 to 20 μm long and ~0.1 μm wide; they stain poorly but can be seen microscopically by dark-field examination and after silver impregnation staining. Leptospires require special media and conditions for growth; it may take weeks for cultures to become positive.

EPIDEMIOLOGY   Leptospirosis is an important zoonosis with a worldwide distribution that affects at least 160 mammalian species. Rodents, especially rats, are the most important reservoir, although other wild mammals as well as domestic and farm animals may also harbor these microorganisms. Leptospires establish a symbiotic relationship with their host and can persist in the renal tubules for years. Some serovars are generally associated with particular animals—e.g., icterohaemorrhagiae/copenhageni with rats, grippotyphosa with voles, hardjo with cattle, canicola with dogs, and pomona with pigs—but may occur in other animals as well.

Transmission of leptospires may follow direct contact with urine, blood, or tissue from an infected animal or exposure to a contaminated environment; human-to-human transmission is rare. Since leptospires are excreted in the urine and can survive in water for many months, water is an important vehicle in their transmission. Epidemics of leptospirosis may result from exposure to flood waters contaminated by urine from infected animals, as has been reported from Nicaragua. Leptospirosis occurs most commonly in the tropics because the climate as well as the sometimes poor hygienic conditions favor the pathogen's survival. In many developing countries, leptospirosis is an underestimated problem. Reliable data on morbidity and mortality from leptospirosis have gradually started to appear. In 1999, more than 500,000 cases were reported from China, with case-fatality rates ranging from 0.9 to 7.9%. In Brazil, more than 28,000 cases were reported in the same year.

Humans are not commonly infected with leptospires. However, in the United States, the 40 to 120 cases reported annually to the Centers for Disease Control and Prevention (CDC) surely represent a significant underestimation of the total number. Certain occupational groups

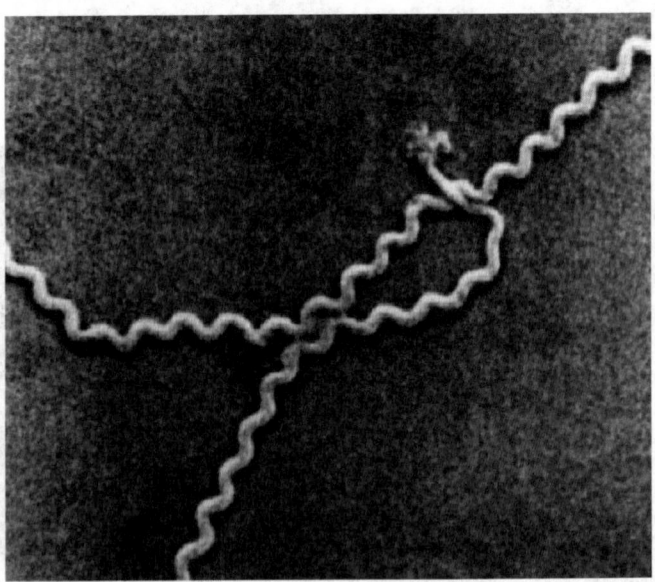

FIGURE 155-1   Scanning electron micrograph of leptospires.

are at especially high risk; included are veterinarians, agricultural workers, sewage workers, slaughterhouse employees, and workers in the fishing industry. Such individuals may acquire leptospirosis through direct exposure to or contact with contaminated water and soil. Leptospirosis has also been recognized in deteriorating inner cities where rat populations are expanding. One report described leptospirosis in urban residents of Baltimore who were sporadically exposed to rat urine.

Recreational exposure and domestic-animal contact are also prominent sources of leptospirosis. Recreational water activities, such as canoeing, windsurfing, swimming, and waterskiing, place persons at risk for leptospirosis. In 1998, a large outbreak occurred among athletes and community residents after a triathlon in Illinois. Among athletes, the ingestion of one or more swallows of lake water was a prominent risk factor for illness. Heavy rains that preceded the triathlon, with consequent agricultural runoff, are likely to have increased the level of leptospiral contamination in the lake water.

Sometimes leptospirosis is acquired during travel abroad. In a study in the Netherlands, 14% of patients with confirmed leptospirosis had acquired the infection while traveling in tropical countries, mostly in Southeast Asia. Transmission via laboratory accidents has been reported but is rare. Leptospirosis develops occasionally after unanticipated immersion in contaminated water (e.g., in an automobile accident) and rarely after an animal bite. Most cases occur in men, with a peak incidence during the summer and fall in Western countries and during the rainy season in the tropics.

PATHOGENESIS The pathogenesis of leptospirosis is incompletely understood. Leptospires may enter the host through abrasions in the skin or through intact mucous membranes, especially the conjunctiva and the lining of the oro- and nasopharynx. Drinking of contaminated water may introduce leptospires through the mouth, throat, or esophagus. After entry of the organisms, leptospiremia develops, with subsequent spread to all organs. Multiplication takes place in blood and in tissues, and leptospires can be isolated from blood and cerebrospinal fluid (CSF) during the first 4 to 10 days of illness. CSF examination during this period documents pleocytosis in the majority of instances, but only a minority of patients develop symptoms and signs of meningitis at this point. All forms of leptospires can damage the wall of small blood vessels; this damage leads to vasculitis with leakage and extravasation of cells, including hemorrhages. The most important known pathogenic properties of leptospires are adhesion to cell surfaces and cellular toxicity.

Vasculitis is responsible for the most important manifestations of the disease. Although leptospires mainly infect the kidneys and liver, any organ may be affected. In the kidney, leptospires migrate to the interstitium, renal tubules, and tubular lumen, causing interstitial nephritis and tubular necrosis. Hypovolemia due to dehydration or altered capillary permeability may contribute to the development of renal failure. In the liver, centrilobular necrosis with proliferation of Kupffer cells may be found. However, severe hepatocellular necrosis is not a feature of leptospirosis. Pulmonary involvement is the result of hemorrhage and not of inflammation. Invasion of skeletal muscle by leptospires results in swelling, vacuolation of the myofibrils, and focal necrosis. In severe leptospirosis, vasculitis may ultimately impair the microcirculation and increase capillary permeability, resulting in fluid leakage and hypovolemia.

When antibodies are formed, leptospires are eliminated from all sites in the host except the eye, the proximal renal tubules, and perhaps the brain, where they may persist for weeks or months. The persistence

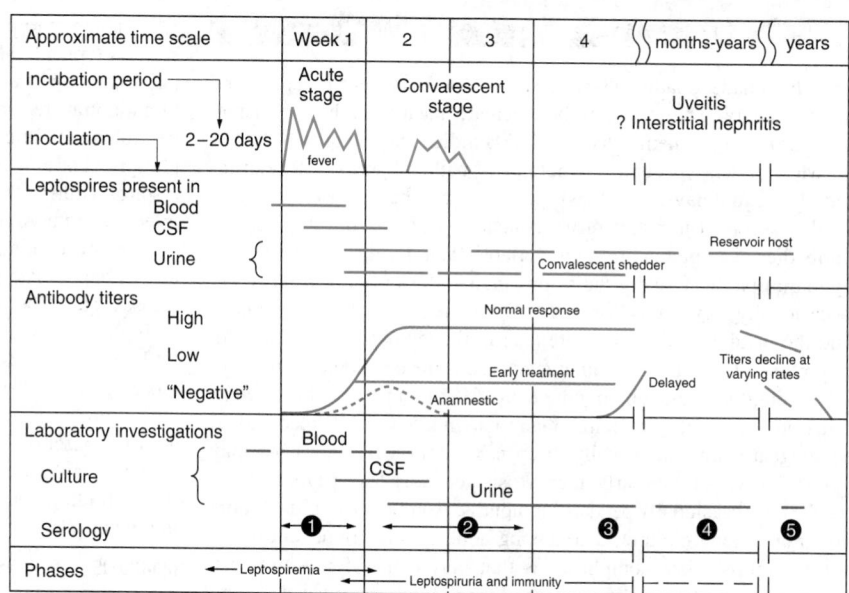

FIGURE 155-2 Biphasic nature of leptospirosis and relevant investigations at different stages of disease. Specimens 1 and 2 for serology are acute-phase serum samples; specimen 3 is a convalescent-phase serum sample that may facilitate detection of a delayed immune response; and specimens 4 and 5 are follow-up serum samples that can provide epidemiologic information, such as the presumptive infecting serogroup. [*Reprinted as adapted by Levett (from Turner LH: Leptospirosis. BMJ 1:231, 1969) with permission from the American Society for Microbiology and the BMJ Publishing Group.*]

of leptospires in the aqueous humor occasionally causes chronic or recurrent uveitis. The systemic immune response is effective in eliminating the organism but may also produce symptomatic inflammatory reactions. A rise in antibody titer coincides with the development of meningitis; this association suggests that an immunologic mechanism is responsible.

After the start of antimicrobial treatment for leptospirosis, a Jarisch-Herxheimer reaction similar to that seen in other spirochetal diseases may develop. Although frequently described in older publications, this reaction seems to be a rare event in leptospirosis and is certainly less frequent in this infection than in other spirochetal diseases.

CLINICAL MANIFESTATIONS (Fig. 155-2) It is important to try to obtain a history of exposure to contaminated materials. Serologic evidence of past inapparent infection is found in 15 to 40% of persons who have been exposed but have not become ill. In symptomatic cases of leptospirosis, clinical manifestations vary from mild to serious or even fatal. More than 90% of symptomatic persons have the relatively mild and usually anicteric form of leptospirosis, with or without meningitis. Severe leptospirosis with profound jaundice (Weil's syndrome) develops in 5 to 10% of infected individuals. The idea that distinct clinical syndromes are associated with specific serogroups has been refuted.

The incubation period is usually 1 to 2 weeks but ranges from 2 to 20 days (Fig. 155-2). Typically, an acute leptospiremic phase is followed by an immune leptospiruric phase. The distinction between the first and second phases is not always clear, and milder cases do not always include the second phase.

Anicteric Leptospirosis Leptospirosis may present as an acute influenza-like illness, with fever, chills, severe headache, nausea, vomiting, and myalgias. Muscle pain, which especially affects the calves, back, and abdomen, is an important feature of leptospiral infection. Less common features include sore throat and rash. The patient usually has an intense headache (frontal or retroorbital) and sometimes develops photophobia. Mental confusion may be evident. Pulmonary involvement, manifested in most cases by cough and chest pain and in a few cases by hemoptysis, is not uncommon.

The most common finding on physical examination is fever with conjunctival suffusion. Less common findings include muscle tenderness, lymphadenopathy, pharyngeal injection, rash, hepatomegaly, and splenomegaly. The rash may be macular, maculopapular, erythematous, urticarial, or hemorrhagic. Mild jaundice may be present.

Most patients become asymptomatic within 1 week. After an interval of 1 to 3 days, the illness recurs in a number of cases. The start of this second (immune) phase coincides with the development of antibodies. Symptoms are more variable than during the first (leptospiremic) phase. Usually the symptoms last for only a few days, but occasionally they persist for weeks. Often the fever is less pronounced and the myalgias are less severe than in the leptospiremic phase. An important event during the immune phase is the development of aseptic meningitis. Although no more than 15% of all patients have symptoms and signs of meningitis, many patients have CSF pleocytosis. Meningeal symptoms usually disappear within a few days but may persist for weeks. Similarly, pleocytosis generally disappears within 2 weeks but occasionally persists for months. Aseptic meningitis is more common among children than among adults. Iritis, iridocyclitis, and chorioretinitis—late complications that may persist for years—can become apparent as early as the third week but often present several months after the initial illness. One epidemic of uveitis among patients with leptospirosis has been reported. Mortality in anicteric leptospirosis is almost nil, although death as a result of pulmonary hemorrhage occurred in 2.4% of cases in a Chinese outbreak.

Severe Leptospirosis (Weil's Syndrome)   Weil's syndrome, the most severe form of leptospirosis, is characterized by jaundice, renal dysfunction, hemorrhagic diathesis, and a mortality rate ranging from 5 to 15%. In Europe, this syndrome is frequently but not exclusively associated with infection due to serovar icterohaemorrhagiae/copenhageni. The onset of illness is no different from that of less severe leptospirosis; however, after 4 to 9 days, jaundice as well as renal and vascular dysfunction generally develop. Although some degree of defervescence may be noted after the first week of illness, a biphasic disease pattern like that seen in anicteric leptospirosis is lacking. The jaundice of Weil's syndrome, which can be profound and give an orange cast to the skin, is usually not associated with severe hepatic necrosis. Death is rarely due to liver failure. Hepatomegaly and tenderness in the right upper quadrant are usually detected. Splenomegaly is found in 20% of cases.

Renal failure may develop, often during the second week of illness. Hypovolemia and decreased renal perfusion contribute to the development of acute tubular necrosis with oliguria or anuria. Dialysis is sometimes required, although a fair number of cases can be managed without dialysis. Renal function may be completely regained.

Pulmonary involvement occurs frequently; in some clusters of cases, it is a major manifestation, resulting in cough, dyspnea, chest pain, and blood-stained sputum and sometimes in hemoptysis or even respiratory failure. Hemorrhagic manifestations are seen in Weil's syndrome: epistaxis, petechiae, purpura, and ecchymoses are found commonly, while severe gastrointestinal bleeding and adrenal or subarachnoid hemorrhage are detected rarely.

Rhabdomyolysis, hemolysis, myocarditis, pericarditis, congestive heart failure, cardiogenic shock, adult respiratory distress syndrome, necrotizing pancreatitis, and multiorgan failure have all been described during severe leptospirosis.

LABORATORY AND RADIOLOGIC FINDINGS   (Fig. 155-2) The kidneys are invariably involved in leptospirosis. Related findings range from urinary sediment changes (leukocytes, erythrocytes, and hyaline or granular casts) and mild proteinuria in anicteric leptospirosis to renal failure and azotemia in severe disease.

The erythrocyte sedimentation rate is usually elevated. In anicteric leptospirosis, peripheral leukocyte counts range from 3000 to 26,000/μL, with a left shift; in Weil's syndrome, leukocytosis is often marked. Mild thrombocytopenia occurs in up to 50% of patients and is associated with renal failure.

In contrast to patients with acute viral hepatitis, those with leptospirosis typically have elevated serum levels of bilirubin and alkaline phosphatase as well as mild increases (up to 200 U/L) in serum levels of aminotransferases. In Weil's syndrome, the prothrombin time may be prolonged but can be corrected with vitamin K. Levels of creatine phosphokinase, which are elevated in up to 50% of patients with leptospirosis during the first week of illness, may help to differentiate this infection from viral hepatitis.

When a meningeal reaction develops, polymorphonuclear leukocytes predominate initially and the number of mononuclear cells increases later. The protein concentration in the CSF may be elevated; CSF glucose levels are normal.

In severe leptospirosis, pulmonary radiographic abnormalities are more common than would be expected on the basis of physical examination. These abnormalities most frequently develop 3 to 9 days after the onset of illness. The most common radiographic finding is a patchy alveolar pattern that corresponds to scattered alveolar hemorrhage. Radiographic abnormalities most often affect the lower lobes in the periphery of the lung fields.

DIAGNOSIS   (Fig. 155-2) A definite diagnosis of leptospirosis is based either on isolation of the organism from the patient or on seroconversion or a rise in antibody titer in the microscopic agglutination test (MAT). In the United States, the MAT is performed only at the CDC. In cases with strong clinical evidence of infection, a single antibody titer of 1:400 to 1:800 (depending on whether the case occurs in a low- or high-endemic area) in the MAT is required. Preferably, a fourfold or greater rise in titer is detected between acute- and convalescent-phase serum specimens. Antibodies generally do not reach detectable levels until the second week of illness. The antibody response can be affected by early treatment.

The MAT, which uses a battery of live leptospiral strains, and the enzyme-linked immunosorbent assay (ELISA), which uses a broadly reacting antigen, are the standard serologic procedures. These tests usually are available only in specialized laboratories and are used for determination of the antibody titer and for tentative identification of the serogroup—and in some cases the serovar—involved (thus the importance of using antigens representative of the serovars prevalent in the particular geographic area). Since cross-reactions occur frequently, however, it is often impossible to identify the infecting serogroup or serovar. Serologic testing cannot be used as the basis for a decision about whether to start treatment.

In addition to the MAT and the ELISA, various other tests with diagnostic value have been developed. Some tests, such as an indirect hemagglutination test and a microcapsule agglutination test, are commercially available. A recent advance is the development of rapid serologic assays that apply lateral flow, latex agglutination, or ELISA methodology with reasonable sensitivity and specificity. These methods do not require culture or MAT facilities. However, in endemic areas, pooled serum samples from the local population are required as positive and negative controls. Polymerase chain reaction (PCR) techniques have been developed but so far have not found widespread use outside research and reference laboratories.

Leptospires can be isolated from blood and/or CSF during the first 10 days of illness and from urine for several weeks beginning at around 1 week. Cultures most often become positive after 2 to 4 weeks, with a range of 1 week to 4 months. Sometimes urine cultures remain positive for months or years after the start of illness. For isolation of leptospires from body fluids or tissues, Ellinghausen-McCullough-Johnson-Harris (EMJH) medium is useful; other possibilities are Fletcher medium and Korthof medium. Specimens can be mailed to a reference laboratory for culture, since leptospires remain viable in anticoagulated blood (heparin, EDTA, or citrate) for up to 11 days. Isolation of leptospires is important since it is the only way the infecting serovar can be correctly identified. Dark-field examination of blood or urine frequently results in misdiagnosis and should not be used.

DIFFERENTIAL DIAGNOSIS   Leptospirosis should be differentiated from other febrile illnesses associated with headache and muscle pain, such as dengue, malaria, enteric fever, viral hepatitis, *Hantavirus* infections, and rickettsial diseases. In light of the strong similarity in epidemiology and clinical presentation between leptospirosis and *Hantavirus* infections and given the reported occurrence of dual infections, it is advisable to conduct serologic testing for *Hantavirus* in cases of suspected leptospirosis. When patients have a flulike disease with disproportionately severe myalgia or aseptic meningitis, a diagnosis of leptospirosis should be considered.

Ⓡ TREATMENT

The effectiveness of antimicrobial therapy for the mild febrile form of leptospirosis is controversial, but such treatment is indicated for more severe forms. Treatment should be initiated as early as possible; nevertheless, contrary to previous reports, treatment started after the first 4 days of illness is effective.

For severe cases of leptospirosis, intravenous administration of penicillin G, amoxicillin, ampicillin, or erythromycin is recommended (Table 155-1). In milder cases, oral treatment with tetracycline, doxycycline, ampicillin, or amoxicillin should be considered. Although several other antibiotics, including newer cephalosporins, are highly active against leptospires in vitro, no clinical experience has yet been gained with these drugs.

In rare cases, a Jarisch-Herxheimer reaction develops within hours after the start of antimicrobial therapy (see "Pathogenesis" above). Although so far the only effective mode of management is supportive, the role of antibodies to tumor necrosis factor in the treatment of this reaction deserves further study. A beneficial effect of the use of such antibodies for the modulation of the reaction has been demonstrated in patients with louse-borne relapsing fever. Patients with severe leptospirosis and renal failure may require dialysis. Those with Weil's syndrome may need transfusions of whole blood and/or platelets. Intensive care may be necessary.

PROGNOSIS Most patients with leptospirosis recover. Mortality is highest among patients who are elderly and those who have Weil's syndrome. Leptospirosis during pregnancy is associated with high fetal mortality. Long-term follow-up of patients with renal failure and hepatic dysfunction has documented good recovery of renal and hepatic function.

PREVENTION Individuals who may be exposed to leptospires through their occupations or their involvement in recreational water activities should be informed about the risks. Measures for controlling leptospirosis include avoidance of exposure to urine and tissues from infected animals, vaccination of animals, and rodent control. The animal

TABLE 155-1 *Treatment and Chemoprophylaxis of Leptospirosis*

Purpose of Drug Administration	Regimen
Treatment	
Mild leptospirosis	Doxycycline, 100 mg orally bid *or* Ampicillin, 500–750 mg orally qid *or* Amoxicillin, 500 mg orally qid
Moderate/severe leptospirosis	Penicillin G, 1.5 million units IV qid *or* Ampicillin, 1 g IV qid *or* Amoxicillin, 1 g IV qid *or* Erythromycin, 500 mg IV qid
Chemoprophylaxis	Doxycycline, 200 mg orally once a week

Note: All regimens used for treatment are administered for 7 days.

vaccine used in a given area should contain the serovars known to be present in that area. Unfortunately, some vaccinated animals still excrete leptospires in their urine. Vaccination of humans against a specific serovar prevalent in an area has been undertaken in some European and Asian countries and has proved effective. Although a large-scale trial of vaccine in humans has been reported from Cuba, no conclusions can be drawn about efficacy and adverse reactions because of insufficient details on study design. Chemoprophylaxis with doxycycline (200 mg once a week) has appeared to be efficacious to some extent but is indicated only in rare instances of sustained short-term exposure (Table 155-1).

FURTHER READING

CHU KM et al: Identification of *Leptospira* species in the pathogenesis of uveitis and determination of clinical ocular characteristics in south India. J Infect Dis 177:1314, 1998

LEVETT PN: Leptospirosis. Clin Microbiol Rev 14: 296, 2001

MORGAN J et al: Outbreak of leptospirosis among triathlon participants and community residents in Springfield, Illinois, 1998. Clin Infect Dis 34:1593, 2002

SEHGAL SC et al: Randomized controlled trial of doxycycline prophylaxis against leptospirosis in an endemic area. Int J Antimicrob Agents 13:249, 2000

TREVEJO RT et al: Epidemic leptospirosis associated with pulmonary hemorrhage—Nicaragua. J Infect Dis 178:1457, 1998

VINETZ JM: Leptospirosis. Curr Opin Infect Dis 14:527, 2001

WORLD HEALTH ORGANIZATION/INTERNATIONAL LEPTOSPIROSIS SOCIETY: *Human Leptospirosis: Guidance for Diagnosis, Surveillance and Control*. Geneva, World Health Organization, 2003, 109 pp

156 RELAPSING FEVER
David T. Dennis, Edward B. Hayes

DEFINITION The term *relapsing fever* describes two distinct diseases. *Tick-borne (endemic)* relapsing fever (TBRF) is a zoonosis that is transmitted principally from rodents to humans by the bite of various soft ticks. *Louse-borne (epidemic)* relapsing fever (LBRF) is a disease of humans that is transmitted from one person to another by the body louse. Both are characterized by recurrent acute episodes of spirochetemia and fever alternating with spontaneous spirochetal clearance and apyrexia.

ETIOLOGY Relapsing fever is caused by infection with spirochetal gram-negative bacteria of the genus *Borrelia* (family Spirochaetaceae). The borreliae are helical in shape and average 0.2 to 0.5 μm in width and 5 to 20 μm in length. They comprise an outer membrane, an intermediate peptidoglycan layer, and an inner cytoplasmic membrane, which encloses the protoplasmic cylinder. A variable number of periplasmic flagella are situated beneath the outer membrane. Relapsing-

fever borreliae are slow-growing and microaerophilic; they grow best at 30° to 35°C in Barbour-Stoenner-Kelly (BSK II) medium.

B. recurrentis is the only species that causes LBRF. Most of the several species of *Borrelia* that cause TBRF are named after the species of *Ornithodoros* tick responsible for their transmission. In North America, *B. hermsii* and *B. turicatae* cause almost all cases of TBRF; *B. duttoni* is the most common cause of TBRF in sub-Saharan Africa, an area of high endemicity. Borreliae are unique among bacteria in having a genome composed of a linear chromosome and a series of linear and circular plasmids. The sequences of both the flagellin and the 16S ribosomal RNA genes are homogeneous among LBRF strains; in contrast, there is considerable heterogeneity of these genes between Old World and New World TBRF strains. A unique process of DNA rearrangement within *vmp* genes located on linear plasmids results in extensive variation in the expression of the surface antigens in relapsing-fever borreliae. These *vmp* genes encode variable major proteins (VMPs) found on the spirochete's outer-membrane surface. The antigenic variation generated by sequential expression of previously silent *vmp* genes allows the borreliae to intermittently escape the immune response of the host and results in the febrile relapses that are characteristic of infection with these organisms.

EPIDEMIOLOGY ■ **Louse-Borne Relapsing Fever**   Body lice (*Pediculus humanus* var. *corporis*) become infected with *B. recurrentis* by feeding on spirochetemic humans, the only reservoirs of infection. In lice, *B. recurrentis* spirochetes are found almost exclusively in the hemolymph; humans acquire infection when infected body lice are crushed and their fluids contaminate mucous membranes or breaks in the skin (such as abrasions caused by scratching of pruritic louse bites). Spirochetes are *not* transmitted directly by the bite of a louse (anterior station transmission) or by inoculation of louse feces (posterior station transmission). Lice have a life span of only a few weeks, feed at frequent intervals, and survive only a few days off the human host. Head lice do not appear to be vectors of LBRF.

LBRF has severely affected military and civilian populations disrupted by war and other disasters. In the nineteenth century, the disease was common among slum dwellers, prisoners, and others living in impoverished, overcrowded, and unhygienic conditions. In the first half of the twentieth century, during periods of war and famine, both LBRF and louse-borne typhus were epidemic in eastern Europe, the Balkans, and the former Soviet Union. The global distribution and incidence of LBRF were substantially reduced following improvements in standards of living, sanitation, and hygiene; LBRF is now an important disease only in northeastern Africa, especially the highlands of Ethiopia, where an estimated 10,000 cases occur annually. In Ethiopia, the disease affects mostly homeless men crowded together in unhygienic circumstances, especially during the cool rainy season, when washing and changing clothing is more difficult. LBRF has repeatedly spilled out of Ethiopia into populations of displaced persons in neighboring Somalia and Sudan. During the Second World War, the spread of LBRF from Ethiopia and the Sudan to western Africa was pandemic.

Short-term visitors to endemic areas (e.g., tourists) are at almost no risk of LBRF, but persons who have close contact with LBRF populations (such as relief workers) can acquire the disease from lice, accidental needle sticks, or other direct contact with contaminated blood.

Tick-Borne Relapsing Fever   Argasid ticks of the genus *Ornithodoros* transmit TBRF through their saliva and excreta when they feed on humans. As a rule, the ticks become infected with TBRF borreliae as part of a zoonotic cycle when they feed on spirochetemic rodents and lagomorphs; the exception to this rule is *O. moubata*, a tick species that acquires *B. duttoni* by feeding on infected humans. Ticks transmit TBRF borreliae vertically from one stage to the next; in some species, infection is transmitted transovarially over several generations. Soft ticks are hardy and can survive for 10 years with only an occasional blood meal. These ticks feed painlessly, relatively quickly (for 20 to 45 min), and usually at night while hosts are sleeping. Thus patients with TBRF are often unaware of tick exposures.

TBRF borreliae are widely distributed throughout the world. Human infection with these organisms is generally underrecognized and underreported. TBRF is most highly endemic in sub-Saharan Africa but is also found in countries of the Mediterranean littoral, Middle Eastern states, southern Russia, the Indian subcontinent, Central Asia, and China and at low frequency in North, Central, and South America. The disease typically occurs sporadically or in small—often familial—clusters. Infected soft ticks may cause repeated infections among persons living or sleeping in the same dwelling. In sub-Saharan Africa, *O. moubata*, the vector of *B. duttoni*, infests native huts and rest houses, hiding in crevices of floors and walls during the day and emerging at night to feed on sleeping inhabitants.

In the United States, TBRF disease occurs west of the Mississippi River, especially in forested mountainous areas of far western states, where *B. hermsii* is the causative agent. Less commonly, persons are infected with *B. turicatae* following exposures in tick-infested caves in semidesert areas of the Southwest. On average, ~35 cases of TBRF are reported annually in the United States. *B. hermsii* infections most often occur during spring and summer months among persons sleeping in rustic mountain cabins and vacation homes and occasionally in permanent residences and in outdoor settings. Infections of humans are sometimes precipitated by the disappearance of rodents (e.g., as a result of epizootic plague) that nest in foundations, wall spaces, and attics and that serve as the usual maintenance hosts for *O. hermsii* ticks. Outbreaks caused by *B. hermsii* have taken place among persons staying in cabins along the north rim of the Grand Canyon and in the mountains of California, Idaho, and Colorado. In North America, most recent cases have been reported from Washington, California, Colorado, Idaho, Oregon, and British Columbia.

PATHOGENESIS AND PATHOLOGY   In humans, relapsing-fever borreliae pass through the skin or mucous membranes, multiply in the blood, and circulate in great numbers during febrile periods. The organisms have also been found in the liver, spleen, bone marrow, and central nervous system and may be sequestered at these sites during periods of remission. The disease tends to be more severe when spirochete density in the blood is high. Even though the pathophysiologic manifestations of the disease resemble responses to endotoxin, and although plasma from some patients with relapsing fever coagulates *Limulus* amebocyte lysates, borreliae and other spirochetes have not been shown to express a true lipopolysaccharide (endotoxin) molecule. Infection with *B. recurrentis* has been shown, however, to activate protein mediators of inflammation, such as Hageman factor (factor XII), prekallikrein, and proteins of the complement system; furthermore, a spirochetal heat-stable pyrogenic factor stimulates mononuclear phagocytes to express increased amounts of leukocyte pyrogen and thromboplastin.

The treatment of relapsing fever with antibiotics may provoke a Jarisch-Herxheimer reaction (see "Treatment," below). In patients with LBRF, this reaction has been associated with a release of various cytokines into the plasma, including interleukin 6, interleukin 8, C-reactive protein, and large amounts of tumor necrosis factor a (TNF-α). Pretreatment of LBRF patients with antibody to TNF-α suppressed Jarisch-Herxheimer reactions following penicillin treatment and reduced the plasma concentrations of certain other cytokines.

Death due to TBRF is rare. In contrast, fatality rates of 20% have been recorded during outbreaks of LBRF in malnourished and stressed populations. Relapsing fever in pregnancy can result in abortion, stillbirth, and fatal neonatal infections. Autopsies of patients with relapsing fever most often reveal hepatosplenomegaly and variable edema and swelling of other organs, including brain, lungs, and kidneys. On microscopic examination, the spleen is congested and contains multiple microabscesses composed of mononuclear cells that replace the white pulp, the myocardium displays diffuse histiocytic inflammation and interstitial edema, and the liver has areas of midzonal necrosis. Petechial hemorrhages are commonly evident over the surfaces of the meninges, pleura, heart, spleen, liver, kidneys, and mesentery. Subcapsular and parenchymal hemorrhagic infarcts of the spleen, heart, liver, and brain are sometimes grossly visible.

CLINICAL MANIFESTATIONS   The clinical manifestations of LBRF and TBRF are similar. The common signs and symptoms of TBRF, as documented in North America, are listed in Table 156-1. The mean incubation period is 7 days (range, 2 to 18 days), and the onset of illness is sudden, with fever, headache, shaking chills, sweats, myalgias, and arthralgias. The arthralgia of relapsing fever can be severe, involving small and large joints, but there is no evidence of arthritis. Dizziness, nausea, and vomiting are common. Sleep may be difficult and is sometimes accompanied by disturbing dreams. The patient is coherent but withdrawn, thirsty, and uninterested in food and other outside stimuli. The fever is high from the first, with temperature usually reaching ≥40°C (≥104°F) and then becoming irregular in pattern. High fever is sometimes accompanied by delirium. Patients are usually

TABLE 156-1 *Manifestations of Tick-Borne Relapsing Fever Acquired in the Northwestern United States and Southwestern British Columbia*

Sign or Symptom	%	Sign or Symptom	%
Headache	94	Photophobia	25
Myalgia	92	Neck pain	24
Chills	88	Rash	18
Nausea	76	Dysuria	13
Arthralgia	73	Jaundice	10
Vomiting	71	Hepatomegaly	10
Abdominal pain	44	Splenomegaly	6
Confusion	38	Conjunctival injection	5
Dry cough	27	Eschar	2
Eye pain	26	Meningitis	2
Diarrhea	25	Nuchal rigidity	2
Dizziness	25		

Source: From a review of 182 cases reported in the period 1980–1995 (Dworkin et al.).

tachycardic and mildly tachypneic and become prostrate as the disease progresses. Some patients have meningismus. The conjunctivae are often injected, and photophobia is common. The sclerae may become icteric, particularly in the later stages of illness. The mucous membranes may be dry, and patients are often dehydrated. Scattered petechiae develop on the trunk, extremities, and mucous membranes in one-third or more of patients with LBRF but in a smaller proportion of patients with TBRF. A nonproductive cough is common, but chest sounds are usually normal; pleuritic pain and an accompanying pleuritic rub are sometimes noted. Cardiac findings are compatible with a high-output state; tachycardia and summation gallop are common. Tender enlargement of the spleen and liver frequently occurs in the acute phase of illness.

Epistaxis and blood-tinged sputum are common complications, and gastrointestinal and central nervous system hemorrhage can occur. Because of this coagulopathy, one LBRF outbreak in southern Sudan was thought to be viral hemorrhagic fever. Other complications of variable incidence include iridocyclitis, optic neuritis, lymphocytic meningitis, coma, isolated cranial-nerve palsy, pneumonitis, myocarditis, and rupture of the spleen. Life-threatening complications are unusual in otherwise healthy persons given supportive care, especially if the illness is diagnosed and treated early. Children generally have a milder course of illness than adults.

Without treatment, symptoms intensify over a 2- to 7-day period (average, 5 days in LBRF and 3 days in TBRF), ending in a spontaneous crisis that coincides with the disappearance of spirochetes from the circulation. The crisis comprises two phases over several hours: a *chill phase*, characterized by rigors, rising temperature, and hypermetabolism, and a *flush phase* of falling temperature, diaphoresis, and a decreased effective circulating blood volume. The pathophysiologic events associated with this crisis are magnified when precipitated by antibiotic treatment and are indistinguishable from the Jarisch-Herxheimer reaction of treated syphilis (see "Treatment," below). The crisis is followed by a period of exhaustion, sleep, and an uneventful recovery. Orthostatic hypotension is typical in the early recovery phase. Not uncommonly, in the first week of convalescence, the patient experiences 1 or 2 days of mild fever unassociated with detectable spirochetemia. In untreated patients, spirochetemia and symptoms may recur after a period of several days or weeks (average interval to first relapse, 9 days in LBRF and 7 days in TBRF). Only one or two relapses characteristically occur in untreated patients with LBRF, whereas as many as 10 (average, three) can occur in untreated patients with TBRF. In most cases, the illness becomes shorter and milder and the afebrile intervals longer with each relapse. Because of the great antigenic variation among *Borrelia* strains, infection confers only partial immunity, and repeated infections of the same individual have been recorded.

Diseases that should be considered in the differential diagnosis of relapsing fever or that may complicate relapsing fever include typhus fever, typhoid fever, nontyphoid salmonellosis, malaria, dengue and other arboviral illnesses, tuberculosis, leptospirosis, and viral hemorrhagic fevers. In the United States, the geographic distribution of Colorado tick fever (Chap. 180) overlaps that of TBRF, and the two diseases have similar manifestations early in their courses.

LABORATORY FINDINGS AND DIAGNOSIS The diagnosis of relapsing fever is confirmed most easily by the detection of spirochetes in blood, bone marrow aspirates, or cerebrospinal fluid. Motile spirochetes can be seen when specimens are examined by dark-field microscopy. Fixed organisms are clearly visible in Wright-, Giemsa-, or acridine orange–stained preparations of thin or dehemoglobinized thick smears of peripheral blood or buffy-coat preparations (Fig. 156-1). Organisms are most numerous in specimens taken during periods of high temperature preceding the crisis; smears of peripheral blood are positive in ≥70% of patients with LBRF and in a lower percentage of patients with TBRF. In reference laboratories, relapsing-fever spirochetes are cultured from blood by the inoculation of BSK II medium or by the intraperitoneal inoculation of immature laboratory mice. Serum antibodies to *Borrelia* can be detected by enzyme immunoassays, indirect fluorescent antibody (IFA) assay, and western immunoblotting using whole-cell sonicates as antigen; however, these tests are unstandardized and subject to insensitivity and cross-reactivity with other spirochetal agents, including *B. burgdorferi* (the agent of Lyme disease) and *Treponema pallidum*. A recently developed western immunoblot test employing species-specific recombinant glycerophosphodiester phosphodiesterase (GlpQ) as antigen has been shown to be more sensitive and specific than the whole-cell sonicate IFA or enzyme-linked immunosorbent assay (ELISA) tests.

Other laboratory findings in relapsing fever are nonspecific. The leukocyte count is normal or moderately elevated, with an unremarkable cell differential. Serum bilirubin levels are generally only slightly elevated. Thrombocytopenia commonly occurs in relapsing-fever patients during the acute phase of the illness; platelet counts rebound during early convalescence. Prothrombin and partial thromboplastin times are often moderately prolonged during acute illness, as are standardized bleeding times. Fibrinogen concentrations in the blood are normal, and fibrinolysis is mild or absent. Results of the Rumpel-

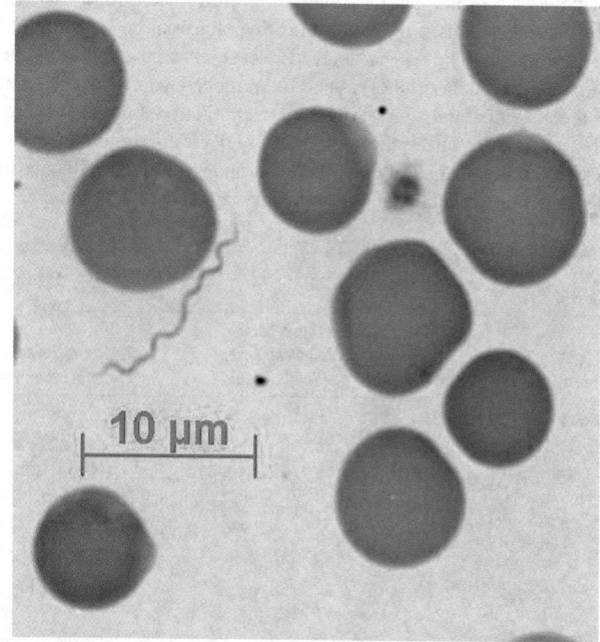

FIGURE 156-1 Photomicrograph of tick-borne relapsing fever spirochete (*B. hermsii*) in a Wright-Giemsa-stained peripheral blood film.

Leede tourniquet test for capillary fragility are negative, despite the presence of petechiae.

Rx TREATMENT

Relapsing-fever borreliae are exquisitely sensitive to antibiotics. Treatment with doxycycline (or another tetracycline), erythromycin, or chloramphenicol produces rapid clearance of spirochetes and a remission of symptoms (Table 156-2). The response to a single dose of penicillin may be delayed and incomplete. Although a single dose of doxycycline (or another tetracycline), erythromycin, or chloramphenicol is highly effective in the treatment of LBRF, less is known about the efficacy of single-dose treatment of TBRF. Empirical treatment of TBRF for 7 days is therefore recommended to reduce the risk of persisting or relapsing borreliosis. For children <8 years of age and for pregnant women, erythromycin or penicillin may be preferred, given the potential adverse effects of tetracyclines.

Treatment of LBRF with a rapidly acting antibiotic regularly precipitates a Jarisch-Herxheimer-like reaction within 1 to 4 h of the first dose. This reaction, which occurs in more than 50% of treated TBRF patients in North America, tends to be more severe when the patient has LBRF rather than TBRF and when high numbers of spirochetes are circulating in the bloodstream. In the chill phase of the reaction, rigors and rising fever are accompanied by an increasing metabolic rate, alveolar hyperventilation, high cardiac output, increasing peripheral vascular resistance, and decreased pulmonary arterial pressure. The body temperature commonly rises to $\geq41°C$ ($\geq105.8°F$). This high fever is accompanied often by agitation and confusion and sometimes by delirium. Fever can be partially controlled by the use of a cooling blanket and ice packs and by sponging of the patient with tepid water and alcohol. The chill phase terminates after 10 to 30 min, giving way to a flush phase characterized by a fall in body temperature, drenching sweats, and sometimes (more commonly in LBRF) a potentially dangerous fall in systemic arterial pressure and rise in pulmonary arterial pressure. Although cardiac output is maintained at high levels, the effective circulating blood volume decreases as peripheral vascular resistance falls. Vital signs must be monitored carefully during this period of the reaction, which usually lasts ≤8 h. Clinical and electrocardiographic evidence of myocarditis and myocardial dysfunction includes a prolonged QT_c interval, a third heart sound (S_3), elevated central venous pressure, arterial hypotension, and rare pulmonary congestion. The use of delayed-release intramuscular penicillin may prolong or delay the clearance of spirochetes and thereby attenuate the accompanying Jarisch-Herxheimer reaction, but this response is not predictable; furthermore, single-dose penicillin treatment sometimes results in relapse of spirochetemia and symptoms. Glucocorticoids and nonsteroidal anti-inflammatory agents do not prevent or significantly modify the cardiopulmonary disturbances of the Jarisch-Herxheimer reaction, although hydrocortisone and acetaminophen given at the same time as antibiotics reduce peak body temperature. Although pretreatment with antibody to TNF-α may moderate the Jarisch-Herxheimer reaction in treated patients with LBRF, its use in LBRF is impractical and its use in TBRF (whose treatment is associated with a relatively mild Jarisch-Herxheimer reaction) is not warranted. Close monitoring of fluid balance, arterial and venous pressures, and myocardial function is advised in supportive management of the Jarisch-Herxheimer reaction in patients with LBRF.

The management of patients with relapsing fever–induced myocardial dysfunction requires caution in the administration of intravenous fluids and, in some cases, use of short-term inotropic therapy. The inability of heparin to control bleeding in LBRF suggests that disseminated intravascular coagulation is not important in its causation. Vitamin K and other soluble vitamins are sometimes given to counter dietary deficiencies in patients with LBRF. Because postural hypotension is often pronounced during the acute phase of relapsing fever and in the early stage of recovery, patients should be assisted when arising from bed.

Untreated LBRF has a high case-fatality rate, especially among persons in otherwise poor health, such as those in famine-affected populations. The fatality rate among treated persons is usually <5%. In general, TBRF is a milder disease than LBRF: the spontaneous crisis and the Jarisch-Herxheimer reactions are less pronounced and the case-fatality rates are lower for TBRF than for LBRF.

PREVENTION AND CONTROL LBRF can be prevented by addressing socioeconomic circumstances that promote louse infestation (crowding, poverty, homelessness), by applying hygienic practices that reduce numbers of body lice (washing clothes, drying clothes in direct sunlight, changing clothes at frequent intervals), and by using acaricides. Spread of infection can be controlled by early case detection and treatment of infected persons and close contacts. Historically, outbreaks of LBRF have been controlled by mass delousing. In situations like those in refugee camps, individuals, their clothes, and their bedding should be deloused with appropriate acaricides, such as 0.5% permethrin dust. Impregnation of clothing with liquid permethrin, a residual acaricide, can provide long-term protection against infestation. In outbreaks of fever that involve louse-infested populations, empirical single-dose treatment with doxycycline will be effective against typhus as well as LBRF. B. recurrentis has a fragile life cycle and is eradicable.

TBRF can be prevented by the avoidance of rodent- and tick-infested dwellings and infested natural sites. Limiting rodent access to the foundations and attics of homes and vacation cabins and eliminating harborage for rodents in and around these dwellings reduce the potential for tick exposure. Rodents and rodent nests should be removed from infested buildings and their surroundings. Tick harborages of infested buildings or other circumscribed sites, such as rodent burrows and nests in hollow logs surrounding dwellings and in rodent-infested caves, can be chemically treated by pest-control specialists using various acaricides, such as carbaryl, diazinon, chlorpyrifos, pyrethrins, and malathion. Persons who enter tick-infested sites can protect themselves by wearing clothing that denies ticks access to the skin, by applying repellents to exposed skin and to clothing, and by applying an acaricide containing permethrin to clothing. Reporting of suspected cases of relapsing fever to public health authorities is important so that an epidemiologic investigation and control measures can be initiated promptly. Prompt diagnosis and treatment of relapsing fever in pregnant women is important in avoiding the potentially severe consequences of fetal or neonatal infection acquired in utero.

FURTHER READING

BARBOUR AG, RESTREPO BI: Antigenic variation in vector-borne pathogens. Emerg Infect Dis 6:449, 2000

TABLE 156-2 *Antibiotic Treatment of Louse-Borne and Tick-Borne Relapsing Fever in Adults*

Medication	Louse-Borne Relapsing Fever (Single Dose)	Tick-Borne Relapsing Fever (7-Day Schedule)
Oral		
Erythromycin	500 mg	500 mg q6h
Tetracycline	500 mg	500 mg q6h
Doxycycline	100 mg	100 mg q12h
Chloramphenicol	500 mg	500 mg q6h
Parenteral[a]		
Erythromycin	500 mg	500 mg q6h
Tetracycline	250 mg	250 mg q6h
Doxycycline	100 mg	100 mg q12h
Chloramphenicol	500 mg	500 mg q6h
Penicillin G (procaine)	600,000 IU	600,000 IU daily

[a]For tick-borne relapsing fever, parenteral therapy is used only until oral treatment is tolerated.

CADAVID D, BARBOUR AG: Neuroborreliosis during relapsing fever: Review of clinical manifestations, pathology, and treatment of infections in humans and experimental animals. Clin Infect Dis 26:151, 1998

CUTLER SJ et al: *Borrelia recurrentis* characterization and comparison with relapsing fever, Lyme-associated, and other *Borrelia* spp. Int J Syst Bacteriol 47:958, 1997

DWORKIN MS et al: Tick-borne relapsing fever in North America. Med Clin North Am 86:417, 2002

HORTON JM, BLASER MJ: The spectrum of relapsing fever in the Rocky Mountains. Arch Intern Med 145:871, 1985

PAUL WS et al: Outbreak of tick-borne relapsing fever at the north rim of the Grand Canyon: Evidence for effectiveness of preventive measures. Am J Trop Med Hyg 66:71, 2002

157 LYME BORRELIOSIS
Allen C. Steere

DEFINITION   Lyme borreliosis is caused by a spirochete, *Borrelia burgdorferi, sensu lato*, that is transmitted by ticks of the *Ixodes ricinus* complex. The infection usually begins with a characteristic expanding skin lesion, erythema migrans (EM; stage 1, localized infection). After several days or weeks, the spirochete may spread hematogenously to many different sites (stage 2, disseminated infection). Possible manifestations of disseminated infection include secondary annular skin lesions, meningitis, cranial or peripheral neuritis, carditis, atrioventricular nodal block, or migratory musculoskeletal pain. Months to years later (usually after periods of latent infection), intermittent or chronic arthritis, chronic encephalopathy or polyneuropathy, or acrodermatitis may develop (stage 3, persistent infection). Most patients experience early symptoms of the illness during the summer, but the infection may not become symptomatic until it progresses to stage 2 or 3. Despite regional variations, the basic stages of the illness are similar worldwide.

Lyme disease was recognized as a separate entity in 1976 because of geographic clustering of children in Lyme, Connecticut, who were thought to have juvenile rheumatoid arthritis. The rural setting of the case clusters and the identification of EM as a feature of the illness suggested that the disorder was transmitted by an arthropod. It became apparent that Lyme disease was a multisystem illness that affected primarily the skin, nervous system, heart, and joints. Epidemiologic studies of patients with EM implicated certain *Ixodes* ticks as vectors of the disease. Early in the twentieth century, EM had been described in Europe and attributed to *I. ricinus* tick bites. In 1982, a previously unrecognized spirochete, now called *Borrelia burgdorferi*, was recovered from *Ixodes scapularis* ticks and then from patients with Lyme disease. The entity is now called Lyme disease or Lyme borreliosis.

ETIOLOGIC AGENT   *B. burgdorferi*, the causative agent of Lyme disease, is a fastidious, microaerophilic bacterium. The spirochete's genome is quite small ($\sim$1.5 Mb) and consists of a highly unusual linear chromosome of 950 kb as well as 9 linear and 12 circular plasmids. *B. burgdorferi* contains many immunogenic proteins, including a number of differentially expressed lipoproteins, most of which are encoded by plasmid DNA. To date, three groups of pathogenic *B. burgdorferi* organisms, together referred to as *B. burgdorferi sensu lato*, have been identified. All North American strains have belonged to the first group, *B. burgdorferi sensu stricto*. Although all three of the identified groups have been found in Europe, most isolates there have been strains of group 2 (*B. garinii*) or group 3 (*B. afzelii*), and only the latter two groups have been found in Asia. These differences may well account for the clinical variations in the disease in different geographic regions.

EPIDEMIOLOGY   Lyme borreliosis in all locations is transmitted by ticks of the *I. ricinus* complex: *I. scapularis* (also called *I. dammini*), *I. pacificus*, *I. ricinus*, and *I. persulcatus*. *I. scapularis* is the principal vector in the northeastern United States from Maine to Maryland and in the midwestern states of Wisconsin and Minnesota. *I. pacificus* is the vector in the western states of California and Oregon. The disease is acquired throughout Europe (from Great Britain to Scandinavia to European Russia), where *I. ricinus* is the vector, and in Asian Russia, China, and Japan, where *I. persulcatus* is the vector. These ticks may transmit other diseases as well. In the United States, *I. scapularis* also transmits babesiosis and human anaplasmosis; in Europe and Asia, *I. ricinus* and *I. persulcatus* also transmit tick-borne encephalitis.

Ticks of the *I. ricinus* complex have larval, nymphal, and adult stages; they require a blood meal at each stage. The risk of infection in a given area depends largely on the density of these ticks as well as their feeding habits and animal hosts, which have evolved differently in different locations. For *I. scapularis* in the northeast, the white-footed mouse is the preferred host of the immature larval and nymphal ticks. It is critical that both of the tick's immature stages feed on the same host, because the life cycle of the spirochete depends on horizontal transmission: in early summer from infected nymphs to mice and in late summer from infected mice to larvae, which then molt to become the infected nymphs that will begin the cycle again the following year. It is the tiny nymphal tick that is primarily responsible for transmission of the disease to humans during the early summer months. White-tailed deer, which are not involved in the life cycle of the spirochete, are the preferred host for the adult stage of *I. scapularis* and seem to be critical to the tick's survival.

Lyme disease is now the most common vector-borne infection in the United States. Since surveillance was begun by the Centers for Disease Control and Prevention (CDC) in 1982, the number of cases has increased dramatically. More than 15,000 new cases are now reported each summer. In Europe, Lyme borreliosis is widely established in forested areas; there, the highest reported frequencies of the disease are in the middle of the continent and in Scandinavia. Cases have occurred in persons who reside in endemic suburban, wooded, or rural areas and in persons who visit, hike, camp, or hunt in these areas.

PATHOGENESIS   To maintain its complex enzootic cycle, *B. burgdorferi* must adapt to two markedly different environments: the tick and the mammalian host. The spirochete expresses outer-surface proteins A and B (OspA and OspB) in the midgut of the tick, whereas OspC is upregulated as the organism travels to the tick's salivary gland and thence to the mammalian host. The tick must usually be attached for at least 24 h for transmission of *B. burgdorferi*.

After injection into the human skin, *B. burgdorferi* may migrate outward, producing EM, and may spread hematogenously to other organs. A number of mechanisms may aid in spirochetal dissemination. For example, the sequences of OspC vary considerably among strains, and only a few groups of sequences are associated with disseminated disease. Spread through the skin and other tissue matrices may be facilitated by the binding of human plasminogen and its activators to the surface of the spirochete. During its dissemination and homing to specific sites, the organism attaches to certain host integrins, matrix glycosaminoglycans, and extracellular matrix proteins. For example, *Borrelia* decorin-binding proteins A and B bind decorin, a glycosaminoglycan on collagen fibrils; this binding may explain why the organism is commonly aligned with collagen fibrils in the extracellular matrix in the heart, nervous system, or joints. The only known virulence factors of *B. burgdorferi* are surface proteins that allow the spirochete to attach to mammalian cells.

Inflammatory innate immune responses are critical in the control of early disseminated infection. Spirochetal lipoproteins, which bind to the CD14 molecule and toll-like receptor 2 on macrophages, are potent activators of the innate immune response, leading to the production of macrophage-derived inflammatory cytokines. After the first several weeks of infection, T cells, which are part of the adaptive immune response, generally exhibit heightened responsiveness to *B.*

burgdorferi antigens, and evidence of B-cell hyperactivity is found, including elevated total serum IgM levels, cryoprecipitates, and circulating immune complexes. Titers of specific IgM antibody to *B. burgdorferi* peak between the third and sixth week after disease onset. The specific IgG response develops gradually over months, with response to an increasing array of at least 12 spirochetal polypeptides and maximal expansion during the period of arthritis. Histologic examination of all affected tissues reveals an infiltration of lymphocytes, macrophages, and plasma cells with some degree of vascular damage (including mild vasculitis or hypervascular occlusion), suggesting that the spirochete may have been present in or around blood vessels.

Despite the innate and adaptive immune responses, *B. burgdorferi* may sometimes survive in certain sites. The ability of the spirochete to downregulate the expression of surface-exposed protein antigens is one important mechanism of immune evasion. In addition, during disseminated infection, a surface-exposed lipoprotein called VlsE undergoes extensive antigenic variation. However, the organism does not have mechanisms that help to protect it from antibiotic therapy. For example, *B. burgdorferi* has only been seen extracellularly in affected tissues; it has not been shown to "hide out" in intracellular locations, thereby evading antibiotic exposure.

CLINICAL MANIFESTATIONS ■ Early Infection: Stage 1 (Localized Infection) After an incubation period of 3 to 32 days, EM, which occurs at the site of the tick bite, usually begins as a red macule or papule that expands slowly to form a large annular lesion. As the lesion increases in size, it often develops a bright red outer border and partial central clearing. Because of the small size of ixodid ticks, most patients do not remember the preceding tick bite. The center of the lesion sometimes becomes intensely erythematous and indurated, vesicular, or necrotic. In other instances, the expanding lesion remains an even, intense red; several red rings are found within an outside ring; or the central area turns blue before the lesion clears. Although EM can be located anywhere, the thigh, groin, and axilla are particularly common sites. The lesion is warm but not often painful. Approximately 20% of patients do not exhibit this characteristic skin manifestation. In Europe, EM is often an indolent localized infection of the skin; in contrast, in the United States, this lesion is associated with more intense inflammation and signs that often suggest dissemination of the spirochete.

Early Infection: Stage 2 (Disseminated Infection) In cases in the United States, *B. burgdorferi* often spreads hematogenously to many sites within days or weeks after the onset of EM. In these cases, patients may develop secondary annular skin lesions similar in appearance to the initial lesion. Skin involvement is commonly accompanied by severe headache, mild stiffness of the neck, fever, chills, migratory musculoskeletal pain, arthralgias, and profound malaise and fatigue. Less common manifestations include generalized lymphadenopathy or splenomegaly, hepatitis, sore throat, nonproductive cough, conjunctivitis, iritis, or testicular swelling. Except for fatigue and lethargy, which are often constant, the early signs and symptoms of Lyme disease are typically intermittent and changing. Even in untreated patients, the early symptoms usually become less severe or disappear within several weeks. In ~15% of patients, the infection presents with these nonspecific systemic symptoms.

Symptoms suggestive of meningeal irritation may develop early in Lyme disease when EM is present but usually are not associated with cerebrospinal fluid (CSF) pleocytosis or an objective neurologic deficit. After several weeks or months, ~15% of untreated patients develop frank neurologic abnormalities, including meningitis, subtle encephalitic signs, cranial neuritis (including bilateral facial palsy), motor or sensory radiculoneuropathy, mononeuritis multiplex, cerebellar ataxia, or myelitis—alone or in various combinations. In the United States, the usual pattern consists of fluctuating symptoms of meningitis accompanied by facial palsy and peripheral radiculoneuropathy. Lymphocytic pleocytosis (~100 cells per μL) is found in CSF, often along with elevated protein levels and normal or slightly low glucose concentrations. In Europe and Asia, the first neurologic sign is characteristically radicular pain, which is followed by the development of CSF pleocytosis (called meningopolyneuritis or *Bannwarth's syndrome*), but meningeal or encephalitic signs are frequently absent. In children, the optic nerve may be affected because of inflammation or increased intracranial pressure, which may lead to blindness. These early neurologic abnormalities usually resolve completely within months, but in rare cases, chronic neurologic disease may occur later.

Within several weeks after the onset of illness, ~8% of patients develop cardiac involvement. The most common abnormality is a fluctuating degree of atrioventricular block (first-degree, Wenckebach, or complete heart block). Some patients have more diffuse cardiac involvement, including electrocardiographic changes indicative of acute myopericarditis, left ventricular dysfunction evident on radionuclide scans, or (in rare cases) cardiomegaly or pancarditis. Cardiac involvement usually lasts for only a few weeks but may recur. Chronic cardiomyopathy caused by *B. burgdorferi* has been reported in Europe.

During this stage, musculoskeletal pain is common. The typical pattern consists of migratory pain in joints, tendons, bursae, muscles, or bones (usually without joint swelling) lasting for hours or days and affecting one or two locations at a time.

Late Infection: Stage 3 (Persistent Infection) Months after the onset of infection, ~60% of patients in the United States who have received no antibiotic treatment develop frank arthritis. The typical pattern comprises intermittent attacks of oligoarticular arthritis in large joints (especially the knees), lasting for weeks to months in a given joint. Small joints and periarticular sites also may be affected, primarily during early attacks. The number of patients who continue to have recurrent attacks decreases each year. However, in a small percentage of cases, involvement of large joints—usually one or both knees—becomes chronic and may lead to erosion of cartilage and bone. These patients have a higher frequency of the class II major histocompatibility complex alleles associated with rheumatoid arthritis, particularly HLA-DRBI*0401 or *0101 alleles, than patients with brief Lyme arthritis. Moreover, they may have persistent arthritis for months or even several years after the apparent eradication of spirochetes from the joints with antibiotic therapy. In these genetically susceptible individuals, it has been postulated that autoimmunity may develop within the proinflammatory milieu of the joints because of molecular mimicry between a dominant T-cell epitope of OspA and a similar sequence in a human protein.

White cell counts in joint fluid range from 500 to 110,000/μL (average, 25,000/μL); most of these cells are polymorphonuclear leukocytes. Tests for rheumatoid factor or antinuclear antibodies usually give negative results. Examination of synovial biopsy samples reveals fibrin deposits, villous hypertrophy, vascular proliferation, microangiopathic lesions, and a heavy infiltration of lymphocytes and plasma cells.

Although less common, chronic neurologic involvement may also become apparent months or years after the onset of infection, sometimes following long periods of latent infection. The most common form of chronic central nervous system involvement is subtle encephalopathy affecting memory, mood, or sleep and often accompanied by axonal polyneuropathy manifested as either distal paresthesia or spinal radicular pain. Patients with encephalopathy frequently have evidence of memory impairment in neuropsychological tests and abnormal results in CSF analyses. In cases with polyneuropathy, electromyography generally shows extensive abnormalities of proximal and distal nerve segments. Encephalomyelitis or leukoencephalitis, a rare manifestation of Lyme borreliosis associated primarily with *B. garinii* infection in Europe, is a severe neurologic disorder that may include spastic paraparesis, upper motor-neuron bladder dysfunction, and lesions in the periventricular white matter. The prolonged course of chronic neuroborreliosis following periods of latent infection is reminiscent of tertiary neurosyphilis.

Acrodermatitis chronica atrophicans, the late skin manifestation of the disorder, has been associated primarily with *B. afzelii* infection in Europe and Asia. It has been observed mostly in elderly women. The skin lesions, which are usually found on the acral surface of an arm or leg, begin insidiously with reddish-violaceous discoloration; they become sclerotic or atrophic over a period of years.

DIAGNOSIS The culture of *B. burgdorferi* in Barbour-Stoenner-Kelly (BSK) medium permits definitive diagnosis, but this complex method has been used only in research studies. Moreover, with a few exceptions, positive cultures have been obtained only early in the illness—primarily from biopsy samples of EM skin lesions, less often from plasma samples, and occasionally from CSF samples. Later in the infection, polymerase chain reaction (PCR) is greatly superior to culture for the detection of *B. burgdorferi* DNA in joint fluid, and this has been the major use for PCR testing in Lyme disease. In one study, *B. burgdorferi* DNA was detected by PCR in synovial fluid samples from 75 (85%) of 88 patients and in none of 64 control samples. However, the sensitivity of PCR determinations in CSF from patients with neuroborreliosis has been much lower. There seems to be little if any role for PCR in the detection of *B. burgdorferi* DNA in blood or urine samples. Moreover, this procedure, which must be carefully controlled to prevent contamination, is not routinely available.

Because of the problems associated with direct detection of *B. burgdorferi*, Lyme disease is usually diagnosed by the recognition of a characteristic clinical picture with serologic confirmation. Although serologic testing may yield negative results during the first several weeks of infection, most patients have a positive antibody response to *B. burgdorferi* after that time. The limitation of serologic tests is that they do not clearly distinguish between active and inactive infection. Patients with previous Lyme disease—particularly in cases progressing to late stages—often remain seropositive for years, even after adequate antibiotic treatment. In addition, about 10% of patients are seropositive because of asymptomatic infection. If these individuals subsequently develop another illness, the positive serologic test for Lyme disease may cause diagnostic confusion. Conversely, in rare instances, patients who receive inadequate antibiotic therapy during the first several weeks of infection may subsequently develop subtle joint or neurologic symptoms but are seronegative. The important point is that seronegative Lyme disease is usually a mild, attenuated illness that responds well to standard courses of antibiotic therapy. According to an algorithm published by the American College of Physicians (Table 157-1), serologic testing for Lyme disease is recommended only for patients with at least an intermediate pretest probability of Lyme disease, such as those with oligoarticular arthritis. It should not be used as a screening procedure in patients with pain or fatigue syndromes. In such patients, the probability of a false-positive serologic result is higher than that of a true-positive result.

For serologic analysis of Lyme disease in the United States, the CDC recommends a two-step approach in which samples are first tested by enzyme-linked immunosorbent assay (ELISA) and equivocal or positive results are then tested by western blotting. During the first month of infection, both IgM and IgG responses to the spirochete should be determined, preferably in both acute- and convalescent-phase serum samples. Approximately 20 to 30% of patients have a positive response detectable in acute-phase samples, whereas about 70 to 80% have a positive response during convalescence (2 to 4 weeks later). After 1 month of infection, by which time most patients with active Lyme disease have disseminated infection, the sensitivity and specificity of the IgG response to the spirochete are both very high—in the range of 95% to 99%—as determined by the two-test approach of ELISA and western blot. At this point and thereafter, a single test (that for IgG) is usually sufficient. In persons with illness of >1 month's duration, a positive IgM test result alone is likely to be false-positive and therefore should not be used to support the diagnosis. According to current criteria adopted by the CDC, an IgM western blot is considered positive if two of the following three bands are present: 23, 39, and 41 kDa. However, the combination of the 23- and 41-kDa bands may still represent a false-positive result. An IgG blot is considered positive if 5 of the following 10 bands are present: 18, 23, 28, 30, 39, 41, 45, 58, 66, and 93 kDa. In European cases, there is less expansion of the antibody response, and no single set of criteria for the interpretation of immunoblots results in high levels of sensitivity and specificity in all countries.

Several second-generation tests that use recombinant spirochetal proteins or synthetic peptides have shown promising results. For example, an IgG ELISA employing a 26-mer peptide from invariant region 6 (IR_6) of the VlsE lipoprotein has a sensitivity and a specificity similar to those achieved with the IgM and IgG two-test approach using sonicated whole spirochetes. However, the IR_6 ELISA has a limitation similar to that affecting standard serology, in that a positive test result does not distinguish clearly between active and past infection. The IR_6 ELISA may be of value with regard to European as well as American strains of the spirochete.

DIFFERENTIAL DIAGNOSIS Classic EM is a slowly expanding erythema, often with partial central clearing. If the lesion expands little, it may represent the red papule of an uninfected tick bite. If the lesion expands rapidly, it may represent cellulitis (e.g., streptococcal cellulitis) or an allergic reaction, perhaps to tick saliva. Patients with secondary annular lesions may be thought to have erythema multiforme, but neither the development of blistering mucosal lesions nor the involvement of the palms or soles is a feature of *B. burgdorferi* infection. In the southeastern United States, an EM-like skin lesion, sometimes with mild systemic symptoms, may be associated with *Amblyomma americanum* tick bites, but the cause of this illness has not yet been identified.

In the United States, *I. scapularis* ticks may transmit not only *B. burgdorferi* but also *Babesia microti*, a red blood cell parasite (Chap. 195), or *Anaplasma phagocytophila*, the agent of human anaplasmosis (formerly called the agent of human granulocytotropic ehrlichiosis; Chap. 158). Although babesiosis and anaplasmosis are most often asymptomatic, infection with any of these three agents may cause nonspecific systemic symptoms, and coinfected patients may have more severe or persistent symptoms than patients infected with a single agent. Standard blood counts may yield clues regarding the presence of coinfection. Anaplasmosis may cause leukopenia or thrombocytopenia, and babesiosis may cause thrombocytopenia or (in severe cases) hemolytic anemia. However, IgM serologic responses may confuse the diagnosis. For example, *A. phagocytophila* may elicit a positive IgM response to *B. burgdorferi*. The frequency of coinfection in different studies has been variable. In one prospective study, 4% of patients with EM had evidence of coinfection.

Facial palsy caused by *B. burgdorferi*, which occurs in the early disseminated phase of the infection (often in July, August, or September), is usually recognized by its association with EM. However, facial palsy without EM may be the presenting manifestation of Lyme disease. In such cases, both the IgM and IgG responses to the spirochete are usually positive. The most common infectious agents that cause

TABLE 157-1 *Algorithm for Testing for and Treating Lyme Disease*

Pretest Probability	Example	Recommendation
High	Patients with erythema migrans	Empirical antibiotic treatment without serologic testing
Intermediate	Patients with oligoarticular arthritis	Serologic testing and antibiotic treatment if test results are positive
Low	Patients with nonspecific symptoms (myalgias, arthralgias, fatigue)	Neither serologic testing nor antibiotic treatment

Source: Adapted from the recommendations of the American College of Physicians (G Nichol et al: Ann Intern Med 128:37, 1998, with permission).

facial palsy are herpes simplex virus type 1 (Bell's palsy; Chap. 163) and varicella-zoster virus (Ramsay-Hunt syndrome; Chap. 164).

Later in the infection, oligoarticular Lyme arthritis most resembles reactive arthritis in an adult or the pauciarticular form of juvenile rheumatoid arthritis in a child. Patients with Lyme arthritis usually have the highest IgG antibody responses seen in the infection, with reactivity to many spirochetal proteins.

The most common problem in diagnosis is to mistake Lyme disease for chronic fatigue syndrome (Chap. 370) or fibromyalgia (Chap. 315). This difficulty is compounded by the fact that a small percentage of patients do in fact develop these chronic pain or fatigue syndromes in association with or soon after Lyme disease. Compared with Lyme disease, chronic fatigue syndrome or fibromyalgia tends to produce more generalized and disabling symptoms, including marked fatigue, severe headache, diffuse musculoskeletal pain, multiple symmetric tender points in characteristic locations, pain and stiffness in many joints, diffuse dysesthesia, difficulty with concentration, and sleep disturbances. Patients with chronic fatigue syndrome or fibromyalgia lack evidence of joint inflammation; they have normal results in neurologic tests; and they usually have a greater degree of anxiety and depression than patients with chronic neuroborreliosis.

Rx TREATMENT

As outlined in the algorithm in Fig. 157-1, the various manifestations of Lyme disease can usually be treated successfully with orally administered antibiotics; the exceptions are objective neurologic abnormalities and third-degree atrioventricular heart block, which seem to require intravenous therapy. For early Lyme disease, doxycycline is effective in men and in nonpregnant women. An advantage of this regimen is that it is also effective against *A. phagocytophila*, which is

transmitted by the same tick that transmits the Lyme disease agent. Amoxicillin, cefuroxime axetil, and erythromycin or its congeners are second-, third-, and fourth-choice alternatives, respectively. In children, amoxicillin is effective (not more than 2 g/d); in cases of penicillin allergy, cefuroxime axetil or erythromycin may be used. In contrast to second- or third-generation cephalosporin antibiotics, first-generation cephalosporins, such as cephalexin, are not effective. For patients with infection localized to the skin, a 14-day course of therapy is generally sufficient; in contrast, for patients with disseminated infection, a 21-day course is recommended. Approximately 15% of patients experience a Jarisch-Herxheimer-like reaction during the first 24 h of therapy. In multicenter studies, more than 90% of patients whose early Lyme disease was treated with these regimens had satisfactory outcomes. Although some patients reported symptoms after treatment, objective evidence of persistent infection or relapse was rare, and retreatment was usually unnecessary.

One of these oral antibiotic regimens, when given for 30 to 60 days, or intravenous ceftriaxone, given for 14 to 28 days, is effective for the treatment of Lyme arthritis. Oral therapy is easier to administer, is associated with fewer side effects, and is considerably less expensive. However, the response to oral therapy may be slower than that to intravenous therapy, and some patients given oral therapy have subsequently developed overt neuroborreliosis, which may require intravenous therapy for a successful outcome. In the small percentage of patients with arthritis in whom arthritic symptoms persist for months or even years after the apparent eradication of spirochetes from the joints with antimicrobial therapy, treatment with anti-inflammatory agents or synovectomy may be successful.

For objective neurologic abnormalities (with the possible exception of facial palsy alone), parenteral antibiotic therapy seems to be necessary. Intravenous ceftriaxone, given for 14 to 28 days, is most commonly used for this purpose, but intravenous cefotaxime or intravenous penicillin G for the same duration may also be effective. In patients with high-degree atrioventricular block or a PR interval of >0.3 s, intravenous therapy for at least part of the course and cardiac monitoring are recommended, but the insertion of a permanent pacemaker is not necessary.

It is unclear how and whether asymptomatic infection should be treated, but patients with such infection are often given a course of oral antibiotics. Because maternal-fetal transmission of *B. burgdorferi* seems to occur rarely, if at all, standard therapy for the manifestations of the illness is recommended for pregnant women. Long-term persistence of *B. burgdorferi* has not been documented in any large series of patients after treatment with currently recommended regimens. Therefore, there is no indication for multiple, repeated antibiotic courses in the treatment of Lyme disease.

After appropriately treated Lyme disease, a small percentage of patients continue to have subjective symptoms, primarily musculoskeletal pain, neurocognitive difficulties, or fatigue. This so-called chronic Lyme disease or post–Lyme disease syndrome is a disabling condition that is similar to chronic fatigue syndrome or fibromyalgia. In a large study, one group of patients with post–Lyme disease syndrome received intravenous ceftriaxone for 30 days followed by oral doxycycline for 60 days, while another group received intravenous and oral placebo preparations for the same durations. No significant differences were found between groups in the numbers of patients reporting that their symptoms had improved, become worse, or stayed the same. Such patients are best treated for the relief of symptoms rather than with prolonged courses of antibiotics.

The risk of infection with *B. burgdorferi* after a recognized tick bite is so low that antibiotic prophylaxis is not routinely indicated. However, if an attached, engorged *I. scapularis* nymph is found or if follow-up is anticipated to be difficult, a single 200-mg dose of doxycycline, which effectively prevents Lyme disease when given within 72 h after the tick bite, may be administered.

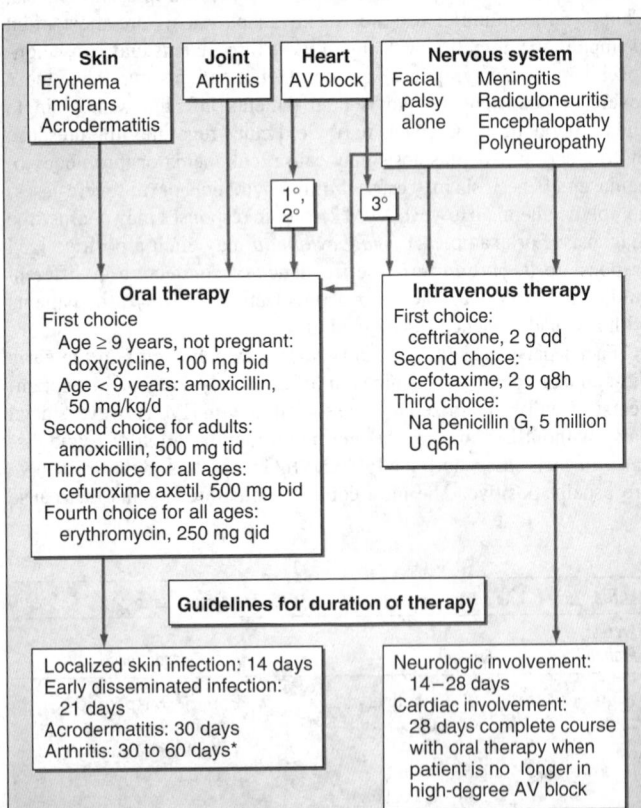

FIGURE 157-1 Algorithm for the treatment of the various acute or chronic manifestations of Lyme borreliosis. AV, atrioventricular. *For Lyme arthritis, intravenous ceftriaxone, 2 g given once a day for 14 to 28 days, is also effective and may elicit a response more quickly than oral therapy; however, compared with oral treatment, this regimen is less convenient to administer, has more side effects, and is more expensive.

PROGNOSIS The response to treatment is best early in the disease. Later treatment of Lyme borreliosis is still effective, but the period of convalescence may be longer. Eventually, most patients recover with minimal or no residual deficits.

REINFECTION Reinfection may occur after EM when patients are treated with antimicrobial agents. In such cases, the immune response is not adequate to provide protection from subsequent infection. However, patients who develop an expanded immune response to the spirochete over a period of months (such as those with Lyme arthritis) have protective immunity for a period of years and do not acquire the infection again.

PREVENTION Protective measures for the prevention of Lyme disease may include the avoidance of tick-infested areas, the use of repellents and acaricides, tick checks, and modification of landscapes in or near residential areas. Although a vaccine for Lyme disease used to be available, the manufacturer has discontinued its production. Therefore, no vaccine is now commercially available for the prevention of this infection.

FURTHER READING

BARBOUR AG, HAYES SF: Biology of *Borrelia* species. Microbiol Rev 50: 381, 1986

KLEMPNER MS et al: Two controlled trials of antibiotic treatment in patients with persistent symptoms and a history of Lyme disease. N Engl J Med 345:85, 2001

LIANG FT et al: Sensitive and specific serodiagnosis of Lyme disease by enzyme-linked immunosorbent assay with a peptide based on an immunodominant conserved region of *Borrelia burgdorferi* VlsE. J Clin Microbiol 37:3990, 1999

NADELMAN RB et al: Prophylaxis with single-dose doxycycline for the prevention of Lyme disease after *Ixodes scapularis* tick bite. N Engl J Med 345:79, 2001

STEERE AC: Lyme disease. N Engl J Med 345:115, 2001

WORMSER GP et al: Guidelines from the Infectious Diseases Society of America: Practice guidelines for the treatment of Lyme disease. Clin Infect Dis 31(Suppl 1):S1, 2000

Section 10   Diseases Caused by Rickettsia, Mycoplasma, and Chlamydia

158   RICKETTSIAL DISEASES
David H. Walker, Didier Raoult, J. Stephen Dumler, Thomas Marrie

The rickettsiae make up a family of gram-negative coccobacilli and short bacilli that grow strictly in eukaryotic cells. Characteristics of these organisms include their obligately intracellular location and persistence. The pathogenic rickettsiae move through mammalian reservoirs; they are transmitted by insect or tick vectors. Except for louse-borne typhus, humans are incidental hosts. Among rickettsiae, *Coxiella burnetii* (the agent of Q fever) is notorious for its ability to survive for an extended period outside of the reservoir or vector and for its extreme infectiousness: inhalation of a single microorganism can cause pneumonia. Clinical infections with rickettsiae can be classified into five general groups: (1) tick-, louse-, flea-, and gamasid mite–borne, spotted fever group (SFG) and typhus group rickettsial diseases; (2) chigger-borne scrub typhus; (3) tick-borne ehrlichioses and anaplasmosis; (4) neorickettsiosis (sennetsu fever); and (5) Q fever. The rickettsiae that cause spotted fevers, typhus, and scrub typhus are listed along with their vectors, geographic ranges, and associated diseases in Table 158-1.

TICK-, MITE-, AND FLEA-BORNE SPOTTED FEVERS

ROCKY MOUNTAIN SPOTTED FEVER Rocky Mountain spotted fever (RMSF), the most severe of the rickettsial diseases, is caused by *Rickettsia rickettsii*. This organism possesses two major immunodominant surface-exposed proteins, OmpA and OmpB, which have species-specific conformational epitopes. OmpA functions as an adhesin for the host cell; OmpB, the most abundant outer-membrane protein, shares genetic sequences and limited antigens with typhus group rickettsiae. This small (0.3 μm by 1.0 μm) bacillus has a gram-negative cell wall

TABLE 158-1 *Features of Selected Rickettsial Infections*

Disease	Organism	Vector(s)	Geographic Range	Incubation Period	Duration
Rocky Mountain spotted fever	*Rickettsia rickettsii*	*Dermacentor andersoni* *D. variabilis* *Amblyomma cajennense* *Rhipicephalus sanguineus*	United States United States Central/South America Mexico	2–14 days	10–20 days
Mediterranean spotted fever[a]	*R. conorii*	*R. sanguineus*	Southern Europe, Africa, Middle East, Central Asia	5–7 days	7–14 days
African tick-bite fever	*R. africae*	*A. hebraeum, A. variegatum*	Sub-Saharan Africa, West Indies	4–10 days	?
Rickettsialpox[a]	*R. akari*	*Liponyssoides sanguineus*	United States, Ukraine, Croatia	10–17 days	3–11 days
Cat-flea typhus	*R. felis*	*Ctenocephalides felis*	North and South America, Europe	8–16 days	8–16 days
Epidemic typhus	*R. prowazekii*	*Pediculus humanus corporis*	Worldwide	7–14 days	10–18 days
Brill-Zinsser disease	*R. prowazekii*	—[b]	Worldwide	Years	7–11 days
Murine typhus	*R. typhi*	*Xenopsylla cheopis*	Worldwide	8–16 days	8–16 days
Scrub typhus[a]	*Orientia tsutsugamushi*	*Leptotrombidium deliense*	Asia, Australia, New Guinea, Pacific Islands	6–21 days	6–21 days

[a] Eschar is usually present at the bite site.

[b] Brill-Zinsser disease represents a recrudescence of latent epidemic typhus.

structure; its lipopolysaccharide shares antigens mainly within the SFG and is not endotoxic in the quantities found in human infections.

Discovered in the American West in the late nineteenth century, RMSF is at present documented in 48 states (with the highest prevalences in the south-central and southeastern states) as well as in Canada, Mexico, Costa Rica, Panama, Colombia, Argentina, and Brazil. It is transmitted by *Dermacentor variabilis*, the American dog tick, in the eastern two-thirds of the United States and in California; by *D. andersoni*, the Rocky Mountain wood tick, in the western United States; by *Rhipicephalus sanguineus* in Mexico; and by *Amblyomma cajennense* in Central and South America. Maintained principally by transovarian transmission from one generation of ticks to the next, *R. rickettsii* can be acquired by uninfected ticks through the ingestion of a blood meal from rickettsemic small mammals.

Humans become infected during the active season of the vector tick species. In northern areas, cases occur mainly in the spring; in warmer southern states, most cases occur from May to September, although some cases are reported in the winter. Although 4% of *D. variabilis* ticks contain rickettsiae, the vast majority of these are nonpathogenic species such as *R. montanensis* and *R. bellii*. The likelihood of an individual tick's containing *R. rickettsii* is remote. From 1971 to 2001, the reported incidence of RMSF was in the range of 0.16 to 0.50 cases per 100,000 population in the United States. In 2001, 0.20 persons per 100,000 in the United States developed RMSF. This rate is probably an underestimate, since the diagnosis is difficult and reporting incomplete. The 5- to 9-year-old age group has the highest incidence. The mortality rate was 20 to 25% in the preantibiotic era and now remains at ~3 to 5% because of delayed diagnosis and treatment. The case-fatality ratio increases with each decade of life above age 20.

Pathogenesis *R. rickettsii* organisms are inoculated into the dermis along with secretions of the tick's salivary glands after ≥6 h of feeding. Rickettsiae spread lymphohematogenously throughout the body, attach via OmpA to the endothelial cell membrane, and induce their own engulfment. Once intracellularly located, they escape rapidly from the phagosome, replicate in the cytosol by binary fission, and spread from cell to cell, propelled by polar polymerization of the host cell's actin. The result is numerous foci of contiguous infected endothelial cells that are extensive enough to manifest clinically after a dose-dependent incubation period of ~1 week (range, 2 to 14 days). *R. rickettsii* is more invasive than other rickettsiae, routinely spreading to infect vascular smooth-muscle cells. Despite frequent statements to the contrary, occlusive thrombosis and ischemic necrosis are not the fundamental pathologic basis for tissue and organ injury in RMSF. Instead, increased vascular permeability, with resulting edema, hypovolemia, and ischemia, is responsible. Indeed, immunohistologic studies of severely infected humans and animals have demonstrated numerous zones of infected endothelium, only a small proportion of which contain thrombi. The thrombi are usually located to one side of the lumen, which is not occluded. These hemostatic plugs appear to be an appropriate host response rather than a pathogenic process. Consumption of platelets results in thrombocytopenia in 32 to 52% of patients, but disseminated intravascular coagulation with hypofibrinogenemia is rare. Activation of platelets, generation of thrombin, and activation of the fibrinolytic system all appear to be homeostatic physiologic responses to endothelial injury.

Clinical Manifestations The incubation period averages 7 days. Early in the illness, when medical attention usually is first sought, RMSF is difficult to distinguish from many self-limiting viral illnesses. Fever, headache, malaise, myalgia, nausea, vomiting, and anorexia are the most frequent symptoms during the first 3 days. The patient becomes progressively more ill as vascular infection and injury advance. In one large series, only one-third of patients were diagnosed with presumptive RMSF early in the clinical course and treated appropriately as outpatients. In the tertiary care setting, RMSF is all too often recog-

nized only when its late severe manifestations, developing at the end of the first week or during the second week of illness in patients without appropriate treatment, prompt admission to the intensive care unit.

The progressive nature of the infection is clearly manifested in the skin. Rash is evident in only 14% of patients on the first day of illness and in only 49% during the first 3 days. Macules (1 to 5 mm) appear first on the wrists and ankles and then on the remainder of the extremities and the trunk. Later, more severe vascular damage results in frank hemorrhage at the center of the maculopapule, a petechia that does not disappear upon compression (Fig. 158-1). This sequence of events is sometimes delayed or aborted by effective treatment. In fact, rash appears on day 6 or later in 20% of cases and does not appear at all in 9 to 16% of cases, including some with severe visceral lesions that result in death. Petechiae occur in 41 to 59% of cases, appearing on or after day 6 in 74% of cases that include a rash. Involvement of the palms and soles, often considered diagnostically important, usually occurs relatively late in the course (after day 5 in 43% of cases) and does not occur at all in 18 to 64% of cases.

The microcirculation, both systemic and pulmonary, is the target of intracellular rickettsial infection, and the clinical manifestations reflect the ensuing vascular changes. Widespread increased vascular permeability results in edema, decreased plasma volume, hypoalbuminemia, reduced serum oncotic pressure, and prerenal azotemia. Hypotension occurs in 17% of cases. Extensive infection of the pulmonary microcirculation is associated with noncardiogenic pulmonary edema. Cardiac involvement is most frequently manifested as dysrhythmia, which is detected in 7 to 16% of cases. Pulmonary involvement, often a major factor in fatal cases, is observed in 17% of cases, of which 12% are considered to represent severe respiratory disease and 8% require mechanical ventilation.

Central nervous system (CNS) involvement is the other important

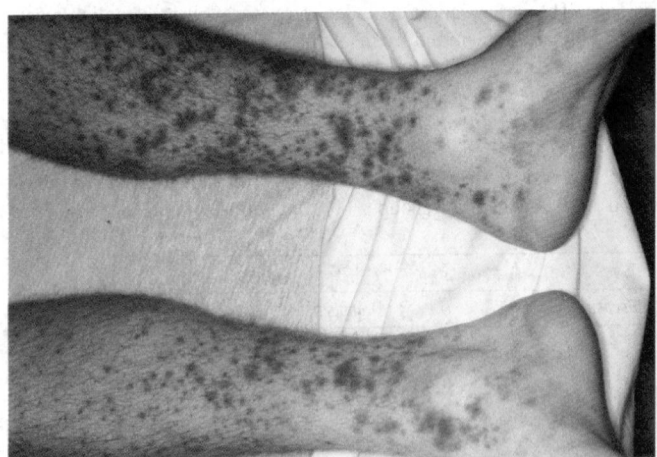

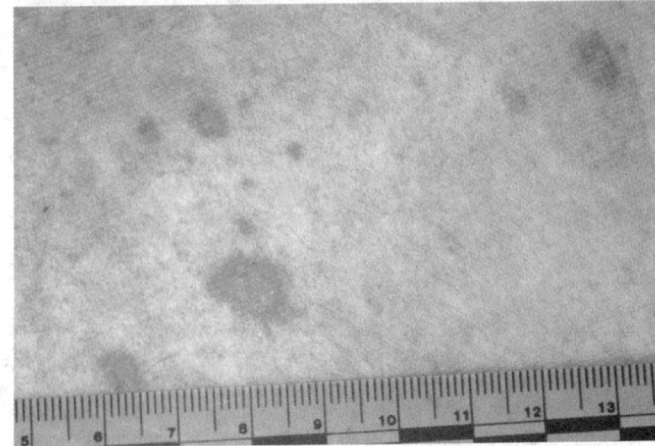

FIGURE 158-1 *Top:* Petechial lesions of Rocky Mountain spotted fever on the lower legs and soles of a young, otherwise-healthy patient. *Bottom:* Close-up of lesions from the same patient. (*Photos courtesy of Dr. Lindsey Baden.*)

determinant of the outcome of RMSF. Encephalitis, presenting as confusion or lethargy, is apparent in 26 to 28% of cases. Progressively severe encephalitis manifests as stupor or delirium in 21 to 26% of cases, as ataxia in 18%, as coma in 9 to 10%, and as seizures in 8%. Cranial nerve palsy, hearing loss, severe vertigo, nystagmus, dysarthria, aphasia, unilateral corticospinal signs, ankle clonus, extensor toe signs, hyperreflexia, spasticity, fasciculations, athetosis, neurogenic bladder, hemiplegia, paraplegia, and complete paralysis have been reported. Meningoencephalitis results in cerebrospinal fluid (CSF) pleocytosis in 34 to 38% of cases; usually there are 10 to 100 cells per microliter with a mononuclear predominance, but occasionally there are more than 100 cells per microliter and a polymorphonuclear predominance. The CSF protein concentration is increased in 30 to 35% of cases, but the CSF glucose concentration is usually normal.

Renal failure, which occurs in more severely ill patients, is often reversible with rehydration. However, in the most severe cases, shock results in acute tubular necrosis–induced renal failure, which often requires hemodialysis.

Hepatic injury is manifested in 38% of cases as mildly or moderately increased serum aminotransferase concentrations and is due to focal death of individual hepatocytes, but hepatic failure does not occur. Jaundice is recognized in 8 to 9% of cases and an elevated serum bilirubin concentration in 18 to 30%. Marked hyperbilirubinemia occasionally occurs, probably as a consequence of both hemolysis and hepatocytic injury.

Bleeding is a potentially life-threatening effect of severe vascular damage. Anemia develops in 30% of cases and is severe enough to require red blood cell transfusions in 11%. Blood is detected in the stools or vomitus of 10% of patients, and death has followed massive upper gastrointestinal hemorrhage.

Other characteristic clinical laboratory findings include a normal white blood cell count with increased numbers of immature myeloid cells, increased plasma levels of proteins of the acute-phase response (C-reactive protein, fibrinogen, ferritin, and others), and hyponatremia (in 56% of cases) due to the appropriate secretion of antidiuretic hormone in response to the hypovolemic state. Skeletal muscle injury, clinically manifested as myositis, has been documented in several individual cases by the detection of marked elevations in serum creatine kinase or of histopathologic evidence of vascular injury in skeletal muscle and multifocal rhabdomyonecrosis. Ocular involvement includes conjunctivitis in 30% of cases and retinal vein engorgement, flame hemorrhages, arterial occlusion, and papilledema with normal CSF pressure in some instances.

In untreated cases, death usually occurs 8 to 15 days after the onset of illness. A rare presentation, fulminant RMSF, is fatal within 5 days after onset. This fulminant presentation has been associated with RMSF in black males who have a glucose-6-phosphate dehydrogenase (G6PD) deficiency and is thought to be related to an undefined effect of hemolysis on the rickettsial infection. Although survivors of RMSF usually appear to return to their previous state of health, permanent sequelae, including neurologic deficits and amputation of gangrenous extremities, may follow severe illness.

Diagnosis The diagnosis of RMSF during the acute stage is more difficult than is generally appreciated. Clinical and epidemiologic considerations are more important than laboratory features early in the illness. The most important epidemiologic factor is a history of exposure within the 12 days preceding disease onset to a potentially tick-infested environment during a season of possible tick activity. However, only 60% of patients actually recall being bitten by a tick during the incubation period.

The differential diagnosis for early clinical manifestations of RMSF (fever, headache, and myalgia without a rash) includes influenza, enteroviral infection, infectious mononucleosis, viral hepatitis, leptospirosis, typhoid fever, gram-negative or gram-positive bacterial sepsis, human monocytotropic or granulocytotropic ehrlichiosis or anaplasmosis, murine typhus, sylvatic flying-squirrel typhus, and rickettsialpox. Enterocolitis may be suggested by nausea, vomiting, and abdominal pain; prominence of abdominal tenderness has resulted in exploratory laparotomy. CNS involvement may masquerade as bacterial and viral meningoencephalitis, with seizures, coma, neurologic signs, and CSF abnormalities. Cough, pulmonary signs, and chest roentgenographic opacities may lead to a diagnostic consideration of bronchitis or pneumonia.

At presentation during the first 3 days of illness, only 3% of patients exhibit the classic triad of fever, rash, and history of tick exposure. When a rash appears, a diagnosis of RMSF should certainly be considered. However, many illnesses considered in the differential diagnosis may also be associated with a rash, including rubeola, rubella, meningococcemia, disseminated gonococcal infection, secondary syphilis, toxic shock syndrome, drug hypersensitivity, idiopathic thrombocytopenic purpura, thrombotic thrombocytopenic purpura, Kawasaki syndrome, and immune complex vasculitis. Conversely, any person in an endemic area with a provisional diagnosis of one of the above illnesses may have RMSF.

The most common serologic test for confirmation of the diagnosis is the indirect immunofluorescence assay. Between 7 and 10 days after onset, a diagnostic titer of ≥1:64 is usually detectable. Latex agglutination and a solid-state enzyme immunoassay are also available commercially. Latex agglutination usually yields a diagnostic titer of ≥1:128 at 7 to 9 days after onset. The sensitivity and specificity of the indirect immunofluorescence assay are 94 to 100% and 100%, respectively, and the latex agglutination test has a sensitivity of 71 to 94% and a specificity of 96 to 99%. The performance of the solid-state immunoassay has not been reported. It is important to understand that serologic tests for RMSF are usually negative at the time of presentation for medical care and that treatment should not be delayed while a positive serologic result is awaited.

The only diagnostic test that is useful during the acute illness is immunohistologic examination (immunofluorescence or immunoenzyme staining) of a cutaneous biopsy of a rash lesion for *R. rickettsii*. Examination of a 3-mm punch biopsy of such a lesion is 70% sensitive and 100% specific. Polymerase chain reaction (PCR) amplification and detection of *R. rickettsii* DNA in peripheral blood is a relatively insensitive approach except in the preterminal state; rickettsiae are present in large quantities in heavily infected foci of endothelial cells but in relatively low quantities in the circulation. Cultivation of rickettsiae in cell culture is technically feasible but is seldom undertaken because of biohazard and technologic concerns.

℞ TREATMENT

The drug of choice for the treatment of both children and adults with RMSF is doxycycline, except when the patient is pregnant or allergic to the drug. Because of the severity of RMSF, immediate empirical administration of doxycycline should be strongly considered in any patient with a consistent clinical presentation in the appropriate epidemiologic setting. Doxycycline is administered orally (or, in the presence of coma or vomiting, intravenously) at 200 mg/d in two divided doses. Patients who are allergic to doxycycline or in whom this drug is contraindicated should receive chloramphenicol (50 to 75 mg/kg daily in four divided oral doses, for 7 days); the complete blood count should be monitored during chloramphenicol treatment. For children with suspected RMSF infection, up to five courses of doxycycline may be administered with minimal risk of dental staining. Other regimens include oral tetracycline (25 to 50 mg/kg per day) in four divided doses. The antirickettsial drug should be administered until the patient has been afebrile and improving clinically for 2 or 3 days. β-Lactam antibiotics, erythromycin, and aminoglycosides have no role in the treatment of RMSF, and sulfa-containing drugs are likely to exacerbate this infection. There is not enough clinical experience to comment on the use of fluoroquinolones in this setting. The most seriously ill patients are managed in intensive care units, with careful administration of fluids to achieve optimal tissue perfusion without precipitating non-

TABLE 158-2 *Laboratory Diagnosis and Treatment of Selected Rickettsial Diseases*

Disease	Laboratory Diagnosis	Treatment
Mediterranean spotted fever, Japanese spotted fever, Queensland tick typhus, Flinders Island spotted fever, African tick-bite fever	Isolation of rickettsiae by shell-vial culture; serology, IFA (IgM, ≥1:64; or IgG, ≥1:128); skin biopsy immunohistochemical detection of rickettsiae; PCR amplification of DNA from tissue specimens	Doxycycline (100 mg bid PO for 1–5 days) *or* Ciprofloxacin (750 mg bid PO for 5 days) *or* Chloramphenicol (500 mg qid PO for 7–10 days) *or* (in pregnancy) Josamycin[a] (3 g/d PO for 5 days)
Rickettsialpox	IFA: seroconversion to a titer of ≥1:64 or a single titer of ≥1:128; cross-adsorption to eliminate antibodies to shared antigens necessary for a specific diagnosis of the spotted fever rickettsial species; skin biopsy immunohistochemistry	Doxycycline (100 mg bid PO for 1–5 days) *or* Ciprofloxacin (750 mg bid PO for 5 days) *or* Chloramphenicol (500 mg qid PO for 7–10 days) *or* (in pregnancy) Josamycin[a] (3 g/d PO for 5 days)
Endemic (murine) typhus	IFA: fourfold rise to a titer of ≥1:64 or a single titer of ≥1:128; immunohistology: skin biopsy; PCR amplification of *R. typhi* or *R. felis* DNA from blood; dot ELISA and immunoperoxidase methods also available	Doxycycline (100 mg bid PO for 7–15 days) *or* Chloramphenicol (500 mg qid PO for 7–15 days)
Epidemic typhus	IFA: titer of ≥1:128; necessary to use clinical and epidemiologic data to distinguish among louse-borne epidemic typhus, flying-squirrel typhus, and Brill-Zinsser disease	Doxycycline (200 mg PO as a single dose or until patient is afebrile for 24 h)
Scrub typhus	IFA: titer of ≥1:200; PCR amplification of *O. tsutsugamushi* DNA from blood of febrile patients	Doxycycline[b] (100 mg bid PO for 7–15 days) *or* Chloramphenicol (500 mg qid PO for 7–15 days *or* (for children) Chloramphenicol (150 mg/kg per day for 5 days)

[a] Not approved by the U.S. Food and Drug Administration.
[b] Azithromycin is more effective than doxycycline in vitro against both doxycycline-susceptible and doxycycline-resistant strains of *O. tsutsugamushi*.

cardiogenic pulmonary edema. In some severely ill patients, hypoxemia requires intubation and mechanical ventilation; oliguric or anuric acute renal failure requires hemodialysis; seizures necessitate the use of antiseizure medication; anemia or severe hemorrhage necessitates transfusions of packed red blood cells; and bleeding with severe thrombocytopenia requires platelet transfusions. Heparin is not a useful component of treatment, and there is no evidence that glucocorticoids, although frequently administered, affect outcome.

Prevention Avoidance of tick bites is the only available preventive approach. Protective clothing and tick repellents, which could reduce the risk, are seldom actually used. After possible tick exposure, it is wise to inspect the body once or twice a day and remove ticks before they can inoculate rickettsiae.

MEDITERRANEAN SPOTTED FEVER (BOUTONNEUSE FEVER) AND OTHER TICK-BORNE SPOTTED FEVERS The etiologic agent of Mediterranean spotted fever, *R. conorii*, is prevalent in southern Europe (below the 45th parallel), all of Africa, and southwestern and south-central Asia. The tick vector and reservoir is *R. sanguineus*, the brown dog tick. The name of this disease varies with the region in which it occurs; examples include Kenya tick typhus, Indian tick typhus, Israeli spotted fever, and Astrakhan spotted fever. Whatever the designation, the disease is characterized by a high fever, rash, and—in most geographic locales—an inoculation eschar (*tâche noire*) at the site of the tick bite. A severe form of the disease, associated with a 50% mortality rate, has been observed in patients with diabetes, alcoholism, or heart failure.

African tick-bite fever, which is caused by *R. africae* and has been recognized since the beginning of the twentieth century, was first doc-

umented in the modern era in Zimbabwe in 1992. The disease occurs in rural areas and follows bites by ticks of cattle and wild animals. *R. africae* is prevalent in *Amblyomma hebraeum* and *A. variegatum* ticks, which readily feed on humans. Cases occur throughout sub-Saharan Africa and in the Caribbean islands. The average incubation period is 7 days (range, 4 to 10 days). The illness is mild and consists of headache, fever, eschar at the tick bite site, and regional lymphadenopathy. *Amblyomma* ticks often feed in groups, and several ticks may be found on one patient, with the subsequent development of multiple eschars. Rash is frequently lacking or transient and may be vesicular. African tick-bite fever is the most prevalent rickettsiosis worldwide, and—because of tourism in sub-Saharan Africa—is the most frequently occurring imported rickettsiosis in Europe and North America.

Rickettsia japonica causes *Japanese spotted fever*. Patients present with fever, cutaneous eruption, and an inoculation eschar. A similar disease in northern Asia is caused by *R. sibirica*. In Australia, two spotted fevers have been described. *Queensland tick typhus* is due to *R. australis* and is transmitted by *Ixodes holocyclus*. The skin rash in this disease is usually maculopapular but is sometimes vesicular, and there is an inoculation eschar. *Flinders Island spotted fever*, observed also on nearby Tasmania, is due to *R. honei*. In Europe, patients infected with *R. slovaca* after a *Dermacentor* tick bite manifest an eschar and regional lymphadenopathy.

Diagnosis The diagnosis of these tick-borne spotted fevers is based on clinical and epidemiologic findings and is confirmed by cell-culture isolation of rickettsiae, by PCR of skin biopsies (a method not available in most laboratories), or by serology. The serologic identification of infection with a specific species requires cross-adsorption (Table 158-2). In an endemic area, patients presenting with fever, rash, and/or a skin lesion consisting of a black necrotic area or a crust surrounded by erythema should be considered to have one of these rickettsial spotted fevers.

Rx TREATMENT

See Table 158-2.

RICKETTSIALPOX Rickettsialpox was first described in 1946 by a general practitioner in New York City and soon afterwards was shown to be caused by a distinct species, *R. akari*. This organism was isolated from mice and their mites (*Liponyssoides sanguineus*), which maintain the organisms by transovarian transmission. *R. akari* shares lipopolysaccharide antigens with other members of the SFG.

Epidemiology More than 100 cases of rickettsialpox were diagnosed annually in the northeastern United States in the late 1940s and the 1950s, and outbreaks occurred in the Ukraine in the 1950s. However, few cases are diagnosed currently. Recently, a culture-confirmed case of rickettsialpox was documented in southern Europe; this case was initially misdiagnosed as Mediterranean spotted fever on the basis of the development of serum antibodies cross-reactive with *R. conorii*. Investigation of eschars suspected to represent bioterrorism-associated cutaneous anthrax has resulted in the diagnosis of cases of rickettsialpox in the United States and has revealed that its occurrence is more widespread than was previously realized. Rickettsialpox is recognized principally in New York City, but cases have also been reported in North Carolina, Virginia, Maryland, Arizona, Utah, and Ohio.

Clinical Manifestations A papule forms at the site of the mite bite. This lesion develops a central vesicle that becomes a 1- to 2.5-cm painless black crusted eschar surrounded by an erythematous halo (Fig. 158-2). Enlargement of the lymph nodes draining the region of the eschar suggests initial lymphogenous spread. After an incubation period of 10 to 17 days, during which the eschar and regional lymphadenopathy frequently go unnoticed, the onset of illness is marked by malaise, chills, fever, headache, and myalgia. A macular rash appears 2 to 6 days after onset and evolves sequentially into papules, vesicles, and crusts that heal without scarring (Fig. 158-3). In some cases the rash remains macular or maculopapular. Some patients suffer nausea, vomiting, abdominal pain, cough, conjunctivitis, or photophobia. Untreated rickettsialpox is not fatal, with fever lasting 6 to 10 days.

Diagnosis and Treatment See Table 158-2.

CAT FLEA–ASSOCIATED RICKETTSIOSIS An emerging rickettsiosis caused by *R. felis* has been documented in North and South America and Europe. Transmitted and maintained transovarially in the geographically widespread cat flea *Ctenocephalides felis*, the infection has been described as moderately severe, with fever, rash, headache, and CNS and gastrointestinal signs. However, the clinical spectrum and frequency of the various clinical manifestations have yet to be determined.

FLEA- AND LOUSE-BORNE TYPHUS GROUP RICKETTSIOSES

ENDEMIC MURINE TYPHUS (FLEA-BORNE) Murine typhus was postulated to be a distinct disease, with rats as the reservoir and fleas as the vector, by Maxcy in 1926. Dyer isolated the etiologic agent, *R. typhi*, from rats and fleas in 1931. By the end of World War II, murine typhus was known to be a global disease.

Epidemiology *R. typhi* is maintained in mammalian host/flea cycles, with rats (*Rattus rattus* and *R. norvegicus*) and the Oriental rat flea (*Xenopsylla cheopis*) as the classic zoonotic niche. Fleas acquire *R. typhi* from rickettsemic rats and carry the organism throughout the rest of their life span. Nonimmune rats and humans are infected when rickettsia-laden flea feces are "scratched" into pruritic bite lesions; less frequently, the flea bite itself transmits the organisms. Yet another possible route of transmission is the inhalation of aerosolized flea feces. Infected rats appear healthy, although they are rickettsemic for ~2 weeks.

Currently, <100 cases of endemic typhus are reported annually in the United States. These cases occur mainly in southern Texas and southern California, where the classic rat/flea cycle is absent and an opossum/cat flea (*C. felis*) cycle is prominent. Cases of endemic typhus occur year-round, mainly in warm (often coastal) areas. This infection has also been reported from Greece, Spain, and Indonesia. The prevalence peaks from April through June in southern Texas and during

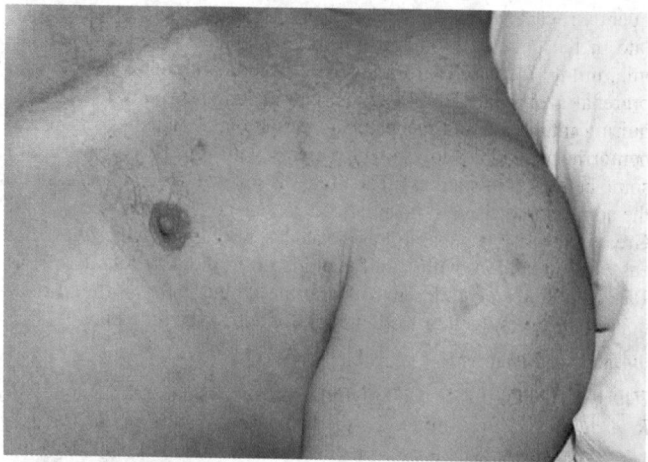

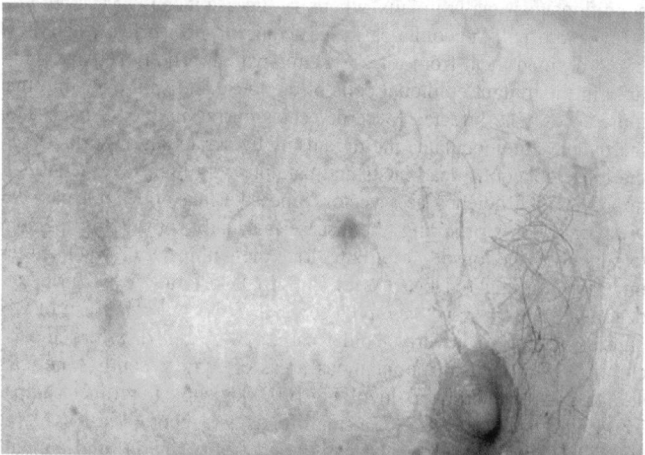

FIGURE 158-3   *Top:* Papulovesicular lesions on the trunk of the patient with rickettsialpox shown in Fig. 158-2. *Bottom:* Close-up of lesions from the same patient. (*Reprinted from A Krusell et al: Emerg Infect Dis 8:727, 2002. Photos obtained by Dr. Kenneth Kaye.*)

the warm months of summer and early fall in other geographic locations. Patients seldom recall a flea bite or exposure to fleas, although exposure to animals such as cats, opossums, raccoons, skunks, and rats is reported by nearly 40% of those who are questioned.

Clinical Manifestations The incubation period of experimental murine typhus in volunteers averages 11 days, with a range of 8 to 16 days. Close observation during this period reveals prodromal symptoms of headache, myalgia, arthralgia, nausea, and malaise developing 1 to 3 days before the abrupt onset of chills and fever. Nearly all patients experience nausea and vomiting early in the illness.

The duration of untreated illness averages 12 days, with a range of 9 to 18 days. Rash is present in only 13% of patients at the time of presentation for medical care (usually ~4 days after onset of symptoms), appearing an average of 2 days later in half of the remaining patients and never appearing in the other half. The initial macular rash is often detected by careful inspection of the axilla or the inner surface of the arm. Subsequently, the rash becomes maculopapular, involving the trunk more often than the extremities; it is seldom petechial and rarely involves the face, palms, or soles. A rash is detected in only 20% of patients with dark brown or black skin.

Pulmonary involvement is frequently prominent in murine typhus; 35% of patients have a hacking, nonproductive cough, and 23% of patients who undergo chest radiography have pulmonary densities due to interstitial pneumonia, pulmonary edema, and pleural effusions. Bibasilar rales are the most common pulmonary sign. Less common clinical symptoms and signs include abdominal pain, confusion, stupor, seizures, ataxia, coma, and jaundice. Clinical laboratory studies fre-

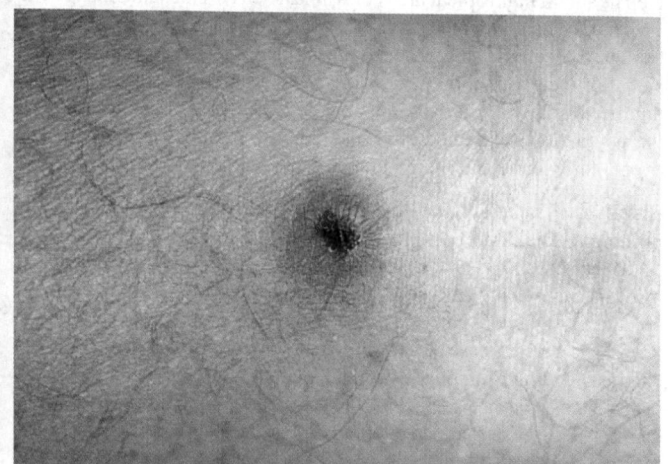

FIGURE 158-2   Eschar at the site of the mite bite in a patient with rickettsialpox. (*Reprinted from A Krusell et al: Emerg Infect Dis 8:727, 2002. Photo obtained by Dr. Kenneth Kaye.*)

quently reveal anemia and leukopenia early in the course, leukocytosis late in the course, thrombocytopenia, hyponatremia, hypoalbuminemia, mildly increased serum levels of hepatic aminotransferases, and prerenal azotemia. Complications may include respiratory failure requiring intubation and mechanical ventilation, hematemesis, cerebral hemorrhage, and hemolysis (in patients with G6PD deficiency and some hemoglobinopathies). The illness is severe enough to necessitate the admission of 10% of hospitalized patients to an intensive care unit. Greater severity is generally associated with old age, underlying disease, and treatment with a sulfonamide drug; the case-fatality rate is 1%. In a study of children with murine typhus, 50% suffered only nocturnal fevers, feeling well enough for active daytime play.

Diagnosis and Treatment   See Table 158-2.

EPIDEMIC TYPHUS (LOUSE-BORNE)   Epidemic typhus due to infection with *R. prowazekii* is transmitted by the human body louse (*Pediculus humanus corporis*), which lives on clothes and is found in poor hygienic conditions (especially in jails, where the disease it causes is called *jail fever*) and usually in cold areas. Lice acquire *R. prowazekii* when they ingest a blood meal from a rickettsemic patient. The rickettsiae multiply in the midgut epithelial cells of the louse and spill over into the louse feces. The infected louse defecates during its blood meal, and the patient autoinoculates the organisms by scratching. The fact that the louse abandons dead hosts and patients with high fever (>40°C) improves its efficiency as a vector. Since the louse does not pass *R. prowazekii* to its offspring, the disease is usually spread from person to person by the louse-borne route. Lice die within 1 to 2 weeks after infection, turning red because of intestinal perforation just prior to death—hence the name *red louse disease*. This epidemic form of typhus is related to poverty, cold weather, war, and disasters and is currently prevalent in mountainous areas of Africa, South America, and Asia. A large outbreak involving 100,000 people in refugee camps in Burundi occurred in 1997, a small focus was reported in Russia in 1998, sporadic cases have been reported from Algeria, and annual outbreaks have occurred in Peru. The global reemergence of the disease is due to proliferation of body lice. In the United States, sporadic cases of epidemic typhus are transmitted by flying-squirrel fleas. Eastern flying-squirrel (*Glaucomys volans*) lice and fleas have been found to be infected with *R. prowazekii*. The flying-squirrel fleas occasionally bite humans.

Brill-Zinsser disease is a recrudescent, mild form of epidemic typhus occurring years after the acute disease, probably as a result of immunosuppression or old age. Nathan Brill first identified recrudescent typhus in New York in 1898. In 1933 Hans Zinsser noted that >90% of patients with recrudescent typhus had emigrated from typhus-endemic areas of Europe. Strains of *R. prowazekii* indistinguishable from classic strains were isolated from patients with recrudescent typhus. Furthermore, *R. prowazekii* was isolated from the lymph nodes of patients undergoing elective surgery who had had typhus years earlier. Thus the typhus rickettsiae can remain dormant for years and can reactivate with waning immunity.

Rickettsiae, particularly *R. prowazekii*, are potential agents of bioterrorism (Chap. 205). *R. prowazekii* and *R. rickettsii* have a high case-fatality ratio, cause diseases that are difficult to diagnose, and can be engineered to display complete antimicrobial resistance. A strain of tetracycline-resistant *R. prowazekii* was developed in the former Soviet Union. *R. prowazekii* and *R. typhi* have dormant forms that survive extracellularly for long periods, and all rickettsiae are highly infectious when inhaled as aerosols.

Clinical Manifestations   After an incubation period of ~1 week (range, 7 to 14 days), the onset of illness is abrupt, with prostration, severe headache, and fever rising rapidly to 38.8° to 40.0°C (102° to 104°F). Cough is frequently prominent, occurring in 70% of patients. Myalgias are usually severe. In the outbreak in Burundi, the disease was referred to as *sutama* ("crouching"), the myalgias being so severe that patients crouched in an attempt to alleviate the pain. A rash begins on the upper trunk, usually on the fifth day, and then becomes generalized, involving all of the body except the face, palms, and soles. Initially, this rash is macular; without treatment, it becomes maculopapular, petechial, and confluent. The rash is frequently absent or not detected on black skin in Africa, where 60% of patients have *spotless epidemic typhus*. Photophobia, with considerable conjunctival injection and eye pain, is frequent. The tongue may be dry, brown, and furred. Confusion and coma are common. Skin necrosis and gangrene of the digits as well as interstitial pneumonia have been noted in severe cases. Untreated disease is fatal in 7 to 40% of cases, with outcome depending primarily on the condition of the host. Patients with untreated infections develop renal insufficiency and multiorgan involvement in which neurologic manifestations are frequently prominent. Overall, 12% of patients with epidemic typhus have neurologic involvement. North American *R. prowazekii* infection transmitted by flying-squirrel ectoparasites is a milder illness; whether this milder disease is due to host factors (e.g., better health status) or organism factors (e.g., attenuated virulence) is unknown.

Diagnosis and Treatment   See Table 158-2. Epidemic typhus is sometimes misdiagnosed as typhoid fever in tropical countries (Chap. 137).

Prevention   Prevention of epidemic typhus involves control of body lice. Clothes should be changed regularly, and insecticides should be used every 6 weeks to control the louse population.

SCRUB TYPHUS

The etiologic agent of scrub typhus is a small, obligately intracellular bacterium of the family Rickettsiaceae that differs substantially from other family members in its genetic makeup and in the composition of its cell wall (which, for example, lacks lipopolysaccharide and peptidoglycan). Consequently, this organism has been classified as a species in a separate genus, *Orientia tsutsugamushi*.

O. tsutsugamushi is maintained in nature by transovarian transmission in trombiculid mites, mainly of the genus *Leptotrombidium*. After hatching, infected larval mites (chiggers, the only stage that feeds on an animal host) inoculate organisms into the skin while feeding. Scrub typhus is found in environments that harbor the infected chiggers, particularly areas of heavy scrub vegetation—e.g., where the forest is regrowing after being cleared and along riverbanks. Infections occur during the wet season, when the mites lay their eggs. The disease is endemic in eastern and southern Asia, northern Australia, and islands of the western Pacific Ocean. Scrub typhus is also found in tropical areas of India, Sri Lanka, Bangladesh, Myanmar, Thailand, Malaysia, Laos, Vietnam, Kampuchea, China, Taiwan, the Philippines, Indonesia, Papua New Guinea, northern Australia, and islands of the South Pacific Ocean; in temperate areas of Japan, Korea, far-eastern Russia, Tadzhikistan, the mountains of northern India, Pakistan, and Nepal; and in nontropical areas of China, such as Tibet and Shangdong Province. Those infected include indigenous rural workers, residents of suburban areas, and westerners visiting endemic areas for professional or recreational purposes. Infections are more prevalent than the number of clinical diagnoses would suggest; in some areas >3% of the population is infected or reinfected each month. Immunity wanes over 1 to 3 years, and there is remarkable antigenic diversity.

Clinical Manifestations   The illness varies in severity from mild and self-limiting to fatal. After an incubation period of 6 to 21 days (usually 8 to 10 days), the onset of disease is characterized by fever, headache, myalgia, cough, and gastrointestinal symptoms. Some patients develop no further signs or symptoms and recover spontaneously after a few days. The classic case description includes an eschar at the site of chigger feeding, regional lymphadenopathy, and a maculopapular rash—signs that are seldom observed in indigenous patients. Fewer than 50% of Westerners develop an eschar, and <40% develop a rash (on day 4 to 6 of illness). Severe cases typically include prominent encephalitis and interstitial pneumonia as key features of vascular injury. Severe illness in persons with G6PD deficiency has been accompanied by hemolysis. The case-fatality rate for untreated classic cases

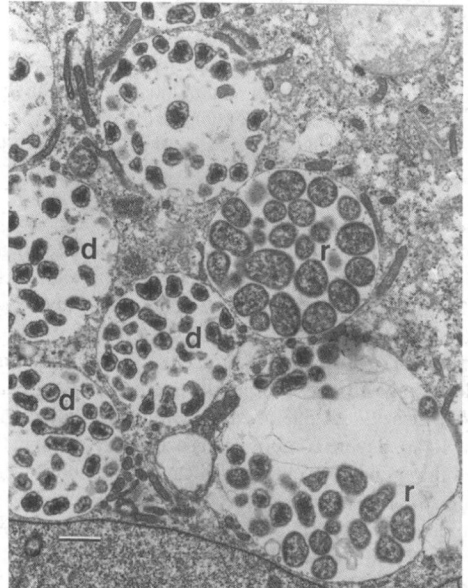

FIGURE 158-4 *Ehrlichia chaffeensis* microcolonies (morulae) within cytoplasmic vacuoles manifest as two morphologic forms: reticulate cells (r) and dense-core cells (d). Bar = 1 μm. *(Photo courtesy of Dr. Vsevolod L. Popov.)*

is 7% but would probably be lower if all relatively mild cases (which are underdiagnosed) were included.

Diagnosis and Treatment See Table 158-2. Some cases of scrub typhus in Thailand are caused by *O. tsutsugamushi* strains that are resistant to doxycycline or chloramphenicol. These strains are susceptible to rifampin, and azithromycin and clarithromycin have been used successfully in small numbers of patients.

EHRLICHIOSES AND ANAPLASMOSIS

Ehrlichiae are small, obligately intracellular bacteria with a gram-negative-type cell wall that grow in cytoplasmic vacuoles to form clusters called *morulae* (Fig. 158-4). Two distinct *Ehrlichia* species and one *Anaplasma* species cause human infections that can be severe and frequent (Table 158-3). *E. chaffeensis*, the agent of human monocytotropic ehrlichiosis (HME), infects predominantly mononuclear phagocytic cells in tissues and blood monocytes. *E. ewingii* and *A. phagocytophila* infect cells of myeloid lineage, particularly neutrophils. Confusion may arise from the facts that *Anaplasma phagocytophila* is the agent of the disease originally designated human granulocytotropic ehrlichiosis (HGE) and *Ehrlichia ewingii* is a human granulocytotropic pathogen. Such confusion can be avoided through use of the terms *human anaplasmosis* and *ehrlichiosis ewingii*, with avoidance of the ambiguous *HGE*. Both *E. chaffeensis* and *E. ewingii* are transmitted mainly by the Lone Star tick *Amblyomma americanum* and cause persistent infections in the same reservoir, the white-tailed deer. *A. phagocytophila* is transmitted, with little geographic overlap, by *Ixodes scapularis* in the northeastern and upper midwestern states and by *I. ricinus* in Europe. In California, both HME and *A. phagocytophila* infection have been documented, with apparent partial overlap of their vectors. In Eurasia, reports of human infection caused by an *I. persulcatus*–transmitted *E. muris*–like agent and of *A. phagocytophila* associated with *I. persulcatus* are beginning to appear. The worldwide prevalence of ehrlichioses and anaplasmoses is an important issue in the field of emerging infectious diseases.

Ehrlichiae were discovered by veterinarians

during the investigation of hemolytic anemia of cattle before 1910. Researchers thereafter discerned that "marginal points" visible within erythrocytes were infectious and named the agent *Anaplasma marginale*. Subsequently, several other species generally considered to be ehrlichiae were detected as veterinary infectious agents, including *E. ruminantium*, *E. canis*, *E. ewingii*, *A. phagocytophila*, and *Neorickettsia risticii*.

The current taxonomic positions are determined by nucleic acid sequences of conserved and unique genes among these species. By analysis of 16S ribosomal RNA and other sequences, the family Anaplasmataceae can be divided into four genera: *Ehrlichia*, *Anaplasma*, *Wolbachia*, and *Neorickettsia*. Given the lack of transovarian transmission in ticks, the natural maintenance of the tick-borne ehrlichiae and anaplasmae clearly depends in part on prolonged or persistent infections in wild and feral mammalian reservoirs. Thus, *Ehrlichia* and *Anaplasma* are propagated by horizontal transmission that relies on a tick-mammal-tick cycle; humans are inadvertently infected when they impinge on the natural habitats occupied by the ticks and the reservoir hosts. Wolbachiae are associated with human diseases caused by filariae, with symbiosis in some instances. The wolbachiae are important for filarial viability and pathogenicity. Treatment of wolbachiae is now a strategy in the control of filariasis. Neorickettsiae parasitize flukes that in turn are parasites of aquatic snails, fish, and insects. Although only a single human neorickettsiosis, *sennetsu fever*, has been described, others may be discovered. Probably in association with the ingestion of raw fish containing *N. sennetsu*–infected flukes, patients develop an infectious mononucleosis–like illness that was first identified in 1953.

HUMAN MONOCYTOTROPIC EHRLICHIOSIS ■ **Epidemiology** More than 1363 cases of infections caused by *E. chaffeensis* had been reported to the Centers for Disease Control and Prevention (CDC) as of September 2002. However, since HME is not a reportable disease in most states, this figure is a gross underestimate. Most *E. chaffeensis* infections have been identified in the south-central, southeastern, and mid-Atlantic states, but cases have also been recognized in California. The vector is the Lone Star tick (*A. americanum*), which in all its life stages feeds on white-tailed deer—a major reservoir host. Dogs and coyotes have been discovered to be subclinically infected and may also be an important reservoir. Tick bites and exposures are reported by patients, frequently in rural areas and especially in the months May through July. The median age of HME patients is 44 years, and 75% of the affected individuals are male; however, severe and fatal infections in children are also well recognized. Active prospective surveillance has revealed that in rural areas inhabited by abundant deer and Lone Star ticks, HME is a common disease, with an incidence as high as 1000 cases per 1 million population.

TABLE 158-3 *Comparison of Three Human Ehrlichioses: Human Monocytotropic Ehrlichiosis (HME), Anaplasmosis, and Human Ehrlichiosis Ewingii*

Variable	HME	Human Anaplasmosis	Ehrlichiosis Ewingii
Etiologic agent	*E. chaffeensis*	*A. phagocytophila*	*E. ewingii*
Tick vector(s)	*Amblyomma americanum*, *Dermacentor variabilis* (dog tick)	*Ixodes scapularis* (deer tick), *I. ricinus*, *I. pacificus*	*A. americanum*
Seasonality	April through September	Year-round (peak: May, June, and July)	April through September
Major target cell	Monocyte	Granulocyte	Neutrophil
Morulae seen	Rarely	Frequently	Rarely
Antigen used in IFA test	*E. chaffeensis*	*A. phagocytophila*	*E. chaffeensis* as surrogate
Diagnostic titer	Fourfold rise or a single titer of ≥1:128; cutoff for negative titer, 1:64	Fourfold rise; cutoff for negative titer, 1:80	No established criteria
Treatment of choice	Doxycycline	Doxycycline	Doxycycline
Mortality	2–3%	<1%	None reported

Note: IFA, indirect immunofluorescence assay.

Clinical Manifestations *E. chaffeensis* is inoculated into the dermal blood pool created by the feeding tick and subsequently disseminates via the blood to tissues. After a median incubation period of 8 days, illness develops. The classic clinical manifestations are not specific and include fever (97% of cases), headache (81%), myalgia (68%), and malaise (84%); less frequently observed are gastrointestinal involvement (nausea, vomiting, diarrhea; 25 to 68%), cough (25%), rash (36% overall, 6% at presentation), and confusion (20%). HME may be severe: 62% of patients with documented cases are hospitalized, and ~3% die. Severe complications include a toxic shock–like or septic shock–like syndrome, respiratory insufficiency and adult respiratory distress, meningoencephalitis, fulminant infection (in immunocompromised patients), severe opportunistic and nosocomial infections, and hemorrhage. Laboratory findings may be of value in the differential diagnosis; 60 to 74% of patients with HME have leukopenia (initially lymphopenia, later neutropenia), 72% have thrombocytopenia, and nearly 90% have elevations in serum levels of hepatic aminotransferases. With effective therapy, rebound lymphocytosis (mainly γ/δ T cells) is common. In spite of abnormal blood counts, examinations reveal hypercellular bone marrow, and noncaseating granulomas may be present. Vasculitis is not a component of HME.

Diagnosis Because HME can be fatal, empirical antibiotic therapy should be instituted on the basis of a clinical diagnosis. This diagnosis may be suggested by fever in the setting of known tick exposure during the preceding 3 weeks, leukopenia and/or thrombocytopenia, and increased aminotransferase concentrations in serum. Morulae are rarely demonstrated in peripheral blood smears unless an intensive examination is performed; even then, an experienced microscopist is required. The active phase of HME may be diagnosed by PCR amplification of *E. chaffeensis* nucleic acids from EDTA-anticoagulated blood obtained before the start of doxycycline therapy. Retrospective serologic diagnosis requires a consistent clinical picture and detection of a fourfold increase in *E. chaffeensis* antibody titer (to ≥1:64) by indirect immunofluorescence in paired serum samples obtained ~3 weeks apart. It must be underscored that separate specific diagnostic tests for HME and HGE are necessary.

EHRLICHIOSIS EWINGII *Ehrlichia ewingii*, originally identified as a neutrophil pathogen that causes febrile lameness in dogs, resembles HME in many respects, including its tick vector (*A. americanum*) and its vertebrate hosts (white-tailed deer and dogs). The illness caused by *E. ewingii* is similar to HME but is somewhat less severe. The majority of cases have been diagnosed in immunocompromised patients.

℞ TREATMENT

Tetracycline is effective therapy for HME or ehrlichiosis ewingii. Either tetracycline (250 to 500 mg given orally every 6 h) or doxycycline (100 mg given orally or intravenously twice daily) is associated with a lowered rate of hospitalization and a shortened duration of fever. The use of chloramphenicol is controversial, and *E. chaffeensis* is not susceptible to this drug in vitro. While a few reports document the persistence of *E. chaffeensis* in patients after the acute phase of illness, such persistence is very infrequent; most infections are cured by relatively short courses of tetracycline therapy (continuing for 3 to 5 days after defervescence).

Prevention HME and ehrlichiosis ewingii are prevented by the avoidance of ticks in endemic areas. The use of protective clothing and tick repellents, careful tick searches after exposures, and prompt removal of attached ticks are practices that markedly diminish risk.

HUMAN ANAPLASMOSIS ■ **Epidemiology** As of 2002, 1278 cases of HGE had been reported to the CDC, most of them from upper midwestern and northeastern states; the distribution of cases was similar to that for Lyme disease. Most cases were identified within the range of various

I. persulcatus–complex ticks, particularly *I. scapularis*. White-footed deer mice and white-tailed deer in the United States as well as red deer in Europe appear to play a role in maintaining HGE in nature. The incidence of HGE peaks in May, June, and July, but the disease may occur throughout the year in conjunction with human exposure to *Ixodes* ticks. HGE affects predominantly males (79%) and older persons (median age, 58 years).

Clinical Manifestations Because of high seroprevalence rates in endemic regions, it seems likely that only a minority of infected individuals develop clinical manifestations. The incubation period for HGE varies between 4 and 8 days, and the disease manifests as fever (94 to 100% of cases), myalgia (78 to 98%), headache (61 to 85%), and malaise (98%)—findings suggestive of an influenza-like illness. A minority of patients develop gastrointestinal involvement, including nausea, vomiting, or diarrhea (22 to 39%); rash (2 to 11%); cough (27%); and confusion (17%). Severe complications occur most often in the elderly, but even children may be severely affected. Respiratory insufficiency, with adult respiratory distress syndrome, a toxic shock–like syndrome, and life-threatening opportunistic infections, are the most worrisome complications. Meningoencephalitis has not yet been conclusively recognized with HGE. The case-fatality rate is probably <1%, but nearly 7% of ill patients may require intensive care. As in HME, laboratory findings are of great assistance; most patients develop leukopenia and/or thrombocytopenia with increased serum levels of hepatic aminotransferases. The pancytopenia observed in HGE presumably relates to sequestration or destruction of platelets and leukocytes, since the bone marrow is ordinarily normo- or hypercellular. Vasculitis is not a component of HGE. Unlike HME, HGE is not associated with granulomas. While clear evidence exists for co-infections with *Borrelia burgdorferi* and *Babesia microti*, which are transmitted by the same tick vector(s), there is little evidence of comorbidity or of a persistent or chronic phase for HGE.

Diagnosis HGE should be included in the differential diagnosis for patients who have been exposed to ticks and who develop an influenza-like illness during the season of *Ixodes* tick activity (May through December). The concurrent detection of thrombocytopenia, leukopenia, and/or elevations in serum aminotransferase activities further increases the likelihood of HGE. A substantial proportion of patients with HGE develop serologic reactions considered diagnostic of Lyme disease in the absence of clear clinical findings consistent with that diagnosis. Thus, HGE should be considered in the differential diagnosis of atypical severe presentations of Lyme disease. Although not highly sensitive, a thorough peripheral blood film examination for morulae in neutrophils may identify 20 to 75% of infections. PCR testing of EDTA-anticoagulated blood collected before the initiation of tetracycline therapy from patients with active disease is a sensitive and specific method for early confirmation. Serodiagnosis is based mostly upon the retrospective demonstration of a fourfold increase in *A. phagocytophila* group antibody titer to a minimum of 1:80 in paired serum samples obtained ~1 month apart. IgM antibodies may be detected in many patients within the first 1.5 months after illness. Approximately 15 to 40% of infected persons have a detectable antibody titer at presentation, but, in regions where seroprevalence is high, a single acute-phase polyvalent titer may be misleading.

℞ TREATMENT

Doxycycline (100 mg by mouth twice daily) is an effective therapeutic agent, while rifampin has been associated with clinical improvement in pregnant patients with HGE. No prospective studies of any therapy for HGE have been conducted. Most treated patients defervesce within 24 to 48 h.

Prevention Prevention of HGE requires tick avoidance. The Lyme disease vaccine offers no protection against HGE, and no other vaccine is available.

Q fever results from infection with *C. burnetii*. This small gram-negative microorganism (0.2 μm by 0.7 μm) exists in two antigenic forms: phase I and phase II. When *C. burnetii* is passaged in cell cultures or embryonated eggs, its lipopolysaccharide undergoes truncation that results in an antigenic change called *phase variation*. The phase I form is extremely infectious and exists in humans and other animals. Passage in cell culture or embryonated eggs results in a shift to the phase II form, which is avirulent. The ability of *C. burnetii* to form spores allows the organism to survive in harsh environments. Indeed, it can survive for >40 months in skim milk at room temperature and is readily recovered from soil up to 1 month after contamination. Three different plasmids have been described in various isolates of *C. burnetii*. Q fever encompasses two broad clinical syndromes: acute and chronic infection. It is likely that the host's immune response (rather than characteristics of the infecting strain) determines whether or not chronic Q fever develops. Attachment of the virulent form (phase I) of *C. burnetii* to monocytes requires $\alpha_v \beta_3$ integrin only, whereas attachment of the avirulent form (phase II) requires both $\alpha_v \beta_3$ and CR_3 integrins. The transendothelial migration of monocytes infected by virulent *C. burnetii* is impaired, while that of monocytes infected by the avirulent form is not. Production of tumor necrosis factor (TNF) by monocytes is initiated by virulent *C. burnetii* through a mechanism involving both $\alpha_v \beta_3$ integrin and interaction with bacterial lipopolysaccharide. *C. burnetii* survives in monocytes from patients with chronic Q fever but not in monocytes from patients with acute Q fever or from seronegative control subjects. Impairment of the bactericidal activity of the *C. burnetii*–infected monocyte seems to be due to dysregulation of the cytokine network, as TNF in monocyte supernatants from these patients depresses the microbicidal activity of monocytes. The soluble TNF receptor TNF-R75 is upregulated in monocytes from patients with chronic Q fever. This upregulation is due to overproduction of interleukin 10, antibodies to which restore the microbicidal activity of these monocytes in vitro. The CD4+/CD8+ ratio is decreased in patients with Q fever endocarditis. All of the above findings translate into the observations that very few organisms and a strong cellular response are seen in patients with acute Q fever, while many organisms and a moderate cellular response are seen in patients with chronic Q fever.

Epidemiology Q fever is a zoonosis. The primary sources of human infection are infected cattle, sheep, and goats. However, infected cats, rabbits, pigeons, and dogs have also been shown to transmit *C. burnetii* to humans. The extensive wildlife reservoir for *C. burnetii* includes mammals, birds, and ticks. In the infected female mammal, *C. burnetii* localizes to the uterus and the mammary glands. Infection is reactivated during pregnancy, and high concentrations of *C. burnetii* are found in the placenta. At parturition, *C. burnetii* is dispersed as an aerosol, and infection follows inhalation of aerosolized organisms by a susceptible host. Soil is contaminated during parturition, and *C. burnetii* aerosols can be generated weeks to months later during wind storms. Individuals up to 18 km from the source may be infected. Infected female animals shed the organism in milk for weeks to months after parturition. In rare instances, human-to-human transmission has followed delivery of an infant to an infected woman or autopsy on an infected individual. *C. burnetii* has been transmitted via blood transfusion. Persons who are at risk for Q fever include abattoir workers, veterinarians, and other individuals who have vocational or avocational contact with infected animals. Exposure to infected newborn animals or to infected products of conception poses the highest risk. Sexual transmission has been demonstrated experimentally in mice, as has transmission during artificial insemination in cattle. Some evidence suggests that *C. burnetii* can be sexually transmitted among humans. The ingestion of contaminated milk in some areas probably represent a major route of transmission to humans, although the experimental evidence on this point is contradictory. In any event, the vast majority of Q fever cases result from inhalation of contaminated

aerosols. Q fever in children is uncommon, accounting for only 1 to 2% of cases.

Infections due to *C. burnetii* occur in most countries. Indeed, the only areas known to be free of *C. burnetii* are New Zealand and Antarctica. The primary manifestation of acute Q fever differs from place to place. For example, the primary manifestation is pneumonia in Nova Scotia (Canada), granulomatous hepatitis in Marseille (France), and both of these conditions in the Basque region of Spain. These differences may reflect the route of infection; i.e., the ingestion of contaminated milk may result in hepatitis and the inhalation of contaminated aerosols in pneumonia.

In New South Wales, Australia, 2351 cases of Q fever were reported in 1991 to 2000, and the number of cases per 100,000 persons varied from 6.7 in 1996 to 1.8 in 2000. Males accounted for 84% of the cases and children for 1.5%. In Australia each year, Q fever costs the meat industry almost $1 million and >1700 weeks of time lost from work.

Clinical Manifestations ■ *ACUTE Q FEVER* The incubation period for acute Q fever ranges from 3 to 30 days. The clinical presentations include flulike syndromes, prolonged fever, pneumonia, hepatitis, pericarditis, myocarditis, meningoencephalitis, and infection during pregnancy. A study of 1383 cases of Q fever from southern France gives an indication of the spectrum of the clinical manifestations of Q fever. Among the 1070 patients with acute Q fever, 40% had hepatitis, 20% had both pneumonia and hepatitis, 17% had pneumonia, 14% had isolated fever, 2% had central nervous system involvement, 1% had pericarditis, and 1% had myocarditis; in 3% of patients, the clinical presentation was not defined.

The symptoms of acute Q fever are nonspecific; common among them are fever, extreme fatigue, and severe headache. Other symptoms include chills, sweats, nausea, vomiting, and diarrhea, which occur in 5 to 20% of patients. Cough develops in about half of patients with Q fever pneumonia. Neurologic manifestations of acute Q fever are uncommon; however, in one outbreak in the West Midlands, United Kingdom, 23% of 102 patients had neurologic signs and symptoms as the major manifestation. A nonspecific rash may be evident in 4 to 18% of patients. The white blood cell count is usually normal. Thrombocytopenia is detected in ~25% of patients, and reactive thrombocytosis [with platelet counts of up to 1 million/μL (1×10^{12}/L)] frequently develops during recovery. This thrombocytosis may account for cases of deep vein thrombophlebitis complicating acute Q fever in some series. Uncommon manifestations of acute Q fever include optic neuritis, extrapyramidal neurologic disease, Guillain-Barré syndrome, inappropriate secretion of antidiuretic hormone, epididymitis, orchitis, priapism, hemolytic anemia, hemolytic-uremic syndrome, mediastinal lymphadenopathy mimicking lymphoma, spontaneous rupture of the spleen, pancreatitis, erythema nodosum, and mesenteric panniculitis. Chest radiography may show an opacity that is indistinguishable from that seen in pneumonia of other etiologies. Multiple rounded opacities are common; in the appropriate epidemiologic setting (e.g., exposure to a parturient cat), they are highly suggestive of Q fever pneumonia. However, right-sided endocarditis resulting in septic pulmonary emboli can produce the same radiographic appearance.

Up to 70% of the uncommon cases of Q fever in children are asymptomatic. Symptomatic cases in children result in a spectrum of disease similar to that in adults, although only a few cases of Q fever endocarditis in children have been reported.

In Australia and the United Kingdom, a prolonged fatigue state (lasting 5 to 10 years) has followed Q fever in some cases. Low levels of *C. burnetii* DNA have been noted in the affected patients 0.75 to 5 years after infection.

CHRONIC Q FEVER Chronic Q fever, which is uncommon, almost always implies endocarditis. This infection usually occurs in patients with previous valvular heart disease, immunosuppression, or chronic renal insufficiency. Fever is usually absent or low grade. Patients may have nonspecific symptoms for up to 1 year before diagnosis. Valvular vegetations have been seen in only 12% of patients with transthoracic echocardiograms, but the rate of detection may be higher with the use of transesophageal echocardiography. The vegetations in chronic Q fever endocarditis are different from those in bacterial endocarditis, manifesting as nodules on the valve. A high index of suspicion is necessary for a correct diagnosis. The disease should be suspected in all patients with culture-negative endocarditis. In addition, all patients with valvular heart disease and an unexplained purpuric eruption, renal insufficiency, stroke, and/or progressive heart failure should be tested for *C. burnetii* infection. Patients with chronic Q fever have hepatomegaly and/or splenomegaly. These two findings, especially in combination with positive rheumatoid factor, high erythrocyte sedimentation rate, high C-reactive protein level, and/or increased γ-globulin concentrations (up to 60 to 70 g/L), suggest this diagnosis. Other manifestations of chronic Q fever include infection of vascular prostheses, aneurysms, and bone and as well as chronic sternal wound infection.

Diagnosis   *C. burnetii* can be isolated from buffy-coat blood samples or tissue specimens by a shell-vial technique; however, most laboratories are not permitted to attempt the isolation of *C. burnetii* since it is considered highly infectious. PCR can be used to amplify *C. burnetii* DNA from tissue or biopsy specimens. This technique can also be used on paraffin-embedded tissues. Serology, however, is the most commonly used diagnostic tool. Three techniques are available: complement fixation, indirect immunofluorescence, and enzyme-linked immunosorbent assay. Indirect immunofluorescence is sensitive and specific and is the method of choice. Rheumatoid factor should be adsorbed from the specimen before testing. An IgG titer of $\geq 1:800$ to phase I antigen is suggestive of chronic Q fever. In almost all instances of chronic Q fever, the antibody titer to phase I antigen is much higher than that to phase II antigen. The reverse is true in acute Q fever. In addition, in acute Q fever, it is usually possible to demonstrate a fourfold rise in titer between acute- and convalescent-phase serum samples.

R̲x̲ **TREATMENT**

Treatment of acute Q fever with doxycycline (100 mg twice daily for 14 days) is usually successful. Quinolones are also effective. If Q fever is diagnosed during pregnancy, treatment with trimethoprim-sulfamethoxazole is recommended for the duration of the pregnancy. Treatment of chronic Q fever should include at least two antibiotics active against *C. burnetii*. Rifampin (300 mg once daily) combined with doxycycline (100 mg twice daily) or ciprofloxacin (750 mg twice daily) has been used with success. The optimal duration of antibiotic therapy for chronic Q fever remains undetermined. We recommend at least 3 years of treatment, with discontinuation only if the phase I IgA antibody titer is $\leq 1:50$ and the IgG phase I titer is $\leq 1:200$. Another therapeutic option under investigation is the combination of doxycycline (100 mg twice daily) with hydroxychloroquine (600 mg once daily). With this combination, therapy can be completed in 18 months. It is necessary to monitor hydroxychloroquine levels and to adjust the dosage to maintain a plasma concentration of 0.8 to 1.2 μg/mL. In vitro, the addition of 1 mg of hydroxychloroquine/mL renders doxycycline bactericidal against *C. burnetii*. Resistance to ciprofloxacin has been associated with substitution of glutamine for lysine at the position corresponding to amino acid 87 in resistant strains of *Escherichia coli*.

Prevention   A vaccine has been shown to be effective in preventing Q fever in abattoir workers in Australia.

FURTHER READING

ARCHIBALD LK, SEXTON DJ: Long-term sequelae of Rocky Mountain spotted fever. Clin Infect Dis 20:1122, 1995

BAKKEN JS et al: Human granulocytic ehrlichiosis in the upper midwest United States. A new species emerging? JAMA 272:212, 1994

BULLER RS et al: *Ehrlichia ewingii*, a newly recognized agent of human ehrlichiosis. N Engl J Med 341:148, 1999

DALTON MJ et al: National surveillance for Rocky Mountain spotted fever, 1981–1982: Epidemiologic summary and evaluation of risk factors for fatal outcome. Am J Trop Med Hyg 52:405, 1995

DUMLER JS, BAKKEN JS: Human ehrlichioses. Newly recognized infections transmitted by ticks. Annu Rev Med 49:201, 1998

RAOULT D et al: Outbreak of epidemic typhus associated with trench fever in Burundi. Lancet 352:353, 1998

———— et al: Treatment of Q fever endocarditis. Comparisons of 2 regimens containing doxycycline and ofloxacin or hydroxychloroquine. Arch Intern Med 159:167, 1999

———— et al: Q fever 1985–1998. Clinical and epidemiologic features of 1,383 infections. Medicine (Baltimore) 79:109, 2000

———— et al: Q fever during pregnancy. Arch Intern Med 162:701, 2002

159   INFECTIONS DUE TO MYCOPLASMAS
William M. McCormack

Mycoplasmas, the smallest free-living organisms known, are prokaryotes that are bounded only by a plasma membrane. Their lack of a cell wall is associated with cellular pleomorphism and resistance to cell wall–active antimicrobial agents, such as penicillins and cephalosporins. The organisms' small genome limits biosynthesis and explains the difficulties encountered with in vitro cultivation. Mycoplasmas typically colonize mucosal surfaces of the respiratory and urogenital tracts of many animal species. Sixteen species of mycoplasmas have been recovered from humans. Most are commensals. *Mycoplasma pneumoniae* causes upper and lower respiratory tract infections. *M. genitalium* and *Ureaplasma urealyticum* are established causes of urethritis and have been implicated in other genital conditions. *M. hominis* and *U. urealyticum* are part of the complex microbial flora of bacterial vaginosis (Chap. 115).

MECHANISMS OF PATHOGENICITY

Adherence of mycoplasmas to the surface of the host cell is necessary for colonization and infection. Some pathogenic mycoplasmas are flask-shaped, with specialized tips that enhance adherence. *M. pneu-* moniae adheres via a network of interactive adhesins and accessory proteins and produces hydrogen peroxide, which may cause injury to host cells. *M. hominis* metabolizes arginine, with the production of potentially cytotoxic amounts of ammonia. Ureaplasmas have been placed in a separate genus because of their unique urease activity; the metabolism of urea also produces ammonia. *M. pneumoniae* may evoke IgM autoantibodies that agglutinate human erythrocytes at 4°C. These cold agglutinins can cause anemia and other complications.

MYCOPLASMA PNEUMONIAE

EPIDEMIOLOGY   *M. pneumoniae* causes upper and lower respiratory tract symptoms in all age groups, with the highest attack rates in 5- to 20-year-olds. The infection is acquired by inhalation of aerosols. The incubation period is 2 to 3 weeks, considerably longer than that of most other respiratory infections. Although epidemics have taken place in closed populations, such as schools and military installations, most cases occur sporadically or in families. In families, cases typically occur serially, with 2- to 3-week intervals between cases. Infections in adults are often the result of contact with children.

Infection with *M. pneumoniae* is worldwide. Cases occur throughout the year, with epidemics every few years. Some studies have noted an increase in the number of cases during the autumn months in temperate climates. Although pneumonia is the classic presentation, non-pneumonic infection is considerably more common. In very young children, most infections result only in upper respiratory symptoms, whereas children >5 years of age and adults may have bronchitis and pneumonia.

CLINICAL PRESENTATION After a prolonged incubation period, fever and constitutional symptoms develop along with headache and cough, both of which can be prominent and distressing. Symptoms typically progress less rapidly than those of viral respiratory tract infections. In the minority (perhaps 5 to 10%) of infected individuals who develop tracheobronchitis or pneumonia, cough becomes more prominent. Sputum, if produced at all, is usually white and may be tinged with blood. The temperature seldom rises above 38.9° to 39.4°C (102° to 103°F). Shaking chills, myalgias, and gastrointestinal symptoms (e.g., nausea, vomiting, and diarrhea) are unusual. Chest muscle soreness may result from frequent and prolonged coughing, but true pleuritic pain is uncommon.

Pharyngeal injection is often noted. Cervical lymph node enlargement is unusual. Ear pain due to bullous myringitis (blisters on the tympanic membrane) is a unique but uncommon manifestation. As in other "atypical" pneumonias, findings on auscultation of the lung may be normal or nearly normal despite striking radiographic abnormalities. Pleural effusions develop in fewer than 20% of patients.

M. pneumoniae infection may be particularly severe in patients who have sickle cell disease and other hemoglobin S–related hemoglobinopathies. The functional asplenia seen in sickle cell disease may contribute to severe mycoplasmal disease as it does in pneumococcal infection. Severe respiratory distress and large pleural effusions may occur.

EXTRAPULMONARY MANIFESTATIONS A broad array of extrapulmonary abnormalities have been associated with *M. pneumoniae* infection. Although these events are unusual, they complicate other respiratory diseases even more rarely and often provide the only clue that an otherwise-unremarkable respiratory infection may be mycoplasmal.

Erythema multiforme (Stevens-Johnson syndrome; see Fig. 46-9) typically occurs in young male patients with *M. pneumoniae* infection. Other dermatologic manifestations, such as maculopapular and vesicular exanthems, erythema nodosum, and urticaria, have been reported, but none is as clearly linked to *M. pneumoniae* as is erythema multiforme. Digital necrosis has been seen in patients with sickle cell disease who develop very high titers of cold agglutinins.

Cardiac abnormalities reported in conjunction with *M. pneumoniae* infection include myocarditis and pericarditis, which may result in abnormalities of conduction. Of the wide variety of neurologic conditions associated with *M. pneumoniae*, most have been documented in case reports, where establishment of a cause-and-effect relationship is problematic. Central nervous system abnormalities that have been associated with *M. pneumoniae* include encephalitis, cerebellar ataxia, Guillain-Barré syndrome, transverse myelitis, and peripheral neuropathies. Arthralgias are not unusual in patients who have mycoplasmal pneumonia; mycoplasmal arthritis is rare except in patients who have hypogammaglobulinemia. Hematologic abnormalities associated with *M. pneumoniae* include hemolytic anemia and coagulopathies.

The pathogenesis of the extrapulmonary manifestations of *M. pneumoniae* infection is controversial. Occasional reports have described the identification of *M. pneumoniae* or its nucleic acids in involved tissues. The fact that most attempts at detection have yielded negative results, however, suggests that these extrapulmonary complications have an immunologic basis. Mycoplasmas, including *M. pneumoniae*, can nonspecifically stimulate B lymphocytes. *M. pneumoniae*–infected individuals can develop autoantibodies, including those reactive with brain, heart, and muscle.

DIAGNOSIS Most infections with *M. pneumoniae* are not diagnosed, as they are indistinguishable from upper and lower respiratory tract infections caused by myriad other viral and bacterial pathogens. When the diagnosis is suspected, it is usually because illness is prolonged or extrapulmonary manifestations develop. The white blood cell count is generally somewhat elevated, with few immature cells. Gram's stain of sputum shows leukocytes without a predominance of any bacterial morphologic type. Since *M. pneumoniae* lacks a cell wall, it cannot be detected on Gram's stain. In patients who have pneumonia, the chest radiograph may show reticulonodular or interstitial infiltration, primarily in the lower lobes. As in other "atypical" pneumonias, radiographic abnormalities may be more prominent than would be predicted by auscultation of the chest.

M. pneumoniae can be grown on artificial media, but the process is exacting, requires special media, and takes upwards of 2 weeks. Thus, mycoplasmal cultures do not provide timely information to aid in patient management. The same, unfortunately, is true of serologic diagnosis. Specific antibodies can be detected by enzyme-linked immunoassays, indirect immunofluorescence, or complement fixation but do not develop early enough to guide decisions regarding treatment. As with most serologic tests, examination of paired acute- and convalescent-phase serum specimens is required for good sensitivity and specificity.

Cold agglutinins are nonspecific but develop within the first 7 to 10 days in more than half of patients with *M. pneumoniae* pneumonia and may be detectable when the patient presents to a health care provider. In a patient with a compatible clinical picture, a cold agglutinin titer of ≥1:32 supports the diagnosis of mycoplasmal pneumonia. Cold agglutinin determinations are readily available from diagnostic laboratories. The test can also be performed at the bedside by the addition of 1 mL of the patient's blood to a tube containing anticoagulant (e.g., a tube used to collect blood for determination of prothrombin activity). Before cooling, the nonaggregated red blood cells coat the sides of the inverted tube. The blood is cooled to 4°C when the tube is placed in an ice bath for 3 to 5 min or in a standard refrigerator. In a positive test, clumps of red blood cells can be observed when the tube is inverted. Rewarming of the sample to 37°C in an incubator or by exposure to body heat should reverse the agglutination. A positive "bedside" cold agglutinin test is equivalent to a laboratory titer of ≥1:64.

The lack of sensitive, specific, and timely diagnostic tests has prompted the development of a variety of antigen detection tests that do not involve serology or the cultivation of live organisms. Such tests include antigen capture, indirect enzyme immunoassays, DNA probing, and nucleic acid amplification. Since many viral and bacterial infections result in clinical presentations similar to that caused by *M. pneumoniae*, examination of specimens for single antigens is unlikely to be useful. Rather, tests that examine an individual specimen for multiple antigens are needed. Multiplex nucleic acid amplification tests that examine a single throat swab or sputum sample for all of the most likely causative microorganisms are feasible with current technology. Prototype multiplex polymerase chain reaction (PCR) assays have already been developed. If such tests become available clinically, more precise etiologic diagnosis of upper and lower respiratory tract infections will be possible.

℞ TREATMENT

Pneumonia due to *M. pneumoniae* is usually self-limited and is seldom life-threatening. Effective antimicrobial agents do shorten the duration of illness and, by reducing coughing, may conceivably render the patient less infectious. Although symptoms are alleviated by antimicrobial treatment, the organism usually is not eradicated. Cultures positive for *M. pneumoniae* may persist for months despite clinically effective antimicrobial therapy. The beneficial effects, if any, of such treatment on extrapulmonary manifestations of *M. pneumoniae* infection are unknown.

Because most mycoplasmal infections are not specifically diagnosed, management is directed at one of two syndromes: upper respiratory tract infection or community-acquired pneumonia. Upper respiratory infections, whether caused by viruses or by *M. pneumoniae*, do not require antimicrobial treatment. Community-acquired pneumonia (Chap. 239) may be caused by bacteria such as *Streptococcus pneumoniae* and *Haemophilus influenzae* or by "atypical" agents such as *Chlamydia pneumoniae*, *Legionella pneumophila*, and *M. pneumoniae*. Recommended treatment regimens are detailed in Tables 159-1 and 159-2. Treatment of documented *M. pneumoniae* pneumonia is usually continued for 14 to 21 days.

GENITAL MYCOPLASMAS (See also Chap. 115)

EPIDEMIOLOGY   *M. hominis* and *U. urealyticum* are the most prevalent genital mycoplasmas. Infants may become colonized with one or both of these organisms during passage through a colonized birth canal. Neonatal colonization tends not to persist. Only ~10% of prepubertal girls and even fewer prepubertal boys are colonized with ureaplasmas. After puberty, colonization occurs mainly as a result of sexual activity. Among adults, disadvantaged populations have higher colonization rates. Ureaplasmas can be cultured from the vaginas of ~80% of women cared for in public clinics and about half of women cared for by private obstetricians and gynecologists. Similarly, vaginal *M. hominis* is found in ~50% of women attending public clinics and in ~20% of private patients. Men have somewhat lower rates of genital colonization than women. In short, both *U. urealyticum* and *M. hominis* are frequently detected in genital specimens from healthy, sexually experienced adults. Evaluation of the role of these organisms in human disease must take into account their high prevalence among healthy people.

M. fermentans colonizes both the respiratory and genital tracts in more than 20% of adults. There is no convincing evidence that *M. fermentans* causes human disease; although it had been implicated as a possible determinant of HIV-1 disease progression, more recent data do not support such a role. *M. genitalium* is a fastidious organism that is difficult to cultivate. PCR studies have identified the organism more successfully. Little is known about the epidemiology of *M. genitalium*.

ASSOCIATION WITH HUMAN DISEASE ■ **Nongonococcal Urethritis (NGU)** *Chlamydia trachomatis* is the organism most firmly implicated in the etiology of NGU. There is no doubt that sexually transmitted *U. urealyticum* and *M. genitalium* also cause some cases of NGU. The ubiquity of ureaplasmas among men who do not have urethritis and the difficulty of identifying *M. genitalium* do not allow precise estimation of the proportion of cases of NGU caused by each of these mycoplasmas. *U. urealyticum* and *M. genitalium* do, however, appear to cause most of the nonchlamydial cases.

Epididymitis and Prostatitis   Ureaplasmas may be an occasional cause of epididymitis. *M. hominis* has not been implicated in this disease. Neither organism has been convincingly associated with prostatitis.

Pelvic Inflammatory Disease (PID)   *M. hominis* and *U. urealyticum* are both prominent components of the complex microbial flora of bacterial vaginosis. Since bacterial vaginosis is associated with PID, it is difficult to determine whether either organism plays an independent role in this condition. Although *M. genitalium* is not associated with bacterial vaginosis, preliminary studies have linked it to PID in women

TABLE 159-1   Oral Antimicrobial Agents for the Treatment of Ambulatory Patients with Community-Acquired Pneumonia

Agent	Dose and Schedule
Doxycycline	100 mg bid
Erythromycin	500 mg qid
Clarithromycin	500 mg bid
Azithromycin	500 mg qd
Levofloxacin	500 mg qd
Gatifloxacin	400 mg qd
Moxifloxacin	400 mg qd

Note: Treatment of documented *M. pneumoniae* pneumonia is usually continued for 14 to 21 days.

TABLE 159-2   Antimicrobial Agents for the Treatment of Hospitalized Patients with Community-Acquired Pneumonia

1. Intravenous ceftriaxone (1.0 g/d) *or*
   Intravenous cefotaxime (1.0 g q8h) *or*
   Intravenous ampicillin/sulbactam (1.5–3.0 g q6h)
        plus
   Intravenous or oral erythromycin (500 mg qid) *or*
   Intravenous or oral azithromycin (500 mg qd) *or*
   Oral clarithromycin (500 mg bid)
2. Intravenous or oral levofloxacin (500 mg qd)
3. Intravenous or oral gatifloxacin (400 mg qd)
4. Intravenous or oral moxifloxacin (400 mg qd)

Note: Treatment of documented *M. pneumoniae* pneumonia is usually continued for 14 to 21 days.

who are not infected with either *Neisseria gonorrhoeae* or *C. trachomatis*.

Disorders of Reproduction   Ureaplasmas have been considered as causes of involuntary infertility in both men and women, but there is no convincing evidence for such an association. These organisms have been associated with chorioamnionitis and late abortion. Given the close association of ureaplasmas with bacterial vaginosis, a condition that is strongly associated with chorioamnionitis and late abortion, it is difficult to define an independent role for ureaplasmas in this condition. In infants of very low birth weight, ureaplasmas have been shown to cause pneumonia and chronic lung disease.

Extragenital Infections   Sexually acquired reactive arthritis and Reiter's syndrome may be triggered by ureaplasmas, although *C. trachomatis* is the usual triggering agent. Patients who have hypogammaglobulinemia may develop chronic arthritis due to ureaplasmas and some other mycoplasmal species. *M. hominis* has been identified in patients with postthoracotomy sternal wound infection and in rare instances of prosthetic heart valve and prosthetic joint infection.

DIAGNOSIS   There is seldom any reason to examine specimens from the lower genital tract (vagina, male urethra) for mycoplasmas. The ubiquity of the organisms among healthy individuals makes a positive result uninterpretable. The organisms should be sought only in specimens from normally sterile areas, such as joint fluid with evidence of inflammation and cultures negative for conventional microorganisms.

M. hominis can replicate in many routine blood culture media without changing the appearance of the media; although it forms nonhemolytic pinpoint colonies on blood agar, organisms cannot be visualized in gram-stained smears of these colonies. Neither *U. urealyticum* nor *M. genitalium* will grow in ordinary microbiologic media.

Microbiologic diagnosis of genital mycoplasmal infection requires specially prepared media and is beyond the capability of all but reference and research laboratories. Nucleic acid amplification tests such as PCR have been developed and may become commercially available.

℞ TREATMENT

Ureaplasmas, *M. genitalium*, and *M. hominis* are usually susceptible to tetracyclines (e.g., doxycycline). Infections caused by tetracycline-resistant ureaplasmas can be treated with erythromycin, while those due to tetracycline-resistant strains of *M. hominis* respond to treatment with clindamycin. As noted above, a specific microbiologic diagnosis of mycoplasmal infection is seldom made. Appropriate treatment provides antimicrobial coverage for the organisms that cause the particular syndrome. Accordingly, NGU is treated with doxycycline (100 mg orally twice a day for 7 days) or azithromycin (1.0 g as a single oral dose) to provide activity against *C. trachomatis*, *U. urealyticum*, and *M. genitalium*. Recommended regimens for the treatment of PID provide antimicrobial activity against gonococci, chlamydiae, and anaerobes as well as genital mycoplasmas.

FURTHER READING

BARTLETT JG et al: Practice guidelines for the management of community-acquired pneumonia in adults. Clin Infect Dis 31:347, 2000

BASEMAN JB, TULLY JG: Mycoplasmas: Sophisticated, reemerging, and burdened by their notoriety. Emerg Infect Dis 3:21, 1997

HAMMERSCHLAG MR: *Mycoplasma pneumoniae* infections. Curr Opin Infect Dis 14:181, 2001

HICKMAN-DAVIS JM: Role of innate immunity in respiratory *Mycoplasma* infection. Front Biosci 7:d1347, 2002

MURRAY HW et al: The protean manifestations of *Mycoplasma pneumoniae* in adults. Am J Med 58:229, 1975

TAYLOR-ROBINSON D: *Mycoplasma genitalium*—an update. Int J STD AIDS 13:145, 2002

———, FURR PM: Update on sexually transmitted mycoplasmas. Lancet 351(Suppl 3):12, 1998

160 CHLAMYDIAL INFECTIONS
Walter E. Stamm

The genus *Chlamydia* contains three species that infect humans: *Chlamydia psittaci*, *C. trachomatis*, and *C. pneumoniae* (formerly the TWAR agent). *C. psittaci* is widely distributed in nature, producing genital, conjunctival, intestinal, or respiratory infections in many mammalian and avian species. Genital infections with *C. psittaci* have been well characterized in several species and cause abortion and infertility. Although mammalian strains of *C. psittaci* are not known to infect humans, avian strains occasionally do so, causing pneumonia and the systemic illness known as *psittacosis*.

C. pneumoniae is a fastidious chlamydial species that appears to be a common cause of upper respiratory tract infection and pneumonia, primarily in children and young adults, and is a cause of recurrent respiratory infections in older adults. Studies have also linked *C. pneumoniae* infection to atherosclerotic cardiovascular disease and perhaps to asthma and sarcoidosis. No animal reservoir has been identified for *C. pneumoniae*; it appears to be an exclusively human pathogen spread via the respiratory route through close personal contact. To date, all strains of *C. pneumoniae* studied have been serologically homologous.

C. trachomatis is also an exclusively human pathogen and was identified as the cause of trachoma in the 1940s. Since then, *C. trachomatis* has been recognized as a major cause of sexually transmitted and perinatal infection.

Chlamydiae are obligate intracellular bacteria that are classified in their own order (Chlamydiales). They possess both DNA and RNA, have a cell wall and ribosomes similar to those of gram-negative bacteria, and are inhibited by antibiotics such as tetracycline.

A unique feature of all chlamydiae is their complex reproductive cycle. Two forms of the microorganism—the extracellular elementary body and the intracellular reticulate body—participate in this cycle. The elementary body is adapted for extracellular survival and is the infective form transmitted from one person to another. Elementary bodies attach to susceptible target cells (usually columnar or transitional epithelial cells) and enter the cells inside a phagosome. Within 8 h of cell entry, the elementary bodies reorganize into reticulate bodies, which are adapted to intracellular survival and multiplication. They undergo binary fission, eventually producing numerous replicates contained within the intracellular membrane-bound "inclusion body," which occupies much of the infected host cell. Chlamydial inclusions resist lysosomal fusion until late in the developmental cycle. After 24 h, the reticulate bodies condense and form elementary bodies still contained within the inclusion. The inclusion then ruptures, releasing elementary bodies from the cell to initiate infection of adjacent cells or transmission to another person.

Studies with monoclonal antibodies to and nucleotide sequencing of the major outer-membrane protein have delineated at least 20 serotypes of *C. trachomatis*. According to the classification of Wang and Grayston, strains associated with trachoma have generally been those of the A, B, Ba, and C serovars, while serovars D through K have largely been associated with sexually transmitted and perinatally acquired infections. Serovars L_1, L_2, and L_3 produce lymphogranuloma venereum (LGV) and hemorrhagic proctocolitis. The LGV strains demonstrate unique biologic behavior in that they are more invasive than the other serovars, produce disease in lymphatic tissue, grow readily in cell culture systems and macrophages, and are lethal when inoculated intracerebrally into mice and monkeys. Non-LGV strains of *C. trachomatis* characteristically produce infections involving the superficial columnar epithelium of the eye, genitalia, and respiratory tract.

C. trachomatis has been reported as an infrequent cause of endocarditis, peritonitis, pleuritis, and possibly periappendicitis and may occasionally cause respiratory infections in older children and adults. Some immunosuppressed patients with pneumonia have had either serologic or cultural evidence of *C. trachomatis* infection, but more data are necessary to define a pathogenic role for *Chlamydia* in these patients.

C. TRACHOMATIS INFECTIONS

C. TRACHOMATIS GENITAL INFECTIONS Genital infections caused by *C. trachomatis* represent the most common bacterial sexually transmitted diseases (STDs) in the United States (Chap. 115). An estimated 4 million cases occur each year. In adults, the clinical spectrum of sexually transmitted *C. trachomatis* infections parallels that of gonococcal infections. Both infections have been associated with urethritis, proctitis, and conjunctivitis in both sexes; with epididymitis in men; and with mucopurulent cervicitis (MPC), acute salpingitis, bartholinitis, and the Fitz-Hugh–Curtis syndrome (perihepatitis) in women. Moreover, both types of infection can be associated with septic arthritis. In general, however, chlamydial infections produce fewer symptoms and signs than corresponding gonococcal infections at the same anatomic site; in fact, chlamydial infections are often totally asymptomatic. Increasing evidence suggests that many chlamydial infections of the genital tract, especially in women, persist for months without producing symptoms. Simultaneous infection with *C. trachomatis* often occurs in women with cervical gonococcal infection and in heterosexual men with gonococcal urethritis.

Epidemiology Infections due to *C. trachomatis* have been reportable in the United States since 1985, and national incidence data show steadily rising numbers of reported infections, undoubtedly reflecting both increased testing and increased reporting. Most testing to date has focused upon women, and thus the reported incidence is severalfold greater among women than among men; this difference likely represents a surveillance artifact.

The age of peak incidence of genital *C. trachomatis* infections, as of other sexually transmitted infections, is the late teens and early twenties. The prevalence of chlamydial urethral infection among young men is at least 3 to 5% for those seen in general medical settings or in urban high schools, >10% for asymptomatic soldiers undergoing routine physical examination, and 15 to 20% for heterosexual men seen in STD clinics. In areas where chlamydial control programs have been implemented, prevalence may be markedly reduced. In short, prevalence varies widely with the population group studied and with the geographic locale. With the newer, more sensitive nucleic acid amplification tests such as polymerase chain reaction (PCR) and ligase chain reaction (LCR), prevalences in most populations have been 10 to 30% higher than those measured with older, less sensitive tests.

The prevalence of cervical infection among women is ~5% for asymptomatic college students and prenatal patients in the United States, >10% for women seen in family planning clinics, and >20% for women seen in STD clinics. As in men, prevalence varies substantially by geographic locale, with the highest rates in the southeast. However, substantial prevalences (~8%) of asymptomatic chlamydial infection have been demonstrated among young female recruits from all parts of the United States. In this country, the prevalence of *C. trachomatis* in the cervix of pregnant women is 5 to 10 times higher than that of *Neisseria gonorrhoeae*. The prevalence of genital infection with either agent is highest among individuals who are between the ages of 18 and 24, single, and non-Caucasian (e.g., African American or Latino). Recurrent chlamydial infections occur frequently in these same risk groups, often acquired from untreated sexual partners. Oral contraceptive pill use and the presence of cervical ectopy also confer an increased risk of chlamydial infection. The proportion of infections that are asymptomatic appears to be higher for *C. trachomatis* than for *N. gonorrhoeae*, and symptomatic *C. trachomatis* infections are clinically less severe. Mild or asymptomatic chlamydial infections of the fallopian tubes nonetheless cause ongoing tubal damage and infertility. Furthermore, because the total number of *C. trachomatis* infections exceeds the total number of *N. gonorrhoeae* infections in industrialized countries, the total morbidity caused by *C. trachomatis* genital infections in these countries equals or exceeds that caused by *N. gonorrhoeae*. The prevalence of *C. trachomatis* is higher than that of *N. gonorrhoeae* in industrialized countries, in part because measures such as treatment of sex partners and routine cultures for case detection in asymptomatic individuals have been applied much longer and more effectively to the control of gonorrhea than to the control of *C. trachomatis* infection.

Pathogenesis　*C. trachomatis* preferentially infects the columnar epithelium of the eye and the respiratory and genital tracts. The infection induces an immune response but often persists for months or years in the absence of antimicrobial therapy. Serious sequelae often occur in association with repeated or persistent infections. The precise mechanism through which repeated infection elicits an inflammatory response that leads to tubal scarring and damage in the female upper genital tract is not yet clear. One antigen, the chlamydial 60-kDa heat-shock protein, may be involved in inducing the pathologic immune response or may elicit antibodies that cross-react with human heat-shock proteins. The recent sequencing of the chlamydial genome may soon offer further insights into the pathogenic mechanisms of *C. trachomatis*.

Clinical Manifestations　■　*NONGONOCOCCAL AND POSTGONOCOCCAL URETHRITIS* Nongonococcal urethritis (NGU) is a diagnosis of exclusion that is applied to men with symptoms and/or signs of urethritis who do not have gonorrhea. Postgonococcal urethritis (PGU) refers to nongonococcal urethritis developing in men 2 to 3 weeks after treatment of gonococcal urethritis with single doses of agents such as amoxicillin or cephalosporins that lack antimicrobial activity against chlamydiae. Since current treatment regimens for gonorrhea also include tetracycline, doxycycline, or azithromycin for possible concomitant chlamydial infection, both the incidence of PGU and the causative role of chlamydiae in this syndrome have declined. *C. trachomatis* causes 20 to 40% of cases of NGU in heterosexual men but is less commonly isolated from homosexual men with this syndrome. The cause of most of the remaining cases is uncertain; considerable evidence suggests that *Ureaplasma urealyticum* and *Mycoplasma genitalium* cause many cases of NGU, while *Trichomonas vaginalis* and herpes simplex virus (HSV) cause some cases.

NGU is diagnosed by documentation of a leukocytic urethral exudate and by exclusion of gonorrhea by Gram's staining or culture. *C. trachomatis* urethritis is generally less severe than gonococcal urethritis, although in an individual patient these two forms of urethritis cannot be reliably differentiated solely on clinical grounds. Symptoms include urethral discharge (often whitish and mucoid rather than frankly purulent), dysuria, and urethral itching. Physical examination may reveal meatal erythema and tenderness and a urethral exudate that is often demonstrable only by stripping of the urethra.

At least one-third of males with *C. trachomatis* urethral infection have no demonstrable signs or symptoms of urethritis. Use of nucleic acid amplification assays on first-void urine specimens to diagnose chlamydial infections in men has facilitated more broadly based testing for asymptomatic infection in males. As a result, asymptomatic chlamydial urethritis has been demonstrated in 5 to 10% of sexually active adolescent males screened in school-based clinics or community centers. Such patients generally have first-glass pyuria ($\geq$15 leukocytes per 400$\times$ microscopic field in the sediment of first-void urine), a positive leukocyte esterase test, or an increased number of leukocytes on Gram-stained smear prepared from a urogenital swab inserted 1 to 2 cm into the anterior urethra. For the enumeration of leukocytes, the smear is first scanned at low power to identify areas of the slide containing the highest concentration of leukocytes. These areas are then examined under oil immersion (1000$\times$). An average of four or more leukocytes in at least three of five 1000$\times$ (oil-immersion) fields is indicative of urethritis and correlates with the recovery of *C. trachomatis*. To differentiate between true urethritis and functional symptoms among symptomatic patients or to make a presumptive diagnosis of *C. trachomatis* infection in "high-risk" but asymptomatic men (e.g., male patients in STD clinics, sex partners of women with nongonococcal salpingitis or MPC, fathers of children with inclusion conjunctivitis), the examination of an endourethral specimen for increased leukocytes is useful if specific diagnostic tests for chlamydiae are not available. Alternatively, noninvasive screening for urethritis can be accomplished by testing of a first-void urine sample for pyuria, either by microscopy or by the leukocyte esterase test. Urine can also be directly tested for chlamydiae or gonococci by DNA amplification methods, as described below.

EPIDIDYMITIS　*C. trachomatis* is the foremost cause of epididymitis in sexually active heterosexual men <35 years of age, accounting for ~70% of cases. *N. gonorrhoeae* causes most of the remaining cases, and some men have simultaneous infections with both pathogens, usually accompanied by asymptomatic urethritis as defined above. In homosexual men, sexually transmitted coliform infection acquired via insertive rectal intercourse may cause epididymitis. Coliform bacteria and *Pseudomonas aeruginosa*, usually in association with preceding urologic instrumentation or surgery, are the most common causes of epididymitis in men over 35. Men with chlamydial epididymitis typically present with unilateral scrotal pain, fever, and epididymal tenderness or swelling on examination. The illness may be mild enough to treat on an outpatient basis with oral antibiotics or severe enough to require hospitalization and parenteral therapy. Testicular torsion should be excluded promptly by radionuclide scan, Doppler flow study, or surgical exploration in a teenager or young adult who presents with acute unilateral testicular pain without urethritis. The possibility of testicular tumor or chronic infection (e.g., tuberculosis) should be excluded when a patient with unilateral intrascrotal pain and swelling does not respond to appropriate antimicrobial therapy.

REITER'S SYNDROME　Reiter's syndrome consists of conjunctivitis, urethritis (or cervicitis in females), arthritis, and characteristic mucocutaneous lesions (Chap. 305). *C. trachomatis* has been recovered from the urethra of up to 70% of men with untreated nondiarrheal Reiter's syndrome and associated urethritis. In the absence of overt urethritis, it is important to exclude subclinical urethritis in the men in whom this diagnosis is suspected.

The pathogenesis of Reiter's syndrome remains obscure. However, since more than 80% of affected patients have the HLA-B27 phenotype and since other mucosal infections (with *Salmonella*, *Shigella*, or *Campylobacter*, for example) produce an identical syndrome, chlamydial infection is thought to initiate an aberrant and hyperactive immune response that produces inflammation at the involved target organs in these genetically predisposed individuals. Evidence of exaggerated cell-mediated and humoral immune responses to chlamydial antigens in Reiter's syndrome supports this hypothesis. The presumptive demonstration of chlamydial elementary bodies and chlamydial DNA in the joint fluid and synovial tissue of patients with Reiter's syndrome suggests that chlamydiae may actually spread from genital to joint tissues in these patients, perhaps in macrophages.

PROCTITIS   *C. trachomatis* strains of either the genital immunotypes D through K or the LGV immunotypes cause proctitis in homosexual men who practice receptive anorectal intercourse. In the United States, the vast majority of cases are due to immunotypes D through K and present either as asymptomatic infection or as mild proctitis not unlike gonococcal proctitis. These infections may develop in heterosexual women as well. Patients present with mild rectal pain, mucous discharge, tenesmus, and (occasionally) bleeding. Nearly all have neutrophils in their rectal Gram's stain. Anoscopy in these non-LGV cases of chlamydial proctitis reveals mild, patchy mucosal friability and mucopurulent discharge, and the disease process is limited to the distal rectum. LGV strains produce more severe ulcerative proctitis or proctocolitis that can be confused clinically with HSV proctitis (severe rectal pain, bleeding, discharge, and tenesmus) and that histologically resembles Crohn's disease in that giant cell formation and granulomas can be seen (Chap. 276). In the United States, these cases occur almost exclusively in homosexual men.

MUCOPURULENT CERVICITIS   Although many women with *C. trachomatis* infection of the cervix have no symptoms or signs, a careful speculum examination reveals evidence of MPC in 30 to 50% of cases. As is discussed more fully in Chap. 115, MPC is associated with yellow mucopurulent endocervical discharge and with ≥20 neutrophils per $1000\times$ microscopic field within strands of cervical mucus on a thinly smeared, Gram-stained preparation of endocervical exudate. Other characteristic findings include edema of the zone of cervical ectopy and a propensity of the mucosa to bleed on minor trauma—e.g., when specimens are collected with a swab. A Pap smear shows increased numbers of neutrophils as well as a characteristic pattern of mononuclear inflammatory cells, including plasma cells, transformed lymphocytes, and histiocytes. Cervical biopsy shows a predominantly mononuclear cell infiltrate of the subepithelial stroma, often with follicular cervicitis.

PELVIC INFLAMMATORY DISEASE (PID) (See also Chap. 115)   In the United States, *C. trachomatis* has been identified in the fallopian tubes or endometrium of up to 50% of women with PID, and its role as an important etiologic agent in this syndrome is well accepted. PID occurs via ascending intraluminal spread of *C. trachomatis* from the lower genital tract. MPC is thus followed by endometritis, endosalpingitis, and finally pelvic peritonitis. Evidence of MPC is usually found in women with laparoscopically verified salpingitis. Similarly, endometritis, demonstrated by endometrial biopsy showing plasma cell infiltration of the endometrial epithelium, is documented in most women with laparoscopically verified chlamydial (or gonococcal) salpingitis. Chlamydial endometritis can also occur in the absence of clinical evidence of salpingitis: ~40 to 50% of women with MPC have plasma cell endometritis. Histologic evidence of endometritis has been correlated with an "endometritis syndrome" consisting of vaginal bleeding, lower abdominal pain, and uterine tenderness in the absence of adnexal tenderness. Chlamydial salpingitis produces milder symptoms than does gonococcal salpingitis and may be associated with less marked adnexal tenderness. Thus mild adnexal or uterine tenderness in sexually active women with cervicitis suggests PID.

Infertility associated with fallopian-tube scarring has been strongly linked to antecedent *C. trachomatis* infection in serologic studies. Since many infertile women with tubal scarring and antichlamydial antibody have no history of PID, it appears that subclinical tubal infection ("silent salpingitis") may produce scarring. Studies in animals and humans with salpingitis and tubal scarring suggest the continuing presence of persistent, slowly replicating chlamydial infection in tubal tissue. While the pathogenesis of *Chlamydia*-induced tubal scarring remains poorly understood, antibodies to the chlamydial 60-kDa heat-shock protein have been correlated with tubal infertility, ectopic pregnancy, and Fitz-Hugh–Curtis syndrome (see below). Thus this antigen may initiate an immune-mediated process that ultimately damages the fallopian tube. Host genetic susceptibility, as defined by HLA type, may also play an important role.

Perihepatitis, or the Fitz-Hugh–Curtis syndrome, was originally described as a complication of gonococcal PID. The syndrome should be suspected whenever a young, sexually active woman presents with an illness resembling cholecystitis (fever and right-upper-quadrant pain of subacute or acute onset). Symptoms and signs of salpingitis may be minimal. Cultural and/or serologic evidence of *C. trachomatis* infection is found in three-quarters of women with this syndrome.

URETHRAL SYNDROME IN WOMEN   In the absence of infection with uropathogens such as coliforms or *Staphylococcus saprophyticus*, *C. trachomatis* is the pathogen most commonly isolated from college women with dysuria, frequency, and pyuria (Chap. 269). *Chlamydia* can also be isolated from the urethra of women without symptoms of urethritis, and up to 25% of female STD clinic patients with chlamydial urogenital infection have cultures positive for *C. trachomatis* from the urethra only.

C. TRACHOMATIS INFECTION IN PREGNANCY AND THE NEONATAL PERIOD   Studies in the United States have demonstrated that 5 to 25% of pregnant women have *C. trachomatis* infections of the cervix. In these studies, approximately one-half to two-thirds of children exposed during birth have acquired *C. trachomatis* infection. Roughly half of the infected infants (or 25% of the group exposed) have developed clinical evidence of inclusion conjunctivitis. In addition to infecting the eye, *C. trachomatis* has been isolated frequently and persistently from the nasopharynx, rectum, and vagina of such infants, occasionally for periods exceeding 1 year in the absence of treatment. Pneumonia develops in ~10% of children infected perinatally, and otitis media may in some cases result from perinatally acquired chlamydial infection.

Neonatal chlamydial conjunctivitis has an acute onset 5 to 14 days after birth and often produces a profuse mucopurulent discharge. However, it is impossible to differentiate chlamydial conjunctivitis from other forms of neonatal conjunctivitis (such as that due to *N. gonorrhoeae*, *Haemophilus influenzae*, *Streptococcus pneumoniae*, or HSV) on clinical grounds; thus laboratory diagnosis is required. Inclusions within epithelial cells are often detected in Giemsa-stained conjunctival smears, but these smears are considerably less sensitive than cultures, antigen detection tests, or nucleic acid hybridization tests for chlamydiae. Gram-stained smears may show gonococci or occasional small gram-negative coccobacilli in *Haemophilus* conjunctivitis, but smears should be accompanied by cultures for these agents.

C. trachomatis causes a distinctive pneumonia syndrome in infants. Recent epidemiologic studies have linked chlamydial pulmonary infection in infants with increased occurrence of subacute lung disease (bronchitis, asthma, wheezing) in later childhood.

Lymphogranuloma Venereum ■ *DEFINITION*   LGV is a sexually transmitted infection caused by *C. trachomatis* strains of the L_1, L_2, and L_3 serovars. In the United States, most cases are caused by L_2 organisms. Acute LGV is characterized by a transient primary genital lesion followed by multilocular suppurative regional lymphadenopathy. Patients exposed via insertive rectal intercourse may develop hemorrhagic proctitis with regional lymphadenitis. Acute LGV is almost always associated with systemic symptoms such as fever and leukocytosis but is rarely associated with systemic complications such as meningoencephalitis. After a period of years, late complications include genital elephantiasis due to lymphatic involvement; strictures; and fistulas of the penis, urethra, and rectum.

EPIDEMIOLOGY   LGV is usually sexually transmitted, but occasional transmission by nonsexual personal contact, fomites, or laboratory accidents has been documented. Laboratory work involving the creation of aerosols of LGV organisms (e.g., sonication, homogenization) must be conducted only with appropriate measures for biologic containment.

The peak incidence of LGV corresponds to the age of greatest sexual activity: the second and third decades of life. The worldwide incidence of LGV is falling, but the disease is still endemic and a major cause of morbidity in Asia, Africa, South America, and parts of the Caribbean. In the Bahamas, an apparent outbreak of LGV has been described in association with a concurrent increase in heterosexual infection with HIV. However, the reported incidence of LGV in the United States has been only 0.1 case per 100,000 persons for more than a decade.

The frequency of infection following exposure is believed to be much lower than that for gonorrhea and syphilis. Early manifestations are recognized far more often in men than in women, who usually present with late complications. In the United States, where the reported male-to-female ratio of cases is 3.4:1, most cases have involved homosexually active men and persons returning from abroad (travelers, sailors, and military personnel). The main reservoir of infection, although it has not been directly demonstrated, is presumed to be asymptomatically infected individuals.

CLINICAL MANIFESTATIONS   A *primary genital lesion* develops from 3 days to 3 weeks after exposure. It is a small, painless vesicle or nonindurated ulcer or papule located on the penis in men and on the labia, posterior vagina, or fourchette in women. The primary lesion is noticed by fewer than one-third of men with LGV and only rarely by women. It heals in a few days without scarring and, even when noticed, is usually recognized as LGV only in retrospect. LGV strains of *C. trachomatis* have occasionally been recovered from genital ulcers and from the urethra of men and the endocervix of women who present with inguinal adenopathy; these areas may be the primary site of infection in some cases.

Primary anal or *rectal infection* develops after receptive anorectal intercourse. In women, rectal infection with LGV (or non-LGV) strains of *C. trachomatis* presumably can also arise by the contiguous spread of infected secretions along the perineum (as in rectal gonococcal infections in women) or perhaps by spread to the rectum via the pelvic lymphatics.

From the site of the primary urethral, genital, anal, or rectal infection, the organism spreads via the regional lymphatics. Penile, vulvar, or anal infection can lead to inguinal and femoral lymphadenitis. Rectal infection produces hypogastric and deep iliac lymphadenitis. Upper vaginal or cervical infection results in enlargement of the obturator and iliac nodes.

The most common presenting picture in heterosexual men is the *inguinal syndrome*, which is characterized by painful inguinal lymphadenopathy beginning 2 to 6 weeks after presumed exposure; in rare instances, the onset comes after a few months. The inguinal adenopathy is unilateral in two-thirds of cases, and palpable enlargement of the iliac and femoral nodes is often evident on the same side as the enlarged inguinal nodes. The nodes are initially discrete, but progressive periadenitis results in a matted mass of nodes that becomes fluctuant and suppurative. The overlying skin becomes fixed, inflamed, and thin and finally develops multiple draining fistulas. Extensive enlargement of chains of inguinal nodes above and below the inguinal ligament ("the sign of the groove") is not specific and, although not uncommon, is documented in only a minority of cases. On histologic examination, infected nodes are initially found to have characteristic small stellate abscesses surrounded by histiocytes. These abscesses coalesce to form large, necrotic, suppurative foci. Spontaneous healing usually takes place after several months; inguinal scars or granulomatous masses of various sizes persist for life. Massive pelvic lymphadenopathy may lead to exploratory laparotomy.

As cultures and serologic tests for *C. trachomatis* are being used more often, increasing numbers of cases of LGV proctitis are being recognized in homosexual men. Such patients present with anorectal pain and mucopurulent, bloody rectal discharge. Although these patients may complain of diarrhea, they are often referring not to diarrhea but rather to frequent, painful, unsuccessful attempts at defecation (tenesmus). Sigmoidoscopy reveals ulcerative proctitis or proctocolitis, with purulent exudate and mucosal bleeding. The histopathologic findings in the rectal mucosa include granulomas with giant cells, crypt

abscesses, and extensive inflammation. These clinical, sigmoidoscopic, and histopathologic findings may closely resemble those of Crohn's disease of the rectum.

Constitutional symptoms are common during the stage of regional lymphadenopathy and, in cases of proctitis, may include fever, chills, headache, meningismus, anorexia, myalgias, and arthralgias. These findings in the presence of lymphadenopathy are sometimes mistakenly interpreted as representing malignant lymphoma. Other systemic complications are infrequent but include arthritis with sterile effusion, aseptic meningitis, meningoencephalitis, conjunctivitis, hepatitis, and erythema nodosum. Chlamydiae have been recovered from the cerebrospinal fluid and in one case were isolated from the blood of a patient with severe constitutional symptoms—a result indicating the dissemination of infection. Laboratory-acquired infections suspected of being due to the inhalation of aerosols have been associated with mediastinal lymphadenitis, pneumonitis, and pleural effusion.

Complications of untreated anorectal infection include perirectal abscess; fistula in ano; and rectovaginal, rectovesical, and ischiorectal fistulas. Secondary bacterial infection probably contributes to these complications. Rectal stricture is a late complication of anorectal infection and usually develops 2 to 6 cm from the anal orifice—i.e., at a site within reach on digital rectal examination. Proximal extension of the stricture for several centimeters may lead to a mistaken clinical and radiographic diagnosis of carcinoma.

A small percentage of cases of LGV in men present as chronic progressive infiltrative, ulcerative, or fistular lesions of the penis, urethra, or scrotum. Associated lymphatic obstruction may produce elephantiasis. When urethral stricture occurs, it usually involves the posterior urethra and causes incontinence or difficulty with urination.

Approach to the Diagnosis and Treatment of *C. trachomatis* Genital Infections
Four types of laboratory procedure are available to confirm *C. trachomatis* infection: direct microscopic examination of tissue scrapings for typical intracytoplasmic inclusions or elementary bodies; isolation of the organism in cell culture; detection of chlamydial antigens or nucleic acid by immunologic or hybridization methods; and detection of antibody in serum or in local secretions.

Except in conjunctivitis, direct microscopic examination of Giemsa-stained cell scrapings for typical inclusions has an unacceptably low degree of sensitivity, and false-positive interpretations by inexperienced observers are common. Even for conjunctivitis, this approach has been replaced by direct fluorescent antibody staining of conjunctival smears to identify chlamydial elementary bodies with specific monoclonal antibodies (see below).

Cell culture techniques for isolation of *C. trachomatis* are available in most large medical centers but not in other clinical settings. In addition to limited availability, other disadvantages of cell culture include its low and variable level of sensitivity (60 to 80%), its requirement for rigorous transport conditions, and its high cost and technically demanding nature. Therefore, nonculture alternatives involving antigen detection or nucleic acid hybridization have been developed. In the direct immunofluorescent antibody (DFA) slide test, potentially infected genital or ocular secretions are smeared onto a slide, fixed, and stained with fluorescein-conjugated monoclonal antibody specific for chlamydial antigens. The observation of fluorescing elementary bodies confirms the diagnosis. Enzyme-linked immunosorbent assay (ELISA) techniques for the detection of chlamydial antigens provide another alternative to culture. The reported sensitivity and specificity of these tests for genital infections (as compared with culture) have been 60 to 80% and 97 to 99%, respectively, in high-risk populations. Assays with nucleic acid probes have also been developed for chlamydial diagnosis. One such test uses DNA-RNA hybridization and appears to be approximately equal to the best ELISAs in terms of sensitivity and specificity. Nucleic acid probes have also been developed for use in amplification assays such as LCR and PCR. These tests are now the most sensitive chlamydial diagnostic methods available, being the first nonculture assays to surpass culture itself in sensitivity. In addition, the ability of these tests to detect chlamydial genes in urine with a high degree of sensitivity and specificity allows—for the first time—the use of urine specimens rather than conventional urethral and cervical swabs. The use of urine specimens is particularly appealing for public-health chlamydial screening programs because of the ease of sample collection, even in community-based settings.

Serologic tests are of limited usefulness in the diagnosis of chlamydial oculogenital infections. The complement fixation test with heat-stable, genus-specific antigen has been used with some success to diagnose LGV but is insensitive in infections due to non-LGV strains of *C. trachomatis*. The microimmunofluorescence (micro-IF) test with *C. trachomatis* antigens is more sensitive but is generally available only in research laboratories. The test measures antibodies by serovar specificity and by immunoglobulin class (IgM, IgG, IgA, secretory IgA) in both serum and local secretions. Serologic diagnosis by the micro-IF test may be useful in infant pneumonia (in which high-titer IgM antibody and/or fourfold rises in titer are often demonstrated), in chlamydial salpingitis (especially Fitz-Hugh–Curtis syndrome), and in LGV. In all of these more invasive syndromes, high antibody levels are present.

Table 160-1 summarizes the diagnostic tests of choice for patients with suspected *C. trachomatis* infection. It is clear that, in most settings and for most purposes, sensitivity and specificity will be greatest with nucleic acid amplification techniques. For patients to whom medicolegal considerations may apply (victims of sexual or child abuse), cultures or nucleic acid amplification methods should always be used. In men with suspected urethritis, PCR or LCR testing of a first-void urine specimen offers a more sensitive and noninvasive diagnostic

method than the use of urethral swabs. For the diagnosis of urogenital (cervical or urethral) infections in women, testing of a first-void urine specimen by nucleic acid amplification methods is at least as sensitive as testing of a cervical swab. Patient-collected vaginal swabs tested by PCR or LCR have also been used successfully. Since chlamydial diagnostic testing has become more widely available and is now more sensitive and specific than in the past, its use for specific diagnosis in patients with suspected chlamydial syndromes (such as MPC, NGU, and PID) and their partners should be promoted. High priority should also be given to the screening of asymptomatic high-risk women who would not otherwise receive treatment for presumptive chlamydial infection, especially those seen in high-risk settings (e.g., STD clinics or abortion clinics) and those with a high-risk profile (e.g., sexually active and ≤21 years of age, new sex partner within the preceding 2 months, or more than one current sex partner). Similar screening programs should be used to detect and treat asymptomatic urethritis in high-risk adolescent males. Where implemented, screening programs of this type have been associated with reductions in the prevalence of chlamydial infection and of its complications, such as PID.

℞ TREATMENT

Until the introduction of azithromycin, chlamydial infections could not be eradicated by single-dose or short-term antimicrobial regimens. In most uncomplicated infections in adults, a 7-day course of treatment

TABLE 160-1 *Diagnostic Tests for Sexually Transmitted and Perinatal Chlamydia trachomatis Infection*

Infection	Suggestive Signs/Symptoms	Presumptive Diagnosis[a]	Confirmatory Test of Choice
MEN			
NGU, PGU	Discharge, dysuria	Gram's stain with >4 neutrophils per oil-immersion field; no gonococci	Urethral culture or nonculture test for *C. trachomatis*; urine or urethral NAAT for *C. trachomatis*
Epididymitis	Unilateral intrascrotal swelling, pain, tenderness; fever; NGU	Gram's stain with >4 neutrophils per oil-immersion field; no gonococci; urinalysis with pyuria	Urethral culture or nonculture test for *C. trachomatis*; urine or urethral NAAT for *C. trachomatis*
WOMEN			
Cervicitis	Mucopurulent cervical discharge, bleeding and edema of the zone of cervical ectopy	Cervical Gram's stain with ≥20 neutrophils per oil-immersion field in cervical mucus	Cervical culture or nonculture test for *C. trachomatis*; urine or cervical NAAT for *C. trachomatis*
Salpingitis	Lower abdominal pain, cervical motion tenderness, adnexal tenderness or masses	*C. trachomatis* always potentially present in salpingitis	Cervical culture or nonculture test for *C. trachomatis*; urine or cervical NAAT for *C. trachomatis*
Urethritis	Dysuria and frequency without urgency or hematuria	MPC; sterile pyuria; negative routine urine culture	Urethral and cervical cultures or nonculture test for *C. trachomatis*; urine NAAT for *C. trachomatis*
ADULTS OF EITHER SEX			
Proctitis	Rectal pain, discharge, tenesmus, bleeding; history of receptive anorectal intercourse	Negative gonococcal culture and Gram's stain; at least 1 neutrophil per oil-immersion field in rectal Gram's stain	Rectal culture or direct immunofluorescence test for *C. trachomatis*
Reiter's syndrome	NGU, arthritis, conjunctivitis, typical skin lesions	Gram's stain with >4 neutrophils per oil-immersion field; lack of gonococci indicative of NGU	Urethral culture or nonculture test for *C. trachomatis*
LGV	Regional adenopathy, primary lesion, proctitis, systemic symptoms	None	Isolation of LGV strain from node or rectum, occasionally from urethra or cervix; LGV CF titer, ≥1:64; micro-IF titer, ≥1:512
NEONATES			
Conjunctivitis	Purulent conjunctival discharge 6 to 18 days postdelivery	Negative culture and Gram's stain for gonococci, *Haemophilus* spp., pneumococci, staphylococci	Conjunctival culture or nonculture test for *C. trachomatis*; FA-stained scraping of conjunctival material
Infant pneumonia	Afebrile, staccato cough, diffuse rales, bilateral hyperinflation, interstitial infiltrates	None	Chlamydial culture of sputum, pharynx, eye, rectum; micro-IF antibody to *C. trachomatis*—fourfold change in IgG or IgM antibody titer

[a] A presumptive diagnosis of chlamydial infection is often made in the syndromes listed when gonococci are not found. A positive test for *Neisseria gonorrhoeae* does not exclude the involvement of *C. trachomatis*, which often is present in patients with gonorrhea.

Note: CF, complement-fixing; FA, fluorescent antibody; LGV, lymphogranuloma venereum; micro-IF, microimmunofluorescence; MPC, mucopurulent cervicitis; NAAT, nucleic acid amplification test; NGU, nongonococcal urethritis; PGU, postgonococcal urethritis.

with doxycycline or tetracycline must be given for genital infections. A 2-week course is recommended for complicated chlamydial infections (e.g., PID, epididymitis) and at least a 3-week course of doxycycline (100 mg orally bid) or erythromycin base (500 mg orally qid) for LGV. Failure of treatment of genital infections with a tetracycline usually indicates poor compliance or reinfection rather than the involvement of a drug-resistant strain. To date, clinically significant drug resistance has not been observed in *C. trachomatis* infection.

Therapy for *C. trachomatis* urethritis is more efficacious than therapy for nonchlamydial NGU. *C. trachomatis* is eradicated from the urethra in nearly all cases by treatment with tetracycline hydrochloride (500 mg qid for 7 days) or doxycycline (100 mg by mouth bid for 7 days).

Eradication of *C. trachomatis* from the cervix by tetracycline and doxycycline, with doses and durations similar to those specified above for urethritis, has been demonstrated. Erythromycin base (500 mg qid for 10 to 14 days) is the regimen of choice for pregnant women with *C. trachomatis* infection. Amoxicillin (500 mg tid for 10 days) has also been used successfully in pregnant women. Tetracycline hydrochloride (500 mg qid) or doxycycline (100 mg bid) for 14 days produces clinical and microbiologic cure of epididymitis and PID associated with *C. trachomatis* infection, but in this situation a tetracycline should always be used together with a drug that is highly effective against gonorrhea.

Azithromycin is highly active against *C. trachomatis*, exhibits prolonged bioavailability, is concentrated intracellularly, and has made possible single-dose therapy for chlamydial infection for the first time. In comparative trials, a 1-g single dose of azithromycin has been as effective as 7 days of doxycycline therapy for uncomplicated chlamydial infection. Azithromycin causes fewer adverse gastrointestinal reactions than do older macrolides such as erythromycin. The single-dose regimen of azithromycin has great appeal for the treatment of patients with uncomplicated chlamydial infection (especially those without symptoms and those with a likelihood of poor compliance) and of sexual partners of infected patients. These advantages must be weighed against the considerably greater cost of azithromycin. Whenever possible, the single 1-g dose should be given as directly observed therapy. Although not approved by the U.S. Food and Drug Administration for the treatment of pregnant women, the 1-g single-dose regimen of azithromycin appears to be safe and effective for this purpose.

Of the newer fluoroquinolones, ofloxacin (300 mg by mouth bid for 7 days) has been shown to be as effective as doxycycline for the treatment of chlamydial infection and appears to be safe and well tolerated. It cannot be used in pregnancy.

Treatment of Sex Partners The continued high prevalence of chlamydial infections in most parts of the United States is due primarily to the failure to diagnose—and therefore treat—patients with symptomatic or asymptomatic infection and their sex partners. *C. trachomatis* urethral or cervical infection has been well documented in a high proportion of the sex partners of patients with NGU, epididymitis, Reiter's syndrome, salpingitis, or endocervicitis. If possible, confirmatory laboratory tests for *Chlamydia* should be undertaken in these individuals, but even those without positive tests or evidence of clinical disease who have recently been exposed to proven or possible chlamydial infection (e.g., NGU) should be offered therapy.

Treatment of Neonates and Infants In neonates with conjunctivitis or infants with pneumonia, erythromycin ethylsuccinate or estolate can be given orally in a dose of 50 mg/kg per day, preferably in four divided doses, for 2 weeks. Careful attention must be given to compliance with therapy—a frequent problem. Relapses of eye infection are common following treatment with topical erythromycin or tetracycline ophthalmic ointment and may also occur after oral erythromycin therapy. Thus follow-up cultures should be performed after treatment. Both parents should be examined for *C. trachomatis* infec-

tion and, if diagnostic testing is not readily available, should be treated with doxycycline or azithromycin.

Prevention Efforts to develop a vaccine for chlamydial infection have not yet been successful. Early diagnosis and treatment shorten the duration of infectiousness and therefore constitute primary prevention of chlamydial infection. By the early 1990s, one of the 10 regions of the United States (Region X, the Pacific Northwest) had formally undertaken a chlamydial control program involving widespread screening of women attending family planning clinics. Approximately 500,000 tests per year were conducted at 150 such clinics throughout the region in women meeting the criteria for high risk. Within 5 years, the prevalence of chlamydial infection had been reduced by >30% in this population. While most regions of the United States have now initiated similar programs, some family planning and STD clinics still do not offer chlamydial testing. The availability of highly sensitive and specific diagnostic tests that can be done with urine specimens and of single-dose therapy makes it feasible to mount an effective chlamydial control program nationwide, with screening of high-risk persons both in traditional health care settings and in novel community- and school-based settings.

TRACHOMA AND ADULT INCLUSION CONJUNCTIVITIS ■ Definition Trachoma is a chronic conjunctivitis associated with infection by *C. trachomatis* serovar A, B, Ba, or C. It has been responsible for an estimated 20 million cases of blindness throughout the world and remains an important cause of preventable blindness. Inclusion conjunctivitis is an acute ocular infection caused by sexually transmitted *C. trachomatis* strains (usually serovars D through K) in adults exposed to infected genital secretions and in their newborn offspring.

Epidemiology In trachoma-endemic areas where the classic eye disease is seen, transmission is from eye to eye via hands, flies, towels, and other fomites and usually involves serovar A, B, Ba, or C. The worldwide incidence and severity of trachoma have decreased dramatically during the past 35 years, mainly as a result of improving hygienic and economic conditions. Endemic trachoma is still the major cause of preventable blindness in northern Africa, sub-Saharan Africa, the Middle East, and parts of Asia. Transmission occurs primarily through close personal contact, particularly among young children in rural communities with limited water supplies. In endemic areas, trachoma is associated with repeated exposure and reinfection, but the infection can also become chronic and persistent. Acute relapse of old trachoma occasionally follows treatment with cortisone eye ointment or develops in very old persons who were exposed in their youth.

Clinical Manifestations Both endemic trachoma and adult inclusion conjunctivitis present initially as a conjunctivitis characterized by small lymphoid follicles in the conjunctiva. In regions with hyperendemic classic blinding trachoma, the disease usually starts insidiously before the age of 2 years. Reinfection is common and probably contributes to the pathogenesis of trachoma. Studies using PCR techniques indicate that chlamydial DNA is often present in the ocular secretions of patients with trachoma, even in the absence of positive cultures. Thus persistent infection may be more common than was previously thought.

The cornea becomes involved, with inflammatory leukocytic infiltrations and superficial vascularization (pannus formation). As the inflammation continues, conjunctival scarring eventually distorts the eyelids, causing them to turn inward so that the inturned lashes constantly abrade the eyeball (trichiasis and entropion); eventually the corneal epithelium is abraded and may ulcerate, with subsequent corneal scarring and blindness. Destruction of the conjunctival goblet cells, lacrimal ducts, and lacrimal gland may produce a "dry-eye" syndrome, with resultant corneal opacity due to drying (xerosis) or secondary bacterial corneal ulcers.

Communities with blinding trachoma often experience seasonal epidemics of conjunctivitis due to *H. influenzae* that contribute to the intensity of the inflammatory process. In such areas the active infectious process usually resolves spontaneously in affected persons between 10 and 15 years of age, but the conjunctival scars continue to shrink, producing trichiasis and entropion and subsequent corneal scarring in adults. In areas with milder and less prevalent disease, the process may be much slower, with active disease continuing into adulthood; blindness is rare in these cases.

Eye infection with genital *C. trachomatis* strains in sexually active young adults presents as the acute onset of unilateral follicular conjunctivitis and preauricular lymphadenopathy similar to that seen in acute adenovirus or herpesvirus conjunctivitis. If untreated, the disease may persist for 6 weeks to 2 years. It is frequently associated with corneal inflammation in the form of discrete opacities ("infiltrates"), punctate epithelial erosions, and minor degrees of superficial corneal vascularization. Very rarely, conjunctival scarring and eyelid distortion occur, particularly in patients treated for many months with topical glucocorticoids. Recurrent eye infections develop most often in patients whose sexual consorts are not treated with antimicrobials.

Diagnosis The clinical diagnosis of classic trachoma can be made if two of the following signs are present: (1) lymphoid follicles on the upper tarsal conjunctiva; (2) typical conjunctival scarring; (3) vascular pannus; or (4) limbal follicles or their sequelae, Herbert's pits.

The clinical diagnosis of endemic trachoma should be confirmed by laboratory tests in children with more marked degrees of inflammation. Intracytoplasmic chlamydial inclusions are found in 10 to 60% of Giemsa-stained conjunctival smears in such populations, but chlamydial PCR or LCR is more sensitive and is often positive when smears or cultures are negative. Follicular conjunctivitis in adult Europeans or Americans living in trachomatous regions is rarely due to trachoma.

℞ TREATMENT

Public health control programs for endemic trachoma have consisted of the mass application of tetracycline or erythromycin ointment to the eyes of all children in affected communities for 21 to 60 days or on an intermittent schedule. These programs also include surgical correction of inturned eyelids by a mobile surgical team that visits each locale. Mass treatment of entire villages with single-dose azithromycin may be an alternative approach.

Adult inclusion conjunctivitis responds well to treatment with full doses of oral tetracycline or erythromycin administered for 3 weeks. Simultaneous treatment of all sexual consorts of the patient is also necessary to prevent ocular reinfection and to avoid genital disease due to chlamydial infection. Topical antibiotic treatment is not required for patients who receive systemic antibiotics.

Prevention Efforts to develop a trachoma vaccine have not yet been successful. General hygienic measures associated with improved living standards are effective in the elimination of endemic trachoma. An adequate water supply for personal cleanliness may be a key factor. In some areas the reduction of numbers of flies in the household is important.

C. PSITTACI INFECTIONS

Definition Psittacosis is primarily an infectious disease of birds and mammals that is caused by *C. psittaci*. Transmission of infection from birds to humans results in a febrile illness characterized by pneumonitis and systemic manifestations. Inapparent infections or mild influenza-like illnesses may also occur. The term *ornithosis* is sometimes applied to infections contracted from birds other than parrots or parakeets, but *psittacosis* is the preferred generic term for all forms of the disease.

Epidemiology Almost any avian species can harbor *C. psittaci*. Psittacine birds (parrots, parakeets, budgerigars) are most commonly infected, but human cases have been traced to contact with pigeons, ducks, turkeys, chickens, and many other birds. Psittacosis may be considered an occupational disease of pet-shop owners, poultry workers, pigeon fanciers, taxidermists, veterinarians, and zoo attendants. During the past 20 years, there has been an increase in incidence, with cases and outbreaks occurring primarily among employees of poultry-

processing plants. It is suspected that many cases go undiagnosed and unreported.

The agent is present in nasal secretions, excreta, tissues, and feathers of infected birds. Although the disease can be fatal, infected birds frequently show only minor evidence of illness, such as ruffled feathers, lethargy, and anorexia. Asymptomatic avian carriers are common, and complete recovery may be followed by continued shedding of the organism for many months.

Psittacosis is almost always transmitted to humans by the respiratory route. On rare occasions the disease may be acquired from the bite of a pet bird. Prolonged contact is not essential for transmission of the disease; a few minutes spent in an environment previously occupied by an infected bird has resulted in human infection. In one outbreak, gardening rather than direct exposure to birds was associated with infection. A psittacosis-like agent has been transmitted among hospital personnel, with severe and sometimes fatal infections. There is evidence that these "human" strains are more virulent than avian organisms. There is no record of infection acquired by the ingestion of poultry products.

Pathogenesis The psittacosis agent gains entrance to the body through the upper part of the respiratory tract, spreads via the bloodstream, and eventually localizes in the pulmonary alveoli and in the reticuloendothelial cells of the spleen and liver. Invasion of the lung probably takes place by way of the bloodstream rather than by direct extension from the upper air passages. A lymphocytic inflammatory response occurs on both the interstitial and the respiratory surfaces of the alveoli as well as in the perivascular spaces. The alveolar walls and interstitial tissues of the lung are thickened, edematous, necrotic, and occasionally hemorrhagic. Histologic examination of the affected areas reveals alveolar spaces filled with fluid, erythrocytes, and lymphocytes. The picture is not pathognomonic of psittacosis unless macrophages containing characteristic cytoplasmic inclusion bodies (Levinthal-Coles-Lillie bodies) can be identified. The respiratory epithelium of the bronchi and bronchioles usually remains intact.

Clinical Manifestations The clinical manifestations and course of psittacosis are extremely variable. After an incubation period of 7 to 14 days or longer, the disease may start abruptly with shaking chills and fever, with temperatures ranging as high as 40.5°C (105°F); however, the onset is often gradual, with fever increasing over a 3- to 4-day period. Headache is almost always a prominent symptom; it is usually diffuse and excruciating and is often the patient's chief complaint.

Many patients present with a dry hacking cough that is usually nonproductive, but small amounts of mucoid or bloody sputum may be raised as the disease progresses. Cough may begin early in the course of the disease or as late as 5 days after the onset of fever. Chest pain, pleurisy with effusion, or a friction rub may all occur but are rare. Pericarditis and myocarditis have been reported. Most patients have a normal or slightly increased respiratory rate; marked dyspnea with cyanosis occurs only in severe psittacosis with extensive pulmonary involvement. In psittacosis, as in mycoplasmal pneumonias, the physical signs of pneumonitis tend to be less prominent than symptoms and x-ray findings would suggest. The initial examination may reveal fine sibilant rales, or clinical evidence of pneumonia may be completely lacking. Rales usually become audible and more numerous as the illness progresses. Signs of frank pulmonary consolidation are usually absent. Symptoms of upper respiratory tract infection are not prominent, although mild sore throat, pharyngitis, and cervical adenopathy are often documented; on occasion, the last may be the only manifestation of illness. Epistaxis is encountered early in the course of nearly one-fourth of cases. Photophobia is also a common complaint.

Patients often report generalized myalgia, and spasm and stiffness of the muscles of the back and neck may lead to an erroneous diagnosis of meningitis. Lethargy, mental depression, agitation, insomnia, and disorientation have been prominent features of the illness in some epidemics but not in others; delirium and stupor develop near the end of the first week in severe cases. Occasional patients are comatose when first seen, and the diagnosis of psittacosis may be elusive in these cases. Gastrointestinal manifestations such as abdominal pain, nausea, vomiting, or diarrhea are noted in some cases; constipation and abdominal distention sometimes occur as late complications. Icterus, the result of severe hepatic involvement, is a rare and ominous finding. A faint macular rash (Horder's spots) resembling the rose spots of typhoid fever has been described.

Patients without cough or other clinical evidence of respiratory involvement present with fever of unknown origin (Chap. 18). The pulse rate is slow in relation to the fever. When splenomegaly is noted in a patient with acute pneumonitis, psittacosis should be considered; the reported incidence of splenomegaly in this disease ranges from 10 to 70%. Nontender hepatic enlargement also occurs, but jaundice is rare. Thrombophlebitis is not unusual during convalescence; indeed, pulmonary infarction is sometimes a late complication and may be fatal.

In untreated cases of psittacosis, sustained or mildly remittent fever persists for 10 days to 3 weeks or occasionally for as long as 3 months. Over this period, the respiratory manifestations gradually abate. Psittacosis contracted from parrots or parakeets is more likely to be a severe, prolonged illness than infection acquired from pigeons or barnyard fowl. Relapses occur but are rare. Occasional patients develop endocarditis, and *C. psittaci* infection should be considered in cases of culture-negative endocarditis. Secondary bacterial infections are uncommon. Immunity to reinfection is probably permanent.

Laboratory Findings   The chest x-ray in psittacosis is nonspecific and may show pneumonic lesions that are usually patchy in appearance but can be hazy, diffuse, homogeneous, lobar, atelectatic, wedge-shaped, nodular, or miliary. The white blood cell count is normal or moderately decreased in the acute phase of the disease but may rise in convalescence. The erythrocyte sedimentation rate frequently is not elevated. Transient proteinuria is common. The cerebrospinal fluid sometimes contains a few mononuclear cells but is otherwise normal. Despite hepatomegaly, the results of liver function tests are generally normal or only mildly elevated.

The diagnosis can be confirmed only by isolation of the causative microorganism or by serologic studies. The agent is present in the blood during the acute phase of the disease and in the bronchial secretions for weeks or sometimes years after infection, but it is difficult to isolate. Further, the organism is hazardous to work with in the laboratory, and most clinical laboratories do not offer culture for *C. psittaci*. Thus psittacosis is most readily diagnosed by the demonstration of a rising titer of complement fixation antibody in the serum of a patient with a compatible clinical syndrome. Both an acute-phase and a convalescent-phase specimen should always be tested. *C. trachomatis*, *C. psittaci*, and *C. pneumoniae* all share a genus-specific "group" antigen, which is the basis of the complement fixation test. Thus acute infections with *C. trachomatis* or *C. pneumoniae* can also produce titer rises in this test. However, these three species have different major outer-membrane proteins that are the principal antigens in the micro-IF test. If there is doubt as to the interpretation of the complement fixation test, the micro-IF test can be used to differentiate among these antigens. The prompt initiation of treatment with tetracycline has been shown to delay an antibody rise in convalescence for several weeks or months.

Differential Diagnosis   A history of exposure to birds may be the only clinical basis for differentiating psittacosis from a variety of infectious and noninfectious febrile disorders. The list of pulmonary diseases that may be confused with psittacosis includes *Mycoplasma* pneumonia, *C. pneumoniae* pneumonia, legionellosis, viral pneumonia, Q fever, coccidioidomycosis, tuberculosis, enterovirus infection, carcinoma of the lung with bronchial obstruction, and common bacterial pneumonias. In the early stages, before pneumonitis appears, psittacosis may

be mistaken for influenza, typhoid fever, miliary tuberculosis, or infectious mononucleosis.

Rx TREATMENT

The tetracyclines are consistently effective in the treatment of psittacosis. Defervescence and alleviation of symptoms usually take place within 24 to 48 h after the institution of therapy with 2 g daily in four divided doses. To avoid relapse, treatment should probably be continued for at least 7 to 14 days after defervescence. In severe cases, hospitalization and pulmonary intensive care may be indicated. Sulfonamides are not active against *C. psittaci*. Erythromycin can be used in patients allergic to or intolerant of tetracyclines.

C. PNEUMONIAE INFECTIONS

Definition   A third chlamydial species that causes disease in humans, *C. pneumoniae*, has been described in the past quarter century. *C. pneumoniae* can be distinguished from the other two species on the basis of DNA hybridization and elementary body morphology. Although *C. pneumoniae* can be grown in a variety of cell cultures, it is considerably more difficult to culture than other chlamydiae, especially from clinical specimens. HL cells appear to be the most effective cell line for isolation of *C. pneumoniae*.

Epidemiology   Knowledge of the epidemiology of *C. pneumoniae* infections has been derived primarily from serologic studies. Infections begin to occur in late childhood, achieve peak incidence in young adults, but continue throughout adult life. Seroprevalence in the many adult populations that have been tested throughout the world exceeds 40%—a figure suggesting that *C. pneumoniae* infections are ubiquitous. Secondary episodes (reinfections) appear to occur commonly in older adults throughout life. *C. pneumoniae* also produces epidemics of pneumonia and respiratory illness, especially in close residential quarters such as military barracks. The incidence of infections outside of epidemics remains poorly defined. Transmission appears to be from person to person, probably primarily in schools and family units.

Pathogenesis   Little is known about the pathogenesis of *C. pneumoniae* infection. The infection begins in the upper respiratory tract and in many persons is a long-lived asymptomatic condition of the upper respiratory mucosal surfaces. However, in at least some individuals, the organism is transported to distant sites—perhaps within macrophages—since evidence exists for replication within arteries and synovial membranes of joints. A *C. pneumoniae* outer-membrane protein may induce host immune responses whose cross-reaction with human proteins results in an autoimmune reaction.

Clinical Manifestations   The clinical spectrum of *C. pneumoniae* infection includes acute pharyngitis, sinusitis, bronchitis, and pneumonitis, primarily in young adults. The clinical manifestations of primary infection appear to be more severe and prolonged than those of reinfection. The pneumonitis resembles that of *M. pneumoniae* pneumonia in that leukocytosis is frequently lacking and patients often have prominent antecedent upper respiratory tract symptoms, fever, nonproductive cough, a mild to moderate degree of illness, minimal findings on chest auscultation, and small segmental infiltrates on chest x-ray. In elderly patients, pneumonia due to *C. pneumoniae* can be especially severe and may necessitate hospitalization and respiratory support.

Epidemiologic studies have demonstrated an association between serologic evidence of *C. pneumoniae* infection and atherosclerotic disease of the coronary and other arteries. In addition, *C. pneumoniae* has been identified in atherosclerotic plaques by electron microscopy, DNA hybridization, and immunocytochemistry. The organism has been recovered in culture from atheromatous plaque—a result indicating the presence of viable replicating bacteria in vessels. Evidence from animal models supports the hypothesis that *C. pneumoniae* infection of the upper respiratory tract is followed by recovery of the organism from atheromatous lesions in the aorta and that the infection accelerates the process of atherosclerosis, especially in hypercholesterolemic animals. Antimicrobial treatment of the infected animals reverses the increased risk of atherosclerosis. In humans, two small trials in patients with unstable angina or recent myocardial infarction also suggested that antibiotics reduce subsequent untoward cardiac events. Larger trials have been initiated to determine more definitively whether antibiotics affect the risk of atherosclerosis.

Diagnosis Diagnosis of *C. pneumoniae* infection is currently difficult because cell culture techniques are not available for routine clinical use and nonculture tests using antigen detection methods or DNA probes have not been developed for commercial use. Acute- and convalescent-phase sera can be tested for chlamydial complement fixation antibody to make a retrospective diagnosis. However, this test does not distinguish *C. pneumoniae* infection from infection due to *C. trachomatis* or *C. psittaci*.

℞ TREATMENT

Although controlled treatment trials have not been conducted, *C. pneumoniae* is inhibited in vitro by erythromycin and tetracycline. Recommended therapy consists of 2 g per day of either agent for 10 to 14 days. Other macrolides, such as azithromycin, and some fluoroquinolones, such as levofloxacin, also appear to be effective.

FURTHER READING

ADIMORA AA: Treatment of uncomplicated genital *Chlamydia trachomatis* infections in adults. Clin Infect Dis 35(Suppl 2):S183, 2002

GILBERT DN, GRAYSTON JT (eds): The potential etiologic role of *Chlamydia pneumoniae* in atherosclerosis: A multidisciplinary meeting to promote collaborative research. J Infect Dis 181(Suppl 3):S383, 2000

GRAYSTON JT: Infections caused by *Chlamydia pneumoniae*, strain TWAR. Clin Infect Dis 15:757, 1992

HOLMES KK, STAMM WE: Lower genital tract infections in women: Cystitis, urethritis, vulvovaginitis, and cervicitis, in *Sexually Transmitted Diseases*, 3d ed, KK Holmes et al (eds). New York, McGraw-Hill, 1999

MARRAZZO JM, STAMM WE: New approaches to the diagnosis, treatment, and prevention of chlamydial infection. Curr Clin Top Infect Dis 18:37, 1998

STAMM WE: Expanding efforts to prevent chlamydial infection. N Engl J Med 339:768, 1998

———: *Chlamydia trachomatis* infections in adults, in *Sexually Transmitted Diseases*, 3d ed, KK Holmes et al (eds). New York, McGraw-Hill, 1999

———: *Chlamydia trachomatis*: The persistent pathogen. Sex Transm Dis 13:684, 2001

US PREVENTIVE SERVICE TASK FORCE: Chlamydial infection. Screening 2001. Guide to clinical preventive services. Alexandria, VA, International Medical Publishing, 2001, pp 325–332

Section 11 Viral Diseases: General Considerations

161 MEDICAL VIROLOGY
Fred Wang, Elliott Kieff

DEFINING A VIRUS

Viruses consist of a nucleic acid surrounded by one or more proteins. Some viruses also have an outer-membrane envelope. Viruses are obligate intracellular parasites: they can replicate only within cells since their nucleic acids do not encode the many enzymes necessary for protein, carbohydrate, or lipid metabolism and for the generation of high-energy phosphates. Typically, viral nucleic acids encode proteins necessary for replicating and packaging the nucleic acids within the biochemical milieu of host cells.

Viruses differ from viroids, prions, and virusoids. *Virusoids* are nucleic acids that depend on helper viruses to package their nucleic acids into virus-like particles. *Viroids* are naked, cyclical, mostly double-stranded, small RNAs. Viroids, which appear to be restricted to plants, spread from cell to cell and are replicated by cellular RNA polymerase II. *Prions* (Chap. 362) are abnormal protein molecules that can spread and change the structure of their normal counterparts (cellular proteins). Prions have been implicated in neurodegenerative conditions such as Creutzfeldt-Jakob disease, Gerstmann-Sträussler disease, kuru, and human bovine spongiform encephalopathy ("mad cow disease").

VIRAL STRUCTURE

Viruses have from a few to several hundred genes. These genes may be in a single-strand or double-strand DNA genome or in a single-strand sense, a single-strand or segmented antisense, or a double-strand segmented RNA genome. Sense-strand RNA genomes can be translated directly into protein. Sense and antisense genomes are also referred to as positive-strand and negative-strand genomes, respectively. The viral nucleic acid is usually associated with one or more virus-encoded nucleoproteins in the core of the viral particle. The viral nucleic acid and nucleoproteins are almost always enclosed in a protein shell called a *capsid*. Because of the limited genetic complexity of viruses, their capsids are usually composed of multimers of identical capsomers. Capsomers are in turn composed of one or a few proteins. Capsids have icosahedral or helical symmetry. Icosahedral structures approximate spheres but have two-, three-, and fivefold axes of sym-

metry, while helical structures have only a twofold axis of symmetry. The entire structural unit of nucleic acid, nucleoprotein(s), and capsid is called a *nucleocapsid*. Many human viruses are simply composed of a core and a capsid. For these viruses, the outer surface of the capsid mediates contact with uninfected cells. Other viruses are more complex and have an outer lipid-containing envelope derived from virus-modified membranes of the infected cell. The piece of infected-cell membrane that becomes the viral envelope has usually been modified during infection by the insertion of virus-encoded glycoproteins. Virus-encoded glycoproteins usually mediate contact of enveloped viruses with uninfected cells. Matrix or tegument proteins fill the space between the nucleocapsid and the envelope in many enveloped viruses. In general, enveloped viruses are sensitive to lipid solvents and nonionic detergents that can dissolve the envelope, while viruses that consist only of nucleocapsids are somewhat resistant. A schematic diagram for large and complex herpesviruses is shown in Fig. 161-1. Prototypical pathogenic human viruses are listed in Table 161-1. The relative sizes and structures of typical pathogenic human viruses are shown in Fig. 161-2.

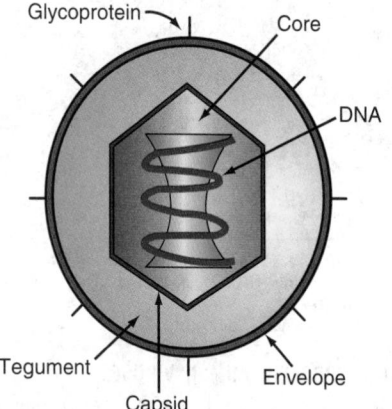

FIGURE 161-1 Schematic diagram of an enveloped herpesvirus with an icosahedral nucleocapsid. The approximate respective dimensions of the nucleocapsid and the enveloped particles are 110 and 180 nm. The capsid is composed of 162 capsomeres: 150 with sixfold and 12 with fivefold axes of symmetry.

TABLE 161-1 *Virus Families Pathogenic for Humans*

Family	Representative Viruses	Type of RNA/DNA	Lipid Envelope
RNA VIRUSES			
Picornaviridae	Poliovirus Coxsackievirus Echovirus Enterovirus Rhinovirus Hepatitis A virus	(+) RNA	No
Caliciviridae	Norwalk agent Hepatitis E virus	(+) RNA	No
Togaviridae	Rubella virus Eastern equine encephalitis virus Western equine encephalitis virus	(+) RNA	Yes
Flaviviridae	Yellow fever virus Dengue virus St. Louis encephalitis virus West Nile virus Hepatitis C virus Hepatitis G virus	(+) RNA	Yes
Coronaviridae	Coronaviruses[a]	(+) RNA	Yes
Rhabdoviridae	Rabies virus Vesicular stomatitis virus	(−) RNA	Yes
Filoviridae	Marburg virus Ebola virus	(−) RNA	Yes
Paramyxoviridae	Parainfluenza virus Respiratory syncytial virus Newcastle disease virus Mumps virus Rubeola (measles) virus	(−) RNA	Yes
Orthomyxoviridae	Influenza A, B, and C viruses	(−) RNA, 8 segments	Yes
Bunyaviridae	Hantavirus California encephalitis virus Sandfly fever virus	(−) RNA, 3 circular segments	Yes
Arenaviridae	Lymphocytic choriomeningitis virus Lassa fever virus South American hemorrhagic fever virus	(−) RNA, 2 circular segments	Yes
Reoviridae	Rotavirus Reovirus Colorado tick fever virus	ds RNA, 10–12 segments	No
Retroviridae	Human T-lymphotropic virus types I and II Human immunodeficiency virus types 1 and 2	(+) RNA, 2 identical segments	Yes
DNA VIRUSES			
Hepadnaviridae	Hepatitis B virus	ds DNA with ss portions	Yes
Parvoviridae	Parvovirus B19	ss DNA	No
Papovaviridae	Human papillomaviruses JC virus BK virus	ds DNA	No
Adenoviridae	Human adenoviruses	ds DNA	No
Herpesviridae	Herpes simplex virus types 1 and 2[b] Varicella-zoster virus[c] Epstein-Barr virus[d] Cytomegalovirus[e] Human herpesvirus 6 Human herpesvirus 7 Kaposi's sarcoma–associated herpesvirus[f]	ds DNA	Yes
Poxviridae	Variola (smallpox) virus Orf virus Molluscum contagiosum virus	ds DNA	Yes

[a] Including the coronavirus causing severe acute respiratory syndrome (SARS).
[b] Also called human herpesvirus (HHV) 1 and 2, respectively; [c] also called HHV-3; [d] also called HHV-4; [e] also called HHV-5; [f] also called HHV-8
Abbreviations: ds, double-strand; ss, single-strand.

TAXONOMY OF PATHOGENIC HUMAN VIRUSES

As is apparent from Table 161-1 and Fig. 161-2, the classification of viruses into orders and families is based on nucleic acid composition, nucleocapsid size and symmetry, and presence or absence of an envelope. Viruses of a single family have similar types of genomes and are often morphologically indistinguishable in electron micrographs.

Further subclassification into genus is dependent on similarities in epidemiology and biologic effects and on the degree of colinear nucleic acid sequence homology. Most human viruses have a common name related to their pathologic effects or the circumstances of their discovery. Formal species names have been assigned by the International Committee on Taxonomy of Viruses. The latter designation consists of the name of the host followed by the family or genus of the virus and a number. This dual terminology has created a confusing situation in which viruses are referred to and referenced by either name—e.g., varicella-zoster virus (VZV) or human herpesvirus (HHV) 3.

VIRAL INFECTION IN VITRO

STAGES OF VIRAL INFECTION AT THE CELLULAR LEVEL

■ **Viral Interactions with the Cell Surface and Cell Entry** Viral infection is initiated by adsorption of the virus to the cell surface. Adsorption results from the molecular interaction of viral surface proteins with receptors on the cell's plasma membrane. For example, a poliovirus capsid protein binds to a cell plasma-membrane protein of the immunoglobulin superfamily type. A rhinovirus capsid protein binds to intracellular adhesion molecule 1. An echovirus capsid protein binds to an integrin. The influenza A virus envelope hemagglutinin protein binds to sialic acid. The HIV envelope glycoprotein binds to CD4 and then engages one of several chemokine receptors that function as coreceptors for the virus. Herpes simplex virus (HSV) envelope glycoproteins bind to heparan sulfate on cell surfaces and then engage one of several immunoglobulin superfamily or tumor necrosis factor (TNF) receptors. Epstein-Barr virus (EBV) glycoprotein gp350 binds to the B lymphocyte complement receptor CD21. Adsorption characteristically proceeds almost as well at 4°C as at 37°C. Adsorbed virus can still be neutralized by antibody. Adsorption frequently initiates changes in virion surface proteins that destabilize the viral surface proteins and prepare the way for the next stage of entry into the cell.

After adsorption, viruses penetrate the cell membrane by fusing with the membrane. The fusion reaction results in the virus's partial decomposition. The virus becomes insensitive to neutralizing antibody as it penetrates, becomes uncoated, and enters the cytoplasm. Penetration and uncoating result in viral nucleocapsid or nucleoprotein entry into the cytoplasm. Penetration and uncoating as well as subsequent steps in viral replication depend on the cell's energy metabolism and on biochemical changes in the cell's plasma membrane and cytoskeleton. Therefore, penetration proceeds slowly at temperatures <37°C. Interaction of viral surface proteins with cell receptors can induce receptor aggregation at the site of adsorption. Receptor aggregation can trigger signaling events within the cytoplasm and changes in the plasma membrane. The cell frequently misperceives that the receptor has encountered its "normal ligand." Aggregated receptor may be internalized with the attached virus in an endocytic process. Viral endocytosis may proceed through clathrin-coated pits. Endocytosis is important in the entry of viruses as diverse as picornaviruses, influenza viruses, HIV, adenoviruses, and herpesviruses. In many cases, entry of the virus into the cytoplasm depends on acidification of the viral endosome.

One of the best-studied examples of the effect of low pH on viral penetration is influenza virus. Influenza hemagglutinin mediates adsorption, receptor aggregation, and endocytosis. In low-pH endosomes, changes in the conformation of the hemagglutinin expose amphipathic domains that interact chemically with the cell membrane and initiate fusion of the viral and cellular membranes. The HIV envelope glycoprotein undergoes similar conformational changes after interaction with CD4 and chemokine receptors. For influenza virus, the M2 membrane protein also plays a key role in the uncoating of the viral envelope by providing an ion channel in the envelope. Fusion of viral and cell membranes results in the mixture of viral envelope lipids and proteins with cell membrane lipids and proteins and the penetration of the influenza nucleocapsid into the cytoplasm. With more complex viruses, such as herpesviruses, different glycoproteins interact with specific receptors on different cell types or on different surfaces of polarized epithelial cells. Viral glycoproteins other than the protein that mediates initial adsorption may be critical in mediating envelope fusion with cell membranes. The fusion of viral proteins with cell membranes is a crucial step in viral infection, which involves hydrophobic interactions. Hydrophobic interactions can be susceptible to chemical inhibition or blockade.

Viral Gene Expression and Replication   After uncoating and release of viral nucleoprotein into the cytoplasm, the viral genome is transported to a site for expression and replication. In order to produce infectious progeny, viruses must (1) produce proteins necessary to replicate their nucleic acid, (2) produce structural proteins, and (3) assemble the nucleic acid and proteins into progeny virions. Different viruses use different strategies and gene repertoires to accomplish these goals. DNA viruses, except for poxviruses, replicate their nucleic acid and assemble into nucleocapsid complexes in the cell nucleus. RNA viruses, except for influenza viruses, transcribe and replicate their nucleic acid and assemble entirely in the cytoplasm. Thus, the replication strategies of DNA and RNA viruses are presented separately below. Positive-strand and negative-strand RNA viruses are discussed separately. Medically important viruses of each group are used for illustrative purposes.

POSITIVE-STRAND RNA VIRUSES   Medically important positive-strand RNA viruses include picornaviruses, flaviviruses, togaviruses, caliciviruses, and coronaviruses. Genomic RNA from positive-strand RNA viruses is released into the cytoplasm without associated enzymes. Cell ribosomes recognize and associate with an internal ribosome entry sequence in the viral genomic RNA and translate a polyprotein that is a fusion of many or all of the viral proteins. The viral RNA polymerase and other viral proteins are cleaved from the polyprotein by protease components of the polyprotein. Antigenomic RNA is then transcribed from the genomic RNA template. Positive-strand genomes and mRNAs are next transcribed from the antigenomic RNA by the viral RNA polymerase. Positive-strand genomic RNA is encapsidated in the cytoplasm.

NEGATIVE-STRAND RNA VIRUSES   Medically important negative-strand RNA viruses include rhabdoviruses, filoviruses, paramyxoviruses, myxoviruses, and bunyaviruses. Negative-strand RNA virus genomes are released into the cytoplasm with an associated RNA polymerase and one or more accessory proteins. Some of these genomes are segmented. Except for influenza viruses, negative-strand RNA viruses replicate entirely in the cytoplasm. The viral RNA polymerase transcribes mes-

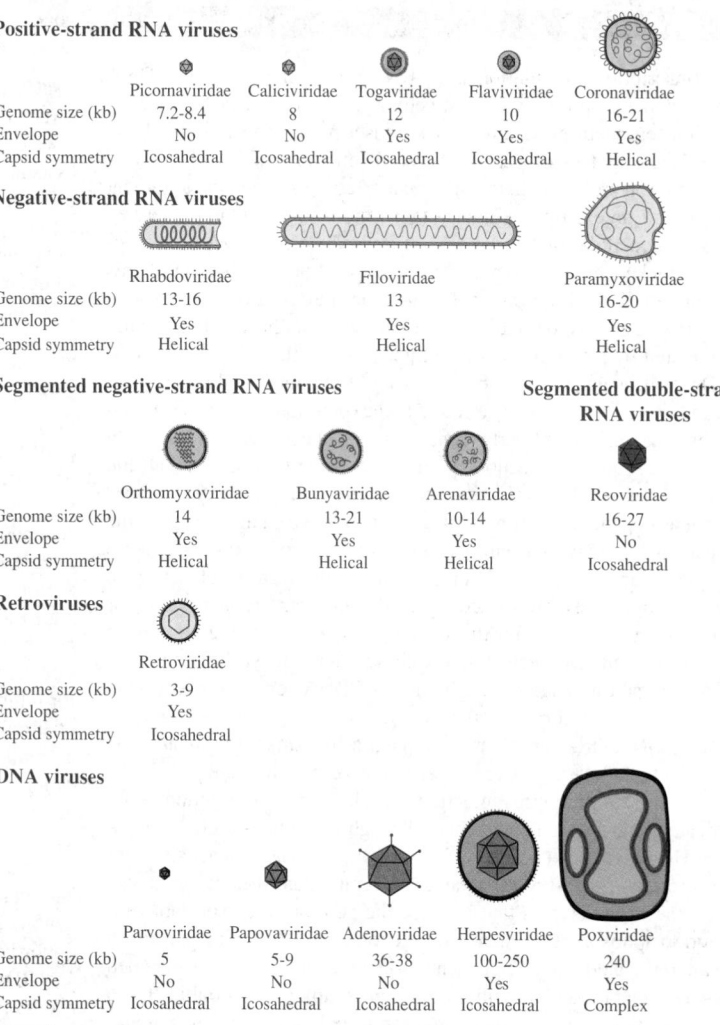

FIGURE 161-2   Schematic diagrams of the major virus families including species that infect humans. The viruses are grouped by genome type and are drawn approximately to scale. Prototype viruses of each family that cause human disease are listed in Table 161-1.

senger RNAs (mRNAs) as well as full-length antigenomic RNA, which is the template for replication of genomic RNA. These mRNAs encode for the viral RNA polymerase and accessory factors as well as for viral structural proteins. Influenza virus is an unusual negative-strand RNA virus that transcribes its mRNAs and antigenomic RNAs in the cell's nucleus. The influenza genome RNA snatches cellular mRNA cap sequences to enhance translation of viral mRNAs and uses cell splicing machinery to encode additional viral mRNAs. All negative-strand RNA viruses, including influenza viruses, assemble in the cytoplasm.

DOUBLE-STRAND SEGMENTED RNA VIRUSES   These viruses, which are taxonomically grouped in the reovirus family, have 10 to 12 RNA segments that make up their genome. The medically important viruses in this group are rotaviruses and Colorado tick fever virus. Reovirus virions include an RNA polymerase complex. Reoviruses replicate and assemble in the cytoplasm.

DNA VIRUSES   Medically important DNA viruses include parvoviruses, papovaviruses (e.g., human papillomaviruses, or HPVs, and polyomaviruses), adenoviruses, herpesviruses, and poxviruses. Other than poxviruses, most DNA viruses must get to the cell's nucleus for DNA transcription by cellular RNA polymerase II. For example, after receptor binding and fusion, herpesvirus nucleocapsids are released into the cytoplasm along with tegument proteins. The complex is then transported along microtubules to nuclear pores, and the DNA is released into the nucleus.

Transcriptional regulation and mRNA processing for nuclear DNA viruses depend on both viral and cellular proteins. For herpesviruses, the viral tegument protein activates transcription of viral immediate-early genes, a class of genes expressed immediately after infection. Transcription of immediate-early genes requires the viral tegument protein and preexisting cellular transcription factors. One of the key preexisting cellular factors for HSV-1 immediate-early gene transcription is docked in the cytoplasm in neurons. Nuclear absence of this critical cell factor important for viral gene transcription may explain why HSV-1 goes into a latent state in neurons and how lytic infection is activated by signaling in a latently infected cell.

DNA virus gene transcription is usually regulated and proceeds in an organized cascade. Transcription and expression of adenovirus and herpesvirus immediate-early genes turn on the promoters for early genes in a sequential fashion, whereas poxvirus virions carry all the factors necessary for early-gene transcription. Smaller DNA viruses are not as dependent on transactivators encoded from the viral genome for early-gene transcription. Most early genes encode proteins that are necessary for viral DNA synthesis and for the turn-on of late-gene transcription. Late genes encode mostly viral structural proteins or viral proteins necessary for the assembly and egress of the virus from the infected cell. Late-gene transcription is continuously dependent on DNA replication. Therefore, inhibitors of DNA replication also stop late-gene transcription.

Each DNA virus family uses unique mechanisms for replicating its DNA. Herpesvirus DNAs are linear in the virion but circularize in the infected cell. In lytic virus infection, circular herpesvirus genomes are replicated into linear concatemers through a "rolling-circle" mechanism. Herpesviruses encode a DNA polymerase and at least six other viral proteins necessary for viral DNA replication; these viruses also encode several enzymes that increase the pool of precursor deoxynucleotide triphosphates. Adenovirus genomes are linear in the virion and are replicated into complementary linear copies by a virus-encoded DNA polymerase and an initiator protein complex. The double-strand circular papovavirus genomes are replicated into progeny circular DNA molecules by cellular DNA replication enzymes. Two viral early proteins contribute to viral DNA replication and to the persistence of papovavirus DNA in latently infected cells. Early papovavirus proteins stimulate cells to remain in cycle, thus facilitating viral DNA replication. Occasionally, HPVs integrate into the host chromosome; overexpression of viral early proteins and excessive stimulation of cellular growth can result. Sometimes the consequence is the development of malignancies such as cervical cancer (see "Persistent Viral Infections and Cancer," below).

Parvoviruses are the smallest DNA viruses: their genomes are half the size of the papovavirus genomes and include only two genes. Parvoviruses have negative single-strand DNA genomes. The replication of autonomous parvoviruses, such as B19, depends on cellular DNA replication and requires the virus-encoded Rep protein. Other parvoviruses, such as adeno-associated virus (AAV), are not autonomous and require helper viruses of the adenovirus or herpesvirus family for their replication. AAV has been touted as a potentially safe human gene therapy vector because its Rep protein causes its integration at a single chromosomal site.

Poxviruses are the largest DNA viruses and are unique among DNA viruses in replicating and assembling in the cytoplasm. Poxviruses encode transcription factors and an RNA polymerase as well as enzymes for RNA capping and polyadenylation and for DNA synthesis. Poxvirus DNA also has a unique structure. The two strands of the double-strand linear DNA are covalently linked at the ends so that the genome is also a covalently closed single-strand circle. In addition, there are inverted repeats at the ends of the DNA. During DNA replication, the genome is cleaved within the terminal inverted repeat, and the inverted repeats self-prime complementary-strand synthesis by the virus-encoded DNA polymerase. Like herpesviruses, poxviruses en-

code several enzymes that increase deoxynucleotide triphosphate precursor levels and thus facilitate viral DNA synthesis.

VIRUSES WITH BOTH RNA AND DNA GENOMES Retroviruses and hepatitis B virus (HBV) are not purely RNA or DNA viruses. Retroviruses are enveloped RNA viruses with two identical sense-strand genomes and associated reverse transcriptase and integrase enzymes. Retroviruses differ from all other viruses in that they reverse-transcribe themselves into partially duplicated double-strand DNA copies and then routinely integrate into the host genome as part of their replication strategy. Cellular RNA polymerase II and transcription factors regulate transcription from the integrated provirus genome. Some retroviruses also encode for regulators of transcription and RNA processing, such as Tax and Rex in human T-lymphotropic virus (HTLV) types I and II and Tat and Rev in HIV-1 and HIV-2. HIV genomes also encode for the additional accessory proteins Vpr, Vpu, and Vif, which are important for efficient infection and immune escape. Full-length proviral transcripts are made from a promoter in the viral terminal repeat and serve as both genomic RNAs that will be packaged in the nucleocapsids and mRNAs that encode for the viral Gag protein, polymerase/integrase protein, and envelope glycoprotein. The Gag protein includes a protease that cleaves it into several components, including a viral matrix protein that coats the viral RNA. Viral RNA polymerase/integrase, matrix protein, and cellular tRNA are key components of the viral nucleocapsid. The HIV Gag protease has been an important target for inhibition of HIV replication. Remnants and even complete copies of simple retroviral DNA in the human genome indicate that there may be replication-competent simple human retroviruses. However, replication has not been documented or associated with any disease. Integrated retroviral DNAs are also present in other animal species, such as pigs. These porcine retroviruses are a potential cause for concern in xenotransplantation because retroviral replication could cause disease in humans. Since the retroviral DNA is integrated into the porcine genome, special pathogen-free breeding practices cannot cleanse the donor herd of retroviral infection.

HBV is unique because virion DNA expression in infected cells results in the packaging of reverse transcriptase and genomic RNA in the virion. The genomic RNA is then copied into an incomplete double-strand circular DNA genome before the virion matures and is released from the infected cell. On entry of HBV into the cytoplasm of an infected cell, the virion reverse transcriptase/DNA polymerase completes DNA synthesis, and the covalently closed circular genome resides in the nucleus. Viral mRNAs are transcribed from the closed circular viral episome by cellular RNA polymerase II. A capped and polyadenylated, full-genome-length, terminally redundant transcript is packaged into virus core particles in the cytoplasm of infected cells. This RNA associates with the viral reverse transcriptase. The reverse transcriptase converts the full-length, terminally redundant, core-particle, encapsidated RNA genome into partially double-strand DNA. HBV is believed to mature by budding through the cell's plasma membrane, which has been modified by the insertion of viral surface antigen protein.

Viral Assembly and Egress For most viruses, nucleic acid and structural protein synthesis are accompanied by the assembly of protein and nucleic acid complexes. The assembly and egress of mature infectious virus mark the end of the eclipse phase of infection, during which infectious virus cannot be recovered from the infected cell. Nucleic acids from RNA viruses and poxviruses assemble into nucleocapsids in the cytoplasm. For all DNA viruses except poxviruses, viral DNA assembles into nucleocapsids in the nucleus. In general, the capsid proteins of viruses with icosahedral nucleocapsids can self-assemble into densely packed and highly ordered capsid structures. Herpesviruses require an assemblin protein as a scaffold for capsid assembly. Viral nucleic acid then spools into the assembled capsid. For herpesviruses, a full unit of the viral DNA genome is packaged into the capsid, and a capsid-associated nuclease cleaves the viral DNA at both ends. In the case of viruses with helical nucleocapsids, the protein component appears to assemble around the nucleic acid, which contributes to capsid organization.

Viruses must egress from the infected cell and not bind back to the outer surface of the plasma membrane. In many cases, enveloped viruses simply egress and acquire their envelope by budding through the cell's plasma membrane. Excess viral membrane glycoproteins are synthesized to saturate cell receptors and facilitate virus separation from the infected cell. Some viruses encode membrane proteins with enzymatic activity for receptor destruction. Influenza virus, for example, encodes a glycoprotein with neuraminidase activity, which destroys sialic acid on the infected cell's plasma membrane. Herpesvirus nucleocapsids acquire their initial envelope by assembling in the nucleus and then budding through the nuclear membrane into the endoplasmic reticular space. The enveloped herpesvirus is then released from the cell either by maturation in cytoplasmic vesicles, which fuse with the plasma membrane and release the virus by exocytosis, or by "de-envelopment" into the cytoplasm and "re-envelopment" at the plasma membrane. In most instances, nonenveloped viruses appear to depend on the death and dissolution of the infected cell for their release.

FIDELITY OF VIRAL REPLICATION   Cells grow by doubling their genome and dividing, whereas viruses typically make large quantities of viral nucleic acid and structural proteins, and thousands of progeny may be produced from a single virus-infected cell. Many particles partially assemble and never mature into virions. Many mature-appearing virions are imperfect and have only incomplete or nonfunctional genomes. Despite the inefficiency of assembly, a typical virus-infected cell releases 10 to 1000 infectious progeny. Some of these progeny may contain genomes that differ from those of the virus that infected the cell. Smaller, "defective" virus genomes have been noted with the replication of many RNA and DNA viruses. Virions with defective genomes can be produced in large numbers through packaging of incompletely synthesized nucleic acid. Adenovirus packaging is notoriously inefficient, and a high particle-to-infectious virus ratio may limit the amount of recombinant adenovirus that can be administered for gene therapy. Mutant viral genomes are also produced and can be of medical significance. In general, viral nucleic acid replication is more error-prone than cellular nucleic acid replication. RNA polymerases and reverse transcriptases are significantly more error-prone than DNA polymerases. Mutant viruses can be virulent and may preferentially cause disease through evasion of the host immune response or through resistance to antiviral drugs. Persistent hepatitis C virus (HCV) infection appears to be due to genome mutation and persistent immune escape. Viral nucleic acids can also mutate by recombination or reassortment between two related viruses in a single cell. While this occurrence is unusual under most circumstances of natural infection, the changes can be substantial and can significantly alter virulence or epidemiology. Reassortment of an avian or mammalian influenza A hemagglutinin gene into a human influenza background is believed to play a role in the emergence of new epidemic influenza A strains.

VIRAL GENES NOT REQUIRED FOR VIRAL REPLICATION   Viruses frequently have genes encoding proteins that are not directly involved in replication or packaging of the viral nucleic acid, in virion assembly, or in regulation of the transcription of viral genes involved in those processes. Most of these proteins fall into five classes: (1) proteins that directly or indirectly alter cell growth; (2) proteins that inhibit cellular RNA or protein synthesis so that viral mRNA can be efficiently transcribed or translated; (3) proteins that promote cell survival or inhibit apoptosis so that progeny virus can mature and escape from the infected cell; (4) proteins that inhibit the host interferon response; and (5) proteins that downregulate host inflammatory or immune responses so that virus infection can proceed in an infected person to the maximum extent consistent with the survival of the virus and its efficient transmission to a new host. More complex viruses of the poxvirus or herpesvirus family encode many proteins that serve these functions. Some of these viral proteins have motifs similar to those of cell pro-

teins, while others are quite novel. Virology has increasingly focused on these more sophisticated strategies evolved by viruses to permit the establishment of long-term infection in humans and other animals. These strategies often provide unique insights into the control of cell growth, cell survival, macromolecular synthesis, proteolytic processing, immune or inflammatory suppression, immune resistance, cytokine mimicry, or cytokine blockade.

HOST RANGE   The concept of host range was originally based on the cell types in which a virus replicated in tissue culture. For the most part, the host range is limited by specific cell-surface proteins required for viral adsorption or penetration. Another common basis for host-range limitation is transcription from viral promoters. Most DNA viruses depend not only on cellular RNA polymerase II and the basal components of the cellular transcription complex but also on activated components and transcriptional accessory factors, both of which differ among differentiated tissues, among cells at various phases of the cell cycle, and between resting and cycling cells.

The concept of host range for virus infection in humans includes these factors and others since (1) most viruses infect more than one cell type in vivo, and (2) the viral life cycle and extent of viral replication can be affected by the differentiation and activation state of a given cell type. This point is particularly relevant for human papovavirus, herpesvirus, and lentivirus infections, in which vigorous replication during initial infection may be followed by quiescent or latent infection—a situation that allows the virus to persist.

VIRAL CYTOPATHIC EFFECTS AND INHIBITORS OF APOPTOSIS   The replication of almost all viruses has adverse effects on the infected cell, inhibiting cellular synthesis of DNA, RNA, or proteins. This inhibitory effect probably stems from the viruses' need to prevent or limit nonspecific, innate host resistance factors, including interferon (IFN). Most commonly, viruses specifically inhibit host protein synthesis by attacking a component of the translational initiation complex—frequently, a component that is not required for efficient translation of viral RNAs. Poliovirus protease 2A, for example, cleaves a cellular component of the complex that ordinarily facilitates translation of cell mRNAs by interacting with their cap structure. Poliovirus RNA is efficiently translated without a cap since it has an internal ribosome entry sequence. Influenza virus inhibits the processing of mRNA by snatching cap structures from nascent cell RNAs and using them as primers in the synthesis of viral mRNA. HSV has a virion tegument protein that inhibits cellular mRNA translation.

Apoptosis is the expected consequence of virus-induced inhibition of cellular macromolecular synthesis and viral nucleic acid replication. While the induction of apoptosis may be important for the release of some viruses (particularly nonenveloped viruses), many viruses have acquired genes or parts of genes that enable them to forestall infected-cell apoptosis. This delay may be advantageous in allowing the completion of viral replication. Adenoviruses and herpesviruses encode analogues of the cellular Bc12 protein, which blocks mitochondrial enhancement of proapoptotic stimuli. Poxviruses and some herpesviruses encode caspase inhibitors. Many viruses, including HPVs and adenoviruses, encode proteins that inhibit p53 or its downstream proapoptotic effects.

VIRAL INFECTION IN VIVO

The capsid and envelope of a virus protect its genome and permit its efficient transmission from cell to cell and to prospective hosts. Most common viral infections are spread by aerosolized particles, by ingestion of contaminated water or food, or by direct contact. In all these situations, infection begins on an epithelial or mucosal surface and spreads along it or from it to deeper tissues. Infection may then spread through the body via the bloodstream, lymphatics, or neural circuits. Parenteral inoculation also serves to transmit some viral infections among humans or from animals, including insects, to humans.

PRIMARY INFECTION The first (primary) episode of viral infection usually lasts from several days to several weeks. During this period, the concentration of virus at sites of infection rises and then falls, usually to unmeasurable levels. The rate at which the intensity of viral infection rises and falls at a given site depends on the accessibility of that organ or tissue to both the virus and systemic immune effectors, the intrinsic ability of the virus to replicate at that site, and endogenous nonspecific and specific resistance. Typically, infections with enterovirus, mumps virus, measles virus, rubella virus, rotavirus, influenza virus, AAV, adenovirus, HSV, and VZV are cleared from almost all sites within 3 to 4 weeks. Some of these viruses are especially proficient in altering or evading the innate and acquired immune responses; thus primary infection with AAV, EBV, or cytomegalovirus (CMV) can last for several months. Characteristically extending beyond several weeks are primary infections due to HBV, HCV, hepatitis D virus (HDV), HIV, HPV, and molluscum contagiosum virus. For some of these viruses (e.g., HPV, HBV, HCV, HDV, and molluscum contagiosum virus), the primary phase of infection is almost indistinguishable from the persistent phase.

Disease manifestations usually arise as a consequence of viral replication and the resultant inflammatory response at a specific site but do not necessarily correlate with levels of replication at that site. For example, the clinical manifestations of limited infection with poliovirus, enterovirus, rabies virus, measles virus, mumps virus, or HSV in neural cells are severe relative to the level of viral replication at mucosal surfaces. Similarly, significant morbidity may accompany in utero fetal infection with rubella virus or CMV.

Primary infections are cleared by nonspecific innate and specific adaptive immune responses. Thereafter, an immunocompetent host is usually immune to the disease manifestations of reinfection by the same virus. Immunity frequently does not prevent transient surface colonization on reexposure, persistent colonization, or even limited deeper infection.

PERSISTENT AND LATENT INFECTIONS Relatively few viruses cause persistent or latent infections. HBV, HCV, rabies virus, measles virus, HIV, HTLV, HPV, HHV, and some poxviruses are notable exceptions. The mechanisms for persistent infection vary widely. In persistent HCV infection and to a lesser extent in HIV infection, the high mutation rates in viral genome replication or reverse transcription significantly facilitate persistent infection, continuously yielding mutant viruses that have lost antigenic determinants to which the host has developed effective immune responses. HIV is also directly immunosuppressive, depleting CD4+ T lymphocytes and compromising CD8+ cytotoxic T-cell immune responsiveness. Moreover, HIV encodes a Nef protein that downmodulates major histocompatibility complex (MHC) class I expression, rendering HIV-infected cells partially resistant to immune CD8+ cytolysis. The high mutation rate and the magnitude of the viral load conspire to promote persistent infection with drug-resistant HIV mutants.

In contrast, DNA viruses have much lower mutation rates. Their persistence is due to their ability to establish latent infection and to reactivate from latency. In this instance, latency is defined as a state of infection in which the virus is not replicating. The complete viral genome is present and may be replicated by cellular DNA polymerase in conjunction with the cell genome replication. Viral genes associated with lytic infection are not expressed and infectious virus is not made. HPVs establish latent infection in basal epithelial cells, which replicate. Some of the progeny cells provide a stable supply of latently infected basal cells, while others go on to squamous differentiation and, in the process, become permissive for lytic viral infection. For herpesviruses, latent infection is established in nonreplicating neural cells (HSV and VZV) or in replicating cells of hematopoietic lineages [EBV and probably CMV, HHV-6, HHV-7, and Kaposi's sarcoma–associated herpesvirus (KSHV, also known as HHV-8)]. Reactivation from neural latency appears to be an intermittent process provoked by external stimuli, whereas reactivation from hematopoietic precursors appears to be a more continuous process. In their latent stage, HPV and herpesvirus genomes are largely hidden from the normal immune response. It is still not fully understood how partially latent and reactivated HPV and herpesvirus infections escape immediate and effective immune responses in highly immune hosts. HPV, HSV, and VZV may be somewhat protected because of their replication in middle and upper layers of the squamous epithelium—sites not routinely visited by immune and inflammatory cells. HSV and CMV are also known to encode proteins that downregulate MHC class I expression and antigenic peptide presentation on infected cells, thereby enabling these cells to escape CD8+ T lymphocyte cytotoxicity. Latent infection and intermittent reactivation perpetuate herpesvirus infections in human populations by allowing the viruses to persist in immune hosts and to be transmitted to the next generation of naive hosts.

Like other poxviruses, molluscum contagiosum virus cannot establish latent infection but rather causes persistent infection in hypertrophic lesions that last for months or years. This virus encodes a chemokine homologue that probably blocks inflammatory responses and an MHC class I analogue that may block cytotoxic T lymphocyte attack.

PERSISTENT VIRAL INFECTIONS AND CANCER Persistent viral infection is estimated to be the root cause of as many as 20% of human malignancies. For the most part, cancer is an accidental and highly unusual or long-term effect of infection with oncogenic human viruses. In these malignancies, viral infection is a critical and ultimately determinative early step, putting infected cells into cycle and enhancing their survival. An unusual virus-infected cell undergoes the subsequent genetic changes that permit the enhanced autonomous growth and survival characteristic of a highly malignant cell.

Most hepatocellular carcinoma is now believed to be caused by chronic inflammatory, immune, and regenerative responses to HBV or HCV infection. Epidemiologic data firmly link HBV and HCV infection to hepatocellular carcinoma. Studies in murine experimental models indicate that chronic liver injury and repair induced by virus-encoded proteins can result in hepatocellular cancer. In rare instances, HBV DNA integrates into cellular DNA—an event that probably contributes to the development of some tumors.

Almost all cervical carcinoma is caused by long-term persistent replication of "high-risk" genital HPV strains. Persistent, high-level HPV replication can result in the integration of a small fragment of the HPV genome encoding the HPV E6 and E7 proteins into chromosomal DNA. Integrations that result in overexpression of HPV type 16 or 18 E6 and E7 cause the loss of at least two major tumor-suppressive functions mediated by pRb and p53. This loss in turn causes profound changes in cell growth and survival. Nevertheless, subsequent chromosomal changes must occur over ensuing cycles of cell growth if a sufficiently malignant cell is to invade the surrounding tissues.

Similarly, long-term EBV infection and expression of the EBV oncogene LMP1 in latently infected epithelial cells appear to be critical early steps in the evolution of anaplastic nasopharyngeal carcinoma, a common malignancy in Chinese and North African populations. High-level LMP1 expression is also a hallmark of many cases of Hodgkin's disease. Among younger age groups, >50% of Hodgkin's disease tumors are clonally derived from an EBV-infected cell. The HTLV-I Tax and Rex proteins appear to be critical to the initiation of cutaneous adult T cell lymphoma/leukemias that may occur long after primary HTLV-I infection.

The EBV-related herpesvirus KSHV was identified in a search for the postulated sexually transmitted etiologic agent of Kaposi's sarcoma in HIV-infected individuals. Molecular data confirm the presence of KSHV DNA in all Kaposi's tumors, including those associated with HIV infection, transplantation, and familial transmission. KSHV infection is also etiologically implicated in pleural-effusion lymphomas and multicentric Castleman's disease, which are more common among HIV-infected than among HIV-uninfected people.

Evidence supporting a causal role of viral infection in these malignancies includes epidemiologic data, the presence of viral DNA in all tumor cells, the ability of the viruses to transform human cells in culture, the results of in vitro assays for transforming effects of specific viral genes on cell growth, and pathologic data indicating the expression of transforming viral genes in premalignant or malignant cells in vivo.

EBV is a unique example of a human virus that relies on the normal immune response to contain the potentially unrestrained growth of infected cells. In the initial stages of normal primary EBV infection, EBV "latently" infects B lymphocytes and expresses at least eight viral proteins that play no role in viral replication but cause the expansion of latently infected cells. These infected cells can grow indefinitely. Most of the viral proteins that cause this proliferative state are highly antigenic. These virus-infected cells, which can transiently constitute 10% of the circulating B lymphocyte population, are met with an overwhelming helper and cytotoxic T cell response during primary infection. The number of virus-infected cells then falls rapidly, and the one EBV-infected cell in a million that persists does not express most of the viral proteins that cause B cell proliferation. These persisting cells are the site of normal latent infection. Breakthrough growth of the EBV-infected B lymphocytes almost never occurs in immunocompetent hosts. However, in immunosuppressed AIDS patients or organ transplant recipients, EBV-infected B lymphocytes expressing the full set of growth-transforming genes may grow and cause self-sustained and potentially fatal lymphoproliferative disease. Clinical investigation has resulted in novel strategies for treating these virus-induced malignancies with EBV-specific T cells or with antibody to B cells.

RESISTANCE TO VIRAL INFECTIONS Resistance to viral infection is initially provided by factors that are not virus-specific. Physical protection is afforded by the cornified layers of the skin and by mucous secretions that continuously sweep over mucosal surfaces. Once the first cell is infected, viral infection induces IFNs, which are important local resistance factors. Viral infection may also trigger the release of other cytokines from infected cells; these cytokines may be chemotactic to inflammatory and immune cells. Viral protein epitopes expressed on the cell surface in the context of MHC class I and II HLA proteins attract T cells with appropriate receptors. Cytokines, inflammatory agents, and antigens released by virus-induced cell death further attract inflammatory cells, dendritic cells, granulocytes, natural killer (NK) cells, and B lymphocytes to the sites of initial infection and to draining lymph nodes. IFNs and NK cells are particularly important in containing viral infection for the first several days. Granulocytes and macrophages are also important in the phagocytosis and degradation of viruses, especially after an initial antibody response.

Some 7 to 10 days after infection, virus-specific antibody responses, virus-specific HLA class II–restricted CD4+ helper T lymphocyte responses, and virus-specific HLA class I–restricted CD8+ cytotoxic T lymphocyte responses emerge. These responses, whose magnitude typically increases over the second and third weeks of infection, are important in rapid recovery. Between the second and third weeks of infection, the antibody type usually changes from IgM to IgG; IgA antibody can then be detected at initially infected mucosal surfaces. Antibody may directly neutralize virus by binding to its surface and preventing its adsorption or penetration. Complement usually enhances antibody-mediated virus neutralization. Antibody and complement can also lyse virus-infected cells that express viral proteins on their surface. A cell infected with an enveloped virus usually expresses viral envelope glycoprotein components on its surface and is subject to destruction by antibodies and complement.

Antibody and CD4+/CD8+ T lymphocyte responses tend to persist for several months after primary infection. Antibody-producing lymphocytes persist in small numbers as memory cells and begin to proliferate rapidly in response to a second infection, providing an early barrier to reinfection with the same virus. Immunologic memory of T cell responses appears to be shorter-lived. Redevelopment of T cell immunity may take longer than secondary antibody responses, particularly when many years have elapsed between primary infection and reexposure. Persistent or latent and reactivating viral infections can result in sustained high-level T cell responses.

Some viruses have genes that alter innate and acquired host defenses. Adenoviruses encode small RNAs that inhibit IFN shutoff of infected-cell protein synthesis. Adenovirus E1A inhibits IFN-mediated changes in cell gene transcription. Adenovirus E3 proteins prevent TNF-induced cytolysis and block HLA class I antigen synthesis by the infected cell. HSV ICP47 and CMV US11 block class I antigen presentation. EBV encodes an interleukin (IL) 10 homologue that inhibits NK and T cell responses. Vaccinia virus B15R is an IL-1 receptor decoy. Vaccinia virus B8R is a soluble TNF receptor that blocks the effects of TNF. Vaccinia virus CrmA inhibits the ability of CD8+ cytotoxic cells to kill virus-infected cells. Some poxviruses and herpesviruses encode blockers of chemokines and thereby inhibit cellular inflammatory responses. The adoption of these strategies by viruses highlights the importance of these host resistance factors in containing viral infection as well as the importance of redundancy in host resistance. The ultimate success of a virus requires a live host to help it disseminate infection.

Much has been written about the role of specific aspects of the host immune response in containment of specific virus infections. Certainly, T lymphocyte disorders and T cell immunosuppression for the purpose of transplantation or as a consequence of HIV infection are associated with severe primary and reactivated herpesvirus infections. Antibody responses are important in most viral infections and may be fully protective in many RNA virus infections. Specific immunoglobulin therapy can ameliorate even herpesvirus infections. T lymphocyte responses may play a significant role in resistance to RNA virus infections. Cytotoxic T cells specific for influenza virus nucleoprotein may provide a measure of protection that is independent of viral changes in hemagglutinin.

Host resistance does not come without a price. Clearly, aspects of the host response contribute to the pathophysiologic manifestations and symptoms of viral infection. Inflammation at sites of viral infection can increase rates of local cell death. Moreover, immune responses to viral infection could, in principle, result in immune attack of related epitopes on normal cells, with consequent autoimmunity. While such effects have been demonstrated in experimental models, their role in the autoimmune manifestations of primary or recurrent human viral infections is uncertain.

INTERFERONS All human cells can synthesize IFN-α or -β in response to viral infection. These IFN responses are usually induced by the presence of double-strand viral RNA, which can be made by both RNA and DNA viruses. IFN-γ is not highly related to IFN-α or -β and is produced mainly by NK cells and by immune T lymphocytes responding to IL-12. IFN-α and -β bind to the IFN-α receptor, while IFN-γ binds to a different but related receptor. Both receptors signal through receptor-associated JAK kinases and other cytoplasmic proteins, including "STAT" proteins. STAT proteins are tyrosine-phosphorylated by JAK kinases, translocate to the nucleus, and transactivate promoters for specific cell genes. Three types of antiviral effects are induced by IFN at the transcriptional level. The first effect is attributable to the induction of 2'-5' oligo(A) synthetases, which require double-strand RNA for their activation. Activated synthetase polymerizes oligo(A) and thereby activates RNAse L, which in turn degrades single-strand RNA. The second effect takes place through the induction of PKR, a serine and threonine kinase that is also activated by double-strand RNA. PKR phosphorylates and negatively regulates the translational initiation factor eIF2-α, shutting down protein synthesis in the infected cell. A third effect is initiated through the induction of Mx proteins, a family of GTPases that is particularly important in inhibiting the replication of influenza virus and vesicular stomatitis virus (VSV). None of these IFN effects is directed specifically against the virus; infected-cell RNA and protein synthesis are globally inhibited by inhibiting cell protein synthesis. IFN probably contributes to the death of the infected cell.

DIAGNOSTIC VIROLOGY A wide variety of methods are now used to diagnose viral infection. Serology and viral isolation in tissue culture remain important standards. Acute- and convalescent-phase sera with rising titers of antibody to virus-specific antigens and a shift from IgM to IgG antibodies are generally accepted as diagnostic of acute viral infection. Traditionally, virus-specific antibodies have been detected by hemadsorption, hemagglutination, or indirect immunofluorescence. Immunofluorescence assays use fixed virus-infected cells as a target for serum antibodies. Hemadsorption and hemagglutination assays measure the ability of serum antibodies to inhibit RNA virus–induced erythrocyte adsorption or agglutination. Serologic diagnosis is based on a greater-than-fourfold rise in IgG antibody concentration when acute- and convalescent-phase serum samples are analyzed at the same time. A simultaneous fall in IgM antibody confirms recent primary viral infection. Immunofluorescence, hemadsorption, and hemagglutination assays for antiviral antibodies are labor-intensive and are being replaced by enzyme-linked immunosorbent assays (ELISAs). ELISAs generally use specific viral proteins purified from virus-infected cells or produced by recombinant DNA technology. These viral antigens are attached to a solid phase, where they can be incubated with serum, washed to eliminate nonspecific antibodies, and reacted with an enzyme-linked reagent to detect human IgG or IgM antibody specifically adhering to the viral antigen on the solid phase. The amount of antibody can then be quantitated by the intensity of a color reaction mediated by the linked enzyme. ELISAs can be sensitive and automated. Western blots can confirm the presence of antibody to multiple specific viral proteins simultaneously. The proteins are separated by size and transferred to an inert membrane, where they are incubated with serum antibodies. Western blots have an internal specificity control, since the level of reactivity for viral proteins can be compared with that for cellular proteins in the same sample. Western blots require individual evaluation and are inherently difficult to quantitate or automate.

Virus isolation in tissue culture is dependent on the infection of susceptible cells and amplification by viral replication in infected cells. Virus growing in tissue culture cells can frequently be identified by its effect under light microscopy. For example, HSV produces a typical cytopathic effect in rabbit kidney cells within 3 days. Other viral cytopathic effects may not be as diagnostically useful. Identification may require confirmation by staining with virus-specific monoclonal antibodies. Viruses growing in tissue culture can also be identified by hemadsorption or by interference; e.g., rubella virus–infected cells resist lysis by echovirus. Electron microscopy can identify the type of virus in tissue or tissue culture (assuming that the specimen has altered cell morphology, as observed by ordinary light microscopy).

The efficiency and speed of virus identification can be enhanced by combining short-term culture with immune detection. In assays with "shell vials" of tissue culture cells growing on a coverslip, viral infection can be detected by staining of the culture with a monoclonal antibody to a specific viral protein expressed early in viral replication. Thus, virus-infected cells can be detected within hours or days of inoculation; several rounds of infection would be required to produce a visible cytopathic effect.

Virus isolation in tissue culture depends on the collection of specimens from the appropriate site and the rapid transport of these specimens in the appropriate medium to the virology laboratory. Rapid transport maintains viral viability and limits bacterial and fungal overgrowth. Lipid-enveloped viruses are generally much more sensitive to freezing and thawing than nonenveloped viruses. The most appropriate site for culture depends on the pathogenesis of the virus in question. Nasopharyngeal, tracheal, or endobronchial aspirates are most appropriate for the identification of respiratory viruses. Sputum cultures generally are less appropriate because bacterial contamination and viscosity threaten tissue-culture cell viability. Aspirates of vesicular fluid are useful for isolation of HSV and VZV. Nasopharyngeal aspirates and stool specimens may be useful when the patient has fever and a rash and an enteroviral infection is suspected. Adenoviruses can be cultured from the urine of patients with hemorrhagic cystitis. CMV can frequently be isolated from cultures of urine or buffy coat. Biopsy material can be effectively cultured when viruses infect major organs, as in HSV encephalitis or adenovirus pneumonia. Virus isolation does not necessarily establish disease causality. Viruses can persistently or intermittently colonize normal human mucosal surfaces. Saliva can be positive for herpesviruses, and normal urine samples can be positive for CMV. Isolations from blood, cerebrospinal fluid (CSF), or tissue are more often diagnostic of significant viral infection.

Another method aimed at increasing the speed of viral diagnosis is direct testing for antigen or cytopathic effects. Virus-infected cells from the patient may be detected by staining with virus-specific monoclonal antibodies; e.g., epithelial cells obtained by nasopharyngeal aspiration can be stained with a variety of monoclonal antibodies to respiratory viruses. The Tzanck preparation can be used to detect multinucleated giant cells in HSV- or VZV-induced lesions. Tzanck preparations can be enhanced by the use of HSV- or VZV-specific monoclonal antibodies. Monoclonal antibodies can also be used in histopathology to identify virus-infected cells.

Advances in nucleic acid technology are revolutionizing diagnostic virology. The speed and sensitivity of tests that directly amplify minute amounts of viral nucleic acids present in specimens mean that detection no longer depends on viable virus and its replication. For example, amplification and detection of HSV nucleic acids in the CSF of patients with HSV encephalitis is a more sensitive detection method than culture of virus from CSF. The extreme sensitivity of these tests can be a problem, since subclinical infection or contamination can lead to false-positive results. Detection of viral nucleic acids does not necessarily indicate virus-induced disease. Herpesviruses can cause persistent asymptomatic infection.

Measurement of the amount of viral RNA or DNA in peripheral blood is becoming an important means for determining which patients are at increased risk for virus-induced disease and for evaluating clinical responses to antiviral chemotherapy. Nucleic acid technologies for RNA quantification are routinely used in AIDS patients to evaluate responses to antiviral agents and to detect resistance to or noncompliance with therapy. Viral-load measurements may also be useful for evaluating the treatment of patients with HBV and HCV infections. Direct staining with CMV-specific monoclonal antibodies to quantitate virus-infected cells in the peripheral blood or CMV antigenemia can be useful in identifying which immunosuppressed patients may be at risk for CMV-induced disease. CMV assays employing nucleic acid technologies for the same purpose have been approved for clinical use.

DRUG TREATMENT FOR VIRAL INFECTIONS Specific antiviral drugs have revolutionized treatment of herpes and HIV infections. Effective drugs have also been developed for influenza A and moderately effective drugs for respiratory syncytial virus and HCV infections. However, the emergence of drug-resistant strains in treated patients can limit therapeutic efficacy. The increased number of antiviral agents with different viral targets has made the identification of drug-resistant viruses clinically relevant, especially for HIV infection. Drug resistance in herpesviruses is a more unusual problem. HIV genotyping is a new method for the rapid identification of drug-resistant viruses. Resistance to reverse transcriptase or protease inhibitors has been associated with specific mutations in the reverse transcriptase or protease genes. Identification of these mutations by polymerase chain reaction amplification and nucleic acid sequencing can be clinically useful for determining which antiviral agents may still be effective. HCV genotyping may also identify patients who can benefit from combination chemotherapy.

IMMUNIZATION FOR THE PREVENTION OF VIRAL INFECTIONS Viral vaccines are among the outstanding accomplishments of medical science. Smallpox has been eradicated except as a potential weapon of biological warfare or bioterrorism (Chap. 205). Poliovirus eradication may soon follow. Measles can be contained or eliminated. Excess mortality due to influenza virus epidemics can be prevented, and the threat of influenza pandemics has decreased. Widespread HBV vaccination has dramatically lessened the frequency of acute and chronic hepatitis and is expected to lead to a dramatic decrease in the incidence of hepatocellular carcinoma. Rubella, mumps, and chickenpox viruses have been attenuated in culture, formulated into vaccines, and widely administered in the developed world. Purified proteins, genetically engineered live virus vaccines, and recombinant DNA-based strategies will make it possible to prevent severe infections with many other viruses. The evolutionary divergence of HIV and HCV and repeated high-level exposure in some populations complicate the development of effective vaccines for these agents. Immunogens that incorporate multiple B and T cell epitopes are likely to be useful for low-level exposures. Concerns about the use of smallpox and other viruses as weapons may create a need to maintain immunity to agents that are not naturally encountered.

VIRUSES AS NOVEL THERAPEUTIC AGENTS Viruses are being experimentally developed for the delivery of biotherapeutics or novel vaccines. Foreign genes can be inserted into viral nucleic acids, and the recombinant virus vectors can be used to infect the patient or the patient's cells ex vivo. Retroviruses integrate into the cell genome and have been used to functionally replace the abnormal gene in T cells of patients with severe combined immunodeficiency (SCID), thereby restoring immune function. Recombinant adenovirus, AAV, and retroviruses are being explored for use in diseases due to single-gene defects, such as cystic fibrosis and hemophilia. Recombinant poxviruses and adeno-

viruses are also being used experimentally as vaccine vectors. Viral vectors are being experimentally tested for expressing cytokines to improve immunity against tumor cells or for expressing proteins that can increase the sensitivity of tumor cells to chemotherapy.

For improved safety, nonreplicating viruses are frequently employed in clinical trial settings. Potential adverse events associated with virus-mediated gene transfer include the induction of inflammatory and antiviral immune responses. Adenoviruses contain many immunogenic proteins, and, since wild-type adenovirus infection is prevalent, immunity to adenovirus infection may reduce the efficacy of or enhance inflammatory responses to adenovirus gene therapy. Integration, another complication of virus-mediated gene therapy, is useful for permanent gene therapy, but integrations can induce disease by enhancing or interrupting the expression of important cellular genes.

FURTHER READING

FIELDS BN et al (eds): *Virology,* 4th ed. New York, Lippincott Williams & Wilkins, 2000

HACEIN-BEY-ABINA S et al: Sustained correction of X-linked severe combined immunodeficiency by ex vivo gene therapy. N Engl J Med 346:1185, 2002

HOLMES KV: SARS-associated coronavirus. N Engl J Med 348:1948, 2003

JOHNSON WE, DESROSIERS RC: Viral persistence: HIV's strategies of immune system evasion. Annu Rev Med 53:499, 2002

KATZE MG et al: Viruses and interferon: A fight for supremacy. Nat Rev Immunol 2:675, 2002

LENNETTE EH, SMITH TF (eds): *Laboratory Diagnosis of Viral Infections.* New York, Marcel Dekker, 1999

ROULSTON A et al: Viruses and apoptosis. Annu Rev Microbiol 53:577, 1999

162 ANTIVIRAL CHEMOTHERAPY, EXCLUDING ANTIRETROVIRAL DRUGS
Lindsey R. Baden, Raphael Dolin

The development of drugs for antiviral chemotherapy and chemoprophylaxis is a relatively recent but extremely active area of biomedical research. Significant progress has been made in recent years on new drugs for several viral infections. Despite these advances, the field of antiviral therapy—both the number of antiviral drugs and our understanding of their optimal use—continues to lag behind the field of antibacterial drug treatment, in which more than 60 years of experience have now been accumulated.

The development of antiviral drugs poses several challenges. Viruses replicate intracellularly and often employ host cell enzymes, macromolecules, and organelles for synthesis of viral particles. Therefore, useful antiviral compounds must discriminate between host and viral functions with a high degree of specificity; agents without such selectivity are likely to be too toxic for clinical use.

The development of laboratory assays to assist clinicians in the appropriate use of antiviral drugs is also in its infancy. Phenotypic and genotypic assays for resistance to antiviral drugs are becoming more widely available, and correlations of laboratory results with clinical outcomes in various settings are beginning to be defined. Of particular note has been the development of highly sensitive and specific methods to measure the concentration of virus in blood (*virus load*), which permit direct assessment of the antiviral effect of a given drug regimen in the host. Virus load measurements have been useful in recognizing the risk of disease progression in patients with certain viral infections and in identifying patients in whom antiviral chemotherapy might be of greatest benefit. Like any in vitro laboratory test, these tests yield results that are highly dependent on (and likely to vary with) the laboratory techniques employed.

Information regarding the pharmacokinetics of some antiviral drugs, particularly in diverse clinical settings, is limited. Assays to measure the concentrations of these drugs, especially of their active moieties within cells, are primarily research procedures and are not

widely available to clinicians. Thus, there are relatively few guidelines for adjusting dosages of antiviral agents to maximize antiviral activity and minimize toxicity. Clinical use of antiviral drugs must therefore be accompanied by particular vigilance with regard to unanticipated adverse effects.

Like that of other infections, the course of viral infections is profoundly affected by an interplay of the pathogen with a complex set of host defenses. The presence or absence of preexisting immunity and the ability to mount humoral and/or cell-mediated immune responses are important determinants of the outcome of viral infections. The state of the host's defenses needs to be considered when antiviral agents are utilized or evaluated.

As with any therapy, the optimal use of antiviral compounds requires a specific and timely diagnosis. For some viral infections, such as herpes zoster, the clinical manifestations are so characteristic that a diagnosis can be made on clinical grounds alone. For other viral infections, such as influenza A, epidemiologic information (e.g., the documentation of a community-wide outbreak) can be used to make a presumptive diagnosis with a high degree of accuracy. However, for most other viral infections, including herpes simplex encephalitis, cytomegaloviral infections other than retinitis, and enteroviral infections, diagnosis on clinical grounds alone cannot be accomplished with certainty. For such infections, rapid viral diagnostic techniques are of great importance. Considerable progress has been made in recent years in the development of such tests, which are now widely available for a number of viral infections.

Despite these complexities, the efficacy of a number of antiviral compounds has been clearly established in rigorously conducted and controlled studies. As summarized in Table 162-1, this chapter reviews the antiviral drugs that are currently approved or are likely to be considered for approval in the near future for use against viral infections other than those caused by HIV. Antiretroviral drugs are reviewed in Chap. 173.

TABLE 162-1 *Antiviral Chemotherapy and Chemoprophylaxis*

Infection	Drug	Route	Dosage	Comment
Influenza A and B				
Prophylaxis	Amantadine[a] or rimantadine[a]	Oral	Adults: 200 mg/d for period at risk Children ≤9 yrs: 5 mg/kg per day (maximum, 150 mg/d) Children ≥13 yrs: 75 mg/d	Therapy must continue for duration of outbreak. Dosage should be reduced for amantadine and rimantadine in patients with renal failure and the elderly. Drugs can be administered along with inactivated vaccine.
Treatment	Oseltamivir Zanamivir	Oral Inhaled orally	10 mg q12h for 5 days in adults and children ≥7 yrs old	Zanamivir and oseltamivir reduce symptoms by 1.0–1.5 and 1.3 days, respectively, in uncomplicated disease when started within 2 days of onset and are under study in complicated disease. Zanamivir may exacerbate bronchospasm in patients with asthma. Oseltamivir's side effects of nausea and vomiting can be reduced in frequency by administration with food. Both amantadine and rimantadine are effective in uncomplicated influenza. None of the above drugs has been thoroughly studied in complicated cases (e.g., pneumonia).
	Oseltamivir	Oral	75 mg bid for 5 days in adults and 2 mg/kg for 5 days up to a total of 45 mg bid in children 1–12 yrs old	
	Amantadine[a]	Oral	100–200 mg/d in adults and dosage for children as above for 5–7 days	
	Rimantadine[a]	Oral	100–200 mg/d for 5–7 days in adults	
RSV infection	Ribavirin	Small-particle aerosol	Administered continuously from reservoir containing 20 mg/mL for 3–6 days	Ribavirin is used for treatment of infants and young children hospitalized with RSV pneumonia and bronchiolitis.
CMV retinitis in immunocompromised host (AIDS)	Ganciclovir	IV	5 mg/kg bid for 14–21 days; then 5 mg/kg per day as maintenance dose	Ganciclovir, valganciclovir, foscarnet, and cidofovir are approved for treatment of CMV retinitis in patients with AIDS. They are also used for colitis, pneumonia, or "wasting" syndromes associated with CMV and for prevention of CMV disease in transplant recipients. Valganciclovir has largely supplanted oral ganciclovir and is frequently used in place of IV ganciclovir. Foscarnet is not myelosuppressive and is active against acyclovir- and ganciclovir-resistant herpesviruses.
		Oral	1 g tid as maintenance dose	
	Valganciclovir	Oral	900 mg bid for 21 days; then 900 mg/d as maintenance dose	
	Foscarnet	IV	60 mg/kg q8h for 14–21 days; then 90–120 mg/kg per day as maintenance dose	
	Cidofovir	IV	5 mg/kg once weekly for 2 weeks, then once every other week; given with probenecid	
Varicella				
Immunocompetent host	Acyclovir	Oral	20 mg/kg (maximum, 800 mg) 4 or 5 times daily for 5 days	Treatment confers modest clinical benefit when administered within 24 h of rash onset.
Immunocompromised host	Acyclovir	IV	500 mg/m^2 q8h for 7 days	A change to oral valacyclovir can be considered once fever has subsided and there is no evidence of visceral involvement.
Herpes simplex encephalitis	Acyclovir	IV	10 mg/kg q8h for 14–21 days	Results are optimal when therapy is initiated early. Some authorities recommend treatment for 21 days to prevent relapses.
Neonatal herpes simplex	Acyclovir	IV	10 mg/kg q8h for 14–21 days	Serious morbidity is frequent despite therapy. Prolonged oral administration of acyclovir after initial IV therapy has been suggested because of long-term sequelae associated with cutaneous recurrences of HSV infection.
Genital herpes simplex				
Primary (treatment)	Acyclovir	IV	5 mg/kg q8h for 5–10 days	The IV route is preferred for infections severe enough to warrant hospitalization or with neurologic complications.
		Oral	200 mg 5 times daily for 10 days	The oral route is preferred for patients whose condition does not warrant hospitalization. Adequate hydration must be maintained.
		Topical	5% ointment; 4–6 applications daily for 7–10 days	Topical use—largely supplemented by oral therapy—may obviate systemic administration to pregnant women. Systemic symptoms and untreated areas are not affected.
	Valacyclovir	Oral	1 g bid for 10 days	Valacyclovir appears to be as effective as acyclovir but can be administered less frequently.
	Famciclovir	Oral	250 mg bid for 5–10 days[b]	Famciclovir appears to be similar in effectiveness to acyclovir.
Recurrent (treatment)	Acyclovir Famciclovir Valacyclovir	Oral Oral Oral	200 mg 5 times daily for 5 days 125 mg bid for 5 days 500 mg bid for 3 days	Clinical effect is modest and is enhanced if therapy is initiated early. Treatment does not affect recurrence rates.

(continued)

TABLE 162-1—*(Continued)*

Infection	Drug	Route	Dosage	Comment
Recurrent (suppression)	Acyclovir	Oral	400 mg bid for ≥12 months	Suppressive therapy is recommended only for patients with at least 6–10 recurrences per year. "Breakthrough" occasionally takes place, and asymptomatic shedding of virus occurs. The need for suppressive therapy should be reevaluated after 1 year. Suppression with valacyclovir reduces transmission of genital HSV among discordant couples.
	Valacyclovir	Oral	500–1000 mg daily	
	Famciclovir	Oral	125–250 mg bid	
Mucocutaneous herpes simplex in immuno-compromised host Treatment	Acyclovir	IV	250 mg/m² q8h for 7 days	Choice of IV or oral route depends on severity of infection and patient's ability to take oral medication. Oral or IV treatment has supplanted topical therapy except for small, easily accessible lesions. Foscarnet is used for acyclovir-resistant viruses.
		Oral	400 mg 5 times daily for 10 days	
		Topical	5% ointment; 4–6 applications daily for 7 days or until healed	
	Valacyclovir	Oral	1 g tid for 7 days[b]	
	Famciclovir	Oral	500 mg bid for 4 days[c]	
Prevention of recurrences during intense immunosuppression	Acyclovir	Oral	200 mg qid	Treatment is administered during periods when intense immunosuppression is expected—e.g., during antitumor chemotherapy or after transplantation—and is usually continued for 2–3 months.
		IV	5 mg/kg q12h	
	Valacyclovir	Oral	1 g tid[b]	
	Famciclovir	Oral	500 mg bid[b]	
Herpes simplex orolabialis (recurrent)	Penciclovir	Topical	1.0% cream applied q2h during waking hours for 4 days	Treatment shortens healing time and symptoms by 0.5–1.0 day (compared with placebo).
	Valacyclovir	Oral	2 g q12h for 1 day	Therapy begun at earliest symptom reduces disease duration by 1 day.
	Famciclovir[b]	Oral	500 mg tid for 5 days	Therapy begun 48 h after UV light exposure decreases time to healing by 2 days.
	Docosanol[d]	Topical	10% cream 5 times daily until healed	Application at initial symptoms reduces healing time by 1 day.
Herpes simplex keratitis	Trifluridine	Topical	1 drop of 1% ophthalmic solution q2h while awake (maximum, 9 drops daily)	Therapy should be undertaken in consultation with an ophthalmologist.
	Vidarabine	Topical	0.5-in. ribbon of 3% ophthalmic ointment 5 times daily	
Herpes zoster Immunocompromised host	Acyclovir	IV	500 mg/m² q8h for 7 days	Effectiveness in localized zoster is most marked when treatment is given early. Foscarnet may be used for VZV infections that are resistant to acyclovir.
		Oral	800 mg 5 times daily for 7 days	
	Famciclovir	Oral	500 mg tid for 10 days[b]	
Immunocompetent host	Valacyclovir	Oral	1 g tid for 7 days	Valacyclovir may be more effective than acyclovir for pain relief; otherwise, it has a similar effect on cutaneous lesions and should be given within 72 h of rash onset.
	Famciclovir	Oral	500 mg q8h for 7 days	The duration of postherpetic neuralgia is shorter than with placebo. Famciclovir showed overall efficacy similar to that of acyclovir in a comparative trial. It should be given ≤72 h of rash onset.
	Acyclovir	Oral	800 mg 5 times daily for 7–10 days	Acyclovir causes faster resolution of skin lesions than placebo and provides some relief of acute symptoms if given within 72 h of rash onset. Combined with tapering doses of prednisone, acyclovir improves quality-of-life outcomes.
Herpes zoster ophthalmicus	Acyclovir	Oral	600 mg 5 times daily for 10 days	Treatment reduces ocular complications, including ocular keratitis and uveitis.
Condyloma acuminatum	IFN-α2b	Intralesional	1 million units per wart (maximum of 5) thrice weekly for 3 weeks)	Intralesional treatment frequently results in regression of warts, but lesions often recur. Parenteral administration may be useful if lesions are numerous.
	IFN-αn3	Intralesional	250,000 units per wart (maximum of 10) twice weekly for up to 8 weeks	
Chronic hepatitis B	IFN-α2b	SC or IM	5 million units daily or 10 million units thrice weekly for 16 weeks	Hepatitis B e antigen and DNA are eliminated in 33–37% of cases. Histopathologic improvement is also seen.
	Lamivudine	Oral	100 mg/d for 12–18 months; 150 mg bid as part of therapy	Efficacy similar to that of IFN but better tolerated. Resistance develops in 24% of recipients.

(continued)

TABLE 162-1 *Antiviral Chemotherapy and Chemoprophylaxis—(Continued)*

Infection	Drug	Route	Dosage	Comment
	Adefovir dipivoxil	Oral	10 mg/d for 12 months	A return of ALT levels to normal is documented in 48–72% of recipients, improved liver histopathology in 53–64%. Adefovir is effective in lamivudine-resistant hepatitis B. Renal functions should be monitored.
Chronic hepatitis C	IFN-α2a or -α2b	SC or IM	3 million units thrice weekly for 12–18 months	A return of ALT levels to normal is documented in 54% of recipients but is sustained in only 28%. Improvement in liver histopathology is seen.
	IFN-α2b/ribavirin	SC or IM (IFN)/ oral (ribavirin)	3 million units thrice weekly (IFN)/1000–1200 mg daily (ribavirin) for 6–12 months	Combination therapy results in sustained responses in up to 40–50% of all recipients.
	Pegylated-IFN-α2b	SC	1 μg/kg weekly for 12–24 months	The slower clearance of pegylated IFNs than of standard IFNs permits once-weekly administration. The pegylated formulations appear to be superior to standard IFNs in tolerability and efficacy, both as monotherapy and in combination with ribavirin. Sustained virologic responses were seen in 42–46% of genotype 1 patients and in 76–82% of those with genotype 2 or 3.
	Pegylated-IFN-α2a	SC	180 μg/kg weekly for 12–24 months	
	Pegylated-IFN-α2b/ribavirin	SC (IFN)/oral (ribavirin)	1 μg/kg weekly (IFN)/800–1200 mg daily (ribavirin) for 12–24 months	
	Pegylated-IFN-α2a/ribavirin	SC (IFN)/oral (ribavirin)	180 μg/kg weekly (IFN)/1000–1200 mg daily (ribavirin) for 12–24 months	
	IFN alfacon	SC	9–15 μg thrice weekly for 6–12 months	Doses of 9 and 15 μg are equivalent to IFN-α2a or -α2b doses of 3 million units and 5 million units, respectively.
Chronic hepatitis D	IFN-α2a or -α2b	SC or IM	9 million units thrice weekly for 12 months	The overall efficacy and the optimal regimen and duration of therapy have not been established. Responses are usually not sustained when therapy is stopped.

[a] Influenza A only.
[b] Not approved for this indication by the U.S. Food and Drug Administration (FDA).
[c] Approved by the FDA for treatment of HIV-infected individuals.

[d] Active ingredient: behenyl alcohol. Available without prescription.
Abbreviations: ALT, alanine aminotransferase; CMV, cytomegalovirus; HSV, herpes simplex virus; IFN, interferon; RSV, respiratory syncytial virus; UV, ultraviolet.

ANTIVIRAL DRUGS ACTIVE AGAINST RESPIRATORY INFECTIONS

AMANTADINE AND RIMANTADINE Amantadine and the closely related compound rimantadine are primary symmetric amines. Their antiviral activity is limited to influenza A viruses, whose replication they inhibit by interfering with the uncoating of virus after infection of the cell. This interference is attributable to the agents' interaction with the influenza A M2 matrix protein, during which the ion channel function of M2 is inhibited. A substitution of a single amino acid at critical sites in the M2 protein can result in a virus that is resistant to amantadine and rimantadine.

Amantadine and rimantadine have been demonstrated to be effective in the prophylaxis of influenza A in large-scale studies of young adults and in less extensive studies of children and elderly subjects. In such studies, efficacy rates of 55 to 80% in the prevention of influenza-like illness were noted, and even higher rates were reported when virus-specific attack rates were calculated. Amantadine and rimantadine have also been demonstrated to be effective in the treatment of influenza A infection in studies involving predominantly young adults and, to a lesser extent, children. Administration of these compounds within 24 to 72 h after the onset of illness has resulted in a reduction of the duration of signs and symptoms by ~50% from that in a placebo-treated group. The effect on signs and symptoms of illness is superior to that of commonly used antipyretic-analgesics. Only anecdotal reports are available concerning the efficacy of amantadine or rimantadine in the prevention or treatment of complications of influenza (e.g., pneumonia).

Amantadine and rimantadine are available only in oral formulations and are ordinarily administered to adults once or twice daily, with a dosage of 100 to 200 mg/d. Despite their structural similarities, the pharmacokinetics of the two compounds are different. Amantadine is not metabolized and is excreted almost entirely by the kidney, with a half-life of 12 to 17 h and peak plasma concentrations of 0.4 μg/mL. Rimantadine is extensively metabolized to hydroxylated derivatives and has a half-life of 30 h. Only 30 to 40% of an orally administered dose is recovered in the urine. The peak plasma levels of rimantadine are approximately half those of amantadine, but rimantadine is concentrated in respiratory secretions to a greater extent than amantadine. For prophylaxis, the compounds must be administered daily for the period at risk (i.e., the peak duration of the outbreak). For therapy, amantadine or rimantadine is generally administered for 5 to 7 days.

Although these compounds are generally well tolerated, 5 to 10% of amantadine recipients experience mild central nervous system side effects consisting primarily of dizziness, anxiety, insomnia, and difficulty in concentrating. These effects are rapidly reversible upon cessation of the drug's administration. At a dose of 200 mg/d, rimantadine is better tolerated than amantadine; in a large-scale study of young adults, adverse effects were no more frequent among rimantadine recipients than among placebo recipients. Seizures and worsening of congestive heart failure have also been reported in patients treated with amantadine, although a causal relationship has not been established. The dosage of amantadine should be reduced to ≤100 mg/d in patients with renal insufficiency [i.e., a creatinine clearance (Cr_{Cl}) rate of <50 mL/min] and in the elderly. A rimantadine dose of 100 mg/d should be used for patients with a Cr_{Cl} of <10 mL/min and in the elderly. Resistance to amantadine and rimantadine can be induced readily in vitro. The emergence and probable transmission of virus resistant to these drugs have also been noted in vivo after their use for the treatment of children or adults. In the United States, both amantadine and rimantadine are approved for the prophylaxis and treatment of influenza A in adults and for prophylaxis in children. Amantadine is also approved for the treatment of influenza A in children.

ZANAMIVIR AND OSELTAMIVIR Influenza viral neuraminidase is essential for release of the virus from infected cells and for its subsequent spread throughout the respiratory tract of the infected host. The enzyme cleaves terminal sialic acid residues, thus destroying the cellular receptors recognized by the viral hemagglutinin. Zanamivir, a sialic acid analogue, is a highly active and specific inhibitor of the neuraminidases of influenza A and B viruses. Oseltamivir is another neuraminidase inhibitor that is a transition-state analogue of sialic acid cleavage. Its antineuraminidase activity is similar to that of zanamivir. Oseltamivir phosphate is an ethyl ester prodrug that is converted to oseltamivir carboxylate by esterases in the liver. Both zanamivir and oseltamivir act through competitive and reversible inhibition of the active site of influenza A and B viral neuraminidases and have relatively little effect on mammalian cell enzymes. As would be expected from their different mechanisms of action, zanamivir and oseltamivir are active against strains of influenza A virus that are resistant to amantadine and rimantadine.

Zanamivir has low oral bioavailability. It is inhaled orally via a hand-held inhaler. By this route, ~15% of the dose is deposited in the lower respiratory tract, and low plasma levels of the drug are detected. Orally administered oseltamivir has a bioavailability of >60% and a plasma half-life of 7 to 9 h. The drug is excreted unmetabolized, primarily by the kidneys.

Intranasal inhaled zanamivir is generally well tolerated, although exacerbations of asthma may occur. The toxicities most frequently encountered with orally administered oseltamivir are nausea, gastrointestinal discomfort, and (less commonly) vomiting. Gastrointestinal discomfort is usually transient and is less likely if the drug is administered with food. No serious clinical or laboratory toxicities have yet been reported with zanamivir or oseltamivir in clinical trials.

Inhaled zanamivir and orally administered oseltamivir have been effective in the treatment of naturally occurring influenza A or B in otherwise-healthy adults. In placebo-controlled studies, illness has been shortened by 1 to 1.5 days of therapy with either of these drugs when administered within 2 days of onset. Once-daily inhaled zanamivir or orally administered oseltamivir provides effective prophylaxis against laboratory-documented influenza A–associated illness. The emergence of viruses resistant to zanamivir or oseltamivir appears to be infrequent in clinical studies carried out thus far.

Zanamivir and oseltamivir have been approved by the U.S. Food and Drug Administration (FDA) for treatment of influenza in adults and in children (those ≥7 years old for zanamivir and those ≥1 year old for oseltamivir) who have been symptomatic for ≤2 days. Oseltamivir is approved for prophylaxis of influenza in individuals ≥13 years of age.

RIBAVIRIN   Ribavirin is a synthetic nucleoside analogue that inhibits a wide range of RNA and DNA viruses. The mechanism of action of ribavirin is not completely defined and may be different for different groups of viruses. Ribavirin-5′-monophosphate blocks the conversion of inosine-5′-monophosphate to xanthosine-5′-monophosphate and interferes with the synthesis of guanine nucleotides as well as that of both RNA and DNA. Ribavirin-5′-monophosphate also inhibits capping of virus-specific messenger RNA in certain viral systems. In studies demonstrating the effectiveness of ribavirin in the treatment of respiratory syncytial virus (RSV) infection in infants, the compound has been administered as a small-particle aerosol. It has been used less extensively to treat parainfluenza virus infections in children and influenza A and B virus infections in young adults. In infants with RSV infection who were given ribavirin by continuous aerosol for 3 to 6 days, illness and lower respiratory tract signs resolved more rapidly and arterial oxygen desaturation was less pronounced than in placebo-treated groups. Ribavirin has also had a beneficial clinical effect in infants with RSV infection who require mechanical ventilation. Aerosolized ribavirin has been administered to older children and adults with severe RSV and parainfluenza virus infections (including immunosuppressed patients), but the benefit of this treatment, if any, is unclear. In RSV infections in immunosuppressed patients, ribavirin is often given in combination with immunoglobulins.

Orally administered ribavirin has not been effective in the treatment of influenza A virus infections. Intravenous or oral ribavirin has reduced mortality among patients with Lassa fever; it has been particularly effective in this regard when given within the first 6 days of illness. Intravenous ribavirin has been reported to be of clinical benefit in the treatment of hemorrhagic fever with renal syndrome caused by Hantaan virus and as therapy for Argentinian hemorrhagic fever. Moreover, oral ribavirin has been recommended for the treatment and prophylaxis of Congo-Crimean hemorrhagic fever. Intravenous ribavirin is being evaluated as therapy for the hemorrhagic fever with pulmonary syndrome caused by newly described hantaviruses in the United States. Oral administration of ribavirin reduces serum aminotransferase levels in patients with chronic hepatitis C virus (HCV) infection; since it appears not to reduce serum HCV RNA levels, the mechanism of this effect is unclear. The drug provides an added beneficial effect when given by mouth in doses of 800 to 1200 mg/d in combination with interferon (IFN) α2b or α2a (see below), and the ribavirin/IFN combination has been approved for the treatment of patients with chronic HCV infection.

Large doses of ribavirin administered orally (800 to 1000 mg/d) have been associated with reversible hematopoietic toxicity. This effect has not been observed with aerosolized ribavirin, apparently because little drug is absorbed systemically. Aerosolized administration of ribavirin is generally well tolerated but occasionally is associated with bronchospasm, rash, or conjunctival irritation. Aerosolized ribavirin has been licensed for treatment of RSV infection in infants and should be administered under close supervision—particularly in the setting of mechanical ventilation, where precipitation of the drug is possible. Health care workers exposed to the drug have experienced minor toxicity, including eye and respiratory tract irritation. Because ribavirin is mutagenic, teratogenic, and embryotoxic, its use is generally contraindicated in pregnancy. Its administration as an aerosol poses a risk to pregnant health care workers.

PLECONARIL   Pleconaril is an investigational drug active in vitro against picornavirus replication, including >90% of the most commonly isolated enterovirus types and 80% of rhinovirus serotypes. Its mechanism of action is through binding to a specific hydrophobic pocket in the viral capsid, which prevents attachment and/or uncoating of the virus. Pleconaril is poorly water soluble and is formulated as an oral suspension. It is generally well tolerated; the most frequently reported adverse effects are headache, nausea, diarrhea, and gastrointestinal discomfort, which have occurred at rates similar to those among placebo recipients. Pleconaril treatment of adults with enterovirus meningitis decreased the overall duration of illness and headache and reduced the use of analgesics from that by placebo recipients. A large-scale clinical study demonstrated a mild therapeutic effect on rhinovirus-associated colds, but pleconaril was deemed to be of insufficient benefit to gain approval by an FDA advisory panel.

ANTIVIRAL DRUGS ACTIVE AGAINST HERPESVIRUS INFECTIONS

ACYCLOVIR AND VALACYCLOVIR   Acyclovir is a highly potent and selective inhibitor of the replication of certain herpesviruses, including herpes simplex virus (HSV) types 1 and 2, varicella-zoster virus (VZV), and Epstein-Barr virus (EBV). It is relatively ineffective in the treatment of human cytomegalovirus (CMV) infections; however, some studies have indicated its effectiveness in the prevention of CMV-associated disease in immunosuppressed patients. Valacyclovir, the L-valyl ester of acyclovir, is converted almost entirely to acyclovir by intestinal and hepatic hydrolysis after oral administration. Valacyclovir has pharmacokinetic advantages over orally administered acyclovir: it exhibits significantly greater oral bioavailability, results in higher blood levels, and can be given less frequently than acyclovir (two or three rather than five times daily).

The high degree of selectivity of acyclovir is related to its mechanism of action, which requires that the compound first be phosphorylated to acyclovir monophosphate. This phosphorylation occurs efficiently in herpesvirus-infected cells by means of a virus-coded thymidine kinase. In uninfected mammalian cells, little phosphorylation of acyclovir occurs, and the drug is therefore concentrated in herpesvirus-infected cells. Acyclovir monophosphate is subsequently converted by host cell kinases to a triphosphate that is a potent inhibitor of virus-induced DNA polymerase but has relatively little effect on host cell DNA polymerase. Acyclovir triphosphate can also be incorporated into viral DNA, with early chain termination.

Acyclovir is available in intravenous, oral, and topical forms, while valacyclovir is available in an oral formulation. Intravenous acyclovir is markedly effective in the treatment of mucocutaneous HSV infections in immunocompromised hosts, reducing time to healing, duration of pain, and virus shedding. When administered prophylactically during periods of intense immunosuppression (e.g., related to chemotherapy for leukemia or transplantation) and before the development of lesions, intravenous acyclovir reduces the frequency of HSV-associated disease. After prophylaxis is discontinued, HSV lesions recur. Intravenous acyclovir is also effective in the treatment of HSV encephalitis; two comparative trials have indicated that acyclovir is more effective than vidarabine for this indication (see below). Because VZV is generally less sensitive to acyclovir than is HSV, higher doses of acyclovir must be used to treat VZV infections. In immunocompromised patients with herpes zoster, intravenous acyclovir reduces the frequency of cutaneous dissemination and visceral complications and—in one comparative trial—was more effective than vidarabine. Acyclovir, administered orally at doses of 800 mg five times a day, had a modest beneficial effect on localized herpes zoster lesions in both immunocompromised and immunocompetent patients. Combination of acyclovir with a tapering regimen of prednisone appeared to be more effective than acyclovir alone in terms of quality-of-life outcomes in immunocompetent herpes zoster patients over age 50. A comparative study of acyclovir (800 mg orally five times daily) and valacyclovir (1 g orally tid) in immunocompetent patients with herpes zoster indicated that the latter drug may be more effective in eliciting the resolution of zoster-associated pain. Orally administered acyclovir (600 mg five times a day) reduced complications of herpes zoster ophthalmicus in a placebo-controlled trial.

In normal children with chickenpox, acyclovir—administered at 20 mg/kg (up to a maximum of 800) four times daily, within 24 h of the onset of rash—resulted in a modest overall clinical benefit. Intravenous acyclovir has also been reported to be effective in the treatment of immunocompromised children with chickenpox.

The most widespread use of acyclovir is in the treatment of genital HSV infections. Intravenous or oral acyclovir or oral valacyclovir has shortened the duration of symptoms, reduced virus shedding, and accelerated healing when employed for the treatment of primary genital HSV infections. Oral acyclovir and valacyclovir have also had a modest effect in treatment of recurrent genital HSV infections. However, the failure of treatment of either primary or recurrent disease to reduce the frequency of subsequent recurrences has indicated that acyclovir is ineffective in eliminating latent infection. Chronic oral administration of acyclovir 1 to 6 years or longer or of valacyclovir for 1 year or longer has reduced the frequency of recurrences markedly during therapy; once the drug is discontinued, lesions recur. In one study, suppressive therapy with valacyclovir (500 mg once daily for 8 months) reduced transmission of HSV-2 genital infections among discordant couples by 50%. A modest effect on herpes labialis (i.e., reduction of disease duration by 1 day) was seen when valacyclovir was administered upon detection of the first symptom of a lesion at a dose of 2 g every 12 h for 1 day. In AIDS patients, chronic or intermittent administration of acyclovir has been associated with the development of HSV and VZV strains resistant to the action of the drug and with clinical failures. The most common mechanism of resistance is a deficiency of the virus-induced thymidine kinase. Patients with HSV or VZV infections resistant to acyclovir have frequently responded to foscarnet.

With the availability of the oral and intravenous forms, there are few indications for topical acyclovir, although treatment with this formulation has been modestly beneficial in primary genital HSV infections and in mucocutaneous HSV infections in immunocompromised hosts.

Overall, acyclovir is remarkably well tolerated and is generally free of toxicity. The most frequently encountered form of toxicity is renal dysfunction, particularly after rapid intravenous administration or with inadequate hydration. Central nervous system changes, including lethargy and tremors, are occasionally reported, primarily in immunosuppressed patients. However, whether these changes are related to acyclovir, to concurrent administration of other therapy, or to underlying infection remains unclear. Acyclovir is excreted primarily unmetabolized by the kidney, via both glomerular filtration and tubular secretion. Approximately 15% of a dose of acyclovir is metabolized to 9-[(carboxymethoxy)methyl]guanine or other minor metabolites. Reduction in dosage is indicated in patients with a Cr_{Cl} of <50 mL/min per 1.73 m^2. The half-life of acyclovir is ~3 h in normal adults, the peak plasma concentration after a 1-h infusion of a dose of 5 mg/kg is 9.8 μg/mL. Approximately 22% of an orally administered acyclovir dose is absorbed, and peak plasma concentrations of 0.3 to 0.9 μg/mL are attained after administration of a 200-mg dose. Acyclovir penetrates relatively well into the cerebrospinal fluid (CSF), with concentrations approaching half of those found in plasma.

Acyclovir causes chromosomal breakage at high doses, but its administration to pregnant women has not been associated with fetal abnormalities. Nonetheless, the potential risks and benefits of acyclovir should be carefully assessed before the drug is used in pregnancy.

Valacyclovir exhibits three to five times greater bioavailability than acyclovir. The concentration-time curve for valacyclovir, given as 1 g by mouth three times daily, is similar to that for acyclovir, given as 5 mg/kg intravenously every 8 h. The safety profiles of valacyclovir and acyclovir are similar, although thrombotic thrombocytopenic purpura/hemolytic-uremic syndrome has been reported in immunocompromised patients who have received high doses (8 g/day) of valacyclovir. Valacyclovir is approved for the treatment of herpes zoster and for initial and recurrent episodes of genital HSV infections in immunocompetent adults as well as for suppressive treatment of genital herpes. Although it has not been extensively studied in other herpesvirus infections, many consultants use valacyclovir rather than oral acyclovir in clinical settings where the latter has been approved because of valacyclovir's superior pharmacokinetics and more convenient dosing schedule.

CIDOFOVIR Cidofovir is a phosphonate nucleotide analogue of cytosine. Its major use is in CMV infections, particularly retinitis, but it is active against a broad range of herpesviruses, including HSV, human herpesvirus (HHV) type 6, HHV-8, and certain other DNA viruses such as polyomaviruses, papillomaviruses, adenoviruses, and poxviruses, including variola (smallpox) and vaccinia. Cidofovir does not require initial phosphorylation by virus-induced kinases; the drug is phosphorylated by host cell enzymes to cidofovir diphosphate, which is a competitive inhibitor of viral DNA polymerases and, to a lesser extent, of host cell DNA polymerases. Incorporation of cidofovir diphosphate slows or terminates nascent DNA chain elongation. Cidofovir is active against HSV isolates that are resistant to acyclovir because of absent or altered thymidine kinase and against CMV isolates that are resistant to ganciclovir because of UL97 mutations. Cidofovir is usually active against foscarnet-resistant CMV, although cross-resistance to foscarnet as well as to ganciclovir has been described.

Cidofovir has poor oral availability and is administered intravenously. It is excreted primarily by the kidney and has a plasma half-life of 2.6 h. Cidofovir diphosphate's intracellular half-life of >48 h is the basis for the recommended dosing regimen of 5 mg/kg once a week for the initial 2 weeks and then 5 mg/kg every other week. The major toxic effect of cidofovir is proximal renal tubular injury, as manifested by elevated serum creatinine levels and proteinuria. The risk of nephrotoxicity can be reduced by vigorous saline hydration and by concomitant oral administration of probenecid. Neutropenia, rashes, and gastrointestinal tolerance may also occur.

Intravenous cidofovir has been approved for the treatment of CMV retinitis in AIDS patients who are intolerant of ganciclovir or foscarnet or in whom those drugs have failed. In a controlled study, a maintenance dosage of 5 mg/kg a week administered to AIDS patients reduced the progression of CMV retinitis from that seen at 3 mg/kg. Intravenous cidofovir has been reported anecdotally to be effective therapy for acyclovir-resistant mucocutaneous HSV infections. Likewise, topically administered cidofovir is reportedly beneficial against these infections in HIV patients; it is also being studied for the treatment of anogenital warts. Intravenous cidofovir is being evaluated as therapy for progressive multifocal leukoencephalopathy and for Kaposi's sarcoma. An ophthalmic formulation is being studied as treatment for adenoviral keratoconjunctivitis. Intravitreal cidofovir has been used to treat CMV retinitis but has been associated with significant toxicity.

FOMIVIRSEN Fomivirsen is the first antisense oligonucleotide approved by the FDA for therapy in humans. This phosphorothioate oligonucleotide, 21 nucleotides in length, inhibits CMV replication through interaction with CMV messenger RNA. Fomivirsen is complementary to messenger transcripts of the major immediate early region 2 (IE2) of CMV, which codes for proteins regulating viral gene expression. In addition to its antisense mechanism of action, fomivirsen may exert activity against CMV through inhibition of viral adsorption to cells as well as direct inhibition of viral replication. Because of its different mechanism of action, fomivirsen is active against CMV isolates that are resistant to nucleoside or nucleotide analogues, such as ganciclovir, foscarnet, or cidofovir.

Fomivirsen has been approved for intravitreal administration in the treatment of CMV retinitis in AIDS patients who have failed to respond to other treatments or cannot tolerate them. Injections of 330 mg every 2 weeks have resulted in significant reductions in the rate of progression of CMV retinitis. The major toxicity is ocular inflammation, including vitritis and iritis, which usually responds to topically administered glucocorticoids.

GANCICLOVIR AND VALGANCICLOVIR An analogue of acyclovir, ganciclovir is active against HSV and VZV and is markedly more active than acyclovir against CMV. Ganciclovir triphosphate inhibits CMV DNA polymerase and can be incorporated into CMV DNA, whose elongation it eventually terminates. In HSV- and VZV-infected cells, ganciclovir is phosphorylated by virus-encoded thymidine kinases; in CMV-infected cells, it is phosphorylated by a viral kinase encoded by the UL97 gene. Ganciclovir triphosphate is present in tenfold higher concentrations in CMV-infected cells than in uninfected cells. Ganciclovir is approved for the treatment of CMV retinitis in immunosuppressed patients and for the prevention of CMV disease in transplant recipients. It is widely used for the treatment of other CMV-associated syndromes, including pneumonia, esophagogastrointestinal infections, hepatitis, and "wasting" illness.

Ganciclovir is available for intravenous or oral administration. Because its oral bioavailability is low (5 to 9%), relatively large doses (1 g three times daily) must be administered by this route. Oral ganciclovir has largely been supplanted by valganciclovir, which is the L-valyl ester of ganciclovir. Valganciclovir is well absorbed orally, with a bioavailability of 60%, and is rapidly hydrolyzed to ganciclovir in the intestine and liver. The area under the curve for a 900-mg dose of valganciclovir is equivalent to that for 5 mg/kg of ganciclovir given intravenously, although peak serum concentrations are ~40% lower for valganciclovir. The serum half-life is 3.5 h after intravenous administration of ganciclovir and 4.0 h after oral administration of valganciclovir. Ganciclovir is excreted primarily by the kidneys in unmetabolized form, and its dosage should be reduced in cases of renal failure. The most commonly employed dosage for initial intravenous therapy is 5 mg/kg every 12 h for 14 to 21 days; this regimen is followed by an intravenous maintenance dose of 5 mg/kg per day or five times per week, possibly for as long as immunosuppression persists. For oral therapy with valganciclovir, the dose is 900 mg twice daily for 21 days followed by 900 mg once a day for maintenance,

with dose adjustment in patients with renal dysfunction. Intraocular ganciclovir, given by either intravitreal injection or intraocular implantation, has also been used to treat CMV retinitis.

Ganciclovir is effective as prophylaxis against CMV-associated disease in organ and bone marrow transplant recipients. Oral ganciclovir administered prophylactically to AIDS patients with CD4+ cell counts of $<100/\mu L$ has provided protection against the development of CMV retinitis. However, the long-term benefits of this approach to prophylaxis in AIDS patients have not been established, and most experts do not recommend the use of oral ganciclovir for this purpose. As already mentioned, valganciclovir has supplanted oral ganciclovir in settings where oral prophylaxis or therapy is considered.

The administration of ganciclovir has been associated with profound bone marrow suppression, particularly neutropenia, which significantly limits the drug's use in many patients. Bone marrow toxicity is potentiated when other bone marrow suppressants, such as zidovudine, are used concomitantly.

Resistance has been noted in CMV isolates obtained after therapy with ganciclovir, especially in patients with AIDS. Such resistance may develop through a mutation in either the viral UL97 gene or the viral DNA polymerase. Ganciclovir-resistant isolates are usually sensitive to foscarnet (see below) or cidofovir (see above).

FAMCICLOVIR AND PENCICLOVIR Famciclovir is the diacetyl 6-deoxyester of the guanosine analogue penciclovir. Famciclovir is well absorbed orally, has a bioavailability of 77%, and is rapidly converted to penciclovir by deacetylation and oxidation in the intestine and liver. Penciclovir's spectrum of activity and mechanism of action are similar to those of acyclovir; thus penciclovir is usually not active against acyclovir-resistant viruses. Penciclovir is phosphorylated initially by a virus-encoded thymidine kinase and subsequently by cellular kinases to penciclovir triphosphate, which inhibits HSV-1, HSV-2, and VZV DNA polymerases as well as hepatitis B virus (HBV). The serum half-life of penciclovir is 2 h, but the intracellular half-life of penciclovir triphosphate is 7 to 20 h—markedly longer than that of acyclovir triphosphate. The latter is the basis for the less frequent (twice-daily) dosing schedule for famciclovir than for acyclovir. Penciclovir is eliminated primarily in the urine by both glomerular filtration and tubular secretion. The usually recommended dosage interval should be adjusted for renal insufficiency.

Clinical trials involving immunocompetent adults with herpes zoster showed that famciclovir was superior to placebo in eliciting the resolution of skin lesions and virus shedding and in shortening the duration of postherpetic neuralgia; moreover, it was at least as effective as acyclovir administered orally at a dose of 800 mg five times daily. Famciclovir was also effective in the treatment of herpes zoster in immunosuppressed patients. Clinical trials have demonstrated its effectiveness in the suppression of genital HSV infections for up to 1 year and in the treatment of initial and recurrent episodes of genital herpes. Famciclovir is effective as therapy for mucocutaneous HSV infections in HIV-infected patients. Application of a 1% penciclovir cream reduces the duration of signs and symptoms of herpes labialis in immunocompetent patients (by 0.5 to 1.0 day) and has been approved for that purpose by the FDA. Famciclovir is generally well tolerated, with occasional headache, nausea, and diarrhea reported in frequencies similar to those among placebo recipients. The administration of high doses of famciclovir for 2 years was associated with an increased incidence of mammary adenocarcinomas in female rats, but the clinical significance of this effect is unknown. Intravenous penciclovir is being investigated for the treatment of mucocutaneous HSV infections in immunosuppressed patients.

FOSCARNET Foscarnet (phosphonoformic acid) is a pyrophosphate-containing compound that potently inhibits herpesviruses, including CMV. This drug inhibits DNA polymerases at the pyrophosphate binding site at concentrations that have relatively little effect on cellular polymerases. Foscarnet does not require phosphorylation to exert its antiviral activity and is therefore active against HSV and VZV isolates that are resistant to acyclovir because of deficiencies in thymidine kinase as well as against most ganciclovir-resistant strains of CMV. Foscarnet also inhibits the reverse transcriptase of HIV and is active against HIV in vivo.

Foscarnet is poorly soluble and must be administered intravenously via an infusion pump in a dilute solution over 1 to 2 h. The plasma half-life of foscarnet is 3 to 5 h and increases with decreasing renal function, since the drug is eliminated primarily by the kidneys. It has been estimated that 10 to 28% of a dose may be deposited in bone, where it can persist for months. The most common initial dosage of foscarnet—60 mg/kg every 8 h for 14 to 21 days—is followed by a maintenance dose of 90 to 120 mg/kg once a day.

Foscarnet is approved for the treatment of CMV retinitis in patients with AIDS and of acyclovir-resistant mucocutaneous HSV infections. In a comparative clinical trial, the drug appeared to be about as efficacious as ganciclovir against CMV retinitis but was associated with a longer survival period, possibly because of its anti-HIV activity. Intraocular foscarnet has been used to treat CMV retinitis. Foscarnet has also been employed to treat acyclovir-resistant HSV and VZV infections as well as ganciclovir-resistant CMV infections, although resistance to foscarnet has been reported in CMV isolates obtained during therapy.

The major form of toxicity associated with foscarnet is renal impairment. Thus renal function should be monitored closely, particularly during the initial phase of therapy. Since foscarnet binds divalent metal ions, hypocalcemia, hypomagnesemia, hypokalemia, and hypo- or hyperphosphatemia can develop. Saline hydration and slow infusion appear to protect the patient against nephrotoxicity and electrolyte disturbances. Although hematologic abnormalities have been documented (most commonly anemia), foscarnet is not generally myelosuppressive and may be administered concomitantly with myelosuppressive medications such as zidovudine.

TRIFLURIDINE Trifluridine is a pyrimidine nucleoside active against HSV-1, HSV-2, and CMV. Trifluridine monophosphate irreversibly inhibits thymidylate synthetase, and trifluridine triphosphate inhibits viral and, to a lesser extent, cellular DNA polymerases. Because of systemic toxicity, its use is limited to topical therapy. Trifluridine is approved for treatment of HSV keratitis, for which trials have shown that it is more effective than topical idoxuridine but similarly effective to topical vidarabine. The drug has benefited some patients with HSV keratitis who have failed to respond to idoxuridine or vidarabine. Topical application of trifluridine to sites of acyclovir-resistant HSV mucocutaneous infections has also been beneficial in some cases.

VIDARABINE Vidarabine is a purine nucleoside analogue with activity against HSV-1, HSV-2, VZV, and EBV. Vidarabine inhibits viral DNA synthesis through its 5′-triphosphorylated metabolite, although its precise molecular mechanisms of action are not completely understood. Intravenously administered vidarabine has been shown to be effective in the treatment of herpes simplex encephalitis, mucocutaneous HSV infections, herpes zoster in immunocompromised patients, and neonatal HSV infections. Its use has been supplanted by that of intravenous acyclovir, which is more effective and easier to administer. Production of the intravenous preparation has been discontinued by the manufacturer, but vidarabine is available as an ophthalmic ointment, which is effective in the treatment of HSV keratitis.

ANTIVIRAL DRUGS ACTIVE AGAINST HEPATITIS VIRUSES

LAMIVUDINE Lamivudine is a pyrimidine nucleoside analogue that is used primarily in combination therapy against HIV infection (Chap. 173). It is also active against HBV through inhibition of the viral DNA polymerase and has been approved for the treatment of chronic HBV infection. At doses of 100 mg/d for 1 year, lamivudine was well tolerated and results in suppression of HBV DNA levels, normalization of serum aminotransferase levels in 50 to 70% of patients, and reduc-

tion of hepatic inflammation and fibrosis in 50 to 60% of patients. Loss of hepatitis B e antigen (HBeAg) occurred in 30% of patients. Resistance to lamivudine develops in 24% of patients treated for 1 year and is associated with changes in the YMDD motif of HBV DNA polymerase. This is an important limitation of monotherapy with the drug. Studies of lamivudine as a component of combination therapy for hepatitis B are under way. Lamivudine also appears to be useful in the prevention or suppression of HBV infection associated with liver transplantation.

ADEFOVIR Adefovir dipivoxil is an acyclic nucleotide analogue of adenosine monophosphate that has activity against HBV, HIV, HSV, and CMV. It is phosphorylated by cellular kinases to the active triphosphate moiety, which is a competitive inhibitor of HBV DNA polymerase and results in chain termination after incorporation into nascent viral DNA. Adefovir is administered orally and is eliminated primarily by the kidneys, with a plasma half-life of 7.5 h. In clinical studies, therapy with adefovir at a dose 10 μg/d for 48 weeks resulted in normalization of alanine aminotransferase (ALT) levels in 48 to 72% of patients and improved liver histology in 53 to 64%; it also resulted in a 3.6-$\log_{10}$ reduction in the number of HBV DNA copies per milliliter of plasma. Adefovir was effective in treatment-naive patients as well as in those infected with lamivudine-resistant HBV. This agent was generally well tolerated. Significant nephrotoxicity attributable to adefovir was uncommon at the dose employed in the treatment of HBV infections (10 μg/d) but was a treatment-limiting adverse effect at the higher doses used in the treatment of HIV infections (30 to 120 μg/d). In any case, renal function should be monitored in patients taking adefovir, even at the lower dose. Adefovir is approved only for treatment of chronic hepatitis B infection.

TENOFOVIR Tenofovir disoproxil fumarate is a nucleotide analogue with activity against both retroviruses and hepadnaviruses. In one small study of patients coinfected with HIV and HBV, tenofovir reduced HBV loads by >10^4 copies/mL at 24 weeks. The drug is approved only for treatment of HIV infection, but its use should be considered in HIV/HBV-coinfected patients. →*For a more detailed discussion of tenofovir, see Chap. 173.*

INTERFERONS

Interferons are cytokines that exhibit a broad spectrum of antiviral activities as well as immunomodulating and antiproliferative properties. The IFNs are not available for oral administration but must be given intramuscularly, subcutaneously, or intravenously. Early studies with human leukocyte IFN demonstrated an effect in the prophylaxis of experimentally induced rhinovirus infections in humans and in the treatment of VZV infections in immunosuppressed patients. DNA recombinant technology has made available highly purified α, β, and γ IFNs that have been evaluated in a variety of viral infections. Results of such trials have confirmed the effectiveness of intranasally administered IFN in the prophylaxis of rhinovirus infections, although its use has been associated with nasal mucosal irritation. Studies have also demonstrated a beneficial effect of intralesionally or systemically administered IFNs on genital warts. The effect of systemic administration consists primarily of a reduction in the size of lesions, and this mode of therapy may be useful in persons who have numerous warts that cannot easily be treated by individual intralesional injections. However, lesions frequently recur after either intralesional or systemic IFN therapy is discontinued.

Interferons have undergone extensive study in the treatment of chronic HBV infection. The administration of IFN-α2b (5 million units daily or 10 million units three times a week for 16 weeks) to patients with stable chronic HBV infection resulted in loss of markers of HBV replication, such as HBeAg and HBV DNA, in 33 to 37% of cases; 8% of patients also became negative for hepatitis B surface antigen. In >80% of patients who lose HBeAg and HBV DNA markers, serum aminotransferases return to normal levels, and both short- and long-term improvements in liver histopathology have been described. Predictors of a favorable response to therapy include low pretherapy levels of HBV DNA, high pretherapy serum levels of ALT, a short duration of chronic HBV infection, and active inflammation in liver histopathology. Poor responses are seen in immunosuppressed patients, including those with HIV infection. Adverse effects of the above dose of IFN are common and include fever, chills, myalgia, fatigue, neurotoxicity (primarily manifested as somnolence and confusion), and leukopenia. Approximately 25% of patients receiving a daily dose of 5 million units require dose reduction, but <5% require discontinuation of therapy.

Several IFN preparations, including IFN-α2a, IFN-α2b, IFN-alfacon-1, and IFN-αm1 (lymphoblastoid), have been studied as therapy for chronic HCV infections. A variety of regimens have been employed, of which the most common is IFN-α2b or -α2a at 3 million units three times per week for 12 to 18 months. The addition of oral ribavirin to IFN-α2b—either as initial therapy or after failure of interferon therapy alone—results in significantly higher rates of sustained virologic and/or serum ALT responses (40 to 50%) than were obtained with monotherapy. *Pegylated* IFN-α2b or -α2a, in which the IFNs are covalently linked with monomethoxy polyethylene glycol, have been approved by the FDA for the treatment of chronic HCV infection. These interferons have a markedly reduced clearance rate and can therefore be administered less frequently than standard IFNs (i.e., once a week). Comparative studies indicate that pegylated IFN therapy may be more effective than standard IFN treatment against chronic HCV infection. The combination of intramuscular pegylated IFN and oral ribavirin appears to be a particularly convenient and effective regimen for treatment of chronic hepatitis C. Prognostic factors for a favorable response include an age of <45 years, a short duration of disease, low levels of HCV RNA, and infection with HCV genotypes other than 1. IFN alfacon, a synthetic "consensus" α interferon, appears to produce response rates similar to those elicited by IFN-α2a or -α2b alone and is also approved in the United States for the treatment of chronic hepatitis C. In early clinical trials, pegylated IFN alfas also appear promising as therapy for hepatitis B.

Treatment of acute hepatitis C with IFN has been investigated relatively little. In one study, the administration of IFN-α2b to patients recently infected with HCV (with a dose of 5 million units per day for 4 weeks followed by 3 million units per week for 20 weeks) resulted in clearance of HCV from blood and normalization of ALT levels in 43 of 44 patients at 48 weeks. Additional studies are required to establish the role of IFN therapy in this setting.

The efficacy of IFN-α treatment for chronic hepatitis D remains unestablished. Anecdotal reports suggested that doses of 5 million units daily to 9 million units three times per week for 12 months elicited biochemical and virologic responses. Results from small controlled trials have been inconsistent, and observed responses have not generally been sustained.

FURTHER READING

BALFOUR HH: Antiviral drugs. N Engl J Med 340:1255, 1999
BEUTNER KR et al: Valaciclovir compared with acyclovir for improved therapy for herpes zoster in immunocompetent adults. Antimicrob Agents Chemother 39:1546, 1995
COUCH RB: Drug therapy: Prevention and treatment of influenza. N Engl J Med 343:1778, 2000
CRUMPACKER CS: Ganciclovir. N Engl J Med 335:721, 1996
DOLIN R et al: A controlled trial of amantadine and rimantadine in the prophylaxis of influenza A infection. N Engl J Med 307:580, 1982
HALL CB et al: Aerosolized ribavirin treatment of infants with respiratory syncytial viral infection: A randomized double-blind study. N Engl J Med 308:1443, 1983
LALEZARI JP et al: Randomized controlled study of the safety and efficacy of intravenous cidofovir for the treatment of relapsing cytomegalovirus retinitis in patients with AIDS. J AIDS 17:339, 1998
LOK AS et al: Management of hepatitis B: 2000—summary of a workshop. Gastroenterology 120:1828, 2001
MARTIN DF et al: A controlled trial of valganciclovir as induction therapy for cytomegalovirus retinitis. N Engl J Med 346:1119, 2002
National Institutes of Health Consensus Development Conference Statement: Management of hepatitis C. September 12, 2002 (available at www.niaid.nih.gov)
WHITLEY RJ et al: Herpes simplex encephalitis: Adenine arabinoside versus acyclovir therapies. N Engl J Med 314:144, 1986

Section 12   Infections Due to DNA Viruses

163 | HERPES SIMPLEX VIRUSES
Lawrence Corey

DEFINITION Herpes simplex viruses (HSV-1, HSV-2; *Herpesvirus hominis*) produce a variety of infections involving mucocutaneous surfaces, the central nervous system (CNS), and—on occasion—visceral organs. Prompt recognition and treatment reduce the morbidity and mortality of HSV infections.

ETIOLOGIC AGENT The genome of HSV is a linear, double-stranded DNA molecule (molecular weight, ~100 × 10⁶ units) that encodes >90 transcription units with 84 identified proteins. The genomic structures of the two HSV subtypes are similar, and the overall sequence homology between HSV-1 and HSV-2 is ~50%. The homologous sequences are distributed over the entire genome map, and most of the polypeptides specified by one viral type are antigenically related to polypeptides of the other viral type. Many type-specific regions unique to HSV-1 and HSV-2 proteins do exist, however, and a number of them appear to be important in host immunity. These type-specific regions have been used to develop serologic assays that distinguish between the two viral subtypes. Either restriction endonuclease analysis of viral DNA or DNA sequencing can be used to distinguish between the two subtypes and among strains of each subtype. The variability of nucleotide sequences from clinical strains of HSV-1 and HSV-2 is such that HSV isolates obtained from two individuals can be differentiated by restriction enzyme patterns or genomic sequences unless the isolates are from epidemiologically related sources, such as sexual partners, mother-infant pairs, or persons involved in a common-source outbreak.

The viral genome is packaged in a regular icosahedral protein shell (capsid) composed of 162 capsomers. The outer covering of the virus is a lipid-containing membrane (envelope) derived from modified cell membrane and acquired as the DNA-containing capsid buds through the inner nuclear membrane of the host cell. Between the capsid and lipid bilayer of the envelope is the tegument. Viral replication has both nuclear and cytoplasmic phases. Attachment and fusion between the viral envelope and the cell membrane involve several ubiquitous heparin-like surface receptors. Replication is highly regulated. After fusion and entry, the nucleocapsid enters the cytoplasm and several viral proteins are released from the virion. Some of these viral proteins shut off host protein synthesis (by increasing cellular RNA degradation), while others "turn on" the transcription of early genes of HSV replication. These early gene products, designated α *genes*, are required for synthesis of the subsequent polypeptide group, the β polypeptides, many of which are regulatory proteins and enzymes required for DNA replication. Most current antiviral drugs interfere with β proteins, such as the viral DNA polymerase enzyme. The third (γ) class of HSV genes requires viral DNA replication for expression and constitutes most of the structural proteins specified by the virus.

After replication of the viral genome and synthesis of structural proteins, nucleocapsids are assembled in the nucleus of the cell. Envelopment occurs as the nucleocapsids bud through the inner nuclear membrane into the perinuclear space. In some cells, viral replication in the nucleus forms two types of inclusion bodies: type A basophilic Feulgen-positive bodies that contain viral DNA and an eosinophilic inclusion body that is devoid of viral nucleic acid or protein and represents a "scar" of viral infection. Virions are then transported via the endoplasmic reticulum and the Golgi apparatus to the cell surface.

HSV infection of some neuronal cells does not result in cell death. Instead, viral genomes are maintained by the cell in a repressed state compatible with survival and normal activities of the cell, a condition called *latency*. Latency is associated with transcription of only a limited number of virus-encoded proteins. Subsequently, the viral genome may become activated; its activation results in the normal pattern of regulated viral gene expression, replication, and release of HSV. The release of virus from the neuron and its subsequent entry into epithelial cells result in viral replication and reappearance of virus on mucosal surfaces. This process is termed *reactivation*. Whereas infectious virus is rarely recovered from sensory or autonomic nervous system ganglia dissected from cadavers, maintenance and growth of the neural cells in tissue culture result in production of infectious virions (*explantation*) and in subsequent permissive infection of susceptible cells (*cocultivation*). The mechanisms by which latency is established, maintained, or recovered are incompletely understood. Two RNA "latency-associated" transcripts that overlap the immediate early (α) gene products, called *ICP-O*, are found in abundance in the nuclei of latently infected neurons. Deletion mutants of this region that can become latent have been made. However, the efficiency of their later reactivation is reduced; thus, the antisense transcripts may play a role in maintaining rather than in establishing latency. Data from animal models suggest that HSV-specific T cell immunity may influence the process of reactivation in neuronal cells. At present, strategies to interrupt latency or to maintain molecular latency in neurons are not available. In experimental animals, ultraviolet light, systemic and local immunosuppression, and trauma to the skin or ganglia are associated with reactivation.

PATHOGENESIS Exposure to HSV at mucosal surfaces or abraded skin sites permits entry of the virus and initiation of its replication in cells of the epidermis and dermis. HSV infections are usually acquired subclinically. Both clinical acquisition and subclinical acquisition are associated with sufficient viral replication to permit infection of either sensory or autonomic nerve endings. On entry into the neuronal cell, the virus—or, more likely, the nucleocapsid—is transported intraaxonally to the nerve cell bodies in ganglia. In humans, the interval from inoculation of virus in peripheral tissue to spread to the ganglia is unknown. During the initial phase of infection, viral replication occurs in ganglia and contiguous neural tissue. Virus then spreads to other mucosal skin surfaces through centrifugal migration of infectious virions via peripheral sensory nerves. This mode of spread helps explain the large surface area involved, the high frequency of new lesions distant from the initial crop of vesicles that is characteristic in patients with primary genital or oral-labial HSV infection, and the recovery of virus from neural tissue distant from neurons innervating the inoculation site. Contiguous spread of locally inoculated virus also may take place and allow further mucosal extension of disease.

Analysis of the DNA from sequentially isolated strains of HSV or from isolates from multiple infected ganglia in any one individual has revealed similar, if not identical, restriction endonuclease or DNA sequence patterns in most persons. Occasionally (most frequently in immunocompromised persons), multiple strains of the same viral subtype are detected in one individual. As exposure to mucosal shedding is relatively common during a person's lifetime, these data suggest that exogenous infection with different strains of the same subtype is possible, albeit very uncommon.

IMMUNITY Host responses to infection with HSV influence the acquisition of disease, the severity of infection, resistance to the develop-

ment of latency, the maintenance of latency, and the frequency of recurrences. Both antibody-mediated and cell-mediated reactions are clinically important. Immunocompromised patients with defects in cell-mediated immunity experience more severe and more extensive HSV infections than those with deficits in humoral immunity, such as agammaglobulinemia. Experimental ablation of lymphocytes indicates that T cells play a major role in preventing lethal disseminated disease, although antibodies help reduce virus titers in neural tissue. Some of the clinical manifestations of HSV disease appear to be related to the host immune response (e.g., stromal opacities associated with recurrent herpetic keratitis). The surface viral glycoproteins have been shown to be antigens recognized by antibodies mediating neutralization and immune-mediated cytolysis (antibody-dependent cell-mediated cytotoxicity). Monoclonal antibodies specific for each of the known viral glycoproteins have, in experimental infections, conferred protection against subsequent neurologic disease or ganglionic latency. However, the use of subunit glycoprotein vaccines in humans has been, up to the present, only partially successful in reducing acquisition of infection. Multiple cell populations, including natural killer cells, macrophages, and a variety of T lymphocytes, play a role in host defenses against HSV infections, as do lymphokines generated by T lymphocytes. In animals, passive transfer of primed lymphocytes confers protection from subsequent challenge. Maximum protection usually requires the activation of multiple T cell subpopulations, including cytotoxic T cells and T cells responsible for delayed hypersensitivity. The latter cells may confer protection by the antigen-stimulated release of lymphokines (e.g., interferons), which may have a direct antiviral effect and may activate and enhance a variety of specific and nonspecific effector cells. Increasing evidence suggests that HSV-specific CD8+ T cell responses are critical for clearance of virus from lesions. In addition, immunosuppressed patients with frequent and prolonged HSV lesions have fewer functional CD8+ T cells directed at HSV. The HSV virion contains a variety of genes that are directed at the inhibition of host responses. These include gene no. 12 (*US-12*), which can bind to the cellular transporter-activating protein TAP-1 and reduce the ability of this protein to bind HSV peptides to HLA class I, thereby reducing recognition of viral proteins by cytotoxic T cells of the host. This effect can be overcome by the addition of interferon γ, but this reversal requires 24 to 48 h; thus, the virus has time to replicate and invade other host cells. Prior HSV-1 infection appears not to reduce the frequency of acquisition of HSV-2, as measured by seroconversion. However, persons with prior HSV-1 infection who acquire HSV-2 appear to have a higher frequency of subclinical acquisition. These data suggest that type-specific immune responses are central to the control of HSV infection.

EPIDEMIOLOGY Seroepidemiologic studies have documented HSV infections worldwide. Serologic assays with whole-virus antigen preparations, such as complement fixation, neutralization, indirect immunofluorescence, passive hemagglutination, radioimmunoassay, and enzyme-linked immunosorbent assay, are useful for differentiating uninfected (seronegative) persons from those with past HSV-1 or HSV-2 infection, but they do not reliably distinguish between the two viral subtypes. Serologic assays that identify antibodies to type-specific surface proteins (epitopes) of the two viral subtypes have been developed and can distinguish reliably between the human antibody responses to HSV-1 and HSV-2. The most commonly used assays are those that measure antibodies to glycoprotein G of HSV-1 (gG1) and HSV-2 (gG2). A western blot assay that can detect several HSV type-specific proteins can also be used.

Infection with HSV-1 is acquired more frequently and earlier than infection with HSV-2. More than 90% of adults have antibodies to HSV-1 by the fifth decade of life. In populations of low socioeconomic status, most persons acquire HSV-1 infection before the third decade of life.

Antibodies to HSV-2 are not detected routinely until puberty. Antibody prevalence rates correlate with past sexual activity and vary greatly among different population groups. Serosurveys indicate that

~20% of the U.S. population has antibodies to HSV-2. In most routine obstetric and family planning clinics, 25% of women have HSV-2 antibodies, although only 10% report a history of genital lesions. As many as 50% of heterosexual adults attending sexually transmitted disease clinics have antibodies to HSV-2. A wide variety of serologic surveys have indicated a similar or even higher seroprevalence of HSV-2 in most parts of Europe, Central and South America, and Africa. Antibody prevalence rates average ~5% higher among women than among men. Several studies suggest that much of this "asymptomatic" infection is largely unrecognized: when "asymptomatic" seropositive persons are shown pictures of genital lesions, more than 60% subsequently identify episodes of symptomatic reactivation. Most important, these asymptomatic seropositive persons with reactivation shed virus on mucosal surfaces as frequently as those with symptomatic disease. The large reservoir of unidentified carriers of HSV-2 and the frequent asymptomatic reactivation of virus from the genital tract have fostered the continued spread of genital herpes throughout the world. HSV-2 infection is an independent risk factor for the acquisition and transmission of infection with HIV type 1. Among coinfected persons, HIV-1 virions can be shed from herpetic lesions of the genital region. This shedding may facilitate the spread of HIV through sexual contact.

HSV infections occur throughout the year. Transmission can result from contact with persons with active ulcerative lesions or with persons without clinical manifestations of infection who are shedding HSV or on whose mucosal surfaces the virus is replicating. Studies using the polymerase chain reaction (PCR) have shown that HSV reactivation on mucosal surfaces is much more frequent than previously recognized. Among immunocompetent adults, HSV-2 can be isolated by culture from the genital tract on 2 to 10% of days, and HSV DNA can be detected on 20 to 30% of days by PCR. Corresponding figures for HSV-1 in oral secretions are similar. Shedding rates are highest during the initial years after acquisition, and viral shedding may occur on as many as 30 to 50% of days during this period. Immunosuppressed patients shed HSV on mucosal sites at even higher frequency (20 to 70% of days). Daily antiviral chemotherapy can markedly reduce shedding rates, as measured by PCR. These data indicate that potential exposure to HSV from sexual or other close contact (kissing, sharing of glasses or silverware) is common, and these high rates of mucosal reactivation are consistent with the continuing spread and high seroprevalence of HSV infections worldwide.

CLINICAL SPECTRUM HSV has been isolated from nearly all visceral and mucocutaneous sites. The clinical manifestations and course of HSV infection depend on the anatomical site involved, the age and immune status of the host, and the antigenic type of the virus. Primary HSV infections (i.e., first infections with either HSV-1 or HSV-2 in which the host lacks HSV antibodies in acute-phase serum) are frequently accompanied by systemic signs and symptoms. Primary infections involve both mucosal and extramucosal sites; compared with recurrent episodes of disease, they are characterized by a longer duration of symptoms and virus isolation from lesions as well as a higher rate of complications. The incubation period ranges from 1 to 26 days (median, 6 to 8 days). Both viral subtypes can cause genital and oral-facial infections, and the infections caused by the two subtypes are clinically indistinguishable. However, the frequency of reactivation of infection is influenced by anatomical site and virus type. Genital HSV-2 infection is twice as likely to reactivate and recurs 8 to 10 times more frequently than genital HSV-1 infection. Conversely, oral-labial HSV-1 infection recurs more frequently than oral-labial HSV-2 infection. Asymptomatic shedding rates follow the same pattern.

Oral-Facial Infections Gingivostomatitis and pharyngitis are the most frequent clinical manifestations of first-episode HSV-1 infection, while recurrent herpes labialis is the most frequent clinical manifestation of reactivation HSV infection. HSV pharyngitis and gingivostomatitis usually result from primary infection and are most commonly seen in children and young adults. Clinical symptoms and signs, which include fever, malaise, myalgias, inability to eat, irritability, and cervical adenopathy, may last from 3 to 14 days. Lesions may involve the hard and soft palate, gingiva, tongue, lip, and facial area. HSV-1 or HSV-2 infection of the pharynx usually results in exudative or ulcerative lesions of the posterior pharynx and/or tonsillar pillars. Lesions of the tongue, buccal mucosa, or gingiva may occur later in the course in one-third of cases. Fever lasting from 2 to 7 days and cervical adenopathy are common. It can be difficult to differentiate HSV pharyngitis clinically from bacterial pharyngitis, *Mycoplasma pneumoniae* infections, and pharyngeal ulcerations of noninfectious etiologies (e.g., Stevens-Johnson syndrome). No substantial evidence suggests that reactivation oral-labial HSV infection is associated with symptomatic recurrent pharyngitis.

Reactivation of HSV from the trigeminal ganglia may be associated with asymptomatic virus excretion in the saliva, development of intraoral mucosal ulcerations, or herpetic ulcerations on the vermilion border of the lip or external facial skin. About 50 to 70% of seropositive patients undergoing trigeminal nerve root decompression and 10 to 15% of those undergoing dental extraction develop oral-labial HSV infection a median of 3 days after these procedures.

In immunosuppressed patients, infection may extend into mucosal and deep cutaneous layers. Friability, necrosis, bleeding, severe pain, and inability to eat or drink may result. The lesions of HSV mucositis are clinically similar to mucosal lesions caused by cytotoxic drug therapy, trauma, or fungal or bacterial infections. Persistent ulcerative HSV infections are among the most common infections in patients with AIDS. HSV and *Candida* infections often occur concurrently. Systemic antiviral therapy speeds the rate of healing and relieves the pain of mucosal HSV infections in immunosuppressed patients. The frequency of HSV reactivation during the early phases of transplantation or induction chemotherapy is high (50 to 90%), and prophylactic systemic antiviral agents such as intravenous acyclovir or penciclovir are used to reduce reactivation rates. Patients with atopic eczema may also develop severe oral-facial HSV infections (eczema herpeticum), which may rapidly involve extensive areas of skin and occasionally disseminate to visceral organs. Extensive eczema herpeticum has resolved promptly with the administration of intravenous acyclovir. Erythema multiforme may also be associated with HSV infections (see Fig. 46-9); some evidence suggests that HSV infection is the precipitating event in ~75% of cases of cutaneous erythema multiforme. HSV antigen has been demonstrated both in circulatory immune complexes and in skin lesion biopsy samples from these cases. Patients with severe HSV-associated erythema multiforme are candidates for chronic suppressive oral antiviral therapy.

HSV-1 and varicella-zoster virus (VZV) have been implicated in the etiology of Bell's palsy (flaccid paralysis of the mandibular portion of the facial nerve). Although uniform recommendations for treatment of this entity are not available, recent evidence suggests that antiviral chemotherapy, usually with a short course of glucocorticoids, may improve outcome.

Genital Infections First-episode primary genital herpes is characterized by fever, headache, malaise, and myalgias. Pain, itching, dysuria, vaginal and urethral discharge, and tender inguinal lymphadenopathy are the predominant local symptoms. Widely spaced bilateral lesions of the external genitalia are characteristic (Fig. 163-1). Lesions may be present in varying stages, including vesicles, pustules, or painful erythematous ulcers. The cervix and urethra are involved in >80% of women with first-episode infections. First episodes of genital herpes in patients who have had prior HSV-1 infection are associated with less frequent systemic symptoms and faster healing than primary genital herpes. The clinical courses of acute first-episode genital herpes among patients with HSV-1 and HSV-2 infections are similar. However, the recurrence rates of genital disease differ with the viral subtype: the 12-month recurrence rates among patients with first-episode HSV-2 and HSV-1 infections are ~90% and ~55%, respectively (median number of recurrences, 4 and <1, respectively). Recurrence rates

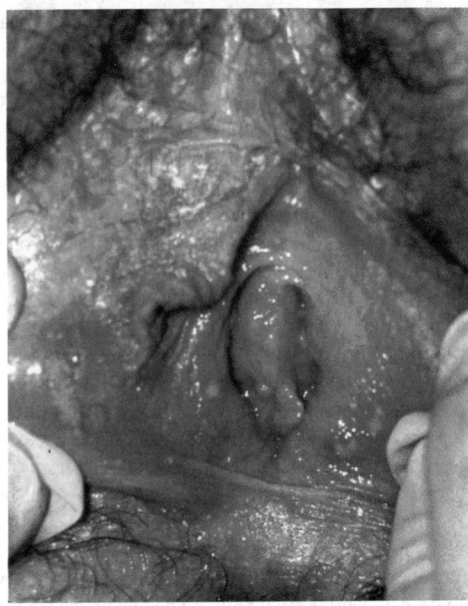

FIGURE 163-1   Bilateral serpiginous ulcerative lesions of the labia minora and majora in a woman with extensive primary genital HSV-2 infection.

for genital HSV-2 infections vary greatly among individuals and over time within the same individual. HSV has been isolated from the urethra and urine of men and women without external genital lesions. A clear mucoid discharge and dysuria are characteristics of symptomatic HSV urethritis. HSV has been isolated from the urethra of 5% of women with the dysuria-frequency syndrome. Occasionally, HSV genital tract disease is manifested by endometritis and salpingitis in women and by prostatitis in men. About 15% of cases of HSV-2 acquisition are associated with these nonlesional clinical syndromes, such as aseptic meningitis, cervicitis, or urethritis. →*A more complete discussion of the differential diagnosis of genital herpes is presented in Chap. 115.*

Both HSV-1 and HSV-2 can cause symptomatic or asymptomatic rectal and perianal infections. HSV proctitis is usually associated with rectal intercourse. However, subclinical perianal shedding of HSV is detected both in heterosexual men and in women who report no rectal intercourse. This phenomenon is due to the establishment of latency in the sacral dermatome from prior genital tract infection, with subsequent reactivation in epithelial cells in the perianal region. Such reactivations are often subclinical. Symptoms of HSV proctitis include anorectal pain, anorectal discharge, tenesmus, and constipation. Sigmoidoscopy reveals ulcerative lesions of the distal 10 cm of the rectal mucosa. Rectal biopsies show mucosal ulceration, necrosis, polymorphonuclear and lymphocytic infiltration of the lamina propria, and (in occasional cases) multinucleated intranuclear inclusion–bearing cells. Perianal herpetic lesions are also found in immunosuppressed patients receiving cytotoxic therapy. Extensive perianal herpetic lesions and/or HSV proctitis is common among patients with HIV infection.

Herpetic Whitlow   Herpetic whitlow—HSV infection of the finger—may occur as a complication of primary oral or genital herpes by inoculation of virus through a break in the epidermal surface or by direct introduction of virus into the hand through occupational or some other type of exposure. Clinical signs and symptoms include the abrupt onset of edema, erythema, and localized tenderness of the infected finger. Vesicular or pustular lesions of the fingertip that are indistinguishable from lesions of pyogenic bacterial infection are seen. Fever, lymphadenitis, and epitrochlear and axillary lymphadenopathy are common. The infection may recur. Prompt diagnosis (to avoid unnecessary and potentially exacerbating surgical therapy and/or transmission) is essential. Antiviral chemotherapy (to speed the healing of the process) is usually recommended (see below).

Herpes Gladiatorum   HSV may infect almost any area of skin. Mucocutaneous HSV infections of the thorax, ears, face, and hands have been described among wrestlers. Transmission of these infections is facilitated by trauma to the skin sustained during wrestling. Several recent outbreaks of this infection have illustrated the importance of prompt diagnosis and therapy, which are required to contain the spread of this infection.

Eye Infections   HSV infection of the eye is the most frequent cause of corneal blindness in the United States. HSV keratitis presents with an acute onset of pain, blurring of vision, chemosis, conjunctivitis, and characteristic dendritic lesions of the cornea. Use of topical glucocorticoids may exacerbate symptoms and lead to involvement of deep structures of the eye. Debridement, topical antiviral treatment, and/or interferon therapy hastens healing. However, recurrences are common, and the deeper structures of the eye may sustain immunopathologic injury. Stromal keratitis due to HSV appears to be related to T cell–dependent destruction of deep corneal tissue. An HSV-1 epitope that is autoreactive with T cell–targeting corneal antigens has been postulated to be a factor in this infection. Chorioretinitis, usually a manifestation of disseminated HSV infection, may occur in neonates or in patients with HIV infection. HSV and VZV can cause acute necrotizing retinitis as an uncommon but severe manifestation.

Central and Peripheral Nervous System Infections   HSV accounts for 10 to 20% of all cases of sporadic viral encephalitis in the United States. The estimated incidence is ~2.3 cases per 1 million persons per year. Cases are distributed throughout the year, and the age distribution appears to be biphasic, with peaks at 5 to 30 and >50 years of age. Subtype 1 virus causes >95% of cases of HSV encephalitis.

The pathogenesis of HSV encephalitis varies. In children and young adults, primary HSV infection may result in encephalitis; presumably, exogenously acquired virus enters the CNS by neurotropic spread from the periphery via the olfactory bulb. However, most adults with HSV encephalitis have clinical or serologic evidence of mucocutaneous HSV-1 infection before the onset of the CNS symptoms. In ~25% of the cases examined, the HSV-1 strains from the oropharynx and brain tissue of the same patient differ; thus some cases may result from reinfection with another strain of HSV-1 that reaches the CNS. Two theories have been proposed to explain the development of actively replicating HSV in localized areas of the CNS in persons whose ganglionic and CNS isolates are similar. Reactivation of latent HSV-1 infection in trigeminal or autonomic nerve roots may be associated with extension of virus into the CNS via nerves innervating the middle cranial fossa. HSV DNA has been demonstrated by DNA hybridization in brain tissue obtained at autopsy—even from healthy adults. Thus, reactivation of long-standing latent CNS infection may be another mechanism for the development of HSV encephalitis.

The clinical hallmark of HSV encephalitis has been the acute onset of fever and focal neurologic symptoms and signs, especially in the temporal lobe (Fig. 163-2). Clinical differentiation of HSV encephalitis from other viral encephalitides, focal infections, or noninfectious processes is difficult. The most sensitive noninvasive method for early diagnosis of HSV encephalitis is the demonstration of HSV DNA in cerebrospinal fluid (CSF) by PCR. Although titers of CSF and serum antibodies to HSV increase in most cases of HSV encephalitis, they rarely do so earlier than 10 days into the illness and therefore, while useful retrospectively, are generally not helpful in establishing an early clinical diagnosis. Demonstration of HSV antigen, HSV DNA, or HSV replication in brain tissue obtained by biopsy is highly sensitive and has a low complication rate; examination of such tissue also provides the best opportunity to identify alternative, potentially treatable causes of encephalitis. Antiviral chemotherapy reduces the rate of death from HSV encephalitis. Intravenous acyclovir is more effective than vidarabine. Even with therapy, however, neurologic sequelae are frequent, especially in persons >50 years of age. Most authorities recommend the administration of intravenous acyclovir to patients with presumed HSV encephalitis until the diagnosis is confirmed or an alternative diagnosis is made. Among proven cases of HSV encephalitis, intravenous therapy is usually recommended until HSV DNA levels in CSF are substantially reduced or at nearly undetectable levels.

HSV DNA has been detected in CSF from 3 to 15% of persons presenting to the hospital with aseptic meningitis. HSV meningitis, which is usually seen in association with primary genital HSV infection, is an acute, self-limited disease manifested by headache, fever, and mild photophobia and lasting from 2 to 7 days. Lymphocytic pleocytosis in the CSF is characteristic. Neurologic sequelae of HSV meningitis are rare. HSV is the most commonly identified cause of recurrent lymphocytic meningitis (Mollaret's meningitis). Demonstration of HSV antibodies in CSF or persistence of HSV DNA in CSF can establish the diagnosis. For persons with frequent recurrences of HSV meningitis, antiviral therapy has been successful in reducing the frequency of such episodes.

Autonomic nervous system dysfunction, especially of the sacral region, has been reported in association with both HSV and VZV infections. Numbness, tingling of the buttocks or perineal areas, urinary retention, constipation, CSF pleocytosis, and (in males) impotence may occur. Symptoms appear to resolve slowly over days to weeks. Occasionally, hypesthesia and/or weakness of the lower extremities may persist for many months. Rarely, transverse myelitis manifested by a rapidly progressive symmetric paralysis of the lower extremities or a Guillain-Barré syndrome may follow HSV infection. Similarly, peripheral nervous system involvement (Bell's palsy) or cranial polyneuritis may also be related to reactivation of HSV-1 infection. Transitory hypesthesia of the area of skin innervated by the trigeminal nerve and vestibular system dysfunction as measured by electronystagmography are the predominant signs of disease. Studies to determine whether antiviral chemotherapy may abort these signs or reduce their frequency and severity are unavailable.

Visceral Infections HSV infection of visceral organs usually results from viremia, and multiple-organ involvement is common. Occasionally, however, the clinical manifestations of HSV infection involve only the esophagus, lung, or liver. HSV esophagitis may result from direct extension of oral-pharyngeal HSV infection into the esophagus or may occur de novo by reactivation and spread of HSV to the esophageal mucosa via the vagus nerve. The predominant symptoms of HSV esophagitis are odynophagia, dysphagia, substernal pain, and weight loss. There are multiple oval ulcerations on an erythematous base with or without a patchy white pseudomembrane. The distal esophagus is most commonly involved. With extensive disease, diffuse friability may spread to the entire esophagus. Neither endoscopic nor barium examination can reliably differentiate HSV esophagitis from *Candida* esophagitis or from esophageal ulcerations due to thermal injury, radiation, or corrosives. Endoscopically obtained secretions for cytologic examination and culture provide the most useful material for diagnosis. Systemic antiviral chemotherapy usually reduces symptoms and heals esophageal ulcerations.

HSV pneumonitis is uncommon except in severely immunosuppressed patients and may result from extension of herpetic tracheobronchitis into lung parenchyma. Focal necrotizing pneumonitis usually ensues. Hematogenous dissemination of virus from sites of oral or genital mucocutaneous disease may also occur and produce bilateral interstitial pneumonitis. Bacterial, fungal, and parasitic pathogens are commonly present in HSV pneumonitis. The mortality rate from untreated HSV pneumonia in immunosuppressed patients is high (>80%). HSV has also been isolated from the lower respiratory tract of persons with adult respiratory distress syndrome. However, the re-

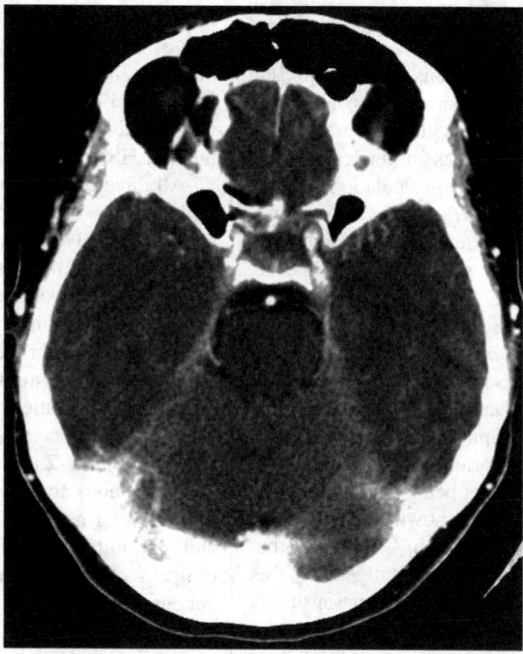
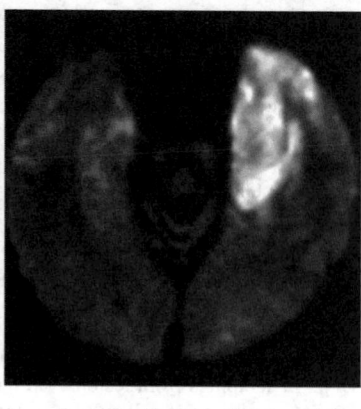

FIGURE 163-2 Computed tomographic and diffusion-weighted magnetic resonance scans of the brain of a patient with left-temporal-lobe HSV encephalitis.

lationship between the isolation of HSV and the pathogenesis of this syndrome is unclear.

HSV is an uncommon cause of hepatitis in immunocompetent patients. HSV infection of the liver is associated with fever, abrupt elevations of bilirubin and serum aminotransferase levels, and leukopenia (<4000 white blood cells per microliter). Disseminated intravascular coagulation may also develop.

Other reported complications of HSV infection include monarticular arthritis, adrenal necrosis, idiopathic thrombocytopenia, and glomerulonephritis. Disseminated HSV infection in immunocompetent patients is rare. In immunocompromised, burned, or malnourished patients, HSV occasionally disseminates to other visceral organs, such as the adrenal glands, pancreas, small and large intestines, and bone marrow. Rarely, primary HSV infection in pregnancy disseminates and may be associated with the death of both mother and fetus. This uncommon event is usually related to the acquisition of primary infection in the third trimester.

Neonatal HSV Infection Of all HSV-infected populations, neonates (infants younger than 6 weeks) have the highest frequency of visceral and/or CNS infection. Without therapy, the overall rate of death from neonatal herpes is 65%; <10% of neonates with CNS infection develop normally. Although skin lesions are the most commonly recognized features of disease, many infants do not develop lesions until well into the course of disease. Neonatal infection is usually acquired perinatally from contact with infected genital secretions at the time of delivery. Congenitally infected infants have been reported. In most series, 30% of neonatal HSV infections are due to HSV-1 and 70% to HSV-2. The risk of developing neonatal HSV infection is 10 times higher for an infant born to a mother who has recently acquired HSV than for other infants. Neonatal HSV-1 infections may also be acquired through postnatal contact with immediate family members who have symptomatic or asymptomatic oral-labial HSV-1 infection or through nosocomial transmission within the hospital. All neonates with presumed neonatal herpes should be treated with intravenous acyclovir (see below). Antiviral chemotherapy has reduced the rate of death from neonatal herpes to 25%. However, the rate of morbidity, especially among infants with HSV-2 infection involving the CNS, is still very high.

DIAGNOSIS Both clinical and laboratory criteria are useful for establishing the diagnosis of HSV infections. A clinical diagnosis can be made accurately when characteristic multiple vesicular lesions on an erythematous base are present. However, it is increasingly being recognized that herpetic ulcerations may clinically resemble skin ulcerations of other etiologies. Mucosal HSV infections may also present as urethritis or pharyngitis without cutaneous lesions. Thus, laboratory studies to confirm the diagnosis and to guide therapy are recommended. While staining of scrapings from the base of the lesions with Wright's, Giemsa's (Tzanck preparation), or Papanicolaou's stain to detect giant cells or intranuclear inclusions of *Herpesvirus* infection is a well-described procedure, few clinicians are skilled in these techniques. Moreover, these cytologic methods do not differentiate between HSV and VZV infections.

HSV infection is best confirmed in the laboratory by isolation of the virus in tissue culture or by demonstration of HSV antigens or DNA in scrapings from lesions. HSV causes a discernible cytopathic effect in a variety of cell culture systems, and this effect can be identified within 48 to 96 h after inoculation. Spin-amplified culture with subsequent staining for HSV antigen has shortened the time needed to identify HSV to <24 h. Increasingly, PCR is being used for the detection of HSV DNA, and several studies have shown this assay to be more sensitive than culture for detection of HSV in CSF and at mucosal sites. The sensitivity of viral isolation and of antigen or DNA detection depends on the stage of the lesions (with higher sensitivity in vesicular than in ulcerative lesions), on whether the patient has a first or a recurrent episode of the disease (with higher sensitivity in first than in recurrent episodes), and on whether the sample is from an immunosuppressed or an immunocompetent patient (with more antigen in immunosuppressed patients). Laboratory confirmation permits subtyping of the virus; information on subtype may be useful epidemiologically and may help to predict the frequency of reactivation after first-episode oral-labial or genital HSV infection.

Acute- and convalescent-phase serum can be useful in demonstrating seroconversion during primary HSV-1 or HSV-2 infection. However, only 5% of patients with recurrent mucocutaneous HSV infections have a fourfold or greater rise in titer of antibody to HSV in the interval between the collection of the first and second samples. Serologic assays, especially type-specific assays, should be used to identify asymptomatic carriers of HSV-1 or HSV-2 infection.

Several studies have shown that persons seropositive for HSV-2 to whom the clinical manifestations of HSV have been explained are able to identify symptomatic reactivations. Individuals seropositive for HSV-2 should be told about the high frequency of subclinical reactivation in mucosal surfaces not visible to the eye (e.g., cervix, urethra, perianal skin) or in microscopic ulcerations that may not be clinically symptomatic. Transmission of infection during such episodes is well established. HSV-2-seropositive persons should be educated about the high likelihood of subclinical shedding and the role condoms (male or female) may play in reducing transmission. Antiviral therapy with the drug valacyclovir (500 mg once daily) has been shown to reduce the transmission of HSV-2 between sexual partners.

℞ TREATMENT

Many aspects of mucocutaneous and visceral HSV infections are amenable to antiviral chemotherapy. For mucocutaneous infections, acyclovir and its congeners famciclovir and valacyclovir have been the mainstay of therapy. Several antiviral agents are available for topical use in HSV eye infections: idoxuridine, trifluorothymidine, topical vidarabine, and cidofovir. For HSV encephalitis and neonatal herpes, intravenous acyclovir is the treatment of choice.

All licensed antiviral agents for use against HSV inhibit the viral DNA polymerase. One class of drugs, typified by the drug acyclovir, is made up of substrates for the HSV enzyme thymidine kinase. Acyclovir, ganciclovir, famciclovir, and valacyclovir are all selectively phosphorylated to the monophosphate form in virus-infected cells. Cellular enzymes convert the monophosphate form of the drug to the triphosphate, which is then incorporated into the viral DNA chain.

Acyclovir is the most frequently used agent for the treatment of HSV infections and is available in intravenous, oral, and topical formulations. Valacyclovir is the valyl ester of acyclovir and offers greater bioavailability than acyclovir. Famciclovir, the oral formulation of penciclovir, is clinically effective in the treatment of a variety of HSV-1 and HSV-2 infections. Ganciclovir is active against both HSV-1 and HSV-2; however, it is more toxic than acyclovir, valacyclovir, and famciclovir and generally is not recommended for the treatment of HSV infections.

All three recommended compounds—acyclovir, valacyclovir, and famciclovir—have proven effective in shortening the duration of symptoms and lesions of mucocutaneous HSV infections in both immunocompromised and immunocompetent patients (Table 163-1). Intravenous and oral formulations prevent reactivation of HSV in seropositive immunocompromised patients during induction chemotherapy or in the period immediately after bone marrow or solid organ transplantation. Chronic daily suppressive therapy reduces the frequency of reactivation disease among patients with frequent genital or oral-labial herpes. Only valacyclovir has been shown to reduce transmission of HSV-2 infection between sexual partners.

Intravenous acyclovir (30 mg/kg per day, given as a 10-mg/kg infusion over 1 h at 8-h intervals) is effective in reducing rates of death and morbidity from HSV encephalitis. Early initiation of therapy is a critical factor in outcome. The major side effect associated with intravenous acyclovir is transient renal insufficiency, usually due to crystallization of the compound in the renal parenchyma. This adverse reaction can be avoided if the medication is given slowly over 1 h and the patient is well hydrated. Because CSF levels of acyclovir average only 30 to 50% of plasma levels, the dosage of acyclovir used for treatment of CNS infection (30 mg/kg per day) is double that used for treatment of mucocutaneous or visceral disease (15 mg/kg per day). Even higher doses of intravenous acyclovir are used for neonatal HSV infection (60 mg/kg per day in 3 divided doses).

Among immunocompetent patients, recent studies have shown the effectiveness of short-course oral therapy to reduce the signs and symptoms of oral and genital HSV infection. These regimens include valacyclovir (1 or 3 days) for oral-labial HSV and acyclovir (2 days) or valacyclovir (3 days) for recurrent-episode genital herpes (Table 163-1).

Suppression of Mucocutaneous Herpes   Recognition of the high frequency of subclinical reactivation has provided an ever-greater rationale for the use of daily antiviral therapy to suppress reactivations of HSV, especially in persons with frequent clinical reactivations (e.g., those with recently acquired genital HSV infection). Immunosuppressed persons, including those with HIV infection, may also benefit from daily antiviral therapy. Of the various regimens used, famciclovir (500 mg twice daily) and valacyclovir (1 g twice daily) are two of the most common; valacyclovir at a dose of 4 g daily was associated with thrombotic thrombocytopenic purpura in one study of HIV-infected persons.

Reduction in Transmission of HSV to Sexual Partners   Once-daily valacyclovir (500 mg) has been shown to reduce transmission of HSV-2 between sexual partners. Transmission rates are higher from males to females and among persons with frequent HSV-2 reactivation. Serologic screening can be used to identify at-risk couples.

Acyclovir Resistance   Acyclovir-resistant strains of HSV have been identified. Most of these strains have an altered substrate specificity for phosphorylating acyclovir. Thus, cross-resistance to famciclovir and valacyclovir is usually found. Occasionally, an isolate with altered thymidine kinase (TK) specificity arises and is sensitive to famciclovir but not to acyclovir. In some patients infected with TK-deficient virus, higher doses of acyclovir are associated with clearing of lesions. In others, clinical disease progresses despite high-dose therapy. Almost all clinically significant acyclovir resistance has been seen in immunocompromised patients, and HSV-2 isolates are more often resistant than HSV-1 strains. A study by the Centers for Disease Control and Prevention indicated that ~5% of HSV-2 isolates from HIV-positive persons exhibit some degree of in vitro resistance to acyclovir. Among immunocompetent patients attending sexually transmitted disease clin-

TABLE 163-1 *Antiviral Chemotherapy for HSV Infection*

I. Mucocutaneous HSV infections
  A. Infections in immunosuppressed patients:
    1. Acute symptomatic first or recurrent episodes: IV acyclovir (5 mg/kg q8h) or oral acyclovir (400 mg qid), famciclovir (500 mg tid), or valacyclovir (500 mg bid). Treatment duration may vary from 7 to 14 days.
    2. Suppression of reactivation disease: IV acyclovir (5 mg/kg q8h) or oral valacyclovir (500 mg bid) or acyclovir (400–800 mg 3–5 times per day) prevents recurrences during the 30-day period immediately after transplantation. Longer-term HSV suppression is often used for persons with continued immunosuppression. In bone marrow and renal transplant recipients, oral valacyclovir (2 g/d) is also effective in preventing cytomegalovirus infection. Oral valacyclovir at a dose of 4 g/d has been associated with thrombotic thrombocytopenic purpura after extended use in HIV-positive persons. In HIV-infected persons, oral famciclovir (500 mg bid) is effective in reducing clinical and subclinical reactivations of HSV-1 and HSV-2.
  B. Genital herpes:
    1. First episodes: Oral acyclovir (200 mg 5 times per day or 400 mg tid), valacyclovir (1 g bid), or famciclovir (250 mg bid) for 10–14 days is effective. IV acyclovir (5 mg/kg q8h for 5 days) is given for severe disease or neurologic complications such as aseptic meningitis.
    2. Symptomatic recurrent genital herpes: Oral acyclovir (200 mg 5 times per day for 5 days, 800 mg tid for 2 days), valacyclovir (500 mg bid for 3 or 5 days), or famciclovir (125 mg bid for 5 days) is effective in shortening lesion duration.
    3. Suppression of recurrent genital herpes: Oral acyclovir (200-mg capsules tid or qid, 400 mg bid, or 800 mg qd), famciclovir (250 mg bid), or valacyclovir (500 mg or 1 g qd or 500 mg bid) prevents symptomatic reactivation. Persons with frequent reactivation but <9 episodes per year can take valacyclovir (500 mg PO daily); those with >9 episodes per year should take 1 g PO daily or 500 mg PO bid.
  C. Oral-labial HSV infections:
    1. First episode: Oral acyclovir (200 mg) is given 4 or 5 times per day. Oral famciclovir (250 mg bid) or valacyclovir (1 g bid) has been used clinically.
    2. Recurrent episodes: Oral valacyclovir (1 g bid for 1 day or 500 mg bid for 3 days) is effective in reducing pain and speeding healing. Self-initiated therapy with 6-times-daily topical penciclovir cream is effective in speeding the healing of oral-labial HSV. Topical acyclovir cream has also been shown to speed healing.
    3. Suppression of reactivation of oral-labial HSV: Oral acyclovir (400 mg bid), if started before exposure and continued for the duration of exposure (usually 5–10 days), will prevent reactivation of recurrent oral-labial HSV infection associated with severe sun exposure.
  D. Herpetic whitlow: Oral acyclovir (200 mg) is given 5 times daily for 7–10 days.
  E. HSV proctitis: Oral acyclovir (400 mg 5 times per day) is useful in shortening the course of infection. In immunosuppressed patients or in patients with severe infection, IV acyclovir (5 mg/kg q8h) may be useful.
  F. Herpetic eye infections: In acute keratitis, topical trifluorothymidine, vidarabine, idoxuridine, acyclovir, penciclovir, and interferon are all beneficial. Debridement may be required; topical steroids may worsen disease.
II. CNS HSV infections
  A. HSV encephalitis: IV acyclovir (10 mg/kg q8h; 30 mg/kg per day) for at least 10 days.
  B. HSV aseptic meningitis: No studies of systemic antiviral chemotherapy exist. If therapy is to be given, IV acyclovir (15–30 mg/kg per day) should be used.
  C. Autonomic radiculopathy: No studies are available. Most authorities recommend a trial of IV acyclovir.
III. Neonatal HSV infections
  Oral acyclovir (60 mg/kg per day, divided into 3 doses) is given. The recommended duration of treatment is 21 days. Monitoring for relapse should be undertaken, and some authorities recommend continued suppression with oral acyclovir suspension for 3 to 4 months.
IV. Visceral HSV infections
  A. HSV esophagitis: IV acyclovir (15 mg/kg per day). In some patients with milder forms of immunosuppression, oral therapy with valacyclovir or famciclovir is effective.
  B. HSV pneumonitis: No controlled studies exist. IV acyclovir (15 mg/kg per day) should be considered.
V. Disseminated HSV infections
  No controlled studies exist. Intravenous acyclovir nevertheless should be tried. No definite evidence indicates that therapy will decrease the risk of death.
VI. Erythema multiforme–associated HSV
  Anecdotal observations suggest that oral acyclovir (400 mg bid or tid) or valacyclovir (500 mg bid) will suppress erythema multiforme.
VII. Surgical prophylaxis
  Several surgical procedures (e.g., laser skin resurfacing, trigeminal nerve root decompression, and lumbar disk surgery) have been associated with HSV reactivation. Intravenous or oral acyclovir (800 mg bid) or oral valacyclovir (500 mg bid) or famciclovir (250 mg bid) is effective in reducing reactivation. Therapy should be initiated 48 h before surgery and continued for 3–7 days.
VIII. Infections due to acyclovir-resistant HSV
  IV foscarnet (40 mg/kg q8h) should be given until lesions heal. The optimal duration of therapy and the usefulness of its continuation to suppress lesions are unclear. Some patients may benefit from cutaneous application of trifluorothymidine or 5% cidofovir gel.

ics, <0.5% of HSV-2 isolates show reduced in vitro sensitivity to acyclovir. The lack of appreciable change in the frequency of detection of such isolates in the past 20 years probably reflects the reduced transmission of TK-deficient mutants. Isolation of HSV from lesions persisting despite adequate dosages and blood levels of acyclovir should raise the suspicion of acyclovir resistance. Therapy with the antiviral drug foscarnet is useful (Chap. 162). Because of its toxicity and cost, this drug is usually reserved for patients with extensive mucocutaneous infections. Cidofovir is a nucleotide analogue and exists as a phosphonate or monophosphate form. Most TK-deficient strains of HSV are sensitive to cidofovir. Cidofovir ointment speeds healing of acyclovir-resistant lesions. No well-controlled trials of systemic cidofovir have been reported. True TK-negative variants of HSV appear to have a reduced capacity to spread because of altered neurovirulence—a feature important in the relatively infrequent presence of such strains in immunocompetent populations, even with increasing use of antiviral drugs.

PREVENTION The success of efforts to control HSV disease on a population basis through suppressive antiviral chemotherapy and/or educational programs will be limited.

Barrier forms of contraception (especially condoms) decrease the likelihood of transmission of HSV infection, particularly during periods of asymptomatic viral excretion. When lesions are present, HSV infection may be transmitted by skin-to-skin contact despite the use of a condom. Nevertheless, the available data suggest that consistent condom use is an effective means of reducing the risk of genital HSV-2 transmission. Recent studies have shown that chronic daily antiviral therapy with valacyclovir can also be partially effective in reducing acquisition of HSV-2, especially among susceptible women. There are no comparative efficacy studies of valacyclovir versus condom use. Most authorities suggest both approaches. Several candidate HSV vaccines are under investigation.

Prevention of neonatal HSV requires the prevention of acquisition of HSV by women in the third trimester of pregnancy. Identification of women or couples susceptible to acquisition of HSV in pregnancy through serologic screening is receiving increasing attention, and such screening is being used with increasing frequency.

FURTHER READING

BROWN ZA et al: The acquisition of herpes simplex virus during pregnancy. N Engl J Med 337:509, 1997

CHILUKURI S, ROSEN T: Management of acyclovir-resistant herpes simplex virus. Dermatol Clin 21:311, 2003

LANGENBERG AGM et al: A prospective study of new infections with herpes simplex virus type 1 and herpes simplex virus type 2. N Engl J Med 341:1532, 1999

LEONE PA et al: Valacyclovir for episodic treatment of genital herpes: A shorter 3-day treatment course compared with 5-day treatment. Clin Infect Dis 34:958, 2002

RABORN GW et al: Effective treatment of herpes simplex labialis with penciclovir cream: Combined results of two trials. J Am Dent Assoc 133:303, 2002

REYES M et al: Acyclovir-resistant genital herpes among persons attending sexually transmitted disease and human immunodeficiency virus clinics. Arch Intern Med 163:76, 2003

SCHACKER T et al: Frequent recovery of HIV-1 from genital herpes simplex virus lesions in HIV-1-infected men. JAMA 280:61, 1998

SPRUANCE SL et al: High-dose, short-duration, early valacyclovir therapy for episodic treatment of cold sores: Results of two randomized, placebo-controlled, multicenter studies. Antimicrob Agents Chemother 47:1072, 2003

WALD A et al: Effect of condoms on reducing the transmission of herpes simplex virus type 2 from men to women. JAMA 285:3100, 2002

——— et al: Frequent genital herpes simplex virus 2 shedding in immunocompetent women: Effect of acyclovir treatment. J Clin Invest 99:1092, 1997

164   VARICELLA-ZOSTER VIRUS INFECTIONS
Richard J. Whitley

DEFINITION   Varicella-zoster virus (VZV) causes two distinct clinical entities: varicella (chickenpox) and herpes zoster (shingles). Chickenpox, a ubiquitous and extremely contagious infection, is usually a benign illness of childhood characterized by an exanthematous vesicular rash. With reactivation of latent VZV (which is most common after the sixth decade of life), herpes zoster presents as a dermatomal vesicular rash, usually associated with severe pain.

ETIOLOGY   A clinical association between varicella and herpes zoster has been recognized for nearly 100 years. Early in the twentieth century, similarities in the histopathologic features of skin lesions resulting from varicella and herpes zoster were demonstrated. Viral isolates from patients with chickenpox and herpes zoster produced similar alterations in tissue culture—specifically, the appearance of eosinophilic intranuclear inclusions and multinucleated giant cells. These results suggested that the viruses were biologically similar. Restriction endonuclease analyses of viral DNA from a patient with chickenpox who subsequently developed herpes zoster verified the molecular identity of the two viruses responsible for these different clinical presentations.

VZV is a member of the family Herpesviridae, sharing with other members such structural characteristics as a lipid envelope surrounding a nucleocapsid with icosahedral symmetry, a total diameter of ~180 to 200 nm, and centrally located double-stranded DNA that is ~125,000 bp in length.

PATHOGENESIS AND PATHOLOGY   ■   Primary Infection   Transmission is most likely to take place by the respiratory route; the subsequent localized replication of the virus at an undefined site (presumably the nasopharynx) leads to seeding of the reticuloendothelial system and ultimately to the development of viremia. Viremia in patients with chickenpox is reflected in the diffuse and scattered nature of the skin lesions and can be verified in selected cases by the recovery of VZV from the blood or routinely by polymerase chain reaction (PCR). Vesicles involve the corium and dermis, with degenerative changes characterized by ballooning, the presence of multinucleated giant cells, and eosinophilic intranuclear inclusions. Infection may involve localized blood vessels of the skin, resulting in necrosis and epidermal hemorrhage. With the evolution of disease, the vesicular fluid becomes cloudy because of the recruitment of polymorphonuclear leukocytes and the presence of degenerated cells and fibrin. Ultimately, the vesicles either rupture and release their fluid (which includes infectious virus) or are gradually reabsorbed.

Recurrent Infection   The mechanism of reactivation of VZV that results in herpes zoster is unknown. Presumably, the virus infects the dorsal root ganglia during chickenpox, where it remains latent until reactivated. Histopathologic examination of representative dorsal root ganglia during active herpes zoster demonstrates hemorrhage, edema, and lymphocytic infiltration.

Active replication of VZV in other organs, such as the lung or the brain, can occur during either chickenpox or herpes zoster but is uncommon in the immunocompetent host. Pulmonary involvement is characterized by interstitial pneumonitis, multinucleated giant cell formation, intranuclear inclusions, and pulmonary hemorrhage. Central nervous system (CNS) infection leads to histopathologic evidence of perivascular cuffing similar to that encountered in measles and other viral encephalitides. Focal hemorrhagic necrosis of the brain, characteristic of herpes simplex virus encephalitis, is uncommon in VZV infection.

EPIDEMIOLOGY AND CLINICAL MANIFESTATIONS   ■   Chickenpox   Humans are the only known reservoir for VZV. Chickenpox is highly contagious, with an attack rate of at least 90% among susceptible (seronegative) individuals. Persons of both sexes and all races are infected equally often. The virus is endemic in the population at large; however, it becomes epidemic among susceptible individuals during seasonal peaks—namely, late winter and early spring in the temperate zone. Historically, children between the ages of 5 and 9 are most commonly affected and account for 50% of all cases. Most other cases involve children aged 1 to 4 and those aged 10 to 14. Approximately 10% of the population of the United States over the age of 15 is susceptible to infection. VZV vaccination during the second year of life is dramatically changing the epidemiology of infection.

The incubation period of chickenpox ranges from 10 to 21 days but is usually between 14 and 17 days. Secondary attack rates in susceptible siblings within a household are between 70 and 90%. Patients are infectious ~48 h prior to the onset of the vesicular rash, during the period of vesicle formation (which generally lasts 4 to 5 days), and until all vesicles are crusted.

Clinically, chickenpox presents as a rash, low-grade fever, and malaise, although a few patients develop a prodrome 1 to 2 days before onset of the exanthem. In the immunocompetent patient, this is usually a benign illness that is associated with lassitude and with body temperatures of 37.8° to 39.4°C (100° to 103°F) of 3 to 5 days' duration. The skin lesions—the hallmark of the infection—include maculopapules, vesicles, and scabs in various stages of evolution (Fig. 164-1). These lesions, which evolve from maculopapules to vesicles over hours to days, appear on the trunk and face and rapidly spread to involve other areas of the body. Most are small and have an erythematous base with a diameter of 5 to 10 mm. Successive crops appear over a 2- to 4-day period. Lesions can also be found on the mucosa of the pharynx and/or the vagina. Their severity varies from one person to another. Some individuals have very few lesions, while others have

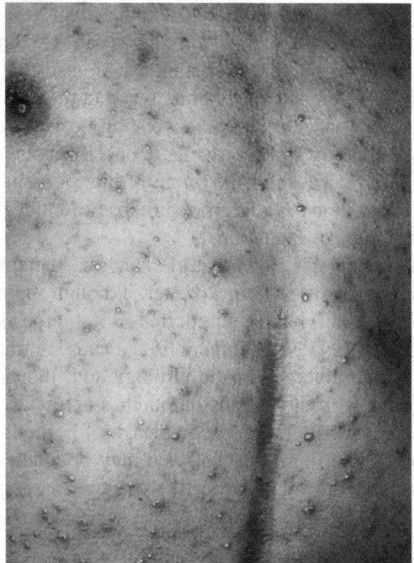

FIGURE 164-1 Numerous varicella lesions at various stages of evolution: vesicles on an erythematous base, umbilical vesicles, and crusts.

as many as 2000. Younger children tend to have fewer vesicles than older individuals. Secondary and tertiary cases within families are associated with a relatively large number of vesicles. Immunocompromised patients—both children and adults, particularly those with leukemia—have lesions (often with a hemorrhagic base) that are more numerous and take longer to heal than those of immunocompetent patients. Immunocompromised individuals are also at greater risk for visceral complications, which occur in 30 to 50% of cases and are fatal 15% of the time in the absence of antiviral therapy.

The most common infectious complication of varicella is secondary bacterial superinfection of the skin, which is usually caused by *Streptococcus pyogenes* or *Staphylococcus aureus*. This complication may result from excoriation of skin lesions after scratching. Gram's staining of skin lesions should help clarify the etiology of unusually erythematous and pustulated lesions.

The most common extracutaneous site of involvement in children is the CNS. The syndrome of acute cerebellar ataxia and meningeal irritation generally appears ~21 days after the onset of the rash and rarely develops in the preeruptive phase. The cerebrospinal fluid (CSF) contains lymphocytes and elevated levels of protein. CNS involvement is a benign complication of VZV infection in children and generally does not require hospitalization. Aseptic meningitis, encephalitis, transverse myelitis, Guillain-Barré syndrome, and Reye's syndrome can also occur. Encephalitis is reported in 0.1 to 0.2% of children with chickenpox. Other than supportive care, no specific therapy is available for patients with CNS involvement.

Varicella pneumonia is the most serious complication following chickenpox, developing more commonly in adults (up to 20% of cases) than in children. It usually has its onset 3 to 5 days into the illness and is associated with tachypnea, cough, dyspnea, and fever. Cyanosis, pleuritic chest pain, and hemoptysis are frequent. Roentgenographic evidence of disease consists of nodular infiltrates and interstitial pneumonitis. Resolution of pneumonitis parallels improvement of the skin rash; however, patients may have persistent fever and compromised pulmonary function for weeks.

Other complications of chickenpox include myocarditis, corneal lesions, nephritis, arthritis, bleeding diatheses, acute glomerulonephritis, and hepatitis. Hepatic involvement, distinct from Reye's syndrome and usually asymptomatic, is common in chickenpox and is generally characterized by elevated levels of liver enzymes, particularly aspartate and alanine aminotransferases.

Perinatal varicella is associated with a high mortality rate when maternal disease develops within 5 days before delivery or within 48 h thereafter. Because the newborn does not receive protective transplacental antibodies and has an immature immune system, the illness may be unusually severe. The reported mortality rate has been as high as 30% in this group. *Congenital varicella*, with clinical manifestations of limb hypoplasia, cicatricial skin lesions, and microcephaly at birth, is extremely uncommon.

Herpes Zoster Herpes zoster, a sporadic disease, is the consequence of reactivation of latent VZV from the dorsal root ganglia. Most patients have no history of recent exposure to other individuals with VZV infection. Herpes zoster occurs at all ages, but its incidence is highest (5 to 10 cases per 1000 persons) among individuals in the sixth decade of life and beyond. Recurrent herpes zoster is exceedingly rare except in immunocompromised hosts, especially those with AIDS.

Herpes zoster, also called shingles, is characterized by a unilateral vesicular eruption within a dermatome, often associated with severe pain. The dermatomes from T3 to L3 are most frequently involved. If the ophthalmic branch of the trigeminal nerve is involved, zoster ophthalmicus results. The factors responsible for the reactivation of VZV are not known. In children reactivation is usually benign, whereas in adults it can be debilitating. The continuum of pain from onset to resolution is known as *zoster-associated pain*. The onset of disease is heralded by pain within the dermatome that may precede lesions by 48 to 72 h; an erythematous maculopapular rash evolves rapidly into vesicular lesions (Fig. 164-2). In the normal host, these lesions may remain few in number and continue to form only for a period of 3 to 5 days. The total duration of disease is generally between 7 and 10 days; however, it may take as long as 2 to 4 weeks for the skin to return to normal. Patients with herpes zoster can transmit infection to seronegative individuals, with consequent chickenpox. In a few patients, characteristic localization of pain to a dermatome with serologic evidence of herpes zoster has been reported in the absence of skin lesions. When branches of the trigeminal nerve are involved, lesions may appear on the face, in the mouth, in the eye, or on the tongue. Zoster ophthalmicus is usually a debilitating condition that can result in blindness in the absence of antiviral therapy. In the Ramsay Hunt syndrome, pain and vesicles appear in the external auditory canal, and patients lose their sense of taste in the anterior two-thirds

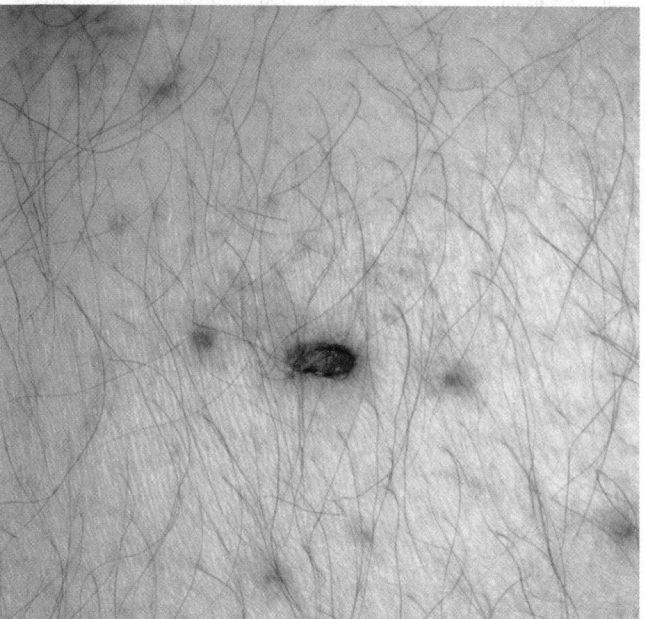

FIGURE 164-2 Close-up of lesions of disseminated zoster. Note lesions at different stages of evolution, including pustules and crusting. (*Photo courtesy of Lindsey Baden.*)

of the tongue while developing ipsilateral facial palsy. The geniculate ganglion of the sensory branch of the facial nerve is involved.

The most debilitating complication of herpes zoster, in both the normal and the immunocompromised host, is pain associated with acute neuritis and postherpetic neuralgia. Postherpetic neuralgia is uncommon in young individuals; however, at least 50% of patients over age 50 with zoster report some degree of pain in the involved dermatome months after the resolution of cutaneous disease. Changes in sensation in the dermatome, resulting in either hypo- or hyperesthesia, are common.

CNS involvement may follow localized herpes zoster. Many patients without signs of meningeal irritation have CSF pleocytosis and moderately elevated levels of CSF protein. Symptomatic meningoencephalitis is characterized by headache, fever, photophobia, meningitis, and vomiting. A rare manifestation of CNS involvement is granulomatous angiitis with contralateral hemiplegia, which can be diagnosed by cerebral arteriography. Other neurologic manifestations include transverse myelitis with or without motor paralysis.

Like chickenpox, herpes zoster is more severe in the immunocompromised host than in the normal individual. Lesions continue to form for over a week, and scabbing is not complete in most cases until 3 weeks into the illness. Patients with Hodgkin's disease and non-Hodgkin's lymphoma are at greatest risk for progressive herpes zoster. Cutaneous dissemination (Fig. 164-3) develops in ~40% of these patients. Among patients with cutaneous dissemination, the risk of pneumonitis, meningoencephalitis, hepatitis, and other serious complications is increased by 5 to 10%. However, even in immunocompromised patients, disseminated zoster is rarely fatal.

Patients who have received a bone marrow transplant are at particularly high risk of VZV infection. Thirty percent of cases of posttransplantation VZV infection occur within 1 year (50% of these within 9 months); 45% of the patients involved have cutaneous or visceral dissemination. The mortality rate in this situation is 10%. Postherpetic neuralgia, scarring, and bacterial superinfection are especially frequent in VZV infections occurring within 9 months of transplantation. Among infected patients, concomitant graft-versus-host disease increases the chance of dissemination and/or death.

DIFFERENTIAL DIAGNOSIS The diagnosis of chickenpox is not difficult. The characteristic rash and a history of recent exposure should lead to a prompt diagnosis. Other viral infections that can mimic chickenpox include disseminated herpes simplex virus infection in patients with atopic dermatitis and the disseminated vesiculopapular lesions sometimes associated with coxsackievirus infection, echovirus infection, or atypical measles. However, these rashes are more commonly morbil-

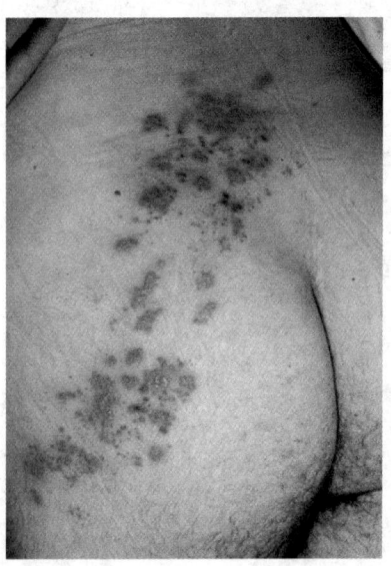

FIGURE 164-3 Herpes zoster is seen in this HIV-infected patient as hemorrhagic vesicles and pustules on an erythematous base grouped in a dermatomal distribution.

liform with a hemorrhagic component rather than vesicular or vesiculopustular. Rickettsialpox (Chap. 158) can be confused with chickenpox; however, it can be distinguished easily by detection of the "herald spot" at the site of the mite bite and the development of a more pronounced headache. Serologic testing is also useful in differentiating rickettsialpox from varicella. Concern about smallpox has recently increased because of the threat of bioterrorism (Chap. 205). The lesions of smallpox are larger than those of chickenpox and are all at the same stage of evolution.

Unilateral vesicular lesions in a dermatomal pattern should lead rapidly to the diagnosis of herpes zoster, although the occurrence of shingles without a rash has been reported. Both herpes simplex virus infections and coxsackievirus infections can cause dermatomal vesicular lesions. Supportive diagnostic virology and fluorescent staining of skin scrapings with monoclonal antibodies are helpful in ensuring the proper diagnosis. In the prodromal stage of herpes zoster, the diagnosis can be exceedingly difficult and may be made only after lesions have appeared or by retrospective serologic assessment.

LABORATORY FINDINGS Unequivocal confirmation of the diagnosis is possible only through the isolation of VZV in susceptible tissue-culture cell lines, the demonstration of either seroconversion or a fourfold or greater rise in antibody titer between convalescent- and acute-phase serum specimens, or the detection of VZV DNA by PCR. A rapid impression can be obtained by a Tzanck smear, with scraping of the base of the lesions in an attempt to demonstrate multinucleated giant cells, although the sensitivity of this method is low (~60%). PCR technology for the detection of viral DNA in vesicular fluid is available in a limited number of diagnostic laboratories. Direct immunofluorescent staining of cells from the lesion base or detection of viral antigens by other assays (such as the immunoperoxidase assay) is also useful, although these tests are not commercially available. The most frequently employed serologic tools for assessing host response are the immunofluorescent detection of antibodies to VZV membrane antigens, the fluorescent antibody to membrane antigen (FAMA) test, immune adherence hemagglutination, and enzyme-linked immunosorbent assay (ELISA). The FAMA test and the ELISA appear to be the most sensitive.

℞ TREATMENT

Medical management of chickenpox in the immunologically normal host is directed toward the prevention of avoidable complications. Obviously, good hygiene includes daily bathing and soaks. Secondary bacterial infection of the skin can be avoided by meticulous skin care, particularly with close cropping of fingernails. Pruritus can be decreased with topical dressings or the administration of antipruritic drugs. Tepid water baths and wet compresses are better than drying lotions for the relief of itching. Aluminum acetate soaks for the management of herpes zoster can be both soothing and cleansing. Administration of aspirin to children with chickenpox should be avoided because of the association of aspirin derivatives with the development of Reye's syndrome. Acyclovir therapy (800 mg by mouth five times daily for 5 to 7 days) is recommended for adolescents and adults with chickenpox of ≤24 h duration. Likewise, acyclovir therapy may be of benefit to children <12 years of age if initiated early in the disease (<24 h) at a dose of 20 mg/kg every 6 h.

Patients with herpes zoster benefit from oral antiviral therapy, as evidenced by accelerated healing of lesions and resolution of zoster-associated pain with acyclovir, valacyclovir, or famciclovir. Acyclovir, now off patent, is administered at a dosage of 800 mg five times daily for 7 to 10 days. Famciclovir, the prodrug of penciclovir, is at least as effective as acyclovir and perhaps more so. One study showed twofold faster resolution of postherpetic neuralgia in famciclovir-treated patients with zoster than in recipients of placebo. The dose is 500 mg by mouth three times daily for 7 days. Valacyclovir, the prodrug of acyclovir, accelerates healing and resolution of zoster-associated pain more promptly than acyclovir. The dose is 1 g by mouth three times daily for 5 to 7 days. Both famciclovir and valacyclovir offer the advantage of a lower dosing frequency than acyclovir.

In the immunocompromised host, both chickenpox and herpes zoster (including disseminated disease) should be treated with intravenous acyclovir, which reduces the occurrence of visceral complications but has no effect on healing of skin lesions or pain. The dose is 10 to 12.5 mg/kg every 8 h for 7 days. Oral acyclovir therapy is not recommended for the treatment of VZV infections in immunocompromised patients. Concomitant with the administration of intravenous acyclovir, it is desirable to attempt to wean these patients from immunosuppressive treatment.

Patients with varicella pneumonia may require removal of bronchial secretions and ventilatory support. Persons with zoster ophthalmicus should be referred immediately to an ophthalmologist. Therapy for this condition consists of the administration of analgesics for severe pain and the use of atropine. Acyclovir accelerates healing.

The management of acute neuritis and/or postherpetic neuralgia can be particularly difficult. In addition to the judicious use of analgesics, ranging from nonnarcotics to narcotic derivatives, drugs such as gabapentin, amitriptyline hydrochloride, lidocaine patches, and fluphenazine hydrochloride have been reported to be beneficial for pain relief. In one study, glucocorticoid therapy administered early in the course of localized herpes zoster significantly accelerated such quality-of-life improvements as a return to usual activity and termination of analgesia. The dose of prednisone administered orally was 60 mg/d on days 1 through 7, 30 mg/d on days 8 through 14, and 15 mg/d on days 15 through 21. This regimen is appropriate only for relatively healthy elderly persons who have moderate or severe pain at presentation. Patients with osteoporosis, diabetes mellitus, glycosuria, or hypertension may not be appropriate candidates. Glucocorticoids should not be used without concomitant antiviral therapy.

PREVENTION　Three methods are used for the prevention of VZV infections. First, a live attenuated varicella vaccine (OKA) is recommended for all children >1 year of age (up to 12 years of age) who have not had chickenpox and for adults known to be seronegative for VZV. A single dose of vaccine is administered to children, whereas adults require two doses. The vaccine is both safe and efficacious. Breakthrough cases are mild and may result in spread of the vaccine virus to susceptible contacts. The universal vaccination of children is resulting in a decreased incidence of chickenpox in sentinel communities. Furthermore, inactivation of the vaccine virus significantly decreases the occurrence of herpes zoster after human stem-cell transplantation. A vaccine study is being performed in individuals >60 years of age to determine its impact on the incidence and severity of shingles.

A second approach is to administer varicella-zoster immune globulin (VZIg) to individuals who are susceptible, are at high risk for developing complications of varicella, and have had a significant exposure. This product should be given within 96 h (preferably within 72 h) of the exposure. Indications for administration of VZIg appear in Table 164-1.

Lastly, antiviral therapy can be given as prophylaxis to individuals at high risk who are ineligible for vaccine or beyond the 96-h window after direct contact. While the initial studies have used acyclovir, similar benefit can be anticipated with either valacyclovir or famciclovir. Therapy is instituted 7 days after intense exposure. At this time, the

TABLE 164-1　*Recommendations for VZIg Administration*

Exposure criteria
1. Exposure to person with chickenpox or zoster
   a. Household: residence in the same household
   b. Playmate: face-to-face indoor play
   c. Hospital
      Varicella: same 2- to 4-bed room or adjacent beds in large ward, face-to-face contact with infectious staff member or patient, visit by a person deemed contagious
      Zoster: intimate contact (e.g., touching or hugging) with a person deemed contagious
   d. Newborn infant: onset of varicella in the mother ≤5 days before delivery or ≤48 h after delivery; VZIg is not indicated if the mother has zoster
2. Patient should receive VZIg as soon as possible but not >96 h after exposure

Candidates (provided they have significant exposure) include:
1. Immunocompromised susceptible children without history of varicella or varicella immunization
2. Susceptible pregnant women
3. Newborn infants whose mother had onset of chickenpox within 5 days before or within 48 h after delivery
4. Hospitalized premature infant (≥28 weeks of gestation) whose mother lacks a reliable history of chickenpox or serologic evidence of protection against varicella
5. Hospitalized premature infant (<28 weeks of gestation or ≤1000-g birth weight), regardless of maternal history of varicella or varicella-zoster virus serologic status

Source: Adapted from American Academy of Pediatrics, *Red Book, Report of the Committee on Infectious Diseases*, G Peter (ed), Elk Grove Village, IL, American Academy of Pediatrics, 2003, pp 678–679; with permission.

host is midway into the incubation period. This approach significantly decreases disease severity, if not totally preventing disease.

FURTHER READING

BEUTNER KR et al: Valacyclovir compared with acyclovir for improved therapy for herpes zoster in immunocompetent adults. Antimicrob Agents Chemother 39:1547, 1995

DUNKLE LM et al: A controlled trial of acyclovir for chickenpox in normal children. N Engl J Med 325:1539, 1991

GNANN JW, WHITLEY RJ: Herpes zoster. N Engl J Med 347:340, 2002

IZURIETA HS et al: Postlicensure effectiveness of varicella vaccine during an outbreak in a child care center. JAMA 278:1495, 1997

ROWBOTHAM M et al: Gabapentin for the treatment of postherpetic neuralgia. A randomized controlled trial. JAMA 280:1837, 1998

SHEPP D et al: Treatment of varicella-zoster virus in severely immunocompromised patients: A randomized comparison of acyclovir and vidarabine. N Engl J Med 314:208, 1987

TYRING S et al: Famciclovir for the treatment of acute herpes zoster. Effects on acute disease and postherpetic neuralgia: A randomized, double-blind, placebo-controlled trial. Ann Intern Med 123:89, 1995

WHITLEY RJ et al: Disseminated herpes zoster in the immunocompromised host: A comparative trial of acyclovir and vidarabine. J Infect Dis 165:450, 1992

——— et al: Acyclovir with and without prednisone for the treatment of herpes zoster: A randomized, placebo-controlled trial. Ann Intern Med 125:376, 1996

WOOD MJ et al: A randomized trial of acyclovir for 7 days or 21 days with and without prednisolone for treatment of acute herpes zoster. N Engl J Med 330:896, 1994

DEFINITION Epstein-Barr virus (EBV) is the cause of heterophile-positive infectious mononucleosis (IM), which is characterized by fever, sore throat, lymphadenopathy, and atypical lymphocytosis. EBV is also associated with several human tumors, including nasopharyngeal carcinoma, Burkitt's lymphoma, Hodgkin's disease, and (in patients with immunodeficiencies) B cell lymphoma. The virus, a member of the family Herpesviridae, consists of a linear DNA core surrounded by a nucleocapsid and an envelope that contains glycoproteins. The two types of EBV that are widely prevalent in nature are not distinguishable by conventional serologic tests.

EPIDEMIOLOGY EBV infections occur worldwide. These infections are most common in early childhood, with a second peak during late adolescence. By adulthood, more than 90% of individuals have been infected and have antibodies to the virus. IM is usually a disease of young adults. In lower socioeconomic groups and in areas of the world with lower standards of hygiene (e.g., developing countries), EBV tends to infect children at an early age, and symptomatic IM is uncommon. In areas with higher standards of hygiene, infection with EBV is often delayed until adulthood, and IM is more prevalent.

EBV is spread by contact with oral secretions. The virus is frequently transmitted from asymptomatic adults to infants and among young adults by transfer of saliva during kissing. Transmission by less intimate contact is rare. EBV has been transmitted by blood transfusion and by bone marrow transplantation. More than 90% of asymptomatic seropositive individuals shed the virus in oropharyngeal secretions.

PATHOGENESIS EBV is transmitted by salivary secretions. The virus infects the epithelium of the oropharynx and the salivary glands and is shed from these cells. While B cells may become infected after contact with epithelial cells, studies suggest that lymphocytes in the tonsillar crypts can be infected directly. The virus then spreads through the bloodstream. The proliferation and expansion of EBV-infected B cells along with reactive T cells during IM result in enlargement of lymphoid tissue. Polyclonal activation of B cells leads to the production of antibodies to host-cell and viral proteins. During the acute phase of IM, up to 1 in every 100 B cells in the peripheral blood is infected by EBV, while after recovery, about 1 in every million B cells is infected. During IM there is an inverted CD4+/CD8+ T cell ratio. The percentage of CD4+ T cells decreases, while there are large clonal expansions of CD8+ T cells; up to 40% of CD8+ T cells are directed against EBV antigens during acute infection. Data suggest that memory B cells, not epithelial cells, are the reservoir for EBV in the body. When patients are treated with acyclovir, shedding of EBV from the oropharynx stops but the virus persists in B cells.

The EBV receptor (CD21), present on the surface of B cells, is also the receptor for the C3d component of complement. EBV infection of epithelial cells results in viral replication and production of virions. When B cells are infected by EBV in vitro, they become transformed and can proliferate indefinitely. During latent infection of B cells, only the EBV nuclear antigens (EBNAs), latent membrane proteins (LMPs), and small EBV RNAs are expressed in vitro. EBV-transformed B cells secrete immunoglobulin; only a small fraction of cells produce virus.

Cellular immunity is more important than humoral immunity in controlling EBV infection. In the initial phase of infection, suppressor T cells, natural killer cells, and nonspecific cytotoxic T cells are important in controlling the proliferation of EBV-infected B cells. Levels of markers of T cell activation and serum interferon γ are elevated. Later in infection, HLA-restricted cytotoxic T cells that recognize EBNAs and LMPs and destroy EBV-infected cells are generated. Studies have shown that one of the late genes expressed during EBV replication, *BCRF1*, is a homologue of interleukin 10 and can inhibit the production of interferon γ by mononuclear cells in vitro.

If T cell immunity is compromised, EBV-infected B cells may begin to proliferate. When EBV is associated with lymphoma, virus-induced proliferation is but one step in a multistep process of neoplastic transformation. In many EBV-containing tumors, LMP-1 mimics members of the tumor necrosis factor receptor family (e.g., CD40), transmitting growth-proliferating signals.

CLINICAL MANIFESTATIONS Most EBV infections in infants and young children either are asymptomatic or present as mild pharyngitis with or without tonsillitis. In contrast, up to 75% of infections in adolescents present as IM.

Signs and Symptoms The incubation period for IM in young adults is ~4 to 6 weeks. A prodrome of fatigue, malaise, and myalgia may last for 1 to 2 weeks before the onset of fever, sore throat, and lymphadenopathy. Fever is usually low-grade and is most common in the first 2 weeks of the illness; however, it may persist for >1 month. Common signs and symptoms are listed along with their frequencies in Table 165-1. Lymphadenopathy and pharyngitis are most prominent during the first 2 weeks of the illness, while splenomegaly is more prominent during the second and third weeks. Lymphadenopathy most often affects the posterior cervical nodes but may be generalized. Enlarged lymph nodes are frequently tender and symmetric but are not fixed in place. Pharyngitis, often the most prominent sign, can be accompanied by enlargement of the tonsils with an exudate resembling that of streptococcal pharyngitis. A morbilliform or papular rash, usually on the arms or trunk, develops in ~5% of cases. Most patients treated with ampicillin develop a macular rash; this rash is not predictive of future adverse reactions to penicillins. Erythema nodosum and erythema multiforme have also been described (Chap. 48). Most patients have symptoms for 2 to 4 weeks, but malaise and difficulty concentrating can persist for months.

Symptomatic IM is uncommon in infants and young children. IM in the elderly presents relatively often as nonspecific symptoms, including prolonged fever, fatigue, myalgia, and malaise; in contrast, pharyngitis, lymphadenopathy, splenomegaly, and atypical lymphocytes are relatively rare in elderly patients.

Laboratory Findings The white blood cell count is usually elevated and peaks at 10,000 to 20,000/μL during the second or third week of illness. Lymphocytosis is usually demonstrable, with >10% atypical lymphocytes. The latter cells are enlarged lymphocytes that have abundant cytoplasm, vacuoles, and indentations of the cell membrane. CD8+ cells predominate among the atypical lymphocytes. Low-grade neutropenia and thrombocytopenia are common during the first month

TABLE 165-1 *Signs and Symptoms of Infectious Mononucleosis*

Manifestation	Median Percentage of Patients (Range)
Symptoms	
Sore throat	75 (50–87)
Malaise	47 (42–76)
Headache	38 (22–67)
Abdominal pain, nausea, or vomiting	17 (5–25)
Chills	10 (9–11)
Signs	
Lymphadenopathy	95 (83–100)
Fever	93 (60–100)
Pharyngitis or tonsillitis	82 (68–90)
Splenomegaly	51 (43–64)
Hepatomegaly	11 (6–15)
Rash	10 (0–25)
Periorbital edema	13 (2–34)
Palatal enanthem	7 (3–13)
Jaundice	5 (2–10)

of illness. Liver function is abnormal in more than 90% of cases. Serum levels of aminotransferases and alkaline phosphatase are usually mildly elevated; the serum concentration of bilirubin is elevated in ~40% of cases.

Complications Most cases of IM are self-limited. Deaths are very rare and most often are due to central nervous system (CNS) complications, splenic rupture, upper airway obstruction, or bacterial superinfection.

When CNS complications develop, they usually do so during the first 2 weeks of EBV infection; in some patients, especially children, they are the only clinical manifestations of IM. Heterophile antibodies and atypical lymphocytes may be absent. Meningitis and encephalitis are the most common neurologic abnormalities, and patients may present with headache, meningismus, or cerebellar ataxia; acute hemiplegia and psychosis have also been described. The cerebrospinal fluid (CSF) contains mainly lymphocytes, with occasional atypical lymphocytes. Most cases resolve without neurologic sequelae. Acute EBV infection has also been associated with cranial nerve palsies (especially ones involving cranial nerve VII), Guillain-Barré syndrome, acute transverse myelitis, and peripheral neuritis.

Autoimmune hemolytic anemia occurs in ~2% of cases during the first 2 weeks. In most cases the anemia is Coombs'-test positive, with cold agglutinins directed against the i red blood cell antigen. Most patients with hemolysis have mild anemia that lasts for 1 or 2 months, but some patients have severe disease with hemoglobinuria and jaundice. Nonspecific antibody responses may also include rheumatoid factor, antinuclear antibodies, anti–smooth muscle antibodies, antiplatelet antibodies, and cryoglobulins. IM has been associated with red-cell aplasia, severe granulocytopenia, thrombocytopenia, pancytopenia, and hemophagocytic syndrome. The spleen ruptures in fewer than 0.5% of cases. Splenic rupture is more common among males than among females and may be manifest as abdominal pain, referred shoulder pain, or hemodynamic compromise.

Hypertrophy of lymphoid tissue in the tonsils or adenoids can result in upper airway obstruction, as can inflammation and edema of the epiglottis, pharynx, or uvula. About 10% of patients with IM develop streptococcal pharyngitis after their initial sore throat resolves.

Other rare complications associated with acute EBV infection include hepatitis (which can be fulminant), myocarditis or pericarditis with electrocardiographic changes, pneumonia with pleural effusion, interstitial nephritis, genital ulcerations, and vasculitis.

OTHER DISEASES ASSOCIATED WITH EBV INFECTION EBV-associated lymphoproliferative disease has been described in patients with congenital or acquired immunodeficiency, including those with severe combined immunodeficiency, AIDS, and recipients of bone marrow or organ transplants who are receiving immunosuppressive drugs (especially cyclosporine). Proliferating EBV-infected B cells infiltrate lymph nodes and multiple organs, and patients present with fever and lymphadenopathy or gastrointestinal symptoms. Pathologic studies show B cell hyperplasia or poly- or monoclonal lymphoma. The X-linked lymphoproliferative syndrome (Duncan's disease) is a recessive disorder of young boys who have a normal response to childhood infections but develop fatal lymphoproliferative disorders after infection with EBV. The gene mutated in this syndrome, *SAP* or *SH2D1A*, has been identified; its product binds to a protein that mediates interactions of B and T cells. Most patients with this syndrome die of acute IM; others develop hypogammaglobulinemia, malignant B cell lymphomas, aplastic anemia, or agranulocytosis. IM has also proved fatal to some patients with no obvious preexisting immune abnormality.

Oral hairy leukoplakia (Fig. 165-1) is an early manifestation of infection with HIV in adults (Chap. 173). Most patients present with raised, white corrugated lesions on the tongue (and occasionally on the buccal mucosa) that contain EBV DNA. Children infected with HIV can develop lymphoid interstitial pneumonitis; EBV DNA is often found in lung tissue from these patients.

Patients with the chronic fatigue syndrome may have titers of antibody to EBV that are elevated but are not significantly different from those in healthy EBV-seropositive adults. While some patients have

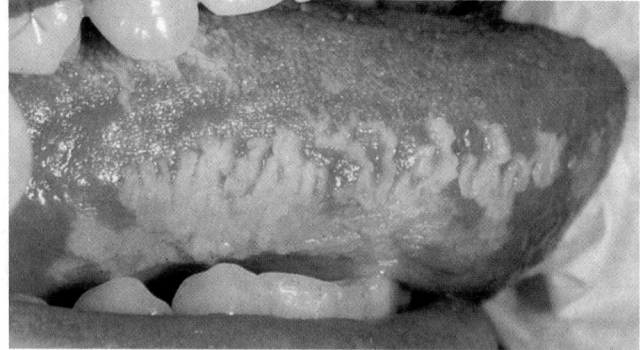

FIGURE 165-1 Oral hairy leukoplakia often presents as white plaques on the lateral surface of the tongue and is associated with Epstein-Barr virus infection.

malaise and fatigue that persist for weeks or months after IM, persistent EBV infection is not a cause of the chronic fatigue syndrome. Chronic active EBV infection is very rare and is distinct from the chronic fatigue syndrome. The affected patients have an illness lasting >6 months with markedly elevated titers of antibody to EBV and evidence of organ involvement, including hepatosplenomegaly, lymphadenopathy, and pneumonitis, uveitis, or neurologic disease.

EBV is associated with several malignancies. About 15% of cases of Burkitt's lymphoma in the United States and ~90% of those in Africa are associated with EBV (Chap. 97). African patients with Burkitt's lymphoma have high levels of antibody to EBV, and their tumor tissue usually contains viral DNA. EBV-containing Burkitt's lymphoma also occurs in patients with AIDS. Anaplastic nasopharyngeal carcinoma is uniformly associated with EBV; the affected tissues contain viral DNA and antigens. Patients with nasopharyngeal carcinoma often have elevated titers of antibody to EBV (Chap. 74).

EBV has been associated with Hodgkin's disease, especially the mixed-cellularity type (Chap. 97). Patients with Hodgkin's disease often have elevated titers of antibody to EBV, and in about half of cases viral DNA and antigens are found in Reed-Sternberg cells. In some cases, EBV DNA has been detected in tonsillar carcinoma, angioimmunoblastic lymphadenopathy, angiocentric nasal NK/T cell immunoproliferative lesions, T cell lymphoma, thymoma, gastric carcinoma, and CNS lymphoma from patients with no underlying immunodeficiency. Studies have demonstrated viral DNA in leiomyosarcomas from AIDS patients and in smooth-muscle tumors from organ transplant recipients. Virtually all CNS lymphomas in AIDS patients are associated with EBV. While serologic studies have shown higher levels of antibodies to EBV before the onset of multiple sclerosis, other studies (including measurement of EBV antibody titers in the CSF) are needed to ascertain a possible causal relationship.

DIAGNOSIS ■ Serologic Testing The heterophile test is used for the diagnosis of IM in children and adults (Table 165-2). In the test for this antibody, human serum is absorbed with guinea pig kidney, and the heterophile titer is defined as the greatest serum dilution that agglutinates sheep, horse, or cow erythrocytes. Although heterophile antibody binds to certain animal erythrocytes, it does not interact with EBV proteins. A titer of 40-fold or greater is diagnostic of acute EBV infection in a patient who has symptoms compatible with IM and atypical lymphocytes. Tests for heterophile antibodies are positive in 40% of patients with IM during the first week of illness and in 80 to 90% during the third week. Therefore, repeated testing may be necessary, especially if the initial test is performed early. Tests usually remain positive for 3 months after the onset of illness, but heterophile antibodies can persist for up to 1 year. These antibodies usually are not detectable in children <5 years of age, in the elderly, or in patients presenting with symptoms not typical of IM. The commercially available monospot test for heterophile antibodies is somewhat more sensitive than the classic heterophile test. The monospot test is ~75%

Condition	Heterophile	Anti-VCA IgM	Anti-VCA IgG	Anti-EA EA-D	Anti-EA EA-R	Anti-EBNA
Acute infectious mononucleosis	+	+	+ +	+	−	−
Convalescence	±	−	+	−	±	+
Past infection	−	−	+	−	−	+
Reactivation with immunodeficiency	−	−	+ +	+	+	±
Burkitt's lymphoma	−	−	+ + +	±	+ +	+
Nasopharyngeal carcinoma	−	−	+ + +	+ +	±	+

[a] VCA, viral capsid antigen; EA, early antigen; EA-D antibody, antibody to early antigen in diffuse pattern in nucleus and cytoplasm of infected cells; EA-R antibody, antibody to early antigen restricted to the cytoplasm; and EBNA, Epstein-Barr nuclear antigen.
Source: Adapted from Okano, 1988.

sensitive and ~90% specific compared with EBV-specific serologies. False-positive monospot results are more common in persons with connective tissue disease, lymphoma, viral hepatitis, and malaria.

EBV-specific antibody testing is used for patients with suspected acute EBV infection who lack heterophile antibodies and for patients with atypical infections (Table 165-2). Serologic tests are particularly useful in young children, who often do not develop heterophile antibodies. Titers of IgM and IgG antibodies to viral capsid antigen (VCA) are elevated in the serum of more than 90% of patients at the onset of disease. IgM antibody to VCA is most useful for the diagnosis of acute IM because it is present at elevated titers only during the first 2 to 3 months of the disease; in contrast, IgG antibody to VCA is usually not useful for diagnosis of IM but is often used to assess exposure to EBV in the past because it persists for life. Seroconversion to EBNA positivity is also useful for the diagnosis of acute infection with EBV. Antibodies to EBNA are detectable relatively late (3 to 6 weeks after the onset of symptoms) in nearly all cases of acute EBV infection and persist for the lifetime of the patient. These antibodies may be lacking in immunodeficient patients and in those with chronic active EBV infection.

Titers of other antibodies may also be elevated in IM; however, these elevations are less useful for diagnosis. Antibodies to early antigens (EAs) are found either in a diffuse pattern in the nucleus and cytoplasm of infected cells (EA-D antibody) or restricted to the cytoplasm (EA-R antibody). These antibodies are detectable 3 to 4 weeks after the onset of symptoms in patients with IM. About 70% of individuals with IM have EA-D antibodies during the course of illness; the presence of EA-D antibodies is especially likely in those with relatively severe disease. These antibodies usually persist for only 3 to 6 months. Levels of EA-D antibodies are also elevated in patients with nasopharyngeal carcinoma or chronic active EBV infection. EA-R antibodies are only occasionally detected in patients with IM but are often found at elevated titers in patients with African Burkitt's lymphoma or chronic active EBV infection. IgA antibodies to EBV antigens have proved useful for the identification of patients with nasopharyngeal carcinoma and of persons at high risk for the disease.

TABLE 165-3 Treatment Options for Posttransplantation EBV Lymphoproliferative Disease

1. Reduction of immunosuppression, when possible
2. Excision of localized lesions
3. Interferon α
4. Monoclonal antibody to CD20 (rituximab)
5. Radiation therapy (especially for CNS lesions)
6. For stem cell transplant recipients: donor lymphocyte infusions or donor EBV-specific cytotoxic T cell infusions[a]
7. For solid organ transplant recipients: autologous or HLA-matched, EBV-specific, cytotoxic T cell infusions[a]
8. Cytotoxic chemotherapy

[a] Infused T cells must be HLA matched; lymphoproliferative lesions are usually of donor origin for stem cell transplant recipients and of recipient origin for solid organ transplant recipients.

Other Studies Detection of EBV DNA, RNA, or proteins has been valuable in demonstrating the association of the virus with various malignancies. The polymerase chain reaction has been used to detect EBV DNA in the CSF of some AIDS patients with lymphomas and to monitor the amount of EBV DNA in the blood of patients with lymphoproliferative disease. Culture of EBV from throat washings or blood is not helpful in the diagnosis of acute infection, since EBV commonly persists in the oropharynx and in B cells for the lifetime of the infected individual.

Differential Diagnosis The differential diagnosis of IM and atypical lymphocytosis includes acute infection with cytomegalovirus, *Toxoplasma*, HIV, human herpesvirus 6, and hepatitis viruses as well as drug hypersensitivity reactions. Cytomegalovirus is the most common cause of heterophile-negative mononucleosis, usually involves older patients, and is associated with a lower frequency of sore throat, splenomegaly, and lymphadenopathy than IM due to EBV. Other diseases that share some of the features of IM include rubella, acute infectious lymphocytosis in children, and lymphoma or leukemia.

Rx TREATMENT

Therapy for IM consists of supportive measures, with rest and analgesia. Excessive physical activity during the first month should be avoided to reduce the possibility of splenic rupture. If splenic rupture occurs, splenectomy is required. Glucocorticoid therapy is not indicated for uncomplicated IM and in fact may predispose to bacterial superinfection. Prednisone (40 to 60 mg/d for 2 to 3 days, with subsequent tapering of the dose over 1 to 2 weeks) has been used for the prevention of airway obstruction in patients with severe tonsillar hypertrophy, for autoimmune hemolytic anemia, and for severe thrombocytopenia. Glucocorticoids have also been used in a few selected patients with severe malaise and fever and in patients with severe CNS or cardiac disease.

Acyclovir has had no significant clinical impact on IM in controlled trials. In one study, the combination of acyclovir and prednisolone had no significant effect on the duration of symptoms of IM. Acyclovir, at a dosage of 400 to 800 mg five times daily, has been effective for the treatment of oral hairy leukoplakia (despite common relapses) and some cases of chronic active EBV disease. The posttransplantation EBV lymphoproliferative syndrome (Chap. 117) generally does not respond to antiviral therapy. When possible, therapy should be directed toward reduction of immunosuppression (Table 165-3). Interferon α or antibody to CD20 has been effective in some cases. Infusions of donor lymphocytes are often effective for stem cell transplant recipients, although graft-versus-host disease can occur. Infusions of EBV-specific cytotoxic T cells have been used to prevent EBV lymphoproliferative disease in high-risk settings as well as to treat the disease.

The isolation of patients with IM is unnecessary. Vaccines directed against the major EBV glycoprotein have been effective in animal studies and are undergoing small-scale clinical trials.

FURTHER READING

AUWAERTER PG: Infectious mononucleosis in middle age. JAMA 281:454, 1999

CHIEN Y-C et al: Serologic markers of Epstein-Barr virus infection and nasopharyngeal carcinoma in Taiwanese men. N Engl J Med 345:1877, 2001

COHEN JI: Epstein-Barr virus infection. N Engl J Med 343:481, 2000

GOTTSCHALK S et al: Treatment of Epstein-Barr virus–associated malignancies with specific T cells. Adv Cancer Res 84:175, 2002

LEVIN LI et al: Multiple sclerosis and Epstein-Barr virus. JAMA 289:1533, 2003

OKANO M et al: Epstein-Barr virus and human diseases: Recent advances in diagnosis. Clin Microbiol Rev 1:300, 1988

PAPADOPOULOS EB et al: Infusions of donor leukocytes to treat Epstein-Barr virus–associated lymphoproliferative disorders after allogeneic bone marrow transplantation. N Engl J Med 330:1185, 1994

PAYA CV et al: Epstein-Barr virus–induced posttransplant lymphoproliferative disorders. Transplantation 68:1517, 1999

RICKINSON AB, KIEFF E: Epstein-Barr virus, in *Fields Virology*, 4th ed, DM Knipe, PM Howley (eds). Philadelphia, Lippincott Williams & Wilkins, 2001

SAYOS J et al: The X-linked lymphoproliferative-disease gene product SAP

regulates signals induced through the co-receptor SLAM. Nature 395:462, 1998

TYNELL E et al: Acyclovir and prednisolone treatment of acute infectious mononucleosis: A multicenter, double-blind, placebo-controlled study. J Infect Dis 174:324, 1996

166 CYTOMEGALOVIRUS AND HUMAN HERPESVIRUS TYPES 6, 7, AND 8
Martin S. Hirsch

CYTOMEGALOVIRUS

DEFINITION Cytomegalovirus (CMV), which was initially isolated from patients with congenital cytomegalic inclusion disease, is now recognized as an important pathogen in all age groups. In addition to inducing severe birth defects, CMV causes a wide spectrum of disorders in older children and adults, ranging from an asymptomatic, subclinical infection to a mononucleosis syndrome in healthy individuals to disseminated disease in immunocompromised patients. Human CMV is one of several related species-specific viruses that cause similar diseases in various animals. All are associated with the production of characteristic enlarged cells—hence the name *cytomegalovirus*.

CMV is a member of the β-herpesvirus group and has double-strand DNA, four species of mRNA, a protein capsid, and a lipoprotein envelope. Like other herpesviruses, CMV demonstrates icosahedral symmetry, replicates in the cell nucleus, and can cause either a lytic and productive or a latent infection. CMV can be distinguished from other herpesviruses by certain biologic properties, such as host range and type of cytopathology induced. Viral replication is associated with the production of large intranuclear inclusions and smaller cytoplasmic inclusions. The virus appears to replicate in a variety of cell types in vivo; in tissue culture it grows preferentially in fibroblasts. Although there is little evidence that CMV is oncogenic in vivo, the virus does transform fibroblasts in rare instances, and genomic transforming fragments have been identified.

EPIDEMIOLOGY CMV has a worldwide distribution. Approximately 1% of newborns in the United States are infected with CMV, and the percentage is higher in many less-developed countries. Communal living and poor personal hygiene facilitate early spread. Perinatal and early childhood infections are common. Virus may be present in breast milk, saliva, feces, and urine. Transmission of CMV has been identified among young children in day-care centers and has been traced from infected toddler to pregnant mother to developing fetus. When an infected child introduces CMV into a household, 50% of susceptible family members seroconvert within 6 months.

The virus is not readily spread by casual contact but requires repeated or prolonged intimate exposure for transmission. In late adolescence and young adulthood, CMV is often transmitted sexually, and asymptomatic viral carriage in semen or cervical secretions is common. CMV antibody is present at detectable levels in nearly 100% of female prostitutes and sexually active homosexual men. Sexually active adults may harbor several strains of CMV simultaneously. Transfusion of whole blood or certain blood products containing viable leukocytes may also transmit CMV, with a frequency of 0.14 to 10% per unit transfused.

Once infected, an individual probably carries CMV for life. The infection usually remains latent. However, CMV reactivation syndromes develop frequently when T lymphocyte–mediated immunity is compromised—for example, after organ transplantation or in association with lymphoid neoplasms and certain acquired immunodeficiencies (in particular, infection with HIV; Chap. 173). Most primary CMV infections in organ transplant recipients (Chap. 117) result from transmission of the virus in the graft itself. In CMV-seropositive transplant recipients, infection results from reactivation of latent virus or, less commonly, from reinfection by a new strain of CMV. CMV infection may be associated with coronary artery stenosis following heart transplantation or coronary angioplasty, but this association requires further validation.

PATHOGENESIS Congenital CMV infection can result from either primary or reactivation infection of the mother. However, clinical disease in the fetus or newborn is almost exclusively related to primary maternal infection (Table 166-1). The factors determining the severity of congenital infection are unknown; a deficient capacity to produce precipitating antibodies and to mount T cell responses to CMV is associated with relatively severe disease.

Primary infection in late childhood or adulthood is often associated with a vigorous T lymphocyte response that may contribute to the development of a mononucleosis syndrome similar to that observed following Epstein-Barr virus (EBV) infection (Chap. 165). The hallmark of such infection is the appearance of atypical lymphocytes in the peripheral blood; these cells are predominantly activated CD8+ T lymphocytes. Polyclonal activation of B cells by the virus contributes to the development of rheumatoid factors and other autoantibodies during CMV mononucleosis.

Once acquired by symptomatic or asymptomatic primary infection,

TABLE 166-1 *CMV in the Immunocompromised Host*

Population	Risk Factors	Principal Syndromes	Treatment	Prevention
Fetus	Primary maternal infection/early pregnancy	Cytomegalic inclusion disease	None (?ganciclovir)	Avoidance of exposure
Organ transplant recipient	Seropositive donor, seronegative recipient; intensive immunosuppression, particularly with antilymphocyte globulins, cyclosporine	Febrile leukopenia; pneumonia; gastrointestinal disease	Ganciclovir or valganciclovir	Donor matching; CMV immuno-globulin; ganciclovir or high-dose acyclovir
Bone marrow transplant recipient	Graft-vs.-host disease; older age; seropositive recipient; viremia	Pneumonia; gastrointestinal disease	Ganciclovir plus CMV immunoglobulin	Ganciclovir or high-dose acyclovir
Person with AIDS	<100 CD4+ cells per microliter; CMV seropositivity	Retinitis; gastrointestinal disease; neurologic disease	Foscarnet, ganciclovir, valganciclovir, or cidofovir	Oral ganciclovir

CMV persists indefinitely in tissues of the host. The sites of persistent or latent infection probably include multiple cell types and various organs. Transmission following blood transfusion or organ transplantation is due to silent infections in these tissues. Autopsy studies suggest that salivary glands and bowel may be areas of latent infection.

If the host's T cell responses become compromised by disease or by iatrogenic immunosuppression, latent virus can be reactivated to cause a variety of syndromes. Chronic antigenic stimulation in the presence of immunosuppression (for example, following tissue transplantation) appears to be an ideal setting for CMV activation and CMV-induced disease. Certain particularly potent suppressants of T cell immunity, such as antithymocyte globulin, are associated with a high rate of clinical CMV syndromes, which may follow either primary or reactivation infection. CMV may itself contribute to further T lymphocyte hyporesponsiveness, which often precedes superinfection with other opportunistic pathogens, such as *Pneumocystis*. CMV and *Pneumocystis* are frequently found together in immunosuppressed patients with severe interstitial pneumonia.

PATHOLOGY Cytomegalic cells in vivo (presumed to be infected epithelial cells) are two to four times larger than surrounding cells and often contain an 8- to 10-μm intranuclear inclusion that is eccentrically placed and is surrounded by a clear halo, producing an "owl's eye" appearance. Smaller granular cytoplasmic inclusions are demonstrated occasionally. Cytomegalic cells are found in a wide variety of organs, including salivary gland, lung, liver, kidney, intestine, pancreas, adrenal gland, and the central nervous system.

The cellular inflammatory response to infection consists of plasma cells, lymphocytes, and monocyte-macrophages. Granulomatous reactions occasionally develop, particularly in the liver. Immunopathologic reactions may contribute to CMV disease. Immune complexes have been detected in infected infants, sometimes in association with CMV-related glomerulopathies. Immune-complex glomerulopathy has been observed in some CMV-infected patients after renal transplantation.

CLINICAL MANIFESTATIONS ■ Congenital CMV Infection Fetal infections range from inapparent to severe and disseminated. Cytomegalic inclusion disease develops in ~5% of infected fetuses and is seen almost exclusively in infants born to mothers who develop primary infections during pregnancy. Petechiae, hepatosplenomegaly, and jaundice are the most common presenting features (60 to 80% of cases). Microcephaly with or without cerebral calcifications, intrauterine growth retardation, and prematurity are reported in 30 to 50% of cases. Inguinal hernias and chorioretinitis are less common. Laboratory abnormalities include elevated alanine aminotransferase levels, thrombocytopenia, conjugated hyperbilirubinemia, hemolysis, and elevated cerebrospinal fluid protein levels. The prognosis for severely infected infants is poor; the mortality rate is 20 to 30%, and few of the patients who survive escape intellectual or hearing difficulties later in childhood. The differential diagnosis of cytomegalic inclusion disease in infants includes syphilis, rubella, toxoplasmosis, infection with herpes simplex virus or enterovirus, and bacterial sepsis.

Most congenital CMV infections are clinically inapparent at birth. Between 5 and 25% of asymptomatically infected infants develop significant psychomotor, hearing, ocular, or dental abnormalities over the next several years.

Perinatal CMV Infection The newborn may acquire CMV at the time of delivery by passage through an infected birth canal or by postnatal contact with breast milk or other maternal secretions. Approximately 40 to 60% of infants who are breast-fed for >1 month by seropositive mothers become infected. Iatrogenic transmission can also result from neonatal blood transfusion. Screening of blood products before they are transfused into low-birth-weight seronegative infants or into seronegative pregnant women decreases the risk of infection.

The great majority of infants infected at or after delivery remain asymptomatic. However, protracted interstitial pneumonitis has been associated with perinatally acquired CMV infection, particularly in premature infants, and occasionally has been accompanied by infection with *Chlamydia trachomatis*, *Pneumocystis*, or *Ureaplasma urealyticum*. Poor weight gain, adenopathy, rash, hepatitis, anemia, and atypical lymphocytosis may also be found, and CMV excretion often persists for months or years.

CMV Mononucleosis The most common clinical manifestation of CMV infection in normal hosts beyond the neonatal period is a heterophil antibody–negative mononucleosis syndrome. This manifestation may develop spontaneously or may follow the transfusion of leukocyte-containing blood products. Although the syndrome occurs at all ages, it most often involves sexually active young adults. Incubation periods range from 20 to 60 days, and the illness generally lasts for 2 to 6 weeks. Prolonged high fevers, sometimes accompanied by chills, profound fatigue, and malaise, characterize this disorder. Myalgias, headache, and splenomegaly are frequent, but in CMV mononucleosis (as opposed to infectious mononucleosis caused by EBV), exudative pharyngitis and cervical lymphadenopathy are rare. Occasional patients develop rubelliform rashes, often after exposure to ampicillin. Less commonly observed are interstitial or segmental pneumonia, myocarditis, pleuritis, arthritis, and encephalitis. In rare cases, Guillain-Barré syndrome complicates CMV mononucleosis. The characteristic laboratory abnormality is relative lymphocytosis in peripheral blood, with more than 10% atypical lymphocytes. Total leukocyte counts may be low, normal, or markedly elevated. Although significant jaundice is uncommon, serum aminotransferase and alkaline phosphatase levels are often moderately elevated. Heterophil antibodies are absent; however, transient immunologic abnormalities are common and may include the presence of cryoglobulins, rheumatoid factors, cold agglutinins, and antinuclear antibodies. Hemolytic anemia, thrombocytopenia, and granulocytopenia complicate recovery in rare instances.

Most patients recover without sequelae, although postviral asthenia may persist for months. The excretion of CMV in urine, genital secretions, and/or saliva often continues for months or years. Rarely, CMV infection is fatal in immunocompetent hosts; even when such patients survive, they can have recurrent episodes of fever and malaise that are sometimes associated with autonomic nervous system dysfunction (e.g., attacks of sweating or flushing).

CMV Infection in the Immunocompromised Host (See also Table 166-1) CMV appears to be the most common and important viral pathogen complicating organ transplantation (Chap. 117). In recipients of kidney, heart, lung, and liver transplants, CMV induces a variety of syndromes, including fever and leukopenia, hepatitis, pneumonitis, esophagitis, gastritis, colitis, and retinitis. CMV disease may be an independent risk factor for both graft loss and death. The period of maximal risk is between 1 and 4 months after transplantation, although retinitis may be a later complication. Disease likelihood and levels of viral replication generally are greater after primary infection than after reactivation. In addition, molecular studies indicate that seropositive transplant recipients are susceptible to reinfection with donor-derived, genotypically variant CMV, and such infection often results in disease. Reactivation infection, although frequent, is less likely than primary infection to be important clinically. The risk of clinical disease is related to various factors, such as the degree of immunosuppression; the use of antibodies to T cell receptors; and co-infection with other pathogens, such as human herpesvirus type 6. The transplanted organ is particularly vulnerable as a target for CMV infection; thus, there is a tendency for CMV hepatitis to follow liver transplantation and for CMV pneumonitis to follow lung transplantation.

CMV pneumonia occurs in 15 to 20% of bone marrow transplant recipients, with a case-fatality rate of 84 to 88%. The risk is greatest between 5 and 13 weeks after transplantation, and the several risk factors identified include certain types of immunosuppressive therapy, acute graft-versus-host disease, older age, viremia, and seropositivity before transplantation.

CMV is recognized as an important pathogen in patients with advanced HIV infection (Chap. 173), in whom it often causes retinitis or disseminated disease, particularly when peripheral-blood CD4+ cell counts fall below 50 to 100/μL. As treatment for underlying HIV infection has improved, the incidence of serious CMV infections (e.g., retinitis) has decreased. However, institution of highly active antiretroviral regimens sometimes leads to acute flare-ups of CMV retinitis during the first few weeks of therapy.

Syndromes produced by CMV in the immunocompromised host often begin with prolonged fever, malaise, anorexia, fatigue, night sweats, and arthralgias or myalgias. Liver function abnormalities, leukopenia, thrombocytopenia, and atypical lymphocytosis may be observed during these episodes. The development of tachypnea, hypoxia, and unproductive cough signals respiratory involvement. Radiologic examination of the lung often reveals bilateral interstitial or reticulonodular infiltrates, which begin in the periphery of the lower lobes and spread centrally and superiorly; localized segmental, nodular, or alveolar patterns are less common. The differential diagnosis includes infection with *Pneumocystis*; infections due to other viral, bacterial, or fungal pathogens; pulmonary hemorrhage; and injury secondary to irradiation or to treatment with cytotoxic drugs.

Gastrointestinal CMV involvement may be localized or extensive and almost exclusively affects compromised hosts. Ulcers of the esophagus, stomach, small intestine, or colon may result in bleeding or perforation. CMV infection may lead to exacerbations of underlying ulcerative colitis. Hepatitis occurs frequently, particularly following liver transplantation, and CMV-associated acalculous cholecystitis and adrenalitis have been described.

CMV rarely causes meningoencephalitis in otherwise-healthy individuals. Two forms of CMV encephalitis are seen in patients with AIDS. One resembles HIV encephalitis and presents as progressive dementia; the other is a ventriculoencephalitis characterized by cranial-nerve deficits, nystagmus, disorientation, lethargy, and ventriculomegaly. In immunocompromised patients, CMV can also cause subacute progressive polyradiculopathy, which is often reversible if recognized and treated promptly.

CMV retinitis is an important cause of blindness in immunocompromised patients, particularly patients with advanced AIDS (Chap. 173). Early lesions consist of small, opaque, white areas of granular retinal necrosis that spread in a centrifugal manner and are later accompanied by hemorrhages, vessel sheathing, and retinal edema (Fig. 166-1). CMV retinopathy must be distinguished from that due to other conditions, including toxoplasmosis, candidiasis, and herpes simplex virus infection.

Fatal CMV infections are often associated with persistent viremia and the involvement of multiple organ systems. Progressive pulmonary infiltrates, pancytopenia, hyperamylasemia, and hypotension are characteristic features that are frequently found in conjunction with a terminal bacterial, fungal, or protozoan superinfection. Extensive ad-

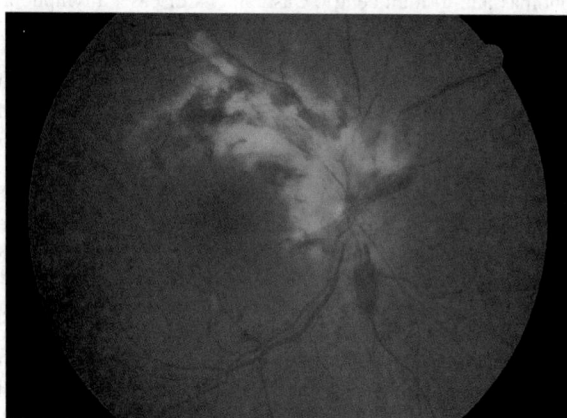

FIGURE 166-1 Cytomegalovirus in a patient with AIDS appears as an arcuate zone of retinitis with hemorrhages and optic disk swelling. Often CMV is confined to the retinal periphery, beyond view of the direct ophthalmoscope.

renal necrosis with CMV inclusions is often documented at autopsy, as is CMV involvement of many other organs.

DIAGNOSIS The diagnosis of CMV infection usually cannot be made reliably on clinical grounds alone. Isolation of the virus or detection of CMV antigens or DNA from appropriate clinical specimens is the preferred diagnostic approach. Virus excretion or viremia is readily detected by culture of appropriate specimens on human fibroblast monolayers. If viral titers are high, as is frequently the case in congenital disseminated infection or in patients with AIDS, characteristic cytopathic effects may be detected within a few days. However, in some situations—such as CMV mononucleosis—viral titers are low, and cytopathic effects may take several weeks to appear. Many laboratories expedite diagnosis with an overnight tissue-culture method (shell vial assay) involving centrifugation and an immunocytochemical detection technique employing monoclonal antibodies to an immediate-early CMV antigen. Isolation of virus from urine or saliva does not, by itself, constitute proof of acute infection, since excretion from these sites may continue for months or years after illness. Detection of CMV viremia is a better predictor of acute infection.

Detection of CMV antigens (pp65) in peripheral-blood leukocytes or of CMV DNA in blood or tissues may hasten the diagnosis of CMV disease in certain populations, including organ transplant recipients and persons with AIDS. Such assays may yield a positive result several days earlier than culture methods. The most sensitive way to detect CMV in blood or other fluids may be by amplifying CMV DNA by polymerase chain reaction (PCR) assays. PCR detection of CMV DNA in blood may predict the risk for disease progression, and PCR detection of CMV DNA in cerebrospinal fluid is useful in the diagnosis of CMV encephalitis or polyradiculopathy.

A variety of serologic assays are available to detect increases in titers of antibody to CMV antigens. An increased antibody level may not be detectable for up to 4 weeks after primary infection, and titers often remain high for years after infection. For this reason, single-sample antibody determinations are of no value in assessing the acuteness of infection. Detection of CMV-specific IgM is sometimes useful in the diagnosis of recent or active infection; circulating rheumatoid factors may result in occasional false-positive IgM tests.

℞ TREATMENT

Several prophylactic measures are useful for the prevention of CMV infection in patients at high risk. The use of blood from seronegative donors or of blood that has been frozen, thawed, and deglycerolized greatly decreases the rate of transfusion-associated transmission of CMV. Similarly, matching of organ or bone marrow transplants by CMV serology, with exclusive use of organs from seronegative donors in seronegative recipients, reduces rates of primary infection following transplantation. Both live attenuated and CMV subunit vaccines have been evaluated, but neither is close to approval for general use.

CMV immune globulin has been reported to reduce rates of CMV-associated syndromes and of fungal or parasitic superinfections among seronegative renal transplant recipients. Studies in bone marrow transplant recipients have produced conflicting results. Prophylactic acyclovir or valacyclovir may reduce rates of CMV infection and disease in certain seronegative renal transplant recipients, although neither drug is effective in the treatment of active CMV disease.

Ganciclovir is a guanosine derivative that has considerably more activity against CMV than its congener acyclovir. After intracellular conversion by a viral phosphotransferase encoded by CMV gene region UL97, ganciclovir triphosphate is a selective inhibitor of CMV DNA polymerase. Several clinical studies have indicated response rates of 70 to 90% among patients with AIDS given ganciclovir for the treatment of CMV retinitis or colitis. In bone marrow transplant recipients with CMV pneumonia, ganciclovir is less effective when given alone, but it elicits a favorable clinical response 50 to 70% of the time when it is combined with CMV immune globulin. Prophylactic or suppressive ganciclovir may be useful in high-risk bone marrow or organ transplant recipients (e.g., those who are CMV-seropositive before transplantation or who are CMV culture–positive afterward). In many patients with AIDS, persistently low CD4+ cell counts, and CMV disease, clinical and virologic relapses occur promptly if treatment with ganciclovir is discontinued. Therefore, prolonged maintenance regimens are recommended for such patients. Resistance to ganciclovir is common among patients treated for >3 months and is usually related to mutations in the CMV UL97 gene.

Valganciclovir is an orally bioavailable prodrug that is rapidly metabolized to ganciclovir in intestinal tissues and the liver. Approximately 60% of an oral dose of valganciclovir is absorbed. An oral valganciclovir dose of 900 mg results in ganciclovir blood levels similar to those obtained with an intravenous ganciclovir dose of 5 mg/kg. Oral valganciclovir appears to be as effective as intravenous ganciclovir for both CMV retinitis induction and maintenance regimens. Furthermore, the adverse-event profiles and rates of resistance development for the two drugs are similar.

Ganciclovir or valganciclovir therapy for CMV retinitis consists of a 14- to 21-day induction course (5 mg/kg intravenously twice daily for ganciclovir or 900 mg twice daily for valganciclovir) followed by a prolonged maintenance regimen. For parenteral maintenance, the ganciclovir dose is 5 mg/kg daily or 6 mg/kg 5 days per week; for oral maintenance, 900 mg of valganciclovir once daily is recommended. Peripheral-blood neutropenia develops in 16 to 29% of treated patients but may be ameliorated by granulocyte colony-stimulating factor or granulocyte-macrophage colony-stimulating factor. Discontinuation of maintenance therapy should be considered in patients with AIDS who, while receiving antiretroviral therapy, have a sustained (>6-month) increase in CD4 cell counts to >100–150/μL.

Foscarnet (sodium phosphonoformate) also acts against CMV infection by inhibiting viral DNA polymerase. Because this agent does not require phosphorylation to be active, it is also effective against most ganciclovir-resistant CMV isolates. Foscarnet is less well tolerated than ganciclovir and causes considerable toxicity, including renal dysfunction, hypomagnesemia, hypokalemia, hypocalcemia, genital ulcers, dysuria, nausea, and paresthesia. Moreover, foscarnet administration requires the use of an infusion pump and close clinical monitoring. With aggressive hydration and dose adjustments for renal dysfunction, the toxicity of foscarnet can be reduced. The use of foscarnet should be avoided when a saline load cannot be tolerated (e.g., in cardiomyopathy). The approved induction regimen is 60 mg/kg every 8 h for 2 weeks, although 90 mg/kg every 12 h is equally effective and no more toxic. Maintenance infusions should deliver 90 to 120 mg/kg once daily; no oral preparation is available. Foscarnet-resistant viruses may emerge during extended therapy.

Ganciclovir may also be administered via a slow-release pellet sutured into the eye. Although this intraocular device provides good local protection, contralateral eye disease and disseminated disease are not affected, and early retinal detachment is possible. A combination of intraocular and systemic therapy may be better than the intraocular implant alone.

Cidofovir is a nucleotide analogue with a long intracellular half-life that allows intermittent intravenous administration. Induction regimens of 5 mg/kg weekly for 2 weeks are followed by maintenance regimens of 3 to 5 mg/kg every 2 weeks. Cidofovir can cause severe nephrotoxicity through dose-dependent proximal tubular cell injury; however, this adverse effect can be ameliorated somewhat by saline hydration and probenecid.

It is still not clear whether universal prophylaxis or preemptive therapy in immunocompromised hosts with CMV seropositivity is the preferable approach. For patients with advanced HIV infection (CD4 cell counts of <50/μL), some authorities have advocated prophylaxis with oral ganciclovir or valganciclovir. However, side effects, lack of proven benefit, possible induction of viral resistance, and cost have precluded the wide acceptance of this practice. Similar questions have arisen concerning prophylaxis in organ transplant recipients. As techniques for identifying individuals at risk improve (e.g., quantification of CMV DNA by PCR), it may become possible to preemptively treat those at highest risk to prevent end-organ disease.

HUMAN HERPESVIRUS TYPES 6, 7, AND 8

Human herpesvirus (HHV) type 6 was first isolated in 1986 from peripheral-blood leukocytes of six persons with various lymphoproliferative disorders. The virus has a worldwide distribution, and two genetically distinct variants (HHV-6A and HHV-6B) are now recognized.

Infection with HHV-6 frequently develops during infancy as maternal antibody wanes. Congenital infections have also been described. HHV-6 (mostly variant B) can cause exanthem subitum (roseola infantum), a common illness characterized by fever with subsequent rash. This virus is also a major cause of febrile seizures without rash during infancy. In older age groups, HHV-6 has been associated with mononucleosis syndromes, focal encephalitis, and (in immunocompromised hosts) pneumonitis and disseminated disease. In transplant recipients, HHV-6 infection may be associated with graft dysfunction. As many as 80% of adults are seropositive for HHV-6. The virus may be transmitted by saliva and possibly by genital secretions. Like many other viruses, HHV-6 has been implicated in the pathogenesis of multiple sclerosis, although further study is needed to distinguish between association and etiology.

HHV-7 was isolated in 1990 from T lymphocytes from the peripheral blood of a healthy 26-year-old man. Other isolates have since been obtained. It appears that the virus is frequently acquired during childhood and is commonly present in the saliva of healthy adults. No human disease has yet been definitively linked to HHV-7, although some cases of exanthem subitum, other childhood febrile illnesses, and neurologic syndromes (encephalitis, flaccid paralysis) have been associated with HHV-7 infection. An association has been made between HHV-7 and pityriasis rosea, but further studies must confirm this relationship.

HHV-6, HHV-7, and CMV infections may cluster in transplant recipients, making it difficult to sort out the roles of the various agents in individual clinical syndromes. HHV-6 and HHV-7 appear to be susceptible to ganciclovir and foscarnet, although definitive evidence of clinical responses is lacking.

Unique herpesvirus-like DNA sequences were reported during 1994 and 1995 in tissues derived from Kaposi's sarcoma (KS) and body cavity–based lymphoma occurring in patients with AIDS. The virus from which these sequences were derived has now been cultured and is designated HHV-8 or Kaposi's sarcoma–associated herpesvirus (KSHV). HHV-8, which infects certain B lymphocytes and endothelium-derived spindle cells, appears to be causally related not only to KS but also to a subgroup of AIDS-related B-cell body-cavity-based lymphomas and to multicentric Castleman's disease, a lymphoproliferative disorder of B cells.

Unlike other herpesvirus infections, HHV-8 infection is more common in some geographic areas (e.g., central and southern Africa) than in others (North America, Asia, northern Europe). Concurrent epidemics of HIV-1 and HHV-8 infections among certain populations (e.g., homosexual and bisexual men) in the late 1970s and early 1980s appear to have resulted in the frequent association of AIDS and KS. Both viruses appear to be sexually transmitted, and HHV-8 may be transmitted in saliva as well. Transmission of HHV-8 may also be associated with organ transplantation and injection drug use. Among individuals with intact immunity, asymptomatic infection is the rule, and neoplastic disorders develop only after immunocompromise. Effective antiretroviral therapy for HIV-infected individuals has led to a marked reduction in rates of KS among individuals dually infected with HHV-8 and HIV in resource-rich areas. HHV-8 itself is susceptible in vitro to ganciclovir, foscarnet, and cidofovir, although clinical evidence for benefit of these agents is lacking.

FURTHER READING

CANNON MJ et al: Blood-borne and sexual transmission of human herpesvirus 8 in women with or at risk for human immunodeficiency virus infection. N Engl J Med 344:637, 2001

CENTERS FOR DISEASE CONTROL AND PREVENTION: Guidelines for preventing opportunistic infections among HIV-infected persons—2002. MMWR 51(RR-8):1, 2002

GOODMAN AD et al: Human herpesvirus 6 genome and antigen in acute multiple sclerosis lesions. J Infect Dis 187:1365, 2003

LUPPI M et al: Bone marrow failure associated with human herpesvirus 8 infection after transplantation. N Engl J Med 343:1378, 2000

LURAIN NS et al: Analysis and characterization of antiviral drug-resistant cytomegalovirus isolates from solid organ transplant recipients. J Infect Dis 186:760, 2002

MARTIN DF et al: A controlled trial of valganciclovir as induction therapy for cytomegalovirus retinitis. N Engl J Med 346:1119, 2002

NOKTA MA et al: Cytomegalovirus (CMV) polymerase chain reaction profiles in individuals with advanced human immunodeficiency virus infection: Relationship to CMV disease. J Infect Dis 185:1717, 2002

PAUK J et al: Mucosal shedding of human herpesvirus 8 in men. N Engl J Med 343:1369, 2000

PAYA CV: Prevention of cytomegalovirus disease in recipients of solid-organ transplants. Clin Infect Dis 32:596, 2001

RENWICK N et al: Seroconversion for human herpesvirus 8 during HIV infection is highly predictive of Kaposi's sarcoma. AIDS 12:2481, 1998

WALSH JC et al: Increasing survival in AIDS patients with cytomegalovirus retinitis treated with combination antiretroviral therapy including protease inhibitors. AIDS 12:613, 1998

167 | MOLLUSCUM CONTAGIOSUM AND OTHER POXVIRUSES, EXCLUDING SMALLPOX VIRUS
Fred Wang

The poxviruses include a large number of related DNA viruses that infect various vertebrate hosts. The poxviruses responsible for infections in humans, along with the main manifestations of these infections, are listed in Table 167-1. Systemic human disease can result from infection with smallpox (variola major) virus, a poxvirus that infects only humans (Chap. 205), or from zoonotic infection with monkeypox virus. Other poxvirus infections cause primarily localized skin disease in humans. Molluscum contagiosum virus (MCV) is an obligate human pathogen that causes distinctive proliferative skin lesions; molluscum contagiosum is the most frequent human disease resulting from poxvirus infection. Exposure to animals infected with other poxviruses can also cause localized skin disease in humans.

MOLLUSCUM CONTAGIOSUM

Molluscum contagiosum is generally a benign disease consisting of pearly, flesh-colored, umbilicated skin lesions 2 to 5 mm in diameter with a characteristic dimple at the center (Fig. 167-1). A relative lack of inflammation and necrosis distinguishes these proliferative lesions from other poxvirus lesions. The lesions occur singly or in clusters. MCV is a human poxvirus that is transmitted by close contact, including sexual intercourse. Swimming pools are a common vector for transmission. Atopy and compromise of skin integrity increase the risk of infection. Lesions may be found anywhere on the body except the palms and soles and may be associated with an eczematous rash. The incubation period ranges from 2 weeks to 6 months, with an average of 2 to 7 weeks. In most cases, the disease is self-limited and regresses spontaneously after 3 to 4 months in immunocompetent hosts. There are no systemic complications, but skin lesions may persist for 3 to 5 years. Molluscum contagiosum develops especially often in association with the advanced stages of HIV infection, with a prevalence of

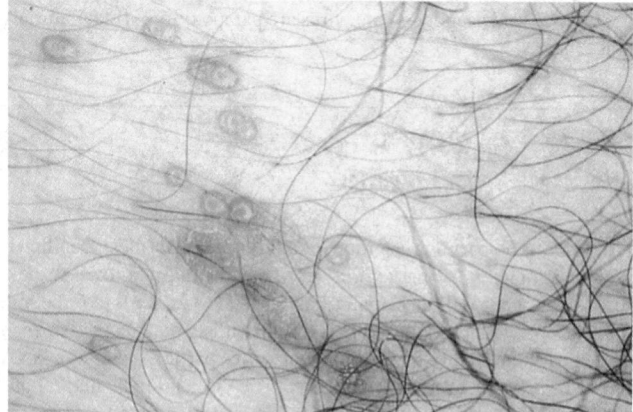

FIGURE 167-1   Molluscum contagiosum is a cutaneous poxvirus infection characterized by multiple umbilicated flesh-colored or hypopigmented papules.

5 to 18% among HIV-infected patients (Chap. 173). The disease is often more generalized, severe, and persistent in AIDS patients than in other groups, frequently involving the face and upper body. Extensive molluscum contagiosum has also been reported in conjunction with other types of immunodeficiency.

The diagnosis of molluscum contagiosum is typically made by its clinical presentation and can be confirmed by histologic demonstration of the cytoplasmic eosinophilic inclusions, or *molluscum bodies*, that are characteristic of poxvirus replication. MCV cannot be propagated in vitro, but electron microscopy and molecular studies can be used for its identification.

There is no specific systemic treatment for molluscum contagiosum, but a variety of techniques for physical ablation have been used. Molluscum contagiosum may respond to effective control of HIV infection with highly active antiretroviral therapy. Cidofovir displays in vitro activity against many poxviruses, including smallpox virus and MCV, and case reports suggest that parenteral or topical cidofovir may have some efficacy in the treatment of recalcitrant molluscum contagiosum in immunosuppressed hosts.

ZOONOTIC POXVIRUS INFECTIONS

Monkeypox virus naturally infects nonhuman primates in the tropical rain forests of western and central Africa and can infect humans who come into direct contact with infected animals. Human disease is rare and is characterized by a systemic illness and vesicular rash similar to those of variola. A large outbreak of monkeypox occurred between February 1996 and October 1997 in central Africa, with a case-fatality ratio of 3%. The prolonged period of active cases suggested a potential

TABLE 167-1   *Poxviruses and Human Infections*

Genus	Species	Human Disease
Orthopoxvirus	Variola[a]	Smallpox, systemic
	Monkeypox	Smallpox-like, systemic
	Vaccinia	Local pox lesion, occasionally systemic
	Cowpox	Local pox lesions
Molluscipoxvirus	Molluscum contagiosum	Molluscum contagiosum, multiple cutaneous lesions
Parapoxvirus	Orf	Contagious pustular dermatitis, local pox lesions
	Pseudocowpox	Milker's nodule, local pox lesions
Yatapoxvirus	Tanapox	Local pox lesions

[a] See Chap. 205.

for sustained person-to-person transmission, and the higher proportion of younger case-patients suggested the possible consequences of discontinued smallpox vaccination. Clinical presentations were occasionally confused with the more common varicella-zoster virus infection. Compared with the lesions of this herpesvirus infection, monkeypox lesions tend to be more uniform (i.e., in the same stage of development at the same time), diffuse, and peripheral in distribution.

The first outbreak of monkeypox infection in the Western Hemisphere occurred in the midwestern United States during May and June 2003. Monkeypox virus infections were diagnosed in several people who had close contact with ill prairie dogs, a Gambian rat, and a rabbit purchased as pets from a common animal distributor. Patients presented most frequently with fever, respiratory symptoms, and lymphadenopathy ~12 days after exposure. The typical vesicular rash developed with or shortly (1 to 3 days) after the fever. The Centers for Disease Control and Prevention recommended smallpox vaccination for persons having close or intimate contact with a documented case of human or animal monkeypox infection in order to reduce the risk of spread. Vaccination can be given up to 14 days after exposure.

Orf virus and pseudocowpox virus are parapoxviruses that naturally infect sheep and cattle. Direct contact with infected animals can result in infections in humans, typically on the hands, with the development of a nodular, highly vascular proliferative lesion that may ulcerate. Human orf virus infection is also called *ecthyma contagiosum*, and human pseudocowpox virus infection causes "milker's nodules." Zoonotic infection with cowpox virus, an orthopoxvirus, causes painful hemorrhagic lesions, mostly on the hands or face, with fever or flulike symptoms and lymphadenitis. Lesions generally resolve in 6 to 8 weeks. Human infection with tanapox virus occurs after contact with infected monkeys. In most cases, a febrile prodrome is followed by eruption of a single nodular lesion on the exposed area, but multiple lesions have also been reported. The lesions are relatively large, often break down to form an ulcer, and resolve in 5 to 6 weeks.

FURTHER READING

BERTHISTLE K, CARRINGTON D: Molluscum contagiosum virus. J Infect 34: 21, 1997
CENTERS FOR DISEASE CONTROL AND PREVENTION: Human monkeypox—Kasai Oriental, Zaire, 1996–1997. MMWR 46:304, 2002
———: Update: Multistate outbreak of monkeypox—Illinois, Indiana, Kansas, Missouri, Ohio, and Wisconsin, 2003. MMWR 52:642, 2003
DECLERCQ E: Cidofovir in the treatment of poxvirus infections. Antiviral Res 55:1, 2002

168 PARVOVIRUS
Neil R. Blacklow

DEFINITION The parvovirus group includes several species-specific viruses of animals. One parvovirus, designated B19, is known to be a human pathogen. B19 is a small (diameter, 20 to 25 nm), icosahedral, nonenveloped, single-stranded DNA virus with an outer capsid formed by two structural proteins. Individual virus particles contain DNA strands of positive or negative polarity. The virus is stable and retains infectivity after incubation at 60°C for 16 h. It has failed to grow in conventional cell culture lines and animal model systems but does replicate in vitro in erythroid progenitor cells derived from human bone marrow, umbilical cord, peripheral blood, or fetal liver sources.

During the 1980s, it was discovered that B19 causes a variety of disorders ranging from erythema infectiosum and acute arthropathy in otherwise healthy hosts to transient aplastic crisis and chronic anemia in compromised patients to fetal infection manifested by death or hydrops fetalis. Many of the severe manifestations of B19 viremia relate to the propensity of the virus to infect and lyse erythroid precursor cells in the bone marrow. The name B19 is derived from the code number of the human serum in which the virus was discovered.

PATHOGENESIS Two studies of adult volunteers have provided a basis for understanding the pathogenesis of B19 infection, which has two phases. The first phase is characterized by viremia that develops approximately 6 days after intranasal inoculation of B19 into susceptible individuals who lack serum antibodies to the virus (Fig. 168-1). The viremia lasts about 1 week; its clearance is correlated with the development of IgM antibodies to B19, which remain detectable for up to a few months. IgG antibodies develop several days later and persist indefinitely. Nonspecific systemic symptoms lasting 2 or 3 days occur early during the viremic phase; these symptoms include headache, malaise, myalgia, fever, chills, and pruritus and are accompanied by reticulocytopenia and excretion of the virus from the respiratory tract. Several days after the onset of symptoms, a clinically insignificant decline in hemoglobin concentration is noted; the decreased level is maintained for 7 to 10 days, during which time examination of bone marrow samples reveals a marked depletion of erythroid precursor cells. Transient mild lymphopenia, neutropenia, and a drop in platelet count also may be found. A second phase of illness begins around 17 or 18 days after virus inoculation (after the clearance of viremia, the cessation of viral shedding in throat secretions, and the resolution of reticulocytopenia). This illness mimics erythema infectiosum in adults, with 2 or 3 days of fine maculopapular rash accompanied by arthralgias and arthritis that last another 1 or 2 days. This phase occurs in the presence of rising serum titers of antibody to B19.

The studies just described indicate that B19 disease in the otherwise *healthy host*, manifested by self-limited erythema infectiosum and/or arthropathy, is almost certainly an immune-complex disorder. This concept is supported by the induction of erythema infectiosum through the infusion of immunoglobulins into chronically viremic patients. In contrast, B19 disease in the *compromised host* (chronic hemolytic disease or immunodeficiency syndromes) is often serious, resulting from the destruction by B19 of erythroid precursor cells. Normal hosts can tolerate 7 to 10 days of shutoff of erythropoiesis; however, patients with hemolytic disease who require increased production of erythrocytes do not tolerate erythroid cell destruction and thus usually develop severe transient aplastic crisis. Patients who are immunodeficient may fail to clear B19 viremia, the results being persistent infection of red blood cells and chronic severe anemia. The fetus requires a higher level of red cell production than do adults and has an immature immune system; both these factors could explain B19-induced hydrops fetalis.

B19 binds specifically to a cellular receptor, erythrocyte P antigen; this specific binding explains the tropism of B19 for erythroid progenitor cells, particularly pronormoblasts and normoblasts. The few persons who lack P antigen cannot be infected with B19.

EPIDEMIOLOGY Although B19 infections occur year-round, they appear most commonly as outbreaks of erythema infectiosum in schools during winter and spring months. Between 20 and 60% of children in outbreaks are symptomatic, and many are asymptomatically infected. Seroepidemiologic studies indicate that approximately half of adults possess serum antibodies to B19. Antibody prevalence (reflecting prior exposure and probable immunity to the virus) rises rapidly between the ages of 5 and 18 years and continues to increase with age—a pattern probably indicating ongoing exposure during adulthood. B19 can be detected in throat swabbings, respiratory tract secretions, and serum, and its detection at these sites probably correlates with infectiousness. Patients with transient aplastic crisis have viremia and shed virus and therefore are highly infectious. Their infectivity has been firmly documented as the source of one well-defined nosocomial outbreak of erythema infectiosum among nurses. In contrast, individuals with erythema infectiosum are much less infectious. The usual route of viral transmission under natural conditions is unknown but may be respiratory or through direct contact. B19 can be transmitted during therapy with clotting factor concentrate and other plasma derivatives, even after exposure to detergent, steam, or dry heat. It has been recommended that polymerase chain reaction (PCR) testing for B19 be used for screening and that potentially infectious material be discarded.

CLINICAL MANIFESTATIONS ■ Erythema Infectiosum

Erythema infectiosum is the most common manifestation of B19 infection and occurs predominantly in children. This entity is also called *fifth disease* because it was classified in the late nineteenth century as the fifth in a series of six exanthems of childhood. Normally a mild illness, erythema infectiosum typically presents as a facial rash with a "slapped-cheek" appearance that is sometimes preceded by low-grade fever. The rash may develop quickly on the arms and legs and usually has a lacy, reticular, erythematous appearance (Fig. 168-2). The trunk, palms, and soles are less commonly involved. Occasionally, the rash appears with maculopapular, morbilliform, vesicular, purpuric, or pruritic characteristics. The typical rash resolves in about a week but can recur intermittently for several weeks, particularly after stress, exercise, exposure to sunlight, bathing, or change in environmental temperature. Arthralgia and arthritis are uncommon among children but are frequent among adults, in whom the rash is often absent or nonspecific, with a lack of the characteristic facial erythema.

Arthropathy B19 infection in adults most commonly presents as acute arthralgias and arthritis, sometimes accompanied by rash. The arthritis is characteristically symmetric and peripheral, involving the wrists, hands, and knees most frequently. It normally resolves in about 3 weeks and is nondestructive. However, a small percentage of patients have arthritis persisting for months or even (in rare cases) for years. It is not known whether these individuals have persistent infection or an abnormal immune response to the virus.

Transient Aplastic Crisis B19 infection is the cause in most instances of transient aplastic crisis developing suddenly in patients with chronic hemolytic disease. Nearly all hemolytic conditions can be affected by B19 infection, including sickle cell disease, erythrocyte enzyme deficiencies, hereditary spherocytosis, thalassemias, paroxysmal nocturnal hemoglobinuria, and autoimmune hemolysis. B19-induced aplastic crisis can also occur in the setting of acute blood loss. Patients present with weakness, lethargy, pallor, and severe anemia, a syndrome often preceded by a few days of nonspecific symptoms. These patients have intense reticulocytopenia lasting 7 to 10 days, and their bone marrow contains no erythroid precursor cells despite a normal myeloid series. Transient aplastic crisis can produce life-threatening anemia and may require urgent transfusion therapy. Unlike patients with erythema infectiosum or arthropathy, those with transient aplastic crisis are viremic and can readily transmit B19 infection to other people.

Chronic Anemia in Immunodeficient Patients Immunodeficient patients may be unable to eliminate B19 infection, probably because they cannot produce adequate levels of virus-specific IgG antibodies. The result is persistent infection with destruction of erythroid precursor cells in the bone marrow and chronic transfusion-dependent anemia. This condition has been described occasionally in patients with immunodeficiency related to infection with HIV, congenital immunodeficiencies, and acute lymphoblastic leukemia during maintenance chemotherapy

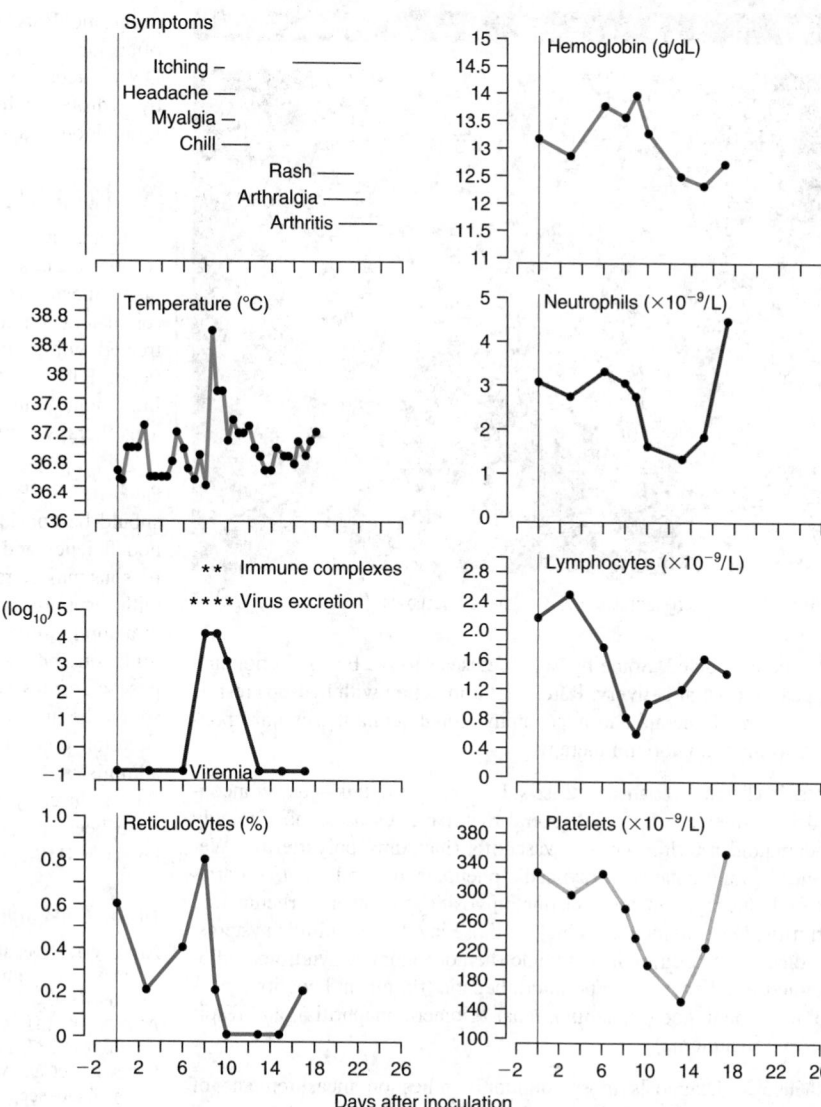

FIGURE 168-1 Features of primary parvovirus infection in a seronegative volunteer inoculated with B19 virus intranasally on day 0. Asterisks indicate days on which immune complexes and virus excretion are detected. Lines refer to the time frame in which the symptoms are detected. *(From Anderson et al, with permission.)*

as well as in recipients of bone marrow, heart, liver, lung, and kidney transplants. In addition, some cases of idiopathic pure red-cell aplasia probably are caused by persistent B19 infection. B19-induced chronic anemia may be the presenting finding of an otherwise unrecognized immunodeficiency. Chronic anemia may fluctuate in intensity over time and may be cured or controlled by immunoglobulin therapy. Both the spectrum of immunodeficiencies associated with B19-induced chronic anemia and the frequency of the association remain to be determined.

Fetal and Congenital Infection Maternal B19 infections usually do not adversely affect the fetus. More often than not, in fact, the fetus remains uninfected. Therefore, couples in which the pregnant woman is infected should be counseled as to the relatively low risk of fetal infection. It is estimated that fewer than 10% of maternal B19 infections in the first 20 weeks of pregnancy lead to fetal death; when fetal death does occur, it is usually attributable to the development of nonimmune hydrops fetalis, wherein the fetus succumbs to severe anemia and congestive heart failure. In these instances, B19 can be detected in fetal tissues, with predominant infection of erythroblasts. One unconfirmed report suggests that B19 causes late second-trimester and third-trimester nonhydropic fetal deaths. Pregnant women with known exposure to B19 should have their serum monitored for IgM antibodies to the virus and for elevated levels of α-fetoprotein and human chorionic gonadotropin; ultrasonic examinations of the fetus for hydrops should

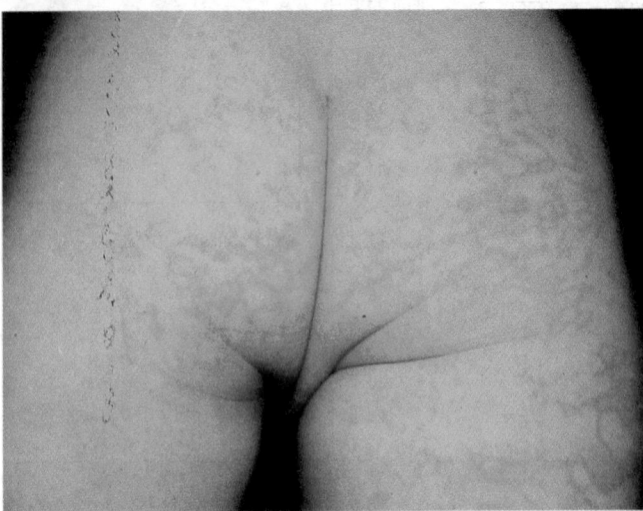

FIGURE 168-2 Lacy reticular rash of erythema infectiosum (fifth disease).

also be conducted. Some hydropic fetuses survive B19 infection and appear normal at delivery. Rarely, fetal infection with hydrops results in congenital anemia and hypogammaglobulinemia that is unresponsive to immunoglobulin therapy.

Possible Clinical Associations Case studies suggest a link—as yet inconclusive—between B19 and several rheumatic diseases, most notably rheumatoid arthritis but also vasculitis (including polyarteritis, Wegener's granulomatosis, Raynaud's phenomenon, and giant cell arteritis), lupus erythematosus, dermatomyositis, and juvenile rheumatoid arthritis. Other associations include those involving multiple systems: cardiac (myocarditis), hematologic (hemophagocytic syndrome, idiopathic thrombocytopenic purpura), hepatic (fulminant hepatitis), neurologic (meningoencephalitis), renal (glomerulonephritis), and respiratory (pneumonia).

DIAGNOSIS Diagnosis most commonly relies on measurements of B19-specific IgM and IgG antibodies, which can be detected with commercially available immunoassay kits. The virus, its DNA, or its antigens are also detected in the serum or infected tissues of some patients. Acute infection can be proven by B19-compatible symptoms and the presence of IgM antibodies or virus itself, whereas past infection is documented by IgG antibodies. Individuals with erythema infectiosum and acute arthropathy usually have IgM antibodies without detectable virus in serum. Those with transient aplastic crisis may have IgM antibodies but typically possess high titers of virus and its DNA in serum; the bone marrow of these patients shows characteristic giant

pronormoblasts and hypoplasia. Immunodeficient patients with anemia often lack readily detectable antibodies but have viral particles and DNA detectable by PCR in serum. Fetal infection may be recognized by hydrops fetalis and the presence of B19 DNA in amniotic fluid or fetal blood in association with maternal IgM antibodies to B19.

℞ TREATMENT

Erythema infectiosum usually requires no treatment; the same is true for many cases of arthropathy. More severe cases of arthritis, particularly those involving chronic symptoms, can be treated with nonsteroidal anti-inflammatory agents. Transient aplastic crisis is usually treated with erythrocyte transfusions. In immunodeficient anemic patients, B19 infection should be treated with commercial intravenous immunoglobulin, which is known to contain IgG antibodies to B19. This therapy controls and may cure B19 infection.

PROPHYLAXIS Prophylaxis of B19 infection with immunoglobulin should be considered for patients with chronic hemolysis or immunodeficiency and for pregnant women. The risk of infection for these persons may be reduced by hand washing before eating or after contact with respiratory or other secretions when B19 is known to be present in a community. Patients with transient aplastic crisis or chronic B19 infection (but not those with erythema infectiosum or arthropathy) pose a serious risk for nosocomial transmission of infection. They should be hospitalized in a private room with contact and respiratory isolation precautions. It is not known whether pre- or postexposure administration of immunoglobulin prevents infection. No vaccine for B19 is currently available; however, noninfectious B19 capsid proteins have been given safely to healthy volunteers, who developed high levels of B19-specific neutralizing antibodies.

FURTHER READING

ABKOWITZ JL et al: Clinical relevance of parvovirus B19 as a cause of anemia in patients with human immunodeficiency virus infection. J Infect Dis 176: 269, 1997

ANDERSON MJ et al: Experimental parvoviral infection in humans. J Infect Dis 152:257, 1985

BARAH F et al: Association of human parvovirus B19 infection with acute meningoencephalitis. Lancet 358:729, 2001

HAREL L et al: Raynaud's phenomenon as a manifestation of parvovirus B19 infection: Case reports and review of parvovirus B19 rheumatic and vasculitic syndromes. Clin Infect Dis 30:500, 2000

MILLER E et al: Immediate and long term outcome of human parvovirus B19 infection in pregnancy. Br J Obstet Gynaecol 105:174, 1998

MORI Y et al: Association of parvovirus B19 infection with acute glomerulonephritis in healthy adults: Case report and review of the literature. Clin Nephrol 57:69, 2002

WEIGEL-KELLEY KA et al: Recombinant human parvovirus B19 vectors: Erythrocyte P antigen is necessary but not sufficient for successful transduction of human hematopoietic cells. J Virol 75:4110, 2001

169 HUMAN PAPILLOMAVIRUS INFECTIONS
Richard C. Reichman

DEFINITION Human papillomaviruses (HPVs) selectively infect the epithelium of skin and mucous membranes. These infections may be asymptomatic, produce warts, or be associated with a variety of both benign and malignant neoplasias.

ETIOLOGIC AGENT Papillomaviruses are members of the family Papillomaviridae. They are nonenveloped, measure 50 to 55 nm in diameter, have icosahedral capsids composed of 72 capsomeres, and contain a double-stranded circular DNA genome of ~7900 base pairs. The genomic organization of all papillomaviruses is similar and consists of an early (E) region, a late (L) region, and a noncoding upstream regulatory region (URR). Oncogenic HPV types can immortalize human

keratinocytes, and this activity has been mapped to products of early genes E6 and E7. E6 protein facilitates the degradation of the p53 tumor-suppressor protein, and E7 protein binds the retinoblastoma gene product and related proteins. The E1 and E2 proteins modulate viral DNA replication and regulate gene expression. The L1 gene codes for the major capsid protein, which makes up 80% of the virion mass. L2 codes for a minor capsid protein. Type-specific conformational antigenic determinants are located on the virion surface. Papillomavirus types are distinguished from one another by the degree of nucleic acid sequence homology. Distinct types share <90% of their DNA sequences in L1. More than 100 HPV types are recognized, and individual types are associated with specific clinical manifestations. For example, HPV-1 causes plantar warts, HPV-6 causes anogenital warts, and HPV-16 infection can produce cervical dysplasia and invasive cervical cancer. HPVs are species-specific and have not been propagated in tissue culture or in common experimental animals. However, some HPV types have been produced in human tissues implanted in immunodeficient mice.

EPIDEMIOLOGY There are few good studies of the incidence or prevalence of human warts in well-defined populations. Common warts (verruca vulgaris) are found in as many as 25% of some groups and are most prevalent among young children. Plantar warts (verruca plantaris) are also widely prevalent; they occur most often among adolescents and young adults. Condyloma acuminatum (anogenital warts) is one of the most common sexually transmitted diseases in the United States. HPV infection of the uterine cervix produces the squamous cell abnormalities most frequently detected on Papanicolaou smears.

Most anogenital HPV infections are transmitted through direct contact with infectious lesions. However, characteristics of infectious lesions, including appearance, have not been defined, and individuals without obvious disease may transmit infection. Close personal contact is also assumed to play a role in the transmission of most cutaneous warts; the importance of fomites in this setting is not clear. Minor trauma at the site of inoculation may facilitate transmission. Recurrent respiratory papillomatosis in young children is an uncommon disease that is acquired from maternal genital tract infection; in adults, orogenital sexual contact may transmit the disease.

According to a consensus panel gathered by the World Health Organization, a large body of epidemiologic and biologic data has established that some HPV infections cause cervical cancer. For example, >95% of cervical cancers contain HPV DNA of oncogenic (high-risk) types, such as 16, 18, 31, 33, and 45. HPV DNA is also present in the precursor lesions of cervical cancer (cervical intraepithelial neoplasias). Such lesions containing DNA of oncogenic types are more likely to progress than those associated with low-risk HPV types, such as 6 and 11. HPV DNA is transcribed in tumor tissues, and many epidemiologic studies have confirmed a strong relationship between HPV infection (with or without cofactors) and the development of cervical cancer. However, it is important to realize that most cervical HPV infections, including those caused by high-risk types, are self-limited. Infection with specific HPV types has also been associated with squamous cell carcinomas and dysplasias of the penis, anus, vagina, and vulva. In patients with epidermodysplasia verruciformis, squamous cell cancers develop frequently at sites infected with specific HPV types, including 5 and 8.

Serologic studies employing virus-like particles as antigens have demonstrated type-specific antibodies in most patients with HPV genital tract infections.

CLINICAL MANIFESTATIONS The clinical manifestations of HPV infection depend on the location of lesions and the type of virus. Common warts usually occur on the hands as flesh-colored to brown, exophytic, and hyperkeratotic papules. Plantar warts may be quite painful; they can be differentiated from calluses by paring of the surface to reveal thrombosed capillaries. Flat warts (verruca plana) are most common among children and occur on the face, neck, chest, and flexor surfaces of the forearms and legs.

Anogenital warts develop on the skin and mucosal surfaces of external genitalia and perianal areas (Fig. 169-1). Among circumcised men, warts are most commonly found on the penile shaft. Lesions frequently occur at the urethral meatus and may extend proximally. Receptive anal intercourse predisposes both men and women to the development of perianal warts, but such lesions occasionally develop without such a history. In women, warts appear first at the posterior introitus and adjacent labia. They then spread to other parts of the vulva and commonly involve the vagina and cervix. External warts in both sexes are suggestive of the presence of internal lesions, although internal lesions may be present without external warts, particularly among women. The differential diagnosis of anogenital warts includes condylomata lata of secondary syphilis, molluscum contagiosum, hirsutoid papillomatosis (pearly penile papules), fibroepitheliomas, and a variety of benign and malignant mucocutaneous neoplasms. Respiratory papillomatosis in young children, which may be life-threaten-

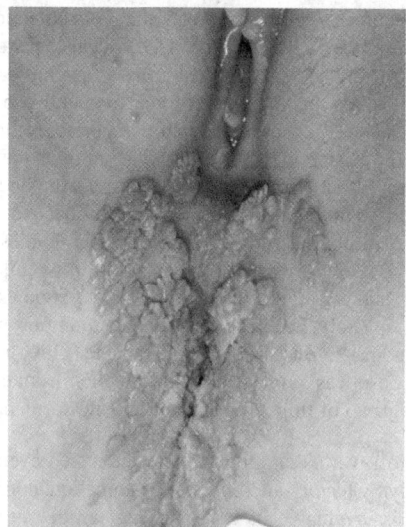

FIGURE 169-1 Condylomata acuminata are lesions produced by human papillomavirus and in this patient are seen as multiple verrucous papules coalescing into plaques.

ing, presents as hoarseness, stridor, or respiratory distress. The disease in adults is usually milder.

Immunosuppressed patients, particularly those undergoing organ transplantation, often develop pityriasis versicolor–like lesions, from which DNA of several HPV types has been extracted. Occasionally, such lesions appear to undergo malignant transformation. Patients infected with HIV frequently have severe clinical manifestations of HPV infection and appear to be at unusually high risk for cervical and anal dysplasia as well as for potentially invasive cancer. HPV disease in patients with HIV infection is difficult to treat and often recurs.

Epidermodysplasia verruciformis is a rare autosomal recessive disease characterized by an inability to control HPV infection. Patients are often infected with unusual HPV types and frequently develop cutaneous squamous cell malignancies, particularly in sun-exposed areas. The lesions resemble flat warts or macules similar to those of pityriasis versicolor.

The complications of warts include itching and occasionally bleeding. In rare cases warts become secondarily infected with bacteria or fungi. Large masses of warts may cause mechanical problems, such as obstruction of the birth canal. Dysplasias of the uterine cervix are generally asymptomatic until frank carcinoma develops. Patients with anogenital HPV disease may develop serious psychological symptoms due to anxiety and depression over this condition.

PATHOGENESIS The incubation period of HPV disease is usually 3 to 4 months (range, 1 month to 2 years). All types of squamous epithelium can be infected by HPV, and the gross and histologic appearances of individual lesions vary with the site of infection and the type of virus. The replication of HPV begins with the infection of basal cells. As cellular differentiation proceeds, HPV DNA replicates and is transcribed. Ultimately, virions are assembled in the nucleus and released when keratinocytes are shed. This process is associated with proliferation of all epidermal layers except the basal layer and produces acanthosis, parakeratosis, and hyperkeratosis. Koilocytes—large round cells with pyknotic nuclei—appear in the granular layer. Histologically normal epithelium may contain HPV DNA, and residual DNA after treatment can be associated with recurrent disease.

Episomal HPV DNA is present in the nuclei of infected cells in benign lesions caused by HPV. However, in severe dysplasias and cancers, HPV DNA is generally integrated, with disruption of the E1/E2 open reading frames. This disruption leads to upregulation of E6 and E7 and subsequent interference with cellular tumor-suppressor proteins.

Host defense responses to HPV infection are incompletely understood, and immune correlates of protection from infection and resolution of disease have not been established. Because patients with defects in cell-mediated immune responses, including transplant recipients and patients with HIV infection, frequently develop severe HPV disease, such responses are probably important for the control of virus replication. Histologic studies demonstrating an epidermal lymphomonocytic infiltrate in resolving warts suggest that local immunity may be of particular importance in the resolution of disease. HPV infection can also elicit a serologic response; antibodies to the viral capsid have been found in sera of patients with anogenital warts, cutaneous warts, and respiratory papillomatosis. Antibodies to E-region proteins, most notably E7, have been detected among patients with cervical carcinoma. In one prophylactic vaccine study, induction of a serologic response was associated with protection from cervical HPV infection in a group of immunocompetent young women.

DIAGNOSIS   Most warts that are visible to the naked eye can be diagnosed correctly by history and physical examination alone. The use of a colposcope is invaluable in assessing vaginal and cervical lesions and is helpful in the diagnosis of oral and cutaneous HPV disease as well. Application of 3 to 5% solutions of acetic acid may aid in the visualization of lesions, although the sensitivity and specificity of this procedure are unknown. Papanicolaou smears prepared from cervical or anal scrapings often show cytologic evidence of HPV infection. Persistent or atypical lesions should be biopsied and examined by routine histologic methods. The most sensitive and specific methods of virologic diagnosis entail the use of techniques such as the polymerase chain reaction or the hybrid capture assay to detect HPV nucleic acids and to identify specific virus types. Such tests may be useful in the diagnosis and management of cervical HPV disease, although their utility may vary according to the prevalence of disease and the availability of traditional cytologic and histologic testing. Serologic techniques to diagnose HPV infection are not helpful in individual cases and are not widely available.

R̲x̲ **TREATMENT** (Table 169-1)

Decisions regarding the initiation of therapy should be made with the knowledge that currently available modes of treatment are not completely effective and some have significant side effects. In addition, treatment may be expensive, and many HPV lesions resolve spontaneously. Frequently used therapies include cryosurgery, application of caustic agents, electrodesiccation, surgical excision, and ablation with a laser. Topical antimetabolites such as 5-fluorouracil have also been used. Both failure and recurrence have been well documented with all of these methods of treatment. Cryosurgery is the initial treatment of choice for condyloma acuminatum. Topically applied podophyllum preparations as well as podofilox may also be used. Various interferon preparations have been employed with modest success in the treatment of respiratory papillomatosis and condyloma acuminatum. A topically applied interferon inducer, imiquimod, is also of benefit in the treatment of condyloma acuminatum. The diagnosis and management of

TABLE 169-1   Treatment of External, Exophytic Anogenital Warts

I. Administered by provider
   A. Cryotherapy with liquid nitrogen or cryoprobe weekly
   B. Podophyllin resin, 10–25% weekly for up to 4 weeks
   C. Trichloroacetic acid or bichloroacetic acid, 80–90% weekly
   D. Surgical excision
   E. Other regimens
      1. Intralesionally administered interferon
      2. Laser surgery
II. Administered by patient
   A. Podofilox, 0.5% solution or gel twice daily for 3 days, followed by 4 days without therapy. This cycle may be repeated four times.
   B. Imiquimod, 5% cream 3 times per week for up to 16 weeks

Source: Modified from Centers for Disease Control and Prevention: MMWR 51(RR-6):1, 2002 (*http://www.cdc.gov/mmwr/PDF/RR/RR5106.pdf*).

anogenital dysplasias and of internal anogenital warts require special skills and resources, and patients with such lesions should be referred to a qualified specialist.

PREVENTION   Apart from the avoidance of contact with infectious lesions, no effective methods for the prevention of HPV infections are available at present. Barrier methods of contraception may be helpful in preventing transmission of condyloma acuminatum and other anogenital HPV-associated diseases. Vaccines consisting of virus-like particles (VLPs) can prevent papillomavirus disease in animal models. One study of an HPV-16 VLP vaccine in uninfected women has shown protection from cervical infection with the homologous virus. More extensive clinical trials of these preparations are likely to demonstrate reductions in rates of cervical HPV disease.

FURTHER READING

BALDWIN SB et al: Human papillomavirus infection in men attending a sexually transmitted disease clinic. J Infect Dis 187:1064, 2003

BONNEZ W, REICHMAN RC: Papillomaviruses, in *Principles and Practice of Infectious Diseases*, 6th ed, GL Mandell et al (eds). Churchill Livingstone, New York, 2004

BOSCH FX et al: The causal relationship between human papillomavirus and cervical cancer. J Clin Pathol 55:244, 2002

CENTERS FOR DISEASE CONTROL AND PREVENTION: Sexually transmitted diseases treatment guidelines—2002. MMWR 51(RR-6):1, 2002

EVANS TG et al: A phase I study of a recombinant virus-like particle vaccine against human papillomavirus type 11 in healthy adult volunteers. J Infect Dis 183:1485, 2001

FRISCH M et al: Human papillomavirus–associated cancers in patients with human immunodeficiency virus infection and acquired immunodeficiency syndrome. J Natl Cancer Inst 92:1500, 2000

KOUTSKY LA et al: A controlled trial of a human papillomavirus type 16 vaccine. N Engl J Med 347:1645, 2002

LUQUE AE et al: Association of human papillomavirus infection and disease with magnitude of human immunodeficiency virus type 1 (HIV-1) RNA plasma level among women with HIV-1 infection. J Infect Dis 179:1405, 1999

MUNOZ N et al: Epidemiologic classification of human papillomavirus types associated with cervical cancer. N Engl J Med 348:518, 2003

WRIGHT TC JR et al: ASCCP-Sponsored Consensus Conference: 2001 consensus guidelines for the management of women with cervical cytological abnormalities. JAMA 287:2120, 2002

170 COMMON VIRAL RESPIRATORY INFECTIONS AND SEVERE ACUTE RESPIRATORY SYNDROME (SARS)
Raphael Dolin

GENERAL CONSIDERATIONS Acute viral respiratory illnesses are among the most common of human diseases, accounting for one-half or more of all acute illnesses. The incidence of acute respiratory disease in the United States is from 3 to 5.6 cases per person per year. The rates are highest among children <1 year old (6.1 to 8.3 cases per year) and remain high until age 6, when a progressive decrease begins. Adults have 3 to 4 cases per person per year. Morbidity from acute respiratory illnesses accounts for 30 to 50% of time lost from work by adults and for 60 to 80% of time lost from school by children. The use of anti-bacterial agents to treat viral respiratory infections represents a major source of abuse of that category of drugs.

It has been estimated that two-thirds to three-fourths of cases of acute respiratory illnesses are caused by viruses. More than 200 antigenically distinct viruses from 9 different genera have been reported to cause acute respiratory illness, and it is likely that additional agents will be described in the future. The vast majority of these viral infections involve the upper respiratory tract, but lower respiratory tract disease can also develop, particularly in younger age groups and in certain epidemiologic settings.

The illnesses caused by respiratory viruses traditionally have been divided into multiple distinct syndromes, such as the "common cold," pharyngitis, croup (laryngotracheobronchitis), tracheitis, bronchiolitis, bronchitis, and pneumonia. Each of these general categories of illness has a certain epidemiologic and clinical profile; for example, croup occurs exclusively in very young children and has a characteristic-clinical course. Some types of respiratory illness are more likely to be associated with certain viruses (e.g., the common cold with rhinoviruses), while others occupy characteristic epidemiologic niches (e.g., adenovirus infections in military recruits). The syndromes most commonly associated with infections with the major respiratory virus groups are summarized in Table 170-1. Most respiratory viruses clearly have the potential to cause more than one type of respiratory illness, and frequently features of several types of illness are found in the same patient. Moreover, the clinical illnesses induced by these viruses are rarely sufficiently distinctive to permit an etiologic diagnosis on clinical grounds alone, although the epidemiologic setting increases the likelihood that one group of viruses rather than another is involved. In general, laboratory methods must be relied on to establish a specific viral diagnosis.

This chapter reviews viral infections caused by six of the major groups of respiratory viruses:

rhinoviruses, coronaviruses, respiratory syncytial viruses, metapneumoviruses, parainfluenza viruses, and adenoviruses. The recent extraordinary outbreaks of lower respiratory tract disease associated with coronaviruses (severe acute respiratory syndrome, or SARS) are also discussed. Influenza viruses, which are a major cause of mortality as well as morbidity, are reviewed in Chap. 171. Herpesviruses, which occasionally cause pharyngitis and which also cause lower respiratory tract disease in immunosuppressed patients, are reviewed in Chap. 163. Enteroviruses, which account for occasional respiratory illnesses during the summer months, are reviewed in Chap. 175.

RHINOVIRUS INFECTIONS

ETIOLOGIC AGENT Rhinoviruses are members of the Picornaviridae family, small (15 to 30 nm) nonenveloped viruses that contain a single-stranded RNA genome. In contrast to other members of the picornavirus family, such as enteroviruses, rhinoviruses are acid-labile and are almost completely inactivated at pH ≤ 3. Rhinoviruses grow preferentially at 33° to 34°C—the temperature of the human nasal passages—rather than at the higher temperature (37°C) of the lower respiratory tract. A total of 102 distinct serotypes of rhinovirus are recognized. Of these serotypes, 91 use intercellular adhesion molecule 1 (ICAM-1) as a cellular receptor and comprise the "major" receptor

TABLE 170-1   *Illnesses Associated with Respiratory Viruses*

Virus	Frequency of Respiratory Syndromes		
	Most Frequent	**Occasional**	**Infrequent**
Rhinoviruses	Common cold	Exacerbation of chronic bronchitis and asthma	Pneumonia in children
Coronaviruses[a]	Common cold	Exacerbation of chronic bronchitis and asthma	Pneumonia and bronchiolitis
Respiratory syncytial virus	Pneumonia and bronchiolitis in young children	Common cold in adults	Pneumonia in elderly and immunosuppressed patients
Parainfluenza viruses	Croup and lower respiratory tract disease in young children	Pharyngitis and common cold	Tracheobronchitis in adults; lower respiratory tract disease in immuno-suppressed patients
Adenoviruses	Common cold and pharyngitis in children	Outbreaks of acute respiratory disease in military recruits[b]	Pneumonia in children; lower respiratory tract and disseminated disease in immunosuppressed patients
Influenza A viruses	Influenza[c]	Pneumonia and excess mortality in high-risk patients	Pneumonia in healthy individuals
Influenza B viruses	Influenza[c]	Rhinitis and pharyngitis alone	Pneumonia
Enteroviruses	Acute undifferentiated febrile illnesses[d]	Rhinitis and pharyngitis	Pneumonia
Herpes simplex viruses	Gingivostomatitis in children; pharyngoton-sillitis in adults	Tracheitis and pneumonia in immunocompromised patients	Disseminated infection in immunocompromised patients
Human metapneumoviruses[e]	—		

[a] SARS-associated coronavirus (SARS-CoV) caused epidemics of pneumonia from November 2002 to July 2003 (see text).
[b] Serotypes 4 and 7.
[c] Fever, cough, myalgia, malaise.
[d] May or may not have a respiratory component.
[e] Newly recognized human metapneumoviruses that cause upper and lower respiratory tract illnesses; their relative frequency has not yet been established.

group, 10 use the low-density lipoprotein receptor and comprise the "minor" receptor group, and 1 uses a sialoprotein cellular receptor.

EPIDEMIOLOGY Rhinoviruses are a major cause of the common cold and have been isolated from 15 to 40% of adults with common cold–like illnesses. Overall rates of infection with rhinoviruses are higher among infants and young children and decrease with increasing age. Rhinovirus infections occur throughout the year, with seasonal peaks in early fall and spring in temperate climates. These infections are most often introduced into families by preschool or grade-school children <6 years old. Between 25 and 70% of initial illnesses in family settings are followed by secondary cases, with the highest attack rates among the youngest siblings at home. Attack rates also increase with family size.

Rhinoviruses appear to spread through direct contact with infected secretions, usually respiratory droplets. In some studies of volunteers, transmission was most efficient by hand-to-hand contact, with subsequent self-inoculation of the conjunctival or nasal mucosa. In other studies, transmission by large- or small-particle aerosol was demonstrated. Virus can also be recovered from plastic surfaces inoculated 1 to 3 h previously; this observation suggests that environmental surfaces contribute to transmission. In studies of married couples in which neither partner had detectable serum antibody, transmission was associated with prolonged contact ($\geq$122 h) during a 7-day period. Transmission was infrequent unless virus was recoverable from the donor's hands and nasal mucosa, at least 1000 $TCID_{50}$ of virus was present in nasal washes from the donor, and the donor was at least moderately symptomatic with the "cold." Despite anecdotal observations, exposure to cold temperatures, fatigue, or sleep deprivation has not been associated with increased rates of rhinovirus-induced illness in volunteers, although some studies have suggested that psychologically defined "stress" may contribute to development of symptoms.

Infection with rhinoviruses is worldwide in distribution. By the time they reach adulthood, nearly all individuals have neutralizing antibodies to multiple serotypes, although the prevalence of antibody to any one serotype varies widely. Multiple serotypes circulate simultaneously, and generally no single serotype or group of serotypes has been more prevalent than the others.

PATHOGENESIS Rhinoviruses infect cells through attachment to specific cellular receptors; as mentioned above, most serotypes attach to ICAM-1, while a few use the low-density lipoprotein receptor. Relatively limited information is available on the histopathology and pathogenesis of acute rhinovirus infections in humans. Examination of biopsy specimens obtained during experimentally induced and naturally occurring illness indicates that the nasal mucosa is edematous, is often hyperemic, and—during acute illness—is covered by a mucoid discharge. There is a mild infiltrate with inflammatory cells, including neutrophils, lymphocytes, plasma cells, and eosinophils. Mucus-secreting glands in the submucosa appear hyperactive; the nasal turbinates are engorged, a condition that may lead to obstruction of nearby openings of sinus cavities. Several mediators, such as bradykinin, lysylbradykinin, prostaglandins, histamine, and interleukins 1, 6, and 8, have been linked to the development of signs and symptoms in rhinovirus-induced colds.

The incubation period for rhinovirus illness is short, generally 1 or 2 days. Virus shedding coincides with the onset of illness or may begin shortly before symptoms develop. The mechanisms of immunity to rhinovirus are not well worked out. In some studies, the presence of homotypic antibody has been associated with significantly reduced rates of subsequent infection and illness, but data conflict regarding the relative importance of serum and local antibody in protection from rhinovirus infection.

CLINICAL MANIFESTATIONS The most common clinical manifestations of rhinovirus infections are those of the common cold. Illness usually begins with rhinorrhea and sneezing accompanied by nasal congestion. The throat is frequently sore, and in some cases sore throat is the initial complaint. Systemic signs and symptoms, such as malaise and headache, are mild or absent, and fever is unusual. Illness generally lasts for 4 to 9 days and resolves spontaneously without sequelae. In children, bronchitis, bronchiolitis, and bronchopneumonia have been reported; nevertheless, it appears that rhinoviruses are not major causes of lower respiratory tract disease in children. Rhinoviruses may cause exacerbations of asthma and chronic pulmonary disease in adults. The vast majority of rhinovirus infections resolve without sequelae, but complications related to obstruction of the eustachian tubes or sinus ostia, including otitis media or acute sinusitis, can develop. In immunosuppressed patients, particularly bone marrow transplant recipients, severe and even fatal pneumonias have been associated with rhinovirus infections.

DIAGNOSIS Although rhinoviruses are the most frequently recognized cause of the common cold, similar illnesses are caused by a variety of other viruses, and the etiologic diagnosis cannot be made on clinical grounds alone. Rather, rhinovirus infection is diagnosed by isolation of the virus from nasal washes or nasal secretions in tissue culture. In practice, this procedure is rarely undertaken because of the benign, self-limited nature of the illness. In most settings, detection of rhinovirus RNA by polymerase chain reaction (PCR) is more sensitive than that by tissue culture; however, this PCR is largely a research procedure. Given the many serotypes of rhinovirus, diagnosis by serum antibody tests is currently impractical. Likewise, common laboratory tests, such as white cell count and sedimentation rate, are not helpful.

R_X TREATMENT

Rhinovirus infections are generally mild and self-limited, so treatment is not usually necessary. Therapy in the form of first-generation antihistamines and nonsteroidal anti-inflammatory drugs may be beneficial in patients with particularly pronounced symptoms, and an oral decongestant may be added if nasal obstruction is particularly troublesome. Reduction of activity is prudent in instances of significant discomfort or fatigability. Antibacterial agents should be used only if bacterial complications such as otitis media or sinusitis develop. Specific antiviral therapy is not available.

PREVENTION Application of interferon sprays intranasally has been effective in the prophylaxis of rhinovirus infections but is also associated with local irritation of the nasal mucosa. Studies of the prevention of rhinovirus infection by administration of antibodies to ICAM-1 or by the soluble purified receptors themselves have yielded disappointing results. Experimental vaccines to certain rhinovirus serotypes have been generated, but their usefulness is questionable because of the myriad serotypes and the uncertainty about mechanisms of immunity. Thorough hand washing, environmental decontamination, and protection against autoinoculation may help to reduce rates of transmission of infection.

CORONAVIRUS INFECTIONS, INCLUDING SARS

ETIOLOGIC AGENT Coronaviruses are pleomorphic, single-strand RNA viruses that measure 100 to 150 nm in diameter. The name derives from the crownlike appearance produced by the club-shaped projections that stud the viral envelope. Coronaviruses infect a wide variety of animal species and have been divided into three antigenic groups. Previously recognized coronaviruses that infect humans fell into two of these groups (I and II), which are represented by prototype isolates HCoV-229E and HCoV-OC43, respectively. The coronavirus associated with SARS (SARS-CoV) appears to be of a novel and distinct group (Fig. 170-1). To date, the SARS-CoV strains that have been fully sequenced have shown only minimal variation.

In general, human coronaviruses have been difficult to cultivate in vitro, and some strains grow only in human tracheal organ cultures rather than in tissue culture. SARS-CoV is an exception whose ready growth in African green monkey kidney (Vero E6) cells greatly facilitates its study.

EPIDEMIOLOGY Generally, human coronavirus infections are present throughout the world. Seroprevalence studies of strains HCoV-229E and HCoV-OC43 have demonstrated that serum antibodies are acquired early in life and increase in prevalence with advancing age, so that >80% of adult populations have antibodies as measured by enzyme-linked immunosorbent assay (ELISA). Overall, coronaviruses account for 10 to 35% of common colds, depending on the season. Coronavirus infections appear to be particularly prevalent in late fall, winter, and early spring—times when rhinovirus infections are less common.

The epidemic of the coronavirus-associated illness known as SARS apparently began in Guangdong Province of China in November 2002 and possibly originated from contact with semidomesticated animals such as the palm civet or the dog raccoon. These animals are prized as edible delicacies in the area and harbor infections with coronaviruses related to SARS-CoV. Between November 16, 2002, and February 28, 2003, 792 cases of apparent SARS were noted in Guangdong, and it was recognized that health care workers and their contacts accounted for many of the cases. A physician from Guangdong who traveled to Hong Kong to visit his family 5 days after the onset of his illness may represent the index case that introduced SARS into Hong Kong. In March 2003, a large number of cases of severe respiratory disease were reported to the World Health Organization (WHO) from Hong Kong. Many of the patients had had contact with the putative index case, had stayed at the hotel where he resided, or had had contact with secondary cases. At nearly the same time, similar cases were noted in Singapore, Thailand, Vietnam, Taiwan, and Toronto (Canada), initially in travelers from Hong Kong or Guangdong. Ultimately, 8422 cases were identified by WHO in 28 countries of Asia, Europe, and North America, although ~90% of cases occurred in China and Hong Kong. Case-fatality rates varied among the outbreaks, with an overall figure of ~11%. The disease appeared to be somewhat milder in cases in the United States and was clearly less severe among children (see below).

The mechanisms of transmission of SARS are incompletely understood. Clusters of cases suggest that spread may occur by both large and small aerosols and perhaps by the fecal-oral route as well. The outbreak of illness in a large apartment complex in Hong Kong suggested that environmental sources, such as sewage or water, may also play a role in transmission. Some ill individuals appeared to be hyperinfectious ("super-spreaders") and were capable of transmitting infection to 10 to 40 contacts, although most infections resulted in spread either to no one or to up to three individuals.

PATHOGENESIS Coronaviruses that cause the common cold (e.g., strains HCoV-229E and HCoV-OC43) infect ciliated epithelial cells in the nasopharynx. Viral replication leads to damage of ciliated cells and induction of chemokines and interleukins, which result in common-cold symptoms similar to those induced by rhinoviruses.

The pathogenesis of SARS is that of a systemic illness in which virus likely enters and infects cells of the respiratory tract but is also found in the bloodstream, in the urine, and (for up to 2 months) in the stool. Virus persists in the respiratory tract for 2 to 3 weeks, and titers peak ~10 days after the onset of systemic illness. Pulmonary pathology consists of hyaline membrane formation, desquamation of pneumocytes in alveolar spaces, and an interstitial infiltrate consisting of lymphocytes and mononuclear cells. Giant cells are frequently seen, and coronavirus particles have been detected in type II pneumocytes.

CLINICAL MANIFESTATIONS After an incubation period that generally lasts 2 to 7 days (range, 1 to 10 days), SARS usually begins as a systemic illness marked by the onset of fever, which is often accompanied by malaise, headache, and myalgias and is followed in 1 to 2 days by a nonproductive cough and dyspnea. Approximately 25% of patients have diarrhea. Chest x-rays can show a variety of infiltrates, including patchy areas of consolidation—most frequently in peripheral and lower lung fields—or interstitial infiltrates, which can progress to diffuse involvement (Fig. 170-2).

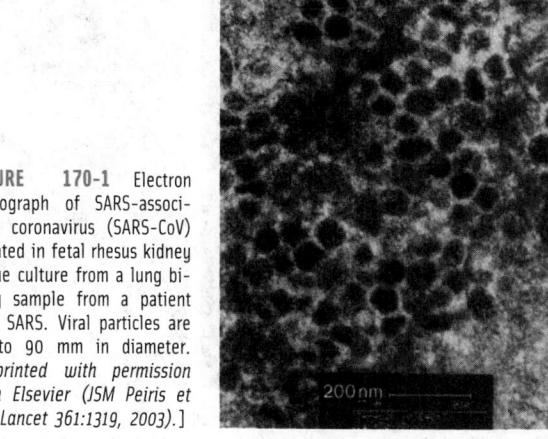

FIGURE 170-1 Electron micrograph of SARS-associated coronavirus (SARS-CoV) isolated in fetal rhesus kidney tissue culture from a lung biopsy sample from a patient with SARS. Viral particles are 55 to 90 mm in diameter. [Reprinted with permission from Elsevier (JSM Peiris et al., Lancet 361:1319, 2003).]

In severe cases, respiratory function may worsen during the second week of illness and progress to frank adult respiratory distress syndrome (ARDS) accompanied by multiorgan dysfunction. Risk factors for severity of disease include an age of >50 and comorbidities such as cardiovascular disease, diabetes, or hepatitis. Illness in pregnant women may be particularly severe, but SARS-CoV infection appears to be milder in children than in adults.

The clinical features of common colds caused by human coronaviruses are similar to those of illness caused by rhinoviruses. In studies of volunteers, the mean incubation period of colds induced by coronaviruses (3 days) is somewhat longer than that of illness caused by rhinoviruses, and the duration of illness is somewhat shorter (mean, 6 to 7 days). In some studies, the amount of nasal discharge was somewhat greater in colds induced by coronaviruses than in those induced by rhinoviruses. Coronaviruses other than SARS-CoV have been recovered occasionally from infants with pneumonia and from military recruits with lower respiratory tract disease and have been associated with worsening of chronic bronchitis.

LABORATORY FINDINGS AND DIAGNOSIS Laboratory abnormalities in SARS include lymphopenia, which is present in ~50% of cases and which mostly affects CD4+ T cells but also involves CD8+ T cells and NK cells. Total white blood cell counts are normal or slightly low, and thrombocytopenia may develop as the illness progresses. Elevated serum levels of aminotransferases, creatine kinase, and lactate dehydrogenase have been reported.

The WHO and the Centers for Disease Control and Prevention have developed case definitions for diagnosis of SARS. These definitions include clinical, epidemiologic, and laboratory features, which are being refined as additional information on SARS is gathered. SARS-CoV can be grown from respiratory tract samples by inoculation into Vero E6 tissue culture cells, in which a cytopathic effect can be seen within days. A rapid diagnosis can be made by reverse-transcriptase PCR (RT-PCR) of respiratory tract samples and plasma early in illness and of urine and stool later on. RT-PCR appears to be more sensitive than tissue culture, but only around one-third of cases are positive by PCR at initial presentation. Serum antibodies can be detected by ELISA or immunofluorescence, and nearly all patients develop detectable serum antibodies within 28 days after the onset of illness.

Laboratory diagnosis of coronavirus-induced colds is rarely required. Coronaviruses that cause those illnesses are frequently difficult to cultivate in vitro but can be detected in clinical samples by ELISA or immunofluorescence assays or by RT-PCR for viral RNA. These research procedures can be used to detect coronaviruses in unusual clinical settings.

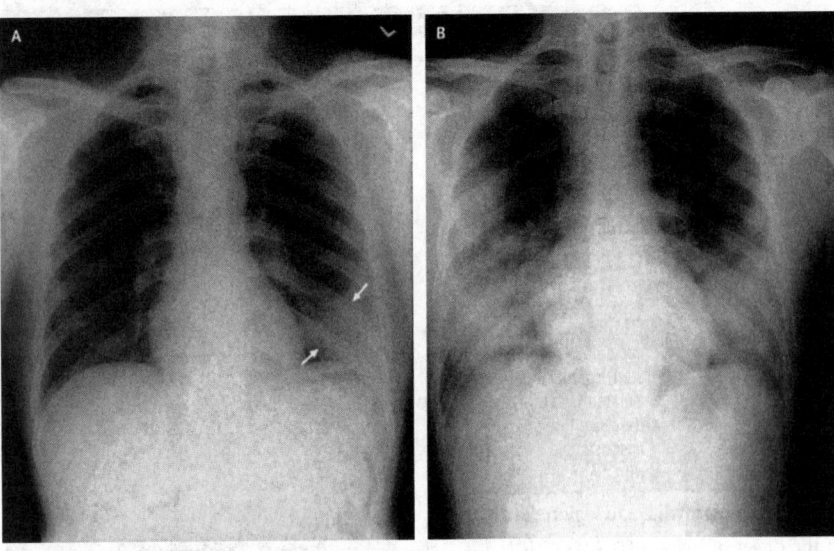

FIGURE 170-2 Chest x-rays of a 46-year-old man with SARS. The left lower lung infiltrate seen initially (*A*) progressed to multiple bilateral opacities (*B*). (*Reprinted with permission from L Lee et al. © 2003 Massachusetts Medical Society.*)

℞ TREATMENT

There is no specific therapy of established efficacy for SARS. Although ribavirin has frequently been used, it has little if any activity against SARS-CoV in vitro, and no beneficial effect on the course of illness has been demonstrated. Because of suggestions that immunopathology may contribute to the disease, glucocorticoids have also been widely used, but their benefit, if any, is likewise unestablished. Supportive care to maintain pulmonary and other organ system functions remains the mainstay of therapy.

The approach to the treatment of common colds caused by coronaviruses is similar to that discussed above for rhinovirus-induced illnesses.

PREVENTION The recognition of SARS led to a worldwide mobilization of public health resources to apply infection control practices and thus to contain the disease. Case definitions were established, travel advisories were proposed, and quarantines were imposed in certain locales. In line with criteria based on the absence of new cases for 30 days (three times the estimated incubation period of 10 days for the disease), all travel advisories have been lifted as of this writing (February 2004). It remains unknown whether the disappearance of cases is a result of the above control measures, whether it is part of a seasonal or otherwise unexplained epidemiologic pattern of SARS, and when or whether SARS might reemerge. The frequent transmission of the disease to health care workers makes it mandatory that strict infection control practices be employed by health care facilities to prevent airborne, droplet, and contact transmission from any suspected cases of SARS in the fruture.

Vaccines have been developed against several animal coronaviruses but not against known human coronaviruses. The emergence of SARS-CoV has emphasized the importance of the development of vaccines against such agents.

RESPIRATORY SYNCYTIAL VIRUS INFECTIONS

ETIOLOGIC AGENT Respiratory syncytial virus (RSV) is a member of the Paramyxoviridae family (genus *Pneumovirus*). RSV, an enveloped virus ~150 to 300 nm in diameter, is so named because its replication in vitro leads to the fusion of neighboring cells into large multinucleated syncytia. The single-stranded RNA genome codes for 11 virus-specific proteins. Viral RNA is contained in a helical nucleocapsid surrounded by a lipid envelope bearing two glycoproteins: the G protein, by which the virus attaches to cells, and the F (fusion) protein, which facilitates entry of the virus into the cell by fusing host and viral

membranes. RSV was once considered to be of a single antigenic type, but two distinct groups (A and B) and multiple subtypes within each group have now been described. Antigenic diversity is reflected by differences in the G protein, while the F protein is highly conserved. Both antigenic groups can circulate simultaneously in outbreaks, although the relative proportions of each vary. Infections with group B viruses may be somewhat milder than those with group A viruses.

EPIDEMIOLOGY RSV is the major respiratory pathogen of young children and the foremost cause of lower respiratory disease in infants. Infection with RSV is seen throughout the world in annual epidemics that occur in late fall, winter, or spring and last up to 5 months. The virus is rarely encountered during the summer. Rates of illness are highest among infants 1 to 6 months of age, peaking between 2 and 3 months of age. The attack rates among susceptible infants and children are extraordinarily high, approaching 100% in settings such as day-care centers where large numbers of susceptible infants are present. By age 2, virtually all children will have been infected with RSV. RSV accounts for 20 to 25% of hospital admissions of young infants and children for pneumonia and for up to 75% of cases of bronchiolitis in this age group. It has been estimated that more than half of infants who are at risk will become infected during an RSV epidemic.

In older children and adults, reinfection with RSV is frequent but disease is milder than in infancy. A common cold–like syndrome is the illness most commonly associated with RSV infection in adults. Severe lower respiratory tract disease with pneumonitis can occur in elderly (often institutionalized) adults and in patients with immunocompromising disorders or treatment, including recipients of bone-marrow and solid-organ transplants. RSV is also an important nosocomial pathogen; during an outbreak, it can infect pediatric patients and up to 25 to 50% of the staff on pediatric wards. The spread of virus among families is efficient: up to 40% of siblings may become infected when RSV is introduced into the family setting.

RSV is transmitted primarily by close contact with contaminated fingers or fomites and by self-inoculation of the conjunctiva or anterior nares. Virus may also be spread by coarse aerosols produced by coughing or sneezing, but it is inefficiently spread by fine-particle aerosols. The incubation period is ~4 to 6 days, and virus shedding may last for ≥2 weeks in children and for shorter periods in adults. In immunosuppressed patients, shedding can be prolonged for multiple weeks.

PATHOGENESIS Little is known about the histopathology of minor RSV infection. Severe bronchiolitis or pneumonia is characterized by necrosis of the bronchiolar epithelium and a peribronchiolar infiltrate of lymphocytes and mononuclear cells. Interalveolar thickening and filling of alveolar spaces with fluid can also be found. The correlates of protective immunity to RSV are incompletely understood. Because reinfection occurs frequently and is often associated with illness, the immunity that develops after single episodes of infection clearly is not complete or long-lasting. However, the cumulative effect of multiple reinfections is to temper subsequent disease and to provide some temporary measure of protection against infection. Studies of experimentally induced disease in healthy volunteers indicate that the presence of nasal IgA neutralizing antibody correlates more closely with protection than does the presence of serum antibody. Studies in infants, however, suggest that maternally acquired antibody provides some protection from lower respiratory tract disease, although illness can be severe even in infants who have moderate levels of maternally derived serum antibody. The relatively severe disease observed in immuno-suppressed patients and experimental animal models indicates that cell-mediated immunity is an important mechanism of host defense against RSV. Evidence suggests that class I MHC-restricted cytotoxic T cells may be particularly important in this regard.

CLINICAL MANIFESTATIONS RSV infection leads to a wide spectrum of respiratory illnesses. In infants, 25 to 40% of infections result in lower respiratory tract involvement, including pneumonia, bronchiolitis, and tracheobronchitis. In this age group, illness begins most frequently with rhinorrhea, low-grade fever, and mild systemic symptoms, often accompanied by cough and wheezing. Most patients recover gradually over 1 to 2 weeks. In more severe illness, tachypnea and dyspnea develop, and eventually frank hypoxia, cyanosis, and apnea can ensue. Physical examination may reveal diffuse wheezing, rhonchi, and rales. Chest radiography shows hyperexpansion, peribronchial thickening, and variable infiltrates ranging from diffuse interstitial infiltrates to segmental or lobar consolidation. Illness may be particularly severe in children born prematurely and in those with congenital cardiac disease, bronchopulmonary dysplasia, nephrotic syndrome, or immunosup-pression. One study documented a 37% mortality rate for infants with RSV pneumonia and congenital cardiac disease.

In adults, the most common symptoms of RSV infection are those of the common cold, with rhinorrhea, sore throat, and cough. Illness is occasionally associated with moderate systemic symptoms such as malaise, headache, and fever. RSV has also been reported to cause lower respiratory tract disease with fever in adults, including severe pneumonia in the elderly—particularly in nursing-home residents, among whom its impact can rival that of influenza. RSV pneumonia can be a significant cause of morbidity and mortality in patients undergoing bone-marrow and solid-organ transplantation, where case-fatality rates of 20 to 80% have been reported. Sinusitis, otitis media, and worsening of chronic obstructive and reactive airway disease have also been associated with RSV infection.

LABORATORY FINDINGS AND DIAGNOSIS The diagnosis of RSV infection can be suspected on the basis of a suggestive epidemiologic setting—that is, severe illness among infants during an outbreak of RSV in the community. Infections in older children and adults cannot be differentiated with certainty from those caused by other respiratory viruses. The specific diagnosis is established by isolation of RSV from respiratory secretions, such as sputum, throat swabs, or nasopharyngeal washes. Virus is isolated in tissue culture and is identified specifically by immunofluorescence, ELISA, or other immunologic techniques. Rapid viral diagnosis is available by immunofluorescence techniques or ELISA of nasopharyngeal washes, aspirates, and (less satisfactorily) nasopharyngeal swabs. In children, these techniques have sensitivities and specificities of 80 to 95%; they are somewhat less sensitive in specimens from adults. Serologic diagnosis may be made by comparison of acute- and convalescent-phase serum specimens by ELISA, neutralization, or complement-fixation tests. These tests may be useful in older children and adults but are less sensitive in children <4 months of age.

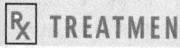 **TREATMENT**

Treatment of upper respiratory tract RSV infection is aimed primarily at the alleviation of symptoms and is similar to that for other viral infections of the upper respiratory tract. For lower respiratory tract infections, respiratory therapy, including hydration, suctioning of secretions, and administration of humidified oxygen and antibronchospastic agents, is given as needed. In severe hypoxia, intubation and ventilatory assistance may be required. Studies of infants with RSV infection who were given aerosolized ribavirin, a nucleoside analogue active in vitro against RSV, have demonstrated a beneficial effect on the resolution of lower respiratory tract illness, including alleviation of blood-gas abnormalities. Treatment with aerosolized ribavirin is recommended for infants who are severely ill or who are at high risk

for complications of RSV infection; included are premature infants and those with bronchopulmonary dysplasia, congenital heart disease, or immunosuppression. The efficacy of ribavirin in older children and adults with RSV pneumonia, including those with immunosuppression, has not been established. Administration of standard immuno-globulin, immunoglobulin with high antibody titers to RSV (RSVIg), or chimeric mouse-human monoclonal IgG against RSV (palivizumab) has not been found to be beneficial in the treatment of RSV pneumonia. Combined therapy with aerosolized ribavirin and palivizumab is being evaluated in the treatment of immunosuppressed patients with RSV pneumonia.

PREVENTION Monthly administration of RSVIg or palivizumab has been approved as prophylaxis against RSV for children <2 years of age who have bronchopulmonary dysplasia or were born prematurely. Considerable interest exists in the development of vaccines against RSV. Inactivated whole-virus vaccines have been ineffective; in one study, they actually potentiated the disease in infants. Other approaches include immunization with purified F and G surface glycoproteins of RSV or generation of stable, live attenuated virus vaccines. In settings such as pediatric wards where rates of transmission are high, barrier methods for the protection of hands and conjunctivae may be useful in reducing the spread of virus.

METAPNEUMOVIRUS INFECTIONS

Human metapneumovirus (HMPV) is a newly described viral respiratory pathogen that has been assigned to the Paramyxoviridae family (genus *Metapneumovirus*). Its morphology and genomic organization are similar to those of avian metapneumoviruses, which are recognized respiratory pathogens of turkeys. HMPV particles may be spherical, filamentous, or pleomorphic in shape and measure 60 to 280 nm in diameter. Particles contain 15-nm projections from the surface that are similar in appearance to those of other Paramyxoviridae. Studies of the RNA genome indicate that there are at least two genetic subgroups or genotypes of HMPV.

HMPV was initially detected in nasal aspirates from 28 children hospitalized with lower respiratory tract illnesses over a 20-year period (1981–2001) in the Netherlands. HMPV infections have since been reported in a wide variety of age groups, including elderly adults, and in both immunocompetent and immunosuppressed hosts. Initial sero-epidemiologic studies suggest that HMPV infections are worldwide in distribution, are most frequent during the winter, and occur early in life, so that serum antibodies to the virus are present in nearly all children by the age of 5. The spectrum of clinical illnesses associated with HMPV is similar to that associated with RSV and includes both upper and lower respiratory tract illnesses, such as bronchiolitis, croup, and pneumonia.

HMPV can be detected in nasal aspirates and respiratory secretions by PCR or by growth in rhesus monkey kidney (LLC-MK2) tissue cultures. Serologic diagnosis can be made by ELISA, which utilizes HMPV-infected tissue culture lysates as sources of antigens.

Preliminary studies indicate that HMPV infections account for 4% of respiratory tract illnesses requiring hospitalization of children and for 2 to 4% of acute respiratory illnesses in ambulatory adults and elderly patients. HMPV has been detected in a few cases of SARS, but its role (if any) in these illnesses has not been established. Assessment of the overall significance of HMPV infections awaits the conduct of large-scale epidemiologic studies.

PARAINFLUENZA VIRUS INFECTIONS

ETIOLOGIC AGENT Parainfluenza viruses belong to the Paramyxoviridae family (genera *Respirovirus* and *Rubulavirus*). They are 150 to 200 nm in diameter, are enveloped, and contain a single-stranded RNA genome. The envelope is studded with two glycoproteins: one possesses both hemagglutinin and neuraminidase activity and the other contains fusion activity. The viral RNA genome is enclosed in a helical nucleocapsid and codes for six structural and several accessory proteins. All four distinct serotypes of parainfluenza viruses share certain antigens with other members of the Paramyxoviridae family, including mumps and Newcastle disease viruses.

EPIDEMIOLOGY Parainfluenza viruses are distributed throughout the world; infection with type 4 (subtypes 4A and 4B) has been reported less widely, probably because type 4 is more difficult to grow in tissue culture. Infection is acquired in early childhood, so that by 5 years of age most children have antibodies to serotypes 1, 2, and 3. Types 1 and 2 cause epidemics during the fall, often occurring in an alternate-year pattern. Type 3 infection has been detected during all seasons of the year, but epidemics have occurred annually in the spring.

The contribution of parainfluenza infections to respiratory disease varies with both the location and the year. In studies conducted in the United States, parainfluenza virus infections have accounted for 4.3 to 22% of respiratory illnesses in children. In adults, parainfluenza infections are generally mild and account for <10% of respiratory illnesses. The major importance of parainfluenza viruses is as a cause of respiratory illness in young children, in whom they rank second only to RSV as causes of lower respiratory tract illness. Parainfluenza virus type 1 is the most frequent cause of croup (laryngotracheobronchitis) in children, while serotype 2 causes similar, although generally less severe, disease. Type 3 is an important cause of bronchiolitis and pneumonia in infants, while illnesses associated with type 4 have generally been mild. Unlike types 1 and 2, type 3 frequently causes illness during the first month of life, when passively acquired maternal antibody is still present. Parainfluenza viruses are spread through infected respiratory secretions, primarily by person-to-person contact and/or by large droplets. The incubation period has varied from 3 to 6 days in experimental infections but may be somewhat shorter for naturally occurring disease in children.

PATHOGENESIS Immunity to parainfluenza viruses is incompletely understood, but evidence suggests that immunity to infections with serotypes 1 and 2 is mediated by local IgA antibodies in the respiratory tract. Passively acquired serum neutralizing antibodies also confer some protection against infection with types 1, 2, and—to a lesser degree—3. Studies in experimental animal models and in immunosuppressed patients suggest that T cell–mediated immunity may also be important in parainfluenza virus infections.

CLINICAL MANIFESTATIONS Parainfluenza virus infections occur most frequently among children, in whom initial infection with serotype 1, 2, or 3 is associated with an acute febrile illness 50 to 80% of the time. Children may present with coryza, sore throat, hoarseness, and cough that may or may not be croupy. In severe croup, fever persists, with worsening coryza and sore throat. A brassy or barking cough may progress to frank stridor. Most children recover over the next 1 or 2 days, although progressive airway obstruction and hypoxia ensue occasionally. If bronchiolitis or pneumonia develops, progressive cough accompanied by wheezing, tachypnea, and intercostal retractions may occur. In this setting, sputum production increases modestly. Physical examination shows nasopharyngeal discharge and oropharyngeal injection, along with rhonchi, wheezes, or coarse breath sounds. Chest x-rays can show air trapping and occasionally interstitial infiltrates.

In older children and adults, parainfluenza infections tend to be milder, presenting most frequently as a common cold or as hoarseness, with or without cough. Lower respiratory tract involvement in older children and adults is uncommon, but tracheobronchitis in adults has been reported. Severe, prolonged, and even fatal parainfluenza infection has been reported in children and adults with severe immunosuppression, including bone-marrow and solid-organ transplant recipients.

LABORATORY FINDINGS AND DIAGNOSIS The clinical syndromes caused by parainfluenza viruses (with the possible exception of croup in young children) are not sufficiently distinctive to be diagnosed on clinical grounds alone. A specific diagnosis is established by detection of virus in respiratory tract secretions, throat swabs, or nasopharyngeal washings. Viral growth in tissue culture is detected either by hemagglutination or by a cytopathic effect. Rapid viral diagnosis may be made by identification of parainfluenza antigens in exfoliated cells from the respiratory tract with immunofluorescence or ELISA, although these techniques appear to be less sensitive than tissue culture. Highly specific and sensitive PCR assays have also been described. Serologic diagnosis can be established by hemagglutination inhibition, complement-fixation, or neutralization tests of acute- and convalescent-phase specimens. However, as frequent heterotypic responses occur among the parainfluenza serotypes, the serotype causing illness often cannot be identified by serologic techniques alone.

Acute epiglottitis caused by *Haemophilus influenzae* type b must be differentiated from viral croup. Influenza A virus is also a common cause of croup during epidemic periods.

℞ TREATMENT

For upper respiratory tract illness, symptoms can be treated as discussed for other viral respiratory tract illnesses. If complications such as sinusitis, otitis, or superimposed bacterial bronchitis develop, appropriate antibiotics should be administered. Mild cases of croup should be treated with bed rest and moist air generated by vaporizers. More severe cases require hospitalization and close observation for the development of respiratory distress. If acute respiratory distress develops, humidified oxygen and intermittent racemic epinephrine are usually administered. Aerosolized or systemically administered glucocorticoids are beneficial; the latter have a more profound effect. No specific antiviral therapy is available, although ribavirin is active against parainfluenza viruses in vitro and anecdotal reports describe its use clinically, particularly in immunosuppressed patients. Effective vaccines against parainfluenza viruses have not been developed.

ADENOVIRUS INFECTIONS

ETIOLOGIC AGENT Adenoviruses are complex DNA viruses that measure 70 to 80 nm in diameter. Human adenoviruses belong to the genus *Mastadenovirus*, which includes 51 serotypes. Adenoviruses have a characteristic morphology consisting of an icosahedral shell composed of 20 equilateral triangular faces and 12 vertices. The protein coat (capsid) consists of hexon subunits with group-specific and type-specific antigenic determinants and penton subunits at each vertex primarily containing group-specific antigens. A fiber with a knob at the end projects from each penton; this fiber contains type-specific and some group-specific antigens. Human adenoviruses have been divided into six subgenera (A through F) on the basis of the homology of DNA genomes and other properties. The adenovirus genome is a linear double-stranded DNA that codes for structural and nonstructural polypeptides. The replicative cycle of adenovirus may result either in lytic infection of cells or in the establishment of a latent infection (primarily involving lymphoid cells). Some adenovirus types can induce oncogenic transformation, and tumor formation has been observed in rodents; however, despite intensive investigation, adenoviruses have not been associated with tumors in humans.

EPIDEMIOLOGY Adenovirus infections most frequently affect infants and children. Infections occur throughout the year but are most common from fall to spring. Adenoviruses account for ~10% of acute respiratory infections in children but for <2% of respiratory illnesses in civilian adults. Nearly 100% of adults have serum antibody to multiple serotypes—a finding indicating that infection is common in childhood. Types 1, 2, 3, and 5 are the most frequent isolates from children. Certain adenovirus serotypes—particularly 4 and 7 but also 3, 14, and 21—are associated with outbreaks of acute respiratory disease in military recruits in winter and spring. Adenovirus infection can be transmitted by inhalation of aerosolized virus, by inoculation of virus into conjunctival sacs, and probably by the fecal-oral route as well. Type-specific antibody generally develops after infection and is associated with protection, albeit incomplete, against infection with the same serotype.

CLINICAL MANIFESTATIONS In children, adenoviruses cause a variety of clinical syndromes. The most common is an acute upper respiratory tract infection, with prominent rhinitis. On occasion, lower respiratory tract disease, including bronchiolitis and pneumonia, also develops. Adenoviruses, particularly types 3 and 7, cause pharyngoconjunctival fever, a characteristic acute febrile illness of children that occurs in outbreaks, most often in summer camps. The syndrome is marked by bilateral conjunctivitis in which the bulbar and palpebral conjunctivae have a granular appearance. Low-grade fever is frequently present for the first 3 to 5 days, and rhinitis, sore throat, and cervical adenopathy develop. The illness generally lasts for 1 to 2 weeks and resolves spontaneously. Febrile pharyngitis without conjunctivitis has also been associated with adenovirus infection. Adenoviruses have been isolated from cases of whooping cough with or without *Bordetella pertussis*; the significance of adenovirus in that disease is unknown.

In adults, the most frequently reported illness has been acute respiratory disease caused by adenovirus types 4 and 7 in military recruits. This illness is marked by a prominent sore throat and the gradual onset of fever, which often reaches 39°C (102.2°F) on the second or third day of illness. Cough is almost always present, and coryza and regional lymphadenopathy are frequently seen. Physical examination may show pharyngeal edema, injection, and tonsillar enlargement with little or no exudate. If pneumonia has developed, auscultation and x-ray of the chest may indicate areas of patchy infiltration.

Adenoviruses have been associated with a number of non–respiratory tract diseases, including acute diarrheal illness caused by types 40 and 41 in young children and hemorrhagic cystitis caused by types 11 and 21. Epidemic keratoconjunctivitis, caused most frequently by types 8, 19, and 37, has been associated with contaminated common sources such as ophthalmic solutions and roller towels. Adenoviruses have also been implicated in disseminated disease and pneumonia in immunosuppressed patients, including recipients of solid-organ or bone-marrow transplants. In bone-marrow transplant recipients, adenovirus infections have manifested as pneumonia, hepatitis, nephritis, colitis, encephalitis, and hemorrhagic cystitis. In solid-organ transplant recipients, adenovirus infection may involve the organ transplanted (e.g., hepatitis in liver transplants, nephritis in renal transplants) but can disseminate to other organs as well. In patients with AIDS, high-numbered and intermediate adenovirus serotypes have been isolated, usually in the setting of low CD4+ cell counts, but their isolation frequently has not been clearly linked to disease manifestations. Adenovirus nucleic acids have been detected in myocardial cells from patients with "idiopathic" myocardiopathies, and adenoviruses have been suggested as causative agents in some cases.

LABORATORY FINDINGS AND DIAGNOSIS Adenovirus infection should be suspected in the epidemiologic setting of acute respiratory disease in military recruits and in certain of the clinical syndromes (such as pharyngoconjunctival fever or epidemic keratoconjunctivitis) in which outbreaks of characteristic illnesses occur. In most cases, however, illnesses caused by adenovirus infection cannot be differentiated from those caused by a number of other viral respiratory agents and *Mycoplasma pneumoniae*. A definitive diagnosis of adenovirus infection is established by detection of the virus in tissue culture (as evidenced by cytopathic changes) and by specific identification with immunoflu-

orescence or other immunologic techniques. Rapid viral diagnosis can be established by immunofluorescence or ELISA of nasopharyngeal aspirates, conjunctival or respiratory secretions, urine, or stool. Highly sensitive and specific PCR assays or nucleic acid hybridization is also available. Adenovirus types 40 and 41, which have been associated with diarrheal disease in children, require special tissue-culture cells for isolation, and these serotypes are most commonly detected by direct ELISA of stool. Serum antibody rises can be demonstrated by complement-fixation or neutralization tests, ELISA, radioimmunoassay, or (for those adenoviruses that hemagglutinate red cells) hemagglutination inhibition tests.

℞ TREATMENT

Only symptom-based treatment and supportive therapy are available for adenovirus infections, and no clinically useful antiviral compounds have been identified. Ribavirin and cidofovir have activity in vitro against adenoviruses, and anecdotes of their use in disseminated infection have been reported.

PREVENTION Live vaccines have been developed against adenovirus types 4 and 7 and have been used to control illness in military recruits. These vaccines consist of live, unattenuated virus administered in enteric-coated capsules. Infection of the gastrointestinal tract with types 4 and 7 does not cause disease but stimulates local and systemic antibodies that are protective against subsequent acute respiratory disease due to those serotypes. This vaccine has not been produced since 1999, and outbreaks of acute respiratory illness caused by adenovirus types 4 and 7 have emerged again among military recruits. Vaccines prepared from purified subunits of adenovirus are being investigated. Adenoviruses are also being studied as live-virus vectors for the delivery of vaccine antigens and for gene therapy.

FURTHER READING

BAUM SG: Adenoviruses, in *Principles and Practice of Infectious Diseases*, 5th ed, GF Mandell et al (eds). New York, Saunders, 2000, pp 1624–1629

COMMITTEE ON INFECTIOUS DISEASES: Use of ribavirin in the treatment of respiratory syncytial virus infection. Pediatrics 92:501, 1993

CRAWFORD-MIKSZU XX et al: Seroepidemiology of new AIDS-associated adenoviruses among the San Francisco Men's Health Study. J Med Virol 50:230, 1996

ENGLUND JA et al: Respiratory syncytial virus infection in immunocompromised adults. Ann Intern Med 109:203, 1988

GLEZEN WP et al: Impact of respiratory virus infections on persons with chronic underlying conditions. JAMA 283:499, 2000

GRAHAM BS et al: Respiratory syncytial virus immunobiology and pathogenesis. Virology 297:1, 2002

GWALTNEY JM: Rhinoviruses, in *Principles and Practice of Infectious Diseases*, 5th ed, GF Mandell et al (eds). New York, Saunders, 2000, pp 1940–1948

HOLMES KH: Coronaviruses, in *Virology*, 4th ed, DN Knipe, PM Howley (eds). Philadelphia, Lippincott Williams & Wilkins, 2001, pp 1187–1204

LEE N et al: A major outbreak of severe acute respiratory syndrome in Hong Kong. N Engl J Med 348:1986, 2003

PEIRIS JSM et al: Coronavirus as a possible cause of severe acute respiratory syndrome. Lancet 361:1319, 2003

PERET T et al: Characterization of human metapneumoviruses isolated from patients in North America. J Infect Dis 185:1660, 2002

STOCKTON J et al: Human metapneumovirus as a cause of community-acquired respiratory illness. Emerg Infect Dis 8:897, 2002

WRIGHT PF: Parainfluenza viruses, in *Viral Infections of the Respiratory Tract*, R Dolin, PF Wright (eds). New York, Marcel Dekker, 1999

DEFINITION   Influenza is an acute respiratory illness caused by infection with influenza viruses. The illness affects the upper and/or lower respiratory tract and is often accompanied by systemic signs and symptoms such as fever, headache, myalgia, and weakness. Outbreaks of illness of variable extent and severity occur nearly every winter. Such outbreaks result in significant morbidity in the general population and in increased mortality rates among certain high-risk patients, mainly as a result of pulmonary complications.

ETIOLOGIC AGENT   Influenza viruses are members of the Orthomyxoviridae family, of which influenza A, B, and C viruses constitute three separate genera. The designation of influenza viruses as type A, B, or C is based on antigenic characteristics of the nucleoprotein (NP) and matrix (M) protein antigens. Influenza A viruses are further subdivided (subtyped) on the basis of the surface hemagglutinin (H) and neuraminidase (N) antigens (see below); individual strains are designated according to the site of origin, isolate number, year of isolation, and subtype—for example, influenza A/Moscow/10/99 (H3N2). Influenza A has 15 distinct H and 9 distinct N subtypes, of which only H1, H2, H3, N1, and N2 have been associated with extensive outbreaks of disease in humans. Influenza B and C viruses are similarly designated, but H and N antigens from these viruses do not receive subtype designations, since intratypic variations in influenza B antigens are less extensive than those in influenza A viruses and may not occur with influenza C virus.

Influenza A and B viruses are major human pathogens and the most extensively studied of the Orthomyxoviridae. The type A and type B viruses are morphologically similar. The virions are irregularly shaped spherical particles, 80 to 120 nm in diameter, and have a lipid envelope from the surface of which the H and N glycoproteins project (Fig. 171-1). The hemagglutinin is the site by which virus binds to cell receptors, whereas the neuraminidase degrades the receptor and plays a role in the release of virus from infected cells after replication has taken place. Influenza viruses enter cells by receptor-mediated endocytosis, forming a virus-containing endosome. The viral hemagglutinin mediates fusion of the endosomal membrane with the virus envelope, and viral nucleocapsids are subsequently released into the cytoplasm. Antibodies to the H antigen are the major determinants of immunity to influenza virus, while those to the N antigen limit viral spread and contribute to reduction of the infection. The inner surface of the lipid envelope contains the M proteins M1 and M2, which are involved in stabilization of the lipid envelope and in virus assembly. The virion also contains the NP antigen, which is associated with the viral genome, as well as three polymerase (P) proteins that are essential for transcription and synthesis of viral RNA. Two nonstructural proteins function as an interferon antagonist and posttranscriptional regulator (NS1) and a nuclear export factor (NS2 or NEP).

The genomes of influenza A and B viruses consist of eight single-stranded RNA segments, which code for the structural and nonstructural proteins. Because the genome is segmented, the opportunity for gene reassortment during infection is high; reassortment often occurs during infection of cells with more than one influenza A virus.

EPIDEMIOLOGY   Influenza outbreaks are recorded virtually every year, although their extent and severity vary widely. Localized outbreaks take place at variable intervals, usually every 1 to 3 years. Except in the past 25 years, global epidemics or pandemics have occurred approximately every 10 to 15 years since the 1918–1919 pandemic (Table 171-1).

The most extensive and severe outbreaks are caused by influenza A viruses, in part because of the remarkable propensity of the H and N antigens of these viruses to undergo periodic antigenic variation. Major antigenic variations, called *antigenic shifts*, may be associated with pandemics and are restricted to influenza A viruses. Minor variations are called *antigenic drifts*. These types of antigenic variation may involve the hemagglutinin alone or both the hemagglutinin and the neuraminidase. An example of an antigenic shift involving both the hemagglutinin and the neuraminidase is that of 1957, when the predominant influenza A virus subtype shifted from H1N1 to H2N2; this shift resulted in a severe pandemic, with an estimated 70,000 excess deaths (i.e., deaths in excess of the number expected without an influenza epidemic) in the United States alone. In 1968, an antigenic shift involving only the hemagglutinin occurred (H2N2 to H3N2); the subsequent pandemic was less severe than that of 1957. In 1977, an H1N1 virus emerged and caused a pandemic that primarily affected younger individuals (i.e., those born after 1957). As can be seen in Table 171-1, H1N1 viruses circulated from 1918 to 1956; thus, individuals born prior to 1957 would be expected to have some degree of immunity to H1N1 viruses. During most outbreaks of influenza A, a single subtype has circulated at a time. However, since 1977, H1N1 and H3N2 viruses have circulated simultaneously, resulting in outbreaks of varying severity. In some outbreaks, influenza B viruses have also circulated simultaneously with influenza A viruses.

The origin of pandemic strains is unknown. Given the marked differences between the primary structures of the hemagglutinins of different subtypes of influenza A viruses (H1, H2, and H3), it seems unlikely that antigenic shifts result from spontaneous mutations in the hemagglutinin gene. Because the segmented genome of influenza viruses may result in high rates of reassortment, it has been suggested that pandemic strains may emerge by reassortment of genes between human and animal influenza A viruses that are known to have a broad host range of infection. There was concern that such reassortment might have occurred in 1997 in Hong Kong, where cases of infection caused by influenza virus A/H5N1 were detected in humans during an extensive outbreak of avian influenza A/H5N1 in poultry. However, only a few cases of A/H5N1 influenza in humans were documented, and the infection did not spread into the community. Recently, H9N2 viruses, which circulate in poultry and swine, have also been associated with limited infections in humans. Influenza B viruses have a much more restricted host range and do not undergo antigenic shifts, although they do undergo antigenic drift.

TABLE 171-1   *Emergence of Antigenic Subtypes of Influenza A Virus Associated with Pandemic or Epidemic Disease*

Years	Subtype	Extent of Outbreak
1889–90	H2N8[a]	Severe pandemic
1900–03	H3N8[a]	?Moderate epidemic
1918–19	H1N1[b] (formerly HswN1)	Severe pandemic
1933–35	H1N1[b] (formerly H0N1)	Mild epidemic
1946–47	H1N1	Mild epidemic
1957–58	H2N2	Severe pandemic
1968–69	H3N2	Moderate pandemic
1977–78[c]	H1N1	Mild pandemic

[a] As determined by retrospective serologic survey of individuals alive during those years ("seroarcheology").
[b] Hemagglutinins formerly designated as Hsw and H0 are now classified as variants of H1.
[c] From this time until the present (2002–2003), viruses of the H1N1 and H3N2 subtypes have circulated either in alternating years or concurrently.

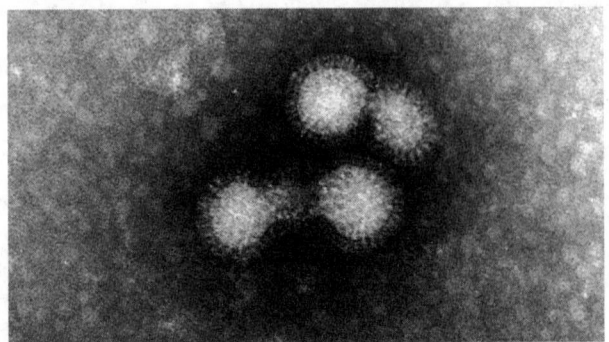

FIGURE 171-1   An electron micrograph of influenza A virus (×140,000).

Pandemics provide the most dramatic evidence of the impact of influenza. However, illnesses that occur between pandemics account for greater total mortality and morbidity, albeit over a longer period. From 1972 through the present, influenza has been associated with at least 20,000 excess deaths during more than half of the interpandemic epidemics in the United States; >40,000 influenza-associated deaths occurred in each of six of these epidemics. Influenza A viruses that circulate between pandemics demonstrate antigenic drifts in the H antigen. These antigenic drifts apparently result from point mutations involving the RNA segment that codes for the hemagglutinin, which occurs most frequently in five hypervariable regions. Epidemiologically significant strains—that is, those with the potential to cause widespread outbreaks—exhibit changes in amino acids in at least two of the major antigenic sites in the hemagglutinin molecule. Since two point mutations are unlikely to occur simultaneously, it is believed that antigenic drifts result from point mutations occurring sequentially during the spread of virus from person to person. Antigenic drifts have been reported nearly annually since 1977 for H1N1 viruses and since 1968 for H3N2 viruses.

Influenza A epidemics begin abruptly, peak over a 2- to 3-week period, generally last for 2 to 3 months, and often subside almost as rapidly as they began. The first indication of influenza activity in a community is an increase in the number of children with febrile respiratory illnesses who present for medical attention. This increase is followed by increases in rates of influenza-like illnesses among adults and eventually by an increase in hospital admissions for patients with pneumonia, worsening of congestive heart failure, and exacerbations of chronic pulmonary disease. Rates of absence from work and school also rise at this time. An increase in the number of deaths caused by pneumonia and influenza is generally a late observation in an outbreak. Attack rates have been highly variable from outbreak to outbreak but most commonly are in the range of 10 to 20% of the general population. During the pandemic of 1957, it was estimated that the attack rate of clinical influenza exceeded 50% in urban populations and that an additional 25% or more of individuals in these populations may have been subclinically infected with influenza A virus. Among institutionalized populations and in semiclosed settings with many susceptible individuals, even higher attack rates have been reported.

Epidemics of influenza occur almost exclusively during the winter months in the temperate zones of the northern and southern hemispheres. In those locations, it is highly unusual to detect influenza A virus at other times, although serologic rises or even outbreaks have been noted rarely during warm-weather months. In contrast, influenza virus infections occur throughout the year in the tropics. Where or how influenza A virus persists between outbreaks in temperate zones is unknown. It is possible that influenza A viruses are maintained in the human population on a worldwide basis by person-to-person transmission and that large population clusters support a low level of interepidemic transmission. Alternatively, human strains may persist in animal reservoirs. Convincing evidence to support either explanation is not available. In the modern era, rapid transportation may contribute to the transmission of viruses among widespread geographic locales.

The factors that result in the inception and termination of outbreaks of influenza are incompletely understood. A major determinant of the extent and severity of an outbreak is the level of immunity in the population at risk. With the emergence of an antigenically novel influenza virus to which little or no antibody is present in a community, extensive outbreaks may occur. When the absence of antibody is worldwide, epidemic disease may spread around the globe, resulting in a pandemic. Such pandemic waves can continue for several years, until immunity in the population reaches a high level. In the years following pandemic influenza, antigenic drifts among influenza viruses result in outbreaks of variable severity in populations with high levels of immunity to the pandemic strain that circulated earlier. This situation persists until another antigenically novel pandemic strain emerges. On the other hand, outbreaks sometimes end despite the persistence of a large pool of susceptible individuals in the population.

Occasionally, the emergence of a significantly different antigenic

variant will result only in a localized outbreak. The swine influenza outbreak of 1976 in the United States, caused by an A/H1N1 virus antigenically similar to the virus that circulated in 1918–1919, may be an example, although this outbreak may have represented simply the introduction of a swine influenza virus into a crowded human population without spread beyond that setting. The cluster of human infections with influenza A/H5N1 in Hong Kong in 1997 may also be an example of this phenomenon. It has been suggested that certain viruses, such as recently circulating A/H1N1 strains, may be intrinsically less virulent and cause less severe disease than other variants, even in immunologically virgin subjects. If so, then other (undefined) factors besides the level of preexisting immunity must play a role in the epidemiology of influenza.

Influenza B virus causes outbreaks that are generally less extensive and are associated with less severe disease than those caused by influenza A virus. The hemagglutinin and neuraminidase of influenza B virus undergo less frequent and less extensive variation than those of influenza A viruses; this characteristic may account, in part, for the lesser extent of disease. Influenza B outbreaks are seen most frequently in schools and military camps, although outbreaks in institutions in which elderly individuals reside have also been noted on occasion. The most serious complication of influenza B virus infection is Reye's syndrome (Chap. 290). In contrast to influenza A and B viruses, influenza C virus appears to be a relatively minor cause of disease in humans. It has been associated with common cold–like symptoms and occasionally with lower respiratory tract illness. The wide prevalence of serum antibody to this virus indicates that asymptomatic infection may be common.

The morbidity and mortality caused by influenza outbreaks continue to be substantial. Most individuals who die in this setting have underlying diseases that place them at high risk for complications of influenza. Excess hospitalizations for adults and children with high-risk medical conditions have ranged from 56 to 1900 per 100,000 during recent outbreaks of influenza. The most prominent high-risk conditions are chronic cardiac and pulmonary diseases and old age. Mortality among individuals with chronic metabolic, renal, and certain immunosuppressive diseases has also been elevated, although lower than that among patients with chronic cardiopulmonary diseases. The morbidity attributable to influenza in the general population is considerable. It is estimated that interpandemic outbreaks of influenza currently incur annual costs of $12 billion in the United States. If a pandemic were to occur, it is estimated that annual costs would range from $71 to $167 billion for attack rates of 15 to 35%.

PATHOGENESIS AND IMMUNITY The initial event in influenza is infection of the respiratory epithelium with influenza virus acquired from respiratory secretions of acutely infected individuals. In all likelihood, transmission occurs via aerosols generated by coughs and sneezes, although hand-to-hand contact, other personal contact, and even fomite transmission may take place. Experimental evidence suggests that infection by a small-particle aerosol (particle diameter <10 μm) is more efficient than that by larger droplets. Initially, viral infection involves the ciliated columnar epithelial cells, but it may also involve other respiratory tract cells, including alveolar cells, mucous gland cells, and macrophages. In infected cells, virus replicates within 4 to 6 h, after which infectious virus is released to infect adjacent or nearby cells. In this way, infection spreads from a few foci to a large number of respiratory cells over several hours. In experimentally induced infection, the incubation period of illness has ranged from 18 to 72 h, depending on the size of the viral inoculum. Histopathologic study reveals degenerative changes, including granulation, vacuolization, swelling, and pyknotic nuclei, in infected ciliated cells. The cells eventually become necrotic and desquamate; in some areas, previously columnar epithelium is replaced by flattened and metaplastic epithelial cells. The severity of illness is correlated with the quantity of virus shed in secretions; thus, the degree of viral replication itself may be an important factor in pathogenesis. Despite the frequent development of systemic signs and symptoms such as fever, headache, and myalgias, influenza virus has only rarely been detected in extrapulmonary sites (including the bloodstream). Evidence suggests that the pathogenesis of systemic symptoms in influenza may be related to the induction of certain cytokines, particularly tumor necrosis factor α, interferon α, and interleukin 6, in respiratory secretions and in the bloodstream.

The host response to influenza infections involves a complex interplay of humoral antibody, local antibody, cell-mediated immunity, interferon, and other host defenses. Serum antibody responses, which can be detected by the second week after primary infection, are measured by a variety of techniques: hemagglutination inhibition (HI), complement fixation (CF), neutralization, enzyme-linked immunosorbent assay (ELISA), and antineuraminidase antibody assay. Antibodies directed against the hemagglutinin appear to be the most important mediators of immunity; in several studies, HI titers of ≥ 40 have been associated with protection from infection. Secretory antibodies produced in the respiratory tract are predominantly of the IgA class and also play a major role in protection against infection. Secretory antibody neutralization titers of ≥ 4 have also been associated with protection. A variety of cell-mediated immune responses, both antigen-specific and antigen-nonspecific, can be detected early after infection and depend on the prior immune status of the host. These responses include T-cell proliferative, T-cell cytotoxic, and natural killer cell activity. In humans, CD8+, HLA class I–restricted cytotoxic T cells (CTLs) are directed at conserved regions of internal proteins (NP, M, and polymerases) as well as against the surface proteins (H and N). Interferons can be detected in respiratory secretions shortly after the shedding of virus has begun, and rises in interferon titers coincide with decreases in virus shedding.

The host defense factors responsible for cessation of virus shedding and resolution of illness have not been defined specifically. Virus shedding generally stops within 2 to 5 days after symptoms first appear, at a time when serum and local antibody responses often are not detectable by conventional techniques (although antibody rises may be detected earlier by use of highly sensitive techniques, particularly in individuals with previous immunity to the virus). It has been suggested that interferon, cell-mediated immune responses, and/or nonspecific inflammatory responses all contribute to the resolution of illness. CTL responses may be particularly important in that regard.

MANIFESTATIONS Influenza has most frequently been described as an illness characterized by the abrupt onset of systemic symptoms, such as headache, feverishness, chills, myalgia, or malaise, and accompanying respiratory tract signs, particularly cough and sore throat. In many cases, the onset is so abrupt that patients can recall the precise time they became ill. However, the spectrum of clinical presentations is wide, ranging from a mild, afebrile respiratory illness similar to the common cold (with either a gradual or an abrupt onset) to severe prostration with relatively few respiratory signs and symptoms. In most of the cases that come to a physician's attention, the patient has a fever, with temperatures of 38° to 41°C (100.4° to 105.8°F). A rapid temperature rise within the first 24 h of illness is generally followed by a gradual defervescence over a 2- to 3-day period, although, on occasion, fever may last for as long as a week. Patients report a feverish feeling and chilliness, but true rigors are rare. Headache, either generalized or frontal, is often particularly troublesome. Myalgias may involve any part of the body but are most common in the legs and lumbosacral area. Arthralgias may also develop.

Respiratory complaints often become more prominent as systemic symptoms subside. Many patients have a sore throat or persistent cough, which may last for a week or more and which is often accompanied by substernal discomfort. Ocular signs and symptoms include pain on motion of the eyes, photophobia, and burning of the eyes.

Physical findings are usually minimal in cases of uncomplicated influenza. Early in the illness, the patient appears flushed and the skin is hot and dry, although diaphoresis and mottled extremities are sometimes evident, particularly in older patients. Examination of the pharynx may yield surprisingly unremarkable results despite a severe sore throat, but injection of the mucous membranes and postnasal discharge are apparent in some cases. Mild cervical lymphadenopathy may be noted, especially in younger individuals. The results of chest examination are largely negative in uncomplicated influenza, although rhonchi, wheezes, and scattered rales have been reported with variable frequency in different outbreaks. Frank dyspnea, hyperpnea, cyanosis, diffuse rales, and signs of consolidation are indicative of pulmonary complications. Patients with apparently uncomplicated influenza have been reported to have a variety of mild ventilatory defects and increased alveolar-capillary diffusion gradients; thus, subclinical pulmonary involvement may be more frequent than is appreciated.

In uncomplicated influenza, the acute illness generally resolves over a 2- to 5-day period, and most patients have largely recovered in 1 week, although cough may persist for 1 to 2 weeks longer. In a significant minority (particularly the elderly), however, symptoms of weakness or lassitude (postinfluenzal asthenia) may persist for several weeks and may prove troublesome for persons who wish to resume their full level of activity promptly. The pathogenetic basis for this asthenia is unknown, although pulmonary function abnormalities may persist for several weeks after uncomplicated influenza.

COMPLICATIONS Complications of influenza occur most frequently in patients >64 years old and in those with certain chronic disorders, including cardiac or pulmonary diseases, diabetes mellitus, hemoglobinopathies, renal dysfunction, and immunosuppression. Pregnancy in the second or third trimester also predisposes to complications with influenza. The most significant complication of influenza is pneumonia: "primary" influenza viral pneumonia, secondary bacterial pneumonia, or mixed viral and bacterial pneumonia. Primary influenza viral pneumonia is the least common but most severe of the pneumonic complications. It presents as acute influenza that does not resolve but instead progresses relentlessly, with persistent fever, dyspnea, and eventual cyanosis. Sputum production is generally scanty, but the sputum can contain blood. Few physical signs may be evident early in the illness. In more advanced cases, diffuse rales may be noted, and chest x-ray findings consistent with diffuse interstitial infiltrates and/or acute respiratory distress syndrome may be present. In such cases, arterial blood-gas determinations show marked hypoxia. Viral cultures of respiratory secretions and lung parenchyma, especially if samples are taken early in illness, yield high titers of virus. In fatal cases of primary viral pneumonia, histopathologic examination reveals a marked inflammatory reaction in the alveolar septa, with edema and infiltration by lymphocytes, macrophages, occasional plasma cells, and variable numbers of neutrophils. Fibrin thrombi in alveolar capillaries, along with necrosis and hemorrhage, have also been noted. Eosinophilic hyaline membranes can be found lining alveoli and alveolar ducts.

Primary influenza viral pneumonia has a predilection for individuals with cardiac disease, particularly those with mitral stenosis, but has also been reported in otherwise-healthy young adults as well as in older individuals with chronic pulmonary disorders. In some epidemics of influenza (notably those of 1918 and 1957), pregnancy increased the risk of primary influenza pneumonia. Subsequent epidemics of influenza have been associated with increased rates of hospitalization among pregnant women.

Secondary bacterial pneumonia follows acute influenza. Improvement of the patient's condition over 2 to 3 days is followed by a reappearance of fever along with clinical signs and symptoms of bacterial pneumonia, including cough, production of purulent sputum, and physical and x-ray signs of consolidation. The most common bacterial pathogens in this setting are *Streptococcus pneumoniae*, *Staphylococcus aureus*, and *Haemophilus influenzae*—organisms that can colonize the nasopharynx and that cause infection in the wake of changes in bronchopulmonary defenses. The etiology can often be determined by Gram's staining and culture of an appropriately obtained sputum specimen. Secondary bacterial pneumonia occurs most frequently in high-risk individuals with chronic pulmonary and cardiac disease and in elderly individuals. Patients with secondary bacterial pneumonia often respond to antibiotic therapy when it is instituted promptly.

Perhaps the most common pneumonic complications during outbreaks of influenza have mixed features of viral and bacterial pneumonia. Patients may experience a gradual progression of their acute illness or may show transient improvement followed by clinical exacerbation, with eventual manifestation of the clinical features of bacterial pneumonia. Sputum cultures may contain both influenza A virus and one of the bacterial pathogens described above. Patchy infiltrates or areas of consolidation may be detected by physical examination and chest x-ray. Patients with mixed viral and bacterial pneumonia generally have less widespread involvement of the lung than those with primary viral pneumonia, and their bacterial infections may respond to appropriate antibiotics. Mixed viral and bacterial pneumonia occurs primarily in patients with chronic cardiovascular and pulmonary diseases.

Other pulmonary complications associated with influenza include worsening of chronic obstructive pulmonary disease and exacerbation of chronic bronchitis and asthma. In children, influenza infection may present as croup. Sinusitis as well as otitis media (the latter occurring particularly often in children) may also be associated with influenza.

In addition to the pulmonary complications of influenza, a number of extrapulmonary complications may occur. These include *Reye's syndrome* (Chap. 290), a serious complication in children that is associated with influenza B and to a lesser extent with influenza A virus infection as well as with varicella-zoster virus infection. An epidemiologic association between Reye's syndrome and aspirin therapy for the antecedent viral infection has been noted, and the syndrome's incidence has decreased markedly with widespread warnings regarding aspirin use by children with acute viral respiratory infections.

Myositis, rhabdomyolysis, and myoglobinuria are occasional complications of influenza infection. Although myalgias are exceedingly common in influenza, true myositis is rare. Patients with acute myositis have exquisite tenderness of the affected muscles, most commonly in the legs, and may not be able to tolerate even the slightest pressure, such as the touch of bedsheets. In the most severe cases, there is frank swelling and bogginess of muscles. Serum levels of creatine phosphokinase and aldolase are markedly elevated, and an occasional patient has developed renal failure from myoglobinuria. The pathogenesis of influenza-associated myositis is also unclear, although the presence of influenza virus in affected muscles has been reported.

Myocarditis and pericarditis were reported in association with influenza virus infection during the 1918–1919 pandemic; these reports were based largely on histopathologic findings, and these complications have been reported only infrequently since that time. Electrocardiographic changes during acute influenza are common among patients who have cardiac disease but have been ascribed most often to exacerbations of the underlying cardiac disease rather than to direct involvement of the myocardium with influenza virus.

Central nervous system (CNS) diseases, including encephalitis, transverse myelitis, and Guillain-Barré syndrome, have been reported during influenza. The etiologic relationship of influenza virus to such CNS illnesses remains uncertain. Toxic shock syndrome associated with *S. aureus* or group A streptococcal infection following acute influenza infection has also been reported (Chaps. 120 and 121).

In addition to complications involving the specific organ systems described above, influenza outbreaks include a number of cases in which elderly and other high-risk individuals develop influenza and subsequently experience a gradual deterioration of underlying cardiovascular, pulmonary, or renal function—changes that occasionally are irreversible and lead to death. These fatalities contribute to the overall excess mortality associated with influenza A outbreaks.

LABORATORY FINDINGS AND DIAGNOSIS Influenza virus may be isolated during acute influenza from throat swabs, nasopharyngeal washes, or sputum. Virus is usually detected by use of tissue culture or, less commonly, chick embryos within 48 to 72 h after inoculation. Most com-

monly, the diagnosis is established by the use of rapid viral tests that detect viral nucleoprotein or neuraminidase with high sensitivity and a specificity of 60 to 90% compared with that of tissue culture. Viral nucleic acids can be detected in clinical samples by reverse transcriptase polymerase chain reaction. The type of influenza virus (A or B) may be determined by either immunofluorescence or HI techniques, and the hemagglutinin subtype of influenza A virus (H1, H2, or H3) may be identified by HI with use of subtype-specific antisera. Serologic methods for diagnosis require comparison of antibody titers in sera obtained during the acute illness with those in sera obtained 10 to 14 days after the onset of illness and are useful primarily in retrospect. Fourfold or greater titer rises as detected by HI or CF or significant rises as measured by ELISA are diagnostic of acute infection. CF tests are generally less sensitive than other serologic techniques, but, as they detect type-specific antigens, they may be particularly useful when subtype-specific reagents are not available.

Other laboratory tests are generally not helpful in making a specific diagnosis of influenza virus infection. Leukocyte counts are variable, frequently being low early in illness and normal or slightly elevated later. Severe leukopenia has been described in overwhelming viral or bacterial infection, while leukocytosis with >15,000 cells/μL raises the suspicion of secondary bacterial infection.

DIFFERENTIAL DIAGNOSIS During a community-wide outbreak of influenza, a clinical diagnosis of influenza can be made with a high degree of certainty in patients who present to a physician's office with the typical febrile respiratory illness described above. In the absence of an outbreak (i.e., in sporadic or isolated cases), influenza may be difficult to differentiate on clinical grounds alone from an acute respiratory illness caused by any of a variety of respiratory viruses or by *Mycoplasma pneumoniae*. Severe streptococcal pharyngitis or early bacterial pneumonia may mimic acute influenza, although bacterial pneumonias generally do not run a self-limited course. Purulent sputum in which a bacterial pathogen can be detected by Gram's staining is an important diagnostic feature in bacterial pneumonia.

℞ TREATMENT

In uncomplicated cases of influenza, symptom-based therapy with acetaminophen for the relief of headache, myalgia, and fever may be considered, but the use of salicylates should be avoided in children <18 years of age because of the possible association of salicylates with Reye's syndrome. Since cough is ordinarily self-limited, treatment with cough suppressants generally is not indicated, although codeine-containing compounds may be employed if the cough is particularly troublesome. Patients should be advised to rest and maintain hydration during acute illness and to return to full activity only gradually after illness has resolved, especially if it has been severe.

Specific antiviral therapy is available for influenza: amantadine and rimantadine for influenza A and the neuraminidase inhibitors zanamivir and oseltamivir for both influenza A and influenza B. If begun within 48 h of the onset of illness, treatment with amantadine or rimantadine has reduced the duration of systemic and respiratory symptoms of influenza by ~50%. From 5 to 10% of individuals who receive amantadine experience mild CNS side effects, primarily jitteriness, anxiety, insomnia, or difficulty in concentrating. These side effects disappear promptly upon cessation of the drug. Rimantadine appears to be equally efficacious and is associated with less frequent CNS side effects than is amantadine. In adults, the usual dose of amantadine or rimantadine is 200 mg/d for 3 to 7 days. Since both drugs are excreted via the kidney, the dose should be reduced to ≤100 mg/d in elderly patients and in patients with renal insufficiency. Zanamivir, inhaled orally at a dose of 10 mg twice a day for 5 days, or oseltamivir, ingested orally at a dose of 75 mg twice a day for 5 days, has reduced the duration of signs and symptoms of influenza by 1 to 1.5 days if treatment is started within 2 days of the onset of illness. Zanamivir may exacerbate bronchospasm in asthmatic patients, and oseltamivir has been associated with nausea and vomiting, whose frequency can be reduced by drug administration with food. Resistant viruses emerge frequently during treatment with amantadine or rimantadine and can be transmitted among family members. The development of resistance appears to be infrequent with zanamivir or oseltamivir. Treatment of children is approved for amantadine and oseltamivir (≥ 1 year of age) and for zanamivir (≥ 7 years of age). Ribavirin is a nucleoside analogue with activity against influenza A and B viruses in vitro. It has been reported to be variably effective against influenza when administered as an aerosol but ineffective when administered orally. Its efficacy in the treatment of influenza A or B is unestablished.

Studies demonstrating the therapeutic efficacy of antiviral compounds in influenza have primarily involved young adults with uncomplicated disease; it is not known whether such compounds are effective in the treatment of influenza pneumonia or of other complications of influenza. Therapy for primary influenza pneumonia is directed at maintaining oxygenation and is most appropriately undertaken in an intensive care unit, with aggressive respiratory and hemodynamic support as needed. Bypass membrane oxygenators have been employed in this setting with variable results. When an acute respiratory distress syndrome develops, fluids must be administered cautiously, with close monitoring of blood gases and hemodynamic function.

Antibacterial drugs should be reserved for the treatment of bacterial complications of acute influenza, such as secondary bacterial pneumonia. The choice of antibiotics should be guided by Gram's staining and culture of appropriate specimens of respiratory secretions, such as sputum or transtracheal aspirates. If the etiology of a case of bacterial pneumonia is unclear from an examination of respiratory secretions, empirical antibiotics effective against the most common bacterial pathogens in this setting (*S. pneumoniae*, *S. aureus*, and *H. influenzae*) should be selected (Chaps. 119, 120, and 130).

PROPHYLAXIS The major public health measure for prevention of influenza has been the use of inactivated influenza vaccines derived from influenza A and B viruses that circulated during the previous influenza season. If the vaccine virus and the currently circulating viruses are closely related, 50 to 80% protection against influenza would be expected. Presently available inactivated vaccines have been highly purified and are associated with few reactions. Up to 5% of individuals experience low-grade fever and mild systemic symptoms 8 to 24 h after vaccination, and up to one-third develop mild redness or tenderness at the vaccination site. Since the vaccine is produced in eggs, individuals with true hypersensitivity to egg products either should be desensitized or should not be vaccinated. Although the 1976 swine influenza vaccine appears to have been associated with an increased frequency of Guillain-Barré syndrome, influenza vaccines administered since 1976 generally have not been. Possible exceptions were noted during the 1992–1993 and 1993–1994 influenza seasons, when there may have been an excess risk of Guillain-Barré syndrome of slightly more than one case per million among vaccine recipients. However, the overall health risk following influenza outweighs the potential risk associated with vaccination.

The U.S. Public Health Service recommends influenza vaccination for any individual >6 months of age who is at an increased risk for complications of influenza, as noted earlier (Table 171-2). Since commercially available vaccines are inactivated ("killed"), they may be administered safely to immunocompromised patients. Influenza vaccination is not associated with exacerbations of chronic nervous-system diseases such as multiple sclerosis. Vaccine should be administered early in the autumn before influenza outbreaks occur and should then be given annually to maintain immunity against the most current influenza virus strains.

Recently, an advisory committee of the U.S. Food and Drug Administration recommended approval of a live attenuated influenza vaccine that is administered by intranasal spray. The vaccine is gen-

TABLE 171-2 *Recommendations for Influenza Vaccination*[a]

Persons at increased risk for complications
  Persons ≥ 65 years of age
  Residents of nursing homes and other chronic-care facilities that house persons of any age who have chronic medical conditions
  Adults and children (≥ 6 months) who have chronic disorders of the pulmonary or cardiovascular systems, including asthma
  Adults and children (≥ 6 months) who have required regular medical follow-up or hospitalization during the preceding year because of chronic metabolic diseases (including diabetes mellitus), renal dysfunction, hemoglobinopathies, or immunosuppression (including immunosuppression caused by medications or by HIV)
  Children and adolescents (6 months to 18 years old) who are receiving long-term aspirin therapy and therefore may be at risk for developing Reye's syndrome after influenza infection
  Women who will be in the second or third trimester of pregnancy during the influenza season
Persons 50 to 64 years of age
  Included because of increased prevalence of high-risk conditions
Persons who can transmit influenza to those at high risk
  Physicians, nurses, and other personnel in both hospital and outpatient-care settings, including medical emergency response workers (e.g., paramedics and emergency medical technicians)
  Employees of nursing homes and chronic-care facilities who have contact with patients or residents
  Employees of assisted-living and other residences for persons in groups at high risk
  Persons who provide home care to individuals in groups at high risk
  Household members (including children) of persons in groups at high risk

[a] Vaccination of healthy children 6 to 23 months of age is encouraged.
Source: Centers for Disease Control and Prevention.

erated by reassortment of currently circulating strains of influenza A and B virus with a cold-adapted, attenuated master strain. The cold-adapted vaccine is well tolerated and highly efficacious (92% protective) in young children; in one study, it provided protection against a circulating influenza virus that had drifted antigenically away from the vaccine strain. The committee recommended approval of the cold-adapted vaccine for use in healthy children and adults from 5 to 49 years of age.

Chemoprophylaxis with amantadine or rimantadine, at dosages of 100 to 200 mg/d, has efficacy rates of 70 to 100% against illness associated with influenza A infection. Chemoprophylaxis with oseltamivir (75 mg/d by mouth) or zanamivir (10 mg/d inhaled) has resulted in efficacy rates of 84 to 89% against influenza A and B. Chemoprophylaxis is most likely to be used for high-risk individuals who have not received influenza vaccine or in a situation where the vaccines previously administered are relatively ineffective because of antigenic changes in the circulating virus. During an outbreak, antiviral chemoprophylaxis can be administered simultaneously with inactivated vaccine, since the drugs do not interfere with an immune response to the vaccine. In fact, there is evidence that the protective effects of chemoprophylaxis and vaccine may be additive. However, concurrent administration of chemoprophylaxis and the live attenuated vaccine may interfere with the immune response to the latter. Chemoprophylaxis may also be employed to control nosocomial outbreaks of influenza. For prophylaxis, administration should be instituted promptly when influenza activity is detected and must be continued daily for the duration of the outbreak. Amantadine and rimantadine are approved for prophylaxis in adults and in children ≥ 1 year old; oseltamivir is approved for prophylaxis in adults and in children ≥ 13 years old.

FURTHER READING

CENTERS FOR DISEASE CONTROL AND PREVENTION: Prevention and control of influenza. MMWR 51(RR–3):1, 2002
DOLIN R et al: A controlled trial of amantadine and rimantadine in the prophylaxis of influenza A infection. N Engl J Med 307:580, 1982

GROSS PA et al: Association of influenza immunization with reduction in mortality in an elderly population: A prospective study. Arch Intern Med 148: 562, 1988

HAYDEN FG et al: Use of the selective oral neuraminidase inhibitor oseltamivir to prevent influenza. N Engl J Med 341:1336, 1999

MIST [MANAGEMENT OF INFLUENZA IN THE SOUTHERN HEMISPHERE TRIALISTS] STUDY GROUP: Randomized trial of efficacy and safety of inhaled zanamivir in treatment of influenza A and B infections. Lancet 352: 1871, 1998

NEUZIL KM et al: Influenza-associated morbidity and mortality in young and middle-aged women. JAMA 281:901, 1999

NICHOL KL et al: Effectiveness of live, attenuated intranasal influenza virus vaccine in healthy, working adults. JAMA 282:137, 1999

SIMONSEN L et al: Pandemic vs epidemic mortality: A pattern of changing age distribution. J Infect Dis 178:53, 1998

WRIGHT DF, WEBSTER RG: Orthomyxoviruses, in Virology, 4th ed, DM Knipe, PM Howley (eds). Philadelphia, Lippincott Williams & Wilkins, 2001, pp 1533–1580

Section 14 Infections Due to Human Immunodeficiency Virus and Other Human Retroviruses

172 THE HUMAN RETROVIRUSES
Dan L. Longo, Anthony S. Fauci

The retroviruses, which make up a large family (Retroviridae), infect mainly vertebrates. They have a unique replication cycle whereby their genetic information is encoded by RNA rather than DNA. Retroviruses contain an RNA-dependent DNA polymerase (a reverse transcriptase) that directs the synthesis of a DNA form of the viral genome after infection of a host cell. The designation *retrovirus* denotes that information in the form of RNA is transcribed into DNA in the host cell—a sequence that overturned a central dogma of molecular biology: that information passes unidirectionally from DNA to RNA to protein. The observation that RNA was the source of genetic information in the causative agents of certain animal tumors led to a number of paradigm-shifting biologic insights regarding not only the direction of genetic-information passage but also the viral etiology of certain cancers and the concept of oncogenes as normal host genes scavenged and altered by a viral vector.

The family Retroviridae includes three subfamilies (Table 172-1): Oncovirinae, of which human T-cell lymphotropic virus (HTLV) type I is the most important in humans; Lentivirinae, of which HIV is the most important in humans; and Spumavirinae, the "foamy" viruses, named for the pathologic appearance of infected cells. A number of spumaviruses have been isolated from humans; however, they are not associated with any known disease and therefore are not discussed further in this chapter.

The wide variety of interactions of a retrovirus with its host range from completely benign events (e.g., silent carriage of endogenous retroviral sequences in the germ-line genome of many animal species) to rapidly fatal infections (e.g., exogenous infection with an oncogenic virus such as Rous sarcoma virus in chickens). The ability of retroviruses to acquire and alter the structure and function of host cell sequences has revolutionized our understanding of molecular carcinogenesis. The viruses can insert into the germ-line genome of the host cell and behave as a transposable or movable genetic element. They can activate or inactivate genes near the site of integration into the genome. They can rapidly alter their own genome by recombination and mutation under selective environmental stimuli.

Most human viral diseases occur as a consequence of either tissue destruction by the virus itself or the host's response to the virus. Although these mechanisms are operative in retroviral infections, retroviruses have addi-tional mechanisms of inducing disease, including the malignant transformation of an infected cell and the induction of an immunodeficiency state that leads to opportunistic diseases (infections and neoplasms; Chap. 173).

STRUCTURE AND LIFE CYCLE Despite the wide range of biologic consequences of retroviral infection, all retroviruses are similar in structure, genome organization, and mode of replication. Retroviruses are 70 to 130 nm in diameter and have a lipid-containing envelope surrounding an icosahedral capsid with a dense inner core. The core contains two identical copies of the single-strand RNA genome. The RNA molecules are 8 to 10 kb long and are complexed with reverse transcriptase and tRNA. Other viral proteins, such as integrase, are also components of the virion particle. The RNA has features usually found in mRNA: a cap site at the 5' end of the molecule, which is important in the initiation of mRNA translation, and a polyadenylation site at the 3' end, which influences mRNA turnover (i.e., messages with shorter polyA tails turn over faster than messages with longer polyA tails). However, the retroviral RNA is not translated; instead it is transcribed into DNA. The DNA form of the retroviral genome is called a *provirus*.

The replication cycle of retroviruses proceeds in two phases (Fig. 172-1). In the first phase, the virus enters the cytoplasm after binding to a specific cell-surface receptor (with HIV, a cell-surface co-receptor is also utilized for binding and entry); the viral RNA and reverse transcriptase synthesize a double-strand DNA version of the RNA template; and the provirus moves into the nucleus and integrates into the host cell genome. This proviral integration is permanent. Although some animal retroviruses integrate into a single specific site of the host

TABLE 172-1 *Classification of Retroviruses: the Family Retroviridae*

Subfamily, Group[a]	Example	Feature
Oncovirinae (oncogenic viruses)		
Avian leukosis	Rous sarcoma virus	Contains *src* oncogene
Mammalian C-type	Abelson leukemia virus	Contains *abl* oncogene
B-type	Murine mammary tumor virus	Can be endogenous or exogenous
D-type	Mason-Pfizer monkey virus	—
HTLV-BLV	HTLV-I	Causes T-cell lymphoma and neurologic disease
Lentivirinae (slow viruses)	HIV-1, HIV-2	Causes AIDS
	Visna virus	Causes lung and brain diseases in sheep
	Feline immunodeficiency virus	Causes immunodeficiency in cats
Spumavirinae (foamy viruses)	Simian foamy virus, human foamy virus	Causes no known disease

[a] The Oncovirinae were originally grouped into types A–D on the basis of morphologic features (size, core location, budding) under electron microscopy; however, this system has been replaced by groupings based on relationships of genome structure and sequence.

Note: HTLV, human T-lymphotropic virus; BLV, bovine leukemia virus.

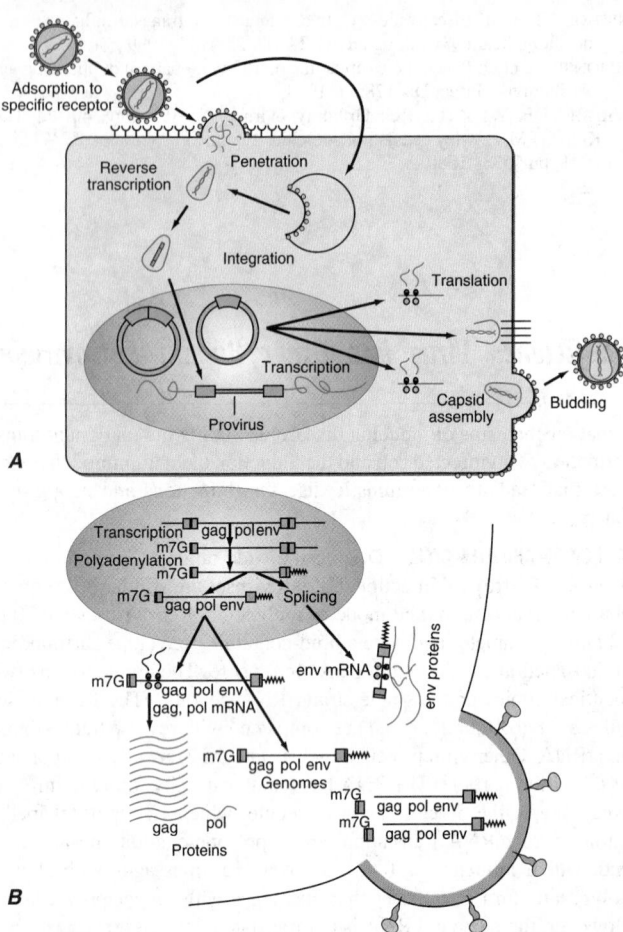

FIGURE 172-1 The life cycle of retroviruses. *A.* Overview of virus replication. The retrovirus enters a target cell by binding to a specific cell-surface receptor; once the virus is internalized, its RNA is released from the nucleocapsid and is reverse-transcribed into proviral DNA. The provirus is inserted into the genome and then transcribed into RNA; the RNA is translated; and virions assemble and are extruded from the cell membrane by budding. *B.* Overview of retroviral gene expression. The provirus is transcribed, capped, and polyadenylated. Viral RNA molecules then have one of three fates: They are exported to the cytoplasm, where they are packaged as the viral RNA in infectious viral particles; they are spliced to form the message for the envelope polyprotein; or they are translated into Gag and Pol proteins. Most of the messages for the Pol protein fail to initiate Pol translation because of a stop codon before its initiation; however, in a fraction of the messages, the stop codon is missed and the Pol proteins are translated. [*Modified from JM Coffin, in BN Fields, DM Knipe (eds): Fields Virology. New York, Raven, 1990, with permission.*]

genome in every infected cell, the four known human retroviruses (HTLV-I, HTLV-II, HIV-1, and HIV-2) integrate randomly. This first phase of replication depends entirely on gene products in the virus. The second phase includes the synthesis and processing of viral genomes, mRNAs, and proteins using host cell machinery, often under the influence of viral gene products. Virions are assembled and released from the cell by budding from the membrane; host cell membrane proteins are frequently incorporated into the envelope of the virus. Proviral integration occurs during the S-phase of the cell cycle; thus, in general, nondividing cells are resistant to retroviral infection. Only the lentiviruses are able to infect nondividing cells. Once a host cell is infected, it is infected for the life of the cell.

Retroviral genomes include both coding and noncoding sequences (Fig. 172-2). In general, noncoding sequences are important recognition signals for DNA or RNA synthesis or processing events and are located in the 5′ and 3′ terminal regions of the genome. All retroviral genomes are terminally redundant, containing identical sequences called *long terminal repeats* (LTRs). The ends of the retroviral RNA genome differ slightly in sequence from the integrated retroviral DNA.

In the latter, the LTR sequences are repeated in both the 5′ and the 3′ terminus of the virus. The LTRs contain sequences involved in initiating the expression of the viral proteins, the integration of the provirus, and the polyadenylation of viral RNAs. The primer binding site, which is critical for the initiation of reverse transcription, and the viral packaging sequences are located outside the LTR sequences. The coding regions include the *gag* (group-specific antigen, core protein), *pol* (RNA-dependent DNA polymerase), and *env* (envelope) genes. The *gag* gene encodes a precursor polyprotein that is cleaved to form three to five capsid proteins; a fraction of the Gag precursor proteins also contain a protease responsible for cleaving the Gag and Pol polyproteins. A Gag-Pol polyprotein gives rise to the protease that is responsible for cleaving the Gag-Pol polyprotein. The *pol* gene encodes three proteins: the reverse transcriptase, the integrase, and the protease. The reverse transcriptase functions to copy the viral RNA into the double-strand DNA provirus, which can attach to the host cell DNA via the action of integrase. The protease functions to cleave the Gag-Pol polyprotein into smaller protein products. The *env* gene encodes the envelope glycoproteins: one protein that binds to specific surface receptors and determines what cell types can be infected and a smaller transmembrane protein that anchors the complex to the envelope. The cartoon in Fig. 172-3 shows how the retroviral gene products make up the virus structure.

HTLVs have a region between *env* and the 3′ LTR that encodes at least two proteins in overlapping reading frames: Tax, a 40-kDa protein that does not bind to DNA but induces the expression of host cell transcription factors that alter host cell gene expression; and Rex, a 27-kDa protein that regulates the expression of viral mRNAs. These two proteins are produced from messages that are similar but that are spliced differently from overlapping but distinct exons.

The lentiviruses in general, and HIV-1 and -2 in particular, contain a larger genome than other pathogenic retroviruses. They contain an untranslated region between *pol* and *env* that encodes portions of several proteins, varying with the reading frame into which the mRNA is spliced. Tat is a 14-kDa protein that augments the expression of virus from the LTR. The Rev protein of HIV-1, similar to the Rex protein of HTLV, regulates RNA splicing and/or RNA transport. The Nef protein downregulates CD4, the cellular receptor for HIV; alters host T cell activation pathways; and enhances viral infectivity. The Vif protein is necessary for the proper assembly of the HIV nucleoprotein core in many types of cells; without Vif, proviral DNA is not efficiently produced in these infected cells. Vpr, Vpu (HIV-1 only), and Vpx (HIV-2 only) are viral proteins encoded by translation of the same message in different reading frames. As noted above, oncogenic retroviruses depend on cell proliferation for their replication; lentiviruses can infect nondividing cells, largely owing to effects mediated by Vpr. Vpr facilitates transport of the provirus into the nucleus and can induce other cellular changes, such as G_2 growth arrest and differentiation of some target cells. Vpx is structurally related to Vpr, but its functions are not fully defined. Vpu promotes the degradation of CD4 in the endoplasmic reticulum and stimulates the release of virions from infected cells.

Retroviruses can be either exogenously acquired by infection with a virion capable of replication or transmitted in the germ line as endogenous virus. Endogenous retroviruses are often replication-defective. The human genome contains endogenous retroviral sequences, but there are no known replication-competent endogenous retroviruses in humans.

In general, viruses that contain only the *gag*, *pol*, and *env* genes either are not pathogenic or take a long time to induce disease; these observations indicate the importance of the other regulatory genes in viral disease pathogenesis. The pathogenesis of neoplastic transformation by retroviruses relies on the chance integration of the provirus at a spot in the genome that will result in the expression of a cellular gene (proto-oncogene) that becomes transforming by virtue of its unregulated expression. For example, avian leukosis virus causes B cell leukemia by inducing the expression of *myc*. Some retroviruses possess captured and altered cellular genes near their integration site, and these viral oncogenes are capable of transforming the infected host cell. Viruses that have oncogenes often have lost a portion of their genome that is required for replication. Such viruses need helper viruses to reproduce, a feature that may explain why these acute transforming retroviruses are rare in nature. All human retroviruses identified to date are exogenous and are not acutely transforming (i.e., they lack a transforming oncogene).

These remarkable properties of retroviruses have led to experimental efforts to use them as vectors to insert specific genes into particular cell types, a process known as *gene therapy* or *gene transfer*. The process could be used to repair a genetic defect or to introduce a new property that could be used therapeutically; for example, a gene (e.g., thymidine kinase) that would make a tumor cell susceptible to killing by a drug (e.g., ganciclovir) could be inserted. One source of concern about the use of retroviral vectors in humans is that replication-competent viruses might rescue endogenous retroviral replication, with unpredictable results. This concern is not merely hypothetical: The detection of proteins encoded by endogenous retroviral sequences on the surface of cancer cells implies that the genetic events leading to the cancer were able to activate the synthesis of these usually silent genes.

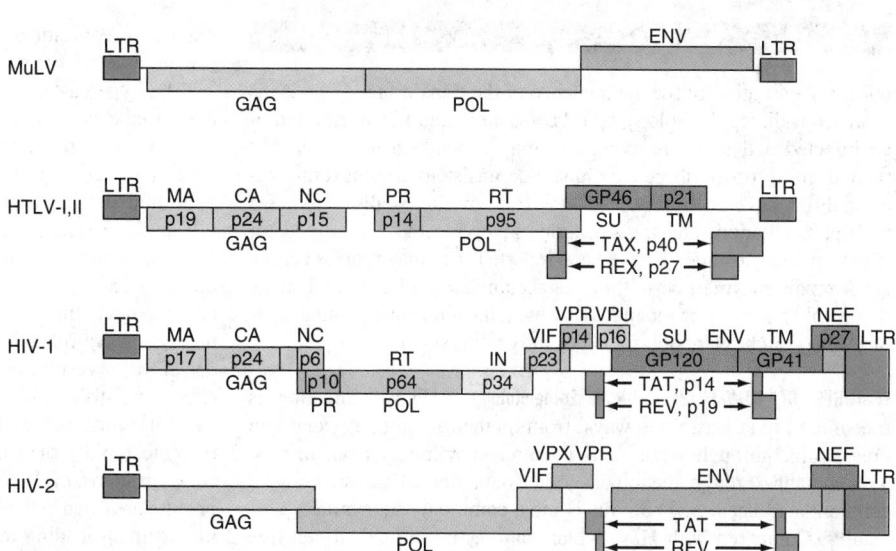

FIGURE 172-2 Genomic structure of retroviruses. The murine leukemia virus MuLV has the typical three structural genes: *gag*, *pol*, and *env*. The *gag* region gives rise to three proteins: matrix (MA), capsid (CA), and nucleic acid–binding (NC) proteins. The *pol* region encodes both a protease (PR) responsible for cleaving the viral polyproteins and a reverse transcriptase (RT). In addition, HIV *pol* encodes an integrase (IN). The *env* region encodes a surface protein (SU) and a small transmembrane protein (TM). The human retroviruses have additional gene products translated in each of the three possible reading frames. HTLV-I and HTLV-II have *tax* and *rex* genes with exons on either side of the *env* gene. HIV-1 and HIV-2 have six accessory gene products: *tat*, *rev*, *vif*, *nef*, *vpr*, and either *vpu* (in HIV-1) or *vpx* (in HIV-2). The genes for these proteins are located mainly between the *pol* and *env* genes.

HUMAN T-CELL LYMPHOTROPIC VIRUS

HTLV-I was isolated in 1980 from a T-cell lymphoma cell line from a patient originally thought to have cutaneous T cell lymphoma. Later it became clear that the patient had a distinct form of lymphoma (originally reported in Japan) called *adult T-cell leukemia/lymphoma* (ATL). Serologic data have determined that HTLV-I is the cause of at least two important diseases: ATL and tropical spastic paraparesis, also called *HTLV-I-associated myelopathy* (HAM). HTLV-I may also play a role in infective dermatitis and uveitis syndromes.

Two years after the isolation of HTLV-I, HTLV-II was isolated from a patient with an unusual form of hairy cell leukemia that affected T cells. Although early epidemiologic studies of HTLV-II failed to reveal a consistent disease association, more recent studies suggest an association of HTLV-II with human disease (see "Associated Diseases" under "Features of HTLV-II Infection," below), particularly among injection drug users.

BIOLOGY AND MOLECULAR BIOLOGY Because the biology of HTLV-I and that of HTLV-II are similar, the following discussion will focus on HTLV-I.

The cellular receptor for HTLV-I has not yet been identified, but it maps to chromosome 17. Generally, only T cells are productively infected, but infection of B cells and other cell types is occasionally detected. The most common outcome of HTLV-I infection is latent carriage of randomly integrated provirus in CD4+ T cells. HTLV-I does not contain an oncogene and does not insert into a unique site in the genome. Indeed, most infected cells express no viral gene products. The only viral gene product that is routinely expressed in tumor cells transformed by HTLV-I in vivo is *tax*, and even *tax* is not expressed in the tumor cells of many ATL patients. Cells transformed in vitro, by contrast, actively transcribe HTLV-I RNA and produce infectious virions. Most HTLV-I-transformed cell lines are the result of the infection of a normal host T cell in vitro. It is difficult to establish cell lines derived from authentic ATL cells.

Although *tax* does not itself bind to DNA, it does induce the expression of a wide range of host cell gene products, including transcription factors (especially c-*rel*, *ets*-1 and -2, and members of the *fos/jun* family), cytokines [e.g., interleukin (IL) 2, granulocyte-macrophage colony-stimulating factor, and tumor necrosis factor (TNF)], and membrane proteins and receptors [major histocompatibility (MHC) molecules and IL-2 receptor α]. The genes activated by *tax* are generally controlled by transcription factors of the c-*rel* and cyclic AMP response element binding (CREB) protein families. It is unclear how this induction of host gene expression leads to neoplastic transformation; *tax* can interfere with G_1 and mitotic cell-cycle checkpoints, block apoptosis, and promote antigen-independent T cell proliferation. Induction of a cytokine-autocrine loop has been proposed; however, IL-2 is not the crucial cytokine. The involvement of IL-4, IL-7, and IL-15 has been proposed.

In light of the irregular expression of *tax* in ATL cells, it has been suggested that *tax* is important in the early phases of transformation

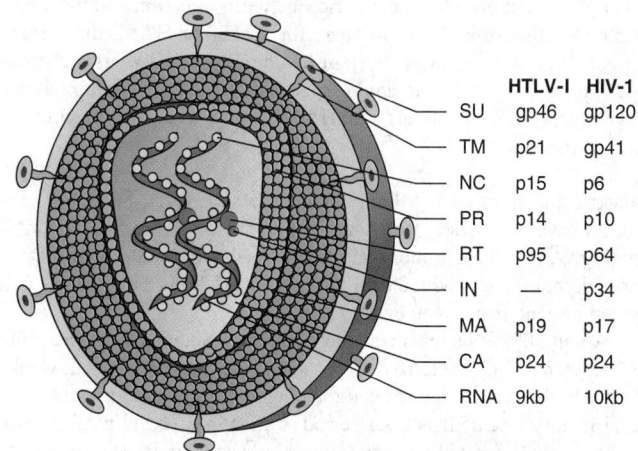

FIGURE 172-3 Schematic structure of human retroviruses. The surface glycoprotein (SU) is responsible for binding to receptors of host cells. The transmembrane protein (TM) anchors SU to the virus. NC is a nucleic acid–binding protein found in association with the viral RNA. A protease (PR) cleaves the polyproteins encoded by the *gag*, *pol*, and *env* genes into their functional components. RT is reverse transcriptase, and IN is an integrase present in some retroviruses (e.g., HIV-1) that facilitates insertion of the provirus into the host genome. MA is a Gag protein closely associated with the lipid of the envelope. The capsid protein (CA) forms the major internal structure of the virus, the core shell.

but is not essential for the maintenance of the transformed state. As is clear from the epidemiology of HTLV-I infection, transformation of an infected cell is a rare event and may depend on heterogeneous second, third, or fourth genetic hits. No consistent chromosomal abnormalities have been described in ATL; however, individual cases with p53 mutations and translocations involving the T cell receptor genes on chromosome 14 have been reported. *Tax* may repress certain DNA repair enzymes, permitting the accumulation of genetic damage that would normally be repaired. However, the molecular pathogenesis of HTLV-I-induced neoplasia is not fully understood.

FEATURES OF HTLV-I INFECTION ■ Epidemiology HTLV-I infection is transmitted in at least three ways: from mother to child, especially in breast milk; through sexual activity, more commonly from men to women; and through the blood—via contaminated transfusions or contaminated needles. The virus is most commonly transmitted perinatally. Compared with HIV, which can be transmitted in cell-free form, HTLV-I is less infectious, and its transmission usually requires cell-to-cell contact.

HTLV-I is endemic in southwestern Japan and Okinawa, where >1 million persons are infected. Antibodies to HTLV-I are present in the serum of up to 35% of Okinawans, 10% of residents of the Japanese island of Kyushu, and <1% of persons in nonendemic regions of Japan. Despite this high prevalence of infection, only ~500 cases of ATL are diagnosed in this area each year. Clusters of infection have been noted in other areas of the Orient, such as Taiwan; in the Caribbean basin, including northeastern South America; in central Africa; in Italy; in Israel; in the Arctic; and in the southeastern part of the United States.

A progressive spastic or ataxic myelopathy that develops in an individual who is HTLV-I positive (i.e., who has serum antibodies to HTLV-I) is likely to be due to direct nervous system infection with the virus; a similar disorder may result from infection with HIV or HTLV-II. In rare instances, patients with HAM are seronegative but have detectable antibody to HTLV-I in the cerebrospinal fluid (CSF).

The cumulative lifetime risk of developing ATL is 3% among HTLV-I-infected patients (the risk is three times greater in men than in women); a similar cumulative risk is projected for HAM. The distribution of the two diseases overlaps the distribution of HTLV-I, with >95% of affected patients showing serologic evidence of HTLV-I infection. The latent period between infection and the emergence of disease is 20 to 30 years for ATL. For HAM, the median latency period is ~3.3 years (range, 4 months to 30 years). The development of ATL is rare among persons infected by blood products; however, ~20% of patients with HAM acquire HTLV-I from contaminated blood.

Associated Diseases ■ *ATL* Four clinical types of HTLV-I-induced neoplasia have been described: acute, lymphomatous, chronic, and smoldering. All of these tumors are monoclonal proliferations of CD4+ post-thymic T cells with clonal proviral integrations and clonal T cell receptor gene rearrangements.

About 60% of patients who develop malignancy have classic acute ATL, which is characterized by a short clinical prodrome (~2 weeks between the first symptoms and the diagnosis) and an aggressive natural history (median survival period, 6 months). The clinical picture is dominated by rapidly progressive skin lesions, pulmonary involvement, hypercalcemia, and lymphocytosis with cells containing lobulated or "flower-shaped" nuclei (see Fig. 97-10). The malignant cells have monoclonal proviral integrations and express CD4, CD3, and CD25 (low-affinity IL-2 receptors) on their surface. Serum levels of CD25 can be used as a tumor marker. Anemia and thrombocytopenia are rare. The skin lesions may be difficult to distinguish from those in mycosis fungoides. Lytic bone lesions, which are common, do not contain tumor cells but rather are composed of osteolytic cells, usually

without osteoblastic activity. Despite the leukemic picture, bone marrow involvement is patchy in most cases.

The hypercalcemia of ATL is multifactorial; the tumor cells produce osteoclast-activating factors (TNF-α, IL-1, lymphotoxin) and can also produce a parathyroid hormone–like molecule. Affected patients have an underlying immunodeficiency that makes them susceptible to opportunistic infections similar to those seen in patients with AIDS (Chap. 173). The pathogenesis of the immunodeficiency is unclear. Pulmonary infiltrates in ATL patients reflect leukemic infiltration half the time and opportunistic infections with organisms such as *Pneumocystis* and other fungi the other half. Gastrointestinal symptoms are nearly always related to opportunistic infection. *Strongyloides stercoralis* is a gastrointestinal parasitic infection that has a pattern of endemic distribution similar to that of HTLV-I. HTLV-I-infected persons also infected with the parasite may develop ATL more often or more rapidly than those without *Strongyloides* infections. Serum concentrations of lactate dehydrogenase (LDH) and alkaline phosphatase are often elevated. About 10% of patients have leptomeningeal involvement leading to weakness, altered mental status, paresthesia, and/or headache. Unlike other forms of central nervous system (CNS) lymphoma, ATL may be accompanied by normal CSF protein levels. The diagnosis depends on finding ATL cells in the CSF (Chap. 97).

The lymphomatous type of ATL occurs in ~20% of patients and is similar to the acute form in its natural history and clinical course, except that circulating abnormal cells are rare and lymphadenopathy is evident. The histology of the lymphoma is variable but does not influence the natural history. In general, the diagnosis is suspected on the basis of the patient's birthplace and the presence of skin lesions and hypercalcemia. The diagnosis is confirmed by the detection of antibodies to HTLV-I in serum.

Patients with the chronic form of ATL generally have normal serum levels of calcium and LDH and no involvement of the CNS, bone, or gastrointestinal tract. The median duration of survival for these patients is 2 years. In some cases, chronic ATL progresses to the acute form of the disease.

Fewer than 5% of patients have the smoldering form of ATL. In this form, the malignant cells have monoclonal proviral integration; <5% of peripheral blood cells exhibit typical morphologic abnormalities; hypercalcemia, adenopathy, and hepatosplenomegaly do not develop; the CNS, the bones, and the gastrointestinal tract are not involved; and skin and pulmonary lesions may be present. The median survival period of this small subset of patients appears to be ≥5 years.

HAM (TROPICAL SPASTIC PARAPARESIS) In contrast to ATL, in which there is a slight predominance of male patients, HAM affects females disproportionately. HAM resembles multiple sclerosis in certain ways (Chap. 359). The onset is insidious. Symptoms include weakness or stiffness in one or both legs, back pain, and urinary incontinence. Sensory changes are usually mild, but peripheral neuropathy may develop. The disease generally takes the form of slowly progressive and unremitting thoracic myelopathy; one-third of patients are bedridden within 10 years of diagnosis, and one-half are unable to walk unassisted by this point. Patients display spastic paraparesis or paraplegia with hyperreflexia, ankle clonus, and extensor plantar responses. Cognitive function is usually spared; cranial nerve abnormalities are unusual.

Magnetic resonance imaging (MRI) reveals lesions in both the white matter and the paraventricular regions of the brain as well as in the spinal cord. Pathologic examination of the spinal cord shows symmetric degeneration of the lateral columns, including the corticospinal tracts; some cases involve the posterior columns as well. The spinal meninges and cord parenchyma contain an inflammatory infiltrate with myelin destruction.

HTLV-I is not usually found in cells of the CNS but may be detected in a small population of lymphocytes present in the CSF. In general, HTLV-I replication is greater in HAM than in ATL, and patients with HAM have a stronger immune response to the virus. Antibodies to HTLV-I are present in the serum and appear to be produced in the CSF of HAM patients, where titers are often higher than in the serum. The pathophysiology of HAM may involve the induction of autoimmune destruction of neural cells by T cells with specificity for viral components such as Tax or Env proteins. One theory is that susceptibility to HAM may be related to the presence of human leukocyte antigen (HLA) alleles capable of presenting viral antigens in a fashion that leads to autoimmunity. Insufficient data are available to confirm an HLA association.

It is unclear what factors influence whether HTLV-I infection will cause disease and, if it does, whether it will induce a neoplasm (ATL) or an autoimmune disorder (HAM). Differences in viral strains, in the susceptibility of particular MHC haplotypes, in the route of HTLV-I infection, in the viral load, and in the nature of the HTLV-I-related immune response are putative factors, but few definitive data are available.

OTHER PUTATIVE HTLV-I-RELATED DISEASES In areas where HTLV-I is endemic, diverse inflammatory and autoimmune diseases have been attributed to the virus, including uveitis, dermatitis, pneumonitis, rheumatoid arthritis, and polymyositis. However, a causal relationship between HTLV-I and these illnesses has not been rigorously established.

Prevention Women in endemic areas should not breast-feed their children, and blood donors should be screened for serum antibodies to HTLV-I. As in the prevention of HIV infection, the practice of safe sex and the avoidance of needle sharing are important.

℞ TREATMENT

For the small number of patients who develop HTLV-I-related disease, therapies are not curative. In patients with the acute and lymphomatous types of ATL, the disease progresses rapidly. Hypercalcemia is generally controlled by glucocorticoid administration and cytotoxic therapy directed against the neoplasm. The tumor is highly responsive to combination chemotherapy that is employed against other forms of lymphoma; however, patients are susceptible to overwhelming bacterial and opportunistic infections, and ATL relapses within 4 to 10 months after remission in most patients. The combination of interferon α and zidovudine may extend survival. Because viral replication is not clearly associated with ATL progression, zidovudine is probably effective through its cytotoxic effects (as a chain-terminating thymidine analogue) rather than its antiviral effects. An experimental approach using an yttrium 90–labeled or toxin-conjugated antibody to the IL-2 receptor appears promising but is not widely available. Patients with the chronic or smoldering form of ATL may be managed with an expectant approach: Treat any infections, and watch and wait for signs of progression to acute disease.

Patients with HAM may obtain some benefit from the use of glucocorticoids to reduce inflammation. Antiretroviral regimens have not been effective. In one study, danazol (200 mg three times daily) produced significant neurologic improvement in five of six treated patients, with resolution of urinary incontinence in two cases, decreased spasticity in three, and restoration of the ability to walk after confinement to a wheelchair in two. Physical therapy and rehabilitation are important components of management.

FEATURES OF HTLV-II INFECTION ■ **Epidemiology** HTLV-II is endemic in certain Native American tribes and in Africa. It is generally considered to be a New World virus that was brought from Asia to the Americas 10,000 to 40,000 years ago during the migration of infected populations across the Bering land bridge.

The mode of transmission of HTLV-II is probably the same as that of HTLV-I (see above). HTLV-II may be less readily transmitted sexually than HTLV-I.

Studies of large cohorts of injection drug users with serologic assays that reliably distinguish HTLV-I from HTLV-II indicate that the vast majority of HTLV-positive subjects are infected with HTLV-II. The seroprevalence of HTLV in a cohort of 7841 injection drug users from drug treatment centers in Baltimore, Chicago, Los Angeles, New Jersey (Asbury Park and Trenton), New York City (Brooklyn and Harlem), Philadelphia, and San Antonio was 20.9%, with >97% of cases due to HTLV-II. The seroprevalence of HTLV-II was higher in the Southwest and the Midwest than in the Northeast. In contrast, the seroprevalence of HIV-1 was higher in the Northeast than in the Southwest or the Midwest. Approximately 3% of the cohort members were infected with both HTLV-II and HIV-1. The seroprevalence of HTLV-II increased linearly with age. Women were significantly more likely to be infected with HTLV-II than were men; the virus is thought to be more efficiently transmitted from male to female than from female to male.

Associated Diseases Although HTLV-II was isolated from a patient with a T cell variant of hairy cell leukemia, this virus has not been consistently associated with a particular disease and in fact has been thought of as "a virus searching for a disease." However, evidence is accumulating that HTLV-II may play a role in certain neurologic, hematologic, and dermatologic diseases. These data require confirmation, particularly in light of the previous confusion regarding the relative prevalences of HTLV-I and HTLV-II among injection drug users.

Prevention Avoidance of needle sharing, safe-sex practices, screening of blood (by assays for HTLV-I, which also detect HTLV-II), and avoidance of breast-feeding by infected women are important principles in the prevention of spread of HTLV-II.

HUMAN IMMUNODEFICIENCY VIRUS

HIV-1 and HIV-2 are members of the lentivirus subfamily of Retroviridae and are the only lentiviruses known to infect humans. The lentiviruses are slow-acting by comparison with viruses that cause acute infection (e.g., influenza virus) but not by comparison with other retroviruses. The features of acute primary infection with HIV resemble those of more classic acute infections. The characteristic chronicity of HIV disease is consistent with the designation lentivirus. →*For a detailed discussion of HIV, see Chap. 173.*

FURTHER READING

BARNAK K et al: Human T cell leukemia virus type I–induced disease: Pathways to cancer and neurodegeneration. Virology 308:1, 2003

GALLO RC: Human retroviruses after 20 years: A perspective from the past and prospects for their future control. Immunol Rev 185:236, 2002

GATZA ML et al: Cellular transformation by the HTLV-I Tax protein, a jack-of-all-trades. Oncogene 22:5141, 2003

JACOBSON S: Immunopathogenesis of human T cell lymphotropic virus type-I–associated neurologic disease. J Infect Dis 186(Suppl 2):S187, 2002

LOWIS GW et al: Epidemiologic features of HTLV-II: Serologic and molecular evidence. Ann Epidemiol 12:46, 2001

POIESZ BJ et al: The human T-cell lymphoma/leukemia viruses. Cancer Invest 21:253, 2003

AIDS was first recognized in the United States in the summer of 1981, when the U.S. Centers for Disease Control and Prevention (CDC) reported the unexplained occurrence of *Pneumocystis carinii* pneumonia in five previously healthy homosexual men in Los Angeles and of Kaposi's sarcoma (KS) in 26 previously healthy homosexual men in New York and Los Angeles. Within months, the disease became recognized in male and female injection drug users (IDUs) and soon thereafter in recipients of blood transfusions and in hemophiliacs. As the epidemiologic pattern of the disease unfolded, it became clear that a microbe transmissible by sexual (homosexual and heterosexual) contact and blood or blood products was the most likely etiologic agent of the epidemic.

In 1983, human immunodeficiency virus (HIV) was isolated from a patient with lymphadenopathy, and by 1984 it was demonstrated clearly to be the causative agent of AIDS. In 1985, a sensitive enzyme-linked immunosorbent assay (ELISA) was developed, which led to an appreciation of the scope and evolution of the HIV epidemic at first in the United States and other developed nations and ultimately among developing nations throughout the world (see below). The staggering worldwide growth of the HIV pandemic has been matched by an explosion of information in the areas of HIV virology, pathogenesis (both immunologic and virologic) and treatment of HIV disease, treatment and prophylaxis of the opportunistic diseases associated with HIV infection, and vaccine development. The information flow related to HIV disease is enormous and continues to expand, and it has become almost impossible for the health care generalist to stay abreast of the literature. The purpose of this chapter is to present the most current information available on the scope of the epidemic; on its pathogenesis, treatment, and prevention; and on prospects for vaccine development. Above all, the aim is to provide a solid scientific basis and practical clinical guidelines for a state-of-the-art approach to the HIV-infected patient.

DEFINITION With the identification of HIV in 1983 and its proof as the etiologic agent of AIDS in 1984, and with the availability of sensitive and specific diagnostic tests for HIV infection, the case definition of AIDS has undergone several revisions over the years. The current CDC classification system for HIV-infected adolescents and adults categorizes persons on the basis of clinical conditions associated with HIV infection and CD4+ T lymphocyte counts. The system is based on three ranges of CD4+ T lymphocyte counts and three clinical categories and is represented by a matrix of nine mutually exclusive categories (Tables 173-1 and 173-2). Using this system, any HIV-infected individual with a CD4+ T cell count of <200/μL has AIDS by definition, regardless of the presence of symptoms or opportunistic diseases (Table 173-1). Once individuals have had a clinical condition in category B, their disease cannot again be classified as category A, even if the condition resolves; the same holds true for category C in relation to category B.

The definition of AIDS is indeed complex and comprehensive; however, the clinician should not focus on whether AIDS is present but should view HIV disease as a spectrum ranging from primary infection, with or without the acute syndrome, to the asymptomatic stage, to advanced disease (see below). The definition of AIDS was established not for the practical care of patients but for surveillance purposes.

TABLE 173-2 *Clinical Categories of HIV Infection*

Category A: Consists of one or more of the conditions listed below in an adolescent or adult (>13 years) with documented HIV infection. Conditions listed in categories B and C must not have occurred.
  Asymptomatic HIV infection
  Persistent generalized lymphadenopathy
  Acute (primary) HIV infection with accompanying illness or history of acute HIV infection
Category B: Consists of symptomatic conditions in an HIV-infected adolescent or adult that are not included among conditions listed in clinical category C and that meet at least one of the following criteria: (1) The conditions are attributed to HIV infection or are indicative of a defect in cell-mediated immunity; or (2) the conditions are considered by physicians to have a clinical course or to require management that is complicated by HIV infection. Examples include, but are not limited to, the following:
  Bacillary angiomatosis
  Candidiasis, oropharyngeal (thrush)
  Candidiasis, vulvovaginal; persistent, frequent, or poorly responsive to therapy
  Cervical dysplasia (moderate or severe)/cervical carcinoma in situ
  Constitutional symptoms, such as fever (38.5°C) or diarrhea lasting >1 month
  Hairy leukoplakia, oral
  Herpes zoster (shingles), involving at least two distinct episodes or more than one dermatome
  Idiopathic thrombocytopenic purpura
  Listeriosis
  Pelvic inflammatory disease, particularly if complicated by tuboovarian abscess
  Peripheral neuropathy
Category C: Conditions listed in the AIDS surveillance case definition.
  Candidiasis of bronchi, trachea, or lungs
  Candidiasis, esophageal
  Cervical cancer, invasive[a]
  Coccidioidomycosis, disseminated or extrapulmonary
  Cryptococcosis, extrapulmonary
  Cryptosporidiosis, chronic intestinal (>1 month's duration)
  Cytomegalovirus disease (other than liver, spleen, or nodes)
  Cytomegalovirus retinitis (with loss of vision)
  Encephalopathy, HIV-related
  Herpes simplex: chronic ulcer(s) (>1 month's duration); or bronchitis, pneumonia, or esophagitis
  Histoplasmosis, disseminated or extrapulmonary
  Isosporiasis, chronic intestinal (>1 month's duration)
  Kaposi's sarcoma
  Lymphoma, Burkitt's (or equivalent term)
  Lymphoma, primary, of brain
  Mycobacterium avium complex or *M. kansasii*, disseminated or extrapulmonary
  Mycobacterium tuberculosis, any site (pulmonary[a] or extrapulmonary)
  Mycobacterium, other species or unidentified species, disseminated or extrapulmonary
  Pneumocystis carinii pneumonia
  Pneumonia, recurrent[a]
  Progressive multifocal leukoencephalopathy
  Salmonella septicemia, recurrent
  Toxoplasmosis of brain
  Wasting syndrome due to HIV

[a] Added in the 1993 expansion of the AIDS surveillance case definition.
Source: MMWR 42(No. RR-17), December 18, 1992.

TABLE 173-1 *1993 Revised Classification System for HIV Infection and Expanded AIDS Surveillance Case Definition for Adolescents and Adults[a]*

CD4+ T Cell Categories	Clinical Categories		
	A Asymptomatic, Acute (Primary) HIV or PGL[b]	B Symptomatic, Not A or C Conditions	C AIDS-Indicator Conditions
>500/μL	A1	B1	C1
200–499/μL	A2	B2	C2
<200/μL	A3	B3	C3

[a] The shaded areas indicate the expanded AIDS surveillance case definition.
[b] PGL, progressive generalized lymphadenopathy.
Source: MMWR 42(No. RR-17), December 18, 1992.

The etiologic agent of AIDS is HIV, which belongs to the family of human retroviruses (Retroviridae) and the subfamily of lentiviruses (Chap. 172). Nononcogenic lentiviruses cause disease in other animal species, including sheep, horses, goats, cattle, cats, and monkeys. The four recognized human retroviruses belong to two distinct groups: the human T lymphotropic viruses (HTLV) I and HTLV-II, which are transforming retroviruses; and the human immunodeficiency viruses, HIV-1 and HIV-2, which are cytopathic viruses (Chap. 172). The most common cause of HIV disease throughout the world, and certainly in the United States, is HIV-1, which comprises several subtypes with different geographic distributions (see below). HIV-2 was first identified in 1986 in West African patients and was originally confined to West Africa. However, a number of cases that can be traced to West Africa or to sexual contacts with West Africans have been identified throughout the world. Both HIV-1 and HIV-2 are zoonotic infections. HIV-2 is more closely related phylogenetically to the simian immunodeficiency virus (SIV) found in sooty mangabeys than it is to HIV-1. HIV-1 likely originated from the *Pan troglodytes troglodytes* species of chimpanzees in whom the virus had co-evolved over centuries. The taxonomic relationship among primate lentiviruses is shown in Fig. 173-1.

MORPHOLOGY OF HIV Electron microscopy shows that the HIV virion is an icosahedral structure (Fig. 173-2A) containing numerous external spikes formed by the two major envelope proteins, the external gp120 and the transmembrane gp41. The virion buds from the surface of the infected cell and incorporates a variety of host proteins, including major histocompatibility complex (MHC) class I and II antigens (Chap. 296), into its lipid bilayer. The structure of HIV-1 is schematically diagrammed in Fig. 173-2B (Chap. 172).

REPLICATION CYCLE OF HIV HIV is an RNA virus whose hallmark is the reverse transcription of its genomic RNA to DNA by the enzyme *reverse transcriptase*. The replication cycle of HIV begins with the high-affinity binding of the gp120 protein via a portion of its V1 region near the N terminus to its receptor on the host cell surface, the CD4 molecule (Fig. 173-3). The CD4 molecule is a 55-kDa protein found predominantly on a subset of T lymphocytes that are responsible for helper or inducer function in the immune sys tem (Chap. 295). It is also expressed on the surface of monocytes/macrophages and dendritic/Langerhans cells. Once gp120 binds to CD4, the gp120 undergoes a conformational change that facilitates binding to one of a group of co-receptors. The two major co-receptors for HIV-1 are CCR5 and CXCR4. Both receptors belong to the family of seven-transmembrane-domain G protein–coupled cellular receptors, and the use of one or the other or both receptors by the virus for entry into the cell is an important determinant of the cellular tropism of the virus (see below for details). Certain dendritic cells express a diversity of C-type lectin receptors on their surface, one of which is called *DC-SIGN*, that bind with high affinity to the HIV gp120 envelope protein, allowing the dendritic cell to facilitate the binding of virus to the CD4+ T cell upon engagement of dendritic cells with CD4+ T cells. Following binding of the envelope protein to the CD4 molecule, the conformation of the viral envelope changes dramatically, and fusion with the host cell membrane occurs via the newly exposed gp41 molecule penetrating the plasma membrane of the target cell and then coiling upon itself to bring the virion and target cell together. Following fusion (Fig. 173-4), the HIV ge-

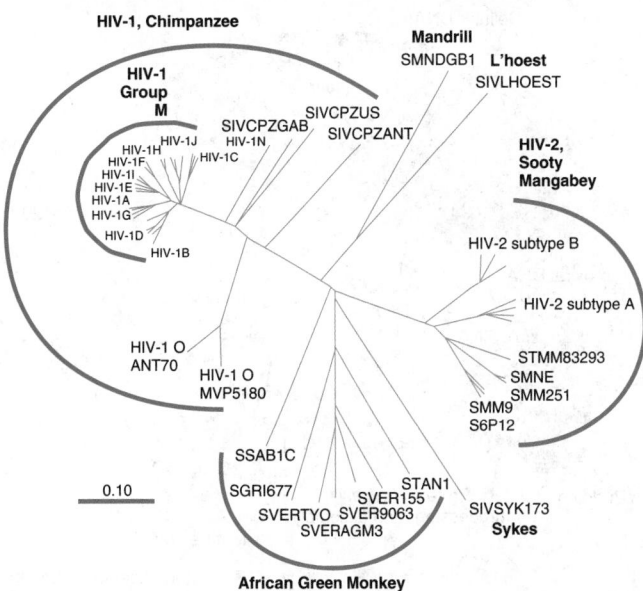

FIGURE 173-1 A phylogenetic tree, based on the complete genomes of primate immunodeficiency viruses. The scale at the bottom (0.10) indicates a 10% difference at the nucleotide level. (*Prepared by Brian Foley, PhD, of the HIV Sequence Database, Theoretical Biology and Biophysics Group, Los Alamos National Laboratory.*)

nomic RNA is uncoated and internalized into the target cell (Fig. 173-3). The reverse transcriptase enzyme, which is contained in the infecting virion, then catalyzes the reverse transcription of the genomic RNA into double-strand DNA. The DNA translocates to the nucleus, where it is integrated in a somewhat, but not completely, random fashion into the host cell chromosomes through the action of another virally encoded enzyme, *integrase*. Sites of HIV integration into the nuclear DNA are preferential for active genes and regional hotspots. This provirus may remain transcriptionally inactive (latent) or it may manifest varying levels of gene expression, up to active production of virus.

Cellular activation plays an important role in the life cycle of HIV and is critical to the pathogenesis of HIV disease (see below). Following initial binding and internalization of virions into the target cell, incompletely reverse-transcribed DNA intermediates are labile in quiescent cells and will not integrate efficiently into the host cell genome

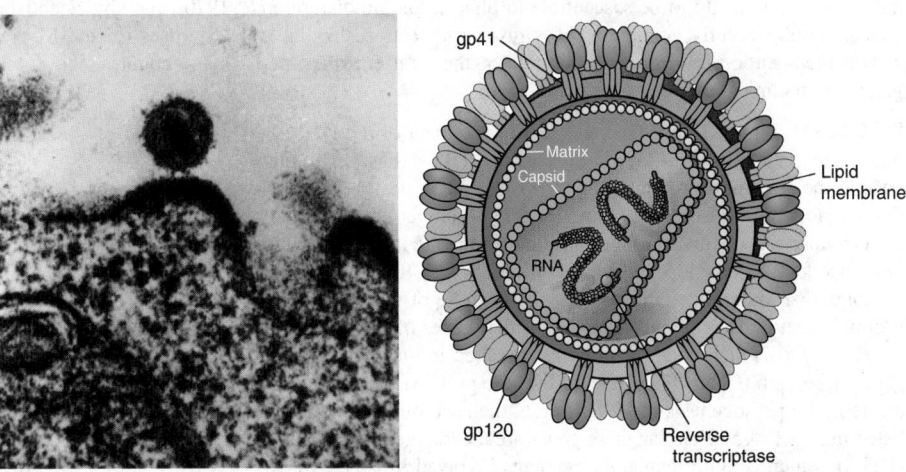

FIGURE 173-2 A. Electron micrograph of HIV. Figure illustrates a typical virion following budding from the surface of a CD4+ T lymphocyte, together with two additional incomplete virions in the process of budding from the cell membrane. B. Structure of HIV-1, including the gp120 outer membrane, gp41 transmembrane components of the envelope, genomic RNA, enzyme reverse transcriptase, p18(17) inner membrane (matrix), and p24 core protein (capsid) (copyright by George V. Kelvin). (*Adapted from RC Gallo: Sci Am 256:46, 1987.*)

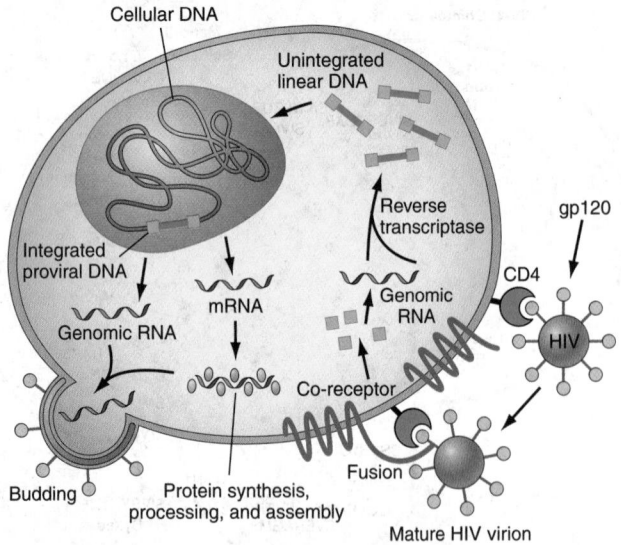

FIGURE 173-3   The replication cycle of HIV. See text for description. (*Adapted from Fauci, 1996.*)

unless cellular activation occurs shortly after infection. Furthermore, some degree of activation of the host cell is required for the initiation of transcription of the integrated proviral DNA into either genomic RNA or mRNA. This latter process may not necessarily be associated with the obvious expression of the classic cell surface markers of activation. In this regard, activation of HIV expression from the latent state depends on the interaction of a number of cellular and viral factors. Following transcription, HIV mRNA is translated into proteins that undergo modification through glycosylation, myristylation, phosphorylation, and cleavage. The viral particle is formed by the assembly of HIV proteins, enzymes, and genomic RNA at the plasma membrane of the cells. Budding of the progeny virion occurs through specialized regions in the lipid bilayer of the host cell membrane known as *lipid rafts*, where the core acquires its external envelope (Chap. 172). The virally encoded protease then catalyzes the cleavage of the gag-pol precursor (see below) to yield the mature virion. Progression through the virus replication cycle is profoundly influenced by a variety of viral regulatory gene products. Likewise, each point in the replication cycle of HIV is a real or potential target for therapeutic intervention (see below). Thus far, the reverse transcriptase and protease enzymes have proven clinically to be susceptible to pharmacologic disruption (see below). Recently, inhibitors of virus–target cell fusion have shown therapeutic promise, and inhibitors of the viral enzyme integrase are in clinical trials.

HIV GENOME   Figure 173-5 illustrates the arrangement of the HIV genome schematically. Like other retroviruses, HIV-1 has genes that encode the structural proteins of the virus: *gag* encodes the proteins that form the core of the virion (including p24 antigen); *pol* encodes the enzymes responsible for reverse transcription and integration; and *env* encodes the envelope glycoproteins. However, HIV-1 is more complex than other retroviruses, particularly those of the nonprimate group, in that it also contains at least six other genes (*tat, rev, nef, vif, vpr,* and *vpu*), which code for proteins involved in the regulation of gene expression (Chap. 172). Several of these proteins are felt to play a role in the pathogenesis of HIV disease; their various functions are listed in Fig. 173-5. Flanking these genes are the long terminal repeats (LTRs), which contain regulatory elements involved in gene expression (Fig. 173-5). The major difference between the genomes of HIV-1 and HIV-2 is the fact that HIV-2 lacks the *vpu* gene and has a *vpx* gene not contained in HIV-1.

MOLECULAR HETEROGENEITY OF HIV-1   Molecular analyses of various HIV isolates reveal sequence variations over many parts of the viral ge-

nome. For example, in different isolates, the degree of difference in the coding sequences of the viral envelope protein ranges from a few percent (very close) to 50%. These changes tend to cluster in hypervariable regions. HIV can evolve by several means, including simple base substitution, insertions and deletions, recombination, and gain and loss of glycosylation sites. The balance of immune pressure and functional constraints on proteins influences the regional level of variation within proteins. For example, Envelope, which is exposed on the surface of the virion and is under immune selective pressure from both antibodies and cytolytic T lymphocytes, is extremely variable, with clusters of mutations in hypervariable domains. In contrast, Reverse Transcriptase, with important enzymatic functions, is relatively conserved, particularly around the active site. The extraordinary variability of HIV-1 is in marked contrast to the relative stability of HTLV-I and -II.

There are three groups of HIV-1: group M (major), which is responsible for most of the infections in the world; group O (outlier), a relatively rare viral form found originally in Cameroon, Gabon, and France; and group N first identified in a Cameroonian woman with AIDS; only a few cases of the latter have been identified. Among primate lentiviruses, HIV-1 is most closely related to viruses isolated from chimpanzees. The M group comprises nine subtypes, or *clades*, designated A, B, C, D, F, G, H, J, and K, as well as a growing number of major circulating recombinant forms (CRFs). These CRFs range from highly prevalent forms such as the AE virus, CRF 01, which is predominant in southeast Asia and often referred to simply as E, despite the fact that the parental E virus has never been found, and AG from west and central Africa, to a large number of CRFs that are more or less rare. The subtypes and CRFs create the major lineages of the M group of HIV-1. The picture has been complicated somewhat when it was found that some subtypes are not equidistant from one another, while others contained sequences so diverse that they could not properly be considered to be the same subtype. Thus, the sub-subtype was introduced, and subtypes A and F are now subdivided into A1 and A2, F1 and F2. It has also been argued that subtypes B and D are really too close to be separate subtypes and should be considered sub-subtypes; it was decided, however, not to increase the confusion by renaming the clades (Fig. 173-6).

The global patterns of HIV-1 variation likely result from accidents of viral trafficking. Subtype B viruses, which now differ by up to 17% in their *env* coding sequences, are the overwhelmingly predominant viruses seen in the United States, Canada, certain countries in South America, western Europe, and Australia. Other subtypes are also present in these countries to varying degrees. It is thought that, purely by chance, subtype B was seeded into the United States in the late 1970s, thereby establishing an overwhelming founder effect. Subtype C viruses (of the M group) are the most common form worldwide; many countries have cocirculating viral subtypes that are giving rise

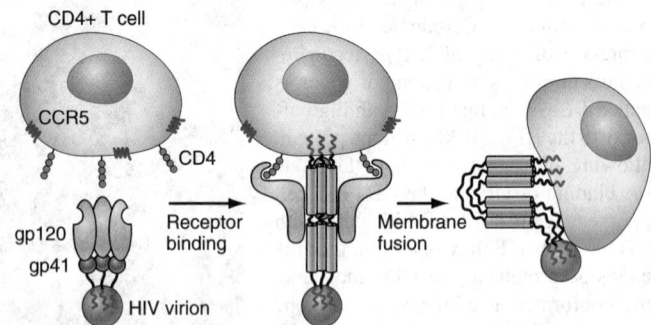

FIGURE 173-4   Binding and fusion of HIV-1 with its target cell. HIV-1 binds to its target cell via the CD4 molecule, leading to a conformational change in the gp120 molecule that allows it to bind to the co-receptor CCR5 (for R5-using viruses). The virus then firmly attaches to the host cell membrane in a coiled-spring fashion via the newly exposed gp41 molecule. Virus-cell fusion occurs as the transitional intermediate of gp41 undergoes further changes to form a hairpin structure that draws the two membranes into close proximity (see text for details). (*Adapted from D Montefiori, JP Moore: Science 283:336, 1999; with permission.*)

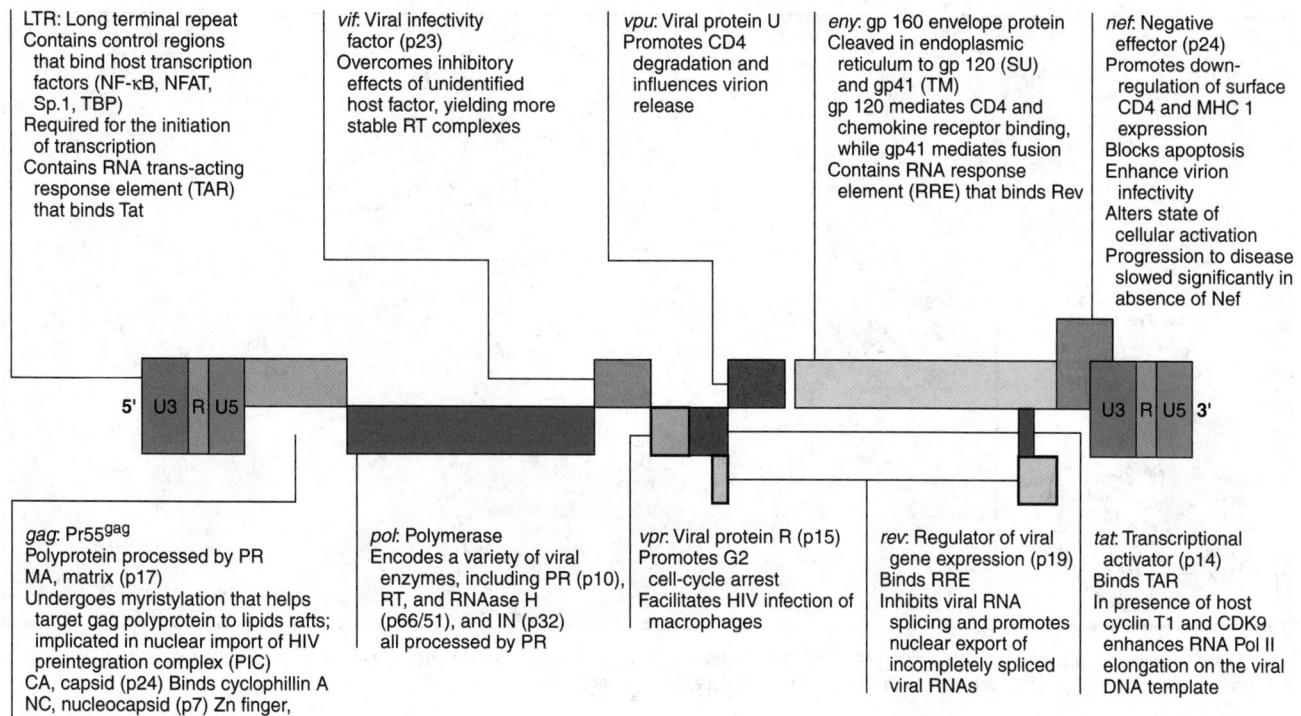

LTR: Long terminal repeat
Contains control regions
 that bind host transcription
 factors (NF-κB, NFAT,
 Sp.1, TBP)
Required for the initiation
 of transcription
Contains RNA trans-acting
 response element (TAR)
 that binds Tat

vif: Viral infectivity
 factor (p23)
Overcomes inhibitory
 effects of unidentified
 host factor, yielding more
 stable RT complexes

vpu: Viral protein U
Promotes CD4
 degradation and
 influences virion
 release

eny: gp 160 envelope protein
Cleaved in endoplasmic
 reticulum to gp 120 (SU)
 and gp41 (TM)
gp 120 mediates CD4 and
 chemokine receptor binding,
 while gp41 mediates fusion
Contains RNA response
 element (RRE) that binds Rev

nef: Negative
 effector (p24)
Promotes down-
 regulation of surface
 CD4 and MHC 1
 expression
Blocks apoptosis
Enhance virion
 infectivity
Alters state of
 cellular activation
Progression to disease
 slowed significantly in
 absence of Nef

gag: Pr55^{gag}
Polyprotein processed by PR
MA, matrix (p17)
Undergoes myristylation that helps
 target gag polyprotein to lipids rafts;
 implicated in nuclear import of HIV
 preintegration complex (PIC)
CA, capsid (p24) Binds cyclophillin A
NC, nucleocapsid (p7) Zn finger,
 RNA-binding protein
p6
Interacts with Vpr; contain slate domain
 (PTAP) that binds TSG101 and
 participates in terminal stops of virion
 budding

pol: Polymerase
Encodes a variety of viral
 enzymes, including PR (p10),
 RT, and RNAase H
 (p66/51), and IN (p32)
 all processed by PR

vpr: Viral protein R (p15)
Promotes G2
 cell-cycle arrest
Facilitates HIV infection of
 macrophages

rev: Regulator of viral
 gene expression (p19)
Binds RRE
Inhibits viral RNA
 splicing and promotes
 nuclear export of
 incompletely spliced
 viral RNAs

tat: Transcriptional
 activator (p14)
Binds TAR
In presence of host
 cyclin T1 and CDK9
 enhances RNA Pol II
 elongation on the viral
 DNA template

FIGURE 173-5 *Organization of the genome of the HIV provirus together with a summary description of its nine genes encoding 15 proteins.* (*From Greene and Peterlin.*)

to CRFs. Figure 173-7 schematically diagrams the worldwide distribution of HIV-1 subtypes by region. The predominant subtype in Europe and the Americas is subtype B. In Africa, >75% of strains recovered to date have been of subtypes A, C, and D, with C being the most common. In Asia, HIV-1 isolates of the CRF01 (AE) lineage and subtypes C and B predominate. CRF01 (AE) accounts for most infections in southeast Asia, while subtype C is prevalent in India (see "HIV Infection and AIDS Worldwide," below). Sequence analyses of HIV-1 isolates from infected individuals indicate that recombination among viruses of different clades likely occurs as a result of infection of an individual with viruses of more than one subtype, particularly in geographic areas where subtypes overlap.

TRANSMISSION

HIV is transmitted by both homosexual and heterosexual contact; by blood and blood products; and by infected mothers to infants either intrapartum, perinatally, or via breast milk. After >20 years of scrutiny, there is no evidence that HIV is transmitted by casual contact or that the virus can be spread by insects, such as by a mosquito bite.

SEXUAL TRANSMISSION HIV infection is predominantly a sexually transmitted disease (STD) worldwide. Although in the United States ~42% of new HIV infections are among men who have sex with men and ~33% of new HIV infections are by heterosexual transmission, the most common mode of infection worldwide, particularly in developing countries, is clearly heterosexual transmission. Furthermore, the yearly incidence of new cases of AIDS attributed to heterosexual transmission of HIV is steadily increasing in the United States, mainly among minorities, particularly women in minority groups (Fig. 173-8).

HIV has been demonstrated in seminal fluid both within infected mononuclear cells and in the cell-free state. The virus appears to concentrate in the seminal fluid, particularly in situations where there are increased numbers of lymphocytes and monocytes in the fluid, as in genital inflammatory states such as urethritis and epididymitis, con-

ditions closely associated with other STDs (see below). The virus has also been demonstrated in cervical smears and vaginal fluid. There is a strong association of transmission of HIV with receptive anal intercourse, probably because only a thin, fragile rectal mucosal membrane separates the deposited semen from potentially susceptible cells in and beneath the mucosa and trauma may be associated with anal intercourse. Anal douching and sexual practices that traumatize the rectal mucosa also increase the likelihood of infection. It is likely that anal intercourse provides at least two modalities of infection: (1) direct inoculation into blood in cases of traumatic tears in the mucosa; and (2) infection of susceptible target cells, such as Langerhans cells, in the mucosal layer in the absence of trauma (see below). Although the vaginal mucosa is several layers thicker than the rectal mucosa and less likely to be traumatized during intercourse, it is clear that the virus can be transmitted to either partner through vaginal intercourse. In a 10-year prospective study in the United States of heterosexual transmission of HIV, male-to-female transmission was approximately eight times more efficient than female-to-male transmission. This difference may be due in part to the prolonged exposure to infected seminal fluid of the vaginal and cervical mucosa, as well as the endometrium (when

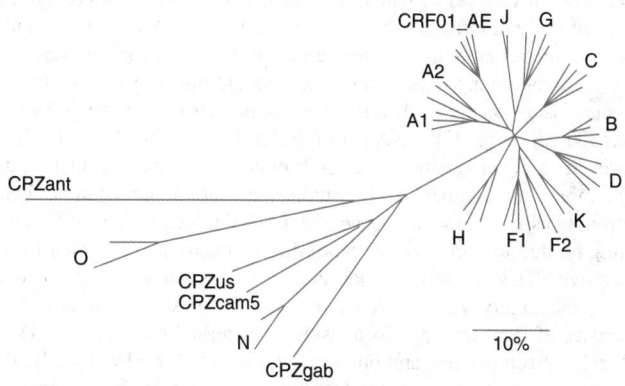

FIGURE 173-6 *Phylogenetic tree constructed from representative viral envelope sequences of the subtypes and circulating recombinant forms (CRFs) in group M and some isolates from groups N and O (human) and CPZ (chimpanzee). The scale bar at the bottom indicates the genetic distances between the sequences. A1 and A2, F1 and F2 are subtypes; CRF01_AE is unique in the envelope gene, but similar to subtype A in the rest of the genome.* (*Courtesy of Bette Korber, PhD, and Carla Kuiken, PhD, HIV Database, Los Alamos National Laboratory*).

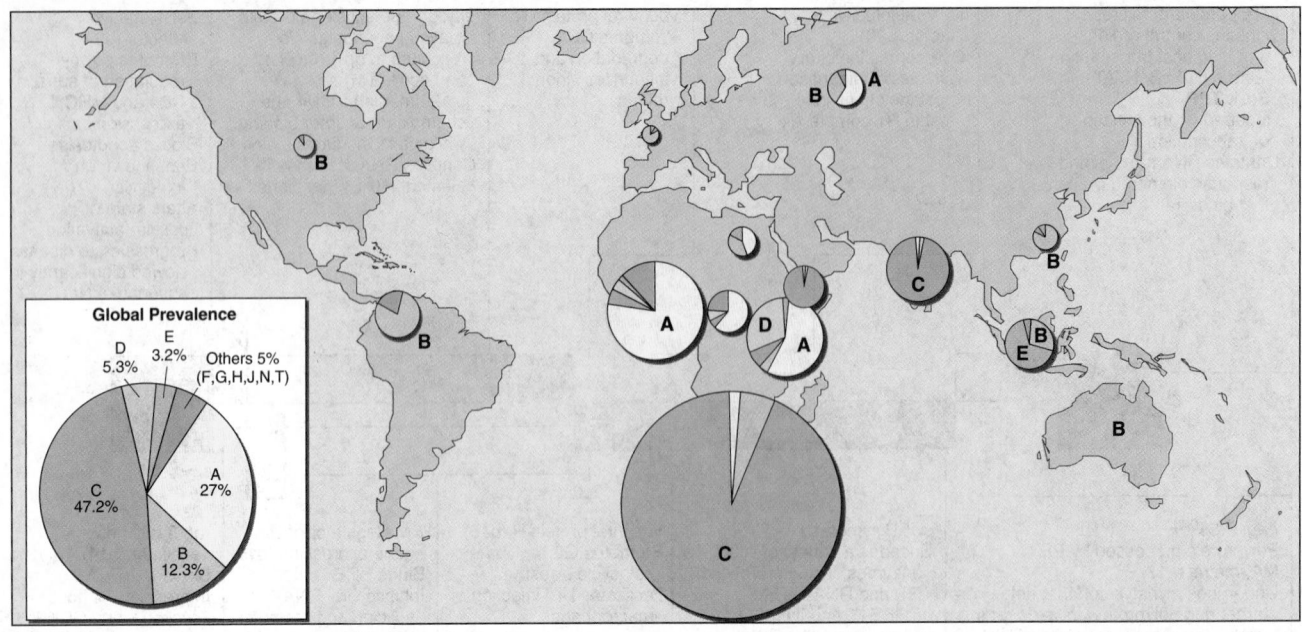

FIGURE 173-7 Geographic distribution of HIV-1 subtypes, 2001. The prevalence of HIV-1 genetic subtypes varies by geographic region. The proportions of subtypes in different regions are indicated by pie charts. (*From S Osmanov et al: J Acquir Imm Def Syndr 29:184, 2002.*)

semen enters through the cervical os). By comparison, the penis and urethral orifice are exposed relatively briefly to infected vaginal fluid. Among various cofactors examined in this study, a history of STDs (see below) was most strongly associated with HIV transmission. In this regard, there is a close association between genital ulcerations and transmission, from the standpoints of both susceptibility to infection and infectivity. Infections with microorganisms such as *Treponema pallidum* (Chap. 153), *Haemophilus ducreyi* (Chap. 130), and herpes simplex virus (HSV; Chap. 163) are important causes of genital ulcerations linked to transmission of HIV. In addition, pathogens responsible for nonulcerative inflammatory STDs such as those caused by *Chlamydia trachomatis* (Chap. 160), *Neisseria gonorrhoeae* (Chap. 128), and *Trichomonas vaginalis* (Chap. 199) are also associated with an increased risk of transmission of HIV infection. Bacterial vaginosis, an infection related to sexual behavior, but not strictly an STD, may also be linked to an increased risk of transmission of HIV infection. Several studies suggest that treating other STDs and genital tract syndromes may help prevent transmission of HIV. This effect is most prominent in populations in which the prevelance of HIV infection is relatively low. In studies conducted in Uganda, the chief predictor of heterosexual transmission of HIV was the level of plasma viremia. In a cohort of couples in which one partner was HIV-infected and one was initially uninfected, the mean serum HIV RNA level was significantly higher among HIV-infected subjects whose partners seroconverted than among those whose partners did not seroconvert. In fact transmission was rare when the infected partner had a plasma level of <1500 copies of HIV RNA per milliliter. Of note, in that study, there were no seroconversions among 50 circumcised male partners. Furthermore, in a number of other studies, lack of circumcision has been strongly associated with a higher risk of HIV infection. This difference may be due to increased susceptibility of uncircumcised men to ulcerative STDs, as well as other factors such as microtrauma. In addition, the highly vascularized inner foreskin tissue contains a high density of Langerhans cells as well as increased numbers of CD4+ T cells, macrophages, and other cellular targets for HIV. Finally, the moist environment under the foreskin may promote the presence or persistence of microbial flora which, via inflammatory changes, may lead to even higher concentrations of target cells for HIV in the foreskin. In some studies the use of oral contraceptives was associated with an increase in incidence of HIV infection over and above that which might be expected by not using a condom for birth control.

Oral sex is a much less efficient mode of transmission of HIV than is receptive anal intercourse. A number of studies have reported that the incidence of transmission of infection by oral sex among couples discordant for HIV was extremely low; indeed, one study reported no cases among 239 men whose only risk was receptive oral intercourse where 28% knew that their partner was HIV-infected. However, there have been several reports of documented HIV transmission resulting solely from receptive fellatio and insertive cunnilingus. There are probably many more cases that go unreported because of the frequent practice of both oral sex and receptive anal intercourse by the same person. Therefore, the assumption that receptive oral sex is com-

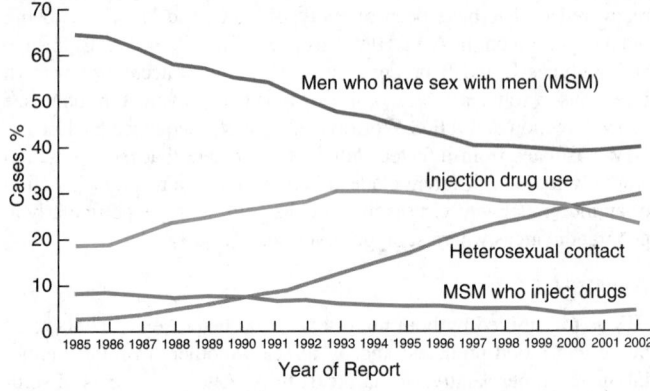

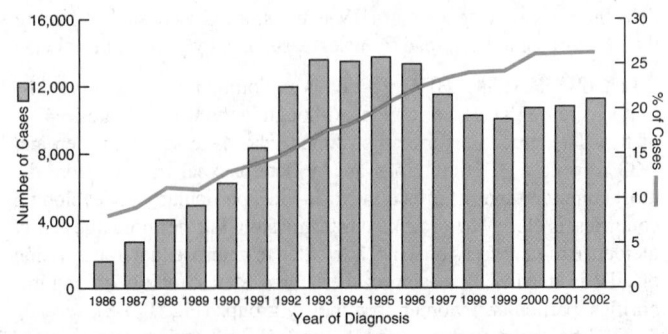

FIGURE 173-8 The changing face of the HIV/AIDS epidemic in the United States *Upper*. Proportion of AIDS cases among U.S. adults and adolescents, by exposure category and year of diagnosis. *Lower*. The proportion of AIDS cases among women and adolescent girls (aged >13 years) increased from 8% in 1986 to 26% in 2002. (*From the Centers for Disease Control and Prevention, 2003.*)

pletely safe is not warranted. The association of alcohol consumption and illicit drug use with unsafe sexual behavior, both homosexual and heterosexual, leads to an increased risk of sexual transmission of HIV.

TRANSMISSION BY BLOOD AND BLOOD PRODUCTS   HIV can be transmitted to individuals who receive HIV-tainted blood transfusions, blood products, or transplanted tissue as well as to IDUs who are exposed to HIV while sharing injection paraphernalia such as needles, syringes, the water in which drugs are mixed, or the cotton through which drugs are filtered. Parenteral transmission of HIV during injection drug use does not require intravenous puncture; subcutaneous ("skin popping") or intramuscular ("muscling") injections can transmit HIV as well, even though these behaviors are sometimes erroneously perceived as low-risk. Among IDUs, the risk of HIV infection increases with the duration of injection drug use; the frequency of needle sharing; the number of partners with whom paraphernalia are shared, particularly in the setting of "shooting galleries" where drugs are sold and large numbers of IDUs may share a limited number of "works"; comorbid psychiatric conditions such as antisocial personality disorder; the use of cocaine in injectable form or smoked as "crack"; and the use of injection drugs in a geographic location with a high prevalence of HIV infection, such as certain inner-city areas in the United States.

From the late 1970s until the spring of 1985, when mandatory testing of donated blood for HIV-1 was initiated, it has been estimated that >10,000 individuals in the United States were infected through transfusions of blood or blood products (Chap. 99). Approximately 9300 individuals in the United States who survived the illness for which they received HIV-contaminated blood transfusions, blood components, or transplanted tissue have developed AIDS. It is estimated that 90 to 100% of individuals who were exposed to such HIV-contaminated products became infected. Transfusions of whole blood, packed red blood cells, platelets, leukocytes, and plasma are all capable of transmitting HIV infection. In contrast, hyperimmune γ globulin, hepatitis B immune globulin, plasma-derived hepatitis B vaccine, and Rh_o immune globulin have not been associated with transmission of HIV infection. The procedures involved in processing these products either inactivate or remove the virus.

In addition to the above, several thousand individuals in the United States with hemophilia or other clotting disorders were infected with HIV by receipt of HIV-contaminated fresh-frozen plasma or concentrates of clotting factors; ~5470 of these individuals have developed AIDS. Currently, in the United States and in most developed countries, the following measures have made the risk of transmission of HIV infection by transfused blood or blood products extremely small: (1) the screening of all blood for HIV nucleic acid, p24 antigen, and/or anti-HIV antibodies; (2) the self-deferral of donors on the basis of risk behavior; (3) the screening out of HIV-negative individuals with positive surrogate laboratory parameters of HIV infection, such as hepatitis B and C; and (4) serologic testing for syphilis. It is currently estimated that the risk of infection with HIV in the United States via transfused screened blood is approximately 1 in 725,000 to 1 in 835,000 donations. Therefore, among the 12 million donations collected in the United States each year, an estimated 16 infectious donations are available for transfusion. Thus, despite the best efforts of science, one cannot completely eliminate the risk of tranfusion-related transmission of HIV since current technology cannot detect HIV RNA for the first 1 to 2 weeks following infection due to the low levels of viremia. In this regard, two individuals in Florida recently contracted HIV from a single donor who had recently become infected; the blood collection system in question had used nucleic acid amplification testing to screen the blood. There have been several reports of sporadic breakdowns in routinely available screening procedures in certain countries, where contaminated blood was allowed to be transfused, resulting in small clusters of patients becoming infected. In China, a disturbingly large number of people have become infected by selling blood in situations where the collectors reused needles that were con-

taminated and in some instances mixed blood products from a number of people, separated the plasma, and re-infused red blood cells back into individual donors. It is estimated that >6% of China's HIV-infected population were infected while selling blood. There have been no reported cases of transmission of HIV-2 in the United States via donated blood, and, currently, donated blood is screened for both HIV-1 and HIV-2 antibodies. The chance of infection of a hemophiliac via clotting factor concentrates has essentially been eliminated because of the added layer of safety resulting from heat treatment of the concentrates.

Prior to the screening of donors, a small number of cases of transmission of HIV via semen used in artificial insemination and tissues used in organ transplantation were well documented. At present, donors of such tissues are prescreened for HIV infection.

OCCUPATIONAL TRANSMISSION OF HIV: HEALTH CARE WORKERS AND LABORATORY WORKERS   There is a small, but definite, occupational risk of HIV transmission to health care workers and laboratory personnel and potentially others who work with HIV-containing materials, particularly when sharp objects are used. An estimated 600,000 to 800,000 health care workers are stuck with needles or other sharp medical instruments in the United States each year. Large, multi-institutional studies have indicated that the risk of HIV transmission following skin puncture from a needle or a sharp object that was contaminated with blood from a person with documented HIV infection is ~0.3% and after a mucous membrane exposure it is 0.09% (see "HIV and the Health Care Worker," p. 1136). HIV transmission after non-intact skin exposure has been documented, but the average risk for transmission by this route has not been precisely determined; however, it is estimated to be less than the risk for mucous membrane exposure. Transmission of HIV through intact skin has not been documented. An increased risk for HIV infection following percutaneous exposures to HIV-infected blood is associated with exposures involving a relatively large quantity of blood, as in the case of a device visibly contaminated with the patient's blood, a procedure that involves a needle placed directly in a vein or artery, or a deep injury. Factors that might be associated with mucocutaneous transmission of HIV include exposure to an unusually large volume of blood, prolonged contact, and a potential portal of entry. In addition, the risk increases for exposures to blood from patients with advanced-stage disease, probably owing to the higher titer of HIV in the blood as well as to other factors, such as the presence of more virulent strains of virus. The use of antiretroviral drugs as postexposure prophylaxis decreases the risk of infection compared to historic controls in occupationally exposed health care workers (see "HIV and the Health Care Worker"). The risk of hepatitis B virus (HBV) infection following a similar type of exposure is 6 to 30% in nonimmune individuals; if a susceptible worker is exposed to HBV, postexposure prophylaxis with hepatitis B immune globulin and initiation of HBV vaccine is >90% effective in preventing HBV infection. The risk of hepatitis C virus (HCV) infection following percutaneous injury is ~1.8% (Chap. 285).

Since the beginning of the HIV epidemic, there have been at least three reported instances in which transmission of infection from a health care worker to patients seemed highly probable. The first involved a dentist in Florida who apparently infected six of his patients, most likely through contaminated instruments. Another case involved an orthopedic surgeon in France who apparently infected a patient during placement of a total hip prosthesis. A third case involved the apparent transmission of HIV from a nurse to a surgical patient in France. An additional situation involved the apparent infection of four patients by an HIV-negative general surgeon in Australia during routine outpatient surgery. The cause of the transmission was felt to be a failure on the part of the surgeon to sterilize instruments properly between procedures following prior surgery on an infected patient. Despite these few cases, the risk of transmission from an infected health care worker to patients is extremely low; in fact, too low to be measured accurately. Indeed several epidemiologic studies have been performed tracing thousands of patients of HIV-infected dentists, physicians, surgeons, obstetricians, and gynecologists, and no other cases of HIV infection that could be linked to the health care providers were identified. The very occurrence of transmission of HIV as well as HBV and HCV to and from health care workers in the workplace underscores the importance of the use of universal precautions when caring for all patients (see below and Chap. 116).

MATERNAL-FETAL/INFANT TRANSMISSION   HIV infection can be transmitted from an infected mother to her fetus during pregnancy, during delivery, or by breast-feeding. This is an extremely important form of transmission of HIV infection in developing countries, where the proportion of infected women to infected men is ~1:1. Virologic analysis of aborted fetuses indicate that HIV can be transmitted to the fetus as early as the first and second trimester of pregnancy. However, maternal transmission to the fetus occurs most commonly in the perinatal period. This conclusion is based on a number of considerations, including the time frame of identification of infection by the sequential appearance of classes of antibodies to HIV (i.e., the appearance of HIV-specific IgA antibody within 3 to 6 months after birth); a positive viral culture; the appearance of p24 antigenemia weeks to months after delivery, but not at the time of delivery; a polymerase chain reaction (PCR) assay of infant blood following delivery that is negative at birth and positive several months later; the demonstration that the firstborn twin of an infected mother is more commonly infected than is the second twin; and the evidence that cesarean section results in decreased transmission to the infant. Two studies performed in Rwanda and the former Zaire indicated that the relative proportions of mother-to-child transmissions were 23 to 30% before birth, 50 to 65% during birth, and 12 to 20% via breast-feeding.

In the absence of prophylactic antiretroviral therapy to the mother during pregnancy, labor, and delivery, and to the fetus following birth (see below), the probability of transmission of HIV from mother to infant/fetus ranges from 15 to 25% in industrialized countries and from 25 to 35% in developing countries. These differences may relate to the adequacy of prenatal care as well as to the stage of HIV disease and the general health of the mother during pregnancy. Higher rates of transmission have been reported to be associated with many factors; some of these are well proven by a number of studies, while others are considered to be potential factors since various studies may have given divergent results. The best-documented factor that is associated with higher rates of transmission is the presence of high maternal levels of plasma viremia. Low maternal CD4+ T cell counts have also been associated with higher rates of transmission; however, since low CD4+ T cell counts are often associated with high levels of plasma viremia, in one study using multivariate analysis including plasma viral load and CD4+ T cell count, only the level of plasma HIV RNA was significant. A prolonged interval between membrane rupture and delivery is another well-documented risk factor for transmission. Other conditions that are potential risk factors, but which have not been consistently demonstrated, are the presence of chorioamnionitis at delivery; STDs during pregnancy; hard drug use during pregnancy; cigarette smoking; preterm delivery; and obstetric procedures such as amniocentesis, amnioscopy, fetal scalp electrodes, and episeotomy. Vitamin A deficiency had been reported to be associated with higher transmission rates; however, vitamin A supplementation during pregnancy resulted in improved birth weight and neonatal growth and reduced anemia but did not affect perinatal transmission of HIV. With regard to levels of viremia, several studies indicate that the risk of transmission increases with the maternal plasma HIV RNA level. In one series of 552 singleton pregnancies in the United States, the rate of mother-to-baby transmission was 0% among women with <1000 copies of HIV RNA per milliliter of blood, 16.6% among women with 1000 to 10,000/mL, 21.3% among women with 10,001 to 50,000/mL, 30.9% among women with 50,001 to 100,000/mL, and 40.6% among women with >100,000/mL. However, there may be no lower "threshold" below which transmission never occurs, since other studies have reported transmission by women with viral RNA levels <50 copies per milliliter. Finally, it has been speculated that if the mother experiences acute primary infection during pregnancy, there is a higher rate of transmission to the fetus, owing to the high levels of viremia that occur during primary infection. However, a study from Thailand reported no increased risk of transmission of HIV from mother-to-child in women who seroconverted during pregnancy. In that study, maternal viral loads at delivery were no different among women who seroconverted during pregnancy and those who were seropositive when first tested. In a study conducted in the United States, zidovudine treatment of HIV-infected pregnant women from the beginning of the second trimester through delivery and of the infant for 6 weeks following birth dramatically decreased the rate of intrapartum and perinatal transmission of HIV infection from 22.6% in the untreated group to <5%. The rate of mother-to-child transmission is approaching 1% or less in pregnant women who are receiving combination antiretroviral therapy for their HIV infection. Such treatment, combined with cesarean section delivery, has rendered mother-to-child transmission of HIV an unusual event in the United States and other developed nations. In developed countries, current recommendations to reduce perinatal transmission of HIV include universal voluntary HIV testing and counseling of pregnant women, antiretroviral prophylaxis with one or more drugs in cases in which the mother does not require therapy for her HIV infection, combination therapy for women who do require therapy, obstetric management that attempts to minimize exposure of the infant to maternal blood and genital secretions, and avoidance of breast-feeding. It is recommended that the choice of antiretroviral therapy for pregnant women should be based on the same considerations used for women who are not pregnant, with discussion of the recognized and unknown risks and benefits of such therapy during pregnancy. The cost and logistics of the above protocol are not currently feasible for developing countries, particularly those in sub-Saharan Africa where the per capita health care delivery allocation is often only a few dollars per year. Studies have demonstrated that truncated regimens of zidovudine alone or in combination with lamivudine given to the mother during the last few weeks of pregnancy or even only during labor and delivery, and to the infant for a week or less, reduced transmission to the infant by 50% compared to placebo. One important study in Uganda demonstrated that a single dose of nevirapine given to the mother at the onset of labor followed by a single dose to the newborn within 72 h of birth decreased transmission by 50% compared with a regimen of zidovudine to the mother that began at the onset of labor and continued throughout labor and to the infant for 1 week following birth. The cost of the nevirapine for the mother and infant was $4.00, thus making this regimen more affordable. Indeed, short-course nevirapine regimens increasingly are being utilized in developing nations for the prevention of mother-to-child transmission. It is estimated that the successful implementation of such regimens could potentially save 1000 babies per day from becoming infected with HIV, the vast majority of whom are in sub-Saharan Africa.

Breast-feeding is an important modality of transmission of HIV infection in developing countries, particularly where mothers continue to breast feed for prolonged periods. The risk factors for mother-to-child transmission of HIV via breast-feeding are not fully understood; factors that increase the likelihood of transmission include detectable levels of HIV in breast milk, the presence of mastitis, low maternal CD4+ T cell counts, and maternal vitamin A deficiency. The risk of HIV infection via breast-feeding is highest in the early months of breast-feeding. In addition, exclusive breast-feeding has been reported to carry a lower risk of HIV transmission than mixed feeding. Certainly, in developed countries breast-feeding by an infected mother should be avoided. However, there is disagreement regarding recommendations for breast-feeding in certain developing countries, where breast milk is the only source of adequate nutrition as well as immunity against potentially serious infections for the infant. Studies are being conducted to determine whether intermittent administration of nevirapine, which has a relatively long half-life, to uninfected babies born of infected mothers decreases the incidence of infection via breast-feeding. The optimal approach to prevent transmission by infected mothers who choose to breast-feed would be to provide continual treatment to the infected mother where feasible.

TRANSMISSION BY OTHER BODY FLUIDS Although HIV can be isolated typically in low titers from saliva of a small proportion of infected individuals, there is no convincing evidence that saliva can transmit HIV infection, either through kissing or through other exposures, such as occupationally to health care workers. Saliva contains endogenous antiviral factors; among these factors, HIV-specific immunoglobulins of IgA, IgG, and IgM isotypes are detected readily in salivary secretions of infected individuals. It has been suggested that large glycoproteins such as mucins and thrombospondin-1 sequester HIV into aggregates for clearance by the host. In addition, a number of soluble salivary factors inhibit HIV to various degrees in vitro, probably by targeting host cell receptors rather than the virus itself. Perhaps the best-studied of these, secretory leukocyte protease inhibitor (SLPI), blocks HIV infection in several cell culture systems, and it is found in saliva at levels that approximate those required for inhibition of HIV in vitro. In this regard, higher salivary levels of SLPI in breast-fed infants were associated with a decreased risk of HIV transmission through breast milk. It has also been suggested that submandibular saliva reduces HIV infectivity by stripping gp120 from the surface of virions, and that saliva-mediated disruption and lysis of HIV-infected cells occurs because of the hypotonicity of oral secretions. There have been outlier cases of suspected transmission by saliva, but these have probably been blood-to-blood transmissions. Transmission of HIV by a human bite can occur but is a rare event; at least four cases of such transmission have been reported. In addition, a most unusual form of HIV transmission from infected children to mothers in the former Soviet Union has been identified. In those cases, the children (infected through transfusion) were said to have bleeding sores in the mouth, and the mothers were said to have lacerations and abrasions on and around the nipples of the breast resulting from trauma from the children's teeth. Breast-feeding had been continued until the children were older than is usual in other developed countries.

Although virus can be identified, if not isolated, from virtually any body fluid, there is no evidence that HIV transmission can occur as a result of exposure to tears, sweat, and urine. However, there have been isolated cases of transmission of HIV infection by body fluids that may or may not have been contaminated with blood. Most of these situations occurred in the setting of a close relative providing intensive nursing care for an HIV-infected person without observing universal precautions. These cases underscore the importance of observing universal precautions in the handling of body fluids and wastes from HIV-infected individuals (see below).

EPIDEMIOLOGY

HIV INFECTION AND AIDS WORLDWIDE HIV infection/AIDS is a global pandemic, with cases reported from virtually every country. The current estimate of the number of cases of HIV infection among adults worldwide is ~37 million, two-thirds of whom are in sub-Saharan Africa; 50% of cases are women. In addition, an estimated 2.5 million children younger than age 15 are living with HIV/AIDS. The global distribution of these cases is illustrated in Fig. 173-9. According to the Joint United Nations Programme on HIV/AIDS (UNAIDS), in 2003 alone there were an estimated 5 million new cases of infection worldwide (>14,000 new infections each day) and 3 million deaths from AIDS, making it the fourth leading cause of mortality worldwide. The cumulative number of AIDS-related deaths worldwide through the year 2003 exceeds 20 million. The HIV epidemic has occurred in "waves" in different regions of the world, each wave having somewhat different characteristics depending on the demographics of the country and region in question and the timing of the introduction of HIV into the population. As noted above, different subtypes, or clades, of HIV-1 are prevalent in different regions of the world (see above and Fig. 173-7), increasing the difficulty in the development of vaccines and perhaps accounting for different degrees of virulence. It is unlikely that a single vaccine will be applicable to all regions of the world. In this regard, in addition to HIV-1 subtype B, the predominant subtype in the United States, HIV-1 subtypes A, AE, AG, C, D, and O have been detected in individuals in the United States, as might be expected given the degree of international travel that occurs.

Table 173-3 provides the statistics and demographic features of HIV/AIDS in different regions of the world. Although the epidemic was first recognized in the United States and shortly thereafter in western Europe, it very likely began in sub-Saharan Africa (see above), which has been particularly devastated by the epidemic, with the prevalence of infection in many cities in the double digits. In certain sub-Saharan African countries, such as Zimbabwe and Botswana, available seroprevalence data indicate >30% of the adult population aged 15 to 49 is HIV-infected. In addition, among high-risk individuals (e.g., commercial sex workers, patients attending STD clinics) who live in urban areas of sub-Saharan Africa, seroprevalence is now >50% in many countries. According to projections of the United Nations Pop-

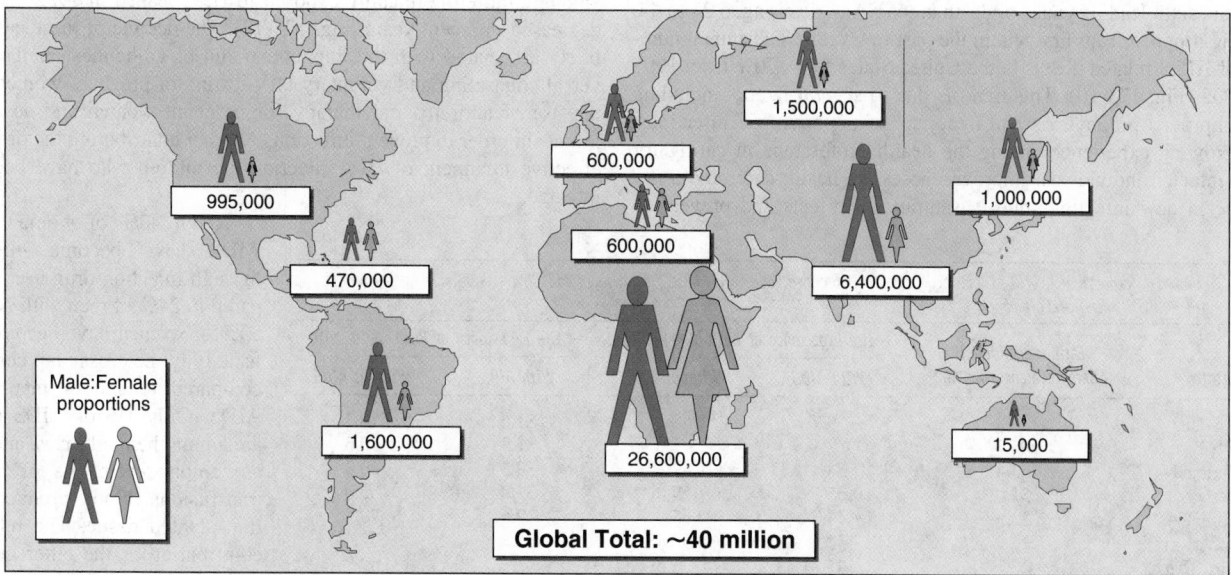

FIGURE 173-9 Estimated number of adults and children living with HIV infection as of December, 2003. (*From Joint United Nations Programme on HIV/AIDS.*)

TABLE 173-3   Regional HIV/AIDS Statistics and Features, December, 2003

Region	Epidemic Started	Adults and Children Living with HIV/AIDS	Adults and Children Newly Infected with HIV in 2003	Adult Prevalence Rate[a]	Adults and Child Deaths due to AIDS in 2003
Sub-Saharan Africa	Late '70s–Early '80s	26.6 million	3.2 million	8.0%	2.3 million
North Africa & Middle East	Late '80s	600,000	55,000	0.3%	42,500
South & Southeast Asia	Late '80s	6.4 million	855,000	0.6%	460,000
East Asia & Pacific	Late '80s	1.0 million	210,000	0.1%	45,000
Latin America	Late '70s–Early '80s	1.6 million	150,000	0.6%	59,500
Caribbean	Late '70s–Early '80s	470,000	62,500	2.5%	40,000
Eastern Europe & Central Asia	Early '90s	1.5 million	230,000	0.7%	30,000
Western Europe	Late '70s–Early '80s	600,000	35,000	0.3%	3,000
North America	Late '70s–Early '80s	995,000	45,000	0.6%	15,000
Australia & New Zealand	Late '70s–Early '80s	15,000	850	0.1%	<100
Total		**40 million**	**5 million**	**1.1%**	**3 million**

[a] The estimated proportion of adults (15–49 years) living with HIV/AIDS in December 2003.

Source: Joint United Nations Programme on HIV/AIDS (UNAIDS).

ulation Division, by the year 2015 life expectancy at birth in the seven countries in Africa with adult HIV prevalence rates >20% will be 32 years lower on average than the projected life expectancy in the absence of AIDS (Table 173-4). The epidemic in Asian countries, particularly India and China, has lagged temporally behind that in Africa; however, the number of new cases in this region is accelerating rapidly, and the magnitude of the epidemic is projected to exceed that of sub-Saharan Africa in the early part of the twenty-first century. The epidemic is also expanding rapidly in the Baltic States, the Russian Federation, and several Central Asian Republics. The major mode of transmission of HIV worldwide is unquestionably heterosexual sex; this is particularly true and has been so since the beginning of the epidemic in developing countries, where the numbers of infected men and women are approximately equal. The epidemic in most developed countries was first introduced among homosexual men and, to a greater or lesser degree (depending on the individual country), among IDUs. In this regard, the total numbers of AIDS cases in those countries still reflect a high proportion of cases among these high-risk groups. However, in most developed countries, including the United States (see below), there has been a gradual shift such that among new cases of AIDS, there is a greater total prevalence among heterosexuals and IDUs than among homosexual men.

AIDS IN THE UNITED STATES   AIDS has had and will continue to have an extraordinary public health impact in the United States. As of January 1, 2003, an estimated 886,575 cumulative cases of AIDS had been diagnosed in adults and adolescents in the United States (Table 173-5) and ~502,000 AIDS-related deaths had occurred. In 2002, AIDS was the sixth leading cause of death among Americans aged 25 to 44, having dropped from first within the past few years. The annual number of AIDS-related deaths in the United States fell ~70% from 1995 to 2002 (Fig. 173-10). This trend is due to several factors including the improved prophylaxis and treatment of opportunistic infections, the growing experience among the health professions in caring for HIV-infected individuals, improved access to health care, and a decrease in new infections due to saturational effects and prevention efforts. However, the most influential factor clearly has been the increased use of potent antiretroviral drugs, generally administered in a combination of three or four agents (see below). When one looks at the totality of data collected from the beginning of the epidemic, ~47% of all cases are among men who have had sex with men. However, since the mid-1980s the proportion of newly reported cases of AIDS in this population has declined from 65% of cases diagnosed in 1985 to 40% of cases diagnosed in 2002. Meanwhile, the proportion of new AIDS cases attributed to heterosexual contact has increased dramatically, from 3% in 1985 to 29% in 2002 (Fig. 173-8). Women are increasingly affected; the proportion of AIDS cases in the United States reported among adult and adolescent females has increased from <5% to 26% from 1985 to 2002 (Fig. 173-8). Most cases of transmission by injection drug use and heterosexual contact are reported from the northeast and southeast regions of the country, particularly among minorities. HIV infection and AIDS have disproportionately affected minority populations in the United States. The estimated rates of AIDS diagnoses per 100,000 population among adults and adolescents in 2002 were 76.4 for African Americans, 26.0 for Hispanics, 7.0 for whites, 11.2 for American Indians/Alaska Natives, and 4.9 for Asian/Pacific Islanders (Fig. 173-11).

As of January 1, 2003, an estimated 9,300 cases of AIDS in children ≤13 years old had been diagnosed, and ~55% of these children have died. Approximately 90% of these children were born to mothers who were HIV-infected or who were at risk for HIV infection and, in ~60% of those cases, the mother was either an IDU or the heterosexual partner of an IDU. The estimated number of AIDS cases diagnosed among children perinatally exposed to HIV peaked in 1992 and has decreased in recent years (Fig. 173-12). The decline of these cases is likely associated with the implementation of guidelines for the universal counseling and voluntary HIV testing of pregnant women and the use of antiretroviral therapy for pregnant women and newborn infants in order to prevent infection. Another contributing factor is the effective treatment of HIV infection in children who have become infected.

About 43% of women with AIDS have become infected through injection drug use, compared to 24% of men with AIDS; 53% of women have become infected by heterosexual contact, compared to 7% of men with AIDS. Only 1% of AIDS cases are among hemophiliacs, and 1% are among recipients of blood transfusions, blood products, or transplanted tissue. The relative contribution of the latter groups will gradually decrease, even though individuals infected pre-

Country	Estimated Adult HIV Seroprevalence, % 2002[a]	Life Expectancy at Birth, 2000–2005		Life Expectancy at Birth, 2010–2015	
		With AIDS	Without AIDS	With AIDS	Without AIDS
Botswana	38.8	39.7	68.1	31.6	70.7
Zimbabwe	33.7	33.1	67.6	31.8	70.5
Swaziland	33.4	34.4	62.2	30.3	66.3
Lesotho	31.0	35.1	59.0	32.2	63.0
Namibia	22.5	44.3	65.4	39.6	78.9
Zambia	21.5	32.4	53.4	35.3	57.4
South Africa	20.1	47.7	66.6	41.5	69.9

[a] Individuals ages 15–49.

Source: United Nations: *World Population Prospects: The 2002 Revision*; UNAIDS.

TABLE 173-5 *Estimated Numbers of AIDS Diagnoses, 2002 and Cumulative Through 2002, by Age at Diagnosis, Race/Ethnicity, and Exposure Category, United States*

	2002	Cumulative 1981–2002
Age at diagnosis (yrs)		
<13	92	9300
13–14	76	839
15–24	1833	35,460
25–34	9688	301,278
35–44	17,398	347,860
45–54	9488	138,386
55–64	2773	40,584
≥65	789	12,868
Race/ethnicity		
White, not Hispanic	11,929	364,458
Black, not Hispanic	21,169	347,491
Hispanic	8242	163,940
Asian/Pacific Islander	478	6924
American Indian/Alaska Native	206	2875
Exposure category		
Male adult or adolescent (≥13 years)		
Male-to-male sexual contact	16,944	420,790
Injection drug use	6945	172,351
Male-to-male sexual contact and injection drug use	1898	59,719
Heterosexual contact	4937	50,793
Other[a]	365	14,350
Subtotal	31,089	718,002
Female adult or adolescent (≥13 years)		
Injection drug use	3180	67,917
Heterosexual contact	7476	84,835
Other[a]	299	6519
Subtotal	10,955	159,271
Child (<13 years)		
Perinatal	90	8629
Other[b]	2	671
Subtotal	92	9300
Total[c]	42,136	886,575

[a] Includes hemophilia, blood transfusion, perinatal transmission, and risk not reported or identified.
[b] Includes hemophilia, blood transfusion, and risk not reported or identified.
[c] Cumulative total includes 887 persons of unknown or multiple race and 2 persons of unknown sex.
Source: Centers for Disease Control and Prevention, 2003.

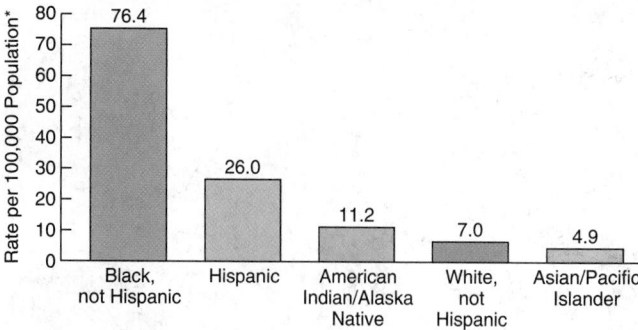

FIGURE 173-11 Rates of adult/adolescent AIDS cases per 100,000 population diagnosed in 2001 in various racial/ethnic groups in the United States. (*From Centers for Disease Control and Prevention, 2003.*)

the course of HIV infection (see below). Also, the demography of newly infected individuals has changed considerably since the mid-1980s (see below).

HIV PREVALENCE AND INCIDENCE IN THE UNITED STATES It is estimated that between 850,000 and 950,000 adults and adolescents in the United States are living with HIV infection, one-quarter of whom are unaware of their infection. This estimate results in an overall nationwide prevalence of HIV infection of ~0.3%. Prevalence is highest among young adults in their late twenties and thirties and among minorities. An estimated 3% of black men and 1% of black women in their thirties are living with HIV infection. The number of new infections per year is estimated to be ~40,000, and this number has remained stable for more than a decade. The estimated proportion of HIV infections has declined among white males, especially those >30, while the proportion of new HIV infections appears to have increased among young homosexual men and heterosexual women, especially in minority groups. Among newly infected persons in the United States, ~70% are men and ~30% are women (Fig. 173-13). Of these newly infected individuals, half are <25 years. Of new infections among men, the CDC estimates that ~60% were infected through homosexual sex, 25% through injection drug use, and 15% through heterosexual sex. Of new infections among women, ~75% were infected through heterosexual sex and 25% through injection drug use.

HIV infection and AIDS are widespread in the United States; although the epidemic on the whole is plateauing, it is spreading rapidly among certain populations, stabilizing in others, and decreasing in others. Similar to other STDs, HIV infection will not spread homogeneously throughout the population of the United States. However, it is clear that anyone who practices high-risk behavior is at risk for HIV infection. In addition, the increase in infections and AIDS cases among young homosexual men, heterosexuals (particularly sexual partners of IDUs, women, and adolescents) as well as the spread in

viously through this mode of transmission will continue to develop AIDS. The risk of additional infections via this mode of transmission in the United States is extremely small (see above). In recent years, the incidence of AIDS has decreased considerably, with ~42,000 new cases in 2002 compared to ~60,000 in 1996 (Fig. 173-10). This trend likely reflects both reduced infection rates since the mid-1980s; more widespread use of prophylactic therapies, which delay the onset of AIDS; and the use of highly effective antiretroviral therapy early in

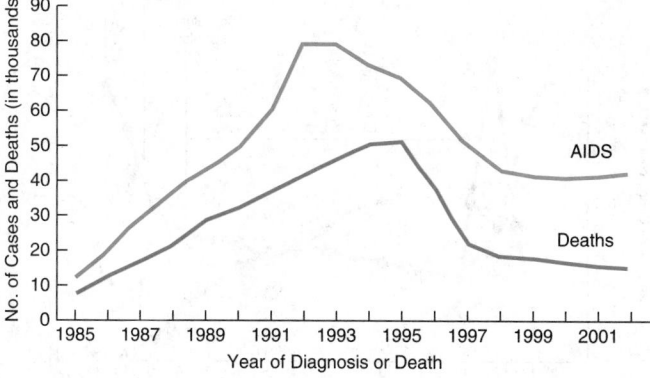

FIGURE 173-10 Estimated incidence of AIDS and deaths of adults and adolescents with AIDS, 1985–2002, United States. (*From the Centers for Diseases Control and Prevention, 2003.*)

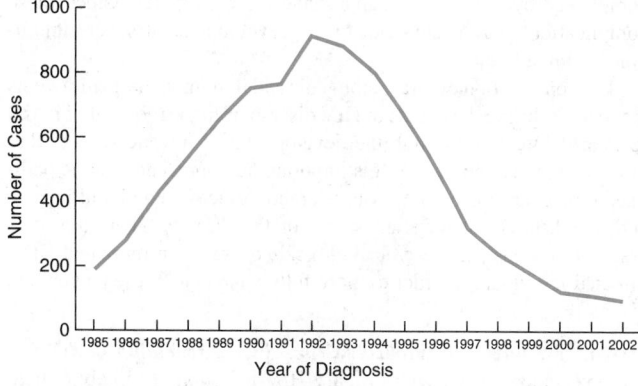

FIGURE 173-12 Perinatally acquired AIDS cases by year of diagnosis, 1985–2002, United States. (*From the Centers for Disease Control and Prevention, 2003.*)

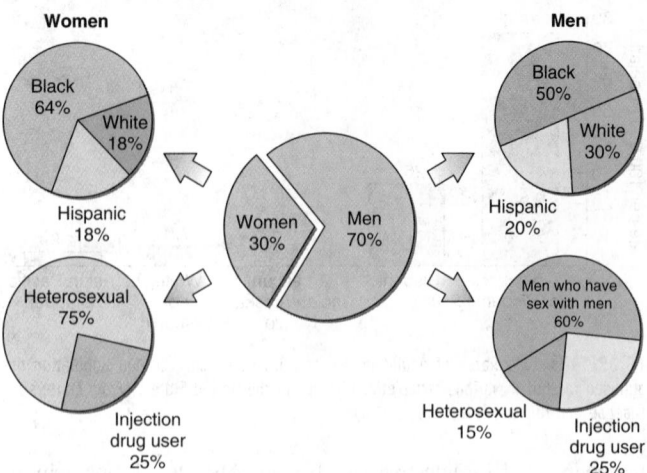

Women   **Men**

Black 64% / White 18%

Hispanic 18%

Heterosexual 75%

Injection drug user 25%

Women 30% / Men 70%

Black 50% / White 30%

Hispanic 20%

Men who have sex with men 60%

Heterosexual 15%

Injection drug user 25%

FIGURE 173-13   Estimated new HIV infections annually by race and risk in the United States. (*From the Centers for Disease Control and Prevention.*)

pockets of poverty in both urban and rural regions (particularly among underserved minority populations with inadequate access to health care) testifies to the fact that the epidemic of HIV infection in the United States is a public health problem of major proportions.

PATHOPHYSIOLOGY AND PATHOGENESIS

The hallmark of HIV disease is a profound immunodeficiency resulting primarily from a progressive quantitative and qualitative deficiency of the subset of T lymphocytes referred to as *helper T cells*, or *inducer T cells*. This subset of T cells is defined phenotypically by the presence on its surface of the CD4 molecule (Chap. 295), which serves as the primary cellular receptor for HIV. A co-receptor must also be present together with CD4 for efficient fusion and entry of HIV-1 into its target cells (Figs. 173-3 and 173-4). HIV uses two major co-receptors for fusion and entry; these co-receptors are also the primary receptors for certain chemoattractive cytokines termed *chemokines* and belong to the seven-transmembrane-domain G protein–coupled family of receptors. CCR5 and CXCR4 are the major co-receptors used by HIV (see above and below). Although a number of mechanisms responsible for cytopathicity and immune dysfunction of CD4+ T cells have been demonstrated in vitro, particularly direct infection and destruction of these cells by HIV and activation-induced cell death (see below), it remains unclear which mechanisms or combination of mechanisms are primarily responsible for their progressive depletion and functional impairment in vivo. When the number of CD4+ T cells declines below a certain level (see below), the patient is at high risk of developing a variety of opportunistic diseases, particularly the infections and neoplasms that are AIDS-defining illnesses. Some features of AIDS, such as KS and neurologic abnormalities (see below), cannot be explained completely by the immunosuppressive effects of HIV, since these complications may occur prior to the development of severe immunologic impairment.

The combination of viral pathogenic and immunopathogenic events that occurs during the course of HIV disease from the moment of initial (primary) infection through the development of advanced-stage disease is complex and varied. It is important to appreciate that the pathogenic mechanisms of HIV disease are multifactorial and multiphasic and are different at different stages of the disease. Therefore, it is essential to consider the typical clinical course of an untreated HIV-infected individual in order to more fully appreciate these pathogenic events (Fig. 173-14).

PRIMARY HIV INFECTION, INITIAL VIREMIA, AND DISSEMINATION OF VIRUS

The events associated with primary HIV infection are likely critical determinants of the subsequent course of HIV disease. In particular, the dissemination of virus to lymphoid organs is a major factor in the

establishment of a chronic and persistent infection (see below). The initial infection of susceptible cells may vary somewhat with the route of infection. Virus that enters directly into the bloodstream via infected blood or blood products (i.e., transfusions, use of contaminated needles for injecting drugs, sharp-object injuries, maternal-to-fetal transmission either intrapartum or perinatally, or sexual intercourse where there is enough trauma to cause bleeding) is likely cleared from the circulation to the spleen and other lymphoid organs, where it replicates to a critical level and then leads to a burst of viremia that disseminates virus throughout the body. Dendritic cells play an important role in the initiation of HIV infection. These cells express a diversity of C-type lectin receptors on their surface, one of which is called *DC-SIGN* (see above). DC-SIGN binds with high affinity to the HIV envelope gp120 and can retain infectious particles for days in vitro. Certain studies have demonstrated that following binding to DC-SIGN, HIV is internalized into a low pH nonlysosomal compartment that allows for the retention of infectivity. Upon encountering a susceptible CD4+ T cell target, the dendritic cell markedly enhances the infectivity of the virus for the target cell. This mechanism likely operates in humans when HIV enters "locally" (as opposed to directly into the blood) and encounters mucosal dendritic cells via the vagina, rectum, or urethra during intercourse or via the upper gastrointestinal tract from swallowed infected semen, vaginal fluid, or breast milk. In primary HIV infection, virus replication in CD4+ T cells intensifies prior to the initiation of an HIV-specific immune response (see below), leading to a burst of viremia (Fig. 173-14) and then to a rapid dissemination of virus to other lymphoid organs, the brain, and other tissues. Individuals who experience the "acute HIV syndrome," which occurs to varying degrees in ~50% of individuals with primary infection, have high levels of viremia measured in millions of copies of HIV RNA per milliliter that last for several weeks (see below). The acute mononucleosis-like symptoms are well correlated with the presence of viremia. Virtually all patients appear to develop some degree of viremia during primary infection, which contributes to virus dissemination throughout the lymphoid tissue, even though they may remain asymptomatic or not recall experiencing symptoms. A more detailed description of the role of lymphoid tissue in the immunopathogenesis of HIV disease is given below. It appears that the initial level of plasma viremia in primary HIV infection does not necessarily determine the rate of disease progression; however, the set point of the level of steady-state plasma viremia after ~1 year does seem to correlate with the rapidity of disease progression (see below).

ESTABLISHMENT OF CHRONIC AND PERSISTENT INFECTION ■ **Persistent Virus Replication** HIV infection is unique among human viral infections. Despite the robust cellular and humoral immune responses that are mounted following primary infection (see below), once infection has been established the virus succeeds in escaping immune-mediated

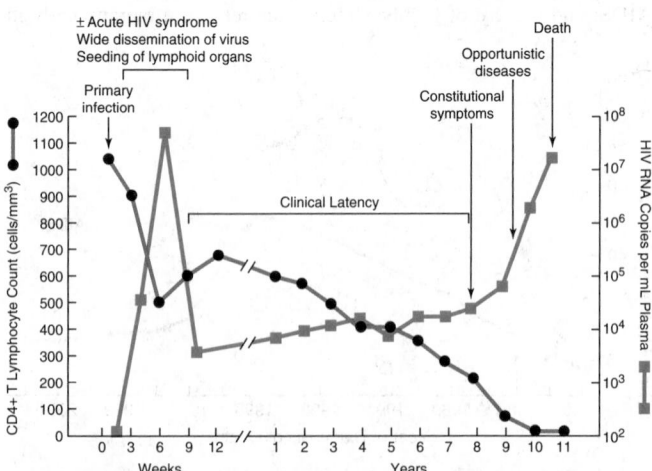

FIGURE 173-14   Typical course of an HIV-infected individual. See text for detailed description. (*From A Fauci et al: Ann Intern Med 124:654, 1996.*)

clearance (see below) and is virtually never eliminated completely from the body. Rather, a chronic infection develops that persists with varying degrees of virus replication in the untreated patient for a median of ~10 years before the patient becomes clinically ill (see below). It is this establishment of a chronic, persistent infection that is the hallmark of HIV disease. Throughout the often protracted course of chronic infection, virus replication can almost invariably be detected in untreated patients, both by highly sensitive assays for plasma viremia as well as by demonstration of cell-associated HIV RNA in immunocompetent cells (predominantly CD4+ T cells and macrophages) in the circulation and in lymphoid tissue. In other human viral infections, with very few exceptions, if the host survives, the virus is completely cleared from the body and a state of immunity against subsequent infection develops. HIV infection very rarely kills the host during primary infection. Certain viruses, such as HSV (Chap. 163), are not completely cleared from the body after infection but instead enter a latent state; in these cases, clinical latency is accompanied by microbiologic latency. This is not the case with HIV infection, in which some degree of virus replication invariably occurs during the period of clinical latency (see below). Chronicity associated with persistent virus replication can also be seen in certain cases of HBV and HCV infections (Chap. 287); however, in these infections the immune system is not a target of the virus.

Evasion of Immune System Control Inherent to the establishment of chronicity of HIV infection is the ability of the virus to evade elimination and control by the immune system. There are a number of mechanisms whereby the virus accomplishes this evasion. Paramount among these is the ability of the virus to mutate, which becomes particularly relevant after the establishment of chronic infection and which contributes to the maintenance of chronicity. The evolution of mutants that escape control by CD8+ cytolytic T lymphocytes (CTLs) is critical to the propagation and progression of HIV infection. The high rate of virus replication and the continual mutation of virus also contribute to the inability of neutralizing antibody to contain the virus quasispecies present in an individual at any given time. Molecular analysis of clonotypes has demonstrated that clones of CD8+ CTLs that expand greatly during primary HIV infection, and likely represent the high-affinity clones that would be expected to be most efficient in eliminating virus-infected cells, are no longer detectable after their initial burst of expansion. It is thought that the initially expanded clones may have been deleted owing to the overwhelming exposure to viral antigens during the initial burst of viremia, similar to the exhaustion of CD8+ CTLs that has been reported in the murine model of lymphocytic choriomeningitis virus (LCMV) infection. To compound this phenomenon, virus replication and thus saturation of antigen-presenting cells with viral antigen take place in the lymphoid tissue (see below), which is also the site of generation of HIV-specific CTLs. Another mechanism of evasion by HIV of immune system control is the downregulation of HLA class I molecules on the surface of HIV-infected cells by the Nef protein of HIV, resulting in the lack of ability of the CD8+ CTL to recognize and kill the infected target cell. Although this downregulation of HLA class I molecules would favor elimination of HIV-infected cells by natural killer (NK) cells, this latter mechanism does not seem to effectively remove HIV-infected cells (see below). An important mechanism of evasion of the humoral immune response is the avoidance by the virus of antibody-mediated neutralization through its conformational masking of receptor-binding sites.

CD4+ T cell help is critical for the integrity of antigen-specific immune responses, both humoral and cell-mediated. HIV preferentially infects HIV-specific CD4+ T cells, and so this loss of viral-specific helper T cell responses has potentially profound negative consequences for the immunologic control of HIV replication. Other means of escape of HIV-infected cells from elimination by CD8+ CTLs are the sequestration of infected cells in immunologically privileged sites such as the central nervous system (CNS) as well as the segregation of HIV-specific CTLs and CTL precursors in the peripheral blood where relatively little active virus replication takes place, rather than in the lymphoid tissue, which is the major site of virus replication and spread.

Finally, the escape of HIV from elimination during primary infection allows the formation of a large pool of latently infected cells that cannot be eliminated by virus-specific CTLs (see below). Thus, despite a potent immune response and the marked downregulation of virus replication following primary HIV infection, HIV succeeds in establishing a state of chronic infection with a variable degree of persistent virus replication. In most cases, during this period the patient makes the clinical transition from acute primary infection to a relatively prolonged state of clinical latency (see below).

Latent Reservoir of HIV-Infected Cells: Obstacle to the Eradication of Virus
There exists in virtually all HIV-infected individuals a pool of latently infected, resting CD4+ T cells that serves as at least one component of the persistent reservoir of virus. Such cells manifest postintegration latency in that the HIV provirus integrates into the genome of the cell and can remain in this state until an activation signal drives the expression of HIV transcripts and ultimately replication-competent virus. This form of latency is to be distinguished from preintegration latency, in which HIV enters a resting CD4+ T cell and, in the absence of an activation signal, only a limited degree of reverse transcription of the HIV genome occurs. This period of preintegration latency may last hours to days, and if no activation signal is delivered to the cell, the proviral DNA loses its capacity to initiate a productive infection. If these cells do become activated, reverse transcription proceeds to completion and the virus continues along its replication cycle (see above and Fig. 173-15). The pool of cells that are in the postintegration state of latency is established early during the course of primary HIV infection. Despite the suppression of plasma viremia to <50 copies of

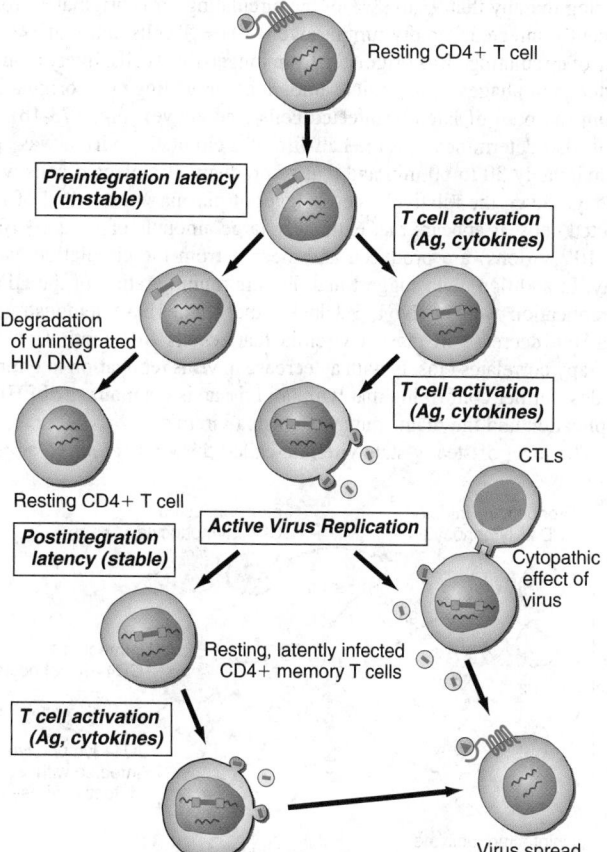

FIGURE 173-15 Generation of latently infected, resting CD4+ T cells in HIV-infected individuals. See text for details. Ag, antigen; CTLs, cytolytic T lymphocytes. (*Courtesy of TW Chun.*)

HIV RNA per milliliter by potent combinations of several antiretroviral drugs for as long as 5 years, this pool of latently infected cells persists and can give rise to replication-competent virus. Modeling studies built on projections of decay curves (see below) have estimated that in a setting of prolonged suppression of plasma viremia to <50 copies of HIV RNA per milliliter by antiretroviral therapy (a goal that is difficult to maintain consistently over years), it would require from 7 to 70 years for the pool of latently infected cells to be completely eliminated. Furthermore, the reservoir of latently infected cells is replenished during minor rebounds of virus replication that may occur intermittently, even in patients who for the most part are treated successfully, and certainly during major rebounds of viremia in patients whose therapy is interrupted for a period of weeks or longer. Thus, this persistent pool of latently infected cells is a major obstacle to any goal of eradication of virus from infected individuals, despite the favorable clinical outcomes that have resulted from antiretroviral therapy (see below).

Viral Dynamics   The dynamics of viral production and turnover have been quantified using mathematical modeling in the setting of the administration of reverse transcriptase and protease inhibitors to HIV-infected individuals in clinical studies. Treatment with these drugs resulted in a precipitous decline in the level of plasma viremia, which typically fell by well over 90% within 2 weeks. The number of CD4+ T cells in the blood increased concurrently, which suggested that the killing of CD4+ T cells was linked directly to the levels of replicating virus. However, it is generally agreed that a significant component of the early rise in CD4+ T cell numbers following the initiation of therapy is due to the redistribution of cells into the peripheral blood from other body compartments as a consequence of alterations in immune system activation. It was determined on the basis of modeling the kinetics of viral decline and the emergence of resistant mutants during therapy that 93 to 99% of the circulating virus originated from recently infected, rapidly turning over CD4+ T cells and that ~1 to 7% of circulating virus originated from longer-lived cells, likely monocyte/macrophages. A negligible amount of circulating virus originated from the pool of latently infected cells (see above) (Fig. 173-16). It was also determined that the half-life of a circulating virion was approximately 30 to 60 min and that of productively infected cells was 1 day. Given the relatively steady level of plasma viremia and of infected cells, it appears that extremely large amounts of virus (~10^{10} to 10^{11} virions) are produced and cleared from the circulation each day. In addition, data suggest that the minimum duration of the HIV-1 replication cycle in vivo is ~2 days. Other studies have demonstrated that the decrease in plasma viremia that results from antiretroviral therapy correlates closely with a decrease in virus replication in lymph nodes, further confirming that lymphoid tissue is the main site of HIV replication and the main source of plasma viremia.

The level of steady-state viremia, called the viral *set point*, at ~1 year has important prognostic implications for the progression of HIV disease. It has been demonstrated that HIV-infected individuals who have a low set point at 6 months to 1 year progress to AIDS much more slowly than individuals whose set point is very high at that time (Fig. 173-17). Levels of viremia generally increase as disease progresses. Measurement of the level of viremia is critical in guiding therapeutic decisions in HIV-infected individuals (see below).

Clinical Latency versus Microbiologic Latency   With the exception of long-term nonprogressors (see below), the level of CD4+ T cells in the blood decreases progressively in HIV-infected individuals. The slope of this decline is usually a good predictor of the pattern of the clinical course and the development of advanced disease. The decline in CD4+ T cells may be gradual or abrupt, the latter usually reflecting a significant spike in the level of plasma viremia. Most patients are entirely asymptomatic while this progressive decline is taking place (see below) and are often described as being in a state of *clinical latency*. However, this term is misleading; it does not mean disease latency, since progression is generally relentless during this period. Furthermore, clinical latency should not be confused with microbiologic latency, since virus replication manifested by low-level viremia is present in the vast majority of patients during the period of clinical latency. Even in those rare patients who have <50 copies of HIV RNA per milliliter in the absence of therapy, there is virtually always some degree of ongoing virus replication, as determined by sensitive molecular methods such as PCR techniques that detect cell-associated viral RNA or that concentrate virus from large volumes of blood.

ADVANCED HIV DISEASE   In untreated patients or in patients in whom therapy has not adequately controlled virus replication (see below), after a variable period, usually measured in years, the CD4+ T cell count falls below a critical level (<200/μL) and the patient becomes highly susceptible to opportunistic disease (Fig. 173-14). For this reason, the CDC case definition of AIDS includes all HIV-infected individuals with CD4+ T cell counts below this level (Table 173-1). Patients may experience constitutional signs and symptoms or may develop an opportunistic disease abruptly without any prior symptoms, although the latter scenario is unusual. The depletion of CD4+ T cells continues to be progressive and unrelenting in this phase. It is not uncommon for CD4+ T cell counts to drop as low as 10/μL or even to zero, yet such patients may survive for months or even years. This situation has become increasingly common as patients are treated more aggressively and are given prophylaxis against the common life-threatening opportunistic infections (see below). In this regard, control of plasma viremia by antiretroviral therapy, even in individuals with extremely low CD4+ T cell counts, has increased survival in these patients despite the fact that their CD4+ T cell counts may not significantly increase as a result of therapy. Ultimately, patients who

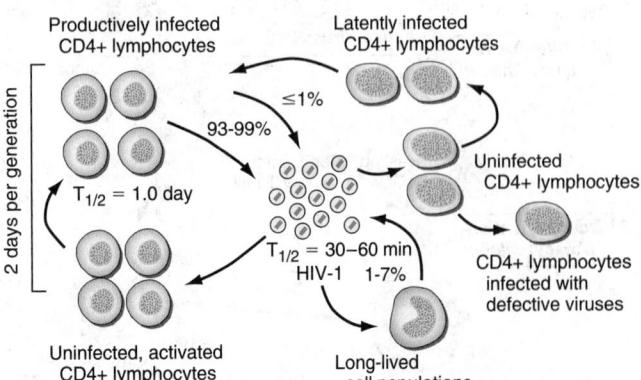

FIGURE 173-16   Dynamics of HIV infection in vivo. See text for detailed description. (*From AS Perelson et al: Science 271:1582, 1996.*)

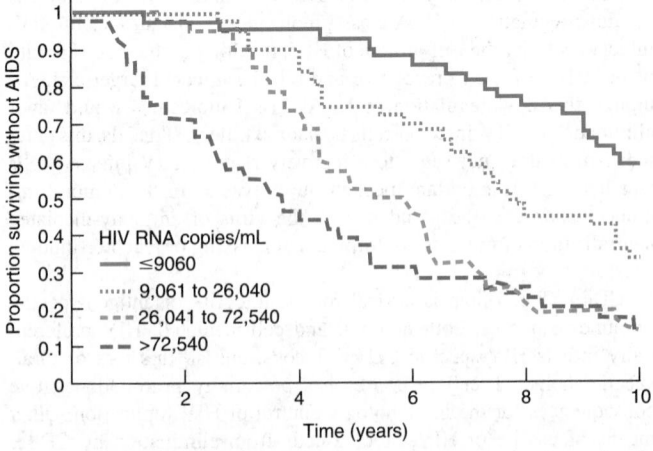

FIGURE 173-17   Relationship between levels of virus and rates of disease progression. Kaplan-Meier curves for AIDS-free survival stratified by baseline HIV-1 RNA categories (copies per milliliter). (*From Mellors et al.*)

progress to this severest form of immunodeficiency usually succumb to opportunistic infections or neoplasms (see below).

LONG-TERM SURVIVORS AND LONG-TERM NONPROGRESSORS The prognosis for HIV-infected individuals who have access to health care and antiretroviral therapy has improved greatly since the beginning of the epidemic. The median time from primary HIV infection to the development of AIDS in untreated individuals in the developed world is ~10 years. This period has been markedly extended by the wide availability of combinations of antiretroviral drugs in the developed world; the full extent of this benefit has yet to be realized. It is important to distinguish between the terms *long-term survivor* and *long-term nonprogressor*. Long-term nonprogressors are by definition long-term survivors; however, the reverse is not always true. The definitions of these categories are empirical and continue to change as more data are collected from prospective cohort studies. Predictions from one study that antedated the availability of effective antiretroviral therapy estimated that ~13% of homosexual/bisexual men who were infected at an early age may remain free of clinical AIDS for >20 years. Originally, individuals were considered to be long-term survivors if they remained alive for 10 to 15 years after initial infection. Currently, individuals are considered to be long-term survivors if they remain alive for ≥20 years after initial infection. In most such individuals the disease has progressed, in that they have significant immunodeficiency, and many have experienced opportunistic diseases. Some of these individuals have CD4+ T cell counts that have decreased to ≤200/μL but have remained stable at that level for years. The mechanisms of this stabilization are not entirely clear but may relate to the beneficial effects of antiretroviral therapy and prophylaxis against opportunistic infections. In addition, a number of viral and/or host determinants likely contribute to the long-term survival of these individuals. Quantitative and qualitative aspects of the HIV-specific immune response, as well as recognized and unrecognized genetic factors (see below), may also contribute to the long-term survival of these individuals.

Definitions of long-term nonprogressors have varied considerably over the years, and so such individuals constitute a heterogeneous group. Originally, individuals considered to be long-term nonprogressors were those who had been infected with HIV for a long period (≥10 years), whose CD4+ T cell counts were in the normal range and remained stable over years, and who had not received antiretroviral therapy. Such patients had low, but usually detectable, levels of plasma viremia, generally normal immune function according to commonly measured parameters (skin tests, in vitro lymphocyte responses to various mitogens and antigens), and normal-appearing lymphoid tissue architecture as determined on lymph node biopsy. The definition rested more on the status of the immune system than on the absolute control of plasma viremia. In general, long-term nonprogressors manifested robust HIV-specific immune responses, both humoral (neutralizing antibodies) and cell-mediated (HIV-specific CTLs). However, this may also be true of some individuals early in the course of disease who ultimately progress to advanced disease. No qualitative abnormalities in the virus were detected in most of these patients. However, a small subset of patients did have defective virus; in particular, in one cohort of five long-term nonprogressors, the virus had a defect in the *nef* gene. In another report, a blood donor in Australia who was HIV-infected and a group of seven individuals who were infected by blood or blood products from that donor remained free of HIV-related disease and maintained normal and stable CD4+ T cell counts for several years after infection. Sequence analysis of viruses isolated from the donor and recipients revealed similar deletions in the *nef* gene and the region of overlap of *nef* and the U3 region of the HIV LTR (Fig. 173-5). The vast majority of these originally reported long-term nonprogressors have now gone on to progressive disease. More recently, cohorts of rare long-term nonprogressors have been described who have been infected for 20 years with normal CD4+ T cell counts and who typically maintain plasma viral RNA <50 copies per milliliter without antiretroviral therapy. When these more stringent definitions based

predominantly on levels of plasma viremia are applied, very strong associations with HLA B*5701 or HLA B*2705 alleles have been found. In addition, the HIV-specific CD8+ T cell response in these patients is highly focused on B5701-restricted peptides, suggesting that the B5701 molecule plays a direct role in restriction of virus replication in these individuals, although the precise mechanisms of this effect remain unclear.

A number of other host genetic factors exert more modest effects on restriction of HIV replication, yet they also may be associated with slower progression of disease (see "Genetic Factors in HIV Pathogenesis," below). The precise role of host factors in long-term nonprogression remains unclear. There is no obvious and consistent genetic determinant for nonprogression. However, several genetic mutations have been demonstrated to result in a delay in the progression of HIV disease. These include heterozygosity for the *CCR5*-Δ32 deletion, heterozygosity for the *CCR2*-64I mutation, homozygosity for the *SDF1*-3′A mutation, and heterozygosity for the *RANTES*-28G mutation (see "Genetic Factors in HIV Pathogenesis," below). Since CCR5 is the major co-receptor for R5 or macrophage-tropic strains of HIV and since individuals who are homozygous for the *CCR5*-Δ32 deletion are, with rare exceptions, protected against HIV infection, the potential mechanism for slow progression in heterozygotes is clear. In addition, certain single nucleotide polymorphisms in the *CCR5* promoter have been shown to be associated with slower progression of disease. The reason for the slowing of progression of HIV disease in individuals who are heterozygous for the *CCR2*-64I mutation is less clear; however, it has been demonstrated that CXCR4 can dimerize with the CCR2-64I mutant but not with wild-type CCR2. This dimerization may reduce the amount of CXCR4 on the cell surface and as a result inhibit infection with X4 viruses. Homozygosity for the *SDF1*-3′A mutation may upregulate the *SDF1* gene enabling SDF-1, which is the natural ligand for CXCR4, to compete more effectively with X4 or T cell tropic virus for the CXCR4 coreceptor. The *RANTES*-28G mutation increases RANTES expression, which is the natural ligand for CCR5 and may thus inhibit infection with R5 viruses. Finally, maximal HLA heterozygosity of class I loci (A, B, and C) has been shown to be associated with delayed progression of HIV disease. Although long-term nonprogressors have robust HIV-specific immune responses as well as competent CD8+ T cell suppressors of HIV replication, it is unclear whether these factors are directly responsible for the state of nonprogression. A substantial proportion of HIV-infected individuals manifest comparable immune responses early in the course of their disease and still experience disease progression. As noted above, long-term nonprogressors likely represent a heterogeneous group. The lack of disease progression may be explained in some by a defect in the virus; in others by any of a variety of host factors, including recognized and as yet unrecognized genetic factors; and in others by a combination of both.

LYMPHOID ORGANS AND HIV PATHOGENESIS Regardless of the portal of entry of HIV, lymphoid tissues are the major anatomic sites for the establishment and propagation of HIV infection (see above) Despite the use of measurements of plasma viremia to determine the level of disease activity, virus replication occurs mainly in lymphoid tissue and not in blood; indeed, the level of plasma viremia directly reflects virus production in lymphoid tissue.

Some patients experience progressive generalized lymphadenopathy (see below) early in the course of the infection; others experience varying degrees of transient lymphadenopathy. Lymphadenopathy reflects the cellular activation and immune response to the virus in the lymphoid tissue, which is generally characterized by follicular or germinal center hyperplasia. Lymphoid tissue involvement is a common denominator of virtually all patients with HIV infection, even those without easily detectable lymphadenopathy.

Simultaneous examinations of lymph tissue and peripheral blood in patients and monkeys during various stages of HIV and SIV infection, respectively, have led to substantial insight into the pathogenesis of HIV disease. Using a combination of PCR techniques for HIV DNA and HIV RNA in tissue and HIV RNA in plasma, in situ hybridization for HIV RNA, and light and electron microscopy, the following picture has emerged. During acute HIV infection, a high level of viral replication in individual cells is demonstrated in lymphoid tissue and is associated with a burst of plasma viremia. A profound degree of cellular activation occurs (see below) and is reflected in follicular or germinal center hyperplasia. At this time copious amounts of extracellular virions are trapped on the processes of the follicular dendritic cells (FDCs) in the germinal centers of the lymph nodes (Fig. 173-18A). Virions that have bound complement components on their surfaces attach to the surface of FDCs via interactions with complement receptors and likely via Fc receptors that bind to antibodies that are attached to the virions. In situ hybridization reveals expression of virus in individual cells of the paracortical area and, to a lesser extent, the germinal center (Fig. 173-18B). The persistence of trapped virus after the transition from acute to chronic infection likely reflects a steady state whereby trapped virus turns over and is replaced by fresh virions, which are continually produced to a greater or lesser degree in individual patients.

During early-stage HIV disease, the architecture of the germinal centers is generally preserved and may even be hyperplastic owing to in situ proliferation of cells (mostly B lymphocytes) and recruitment to the lymph nodes of a number of cell types (B cells, CD4+ and CD8+ T cells). Electron microscopy demonstrates a fine network of FDCs with many long, finger-like processes that envelop virtually every lymphocyte in the germinal center (Fig. 173-18C). Extracellular virions can be seen attached to the processes, yet the FDCs appear to be relatively healthy. The trapping of antigen is a physiologically normal function for the FDCs, which present antigen to B cells and contribute to the generation of B cell memory. However, in the case of HIV, the trapped virions serve as a persistent source of cellular activation, resulting in the secretion of proinflammatory cytokines such as interleukin (IL) 1β, tumor necrosis factor (TNF) α, and IL-6, which can upregulate virus replication in infected cells (see below). Furthermore, although trapped virus is coated by neutralizing antibodies, it has been demonstrated that these virions remain infectious for CD4+ T cells while attached to the processes of the FDCs. CD4+ T cells that migrate into the germinal center to provide help to B cells in the generation of an HIV-specific immune response are susceptible to infection by these trapped virions. Thus, in HIV infection, a normal physiologic function of the immune system, which contributes to the clearance of virus as well as to the generation of a specific immune response, can also have deleterious consequences. It is difficult to demonstrate infection of the FDCs at this point, or even in advanced disease; however, rare examples of virus budding off FDCs have been reported.

As the disease progresses, the architecture of the germinal centers begins to show disruption, and the trapping efficiency of the lymph node diminishes. Electron microscopy reveals swollen organelles, and the FDCs begin to undergo cell death. The mechanisms of FDC death remain unclear; there is no indication by electron microscopy of copious virus replication or budding of virions off the cell in great quantities. As the disease progresses to an advanced stage, there is complete disruption of the architecture of the germinal centers, accompanied by

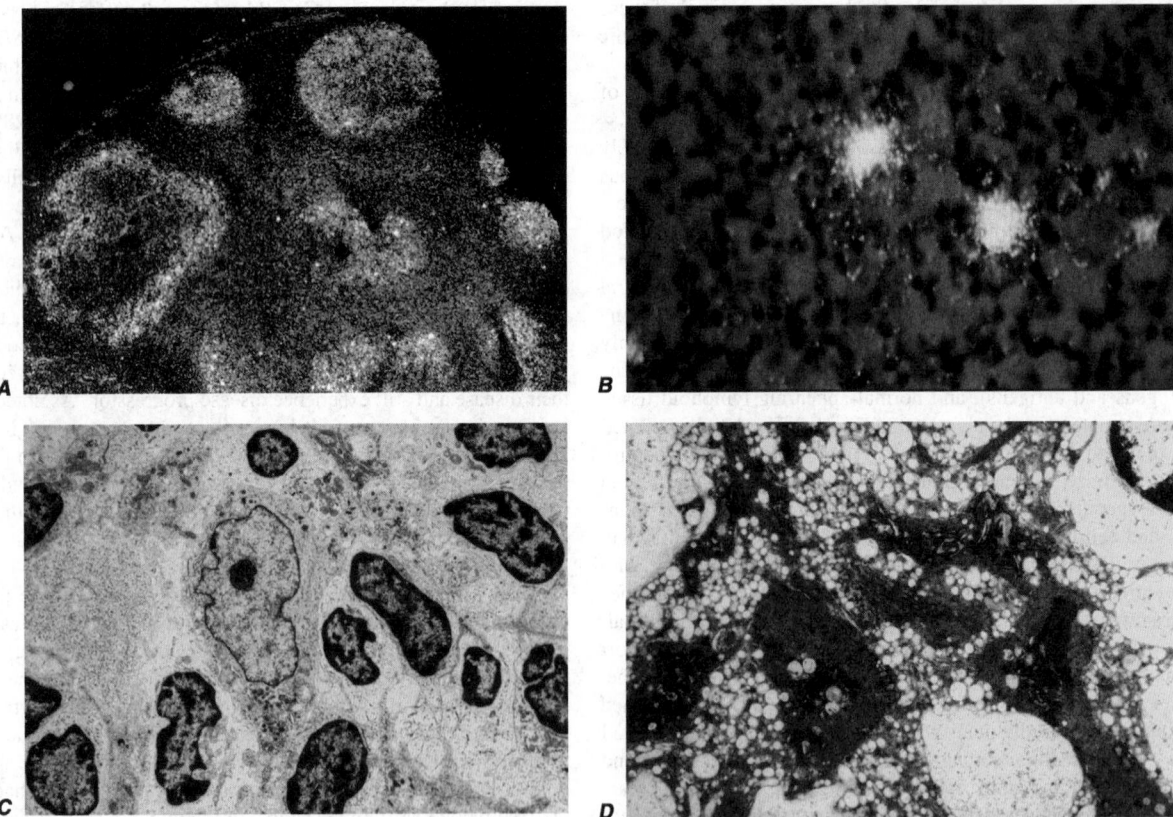

FIGURE 173-18   HIV in the lymph nodes of HIV-infected individuals. *A.* Cervical lymph node from an asymptomatic individual with very low levels of plasma viremia. In situ hybridization using a molecular probe for HIV RNA reveals copious virus demarcating the numerous germinal centers (bright areas) of the node. The virus was extracellular and bound to the processes of the follicular dendritic cells (FDCs), which form a matrix within the confines of the germinal centers. Original ×25. *B.* Individual cells infected with HIV. Two cells in the paracortical area of the lymph node are shown expressing HIV RNA by in situ hybridization using a radiolabeled molecular probe. Original ×250. *C.* FDCs in cervical node of an asymptomatic HIV-infected individual.

Electron microscopy reveals an FDC with a prominent nucleolus surrounded by several lymphocytes within the germinal center of the node. Higher magnification of several fields indicates that multiple processes of the FDCs are in contact with several lymphocytes. Original ×1920. *D.* Dissolution of FDCs in the germinal center of a cervical lymph node from a patient with advanced HIV disease. Widespread death of FDCs is associated with a loss of ability of the lymph node to trap virus late in the course of HIV disease. Original ×3744. (*A and B courtesy of Dr. Cecil Fox; C and D courtesy of Dr. Jan Orenstein. Adapted from G Pantaleo et al: N Engl J Med 328:327, 1993.*)

dissolution of the FDC network and massive dropout of FDCs (Fig. 173-18*D*). At this point, the lymph nodes are "burnt out." This destruction of lymphoid tissue compounds the immunodeficiency of HIV disease and contributes both to the inability to control HIV replication (leading usually to high levels of plasma viremia in the untreated or inadequately treated patient) and to the inability to mount adequate immune responses against opportunistic pathogens. The events from primary infection to the ultimate destruction of the immune system are illustrated in Fig. 173-19.

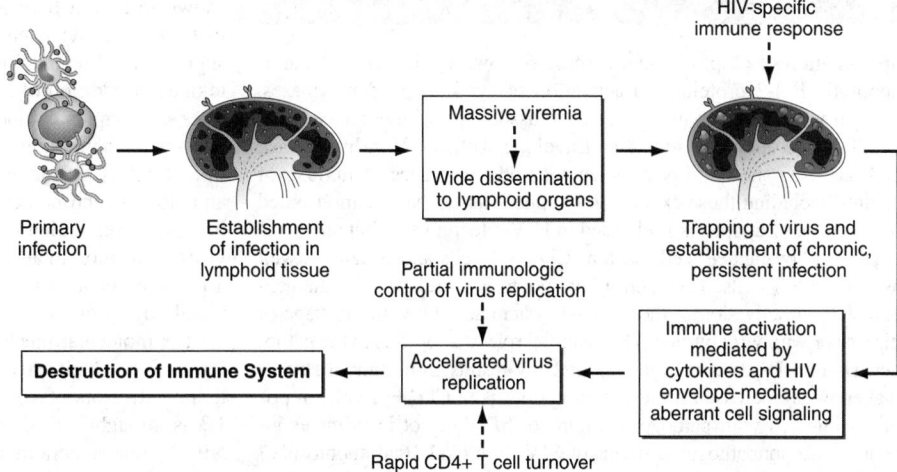

FIGURE 173-19   Events that transpire from primary HIV infection through the establishment of chronic persistent infection to the ultimate destruction of the immune system. See text for details; CTLs, cytolytic T lymphocytes.

CELLULAR ACTIVATION AND HIV PATHOGENESIS

Activation of the immune system is an essential component of an appropriate immune response to a foreign antigen. The immune system is normally in a state of homeostasis, awaiting perturbation by foreign antigenic stimuli. Once the immune response deals with and clears the antigen, the system returns to relative quiescence (Chap. 295). In HIV infection, however, the immune system is chronically activated owing to the persistence of virus replication throughout the course of HIV disease, particularly in the untreated patient (see above) and to variable degrees even in certain patients receiving antiretroviral therapy whose level of plasma viremia is suppressed to below the level of detection by standard assays (see below). Aberrant immune activation is the hallmark of HIV infection and is a critical component of the pathogenesis of HIV disease. This activated state is reflected by hyperactivation of B cells leading to hypergammaglobulinemia; spontaneous lymphocyte proliferation; activation of monocytes; expression of activation markers on CD4+ and CD8+ T cells; lymph node hyperplasia, particularly early in the course of disease (see above); increased secretion of proinflammatory cytokines (see below); elevated levels of neopterin, β_2-microglobulin, acid-labile interferon, and soluble IL-2 receptors; and autoimmune phenomena (see below). Even in the absence of direct infection of a target cell, HIV envelope proteins can interact with cellular receptors (CD4 molecules and chemokine receptors) to deliver potent activation signals resulting in calcium flux, the phosphorylation of certain proteins involved in signal transduction, co-localization of cytoplasmic proteins including those involved in cell trafficking, immune dysfunction, and under certain circumstances, apoptosis (see below). The secretion of certain proinflammatory and immunoregulatory cytokines is both a consequence of the aberrant immune activation associated with HIV infection and a mechanism of propagation of the process of aberrant cellular activation (see below).

In addition to endogenous factors such as cytokines, a number of exogenous factors such as other microbes that are associated with heightened cellular activation can enhance HIV replication and thus may have important effects on HIV pathogenesis. Co-infection or simultaneous cotransfection of cells with HIV and other viruses or viral genes has demonstrated that certain viruses, such as HSV type 1, cytomegalovirus (CMV), human herpesvirus (HHV) 6, Epstein-Barr virus (EBV), HBV, adenovirus, pseudorabies virus, and HTLV-I can upregulate HIV expression. Other microbes, such as *Mycoplasma*, have been reported to contribute to the induction of HIV expression. In addition, infestation with nematodes has been shown to be associated with a heightened state of immune activaton that facilitates HIV replication; de-worming of the infected host results in a decrease in plasma viremia. *Mycobacterium tuberculosis* is a common opportunistic infection in HIV-infected individuals (see below and Chap. 150). In addition to the fact that HIV-infected individuals are more likely to develop active tuberculosis (TB) after exposure, it has been demonstrated that active TB can accelerate the course of HIV infection. It has also been shown that levels of plasma viremia are greatly elevated in HIV-infected individuals with active TB, compared to pre-TB levels

and levels of viremia after successful treatment of the active TB. In vitro studies demonstrated that virus replication was markedly enhanced in lymphocytes of HIV-infected individuals who were skin test–positive for purified protein derivative (PPD) when PPD antigen was added to culture, resulting in cellular activation. Confirmatory evidence that antigen-induced activation was a major contributor to the accelerated viremia in HIV-infected individuals with active TB was provided by studies in which HIV-infected individuals were immunized with common recall antigens such as tetanus toxoid, influenza, or pneumococcal polysaccharide. Under these circumstances, a transient elevation of plasma viremia accompanied the cellular activation induced by the immunization. A greater degree of induction of virus was seen in those individuals with early-stage as opposed to advanced stage HIV disease, and the degree of virus induction correlated with the level of immune system activation.

Persistent immune activation may have several deleterious consequences. From a virologic standpoint, although quiescent CD4+ T cells can be infected with HIV, reverse transcription, integration, and virus spread are much more efficient in activated cells. Furthermore, cellular activation induces expression of virus in cells latently infected with HIV (see above). From an immunologic standpoint, chronic exposure of the immune system to a particular antigen over an extended period may ultimately lead to an inability to sustain an adequate immune response to the antigen in question. Furthermore, the ability of the immune system to respond to a broad spectrum of antigens may be compromised if immunocompetent cells are maintained in a state of chronic activation. In addition, activation of the immune system may favor the elimination of cells via programmed cell death (apoptosis) (see below) as well as the secretion of certain cytokines that can induce HIV expression (see below).

Apoptosis   *Apoptosis* is a form of programmed cell death that is a normal mechanism for the elimination of effete cells in organogenesis as well as in the cellular proliferation that occurs during a normal immune response (Chap. 295). Apoptosis is strictly dependent on cellular activation, and the aberrant cellular activation associated with HIV disease (see above) is correlated with a heightened state of apoptosis. It has been hypothesized that, in HIV infection, sequential activation signals delivered to CD4+ T cells induce apoptosis. Cross-linking of the CD4 molecule by gp120 or gp120/anti-gp120 complexes delivers the first of two signals required for apoptosis. The second signal supposedly leading to cell death is delivered via the T cell receptor by antigen. According to this hypothesis, direct infection of CD4+ T cells is not required for apoptosis to occur, although it has been demonstrated that alterations in tyrosine kinase activity of HIV-infected cells may induce the cell to undergo apoptosis. HIV can trigger both Fas-dependent and Fas-independent pathways of apoptosis. Mechanisms involved in this process include upregulation of Fas and Fas ligand, upregulation of caspase-1 and caspase-6, downregulation of the anti-apoptotic Bcl-2 protein, and activation of cyclin-dependent kinases. Certain viral gene products have been associated with enhanced susceptibility to apoptosis including Envelope, Tat, and Vpr. In contrast, Nef has been shown to possess antiapoptotic properties. A number of studies, including those examining lymphoid tissue, have demonstrated that the rate of apoptosis is elevated in HIV infection and that apoptosis is seen in "bystander" cells such as CD8+ T cells and B cells as well as in CD4+ T cells. The intensity of apoptosis correlates with the general state of activation of the immune system and not with the stage of disease or with viral burden. The potential role of apoptosis in the pathogenesis of HIV disease is underscored by results from animal studies that show an increased frequency of apoptosis in CD4+ T cells in primates infected with pathogenic strains of SIV but not in primates infected with nonpathogenic strains of SIV. It is likely that apoptosis of immunocompetent cells contributes to the immune abnormalities in HIV disease; however, this is probably a nonspecific mechanism that merely reflects the aberrant state of immune activation.

Autoimmune Phenomena The autoimmune phenomena that are common in HIV-infected individuals reflect, at least in part, chronic immune system activation as well as molecular mimickry by viral components. Although these phenomena usually occur in the absence of autoimmune disease, a wide spectrum of clinical manifestations that may be associated with autoimmunity have been described (see below). Autoimmune phenomena include antibodies to lymphocytes and, less commonly, to platelets and neutrophils. Antiplatelet antibodies have some clinical relevance, in that they may contribute to the thrombocytopenia of HIV disease (see below). Antibodies to nuclear and cytoplasmic components of cells have been reported, as have antibodies to cardiolipin; CD4 molecules; CD43 molecules, C1q-A; variable regions of the T cell receptor α, β, and γ chains; Fas; denatured collagen; and IL-2. In addition, autoantibodies to a range of serum proteins, including albumin, immunoglobulin, and thyroglobulin, have been reported. There is antigenic cross-reactivity between HIV viral proteins (gp120 and gp41) and MHC class II determinants, and anti-MHC class II antibodies have been reported in HIV infection. These antibodies could potentially lead to the elimination of MHC class II–bearing cells via antibody-dependent cellular cytotoxicity (ADCC) (Chap. 295). In addition, regions of homology exist between HIV envelope glycoproteins and IL-2 as well as MHC class I molecules.

THE CYTOKINE NETWORK IN HIV PATHOGENESIS The immune system is homeostatically regulated by a complex network of immunoregulatory cytokines, which are pleiotropic and redundant and operate in an autocrine and paracrine manner. They are expressed continuously, even during periods of apparent quiescence of the immune system. On perturbation of the immune system by antigenic challenge, the expression of cytokines increases to varying degrees (Chap. 295). Cytokines that are important components of this immunoregulatory network have been demonstrated to play a major role in the regulation of HIV expression in vitro. Potent modulation of HIV expression has been demonstrated either by manipulating endogenous cytokines or by adding exogenous cytokines to culture. Cytokines that induce HIV expression in one or more of these systems include IL-1, IL-2, IL-3, IL-6, IL-12, TNF-α, TNF-β, macrophage colony-stimulating factor (M-CSF), and granulocyte-macrophage colony-stimulating factor (GM-CSF). Among these cytokines, the most consistent and potent inducers of HIV expression are the *proinflammatory cytokines* TNF-α, IL-1β, and IL-6. Interferon (IFN)-α and -β suppress HIV replication, whereas transforming growth factor (TGF) β, IL-4, IL-10, and IFN-γ can either induce or suppress HIV expression, depending on the system involved. The *CC-chemokines* RANTES, macrophage inflammatory protein (MIP) 1α, and MIP-1β (Chap. 295) inhibit infection by and spread of R5 (macrophage-tropic) HIV-1 strains, while *stromal cell–derived factor* (SDF) 1 inhibits infection by and spread of X4 (T cell–tropic) strains (see below). The alpha defensin family of cytokines has been

shown to inhibit both R5 and X4 viruses, and other soluble factors that have not yet been fully characteized have also been shown to suppress HIV replication. Blocking of endogenous HIV-inducing cytokines or addition of inhibitors of HIV suppressor cytokines in cultures of peripheral blood and lymph node mononuclear cells from HIV-infected individuals has demonstrated that HIV replication is controlled tightly by endogenous cytokines that act synergistically and in an autocrine and paracrine manner, similar to their physiologic function in the regulation of the immune system. Indeed, the net level of virus replication in an HIV-infected individual reflects at least in part a balance between inductive and suppressive host factors, mediated mainly by cytokines.

The molecular mechanisms of HIV regulation are best understood for TNF-α, which activates NF-κB proteins that function as transcriptional activators of HIV expression. The HIV-inducing effect of IL-1β is thought to occur at the level of viral transcription in an NF-κB-independent manner. IL-6, GM-CSF, and IFN-γ regulate HIV expression mainly by posttranscriptional mechanisms. Elevated levels of TNF-α and IL-6 have been demonstrated in plasma and cerebrospinal fluid (CSF), and increased expression of TNF-α, IL-1β, IFN-γ, and IL-6 has been demonstrated in the lymph nodes of HIV-infected individuals. The mechanisms whereby the CC-chemokines RANTES, MIP-1α, and MIP-1β inhibit infection of R5 strains of HIV involve blocking of the binding of the virus to its co-receptor, the CC-chemokine receptor CCR5 (see above and below). Of note is the fact that CC-chemokines that inhibit infection by R5 strains of virus actually enhance infection by X4 strains of virus by inducing intracellular signal transduction through the CCR5 and CD4 molecules. The mechanisms whereby other less well characterized factors (see above) inhibit HIV replication are not completely understood.

LYMPHOCYTE TURNOVER IN HIV INFECTION The immune systems of patients with HIV infection are characterized by a profound increase in lymphocyte turnover that is immediately reduced with effective antiretroviral therapy. Studies utilizing in vivo or in vitro labelling of lymphocytes in the S-phase of the cell cycle have demonstrated a tight correlation between the degree of lymphocyte turnover and plasma levels of HIV RNA. This increase in turnover is seen in CD4+ and CD8+ T lymphocytes as well as B lymphocytes and can be observed in peripheral blood and lymphoid tissue. Mathematical models derived from these data suggest that one can view the lymphoid pool as consisting of dynamically distinct subpopulations of cells that are differentially affected by HIV infection. A major consequence of HIV infection appears to be a shift in cells from a more quiescent pool to a pool with a higher turnover rate. It is likely that a consequence of a higher rate of turnover is a higher rate of death. The role of the thymus in adult human T cell homeostasis and HIV pathogenesis is an area of controversy. While some data point to an important role for the thymus in maintaining T cell numbers and suggest that impairment of thymic function may be responsible for the declines in CD4+ T cells seen in the setting of HIV infection, other studies have concluded that the thymus plays a minor role in HIV pathogenesis. Among the data supporting an important role for the thymus are those that demonstrate an increase in the levels of T cell receptor excision circles (TRECs) following initiation of antiretroviral therapy. TRECs are a byproduct of T cell development and represent episomal fragments of DNA that are excised during T cell receptor gene rearrangement (Chap. 295). Levels of TRECs will be the net result of changes in thymic output and changes in T cell turnover. An increase in thymic output and/or a decrease in T cell turnover will lead to an increase in levels of TRECs. While it is clear that levels of TRECs increase following initiation of antiretroviral therapy, it is not clear whether this is a consequence of increased thymic output or decreased T cell turnover.

CELLULAR TROPISM FOR HIV: ROLE OF CO-RECEPTORS HIV-1 utilizes two major co-receptors along with CD4 to bind to, fuse with, and enter target cells; these co-receptors are CCR5 and CXCR4, which are receptors for certain endogenous chemokines and belong to the seven-transmembrane-domain G protein–coupled family of receptors (see above). Strains of HIV that utilize CCR5 as a co-receptor are referred to as *R5 viruses*. Strains of HIV that utilize CXCR4 are referred to as *X4 viruses*. Many virus strains are *dual tropic* in that they utilize both CCR5 and CXCR4; these are referred to as *R5X4 viruses*. Other terminology that has been associated with R5 versus X4 viruses is *non-syncytium-inducing viruses* versus *syncytium-inducing viruses*, respectively, based on the observation that R5 viruses generally do not form syncytia in culture with certain T cell lines, whereas X4 viruses readily form syncytia. In reality, under certain conditions both R5 and X4 viruses are capable of forming syncytia in culture.

The natural chemokine ligands for the major HIV co-receptors can readily block entry of HIV. For example, the CC-chemokines RANTES, MIP-1α, and MIP-1β, which are the natural ligands for CCR5, block entry of R5 viruses, whereas SDF-1, the natural ligand for CXCR4, blocks entry of X4 viruses. The mechanism of inhibition of viral entry is a steric inhibition of binding that is not dependent on signal transduction (Fig. 173-20).

The transmitting virus is almost invariably an R5 virus that predominates during the early stages of HIV disease. In ~40% of HIV-infected individuals, there is a transition to a predominantly X4 virus that is associated with a relatively rapid progression of disease. However, at least 60% of infected individuals progress in their disease while maintaining predominance of an R5 virus. Other chemokine receptor family members may function as coreceptors for HIV and SIV entry, but to a much lesser extent than do CCR5 and CXCR4; these include CCR3, BOB/GPR15, Bonzo/STRL33/TYMSTR, CCR2, CCR8, CX₃CR1(V28), and GPR1.

The basis for the tropism of different envelope glycoproteins for either CCR5 or CXCR4 relates to the ability of the HIV envelope, particularly the third variable region (V3 loop) of gp120, to interact with these co-receptors. In this regard, binding of gp120 to CD4 induces a conformational change in gp120 that increases its affinity for CCR5. It appears that the interaction of gp120 with CXCR4 is less

dependent on the conformational change induced in gp120 by CD4. In fact, there are X4 strains of HIV that bind to CXCR4 in the absence of surface-bound or soluble CD4. Finally, R5 viruses are more efficient in infecting monocyte/macrophages and microglial cells of the brain (see "Neuropathogenesis," below).

CELLULAR TARGETS OF HIV Although the CD4+ T lymphocytes and CD4+ cells of monocyte lineage are the principal targets of HIV, virtually any cell that expresses the CD4 molecule together with co-receptor molecules (see above and below) can potentially be infected with HIV. Circulating dendritic cells have been reported to express low levels of CD4, and depending on their stage of maturation, these cells can be infected with HIV (see below). Epidermal Langerhans cells express CD4 and have been infected by HIV in vivo. In vitro, HIV has been reported also to infect a wide range of cells and cell lines that express low levels of CD4, no detectable CD4, or only CD4 mRNA; among these are FDCs; megakaryocytes; eosinophils; astrocytes; oligodendrocytes; microglial cells; CD8+ T cells; B cells; NK cells; renal epithelial cells; cervical cells; rectal and bowel mucosal cells such as enterochromaffin, goblet, and columnar epithelial cells; trophoblastic cells; and cells from a variety of organs, such as liver, lung, heart, salivary gland, eye, prostate, testis, and adrenal gland. Since the only cells that have been shown unequivocally to be infected with HIV and to support replication of the virus are CD4+ T lymphocytes and cells of monocyte/macrophage lineage, the relevance of the in vitro infection of these other cell types is questionable.

Of potentially important clinical relevance is the demonstration that thymic precursor cells, which were assumed to be negative for CD3, CD4, and CD8 molecules, actually do express low levels of CD4 and can be infected with HIV in vitro. In addition, human thymic epithelial cells transplanted into an immunodeficient mouse can be infected with HIV by direct inoculation of virus into the thymus. Since these cells may play a role in the normal regeneration of CD4+ T cells, it is possible that their infection and depletion contribute, at least in part, to the impaired ability of the CD4+ T cell pool to completely reconstitute itself in certain infected individuals in whom antiretroviral therapy has suppressed viral replication to <50 copies of HIV RNA per milliliter (see below). In addition, CD34+ monocyte precursor cells have been shown to be infected in vivo in patients with advanced HIV disease. It is likely that these cells express low levels of CD4, and therefore it is not essential to invoke CD4-independent mechanisms to explain the infection.

ABNORMALITIES OF MONONUCLEAR CELLS ■ CD4+ T Cells The range of T cell abnormalities in advanced HIV infection is broad. The defects are both quantitative and qualitative and affect virtually every limb of the immune system (see below), indicating the critical dependence of the integrity of the immune system on the inducer/helper function of CD4+ T cells. In advanced HIV disease, virtually all of the observed immune defects can ultimately be explained by the quantitative depletion of CD4+ T cells. However, T cell dysfunction (see below) can be demonstrated in patients early in the course of infection, even when the CD4+ T cell count is in the low-normal range. The degree and spectrum of dysfunctions increase as the disease progresses. One of the first abnormalities to be detected is a defect in response to remote recall antigens, such as tetanus toxoid and influenza, at a time when mononuclear cells can still respond normally to mitogenic stimulation. Defects in responses to soluble antigens are followed in time by the loss of T cell proliferative responses to alloantigens, and subsequently to mitogens. Essentially every T cell function has been reported to be abnormal at some stage of HIV infection. These abnormalities include defective T cell cloning and colony-forming efficiencies, impaired expression of IL-2 receptors, defective IL-2 production, and decreased IFN-γ production in response to antigens. The proportion of CD4+ T cells that express CD28, which is a major co-stimulatory molecule necessary for the normal activation of T cells, is reduced during HIV infection. Cells lacking expression of CD28 do not respond normally

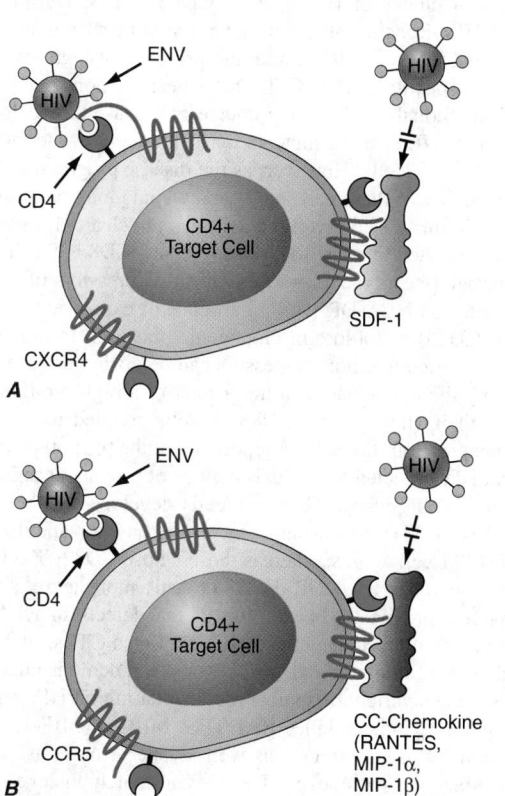

FIGURE 173-20 Model for the role of co-receptors CXCR4 and CCR5 in the efficient binding and entry of X4 (*A*) and R5 (*B*) strains of HIV-1, respectively, into CD4+ target cells. Blocking of this initial event in the virus life cycle can be accomplished by inhibition of binding to the co-receptor by the normal ligand for the receptor in question. The ligand for CXCR4 is stromal cell–derived factor (SDF-1); the ligands for CCR5 are RANTES, MIP-1α, and MIP-1β.

to activation signals and may express markers of terminal activation including HLA-DR, CD38, and CD45RO. CD4+ T cells from HIV-infected individuals express abnormally low levels of CD40 ligand, which may contribute to the dysregulation of B cell function observed in HIV disease.

It is difficult to explain completely the profound immunodeficiency noted in HIV-infected individuals solely on the basis of direct infection and quantitative depletion of CD4+ T cells. This is particularly apparent during the early stages of HIV disease, when CD4+ T cell numbers may be only marginally decreased. In this regard, it is likely that CD4+ T cell dysfunction results from a combination of depletion of cells due to direct infection of the cell and a number of virus-related but indirect effects on the cell (Table 173-6). Indeed, it has been demonstrated that patients with high levels of plasma viremia have a variety of subtle abnormalities of CD4+ T cell function, particularly involving aberrancies in signal transduction pathways. These abnormalities could be due either to aberrant activation induced by the cascade of cytokines that are expressed in viremic patients or by the direct effect of virus on the cell. In this regard, certain of these abnormalities can be reproduced by exposing CD4+ T cells of normal individuals to oligomeric HIV envelope proteins in vitro (see below).

Single-cell killing and the formation of syncytia between infected and uninfected cells have been demonstrated clearly in vitro, although the precise mechanisms of cell death in vivo have not been determined. Cytopathicity in an infected cell in vitro may result from a number of mechanisms, including copious budding of virions from the cell surface with resulting disruption of the integrity of the cell membrane; interference with cellular RNA processing or the accumulation of high levels of heterodisperse RNA molecules; disruption of cellular protein synthesis owing to high levels of viral RNA; accumulation of high levels of unintegrated viral DNA in the cell cytoplasm; induction of aberrant patterns of protein tyrosine phosphorylation; and the interaction between HIV gp120 and CD4 intracellularly. Strain differences in single-cell killing are determined largely by gp120 sequences, which supports the importance of the viral envelope in this process. *Syncytia formation* involves fusion of the cell membrane of an infected cell with the cell membranes of variable numbers of uninfected CD4+ cells. Although cell fusion has not been shown to be an important pathogenic process in vivo, a direct relationship between the presence of syncytia and the degree of cytopathic effect has been demonstrated in vitro, and a correlation has been reported between the presence of virus isolates that readily induce syncytia in vitro and a more aggressive clinical course in the patient. Humoral and cellular immune responses to HIV may contribute to protective immunity by eliminating virus and virus-infected cells (see below). However, since the main targets of HIV infection are immunocompetent cells, these responses may contribute to immune cell depletion and immunologic dysfunction by eliminating both infected cells and "innocent bystander" cells. Soluble viral proteins, particularly gp120, can bind with high affinity to the CD4 molecules on uninfected T cells and monocytes; in addition, virus and/or viral proteins can bind to dendritic cells or FDCs. HIV-specific antibody can recognize these bound molecules and potentially collaborate in the elimination of the cells by ADCC.

Nonpolymorphic determinants of MHC class I products share a degree of homology with gp120 and gp41 proteins of HIV. Such similarities may lead to the generation of autoantibodies to self-MHC determinants. In fact, anti-HLA-DR antibodies have been demonstrated in the sera of HIV-infected individuals (see "Autoimmune Phenomena," above). These antibodies could contribute to the elimination of HLA-DR–expressing cells by ADCC; in addition, it has been suggested that these antibodies may inhibit certain T cell functions that involve HLA-DR molecules.

HIV envelope glycoproteins gp120 and gp160 manifest high-affinity binding to CD4 as well as to various chemokine receptors (see above). Intracellular signals transduced by gp120 have been associated with a number of immunopathogenic processes including anergy, apoptosis, and abnormalities of cell trafficking. The molecular mechanisms responsible for these abnormalities include dysregulation of the T cell receptor–phosphoinositide pathway, p56lck activation, phosphorylation of focal adhesion kinase, activation of the MAP kinase and ras signaling pathways, and downregulation of the co-stimulatory molecules CD40 ligand and CD80.

Finally, the inexorable decline in CD4+ T cell counts that occurs in most HIV-infected individuals may result in part from the inability of the immune system to regenerate the rapidly turning over CD4+ T cell pool efficiently enough to compensate for both HIV-mediated and naturally occurring attrition of cells. At least two major mechanisms may contribute to the failure of the CD4+ T cell pool to reconstitute itself adequately over the course of HIV infection. The first is the destruction of lymphoid precursor cells, including thymic and bone marrow progenitor cells (see above); the other is the gradual disruption of the lymphoid tissue microenvironment, which is essential for efficient regeneration of immunocompetent cells (see above).

CD8+ T Cells   A relative C8+ T lymphocytosis is generally associated with high levels of HIV plasma viremia and may in part reflect the expansion of clones of HIV-specific CD8+ CTLs. During the late stages of HIV infection, there may be a significant reduction in the numbers of CD8+ T cells despite the presence of high levels of viremia. HIV-specific CD8+ CTLs have been demonstrated in HIV-infected individuals early in the course of disease (see below). The emergence of HIV escape mutants may ultimately evade these HIV-specific CD8+ T cells. However, as the disease progresses, the functional capability of these cells may decrease and may be lost entirely. The cause of this loss of cytolytic activity is unclear. However, it has been demonstrated that, as disease progresses, CD8+ T cells assume an abnormal phenotype characterized by expression of activation markers such as HLA-DR with an absence of expression of the IL-2 receptor (CD25) and a loss of clonogenic potential. In this regard, it has been reported that nonprogressors can be distinguished from progressors by the maintenance in the former of a high proliferative capacity of their HIV-specific CD8+ T cells coupled to increases in perforin expression. It has been reported that the phenotype of CD8+ T cells in HIV-infected individuals may be of prognostic significance. Those individuals whose CD8+ T cells developed a phenotype of HLA-DR+/CD38− following seroconversion had stabilization of their CD4+ T cell counts, whereas those whose CD8+ T cells developed a phenotype of HLA-DR+/CD38+ had a more aggressive course and a poorer prognosis. In addition to the defects in HIV-specific CTLs, functional defects in other MHC-restricted CTLs, such as those directed against influenza and CMV, have been demonstrated. CD8+ T cells secrete a variety of soluble factors that inhibit HIV replication including the CC-chemokines RANTES, MIP-1α, MIP-1β, and the alpha defensins -1, -2, and -3, as well as one or more as yet poorly identified factors (see above). The presence of high levels of HIV viremia in vivo as well as exposure of CD8+ T cells in vitro to HIV envelope has been shown to be associated with a variety of cellular functional abnormalities. Finally, since the integrity of CD8+ T cell function depends in part on adequate inductive signals from CD4+ T cells, the defect in CD8+ CTLs is likely compounded by the quantitative loss and qualitative dysfunction of CD4+ T cells.

TABLE 173-6   *Mechanisms of CD4+ T Cell Dysfunction and Depletion*

Direct Mechanisms	Indirect Mechanisms
Loss of plasma membrane integrity due to viral budding	Aberrant intracellular signaling events
Accumulation of unintegrated viral DNA	Autoimmunity
Interference with cellular RNA processing	Innocent bystander killing of viral antigen–coated cells
Intracellular gp120-CD4 autofusion events	Apoptosis
Syncytia formation	Inhibition of lymphopoiesis
	Activation-induced cell death
	Elimination of HIV-infected cells by virus-specific immune responses

B Cells The predominant defect in B cells from HIV-infected individuals is one of aberrant cellular activation, which is reflected by spontaneous proliferation and immunoglobulin secretion and by increased spontaneous secretion of TNF-α and IL-6. In addition, B cells from HIV viremic patients manifest a decreased capacity to mount a proliferative response to ligation of the B cell antigen receptor (surface IgM) at the same time as they are capable of robust differentiation in response to a variety of stimuli. B cells from HIV-infected individuals manifest enhanced spontaneous in vitro transformation with EBV, a process that is likely due to defective T cell immune surveillance. The in vivo counterpart of this phenomenon is an increase in the incidence of EBV-related B cell lymphomas. Untransformed B cells cannot be infected with HIV. However, HIV or its products can activate B cells directly; portions of the HIV gp41 envelope protein have been reported to induce polyclonal B cell activation. In addition, it has been reported that products of the VH$_3$ genes on the surface of B cells can serve as a receptor for HIV. B cells from patients with high levels of viremia bind virions to their surface via the CD21 complement receptor. It is likely that in vivo activation of B cells by virus products during the viremic state accounts at least in part for the spontaneous activation of these cells noted ex vivo. B cells from HIV-infected individuals express abnormally low levels of HLA-DR and CD21 on their surface. Cognate B cell–CD4+ T cell interactions are abnormal in viremic HIV-infected individuals. B cells respond poorly to CD4+ T cell help; this is due at least in part to an intrinsic defect in responder B cells with regard to their inability to normally upregulate CD25 (IL-2 receptor) and thus to proliferate normally in response to IL-2; in addition, B cells fail to adequately upregulate CD80 and CD86 following stimulation with activated T cells. In vivo, the aberrant activated state of B cells manifests itself by hypergammaglobulinemia and by the presence of circulating immune complexes and autoantibodies (see above). HIV-infected individuals respond poorly to primary and secondary immunizations with protein and polysaccharide antigens. These B cell defects are likely responsible in part for the increase in certain bacterial infections seen in advanced HIV disease in adults, as well as for the important role of bacterial infections in the morbidity and mortality of HIV-infected children, who cannot mount an adequate humoral response to common bacterial pathogens. The absolute number of circulating B cells may be depressed in primary HIV infection; however, this phenomenon is usually transient and likely reflects in part a redistribution of cells out of the circulation and into the lymphoid tissue. In certain patients, the number of circulating B cells decreases in advanced-stage disease.

Monocyte/Macrophages Circulating monocytes are generally normal in number in HIV-infected individuals. Monocytes express the CD4 molecule and several co-receptors for HIV on their surface, including CCR5, CXCR4, and CCR3, and thus are targets of HIV infection. Of note is the fact that the degree of cytopathicity of HIV for cells of the monocyte lineage is low, and HIV can replicate extensively in cells of the monocyte lineage with little cytopathic effect. Hence, monocyte-lineage cells may play a role in the dissemination of HIV in the body and can serve as reservoirs of HIV infection, thus representing an obstacle to the eradication of HIV by antiretroviral drugs. In vivo infection of circulating monocytes is difficult to demonstrate; however, infection of tissue macrophages and macrophage-lineage cells in the brain (infiltrating macrophages or resident microglial cells) and lung (pulmonary alveolar macrophages) can be demonstrated easily. Tissue macrophages are an important source of HIV during opportunistic infections. Infection of monocyte precursors in the bone marrow may directly or indirectly be responsible for certain of the hematologic abnormalities in HIV-infected individuals. A number of abnormalities of circulating monocytes have been reported in HIV-infected individuals, including decreased secretion of IL-1 and IL-12; increased secretion of IL-10; defects in antigen presentation and induction of T cell responses due to decreased MHC class II expression; and abnormalities of Fc receptor function, C3 receptor–mediated clearance, oxidative burst responses, and certain cytotoxic functions such as ADCC,

possibly related to low levels of expression of Fc and complement receptors. Exposure of monocytes to viral proteins such as gp120 and Tat, as well as to certain cytokines, can cause abnormal activation, and this may play a role in cellular dysfunction (see above).

Dendritic and Langerhans Cells Dendritic cells play an important role in the initiation of HIV infection by virtue of the ability of HIV to bind to cell surface C-type lectin receptors, particularly DC-SIGN (see above). This allows efficient presentation of virus to CD4+ T cell targets that become infected; complexes of infected CD4+ T cells and dendritic cells provide an optimal microenvironment for virus replication. There has been considerable disagreement regarding the HIV infectibility and hence the depletion as well as the dysfunction of dendritic cells themselves. Depending on their state of maturation, dendritic cells express varying levels of CD4 as well as several chemokine receptors. In this regard, it appears that the ability of a dendritic cell to become infected depends in part on its state of maturation. Mature dendritic cells have been demonstrated to be infectable by both R5 and X4 isolates of HIV-1. Immature tissue dendritic cells have been less well studied in their native state. Even in those dendritic cells in which infection occurs, the efficiency of infection and level of productivity of infection is quite low compared to CD4+ T cells.

Natural Killer Cells The role of NK cells is to provide immunosurveillance against virus-infected cells, certain tumor cells, and allogeneic cells (Chap. 295). Functional abnormalities in NK cells have been observed throughout the course of HIV disease, and the severity of these abnormalities increases as disease progresses. Most studies report that NK cells are normal in number and phenotype in HIV-infected individuals; however, a numerical decrease in the CD16+/CD56+ subpopulation of NK cells has been reported together with an increase in activation markers. The abnormality in NK cell function is thought to result from a defect in postbinding lysis. However, the lytic machinery does not appear to be impaired, since NK cells from HIV-infected individuals mediate ADCC normally. The addition of either IL-2, IL-12, IL-15, or IFN-α to cultures improves the defective in vitro NK cell function of HIV-infected individuals. HIV-mediated downregulation of HLA-A and -B, but not HLA-C and -D molecules may inhibit NK-mediated killing of HIV-infected target cells. NK cells serve as important sources of HIV-inhibitory CC-chemokines. NK cells isolated from HIV-infected individuals constitutively produce high levels of MIP-1α, MIP-1β, and RANTES. In addition, high levels of these chemokines are seen when NK cells are stimulated with IL-2 or IL-15 or when CD16 is cross-linked or during the process of lytic killing of target cells. HIV-infected patients with high levels of plasma viremia manifest a decreased ability, compared to HIV-infected individuals who are aviremic, of their NK cells to block HIV replication in vitro in assays of both cell contact and supernatant-mediated suppression of virus. In addition, viremic patients have a decrease in expression of activating receptors (responsible for killer activity) and an increase in certain inhibitory receptors (responsible for inhibition of killer activity) on NK cells, suggesting one potential mechanism whereby viremia might inhibit the ability of NK cells to kill HIV-infected target cells.

GENETIC FACTORS IN HIV PATHOGENESIS Several reports have described MHC alleles and other host factors that may influence the pathogenesis and course of HIV disease. These include associations with certain HIV-related manifestations, such as KS and diffuse lymphadenopathy, or with the type of clinical course, such as long-term survival or rapid progression (Table 173-7). A number of mechanisms have been proposed whereby MHC-encoded molecules might predispose an individual either to rapid progression or to nonprogression to AIDS. These proposed mechanisms include the ability to present certain immunodominant HIV T helper or CTL epitopes, leading to a relatively protective immune response against HIV and hence to slow progression of disease. In contrast, certain MHC class I or class II alleles might predispose an individual to an immunopathogenic response against

Factor	Association
MAJOR HISTOCOMPATIBILITY LOCI-ENCODED GENES	
B35, C4, DR1, DQ1	Kaposi's sarcoma
DR1	Kaposi's sarcoma
DR2, DR5	Kaposi's sarcoma
DR5	Kaposi's sarcoma
Aw23, Bw49	Kaposi's sarcoma
B62	Fever, skin rash in primary HIV infection
Aw19	HIV seropositivity in individuals multiply exposed to HIV
A1, A24, C7, B8, DR3	Rapid progression to AIDS
DR4, DQB1*0302	Rapid progression to AIDS
DR3, DQ1	Rapid progression to AIDS
B*35	Rapid progression to AIDS
Cw*04	Rapid progression to AIDS
TAP2.1	Promotes HIV progression to AIDS
DR5	Thrombocytopenia and lymphadenopathy in HIV infection
DR5, DR6	Diffuse infiltrative CD8+ lymphocytosis with Sjögren-like syndrome in HIV infection
Bw4	Slow decline in CD4+ T cell count
B13, B27, B51, B57, DQB1*0302,0303	Protects from progression to AIDS
B*5701	Strong protection from progression to AIDS
A26, B38, TAP1.4, TAP2.3	Ability to clear HIV infection in transiently infected seronegative individuals
A28, Bw70, Aw69, B18	Protection from HIV infection
A32, B4, C2	Long-term survival in HIV infection
A11, A32, B13, C2, DQA1*0301, DQB1*0302, DRB1*0400, DRB4*0101	Long-term survival in HIV infection
Heterozygosity for class I loci (A, B, and C)	Delayed onset to AIDS
Homozygosity for class I loci (A, B, and C)	Rapid onset to AIDS and death
OTHER GENES	
p53 tumor-suppressor gene	Controls HIV replicative patterns and determinant of viral latency
CCR5 gene	Homozygous defect involving a 32-bp deletion corresponding to the second extracellular loop of the receptor results in resistance to infection; heterozygous defect appears to result in partial protection against disease progression. Also, several single nucleotide polymorphisms (SNPs) in the CCR5 promoter have been shown to be associated with variable rates of progression in AIDS.
CCR2 gene	Heterozygosity for CCR2-64I mutation is associated with delay in progression of HIV disease
CX3CR1 gene	Mutations in I249 and M280 associated with rapid progression to AIDS
RANTES gene	A mutation of the RANTES gene (RANTES-28G) results in increased transcription and expression of RANTES on mononuclear cells with resulting inhibition of infection with R5 strains of HIV and delay of disease progression. Three SNPs; 403A in the RANTES promoter, In1.1C in the first intron, and 3'222C in the 3' untranslated region of the gene are associated with increased frequency of HIV-1 infection. The SNP In1.1C allele results in decreased RANTES production and correlates with rapid progression to AIDS.
IL-10 gene	Individuals carrying the IL10-5'-592A promoter allele were at increased risk for HIV infection and, once infected, progressed more rapidly than homozygotes for the alternative IL10-5'-592 C/C genotype
VDR gene	Homozygosity for vitamin D receptor gene polymorphism B (VDR-BB) correlates with rapid progression to AIDS
IL-4 gene	SNP IL-4-589T causes higher levels of IL-4 production in vivo, resulting in downregulation of CCR5. The presence of SNP IL-4-589T is modestly associated with protection from acquisition of HIV-1 by heterosexual contact. This SNP also correlates with slower disease progression and decreased viral load early in infection.
IL-1ra gene	Homozygosity IL-1ra gene*2 correlates with significantly lower viral loads.
TNF-α gene	SNP TNF-α-238A, but not the -308A allele correlates with a higher frequency of lipodystrophy.
IL-6 gene	Among HIV-positive men, homozygosity for SNP IL-6-174G carries an increased risk of development of Kaposi sarcoma; men with homozygosity for SNP IL-6-174C were less likely to develop Kaposi sarcoma.
GENE INTERACTIONS	
KIR gene with HLA-B	In the absence of HLA-B Bw4-80I, KIR3DS1 is strongly associated with rapid progression to AIDS. This effect is reversed by the presence of HLA-B Bw4-80I. Individuals carrying both genes have a delayed progression to AIDS; in the absence of KIR3DS1, HLA-B Bw4-80I has no effect on disease progression.

Sources: Adapted from BF Haynes et al: Science 271:324, 1996; O'Brien and Moore.

viral epitopes in certain tissues, such as the CNS or lungs, or against certain HIV-infected cell types, such as macrophages or dendritic cells/Langerhans cells. In addition, certain rare MHC class I and class II alleles might facilitate rapid recognition of HIV-infected cells from the infecting partner in primary HIV infection and promote rejection of these cells by alloreactive responses. Similarly, common MHC alleles could lead to less effective removal of HIV-infected allogeneic cells. It has been clearly demonstrated that maximal *HLA* heterozygosity for class I loci (A, B, and C) is associated with a delayed onset of AIDS among HIV-infected individuals, whereas homozygosity for these loci was associated with a more rapid progression to AIDS and death. This observation is likely due to the fact that individuals who

are heterozygous at *HLA* loci are able to present a greater variety of antigenic peptides to cytotoxic T lymphocytes than are homozygotes, resulting in a more effective immune response against a number of pathogens including HIV. Of particular note is the fact that the HLA class I alleles B*35 and Cw*04 were consistently associated with rapid development of AIDS. Other data have indicated that transporter associated with antigen-presenting (TAP) genes play a role in determining the outcome of HIV infection. HLA profiles that reflect certain combinations of MHC-encoded TAP and class I and class II genes are strongly associated with different rates of progression to AIDS. A recent finding of genetic association with HIV disease progression has highlighted the role for NK cells in HIV disease. A single nucleotide polymorphism (SNP) in the killer immunoglobulin-like receptor (KIR) gene was shown to be strongly associated with rapid progression to AIDS. However, when the KIR3 DS1 SNP was present with HLA-B Bw4-80I, the resultant phenotype was delayed progression to AIDS, even though this HLA-B allele alone has no effect on HIV disease progression. Furthermore, the KIR3 DS1/HLA-B Bw4-80I-carrying individuals had a significantly reduced viral load, beginning early in the course of infection. This points to the potential role of NK cells in the maintenance of the viral set point, strongly suggesting that HLA-B Bw4-80I serves as the ligand activating this KIR receptor, resulting in the death of the target cell.

The most dramatic example of a genetic factor influencing HIV infection and/or pathogenesis relates to the gene that codes for the HIV cellular co-receptor CCR5. Rare individuals have been reported who had had repetitive sexual exposure to HIV in high-risk situations but remained uninfected. The peripheral blood mononuclear cells of two such individuals were found to be highly resistant to infection in vitro with R5 strains of HIV-1, but they were readily infected with X4 strains. Genetic analysis revealed that these two individuals inherited a homozygous defect in the gene that codes for CCR5, the cellular co-receptor for R5 strains of HIV-1. The defective *CCR5* allele contained a 32-bp deletion corresponding to the second extracellular loop of the receptor. The encoded protein was severely truncated, and the receptor was nonfunctional, explaining the refractoriness to infection with R5 strains of HIV-1. Population studies revealed that ~1% of the Caucasian population of western European ancestry possessed the homozygous defect. Up to 20% of this group had the heterozygous defect. Of note, cohort studies of hundreds of DNA samples originating from western and central Africa and Japan did not reveal a single mutant allele, suggesting that the allele is either absent or extremely rare in Africa and Japan. In a cohort of 1400 HIV-1–infected Caucasian individuals, no subject homozygous for the mutation was found, strongly supporting the concept that the homozygous defect confers protection against infection. This finding is particularly compelling in light of the fact that transmitting viruses are strongly biased towards R5 strains of HIV-1 (see above). Furthermore, there was a higher frequency of individuals heterozygous for the genetic defect among HIV-infected patients who were long-term nonprogressors compared to HIV-infected individuals who progressed more rapidly (see above). Of note, several individuals have been identified who were homozygous for the *CCR5*-Δ32 defect who in fact did become infected with HIV. These individuals were found to have an X4 strain of HIV that was associated in some cases with an accelerated course of disease. Slow progression of HIV disease is also seen in individuals who are heterozygous for the *CCR2-64I* mutation or SNP; this is felt to be due to dimerization of CXCR4 with the mutated CCR2-64I resulting in a decreased expression of CXCR4 on the cell surface. Delayed progression of disease is also seen in those individuals who have any of a number of SNPs in the *CCR5* promoter. In addition, individuals who carry a certain allele (IL-10-5-592A) of the IL-10 promoter are at increased risk of infection and, once infected, progress more rapidly than homozygotes for the alternative genotype. The mechanism of this effect is felt to be a downregulation of the inhibitory cytokine IL-10 resulting in facilitation of HIV replication. The SNP, IL-4-589T, increases IL-4 production. This allele associates with a slower progression to AIDS, presumably through the downregulation of CCR5 by higher and more sustained levels of IL-4. Separate SNPs have been found in the RANTES gene that correlate with either an increased or decreased expression of this chemokine (Table 173-7). As expected, based upon the effect of RANTES as an inhibitor of R5 HIV, RANTES-28G SNP upregulates RANTES and is associated with delayed progression to AIDS. The opposite effects are seen with SNP RANTES In1.1C. This SNP decreases RANTES expression and correlates strongly with rapid progression to AIDS. Other SNPs that decrease RANTES expression are associated with a higher rate of HIV infection, reinforcing the central role for R5 viruses in the establishment of HIV infection.

Additional genes have been found that are associated with rapid progression to AIDS or susceptibility to significant AIDS complication. Homozygosity for the vitamin D receptor form B correlates with rapid progression to AIDS. The mechanism is thought to relate to the known effects of vitamin D on immune modulation. The TNF-α SNP-238A is associated with a higher frequency of lipodystrophy. The underlying causes of this complication of AIDS remain to be defined, including the role of combination antiretroviral therapy. Finally, SNP IL-6-174G has been shown to lead to higher levels of IL-6. Homozygosity at this locus correlates with an increased risk of development of KS. Not surprisingly, homozygosity for SNP IL-6-174C, which results in lower levels of IL-6, was protective, correlating with significantly lower levels of KS.

NEUROPATHOGENESIS HIV-infected individuals can experience a variety of neurologic abnormalities due either to opportunistic infections and neoplasms (see below) or to direct effects of HIV or its products. With regard to the latter, HIV has been demonstrated in the brain and CSF of infected individuals with and without neuropsychiatric abnormalities. The main cell types that are infected in the brain in vivo are the perivascular macrophages and the microglial cells; monocytes that have already been infected in the blood can migrate into the brain, where they then reside as macrophages, or macrophages can be directly infected within the brain. The precise mechanisms whereby HIV enters the brain are unclear; however, they are felt to relate, at least in part, to the ability of virus-infected and immune-activated macrophages to induce adhesion molecules such as E-selectin and vascular cell adhesion molecule-1 (VCAM-1) on brain endothelium. Other studies have demonstrated that HIV gp120 enhances the expression of intercellular adhesion molecule-1 (ICAM-1) in glial cells; this effect may facilitate entry of HIV-infected cells into the CNS and may promote syncytia formation. Virus isolates from the brain are preferentially R5 strains as opposed to X4 strains (see above); in this regard, HIV-infected individuals who are heterozygous for *CCR5-δ32* appear to be relatively protected against the development of HIV encephalopathy compared to wild-type individuals. Distinct HIV envelope sequences are associated with the clinical expression of the AIDS dementia complex (see below). Although there have been reports of infrequent HIV infection of neuronal cells and astrocytes, there is no convincing evidence that brain cells other than those of monocyte/macrophage lineage can be productively infected in vivo.

HIV-infected individuals may manifest white matter lesions as well as neuronal loss. Given the relative absence of evidence of HIV infection of neurons either in vivo or in vitro, it is unlikely that direct infection of these cells accounts for their loss. Rather, the HIV-mediated effects on neurons and oligodendrocytes are felt to involve indirect pathways whereby viral proteins, particularly gp120 and Tat, trigger the release of endogenous neurotoxins from macrophages and to a lesser extent from astrocytes. In addition, it has been demonstrated that both HIV-1 Nef and Tat can induce chemotaxis of leukocytes, including monocytes, into the CNS. Neurotoxins can be released from monocytes as a consequence of infection and/or immune activation. Monocyte-derived neurotoxic factors have been reported to kill neurons via the N-methyl-D-aspartate (NMDA) receptor. In addition, HIV gp120 shed by virus-infected monocytes could cause neurotoxicity by antagonizing the function of vasoactive intestinal peptide (VIP), by elevating intracellular calcium levels, and by decreasing nerve growth factor levels in the cerebral cortex. A variety of monocyte-derived cytokines can contribute directly or indirectly to the neurotoxic effects in HIV infection; these include TNF-α, IL-1, IL-6, TGF-β, IFN-γ, platelet-activating factor, and endothelin. Furthermore, among the CC-chemokines, elevated levels of monocyte chemotactic protein (MCP)1 in the brain and CSF have been shown to correlate best with the presence and degree of HIV encephalopathy. In addition, infection and/or activation of monocyte-lineage cells can result in increased production of eicosanoids, nitric oxide, and quinolinic acid, which may contribute to neurotoxicity. Astrocytes may play diverse roles in HIV neuropathogenesis. Reactive gliosis or astrocytosis has been demonstrated in the brains of HIV-infected individuals, and TNF-α and IL-6 have been shown to induce astrocyte proliferation. In addition, astrocyte-derived IL-6 can induce HIV expression in infected cells in vitro. Furthermore, it has been suggested that astrocytes may downregulate macrophage-produced neurotoxins. It has been reported that HIV-infected individuals with the E4 allele for apolipoprotein E (apo E) are at increased risk for AIDS encephalopathy and peripheral neuropathy. The likelihood that HIV or its products are involved in neuropathogenesis is supported by the observation that neuropsychiatric abnormalities may undergo remarkable and rapid improvement upon the initiation of antiretroviral therapy; this is true of HIV-infected children as well as adults. In fact, there has been a remarkable decrease in the incidence of HIV encephalopathy in the era of successful combination antiretroviral therapy.

PATHOGENESIS OF KAPOSI'S SARCOMA There are at least four distinct epidemiologic forms of KS: (1) the classic form that occurs in older men of predominantly Mediterranean or eastern European Jewish backgrounds with no recognized contributing factors; (2) the equatorial African form that occurs in all ages, also without any recognized precipitating factors; (3) the form associated with organ transplantation and its attendant iatrogenic immunosuppressed state; and (4) the form associated with HIV-1 infection. In the latter two forms, KS is an opportunistic disease; in HIV-infected individuals, unlike typical opportunistic infections, its occurrence is not strictly related to the level of depression of CD4+ T cell counts (see below). The pathogenesis of KS is complex; fundamentally, it is an angioproliferative disease that is not a true neoplastic sarcoma, at least not in its early stages. It is a manifestation of excessive proliferation of spindle cells that are believed to be of vascular origin and have features in common with endothelial and smooth-muscle cells. In HIV disease the development of KS is dependent on the interplay of a variety of factors including HIV-1 itself, human herpes virus 8 (HHV-8), immune activation, and cytokine secretion. A number of epidemiologic and virologic studies have clearly linked HHV-8, which is also referred to as *Kaposi's sarcoma–associated herpesvirus* (KSHV), to KS not only in HIV-infected individuals but also in individuals with the other forms of KS. HHV-8 is a γ-herpesvirus related to EBV and herpesvirus saimiri. It encodes a homologue to human IL-6 and in addition to KS has been implicated in the pathogenesis of body cavity lymphoma, multiple myeloma, and monoclonal gammopathy of undetermined significance. Sequences of HHV-8 are found universally in the lesions of KS, and patients with KS are virtually all seropositive for HHV-8. HHV-8 DNA sequences can be found in the B cells of 30 to 50% of patients with KS and 7% of patients with AIDS without clinically apparent KS.

Between 1 and 2% of eligible blood donors are positive for antibodies to HHV-8, while the prevalence of HHV-8 seropositivity in HIV-infected men is 30 to 35%. The prevalence in HIV-infected women is ~4%. This finding is reflective of the lower incidence of KS in women. It has been debated whether HHV-8 is actually the transforming agent in KS; the bulk of the cells in the tumor lesions of KS are not neoplastic cells. However, it has been demonstrated that endothelial cells can be transformed in vitro by HHV-8. In this regard, HHV-8 possesses a number of genes including homologues of the IL-8 receptor, Bcl-2, and cyclin D, which can potentially transform the host cell. Despite the complexity of the pathogenic events associated with the development of KS in HIV-infected individuals, it is generally agreed that HHV-8 is indeed the etiologic agent of this disease. The initiation and/or propagation of KS requires an activated state and is mediated, at least in part, by cytokines. A number of factors, including TNF-α, IL-1β, IL-6, GM-CSF, basic fibroblast growth factor, and oncostatin M, function in an autocrine and paracrine manner to sustain the growth and chemotaxis of the KS spindle cells. In this regard, KSHV-derived IL-6 has been demonstrated to induce proliferation of lymphoma cells and to inhibit the cytostatic effects of INF-α on

KSHV-infected lymphoma cells. It has been suggested that the HIV Tat protein plays a major role in the pathogenesis of KS. In this regard, it has been demonstrated that IFN-γ can induce endothelial cells to proliferate and to invade the extracellular matrix in response to HIV Tat. This occurs as a result of the upregulation by IFN-γ of the expression and activity of the receptors for Tat, which are the integrins $\alpha_5\beta_1$ and $\alpha_v\beta_3$. In addition, the HIV-1 Tat protein has been shown to act synergistically with basic fibroblast growth factor in the induction of lesions resembling KS lesions in mice by increasing matrix-metalloproteinase-2 secretion and activation in endothelial cells. Glucocorticoids have been shown to have a stimulatory effect, and human chorionic gonadotropin an inhibitory effect, on KS spindle cells, suggesting that modulation of the balance of autocrine factors may have therapeutic potential in KS. It has been demonstrated that HIV protease inhibitors have potent anti-angiogenic properties and, as such, promote regression of KS.

IMMUNE RESPONSE TO HIV

As detailed above and below, following the initial burst of viremia during primary infection, HIV-infected individuals mount a robust immune response that usually substantially curtails the levels of plasma viremia and likely contributes to delaying the ultimate development of clinically apparent disease for a median of 10 years. This immune response contains elements of both humoral and cell-mediated immunity (Table 173-8; Fig. 173-21). It is directed against multiple antigenic determinants of the HIV virion as well as against viral proteins expressed on the surface of infected cells. Ironically, those CD4+ T cells with T cell receptors specific for HIV are theoretically those CD4+ T cells most likely to bind to infected cells and themselves be infected and destroyed. Thus, an early consequence of HIV infection may be interference with the generation of an effective immune response through the elimination or compromise of HIV-specific CD4+ T lymphocytes.

Although a great deal of investigation has been directed toward delineating and better understanding the components of this immune response, it remains unclear which of these phenomena are most important in delaying progression of infection and which, if any, play a role in the pathogenesis of HIV disease. This lack of knowledge has also hampered the ability to develop an effective vaccine for HIV disease.

HUMORAL IMMUNE RESPONSE Antibodies to HIV usually appear within 6 weeks and almost invariably within 12 weeks of primary infection (Fig. 173-22); rare exceptions are individuals who have defects in the ability to produce HIV-specific antibodies. Detection of these antibodies forms the basis of most diagnostic screening tests for HIV infection. The appearance of HIV-binding antibodies detected by ELISA and western blot assays occurs prior to the appearance of neutralizing antibodies; the latter generally appear following the initial decreases in plasma viremia, which is more closely related to the appearance of HIV-specific CD8+ T lymphocytes. The first antibodies detected are

---

TABLE 173-8 *Elements of the Immune Response to HIV*

Humoral immunity
  Binding antibodies
  Neutralizing antibodies
    Type specific
    Group specific
  Antibodies participating in antibody-dependent cellular cytotoxicity (ADCC)
    Protective
    Pathogenic (bystander killing)
  Enhancing antibodies
Cell-mediated immunity
  Helper CD4+ T lymphocytes
  Class I MHC–restricted cytotoxic CD8+ T lymphocytes
  CD8+ T cell–mediated inhibition (noncytolytic)
  ADCC
  Natural killer cells

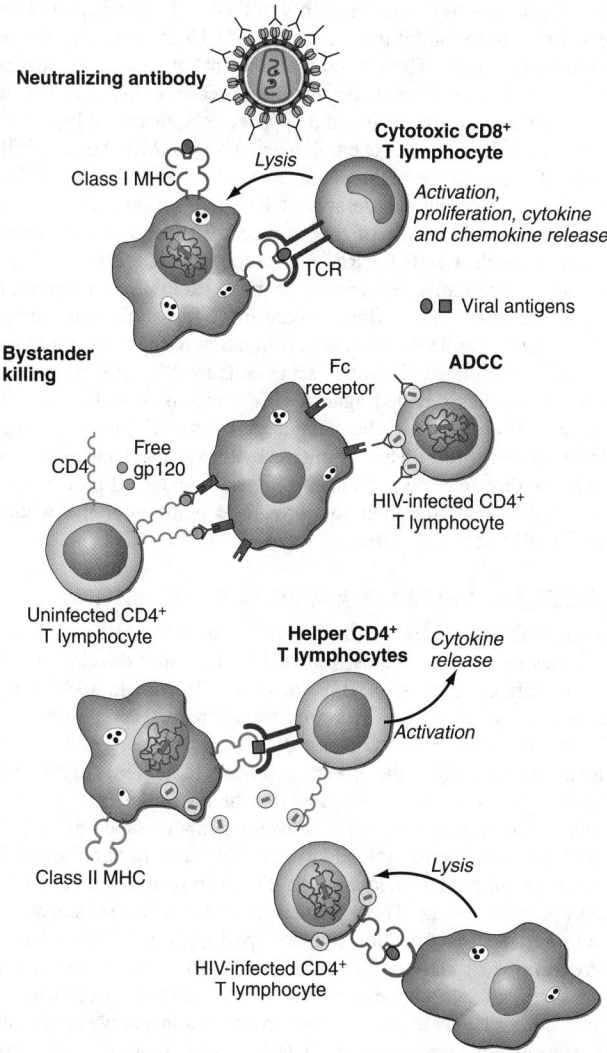

FIGURE 173-21 Schematic representation of the different immunologic effector mechanisms felt to be active in the setting of HIV infection. Detailed descriptions are given in the text. TCR, T cell receptor; ADCC, antibody dependent cellular cytotoxicity; MHC, major histocompatibility complex.

those directed against the structural or gag proteins of HIV, p24 and p17, and the gag precursor p55. The development of antibodies to p24 is associated with a decrease in the serum levels of free p24 antigen. Antibodies to the gag proteins are followed by the appearance of antibodies to the envelope proteins (gp160, gp120, p88, and gp41) and to the products of the *pol* gene (p31, p51, and p66). In addition, one may see antibodies to the low-molecular-weight regulatory proteins encoded by the HIV genes *vpr*, *vpu*, *vif*, *rev*, *tat*, and *nef*.

While antibodies to multiple antigens of HIV are produced, the precise functional significance of these different antibodies is unclear. The best studied have been the antibodies directed toward the envelope proteins of the virus. As noted above, the envelope of HIV consists of an outer envelope glycoprotein with a molecular mass of 120 kDa and a transmembrane glycoprotein with a molecular mass of 41 kDa. These are initially synthesized as a 160-kDa precursor that is cleaved by cellular proteases. Most of the antienvelope antibodies are directed either toward an epitope in the gp41 region comprising amino acids 579 to 613 or toward a hypervariable region in the gp120 molecule, known as the *V3 loop region*, comprising amino acids 303 through 338. This V3 region is a major site for the development of mutations that lead to variants of HIV that are not well recognized by the immune system.

Antibodies directed toward the envelope proteins of HIV have been characterized both as being protective and as possibly contributing to

the pathogenesis of HIV disease. Among the protective antibodies are those that function to neutralize HIV directly and prevent the spread of infection to additional cells, as well as those that participate in ADCC. *Neutralizing antibodies* may be a component of primary HIV infection, and some long-term nonprogressors have been reported to have increased titers of neutralizing antibodies. Neutralizing antibodies appear to be of two forms, type-specific and group-specific. *Type-specific neutralizing antibodies* are generally directed to the V3 loop region. These antibodies neutralize only viruses of a given strain and are present in low titer in most infected individuals. *Group-specific neutralizing antibodies* are capable of neutralizing a wide variety of HIV isolates. At least two forms of group-specific antibodies have been identified: those binding to amino acids 423 to 437 of gp120 and those binding to amino acids 728 to 745 of gp41. The other major class of protective antibodies are those that participate in ADCC, which is actually a form of cell-mediated immunity (Chap. 295) in which NK cells that bear Fc receptors are armed with specific anti-HIV antibodies that bind to the NK cells via their Fc portion. These armed NK cells then bind to and destroy cells expressing HIV antigens. Antibodies to both gp120 and gp41 have been shown to participate in ADCC-mediated killing of HIV-infected cells. The levels of antienvelope antibodies capable of mediating ADCC are highest in the earlier stages of HIV infection. In vitro, IL-2 can augment ADCC-mediated killing.

In addition to playing a role in host defense, HIV-specific antibodies have also been implicated in disease pathogenesis. Antibodies directed to gp41, when present in low titer, have been shown in vitro to be capable of facilitating infection of cells through an Fc receptor–mediated mechanism known as *antibody enhancement*. Thus, the same regions of the envelope protein of HIV that give rise to antibodies capable of mediating ADCC also elicit the production of antibodies that can facilitate infection of cells in vitro. In addition, it has been postulated that anti-gp120 antibodies that participate in the ADCC killing of HIV-infected cells might also kill uninfected CD4+ T cells if the uninfected cells had bound free gp120, a phenomenon referred to as *bystander killing*.

CELLULAR IMMUNE RESPONSE Given the fact that T cell–mediated immunity is known to play a major role in host defense against most viral infections (Chap. 295), it is generally thought to be an important component of the host immune response to HIV. T cell immunity can be divided into two major categories, mediated respectively by the *helper/inducer CD4+ T cells* and the *cytotoxic/immunoregulatory CD8+ T cells*.

HIV-specific CD4+ T cells can be detected in the majority of HIV-infected patients through the use of flow cytometry to measure single-

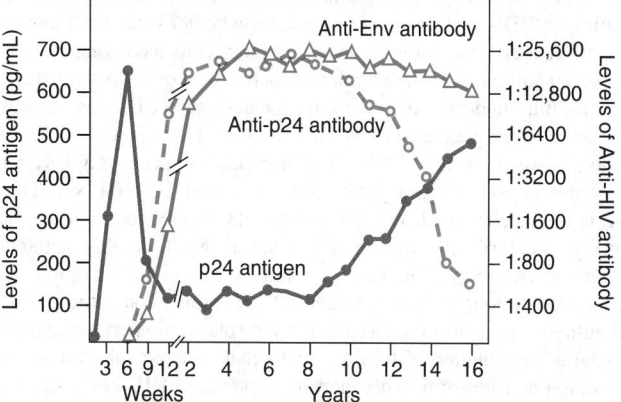

FIGURE 173-22 Relationship between antigenemia and the development of antibodies to HIV. Antibodies to HIV proteins are generally seen 6 to 12 weeks following infection and 3 to 6 weeks after the development of plasma viremia. Late in the course of illness, antibody levels to p24 decline, generally in association with a rising titer of p24 antigen.

cell IFN-γ production in response to HIV antigens, binding to MHC class II tetramers, or HIV p24 lymphocyte proliferation assays. Although these cells, with their high affinity for binding to HIV-infected cells, may be among the first to be infected and destroyed during HIV infection, they also are likely to undergo clonal expansions in response to HIV antigens and thus survive as a population of cells. No clear correlations exist between levels of HIV-specific CD4+ T lymphocytes and plasma HIV RNA levels; however, in the setting of high viral loads, CD4+ T cell responses to HIV antigens appear to shift from one of proliferaton to one of IFN-γ production. Thus, while a reverse correlation exists between the level of p24-specific proliferation and levels of plasma HIV viremia, the nature of the causal relationship between these parameters is unclear. Through the use of computer modeling, several regions of the HIV-1 envelope molecule have been identified that are structurally analogous to other known T cell epitopes by virtue of having structures known as *amphipathic helices*. Peptides from these envelope regions have been used to identify the presence of CD4+ T cells specific for these regions in the peripheral blood of HIV-infected individuals. Other studies have demonstrated that peripheral blood T cells of some healthy, HIV-negative individuals also react to the envelope proteins of HIV. It is unclear whether or not this represents the presence of a degree of protective immunity in these individuals.

MHC class I–restricted, HIV-specific CD8+ T cells have been identified in the peripheral blood of patients with HIV-1 infection. These cells include CTLs and T cells that can be induced by HIV antigens to express cytokines such as IFN-γ. CTLs have been identified in the peripheral blood of patients within weeks of HIV infection. These CD8+ T lymphocytes, through their HIV-specific antigen receptors, bind to and cause the lytic destruction of target cells bearing autologous MHC class I molecules associated with HIV antigens. Two types of CTL activity can be demonstrated in the peripheral blood or lymph node mononuclear cells of HIV-infected individuals. The first type directly lyses appropriate target cells in culture without prior in vitro stimulation (*spontaneous CTL activity*). The other type of CTL activity reflects the *precursor frequency of CTLs* (CTLp); this type of CTL activity can be demonstrated by stimulation of CD8+ T cells in vitro with a mitogen such as phytohemagglutinin or anti-CD3 antibody. Following primary HIV infection, the qualitative nature of the HIV-specific CTL response is an important predictor of eventual clinical outcome. Patients who mount a broad CD8+ CTL response generally have a more favorable clinical course than do patients who mount a more restricted CTL response. These data are consistent with studies in the SIV model where deletion of CD8+ T cells leads to a more accelerated clinical course.

In addition to CTLs, CD8+ T cells capable of being induced by HIV antigens to express cytokines such as IFN-γ also appear in the setting of HIV-1 infection. It is not clear whether these are the same or different effector pools compared to those cells mediating cytotoxicity; in addition, the relative roles of each in host defense against HIV are not fully understood. It does appear that these CD8+ T cells are driven to in vivo expansion by HIV antigen. There is a direct correlation between levels of CD8+ T cells capable of producing IFN-γ in response to HIV antigens and plasma levels of HIV-1 RNA. Thus, while these cells are clearly induced by HIV-1 infection, their overall ability to control infection remains unclear. Multiple HIV antigens, including Gag, Env, Pol, Tat, Rev, and Nef, can elicit CD8+ T cell responses. Among patients who control viral replication in the absence of antiretroviral drugs are a subset of patients whose peripheral blood contains a population of CD8+ T cells that undergo substantial proliferation and perforin expression in response to HIV antigens. It is possible that these cells play an important role in HIV-specific host defense.

At least three other forms of cell-mediated immunity to HIV have been described: CD8+ T cell–mediated suppression of HIV replication, ADCC, and NK cell activity. *CD8+ T cell–mediated suppression of HIV replication* refers to the ability of CD8+ T cells from an HIV-infected patient to inhibit the replication of HIV in tissue culture in a noncytolytic manner. There is no requirement for HLA compatibility between the CD8+ T cells and the HIV-infected cells. This effector mechanism is thus nonspecific and appears to be mediated by soluble factor(s) including the CC-chemokines RANTES, MIP-1α, and MIP-1β (see above) and the alpha defensin family of cytokines. The CC-chemokines are potent suppressors of HIV replication and operate at least in part via blockade of the co-receptor (CCR5) on peripheral blood mononuclear cells for R5 or macrophage-tropic strains of HIV (see above). The alpha defensins appear able to inhibit replication of either R5 or X4 viruses. The mechanism of this inhibition remains unclear. *ADCC*, as described above in relation to humoral immunity, involves the killing of HIV-expressing cells by NK cells armed with specific antibodies directed against HIV antigens. Finally, *NK cells* alone have been shown to be capable of killing HIV-infected target cells in tissue culture. This primitive cytotoxic mechanism of host defense is directed toward nonspecific surveillance for neoplastic transformation and viral infection through recognition of altered class I MHC molecules.

DIAGNOSIS AND LABORATORY MONITORING OF HIV INFECTION

The establishment of HIV as the causative agent of AIDS and related syndromes early in 1984 was followed by the rapid development of sensitive screening tests for HIV infection. By March, 1985, blood donors in the United States were routinely screened for antibodies to HIV. In June 1996, blood banks in the United States added the p24 antigen capture assay to the screening process to help identify the rare infected individuals who were donating blood in the time (up to 3 months) between infection and the development of antibodies. In 2002 the ability to detect early infection with HIV was further enhanced by the licensure of nucleic acid amplification testing as a routine part of blood donor screening. These refinements decreased the interval between infection and detection (window period) from 22 days for antibody testing to 16 days with p24 antigen testing and subsequently to 12 days with nucleic acid testing. The development of sensitive assays for monitoring levels of plasma viremia ushered in a new era of being able to monitor the progression of HIV disease more closely. Utilization of these tests, coupled with the measurement of levels of CD4+ T lymphocytes in peripheral blood, is essential in the management of patients with HIV infection.

DIAGNOSIS OF HIV INFECTION The diagnosis of HIV infection depends upon the demonstration of antibodies to HIV and/or the direct detection of HIV or one of its components. As noted above, antibodies to HIV generally appear in the circulation 2 to 12 weeks following infection.

The standard screening test for HIV infection is the ELISA, also referred to as an enzyme immunoassay (EIA). This solid-phase assay is an extremely good screening test with a sensitivity of >99.5%. Most diagnostic laboratories use a commercial EIA kit that contains antigens from both HIV-1 and HIV-2 and thus are able to detect either. These kits use both natural and recombinant antigens and are continuously updated to increase their sensitivity to newly discovered species, such as group O viruses (Fig. 173-6). EIA tests are generally scored as positive (highly reactive), negative (nonreactive), or indeterminate (partially reactive). While the EIA is an extremely sensitive test, it is not optimal with regard to specificity. This is particularly true in studies of low-risk individuals, such as volunteer blood donors. In this latter population, only 10% of EIA-positive individuals are subsequently confirmed to have HIV infection. Among the factors associated with false-positive EIA tests are antibodies to class II antigens, autoantibodies, hepatic disease, recent influenza vaccination, and acute viral infections. For these reasons, anyone suspected of having HIV infection based upon a positive or inconclusive EIA result must have the result confirmed with a more specific assay. One can estimate whether or not an indivdual has a recent infection with HIV-1 by comparing the results on a standard assay that will score positive for all infected individuals to the results on an assay modified to be less sensitive ("detuned assay") that will only score positive for individuals with established HIV infection.

The most commonly used confirmatory test is the western blot (Fig. 173-23). This assay takes advantage of the fact that multiple HIV antigens of different, well-characterized molecular weights elicit the production of specific antibodies. These antigens can be separated on the basis of molecular weight, and antibodies to each component can be detected as discrete bands on the western blot. A negative western blot is one in which no bands are present at molecular weights corresponding to HIV gene products. In a patient with a positive or indeterminate EIA and a negative western blot, one can conclude with certainty that the EIA reactivity was a false positive. On the other hand, a western blot demonstrating antibodies to products of all three of the major genes of HIV (*gag*, *pol*, and *env*) is conclusive evidence of infection with HIV. Criteria established by the U.S. Food & Drug Administration (FDA) in 1993 for a positive western blot state that a result is considered positive if antibodies exist to two of the three HIV proteins: p24, gp41, and gp120/160. Using these criteria, ~10% of all blood donors deemed positive for HIV-1 infection lacked an antibody band to the *pol* gene product p31. Some 50% of these blood donors were subsequently found to be false positives. Thus, the absence of the p31 band should increase the suspicion that one may be dealing with a false-positive test result. In this setting it is prudent to obtain additional confirmation with an RNA-based test and/or a follow-up western blot. By definition, western blot patterns of reactivity that do not fall into the positive or negative categories are considered "indeterminate." There are two possible explanations for an indeterminate western blot result. The most likely explanation in a low-risk individual is that the patient being tested has antibodies that cross-react with one of the proteins of HIV. The most common patterns of cross-reactivity are antibodies that react with p24 and/or p55. The least likely explanation in this setting is that the individual is infected with HIV and is in the process of mounting a classic antibody response. In either instance, the western blot should be repeated in 1 month to determine whether or not the indeterminate pattern is a pattern in evolution. In addition, one may attempt to confirm a diagnosis of HIV infection with the p24 antigen capture assay or one of the tests for HIV RNA (discussed below). While the western blot is an excellent confirmatory test for HIV infection in patients with a positive or indeterminate EIA, it is a poor screening test. Among individuals with a negative EIA and PCR for HIV, 20 to 30% may show one or more bands on western blot. While these bands are usually faint and represent cross-reactivity, their presence creates a situation in which other diagnostic modalities [such as DNA PCR, RNA PCR, the (b)DNA assay, or p24 antigen capture] must be employed to ensure that the bands do not indicate early HIV infection.

A guideline for the use of these serologic tests in attempting to make a diagnosis of HIV infection is depicted in Fig. 173-24. In patients in whom HIV infection is suspected, the appropriate initial test is the EIA. If the result is negative, unless there is strong reason to suspect early HIV infection (as in a patient exposed within the previous 3 months), the diagnosis is ruled out and retesting should be performed only as clinically indicated. If the EIA is indeterminate or positive, the test should be repeated. If the repeat is negative on two occasions, one can assume that the initial positive reading was due to a technical error in the performance of the assay and that the patient is negative. If the repeat is indeterminate or positive, one should proceed to the HIV-1 western blot. If the western blot is positive, the diagnosis is HIV-1

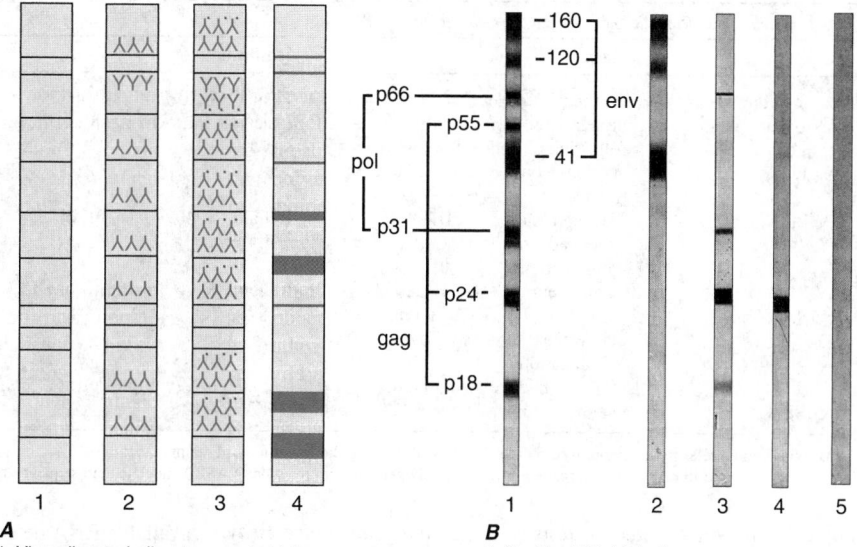

A
1. Virus digested: digest separated into components by molecular weight
2. Proteins transferred to filter paper: reaction with test serum
3. Enzyme-conjugated antihuman antibody added
4. Substrate added and color noted

B
1. Positive HIV-1 infection
2. gp 160 immunization
3. Indeterminate (HIV-2 infection)
4. Indeterminate (cross-reacting antibody to p24)
5. Negative

FIGURE 173-23 *A.* Schematic representation of how a western blot is performed. *B.* Examples of patterns of western blot reactivity. In each instance the western blot strip contains antigens to HIV-1. The sera from the patient immunized to the HIV-1 envelope only contains antibodies to the HIV-1 envelope proteins. The sera from the patient with HIV-2 infection cross-reacts with both *reverse transcriptase* and *gag* gene products of HIV-1.

infection. If the western blot is negative, the EIA can be assumed to have been a false positive for HIV-1 and the diagnosis of HIV-1 infection is ruled out. It would be prudent at this point to perform specific serologic testing for HIV-2 following the same type of algorithm. If the western blot for HIV-1 is indeterminate, it should be repeated in 4 to 6 weeks; in addition, one may proceed to a p24 antigen capture assay, HIV-1 RNA assay, or HIV-1 DNA PCR and specific serologic testing for HIV-2. If the p24 and HIV RNA assays are negative and there is no progression in the western blot, a diagnosis of HIV-1 is ruled out. If either the p24 or HIV-1 RNA assay is positive and/or the HIV-1 western blot shows progression, a tentative diagnosis of HIV-1 infection can be made and later confirmed with a follow-up western blot demonstrating a positive pattern.

As mentioned above, a variety of laboratory tests are available for the direct detection of HIV or its components (Table 173-9; Fig. 173-25). These tests may be of considerable help in making a diagnosis of HIV infection when the western blot results are indeterminate. In addition, the tests detecting levels of HIV RNA can be used to determine prognosis and to assess the response to antiretroviral therapies. The

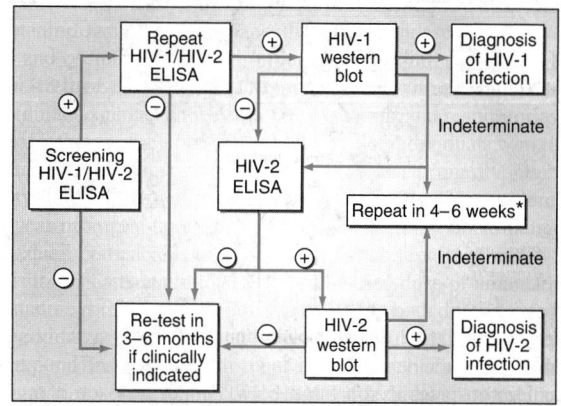

FIGURE 173-24 Algorithm for the use of serologic tests in the diagnosis of HIV-1 or HIV-2 infection. * Stable indeterminate western blot 4 to 6 weeks later makes HIV infection unlikely. However, it should be repeated twice at 3-month intervals to rule out HIV infection. Alternatively, one may test for HIV-1 p24 antigen or HIV RNA.

TABLE 173-9 *Characteristics of Tests for Direct Detection of HIV*

Test	Technique	Sensitivity[a]	Cost/Test
Immune complex–dissociated p24 antigen capture assay	Measurement of levels of HIV-1 core protein in an ELISA-based format following dissociation of antigen-antibody complexes by weak acid treatment	Positive in 50% of patients; detects down to 15 pg/mL of p24 protein	$1–2
HIV RNA by PCR	PCR amplification of cDNA generated from viral RNA (target amplification)	Reliable to 40 copies/mL of HIV RNA	$75–150
HIV RNA by bDNA	Measurement of levels of particle-associated HIV RNA in a nucleic acid capture assay employing signal amplification	Reliable to 75 copies/mL of HIV RNA	$75–150
HIV RNA by NASBA	Isothermic nucleic acid amplification with internal controls	Reliable to 176 copies/mL of HIV RNA	$75–150

[a] Sensitivity figures refer to those approved by the US FDA. Prices may be lower in large volume settings.
Note: ELISA, enzyme-linked immunosorbent assay; PCR, polymerase chain reaction; NASBA, nucleic acid sequence based assay.

simplest of the direct detection tests is the *p24 antigen capture assay*. This is an EIA-type assay in which the solid phase consists of antibodies to the p24 antigen of HIV. It detects the viral protein p24 in the blood of HIV-infected individuals where it exists either as free antigen or complexed to anti-p24 antibodies. Overall, ~30% of individuals with untreated HIV infection have detectable levels of free p24 antigen. This increases to about 50% when samples are treated with a weak acid to dissociate antigen-antibody complexes. Throughout the course of HIV infection, an equilibrium exists between p24 antigen and anti-p24 antibodies. During the first few weeks of infection, before an immune response develops, there is a brisk rise in p24 antigen levels (Fig. 173-22). After the development of anti-p24 antibodies, these levels decline. Late in the course of infection, when circulating levels of virus are high, p24 antigen levels also increase, particularly when detected by techniques involving dissociation of antigen-antibody complexes. This assay has its greatest use as a screening test for HIV infection in patients suspected of having the acute HIV syndrome, as high levels of p24 antigen are present prior to the development of antibodies. In addition, it is currently used routinely along with the HIV EIA and nucleic acid test to screen blood donors in the United States for evidence of HIV infection. The ability to measure and monitor levels of HIV RNA in the plasma of patients with HIV infection has been of extraordinary value in furthering our understanding of the pathogenesis of HIV infection and in providing a diagnostic tool in settings where measurements of anti-HIV antibodies may be misleading, such as in acute infection and neonatal infection. Three assays are predominantly used for this purpose. They are the reverse transcriptase PCR (*RT-PCR*; Amplicor); the branched DNA (*bDNA*; VERSANT); and the nucleic acid sequenced based assay (*NASBA*; NucliSens).

While routinely used in the past, along with testing for HIV antibodies, to screen blood donors for HIV infection, this use of the p24 assay has been replaced by the use of nucleic acid testing. These tests are of value in making a diagnosis of HIV infection, in establishing intial prognosis and determining the need for therapy, and for monitoring the effects of therapy. In addition to these three commercially available tests, the *DNA PCR* is also employed by research laboratories for making a diagnosis of HIV infection by amplifying HIV proviral DNA from peripheral blood mononuclear cells. The commercially available RNA detection tests have a sensitivity of 50 to 75 copies of HIV RNA per milliliter of plasma, while the DNA PCR tests can detect proviral DNA at a frequency of one copy per 10,000 to 100,000 cells. Thus, these tests are extremely sensitive. One frequent consequence of a high degree of sensitivity is some loss of specificity, and false-positive results have been reported with each of these techniques. For this reason, a positive EIA with a confirmatory western blot remains the "gold standard" for a diagnosis of HIV infection, and the interpretation of other test results must be done with this in mind.

In the RT-PCR technique, following DNase treatment, a cDNA copy is made of all RNA species present in plasma. Insofar as HIV is an RNA virus, this will result in the production of DNA copies of the HIV genome in amounts proportional to the amount of HIV RNA present in plasma. This cDNA is then amplified and characterized using standard PCR techniques, employing primer pairs that can distinguish genomic cDNA from messenger cDNA. The bDNA assay involves the use of a solid-phase nucleic acid capture system and signal amplification through successive nucleic acid hybridizations to detect small quantities of HIV RNA. Both tests can achieve a tenfold increase in sensitivity to 40 to 50 copies of HIV RNA per milliliter with a preconcentration step in which plasma undergoes ultracentrifugation to pellet the viral particles. The NASBA technique involves the isothermal amplification of a sequence within the gag region of HIV in the presence of internal standards and employs the production of multiple RNA copies through the action of T7-RNA polymerase. The lower limit of detection for the NASBA is 176 copies/mL.

In addition to being a diagnostic and prognostic tool, RT-PCR is also useful for amplifying defined areas of the HIV genome for sequence analysis and has become an important technique for studies of sequence diversity and microbial resistance to antiretroviral agents. In patients with a positive or indeterminate EIA test and an indeterminate western blot, and in patients in whom serologic testing may be unreliable (such as patients with hypogammaglobulinemia or advanced HIV disease), these tests for quantitating HIV RNA in plasma provide valuable tools for making a diagnosis of HIV infection; however, they should be used for diagnosis only when standard serologic testing has failed to provide a definitive result.

LABORATORY MONITORING OF PATIENTS WITH HIV INFECTION The epidemic of HIV infection and AIDS has provided the clinician with new challenges for integrating clinical and laboratory data to effect optimal patient management.

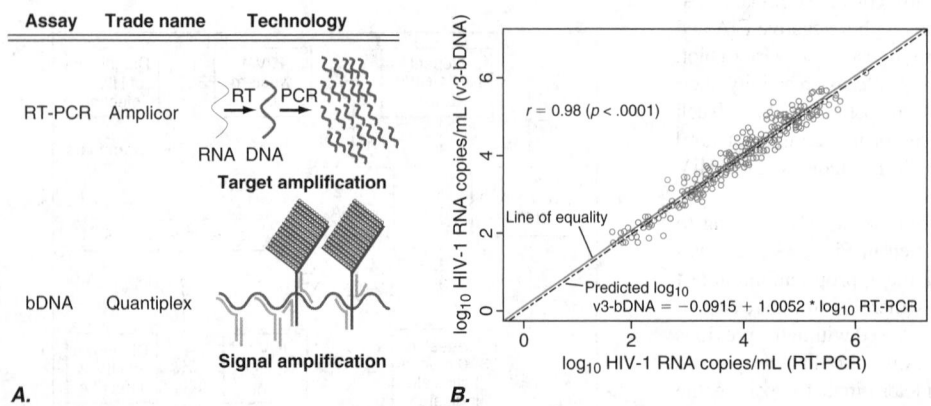

FIGURE 173-25 Comparison of RT-PCR and bDNA assays. *A.* Schematic representation of reverse transcriptase–polymerase chain reaction (RT-PCR) and bDNA assays. See text for detailed description. *B.* Scatter plot of $\log_{10}$ v3 bDNA versus $\log_{10}$ RT-PCR with the line of equity (solid) and the fitted regression line (hatched). The equation for the fitted regression line is given in the lower-right-hand corner. There is good agreement between the two assays. v3, version 3 of the bDNA assay. (*From HC Highbarger et al: J Clin Microbiol 37:3612, 1999.*)

The close relationship between clinical manifestations of HIV infection and CD4+ T cell count has made measurement of the latter a routine part of the evaluation of HIV-infected individuals. Determinations of CD4+ T cell counts and measurements of the levels of HIV RNA in serum or plasma provide a powerful set of tools for determining prognosis and monitoring response to therapy. While the CD4+ T cell count provides information on the current immunologic status of the patient, the HIV RNA level predicts what will happen to the CD4+ T cell count in the near future, and hence provides an important piece of prognostic information.

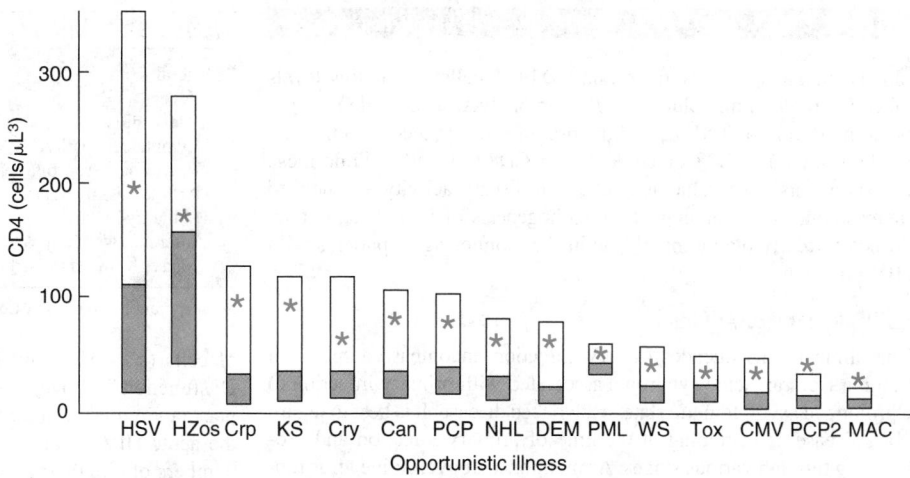

FIGURE 173-26 Relationship between CD4+ T cell counts and the development of opportunistic diseases. Boxplot of the median (line inside the box), first quartile (bottom of the box), third quartile (top of the box), and mean (asterisk) CD4+ lymphocyte count at the time of the development of opportunistic disease. Can, candidal esophagitis; CMV, cytomegalovirus infection; Crp, cryptosporidiosis; Cry, cryptococcal meningitis; DEM, AIDS dementia complex; HSV, herpes simplex virus infection; HZos, herpes zoster; KS, Kaposi's sarcoma; MAC, *Mycobacterium avium* complex bacteremia; NHL, non-Hodgkin's lymphoma; PCP, primary *Pneumocystis carinii* pneumonia; PCP2, secondary *Pneumocystis carinii* pneumonia; PML, progressive multifocal leukoencephalopathy; Tox, *Toxoplasma gondii* encephalitis; WS, wasting syndrome. (*From RD Moore, RE Chaisson: Ann Intern Med 124:633, 1996.*)

CD4+ T Cell Counts The CD4+ T cell count is the laboratory test generally accepted as the best indicator of the immediate state of immunologic competence of the patient with HIV infection. This measurement, which is the product of the percent of CD4+ T cells (determined by flow cytometry) and the total lymphocyte count [determined by the white blood cell count (WBC) and the differential percent] has been shown to correlate very well with the level of immunologic competence. Patients with CD4+ T cell counts <200/μL are at high risk of infection with *P. carinii*, while patients with CD4+ T cell counts <50/μL are at high risk of infection with CMV and mycobacteria of the *M. avium complex* (MAC) (Fig. 173-26). Patients with HIV infection should have CD4+ T cell measurements performed at the time of diagnosis and every 3 to 6 months thereafter. More frequent measurements should be made if a declining trend is noted. According to most guidelines, a CD4 T cell count <350/μL is an indication for consideration of initiating antiretroviral therapy, and a decline in CD4+ T cell count of >25% is an indication for considering a change in therapy. Once the CD4+ T cell count is <200/μL, patients should be placed on a regimen for *P. carinii* prophylaxis, and once the count is <50/μL, primary prophylaxis for MAC infection is indicated. As with any laboratory measurement, one may wish to obtain two determinations prior to any significant changes in patient management based upon CD4+ T cell count alone.

HIV RNA Determinations Facilitated by highly sensitive techniques for the precise quantitation of small amounts of nucleic acids, the measurement of serum or plasma levels of HIV RNA has become an essential component in the monitoring of patients with HIV infection. As discussed under diagnosis of HIV infection, the two most commonly used techniques are the RT-PCR assay and the bDNA assay. Both assays generate data in the form of number of copies of HIV RNA per milliliter of serum or plasma and, by employing a 1:10 concentration step with ultracentrifugation, can detect as few as 50 to 75 copies of HIV RNA per milliliter of plasma. Although earlier versions of the bDNA assay generated values that were ~50% of those of the RT-PCR assay, the more recent versions (version 3 or higher) provide numbers essentially identical to those of the RT-PCR test (Fig. 173-25). While it is common practice to describe levels of HIV RNA below these cut-offs as "undetectable," this is a term that should be avoided as it is imprecise and leaves the false impression that the level of virus is 0. By utilizing more sensitive, nested PCR techniques and by studying tissue levels of virus as well as plasma levels, HIV RNA can be detected in virtually every patient with HIV infection. Measurements of changes in HIV RNA levels over time have been of great value in delineating the relationship between levels of virus and rates of disease progression (Fig. 173-17), the rates of viral turnover, the relationship between immune system activation and viral replication, and the time to development of drug resistance. HIV RNA measurements are greatly influenced by the state of activation of the immune system and may fluctuate greatly in the setting of secondary infections or immunization. For these reasons, decisions based upon HIV RNA levels should never be made on a single determination. Measurements of plasma HIV RNA levels should be made at the time of HIV diagnosis and every 3 to 4 months thereafter in the untreated patient. In general, most guidelines suggest that therapy be considered in patients with >50,000 copies of HIV RNA per milliliter (see below). Following the initiation of therapy or any change in therapy, plasma HIV RNA levels should be monitored approximately every 4 weeks until the effectiveness of the therapeutic regimen is determined by the development of a new steady-state level of HIV RNA. In most instances of effective therapy this will be <50 copies per milliliter. This level of virus is generally achieved within 6 months of the initiation of effective treatment. During therapy, levels of HIV RNA should be monitored every 3 to 4 months to evaluate the continuing effectiveness of therapy.

HIV Resistance Testing The availability of multiple antiretroviral drugs as treatment options has generated a great deal of interest in the potential for measuring the sensitivity of an individual's HIV virus(es) to different antiretroviral agents. HIV resistance testing can be done through either genotypic or phenotypic measurements. In the genotypic assays, sequence analyses of the HIV genomes obtained from patients are compared to sequences of viruses with known antiretroviral resistance profiles. In the phenotypic assays, the in vivo growth of viral isolates obtained from the patient are compared to the growth of reference strains of the virus in the presence or absence of different antiretroviral drugs. A modification of this phenotypic approach utilizes a comparison of the enzymatic activities of the reverse transcriptase or protease genes obtained by molecular cloning of patients' isolates to the enzymatic activities of genes obtained from reference strains of HIV in the presence or absence of different drugs targeted to these genes. These tests are quite good in identifying those antiretroviral agents that have been utilized in the past in a given patient. In the hands of experts, resistance testing enhances the short-term ability to decrease viral load by ~0.5 log compared to changing drugs merely on the basis of drug history. While some have advocated the use of resistance testing in the selection of an intial treatment regimen, the value of resistance testing in this setting is unknown.

Other Tests A variety of other laboratory tests have been studied as potential markers of HIV disease activity. Among these are quantitative culture of replication-competent HIV from plasma, peripheral blood mononuclear cells, or resting CD4+ T cells; circulating levels of β_2-microglobulin, soluble IL-2 receptor, IgA, acid-labile endogenous interferon, or TNF-α; and the presence or absence of activation markers such as CD38 or HLA-DR on CD8+ T cells. While these measurements have value as markers of disease activity and help to increase our understanding of the pathogenesis of HIV disease, they do not currently play a major role in the monitoring of patients with HIV infection.

CLINICAL MANIFESTATIONS

The clinical consequences of HIV infection encompass a spectrum ranging from an acute syndrome associated with primary infection to a prolonged asymptomatic state to advanced disease. It is best to regard HIV disease as beginning at the time of primary infection and progressing through various stages. As mentioned above, active virus replication and progressive immunologic impairment occur throughout the course of HIV infection in most patients. With the exception of the rare true long-term nonprogressors (see above), HIV disease in untreated patients inexorably progresses even during the clinically latent stage. However, antiretroviral therapy has had a major impact on blocking or slowing the progression of disease over extended periods of time in a substantial proportion of adequately treated patients (see below).

THE ACUTE HIV SYNDROME It is estimated that 50 to 70% of individuals with HIV infection experience an acute clinical syndrome approximately 3 to 6 weeks after primary infection (Fig. 173-27). Varying degrees of clinical severity have been reported, and although it has been suggested that symptomatic seroconversion leading to the seeking of medical attention indicates an increased risk for an accelerated course of disease, this has not been shown definitively. In fact, there does not appear to be a correlation between the level of the initial burst of viremia in acute HIV infection and the subsequent course of disease. The typical clinical findings in the acute HIV syndrome are listed in Table 173-10; they occur along with a burst of plasma viremia. It has been reported that several symptoms of the acute HIV syndrome (fever, skin rash, pharyngitis, and myalgia) occur less frequently in those infected by injection drug use versus those infected by sexual contact. The syndrome is typical of an acute viral syndrome and has been likened to acute infectious mononucleosis. Symptoms usually persist for 1 to several weeks and gradually subside as an immune response to HIV develops and the levels of plasma viremia decrease. Opportunistic infections have been reported during this stage of infection, reflecting the immunodeficiency that results from reduced numbers of CD4+ T cells and likely also from the dysfunction of CD4+ T cells owing to viral protein and endogenous cytokine-induced perturbations

TABLE 173-10 Clinical Findings in the Acute HIV Syndrome	
General	Neurologic
Fever	Meningitis
Pharyngitis	Encephalitis
Lymphadenopathy	Peripheral neuropathy
Headache/retroorbital pain	Myelopathy
Arthralgias/myalgias	Dermatologic
Lethargy/malaise	Erythematous maculopapular rash
Anorexia/weight loss	Mucocutaneous ulceration
Nausea/vomiting/diarrhea	

Source: From B Tindall, DA Cooper: AIDS 5:1, 1991.

of cells (see "Mechanisms of CD4+ T Lymphocyte Depletion and Dysfunction," above) associated with the extremely high levels of plasma viremia. A number of immunologic abnormalities accompany the acute HIV syndrome, including multiphasic perturbations of the numbers of circulating lymphocyte subsets. The number of total lymphocytes and T cell subsets (CD4+ and CD8+) are initially reduced. An inversion of the CD4+/CD8+ T cell ratio occurs later because of a rise in the number of CD8+ T cells. In fact, there may be a selective and transient expansion of CD8+ T cell subsets, as determined by T cell receptor analysis (see above). The total circulating CD8+ T cell count may remain elevated or return to normal; however, CD4+ T cell levels usually remain somewhat depressed, although there may be a slight rebound towards normal. Lymphadenopathy occurs in ~70% of individuals with primary HIV infection. Most patients recover spontaneously from this syndrome and many are left with only a mildly depressed CD4+ T cell count that remains stable for a variable period before beginning its progressive decline (see below); in some individuals, the CD4+ T cell count returns to the normal range. Approximately 10% of patients manifest a fulminant course of immunologic and clinical deterioration after primary infection, even after the disappearance of initial symptoms. In most patients, primary infection with or without the acute syndrome is followed by a prolonged period of clinical latency.

THE ASYMPTOMATIC STAGE—CLINICAL LATENCY Although the length of time from initial infection to the development of clinical disease varies greatly, the median time for untreated patients is ~10 years. As emphasized above, HIV disease with active virus replication is ongoing and progressive during this asymptomatic period. The rate of disease progression is directly correlated with HIV RNA levels. Patients with high levels of HIV RNA in plasma progress to symptomatic disease faster than do patients with low levels of HIV RNA (Fig. 173-17). Some patients referred to as long-term nonprogressors show little if any decline in CD4+ T cell counts over extended periods of time. These patients generally have extremely low levels of HIV RNA. Certain other patients remain entirely asymptomatic despite the fact that their CD4+ T cell counts show a steady progressive decline to extremely low levels. In these patients, the appearance of an opportunistic disease may be the first manifestation of HIV infection. During the asymptomatic period of HIV infection, the average rate of CD4+ T cell decline is ~50/μL per year. When the CD4+ T cell count falls to <200/μL, the resulting state of immunodeficiency is severe enough to place the patient at high risk for opportunistic infection and neoplasms, and hence for clinically apparent disease.

SYMPTOMATIC DISEASE Symptoms of HIV disease can appear at any time during the course of HIV infection. Generally speaking, the spectrum of illness that one observes changes as the CD4+ T cell count declines. The more severe and life-threatening complications of HIV infection occur in patients with CD4+ T cells counts <200/μL. A diagnosis of AIDS is made in anyone with HIV infection and a CD4+ T cell count <200/μL and in anyone with HIV infection who develops one of the HIV-associated diseases considered to be indicative of a severe defect in cell-mediated immunity (category C, Table 173-2). While the causative agents of the secondary infections are characteristically opportunistic organisms such as *P. carinii*, atypical mycobacteria, CMV, and other organisms that do not ordinarily cause disease

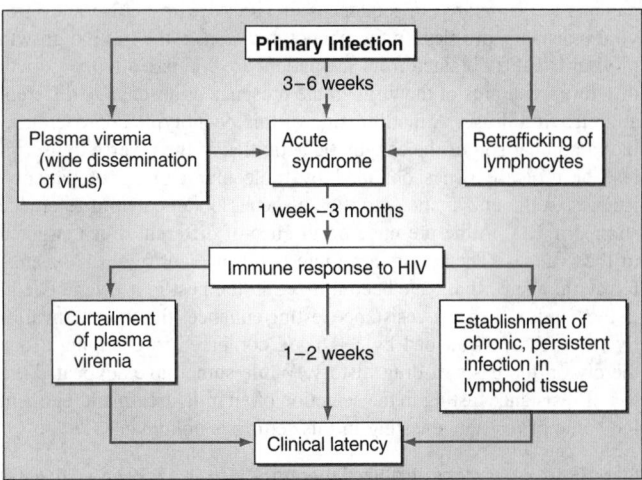

FIGURE 173-27   The acute HIV syndrome. See text for detailed description. (*Adapted from G Pantaleo et al: N Engl J Med 328:327, 1993.*)

in the absence of a compromised immune system, they also include common bacterial and mycobacterial pathogens. Approximately 60% of deaths among AIDS patients are as a direct result of an infection other than HIV, with *P. carinii*, viral hepatitis, and non-AIDS-defining bacterial infections heading the list. Following the widespread use of combination antiretroviral therapy and implementation of guidelines for the prevention of opportunistic infections (Table 173-11), the incidence of secondary infections has decreased dramatically (Fig. 173-28). Overall, the clinical spectrum of HIV disease is constantly changing as patients live longer and new and better approaches to treatment and prophylaxis are developed. In general, it should be stressed that a key element of treatment of symptomatic complications of HIV disease, whether they are primary or secondary, is achieving good control of HIV replication through the use of combination antiretroviral therapy and instituting primary and secondary prophylaxis as indicated.

Disease of the Respiratory System Acute bronchitis and sinusitis are prevalent during all stages of HIV infection. The most severe cases tend to occur in patients with lower CD4+ T cell counts. Sinusitis presents as fever, nasal congestion, and headache. The diagnosis is made by computed tomography (CT) or magnetic resonance imaging (MRI). The maxillary sinuses are most commonly involved; however, disease is also frequently seen in the ethmoid, sphenoid, and frontal sinuses. While some patients may improve without antibiotic therapy, radiographic improvement is quicker and more pronounced in patients who have received antimicrobial therapy. It is postulated that this high incidence of sinusitis results from an increased frequency of infection with encapsulated organisms such as *H. influenzae* and *Streptococcus pneumoniae*. In patients with low CD4+ T cell counts one may see mucormycosis infections of the sinuses. In contrast to the course of this infection in other patient populations, mucormycosis of the sinuses in patients with HIV infection may progress more slowly. In this setting aggressive, frequent local debridement in addition to local and systemic amphotericin B may be needed for effective treatment.

Pulmonary disease is one of the most frequent complications of HIV infection. The most common manifestation of pulmonary disease is pneumonia. The two most common causes of pneumonia are bacterial infections and *P. carinii* infection. Other major causes of pulmonary infiltrates include mycobacterial infections, fungal infections, nonspecific interstitial pneumonitis, KS, and lymphoma.

Pneumonia is seen with an increased frequency in patients with HIV infection; they appear to be particularly prone to infections with encapsulated organisms. *S. pneumoniae* (Chap. 119) and *H. influenzae* (Chap. 130) are responsible for most cases of bacterial pneumonia in patients with AIDS. This may be a consequence of altered B cell function and/or defects in neutrophil function that may be secondary to HIV disease (see above). Pneumococcal infection may be the earliest serious infection to occur in patients with HIV disease. This can present as pneumonia, sinusitis, and/or bacteremia. Patients with HIV infection have a sixfold increase in the incidence of pneumococcal pneumonia and a 100-fold increase in the incidence of pneumococcal bacteremia. Pneumococcal disease may be seen in patients with relatively intact immune systems. In one study, the baseline CD4+ T cell count at the time of a first episode of pneumococcal pneumonia was ~300/μL. Of interest is the fact that the inflammatory response to pneumococcal infection appears proportional to the CD4+ T cell count. Due to this high risk of pneumococcal disease, immunization with pneumococcal polysaccharide is one of the generally recommended prophylactic measures for patients with HIV infection and CD4+ T cell counts >200/μL. It is less clear if this intervention is of benefit in patients with more advanced disease and high viral loads.

P. carinii pneumonia (PCP), once the hallmark of AIDS, has dramatically declined in incidence following the development of effective prophylactic regimens and the widespread use of combination antiretroviral therapy. It is, however, the single most common cause of pneumonia in patients with HIV infection in the United States and can be identified as a likely etiologic agent in 25% of cases of pneumonia in patients with HIV infection. Approximately 25% of cases of HIV-associated PCP occur in patients who are unaware of their HIV status. The risk of PCP is greatest among those who have experienced a previous bout of PCP and those who have CD4+ T cell counts of <200/μL. Overall, 79% of patients with PCP have CD4+ T cell counts <100/μL and 95% of patients have CD4+ T cell counts <200/μL. Recurrent fever, night sweats, thrush, and unexplained weight loss are also associated with an increased incidence of PCP. For these reasons, it is strongly recommended that all patients with CD4+ T cell counts <200/μL (or a CD4 percentage <15) receive some form of PCP prophylaxis. At present the incidence of PCP is approaching zero in patients with known HIV infection receiving appropriate antiretroviral therapy and prophylaxis. In the United States, primary PCP is now occurring at a median CD4+ T cell count of 36/μL, while secondary PCP is occurring at a median CD4+ T cell count of 10/μL. Patients with PCP generally present with fever and a cough that is usually nonproductive or productive of only scant amounts of white sputum. They may complain of a characteristic retrosternal chest pain that is worse on inspiration and is described as sharp or burning. HIV-associated PCP may have an indolent course characterized by weeks of vague symptoms and should be included in the differential diagnosis of fever, pulmonary complaints, or unexplained weight loss in any patient with HIV infection and <200 CD4+ T cells/μL. The most common finding on chest x-ray is either a normal film, if the disease is suspected early, or a faint bilateral interstitial infiltrate. The classic finding of a dense perihilar infiltrate is unusual in patients with AIDS. In patients with PCP who have been receiving aerosolized pentamidine for prophylaxis, one may see an x-ray picture of upper lobe cavitary disease, reminiscent of TB. Other less common findings on chest x-ray include lobar infiltrates and pleural effusions. Routine laboratory evaluation is usually of little help in the differential diagnosis of PCP. A mild leukocytosis is common, although this may not be obvious in patients with prior neutropenia. Arterial blood gases may indicate hypoxemia with a decline in Pa_{O_2} and an increase in the arterial-alveolar (a − A) gradient. Arterial blood gas measurements not only aid in making the diagnosis of PCP but also provide important information for staging the severity of the disease and directing treatment (see below). A definitive diagnosis of PCP requires demonstration of the trophozoite or cyst form of the organism in samples obtained from induced sputum, bronchoalveolar lavage, transbronchial biopsy, or open lung biopsy. PCR has been used to detect specific DNA sequences for *P. carinii* in clinical specimens where histologic examinations have failed to make a diagnosis.

In addition to pneumonia, a number of other clinical problems have been reported in HIV-infected patients as a result of infection with *P. carinii*. Otic involvement may be seen as a primary infection, presenting as a polypoid mass involving the external auditory canal. In patients receiving aerosolized pentamidine for prophylaxis against PCP one may see a variety of extrapulmonary manifestations of *P. carinii*. These include ophthalmic lesions of the choroid, a necrotizing vasculitis that resembles Burger's disease, bone marrow hypoplasia, and intestinal obstruction. Other organs that have been involved include lymph nodes, spleen, liver, kidney, pancreas, pericardium, heart, thyroid, and adrenals. Organ infection may be associated with cystic lesions that may appear calcified on CT or ultrasound.

The standard treatment for PCP or disseminated pneumocystosis is trimethoprim/sulfamethoxazole (TMP/SMX). A high incidence of side effects, particularly skin rash and bone marrow suppression, is seen with TMP/SMX in patients with HIV infection. Alternative treatments for mild to moderate PCP include dapsone/trimethoprim and clindamycin/primaquine. Intravenous pentamidine is the treatment of choice for severe disease in the patient unable to tolerate TMP/SMX. For patients with a Pa_{O_2} < 70 mmHg or with an a − A gradient >35 mmHg, adjunct glucocorticoid therapy should be used in addition to specific antimicrobials. Overall, treatment should be for 21 days and followed by secondary prophylaxis. Prophylaxis for PCP is indicated for any HIV-infected individual who has experienced a prior bout of

Pathogen	Indications	First Choice(s)	Alternatives
STRONGLY RECOMMENDED AS STANDARD OF CARE FOR PRIMARY AND SECONDARY PROPHYLAXIS			
Pneumocystis carinii	CD4 count <200/μL or Oropharyngeal candidiasis or Unexplained fever >2 weeks or Prior bout of PCP	Trimethoprim/sulfamethoxazole (TMP/SMZ), 1 DS tablet qd	Dapsone 50 mg bid PO or 100 mg/d PO Dapsone 50 mg/d PO+ Pyrimethamine 50 mg/wk PO+ Leucovorin 25 mg/wk PO
	May stop prophylaxis if CD4+ T cell count > 200/μL for 6 mo	TMP/SMZ, 1 SS tablet qd	Dapsone 200 mg PO+ Pyrimethamine 75 mg + Leucovorin 25 mg PO weekly Aerosolized pentamidine, 300 mg qm via Respirgard II nebulizer Atovoquone 1500 mg/d PO TMP/SMZ 1 DS tablet PO 3×/wk
Mycobacterium tuberculosis			
Isoniazid sensitive	Skin test >5 mm or Prior positive test without treatment or Contact with case of active TB	Isoniazid 300 mg PO+ Pyridoxine 50 mg/d PO ×9 mo	Rifampin 600 mg/d PO or Rifabutin 300 mg/d PO+ Pyrazinamide 20 (mg/kg)/d PO ×2 mo
		Isoniazid 900 mg PO+ Pyridoxine 100 mg PO 2 ×/wk ×9 mo	Rifampin 600 mg/d PO or Rifabutin 300 mg/d PO ×4 mo
Isoniazid resistant	Same with high probability of exposure to isoniazid-resistant TB	Rifabutin 300 mg or Rifampin 600 mg; PO qd ×4 mo	Pyrazinamide 20 (mg/kg)/d PO ×2 mo + either Rifampin 600 mg/d or Rifabutin 300 mg/d PO ×4 mo
Multidrug resistant	Same with high probability of exposure to multidrug resistant TB	Consult local public health authorities	
Mycobacterium-avium complex	CD4 count <50/μL Prior documented disseminated disease	Azithromycin 1200 mg weekly PO Clarithromycin 500 mg bid PO	Rifabutin 300 mg/d PO Azithromycin 1200 mg weekly PO + Rifabutin 300 mg/d PO
	May stop prophylaxis if CD4+ T cell count > 100/μL for 6 mo	Clarithromycin 500 mg bid PO + Ethambutol 15 (mg/kg)/d PO +/− Rifabutin 300 mg/d PO	Azithromycin 500 mg/d PO + Ethambutol 15 (mg/kg)/d PO +/− Rifabutin 300 mg/d PO
Toxoplasma gondii	IgG antibody and CD4 count <100/μL	TMP/SMZ 1 DS tablet qd	TMP/SMZ 1 SS tablet qd Dapsone 50 mg/d PO + Pyrimethamine 50 mg weekly PO + Leucovorin 25 mg weekly PO Dapsone 200 mg PO + Pyrimethamine 75 mg PO + Leucovorin 25 mg PO weekly Atovaquone 1500 mg PO + Pyrimethamine 25 mg PO + Leucovorin 10 mg PO daily
	Prior toxoplasmic encephalitis	Sulfadiazine 500–1000 mg qid PO+ Pyrimethamine 25–50 mg/d PO+ Leucovorin 10–25 mg/d PO Atovaquone 750 mg PO q6–12 h +/− Pyrimethamine 25 mg/d + Leucovorin 10 mg/d PO	Clindamycin 300–450 mg q6–8h PO+ Pyrimethamine 25–75 mg/d PO+ Leucovorin 10–25 mg/d PO
Varicella zoster virus	Significant exposure to chickenpox or shingles in a patient with no history of immunization or prior exposure to either	Varicella zoster immune globulin 6.25 mL, IM, within 96 h	
Cryptococcus neoformans	Prior documented disease	Fluconazole 200 mg/d PO	Amphotericin B 0.6–1.0 mg/kg 3 ×/wk IV Itraconazole 200 mg/d PO
Histoplasma capsulatum	Prior documented disease	Itraconazole 200 mg bid PO	Amphotericin B 1.0 (mg/kg)/wk IV
Coccidioides immitis	Prior documented disease	Fluconazole 400 mg/d PO	Amphotericin B 1.0 (mg/kg)/wk IV Itraconazole 200 mg/d PO
Salmonella species	Prior bacteremia	Ciprofloxacin 500 mg bid PO for several months	
Cytomegalovirus	Prior end-organ disease May stop prophylaxis if CD4+ T cell count > 100/μL for 6 mo	Ganciclovir, 5–6 mg/kg 5–7 d/wk IV Ganciclovir 1000 mg tid PO Foscarnet 90–120 (mg/kg)/d IV	Cidofovir 5 mg/kg every other week IV + Probenecid Formivirsen 330 μg intravitreal q2–4 wk
	Prior retinitis	Ganciclovir implant q6–9 mo + Ganciclovir 1–1.5 g PO tid Ganciclovir sustained-release implant q6–9mo + Ganciclovir 1– 1.5 g tid PO	Valganciclovir 900 mg PO daily Fomivirsen, 1 vial injected into the vitreous q2–4wk

(continued)

TABLE 173-11—(Continued)

Pathogen	Indications	First Choice(s)	Alternatives
IMMUNIZATIONS GENERALLY RECOMMENDED			
Hepatitis B virus	All susceptible (anti-HBc and anti-HBs negative) patients	Hepatitis B vaccine: 3 doses	
Hepatitis A virus	All susceptible (anti-HAV negative) patients with chronic hepatitis C or at increased risk for hepatitis A	Hepatitis A vaccine: 2 doses	
Influenza virus	All patients annually	Inactivated trivalent influenza virus vaccine 1 dose yearly Oseltamivir 75 mg PO qd Rimantadine or amantadine 100 mg PO qd	
Streptococcus pneumoniae	All patients	Pneumoccal vaccine 0.5 mL IM ×1 if CD4 count >200/µL Reimmunize patients initially immunized at a CD4 count <200/µL whose CD4 count then increases to >200/µL	
RECOMMENDED FOR PREVENTION OF SEVERE OR FREQUENT RECURRENCES			
Herpes simplex	Frequent/severe recurrences	Acyclovir 200 mg tid PO Acyclovir 400 mg bid PO Famciclovir 250 mg bid PO	Valacyclovir 500 mg PO bid
Candida	Frequent/severe recurrences	Fluconazole 100–200 mg/d PO	Itraconazole solution 200 mg/d PO

Note: DS, double strength; SS, single strength; PCP, *Pneumocystis carinii* pneumonia; TB, tuberculosis

PCP, any patient with a CD4+ T cell count of <200/µL or a CD4 percentage <15, any patient with unexplained fever for >2 weeks, and any patient with a history of oropharyngeal candidiasis. The preferred regimen for prophylaxis is TMP/SMX, one double-strength tablet daily. This regimen also provides protection against toxoplasmosis and some bacterial respiratory pathogens. For patients who cannot

tolerate TMP/SMX, alternatives include dapsone plus pyrimethamine plus leucovorin, aerosolized pentamidine administered by the Respirgard II nebulizer, and atovaquone. Primary or secondary prophylaxis for PCP can be discontinued in those patients treated with combination antiretroviral therapy who maintain good suppression of HIV (<500 copies per milliliter) and CD4+ T cell counts >200/µL for at least 3 to 6 months.

M. tuberculosis, once thought to be on its way to extinction in the United States, experienced a resurgence associated with the HIV epidemic (Chap. 150). Worldwide, approximately one-third of all AIDS-related deaths are associated with TB. In the United States ~5% of AIDS patients have active TB. HIV infection increases the risk of developing active TB by a factor of 100. For the patient with untreated HIV infection and a positive PPD skin test, the rate of reactivation TB is 7 to 10% per year. Untreated TB can accelerate the course of HIV infection. Levels of plasma HIV RNA increase in the setting of active TB and decline in the setting of successful TB treatment. Active TB is most common in patients 25 to 44 years of age, in African Americans and Hispanics, in patients in New York City and Miami, and in patients in developing countries. In these demographic groups, 20 to 70% of the new cases of active TB are in patients with HIV infection. The epidemic of TB embedded in the epidemic of HIV infection probably represents the greatest health risk to the general public and the health care profession associated with the HIV epidemic. In contrast to infection with atypical mycobacteria such as MAC, active TB often develops relatively early in the course of HIV infection and may be an early clinical sign of HIV disease. In one study, the median CD4+ T cell count at presentation of TB was 326/µL. The clinical manifestations of TB in HIV-infected patients are quite varied and generally show different patterns as a function of the CD4+ T cell count. In patients with relatively high CD4+ T cell counts, the typical pattern of pulmonary reactivation occurs in which patients present with fever, cough, dyspnea on exertion, weight loss, night sweats, and a chest x-ray revealing cavitary apical disease of the upper lobes. In patients with lower CD4+ T cell counts, disseminated disease is more common. In these patients the chest x-ray may reveal diffuse or lower lobe bilateral reticulonodular infiltrates consistent with miliary spread, pleural effusions, and hilar and/or mediastinal adenopathy. Infection may be present in bone, brain, meninges, gastrointestinal tract, lymph nodes (particularly cervical lymph nodes), and viscera. Approximately 60 to 80% of patients have pulmonary disease, and 30 to 40% have extrapulmonary disease. Respiratory isolation and a negative-pressure room should be used for patients in whom a diagnosis of pulmonary

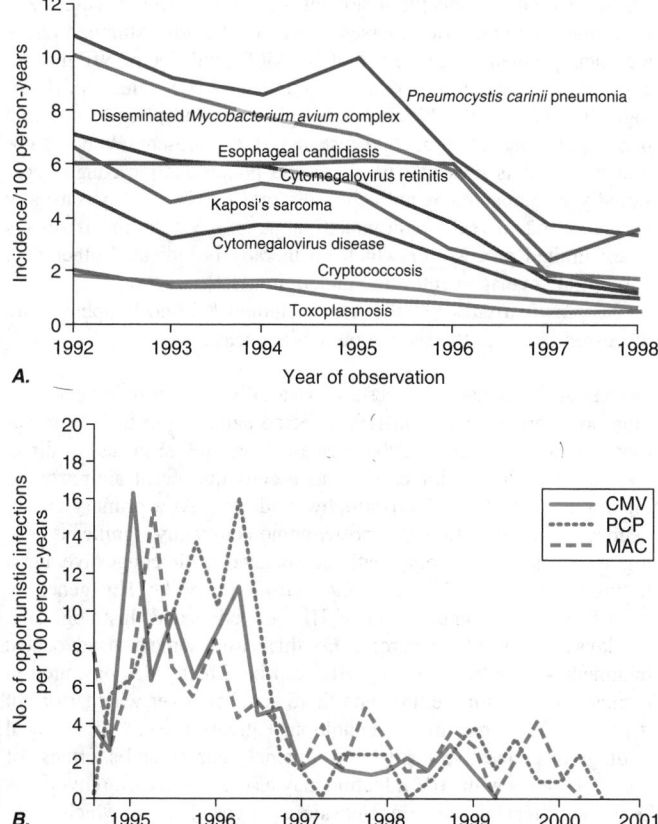

FIGURE 173-28 *A.* Decrease in the incidence of opportunistic infections and Kaposi's sarcoma in HIV-infected individuals with CD4+ T cell counts <100/µL from 1992 through 1998. [*Adapted and updated from Palella et al, and JE Kaplan et al: Clin Infect Dis 30(S1):S5, 2000, with permission.*] *B.* Quarterly incidence rates of cytomegalovirus (CMV), *Pneumocystis carinii* pneumonia (PCP), and *Mycobacterium avium* complex (MAC) from 1995–2001. (*From FJ Palella et al: AIDS 16:1617, 2002.*)

TB is being considered. This approach is critical to limit nosocomial and community spread of infection. Culture of the organism from an involved site provides a definitive diagnosis. Blood cultures are positive in 15% of patients. In the setting of fulminant disease one cannot rely upon the accuracy of a negative PPD skin test to rule out a diagnosis of TB. TB is one of the conditions associated with HIV infection for which cure is possible. Therapy for TB is generally the same in the HIV-infected patient as in the HIV-negative patient (Chap. 150). Due to pharmacokinetic interactions, rifabutin should be substituted for rifampin in patients receiving the HIV protease inhibitors or nonnucleoside reverse transcriptase inhibitors; both drugs should be avoided in patients receiving ritonavir. Treatment is most effective in programs that involve directly observed therapy. Effective prevention of active TB can be a reality if the health care professional is aggressive in looking for evidence of latent TB by making sure that all patients with HIV infection receive a PPD skin test. Anergy testing is not of value in this setting. HIV-infected individuals with a skin test reaction of >5 mm or those who are close household contacts of persons with active TB should receive treatment with 9 months of isoniazid.

Atypical mycobacterial infections are also seen with an increased frequency in patients with HIV infection. Infections with at least 12 different mycobacteria have been reported, including *M. bovis* and representatives of all four Runyon groups. The most common atypical mycobacterial infection is with *M. avium* or *M. intracellulare* species—MAC. Infections with MAC are seen mainly in patients in the United States and are rare in Africa. It has been suggested that prior infection with *M. tuberculosis* decreases the risk of MAC infection. MAC infections probably arise from organisms that are ubiquitous in the environment, including both soil and water. The presumed portals of entry are the respiratory and gastrointestinal tract. MAC infection is a late complication of HIV infection, predominantly occurring in patients with CD4+ T cell counts of <50/μL. The average CD4+ T cell count at the time of diagnosis is 10/μL. The most common presentation is disseminated disease with fever, weight loss, and night sweats. At least 85% of patients with MAC infection are mycobacteremic, and large numbers of organisms can often be demonstrated on bone marrow biopsy. The chest x-ray is abnormal in ~25% of patients, with the most common pattern being that of a bilateral, lower lobe infiltrate suggestive of miliary spread. Alveolar or nodular infiltrates and hilar and/or mediastinal adenopathy can also occur. Other clinical findings include endobronchial lesions, abdominal pain, diarrhea, and lymphadenopathy. The diagnosis is made by the culture of blood or involved tissue. The finding of two consecutive sputum samples positive for MAC is highly suggestive of pulmonary infection. Cultures may take 2 weeks to turn positive. Therapy consists of a macrolide, usually clarithromycin, with ethambutol. Some physicians elect to add a third drug from among rifabutin, ciprofloxacin, or amikacin in patients with extensive disease. Therapy is generally for life; however, with the advent of highly active antiretroviral therapy (HAART), it may be possible to discontinue therapy in patients with sustained suppression of HIV replication and CD4+ T cell counts >100/μL for >6 months. Primary prophylaxis for MAC is indicated in patients with HIV infection and CD4+ T cell counts <50/μL. This may be discontinued in patients in whom HAART induces a sustained suppression of viral replication and increases in CD4+ T cell counts to >100/μL for 3 to 6 months.

Rhodococcus equi is a gram-positive pleomorphic acid-fast non-spore-forming bacillus that can cause pulmonary and/or disseminated infection in patients with HIV infection. Fever and cough are the most common presenting signs. Radiographically one may see cavitary lesions and consolidation. Blood cultures are often positive. Treatment is based upon antimicrobial sensitivity testing.

Fungal infections of the lung, in addition to PCP, can be seen in patients with AIDS. Patients with pulmonary cryptococcal disease present with fever, cough, dyspnea, and in some cases, hemoptysis. A focal or diffuse interstitial infiltrate is seen on chest x-ray in >90% of patients. In addition, one may see lobar disease, cavitary disease, pleural effusions, and hilar or mediastinal adenopathy. Over half of patients are fungemic, and 90% of patients have concomitant CNS infection. *Coccidioides immitis* is a mold that is endemic in the southwest United States. It can cause a reactivation pulmonary syndrome in patients with HIV infection. Most patients with this condition will have CD4+ T cell counts <250/μL. Patients present with fever, weight loss, cough, and extensive, diffuse reticulonodular infiltrates on chest x-ray. One may also see nodules, cavities, pleural effusions, and hilar adenopathy. While serologic testing is of value in the immunocompetent host, serologies are negative in 25% of HIV-infected patients with coccidioidal infection. Invasive aspergillosis is not an AIDS-defining illness and is generally not seen in patients with AIDS in the absence of neutropenia or administration of glucocorticoids. *Aspergillus* infection may have an unusual presentation in the respiratory tract of patients with AIDS where it gives the appearance of a pseudomembranous tracheobronchitis. Primary pulmonary infection of the lung may be seen with *histoplasmosis*. The most common pulmonary manifestation of histoplasmosis, however, is in the setting of disseminated disease, presumably due to reactivation. In this setting respiratory symptoms are usually minimal, with cough and dyspnea occurring in 10 to 30% of patients. The chest x-ray is abnormal in ~50% of patients, showing either a diffuse interstitial infiltrate or diffuse small nodules.

Two forms of *idiopathic interstitial pneumonia* have been identified in patients with HIV infection: lymphoid interstitial pneumonitis (LIP) and nonspecific interstitial pneumonitis (NIP). LIP, a common finding in children, is seen in about 1% of adult patients with HIV infection. This disorder is characterized by a benign infiltrate of the lung and is felt to be part of the polyclonal activation of lymphocytes seen in the context of HIV and EBV infections. Transbronchial biopsy is diagnostic in 50% of the cases, with an open-lung biopsy required for diagnosis in the remainder of cases. This condition is generally self-limited and no specific treatment is necessary. Severe cases have been managed with brief courses of glucocorticoids. Although rarely a clinical problem since the use of HAART, evidence of NIP may be seen in up to half of all patients with untreated HIV infection. Histologically, interstitial infiltrates of lymphocytes and plasma cells in a perivascular and peribronchial distribution are present. When symptomatic, patients present with fever and nonproductive cough occasionally accompanied by mild chest discomfort. Chest x-ray is usually normal or may reveal a faint interstitial pattern. Similar to LIP, this is a self-limited process for which no therapy is indicated other than appropriate management of the underlying HIV infection.

Neoplastic diseases of the lung including KS and lymphoma are discussed below in the section on malignancies.

Diseases of the Cardiovascular System   Heart disease is a relatively common postmortem finding in HIV-infected patients (25 to 75% in autopsy series). Cardiovascular disease may be seen as a direct consequence of HIV infection or as a consequence of antiretroviral therapy as part of the lipodystrophy syndrome. As a primary consequence of HIV infection, the most common clinically significant finding is a dilated cardiomyopathy associated with congestive heart failure referred to as *HIV-associated cardiomyopathy*. This generally occurs as a late complication of HIV infection and, histologically, displays elements of myocarditis. For this reason some have advocated treatment with intravenous Ig. HIV can be directly demonstrated in cardiac tissue in this setting, and there is debate over whether or not it plays a direct role in this condition. Patients present with typical findings of congestive heart failure, namely edema and shortness of breath. Patients with HIV infection may also develop cardiomyopathy as a side effect of IFN-α nucleoside analogue therapy, which is reversible once therapy is stopped. KS, cryptococcosis, Chagas disease, and toxoplasmosis can involve the myocardium, leading to cardiomyopathy. In one series, most patients with HIV infection and a treatable myocarditis were found to have myocarditis associated with toxoplasmosis. Most of these patients also had evidence of CNS toxoplasmosis. Thus, MRI or double-dose contrast CT scan of the brain should be included in the workup of any patient with advanced HIV infection and cardiomyopathy.

A variety of other cardiovascular problems are found in patients with HIV infection. Pericardial effusions may be seen in the setting of advanced HIV infection. Predisposing factors include TB, congestive heart failure, mycobacterial infection, cryptococcal infection, pulmonary infection, lymphoma, and KS. While pericarditis is quite rare, in one series 5% of patients with HIV disease had pericardial effusions that were considered to be moderate or severe. Tamponade and death have occurred in association with pericardial KS, presumably owing to acute hemorrhage. Nonbacterial thrombotic endocarditis has been reported and should be considered in patients with unexplained embolic phenomena. Intravenous pentamidine, when given rapidly, can result in hypotension as a consequence of cardiovascular collapse. A high percentage of patients have hypertriglyceridemia and elevations in serum cholesterol, and coronary artery disease has been a relatively frequent finding at autopsy. This problem appears to becoming even more prevalent as a side effect of HAART. While the clinical significance of these findings has not been precisely defined, recent data suggest a linear relationship between time on HAART and development of ischemic heart disease. In one large series the overall rate of myocardial infarction was 3.5/1000 years, 28% of these events were fatal, and myocardial infarction was responsible for 7% of all deaths in the cohort. The risk of myocardial infarction increased by 26% per year of HAART. This small increase in the risk of death from myocardial infarction in the setting of HAART has to be balanced against the marked increase in overall survival brought about by HAART.

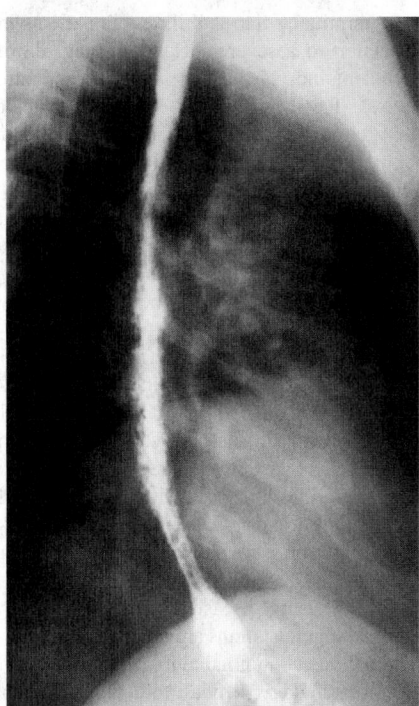

FIGURE 173-29 Barium swallow of a patient with *Candida* esophagitis. The flow of barium along the mucosal surface is grossly irregular.

Diseases of the Oropharynx and Gastrointestinal System
Oropharyngeal and gastrointestinal diseases are common features of HIV infection. They are most frequently due to secondary infections. In addition, oral and gastrointestinal lesions may occur with KS and lymphoma.

Oral lesions, including *thrush*, *hairy leukoplakia*, and *aphthous ulcers*, are particularly common in patients with untreated HIV infection. Thrush, due to *Candida* infection, and oral hairy leukoplakia, presumed due to EBV, are usually indicative of fairly advanced immunologic decline; they generally occur in patients with CD4+ T cell counts of <300/μL. In one study, 59% of patients with oral candidiasis went on to develop AIDS in the next year. Thrush appears as a white, cheesy exudate, often on an erythematous mucosa in the posterior oropharynx (see Fig. 187-1). While most commonly seen on the soft palate, early lesions are often found along the gingival border. The diagnosis is made by direct examination of a scraping for pseudohyphal elements. Culturing is of no diagnostic value, as most patients with HIV infection will have a positive throat culture for *Candida* even in the absence of thrush. Oral hairy leukoplakia presents as white, frondlike lesions, generally along the lateral borders of the tongue and sometimes on the adjacent buccal mucosa (see Fig. 165-1). Despite its name, oral hairy leukoplakia is not considered a premalignant condition. Lesions are associated with florid replication of EBV. While usually more disconcerting as a sign of HIV-associated immunodeficiency than a clinical problem in need of treatment, severe cases have been reported to respond to topical podophyllin or systemic therapy with anti-herpesvirus agents. Aphthous ulcers of the posterior oropharynx are also seen with regularity in patients with HIV infection. These lesions are of unknown etiology and can be quite painful and interfere with swallowing. Topical anesthetics provide immediate symptomatic relief of short duration. The fact that thalidomide is an effective treatment for this condition suggests that the pathogenesis may involve the action of tissue-destructive cytokines. Palatal, glossal, or gingival ulcers may also result from cryptococcal disease or histoplasmosis.

Esophagitis (Fig. 173-29) may present with odynophagia and retrosternal pain. Upper endoscopy is generally required to make an accurate diagnosis. Esophagitis may be due to *Candida*, CMV, or HSV. While CMV tends to be associated with a single large ulcer, HSV infection is more often associated with multiple small ulcers. The esophagus may also be the site of KS and lymphoma. Like the oral mucosa, the esophageal mucosa may have large, painful ulcers of unclear etiology that may respond to thalidomide. While achlorhydria is a common problem in patients with HIV infection, other gastric problems are generally rare. Among the conditions involving the stomach are KS and lymphoma. Infections of the small and large intestine leading to diarrhea, abdominal pain, and occasionally fever are among the most significant gastrointestinal problems in the HIV-infected patients. They include infections with bacteria, protozoa, and viruses.

Bacteria may be responsible for secondary infections of the gastrointestinal tract. Infections with enteric pathogens such as *Salmonella*, *Shigella*, and *Campylobacter* are more common in homosexual men and are often more severe and more apt to relapse in patients with HIV infection. Patients with untreated HIV have approximately a 20-fold increased risk of infection with *S. typhimurium*. They may present with a variety of nonspecific symptoms including fever, anorexia, fatigue, and malaise of several weeks' duration. Diarrhea is common but may be absent. Diagnosis is made by culture of blood and stool. Long-term therapy with ciprofloxacin is the recommended treatment. HIV-infected patients also have an increased incidence of *S. typhi* infection in areas of the world where typhoid is a problem. *Shigella* spp., particularly *S. flexneri*, can cause severe intestinal disease in HIV-infected individuals. Up to 50% of patients will develop bacteremia. *Campylobacter* infections occur with an increased frequency in patients with HIV infection. While *C. jejuni* is the strain most frequently isolated, infections with many other strains have been reported. Patients usually present with crampy abdominal pain, fever, and bloody diarrhea. Infection may present as proctitis. Stool examination reveals the presence of fecal leukocytes. Systemic infection can occur, with up to 10% of infected patients exhibiting bacteremia. Most strains are sensitive to erythromycin. Abdominal pain and diarrhea may be seen with MAC infection.

Fungal infections may also be a cause of diarrhea in patients with HIV infection. Histoplasmosis, coccidioidomycosis, and penicilliosis have all been identified as a cause of fever and diarrhea in patients with HIV infection. Peritonitis has been seen with *C. immitis*.

Cryptosporidia, microsporidia, and *Isospora belli* (Chap. 199) are the most common opportunistic protozoa that infect the gastrointestinal tract and cause diarrhea in HIV-infected patients. Cryptosporidial infection may present in a variety of ways, ranging from a self-limited or intermittent diarrheal illness in patients in the early stages of HIV infection to a severe, life-threatening diarrhea in severely immunodeficient individuals. In patients with untreated HIV infection and CD4+ T cell counts of <300/μL, the incidence of cryptosporidiosis is ~1% per year. In 75% of cases the diarrhea is accompanied by crampy abdominal pain, and 25% of patients have nausea and/or vomiting. Cryptosporidia may also cause biliary tract disease in the HIV-infected patient, leading to cholecystitis with or without accompanying cholangitis. The diagnosis of cryptosporidial diarrhea is made by stool examination. The diarrhea is noninflammatory, and the characteristic finding is the presence of oocysts that stain with acid-fast dyes. Therapy is predominantly supportive, and marked improvements have been reported in the setting of effective antiretroviral therapy. Treatment with up to 2000 mg/d of nitazoxanide (NTZ) is associated with improvement in symptoms or a decrease in shedding of organisms in about half of patients. Its overall role in the management of this condition remains unclear. Patients can minimize their risk of developing cryptosporidiosis by avoiding contact with human and animal feces and by not drinking untreated water from lakes or rivers.

Microsporidia are small, unicellular, obligate intracellular parasites that reside in the cytoplasm of enteric cells (Chap. 199). The main species causing disease in humans is *Enterocytozoon bieneusi*. The clinical manifestations are similar to those described for cryptosporidia and include abdominal pain and diarrhea. The small size of the organism may make it difficult to detect; however, with the use of chromotrope-based stains, organisms can be identified in stool samples by light microscopy. Definitive diagnosis generally depends on electron microscopic examination of a stool specimen, intestinal aspirate, or intestinal biopsy specimen. In contrast to cryptosporidia, microsporidia have been noted in a variety of extraintestinal locations, including the eye, muscle, and liver, and have been associated with conjunctivitis and hepatitis. Albendazole, 400 mg bid, has been reported to be of benefit in some patients.

I. belli is a coccidian parasite (Chap. 199) most commonly found as a cause of diarrhea in patients from the Caribbean and Africa. Its cysts appear in the stool as large, acid-fast structures that can be differentiated from those of cryptosporidia on the basis of size, shape, and number of sporocysts. The clinical syndromes of *Isospora* infection are identical to those caused by cryptosporidia. The important distinction is that infection with *Isospora* is generally relatively easy to treat with TMP/SMX. While relapses are common, a thrice-weekly regimen, similar to that used to provide prophylaxis against PCP, appears adequate to prevent recurrence.

CMV colitis was once seen in 5 to 10% of patients with AIDS. It is much less common with the advent of HAART. CMV colitis presents as diarrhea, abdominal pain, weight loss, and anorexia. The diarrhea is usually nonbloody, and the diagnosis is achieved through endoscopy and biopsy. Multiple mucosal ulcerations are seen at endoscopy, and biopsies reveal characteristic intranuclear inclusion bodies. Secondary bacteremias may result as a consequence of thinning of the bowel wall. Treatment is with either ganciclovir or foscarnet for 3 to 6 weeks. Relapses are common, and maintenance therapy is typically necessary in patients whose HIV infection is poorly controlled. Patients with CMV disease of the gastrointestinal tract should be carefully monitored for evidence of retinitis.

In addition to disease caused by specific secondary infections, patients with HIV infection may also experience a chronic diarrheal syndrome for which no etiologic agent other than HIV can be identified. This entity is referred to as *AIDS enteropathy* or *HIV enteropathy*. It is most likely a direct result of HIV infection in the gastrointestinal tract. Histologic examination of the small bowel in these patients reveals low-grade mucosal atrophy with a decrease in mitotic figures, suggesting a hyporegenerative state. Patients often have decreased or absent small-bowel lactase and malabsorption with accompanying weight loss.

The initial evaluation of a patient with HIV infection and diarrhea

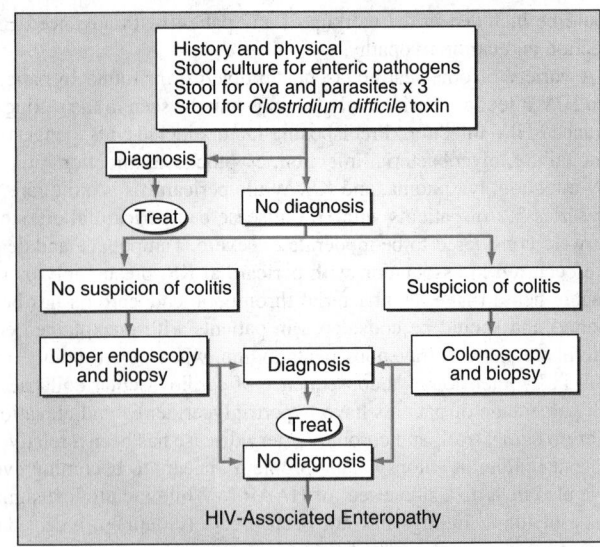

FIGURE 173-30 Algorithm for the evaluation of diarrhea in a patient with HIV infection. HIV-associated enteropathy is a diagnosis of exclusion and can be made only after other, generally treatable, forms of diarrheal illness have been ruled out.

should include a set of stool examinations, including culture, examination for ova and parasites, and examination for *Clostridium difficile* toxin. Approximately 50% of the time this workup will demonstrate infection with pathogenic bacteria, mycobacteria, or protozoa. If the initial stool examinations are negative, additional evaluation, including upper and/or lower endoscopy with biopsy, will yield a diagnosis of microsporidial or mycobacterial infection of the small intestine ~30% of the time. In patients for whom this diagnostic evaluation is nonrevealing, a presumptive diagnosis of HIV enteropathy can be made if the diarrhea has persisted for >1 month. An algorithm for the evaluation of diarrhea in patients with HIV infection is given in Fig. 173-30.

Rectal lesions are common in HIV-infected patients, particularly the perirectal ulcers and erosions due to the reactivation of HSV (Fig. 173-31). These may appear quite atypical, as denuded skin without vesicles, and they respond well to treatment with acyclovir, famciclovir, or foscarnet. Other rectal lesions encountered in patients with HIV infection include condylomata acuminata, KS, and intraepithelial neoplasia (see below).

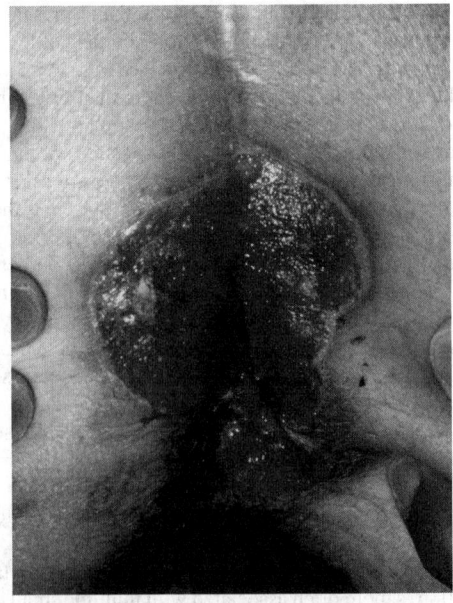

FIGURE 173-31 Severe, erosive perirectal herpes simplex in a patient with AIDS.

Hepatobiliary Disease Diseases of the hepatobiliary system are a major problem in patients with HIV infection. It has been estimated that approximately one-third of the deaths of patients with HIV infection are in some way related to liver disease. While this is predominantly a reflection of the problems encountered in the setting of co-infection with hepatitis B or C, it is also a reflection of the hepatic injury, ranging from hepatic steatosis to hypersensitivity reactions to immune reconstitution, that can be seen in the context of antiretroviral therapy.

Approximately 95% of HIV-infected individuals have evidence of infection with HBV; 5 to 40% of patients are co-infected with HCV; and co-infection with hepatitis D, E, and/or G viruses is common. HIV infection has a significant impact on the course of hepatitis virus infection. It is associated with approximately a threefold increase in the development of persistent hepatitis B surface antigenemia. Patients infected with both HBV and HIV have decreased evidence of inflammatory liver disease. The presumption that this is due to the immunosuppressive effects of HIV infection is supported by the observations that this situation can be reversed, and one may see the development of more severe hepatitis following the initiation of effective antiretroviral therapy. In a study of the impact of HIV on hepatitis B infection a tenfold increase in liver-related mortality was noted in patients with HIV and active HBV infection compared to rates in patients with either infection alone. IFN-α is less successful as a treatment of HBV in patients with HIV co-infection, and lamivudine or adefovir/tenofovir is the treatment of choice. It is important to remember that these drugs are also potent antiretroviral agents in the setting of combination antiretroviral therapy. They should not be used as single agents in patients with HIV infection, even if it is only being used to treat HBV, in order to avoid the rapid development of resistant quasispecies of HIV. In contrast to the situation with HBV, HCV infection is more severe in the patient with HIV infection; however, it does not appear to affect overall mortality when other variables such as age, baseline CD4+ T cell count, and use of HAART are taken into account. In the setting of HIV and HCV co-infection, levels of HCV are approximately tenfold higher than in the HIV-negative patient with HCV infection and there is an increased rate of progression to cirrhosis. Treatment for HCV infection consists of pegylated IFN-α and ribavirin. If a 2-log drop in levels of HCV RNA is not seen within 12 weeks, it is unlikely that therapy will be of value. Hepatitis A virus infection is not seen with an increased frequency in patients with HIV infection. It is recommended that all patients with HIV infection who have not experienced natural infection be immunized with hepatitis A and/or hepatitis B vaccines. Infection with hepatits G virus, also known as GB virus C, is seen in ~50% of patients with HIV infection. For reasons that are currently unclear there are data to suggestion that patients with HIV infection co-infected with this virus have a decreased rate of progression to AIDS.

A variety of other infections may also involve the liver. Granulomatous hepatitis may be seen as a consequence of mycobacterial or fungal infections, particularly MAC infection. Hepatic masses may be seen in the context of TB, peliosis hepatis, or fungal infection. Among the fungal opportunistic infections *C. immitis* and *Histoplasma capsulatum* are those most likely to involve the liver. Biliary tract disease in the form of papillary stenosis or sclerosing cholangitis has been reported in the context of cryptosporidiosis, CMV infection, and KS.

Many of the drugs used to treat HIV infection are metabolized by the liver and can cause liver injury. Fatal hepatic reactions have been reported with a wide array of antiretrovirals including nucleoside analogues, nonnucleoside analogues, and protease inhibitors. Nucleoside analogues work by inhibiting DNA synthesis. This can result in toxicity to mitochondria, which can lead to disturbances in oxidative metabolism. This may be manifest as hepatic steatosis and, in severe cases, lactic acidosis and fulminant liver failure. It is important to be aware of this condition and to watch for it in patients with HIV infection receiving nucleoside analogues. It is reversible if diagnosed early and the offending agent(s) discontinued. Nevirapine has been associated with at times fatal fulminant and cholestatic hepatitis, hepatic necrosis, and hepatic failure. Indinavir may cause mild to moderate

elevations in serum bilirubin in 10 to 15% of patients in a syndrome similar to Gilbert's syndrome. A similar pattern of hepatic injury may be seen with atazanavir. In the patient receiving HAART with an unexplained increase in hepatic transaminases, strong consideration should be given to drug toxicity. *Pancreatic injury* is most commonly a consequence of drug toxicity, notably that secondary to pentamidine or dideoxynucleosides. While up to half of patients in some series have biochemical evidence of pancreatic injury, <5% of patients show any clinical evidence of pancreatitis that is not linked to a drug toxicity.

Diseases of the Kidney and Genitourinary Tract Diseases of the kidney or genitourinary tract may be a direct consequence of HIV infection, due to an opportunistic infection or neoplasm, or related to drug toxicity. *HIV-associated nephropathy* was first described in IDUs and was initially thought to be IDU nephropathy in patients with HIV infection; it is now recognized as a true direct complication of HIV infection. HIV-associated nephropathy can be an early manifestation of HIV infection and is also seen in children. Over 90% of reported cases have been in African-American or Hispanic individuals; the disease is not only more prevalent in these populations but also more severe. Proteinuria is the hallmark of this disorder. Overall, microalbuminuria is seen in ~20% of untreated HIV-infected patients; significant proteinuria is seen in closer to 2%. Edema and hypertension are rare. Ultrasound examination reveals enlarged, hyperechogenic kidneys. A definitive diagnosis is obtained through renal biopsy. Histologically, focal segmental glomerulosclerosis is present in 80%, and mesangial proliferation in 10 to 15% of cases. Prior to effective antiretroviral therapy, this disease was characterized by relatively rapid progression to end-stage renal disease. Treatment with prednisone, 60 mg/d, has been reported to be of benefit in some cases. The incidence of this disease in patients receiving adequate antiretroviral therapy has not been well defined; however, the impression is that it has decreased in frequency. It is the leading cause of end-stage renal disease in patients with HIV infection.

Among the drugs commonly associated with renal damage in patients with HIV disease are pentamidine, amphotericin, adefovir, cidofovir, and foscarnet. TMP/SMX may compete for tubular secretion with creatinine and cause an increase in the serum creatinine level. Sulfadiazine may crystallize in the kidney and result in an easily reversible form of renal shutdown. One of the most common drug-induced renal complications is indinavir-associated renal calculi. This condition is seen in ~10% of patients receiving this HIV protease inhibitor. It may present with a variety of manifestations, ranging from asymptomatic hematuria to renal colic. Adequate hydration is the mainstay of treatment and prevention for this condition.

Genitourinary tract infections are seen with a high frequency in patients with HIV infection; they present with dysuria, hematuria, and/or pyuria and are managed in the same fashion as in patients without HIV infection. Infections with *T. pallidum*, the etiologic agent of *syphilis*, play an important role in the HIV epidemic (Chap. 172). In HIV-negative individuals, genital syphilitic ulcers as well as the ulcers of chancroid are major predisposing factors for heterosexual transmission of HIV infection. While most HIV-infected individuals with syphilis have a typical presentation, a variety of formerly rare clinical problems may be encountered in the setting of dual infection. Among them are *lues maligna*, an ulcerating lesion of the skin due to a necrotizing vasculitis; unexplained fever; nephrotic syndrome; and neurosyphilis. The most common presentation of syphilis in the HIV-infected patient is that of *condylomata lata*, a form of secondary syphilis. Neurosyphilis may be asymptomatic or may present as acute meningitis, neuroretinitis, deafness, or stroke. The rate of neurosyphilis may be as high as 1% in patients with HIV infection. As a consequence of the immunologic abnormalities seen in the setting of HIV infection, diagnosis of syphilis through standard serologic testing may be challenging. On the one hand, a significant number of patients have false-positive Venereal Disease Research Laboratory (VDRL) tests

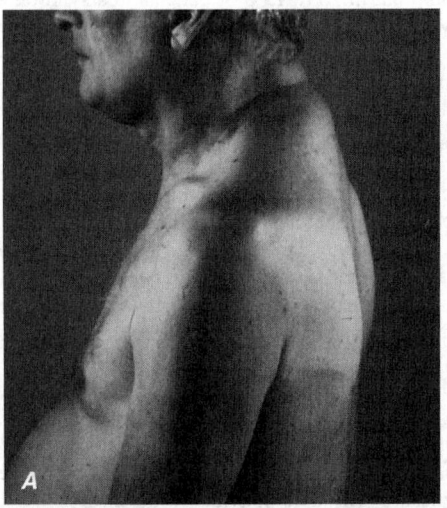

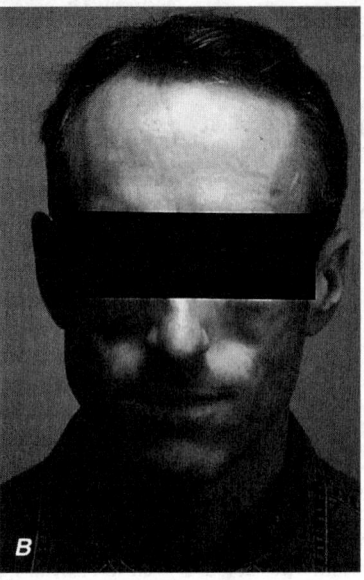

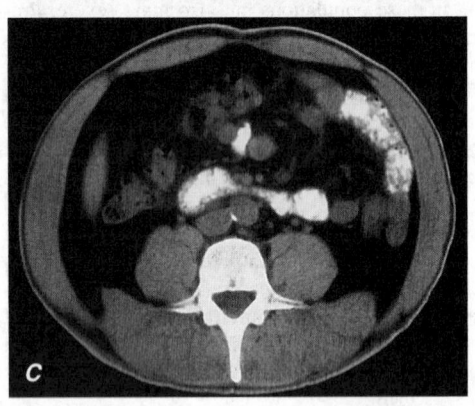

FIGURE 173-32 Characteristics of lipodystrophy. *A.* Truncal obesity and buffalo hump. *B.* Facial wasting. *C.* Accumulation of intraabdominal fat on CT scan.

due to polyclonal B cell activation. On the other hand, the development of a new positive VDRL may be delayed in patients with new infections, and the anti-fluorescent treponema antibody (anti-FTA) test may be negative due to immunodeficiency. Thus, dark-field examination of appropriate specimens should be performed in any patient in whom syphilis is suspected, even if the patient has a negative VDRL. Similarly, any patient with a positive serum VDRL test, neurologic findings, and an abnormal spinal fluid examination should be considered to have neurosyphilis, regardless of the CSF VDRL result. In any setting, patients treated for syphilis need to be carefully monitored to ensure adequate therapy.

Vulvovaginal candidiasis is a common problem in women with HIV infection. Symptoms include pruritus, discomfort, dyspareunia, and dysuria. Vulvar infection may present as a morbilliform rash that may extend to the thighs. Vaginal infection is usually associated with a white discharge, and plaques may be seen along an erythematous vaginal wall. Diagnosis is made by microscopic examination of the discharge for pseudohyphal elements in a 10% potassium hydroxide solution. Mild disease can be treated with topical therapy. More serious disease can be treated with fluconazole. Other causes of vaginitis include *Trichomonas* and mixed bacteria.

Diseases of the Endocrine System and Metabolic Disorders A variety of endocrine and metabolic disorders are seen in the context of HIV infection. Between 33 and 75% of patients with HIV infection receiving HAART develop a syndrome often referred to as *lipodystrophy*, consisting of elevations in plasma triglycerides, total cholesterol, and apolipoprotein B, as well as hyperinsulinemia and hyperglycemia. Many of these patients have been noted to have a characteristic set of body habitus changes associated with fat redistribution, consisting of truncal obesity coupled with peripheral wasting (Fig. 173-32). Truncal obesity is apparent as an increase in abdominal girth related to increases in

mesenteric fat, a dorsocervical fat pad ("buffalo hump") reminiscent of patients with Cushing's syndrome, and enlargement of the breasts. The peripheral wasting or lipoatrophy is particularly noticeable in the face and buttocks and by the prominence of the veins in the legs. These changes may develop at any time ranging from ~6 weeks to several years following the initiation of HAART. The syndrome has been reported in association with regimens containing a variety of different drugs, and while initially reported in the setting of protease inhibitor therapy, it appears similar changes can also be induced by potent protease-sparing regimens. It has been suggested that the lipoatrophy changes are particularly severe in patients receiving thymidine analogues. National Cholesterol Education Program (NCEP) guidelines should be followed in the management of these lipid abnormalities (Chap. 225). Due to concerns regarding drug interactions, the most commonly utilized agents in this setting are gemfibrozil and atorvostatin. In addition to these abnormalities, patients with HIV infection treated with HAART have been found to have an increased incidence of osteonecrosis or avascular necrosis of the hip and shoulders. In a study of asymptomatic patients, 4.4% were found to have evidence of osteonecrosis on MRI. This complication was associated with the use of lipid-lowering agents, systemic glucocorticoids or testosterone; bodybuilding exercise; and the presence of anticardiolipin antibodies. Lactic acidosis is also associated with antiretroviral therapy. This is most commonly seen with nucleoside reverse transcriptase inhibitors and can be fatal (see below).

Patients with advanced HIV disease may develop hyponatremia due to the syndrome of inappropriate antidiuretic hormone (vasopressin) secretion (SIADH) as a consequence of increased free water intake and decreased free water excretion. SIADH is usually seen in conjunction with pulmonary or CNS disease. Low serum sodium may also be due to adrenal insufficiency; concomitant high serum potassium should alert one to this possibility. Adrenal gland disease may be due to mycobacterial infections, CMV disease, cryptococcal disease, histoplasmosis, or ketoconazole toxicity.

Thyroid function is generally normal in patients with HIV infection although ~2 to 3% of patients may have elevations in thyroid-stimulating hormone (TSH). In the setting of HAART up to 10% of patients have been noted to have elevated TSH levels, suggesting that this may be a manifestation of immune reconstitution. In advanced HIV disease, infection of the thyroid gland may occur with opportunistic pathogens, including *P. carinii*, CMV, mycobacteria, *Toxoplasma gondii*, and *Cryptococcus neoformans*. These infections are generally associated with a nontender, diffuse enlargement of the thyroid gland. Thyroid function is usually normal. Diagnosis is made by fine-needle aspirate or open biopsy.

Advanced HIV disease is associated with *hypogonadism* in ~50% of men. While this is generally a complication of underlying illness, testicular dysfunction may also be a side effect of ganciclovir therapy. In some surveys, up to two-thirds of patients report decreased libido and one-third complain of impotence. Androgen replacement therapy should be considered in patients with symptomatic hypogonadism. HIV infection does not seem to have a significant effect on the menstrual cycle outside the setting of advanced disease.

Rheumatologic Diseases Immunologic and rheumatologic disorders are common in patients with HIV infection and range from excessive immediate-type hypersensitivity reactions (Chap. 298) to an increase in the incidence of reactive arthritis (Chap. 305) to conditions characterized by a diffuse infiltrative lymphocytosis. The occurrence of these phenomena is an apparent paradox in the setting of the profound immunodeficiency and immunosuppression that characterizes HIV infection. In addition, following the initiation of antiretroviral therapy, one may see a variety of exaggerated immune responses to existing opportunistic infections referred to as *immune reactivation syndromes.*

Drug allergies are the most significant allergic reactions occurring in HIV-infected patients and appear to become more common as the disease progresses. They occur in 65% of patients who receive therapy with TMP/SMX for PCP. In general, these drug reactions are characterized by erythematous, morbilliform eruptions that are pruritic, tend to coalesce, and are often associated with fever. Nonetheless, ~33% of patients can be maintained on the offending therapy, and thus these reactions are not an immediate indication to stop the drug. Anaphylaxis is extremely rare in patients with HIV infection, and patients who have a cutaneous reaction during a single course of therapy can still be considered candidates for future treatment or prophylaxis with the same agent. The one exception to this is the nucleoside analogue abacavir, where fatal hypersensitivity reactions have been reported with rechallenge. A hypersensitivity reaction to abacavir is an absolute contraindication to future therapy. For other agents, including TMP/SMX, desensitization regimens are moderately successful. While the mechanisms underlying these allergic-type reactions remain unknown, patients with HIV infection have been noted to have elevated IgE levels that increase as the CD4+ T cell count declines. The numerous examples of patients with multiple drug reactions suggest that a common pathway is involved.

HIV infection shares many similarities with a variety of autoimmune diseases, including a substantial polyclonal B cell activation that is associated with a high incidence of antiphospholipid antibodies, such as anticardiolipin antibodies, VDRL antibodies, and lupus-like anticoagulants. In addition, HIV-infected individuals have an increased incidence of antinuclear antibodies. Despite these serologic findings, there is no evidence that HIV-infected individuals have an increase in two of the more common autoimmune diseases, i.e., systemic lupus erythematosus and rheumatoid arthritis. In fact, it has been observed that these diseases may be somewhat ameliorated by the concomitant presence of HIV infection, suggesting that an intact CD4+ T cell limb of the immune response plays an integral role in the pathogenesis of these conditions. Similarly, there are anecdotal reports of patients with common variable immunodeficiency (Chap. 297), characterized by hypogammaglobulinemia, who have had a normalization of Ig levels following the development of HIV infection, suggesting a possible role for overactive CD4+ T cell immunity in certain forms of that syndrome. The one autoimmune disease that may occur with an increased frequency in patients with HIV infection is a variant of primary Sjögren's syndrome (Chap. 304). Patients with HIV infection may develop a syndrome consisting of parotid gland enlargement, dry eyes, and dry mouth that is associated with lymphocytic infiltrates of the salivary gland and lung. In contrast to Sjögren's syndrome, in which these infiltrates are composed predominantly of CD4+ T cells, in patients with HIV infection the infiltrates are composed predominantly of CD8+ T cells. In addition, while patients with Sjögren's syndrome are mainly women who have autoantibodies to Ro and La and who frequently have HLA-DR3 or -B8 MHC haplotypes, HIV-infected individuals with this syndrome are usually African-American men who do not have anti-Ro or anti-La and who most often are HLA-DR5. This syndrome appears to be less common with the increased use of effective antiretroviral therapy. The term *diffuse infiltrative lymphocytosis syndrome* (DILS) has been proposed to describe this entity and to distinguish it from Sjögren's syndrome.

Approximately one-third of HIV-infected individuals experience arthralgias; furthermore, 5 to 10% are diagnosed as having some form of reactive arthritis, such as Reiter's syndrome or psoriatic arthritis (Chap. 305). These syndromes occur with increasing frequency as the competency of the immune system declines. This association may be related to an increase in the number of infections with organisms that

may trigger a reactive arthritis with progressive immunodeficiency or to a loss of important regulatory T cells. Reactive arthritides in HIV-infected individuals generally respond well to standard treatment; however, therapy with methotrexate has been associated with an increase in the incidence of opportunistic infections and should be used with caution and only in severe cases.

HIV-infected individuals also experience a variety of joint problems without obvious cause that are referred to generically as *HIV- or AIDS-associated arthropathy*. This syndrome is characterized by subacute oligoarticular arthritis developing over a period of 1 to 6 weeks and lasting 6 weeks to 6 months. It generally involves the large joints, predominantly the knees and ankles, and is nonerosive with only a mild inflammatory response. X-rays of the joint are nonrevealing. Nonsteroidal anti-inflammatory drugs are only marginally helpful; however, relief has been noted with the use of intraarticular glucocorticoids. A second form of arthritis also thought to be secondary to HIV infection is called *painful articular syndrome*. This condition, found in as many as 10% of AIDS patients, presents as an acute, severe, sharp pain in the affected joint. It affects primarily the knees, elbows, and shoulders; lasts 2 to 24 h; and may be severe enough to require narcotic analgesics. The cause of this arthropathy is unclear; however, it is thought to result from a direct effect of HIV on the joint. This condition is reminiscent of the fact that other lentiviruses, in particular the caprine arthritis-encephalitis virus, are capable of directly causing arthritis.

A variety of other immunologic or rheumatologic diseases have been reported in HIV-infected individuals, either de novo or in association with opportunistic infections or drugs. Using the criteria of widespread musculoskeletal pain of at least 3 months' duration and the presence of at least 11 of 18 possible tender points by digital palpation, 11% of an HIV-infected cohort containing 55% IDUs were diagnosed as having *fibromyalgia* (Chap. 315). While the incidence of frank arthritis was less in this population than in other studied populations that consisted predominantly of homosexual men, these data support the concept that there are musculoskeletal problems that occur as a direct result of HIV infection. In addition there have been reports of leukocytoclastic vasculitis in the setting of zidovudine therapy. CNS angiitis and polymyositis have also been reported in HIV-infected individuals. Septic arthritis is surprisingly rare, especially given the increased incidence of staphylococcal bacteremias seen in this population. When septic arthritis has been reported, it has usually been due to systemic fungal infections with *C. neoformans, Sporothrix schenckii*, or *H. capsulatum*, or to systemic mycobacterial infection with *M. haemophilum*.

Following the initiation of effective antiretroviral therapy, a paradoxical worsening of preexisting, untreated, or partially treated opportunistic infections may be noted. These *immune reactivation syndromes* are particularly common in patients with underlying untreated mycobacterial infections. They appear to be related to a phenomenon similar to type IV hypersensitivity reactions and reflect the immediate improvements in immune function that occur as levels of HIV RNA drop and the immunosuppressive effects of HIV infection are controlled. In severe cases the use of immunosuppressive drugs such as glucocorticoids may be required to blunt the inflammatory component of these reactions while specific antimicrobial therapy takes effect.

Diseases of the Hematopoietic System Disorders of the hematopoietic system including lymphadenopathy, anemia, leukopenia, and/or thrombocytopenia are common throughout the course of HIV infection and may be the direct result of HIV, manifestations of secondary infections and neoplasms, or side effects of therapy (Table 173-12). Direct histologic examination and culture of lymph node or bone marrow tissue are often diagnostic. A significant percentage of bone marrow aspirates from patients with HIV infection have been reported to contain lymphoid aggregates, the precise significance of which is un-

TABLE 173-12 Causes of Bone Marrow Suppression in Patients with HIV Infection

HIV infection	Medications
Mycobacterial infections	Zidovudine
Fungal infections	Dapsone
B19 parvovirus infection	Trimethoprim/sulfamethoxazole
Lymphoma	Pyrimethamine
	5-Flucytosine
	Ganciclovir
	Interferon-α
	Trimetrexate
	Foscarnet

known. Initiation of HAART will lead to reversal of most hematologic complications that are the direct result of HIV infection.

Some patients, otherwise asymptomatic, may develop *persistent generalized lymphadenopathy* as an early clinical manifestation of HIV infection. This condition is defined as the presence of enlarged lymph nodes (>1 cm) in two or more extrainguinal sites for >3 months without an obvious cause. The lymphadenopathy is due to marked follicular hyperplasia in the node in response to HIV infection. The nodes are generally discrete and freely movable. This feature of HIV disease may be seen at any point in the spectrum of immune dysfunction and is not associated with an increased likelihood of developing AIDS. Paradoxically, a loss in lymphadenopathy or a decrease in lymph node size outside the setting of antiretroviral therapy may be a prognostic marker of disease progression. In patients with CD4+ T cell counts >200/μL, the differential diagnosis of lymphadenopathy includes KS, TB, and lymphoma. In patients with more advanced disease, lymphadenopathy may also be due to atypical mycobacterial infection, toxoplasmosis, systemic fungal infection, or bacillary angiomatosis. While indicated in patients with CD4+ T cell counts <200/μL, lymph node biopsy is not indicated in patients with early-stage disease unless there are signs and symptoms of systemic illness, such as fever and weight loss, or unless the nodes begin to enlarge, become fixed, or coalesce.

Anemia is the most common hematologic abnormality in HIV-infected patients. While generally mild, anemia can be quite severe and require chronic blood transfusions. Among the specific reversible causes of anemia in the setting of HIV infection are drug toxicity, systemic fungal and mycobacterial infections, nutritional deficiencies, and parvovirus B19 infections. Zidovudine may block erythroid maturation, prior to its effects on other marrow elements. A characteristic feature of zidovudine therapy is an elevated mean corpuscular volume (MCV). Another drug used in patients with HIV infection that has a selective effect on the erythroid series is dapsone. This drug can cause a serious hemolytic anemia in patients who are deficient in glucose-6-phosphate dehydrogenase and can create a functional anemia in others through induction of methemoglobinemia. Folate levels are usually normal in HIV-infected individuals; however, vitamin B_{12} levels may be depressed as a consequence of achlorhydria or malabsorption. True autoimmune hemolytic anemia is rare, although ~20% of patients with HIV infection may have a positive direct antiglobulin test as a consequence of polyclonal B cell activation. Infection with parvovirus B19 may also cause anemia. It is important to recognize this possibility given the fact that it responds well to treatment with intravenous immunoglobulin. Erythropoietin levels in patients with HIV infection and anemia are generally less than expected given the degree of anemia. Treatment with erythropoietin at doses of 100 μg/kg three times a week may result in an increase in hemoglobulin levels. An exception to this is a subset of patients with zidovudine-associated anemia in whom erythropoietin levels may be quite high.

During the course of HIV infection, neutropenia may be seen in approximately half of patients. In most instances it is mild; however, it can be severe and can put patients at risk of spontaneous bacterial infections. This is most frequently seen in patients with severely advanced HIV disease and in patients receiving any of a number of potentially myelosuppressive therapies. In the setting of neutropenia, diseases that are not commonly seen in HIV-infected patients, such as aspergillosis or mucormycosis, may occur. The potential role of colony-stimulating factors in the management of patients with HIV infection has undergone extensive evaluation. Both granulocyte colony-stimulating factor (G-CSF) and GM-CSF increase neutrophil counts in patients with HIV infection regardless of the cause of the neutropenia. Earlier concerns about the potential of these agents to also increase levels of HIV were not confirmed in controlled clinical trials.

Thrombocytopenia may be an early consequence of HIV infection. Approximately 3% of patients with untreated HIV infection and CD4+ T cell counts ≥400/μL have platelet counts <150,000/μL. For untreated patients with CD4+ T cell counts <400/μL, this incidence increases to 10%. Thrombocytopenia is rarely a serious clinical problem in patients with HIV infection and generally responds well to antiretroviral therapy. Clinically, it resembles the thrombocytopenia seen in patients with idiopathic thrombocytopenic purpura (Chap. 101). Immune complexes containing anti-gp120 antibodies and anti-anti-gp120 antibodies have been noted in the circulation and on the surface of platelets in patients with HIV infection. Patients with HIV infection have also been noted to have a platelet-specific antibody directed towards a 25-kDa component of the surface of the platelet. Other data suggest that the thrombocytopenia in patients with HIV infection may be due to a direct effect of HIV on megakaryocytes. Whatever the cause, it is very clear that the most effective medical approach to this problem has been the use of HAART. For patients with platelet counts <20,000/μL a more aggressive approach combining intravenous Ig or anti-Rh Ig for an immediate response with antiretroviral therapy for a more lasting response is appropriate. Splenectomy is a rarely needed option and is reserved for patients refractory to medical management. Because of the risk of serious infection with encapsulated organisms, all patients with HIV infection about to undergo splenectomy should be immunized with pneumococcal polysaccharide. It should be noted that, in addition to causing an increase in the platelet count, removal of the spleen will result in an increase in the peripheral blood lymphocyte count, making CD4+ T cell counts unreliable. In this setting, the clinician should rely on the CD4+ T cell percent for making diagnostic decisions with respect to the likelihood of opportunistic infections. A CD4+ T cell percent of 15 is approximately equivalent to a CD4+ T cell count of 200/μL. In patients with early HIV infection, thrombocytopenia has also been reported as a consequence of classic thrombotic thrombocytopenic purpura (Chap. 101). This clinical syndrome, consisting of fever, thrombocytopenia, hemolytic anemia, and neurologic and renal dysfunction, is a rare complication of early HIV infection. As in other settings, the appropriate management is the use of salicylates and plasma exchange. Other causes of thrombocytopenia include lymphoma, mycobacterial infections, and fungal infections.

Dermatologic Diseases Dermatologic problems occur in >90% of patients with HIV infection. From the macular, roseola-like rash seen with the acute seroconversion syndrome to extensive end-stage KS, cutaneous manifestations of HIV disease can be seen throughout the course of HIV infection. Among the more common nonneoplastic problems are seborrheic dermatitis, eosinophilic pustular folliculitus, and opportunistic infections. Extrapulmonary pneumocystosis may cause a necrotizing vasculitis. Neoplastic conditions are covered below in the section on malignant diseases.

Seborrheic dermatitis occurs in 3% of the general population and in up to 50% of patients with HIV infection. Seborrheic dermatitis increases in prevalence and severity as the CD4+ T cell count declines. In HIV-infected patients, seborrheic dermatitis may be aggravated by concomitant infection with *Pityrosporum*, a yeastlike fungus; use of topical antifungal agents has been recommended in cases refractory to standard topical treatment.

Eosinophilic pustular folliculitis is a rare dermatologic condition that is seen with increased frequency in patients with HIV infection.

It presents as multiple, urticarial perifollicular papules that may coalesce into plaquelike lesions. Skin biopsy reveals an eosinophilic infiltrate of the hair follicle, which in certain cases has been associated with the presence of a mite. Patients typically have an elevated serum IgE level and may respond to treatment with topical anthelminthics. Patients with HIV infection have also been reported to develop a severe form of *Norwegian scabies* with hyperkeratotic psoriasiform lesions.

Both *psoriasis* and *ichthyosis*, although they are not reported to be increased in frequency, may be particularly severe when they occur in patients with HIV infection. Preexisting psoriasis may become guttate in appearance and more refractory to treatment in the setting of HIV infection.

Reactivation herpes zoster (*shingles*) is seen in 10 to 20% of patients with HIV infection. This reactivation syndrome of varicella-zoster virus indicates a modest decline in immune function and may be the first indication of clinical immunodeficiency. In one series, patients who developed shingles did so an average of 5 years after HIV infection. In a cohort of patients with HIV infection and localized zoster, the subsequent rate of the development of AIDS was 1% per month. In that study, AIDS was more likely to develop if the outbreak of zoster was associated with severe pain, extensive skin involvement, or involvement of cranial or cervical dermatomes. The clinical manifestations of reactivation zoster in HIV-infected patients, although indicative of immunologic compromise, are not as severe as those seen in other immunodeficient conditions. Thus, while lesions may extend over several dermatomes (see Fig. 164-3) and frank cutaneous dissemination may be seen, visceral involvement has not been reported. In contrast to patients without a known underlying immunodeficiency state, patients with HIV infection tend to have recurrences of zoster with a relapse rate of ~20%. Acyclovir or famciclovir is the treatment of choice. Foscarnet is of value in patients with acyclovir-resistant virus.

Infection with *herpes simplex virus* in HIV-infected individuals is associated with recurrent orolabial, genital, and perianal lesions as part of recurrent reactivation syndromes (Chap. 163). As HIV disease progresses and the CD4+ T cell count declines, these infections become more frequent and severe. Lesions often appear as beefy red, are exquisitely painful, and have a tendency to occur high in the gluteal cleft (Fig. 173-31). Perirectal HSV may be associated with proctitis and anal fissures. HSV should be high in the differential diagnosis of any HIV-infected patient with a poorly healing, painful perirectal lesion. In addition to recurrent mucosal ulcers, recurrent HSV infection in the form of *herpetic whitlow* can be a problem in patients with HIV infection, presenting with painful vesicles or extensive cutaneous erosion. Acyclovir or famciclovir is the treatment of choice in these settings. Of note is the fact that even subclinical reactivation of herpes simplex may be associated with increases in plasma HIV RNA levels. Consideration should be given to chronic suppressive therapy in patients with recurrent outbreaks of herpesvirus.

Diffuse skin eruptions due to *Molluscum contagiosum* may be seen in patients with advanced HIV infection. These flesh-colored, umbilicated lesions may be treated with local therapy. They tend to regress with effective antiretroviral therapy. Similarly, *condyloma acuminatum* lesions may be more severe and more widely distributed in patients with low CD4+ T cell counts. Atypical mycobacterial infections may present as erythematous cutaneous nodules as may fungal infections, *Bartonella*, *Acanthamoeba*, and KS.

The skin of patients with HIV infection is often a target organ for drug reactions (Chap. 50). Although most skin reactions are mild and not necessarily an indication to discontinue therapy, patients may have particularly severe cutaneous reactions, including erythroderma and *Stevens-Johnson syndrome*, as a reaction to drugs, particularly sulfa drugs, the nonnucleoside reverse transcriptase inhibitors, abacavir, and amprenavir. Similarly, patients with HIV infection are often quite photosensitive and burn easily following exposure to sunlight or as a side effect of radiation therapy (Chap. 51).

HIV infection and its treatment may be accompanied by cosmetic changes of the skin that are not of great clinical importance but may be troubling to patients. Yellowing of the nails and straightening of the hair, particularly in African-American patients, have been reported as a consequence of HIV infection. Zidovudine therapy has been associated with elongation of the eyelashes and the development of a bluish discoloration to the nails, again more common in African-American patients. Therapy with clofazimine may cause a yellow-orange discoloration of the skin.

Neurologic Diseases Clinical disease of the nervous system accounts for a significant degree of morbidity in a high percentage of patients with HIV infection (Table 173-13). The neurologic problems that occur in HIV-infected individuals may be either primary to the pathogenic processes of HIV infection or secondary to opportunistic infections or neoplasms (see above). Among the more frequent opportunistic diseases that involve the CNS are toxoplasmosis, cryptococcosis, progressive multifocal leukoencephalopathy, and primary CNS lymphoma. Other less common problems include mycobacterial infections; syphilis; and infection with CMV, HTLV-I, *T. cruzi*, or *Acanthamoeba*. Overall, secondary diseases of the CNS occur in approximately one-third of patients with AIDS. These data antedate the widespread use of combination antiretroviral therapy, and this frequency is considerably less in patients receiving effective antiretroviral drugs. Primary processes related to HIV infection of the nervous system are reminiscent of those seen with other lentiviruses, such as the Visna-Maedi virus of sheep. Neurologic problems occur throughout the course of disease and may be inflammatory, demyelinating, or degenerative in nature. While only one of these, the *AIDS dementia complex*, or *HIV encephalopathy*, is considered an AIDS-defining illness, most HIV-infected patients have some neurologic problem during the course of their disease. As noted in the section on pathogenesis, damage to the CNS may be a direct result of viral infection of the CNS macrophages or glial cells or may be secondary to the release of neurotoxins and potentially toxic cytokines such as IL-1β, TNF-α, IL-6, and TGF-β. It has been reported that HIV-infected individuals with the E4 allele for apolipoprotein E (apo E) are at increased risk for AIDS encephalopathy and peripheral neuropathy. Virtually all patients with HIV infection have some degree of nervous system involvement with the virus. This is evidenced by the fact that CSF findings are abnormal in ~90% of patients, even during the asymptomatic phase of HIV infection. CSF abnormalities include pleocytosis (50 to 65% of patients), detection of viral RNA (~75%), elevated CSF protein (35%), and evidence of intrathecal synthesis of anti-HIV antibodies (90%). It is important to point out that evidence of infection of the CNS with HIV does not imply impairment of cognitive function. The neurologic function of an HIV-infected individual should be considered normal unless clinical signs and symptoms suggest otherwise.

Aseptic meningitis may be seen in any but the very late stages of HIV infection. In the setting of acute primary infection patients may

TABLE 173-13 *Neurologic Diseases in Patients with HIV Infection*

Opportunistic infections	Myelopathy
Toxoplasmosis	Vacuolar myelopathy
Cryptococcosis	Pure sensory ataxia
Progressive multifocal	Paresthesia/dysesthesia
leukoencephalopathy	Peripheral neuropathy
Cytomegalovirus	Acute inflammatory demyelinating
Syphilis	polyneuropathy (Guillain-Barré
Mycobacterium tuberculosis	syndrome)
HTLV-I infection	Chronic inflammatory demyelinating
Neoplasms	polyneuropathy (CIDP)
Primary CNS lymphoma	Mononeuritis multiplex
Kaposi's sarcoma	Distal symmetric polyneuropathy
Result of HIV-1 infection	Myopathy
Aseptic meningitis	
HIV encephalopathy (AIDS	
dementia complex)	

experience a syndrome of headache, photophobia, and meningismus. Rarely, an acute encephalopathy due to encephalitis may occur. Cranial nerve involvement may be seen, predominantly cranial nerve VII but occasionally V and/or VIII. CSF findings include a lymphocytic pleocytosis, elevated protein level, and normal glucose level. This syndrome, which cannot be clinically differentiated from other viral meningitides (Chap. 361), usually resolves spontaneously within 2 to 4 weeks; however, in some patients, signs and symptoms may become chronic. Aseptic meningitis may occur any time in the course of HIV infection; however, it is rare following the development of AIDS. This fact suggests that clinical aseptic meningitis in the context of HIV infection is an immune-mediated disease.

C. neoformans is the leading infectious cause of meningitis in patients with AIDS (Chap. 186). It is the initial AIDS-defining illness in ~2% of patients and generally occurs in patients with CD4+ T cell counts <100/μL. Cryptococcal meningitis is particularly common in patients with AIDS in Africa, occurring in ~20% of patients. Most patients present with a picture of subacute meningoencephalitis with fever, nausea, vomiting, altered mental status, headache, and meningeal signs. The incidence of seizures and focal neurologic deficits is low. The CSF profile may be normal or may show only modest elevations in WBC or protein levels. In addition to meningitis, patients may develop cryptococcomas. Approximately one-third of patients also have pulmonary disease. Uncommon manifestations of cryptococcal infection include skin lesions that resemble *molluscum contagiosum*, lymphadenopathy, palatal and glossal ulcers, arthritis, gastroenteritis, myocarditis, and prostatitis. The prostate gland may serve as a reservoir for smoldering cryptococcal infection. The diagnosis of cryptococcal meningitis is made by identification of organisms in spinal fluid with India ink examination or by the detection of cryptococcal antigen. A biopsy may be needed to make a diagnosis of CNS cryptococcoma. Treatment is with intravenous amphotericin B, at a dose of 0.7 mg/kg daily, with flucytosine, 25 mg/kg qid for 2 weeks, followed by fluconazole, 400 mg/d orally for 10 weeks, and then fluconazole, 200 mg/d until the CD4+ T cell count has increased to >200 cells/μl for 6 months in response to HAART. Symptoms may recur with initiation of HAART as an immune reconstitution syndrome (see above). Other fungi that may cause meningitis in patients with HIV infection are *C. immitis* and *H. capsulatum*. Meningoencephalitis has also been reported due to *Acanthamoeba* or *Naegleria*.

HIV encephalopathy, also called HIV-associated dementia or AIDS dementia complex, consists of a constellation of signs and symptoms of CNS disease. While this is generally a late complication of HIV infection that progresses slowly over months it can be seen in patients with CD4 counts >350 cells/μl. A major feature of this entity is the development of dementia, defined as a decline in cognitive ability from a previous level. It may present as impaired ability to concentrate, increased forgetfulness, difficulty reading, or increased difficulty performing complex tasks. Initially these symptoms may be indistinguishable from findings of situational depression or fatigue. In contrast to "cortical" dementia (such as Alzheimer's disease), aphasia, apraxia, and agnosia are uncommon, leading some investigators to classify HIV encephalopathy as a "subcortical dementia" (see below). In addition to dementia, patients with HIV encephalopathy may also have motor and behavioral abnormalities. Among the motor problems are unsteady gait, poor balance, tremor, and difficulty with rapid alternating movements. Increased tone and deep tendon reflexes may be found in patients with spinal cord involvement. Late stages may be complicated by bowel and/or bladder incontinence. Behavioral problems include apathy and lack of initiative, with progression to a vegetative state in some instances. Some patients develop a state of agitation or mild mania. These changes usually occur without significant changes in level of alertness. This is in contrast to the finding of somnolence in patients with dementia due to toxic/metabolic encephalopathies.

HIV encephalopathy is the initial AIDS-defining illness in ~3% of patients with HIV infection and thus only rarely precedes clinical ev-

idence of immunodeficiency. Clinically significant encephalopathy eventually develops in approximately one-fourth of patients with AIDS. As immunologic function declines, the risk and severity of HIV encephalopathy increases. Autopsy series suggest that 80 to 90% of patients with HIV infection have histologic evidence of CNS involvement. Several classification schemes have been developed for grading HIV encephalopathy; a commonly used clinical staging system is outlined in Table 173-14.

The precise cause of HIV encephalopathy remains unclear, although the condition is thought to be a result of direct effects of HIV on the CNS. HIV has been found in the brains of patients with HIV encephalopathy by Southern blot, in situ hybridization, PCR, and electron microscopy. Multinucleated giant cells, macrophages, and microglial cells appear to be the main cell types harboring virus in the CNS. Histologically, the major changes are seen in the subcortical areas of the brain and include pallor and gliosis, multinucleated giant cell encephalitis, and vacuolar myelopathy. Less commonly, diffuse or focal spongiform changes occur in the white matter.

There are no specific criteria for a diagnosis of HIV encephalopathy, and this syndrome must be differentiated from a number of other diseases that affect the CNS of HIV-infected patients (Table 173-13). The diagnosis of dementia depends upon demonstrating a decline in cognitive function. This can be accomplished objectively with the use of a Mini-Mental Status Examination (MMSE) in patients for whom prior scores are available. For this reason, it is advisable for all patients with a diagnosis of HIV infection to have a baseline MMSE. However, changes in MMSE scores may be absent in patients with mild HIV encephalopathy. Imaging studies of the CNS, by either MRI or CT, often demonstrate evidence of cerebral atrophy (Fig. 173-33). MRI may also reveal small areas of increased density on T2-weighted images. Lumbar puncture is an important element of the evaluation of patients with HIV infection and neurologic abnormalities. It is generally most helpful in ruling out or making a diagnosis of opportunistic infections. In HIV encephalopathy, patients may have the nonspecific findings of an increase in CSF cells and protein level. While HIV RNA can often be detected in the spinal fluid and HIV can be cultured from the CSF, this finding is not specific for HIV encephalopathy. There

TABLE 173-14 *Clinical Staging of HIV Encephalopathy (AIDS Dementia Complex)*

Stage	Definition
Stage 0 (normal)	Normal mental and motor function
Stage 0.5 (equivocal/ subclinical)	Absent, minimal, or equivocal symptoms without impairment of work or capacity to perform activities of daily living. Mild signs (snout response, slowed ocular or extremity movements) may be present. Gait and strength are normal.
Stage 1 (mild)	Able to perform all but the more demanding aspects of work or activities of daily living but with unequivocal evidence (signs or symptoms that may include performance on neuropsychological testing) of functional, intellectual, or motor impairment. Can walk without assistance.
Stage 2 (moderate)	Able to perform basic activities of self-care but cannot work or maintain the more demanding aspects of daily life. Ambulatory, but may require a single prop.
Stage 3 (severe)	Major intellectual incapacity (cannot follow news or personal events, cannot sustain complex conversation, considerable slowing of all output) or motor disability (cannot walk unassisted, usually with slowing and clumsiness of arms as well).
Stage 4 (end-stage)	Nearly vegetative. Intellectual and social comprehension and output are at a rudimentary level. Nearly or absolutely mute. Paraparetic or paraplegic with urinary and fecal incontinence.

Source: Adapted from JJ Sidtis, RW Price, Neurology 40:197, 1990.

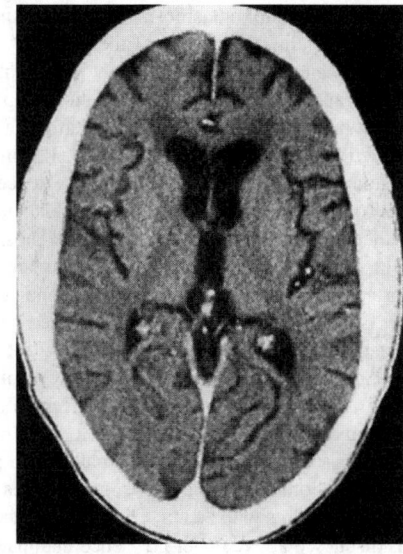

FIGURE 173-33 AIDS dementia complex. Postcontrast CT scan through the lateral ventricles of a 47-year-old man with AIDS, altered mental status, and dementia. The lateral and third ventricles and the cerebral sulci are abnormally prominent. Mild white matter hypodensity is also seen adjacent to the frontal horns of the lateral ventricles.

appears to be no correlation between the presence of HIV in the CSF and the presence of HIV encephalopathy. Elevated levels of β_2-microglobulin, neopterin, and quinolinic acid (a metabolite of tryptophan reported to cause CNS injury) have been noted in the CSF of patients with HIV encephalopathy. These findings suggest that these factors as well as inflammatory cytokines may be involved in the pathogenesis of this syndrome.

Combination antiretroviral therapy is of benefit in patients with HIV encephalopathy. Improvement in neuropsychiatric test scores has been noted for both adult and pediatric patients treated with antiretrovirals. The rapid improvement in cognitive function noted with the initiation of antiretroviral therapy suggests that at least some component of this problem is quickly reversible, again supporting at least a partial role of soluble mediators in the pathogenesis. It should also be noted that these patients have an increased sensitivity to the side effects of neuroleptic drugs. The use of these drugs for symptomatic treatment is associated with an increased risk of extrapyramidal side effects; therefore, patients with HIV encephalopathy who receive these agents must be monitored carefully.

Seizures may be a consequence of opportunistic infections, neoplasms, or HIV encephalopathy (Table 173-15). The seizure threshold is often lower than normal in these patients owing to the frequent presence of electrolyte abnormalities. Seizures are seen in 15 to 40% of patients with cerebral toxoplasmosis, 15 to 35% of patients with primary CNS lymphoma, 8% of patients with cryptococcal meningitis, and 7 to 50% of patients with HIV encephalopathy. Seizures may also be seen in patients with CNS tuberculosis, aseptic meningitis, and progressive multifocal leukoencephalopathy. Seizures may be the presenting clinical symptom of HIV disease. In one study of 100 patients with HIV infection presenting with a first seizure, cerebral mass lesions were the most common cause, responsible for 32 of the 100 new-onset seizures. Of these 32 cases, 28 were due to toxoplasmosis and 4 to lymphoma. HIV encephalopathy accounted for an additional 24 new-onset seizures. Cryptococcal meningitis was the third most common

diagnosis, responsible for 13 of the 100 seizures. In 23 cases, no cause could be found, and it is possible that these cases represent a subcategory of HIV encephalopathy. Of these 23 cases, 16 (70%) had two or more seizures, suggesting that anticonvulsant therapy is indicated in all patients with HIV infection and seizures unless a rapidly correctable cause is found. While phenytoin remains the initial treatment of choice, hypersensitivity reactions to this drug have been reported in >10% of patients with AIDS, and therefore the use of phenobarbital or valproic acid must be considered as alternatives.

Patients with HIV infection may present with *focal neurologic deficits* from a variety of causes. The most common causes are toxoplasmosis, progressive multifocal leukoencephalopathy, and CNS lymphoma. Other causes include cryptococcal infections (discussed above; also Chap. 186), stroke, and reactivation Chagas' disease.

Toxoplasmosis has been one of the most common causes of secondary CNS infections in patients with AIDS, but its incidence is decreasing in the era of HAART. It is most common in patients from the Caribbean and from France. Toxoplasmosis is generally a late complication of HIV infection and usually occurs in patients with CD4+ T cell counts <200/μL. Cerebral toxoplasmosis is thought to represent a reactivation syndrome. It is 10 times more common in patients with antibodies to the organism than in patients who are seronegative. Patients diagnosed with HIV infection should be screened for IgG antibodies to *T. gondii* during the time of their initial workup. Those who are seronegative should be counseled about ways to minimize the risk of primary infection including avoiding the consumption of undercooked meat and careful hand washing after contact with soil or changing the cat litter box. The most common clinical presentation of cerebral toxoplasmosis in patients with HIV infection is fever, headache, and focal neurologic deficits. Patients may present with seizure, hemiparesis, or aphasia as a manifestation of these focal deficits or with a picture more influenced by the accompanying cerebral edema and characterized by confusion, dementia, and lethargy, which can progress to coma. The diagnosis is usually suspected on the basis of MRI findings of multiple lesions in multiple locations, although in some cases only a single lesion is seen. Pathologically, these lesions generally exhibit inflammation and central necrosis and, as a result, demonstrate ring enhancement on contrast MRI (Fig. 173-34) or, if MRI is unavailable or contraindicated, on double-dose contrast CT. There is usually evidence of surrounding edema. In addition to toxoplasmosis, the differential diagnosis of single or multiple enhancing mass lesions in the HIV-infected patient includes primary CNS lymphoma (see below) and, less commonly, TB or fungal or bacterial abscesses.

Disease	Overall Contribution to First Seizure, %	Fraction of Patients Who Have Seizures, %
HIV encephalopathy	24–47	7–50
Cerebral toxoplasmosis	28	15–40
Cryptococcal meningitis	13	8
Primary central nervous system lymphoma	4	15–30
Progressive multifocal leukoencephalopathy	1	

TABLE 173-15 *Causes of Seizures in Patients with HIV Infection*

Source: From DM Holtzman et al: Am J Med 87:173, 1989.

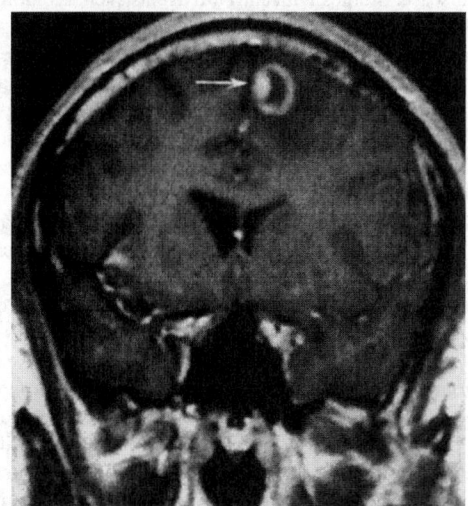

FIGURE 173-34 Central nervous system toxoplasmosis. A coronal postcontrast T1-weighted MR scan demonstrates a peripheral enhancing lesion in the left frontal lobe, associated with an eccentric nodular area of enhancement (*arrow*); this so-called "eccentric target sign" is typical of toxoplasmosis.

The definitive diagnostic procedure is brain biopsy. However, given the morbidity than can accompany this procedure, it is usually reserved for the patient who has failed 2 to 4 weeks of empirical therapy. If the patient is seronegative for *T. gondii*, the likelihood that a mass lesion is due to toxoplasmosis is <10%. In that setting, one may choose to be more aggressive and perform a brain biopsy sooner. Standard treatment is sulfadiazine and pyrimethamine with leucovorin as needed for a minimum of 4 to 6 weeks. Alternative therapeutic regimens include clindamycin in combination with pyrimethamine; atovaquone plus pyrimethamine; and azithromycin plus pyrimethamine plus rifabutin. Relapses are common, and it is recommended that patients with a history of prior toxoplasmic encephalitis receive maintenance therapy with sulfadiazine, pyrimethamine, and leucovorin. Patients with CD4+ T cell counts <100/μL and IgG antibody to *Toxoplasma* should receive primary prophylaxis for toxoplasmosis. Fortunately, the same daily regimen of a single double-strength tablet of TMP/SMX used for *P. carinii* prophylaxis provides adequate primary protection against toxoplasmosis. Secondary prophylaxis for toxoplasmosis may be discontinued in the setting of effective antiretroviral therapy and increases in CD4+ T cell counts to >200/μL for 6 months.

JC virus, a human polyomavirus that is the etiologic agent of *progressive multifocal leukoencephalopathy* (PML), is an important opportunistic pathogen in patients with AIDS (Chap. 361). While ~70% of the general adult population have antibodies to JC virus, indicative of prior infection, <10% of healthy adults show any evidence of ongoing viral replication. PML is the only known clinical manifestation of JC virus infection. It is a late manifestation of AIDS and is seen in ~4% of patients with AIDS. The lesions of PML begin as small foci of demyelination in subcortical white matter that eventually coalesce. The cerebral hemispheres, cerebellum, and brainstem may all be involved. Patients typically have a protracted course with multifocal neurologic deficits, with or without changes in mental status. Ataxia, hemiparesis, visual field defects, aphasia, and sensory defects may occur. MRI typically reveals multiple, nonenhancing white matter lesions that may coalesce and have a predilection for the occipital and parietal lobes. The lesions show signal hyperintensity on T2-weighted images and diminished signal on T1-weighted images. Prior to the availability of potent antiretroviral combination therapy, the majority of patients with PML died within 3 to 6 months of the onset of symptoms. Paradoxical worsening of PML has been seen with initiation of HAART as an immune reactivation syndrome. There is no specific treatment for PML; however, regressions of >2.5 years in duration have been reported in patients with PML treated with HAART for their HIV disease. Studies with antiviral agents such as cidofovir have failed to show clear benefit. Factors influencing a favorable prognosis for PML in the setting of HIV infection include a CD4+ T cell count >100/μL at baseline and the ability to maintain an HIV viral load of <500 copies per milliliter. Baseline viral load does not have independent predictive value of survival. PML is one of the few opportunistic infections that continues to occur with some frequency despite the widespread use of HAART.

Reactivation American trypanosomiasis may present as acute meningoencephalitis with focal neurologic signs, fever, headache, vomiting, and seizures. In South America, reactivation of *Chagas' disease* is considered to be an AIDS-defining condition and may be the initial AIDS-defining condition. Lesions appear radiographically as single or multiple hypodense areas, typically with ring enhancement and edema. They are found predominantly in the subcortical areas, a feature that differentiates them from the deeper lesions of toxoplasmosis. *Trypanosoma cruzi* amastigotes, or trypanosomes, can be identified from biopsy specimens or CSF. Other CSF findings include elevated protein and a mild (<100 cells/μL) lymphocytic pleocytosis. Organisms can also be identified by direct examination of the blood. Treatment consists of benzimidazole (2.5 mg/kg bid) or nifurtimox (2 mg/kg qid) for at least 60 days, followed by maintenance therapy for life with either drug at a dose of 5 mg/kg three times a week. As is the case

with cerebral toxoplasmosis, successful therapy with antiretrovirals may allow discontinuation of therapy for Chagas' disease.

Stroke may occur in patients with HIV infection. In contrast to the other causes of focal neurologic deficits in patients with HIV infection, the symptoms of a stroke are sudden in onset. Among the secondary infectious diseases in patients with HIV infection that may be associated with stroke are vasculitis due to cerebral varicella zoster or neurosyphilis and septic embolism in association with fungal infection. Other elements of the differential diagnosis of stroke in the patient with HIV infection include atherosclerotic cerebral vascular disease, thrombotic thrombocytopenic purpura, and cocaine or amphetamine use.

Primary CNS lymphoma is discussed below in the section on neoplastic diseases.

Spinal cord disease, or myelopathy, is present in ~20% of patients with AIDS, often as part of HIV encephalopathy. In fact, 90% of the patients with HIV-associated myelopathy have some evidence of dementia, suggesting that similar pathologic processes may be responsible for both conditions. Three main types of spinal cord disease are seen in patients with AIDS. The first of these is a vacuolar myelopathy, as discussed above under HIV encephalopathy. This condition is pathologically similar to subacute combined degeneration of the cord such as occurs with pernicious anemia. Although vitamin B$_{12}$ deficiency can be seen in patients with AIDS, it does not appear to be responsible for the myelopathy seen in the majority of patients. Vacuolar myelopathy is characterized by a subacute onset and often presents with gait disturbances, predominantly ataxia and spasticity; it may progress to include bladder and bowel dysfunction. Physical findings include evidence of increased deep tendon reflexes and extensor plantar responses. The second form of spinal cord disease involves the dorsal columns and presents as a pure sensory ataxia. The third form is also sensory in nature and presents with paresthesias and dysesthesias of the lower extremities. In contrast to the cognitive problems seen in patients with HIV encephalopathy, these spinal cord syndromes do not respond well to antiretroviral drugs, and therapy is mainly supportive.

One important disease of the spinal cord that also involves the peripheral nerves is a *myelopathy* and *polyradiculopathy* seen in association with CMV infection. This entity is generally seen late in the course of HIV infection and is fulminant in onset, with lower extremity and sacral paresthesias, difficulty in walking, areflexia, ascending sensory loss, and urinary retention. The clinical course is rapidly progressive over a period of weeks. CSF examination reveals a predominantly neutrophilic pleocytosis, and CMV DNA can be detected by CSF PCR. Therapy with ganciclovir or foscarnet can lead to rapid improvement, and prompt initiation of foscarnet or ganciclovir therapy is important in minimizing the degree of permanent neurologic damage. Combination therapy with both drugs should be considered in patients who have been previously treated for CMV disease. Other diseases involving the spinal cord in patients with HIV infection include HTLV-I-associated myelopathy (HAM) (Chap. 172), neurosyphilis (Chap. 153), infection with herpes simplex (Chap. 163) or varicella-zoster (Chap. 164), TB (Chap. 150), and lymphoma (Chap. 97).

Peripheral neuropathies are common in patients with HIV infection. They occur at all stages of illness and take a variety of forms. Early in the course of HIV infection, an acute inflammatory demyelinating polyneuropathy resembling Guillain-Barré syndrome may occur (Chap. 366). In other patients, a progressive or relapsing-remitting inflammatory neuropathy resembling chronic inflammatory demyelinating polyneuropathy (CIDP) has been noted. Patients commonly present with progressive weakness, areflexia, and minimal sensory changes. CSF examination often reveals a mononuclear pleocytosis, and peripheral nerve biopsy demonstrates a perivascular infiltrate suggesting an autoimmune etiology. Plasma exchange or intravenous immunoglobulin has been tried with variable success. Because of the immunosuppressive effects of glucocorticoids, they should be reserved for severe cases of CIDP refractory to other measures. Another autoimmune peripheral neuropathy seen in patients with AIDS is mononeuritis multiplex (Chaps. 366 and 306) due to a necrotizing arteritis of peripheral nerves. The most common peripheral neuropathy in patients with HIV infection is a *distal sensory polyneuropathy* that may be a direct consequence of HIV infection or a side effect of dideoxynucleoside therapy. Two-thirds of patients with AIDS may be shown by electrophysiologic studies to have some evidence of peripheral nerve disease. Presenting symptoms are usually painful burning sensations in the feet and lower extremities. Findings on examination include a stocking-type sensory loss to pinprick, temperature, and touch sensation and a loss of ankle reflexes. Motor changes are mild and are usually limited to weakness of the intrinsic foot muscles. Response of this condition to antiretrovirals has been variable, perhaps because antiretrovirals are responsible for the problem in some instances. When due to dideoxynucleoside therapy, patients with lower extremity peripheral neuropathy may complain of a sensation that they are walking on ice. Other entities in the differential diagnosis of peripheral neuropathy include diabetes mellitus, vitamin B_{12} deficiency, and side effects from metronidazole or dapsone. For distal symmetric polyneuropathy that fails to resolve following the discontinuation of dideoxynucleosides, therapy is symptomatic; gabapentin, carbamazepine, tricyclics, or analgesics may be effective for dysesthesias. Treatment-naive patients may respond to combination antiretroviral therapy, and preliminary data suggest that nerve growth factor may benefit some cases.

Myopathy may complicate the course of HIV infection; causes include HIV infection itself, zidovudine, and the generalized wasting syndrome. HIV-associated myopathy may range in severity from an asymptomatic elevation in creatine kinase levels to a subacute syndrome characterized by proximal muscle weakness and myalgias. Quite pronounced elevations in creatine kinase may occur in asymptomatic patients, particularly after exercise. The clinical significance of this as an isolated laboratory finding is unclear. A variety of both inflammatory and noninflammatory pathologic processes have been noted in patients with more severe myopathy, including myofiber necrosis with inflammatory cells, nemaline rod bodies, cytoplasmic bodies, and mitochondrial abnormalities. Profound muscle wasting, often with muscle pain, may be seen after prolonged zidovudine therapy. This toxic side effect of the drug is dose-dependent and is related to its ability to interfere with the function of mitochondrial polymerases. It is reversible following discontinuation of the drug. Red ragged fibers are a histologic hallmark of zidovudine-induced myopathy.

Ophthalmologic Disease Ophthalmologic problems occur in approximately half of patients with advanced HIV infection. The most common abnormal findings on funduscopic examination are cotton-wool spots. These are hard white spots that appear on the surface of the retina and often have an irregular edge. They represent areas of retinal ischemia secondary to microvascular disease. At times they are associated with small areas of hemorrhage and thus can be difficult to distinguish from CMV retinitis. In contrast to CMV retinitis, however, these lesions are not associated with visual loss and tend to remain stable or improve over time.

One of the most devastating consequences of HIV infection is CMV retinitis. Patients at high risk of CMV retinitis (CD4+ T cell count <100/μL) should undergo an ophthalmologic examination every 3 to 6 months. The majority of cases of CMV retinitis occur in patients with a CD4+ T cell count <50/μL. Prior to the availability of HAART, this CMV reactivation syndrome was seen in 25 to 30% of patients with AIDS. CMV retinitis usualy presents as a painless, progressive loss of vision. Patients may also complain of blurred vision, "floaters," and scintillations. The disease is usually bilateral, affecting one eye more than the other. The diagnosis is made on clinical grounds by an experienced ophthalmologist. The characteristic retinal appearance is that of perivascular hemorrhage and exudate (see Fig. 25-5). In situations where the diagnosis is in doubt due to an atypical presentation or an unexpected lack of response to therapy, vitreous or aqueous humor sampling with molecular diagnostic techniques may be of value. CMV infection of the retina results in a necrotic inflammatory process, and the visual loss that develops is irreversible. CMV

retinitis may be complicated by rhegmatogenous retinal detachment as a consequence of retinal atrophy in areas of prior inflammation. Therapy for CMV retinitis consists of oral valganciclovir, intravenous ganciclovir, or intravenous foscarnet, with cidofovir as an alternative. Combination therapy with ganciclovir and foscarnet has been shown to be slightly more effective than either ganciclovir or foscarnet alone in the patient with relapsed CMV retinitis. A 3-week induction course is followed by maintenance therapy with oral valganciclovir. If CMV disease is limited to the eye, a ganciclovir-releasing intraocular implant, periodic injections of the antisense nucleic acid preparation formivirsen, or intravitreal injections of ganciclovir or foscarnet may be considered; some choose to combine intraocular implants with oral valganciclovir. Intravitreal injections of cidofovir are generally avoided due to the increased risk of uveitis and hypotony. Maintenance therapy is continued until the CD4+ T cell count remains >100 to 150/μL for >6 months. The majority of patients with HIV infection and CMV disease develop some degree of uveitis with the initiation of antiretroviral therapy. The etiology of this is unknown; however, it has been suggested that this may be due to the generation of an enhanced immune response to CMV as an immune reactivation syndrome. In some instances this has required the use of topical glucocorticoids.

Both HSV and varicella zoster virus can cause a rapidly progressing, bilateral necrotizing retinitis referred to as the *acute retinal necrosis syndrome* or progressive outer retinal necrosis (PORN). This syndrome, in contrast to CMV retinitis, is associated with pain, keratitis, and iritis. It is often associated with orolabial HSV or trigeminal zoster. Ophthalmologic examination reveals widespread pale gray peripheral lesions. This condition is often complicated by retinal detachment. It is important to recognize and treat this condition with intravenous acyclovir as quickly as possible to minimize the loss of vision.

Several other secondary infections may cause ocular problems in HIV-infected patients. *P. carinii* can cause a lesion of the choroid that may be detected as an incidental finding on ophthalmologic examination. These lesions are typically bilateral, are from half to twice the disc diameter in size, and appear as slightly elevated yellow-white plaques. They are usually asymptomatic and may be confused with cotton-wool spots. Chorioretinitis due to toxoplasmosis can be seen alone or, more commonly, in association with CNS toxoplasmosis. Kaposi's sarcoma may involve the eyelid or conjunctiva while lymphoma may involve the retina.

Additional Disseminated Infections and Wasting Syndrome Infections with species of the small, gram-negative rickettsia-like organism *Bartonella* (Chap. 144) are seen with increased frequency in patients with HIV infection. While not considered an AIDS-defining illness by the CDC, many experts view infection with *Bartonella* as indicative of a severe defect in cell-mediated immunity. It is usually seen in patients with CD4+ T cell counts <100/μL. Among the clinical manifestations of *Bartonella* infection are bacillary angiomatosis, cat-scratch disease, and trench fever. *Bacillary angiomatosis* is usually due to infection with *B. henselae*. It is characterized by a vascular proliferation that leads to a variety of skin lesions that have been confused with the skin lesions of KS. In contrast to the lesions of KS, the lesions of bacillary angiomatosis generally blanch, are painful, and typically occur in the setting of systemic symptoms. Infection can extend to the lymph nodes, liver (peliosis hepatis), spleen, bone, heart, CNS, respiratory tract, and gastrointestinal tract. *Cat-scratch disease* generally begins with a papule at the site of inoculation. This is followed several weeks later by the development of regional adenopathy and malaise. Infection with *B. quintana* is transmitted by lice and has been associated with case reports of trench fever, endocarditis, adenopathy, and bacillary angiomatosis. The organism is quite difficult to culture, and diagnosis often relies upon identifying the organism in biopsy specimens using the Warthin-Starry or similar stains. Treatment is with either erythromycin or doxycyline for at least 3 months.

Histoplasmosis is an opportunistic infection that is seen most frequently in patients in the Mississippi and Ohio River valleys, Puerto Rico, the Dominican Republic, and South America. These are all areas in which infection with *H. capsulatum* is endemic (Chap. 183). Because of this limited geographic distribution, the percentage of AIDS cases in the United States with histoplasmosis is only ~0.5. Histoplasmosis is generally a late manifestation of HIV infection; however, it may be the initial AIDS-defining condition. In one study, the median CD4+ T cell count for patients with histoplasmosis and AIDS was 33/μL. While disease due to *H. capsulatum* may present as a primary infection of the lung, disseminated disease, presumably due to reactivation, is the most common presentation in HIV-infected patients. Patients usually present with a 4- to 8-week history of fever and weight loss. Hepatosplenomegaly and lymphadenopathy are each seen in about 25% of patients. CNS disease, either meningitis or a mass lesion, is seen in 15% of patients. Bone marrow involvement is common, with thrombocytopenia, neutropenia, and anemia occurring in 33% of patients. Approximately 7% of patients have mucocutaneous lesions consisting of a maculopapular rash and skin or oral ulcers. Respiratory symptoms are usually mild, with chest x-ray showing a diffuse infiltrate or diffuse small nodules in approximately half of cases. Diagnosis is made by culturing the organisms from blood, bone marrow, or tissue. Treatment is typically with amphotericin B, 0.7 to 1.0 mg/kg daily to a total dose of 1 g followed by maintenance therapy with itraconazole. In the setting of mild infection, it may be appropriate to treat with itraconazole alone.

Following the spread of HIV infection to southeast Asia, disseminated infection with the fungus *Penicillium marneffei* was recognized as a complication of HIV infection and is considered an AIDS-defining condition in those parts of the world where it occurs. *P. marneffei* is the third most common AIDS-defining illness in Thailand, following TB and cryptococcosis. It is more frequently diagnosed in the rainy than the dry season. Clinical features include fever, generalized lymphadenopathy, hepatosplenomegaly, anemia, thrombocytopenia, and papular skin lesions with central umbilication. Treatment is with amphotericin B followed by itraconazole.

Visceral leishmaniasis (Chap. 196) is recognized with increasing frequency in patients with HIV infection who live in or travel to areas endemic for this protozoal infection transmitted by sandflies. The clinical presentation is one of hepatosplenomegaly, fever, and hematologic abnormalities. Lymphadenopathy and other constitutional symptoms may be present. Organisms can be isolated from cultures of bone marrow aspirates. Histologic stains may be negative, and antibody titers are of little help. Patients with HIV infection usually respond well initially to standard therapy with pentavalent antimony compounds. Eradication of the organism is difficult, however, and relapses are common.

Generalized wasting is an AIDS-defining condition; it is defined as involuntary weight loss of >10% associated with intermittent or constant fever and chronic diarrhea or fatigue lasting >30 days in the absence of a defined cause other than HIV infection. It is the initial AIDS-defining condition in ~10% of patients with AIDS in the United States and is an indication for intiation of HAART. A constant feature of this syndrome is severe muscle wasting with scattered myofiber degeneration and occasional evidence of myositis. Glucocorticoids may be of some benefit; however, this approach must be carefully weighed against the risk of compounding the immunodeficiency of HIV infection. Androgenic steroids, growth hormone, and total parenteral nutrition have been used as therapeutic interventions with variable success.

Neoplastic Diseases　The neoplastic diseases clearly seen with an increased frequency in patients with HIV infection are KS and non-Hodgkin's lymphoma. In addition, there also appears to be an increased incidence of Hodgkin's disease; multiple myeloma; leukemia; melanoma; and cervical, brain, testicular, oral, lung, and anal

cancers. Recent years have witnessed a marked reduction in the incidence of KS (Fig. 173-28), felt to be primarily due to the use of potent antiretroviral therapy. Rates of non-Hodgkin's lymphoma have declined as well; however, this decline has not been as dramatic as the decline in rates of KS.

Kaposi's sarcoma is a multicentric neoplasm consisting of multiple vascular nodules appearing in the skin, mucous membranes, and viscera. The course ranges from indolent, with only minor skin or lymph node involvement, to fulminant, with extensive cutaneous and visceral involvement. In the initial period of the AIDS epidemic, KS was a prominent clinical feature of the first cases of AIDS, occurring in 79% of the patients diagnosed in 1981. By 1989 it was seen in only 25% of cases, by 1992 the number had decreased to 9%, and by 1997 the number was <1%. HHV-8 or KSHV has been strongly implicated as a viral cofactor in the pathogenesis of KS (see above).

Clinically, KS has varied presentations and may be seen at any stage of HIV infection, even in the presence of a normal CD4+ T cell count. The initial lesion may be a small, raised reddish-purple nodule on the skin, a discoloration on the oral mucosa, or a swollen lymph node (Fig. 173-35). Lesions often appear in sun-exposed areas, particularly the tip of the nose, and have a propensity to occur in areas of trauma (Koebner phenomenon). Because of the vascular nature of the tumors and the presence of extravasated red blood cells in the lesions, their color ranges from reddish to purple to brown and often take the appearance of a bruise, with yellowish discoloration and tattooing. Lesions range in size from a few millimeters to several centimeters in diameter and may be either discrete or confluent. KS lesions most commonly appear as raised macules; however, they also can be papular, particularly in patients with higher CD4+ T cell counts. Confluent lesions may give rise to surrounding lymphedema and may be disfiguring when they involve the face and disabling when they involve the lower extremities or the surfaces of joints. Apart from skin, lymph nodes, gastrointestinal tract, and lung are the organ systems most commonly affected by KS. Lesions have been reported in virtually every organ, including the heart and the CNS. In contrast to most malignancies, in which lymph node involvement implies metastatic spread and a poor prognosis, lymph node involvement may be seen very early in KS and is of no special clinical significance. In fact, some patients may present with disease limited to the lymph nodes. These are generally patients with relatively intact immune function and thus the patients with the best prognosis. Pulmonary involvement with KS generally presents with shortness of breath. Some 80% of patients with pulmonary KS also have cutaneous lesions. The chest x-ray characteristically shows bilateral lower lobe infiltrates that obscure the margins of the mediastinum and diaphragm (Fig. 173-36). Pleural effusions are seen in 70% of cases of pulmonary KS, a fact that is often helpful in the differential diagnosis. Gastrointestinal involvement is seen in 50% of patients and usually takes one of two forms. The first is mucosal involvement, which may lead to bleeding that can be

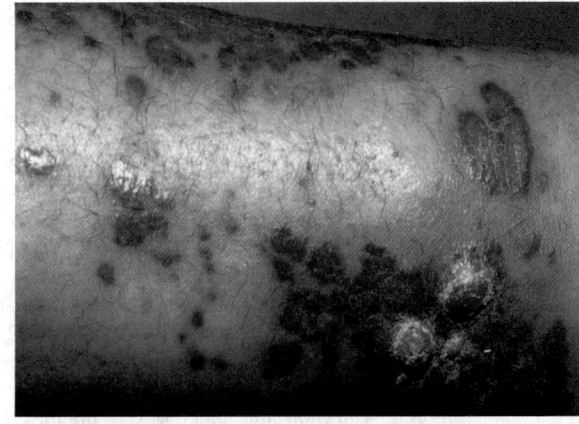

FIGURE 173-35　Kaposi's sarcoma in a patient with AIDS demonstrating patch, plaque, and tumor stages.

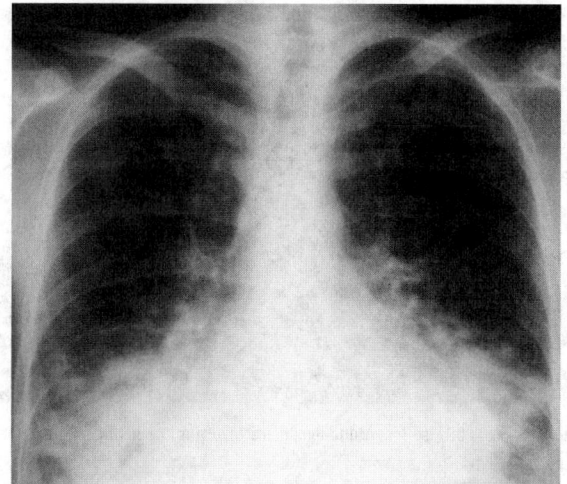

FIGURE 173-36 Chest x-ray of a patient with AIDS and pulmonary Kaposi's sarcoma. The characteristic findings include dense bilateral lower lobe infiltrates obscuring the heart borders and a pleural effusion.

cordingly. The use of systemic therapy, either IFN-α or chemotherapy, should be considered in patients with a large number of lesions or in patients with visceral involvement. The single most important determinant of response appears to be the CD4+ T cell count. This relationship between response rate and baseline CD4+ T cell count is particularly true for IFN-α. The response rate for patients with CD4+ T cell counts >600/μL is ~80%, while the response rate for patients with counts <150/μL is <10%. In contrast to the other systemic therapies, IFN-α provides an added advantage of having antiretroviral activity; thus, it may be the appropriate first choice for single-agent systemic therapy for early patients with disseminated disease. A variety of chemotherapeutic agents have also been shown to have activity against KS. Three of them, liposomal daunorubicin, liposomal doxorubicin, and paclitaxel have been approved by the FDA for this indication. Liposomal daunorubicin is approved as first-line therapy for patients with advanced KS. It has fewer side effects than conventional chemotherapy. In contrast, liposomal doxorubicin and paclitaxel are approved only for KS patients who have failed standard chemotherapy. Response rates vary from 23 to 88%, appear to be comparable to what had been achieved earlier with combination chemotherapy regimens, and are greatly influenced by CD4+ T cell count.

Lymphomas occur with an increased frequency in patients with congenital or acquired T cell immunodeficiencies (Chap. 297). AIDS is no exception; at least 6% of all patients with AIDS develop lymphoma at some time during the course of their illness. This is a 120-fold increase in incidence compared to the general population. In contrast to the situation with KS, primary CNS lymphoma, and most opportunistic infections, the incidence of AIDS-associated systemic lymphomas has not experienced as dramatic a decrease as a consequence of the widespread use of effective antiretroviral therapy. Lymphoma occurs in all risk groups, with the highest incidence in patients with hemophilia and the lowest incidence in patients from the Caribbean or Africa with heterosexually acquired infection. Lymphoma is a late manifestation of HIV infection, generally occurring in patients with CD4+ T cell counts <200/μL. As HIV disease progresses, the risk of lymphoma increases. In contrast to KS, which occurs at a relatively constant rate throughout the course of HIV disease, the attack rate for lymphoma increases exponentially with increasing duration of HIV infection and decreasing level of immunologic function. At 3 years following a diagnosis of HIV infection, the risk of lymphoma is 0.8% per year; by 8 years after infection, it is 2.6% per year. As people with HIV infection live longer as a consequence of improved antiretroviral therapy and better treatment and prophylaxis of opportunistic infections, it is anticipated that the incidence of lymphomas may increase.

Three main categories of lymphoma are seen in patients with HIV infection: grade III or IV immunoblastic lymphoma, Burkitt's lym-

severe. These patients sometimes also develop symptoms of gastrointestinal obstruction if lesions become large. The second gastrointestinal manifestation is due to biliary tract involvement. KS lesions may infiltrate the gallbladder and biliary tree, leading to a clinical picture of obstructive jaundice similar to that seen with sclerosing cholangitis. Several staging systems have been proposed for KS. One in common use was developed by the National Institute of Allergy and Infectious Diseases AIDS Clinical Trials Group; it distinguishes patients on the basis of tumor extent, immunologic function, and presence or absence of systemic disease (Table 173-16).

A diagnosis of KS is based upon biopsy of a suspicious lesion. Histologically one sees a proliferation of spindle cells and endothelial cells, extravasation of red blood cells, hemosiderin-laden macrophages, and, in early cases, an inflammatory cell infiltrate. Included in the differential diagnosis are lymphoma (particularly for oral lesions), bacillary angiomatosis, and cutaneous mycobacterial infections.

Management of KS (Table 173-17) should be carried out in consultation with an expert since definitive treatment guidelines do not exist. In the majority of cases effective antiretroviral therapy will go a long way in achieving control. Indeed, spontaneous regressions have been reported in the setting of HAART. For patients in whom tumor persists or in whom control of HIV replication is not possible, a variety of options exist. In some cases, lesions remain quite indolent, and many of these patients can be managed with no specific treatment. Fewer than 10% of AIDS patients with KS die as a consequence of their malignancy, and death from secondary infections is considerably more common. Thus, whenever possible one should avoid treatment regimens that may further suppress the immune system and increase susceptibility to opportunistic infections. Treatment is indicated under two main circumstances. The first is when a single lesion or a limited number of lesions are causing significant discomfort or cosmetic problems, such as with prominent facial lesions, lesions overlying a joint, or lesions in the oropharynx that interfere with swallowing or breathing. Under these circumstances, treatment with localized radiation, intralesional vinblastine, or cryotherapy may be indicated. It should be noted that patients with HIV infection are particularly sensitive to the side effects of radiation therapy. This is especially true with respect to the development of radiation-induced mucositis; doses of radiation directed at mucosal surfaces, particularly in the head and neck region, should be adjusted ac-

TABLE 173-16 *National Institute of Allergy and Infectious Diseases AIDS Clinical Trials Group TIS Staging System for Kaposi's Sarcoma*

Parameter	Good Risk (stage 0): All of the Following	Poor Risk (stage 1): Any of the Following
Tumor (T)	Confined to skin and/or lymph nodes and/or minimal oral disease	Tumor-associated edema or ulceration Extensive oral lesions Gastrointestinal lesions Nonnodal visceral lesions
Immune system (I) Systemic illness (S)	CD4+ T cell count ≥200/μL No B symptoms[a] Karnofsky performance status >70 No history of opportunistic infection, neurologic disease, lymphoma, or thrush	CD4+ T cell count <200/μL B symptoms[a] present Karnofsky performance status <70 History of opportunistic infection, neurologic disease, lymphoma, or thrush

[a] Defined as unexplained fever, night sweats, >10% involuntary weight loss, or diarrhea persisting for more than 2 weeks.

TABLE 173-17 *Management of AIDS-Associated Kaposi's Sarcoma*

Observation and optimization of antiretroviral therapy
Single or limited number of lesions
  Radiation
  Intralesional vinblastine
  Cryotherapy
Extensive disease
  Initial therapy
    Interferon-α (if CD4+ T cells >150/μL)
    Liposomal daunorubicin
  Subsequent therapy
    Liposomal doxorubicin
    Paclitaxel
Combination chemotherapy with low-dose doxorubicin, bleomycin,
  and vinblastine (ABV)
Radiation treatment

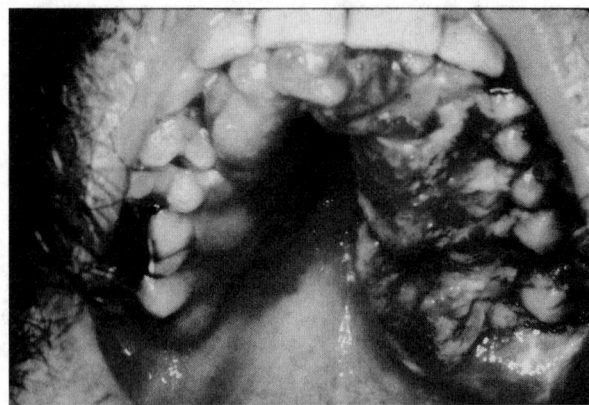

FIGURE 173-37 Diffuse histiocytic lymphoma involving the hard palate of a patient with AIDS.

phoma, and primary CNS lymphoma. Approximately 90% of these lymphomas are B cell in phenotype, and half contain EBV DNA. These tumors may be either monoclonal or oligoclonal in nature and are probably in some way related to the pronounced polyclonal B cell activation seen in patients with AIDS.

Immunoblastic lymphomas account for ~60% of the cases of lymphoma in patients with AIDS. These are generally high grade and would have been classified as diffuse histiocytic lymphomas in earlier classification schemes. This tumor is more common in older patients, increasing in incidence from 0% in HIV-infected individuals <1 year old to >3% in those >50. One variant of immunoblastic lymphoma is body cavity lymphoma. This malignancy presents with lymphomatous pleural, pericardial, and/or peritoneal effusions in the absence of discrete nodal or extranodal masses. The tumor cells do not express surface markers for B cells or T cells. HHV-8 DNA sequences have been found in the genome of the malignant cells (see above).

Small non-cleaved cell lymphoma (Burkitt's lymphoma) accounts for ~20% of the cases of lymphoma in patients with AIDS. It is most frequent in patients 10 to 19 years old and usually demonstrates characteristic c-*myc* translocations from chromosome 8 to chromosomes 14 or 22. Burkitt's lymphoma is not commonly seen in the setting of immunodeficiency other than HIV-associated immunodeficiency, and the incidence of this particular tumor is over 1000-fold higher in the setting of HIV infection than in the general population. In contrast to African Burkitt's lymphoma, where 97% of the cases contain EBV genome, only 50% of HIV-associated Burkitt's lymphomas are EBV-positive.

Primary CNS lymphoma accounts for ~20% of the cases of lymphoma in patients with HIV infection. In contrast to HIV-associated Burkitt's lymphoma, primary CNS lymphomas are usually positive for EBV. In one study, the incidence of Epstein-Barr positivity was 100%. This malignancy does not have a predilection for any particular age group. The median CD4+ T cell count at the time of diagnosis is ~50/μL. Thus, CNS lymphoma generally presents at a later stage of HIV infection than systemic lymphoma. This fact may at least in part explain the poorer prognosis for this subset of patients.

The clinical presentation of lymphoma in patients with HIV infection is quite varied, ranging from focal seizures to rapidly growing mass lesions in the oral mucosa (Fig. 173-37) to persistent unexplained fever. At least 80% of patients present with extranodal disease, and a similar percentage have B-type symptoms of fever, night sweats, or weight loss. Virtually any site in the body may be involved. The most common extranodal site is the CNS, which is involved in approximately one-third of all patients with lymphoma. Approximately 60% of these cases are primary CNS lymphoma. Primary CNS lymphoma generally presents with focal neurologic deficits, including cranial nerve findings, headaches, and/or seizures. MRI or CT generally reveals a limited number (one to three) of 3- to 5-cm lesions (Fig. 173-38). The lesions often show ring enhancement on contrast administra-

tion and may occur in any location. Locations that are most commonly involved with CNS lymphoma are deep in the white matter. Contrast enhancement is usually less pronounced than that seen with toxoplasmosis. The main diseases in the differential diagnosis are cerebral toxoplasmosis and cerebral Chagas' disease. In addition to the 20% of lymphomas in HIV-infected individuals that are primary CNS lymphomas, CNS disease is also seen in HIV-infected patients with systemic lymphoma. Approximately 20% of patients with systemic lymphoma have CNS disease in the form of leptomeningeal involvement. This fact underscores the importance of lumbar puncture in the staging evaluation of patients with systemic lymphoma.

Systemic lymphoma is seen at earlier stages of HIV infection than primary CNS lymphoma. In one series the mean CD4+ T cell count was 189/μL. In addition to lymph node involvement, systemic lymphoma may commonly involve the gastrointestinal tract, bone marrow, liver, and lung. Gastrointestinal tract involvement is seen in ~25% of patients. Any site in the gastrointestinal tract may be involved, and patients may complain of difficulty swallowing or abdominal pain. The diagnosis is usually suspected on the basis of CT or MRI of the abdomen. Bone marrow involvement is seen in ~20% of patients and may lead to pancytopenia. Liver and lung involvement are each seen in ~10% of patients. Pulmonary disease may present as either a mass lesion, multiple nodules, or an interstitial infiltrate.

Both conventional and unconventional approaches have been employed in an attempt to treat HIV-related lymphomas. Systemic lymphoma is generally treated by the oncologist with combination

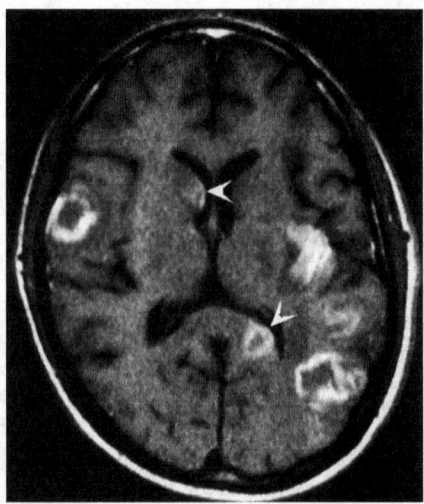

FIGURE 173-38 Central nervous system lymphoma. Postcontrast T1-weighted MR scan in a patient with AIDS, an altered mental status, and hemiparesis. Multiple enhancing lesions, some ring-enhancing, are present. The left Sylvian lesion shows gyral and subcortical enhancement, and the lesions in the caudate and splenium (*arrowheads*) show enhancement of adjacent ependymal surfaces.

chemotherapy. Earlier disappointing figures are being replaced with more optimistic results for the treatment of systemic lymphoma following the availability of more effective combination antiretroviral therapy. As in most situations in patients with HIV disease, those with the higher CD4+ T cell counts tend to do better. Response rates as high as 72% and disease-free intervals >15 months have been reported. Treatment of primary CNS lymphoma remains a significant challenge. Treatment is complicated by the fact that this illness usually occurs in patients with advanced HIV disease. Palliative measures such as radiation therapy provide some relief. The prognosis remains poor in this group, with median survival <1 year.

Evidence of infection with *human papilloma virus* (HPV), associated with *intraepithelial dysplasia of the cervix or anus*, is approximately twice as common in HIV-infected individuals as in the general population and can lead to intraepithelial neoplasia and eventually invasive cancer. In two separate studies, HIV-infected men without anorectal symptoms were studied for evidence of dysplasia, and Papanicolauo (Pap) smears were found to be abnormal in 40%. These changes were persistent at 1 year follow-up, raising the possibility of a subsequent transition to a more malignant condition. While the incidence of an abnormal Pap smear of the cervix is ~5% in otherwise healthy women, the incidence of abnormal cervical smears in women with HIV infection is 60%. Based on this finding, *invasive cervical cancer* was added to the list of AIDS-defining conditions. Thus far, however, only small increases in the incidence of cervical or anal cancer have been seen as a consequence of HIV infection. However, given this high rate of dysplasia, a comprehensive gynecologic and rectal examination, including Pap smear, is indicated at the initial evaluation and 6 months later for all patients with HIV infection. If these examinations are negative at both time points, the patient should be followed with yearly evaluations. If an initial or repeat Pap smear shows evidence of severe inflammation with reactive squamous changes, the next Pap smear should be performed at 3 months. If, at any time, a Pap smear shows evidence of squamous intraepithelial lesions, colposcopic examination with biopsies as indicated should be performed. HAART has been found to reduce the rate of progression and in some instances to induce regression of HPV-induced dysplasia.

IDIOPATHIC CD4+ T LYMPHOCYTOPENIA

A syndrome was recognized in 1992 that was characterized by an absolute CD4+ T cell count of $<300/\mu L$ or $<20\%$ of total T cells on more than one occasion; no evidence of HIV-1, HIV-2, HTLV-I, or HTLV-II on testing; and the absence of any defined immunodeficiency or therapy associated with decreased levels of CD4+ T cells. By mid-1993, ~100 patients had been described. After extensive multicenter investigations, a series of reports were published in early 1993, which together allowed a number of conclusions. Idiopathic CD4+ lymphocytopenia (ICL) is a very rare syndrome, as determined by studies of blood donors and cohorts of HIV-seronegative homosexual men. Cases were clearly identified as early as 1983, and cases remarkably similar to ICL had been identified decades ago. The definition of ICL based on CD4+ T cell counts coincided with the ready availability of testing for CD4+ T cells in patients suspected of being immunosuppressed. Although, as a result of immune deficiency, certain patients with ICL develop some of the opportunistic diseases (particularly cryptococcosis) seen in HIV-infected patients, the syndrome is demographically, clinically, and immunologically unlike HIV infection and AIDS. Fewer than half of the reported ICL patients had risk factors for HIV infection, and there were wide geographic and age distributions. The fact that a significant proportion of patients did have risk factors probably reflects a selection bias, in that physicians who take care of HIV-infected patients are more likely to monitor CD4+ T cells. Approximately one-third of the patients are women, compared to 16% of women among HIV-infected individuals in the United States. Many patients with ICL remained clinically stable, and their condition did not deteriorate progressively as is common with seriously immunodeficient HIV-infected patients. Certain patients with ICL even experienced spontaneous reversal of the CD4+ T lymphocytopenia.

Immunologic abnormalities in ICL are somewhat different from those of HIV infection. ICL patients often also have decreases in CD8+ T cells and in B cells. Furthermore, immunoglobulin levels were either normal or, more commonly, decreased in patients with ICL, compared to the usual hypergammaglobulinemia of HIV-infected individuals. Finally, virologic studies revealed no evidence of HIV-1, HIV-2, HTLV-I, or HTLV-II or of any other mononuclear cell–tropic virus. Furthermore, there was no epidemiologic evidence to suggest that a transmissible microbe was involved. The cases of ICL were widely dispersed, with no clustering. Close contacts and sexual partners who were studied were clinically well and were serologically, immunologically, and virologically negative for HIV. ICL is a heterogeneous syndrome, and it is highly likely that there is no common cause; however, there may be common causes among subgroups of patients that are currently unrecognized.

Patients who present with laboratory data consistent with ICL should be worked up for underlying diseases that could be responsible for the immune deficiency. If no underlying cause is detected, no specific therapy should be initiated. However, if opportunistic diseases occur, they should be treated appropriately (see above). Depending on the level of the CD4+ T cell count, patients should receive prophylaxis for the commonly encountered opportunistic infections.

℞ TREATMENT

General Principles of Patient Management   The treatment of patients with HIV infection requires not only a comprehensive knowledge of the possible disease processes that may occur but also the ability to deal with the problems of a chronic, potentially life-threatening illness. Great advances have been made in the treatment of patients with HIV infection. The appropriate use of potent combination antiretroviral therapy and other treatment and prophylactic interventions is of critical importance in providing each patient with the best opportunity to live a long and healthy life despite the presence of HIV infection. In contrast to the earlier days of this epidemic, a diagnosis of HIV infection need no longer be equated with an inevitably fatal disease. In addition to medical interventions, the health care provider has a responsibility to provide each patient with appropriate counseling and education concerning their disease as part of a comprehensive care plan. Patients must be educated about the potential transmissibility of their infection and about the fact that while health care providers may refer to levels of the virus as "undetectable," this is more a reflection of the sensitivity of the assay being used to measure the virus than a comment on the presence or absence of the virus. It is important for patients to be aware that the virus is still present and capable of being transmitted at all stages of HIV disease. Thus, there need to be frank discussions concerning sexual practices and the sharing of needles. The treating physician must not only be aware of the latest medications available for patients with HIV infection but must also educate patients concerning the natural history of their illness and listen and be sensitive to their fears and concerns. As with other diseases, therapeutic decisions should be made in consultation with the patient, when possible, and with the patient's proxy if the patient is incapable of making decisions. In this regard, it is recommended that all patients with HIV infection, and in particular those with CD4+ T cell counts $<200/\mu L$, designate a trusted individual with durable power of attorney to make medical decisions on their behalf, if necessary.

No matter how well prepared a patient is for adversity, the discovery of a diagnosis of HIV infection is a devastating event. For this reason, it is recommended that anyone about to undergo testing have "pretest counseling" to prepare him or her at least partially should the results demonstrate the presence of HIV infection. Following a diagnosis of HIV infection, the health care provider should be prepared to activate support systems immediately for the newly diagnosed patient. These should include an experienced social worker or nurse who can spend time talking to the person and ensuring that he or she is emotionally stable. Most communities have HIV crisis centers that can be of great help in these difficult situations.

Following a diagnosis of HIV infection, there are several examinations and laboratory studies that should be performed to help determine the extent of disease and provide baseline standards for future reference (Table 173-18). In addition to routine chemistry and hematology screening panels and chest x-ray, one should also obtain a CD4+ T cell count, two separate plasma HIV RNA levels, a VDRL test, and an anti-*Toxoplasma* antibody titer. A PPD test should be done, and a MMSE performed and recorded. Patients should be immunized with pneumococcal polysaccharide and, if seronegative for these viruses, with hepatitis A and hepatitis B vaccines. The status of hepatitis C infection should be determined. In addition, patients should be counseled with regard to sexual practices and needle sharing, and counseling should be offered to those whom the patient knows or suspects may also be infected. Once these baseline activities are performed, short- and long-term medical management strategies should be developed based upon the most recent information available and modified as new information becomes available. The field of HIV medicine is changing rapidly, and it is difficult to remain fully up to date. Fortunately there are a series of excellent sites on the internet that are frequently updated, and they provide the most recent information on a variety of topics, including consensus panel reports on treatment (Table 173-19).

Antiretroviral Therapy Combination antiretroviral therapy, or HAART, is the cornerstone of management of patients with HIV infection. Following the initiation of widespread use of HAART in the United States in 1995 to 1996, marked declines have been noted in the incidence of most AIDS-defining conditions (Fig. 173-28). Suppression of HIV replication is an important component in prolonging life as well as improving the quality of life in patients with HIV infection. Unfortunately, many of the most important questions related to the treatment of HIV disease currently lack definitive answers. Among them are the questions of when should therapy be started, what is the best initial regimen, when should a given regimen be changed, and what should it be changed to when a change is made. Notwithstanding these uncertainties, the physician and patient must come to a mutually agreeable plan based upon the best available data. In an effort to facilitate this process, the United States Department of Health and Human Services has published a series of frequently updated guidelines including the "*Principles of Therapy of HIV Infection*," "*Guidelines for the Use of Antiretroviral Agents in HIV-Infected Adults and Adolescents*," and "*Guidelines for the Prevention of Opportunistic Infections in Persons Infected with Human Immunodeficiency Virus*." At present, an extensive clinical trials network, involving both clinical investigators and patient advocates, is in place attempting to develop improved approaches to therapy. Consortia comprising representatives of academia, industry, and the federal government are involved in the process of drug development, including a wide-ranging series of clinical trials. As a result, new therapies and new therapeutic strategies are contin-

TABLE 173-18 *Initial Evaluation of the Patient with HIV Infection*

History and physical examination
Routine chemistry and hematology
CD4+ T lymphocyte count
Two plasma HIV RNA levels
RPR test
Anti-*Toxoplasma* antibody titer
PPD skin test
Mini-mental status examination
Serologies for hepatitis A, hepatitis B, and hepatitis C
Immunization with pneumococcal polysaccharide; influenza as indicated
Immunization with hepatitis A and hepatitis B if seronegative
Counseling regarding natural history and transmission
Help contacting others who might be infected

Note: VDRL, Venereal Disease Research Laboratory; PPD, purified protein derivative.

TABLE 173-19 *Resources Available on the World Wide Web on HIV Disease*

www.aidsinfo.nih.gov	AIDS info, a service of the U.S. Department of Health and Human Services, posts federally approved treatment guidelines for HIV and AIDS; provides information on federally funded and privately funded clinical trials and CDC publications and data
www.cdcnpin.org	Updates on epidemiologic data from the CDC
www.cc.nih.gov/phar/hiv-mgt	Online images of HIV drugs and information regarding dosing

Note: CDC, Centers for Disease Control and Prevention.

ually emerging. New drugs are often available through expanded access programs prior to official licensure. Given the complexity of this field, decisions regarding antiretroviral therapy are best made in consultation with experts. Currently licensed drugs for the treatment of HIV infection fall into three categories: those that inhibit the viral reverse transcriptase enzyme (Table 173-20, Fig. 173-39), those that inhibit the viral protease enzyme, and those that interfere with viral entry. There are numerous drug-drug interactions that one must take into consideration when using these agents (Table 173-21).

The FDA-approved reverse transcriptase inhibitors include the *nucleoside analogues* zidovudine, didanosine, zalcitabine, stavudine, lamivudine, abacavir, and emtricitabine; the *nucleotide analogue* tenofovir; and the *nonnucleoside reverse transcriptase inhibitors* nevirapine, delavirdine, and efavirenz (Fig. 173-39; Table 173-20). These were the first class of drugs that were licensed for the treatment of HIV infection. They are indicated for this use as part of combination regimens. It should be stressed that none of these drugs should be used as monotherapy for HIV infection. Thus, when lamivudine or tenofovir are used to treat hepatitis B infection in the setting of HIV infection, one should ensure that the patient is also on additional antiretroviral medication. The reverse transcriptase inhibitors block the HIV replication cycle at the point of RNA-dependent DNA synthesis, the reverse transcription step. While the nonnucleoside reverse transcriptase inhibitors are quite selective for the HIV-1 reverse transcriptase, the nucleoside and nucleotide analogues inhibit a variety of DNA polymerization reactions in addition to those of the HIV-1 reverse transcriptase. For this reason, serious side effects are more common with the nucleoside analogues and include mitochondrial damage that can lead to hepatic steatosis and lactic acidosis as well as peripheral neuropathy and pancreatitis. One of the more recently recognized problems that has been encountered with the widespread use of HAART therapy has been a syndrome of hyperlipidemia, glucose intolerance, and fat distribution often referred to as *lipodystrophy syndrome* (discussed above under metabolic abnormalities).

Zidovudine (AZT; 3'-azido-2',3'-dideoxythymidine) was the first drug approved for the treatment of HIV infection and is the prototype nucleoside analogue. These compounds, in which the hydroxyl group in the 3' position of the ribose moiety is substituted with a hydrogen or other chemical group, act as DNA chain terminators owing to their inability to form a 3'-5' phosphodiester linkage with another nucleoside. They bind much more avidly to the active site of the RNA-dependent DNA polymerase of HIV (reverse transcriptase) than to the active site of mammalian cell DNA polymerases; this explains their selective effect on HIV replication. Zidovudine also has a relatively high avidity for the DNA polymerase-γ of human mitochondria. This may contribute to the development of the fatty liver and the myopathy sometimes observed in patients taking zidovudine. As with all the nucleoside analogues, the active form of zidovudine is the triphosphate, and the rate of phosphorylation, a thymidine kinase–dependent pathway, may be different in different cells. This may explain why zidovudine is more effective at inhibiting HIV replication in some cells than others. The clinical efficacy of zidovudine was clearly established in 1986 in a phase II, randomized, placebo-controlled trial in patients

Drug	Status	Indication	Dose as Monotherapy	Dose in Combination	Supporting Data	Toxicity
REVERSE TRANSCRIPTASE INHIBITORS						
Zidovudine (AZT, azidothymidine, Retrovir, 3′azido-3′-deoxythymidine)	Licensed	Treatment of HIV infection in combination with other antiretroviral agents Prevention of maternal-fetal HIV transmission	Not indicated *Mother:* 200 mg tid or 300 mg bid until the start of labor, then 2 mg/kg over 1 h IV, followed by 1 mg/kg per h IV until clamping of umbilical cord; *Infant:* 2 mg/kg q6h PO beginning within 12 h birth, or 1.5 mg/kg q6h IV over 30 min for 6 weeks	200 mg q8h or 300 mg bid	19 vs 1 death in original placebo-controlled trial in 281 patients with AIDS or ARC. Decreased progression to AIDS in patients with CD4+ T cell counts <500/μL, n = 2051 In pregnant women with CD4+ T cell count ≥200/μL, AZT PO beginning at weeks 14–34 of gestation plus IV drug during labor and delivery plus PO AZT to infant for 6 wk decreased transmission of HIV by 67.5% (from 25.5% to 8.3%), n = 363	Anemia, granulocytopenia, myopathy, lactic acidosis, hepatomegaly with steatosis, headache, nausea
Didanosine (Videx, Videx EC, ddI, dideoxyinosine, 2′,3′-dideoxyinosine)	Licensed	For treatment of HIV infection in combination with other antiretroviral agents	Not indicated	Buffered: Requires 2 tablets to achieve adequate buffering of stomach acid; should be administered on an empty stomach ≥60 kg: 200 mg bid <60 kg: 125 mg bid Enteric coated: ≥60 kg: 400 mg qd < 60 kg: 250 mg qd	Clinically superior to AZT as monotherapy in 913 patients with prior AZT therapy. Clinically superior to AZT and comparable to AZT + ddI and AZT + ddC in 1067 AZT-naive patients with CD4+ T cell counts of 200–500/μL	Pancreatitis, peripheral neuropathy, abnormalities on liver function tests, lactic acidosis, hepatomegaly with steatosis
Zalcitabine (ddC, HIVID, 2′3′-dideoxycytidine)	Licensed	In combination with other antiretroviral agents for the treatment of HIV infection	Not indicated	0.75 mg tid	Clinically inferior to AZT monotherapy as initial treatment. Clinically as good as ddI in advanced patients intolerant to AZT. In combination with AZT, was clinically superior to AZT alone in patients with AIDS or CD4+ T cell count <350/μL	Peripheral neuropathy, pancreatitis, lactic acidosis, hepatomegaly with steatosis, oral ulcers
Stavudine (d4T, Zerit, 2′3′-didehydro-3′-dideoxythymidine)	Licensed	Treatment of HIV-infected patients in combination with other antiretroviral agents	Not indicated	≥60 kg: 40 mg bid <60 kg: 30 mg bid	Superior to AZT with respect to changes in CD4+ T cell counts in 359 patients who had received ≥24 wk of AZT. Following 12 wk of randomization, the CD4+ T cell count had decreased in AZT-treated controls by a mean of 22/μL, while in stavudine-treated patients, it had increased by a mean of 22/μL	Peripheral neuropathy, pancreatitis, lactic acidosis, hepatomegaly with steatosis, ascending neuromuscular weakness, lipodystrophy
Lamivudine (Epivir, 2′3′-dideoxy-3′-thiacytidine, 3TC)	Licensed	In combination with other antiretroviral agents for the treatment of HIV infection	Not indicated	150 mg bid 300 mg qd	Superior to AZT alone with respect to changes in CD4 counts in 495 patients who were zidovudine-naive and 477 patients who were zidovudine-experienced. Overall CD4+ T cell counts for the zidovudine group were at baseline by 24 wk, while in the group treated with zidovudine plus lamivudine, they were 10–50 cells/μL above baseline. 54% decrease in progression to AIDS/death compared to AZT alone	

(continued)

Drug	Status	Indication	Dose as Monotherapy	Dose in Combination	Supporting Data	Toxicity
Emtricitabine (FTC, Emtriva)	Licensed	In combination with other antiretroviral agents for the treatment of HIV infection	Not indicated	200 mg qd	Comparable to d4T in combination with ddI and efavirenz in 571 treatment-naive patients. Similar to 3TC in combination with 2DV or d4T + NNRT1 or PI in 440 patients doing well for at least 12 weeks on a 3TC regimen.	
Abacavir (Ziagen)	Licensed	For treatment of HIV infection in combination with other antiretroviral agents	Not indicated	300 mg bid	Abacavir + AZT + 3TC equivalent to indinavir + AZT + 3TC with regard to viral load suppression (~60% in each group with <400 HIV RNA copies/mL plasma) and CD4 cell increase (~100/μL in each group) at 24 weeks	Hypersensitivity reaction (can be fatal); fever, rash, nausea, vomiting, malaise or fatigue, and loss of appetite
Tenofovir (Viread)	Licensed	For use in combination with other antiretroviral agents when treatment is indicated	Not indicated	300 mg qd	Reduction of ~0.6 log in HIV-1 RNA levels when added to background regimen in treatment-experienced patients	Potential for renal toxicity
Delavirdine (Rescriptor)	Licensed	For use in combination with appropriate antiretrovirals when treatment is warranted	Not indicated	400 mg tid	Delavirdine + AZT superior to AZT alone with regard to viral load suppression at 52 weeks	Skin rash, abnormalities in liver function tests
Nevirapine (Viramune)	Licensed	In combination with other antiretroviral agents for treatment of progressive HIV infection	Not indicated	200 mg/d × 14 days then 200 mg bid	Increases in CD4+ T cell count, decrease in HIV RNA when used in combination with nucleosides	Skin rash, hepatotoxicity
Efavirenz (Sustiva)	Licensed	For treatment of HIV infection in combination with other antiretroviral agents	Not indicated	600 mg qhs	Efavirenz + AZT + 3TC comparable to indinavir + AZT + 3TC with regard to viral load suppression (a higher percentage of the efavirenz group achieved viral load <50 copies/mL; however, the discontinuation rate in the indinavir group was unexpectedly high, accounting for most treatment "failures") and CD4 cell increase (~140/μL in each group) at 24 weeks	Rash, dysphoria, elevated liver function tests, drowsiness, abnormal dreams, depression
PROTEASE INHIBITORS						
Saquinavir mesylate (Invirase—hard gel capsule)	Licensed	In combination with other antiretroviral agents when therapy is warranted	Not indicated	600 mg q8h	Increases in CD4+ T cell counts, reduction in HIV RNA most pronounced in combination therapy with ddC. 50% reduction in first AIDS-defining event or death in combination with ddC compared to either agent alone	Diarrhea, nausea, headaches, hyperglycemia, fat redistribution, lipid abnormalities
(Fortovase—soft gel capsule)	Licensed	For use in combination with other antiretroviral agents when treatment is warranted	Not indicated	1200 mg tid	Reduction in the mortality rate and AIDS-defining events for patients who received hard-gel formulation in combination with ddC	Diarrhea, nausea, abdominal pain, headaches, hyperglycemia, fat redistribution, lipid abnormalities
Ritonavir (Norvir)	Licensed	In combination with other antiretroviral agents for treatment of HIV infection when treatment is warranted	Not indicated	600 mg bid	Reduction in the cumulative incidence of clinical progression or death from 34 to 17% in patients with CD4+ T cell count <100/μL treated for a median of 6 months	Nausea, abdominal pain, hyperglycemia, fat redistribution, lipid abnormalities, may alter levels of many other drugs, including saquinavir

(continued)

TABLE 173–20—(Continued)

Drug	Status	Indication	Dose as Monotherapy	Dose in Combination	Supporting Data	Toxicity
Indinavir sulfate (Crixivan)	Licensed	For treatment of HIV infection in combination with other antiretroviral agents when antiretroviral treatment is warranted	Not indicated	800 mg q8h	Increase in CD4+ T cell count by 100/μL and 2-log decrease in HIV RNA levels when given in combination with zidovudine and lamivudine. Decrease of 50% in risk of progression to AIDS or death when given with zidovudine and lamivudine compared with zidovudine and lamivudine alone	Nephrolithiasis, indirect hyperbilirubinemia, hyperglycemia, fat redistribution, lipid abnormalities
Nelfinavir mesylate (Viracept)	Licensed	For treatment of HIV infection in combination with other antiretroviral agents when antiretroviral therapy is warranted	Not indicated	750 mg tid or 1250 mg bid	2.0-log decline in HIV RNA when given in combination with stavudine	Diarrhea, loose stools, hyperglycemia, fat redistribution, lipid abnormalities
Amprenavir (Agenerase)	Licensed	In combination with other antiretroviral agents for treatment of HIV infection	Not indicated	1200 mg bid or 600 mg bid + Ritonavir 100 mg bid or 1200 mg qd + Ritonavir 200 mg qd	In treatment-naïve patients, amprenavir + AZT + 3TC superior to AZT + 3TC with regard to viral load suppression (53% vs 11% with <400 HIV RNA copies/mL plasma at 24 weeks). CD4+ T cell responses similar between treatment groups. In treatment-experienced patients, amprenavir + NRTIs similar to indinavir + NRTIs with regard to viral load suppression (43% vs 53% with <400 HIV RNA copies/mL plasma at 24 weeks). CD4+ T cell responses superior in the indinavir + NRTIs group	Nausea, vomiting, diarrhea, rash, oral paresthesias, elevated liver function tests, hyperglycemia, fat redistribution, lipid abnormalities
Fosamprenavir (Lexiva)	Licensed			1400 mg bid or 700 mg bid + Ritonavir 100 mg bid		
Lopinavir/ritonavir (Kaletra)	Licensed	For treatment of HIV infection in combination with other antiretroviral agents	Not indicated	400 mg/100 mg bid	In treatment of naïve patients, lopinavir/ritonavir + d4T + 3TC superior to nelfinavir + d4T + 3TC with regard to viral load suppression (79% vs 64% with <400 HIV RNA copies/mL at 40 weeks). CD4+ T cell increases similar in both groups.	Diarrhea, hyperglycemia, fat redistribution, lipid abnormalities
Atazanavir (Reyataz)	Licensed	For treatment of HIV infection in combination with other antiretroviral agents	Not indicated	400 mg qd or 300 mg qd + Ritonavir 100 mg qd when given with efavirenz	Comparable to efavirenz when given in combination with AZT + 3TC in a study of 810 treatment-naive patients. Comparable to nelfinavir when given in combination with d4T + 3TC in a study of 467 treatment-naive patients.	Hyperbilirubinemia, PR prolongation, nausea, vomiting, hyperglycemia, fat maldistribution
FUSION INHIBITOR						
Enfuvirtide (Fuzeon)	Licensed	In combination with other agents in treatment-experienced patients with evidence of HIV-1 replication despite ongoing antiretroviral therapy	Not indicated	90 mg SC bid	In treatment of experienced patients, superior to placebo when added to new optimized background (37% vs 16% with <400 HIV RNA copies/mL at 24 weeks; + 71 vs + 35 CD4+ T cells at 24 weeks)	Local injection reactions, hypersensitivity reactions, increased rate of bacterial pneumonia

Note: ARC, AIDS-related complex; NRTIs, nonnucleoside reverse transcriptase inhibitors.

with advanced HIV disease. However, while treatment of patients with early stages of HIV infection was associated with increases in CD4+ T cell count, it was not associated with a better overall outcome than waiting until later to treat. Subsequent trials established the ability of this drug to dramatically decrease the incidence of perinatal transmission of HIV from infected mother to infant. Eventually a series of studies demonstrated the superiority of combination antiretroviral regimens over zidovudine alone, and combination therapy (discussed below) remains the standard of treatment today. Among the side effects of zidovudine at the initiation of therapy are fatigue, malaise, nausea, and headache. These side effects often subside over time. Patients on zidovudine may develop a macrocytic anemia, myopathy, cardiomyopathy, and lactic acidosis associated with fatty infiltration of the liver. As with every antiretroviral drug, HIV has the ability to develop re-

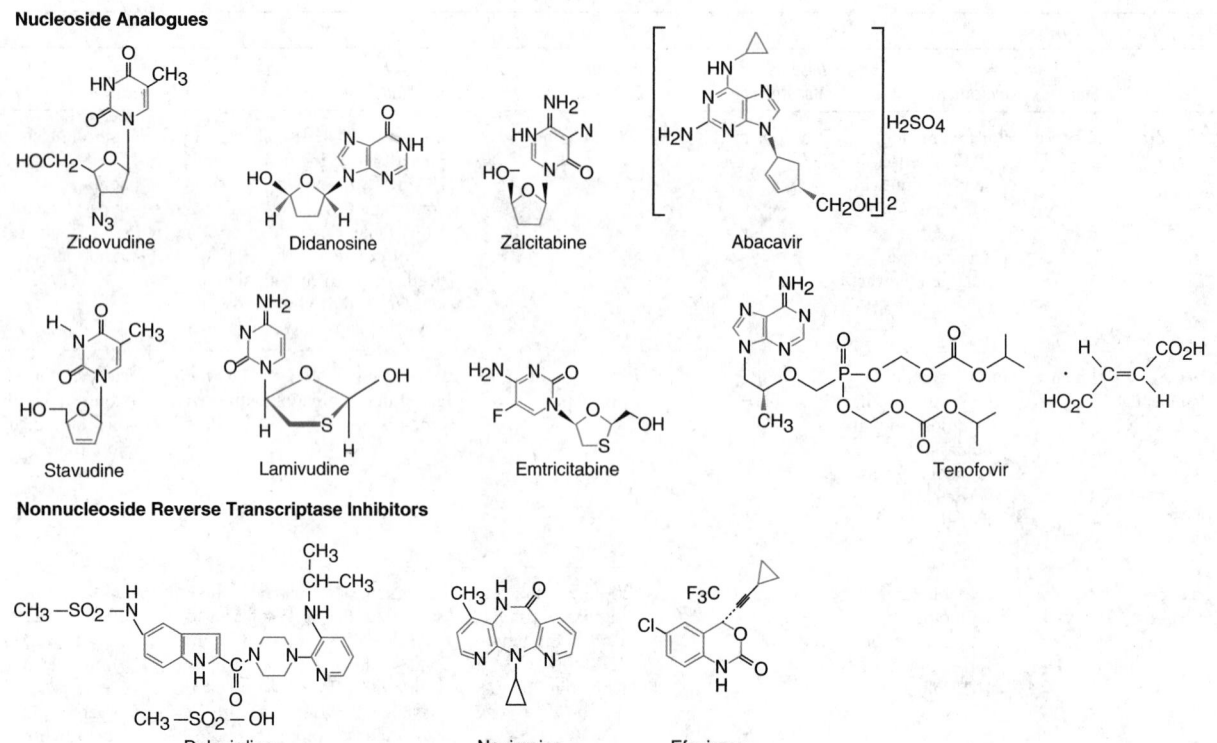

Nucleoside Analogues

Zidovudine Didanosine Zalcitabine Abacavir

Stavudine Lamivudine Emtricitabine Tenofovir

Nonnucleoside Reverse Transcriptase Inhibitors

Delavirdine Nevirapine Efavirenz

FIGURE 173-39 Molecular structures of antiretroviral agents.

sistance to zidovudine. Zidovudine resistance has been reported to occur ~6 months following the initiation of zidovudine monotherapy. More recently, zidovudine-resistant viruses have been noted in patients with acute infection prior to the initiation of therapy, implying that zidovudine-resistant viruses can be transmitted from person to person. Resistance emerges more rapidly in late-stage patients, presumably as a consequence of a greater degree of viral replication and thus a greater opportunity for mutation. A variety of amino acid changes including substitutions, insertions, and deletions have been reported to confer zidovudine resistance (Fig. 173-40). One combination preparation, Combivir, consists of zidovudine and lamivudine, while another, Trizivir, consists of zidovudine, lamivudine, and abacavir.

Didanosine (ddI; 2′,3′-dideoxyinosine) was the second drug licensed for the treatment of HIV infection, followed shortly thereafter by zalcitabine. Didanosine is metabolized to dideoxyadenosine in vivo. It is best absorbed on an empty stomach at a high pH. For this reason, the formulations of didanosine either contain a buffer, and each dose must be administered in no fewer than two tablets to ensure adequate buffering of stomach acid, or are provided as an extended-release enteric-coated capsule. The toxicity profile of didanosine is quite different from that of zidovudine. The most common toxicity is a painful sensory peripheral neuropathy that occurs in ~30% of patients receiving >400 mg/d. It generally resolves with discontinuation of the drug and may not recur if the drug is resumed at a reduced dose. At higher doses than are currently used one may see pancreatitis in ~10% of patients. Pancreatitis associated with didanosine therapy can be fatal. Didanosine should be discontinued if a patient experiences abdominal pain consistent with pancreatitis or if an elevated serum amylase or lipase level is found in association with an edematous pancreas on ultrasound. Didanosine is contraindicated in patients with a prior history of pancreatitis, regardless of etiology.

Zalcitabine (ddC; 2′,3′-dideoxycytidine) is rarely used today in the management of patients with HIV infection. Among the nucleoside analogues licensed for the treatment of HIV infection, it is probably the weakest. The main toxicity of ddC is pancreatitis.

Stavudine (d4T; 2′,3′-didehydro-3′-deoxythymidine) was the fourth drug licensed for the treatment of HIV infection. Like zidovudine, stavudine is a thymidine analogue. These two drugs are antagonistic in vitro and in vivo and should not be given together. Peripheral neuropathy and hepatic steatosis are the main toxicities of stavudine. It is commonly used with lamivudine as part of an initial treatment regimen.

Lamivudine (3TC; 2′,3′-dideoxy-3′-thiacytidine) is the fifth of the nucleoside analogues to be licensed in the United States. It is licensed for use in combination with zidovudine in situations where zidovudine is indicated. In actual practice, lamivudine is a frequent element of many different combination regimens currently in use. It is available either alone or in combination with zidovudine (Combivir). One reason behind the excellent synergy seen between lamivudine and the other nucleoside analogues may be that strains of HIV resistant to lamivudine (M184V substitution) appear to have enhanced sensitivity to other nucleosides, and thus development of dual resistance is quite difficult. In addition, there is a suggestion that 3TC-resistant strains of HIV may be less virulent and are less able to generate new mutants than are strains of HIV that are 3TC-sensitive. Lamivudine is among the best tolerated and least toxic nucleoside analogues.

Emtricitabine (FTC; 5-fluoro-1-(2R,5S)-[2-(hydroxymethyl)-1,3-oxathiolan-5-yl]cytosine) is the negative enantiomer of a thio analogue of cytidine with a fluorine in the 5 position. It is licensed for use in combination with other antiretroviral agents for treatment of HIV-1 infection in adults. Similar in activity to lamivudine, resistance to emtricitabine is associated with the M184V mutation in reverse transcriptase. Viruses showing the K65R mutation in reverse transcriptase may have reduced susceptibility to emtricitabine.

Abacavir {(1S,cis)-4-[2-amino-6-(cyclopropylamino)-9H-purin-9-yl]-2-cyclopentene-1-methanol sulfate (salt)(2:1)} is a synthetic carbocyclic analogue of the nucleoside guanosine. It is licensed to be used in combination with other antiretroviral agents for the treatment of HIV-1 infection. Hypersensitivity reactions have been reported in ~4% of patients treated with this drug, and patients developing signs or symptoms of hypersensitivity such as fever, skin rash, fatigue, and gastrointestinal symptoms should discontinue the drug and not restart it. Fatal hyper-

Protease Inhibitors

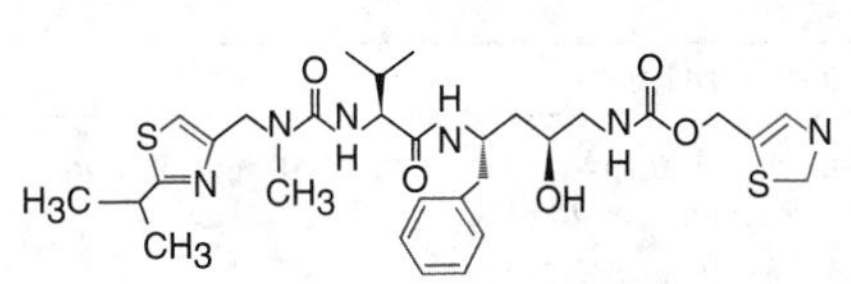

Ritonavir

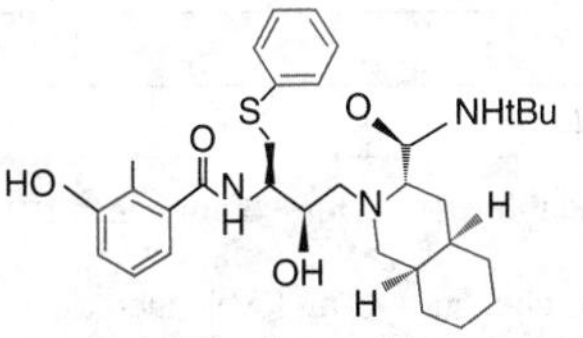

Nelfinavir mesylate

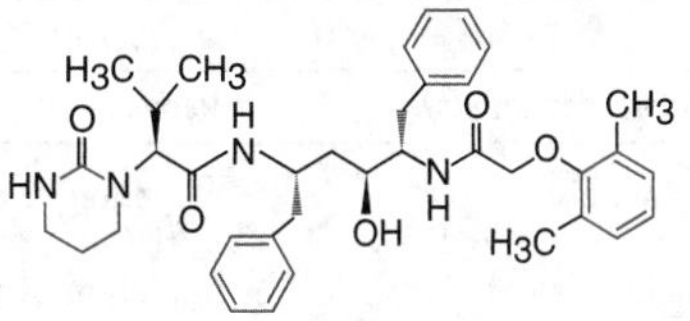

Lopinavir

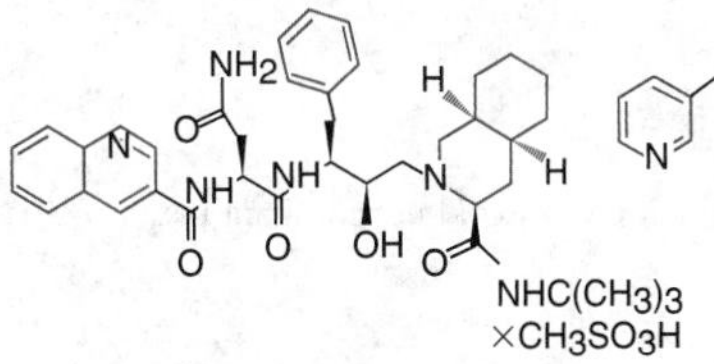

Saquinavir mesylate

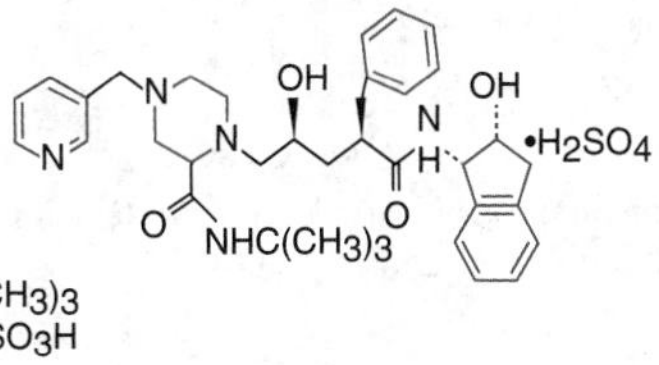

Indinavir sulfate

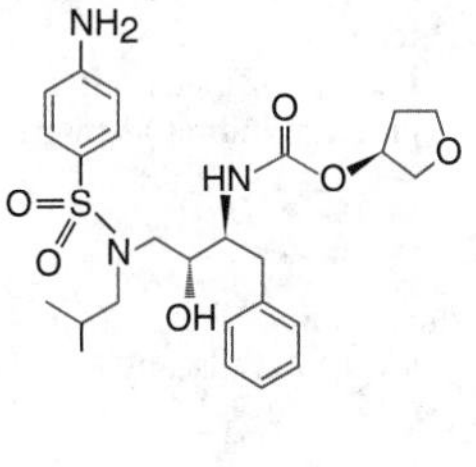

Amprenavir

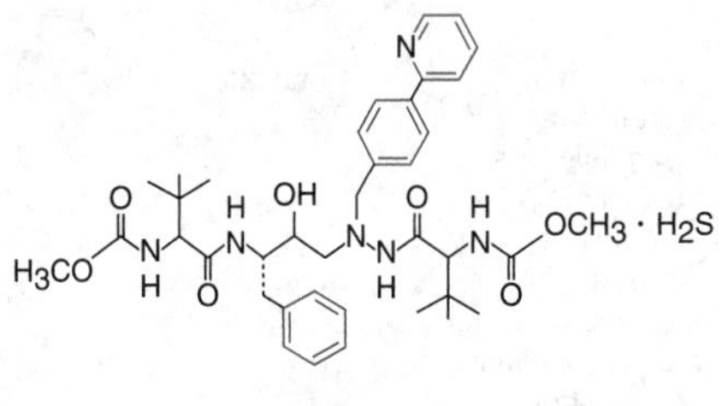

Atazanavir

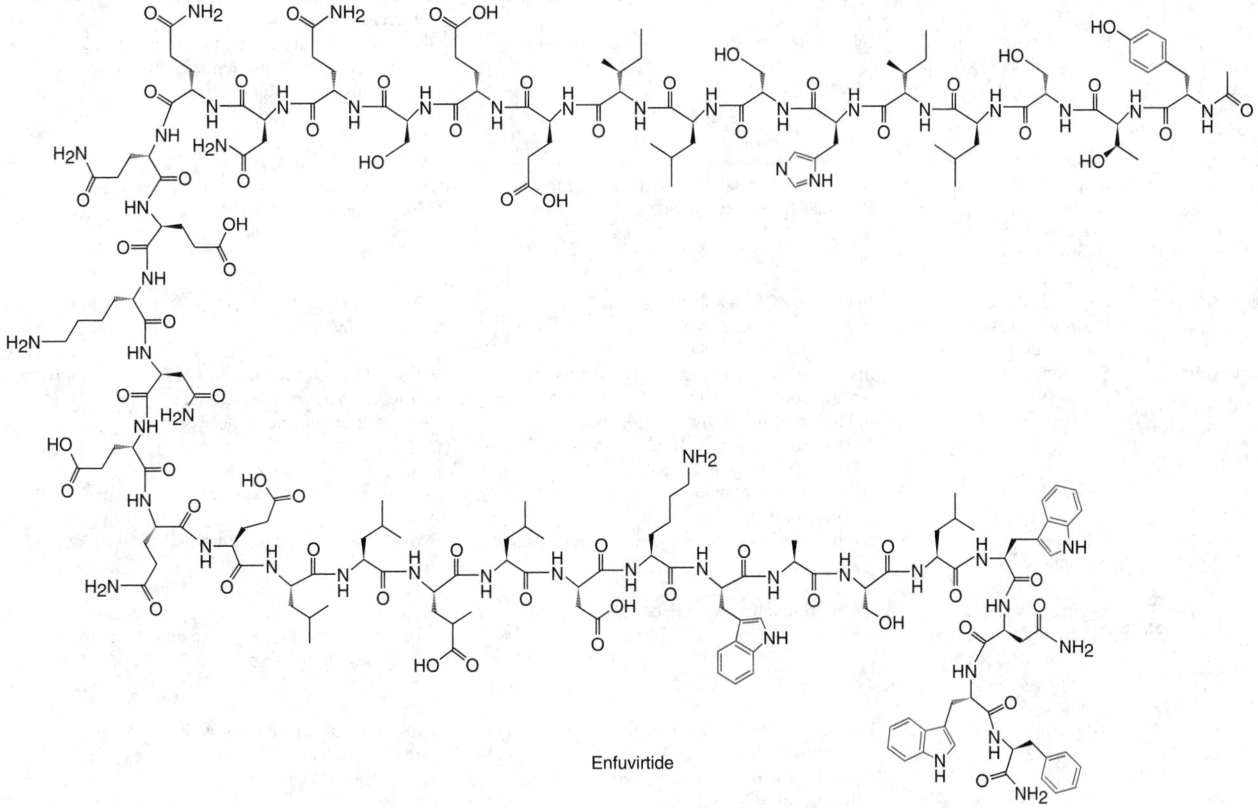

Enfuvirtide

FIGURE 173-39—*(Continued)*

sensitivity reactions have been reported with rechallenge. Abacavir hypersensitiviy appears to occur with a higher frequency in patients who are HLA-B57. Abacavir-resistant strains of HIV are typically also resistant to lamivudine, didanosine, and zalcitabine.

Tenofovir disoproxil fumarate (9-[(R)-2-[[bis[[(isopropoxycarbonyl)oxy]methoxy]phosphinyl]methoxy]propyl]adenine fumarate (1:1)) is an acyclic nucleoside phosphonate diester analogue of adenosine monophosphate. It undergoes diester hydrolysis to form tenofovir and is the first nucleotide analogue to be licensed for treatment of HIV infection. It is indicated in combination with other antiretroviral agents for the treatment of HIV-1 infection. HIV isolates with increased resistance typically express a K65R mutation in reverse transcriptase and a three- to four-fold reduction in sensitivity to tenofovir. Tenofovir is primarily eliminated by the kidneys, and renal impairment with hypophosphatemia may occur. Tenofovir is contraindicated in patients with renal impairment. Coadministration with didanosine leads to a 60% increase in didanosine levels, and thus doses of didanosine need

to be adjusted and patients monitored carefully if these two drugs are used in combination.

Nevirapine, delavirdine, and *efavirenz* are nonnucleoside inhibitors of the HIV-1 reverse transcriptase. They are licensed for use in combination with nucleoside analogues for the treatment of HIV-infected adults. These agents inhibit reverse transcriptase by binding to regions of the enzyme outside the active site and causing conformational changes in the enzyme that render it inactive. Although these agents are active in the nanomolar range, they are also very selective for the reverse transcriptase of HIV-1, have no activity against HIV-2, and, when used as monotherapy, are associated with the rapid emergence of drug-resistant mutants (Table 173-20; Fig. 173-40). Efavirenz is administered once a day, nevirapine twice a day, and delavirdine three times a day. All three drugs are associated with the development of a maculopapular rash, generally seen within the first few weeks of therapy. While it is possible to treat through this rash, it is important to be sure that one is not dealing with a more severe eruption such as

TABLE 173-21 *Drug-Drug Interactions Involving Antiretroviral Agents*

Index Drug	Interacting Drug(s)	Mechanism/Effect	Recommendation
Amprenavir	Efavirenz	Induction of metabolism, decreased amprenavir AUC	Consider dosage increase to 1200 mg tid or add ritonavir 200 mg bid
	Indinavir	Inhibition of metabolism—drug levels increased 33%	No change
	Ritonavir	Inhibition of metabolism—amprenavir AUC increased 2.5-fold	Decrease to 600 mg bid
Amprenavir, indinavir, saquinavir, ritonavir, nelfinavir	Rifampin	Induction of metabolism—marked decrease in protease inhibitor drug levels	Avoid concomitant use
Antiarrhythmics (flecainaide, quinidine, propafenone, amiodarone)	Ritonavir	Inhibition of metabolism—potential for increased levels and toxicity	Use with caution or avoid concomitant use
Atorvastatin	Protease inhibitors	Inhibition of metabolism—increased drug levels	Use with caution
Atovaquone	Rifampin	Induction of metabolism—decreased drug levels	Concentrations may not be therapeutic—avoid or increase dose
Benzodiazepines (flurazepam, diazepam, midazolam, triazolam)	Protease inhibitors, delavirdine, efavirenz	Inhibition of metabolism—increased drug levels	Monitor for toxicity such as increased sedation, decrease dose, or use temazepam, lorazepam Not recommended for use with triazolam
Bepridil	Ritomavir, amprenavir	Inhibition of metabolism—increased drug levels	Avoid concomitant use
Carbamazepine	Indinavir, ritonavir	Inhibition of metabolism—increased toxicity	Avoid concomitant use or monitor levels
Cidofovir	Nephrotoxic drugs (aminoglycosides, amphotericin, foscarnet)	Potential for increased side effects	Monitor renal function
Cisapride	Protease inhibitors, azole antifungals, macrolides, delavirdine, efavirenz	Inhibition of metabolism	Cardiotoxic life-threatening effects possible—avoid concomitant use
Clarithromycin	Efavirenz	Induction of metabolism—40% decrease in clarithromycin AUC	Clinical significance unknown, but clarithromycin effectiveness may be altered
	Nevirapine	Induction of metabolism—decrease in clarithromycin AUC by 30%, increase in 14-OH clarithromycin by 58%	No dosage adjustments necessary
	Delavirdine	Inhibition of metabolism—100% increase in clarithromycin	Adjust dose in renal failure
	Ritonavir Atazanavir	Inhibition of metabolism—drug levels increased 77%	No adjustment needed in normal renal function
	Agents that increase gastric pH—antacids, H₂ blockers, proton pump inhibitors, didanosine	Delavirdine absorption decreased with increased pH	Avoid concomitant use with H₂ blockers and proton pump inhibitors; separate from antacids by at least 2 h
	Rifabutin	Induction of metabolism—50–60% decrease in delavirdine levels	Clinical significance unknown; may require increased delavirdine dose
	Rifampin	Induction of metabolism—marked decrease in drug levels	Avoid concomitant use
Didanosine (ddI)	Allopurinol	Increased ddI AUC by 2-fold	Clinical significance unknown
	Methadone	Decrease in ddI AUC by 52%	No clinical data, but potential for decreased ddI efficacy
	Tenofovir	Increase in ddI AUC by 44%	Consider ddI dose reduction
	Ganciclovir	Increased ddI AUC by 111%	Monitor for ddI toxicity
Efavirenz	Fluconazole	Inhibition of metabolism—efavirenz AUC increased 15%	No dosage adjustment necessary
	Indinavir	Induction of hepatic metabolism—indinavir AUC decreased 35%	Consider increasing indinavir dose to 1000 mg q8h
	Nelfinavir	Nelfinavir AUC increased 21%	No dosage adjustment necessary
	Rifampin	Induction of metabolism—significant reduction in efavirenz AUC	Clinical significance unknown; increase in efavirenz dose may be required
	Rifampin	Induction of metabolism—efavirenz AUC decreased 26%	Clinical significance unknown
	Ritonavir	Inhibition of metabolism—efavirenz AUC increased 21%	No dosage adjustment necessary
Ergot alkaloids (ergotamine, dihydroergotamine, ergoloid mesylates)	Protease inhibitors, azole antifungals, macrolides, delavirdine, efavirenz	Inhibition of metabolism—potential for acute toxicity	Use with caution or avoid concomitant use; monitor for toxicity such as peripheral vasoconstriction, nausea and vomiting, and impaired mental status

(continued)

TABLE 173-21— (Continued)

Index Drug	Interacting Drug(s)	Mechanism/Effect	Recommendation
Ethinyl estradiol	Efavirenz	Inhibition of metabolism—37% increase in estradiol AUC	No dosage adjustment necessary
	Protease inhibitors, nevirapine	Induction of metabolism—decreased levels of oral contraceptive	Use alternative or additional method of contraception
Fluvastatin, lovastatin, simvastatin	Protease inhibitors, azole antifungals, macrolides, delavirdine	Inhibition of metabolism—potential for increased levels and toxicity	Potential for hypolipidemic toxicity (dizziness, headache, GI side effects); monitor patient closely and consider dose reduction or use pravastatin or atorvastatin
Foscarnet	Nephrotoxic drugs (aminoglycosides, amphotericin, cidofovir)	Potential for increased toxicity	Monitor renal function
Ganciclovir	Drugs causing bone marrow suppression (i.e., TMP/SMZ, zidovudine)	Potential for increased hematologic toxicity	Monitor for anemia and neutropenia—adjust/ change doses and drugs if required; consider supportive therapy with G-CSF
	Tenofovir	Competition for tubular secretion	Monitor for renal toxicity
Indinavir, saquinavir, ritonavir, nelfinavir, amprenavir	Anticonvulsants (carbamazepine, phenytoin, phenobarbital)	Induction of metabolism—potential decrease in drug levels	Clinical effects unknown; monitor blood levels, consider dosage increase, or avoid concomitant use
Indinavir	Delavirdine	Increased indinavir levels	Consider reducing indinavir dose to 600 mg q8h
	St. John's wort	Decreased indinavir levels	Avoid use of St. John's wort
	Didanosine, antacids	ddl buffer decreases absorption of indinavir	Separate doses by at least 1 h
	Methadone	Indinavir C_{max} decreased 16–36%; indinavir C_{min} increased by 50–100%	No dosage adjustments necessary
	Nelfinavir	Inhibition of metabolism—indinavir drug levels increased by 51%, nelfinavir drug levels by 83%	Avoid concommitant use
	Nevirapine	Induction of metabolism—decreased drug levels of indinavir by 30%	Consider increasing indinavir dose to 1000 mg q8h
	Ritonavir	Inhibition of metabolism—indinavir AUC increased 3–7-fold	Consider 800 mg indinavir/200 mg ritonavir bid
	Efavirenz	Induction of metabolism—31% decrease in indinavir levels	Dose indinavir at 1000 mg q8h or add ritomavir
Lopinavir/ritonavir	Nevirapine, efavirenz	Induction of metabolism—40–55% decrease in lopinavir levels	Dose lopinavir/ritonavir at 533/133 mg bid
Meperidine	Ritonavir	Likely induction of metabolism—decrease in meperidine AUC 67%, increase in normeperidine 47%	Potential for decreased meperidine effectiveness—may require increased dose; caution with chronic dosing
Methadone	Abacavir	Methadone clearance decreased 22%	Low potential for opiate withdrawal; monitor closely and increase methadone dose as required to control symptoms
	Fluconazole	Inhibition of metabolism—drug levels increased 30%	Monitor for methadone toxicity such as respiratory depression, drop in blood pressure, and mental status changes; consider dosage adjustment
	Nevirapine, efavirenz, ritonavir	Induction of metabolism—substantial decrease in methadone levels	Potential for opiate withdrawal; monitor closely and increase methadone dose as required to control symptoms
Nelfinavir	Ritonavir	Inhibition of metabolism—increased drug levels of nelfinavir by 152%	Consider nelfinavir 500–750 mg bid + ritonavir 200–400 mg bid
Pentamidine	Drugs that cause pancreatitis (didanosine, zalcitabine)	Increased risk of pancreatitis	Monitor amylase, lipase
Quinolone antibiotics (ciprofloxacin, levofloxacin, ofloxaxin, etc)	Didanosine buffered tablet, antacids, iron products, calcium products, sucralfate	Chelation resulting in marked decrease in quinolone drug levels	Administer cation preparations at least 2 h after quinolone
Rifabutin	Amprenavir, atazanavir, ritonavir, indinavir, nelfinavir, lopinavir/ ritonavir	Inhibition of metabolism—marked increase in rifabutin drug levels	Use 150 mg qd with indinavir, nelfinavir, amprenavir; increase nelfinavir to 1000 mg tid Use 150 mg every other day with ritonavir, lopinavir/ritonavir, atazanavir
	Delavirdine	Induction of delavirdine metabolism; inhibition of rifabutin metabolism	Avoid concomitant use
	Efavirenz	Induction of rifabutin metabolism—levels decrease 35%	Increase rifabutin to 450–600 mg qd
	Fluconazole	Inhibition of metabolism—marked increase in rifabutin drug levels	Monitor for rifabutin toxicity such as uveitis, nausea, neutropenia

(continued)

Index Drug	Interacting Drug(s)	Mechanism/Effect	Recommendation
Rifampin	Protease inhibitors, delavirdine, nevirapine	Induction of metabolism—decreased drug levels	Avoid concomitant use
	Efavirenz	Induction of metabolism	Increase efavirenz to 800 mg qd
Ritonavir	Delavirdine	Inhibition of metabolism—70% increase in ritonavir levels	No data to base recommendations
Saquinavir	Nevirapine	Induction of metabolism—drug levels decreased 27%	Clinical significance unknown—consider dosage increase of saquinavir or add ritonavir
	Ritonavir	Inhibition of metabolism—3-fold or higher increase in saquinavir drug levels	Various combinations used to optimize saquinavir therapy including 400 mg saquinavir/400 mg ritonavir
	Delavirdine	Inhibition of metabolism—5-fold increase in saquinavir drug levels	Dose saquinavir at 800 mg tid
	Nelfinavir	Inhibition of metabolism—3–5-fold increase in saquinavir drug levels	Dose saquinavir at 800 mg tid or 1200 mg bid
	Efavirenz	Induction of metabolism—saquinavir AUC decreased 62%	Avoid concomitant use unless saquinavir is administered with ritonavir
Sildenafil	Protease inhibitors, delavirdine	Inhibition of metabolism—sildenafil AUC increased 2–11-fold	Use 25-mg sildenafil dose and do not repeat for 48 h
St. John's Wort	Protease inhibitors, NRT1s	Induction of metabolism—decreased drug levels	Avoid concomitant use
Terfenadine, astemizole	Protease inhibitors, azole antifungals, macrolides, delavirdine, efavirenz	Inhibition of metabolism	Cardiotoxic life-threatening effects possible—avoid concomitant use
Theophylline	Ritonavir	Induction of metabolism—decreased blood levels	Monitor theophylline levels
Tipranavir	Ritonavir	Inhibition of metabolism—tipranavir AUC increased 7–45-fold	Combination under investigation to optimize tipranavir levels
TMP/SMZ	Rifampin	TMP AUC decreased 63%, SMX AUC decreased 23%	Clinical significance unknown
Zalcitabine, stavudine, didanosine	Drugs that cause peripheral neuropathy— INH, d4T, ddI, ddC	Potential for increased risk of peripheral neuropathy	Monitor for signs and symptoms such as numbness and tingling in extremities
Zidovudine	Drugs causing bone marrow suppression (i.e., TMP/SMX, ganciclovir, sulfadiazine)	Increased bone marrow suppression	Monitor for anemia, neutropenia—may require supportive therapy (EPO, G-CSF)

Note: AUC, area under the curve; *C*, concentration; EPO, erythropoietin; G-CSF, granulocyte colony stimulating factor; TMP/SMX, trimethoprim/sulfamethoxazole.

Stevens-Johnson syndrome by looking carefully for signs of mucosal involvement, significant fever, or painful lesions with desquamation. Severe, life-threatening, and in some cases fatal hepatotoxicity, including fulminant and cholestatic hepatitis, hepatic necrosis and hepatic failure, have been reported in patients treated with nevirapine. Many patients treated with efavirenz note a feeling of light-headedness, dizziness, or out of sorts following the initiation of therapy. Some complain of vivid dreams. These symptoms tend to disappear after several weeks of therapy. Aside from difficulties with dreams, taking efavirenz at bedtime may minimize the side effects. Nevirapine and efavirenz are both commonly used as part of initial treatment regimens in combination with two nucleoside analogues. Another common use of these drugs is as part of salvage regimens in patients whose current regimen is inadequate.

The introduction of the HIV-1 protease inhibitors (saquinavir, indinavir, ritonavir, nelfinavir, amprenavir, lopinavir/ritonavir, and atazanavir) to the therapeutic armamentarium of antiretrovirals has had a profound impact on the efficacy of antiretroviral therapy. When used as part of initial regimens in combination with reverse transcriptase inhibitors, these agents have been shown to be capable of suppressing levels of HIV replication to under 50 copies per milliliter in the majority of patients for a minimum of 5 years. HIV protease inhibitors appear to be good substrates for the drug transporters MDR-1 and MRP-2. Whether or not genetic variations in these genes will lead to variability in protease inhibitor activity remains to be determined. As in the case of reverse transcriptase inhibitors, resistance to protease inhibitors can develop rapidly in the setting of monotherapy, and thus these agents should only be used as part of combination therapeutic regimens. A summary of known resistance mutations for protease inhibitors is shown in Fig. 173-40.

Saquinavir was the first of the HIV-1 protease inhibitors to be licensed. Initially provided as a hard gel (Invirase) with poor bioavailability, the soft-gel formulation (Fortavase) provides good plasma levels of drug, particularly when administered in conjunction with ritonavir. Saquinavir is metabolized by the cytochrome P450 system, and ritonavir therapy results in inhibition of cytochrome P450 action. Thus, when both drugs are administered together there is the potential for increases in saquinavir levels. The use of low doses of ritonavir to provide pharmacodynamic boosting of other agents has become a fairly common strategy in HIV therapy. Saquinavir is among the best-tolerated protease inhibitors.

Ritonavir was the first protease inhibitor for which clinical efficacy was demonstrated. In a study of 1090 patients with CD4+ T cell counts $<100/\mu L$ who were randomized to receive either placebo or ritonavir in addition to any other licensed medications, patients receiving ritonavir had a reduction in the cumulative incidence of clinical progression or death from 34% to 17%. Mortality decreased from 10.1% to 5.8%. At full doses, ritonavir is poorly tolerated. Among the main side effects are nausea, diarrhea, abdominal pain, and circumoral paresthesia. Ritonavir has a high affinity for several isoforms of cytochrome P450, and its use can result in large increases in the plasma concentrations of drugs metabolized by this pathway. Among the agents affected in this manner are saquinavir, indinavir, macrolide antibiotics, R-warfarin, ondansetron, rifampin, most calcium channel blockers, glucocorticoids, and some of the chemotherapeutic agents used to treat KS. In addition, ritonavir may increase the activity of glucuronyltransferases, thus decreasing the levels of drugs metabolized by this pathway. Overall, great care must be taken when prescribing additional drugs to patients taking ritonavir. As mentioned above, the pharmacodynamic boosting property of ritonavir, seen with

MUTATIONS IN THE PROTEASE GENE ASSOCIATED WITH RESISTANCE TO PROTEASE INHIBITORS

Protease Inhibitors[18]

Multi-PI Resistance: Accumulation of Mutations[19]

Position	10	32	46	54	82	84	90
Wild-type	L	V	M	I	V	I	L
Substitution	F, I, R, V	I	I, L	V, M, L	A, F, T, S	V, C	M

Indinavir[20]

Position	10	20	24	32	36	46	54	71	73	77	82	84	90
Wild-type	L	K	L	V	M	M	I	A	G	V	V	I	L
Substitution	I, R, V	M, R	I	I	I	I, L	V	V, T	S, A	I	A, F, T	V	M

Ritonavir

Position	10	20	32	33	36	46	54	71	77	82	84	90
Wild-type	L	K	V	L	M	M	I	A	V	V	I	L
Substitution	F, I, R, V	M, R	I	F	I	I, L	V, L	V, T	I	A, F, T, S	V	M

Saquinavir

Position	10	48	54	71	73	77	82	84	90
Wild-type	L	G	I	A	G	V	V	I	L
Substitution	I, R, V	V	V, L	V, T	S	I	A	V	M

Nelfinavir

Position	10	30	36	46	71	77	82	84	88	90
Wild-type	L	D	M	M	A	V	V	I	N	L
Substitution	F, I	N	I	I, L	V, T	I	A, F, T, S	V	D, S	M

Amprenavir

Position	10	32	46	47	50	54	73	84	90
Wild-type	L	V	M	I	I	I	G	I	L
Substitution	F, I, R, V	I	I, L	V	V	L, V, M	S	V	M

Lopinavir/Ritonavir[21,22]

Position	10	20	24	32	33	46	47	50	53	54	(63)	71	73	82	84	90
Wild-type	L	K	L	V	L	M	I	F	I	L	L	A	G	V	I	L
Substitution	F, I, R, V	M, R	I	I	F	I, L	V, A	V	L	V, L, A, M, T, S	P	V, T	S	A, F, T, S	V	M

Atazanavir[23]

Position	10	20	24	32	33	36	46	48	50	54	71	73	82	84	88	90
Wild-type	L	K	L	V	L	M	M	G	I	I	A	G	V	I	N	L
Substitution	I, F, V	R, M, I	I	I	I, F, V	I, L, V	I	V	L	L	V	C, S, T, A	A	V	S	M

Tipranavir/Ritonavir[24] (expanded access)

Position	10	20	33	46	54	82	84	90
Wild-type	L	K	L	M	I	V	I	L
Substitution	I, V	M, L, T	I, F, V	I	V	A, F, L, T	V	M

MUTATIONS IN THE GP41 ENVELOPE GENE ASSOCIATED WITH RESISTANCE TO ENTRY INHIBITORS

Enfuvirtide[25]

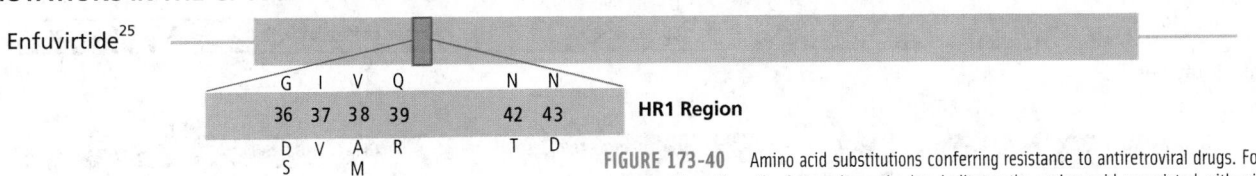

HR1 Region

Position	36	37	38	39	42	43
Wild-type	G	I	V	Q	N	N
Substitution	D, S	V	A, M	R	T	D

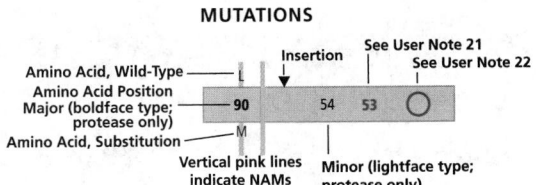

MUTATIONS

Amino Acid, Wild-Type — L
Amino Acid Position
Major (boldface type; protease only) — 90
Amino Acid, Substitution — M
Insertion
See User Note 21
See User Note 22
Minor (lightface type; protease only) — 54 53
Vertical pink lines indicate NAMs

FIGURE 173-40 Amino acid substitutions conferring resistance to antiretroviral drugs. For each amino acid residue, the letter above the bar indicates the amino acid associated with wildtype virus and the letter(s) below indicate the substitution(s) that confer viral resistance. The number shows the position of the mutation in the protein. Mutations selected by protease inhibitors in Gag cleavage sites are not listed because their contribution to resistance is not yet fully defined. HR1 indicates first heptad repeat; NAMs indicates nRTI-associated mutations; nRTI indicates nucleoside reverse transcriptase inhibitor; NNRTI indicates nonnucleoside reverse transcriptase inhibitor; PI indicates protease inhibitor. Amino acid abbreviations: A, alanine; C, cysteine; D, aspartate; E, glutamine; F, phenylalenine; G, glycine; H, histidine; I, isoleucine; K, lysine; L, leucine; M, methionine; N, asparagine; P, proline; Q, glutamine; R, arginine; S, serine; T, threonine; V, valine; W, tryptophan; Y, tyrosine. (*Reprinted with permission from the International AIDS Society-USA. Johnson VA et al: Topics HIV Med 11:215, 2003. Superscript numbers refer to the references cited in their journal. Accompanying usernotes, updates of the figure, and additional information available at http://www.iasusa.org.*)

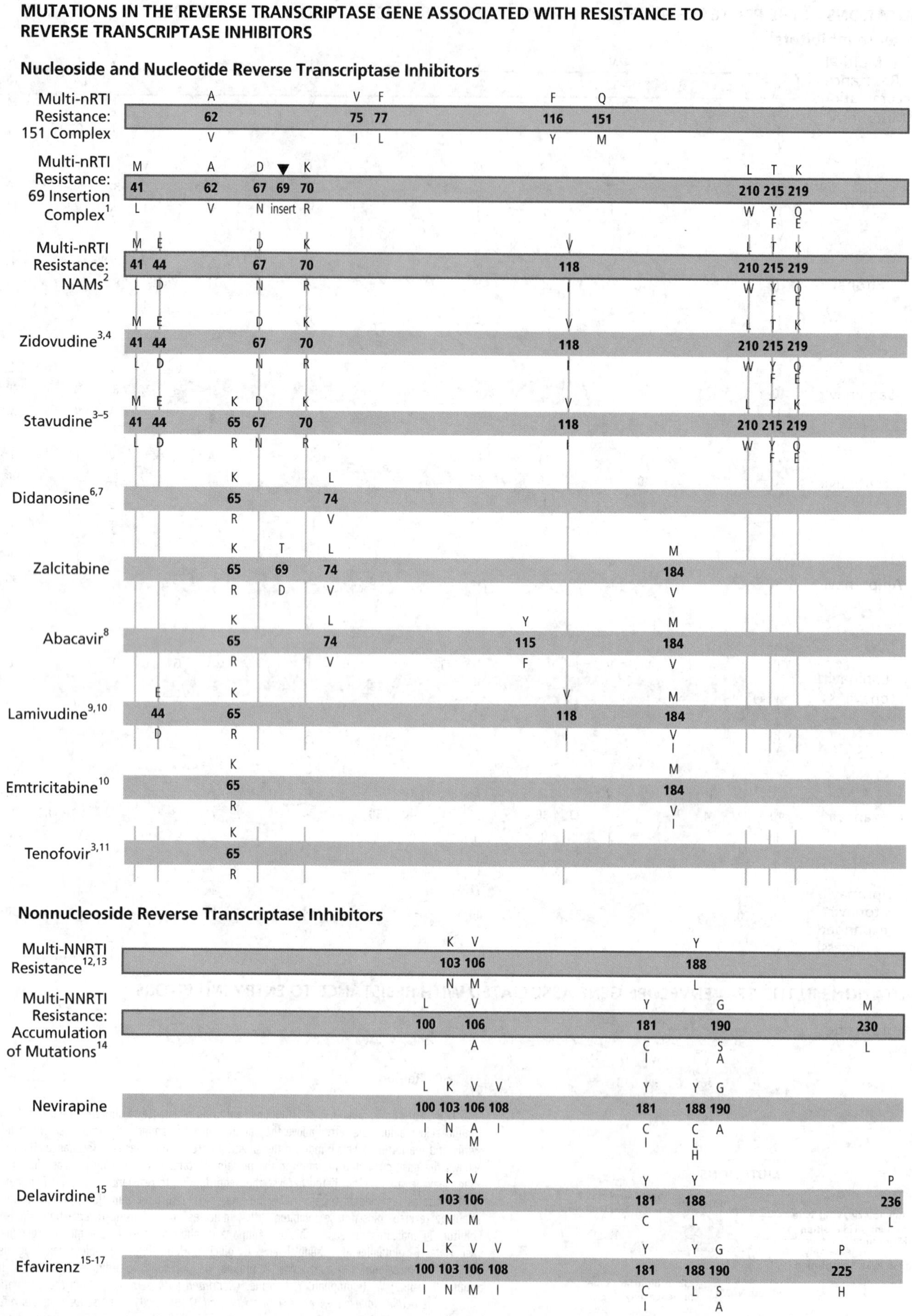
MUTATIONS IN THE REVERSE TRANSCRIPTASE GENE ASSOCIATED WITH RESISTANCE TO REVERSE TRANSCRIPTASE INHIBITORS
Nucleoside and Nucleotide Reverse Transcriptase Inhibitors
Multi-nRTI Resistance: 151 Complex
A 62 V; V 75 I; F 77 L; F 116 Y; Q 151 M
Multi-nRTI Resistance: 69 Insertion Complex[1]
M 41 L; A 62 V; D 67 N; 69 insert; K 70 R; L 210 W; T 215 Y F; K 219 Q E
Multi-nRTI Resistance: NAMs[2]
M 41 L; E 44 D; D 67 N; K 70 R; V 118 I; L 210 W; T 215 Y F; K 219 Q E
Zidovudine[3,4]
M 41 L; E 44 D; D 67 N; K 70 R; V 118 I; L 210 W; T 215 Y F; K 219 Q E
Stavudine[3–5]
M 41 L; E 44 D; K 65 R; D 67 N; K 70 R; V 118 I; L 210 W; T 215 Y F; K 219 Q E
Didanosine[6,7]
K 65 R; L 74 V
Zalcitabine
K 65 R; T 69 D; L 74 V; M 184 V
Abacavir[8]
K 65 R; L 74 V; Y 115 F; M 184 V
Lamivudine[9,10]
E 44 D; K 65 R; V 118 I; M 184 V I
Emtricitabine[10]
K 65 R; M 184 V I
Tenofovir[3,11]
K 65 R
Nonnucleoside Reverse Transcriptase Inhibitors
Multi-NNRTI Resistance[12,13]
K 103 N; V 106 M; Y 188 L
Multi-NNRTI Resistance: Accumulation of Mutations[14]
L 100 I; V 106 A; Y 181 C I; G 190 S A; M 230 L
Nevirapine
L 100 I; K 103 N; V 106 A M; V 108 I; Y 181 C I; Y 188 C L H; G 190 A
Delavirdine[15]
K 103 N; V 106 M; Y 181 C; Y 188 L; P 236 L
Efavirenz[15-17]
L 100 I; K 103 N; V 106 M; V 108 I; Y 181 C I; Y 188 L; G 190 S A; P 225 H

FIGURE 173-40—(Continued)

doses as low as 100 to 200 mg twice a day, is often used in the setting of HIV infection to derive more convenient regimens. For example, when given with low-dose ritonavir, saquinavir and indinavir can both be given on twice-a-day schedules and taken with food.

Indinavir is among the best studied of the HIV-1 protease inhibitors. It was the first protease inhibitor used in combination with dual nucleoside therapy. The combination of zidovudine, lamivudine, and indinavir was the first "triple combination" shown to have a profound effect on HIV replication. The main side effects of indinavir are nephrolithiasis (seen in 4% of patients) and asymptomatic indirect hyperbilirubinemia (seen in 10%). Indinavir is predominantly metabolized by the liver. The dose should be lowered in patients with cirrhosis. Indinavir shares metabolic pathways with terfenadine, astemizole, cisapride, triazolam, and midazolam. To avoid the potential for cardiac arrhythmias or prolonged sedation, these drugs should not be administered to patients taking indinavir. Levels of indinavir are decreased during concurrent therapy with rifabutin or nevirapine and increased during concurrent therapy with ketoconazole, delavirdine, efavirenz, or ritonavir. Dosages should be modified appropriately in these circumstances (Table 173-21).

Nelfinavir was approved in 1997 and *amprenavir* was approved in 1999 for the treatment of adult or pediatric HIV infection when antiretroviral therapy is warranted. As with most of the newer antiretroviral agents, these approvals were based on randomized, controlled trials that demonstrated decreases in plasma HIV RNA levels and increases in CD4+ T cell counts. Both agents have unique resistance profiles. Nelfinavir resistance is associated with a D30N substitution in the protease gene. Viruses harboring this single mutation retain sensitivity to other protease inhibitors, and it has been suggested that for this reason nelfinavir is a good initial protease inhibitor. It is not clear, however, whether this theoretical consideration will be borne out in the results of clinical trials. Protease inhibitor resistance typically involves multiple amino acid substitutions and reduced susceptibility across the class. Amprenavir resistance is associated with a unique substitution at amino acid 50 (I50V), and it has been suggested that amprenavir may be of particular value in salvage regimens. This assumption also awaits verification in controlled clinical trials. Nelfinavir and amprenavir are both associated with gastrointestinal side effects. About 1% of patients receiving amprenavir have experienced severe and life-threatening skin reactions. An additional disadvantage of amprenavir is that the original formulation requires the patient to take 8 large capsules twice a day.

Fosamprenavir (Lexiva) is a recently licensed prodrug of amprenavir that is rapidly converted to amprenavir by cellular phosphatases. It is supplied as a 700-mg tablet. The recommended dosage is 1400 mg bid or 700 mg bid with ritonavir 100 mg bid or 1400 mg once a day with ritonavir 200 mg once a day.

Lopinavir/ritonavir (Kaletra) is a fixed dose combination of the protease inhibitors lopinavir (133.3 mg) and ritonavir (33.3 mg). It is indicated for treatment of HIV-1 infection in combination with other agents. A main advantage of this pill is that it combines the pharmacologic enhancement of low-dose ritonavir with a second protease inhibitor in a single capsule. In a randomized, controlled trial, this combination capsule was found to be superior to nelfinavir.

Atazanavir (Reytaz) is an azapeptide inhibitor of the HIV-1 protease. Initial studies suggest that total cholesterol and triglyceride levels may not increase as much with atazanavir as is seen with other protease inhibitors. Atazanavir is associated with increases in serum bilirubin and prolongations of the PR interval. Atazanavir-resistant isolates emerging in previously treatment-naïve individuals frequently harbor an I50L substitution. This mutation in some instances is associated with increased sensitivity to other protease inhibitors. Atazanavir is an inhibitor of cytochrome P3A and its use may be associated with increased levels of calcium channel blockers, HMB-CoA reductase inhibitors, and sildenafil.

The newest class of antiretroviral compounds are the entry inhibitors. These agents act by interfering with the binding of HIV to its receptor or co-receptor or by interfering with the process of fusion (see above). A variety of small molecules that bind to HIV-1 co-receptors are currently in clinical trials. The first drug in this class to be licensed is the fusion inhibitor enfuvirtide (Fuzeon), or T-20.

Enfuvirtide is a linear 36-amino acid synthetic peptide with the N-terminus acetylated and the C-terminus a carboxamide. It is composed of naturally occurring L-amino acid residues and interferes with the fusion of the viral and cellular membranes by binding to the HR1 region in the gp41 subunit of the HIV-1 envelope. This binding interferes with the coil-coil interaction required to approximate the two membranes. Resistant isolates of HIV exhibit amino acid changes in positions 36 to 45 of gp41. In two independent studies, patients who had persistent viremia despite prior treatment with agents from all three available classes of drugs were randomized to receive an individualized regimen (based upon prior treatment history and resistance profile) with or without enfuvirtide. The change in plasma HIV-1 RNA from baseline was approximately 1 log greater (-1.53 vs. -0.68) in patients randomized to receive enfuvirtide. Among the drawbacks of this agent are the requirement for twice-a-day injection, the occurrence of injection site reactions in 98% of patients, and an increase in bacterial pneumonia in the enfuvirtide-treated patients compared to the patients in the control arm (4.68 vs. 0.61 events per 100 patient years) in the phase III studies.

The principles of therapy for HIV infection have been articulated by a panel sponsored by the U.S. Department of Health and Human Services and the Henry J. Kaiser Family Foundation. These principles are summarized in Table 173-22. As noted in these guidelines, eradication of HIV infection has not yet been possible. Treatment decisions must take into account the fact that one is dealing with a chronic infection. While early therapy is generally the rule in infectious diseases, immediate treatment of every HIV-infected individual upon diagnosis may not be prudent, and therapeutic decisions must take into account the balance between risks and benefits. At present, a reasonable course of action is to initiate antiretroviral therapy in anyone with the acute HIV syndrome; patients with symptomatic disease; patients with asymptomatic disease with CD4+ T cell counts $<250/\mu L$ or with $>50,000$ copies of HIV RNA per milliliter (Table 173-23). In addition, one may wish to administer a 6-week course of therapy to uninfected

---

TABLE 173-22 *Principles of Therapy of HIV Infection*

1. Ongoing HIV replication leads to immune system damage and progression to AIDS.
2. Plasma HIV RNA levels indicate the magnitude of HIV replication and the rate of CD4+ T cell destruction. CD4+ T cell counts indicate the current level of competence of the immune system.
3. Rates of disease progression differ among individuals, and treatment decisions should be individualized based upon plasma HIV RNA levels and CD4+ T cell counts.
4. Maximal suppression of viral replication is a goal of therapy; the greater the suppression the less likely the appearance of drug-resistant quasispecies.
5. The most effective therapeutic strategies involve the simultaneous initiation of combinations of effective anti-HIV drugs with which the patient has not been previously treated and that are not cross-resistant with antiretroviral agents that the patient has already received.
6. The antiretroviral drugs used in combination regimens should be used according to optimum schedules and dosages.
7. The number of available drugs is limited. Any decisions on antiretroviral therapy have a long-term impact on future options for the patient.
8. Women should receive optimal antiretroviral therapy regardless of pregnancy status.
9. The same principles apply to children and adults. The treatment of HIV-infected children involves unique pharmacologic, virologic, and immunologic considerations.
10. Compliance is an important part of ensuring maximal effect from a given regimen. The simpler the regimen, the easier it is for the patient to be compliant.

Source: Modified from, *Principles of Therapy of HIV Infection*, USPHS and the Henry J. Kaiser Family Foundation.

TABLE 173-23 *Indications for the Initiation of Antiretroviral Therapy in Patients with HIV Infection*

I. Acute infection syndrome
II. Chronic infection
   A. Symptomatic disease
   B. Asymptomatic diseases[a]
     1. CD4+ T cell count <350/μL or decreasing
     2. HIV RNA >50,000 copies mL or increasing
III. Postexposure prophylaxis

[a] This is the area of greatest controversy. Some experts would wait until the CD4 cell count declines to 200/μL, whereas others would treat everyone regardless of CD4+ T cell count.

Source: *Guidelines for the Use of Antiretroviral Agents in HIV-Infected Adults and Adolescents.* USPHS.

individuals immediately following a high-risk exposure to HIV (see below).

Once the decision has been made to initiate therapy, the health care provider must decide which drugs to use as the first regimen. The decision regarding choice of drugs not only will affect the immediate response to therapy but also will have implications regarding options for future therapeutic regimens. The initial regimen is usually the most effective insofar as the virus has yet to develop significant resistance. The two options for initial therapy most commonly in use today are two different three-drug regimens. The first regimen utilizes two nucleoside analogues (one of which is usually lamivudine) and a nonnucleoside reverse transcriptase inhibitor. The second regimen utilizes two nucleoside analogues and a protease inhibitor. Unfortunately there are no clear data at present on which to base distinctions between these two approaches. Following the initiation of therapy one should expect a 1 log (tenfold) reduction in plasma HIV RNA levels within 1 to 2 months and eventually a decline in plasma HIV RNA levels to <50 copies per milliliter. During this same time there should be a rise in the CD4+ T cell count of 100 to 150/μL that is particularly brisk during the first month of therapy. Many clinicians feel that failure to achieve this endpoint is an indication for a change in therapy. Other reasons for a change in therapy include a persistently declining CD4+ T cell count, clinical deterioration, or drug toxicity (Table 173-24). As in the case of initiating therapy, changing therapy may have a lasting impact on future therapeutic options. When changing therapy because of treatment failure (clinical progression or worsening laboratory parameters), it is important to attempt to provide a regimen with at least two new drugs. In the patient in whom a change is made for reasons of drug toxicity, a simple replacement of one drug is reasonable. It should be stressed that in attempting to sort out a drug toxicity it may be advisable to hold all therapy for a period of time to distinguish between drug toxicity and disease progression. Drug toxicity will usually begin to show signs of reversal within 1 to 2 weeks. Prior to changing a treatment regimen because of drug failure, it is important to ensure that the patient has been adherent to the prescribed regimen.

TABLE 173-24 *Indications for Changing Antiretroviral Therapy in Patients with HIV Infection[a]*

Less than a 1-log drop in plasma HIV RNA by 4 weeks following the initiation of therapy
A reproducible significant increase (defined as 3-fold or greater) from the nadir of plasma HIV RNA level not attributable to intercurrent infection, vaccination, or test methodology
Persistently declining CD4+ T cell numbers
Clinical deterioration
Side effects

[a] Generally speaking, a change should involve the initiation of at least 2 drugs felt to be effective in the given patient. The exception to this is when change is being made to manage toxicity, in which case a single substitution is reasonable.

Source: *Guidelines for the Use of Antiretroviral Agents in HIV-Infected Adults and Adolescents.* USPHS.

As in the case of initial therapy, the simpler the therapeutic regimen, the easier it is for the patient to be compliant. Plasma HIV RNA levels and CD4+ T lymphocyte counts should be monitored every 3 to 4 months during therapy and more frequently if one is contemplating a change in regimen or immediately following a change in regimen.

In an attempt to determine an optimal therapeutic regimen, one may attempt to measure antiretroviral drug susceptibility through genotyping or phenotyping of HIV quasispecies and determine adequacy of dosing through measurement of drug levels. Genotyping may be done through dideoxynucleotide sequencing, DNA chip hybridization, or line probe assays. Phenotypic assays measure the performance of reverse transcriptase or protease in the presence or absence of different concentrations of different drugs. These assays will generally detect quasispecies present at a frequency of at least 10%. The precise role of resistance testing in the management of patients with HIV infection is not yet clear. While randomized studies have suggested that information regarding HIV resistance profiles may improve virologic outcomes in patients failing their current antiretroviral regimen, the degree of improvement thus far has been small and the duration of the benefit limited. Resistance testing may be of particular value in distinguishing drug-resistant virus from poor patient compliance; it may also be of value to help guide initial therapy in a setting where transmission of a drug-resistant isolate is felt to be likely. Measurement of plasma drug levels can also be used to tailor an individual treatment. The inhibitory quotient, defined as the trough blood level/IC50 of the patient's virus is used by some to determine the adequacy of dosing of a given treatment regimen.

In addition to the licensed medications discussed above, a large number of experimental agents are being evaluated as possible therapies for HIV infection. Therapeutic strategies are being developed that interfere with virtually every step of the replication cycle of the virus (Fig. 173-3). In addition, as more is discovered about the role of the immune system in controlling viral replication, additional strategies, generically referred to as "immune-based therapies," are being developed as a complement to antiviral therapy. Among the antiviral agents in early clinical trials are additional nucleoside and nucleotide analogues, additional protease inhibitors including nonpeptidomimetic compounds, additional fusion inhibitors, receptor and co-receptor antagonists, integrase inhibitors, and antisense nucleic acids. Among the immune-based therapies being evaluated are IFN-α, bone marrow transplantation, adoptive transfer of lymphocytes genetically modified to resist infection or enhance HIV-specific immunity, active immunotherapy with inactivated HIV or its components, and IL-2.

HIV AND THE HEALTH CARE WORKER

Health care workers, especially those who deal with large numbers of HIV-infected patients, have a small but definite risk of becoming infected with HIV as a result of professional activities. As of January 1, 2002, 57 health care workers in the United States had been documented as having seroconverted to HIV following occupational exposure; 26 have developed AIDS. The individuals who seroconverted include 19 laboratory workers (16 of whom were clinical laboratory workers), 24 nurses, 6 physicians, 2 surgical technicians, 1 dialysis technician, 1 respiratory therapist, 1 health aide, 1 embalmer/morgue technician, and 2 housekeeper/maintenance workers. The exposures included 48 percutaneous (puncture/cut injury), 5 mucocutaneous (mucous membrane and/or skin), 2 both percutaneous and mucocutaneous, and 2 unknown route of exposure. Forty-nine exposures were to HIV-infected blood, three to concentrated virus in a laboratory, one to visibly bloody fluid, and four to an unspecified fluid. As of January 1, 2002, there had been 138 other cases of HIV infection or AIDS among health care workers who have not reported other risk factors for HIV infection and who report a history of exposure to blood, body fluids, or HIV-infected laboratory material, but for whom seroconversion after exposure was not documented. The number of these workers who actually acquired their infection through occupational exposures is not known. Taken together, the data from several large studies suggest that the risk of HIV infection following a percutaneous exposure to HIV-contaminated blood is ~0.3%, and after a mucous membrane exposure, approximately 0.09%. Although episodes of HIV transmission after non-intact skin exposure have been documented, the average risk for transmission by this route has not been precisely quantified but is estimated to be less than the risk for mucous membrane exposures. The risk for transmission after exposure to fluids or tissues other than HIV-infected blood also has not been quantified but is probably considerably lower than for blood exposures. A seroprevalence survey of 3420 orthopedic surgeons, 75% of whom practiced in an area with a relatively high prevalence of HIV infection and 39% of whom reported percutaneous exposure to patient blood, usually through an accident involving a suture needle, failed to reveal any cases of possible occupational infection, suggesting that the risk of infection with a suture needle may be considerably less than that with a blood-drawing needle.

Most cases of health care worker seroconversion occur as a result of needle-stick injuries. When one considers the circumstances that result in needle-stick injuries, it is immediately obvious that adhering to the standard guidelines for dealing with sharp objects would result in a significant decrease in this type of accident. In one study, 27% of needle-stick injuries resulted from improper disposal of the needle (over half of these were due to recapping the needle), 23% occurred during attempts to start an intravenous line, 22% occurred during blood drawing, 16% were associated with an intramuscular or subcutaneous injection, and 12% were associated with giving an intravenous infusion.

Recommendations regarding postexposure prophylaxis must take into account that several circumstances determine the risk of transmission of HIV following occupational exposure. In this regard, several factors have been associated with an increased risk for occupational transmission of HIV infection including: deep injury, the presence of visible blood on the instrument causing the exposure, injury with a device that had been placed in the vein or artery of the source patient, terminal illness in the source patient, and lack of postexposure antiretroviral therapy in the exposed health care worker. Other important considerations include pregnancy in the health care worker and the possibility of exposure to drug-resistant virus. Regardless of the decision to use postexposure prophylaxis, the wound should be cleansed immediately and antiseptic applied. If a decision is made to offer postexposure prophylaxis, U.S. Public Health Service guidelines recommend (1) a combination of two nucleoside analogue reverse transcriptase inhibitors given for 4 weeks for routine exposures, or (2) a combination of two nucleoside analogue reverse transcriptase inhibitors plus a third drug given for 4 weeks for high-risk or otherwise complicated exposures, although most clinicians administer the latter regimen in all cases in which a decision is made to treat. Further details are available from the *Updated U.S. Public Health Service Guidelines for the Management of Occupational Exposures to HBV, HCV and HIV and Recommendations for Postexposure Prophylaxis* (CDC, 2001).

Health care workers can minimize their risk of occupational HIV infection by following the CDC guidelines of July 1991, which include adherence to universal precautions, refraining from direct patient care if one has exudative lesions or weeping dermatitis, and disinfecting and sterilizing reusable devices employed in invasive procedures. The premise of universal precautions is that every specimen should be handled as if it came from someone infected with a bloodborne pathogen. All samples should be double-bagged, gloves should be worn when drawing blood, and spills should be immediately disinfected with bleach.

In attempting to put this small but definite risk to the health care worker in perspective, it is important to point out that ~200 health care workers die each year as a result of occupationally acquired hepatitis B infection. The tragedy in this instance is that these infections and deaths due to HBV could be greatly decreased by more extended use of the HBV vaccine. The risk of HBV infection following a needle-stick injury from a hepatitis antigen–positive patient is much higher than the risk of HIV infection (see "Transmission," above). There are

multiple examples of needle-stick injuries where the patient was positive for both HBV and HIV and the health care worker became infected only with HBV. For these reasons, it is advisable, given the high prevalence of HBV infection in HIV-infected individuals, that all health care workers dealing with HIV-infected patients be immunized with the HBV vaccine.

TB is another infection common to HIV-infected patients that can be transmitted to the health care worker. For this reason, all health care workers should know their PPD status, have it checked yearly, and receive 1 year of isoniazid treatment if their skin test converts to positive. In addition, all patients in whom a diagnosis of TB is being entertained should be placed immediately in respiratory isolation, pending results of the diagnostic evaluation. The emergence of drug-resistant organisms has made TB an increasing problem for health care workers. This is particularly true for the health care worker with pre-existing HIV infection.

One of the most charged issues ever to come between health care workers and patients is that of transmission of infection from HIV-infected health care workers to their patients. This is discussed under "Occupational Transmission of HIV: Health Care Workers and Laboratory Workers." Theoretically, the same universal precautions that are used to protect the health care worker from the HIV-infected patient will also protect the patient from the HIV-infected health care worker.

VACCINES

Historically, vaccines have provided a safe, cost-effective, and efficient means of preventing illness, disability, and death from infectious diseases. Given the fact that human behavior, especially human sexual behavior, is extremely difficult to change, the best hope for preventing the spread of HIV infection rests with the development of a safe and effective vaccine. This task is problematic for a number of reasons, including the high mutability of the virus, the fact that the infection can be transmitted by cell-free or cell-associated virus, the likely need for the development of effective mucosal immunity, and the fact that it has been difficult to establish the precise correlates of protective immunity to HIV infection. Some HIV-infected individuals are long-term nonprogressors (see above), and a number of individuals have been exposed to HIV multiple times but remain uninfected; these facts suggest that there are protective elements of an HIV-specific immune response. In addition, studies using animal models, specifically SIV in the monkey and HIV-1 in the chimpanzee, have been encouraging and suggest that an HIV vaccine is possible. It should be pointed out that while the ideal goal of an HIV vaccine is to prevent infection, a vaccine given to an uninfected individual that significantly alters the course of disease or the infectivity of the individual, should that person become infected, could have an impact not only on the individual in question but also on the spread of infection in the community.

A number of clinical trials ranging from several small phase I trials to determine safety to fewer intermediate-sized phase II trials to determine safety and immunogenicity have taken place and are under way. The single completed phase III trial of a recombinant gp120 protein failed to show protection despite evidence of HIV-specific antibodies and CD4+T cells in phase II. These results suggest the potential importance of CD8+ T cell immunity in host defense against HIV-1. The furthest advanced among the current phase II trials involves a combination approach using a live canarypox vector expressing one or multiple HIV epitopes given together with gp120 or using the gp120 as a boost. This approach has resulted in neutralizing antibodies in virtually all recipients and HIV-specific cytolytic T cells in ~30% of individuals at any given time during the course of the trial. Other work is exploring the effects of recombinant adenovirus or naked DNA in combination with protein immunization.

Other approaches currently being tested in phase I and/or phase II trials in humans include vaccines employing vectors such as modified vaccinia Ankara (MVA), salmonella, and Venezuela equine encepha-

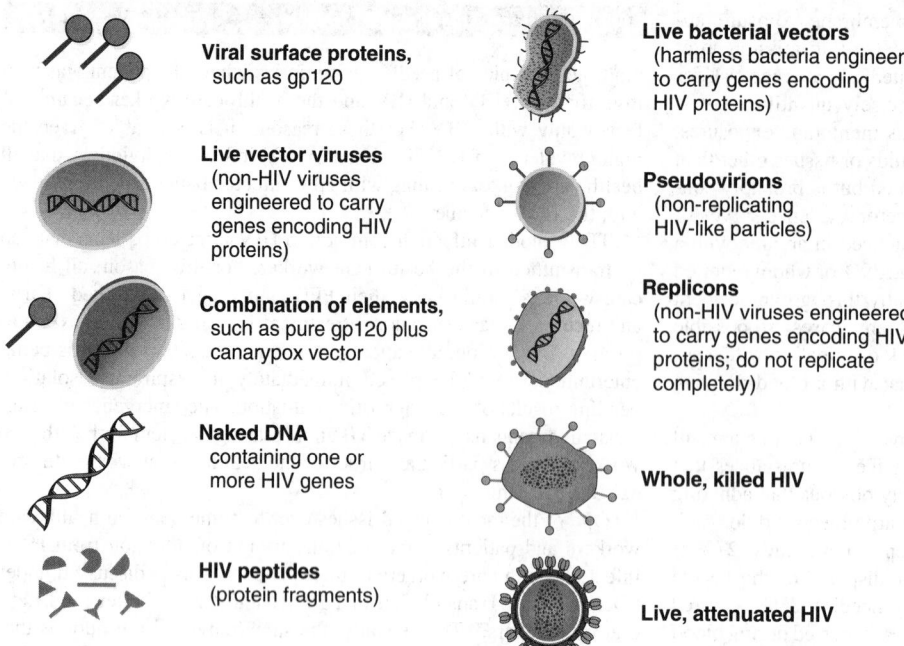

Viral surface proteins, such as gp120

Live vector viruses (non-HIV viruses engineered to carry genes encoding HIV proteins)

Combination of elements, such as pure gp120 plus canarypox vector

Naked DNA containing one or more HIV genes

HIV peptides (protein fragments)

Live bacterial vectors (harmless bacteria engineered to carry genes encoding HIV proteins)

Pseudovirions (non-replicating HIV-like particles)

Replicons (non-HIV viruses engineered to carry genes encoding HIV proteins; do not replicate completely)

Whole, killed HIV

Live, attenuated HIV

FIGURE 173-41 Candidate HIV vaccines. See text for detailed discussion. (*Adapted from D Baltimore, C Heilman: Sci Am 279:98, 1998. Copyright Slim Films.*)

litis (VEE) virus, among others; peptide and subunit vaccines; and pseudovirions (Fig. 173-41). Live attenuated HIV vaccines have not proceeded into human trials at this time because of safety concerns. It is clear that it will take several years of clinical trials to establish the efficacy or lack thereof of a candidate vaccine for HIV.

PREVENTION

Education, counseling, and behavior modification are the cornerstones of an HIV prevention strategy. Widespread voluntary testing of individuals who have practiced or are practicing high-risk behavior, together with counseling of infected individuals, is recommended. Information gathered from such an approach should serve as the basis for behavior-modification programs, both for infected individuals who may be unaware of their HIV status and who could infect others and for uninfected individuals practicing high-risk behavior. The practice of "safer sex" is the most effective way for sexually active uninfected individuals to avoid contracting HIV infection and for infected individuals to avoid spreading infection. Abstinence from sexual relations is the only absolute way to prevent sexual transmission of HIV infection. However, for many people this may not be feasible, and there are a number of relatively safe practices that can markedly decrease the chances of transmission of HIV infection. Partners engaged in monogamous sexual relationships who wish to be assured of safety should both be tested for HIV antibody. If both are negative, it must be understood that any divergence from monogamy puts both partners at risk; open discussion of the importance of honesty in such relationships should be encouraged. When the HIV status of either partner is not known, or when one partner is positive, there are a number of options. Use of condoms can markedly decrease the chance of HIV transmission. It should be remembered that condoms are not 100% effective in preventing transmission of HIV infection, and there is an ~10% failure rate of condoms used for contraceptive purposes. Most condom failures result from breakage or improper usage, such as not wearing the condom for the entire period of intercourse. Latex condoms are preferable, since virus has been shown to leak through natural skin condoms. Petroleum-based gels should never be used for lubrication of the condom, since they increase the likelihood of condom rupture. There has been a tendency among homosexual men to practice fellatio as a "minimal risk" activity compared to receptive anal intercourse. It should be emphasized that receptive fellatio is definitely not safe sex, and although the incidence of transmission via fellatio is

considerably less than that of rectal or vaginal intercourse, there has been documentation of transmission of HIV where receptive fellatio was the only sexual act performed (see "Transmission," above). Topical microbicides for vaginal and anal use are being pursued actively as a means by which individuals could avoid infection when the insertive partner cannot be relied on to use a condom. Kissing is considered safe, although there is a theoretical possibility of transmission via virus in saliva. The low concentration of virus in saliva of infected individuals, as well as the presence in saliva of HIV-inhibitory proteins (see above), lessens any risk of transmission by kissing.

The most effective way to prevent transmission of HIV infection among IDUs is to stop the use of injectable drugs. Unfortunately, that is extremely difficult to accomplish unless the individual enters a treatment program. For those who will not or cannot participate in a drug treatment program and who will continue to inject drugs, the avoidance of sharing of needles and other paraphernalia ("works") is the next best way to avoid transmission of infection. The cultural and social factors that contribute to the sharing of paraphernalia are complex and difficult to overcome. In addition, needles and syringes may be in short supply. Under these circumstances, paraphernalia should be cleaned after each usage with a virucidal solution, such as undiluted sodium hypochlorite (household bleach). Data from a number of studies have indicated that programs that provide sterile needles to addicts in exchange for used needles have resulted in a decrease in HIV transmission without increasing the use of injection drugs. It is important for IDUs to be tested for HIV infection and counseled, to avoid transmission to their sexual partners. Secondary and tertiary spread of HIV infection by the heterosexual route within settings of a high level of injection drug use has increased greatly in the United States (see above).

Transmission of HIV via transfused blood or blood products has been decreased dramatically by a combination of screening of all blood donors for HIV infection by assays for both HIV antibody and p24 antigen and self-deferral of individuals at risk for HIV infection. In addition, clotting factor concentrates are heat-treated, essentially eliminating the risk to hemophiliacs who require these products. Autologous transfusions are preferable to transfusions from another individual. However, logistic constraints as well as the unpredictability of the need for most transfusions limit the feasibility of this approach. At present the risk of becoming HIV-infected from a contaminated blood transfusion is approximately 1 in 725,000 to 1 in 835,000 donations.

Treatment of an HIV-infected mother with antiretroviral therapy during pregnancy and the infant during the first weeks following birth has proven very effective in dramatically decreasing mother to child transmission of HIV. In situations such as that seen in certain developing countries where pregnant women frequently present to a health care system during labor, administration of a short course (as little as a single dose of one drug) of antiretroviral therapy to the mother during labor and to the infant within 48 h of birth has also been successful in decreasing the incidence of mother to child transmission of HIV.

HIV can be transmitted via breast milk and colostrum. The avoidance of breast-feeding may not be practical in developing countries, where nutritional concerns override the risk of HIV transmission. However, it is becoming appreciated that 5 to 15% of infants who were born of HIV-infected mothers and who were fortunate enough not to have been infected intrapartum or peripartum become infected via breast-feeding. Therefore, in developing countries, breast-feeding from an infected mother should be avoided if at all possible. Unfortunately, this is rarely the case, and given the disadvantages of withholding breast-feeding in developing countries (see above), health authorities in most developing countries continue to recommend breast-feeding despite the potential for HIV transmission. Treatment of the infected mother with antiretroviral therapy, in addition to decreasing perinatal mother-to-child transmission can also decrease transmission by breast-feeding. In developed countries such as the United States, where bottled formula and milk are readily accessible, breast-feeding is absolutely contraindicated when a mother is HIV positive.

FURTHER READING

ANTMAN K, CHANG Y: Kaposi's sarcoma. N Engl J Med 342:1027, 2000

AUERBACH JD, COATES TJ: HIV prevention research: Accomplishments and challenges for the third decade of AIDS. Am J Public Health 90:1029, 2000

CARDO DM et al: A case-control study of HIV seroconversion in health care workers after percutaneous exposure. N Engl J Med 337:1485, 1997

CENTERS FOR DISEASE CONTROL AND PREVENTION: HIV/AIDS Surveillance Report, 2002;14, 2003. Available at *http://www.cdc.gov/hiv/stats/ hasrlink.HTM*

———: Updated U.S. Public Health Service guidelines for the management of occupational exposures to HBV, HCV, and HIV and recommendations for postexposure prophylaxis. MMWR 50 (RR11):1, 2001

———: Revised guidelines for HIV counseling, testing, and referral. MMWR Recomm Rep 50(RR-19):1, 2001

———; HEALTH RESOURCES AND SERVICES ADMINISTRATION; NATIONAL INSTITUTES OF HEALTH; HIV MEDICINE ASSOCIATION OF THE INFECTIOUS DISEASES SOCIETY OF AMERICA: Incorporating HIV prevention into the medical care of persons living with HIV. MMWR Recomm Rep 52(RR-12):1–24, 2003

CHUN TW, FAUCI AS: Latent reservoirs of HIV: Obstacles to the eradication of virus. Proc Natl Acad Sci USA 96:10958, 1999

D'AQUILA RT et al: Drug resistance mutations in HIV-1. Top HIV Med 11: 92, 2003

DAVEY RT JR et al: HIV-1 and T cell dynamics after interruption of highly active antiretroviral therapy (HAART) in patients with a history of sustained viral suppression. Proc Natl Acad Sci USA 21:96,15109, 1999

DONG KL et al: Changes in body habitus and serum lipid abnormalities in HIV-positive women on highly active antiretroviral therapy. J Acquir Immune Defic Syndr 21:107, 1999

DYBUL M et al: Guidelines for using antiretroviral agents among HIV-infected adults and adolescents. Recommendations of the Panel on Clinical Practices for Treatment of HIV. MMWR Recomm Rep 51(RR-7):1, 2002. Updates available at *http://www.aidsinfo.nih.gov*

EGGLER M et al: Prognosis of HIV-1 infected patients starting highly active antiretroviral therapy: A collaborative analysis of prospective studies. Lancet 360:119, 2002

FAUCI AS: Host factors and the pathogenesis of HIV-induced disease. Nature 384:529, 1996

———: The AIDS epidemic—considerations for the 21st century. N Engl J Med 341:1046, 1999

GALLO RC: Human retroviruses after 20 years: A perspective from the past and prospects for their future control. Immunol Rev 185:236, 2002

GANDHI RT, WALKER BD: Immunologic control of HIV-1. Annu Rev Med 53:149, 2002

GAO F et al: Origin of HIV-1 in the chimpanzee *Pan troglodytes troglodytes*. Nature 397:436, 1999

GOEDERT JJ et al: Spectrum of AIDS-associated malignant disorders. Lancet 351:1833, 1998

GREENE WC, PETERLIN BM: Charting HIV's remarkable voyage through the cell: Basic science as a passport to future therapy. Nat Med 8:673, 2002

GULICK RM: New antiretroviral drugs. Clin Microbiol Infect 9:186, 2003

HO DD et al: Rapid turnover of plasma virions and CD4 lymphocytes in HIV infection. Nature 373:123, 1995

JOINT UNITED NATIONS PROGRAMME ON HIV/AIDS (UNAIDS): AIDS Epidemic Update, December, 2003.

JONES D, HAVLIR DV: Nontuberculous mycobacteria in the HIV infected patient. Clin Chest Med 3:665, 2002

KAPLAN JE et al: Guidelines for preventing opportunistic infections among HIV-infected persons—2002. Recommendations of the U.S. Public Health Service and the Infectious Diseases Society of America. MMWR Recomm Rep 51(RR-8):1, 2003. Updates available at *http://www.aidsinfo.nih.gov*

KINTER A et al: Chemokines, cytokines and HIV: A complex network of interactions that influence HIV pathogenesis. Immunol Rev 177:88, 2000

LOPEZ BERNALDO DE QUIROS JC et al: A randomized trial of the discontinuation of primary and secondary prophylaxis against *Pneumocystis carinii* pneumonia after highly active antiretroviral therapy in patients with HIV infection. N Engl J Med 344:159, 2001

MELLORS JW et al: Prognosis in HIV-1 infection predicted by the quantity of virus in plasma. Science 272:1167, 1996

MIGUELES SA: et al: HIV-specific CD*+ T cell proliferation is coupled to perforin expression and is maintained in nonprogressors. Nat Immunol 3: 1061, 2002

MILLER KD et al: High prevalence of osteonecrosis of the femoral head in HIV-infected adults. Ann Intern Med 137:17, 2002

MOFENSON LM et al: Risk factors for perinatal transmission of human immunodeficiency virus type 1 in women treated with zidovudine. N Engl J Med 334:385, 1999

——— et al: U.S. Public Health Service Task Force recommendations for use of antiretroviral drugs in pregnant HIV-1-infected women for maternal health and interventions to reduce perinatal HIV-1 transmission in the United States. MMWR Recomm Rep 51(RR-18):1, 2002. Updates available at *http://www.aidsinfo.nih.gov*

NABEL GJ: Challenges and opportunities for development of an AIDS vaccine. Nature 410(6831):1002, 2001

NAKASHIMA AK, FLEMING PL: HIV/AIDS surveillance in the United States, 1981–2001. J Acquir Immune Defic Syndr 32(Suppl 1):S68, 2003

O'BRIEN SJ, MOORE JP: The effect of genetic variation in chemokines and their receptors on HIV transmission and progression to AIDS. Immunol Rev 177:99, 2000

PANTALEO G, FAUCI AS: HIV infection is active and progressive in lymphoid tissue during the clinically latent stage of disease. Nature 362:355, 1993

QUINN TC et al: Viral load and heterosexual transmission of human immunodeficiency virus type 1. Rakai Project Group Study. N Engl J Med 342: 921, 2000

RAMRATNAM B et al: The decay of the latent reservoir of replication-competent HIV-1 is inversely correlated with the extent of residual viral replication during prolonged anti-retroviral therapy. Nat Med 6:82, 2000

ROWLAND-JONES SL: Timeline: AIDS pathogenesis: What have two decades of HIV research taught us? Nat Rev Immunol 3:343, 2002

SMITH KJ et al: Cutaneous findings in HIV-1 positive patients: A 42-month prospective study. J Am Acad Dermatol 31:746, 1994

STEVENSON M: HIV-1 pathogenesis. Nat Med 9:853, 2003

STOVER J et al: Can we reverse the HIV/AIDS pandemic with an expanded response? Lancet 360:73, 2002

TEDALDI EM et al: Influence of coinfection with hepatitis C virus on morbidity and mortality due to human immunodeficiency virus infection in the era of highly active antiretroviral therapy. Clin Infect Dis 36:363, 2003

THIO CL et al: HIV-1, hepatitis B virus, and risk of liver-related mortality in the Multicenter Cohort Study (MACS). Lancet 360:1921, 2002

U.S. PUBLIC HEALTH SERVICE: Updated U.S. Public Health Service Guidelines for the Management of Occupational Exposures to HBV, HCV, and HIV and Recommendations for Postexposure Prophylaxis. MMWR Recomm Rep 50(RR-11):1, 2001. Updates available at *http:// www.aidsinfo.nih.gov*

VALDISERRI RO et al: Accomplishments in HIV prevention science: Implications for stemming the epidemic. Nat Med 9:881, 2003

VIALE P et al: HIV-associated community-acquired pneumonia in the highly active antiretroviral therapy era. AIDS 16:2361, 2002

WEI X et al: Viral dynamics in human immunodeficiency virus type 1 infection. Nature 373:117, 1995

Acute infectious gastroenteritis is a common illness that affects persons of all ages worldwide. It is a leading cause of mortality among children in developing countries, accounting for an estimated 2.4 to 2.9 million deaths each year, and is responsible for up to 10 to 12% of all hospitalizations among children in industrialized countries, such as the United States. Elderly persons, especially those with debilitating health conditions, are also at risk of severe complications and death from acute gastroenteritis. Acute gastroenteritis rarely causes mortality among healthy young adults, but it incurs substantial medical and social costs, including those of time lost from work.

Several enteric viruses have been recognized as important etiologic agents of acute infectious gastroenteritis (Table 174-1). Illness caused by these viruses is characterized by the acute onset of vomiting and/or diarrhea, which may be accompanied by fever, nausea, abdominal cramps, anorexia, and malaise. As shown in Table 174-2, several features can help distinguish gastroenteritis caused by viruses from that caused by bacterial agents. However, the distinction based on clinical and epidemiologic parameters alone is often difficult, and laboratory tests may be required to confirm the diagnosis.

The Norwalk and related human caliciviruses affect both adults and children and are a leading cause of epidemics of gastroenteritis. Rotaviruses are the leading cause of severe childhood gastroenteritis worldwide. Enteric adenoviruses and astroviruses are recognized as less common causes of gastroenteritis, and the role of some viruses, such as toroviruses and picobirnaviruses, remains to be elucidated. A brief discussion of these agents of acute infectious gastroenteritis among humans follows.

NORWALK AND RELATED HUMAN CALICIVIRUSES ■ **Etiologic Agent** The Norwalk virus is the prototype strain of a group of nonenveloped, small (27 to 40 nm), round, icosahedral viruses with relatively amorphous surface features on visualization by electron microscopy. These viruses are usually named after the geographic location of the gastroenteritis outbreak from which they were first identified (e.g., Norwalk virus, Hawaii virus, Toronto virus) and have been difficult to classify because they have not been adapted to cell culture, no animal models are available, and often they are shed in low titers for only a few days. Molecular cloning and characterization have demonstrated that these viruses have a single, positive-strand RNA genome that is ~7.5 kb in length and that they possess a single virion-associated protein with a molecular mass of 60 kDa, similar to that of typical caliciviruses. On the basis of these molecular characteristics, these viruses are presently classified in two genera belonging to the family Caliciviridae: the *noroviruses* and the *sapoviruses* (previously called Norwalk-like viruses and Sapporo-like viruses, respectively).

Epidemiology Infections with the Norwalk and related human caliciviruses are common, and most adults have antibodies to these viruses. Antibody is acquired at an earlier age in developing countries—a pattern consistent with the presumed fecal-oral mode of transmission of these viruses. Infections occur year-round, although, in temperate climates, a distinct increase has been noted in cold-weather months.

Noroviruses may be the most common infectious agents of mild gastroenteritis in the community and affect all age groups, whereas sapoviruses primarily cause gastroenteritis in children. Noroviruses are also a cause of traveler's diarrhea, and outbreaks have occurred among military personnel deployed to various parts of the world. The etiologic role of noroviruses in moderate to severe gastroenteritis requiring a visit to a physician or hospitalization is still being studied, but data from industrialized countries indicate that norovirus may be the second most common viral agent (after rotavirus) among young children and the most common agent among older children and adults.

Noroviruses are also recognized as the major cause of epidemics of gastroenteritis worldwide. In the United States, more than 90% of outbreaks of nonbacterial gastroenteritis are caused by noroviruses. Epidemics occur throughout the year, in all age groups, and in a variety of settings, such as schools, camps and recreational facilities, nursing homes, cruise ships, swimming facilities, and restaurants. Food items contaminated either by infectious food handlers or at the source are often implicated in outbreaks of infection. Because of their capacity to concentrate virus through filtration, shellfish harvested from fecally contaminated waters pose a special risk.

Transmission occurs predominantly by the fecal-oral route, but virus is also present in vomitus. Because an inoculum with very few viruses can be infectious, transmission can occur by aerosolization, by contact with contaminated formites, and by person-to-person contact. Viral shedding and infectivity are greatest during the acute illness, but challenge studies of volunteers with Norwalk virus indicate that viral antigen may be shed by asymptomatically infected persons and also by symptomatic persons prior to the onset of symptoms and for up to 2 weeks after the resolution of illness.

Pathogenesis The exact sites and cellular receptors for attachment of viral particles have not been determined. Data suggest that carbohydrates that are similar to human histo-blood group antigens and are present on the gastroduodenal epithelium of individuals with the secretor phenotype may serve as ligands for the attachment of Norwalk virus. Additional studies must more fully elucidate norovirus-carbohydrate interactions, including potential strain-specific variations. After the infection of volunteers, reversible lesions are noted in the upper jejunum, with broadening and blunting of the villi, shortening of the microvilli, vacuolization of the lining epithelium, crypt hyperplasia, and infiltration of the lamina propria by polymorphonuclear cells and lymphocytes. The lesions persist for at least 4 days after the resolution of symptoms and are associated with malabsorption of carbohydrates and fats and a decreased level of brush-border enzymes. Adenylate cyclase activity is not altered. No histopathologic changes are seen in the stom-

TABLE 174-1 *Viral Causes of Gastroenteritis among Humans*

Virus	Family	Genome	Primary Age Group at Risk	Clinical Severity	Detection Assays[a]
Group A rotavirus	Reoviridae	Double-strand segmented RNA	Children <5 years	+++	EM, EIA (commercial), PAGE, RT-PCR
Norovirus	Caliciviridae	Positive-sense single-strand RNA	All ages	++	EM, EIA, RT-PCR
Sapovirus	Caliciviridae	Positive-sense single-strand RNA	Children <5 years	+	EM, EIA, RT-PCR
Astrovirus	Astroviridae	Positive-sense single-strand RNA	Children <5 years	+	EM, EIA, RT-PCR
Adenovirus (types 40 and 41)	Adenoviridae	Double-strand DNA	Children <5 years	+/++	EM, EIA (commercial), RT-PCR

[a] EIA, enzyme immunoassay; EM, electron microscopy; PAGE, polyacrylamide gel electrophoresis; RT-PCR, reverse-transcriptase polymerase chain reaction.

ach or colon, but gastric motor function is delayed, and this alteration is believed to contribute to the nausea and vomiting that are typical of this illness.

Clinical Manifestations Gastroenteritis caused by Norwalk and related human caliciviruses has a sudden onset, following an average incubation period of 24 h (range, 12 to 72 h). The illness generally lasts 12 to 60 h and is characterized by one or more of the following symptoms: nausea, vomiting, abdominal cramps, and diarrhea. Vomiting is more prevalent among children, whereas a greater proportion of adults develop diarrhea. Constitutional symptoms are common, including headache, fever, chills, and myalgias. Noroviruses appear to cause more severe illness than sapoviruses, although both illnesses are less severe than that due to rotavirus. The stools are characteristically loose and watery, without blood, mucus, or leukocytes. White cell counts are generally normal; rarely, leukocytosis with relative lymphopenia may be observed. Death is a rare outcome and usually results from severe dehydration in vulnerable persons (e.g., elderly patients with debilitating health conditions).

Immunity Approximately 50% of persons challenged with Norwalk virus become ill and acquire short-term immunity against the infecting strain. Immunity to Norwalk virus appears to correlate inversely with level of antibody; i.e., persons with higher levels of preexisting antibody to Norwalk virus are more susceptible to illness. This observation suggests that some individuals have a genetic predisposition to illness. Recent data indicate that specific ABO, Lewis, and secretor blood group phenotypes may influence susceptibility to Norwalk virus infection.

Diagnosis Cloning and sequencing of the genome of Norwalk and several other human caliciviruses have allowed the development of assays based on polymerase chain reaction (PCR) for detection of virus in stool and vomitus. Virus-like particles produced by expression of capsid proteins in a recombinant baculovirus vector have been used to develop enzyme immunoassays (EIAs) for detection of virus in stool or a serologic response to a specific viral antigen. These newer diagnostic techniques are considerably more sensitive than previous detection methods such as electron microscopy, immune electron microscopy, and EIAs based on reagents derived from humans. However, no currently available single assay can detect all human caliciviruses because of their great genetic and antigenic diversity. In addition, the assays are still cumbersome and are available primarily in research laboratories, although they are increasingly being adopted by public health laboratories for routine screening of fecal specimens from patients affected by outbreaks of gastroenteritis.

℞ TREATMENT

Treatment generally is not required because the disease is self-limited. If severe dehydration develops, oral or intravenous fluid therapy is indicated. No specific antiviral therapy is available.

Prevention Epidemic prevention relies on situation-specific measures, such as control of contamination of food and water, exclusion of ill food handlers, and reduction of person-to-person spread through good personal hygiene and disinfection of contaminated fomites. The role

TABLE 174-2	Characteristics of Gastroenteritis Caused by Viral and Bacterial Agents	
Feature	**Viral Gastroenteritis**	**Bacterial Gastroenteritis**
Setting	Incidence similar in developing and developed countries	More common in settings with poor hygiene and sanitation
Infectious dose	Low (10–100 viral particles) for most agents	High (>10^5 bacteria) for *Escherichia coli*, *Salmonella*, *Vibrio*; medium (10^2–10^5 bacteria) for *Campylobacter jejuni*; low (10–100 bacteria) for *Shigella*
Seasonality	In temperate climates, winter seasonality for most agents; year-round occurrence in tropical areas	More common in summer or rainy months, particularly in developing countries with a high disease burden
Incubation period	1–3 days for most agents; can be shorter for norovirus	1–7 days for common agents (e.g., *Campylobacter*, *E. coli*, *Shigella*, *Salmonella*); few hours for bacteria producing preformed toxins (e.g., *Staphylococcus aureus*, *Bacillus cereus*)
Reservoir	Primarily humans	Depending on species, both human (e.g., *Shigella*, *Salmonella*) and animal (e.g., *Campylobacter*, *Salmonella*, *E. coli*) reservoirs exist.
Fever	Common with rotavirus and norovirus; uncommon with other agents	Common with agents causing inflammatory diarrhea (e.g., *Salmonella*, *Shigella*)
Vomiting	Prominent and can be the only presenting feature, especially in children	Common with bacteria producing preformed toxins; less prominent in diarrhea due to other agents
Diarrhea	Common; nonbloody in almost all cases	Prominent and frequently bloody with agents causing inflammatory diarrhea
Duration	1–3 days for norovirus and sapovirus; 2–8 days for other viruses	1–2 days for bacteria producing preformed toxins; 2–8 days for most other bacteria
Diagnosis	This is often a diagnosis of exclusion in clinical practice. Commercial enzyme immunoassays are available for detection of rotavirus and adenovirus, but identification of other agents is limited to research and public health laboratories.	Fecal examination for leukocytes and blood is helpful in differential diagnosis. Culture of stool specimens, sometimes on special media, can identify several pathogens. Molecular techniques are useful epidemiologic tools but are not routinely used in most laboratories.
Treatment	Supportive therapy to maintain adequate hydration and nutrition should be given. Antibiotics and antimotility agents are contraindicated.	Supportive hydration therapy is adequate for most patients. Antibiotics are recommended for patients with dysentery caused by *Shigella* or *Vibrio cholerae* and for some patients with *Clostridium difficile* colitis.

of immunoprophylaxis is not clear, given the lack of long-term immunity from natural disease and the paradoxic inverse association between the level of immune response and protection from disease.

ROTAVIRUS ■ Etiologic Agent Rotaviruses are members of the family Reoviridae. The viral genome consists of 11 segments of double-strand RNA that are enclosed in a triple-layered, nonenveloped, icosahedral capsid 75 nm in diameter. Viral protein 6 (VP6), the major structural protein, is the target of commercial immunoassays and determines the group specificity of rotaviruses. There are seven major groups of rotavirus (A through G); human illness is caused primarily by group A and, to a much lesser extent, by groups B and C. Two outer-capsid proteins, VP7 (G-protein) and VP4 (P-protein), determine serotype specificity, induce neutralizing antibodies, and form the basis of the binary classification of rotaviruses (G and P types). The segmented genome of rotavirus allows genetic reassortment (i.e., exchange of genome segments between viruses) during co-infection—a property that may play a role in viral evolution and has been utilized in the development of reassortant animal-human rotavirus–based vaccines.

Epidemiology Nearly all children are infected with rotavirus by 3 to 5 years of age. Neonatal infections are common but are often asymptomatic or mild, presumably because of protection from maternal antibody or breast-feeding. Nevertheless, rotavirus is known to cause disease in neonates, particularly in those admitted to intensive care units, and some data suggest that the clinical manifestations in full-term infants may differ from those in preterm infants. First infections after 3 months of age are likely to be symptomatic, and the incidence of disease peaks among children 4 to 23 months of age. Reinfections are common, but the severity of disease decreases with each repeat infection. Therefore, severe rotavirus infections are relatively uncommon in older children and adults. However, rotavirus can cause illness in parents and caretakers of children with rotavirus diarrhea, immunocompromised persons, travelers, and elderly individuals and should be considered in the differential diagnosis of gastroenteritis among adults.

In temperate climates, rotavirus disease occurs predominantly during the cooler fall and winter months. In the United States, the annual rotavirus epidemic begins in the Southwest in autumn (October through December) and migrates across the continent, peaking in the Northeast during spring (March through May). In tropical settings, rotavirus disease occurs year-round, with less pronounced seasonal peaks.

Rotavirus gastroenteritis is more frequently associated with dehydration than is gastroenteritis caused by other pathogens. Therefore, the proportion of gastroenteritis cases that are attributable to rotavirus increases with increasing severity of illness, ranging from a median of 8% of cases in the community to 18% of cases in outpatients and 30% of cases in hospitalized patients. Each year, rotavirus is estimated to cause ~500,000 childhood deaths worldwide.

During episodes of rotavirus-associated diarrhea, virus is shed in large quantities (10^7 to 10^{12}/g) in stool. Viral shedding detectable by EIA usually subsides within a week but may persist for >30 days in immunocompromised individuals. Viral shedding may be detected for longer periods by sensitive molecular assays, such as PCR. The virus is transmitted predominantly through the fecal-oral route. Spread through respiratory secretions, person-to-person contact, or contaminated environmental surfaces has also been postulated to explain the rapid acquisition of antibody in the first 3 years of life, regardless of sanitary conditions.

At least 10 different G serotypes of group A rotavirus have been identified in humans, but only 5 types (G1 through G4 and G9) are common. While human rotavirus strains that possess a high degree of genetic homology with animal strains have been identified, animal-to-human transmission appears to be uncommon. Group B rotaviruses have been associated with several large epidemics of severe gastroenteritis among adults in China since 1982 and have recently been identified in India but not in other parts of the world. Group C rotaviruses have been associated with a small proportion of pediatric gastroenteritis cases in several countries worldwide.

Pathogenesis Rotaviruses infect and ultimately destroy the mature enterocytes in the villous epithelium of the proximal small intestine. The loss of absorptive villous epithelium coupled with the proliferation of secretory crypt cells results in secretory diarrhea. Brush-border enzymes characteristic of differentiated cells are reduced, and this change leads to the accumulation of unmetabolized disaccharides and consequent osmotic diarrhea. Studies in mice indicate that a nonstructural rotavirus protein, NSP4, functions as an enterotoxin and contributes to secretory diarrhea by altering epithelial cell function and permeability. In addition, rotavirus may evoke fluid secretion through activation of the enteric nervous system in the intestinal wall. Recent data indicate that rotavirus antigen and RNA are present in serum of children with acute rotavirus infection; further investigations are needed to establish the significance of these findings in the pathogenesis of rotavirus disease.

Clinical Manifestations The clinical spectrum of rotavirus infection ranges from subclinical illness to severe gastroenteritis leading to the development of life-threatening dehydration. After an incubation period of 1 to 3 days, the illness has an abrupt onset, with vomiting frequently preceding the onset of diarrhea. Up to one-third of patients may have a temperature of >39°C. The stools are characteristically loose and watery and only infrequently contain red or white cells. The gastrointestinal symptoms generally resolve in 3 to 7 days.

Respiratory and neurologic features in children with rotavirus infection have been reported, but causal associations have not been proven. Rotavirus infection has been associated with a variety of other clinical syndromes (e.g., sudden infant death syndrome, necrotizing enterocolitis, intussusception, and diabetes mellitus type 1), but no causal relationship has been confirmed with any of these syndromes.

Rotavirus does not appear to be a major opportunistic pathogen in children with HIV infection. In severely immunodeficient children, rotavirus can cause protracted diarrhea with prolonged viral excretion and, in rare instances, can disseminate systemically. Persons who are immunosuppressed for bone marrow transplantation are also at risk for severe, or even fatal, rotavirus disease.

Immunity Protection against rotavirus disease is correlated with the presence of virus-specific secretory IgA antibodies in the intestine and, to some extent, the serum. Because virus-specific IgA production at the intestinal surface is short-lived, complete protection against disease is only temporary. However, each infection and subsequent reinfection confers progressively greater immunity, so severe disease is most common among young children with first or second infections. Immunologic memory is believed to be important in the attenuation of the severity of disease upon reinfection.

Diagnosis Illness caused by rotavirus is difficult to distinguish clinically from that caused by other enteric viruses. Because large quantities of virus are shed in feces, the diagnosis can usually be confirmed by a wide variety of commercially available EIAs or by techniques for detecting viral RNA, such as gel electrophoresis, probe hybridization, or PCR.

℞ TREATMENT

Rotavirus gastroenteritis can lead to severe dehydration. Thus appropriate treatment should be instituted early. Standard oral rehydration therapy is successful in most children who can take oral fluids, but intravenous fluid replacement may be required for patients who are severely dehydrated or are unable to tolerate oral therapy because of frequent vomiting. The therapeutic role of probiotics, bismuth salicylate, and enkephalinase inhibitors has been evaluated in clinical studies but is not clearly defined. Antibiotics and antimotility agents should be avoided. In immunocompromised children with chronic symptomatic rotavirus disease, orally administered immunoglobulins or colostrum may resolve symptoms, but the choice of agents and their doses have not been well studied and are often empirical.

Prevention Efforts to develop rotavirus vaccines were pursued because it was apparent—given the similar rates in less developed and industrialized nations—that improvements in hygiene and sanitation were unlikely to reduce disease incidence. In 1998, a rotavirus vaccine was licensed in the United States and was recommended for routine immunization of infants. However, this vaccine was withdrawn in 1999 because it was causally linked with intussusception, with an estimated 1 case per 11,000 vaccinated infants. Other rotavirus vaccines are being developed, including two leading multinational candidate vaccines whose safety and efficacy are currently being studied in large-scale clinical trials.

OTHER VIRAL AGENTS OF GASTROENTERITIS Enteric adenoviruses of serotypes 40 and 41 belonging to subgroup F are 70- to 80-nm viruses with double-strand DNA that cause ~2 to 12% of all diarrhea episodes in young children. Unlike adenoviruses that cause respiratory illness, enteric adenoviruses are difficult to cultivate in cell lines, but they can be detected with commercially available EIAs.

Astroviruses, 28- to 30-nm viruses with a characteristic icosahedral structure, contain a positive-sense, single-strand RNA. At least seven serotypes have been identified, of which serotype 1 is most common. Astroviruses are primarily pediatric pathogens, causing ~2 to 10% of cases of mild to moderate gastroenteritis in children. The availability of simple immunoassays to detect virus in fecal specimens and of molecular methods to confirm and characterize strains will permit more comprehensive assessment of the etiologic role of these agents.

Toroviruses are 100- to 140-nm, enveloped, positive-strand RNA viruses that are recognized as causes of gastroenteritis in horses (Berne virus) and cattle (Breda virus). Their role as a cause of diarrhea in humans is still unclear, but a study from Canada demonstrated an association between torovirus excretion and nosocomial gastroenteritis in pediatric patients. In this study, more than half of the patients with torovirus in stool also had a demonstrable immune response. Patients with torovirus infection were older and experienced less vomiting and more bloody diarrhea than did those with rotavirus or astrovirus infection. Further studies are required to confirm these findings.

Picobirnaviruses are small, bi-segmented, double-strand RNA viruses that cause gastroenteritis in a variety of animals. Their role as primary causes of gastroenteritis in humans remains unclear, but several studies have found an association between picobirnaviruses and gastroenteritis in HIV-infected adults.

The recently recognized severe acute respiratory syndrome–associated coronavirus (SARS-CoV) has been associated with gastroenteritis in 20 to 66% of affected patients. In one study of 138 SARS patients in Hong Kong, 20.3% presented with watery diarrhea, and up to 38.4% had diarrhea during their illness. Diarrhea was most common during the first week of illness, lasted for an average of 3.7 days, and was self-limiting in most instances. Studies of intestinal biopsy specimens showed minimal architectural disruption but also revealed active viral replication within both the small and the large intestine. SARS-CoV RNA could be detected in the stool of patients for >10 weeks after the onset of symptoms.

Several other viruses (e.g., enteroviruses, reoviruses, pestiviruses, and parvoviruses B) have been identified in the feces of patients with diarrhea, but their etiologic role in gastroenteritis has not been proved.

FURTHER READING

BLUTT SE et al: Rotavirus antigenaemia and viraemia: A common event? Lancet 362:1445, 2003

CUNLIFFE NA et al: Effect of concomitant HIV infection on presentation and outcome of rotavirus gastroenteritis in Malawian children. Lancet 358:550, 2001

FANKHAUSER RL et al: Epidemiologic and molecular trends of "Norwalk-like viruses" associated with outbreaks of gastroenteritis in the United States. J Infect Dis 186:1, 2002

JAMIESON FB et al: Human torovirus: A new nosocomial gastrointestinal pathogen. J Infect Dis 178:1263, 1998

LEUNG WK et al: Enteric involvement of severe acute respiratory syndrome–associated coronavirus infection. Gastroenterology 125:1011, 2003

MURPHY TV et al: Intussusception among infants given an oral rotavirus vaccine. N Engl J Med 344:564, 2001

NAKAJIMA H et al: Winter seasonality and rotavirus diarrhoea in adults. Lancet 357:1950, 2001

PANG XL et al: Human caliciviruses in acute gastroenteritis of young children in the community. J Infect Dis 181:S288, 2000

175 ENTEROVIRUSES AND REOVIRUSES
Jeffrey I. Cohen

ENTEROVIRUSES

CLASSIFICATION AND CHARACTERIZATION Enteroviruses are so named because of their ability to multiply in the gastrointestinal tract. Despite their name, these viruses are not a prominent cause of gastroenteritis. Enteroviruses encompass 64 human serotypes: 3 serotypes of poliovirus, 23 serotypes of coxsackievirus A, 6 serotypes of coxsackievirus B, 28 serotypes of echovirus, and enteroviruses 68 through 71. Enterovirus surveillance conducted in the United States by the Centers for Disease Control and Prevention (CDC) in 2000 and 2001 revealed that echoviruses accounted for >60% of all enterovirus isolates (Table 175-1).

Human enteroviruses contain a single-stranded RNA genome surrounded by an icosahedral capsid comprising four viral proteins. These viruses have no lipid envelope and are stable in acidic environments, including the stomach. They are resistant to inactivation by standard disinfectants (e.g., alcohol, detergents) and can persist for days at room temperature.

PATHOGENESIS AND IMMUNITY Much of what is known about the pathogenesis of enteroviruses has been derived from studies of poliovirus infection. After ingestion, poliovirus is thought to infect epithelial cells in the mucosa of the gastrointestinal tract and then to spread to and replicate in the submucosal lymphoid tissue of the tonsils and Peyer's patches. The virus next spreads to the regional lymph nodes, a viremic phase ensues, and the virus replicates in organs of the reticuloendothelial system. In some cases, a second viremia occurs and the virus replicates further in various tissues, sometimes causing symptomatic disease.

It is uncertain whether poliovirus reaches the central nervous system (CNS) during viremia or whether it also spreads via peripheral nerves. Since viremia precedes the onset of neurologic disease in humans and in experimentally infected chimpanzees, it has been assumed that the virus enters the CNS via the bloodstream. The poliovirus receptor is a member of the immunoglobulin superfamily. Poliovirus infection is limited to primates, largely because of the ability of their cells to express the viral receptor. Studies demonstrating the poliovirus receptor in the end-plate region of muscle at the neuromuscular junction suggest that, if the virus enters the muscle during viremia, it could travel across the neuromuscular junction up the axon to the anterior horn cells. Studies of monkeys or transgenic mice expressing the poliovirus receptor show that, after intramuscular injection, poliovirus does not reach the spinal cord if the sciatic nerve is cut. Taken together, these findings suggest that poliovirus can spread directly from muscle to the CNS by neural pathways. Intercellular adhesion molecule 1 (ICAM-1) is a receptor for coxsackieviruses A13, A18, and A21; CAR for coxsackievirus B; VLA-2 integrin for echovirus types 1 and 8; and CD55 for enterovirus 70 and some serotypes of coxsackievirus B and echovirus.

Poliovirus can usually be cultured from the blood 3 to 5 days after infection, before the development of neutralizing antibodies. While viral replication at secondary sites begins to slow 1 week after infection, it continues in the gastrointestinal tract. Poliovirus is shed from the oropharynx for up to 3 weeks after infection and from the gastrointestinal tract for as long as 12 weeks; immunodeficient patients can shed poliovirus for more than 1 year. During replication in the gastrointestinal tract, attenuated oral poliovirus can mutate, reverting to a more neurovirulent phenotype within a few days. The clinical significance of this increased neurovirulence is unknown.

TABLE 175-1 *Frequency of the Most Common Non-Poliovirus Isolates of Enterovirus in the United States, 2000–2001*

Serotype	Percentage
Echovirus 18	22.0
Echovirus 13	20.8
Coxsackievirus B5	11.9
Coxsackievirus B2	6.3
Echovirus 6	6.1
Echovirus 11	4.5
Coxsackievirus A9	4.0
Echovirus 9	3.3
Coxsackievirus B4	3.2
Echovirus 4	3.1
All others	15.0

Source: Centers for Disease Control and Prevention, 2002.

Humoral and secretory immunity in the gastrointestinal tract is important for the control of enterovirus infections. Enteroviruses induce specific IgM, which usually persists for <6 months, and specific IgG, which persists for life. Capsid protein VP1 is the predominant target of neutralizing antibody, which generally confers lifelong protection against subsequent disease caused by the same serotype but does not prevent infection or virus shedding. Enteroviruses also induce cellular immunity, but the significance of this mechanism in limiting infection is uncertain. Patients with impaired cellular immunity are not known to develop unusually severe disease when infected with enteroviruses. In contrast, the severe infections in patients with agammaglobulinemia emphasize the importance of humoral immunity in controlling enterovirus infections. IgA antibodies are instrumental in reducing poliovirus replication in and shedding from the gastrointestinal tract. Breast milk contains IgA specific for enteroviruses and can protect humans from infection.

EPIDEMIOLOGY   Enteroviruses have a worldwide distribution. More than 50% of nonpoliovirus enterovirus infections and more than 90% of poliovirus infections are subclinical. When symptoms do develop, they are usually nonspecific and occur in conjunction with fever; only a minority of infections are associated with specific clinical syndromes. The incubation period for most enterovirus infections ranges from 2 to 14 days but usually is <1 week.

Enterovirus infection is more common in socioeconomically disadvantaged areas, especially in those where conditions are crowded and in tropical areas where hygiene is poor. Infection is most common among infants and young children; serious illness develops most often during the first few days of life and in older children and adults. In developing countries, where children are infected at an early age, poliovirus infection has less often been associated with paralysis; in countries with better hygiene, older children and adults are more likely to be seronegative, become infected, and develop paralysis. Passively acquired maternal antibody reduces the risk of symptomatic infection in neonates. Young children are the most frequent shedders of enteroviruses and are usually the index cases in family outbreaks. In temperate climates, enterovirus infections occur most often in the summer and fall; no seasonal pattern is apparent in the tropics.

Most enteroviruses are transmitted primarily by the fecal-oral route from fecally contaminated fingers or inanimate objects. Patients are most infectious shortly before and after the onset of symptomatic disease, when virus is present in the stool and throat. The ingestion of virus-contaminated food or water can also cause disease. Certain enteroviruses (such as enterovirus 70, which causes acute hemorrhagic conjunctivitis) can be transmitted by direct inoculation from the fingers to the eye. Airborne transmission is important for some viruses that cause respiratory tract disease, such as coxsackievirus A21. Enteroviruses can be transmitted across the placenta from mother to fetus, causing severe disease in the newborn. The transmission of enteroviruses through blood transfusions or insect bites has not been documented. Nosocomial spread of coxsackievirus and echovirus has taken place in hospital nurseries.

CLINICAL FEATURES OF INFECTION WITH POLIOVIRUS   Most infections with poliovirus are asymptomatic. After an incubation period of 3 to 6 days, ~5% of patients present with a minor illness (abortive poliomyelitis) manifested by fever, malaise, sore throat, anorexia, myalgias, and headache. This condition usually resolves in 3 days. About 1% of patients present with aseptic meningitis (nonparalytic poliomyelitis). Examination of cerebrospinal fluid (CSF) reveals lymphocytic pleocytosis, a normal glucose level, and a normal or slightly elevated protein level; CSF polymorphonuclear leukocytes may be present early. In some patients, especially children, malaise and fever precede the onset of aseptic meningitis.

The least common presentation is that of paralytic disease. After one or several days, signs of aseptic meningitis are followed by severe back, neck, and muscle pain and by the rapid or gradual development of motor weakness. In some cases the disease appears to be biphasic, with aseptic meningitis followed first by apparent recovery but then (1 or 2 days later) by the return of fever and the development of paralysis; this form is more common among children than among adults. Weakness is generally asymmetric, is proximal more than distal, and may involve the legs (most commonly); the arms; or the abdominal, thoracic, or bulbar muscles. Paralysis develops during the febrile phase of the illness and usually does not progress after defervescence. Urinary retention may also occur. Examination reveals weakness, fasciculations, decreased muscle tone, and reduced or absent reflexes in affected areas. Transient hyperreflexia sometimes precedes the loss of reflexes. Patients frequently report sensory symptoms, but objective sensory testing usually yields normal results. Bulbar paralysis may lead to dysphagia, difficulty in handling secretions, or dysphonia. Respiratory insufficiency due to aspiration, involvement of the respiratory center in the medulla, or paralysis of the phrenic or intercostal nerves may develop, and severe medullary involvement may lead to circulatory collapse. Most patients with paralysis recover some function weeks to months after infection. About two-thirds of patients have residual neurologic sequelae.

Paralytic disease is more common among older individuals, pregnant women, and persons exercising strenuously or undergoing trauma at the time of CNS symptoms. Tonsillectomy predisposes to bulbar poliomyelitis, and intramuscular injections increase the risk of paralysis in the involved limb(s).

Until recently, poliomyelitis due to live poliovirus vaccine occurred in the United States. The risk of developing poliomyelitis after oral vaccination is estimated at 1 case per 2.5 million doses. The risk is ~2000 times higher among immunodeficient persons, especially in persons with hypo- or agammaglobulinemia. Before 1997, an average of eight cases of vaccine-associated poliomyelitis occurred—in both vaccinees and their contacts—in the United States each year. With the change in recommendations first to a sequential regimen of inactivated poliovirus vaccine (IPV) and oral poliovirus vaccine (OPV) in 1997 and then to an all-IPV regimen in 2000, the number of cases of vaccine-associated poliovirus declined. From 1997 to 1999, six such cases were reported in the United States; no cases have been reported since 1999.

The *postpolio syndrome* presents as a new onset of weakness, fatigue, fasciculations, and pain with additional atrophy of the muscle group involved during the initial paralytic disease 20 to 40 years earlier. The syndrome is more common among women and with increasing time after acute disease. The onset is usually insidious, and weakness occasionally extends to muscles that were not involved during the initial illness. The prognosis is generally good; progression to further weakness is usually slow, with plateau periods that range from 1 to 10 years. The postpolio syndrome is thought to be due to progressive dysfunction and loss of motor neurons that compensated for the neurons lost during the original infection and not to persistent or reactivated poliovirus infection.

CLINICAL FEATURES OF INFECTION WITH COXSACKIEVIRUS, ECHOVIRUS, AND OTHER ENTEROVIRUSES   An estimated 5 to 10 million cases of symptomatic disease due to enterovirus other than poliovirus occur in the United States each year. Enteroviruses are the most common cause of aseptic meningitis and nonspecific febrile illnesses of neonates. Certain clinical syndromes are more likely to be caused by certain serotypes (Table 175-2), but there is much overlap. In 2000–2001, 85% of enterovirus infections were caused by only 10 of the 64 human serotypes. Echoviruses 13 and 18 accounted for 43% of recognized enterovirus infections (Table 175-1).

Nonspecific Febrile Illness (Summer Grippe)   The most common clinical manifestation of enterovirus infection is a nonspecific febrile illness. After an incubation period of 3 to 6 days, patients present with an acute onset of fever, malaise, and headache. Occasional cases are associated with upper respiratory symptoms, and some cases include nausea and vomiting. Symptoms often last for 3 to 4 days, and most cases resolve in a week. While infections with other respiratory viruses occur more often from late fall to early spring, enterovirus febrile illness frequently occurs in the summer and early fall.

Generalized Disease of the Newborn Most serious enterovirus infections in infants develop during the first week of life, although severe disease can occur up to 3 months of age. Neonates often present with an illness resembling bacterial sepsis, with fever, irritability, and lethargy. Laboratory abnormalities include leukocytosis with a left shift, thrombocytopenia, elevated values in liver function tests, and CSF pleocytosis. The illness can be complicated by myocarditis and hypotension, fulminant hepatitis and disseminated intravascular coagulation, meningitis or meningoencephalitis, or pneumonia. It may be difficult to distinguish enterovirus infection from bacterial sepsis, although a history of a recent virus-like illness in the mother provides a clue.

Aseptic Meningitis and Encephalitis Enteroviruses are the cause of up to 90% of cases of aseptic meningitis in children and young adults in which an etiologic agent can be identified. Patients with aseptic meningitis typically present with an acute onset of fever, chills, headache, photophobia, and pain on eye movement. Nausea and vomiting are also common. Examination reveals meningismus without localizing neurologic signs; drowsiness or irritability may also be apparent. In some cases, a febrile illness may be reported that remits but returns several days later in conjunction with signs of meningitis. Other systemic manifestations may provide clues to an enteroviral cause, including diarrhea, myalgias, rash, pleurodynia, myocarditis, and herpangina. Examination of the CSF invariably reveals pleocytosis; early in the course, polymorphonuclear leukocytes may be present or even predominant, raising the possibility of bacterial or other nonviral causes of meningitis. Partially treated bacterial meningitis may be particularly difficult to exclude in some instances. A useful rule is that the CSF cell count in enteroviral meningitis shows a shift to lymphocytic predominance within 24 h of presentation, and the total count generally does not exceed 1000 cells/μL. Additional CSF findings consist of a normal glucose content and a normal or only slightly elevated (by ≤100 mg/mL) level of protein. Enteroviruses and mumps virus may produce a similar picture of meningitis; a low CSF glucose level suggests mumps, whereas a normal CSF glucose level and transient CSF polymorphonuclear pleocytosis suggest enterovirus infection. Enteroviral meningitis is more frequent in summer and fall in temperate climates, while viral meningitis of other etiologies (e.g., mumps) is more common in winter and spring. Symptoms ordinarily resolve within a week, although CSF abnormalities can persist for several weeks. Enteroviral meningitis is often more severe in adults than in children. Neurologic sequelae are rare, and most patients have an excellent prognosis.

Enteroviral encephalitis is much less common than enteroviral aseptic meningitis. Occasional highly inflammatory cases of enteroviral meningitis may be complicated by a mild form of encephalitis that is recognized on the basis of progressive lethargy, disorientation, and sometimes seizures. Less commonly, severe primary encephalitis may develop. It is estimated that 10 to 20% of cases of viral encephalitis are due to enteroviruses. Immunocompetent patients generally have a good prognosis.

Patients with hypo- or agammaglobulinemia or severe combined immunodeficiency may develop chronic meningitis or encephalitis; about half of these patients have a dermatomyositis-like syndrome, with peripheral edema, rash, and myositis. They may also have chronic hepatitis. Patients may develop neurologic disease while receiving gamma globulin replacement therapy. Echoviruses (especially echovirus 11) are the most common pathogens in this situation.

TABLE 175-2 *Manifestations Commonly Associated with Enterovirus Serotypes*

Manifestation	Serotype(s) of Indicated Virus	
	Coxsackievirus	Echovirus (E) and Enterovirus (Ent)
Acute hemorrhagic conjunctivitis	A24	E70
Aseptic meningitis	A2, 4, 7, 9, 10; B1-5	E4, 6, 7, 9, 11, 13, 16, 18, 19, 30, 33; Ent70, 71
Encephalitis	A9; B1-5	E3, 4, 6, 9, 11, 25, 30; Ent71
Exanthem	A4, 5, 9, 10, 16; B1, 3-5	E4-7, 9, 11, 16-19, 25, 30; Ent71
Generalized disease of the newborn	B2-5	E4-6, 9, 11, 14, 16, 19
Hand-foot-and-mouth disease	A5, 7, 9, 10, 16; B2, 5	Ent71
Herpangina	A1-10, 16, 22; B1-5	E6, 9, 11, 16, 17, 25; Ent71
Myocarditis, pericarditis	A4, 9, 16; B1-5	E6, 9, 11, 22
Paralysis	A4, 7, 9; B1-5	E2, 4, 6, 9, 11, 30; Ent70, 71
Pleurodynia	A1, 2, 4, 6, 9, 10, 16; B1-6	E1-3, 6, 7, 9, 11, 12, 14, 16, 19, 24, 25, 30
Pneumonia	A9, 16; B1-5	E6, 7, 9, 11, 12, 19, 20, 30; Ent68, 71

Paralytic disease due to enteroviruses other than poliovirus occurs sporadically and is usually less severe than poliomyelitis. Most cases are due to enterovirus 70 or 71 or to coxsackievirus A7 or A9. Guillain-Barré syndrome is also associated with enterovirus infection. While some studies have suggested a link between enteroviruses and the chronic fatigue syndrome, most recent studies have not demonstrated such an association.

Pleurodynia (Bornholm Disease) Patients with pleurodynia present with an acute onset of fever and spasms of pleuritic chest or upper abdominal pain. Chest pain is more common in adults, and abdominal pain is more common in children. Paroxysms of severe, knifelike pain usually last 15 to 30 min and are associated with diaphoresis and tachypnea. Fever peaks within an hour after the onset of paroxysms and subsides when pain resolves. The involved muscles are tender to palpation, and a pleural rub may be detected. The white blood cell count and chest x-ray are usually normal. Most cases are due to coxsackievirus B and occur during epidemics. Symptoms resolve in a few days, and recurrences are rare. Treatment includes the administration of nonsteroidal anti-inflammatory agents or the application of heat to the affected muscles.

Myocarditis and Pericarditis Enteroviruses are estimated to cause up to one-third of cases of acute myocarditis. Coxsackievirus B and its RNA have been detected in pericardial fluid and myocardial tissue in some cases of acute myocarditis and pericarditis. Most cases of enteroviral myocarditis or pericarditis occur in newborns, adolescents, or young adults. More than two-thirds of patients are male. Patients often present with an upper respiratory tract infection that is followed by fever, chest pain, dyspnea, arrhythmias, and occasionally heart failure. A pericardial friction rub is documented in half of cases, and the electrocardiogram shows ST segment elevations or ST- and T-wave abnormalities. Serum levels of myocardial enzymes are often elevated. Neonates commonly have severe disease, while most older children and adults recover completely. Up to 10% of cases progress to chronic dilated cardiomyopathy. Chronic constrictive pericarditis may also be a sequela.

Exanthems Enterovirus infection is the leading cause of exanthems in children in the summer and fall. While exanthems are associated with many enteroviruses, certain types have been linked to specific syndromes. Echoviruses 9 and 16 have frequently been associated with exanthem and fever. Rashes may be discrete (rubelliform) or confluent (morbilliform), beginning on the face and spreading to the trunk and extremities. Echovirus 9 is the most common cause of rubelliform rash. Unlike the rash of rubella, the enteroviral rash occurs in the summer and is not associated with lymphadenopathy. Roseola-like rashes develop after defervescence, with macules and papules on the face and trunk. The Boston exanthem, caused by echovirus 16, is a roseola-like rash that often affects multiple members of a family. A variety of other rashes have been associated with enteroviruses, including erythema multiforme and vesicular, urticarial, petechial, or purpuric lesions. Enanthems also occur, including lesions that resemble the Koplik's spots seen with measles.

Hand-Foot-and-Mouth Disease   After an incubation period of 4 to 6 days, patients with hand-foot-and-mouth disease present with fever, anorexia, and malaise; these manifestations are followed by the development of sore throat and vesicles (Fig. 175-1) on the buccal mucosa and often on the tongue and then by the appearance of tender vesicular lesions on the dorsum of the hands, sometimes with involvement of the palms. The vesicles may form bullae and quickly ulcerate. About one-third of patients also have lesions on the palate, uvula, or tonsillar pillars, and one-third have a rash on the feet (including the soles) or on the buttocks. The disease is highly infectious, with attack rates of close to 100% among young children. The lesions usually resolve in 1 week. Most cases are due to coxsackievirus A16 or enterovirus 71.

An epidemic of enterovirus 71 infection in Taiwan in 1998 resulted in thousands of cases of hand-foot-and-mouth disease or herpangina. Severe complications included CNS disease, myocarditis, and pulmonary hemorrhage. About 90% of those who died were children ≤5 years old, and these deaths were associated with pulmonary edema or pulmonary hemorrhage. CNS disease included aseptic meningitis, flaccid paralysis (similar to poliomyelitis), or rhombencephalitis with myoclonus and tremor or ataxia. The mean age of patients with CNS complications was 2.5 years, and magnetic resonance imaging in cases with encephalitis usually showed brain-stem lesions.

Herpangina   Herpangina is usually caused by coxsackievirus A and presents as acute-onset fever, sore throat, dysphagia, and grayish-white papulovesicular lesions on an erythematous base that ulcerate. The lesions can persist for weeks; are present on the soft palate, anterior pillars of the tonsils, and uvula; and are concentrated in the posterior portion of the mouth. In contrast to herpes stomatitis, enteroviral herpangina is not associated with gingivitis. Acute lymphonodular pharyngitis associated with coxsackievirus A10 presents as white or yellow

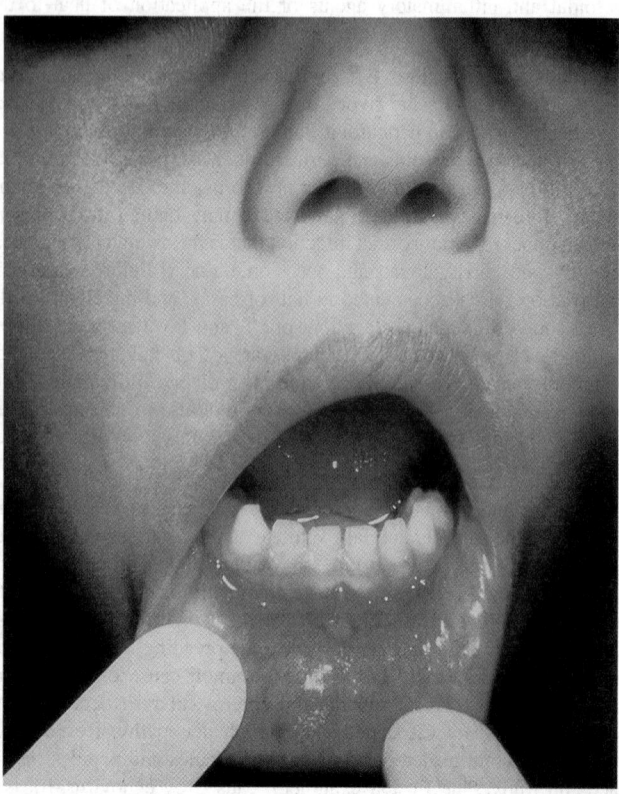

FIGURE 175-1   Tender vesicles and erosions in the mouth of a patient with hand-foot-and-mouth disease.

nodules surrounded by erythema in the posterior oropharynx. The lesions do not ulcerate.

Acute Hemorrhagic Conjunctivitis   Patients with acute hemorrhagic conjunctivitis present with an acute onset of severe eye pain, blurred vision, photophobia, and watery discharge from the eye. Examination reveals edema, chemosis, and subconjunctival hemorrhage and often shows punctate keratitis and conjunctival follicles as well. Preauricular adenopathy is often found. Epidemics and nosocomial spread have been associated with enterovirus 70 and coxsackievirus A24. Systemic symptoms, including headache and fever, develop in 20% of cases, and recovery is usually complete in 10 days. The sudden onset and short duration of the illness help to distinguish acute hemorrhagic conjunctivitis from other ocular infections such as those due to adenovirus and *Chlamydia*. Paralysis has been associated with some cases of acute hemorrhagic conjunctivitis due to enterovirus 70 during epidemics.

Other Manifestations   Enteroviruses are an infrequent cause of childhood pneumonia and the common cold. Coxsackievirus B has been isolated at autopsy from the pancreas of a few children presenting with insulin-dependent diabetes mellitus; however, most attempts to isolate the virus have been unsuccessful. Other diseases that have been associated with enterovirus infection include parotitis, bronchitis, bronchiolitis, croup, infectious lymphocytosis, polymyositis, acute arthritis, and acute nephritis.

DIAGNOSIS   Isolation of enterovirus in cell culture is the most common procedure for the diagnosis of infection. While cultures of stool, nasopharyngeal, or throat samples from patients with enterovirus diseases are often positive, isolation of the virus from these sites does not prove that it is directly associated with disease because these sites are frequently colonized for weeks in patients with subclinical infections. Isolation of virus from the throat is more likely to be associated with disease than isolation from the stool since virus is shed for shorter periods from the throat. Cultures of CSF, serum, fluid from body cavities, or tissues are positive less frequently, but a positive result is indicative of disease caused by enterovirus. In some cases the virus can be isolated only from the blood or only from the CSF; therefore, it is important to culture multiple sites. Cultures are more likely to be positive earlier than later in the course of infection. Most human enteroviruses can be detected within a week after inoculation of cell cultures. Cultures may be negative because of the presence of neutralizing antibody, lack of susceptibility of the cells used, or inappropriate handling of the specimen. Coxsackievirus A may require inoculation into special cell-culture lines or into suckling mice.

Identification of the serotype of an enterovirus is useful primarily for epidemiologic studies and, with a few exceptions, has little clinical utility. It is important to identify serious infections with enterovirus during epidemics and to distinguish the vaccine strain of poliovirus from the other enteroviruses in the throat or in the feces. Stool and throat samples for culture as well as acute- and convalescent-phase serum specimens should be obtained from all patients with suspected poliomyelitis. In the absence of a positive CSF culture, a positive culture of stool obtained within the first 2 weeks after the onset of symptoms is most often used to confirm the diagnosis of poliomyelitis. If poliovirus is isolated, it should be sent to the CDC in Atlanta for identification as either a wild-type or a vaccine virus.

The polymerase chain reaction (PCR) has been used to amplify viral nucleic acid from CSF, serum, urine, throat swabs, and tissues. A single pair of PCR primers can detect more than 92% of the serotypes that infect humans. With the proper controls, PCR of the CSF is highly sensitive (≥95%) and specific (>80%) and is more rapid than culture. PCR of serum is also highly sensitive and specific in the diagnosis of disseminated disease. PCR may be particularly helpful for the diagnosis and follow-up of enterovirus disease in immunodeficient patients receiving immunoglobulin therapy, whose viral cultures may be negative. Antigen detection and hybridization of enterovirus sequences in human tissues with a specific probe are additional options, but these techniques are generally less sensitive than PCR.

Serologic diagnosis of enterovirus infection is limited by the large number of serotypes and the lack of a common antigen. Demonstration of seroconversion may be useful in rare cases for confirmation of culture results, but serologic testing is usually limited to epidemiologic studies. Serum should be collected and frozen soon after the onset of disease and again about 4 weeks later. Measurement of neutralizing titers is the most accurate method for antibody determination; measurement of complement-fixation titers is usually less sensitive. Titers of virus-specific IgM are elevated in both acute and chronic infection.

℞ TREATMENT

Most enterovirus infections are mild and resolve spontaneously; however, intensive supportive care may be needed for cardiac, hepatic, or CNS disease. Intravenous, intrathecal, or intraventricular immunoglobulin has been used with apparent success for the treatment of chronic enterovirus meningoencephalitis and dermatomyositis in patients with hypo- or agammaglobulinemia. The disease may stabilize or resolve during therapy; however, some patients decline inexorably despite therapy. Intravenous administration of immunoglobulin with high titers of antibody to the infecting virus has been used in the treatment of some cases of life-threatening infection in neonates, who may not have maternally acquired antibody. In one trial involving neonates with enterovirus infections, immunoglobulin containing very high titers of antibody to the infecting virus reduced rates of viremia; however, the study was too small to show a substantial clinical benefit. The level of enteroviral antibodies varies with the immunoglobulin preparation. Oral pleconaril, which binds to the enterovirus capsid, reduced symptoms in a placebo-controlled trial of enteroviral aseptic meningitis. In a review of compassionate-release pleconaril therapy in patients with potentially life-threatening enteroviral infections, ~75% of persons were judged to have a clinical response associated with therapy. These individuals included patients with chronic enteroviral meningoencephalitis, neonatal sepsis, myocarditis, and vaccine-associated paralytic poliomyelitis. Further study is needed to confirm these findings. Glucocorticoids are contraindicated.

Good hand-washing practices and the use of gowns and gloves are important in limiting nosocomial transmission of enteroviruses during epidemics. Enteric precautions are indicated for 7 days after the onset of enterovirus infections.

PREVENTION AND ERADICATION OF POLIOVIRUS (See also Chap. 107) After a peak of 57,879 cases of poliomyelitis in the United States in 1952, the introduction of inactivated vaccine in 1955 and of oral vaccine in 1961 ultimately eradicated disease due to wild-type poliovirus in the Western Hemisphere. Such disease has not been documented in the United States since 1979, when cases occurred among religious groups who had declined immunization. In the Western Hemisphere, paralysis due to wild-type poliovirus was last documented in 1991.

In 1988, the World Health Organization adopted a resolution to eradicate poliomyelitis by the year 2000. From 1988 to 2001, the number of cases worldwide decreased by >99%, with fewer than 1000 confirmed cases reported in 2001. In 2002, however, there were ~1900 cases of polio, with ~1500 reported in India. Wild-type poliovirus type 2 has not been detected in the world since 1999. The Americas were certified free of indigenous wild-type poliovirus transmission in 1994, the Western Pacific Region in 2000, and the European Region in 2002. In 2002, there were 8 countries in which indigenous wild-type poliovirus was still being transmitted (Table 175-3). Polio is a source of concern for unimmunized or partially immunized travelers to these regions. Outbreaks of polio in Europe and North America have been traced to cases imported from the Indian subcontinent. Clearly, global eradication of polio is necessary to eliminate the risk of importation of wild-type virus. Outbreaks are thought to have been facilitated by suboptimal rates of vaccination, isolated pockets of unvaccinated children, poor sanitation and crowding, improper vaccine-storage conditions, and a reduced level of response to one of the serotypes in the vaccine.

TABLE 175-3 *Laboratory-Confirmed Cases of Poliomyelitis in Countries Where Wild-Type Poliovirus Was Endemic in 2002*

Country	Virus-Confirmed Cases in 2001
India	1600
Pakistan	202
Nigeria	90
Afghanistan	10
Somalia	7
Niger	3
Egypt	3
Angola, Ethiopia, Sudan, Mauritania	1 case each
Total	1916

Source: World Health Organization.

Outbreaks of poliomyelitis due to circulating vaccine-derived poliovirus have recently occurred. In the Dominican Republic and Haiti, 21 cases of vaccine-derived polio occurred in 2000 and 2001; 32 cases occurred in Egypt from 1988 to 1993, and 3 cases occurred in the Philippines in 2001. These OPV-derived viruses reverted to a more neurovirulent phenotype after undetected circulation (probably for >2 years). The epidemic in Hispaniola was rapidly terminated after intensive vaccination with OPV. These outbreaks emphasize the need for maintaining high levels of vaccine coverage and continued surveillance for circulating virus.

IPV is used in most industrialized countries and OPV in most developing countries, including those in which polio still is or recently was endemic. After several doses of OPV alone, the seropositivity rate for individual poliovirus serotypes may still be suboptimal for children in developing countries; one or more supplemental doses of IPV can increase the rate of seropositivity for these serotypes. While intramuscular injections of other vaccines (live or attenuated) can be given concurrently with OPV, unnecessary intramuscular injections should be avoided during the first month after vaccination because they increase the risk of vaccine-associated paralysis. Since 1988, an enhanced-potency inactivated poliovirus vaccine has been available in the United States.

OPV and IPV induce antibodies that persist for at least 5 years. Both vaccines induce IgG and IgA antibodies. Compared with recipients of IPV, recipients of OPV shed less virus and less frequently develop reinfection with wild-type virus after exposure to poliovirus. Although IPV is safe and efficacious, OPV offers the advantages of ease of administration, lower cost, and induction of intestinal immunity resulting in a reduction in the risk of community transmission of wild-type virus. Because of progress toward global eradication of polio (with a reduced risk of imported cases) and the continued occurrence of cases of vaccine-associated polio, an all-IPV regimen was recommended in 2000 for childhood poliovirus vaccination in the United States, with vaccine administration at 2, 4, and 6 to 18 months and 4 to 6 years of age. OPV will be used only in special circumstances: (1) for mass immunization campaigns to control outbreaks of polio; (2) for vaccination of unimmunized children who will be traveling to a polio-endemic area within 4 weeks; and (3) for children whose parents do not accept an all-IPV regimen. The latter children should receive at least two doses of IPV before receiving OPV. The risk of vaccine-associated polio should be discussed before administering OPV. Recommendations for vaccination of adults are listed in Table 175-4.

While it is hoped that endemic spread of poliovirus may be eliminated during the first decade of the 21st century, there are concerns about stopping vaccination. These include the observations that poliovirus is shed from some immunocompromised persons for several years, that vaccine-derived poliovirus can circulate and cause disease, and that wild-type poliovirus is present in a large number of laboratories. A national survey began in October 2002 to encourage laboratories to dispose of all unneeded wild-type poliovirus materials and to identify laboratories that have wild-type poliovirus or specimens (e.g., feces) that may contain the virus.

1. Routine primary poliovirus vaccination is not indicated for unvaccinated adults residing in the United States, except for:
   a. travelers to areas where poliovirus is or may be epidemic or endemic;
   b. members of communities or population groups with disease caused by wild-type polioviruses;
   c. laboratory workers handling specimens that may contain wild-type polioviruses;
   d. health care workers in close contact with patients who may be excreting wild-type polioviruses.
2. Three doses of IPV are recommended for adults who need to be immunized. The second dose should be given 1 to 2 months after the first dose; the third dose should be given 6 to 12 months after the second dose.
3. Adults who are at increased risk of exposure to wild-type poliovirus and who have previously completed primary immunization should receive a single dose of IPV.

Abbreviation: IPV, inactivated poliovirus vaccine.
Source: Modified from 2003 Redbook, Report of the Committee on Infectious Diseases.

REOVIRUSES

Reoviruses are double-stranded RNA viruses encompassing three serotypes. Serologic studies indicate that most humans are infected with reoviruses during childhood; however, it has been difficult to establish a definite link of reovirus infection with a particular disease. It is likely that most infections either are asymptomatic or cause very mild disease. One outbreak of reovirus infection in children resulted in minor upper respiratory tract symptoms. Reovirus is considered a rare cause of mild gastroenteritis in infants and children. Speculation regarding an association of reovirus type 3 with idiopathic neonatal hepatitis and extrahepatic biliary atresia is based on an elevated prevalence of antibody to reovirus among some of these patients, detection of viral RNA by PCR in hepatobiliary tissues in some studies, and detection of virus in the porta hepatis in one case.

FURTHER READING

CENTERS FOR DISEASE CONTROL AND PREVENTION: Enterovirus surveillance—United States, 2000–2001. MMWR 51:1047, 2002

————: Progress toward global eradication of poliomyelitis, 2001. MMWR 51:253, 2002

HENDERSON DA: Countering the posteradication threat of smallpox and polio. Clin Infect Dis 34:79, 2002

HO M et al: An epidemic of enterovirus 71 infection in Taiwan. N Engl J Med 341:929, 1999

JUBELT B, AGRE JC: Characteristics and management of postpolio syndrome. JAMA 284:412, 2000

KEW O et al: Outbreak of poliomyelitis in Hispaniola associated with circulating type 1 vaccine-derived poliovirus. Science 296:356, 2002

ROTBART HA et al: Treatment of potentially life-threatening enterovirus infections with pleconaril. Clin Infect Dis 32:28, 2001

176 MEASLES (RUBEOLA)
Anne Gershon

DEFINITION   Measles (rubeola) is a highly contagious, acute, exanthematous respiratory disease with a characteristic clinical picture and a pathognomonic enanthem: Koplik's spots, an eruption on the buccal mucous membranes (Fig. 176-1). A successful live attenuated measles vaccine became available in 1963 in the United States and elsewhere, and measles is now an unusual disease in most developed countries where this vaccine is widely used. However, measles continues to occur sporadically in miniepidemics in the United States, and major epidemics in developing nations make this disease a persistent cause of childhood morbidity and mortality.

ETIOLOGIC AGENT   Measles virus is the only member of the genus *Morbillivirus* that infects humans. Part of the family Paramyxoviridae, it is closely related to the viruses causing canine and porcine distemper, rinderpest of cattle, morbilli of certain aquatic mammals, and *peste des petits ruminants* of goats and sheep. There is only one antigenic type. Measles virions are pleomorphic spherical structures having a diameter of 100 to 250 nm and consisting of six proteins. The inner capsid is composed of a coiled helix of RNA and three proteins, and the outer envelope consists of a matrix protein bearing two types of short surface-glycoprotein projections or peplomers. One peplomer is a conical hemagglutinin (H) and the other a dumbbell-shaped fusion (F) protein. Sequencing of the single-stranded genome has made it possible to distinguish vaccine-type measles virus from the wild type. The genetic variability of wild-type measles virus permits the identification of strains that are endemic within a given locale where measles cases have occurred. In all, 20 genotypes have been identified. The cellular receptors for measles virus are the CD46 and CD150 molecules expressed on human lymphocytes and many other human cell types.

EPIDEMIOLOGY   Measles has a worldwide distribution; humans are the only natural hosts, although other primates can be experimentally infected. During the prevaccination era in the United States, measles epidemics occurred every 2 to 5 years in the winter and spring. In an epidemic year, roughly half a million measles cases were reported; 99% of adults had serologic evidence of previous measles infection.

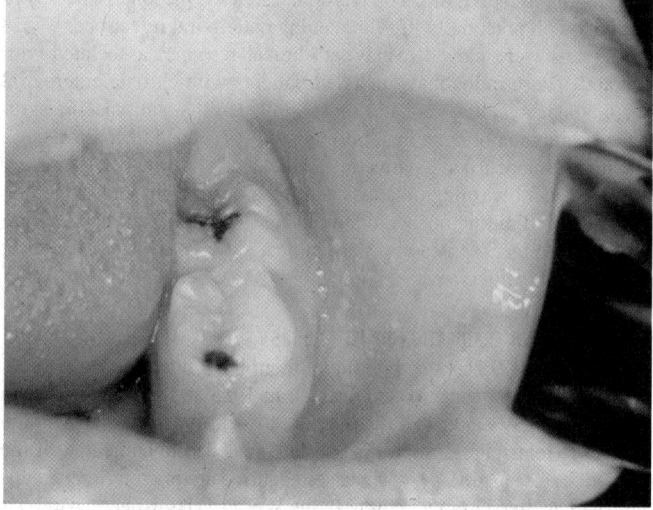

FIGURE 176-1   Koplik's spots, which manifest as white or bluish lesions with an erythematous halo on the buccal mucosa, usually occur in the first 2 days of measles symptoms and may briefly overlap the measles exanthem. The presence of the erythematous halo differentiates Koplik's spots from Fordyce's spots (ectopic sebaceous glands), which occur in the mouths of healthy individuals. (*Source: CDC. Photo selected by Dr. Kenneth Kaye.*)

After the live attenuated vaccine became available, the number of cases reported to the Centers for Disease Control and Prevention (CDC) fell, with a nadir of 1497 cases in 1983. After an upsurge to more than 27,000 cases (with 89 deaths) in 1990, the disease was once more brought under control, in part through the routine administration of two doses of vaccine. The foremost reason for the resurgence of measles was failure to immunize infants and young children, especially in inner-city areas. Primary vaccine failure (documented in about 5% of individuals) and secondary vaccine failure or waning immunity accounted for some cases.

In recent years, the majority of cases of measles have involved preschool children. Between 1993 and 1996, fewer than 1000 cases were reported annually in the United States; 309 cases were reported in 1995 and 116 cases in 2001. Molecular studies indicated interruption of transmission of indigenous measles in 1993. Most cases have since resulted from international importations of the virus. Mortality is highest among children under 2 years of age and among adults. Patients with impaired cell-mediated immunity are at especially high risk for severe or even fatal measles. The measles-associated mortality rate in the United States is about 0.3%; in developing countries, mortality frequently exceeds 1% and sometimes approaches 10%.

Measles virus is transmitted by respiratory secretions, predominantly through exposure to aerosols but also through direct contact with larger droplets. Patients are contagious from 1 or 2 days before the onset of symptoms until 4 days after the appearance of the rash. Infectivity peaks during the prodromal phase. The mean intervals from infection to onset of symptoms and to appearance of rash are 10 and 14 days, respectively.

PATHOGENESIS, IMMUNITY, AND PATHOLOGY   Measles virus invades the respiratory epithelium and spreads via the bloodstream to the reticuloendothelial system, from which it infects all types of white blood cells, thereby establishing infection of the skin, respiratory tract, and other organs. Both viremia and viruria develop. Multinucleated giant cells with inclusion bodies in the nucleus and cytoplasm (Warthin-Finkeldey cells) are found in respiratory and lymphoid tissues and are pathognomonic for measles. Direct invasion of T lymphocytes and increased levels of suppressive cytokines, such as interleukin 4, may play a role in the temporary depression of cellular immunity that accompanies and transiently follows measles. The major infected cell in the blood is the monocyte. Infection of the entire respiratory tract accounts for the characteristic cough and coryza of measles and for the less frequent manifestations of croup, bronchiolitis, and pneumonia. Generalized damage to the respiratory tract, with resultant loss of cilia, predisposes to secondary bacterial infections such as pneumonia and otitis media.

Specific antibodies are not detectable before the onset of rash. Cellular immunity (consisting of cytotoxic T cells and possibly natural killer cells) plays a prominent role in host defense, and patients who are deficient in cellular immunity are at high risk for severe measles. Children with isolated agammaglobulinemia are not at increased risk. Immune reactions to the virus in the endothelial cells of dermal capillaries play a substantial role in the development of Koplik's spots (the pathognomonic enanthem) as well as in that of rash; in immunodeficient hosts, measles may be severe despite the absence of these manifestations. Measles antigens have been demonstrated in involved skin during early stages of the illness.

Pathologic changes in measles encephalitis include focal hemorrhage, congestion, and perivascular demyelination. Measles virus is rarely isolated from cerebrospinal fluid (CSF) in cases of encephalitis, which are thought to be due to the interaction of virus-infected cells with local cellular immune factors.

CLINICAL MANIFESTATIONS   Measles begins with a 2- to 4-day respiratory prodrome of malaise, cough, coryza, conjunctivitis with lacrimation, nasal discharge, and increasing fever [with temperatures as high as 40.6°C (105°F), probably reflecting secondary viremia]. At this stage of the illness, in which the rash has not yet developed, influenza may be suspected. Just before the onset of the rash, Koplik's spots appear as 1- to 2-mm blue-white spots on a bright red background (Fig. 176-1). Without adequate illumination for examination, they may be overlooked. Koplik's spots are typically located on the buccal mucosa alongside the second molars and may be extensive; they are not associated with any other infectious disease. The spots wane after the onset of rash and soon disappear. The entire buccal and inner labial mucosa may be inflamed, and the lips may be reddened.

The characteristic erythematous, nonpruritic, maculopapular rash of measles begins at the hairline and behind the ears, spreads down the trunk and limbs to include the palms and soles, and often becomes confluent (Fig. 176-2). At this time, the patient is at the most severe point of the illness. By the fourth day, the rash begins to fade in the order in which it appeared. Brownish discoloration of the skin and

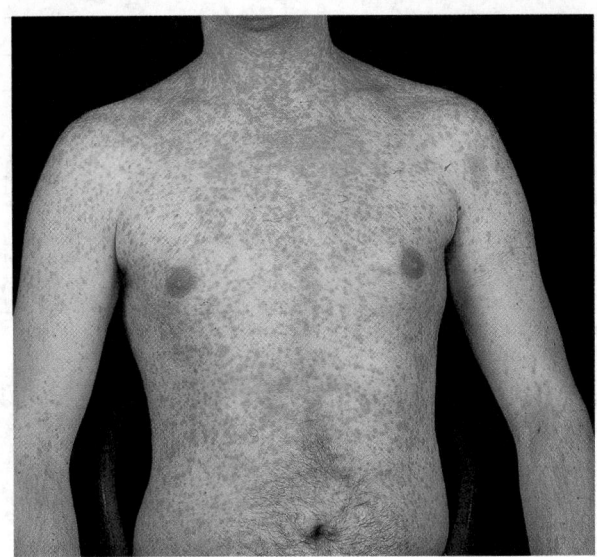

FIGURE 176-2   In measles, discrete erythematous lesions become confluent as the rash spreads downward. *(Reprinted with permission from Fitzpatrick TB et al: Color Atlas & Synopsis of Clinical Dermatology, 4th ed. New York, McGraw-Hill, 2001, p 775.)*

desquamation may occur later. Fever usually resolves by the fourth or fifth day after the onset of rash; prolonged fever suggests a complication of measles. Lymphadenopathy, diarrhea, vomiting, and splenomegaly are common features. The chest x-ray may be abnormal, even in uncomplicated measles, because of the propensity of this virus to invade the respiratory tract. The entire illness usually lasts about 10 days. The disease tends to be more severe in adults than in children, with higher fever, more prominent rash, and a higher incidence of complications.

Milder forms of the illness with less intense symptoms and a milder rash, termed *modified measles*, may occur in individuals with preexisting partial immunity induced by active or passive vaccination. These patients include infants under 1 year of age who retain some proportion of passively acquired maternal antibodies. On occasion, individuals with a history of immunization may develop modified measles.

COMPLICATIONS   The complications of measles (Table 176-1) can conveniently be divided into three groups, according to the site involved: the respiratory tract, the central nervous system (CNS), and the gastrointestinal tract. Respiratory tract involvement, manifested as laryngitis, croup, or bronchitis, occurs in the majority of cases of uncomplicated measles. In young children, otitis media is the most common complication. Pneumonia is a frequent reason for hospitalization, especially of adults. The pneumonia is of viral origin in the majority of cases, but secondary bacterial infection (most commonly caused by streptococci, pneumococci, or staphylococci) also develops with some frequency. Primary giant cell (Hecht's) pneumonia is most often documented in immunocompromised and/or malnourished patients.

Encephalographic abnormalities in the absence of symptoms of CNS disease are extremely frequent in measles. Symptomatic CNS disease may present with fever, headache, drowsiness, coma, and/or seizures. Symptoms usually begin within days after the onset of rash but occasionally appear for the first time several weeks later. About 10% of patients do not survive acute measles encephalitis; a significant percentage of surviving patients develop permanent sequelae, such as mental retardation or epilepsy. Most cases appear to result from an immune-mediated response to myelin proteins (postinfectious encephalomyelitis) and not directly from viral infection of the CNS (Chap. 359). Rarely, transverse myelitis follows measles. Immunocompromised patients are at risk for progressive fatal encephalitis 1 to 6 months after measles; in some cases, even though prior measles has

TABLE 176-1 *Complications of Measles*

Complication	Comments
Otitis media	Very common in infants with measles
Pneumonia	May be primary viral pneumonia or bacterial superinfection; frequent reason for hospitalization of adults; measles rash sometimes lacking in immunocompromised patients with measles pneumonia
Croup	Occasionally severe, requiring intubation in infants
Gastroenteritis	Diarrhea can be life threatening in infants
Cervical adenitis	Due to lymphoid hyperplasia as host response to virus; common
Acute encephalitis	May be mild to severe/fatal; occurs in 1 in 1000 cases of measles; cerebral and cerebellar forms; immune-mediated pathogenesis
Subacute sclerosing panencephalitis (SSPE)	In 1 in 100,000 cases of measles, usually when measles occurred in infancy; seen 5–10 years later. In United States, most children with SSPE were born in another country where measles vaccine is not routinely used.

not been recognized, the virus is identified at autopsy. Subacute sclerosing panencephalitis (SSPE)—a protracted, chronic, extremely rare form of measles encephalitis—sometimes follows measles and is particularly common among children who have measles before the age of 2 years (Chap. 360). SSPE has virtually disappeared in the United States as a result of widespread vaccination. Typically, progressive dementia evolves over several months. SSPE is thought to be due to a complex interaction of the host with defective measles virus. It is associated with extremely high levels of antibodies to measles virus in the blood and CSF.

Gastrointestinal complications of measles include gastroenteritis, hepatitis, appendicitis, ileocolitis, and mesenteric adenitis. It is not uncommon to detect high levels of alanine and aspartate aminotransferases in the absence of gastrointestinal signs such as jaundice.

Other, rare complications include myocarditis, glomerulonephritis, and postinfectious thrombocytopenic purpura. Measles can exacerbate preexisting tuberculosis, presumably through depression of cellular immunity induced by the virus. Natural measles and immunization against measles can result in tuberculin skin-test anergy lasting for about 1 month.

ATYPICAL MEASLES An atypical form of measles has been reported in individuals who received formalin-inactivated measles vaccine (used in the United States from 1963 through 1967 and in Canada until 1970) and subsequently were exposed to measles virus. After a several-day prodrome of fever, myalgia, and headache, the rash appears (Fig. 176-3). Unlike the rash of typical measles, that of atypical measles begins peripherally and moves centrally; it can be urticarial, maculopapular, hemorrhagic, and/or vesicular. Fever is usually high and is accompanied by edema of the extremities, interstitial pulmonary infiltrates, hepatitis, and (on occasion) pleural effusion. The differential diagnosis often includes Rocky Mountain spotted fever, Henoch-Schönlein purpura, meningococcemia, drug allergy, toxic shock syndrome, and varicella. Despite the severity of atypical measles, patients invariably recover after a convalescence that may be prolonged. Measles virus is not isolated from these patients, and they do not spread the virus to others. This disease is believed to be due to hypersensitivity to measles virus induced by the inactivated vaccine. Formalin inactivation destroys the antigenicity of the F protein, antibodies to which are important in preventing spread of the virus from one cell to another. The role of cellular immunity in this process is unknown. Extremely high convalescent titers of antibody to measles virus (e.g., 1:1,000,000) are diagnostic of atypical measles. To prevent this syndrome, adults who

received formalin-inactivated measles vaccine should be reimmunized with at least one dose of live attenuated measles vaccine. Because inactivated measles vaccine has not been available for more than 25 years, atypical measles has now virtually disappeared.

MEASLES IN THE IMMUNOCOMPROMISED HOST Patients with defects in cell-mediated immunity are at risk for severe protracted and fatal measles. Included in this category are patients with congenital cellular immune defects or malignancy, recipients of immunosuppressive therapy, or persons infected with HIV. In these patients, measles may not be accompanied by a rash. Complications are primary measles (giant cell) pneumonia, progressive encephalitis beginning weeks to months after initial infection, and (in HIV-infected patients) progression to AIDS.

MEASLES IN ADULTS Measles is naturally a disease of childhood and, like many other viral infections, is more severe in adults than in children. About 3% of young adults with measles develop primary viral pneumonia and require hospitalization. Hepatitis and bronchospasm are more common among adults with measles than among children, and the rash is more severe and more confluent in adults. Bacterial superinfection is more common among adults, more than one-third of whom develop respiratory complications such as otitis media, sinusitis, and pneumonia. Adults may develop measles because they were never immunized or (more rarely) because their vaccine-induced immunity has waned. Very low titers of antibody to measles virus have been associated with lack of protection.

LABORATORY FINDINGS Lymphopenia and neutropenia are common in measles and may be due to invasion of leukocytes by the virus, with subsequent cell death. Leukocytosis may herald a bacterial superinfection. Patients with measles encephalitis usually have an elevated protein concentration in CSF as well as lymphocytosis.

DIAGNOSIS A specific diagnosis of measles can be made quickly by immunofluorescent staining of a smear of respiratory secretions for measles antigen; monoclonal antibodies conjugated to fluorescein are commercially available for this purpose. Secretions can also be examined microscopically for multinucleated giant cells. Measles virus can be isolated from respiratory secretions or urine and rapidly identified in tissue culture with fluorescein-labeled monoclonal antibodies. The presence of measles virus RNA has been demonstrated by diagnostic reverse-transcription polymerase chain reaction. A number of serologic tests are available for the diagnosis of measles; however, a serologic diagnosis cannot necessarily be made quickly because both acute- and convalescent-phase sera are usually tested, ideally at the same time. The older hemagglutination inhibition test has been re-

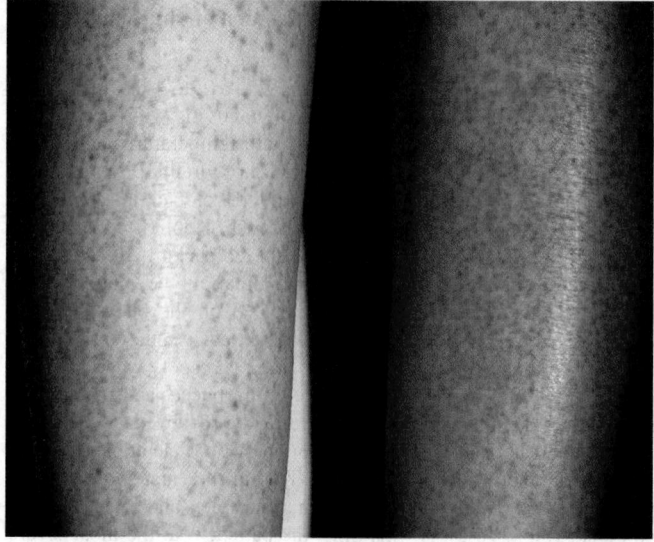

FIGURE 176-3 Petechial lesions in a patient with atypical measles. *(Photo courtesy of Stephen E. Gellis, MD.)*

placed by enzyme immunoassay (EIA), which is more sensitive and simpler to perform. EIA can be used to measure specific IgM and thus to diagnose measles on the basis of an acute-phase serum sample alone. Specific IgM antibodies are detectable within 1 to 2 days after the appearance of rash, and the IgG titer rises significantly after 10 days. As already mentioned, atypical measles and SSPE are associated with extremely high titers of antibody.

DIFFERENTIAL DIAGNOSIS Classic measles—with Koplik's spots, cough, coryza, conjunctivitis, and a rash beginning on the head—is easily diagnosed on clinical grounds. Modified measles is more difficult to diagnose clinically because one or more characteristic signs may be lacking. The differential diagnosis of measles includes Kawasaki disease, scarlet fever, infectious mononucleosis, toxoplasmosis, drug eruption, and *Mycoplasma pneumoniae* infection. Most of these conditions can be identified by either culture or serologic assay. In the differential diagnosis of measles, attention should be paid to the current epidemiology of the disease in the community and to the patient's history of measles vaccination and foreign travel.

PREVENTION The development of live attenuated measles vaccine by Enders and colleagues was a milestone in American medicine. This vaccine, used in the United States for the routine immunization of children since 1963, induces seroconversion in about 95% of recipients and probably confers lifelong protection. Waning immunity to measles after immunization has been documented only on rare occasions. For the past three decades, measles vaccine has been available as the combination vaccine measles-mumps-rubella (MMR); MMR vaccine should be administered to children between the ages of 12 and 15 months. (Vaccination at 12 months is preferred for infants whose mothers were immunized against measles in childhood. These mothers have lower antibody titers than women who have had natural measles, and their infants correspondingly have transplacental antibodies of lower titer and shorter duration.) A second dose of MMR vaccine is recommended for school-age children at 4 to 12 years of age. This two-dose policy was developed in the late 1980s in response to measles outbreaks in the United States. Since the institution of the two-dose regimen and the increased effort to immunize all children, measles has again become an unusual disease in the United States. Regional guidelines that reflect the current local epidemiology of measles should be followed.

Older susceptible persons should also be immunized. Individuals should be considered susceptible to measles unless they have documentation of physician-diagnosed measles or of the receipt of two doses of vaccine, have laboratory evidence of measles immunity, or were born before 1957. Rarely, individuals born before 1957 develop measles, and those who are at risk of exposure to measles (e.g., health care workers, teachers, and international travelers) should be tested for measles antibody and immunized if necessary. Approximately 10% of healthy vaccinees develop a fever, with temperatures up to 39.4°C (103°F), 5 to 7 days after vaccination; this fever lasts 1 to 5 days and is accompanied by a transient rash. Individuals previously immunized only with killed vaccine are considered susceptible and should receive at least one dose—preferably two doses—of MMR vaccine. Transient adverse reactions in these individuals include fever, malaise, and redness and swelling at the injection site.

Because of the severity of measles in this group and the lack of reported problems following vaccination, children with asymptomatic HIV infection should receive MMR vaccine; those with severe immunosuppression (<15% CD4 lymphocytes) should not. A case of fatal measles due to vaccine-type virus was reported in a college student with AIDS. Measles vaccine is contraindicated for persons with impaired cell-mediated immunity, for pregnant women, and for persons with a history of anaphylaxis due to egg protein or neomycin. Minor illnesses, with or without fever and a history of convulsions, are not contraindications to vaccination. Vaccination should be deferred for 6 to 11 months after the receipt of immune globulin or of blood products containing antibodies and for at least 3 months after the discontinuation of immunosuppressive treatment. Vaccine failures

have been ascribed to faulty storage of the preparation used, immunization of infants with preexisting (maternally derived) antibodies, and simultaneous administration of measles vaccine and immune globulin.

The only temporally related apparent complications of measles vaccination that are thought to be causal are febrile seizures, which rarely have long-term sequelae; thrombocytopenia, which is self-limited; and anaphylaxis, which is very rare. An exhaustive analysis conducted in 2000 by a number of official committees, including those of the American Academy of Pediatrics and the Institute of Medicine, found no causal relationship between MMR vaccination and development of autism.

Children and adults who are susceptible to measles and are exposed to the disease should receive postexposure prophylaxis. Standard immune globulin, given intramuscularly within 6 days of exposure, can exert a protective or modifying effect; the earlier it is given, the better the outcome. The dose is 0.25 mL/kg for healthy persons and 0.5 mL/kg for immunocompromised persons, with a maximum dose of 15 mL. Immune globulin is particularly strongly indicated for susceptible household contacts, especially those <1 year of age, and for immunocompromised persons. HIV-infected persons, particularly those with severe immunosuppression, should be given immune globulin after exposure, regardless of their measles immune status and whether or not they are receiving intravenous immune globulin. Vaccination within 72 h of exposure may also provide protection against clinical measles, but this strategy is contraindicated as postexposure prophylaxis for immunocompromised individuals. Vaccine and immune globulin should not be given concurrently.

℞ TREATMENT

Therapy for measles is largely supportive and symptom based. Patients with otitis media and pneumonia should be given standard antibiotics. Patients with encephalitis need supportive care, including observation for increased intracranial pressure. Controlled trials suggest clinical benefit from high doses of vitamin A in severe or potentially severe measles, especially in children under the age of 2 years who are or may be malnourished. On the basis of limited data, a dose of 50,000 IU is used for infants 1 to 6 months old; a dose of 100,000 IU is recommended for infants 7 to 12 months old; and a dose of 200,000 IU is recommended for children >1 year old. A single dose is administered on two consecutive days. In the United States, vitamin A treatment is recommended for young children hospitalized for measles and for pediatric measles patients with immunodeficiency, clinical evidence of vitamin A deficiency, impaired intestinal absorption, moderate to severe malnutrition, or recent immigration from an area where there is high mortality from measles. Transient vomiting and headache may be associated with the administration of vitamin A. Ribavirin is effective against measles virus in vitro and may be considered for use in immunocompromised individuals.

FURTHER READING

CENTERS FOR DISEASE CONTROL AND PREVENTION: Measles, mumps, and rubella—vaccine use and strategies for elimination of measles, rubella, and congenital rubella syndrome and control of mumps. MMWR 47:1, 1998

D'SOUZA RM, D'SOUZA R: Vitamin A for preventing secondary infections in children with measles—a systematic review. J Trop Pediatr 48:72, 2002

FOMBONE E et al: No evidence for a new variant of MMR-induced autism. Pediatrics 108:E58, 2001

FORNI AL et al: Severe measles pneumonitis in adults: Evaluation of clinical characteristics and therapy with intravenous ribavirin. Clin Infect Dis 19: 454, 1994

KAPLAN LJ et al: Severe measles in immunocompromised patients. JAMA 267:1237, 1992

PELTOLA H et al: The elimination of indigenous measles, mumps, and rubella from Finland by a 12-year, two-dose vaccination program. N Engl J Med 331:1397, 1994

STALKUP JR: A review of measles virus. Dermatol Clin 20:209, 2002

DEFINITION   Rubella is an acute viral infection of children and adults that characteristically includes rash, fever, and lymphadenopathy and has a broad spectrum of other possible manifestations. However, a high percentage of rubella infections in both children and adults are subclinical. In addition, the illness can resemble a mild attack of measles (rubeola) and can cause arthritis, especially in adults. Rubella was formerly known as *German measles* because it was first described clinically as distinct from rubeola in Germany, where it generated much medical interest in the mid-eighteenth and early nineteenth centuries. Rubella during pregnancy can lead to fetal infection, with the production of a significant constellation of malformations (*congenital rubella syndrome*) in a high proportion of infected fetuses. Rubella virus was first isolated in cell culture just before the last pandemic of the disease began in 1962. Since the licensing of rubella vaccine in the United States in 1969, there have been no further epidemics in this country.

ETIOLOGIC AGENT   Rubella virus, a togavirus, is the only member of the *Rubivirus* genus and is closely related to the alphaviruses. Unlike these agents, however, it does not require a vector for transmission. Moreover, there is no RNA sequence homology between rubella virus and the alphaviruses.

The rubella virion is composed of an inner icosahedral capsid of RNA and protein that is surrounded by a lipid-containing envelope with glycoprotein spikes and a diameter of about 60 nm. The structural proteins associated with rubella virus are E1 and E2 (transmembrane envelope glycoproteins) and C (the capsid protein that surrounds the viral RNA). Only one serotype has been identified.

EPIDEMIOLOGY   In the United States during the prevaccine era, rubella was most common in the spring and most often affected school-age children; only 80 to 90% of adults were immune; and major epidemics occurred every 6 to 9 years. The most recent epidemic in the United States occurred in 1964 to 1965, when more than 12 million cases of postnatal rubella and more than 20,000 cases of the congenital rubella syndrome were reported. Although there have been no epidemics since the introduction of live attenuated rubella vaccine in 1969, limited outbreaks have been reported in settings where susceptible individuals come into close contact with one another (e.g., schools and workplaces). In 2001, only 23 cases of postnatally acquired rubella—most of them in young adults—and 3 confirmed cases of congenital rubella syndrome were reported to the Centers for Disease Control and Prevention (CDC).

Whether symptomatic or subclinical, rubella is contagious, albeit less so than measles. Its incubation period is 18 days on average, with a range of 12 to 23 days. The virus, which is spread in droplets shed in respiratory secretions, infects the respiratory tract and then the bloodstream. In postnatally acquired infections, rubella virus is shed during the prodromal phase of the illness, and shedding from the pharynx can continue for about a week after onset. Despite high titers of specific neutralizing antibodies, infants with congenital rubella may excrete rubella virus from the respiratory tract and in the urine until the age of 2 years. This excretion raises important issues related to infection control in hospital and day-care settings. Persons recently immunized with live attenuated rubella vaccine do not transmit the vaccine virus to others, although low titers of rubella virus may be detected transiently in the pharynx.

After an attack of rubella, specific antibodies and cell-mediated immunity develop and probably play a significant role in protection against future disease. Asymptomatic reinfection at the level of the respiratory tract is common upon re-exposure to the virus but is rarely, if ever, associated with viremia.

Rubella virus has been cultured from respiratory secretions during reinfection. Fetal infection may occur during maternal reinfection but

is acknowledged to be extremely rare because of the absence of maternal viremia under these circumstances. Viremia following reinfection of individuals immunized against rubella is also rare. Thus the current level of congenital rubella in the United States is exceedingly low. Recently, however, it has been observed that young immigrants to the United States from countries in Latin America and the Caribbean, where rubella vaccine is not routinely given to children, are at increased risk for rubella susceptibility. Because infants with the congenital rubella syndrome have been born to immigrant Hispanic women, increasing efforts are being made to identify and vaccinate such women before they become pregnant.

PATHOGENESIS AND PATHOLOGY   Little is known about the microscopic pathology of postnatally acquired rubella because the disease is invariably self-limited. Like that of measles, the rash of rubella is immunologically mediated; its onset coincides with the development of specific antibodies. Viremia can be demonstrated for about a week before and ends within a few days after the onset of rash.

The cause of the damage to cells and organs in congenital rubella is not well understood. Proposed mechanisms of fetal damage include mitotic arrest of cells, tissue necrosis without inflammation, and chromosomal damage. The growth of the fetus may be retarded. Other findings may include decreased numbers of megakaryocytes in the bone marrow, extramedullary hematopoiesis, and interstitial pneumonia.

CLINICAL MANIFESTATIONS ■ Postnatally Acquired Rubella   Infection acquired after birth usually results in an extremely mild or subclinical illness. A prodromal phase is uncommon in children; adults may have more severe disease, with a brief prodrome of malaise, fever, and anorexia. The foremost symptoms of postnatally acquired rubella include posterior auricular, cervical, and suboccipital lymphadenopathy; fever; and rash. The rash often begins on the face (Fig. 177-1) and spreads down the body. It is maculopapular but not confluent, is sometimes accompanied by mild coryza and conjunctivitis, and generally lasts for 3 to 5 days. A petechial enanthem on the soft palate, designated *Forschheimer spots*, may occur but is not specific for rubella. Fever may be absent entirely or may be present for only several days in the early phase of the illness.

Complications of postnatally acquired rubella are uncommon; bacterial superinfection is rare. One particularly troublesome complication

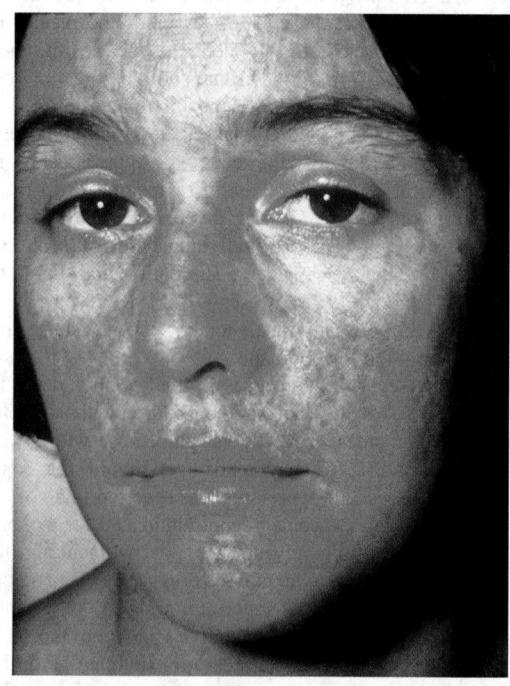

FIGURE 177-1   In rubella, an erythematous exanthem spreads from the hairline downward and clears as it spreads. (*Photo courtesy of Stephen E. Gellis, MD.*)

is seen almost exclusively in women: arthritis, most frequently involving the fingers, wrists, and/or knees. Arthritis develops as the rash is appearing and may take several weeks to resolve. Chronic arthritis resulting from rubella is extremely rare. Rubella virus has been isolated from joint fluid during acute rubella arthritis and from peripheral blood in chronic rubella arthritis.

Another complication of postnatally acquired rubella is hemorrhage due to both thrombocytopenia and vascular damage; this complication occurs in 1 of every 3000 patients. Thrombocytopenia may last for weeks or months; it can have long-term consequences if there is bleeding into organs such as the eye or the brain.

Both children and adults may develop encephalitis after rubella; the incidence is about five times lower than that of encephalitis following measles. Adults are more likely than children to develop encephalitis; the mortality rate from this complication is 20 to 50%. Mild hepatitis is an unusual complication. Immunosuppressed patients are not at increased risk for rubella as they are for measles.

Congenital Rubella   Maternal infection in early pregnancy can lead to fetal infection, with resultant congenital rubella. The classic signs of congenital rubella are cataract, heart disease, deafness, and myriad other defects (Table 177-1). The most important factor in the pathogenicity of rubella virus for the fetus is gestational age at the time of infection. Maternal infection during the first trimester leads to fetal infection in about 50% of cases; maternal infection early in the second trimester leads to fetal infection in about one-third of cases. Fetal malformations not only are more common after maternal infection in the first trimester but also tend to be more severe and to involve more organ systems. Whereas a fetus infected in the fourth week of gestation may develop many problems, one infected later (e.g., in the twentieth week) may have isolated deafness as the only symptom.

DIAGNOSIS   Because postnatally acquired rubella is often a mild disease and because many cases are subclinical, diagnosis on clinical grounds can be difficult. Other diseases that may mimic rubella include toxoplasmosis, scarlet fever, modified measles, roseola, fifth disease (erythema infectiosum due to parvovirus B19), and enteroviral infection. Routine laboratory tests usually reveal leukopenia and atypical lymphocytes.

The isolation of rubella virus in cell cultures of throat samples, urine, or other secretions is difficult and expensive but is sometimes undertaken. This technique is most useful when congenital rubella is suspected. A laboratory diagnosis is more often made serologically. The most commonly used test is an enzyme-linked immunosorbent assay (ELISA) for IgG and IgM antibodies. Acute rubella is diagnosed by the documentation of a fourfold or greater rise in the titer of IgG antibodies in paired acute- and convalescent-phase serum specimens or by the detection of rubella-specific IgM antibodies in one serum specimen. However, false-negative and false-positive IgM reactions are sometimes obtained. Moreover, true-positive IgM reactions can occur in both primary infection and reinfection. Congenital rubella is diagnosed by the isolation of rubella virus, the detection of IgM antibodies in a single serum sample, and/or the documentation of either the persistence of rubella antibodies in serum beyond 1 year of age or a rising antibody titer anytime during infancy in an unvaccinated child. Biopsied tissues and/or blood and cerebrospinal fluid have also been used for the demonstration of rubella antigens with monoclonal antibodies and for the detection of rubella RNA by in situ hybridization and polymerase chain reaction.

PREVENTION   Live attenuated rubella vaccine was licensed in 1969, 7 years after the virus was first isolated in culture. This vaccine was developed as a strategy to prevent congenital rubella by ensuring that very few pregnant women would be susceptible and that there would be little circulating wild-type virus. Rubella vaccine induces seroconversion in more than 95% of recipients. Since its licensure, there have been no major epidemics in the United States, and the number of cases has declined by 98%. The vaccine currently licensed in the United States, RA 27/3, is propagated in human diploid cells and is more immunogenic (particularly with regard to the stimulation of secretory immunity) than previously licensed vaccines. The present vaccination strategy, developed in part when measles was not being adequately controlled, is to immunize all infants at 12 to 15 months of age with measles-mumps-rubella (MMR) vaccine and to administer a second dose in early childhood. Rubella vaccine may also be administered to anyone who is thought to be susceptible to the infection and is not pregnant; it is particularly important that hospital workers of either sex be immune to rubella so that nosocomial transmission is avoided. Although there has been little change in the prevalence of immunity to rubella among women of childbearing age (about 80%), the incidence of congenital rubella is extremely low—fewer than 10 cases annually. It is likely that, although antibody may be undetectable years after immunization, protection against infection—possibly due to cell-mediated immunity—is the rule. At present, there is little if any evidence of significant waning of clinically important immunity to rubella with time.

On occasion, rubella vaccine may cause arthralgia or arthritis, especially in young women. Very rarely, rubella vaccination results in chronic arthritis; however, even cases of frank arthritis in vaccinees are self-limited, lasting only about 1 week.

After investigation of a series of more than 400 women who were inadvertently immunized during pregnancy and who carried their infants to term, the CDC has concluded that vaccine-type rubella virus either does not cause the congenital rubella syndrome at all or does so at an incidence too low to be detected. Nonetheless, rubella vaccine is contraindicated for use in pregnant women, and it is recommended that pregnancy be avoided for at least 3 months after rubella vaccination. It is acceptable for rubella-susceptible children whose mothers are also susceptible to be immunized, as vaccinated individuals do not shed rubella virus or transmit it to susceptible individuals. Although it is recommended that rubella vaccine not be given to immunosuppressed persons, the vaccine is given to children infected with HIV. No adverse effects of rubella vaccine have been reported in immunocompromised patients.

TABLE 177-1 *Clinical Problems Associated with the Congenital Rubella Syndrome*	
Transient Signs/Symptoms (at Birth Only)	**Permanent Signs/Symptoms (Developmental)**
Bony abnormalities	Autism
Cloudy cornea	Behavioral disorders
Hemolytic anemia	Congenital heart disease (patent ductus
Hepatitis	arteriosus, pulmonic stenosis)
Hepatosplenomegaly	Cryptorchidism
Jaundice	Deafness
Low birth weight	Degenerative brain disease
Lymphadenopathy	Diabetes mellitus
Meningoencephalitis	Glaucoma
Rubella viral pneumonia	Inguinal hernia
Thrombocytopenic purpura	Mental retardation
	Microcephaly
	Myopia
	Precocious puberty
	Retinopathy
	Seizures
	Spastic diplegia
	Thyroid disorders

℞ TREATMENT

There is no specific therapy for rubella. At one time, immune globulin was used in an effort to prevent congenital rubella when pregnant women became infected. However, because administration of immune globulin did not prevent maternal viremia, this approach was discarded. Symptom-based treatment is given for manifestations such as fever, arthralgia, and arthritis.

FURTHER READING

CENTERS FOR DISEASE CONTROL AND PREVENTION: Measles, mumps, and rubella—vaccine use and strategies for elimination of measles, rubella, and congenital rubella syndrome and control of mumps. MMWR 47:1, 1998

————: Control and prevention of rubella: Evaluation and management of suspected outbreaks, rubella in pregnant women, and surveillance for congenital rubella syndrome. MMWR 50:1, 2001

DANAVARO-HOLLIDAY MC et al: A large rubella outbreak with spread from the workplace to the community. JAMA 284:2733, 2000

DYKEWICZ C et al: Rubella seropositivity in the United States, 1988–1994. Clin Infect Dis 233:1279, 2001

MELLINGER AK et al: High incidence of congenital rubella syndrome after a rubella outbreak. Pediatr Infect Dis J 14:573, 1995

REEF SE et al: The changing epidemiology of rubella in the 1990s: On the verge of elimination and new challenges for control and prevention. JAMA 287:464, 2002

SHERIDAN E: Congenital rubella syndrome: A risk in immigrant populations. Lancet 359:674, 2002

178 MUMPS
Anne Gershon

DEFINITION   Mumps is an acute, systemic, communicable viral infection whose most distinctive feature is swelling of one or both parotid glands. Involvement of other salivary glands, the meninges, the pancreas, and the gonads is also common.

ETIOLOGIC AGENT   Mumps virus, a paramyxovirus, is pleomorphic and has a diameter ranging from 100 to 300 nm. The virion is composed of RNA and seven proteins. The RNA is surrounded by an envelope with glycoprotein projections. There are two envelope glycoproteins—a hemagglutinin-neuraminidase (HN) and a hemolysis cell fusion antigen (F)—as well as a matrix envelope protein (M). A fourth protein (SH) may also be membrane-associated. There are three internal components: a nucleocapsid protein (NP), a phosphoprotein (P), and a large protein (L). There is only one antigenic type of mumps virus. The polymerase chain reaction (PCR) has detected geographic differences among mumps viruses from different locales.

EPIDEMIOLOGY   After the introduction of mumps vaccine in 1967, the incidence of clinical mumps declined significantly in the United States. In 1968 (before widespread immunization), 185,691 cases of mumps were reported in this country. The 266 cases reported in 2001 represent a reduction in the number of cases by >99% from prevaccine levels; this is the lowest number of cases ever reported in a year. Before widespread vaccination, the incidence of mumps was highest in the winter and spring, with epidemics every 2 to 5 years. At that time, mumps was principally a disease of childhood, although today more than 50% of cases occur in young adults. Epidemics tended to occur in confined populations, such as those in schools and the military services.

The incubation period of mumps generally ranges from 14 to 18 days, with extremes of 7 and 23 days. However, because a contact may be shedding virus before the onset of clinical disease or (like one-third of patients) may have subclinical infection, the incubation period in individual cases is often uncertain. One attack of mumps usually confers lifelong immunity. Long-term immunity is also associated with immunization.

PATHOGENESIS   Mumps virus is transmitted by droplet nuclei, saliva, and fomites. Replication of the virus in the epithelium of the upper respiratory tract leads to viremia, which is followed by infection of glandular tissues and/or the central nervous system (CNS).

Little is known of the pathology of mumps since the disease is rarely fatal. The affected glands contain perivascular and interstitial mononuclear cell infiltrates with prominent edema. Necrosis of acinar and epithelial duct cells is evident in the salivary glands and in the germinal epithelium of the seminiferous tubules.

CLINICAL MANIFESTATIONS   The prodrome of mumps consists of fever, malaise, myalgia, and anorexia. Parotitis, if it develops, usually does so within the next 24 h but may be delayed for as long as a week; it is generally bilateral, although the onset on the two sides may not be synchronous and at times only one side is affected. The submaxillary and sublingual glands are involved less often than the parotid and are almost never involved alone. Swelling of the parotid is accompanied by tenderness and obliteration of the space between the ear lobe and the angle of the mandible. The patient frequently reports an earache and finds it difficult to eat, swallow, or talk. Glandular swelling increases for a few days and then gradually subsides, disappearing within a week. The orifice of Stensen's duct is commonly red and swollen. Presternal pitting edema has been described in about 5% of mumps cases, often in association with submandibular adenitis.

Other than parotitis, orchitis is the most common manifestation of mumps among postpubertal males, developing in about 20% of cases. The testis is painful and tender and is enlarged to several times its normal size; accompanying fever is common. Later, testicular atrophy develops in half of the affected men. Since orchitis is bilateral in fewer than 15% of cases, sterility after mumps is rare. Oophoritis in women—far less common than orchitis in men—may cause lower abdominal pain but does not lead to sterility.

Aseptic meningitis, which may develop before, during, after, or in the absence of parotitis, is a common manifestation of mumps in both children and adults. Symptoms include stiff neck, headache, and drowsiness. Pleocytosis of the cerebrospinal fluid (CSF), with up to 1000 cells/μL, may develop in up to 50% of cases of clinical mumps, but clinical signs of meningeal irritation are documented in only 5 to 25% of cases. Within the first 24 h, polymorphonuclear leukocytes may predominate in CSF, but by the second day nearly all the cells are lymphocytes. The glucose level in CSF may be abnormally low, and this finding may arouse suspicion of bacterial meningitis. Aseptic meningitis due to mumps without parotitis is indistinguishable clinically from that caused by other viruses. Mumps meningitis is almost invariably self-limited, although cranial nerve palsies have occasionally led to permanent sequelae, particularly deafness. More rarely, mumps virus may cause encephalitis, which presents as high fever with marked changes in the level of consciousness and frequently results in permanent sequelae in survivors. Other CNS problems occasionally associated with mumps include cerebellar ataxia, facial palsy, transverse myelitis, Guillain-Barré syndrome, and aqueductal stenosis leading to hydrocephalus.

Mumps pancreatitis, which may present as abdominal pain, is difficult to diagnose because an elevated serum amylase level can be associated with either parotitis or pancreatitis. Other unusual complications of mumps include myocarditis, mastitis, thyroiditis, nephritis, arthritis, and thrombocytopenic purpura. An excessive number of spontaneous abortions are associated with gestational mumps when the disease occurs during the first trimester. Mumps in pregnancy does not lead to premature birth or fetal malformations.

DIFFERENTIAL DIAGNOSIS   The diagnosis of mumps is made easily in patients with acute bilateral parotitis and a history of recent exposure, but mumps is currently a rare disease in the United States due to widespread vaccination. When parotitis is unilateral or absent or when sites other than the parotid gland are involved, laboratory diagnosis may be required. The differential diagnosis of parotitis is presented in Table 178-1.

Other entities should be considered when manifestations consistent with mumps appear in organs other than the parotid. Testicular torsion may produce a painful scrotal mass resembling that seen in mumps

TABLE 178-1 *Differential Diagnosis of Parotitis*	
Etiology	Comments
SYSTEMIC INFECTIONS	
Mumps	Rare in countries with vaccination programs
Coxsackievirus infection	Particularly likely in children
HIV infection	In HIV-positive children receiving no antiretroviral therapy; additional disease manifestations likely
Parainfluenza virus type 3 infection	Particularly likely in children, associated with acute respiratory tract symptoms
Influenza A virus infection	Seasonal (winter, spring), associated with acute respiratory tract symptoms
Cat-scratch disease	Unusual but described
Epstein-Barr virus infection	Unusual but described
SYSTEMIC NONINFECTIOUS CAUSES	
Sarcoidosis	Additional manifestations of disease likely
Sjögren's syndrome	Additional manifestations of disease likely
Uremia	Additional manifestations of disease likely
Diabetes mellitus	Additional manifestations of disease likely
Drugs	Phenylbutazone, thiouracil
UNILATERAL PAROTITIS	
Ductal obstruction due to stones or strictures	Unilateral, gradual onset, suppurative
Parotid cyst	Unilateral, gradual onset
Parotid tumor	Unilateral, gradual onset
ACUTE SUPPURATIVE PAROTITIS	
Staphylococcus aureus, *Streptococcus* species, and (rarely) gram-negative bacteria, anaerobes	

orchitis. Other viruses (e.g., enteroviruses) may cause aseptic meningitis that is clinically indistinguishable from that due to mumps virus.

Myocarditis as a severe but usually self-limited complication of mumps has been described. Molecular diagnostic assays have implicated mumps virus in some cases of endocardial fibroelastosis following myocarditis.

LABORATORY DIAGNOSIS Mumps virus is readily isolated after inoculation of appropriate clinical specimens into a variety of host systems, such as rhesus monkey kidney cells and human embryonic lung fibroblasts. The virus can be rapidly identified by inoculation of cells grown in shell vials and subsequent staining with fluorescein-labeled monoclonal antibodies to detect viral growth. Mumps virus may be recovered from saliva, throat, and urine during the first few days of illness and from the CSF of patients with mumps meningitis. Shedding of virus in the urine may persist for as long as 2 weeks. PCR is also used to detect mumps virus in clinical specimens. No particular peripheral blood cell count is characteristic of mumps.

Highly sensitive enzyme-linked immunosorbent assays are useful for serologic diagnosis of mumps and for determination of susceptibility to the disease. Acute mumps can be diagnosed either by the examination of acute- and convalescent-phase sera for a significant increase in IgG antibody titer or by the demonstration of specific IgM in one serum specimen. Use of a skin-test antigen to assess immunity to mumps has been replaced by serologic testing.

PREVENTION Live attenuated mumps vaccine (Jeryl Lynn strain) induces antibodies that protect the recipient against infection in more than 95% of cases. The subcutaneously administered vaccine may be given to children older than 1 year but is not recommended for younger infants because of the potential for interference by passive maternal antibodies. Mumps vaccine is usually administered as part of the measles-mumps-rubella (MMR) vaccine at the age of 12 to 15 months and again at 4 to 12 years of age. This MMR vaccine is also recommended for susceptible older children, adolescents, and adults, particularly adolescent males who have not had mumps. For these patients, either MMR or monovalent mumps vaccine may be given; two doses are preferred. Inadvertent immunization of individuals who are already immune is not associated with significant adverse reactions. Mumps vaccine is not recommended for pregnant women, for patients receiving glucocorticoids, or for other immunocompromised hosts. However, children with HIV infection who are not severely immunocompromised can safely be immunized against mumps; MMR vaccine is usually used for this purpose (Chap. 107). Occasionally, febrile reactions and parotitis have been reported soon after mumps vaccination. Allergic reactions after vaccination, such as rash and pruritus, occur uncommonly and are usually mild and self-limited. In the United States, the incidence of encephalitis during the month after mumps vaccination is no greater than the background incidence rate of encephalitis in the population.

℞ TREATMENT

Therapy for parotitis and other manifestations of mumps is symptom-based. The administration of analgesics and the application of warm or cold compresses to the parotid area may be helpful. Mumps immune globulin is of no value in prophylaxis or treatment of established disease. Testicular pain may be minimized by the local application of cold compresses and gentle support for the scrotum. Anesthetic blocks may also be used. Neither the administration of glucocorticoids nor incision of the tunica albuginea is of proven value for the treatment of severe orchitis. Anecdotal information on a small number of patients with orchitis suggests that administration of interferon α may be helpful.

FURTHER READING

Briss PA et al: Sustained transmission of mumps in a highly vaccinated population: Assessment of primary vaccine failure and waning vaccine-induced immunity. J Infect Dis 169:77, 1994

Centers for Disease Control and Prevention: Notice to readers: Final 2001 reports of notifiable diseases. MMWR 51:710, 2002

———: Measles, mumps, and rubella—vaccine use and strategies for elimination of measles, rubella, and congenital rubella syndrome and control of mumps. MMWR 47:1, 1998

Chaudary S et al: Fulminant mumps myocarditis. Ann Intern Med 110:569, 1989

Gut JP et al: Symptomatic mumps reinfections. J Med Virol 45:17, 1995

McDonald JC et al: Clinical and epidemiologic features of mumps encephalitis and possible causes of vaccine-related disease. Pediatr Infect Dis J 8:751, 1989

Swierkosz EM et al: Mumps, in *Manual of Clinical Virology*, 8th ed, PR Murray (ed). Washington, DC, ASM Press, 2002 (in press)

179 RABIES VIRUS AND OTHER RHABDOVIRUSES
Cathleen A. Hanlon, Lawrence Corey

RABIES VIRUS

DEFINITION Rabies is an invariably lethal, acute viral disease of the central nervous system (CNS) that affects all mammals and that is transmitted by infected secretions. Most commonly, transmission to humans takes place through exposure to saliva during a bite by an infected animal.

ETIOLOGY The rabies and rabies-related viruses are in the family Rhabdoviridae, with at least seven distinct types within the genus *Lyssa-*

virus. Isolates of rabies virus from different animal species and locales differ in their antigenic and biologic properties. These variations may account for differences in virulence between isolates. The bullet-shaped, enveloped viruses are single-strand RNA viruses of negative polarity. The rabies virus genome encodes five proteins: the nucleoprotein, the matrix protein, the glycoprotein, the phosphorylated protein, and a large polymerase protein. In immunofluorescence and complement fixation studies, broadly cross-reacting antigenic sites on the nucleoprotein are used to determine placement within the genus. The relatedness of a viral isolate to rabies and rabies-related viruses is determined by the comparison of specific antigenic sites or, more recently, by examination of RNA sequences. Cross-neutralization by rabies virus antisera ranges from moderate to very low. Only one serogroup is recognized within the genus. Recently, four new lyssaviruses have been described that expand current knowledge, classification, and taxonomy of rabies and rabies-related viruses.

EPIDEMIOLOGY An understanding of the epizootiology of rabies is necessary in evaluating the risk of exposure and the need for rabies postexposure prophylaxis (PEP) in humans. Rabies is found in mammals in all regions of the world except Antarctica. The susceptibility of mammals varies greatly and most likely is related to differences in cell surface receptor characteristics (e.g., type and abundance) and the impact of these differences on receptor-virus interactions. Rabies exists in two forms: *urban rabies,* propagated chiefly by unimmunized domestic dogs, and *sylvatic rabies,* propagated by skunks, foxes, raccoons, mongooses, wolves, and bats. Infection in domestic animals usually represents a "spillover" from sylvatic reservoirs of infection. Human infection occurs through contact with unimmunized domestic animals or from exposure to wild animals in locales where rabies is enzootic or epizootic. The worldwide incidence of human rabies is estimated at more than 30,000 cases per year. Southeast Asia, the Philippines, Africa, the Indian subcontinent, and tropical South America are areas where the disease is especially common. In some endemic areas, 1 to 2% of autopsies yield evidence of rabies. Increased travel of humans, along with intentional and unintentional translocation of animals (including known potential rabies-reservoir species), has made the recognition of clinical rabies and its prevention of increasing importance.

Although there are island countries and whole continents that consider themselves rabies-free, the designation is relative and should take into account potential animal translocation events, the capacity of rabies reservoir hosts (e.g., bats) for long-distance flight, the lack of adequate rabies diagnostic capacity and expertise, and the reluctance of national authorities to change official designations despite the identification of lyssaviruses among volant hosts (i.e., those capable of flight) and the identification of associated human rabies deaths.

The main reservoir of rabies throughout the world is the domestic dog. In developed countries, control of stray dogs and mandatory vaccination of owned dogs have resulted in the virtual elimination of this problem across large geographic areas (e.g., most of North America). With the virtual elimination of dog rabies in the United States since the 1960s, a dog bite now poses a dramatically reduced risk of rabies exposure that is appropriately managed by a 10-day observation of the dog. Tremendous advances in the control of dog rabies have recently been made in Latin and South American countries. However, dog rabies remains largely uncontrolled in most of Asia and Africa.

In addition to rabies in dogs, diverse rabies virus variants occur among other mammalian hosts. For example, the disease is found in the several species of mongoose in Asia and Africa and has been translocated to several Caribbean Islands. In Canada, rabies occurs among skunks and foxes, and raccoon rabies has invaded Ontario from New York. In Eastern Europe, rabies occurs among raccoon dogs. Coyotes, jackals, and other wild canids may serve as reservoirs or vectors in North America, Asia, and Africa. The major rabies virus variants in the United States occur among raccoons, skunks, red and gray foxes,

coyotes, and multiple insectivorous bat species. The most recent outbreak—and the most intense to date—affects raccoons in the eastern states from Florida to Maine and westward to the Appalachians and eastern Ohio. At the epizootic front in Ohio, New York, Pennsylvania, and West Virginia, the largest evaluation of oral rabies vaccination of free-ranging raccoons is in progress and represents an attempt to contain the westward spread of raccoon rabies. The vaccine, which is contained in baits and distributed primarily by air, is a vaccinia-rabies glycoprotein recombinant virus. Although highly attenuated by the lack of a critical enzyme (thymidine kinase), the vaccine is a live vaccinia virus and can infect humans, as demonstrated by at least one accidental human infection. In the United States, the domestic animal most commonly infected with rabies is the cat (~300 cases per year vs. ~100 cases in dogs). All other domestic animals combined (i.e., cattle, horses, sheep, goats, and pigs) account for a total of 150 to 200 cases per year.

Rabies in insectivorous bats occurs in the United States, Canada, Europe, Asia, Australia, and Africa—i.e., in essentially every locality where these bats are found. The epidemiology of rabies in bats is not well understood. In the United States, multiple rabies virus variants are generally associated with particular bat species, but variants may infect bat species other than their primary reservoir and may also infect terrestrial mammals, including other wildlife, domestic animals, and humans. Because migratory bat species travel widely and aggregate in large numbers, the rabies virus variants associated with these species are relatively homogeneous. In contrast, variants associated with nonmigratory bat species may demonstrate more genetic variation, such that isolates from particular geographic areas form distinct lineages. In general, the rate of rabies among seemingly healthy captured bats is low (1 in 100 to 1000). However, the rate of rabies among dead and dying bats in high-density colonies may be >50%. Rabies cannot be ruled out definitively in an individual bat or in any other animal except by direct fluorescent antibody testing of brain tissue.

The "bat" category in rabies surveillance reports includes a wide variety of species as well as many individual bats whose species is never identified. For surveillance purposes, it is uninformative to lump all bats together by order, as is the current practice in many states. Nevertheless, the total of rabid bats is second only to the number of rabid raccoons and skunks. In contrast to a single human case due to the raccoon rabies virus variant, a single human case of skunk-associated rabies, and two human cases of dog/coyote-associated rabies since 1980, the 30 human rabies cases due to bats account for >90% of all human rabies cases in the United States since that date. It is intriguing that a particular bat-associated rabies virus is implicated in most human cases: Ln/Ps, which is associated with silver-haired and eastern pipistrelle bats. Several factors may be involved in this observation. One possibility is that the teeth of these bats are so small that a bite may be dismissed (e.g., if the victim is unaware of the potential for rabies in these animals) or even go unrecognized (e.g., if the victim is asleep or under the influence of drugs or alcohol). Another possibility is that this virus variant may be better than others at replicating in cells of epidermal origin and at cooler temperatures. Perhaps a unique viral adaptation coupled with a relatively nontraumatic bite introduction is facilitating the emergence of this source of rabies in humans in the United States.

Human rabies is rare in the United States. The disease can be prevented if the exposure is recognized and appropriate local wound care and human rabies PEP are administered. From 1980 to 2002, most human rabies cases in the United States were acquired indigenously, with no apparent geographic trends. Two indigenously acquired human cases were associated with a localized outbreak of rabies among coyotes and dogs at the U.S.–Mexico border; however, this was a small outbreak in terms of relative animal case numbers.

A comparison of the epidemiology of animal rabies, human rabies PEP, and human rabies cases in the United States presents an interesting conundrum. Raccoons are the leading rabies reservoir, but only one human death from the raccoon-associated rabies virus variant has been documented. Since human rabies PEP is not reportable, there are few epidemiologic data on exposure to this reservoir. However, according to limited studies, most human rabies PEP is administered because of potential exposure to domestic cats and dogs in which rabies is suspected rather than because of direct exposure to raccoons or skunks—the first and second most commonly rabid animals in the United States.

PATHOGENESIS The first event in rabies is the inoculation of virus through the skin, usually through a bite that delivers virus-laden saliva. Initial viral replication appears to occur within striated muscle cells at the site of inoculation. The peripheral nervous system is exposed at the neuromuscular and/or neurotendinous spindles of unmyelinated sensory nerve cell endings, with neurotransmitter receptors such as acetylcholine implicated in viral attachment and internalization. The virus then spreads centripetally up the nerve to the CNS, probably via peripheral nerve axoplasm, at a rate of ~3 mm/h. Viremia has been documented in experimental conditions but is not thought to play a role in naturally acquired disease. Once the virus reaches the CNS, it replicates almost exclusively within the gray matter and then passes centrifugally along autonomic nerves to other tissues—the salivary glands, adrenal medulla, kidneys, lungs, liver, skeletal muscles, skin, and heart. Passage of the virus into the salivary glands and viral replication in mucinogenic acinar cells facilitate further transmission via infected saliva. The incubation period of rabies is exceedingly variable, ranging from 7 days to >1 year (mean, 1 to 2 months) and apparently depending on the amount of virus introduced, the amount of tissue involved, host defense mechanisms, and the actual distance that the virus has to travel from the site of inoculation to the CNS. Rates of infection and mortality are highest from bites on the face, intermediate from bites on the hands and arms, and lowest from bites on the legs. Cases of human rabies with an extended incubation period (2 to 7 years) have been reported, but they are rare. Host immune responses and viral strains also influence disease expression.

The neuropathology of rabies resembles that of other viral diseases of the CNS: hyperemia, varying degrees of chromatolysis, nuclear pyknosis, and neuronophagia of the nerve cells; infiltration by lymphocytes and plasma cells of the Virchow-Robin space; microglial infiltration; and parenchymal areas of nerve cell destruction. In experimental animal models, adenohypophyseal infection with rabies virus, with reduction in growth hormone and vasopressin release, is common. The most characteristic pathologic finding of rabies in the CNS is the formation of cytoplasmic inclusions called *Negri bodies* within neurons. Each eosinophilic mass measures ~10 nm and is made up of a finely fibrillar matrix and rabies virus particles. Negri bodies are distributed throughout the brain, particularly in Ammon's horn, the cerebral cortex, the brainstem, the hypothalamus, the Purkinje cells of the cerebellum, and the dorsal spinal ganglia. Negri bodies are not demonstrated in at least 20% of cases of rabies, and their absence from brain material does not rule out the diagnosis.

CLINICAL MANIFESTATIONS (See also Table 179-1) The clinical manifestations of rabies can be divided into four stages: (1) a nonspecific prodrome; (2) an acute encephalitis similar to other viral encephalitides; (3) a profound dysfunction of brainstem centers that produces the classic features of rabies encephalitis; and (4) death or, in rare cases, recovery.

The prodromal period usually lasts 1 to 4 days and is marked by fever, headache, malaise, myalgias, increased fatigability, anorexia, nausea and vomiting, sore throat, and a nonproductive cough. The prodromal symptom suggestive of rabies is the complaint of paresthesia and/or fasciculations at or around the site of inoculation of virus. These sensations, which may be related to the multiplication of virus in the dorsal root ganglion of the sensory nerve supplying the area of the bite, are reported by 50 to 80% of patients.

The encephalitic phase is usually ushered in by periods of excessive motor activity, excitation, and agitation. Confusion, hallucinations, combativeness, bizarre aberrations of thought, muscle spasms, meningismus, opisthotonic posturing, seizures, and focal paralysis soon appear. Characteristically, the periods of mental aberration are inter-

TABLE 179-1 *General Clinical Course of Human Rabies*

Phase	Duration	Features/Comments
Exposure	—	Often unrecognized, particularly if of bat origin
Incubation period	3–4 weeks to 3–4 months in 95% of cases; 1–7 years in 1% of cases	—
Prodrome	1–2 days to 1 week	Fever, headache, anorexia, nausea, vomiting, malaise, lethargy, focal pain, paresthesia, anxiety, agitation, depression
Acute neurologic (encephalitic) phase	1–2 days to <1 week	Confusion, delirium, hallucinations, dysphagia, hypersalivation, aphasia, incoordination, marked hyperactivity, pharyngeal spasms, hydrophobia, aerophobia, hyperventilation, hypoxia, seizures
Coma, death	Several days to 1 week	Autonomic instability, hypoventilation, apnea, respiratory arrest, hypo-/hyperthermia, hypotension, pituitary dysfunction, rhabdomyolysis, cardiac arrhythmia, cardiac arrest

spersed with completely lucid periods, but as the disease progresses the lucid periods get shorter until the patient lapses into coma. Hyperesthesia, with excessive sensitivity to bright light, loud noise, touch, and even gentle breezes, is very common. On physical examination, the temperature may be found to be as high as 40.6°C (105°F). Abnormalities of the autonomic nervous system include dilated irregular pupils; increased lacrimation, salivation, and perspiration; and postural hypotension. Evidence of upper motor neuron paralysis, with weakness, increased deep tendon reflexes, and extensor plantar responses, is the rule. Paralysis of the vocal cords is common. Unfortunately, the presenting signs and symptoms of rabies are indistinguishable from those of other viral and neurologic diseases. Thus delays in diagnosis are frequent. The presence of hydrophobia or aerophobia (seen in about two-thirds of recent cases) increases the likelihood of antemortem diagnosis.

The manifestations of brainstem dysfunction begin shortly after the onset of the encephalitic phase. Cranial nerve involvement causes diplopia, facial palsies, optic neuritis, and the characteristic difficulty with deglutition. The combination of excessive salivation and difficulty in swallowing produces the traditional picture of "foaming at the mouth." Hydrophobia—the painful, violent, involuntary contraction of the diaphragmatic, accessory respiratory, pharyngeal, and laryngeal muscles initiated by swallowing liquids—is seen in ~50% of cases. Involvement of the amygdaloid nucleus may result in priapism and spontaneous ejaculation. The patient lapses into coma, and involvement of the respiratory center produces an apneic death. The prominence of early brainstem dysfunction distinguishes rabies from other viral encephalitides and accounts for the rapid downhill course. The median period of survival after the onset of symptoms is 4 days, with a maximum of 20 days, unless artificial supportive measures are instituted.

If intensive respiratory support is used, a number of late complications may appear. These include inappropriate secretion of antidiuretic hormone, diabetes insipidus, cardiac arrhythmias, vascular instability, adult respiratory distress syndrome, gastrointestinal bleeding, thrombocytopenia, and paralytic ileus. Recovery is very rare and, when it occurs, gradual.

Rabies may also present as an ascending paralysis resembling the Landry/Guillain-Barré syndrome (dumb rabies, *rage tranquille*). Initially, this clinical pattern was reported most frequently among persons given PEP after being bitten by vampire bats. Paralytic rabies also occurs in Southeast Asia among persons with canine exposures. The difficulty of diagnosing rabies associated with ascending paralysis is illustrated by cases of person-to-person transmission of the virus by tissue transplantation. Corneal transplants from donors who died of presumed Landry/Guillain-Barré syndrome produced clinical rabies in and caused the deaths of the recipients. Retrospective pathologic examinations of the brains of recipients demonstrated Negri bodies, and rabies virus was subsequently isolated from each donor's frozen eye.

LABORATORY FINDINGS During the early clinical period of rabies infection, laboratory findings—like signs and symptoms—are nonspecific. Complete blood cell counts and differentials are compatible with an acute viral illness. As with encephalitis or meningitis of any viral etiology, there is mild pleocytosis (>5 cells/μL) in the cerebrospinal fluid (CSF), with lymphocytosis. The CSF protein level may be mildly elevated, but the glucose level is generally normal. A decreased level of glucose in the CSF suggests the possibility of fungal, tuberculous, parasitic, leptospiral, syphilitic, sarcoid, or neoplastic meningitis. Severe pleocytosis (>1000 cells/μL) is compatible with nonviral and other inflammatory etiologies. The presence of large numbers of polymorphonuclear cells is indicative of bacterial infection, leptospirosis, amebic infection, and some noninfectious processes.

The most critical laboratory findings in suspected cases of human rabies are those that permit the exclusion of other etiologies (i.e., the most common sources of encephalitis) and that document a rapidly deteriorating clinical course compatible with rabies (see "Differential Diagnosis," below). Antemortem diagnosis of human rabies can be arranged through consultation with the relevant state health department and the Centers for Disease Control and Prevention (CDC). Such a diagnosis requires samples of the patient's CSF and serum (preferably paired), fresh saliva, and a full-thickness skin biopsy sample from the nape of the neck. If a patient dies during the effort to rule out rabies, fresh brain material is the optimal sample for a definitive postmortem diagnosis.

Rabies Virus–Specific Antibodies in Serum and CSF Since rabies virus remains in the "immunologically privileged" CNS (with no viremia), the infection is largely undetected by the immune system until late in the clinical course. Once encephalitis develops, immune surveillance within the CNS is substantially heightened and viral antigen is widespread, resulting in the development of an antibody response and the influx of cytotoxic T cells. Thus, rabies virus–specific antibodies in serum and CSF develop relatively late in the clinical course and, when the patient dies during the acute phase, may be undetectable.

Two laboratory methods are commonly used to detect rabies virus–specific antibodies. The *indirect fluorescent antibody test* involves the addition of dilutions of test serum to plates with wells containing rabies virus–infected cells. If rabies antigen–specific antibodies are present in the serum, they bind to infected cells. The bound antibody is then detected with fluorescein-tagged antihuman antibodies. This rapid test predominantly detects antibodies to the rabies virus nucleoprotein. The *rapid fluorescent focus inhibition test* (RFFIT) is a valuable but labor-intensive method that takes 1 day to complete. The RFFIT requires that a fixed amount of live rabies virus and dilutions of test serum be added to cell monolayers and allowed to incubate for 20 h. If neutralizing antibodies to the rabies virus glycoprotein are present in the patient's serum, few or no infected foci are seen when the direct fluorescent antibody (DFA) test is applied to the cell monolayer, because the viral particles will have been neutralized by antibodies and prevented from infecting cells. Rabies virus–specific antibodies may be found in serum as a result of previous vaccination against rabies. In contrast, the occurrence of rabies virus antibodies in the CSF is diagnostic for rabies (or, in extremely rare cases, indicative of previous exposure to and survival of rabies virus), since antibodies from vaccination do not cross an intact blood-brain barrier.

Reverse-Transcription Polymerase Chain Reaction (RT-PCR) on Fresh Saliva Viral shedding in the saliva directly precedes and accompanies the development of clinical signs in animals and probably in humans as well. During early CNS infection, the host may appear normal, but virus may already be present in the saliva as a result of centrifugal spread. With the exquisitely sensitive RT-PCR, the presence of rabies virus nucleic acid in fresh saliva can be confirmed or ruled out. If testing is performed very early in the clinical course, additional samples may need to be evaluated, because viral shedding may be intermittent at this time.

DFA Testing and RT-PCR on a Skin Biopsy Sample As a result of wide centrifugal spread, the rabies virus genome and antigen may be detectable in a skin biopsy from the nape of the patient's neck during the clinical course of suspected rabies. With the DFA test, viral antigen may be demonstrated in peripheral nerves associated with hair follicles in the skin sample. RT-PCR has shown greater sensitivity for detection of rabies genomic material in skin samples.

Other Tests Although patients with encephalitis are invariably evaluated with advanced tests (e.g., magnetic resonance imaging, computed tomography, electroencephalography, evoked response studies, electromyography, and nerve conduction studies), the results are nondiagnostic for rabies.

DIFFERENTIAL DIAGNOSIS The differential diagnosis in a case of suspected human rabies may initially include any cause of encephalitis, particularly infection with viruses such as herpesviruses, enteroviruses, and arboviruses (e.g., West Nile virus). The most important viruses to rule out are herpes simplex virus type 1, varicella-zoster virus, and (less commonly) enteroviruses, including coxsackieviruses, echoviruses, polioviruses, and human enteroviruses 68 to 71. A specific diagnosis may be made by a variety of diagnostic techniques, including CSF PCR testing, culture, and serology. In addition, consideration should be given to the local epidemiology of encephalitis caused by arboviruses belonging to several taxonomic groups, including eastern and western equine encephalitis viruses, St. Louis encephalitis virus, Powassan virus, the California encephalitis virus serogroup, and La Crosse virus.

New causes of viral encephalitis are also possible, as was evidenced by the recent outbreak in Malaysia of ~300 cases of encephalitis (mortality rate, 40%) caused by Nipah virus, a new paramyxovirus. Similarly, well-known viruses may be introduced into new locations, as is illustrated by the recent outbreak of encephalitis due to West Nile virus in the eastern United States. Epidemiologic factors (e.g., season, geographic location, and the patient's age, travel history, and possible exposure to animal bites, rodents, and ticks) may help direct the diagnostic workup.

℞ TREATMENT

There is no specific treatment for clinical rabies. Death is virtually inevitable once clinical signs develop. Medical management is supportive and palliative.

POSTEXPOSURE PROPHYLAXIS When an exposure to rabies is recognized, immediate and thorough wound cleansing and the prompt administration of PEP (Table 179-2) are extremely effective in preventing infection. With regard to the prevention of human rabies in developed countries, recognition of a potential exposure and its distinction from circumstances in which no exposure has occurred are key steps in the judicious administration of rabies biologics. In developing countries, the prevention of rabies is hindered by economic conditions and inadequate access to modern biologics.

Unprovoked bites, especially if severe and multiple, by a confirmed rabid animal constitute the most obvious and highest-risk route of exposure to rabies. As stated in the recommendations of the Advisory Committee on Immunization Practices (ACIP, Table 179-2), simply touching a rabid animal (or person) does not constitute an exposure to rabies. Rabies virus forms an infectious aerosol only under intentional

TABLE 179-2 *Rabies Postexposure Prophylaxis Guide—United States*

Animal Type	Evaluation and Disposition of Animal	Postexposure Prophylaxis Recommendations
Dogs, cats, and ferrets	Healthy and available for 10 days observation	No treatment is necessary unless animal develops clinical signs of rabies.[a]
	Rabid or suspected rabid	Begin PEP.
	Unknown (e.g., escaped)	Consult public health officials.
Skunks, raccoons, foxes, and most other carnivores; bats	Regarded as rabid unless animal proven negative by laboratory tests[b]	Consider immediate vaccination.
Livestock, small rodents, lagomorphs (rabbits and hares), large rodents (woodchucks and beavers), and other mammals	Consider individually	Consult public health officials. Bites of squirrels, hamsters, guinea pigs, gerbils, chipmunks, rats, mice, other small rodents, small rodents, rabbits, and hares almost never require antirabies postexposure prophylaxis.

[a] During the 10-day observation period, begin postexposure prophylaxis at the first sign of rabies in a dog, cat, or ferret that has bitten someone. If the animal exhibits clinical signs of rabies, it should be euthanized immediately and tested.

[b] The animal should be euthanized and tested as soon as possible. Holding for observation is not recommended. Discontinue vaccine if immunofluorescence test results of the animal are negative.

Source: Human rabies prevention—United States, 1999. Recommendations of the Advisory Committee on Immunization Practices (ACIP). MMWR Recomm Rep 48(RR-1): 1-21, 1999; erratum in MMWR 48(1):16, 1999; MMWR 49(32):737, 2000.

or highly unnatural conditions. The only cases in which the aerosol route has been implicated are laboratory accidents and the Frio cave incidents of 50 years ago; in the latter situation, other routes of exposure for the bat biologists (e.g., bat bites or—in one person—contamination of an excoriated area of eczema) could not be ruled out. Contamination of mucous membranes with infectious material is considered an exposure to rabies because of observations in various species of occasional rabies cases resulting from intentional oral or intranasal exposure to high titers of virus; however, the majority of animals so exposed are unaffected, and a few such animals even develop immunity to rabies. Limited laboratory experiments with direct ocular exposure to rabies in one animal species did not result in viral infection; nevertheless, ocular contact with potentially contaminated material is considered an exposure because of the historic occurrence of human rabies cases after the transplantation of corneas from donors retrospectively diagnosed with rabies. Contamination of a fresh wound with infectious material (brain, salivary gland, or other innervated tissue from a rabid animal) constitutes an exposure to rabies.

Once the possibility of exposure has been identified, the wound should be thoroughly scrubbed with soap and then flushed with water. Both mechanical cleansing and chemical cleansing are important. Quaternary ammonium compounds such as 1 to 4% benzalkonium chloride, 1% cetrimonium bromide, or povidone-iodine solutions should be used. Tetanus toxoid and antibiotic prophylaxis should be administered as needed.

With an established exposure, the decision to administer human rabies biologics is straightforward if the animal is available for rabies diagnosis (i.e., euthanasia, brain removal, and laboratory testing). In dogs, cats, and ferrets in the United States, the potential shedding period indicates the adequacy of observation of the animal for 10 days after a bite to a human. If the animal remains clinically normal, laboratory and epidemiologic data indicate no risk of rabies exposure through the bite (although clearly, if unvaccinated, the animal may develop rabies in the future). If the animal develops signs suggestive

of rabies, it should be euthanized and tested immediately, and the human victim should be treated according to the laboratory test result. If the animal is unavailable, the decision to treat depends upon the risk of rabies in the individual animal, the local epizootiology of rabies and the consequent risk to the individual animal, the potential route of exposure (i.e., multiple severe bites vs. potential contamination of mucous membranes with infectious material), and other factors. This decision may best be made in consultation with local, state, and federal public health professionals who have specialized knowledge of these variables.

Human rabies PEP consists of five doses of a modern cell culture vaccine, of which two types are commonly available for use in the United States (Table 179-3). The current cell culture vaccines are virtually equivalent in their unfailing potency and relative paucity of adverse effects. A reaction compatible with delayed-type hypersensitivity may occur in up to 12% of patients receiving human diploid cell vaccine; continuation of the pre- or postexposure series with an alternative vaccine may be sufficient for the resolution of this reaction. Doses are administered on a schedule of 0, 3, 7, 14, and 28 days. In addition to vaccine on day 0, one dose of human rabies immune globulin (20 IU/kg) should be given; as much of the dose as is anatomically feasible should be administered at the site of the bite, with any excess administered intramuscularly at a distant site—e.g., in the deltoid opposite the vaccine site. Periodically, human rabies immune globulin is in short supply. If it is not immediately available, the vaccine series should be initiated and the rabies immune globulin may be added at any point through day 7. After day 7, it is not necessary to add rabies immune globulin to the patient's regimen because endogenous antibodies are being produced and exogenous antibodies may actually be counterproductive. If a patient presents at a long interval after a potential exposure, it is not too late to initiate full human PEP unless clinical signs are present.

PREEXPOSURE RABIES VACCINATION Preexposure rabies vaccination is available to persons at risk of rabies exposure. The ACIP recommends a series of 1-mL doses of modern cell culture vaccine administered intramuscularly on days 0, 7, and 21 or 28. Once immunized against rabies with potent vaccines, individuals are primed against rabies for the rest of their lives. If an exposure occurs, a previously immunized

TABLE 179-3 *Commonly Available Human Rabies Biologics*

Vaccine Type	Product	Source
AVAILABLE IN UNITED STATES		
Human rabies vaccine		
Rabies vaccine, human diploid cell (HDCV), IM	Imovax Rabies	Aventis-Pasteur[a]
Rabies vaccine, purified chick embryo cell (PCEC), IM	RabAvert	Chiron Behring GmbH[b]
Rabies immune globulin, human (RIG)	Imogam Rabies-HT	Aventis-Pasteur[a]
	BayRab	Bayer Corporation Pharmaceutical Division[c]
CELL CULTURE RABIES VACCINES WIDELY AVAILABLE OUTSIDE UNITED STATES		
Purified chick embryo cell vaccine (PCEC)	Rabipur	
Purified Vero cell vaccine (PVRV)	Verorab Imovax-Rabies Vero TRC Verorab	
Human diploid cell vaccine (HDCV)	Rabivac	
Purified duck embryo vaccine (PDEV)	Lyssavac N	

[a] Phone: 1-800-VACCINE.
[b] Phone: 1-800-CHIRON8.
[c] Phone: 1-800-288-8370.

person should receive postexposure boosters consisting of two doses 3 days apart. Persons in the high-risk and moderate-risk rabies exposure categories should have their rabies virus–neutralizing antibody titers monitored every 6 months and every 2 years, respectively. Persons in the low-exposure category do not require serologic monitoring but, like all previously immunized persons, must receive the two booster vaccinations upon exposure to rabies. Moreover, appropriate wound care (i.e., copious flushing and the use of soap or detergent) remains critical.

MOKOLA VIRUS

Mokola virus was first isolated from wild shrews captured in Nigeria and was shown to be related morphologically and serologically to rabies virus. The subsequent isolation of the virus from cats in South Africa suggested a wider prevalence of the agent than had previously been expected. Only two cases of clinical infection have been reported; both were in children. One patient had a nonfatal illness characterized by fever, pharyngitis, and convulsions; Mokola virus was recovered from CSF. In the second patient, fever with cough and vomiting was followed within several days by drowsiness, confusion, and generalized flaccid weakness. The CSF was normal. The patient progressed to deep coma and died within 10 days of onset. Mokola virus was isolated from the brain, and examination of histopathologic sections revealed finely granular cytoplasmic inclusions that were distinguishable from Negri bodies in many neurons.

VESICULAR STOMATITIS VIRUS

Vesicular stomatitis is a viral illness of animals that occasionally affects humans. It presents as an acute, self-limited, influenza-like disease. The disease in animals is found in the United States and South America and affects chiefly domestic cattle, horses, swine, wild deer, raccoons, skunks, and bobcats.

In animals, vesicular stomatitis is characterized by the development of vesicles on the oral mucosa, particularly the tongue; the udders; and the heels. The mode of spread is probably by direct contact; however, epidemics tend to occur in warm weather, and isolation of the virus from *Phlebotomus* sandflies in Panama and *Aedes* mosquitoes in New Mexico suggests that these insects may be vectors. Two distinct types, New Jersey and Indiana, have been recognized, and most outbreaks in North America have been attributed to the New Jersey strain.

In humans, vesicular stomatitis is most common among laboratory workers. In one report, three-fourths of laboratory personnel handling experimentally infected animals or manipulating the virus developed neutralizing antibodies. The disease is also transmissible, however, under natural conditions among workers having direct contact with infected animals, especially cattle. An incubation period ranging from 1 to 6 days is followed by the sudden onset of fever [with temperatures of up to 40°C (104°F)], chills, profuse sweating, myalgias, malaise, headache, and pain on ocular movement. One-third to one-half of patients have a sore throat and cervical and/or submandibular adenopathy. Small raised vesicular lesions may appear on the buccal mucosa. Conjunctivitis and coryza are evident in ~20% of cases. Small subcorneal, intraepithelial vesicles occasionally appear on the fingers, usually in association with direct inoculation of the virus. Symptoms generally last 3 to 4 days, but occasionally the course is diphasic. Inapparent infection is common: among laboratory workers with serologic evidence of infection, only about one-half report symptoms. In some areas of Panama, 17 to 35% of the population have neutralizing antibodies to vesicular stomatitis virus.

The differential diagnosis includes hand-foot-and-mouth disease, herpangina, primary herpetic pharyngitis and other mucocutaneous syndromes, and influenza. The virus is not commonly isolated from patients. However, a rise in titer of complement-fixation and/or neutralizing antibody to vesicular stomatitis virus between acute- and convalescent-phase sera helps to confirm the diagnosis. Treatment is nonspecific.

FURTHER READING

CENTERS FOR DISEASE CONTROL AND PREVENTION: Human rabies—Iowa, 2002. MMWR 52:47, 2003

———: First human rabies case associated with raccoon rabies—Virginia, 2003. MMWR 52:1102, 2003

———: Human rabies prevention—United States, 1999: Recommendations of the Advisory Committee on Immunization Practices (ACIP). MMWR 48(RR-1), 1999

CONSTANTINE DG: Geographic translocation of bats: Known and potential problems. Emerg Infect Dis 9:17, 2003

JACKSON AC et al: Management of rabies in humans. Clin Infect Dis 36:60, 2003

KREBS JW et al: Rabies surveillance in the United States during 2002. J Am Vet Med Assoc 223:1736, 2003

KUZMIN IV et al: Bat lyssaviruses (Aravan and Khujand) from Central Asia: Phylogenetic relationships according to N, P, and G gene sequences. Virus Res 97:65, 2003

——— et al: Novel lyssaviruses isolated from bats in Russia. Emerg Infect Dis 9:1623, 2003

MESSENGER SL et al: Emerging epidemiology of bat-associated cryptic cases of rabies in the United States. Clin Infect Dis 35:738, 2002

NOAH DL et al: Epidemiology of human rabies in the United States, 1980 to 1996. Ann Intern Med 128:922, 1998

Some viruses are transmitted in nature without regard to humans and only incidentally infect and produce disease in humans; in addition, a few agents are regularly spread among humans by arthropods. Most of these viruses either are maintained by arthropods or chronically infect rodents. Obviously, the mode of transmission is not a rational basis for taxonomic classification. Indeed, zoonotic viruses from at least seven virus families act as significant human pathogens (Table 180-1). The virus families differ fundamentally from one another in terms of morphology, replication mechanisms, and genetics. Information on a virus's membership in a family or genus is enlightening with regard to maintenance strategies, sensitivity to antivirals, and some aspects of pathogenesis but does not necessarily predict which clinical syndromes—if any—the virus will cause in humans.

FAMILIES OF ARTHROPOD- AND RODENT-BORNE VIRUSES (Table 180-1)

■ **The Arenaviridae** The Arenaviridae are spherical, 110- to 130-nm particles that bud from the cell's plasma membrane and utilize ambisense RNA genomes with two segments for replication. There are two main phylogenetic branches of Arenaviridae: the Old World viruses, such as Lassa fever and lymphocytic choriomeningitis (LCM) viruses, and the New World viruses, including those causing the South American hemorrhagic fevers (HFs). Arenaviruses persist in nature by chronically infecting rodents with a striking one-virus–one-rodent species relationship. These rodent infections result in long-term virus excretion and perhaps in lifelong viremia; vertical infection is common with some arenaviruses. Humans become infected through the inhalation of aerosols containing arenaviruses, which are then deposited in the terminal air passages, and probably also through close contact with

rodents and their excreta, which results in the contamination of mucous membranes or breaks in the skin.

The Bunyaviridae The family Bunyaviridae includes four medically significant genera. All of these spherical viruses have three negative-sense RNA segments maturing into 90- to 120-nm particles in the Golgi complex and exiting the cell by exocytosis. Viruses of the genus *Bunyavirus* are largely mosquito-borne and have a viremic vertebrate intermediate host; many are also transovarially transmitted in their specific mosquito host. One serologic group also uses biting midges as vectors. Sandflies or mosquitoes are the vectors for the genus *Phlebovirus* (named after phlebotomus fever or sandfly fever, the best-known disease associated with the genus), while ticks serve as vectors for the genus *Nairovirus*. Viruses of both of these genera are also associated with vertical transmission in the arthropod host and with horizontal spread through viremic vertebrate hosts. The genus *Hantavirus* is unique among the Bunyaviridae in that it is not transmitted by arthropods but is maintained in nature by rodent hosts that chronically shed virus. Like the arenaviruses, the hantaviruses usually display striking virus-rodent species specificity. Hantaviruses do not cause chronic viremia in their rodent hosts and are transmitted only horizontally from rodent to rodent.

Other Families The Flaviviridae are positive-sense, single-strand RNA viruses that form particles of 40 to 50 nm in the endoplasmic reticulum. The flaviviruses discussed here are from the genus *Flavivirus* and make up two phylogenetically and antigenically distinct divisions transmitted among vertebrates by mosquitoes and ticks, respectively.

TABLE 180-1 *Major Zoonotic Virus Families and Some Characteristics of Typical Members*

Family	Genus or Group	Syndrome(s): Typical Viruses	Maintenance Strategy
Arenaviridae	Old World complex	FM, E: Lymphocytic choriomeningitis virus HF: Lassa fever virus	Chronic infection of rodents, often with persistent viremia; vertical transmission common
	New World or Tacaribe complex	HF: South American HF viruses (Machupo, Junin, Guanarito, Sabia)	Chronic infection of rodents, sometimes with persistent viremia; vertical infection may occur
Bunyaviridae	*Bunyavirus*	E: California serogroup viruses (La Crosse, Jamestown Canyon, California encephalitis) FM: Bunyamwera, group C, Tahyna viruses	Mosquito-vertebrate cycle; transovarial transmission in mosquito common
		FM: Oropouche virus	Transmitted by *Culicoides*
	Phlebovirus	FM: Sandfly fever, Toscana viruses FM: Punta Toro virus	Sandfly transmission between vertebrates, with prominent transovarial component in sandfly
		HF, FM, E: Rift Valley fever virus	Mosquito-vertebrate transmission, with transovarial component in mosquito
	Nairovirus	HF: Crimean-Congo HF virus	Tick-vertebrate, with transovarial transmission in tick
	Hantavirus	HF: Hantaan, Dobrava, Puumala viruses	Rodent reservoir; chronic virus shedding, but chronic viremia unknown
		HF: Sin Nombre and related hantaviruses	Sigmodontine rodent reservoir
Filoviridae[a]		HF: Marburg viruses, Ebola viruses (4 subtypes)	Unknown
Flaviviridae	*Flavivirus* (mosquito-borne)	HF: Yellow fever virus	Mosquito-vertebrate; transovarial rare
		FM, HF: Dengue viruses (4 subtypes)	
		E: St. Louis, Japanese, West Nile, and Murray Valley encephalitis viruses; Rocio viruses	
	Flavivirus (tick-borne)	E: Central European tick-borne encephalitis, Russian spring-summer encephalitis, Powassan viruses	Tick-vertebrate
		HF: Omsk HF, Kyasanur Forest disease viruses	
Reoviridae	*Coltivirus*	FM, E: Colorado tick fever virus	Tick-vertebrate
	Orbivirus	FM, E: Orungo, Kemerova viruses	Arthropod-vertebrate
Rhabdoviridae[b]	*Vesiculovirus*	FM: Vesicular stomatitis virus (Indiana, New Jersey); Chandipura, Piry viruses	Sandfly-vertebrate, with prominent transovarial component in sandfly
Togaviridae	*Alphavirus*	AR: Sindbis, chikungunya, Mayaro, Ross River, Barmah Forest viruses	Mosquito-vertebrate
		E: Eastern, western, and Venezuelan equine encephalitis viruses	

[a] The Filoviridae are discussed in Chap. 181.
[b] The Rhabdoviridae are discussed in Chap. 179.

Note: Abbreviations refer to the disease syndrome most commonly associated with the virus: FM, fever, myalgia; AR, arthritis, rash; E, encephalitis; HF, hemorrhagic fever.

The mosquito-borne viruses fall into phylogenetic groups that include yellow fever virus, the four dengue viruses, and encephalitis viruses, while the tick-borne group encompasses a geographically varied spectrum of species, some of which are responsible for encephalitis or for hemorrhagic disease with encephalitis. The Reoviridae are double-strand RNA viruses with multisegmented genomes. These 80-nm particles are the only viruses discussed in this chapter that do not have a lipid envelope and thus are insensitive to detergents. The Togaviridae have a single positive-strand RNA genome and bud particles of ~60 to 70 nm from the plasma membrane. The togaviruses discussed here are all members of the genus *Alphavirus* and are transmitted among vertebrates by mosquitoes in their natural cycle. →*The Filoviridae and the Rhabdoviridae are discussed in Chaps. 181 and 179, respectively.*

PROMINENT FEATURES OF ARTHROPOD- AND RODENT-BORNE VIRUSES Although this chapter discusses the major features of selected arthropod- and rodent-borne viruses, it does not deal with >500 other distinct recognized zoonotic viruses, about one-fourth of which infect humans. Zoonotic viruses are undergoing genetic evolution, "new" zoonotic viruses are being discovered, and the epidemiology of zoonotic viruses is continuing to evolve through environmental changes affecting vectors, reservoirs, and humans. These zoonotic viruses are most numerous in the tropics but are also found in temperate and frigid climates. Their distribution and seasonal activity may be variable and often depend largely on ecologic conditions such as rainfall and temperature, which in turn affect the density of vectors and reservoirs and the development of infection therein.

Maintenance and Transmission Arthropod-borne viruses infect their vectors after the ingestion of a blood meal from a viremic vertebrate. The vectors then develop chronic, systemic infection as the viruses penetrate the gut and spread throughout the body. The viruses eventually reach the salivary glands during a period that is referred to as *extrinsic incubation* and that typically lasts 1 to 3 weeks in mosquitoes. At this point an arthropod is competent to continue the chain of transmission by infecting another vertebrate when a subsequent blood meal is taken.

The arthropod generally is unharmed by the infection, and the natural vertebrate partner usually has only transient viremia with no overt disease. An alternative mechanism for virus maintenance in its arthropod host is transovarial transmission, which is common among members of the family Bunyaviridae.

Rodent-borne viruses such as the hantaviruses and arenaviruses are maintained in nature by chronic infection transmitted between rodents. As in arthropod-borne virus cycles, there is usually a high degree of rodent-virus specificity, and there is no overt disease in the reservoir/vector.

Epidemiology The distribution of arthropod- and rodent-borne viruses is restricted by the areas inhabited by their reservoir/vectors and provides an important clue in the differential diagnosis. Table 180-2 shows the approximate geographic distribution of the most important of these viruses. Members of each family, each genus, and even each serologically related group usually occur in each area but may not be pathogenic in all areas or may not be a commonly recognized cause of disease in all areas and so may not be included in the table.

Most of these diseases are acquired in a rural setting; a few have urban vectors. Seoul, sandfly fever, and Oropouche viruses are examples of urban viruses, but the most notable are yellow fever, dengue, and chikungunya viruses. A history of mosquito bite has little diagnostic significance in the individual; a history of tick bite is more diagnostically specific. Rodent exposure is often reported by persons infected with an arenavirus or a hantavirus but again has little specificity. Indeed, aerosols may infect persons who have no recollection of having even seen rodents.

Syndromes Human disease caused by arthropod- and rodent-borne viruses is often subclinical. The spectrum of possible responses to infection is wide, and our knowledge of the outcome of most of these infections is limited. The usual disease syndromes associated with these viruses have been grouped into four categories: fever and myalgia, arthritis and rash, encephalitis, and hemorrhagic fever. Although for the purposes of this discussion most viruses have been placed in a single group, the categories often overlap. For example, West Nile and Venezuelan equine encephalitis viruses are discussed as encephalitis viruses, but during epidemics they may cause many cases of milder

TABLE 180-2 *Geographic Distribution of Some Important and Commonly Encountered Human Zoonotic Viral Diseases*

Area	Arenaviridae	Bunyaviridae	Flaviviridae	Rhabdoviridae	Togaviridae
North America	Lymphocytic choriomeningitis	La Crosse, Jamestown Canyon, California encephalitis; hantavirus pulmonary syndrome	St. Louis, Powassan, West Nile encephalitis; dengue	Vesicular stomatitis	Eastern, western equine encephalitis
South America	Bolivian, Argentine, Venezuelan, and Brazilian HF; lymphocytic choriomeningitis	Oropouche, group C, Punta Toro infection; hantavirus pulmonary syndrome	Yellow fever, dengue, Rocio virus infection	Vesicular stomatitis, Piry virus infection	Mayaro virus infection, Venezuelan equine encephalitis
Europe	Lymphocytic choriomeningitis	Tahyna, Toscana, sandfly fever, HF with renal syndrome	West Nile, Central European tick-borne, Russian spring-summer encephalitis	—	Sindbis virus infection
Middle East	—	Sandfly fever, Crimean-Congo HF	West Nile encephalitis, dengue	—	—
Eastern Asia	—	Sandfly fever; Hantaan, Seoul virus infection	Dengue; Japanese, Russian spring-summer encephalitis; Omsk HF	Chandipura virus infection	—
Southwestern Asia	—	Sandfly fever, Crimean-Congo HF	West Nile, Japanese encephalitis; dengue; Kyasanur Forest disease	—	Chikungunya
Southeast Asia	—	Seoul virus infection	Japanese encephalitis, dengue	—	Chikungunya
Africa	Lassa fever	Bunyamwera virus infection, Rift Valley fever	Yellow fever, dengue	—	Sindbis virus infection, chikungunya
Australia	—	—	Murray Valley encephalitis, dengue	—	Ross River, Barmah Forest virus infection

Note: HF, hemorrhagic fever.

febrile syndromes and relatively uncommon cases of encephalitis. Similarly, Rift Valley fever virus is best known as a cause of HF, but the attack rates for febrile disease are far higher, and encephalitis is occasionally seen as well. LCM virus is classified as a cause of fever and myalgia because this syndrome is its most common disease manifestation and because, even when central nervous system (CNS) disease occurs, it is usually mild and is preceded by fever and myalgia. Dengue virus infection is considered as a cause of fever and myalgia (dengue fever) because this is by far the most common manifestation worldwide and is the syndrome most likely to be seen in the United States; however, dengue HF is also discussed in the HF section because of its complicated pathogenesis and importance in pediatric practice in certain areas of the world.

Diagnosis Laboratory diagnosis is required in any given case, although epidemics occasionally provide clinical and epidemiologic clues on which an educated guess as to etiology can be based. For most arthropod- and rodent-borne viruses, acute-phase serum samples (collected within 3 or 4 days of onset) have yielded isolates, and paired sera have been used to demonstrate rising antibody titers by a variety of tests. Intensive efforts to develop rapid tests for HF have resulted in an antigen-detection enzyme-linked immunosorbent assay (ELISA) and an IgM-capture ELISA that can provide a diagnosis based on a single serum sample within a few hours and are particularly useful in severe cases. More sensitive reverse-transcription polymerase chain reaction (RT-PCR) tests may yield diagnoses based on samples without detectable antigen and may also provide useful genetic information about the virus. Hantavirus infections differ from others discussed here in that severe acute disease is immunopathologic; patients present with serum IgM that serves as the basis for a sensitive and specific test.

At diagnosis, patients with encephalitis are generally no longer viremic or antigenemic and usually do not have virus in cerebrospinal fluid (CSF). In this situation, the value of serologic methods and RT-PCR is being validated. IgM capture is increasingly being used for the simultaneous testing of serum and CSF. IgG ELISA or classic serology is useful in the evaluation of past exposure to the viruses, many of which circulate in areas with a minimal medical infrastructure and sometimes cause mild or subclinical infection.

The remainder of this chapter offers general descriptions of the broad syndromes caused by arthropod- and rodent-borne viruses. Most of the diseases under consideration have not been studied in detail with modern medical approaches; thus available data may be incomplete or biased.

FEVER AND MYALGIA

Fever and myalgia constitute the syndrome most commonly associated with zoonotic virus infection. Many of the numerous viruses belonging to the families listed in Table 180-1 probably cause this syndrome, but several viruses have been selected for inclusion in the table because of their prominent associations with the syndrome and their biomedical importance.

The syndrome typically begins with the abrupt onset of fever, chills, intense myalgia, and malaise. Patients may also report joint pains, but no true arthritis is detectable. Anorexia is characteristic and may be accompanied by nausea or even vomiting. Headache is common and may be severe, with photophobia and retroorbital pain. Physical findings are minimal and are usually confined to conjunctival injection with pain on palpation of muscles or the epigastrium. The duration of symptoms is quite variable but generally is 2 to 5 days, with a biphasic course in some instances. The spectrum of disease varies from subclinical to temporarily incapacitating.

Less constant findings include a maculopapular rash. Epistaxis may occur but does not necessarily indicate a bleeding diathesis. A minority of the cases caused by some viruses are known or suspected to include aseptic meningitis, but this diagnosis is difficult in remote areas, given the patients' photophobia and myalgia as well as the lack of opportunity to examine the CSF. Although pharyngitis may be noted or radiographic evidence of pulmonary infiltrates found in some cases,

these viruses are not primary respiratory pathogens. The differential diagnosis includes anicteric leptospirosis, rickettsial diseases, and the early stages of other syndromes discussed in this chapter. These diseases are often described as "flulike," but the usual absence of cough and coryza makes influenza an unlikely confounder except at the earliest stages.

Complete recovery is generally the outcome in this syndrome, although prolonged asthenia and nonspecific symptoms have been described in some cases, particularly after infection with LCM or dengue virus. Treatment is supportive, with aspirin avoided because of the potential for exacerbated bleeding and Reye's syndrome. Efforts at prevention are best based on vector control, which, however, may be expensive or impossible. For mosquito control, destruction of breeding sites is generally the most economically and environmentally sound approach. Measures taken by the individual to avoid the vector can be valuable. Avoiding the vector's habitat and times of peak activity, preventing the vector from entering dwellings by using screens or other barriers, judiciously applying arthropod repellents such as diethyltoluamide (DEET) to the skin, and wearing permethrin-impregnated clothing are all possible approaches, depending on the vector and its habits.

LYMPHOCYTIC CHORIOMENINGITIS LCM is transmitted from the common house mouse (*Mus musculus*) to humans by aerosols of excreta and secreta. LCM virus, an arenavirus, is maintained in the mouse mainly by vertical transmission from infected dams. The vertically infected mouse remains viremic for life, with high concentrations of virus in all tissues. Infected colonies of pet hamsters have also served as a link to humans. LCM virus is widely used in immunology laboratories as a model of T cell function and can silently infect cell cultures and passaged tumor lines, resulting in infections among scientists and animal caretakers. Patients with LCM may have a history of residence in rodent-infested housing or other exposure to rodents. An antibody prevalence of ~5 to 10% has been reported among adults from the United States, Argentina, and endemic areas of Germany.

LCM differs from the general syndrome of fever and myalgia in that its onset is gradual. Among the conditions occasionally associated with LCM are orchitis, transient alopecia, arthritis, pharyngitis, cough, and maculopapular rash. An estimated one-fourth of patients or fewer suffer a febrile phase of 3 to 6 days and then, after a brief remission, develop renewed fever accompanied by severe headache, nausea and vomiting, and meningeal signs lasting for about a week. These patients virtually always recover fully, as do the uncommon patients with clearcut signs of encephalitis. Recovery may be delayed by transient hydrocephalus.

During the initial febrile phase, leukopenia and thrombocytopenia are common and virus can usually be isolated from blood. During the CNS phase of the illness, virus may be found in the CSF, but antibodies are present in blood. The pathogenesis of LCM is thought to resemble that following direct intracranial inoculation of the virus into adult mice; the onset of the immune response leads to T cell–mediated immunopathologic meningitis. During the meningeal phase, CSF mononuclear-cell counts range from the hundreds to the low thousands per microliter, and hypoglycorrhachia is found in one-third of cases. The IgM-capture ELISA of serum and CSF is usually positive; RT-PCR assays have been developed for application to CSF.

Infection with LCM virus should be suspected in acutely ill febrile patients with marked leukopenia and thrombocytopenia. In cases of aseptic meningitis, any of the following should suggest LCM: well-marked febrile prodrome, adult age, autumn seasonality, low CSF glucose levels, or CSF mononuclear cell counts of $>1000/\mu L$.

In pregnant women, LCM virus infection may lead to fetal invasion with consequent congenital hydrocephalus and chorioretinitis. Since the maternal infection may be mild, consisting of only a short febrile illness, antibodies to the virus should be sought in both the mother and the fetus in suspicious circumstances, particularly TORCH-negative neonatal hydrocephalus. [TORCH is a battery of tests encompassing toxoplasmosis, other conditions (congenital syphilis and viruses), rubella, cytomegalovirus, and herpes simplex virus.]

SANDFLY FEVER   The sandfly *Phlebotomus papatasi* transmits sandfly fever. Female sandflies may be infected by the oral route as they take a blood meal and may transmit the virus to offspring when they lay their eggs after a second blood meal. This prominent transovarial pattern was the first to be recognized among dipterans and complicates virus control. A previous designation for sandfly fever, "3-day fever," instructively describes the brief, debilitating course associated with this essentially benign infection. There is neither a rash nor CNS involvement, and complete recovery is the rule.

Sandfly fever is found in the circum-Mediterranean area, extending to the east through the Balkans into China as well as into the Middle East and southwestern Asia. The vector is found in both rural and urban settings and is known for its small size, which enables it to penetrate standard mosquito screens and netting, and for its short flight range. Epidemics have been described in the wake of natural disasters and wars. In parts of Europe, sandfly populations and virus transmission were greatly reduced by the extensive residual spraying conducted after World War II to control malaria, and the incidence continues to be low. A common pattern of disease in endemic areas consists of high attack rates among travelers and military personnel with little or no disease in the local population, who are protected after childhood infection. More than 30 related phleboviruses are transmitted by sandflies and mosquitoes, but most are of unknown significance in terms of human health.

DENGUE FEVER   All four distinct dengue viruses (dengue 1–4) have *Aedes aegypti* as their principal vector, and all cause a similar clinical syndrome. In rare cases, second infection with a serotype of dengue virus different from that involved in the primary infection leads to dengue HF with severe shock (see below). Sporadic cases are seen in the settings of endemic transmission and epidemic disease. Year-round transmission between latitudes 25°N and 25°S has been established, and seasonal forays of the viruses to points as far north as Philadelphia are thought to have taken place in the United States. Dengue fever is seen in the Caribbean region, including Puerto Rico. With increasing spread of the vector mosquito throughout the tropics and subtropics, large areas of the world have become vulnerable to the introduction of dengue viruses, particularly through air travel by infected humans, and both dengue fever and the related dengue HF are becoming increasingly common. Conditions favorable to dengue transmission exist in the southern United States, and bursts of dengue fever activity are to be expected in this region, particularly along the Mexican border, where water may be stored in containers and *A. aegypti* numbers may therefore be greatest: this mosquito, which is also an efficient vector of the yellow fever and chikungunya viruses, typically breeds near human habitation, using relatively fresh water from sources such as water jars, vases, discarded containers, coconut husks, and old tires. *A. aegypti* usually inhabits dwellings and bites during the day.

After an incubation period of 2 to 7 days, the typical patient experiences the sudden onset of fever, headache, retroorbital pain, and back pain along with the severe myalgia that gave rise to the colloquial designation "break-bone fever." There is often a macular rash on the first day as well as adenopathy, palatal vesicles, and scleral injection. The illness may last a week, with additional symptoms usually including anorexia, nausea or vomiting, marked cutaneous hypersensitivity, and—near the time of defervescence—a maculopapular rash beginning on the trunk and spreading to the extremities and the face. Epistaxis and scattered petechiae are often noted in uncomplicated dengue, and preexisting gastrointestinal lesions may bleed during the acute illness.

Laboratory findings include leukopenia, thrombocytopenia, and, in many cases, serum aminotransferase elevations. The diagnosis is made by IgM ELISA or paired serology during recovery or by antigen-detection ELISA or RT-PCR during the acute phase. Virus is readily isolated from blood in the acute phase if mosquito inoculation or mosquito cell culture is used.

COLORADO TICK FEVER   Several hundred cases of Colorado tick fever are reported annually in the United States. The infection is acquired between March and November through the bite of an infected *Dermacentor andersoni* tick in mountainous western regions at altitudes of 1200 to 3000 m (4000 to 10,000 ft). Small mammals serve as the amplifying host. The most common presentation consists of fever and myalgia; meningoencephalitis is not uncommon, and hemorrhagic disease, pericarditis, myocarditis, orchitis, and pulmonary presentations are also reported. Rash develops in a substantial minority of cases. The disease usually lasts 7 to 10 days and is often biphasic. The most important differential diagnostic considerations since the beginning of the twentieth century have been Rocky Mountain spotted fever and tularemia. In Colorado, Colorado tick fever is much more common than Rocky Mountain spotted fever.

Infection of erythroblasts and other marrow cells by Colorado tick fever virus results in the appearance and persistence (for several weeks) of erythrocytes containing the virus. This feature, detected in smears stained by immunofluorescence, can be diagnostically helpful. The clinical laboratory detects leukopenia and thrombocytopenia.

OTHER VIRUSES CAUSING FEVER AND MYALGIA   For a discussion of additional zoonotic viral infections presenting with fever and myalgia, see Chap. 180 in *Harrison's Online* (*www.harrisonsonline.com*).

ENCEPHALITIS

Arboviral encephalitis is a seasonal disease, commonly occurring in the warmer months. Its incidence varies markedly with time and place, depending on ecologic factors. The causative viruses differ substantially in terms of case-infection ratio (i.e., the ratio of clinical to subclinical infections), mortality, and residua (Table 180-3). Humans are not an important amplifier of these viruses.

All the viral encephalitides discussed in this section have a similar pathogenesis as far as is known. An infected arthropod ingests a blood meal from a human and infects the host. The initial period of viremia is thought to originate most commonly from the lymphoid system. Viremia leads to CNS invasion, presumably through infection of olfactory neuroepithelium with passage through the cribriform plate or through infection of brain capillaries and multifocal entry into the CNS. During the viremic phase, there may be little or no recognized disease except in the case of tick-borne flaviviral encephalitis, in which there may be a clearly delineated phase of fever and systemic illness. The disease process in the CNS arises partly from direct neuronal infection and subsequent damage and partly from edema, inflammation, and other indirect effects. The usual pathologic picture is one of focal necrosis of neurons, inflammatory glial nodules, and perivascular lymphoid cuffing; the severity and distribution of these abnormalities vary with the infecting virus. Involved areas display the "luxury perfusion" phenomenon, with normal or increased total blood flow and low oxygen extraction.

The typical patient presents with a prodrome of nonspecific constitutional symptoms, including fever, abdominal pain, vertigo, sore throat, and respiratory symptoms. Headache, meningeal signs, photophobia, and vomiting follow quickly. Involvement of deeper structures may be signaled by lethargy, somnolence, and intellectual deficit (as disclosed by the mental status examination or failure at serial 7 subtraction); more severely affected patients will be obviously disoriented and may be comatose. Tremors, loss of abdominal reflexes, cranial nerve palsies, hemiparesis, monoparesis, difficulty in swallowing, and frontal lobe signs are all common. Spinal and motor neuron diseases are documented with West Nile and Japanese encephalitis viruses. Convulsions and focal signs may be evident early or may appear during the course of the disease. Some patients present with an abrupt onset of fever, convulsions, and other signs of CNS involvement. The results of human infection range from no significant symptoms through febrile headache to aseptic meningitis and finally to

TABLE 180-3 Prominent Features of Arboviral Encephalitis

Virus	Natural Cycle	Incubation Period, Days	Annual No. of Cases	Case-to-Infection Ratio	Age of Cases	Case-Fatality Rate, %	Residua
La Crosse	*Aedes triseriatus–*chipmunk (transovarial component in mosquito also important)	~3–7	70 (U.S.)	<1:1000	<15 years	<0.5	Recurrent seizures in ~10%; severe deficits in rare cases; decreased school performance and behavioral change suspected in small proportion
St. Louis	*Culex tarsalis, C. pipiens, C. quinquefasciatus–*birds	4–21	85, with hundreds to thousands in epidemic years (U.S.)	<1:200	Milder cases in the young; more severe cases in adults >40 years old, particularly the elderly	7	Common in the elderly
Japanese	*Culex tritaeniorhyncus–*birds	5–15	>25,000	1:200–300	All ages; children in highly endemic areas	20–50	Common (approximately half of cases); may be severe
West Nile	*Culex* mosquitoes–birds	3–6	?	Very low	Mainly the elderly	5–10	Uncommon
Central European	*Ixodes ricinus–*rodents, insectivores	7–14	Thousands	1:12	All ages; milder in children	1–5	20%
Russian spring-summer	*I. persulcatus–*rodents, insectivores	7–14	Hundreds	—	All ages; milder in children	20	Approximately half of cases; often severe; limb-girdle paralysis
Powassan	*I. cookei–*wild mammals	~10	~1 (U.S.)	—	All ages; some predilection for children	~10	Common (approximately half of cases)
Eastern equine	*Culiseta melanura–*birds	~5–10	5 (U.S.)	1:40 adult 1:17 child	All ages; predilection for children	50–75	Common
Western equine	*Culex tarsalis–*birds	~5–10	~20 (U.S.)	1:1000 adult 1:50 child 1:1 infant	All ages; predilection for children <2 years old (increased mortality in elderly)	3–7	Common only among infants <1 year old
Venezuelan equine (epidemic)	Unknown (multiple mosquito species and horses in epidemics)	1–5	?	1:250 adult 1:25 child (approximate)	All ages; predilection for children	~10	—

full-blown encephalitis; the proportions and severity of these manifestations vary with the infecting virus.

The acute encephalitis usually lasts from a few days to as long as 2 to 3 weeks, but recovery may be slow, with weeks or months required for the return of maximal recoupable function. Common complaints during recovery include difficulty concentrating, fatigability, tremors, and personality changes. The acute illness requires management of a comatose patient who may have intracranial pressure elevations, inappropriate secretion of antidiuretic hormone, respiratory failure, and convulsions. There is no specific therapy for these viral encephalitides. The only practical preventive measures are vector management and personal protection against the arthropod transmitting the virus; for Japanese encephalitis or tick-borne encephalitis, vaccination should be considered in certain circumstances (see relevant sections below).

The diagnosis of arboviral encephalitis depends on the careful evaluation of a febrile patient with CNS disease, with rapid identification of treatable herpes simplex encephalitis, ruling out of brain abscess, exclusion of bacterial meningitis by serial CSF examination, and performance of laboratory studies to define the viral etiology. Leptospirosis, neurosyphilis, Lyme disease, cat-scratch fever, and newer viral encephalitides such as Nipah virus infection from Malaysia should be considered. The CSF examination usually shows a modest cell count—in the tens or hundreds or perhaps a few thousand. Early in the process, a significant proportion of these cells may be polymorphonuclear leukocytes, but usually there is a mononuclear cell predominance. CSF glucose levels are usually normal. There are exceptions to this pattern of findings. In eastern equine encephalitis, for example, polymorphonuclear leukocytes may predominate during the first 72 h of disease and hypoglycorrhachia may be detected. In LCM, lymphocyte counts may be in the thousands, and the glucose concen-

tration may be diminished. Experience with imaging studies is still evolving; clearly, however, both computed tomography (CT) and magnetic resonance imaging (MRI) may be normal, except for evidence of preexisting conditions, or sometimes may suggest diffuse edema. Several patients with eastern equine encephalitis have had focal abnormalities, and individuals with severe Japanese encephalitis have presented with bilateral thalamic lesions that have often been hemorrhagic. Electroencephalography usually shows diffuse abnormalities and is not directly helpful.

A humoral immune response is usually detectable at or near the onset of disease. Both serum and CSF should be examined for IgM antibodies. Virus generally cannot be isolated from blood or CSF, although Japanese encephalitis virus has been recovered from CSF in severe cases. Virus can be obtained from and viral antigen is present in brain tissue, although its distribution may be focal.

CALIFORNIA, LA CROSSE, AND JAMESTOWN CANYON VIRUS ENCEPHALITIS The isolation of California encephalitis virus established the California serogroup of viruses as a cause of encephalitis, and its use as a diagnostic antigen led to the description of many cases of "California encephalitis." In fact, however, this virus has been implicated in only a few cases of encephalitis, and the serologically related La Crosse virus is the major cause of encephalitis among viruses in the California serogroup. "California encephalitis" due to La Crosse virus infection is most commonly reported from the upper Midwest but is also found in other areas of the central and eastern United States, most often in West Virginia, Tennessee, North Carolina, and Georgia. The serogroup includes 13 other viruses, some of which may also be involved in human disease that is misattributed because of the complexity of the group's serology; these viruses include the Jamestown Canyon, snowshoe hare, Inkoo, and Trivittatus viruses, all of which have *Aedes* mosquitoes as their vector and all of which have a strong element of transovarial transmission in their natural cycles.

The mosquito vector of La Crosse virus is *A. triseriatus*. In addition to a prominent transovarial component of transmission, a mosquito can also become infected through feeding on viremic chipmunks and other mammals as well as through venereal transmission from another mosquito. The mosquito breeds in sites such as tree holes and abandoned tires and bites during daylight hours; these findings correlate with the risk factors for cases: recreation in forested areas, residence at the forest's edge, and the presence of abandoned tires around the home. Intensive environmental modification based on these findings has reduced the incidence of disease in a highly endemic area in the Midwest. Most cases occur from July through September. The Asian tiger mosquito, *A. albopictus*, efficiently transmits the virus to mice and also transmits the agent transovarially in the laboratory; this aggressive anthropophilic mosquito has the capacity to urbanize, and its possible impact on transmission to humans is of concern.

An antibody prevalence of ≥20% in endemic areas indicates that infection is common, but CNS disease has been recognized primarily in children <15 years of age. The illness varies from a picture of aseptic meningitis accompanied by confusion to severe and occasionally fatal encephalitis. Although there may be prodromal symptoms, the onset of CNS disease is sudden, with fever, headache, and lethargy often joined by nausea and vomiting, convulsions (in one-half of patients), and coma (in one-third of patients). Focal seizures, hemiparesis, tremor, aphasia, chorea, Babinski's sign, and other evidence of significant neurologic dysfunction are common, but residua are not. Perhaps 10% of patients have recurrent seizures in the succeeding months. Other serious sequelae are rare, although a decrease in scholastic standing has been reported and mild personality change has occasionally been suggested. Treatment is supportive over a 1- to 2-week acute phase during which status epilepticus, cerebral edema, and inappropriate secretion of antidiuretic hormone are important concerns. Ribavirin has been used in severe cases, and a clinical trial of this drug is under way.

The blood leukocyte count is commonly elevated, sometimes reaching levels of 20,000/μL, and there is usually a left shift. CSF cell counts are typically 30 to 500/μL with a mononuclear cell predominance (although 25 to 90% of cells are polymorphonuclear in some cases). The protein level is normal or slightly increased, and the glucose level is normal. Specific virologic diagnosis based on IgM-capture assays of serum and CSF is efficient. The only human anatomical site from which virus has been isolated is the brain.

Jamestown Canyon virus has been implicated in several cases of encephalitis in adults; in these cases the disease was usually associated with a significant respiratory illness at onset. Human infection with this virus has been documented in New York, Wisconsin, Ohio, Michigan, Ontario, and other areas of North America where the vector mosquito, *A. stimulans*, feeds on its main host, the white-tailed deer.

ST. LOUIS ENCEPHALITIS   St. Louis encephalitis virus is transmitted between *Culex* mosquitoes and birds. This virus causes low-level endemic infection among rural residents of the western and central United States, where *C. tarsalis* is the vector (see "Western Equine Encephalitis," below), but the more urbanized mosquito species *C. pipiens* and *C. quinquefasciatus* have been responsible for epidemics resulting in hundreds or even thousands of cases in cities of the central and eastern United States. Most cases occur in June through October. The urban mosquitoes breed in accumulations of stagnant water and sewage with high organic content and readily bite humans in and around houses at dusk. The elimination of open sewers and trash-filled drainage systems is expensive and may not be possible, but screening of houses and implementation of personal protective measures may be an effective approach for individuals. The rural vector is most active at dusk and outdoors; its bites can be avoided by modification of activities and use of repellents.

Disease severity increases with age: infections that result in aseptic meningitis or mild encephalitis are concentrated in children and young adults, while severe and fatal cases primarily affect the elderly. Infection rates are similar in all age groups; thus the greater susceptibility of older persons to disease is a biologic consequence of aging. The disease has an abrupt onset, sometimes following a prodrome, and begins with fever, lethargy, confusion, and headache. In addition, nuchal rigidity, hypotonia, hyperreflexia, myoclonus, and tremor are common. Severe cases can include cranial nerve palsies, hemiparesis, and convulsions. Patients often complain of dysuria and may have viral antigen in urine as well as pyuria. The overall mortality is generally ~7% but may reach 20% among patients over the age of 60. Recovery is slow. Emotional lability, difficulties in concentration and memory, asthenia, and tremor are commonly prolonged in older patients.

The CSF of patients with St. Louis encephalitis usually contains tens to hundreds of cells, with a lymphocytic predominance and a normal glucose level. Leukocytosis with a left shift is often documented.

JAPANESE ENCEPHALITIS   Japanese encephalitis virus is found throughout Asia, including far eastern Russia, Japan, China, India, Pakistan, and Southeast Asia, and causes occasional epidemics on western Pacific islands. The virus has been detected in the Torres Strait islands, and a human encephalitis case has been identified on the nearby Australian mainland. This flavivirus is particularly common in areas where irrigated rice fields attract the natural avian vertebrate hosts and provide abundant breeding sites for mosquitoes such as *C. tritaeniorhyncus*, which transmit the virus to humans. Additional amplification by pigs, which suffer abortion, and horses, which develop encephalitis, may be significant as well. Vaccination of these additional amplifying hosts may reduce the transmission of the virus. An effective, formalin-inactivated vaccine purified from mouse brain is produced in Japan and licensed for human use in the United States. It is given on days 0, 7, and 30 or—with some sacrifice in serum neutralizing titer—on days 0, 7, and 14. Vaccination is indicated for summer travelers to rural Asia, where the risk of clinical disease may be 0.05 to 2.1/10,000 per week (Table 107-5). The severe and often fatal disease reported in expatriates must be balanced against the 0.1 to 1% chance of a late systemic or cutaneous allergic reaction. These reactions are rarely fatal but may be severe and have been known to begin 1 to 9 days after vaccination, with associated pruritus, urticaria, and angioedema. Live attenuated vaccines are being used in China but are not recommended in the United States at this time.

WEST NILE VIRUS INFECTION   West Nile virus is transmitted among wild birds by *Culex* mosquitoes in Africa, the Middle East, southern Europe, and Asia. It is a frequent cause of febrile disease without CNS involvement, but it occasionally causes aseptic meningitis and severe encephalitis; these serious infections are particularly common among the elderly. The febrile-myalgic syndrome caused by West Nile virus differs from many others by the frequent appearance of a maculopapular rash concentrated on the trunk and lymphadenopathy. Headache, ocular pain, sore throat, nausea and vomiting, and arthralgia (but not arthritis) are common accompaniments. In addition, the virus has been implicated in severe and fatal hepatic necrosis in Africa.

In 1996 West Nile virus caused >300 cases of CNS disease, with 10% mortality, in the Danube flood plain, including Bucharest. In 1999 the virus appeared in New York City and other areas of the northeastern United States, causing >60 cases of aseptic meningitis or encephalitis among humans as well as die-offs among crows, exotic zoo birds, and other avians. The encephalitis was most severe among the elderly and was often associated with notable muscle weakness and even with flaccid paralysis. The virus, thought to have been transmitted in New York City by the ubiquitous *C. pipiens* mosquito, spread as far west as Minnesota and Texas as well as north into Canada by 2002. It seems likely that further spread will occur, and involvement of new vectors may enhance transmission to humans.

West Nile virus falls into the same phylogenetic group of flaviviruses as St. Louis and Japanese encephalitis viruses, as do Murray

Valley and Rocio viruses. The latter two viruses are both maintained in mosquitoes and birds and produce a clinical picture resembling that of Japanese encephalitis. Murray Valley virus has caused occasional epidemics and sporadic cases in Australia. Rocio virus caused recurrent epidemics in a focal area of Brazil in 1975 to 1977 and then virtually disappeared.

CENTRAL EUROPEAN TICK-BORNE ENCEPHALITIS AND RUSSIAN SPRING-SUMMER ENCEPHALITIS A spectrum of tick-borne flaviviruses has been identified across the Eurasian land mass. Many are known mainly as agricultural pathogens (e.g., louping ill virus in the United Kingdom). From Scandinavia to the Urals, central European tick-borne encephalitis is transmitted by *Ixodes ricinus*. Human cases occur between April and October, with a peak in June and July. A related and more virulent virus is that of Russian spring-summer encephalitis, which is associated with *I. persulcatus* and is distributed from Europe across the Urals to the Pacific Ocean. The ticks transmit the disease primarily in the spring and early summer, with a lower rate of transmission later in summer. Small mammals are the vertebrate amplifiers for both viruses. The risk varies by geographic area and can be highly localized within a given area; human cases usually follow outdoor activities or consumption of raw milk from infected goats or other infected animals.

After an incubation period of 7 to 14 days or perhaps longer, the central European viruses classically result in a febrile-myalgic phase that lasts for 2 to 4 days and is thought to correlate with viremia. A subsequent remission for several days is followed by the recurrence of fever and the onset of meningeal signs. The CNS phase varies from mild aseptic meningitis, which is more common among younger patients, to severe encephalitis with coma, convulsions, tremors, and motor signs lasting for 7 to 10 days before improvement begins. Spinal and medullary involvement can lead to typical limb-girdle paralysis and to respiratory paralysis. Most patients recover, only a minority with significant deficits. Infections with the far eastern viruses generally run a more abrupt course. The encephalitic syndrome caused by these viruses sometimes begins without a remission and has more severe manifestations than the European syndrome. Mortality is high, and major sequelae—most notably, lower motor neuron paralyses of the proximal muscles of the extremities, trunk, and neck—are common.

In the early stage of the illness, virus may be isolated from the blood. In the CNS phase, IgM antibodies are detectable in serum and/or CSF. Thrombocytopenia sometimes develops during the initial febrile illness, which resembles the early hemorrhagic phase of some other tick-borne flaviviral infections, such as Kyasanur Forest disease. Other tick-borne flaviviruses are less common causes of encephalitis, including louping ill virus in the United Kingdom and Powassan virus.

There is no specific therapy for infection with these viruses. However, effective alum-adjuvanted, formalin-inactivated vaccines are produced in Austria, Germany, and Russia. Two doses of the Austrian vaccine separated by an interval of 1 to 3 months appear to be effective in the field, and antibody responses are similar when vaccine is given on days 0 and 14. Other vaccines have elicited similar neutralizing antibody titers. Since rare cases of postvaccination Guillain-Barré syndrome have been reported, vaccination should be reserved for persons likely to experience rural exposure in an endemic area during the season of transmission. Cross-neutralization for the central European and far eastern strains has been established, but there are no published field studies on cross-protection of formalin-inactivated vaccines. Because 0.2 to 4% of ticks in endemic areas may be infected, tick bites raise the issue of immunoglobulin prophylaxis. Prompt administration of high-titered specific preparations should probably be undertaken, although no controlled data are available to prove the efficacy of this measure. Immunoglobulin should not be administered late because of the risk of antibody-mediated enhancement.

POWASSAN ENCEPHALITIS Powassan virus is a member of the tick-borne encephalitis virus complex and is transmitted by *I. cookei* among small mammals in eastern Canada and the United States, where it has been responsible for 20 recognized cases of human disease. Other ticks may

transmit the virus in a wider geographic area, and there is some concern that *I. scapularis* (also called *I. dammini*), a competent vector in the laboratory, may become involved as it becomes more prominent in the United States. Patients with Powassan encephalitis—often children—present in May through December after outdoor exposure and an incubation period thought to be ~1 week. Powassan encephalitis is severe, and sequelae are common.

EASTERN EQUINE ENCEPHALITIS Eastern equine encephalitis is found primarily within endemic swampy foci along the eastern coast of the United States, with a few inland foci as far removed as Michigan. Human cases present from June through October, when the bird–*Culiseta* mosquito cycle spills over into other mosquito species such as *A. sollicitans* or *A. vexans*, which are more likely to bite mammals. There is concern over the potential role of the introduced anthropophilic mosquito species *A. albopictus*, which has been found to be naturally infected and is an effective vector in the laboratory. Horses are a common target for the virus; contact with unvaccinated horses may be associated with human disease, but horses probably do not play a significant role in amplification of the virus.

Eastern equine encephalitis is one of the most destructive of the arboviral conditions, with a brusque onset, rapid progression, high mortality, and frequent residua. This severity is reflected in the extensive necrotic lesions and polymorphonuclear infiltrates found at postmortem examination of the brain and the acute polymorphonuclear CSF pleocytosis often occurring during the first 1 to 3 days of disease. In addition, leukocytosis with a left shift is a common feature. A formalin-inactivated vaccine has been used to protect laboratory workers but is not generally available or applicable.

WESTERN EQUINE ENCEPHALITIS The primary maintenance cycle for western equine encephalitis virus in the United States is between *C. tarsalis* and birds, principally sparrows and finches. Equines and humans become infected, and both species suffer encephalitis without amplifying the virus in nature. St. Louis encephalitis is transmitted in a similar cycle in the same region but causes human disease about a month earlier than the period (July through October) in which western equine encephalitis virus is active. Large epidemics of western equine encephalitis took place in the western and central United States and Canada during the 1930s to 1950s, but in recent years the disease has been uncommon. There were 41 reported cases in the United States in 1987 but only 5 reported cases from 1988 to 2001. This decline in incidence may reflect in part the integrated approach to mosquito management that has been employed in irrigation projects and the increasing use of agricultural pesticides; it almost certainly reflects the increased tendency for humans to be indoors behind closed windows at dusk, the peak period of biting by the major vector.

Western equine encephalitis virus causes a typical diffuse viral encephalitis with an increased attack rate and increased morbidity in the young, particularly children <2 years old. In addition, mortality is high among the young and the very elderly. One-third of individuals who have convulsions during the acute illness have subsequent seizure activity. Infants <1 year old—particularly those in the first months of life—are at serious risk of motor and intellectual damage. Twice as many males as females develop clinical encephalitis after 5 to 9 years of age; this difference may be related to greater outdoor exposure of boys to the vector but is also likely to be due in part to biologic differences. A formalin-inactivated vaccine has been used to protect laboratory workers but is not generally available or applicable.

VENEZUELAN EQUINE ENCEPHALITIS There are six known types of virus in the Venezuelan equine encephalitis complex. An important distinction is between the "epizootic" viruses (subtypes IAB and IC) and the "enzootic" viruses (subtypes ID to IF and types II to VI). The epizootic viruses have an unknown natural cycle but periodically cause extensive epidemics in equines and humans in the Americas. These epidemics rely on the high-level viremia in horses and mules that results in the infection of several species of mosquitoes, which in turn infect humans and perpetuate virus transmission. Humans also have high-level viremia but probably are not important in virus transmission. Enzootic viruses are found primarily in humid tropical forest habitats and are maintained between *Culex* mosquitoes and rodents; these viruses cause human disease but are not pathogenic for horses and do not cause epizootics.

Epizootics of Venezuelan equine encephalitis occurred repeatedly in Venezuela, Colombia, Ecuador, Peru, and other South American countries at intervals of ≤10 years from the 1930s until 1969, when a massive epizootic spread throughout Central America and Mexico, reaching southern Texas in 1972. Genetic sequencing of the virus from the 1969 to 1972 outbreak suggested that it originated from residual "un-inactivated" virus in veterinary vaccines. The outbreak was terminated in Texas with the use of a live attenuated vaccine (TC-83) originally developed for human use by the U.S. Army; this virus was then used for further production of inactivated veterinary vaccines. No further epizootic disease was identified until 1995 and subsequently, when additional epizootics took place in Colombia, Venezuela, and Mexico. The viruses involved in these epizootics as well as previously epizootic subtype IC viruses have been shown to be close phylogenetic relatives of known enzootic subtype ID viruses. This finding suggests that active evolution and selection of epizootic viruses are under way in northern South America.

During epizootics, extensive human infection is the rule, with clinical disease in 10 to 60% of infected individuals. Most infections result in notable acute febrile disease, while relatively few result in encephalitis. A low rate of CNS invasion is supported by the absence of encephalitis among the many infections resulting from exposure to aerosols in the laboratory or from vaccine accidents. The most recent large epizootic of Venezuelan equine encephalitis occurred in Colombia and Venezuela in 1995; of the >85,000 clinical cases, 4% (with a higher proportion among children than adults) included neurologic symptoms and 300 ended in death.

Enzootic strains of Venezuelan equine encephalitis virus are common causes of acute febrile disease, particularly in areas such as the Florida Everglades and the humid Atlantic coast of Central America. Encephalitis has been documented only in the Florida infections; the three cases were caused by type II enzootic virus, also called *Everglades virus*. All three patients had preexisting cerebral disease. Extrapolation from the rate of genetic change suggests that Everglades virus may have been introduced into Florida <200 years ago and that it is most closely related to the ID subtypes that appear to have given evolutionary rise to the epizootic strains active in South America.

The prevention of epizootic Venezuelan equine encephalitis depends on vaccination of horses with the attenuated TC-83 vaccine or with an inactivated vaccine prepared from that strain. Humans can be protected with similar vaccines, but the use of such products is restricted to laboratory personnel because of reactogenicity and limited availability. In addition, wild-type virus and perhaps TC-83 vaccine may have some degree of fetal pathogenicity. Enzootic viruses are genetically and antigenically different from epizootic viruses, and protection against the former with vaccines prepared from the latter is relatively ineffective.

ARTHRITIS AND RASH

True arthritis is a common accompaniment of several viral diseases, such as rubella (caused by a non-alphavirus togavirus), parvovirus B19 infection, and hepatitis B; it is an occasional accompaniment of infection due to mumps virus, enteroviruses, herpesviruses, and adenoviruses. It is not generally appreciated that the alphaviruses are also common causes of arthritis. In fact, the alphaviruses discussed below all cause acute febrile diseases accompanied by the development of true arthritis and a maculopapular rash. Rheumatic involvement includes arthralgia alone, periarticular swelling, and (less commonly) joint effusions. Most of these diseases are less severe and have fewer articular manifestations in children than in adults. In temperate cli-

mates, these are summer diseases. No specific therapy or licensed vaccines exist.

SINDBIS VIRUS INFECTION   Sindbis virus is transmitted among birds by mosquitoes. Infections with the northern European strains of this virus (which cause, for example, Pogosta disease in Finland, Karelian fever in the independent states of the former Soviet Union, and Okelbo disease in Sweden) and with the genetically related southern African strains are particularly likely to result in the arthritis-rash syndrome. Exposure to a rural environment is commonly associated with this infection, which has an incubation period of <1 week.

The disease begins with rash and arthralgia. Constitutional symptoms are not marked, and fever is modest or lacking altogether. The rash, which lasts about a week, begins on the trunk, spreads to the extremities, and evolves from macules to papules that often vesiculate. The arthritis of this condition is multiarticular, migratory, and incapacitating, with resolution of the acute phase in a few days. Wrists, ankles, phalangeal joints, knees, elbows, and—to a much lesser extent—proximal and axial joints are involved. Persistence of joint pains and occasionally of arthritis is a major problem and may go on for months or even years despite a lack of deformity.

CHIKUNGUNYA VIRUS INFECTION   It is likely that chikungunya virus ("that which bends up") is of African origin and is maintained among non-human primates on that continent by *Aedes* mosquitoes of the subgenus *Stegomyia* in a fashion similar to yellow fever virus. Like yellow fever virus, chikungunya virus is readily transmitted among humans in urban areas by *A. aegypti*. The *A. aegypti*–chikungunya virus transmission cycle has also been introduced into Asia, where it poses a prominent health problem. The disease is endemic in rural areas of Africa, and intermittent epidemics take place in towns and cities of Africa and Asia. Chikungunya is one more reason (in addition to dengue and yellow fever) that *A. aegypti* must be controlled.

Full-blown disease is most common among adults, in whom the clinical picture may be dramatic. The abrupt onset follows an incubation period of 2 to 3 days. Fever and severe arthralgia are accompanied by chills and constitutional symptoms such as headache, photophobia, conjunctival injection, anorexia, nausea, and abdominal pain. Migratory polyarthritis mainly affects the small joints of the hands, wrists, ankles, and feet, with lesser involvement of the larger joints. Rash may appear at the outset or several days into the illness; its development often coincides with defervescence, which takes place around day 2 or day 3 of disease. The rash is most intense on the trunk and limbs and may desquamate. Petechiae are occasionally seen, and epistaxis is not uncommon, but this virus is not a regular cause of the HF syndrome, even in children. A few patients develop leukopenia. Elevated levels of aspartate aminotransferase (AST) and C-reactive protein have been described, as have mildly decreased platelet counts. Recovery may require weeks. Some older patients continue to suffer from stiffness, joint pain, and recurrent effusions for several years; this persistence may be especially common in HLA-B27 patients. An investigational live attenuated vaccine has been developed but requires further testing.

A related virus, O'nyong-nyong, caused a major epidemic of arthritis and rash involving at least 2 million people as it moved across eastern and central Africa in the 1960s. After its mysterious emergence, the virus virtually disappeared, leaving only occasional evidence of its persistence in Kenya until a transient resurgence of epidemic activity in 1997.

EPIDEMIC POLYARTHRITIS (ROSS RIVER VIRUS INFECTION)   Ross River virus has caused epidemics of distinctive clinical disease in Australia since the beginning of the twentieth century and continues to be responsible for thousands of cases in rural and suburban areas annually. The virus is transmitted by *A. vigilax* and other mosquitoes, and its persistence is thought to involve transovarial transmission. No definitive vertebrate host has been identified, but several mammalian species, including wallabies, have been suggested. Endemic transmission has also been documented in New Guinea, and in 1979 the virus swept through the eastern Pacific Islands, causing hundreds of thousands of illnesses.

The virus was carried from island to island by infected humans and was believed to have been transmitted among humans by *A. polynesiensis* and *A. aegypti*.

The incubation period is 7 to 11 days long, and the onset of illness is sudden, with joint pain usually ushering in the disease. The rash generally develops coincidentally or follows shortly but in some cases precedes joint pains by several days. Constitutional symptoms such as low-grade fever, asthenia, myalgia, headache, and nausea are not prominent and indeed are absent in many cases. Most patients are incapacitated for considerable periods by joint involvement, which interferes with sleeping, walking, and grasping. Wrist, ankle, metacarpophalangeal, interphalangeal, and knee joints are the most commonly involved, although toes, shoulders, and elbows may be affected with some frequency. Periarticular swelling and tenosynovitis are common, and one-third of patients have true arthritis. Only half of all arthritis patients can resume normal activities within 4 weeks, and 10% still must limit their activity at 3 months. Occasional patients are symptomatic for 1 to 3 years but without progressive arthropathy. Aspirin and nonsteroidal anti-inflammatory drugs are effective for the treatment of symptoms.

Clinical laboratory values are normal or variable in Ross River virus infection. Tests for rheumatoid factor and antinuclear antibodies are negative, and the erythrocyte sedimentation rate is acutely elevated. Joint fluid contains 1000 to 60,000 mononuclear cells per microliter, and Ross River virus antigen is demonstrable in macrophages. IgM antibodies are valuable in the diagnosis of this infection, although they occasionally persist for years. The isolation of the virus from blood by mosquito inoculation or mosquito cell culture is possible early in the illness. Because of the great economic impact of annual epidemics in Australia, an inactivated vaccine is being developed and has been found to be protective in mice.

Perhaps because of the local interest in arboviruses in general and in Ross River virus in particular, other arthritogenic arboviruses have been identified in Australia, including Gan Gan virus, a member of the family Bunyaviridae; Kokobera virus, a flavivirus; and Barmah Forest virus, an alphavirus. The last virus is a common cause of infection and must be differentiated from Ross River virus by specific testing.

HEMORRHAGIC FEVERS

The viral HF syndrome is a constellation of findings based on vascular instability and decreased vascular integrity. An assault, direct or indirect, on the microvasculature leads to increased permeability and (particularly when platelet function is decreased) to actual disruption and local hemorrhage. Blood pressure is decreased, and in severe cases shock supervenes. Cutaneous flushing and conjunctival suffusion are examples of common, observable abnormalities in the control of local circulation. The hemorrhage is inconstant and is in most cases an indication of widespread vascular damage rather than a life-threatening loss of blood volume. Disseminated intravascular coagulation (DIC) is occasionally found in any severely ill patient with HF but is thought to occur regularly only in the early phases of HF with renal syndrome, Crimean-Congo HF, and perhaps some cases of filovirus HF. In some viral HF syndromes, specific organs may be particularly impaired, such as the kidney in HF with renal syndrome, the lung in hantavirus pulmonary syndrome, or the liver in yellow fever, but in all these diseases the generalized circulatory disturbance is critically important.

The pathogenesis of HF is poorly understood and varies among the viruses regularly implicated in the syndrome, which number more than a dozen. In some cases direct damage to the vascular system or even to parenchymal cells of target organs is important, whereas in others soluble mediators are thought to play the major role. The acute phase in most cases of HF is associated with ongoing virus replication and viremia. Exceptions are the hantavirus diseases and dengue HF/dengue shock syndrome (DHF/DSS), in which the immune response plays a major pathogenic role.

The HF syndromes all begin with fever and myalgia, usually of abrupt onset. Within a few days the patient presents for medical atten-

tion because of increasing prostration that is often accompanied by severe headache, dizziness, photophobia, hyperesthesia, abdominal or chest pain, anorexia, nausea or vomiting, and other gastrointestinal disturbances. Initial examination often reveals only an acutely ill patient with conjunctival suffusion, tenderness to palpation of muscles or abdomen, and borderline hypotension or postural hypotension, perhaps with tachycardia. Petechiae (often best visualized in the axillae), flushing of the head and thorax, periorbital edema, and proteinuria are common. Levels of AST are usually elevated at presentation or within a day or two thereafter. Hemoconcentration from vascular leakage, which is usually evident, is most marked in hantavirus diseases and in DHF/DSS. The seriously ill patient progresses to more severe symptoms and develops shock and other findings typical of the causative virus. Shock, multifocal bleeding, and CNS involvement (encephalopathy, coma, convulsions) are all poor prognostic signs.

One of the major diagnostic clues is travel to an endemic area within the incubation period for a given syndrome (Table 180-4). Except for Seoul, dengue, and yellow fever virus infections, which have urban vectors, travel to a rural setting is especially suggestive of a diagnosis of HF.

Early recognition is important because of the need for virus-specific therapy and supportive measures, including prompt, atraumatic hospitalization; judicious fluid therapy that takes into account the patient's increased capillary permeability; administration of cardiotonic drugs; use of pressors to maintain blood pressure at levels that will support renal perfusion; treatment of the relatively common secondary bacterial infections; replacement of clotting factors and platelets as indicated; and the usual precautionary measures used in the treatment of patients with hemorrhagic diatheses. DIC should be treated only if clear laboratory evidence of its existence is found and if laboratory monitoring of therapy is feasible; there is no proven benefit of such therapy. The available evidence suggests that HF patients have a decreased cardiac output and will respond poorly to fluid loading as it is often practiced in the treatment of shock associated with bacterial sepsis. Specific therapy is available for several of the HF syndromes. In addition, several diseases considered in the differential diagnosis—malaria, shigellosis, typhoid, leptospirosis, relapsing fever, and rickettsial disease—are treatable and potentially lethal. Strict barrier nursing and other precautions against infection of medical staff and visitors are indicated in HF except that due to hantaviruses, yellow fever, Rift Valley fever, and dengue.

LASSA FEVER   Lassa virus is known to cause endemic and epidemic disease in Nigeria, Sierra Leone, Guinea, and Liberia, although it is probably more widely distributed in West Africa. This virus and its relatives exist elsewhere in Africa, but their health significance is unknown. Like other arenaviruses, Lassa virus is spread to humans by small-particle aerosols from chronically infected rodents and may also be acquired during the capture or eating of these animals. It can be transmitted by close person-to-person contact. The virus is often present in urine during convalescence and is suspected to be present in seminal fluid early in recovery. Nosocomial spread has occurred but is uncommon if proper sterile parenteral techniques are used. Individuals of all ages and both sexes are affected; the incidence of disease is highest in the dry season, but transmission takes place year-round. In countries where Lassa virus is endemic, Lassa fever can be a prominent cause of febrile disease. For example, in one hospital in Sierra Leone, laboratory-confirmed Lassa fever is consistently responsible for one-fifth of admissions to the medical wards. There are probably tens of thousands of Lassa fever cases annually in West Africa alone.

The average case has a gradual onset (among the HF agents, only the arenaviruses are typically associated with a gradual onset) that gives way to more severe constitutional symptoms and prostration. Bleeding is seen in only ~15 to 30% of cases. A maculopapular rash is often noted in light-skinned Lassa patients. Effusions are common,

Disease	Incubation Period, Days	Case-Infection Ratio	Case-Fatality Rate, %	Geographic Range	Target Population
Lassa fever	5–16	Mild infections probably common	15	West Africa	All ages, both sexes
South American HF	7–14	Most infections (more than half) result in disease	15–30	Selected rural areas of Bolivia, Argentina, Venezuela, and Brazil	Bolivia: Men in countryside; all ages, both sexes in villages Argentina: All ages, both sexes; excess exposure and disease in men Venezuela: All ages, both sexes
Rift Valley fever	2–5	~1:100[a]	~50	Sub-Saharan Africa, Madagascar, Egypt	All ages, both sexes; more often diagnosed in men; preexisting liver disease may predispose
Crimean-Congo HF	3–12	≥1:5	15–30	Africa, Middle East, Balkans, southern region of former Soviet Union, western China	All ages, both sexes; men more exposed in some settings
HF with renal syndrome	9–35	Hantaan, >1:1.25; Puumala, 1:20	5–15, Hantaan; <1, Puumala	Worldwide, depending on rodent reservoir	Excess of male patients (partly due to greater exposure); mainly adults
Hantavirus pulmonary syndrome	~7–28	Very high	40–50	Americas	Excess of male patients due to some occupational exposure; mainly adults
Marburg or Ebola HF	3–16	High	25–90	Sub-Saharan Africa	All ages, both sexes; children less exposed
Yellow fever	3–6	1:2–1:20	20	Africa, South America	All ages, both sexes; adults more exposed in jungle setting; preexisting flavivirus immunity may cross-protect
Dengue HF/dengue shock syndrome	2–7	1:10,000, nonimmune; 1:100, heterologous immune	<1 with supportive treatment	Tropics and subtropics worldwide	Predominantly children; previous heterologous dengue infection predisposes to HF
Kyasanur Forest/ Omsk HF	3–8	Variable	0.5–10	Mysore State, India/ western Siberia	Variable

[a] Figure is for HF cases only. Most infections with Rift Valley fever virus result in fever and myalgia rather than HF.

and male-dominant pericarditis may develop late. The fetal death rate is 92% in the last trimester, when maternal mortality is also increased from the usual 15% to 30%; these figures suggest that interruption of the pregnancy of infected women should be considered. White blood cell counts are normal or slightly elevated, and platelet counts are normal or somewhat low. Deafness coincides with clinical improvement in ~20% of cases and is permanent and bilateral in some. Reinfection may occur but has not been associated with severe disease.

High-level viremia or a high serum concentration of AST statistically predicts a fatal outcome. Thus patients with an AST level of >150 IU/mL should be treated with intravenous ribavirin. This antiviral nucleoside analogue appears to be effective in reducing mortality from rates among retrospective controls, and its only major side effect is reversible anemia that usually does not require transfusion. The drug should be given by slow intravenous infusion in a dose of 32 mg/kg; this dose should be followed by 16 mg/kg every 6 h for 4 days and then by 8 mg/kg every 8 h for 6 days.

SOUTH AMERICAN HF SYNDROMES (ARGENTINE, BOLIVIAN, VENEZUELAN, AND BRAZILIAN) These diseases are similar to one another clinically, but their epidemiology differs with the habits of their rodent reservoirs and the interactions of these animals with humans (Table 180-4). Person-to-person or nosocomial transmission is rare but has occurred.

The basic disease resembles Lassa fever, with two marked differ-

ences. First, thrombocytopenia—often marked—is the rule, and bleeding is quite common. Second, CNS dysfunction is much more common than in Lassa fever and is often manifest by marked confusion, tremors of the upper extremities and tongue, and cerebellar signs. Some cases follow a predominantly neurologic course, with a poor prognosis. The clinical laboratory is helpful in diagnosis since thrombocytopenia, leukopenia, and proteinuria are typical findings.

Argentine HF is readily treated with convalescent-phase plasma given within the first 8 days of illness. In the absence of passive antibody therapy, intravenous ribavirin in the dose recommended for Lassa fever is likely to be effective in all the South American HF syndromes. The transmission of the disease from men convalescing from Argentine HF to their wives suggests the need for counseling of arenavirus HF patients concerning the avoidance of intimate contacts for several weeks after recovery. A safe, effective, live attenuated vaccine exists for Argentine HF. In experimental animals, this vaccine is cross-protective against the Bolivian HF virus.

RIFT VALLEY FEVER The mosquito-borne Rift Valley fever virus is also a pathogen of domestic animals such as sheep, cattle, and goats. It is maintained in nature by transovarial transmission in floodwater *Aedes* mosquitoes and presumably also has a vertebrate amplifier. Epizootics and epidemics occur when sheep or cattle become infected during particularly heavy rains; developing high-level viremia, these animals infect many different species of mosquitoes. Remote sensing via satellite can detect the ecologic changes associated with high rainfall that predict the likelihood of Rift Valley fever transmission; it can also detect the special depressions from which the floodwater *Aedes* mosquito vectors emerge. In addition, the virus is infectious when transmitted by contact with blood or aerosols from domestic animals or their abortuses. The slaughtered meat is not infectious; anaerobic glycolysis in postmortem tissues results in an acidic environment that rapidly inactivates Bunyaviridae such as Rift Valley fever virus and Crimean-Congo HF virus. The natural range of Rift Valley fever virus is confined to sub-Saharan Africa, where its circulation is markedly enhanced by substantial rainfall such as that which occurred during the El Niño phenomenon of 1997; subsequent spread to the Arabian Peninsula caused epidemic disease in 2000. The virus has also been found in Madagascar and has been introduced into Egypt, where it caused major epidemics in 1977 to 1979, 1993, and subsequently. Neither person-to-person nor nosocomial transmission has been documented.

Rift Valley fever virus is unusual in that it causes at least four different clinical syndromes. Most infections are manifested as the febrile-myalgic syndrome. A small proportion result in HF with especially prominent liver involvement. Perhaps 10% of otherwise mild infections lead to retinal vasculitis; funduscopic examination reveals edema, hemorrhages, and infarction, and some patients have permanently impaired vision. A small proportion of cases (<1 in 200) are followed by typical viral encephalitis. One of the complicated syndromes does not appear to predispose to another.

There is no proven therapy for any of the syndromes described above. The sensitivity of animal models of Rift Valley fever to antibody or ribavirin therapy suggests that either could be given intravenously to persons with HF. Both retinal disease and encephalitis occur after the acute febrile syndrome has ended and serum neutralizing antibody has developed—events suggesting that only supportive care need be given. Epidemic disease is best prevented by vaccination of livestock. The established ability of this virus to propagate after an introduction into Egypt suggests that other potentially receptive areas, including the United States, should have a response ready for such an eventuality. It seems likely that this disease, like Venezuelan equine encephalitis, can be controlled only with adequate stocks of an effective live attenuated vaccine, and there are no such global stocks. A formalin-inactivated vaccine confers immunity to humans, but quantities are limited and three injections are required; this vaccine is recommended for exposed laboratory workers and for veterinarians working in sub-Saharan Africa.

CRIMEAN-CONGO HF This severe HF syndrome has a wide geographic distribution, potentially being found wherever ticks of the genus *Hyalomma* occur (Table 180-4). The propensity of these ticks to feed on domestic livestock and certain wild mammals means that veterinary serosurveys are the most effective mechanism for the surveillance of virus circulation in a region. Human infection is acquired via a tick bite or during the crushing of infected ticks. Domestic animals do not become ill but do develop viremia; thus there is danger of infection at the time of slaughter and for a brief interval thereafter (through contact with hides or carcasses). Cases have followed sheep shearing. An epidemic in South Africa was associated with slaughter of tick-infested ostriches. Nosocomial epidemics are common and are usually related to extensive blood exposure or needle sticks.

Although generally similar to other HF syndromes, Crimean-Congo HF causes extensive liver damage, resulting in jaundice in some cases. Clinical laboratory values indicate DIC and show elevations in AST, creatine phosphokinase, and bilirubin. Patients with fatal cases generally have more marked changes, even in the early days of illness, and also develop leukocytosis rather than leukopenia. Thrombocytopenia is also more marked and develops earlier in cases with a fatal outcome.

No controlled trials have been performed with intravenous ribavirin, but clinical experience and retrospective comparison of patients with ominous clinical laboratory values suggest that ribavirin is efficacious and should be given. No human or veterinary vaccines are recommended.

HF WITH RENAL SYNDROME This disease, the first to be identified as an HF, is widely distributed over Europe and Asia; the major causative viruses and their rodent reservoirs on these two continents are Puumala virus (bank vole, *Clethrionomys glareolus*) and Hantaan virus (striped field mouse, *Apodemus agrarius*), respectively. Other potential causative viruses exist, including Dobrava virus (yellow-necked field mouse, *A. flavicollus*), which causes severe HF with renal syndrome in the Balkans. Seoul virus is associated with the Norway or sewer rat, *Rattus norvegicus*, and has a worldwide distribution through the migration of the rodent; it is associated with mild or moderate HF with renal syndrome in Asia, but in many areas of the world the human disease has been difficult to identify. Most cases occur in rural residents or vacationers; the exception is Seoul virus disease, which may be acquired in an urban or rural setting or from contaminated laboratory rat colonies. Classic Hantaan disease in Korea (Korean HF) and in rural China (epidemic HF) is most common in spring and fall and is related to rodent density and agricultural practices. Human infection is acquired primarily through aerosols of rodent urine, although virus is also present in saliva and feces. Patients with hantavirus diseases are not infectious. HF with renal syndrome is the most important form of HF today, with >100,000 cases of severe disease in Asia annually and milder Puumala infections numbering in the thousands as well.

Severe cases of HF with renal syndrome caused by Hantaan virus evolve in identifiable stages: the febrile stage with myalgia, lasting 3 to 4 days; the hypotensive stage, often associated with shock and lasting from a few hours to 48 h; the oliguric stage with renal failure, lasting 3 to 10 days; and the polyuric stage with diuresis and hyposthenuria.

The *febrile period* is initiated by the abrupt onset of fever, headache, severe myalgia, thirst, anorexia, and often nausea and vomiting. Photophobia, retroorbital pain, and pain on ocular movement are common, and the vision may become blurred with ciliary body inflammation. Flushing over the face, the V area of the neck, and the back are characteristic, as are pharyngeal injection, periorbital edema, and conjunctival suffusion. Petechiae often develop in areas of pressure, the conjunctivae, and the axillae. Back pain and tenderness to percussion at the costovertebral angle reflect massive retroperitoneal edema. Laboratory evidence of mild to moderate DIC is present. Other laboratory findings include proteinuria and an active urinary sediment.

The *hypotensive phase* is ushered in by falling blood pressure and sometimes by shock. The relative bradycardia typical of the febrile phase is replaced by tachycardia. Kinin activation is marked. The rising hematocrit reflects increasing vascular leakage. Leukocytosis with a left shift develops, and thrombocytopenia continues. Atypical lymphocytes—which in fact are activated CD8+ and to a lesser extent CD4+ T cells—circulate. Proteinuria is marked, and the urine's specific gravity falls to 1.010. The renal circulation is congested and compromised from local and systemic circulatory changes resulting in necrosis of tubules, particularly at the corticomedullary junction, and oliguria.

During the *oliguric phase*, hemorrhagic tendencies continue, probably in large part because of uremic bleeding defects. The oliguria persists for 3 to 10 days before renal function returns and marks the onset of the *polyuric stage*, which carries the danger of dehydration and electrolyte abnormalities.

Mild cases of HF with renal syndrome may be much less stereotypical. The presentation may include only fever, gastrointestinal abnormalities, and transient oliguria followed by hyposthenuria.

HF with renal syndrome should be suspected in patients with rural exposure in an endemic area. Prompt recognition of the disease will permit rapid hospitalization and expectant management of shock and renal failure. Useful clinical laboratory parameters include leukocytosis, which may be leukemoid and is associated with a left shift; thrombocytopenia; and proteinuria. Mainstays of therapy are the management of shock, reliance on pressors, modest crystalloid infusion, intravenous use of human serum albumin, and treatment of renal failure with prompt dialysis for the usual indications. Hydration may result in pulmonary edema, and hypertension should be avoided because of the possibility of intracranial hemorrhage. Use of intravenous ribavirin has reduced mortality and morbidity in severe cases provided treatment is begun within the first 4 days of illness. The case-fatality ratio may be as high as 15% but with proper therapy should be <5%. Sequelae have not been definitely established, but there is a correlation in the United States between chronic hypertensive renal failure and the presence of antibodies to Seoul virus.

Infections with Puumala virus, the most common cause of HF with renal syndrome in Europe, result in a much attenuated picture but the same general presentation. The syndrome may be referred to by its former name, *nephropathia epidemica*. Bleeding manifestations are found in only 10% of cases, hypotension rather than shock is usually seen, and oliguria is present in only about half of patients. The dominant features may be fever, abdominal pain, proteinuria, mild oliguria, and sometimes blurred vision or glaucoma followed by polyuria and hyposthenuria in recovery. Mortality is <1%.

The diagnosis is readily made by IgM-capture ELISA, which should be positive at admission or within 24 to 48 h thereafter. The isolation of virus is difficult, but RT-PCR of a blood clot collected early in the clinical course or of tissues obtained postmortem will give positive results. Such testing is usually undertaken only if definitive identification of the infecting viral species is required or if molecular epidemiologic questions exist.

HANTAVIRUS PULMONARY SYNDROME   Hantavirus pulmonary syndrome was discovered in 1993, but retrospective identification of cases by immunohistochemistry (1978) and serology (1959) support the idea that it is a recently discovered rather than a truly new disease. The causative viruses are hantaviruses of a distinct phylogenetic lineage that is associated with the rodent subfamily Sigmodontinae. Sin Nombre virus chronically infects the deer mouse (*Peromyscus maniculatus*) and is the most important virus causing hantavirus pulmonary syndrome in the United States. The disease is also caused by a Sin Nombre virus variant from the white-footed mouse (*P. leucopus*), by Black Creek Canal virus (*Sigmodon hispidus*, the cotton rat), and by Bayou virus (*Oryzomys palustris*, the rice rat). Several other related viruses cause the disease in South America, but Andes virus is unusual in that it, alone among hantaviruses, has been implicated in human-to-human transmission. The disease is linked to rodent exposure and particularly affects rural residents living in dwellings permeable to rodent entry or working at occupations that pose a risk of rodent exposure. Each rodent species has its own particular habits; in the case of the deer mouse, these behaviors include living in and around human habitation.

The disease begins with a prodrome of about 3 to 4 days (range, 1 to 11 days) comprising fever, myalgia, malaise, and often gastrointestinal disturbances such as nausea, vomiting, and abdominal pain. Dizziness is common and vertigo occasional. Severe prodromal symptoms bring some individuals to medical attention, but patients are usually recognized as the cardiopulmonary phase begins. Typically, there is slightly lowered blood pressure, tachycardia, tachypnea, mild hypoxemia, and early radiographic signs of pulmonary edema. Physical findings in the chest are often surprisingly scant. The conjunctival and cutaneous signs of vascular involvement seen in other types of HF are absent. During the next few hours, decompensation may progress rapidly to severe hypoxemia and respiratory failure. Most patients surviving the first 48 h of hospitalization are extubated and discharged within a few days, with no apparent residua.

Management during the first few hours after presentation is critical. The goal is to prevent severe hypoxemia by oxygen therapy and, if needed, intubation and intensive respiratory management. During this period, hypotension and shock with increasing hematocrit invite aggressive fluid administration, but this intervention should be undertaken with great caution. Because of low cardiac output with myocardial depression and increased pulmonary vascular permeability, shock should be managed expectantly with pressors and modest infusion of fluid guided by the pulmonary capillary wedge pressure. Mild cases can be managed by frequent monitoring and oxygen administration without intubation. Many patients require intubation to manage hypoxemia and also develop shock. Mortality remains at ~30 to 40% with good management. The antiviral drug ribavirin inhibits the virus in vitro but did not have a marked effect on patients treated in an open-label study.

During the prodrome, the differential diagnosis of hantavirus pulmonary syndrome is difficult, but by the time of presentation or within 24 h thereafter, a number of diagnostically helpful clinical features become apparent. Cough is not usually present at the outset but may develop later. Interstitial edema is evident on the chest x-ray. Later, bilateral alveolar edema with a central distribution develops in the setting of a normal-sized heart; occasionally, the edema is initially unilateral. Pleural effusions are often visualized. Thrombocytopenia, circulating atypical lymphocytes, and a left shift (often with leukocytosis) are almost always evident; thrombocytopenia has been a particularly important early clue. Hemoconcentration, proteinuria, and hypoalbuminemia should also be sought. Although thrombocytopenia virtually always develops and prolongation of the partial thromboplastin time is the rule, clinical evidence for coagulopathy or laboratory indications of DIC are found in only a minority of cases, usually in severely ill patients. Severely ill patients also have acidosis and elevated serum levels of lactate. Mildly increased values in renal function tests are common, but patients with severe cases often have markedly elevated concentrations of serum creatinine; some of the viruses other than Sin Nombre virus have been associated with more kidney involvement, but few such cases have been studied. The differential diagnosis includes abdominal surgical conditions and pyelonephritis as well as rickettsial disease, sepsis, meningococcemia, plague, tularemia, influenza, and relapsing fever.

A specific diagnosis is best made by IgM testing of acute-phase serum, which has yielded positive results even in the prodrome. Tests using a Sin Nombre virus antigen detect the related hantaviruses causing the pulmonary syndrome in the Americas. Occasionally, heterologous viruses will react only in the IgG ELISA, but this finding is highly suspicious given the very low seroprevalence of these viruses in normal populations. RT-PCR is usually positive when used to test blood clots obtained in the first 7 to 9 days of illness as well as tissues; this test is useful in identifying the infecting virus in areas outside the home range of the deer mouse and in atypical cases.

YELLOW FEVER   Yellow fever virus caused major epidemics in the Americas, Africa, and Europe before the discovery of mosquito transmission in 1900 led to its control through attacks on its urban vector, *A. aegypti*. Only then was it found that a jungle cycle also existed in Africa, involving other *Aedes* mosquitoes and monkeys, and that colonization of the New World with *A. aegypti*, originally an African species, had established urban yellow fever as well as an independent sylvatic yellow fever cycle in American jungles involving *Haemagogus* mosquitoes and New World monkeys. Today, urban yellow fever transmission occurs only in some African cities, but the threat exists in the great cities of South America, where reinfestation by *A. aegypti* has taken place and dengue transmission by the same mosquito is common. As late as 1905, New Orleans suffered >3000 cases with 452 deaths from "yellow jack." Despite the existence of a highly effective and safe vaccine, several hundred jungle yellow fever cases occur annually in South America, and thousands of jungle and urban cases occur each year in Africa.

Yellow fever is a typical HF accompanied by prominent hepatic necrosis. A period of viremia, typically lasting 3 or 4 days, is followed by a period of "intoxication." During the latter phase in severe cases, the characteristic jaundice, hemorrhages, black vomit, anuria, and terminal delirium occur, perhaps related in part to extensive hepatic involvement. Blood leukocyte counts may be normal or reduced and are often high in terminal stages. Albuminuria is usually noted and may be marked; as renal function fails in terminal or severe cases, the level of blood urea nitrogen rises proportionately. Abnormalities detected in liver function tests range from modest elevations of AST levels in mild cases to severe derangement.

Urban yellow fever can be prevented by the control of *A. aegypti*. The continuing sylvatic cycle requires vaccination of all visitors to areas of potential transmission. With few exceptions (in the very young and the elderly), reactions to vaccine are minimal; immunity is provided within 10 days and lasts for at least 10 years. An egg allergy dictates caution in vaccine administration. Although there are no documented harmful effects of the vaccine on the fetus, pregnant women should be immunized only if they are definitely at risk of yellow fever exposure. Since vaccination has been associated with several cases of encephalitis in children <6 months of age, it should be delayed until after 12 months of age unless the risk of exposure is very high. Timely information on changes in yellow fever distribution and yellow fever vaccine requirements can be obtained from Health Information for Travelers, Centers for Disease Control and Prevention, Atlanta, GA 30333; by fax request (404-332-4565; document number 220022#); by phone (404-332-4559); or via the Internet (*www.cdc.gov*).

DENGUE HEMORRHAGIC FEVER/DENGUE SHOCK SYNDROME   A syndrome of HF noted in the 1950s among children in the Philippines and Southeast Asia was soon associated with dengue virus infections, particularly those occurring against a background of previous exposure to another serotype. The transient heterotypic protection after dengue virus infection is replaced within several weeks by the potential for heterotypic infection resulting in typical dengue fever (see above) or—uncommonly—for enhanced disease (secondary DHF/DSS). In rare instances, primary dengue infections lead to an HF syndrome, but much less is known about pathogenesis in this situation. In the past 20 years, *A. aegypti* has progressively reinvaded Latin America and other areas, and frequent travel by infected individuals has introduced multiple strains of dengue virus from many geographic areas. Thus the pattern of hyperendemic transmission of multiple dengue serotypes has now been established in the Americas and the Caribbean and has led to the emergence of DHF/DSS as a major problem there as well. Millions of dengue infections, including many thousands of cases of DHF/DSS, occur annually. The severe syndrome is unlikely to be seen in U.S. citizens since few children have the dengue antibodies that can trigger the pathogenetic cascade when a second infection is acquired.

Macrophage/monocyte infection is central to the pathogenesis of dengue fever and to the origin of DHF/DSS. Previous infection with a heterologous dengue-virus serotype may result in the production of nonprotective antiviral antibodies that nevertheless bind to the virion's surface and through interaction with the Fc receptor focus secondary dengue viruses on the target cell, the result being enhanced infection. The host is also primed for a secondary antibody response when viral antigens are released and immune complexes lead to activation of the classic complement pathway, with consequent phlogistic effects. Cross-reactivity at the T cell level results in the release of physiologically active cytokines, including interferon γ and tumor necrosis factor α. The induction of vascular permeability and shock depends on multiple factors, including the following:

1. *Presence of enhancing and nonneutralizing antibodies*—Transplacental maternal antibody may be present in infants <9 months old, or antibody elicited by previous heterologous dengue infection may be present in older individuals. T cell reactivity is also intimately involved.
2. *Age*—Susceptibility to DHF/DSS drops considerably after 12 years of age.
3. *Sex*—Females are more often affected than males.

4. *Race*—Caucasians are more often affected than blacks.
5. *Nutritional status*—Malnutrition is protective.
6. *Sequence of infection*—For example, serotype 1 followed by serotype 2 seems to be more dangerous than serotype 4 followed by serotype 2.
7. *Infecting serotype*—Type 2 is apparently more dangerous than other serotypes.

In addition, there is considerable variation among strains of a given serotype, with Southeast Asian serotype 2 strains having more potential to cause DHF/DSS than others.

Dengue HF is identified by the detection of bleeding tendencies (tourniquet test, petechiae) or overt bleeding in the absence of underlying causes such as preexisting gastrointestinal lesions. Dengue shock syndrome, usually accompanied by hemorrhagic signs, is much more serious and results from increased vascular permeability leading to shock. In mild DHF/DSS, restlessness, lethargy, thrombocytopenia (<100,000/μL), and hemoconcentration are detected 2 to 5 days after the onset of typical dengue fever, usually at the time of defervescence. The maculopapular rash that often develops in dengue fever may also appear in DHF/DSS. In more severe cases, frank shock is apparent, with low pulse pressure, cyanosis, hepatomegaly, pleural effusions, ascites, and in some cases severe ecchymoses and gastrointestinal bleeding. The period of shock lasts only 1 or 2 days, and most patients respond promptly to close monitoring, oxygen administration, and infusion of crystalloid or—in severe cases—colloid. The case-fatality rates reported vary greatly with case ascertainment and the quality of treatment; however, most DHF/DSS patients respond well to supportive therapy, and overall mortality in an experienced center in the tropics is probably as low as 1%.

A virologic diagnosis can be made by the usual means, although multiple flavivirus infections lead to a broad immune response to several members of the group, and this situation may result in a lack of virus specificity of the IgM and IgG immune responses. A secondary antibody response can be sought with tests against several flavivirus antigens to demonstrate the characteristic wide spectrum of reactivity.

The key to control of both dengue fever and DHF/DSS is the control of *A. aegypti*, which also reduces the risk of urban yellow fever and chikungunya virus circulation. Control efforts have been handicapped by the presence of nondegradable tires and long-lived plastic containers in trash repositories, insecticide resistance, urban poverty, and an inability of the public health community to mobilize the populace to respond to the need to eliminate mosquito breeding sites. Live attenuated dengue vaccines are in the late stages of development and have produced promising results in early tests. Whether vaccines can provide safe, durable immunity to an immunopathologic disease such as DHF/DSS in endemic areas is an issue that will have to be tested, but it is hoped that vaccination will reduce transmission to negligible levels.

KYASANUR FOREST DISEASE AND OMSK HEMORRHAGIC FEVER   See Chap. 180 in *Harrison's Online* (*www.harrisonsonline.com*).

FILOVIRUS HEMORRHAGIC FEVER   See Chap. 181.

FURTHER READING

BRUNO P et al: The protean manifestations of hemorrhagic fever with renal syndrome. A retrospective review of 26 cases from Korea. Ann Intern Med 113:385, 1990

CALISHER CH: Medically important arboviruses of the United States and Canada. Clin Microbiol Rev 7:89, 1994

CENTERS FOR DISEASE CONTROL AND PREVENTION: Update: Management of patients with suspected viral hemorrhagic fever—United States. MMWR 44:475, 1995 (*http://www.cdc.gov/mmwr/preview/mmwrhtml/00038033.htm*)

DERESIEWICZ RL et al: Clinical and neuroradiographic manifestations of east-ern equine encephalitis. N Engl J Med 336:1867, 1997

ENRIA D et al: Arenaviruses, in *Tropical Infectious Diseases: Principles, Pathogens, & Practice*, RL Guerrant et al (eds). New York, Saunders, 1999, pp 1189–1212

PETERS CJ, KHAN AS: Hantavirus pulmonary syndrome: The new American hemorrhagic fever. Clin Infect Dis 34:1224, 2002

RIVAS F et al: Epidemic Venezuelan equine encephalitis in La Guajira, Colombia, 1995. J Infect Dis 175:828, 1997

SOLOMON SR, VAUGHN DW: Pathogenesis and clinical features of Japanese encephalitis and West Nile virus infections. Curr Top Microbiol Immunol 267:171, 2002

SOLOMON T et al: West Nile encephalitis. BMJ 326:865, 2003

WURTZ R, PALEOLOGOS N: La Crosse encephalitis presenting like herpes simplex encephalitis in an immunocompromised adult. Clin Infect Dis 31:1113, 2000

181 | EBOLA AND MARBURG VIRUSES
Clarence J. Peters

DEFINITION Both Marburg virus and Ebola virus cause an acute febrile illness associated with high mortality. This illness is characterized by multisystem involvement that begins with the abrupt onset of headache, myalgias, and fever and proceeds to prostration, rash, and shock and often to bleeding manifestations. Epidemics usually begin with a single case acquired from an unknown reservoir in nature and spread mainly through close contact with sick persons or their body fluids, either in the home or at the hospital.

ETIOLOGY The family Filoviridae comprises two antigenically and genetically distinct viruses: Marburg virus and Ebola virus. Ebola virus has four readily distinguishable subtypes named for their original sites of recognition (Zaire, Sudan, Cote d'Ivoire, and Reston). Except for Ebola virus subtype Reston, all the Filoviridae are African viruses that cause severe and often fatal disease in humans. The Reston virus, which has been exported from the Philippines on several occasions, has caused fatal infections in monkeys but only subclinical infections in humans. Different isolates of the four Ebola subtypes made over time and space exhibit remarkable sequence conservation, indicating marked genetic stability in their selective niche. Typical filovirus particles contain a single linear, negative-sense, single-stranded RNA arranged in a helical nucleocapsid. The virions are 790 to 970 nm in length; they may also appear in elongated, contorted forms. The lipid envelope confers sensitivity to lipid solvents and common detergents. The viruses are largely destroyed by heat (60°C, 30 min) and by acidity but may persist for weeks in blood at room temperature. The surface glycoprotein self-associates to form the virion surface spikes, which presumably mediate attachment to cells and fusion. The glycoprotein's high sugar content may contribute to its low capacity to elicit neutralizing antibodies. A smaller form of the glycoprotein, bearing many of its antigenic determinants, is produced by in vitro–infected cells and is found in the circulation in human disease; it has been speculated that this circulating soluble protein may suppress the immune response to the virion surface protein or block antiviral effector mechanisms. Both Marburg virus and Ebola virus are biosafety level 4 pathogens because of their high associated mortality rate and aerosol infectivity.

EPIDEMIOLOGY Marburg virus was first identified in Germany in 1967, when infected African green monkeys (*Cercopithecus aethiops*) imported from Uganda transmitted the agent to vaccine-laboratory workers. Of the 25 human cases acquired from monkeys, 7 ended in death. The six secondary cases were associated with close contact or parenteral exposure. Secondary spread to the wife of one patient was documented, and virus was isolated from the husband's semen despite the presence of circulating antibodies. Subsequently, isolated cases of Marburg virus infection have been reported from eastern and southern Africa, with limited spread.

In 1999, repeated transmission of Marburg virus to workers in a gold mine in eastern Democratic Republic of Congo was documented. The secondary spread of the virus among patients' families was more extensive than previously noted, resembling that of Ebola virus and emphasizing the importance of hygiene and proper barrier nursing in the epidemiology of these viruses in Africa.

In 1976, epidemics of severe hemorrhagic fever (550 human cases) occurred simultaneously in Zaire and Sudan, and Ebola virus was found to be the etiologic agent. Later, it was shown that different subtypes of virus—associated with 90 and 50% mortality, respectively—caused the two epidemics. Both epidemics were associated with interhuman spread (particularly in the hospital setting) and the use of unsterilized needles and syringes, a common practice in developing-country hospitals. The epidemics dwindled as the clinics were closed and people in the endemic area increasingly shunned affected persons and avoided traditional burial practices.

The Zaire subtype of Ebola virus recurred in a major epidemic (317 cases, 88% mortality) in Democratic Republic of Congo in 1995 and in smaller epidemics in Gabon in 1994–1996. Mortality was high, transmission to caregivers and others who had direct contact with body fluids was common, and poor hygiene in hospitals exacerbated spread. In the Congo epidemic, an index case was infected in Kikwit in January 1995. The epidemic smoldered until April, when intense nosocomial transmission forced closure of the hospitals; samples were finally sent to the laboratory for Ebola testing, which yielded positive results within a few hours. International assistance, with barrier nursing instruction and materials, was provided; nosocomial transmission ceased, hospitals reopened, and patients were segregated to prevent intrafamilial spread. The last case was reported in June 1995.

Separate emergences of Ebola virus (subtype Zaire) were detected in Gabon from 1994 through 2003, usually in association with deep forest exposure and subsequent familial and nosocomial transmission. Nonhuman primates sometimes exhibited die-offs, and Ebola infection was confirmed in at least some animals. In a 1996 episode, a physician exposed to Ebola-infected patients traveled to South Africa with a fever; a nurse who assisted in a cutdown on the physician developed Ebola hemorrhagic fever and died despite intensive care. The index patient was identified retrospectively on the basis of serum antibodies and virus isolation from semen. Thus, distant transport of Ebola virus is an established risk, but limited nosocomial spread occurs under proper hygienic conditions.

In 2000–2001, an indolent outbreak of the Sudan subtype claimed the lives of 224 (53%) of 425 patients with presumptive cases in Uganda.

The Reston subtype of Ebola virus was first seen in the United States in 1989, when it caused a fatal, highly transmissible disease among cynomolgus macaques imported from the Philippines and quarantined in Reston, VA, pending distribution to biomedical researchers. This and other appearances of the Reston virus have been traced to a single export facility in the Philippines, but no source in nature has been established.

Epidemiologic studies (including a specific search in the Kikwit epidemic) have failed to yield evidence for an important role of airborne particles in human disease. This lack of epidemiologic evidence is surprising and seems to conflict with the viruses' classification as biosafety level 4 pathogens based in part on their aerosol infectivity and with formal laboratory assessments showing a high degree of aerosol infectivity for monkeys. Sick humans apparently do not usually generate sufficient amounts of infectious aerosols to pose a significant hazard to those around them.

Available evidence points to a nonprimate reservoir for these viruses, but an intensive search has failed to elucidate what this reservoir might be. Speculation has centered on a possible role for bats, but that hypothesis has risen in part merely because of the ubiquity of bats when sought in affected areas and the frustration of researchers in identifying a source of virus.

PATHOLOGY AND PATHOGENESIS In humans and in animal models, Ebola and Marburg viruses replicate well in virtually all cell types, including endothelial cells, macrophages, and parenchymal cells of multiple organs. The earliest involvement is that of the mononuclear phagocyte system, and this is responsible for initiation of the disease process. Viral replication is associated with cellular necrosis both in vivo and in vitro. Significant findings at the light-microscopic level include liver necrosis with Councilman bodies (intracellular inclusions that correlate with extensive collections of viral nucleocapsids), interstitial pneumonitis, cerebral glial nodules, and small infarcts. Antigen and virions are abundant in fibroblasts, interstitium, and (to a lesser extent) the appendages of the subcutaneous tissues in fatal cases; escape through small breaks in the skin or possibly through sweat glands may occur and, if so, may be correlated with the established epidemiologic risk of close contact with patients and the touching of the deceased. Inflammatory cells are not prominent, even in necrotic areas.

In addition to sustaining direct damage from viral infection, patients infected with Ebola virus (Zaire subtype) have high circulating levels of proinflammatory cytokines, which presumably contribute to the severity of the illness. In fact, the virus interacts intimately with the cellular cytokine system. It is resistant to the antiviral effects of interferon α, although this mediator is amply induced. Viral infection of endothelial cells selectively inhibits the expression of MHC class I molecules and blocks the induction of several genes by the interferons. In addition, glycoprotein expression inhibits αV integrin expression, an effect that has been shown in vitro to lead to detachment and subsequent death of endothelial cells.

Acute infection is associated with high levels of circulating virus and viral antigen. Clinical improvement takes place when viral titers decrease concomitantly with the onset of a virus-specific immune response, as detected by enzyme-linked immunosorbent assay (ELISA) or fluorescent antibody test. In fatal cases, there is usually little evidence of an antibody response and there is extensive depletion of spleen and lymph nodes. Recovery is apparently mediated by the cellular immune response: convalescent-phase plasma has little in vitro virus-neutralizing capacity and is not protective in passive transfer experiments in monkey and guinea pig models.

CLINICAL MANIFESTATIONS After an incubation period of ~7 to 10 days (range, 3 to 16 days), the patient abruptly develops fever, severe headache, malaise, myalgia, nausea, and vomiting. Continued fever is joined by diarrhea (often severe), chest pain (accompanied by cough), prostration, and depressed mentation. In light-skinned patients (and less often in dark-skinned individuals), a maculopapular rash appears around day 5 to 7 and is followed by desquamation. Bleeding may begin about this time and is apparent from any mucosal site and into the skin. In some epidemics, fewer than half of patients have had overt bleeding, and this manifestation has been absent even in some fatal cases. Additional findings include edema of the face, neck, and/or scrotum; hepatomegaly; flushing; conjunctival injection; and pharyngitis. Around 10 to 12 days after the onset of disease, the sustained fever may break, with improvement and eventual recovery of the patient. Recrudescence of fever may be associated with secondary bacterial infections or possibly with localized virus persistence. Late hepatitis, uveitis, and orchitis have been reported, with isolation of virus from semen or detection of polymerase chain reaction (PCR) products in vaginal secretions for several weeks.

LABORATORY FINDINGS Leukopenia is common early on; neutrophilia has its onset later. Platelet counts fall below (sometimes much below) 50,000/μL. Laboratory evidence of disseminated intravascular coagulation may be found, but its clinical significance and the need for therapy are controversial. Serum levels of alanine and aspartate aminotransferases (particularly the latter) rise progressively, and jaundice develops in some cases. The serum amylase level may be elevated, and this elevation may be associated with abdominal pain suggesting pancreatitis. Proteinuria is usual; decreased kidney function is proportional to shock.

DIAGNOSIS Most patients acutely ill as a result of infection with Ebola or Marburg viruses have high concentrations of virus in blood. Antigen-detection ELISA is a sensitive, robust diagnostic modality. Virus isolation and reverse-transcriptase PCR are also effective and provide additional sensitivity in some cases. Patients who are recovering develop IgM and IgG antibodies that are best detected by ELISA but are also reactive in the less specific fluorescent antibody test. Skin biopsies are an extremely useful adjunct in postmortem diagnosis of Ebola (and, to a lesser extent, Marburg) virus infections because of the presence of large amounts of viral antigen, the relative safety of obtaining the sample, and the freedom from cold-chain requirements for formalin-fixed tissues.

℞ TREATMENT

No virus-specific therapy is available, and, given the extensive viral involvement in fatal cases, supportive treatment may not be as useful as was once hoped. However, recent studies in rhesus monkeys have shown improved survival among animals treated with an inhibitor of factor VIIa/tissue factor. Vigorous treatment of shock should take into account the likelihood of vascular leak in the pulmonary and systemic circulation and of myocardial functional compromise. The membrane fusion mechanism of Ebola resembles that of retroviruses, and the identification of "fusogenic" sequences suggests that inhibitors of cell entry may be developed. Despite the poor neutralizing capacity of polyclonal convalescent-phase sera, phage display of immunoglobulin mRNA from convalescent bone marrow has produced monoclonal antibodies that have in vitro neutralizing capacity and mediate protection in guinea pig—but, unfortunately, not in monkey—models.

PREVENTION No vaccine or antiviral drug is currently available, but barrier nursing precautions in African hospitals can greatly decrease the spread of the virus beyond the index case and thus prevent epidemics of filoviruses and other agents as well. An adenovirus-vectored Ebola glycoprotein gene has proved protective in nonhuman primates and is undergoing phase 1 trials in humans.

FURTHER READING

CENTERS FOR DISEASE CONTROL AND PREVENTION: Outbreak of Ebola hemorrhagic fever—Uganda, August 2000–January 2001. JAMA 285: 1010, 2001

GEISBERT TW et al: Treatment of Ebola virus infection with a recombinant inhibitor of factor VIIa/tissue factor: A study in rhesus monkeys. Lancet 362:1953, 2003

PETERS CJ, LEDUC JW: An introduction to Ebola: The virus and the disease. J Infect Dis 179(Suppl 1):ix, 1999 (Also available at *www.journals.uchicago.edu/JID/*)

SULLIVAN NT: Accelerated vaccination for Ebola virus haemorrhagic fever in non-human primates. Nature 424:681, 2003

WORLD HEALTH ORGANIZATION: Outbreak(s) of Ebola haemorrhagic fever in the Republic of the Congo, January–April 2003. Wkly Epidemiol Rec 78:285, 2003

182 DIAGNOSIS AND TREATMENT OF FUNGAL INFECTIONS
John E. Bennett

MYCOLOGY FUNDAMENTALS

Fungi can appear microscopically as either rounded, budding forms (yeastlike organisms) or hyphae (molds). Yeastlike colonies are smooth, while mold colonies are fuzzy; fungi that grow as yeasts include species of *Candida* and *Cryptococcus*, while fungi that grow as molds include species of *Aspergillus*, *Rhizopus*, and dermatophytes (ringworm fungi). The fungi that cause histoplasmosis, blastomycosis, sporotrichosis, coccidioidomycosis, and paracoccidioidomycosis are called *dimorphic* ("having two forms") because they are spherical in tissue but grow like molds when cultured at room temperature. *Candida* species other than *Candida glabrata* appear in tissue as both budding yeasts and tubular elements called *pseudohyphae*. Pseudohyphae, unlike true hyphae, have constrictions in the cell wall where septa are located and have septa at branching points. *Pneumocystis* (Chap. 191) is closer to fungi than to parasites by ribosomal sequences. Because the drugs used to treat *Pneumocystis* pneumonia are also used to treat parasitic or bacterial infections (see Chaps. 118 and 193), those drugs will not be discussed in this chapter.

Many fungi can form two different types of spores and are given different names, depending on the spore-bearing structures. When the spores are produced by mitosis, the fungus is said to be an *anamorph*, or to be in the imperfect state. Many fungi can have different sporulating structures in which genetic recombination occurs, often as a result of coculture with a strain of the opposite mating type. A fungus producing those distinctive spores is said to be a *teleomorph*, or to be in the perfect state. Diagnostic laboratories usually use the name of the anamorph because they do not use culture conditions that would produce the teleomorph. One exception is *Scedosporium apiospermum*, which is often observed as a teleomorph in the diagnostic laboratory and identified as *Pseudallescheria boydii*.

Most fungi that are pathogenic for humans are saprophytes in nature; they cause infection when airborne spores reach the lung or paranasal sinus or when hyphae or spores are accidentally inoculated into the skin or cornea. Acquisition of infection from another person or an animal has been reported in the case of ringworm but is very rare in other mycoses. Thus, hospitalized patients with fungal infections do not require special isolation. Most fungi infect hosts preferentially by one route and only infrequently by other routes. For example, the agents of ringworm, pityriasis versicolor, and piedra infect the epidermis and its appendages. Sporotrichosis and mycetoma usually arise from subcutaneous inoculation. Inhalation is the route of inoculation for the agents of most deep mycoses. Ingestion of fungi rarely causes infection; *Candida albicans*, a normal commensal in the mouth and intestine, reaches deeper tissues only when mucosal or cutaneous barriers are breached by disease, surgery, trauma, or catheterization. Histoplasmosis, blastomycosis, coccidioidomycosis, and paracoccidioidomycosis have been called "endemic" mycoses to emphasize their restricted geographic distribution. Some fungi, such as *Aspergillus* and *Fusarium*, are said to be opportunists in that they usually infect hosts with compromised immunity. This distinction is relative, not absolute.

Immunity after exposure to fungi may confer partial protection against reinfection. Residents of areas in which mycoses are endemic are less subject to infection than are newcomers. Predisposing factors are helpful in defining host defense. Immunoglobulin deficiencies do not appear to predispose to any mycosis, whereas neutropenia is common among patients who develop invasive mold infections or deep candidiasis. Cell-mediated immunity appears to be of paramount importance in cryptococcosis, histoplasmosis, and coccidioidomycosis.

DIAGNOSIS

Many fungi can be identified to the genus or even the species level by microscopic examination of smears or biopsy specimens. Calcofluor white staining with fluorescence microscopy is a sensitive technique for smears of sputum, bronchoalveolar lavage fluid, or pus. India ink smear remains the method of choice for detecting cryptococci in cerebrospinal fluid (CSF). *Candida* yeast cells and pseudohyphae are the only fungi that are usually gram-positive on smears. For other fungi, Gram's staining is distinctly suboptimal. For histopathology slides, Gomori methenamine silver and a neutral counterstain are preferred.

The method used has a marked effect on the rapidity and sensitivity of blood cultures for fungi except in the case of *Candida* species, which are relatively easy to grow. For most other fungi, concentration of the blood by lysis centrifugation and culture on solid medium constitute the optimal technique. Commercially available nucleic acid hybridization techniques can speed the identification of slow-growing molds, such as *Histoplasma capsulatum* and *Coccidioides immitis*. Serology has limited value, but testing of serum or CSF for cryptococcal antigen or antibody to *C. immitis* can be diagnostic. Detection of *Histoplasma* antigen in urine or serum is helpful in diagnosis and in following the results of treatment for disseminated histoplasmosis. Skin testing with fungal antigens is not useful in detecting active infection.

ANTIFUNGAL THERAPY

TOPICAL AGENTS ■ Imidazoles and Triazoles (See also "Systemic Antifungals") These synthetic compounds act by inhibiting ergosterol synthesis in the fungal cell wall and, when given topically, may cause direct damage to the fungal cytoplasmic membrane. The imidazoles available for cutaneous application include clotrimazole, econazole, ketoconazole, sulconazole, oxiconazole, and miconazole. Vaginal formulations include four imidazoles (miconazole, clotrimazole, tioconazole, and butoconazole) and one triazole (terconazole). As yet, no substantial differences in the efficacy of or local intolerance to the various topical azoles have become apparent. All are effective in the treatment of cutaneous candidiasis, tinea (pityriasis) versicolor, and mild to moderately severe ringworm of the glabrous skin. Vaginal formulations are effective for vulvovaginal candidiasis. Clotrimazole is poorly absorbed from the gastrointestinal tract, but the oral troche is useful as a topical treatment for oral and esophageal candidiasis.

Polyene Macrolide Antibiotics These broad-spectrum antifungal agents combine with sterol in the fungal cytoplasmic membrane, increasing membrane permeability. Topically, they are not active against ringworm but are effective against candidiasis of the skin and mucous membranes. Nystatin and amphotericin B suspensions are effective in oral thrush, and vaginal troches are effective in vulvovaginal candidiasis. Both nystatin and amphotericin B are available in topical preparations for cutaneous candidiasis.

Other Topical Antifungals Ciclopirox olamine, haloprogin, terbinafine, and naftifine have the same clinical spectrum among the cutaneous mycoses as the imidazoles. Tolnaftate and undecylenic acid are effective against ringworm but not candidiasis. Keratolytic agents, such as salicylic acid, are helpful as accessory drugs for some hyperkeratotic skin lesions.

SYSTEMIC ANTIFUNGALS ■ Griseofulvin Griseofulvin is a useful drug in the treatment of certain kinds of ringworm; however, it is ineffective in the treatment of candidiasis. The microcrystalline and ultramicrocrystalline preparations differ in dose but not in efficacy. Absorption of both is enhanced when the drug is ingested with fat-containing foods. Griseofulvin interacts with phenobarbital and warfarin.

Terbinafine Oral terbinafine (250 mg once daily) is at least as effective as itraconazole and more effective than griseofulvin in onychomycosis and ringworm. Treatment duration ranges from 3 months for fingernails to 6 months for toenails. Gastrointestinal distress is the most common side effect. Rash, hepatitis, and pancytopenia have occurred, but serious adverse effects have been uncommon. Terbinafine decreases cyclosporine levels. Cimetidine increases and rifampin decreases terbinafine levels in blood.

Imidazoles and Triazoles ■ *GENERAL FEATURES* The azole antifungals include imidazoles and triazoles. Fluconazole, itraconazole, voriconazole, and the investigational azoles posaconazole and ravuconazole are all triazoles, so named because they have three nitrogens in the ring structure. This class has less impact on human hormonal synthesis and less hepatotoxicity than the only widely used systemic imidazole, ketoconazole. Itraconazole has many structural features in common with ketoconazole; however, it has a broader spectrum of activity and has largely replaced ketoconazole.

Interactions between azoles and other drugs can increase the plasma concentrations of the other drugs to toxic levels or decrease the azole plasma concentrations to subtherapeutic levels. A few drugs can increase the plasma concentrations of azoles, but the effect is modest. Drug-drug interactions are most numerous with itraconazole and ketoconazole; some drugs are contraindicated for concomitant use with these agents. Azole interactions with any one class of drugs, such as benzodiazepines, HMG-CoA reductase inhibitors, or drugs that decrease gastric acidity, should be considered to apply to all drugs of that class until proven otherwise. Fluconazole differs substantially from itraconazole: unlike that of itraconazole, the absorption of fluconazole is independent of food or gastric acid, and fluconazole has much less effect on the hepatic metabolism of other drugs than does itraconazole. High fluconazole blood levels engendered by azotemia or by dosages above those used in pharmacologic studies may lead to new and profound drug interactions.

All azoles have the potential for embryotoxicity and teratogenicity. In fact, it seems likely that azoles should not be given during pregnancy without a discussion of the serious risks and possible benefits with the mother. Four infants born to mothers taking at least 400 mg of fluconazole daily for coccidioidal meningitis have had severe bone, craniofacial, or cardiac abnormalities. Similarity of these abnormalities to those in pregnant animals given fluconazole suggests that fluconazole caused the defects.

ITRACONAZOLE Itraconazole is useful in the treatment of blastomycosis, histoplasmosis, cutaneous candidiasis, coccidioidomycosis, sporotrichosis, pseudallescheriasis, onychomycosis, ringworm, tinea versicolor, and indolent cases of aspergillosis. The drug is metabolized in the liver, with the hydroxy metabolite accounting for at least half of the antifungal activity in serum. The sum of the blood levels of the native drug and its hydroxylated metabolite is usually at least 2 μg/mL a few hours after oral administration. Almost no bioactive drug appears in urine or CSF.

Itraconazole is available as a 100-mg capsule, an oral solution, and an intravenous formulation. Although itraconazole capsules are less expensive and cause less gastrointestinal distress than the oral solution, their absorption is sometimes problematic. Cyclodextrin, which is used to formulate both the oral solution and the intravenous formulation, is renally excreted but is not absorbed from the gastrointestinal tract. Food increases the absorption of itraconazole capsules by about threefold but substantially reduces the absorption of the cyclodextrin suspension.

The oral solution is effective in oropharyngeal and esophageal candidiasis at a dose of 100 mg (10 mL) twice daily and has also been used at twice that dose for the treatment of deep mycoses in patients who absorb itraconazole capsules poorly. The efficacy of itraconazole in mycoses of the central nervous system has been modest at best, given the drug's inability to reach the CSF. For deep infections, itraconazole capsules are given at an initial dosage of 600 to 800 mg daily for 3 days and a subsequent dosage of 200 to 400 mg once daily

continued for 6 to 12 months. Itraconazole blood levels (see above) are helpful in documenting absorption when the oral drug is used for the treatment of deep mycoses. The commercially available intravenous formulation should be considered for initial therapy in hospitalized patients whose itraconazole absorption from the gastrointestinal tract may be suboptimal and whose creatinine clearance rate exceeds 30 mL/min. The dose is 200 mg twice daily for four doses followed by 200 mg daily for up to 2 weeks. Intravenous itraconazole, followed by the oral solution, is approved for the treatment of fever of unknown origin in neutropenic patients not responding to at least 96 h of therapy with antibacterial antibiotics.

Except for gastrointestinal distress from the oral solution, the toxicity of itraconazole is generally low, although life-threatening hepatotoxicity, congestive heart failure, edema, cardiac dysrhythmias, and peripheral neuropathy have been reported.

FLUCONAZOLE This triazole can be administered in tablet form, as a suspension, or as an intravenous infusion. With a half-life of about 31 h, fluconazole can be given once a day. Approximately 80% of the drug is excreted unchanged in the urine. Patients with creatinine clearance rates of 21 to 50 mL/min and 11 to 20 mL/min should have their fluconazole doses reduced by 50 and 75%, respectively. The drug penetrates the CSF and other body fluids very well.

Nausea and abdominal distress are the most common forms of dose-limiting fluconazole toxicity. An allergic rash may develop and is particularly common among patients infected with HIV. Fatal cases of Stevens-Johnson syndrome have been described in the HIV-infected population. Alopecia commonly follows prolonged administration of ≥400 mg daily but resolves when therapy is discontinued. Rare cases of anaphylaxis, hepatic necrosis, and neutropenia have been described.

Fluconazole is useful in the treatment of oropharyngeal and esophageal candidiasis in adults. A single 150-mg tablet is effective in vulvovaginal candidiasis. Catheter-acquired candidemia in the immunocompetent host responds to 400 mg of fluconazole daily in conjunction with the removal of the infected catheter. Treatment should be continued for 10 to 14 days after the patient has become afebrile. Fluconazole is also effective in initial and maintenance therapy for cryptococcal meningitis in patients with AIDS, although most of these patients should initially receive a 2-week course of intravenous amphotericin B. Fluconazole is the drug of choice for coccidioidal meningitis.

The incidence of deep candidiasis among recipients of allogeneic bone marrow transplants can be reduced by the administration of fluconazole (400 mg daily) for 75 days after initiation of the transplantation-preparative regimen. Prophylaxis in other neutropenic patients has not appeared useful. Fluconazole (200 mg daily) reduced the incidence of cryptococcosis and mucosal candidiasis among AIDS patients whose CD4+ cell counts were <200/μL and was particularly effective among those with counts of <50/μL. However, this regimen is not recommended because it does not reduce mortality, is expensive, and can lead to drug resistance.

Fluconazole is less effective than itraconazole in blastomycosis, histoplasmosis, and sporotrichosis. The drug is not active in aspergillosis, pseudallescheriasis, or mucormycosis.

VORICONAZOLE This recently marketed triazole is available as 50- and 200-mg tablets and as vials of 200 mg for intravenous administration. The average-sized adult is given 6 mg/kg intravenously every 12 h for two doses followed by maintenance doses of 4 mg/kg intravenously every 12 h. In patients whose condition is improving, the regimen can be changed to 200 mg twice daily by mouth. Up to 300 mg twice daily by mouth can be given to patients who do not respond adequately to the lower dose.

Voriconazole is well absorbed from the gastrointestinal tract and is metabolized completely by the liver by way of CYP2C9, CYP2C19, and CYP3A4. Genetic polymorphisms in CYP2C19 activity cause substantial variation in voriconazole metabolism. Dose adjustment for azotemia is not necessary, but the dose should be reduced by half in patients with moderate liver disease. Because the cyclodextrin used in the intravenous formulation is renally excreted, oral—not intravenous—voriconazole should be used in patients with creatinine clearance rates below 50 mL/min. Penetration into the CSF is good. Concurrent use of sirolimus is contraindicated because its serum levels are markedly increased in the presence of voriconazole. Until more complete data are available, the drug interactions for voriconazole should be considered to be similar to those for itraconazole. The toxic effects of voriconazole include transient visual disturbances (color changes, blurring) in 30% of patients, hepatotoxicity in 10%, and rash in 5%.

The spectrum of voriconazole includes all the fungi against which itraconazole and fluconazole are active. Voriconazole is indicated for initial treatment of invasive aspergillosis, pseudallescheriasis, and fusariosis. The drug is also useful as empirical therapy in febrile neutropenic patients who do not respond to at least 96 h of treatment with antibacterial antibiotics and who are at high risk of invasive mold infections.

INVESTIGATIONAL TRIAZOLES Posaconazole and ravuconazole, which are undergoing early clinical trials, have antifungal spectra similar to that of voriconazole. Ravuconazole is notable for a half-life of ~1 week.

Echinocandins One echinocandin (caspofungin) is on the market, and two others (micafungin and anidulafungin) are being assessed in clinical trials. All are administered intravenously and act by inhibiting synthesis of $(1,3)\beta$-D-glucan in the cell wall. The in vitro activity of these drugs against nearly all *Candida* species is similar and is independent of azole resistance. The possible exception is *Candida parapsilosis*, a species whose susceptibility varies with the isolate and the particular echinocandin. Activity against *Aspergillus* species is more obvious in experimentally infected animals than in vitro, where changes in hyphal shape are more obvious than decreased growth. The recommended regimen is a 70-mg loading dose followed by 50 mg daily. Toxicity is low and includes histamine-like acute infusion reactions and hepatotoxicity. Cyclosporine elevates caspofungin blood levels, but other drug-drug interactions have been minor so far. No dosage adjustment is needed in patients with azotemia or hemodialysis, but the dose should be reduced for moderate hepatic insufficiency. Penetration into CSF is negligible. On the basis of an open trial in 63 patients, caspofungin has been approved for salvage therapy in aspergillosis. Data on candidemia in nonneutropenic patients indicate an efficacy equivalent to that of fluconazole or amphotericin B.

Amphotericin B A colloidal deoxycholate complex of the polyene drug amphotericin B is available for intravenous or intrathecal administration. The catabolism of amphotericin B is extremely slow and is not influenced by renal failure, hepatic failure, or hemodialysis. The drug's penetration into CSF and vitreous humor is poor; however, the concentrations in pleural, peritoneal, and articular exudates are adequate for many mycoses. Histoplasmosis, blastomycosis, paracoccidioidomycosis, candidiasis, and cryptococcosis are the most responsive mycoses; coccidioidomycosis, extraarticular sporotrichosis, aspergillosis, and mucormycosis are less responsive; and chromoblastomycosis, mycetoma, and pseudallescheriasis respond little, if at all. The usual course is 0.5 to 0.7 mg/kg daily for 8 to 10 weeks. Infusions are generally given in 5% dextrose over 2 to 4 h.

Initial doses of amphotericin B occasionally cause marked febrile reactions that may be poorly tolerated by adult patients with limited cardiac or pulmonary function. It may be prudent to give such patients an initial 1-mg test dose followed by rapidly escalating doses, depending on tolerance. Premedication with aspirin or acetaminophen or the addition of hydrocortisone (25 mg) to the infusion decreases chills and fever. Azotemia during treatment is usual, the extent depending on the daily dose, underlying renal disease, and concomitant nephrotoxic agents. Saline infusions have been advocated to reduce azotemia. Continuous amphotericin B infusions may reduce nephrotoxicity, but the impact on efficacy is unknown. Other side effects include anemia,

hypokalemia, renal tubular acidosis, nausea, anorexia, weight loss, phlebitis, and occasionally hypomagnesemia. Intrathecal amphotericin B has been used in coccidioidal meningitis and refractory cryptococcal meningitis, although this therapy is associated with transient fever, headache, nausea, and vomiting.

Three lipid formulations of intravenous amphotericin B are commercially available in the United States. These formulations and their usual once-daily doses are amphotericin B lipid complex (ABLC), 5 mg/kg; amphotericin B colloidal dispersion (ABCD), 6 mg/kg; and liposomal amphotericin B (L-AB), 4–5 mg/kg. The most nephrotoxic lipid formulation is ABLC; ABCD causes less azotemia; and L-AB is the least nephrotoxic. Acute, febrile, infusion-related reactions occur with all amphotericin B formulations; their degree of severity is greatest with ABCD and lesser with ABLC and L-AB. The recommended duration for initial infusions of ABCD is 6 h for 6 mg/kg, slower than the 2-h duration of ABLC or L-AB infusions. Infusions of ABCD given more rapidly than 1 mg/kg per hour have caused severe reactions with fever and hypoxia. Use of these remarkably expensive formulations should be restricted to patients who cannot tolerate the nephrotoxicity of the deoxycholate formulation (ABD). Although the lipid formulations are also approved for patients with mycoses failing to respond to ABD, there is no indication that these formulations are more effective than ABD for any mycosis. ABLC and L-AB are probably equivalent in efficacy to ABD for most mycoses. Data on the efficacy of ABCD are largely confined to aspergillosis, in which the efficacy of this lipid formulation was equivalent to that of conventional amphotericin B.

Flucytosine Flucytosine (5-fluorocytosine) is a synthetic oral drug useful in cryptococcosis, candidiasis, and chromoblastomycosis. Within the fungal cell, flucytosine is converted to the antimetabolite 5-fluorouracil. Drug resistance appears rather rapidly when flucytosine is used alone. For this reason, the drug is generally used in combination with amphotericin B. The usual dose of flucytosine is 25 to 37.5 mg/kg every 6 h. Flucytosine is well absorbed from the gastrointestinal tract. The drug penetrates well into the CSF and is excreted unchanged in the urine. Even modest reductions in renal function may elevate flucytosine blood levels into the toxic range ($\geq$100 to 125 μg/mL). Elevated levels are associated with a significant incidence of neutropenia and thrombocytopenia and also seem to predispose to colitis, the other major toxic effect of this drug. Hepatotoxicity is idiosyncratic and uncommon. An allergic rash may develop.

FURTHER READING

BOWDEN R et al: A double-blind, randomized, controlled trial of amphotericin B colloidal dispersion versus amphotericin B for treatment of invasive aspergillosis in immunocompromised patients. Clin Infect Dis 35:359, 2002

HERBRECHT R et al: Voriconazole versus amphotericin B for primary therapy of invasive aspergillosis. N Engl J Med 347:408, 2002

HOSPENTHAL DR et al: Flucytosine monotherapy for cryptococcosis. Clin Infect Dis 27:260, 1998

MANGINO JE, PAPPAS PG: Itraconazole for the treatment of histoplasmosis and blastomycosis. Int J Antimicrob Agents 5:219, 1995

MORA-DUARTE J et al: Comparison of caspofungin and amphotericin B in invasive candidiasis. N Engl J Med 347:2070, 2002

SOBEL JD: Practice guidelines for the treatment of fungal infections. Clin Infect Dis 30:652, 2000

VAN DER HORST CM et al: Treatment of cryptococcal meningitis associated with the acquired immunodeficiency syndrome. N Engl J Med 337:15, 1997

VILLANUEVA A et al: A randomized double-blind study of caspofungin versus amphotericin for the treatment of candidal esophagitis. Clin Infect Dis 33:1529, 2001

WALSH TJ et al: Voriconazole compared with liposomal amphotericin B for empirical antifungal therapy in patients with neutropenia and persistent fever. N Engl J Med 346:225, 2002

——— et al: Liposomal amphotericin B for empirical therapy in patients with persistent fever and neutropenia. N Engl J Med 340:764, 1999

WINGARD J et al: A randomized, double-blind comparative trial evaluating the safety of liposomal amphotericin B versus amphotericin B lipid complex in the empirical treatment of febrile neutropenia. LAmph/ABLC Collaborative Study Group. Clin Infect Dis 31:1155, 2000

183 HISTOPLASMOSIS
John E. Bennett

ETIOLOGIC AGENT *Histoplasma capsulatum* var. *capsulatum* is a dimorphic fungus that grows as a mold in nature or on Sabouraud's agar at room temperature. Hyphae bear both large and small spores, which are used for identification. Nucleic acid hybridization can also be used to identify the organism in culture. *H. capsulatum* var. *capsulatum* grows as a small budding yeast in host tissue and on enriched agar, such as blood cysteine glucose, at 37°C. Despite its name, the fungus is unencapsulated. Coculture of isolates with opposite mating types can produce different sporulating structures in which genetic recombination occurs. When these structures, referred to as a *teleomorph* or the *perfect state*, are seen in culture, the name *Ajellomyces capsulatus* is used. *H. capsulatum* var. *duboisii* is a rare cause of infection, with most cases originating in Africa. The yeast cells of the *duboisii* variant are larger than those of *H. capsulatum* var. *capsulatum*, but the mold forms of the two appear identical.

EPIDEMIOLOGY Infection with *H. capsulatum* has been encountered in many areas of the world but is much more frequent in certain areas. Within the United States, infection is most common in the southeastern, mid-Atlantic, and central states. Infection has been reported in travelers returning from Latin America and other endemic areas overseas. Endemicity is contingent on the availability of proper conditions in nature for growth of the fungus. *H. capsulatum* prefers moist surface soil, particularly soil enriched by droppings of certain birds and bats. The fungus persists in contaminated soil for years and becomes airborne when the soil is disturbed. Acute infection is usually recognized as case clusters occurring 5 to 18 days after the exposure of groups of people to dust while (for example) cleaning dirt-floored chicken coops; raking or rototilling soil; exploring caves; and cleaning, remodeling, or demolishing old buildings. Skin-test reactivity in many endemic areas indicates that ≥80% of residents over age 16 have been exposed.

PATHOGENESIS AND PATHOLOGY Microconidia, or small spores, of *H. capsulatum* are small enough to reach the alveoli on inhalation and are transformed there to budding forms. With time, an intense granulomatous reaction occurs. Caseation necrosis or calcification may mimic tuberculosis. In children, the primary infection usually heals completely but may leave spotty calcification in the hilar nodes or lung. Transient dissemination may leave calcified granulomas in the spleen. In adults, a rounded mass of scar tissue, with or without central calcification, may remain in the lung. This mass has been called a *histoplasmoma*. Previous exposure is thought to confer some protection against reinfection, but infection in persons with prior positive skin tests clearly has occurred.

In a small proportion of patients, histoplasmosis becomes a progressive, potentially fatal infection. The disease occurs either as chronic fibrocavitary pneumonia or, less commonly, as disseminated infection. Patients with either form lack a history of acute primary pulmonary histoplasmosis. Chronic pulmonary infection favors otherwise-healthy males over the age of 40. A history of cigarette use or the presence of emphysema is elicited from nearly all patients with chronic progressive pulmonary histoplasmosis. An acute, rapidly fatal disseminated infection is most likely to be encountered among young children and immunosuppressed patients, including those with AIDS. Use of tumor necrosis factor α antagonists, particularly infliximab, also appears to predispose to severe disseminated histoplasmosis. A more chronic but equally lethal disseminated infection is more common among previously healthy adults.

CLINICAL MANIFESTATIONS The vast majority of infections are either asymptomatic or mild, and the diagnosis is elusive. Cough, fever, malaise, and chest x-ray findings of hilar adenopathy with or without one or more areas of pneumonitis are typical features. Erythema nodosum and erythema multiforme have been reported in a few outbreaks. Hilar adenopathy may cause temporary compression of the right-middle-lobe bronchus in children and young adults. Subacute pericarditis may develop, probably by extension from contiguous lymph nodes. Rarely, hilar nodes undergo a caseous, granulomatous reaction with perinodal fibrosis. Mediastinal structures become encased by progressive fibrosis, and compression of the pulmonary veins, superior vena cava, pulmonary arteries, and esophagus may take place over many years. Late in mediastinal disease, only rare nonviable *Histoplasma* cells can be found in caseous residua of lymph nodes.

Chronic pulmonary histoplasmosis is characterized by a gradual onset (over weeks or months) of increasing productive cough, weight loss, and sometimes night sweats. Chest x-ray reveals uni- or bilateral fibronodular apical infiltrates. Approximately one-third of cases stabilize or improve spontaneously early in the course. The remainder progress insidiously. Retraction and cavitation of the upper lobes occur, with spread to the apex of the lower lobes and other areas of the lung. Emphysema and bulla formation further compromise pulmonary function. Death from cor pulmonale, bacterial pneumonia, or histoplasmosis occurs after months or years.

Disseminated histoplasmosis has many features in common with hematogenously disseminated tuberculosis (Chap. 150). Common findings include fever, emaciation, hepatosplenomegaly, lymphadenopathy, abnormal liver function, anemia, leukopenia, and thrombocytopenia. Although skin lesions are uncommon in histoplasmosis, patients with far-advanced HIV infection may present with one or more discrete erythematous skin papules. Diffuse pulmonary disease may be mistaken for *Pneumocystis* pneumonia in patients infected with HIV. HIV-infected patients responding to highly active antiretroviral therapy may experience a return of the symptoms of histoplasmosis as a result of immune reconstitution. Previously normal patients usually have a much more indolent disease that progresses over weeks or months. Disease tends to be more focal, with one or more indurated ulcers of the mouth, tongue, nose, or larynx in about one-fourth of cases. Other focal findings include granulomatous hepatitis, Addison's disease, gastrointestinal ulcers, endocarditis, and chronic meningitis. Chest x-ray abnormalities are evident in half of cases and characteristically have a miliary pattern.

Infection with *H. capsulatum* var. *duboisii* is rare but should be considered in previous residents of Africa. Clinical manifestations resemble those of blastomycosis more than those of histoplasmosis in that skin and bone lesions are very common.

Presumed ocular histoplasmosis syndrome (POHS) is a clinical syndrome characterized by discrete atrophic choroidal scars in the macula or midperiphery, peripapillary atrophy, and choroidal neovascularization. These changes lead to a severe loss of central vision. It is unclear whether POHS represents an immune response to prior histoplasmosis, but there is no evidence of active infection. Susceptibility may be correlated with certain HLA types.

DIAGNOSIS Culture of the etiologic organism is the preferred method for diagnosis of histoplasmosis but is often difficult. Blood cultures are best performed by the lysis-centrifugation technique, with plates held at 30°C for at least 2 weeks. Approximately 15 mL of blood should be cultured from adults. Routine blood cultures in broth are generally unsuitable. Cultures of bone marrow, mucosal lesions, liver, and bronchoalveolar lavage fluid are diagnostically useful in disseminated histoplasmosis. Sputum culture is the preferred method for the diagnosis of chronic pulmonary histoplasmosis. However, growth may require 2 to 4 weeks to become visible, and other organisms may overgrow the plate. Diagnosis based on Giemsa-stained smears of blood or bronchoalveolar lavage fluid or on methenamine silver staining of infected lung, bone marrow, lymph node, or mucosal lesions requires considerable expertise, although these techniques yield results rapidly and provide specimens that can easily be sent to a referral laboratory. Organisms may be very scanty in lesions with marked caseous necrosis. An assay for *Histoplasma* antigen in blood or urine is commercially available and is useful both for diagnosis and for monitoring the response to therapy in patients with disseminated infection.

Antigen is detected occasionally in acute pulmonary histoplasmosis but rarely in chronic pulmonary disease. Diagnosis by antigen detection requires confirmation by culture or histopathology because false-positive results have occasionally been obtained. Tests for antibody to *H. capsulatum* have been of limited value in diagnosis. Histoplasmin skin testing has proven useful in epidemiologic studies but is no longer commercially available.

℞ TREATMENT

See also Table 183-1. Acute pulmonary histoplasmosis requires no therapy. Oral itraconazole (200 mg/d) can be given in the hope of shortening the course of illness, although this effect has not been proven. Patients with mediastinal fibrosis may benefit from vascular stent placement, but their ultimate prognosis is poor. All patients with disseminated or chronic pulmonary histoplasmosis should receive antifungal therapy. Intravenous amphotericin B (conventional or lipid formulation) is the drug of choice for the initial treatment of patients with disseminated histoplasmosis who are severely ill or immunosuppressed or whose infection involves the central nervous system; the regimen can be changed to itraconazole (200 mg twice daily) once clinical improvement is evident, and the latter regimen can be used as the initial therapy in less severely ill patients. Fluconazole at doses up to 400 mg/d has been less effective. Patients with AIDS whose disseminated histoplasmosis has responded to 10 weeks of therapy should receive itraconazole (200 mg/d) for life to prevent relapse. Lifelong maintenance therapy may not be necessary for HIV-infected patients who have received prolonged itraconazole treatment, have had a sustained response to highly active antiretroviral therapy, and no longer have detectable *Histoplasma* antigen in serum.

Immunocompetent patients with disseminated or chronic pulmonary histoplasmosis are given itraconazole (200 mg twice daily) and are generally treated for 6 to 12 months. Alternatively, immunocompetent patients can be given a 10-week course of amphotericin B (0.5 mg/kg daily).

Long-term maintenance therapy with an azole is not recommended for patients other than those with AIDS. However, relapse of chronic

TABLE 183-1 *Treatment of Histoplasmosis[a]*

Type of Disease	Preferred Treatment	Alternatives
Acute pulmonary	None	. . .
Chronic pulmonary	Itraconazole	Amphotericin B
Disseminated		
Immunocompetent patient, less severe illness	Itraconazole	Amphotericin B
Rapid progression, severe illness, CNS involvement, HIV infection or other immunocompromise	Amphotericin B	Switch to itraconazole after 2 weeks if patient is improved and clinically stable.

[a] Amphotericin B is given as 0.5 mg/kg daily for 10 to 12 weeks. Liposomal amphotericin B (3–5 mg/kg daily) can also be used. Itraconazole is given as 200 mg twice daily for 6 to 12 months except in AIDS patients, in whom therapy is lifelong.

pulmonary and disseminated histoplasmosis is not rare and warrants careful follow-up for 1 year after therapy.

FURTHER READING

CANO MV et al: The epidemiology of histoplasmosis. A review. Semin Respir Infect 16:109, 2001

HECHT FM et al: Itraconazole maintenance treatment for histoplasmosis in AIDS: A prospective, multicenter trial. J Acquir Immune Defic Syndr 16: 100, 1997

LEE JH et al: Life-threatening histoplasmosis complicating immunotherapy with tumor necrosis factor alpha antagonists infliximab and etanercept. Arthritis Rheum 46:2565, 2002

ONGKOSUWITO JV et al: Amino acid residue 67 (isoleucine) of HLA-DRB is associated with POHS. Invest Ophthalmol Vis Sci 43:1725, 2002

WHEAT J et al: Antigen clearance during treatment of disseminated histoplasmosis with itraconazole versus fluconazole in patients with AIDS. Antimicrob Agents Chemother 46:248, 2002

——— et al: Practice guidelines for the management of patients with histoplasmosis. Clin Infect Dis 30:688, 2000

———: Histoplasmosis. Experience during outbreaks in Indianapolis and review of the literature. Medicine (Baltimore) 76:339, 1997

——— et al: Disseminated histoplasmosis in the acquired immune deficiency syndrome: Clinical findings, diagnosis and treatment, and review of the literature. Medicine 69:361, 1990

184   COCCIDIOIDOMYCOSIS
John E. Bennett

ETIOLOGIC AGENT   *Coccidioides immitis* has two forms, growing as a white fluffy mold on most culture media but as a nonbudding spherical form (a spherule) in host tissue or under special conditions. Solely on the basis of DNA evidence, isolates from outside the San Joaquin Valley of California have been designated *Coccidioides posadasii* by some authorities. *C. immitis* reproduces in host tissue by forming small endospores within mature spherules. After rupture of the spherule, the released endospores enlarge, become spherules, and repeat the cycle. The fungus is identified by its appearance and by the formation of thick-walled, barrel-shaped spores, called *arthrospores*, in the hyphae of the mold form. Nucleic acid hybridization is a highly accurate and relatively safe way to identify this biohazard level 3 fungus.

EPIDEMIOLOGY, PATHOGENESIS, AND PATHOLOGY   *C. immitis* is a soil saprophyte found in certain arid regions of the United States, Mexico, Central America, and South America. Within the United States, most cases of infection with *C. immitis* are acquired in California, Arizona, and western Texas (Fig. 184-1). A few cases are acquired by exposure to fomites from endemic areas (e.g., in cotton bales). Use of *C. immitis* by bioterrorists should be kept in mind should large outbreaks occur (Chap. 205).

Infection in humans and animals results from inhalation of wind-borne arthrospores from soil sites. This primary pulmonary infection is symptomatic in only 40% of cases, with symptoms ranging from a mild influenza-like illness to severe pneumonia. Mild self-limited infections may come to medical attention because of case clusters or hypersensitivity reactions: erythema nodosum, erythema multiforme, toxic erythema, arthralgia, arthritis, conjunctivitis, or episcleritis. Case clusters occur 10 to 14 days after a group of susceptible individuals is exposed to dust in an endemic area through such activities as archaeologic excavation, rock hunting, military maneuvers, model airplane contests, or construction work. Windstorms can carry spores to adjacent nonendemic areas and cause case clusters. The usual course of primary pneumonia is complete healing, although an area of pneumonitis (detected on radiographs) may heal by the formation of a coin-like lesion called a *coccidioidoma*. Less commonly, a single thin-walled cavity remains as a chronic sequela in the area of consolidation. Alternatively, an area of consolidation may persist as chronic pneumonia or progress to fibronodular cavitary disease.

Pleural effusion may be the only manifestation of primary infection. Spontaneous healing of this form is common.

An uncommon but dreaded complication of coccidioidomycosis is dissemination beyond the lung and hilar lymph nodes. Dissemination is especially frequent among blacks, Filipinos, Native Americans, Mexican Americans, pregnant women, and immunosuppressed patients, including those with AIDS.

C. immitis incites a chronic pyogranuloma in host tissue, often with areas of caseation necrosis. Lung and hilar node lesions may show

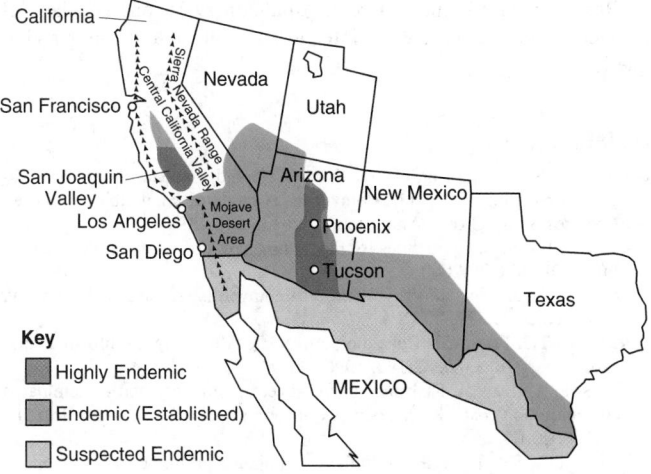

California

San Francisco

San Joaquin
Valley
Los Angeles
San Diego

Nevada

Utah

Arizona

New Mexico

Phoenix

Tucson

Texas

MEXICO

Key
- Highly Endemic
- Endemic (Established)
- Suspected Endemic

FIGURE 184-1 Geographic distribution of coccidioidomycosis. *(From Emerg Infect Dis 2:192, 1996)*

calcification. Both IgM and IgG antibodies to *C. immitis* are induced by infection, but neither type of antibody appears to be protective. The amount of specific IgG antibody is a rough measure of the antigenic mass (i.e., of the intensity of infection), and a high titer is a poor prognostic sign. Appearance of delayed hypersensitivity to antigens of *C. immitis* is most common in clinical forms of disease with a good prognosis, such as self-limited primary pulmonary disease.

CLINICAL MANIFESTATIONS Symptomatic primary pulmonary infection begins 10 to 14 days after exposure and is manifested by fever, cough, chest pain, malaise, and sometimes the hypersensitivity reactions listed above. Chest radiographs may show an infiltrate, hilar adenopathy, or pleural effusion. Mild peripheral-blood eosinophilia may be found. Spontaneous improvement begins after several days to 2 weeks of illness and usually culminates in complete recovery.

The symptoms of a chronic thin-walled cavity include cough or hemoptysis in half of cases; the other half are asymptomatic. The cavity contracts to a nodule during the first year in about half of cases. Chronic fibrocavitary pulmonary coccidioidomycosis causes cough, sputum production, variable degrees of fever, and weight loss. The first indications of dissemination usually appear during primary infection. Reactivation with dissemination in later years occurs occasionally, especially if Hodgkin's disease, non-Hodgkin's lymphoma, renal transplantation, AIDS, or immunosuppression of some other etiology has supervened. Dissemination should be suspected when fever, malaise, hilar or paratracheal lymphadenopathy, elevated sedimentation rate, and high complement fixation titers signal abnormal persistence in patients with primary pulmonary coccidioidomycosis. With time, lesions appear in the bone, skin, subcutaneous tissue, meninges, joints, and other sites. Chronic meningitis presents as headache of indolent onset, with or without other signs of disseminated coccidioidomycosis. Cultures and smears of cerebrospinal fluid (CSF) are most often negative, but antibody is usually detectable in CSF by complement fixation. Skin lesions are indolent and maculopapular. Soft tissue and bony lesions contain pus and may present as a draining sinus. Without treatment, disseminated coccidioidomycosis progresses to death over weeks to years.

Disseminated coccidioidomycosis can progress rapidly in patients with advanced HIV infection. Fever with skin or bone lesions may be the first sign. Those who present with diffuse pulmonary infiltrates have a poor prognosis. Blood cultures are positive late in the disease, if at all.

DIAGNOSIS When coccidioidomycosis is suspected, sputum, urine, and pus should be examined for *C. immitis* by wet smear and culture. *The laboratory request should indicate clearly that coccidioidomycosis is suspected, because the mold form must be handled with extreme care to prevent infection of laboratory personnel.* On biopsy, smaller spherules must be distinguished from nonbudding forms of *Blastomyces* and *Cryptococcus*, but the appearance of the mature spherule is diagnostic.

Serologic tests are very helpful in the diagnosis of coccidioidomycosis. Latex agglutination and agar gel diffusion tests are useful in screening sera for antibody to *Coccidioides*. The complement fixation test is used for CSF determinations and for the confirmation and quantitation of serum antibody detected by screening tests. The number of cases with a positive complement fixation test depends on the severity of disease and on the laboratory performing the test. Positive tests are least common among patients with solitary pulmonary cavities or primary pulmonary infection, while sera from patients with disseminated disease in multiple organs are nearly all positive. Seroconversion is helpful in diagnosing primary pulmonary coccidioidomycosis but may not occur for up to 8 weeks after onset. A positive complement fixation test of unconcentrated CSF is diagnostic of meningitis. Rarely, a parameningeal focus causes a positive complement fixation test of CSF.

Conversion of the skin test from negative to positive (≥5 mm of induration at 24 or 48 h) with spherulin may take place between days 3 and 21 of symptoms in primary pulmonary coccidioidomycosis. Spherulin is not currently available commercially, but skin testing can be helpful in epidemiologic studies, such as investigations of case clusters or the definition of endemic areas. The utility of skin testing as a diagnostic tool is limited by the persistence of positive tests resulting from remote exposures to *Coccidioides* and by the frequency of negative skin tests among patients with either thin-walled cavities or disseminated coccidioidomycosis. A positive skin test has not predicted dissemination in HIV-infected patients. The presence of complement-fixing antibody to *C. immitis* in AIDS patients should prompt a search for active infection.

℞ TREATMENT

See also Table 184-1. Primary pulmonary coccidioidomycosis usually resolves spontaneously. Some physicians give a few weeks of treatment with intravenous amphotericin B followed by oral itracon-

TABLE 184-1 *Treatment of Coccidioidomycosis*

Type of Disease	Preferred Treatment	Alternatives
Asymptomatic pulmonary nodule	None	...
Solitary pulmonary cavity	None; excision with persistence for >1 year	Itraconazole or fluconazole
Chronic fibrocavitary pneumonia	Itraconazole or fluconazole[a]	Amphotericin B[b]; excision if refractory
Acute pneumonia		
No risk factors[c]	Itraconazole or fluconazole	Observation
Risk factors, severe illness, rapid progression, or diffuse pulmonary infiltrates	Amphotericin B	Switch to itraconazole or fluconazole after 2–3 months if patient's condition improves.
Chronic dissemination (no CNS disease)	Itraconazole or fluconazole[d]	Amphotericin B
Meningitis	Fluconazole[e]	Intrathecal amphotericin B

[a] Itraconazole is given as 200 mg twice daily by mouth and fluconazole as 400 mg/d by mouth.
[b] Amphotericin B is given as 0.5–0.7 mg/kg daily or as a lipid formulation (5 mg/kg daily).
[c] Risk factors include HIV infection, organ transplantation, treatment with high-dose glucocorticoids, and pregnancy.
[d] The optimal duration of therapy for disseminated infection is unclear but should probably be lifelong in both immunocompetent and immunocompromised patients.
[e] Patients in whom fluconazole therapy fails at the 400-mg dose may be advanced to 600 or 800 mg daily. Lifelong therapy for meningitis is recommended.

azole or fluconazole to patients with unusually severe or protracted primary infection in the hope of aborting disseminated or chronic pulmonary disease. Solitary pulmonary cavities that do not close spontaneously over the first year can be excised electively, particularly if complicated by hemoptysis or recurrent bacterial infection. Response to systemic antifungal therapy is poor.

Patients with severe or rapidly progressing disseminated coccidioidomycosis are first given intravenous amphotericin B at a dose of 0.5 to 0.7 mg/kg daily. Patients whose condition improves after 2 to 3 months of amphotericin B treatment or who have more indolent disseminated infection are given itraconazole (200 mg twice daily) or fluconazole (400 mg/d). These oral agents are useful for long-term suppression of infection, and treatment should be continued for years. Patients with coccidioidal meningitis usually are initially given fluconazole (400 to 800 mg/d) but may require intrathecal amphotericin B. Hydrocephalus is a frequent complication of uncontrolled meningitis. Surgical debridement of bone lesions or drainage of abscesses can be helpful. The prognosis for ultimate cure of disseminated coccidioidomycosis is guarded.

Resection of chronic progressive pulmonary lesions is a helpful adjunct to chemotherapy when infection is confined to the lung and to one lobe.

FURTHER READING

GALGIANI JN: Comparison of oral fluconazole and itraconazole for progressive, nonmeningeal coccidioidomycosis. A randomized, double-blind trial. Mycoses Study Group. Ann Intern Med 133:676, 2000

———— et al: Practice guidelines for the treatment of coccidioidomycosis. Clin Infect Dis 30:658, 2000

HOLLEY K et al: *Coccidioides immitis* osteomyelitis: A case series review. Orthopedics 25:827, 2002

KIRKLAND TN, FIERER J: Coccidioidomycosis: A reemerging infectious disease. Emerg Infect Dis 2:192, 1996

ROSENSTEIN NE et al: Risk factors for severe pulmonary and disseminated coccidioidomycosis: Kern County, California, 1995–1996. Clin Infect Dis 32:708, 2001

STEVENS DA, SHATSKY SA: Intrathecal amphotericin in the management of coccidioidal meningitis. Semin Respir Infect 16:263, 2001

WHEAT LJ et al: State-of-the-art review of pulmonary fungal infections. Semin Respir Infect 17:158, 2002

185   BLASTOMYCOSIS
John E. Bennett

ETIOLOGIC AGENT   *Blastomyces dermatitidis* is a dimorphic fungus that grows at room temperature as a white or tan mold but grows within the host or at 37°C as budding, round yeastlike cells. The fungus can be identified on the basis of its appearance, its dimorphism, the small spores borne on hyphae of the mold form, or the results of nucleic acid hybridization. When isolates of the two opposite mating types are grown close together on special culture medium, such as yeast extract or soil extract agar, sporulating structures that characterize the perfect state (*teleomorph*), called *Ajellomyces dermatitidis*, appear.

EPIDEMIOLOGY   The infection is restricted by geography and age. Blastomycosis is uncommon in any locality, but most cases occur in the southeastern, central, and mid-Atlantic areas of the United States and in the Canadian provinces of Ontario and Manitoba. Mississippi, Kentucky, Arkansas, Tennessee, North Carolina, Wisconsin, and Illinois typically report the most cases. Cases have also been encountered in Africa, Mexico, Central America, and (rarely) South America. Most patients are between 20 and 69 years old. The male-to-female ratio is about 10:1. There is no occupational predisposition to the development of blastomycosis.

PATHOGENESIS AND PATHOLOGY   Infection with *B. dermatitidis* appears to be acquired by inhalation of the fungus from soil, decomposed vegetation, or rotting wood. Several case clusters have resulted from participation in recreational activities in wooded areas along waterways. Infection is not transmissible from person to person. The initial pulmonary infection may either heal spontaneously or become chronic. Spread to other portions of the lung, cavitation, or endobronchial lesions may be found in patients with chronic disease. Whether or not the lung lesion resolves spontaneously, infection commonly spreads hematogenously to the skin, subcutaneous tissue, bone, prostate, epididymis, or mucosa of the nose, mouth, or larynx. Less commonly, infection spreads to the brain, meninges, liver, lymph nodes, or spleen. Dissemination may not be evident for weeks or years after the appearance of the lung lesion. Progressive infection is only rarely attributable to an underlying disease, to HIV infection, or to immunosuppressive treatment. The inflammatory response includes lymphocytes, giant cells, and neutrophils. Pseudoepitheliomatous hyperplasia may be striking and may lead to a mistaken diagnosis of squamous cell carcinoma of the skin, lung, or larynx.

CLINICAL MANIFESTATIONS   A few patients have acute, self-limited pneumonia. Fever, productive cough, myalgia, and malaise usually resolve within a month. Pulmonary infiltrates clear slowly as *B. dermatitidis* disappears from the sputum.

In the vast majority of patients, blastomycosis has an indolent onset and a chronically progressive course. Fever, cough, weight loss, lassitude, skin lesions, and chest ache are common. Skin lesions favor exposed areas and enlarge over many weeks from pimples to well-circumscribed, verrucous, crusted, or ulcerated lesions. Pain and regional lymphadenopathy are minimal. Large chronic lesions may undergo central healing with scarring and contracture. Mucous membrane and laryngeal lesions present as an indurated, nontender, sharply circumscribed hypertrophic plaque, often mistaken for squamous cell carcinoma. Chest x-ray findings are abnormal in two-thirds of patients, with one or more densely consolidated areas of pneumonia or nodular infiltrates that occasionally include areas of cavitation. Pleural thickening or small pleural effusions develop occasionally, but large pleural effusions are rare, as is calcification of the lung or hilar nodes. Patients may present with an acute respiratory distress syndrome (ARDS), although indolent symptoms usually precede this syndrome. The lungs of ARDS patients are filled with myriad organisms, and the patient often dies within a few days of admission to the hospital. Calcification, hilar adenopathy, and large pleural effusions are rare. Osteolytic lesions occur in one-fourth of patients and may involve nearly any bone. Osseous lesions, which appear radiologically as circumscribed osteolytic areas, present clinically as a cold abscess or a draining sinus or extend to a contiguous joint and cause an indolent arthritis yielding pus on aspiration. Prostatic and epididymal lesions present as an indurated nontender mass. Hydrocele or a draining sinus may accompany blastomycotic epididymitis.

DIAGNOSIS   The diagnosis of blastomycosis is made by demonstration of the fungus in a culture of sputum, pus, or urine. An expert can diagnose blastomycosis by the appearance of the organism in wet smear or histopathologic section. The fungus may be visible in a sputum cytology smear but is easily overlooked.

℞ TREATMENT

See also Table 185-1. A few patients have developed only transitory lung lesions, but no guidelines are known to distinguish these patients from those whose disease will progress locally or disseminate. Therefore, every patient should receive treatment. Intravenous amphotericin B is the drug of choice for patients with rapidly progressive infections, severe illness, or central nervous system lesions. Because the clinical

TABLE 185-1 *Treatment of Blastomycosis*

Type of Disease	Preferred Treatment[a]	Alternatives
Rapid progression or severe illness	Amphotericin B for 10–12 weeks	Switch to itraconazole (400 mg/d) when condition stabilizes; continue for 6–12 months.
CNS disease	Amphotericin B for 10–12 weeks	Give fluconazole (800 mg/d) if patient improves and cannot tolerate amphotericin B; continue for 6–12 months.
Indolent infection, mild to moderate illness, no CNS disease	Itraconazole (400 mg/d) for 6–12 months	. . .

[a] See text for dosage of amphotericin B.

response to amphotericin B is more rapid than that to an azole, intravenous itraconazole is less appropriate. However, therapy may be switched to itraconazole when the patient's condition stabilizes. Skin and noncavitary lung lesions should be treated for about 8 to 10 weeks when amphotericin B alone is used. The recommended total dose for an adult is ~2 g. Cavitary lung disease or infection extending beyond the lung and skin is more likely to relapse after 10 weeks of amphotericin B administration at this total dose; thus it should be treated for about 10 to 12 weeks with a total dose of ≥2.5 g, or the patient should be switched to itraconazole for prolonged therapy. Experience with lipid amphotericin B formulations is limited, but they are likely to prove effective.

Oral itraconazole (200 mg twice daily with food) is the drug of choice for the treatment of patients who have indolent nonmeningeal blastomycosis of mild to moderate severity and who take the drug reliably. Therapy with itraconazole is continued for 6 to 12 months, whether given initially or after a short course of amphotericin B. HIV-infected patients should probably receive lifelong therapy, but relevant experience is limited. Fluconazole is less effective than itraconazole; however, because of its good penetration into the central nervous system, treatment with 400 to 800 mg daily may be considered to follow amphotericin B therapy in CNS blastomycosis. The mortality rate in appropriately treated cases of blastomycosis is ≤15% but exceeds 50% in cases presenting as ARDS.

FURTHER READING

BAUMGARDNER DJ et al: Epidemiology of blastomycosis in a region of high endemicity in north-central Wisconsin. Clin Infect Dis 15:629, 1992

CHAPMAN SW et al: Endemic blastomycosis in Mississippi: Epidemiological and clinical studies. Semin Respir Infect 12:219, 1997

CRAMPTON TL et al: Epidemiology and clinical spectrum of blastomycosis diagnosed at Manitoba hospitals. Clin Infect Dis 34:1310, 2002

LEMOS LB et al: Acute respiratory distress syndrome and blastomycosis: Presentation of nine cases and review of the literature. Ann Diagn Pathol 5:1, 2001

MANGINO JE, PAPPAS PG: Itraconazole for the treatment of histoplasmosis and blastomycosis. Int J Antimicrob Agents 5:219, 1995

PAPPAS PG et al: Blastomycosis in immunocompromised patients. Medicine 72:311, 1993

SACCENTE M et al: Vertebral blastomycosis with paravertebral abscess: Report of eight cases and review of the literature. Clin Infect Dis 26:413, 1998

WINER-MURAM HT et al: Blastomycosis of the lung: CT features. Radiology 182:829, 1992

186 CRYPTOCOCCOSIS
John E. Bennett

ETIOLOGIC AGENT Cryptococcosis is an infection caused by the yeastlike fungus *Cryptococcus neoformans*. This fungus reproduces by budding and forms round, yeastlike cells. Within the host and on certain culture media, a large polysaccharide capsule surrounds each yeast cell. The fungus grows well in smooth, creamy-white colonies on Sabouraud's or other simple media at 20° to 37°C. Identification of the organism is based on gross and microscopic appearance, biochemical test results, and growth at 37°C. The results of nucleic acid hybridization or the formation of brown pigment on Niger seed agar can also be used for identification.

The fungus has four capsular serotypes, designated A, B, C, and D. There are also two mating types. Coculture of opposite mating types creates a transient diploid state called *Filobasidiella neoformans* var. *neoformans* for serotypes A and D and *F. neoformans* var. *bacillispora* for serotypes B and C. Organisms not cultured under mating conditions are designated *C. neoformans* var. *neoformans* for serotypes A and D and *C. neoformans* var. *gattii* for serotypes B and C; a simple color medium distinguishes the two varieties. Some authorities have called serotype A *C. neoformans* var. *grubii*.

EPIDEMIOLOGY Weathered pigeon droppings commonly contain serotype A or D (*C. neoformans* var. *neoformans*). *C. neoformans* var. *gattii* has been isolated from the litter around trees of the species *Eucalyptus camaldulensis* and *E. tereticornis*. Eucalyptus isolates have so far typed as serotype B. The distribution of these eucalyptus species in Australia corresponds to the distribution of infections due to *C. neoformans* var. *gattii* in that country. The high prevalence of these trees in other subtropical climates has been postulated to explain the relative restriction of such infections to warm climates. A notable exception is the cluster of clinical cases and environmental isolates *not* from eucalyptus trees on the eastern coast of Vancouver Island in British Columbia, Canada.

The most common predisposing factor to cryptococcosis worldwide is currently AIDS. CD4+ cell counts are usually below 200/μL in AIDS patients who develop cryptococcal infection. The incidence of cryptococcosis has been declining in the United States since the advent of highly active antiretroviral therapy (HAART). More than half of non-AIDS patients with cryptococcosis have been receiving glucocorticoids or other immunosuppressive drugs prior to the onset of the fungal infection. Solid organ transplantation, lymphoma, sarcoidosis, and idiopathic CD4+ lymphocytopenia also predispose to infection by *C. neoformans* var. *neoformans*. Most infections in immunocompromised patients are caused by serotype A, although serotype D occurs in up to 20% of cases in Western Europe. Infections with var. *gattii* have been rare among AIDS patients and other immunocompromised patients, even in subtropical climates where var. *gattii* infection occurs in previously healthy individuals.

Animals, particularly cats, can acquire cryptococcosis but have not been known to transmit the infection to other animals or to humans. The source from which humans acquire the infection is unknown, with the rare exception of cases acquired through a transplanted cornea, kidney, or other solid organ. Cryptococcosis is rare before puberty.

PATHOGENESIS AND PATHOLOGY Cryptococcal infection is thought to be acquired by inhalation of the fungus into the lungs, although rare cases of cutaneous cryptococcosis appear to arise by minor trauma. Pulmonary infection has a tendency toward spontaneous resolution and is frequently asymptomatic. Silent hematogenous spread to the brain leads to clusters of cryptococci in the perivascular areas of cortical gray matter, in the basal ganglia, and, to a lesser extent, in other areas of the central nervous system. The inflammatory response around these foci is usually scant. In the more chronic cases, a dense basilar arachnoiditis is typical. Lung lesions are characterized by intense granulomatous inflammation. Cryptococci are best seen in tissue by staining with methenamine silver or periodic acid–Schiff. Although a strongly positive result on mucicarmine staining of tissue is diagnostic, staining varies from intense to absent.

CLINICAL MANIFESTATIONS Most patients have *meningoencephalitis* at the time of diagnosis. This form of cryptococcosis is invariably fatal without appropriate therapy; death occurs anytime from 2 weeks to several years after the onset of symptoms. Early manifestations include headache, nausea, staggering gait, dementia, irritability, confusion, and blurred vision. Both fever and nuchal rigidity are often mild or lacking. Papilledema is evident in one-third of cases at the time of diagnosis. Rapid and permanent loss of vision may occur, leaving a central scotoma or optic atrophy. Cranial nerve palsies, typically asymmetric, occur in about one-fourth of cases. Other lateralized signs are rare. With progression of the infection, deepening coma and signs of brainstem compression appear. Autopsy often reveals cerebral edema in more acute cases and hydrocephalus in more chronic cases. Neuroimaging is most often normal. Focal lesions called *cryptococcomas* are more common in previously normal patients, particularly those with var. *gattii* infections, than in immunosuppressed patients. These lesions are commonly located in the basal ganglia or the head of the caudate nucleus. Cryptococcomas are best seen on magnetic resonance imaging (MRI) with T2 or FLARE imaging and gadolinium enhancement. Edema around the mass disappears with successful therapy, but the cryptococcoma can persist for years.

Pulmonary cryptococcosis causes chest pain in ~40% of patients and cough in ~20%. Fever is modest or absent. The chest x-ray shows one or more dense infiltrates, which are often well circumscribed. Cavitation, pleural effusions, and hilar adenopathy are infrequent. Calcification is not evident, and fibrotic stranding is rarely noticeable.

Some 10% of patients with cryptococcosis have skin lesions, and the vast majority of patients with skin lesions have disseminated infection (Fig. 186-1). One or a few asymptomatic tiny papular lesions appear and slowly enlarge; they display a tendency toward central softening leading to ulceration. Osteolytic lesions occur in 4% of cases and usually present as a cold abscess. Rare manifestations of cryptococcosis include prostatitis, endophthalmitis, hepatitis, pericarditis, endocarditis, and renal abscess.

Cryptococcosis in AIDS patients is notable for the relative paucity of symptoms and signs, even in severe disease. Headache is present in ~90% of cases and fever in ~75%. Blurred vision, cranial nerve

palsies, lethargy, and confusion signal advanced infection. Cerebrospinal fluid (CSF) abnormalities in protein and glucose levels and in cell count are modest (see "Diagnosis"). A CSF leukocyte count of <10/μL and an opening pressure of >250 mm are bad prognostic signs. Immune reconstitution during a response to HAART can lead to a return of fever and headache, suppuration of mediastinal lymph nodes, or meningeal enhancement on MRI.

DIAGNOSIS Fever and headache in a patient with AIDS or with risk factors for HIV infection suggest the possibility of cryptococcosis, toxoplasmosis, or central nervous system lymphoma. Evidence of a focal lesion on MRI is unusual in cryptococcosis. Most cryptococcal cerebral mass lesions occur in patients infected with *C. neoformans* var. *gattii* who also have meningitis. In patients without AIDS, meningitis due to *C. neoformans* resembles that due to *Mycobacterium tuberculosis*, *Histoplasma capsulatum*, *Coccidioides immitis*, or metastatic cancer. Lumbar puncture is the single most useful diagnostic test. An india ink smear of centrifuged CSF sediment reveals encapsulated yeast in more than half of cases, although artifacts can cause confusion. In patients without AIDS, levels of glucose in CSF are reduced in half of all cases; protein levels are usually increased; and lymphocytic pleocytosis is usually found. CSF abnormalities are less pronounced in patients with AIDS, although india ink smear and serum antigen tests are more often positive.

Approximately 90% of patients with cryptococcal meningoencephalitis, including all those with a positive CSF smear and nearly all AIDS patients, have capsular antigen detectable in CSF or serum by latex agglutination. An enzyme immunoassay for cryptococcal antigen does not offer useful quantitative results but more clearly establishes positivity. Occasional false-positive results in both antigen tests make culture the definitive diagnostic test and have prevented serum antigen from being a useful screening test in asymptomatic patients with AIDS. Testing for serum antigen in AIDS patients with headache or fever is helpful. *C. neoformans* can often be cultured from the urine of patients with meningoencephalitis. Fungemia occurs in 10 to 30% of non-AIDS patients and in 60% of AIDS patients.

Pulmonary cryptococcosis appears on computed tomography (CT) as nodules with smooth or relatively undefined margins and homogeneous attenuation. In rare instances, ground-glass opacification is seen. Sputum culture is positive in only 10% of cases, and serum antigen tests are positive in only one-third. Occasionally, *C. neoformans* appears in one or more sputum specimens as an endobronchial saprophyte. Biopsy is usually required for diagnosis.

Cutaneous cryptococcosis may be mistaken for a comedo, basal cell carcinoma, or sarcoidosis. In patients with AIDS, skin lesions may be numerous and are sometimes mistaken for molluscum contagiosum (as shown for a liver transplant recipient in Fig. 186-1). Biopsy reveals myriad cryptococci. Osseous cryptococcosis is diagnosed by examination of bone or an adjacent soft tissue abscess.

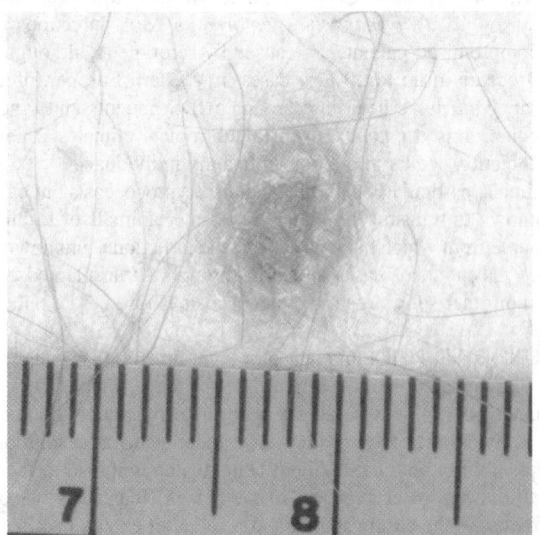

FIGURE 186-1 Disseminated fungal infection. A liver transplant recipient developed six cutaneous lesions similar to the one shown. Biopsy and serum antigen testing demonstrated *Cryptococcus*. Important features of the lesion include a benign-appearing fleshy papule with central umbilication resembling molluscum contagiosum. (*Photo courtesy of Dr. Lindsey Baden.*)

Rx TREATMENT

See also Table 186-1. Patients with AIDS and cryptococcosis are treated initially with intravenous amphotericin B (0.7 to 1.0 mg/kg daily) for at least 2 weeks and until their clinical condition is stable; thereafter, they receive fluconazole. The addition of flucytosine (25 mg/kg every 6 h) to amphotericin B for 2 weeks has minimal impact on morbidity and mortality. After treatment with amphotericin B, fluconazole (400 mg) is given once daily; daily doses of 800 mg have been used with marginal changes in toxicity or efficacy. The addition of flucytosine to fluconazole increases gastrointestinal intolerance. Serum and CSF antigen have not been helpful in determining the efficacy of therapy, but CSF cultures should convert to negative. After at least 10 weeks of treatment and when the patient is asymptomatic, treatment with fluconazole (200 mg/d) is continued indefinitely. Itraconazole is less effective than fluconazole in cryptococcal meningitis but can be used. Patients with incapacitating symptoms of immune reconstitution improve with glucocorticoid therapy; it is unclear whether amphotericin B should be restarted until the glucocorticoid dose has been tapered. AIDS patients who have negative antigen and fungal cultures of CSF after prolonged fluconazole treatment and who have a sustained (≥6-month) CD4+ response to HAART (with counts of at least 100 to 200/μL) may be candidates for discontinuation of maintenance therapy. Should CD4+ cell counts fall again, resumption of maintenance therapy would be reasonable.

In patients without AIDS, the therapeutic goal is to cure cryptococcal meningitis, not merely to control its symptoms. A single intensive course of amphotericin B is given for at least 10 weeks until cultures from all previously positive sites (particularly CSF) become convincingly negative. Normalization

TABLE 186-1 Treatment of Cryptococcosis

Type of Disease	Preferred Treatment	Alternatives
Disease in AIDS patient	Amphotericin B (0.7–1.0 mg/kg daily) or liposomal amphotericin B (4–5 mg/kg daily) for 2 weeks and until symptoms improve; then fluconazole (400 mg/d) for 8 weeks; then fluconazole (200 mg/d) for life	Itraconazole (400 mg/d) for 8 weeks after amphotericin B; then 200 mg/d maintenance
Disease in non-AIDS patient		
Meningitis	Amphotericin B (0.6–0.7 mg/kg daily) or liposomal amphotericin B (4–5 mg/kg daily) for 10 weeks[a]	Switch to fluconazole (400 mg/d) when patient's condition has improved; continue for 6–12 months
Pulmonary disease	Treat immunosuppressed patients as for meningitis; previously normal patients may respond to fluconazole (400 mg/d) for 6–12 months.	Itraconazole (400 mg/d) for previously normal patients

[a] CSF culture should be negative, antigen titer falling, and glucose level normal.

of the glucose level in lumbar CSF is important. The CSF antigen titer should fall by the end of therapy, but complete clearance of CSF or serum antigen during therapy is not essential. Amphotericin B (0.6 to 0.7 mg/kg daily for 10 weeks) is the best-studied regimen, but liposomal amphotericin B (4 to 5 mg/kg daily) is probably equivalent. Amphotericin B lipid complex and amphotericin B colloidal dispersion are not recommended pending further study. Flucytosine has been added to amphotericin B to accelerate the culture response, but grave toxicity can result unless flucytosine blood levels are kept below 100 μg/mL. Fluconazole (400 mg daily), given initially or begun after a course of amphotericin B, has cured cryptococcal meningitis or pulmonary cryptococcosis in some less immunosuppressed patients. Useful parameters for deciding when to discontinue therapy are unknown, but culture conversion, normalization of CSF glucose levels, and a fall in CSF antigen titer are minimal end points. A 6- to 12-month course of treatment is often used. Routine follow-up CSF cultures for the next year are useful in detecting relapse before symptoms supervene. Lung lesions on CT may take 6 weeks to improve and many months to resolve, if they ever do. Some immunosuppressed patients are treated as described above for AIDS patients, with indefinite fluconazole maintenance therapy.

Hydrocephalus may be the presenting manifestation or a later complication of cryptococcosis. Blindness, dementia, and personality change are among the other sequelae. Cerebral edema (in the absence of a cryptococcoma) causing headache, confusion, or blurred vision should be treated by daily lumbar puncture or CSF shunting to avert blindness. The shunt does not act as a nidus of persistent infection.

PROPHYLAXIS Fluconazole (200 mg/d) has been shown to decrease the incidence of cryptococcosis in HIV-infected patients with CD4+ cell counts of <200/μL and particularly in those with counts of <50/μL. Weekly fluconazole has not provided this protection. Daily fluconazole has not conferred a survival advantage; in light of its cost and the currently low incidence of cryptococcosis in patients with AIDS in the United States, prophylaxis is strongly discouraged.

FURTHER READING

HOSPENTHAL DR, BENNETT JE: Persistence of cryptococcomas on neuroimaging. Clin Infect Dis 31:1303, 2000
KIRK O et al: Safe interruption of maintenance therapy against previous infection with four common HIV-associated opportunistic infections during potent antiretroviral therapy. Ann Intern Med 137:239, 2002
LILIANG P et al: Use of ventriculoperitoneal shunts to treat uncontrollable intracranial hypertension in patients who have cryptococcal meningitis without hydrocephalus. Clin Infect Dis 34:E64, 2002
MASUR H et al: Guidelines for preventing opportunistic infections among HIV-infected persons—2002. Ann Intern Med 137:435, 2002
NEWTON PN et al: A randomized, double-blind, placebo-controlled trial of acetazolamide for the treatment of elevated intracranial pressure in cryptococcal meningitis. Clin Infect Dis 35:769, 2002
SAAG MS et al: Practice guidelines for the management of cryptococcal disease. Clin Infect Dis 30:710, 2000
——— et al: A comparison of itraconazole versus fluconazole as maintenance therapy for AIDS-associated cryptococcal meningitis. Clin Infect Dis 28:291, 1999
ZINCK SE et al: Pulmonary cryptococcosis: CT and pathologic findings. J Comput Assist Tomogr 26:330, 2002

187 CANDIDIASIS
John E. Bennett

ETIOLOGIC AGENTS *Candida albicans* is the most common cause of mucosal candidiasis and is responsible for about half of all cases of candidemia in hospitalized patients. A small proportion of isolates previously identified as *C. albicans* have been transferred to a new species, *C. dubliniensis*. *C. tropicalis*, *C. parapsilosis*, *C. guilliermondii*, *C. glabrata* (formerly *Torulopsis glabrata*), *C. krusei*, and a few other *Candida* species account for the other half of candidemia cases; all can cause potentially lethal septic shock. The majority of these non-*albicans* species enter the bloodstream through intravascular catheters. *Candida* species, taken together, are the fourth or fifth most common cause of nosocomial bloodstream infections in the United States.

All *Candida* species pathogenic for humans are also encountered as commensals of humans, particularly in the mouth, stool, and vagina. These species grow rapidly at 25° to 37°C on simple media as oval, budding cells. In tissue, both yeasts and pseudohyphae are present. The latter are elongated branching structures with constrictions at the septae. Budding yeasts may be seen as separate structures or as projections from pseudohyphae. *C. glabrata* differs from other members of the genus in that it forms no true hyphae or pseudohyphae in vitro or in infected tissue. *C. albicans* and *C. dubliniensis* can be identified preliminarily by their ability to form germ tubes in serum—a test that requires only a few hours. These two species can be more accurately identified by the formation in special culture medium of thick-walled large spores called *chlamydospores*. Culture media now available for primary inoculation allow preliminary identification of *Candida* species by colony color. Accurate identification of *Candida* species other than *C. albicans* requires biochemical tests.

PATHOGENESIS Deeply invasive candidiasis is often preceded by increased colonization of the mouth, vagina, and stool with *Candida* due to broad-spectrum antibiotic therapy. Additional local and systemic factors favor infection. Oropharyngeal thrush is particularly likely to occur in neonates and in patients with diabetes mellitus, HIV infection, or dentures. Vulvovaginal candidiasis (Chap. 115) is especially common in the third trimester of pregnancy. *Candida* from the perineum can enter the urinary tract via an indwelling bladder catheter. Cutaneous candidiasis most often involves macerated skin, such as that in the diapered area of infants, under pendulous breasts, or on hands constantly in water or covered by occlusive gloves. *Candida* can pass from the colonized surface into deep tissue when the integrity of the mucosa or skin is violated, as, for example, by perforation of the gastrointestinal tract through trauma, surgery, or peptic ulceration or by mucosal damage due to cytotoxic agents used for cancer chemotherapy. Although *Candida* is not normally a resident of the skin, secretions from the mouth, rectum, or vagina as well as drainage from surgical wounds or tracheostomy sites can contaminate the hub or skin site of a catheter in an umbilical or central vein. Intravenous drug abuse or third-degree burns can also provide a skin portal for *Candida* that can lead to deep candidiasis. Once *Candida* has passed the integumentary barrier, very low birth weight (in neonates) and neutropenia or glucocorticoid therapy (in any patient) markedly compromise host defense. Hematogenous seeding is particularly evident in the retina, kidney, spleen, and liver.

CLINICAL MANIFESTATIONS ■ Mucocutaneous Candidiasis

Oral thrush presents as discrete and confluent adherent white plaques on the oral and pharyngeal mucosa, particularly in the mouth and on the tongue. These lesions are usually painless, but fissuring at the corners of the mouth can be painful. Unexplained oropharyngeal thrush raises the possibility of HIV infection. Oral thrush is common in acute HIV infection and becomes increasingly common late in disease as the CD4+ cell count falls. At CD4+ counts of <50/μL, esophageal thrush also becomes common. HIV infection appears not to be an independent risk factor for vulvovaginal thrush.

Cutaneous candidiasis presents as red macerated intertriginous areas, paronychia, balanitis, or pruritus ani. Candidiasis of the perineal and scrotal skin may be accompanied by discrete pustular lesions on the inner aspects of the thighs. *Chronic mucocutaneous candidiasis* (*CMC*) or *candidal granuloma* typically presents as circumscribed hyperkeratotic skin lesions, crumbling dystrophic nails, partial alopecia in areas of scalp lesions, and both oral and vaginal thrush. Other findings may include chronic ringworm, dental dysplasia, and hypofunction of the parathyroid, adrenal, or thyroid gland. CMC is a major component of the immune polyendocrinopathy syndrome caused by a mutation in the autoimmune regulator gene (*AIRE*) on chromosome 21q22,3 (Chap. 330). CMC can begin in childhood as an autosomal dominant or recessive disorder or in association with Job's syndrome and can occur in adults in association with thymoma. Systemic infection is very rare in CMC, but permanent alopecia and disfigurement of the face and hands can be severe. Vulvovaginal thrush (Chap. 115) causes pruritus, discharge, and sometimes pain on intercourse or urination. Speculum examination reveals an inflamed mucosa and a thin exudate, often with white curds. Excessive colonization of the gastrointestinal tract has been associated with diarrhea and with chronic fatigue syndrome, but the linkage is unconvincing.

Esophageal candidiasis is often asymptomatic but can cause substernal pain or a sense of obstruction on swallowing. The pain of esophageal candidiasis may be mistaken for pain of cardiac origin. Most lesions are in the distal third of the esophagus and appear on endoscopy as areas of redness and edema, focal white patches, or ulcers. Biopsy or brushing is required for diagnosis and for detection of concomitant infections, particularly herpes simplex in patients with hematologic malignancies and cytomegalovirus infection in AIDS patients. *Candida* esophagitis can cause bleeding and impaired alimentation. Hematogenous dissemination from the esophagus probably occurs in some neutropenic patients but is rarely reported in HIV-infected patients.

Deeply Invasive Candidiasis

In the obstructed *urinary tract*, *Candida* can cause cystitis, pyelitis, or renal papillary necrosis. When a colonized urinary tract is operated on or instrumented, candidemia may result. However, most patients with *Candida* cultured from the urine simply have bladder colonization from a Foley catheter or a sizable volume of residual urine. Contamination of a voided midstream specimen by vaginal *Candida* is also common.

Candidemia originating from an intravascular catheter may clear in the immunocompetent patient when the catheter is removed. Focal seeding of the retina can take place even if candidemia clears and the patient becomes afebrile. Unilateral or bilateral small white retinal exudates appear within 2 weeks of the onset of candidemia. Lesions may regress spontaneously or enlarge slowly. The vitreous humor becomes cloudy, and the patient notices blurring, ocular pain, or a scotoma. Retinal detachment, vitreous abscess, and extension to the anterior chamber can occur over the ensuing weeks. These retinal lesions, present in ~10% of nonneutropenic patients with candidemia, are the principal reason that systemic antifungal therapy is recommended for all patients with candidemia. Funduscopy should be performed to ensure that retinal lesions, if present, resolve completely. Most cases with ocular involvement have occurred in nonneutropenic patients. In contrast, so-called *hepatosplenic candidiasis* is usually recognized in patients with acute leukemia who are recovering from profound neutropenia. This entity, better called *chronic disseminated candidiasis*, originates from intestinal seeding of the portal and venous circulation. Fever, modestly elevated serum concentrations of alkaline phosphatase, and multiple small abscesses evident on ultrasonography, magnetic resonance imaging, or computed tomography (CT) of the liver, spleen, or kidney suggest the diagnosis. During acute candidemia in neutropenic patients, small erythematous papules may appear anywhere on the skin (Fig. 187-1). If the patient does not expire promptly from disseminated candidiasis, the lesions will develop a necrotic center. Painful muscle lesions may also be found. Punch biopsy of a skin lesion helps distinguish this extremely grave condition from *Malassezia* folliculitis, a similar-appearing but benign condition that can involve the cape area of the chest or the extremities of a sweaty febrile patient.

Hematogenous seeding in the neutropenic patient is occasionally visible radiologically as tiny pulmonary nodules. *Candida pneumonia*, apart from hematogenous candidiasis, is very rare. *Candida endocarditis* can be caused by any *Candida* species and favors previously damaged or prosthetic heart valves. The source is often an intravascular catheter or contaminated equipment used for illicit intravenous drug injection. An interval of weeks or even months between candidemia and discovery of endocarditis is common. Emboli to large arteries, such as the iliac or femoral artery, are characteristic. Intravenous injection of impure brown heroin has caused a clinical syndrome consisting of *Candida endophthalmitis* and purulent *folliculitis*, sometimes accompanied by vertebral *osteomyelitis*.

Candida can cause indolent *arthritis*, most commonly of the knee, in patients who have received glucocorticoid injections into the joint, in patients who are immunosuppressed, and in low-birth-weight neonates. Prosthetic joints may become infected during implantation. Scanty growth of *Candida* from joint fluid can cause the laboratory to

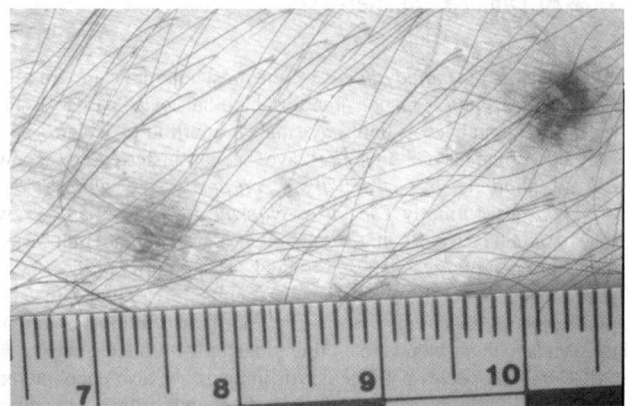

FIGURE 187-1 Disseminated candidiasis. Tender, erythematous, nodular lesions developed in a neutropenic patient with leukemia who was undergoing induction chemotherapy. (Photo courtesy of Dr. Lindsey Baden.)

incorrectly dismiss the organism as a contaminant. *Candida* can cause subacute *peritonitis* arising either from a perforated viscus or from a peritoneal dialysis catheter.

Hematogenous dissemination can lead to *brain abscess* or chronic *meningitis*. Diagnosis of infections of ventriculoperitoneal shunts is difficult because symptoms are indolent and cultures of lumbar fluid are usually sterile.

DIAGNOSIS Demonstration of pseudohyphae on wet smear with confirmation by culture is the procedure of choice for diagnosing superficial candidiasis. Scrapings for the smear may be obtained from skin, nails, and oral and vaginal mucosa. A culture of urine, sputum, existing abdominal drains, endotracheal aspirates, or the vagina is not diagnostic; however, recovery of *Candida* species from multiple superficial sites has been identified as a risk factor for deeply invasive candidiasis in some studies of patients with prolonged neutropenia or complicated abdominal surgery.

Deeper lesions due to *Candida* may be diagnosed by histologic section of biopsies or by culture of cerebrospinal fluid, blood, joint fluid, CT-guided needle aspirates, or surgical specimens. Blood cultures are useful in the diagnosis of *Candida* endocarditis and intravenous catheter–induced sepsis but are positive less often in other forms of disseminated disease. Serologic tests for antibody or antigen are not useful.

TABLE 187-1 Treatment of Candidiasis		
Type of Disease	**Preferred Treatment[a]**	**Alternatives**
Mucocutaneous		
Cutaneous	Topical azole	Topical nystatin
Vulvovaginal	Azole cream or suppository or oral fluconazole (150 mg)	Nystatin suppository
Oropharyngeal	Clotrimazole troche or fluconazole tablet (100 mg/d) or itraconazole solution (200 mg/d)	Nystatin suspension; for azole-unresponsive disease: caspofungin (50 mg/d) or amphotericin B (0.3–0.5 mg/kg daily)
Esophageal	Fluconazole tablet (100–200 mg/d) or itraconazole solution (200 mg/d)	For azole-unresponsive disease: caspofungin (70 mg once, then 50 mg/d) or amphotericin B (0.3–0.5 mg/kg daily)
Deeply invasive		
Nonneutropenic	Fluconazole (400 mg/d) or amphotericin B[b] or caspofungin (70 mg once, then 50 mg/d)	
Neutropenic	Amphotericin B[b]	

[a] Removal of foreign bodies is critical, including plastic catheters for intravenous fluids, peritoneal dialysis or cerebrospinal fluid shunts, prosthetic cardiac valves, and prosthetic joints.
[b] The dosage of amphotericin B for deeply invasive candidiasis is 0.5 mg/kg daily, although initial doses of 0.7–1.0 mg/kg daily may be appropriate for severely immunosuppressed patients. Amphotericin B lipid complex and liposomal amphotericin B are given as 5 mg/kg daily.

RX TREATMENT

(See also Table 187-1.) Cutaneous candidiasis of macerated areas responds to measures that reduce moisture and chafing plus topical application of an antifungal agent in a nonocclusive base. Nystatin powder or a cream containing ciclopirox or an azole is useful. Clotrimazole, miconazole, econazole, ketoconazole, sulconazole, and oxiconazole are available as creams or lotions. *Candida* vulvovaginitis responds better to an azole than to nystatin suppositories. There is little difference in efficacy among miconazole, clotrimazole, tioconazole, butoconazole, and terconazole vaginal formulations. Systemic treatment of *Candida* vulvovaginitis with a single 150-mg capsule of fluconazole is more convenient than topical treatment; however, this option is contraindicated in pregnancy, is less effective in patients with multiple relapses, and poses a higher risk of adverse effects. Clotrimazole troches, used five times a day, are more effective in oral candidiasis than nystatin suspension and are approximately as effective as oral fluconazole (100 mg daily). Oral fluconazole (100 to 200 mg once daily) is more convenient and more effective in esophagitis than clotrimazole troches. Esophagitis not responding to fluconazole may warrant repeat endoscopy to exclude other conditions. Itraconazole suspension (100 mg twice daily) alleviates *Candida* esophagitis in some patients in whom fluconazole treatment fails. Nearly all patients with azole-resistant oropharyngeal or esophageal candidiasis respond to a 2-week course of intravenous amphotericin B (0.3 to 0.5 mg/kg daily) or caspofungin (70 mg for one dose, then 50 mg daily). Relapse is usual.

Management of recurrent oropharyngeal candidiasis in the HIV-infected patient presents special problems. Patients with CD4+ cell counts of <100/μL who have received prolonged fluconazole therapy are at risk of developing azole resistance, requiring an increased dose to mount a response, relapsing early, and eventually failing to respond well to any dose of fluconazole. The increasing azole resistance in this population suggests that HIV-infected patients with oropharyngeal or esophageal candidiasis should be treated for each individual episode and that only when episodes become intolerably frequent or severe should prophylaxis be given.

Bladder thrush responds to bladder irrigations with amphotericin B (50 μg/mL for 5 days). If no bladder catheter is in place, oral fluconazole can be used to control candiduria. Most patients with candiduria do not have unrelieved urinary tract obstruction and do not benefit from therapy.

Intravenous amphotericin B is the drug of choice for deeply invasive candidiasis in neutropenic or seriously immunosuppressed patients. The deoxycholate formulation is usually given at a dosage of 0.5 to 0.7 mg/kg daily. Open, noncomparative studies of amphotericin B lipid complex and liposomal amphotericin B indicate that either preparation is effective in deeply invasive candidiasis. The usual dose of either formulation is 5 mg/kg daily by the intravenous route.

Candida endocarditis on prosthetic or native valves usually relapses unless the valve is replaced. Long-term fluconazole administration has been used to prevent recurrence after valve replacement.

In immunocompetent patients with intravenous catheter–acquired *C. albicans* fungemia, the catheter should be removed in conjunction with the administration of fluconazole (400 mg/d), amphotericin B (0.5 mg/kg daily), or caspofungin (one 70-mg dose followed by 50 mg daily by the intravenous route). Amphotericin B (0.7 to 1.0 mg/kg daily) may be appropriate as initial therapy in severely neutropenic patients. Candidemia from suppurative phlebitis of a peripheral vein may not respond until the infected portion of the vein is excised. Therapy for candidemia is continued for 2 weeks after the patient becomes afebrile. The *Candida* species involved should be considered in choosing a drug for candidemia. *C. krusei* and *C. inconspicua* are rare causes of candidemia but are resistant to fluconazole in vitro. *C. glabrata* exhibits intermediate susceptibility to fluconazole. Thus either increasing the daily fluconazole dose to 800 mg or using amphotericin B or caspofungin may be appropriate. Caspofungin displays approximately equal activity in vitro against all *Candida* species, including azole-resistant strains. Strains of *C. lusitaniae* resistant to amphotericin B but susceptible to azoles or caspofungin have been encountered. Intravenous amphotericin B, with or without flucytosine, is the preferred treatment for *Candida* endophthalmitis, although cures have been reported with fluconazole. Pars plana vitrectomy may facilitate diagnosis and cure when a *Candida* vitreous abscess is present. Injection of amphotericin B into the vitreous humor can also be helpful.

Because amphotericin B and fluconazole penetrate reasonably well into an infected joint, the pleural cavity, and the peritoneum, local injection is not indicated. Removal of prostheses (including prosthetic joints and cardiac valves), peritoneal dialysis catheters, and central venous catheters is usually essential. Debridement, along with antifungal therapy, is beneficial in *Candida* osteomyelitis. All collections of pus, such as those in the postoperative abdomen, need to be drained surgically or by percutaneous, CT-guided catheterization; an exception relates to the numerous small abscesses in liver, spleen, or kidney in chronic disseminated candidiasis, which cannot be drained effectively and require prolonged antifungal therapy. In general, treatment should continue until the patient with chronic disseminated candidiasis has been afebrile and nonneutropenic for at least 2 weeks. Defects may persist on imaging studies long after cure. Relapse during another episode of neutropenia is common unless the patient is receiving amphotericin B. Repeat cytotoxic therapy or even bone marrow transplantation can be undertaken in patients with prior chronic disseminated candidiasis, but amphotericin B should be given empirically during neutropenia.

PROPHYLAXIS Fluconazole can decrease the incidence of deeply invasive candidiasis in recipients of allogeneic bone marrow transplants when 400 mg is given daily. Some centers continue such prophylaxis for 70 days; others discontinue it after engraftment. Studies of leukemic and other neutropenic patients have found no significant reduction in the incidence of deeply invasive candidiasis associated with prophylactic use of fluconazole or itraconazole oral suspension, although this topic remains controversial. Prophylaxis against recurrent oropharyngeal or esophageal candidiasis in HIV-infected patients is no longer recommended unless recurrences are very frequent or severe. Fluconazole (3 to 6 mg/kg) or itraconazole solution (5 mg/kg) is the recommended daily oral dose. Fluconazole prophylaxis at 400 mg daily may be useful in preventing deeply invasive candidiasis in some high-risk postoperative patients. Definition of groups at sufficient risk to benefit from fluconazole depends on the intensive care unit but likely includes patients undergoing repeat, complicated abdominal surgery and patients who are both heavily colonized with *Candida* and immunosuppressed at the time of complicated surgery. The presence of intravenous catheters, prolonged stays in the intensive care unit, and renal failure increase the risk of candidemia.

FURTHER READING

BENOIT D et al: Management of candidal thrombophlebitis of the central veins: Case report and review. Clin Infect Dis 26:393, 1998

MARR KA et al: Prolonged fluconazole prophylaxis is associated with persistent protection against candidiasis-related death in allogeneic marrow transplant recipients: Long-term follow-up of a randomized, placebo-controlled trial. Blood 96:2055, 2000

MASUR H et al: Guidelines for preventing opportunistic infections among HIV-infected persons—2002. Recommendations of the U.S. Public Health Service and the Infectious Diseases Society of America. Ann Intern Med 137:435, 2002

MELGAR GR et al: Fungal prosthetic valve endocarditis in 16 patients. An 11-year experience in a tertiary care hospital. Medicine 76:94, 1997

PELZ RK et al: Double-blind placebo-controlled trial of fluconazole to prevent candidal infections in critically ill surgical patients. Ann Surg 233:542, 2001

REX JH et al: Practice guidelines for the treatment of candidiasis. Clin Infect Dis 30:662, 2000

ZUCCARELLO D et al: Familial chronic nail candidiasis with ICAM-1 deficiency: A new form of chronic mucocutaneous candidiasis. J Med Genet 39:671, 2002

188 | ASPERGILLOSIS
John E. Bennett

ETIOLOGIC AGENTS *Aspergillus fumigatus* is the most common cause of aspergillosis, but *A. flavus*, *A. niger*, *A. nidulans*, *A. terreus*, and several other species can also cause disease. *Aspergillus* is a mold with septate branching hyphae ~2 to 4 μm in diameter. The fungus is identified by its gross and microscopic appearance in culture.

PATHOGENESIS AND PATHOLOGY All the common species of *Aspergillus* that cause disease in humans are ubiquitous in the environment, growing on dead leaves, stored grain, compost piles, hay, and other decaying vegetation. The fungus can also be isolated from potable water, although the clinical significance of this observation is unknown. Inhalation of *Aspergillus* spores must be extremely common, but disease is rare. Invasion of lung tissue is confined almost entirely to immunosuppressed patients, in roughly 90% of whom two of the following three conditions will be operative: a granulocyte count in peripheral blood of <500/μL, treatment with supraphysiologic doses of adrenal glucocorticoids, and a history of treatment with other immunosuppressive drugs such as cyclosporine. Invasive aspergillosis is an occasional complication of AIDS. *Aspergillus* infection in the neutropenic patient is characterized by hyphal invasion of blood vessels, thrombosis, necrosis, and hemorrhagic infarction. Chronic granulomatous disease of childhood also predisposes to invasive pulmonary aspergillosis, but in that situation the inflammatory response is a pyogranuloma and blood vessel invasion is rare.

Massive inhalation of *Aspergillus* spores by healthy persons can lead to acute, diffuse, self-limited pneumonitis. Epithelioid granulomas with giant cells and central pyogenic areas containing hyphae are detected in these cases. Spontaneous recovery taking several weeks is the usual course. Such patients should be tested for underlying chronic granulomatous disease.

Aspergillus can colonize the damaged bronchial tree, pulmonary cysts, or cavities of patients with underlying lung disease. Balls of hyphae within cysts or cavities (aspergillomas), usually in the upper lobe, may reach several centimeters in diameter and may be visible on chest x-ray. Tissue invasion does not occur.

CLINICAL MANIFESTATIONS *Allergic bronchopulmonary aspergillosis* occurs in patients with preexisting asthma (particularly glucocorticoid-dependent asthma) or cystic fibrosis and causes intermittent episodes of wheezing, pulmonary infiltrates from transient bronchial plugging, sputum and blood eosinophilia, low-grade fever, and brownish or greenish flecks in the sputum. These flecks contain *Aspergillus* hyphae, thick mucus, eosinophils, and Charcot-Leyden crystals. Some patients with repeated exacerbations develop central bronchiectasis and progressive loss of pulmonary function.

Endobronchial saprophytic pulmonary aspergillosis presents as chronic productive cough, often with hemoptysis, in a patient with prior chronic lung disease, such as tuberculosis, sarcoidosis, bronchiectasis, or histoplasmosis. *Aspergillus* may be spread from its endocavitary or endobronchial site to the pleura during the course of bacterial lung abscess or surgery. Patients reported to have chronic necrotizing *Aspergillus* pneumonia appear in most instances to have had saprophytic endobronchial colonization and a pulmonary process attributable to another disease, with or without superimposed bacterial infections. Patients with chronic pneumonia and *Aspergillus* in the sputum should be assumed to have either pneumonia of a different etiology (e.g., histoplasmosis) or *Aspergillus* pneumonia with underlying immunosuppression (e.g., chronic granulomatous disease or infection with HIV).

Invasive aspergillosis in the immunocompromised host presents as an acute, rapidly progressive, densely consolidated pulmonary infiltrate and is most common among patients with acute leukemia and recipients of tissue transplants. Infection progresses by direct extension across tissue planes and by hematogenous dissemination to lung, brain, and other organs. Computed tomography (CT) has been particularly valuable in suggesting the diagnosis of invasive pulmonary aspergillosis in patients with neutropenia. The earliest CT finding is one or more small pulmonary nodules. As a nodule enlarges, the dense central core of infarcted tissue becomes surrounded by edema or hemorrhage, forming a hazy rim called the *halo sign*. This rim disappears in a few days as the dense core enlarges. When bone marrow function recovers, the infarcted central core cavitates, creating the *crescent sign*. *Aspergillus* may invade immunosuppressed patients through the skin at a site of minor trauma or through the upper airway mucosa. Early lesions in the nose should be sought in patients with neutropenia who have fever and minimal epistaxis. Scarlet-red patches of the mucosa rapidly become necrotic and white, then black. Rapid extension into the adjacent paranasal sinus, orbit, or face is usual, with or without the appearance of lung lesions.

Aspergillus sinusitis in immunocompetent patients may take three forms. A ball of hyphae may form in a chronically obstructed paranasal sinus, without tissue invasion. Much less commonly, a chronic, fibrosing granulomatous inflammation associated with *Aspergillus* hyphae within tissue may begin in the sinus and spread slowly to the orbit and the brain. *Aspergillus* is also a cause of allergic fungal sinusitis, but dark-walled fungi (e.g., *Curvularia*, *Alternaria*) are more common in this setting. Patients usually have a history of chronic allergic rhinitis, sometimes with nasal polyps, but are otherwise healthy, presenting with painless proptosis, nasal obstruction, or dull aching pain. On CT or magnetic resonance imaging, a solid soft-tissue mass pushing out the lateral wall of the ethmoid sinus or the medial wall of the maxillary sinus may be detected. On sinus exploration, the mucosa is found to be thickened and inflamed but intact. Within the sinus cavity, sticky mucopus with strands of neutrophils, eosinophils, Charcot-Leyden crystals, and occasional hyphae can be found.

Aspergillosis in HIV-infected patients most commonly involves the lung, presenting as fever, cough, and dyspnea. Typically, the CD4+ cell count is <50/μL. Roughly half of these patients have neutropenia or have recently been treated with glucocorticoids. Bilateral diffuse or focal pulmonary infiltrates with a tendency to cavitate constitute the most common radiologic manifestation. Well-localized, white, necrotic pseudomembranes full of hyphae or ulcers may develop in the trachea or the major bronchi. Progression of bronchitis to pneumonia is usual, but hematogenous dissemination is uncommon. Either allergic or invasive *Aspergillus* sinusitis can occur in HIV-infected patients; the allergic form can develop even at CD4+ cell counts of >50/μL.

The growth of *Aspergillus* on cerumen and detritus within the external auditory canal is termed *otomycosis*. Trauma to the cornea may cause *Aspergillus* keratitis. Endophthalmitis follows the introduction of *Aspergillus* into the globe by trauma or surgery. *Aspergillus* may infect intracardiac or intravascular prostheses.

DIAGNOSIS The repeated isolation of *Aspergillus* from sputum or the demonstration of hyphae in sputum or bronchoalveolar lavage fluid suggests endobronchial colonization or infection. Even a single isolation of *Aspergillus* from the sputum of a neutropenic patient or a hematopoietic stem-cell transplant recipient with pneumonia, particularly a child or a nonsmoker, suggests the diagnosis of invasive aspergillosis. In patients with advanced AIDS, fever, and cough, the isolation of *Aspergillus* from respiratory secretions raises the possibility of aspergillosis and thus should prompt bronchoscopy. Fungus ball of the lung is usually detectable by chest x-ray. IgG antibody to *Aspergillus* antigens is demonstrable in the serum of many colonized patients and of virtually all patients with fungus ball. Patients with allergic bronchopulmonary aspergillosis have specific serum IgE antibody to *Aspergillus* antigens and often have IgG antibody as well. No standardized test for these antibodies exists. Serum IgE concentrations are often >1000 ng/mL.

Biopsy is usually required for the diagnosis of invasive aspergillosis of the lung, nose, paranasal sinus, bronchi, or sites of dissemination. Blood cultures are rarely positive, even in patients with infected cardiac valves (native or prosthetic). Detection of galactomannan antigen in serum suggests the diagnosis, but sensitivity is low early in the disease and false-positive results occur, particularly in children. *Aspergillus* hyphae can be identified presumptively by histology, but culture is required for confirmation and for identification of the species. Only culture can reliably distinguish aspergillosis from pseudallescheriasis; drug therapy for these two diseases differs.

℞ TREATMENT

(See also Table 188-1.) Patients with severe hemoptysis due to fungus ball of the lung may benefit from lobectomy. Poor pulmonary function in residual lung and dense pleural adhesions around the lesion can complicate the resection. Bead embolization directed to the bronchial arterial supply has been used as a temporizing measure. Systemic chemotherapy is of no value in endobronchial or endocavitary aspergillosis. Short courses of oral adrenal glucocorticoids have been used to treat acute bronchial plugging in patients with allergic bronchopulmonary aspergillosis. Two small studies have indicated that patients with allergic bronchopulmonary aspergillosis require less glucocorticoid therapy and have fewer exacerbations when given prophylaxis with oral itraconazole (200 mg twice daily). Itraconazole has also been used with glucocorticoids to treat exacerbations.

Treatment with intravenous amphotericin B (1.0 to 1.5 mg/kg daily) has elicited a response in 30 to 40% of patients with invasive aspergillosis. Intravenous voriconazole (6 mg/kg every 12 h for two doses, then 4 mg/kg every 12 h) is better tolerated and more efficacious than a regimen starting with conventional amphotericin B. Once the patient has begun to respond, voriconazole can be given orally as 200 mg twice daily. Liposomal amphotericin B at daily doses of 5 mg/kg is probably comparable to voriconazole, but no comparative study is available. Compared with conventional amphotericin B, amphotericin B colloidal dispersion shows equivalent efficacy in aspergillosis, is less nephrotoxic, and more often causes infusion-related chills and fever. Itraconazole (200 mg twice daily) is useful in some less immunosuppressed patients with indolent or slowly progressive invasive aspergillosis. Over the first 2 weeks, itraconazole can be given intravenously as 200 mg twice daily for four doses and then 200 mg daily to patients who are unable to take or unlikely to absorb oral itraconazole. The intravenous formulation is contraindicated in patients with a creatinine clearance rate of <30 mL/min. Itraconazole capsules are given as 200 mg twice daily. Intravenous caspofungin (70 mg once, then 50 mg daily) can be considered for patients in whom therapy with other drugs fails. Surgery is the only treatment needed for fungus ball of the sinus and for allergic fungal sinusitis. Antifungal therapy has little effect on either entity if used alone, but chronic suppressive therapy has been begun postoperatively for relapse of allergic fungal si-

TABLE 188-1 *Treatment of Aspergillosis*

Type of Disease	Preferred Treatment	Alternatives
Fungus ball of the lung	Surgical resection	Bead embolization for hemoptysis
Allergic broncho-pulmonary aspergillosis	Short courses of glucocorticoids	Itraconazole prophylaxis
Invasive aspergillosis[a]	Voriconazole, liposomal or conventional amphotericin B	Amphotericin B colloidal dispersion or lipid complex, itraconazole, or caspofungin

[a] Voriconazole dose: 6 mg/kg twice daily for two doses; then 4 mg/kg twice daily; for later oral administration, 200 mg twice daily. Liposomal amphotericin B dose: 5 mg/kg daily. Conventional amphotericin B dose: 1.0 to 1.5 mg/kg daily. Amphotericin B colloidal dispersion dose: 6 mg/kg daily. Amphotericin B lipid complex dose: 5 mg/kg daily. Intravenous itraconazole dose: 200 mg twice daily for four doses, then 200 mg daily. Intravenous caspofungin dose: 70 mg once, then 50 mg daily.

nusitis. The prognosis for cure of invasive aspergillosis in the paranasal sinus is very poor when the patient has profound and unremitting neutropenia. The prognosis is better in less immunosuppressed patients.

FURTHER READING

BOWDEN R et al: A double-blind, randomized, controlled trial of amphotericin B colloidal dispersion versus amphotericin B for treatment of invasive aspergillosis in immunocompromised patients. Clin Infect Dis 35:359, 2002

CAILLOT D et al: Increasing volume and changing characteristics of invasive pulmonary aspergillosis on sequential thoracic computed tomography scans in patients with neutropenia. J Clin Oncol 19:253, 2001

DENNING DW: Invasive aspergillosis. Clin Infect Dis 26:781, 1998

HERBRECHT R et al: Voriconazole versus amphotericin B for primary therapy of invasive aspergillosis. N Engl J Med 347:408, 2002

MAERTENS J et al: Use of circulating galactomannan screening for early diagnosis of invasive aspergillosis in allogeneic stem cell transplant recipients. J Infect Dis 186:1297, 2002

MARR KA: Invasive aspergillosis in allogeneic stem cell transplant recipients: Changes in epidemiology and risk factors. Blood 102:827, 2003

MOSS RB: Allergic bronchopulmonary aspergillosis. Clin Rev Allergy Immunol 23:87, 2002

SHIRAKUSA T et al: Surgical treatment of pulmonary aspergilloma and *Aspergillus* empyema. Ann Thorac Surg 48:779, 1989

STEVENS DA et al: Practice guidelines for diseases caused by *Aspergillus*. Clin Infect Dis 30:696, 2000

189 | MUCORMYCOSIS
John E. Bennett

ETIOLOGIC AGENTS Species of *Rhizopus*, *Rhizomucor*, and *Cunninghamella* are the most common causes of mucormycosis, but species of *Apophysomyces*, *Saksenaea*, *Mucor*, and *Absidia* also are occasionally responsible for this infection. The etiologic organism in tissue is composed of broad, rarely septate hyphae of uneven diameter (6 to 15 μm). The organisms are inexplicably difficult to grow from infected tissue. When growth does take place, it is rapid and profuse on most media at room temperature. Identification is based on the gross and microscopic appearance of the mold.

Zygomycosis is a term that includes mucormycosis and entomophthoramycosis. The latter is a tropical infection of the subcutaneous tissue or paranasal sinuses caused by species of *Basidiobolus* and *Conidiobolus*, respectively.

EPIDEMIOLOGY AND PATHOLOGY *Rhizopus* and *Rhizomucor* species are ubiquitous, appearing on decaying vegetation, dung, and foods of high sugar content. Mucormycosis is uncommon and is largely confined to patients with serious preexisting diseases. Mucormycosis originating in the paranasal sinuses and nose predominantly affects patients with poorly controlled diabetes mellitus. Patients who have undergone organ transplantation, who have a hematologic malignancy, or who are receiving long-term deferoxamine therapy are predisposed to mucormycosis of either sinus or lung. Deferoxamine chelates iron in a form that the fungus can utilize. Gastrointestinal mucormycosis occurs in a variety of conditions, including uremia, severe malnutrition, and diarrheal diseases. The infection is acquired from nature, with no person-to-person spread. In all forms of mucormycosis, vascular invasion by hyphae is a prominent feature. Ischemic or hemorrhagic necrosis is the foremost histologic finding.

CLINICAL MANIFESTATIONS Mucormycosis originating in the nose and paranasal sinuses produces a characteristic clinical picture. Low-grade fever, dull sinus pain, and sometimes nasal congestion or a thin, bloody nasal discharge are followed in a few days by double vision, increasing fever, and obtundation. Examination reveals a unilateral generalized reduction of ocular motion, chemosis, and proptosis. The nasal turbinates on the involved side may be dusky red or necrotic. A sharply delineated area of necrosis, strictly respecting the midline, may appear in the hard palate. Facial skin adjacent to paranasal sinuses may be invaded by direct extension, turning progressively red, purple, and black. Fungal invasion of the globe or ophthalmic artery leads to blindness. Opacification of one or more sinuses is detected by computed tomography (CT) or magnetic resonance imaging (MRI). Magnetic resonance angiography (MRA) with gadolinium enhancement may show invasion or obstruction of the carotid siphon. Coma is due to direct invasion of the frontal lobe. Early symptoms mimic those of bacterial sinusitis. Clouding of the sensorium may be attributed to diabetic acidosis. Cavernous sinus thrombosis may be considered when orbital invasion occurs. Without treatment, the patient may die after an interval ranging from a few days to a few weeks.

Pulmonary mucormycosis manifests as progressive severe pneumonia accompanied by high fever and toxicity. The necrotic center of large infiltrates may cavitate. Fatal hemoptysis may occur from cavities formed near the hilum. Hematogenous spread to other areas of the lung, as well as to the brain and other organs, is common. Survival beyond 2 weeks is unusual. Gastrointestinal invasion presents as one or more ulcers that tend to perforate. Hematogenous dissemination can originate from the gastrointestinal tract, lung, or paranasal sinuses. Sometimes no portal of entry can be found. Primary cutaneous inoculation is uncommon but occurs in burn eschars, underneath occlusive dressings, and at sites of minor trauma in immunocompromised adults and low-birth-weight neonates. Several reported infections with *Apophysomyces elegans* have manifested as cellulitis in diabetics or previously normal patients.

DIAGNOSIS CT or MRI is very helpful in assessing the extent of sinusitis before surgery and in evaluating the patient afterward. CT is better for detecting bony erosion; MRI better visualizes extension into the frontal lobe or carotid artery in the siphon. Lesions of the lung and craniofacial structures are best diagnosed by biopsy and histologic section. Cultural confirmation should be attempted. Wet smear of crushed tissue can provide a rapid diagnosis. Cultures of blood and cerebrospinal fluid are negative. Smear and culture of sputum may be positive during cavitation of a lung lesion.

℞ TREATMENT

Regulation of diabetes mellitus and a decrease in the dose of immunosuppressive drugs facilitate the treatment of mucormycosis. Extensive debridement of craniofacial lesions appears to be very important. Orbital exenteration may be required. Intravenous amphotericin B is clearly of value in craniofacial mucormycosis and should be employed in the other forms of mucormycosis as well. The maximal tolerated doses are given until progression is halted. Endoscopic examination of paranasal sinuses can help assess progression. With the deoxycholate formulation, a dosage of 1 to 1.5 mg/kg daily is indicated. Amphotericin B lipid complex or liposomal amphotericin B, each at 5 mg/kg daily, appears to be as effective as and less toxic than conventional amphotericin B. Therapy is continued for a total of 10 to 12 weeks. Voriconazole and itraconazole are of no value. Results of hyperbaric oxygen therapy have been unimpressive. Appropriate management results in cure of about half of craniofacial infections. Primary cutaneous lesions benefit from debridement; extensive plastic surgical repair may be required, but the prognosis is good. Survival is rare among patients who have received deferoxamine and among those with pulmonary, gastrointestinal, or disseminated mucormycosis.

FURTHER READING

BLAIR JE et al: Locally invasive cutaneous *Apophysomyces elegans* infection acquired from snapdragon patch test. A review. Mayo Clin Proc 77:717, 2002

HOLLAND J: Emerging zygomycoses of humans: *Saksenaea vasiformis* and *Apophysomyces elegans*. Curr Top Med Mycol 8:27, 1997

MCADAMS HP et al: Pulmonary mucormycosis: Radiologic findings in 32 cases. Am J Radiol 168:1541, 1997

OH D, NOTRICA D: Primary cutaneous mucormycosis in infants and neonates: Case report and review of the literature. J Pediatr Surg 37:1607, 2002

RICKERTS V et al: Cluster of pulmonary infections caused by *Cunninghamella bertholletiae* in immunocompromised patients. Clin Infect Dis 31:910, 2000

TEDDER M et al: Pulmonary mucormycosis: Results of medical and surgical therapy. Ann Thorac Surg 57:1044, 1994

WARWAR RE, BULLOCK JD: Rhino-orbital-cerebral mucormycosis: A review. Orbit 17:237, 1998

190 MISCELLANEOUS MYCOSES AND ALGAL INFECTIONS
John E. Bennett

CHROMOBLASTOMYCOSIS (CHROMOMYCOSIS) This chronic subcutaneous mycosis, rarely seen in the United States, presents as nodular or verrucoid, ulcerated, or crusted skin lesions on exposed areas of skin, particularly on the lower extremities. Over months and years, lesions extend to contiguous skin; they may be tender or itchy. Pain is not a prominent symptom. The disease, which in fact causes few symptoms, follows the introduction of any of several fungi into subcutaneous tissue by thorns or bits of vegetation. The appearance of thick-walled, dark-colored, rounded forms ("copper pennies") in a histopathologic section of the dermis is diagnostic. Dark-walled hyphae may be seen in the stratum corneum. Surgical excision is the treatment of choice for small lesions. Cryotherapy and itraconazole with or without flucytosine have ameliorated larger lesions. Repeated treatments may be necessary.

DERMATOPHYTOSIS ■ Definition Dermatophytosis, also known as ringworm or tinea, is a chronic fungal infection of the skin, hair, or nails.

Etiology Species of *Trichophyton*, *Microsporum*, and *Epidermophyton* are called *dermatophytes*. These organisms grow in and remain confined to the keratinous structures of the body. Other mycoses, such as candidiasis, pityriasis versicolor, and tinea nigra, may include fungal invasion of keratinous structures but traditionally are not called dermatophytoses.

Pathology and Pathogenesis Dermatophyte species are referred to as *anthropophilic*, *zoophilic*, or *geophilic*, depending on whether their usual reservoir in nature appears to be humans, animals, or soil, respectively. The infectivity of organisms from all these sources is low, and outbreaks are largely confined to occasional clusters of cases of scalp infection in children. Acquisition of a dermatophytosis appears to be favored by minor trauma (including that incurred during wrestling), maceration, and poor hygiene of the skin. Infection does not seem to confer solid immunity: repeated infection with the same species is common, particularly with anthropophilic species. The infrequency of scalp infection among adults has been attributed to local factors rather than immunity.

Invasion of the stratum corneum by dermatophytes may cause inflammation that is either mild or (particularly with zoophilic fungi) intense. Shedding of the stratum corneum is increased by inflammation. To the extent that fungal growth cannot keep up with shedding, inflammation may help terminate infection. Conversely, infection is probably favored when shedding is reduced by treatment with glucocorticoids and cytotoxic drugs. Antifungal drugs interfere with the ability of fungal growth to keep up with shedding.

Clinical Manifestations The disease varies with the site of infection and the fungal species involved. Foot infection (athlete's foot, tinea pedis) may present as fissuring of the toe webs, scaling of the plantar surfaces, or vesicles around the toe webs and soles. Interdigital lesions may be pruritic or, when bacterial superinfection occurs, may be painful. Hand infection is less common but resembles foot infection.

Scalp dermatophytosis (tinea capitis) is characterized by areas of alopecia and scaling. In so-called endothrix infection, the hair shaft breaks off at the skin surface, leaving the hairs visible as black dots in the scalp. Some forms of scalp infection include an area of intense boggy suppuration called a *kerion*.

Dermatophytosis of the glabrous skin (Fig. 190-1) presents as circumscribed lesions with a wide variety of appearances, including scales, vesicles, and pustules. Inflammation may be minimal or intense. Central healing of less inflamed lesions may take place. The serpiginous border of inflammation is the source of the name *ringworm*.

Dermatophytosis of the bearded area (tinea barbae) appears as a pustular folliculitis. Onychomycosis (tinea unguium) presents as a white discoloration of the nails or as thickening, chalkiness, and crumbling of the nails. Peeling and fissuring of paronychial nail folds or keratotic debris under the nail edge also may be evident.

Diagnosis Discolored hairs, scales, and keratotic debris under infected nails should be collected for KOH or calcofluor smear and culture. In the scraping of skin lesions, a drop of water on the skin site may keep the removed scales from flying off and thus may aid in their collection. Culture is important in distinguishing dermatophytes from *Candida* and fungal saprophytes growing in keratinaceous debris.

℞ TREATMENT

Noninflammatory lesions of the trunk, groin, hands, and feet usually respond to twice-daily applications of clotrimazole, miconazole, ketoconazole, econazole, naftifine, terbinafine, or ciclopirox olamine cream. Hyperkeratotic lesions of the palms and soles respond slowly to these agents and may benefit from the initial application of Whitfield's ointment to thin the keratin. Ointment should not be used between the toes, in the groin, or in the gluteal crease because maceration promotes bacterial infection.

Ringworm that is moderately severe, that is unresponsive to topical

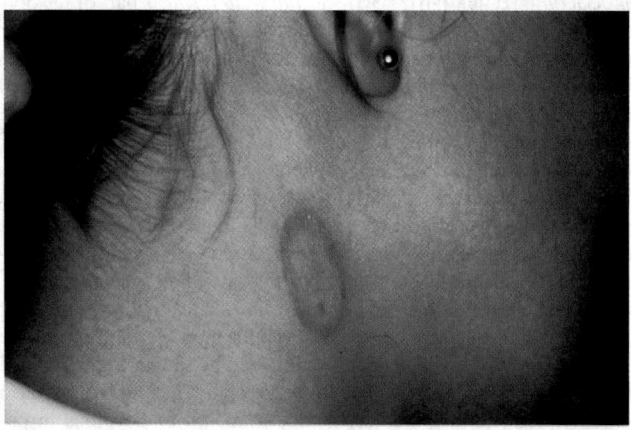

FIGURE 190-1 Tinea corporis is a superficial fungal infection, seen here as an erythematous annular scaly plaque with central clearing.

therapy, or that involves the scalp, nails, or bearded area should be treated systemically. Once-daily therapy with itraconazole (200 mg), terbinafine (250 mg), microcrystalline griseofulvin (500 mg), or ultramicrocrystalline griseofulvin (375 mg) is effective. Treatment must be continued until all infected keratin is gone. Cutting off infected hair and cleansing interdigital webs can expedite cure. Secondary bacterial infection of the foot may require soaks or antibacterial agents. The likelihood of relapse of dermatophyte foot infections may be decreased by keeping the feet clean and dry. For nail infections, itraconazole or terbinafine is preferred. In distal subungual onychomycosis, a single course of either drug results in initial improvement in half of patients, of whom half relapse. Results are better with fingernails than with toenails and for more distal rather than proximal nail involvement. To save money, itraconazole can be given as a double dose (400 mg) for 1 week each month with only marginal loss of efficacy. The rare but life-threatening complications of itraconazole must be weighed against the patient's desire to have normal-appearing nails. The duration of therapy with itraconazole or terbinafine is 2 to 3 months for fingernails and 4 to 6 months for toenails.

PROTOTHECOSIS *Prototheca* species are ubiquitous achlorophyllic algae that enter exposed areas of skin through contaminated wounds and cause localized infections in the skin, olecranon bursa, and, rarely, tendon sheaths or deeper tissue. Diagnosis is based on culture or histopathologic demonstration of morula-like sporangia containing endospores in tissue. *Prototheca wickerhamii*, the usual agent, grows readily on fungal culture medium. Surgical debridement and treatment with itraconazole or intravenous amphotericin B are useful.

FUSARIOSIS *Fusarium* species can cause localized or hematogenously disseminated infection. Indolent cellulitis or soft-tissue necrosis can occur in immunocompetent patients at the site of trauma (including burns) or adjacent to onychomycosis. Immunocompromised patients may develop skin lesions at the site of minor trauma or, more often, as a result of hematogenous dissemination. Two-thirds of patients with disseminated infection who are severely immunosuppressed, particularly those who are profoundly neutropenic, develop skin lesions. One or more tender erythematous papules enlarge rapidly, may develop a surrounding rim of erythema, and may become necrotic or ulcerated in the center. A portal of infection is not usually apparent. Blood cultures have been positive in 59% of cases. The presence of a mold growing in a culture of blood from a neutropenic patient suggests fusariosis. Blood cultures are rarely positive in aspergillosis or mucormycosis. Voriconazole or amphotericin B is the drug of choice for fusariosis, but survival from disseminated infection depends on the diminution of neutropenia. Debridement of localized lesions in immunocompetent patients is useful.

MALASSEZIA INFECTION (PITYRIASIS) *Malassezia furfur* is part of the normal flora of the human skin but can cause tinea (pityriasis) versicolor or catheter-acquired sepsis. Tinea versicolor appears as asymptomatic, well-delineated, hyperpigmented or hypopigmented macules centered on the upper trunk and upper arms. Confluent lesions may cover large areas, making the border difficult to find. A fine "branny" scale or folliculitis is sometimes visible. When examined microscopically by KOH mount, skin sections are seen to contain characteristic round and elongated cells. On inspection with Wood's light, lesions either do not fluoresce or appear yellow-green. *Erythrasma* resembles tinea versicolor but is characterized by gram-positive bacilli on smear and coral-red fluorescence. Azole creams are effective for the treatment of small areas of tinea versicolor; however, the application of selenium sulfide shampoo (Selsun) for 10 min daily, followed by showering to remove the shampoo, is more practical for large areas. Itraconazole is also effective. Catheter-acquired sepsis due to *M. furfur* develops in patients (particularly neonates) receiving intravenous lipid. The organism requires special culture conditions for growth, and the infection is cured by catheter removal.

MYCETOMA ■ Etiology *Actinomycetoma* refers to infection by actinomycetes of the genera *Nocardia* (Chap. 146), *Nocardiopsis*, *Streptomyces*, and *Actinomadura*. *Eumycetoma* is caused by true fungi of many different genera. The predominant agent varies with the locality.

Pathogenesis and Pathology The pathogens live in the soil and enter the skin through minor trauma. The most common site of infection is the foot. The infection runs a relentless course over many years, with destruction of contiguous bone and fascia. Grains are found in purulent foci surrounded by fibrosis and a mononuclear cell inflammatory response.

Clinical Manifestations Mycetoma is a chronic suppurative infection originating in subcutaneous tissue and characterized by the presence of grains, which are tightly clumped colonies of the causative agent. The infected site is characterized by painless swelling, woody induration, and sinus tracts that discharge pus intermittently. Systemic symptoms do not develop, and spread to distant sites in the body does not take place.

Diagnosis Although the clinical picture is characteristic, mycetoma is sometimes confused with chronic osteomyelitis or botryomycosis. The diagnosis requires demonstration of grains in pus from the draining sinus or in biopsy sections. Many histologic sections may need to be examined to locate a grain.

℞ TREATMENT

Actinomycetoma may respond to prolonged combination chemotherapy—e.g., with streptomycin and either dapsone or trimethoprim-sulfamethoxazole. Eumycetoma rarely responds to chemotherapy; some cases caused by *Madurella mycetomatis* have appeared to respond to ketoconazole or itraconazole.

PARACOCCIDIOIDOMYCOSIS ■ Etiology Formerly called *South American blastomycosis*, this mycosis is caused by *Paracoccidioides brasiliensis*. A dimorphic fungus, *P. brasiliensis* grows as a budding yeast in tissue and as either a yeast or a mold on culture medium. The organism is identified by its gross and microscopic appearance.

Pathogenesis and Pathology Infection is thought to be acquired by inhalation of spores from environmental sources, possibly soil. Pulmonary infection produces few symptoms initially. Hematogenous spread to the mucous membranes of the mouth and nose, the lymph nodes, and other sites causes patients to seek medical attention. In fatal cases, the infection spreads to the adrenals, the gastrointestinal tract, and many other viscera.

Clinical Manifestations Common signs include indurated ulcers of the mouth, oropharynx, larynx, and nose; enlarged and draining lymph nodes; lesions of the skin and genitalia; and productive cough, weight loss, dyspnea, and sometimes fever. Paracoccidioidomycosis is acquired only in South America, Central America, and Mexico, but its extreme indolence may delay its recognition until many years after the patient has left the endemic area. Chest radiography most often shows bilateral patchy pneumonia.

Diagnosis Cultures of sputum, pus, and mucosal lesions are often diagnostic. The diagnosis can be made by smear or histologic section, although confirmation by culture is preferable. Serologic tests are useful in suggesting the diagnosis and monitoring the response to therapy.

℞ TREATMENT

Relatively mild cases of paracoccidioidomycosis may be cured by 1 year of treatment with oral itraconazole (200 to 400 mg daily). More advanced cases are treated with intravenous amphotericin B followed by itraconazole.

PENICILLIOSIS MARNEFFEI *Penicillium marneffei* has emerged as a leading cause of opportunistic infection in patients in the late stages of HIV infection in Southeast Asia—notably, northern Thailand and southern China. Infection is probably acquired by the inhalation of spores from an unknown site in nature. At the time of diagnosis, infection has usually disseminated to bone marrow, liver, spleen, skin, or bone. Clinical manifestations and histopathologic findings resemble those of histoplasmosis. Both *P. marneffei* and *Histoplasma* are dimorphic fungi, appearing as small yeast cells in tissue and as a mold in culture. Unlike *Histoplasma*, the yeastlike cells of *P. marneffei* do not bud but divide by longitudinal fission. During growth as a mold, a red pigment forming in the agar underneath *P. marneffei* colonies can aid in the organism's identification. Treatment consists of amphotericin B administration for 2 weeks or until improvement is documented, with subsequent administration of itraconazole (400 mg daily for 8 weeks, then 200 mg daily as maintenance therapy). A few patients with a sustained response to highly active antiretroviral therapy and prolonged maintenance therapy have had itraconazole discontinued, with no subsequent relapse.

PHAEOHYPHOMYCOSIS This is the name given to infections caused by fungi with dark-walled hyphae, excluding those given conventional names like chromoblastomycosis. Although an extraordinary variety of fungi and clinical syndromes are encompassed by this definition, most patients have brain abscess, subcutaneous abscess, or allergic fungal sinusitis. Most of the brain abscesses are due to *Cladophialophora bantiana*, *Ochroconis gallopavum*, *Exophiala dermatitidis*, *Bipolaris* species, and *Ramichloridium mackenziei (obovoideum)*. Patients are previously healthy. Subcutaneous abscesses are usually single, arise at the site of minor trauma, and occur in both immunosuppressed and immunocompetent individuals. A large number of dematiaceous (dark-walled) mold species cause subcutaneous phaeohyphomycosis as well as allergic fungal sinusitis. The latter entity develops in patients with allergic rhinitis and presents as an expanding mucoid mass in one or more paranasal sinuses. The tenacious mucus contains eosinophils, Charcot-Leyden crystals, and occasional hyphae. Surgical excision of phaeohyphomycotic lesions is important. Antifungal therapy may retard recurrences but is of little value without surgical excision.

PSEUDALLESCHERIASIS ■ **Etiology** Also called *Petriellidium boydii*, *Pseudallescheria boydii* is a mold frequently found in soil. When isolated in the imperfect state, the anamorph is called *Scedosporium apiospermum*. *Scedosporium prolificans* is a closely related species.

Pathogenesis and Pathology Wind-borne spores of *P. boydii*, arising from the soil, are the presumed source of infection. The fungus grows as a mold within tissue, causing necrosis and abscess formation.

Clinical Manifestations *P. boydii* resembles *Aspergillus* in its ability to colonize the endobronchial tree, to form fungus balls in the lungs or paranasal sinuses, and to invade the cornea or globe of the eye, the soft tissues, the joints, or the bones after trauma or surgery and in its propensity to invade the lungs and paranasal sinuses of immunosuppressed hosts, including patients with AIDS. Hematogenous dissemination to the eye, brain, soft tissues, and other sites is common. Severe pneumonia, often with hematogenous dissemination and brain abscesses, has followed near-drowning in stagnant water. Hyphae of *P. boydii* in tissue may be difficult to distinguish from those of *Aspergillus*. Intravascular hyphae, a hallmark of invasive aspergillosis, are also found in pseudallescheriasis in neutropenic patients.

S. prolificans has caused infections in bones, joints, and soft tissue, usually after trauma.

Diagnosis Demonstration of hyphae in tissue and culture confirmation are required for diagnosis.

℞ TREATMENT

Soft-tissue infections in previously normal patients respond well to surgical debridement and treatment with itraconazole or voriconazole. Immunosuppressed patients respond poorly, and those with disseminated infection usually die. Surgical drainage is useful in brain abscesses. Voriconazole is the drug of choice for immunosuppressed individuals, and itraconazole is a suitable alternative. *P. boydii* appears to be unresponsive to systemic amphotericin B therapy, although injection of amphotericin B into an infected joint has been helpful in a

few cases. In previously normal patients with *S. prolificans* soft-tissue infection, surgical debridement has been useful. The response to all antifungal agents has been poor in immunosuppressed patients, but voriconazole treatment has resulted in cure in a few cases.

SPOROTRICHOSIS ■ **Etiology** *Sporothrix schenckii* lives as a saprophyte on plants in many areas of the world. In nature and on culture at room temperature, the fungus grows as a mold; within host tissue or at 37°C on enriched media, it grows as a budding yeast. It is identified by its appearance in mold and yeast forms.

Pathogenesis and Pathology Infection results from the inoculation of *S. schenckii* into subcutaneous tissue through minor trauma. Nursery workers, florists, and gardeners acquire the illness from roses, sphagnum moss, and other plants. Infection may be limited to the site of inoculation (plaque sporotrichosis) or extend along proximal lymphatic channels (lymphangitic sporotrichosis). Spread beyond an extremity—the usual site of infection—is rare, and hematogenous dissemination from the skin remains unproven. The portal for osteoarticular, pulmonary, and other extracutaneous forms of sporotrichosis is unknown but is probably the lung. Untreated sporotrichosis persists for months. The inflammatory response includes neutrophil clustering and a marked granulomatous response with epithelioid and giant cells.

Clinical Manifestations In lymphangitic sporotrichosis, which is by far the most common manifestation, a nearly painless red papule forms at the site of inoculation. Over the next several weeks, similar nodules form along proximal lymphatic channels. The nodules intermittently discharge small amounts of pus. Ulceration may occur. The proximal extension of these lesions, often with skip areas, is quite distinctive but may be mimicked by lesions of *Nocardia brasiliensis*, *Mycobacterium marinum*, or (in rare cases) *Leishmania brasiliensis* or *Mycobacterium kansasii*.

Plaque sporotrichosis manifests as a nontender red maculopapular granuloma confined to the site of inoculation. Osteoarticular sporotrichosis presents as mono- or polyarticular arthritis of indolent onset and progression over months or years, involving the elbows, knees, wrists, ankles, and (rarely) smaller joints of the extremities. Periarticular bone develops areas of demineralization detectable on x-ray, and draining sinuses may appear over joints and bursae. Hematogenous spread to the skin may take place during polyarticular disease, but none of the skin lesions shows lymphangitic spread. Immunosuppression, including that due to advanced infection with HIV, predisposes to hematogenous spread. Pulmonary sporotrichosis usually presents as a single chronic cavitary upper-lobe lung lesion. Chronic meningitis can develop in the absence of skin or lung lesions. *S. schenckii* is difficult to recover from cerebrospinal fluid.

Diagnosis Culture of pus, joint fluid, sputum, or a skin biopsy specimen is preferred. The appearance of *S. schenckii* in tissue is variable. In skin lesions, the organisms are hard to find.

℞ TREATMENT

Itraconazole (100 to 200 mg daily) is the drug of choice for the treatment of cutaneous sporotrichosis. A saturated solution of potassium iodide given orally is also effective, but side effects often prevent the effective use of this regimen. Therapy should be continued for 1 month after the resolution of all lesions. Fluconazole is less effective. Extracutaneous sporotrichosis may be cured by itraconazole (200 mg twice daily), but the response is slow and may be incomplete. Prolonged courses of intravenous amphotericin B are more effective. Cavitary pulmonary sporotrichosis may require resection for cure.

TRICHOSPORONOSIS A change in the taxonomy of the genus *Trichosporon* moved most of the agents causing deep infections from *T. beigelii* into the species *T. asahii*, with a few categorized as *T. mucoides*. White piedra of the scalp is caused by *T. ovoides* and that of the pubic hair by *T. inkin*. *T. cutaneum* and *T. asteroides* cause superficial infections. Most of what is currently known about *Trichosporon* infections is not species specific, so the following description refers to *T. beigelii*. *T. capitatum*, which causes disseminated infection in patients with neutropenia, was previously reclassified as *Blastoschizomyces capitatus* and will not be covered here.

T. beigelii can be isolated from soil, the human gastrointestinal tract, and skin. The organism can enter the bloodstream of patients with severe neutropenia through an inapparent source. Hematogenously disseminated infection is manifested by fever and often by the development of several erythematous or purpuric tender papules anywhere on the body. Lesions can form large, tense hemorrhagic bullae. In some patients, native or prosthetic cardiac valves become infected. In tissue, hyphae and yeastlike cells are seen. Amphotericin B is probably the drug of choice for treatment, but recovery depends on the return of bone marrow function.

***PFIESTERIA* INFECTION**   See Chap. 378.

FURTHER READING

BONIFAZ A et al: Chromoblastomycosis: Clinical and mycologic experience of 51 cases. Mycoses 44:1, 2001

CASTIGLIONI B et al: *Pseudallescheria boydii* (anamorph *Scedosporium apiospermum*). Infection in solid organ transplant recipients in a tertiary medical center and review of the literature. Medicine 81:333, 2002

CHAO SC et al: Cutaneous protothecosis: Report of five cases. Br J Dermatol 146:688, 2002

HAUGH M et al: Terbinafine in fungal infections of the nails: A meta-analysis of randomized clinical trials. Br J Dermatol 47:118, 2002

KAUFFMAN CA et al: Practice guidelines for the management of patients with sporotrichosis. Clin Infect Dis 30:684, 2000

MELLINGHOFF IK et al: Treatment of *Scedosporium apiospermum* brain abscesses with posaconazole. Clin Infect Dis 34:1648, 2002

NUCCI M, ANAISSIE E: Cutaneous infection by *Fusarium* species in healthy and immunocompromised hosts: Implications for diagnosis and management. Clin Infect Dis 35:909, 2002

SUPPARATPINYO K et al: A controlled trial of itraconazole to prevent relapse of *Penicillium marneffei* infection in patients infected with the human immunodeficiency virus. N Engl J Med 339:1739, 1998

191 | *PNEUMOCYSTIS* INFECTION
Peter D. Walzer

DEFINITION AND DESCRIPTION   *Pneumocystis* is an opportunistic fungal pulmonary pathogen that is an important cause of pneumonia (pneumocystosis) in the immunocompromised host. The taxonomic classification of *Pneumocystis* as a fungus is based on factors such as analysis of gene sequences for ribosomal RNA, mitochondrial proteins, and major enzymes; the presence of β-1,3 glucan in the cell wall; and the efficacy of antifungal drugs that inhibit β-glucan synthesis in animal models. However, in contrast to most fungi, *Pneumocystis* lacks ergosterol and is not susceptible to antifungal drugs that inhibit ergosterol synthesis.

Although *Pneumocystis* organisms obtained from different sources are morphologically very similar, they are genetically diverse and host specific. New nomenclature, which is still evolving, has established that organisms derived from rats and humans are separate species termed *P. carinii* and termed *P. jiroveci*, respectively. For the purpose of clarity, only the genus designation, *Pneumocystis*, will be used in this chapter.

Research on *Pneumocystis* has been limited by the lack of a reliable in vitro culture system. Developmental stages of the organism include the small (1- to 4-μm) pleomorphic trophic form; the 5- to 8-μm cyst, which has a thick cell wall and contains up to eight intracystic bodies; and the precyst, an intermediate stage. The life cycle of *Pneumocystis* probably involves sexual and asexual reproduction. *Pneumocystis* contains several different antigen groups, the most prominent of which is the 95- to 140-kDa major surface glycoprotein (MSG). MSG represents a multigene family of proteins, and the ability of MSG to undergo antigenic variation may represent a mechanism by which *Pneumocystis* evades host defenses. MSG is highly immunogenic, contains protective epitopes, and facilitates adherence of the organism to host cells via extracellular matrix proteins, surfactant proteins, and the mannose receptor.

EPIDEMIOLOGY   Serologic surveys have demonstrated that *Pneumocystis* has a worldwide distribution and that most healthy children have been exposed to the organism by 3 to 4 years of age. Airborne transmission of *Pneumocystis* has been documented in animal studies; person-to-person transmission has been suggested by hospital outbreaks of pneumocystosis and by molecular analysis of isolates from patients and their close contacts. Geography has also emerged as a contributory factor in the epidemiology of *Pneumocystis* infection.

PATHOGENESIS AND PATHOLOGY   The host factors that predispose to the development of pneumocystosis include defects in cellular and humoral immunity. The risk of developing *Pneumocystis* pneumonia among HIV patients rises markedly when circulating CD4+ cell counts fall below 200/μL. The frequency of serum antibodies to a specific segment of MSG is significantly higher in HIV patients who have recovered from an episode of pneumocystosis than in HIV patients who have never had the disease. Other persons at risk for *Pneumocystis* pneumonia are patients receiving immunosuppressive therapy (particularly glucocorticoids) for cancer, organ transplantation, and other disorders; children with primary immunodeficiency diseases; and premature malnourished infants.

The principal host effector cells against *Pneumocystis* are alveolar macrophages, which ingest and kill the organism, releasing a variety of inflammatory mediators. Tumor necrosis factor α and interleukin (IL) 1, interferon γ, and granulocyte-macrophage colony-stimulating factor contribute to host defenses against *Pneumocystis*. HIV reduces the mannose receptor–mediated binding and phagocytosis of *Pneumocystis* and alters the cytokine responses to the organism.

After being inhaled, *Pneumocystis* takes up residence in the alveoli, where it attaches tightly to type I cells but maintains an extracellular existence. It was formerly thought that the organism remains latent in the host for long periods, but more recent data suggest that pneumonia can arise from a new bout of infection. As the immune system of the host becomes compromised, *Pneumocystis* organisms propagate and gradually fill the alveoli. This scenario is accompanied by a complex series of events that result in increased alveolar-capillary permeability and damage to alveolar type I cells. Surfactant abnormalities include a fall in bronchoalveolar lavage (BAL) fluid phospholipids and an increase in surfactant proteins A and D. Contributions of the host inflammatory response to lung injury are suggested by the correlation of increased IL-8 levels and neutrophil counts in BAL fluid from patients with severe disease. In addition, immune reconstitution with the start of highly potent anti-HIV drugs and treatment of pneumocystosis is sometimes associated with new pulmonary infiltrates.

On lung sections stained with hematoxylin and eosin, the alveoli are filled with a typical foamy, vacuolated exudate. Severe disease may include interstitial edema, fibrosis, and hyaline membrane formation. The host inflammatory changes usually consist of hypertrophy of alveolar type II cells, a typical reparative response, and a mild mononuclear cell interstitial infiltrate. Malnourished infants display an intense plasma cell infiltrate that gave the disease its early name: interstitial plasma cell pneumonia.

CLINICAL FEATURES   Patients with pneumocystosis develop dyspnea, fever, and nonproductive cough. Symptoms in non-HIV-infected patients often begin after the glucocorticoid dose has been tapered and typically last 1 to 2 weeks. HIV-infected patients are usually ill for several weeks or longer and have relatively subtle manifestations. The clinical picture in individual patients is variable. A high index of suspicion and a thorough history are key factors in early detection.

Physical findings include tachypnea, tachycardia, and cyanosis, but lung auscultation reveals few abnormalities. The white blood cell count is variable and is usually governed by the patient's underlying disease. Reduced arterial oxygen pressure (Pa_{O_2}), increased alveolar-arterial oxygen gradient ($PA_{O_2} - Pa_{O_2}$), and respiratory alkalosis are evident. There also may be changes in pulmonary function test values (diffusing capacity) and heightened uptake with nonspecific nuclear imaging techniques (gallium scan). Elevated serum concentrations of lactate dehydrogenase (LDH) have been reported; the increase probably reflects lung parenchymal damage but is not specific to *Pneumocystis* infection. In general, laboratory abnormalities are less severe in HIV-infected patients than in non-HIV-infected patients.

The classic findings on chest radiography consist of bilateral diffuse infiltrates beginning in the perihilar regions (Fig. 191-1), but various atypical manifestations (nodular densities, cavitary lesions) have also been reported. Patients who receive aerosolized pentamidine have an increased frequency of upper-lobe infiltrates. Pneumothorax also occurs, and management is often difficult. Early in the course of pneumocystosis, the chest radiograph may be normal.

Although *Pneumocystis* usually remains confined to the lungs, cases of disseminated infection have occurred in both HIV-infected and non-HIV-infected patients. One risk factor for extrapulmonary spread in patients with HIV is the administration of aerosolized pentamidine. The most common sites of involvement are the lymph nodes, spleen, liver, and bone marrow. Eye lesions (choroiditis) also occur and must be distinguished from retinitis caused by cytomegalovirus. Clinical manifestations range from incidental findings at autopsy to specific organ involvement. Histopathologic examination reveals *Pneumocystis* and the characteristic associated foamy material.

DIAGNOSIS Because the clinical picture of *Pneumocystis* infection can be produced by many other infectious and noninfectious agents, the diagnosis must be based on specific identification of the organism. A definitive diagnosis is made by histopathologic staining. Traditional stains have included reagents such as methenamine silver, toluidine blue, and cresyl echt violet, which selectively stain the wall of *Pneumocystis* cysts, and reagents such as Wright-Giemsa, which stain the nuclei of all developmental stages. Other reagents include nonspecific fluorochrome stains (calcofluor white) and Papanicolaou's stain. Immunofluorescence with monoclonal antibodies is more sensitive than histologic staining but is also more expensive. DNA amplification by the polymerase chain reaction (PCR) is most sensitive and should be part of routine diagnosis if commercial kits become available.

The successful diagnosis of pneumocystosis depends upon the collection of proper specimens. In general, the yield from different diagnostic procedures is higher in HIV-infected patients than in non-HIV-infected patients because of the higher organism burden in the

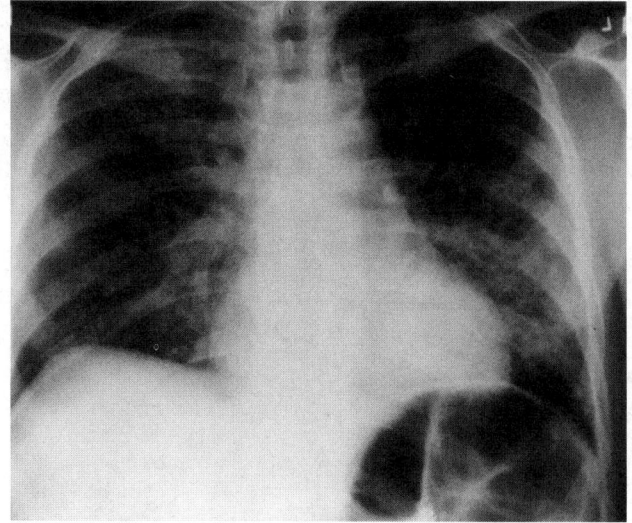

FIGURE 191-1 Chest radiograph depicting diffuse infiltrates in an HIV-infected patient with pneumocystosis.

former group. Sputum induction has gained popularity as a simple, noninvasive technique; this procedure requires trained and dedicated personnel, and its success has varied at different institutions. Oral washes, combined with PCR, have also shown promise. Fiberoptic bronchoscopy with BAL, which is more sensitive than sputum induction, remains the mainstay of *Pneumocystis* diagnosis. This procedure also provides information about the organism burden, the host inflammatory response, and the presence of other opportunistic infections. Transbronchial biopsy and open lung biopsy, the most invasive procedures, are used only when a diagnosis cannot be made by BAL.

COURSE AND PROGNOSIS In the typical case of untreated *Pneumocystis* pneumonia, progressive respiratory embarrassment leads to death. Therapy is most effective when instituted early in the course of the disease, before there is extensive alveolar damage. If induced sputum is nondiagnostic and BAL cannot be performed in a timely manner, it is reasonable to begin empirical therapy with drugs active against *Pneumocystis*. However, this practice does not obviate a specific etiologic diagnosis. With improved management of HIV and its complications, mortality from pneumocystosis is 15 to 20% at 1 month and 50 to 55% at 1 year. Rates of early death remain high among people who require mechanical ventilation (60%) and among non-HIV patients (40%). The most widely used prognostic factor is the degree of hypoxemia. Other factors include pneumocystosis history, age, CD4+ count, neutrophil and IL-8 levels in BAL fluid, albumin and LDH levels in serum, and the degree of expertise with which HIV infection is managed.

℞ TREATMENT

For decisions about therapy (see also Chaps. 118 and 193), pneumocystosis has been classified as mild (a Pa_{O_2} of >70 mmHg or a $PA_{O_2} - Pa_{O_2}$ of <35 mmHg) or as moderate to severe (a Pa_{O_2} of ≤70 mmHg or a $PA_{O_2} - Pa_{O_2}$ of ≥35 mmHg) on breathing room air. Trimethoprim-sulfamethoxazole (TMP-SMX), which acts by inhibiting folic acid synthesis, is considered the drug of choice for all forms of pneumocystosis (Table 191-1). Treatment for extrapulmonary disease is the same as that for pneumonia. Therapy is continued for 14 days in non-HIV-infected patients and for 21 days in persons infected with HIV. Since HIV-infected patients respond more slowly than non-HIV-infected patients, it is prudent to wait at least 7 days after the initiation of treatment before concluding that therapy has failed. Adding drugs to an existing regimen is no more effective than switching regimens and may increase the risk of toxicity. TMP-SMX is well tolerated by non-HIV-infected patients, whereas more than half of HIV-infected patients experience serious adverse reactions.

Several alternative regimens are available for the treatment of mild to moderate cases of pneumocystosis. TMP plus dapsone and clindamycin plus primaquine are about as effective as TMP-SMX. Dapsone and primaquine should not be used in patients with glucose-6-phosphate dehydrogenase (G6PD) deficiency. Atovaquone is less effective than TMP-SMX but is better tolerated. Atovaquone should be given with food to enhance absorption.

One alternative regimen for the treatment of moderate to severe *Pneumocystis* pneumonia is parenteral pentamidine. Pentamidine is about as effective as TMP-SMX but is highly toxic to both HIV-infected and non-HIV-infected patients. Other regimens include parenteral clindamycin plus primaquine and trimetrexate plus leucovorin (with leucovorin administered to prevent bone marrow suppression).

In recent years, molecular evidence of resistance to sulfonamides—and, to a lesser extent, atovaquone—has emerged among human *Pneumocystis* isolates. Although prior sulfonamide exposure has been a risk factor, this resistance has also occurred in HIV-infected patients who never used sulfonamides. Some studies have found an association of sulfonamide resistance with a poor response to therapy, whereas other studies have not.

Patients infected with HIV frequently experience deterioration in respiratory function shortly after receiving anti-*Pneumocystis* drugs. The adjunctive administration of tapering doses of glucocorticoids to patients with HIV infection and moderate to severe pneumocystosis can prevent this problem and improve the rate of survival (Table 191-1). For maximal benefit, this adjunctive therapy should be started early in the course of the illness (usually when antimicrobial drugs are begun). This regimen has generally proved to be safe despite concern about its effects on other opportunistic infections. The use of steroids as adjunctive therapy in HIV-infected patients with mild pneumocystosis or in non-HIV-infected patients remains to be evaluated.

PREVENTION   Primary prophylaxis is indicated for HIV-infected patients with CD4+ cell counts of <200/μL or a history of oropharyngeal candidiasis. Primary prophylaxis guidelines for other immunocompromised hosts are less clear. Secondary prophylaxis is indicated for both HIV-infected and non-HIV-infected patients who have recovered from pneumocystosis. Primary and secondary prophylaxis may be discontinued in HIV-infected persons once CD4+ counts have risen to >200/μL and remained at that level for ≥3 months.

TABLE 191-1   *Treatment of Pneumocystosis*

Drug(s), Dose, Route	Adverse Effects
FIRST CHOICE[a]	
TMP-SMX (5 mg/kg TMP, 25 mg/kg SMX[b]) q6–8 h PO or IV	Fever, rash, cytopenias, hepatitis, hyperkalemia, GI disturbances
OTHER AGENTS[a]	
TMP, 5 mg/kg q6–8h, plus dapsone, 100 mg qd PO	Hemolysis (G6PD deficiency), methemoglobinemia, fever, rash, GI disturbances
Atovaquone, 750 mg bid PO	Rash, fever, GI and hepatic disturbances
Clindamycin, 300–450 mg q6h PO or 600 mg q6–8h IV, plus primaquine, 15–30 mg qd PO	Hemolysis (G6PD deficiency), methemoglobinemia, rash, colitis, neutropenia
Pentamidine, 3–4 mg/kg qd IV	Hypotension, azotemia, cardiac arrhythmias, pancreatitis, dysglycemias, hypocalcemia, neutropenia, hepatitis
Trimetrexate, 45 mg/m² qd IV, plus leucovorin[c], 20 mg/kg q6h PO or IV	Cytopenias, peripheral neuropathy, hepatic disturbances
ADJUNCTIVE AGENT	
Prednisone, 40 mg bid × 5 d, 40 mg qd × 5 d, 20 mg qd × 11 d; PO or IV	Immunosuppression, peptic ulcer, hyperglycemia, mood changes, hypertension

[a] Therapy is administered for 14 days to non-HIV-infected patients and for 21 days to HIV-infected patients.
[b] Equivalent of 2 double-strength (DS) tablets. (One DS tablet contains 160 mg of TMP and 800 mg of SMX.)
[c] Leucovorin prevents bone marrow toxicity from trimetrexate.
Note: GI, gastrointestinal; G6PD, glucose-6-phosphate dehydrogenase; TMP-SMX, trimethoprim-sulfamethoxazole.

TABLE 191-2   *Prophylaxis of Pneumocystosis*[a]

Drug, Dose, Route	Comments
FIRST CHOICE	
TMP-SMX, 1 DS tablet or 1 SS tablet qd PO[b]	TMP-SMX can be safely reintroduced in some patients who have experienced mild to moderate side effects.
OTHER AGENTS	
Dapsone, 50 mg bid or 100 mg qd PO	—
Dapsone, 50 mg qd PO, plus pyrimethamine, 50 mg weekly PO, plus leucovorin, 25 mg weekly PO	Leucovorin prevents bone marrow toxicity from pyrimethamine.
Dapsone, 200 mg weekly PO, plus pyrimethamine, 75 mg weekly PO, plus leucovorin, 25 mg weekly PO	Leucovorin prevents bone marrow toxicity from pyrimethamine.
Pentamidine, 300 mg monthly via Respirgard II nebulizer	Adverse reactions include cough, bronchospasm.
Atovaquone, 1500 mg qd PO	—
TMP-SMX, 1 DS tablet three times weekly PO	TMP-SMX can be safely reintroduced in some patients who have experienced mild to moderate side effects.

[a] For list of adverse effects, see Table 191-1.
[b] One DS tablet contains 160 mg of TMP and 800 mg of SMX.
Note: DS, double-strength; SS, single-strength; TMP-SMX, trimethoprim-sulfamethoxazole.

TMP-SMX is the drug of choice for primary and secondary prophylaxis (Table 191-2). This agent also provides protection against toxoplasmosis and some bacterial infections. Alternative regimens include dapsone, dapsone plus pyrimethamine plus leucovorin, aerosolized pentamidine, and atovaquone. Although there are no specific recommendations for preventing the spread of *Pneumocystis* infection in health care facilities, it seems prudent to prevent direct contact between patients with pneumocystosis and other susceptible hosts.

FURTHER READING

BARRY SM et al: *Pneumocystis carinii* pneumonia: A review of current issues in diagnosis and management. HIV Medicine 2:123, 2001

CENTERS FOR DISEASE CONTROL AND PREVENTION: Guidelines for preventing opportunistic infections among HIV-infected persons—2002 recommendations of the U.S. Public Health Service and the Infectious Diseases Society of America. MMWR 51(RR-8):1, 2002

DWORKIN MS et al: Survival of patients with AIDS, after diagnosis of *Pneumocystis carinii* pneumonia, in the United States. J Infect Dis 183:1409, 2001

LEOUNG GS et al: Trimethoprim-sulfamethoxazole (TMP-SMX) dose escalation versus direct rechallenge for *Pneumocystis carinii* pneumonia prophylaxis in human immunodeficiency virus–infected patients with previous adverse reaction to TMP-SMX. J Infect Dis 184:992, 2001

STRINGER JR et al: A new name (*Pneumocystis jiroveci*) for *Pneumocystis* from humans. Emerg Infect Dis 8:891, 2002

WALZER PD: Immunological features of *Pneumocystis carinii* infection in humans. Clin Diagn Lab Immunol 6:149, 1999

192 | LABORATORY DIAGNOSIS OF PARASITIC INFECTIONS
Charles E. Davis

The cornerstone for the diagnosis of parasitic infections is a thorough history of the patient's illness. Epidemiologic aspects of the illness are especially important because the risks of acquiring many parasites are closely related to occupation, recreation, or travel to areas of high endemicity. Without a basic knowledge of the epidemiology and life cycles of the major parasites, it is difficult to approach the diagnosis of parasitic infections systematically. Accordingly, the medical classification of important human parasites in this chapter emphasizes their

TABLE 192-1   *Flatworm Infections*

| Parasite | Geographic Distribution | Life-Cycle Hosts | | Diagnosis | | | |
		Intermediate (Transmission)	Definitive	Parasite Stage	Body Fluid or Tissue	Serologic Tests	Other
TAPEWORMS (CESTODES)							
Intestinal tapeworms							
Taenia saginata (beef tapeworm)	Worldwide	Beef	Humans	Ova, segments	Feces	—	Motile segments
Hymenolepis nana (dwarf tapeworm)	Worldwide	Grain beetles	Humans, mice[a]	Ova	Feces	—	
Diphyllobothrium latum (fish tapeworm)	Worldwide	Copepods–fish[c]	Humans, other mammals	Ova, segments	Feces	—	Megaloblastic anemia in 1%
T. solium[b] (pork tapeworm)	Worldwide	Swine	Humans	Ova, segments	Feces	WB	Especially Mexico, Central and South America, Africa
Somatic tapeworms							
Echinococcus granulosus (hydatid disease)	Sheep-raising and hunting areas	Sheep, camels, humans, others	Dogs	Hydatid	Lung, liver	WB, EIA	Chest radiography, CT, MRI
E. multilocularis (hydatid disease)	Subarctic areas	Rodents, humans	Foxes, dogs, cats	Hydatid	Liver	—	May resemble cholangio-cellular carcinoma
T. solium[b] (pork tapeworm)	Worldwide	Swine, humans	Humans	Cysticercus	Muscles, CNS	WB	CT, MRI, radiography
FLUKES (TREMATODES)							
Intestinal flukes							
Fasciolopsis buski	China, India	Snails–water chestnuts	Humans	Ova	Feces	—	—
Heterophyes heterophyes	Far East, India	Snails–fish	Humans	Ova	Feces	—	—
Metagonimus yokogawai	Focal in Europe and North Africa	Snails–fish	Humans	Ova	Feces	—	—
Liver flukes							
Clonorchis sinensis	China, Southeast Asia	Snails–fish	Humans	Ova	Feces, bile	—	Recurrent bacterial cholangitis
Fasciola hepatica	Sheep-raising areas	Snails–watercress	Humans, sheep	Ova	Feces,[d] bile	EIA	Cirrhosis, portal hypertension
Lung flukes							
Paragonimus spp.	Orient, Africa, South America	Snails–crabs/crayfish	Humans, other mammals	Adults, ova	Lung, sputum, feces	WB	Chest radiography, CT, MRI
Blood flukes							
Schistosoma mansoni	Africa, Central and South America, West Indies	Snails	Humans	Ova, adults	Feces	EIA, WB	Rectal snips, liver biopsy
S. haematobium	Africa	Snails	Humans	Ova, adults	Urine	WB	Liver, urine, or bladder biopsy
S. japonicum	Far East	Snails	Humans	Ova, adults	Feces	WB	Liver biopsy

[a] Larvae also can mature in intestinal villi of humans and mice.
[b] *T. solium* can cause either intestinal infections or cysticercosis. Its ova are identical to those of *T. saginata*; scolices and segments of the two species differ.
[c] When there are two intermediate hosts, the first is separated from the second by a dash. Definitive hosts are infected by the second intermediate host.
[d] Ova seldom reach the fecal stream during acute disease.
Note: WB, western blot; CT, computed tomography; MRI, magnetic resonance imaging; CNS, central nervous system; EIA, enzyme immunoassay. Serologic tests listed in Tables 192-1, 192-2, and 192-3 are available commercially or from the Centers for Disease Control and Prevention, Atlanta, GA.

TABLE 192-2 *Roundworm Infections*

| Parasite | Geographic Distribution | Life-Cycle Hosts | | Diagnosis | | | |
		Intermediate (Transmission)	Definitive	Parasite Stage	Body Fluid or Tissue	Serologic Tests	Other
INTESTINAL ROUNDWORMS							
Enterobius vermicularis (pinworm)	Temperate and tropical zones	Fecal-oral	Humans	Ova	Perianal skin	—	"Scotch tape" test
Trichuris trichiura (whipworm)	Temperate and tropical zones	Soil, fecal-oral	Humans	Ova	Feces	—	Rectal prolapse
Ascaris lumbricoides (roundworm of humans)	Temperate and tropical zones	Soil, fecal-oral	Humans	Ova	Feces	—	Sx of pulmonary migration
Ancylostoma duodenale (Old World hookworm)	Eurasia, Africa, Pacific	Soil→skin	Humans	Ova/larvae	Feces	—	Sx of pulmonary migration, anemia
Necator americanus (New World hookworm)	U.S., Africa, worldwide	Soil→skin	Humans	Ova/larvae	Feces	—	Sx of pulmonary migration, anemia
Strongyloides stercoralis (strongyloidiasis)	Moist tropics and subtropics	Soil→skin	Humans	Larvae	Feces, sputum, duodenal fluid	EIA	Dissemination in immunodeficiency
TISSUE ROUNDWORMS							
Trichinella spiralis (trichinosis)	Worldwide	Swine/humans	Swine/humans	Larvae	Muscle	EIA	Muscle biopsy
Wuchereria bancrofti (filariasis)	Coastal areas in tropics and subtropics	Mosquitoes	Humans	Microfilariae	Blood, lymph nodes	EIA	Nocturnal periodicity[a]
Brugia malayi (filariasis)	Asia, Indian subcontinent	Mosquitoes	Humans	Microfilariae	Blood	EIA	Nocturnal
Loa loa (African eye worm)	West and Central Africa	Mango flies (*Chrysops*)	Humans	Microfilariae	Blood	—	May be visible in eye, diurnal
Onchocerca volvulus (river blindness)	Africa, Mexico, Central and South America	Blackflies	Humans	Adults/larvae	Skin/eye	—	Examine nodules or skin snips
Dracunculus medinensis (guinea worm)	Africa	*Cyclops*	Humans	Adults/larvae	Skin	—	May be visible in lesion
LARVA MIGRANS SYNDROMES							
Ancylostoma braziliense (creeping eruption)	Tropical and temperate zones	Soil→skin	Dogs/cats, humans	Larvae	Skin	—	Dog and cat hookworm
Toxocara canis and *cati* (visceral larva migrans)	Tropical and temperate zones	Soil, fecal-oral	Dogs/cats, humans	Larvae	Viscera, CNS, eye	EIA[b]	Also caused by roundworms of other species

[a] Blood should be drawn at midnight, except for infection acquired in the South Pacific.
[b] The presence of hemagglutinins is a useful clue.

Note: Sx, signs/symptoms; EIA, enzyme immunoassay; CNS, central nervous system.

geographic distribution, their transmission, and the anatomic location and stages of their life cycle in humans. The text and tables are intended to serve as a guide to the correct diagnostic procedures for the major parasitic infections and to direct the reader to other chapters that contain more comprehensive information about each infection. Tables 192-1, 192-2, and 192-3 summarize the geographic distributions, the anatomic locations, and the methods employed for the diagnosis of flatworm, roundworm, and protozoal infections, respectively.

In addition to selecting the correct diagnostic procedures, physicians must counsel their patients to ensure that specimens are collected properly and arrive at the laboratory promptly. For example, the diagnosis of bancroftian filariasis is unlikely to be confirmed by the laboratory unless blood is drawn near midnight, when the nocturnal microfilariae are active. Laboratory personnel and surgical pathologists should be notified in advance when a parasitic infection is suspected. Continuing interaction with the laboratory staff and the sur-

gical pathologists increases the likelihood that parasites in body fluids or biopsy specimens will be examined carefully by the most capable individuals.

INTESTINAL PARASITES Most helminths and protozoa exit the body in the fecal stream. The patient should be instructed to collect feces in a clean cardboard container and to record the time of collection on the container. Contamination with water (which could contain free-living protozoa) or with urine should be avoided. Fecal samples should be collected before ingestion of barium or other contrast agents for radiologic procedures and before treatment with antidiarrheal agents and antacids, because these substances change the consistency of the feces and interfere with microscopic detection of parasites. Because of the cyclic shedding of most parasites in the feces, a minimum of three samples collected on alternate days should be examined. When delays in transport to the laboratory are unavoidable, fecal samples should be kept in polyvinyl alcohol to preserve protozoal trophozoites. Refrig-

TABLE 192-3 Protozoal Infections

| Parasite | Geographic Distribution | Life-Cycle Hosts | | Diagnosis | | | |
		Intermediate (Transmission)	Definitive	Parasite Stage	Body Fluid or Tissue	Serologic Tests	Other
INTESTINAL PROTOZOANS							
Entamoeba histolytica (amebiasis)	Worldwide, especially tropics	Fecal-oral	Humans	Troph, cyst	Feces, liver	EIA, antigen detection	Ultrasound, liver CT, PCR
Giardia lamblia (giardiasis)	Worldwide	Fecal-oral	Humans	Troph, cyst	Feces	Antigen detection	String test
Isospora belli	Worldwide	Fecal-oral	Humans	Oocyst	Feces	—	Acid-fast
Cryptosporidium	Worldwide	Fecal-oral	Humans, other animals	Oocyst	Feces	Antigen detection	Acid-fast, biopsy, PCR
Cyclospora cayetanensis	Worldwide?	Fecal-oral	Humans, other animals?	Oocyst	Feces	—	Modified safranin, epifluorescence, PCR
Enterocytozoon bieneusi (microsporidiosis)	Worldwide?	?	Animals, humans	Spore	Feces	—	Modified trichrome, biopsy, PCR
FREE-LIVING AMEBAS							
Naegleria	Worldwide	Warm water	Humans	Troph, cyst	CNS, nares	—	Biopsy, nasal swab
Acanthamoeba	Worldwide	Soil, water	Humans	Troph, cyst	CNS, skin, cornea	—	Biopsy, scrapings
BLOOD AND TISSUE PROTOZOANS							
Plasmodium spp. (malaria)	Subtropics and tropics	Mosquitoes	Humans	Asexual	Blood	Limited use	PCR
Babesia microti (babesiosis)	U.S., especially New England	Ticks	Rodents, humans	Asexual	Blood	IIF	Animal spp. in asplenia, PCR
Trypanosoma rhodesiense (African sleeping sickness)	Sub-Saharan East Africa	Tsetse flies	Humans, herbivores	Tryp	Blood, CSF	Card agglutination, IIF[a]	Also chancre, lymph nodes
T. gambiense (African sleeping sickness)	Sub-Saharan West Africa	Tsetse flies	Humans, swine	Tryp	Blood, CSF	Card agglutination, IIF[a]	Also chancre, lymph nodes
T. cruzi (Chagas' disease)	Mexico→South America	Reduviid bugs (triatomes)	Humans, dogs, wild animals	Amastigote, tryp	Multiple organs/ blood	IIF, EIA	Reactivation in immunosuppression
Leishmania tropica, etc.	Widespread in tropics and subtropics	Sandflies (*Phlebotomus*)	Humans, dogs, rodents	Amastigote	Skin	IFA, EIA[b]	Biopsy, scraping, culture
L. braziliensis (mucocutaneous)	Mexico→South America	Sandflies (*Lutzomyia*)	Humans, dogs, rodents	Amastigote	Skin, mucous membranes	IFA[b], EIA	Biopsy, scraping, culture
L. donovani (kala-azar)	Widespread in tropics and subtropics	Sandflies (*Phlebotomus*)	Humans, dogs, wild animals	Amastigote	RE system	IFA[b], EIA	Biopsy, culture, PCR
Toxoplasma gondii (toxoplasmosis)	Worldwide	Humans, other mammals	Cats	Cyst, troph	CNS, eye, muscles, other	EIA, IIF	PCR

[a] Card agglutination provided to endemic countries by the World Health Organization; contact the CDC at 770-488-7760.

[b] Limited specificity. Most sensitive for *L. donovani* (kala-azar).

Note: CT, computed tomography; troph, trophozoite; tryp, trypomastigote form; IIF, indirect immunofluorescence; RE, reticuloendothelial; PCR, polymerase chain reaction; EIA, enzyme immunoassay; CNS, central nervous system; IFA, indirect fluorescent antibody; CSF, cerebrospinal fluid.

eration will also preserve trophozoites for a few hours and protozoal cysts and helminthic ova for several days.

Analysis of fecal samples consists of both a macroscopic and a microscopic examination. Watery or loose stools are more likely to contain protozoal trophozoites, but protozoal cysts and all stages of helminths may be found in formed feces. If adult worms or tapeworm segments are observed, they should be transported promptly to the laboratory or washed and preserved in fixative for later examination. The only tapeworm with motile segments is *Taenia saginata*, the beef tapeworm, which patients sometimes bring to the physician. Motility is an important distinguishing characteristic, because the ova of *T. saginata* and *Taenia solium*, the cause of cysticercosis, are morphologically indistinguishable.

Microscopic examination of feces (Table 192-4) is not complete until direct wet mounts have been evaluated and concentration techniques as well as permanent stains have been applied. Before accepting a report of negativity for ova and parasites as final, the physician

should insist that the laboratory undertake each of these procedures. Some intestinal parasites are more readily detected in material other than feces. For example, use of the string test to sample duodenal contents is sometimes necessary to detect *Giardia lamblia*, *Cryptosporidium*, and *Strongyloides* larvae. Use of the "Scotch tape" technique to detect pinworm ova on the perianal skin sometimes also reveals ova of *T. saginata* deposited perianally when the motile segments disintegrate (Table 192-4).

Two routine solutions are used to make wet mounts for the identification of the various life stages of helminths and protozoa: physiologic saline for trophozoites, cysts, ova, and larvae and dilute iodine solution for protozoal cysts and ova. Iodine solution must never be used to examine specimens for trophozoites because it kills the parasites and thus eliminates their characteristic motility.

The two most common concentration procedures for detecting small numbers of cysts and ova are formalin-ether sedimentation and zinc sulfate flotation. The formalin-ether technique is preferable, be-

TABLE 192-4 *Alternative Procedures for Laboratory Diagnosis of Parasites Found in Feces*[a]

Parasites and Fecal Stages	Alternative Diagnostic Procedures
TAPEWORMS (CESTODES)	
Taenia saginata ova and segments	Perianal "Scotch tape" test for ova
T. solium ova and segments	Serology; brain biopsy for neurocysticercosis
FLUKES (TREMATODES)	
Clonorchis (Opisthorchis) sinensis ova	Examination of bile for ova and adults in cholangitis
Fasciola hepatica ova	Examination of bile for ova and adults in cholangitis
Paragonimus spp. ova	Serology; sputum; biopsy of lung or brain for ova
Schistosoma ova	Serology for all; rectal snips (especially for *S. mansoni*), urine (*S. haematobium*), liver biopsy and liver ultrasound
ROUNDWORMS	
Enterobius vermicularis ova and adults	Perianal "Scotch tape" test for ova and adults
Trichuris trichiura ova	None
Ascaris lumbricoides ova and adults	Examination of sputum for larvae in lung disease
Hookworm ova and occasional larvae	Examination of sputum for larvae in lung disease
Strongyloides larvae	Duodenal aspirate or jejunal biopsy; serology; sputum or lung biopsy for filariform larvae in disseminated disease
PROTOZOANS	
Entamoeba histolytica trophozoites and cysts	Serology; liver biopsy for trophozoites
Giardia lamblia trophozoites and cysts	Duodenal aspirate or jejunal biopsy[b]
Isospora belli oocysts	Duodenal aspirate or jejunal biopsy[b]
Cryptosporidium oocysts	Duodenal aspirate or jejunal biopsy[b]
Enterocytozoon bieneusi spores	Duodenal aspirate or jejunal biopsy[b]

[a] Stains and concentration techniques are discussed in the text.
[b] Commercial string test is satisfactory; *Isospora* and *Cryptosporidium* are acid-fast.

cause all parasites sediment but not all float. Slides permanently stained for trophozoites should be prepared before concentration. Additional slides stained for cysts and ova may be made from the concentrate.

In many instances, especially in the differentiation of *Entamoeba histolytica* from other amebas, identification of parasites from wet mounts or concentrates must be considered tentative. Permanently stained smears allow study of the cellular detail necessary for definitive identification. The iron-hematoxylin stain is excellent for critical work, but trichrome staining, which can be completed in 1 h, is a satisfactory alternative that also reveals parasites in specimens preserved in polyvinyl alcohol fixative.

BLOOD AND TISSUE PARASITES Invasion of tissue by protozoa and helminths renders the choice of diagnostic techniques more difficult. For example, physicians must understand that aspiration of an amebic liver abscess rarely reveals *E. histolytica* because the trophozoites are located primarily in the abscess wall. They must remember that the urine sediment offers the best opportunity to detect *Schistosoma haematobium* in the Ethiopian youngster or the American traveler who returns from Africa with hematuria (Table 192-5). Tables 192-1, 192-2, and 192-3, which offer a quick guide to the geographic distribution and anatomic locations of the major tissue parasites, should help the physician to select the appropriate body fluid or biopsy site for microscopic examination. Tables 192-5 and 192-6 provide additional information about the identification of parasites in samples from specific anatomic locations. The laboratory procedures for detection of parasites in other body fluids are similar to those used in the examination of feces. The physician should insist on wet mounts, concentration techniques, and permanent stains for all body fluids. The trichrome or iron-hematoxylin stain is satisfactory for all tissue helminths in body fluids other than blood, but microfilarial worms and blood protozoa are more easily visualized when stained with Giemsa or Wright's stain.

The most common parasites detected in Giemsa-stained blood smears are the plasmodia, microfilariae, and African trypanosomes (Table 192-5). Most patients with Chagas' disease present in the chronic phase, when *Trypanosoma cruzi* is no longer microscopically detectable in blood smears. Wet mounts are sometimes more sensitive than stained smears for the detection of microfilariae and African trypanosomes because these active parasites cause noticeable movement of the erythrocytes in the microscopic field. Nuclepore filtration of blood facilitates the detection of microfilariae. The intracellular amastigote forms of *Leishmania* spp. and *T. cruzi* can sometimes be visualized in stained smears of peripheral blood, but aspirates of the bone marrow, liver, and spleen are the best sources for microscopic detection and culture of *Leishmania* in kala-azar and of *T. cruzi* in chronic Chagas' disease. The diagnosis of malaria and the critical distinction among the various *Plasmodium* species are made by microscopic examination of stained thick and thin blood films (Chap. 195).

TABLE 192-5 *Identification of Parasites in Blood and Other Body Fluids*

Body Fluid, Parasite	Enrichment/Stain	Culture Technique
BLOOD		
Plasmodium spp.	Thick and thin smears/Giemsa or Wright's	Not useful for diagnosis
Leishmania spp.	Buffy coat/Giemsa	Media available from CDC
African trypanosomes[a]	Buffy coat, anion column/wet mount and Giemsa	Mouse or rat inoculation[b]
Trypanosoma cruzi[c]	As for African species	As above and xenodiagnosis
Toxoplasma gondii	Buffy coat/Giemsa	Fibroblast cell lines
Microfilariae[d]	Nuclepore filtration/wet mount and Giemsa	None
URINE		
Schistosoma haematobium	Centrifugation/wet mount	None
Microfilariae (in chyluria)	As for blood	None
SPINAL FLUID		
African trypanosomes	Centrifugation, anion column/wet mount and Giemsa	As for blood
Naegleria fowleri	Centrifugation/wet mount and Giemsa or trichrome	Nonnutrient agar overlaid with *Escherichia coli*

[a] *Trypanosoma rhodesiense* and *T. gambiense*.
[b] Inject mice intraperitoneally with 0.2 mL of whole heparinized blood (0.5 mL for rats). After 5 days, tail blood should be checked daily for trypanosomes as described above.
[c] Detectable in blood by conventional techniques only during acute disease. Xenodiagnosis is successful in ~ 50% of patients with chronic Chagas' disease.
[d] Day (1000–1400 h) and night (2200–0200 h) blood should be drawn to maximize the chance of detecting *Wuchereria* (nocturnal except for Pacific strains), *Brugia* (nocturnal), and *Loa loa* (diurnal).

Although most tissue parasites stain with the traditional hematoxylin and eosin, surgical biopsy specimens should also be stained with appropriate special stains. The surgical pathologist who is accustomed to applying silver stains for *Pneumocystis carinii* to induced sputum and transbronchial biopsies may have to be reminded to examine wet mounts and iron-hematoxylin–stained preparations of pulmonary specimens for helminthic ova and *E. histolytica*. The clinician should also be able to advise the surgeon and pathologist about optimal techniques for the identification of parasites in specimens obtained by certain specialized minor procedures (Table 192-6). For example, the excision of skin snips for the diagnosis of onchocerciasis, the collection of rectal snips for the diagnosis of schistosomiasis, and punch biopsy of skin lesions for the identification and culture of cutaneous and mucocutaneous species of *Leishmania* are simple procedures, but the diagnosis can be missed if the specimens are improperly obtained or processed.

TABLE 192-6 *Minor Procedures for Diagnosis of Parasitic Infections*

Parasite(s) and Stage	Procedure
Onchocerca volvulus and *Mansonella streptocerca* microfilariae	*Skin snips:* Lift skin with a needle and excise ~ 1 mg to a depth of 0.5 mm from several sites. Weigh each sample, place it in 0.5 mL of saline for 4 h, and examine wet mounts and Giemsa stains of the saline either directly or after filtration. Count microfilariae.[a]
Loa loa adults and *O. volvulus* adults and microfilariae	*Biopsies of subcutaneous nodules:* Stain routine histopathologic sections and impression smears with Giemsa.
Trichinella spiralis larvae (and perhaps *Taenia solium* cysticerci)	*Muscle biopsies:* Excise about 1.0 g of deltoid or gastrocnemius muscle and squash between two glass slides for direct microscopic examination.
Schistosoma ova of all species, but especially *S. mansoni*	*Rectal snips:* From four areas of mucosa, take 2-mg snips, tease onto a glass slide, and flatten with a second slide before examining directly at 10×. Preparations may be fixed in alcohol or stained.
Trypanosoma gambiense and *T. rhodesiense* trypomastigotes	*Aspirate of chancre or lymph node[b]:* Aspirate center with 18-gauge needle, place a drop on a slide, and examine for motile forms. An otherwise insufficient volume of material may be stained with Giemsa.
Acanthamoeba spp. trophozoites or cysts	*Corneal scrapings:* Obtain sample from ophthalmologist for immediate Giemsa staining and culture on nutrient agar overlaid with *Escherichia coli*.
Cutaneous and mucocutaneous *Leishmania* spp.	*Swabs, aspirates, or punch biopsies of skin lesions:* Obtain specimen from margin of lesion for Giemsa staining of impression smears, and section and culture on special media from CDC.

[a] Counts of >100/mg are associated with significant risk of complications.
[b] Lymph node aspiration is contraindicated in some infections and should be used judiciously.

NONSPECIFIC TESTS Eosinophilia is a common accompaniment of infections with most of the tissue helminths; absolute numbers of eosinophils may be high in trichinosis and the migratory phases of filariasis (Table 192-7). Intestinal helminths provoke eosinophilia only during pulmonary migration of the larval stages. Eosinophilia is not a manifestation of protozoal infections, with the possible exceptions of those due to *Isospora* and *Dientamoeba fragilis*.

Like the hypochromic, microcytic anemia of heavy hookworm infections, other nonspecific laboratory abnormalities may suggest parasitic infection in patients with appropriate geographic and/or environmental exposures. Biochemical evidence of cirrhosis or an abnormal urine sediment in an African immigrant certainly raises the possibility of schistosomiasis, and anemia and thrombocytopenia in a febrile traveler or immigrant are among the hallmarks of malaria. Computed tomography and magnetic resonance imaging also contribute to the diagnosis of infections with many tissue parasites and have become invaluable adjuncts in the diagnosis of neurocysticercosis and cerebral toxoplasmosis.

ANTIBODY AND ANTIGEN DETECTION Useful antibody assays for many of the important tissue parasites are available; most of those listed in Table 192-8 can be obtained from the Centers for Disease Control and Prevention (CDC) in Atlanta. The results of serologic tests not listed in the tables should be interpreted with caution.

The value of antibody assays is limited by several factors. For example, the preparation of thick and thin blood smears remains the procedure of choice for the diagnosis of malaria in individual patients because diagnostic titers to plasmodia develop slowly. Filarial antigens cross-react with those from other nematodes; as in assays for antibody to most parasites, the presence of antibody in the filarial assay fails to distinguish between past and current infection. Despite these specific limitations, the restricted geographic distribution of many tropical parasites increases the diagnostic usefulness of both the presence and the absence of antibody in travelers from industrialized countries. In contrast, a large proportion of the world's population has been exposed to *Toxoplasma gondii*, and the presence of IgG antibody to *T. gondii* does not constitute proof of active disease.

Fewer antibody assays are available for the diagnosis of infection with intestinal parasites. *E. histolytica* is the major exception. Sensi-

tive, specific serologic tests are invaluable in the diagnosis of amebiasis. Commercial kits for the detection of antigen by enzyme-linked immunosorbent assay or of whole organisms by fluorescent antibody assay are now available for several protozoan parasites (Table 192-8).

MOLECULAR TECHNIQUES DNA hybridization with probes that are repeated many times in the genome of a specific parasite and amplifi-

TABLE 192-7 *Parasites Frequently Associated with Eosinophilia[a]*

Parasite	Comment
TAPEWORMS (CESTODES)	
Echinococcus granulosus	When hydatid cyst leaks
Taenia solium	During muscle encystation and in CSF with neurocysticercosis
FLUKES (TREMATODES)	
Paragonimus spp.	Uniformly high in acute stage
Fasciola hepatica	May be high in acute stage
Clonorchis (Opisthorchis) sinensis	Variable
Schistosoma mansoni	50% of infected travelers
S. haematobium	25% of infected travelers
S. japonicum	Up to 6000/μL in acute infection
ROUNDWORMS	
Ascaris lumbricoides	During larval migration
Hookworm species	During larval migration
Strongyloides stercoralis	Profound during migration and early years of infection
Trichinella spiralis	Up to 7000/μL
Filarial species[b]	Varies but can reach 5000 to 8000/μL
Toxocara spp.	>3000/μL
Ancylostoma braziliense	With extensive cutaneous eruption
Gnathostoma spinigerum	In visceral larva migrans and eosinophilic meningitis
Angiostrongylus cantonensis	In eosinophilic meningitis
A. costaricensis	During larval migration in mesenteric vessels

[a] Virtually every helminth has been associated with eosinophilia. This table includes both common and uncommon parasites that frequently elicit eosinophilia during infection.
[b] *Wuchereria bancrofti*, *Brugia* spp., *Loa loa*, and *Onchocerca volvulus*.

TABLE 192-8 *Serologic and Molecular Tests for Parasitic Infections*

Parasite, Infection	Antibody	Antigen or DNA/RNA
TAPEWORMS		
Echinococcosis	WB, EIA	
Cysticercosis	WB	
FLUKES		
Paragonimiasis	WB, EIA	
Schistosomiasis	EIA, WB	
Fascioliasis	EIA[a]	
ROUNDWORMS		
Strongyloidiasis	EIA	
Trichinellosis	EIA	
Toxocariasis	EIA	
Filariasis	EIA[b]	
PROTOZOANS		
Amebiasis	EIA	EIA, PCR
Giardiasis	—	EIA, IIF, DFA
Cryptosporidiosis	—	IIF, EIA, DFA, PCR
Malaria (all species)	IIF[c]	PCR
Babesiosis	IIF	PCR
Chagas' disease	IIF, EIA	PCR
Leishmaniasis	IIF, EIA	PCR
Toxoplasmosis	IIF, EIA (IgM)	PCR
Microsporidiosis	—	PCR
Cyclosporiasis	—	PCR

[a] Commercial laboratories only.
[b] Available at the NIH (301-496-5398) and commercially.
[c] Of limited use for management of acute disease.
Note: WB, western blot; EIA, enzyme immunoassay; IIF, indirect immunofluorescence; DFA, direct fluorescent antibody; PCR, polymerase chain reaction. Unless specified, antibody tests listed are available from the CDC. Antigen and parasite detection kits are available commercially. The PCRs listed are available in commercial or research laboratories. The CDC currently uses PCRs as research tools and in selected diagnostic situations (contact Dr. Alexandre da Silva 770-488-4072).

cation of a specific DNA fragment by the polymerase chain reaction (PCR) are promising techniques for the diagnosis of parasitic infections. Although molecular techniques for the detection of many parasites are already being used in insect vectors, animal models, and human trials, relatively few are available for routine use in patients at this time. Several commercial laboratories now perform PCRs for detection of the nucleic acid of a few specific parasites in stool, biopsy, bronchoalveolar lavage, and blood samples (Table 192-8). Because their roles in the diagnosis and management of individual patients are still being defined, the CDC currently uses PCRs as research tools and in selected diagnostic situations (contact Dr. Alexandre da Silva, 770-488-4072).

FURTHER READING

FLECK SL, MOODY AH: *Diagnostic Techniques in Medical Parasitology.* London, Wright, 1988

GARCIA LS: Laboratory identification of the microsporidia. J Clin Microbiol 40:1892, 2002

———— et al: Algorithms for detection and identification of parasites, in *Manual of Clinical Microbiology*, 7th ed, PR Murray et al (eds). Washington, DC, ASM Press, 1999, pp. 1336–1354

HAQUE R et al: Comparison of PCR, isoenzyme analysis, and antigen detection for diagnosis of *Entamoeba histolytica* infection. J Clin Microbiol 36:449, 1998

HERWALDT BL: *Cyclospora cayetanensis*: A review, focusing on the outbreaks of cyclosporiasis in the 1990s. Clin Infect Dis 31:1040, 2000

SHULTE C (ed): et al: Diagnostic significance of blood eosinophilia in returning travelers. Clin Infect Dis 34:407, 2002

WILSON M et al: Evaluation of six commercial kits for detection of human immunoglobulin M antibodies to *Toxoplasma gondii*. J Clin Microbiol 35: 3112, 1997

———— et al: Clinical immunoparasitology, in *Manual of Clinical Laboratory Immunology,* 6th ed, NR Rose et al (eds). Washington, DC, ASM Press, 2002, pp. 547–558

---

193 AGENTS USED TO TREAT INFECTIONS DUE TO PARASITES AND *PNEUMOCYSTIS*
Thomas A. Moore

Parasitic infections afflict more than half of the world's population and impose a substantial health burden, particularly in underdeveloped nations, where they are most prevalent. The remarkable success of global campaigns aimed at controlling or eliminating ancient scourges such as dracunculiasis and onchocerciasis has been offset by the spread of other diseases such as trypanosomiasis due to crumbling infrastructures in settings of HIV infection, civil war, and unstable government. The reach of some parasitic diseases, including malaria, has expanded over the past few decades as a result of factors such as deforestation, population shifts, global warming, and other climatic events. Despite major efforts at vaccine development, chemotherapy remains the single most effective means of controlling parasitic infections. However, efforts to combat the spread of some diseases are hindered by the development and spread of drug resistance and the limited introduction of new antiparasitic agents. Since the last edition of this text was published, new and significant obstacles have arisen. The most serious problems include the discontinued production of inexpensive agents that appear on the essential medicine list of the World Health Organization (WHO)—e.g., amphotericin B deoxycholate, eflornithine, metrifonate, and praziquantel—and the introduction in some areas of counterfeit antiparasitic agents.

Significant advances toward the reduction of the burden of parasitic disease have nevertheless been made. The continued generous donation of ivermectin and albendazole for global eradication programs has improved the health of countless individuals and offers the promise of eradication of some diseases (e.g., the filariases). Shortages of some drugs have prompted a fresh look at currently available agents (e.g., high-dose metronidazole for schistosomiasis). The broader use of newer agents, either alone (e.g., fumagillin, metrifonate, nitazoxanide) or in combination (e.g., lumefantrine with artemether), also appears promising.

This chapter deals exclusively with the agents used to treat infections due to parasites and the fungus *Pneumocystis* (Chap. 191). Specific treatment recommendations for the parasitic diseases of humans are listed in subsequent chapters. Table 193-1 presents a brief overview of each agent (including some that are not discussed in the text but are covered in other chapters), along with its major toxicities, spectrum of activity, and safety for use during pregnancy and lactation. Many of the agents are approved by the U.S. Food and Drug Administration (FDA) but are considered investigational for the treatment of certain infections; these drugs are marked accordingly in Table 193-1. Drugs marked in the text with an asterisk (*) are available only through the Centers for Disease Control and Prevention (CDC) Drug Service (telephone: 404-639-3670 or 404-639-2888; *www.cdc.gov/ncidod/dpd/professional/drug_service.htm*). Other drugs, marked with a dagger (†), are available only through their manufacturers; contact information for these manufacturers may be available from the CDC.

Albendazole Like all benzimidazoles, albendazole acts by binding to free β-tubulin, inhibiting the polymerization of tubulin and the microtubule-dependent uptake of glucose. This fundamental disruption of

Drug	Infection(s)	Adverse Effects	Major Drug Interactions	Pregnancy Class[a]	Breast Milk
Albendazole	Ascariasis, capillariasis, clonorchiasis, cutaneous larva migrans, cysticercosis,[b] echinococcosis,[b] enterobiasis, eosinophilic enterocolitis, gnathostomiasis, hookworm, microsporidiosis, strongyloidiasis, trichinellosis, trichostrongyliasis, trichuriasis, visceral larva migrans	Occasional: nausea, vomiting, abdominal pain, headache, reversible alopecia, elevated aminotransferases. Rare: leukopenia, rash	Dexamethasone, praziquantel: increase plasma level of albendazole sulfoxide by ~50%	C	Yes[c]
Amphotericin B [amphotericin B deoxycholate, Amphotec (InterMune), amphotericin B lipid complex (ABLC, Abelcet), liposomal amphotericin B (AmBisome)]	Leishmaniasis,[d] amebic meningoencephalitis	Frequent: fever, chills, hypokalemia, hypomagnesemia, nephrotoxicity. Occasional: vomiting, dyspnea, hypotension	Antineoplastic agents: renal toxicity, bronchospasm, hypotension Glucocorticoids, ACTH, digitalis: hypokalemia Zidovudine: increased myelo- and nephrotoxicity (ABLC only)	B	No information
Antimonials [pentavalent antimony (Pentostam), meglumine antimonate (Glucantime)]	Leishmaniasis	Frequent: arthralgias/myalgias, pancreatitis, ECG changes (QT prolongation, T wave flattening or inversion)	Antiarrhythmics and tricyclic antidepressants: increased risk of cardiotoxicity (meglumine antimonate only)	Not assigned	Yes (pentavalent antimony); unknown (meglumine antimonate)
Artemisinin derivatives	Malaria	Occasional: neurotoxicity (ataxia, convulsions), nausea, vomiting, anorexia, contact dermatitis	Mefloquine: levels decreased and clearance accelerated by artesunate	Not assigned	Yes
Atovaquone	Malaria,[b] pneumocystosis,[b] babesiosis	Frequent: nausea, vomiting. Occasional: abdominal pain, headache	Plasma levels decreased by rifampin, tetracycline; bioavailability decreased by metoclopramide	C	No information
Azithromycin	Babesiosis	Occasional: nausea, vomiting, diarrhea, abdominal pain. Rare: angioedema, cholestatic jaundice	Cyclosporine and digoxin: levels increased by azithromycin. Nelfinavir: increases levels of azithromycin	B	
Azoles (fluconazole, itraconazole, ketoconazole)	Leishmaniasis	Occasional: hepatotoxicity. Rare: exfoliative skin disorders, anaphylaxis	Warfarin, oral hypoglycemics, phenytoin, cyclosporine, theophylline, digoxin, dofetilide, quinidine, carbamazepine, rifabutin, busulfan, docetaxel, vinca alkaloids, pimozide, alprazolam, diazepam, midazolam, triazolam, verapamil, atorvastatin, cerivastatin, lovastatin, simvastatin, tacrolimus, sirolimus, indinavir, ritonavir, saquinavir, alfentanil, buspirone, methylprednisolone, trimetrexate: plasma levels increased by azoles. Carbamazepine, phenobarbital, phenytoin, isoniazid, rifabutin, rifampin, antacids, H2-receptor antagonists, proton pump inhibitors, nevirapine: decrease plasma levels of azoles. Clarithromycin, erythromycin, indinavir, ritonavir: increase plasma levels of azoles	C	Yes
Benznidazole	Chagas' disease	Frequent: rash, pruritus, nausea, leukopenia, paresthesias	No major interactions	Not assigned	No information

(continued)

Drug	Infection(s)	Adverse Effects	Major Drug Interactions	Pregnancy Class[a]	Breast Milk
Chloroquine	Malaria[b]	Occasional: pruritus, nausea, vomiting, headache, hair depigmentation, exfoliative dermatitis, reversible corneal opacity. Rare: irreversible retinal injury, nail discoloration, blood dyscrasias	Antacids and kaolin: reduce absorption of chloroquine. Ampicillin: bioavailability reduced by chloroquine. Cimetidine: increases serum levels of chloroquine. Cyclosporine: serum levels increased by chloroquine	Not assigned[e]	Yes
Ciprofloxacin	Cyclosporiasis, isosporiasis	Occasional: nausea, diarrhea, vomiting, abdominal pain/discomfort, headache, restlessness, rash. Rare: myalgias/arthralgias, tendon rupture, CNS symptoms (nervousness, agitation, insomnia, anxiety, nightmares, or paranoia), convulsions	Probenecid: increases serum levels of ciprofloxacin. Theophylline, warfarin: serum levels increased by ciprofloxacin	C	Yes
Clindamycin	Babesiosis, malaria, toxoplasmosis, pneumocystosis	Occasional: pseudomembranous colitis, abdominal pain, diarrhea, nausea/vomiting. Rare: pruritus, skin rashes	No major interactions	B	Yes[c]
Dapsone	Leishmaniasis, malaria, pneumocystosis, toxoplasmosis	Frequent: rash, anorexia. Occasional: hemolysis, methemoglobinemia, neuropathy, allergic dermatitis, anorexia, nausea, vomiting, tachycardia, headache, insomnia, psychosis, hepatitis. Rare: agranulocytosis	Rifampin: lowers plasma levels of dapsone	C	Yes
Diethylcarbamazine	Lymphatic filariasis, loiasis	Frequent: dose-related nausea, vomiting. Rare: fever, chills, arthralgias, headaches	None reported	Not assigned[e]	No information
Diloxanide furoate	Amebiasis	Frequent: flatulence. Occasional: nausea, vomiting, diarrhea. Rare: pruritus	None reported	Contraindicated	No information
Eflornithine (difluoromethylornithine, DFMO)	Trypanosomiasis	Frequent: pancytopenia. Occasional: diarrhea, seizures. Rare: transient hearing loss	No major interactions	Contraindicated	No information
Fumagillin	Microsporidiosis	Rare: neutropenia, thrombocytopenia	None reported	No information	No information
Furazolidone	Giardiasis	Frequent: nausea/vomiting, brown urine. Occasional: rectal itching, headache. Rare: hemolytic anemia, disulfiram-like reactions, MAO-inhibitor interactions	Risk of hypertensive crisis when administered >5 days with MAO inhibitors	No information	No information
Halofantrine	Malaria[b]	Frequent: abdominal pain, diarrhea. Occasional: ECG disturbances (dose-related prolongation of QTc and PR interval), nausea, pruritus. Contraindicated in persons who have cardiac disease or who have taken mefloquine in preceding 3 weeks	Concomitant use of agents that prolong QTc interval contraindicated	C	No information
Iodoquinol	Amebiasis,[b] balantidiasis, *Dientamoeba fragilis* infection	Occasional: headache, rash, pruritus, thyrotoxicosis, nausea, vomiting, abdominal pain, diarrhea. Rare: optic neuritis, peripheral neuropathy, seizures, encephalopathy	No major interactions	No information	No information
Ivermectin	Ascariasis, cutaneous larva migrans, enterobiasis, gnathostomiasis, loiasis, lymphatic filariasis, onchocerciasis,[b] scabies, strongyloidiasis[b]	Occasional: fever, pruritus, headache, myalgias. Rare: hypotension	No major interactions	C	Yes[c]

(continued)

TABLE 193-1— (Continued)

Drug	Infection(s)	Adverse Effects	Major Drug Interactions	Pregnancy Class[a]	Breast Milk
Lumefantrine	Malaria	Occasional: nausea, vomiting, diarrhea, abdominal pain, anorexia, headache, dizziness	No major interactions	Not assigned	No information
Mebendazole	Ascariasis,[b] capillariasis, eosinophilic enterocolitis, enterobiasis,[b] hookworm,[b] trichinellosis, trichostrongyliasis, trichuriasis,[b] visceral larva migrans	Occasional: diarrhea, abdominal pain, elevated aminotransferases. Rare: agranulocytosis, thrombocytopenia, alopecia	Cimetidine: inhibits mebendazole metabolism	C	No information
Mefloquine	Malaria[b]	Frequent: light-headedness, nausea, headache. Occasional: confusion, nightmares, insomnia, visual disturbances, transient and clinically silent ECG abnormalities (including sinus bradycardia, sinus arrhythmia, first-degree AV block, prolongation of QTc interval, and abnormal T waves). Rare: psychosis, convulsions, hypotension	Administration of halofantrine <3 weeks after mefloquine use may produce fatal QTc prolongation. Mefloquine may lower plasma levels of anticonvulsants. Mefloquine levels decreased and clearance accelerated by artesunate	C	Yes
Melarsoprol	Trypanosomiasis	Frequent: myocardial injury, encephalopathy, peripheral neuropathy, hypertension. Occasional: G6PD-induced hemolysis, erythema nodosum leprosum. Rare: hypotension	No major interactions	Not assigned	No information
Metrifonate	Schistosomiasis	Frequent: abdominal pain, nausea, vomiting, diarrhea, headache, vertigo, bronchospasm. Rare: cholinergic symptoms	No major interactions	Not assigned	No information
Metronidazole	Amebiasis,[b] balantidiasis, dracunculiasis, giardiasis, trichomoniasis,[b] D. fragilis infection	Frequent: nausea, headache, anorexia, metallic aftertaste. Occasional: vomiting, insomnia, vertigo, paresthesias, disulfiramlike effects. Rare: seizures, peripheral neuropathy	Warfarin: effect enhanced by metronidazole. Disulfiram: psychotic reaction. Phenobarbital, phenytoin: accelerate elimination of metronidazole. Lithium: serum levels elevated by metronidazole. Cimetidine: prolongs half-life of metronidazole	B	Yes
Miltefosine	Leishmaniasis	Frequent: mild and transient (1-2 days) gastrointestinal disturbances within first 2 weeks of therapy (resolve after treatment completion), motion sickness. Occasional: reversible elevations of creatinine and aminotransferases	No major interactions	Not assigned	No information
Niclosamide	Intestinal cestodes[b]	Occasional: nausea, vomiting, dizziness, pruritus	No major interactions	Not assigned	No information
Nifurtimox	Chagas' disease	Frequent: nausea, vomiting, abdominal pain, insomnia, paresthesias, weakness, tremors. Rare: seizures. All effects reversible and dose-related	No major interactions	Not assigned	No information
Nitazoxanide	Cryptosporidiosis,[b] giardiasis[b]	Occasional: abdominal pain, diarrhea. Rare: vomiting, headache	No major interactions	B	No information
Oxamniquine	Schistosomiasis	Occasional: dizziness, drowsiness, headache, orange urine, elevated aminotransferases. Rare: seizures	No major interactions	Not assigned	No information

(continued)

Drug	Infection(s)	Adverse Effects	Major Drug Interactions	Pregnancy Class[a]	Breast Milk
Paromomycin	Amebiasis,[b] *D. fragilis* infection, giardiasis, leishmaniasis	Frequent: gastrointestinal disturbances (oral dosing only). Occasional: nephrotoxicity, ototoxicity, vestibular toxicity (parenteral dosing only)	No major interactions	Not assigned[e]	No information
Pentamidine isethionate	Pneumocystosis,[b] leishmaniasis, trypanosomiasis	Frequent: hypotension, hypoglycemia, pancreatitis, sterile abscesses at intramuscular injection sites, gastrointestinal disturbances, reversible renal failure. Occasional: hepatotoxicity, cardiotoxicity, delirium. Rare: pancreatitis, anaphylaxis	No major interactions	C	No information
Praziquantel	Clonorchiasis,[b] cysticercosis, diphyllobothriasis, hymenolepiasis, taeniasis, opisthorchiasis, intestinal trematodes, paragonimiasis, schistosomiasis[b]	Frequent: abdominal pain, diarrhea, dizziness, headache, malaise. Occasional: fever, nausea. Rare: pruritus, singultus	No major interactions	B	Yes
Primaquine phosphate	Malaria,[b] pneumocystosis	Frequent: hemolytic anemia in patients with G6PD deficiency. Occasional: methemoglobinemia, gastrointestinal disturbances. Rare: CNS symptoms	Quinacrine: potentiates toxicity of primaquine	Contraindicated	No information
Proguanil (chloroguanide)	Malaria	Occasional: urticaria. Rare: hematuria, gastrointestinal disturbances	No major interactions	C	Yes
Pyrantel pamoate	Ascariasis, eosinophilic enterocolitis, enterobiasis,[b] hookworm, trichostrongyliasis	Occasional: gastrointestinal disturbances, headache, dizziness, elevated aminotransferases	No major interactions	C	No information
Pyrimethamine	Malaria,[b] pneumocystosis, toxoplasmosis[b]	Occasional: folate deficiency. Rare: rash, seizures, severe skin reactions (toxic epidermal necrolysis, erythema multiforme, Stevens-Johnson syndrome)	Sulfonamides, proguanil, zidovudine: increased risk of bone marrow suppression when used concomitantly	C	Yes
Quinacrine	Giardiasis[b]	Frequent: headache, nausea, vomiting, bitter taste. Occasional: yellow-orange discoloration of skin, sclerae, urine (begins after 1 week of treatment and lasts up to 4 months after drug discontinuation). Rare: psychosis, exfoliative dermatitis, retinopathy, G6PD-induced hemolysis, exacerbation of psoriasis, disulfiram-like effects	Primaquine: toxicity potentiated by quinacrine	Contraindicated	No information
Quinine and quinidine	Malaria, babesiosis	Frequent: cinchonism (tinnitus, high-tone deafness, headache, dysphoria, nausea, vomiting, abdominal pain, visual disturbances, postural hypotension), hyperinsulinemia resulting in life-threatening hypoglycemia. Occasional: deafness, hemolytic anemia, arrhythmias, hypotension due to rapid intravenous infusion	Carbonic-anhydrase inhibitors, thiazide diuretics: reduce renal elimination of quinidine. Amiodarone, cimetidine: increase quinidine levels. Nifedipine: decreases quinidine levels; quinidine slows metabolism of nifedipine. Phenobarbital, phenytoin, rifampin: accelerate hepatic elimination of quinidine. Verapamil: reduces hepatic clearance of quinidine. Diltiazem: decreases clearance of quinidine	X	Yes[c]

(continued)

TABLE 193-1— (Continued)

Drug	Infection(s)	Adverse Effects	Major Drug Interactions	Pregnancy Class[a]	Breast Milk
Spiramycin	Toxoplasmosis	Occasional: gastrointestinal disturbances, transient skin eruptions. Rare: thrombocytopenia, QT prolongation in an infant, cholestatic hepatitis	No major interactions	Not assigned[e]	Yes[c]
Sulfonamides	Malaria,[b] pneumocystosis,[b] toxoplasmosis[b]	Frequent: gastrointestinal disturbances, allergic skin reactions. Rare: severe skin reactions (toxic epidermal necrolysis, erythema multiforme, Stevens-Johnson syndrome), agranulocytosis, aplastic anemia, hypersensitivity of respiratory tract, hepatitis, interstitial nephritis, hypoglycemia, aseptic meningitis	Thiazide diuretics: increased risk of thrombocytopenia in elderly patients. Warfarin: effect prolonged by sulfonamides. Methotrexate: levels increased by sulfonamides. Phenytoin: metabolism impaired by sulfonamides	B	Yes
Suramin	Trypanosomiasis	Frequent, immediate: fever, urticaria, nausea, vomiting, hypotension. Frequent, delayed (up to 24 h): exfoliative dermatitis, stomatitis, paresthesias, photophobia, renal dysfunction. Occasional: nephrotoxicity, adrenal toxicity, optic atrophy, anaphylaxis	No major interactions	Not assigned	No information
Tetracyclines	Balantidiasis, *D. fragilis* infection, malaria	Frequent: gastrointestinal disturbances. Occasional: photosensitivity dermatitis. Rare: exfoliative dermatitis, esophagitis, hepatotoxicity	Warfarin: effect prolonged by tetracyclines	D	Yes
Thiabendazole	Strongyloidiasis,[b] cutaneous larva migrans,[b] visceral larva migrans[b]	Frequent: anorexia, nausea, vomiting, diarrhea, headache, dizziness, asparagus-like urine odor. Occasional: drowsiness, giddiness, crystalluria, elevated aminotransferases, psychosis. Rare: hepatitis, seizures, angioneurotic edema, Stevens-Johnson syndrome, tinnitus	Theophylline: serum levels increased by thiabendazole	C	No information
Tinidazole	Amebiasis,[b] giardiasis, trichomoniasis	Occasional: nausea, vomiting, metallic taste	See metronidazole	Not assigned	No information
Triclabendazole	Fascioliasis, paragonimiasis	Occasional: abdominal cramps, diarrhea, biliary colic, transient headache	No information	Not assigned	Yes
Trimethoprim-sulfamethoxazole	Cyclosporiasis, isosporiasis, pneumocystosis	See sulfonamides	See sulfonamides	C	Yes

[a] Based on U.S. Food and Drug Administration (FDA) pregnancy categories A through D and X.

[b] Approved by the FDA for this indication.

[c] Not believed to be harmful.

[d] Only AmBisome has been approved for this indication.

[e] Use in pregnancy is recommended by international organizations outside the United States.

Abbreviations: ACTH, adrenocorticotropic hormone; AV, atrioventricular; CNS, central nervous system; ECG, electrocardiogram; G6PD, glucose 6-phosphate dehydrogenase; MAO, monoamine oxidase.

cellular metabolism offers treatment for a wide range of parasitic diseases.

Albendazole is poorly absorbed from the gastrointestinal tract. Administration with a fatty meal increases its absorption by two- to sixfold. While poor absorption may be advantageous for the treatment of intestinal helminths, successful treatment of tissue helminth infections such as hydatid disease or neurocysticercosis requires that a sufficient quantity of active drug reach the site of infection. The metabolite albendazole sulfoxide is responsible for the drug's therapeutic effect outside the gut lumen. Significant quantities of this metabolite are measurable in lung and liver tissues and in hydatid cyst fluid obtained at surgery. Cyst concentrations are considerably higher than those obtained with mebendazole. Albendazole sulfoxide crosses the blood-brain barrier, reaching a level significantly higher than that achieved in plasma. The high concentrations of albendazole sulfoxide attained in cerebrospinal fluid (CSF) probably explain the efficacy of albendazole in the treatment of neurocysticercosis.

Albendazole is extensively metabolized in the liver, but there are few data regarding the drug's use in patients with significant hepatocellular disease. Prolonged therapy with full-dose albendazole (800 mg/d) should be approached cautiously in patients also receiving drugs with known effects on the cytochrome P450 system. A single dose of 400 mg is generally recommended for clearance of gastrointestinal nematode infection in both adults and children >2 years of age.

Single-dose albendazole therapy in humans is largely without side effects (overall frequency, ≤1%). More prolonged courses (e.g., as administered for cystic and alveolar echinococcal disease) have been associated with liver function abnormalities and bone marrow toxicity. Thus, when prolonged use is anticipated, the drug should be administered in treatment cycles of 28 days interrupted by 14 days off therapy.

Amphotericin B   See Table 193-1 and Chap. 182.

Antimonials*   Despite associated adverse reactions and the need for prolonged parenteral treatment, the pentavalent antimonial compounds (designated Sb^v) have remained the first-line therapy for all forms of leishmaniasis throughout the world, primarily because they are affordable, are effective, and have survived the test of time. Although they have been used for almost 100 years, their mechanism of action against *Leishmania* spp. remains unknown. Presumably, the compounds interfere with parasite metabolism. The drugs are taken up by the reticuloendothelial system, and their activity against *Leishmania* spp. may be enhanced by this localization. Sodium stibogluconate is the only pentavalent antimonial available in the United States; meglumine antimonate is principally used in francophone countries.

Resistance is a major problem in some areas. Although low-level unresponsiveness to Sb^v was identified in India in the 1970s, incremental increases in both the recommended daily dosage (to 20 mg/kg) and the duration of treatment (to 28 days) satisfactorily compensated for the growing resistance until around 1990. Since that time, there has been steady erosion in the capacity of Sb^v to induce long-term cure in patients with kala-azar who live in eastern India. Foremost among the many factors that have probably contributed to this failure is the provision of suboptimal treatment for years, which led to the development of drug resistance among parasites. Co-infection with HIV impairs the response to therapy.

Sodium stibogluconate is available in aqueous solution and is administered parenterally. Antimony appears to have two elimination phases. When administered intravenously, the mean half-life of the first phase is <2 h; the mean half-life of the terminal elimination phase is nearly 36 h. This slower phase may be due to conversion of pentavalent antimony to a trivalent form that is the likely cause of the side effects often seen with prolonged therapy.

Artemisinin Derivatives   Artesunate, artemether, arteether, and the parent compound artemisinin are sesquiterpene lactones derived from the wormwood plant *Artemisia annua*. These agents are at least ten-fold more potent in vivo than other antimalarial drugs and presently show no cross-resistance with known antimalarials; thus they have become first-line treatments for severe falciparum malaria in some areas where multidrug resistance is a major problem. They are rapidly effective against the asexual blood forms of *Plasmodium* spp., including multidrug-resistant *Plasmodium falciparum*, but they are not active against intrahepatic forms. A combined formulation of artemether and lumefantrine has been developed for the treatment of acute uncomplicated falciparum malaria in areas where *P. falciparum* is resistant to chloroquine and antifolates. Artemether appears to be effective for the treatment of schistosomiasis and is being evaluated for community-based treatment programs.

The antimalarial effect of artemisinin compounds results primarily from dihydroartemisinin, a compound to which artemether and artesunate are both converted. In the presence of antiparasitic iron, dihydroartemisinin produces superoxide radicals, resulting in damage to parasite proteins. Long treatment courses are required. When these agents are used alone, recrudescence may occur. The compounds are available for oral, rectal, intravenous, or intramuscular administration, depending on the derivative. Artemisinin and its derivatives are cleared rapidly from the circulation. Their short half-lives limit their value for prophylaxis. These drugs are not available in the United States.

Atovaquone   Atovaquone is a hydroxynaphthoquinone that exerts broad-spectrum antiprotozoal activity via selective inhibition of parasite mitochondrial electron transport. Atovaquone is an alternative to trimethoprim-sulfamethoxazole for the treatment of *Pneumocystis* pneumonia. This agent exhibits potent activity against toxoplasmosis when used with pyrimethamine. It is active against the erythrocytic and exoerythrocytic stages of *Plasmodium* spp.; when combined with proguanil or doxycycline, it is effective for both treatment and prophylaxis of malaria. Malarone is a fixed-dose combination of atovaquone and proguanil used for malaria prophylaxis as well as for the treatment of acute, uncomplicated *P. falciparum* malaria. Malarone has been shown to be effective in regions with multidrug-resistant *P. falciparum*. Resistance to atovaquone has yet to be reported, although strains of *P. falciparum* with diminished susceptibility to atovaquone alone can be selected both in vitro and in vivo. The drug does not eradicate hypnozoites from the liver; thus patients with *P. vivax* or *P. ovale* infections must be given radical prophylaxis.

The bioavailability of atovaquone varies considerably. Absorption after a single oral dose is slow, increases two- to three-fold with a fatty meal, and is dose-limited above 750 mg. The elimination half-life is increased in patients with moderate hepatic impairment. Because of the potential for drug accumulation, the use of atovaquone is contraindicated in persons with severe renal impairment (creatinine clearance rate <30 mL/min). No dosage adjustments are needed in patients with mild to moderate renal impairment. It is unknown if atovaquone is dialyzable.

Azithromycin   See Table 193-1 and Chap. 118.

Azoles   See Table 193-1 and Chap. 182.

Benznidazole   This oral nitroimidazole derivative is used to treat Chagas' disease, with cure rates of 80 to 90% recorded in acute infections. Benznidazole exerts its trypanocidal effects by generating oxygen radicals to which the parasite is more sensitive than mammalian cells because of a relative deficiency in antioxidant enzymes. Benznidazole also appears to alter the balance between pro- and anti-inflammatory mediators by downregulating the synthesis of nitrite, interleukin (IL) 6, and IL-10 in macrophages.

Benznidazole is highly lipophilic and readily absorbed. The drug is extensively metabolized; only 5% of the dose is excreted unchanged in the urine. Benznidazole is currently unavailable in the United States.

Chloroquine   This 4-aminoquinoline has marked, rapid schizontocidal and gametocidal activity against blood forms of *P. ovale* and *Plasmodium malariae* and against susceptible strains of *P. vivax* and *P. falciparum*. It is not active against intrahepatic forms (*P. vivax* and *P. ovale*). Chloroquine is concentrated in the acidic food vacuoles of intraerythrocytic parasites, reaching levels at this site that are 600-fold higher than plasma levels. The drug inhibits a parasite heme polymerase; as a result, the parasite is effectively killed with its own metabolic waste. Compared with susceptible strains, chloroquine-resistant plasmodia transport chloroquine out of intraparasitic compartments more rapidly and maintain lower chloroquine concentrations in their acid vesicles. Hydroxychloroquine, a congener of chloroquine, is equivalent to chloroquine in its antimalarial efficacy but is preferred to chloroquine for the treatment of autoimmune disorders because it produces less ocular toxicity when used in high doses.

Chloroquine is well absorbed. However, because it exhibits extensive tissue binding, a loading dose is required to yield effective plasma concentrations. A therapeutic drug level in plasma is reached 2 to 3 h after oral administration (the preferred route). Chloroquine can be administered intravenously, but excessively rapid parenteral administration can result in seizures and death from cardiovascular collapse. The mean half-life of chloroquine is 4 days, but the rate of excretion decreases as plasma levels decline, making once-weekly administration possible for prophylaxis in areas with sensitive strains. About half of the parent drug is excreted in urine, but the dose should not be reduced for persons with acute malaria and renal insufficiency.

Ciprofloxacin   See Table 193-1 and Chap. 118.

Clindamycin See Table 193-1 and Chap. 118.

Dapsone See Table 193-1 and Chap. 149.

Diethylcarbamazine* A derivative of the antihelminthic agent piperazine with a long history of successful use, diethylcarbamazine (DEC) remains the treatment of choice for lymphatic filariasis and loiasis and has also been used for visceral larva migrans. While piperazine itself has no antifilarial activity, the piperazine ring of DEC is essential for activity of the drug. DEC exerts various effects on helminths, including immobilization due to a decrease in muscle activity, disruption of microtubule formation, and alteration of helminthic surface membranes resulting in enhanced killing by the host's immune system. In addition, this agent enhances adherence properties of eosinophils. The development of resistance under drug pressure (i.e., a progressive decrease in efficacy when the drug is used widely in human populations) has not been observed, although the drug's effect is variable when administered to persons with filariasis. Monthly administration provides effective prophylaxis against both bancroftian filariasis and loiasis.

DEC is well absorbed after oral administration, with peak plasma concentrations reached within 1 to 2 h. No parenteral form is available. The drug is eliminated largely by renal excretion, with <5% found in feces. If more than one dose is to be administered to an individual with renal dysfunction, the dose should be reduced commensurate with the reduction in creatinine clearance rate. Alkalinization of the urine prevents renal excretion and increases the half-life of the drug. Use in patients with onchocerciasis can precipitate a Mazzotti reaction, with pruritus, fever, and arthralgias.

Diloxanide Furoate Diloxanide furoate, a substituted acetanilide, is a luminally active agent used to eradicate the cysts of *Entamoeba histolytica*. After ingestion, diloxanide furoate is hydrolyzed by enzymes in the lumen or mucosa of the intestine, releasing furoic acid and the ester diloxanide, the latter of which acts directly as an amebicide.

Diloxanide furoate is given alone in asymptomatic cyst passers. For patients with active amebic infections, diloxanide is generally administered in combination with a 5-nitroimidazole such as metronidazole or tinidazole. Diloxanide furoate is rapidly absorbed after oral administration. When coadministered with a 5-nitroimidazole, only diloxanide appears in the systemic circulation; levels peak within 1 h and disappear within 6 h. About 90% of an oral dose is excreted in the urine within 48 h, chiefly as the glucuronide metabolite. Diloxanide furoate is contraindicated in pregnant and breast-feeding women and in children <2 years of age. The drug is not currently available in the United States.

Eflornithine† Eflornithine (difluoromethylornithine, or DFMO) is a fluorinated analogue of the amino acid ornithine. Although originally designed as an antineoplastic agent, eflornithine has proven effective against some trypanosomatids as well as *Pneumocystis*. At one point, the production of this effective agent ceased despite the increasing incidence of human African trypanosomiasis; however, production resumed after eflornithine was discovered to be an effective cosmetic depilatory agent.

Eflornithine has specific activity against all stages of infection with *Trypanosoma brucei gambiense*; however, it is inactive against *T. b. rhodesiense*. The drug acts by irreversibly inhibiting ornithine decarboxylase—an enzyme critical to the formation of polyamines, which are essential to the growth, differentiation, and replication of the trypanosomatids. The diminished effectiveness of eflornithine against *T. b. rhodesiense* appears to be due to the parasite's ability to replace the inhibited enzyme more rapidly than *T. b. gambiense*. Eflornithine is less toxic but more costly than conventional therapy. Supplies of the drug are very limited due to the aforementioned halt in production.

Eflornithine HCl can be administered intravenously or orally; however, its bioavailability after oral administration is only 54%. Eflornithine readily crosses the blood-brain barrier; CSF levels are highest in persons with the most severe central nervous system involvement.

The kidney excretes >80% of the drug; therefore, the dosage should be reduced in patients with renal failure.

Fumagillin Fumagillin, an antibiotic derived from the fungus *Aspergillus fumigatus*, has been used to treat microsporidiosis in honeybees and has been effective against other microsporidia in vitro. This agent was used >40 years ago for the treatment of intestinal amebiasis, and it is effective when used topically in the treatment of microsporidial keratoconjunctivitis.

Fumagillin is being investigated as an angiogenesis inhibitor for the treatment of solid tumors.

Fumagillin exerts its antineoplastic action by inhibiting endothelial cell proliferation and angiogenesis. However, the mechanisms by which fumagillin inhibits microsporidial replication are poorly understood. Fumagillin is not yet available in the United States.

Furazolidone This nitrofuran derivative is an effective alternative agent for the treatment of giardiasis and exhibits activity against *Isospora belli*. Like other nitrofurans, it acts by damaging DNA. Since it is the only agent active against *Giardia* that is available in liquid form, it is often used to treat young children. Although furazolidone had been thought to be largely unabsorbed when administered orally, the occurrence of systemic adverse reactions indicates that this is not the case. More than 65% of the drug can be recovered from the urine as colored metabolites.

Furazolidone is a monoamine oxidase (MAO) inhibitor; thus caution should be used in its concomitant administration with other drugs (especially indirectly acting sympathomimetic amines) and in the consumption of food and drink containing tyramine during treatment. However, hypertensive crises have not been reported in patients receiving furazolidone, and it has been suggested that—since furazolidone inhibits MAO gradually over several days—the risks are small if treatment is limited to a 5-day course. Because hemolytic anemia can occur in patients with glucose-6-phosphate dehydrogenase (G6PD) deficiency and glutathione instability, furazolidone treatment is contraindicated in mothers who are breast-feeding and in neonates.

Halofantrine This 9-phenanthrenemethanol is one of three classes of arylaminoalcohols first identified as potential antimalarial agents by the World War II Malaria Chemotherapy Program. Its activity is believed to be similar to that of chloroquine, although it is an oral alternative for the treatment of malaria due to chloroquine-resistant *P. falciparum*. The mechanism of action is poorly understood.

Halofantrine exhibits erratic bioavailability, but its absorption is significantly enhanced when it is taken with a fatty meal. The elimination half-life of halofantrine is 1 to 2 days; it is excreted mainly in feces. Halofantrine is metabolized into *N*-debutyl-halofantrine by the cytochrome P450 enzyme CYP3A4. Grapefruit juice should be avoided during treatment because it increases both halofantrine's bioavailability and halofantrine-induced QT interval prolongation by inhibiting CYP3A4 at the enterocyte level. Halofantrine is currently unavailable in the United States.

Iodoquinol Iodoquinol (diiodohydroxyquin), a hydroxyquinoline, is an effective luminal agent for the treatment of amebiasis, balantidiasis, and infection with *Dientamoeba fragilis*. Its mechanism of action is unknown. It is poorly absorbed. Because the drug contains 64% organically bound iodine, it should be used with caution in patients with thyroid disease. Iodine dermatitis occurs occasionally during iodoquinol treatment. Protein-bound serum iodine levels may be increased during treatment and can interfere with certain tests of thyroid function. These effects may persist for as long as 6 months after discontinuation of therapy. Iodoquinol is contraindicated in patients with liver disease. Most serious are the reactions related to prolonged high-dose therapy (optic neuritis, peripheral neuropathy), which should not occur if the recommended dosage regimens are followed.

Ivermectin Ivermectin (22,23 dihydroavermectin) is a derivative of the macrocyclic lactone avermectin produced by the soil-dwelling actinomycete *Streptomyces avermitilis*. Ivermectin is active at low doses against a wide range of helminths and ectoparasites. It is the drug of choice for the treatment of onchocerciasis, strongyloidiasis, cutaneous larva migrans, and scabies. Ivermectin is highly active against microfilariae of the lymphatic filariases but has no macrofilaricidal activity. When ivermectin is used in combination with other agents such as diethylcarbamazine or albendazole for treatment of lymphatic filariasis, synergistic activity is seen. While active against the intestinal helminths *Ascaris lumbricoides* and *Enterobius vermicularis*, ivermectin is only variably effective in trichuriasis and is ineffective against hookworms. Widespread use of ivermectin for treatment of intestinal nematode infections in sheep and goats has led to the emergence of drug resistance in veterinary practice; this development may portend problems in human medical use.

Recent data suggest that ivermectin acts by opening the neuromuscular membrane–associated, glutamate-dependent chloride channels that are unique to nematodes and arthropods. In this proposed scenario, the result is an influx of chloride ions followed by worm paralysis and subsequent death (via immune or other mechanisms).

Because of its low water solubility, ivermectin is available only as an oral formulation. The drug is highly protein bound; it is almost completely excreted in feces. The effect of food on bioavailability is unknown. Ivermectin is distributed widely throughout the body; animal studies indicate that it accumulates at the highest concentration in adipose tissue and liver, with little accumulation in the brain. Few data exist to guide therapy in hosts with conditions that may influence drug pharmacokinetics.

Ivermectin is generally administered as a single dose of 150 to 200 μg/kg. In the absence of parasitic infection, the adverse effects of ivermectin in therapeutic doses are minimal. Adverse effects in patients with filarial infections include fever, myalgia, malaise, lightheadedness, and (occasionally) postural hypotension. The severity of such side effects is related to the intensity of parasite infection, with more symptoms in individuals with a heavy parasite burden. In onchocerciasis, skin edema, pruritus, and mild eye irritation may also occur. The adverse effects are generally self-limiting and only occasionally require symptom-based treatment with antipyretics or antihistamines. More severe complications of ivermectin therapy for onchocerciasis include encephalopathy in patients heavily infected with *Loa loa*. This reaction has led to the suspension of ivermectin distribution for this indication in regions where the two filarial infections are coendemic.

Lumefantrine   Lumefantrine (benflumetol), a fluorene (benzindene) derivative synthesized in the 1970s by the Chinese Academy of Military Medical Sciences (Beijing), has marked blood schizontocidal activity against a wide range of plasmodia. This agent conforms structurally and in mode of action to the arylaminoalcohol group of antimalarial drugs, including quinine, mefloquine, and halofantrine. Lumefantrine exerts its antimalarial effect as a consequence of its interaction with heme, a degradation product of hemoglobin metabolism. Its antimalarial activity is slower than that of the artemisinin-based drugs, but at the recommended dose regimen the recrudescence rate with lumefantrine is lower. The pharmacokinetic properties of lumefantrine are reminiscent of those of halofantrine, with variable oral bioavailability, considerable augmentation of oral bioavailability by concomitant fat intake, and a terminal elimination half-life of ~4 to 5 days in patients with malaria.

Artemether and lumefantrine have synergistic activity, and clinical studies in China on several hundred patients show the combination to be safe and well tolerated. The combined formulation of artemether and lumefantrine has been developed for the treatment of falciparum malaria in areas where *P. falciparum* is resistant to chloroquine and antifolates. Neither drug is available in the United States.

Mebendazole   This benzimidazole is a broad-spectrum antiparasitic agent widely used to treat intestinal helminthiases. Its mechanism of action is similar to that of albendazole.

Mebendazole is available only in oral form but is poorly absorbed from the gastrointestinal tract; only 5 to 10% of a standard dose is measurable in plasma. The proportion absorbed from the gastrointestinal tract is extensively metabolized in the liver. Metabolites appear in the urine and bile; impaired liver or biliary function results in higher plasma mebendazole levels in treated patients. No dose reduction is warranted in patients with renal function impairment. Because mebendazole is poorly absorbed, its incidence of side effects is low. Transient abdominal pain and diarrhea sometimes occur, usually in persons with massive parasite burdens.

Mefloquine   Like quinine and chloroquine, this quinoline is active only against the asexual erythrocytic stages of malarial parasites. It is the preferred drug for prophylaxis of chloroquine-resistant malaria; high doses can be used for treatment. Despite the recent development of drug-resistant strains of *P. falciparum* in parts of Africa and Southeast Asia, mefloquine is an effective drug throughout most of the world. Cross-resistance of mefloquine with halofantrine and with quinine has been documented in limited areas. Mefloquine's mode of action is similar to that of chloroquine, but mefloquine is not concentrated so extensively in the food vacuole and may act on alternative targets in the parasite.

Mefloquine HCl is available as 250-mg tablets (equivalent to 228.0 mg of the free base). The presence of food significantly enhances the rate and extent of absorption. About 98% of the drug binds to protein. Mefloquine is excreted mainly in the bile and feces; therefore, no dose adjustment is needed in persons with renal insufficiency. The drug and its main metabolite are not appreciably removed by hemodialysis. No special chemoprophylactic dosage adjustments are indicated for dialysis patients to achieve plasma concentrations similar to those in healthy persons. Pharmacokinetic differences have been detected between various ethnic populations. In practice, however, these are of minor importance compared with host immune status and parasite sensitivity. In patients with impaired liver function, the elimination of mefloquine may be prolonged, leading to higher plasma levels.

Mefloquine should be used with caution in individuals participating in activities requiring alertness and fine-motor coordination (e.g., driving, piloting aircraft, operating machinery, and deep-sea diving). If the drug is to be administered for a prolonged period, periodic evaluations are recommended, including liver function tests and ophthalmic examinations. Sleep abnormalities (insomnia, abnormal dreams) have occasionally been reported. Psychosis and seizures occur rarely; mefloquine should not be prescribed to patients with neuropsychiatric conditions, including depression, generalized anxiety disorder, psychosis, schizophrenia, and seizure disorder. If acute anxiety, depression, restlessness, or confusion develops during prophylaxis, these psychiatric symptoms may be considered prodromal to a more serious event, and the drug should be discontinued.

Concomitant use of quinine, quinidine, or drugs producing β-adrenergic blockade may cause significant electrocardiographic abnormalities or cardiac arrest. Halofantrine must not be given simultaneously with or <3 weeks after mefloquine because a potentially fatal prolongation of the QTc interval on electrocardiography may occur. No data exist on mefloquine use after halofantrine use. Administration of mefloquine with quinine or chloroquine may increase the risk of convulsions. Mefloquine may lower plasma levels of anticonvulsants. Caution should be exercised with regard to concomitant antiretroviral therapy, since mefloquine has been shown to exert variable effects on ritonavir pharmacokinetics that are not explained by hepatic CYP3A4 activity or ritonavir protein binding. Vaccinations with attenuated live bacteria should be completed at least 3 days before the first dose of mefloquine.

Women of childbearing age who are traveling to areas where malaria is endemic should be warned against becoming pregnant and encouraged to practice contraception during malaria prophylaxis with mefloquine and for up to 3 months thereafter. However, in the case of unplanned pregnancy, use of mefloquine is not considered an indication for pregnancy termination.

Melarsoprol* This trivalent arsenical compound has been used outside the United States since 1949 for the treatment of human African trypanosomiasis (HAT). It is considered investigational in the United States and is indicated for the treatment of HAT with neurologic involvement and for the treatment of early HAT that is resistant to suramin or pentamidine. The drug enters the parasite via an adenosine transporter; resistant strains lack this transport system. Arsenicals react avidly with sulfhydryl groups on proteins, inhibiting their function. This is the likely mechanism of action and the cause of the severe adverse reactions that commonly occur. Resistance to melarsoprol is attributed to the expression of an unusual purine transporter, resulting in altered drug uptake.

Melarsoprol is always administered intravenously. The most common treatment protocol consists of three or four series of three or four injections each (one intravenous injection per day) separated by rest periods. A recently proposed alternative protocol for *T. b. gambiense* HAT appears to be similarly efficacious and consists of 10 consecutive injections of 2.2 mg/kg per day. A small but therapeutically significant amount of the drug enters the CSF. The compound is excreted rapidly, with ~80% of the arsenic found in feces.

Melarsoprol is highly toxic. The most serious adverse reaction is reactive encephalopathy, which affects 6% of treated individuals and usually develops within 4 days of the start of therapy, with an average case-fatality rate of 50%. Glucocorticoids are administered with melarsoprol to prevent this development. Because melarsoprol is intensely irritating, care must be taken to avoid infiltration of the drug.

Metrifonate This organophosphorous compound has selective activity against *Schistosoma haematobium*. Metrifonate is a prodrug; it is converted nonenzymatically to dichlorvos (2,2-dichlorovinyl dimethylphosphate, DDVP), a highly active chemical that irreversibly inhibits the acetylcholinesterase enzyme. Schistosomal cholinesterase is more susceptible to dichlorvos than is the corresponding human enzyme. The exact mechanism of action of metrifonate is uncertain, but it is believed to inhibit tegumental acetylcholine receptors that mediate glucose transport.

Metrifonate is administered in a series of three doses at 2-week intervals. After a single oral dose, metrifonate produces a 95% decrease in plasma cholinesterase activity within 6 h, with a fairly rapid return to normal. However, 2.5 months are required for erythrocyte cholinesterase levels to return to normal. Treated persons should not be exposed to neuromuscular blocking agents or organophosphate insecticides for at least 48 h after treatment. Metrifonate is currently unavailable in the United States.

Metronidazole and Other Nitroimidazoles See Table 193-1 and Chap. 118.

Miltefosine Miltefosine (hexadecylphosphocholine), originally developed as an antineoplastic agent, was discovered to have significant antiproliferative activity against *Leishmania* spp., *Trypanosoma cruzi*, and *T. brucei* parasites in vitro and in experimental animal models in the early 1990s. In 1995, Tropical Disease Research, a program sponsored by the WHO and other international groups, entered into an agreement with the company now known as ASTA Medica/Zentaris to develop miltefosine for the treatment of visceral leishmaniasis in India. Miltefosine is the first oral drug that has proved to be highly effective and comparable to amphotericin B against visceral leishmaniasis in India, where antimonial-resistant cases are now prevalent. Miltefosine exerts activity in both previously untreated and pentavalent antimonial–unresponsive visceral infections. A recently concluded study in Colombia demonstrated miltefosine cure rates comparable to those for antimony against cutaneous leishmaniasis.

The activity of miltefosine is attributed to interaction with cell signal transduction pathways and inhibition of phospholipid and sterol biosynthesis.

Resistance to miltefosine has not been observed clinically.

Miltefosine is readily absorbed from the gastrointestinal tract, is widely distributed, and accumulates in several tissues. The efficacy of a 28-day treatment course in Indian visceral leishmaniasis is equivalent

to that of amphotericin B therapy; however, it appears that a shortened course of 21 days may be equally efficacious.

General recommendations for the use of miltefosine are limited by the exclusion of specific groups from the published clinical trials: persons <12 or >65 years of age, persons with the most advanced disease, breast-feeding women, HIV-infected patients, and individuals with significant renal or hepatic insufficiency. Miltefosine is currently unavailable in the United States.

Niclosamide Niclosamide is active against a wide variety of adult tapeworms but not against tissue cestodes. It is also a molluscacide and is used in snail-control programs. The drug acts by inhibiting oxidative phosphorylation in worm mitochondria, with consequent energy depletion. Use of the drug is limited by side effects, necessary duration of therapy, the recommended use of purgatives, and—most important—limited availability (i.e., availability on a named-patient basis from the manufacturer).

Niclosamide is poorly absorbed. Tablets are given on an empty stomach in the morning after a liquid meal the night before, and this dose is followed by another 1 h later. For treatment of hymenolepiasis, the drug is administered for 7 days. A second course is often prescribed. The scolex and proximal segments of the tapeworms are killed on contact with niclosamide and may be digested in the gut. However, disintegration of the adult tapeworm results in the release of viable ova, which theoretically can result in autoinfection. Although fears of the development of cysticercosis in patients with *Taenia solium* infections have proved unfounded, it is still recommended that a brisk purgative be given 2 h after the first dose. Niclosamide is no longer approved for use in the United States.

Nifurtimox* This nitrofuran compound is a cheap and effective oral agent for the treatment of acute Chagas' disease. Intracellular reduction followed by auto-oxidation yielding oxygen radicals has been suggested as the mode of action of nifurtimox on *T. cruzi* and as the basis of the drug's toxicity to humans. Prolonged use is required, but the course may have to be interrupted because of drug toxicity, which develops in 40 to 70% of recipients.

Nifurtimox is well absorbed and undergoes rapid and extensive biotransformation: <0.5% of the original drug is excreted in urine.

Nitazoxanide† Nitazoxanide is a 5-nitrothiazole compound used for the treatment of cryptosporidiosis and giardiasis; it is active against other intestinal protozoa as well. The drug is approved for use in children 1 through 11 years of age.

The antiprotozoal activity of nitazoxanide is believed to be due to interference with the pyruvate-ferredoxin oxidoreductase (PFOR) enzyme–dependent electron transfer reaction that is essential to anaerobic energy metabolism. Studies have shown that the PFOR enzyme from *Giardia lamblia* directly reduces nitazoxanide by transfer of electrons in the absence of ferredoxin. The DNA-derived PFOR protein sequence of *Cryptosporidium parvum* appears to be similar to that of *G. lamblia*. Interference with the PFOR enzyme–dependent electron transfer reaction may not be the only pathway by which nitazoxanide exerts antiprotozoal activity.

Nitazoxanide is currently available only as an oral suspension. After oral administration, nitazoxanide is rapidly hydrolyzed to an active metabolite, tizoxanide (desacetyl-nitazoxanide). Tizoxanide then undergoes conjugation, primarily by glucuronidation. It is recommended that nitazoxanide be taken with food; however, no studies have been conducted to determine whether the pharmacokinetics of tizoxanide and tizoxanide glucuronide differ in fasted versus fed subjects. Tizoxanide is excreted in urine, bile, and feces, and tizoxanide glucuronide is excreted in urine and bile. The pharmacokinetics of nitazoxanide in patients with impaired hepatic and/or renal function have not been studied. Tizoxanide is highly bound to plasma protein (>99.9%). Therefore, caution should be used when administering this agent concurrently with other highly plasma protein–bound drugs with narrow therapeutic indices, as competition for binding sites may occur.

Oxamniquine This tetrahydroquinoline derivative is an effective alternative agent for the treatment of *Schistosoma mansoni*, although susceptibility to this drug exhibits regional variation. Oxamniquine exhibits anticholinergic properties, but its primary mode of action seems to rely on ATP-dependent enzymatic drug activation generating an intermediate that alkylates essential macromolecules, including DNA. In treated adult schistosomes, oxamniquine produces marked tegumental alterations similar to those seen with praziquantel but developing less rapidly (i.e., evident 4 to 8 days after treatment).

Oxamniquine is administered orally as a single dose and is well absorbed. Food retards absorption and reduces bioavailability. About 70% of an administered dose is excreted in urine as a mixture of pharmacologically inactive metabolites. Patients should be warned that their urine might have an intense orange-red color. Side effects are uncommon and usually mild, although hallucinations and seizures have been reported. Oxamniquine remains unavailable in the United States.

Paromomycin (Aminosidine) First isolated in 1956, this aminoglycoside is an effective oral agent for the treatment of infections due to intestinal protozoa. Parenteral paromomycin appears to be effective against visceral leishmaniasis in India.

Paromomycin inhibits protozoan protein synthesis by binding to the 30S ribosomal RNA in the aminoacyl-tRNA site, causing misreading of mRNA codons. Paromomycin is less active against *G. lamblia* than standard agents; however, like other aminoglycosides, paromomycin is poorly absorbed from the intestinal lumen, and the high levels of drug in the gut compensate for this relatively weak activity. If absorbed or administered systemically, paromomycin can cause ototoxicity and nephrotoxicity. However, systemic absorption is very limited, and toxicity should not be a concern in persons with normal kidneys. Topical formulations are not generally available.

Pentamidine Isethionate This diamidine is an effective alternative agent for *Pneumocystis* pneumonia and for some forms of leishmaniasis and trypanosomiasis. It is available for parenteral and aerosolized administration. While its mechanism of action remains undefined, it is known to exert a wide range of effects, including interaction with trypanosomal kinetoplast DNA; interference with polyamine synthesis by a decrease in the activity of ornithine decarboxylase; and inhibition of RNA polymerase, ribosomal function, and the synthesis of nucleic acids and proteins.

Pentamidine isethionate is well absorbed, is highly tissue bound, and is excreted slowly over several weeks, with an elimination half-life of 12 days. No steady-state plasma concentration is attained in persons given daily injections; the result is extensive accumulation of pentamidine in tissues, primarily the liver, kidney, adrenal, and spleen. Pentamidine does not penetrate well into the central nervous system. Pulmonary concentrations of pentamidine are increased when delivered in aerosolized form.

Praziquantel This heterocyclic pyrazinoisoquinoline derivative is highly active against a broad spectrum of trematodes and cestodes. It is the mainstay of treatment for schistosomiasis and is a critical part of community-based control programs.

All of the effects of praziquantel can be attributed either directly or indirectly to an alteration of intracellular calcium concentrations. Although the exact mechanism of action remains unclear, the major mechanism is disruption of the parasite tegument, causing tetanic contractures with loss of adherence to host tissues and, ultimately, disintegration or expulsion. Praziquantel induces changes in the antigenicity of the parasite by causing the exposure of concealed antigens. Praziquantel also produces alterations in schistosomal glucose metabolism, including decreases in glucose uptake, lactate release, glycogen content, and ATP levels.

Praziquantel exerts its parasitic effects directly and does not need to be metabolized to be effective. It is well absorbed but undergoes extensive first-pass hepatic clearance. Levels of the drug are increased when it is taken with food, particularly carbohydrates, or with cimetidine. Serum levels are reduced by glucocorticoids, chloroquine, carbamazepine, and phenytoin. Praziquantel is completely metabolized in humans, with 80% of the dose recovered as metabolites in urine within 4 days. It is not known to what extent praziquantel crosses the placenta.

Patients with schistosomiasis who have heavy parasite burdens may develop abdominal discomfort, nausea, headache, dizziness, and drowsiness. Symptoms begin 30 min after ingestion, may require spasmolytics for relief, and usually disappear spontaneously after a few hours.

Primaquine Phosphate This drug is the only agent available for eradication of the hepatic stage of malarial parasites. Primaquine must be metabolized by the host to be effective. It is, in fact, rapidly metabolized; only a small fraction of the dose of the parent drug is excreted unchanged. Although the parasiticidal activity of the three oxidative metabolites remains unclear, they are believed to affect both pyrimidine synthesis and the mitochondrial electron transport chain. The metabolites appear to have significantly less antimalarial activity than primaquine; however, their hemolytic activity is greater than that of the parent drug.

Primaquine causes marked hypotension after parenteral administration and therefore is given only by the oral route. It is rapidly and almost completely absorbed from the gastrointestinal tract.

Patients should be tested for G6PD deficiency before they receive primaquine. Primaquine is otherwise well tolerated.

Proguanil (Chloroguanide) Proguanil inhibits plasmodial dihydrofolate reductase and is used with atovaquone for oral treatment of uncomplicated malaria or with chloroquine for malaria prophylaxis in parts of Africa without widespread chloroquine-resistant *P. falciparum*.

Proguanil primarily exerts its effect by means of the metabolite cycloguanil, whose inhibition of dihydrofolate reductase in the parasite disrupts deoxythymidylate synthesis, thus interfering with a key pathway involved in the biosynthesis of pyrimidines required for nucleic acid replication. There are no clinical data indicating that folate supplementation diminishes drug efficacy; women of childbearing age for whom atovaquone/proguanil is prescribed should continue taking folate supplements to prevent neural-tube birth defects.

Proguanil is extensively absorbed regardless of food intake. The drug is 75% protein-bound. The main routes of elimination are hepatic biotransformation and renal excretion. Between 40 and 60% of proguanil is excreted by the kidneys. Drug levels are increased and elimination is impaired in patients with hepatic impairment. Proguanil is not available in the United States.

Pyrantel Pamoate Pyrantel is a tetrahydropyrimidine formulated as pamoate. This safe, well-tolerated, inexpensive drug is used to treat a variety of intestinal nematode infections but is ineffective in trichuriasis. Pyrantel pamoate is usually effective in a single dose. It depolarizes the neuromuscular junctions of most intestinal nematodes, resulting in their irreversible paralysis and allowing natural expulsion of the worms with the host's feces.

Pyrantel pamoate is poorly absorbed from the intestine; >85% of the dose is passed unaltered in feces. The absorbed portion is metabolized and excreted in urine. Piperazine, which produces hyperpolarization of muscle cells in intestinal helminths, is antagonistic to pyrantel pamoate and should not be used concomitantly.

Pyrantel pamoate has minimal toxicity at the oral doses used to treat intestinal helminthic infection. It is not recommended for pregnant women or children <12 months old.

Pyrimethamine When combined with short-acting sulfonamides, this diaminopyrimidine is effective in malaria, toxoplasmosis, and isosporiasis. Unlike mammalian cells, the parasites that cause these infections cannot utilize preformed pyrimidines obtained through salvage pathways but rather rely completely on de novo pyrimidine synthesis, for which folate derivatives are essential cofactors. The efficacy of pyrimethamine is increasingly limited by the development of resistant strains of *P. falciparum* and *P. vivax*. Single amino acid substitutions to parasite dihydrofolate reductase confer resistance to pyrimethamine by decreasing the enzyme's binding affinity for the drug.

Pyrimethamine is well absorbed; the drug is 87% bound to human plasma proteins. In healthy volunteers, drug concentrations remain at therapeutic levels for up to 2 weeks; drug levels are lower in patients with malaria. Pyrimethamine is extensively metabolized; <3% is excreted unchanged in urine.

At the usual dosage, pyrimethamine alone causes little toxicity except for occasional skin rashes and blood dyscrasias. Bone marrow suppression sometimes occurs at the higher doses used for toxoplasmosis; at these doses, the drug should be administered with folinic acid.

Quinacrine* First introduced as an antimalarial agent in 1930, quinacrine is the only drug approved by the FDA for the treatment of giardiasis. Its production was discontinued in 1992. Although not commercially available, quinacrine can be obtained from alternative sources through the CDC Drug Service. The antiprotozoal mechanism of quinacrine has not been fully elucidated. Quinacrine, a substituted acridine, intercalates into parasite DNA, and it is this interaction that is thought to cause an inhibition of nucleic acid synthesis. The drug inhibits NADH oxidase—the same enzyme that activates furazolidone. The differing relative quinacrine uptake rate between human cells and *G. lamblia* may explain the selective toxicity of the drug. Resistance correlates with decreased drug uptake.

Quinacrine is rapidly absorbed from the intestinal tract and is widely distributed in body tissues. Alcohol is best avoided due to a disulfiram-like effect.

Quinine and Quinidine When combined with another agent, the cinchona alkaloid quinine is effective for the oral treatment of both uncomplicated, chloroquine-resistant malaria and babesiosis. Quinine acts rapidly against the asexual blood stages of all forms of human malaria. For severe malaria, only quinidine (the dextroisomer of quinine) is available in the United States. Quinine concentrates in the acidic food vacuoles of *Plasmodium* spp. The drug inhibits the nonenzymatic polymerization of the highly reactive, toxic heme molecule into a nontoxic polymer pigment called *hemozoin*.

Quinine is readily absorbed when given orally. In patients with malaria, the elimination half-life of quinine increases according to the severity of the infection. However, toxicity is avoided by an increase in the concentration of plasma glycoproteins. The cinchona alkaloids are extensively metabolized, particularly by CYP3A4; only 20% of the dose is excreted unchanged in urine. The drug's metabolites are also excreted in urine and may be responsible for toxicity in patients with renal failure. Renal excretion of quinine is decreased when cimetidine is taken and increased when the urine is acidic. The drug readily crosses the placenta.

Quinidine is both more potent as an antimalarial and more toxic than quinine. Its use requires cardiac monitoring. Dose reduction is necessary in persons with severe renal impairment.

Spiramycin† This macrolide is used to treat acute toxoplasmosis in pregnancy and congenital toxoplasmosis. While the mechanism of action is similar to that of other macrolides, the efficacy of spiramycin in toxoplasmosis appears to stem from its rapid and extensive intracellular penetration, resulting in macrophage drug concentrations 10 to 20 times greater than serum concentrations.

Spiramycin is rapidly and widely distributed throughout the body and reaches concentrations in the placenta up to five times those in serum. This agent is excreted mainly in bile. Indeed, in humans, the urinary excretion of active compounds represents only 20% of the administered dose.

Serious reactions to spiramycin are rare. Of the available macrolides, spiramycin appears to have the lowest risk of drug interactions. Complications of treatment are rare but, in neonates, can include life-threatening ventricular arrhythmias that disappear with drug discontinuation. Although not yet licensed in the United States, spiramycin is available through the FDA.

Sulfonamides See Table 193-1 and Chap. 118.

Suramin* This derivative of urea is the drug of choice for the early stage of African trypanosomiasis. The drug is polyanionic and acts by forming stable complexes with proteins, inhibiting multiple enzymes essential to parasite energy metabolism.

Suramin is parenterally administered. It binds to plasma proteins and persists at low levels for several weeks after infusion. Its metabolism is negligible. This drug does not penetrate the central nervous system.

Tetracyclines See Table 193-1 and Chap. 118.

Thiabendazole Discovered in 1961, thiabendazole remains one of the most potent of the numerous benzimidazole derivatives. However, its use has declined significantly because of a higher frequency of adverse effects than is seen with other, equally effective agents.

Thiabendazole is available in tablet form and as an oral suspension. The drug is rapidly absorbed from the gastrointestinal tract but can also be absorbed through the skin. Thiabendazole should be taken after meals. This agent is extensively metabolized in the liver before ultimately being excreted, principally as glucuronide or sulfate conjugates of 5-hydroxythiabendazole. Within 48 h, 87% of an oral dose of thiabendazole is excreted in urine, and 5% is excreted in feces; most of the dose is excreted within the first 24 h. The usual dose of thiabendazole is determined by the patient's weight, but some treatment regimens are parasite-specific. No specific adjustments are recommended in patients with renal or hepatic failure; only cautious use is advised.

Thiabendazole is active against most intestinal nematodes that infect humans. Although the exact mechanism of its antihelminthic activity has not been fully elucidated, it is likely to be similar to that of other benzimidazole drugs: namely, inhibition of polymerization of parasite β-tubulin. The drug also inhibits the helminth-specific enzyme fumarate reductase. In animals, thiabendazole has anti-inflammatory, antipyretic, and analgesic effects, which may explain its usefulness in dracunculiasis and trichinosis. Thiabendazole also suppresses egg and/or larval production by some nematodes and may inhibit the subsequent development of eggs or larvae passed in feces. Despite the emergence and global spread of thiabendazole-resistant trichostrongyliasis among sheep, there have been no reports of drug resistance in humans.

Coadministration of thiabendazole in patients taking theophylline can result in an increase in theophylline levels by >50%. Therefore, serum levels of theophylline should be monitored closely in this situation.

Tinidazole This nitroimidazole is effective for the treatment of amebiasis, giardiasis, and trichomoniasis. Its mechanism of action and side effects are similar to those of metronidazole, but adverse events appear to be less frequent and severe with tinidazole. In addition, the significantly longer half-life of tinidazole (>12 h) offers potential cure with a single dose. This agent is currently unavailable in the United States.

Triclabendazole This narrow-spectrum benzimidazole is effective against paragonimiasis and all stages of *Fasciola hepatica*, a trematode with inherent resistance to praziquantel. Triclabendazole was originally introduced into veterinary practice in 1983 for the treatment of fascioliasis and was first used in humans in Iran in 1989 during an epidemic of fascioliasis near the Caspian Sea. In 1990, the WHO Division of Control of Tropical Diseases and the pharmaceutical company Ciba-Geigy (now Novartis) agreed to conduct additional clinical trials of triclabendazole for the treatment of fascioliasis and paragonimiasis. In light of the remarkable success of these trials, the WHO Expert Committee on the Use of Essential Drugs recommended in 1997 that the drug be put on the essential drug list. The manufacturer has initiated the process of registering triclabendazole for human use in countries where fascioliasis is endemic. The FDA has not yet approved triclabendazole for use in humans.

While most benzimidazoles have broad-spectrum antihelminthic activity, they exhibit minimal or no activity against *F. hepatica*. In contrast, the antihelminthic activity of triclabendazole is highly specific for *Fasciola* spp. and *Paragonimus* spp., with little activity against nematodes, cestodes, and other trematodes. Triclabendazole is effective against all stages of *Fasciola* spp. The active sulfoxide metabolite of triclabendazole binds to fluke tubulin by assuming a unique nonplanar configuration and disrupts microtubule-based processes. Resistance to triclabendazole in veterinary use has been reported in Australia and Europe; however, no resistance has been documented in humans.

Triclabendazole is rapidly absorbed after oral ingestion and undergoes extensive first-pass metabolism in the liver. Its administration with food enhances its absorption and shortens the elimination half-life of the active metabolite. Both the sulfoxide and sulfone metabolites are highly protein-bound (>99%). Treatment with triclabendazole is typically given in one or two doses. No clinical data are available regarding dose adjustment in renal or hepatic insufficiency; however, given the short course of therapy and extensive hepatic metabolism of triclabendazole, dose adjustment is unlikely to be necessary. No information exists on drug interactions. Triclabendazole is currently unavailable in the United States.

Trimethoprim-Sulfamethoxazole   See Table 193-1 and Chap. 118.

FURTHER READING

ABRAMOWICZ M (ed): Drugs for parasitic infections. Med Lett Drugs Ther 40:1, 2000

MOORE TA, NASH TE: Tissue nematodes, in *Current Therapy of Infectious Disease*, 2d ed, D Schlossberg (ed). St. Louis, Mosby, 2000, pp 660–665

ROSENBLATT JE: Antiparasitic agents. Mayo Clin Proc 74:1161, 1999

TRACY JW, WEBSTER LT: Drugs used in the chemotherapy of protozoal infections: Malaria, in *Goodman and Gilman's The Pharmacological Basis of Therapeutics*, 10th ed, JG Hardman, LE Limbird (eds). New York, McGraw-Hill, 2001, pp 1069–1140

WORLD HEALTH ORGANIZATION: *Model Prescribing Information: Drugs Used in Parasitic Diseases*, 2d ed. Geneva, WHO, 1995

Section 18   Protozoal Infections

194   AMEBIASIS AND INFECTION WITH FREE-LIVING AMEBAS
Sharon L. Reed

AMEBIASIS

DEFINITION   Amebiasis is an infection with the intestinal protozoan *Entamoeba histolytica*. About 90% of infections are asymptomatic, and the remaining 10% produce a spectrum of clinical syndromes ranging from dysentery to abscesses of the liver or other organs.

LIFE CYCLE AND TRANSMISSION   *E. histolytica* is acquired by ingestion of viable cysts from fecally contaminated water, food, or hands. Foodborne exposure is most prevalent and is particularly likely when food handlers are shedding cysts or food is being grown with feces-contaminated soil, fertilizer, or water. Less common means of transmission include contaminated water, oral and anal sexual practices, and—in rare instances—direct rectal inoculation through colonic irrigation devices. Motile trophozoites are released from cysts in the small intestine and, in most patients, remain as harmless commensals in the large bowel. After encystation, infectious cysts are shed in the stool and can survive for several weeks in a moist environment. In some patients, the trophozoites invade either the bowel mucosa, causing symptomatic colitis, or the bloodstream, causing distant abscesses of the liver, lungs, or brain. The trophozoites may not encyst in patients with active dysentery, and motile hematophagous trophozoites are frequently present in fresh stools. Trophozoites are rapidly killed by exposure to air or stomach acid, however, and therefore cannot cause infection.

EPIDEMIOLOGY   About 10% of the world's population is infected with *Entamoeba*, the majority with noninvasive *Entamoeba dispar*. Amebiasis results from infection with *E. histolytica* and is the third most common cause of death from parasitic disease (after schistosomiasis and malaria). Areas of highest incidence (due to inadequate sanitation and crowding) include most developing countries in the tropics, particularly Mexico, India, and nations of Central and South America, tropical Asia, and Africa. The main groups at risk in developed countries are travelers, recent immigrants, homosexual men, and inmates of institutions.

The wide spectrum of clinical disease is caused in part by infection with the two different species of *Entamoeba*. Isolates of *E. histolytica* from patients with invasive amebiasis have unique isoenzymes, surface antigens, DNA markers, and virulence properties and now are recognized as a distinct species from the noninvasive *E. dispar* (Table 194-1).

TABLE 194-1   *E. histolytica and E. dispar, Compared and Contrasted*

SIMILARITIES
1. Both species are spread through ingestion of infectious cysts.
2. Cysts of the two species are morphologically identical.
3. Both species colonize the large intestine.

DIFFERENCES
1. Only *E. histolytica* causes invasive disease.
2. Only *E. histolytica* infections elicit a positive amebic serology.
3. The two species have distinct rRNA sequences.
4. The two species have distinct surface antigens and isoenzyme markers.
5. Gal/GalNAc lectin can be used to differentiate the two species in stool ELISA.

Note: ELISA, enzyme-linked immunosorbent assay; Gal/GalNAc, galactose *N*-acetylgalactosamine. See text.

Most asymptomatic carriers, including homosexual men and AIDS patients, harbor *E. dispar* and have self-limited infections. These observations suggest that *E. dispar* is incapable of causing invasive disease, since *Cryptosporidium* and *Isospora belli*, which also cause only self-limited illnesses in immunocompetent people, cause devastating diarrhea in patients with AIDS. However, host factors play a role as well. In one study, 10% of asymptomatic patients who were colonized with *E. histolytica* went on to develop amebic colitis, while the rest remained asymptomatic and cleared the infection within 1 year.

PATHOGENESIS AND PATHOLOGY   Both trophozoites (Fig. 194-1) and cysts (Fig. 194-2) are found in the intestinal lumen, but only trophozoites of *E. histolytica* invade tissue. The trophozoite is 20 to 60 μm in diameter and contains vacuoles and a nucleus with a characteristic central nucleolus. In animals, depletion of intestinal mucus, diffuse inflammation, and disruption of the epithelial barrier occur before trophozoites actually come into contact with the colonic mucosa. Trophozoites attach to colonic mucus and epithelial cells by galactose *N*-acetylgalactosamine (Gal/GalNAc) lectin. The earliest intestinal lesions are microulcerations of the mucosa of the cecum, sigmoid colon, or rectum that release erythrocytes, inflammatory cells, and epithelial cells. Proctoscopy reveals small ulcers with heaped up margins and normal intervening mucosa. Submucosal extension of ulcerations under viable-appearing surface mucosa causes the classic "flask-shaped"

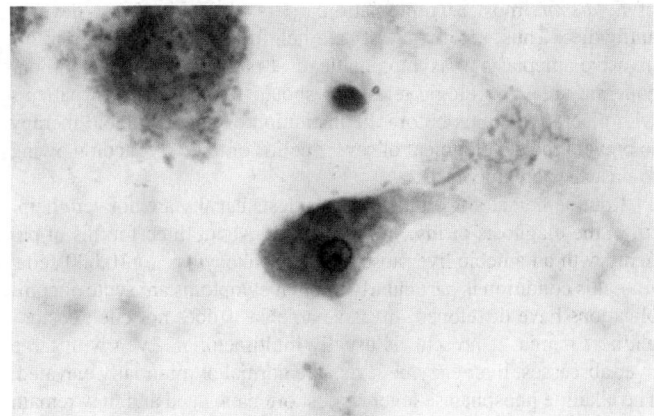

FIGURE 194-1　Trophozoite of *E. histolytica* demonstrating a single nucleus with a central, dotlike nucleolus (trichrome stain).

ulcer containing trophozoites at the margins of dead and viable tissues. Although neutrophilic infiltrates may accompany the early lesions in animals, human intestinal infection is marked by a paucity of inflammatory cells, probably in part because of the killing of neutrophils by trophozoites. Treated ulcers characteristically heal with little or no scarring. Occasionally, however, full-thickness necrosis and perforation occur.

Rarely, intestinal infection results in the formation of a mass lesion, or *ameboma*, in the bowel lumen. The overlying mucosa is usually thin and ulcerated, while other layers of the wall are thickened, edematous, and hemorrhagic; this condition results in exuberant formation of granulation tissue with little fibrous-tissue response.

A number of virulence factors have been linked to the ability of *E. histolytica* to invade through the interglandular epithelium. One consists of the extracellular cysteine proteinases that degrade collagen, elastin, IgA, IgG, and the anaphylatoxins C3a and C5a. Other enzymes may disrupt glycoprotein bonds between mucosal epithelial cells in the gut. Amebas can lyse neutrophils, monocytes, lymphocytes, and cells of colonic and hepatic cell lines. The cytolytic effect of amebas appears to require direct contact with target cells and may be linked to the release of phospholipase A and pore-forming peptides.

Liver abscesses are always preceded by intestinal colonization, which may be asymptomatic. Blood vessels may be compromised early by lysis of the wall and thrombus formation. Trophozoites invade veins to reach the liver through the portal venous system. *E. histolytica* is resistant to complement-mediated lysis, a property critical to survival in the bloodstream. In contrast, *E. dispar* is rapidly lysed by complement and is thus restricted to the bowel lumen. Inoculation of amebas into the portal system of hamsters results in an acute cellular infiltrate consisting predominantly of neutrophils. Later, the neutro-

phils are lysed by contact with amebas, and the release of neutrophil toxins may contribute to necrosis of hepatocytes. The liver parenchyma is replaced by necrotic material that is surrounded by a thin rim of congested liver tissue. The necrotic contents of a liver abscess are classically described as "anchovy paste," although the fluid is variable in color and is composed of bacteriologically sterile granular debris with few or no cells. Amebas, if seen, tend to be found near the capsule of the abscess.

A recent study in Bangladeshi schoolchildren revealed that an intestinal IgA response to the Gal/GalNAc lectin reduced the risk of new *E. histolytica* infection by 64%. Serum IgG antibody is not protective; titers correlate with the length of illness rather than with the severity of disease. Indeed, Bangladeshi children with a serum IgG response were more likely than those without such a response to develop new *E. histolytica* infection. Studies of animals suggest that cell-mediated immunity may be important for protection, although patients with AIDS appear not to be predisposed to more severe disease.

CLINICAL SYNDROMES ▪ Intestinal Amebiasis　The most common type of amebic infection is asymptomatic cyst passage. Even in highly endemic areas, most patients harbor *E. dispar*.

Symptomatic amebic colitis develops 2 to 6 weeks after the ingestion of infectious cysts. Lower abdominal pain and mild diarrhea develop gradually and are followed by malaise, weight loss, and diffuse lower abdominal or back pain. Cecal involvement may mimic acute appendicitis. Patients with full-blown dysentery may pass 10 to 12 stools per day. The stools contain little fecal material and consist mainly of blood and mucus. In contrast to those with bacterial diarrhea, fewer than 40% of patients with amebic dysentery are febrile. Virtually all patients have heme-positive stools.

More fulminant intestinal infection, with severe abdominal pain, high fever, and profuse diarrhea, is rare and occurs predominantly in children. Patients may develop toxic megacolon, in which there is severe bowel dilation with intramural air. Patients receiving glucocorticoids are at risk for severe amebiasis. Uncommonly, patients develop a chronic form of amebic colitis, which can be confused with inflammatory bowel disease. The association between severe amebiasis complications and glucocorticoid therapy emphasizes the importance of excluding amebiasis when inflammatory bowel disease is suspected. An occasional patient presents with only an asymptomatic or tender abdominal mass caused by an ameboma, which is easily confused with cancer on barium studies. A positive serologic test or biopsy can prevent unnecessary surgery in this setting. The syndrome of postamebic colitis—persistent diarrhea following documented cure of amebic colitis—is controversial; no evidence of recurrent amebic infection can be found, and re-treatment usually has no effect.

Amebic Liver Abscess　Extraintestinal infection by *E. histolytica* most often involves the liver. Of travelers who develop an amebic liver abscess after leaving an endemic area, 95% do so within 5 months. Young patients with an amebic liver abscess are more likely than older patients to present in the acute phase with prominent symptoms of <10 days' duration. Most patients are febrile and have right-upper-quadrant pain, which may be dull or pleuritic in nature and radiate to the shoulder. Point tenderness over the liver and right-sided pleural effusion are common. Jaundice is rare. Although the initial site of infection is the colon, fewer than one-third of patients with an amebic abscess have active diarrhea. Older patients from endemic areas are more likely to have a subacute course lasting 6 months, with weight loss and hepatomegaly. About one-third of patients with chronic presentations are febrile. Thus, the clinical diagnosis of an amebic liver abscess may be difficult to establish because the symptoms and signs are often nonspecific. Since 10 to 15% of patients present only with fever, amebic liver abscess must be considered in the differential diagnosis of fever of unknown origin (Chap. 18).

Complications of Amebic Liver Abscess　Pleuropulmonary involvement, which is reported in 20 to 30% of patients, is the most frequent com-

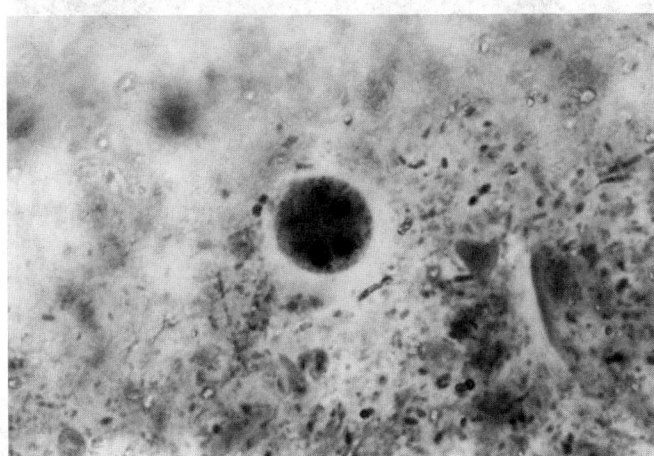

FIGURE 194-2　Cyst of *E. histolytica* showing three of the four nuclei (trichrome stain).

plication of amebic liver abscess. Manifestations include sterile effusions, contiguous spread from the liver, and rupture into the pleural space. Sterile effusions and contiguous spread usually resolve with medical therapy, but frank rupture into the pleural space requires drainage. A hepatobronchial fistula may cause cough productive of large amounts of necrotic material that may contain amebas. This dramatic complication carries a good prognosis. Abscesses that rupture into the peritoneum may present as an indolent leak or an acute abdomen and require both percutaneous catheter drainage and medical therapy. Rupture into the pericardium, usually from abscesses of the left lobe of the liver, carries the gravest prognosis; it can occur during medical therapy and requires surgical drainage.

Other Extraintestinal Sites   The genitourinary tract may become involved by direct extension of amebiasis from the colon or by hematogenous spread of the infection. Painful genital ulcers, characterized by a punched-out appearance and profuse discharge, may develop secondary to extension from either the intestine or the liver. Both these conditions respond well to medical therapy. Cerebral involvement has been reported in fewer than 0.1% of patients in large clinical series. Symptoms and prognosis depend on the size and location of the lesion.

DIAGNOSTIC TESTS ■ Laboratory Diagnosis   Stool examinations, serologic tests, and noninvasive imaging of the liver are the most important procedures in the diagnosis of amebiasis. Fecal findings suggestive of amebic colitis include a positive test for heme, a paucity of neutrophils, and amebic cysts or trophozoites. The definitive diagnosis of amebic colitis is made by the demonstration of hematophagous trophozoites of *E. histolytica* (Fig. 194-1). Because trophozoites are killed rapidly by water, drying, or barium, it is important to examine at least three fresh stool specimens. Examination of a combination of wet mounts, iodine-stained concentrates, and trichrome-stained preparations of fresh stool and concentrates for cysts (Fig. 194-2) or trophozoites (Fig. 194-1) confirms the diagnosis in 75 to 95% of cases. Cultures of amebas are more sensitive but are not routinely available. If stool examinations are negative, sigmoidoscopy with biopsy of the edge of ulcers may increase the yield, but this procedure is dangerous during fulminant colitis because of the risk of perforation. Trophozoites in a biopsy specimen from a colonic mass confirm the diagnosis of ameboma, but trophozoites are rare in liver aspirates because they are found in the abscess capsule and not in the readily aspirated necrotic center. Accurate diagnosis requires experience, since the trophozoites may be confused with neutrophils and the cysts must be differentiated morphologically from *Entamoeba hartmanni*, *Entamoeba coli*, and *Endolimax nana*, which do not cause clinical disease and do not warrant therapy. Unfortunately, the cysts of *E. histolytica* cannot be distinguished microscopically from those of *E. dispar*. Therefore, the microscopic diagnosis of *E. histolytica* can be made only by the detection of *Entamoeba* trophozoites that have ingested erythrocytes (Fig. 194-1). In terms of sensitivity, stool diagnostic tests based on the detection of the Gal/GalNAc lectin of *E. histolytica* compare favorably with the polymerase chain reaction and with isolation in culture followed by isoenzyme analysis.

Serology is an important addition to the methods used for the parasitologic diagnosis of invasive amebiasis. Enzyme-linked immunosorbent assays (ELISAs) and agar gel diffusion assays are positive in more than 90% of patients with colitis, amebomas, or liver abscess. Positive results in conjunction with the appropriate clinical syndrome suggest active disease because serologic findings usually revert to negative within 6 to 12 months. Even in highly endemic areas such as South Africa, fewer than 10% of asymptomatic individuals have a positive amebic serology. The interpretation of the indirect hemagglutination test is more difficult because titers may remain positive for as long as 10 years.

Up to 10% of patients with acute amebic liver abscess may have negative serologic findings; in suspected cases with an initially negative result, testing should be repeated in a week. In contrast to carriers of *E. dispar*, most asymptomatic carriers of *E. histolytica* develop antibodies. Thus, serologic tests are helpful in assessing the risk of invasive amebiasis in asymptomatic, cyst-passing individuals in nonendemic areas. Serologic tests also should be performed in patients with ulcerative colitis before the institution of glucocorticoid therapy to prevent the development of severe colitis or toxic megacolon owing to unsuspected amebiasis.

Routine hematology and chemistry tests usually are not very helpful in the diagnosis of invasive amebiasis. About three-fourths of patients with an amebic liver abscess have leukocytosis (>10,000 cells/μL); this condition is particularly likely if symptoms are acute or complications have developed. Invasive amebiasis does not elicit eosinophilia. Anemia, if present, is usually multifactorial. Even with large liver abscesses, liver enzyme levels are normal or minimally elevated. The alkaline phosphatase level is most often elevated and may remain so for months. Aminotransferase elevations suggest acute disease or a complication.

Radiographic Studies   Radiographic barium studies are potentially dangerous in acute amebic colitis. Amebomas are usually identified first by a barium enema, but biopsy is necessary for differentiation from carcinoma.

Radiographic techniques such as ultrasonography, computed tomography (CT) (Fig. 194-3), and magnetic resonance imaging are all useful for detection of the round or oval hypoechoic cyst. More than 80% of patients who have had symptoms for >10 days have a single abscess of the right lobe of the liver. Approximately 50% of patients who have had symptoms for <10 days have multiple abscesses. Findings associated with complications include large abscesses (>10 cm) in the superior part of the right lobe, which may rupture into the pleural space; multiple lesions, which must be differentiated from pyogenic abscesses; and lesions of the left lobe, which may rupture into the pericardium. Because abscesses resolve slowly and may increase in size in patients who are responding clinically to therapy, frequent follow-up ultrasonography may prove confusing. Complete resolution of a liver abscess within 6 months can be anticipated in two-thirds of patients, but 10% may have persistent abnormalities for a year.

DIFFERENTIAL DIAGNOSIS   The differential diagnosis of intestinal amebiasis includes bacterial diarrheas caused by *Campylobacter*; enteroinvasive *Escherichia coli*; and *Shigella*, *Salmonella*, and *Vibrio* species. Although the typical patient with amebic colitis has less prominent fever than in these other conditions as well as heme-positive stools with few neutrophils, correct diagnosis requires bacterial cultures, microscopic examination of stools, and amebic serologic testing. As has already been mentioned, amebiasis must be ruled out in any patient thought to have inflammatory bowel disease.

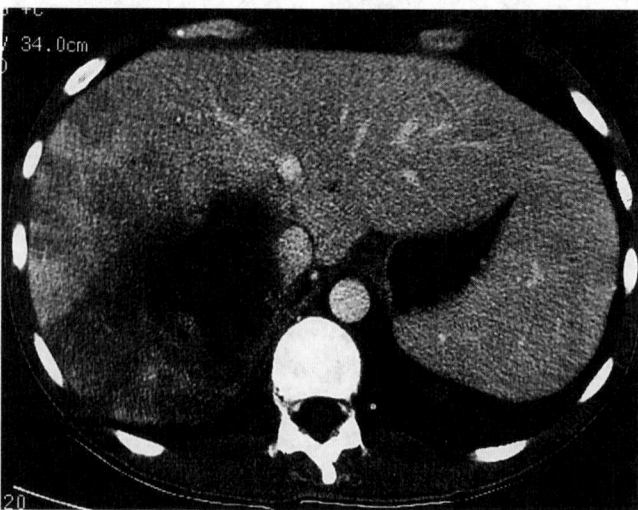

FIGURE 194-3   Abdominal computed tomography scan of a large amebic abscess of the right lobe of the liver. (*Courtesy of the Department of Radiology, UCSD Medical Center, San Diego.*)

Because of the variety of presenting signs and symptoms, amebic liver abscess can easily be confused with pulmonary or gallbladder disease or with any febrile illness with few localizing signs, such as malaria or typhoid fever. The diagnosis should be considered in members of high-risk groups who have recently traveled outside the United States and in inmates of institutions. Once radiographic studies have identified an abscess in the liver, the most important differential diagnosis is between amebic and pyogenic abscess. Patients with pyogenic abscess typically are older and have a history of underlying bowel disease or recent surgery. Amebic serology is helpful, but aspiration of the abscess, with Gram's staining and culture of the material, may be required for differentiation of the two diseases.

℞ TREATMENT

Intestinal Disease The drugs used to treat amebiasis can be classified according to their primary site of action. Luminal amebicides are poorly absorbed and reach high concentrations in the bowel, but their activity is limited to cysts and trophozoites close to the mucosa. Only two luminal drugs are available in the United States: iodoquinol and paromomycin (Table 194-2). Indications for the use of luminal agents include eradication of cysts in patients with colitis or a liver abscess and treatment of asymptomatic carriers. The majority of asymptomatic individuals who pass cysts are colonized with *E. dispar*, which does not warrant specific therapy. However, it is prudent to treat asymptomatic individuals who pass cysts unless *E. dispar* colonization can be definitively demonstrated by specific antigen-detection tests.

Tissue amebicides reach high concentrations in the blood and tissue after oral or parenteral administration. The development of nitroimidazole compounds, especially metronidazole, was a major advance in the treatment of invasive amebiasis. Patients with amebic colitis should be treated with intravenous or oral metronidazole (750 mg three times daily for 5 to 10 days). Side effects include nausea, vomiting, abdominal discomfort, and a disulfiram-like reaction. Other imidazole compounds, such as tinidazole and ornidazole, are as effective but are not available in the United States. All patients should also receive a full course of therapy with a luminal agent, since metronidazole does not eradicate cysts. Resistance to metronidazole has not been identified. Relapses are not uncommon and probably represent reinfection or failure to eradicate amebas from the bowel because of an inadequate dosage or duration of therapy.

Amebic Liver Abscess Metronidazole is the drug of choice for amebic liver abscess. Longer-acting nitroimidazoles (tinidazole and ornidazole) have been shown to be effective as single-dose therapy in developing countries. With early diagnosis and therapy, mortality from uncomplicated amebic liver abscess is <1%. The second-line therapeutic agents emetine and chloroquine should be avoided if possible because of the potential cardiovascular and gastrointestinal side effects of the former and the higher relapse rates with the latter. There is no

evidence that combined therapy with two drugs is more effective than the single-drug regimen. Studies of South Africans with liver abscesses demonstrated that 72% of patients without intestinal symptoms had bowel infection with *E. histolytica*; thus, all treatment regimens should include a luminal agent to eradicate cysts and prevent further transmission. Amebic liver abscess recurs rarely.

Aspiration of Liver Abscesses More than 90% of patients respond dramatically to metronidazole therapy with decreases in both pain and fever within 72 h. Indications for aspiration of liver abscesses are (1) the need to rule out a pyogenic abscess, particularly in patients with multiple lesions; (2) the failure to respond clinically in 3 to 5 days; (3) the threat of imminent rupture; and (4) the prevention of rupture of left-lobe abscesses into the pericardium. There is no evidence that aspiration, even of large abscesses (up to 10 cm), accelerates healing. Percutaneous drainage may be successful even if the liver abscess has already ruptured. Surgery should be reserved for instances of bowel perforation and rupture into the pericardium.

PREVENTION Amebic infection is spread by ingestion of food or water contaminated with cysts. Since an asymptomatic carrier may excrete up to 15 million cysts per day, prevention of infection requires adequate sanitation and eradication of cyst carriage. In high-risk areas, infection can be minimized by the avoidance of unpeeled fruits and vegetables and the use of bottled water. Because cysts are resistant to readily attainable levels of chlorine, disinfection by iodination (tetraglycine hydroperiodide) is recommended. There is no effective prophylaxis.

INFECTION WITH FREE-LIVING AMEBAS

EPIDEMIOLOGY Free-living amebas of the genera *Acanthamoeba, Naegleria*, and *Balamuthia* are distributed throughout the world and have been isolated from a wide variety of fresh and brackish water, including that from lakes, taps, hot springs, swimming pools, and heating and air-conditioning units, and even from the nasal passages of healthy children. Encystation may protect the protozoa from desiccation and food deprivation. The persistence of *Legionella pneumophila* in water supplies may be attributable in part to chronic infection of free-living amebas, particularly *Naegleria*.

NAEGLERIA INFECTIONS Primary amebic meningoencephalitis caused by *Naegleria fowleri* follows the aspiration of water contaminated with trophozoites or cysts or the inhalation of contaminated dust, leading to invasion of the olfactory neuroepithelium. After an incubation period of 2 to 15 days, severe headache, high fever, nausea, vomiting, and meningismus develop. Photophobia and palsies of the third, fourth, and sixth cranial nerves are common. Rapid progression to seizures and coma may follow, and most patients die within a week. Infection is most common in otherwise-healthy children or young adults, who often report recent swimming in lakes or heated swimming pools.

Diagnosis depends on the detection of motile trophozoites in wet mounts of fresh spinal fluid. Other laboratory findings resemble those for fulminant bacterial meningitis, with elevated intracranial pressure, high white blood cell counts (up to 20,000 cells/μL), and elevated protein concentrations and low glucose levels in cerebrospinal fluid. The diagnosis should be considered in any patient who has purulent meningitis without evidence of bacteria on Gram's staining, antigen detection assay, and culture. The prognosis is uniformly poor. Only a few survivors, treated with high-dose amphotericin B and rifampin, have been reported. Antibodies to *Naegleria* spp. have been detected in normal adults; serologic testing is not useful in the diagnosis of acute infection.

ACANTHAMOEBA INFECTIONS ■ **Granulomatous Amebic Encephalitis** Infection with *Acanthamoeba* species follows a more indolent course and occurs typically in chronically ill or debilitated patients. Risk factors include lymphoproliferative disorders, chemotherapy, glucocorticoid

TABLE 194-2 *Drug Therapy for Amebiasis*

Drug	Dosage
ASYMPTOMATIC CARRIER (LUMINAL AGENTS)	
Iodoquinol (650-mg tablets)	650 mg tid for 20 days
Paromomycin (250-mg tablets)	500 mg tid for 10 days
ACUTE COLITIS	
Metronidazole (250- or 500-mg tablets) *plus* Luminal agent as above	750 mg PO or IV tid for 5 to 10 days
AMEBIC LIVER ABSCESS	
Metronidazole	750 mg PO or IV tid for 5 to 10 days
Tinidazole[a]	2 g PO
Ornidazole[a] *plus* Luminal agent as above	2 g PO

[a] Not available in the United States.

therapy, lupus erythematosus, and AIDS. Infection usually reaches the central nervous system hematogenously from a primary focus in the sinuses, skin, or lungs. In the central nervous system, the onset is insidious, and the syndrome often mimics a space-occupying lesion. Altered mental status, headache, and stiff neck may be accompanied by focal findings such as cranial nerve palsies, ataxia, and hemiparesis. Cutaneous ulcers or hard nodules containing amebas are frequently detected in AIDS patients with disseminated *Acanthamoeba* infection.

Examination of the cerebrospinal fluid for trophozoites may be diagnostically helpful, but lumbar puncture may be contraindicated because of increased intracerebral pressure. CT frequently reveals cortical and subcortical lesions of decreased density consistent with embolic infarcts. In other patients, multiple enhancing lesions with edema may mimic the computed tomographic appearance of toxoplasmosis. Demonstration of the trophozoites and cysts of *Acanthamoeba* on wet mounts or in biopsy specimens establishes the diagnosis. Culture on nonnutrient agar plates seeded with *Escherichia coli* may also be helpful. Fluorescein-labeled antiserum is available from the Centers for Disease Control and Prevention (CDC) for the detection of protozoa in biopsy specimens. Granulomatous amebic encephalitis in patients with AIDS may have an accelerated course (with survival for only 3 to 40 days) because of the difficulty these individuals have in forming granulomas. Although studies in animals suggest that rifampin may be useful, the infection is almost uniformly fatal.

Keratitis The incidence of keratitis caused by *Acanthamoeba* has increased in the past 20 years, in part as a result of improved diagnosis. The first of these infections to be recognized were associated with trauma to the eye and exposure to contaminated water. At present, most infections are linked to extended-wear contact lenses. Risk factors include the use of homemade saline, the wearing of lenses while swimming, and inadequate disinfection. Since contact lenses presumably cause microscopic trauma, the early corneal findings may be nonspecific. The first symptoms usually include tearing and the painful sensation of a foreign body. Once infection is established, progression is rapid; the characteristic clinical sign is an annular, paracentral corneal ring representing a corneal abscess. Deeper corneal invasion and loss of vision may follow.

The differential diagnosis includes bacterial, mycobacterial, and herpetic infection. The irregular polygonal cysts of *Acanthamoeba* (Fig. 194-4) may be identified in corneal scrapings or biopsy material, and trophozoites can be grown on special media. Cysts are resistant to available drugs, and the results of medical therapy have been disappointing. Some reports have suggested partial responses to propamidine isethionate eyedrops. Severe infections usually require keratoplasty.

BALAMUTHIA INFECTIONS *Balamuthia mandrillaris*, a free-living ameba previously referred to as a leptomyxid ameba, is an important etiologic agent of amebic meningoencephalitis in immunocompetent hosts. The course is typically subacute, with focal neurologic signs, fever, sei-

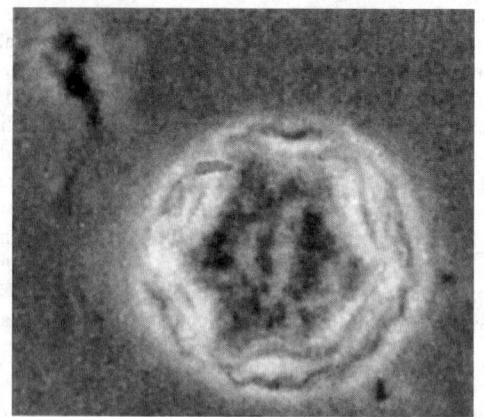

FIGURE 194-4 Double-walled cyst of *Acanthamoeba castellani*, as seen by phase-contrast microscopy. [From DJ Krogstad et al, in A Balows et al (eds): Manual of Clinical Microbiology, 5th ed. Washington, DC, American Society for Microbiology, 1991.]

zures, and headaches leading to death within 1 week to several months after onset. Examination of cerebrospinal fluid reveals mononuclear pleocytosis, elevated protein levels, and normal to low glucose concentrations. Multiple hypodense lesions are usually detected with imaging studies. The diagnosis is almost always made post-mortem, and specific identification may require immunofluorescence with antibodies from the CDC to differentiate the trophozoites from *Acanthamoeba*.

FURTHER READING

DENNEY CF et al: Amebic meningoencephalitis caused by *Balamuthia mandrillaris*: Case report and review. Clin Infect Dis 25:1354, 1997

HAQUE R et al: Innate and acquired resistance to amebiasis in Bangladeshi children. J Infect Dis 186:547, 2002

——— et al: Comparison of PCR, isoenzyme analysis, and antigen detection for diagnosis of *Entamoeba histolytica* infection. J Clin Microbiol 36:449, 1998

KUMAR R, LLOYD D: Recent advances in the treatment of *Acanthamoeba* keratitis. Clin Infect Dis 35:434, 2002

MARTINEZ AJ, VISVESVARA GS: Free-living, amphizoic and opportunistic amebas. Brain Pathol 7:583, 1997

PETRI WA et al: The bittersweet interface of parasite and host lectin-carbohydrate interactions during human invasion by the parasite *Entamoeba histolytica*. Annu Rev Microbiol 56:39, 2002

———, SINGH U: Diagnosis and management of amebiasis. Clin Infect Dis 29:1117, 1999

QUE X, REED SL: Cysteine proteinases and the pathogenesis of amebiasis. Clin Microbiol Rev 13:196, 2002

SISON P et al: Disseminated acanthamoeba infection in patients with AIDS: Case reports and review. Clin Infect Dis 20:1207, 1995

STANLEY SL, REED SL: Microbes and microbial toxins: Paradigms for microbial-mucosal interactions. VI. *Entamoeba histolytica*: Parasite-host interactions. Am J Physiol Gastrointest Liver Physiol 280:G1049, 2001

———: Protective immunity to amebiasis: New insights and new challenges. J Infect Dis 184:504, 2001

---

195 | MALARIA AND BABESIOSIS: DISEASES CAUSED BY RED BLOOD CELL PARASITES
Nicholas J. White, Joel G. Breman

"Humanity has but three great enemies: Fever, famine and war; of these by far the greatest, by far the most terrible, is fever."

William Osler

MALARIA

Malaria is a protozoan disease transmitted by the bite of infected *Anopheles* mosquitoes. It is the most important of the parasitic diseases of humans, with transmission in 103 countries affecting >1 billion people and causing between 1 and 3 million deaths each year. Malaria

has now been eliminated from North America, Europe, and Russia but, despite enormous control efforts, has resurged in many parts of the tropics. Added to this resurgence are the increasing problems of drug resistance of the parasite and insecticide resistance of the vectors. Occasional local transmission following importation of malaria has occurred recently in several southern and eastern areas of the United States and in Europe, indicating the continual danger to nonmalarious countries. Malaria remains today, as it has been for centuries, a heavy burden on tropical communities, a threat to nonendemic countries, and a danger to travelers.

ETIOLOGY AND PATHOGENESIS Four species of the genus *Plasmodium* cause nearly all malarial infections in humans (although rare infections involve species normally affecting other primates). These are *P. falciparum*, *P. vivax*, *P. ovale*, and *P. malariae* (Table 195-1). Almost all deaths are caused by falciparum malaria. Human infection begins when a female anopheline mosquito inoculates plasmodial *sporozoites* from its salivary gland during a blood meal (Fig. 195-1). These microscopic motile forms of the malarial parasite are carried rapidly via the bloodstream to the liver, where they invade hepatic parenchymal cells and begin a period of asexual reproduction. By this amplification process (known as intrahepatic or preerythrocytic *schizogony* or *merogony*), a single sporozoite eventually may produce 10,000 to >30,000 daughter merozoites. The swollen liver cell eventually bursts, discharging motile *merozoites* into the bloodstream. These then invade the red blood cells (RBCs) and multiply 6- to 20-fold every 48 to 72 h. When the parasites reach densities of ~50/μL of blood, the symptomatic stage of the infection begins. In *P. vivax* and *P. ovale* infections, a proportion of the intrahepatic forms do not divide immediately but remain dormant for a period ranging from 3 weeks to a year or longer before reproduction begins. These dormant forms, or *hypnozoites*, are the cause of the relapses that characterize infection with these two species.

After entry into the bloodstream, merozoites rapidly invade erythrocytes and become *trophozoites*. Attachment is mediated via a specific erythrocyte surface receptor. In the case of *P. vivax*, this receptor is related to the Duffy blood-group antigen Fy^a or Fy^b. Most West Africans and people with origins in that region carry the Duffy-negative FyFy phenotype and are therefore resistant to *P. vivax* malaria. During the early stage of intraerythrocytic development, the small "ring forms" of the four parasitic species appear similar under light microscopy. As the trophozoites enlarge, species-specific characteristics become evident, pigment becomes visible, and the parasite assumes an irregular or ameboid shape. By the end of the 48-h intraerythrocytic life cycle (72 h for *P. malariae*), the parasite has consumed nearly all the hemoglobin and grown to occupy most of the RBC. It is now called a *schizont*. Multiple nuclear divisions have taken place (*shizogony* or *merogony*), and the RBC ruptures to release 6 to 30 daughter merozoites, each potentially capable of invading a new RBC and repeating the cycle. The disease in human beings is caused by the direct effects of RBC invasion and destruction by the asexual parasite and the host's reaction. After a series of asexual cycles (*P. falciparum*) or immediately after release from the liver (*P. vivax*, *P. ovale*, *P. malariae*), some of the parasites develop into morphologically distinct, long-lived sexual forms (*gametocytes*) that can transmit malaria.

After being ingested in the blood meal of a biting female anopheline mosquito, the male and female gametocytes form a zygote in the insect's midgut. This zygote matures into an ookinete, which penetrates and encysts in the mosquito's gut wall. The resulting oocyst expands by asexual division until it bursts to liberate myriad motile sporozoites, which then migrate in the hemolymph to the salivary gland of the mosquito to await inoculation into another human at the next feeding.

EPIDEMIOLOGY Malaria occurs throughout most of the tropical regions of the world (Fig. 195-2). *P. falciparum* predominates in Africa, New Guinea, and Haiti; *P. vivax* is more common in Central America and the Indian subcontinent. The prevalence of these two species is approximately equal in South America, eastern Asia, and Oceania. *P. malariae* is found in most endemic areas, especially throughout sub-Saharan Africa, but is much less common. *P. ovale* is relatively unusual outside of Africa and, where it is found, comprises <1% of isolates.

The epidemiology of malaria is complex and may vary considerably even within relatively small geographic areas. Endemicity tradi-

TABLE 195-1 *Characteristics of Plasmodium Species Infecting Humans^a*

Characteristic	Finding for Indicated Species			
	P. falciparum	*P. vivax*	*P. ovale*	*P. malariae*
Duration of intrahepatic phase (days)	5.5	8	9	15
Number of merozoites released per infected hepatocyte	30,000	10,000	15,000	15,000
Duration of erythrocytic cycle (hours)	48	48	50	72
Red cell preference	Younger cells (but can invade cells of all ages)	Red cells up to 14 days old	Reticulocytes	Older cells
Morphology	Usually only ring forms; banana-shaped gametocytes	Irregularly shaped large rings and trophozoites; enlarged erythrocytes; Schüffner's dots	Infected erythrocytes, enlarged and oval with tufted ends; Schüffner's dots	Band or rectangular forms of trophozoites common
Pigment color	Black	Yellow-brown	Dark brown	Brown-black
Ability to cause relapses	No	Yes	Yes	No

^{a} Parasitemias of >2% are suggestive of *P. falciparum* infection.

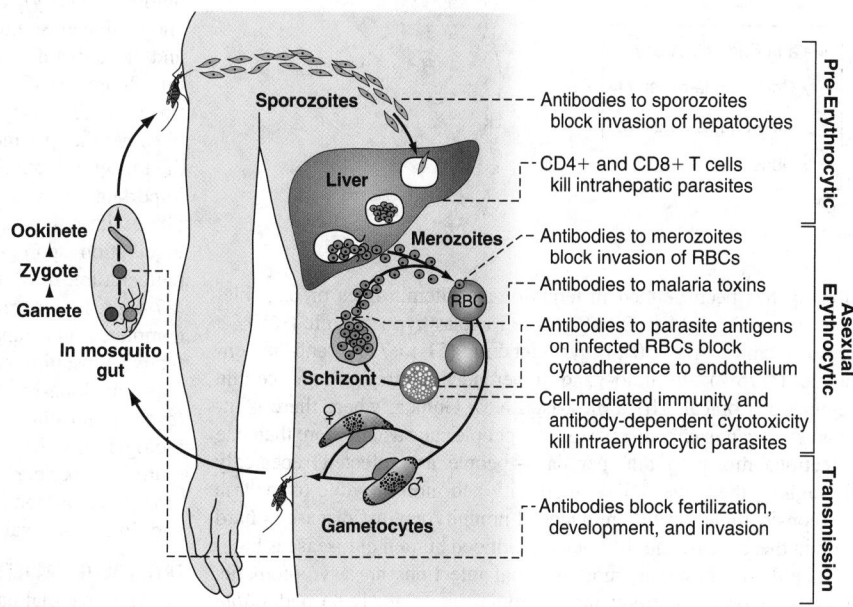

FIGURE 195-1 The malaria transmission cycle from mosquito to human. RBC, red blood cell.

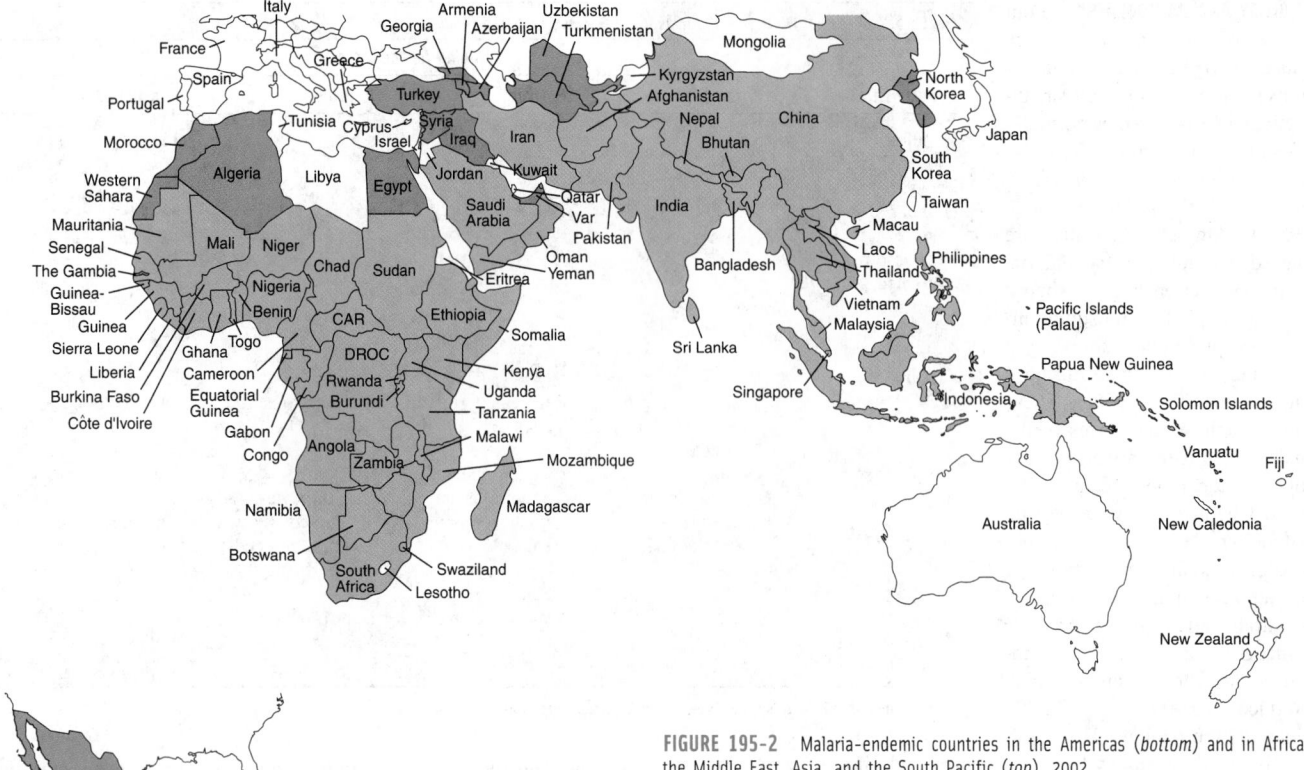

FIGURE 195-2 Malaria-endemic countries in the Americas (*bottom*) and in Africa, the Middle East, Asia, and the South Pacific (*top*), 2002.

Malaria-Endemic Areas

- ⬤ Chloroquine-resistant
- ⬤ Chloroquine-sensitive
- ◯ None

protective immunity is not acquired, and symptomatic disease may occur at all ages. This situation usually exists in hypoendemic areas and is termed *unstable transmission*. Even in areas with stable transmission, there is often an increased incidence of symptomatic malaria coinciding with increased mosquito breeding and transmission during the rainy season. Malaria behaves like an epidemic disease in some areas, particularly those with unstable malaria, such as northern India, Sri Lanka, Southeast Asia, Ethiopia, southern Africa, and Madagascar. An epidemic can develop when there are changes in environmental, economic, or social conditions, such as heavy rains following drought or migrations (usually of refugees or workers) from a nonmalarious region to an area of high transmission; a breakdown in malaria control and prevention services can intensify epidemic conditions. This situation usually results in considerable mortality among all age groups.

The principal determinants of the epidemiology of malaria are the number (density), the human-biting habits, and the longevity of the anopheline mosquito vectors. Not all anophelines can transmit malaria, and those that do vary considerably in their efficiency as malaria vectors. More specifically, the transmission of malaria is directly proportional to the density of the vector, the square of the number of human bites per day per mosquito, and the tenth power of the probability of the mosquito's surviving for 1 day. Mosquito longevity is particularly important, because the portion of the parasite's life cycle that takes place within the mosquito—from gametocyte ingestion to subsequent inoculation (sporogony)—lasts for 8 to 30 days, depending on ambient temperature; thus, to transmit malaria, the mosquito must survive for >7 days. In general, at temperatures <16° to 18°C, sporogony is not completed and transmission does not occur. Therefore, the most effective mosquito vectors of malaria are those such as *A. gambiae*, which are long-lived, occur in high densities in tropical climates, breed readily, and bite humans in preference to other animals. The entomologic inoculation rate—the number of sporozoite-positive mosquito bites per person per year—is the most common measure of malarial transmission and varies from <1 in some parts of Latin America and Southeast Asia to >300 in parts of tropical Africa.

ERYTHROCYTE CHANGES IN MALARIA   After invading an erythrocyte, the growing malarial parasite progressively consumes and degrades intracellular proteins, principally hemoglobin. The potentially toxic heme

tionally has been defined in terms of parasitemia rates or palpable-spleen rates in children 2 to 9 years of age as hypoendemic (<10%), mesoendemic (11 to 50%), hyperendemic (51 to 75%), and holoendemic (>75%). In holo- and hyperendemic areas—e.g., certain regions of tropical Africa or coastal New Guinea, where there is intense *P. falciparum* transmission and people can sustain more than one infectious mosquito bite per day—people are infected repeatedly throughout their lives. Here, morbidity and mortality due to malaria are considerable during childhood. Immunity against disease is hard won in these areas, and the young-childhood burden of disease is high; by adulthood, however, most malarial infections are asymptomatic. This situation, with frequent year-round infection, is termed *stable transmission*. In areas where transmission is low, erratic, or focal, full

is polymerized to biologically inert hemozoin, or malaria pigment. The parasite also alters the RBC membrane by changing its transport properties, exposing cryptic surface antigens, and inserting new parasite-derived proteins. The RBC becomes more irregular in shape, more antigenic, and less deformable.

In *P. falciparum* infections, membrane protuberances appear on the erythrocyte's surface toward the end of the first 24 h of the asexual cycle. These "knobs" extrude a high-molecular-weight, antigenically variant, strain-specific, adhesive protein (PfEMP1) that mediates attachment to receptors on venular and capillary endothelium—an event termed *cytoadherence*. Several vascular receptors have been identified, of which intercellular adhesion molecule 1 is probably the most important in the brain, chondroitin sulfate B in the placenta, and CD36 in most other organs. Thus the infected erythrocytes stick inside the small blood vessels. At the same stage, these *P. falciparum*–infected RBCs may also adhere to uninfected RBCs to form rosettes and to other parasitized erythrocytes (agglutination). The processes of cytoadherence, rosetting, and agglutination are central to the pathogenesis of falciparum malaria. They result in the sequestration of RBCs containing mature forms of the parasite in vital organs (particularly the brain), where they interfere with microcirculatory flow and metabolism. Sequestered parasites continue to develop out of reach of the principal host defense mechanism: splenic processing and filtration. As a consequence, only the younger ring forms of the asexual parasites are seen circulating in the peripheral blood in falciparum malaria, and the level of peripheral parasitemia underestimates the true number of parasites within the body. Severe malaria is also associated with reduced deformability of the uninfected erythrocytes, which compromises their passage through the partially obstructed capillaries and venules and shortens RBC survival.

In the other three ("benign") malarias, sequestration does not occur, and all stages of the parasite's development are evident on peripheral blood smears. Whereas *P. vivax*, *P. ovale*, and *P. malariae* show a marked predilection for either young RBCs (*P. vivax*, *P. ovale*) or old cells (*P. malariae*) and produce a level of parasitemia seldom >2%, *P. falciparum* can invade erythrocytes of all ages and may be associated with very high levels of parasitemia.

HOST RESPONSE Initially, the host responds to plasmodial infection by activating nonspecific defense mechanisms. Splenic immunologic and filtrative clearance functions are augmented in malaria, and the removal of both parasitized and uninfected erythrocytes is accelerated. The parasitized cells escaping splenic removal are destroyed when the schizont ruptures. The material released induces the activation of macrophages and the release of proinflammatory mononuclear cell–derived cytokines, which cause fever and exert other pathologic effects. Temperatures of ≥40°C damage mature parasites; in untreated infections, the effect of such temperatures is to further synchronize the parasitic cycle, with eventual production of the regular fever spikes and rigors that originally served to characterize the different malarias. These regular fever patterns (tertian, every 2 days; quartan, every 3 days) are seldom seen today in patients who receive prompt and effective antimalarial treatment.

The geographic distributions of sickle cell disease, thalassemia, and glucose-6-phosphate dehydrogenase (G6PD) deficiency closely resemble that of malaria before the introduction of control measures. This observation suggests that these genetic disorders confer protection against death from falciparum malaria. For example, HbA/S heterozygotes (sickle cell trait) have a sixfold reduction in the risk of dying from severe falciparum malaria. This decrease in risk appears to be related to impaired parasite growth at low oxygen tensions. Parasite multiplication in HbA/E heterozygotes is reduced at high parasite densities. In Melanesia, children with α-thalassemia appear to have more frequent malaria (both vivax and falciparum) in the early years of life, and this pattern of infection appears to protect against severe disease. In Melanesian ovalocytosis, rigid erythrocytes resist merozoite invasion, and the intraerythrocytic milieu is hostile.

The specific immune response to malaria eventually controls the

infection and, with exposure to sufficient strains, confers protection from high-level parasitemia and disease but not from infection. As a result of this state of infection without illness (*premunition*), asymptomatic parasitemia is common among adults and older children living in regions with stable and intense transmission (i.e., holo- or hyperendemic areas). Immunity is mainly specific for both the species and the strain of infecting malarial parasite. Both humoral immunity and cellular immunity are necessary for protection, but the mechanisms of each are incompletely understood (Fig. 195-1). Immune individuals have a polyclonal increase in serum levels of IgM, IgG, and IgA, although much of this antibody is unrelated to protection. Antibodies to a variety of parasitic antigens presumably act in concert to limit in vivo replication of the parasite. In the case of falciparum malaria, the most important of these antigens is the variant protein PfEMP1 mentioned above. Passively transferred IgG from immune adults has been shown to reduce levels of parasitemia in children, and passive transfer of maternal antibody contributes to the relative protection of infants from severe malaria in the first months of life. This complex immunity to disease declines when a person lives outside an endemic area for several months or longer.

Several factors retard the development of cellular immunity to malaria. These factors include the absence of major histocompatibility antigens on the surface of infected RBCs, which precludes direct T cell recognition; malaria antigen–specific immune unresponsiveness; and the enormous strain diversity of malarial parasites along with the ability of the parasites to express variant immunodominant antigens on the erythrocyte surface that change during the period of infection. Strain diversity also has an impact on the heterogeneity of the humoral antibody response. Immunity to all strains is never achieved. Parasites may persist in the blood for months (or, in the case of *P. malariae*, for many years) if treatment is not given. The complexity of the immune response in malaria, the sophistication of the parasites' evasion mechanisms, and the lack of a good in vitro correlate with clinical immunity have all slowed progress toward an effective vaccine.

CLINICAL FEATURES Malaria is a very common cause of fever in tropical countries. The first symptoms of malaria are nonspecific; the lack of a sense of well-being, headache, fatigue, abdominal discomfort, and muscle aches followed by fever are all similar to the symptoms of a minor viral illness. In some instances, a prominence of headache, chest pain, abdominal pain, arthralgia, myalgia, or diarrhea may suggest another diagnosis. Although headache may be severe in malaria, there is no neck stiffness or photophobia resembling that in meningitis. While myalgia may be prominent, it is not usually as severe as in dengue fever, and the muscles are not tender as in leptospirosis or typhus. Nausea, vomiting, and orthostatic hypotension are common. The classic malarial paroxysms, in which fever spikes, chills, and rigors occur at regular intervals, are relatively unusual and suggest infection with *P. vivax* or *P. ovale*. The fever is irregular at first (that of falciparum malaria may never become regular); the temperature of nonimmune individuals and children often rises above 40°C in conjunction with tachycardia and sometimes delirium. Although childhood febrile convulsions may occur with any of the malarias, generalized seizures are specifically associated with falciparum malaria and may herald the development of cerebral disease. Many clinical abnormalities have been described in acute malaria, but most patients with uncomplicated infections have few abnormal physical findings other than fever, malaise, mild anemia, and (in some cases) a palpable spleen. Anemia is quite common among young children living in areas with stable transmission, particularly where there is parasite resistance to chloroquine or other drugs. Splenic enlargement is very common among otherwise-healthy individuals in malaria-endemic areas and reflects repeated infections; however, in nonimmune individuals with malaria, the spleen takes several days to become palpable. Slight enlargement of the liver is also common, particularly among young children. Mild jaundice is common among adults; it may develop in patients with otherwise-uncomplicated falciparum malaria and usually resolves over 1 to 3 weeks. Malaria is not associated with a rash like those seen in meningococcal septicemia, typhus, enteric fever, viral exanthems, and drug reactions. Petechial hemorrhages in the skin or mucous membranes—features of viral hemorrhagic fevers and leptospirosis—develop only rarely in severe falciparum malaria.

Severe Falciparum Malaria Appropriately treated, uncomplicated falciparum malaria carries a mortality rate of ~0.1%. However, once vital-organ dysfunction occurs or the proportion of erythrocytes infected increases to >3%, mortality rises steeply. The major manifestations of severe falciparum malaria are shown in Table 195-2, and features indicating a poor prognosis are listed in Table 195-3.

CEREBRAL MALARIA Coma is a characteristic and ominous feature of falciparum malaria and, despite treatment, is associated with death rates of ~20% among adults and 15% among children. Lesser degrees of obtundation, delirium, and abnormal behavior should also be taken very seriously. The onset may be gradual or sudden following a convulsion.

Cerebral malaria manifests as diffuse symmetric encephalopathy; focal neurologic signs are unusual. Although some passive resistance to head flexion may be detected, signs of meningeal irritation are lack-

TABLE 195-2 *Manifestations of Severe Falciparum Malaria*

Signs	Manifestations
Major	
Unarousable coma/ cerebral malaria	Failure to localize or respond appropriately to noxious stimuli; coma persisting for >30 min after generalized convulsion
Acidemia/acidosis	Arterial pH <7.25 or plasma bicarbonate level of <15 mmol/L; venous lactate level of >5 mmol/L manifests as labored deep breathing, often termed "respiratory distress"
Severe normochromic, normocytic anemia	Hematocrit of <15% or hemoglobin level of <50 g/L (<5 g/dL) with parasitemia of >100,000/μL
Renal failure	Urine output (24 h) of <400 mL in adults or <12 mL/kg in children; no improvement with rehydration; serum creatinine level of >265 μmol/L (>3.0 mg/dL)
Pulmonary edema/ adult respiratory distress syndrome	Noncardiogenic pulmonary edema, often aggravated by overhydration
Hypoglycemia	Plasma glucose level of <2.2 mmol/L (<40 mg/dL)
Hypotension/shock	Systolic blood pressure of <50 mmHg in children 1–5 years or <80 mmHg in adults; core/skin temperature difference of >10°C
Bleeding/ disseminated intravascular coagulation	Significant bleeding and hemorrhage from the gums, nose, and gastrointestinal tract and/or evidence of disseminated intravascular coagulation
Convulsions	More than two generalized seizures in 24 h
Hemoglobinuria[a]	Macroscopic black, brown, or red urine; not associated with effects of oxidant drugs and red blood cell enzyme defects (such as G6PD deficiency)
Other	
Impaired consciousness	Obtunded but arousable
Extreme weakness	Prostration; inability to sit unaided[b]
Hyperparasitemia	Parasitemia level of >5% in nonimmune patients (>20% in any patient)
Jaundice	Serum bilirubin level of >50 mmol/L (>3.0 mg/dL) if combined with other evidence of vital-organ dysfunction

[a] Hemoglobinuria may occur in uncomplicated malaria.
[b] In a child who is normally able to sit.
Note: G6PD, glucose-6-phosphate dehydrogenase.

TABLE 195-3 *Features Indicating a Poor Prognosis in Severe Falciparum Malaria*

Clinical
  Marked agitation
  Hyperventilation (respiratory distress)
  Hypothermia (<36.5°C)
  Bleeding
  Deep coma
  Repeated convulsions
  Anuria
  Shock
Laboratory
  Biochemistry
    Hypoglycemia (<2.2 mmol/L)
    Hyperlactatemia (>5 mmol/L)
    Acidosis (arterial pH <7.3, serum HCO₃ <15 mmol/L)
    Elevated serum creatinine (>265 μmol/L)
    Elevated total bilirubin (>50 μmol/L)
    Elevated liver enzymes (AST/ALT 3 times upper limit of normal, 5-nucleotidase ↑)
    Elevated muscle enzymes (CPK ↑, myoglobin ↑)
    Elevated urate (>600 μmol/L)
  Hematology
    Leukocytosis (>12,000/μL)
    Severe anemia (PCV <15%)
    Coagulopathy
      Decreased platelet count (<50,000/μL)
      Prolonged prothrombin time (>3 s)
      Prolonged partial thromboplastin time
      Decreased fibrinogen (<200 mg/dL)
  Parasitology
    Hyperparasitemia
      Increased mortality at >100,000/μL
      High mortality at >500,000/μL
      >20% of parasites identified as pigment-containing trophozoites and schizonts
      >5% of neutrophils with visible pigment

Note: ALT, alanine aminotransferase; AST, aspartate aminotransferase; CPK, creatine phosphokinase; PCV, packed cell volume.

ing. The eyes may be divergent and a pout reflex is common, but other primitive reflexes are usually absent. The corneal reflexes are preserved except in deep coma. Muscle tone may be either increased or decreased. The tendon reflexes are variable, and the plantar reflexes may be flexor or extensor; the abdominal and cremasteric reflexes are absent. Flexor or extensor posturing may be documented. Approximately 15% of patients have retinal hemorrhages; with pupillary dilatation and indirect ophthalmoscopy, this figure increases to 30 to 40%. Other funduscopic abnormalities include discrete spots of retinal opacification (30 to 60%), papilledema (8% among children, rare among adults), cotton wool spots (<5%), and decolorization of a retinal vessel or segment of vessel (occasional cases). Convulsions, usually generalized and often repeated, occur in up to 50% of children with cerebral malaria. More covert seizure activity is also common, particularly among children, and may manifest as repetitive tonic-clonic eye movements. Whereas adults rarely (i.e., in <3% of cases) suffer neurologic sequelae, ~15% of children surviving cerebral malaria—especially those with hypoglycemia, severe anemia, repeated seizures, and deep coma—have some residual neurologic deficit when they regain consciousness; hemiplegia, cerebral palsy, cortical blindness, deafness, and impaired cognition and learning—all of varying duration—have been reported.

HYPOGLYCEMIA An important and common complication of severe malaria, hypoglycemia is associated with a poor prognosis and is particularly problematic in children and pregnant women. Hypoglycemia in malaria results from a failure of hepatic gluconeogenesis and an increase in the consumption of glucose by both host and—to a lesser extent—the malaria parasites. To compound the situation, quinine and quinidine—drugs commonly used for the treatment of severe chloroquine-resistant malaria—are powerful stimulants of pancreatic insulin secretion. Hyperinsulinemic hypoglycemia is especially troublesome in pregnant women receiving quinine treatment. In severe disease, the clinical diagnosis of hypoglycemia is difficult: the usual physical signs (sweating, gooseflesh, tachycardia) are absent, and the neurologic impairment caused by hypoglycemia cannot be distinguished from that caused by malaria.

LACTIC ACIDOSIS Lactic acidosis commonly coexists with hypoglycemia and is an important contributor to death from severe malaria. In adults, coexisting renal impairment often compounds the acidosis; in children, ketoacidosis may also contribute. Acidotic breathing, sometimes called respiratory distress, is a sign of poor prognosis. It is often followed by circulatory failure refractory to volume expansion or inotropic drugs or by respiratory arrest. The plasma concentrations of bicarbonate or lactate are the best biochemical prognosticators in severe malaria. Lactic acidosis is caused by the combination of anaerobic glycolysis in tissues where sequestered parasites interfere with microcirculatory flow, hypovolemia, lactate production by the parasites, and a failure of hepatic and renal lactate clearance. The prognosis of severe lactic acidosis is poor.

NONCARDIOGENIC PULMONARY EDEMA Adults with severe falciparum malaria may develop noncardiogenic pulmonary edema even after several days of antimalarial therapy. The pathogenesis of this variant of the adult respiratory distress syndrome is unclear. The mortality rate is >80%. This condition can be aggravated by overly vigorous administration of intravenous fluid. Noncardiogenic pulmonary edema can also develop in otherwise-uncomplicated vivax malaria, where recovery is usual.

RENAL IMPAIRMENT Renal impairment is common among adults with severe falciparum malaria but rare among children. The pathogenesis of renal failure is unclear but may be related to erythrocyte sequestration interfering with renal microcirculatory flow and metabolism. Clinically and pathologically, this syndrome manifests as acute tubular necrosis, although renal cortical necrosis never develops. Acute renal failure may occur simultaneously with other vital-organ dysfunction (in which case mortality is high) or may progress as other disease manifestations resolve. In survivors, urine flow resumes in a median of 4 days, and serum creatinine levels return to normal in a mean of 17 days (Chap. 260). Early dialysis or hemofiltration considerably enhances the likelihood of a patient's survival, particularly in acute hypercatabolic renal failure.

HEMATOLOGIC ABNORMALITIES Anemia results from accelerated RBC destruction and removal by the spleen in conjunction with ineffective erythropoiesis. In severe malaria, both infected and uninfected RBCs show reduced deformability, which correlates with prognosis and development of anemia. Splenic clearance of RBCs is increased. In nonimmune individuals and in areas with unstable transmission, anemia can develop rapidly and transfusion is often required. As a consequence of repeated malarial infections, children in many areas of Africa may develop severe anemia resulting from both shortened RBC survival and masked dyserythropoiesis. Anemia is a common consequence of antimalarial drug resistance, which results in repeated or continued infection.

Slight coagulation abnormalities are common in falciparum malaria, and mild thrombocytopenia is usual. As mentioned above, <5% of patients with severe malaria have significant bleeding with evidence of disseminated intravascular coagulation. Hematemesis from stress ulceration or acute gastric erosions may also occur.

LIVER DYSFUNCTION Mild hemolytic jaundice is common in malaria. Severe jaundice is associated with *P. falciparum* infections, is more common among adults than among children, and results from hemolysis, hepatocyte injury, and cholestasis. When accompanied by other vital-organ dysfunction (often renal impairment), liver dysfunction carries a poor prognosis. Hepatic dysfunction contributes to hypoglycemia, lactic acidosis, and impaired drug metabolism. Occasional patients with falciparum malaria may develop deep jaundice (with hemolytic, hepatitic, and cholestatic components) without evidence of other vital-organ dysfunction.

TABLE 195-4 *Relative Incidence of Severe Complications of Falciparum Malaria*

Complication	Nonpregnant Adults	Pregnant Women	Children
Anemia	+	++	+++
Convulsions	+	+	+++
Hypoglycemia	+	+++	+++
Jaundice	+++	+++	+
Renal failure	+++	+++	−
Pulmonary edema	++	+++	+

Key: −, rare; +, infrequent; ++, frequent; +++, very frequent.

OTHER COMPLICATIONS Aspiration pneumonia following convulsions is an important cause of death in cerebral malaria. Chest infections and catheter-induced urinary tract infections are common among patients who are unconscious for >3 days. Septicemia may complicate severe malaria, particularly in children; in endemic areas, *Salmonella* bacteremia has been associated specifically with *P. falciparum* infections. The frequency of complications of severe falciparum malaria is summarized in Table 195-4.

Malaria in Pregnancy In hyper- and holoendemic areas, falciparum malaria in primi- and secundigravid women is associated with low birth weight (average reduction, ~170 g) and consequently increased infant and childhood mortality. In general, infected mothers in areas of stable transmission remain asymptomatic despite intense accumulation of parasitized erythrocytes in the placental microcirculation. Maternal HIV infection predisposes pregnant women to malaria and predisposes their newborns to congenital malaria infection and low birth weight.

In areas with unstable transmission of malaria, pregnant women are prone to severe infections and are particularly vulnerable to high-level parasitemia with anemia, hypoglycemia, and acute pulmonary edema. Fetal distress, premature labor, and stillbirth or low birth weight are common results. Fetal death is usual in severe malaria. Congenital malaria occurs in <5% of newborns whose mothers are infected and is related directly to the parasite density in maternal blood and in the placenta. *P. vivax* malaria in pregnancy is also associated with a reduction in birth weight (average, 100 g), but, in contrast to the situation in falciparum malaria, this effect is more pronounced in multigravid than in primigravid women.

Malaria in Children Most of the estimated 1 to 3 million persons who die of falciparum malaria each year are young African children. Convulsions, coma, hypoglycemia, metabolic acidosis, and severe anemia are relatively common among children with severe malaria, whereas deep jaundice, acute renal failure, and acute pulmonary edema are unusual. Severely anemic children may present with labored deep breathing, which in the past has been attributed incorrectly to "anemic congestive cardiac failure" but in fact is usually caused by metabolic acidosis, often compounded by hypovolemia. In general, children tolerate antimalarial drugs well and respond rapidly to treatment.

Transfusion Malaria Malaria can be transmitted by blood transfusion, needle-stick injury, sharing of needles by infected drug addicts, or organ transplantation. The incubation period in these settings is often short because there is no preerythrocytic stage of development. The clinical features and management of these cases are the same as for naturally acquired infections. Radical chemotherapy with primaquine is unnecessary for transfusion-transmitted *P. vivax* and *P. ovale* infections.

CHRONIC COMPLICATIONS OF MALARIA ■ **Tropical Splenomegaly (Hyperreactive Malarial Splenomegaly)** Chronic or repeated malarial infections produce hypergammaglobulinemia; normochromic, normocytic anemia; and, in certain situations, splenomegaly. Some residents of malaria-endemic areas in tropical Africa and Asia exhibit an abnormal immunologic response to repeated infections that is characterized by massive splenomegaly, hepatomegaly, marked elevations in serum titers of IgM and malarial antibody, hepatic sinusoidal lymphocytosis, and (in Af-

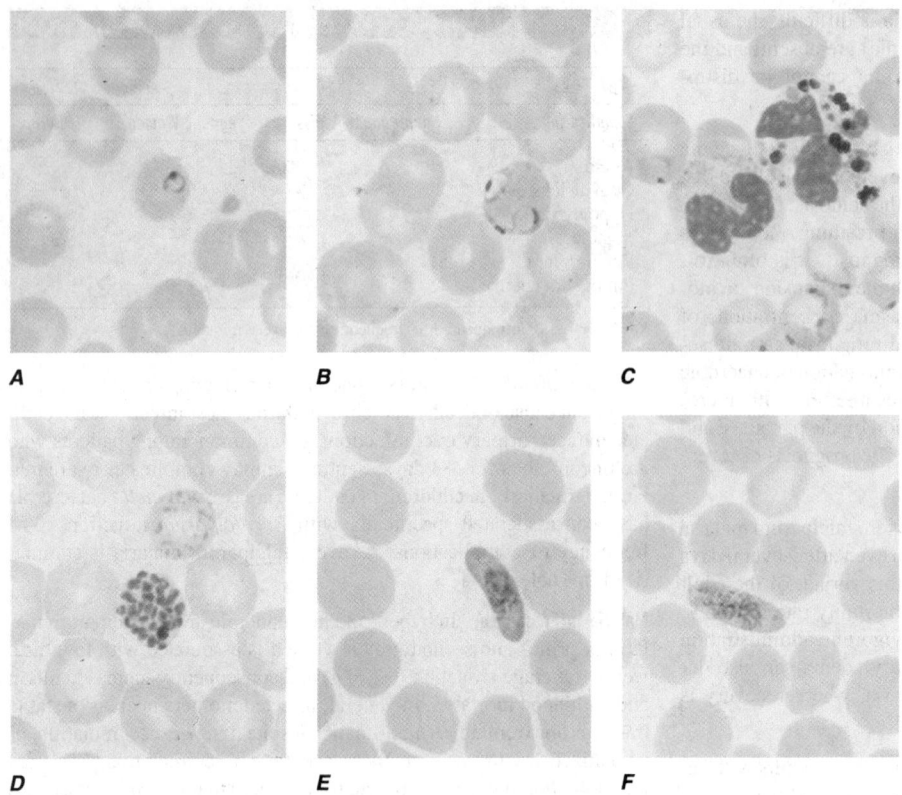

rica) peripheral B cell lymphocytosis. This syndrome has been associated with the production of cytotoxic IgM antibodies to CD8+ T lymphocytes, antibodies to CD5+ T lymphocytes, and an increase in the ratio of CD4+ T cells to CD8+ T cells. These events may lead to uninhibited B cell production of IgM and the formation of cryoglob-

ulins (IgM aggregates and immune complexes). This immunologic process stimulates reticuloendothelial hyperplasia and clearance activity and eventually produces splenomegaly. Patients with hyperreactive malarial splenomegaly (HMS) present with an abdominal mass or a dragging sensation in the abdomen and occasional sharp abdominal pains suggesting perisplenitis. Anemia and some degree of pancytopenia are usually evident, but in many cases malarial parasites cannot be found in peripheral-blood smears. Vulnerability to respiratory and skin infections is increased; many patients die of overwhelming sepsis. Persons with HMS who are living in endemic areas should receive antimalarial chemoprophylaxis: the results are usually good. In nonendemic areas, antimalarial treatment is advised. In some cases refractory to therapy, clonal lymphoproliferation may develop and then evolve into a malignant lymphoproliferative disorder.

Quartan Malarial Nephropathy Chronic or repeated infections with *P. malariae* (and possibly with other malarial species) may cause soluble immune-complex injury to the renal glomeruli, resulting in the nephrotic syndrome. Other, unidentified factors must contribute to this process since only a very small proportion of infected patients develop renal disease. The histologic appearance is that of focal or segmental glomerulonephritis with splitting of the capillary basement membrane. Subendothelial dense deposits are seen on electron microscopy, and immunofluorescence reveals deposits of complement and immunoglobulins; in samples of renal tissue from children, *P. malariae* antigens are often visible. A coarse-granular pattern of basement-membrane immunofluorescent deposits (predominantly IgG3) with selective proteinuria carries a better prognosis than a fine-granular, predominantly IgG2 pattern with nonselective proteinuria. Quartan nephropathy usually responds poorly to treatment with either antimalarial agents or glucocorticoids and cytotoxic drugs.

Burkitt's Lymphoma and Epstein-Barr Virus Infection It is possible that malaria-related immunosuppression provokes infection with lymphoma viruses. Burkitt's lymphoma is strongly associated with Epstein-Barr virus. The prevalence of this childhood tumor is high in malarious areas of Africa.

DIAGNOSIS ■ Demonstration of the Parasite
The diagnosis of malaria rests on the demonstration of asexual forms of the parasite in stained peripheral-blood smears. After a negative blood smear, repeat smears should be made if there is a high degree of suspicion. Of the Romanowsky stains, Giemsa at pH 7.2 is preferred; Wright's, Field's, or Leishman's stain can also be used. Both thin (Fig. 195-3 through Fig. 195-6) and thick (Fig. 195-7 through Fig. 195-10) blood smears should be examined.

The thin blood smear should be rapidly

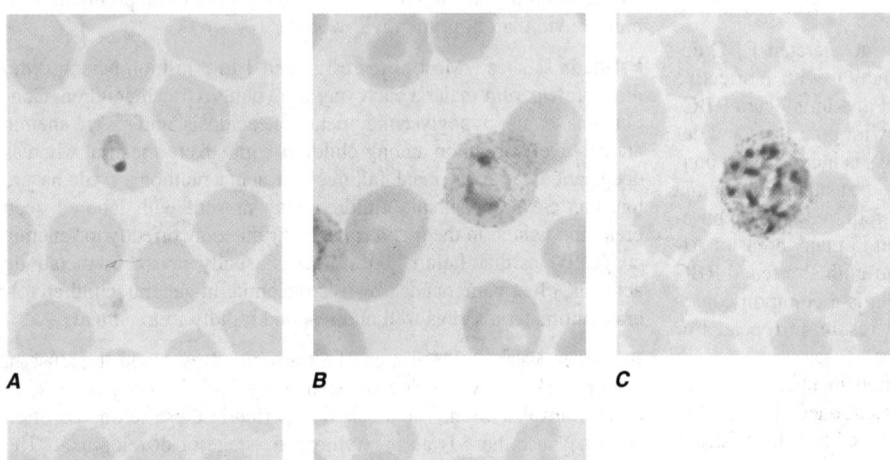

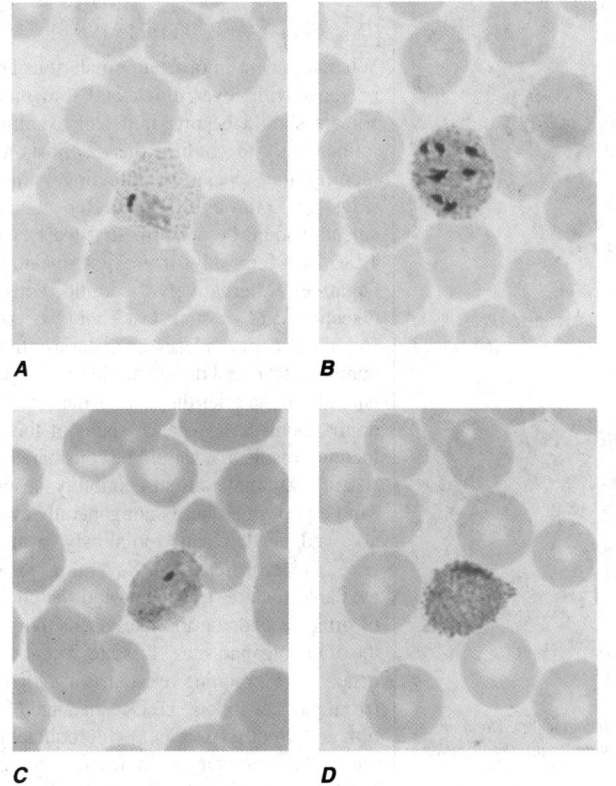

FIGURE 195-5 Thin blood films of *Plasmodium ovale*. *A.* Old trophozoites. *B.* Mature schizonts. *C.* Male gametocytes. *D.* Female gametocytes. (*Reproduced from Benchaids for the Diagnosis of Malaria Infections, 2d ed, with the permission of the World Health Organization.*)

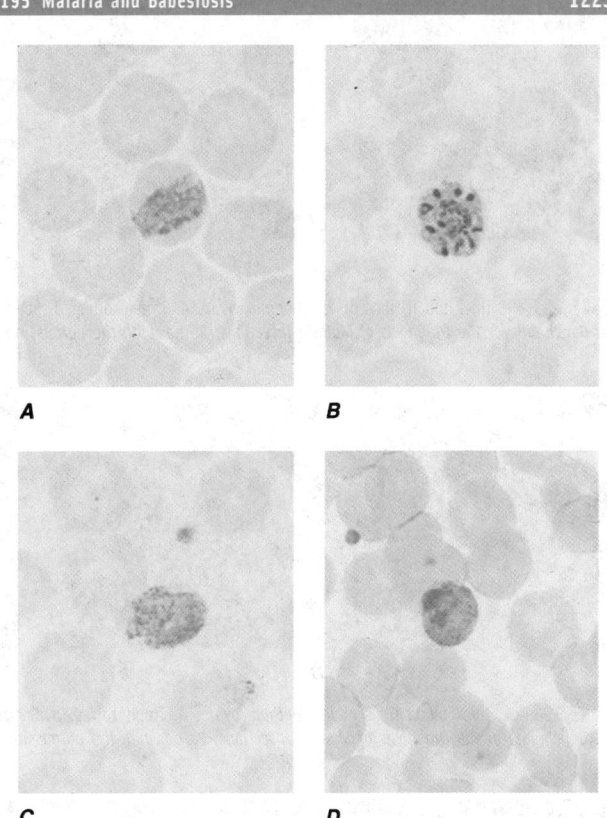

FIGURE 195-6 Thin blood films of *Plasmodium malariae*. *A.* Old trophozoites. *B.* Mature schizonts. *C.* Male gametocytes. *D.* Female gametocytes. (*Reproduced from Benchaids for the Diagnosis of Malaria Infections, 2d ed, with the permission of the World Health Organization.*)

air-dried, fixed in anhydrous methanol, and stained, and the RBCs in the tail of the film should then be examined under oil immersion (×1000 magnification). The level of parasitemia is expressed as the number of parasitized erythrocytes per 1000 RBCs, or per 200 white blood cells (WBCs), and this figure is converted to the number of parasitized erythrocytes per microliter. In high-transmission areas, the presence of up to 10,000 parasites per microliter of blood may be tolerated without symptoms or signs in partially immune individuals. Rapid, simple, sensitive, and specific antibody-based diagnostic stick or card tests that detect *P. falciparum*–specific, histidine-rich protein 2 (PfHRP2) or lactate dehydrogenase antigens in finger-prick blood samples have been introduced (Table 195-5). Some of these tests carry a second antibody, which allows falciparum malaria to be distinguished from the less dangerous malarias. PfHRP2-based tests may remain positive for several weeks after acute infection. This feature is a disadvantage in high-transmission areas where infections are frequent but is of value in the diagnosis of severe malaria in patients who have taken antimalarial drugs and cleared peripheral parasitemia (but in whom the PfHRP2 test remains strongly positive) or where malaria is alleged to have been eliminated. The relationship between parasitemia and prognosis is complex; in general, patients with >10⁵ parasites per microliter are at increased risk of dying, but nonimmune patients may die with much lower counts, and semi-immune persons may tolerate parasitemia levels many times higher with only minor symptoms. In severe malaria, a poor prognosis is indicated by a predominance of more mature *P. falciparum* parasites (i.e., >20% of parasites with visible pigment) in the peripheral blood film or by the presence of phagocytosed malarial pigment in >5% of neutrophils. In *P. falciparum* infections, gametocytemia peaks 1 week after the peak of asexual parasites. Because the mature gametocytes of *P. falciparum* are not affected by most antimalarial drugs, their persistence does not constitute evidence of drug resistance.

The thick blood film should be of uneven thickness. The smear should be dried thoroughly and stained without fixing. As many layers of erythrocytes overlie one another and are lysed during the staining procedure, the thick film has the advantage of concentrating the parasites (by 20- to 40-fold compared with a thin blood film) and thus increasing diagnostic sensitivity. Both parasites and WBCs are counted, and the number of parasites per unit volume is calculated from the total leukocyte count. Alternatively, a WBC count of 8000/μL is assumed. A minimum of 200 WBCs should be counted under oil immersion. Interpretation of blood smear films requires some experience because artifacts are common. Before a thick smear is judged to be negative, 100 to 200 fields should be examined under oil immersion. Phagocytosed malarial pigment is sometimes seen inside peripheral-blood monocytes or polymorphonuclear leukocytes and may provide a clue to recent infection if malaria parasites are not detectable. After the clearance of the parasites, this intraphagocytic malarial pigment is often evident for several days in the peripheral blood or for longer in bone marrow aspirates or smears of fluid expressed after

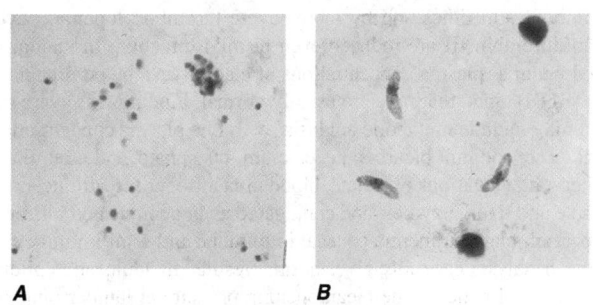

FIGURE 195-7 Thick blood films of *Plasmodium falciparum*. *A.* Trophozoites. *B.* Gametocytes. (*Reproduced from Benchaids for the Diagnosis of Malaria Infections, 2d ed, with the permission of the World Health Organization.*)

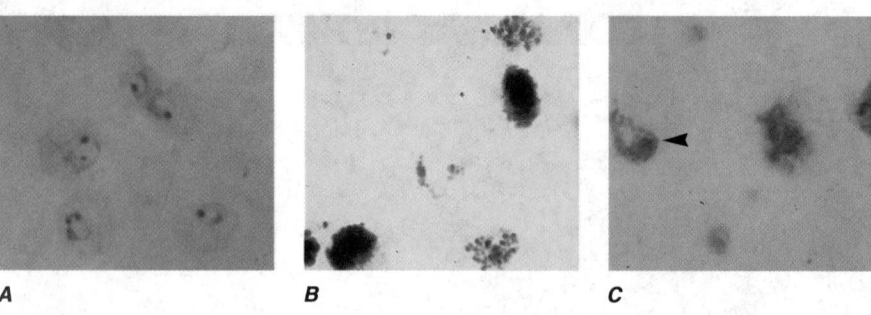

FIGURE 195-8 Thick blood films of *Plasmodium vivax*. A. Trophozoites. B. Schizonts. C. Gametocytes. (*Reproduced from Benchaids for the Diagnosis of Malaria Infections, 2d ed, with the permission of the World Health Organization.*)

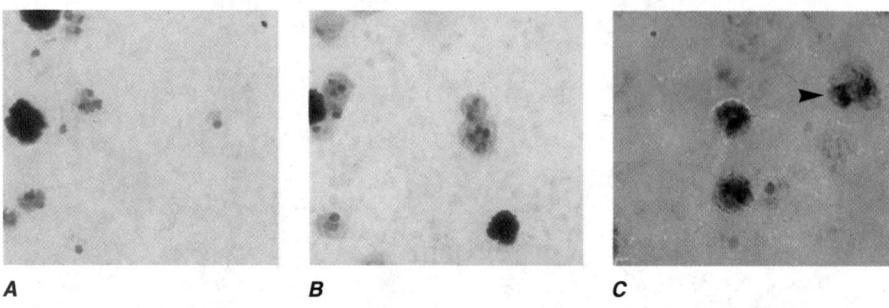

FIGURE 195-9 Thick blood films of *Plasmodium ovale*. A. Trophozoites. B. Schizonts. C. Gametocytes. (*Reproduced from Benchaids for the Diagnosis of Malaria Infections, 2d ed, with the permission of the World Health Organization.*)

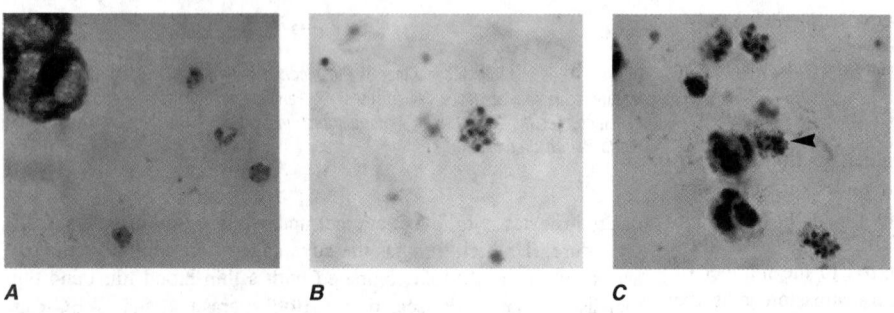

FIGURE 195-10 Thick blood films of *Plasmodium malariae*. A. Trophozoites. B. Schizonts. C. Gametocytes. (*Reproduced from Benchaids for the Diagnosis of Malaria Infections, 2d ed, with the permission of the World Health Organization.*)

intradermal puncture. Staining of parasites with the fluorescent dye acridine orange allows more rapid diagnosis of malaria (but not speciation of the infection) in patients with low-level parasitemia.

Laboratory Findings Normochromic, normocytic anemia is usual. The leukocyte count is generally normal, although it may be raised in very severe infections. The erythrocyte sedimentation rate, plasma viscosity, and levels of C-reactive protein and other acute-phase proteins are high. The platelet count is usually reduced to $\sim 10^5/\mu L$. Severe infections may be accompanied by prolonged prothrombin and partial thromboplastin times and by more severe thrombocytopenia. Levels of antithrombin III are reduced even in mild infection. In uncomplicated malaria, plasma concentrations of electrolytes, blood urea nitrogen (BUN), and creatinine are usually normal. Findings in severe malaria may include metabolic acidosis, with low plasma concentrations of glucose, sodium, bicarbonate, calcium, phosphate, and albumin together with elevations in lactate, blood urea nitrogen, creatinine, urate, muscle and liver enzymes, and conjugated and unconjugated bilirubin. Hypergammaglobulinemia is usual in immune and semi-immune subjects. Urinalysis generally gives normal results. In adults and children with cerebral malaria, the mean opening pressure at lumbar puncture is ~ 160 mm of cerebrospinal fluid (CSF); usually the CSF is normal or has a slightly elevated total protein level [<1.0 g/L (<100 mg/dL)] and cell count (<20/μL).

1226

Rx TREATMENT (Table 195-6)

When a patient in or from a malarious area presents with fever, thick and thin blood smears should be prepared and examined immediately to confirm the diagnosis and identify the species of infecting parasite (Figs. 195-3 through 195-10). Repeat blood smears should be performed at least every 12 to 24 h for 2 days if the first smears are negative. Alternatively, a rapid antigen detection card or stick test should be performed. Patients with severe malaria or those unable to take oral drugs should receive parenteral antimalarial therapy. If there is any doubt about the resistance status of the infecting organism, it should be considered resistant. Antimalarial susceptibility testing can be performed but is not generally available and yields results too slowly to influence choice of treatment. Several drugs are available for oral treatment, and the choice of drug depends on the likely sensitivity of the infecting parasites. Despite recent evidence of chloroquine resistance in *P. vivax* (from parts of Indonesia, Oceania, and Central and South America), chloroquine remains the treatment of choice for the "benign" human malarias (*P. vivax, P. ovale, P. malariae*). Characteristics of various antimalarial agents are shown in Table 195-7, and drug regimens approved by the U.S. Food and Drug Administration are detailed in Table 195-6. The availability of antimalarial drugs varies considerably between countries. Many of the drugs used to treat malaria in endemic areas are not available in temperate countries such as the United States. Fake or adulterated drugs, including antimalarial agents, are being sold in many low-income countries; thus careful attention is required at purchase, especially when the patient fails to respond as expected.

Severe Malaria Because of resistance, chloroquine can no longer be relied upon in most countries for the treatment of severe malaria. The antiarrhythmic quinidine gluconate is as effective as quinine and, as it is more readily available, has replaced quinine for the treatment of malaria in the United States. The administration of quinidine must be closely monitored if dysrrhythmias and hypotension are to be avoided. Total plasma levels >8 $\mu g/mL$, a QT$_c$ interval >0.6 s, or QRS widening beyond 25% of baseline are indications for slowing infusion rates. If arrhythmia or saline-unresponsive hypotension develops, treatment with this drug should be discontinued. Quinine is safer than quinidine; cardiovascular monitoring is not required except when the recipient has cardiac disease. Quinine is the most widely used drug for the treatment of severe malaria worldwide. In some areas, the Chinese drugs derived from artemisinin (artemether and artesunate) have become first-line treatments for severe malaria. These agents are rapidly effective against multidrug-resistant falciparum malaria and are at least as effective as and considerably safer than quinine or quinidine. Artesunate, a water-soluble derivative, can be given by intravenous or intramuscular injection or in a rectal formulation for use primarily in the rural tropics. Artemether and the closely related drug arteether are oil-based formulations given by intramuscular injection. They are not yet available in the United States.

Severe falciparum malaria constitutes a medical emergency re-

TABLE 195-5 *Methods for the Diagnosis of Malaria*ᵃ

Method	Procedure	Advantages	Disadvantages
Thick blood film[b]	Blood should be uneven in thickness but sufficiently thin to read watch hands through part of the spot. Stain dried, unfixed blood spot with Giemsa, Field's, or other Romanowsky stain. Count number of asexual parasites per 200 WBCs (or per 500 at low densities). Count gametocytes separately.[c]	Sensitive (0.001% parasitemia); species specific; inexpensive	Requires experience (artifacts may be misinterpreted as low-level parasitemia); underestimates true count
Thin blood film[d]	Stain fixed smear with Giemsa, Field's, or other Romanowsky stain. Count number of RBCs containing asexual parasites per 1000 RBCs. In severe malaria, assess stage of parasite development and count neutrophils containing malaria pigment.[e] Count gametocytes separately.[c]	Rapid; species specific; inexpensive; in severe malaria, provides prognostic information[e]	Insensitive (>0.05% parasitemia); uneven distribution of *P. vivax*, as enlarged infected red cells concentrate at leading edge
PfHRP2 dipstick or card test	A drop of blood is placed on the stick or card, which is then immersed in washing solutions. Monoclonal antibody captures the parasite antigen and reads out as a colored band.	Rapid; sensitivity similar to or slightly lower than that of thick films (~0.001% parasitemia)	Detects only *Plasmodium falciparum*; remains positive for weeks after infection[f]; does not quantitate *P. falciparum* parasitemia
Plasmodium LDH dipstick or card test	A drop of blood is placed on the stick or card, which is then immersed in washing solutions. Monoclonal antibodies capture the parasites and read out as colored bands. One band is genus specific (all malarias), and the other is specific for *P. falciparum*.	Rapid; sensitivity similar to or slightly lower than that of thick films for *P. falciparum* (~0.001% parasitemia); provides less sensitive diagnosis for other malarias (*P. vivax*, *P. ovale*, *P. malariae*) and does not speciate these organisms	Slightly more difficult preparation than PfHRP2 tests; may miss low-level parasitemia with *P. vivax*, *P. ovale*, and *P. malariae*; does not quantitate *P. falciparum* parasitemia
Microtube concentration methods with acridine orange staining	Blood is collected in a specialized tube containing acridine orange, anticoagulant, and a float. After centrifugation, which concentrates the parasitized cells around the float, fluorescence microscopy is performed.	Sensitivity similar or superior to that of thick films (~0.001% parasitemia); ideal for processing large numbers of samples rapidly	Does not speciate or quantitate; requires fluorescence microscopy

ᵃ Malaria cannot be diagnosed clinically with accuracy, but treatment should be started on clinical grounds if the laboratory confirmation is likely to be delayed. In areas of the world where malaria is endemic and transmission is high, low-level asymptomatic parasitemia is common in otherwise-healthy people. Thus malaria may not be the cause of a fever, although in this context the presence of >10,000 parasites/μL (~0.2%) *does* indicate that malaria is the cause. Antibody and polymerase chain reaction tests have no role in the diagnosis of malaria.

[b] Asexual parasites/200 WBCs × 40 = parasite count/μL (assumes a WBC count of 8000/μL). See Figs. 195-7 through 195-10.

[c] Gametocytemia may persist for days or weeks after clearance of asexual parasites. Gametocytemia without asexual parasitemia does not indicate active infection.

[d] Parasitized RBCs (%) × hematocrit × 1256 = parasite count/μL. See Figs. 195-3 through 195-6.

[e] The presence of >100,000 parasites/μL (~2%) is associated with an increased risk of severe malaria, but some patients have severe malaria with lower counts. At any level of parasitemia, the finding that >50% of parasites are tiny rings (cytoplasm width less than half of nucleus width) carries a relatively good prognosis. The presence of visible pigment in >20% of parasites or in >5% of polymorphonuclear leukocytes (indicating massive recent schizogony) carries a worse prognosis.

[f] Persistence of PfHRP2 is a disadvantage in high-transmission settings, where many asymptomatic people have positive tests, but can be used to diagnostic advantage in low-transmission settings when a sick patient has received previous unknown treatment (which, in endemic areas, often consists of antimalarial drugs). A positive PfHRP2 test indicates that the illness is falciparum malaria, even if the blood smear is negative.

Note: LDH, lactate dehydrogenase; PfHRP2, *P. falciparum* histidine-rich protein 2; RBCs, red blood cells; WBCs, white blood cells.

quiring intensive nursing care and careful management. The patient should be weighed and, if comatose, placed on his or her side or prone. Frequent evaluation of the patient's condition is essential. Ancillary drugs such as high-dose glucocorticoids, urea, heparin, dextran, desferrioxamine, antibody to tumor necrosis factor α, and high-dose phenobarbital (20 mg/kg) have proved either ineffective or harmful in clinical trials and should not be used. In acute renal failure or severe metabolic acidosis, hemofiltration or hemodialysis should be started as early as possible.

Parenteral antimalarial treatment should be started as soon as possible. An initial loading dose must be given so that therapeutic concentrations are reached as soon as possible. Both quinine and quinidine will cause dangerous hypotension if injected rapidly; when given intravenously, they must be administered carefully by rate-controlled infusion only. The optimal therapeutic range for quinine and quinidine in severe malaria is not known with certainty, but total plasma concentrations of 8 to 15 mg/mL for quinine and 3.5 to 8.0 mg/mL for quinidine are effective and do not cause serious toxicity. The systemic clearance and apparent volume of distribution of these alkaloids are markedly reduced and plasma protein binding is increased in severe malaria, so that the blood concentrations attained with a given dose are higher. If the patient remains seriously ill or in acute renal failure for >2 days, the maintenance doses of quinine or quinidine should be reduced by 30 to 50% to prevent toxic accumulation of the drugs. The initial doses should never be reduced. If one of the artemisinin derivatives or chloroquine is given, dose reductions are unnecessary, even in renal failure. Exchange transfusion should be considered for severely ill patients, although the precise indications for this procedure have not been agreed upon. It has been recommended that—if safe and feasible—exchange should be considered for patients with severe malaria and parasitemia levels of 5 to 15% and is indicated for parasitemia levels of >15%. The role of prophylactic anticonvulsants is uncertain. If respiratory support is not available, then a full loading dose of phenobarbital (20 mg/kg) to prevent convulsions should not be given as it may cause respiratory arrest.

When the patient is unconscious, the blood glucose level should be measured every 4 to 6 h, and values <2.2 mmol/L (40 mg/dL) should mandate treatment with intravenous dextrose. All patients treated with intravenous quinine or quinidine should receive a continuous infusion of 5 to 10% dextrose. The parasite count and hematocrit level should be measured every 6 to 12 h. Anemia develops rapidly; if the hematocrit falls to <20%, then whole blood (preferably fresh) or packed cells should be transfused slowly, with careful attention to circulatory status. Renal function should be checked daily. Children presenting with severe anemia and acidotic breathing are often hypovolemic; in this situation, resuscitation with crystalloids or blood is

TABLE 195-6 *Recommended Therapeutic Doses of Antimalarial Drugs*

Drug	Uncomplicated Malaria (Oral)	Severe Malaria[a] (Parenteral)
Chloroquine[b]	10 mg of base/kg followed by 10 mg/kg at 24 h and 5 mg/kg at 48 h *or* by 5 mg/kg at 12, 24, and 36 h (total dose, 25 mg/kg); for *P. vivax* or *P. ovale*, primaquine (0.25 mg of base/kg per day for 14 days[d]) added for radical cure	10 mg of base/kg by constant-rate infusion over 8 h followed by 15 mg/kg over 24 h *or* by 3.5 mg of base/kg by IM or SC injection every 6 h (total dose, 25 mg/kg)[c]
Amodiaquine[b]	15 mg of base/kg followed by 10 mg per day at 24 and 48 h (total dose, 35 mg/kg)	—
Sulfadoxine/ pyrimethamine[b]	25/1.25 mg/kg, single oral dose (3 tablets for adults)	—
Mefloquine[b]	15 mg/kg followed 8–12 h later by second dose of 10 mg/kg	—
Quinine	10 mg of salt/kg q8h for 7 days combined with tetracycline[e] (4 mg/kg qid) or doxycycline (3 mg/kg once daily) or clindamycin (10 mg/kg bid) for 7 days	20 mg of salt/kg by IV infusion over 4 h[f] followed by 10 mg/kg infused over 2–8 h every 8 h
Quinidine gluconate	—	10 mg of base/kg by constant-rate infusion over 1–2 h followed by 0.02 mg/kg per min, with ECG monitoring[g]
Artesunate	In combination with 25 mg of mefloquine/kg, 12 mg/kg given in divided doses over 3–5 days (e.g., 4 mg/kg for 3 days or 4 mg/kg followed by 2 mg/kg per day for 4 days); if used alone or in combination with clindamycin or doxycycline, give for 7 days (usually 4 mg/kg initially followed by 2 mg/kg daily)	2.4 mg/kg IV or IM stat followed by 1.2 mg/kg at 12 and 24 h and then daily (or 2.4 mg/kg once daily)
Artemether	Same regimen as for artesunate	3.2 mg/kg IM stat followed by 1.6 mg/kg per day
Atovaquone- proguanil (Malarone)	For adults >40 kg, each dose comprises 4 tablets (each tablet containing atovaquone 250 mg and proguanil 100 mg) taken once daily for 3 days with food	—
Artemether- lumefantrine	For adults ≥35 kg, each dose comprises 4 tablets (each tablet containing artemether 20 mg and lumefantrine 120 mg) at 0, 8, 24, 36, 48, and 60 h, taken after food	—

[a] Oral treatment should be substituted for parenteral therapy as soon as the patient can take tablets by mouth.

[b] These drugs should be combined with either artesunate or artemether when used to treat falciparum malaria. Where there is full susceptibility to both drugs, chloroquine or amodiaquine can be combined with sulfadoxine/pyrimethamine.

[c] Chloroquine-resistant *P. falciparum* is now very widespread, so this regimen should not be used unless there is confirmed full susceptibility in the area.

[d] In Oceania and Southeast Asia, the dose should be 0.33 to 0.5 mg of base/kg. This regimen should not be used in patients with severe variants of G6PD deficiency.

[e] Neither tetracycline nor doxycycline should be given to pregnant women or to children <8 years old.

[f] Alternatively, infusion of 7 mg of salt/kg over 30 min can be followed by 10 mg of salt/kg over 4 h.

[g] Some authorities recommend a lower dose of intravenous quinidine: 6.2 mg of base/kg over 1–2 h followed by 0.0125 mg/kg per min.

Note: In severe malaria, quinine or quinidine should be used if there is any doubt about the infecting strain's sensitivity to chloroquine.

Abbreviations: IM, intramuscular; SC, subcutaneous; IV, intravenous; ECG, electrocardiogram; G6PD, glucose-6-phosphate dehydrogenase.

indicated. Accurate assessment is vital. Management of fluid balance is difficult in severe malaria, particularly in adults, because of the thin dividing line between overhydration (leading to pulmonary edema) and underhydration (contributing to renal impairment). If necessary, pulmonary artery occlusion pressures should be measured and maintained in the low-normal range. As soon as the patient can take fluids, oral therapy should be substituted for parenteral treatment.

Uncomplicated Malaria Infections due to *P. vivax*, *P. malariae*, *P. ovale*, and known sensitive strains of *P. falciparum* should be treated with oral chloroquine (total dose, 25 mg of base/kg). Chloroquine-resistant *P. falciparum* is now widespread. Chloroquine-resistant strains may be sensitive to sulfadoxine/pyrimethamine in some areas. Where there is resistance to the latter combination, either (1) quinine plus tetracycline or doxycycline (or clindamycin) or (2) mefloquine should be used; tetracycline and doxycycline cannot be given to pregnant women

or to children <8 years of age. Oral quinine is extremely bitter and regularly produces cinchonism comprising tinnitus, high-tone deafness, nausea, vomiting, and dysphoria. Compliance is poor with the required 5- to 7-day regimens of this drug. Mefloquine should be given at a total dosage of 25 mg/kg (15 mg/kg followed 8 to 12 h later by 10 mg/kg) and, where available and approved for use, combined with artesunate or artemether (4 mg/kg per day for 3 days). Although significant resistance to mefloquine has been documented in Thailand, Myanmar, Vietnam, and Cambodia (Fig. 195-11), mefloquine is usually effective against multidrug-resistant strains of *P. falciparum* outside these areas. Artemether-lumefantrine and atovaquone-proguanil (Malarone) are recently introduced, well-tolerated antimalarial drugs used in 3-day regimens. They are both highly effective against multidrug-resistant falciparum malaria.

Patients should be monitored for vomiting for 1 h after the administration of any oral antimalarial drug. If there is vomiting, the dose should be repeated. Symptom-based treatment, with tepid sponging and acetaminophen administration, lowers fever and thereby reduces the patient's propensity to vomit these drugs. Minor central nervous system reactions (nausea, dizziness, sleep disturbances) are common. The incidence of serious adverse neuropsychiatric reactions to mefloquine treatment is ~1 in 1000 in Asia but may be as high as 1 in 200 among Africans and Caucasians. All the antimalarial quinolines (chloroquine, mefloquine, and quinine) exacerbate the orthostatic hypotension associated with malaria, and all are tolerated better by children than by adults. Pregnant women, young children, patients unable to tolerate oral therapy, and nonimmune subjects (e.g., travelers) with suspected malaria should be evaluated carefully and hospitalization considered. If there is any doubt as to the identity of the infecting malarial species, treatment for falciparum malaria should be given. A negative blood smear does not rule out malaria; thick blood films should be checked 1 and 2 days later to exclude the diagnosis. Nonimmune subjects receiving treatment for malaria should have daily parasite counts performed until negative thick films indicate clearance of the parasite. If the level of parasitemia does not fall below 25% of the admission value in 48 h or if parasitemia has not cleared by 7 days (and adherence is assured), drug resistance is likely and the regimen should be changed. If treatment failures occur with commonly used antimalarial agents, alternative drugs should be used (Table 195-8).

To eradicate persistent liver stages and prevent relapse (radical treatment), primaquine (0.3 mg of base/kg; 15 mg of base, adult dose) should be given daily for 14 days to patients with *P. vivax* or *P. ovale* infections after laboratory tests for G6PD deficiency have proved negative. A dose of 22.5 to 30 mg for an adult is recommended for infections acquired in Southeast Asia and Oceania. If the patient has a mild variant of G6PD deficiency, primaquine can be given in a dose of 0.6 mg of base/kg (45 mg maximum) once weekly for 8 weeks.

PREVENTING DRUG RESISTANCE In much of the tropics, drug-resistant *P. falciparum* is increasing in distribution, frequency, and intensity.

TABLE 195-7 Properties of Antimalarial Drugs

Drug(s)	Pharmacokinetic Properties	Antimalarial Activity	Minor Toxicity	Major Toxicity
Quinine, quinidine	Good oral and IM absorption (quinine); Cl and V_d reduced, but plasma protein binding (principally to $\propto 1$ acid glycoprotein) increased (90%) in malaria; quinine $t_{1/2}$: 16 h in malaria, 11 h in healthy persons; quinidine $t_{1/2}$: 13 h in malaria, 8 h in healthy persons	Acts mainly on trophozoite blood stage; kills gametocytes of *P. vivax*, *P. ovale*, and *P. malariae* (but not *P. falciparum*); no action on liver stages	*Common:* "Cinchonism": tinnitus, high-tone hearing loss, nausea, vomiting, dysphoria, postural hypotension; ECG QT_c interval prolongation (quinine usually by <10% but quinidine by up to 25%) *Rare:* Diarrhea, visual disturbance, rashes *Note:* Very bitter taste	*Common:* Hypoglycemia *Rare:* Hypotension, blindness, deafness, cardiac arrhythmias, thrombocytopenia, hemolysis, hemolytic-uremic syndrome, vasculitis, cholestatic hepatitis, neuromuscular paralysis *Note:* Quinidine more cardiotoxic
Chloroquine	Good oral absorption, very rapid IM and SC absorption; complex pharmacokinetics; enormous Cl and V_d (unaffected by malaria); blood concentration profile determined by distribution processes in malaria; $t_{1/2}$: 1–2 months	As for quinine but acts slightly earlier in asexual cycle	*Common:* Nausea, dysphoria, pruritus in dark-skinned patients, postural hypotension *Rare:* Accommodation difficulties, keratopathy, rash *Note:* Bitter taste, well tolerated	*Acute:* Hypotensive shock (parenteral), cardiac arrhythmias, neuropsychiatric reactions *Chronic:* Retinopathy (cumulative dose, >100 g), skeletal and cardiac myopathy
Amodiaquine	Good oral absorption; largely converted to active metabolite desethylamodiaquine	As for chloroquine	Nausea (tastes better than chloroquine)	Agranulocytosis; hepatitis, mainly with prophylactic use
Mefloquine	Adequate oral absorption; no parenteral preparation; $t_{1/2}$: 14–20 days (shorter in malaria)	As for quinine	Nausea, giddiness, dysphoria, fuzzy thinking, sleeplessness, nightmares, sense of dissociation	Neuropsychiatric reactions, convulsions, encephalopathy
Tetracycline, doxycycline[a]	Excellent absorption; $t_{1/2}$: 8 h for tetracycline, 18 h for doxycycline	Weak antimalarial activity; should not be used alone for treatment	Gastrointestinal intolerance, deposition in growing bones and teeth, photosensitivity, moniliasis, benign intracranial hypertension	Renal failure in patients with impaired renal function (tetracycline)
Halofantrine[b]	Highly variable absorption related to fat intake; $t_{1/2}$: 1–3 days (active desbutyl metabolite $t_{1/2}$: 3–7 days)	As for quinine	Diarrhea	Cardiac conduction disturbances; atrioventricular block; ECG QT_c interval prolongation; potentially lethal ventricular tachyarrhythmias
Artemisinin and derivatives (artemether, artesunate)	Good oral absorption, slow and variable absorption of IM artemether; artesunate and artemether biotransformed to active metabolite dihydroartemisinin; all drugs eliminated very rapidly; $t_{1/2}$: <1 h	Broader stage specificity and more rapid than other drugs; no action on liver stages; kills all but fully mature gametocytes of *P. falciparum*	Reduction in reticulocyte count (but not anemia)	Anaphylaxis, urticaria, fever
Pyrimethamine	Good oral absorption, variable IM absorption; $t_{1/2}$: 4 days	For blood stages, acts mainly on mature forms; causal prophylactic	Well tolerated	Megaloblastic anemia, pancytopenia, pulmonary infiltration
Proguanil (chloroguanide)	Good oral absorption; biotransformed to active metabolite cycloguanil; $t_{1/2}$: 16 h; biotransformation reduced by oral contraceptive use and in pregnancy	Causal prophylactic; not used alone for treatment	Well tolerated; mouth ulcers and rare alopecia	Megaloblastic anemia in renal failure
Primaquine	Complete oral absorption; active compound not known; $t_{1/2}$: 7 h	Radical cure; eradicates hepatic forms of *P. vivax* and *P. ovale*; kills all stages of gametocyte development of *P. falciparum*	Nausea, vomiting, diarrhea, abdominal pain, hemolysis, methemoglobinemia	Massive hemolysis in subjects with severe G6PD deficiency
Atovaquone	Highly variable absorption related to fat intake; $t_{1/2}$: 30–70 h	Acts mainly on trophozoite blood stage	None identified	None identified
Lumefantrine	Highly variable absorption related to fat intake; $t_{1/2}$: 3–4 days	As for quinine	None identified	None identified

[a] Tetracycline and doxycycline should not be given to pregnant women or to children <8 years of age.

[b] Halofantrine should not be used by patients with long ECG QT_c intervals or known conduction disturbances or by those taking drugs that may affect ventricular repolarization, e.g., quinidine, quinine, mefloquine, chloroquine, neuroleptics, antiarrhythmics, tricyclic antidepressants, terfenadine, or astemizole.

Abbreviations: Cl, systemic clearance; V_d, total apparent volume of distribution; IM, intramuscular; SC, subcutaneous; ECG, electrocardiogram; G6PD, glucose-6-phosphate dehydrogenase.

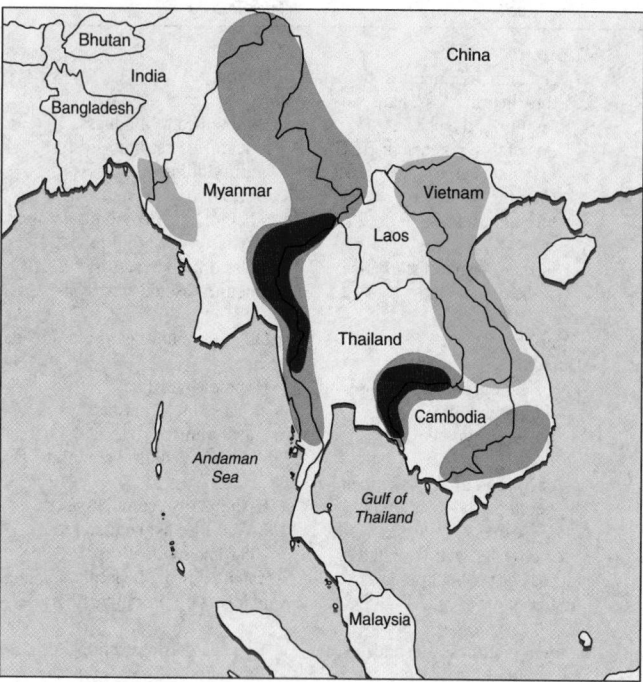

FIGURE 195-11   Mefloquine resistance in *Plasmodium falciparum* in Southeast Asia: high-level mefloquine resistance (*brown*), low-level mefloquine resistance (*red*), and mefloquine sensitivity (failure rate, <20%; *green*). There is insufficient information for the other areas.

There is a growing belief among malariologists that, to prevent resistance, falciparum malaria should be treated with drug combinations and should no longer be treated with single drugs in endemic areas; the same rationale has been applied successfully in the treatment of tuberculosis and HIV/AIDS. This combination strategy is based upon simultaneous use of two or more drugs with different modes of action: one, usually an artemisinin derivative (artesunate, artemether, or dihydroartemisinin), given for 3 days; and the other, a slower-acting antimalarial to which *P. falciparum* is sensitive. Where the malaria parasites are fully sensitive, either amodiaquine or sulfadoxine/pyrimethamine can be used in combination with the artemisinin derivative, or amodiaquine can be combined with sulfadoxine/pyrimethamine. Where there is also resistance to sulfadoxine/pyrimethamine or amodiaquine, a combination of artesunate plus mefloquine, artemether plus lumefantrine, or quinine plus tetracycline or clindamycin can be considered (although tetracycline cannot be given to pregnant women or to children <8 years of age). Atovaquone-proguanil, which is also effective against drug-resistant malaria, can also be combined with artesunate to prevent the emergence of resistance. While there is significant resistance to mefloquine in parts of Southeast Asia, the mefloquine/artesunate combinations are still reliably effective in these areas. The artemisinin derivatives and lumefantrine (all unlicensed in the United States) as well as atovaquone-proguanil are all very well tolerated, with no significant adverse effects.

COMPLICATIONS ■ Acute Renal Failure   If the level of BUN or creatinine rises despite adequate rehydration, fluid administration should be restricted to prevent volume overload. As in other forms of hypercatabolic acute renal failure, renal replacement is best performed early (Chap. 260). Hemofiltration and hemodialysis are more effective than peritoneal dialysis and are associated with lower mortality. Some patients with renal impairment pass small volumes of urine sufficient to allow control of fluid balance; these cases can be managed conservatively if other indications for dialysis do not arise. Renal function usually improves within days, but full recovery may take weeks.

Acute Pulmonary Edema   Patients should be positioned at 45° and given oxygen and intravenous diuretics. Pulmonary artery occlusion pressures may be normal, indicating increased pulmonary capillary permeability. Positive-pressure ventilation should be started early if the immediate measures fail (Chap. 217).

Hypoglycemia   An initial slow injection of 50% dextrose (0.5 g/kg) should be followed by an infusion of 10% dextrose (0.10 g/kg per hour). The blood glucose level should be checked regularly thereafter, as recurrent hypoglycemia is common, particularly in patients receiving quinine or quinidine. In severely ill patients, hypoglycemia commonly occurs together with metabolic (lactic) acidosis and carries a poor prognosis.

Other Complications   Patients who develop spontaneous bleeding should be given fresh blood and intravenous vitamin K. Convulsions should be treated with intravenous or rectal benzodiazepines and, if necessary, respiratory support. Aspiration pneumonia should be suspected in any unconscious patient with convulsions, particularly with persistent hyperventilation; intravenous antimicrobial agents and oxygen should be administered, and pulmonary toilet should be undertaken. Hypoglycemia or gram-negative septicemia should be suspected when the condition of any patient suddenly deteriorates for no obvious reason during antimalarial treatment. Systemic *Salmonella* infections are common complications among African children with falciparum malaria.

PREVENTION   In most of the tropics, the eradication of malaria is not yet feasible because of the widespread distribution of *Anopheles* breeding sites; the great number of infected persons; the use of ineffective antimalarial drugs; and inadequacies in resources, infrastructure, and control programs. Malaria may be contained by judicious use of insecticides to kill the mosquito vector, rapid diagnosis and appropriate patient management, and—where effective and feasible—administration of chemoprophylaxis to high-risk groups. Malaria researchers are intensifying their efforts to understand parasite-human-mosquito interactions better and to develop more effective control and prevention interventions. Despite the enormous investment in efforts to develop a malaria vaccine, no safe, effective, long-lasting vaccine is likely to be available for general use in the near future (Chap. 107). While there is promise for one or more malaria vaccines on the more distant horizon, prevention and control measures continue to rely on antivector and drug use strategies.

Personal Protection Against Malaria   Simple measures to reduce the frequency of mosquito bites in malarious areas are very important. These measures include the avoidance of exposure to mosquitoes at their peak feeding times (usually dusk and dawn), but also throughout the night and the use of insect repellents containing DEET (10 to 35%), suitable clothing, and insecticide-impregnated bed nets or other materials. Widespread use of bed nets treated with residual pyrethroids reduces the incidence of malaria in areas where vectors bite indoors at night and has been shown to reduce mortality in western and eastern Africa.

Chemoprophylaxis (Table 195-9)   Few areas of therapeutics are as controversial as antimalarial drug prophylaxis. Recommendations for prophylaxis depend on knowledge of local patterns of plasmodial drug sensitivity and the likelihood of acquiring malarial infection. When there is uncertainty, drugs effective against resistant *P. falciparum* should be used [mefloquine, atovaquone-proguanil (Malarone), doxy-

TABLE 195-8	*Alternative Drugs for Use When Initial Malaria Treatment Fails*
Drug Used Initially	**Drug Used to Treat Recrudescence**
Chloroquine	→ Sulfadoxine/pyrimethamine[a] ↘
Sulfadoxine/pyrimethamine	→ Artesunate-mefloquine[a]
Mefloquine ± artesunate	→ Quinine ± tetracycline (or doxycycline) for 7 days ↘ Artesunate + doxycycline or clindamycin for 7 days

[a] Or artemether-lumefantrine.

cycline, or primaquine]. Chemoprophylaxis is never entirely reliable, and malaria should always be considered in the differential diagnosis of fever in patients who have traveled to endemic areas, even if they are taking prophylactic antimalarial drugs.

Pregnant women traveling to malarious areas should be warned about the potential risks. All pregnant women at risk in endemic areas should be encouraged to attend regular antenatal clinics and should receive either prophylaxis with chloroquine (300 mg of base weekly) alone or with proguanil (chloroguanide, 200 mg daily) or intermittent preventive treatment (IPT) with sulfadoxine/pyrimethamine, provided there is not high-level resistance to these drugs. The safety of other prophylactic antimalarial agents in pregnancy has not been established. In addition, antimalarial prophylaxis should be considered for children between the ages of 3 months and 4 years in areas where malaria causes high childhood mortality; such prophylaxis may not be logistically or economically feasible in many countries. Research on IPT for infants and young children shows promise for more widespread use. Children born to nonimmune mothers in endemic areas (usually expatriates moving to these areas) should receive prophylaxis from birth.

Travelers should start taking antimalarial drugs at least 1 week before departure so that any untoward reactions can be detected and therapeutic antimalarial blood concentrations will be present when needed. Antimalarial prophylaxis should continue for 4 weeks after the traveler has left the endemic area, except if atovaquone-proguanil or primaquine has been taken; these drugs have significant activities against the liver stage of the infection (causal prophylaxis) and can be discontinued 1 week after departure from the endemic area.

Mefloquine (250 mg of salt weekly, adult dose) has been the antimalarial prophylactic agent of choice for much of the tropics because it is usually effective against multidrug-resistant falciparum malaria and is reasonably well tolerated. Mild nausea, dizziness, fuzzy thinking, disturbed sleep patterns, vivid dreams, and malaise are relatively common. Approximately 1 in every 10,000 recipients develops an acute reversible neuropsychiatric reaction manifested by confusion, psychosis, convulsions, or encephalopathy. The role of mefloquine prophylaxis during pregnancy remains uncertain; in studies in Africa, mefloquine prophylaxis was found to be effective and safe during pregnancy. However, in one study from Thailand, treatment of malaria with mefloquine was associated with an increased risk of stillbirth.

Atovaquone-proguanil (Malarone; 3.75/1.5 mg per kg or 250/100 mg, daily adult dose) is a fixed-combination once-daily prophylactic agent that is very well tolerated by adults and children, with fewer adverse gastrointestinal effects than chloroquine-proguanil and fewer adverse central nervous system effects than mefloquine. It is proguanil itself, rather than the antifolate metabolite cycloguanil, that acts synergistically with atovaquone. This combination is effective against all types of malaria, including multidrug-resistant falciparum malaria, and, because of its causal activity, may be discontinued 1 week after departure from the endemic area. Atovaquone-proguanil is best taken with food or a milky drink to optimize absorption. There are insufficient data on the safety of this regimen in pregnancy.

Daily administration of doxycycline (100 mg daily, adult dose) is an effective alternative to mefloquine. Doxycycline is generally well tolerated but may cause vulvovaginal thrush, diarrhea, and photosensitivity and cannot be used by children <8 years old or by pregnant women.

Chloroquine remains the drug of choice for the prevention of infection with drug-sensitive *P. falciparum* and with the other human malarial species (although chloroquine-resistant *P. vivax* has been reported from parts of eastern Asia, Oceania, and Central and South America). Unfortunately, there are now few areas of the world with chloroquine-sensitive *P. falciparum*. Chloroquine is generally well tol-

TABLE 195-9 *Prophylaxis and Self-Treatment for Malaria*

Drug	Usage	Adult Dosage	Child Dosage
Prophylaxis			
Mefloquine	Used in areas where chloroquine-resistant malaria has been reported	228 mg of base (250 mg of salt) orally, once/week[a]	<15 kg: 4.6 mg of base/kg (5 mg of salt/kg) 15–19 kg: ¼ tablet/week 20–30 kg: ½ tablet/week 31–45 kg: ¾ tablet/week >45 kg: 1 tablet/week
Doxycycline[b]	Used as alternative to mefloquine or atovaquone-proguanil	100 mg orally, once/day	>8 years of age: 2 mg/kg per day orally; maximum dose, 100 mg/d
Atovaquone-proguanil (Malarone)[c]	Used as alternative to mefloquine or doxycycline	250/100 mg orally once/day	11–20 kg: 62.5 mg/25 mg 21–30 kg: 125 mg/50 mg 31–40 kg: 187.5 mg/75 mg >40 kg: 250 mg/100 mg
Chloroquine	Used in areas where chloroquine-resistant malaria has *not* been reported	300 mg of base (500 mg of salt) orally, once/week	5 mg of base/kg (8.3 mg of salt/kg) orally, once/week; maximum dose, 300 mg of base
Proguanil (not available in U.S.)	Used simultaneously *with* chloroquine as alternative to mefloquine or doxycycline	200 mg orally, once/day, in combination with weekly chloroquine	<2 years: 50 mg/d 2–6 years: 100 mg/d 7–10 years: 150 mg/d >10 years: 200 mg/d
Primaquine[c]	Used for travelers only after testing for G6PD deficiency; postexposure prevention for relapsing malaria or prophylaxis	Postexposure: 15 mg of base (26.3 mg of salt) orally, once/day for 14 days Prophylaxis: 30 mg of base daily	0.3 mg of base/kg (0.5 mg of salt/kg) orally, once/day for 14 days
Self-treatment			
Atovaquone-proguanil (Malarone)[d]	In areas with chloroquine-resistant malaria, should be carried during travel to very remote areas by persons taking mefloquine or doxycycline	4 tablets (1000 mg of atovaquone and 400 mg of proguanil) orally, as a single daily dose for 3 consecutive days	11–20 kg: 1 adult tablet 21–30 kg: 2 adult tablets 31–40 kg: 3 adult tablets >40 kg: 4 adult tablets
Sulfadoxine/pyrimethamine[e]	Used as alternative to atovaquone-proguanil for self-treatment	3 tablets (75 mg of pyrimethamine and 1500 mg of sulfadoxine) orally, as a single dose	5–10 kg: ½ tablet 11–20 kg: 1 tablet 21–30 kg: 1½ tablets 31–45 kg: 2 tablets >45 kg: 3 tablets

[a] Tablets manufactured outside the United States contain 250 mg of base.
[b] Not in pregnant women or children <8 years old.
[c] Primaquine and atovaquone-proguanil have both proved safe and effective for antimalarial chemoprophylaxis in areas with chloroquine-resistant falciparum malaria, but more data are needed, particularly in children. These drugs should not be used in pregnancy.
[d] Not for patients on atovaquone-proguanil prophylaxis.
[e] Regimen is used for treatment only (*not* prophylaxis) in areas with known susceptibility.

erated, although some patients are unable to take the drug because of malaise, headache, visual symptoms (from reversible keratopathy), gastrointestinal intolerance, or (in dark-skinned patients) pruritus. A concomitant filarial infection may provoke or aggravate chloroquine-induced pruritus. Chloroquine is considered safe in pregnancy. With chronic administration for >5 years, a characteristic dose-related retinopathy may develop, but this condition is rare at the doses used for antimalarial prophylaxis. Idiosyncratic or allergic reactions are also rare. Skeletal and cardiac myopathy are potential problems with protracted prophylactic use; they are more likely to occur with the high doses used in the treatment of rheumatoid arthritis. Neuropsychiatric reactions and skin rashes are unusual. When used continuously, amodiaquine, a related aminoquinoline, is associated with a high risk of agranulocytosis (~1 person in 2000) and also hepatotoxicity (~1 person in 16,000) and should not be used for prophylaxis.

Primaquine (0.5 mg of base/kg or 30 mg, daily adult dose) has proved safe and effective in the prevention of drug-resistant falciparum and vivax malaria in adults. Abdominal pain and oxidant hemolysis, the principal adverse effects, are not common as long as the drug is taken with food and is not given to G6PD-deficient persons. Primaquine should not be given to pregnant women or neonates.

In the past, the dihydrofolate reductase inhibitors pyrimethamine and proguanil (chloroguanide) have been administered widely, but the rapid selection of resistance in both *P. falciparum* and *P. vivax* has limited their use. Whereas antimalarial quinolines such as chloroquine act on the erythrocyte stage of parasitic development, the dihydrofolate reductase inhibitors also inhibit preerythrocytic growth in the liver (causal prophylaxis) and development in the mosquito (sporontocidal activity). Proguanil is safe and well tolerated, although mouth ulceration occurs in ~8% of persons using this drug; it is considered safe for antimalarial prophylaxis in pregnancy. The prophylactic use of the combination of pyrimethamine and sulfadoxine is not recommended because of an unacceptable incidence of severe toxicity, principally exfoliative dermatitis and other skin rashes, agranulocytosis, hepatitis, and pulmonary eosinophilia (incidence, 1:7000; fatal reactions, 1:18,000). The combination of pyrimethamine with dapsone (0.2/1.5 mg/kg weekly; 12.5/100 mg, adult dose) is a second-line alternative available in some countries. Dapsone may cause methemoglobinemia and allergic reactions and (at higher doses) may pose a significant risk of agranulocytosis. Proguanil and the pyrimethamine-dapsone combination are not available in the United States.

Because of the increasing spread and intensity of antimalarial drug resistance (Figs. 195-2 and 195-11), the Centers for Disease Control and Prevention (CDC; *www.cdc.gov/travel/index.htm*), which recommends a weekly dose of mefloquine for all travelers, maintains an updated 24-h travel and malaria information audiotape that can be accessed by touch-tone telephone (888-232-3228). Regional and disease-specific documents may be requested from the CDC Fax Information Service (888-232-3299). Consultation for the evaluation of prophylaxis failures or treatment of malaria can be obtained from state and local health departments and the CDC Malaria Hotline (770-488-7788).

BABESIOSIS

Babesiosis is a worldwide protozoan disease of animals that is transmitted by ticks; humans are infected incidentally and initially develop a nonspecific febrile illness that can lead to hemolytic anemia. *Babesia* organisms enter RBCs and resemble malarial parasites morphologically, thus posing a diagnostic problem.

ETIOLOGY AND NATURAL CYCLE   Of the >100 species of *Babesia*, *B. microti* and *B. divergens* are the two that cause most human infections. *Babesia* species infect many mammalian hosts. The majority of species are from rodents and birds; however, almost any mammal serving as a host for *Babesia*-infected ticks can be a reservoir. Ixodid (hard-bodied) ticks, in particular *Ixodes scapularis* (*I. dammini*) and *I. ricinus*, are the vectors of the parasite. Ticks ingest *Babesia* while feeding, and the parasite multiplies within the tick's gut wall. The organisms then spread to the salivary glands; their inoculation into a vertebrate host by a tick larva, nymph, or adult completes the cycle of transmission. Asexual reproduction of *Babesia* within RBCs produces two or four parasites.

EPIDEMIOLOGY   While *Babesia* infections in wild and domestic animals are distributed globally, almost all of the >300 *B. microti* infections in the United States have occurred along the northeastern coast, including Nantucket Island, Martha's Vineyard, and Cape Cod in Massachusetts; Block Island in Rhode Island; Long Island, Shelter Island, and Fire Island in New York; and the nearby mainland, including eastern Connecticut and areas of Westchester County in New York. In Nantucket, 60% of deer mice are infected with *B. microti*. Cases have also been reported from Wisconsin, Minnesota, Virginia, Maryland, Georgia, and Mexico. *Babesia* isolates from patients in Washington (WA-1) and California (CA-1) are structurally similar but genetically and antigenically distinct from *B. microti*. A strain isolated in Japan and another in Missouri (MO-1) differ from these isolates, suggesting that babesiosis may be an "emerging infection." The vast majority of *Babesia* infections are not clinically apparent. The deer tick, *I. scapularis*, is the vector associated with *B. microti*. In Europe, *B. divergens* has been responsible for the majority of the 30 reported cases of babesiosis; Yugoslavia, Russia, France, the United Kingdom, and Ireland have accounted for most of these infections.

Transfusions are another source of babesiosis. In the >20 transfusion-associated cases reported, parasites were uncommonly detected in blood donors, but serologic testing of their blood for *Babesia* gave positive results.

Infections with *B. divergens* have occurred sporadically in previously splenectomized patients in several countries in Europe. *I. ricinus* is probably the vector in these cases, as it is for the transmission of this organism among cattle. The infected persons were predisposed to illness by their asplenic status.

I. scapularis feeds on rodents as a larva and a nymph and on deer as an adult; nymphs are abundant during the spring and summer and feed on humans readily. In some endemic areas, the seroprevalence in the human population may be >2%; residents of Shelter Island and Nantucket have had a 4 to 7% seroconversion rate. These figures indicate that asymptomatic infection is more frequent than is generally thought and that *Babesia* can be a peril for persons being transfused.

CLINICAL PRESENTATION   The incubation period for *B. microti* infection is ~1 to 4 weeks. Immunosuppressed patients, splenectomized individuals, and the elderly have the most severe illness. The clinical presentation varies widely and resembles malaria or rickettsiosis; symptoms and signs include a gradual onset of irregular fever, chills, sweating, muscle pain, and fatigue. Mild hepatosplenomegaly and mild hemolytic anemia may develop, but a rash is not present. The level of parasitemia may range from 1 to 50%. The illness may continue for weeks or months, particularly in patients with HIV infection or AIDS.

Patients infected with *B. divergens* have usually been splenectomized and have a more severe illness, with a rapid onset of chills,

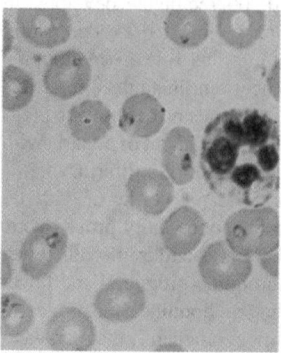

FIGURE 195-12   Thin blood film showing trophozoites of *Babesia*. (*Reproduced from Benchaids for the Diagnosis of Malaria Infections, 2d ed, with the permission of the World Health Organization.*)

fever, nausea, vomiting, and hemolytic anemia progressing to jaundice, hemoglobinemia, and renal failure. *B. divergens* infections are often fatal.

DIAGNOSIS Whether or not they have a history of exposure to ticks or tick bites, febrile persons living in endemic areas should have Giemsa-stained thick and thin blood films (Fig. 195-12) examined for small intraerythrocytic parasites. *B. microti* appears as a small ring form resembling *P. falciparum*. Unlike infection with *Plasmodium*, however, that with *Babesia* does not cause the production of pigment in parasites, nor are schizonts or gametocytes formed. Dividing within RBCs, *B. microti* can form four daughter parasites attached by strands of cytoplasm; these "tetrad" forms are seen infrequently in human blood films but are a distinguishing feature. A sensitive and specific indirect immunofluorescence antibody test is useful for the diagnosis of infection with *B. microti* and exists for *B. divergens* and WA-1 but does not replace the blood smear. The serum antibody titer rises 2 to 4 weeks after the onset of illness and then wanes over 6 to 12 months; cross-reactions can occur with other species of *Babesia* and with *Plasmodium*. A species-specific polymerase chain reaction test using the RNA gene has been used to show parasite persistence when the blood smear is negative.

About 50% of patients infected with *B. microti* have antibody to *Borrelia burgdorferi*, the agent of Lyme disease (Chap. 157); this figure varies with the geographic area. The occurrence of mixed infections is not surprising since both organisms are transmitted by *I. scapularis*. This tick species is also a potential vector of human granulocytotropic ehrlichiosis; the same tick may carry more than one tick-borne disease. Intraperitoneal inoculation of blood from patients with babesiosis into hamsters or gerbils results in detectable parasitemia within 2 to 4 weeks.

℞ **TREATMENT** (See Table 195-10)

B. microti infections in patients with intact spleens are often self-limiting without treatment, although symptoms may persist for months with or without treatment. Because silent parasitemia may have prolonged symptoms and signs, treatment is advised for all patients infected with *Babesia*. Patients infected with *B. divergens* or other *Babesia* species (including MO-1, WA-1, and CA-1) should receive quinine, clindamycin, and atovaquone; in addition, exchange transfusion or apheresis should be strongly considered. Treatment with the combination of quinine sulfate (650 mg of salt orally three times daily)

TABLE 195-10 *Treatment of Babesiosis*

Organism	Adults	Children
Babesia microti	Atovaquone 750 mg bid PO *plus* azithromycin 600 mg/d PO *or*	Atovaquone 40 mg/kg/d PO *plus* azithromycin 12 mg/kg/d PO *or*
	Quinine 650 mg tid PO *plus* clindamycin 1200 mg bid IV (or 600 mg tid PO)	Quinine 25 mg/kg tid PO *plus* clindamycin 20–40 mg/kg tid PO
Babesia divergens and other *Babesia* species, including MO-1, WA-1, and CA-1	Quinine 650 mg tid PO *plus* clindamycin 1200 mg bid IV (or 600 mg tid PO) *plus* atovaquone 750 mg bid PO[a]	Quinine 25 mg/kg tid PO *plus* clindamycin 20–40 mg/kg tid PO *plus* atovaquone 40 mg/kg per day PO[a]

[a] Consider exchange transfusion or apheresis.

plus clindamycin (600 mg orally three times daily or 1.2 g parenterally twice daily) for 7 to 10 days is usually effective but may not always eliminate parasites. Especially severe infections with high-level *B. microti* parasitemia in asplenic patients have been successfully treated with exchange transfusions in addition to quinine and clindamycin. The current view is that the combination of atovaquone (750 mg twice daily for adults) and azithromycin (600 mg/d for adults) for 7 to 10 days offers optimal therapy.

FURTHER READING

ARTEMETHER–QUININE META-ANALYSIS STUDY GROUP: A meta-analysis using individual patient data of trials comparing artemether with quinine in the treatment of severe falciparum malaria. Trans R Soc Trop Med Hyg 95:637, 2001

CENTERS FOR DISEASE CONTROL AND PREVENTION: *Health Information for International Travel, 1999–2000*. Atlanta, Department of Health and Human Services, 2000

GUERIN PJ et al: Malaria: Current status of control, diagnosis, treatment, and a proposed agenda for research and development. Lancet Infect Dis 2:564, 2002

HOGH B: Atovaquone-proguanil versus chloroquine-proguanil for malaria prophylaxis in non-immune travellers: A randomised, double-blind study. Lancet 356:1888, 2000

NEWTON P, WHITE NJ: Malaria: New developments in treatment and prevention. Annu Rev Med 50:179, 1999

PHU NH et al: Hemofiltration and peritoneal dialysis in infection-associated acute renal failure in Vietnam. N Engl J Med 347:895, 2002

VAN VUGT M et al: Treatment of uncomplicated multidrug-resistant falciparum malaria with artesunate-atovaquone-proguanil. Clin Infect Dis 35:1498, 2002

WEISS LM: Babesiosis in humans: A treatment review. Expert Opin Pharmacother 3:1109, 2002

WHITE NJ: The assessment of antimalarial drug efficacy. Trends Parasitol 18:865, 2002

WORLD HEALTH ORGANIZATION: Severe falciparum malaria. Trans R Soc Trop Med Hyg 94(Suppl 1):51, 2000

196 LEISHMANIASIS
Barbara L. Herwaldt

OVERVIEW

DEFINITION The term *leishmaniasis* refers collectively to various clinical syndromes caused by obligate intracellular protozoa of the genus *Leishmania* (order Kinetoplastida). Leishmaniasis is endemic in diverse ecologic settings in the tropics, the subtropics, and southern Europe that range from deserts to rain forests and from rural to periurban areas. It is typically a vector-borne zoonosis, with rodents and canids as common reservoir hosts and humans as incidental hosts. In humans, visceral, cutaneous, and mucosal leishmaniasis result from infection of macrophages throughout the reticuloendothelial system, in the skin, and in the naso-oropharyngeal mucosa, respectively. Current challenges include the emergence of leishmaniasis in new geographic areas

and host populations (e.g., visceral leishmaniasis in persons infected with HIV) as well as the need for field-applicable, rapid diagnostic tests and for effective, safe, and affordable oral therapies, control measures, and vaccines.

ETIOLOGY The organisms that cause the various forms of leishmaniasis in humans (Table 196-1) are in the subgenus *Leishmania* or the subgenus *Viannia*. Visceral leishmaniasis is typically but not exclusively caused by organisms of the *Leishmania donovani* complex; Old World cutaneous leishmaniasis by *L. tropica*, *L. major*, and *L. aethiopica*; and New World (or American) cutaneous leishmaniasis by organisms of the *L. mexicana* complex and the *Viannia* subgenus. Mucosal leishmaniasis is caused primarily by some organisms in the *Viannia* subgenus and also by *L. amazonensis*.

LIFE CYCLE *Leishmania* parasites are transmitted by the bite of female phlebotomine sandflies [genus *Phlebotomus* (Old World) or *Lutzomyia* (New World)]. As the flies attempt to feed, they regurgitate the para-

TABLE 196-1 *Major Leishmania Species That Cause Disease in Humans*

Species[a]	Clinical Syndrome[b]	Geographic Distribution
SUBGENUS LEISHMANIA		
L. donovani complex		
L. donovani sensu stricto	VL (PKDL, OWCL)	China, Indian subcontinent, southwestern Asia, Ethiopia,[c] Kenya, Sudan, Uganda; possibly sporadic in sub-Saharan Africa
L. infantum sensu stricto[d]	VL (OWCL)	China, central and southwestern Asia, Middle East, southern Europe, North Africa, Ethiopia,[c] Sudan; sporadic in sub-Saharan Africa
L. chagasi[d]	VL (NWCL)	Central and South America
L. mexicana complex		
L. mexicana	NWCL (DCL)	Texas, Mexico, Central and South America
L. amazonensis	NWCL (ML, DCL, VL)	Panama and South America
L. tropica	OWCL (VL)[e]	Central Asia, India, Pakistan, southwestern Asia, Middle East, Turkey, Greece, North Africa, Ethiopia,[c] Kenya, Namibia
L. major	OWCL[f]	Central Asia, India, Pakistan, southwestern Asia, Middle East, Turkey, North Africa, Sahel region of north-central Africa, Ethiopia,[c] Sudan, Kenya
L. aethiopica	OWCL (DCL, ML)	Ethiopia,[c] Kenya, Uganda
SUBGENUS VIANNIA		
L. (V.) braziliensis	NWCL (ML)	Central and South America
L. (V.) guyanensis	NWCL (ML)	South America
L. (V.) panamensis	NWCL (ML)	Central America, Venezuela, Colombia, Ecuador, Peru
L. (V.) peruviana	NWCL[g]	Peru (western slopes of Andes)

[a] Species other than those listed here have been reported to infect humans.
[b] **Abbreviations**: VL, visceral leishmaniasis; PKDL, post–kala-azar dermal leishmaniasis; OWCL, Old World cutaneous leishmaniasis; NWCL, New World (American) cutaneous leishmaniasis; DCL, diffuse cutaneous leishmaniasis; ML, mucosal leishmaniasis. Clinical syndromes less frequently associated with the various species are shown in parentheses.
[c] Cutaneous and visceral leishmaniasis also are endemic in parts of Eritrea, but the causative species have not been well established.
[d] "*L. infantum*" and "*L. chagasi*" are synonymous.
[e] *L. tropica* also causes leishmaniasis recidivans and viscerotropic leishmaniasis.
[f] *L. major*–like organisms also cause New World cutaneous leishmaniasis.
[g] The cutaneous leishmaniasis syndrome caused by this species is called *uta*.

site's flagellated promastigote stage into the skin of mammalian hosts. Components of sandfly saliva can affect the host's response to the parasite. Promastigotes attach to receptors on macrophages, are phagocytized, and transform within phagolysosomes into the nonflagellated amastigote stage, which multiplies by binary fission. After rupture of infected macrophages, amastigotes are phagocytized by other macrophages. If ingested by feeding sandflies, amastigotes transform back into promastigotes, which require at least 7 days to become infective.

IMMUNOLOGY Advances in the understanding of the immunology of leishmaniasis have made this parasitic disease the paradigm for studies of the T cell subsets and cytokines that govern resistance and susceptibility to intracellular pathogens. The paradigm is best demonstrated in murine *L. major* infection. In inbred mice, production of interferon γ (IFN-γ) by T_H1 and natural killer cells confers resistance. Interleukin (IL)12 induces naive T cells to differentiate into T_H1 cells and induces T cells and natural killer cells to produce IFN-γ. In contrast, expansion of IL-4-producing T_H2 cells and IL-10 mediate susceptibility.

Not all aspects of leishmaniasis in mice, whose susceptibility to leishmanial infection is genetically determined, apply to human infection, for which the genetic determinants are being investigated. However, a consistent principle is that healing and resistance to reinfection are associated with an intact T_H1 cell response, production of IFN-γ, and activation of macrophages to kill intracellular amastigotes. In human visceral leishmaniasis, IL-10, which deactivates the T_H1 cell response, appears particularly important in the progression of disease.

GENERAL DIAGNOSTIC PRINCIPLES Definitive diagnosis of leishmaniasis requires demonstration of the parasite. To identify amastigotes by light-microscopic examination, the specimen obtained from an infected site (e.g., thin smear, histologic section) should be stained with Giemsa or another Romanovsky stain and presumptive amastigotes (2 to 4 μm in diameter) examined under oil immersion for the presence of a nucleus and a rod-shaped kinetoplast (Fig. 196-1); the latter is a specialized mitochondrial structure that contains extranuclear DNA. Other means of parasitologic confirmation include in vitro culture

(e.g., on Novy-MacNeal-Nicolle medium), animal inoculation, and use of investigational molecular techniques [e.g., polymerase chain reaction (PCR)].

The *Leishmania* species that infect humans are morphologically similar. They can be distinguished by isoenzyme analysis of cultured promastigotes, determination of monoclonal antibody specificity, or various molecular methods.

Indirect immunologic methods for diagnosis include serologic assays and tests for *Leishmania*-specific cell-mediated immunity (e.g., skin testing for delayed-type hypersensitivity reactions). The usefulness of such methods depends in part on the clinical syndrome (see below). Traditional serologic assays (e.g., indirect fluorescent antibody testing) do not reliably distinguish past from current infection, and no leishmanin skin-test preparation has been approved for use in the United States. Advances in molecular methods (e.g., production of recombinant/synthetic antigens) are leading to the development of better diagnostic techniques.

GENERAL THERAPEUTIC PRINCIPLES For a given case of leishmaniasis, it is important to consider whether the patient's illness could result in substantial morbidity or in death and therefore requires expeditious treatment with a regimen that generally is highly effective. For more than half a century the pentavalent antimonial (Sb^V) compounds sodium stibogluconate and meglumine antimonate have been the mainstays of antileishmanial therapy (Table 196-2). Toxicity (such as myalgia, arthralgia, fatigue

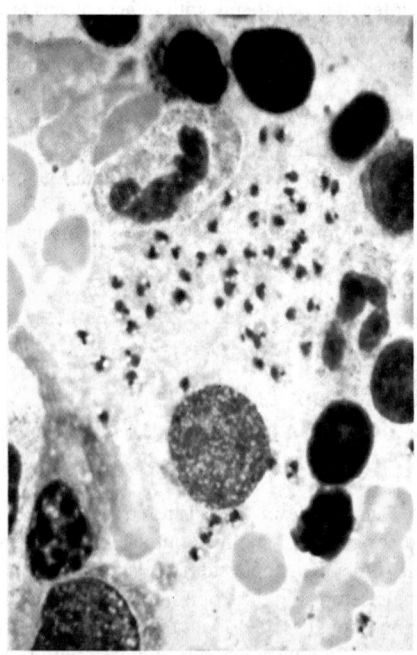

FIGURE 196-1 Amastigotes (the tissue form of the *Leishmania* parasite) in a bone marrow specimen from a patient with visceral leishmaniasis. Each amastigote has a nucleus and kinetoplast. Visualization of the kinetoplast is essential in differentiating leishmaniasis from diseases such as histoplasmosis. The extracellular amastigotes probably were released from mononuclear phagocytes during specimen collection and processing. (*Photograph courtesy of Dr. R. Hamill.*)

TABLE 196-2 *Parenteral and Oral Drug Regimens for Treatment of Leishmaniasis*[a]

Clinical Syndrome, Drug	Route of Administration	Regimen
VISCERAL LEISHMANIASIS		
First-line therapy		
Pentavalent antimony[b]	IV, IM	20 mg Sb^V/kg qd for 28 days
Amphotericin B, lipid formulation[c]	IV	2–5 mg/kg qd (total: usually ~15–21 mg/kg)
Alternatives		
Amphotericin B (deoxycholate)	IV	0.5–1 mg/kg qod or qd (total: usually ~15–20 mg/kg)
Paromomycin sulfate[d]	IV, IM	15–20 mg/kg qd for ~21 days
Pentamidine isethionate	IV, IM	4 mg/kg qod or thrice weekly for ~15–30 doses
Miltefosine	PO	See text
CUTANEOUS LEISHMANIASIS		
First-line therapy		
Pentavalent antimony[b]	IV, IM	20 mg Sb^V/kg qd for 10–20 days (standard recommendation is 20 days)
Parenteral alternatives		
Pentamidine isethionate	IV, IM	3 mg/kg qod for 4 doses or 2 mg/kg qod for 7 doses
Amphotericin B (deoxycholate)	IV	0.5–1 mg/kg qod or qd (total: up to ~20 mg/kg)[e]
Oral alternatives		
Fluconazole	PO	200 mg qd or bid for 6 weeks[f]
Ketoconazole	PO	600 mg/d for 28 days[f]
Itraconazole	PO	200 mg bid for 28 days[f]
Dapsone	PO	100 mg bid for 6 weeks[f]
MUCOSAL LEISHMANIASIS		
First-line therapy		
Pentavalent antimony[b]	IV, IM	20 mg Sb^V/kg qd for 28 days
Amphotericin B (deoxycholate)	IV	1 mg/kg qod or qd (total: usually ~20–40 mg/kg)
Alternative		
Pentamidine isethionate	IV, IM	2–4 mg/kg qod or thrice weekly for ≥15 doses

[a] See text for additional details. Some of the listed drugs are effective only against certain *Leishmania* species and only in certain areas of the world. To maximize effectiveness and minimize toxicity, the listed regimens should be individualized according to the particularities of the case and in consultation with an expert. Children may need different dosage regimens. Except for liposomal amphotericin B (see footnote[c]), none of the drugs listed are licensed by the U.S. Food and Drug Administration (FDA) for the treatment of leishmaniasis per se.

[b] The Centers for Disease Control and Prevention (CDC) provides the pentavalent antimonial (Sb^V) compound sodium stibogluconate (Pentostam; GlaxoSmithKline Export Limited, Middlesex, United Kingdom; 100 mg Sb^V/mL) to U.S.-licensed physicians through the CDC Drug Service (404-639-3670) under an IND mechanism with the FDA. The other widely used pentavalent antimonial compound, meglumine antimonate (Glucantime; Aventis Pharma Venezuela, Caracas; 85 mg Sb^V/mL), is available primarily in Spanish- and French-speaking areas of the world. Locally made Sb^V preparations may have different Sb^V concentrations and may vary in quality and safety.

[c] The lipid formulations of amphotericin B include liposomal amphotericin B and amphotericin B lipid complex. The FDA has approved the following regimen of liposomal amphotericin B for immunocompetent patients: 3 mg/kg qd on days 1–5, 14, and 21, for a total of 21 mg/kg. For immunosuppressed patients, the approved regimen is 4 mg/kg qd on days 1–5, 10, 17, 24, 31, and 38, for a total of 40 mg/kg. Alternative regimens that have been proposed for immunocompetent patients include treatment on days 1–5 and 10 with 3–4 mg/kg for cases from Europe or Brazil, with 3 mg/kg qd for cases from Africa, and with 2–3 mg/kg qd for cases from India.

[d] Not commercially available as of this writing.

[e] No dosage regimen has been established for use of this drug to treat cutaneous leishmaniasis.

[f] Adult dosage.

elevated aminotransferase levels, chemical pancreatitis, and electrocardiographic abnormalities) becomes increasingly common as the course of treatment progresses but usually does not limit therapy and is reversible.

The traditional parenteral alternatives to Sb^V—amphotericin B and pentamidine isethionate—are generally considered more apt to induce serious or irreversible toxicity (e.g., nephrotoxicity or diabetes). However, these agents, especially amphotericin B, are being advocated for use in some situations (see below; Table 196-2), in part because of the benefits of new formulations (e.g., lipid formulations of amphotericin B) and the decreasing effectiveness of Sb^V in some settings. Many other agents have been touted as alternatives or adjuncts to Sb^V, often on the basis of suboptimal data. Some of these agents may be useful in certain situations, with the caveat that even the results of well-conducted clinical trials are not always generalizable to the treatment of patients infected with other leishmanial species acquired in other settings. With the apparent exception of miltefosine, the other oral agents evaluated to date typically have at best modest activity against some of the *Leishmania* species.

PREVENTION AND CONTROL The transmission of *Leishmania* species typically is focal, in part because of the limited flight range of sandflies; these insects usually remain within a few hundred meters of their breeding site. They rest in dark, moist places in habitats ranging from deserts to rain forests; peridomestic sandflies rest in debris or rubble near buildings. Vector control may be useful in some settings.

Personal protective measures include avoiding outdoor activities when sandflies are most active (dusk to dawn); using mechanical barriers such as screens and bed-nets that keep out sandflies, which typically are about one-third the size of mosquitoes; wearing protective clothing; and applying insect repellent to exposed skin. Impregnating clothing, bed-nets, and screens with permethrin may also be useful, as may spraying dwellings with residual-action insecticide, if transmission of infection is intra- or peridomiciliary. If dogs are important reservoir hosts, use of insecticide-impregnated dog collars might be helpful. Vaccine strategies are being investigated. Treating human cases is an effective control measure only where humans are the primary reservoir hosts of infection (e.g., of *L. donovani* infection in India).

VISCERAL LEISHMANIASIS

More than 90% of the world's cases of visceral leishmaniasis occur in Bangladesh, northeastern India (particularly Bihar State), Nepal, Sudan, and northeastern Brazil. The causative species typically are those of the *L. donovani* complex (Table 196-1). The organisms can be transmitted not only by sandflies but also congenitally and parenterally (e.g., through blood transfusions or needle sharing). Infection begins in macrophages at the inoculation site (e.g., in dermal macrophages at the site of a sandfly bite) and disseminates throughout the reticuloendothelial system.

CLINICAL MANIFESTATIONS Visceral infection often remains subclinical but can become symptomatic, with an acute, subacute, or chronic course. In some settings, inapparent infections far outnumber clinically apparent ones; malnutrition is among the risk factors for the development of disease. The incubation period usually ranges from weeks to months but can be as long as years. Whereas the general term *visceral leishmaniasis* covers a broad spectrum of severity and manifestations, the term *kala-azar* (Hindi for "black fever," indicating that the skin of some patients turns gray) generally conjures up the classic image of profoundly cachectic, febrile patients who are heavily infected with parasites and have life-threatening disease. Splenomegaly (with the spleen most often soft and nontender) typically is more impressive than hepatomegaly, and the spleen can be massive. Peripheral lymphadenopathy is common in some settings, including Sudan.

The abnormal laboratory findings associated with advanced disease include pancytopenia—anemia, leukopenia (neutropenia, marked eosinopenia, relative lymphocytosis and monocytosis), and thrombocytopenia—as well as hypergammaglobulinemia (chiefly involving IgG, from polyclonal B cell activation) and hypoalbuminemia. Causes of anemia can include bone-marrow infiltration, hypersplenism, autoimmune hemolysis, and bleeding.

Some patients develop post-kala-azar dermal leishmaniasis. This syndrome is manifested by skin lesions (including macules, papules, nodules, and patches) that typically are most prominent on the face. These lesions can develop during therapy or within a few months thereafter (e.g., in East Africa) or can develop years later (e.g., in India); relapse of visceral infection can occur. Persons in India (i.e., in areas where humans are the primary reservoir hosts of infection) who have persistent skin lesions can serve as reservoir hosts who maintain transmission of infection.

Viscerotropic leishmaniasis caused by *L. tropica*, which is thought typically to be dermotropic, was parasitologically confirmed in 12 U.S. soldiers who participated in Operation Desert Storm in the Persian Gulf in the early 1990s. The affected persons had light parasite burdens and nonspecific manifestations of visceral infection (e.g., fatigue, fever, and gastrointestinal symptoms).

DIAGNOSIS Although molecular techniques are under investigation, parasitologic diagnosis of visceral leishmaniasis has traditionally been accomplished by demonstration of the parasite on stained slides (Fig. 196-1) or in cultures of a tissue aspirate or a biopsy specimen (e.g., of spleen, liver, bone marrow, or lymph node). The diagnostic yield is highest for splenic aspiration (specifically, as high as 98% vs. <90% for other specimens), but this procedure can cause hemorrhage.

Patients with florid kala-azar commonly have relatively heavy parasite burdens, develop high titers of antibody to *Leishmania* (diagnostically useful but not protective), and have undetectable *Leishmania*-specific cell-mediated immunity. (Leishmanin skin-test reactivity as well as lymphocyte proliferation and IFN-γ responses to leishmanial antigens develop after recovery.) Promising noninvasive serologic methods for diagnosing kala-azar use recombinant leishmanial antigens or synthetic peptides (e.g., K39); these techniques are being field-tested.

DIFFERENTIAL DIAGNOSIS The differential diagnosis of visceral leishmaniasis includes other tropical and infectious diseases that cause fever or organomegaly (e.g., typhoid fever, miliary tuberculosis, brucellosis, histoplasmosis, malaria, tropical splenomegaly syndrome, and schistosomiasis) as well as diseases such as leukemia and lymphoma. Post-kala-azar dermal leishmaniasis should be differentiated from syphilis, yaws, and leprosy.

℞ TREATMENT (Table 196-2)

Because persons who have kala-azar generally die if not appropriately treated, highly effective therapy is essential, as is close monitoring for bleeding and intercurrent infectious conditions such as pneumonia and diarrhea. Outside of India, treatment with a pentavalent antimonial compound still is usually effective. The use of an alternative parenteral agent should be considered even for first-line therapy if unresponsiveness to Sb^V therapy is prevalent, as it is in India, or if nonantimonial therapy would be advantageous for other reasons (e.g., toxicity profile or duration of therapy).

A major advance has been the advent of lipid formulations of amphotericin B, in which various lipids have replaced deoxycholate. These formulations, which passively target amphotericin to macrophage-rich organs, are much more costly than conventional amphotericin B (cost-prohibitive in poor countries) but are associated with less nephrotoxicity and can be given in considerably shorter courses. Other parenteral alternatives that have merit in some settings include the aminoglycoside paromomycin (identical to aminosidine; not commercially available at present), which has been used as monotherapy (in India) or as an adjunct to Sb^V, and pentamidine. As judged by clinical trials in India, miltefosine (not currently available in the United States) is the first highly effective oral agent for this infection. In the phase 3 trial, the dosage regimen for adults was 50 or 100 mg (~2.5 mg/kg) daily for 28 days. Sitamaquine, another oral agent, is also being field-tested.

VISCERAL LEISHMANIASIS IN PERSONS INFECTED WITH HIV Visceral leishmaniasis is an important opportunistic infection among persons in-

fected with HIV-1 in geographic areas in which both infections are endemic. Although most dual infections have been reported from southern Europe, where *L. infantum* (of the *L. donovani* complex) is endemic, co-infection is becoming increasingly common elsewhere. Most (95%) of the co-infected cases reported to the World Health Organization have been cases of visceral leishmaniasis. (The remaining 5% have been cases of cutaneous disease.) In patients infected with HIV, even relatively avirulent *Leishmania* strains can disseminate to the viscera. Clinical leishmaniasis in co-infected patients can represent newly acquired or reactivated infection; most co-infected patients with clinically evident leishmaniasis have fewer than 200 CD4+ T lymphocytes per microliter. The use of highly active antiretroviral therapy (HAART) decreases the incidence of clinical leishmaniasis. The diagnosis of visceral leishmaniasis should be considered for HIV-infected patients who have ever been in leishmaniasis-endemic areas and who have manifestations such as unexplained fever, organomegaly, anemia, or pancytopenia. Co-infected patients can develop unusual manifestations of visceral leishmaniasis, in part because of atypical localization of the parasite (e.g., in the gastrointestinal tract).

The diagnostic sensitivity of classic serologic methods is lower in co-infected than in immunocompetent patients (~50% vs. >90%), especially if the HIV infection preceded the leishmanial infection. However, parasitologic diagnosis by noninvasive means is easier in co-infected patients. Parasites are more commonly found in the circulating blood monocytes of these patients; the sensitivities are ~50% for a Giemsa-stained peripheral-blood smear and ~70% for culture of a buffy-coat preparation. Invasive methods of parasitologic diagnosis (e.g., microscopic examination or culture of a bone marrow aspirate) typically are highly sensitive, especially for previously untreated patients, who commonly have heavy parasite burdens.

Co-infected patients may initially respond well to standard antileishmanial therapy, albeit with more drug toxicity than is experienced by most immunocompetent persons. However, relapses are common and can occur despite the use of HAART. No standard approach to secondary prophylaxis has been established. Various drug regimens are being evaluated.

CUTANEOUS LEISHMANIASIS

Cutaneous leishmaniasis has traditionally been classified as New World (American) or Old World disease. More than 90% of the world's cases of cutaneous leishmaniasis occur in Afghanistan (Fig. 196-2), Algeria, Iran, Iraq, Saudi Arabia, Syria, Brazil, and Peru. In the Americas, the leishmaniasis-endemic area extends from southern Texas to northern Argentina; the etiologic agents typically are those of the *L. mexicana* complex and the *Viannia* subgenus (Table 196-1) but also include *L. major*–like organisms and *L. chagasi* (which is synonymous with *L. infantum*). Old World cutaneous leishmaniasis is caused by *L. tropica*, *L. major*, and *L. aethiopica* as well as by *L. infantum* and *L. donovani*.

CLINICAL MANIFESTATIONS The incubation period for clinically evident disease typically ranges from weeks to months. The first manifestation is usually a papule at the site of the sandfly bite but can be regional lymphadenopathy (sometimes bubonic) in *L. (V.) braziliensis* infection. Most skin lesions evolve from papular to nodular to ulcerative, with a central depression (which can be several centimeters in diameter) surrounded by a raised indurated border (Fig. 196-2). Some lesions persist as nodules or plaques. The skin lesions can cause considerable morbidity (Fig. 196-3). Multiple primary lesions, satellite lesions, regional adenopathy, sporotrichoid subcutaneous nodules, lesion pain or pruritus, and secondary bacterial infection are variably present. The infecting species, the location of the lesion, and the host's immune response are among the determinants of the clinical manifestations and chronicity of untreated lesions. For example, in the New World, lesions caused by *L. mexicana* tend to be smaller and less chronic than those caused by *L. (V.) braziliensis*; in the Old World, *L. major* tends to cause "wet" exudative lesions that are less chronic than

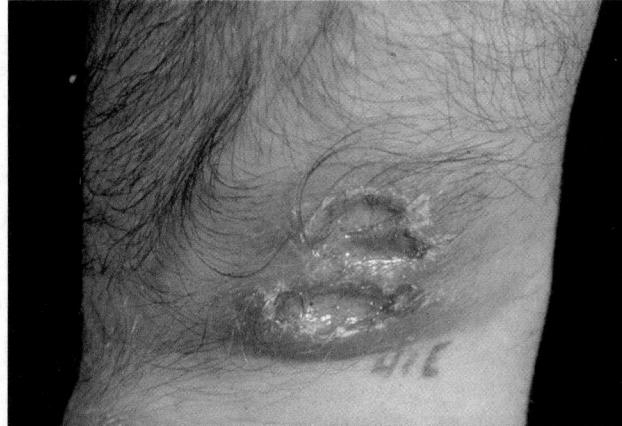

FIGURE 196-2 Ulcerative skin lesions with raised outer borders on the arm of a patient with New World (American) cutaneous leishmaniasis acquired in Costa Rica. *(Photograph courtesy of Dr. A. Wright.)*

the "dry" lesions with central crusting caused by *L. tropica*. The spontaneous resolution of lesions does not preclude reactivation or reinfection.

The polyparasitic and oligoparasitic ends of the spectrum of cutaneous leishmaniasis are respectively represented by the rare syndromes of diffuse cutaneous leishmaniasis (DCL) and leishmaniasis recidivans, both of which are notoriously difficult to treat. DCL, caused by *L. aethiopica* (Old World) or by the *L. mexicana* complex (New World), develops in the context of *Leishmania*-specific anergy and is manifested by chronic, disseminated, nonulcerative skin lesions; on histopathologic examination of specimens from these lesions, abundant parasites but few lymphocytes are noted. Leishmaniasis recidivans, a hyperergic variant with scarce parasites, is usually caused by *L. tropica* and manifested by a chronic solitary lesion on the cheek that expands slowly despite central healing.

DIAGNOSIS Although examination of histologic sections of biopsy specimens with special stains can help exclude other diagnoses (see below), amastigotes appear larger and are more easily recognizable on Giemsa-stained thin smears (e.g., smears of dermal scrapings, touch preparations of biopsy specimens). Aspirates of skin lesions and lymph nodes are useful for in vitro culture, and biopsy specimens are useful for histologic examination, culture, and PCR. As lesions age, amastigotes become scarcer, and parasitologic confirmation becomes more difficult. Species identification (see above) can be important in guiding therapy.

Serologic testing currently is an insensitive means for diagnosing cutaneous leishmaniasis; antibody titers usually are at most minimally elevated except in patients who have DCL. In contrast, leishmanin skin-test reactivity usually develops during active infection in persons who have simple cutaneous leishmaniasis or leishmaniasis recidivans but not in those who have DCL.

DIFFERENTIAL DIAGNOSIS Cutaneous leishmaniasis is frequently confused with tropical, traumatic, and venous-stasis ulcers; foreign-body reactions; superinfected insect bites; myiasis; impetigo; fungal infections (e.g., sporotrichosis); mycobacterial infections; and other diseases (e.g., sarcoidosis, neoplasms). DCL and leishmaniasis recidivans should be differentiated from lepromatous leprosy and lupus vulgaris, respectively.

℞ TREATMENT (Table 196-2)

Decisions about whether and how to treat cutaneous leishmaniasis should take into account the species, if known, and therefore whether mucosal dissemination is possible (as it is to variable degrees in the Americas with some organisms in the *Viannia* subgenus; Table 196-1) as well as the likelihood of rapid self-healing and the location (e.g., on the face), number, size, evolution, and chronicity of the cutaneous

lesions. When optimal effectiveness is important, intravenous or intramuscular Sb^V therapy is generally recommended. In studies in Colombia (predominantly with the *Viannia* subgenus), relatively short courses of treatment with pentamidine were effective (cure rate, 96%) and quite well tolerated. However, preliminary data from a clinical trial in Peru with *L. (V.) braziliensis* are not looking as promising. No controlled clinical trials have been conducted for cutaneous leishmaniasis with conventional or lipid formulations of amphotericin B. Some data suggest that conventional amphotericin B is likely to be effective. The data for the lipid formulations are too few and too conflicting for this therapy to be recommended at this time. In general, the clinical response to antileishmanial therapy begins with lessening induration; the process of healing often continues after the end of therapy. Relapse typically is manifested by clinical reactivation at the margin of the lesion.

Although many oral agents have been touted for treatment of leishmaniasis, even those that are the most effective typically are moderately active at best and are effective only against some *Leishmania* species or strains. The oral agent miltefosine is being evaluated. In the New World, ketoconazole has some activity against *L. mexicana* and *L. (V.) panamensis* and may be more active than itraconazole (at least against the *Viannia* subgenus), which is better tolerated. Fluconazole led to more rapid healing of *L. major* infection in a clinical trial in Saudi Arabia. Dapsone has looked promising in India but not in Colombia. Adjunctive immunotherapy remains highly investigational. Local or topical therapy can be considered for some cases of infection without risk for mucosal dissemination (e.g., for relatively benign lesions caused by *L. mexicana* or *L. major*). Examples of local approaches include the application of an ointment containing paromomycin and methylbenzethonium chloride (not licensed in the United States), the intralesional administration of Sb^V, heat therapy, and cryotherapy.

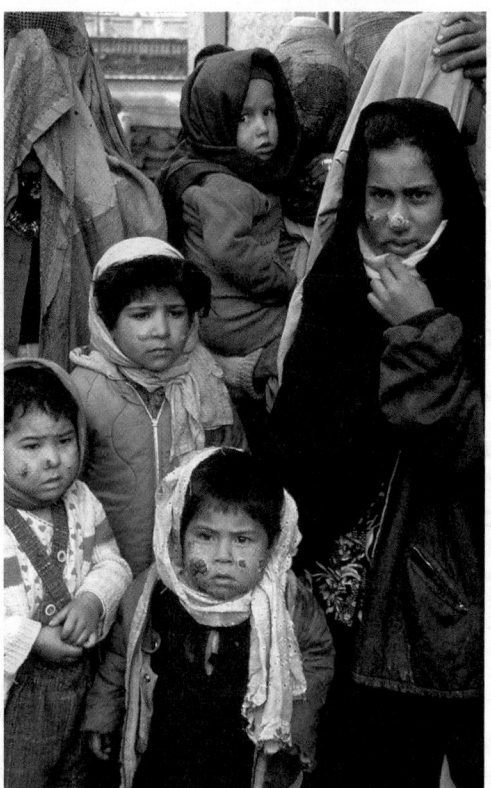

FIGURE 196-3 People in Kabul, Afghanistan, infected with *Leishmania tropica*, standing in line for hours on a bitterly cold day in February 1997 at a treatment center for cutaneous leishmaniasis. *[Photograph courtesy of Dr. R. Ashford and reprinted with permission from Elsevier Science (Lancet 354:1193, 1999).]*

MUCOSAL LEISHMANIASIS

Clinically evident leishmanial infection of the naso-oropharyngeal mucosa is a relatively rare but potentially disfiguring metastatic complication of cutaneous leishmaniasis. Mucosal disease develops despite antileishmanial cell-mediated immunity; most commonly is caused by organisms of the *Viannia* subgenus, typically *L. (V.) braziliensis* but also *L. (V.) panamensis* and occasionally *L. (V.) guyanensis*; and is more common in South America than in Central America. Although mucosal disease usually becomes clinically evident within several years after the healing of the original cutaneous lesions, cutaneous and mucosal lesions can coexist or appear decades apart; the potential for long delay is one of the reasons that the risk for mucosal leishmaniasis in particular settings is so difficult to determine. Typically, the original cutaneous lesions of patients who develop mucosal disease were not treated or were suboptimally treated.

Mucosal involvement generally is manifested first by persistent unusual nasal symptoms (e.g., epistaxis), with erythema and edema of the nasal mucosa, and then by progressive, ulcerative, naso-oropharyngeal destruction. Supportive laboratory data (e.g., a positive serologic or PCR result) are useful, but the scarcity of amastigotes makes parasitologic confirmation difficult. The differential diagnosis includes sarcoidosis, neoplasms, midline granuloma, rhinoscleroma, paracoccidioidomycosis, histoplasmosis, leprosy, syphilis, and tertiary yaws.

℞ **TREATMENT** (Table 196-2)

Treatment with a pentavalent antimonial compound is moderately ef-
fective for mild mucosal disease, whereas advanced disease may not respond to such treatment or may relapse repeatedly. Amphotericin B (deoxycholate) can also be considered first-line therapy. Conflicting and limited data have been obtained for lipid formulations of amphotericin B, which therefore are not generally recommended at this time. Patients who develop respiratory compromise after initiation of therapy (e.g., because of an inflammatory reaction) may benefit from the concomitant administration of glucocorticoids.

FURTHER READING

BERMAN JD: Human leishmaniasis: Clinical, diagnostic, and chemotherapeutic developments in the last 10 years. Clin Infect Dis 24:684, 1997

DAVIES CR et al: Leishmaniasis: New approaches to disease control. BMJ 326:377, 2003

DE LA ROSA R et al: Incidence of and risk factors for symptomatic visceral leishmaniasis among human immunodeficiency virus type 1–infected patients from Spain in the era of highly active antiretroviral therapy. J Clin Microbiol 40:762, 2002

HERWALDT BL: Leishmaniasis. Lancet 354:1191, 1999

——, BERMAN JD: Recommendations for treating leishmaniasis with sodium stibogluconate (Pentostam) and review of pertinent clinical studies. Am J Trop Med Hyg 46:296, 1992

MURRAY HW: Clinical and experimental advances in treatment of visceral leishmaniasis. Antimicrob Agents Chemother 45:2185, 2001

SUNDAR S, RAI M: Laboratory diagnosis of viseral leishmaniasis. Clin Diagn Lab Immunol 9:951, 2002

—— et al: Oral miltefosine for Indian visceral leishmaniasis. N Engl J Med 347:1739, 2002

WEIGLE K, SARAVIA NG: Natural history, clinical evolution, and the host-parasite interaction in New World cutaneous leishmaniasis. Clin Dermatol 14:433, 1996

197 TRYPANOSOMIASIS
Louis V. Kirchhoff

The genus *Trypanosoma* contains many species of protozoans. *Trypanosoma cruzi*, the cause of Chagas' disease in the Americas, and the two trypanosome subspecies that cause human African trypanosomiasis, *Trypanosoma brucei gambiense* and *T. brucei rhodesiense*, are the only members of the genus that cause disease in humans.

CHAGAS' DISEASE

DEFINITION Chagas' disease, or American trypanosomiasis, is a zoonosis caused by the protozoan parasite *T. cruzi*. Acute Chagas' disease is usually a mild febrile illness that results from initial infection with the organism. After spontaneous resolution of the acute illness, most infected persons remain for life in the indeterminate phase of chronic Chagas' disease, which is characterized by subpatent parasitemia, easily detectable antibodies to *T. cruzi*, and an absence of symptoms. In a minority of chronically infected patients, cardiac and gastrointestinal lesions develop that can result in serious morbidity and even death.

LIFE CYCLE AND TRANSMISSION *T. cruzi* is transmitted among its mammalian hosts by hematophagous triatomine insects, often called *reduviid bugs*. The insects become infected by sucking blood from animals or humans who have circulating parasites. Ingested organisms multiply in the gut of the triatomines, and infective forms are discharged with the feces at the time of subsequent blood meals. Transmission to a second vertebrate host occurs when breaks in the skin, mucous membranes, or conjunctivae become contaminated with bug feces that contain infective parasites. *T. cruzi* can also be transmitted by the transfusion of blood donated by infected persons, by organ transplantation, from mother to fetus, and in laboratory accidents.

PATHOLOGY An indurated inflammatory lesion called a *chagoma* often appears at the parasites' portal of entry. Local histologic changes include the presence of parasites within leukocytes and cells of subcu-
taneous tissues and the development of interstitial edema, lymphocytic infiltration, and reactive hyperplasia of adjacent lymph nodes. After dissemination of the organisms through the lymphatics and the bloodstream, muscles (including the myocardium) may become heavily parasitized. The characteristic pseudocysts present in sections of infected tissues are intracellular aggregates of multiplying parasites.

In the minority of persons with chronic *T. cruzi* infections who develop related clinical manifestations, the heart is the organ most commonly affected. Changes include thinning of the ventricular walls, biventricular enlargement, apical aneurysms, and mural thrombi. Widespread lymphocytic infiltration, diffuse interstitial fibrosis, and atrophy of myocardial cells are often apparent, but parasites are difficult to find in myocardial tissue. Conduction-system involvement often affects the right branch and the left anterior branch of the bundle of His. In chronic Chagas' disease of the gastrointestinal tract (megadisease), the esophagus and colon may exhibit varying degrees of dilatation. On microscopic examination, focal inflammatory lesions with lymphocytic infiltration are seen, and the number of neurons in the myenteric plexus may be markedly reduced. Accumulating experimental evidence implicates the persistence of parasites and the accompanying chronic inflammation—rather than autoimmune mechanisms—as the basis for the pathology in patients with chronic *T. cruzi* infection.

EPIDEMIOLOGY *T. cruzi* is found only in the Americas. Wild and domestic mammals harboring *T. cruzi* and infected triatomines are found in spotty distributions from the southern United States to southern Argentina. Humans become involved in the cycle of transmission when infected vectors take up residence in the primitive wood, adobe, and stone houses common in much of Latin America. Thus human *T. cruzi* infection is a health problem primarily among the poor in rural areas of Mexico and Central and South America. Most new *T. cruzi* infections in rural settings occur in children, but the incidence is unknown because most cases go undiagnosed. Historically, transfusion-associated transmission of *T. cruzi* has been a serious public health problem in many endemic countries. However, with some notable exceptions, transmission by this route has been markedly reduced as effective programs for the screening of donated blood have been implemented. Several dozen patients with HIV and chronic *T. cruzi* infections who underwent acute recrudescence of the latter have been described. These patients generally presented with *T. cruzi* brain abscesses, a manifestation of the illness that does not occur in immunocompetent persons. Currently, it is estimated that 16 to 18 million people are chronically infected with *T. cruzi* and that 45,000 deaths due to the illness occur each year. Of chronically infected persons, 10 to 30% eventually develop symptomatic cardiac lesions or gastrointestinal disease. The resulting morbidity and mortality make Chagas' disease the most important parasitic disease burden in Latin America.

In recent years, the rate of *T. cruzi* transmission has decreased markedly in several endemic countries as a result of successful programs involving vector control, blood-bank screening, and education of at-risk populations. A major program begun in 1991 in the "southern cone" nations of South America (Uruguay, Paraguay, Bolivia, Brazil, Chile, and Argentina) has provided the framework for much of this progress. Uruguay and Chile were certified transmission-free in the late 1990s, and Argentina and Brazil are expected to follow suit shortly. Similar control programs have been initiated in the countries of northern South America and in the Central American nations.

Acute Chagas' disease is rare in the United States. Five cases of autochthonous transmission and six instances of transmission by blood transfusion have been reported. *T. cruzi* was recently transmitted to three recipients of organs from a single *T. cruzi*–infected donor from Central America. In the past 30 years, more than a dozen instances of laboratory-acquired infection and imported cases of acute Chagas' disease were reported to the Centers for Disease Control and Prevention (CDC). Acute Chagas' disease has not been reported in tourists returning to the United States from Latin America. In contrast, the prevalence of chronic *T. cruzi* infections in the United States has increased considerably in recent years. Data from the 2000 census indicate that >12 million immigrants from Chagas'-endemic countries currently live in the United States, ~8 million of whom are Mexicans. The prevalence of *T. cruzi* infection in Mexico is 0.5 to 1.0%, and most of the 4 million immigrants from Chagas'-endemic nations who are not Mexicans come from countries in which the prevalence of *T. cruzi* infection is greater than it is in Mexico. The total number of *T. cruzi*–infected persons living in the United States can be estimated reasonably to be 80,000 to 120,000. The number of instances of transfusion-associated transmission in this country is likely to be considerably greater than the number reported.

CLINICAL COURSE   The first signs of acute Chagas' disease develop at least 1 week after invasion by the parasites. When the organisms enter through a break in the skin, an indurated area of erythema and swelling (the chagoma), accompanied by local lymphadenopathy, may appear. *Romaña's sign*—the classic finding in acute Chagas' disease, which consists of unilateral painless edema of the palpebrae and periocular tissues—can result when the conjunctiva is the portal of entry (Fig. 197-1). These initial local signs may be followed by malaise, fever, anorexia, and edema of the face and lower extremities. A morbilliform rash may also appear. Generalized lymphadenopathy and hepatosplenomegaly may develop. Severe myocarditis develops rarely; most deaths in acute Chagas' disease are due to heart failure. Neurologic signs are not common, but meningoencephalitis occurs occasionally. The acute symptoms resolve spontaneously in virtually all patients, who then enter the asymptomatic or indeterminate phase of chronic *T. cruzi* infection.

Symptomatic chronic Chagas' disease becomes apparent years or even decades after the initial infection. The heart is commonly involved, and symptoms are caused by rhythm disturbances, dilated cardiomyopathy, and thromboembolism. Right bundle-branch block is a common electrocardiographic abnormality, but other types of atrioventricular block, premature ventricular contractions, and tachy- and bradyarrhythmias occur frequently. Cardiomyopathy often results in right-sided or biventricular heart failure. Embolization of mural

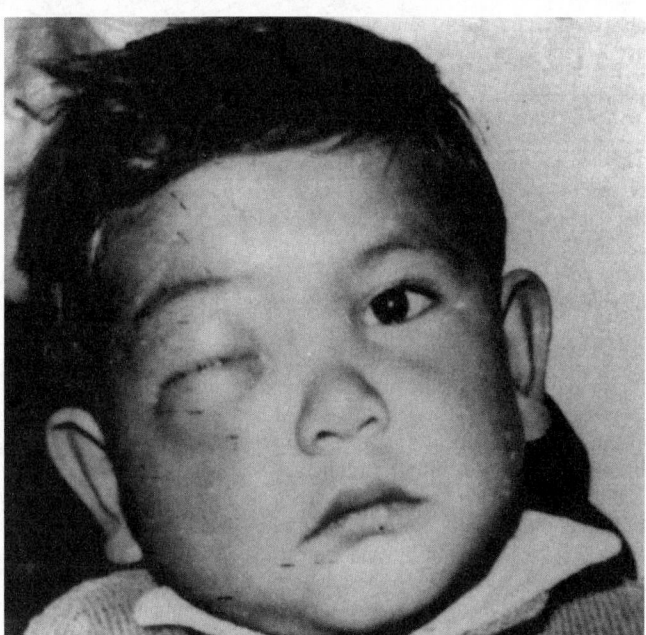

FIGURE 197-1   Romaña's sign in an Argentinean patient with acute *T. cruzi* infection. (*Courtesy of Dr. Humberto Lugones, Centro de Chagas, Santiago del Estero, Argentina.*)

thrombi to the brain or other areas may take place. Patients with megaesophagus suffer from dysphagia, odynophagia, chest pain, and regurgitation. Aspiration can occur (especially during sleep) in patients with severe esophageal dysfunction, and repeated episodes of aspiration pneumonitis are common. Weight loss, cachexia, and pulmonary infection can result in death. Patients with megacolon are plagued by abdominal pain and chronic constipation, and advanced megacolon can cause obstruction, volvulus, septicemia, and death.

DIAGNOSIS   The diagnosis of acute Chagas' disease requires the detection of parasites. Microscopic examination of fresh anticoagulated blood or of the buffy coat is the simplest way to see the motile organisms. Parasites also can be seen in Giemsa-stained thin and thick blood smears. Microhematocrit tubes containing acridine orange as a stain can be used for the same purpose. When repeated attempts to visualize the organisms are unsuccessful, polymerase chain reaction (PCR) or hemoculture in specialized media can be performed. When used by experienced personnel, all of these methods yield positive results in a high proportion of patients with acute Chagas' disease. Hemoculture has the disadvantage of taking several weeks to give positive results. Serologic testing plays no role in diagnosing acute Chagas' disease.

Chronic Chagas' disease is diagnosed by the detection of specific antibodies that bind to *T. cruzi* antigens. Demonstration of the parasite is not of primary importance. In Latin America, ~20 assays are commercially available, including several based on recombinant antigens. Unfortunately, these tests have varying levels of sensitivity and specificity, and false-positive reactions are a particular problem—typically with samples from patients who have other infectious and parasitic diseases or autoimmune disorders. In addition, confirmatory testing has presented a persistent challenge. For these reasons, it is generally recommended that specimens be tested in at least two assays and that well-characterized positive and negative comparison samples be included in each run. A highly sensitive and specific confirmatory method for detecting antibodies to *T. cruzi* [approved under the Clinical Laboratory Improvement Amendment (CLIA) and available in the author's laboratory] employs immunoprecipitation of radiolabeled *T. cruzi* antigens and electrophoresis. The use of PCR assays to detect *T. cruzi* DNA in chronically infected persons has been studied extensively. The sensitivity of this approach has not been shown to be reliably greater than that of serology, and no PCR assays are commercially available.

℞ TREATMENT

Therapy for Chagas' disease is unsatisfactory. For many years, only two drugs—nifurtimox and benznidazole—have been available for this purpose. Unfortunately, both drugs lack efficacy and often cause severe side effects.

In acute Chagas' disease, nifurtimox markedly reduces the duration of symptoms and parasitemia and decreases the mortality rate. Nevertheless, limited studies have shown that only ~70% of acute infections are cured parasitologically by a full course of treatment. Despite its limitations, treatment with nifurtimox should be initiated as early as possible in acute Chagas' disease. Moreover, when laboratory accidents occur in which it appears likely that *T. cruzi* infection could become established, nifurtimox therapy should be initiated without waiting for clinical or parasitologic indications of infection.

Common adverse effects of nifurtimox include abdominal pain, anorexia, nausea, vomiting, and weight loss. Neurologic reactions to the drug may include restlessness, disorientation, insomnia, twitching, paresthesia, polyneuritis, and seizures. These symptoms usually disappear when the dosage is reduced or treatment is discontinued. The recommended daily dosage is 8 to 10 mg/kg for adults, 12.5 to 15 mg/kg for adolescents, and 15 to 20 mg/kg for children 1 to 10 years of age. The drug should be given orally in four divided doses each day, and therapy should be continued for 90 to 120 days. Nifurtimox is available from the Drug Service of the CDC in Atlanta (telephone number, 770-639-3670).

The efficacy of benznidazole is similar to that of nifurtimox; a cure rate of 90% among congenitally infected infants treated before their first birthday has been reported. Adverse effects include peripheral neuropathy, rash, and granulocytopenia. The recommended oral dosage is 5 mg/kg per day for 60 days. Benznidazole is generally considered the drug of choice in Latin America.

The question of whether patients in the indeterminate or chronic symptomatic phase of Chagas' disease should be treated with nifurtimox or benznidazole has been debated for years. The fact that parasitologic cure rates in chronically infected persons are <20% is central to this controversy. Limited studies of *T. cruzi*–infected laboratory animals and humans suggest that elimination of the parasites reduces the appearance or progression of cardiac pathology. In view of these findings, an international panel of experts recommended that all patients infected with *T. cruzi* be treated with one drug or the other, regardless of their clinical status or the duration of infection. Considerable debate has followed this recommendation, and the issue remains unresolved.

The usefulness of allopurinol, fluconazole, and itraconazole for the treatment of acute Chagas' disease has been studied in laboratory animals and to a lesser extent in humans. None of these drugs has exhibited a level of anti–*T. cruzi* activity that warrants its use in patients. Several newer antifungal azoles have shown promise in animal studies but have not yet been tested in humans. Studies in mice have shown that recombinant interferon γ decreases the duration and severity of acute *T. cruzi* infection; however, its usefulness in persons with acute Chagas' disease has not been evaluated systematically.

Patients who develop cardiac and/or gastrointestinal disease in association with *T. cruzi* infection should be referred to appropriate subspecialists for further evaluation and treatment. Cardiac transplantation is an option for patients with end-stage chagasic cardiopathies, and >100 such transplantations have been done in Brazil and the United States. The survival rate among Chagas' disease cardiac transplant recipients is higher than that among persons receiving cardiac transplants for other reasons. This better outcome may be due to the fact that lesions are limited to the heart in most patients with symptomatic chronic Chagas' disease.

PREVENTION Since drug therapy is unsatisfactory and vaccines are not available, the control of *T. cruzi* transmission in endemic countries must depend on reduction of domiciliary vector populations by spraying of insecticides, improvements in housing, and education of at-risk persons. As noted above, these measures, coupled with serologic screening of blood donors, have markedly reduced transmission of the parasite in many endemic countries. Tourists would be wise to avoid sleeping in dilapidated houses in rural areas in endemic countries. Mosquito nets and insect repellent provide additional protection.

The question of whether blood donated in the United States should be screened for antibodies to *T. cruzi* has been considered by both public and private blood banking authorities for more than a decade. Since no assay for this purpose has been cleared by the U.S. Food and Drug Administration (FDA), serologic testing is not yet an option. Some blood-donor centers currently use a questionnaire to identify and defer donors at high risk for *T. cruzi* infection. The efficacy of this approach has not been assessed specifically, and it is important to bear in mind that approaches based solely on questionnaires have not been entirely successful at eliminating transfusion-associated transmission of other infectious agents.

In view of the possibly serious consequences of chronic *T. cruzi* infection, it would be prudent for all immigrants from endemic regions living in the United States to be tested for evidence of infection. Identification of persons harboring the parasite would permit periodic electrocardiographic monitoring, which can be important because pacemakers benefit some patients who develop ominous rhythm disturbances. The possibility of congenital transmission is yet another justification for screening.

Laboratory personnel should wear gloves and eye protection when working with *T. cruzi* and infected vectors.

SLEEPING SICKNESS

DEFINITION Sleeping sickness, or human African trypanosomiasis (HAT), is caused by flagellated protozoan parasites that belong to the *T. brucei* complex and are transmitted to humans by tsetse flies. In untreated patients, the trypanosomes first cause a febrile illness that is followed months or years later by progressive neurologic impairment and death.

THE PARASITES AND THEIR TRANSMISSION The East African (*rhodesiense*) and the West African (*gambiense*) forms of sleeping sickness are caused, respectively, by two trypanosome subspecies: *T. brucei rhodesiense* and *T. brucei gambiense*. These subspecies are morphologically indistinguishable but cause illnesses that are epidemiologically and clinically distinct (Table 197-1). The parasites are transmitted by blood-sucking tsetse flies of the genus *Glossina*. The insects acquire the infection when they ingest blood from infected mammalian hosts. After many cycles of multiplication in the midgut of the vector, the

TABLE 197-1 *Comparison of West African and East African Trypanosomiases*

Point of Comparison	West African (Gambiense)	East African (Rhodesiense)
Organism	*T. b. gambiense*	*T. b. rhodesiense*
Vectors	Tsetse flies (palpalis group)	Tsetse flies (morsitans group)
Primary reservoir	Humans	Antelope and cattle
Human illness	Chronic (late CNS disease)	Acute (early CNS disease)
Duration of illness	Months to years	<9 months
Lymphadenopathy	Prominent	Minimal
Parasitemia	Low	High
Diagnosis by rodent inoculation	No	Yes
Epidemiology	Rural populations	Workers in wild areas, rural populations, tourists in game parks

Abbreviation: CNS, central nervous system.
Source: Reprinted with permission from LV Kirchhoff in GL Mandell et al (eds): *Principles and Practice of Infectious Diseases*, 5th ed. Philadelphia, Churchill Livingstone, 2000.

parasites migrate to the salivary glands. Their transmission takes place when they are inoculated into a mammalian host during a subsequent blood meal. The injected trypanosomes multiply in the blood and other extracellular spaces and evade immune destruction for long periods by undergoing antigenic variation, a process whereby the antigenic structure of their surface coat of glycoproteins changes periodically.

PATHOGENESIS AND PATHOLOGY A self-limited inflammatory lesion (trypanosomal chancre) may appear a week or so after the bite of an infected tsetse fly. A systemic febrile illness then evolves as the parasites are disseminated through the lymphatics and bloodstream. Systemic HAT without central nervous system (CNS) involvement is generally referred to as *stage I disease*. In this stage, widespread lymphadenopathy and splenomegaly reflect marked lymphocytic and histiocytic proliferation and invasion of morular cells, which are plasmacytes that may be involved in the production of IgM. Endarteritis, with perivascular infiltration of both parasites and lymphocytes, may develop in lymph nodes and spleen. Myocarditis develops frequently in patients with stage I disease and is especially common in *T. b. rhodesiense* infections.

Hematologic manifestations that accompany stage I HAT include moderate leukocytosis, thrombocytopenia, and anemia. High levels of immunoglobulins, consisting primarily of polyclonal IgM, are a constant feature, and heterophile antibodies, antibodies to DNA, and rheumatoid factor are often detected. High levels of antigen-antibody complexes may play a role in the tissue damage and increased vascular permeability that facilitate dissemination of the parasites.

Stage II disease involves invasion of the CNS. The presence of trypanosomes in perivascular areas is accompanied by intense infiltration of mononuclear cells. Abnormalities in cerebrospinal fluid (CSF) include increased pressure, elevated total protein concentration, and pleocytosis. In addition, trypanosomes are frequently found in CSF.

EPIDEMIOLOGY The trypanosomes that cause sleeping sickness are found only in Africa. Approximately 50 million persons are at risk of acquiring HAT, and tens of thousands of new cases occur every year. Precise data are not available because health statistics are often incomplete in the developing countries where HAT is endemic. Sleeping sickness has undergone a resurgence in recent years, with major epidemics in the Sudan, Ivory Coast, Chad, the Central African Republic, and several other endemic countries.

Humans are the only reservoir of *T. b. gambiense*, which occurs in widely distributed foci in tropical rain forests of Central and West Africa. *Gambiense* trypanosomiasis is primarily a problem in rural populations; tourists rarely become infected. Trypanotolerant antelope species in savanna and woodland areas of Central and East Africa are the principal reservoir of *T. b. rhodesiense*. Cattle can also be infected with *T. b. rhodesiense* and other trypanosome species but generally succumb to the infection. Since risk results for the most part from contact with tsetse flies that feed on wild animals, humans acquire *T. b. rhodesiense* infection only incidentally, usually while visiting or working in areas where infected game and vectors are present. Roughly one or two patients with HAT acquired in East African game parks (and typically caused by *T. b. rhodesiense*) are reported to the CDC each year.

CLINICAL COURSE A painful trypanosomal chancre appears in some patients at the site of inoculation of the parasite. Hematogenous and lymphatic dissemination (stage I disease) is marked by the onset of fever. Typically, bouts of high temperatures lasting several days are separated by afebrile periods. Lymphadenopathy is prominent in *T. b. gambiense* trypanosomiasis. The nodes are discrete, movable, rubbery, and nontender. Cervical nodes are often visible, and enlargement of the nodes of the posterior cervical triangle, or *Winterbottom's sign*, is a classic finding. Pruritus and maculopapular rashes are common. Inconstant findings include malaise, headache, arthralgias, weight loss, edema, hepatosplenomegaly, and tachycardia. The differential diagnosis of stage I HAT includes many diseases that are common in the tropics and are associated with fevers. HIV infection, malaria, and

typhoid fever are common in populations at risk for HAT and need to be considered.

CNS invasion (stage II disease) is characterized by the insidious development of protean neurologic manifestations that are accompanied by progressive abnormalities in the CSF. A picture of progressive indifference and daytime somnolence develops (hence the designation "sleeping sickness"), sometimes alternating with restlessness and insomnia at night. A listless gaze accompanies a loss of spontaneity, and speech may become halting and indistinct. Extrapyramidal signs may include choreiform movements, tremors, and fasciculations. Ataxia is frequent, and the patient may appear to have Parkinson's disease, with a shuffling gait, hypertonia, and tremors. In the final phase, progressive neurologic impairment ends in coma and death.

The most striking difference between the West African and East African trypanosomiases is that the latter illness tends to follow a more acute course. Typically, in tourists with *T. b. rhodesiense* disease, systemic signs of infection, such as fever, malaise, and headache, appear before the end of the trip or shortly after the return home. Persistent tachycardia unrelated to fever is common early in the course of *T. b. rhodesiense* trypanosomiasis, and death may result from arrhythmias and congestive heart failure before CNS disease develops. In general, untreated *T. b. rhodesiense* trypanosomiasis leads to death in a matter of weeks to months, often without a clear distinction between the hemolymphatic and CNS stages. In contrast, *T. b. gambiense* disease can smolder for many months or even for years.

DIAGNOSIS A definitive diagnosis of HAT requires detection of the parasite. If a chancre is present, fluid should be expressed and examined directly by light microscopy for the highly motile trypanosomes. The fluid also should be fixed and stained with Giemsa. Material obtained by needle aspiration of lymph nodes early in the illness should be examined similarly. Examination of wet preparations and Giemsa-stained thin and thick films of serial blood samples is also useful. If parasites are not seen initially in blood, efforts should be made to concentrate the organisms; the simplest method involves the use of microhematocrit tubes containing acridine orange. In these tubes the parasites are separated from blood cells by centrifugation and are easily seen under light microscopy because of the stain. Alternatively, the buffy coat from 10 to 15 mL of anticoagulated blood can be examined directly under a microscope. The likelihood of finding parasites in blood is higher in stage I than in stage II disease and in patients infected with *T. b. rhodesiense* rather than *T. b. gambiense*. Trypanosomes may also be seen in material aspirated from the bone marrow; the aspirate can be inoculated into liquid culture medium, as can blood, buffy coat, lymph node aspirates, and CSF. Finally, *T. b. rhodesiense* infection can be detected by inoculation of these specimens into mice or rats, which—when positive—results in patent parasitemias in a week or two. Although this method is highly sensitive for the detection of *T. b. rhodesiense*, it does not detect *T. b. gambiense* because of host specificity.

It is essential to examine CSF from all patients in whom HAT is suspected. Abnormalities in the CSF that may be associated with stage II disease include an increase in the CSF mononuclear cell count as well as increases in opening pressure and in levels of total protein and IgM. Trypanosomes may be seen in the sediment of centrifuged CSF. Any CSF abnormality in a patient in whom trypanosomes have been found at other sites must be viewed as pathognomonic for CNS involvement and thus must prompt specific treatment for CNS disease. In patients with CSF pleocytosis in whom parasites are not found, tuberculous meningitis and HIV-associated CNS infections such as cryptococcosis should be considered in the differential diagnosis.

A number of serologic assays are available to aid in the diagnosis of HAT, but their variable sensitivity and specificity mandate that decisions about treatment be based on demonstration of the parasite. These tests are of value for epidemiologic surveys. PCR assays for detecting African trypanosomes in humans have been developed, but none is commercially available.

℞ TREATMENT

The drugs traditionally used for treatment of HAT are suramin, pentamidine, and organic arsenicals. An addition to this list is eflornithine (difluoromethylornithine), which was approved by the FDA in November 1990 for the treatment of West African trypanosomiasis. In the United States these drugs can be obtained from the CDC. Therapy for HAT must be individualized on the basis of the infecting subspecies, the presence or absence of CNS disease, adverse reactions, and occasionally drug resistance. The choices of drugs for the treatment of HAT are summarized in Table 197-2.

Suramin is highly effective against stage I disease. However, it can cause serious adverse effects and must be administered under the close supervision of a physician. A 100- to 200-mg intravenous test dose should be administered to detect hypersensitivity. The dosage for adults is 1 g on days 1, 3, 7, 14, and 21. The regimen for children is 20 mg/kg (maximum, 1 g) on days 1, 3, 7, 14, and 21. The drug is given by slow intravenous infusion of a freshly prepared 10% aqueous solution. Approximately 1 patient in 20,000 has an immediate, severe, and potentially fatal reaction to the drug, developing nausea, vomiting, shock, and seizures. Less severe reactions include fever, photophobia, pruritus, arthralgias, and skin eruptions. Renal damage is the most common important adverse effect of suramin. Transient proteinuria often appears during treatment. A urinalysis should be done before each dose, and treatment should be discontinued if proteinuria increases or if casts and red cells appear in the sediment. Suramin should not be given to patients with renal insufficiency.

Eflornithine is highly effective for treatment of both stages of West African trypanosomiasis. In the trials on which the FDA based its approval, this agent cured >90% of 600 patients with stage II disease. The recommended treatment schedule is 400 mg/kg per day, given intravenously in four divided doses, for 2 weeks. Adverse reactions include diarrhea, anemia, thrombocytopenia, seizures, and hearing loss. The high dosage and duration of therapy required are disadvantages that make widespread use of eflornithine difficult.

Pentamidine is the alternative drug for patients with stage I HAT, although some *T. b. rhodesiense* infections are unresponsive to this agent. The dose for both adults and children is 4 mg/kg per day, given intramuscularly or intravenously, for 10 days. Frequent, immediate adverse reactions include nausea, vomiting, tachycardia, and hypotension. These reactions are usually transient and do not warrant cessation of therapy. Other adverse reactions include nephrotoxicity, abnormal liver function tests, neutropenia, rashes, hypoglycemia, and sterile abscesses.

The arsenical melarsoprol is the drug of choice for the treatment of East African trypanosomiasis with CNS involvement. Melarsoprol cures both stages of the disease and therefore is also indicated for the treatment of stage I disease in patients who fail to respond to or cannot tolerate suramin and/or pentamidine. However, because of its relatively high toxicity, melarsoprol is never the first choice for the treatment of stage I disease. The drug should be given to adults in three courses of 3 days each. The dosage is 2 to 3.6 mg/kg per day, given intravenously in three divided doses for 3 days, followed 1 week later by 3.6 mg/kg per day, also in three divided doses and for 3 days. The latter course is repeated 10 to 21 days later. In debilitated patients, suramin is administered for 2 to 4 days before therapy with melarsoprol is initiated; an 18-mg initial dose of the latter drug, followed by progressive increases to the standard dose, has been recommended. For children, a total of 18 to 25 mg/kg should be given over 1 month. An intravenous starting dose of 0.36 mg/kg should be increased gradually to a maximum of 3.6 mg/kg at 1- to 5-day intervals, for a total of 9 or 10 doses.

Melarsoprol is highly toxic and should be administered with great care. The incidence of reactive encephalopathy has been reported to be as high as 18% in some series. Clinical manifestations of reactive encephalopathy include high fever, headache, tremor, impaired speech, seizures, and even coma and death. Treatment with melarsoprol should be discontinued at the first sign of encephalopathy but may be restarted cautiously at lower doses a few days after signs have resolved. Extravasation of the drug results in intense local reactions. Vomiting, abdominal pain, nephrotoxicity, and myocardial damage can occur.

The treatment of patients with stage II East African disease who cannot tolerate melarsoprol is problematic. The combination of the arsenical tryparsamide and suramin is one possible approach, but its efficacy is limited because suramin does not penetrate the CNS well and tryparsamide is much less effective against *T. b. rhodesiense* than it is against *T. b. gambiense*. The schedule for tryparsamide therapy is 30 mg/kg (maximum, 2 g) in a single intravenous dose every 5 days for a total of 12 doses; that for suramin treatment is 10 mg/kg intravenously every 5 days, also for a total of 12 injections. Tryparsamide can cause encephalopathy, fever, vomiting, abdominal pain, rash, tinnitus, and a variety of ocular symptoms. Alternatively, eflornithine can be administered as outlined above to patients who cannot tolerate melarsoprol; however, the effectiveness of eflornithine against *T. b. rhodesiense* is variable.

PREVENTION HAT poses complex public-health and epizootic problems in Africa. Considerable progress has been made in some areas through control programs that focus on eradication of vectors and drug treatment of infected humans; however, there is no consensus on the best approach to solving the overall problem, and major epidemics continue to occur. Individuals can reduce their risk of acquiring trypanosomiasis by avoiding areas known to harbor infected insects, by wearing protective clothing, and by using insect repellent. Chemoprophylaxis is not recommended, and no vaccine is available to prevent transmission of the parasites.

FURTHER READING

BOCCHI EA, FIORELLI A: The paradox of survival results after heart transplantation for cardiomyopathy caused by *Trypanosoma cruzi*. First Guidelines Group for Heart Transplantation of the Brazilian Society of Cardiology. Ann Thorac Surg 71:1833, 2001

HUTCHINSON OC et al: Lessons learned from the emergence of a new *Trypanosoma brucei rhodesiense* sleeping sickness focus in Uganda. Lancet Infect Dis 3:42, 2003

JELINEK T et al: Cluster of African trypanosomiasis in travelers to Tanzanian national parks. Emerg Infect Dis 8:634, 2002

KIERSZENBAUM F: Views on the autoimmunity hypothesis for Chagas' disease pathogenesis. FEMS Immunol Med Microbiol 37:1, 2003

KIRCHHOFF LV et al: Transfusion-associated Chagas' disease (American trypanosomiasis) in Mexico: Implications for transfusion medicine in the United States. Submitted 2004

SARTORI AM et al: Exacerbation of HIV viral load simultaneous with asymptomatic reactivation of chronic Chagas' disease. Am J Trop Med Hyg 67: 521, 2002

TABLE 197-2 *Treatment of Human African Trypanosomiases*[a]

Causative Organism	Clinical Stage	
	I (Normal CSF)	II (Abnormal CSF)
T. brucei gambiense (West African)	Suramin or eflornithine Alternative: Pentamidine	Eflornithine Alternative: Tryparsamide plus suramin
T. brucei rhodesiense (East African)	Suramin Alternative: Pentamidine	Melarsoprol

[a] For doses and duration, see text.
Note: CSF, cerebrospinal fluid.

DEFINITION Toxoplasmosis is the disease caused by infection with the obligate intracellular parasite *Toxoplasma gondii*. Acute infection acquired after birth may be asymptomatic but frequently results in the chronic persistence of cysts within the tissues of the host. Both acute and chronic toxoplasmosis are conditions in which the parasite is responsible for the development of clinically evident disease, including lymphadenopathy, encephalitis, myocarditis, and pneumonitis. Congenital toxoplasmosis is an infection of newborns that results from the transplacental passage of parasites from an infected mother to the fetus. These infants usually are asymptomatic at birth but later manifest a wide range of signs and symptoms, including chorioretinitis, strabismus, epilepsy, and psychomotor retardation.

ETIOLOGY *T. gondii* is an intracellular coccidian that infects both birds and mammals. There are two distinct stages in the life cycle of *T. gondii*: the nonfeline and feline stages (Fig. 198-1). In the nonfeline stage, tissue cysts that contain bradyzoites or sporulated oocysts are ingested by an intermediate host (e.g., a human, mouse, sheep, or pig). The cyst is rapidly digested by the acidic-pH gastric secretions. Bradyzoites or sporozoites are released, enter the small-intestinal epithelium, and transform into rapidly dividing tachyzoites. The tachyzoites can infect and replicate in all mammalian cells except red blood cells. Once attached to the host cell, the parasite penetrates the cell and forms a parasitophorous vacuole within which it divides. Parasite replication continues until the number of parasites within the cell approaches a

critical mass and the cell ruptures, releasing parasites that infect adjoining cells.

As a result of this process, an infected organ soon shows evidence of cytopathology. Most tachyzoites are eliminated by means of the host's humoral and cell-mediated immune responses. Tissue cysts containing many bradyzoites develop 7 to 10 days after the systemic tachyzoite infection. These tissue cysts occur in a variety of host organs but persist principally within the central nervous system (CNS) and muscle. The development of this chronic stage completes the nonfeline portion of the life cycle. Active infection in the immunocompromised host is most likely due to the spontaneous release of encysted parasites that undergo rapid transformation into tachyzoites within the CNS.

The principal stage in the life cycle of the parasite takes place in the cat (the definitive host) and its prey. The parasite's sexual phase is defined by the formation of oocysts within the feline host. This enteroepithelial cycle begins with the ingestion of the bradyzoite tissue cysts and culminates after several intermediate stages in the production of gametes. Gamete fusion produces a zygote, which envelops itself in a rigid wall and is secreted in the feces as an unsporulated oocyst. After 2 to 3 days of exposure to air at ambient temperature, the noninfectious oocyst sporulates to produce eight sporozoite progeny. The sporulated oocyst can be ingested by an intermediate host, such as a person emptying a cat's litter box, a pig rummaging in a barnyard, or perhaps a mouse. It is in the intermediate host that the parasite completes its life cycle.

EPIDEMIOLOGY *T. gondii* infects a wide range of mammals and birds. Its seroprevalence depends on the locale and the age of the population. Generally, hot arid climatic conditions are associated with a low prevalence of infection. In the United States and most European countries, the prevalence of seroconversion increases with age and exposure. For example, in the United States, 5 to 30% of individuals 10 to 19 years old and 10 to 67% of those over the age of 50 years show serologic evidence of exposure; seroprevalence increases by ~1% per year. In Central America, France, Turkey, and Brazil, the seroprevalence is higher. There may be as many as 2100 cases of toxoplasmic encephalitis each year in the United States.

TRANSMISSION ■ **Oral Transmission** The principal source of human *Toxoplasma* infection remains uncertain. Transmission usually takes place by the oral route and can be attributable to ingestion of either sporulated oocysts from contaminated soil or bradyzoites from undercooked meat. During acute feline infection, a cat may excrete as many as 100 million parasites per day. These very stable sporozoite-containing oocysts are highly infectious and may remain viable for many years in the soil. Humans infected during a well-documented outbreak of oocyst-transmitted infection develop stage-specific antibodies to the oocyst/sporozoite.

Children and adults also can acquire infection from tissue cysts containing bradyzoites. The ingestion of a single cyst is all that is required for human infection. Undercooking or insufficient freezing of meat is an important source of infection in the developed world. In the United States, 10 to 20% of lamb products and 25 to 35% of pork products show evidence of cysts that contain bradyzoites. The incidence in beef is much lower—perhaps as low as 1%. Direct ingestion of bradyzoite cysts in these various meat products leads to acute infection.

Transmission via Blood or Organs In addition to oral transmission, direct transmission of the parasite by blood or organ products during transplantation takes place at a low rate. Viable parasites can be cultured from refrigerated anticoagulated blood, which may be a source of infection in individuals receiving blood transfusions. *T. gondii* infection also has been reported in kidney and heart transplant recipients who were uninfected before transplantation.

Transplacental Transmission About one-third of all women who acquire infection with *T. gondii* during pregnancy transmit the parasite to the

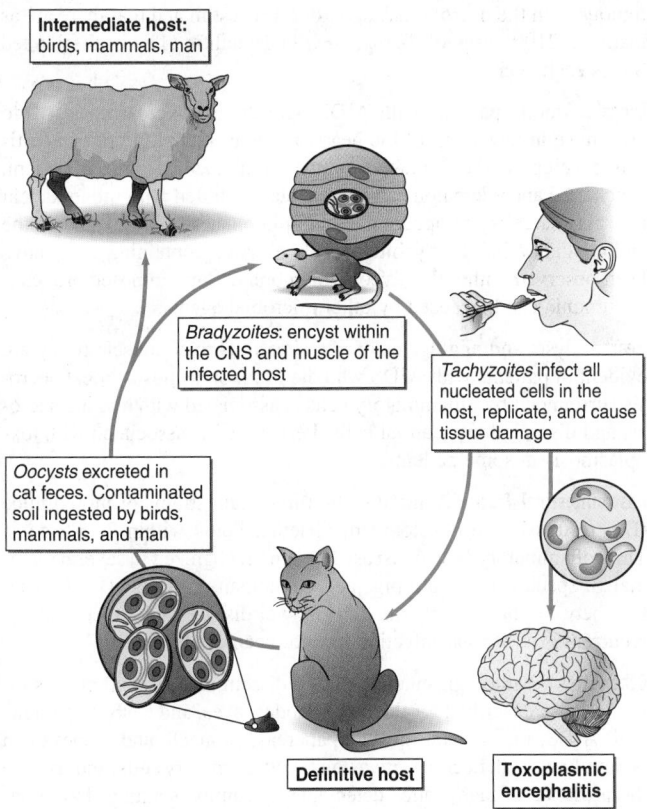

Intermediate host: birds, mammals, man

Bradyzoites: encyst within the CNS and muscle of the infected host

Tachyzoites infect all nucleated cells in the host, replicate, and cause tissue damage

Oocysts excreted in cat feces. Contaminated soil ingested by birds, mammals, and man

Definitive host

Toxoplasmic encephalitis

FIGURE 198-1 Life cycle of *Toxoplasma gondii*. The cat is the definitive host in which the sexual phase of the cycle is completed. Oocysts shed in cat feces can infect a wide range of animals, including birds, rodents, grazing domestic animals, and humans. The bradyzoites found in the muscle of food animals may infect humans who eat insufficiently cooked meat products, particularly lamb and pork. Although human disease can take many forms, congenital infection and encephalitis from reactivation of latent infection in the brains of immunosuppressed persons are the most important manifestations. CNS, central nervous system. (*Courtesy of Dominique Buzoni-Gatel, Institut Pasteur, Paris.*)

fetus; the remainder give birth to normal, uninfected babies. Of the various factors that influence fetal outcome, gestational age at the time of infection is the most critical (see below). Few data support a role for recrudescent maternal infection as the source of congenital disease. Thus, women who are seropositive before pregnancy usually are protected against acute infection and do not give birth to congenitally infected neonates.

The following general guidelines can be used to evaluate congenital infection. There is essentially no risk if the mother becomes infected ≥6 months before conception. If infection is acquired <6 months before conception, the likelihood of transplacental infection increases as the interval between infection and conception decreases. In pregnancy, if the mother becomes infected during the first trimester, the incidence of transplacental infection is lowest (~15%), but the disease in the neonate is most severe. If maternal infection occurs during the third trimester, the incidence of transplacental infection is greatest (65%), but the infant is usually asymptomatic at birth. Infected infants who are normal at birth may have a higher incidence of learning disabilities and chronic neurologic sequelae than uninfected children. Only a small proportion (20%) of women infected with *T. gondii* develop clinical signs of infection. Often the diagnosis is first appreciated when routine postconception serologic tests show evidence of specific antibody.

PATHOGENESIS Upon the host's ingestion of either tissue cysts containing bradyzoites or oocysts containing sporozoites, the parasites are released from the cysts by a digestive process. Bradyzoites are resistant to the effect of pepsin and invade the host's gastrointestinal tract. Within enterocytes (or other gut-associated cells), the parasites undergo morphologic transformation, giving rise to invasive tachyzoites. These tachyzoites induce a parasite-specific secretory IgA response. From the gastrointestinal tract, parasites are disseminated to a variety of organs, particularly lymphatic tissue, skeletal muscle, myocardium, retina, placenta, and the CNS. At these sites, the parasite infects host cells, replicates, and invades the adjoining cells. In this fashion, the hallmarks of the infection develop: cell death and focal necrosis surrounded by an acute inflammatory response.

In the normal immune host, both the humoral and the cellular immune responses control infection; parasite virulence and tissue tropism may be strain specific. Tachyzoites are sequestered by a variety of immune mechanisms, including induction of parasiticidal antibody, activation of macrophages with radical intermediates, production of interferon γ (IFN-γ), and stimulation of cytotoxic T lymphocytes of the CD8+ phenotype. These antigen-specific lymphocytes are capable of killing both extracellular parasites and target cells infected with parasites. As tachyzoites are cleared from the acutely infected host, tissue cysts containing bradyzoites begin to appear, usually within the CNS and the retina. In the immunocompromised or fetal host, the immune factors necessary to control the spread of tachyzoite infection are lacking. This altered immune state allows the persistence of tachyzoites and gives rise to the progressive focal destruction that results in organ failure (i.e., necrotizing encephalitis, pneumonia, and myocarditis).

Persistence of infection with cysts containing bradyzoites is common in the immunocompetent host. This lifelong infection usually remains subclinical. Although bradyzoites are in a slow metabolic phase, cysts do degenerate and rupture within the CNS. This degenerative process, with the development of new bradyzoite-containing cysts, is the most probable source of recrudescent infection in immunocompromised individuals and the most likely stimulus for the persistence of antibody titers in the immunocompetent host.

PATHOLOGY Cell death and focal necrosis due to replicating tachyzoites induce an intense mononuclear inflammatory response in any tissue or cell type infected. Tachyzoites rarely can be visualized by routine histopathologic staining of these inflammatory lesions. However, immunofluorescence staining with parasitic antigen-specific antibodies can reveal either the organism itself or evidence of antigen. In contrast to this inflammatory process caused by tachyzoites, bradyzoite-containing cysts cause inflammation only at the early stages of development, and even this inflammation may be a response to the presence of tachyzoite antigens. Once the cysts reach maturity, the inflammatory process can no longer be detected, and the cysts remain immunologically quiescent within the brain matrix until they rupture.

Lymph Nodes During acute infection, lymph node biopsy demonstrates characteristic findings, including follicular hyperplasia and irregular clusters of tissue macrophages with eosinophilic cytoplasm. Granulomas rarely are evident in these specimens. Although tachyzoites are not usually visible, they can be sought either by subinoculation of infected tissue into mice, with resultant disease, or by polymerase chain reaction (PCR). PCR amplification of DNA fragments representing either p30 (SAG-1) or p22 (SAG-2) surface antigen or B1 antigen is an effective and sensitive assay for establishing infection of lymph node tissue by tachyzoites.

Eyes In the eye, infiltrates of monocytes, lymphocytes, and plasma cells may produce uni- or multifocal lesions. Granulomatous lesions and chorioretinitis can be observed in the posterior chamber following acute necrotizing retinitis. Other ocular complications of infection include iridocyclitis, cataracts, and glaucoma.

Central Nervous System During CNS involvement, both focal and diffuse meningoencephalitis can be documented, with evidence of necrosis and microglial nodules. Necrotizing encephalitis in patients without AIDS is characterized by small diffuse lesions with perivascular cuffing in contiguous areas. In the AIDS population, polymorphonuclear leukocytes may be present in addition to monocytes, lymphocytes, and plasma cells. Cysts containing bradyzoites frequently are found contiguous with the necrotic tissue border. It is estimated that there are as many as 2100 cases of *Toxoplasma* encephalitis (TE) in the United States each year.

Lungs Among patients with AIDS who die of toxoplasmosis, 40 to 70% have involvement of the heart and lung. Interstitial pneumonitis can develop in the neonate and the immunocompromised patient. Thickened and edematous alveolar septa infiltrated with mononuclear and plasma cells are apparent. This inflammation may extend to the endothelial walls. Tachyzoites and bradyzoite-containing cysts have been observed within the alveolar membrane. Superimposed bronchopneumonia can be caused by other microbial agents.

Heart Cysts and aggregates of parasites in cardiac muscle tissue are evident in patients with AIDS who die of toxoplasmosis. Focal necrosis surrounded by inflammatory cells is associated with hyaline necrosis and disrupted myocardial cells. Pericarditis is associated with toxoplasmosis in some patients.

Gastrointestinal Tract Acute infection in certain strains of inbred mice (B6) results in the development of lethal ileitis within 7 to 9 days. This inflammatory bowel disease has been recognized in several mammalian species, including pigs and nonhuman primates. The association between human inflammatory bowel disease and either acute or recurrent *Toxoplasma* infection has not been established.

Other Sites Pathologic changes during disseminated infection are similar to those described for the lymph nodes, eyes, and CNS. In patients with AIDS, the skeletal muscle, pancreas, stomach, and kidneys can be involved, with necrosis, invasion by inflammatory cells, and (rarely) the presence of tachyzoites detectable by routine staining. Large necrotic lesions may cause direct tissue destruction. In addition, secondary effects from acute infection of these various organs, including pancreatitis, myositis, and glomerulonephritis, have been reported.

HOST IMMUNE RESPONSE Acute *Toxoplasma* infection evokes a cascade of protective immune responses in the normal host. *Toxoplasma* enters the host at the gut mucosal level and evokes a mucosal immune response that includes the production of antigen-specific secretory IgA. Titers of serum IgA antibody directed at p30 (SAG-1) have been shown to be a useful marker of congenital and acute toxoplasmosis. Milk-whey IgA from acutely infected mothers contains a high titer of antibody to *T. gondii* and can block infection of enterocytes in vitro. In mice, IgA intestinal secretions directed at the parasite are abundant and are associated with the induction of mucosal T cells.

Within the host, *T. gondii* rapidly induces detectable levels of both IgM and IgG serum antibodies. Monoclonal gammopathy of the IgG class can occur in congenitally infected infants. IgM levels may be increased in newborns with congenital infection. The polyclonal IgG antibodies evoked by infection are parasiticidal in vitro in the presence of serum complement and are the basis for the Sabin-

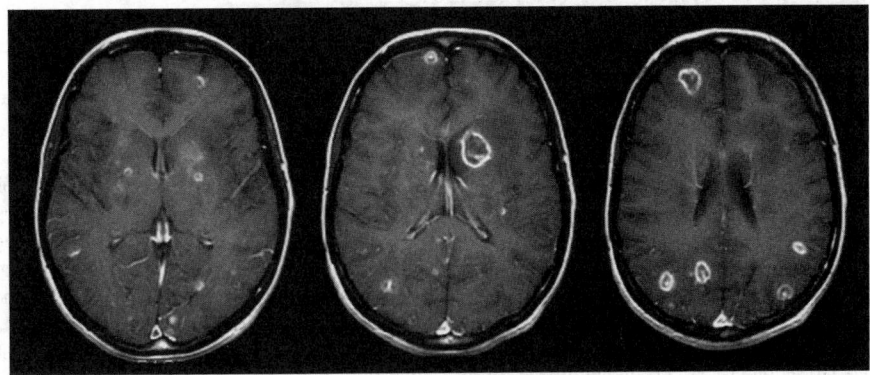

FIGURE 198-2 Toxoplasmic encephalitis in a 36-year-old patient with AIDS. The multiple lesions are demonstrated by magnetic resonance scanning (T1 weighted with gadolinium enhancement). (*Courtesy of Clifford Eskey, Dartmouth Hitchcock Medical Center, Hanover, NH.*)

Feldman dye test. However, cell-mediated immunity is the major protective response evoked by the parasite during host infection. Macrophages are activated following phagocytosis of antibody-opsonized parasites. This activation can lead to death of the parasite by either an oxygen-dependent or an oxygen-independent process. If the parasite is not phagocytosed and enters the macrophage by active penetration, it continues to replicate, and this replication may represent the mechanism for transport and dissemination to distant organs. *Toxoplasma* stimulates a robust interleukin (IL) 12 response by human dendritic cells. The requirement for costimulation via CD40/154 has been established. The CD4+ and CD8+ T cell responses are antigen-specific and further stimulate the production of a variety of important lymphokines that expand the T cell and natural killer cell repertoire. *T. gondii* is a potent inducer of a T_H1 phenotype, with IL-12 and IFN-γ playing an essential role in the control of the parasites' growth in the host. Regulation of the inflammatory response is at least partially under the control of a T_H2 response that includes the production of IL-4 and IL-10 in seropositive individuals. Both asymptomatic patients and those with active infection may show a depression in the ratio of CD4+ to CD8+ lymphocytes. This shift may be correlated with a disease syndrome but is not necessarily correlated with disease outcome. Human T cell clones of both the CD4+ and the CD8+ phenotypes are cytolytic against parasite-infected macrophages. These T cell clones produce cytokines that are "microbistatic." IL-18, IL-7, and IL-15 upregulate the production of IFN-γ and may be important during acute and chronic infection. The effect of IFN-γ may be paradoxical, with stimulation of a host downregulatory response as well.

Although in patients with AIDS *T. gondii* infection is believed to be recrudescent, determination of antibody titers is not helpful in establishing reactivation. Because of the severe depletion in CD4+ T cells, quite frequently there is no observed increase in antibody titer during exacerbation of infection. T cells from AIDS patients with reactivation of toxoplasmosis fail to secrete both IFN-γ and IL-2. This alteration in the production of these critical immune cytokines contributes to the persistence of infection. *Toxoplasma* infection frequently develops late in the course of AIDS, when the loss of T cell–dependent protective mechanisms, particularly CD8+ T cells, becomes most pronounced.

CLINICAL MANIFESTATIONS In persons whose immune systems are intact, acute toxoplasmosis is usually asymptomatic and self-limited. This condition can go unrecognized in 80 to 90% of adults and children with acquired infection. The asymptomatic nature of this infection makes diagnosis difficult in mothers infected during pregnancy. In contrast, the wide range of clinical manifestations in congenitally infected children includes severe neurologic complications such as hydrocephalus, microcephaly, mental retardation, and chorioretinitis. If prenatal infection is severe, multiorgan failure and subsequent intrauterine fetal death can occur. In children and adults, chronic infection can persist throughout life, with little consequence to the immunocompetent host.

Toxoplasmosis in Immunocompetent Patients The most common manifestation of acute toxoplasmosis is cervical lymphadenopathy. The nodes may be single or multiple, are usually nontender, are discrete, and vary in firmness. Lymphadenopathy also may be found in suboccipital, supraclavicular, inguinal, and mediastinal areas. Generalized lymphadenopathy occurs in 20 to 30% of symptomatic patients. Between 20 and 40% of patients with lymphadenopathy also have headache, malaise, fatigue, and fever [usually with a temperature of <40°C (<104°F)]. A smaller proportion of symptomatic individuals have myalgia, sore throat, abdominal pain, maculopapular rash, meningoencephalitis, and confusion. Rare complications associated with infection in the normal immune host include pneumonia, myocarditis, encephalopathy, pericarditis, and polymyositis. Symptoms associated with acute infection usually resolve within several weeks, although the lymphadenopathy may persist for some months. In one epidemic, toxoplasmosis was diagnosed correctly in only 3 of the 25 patients who consulted physicians. If toxoplasmosis is considered in the differential diagnosis, routine laboratory and serologic screening should be performed before node biopsy.

The results of routine laboratory studies are usually unremarkable except for minimal lymphocytosis, an elevated sedimentation rate, and a nominal increase in liver aminotransferases. Evaluation of cerebrospinal fluid (CSF) in cases with evidence of encephalopathy or meningoencephalitis shows an elevation of intracranial pressure, mononuclear pleocytosis (10 to 50 cells/mL), a slight increase in protein concentration, and (occasionally) an increase in the gamma globulin level. PCR amplification of the *Toxoplasma* DNA target sequence in the CSF may be beneficial. The CSF of chronically infected individuals is normal.

Infection of Immunocompromised Patients Patients with AIDS and those receiving immunosuppressive therapy for lymphoproliferative disorders are at greatest risk for developing acute toxoplasmosis. This predilection may be due either to reactivation of latent infection or to acquisition of parasites from exogenous sources such as blood or transplanted organs. In individuals with AIDS, more than 95% of cases of TE are believed to be due to recrudescent infection. In most of these cases, encephalitis develops when the CD4+ cell count falls below $100/\mu L$. In the immunocompromised individual, the disease may be rapidly fatal if untreated. Thus accurate diagnosis and initiation of appropriate therapy are necessary to prevent fulminant infection.

Toxoplasmosis is a principal opportunistic infection of the CNS in persons with AIDS. Although geographic origin may be related to frequency of infection, it has no correlation with the severity of disease in the immunocompromised host. Individuals with AIDS who are seropositive for *T. gondii* are at a very high risk for developing encephalitis. In the United States, about one-third of the 15 to 40% of adult patients with AIDS who are latently infected with the parasite develop TE.

The signs and symptoms of acute toxoplasmosis in the immunocompromised patient principally involve the CNS (Fig. 198-2). More than 50% of patients with clinical manifestations have intracerebral involvement. Clinical findings at the time of presentation range from nonfocal to focal dysfunction. CNS findings include encephalopathy, meningoencephalitis, and mass lesions. Patients may present with altered mental status (75%), fever (10 to 72%), seizures (33%), headaches (56%), and focal neurologic findings (60%), including motor deficits, cranial nerve palsies, movement disorders, dysmetria, visual-field loss, and aphasia. Patients who present with evidence of diffuse cortical dysfunction develop evidence of focal neurologic disease as the infection progresses. This altered condition is due not only to the necrotizing encephalitis caused by direct invasion of the parasite but also to secondary effects, including vasculitis, edema, and hemorrhage. The onset of infection can range from an insidious process over several weeks to an acute confusional state with fulminant focal deficits, including hemiparesis, hemiplegia, visual-field defects, localized headache, and focal seizures.

Although lesions can occur anywhere within the CNS, the areas most involved appear to be the brainstem, basal ganglia, pituitary gland, and corticomedullary junction. Brainstem involvement gives rise to a variety of neurologic dysfunctions, including cranial nerve palsy, dysmetria, and ataxia. With basal ganglionic infection, patients may develop hydrocephalus, choreiform movements, and choreoathetosis. Because *Toxoplasma* usually causes encephalitis, meningeal involvement is uncommon, and thus CSF findings may be unremarkable or may include a modest increase in cell count and in protein—but not glucose—concentration.

Cerebral toxoplasmosis needs to be differentiated from other opportunistic infections or tumors within the CNS of those afflicted with AIDS. The differential diagnosis includes herpes simplex encephalitis, cryptococcal meningitis, progressive multifocal leukoencephalopathy, and primary CNS lymphoma. Involvement of the pituitary gland can give rise to panhypopituitarism and hyponatremia from inappropriate secretion of vasopressin (antidiuretic hormone). AIDS-dementia complex may present as cognitive impairment, attention loss, and altered memory. Brain biopsy in those patients who have been treated for TE but who continue to exhibit neurologic dysfunction often fails to identify organisms.

Autopsies of patients infected with *Toxoplasma* have demonstrated the involvement of multiple organs, including the lungs, gastrointestinal tract, pancreas, skin, eyes, heart, and liver. *Toxoplasma* pneumonia can occur and can be confused with *Pneumocystis carinii* infection. Respiratory involvement usually presents as dyspnea, fever, and a nonproductive cough and may rapidly progress to acute respiratory failure with hemoptysis, metabolic acidosis, hypotension, and (occasionally) disseminated intravascular coagulation. Histopathologic studies demonstrate necrosis and a mixed cellular infiltrate. The presence of organisms is a helpful diagnostic indicator, but organisms can also be found in healthy tissue. Infection of the heart is usually asymptomatic but can be associated with cardiac tamponade or biventricular failure. Infections of the gastrointestinal tract and the liver have been documented.

Congenital Toxoplasmosis Between 400 and 4000 infants born each year in the United States are affected by congenital toxoplasmosis. Infection of the placenta leads to hematogenous infection of the fetus. As has already been stated, the proportion of fetuses that become infected increases but the clinical severity of the infection declines as gestation proceeds. Persistence of the parasite can ultimately result in reactivation and further damage decades later. Factors associated with relatively severe disabilities include delayed diagnosis and initiation of therapy, neonatal hypoxia and hypoglycemia, profound visual impairment (see "Ocular Infection," below), uncorrected hydrocephalus, and increased intracranial pressure. If treated appropriately, upwards of 70% of children have normal developmental, neurologic, and ophthalmologic findings at follow-up evaluations. Treatment for 1 year with pyrimethamine and a sulfonamide is tolerated with minimal toxicity (see "Treatment," below).

Ocular Infection Infection with *T. gondii* is estimated to cause 35% of all cases of chorioretinitis in the United States and Europe. Most ocular involvement is believed to be due to congenital infection, with a very low incidence following acquired infection. Between 1 and 3% of all patients with AIDS develop debilitating chorioretinitis due to *T. gondii*. A variety of ocular manifestations are documented, including blurred vision, scotoma, photophobia, and eye pain. Macular involvement occurs with loss of central vision, and nystagmus is secondary to poor fixation. Involvement of the extraocular muscles may lead to disorders of convergence and to strabismus. Ophthalmologic examination should be undertaken in newborns with suspected congenital infection. As the inflammation resolves, vision improves, but episodic flare-ups of chorioretinitis, which progressively destroy retinal tissue and lead to glaucoma, are common.

The ophthalmologic examination reveals yellow-white, cotton-like patches with indistinct margins of hyperemia. As the lesions age, white plaques with distinct borders and black spots within the retinal pigment become more apparent. Lesions usually are located near the posterior pole of the retina; they may be single but are more commonly multiple. Congenital lesions may be unilateral or bilateral and show evidence of massive chorioretinal degeneration with extensive fibrosis. Surrounding these areas of involvement are a normal retina and vasculature. In patients with AIDS, retinal lesions are often large, with diffuse retinal necrosis, and include both free tachyzoites and cysts containing bradyzoites. Toxoplasmic chorioretinitis may be a prodrome to the development of encephalitis.

DIAGNOSIS ■ Tissue and Body Fluids The differential diagnosis of acute toxoplasmosis can be made by appropriate culture, serologic testing, and PCR (Table 198-1). Although difficult, the isolation of *T. gondii* from blood or other body fluids can be accomplished after subinoculation of the sample into the peritoneal cavity of mice. Mice should be tested for organisms in the peritoneal fluid 6 to 10 days after inoculation. If no parasites are found in the mouse's peritoneal fluid, its anti-*Toxoplasma* serum titer can be evaluated 4 to 6 weeks after inoculation. Isolation of *T. gondii* from the patient's body fluids reflects acute infection, whereas isolation from biopsied tissue is an indication only of the presence of tissue cysts and should not be misinterpreted as evidence of acute toxoplasmosis. Persistent parasitemia in patients with latent, asymptomatic infection is rare. Histologic examination of lymph nodes may suggest the characteristic changes described above.

TABLE 198-1 *Differential Laboratory Diagnosis of Toxoplasmosis*

Clinical Setting	Alternative Diagnosis	Distinguishing Characteristics
Mononucleosis syndrome	Epstein-Barr virus	Serologic test
	Cytomegalovirus	Serologic test
	HIV	Serologic test
Congenital infection	Cytomegalovirus	Viral culture
	Herpes simplex virus	Viral culture
	Rubella virus	Viral culture/serologic test
	Syphilis	Serologic test
	Listeriosis	Bacterial culture
Retinochoroiditis in immunocompetent individual	Tuberculosis	Bacterial culture
	Syphilis	Serologic test
	Histoplasmosis	Serologic test/culture
Retinochoroiditis in AIDS	Cytomegalovirus	Viral culture/PCR
	Syphilis	Serologic test
	Herpes simplex virus	Viral culture/PCR
	Varicella-zoster virus	Viral culture/PCR
	Fungal infection	Culture
CNS lesions in AIDS	Lymphoma or metastatic tumor	Tissue biopsy
	Brain abscess	Bacterial culture
	Progressive multifocal leukoencephalopathy	PCR
	Fungal/mycobacterial infection	Biopsy and culture

Source: Adapted from Schwartzman JD: Toxoplasmosis, in *Principles and Practice of Clinical Parasitology*. Hoboken, Wiley, 2001.

Demonstration of tachyzoites in lymph nodes establishes the diagnosis of acute toxoplasmosis. Like subinoculation into mice, histologic demonstration of cysts containing bradyzoites confirms prior infection with *T. gondii* but is nondiagnostic for acute infection.

Serology The procedures just described have great diagnostic value but are limited by difficulties encountered either in the growth of parasites in vivo or in the identification of tachyzoites by histochemical methods. Serologic testing has become the routine method of diagnosis. A wide range of serologic tests that can be used to measure antibody to *T. gondii* are available commercially.

Diagnosis of acute infection with *T. gondii* can be established by detection of the simultaneous presence of IgG and IgM antibody to *Toxoplasma* in serum. The presence of circulating IgA favors the diagnosis of an acute infection. The Sabin-Feldman dye test, the indirect fluorescent antibody test, and the enzyme-linked immunosorbent assay (ELISA) all satisfactorily measure circulating IgG antibody to *Toxoplasma*. Positive IgG titers (>1:10) can be detected as early as 2 to 3 weeks after infection. These titers usually peak at 6 to 8 weeks and decline slowly to a new baseline level that persists for life. It is necessary to measure the serum IgM titer in concert with the IgG titer to better establish the time of infection. The methods currently available for this determination are the double-sandwich IgM-ELISA and the IgM-immunosorbent assay (IgM-ISAGA). Both of these assays are specific and sensitive, and their use precludes the false-positive results associated with tests for rheumatoid factor and antinuclear antibody. The double-sandwich IgA-ELISA is more sensitive than the IgM-ELISA for detecting congenital infection in the fetus and newborn.

Recently, the results obtained with PCR have suggested high sensitivity, specificity, and clinical utility in the diagnosis of TE in a resource-poor setting.

The Immunocompetent Adult or Child For the patient who presents with lymphadenopathy only, a positive IgM titer is an indication of acute infection—and an indication for therapy, if that is clinically warranted (see "Treatment," below). The serum IgM titer should be determined again in 3 weeks. An elevation in the IgG titer without an increase in the IgM titer suggests that infection is present but that it is not acute. If there is a borderline increase in either IgG or IgM, the titers should be assessed again in 3 to 4 weeks.

The Immunocompromised Host A presumptive clinical diagnosis of TE in patients with AIDS is based on clinical presentation, history of exposure as evidenced by positive serology, and radiologic evaluation. To detect latent infection with *T. gondii*, HIV-infected persons should be tested for IgG antibody to *Toxoplasma* soon after the diagnosis of HIV infection. When these criteria are used, the predictive value is as high as 80%. More than 97% of patients with AIDS and toxoplasmosis have IgG antibody to the parasite in their sera. IgM serum antibody is usually not demonstrable. Attempts to evaluate rising IgG titers or to determine whether IgM is present are not productive. Serologic evidence of infection virtually always precedes the development of TE. It is therefore important to determine the *Toxoplasma* antibody status of all patients infected with HIV. Antibody titers may range from negative to 1:1024 in patients with AIDS and TE. Fewer than 3% of patients have no demonstrable antibody to *Toxoplasma* at the time of diagnosis. Intrathecal antibody to *T. gondii* may be present; determination of the intrathecal antibody titer may be useful in identifying prior infection.

Patients with TE have focal or multifocal abnormalities demonstrable by computed tomography (CT) or magnetic resonance imaging (MRI). Neuroradiologic evaluation should include double-dose contrast CT of the head. By this test, single and frequently multiple contrast-enhancing lesions (<2 cm) may be identified. MRI usually demonstrates multiple lesions located in both hemispheres, with the basal ganglia and corticomedullary junction most commonly involved; MRI provides a more sensitive evaluation of the efficacy of therapy than does CT (Fig. 198-2). These findings are not pathognomonic of *Toxoplasma* infection since 40% of CNS lymphomas are multifocal and 50% are ring-enhancing. For both MRI and CT scans, the rate of false-

negative results is ~10%. The finding of a single lesion on an MRI scan increases the suspicion of primary CNS lymphoma (in which solitary lesions are four times more likely than in TE) and strengthens the argument for the performance of a brain biopsy. A therapeutic trial of anti-*Toxoplasma* medications is frequently used to assess the diagnosis. Treatment of presumptive TE with pyrimethamine clindamycin results in quantifiable clinical improvement in more than 50% of patients by day 3. By day 7, more than 90% of treated patients show evidence of improvement. In contrast, if patients fail to respond or have lymphoma, clinical signs and symptoms worsen by day 7. Patients in this category require brain biopsy with or without a change in therapy. This procedure can now be performed by a stereotactic CT-guided method that reduces the potential for complications. Brain biopsy for *T. gondii* identifies organisms in 50 to 75% of cases. PCR amplification of genetic material of the parasite found in the CSF may prove diagnostically beneficial in the future.

Now used in some centers, single-photon emission CT (SPECT) has been touted as a definitive means of detecting or ruling out *Toxoplasma* infection when a CNS lesion is suspected. In the future, SPECT may well be widely used for this purpose.

As in other conditions, the radiologic response may lag behind the clinical response. Resolution of lesions may take from 3 weeks to 6 months. Some patients show clinical improvement despite worsening radiographic findings.

Congenital Infection The issue of concern when a pregnant woman has evidence of recent *T. gondii* infection is obviously whether the fetus is infected. PCR of the amniotic fluid to detect the B1 gene of the parasite has replaced fetal blood sampling. Serologic diagnosis is based on the persistence of IgG antibody or a positive IgM titer after the first week of life (a time frame that excludes placental leak). The IgG determination should be repeated every 2 months. An increase in IgM beyond the first week of life is indicative of acute infection. However, up to 25% of infected newborns may be seronegative and have normal routine physical examinations. Thus assessment of the eye and the brain, with ophthalmologic testing, CSF evaluation, and radiologic studies, is important in establishing the diagnosis.

Ocular Toxoplasmosis Because of the congenital nature of ocular toxoplasmosis, the serum antibody titer may not correlate with the presence of active lesions in the fundus. In general, a positive IgG titer (measured in undiluted serum if necessary) in conjunction with typical lesions establishes the diagnosis. If lesions are atypical and the titer is in the low-positive range, the diagnosis is presumptive. The parasitic antigen-specific polyclonal IgG assay as well as the parasitic antigen-specific PCR may facilitate the diagnosis.

℞ TREATMENT

Congenital Infection Congenitally infected neonates are treated with daily oral pyrimethamine (0.5 to 1 mg/kg) and sulfadiazine (100 mg/kg) for 1 year. In addition, therapy with spiramycin (100 mg/kg per day) plus prednisone (1 mg/kg per day) has been shown to be efficacious for congenital infection.

Infection in Immunocompetent Patients Immunologically competent adults and older children who have only lymphadenopathy do not require specific therapy unless they have persistent, severe symptoms. Patients with ocular toxoplasmosis should be treated for 1 month with pyrimethamine plus either sulfadiazine or clindamycin. Prenatal antibiotic therapy can reduce the number of infants severely affected by *Toxoplasma* infection.

Infection in Immunocompromised Patients ■ *PRIMARY PROPHYLAXIS* Patients with AIDS should be treated for acute toxoplasmosis; in the immunocompromised patient, toxoplasmosis is rapidly fatal if untreated. AIDS patients who are seropositive for *T. gondii* and have a CD4+ T lymphocyte count of <100/μL should receive prophylaxis against TE. The daily dose of trimethoprim-sulfamethoxazole (TMP-SMX) recommended as the preferred regimen for *P. carinii* pneumonia (PCP) prophylaxis (one double-strength tablet) is effective against TE. If patients cannot tolerate TMP-SMX, the recommended alternative is dapsone-pyrimethamine, which is also effective against PCP. Atovaquone with or without pyrimethamine also can be considered. Prophylactic monotherapy with dapsone, pyrimethamine, azithromycin, clarithromycin, or aerosolized pentamidine is probably insufficient. AIDS patients who are seronegative for *Toxoplasma* and are not receiving prophylactic medication for PCP should be retested for IgG antibody to *Toxoplasma* if their CD4+ T cell count drops to <100/μL. If seroconversion has taken place, then the patient should be given prophylactic medication as described above.

DISCONTINUING PRIMARY PROPHYLAXIS Some current studies indicate that prophylaxis against TE can be discontinued in patients who have responded to highly active antiretroviral therapy (HAART) and whose CD4+ T lymphocyte count has been >200/μL for 3 months. Although patients with CD4+ T lymphocyte counts of <100/μL are at greatest risk for developing TE, the risk that this condition will develop when the CD4+ T lymphocyte count has increased to 100–200/μL has not been established. Thus, prophylaxis should be discontinued only when the CD4+ T cell count has increased to >200/μL. Continued prophylaxis when the CD4+ count is >200/μL has only a limited preventive effect against TE. Discontinuation of therapy reduces pill burden, potential for drug toxicity, drug interaction, selection of drug-resistant pathogens, and cost. Prophylaxis should be reintroduced if the CD4+ T lymphocyte count decreases to <100–200/μL.

Individuals who have completed initial therapy for TE should continue treatment indefinitely unless immune reconstitution, with a CD4+ T cell count of >200/μL, occurs as a consequence of HAART. Combination therapy with pyrimethamine plus sulfadiazine plus leucovorin is effective for this purpose. An alternative to sulfadiazine in this regimen is clindamycin. Unfortunately, only the combination of pyrimethamine plus sulfadiazine provides protection against PCP as well.

DISCONTINUING SECONDARY PROPHYLAXIS (CHRONIC MAINTENANCE THERAPY) Patients receiving secondary prophylaxis for TE are at low risk for recurrence when they have completed initial therapy for TE, remain asymptomatic, and have a CD4+ T lymphocyte count of >200/μL for at least 6 months after HAART. This recommendation is based on limited patient assessment and is consistent with more extensive data indicating the safety of discontinuing secondary prophylaxis for other opportunistic infections during advanced HIV disease. Discontinuation of chronic maintenance therapy among these patients appears rea-

sonable. A repeat MRI scan of the brain is recommended to determine whether discontinuing therapy is appropriate. Secondary prophylaxis should be reintroduced if the CD4+ T lymphocyte count decreases to <200/μL.

PREVENTION All HIV-infected persons, including those who lack IgG antibody to *Toxoplasma*, should be counseled regarding sources of *Toxoplasma* infection. The chances of primary infection with *Toxoplasma* can be reduced by not eating undercooked meat and by avoiding oocyst-contaminated material (i.e., a cat's litter box). Specifically, lamb, beef, and pork should be cooked to an internal temperature of 165° to 170°F; from a more practical perspective, meat cooked until it is no longer pink inside usually satisfies this requirement. Hands should be washed thoroughly after work in the garden, and all fruits and vegetables should be washed. If the patient owns a cat, the litter box should be cleaned or changed daily, preferably by an HIV-negative, nonpregnant person; alternatively, patients should wash their hands thoroughly after changing the litter box. Patients should be encouraged to keep their cats inside and not to adopt or handle stray cats. Cats should be fed only canned or dried commercial food or well-cooked table food, not raw or undercooked meats. Patients need not be advised to part with their cats or to have their cats tested for toxoplasmosis. Blood intended for transfusion into *Toxoplasma*-seronegative immunocompromised individuals should be screened for antibody to *T. gondii*. Although such serologic screening is not routinely performed, seronegative women should be screened for evidence of infection several times during pregnancy if they are exposed to environmental conditions that put them at risk for infection with *T. gondii*. HIV-positive individuals should adhere closely to these preventive measures.

FURTHER READING

DWORKIN MS et al: Risk for preventable opportunistic infections in persons with AIDS after antiretroviral therapy increases CD4+ T lymphocyte counts above prophylaxis thresholds. J Infect Dis 182:611, 2000

FOULON W et al: Treatment of toxoplasmosis during pregnancy. Am J Obstet Gynecol 180:410, 1999

FURRER H et al: Stopping primary prophylaxis in HIV-1-infected patients at high risk of *toxoplasma* encephalitis. Swiss HIV Cohort Study (letter). Lancet 355:2217, 2000

MASUR H et al: Guidelines for preventing opportunistic infections among HIV-infected persons—2002. Ann Intern Med 137:435, 2002

MUSSINI C et al: Discontinuation of primary prophylaxis for *Pneumocystis carinii* pneumonia and toxoplasmic encephalitis in human immunodeficiency virus type I–infected patients: The Changes in Opportunistic Prophylaxis Study. J Infect Dis 181:1635, 2000

VILLENA I et al: Pyrimethamine-sulfadoxine treatment of congenital toxoplasmosis. Scand J Infect Dis 30:295, 1999

199 PROTOZOAL INTESTINAL INFECTIONS AND TRICHOMONIASIS
Peter F. Weller

PROTOZOAL INFECTIONS

GIARDIASIS *Giardia lamblia* (also known as *G. intestinalis*) is a cosmopolitan protozoal parasite that inhabits the small intestines of humans and other mammals. Giardiasis is one of the most common parasitic diseases worldwide and causes both endemic and epidemic intestinal disease and diarrhea.

Life Cycle and Epidemiology (Fig. 199-1) Infection follows the ingestion of the environmentally hardy cysts, which excyst in the small intestine, releasing flagellated trophozoites (Fig. 199-2) that multiply by binary fission. *Giardia* remains a pathogen of the proximal small bowel and does not disseminate hematogenously. Trophozoites remain free in the lumen or attach to the mucosal epithelium by means of a ventral sucking disk. As a trophozoite encounters altered conditions, it forms a morphologically distinct cyst, which is the stage of the parasite usually

found in the feces. Trophozoites may be present and even predominate in loose or watery stools, but it is the resistant cyst that survives outside the body and is responsible for transmission. Cysts do not tolerate heating, desiccation, or continued exposure to feces but do remain viable for months in cold fresh water. The number of cysts excreted varies widely but can approach 10^7 per gram of stool.

Giardia infections are common in both developed and developing countries. Ingestion of as few as 10 cysts is sufficient to cause infection in humans. Because cysts are infectious when excreted or shortly thereafter, person-to-person transmission occurs where fecal hygiene is poor. Giardiasis, as a symptomatic or an asymptomatic infection, is especially prevalent in day-care centers; person-to-person spread also takes place in other institutional settings with poor fecal hygiene and during anal-oral contact. If food is contaminated with *Giardia* cysts after cooking or preparation, food-borne transmission can occur. Wa-

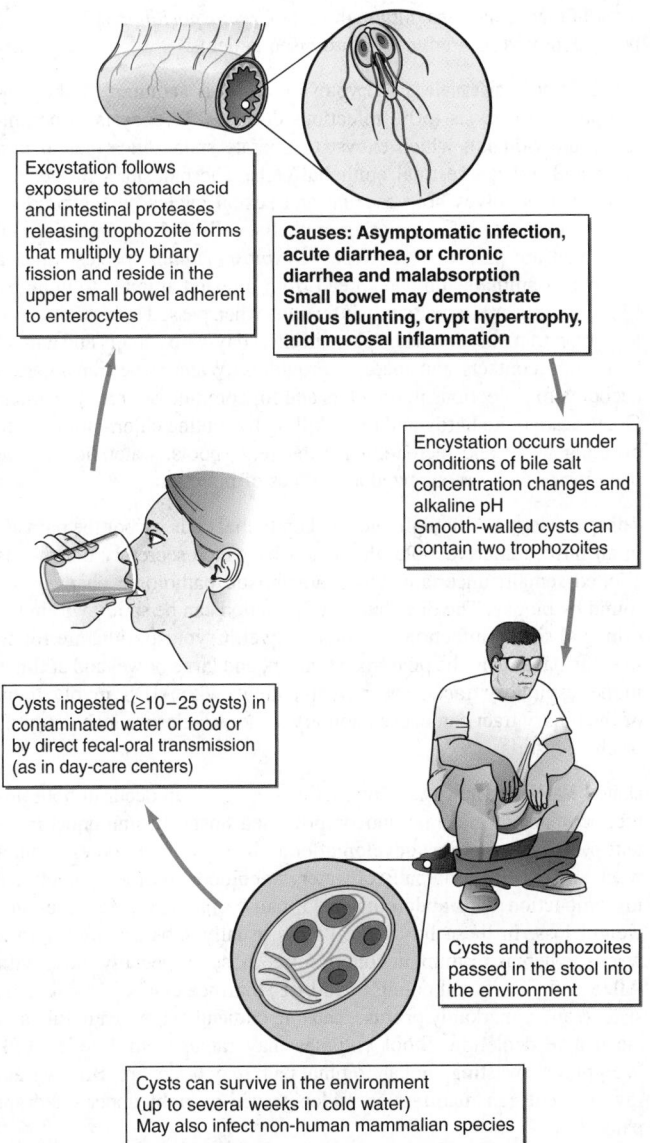

Excystation follows exposure to stomach acid and intestinal proteases releasing trophozoite forms that multiply by binary fission and reside in the upper small bowel adherent to enterocytes

Causes: Asymptomatic infection, acute diarrhea, or chronic diarrhea and malabsorption Small bowel may demonstrate villous blunting, crypt hypertrophy, and mucosal inflammation

Encystation occurs under conditions of bile salt concentration changes and alkaline pH Smooth-walled cysts can contain two trophozoites

Cysts ingested (≥10–25 cysts) in contaminated water or food or by direct fecal-oral transmission (as in day-care centers)

Cysts and trophozoites passed in the stool into the environment

Cysts can survive in the environment (up to several weeks in cold water) May also infect non-human mammalian species

FIGURE 199-1 Life cycle of *Giardia*. (*Reprinted from RL Guerrant et al: Essentials of Tropical Infectious Diseases, 2001, p 330, with permission from Elsevier Science.*)

terborne transmission accounts for episodic infections (e.g., in campers and other travelers) and for massive epidemics in metropolitan areas. Surface water, ranging from mountain streams to large municipal reservoirs, can become contaminated with fecally derived *Giardia* cysts; outmoded water systems are subject to cross-contamination from leaking sewer lines. The efficacy of water as a means of transmission is enhanced by the small infectious inoculum of *Giardia*, the prolonged

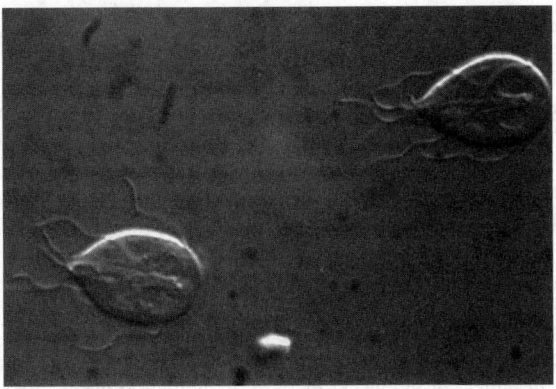

FIGURE 199-2 Flagellated, binucleate *Giardia* trophozoite.

survival of cysts in cold water, and the resistance of cysts to killing by routine chlorination methods that are adequate for controlling bacteria. Viable cysts can be eradicated from water by either boiling or filtration. In the United States, *Giardia* is a common agent identified in waterborne epidemics of gastroenteritis; it is also common in developing countries.

The importance of animal reservoirs as sources of infection for humans is unclear. *Giardia* parasites morphologically similar to those in humans are found in a large number of mammals, including beavers from reservoirs implicated in epidemics, dogs, cats, and ruminants.

Giardiasis, like cryptosporidiosis (see below), creates a significant economic burden because of the costs incurred in the installation of water filtration systems required to prevent waterborne epidemics, in the management of epidemics that involve large communities, and in the evaluation and treatment of endemic infections.

Pathophysiology The reasons that some, but not all, infected patients develop clinical manifestations and the mechanisms by which *Giardia* causes alterations in small-bowel function are largely unknown. Although trophozoites adhere to the epithelium, they do not cause invasive or locally destructive alterations. The lactose intolerance and significant malabsorption that develop in a minority of infected adults and children are clinical signs of the loss of brush border enzyme activities. In most infections the morphology of the bowel is unaltered, but in a few cases—usually in chronically infected, symptomatic patients—the histopathologic findings (including flattened villi) and the clinical manifestations resemble those of tropical sprue and gluten-sensitive enteropathy. The pathogenesis of diarrhea in giardiasis is not known.

The natural history of *Giardia* infection varies markedly. Infections may be aborted, transient, recurrent, or chronic. Parasite as well as host factors may be important in determining the course of infection and disease. Both cellular and humoral responses develop in human infections, but their precise roles in the control of infection and/or disease are unknown. Because patients with hypogammaglobulinemia commonly suffer from prolonged, severe infections that are poorly responsive to treatment, humoral immune responses appear to be important. The greater susceptibility of the young than of the old and of newly exposed persons than of chronically exposed populations also suggests that at least partial protective immunity may develop. Although no strains of the parasite that are clearly nonpathogenic have been identified, *Giardia* isolates vary genotypically, biochemically, and biologically. The marked biochemical differences among some isolates may help account for the different courses of infection in experimentally infected humans and animals.

Clinical Manifestations Disease manifestations of giardiasis range from asymptomatic carriage to fulminant diarrhea and malabsorption. Most infected persons are asymptomatic, but in epidemics the proportion of symptomatic cases may be higher. Symptoms may develop suddenly or gradually. In persons with acute giardiasis, symptoms develop after an incubation period that lasts at least 5 to 6 days and usually 1 to 3 weeks. Prominent early symptoms include diarrhea, abdominal pain, bloating, belching, flatus, nausea, and vomiting. Although diarrhea is common, upper intestinal manifestations such as nausea, vomiting, bloating, and abdominal pain may predominate. The duration of acute giardiasis is usually >1 week, although diarrhea often subsides. Individuals with chronic giardiasis may present with or without having experienced an antecedent acute symptomatic episode. Diarrhea is not necessarily prominent, but increased flatus, loose stools, sulfurous burping, and (in some instances) weight loss occur. Symptoms may be continual or episodic and can persist for years. Some persons who have relatively mild symptoms for long periods recognize the extent of their discomfort only in retrospect. Fever, the presence of blood and/or mucus in the stools, and other signs and symptoms of colitis are uncommon and suggest a different diagnosis or a concomitant illness. Symptoms tend to be intermittent yet recurring and gradually debilitating, in contrast with the acute disabling symptoms associated with many enteric bacterial infections. Because of the less severe illness and the propensity for chronic infections, patients may seek medical advice late in the course of the illness; however, disease can be severe, resulting in malabsorption, weight loss, growth retardation, dehydration, and (in rare cases) death. A number of extraintestinal manifestations have been described, such as urticaria, anterior uveitis, and arthritis; whether these are caused by giardiasis or concomitant processes is unclear.

Giardiasis can be life-threatening in patients with hypogammaglobulinemia and is typically difficult to treat and eradicate. *Giardia* infections can complicate other preexisting intestinal diseases, such as cystic fibrosis. Although *Giardia* can cause enteric illness in patients with AIDS, neither the course of infection nor the response to treatment differs for patients with and without AIDS.

Diagnosis   Giardiasis is diagnosed by the detection of parasite antigen in the feces or by the identification of cysts in the feces or of trophozoites in the feces or small intestines. Cysts are oval, measure 8 to 12 μm $\times$ 7 to 10 μm, and characteristically contain four nuclei. Trophozoites are pear-shaped, dorsally convex, flattened parasites with two nuclei and four pairs of flagella. The diagnosis is sometimes difficult to establish. Direct examination of fresh or properly preserved stools as well as concentration methods should be used. Because cyst excretion is variable and may be undetectable at times, repeated examination of stool, sampling of duodenal fluid, and biopsy of the small intestine may be required to detect the parasite. Tests for parasitic antigen in stool are at least as sensitive and specific as good microscopic examinations and are easier to perform. All of these methods occasionally yield false-negative results.

Rx TREATMENT

Cure rates with metronidazole (250 mg thrice daily for 5 days) are usually >90%. Alternatively, quinacrine (100 mg thrice daily for 5 days) is effective but is available from only a limited number of compounding pharmacies. Tinidazole, which is not available in the United States, is more effective than metronidazole or quinacrine. Furazolidone (6 mg/kg daily in four doses for 7 to 10 days) is used principally for children because it is available as a palatable elixir that is not bitter. Nitazoxanide, currently available in the United States as an oral suspension, is approved by the U.S. Food and Drug Administration (FDA) for the treatment of giardiasis in children. Paromomycin, an oral aminoglycoside that is not well absorbed, can be given to symptomatic pregnant patients, although information is limited on how effectively this agent eradicates infection.

Patients in whom initial treatment fails can be re-treated with a longer course. Almost all patients respond to therapy and are cured, although some with chronic giardiasis experience delayed resolution of symptoms after eradication of *Giardia*. Those who remain infected after repeated treatments should be evaluated for reinfection through family members, close personal contacts, and environmental sources as well as for hypogammaglobulinemia. In cases refractory to multiple treatment courses, prolonged therapy with metronidazole (750 mg thrice daily for 21 days), alone or in combination with quinacrine, has been successful. When children attending day-care centers infect an entire family, treatment of all infected family members, including asymptomatic carriers, may be required to prevent reinfection.

Prevention   Although *Giardia* is extremely infectious, disease can be prevented by the exclusive consumption of noncontaminated food and water. Cooking food adequately and boiling or filtering potentially contaminated water prevent infection.

CRYPTOSPORIDIOSIS   The coccidian parasite *Cryptosporidium* causes diarrheal disease that is self-limited in immunocompetent human hosts but can be severe in persons with AIDS or other forms of immunodeficiency. Two distinct genotypes of *Cryptosporidium parvum* cause

most human infections, although other *Cryptosporidium* species have been identified in immunocompromised patients.

Life Cycle and Epidemiology   Cryptosporidiosis is acquired by the consumption of oocysts (50% infectious dose: ~132 oocysts in nonimmune individuals), which excyst to liberate sporozoites that in turn enter and infect intestinal epithelial cells. The parasite's further development involves both asexual and sexual cycles, which produce forms capable of infecting other epithelial cells and of generating oocysts that are passed in the feces. *Cryptosporidium* species infect a number of animals and can spread from infected animals to humans. Since oocysts are immediately infectious when passed in feces, person-to-person transmission takes place in child day-care centers and among household contacts and medical providers. Waterborne transmission accounts for infections in travelers and for common-source epidemics. Oocysts are quite hardy and resist killing by routine chlorination. Both drinking water and recreational water (e.g., pools, waterslides) have been increasingly recognized as sources of infection.

Pathophysiology   Although intestinal epithelial cells harbor the parasite in an intracellular vacuole, the means by which secretory diarrhea is elicited remain uncertain. No characteristic pathologic changes are found by biopsy. The distribution of infection can be spotty within the principal site of infection, the small bowel. Cryptosporidia are found in some patients in the pharynx, stomach, and large bowel and at times in the respiratory tract. Especially in patients with AIDS, involvement of the biliary tract can cause papillary stenosis, sclerosing cholangitis, or cholecystitis.

Clinical Manifestations   Asymptomatic infections can occur in both immunocompetent and immunocompromised hosts. In immunocompetent persons, symptoms develop after an incubation period of about a week and consist principally of watery nonbloody diarrhea, sometimes in conjunction with abdominal pain, nausea, anorexia, fever, and/or weight loss. In these hosts, the illness usually subsides after 1 to 2 weeks, whereas in immunocompromised hosts, especially those with AIDS and CD4+ cell counts <100/μL, diarrhea can be chronic, persistent, and remarkably profuse, causing clinically significant fluid and electrolyte depletion. Stool volumes may range from 1 to 25 L/d. Weight loss, wasting, and abdominal pain may be severe. Biliary tract involvement can manifest as midepigastric or right upper quadrant pain.

Diagnosis   Evaluation usually starts with fecal examination for small oocysts, which are 4 to 5 μm in diameter and are smaller than the fecal stages of most other parasites. Because conventional stool examination for ova and parasites will not detect *Cryptosporidium*, specific testing must be requested. Detection is enhanced by evaluation of stools (obtained on multiple days) by several techniques, including modified acid-fast and direct immunofluorescent stains and enzyme immunoassays. Cryptosporidia also can be identified by light and electron microscopy at the apical surfaces of intestinal epithelium from biopsy specimens of the small bowel and, less frequently, the large bowel.

Rx TREATMENT

Until recently, no chemotherapeutic agents effective against *Cryptosporidium* had been identified, although paromomycin (500 to 750 mg four times daily) was thought to be partially effective for some patients infected with HIV. Nitazoxanide, currently available in the United States as an oral suspension, is FDA-approved for the treatment of cryptosporidiosis in children. In addition, improvement in immune status with antiretroviral therapy often leads to amelioration of cryptosporidiosis. Otherwise, treatment includes supportive care with replacement of fluids and electrolytes and administration of antidiarrheal agents. Biliary tract obstruction may require papillotomy or T-tube placement. Prevention requires minimizing exposure to infectious oocysts in human or animal feces. Use of submicron water filters may minimize acquisition of infection from drinking water.

ISOSPORIASIS The coccidian parasite *Isospora belli* causes human intestinal disease. Infection is acquired by the consumption of oocysts, after which the parasite invades intestinal epithelial cells and undergoes both sexual and asexual cycles of development. Oocysts excreted in stool are not immediately infectious but must undergo further maturation. Although *I. belli* infects many animals, little is known about the epidemiology or prevalence of this parasite in humans. It appears to be most common in tropical and subtropical countries. Acute infections can begin abruptly with fever, abdominal pain, and watery nonbloody diarrhea and can last for weeks or months. In patients who have AIDS or are immunocompromised for other reasons, infections often are not self-limited but rather resemble cryptosporidiosis, with chronic, profuse watery diarrhea. Eosinophilia, which is not found in other enteric protozoan infections, may be detectable. The diagnosis is usually made by detection of the large (~25-μm) oocysts in stool by modified acid-fast staining. Oocyst excretion may be low-level and intermittent; if repeated stool examinations are unrevealing, sampling of duodenal contents by aspiration or small-bowel biopsy (often with electron-microscopic examination) may be necessary.

℞ **TREATMENT**

In contrast to cryptosporidiosis, isosporiasis responds to chemotherapy. Trimethoprim-sulfamethoxazole (160/800 mg four times daily for 10 days and then three times daily for 3 weeks) has been effective; for patients intolerant of sulfonamides, pyrimethamine (50 to 75 mg/d) or ciprofloxacin (500 mg twice daily for 7 days) can be used. Relapses can occur in persons with AIDS and necessitate maintenance therapy with trimethoprim-sulfamethoxazole (160/800 mg three times a week) or combined sulfadoxine (500 mg) and pyrimethamine (25 mg) once weekly.

CYCLOSPORIASIS Coccidian parasites of the genus *Cyclospora* have been identified as the causative organisms in diarrheal illness formerly ascribed to blue-green algae or *Cyanobacteria*-like forms. This parasite is globally distributed: illness due to *Cyclospora cayetanensis* has been reported in the United States, Asia, Africa, Latin America, and Europe. The epidemiology of this parasite has not yet been fully defined, but waterborne transmission and food-borne transmission by basil and imported raspberries have been recognized. The full spectrum of illness attributable to *Cyclospora* has not been delineated. Some patients may harbor the infection without symptoms, but many with cyclosporiasis have diarrhea, flulike symptoms, and flatulence and burping. The illness can be self-limited, can wax and wane, or (in many cases) can involve prolonged diarrhea, anorexia, and upper gastrointestinal symptoms, with sustained fatigue and weight loss in some instances. Diarrheal illness may persist for longer than a month. *Cyclospora* can cause enteric illness in patients infected with HIV, albeit at an unknown frequency.

The parasite is detectable in epithelial cells of small-bowel biopsy samples and elicits secretory diarrhea by an unknown means. The absence of fecal blood and leukocytes indicates that disease due to *Cyclospora* is not caused by destruction of the small-bowel mucosa. The diagnosis can be made by detection of spherical 8- to 10-μm oocysts in the stool, although routine stool O and P examinations are not sufficient. Specific fecal examinations must be requested to detect the oocysts, which are variably acid-fast and are fluorescent when viewed with ultraviolet light microscopy. Cyclosporiasis should be considered in the differential diagnosis of prolonged diarrhea, with or without a history of travel by the patient to other countries.

℞ **TREATMENT**

Cyclosporiasis is effectively treated with trimethoprim-sulfamethoxazole (160/800 mg twice daily for 7 days). For patients intolerant of sulfonamides, ciprofloxacin (500 mg twice daily for 7 days) may be used. Patients infected with HIV, however, may experience relapses after such treatment and thus may require longer-term suppressive maintenance therapy.

MICROSPORIDIOSIS Microsporidia are obligate intracellular spore-forming protozoa that infect many animals and cause disease in humans, especially as opportunistic pathogens in AIDS. Microsporidia are members of a distinct phylum, Microspora, which contains dozens of genera and hundreds of species. The various microsporidia are differentiated by their developmental life cycles, by ultrastructural features, and by molecular taxonomy based on ribosomal RNA. The complex life cycles of the organisms result in the production of infectious spores. Currently, seven genera of microsporidia—*Encephalitozoon*, *Pleistophora*, *Nosema*, *Vittaforma*, *Trachipleistophora*, *Brachiola*, and *Enterocytozoon*—are recognized as causes of human disease; an eighth genus—*Microsporidium*, which includes organisms of uncertain taxonomic status—also causes disease in humans. Although some microsporidia are probably prevalent causes of self-limited or asymptomatic infections in immunocompetent patients, little is known of how microsporidiosis is acquired.

Microsporidiosis is most common among patients with AIDS, less common among patients with other types of immunocompromise, and rare among immunocompetent hosts. In patients with AIDS, intestinal infections with *Enterocytozoon bieneusi* and *Encephalitozoon* (formerly *Septata*) *intestinalis* are increasingly recognized to contribute to chronic diarrhea and wasting; these infections are found in 10 to 40% of patients with chronic diarrhea. Both organisms have been found in the biliary tracts of patients with cholecystitis. *E. intestinalis* may also disseminate to cause fever, diarrhea, sinusitis, cholangitis, and bronchiolitis. In patients with AIDS, *Encephalitozoon hellem* has caused superficial keratoconjunctivitis as well as sinusitis, respiratory tract disease, and disseminated infection. Myositis due to *Pleistophora* has been documented. *Nosema*, *Vittaforma*, and *Microsporidium* have caused stromal keratitis associated with trauma in immunocompetent patients.

Microsporidia are small gram-positive organisms with mature spores measuring 0.5 to 2 μm $\times$ 1 to 4 μm. Diagnosis of microsporidial infections in tissue often requires electron microscopy, although intracellular spores can be visualized by light microscopy with hematoxylin and eosin, Giemsa, or tissue Gram's stains. For the diagnosis of intestinal microsporidiosis, modified trichrome or chromotrope 2R-based staining and Uvitex 2B or calcofluor fluorescent staining reveal spores in smears of feces or duodenal aspirates. Definitive therapies for microsporidial infections remain to be established. For superficial keratoconjunctivitis due to *E. hellem*, topical therapy with fumagillin suspension has shown promise (Chap. 193). For enteric infections with *E. bieneusi* and *E. intestinalis* in HIV-infected patients, therapy with albendazole may be efficacious (Chap. 193).

OTHER INTESTINAL PROTOZOA ■ Balantidiasis *Balantidium coli* is a large ciliated protozoal parasite that can produce a spectrum of large-intestinal disease analogous to amebiasis. The parasite is widely distributed in the world. Since it infects pigs, cases in humans are more common where pigs are raised; in Muslim countries, rodents may be important carriers. Infective cysts can be transmitted from person to person and through water, but many cases are due to the ingestion of cysts derived from porcine feces in association with slaughtering, with use of pig feces for fertilizer, or with contamination of water supplies by pig feces.

Ingested cysts liberate trophozoites, which reside and replicate in the large bowel. Many patients remain asymptomatic, but some have persisting intermittent diarrhea, and a few develop more fulminant dysentery. In symptomatic individuals, the pathology in the bowel—both gross and microscopic—is similar to that seen in amebiasis, with varying degrees of mucosal invasion, focal necrosis, and ulceration. Balantidiasis, unlike amebiasis, does not spread hematogenously to other organs. The diagnosis is usually made by detection of the trophozoite stage in stool or sampled colonic tissue. Tetracycline (500 mg four times daily for 10 days) is an effective therapeutic agent.

***Blastocystis hominis* Infection** *B. hominis*, long considered a nonpathogenic yeast, is believed by some to be a protozoan capable of causing intestinal disease, although its taxonomy and inherent pathogenicity remain uncertain. Some patients who pass *B. hominis* in their stools are asymptomatic, whereas others have diarrhea and associated intestinal symptoms. Diligent evaluation reveals other potential bacterial, viral, or protozoal causes of diarrhea in some but not all patients with symptoms. Because the pathogenicity of *B. hominis* is uncertain and because therapy for *Blastocystis* infection is neither specific nor uniformly effective, patients with prominent intestinal symptoms should be fully evaluated for other infectious causes of diarrhea. If diarrheal symptoms associated with *Blastocystis* are prominent, either metronidazole (750 mg thrice daily for 10 days) or iodoquinol (650 mg thrice daily for 20 days) can be used.

Dientamoeba fragilis **Infection**   *D. fragilis* is unique among intestinal protozoa in that it has a trophozoite stage but not a cyst stage. How trophozoites survive to transmit infection is not known, but the unusually high prevalence of *D. fragilis* infection among persons with pinworm infection raises the possibility that eggs or larvae of *Enterobius* facilitate the transmission of *D. fragilis*. When symptoms develop in patients with *D. fragilis* infection, they are generally mild and include intermittent diarrhea, abdominal pain, and anorexia. The diagnosis is made by the detection of trophozoites in stool; the lability of these forms accounts for the greater yield when fecal samples are preserved immediately after collection. Since fecal excretion rates vary, examination of several samples obtained on alternate days increases the rate of detection. Iodoquinol (650 mg three times daily for 20 days), paromomycin (25 to 30 mg/kg per day in three doses for 7 days), metronidazole (500 to 750 mg three times daily for 10 days), or tetracycline (500 mg four times daily for 10 days) is appropriate for treatment.

Sarcosporidiosis   Various *Sarcocystis* species of coccidian parasites are widely distributed agents of infection in numerous animals. These parasites have an obligatory cycle of development involving two hosts. Sexual reproduction occurs in the intestine, with sporocysts passed in the feces; asexual multiplication leads to the development of muscle cysts. Humans can develop intestinal infections—although they apparently do so infrequently—by ingesting muscle-stage cysts in undercooked pork or beef. While the full spectrum of the intestinal disease is not defined, a diarrheal illness can ensue, and sporocysts are found in the stool. Alternatively, ingestion of fecally derived sporocysts can lead to the development of cysts in striated or cardiac muscle. Some patients experience muscle pain and swelling, but the frequency and nature of symptoms elicited by muscle involvement are not clear, and these cysts, measuring 100 to 325 μm, also have been found incidentally in muscle specimens. Muscle-stage infections are not followed by further spread in humans. No specific therapy exists for either intestinal or muscle-stage *Sarcocystis* infections in humans.

TRICHOMONIASIS

Various species of trichomonads can be found in the mouth (in association with periodontitis) and occasionally in the gastrointestinal tract. *Trichomonas vaginalis*—one of the most prevalent protozoal parasites in the United States—is a pathogen of the genitourinary tract and a major cause of symptomatic vaginitis.

Life Cycle and Epidemiology   *T. vaginalis* is a pear-shaped, actively motile organism that measures about 10 by 7 μm, replicates by binary fission, and inhabits the lower genital tract of females and the urethra and prostate of males. In the United States, it accounts for ~3 million infections per year in women. While the organism can survive for a few hours in moist environments and could be acquired by direct contact, person-to-person venereal transmission accounts for virtually all cases of trichomoniasis. Its prevalence is greatest among persons with multiple sexual partners and among those with other sexually transmitted diseases (Chap. 115).

Clinical Manifestations   Most men infected with *T. vaginalis* are asymptomatic, although some develop urethritis and a few have epididymitis or prostatitis. In contrast, infection in women, which has an incubation period of 5 to 28 days, is usually symptomatic and manifests with malodorous vaginal discharge (often yellow), vulvar erythema and itching, dysuria or urinary frequency (in 30 to 50% of patients), and dyspareunia. These manifestations, however, do not clearly distinguish trichomoniasis from other types of infectious vaginitis.

Diagnosis   Detection of motile trichomonads by microscopy of wet mounts of vaginal or prostatic secretions has been the conventional means of diagnosis. Although such microscopy provides an immediate diagnosis, its sensitivity for the detection of *T. vaginalis* is only ~50 to 60% in routine evaluations of vaginal secretions. Direct immunofluorescent antibody staining is more sensitive (70 to 90%) than wet-mount examinations. *T. vaginalis* can be recovered from the urethra of both males and females and is detectable in males after prostatic massage. Culture of the parasite is the most sensitive means of detection; however, the facilities for culture are not generally available, and detection of the organism takes 3 to 7 days.

R_x TREATMENT

Metronidazole is the mainstay of treatment and may be given either as a single 2-g dose or as 500 mg twice daily for 7 days. Tinidazole (a single 2-g dose or 500 mg twice daily) is also effective but is not available in the United States. All sexual partners must be treated concurrently to prevent reinfection, especially from asymptomatic males. In males with persistent symptomatic urethritis after therapy for nongonococcal urethritis, metronidazole therapy should be considered for possible trichomoniasis. Alternatives to metronidazole for treatment during pregnancy are not readily available, although use of 100-mg clotrimazole vaginal suppositories nightly for 2 weeks may cure some infections in pregnant women. Reinfection often accounts for apparent treatment failures, but strains of *T. vaginalis* exhibiting high-level resistance to metronidazole have been encountered. Treatment of these resistant infections with higher oral doses, parenteral doses, or concurrent oral and vaginal doses of metronidazole has been successful.

FURTHER READING

CHEX XM et al: Cryptosporidiosis. N Engl J Med 346:1723, 2002

FURNESS BW et al: Giardiasis surveillance—United States, 1992–1997. MMWR Surveill Summ 49(SS-07):1, 2000

GARNER TB, HILL DR: Treatment of giardiasis. Clin Microbiol Rev 14:114, 2001

HO AY et al: Outbreak of cyclosporiasis associated with imported raspberries, Philadelphia, Pennsylvania, 2000. Emerg Infect Dis 8:783, 2002

KAPLAN JE et al: Guidelines for preventing opportunistic infections among HIV-infected persons—2002. Recommendations of the U.S. Public Health Service and the Infectious Diseases Society of America, MMWR Recomm Rep 51(RR-8):1, 2002

LEE SH et al: Surveillance for waterborne-disease outbreaks—United States, 1999–2000. MMWR Surveill Summ 51(SS-8):1, 2002

NASH TE et al: Treatment of patients with refractory giardiasis. Clin Infect Dis 33:22, 2001

VERDIER RI et al: Trimethoprim-sulfamethoxazole compared with ciprofloxacin for treatment and prophylaxis of *Isospora belli* and *Cyclospora cayetanensis* infection in HIV-infected patients. A randomized, controlled trial. Ann Intern Med 132:885, 2000

200 | TRICHINELLA AND OTHER TISSUE NEMATODES
Peter F. Weller

Nematodes are elongated, symmetric roundworms. Parasitic nematodes of medical significance may be broadly classified as either predominantly intestinal or tissue nematodes. This chapter covers trichinellosis, visceral and ocular larva migrans, cutaneous larva migrans, cerebral angiostrongyliasis, and gnathostomiasis. All are zoonotic infections caused by incidental exposure to infectious nematodes. The clinical symptoms of these infections are due largely to invasive larval stages that (except in the case of *Trichinella*) do not reach maturity in humans.

TRICHINELLOSIS Trichinellosis develops after the ingestion of meat containing cysts of *Trichinella*—for example, pork or other meat from a carnivore. Although most infections are mild and asymptomatic, heavy infections can cause severe enteritis, periorbital edema, myositis, and (infrequently) death.

Life Cycle and Epidemiology Seven species of *Trichinella* are now recognized as causes of infection in humans. Two species are distributed worldwide: *T. spiralis*, which is found in a great variety of carnivorous and omnivorous animals, and *T. pseudospiralis*, which is found in mammals and birds. *T. nativa* is present in Arctic regions and infects bears; *T. nelsoni* is found in equatorial Africa, where it is common among felid predators and scavengers such as hyenas and bush pigs; and *T. britovi* is found in temperate areas of Europe and western Asia among carnivores but not among domestic swine. *T. murrelli* is present in North American game animals, and *T. papuae* is found in pigs and game animals in Papua New Guinea.

After the consumption of trichinous meat by the host, encysted larvae are liberated by digestive acid and pepsin (Fig. 200-1). The larvae invade the small-bowel mucosa and mature rapidly into adult worms. After ~1 week, female worms release newborn larvae that migrate via the circulation to striated muscle. The larvae of all species except *T. pseudospiralis* and *T. papuae* then encyst by inducing a radical transformation in the muscle cell architecture. Although host immune responses may help to expel adult worms, they have little effect on muscle-dwelling larvae.

Human trichinellosis is most often caused by the ingestion of infected pork products and thus can occur in almost any location where the meat of domestic or wild swine is eaten. Human trichinellosis also may be acquired from the meat of other animals, including dogs (in parts of Asia and Africa), horses (in Italy and France), and bears and walruses (in northern regions). Although cattle (being herbivores) are not natural hosts of *Trichinella*, beef has been implicated in outbreaks when contaminated or adulterated with trichinous pork. Laws that prohibit the feeding of uncooked garbage to pigs have greatly reduced the transmission of trichinellosis in the United States. About 40 cases of trichinellosis are reported annually in this country, but most mild cases probably remain undiagnosed. Recent U.S. outbreaks have been attributable to undercooked ethnic pork dishes, homemade and commercial sausage, wild boar meat, and walrus meat.

Pathogenesis and Clinical Features Clinical symptoms of trichinellosis arise from the successive phases of parasite enteric invasion, larval migration, and muscle encystment (Fig. 200-1). Most light infections (those with <10 larvae per gram of muscle) are asymptomatic, whereas heavy infections (which can involve >50 larvae per gram of muscle) can be life-threatening. Invasion of the gut by large numbers of parasites occasionally provokes diarrhea during the first week after infection. Abdominal pain, constipation, nausea, or vomiting also may be prominent.

Symptoms due to larval migration and muscle invasion begin to appear in the second week after infection. The migrating *Trichinella* larvae provoke a marked local and systemic hypersensitivity reaction, with fever and hypereosinophilia. Periorbital and facial edema is common, as are hemorrhages in the subconjunctivae, retina, and nail beds ("splinter" hemorrhages). A maculopapular rash, headache, cough, dyspnea, or dysphagia sometimes develops. Myocarditis with tachyarrhythmias or heart failure—and, less commonly, encephalitis or pneumonitis—may develop and accounts for most deaths of patients with trichinellosis.

Upon onset of larval encystment in muscle 2 to 3 weeks after in-

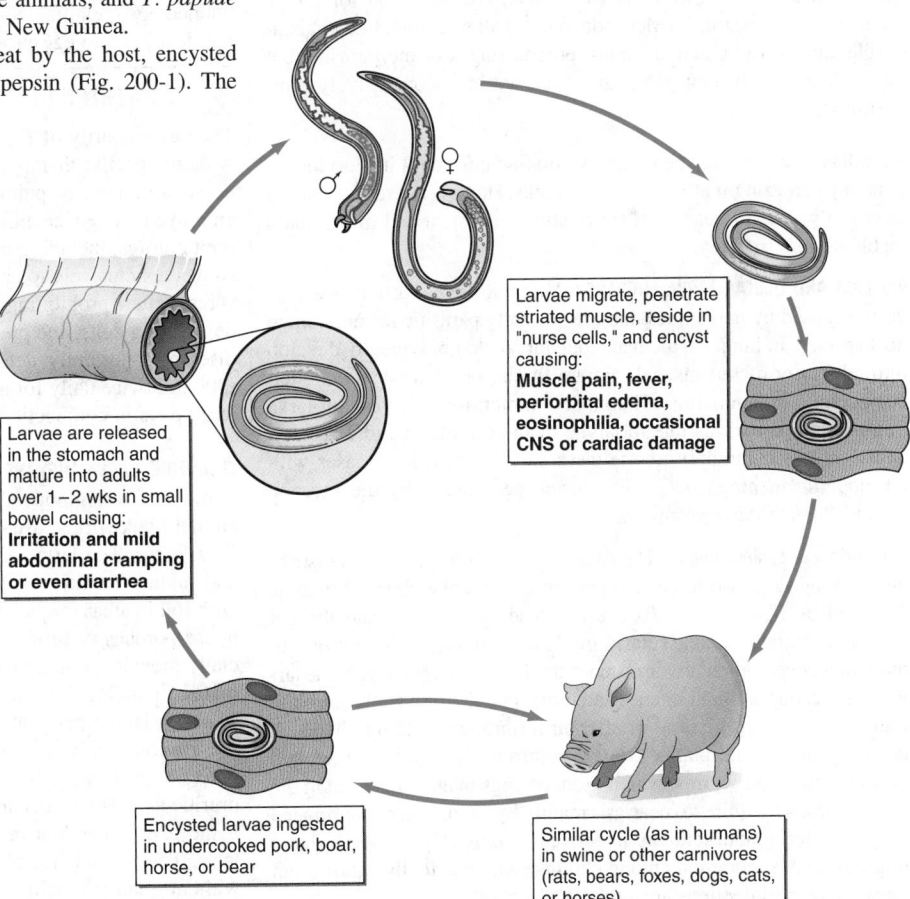

Larvae migrate, penetrate striated muscle, reside in "nurse cells," and encyst causing:
Muscle pain, fever, periorbital edema, eosinophilia, occasional CNS or cardiac damage

Larvae are released in the stomach and mature into adults over 1–2 wks in small bowel causing:
Irritation and mild abdominal cramping or even diarrhea

Encysted larvae ingested in undercooked pork, boar, horse, or bear

Similar cycle (as in humans) in swine or other carnivores (rats, bears, foxes, dogs, cats, or horses)

FIGURE 200-1 Life cycle of *Trichinella spiralis* (cosmopolitan); *nelsoni* (Africa); *britovi* (S. Europe); *nativa* (Arctic); and *pseudospiralis* (New Zealand). (*Reprinted from Guerrant RL et al: Essentials of Tropical Infectious Diseases, p 434. © 2001, with permission from Elsevier Science.*)

fection, symptoms of myositis with myalgias, muscle edema, and weakness develop, usually overlapping with the inflammatory reactions to migrating larvae. The most commonly involved muscle groups include the extraocular muscles; the biceps; and the muscles of the jaw, neck, lower back, and diaphragm. Peaking ~3 weeks after infection, symptoms subside only gradually during a prolonged convalescence.

Laboratory Findings and Diagnosis   Blood eosinophilia develops in >90% of patients with symptomatic trichinellosis and may peak at a level of >50% between 2 and 4 weeks after infection. Serum levels of IgE and muscle enzymes, including creatine phosphokinase, are elevated in most symptomatic patients. Patients should be questioned thoroughly about their consumption of pork or wild-animal meat and about illness in other individuals who ate the same meat. A presumptive clinical diagnosis can be based on fevers, eosinophilia, periorbital edema, and myalgias after a suspect meal. A rise in the titer of parasite-specific antibody, which usually does not occur until after the third week of infection, confirms the diagnosis. Alternatively, a definitive diagnosis requires surgical biopsy of at least 1 g of involved muscle; the yields are highest near tendon insertions. The fresh muscle tissue should be compressed between glass slides and examined microscopically, because larvae may be overlooked by examination of routine histopathologic sections alone.

℞ TREATMENT

Current anthelmintic drugs are ineffective against *Trichinella* larvae in muscle. Fortunately, most lightly infected patients recover uneventfully with bed rest, antipyretics, and analgesics. Glucocorticoids like prednisone (1 mg/kg daily for 5 days) are beneficial for severe myositis and myocarditis. Mebendazole and albendazole, like thiabendazole, appear to be active against enteric stages of the parasite, but their efficacy against encysted larvae has not been conclusively demonstrated.

Prevention   Larvae may be killed by cooking pork until it is no longer pink or by freezing it at −15°C for 3 weeks. However, Arctic *T. nativa* larvae in walrus or bear meat are relatively resistant and may remain viable despite freezing.

VISCERAL AND OCULAR LARVA MIGRANS   Visceral larva migrans is a syndrome caused by nematodes that are normally parasitic for nonhuman host species. In humans, the nematode larvae do not typically develop into adult worms but instead migrate through host tissues and elicit eosinophilic inflammation. The most common form of visceral larva migrans is toxocariasis due to larvae of the canine ascarid *Toxocara canis* or, less commonly, the feline ascarid *T. cati*. Rare cases with eosinophilic meningoencephalitis have been caused by the raccoon ascarid *Baylisascaris procyonis*.

Life Cycle and Epidemiology   The canine roundworm *T. canis* is distributed among dogs worldwide. Ingestion of infective eggs by dogs is followed by liberation of *Toxocara* larvae, which penetrate the gut wall and migrate intravascularly into canine tissues, where most remain in a developmentally arrested state. During pregnancy, some larvae resume migration in bitches and infect puppies prenatally (through transplacental transmission) or after birth (through suckling). Thus, in lactating bitches and puppies, larvae return to the intestinal tract and develop into adult worms, which produce eggs that are released in the feces. Humans acquire toxocariasis mainly by eating soil contaminated by puppy feces that contains infective *T. canis* eggs. Visceral larva migrans is most common among children who habitually eat dirt, but most toxocaral infections are subclinical.

Pathogenesis and Clinical Features   Clinical disease most commonly afflicts preschool children. After humans ingest *Toxocara* eggs, the larvae hatch and penetrate the intestinal mucosa, from which they are carried by the circulation to a wide variety of organs and tissues. The larvae invade the liver, lungs, central nervous system, and other sites, releasing toxic products and provoking intense local eosinophilic granulomatous responses. The degree of clinical illness depends on larval number and tissue distribution, reinfection, and host immune responses. Most light infections are asymptomatic and may be manifest only by blood eosinophilia. Characteristic symptoms of visceral larva migrans include fever, malaise, anorexia and weight loss, cough, wheezing, and rashes. Hepatosplenomegaly is common. These features are often accompanied by extraordinary peripheral eosinophilia, which may approach 90%. Uncommonly, seizures or behavioral disorders develop. Rare deaths are due to severe neurologic, pneumonic, or myocardial involvement.

The ocular form of the larva migrans syndrome occurs when *Toxocara* larvae invade the eye. An eosinophilic granulomatous mass, most commonly in the posterior pole of the retina, develops around the entrapped larva. The retinal lesion can mimic retinoblastoma in appearance, and mistaken diagnosis of the latter condition can lead to unnecessary enucleation. The spectrum of eye involvement also includes endophthalmitis, uveitis, and chorioretinitis. Unilateral visual disturbances, strabismus, and eye pain are the most common presenting symptoms. In contrast to visceral larva migrans, ocular toxocariasis usually develops in older children or young adults with no history of pica; these patients seldom have eosinophilia or visceral manifestations.

Diagnosis   In addition to eosinophilia, leukocytosis and hypergammaglobulinemia may be evident. Transient pulmonary infiltrates are apparent on chest x-rays of about half of patients with symptoms of pneumonitis. The clinical diagnosis can be confirmed by an enzyme-linked immunosorbent assay for toxocaral antibodies. Stool examination for parasite eggs, while important in the evaluation of unexplained eosinophilia, is worthless for toxocariasis, since the larvae do not develop into egg-producing adults in humans.

℞ TREATMENT

The vast majority of *Toxocara* infections are self-limited and resolve without specific therapy. In patients with severe myocardial, central nervous system, or pulmonary involvement, glucocorticoids may be employed to reduce inflammatory complications. Available anthelmintic drugs, including mebendazole, and albendazole, have not been shown conclusively to alter the course of larva migrans. Control measures include prohibiting dog excreta in public parks and playgrounds, deworming dogs, and preventing pica in children. Treatment of ocular disease is not fully defined, but the administration of albendazole (800 mg twice daily for adults; 400 mg twice daily for children) for 5 to 20 days in conjunction with glucocorticoids has been effective.

CUTANEOUS LARVA MIGRANS   Cutaneous larva migrans ("creeping eruption") is a serpiginous skin eruption caused by burrowing larvae of animal hookworms, usually the dog and cat hookworm *Ancylostoma braziliense*. The larvae hatch from eggs passed in dog and cat feces and mature in the soil. Humans become infected after skin contact with soil in areas frequented by dogs and cats, such as areas underneath house porches or scrub vegetation. Cutaneous larva migrans is especially prevalent among children and in regions with warm humid climates, including the southeastern United States.

After larvae penetrate the skin, erythematous lesions form along the tortuous tracks of their migration through the dermal-epidermal junction; the larvae advance several centimeters in a day. The intensely pruritic lesions may occur anywhere on the body and can be numerous if the patient has lain on the ground. Vesicles and bullae may form later. The animal hookworm larvae do not mature in humans and, without treatment, will die out after several weeks, with resolution of skin lesions. The diagnosis is made readily on clinical grounds, and a skin biopsy only rarely yields diagnostic parasite material. Symptoms can be alleviated by ivermectin (a single dose of 200 μg/kg) or albendazole (200 mg twice daily for 3 days).

ANGIOSTRONGYLUS CANTONENSIS INFECTION *A. cantonensis*, the rat lungworm, is the most common cause of human eosinophilic meningitis (Fig. 200-2).

Life Cycle and Epidemiology This infection occurs principally in Southeast Asia and the Pacific Basin but has spread to other areas of the world. *A. cantonensis* larvae produced by adult worms in the rat lung migrate to the gastrointestinal tract and are expelled with the feces. They develop into infective larvae in land snails and slugs. Humans acquire the infection by ingesting raw infected mollusks; vegetables contaminated by mollusk slime; or crabs, freshwater shrimp, and certain marine fish that have themselves eaten infected mollusks. The larvae then migrate to the brain.

Pathogenesis and Clinical Features The parasites eventually die in the central nervous system, but not before initiating pathologic consequences that, in heavy infections, can result in permanent neurologic sequelae or death. Migrating larvae cause proteolytic damage and marked local eosinophilic inflammation and hemorrhage, with subsequent necrosis and granuloma formation around dying worms. Clinical symptoms develop between 2 and 35 days after the ingestion of larvae. Patients usually present with an insidious or abrupt excruciating frontal, occipital, or bitemporal headache. Neck stiffness, nausea and vomiting, and paresthesias are also common. Fever, cranial and extraocular nerve palsies, seizures, paralysis, and lethargy are uncommon.

Laboratory Findings Examination of the cerebrospinal fluid is mandatory in suspected cases and usually reveals an elevated opening pressure, a white blood cell count of 150 to 2000/μL, and an eosinophilic pleocytosis of >20%. The protein concentration is usually elevated and the glucose level normal. The motile larvae of *A. cantonensis* are only rarely seen in the cerebrospinal fluid. Peripheral-blood eosinophilia may be mild. The diagnosis is generally based on the clinical presentation of eosinophilic meningitis together with a compatible epidemiologic history.

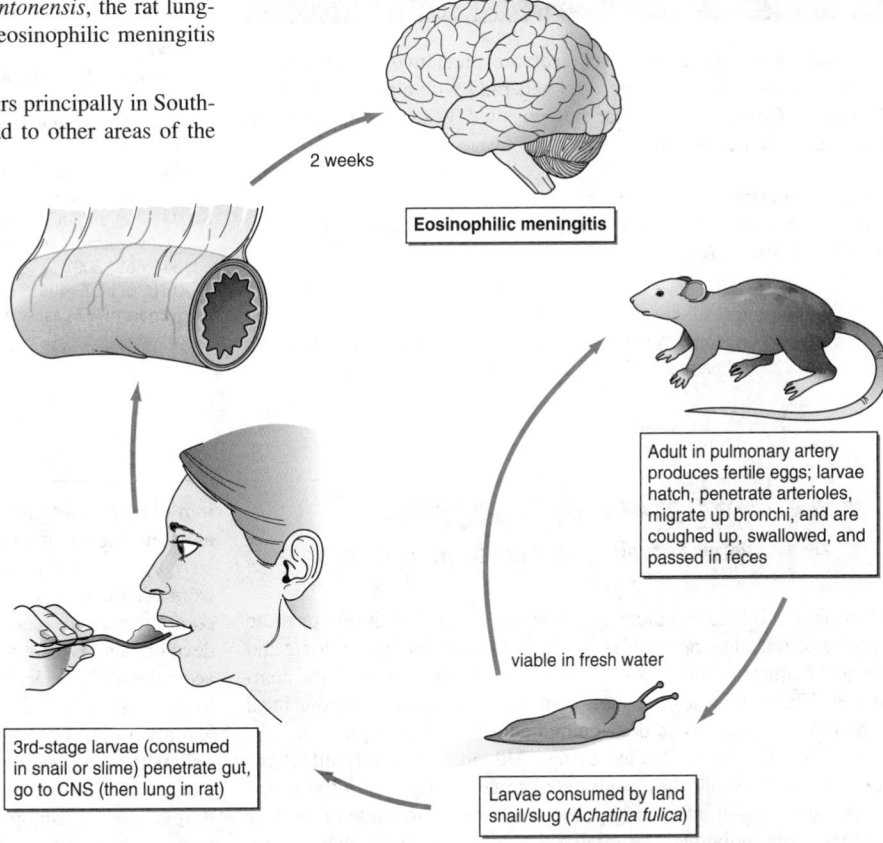

2 weeks

Eosinophilic meningitis

Adult in pulmonary artery produces fertile eggs; larvae hatch, penetrate arterioles, migrate up bronchi, and are coughed up, swallowed, and passed in feces

viable in fresh water

3rd-stage larvae (consumed in snail or slime) penetrate gut, go to CNS (then lung in rat)

Larvae consumed by land snail/slug (*Achatina fulica*)

FIGURE 200-2 Life cycle of *Angiostrongylus cantonensis* (rat lung worm). Also found in Southeast Asia, Pacific Islands, and in U.S. ports, Cuba, Australia, Japan, China, and Mauritius. *(Reprinted from Guerrant RL et al: Essentials of Tropical Infectious Diseases, p 439. © 2001, with permission from Elsevier Science.)*

℞ TREATMENT

Specific chemotherapy is not of benefit in angiostrongyliasis; larvicidal agents may actually exacerbate inflammatory brain lesions. Management consists of supportive measures, including the administration of analgesics, sedatives, and—in severe cases—glucocorticoids. In most patients, cerebral angiostrongyliasis has a self-limited course, and recovery is complete. The infection may be prevented by adequately cooking snails, crabs, and prawns and inspecting vegetables for mollusk infestation. Other parasitic or fungal causes of eosinophilic meningitis in endemic areas may include gnathostomiasis, paragonimiasis, schistosomiasis, neurocysticercosis, and coccidioidomycosis.

GNATHOSTOMIASIS Infection of human tissues with larvae of *Gnathostoma spinigerum* can cause eosinophilic meningoencephalitis, migratory cutaneous swellings, or invasive masses of the eye and visceral organs.

Life Cycle and Epidemiology Human gnathostomiasis occurs in many countries and is notably endemic in Southeast Asia and parts of China and Japan. In nature, the mature adult worms parasitize the gastrointestinal tract of dogs and cats. First-stage larvae hatch from eggs passed into water and are ingested by *Cyclops* species (water fleas). Infective third-stage larvae develop in the flesh of many animal species (including fish, frogs, eels, snakes, chickens, and ducks) that have eaten either infected *Cyclops* or another infected second intermediate host. Humans typically acquire the infection by eating raw or undercooked fish or poultry. Raw fish dishes, such as *somfak* in Thailand and *sashimi* in Japan, account for many cases of human gnathostomiasis. Some cases in Thailand result from the local practice of applying frog or snake flesh as a poultice.

Pathogenesis and Clinical Features Clinical symptoms are due to the aberrant migration of a single larva into cutaneous, visceral, neural, or ocular tissues. After invasion, larval migration may cause local inflammation, with pain, cough, or hematuria accompanied by fever and eosinophilia. Painful, itchy, migratory swellings may develop in the skin, particularly in the distal extremities or periorbital area. Cutaneous swellings usually last about a week but often recur intermittently over many years. Larval invasion of the eye can provoke a sight-threatening inflammatory response. Finally, invasion of the central nervous system results in eosinophilic meningitis with myeloencephalitis, a serious complication due to ascending larval migration along a large nerve track. Patients characteristically present with agonizing radicular pain and paresthesias in the trunk or a limb, which are followed shortly by paraplegia. Cerebral involvement, with focal hemorrhages and tissue destruction, is often fatal.

Diagnosis and Treatment Cutaneous migratory swellings with marked peripheral eosinophilia, supported by an appropriate geographic and dietary history, generally constitute an adequate basis for a clinical diagnosis of gnathostomiasis. However, patients may present with ocular or cerebrospinal involvement without antecedent cutaneous swellings. In the latter case, eosinophilic pleocytosis is demonstrable (usually along with hemorrhagic or xanthochromic cerebrospinal fluid), but worms are almost never recovered from the cerebrospinal fluid. Surgical removal of the parasite from subcutaneous or ocular tissue, though rarely feasible, is both diagnostic and therapeutic. Albendazole (400 mg twice daily for 21 days) or ivermectin (200 μg/kg daily for

2 days) may be helpful. At present, cerebrospinal involvement is managed with supportive measures and generally with a course of glucocorticoids. Gnathostomiasis can be prevented by adequate cooking of fish and poultry in endemic areas.

ACKNOWLEDGMENT

The contributions of Leo X. Liu, M.D., to earlier editions of this chapter are gratefully acknowledged.

FURTHER READING

BARISANI-ASENBAUER T et al: Treatment of ocular toxocariasis with albendazole. J Ocul Pharmacol Ther 17:287, 2001

BOUCHARD O et al: Cutaneous larva migrans in travelers: A prospective study, with assessment of therapy with ivermectin. Clin Infect Dis 31:493, 2000

BRUSCHI F, MURRELL KD: New aspects of human trichinellosis: The impact of new *Trichinella* species. Postgrad Med J 78:15, 2002

CAUMES E: Treatment of cutaneous larva migrans. Clin Infect Dis 30:811, 2000

MOOREHEAD A et al: Trichinellosis in the United States, 1991–1996: Declining but not gone. Am J Trop Med Hyg 60:66, 1999

SLOM TJ et al: An outbreak of eosinophilic meningitis caused by *Angiostrongylus cantonensis* in travelers returning from the Caribbean. N Engl J Med 346:668, 2002

TSAI HC et al: Eosinophilic meningitis caused by *Angiostrongylus cantonensis*: Report of 17 cases. Am J Med 111:109, 2001

201 INTESTINAL NEMATODES
Peter F. Weller, Thomas B. Nutman

More than a billion people worldwide are infected with one or more species of intestinal nematodes. Table 201-1 summarizes biologic and clinical features of infections due to the major intestinal parasitic nematodes. These parasites are most common in regions with poor fecal sanitation, particularly in developing countries in the tropics and subtropics but also in the United States. Although nematode infections are not usually fatal, they contribute to malnutrition and diminished work capacity. An interesting point is that these same infections may protect some individuals from allergic disease. Humans may on occasion be infected with nematode parasites that ordinarily infect animals; these zoonotic infections include trichostrongyliasis, anisakiasis, capillariasis, and abdominal angiostrongyliasis.

Intestinal nematodes are roundworms; they range in length from 1 mm to many centimeters when mature (Table 201-1). Their life cycles are complex and highly varied; some species, including *Strongyloides stercoralis* and *Enterobius vermicularis*, can be transmitted directly from person to person, while others, such as *Ascaris lumbricoides*, *Necator americanus*, and *Ancylostoma duodenale*, require a soil phase for development. Because most helminth parasites do not self-replicate, the acquisition of a heavy burden of adult worms requires repeated exposure to the parasite in its infectious stage, whether larva or egg. Hence, clinical disease, as opposed to asymptomatic infection, generally develops only with prolonged residence in an endemic area. In persons with marginal nutrition, intestinal helminth infections may impair growth and development. Eosinophilia and elevated serum IgE levels are features of many helminthic infections and, when unexplained, should always prompt a search for occult helminthiasis. Significant protective immunity to intestinal nematodes appears not to develop in humans, although mechanisms of parasite immune evasion and host immune responses to these infections have not been elucidated in detail.

TABLE 201-1 *Major Human Intestinal Parasitic Nematodes*

	Parasitic Nematode				
Feature	*Ascaris lumbricoides* (Roundworm)	*Necator americanus, Ancylostoma duodenale* (Hookworm)	*Strongyloides stercoralis*	*Trichuris trichiura* (Whipworm)	*Enterobius vermicularis* (Pinworm)
Global prevalence in humans (millions)	1273	1277	50	902	300
Endemic areas	Worldwide	Hot, humid regions	Hot, humid regions	Worldwide	Worldwide
Infective stage	Egg	Filariform larva	Filariform larva	Egg	Egg
Route of infection	Oral	Percutaneous	Percutaneous or autoinfection	Oral	Oral
Gastrointestinal location of worms	Jejunal lumen	Jejunal mucosa	Small-bowel mucosa	Cecum, colonic mucosa	Cecum, appendix
Adult worm size	15–40 cm	7–12 mm	2 mm	30–50 mm	8–13 mm (female)
Pulmonary passage of larvae	Yes	Yes	Yes	No	No
Incubation period[a] (days)	60–75	40–100	17–28	70–90	35–45
Longevity	1 y	*N. americanus*: 2–5 y; *A. duodenale*: 6–8 y	Decades (owing to autoinfection)	5 y	2 months
Fecundity (eggs/day/worm)	240,000	*N. americanus*: 4000–10,000; *A. duodenale*: 10,000–25,000	5000–10,000	3000–7000	2000
Principal symptoms	Rarely gastrointestinal or biliary obstruction	Iron-deficiency anemia in heavy infection	Gastrointestinal symptoms; malabsorption or sepsis in hyperinfection	Gastrointestinal symptoms, anemia	Perianal pruritus
Diagnostic stage	Eggs in stool	Eggs in fresh stool, larvae in old stool	Larvae in stool or duodenal aspirate; sputum in hyperinfection	Eggs in stool	Eggs from perianal skin on cellulose acetate tape
Treatment	Mebendazole Albendazole Pyrantel pamoate	Mebendazole Pyrantel pamoate Albendazole	1. Ivermectin 2. Albendazole 3. Thiabendazole	Mebendazole Albendazole	Mebendazole Pyrantel pamoate Albendazole

[a] Time from infection to egg production by mature female worm.

ASCARIASIS *A. lumbricoides* is the largest intestinal nematode parasite of humans, reaching up to 40 cm in length. Most infected individuals have low worm burdens and are asymptomatic. Clinical disease arises from larval migration in the lungs or effects of the adult worms in the intestines.

Life Cycle Adult worms live in the lumen of the small intestine. Mature female *Ascaris* worms are extraordinarily fecund, each producing up to 240,000 eggs a day, which pass with the feces. Ascarid eggs, which are remarkably resistant to environmental stresses, become infective after several weeks of maturation in the soil and can remain infective for years. After infective eggs are swallowed, larvae hatched in the intestine invade the mucosa, migrate through the circulation to the lungs, break into the alveoli, ascend the bronchial tree, and return via swallowing to the small intestine, where they develop into adult worms. Between 2 and 3 months elapse between initial infection and egg production. The adult worms live for 1 to 2 years.

Epidemiology *Ascaris* is widely distributed in tropical and subtropical regions as well as in other humid areas, including the rural southeastern United States. Transmission typically occurs through fecally contaminated soil and is due either to a lack of sanitary facilities or to the use of human manure ("night soil") as fertilizer. With their propensity for hand-to-mouth fecal carriage, younger children in impoverished rural areas are most affected. Infection outside endemic areas, though uncommon, can occur from eggs borne on transported vegetables.

Clinical Features During the lung phase of larval migration, about 9 to 12 days after egg ingestion, patients may develop an irritating nonproductive cough and burning substernal discomfort that is aggravated by coughing or deep inspiration. Dyspnea and blood-tinged sputum are less common. Fever is usually reported, with temperatures sometimes exceeding 38.5°C (101.3°F). Eosinophilia develops during this symptomatic phase and subsides slowly over weeks. Chest x-rays may reveal evidence of eosinophilic pneumonitis (Löffler's syndrome), with round or oval infiltrates a few millimeters to several centimeters in size. These infiltrates may be transient and intermittent, clearing after several weeks. Where there is seasonal transmission of the parasite, seasonal pneumonitis with eosinophilia may develop in previously infected and sensitized hosts.

In established infections, adult worms in the small intestine usually cause no symptoms. In heavy infections, particularly in children, a large bolus of entangled worms can cause pain and small-bowel obstruction, sometimes complicated by perforation, intussusception, or volvulus. Single worms may cause disease when they migrate into aberrant sites. A large worm can enter and occlude the biliary tree, causing biliary colic, cholecystitis, cholangitis, pancreatitis, or (rarely) intrahepatic abscesses. Migration of an adult worm up the esophagus can provoke coughing and oral expulsion of the worm. In highly endemic areas, intestinal and biliary ascariasis can rival acute appendicitis and gallstones as causes of surgical acute abdomen.

Laboratory Findings Most cases of ascariasis can be diagnosed by the microscopic detection of characteristic mamillated *Ascaris* eggs (65 by 45 μm) in fecal samples. Occasionally, patients present after passing an adult worm—identifiable by its large size and smooth cream-colored surface—in the stool or through the mouth or nose. During the early transpulmonary migratory phase, when eosinophilic pneumonitis occurs, larvae can be found in sputum or gastric aspirates before diagnostic eggs appear in the stool. The eosinophilia that is prominent during this early stage usually decreases to minimal levels in established infection. The large adult worms may be visualized, occasionally serendipitously, on contrast studies of the gastrointestinal tract. A plain abdominal film may reveal masses of worms in gas-filled loops of bowel in patients with intestinal obstruction. Pancreaticobiliary worms can be detected by ultrasound and endoscopic retrograde cholangiopancreatography; the latter method also has been used to extract biliary *Ascaris* worms.

℞ TREATMENT

Ascariasis should always be treated to prevent potentially serious complications. Albendazole (400 mg once), which is considered an investigational drug by the Food and Drug Administration for this indication, or mebendazole (500 mg once) is effective. These benzimidazoles are contraindicated in pregnancy, however. Pyrantel pamoate (11 mg/kg once; maximum, 1 g) is safe in pregnancy. Mild diarrhea and abdominal pain are uncommon side effects of these agents. Partial intestinal obstruction should be managed with nasogastric suction, intravenous fluid administration, and instillation of piperazine through the nasogastric tube, but complete obstruction and its severe complications require immediate surgical intervention.

HOOKWORM One-fourth of the world's population is infected with one of the two hookworm species (*A. duodenale* and *N. americanus*). Most infected individuals are asymptomatic. Hookworm disease develops from a combination of factors—a heavy worm burden, a prolonged duration of infection, and an inadequate iron intake—and results in iron-deficiency anemia and, on occasion, hypoproteinemia.

Life Cycle Adult hookworms, which are ~1 cm long, use buccal teeth (*Ancylostoma*) or cutting plates (*Necator*) to attach to the small-bowel mucosa and suck blood (0.2 mL/d per *Ancylostoma* adult) and interstitial fluid. The adult hookworms produce thousands of eggs daily. The eggs are deposited with feces in soil, where rhabditiform larvae hatch and develop over a 1-week period into infectious filariform larvae. Infective larvae penetrate the skin and reach the lungs by way of the bloodstream. There they invade alveoli and ascend the airways before being swallowed and reaching the small intestine. The prepatent period from skin invasion to appearance of eggs in the feces is about 6 to 8 weeks, but it may be longer with *A. duodenale*. Larvae of *A. duodenale*, if swallowed, can survive and develop directly in the intestinal mucosa. Adult hookworms may survive over a decade but usually live about 6 to 8 years for *A. duodenale* and 2 to 5 years for *N. americanus*.

Epidemiology *A. duodenale* is prevalent in southern Europe, North Africa, and northern Asia, and *N. americanus* is the predominant species in the western hemisphere and equatorial Africa. The two species overlap in many tropical regions, particularly Southeast Asia. In most areas, older children have the greatest incidence and intensity of hookworm infection. In rural areas where fields are fertilized with night soil, older working adults also may be heavily affected.

Clinical Features Most hookworm infections are asymptomatic. Infective larvae may provoke pruritic maculopapular dermatitis ("ground itch") at the site of skin penetration as well as serpiginous tracks of subcutaneous migration (similar to cutaneous larva migrans) in previously sensitized hosts. Larvae migrating through the lungs occasionally cause mild transient pneumonitis, but this condition develops less frequently in hookworm infection than in ascariasis. In the early intestinal phase, infected persons may develop epigastric pain (often with postprandial accentuation), inflammatory diarrhea, or other abdominal symptoms accompanied by eosinophilia. The major consequence of chronic hookworm infection is iron deficiency. Symptoms are minimal if iron intake is adequate, but marginally nourished individuals develop symptoms of progressive iron-deficiency anemia and hypoproteinemia, including weakness, shortness of breath, and skin depigmentation.

Laboratory Findings The diagnosis is established by the finding of characteristic 40- by 60-μm oval hookworm eggs in the feces. Stool-concentration procedures may be required to detect light infections. Eggs of the two species are indistinguishable by light microscopy. In a stool sample that is not fresh, the eggs may have hatched to release rhabditiform larvae, which need to be differentiated from those of *S. ster-*

coralis. Hypochromic microcytic anemia, occasionally with eosinophilia or hypoalbuminemia, is characteristic of hookworm disease.

Rx TREATMENT

Hookworm infection can be eradicated with several safe and highly effective anthelmintic drugs, including albendazole (400 mg once), mebendazole (500 mg once), and pyrantel pamoate (11 mg/kg for 3 days). Mild iron-deficiency anemia can often be treated with oral iron alone. Severe hookworm disease with protein loss and malabsorption necessitates nutritional support and oral iron replacement along with deworming.

Ancylostoma caninum* and *Ancylostoma braziliense   *A. caninum*, the canine hookworm, has been identified as a cause of human eosinophilic enteritis, especially in northeastern Australia. In this zoonotic infection, adult hookworms attach to the small intestine (where they may be visualized by endoscopy) and elicit abdominal pain and intense local eosinophilia. Treatment with mebendazole (100 mg twice daily for 3 days) or albendazole (400 mg once) is effective. Both of these animal hookworm species can cause cutaneous larva migrans ("creeping eruption"; Chap. 200).

STRONGYLOIDIASIS   *S. stercoralis* is distinguished by its ability—unusual among helminths—to replicate in the human host. This capacity permits ongoing cycles of autoinfection as infective larvae are internally produced. Strongyloidiasis can thus persist for decades without further exposure of the host to exogenous infective larvae. In immunocompromised hosts, large numbers of invasive *Strongyloides* larvae can disseminate widely and can be fatal.

Life Cycle   In addition to a parasitic cycle of development, *Strongyloides* can undergo a free-living cycle of development in the soil. This adaptability facilitates the parasite's survival in the absence of mammalian hosts. Rhabditiform larvae passed in feces can transform into infectious filariform larvae either directly or after a free-living phase of development. Humans acquire strongyloidiasis when filariform larvae in fecally contaminated soil penetrate the skin or mucous membranes. The larvae then travel through the bloodstream to the lungs, where they break into the alveolar spaces, ascend the bronchial tree, are swallowed, and thereby reach the small intestine. There the larvae mature into adult worms that penetrate the mucosa of the proximal small bowel. The minute (2-mm-long) parasitic adult female worms reproduce by parthenogenesis; parasitic adult males do not exist. Eggs hatch locally in the intestinal mucosa, releasing rhabditiform larvae that migrate to the lumen and pass with the feces into soil. Alternatively, rhabditiform larvae in the bowel can develop directly into filariform larvae that penetrate the colonic wall or perianal skin and enter the circulation to repeat the migration that establishes ongoing internal reinfection. This autoinfection cycle allows strongyloidiasis to persist for decades after the host has left an endemic area.

Epidemiology   *S. stercoralis* is spottily distributed in tropical areas and other hot, humid regions and is particularly common in Southeast Asia, sub-Saharan Africa, and Brazil. In the United States, the parasite is endemic in parts of the South and is found in institutionalized patients who practice poor hygiene and in immigrants and military veterans who have lived in endemic areas abroad.

Clinical Features   In uncomplicated strongyloidiasis, many patients are asymptomatic or have mild cutaneous and/or abdominal symptoms. Recurrent urticaria, often involving the buttocks and wrists, is the most common cutaneous manifestation. Migrating larvae can elicit a pathognomonic serpiginous eruption, *larva currens* ("running larva")—a pruritic, raised, erythematous lesion that advances as rapidly as 10 cm/h along the course of larval migration. Adult parasites burrow into the duodenojejunal mucosa and can cause abdominal (usually midepigastric) pain, which resembles peptic ulcer pain except that it is aggravated by food ingestion. Nausea, diarrhea, gastrointestinal bleed-

ing, mild chronic colitis, and weight loss can occur. Small-bowel obstruction may develop with early, heavy infection. Pulmonary symptoms are rare in uncomplicated strongyloidiasis. Eosinophilia is common, with levels fluctuating over time.

The ongoing autoinfection cycle of strongyloidiasis is normally contained by unknown factors of the host's immune system. Abrogation of host immunity, especially with glucocorticoid therapy and much less commonly with other immunosuppressive medications, leads to hyperinfection, with the generation of large numbers of filariform larvae. Colitis, enteritis, or malabsorption may develop. In disseminated strongyloidiasis, larvae may invade not only gastrointestinal tissues and the lungs but also the central nervous system, peritoneum, liver, and kidney. Moreover, bacteremia may develop because of the entry of enteric flora through disrupted mucosal barriers. Gram-negative sepsis, pneumonia, or meningitis may complicate or dominate the clinical course. Eosinophilia is often absent in severely infected patients. Disseminated strongyloidiasis, particularly in patients with unsuspected infection who are given glucocorticoids, can be fatal. Strongyloidiasis is a frequent complication of infection with human T cell lymphotropic virus type I, but disseminated strongyloidiasis is not common among patients infected with HIV.

Diagnosis   In uncomplicated strongyloidiasis, the finding of rhabditiform larvae in feces is diagnostic. The eggs are almost never detectable because they hatch in the intestine. Rhabditiform larvae are 200 to 250 μm long, with a short buccal cavity that distinguishes them from hookworm rhabditiform larvae. Single stool examinations detect only about one-third of uncomplicated infections, in which few larvae are passed. Serial examinations and the use of the agar plate detection method improve the sensitivity of stool diagnosis. In uncomplicated—but not hyperinfection—strongyloidiasis, stool examinations may be repeatedly negative. If stool examinations are negative, *Strongyloides* can be assayed by sampling of the duodenojejunal contents by aspiration or biopsy. An enzyme-linked immunosorbent assay for antibodies to excretory-secretory or somatic antigens of *Strongyloides* is a sensitive method of diagnosing uncomplicated infections. In disseminated strongyloidiasis, filariform larvae (550 μm long) should be sought in stool as well as in samples obtained from sites of potential larval migration, including sputum, bronchoalveolar lavage fluid, or surgical drainage fluid.

Rx TREATMENT

Even in the asymptomatic state, strongyloidiasis must be treated because of the potential for fatal hyperinfection. Ivermectin (200 μg/kg daily for 1 or 2 days) is more effective than albendazole (400 mg daily for 3 days, repeated at 2 weeks) and is better tolerated than thiabendazole (25 mg/kg twice daily for 2 days), whose common adverse effects include nausea, vomiting, diarrhea, dizziness, and neuropsychiatric disturbances. Because thiabendazole is not uniformly effective, stool examinations, eosinophil counts, and monitoring of clinical symptoms should be continued after treatment. For disseminated strongyloidiasis, treatment with ivermectin should be extended for at least 5 to 7 days or until the parasites are eradicated.

Strongyloides fülleborni   This unusual species, which has been encountered in Africa and Papua New Guinea, is thought to be transmitted from person to person and through maternal milk. *S. fülleborni* releases membranous sacs filled with eggs into the stool. Most commonly affected are infants and young children, who present with abdominal distention, respiratory distress, vomiting, or diarrhea.

TRICHURIASIS   Most infections with the whipworm *Trichuris trichiura* are asymptomatic, but heavy infections may cause gastrointestinal symptoms. Like the other soil-transmitted helminths, whipworm is distributed globally in the tropics and subtropics and is most common among poor children.

Life Cycle   A broad posterior section and a thin anterior portion give *Trichuris* its characteristic whiplike shape. The adult worms reside in the colon and cecum, the anterior portions threaded into the superficial mucosa. Thousands of eggs laid daily by adult female worms pass with the feces and mature in the soil. After ingestion, infective eggs hatch in the duodenum, releasing larvae that mature before migrating to the large bowel. The entire cycle takes about 3 months, and adult worms may live for several years.

Clinical Features Tissue reactions to whipworms are mild. Most infected individuals have no symptoms or eosinophilia. Heavy infections may result in abdominal pain, anorexia, and bloody or mucoid diarrhea resembling inflammatory bowel disease. Rectal prolapse can result from massive infections in children, who often suffer from malnourishment and other diarrheal illnesses. Moderately heavy whipworm burdens also contribute to growth retardation.

Diagnosis and Treatment The characteristic 50- by 20-μm lemon-shaped whipworm eggs are readily detected on stool examination. Adult worms, which are 3 to 5 cm long, occasionally can be seen on proctoscopy. Mebendazole (500 mg once) or albendazole (400 mg daily for 3 doses) is safe and effective for treatment.

ENTEROBIASIS (PINWORM) *E. vermicularis* is more common in temperate countries than in the tropics. In the United States, >40 million people are estimated to be infected with pinworms; schoolchildren account for a disproportionate number of cases.

Life Cycle and Epidemiology *Enterobius* adult worms are ~1 cm long and dwell in the bowel lumen. The gravid female worm migrates nocturnally out into the perianal region and releases up to 10,000 immature eggs. The eggs become infective within hours and are transmitted by hand-to-mouth passage. The larvae hatch and mature entirely within the intestine. This life cycle takes ~1 month, and adult worms survive for ~2 months. Self-infection results from perianal scratching and transport of infective eggs on the hands or under the nails to the mouth. Because of the ease of person-to-person spread, pinworm infections are common among family members and institutionalized populations.

Clinical Features Most pinworm infections are asymptomatic. Perianal pruritus is the cardinal symptom. The itching, which is often worse at night as a result of the nocturnal migration of the female worms, may lead to excoriation and bacterial superinfection. Heavy infections have been claimed to cause abdominal pain and weight loss. On rare occasions, pinworms invade the female genital tract, causing vulvovaginitis and pelvic or peritoneal granulomas. Eosinophilia or elevated levels of serum IgE are rare.

Diagnosis Since pinworm eggs are not usually released in the bowel, the diagnosis cannot be made by looking for eggs in the feces. Instead, eggs deposited in the perianal region are detected by the application of clear cellulose acetate tape to the perianal region in the morning. After the tape is transferred to a microscope slide, low-power examination will reveal the characteristic pinworm eggs, which are oval, measure 55 by 25 μm, and are flattened along one side.

℞ TREATMENT

All affected individuals should be given a dose of mebendazole (100 mg once), albendazole (400 mg once), or pyrantel pamoate (11 mg/kg base once; maximum, 1 g), with the same treatment repeated after 10 to 14 days. Treatment of household members is also advocated to eliminate asymptomatic reservoirs of potential reinfection.

TRICHOSTRONGYLIASIS *Trichostrongylus* species, which are normally parasites of herbivorous animals, occasionally infect humans, particularly in Asia and Africa. This parasite has been termed *pseudohookworm* because of similarities to the hookworms in life cycle and egg morphology. Humans acquire the infection by accidentally ingesting *Trichostrongylus* larvae on contaminated leafy vegetables. The larvae do not migrate in humans but mature directly into adult worms in the small bowel. These worms ingest far less blood than hookworms; most infected people are asymptomatic, but heavy infections may give rise to mild anemia and eosinophilia. *Trichostrongylus* eggs encountered

on stool examination resemble those of hookworms but are larger (85 by 115 μm). Appropriate treatment consists of mebendazole or albendazole (Chap. 193).

ANISAKIASIS Anisakiasis is a gastrointestinal infection caused by the accidental ingestion in uncooked saltwater fish of nematode larvae belonging to the family Anisakidae. The incidence of anisakiasis in the United States has increased as a result of the growing popularity of raw fish dishes. Most cases occur in Japan, the Netherlands, and Chile, where raw fish—sushi, pickled green herring, and seviche, respectively—are national culinary staples. Anisakid nematodes parasitize large sea mammals such as whales, dolphins, and seals. As part of a complex parasitic life cycle involving marine food chains, infectious larvae migrate to the musculature of a variety of fish. Both *Anisakis simplex* and *Pseudoterranova decipiens* have been implicated in human anisakiasis, but an identical gastric syndrome may be caused by the red larvae of eustrongylid parasites of fish-eating birds.

When humans consume infected raw fish, live larvae may be coughed up within 48 h. Alternatively, larvae may immediately penetrate the mucosa of the stomach. Within hours, violent upper abdominal pain accompanied by nausea and occasionally vomiting ensues, mimicking an acute abdomen. The diagnosis can be established by direct visualization on upper endoscopy, outlining of the worm by contrast radiographic studies, or histopathologic examination of extracted tissue. In experienced hands, the first technique is preferable because extraction of the burrowing larvae by endoscopic technique is curative. In addition, larvae may pass to the small bowel, where they penetrate the mucosa and provoke a vigorous eosinophilic granulomatous response. Symptoms may appear 1 or 2 weeks after the infective meal, with intermittent abdominal pain, diarrhea, nausea, and fever resembling the manifestations of Crohn's disease. The diagnosis may be suggested by barium studies and confirmed by curative surgical resection of a granuloma in which the worm is embedded. Anisakid eggs are not found in the stool, since the larvae do not mature in humans. Anisakid larvae in saltwater fish are killed by cooking to 60°C, freezing at −20°C for 3 days, or commercial blast freezing, but not usually by salting, marinating, or cold smoking. No medical treatment is available; if possible, surgical or endoscopic removal should be undertaken.

CAPILLARIASIS Intestinal capillariasis is caused by ingestion of raw fish infected with *Capillaria philippinensis*. Subsequent autoinfection can lead to a severe wasting syndrome. The disease occurs in the Philippines and Thailand and, on occasion, elsewhere in Asia. The natural cycle of *C. philippinensis* involves fish from fresh and brackish water. When humans eat infected raw fish, the larvae mature in the intestine into adult worms, which produce invasive larvae that cause intestinal inflammation and villus loss. Capillariasis has an insidious onset with nonspecific abdominal pain and watery diarrhea. If untreated, progressive autoinfection can lead to protein-losing enteropathy and severe malabsorption and ultimately to death from cachexia, cardiac failure, or superinfection. The diagnosis is established by identification of the characteristic peanut-shaped (20- by 40-μm) eggs on stool examination. Severely ill patients require hospitalization and supportive therapy in addition to prolonged anthelmintic treatment with mebendazole or albendazole (Chap. 193).

ABDOMINAL ANGIOSTRONGYLIASIS Abdominal angiostrongyliasis is found in Latin America and Africa. The zoonotic parasite *Angiostrongylus costaricensis* causes eosinophilic ileocolitis after the ingestion of contaminated vegetation. *A. costaricensis* normally parasitizes the cotton rat and other rodents, with slugs and snails serving as intermediate hosts. Humans become infected by accidentally ingesting infective larvae in mollusk slime deposited on fruits and vegetables; children are at highest risk. The larvae penetrate the gut wall and migrate to the mesenteric artery, where they develop into adult worms. Eggs deposited in the gut wall provoke an intense eosinophilic granulomatous reaction, and adult worms may cause mesenteric arteritis, thrombosis, or frank bowel infarction. Symptoms may mimic those of appendicitis, including abdominal pain and tenderness, fever, vomiting, and a palpable mass in the right iliac fossa. Leukocytosis and eosinophilia are prominent. A barium enema may reveal ileocecal filling defects, but a definitive diagnosis is usually made surgically with partial bowel resection. Pathologic study reveals a thickened bowel wall with eosinophilic granulomas surrounding the *Angiostrongylus* eggs. In nonsurgical cases, the diagnosis rests solely on clinical grounds because larvae and eggs cannot be detected in the stool. Medical therapy for abdominal angiostrongyliasis (thiabendazole; Chap. 193) is of uncertain efficacy. Careful observation and surgical resection for severe symptoms are the mainstays of treatment.

FURTHER READING

BECKINGHAM IJ et al: Management of hepatobiliary and pancreatic *Ascaris* infestation in adults after failed medical treatment. Br J Surg 85:907, 1998

COWDEN J et al: Mebendazole and albendazole treatment of geohelminth infections in children and pregnant women. Pediatr Infect Dis J 19:659, 2000

CROESE J et al: Human enteric infection with canine hookworms. Ann Intern Med 120:369, 1994

CROSS JH: Intestinal capillariasis. Clin Microbiol Rev 5:120, 1992

GOTUZZO E et al: *Strongyloides stercoralis* hyperinfection associated with human T cell lymphotropic virus type-1 infection in Peru. Am J Trop Med Hyg 60:146, 1999

HORTON J: Albendazole: A broad spectrum anthelminthic for treatment of individuals and populations. Curr Opin Infect Dis 15:599, 2002

KEISER PB et al: *Strongyloides stercoralis* in the immunocompromised population. Clin Microbiol Rev (in press)

REEDER MM: The radiological and ultrasound evaluation of ascariasis of the gastrointestinal, biliary, and respiratory tracts. Semin Roentgenol 33:57, 1998

202 FILARIAL AND RELATED INFECTIONS
Thomas B. Nutman, Peter F. Weller

Filarial worms are nematodes that dwell in the subcutaneous tissues and the lymphatics. Eight filarial species infect humans (Table 202-1); of these, four—*Wuchereria bancrofti*, *Brugia malayi*, *Onchocerca volvulus*, and *Loa loa*—are responsible for most serious filarial infections. Filarial parasites, which infect an estimated 170 million persons worldwide, are transmitted by specific species of mosquitoes or other arthropods and have a complex life cycle including infective larval stages carried by insects and adult worms that reside in either lymphatic or subcutaneous tissues of humans. The offspring of adults are microfilariae, which, depending on their species, are 200 to 250 μm long and 5 to 7 μm wide, may or may not be enveloped in a loose sheath, and either circulate in the blood or migrate through the skin (Table 202-1). To complete the life cycle, microfilariae are ingested by the arthropod vector and develop over 1 to 2 weeks into new infective larvae. Adult worms live for many years, whereas microfilariae survive from 3 to 36 months. There has been a resurgence of interest in the rickettsia-like endosymbiont of *Wolbachia* that has been found intracellularly in all stages of *Brugia*, *Wuchereria*, *Mansonella*, and *Onchocerca*. These intracellular bacteria have recently been viewed as possible targets for antifilarial chemotherapy.

Usually, infection is established only with repeated and prolonged exposures to infective larvae. Since the clinical manifestations of filarial diseases develop relatively slowly, these infections should be considered chronic diseases with possible long-term debilitating effects. In terms of the nature, severity, and timing of clinical manifestations, patients with filarial infections who are native to endemic areas and undergo lifelong exposure may differ significantly from those who are travelers or who have recently moved to these areas. Characteristically, the disease is more acute and intense in newly exposed individuals than in natives of endemic areas.

LYMPHATIC FILARIASIS

Lymphatic filariasis is caused by *W. bancrofti*, *B. malayi*, or *B. timori*. The threadlike adult parasites reside in lymphatic channels or lymph nodes, where they may remain viable for more than two decades.

EPIDEMIOLOGY *W. bancrofti*, the most widely distributed human filarial parasite, affects an estimated 115 million people and is found throughout the tropics and subtropics, including Asia and the Pacific Islands, Africa, areas of South America, and the Caribbean basin. Humans are the only definitive host for the parasite. Generally, the subperiodic form is found only in the Pacific Islands; elsewhere, *W. bancrofti* is nocturnally periodic. (Nocturnally periodic forms of microfilariae are scarce in peripheral blood by day and increase at night, whereas sub-

TABLE 202-1 *Characteristics of the Filariae*

Organism	Periodicity	Distribution	Vector	Location of Adult	Microfilarial Location	Sheath
Wuchereria bancrofti	Nocturnal	Cosmopolitan areas worldwide, including South America and Africa	*Culex* (mosquitoes)	Lymphatic tissue	Blood	+
		Mainly India	*Anopheles* (mosquitoes)			
		China, Indonesia	*Aedes* (mosquitoes)			
	Subperiodic	Eastern Pacific	*Aedes* (mosquitoes)	Lymphatic tissue	Blood	+
Brugia malayi	Nocturnal	Southeast Asia, Indonesia, India	*Mansonia, Anopheles* (mosquitoes)	Lymphatic tissue	Blood	+
	Subperiodic	Indonesia, Southeast Asia	*Coquillettidia, Mansonia* (mosquitoes)	Lymphatic tissue	Blood	+
B. timori	Nocturnal	Indonesia	*Anopheles* (mosquitoes)	Lymphatic tissue	Blood	+
Loa loa	Diurnal	West and Central Africa	*Chrysops* (deerflies)	Subcutaneous tissue	Blood	+
Onchocerca volvulus	None	South and Central America, Africa	*Simulium* (blackflies)	Subcutaneous tissue	Skin, eye	−
Mansonella ozzardi	None	South and Central America Caribbean	*Culicoides* (midges) *Simulium* (blackflies)	Undetermined site	Blood	−
M. perstans	None	South and Central America, Africa	*Culicoides* (midges)	Body cavities, mesentery, perirenal tissue	Blood	−
M. streptocerca	None	West and Central Africa	*Culicoides* (midges)	Subcutaneous tissue	Skin	−

periodic forms are present in peripheral blood at all times and reach maximal levels in the afternoon.) Natural vectors for *W. bancrofti* are *Culex fatigans* mosquitoes in urban settings and anopheline or aedean mosquitoes in rural areas.

Brugian filariasis due to *B. malayi* occurs primarily in China, India, Indonesia, Korea, Japan, Malaysia, and the Philippines. *B. malayi* also has two forms distinguished by the periodicity of microfilaremia. The more common nocturnal form is transmitted in areas of coastal rice fields, while the subperiodic form is found in forests. *B. malayi* naturally infects cats as well as humans. *B. timori* exists only on islands of the Indonesian archipelago.

PATHOLOGY The principal pathologic changes result from inflammatory damage to the lymphatics, which is caused by adult worms and not by microfilariae. Adult worms live in afferent lymphatics or sinuses of lymph nodes and cause lymphatic dilatation and thickening of the vessel walls. The infiltration of plasma cells, eosinophils, and macrophages in and around the infected vessels, along with endothelial and connective tissue proliferation, leads to tortuosity of the lymphatics and damaged or incompetent lymph valves. Lymphedema and chronic-stasis changes with hard or brawny edema develop in the overlying skin. These consequences of filariasis are due both to direct effects of the worms and to the inflammatory response of the host to the parasite. These inflammatory responses are believed to cause the granulomatous and proliferative processes that precede total lymphatic obstruction. It is thought that the lymphatic vessel remains patent as long as the worm remains viable and that death of the worm leads to enhanced granulomatous reaction and fibrosis. Lymphatic obstruction results, and, despite collateralization of the lymphatics, lymphatic function is compromised.

CLINICAL FEATURES The most common presentations of the lymphatic filariases are asymptomatic (or subclinical) microfilaremia, hydrocele (Fig. 202-1), acute adenolymphangitis (ADL), and chronic lymphatic disease. In areas where *W. bancrofti* or *B. malayi* is endemic, the overwhelming majority of infected individuals have few overt clinical manifestations of filarial infection despite large numbers of circulating microfilariae in the peripheral blood. Although they may be clinically asymptomatic, virtually all persons with *W. bancrofti* or *B. malayi* microfilaremia have some degree of subclinical disease that includes microscopic hematuria and/or proteinuria, dilated (and tortuous) lymphatics (visualized by imaging), and—in men—scrotal lymphangiectasia (detectable by ultrasound). In spite of these findings, the majority of individuals appear to remain clinically asymptomatic for years; relatively few progress to the acute and chronic stages of infection.

ADL is characterized by high fever, lymphatic inflammation (lymphangitis and lymphadenitis), and transient local edema. The lymphangitis is retrograde, extending peripherally from the lymph node draining the area where the adult parasites reside. Regional lymph nodes are often enlarged, and the entire lymphatic channel can become indurated and inflamed. Concomitant local thrombophlebitis can occur as well. In brugian filariasis, a single local abscess may form along the involved lymphatic tract and subsequently rupture to the surface. The lymphadenitis and lymphangitis can involve both the upper and lower extremities in both bancroftian and brugian filariasis, but involvement of the genital lymphatics occurs almost exclusively with *W. bancrofti* infection. This genital involvement can be manifested by funiculitis, epididymitis, and scrotal pain and tenderness. In endemic areas, another type of acute disease—dermatolymphangioadenitis (DLA)—is recognized as a syndrome that includes high fever, chills, myalgias, and headache. Edematous inflammatory plaques clearly demarcated from normal skin are seen. Vesicles, ulcers, and hyperpigmentation may also be noted. There is often a history of trauma, burns, radiation, insect bites, punctiform lesions, or chemical injury. Entry lesions, especially in the interdigital area, are common. DLA is often diagnosed as cellulitis.

If lymphatic damage progresses, transient lymphedema can develop into lymphatic obstruction and the permanent changes associated with elephantiasis (Fig. 202-2). Brawny edema follows early pitting edema, and thickening of the subcutaneous tissues and hyperkeratosis occur. Fissuring of the skin develops, as do hyperplastic changes. Superinfection of these poorly vascularized tissues becomes a problem. In bancroftian filariasis, in which genital involvement is common, hydroceles may develop; in advanced stages, this condition may evolve into scrotal lymphedema and scrotal elephantiasis. Furthermore, if there is obstruction of the retroperitoneal lymphatics, the increased renal lymphatic pressure leads to rupture of the renal lymphatics and the development of chyluria, which is usually intermittent and most prominent in the morning.

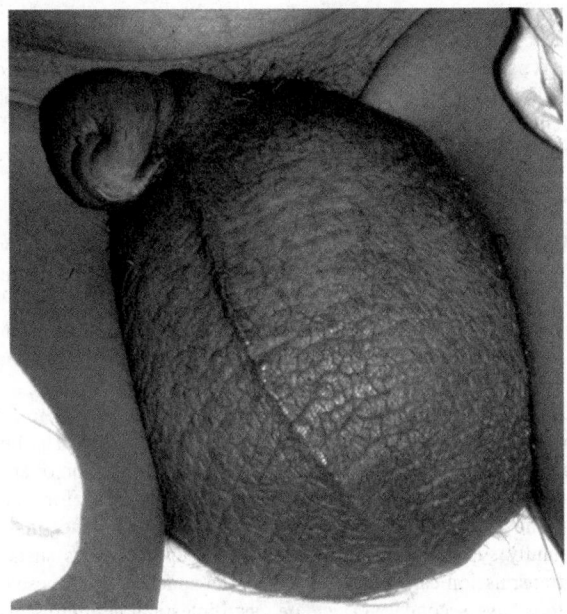

FIGURE 202-1 Hydrocele associated with *Wuchereria bancrofti* infection.

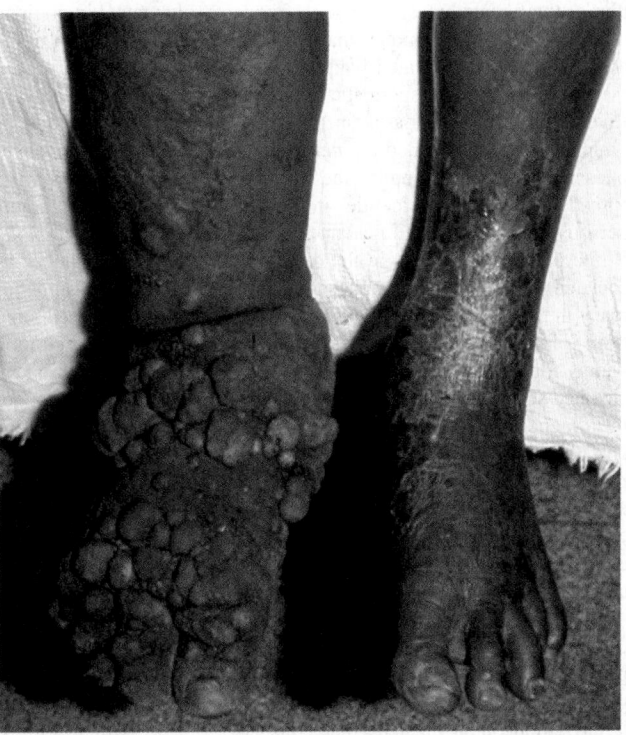

FIGURE 202-2 Elephantiasis of the lower extremity associated with *Wuchereria bancrofti* infection.

The clinical manifestations of filarial infections in travelers or transmigrants who have recently entered an endemic region are distinctive. Given a sufficient number of bites by infected vectors, usually over a 3- to 6-month period, recently exposed patients can develop acute lymphatic or scrotal inflammation with or without urticaria and localized angioedema. Lymphadenitis of epitrochlear, axillary, femoral, or inguinal lymph nodes is often followed by retrogradely evolving lymphangitis. Acute attacks are short-lived and, in contrast to filarial fevers in patients native to endemic areas, are usually not accompanied by fever. With prolonged exposure to infected mosquitoes, these attacks, if untreated, become more severe and lead to permanent lymphatic inflammation and obstruction.

DIAGNOSIS A definitive diagnosis can be made only by detection of the parasites and hence can be difficult. Adult worms localized in lymphatic vessels or nodes are largely inaccessible. Microfilariae can be found in blood, in hydrocele fluid, or (occasionally) in other body fluids. Such fluids can be examined microscopically, either directly or—for greater sensitivity—after concentration of the parasites by the passage of fluid through a polycarbonate cylindrical pore filter (pore size, 3 μm) or by the centrifugation of fluid fixed in 2% formalin (Knott's concentration technique). The timing of blood collection is critical and should be based on the periodicity of the microfilariae in the endemic region involved. Many infected individuals do not have microfilaremia, and definitive diagnosis in such cases can be difficult. Assays for circulating antigens of *W. bancrofti* permit the diagnosis of microfilaremic and cryptic (amicrofilaremic) infection. Two tests are commercially available: one is an enzyme-linked immunosorbent assay (ELISA) and the other a rapid-format immunochromatographic card test. Both assays have sensitivities that range from 96 to 100% and specificities that approach 100%. There are currently no tests for circulating antigens in brugian filariasis.

Polymerase chain reaction (PCR)–based assays for DNA of *W. bancrofti* and *B. malayi* in blood have been developed. A number of studies indicate that this diagnostic method is of equivalent or greater sensitivity compared with parasitologic methods, detecting patent infection in almost all infected subjects.

In cases of suspected lymphatic filariasis, examination of the scrotum or the female breast using high-frequency ultrasound in conjunction with Doppler techniques may result in the identification of motile adult worms within dilated lymphatics. Worms may be visualized in the lymphatics of the spermatic cord in up to 80% of infected men. Live adult worms have a distinctive pattern of movement within the lymphatic vessels (termed the *filaria dance sign*). Radionuclide lymphoscintigraphic imaging of the limbs reliably demonstrates widespread lymphatic abnormalities in both asymptomatic microfilaremic persons and those with clinical manifestations of lymphatic pathology. While of potential utility in the delineation of anatomic changes associated with infection, lymphoscintigraphy is unlikely to assume primacy in the diagnostic evaluation of individuals with suspected infection; it is principally a research tool, although it has been used more widely for assessment of lymphedema of all causes. Eosinophilia and elevated serum concentrations of IgE and antifilarial antibody support the diagnosis of lymphatic filariasis. There is, however, extensive cross-reactivity between filarial antigens and antigens of other helminths, including the common intestinal roundworms; thus, interpretations of serologic findings can be difficult. In addition, residents of endemic areas can become sensitized to filarial antigens through exposure to infected mosquitoes without having patent filarial infections.

In acute episodes, lymphatic filariasis must be distinguished from thrombophlebitis, infection, and trauma. Retrogradely evolving lymphangitis is a characteristic feature that helps distinguish filarial lymphangitis from typically ascending bacterial lymphangitis. Chronic filarial lymphedema must be distinguished from the lymphedema of malignancy, postoperative scarring, trauma, chronic edematous states, and congenital lymphatic system abnormalities.

R_x TREATMENT

With newer definitions of clinical syndromes in lymphatic filariasis and new tools to assess clinical status (e.g., ultrasound, lymphoscintigraphy, circulating filarial antigen assays, PCR), approaches to treatment based on infection status can be considered. Diethylcarbamazine (DEC, 6 mg/kg daily for 12 days), which has both macro- and microfilaricidal properties, remains the treatment of choice for the individual with active lymphatic filariasis (microfilaremia, antigen positivity, or adult worms on ultrasound), although albendazole (400 mg twice daily for 21 days) has also demonstrated macrofilaricidal efficacy.

As has already been mentioned, a growing body of evidence indicates that, although they may be asymptomatic, virtually all persons with *W. bancrofti* or *B. malayi* microfilaremia have some degree of subclinical disease (hematuria, proteinuria, abnormalities on lymphoscintigraphy). Thus, early treatment of asymptomatic persons is recommended to prevent further lymphatic damage. For ADL, supportive treatment (including the administration of antipyretics and analgesics) is recommended, as is antibiotic therapy if secondary bacterial infection is likely. Similarly, because lymphatic disease is associated with the presence of adult worms, treatment with DEC is recommended for microfilaria-negative adult-worm carriers.

In persons with chronic manifestations of lymphatic filariasis, treatment regimens that emphasize hygiene, prevention of secondary bacterial infections, and physiotherapy have gained wide acceptance for morbidity control. These regimens are similar to those recommended for lymphedema of most nonfilarial causes and known by a variety of names, including *complex decongestive physiotherapy* and *complex lymphedema therapy*. Hydroceles can be drained repeatedly or managed surgically. With chronic manifestations of lymphatic filariasis, drug treatment should be reserved for individuals with evidence of active infection; therapy has been associated with clinical improvement and, in some cases, reversal of lymphedema.

The recommended course of DEC treatment (12 days; total dose, 72 mg/kg) has remained standard for many years; however, data indicate that single-dose DEC treatment with 6 mg/kg may be equally efficacious. The 12-day course provides more rapid short-term microfilarial suppression. Regimens that utilize single-dose DEC or ivermectin or combinations of single doses of albendazole and either DEC or ivermectin have all been demonstrated to have a sustained microfilaricidal effect.

Side effects of DEC treatment include fever, chills, arthralgias, headaches, nausea, and vomiting. Both the development and the severity of these reactions are directly related to the number of microfilariae circulating in the bloodstream and may represent either an acute hypersensitivity reaction to the antigens being released by dead and dying parasites or an inflammatory reaction induced by lipopolysaccharides from the intracellular *Wolbachia* endosymbionts freed from their intracellular niche. Ivermectin has a side effect profile similar to that of DEC when used in lymphatic filariasis.

PREVENTION AND CONTROL Avoidance of mosquito bites is usually not feasible for residents of endemic areas, but visitors should make use of insect repellent and mosquito nets. Impregnated bednets have been shown to have a salutary effect. DEC can kill developing forms of filarial parasites and has been shown to be useful as a prophylactic agent in humans.

Community-based intervention is the current approach to elimination of lymphatic filariasis as a public health problem. The underlying tenet of this approach is that mass annual distribution of antimicrofilarial chemotherapy—albendazole with either DEC (for all areas except those where onchocerciasis is coendemic) or ivermectin—will profoundly suppress microfilaremia. If the suppression is sustained, then transmission can be interrupted. As an added benefit, these combinations have secondary effects on gastrointestinal helminths. An alternative approach to the control of lymphatic filariasis is the use of salt fortified with DEC. Community use of DEC-fortified salt dramatically reduces microfilarial density with no apparent adverse reactions. Community education and clinical care for persons already suffering from the chronic sequelae of lymphatic filariasis are important components of filariasis control and elimination programs.

TROPICAL PULMONARY EOSINOPHILIA

Tropical pulmonary eosinophilia (TPE) is a distinct syndrome that develops in some individuals infected with lymphatic filarial species. This syndrome affects males and females in a ratio of 4:1, often during the third decade of life. The majority of cases have been reported from India, Pakistan, Sri Lanka, Brazil, Guyana, and Southeast Asia.

CLINICAL FEATURES The main features include a history of residence in filarial-endemic regions, paroxysmal cough and wheezing that are usually nocturnal (and probably related to the nocturnal periodicity of microfilariae), weight loss, low-grade fever, adenopathy, and pronounced blood eosinophilia (>3000 eosinophils/μL). Chest x-rays may be normal but generally show increased bronchovascular markings; diffuse miliary lesions or mottled opacities may be present in the middle and lower lung fields. Tests of pulmonary function show restrictive abnormalities in most cases and obstructive defects in half. Total serum IgE levels (10,000 to 100,000 ng/mL) and antifilarial antibody titers are characteristically elevated.

PATHOLOGY In TPE there is rapid clearance of microfilariae and parasite antigens from the bloodstream by the lungs, and the clinical symptoms result from allergic and inflammatory reactions elicited by the cleared parasites. In some patients, trapping of microfilariae in other reticuloendothelial organs can cause hepatomegaly, splenomegaly, or lymphadenopathy. A prominent, eosinophil-enriched, intraalveolar infiltrate is often reported, and with it comes the release of cytotoxic proinflammatory granular proteins that may mediate some of the pathology seen in TPE. In the absence of successful treatment, interstitial fibrosis can lead to progressive pulmonary damage.

DIFFERENTIAL DIAGNOSIS TPE must be distinguished from asthma, Löffler's syndrome, allergic bronchopulmonary aspergillosis, allergic granulomatosis with angiitis (Churg-Strauss syndrome), the systemic vasculitides (most notably periarteritis nodosa and Wegener's granulomatosis), chronic eosinophilic pneumonia, and the idiopathic hypereosinophilic syndrome. In addition to a geographic history of filarial exposure, useful features for distinguishing TPE include wheezing that is solely nocturnal, very high levels of antifilarial antibodies, and a rapid initial response to treatment with DEC.

℞ TREATMENT

DEC is used at a dosage of 4 to 6 mg/kg of body weight per day for 14 days. Symptoms usually resolve within 3 to 7 days after the initiation of therapy. Relapse, which occurs in ~12 to 25% of cases (sometimes after an interval of years), requires re-treatment.

ONCHOCERCIASIS

Onchocerciasis ("river blindness") is caused by the filarial nematode *O. volvulus*, which infects an estimated 13 million individuals. The majority of individuals infected with *O. volvulus* live in the equatorial region of Africa extending from the Atlantic coast to the Red Sea. About 70,000 persons are infected in Guatemala and Mexico, with smaller foci in Venezuela, Colombia, Brazil, Ecuador, Yemen, and Saudi Arabia. Onchocerciasis is the second leading cause of infectious blindness worldwide.

ETIOLOGY AND EPIDEMIOLOGY Infection in humans begins with the deposition of infective larvae on the skin by the bite of an infected blackfly. The larvae develop into adults, which are typically found in subcutaneous nodules. About 7 months to 3 years after infection, the gravid female releases microfilariae that migrate out of the nodule and throughout the tissues, concentrating in the dermis. Infection is transmitted to other persons when a female fly ingests microfilariae from the host's skin and these microfilariae then develop into infective lar-

vae. Adult *O. volvulus* females and males are about 40 to 60 cm and 3 to 6 cm in length, respectively. The life span of adults can be as long as 18 years, with an average of ~9 years. Because the blackfly vector breeds along free-flowing rivers and streams (particularly in rapids) and generally restricts its flight to an area within several kilometers of these breeding sites, both biting and disease transmission are most intense in these locations.

PATHOLOGY Onchocerciasis affects primarily the skin, eyes, and lymph nodes. In contrast to that in lymphatic filariasis, the damage in onchocerciasis is elicited by microfilariae and not by adult parasites. In the skin, there are mild but chronic inflammatory changes that can result in loss of elastic fibers, atrophy, and fibrosis. The subcutaneous nodules, or onchocercomata, consist primarily of fibrous tissues surrounding the adult worm, often with a peripheral ring of inflammatory cells. In the eye, neovascularization and corneal scarring lead to corneal opacities and blindness. Inflammation in the anterior and posterior chambers frequently results in anterior uveitis, chorioretinitis, and optic atrophy. Although punctate opacities are due to an inflammatory reaction surrounding dead or dying microfilariae, the pathogenesis of most manifestations of onchocerciasis is still unclear.

CLINICAL FEATURES ■ **Skin** Pruritus and rash are the most frequent manifestations of onchocerciasis. The pruritus can be incapacitating; the rash is typically a papular eruption (Fig. 202-3) that is generalized rather than localized to a particular region of the body. Long-term infection results in exaggerated and premature wrinkling of the skin, loss of elastic fibers, and epidermal atrophy that can lead to loose, redundant skin and hypo- or hyperpigmentation. Localized eczematoid dermatitis can cause hyperkeratosis, scaling, and pigmentary changes. Such lesions are often seen in the lower extremities but can be distributed more extensively.

Onchocercomata These subcutaneous nodules, which can be palpable and/or visible, contain the adult worm. In African patients, they are common over the coccyx and sacrum, the trochanter of the femur, the lateral anterior crest, and other bony prominences; in Latin American patients, nodules tend to develop preferentially in the upper part of the body, particularly on the head, neck, and shoulders. Nodules vary in size and characteristically are firm and not tender. It has been estimated that, for every palpable nodule, there are four deeper nonpalpable ones.

Ocular Tissue Visual impairment is the most serious complication of onchocerciasis and usually affects only those persons with moderate or heavy infections. Lesions may develop in all parts of the eye. The most common early finding is conjunctivitis with photophobia. In the

FIGURE 202-3 Papular eruption as a consequence of onchocerciasis.

cornea, punctate keratitis—consisting of acute inflammatory reactions surrounding dying microfilariae manifested as "snowflake" opacities—is frequent in younger patients and resolves without apparent complications. Sclerosing keratitis occurs in 1 to 5% of infected persons and is the leading cause of onchocercal blindness in Africa. Anterior uveitis and iridocyclitis develop in ~5% of infected persons in Africa. In Latin America, complications of the anterior uveal tract (pupillary deformity) may cause secondary glaucoma. Characteristic chorioretinal lesions develop as a result of atrophy and hyperpigmentation of the retinal pigment epithelium. Constriction of the visual field and frank optic atrophy may occur.

Lymph Nodes   Mild to moderate lymphadenopathy is frequent, particularly in the inguinal and femoral areas, where the enlarged nodes may hang down in response to gravity ("hanging groin"), sometimes predisposing to inguinal and femoral hernias.

Systemic Manifestations   Some heavily infected individuals develop cachexia with loss of adipose tissue and muscle mass. Among adults who become blind, there is a three- to fourfold increase in the mortality rate.

DIAGNOSIS   Definitive diagnosis depends on the detection of an adult worm in an excised nodule or, more commonly, of microfilariae in a skin snip. Skin snips are obtained with a corneal-scleral punch, which collects a blood-free skin biopsy sample extending to just below the epidermis, or by lifting of the skin with the tip of a needle and excision of a small (1- to 3-mm) piece with a sterile scalpel blade. The biopsy tissue is incubated in tissue culture medium or in saline on a glass slide or flat-bottomed microtiter plate. After incubation for 2 to 4 h (or occasionally overnight in light infections), microfilariae emergent from the skin can be visualized by low-power microscopy.

Eosinophilia and elevated serum IgE levels are common but, because they occur in many parasitic infections, are not diagnostic in themselves. Assays to detect specific antibodies to *Onchocerca* and PCR to detect onchocercal DNA in skin snips are now in use in specialized laboratories and are highly sensitive and specific.

The *Mazzotti test* is a provocative technique that can be used in cases where the diagnosis of onchocerciasis is still in doubt (i.e., when skin snips and ocular examination reveal no microfilariae). A small dose of DEC (0.5 to 1.0 mg/kg) is given orally; the development or exacerbation of pruritus or dermatitis within hours is highly suggestive of onchocerciasis.

℞ TREATMENT

The main goals of therapy are to prevent the development of irreversible lesions and to alleviate symptoms. Surgical excision is recommended when nodules are located on the head (because of the proximity of microfilaria-producing adult worms to the eye), but chemotherapy is the mainstay of management. Ivermectin, a semisynthetic macrocyclic lactone active against microfilariae, is the first-line agent for the treatment of onchocerciasis. It is given orally in a single dose of 150 μg/kg, either yearly or semiannually. Recently, more frequent ivermectin administration (every 3 months) has been suggested to ameliorate pruritus and skin disease; moreover, quadrennial administration of ivermectin has been demonstrated to have some macrofilaricidal activity. After treatment, most individuals have few or no reactions. Pruritus, cutaneous edema, and/or maculopapular rash occurs in ~1 to 10% of treated individuals. In areas of Africa coendemic for *O. volvulus* and *L. loa*, however, ivermectin is contraindicated (as it is for pregnant or breastfeeding women) because of severe posttreatment encephalopathy seen in patients, especially children, who are heavily microfilaremic for *L. loa* (2000 to 5000 microfilariae per milliliter). Although ivermectin treatment results in a marked drop in microfilarial density, its effect can be short-lived (<3 months in some cases). Thus, it is occasionally necessary to give ivermectin more frequently for persistent symptoms. A 6-week course of doxycycline has

been demonstrated to be macrofilaristatic (rendering the female adult worms sterile for long periods). Because this regimen targets the *Wolbachia* endosymbiont of the filarial parasite, new options for definitive treatment may become available.

PREVENTION   Vector control has been beneficial in highly endemic areas in which breeding sites are vulnerable to insecticide spraying, but most areas endemic for onchocerciasis are not suited to this type of control. Community-based administration of ivermectin every 6 to 12 months is now being used to interrupt transmission in endemic areas. This measure, in conjunction with vector control, has already helped reduce the prevalence of disease in endemic foci in Africa and Latin America. No drug has proven useful for prophylaxis of *O. volvulus* infection.

LOIASIS

ETIOLOGY AND EPIDEMIOLOGY   Loiasis is caused by *L. loa* (the African eye worm), which is present in the rain forests of West and Central Africa. Adult parasites (females, 50 to 70 mm long and 0.5 mm wide; males, 25 to 35 mm long and 0.25 mm wide) live in subcutaneous tissues; microfilariae circulate in the blood with a diurnal periodicity that peaks between 12:00 noon and 2:00 P.M.

CLINICAL FEATURES   Manifestations of loiasis in natives of endemic areas may differ from those in temporary residents or visitors. Among the indigenous population, loiasis is often an asymptomatic infection with microfilaremia. Infection may be recognized only after subconjunctival migration of an adult worm (Fig. 202-4) or may be manifested by episodic Calabar swellings—evanescent localized areas of angioedema and erythema developing on the extremities and less frequently at other sites. Nephropathy, encephalopathy, and cardiomyopathy are rare. In patients who are not residents of endemic areas, allergic symptoms predominate, episodes of Calabar swelling tend to be more frequent and debilitating, microfilaremia is rare, and eosinophilia and increased levels of antifilarial antibodies are characteristic.

PATHOLOGY   The pathogenesis of the manifestations of loiasis is poorly understood. Calabar swellings are thought to result from a hypersensitivity reaction to the adult worm.

DIAGNOSIS   Definitive diagnosis of loiasis requires the detection of microfilariae in the peripheral blood or the isolation of the adult worm from the eye or from a subcutaneous biopsy specimen from a site of swelling developing after treatment. PCR-based assays for the detection of *L. loa* DNA in blood are now available in specialized laboratories and are highly sensitive and specific. In practice, the diagnosis must often be based on a characteristic history and clinical presentation, blood eosinophilia, and elevated levels of antifilarial antibodies,

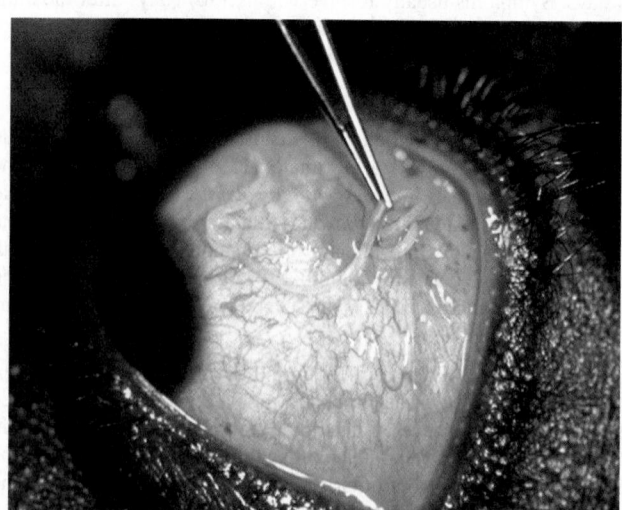

FIGURE 202-4 Adult *Loa loa* in the process of surgical removal after its subconjunctival migration.

particularly in travelers to an endemic region, who are usually amicrofilaremic. Other clinical findings in the latter individuals include hypergammaglobulinemia, elevated levels of serum IgE, and elevated leukocyte and eosinophil counts.

℞ TREATMENT

DEC (8 to 10 mg/kg per day for 21 days) is effective against both the adult and the microfilarial forms of *L. loa*, but multiple courses are frequently necessary before the disease resolves completely. In cases of heavy microfilaremia, allergic or other inflammatory reactions can take place during treatment, including central nervous system involvement with coma and encephalitis. Heavy infections can be treated initially with apheresis to remove the microfilariae and with glucocorticoids (40 to 60 mg of prednisone per day) followed by doses of DEC (0.5 mg/kg per day). If antifilarial treatment has no adverse effects, the prednisone dose can be rapidly tapered and the dose of DEC gradually increased to 8 to 10 mg/kg per day.

Albendazole or ivermectin (although neither is approved for this use by the Food and Drug Administration) has been shown to be effective in reducing microfilarial loads. DEC (300 mg weekly) is an effective prophylactic regimen for loiasis.

STREPTOCERCIASIS

Mansonella streptocerca, found mainly in the tropical forest belt of Africa from Ghana to Zaire, is transmitted by biting midges. The major clinical manifestations involve the skin and include pruritus, papular rashes, and pigmentation changes. Many infected individuals have inguinal adenopathy, although most are asymptomatic. The diagnosis is made by detection of the characteristic microfilariae in skin snips. DEC (6 mg/kg per day in divided doses for 14 to 21 days) is effective in killing both microfilariae and adult worms. As in onchocerciasis, treatment is sometimes accompanied by urticaria, arthralgias, myalgias, headaches, and abdominal discomfort. Ivermectin at a single dose of 150 μg/kg leads to sustained suppression of microfilariae in the skin and is likely to assume primacy in the treatment of streptocerciasis.

MANSONELLA PERSTANS INFECTION

Mansonella perstans, distributed across the center of Africa and in northeastern South America, is transmitted by midges. Adult worms reside in serous cavities—pericardial, pleural, and peritoneal—as well as in the mesentery and the perirenal and retroperitoneal tissues. Microfilariae circulate in the blood without periodicity. The clinical and pathologic features of the infection are poorly defined. Most patients appear to be asymptomatic, but manifestations may include transient angioedema and pruritus of the arms, face, or other parts of the body (analogous to the Calabar swellings of loiasis); fever; headache; arthralgias; and right-upper-quadrant pain. Occasionally, pericarditis and hepatitis occur. The diagnosis is based on the demonstration of microfilariae in blood or serosal effusions. Perstans filariasis is often associated with peripheral-blood eosinophilia and antifilarial antibody elevations. Although DEC (8 to 10 mg/kg per day for 21 days) is the standard therapeutic agent, there is little evidence that it is effective. Cure is indicated by the disappearance of symptoms and eosinophilia; multiple courses of therapy are usually required. Ivermectin, used in frequent repeated doses, has been shown to be capable of reducing blood microfilarial levels. Both mebendazole (100 mg twice daily for 30 days) and albendazole (400 mg twice daily for 10 days) have been reported occasionally to be effective.

MANSONELLA OZZARDI INFECTION

The distribution of *Mansonella ozzardi* is restricted to Central and South America and certain Caribbean islands. Adult worms are rarely recovered from humans. Microfilariae circulate in the blood without periodicity. Although this organism has often been considered nonpathogenic, headache, articular pain, fever, pulmonary symptoms, adenopathy, hepatomegaly, pruritus, and eosinophilia have been ascribed to *M. ozzardi* infection. Diagnosis is made by the detection of micro-

filariae in peripheral blood. Ivermectin (a single dose of 6 mg) has been shown to be effective in treating this infection.

DRACUNCULIASIS (GUINEA WORM INFECTION)

ETIOLOGY AND EPIDEMIOLOGY Dracunculiasis, caused by *Dracunculus medinensis*, is a parasitic infection whose incidence has declined dramatically because of global eradication efforts. Current estimates suggest that there are 56,000 cases worldwide, the majority in Sudan. Humans acquire this infection when they ingest water containing infective larvae derived from *Cyclops*, a crustacean that is the intermediate host. Larvae penetrate the stomach or intestinal wall, mate, and mature. The adult male probably dies; the female *Dracunculus* develops over a year and migrates to subcutaneous tissues, usually in the lower extremity. As the thin female *Dracunculus*, ranging in length from 300 cm to 1 m, approaches the skin, a blister forms that, over days, breaks down and forms an ulcer. When the blister opens, large numbers of motile, rhabditiform larvae can be released into stagnant water; ingestion by *Cyclops* completes the life cycle.

CLINICAL FEATURES Few or no clinical manifestations of dracunculiasis are evident until just before the blister forms, when there is an onset of fever and generalized allergic symptoms, including periorbital edema, wheezing, and urticaria. The emergence of the worm is associated with local pain and swelling. When the blister ruptures (usually as a result of immersion in water), the adult worm releases larva-rich fluid, and this release is associated with a relief of symptoms. The shallow ulcer surrounding the emerging adult worm heals over weeks to months. Such ulcers, however, can become secondarily infected, the result being cellulitis, local inflammation, abscess formation, or (uncommonly) tetanus. Occasionally, the adult worm does not emerge but becomes encapsulated and calcified.

DIAGNOSIS The diagnosis is based on the findings developing with the emergence of the adult worm, as described above.

℞ TREATMENT

Gradual extraction of the worm by winding of a few centimeters on a stick each day remains the common and effective practice. Worms may be excised surgically. The administration of metronidazole (250 mg three times daily for 10 days) may relieve symptoms but has no proven activity against the worm.

PREVENTION Prevention, which remains the only real control measure, depends on the provision of safe drinking water.

ZOONOTIC FILARIAL INFECTIONS

Dirofilariae that affect primarily dogs, cats, and raccoons occasionally infect humans incidentally, as do *Brugia* and *Onchocerca* parasites that affect small mammals. Because humans are an abnormal host, the parasites never develop fully. Pulmonary dirofilarial infection caused by the canine heartworm *Dirofilaria immitis* generally presents in humans as a solitary pulmonary nodule. Chest pain, hemoptysis, and cough are uncommon. Infections with *D. repens* (from dogs) or *D. tenuis* (from raccoons) can cause local subcutaneous nodules in humans. Zoonotic *Brugia* infection can produce isolated lymph node enlargement, whereas zoonotic *Onchocerca* can cause subconjunctival masses. Eosinophilia levels and antifilarial antibody titers are not commonly elevated. Excisional biopsy is both diagnostic and curative; these infections usually do not respond to chemotherapy.

FURTHER READING

ADDISS DA, DREYER G: Treatment of lymphatic filariasis, in *Lymphatic Filariasis*, TB Nutman (ed). London, Imperial College Press, 1999, pp 151–199

BOCKARIE MJ et al: Mass treatment to eliminate filariasis in Papua New Guinea. N Engl J Med 347:1841, 2002

DREYER G et al: Acute attacks in the extremities of persons living in an area endemic for bancroftian filariasis: Differentiation of two syndromes. Trans R Soc Trop Med Hyg 93:413, 1999

GARDON J et al: Serious reactions after mass treatment of onchocerciasis with ivermectin in an area endemic for *Loa loa* infection. Lancet 350:18, 1997

———— et al: Effects of standard and high doses of ivermectin on adult worms of *Onchocerca volvulus*: A randomised controlled trial. Lancet 360:203, 2002

HOERAUF A et al: Depletion of *Wolbachia* endobacteria in *Onchocerca vol-*

vulus by doxycycline and microfilaridermia after ivermectin treatment. Lancet 357:1415, 2001

———— et al: Onchocerciasis. BMJ 326:207, 2003

HOPKINS DR et al: Dracunculiasis eradication: And now, Sudan. Am J Trop Med Hyg 67:415, 2002

MCCARTHY JS: Diagnosis of lymphatic filarial infections, in *Lymphatic Filariasis*, TB Nutman (ed). London, Imperial College Press, 1999, pp 127–149

WHO EXPERT COMMITTEE ON ONCHOCERCIASIS: Onchocerciasis and its control: Fourth report. Tech Rep Ser No 852. Geneva, World Health Organization, 1995

203 SCHISTOSOMIASIS AND OTHER TREMATODE INFECTIONS
Adel A.F. Mahmoud

Trematodes, or flatworms, are a group of morphologically and biologically heterogeneous organisms that belong to the phylum Platyhelminthes. Human infection with trematodes occurs in many geographic areas and can cause considerable morbidity and mortality. For clinical purposes, the significant trematode infections of humans may be divided according to the tissues invaded by adult flukes: blood, biliary tree, intestines, and lungs (Table 203-1).

Trematodes share some common morphologic features, including macroscopic size (from 1 cm to several cm); dorsoventral, flattened, bilaterally symmetric bodies (adult worms); and the prominence of two suckers. Except for the schistosomes, all trematodes that parasitize humans are hermaphroditic. The life cycle of trematodes involves a definitive host (mammalian/human), in which adult worms initiate sexual reproduction, and an intermediate host (snails), in which asexual multiplication of the larval forms occurs. More than one intermediate host may be necessary for some species of trematodes. Human infection is initiated either by direct penetration of intact skin or by ingestion. Upon maturation within the human host, adult flukes initiate sexual reproduction that results in egg production. Helminth ova leave the definitive host in excreta or sputum and, upon reaching suitable environmental conditions, they hatch, releasing free-living miracidia that must find a specific snail intermediate host. After asexual reproduction, cercariae are released from infected snails; these organisms either infect humans or must find another intermediate host to allow encystment into metacercariae—the infective stage in these species.

The host-parasite relationship in trematode infections is a product of the biologic features of these organisms: they are multicellular, undergo several developmental changes within the host, and usually result in chronic infections. In general, the distribution of worm infections in human populations is *overdispersed*; i.e., it follows a negative binomial mathematical relationship in which most infected individuals harbor low worm burdens while a small percentage are heavily infected. It is the heavily infected minority who are particularly prone to disease sequelae and who constitute an epidemiologically significant reservoir of infection in endemic areas. It is also important to appreciate that worms do not multiply within the definitive host and that they have a relatively long life span, ranging from a few months to a few years. Morbidity and mortality due to trematode infections reflect a multifactorial process that results from the tipping of a delicate balance based on the intensity of infection and the host reactions that initiate and modulate pathologic outcome. Furthermore, the genetics of the parasite and the human host contribute to the outcome of infection and disease. Infections with trematodes that migrate through or reside in host tissues are associated with a moderate to high degree of peripheral blood eosinophilia; this association is of significance in protective and immunopathologic sequelae and is a useful clinical indicator of infection.

APPROACH TO THE PATIENT

The approach to individuals with suspected trematode infection begins with a question: Where have you been? Details of geographic history, exposure to freshwater bodies, and indulgence in local eating habits without ensuring safety of food and drink are all essential elements in the history. The workup plan must include a detailed physical examination and tests appropriate for the suspected infection. Diagnosis is based either on detection of the relevant stage of the parasite in excreta, sputum, or (rarely) tissue samples or on sensitive and specific serologic tests. Consultation with physicians familiar with these infections or with the U.S. Centers for Disease Control and Prevention (CDC) is helpful in guiding diagnosis and selecting therapy.

BLOOD FLUKES: SCHISTOSOMIASIS

Human schistosomiasis is caused by five species of this parasitic trematode: the intestinal species *Schistosoma mansoni*, *S. japonicum*, *S. mekongi*, and *S. intercalatum* and the urinary species *S. haematobium*. Infection may cause considerable morbidity in the intestines, liver, and urinary tract, and a proportion of affected individuals die. Other schistosome species (e.g., avian species) may invade human skin but then die in subcutaneous tissue, producing only self-limiting cutaneous manifestations.

Information on the prevalence and geographic distribution of human schistosomiasis is inexact. The five species are estimated to infect 200 to 300 million people in South America, the Caribbean, Africa, the Middle East, and Southeast Asia. The total population living under conditions favoring transmission approximates double or triple that number—a fact reflecting the public health significance of schistosomiasis.

ETIOLOGY Human infection is initiated by penetration of intact skin with infective cercariae. These organisms are released from infected snails in freshwater bodies; they measure ~2 mm in length and possess an anterior and a ventral sucker that attach to the skin surface and facilitate penetration. Once in the subcutaneous tissue, the organism transforms into the next stage: the schistosomula. This transformation involves morphologic, membrane, and immunologic changes, prominent among which is the transformation of the cercarial outer membrane from a trilaminar to a heptalaminar membrane that is then maintained throughout the life span of the worms in humans. The transformation to a heptalaminar structure is thought to be the schistosome's main adaptive mechanism for survival in humans. Schistosomulae begin their migration within 2 to 4 days via venous or lymphatic vessels, reaching the lungs and finally the liver parenchyma. Sexually mature worms descend into the venous system at specific anatomical locations: intestinal veins (*S. mansoni*, *S. japonicum*, *S. mekongi*, and *S. intercalatum*) and vesical veins (*S. haematobium*). After mating, adult gravid females travel against venous blood flow to small tributaries, where they deposit their ova intravascularly. Schistosome ova (Fig. 203-1) have specific morphologic features that can be used to differentiate species. Aided by enzymatic secretions through minipores in eggshells, ova move through the venous wall, traversing host tissues to reach the lumen of the intestinal or urinary tract, and are voided with stools or urine. Approximately 50% of ova are retained in host tissues locally (intestines or urinary tract) or are carried by venous blood flow to the liver and other organs. Schistosome ova that reach freshwater bodies hatch, releasing free-living miracidia that seek the snail intermediate host to undergo several asexual multiplication cycles. Finally, infective cercariae are shed from snails.

Adult schistosome worms measure ~1 to 2 cm in length. The male is slightly shorter, with a flattened body; its edges curve anteriorly to form the gynecophoral canal, in which mature adult females are usually held. The females are longer, slender, and rounded in cross-section. The precise nature of biochemical and reproductive exchanges between the two sexes is unknown, as are the regulatory mechanisms for pairing. Adult schistosomes parasitize specific sites in the host venous system. What guides adult intestinal schistosomes to branches of the superior or inferior mesenteric veins or adult *S. haematobium* worms to the vesical plexus is unknown. In addition, the evasion mechanisms by which adult worms inhibit the coagulation cascade and the effector arms of the host immune responses are not fully understood. The genome of schistosomes is made of 16 chromosomes; its DNA sequence is currently being determined.

EPIDEMIOLOGY The distribution of schistosome infection and related disease syndromes in human populations (Fig. 203-2) is dependent on both parasite and host factors. In endemic areas, the rate of yearly onset of new infection, or incidence, is generally low. Prevalence, on the other hand, starts to be appreciable by the age of 3 to 4 years and builds to a maximum that varies by endemic region (up to 100%) in the 15- to 20-year age group. Prevalence then stabilizes or decreases slightly in older age groups (>40 years). Intensity of infection (as measured by fecal or urinary egg counts, which correlate with adult worm burdens in most circumstances) follows the increase in prevalence up to the age of 15 to 20 years and then declines markedly in older age groups. This decline may reflect acquisition of resistance, or it may be due to changes in water contact patterns, since older people are exposed less. Furthermore, the unique distribution of schistosomes in human populations (i.e., an overdispersed distribution) may be due to the heterogeneity of worm populations, with some more invasive than others; alternatively, it may be due to differences in the genetic susceptibility of host populations, as has recently been demonstrated.

Disease due to schistosome infection is the outcome of parasitologic, host, and additional infectious, nutritional, and environmental factors. Most of the disease syndromes relate to the presence of one or more of the parasite stages in the human host. The distribution of disease manifestations in the populations of endemic areas correlates, in general, with the intensity and duration of infection as well as with the age and genetic susceptibility of the host. Overall, disease manifestations are clinically relevant in only a small proportion of persons infected with any of the intestinal schistosomes. In contrast, urinary schistosomiasis manifests clinically in most infected individuals.

Patients with both HIV infection and schistosomiasis have been found to excrete far fewer eggs in their stools than those infected with *S. mansoni* alone; the mechanism underlying this difference is unknown. The two groups, however, respond equally to treatment with praziquantel.

PATHOGENESIS AND IMMUNITY During the invasive stage, cercaria-associated dermatitis reflects dermal and subdermal inflammatory responses—both humoral and cell-mediated. As the parasites approach

TABLE 203-1	*Major Human Trematode Infections*	
Trematode	Transmission	Endemic Area(s)
BLOOD FLUKES		
Schistosoma mansoni	Skin penetration by cercariae released from snails	Africa, South America, Middle East
S. japonicum	Skin penetration by cercariae released from snails	China, Philippines, Indonesia
S. intercalatum	Skin penetration by cercariae released from snails	West Africa
S. mekongi	Skin penetration by cercariae released from snails	Southeast Asia
S. haematobium	Skin penetration by cercariae released from snails	Africa, Middle East
BILIARY (HEPATIC) FLUKES		
Clonorchis sinensis	Ingestion of metacercariae in freshwater fish	Far East
Opisthorchis viverrini	Ingestion of metacercariae in freshwater fish	Far East, Thailand
O. felineus	Ingestion of metacercariae in freshwater fish	Far East, Europe
Fasciola hepatica	Ingestion of metacercariae on aquatic plants or in water	Worldwide
F. gigantica	Ingestion of metacercariae on aquatic plants or in water	Sporadic, Africa
INTESTINAL FLUKES		
Fasciolopsis buski	Ingestion of metacercariae on aquatic plants	Southeast Asia
Heterophyes heterophyes	Ingestion of metacercariae in freshwater or brackish-water fish	Far East, North Africa
LUNG FLUKES		
Paragonimus westermani	Ingestion of metacercariae in crayfish or crabs	Global except North America and Europe

sexual maturity and the commencement of oviposition, acute schistosomiasis or Katayama fever (a serum sickness–like illness; see "Clinical Features," below) may occur. The associated antigen excess results in the formation of soluble immune complexes, which may be deposited in several tissues, initiating the sequence of pathologic events. In chronic schistosomiasis, most disease manifestations are due to eggs retained in host tissues. The granulomatous response around these ova is cell-mediated and is regulated both positively and negatively by a cascade of cytokine, cellular, and humoral responses. Granuloma formation begins with recruitment of a host of inflammatory cells in response to antigens secreted by the living organism within the ova. Cells recruited initially include phagocytes, antigen-specific T cells, and eosinophils. Fibroblasts, giant cells, and B lymphocytes predominate later. Once activated, T cells produce cytokines [such as tumor necrosis factor α (TNF-α), interleukin (IL) 2, IL-4, and IL-5, which in turn activate endothelial cells] as well as specific chemokines [such as monocyte chemotactic protein 1 (MCP-1)]. The result is recruitment of the cellular elements that organize in the form of granulomas around parasite eggs. These lesions reach a size many times that of the eggs, thus inducing organomegaly and obstruction. Immunomodulation or downregulation of host responses to schistosome eggs plays a significant role in limiting the extent of the granulomatous lesions—and consequently disease—in chronically infected experimental animals or humans. The underlying mechanisms involve another cascade of regulatory cytokines (IL-10, IL-12) and idiotypic antibodies. Subsequent to the granulomatous response, fibrosis sets in, resulting in more permanent disease sequelae. Because schistosomiasis is a chronic infection, the accumulation of antigen-antibody complexes results in deposits in renal glomeruli and may cause significant kidney disease.

The better-studied pathologic sequelae in schistosomiasis are those observed in liver disease. Ova that are carried by portal blood embolize to the liver. Because of their size (~150 × 60 μm in the case of *S. mansoni*), they lodge at presinusoidal sites, where granulomas are formed. The granulomas contribute to the liver enlargement observed in infected individuals. Schistosomal hepatomegaly is also associated

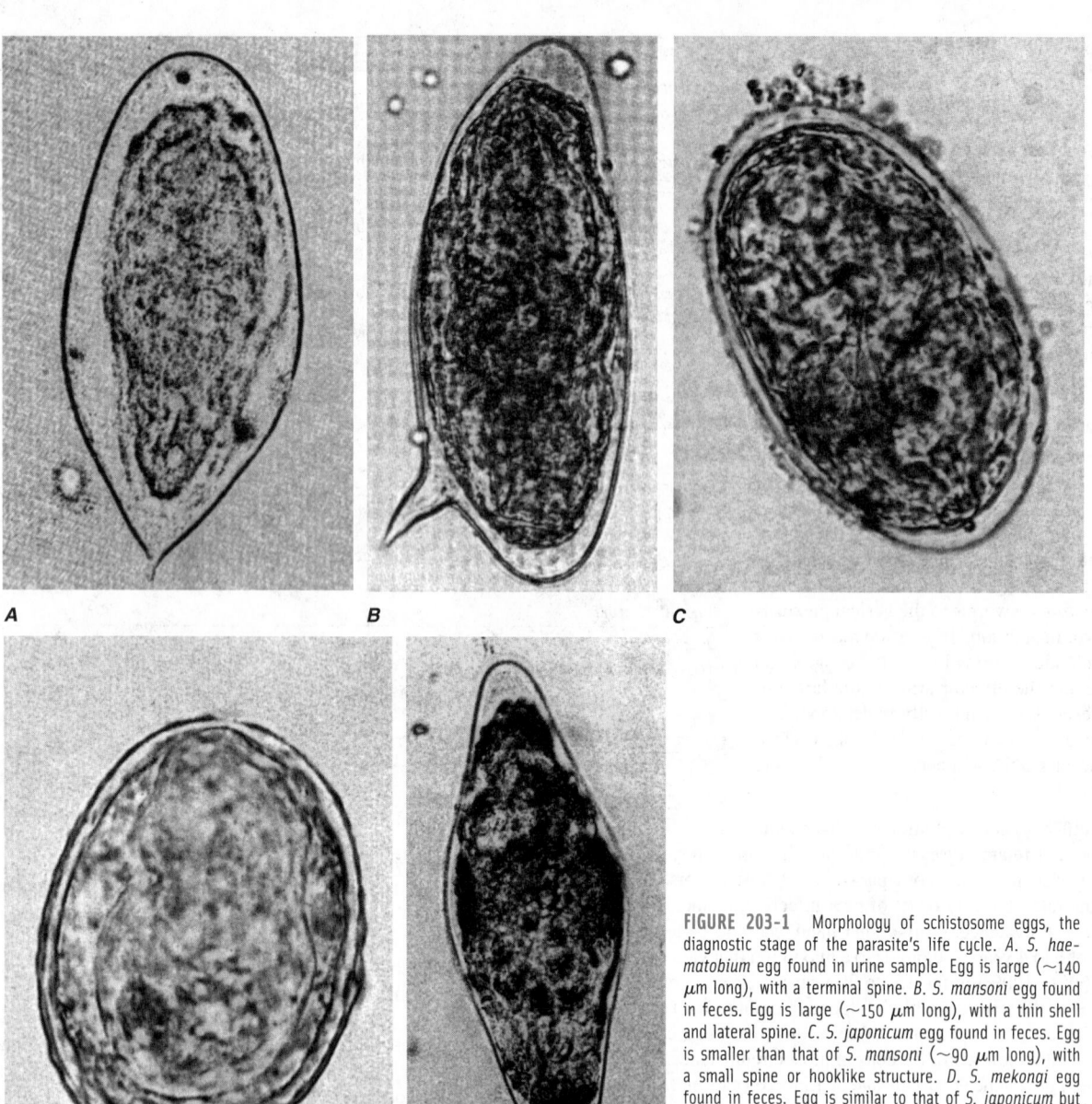

FIGURE 203-1 Morphology of schistosome eggs, the diagnostic stage of the parasite's life cycle. *A. S. haematobium* egg found in urine sample. Egg is large (~140 μm long), with a terminal spine. *B. S. mansoni* egg found in feces. Egg is large (~150 μm long), with a thin shell and lateral spine. *C. S. japonicum* egg found in feces. Egg is smaller than that of *S. mansoni* (~90 μm long), with a small spine or hooklike structure. *D. S. mekongi* egg found in feces. Egg is similar to that of *S. japonicum* but smaller (~65 μm long). *E. S. intercalatum* egg found in feces. Egg is larger than that of *S. haematobium* (~190 μm long), with a longer, sharply pointed spine. *(From LR Ash, TC Orihel: Atlas of Human Parasitology, 3d ed. Chicago, ASCP Press, 1990; with permission.)*

with certain class I and class II human leukocyte antigen (HLA) markers; its genetic basis appears to be multigenic. Presinusoidal portal blockage causes several hemodynamic changes, including portal hypertension and associated development of portosystemic collaterals at the esophagogastric junction and other sites. Esophageal varices are most likely to break and cause repeated episodes of hematemesis. Because changes in liver hemodynamics in schistosomiasis are slow, compensatory arterialization of blood flow through the liver is established. While this compensatory mechanism may be associated with certain metabolic side effects, the retention of hepatocyte perfusion permits the maintenance of normal liver function for several years.

After granuloma formation, the second most significant pathologic change in the liver relates to the onset of fibrosis. It is characteristically periportal (Symmers' clay pipe–stem fibrosis) but may be diffuse. Fibrosis, when diffuse, may be seen in areas of egg deposition and granuloma formation, but it is also seen in distant locations such as portal tracts. Schistosomiasis alone results in pure fibrotic lesions in the liver; cirrhosis occurs when other nutritional or infectious agents (e.g., hepatitis B or C virus) are involved. In recent years, it has been recognized that deposition of fibrotic tissue in the extracellular matrix

results from the interaction of T lymphocytes with cells of the fibroblast series; several cytokines, such as IL-2, IL-4, IL-1, and transforming growth factor β (TGF-β), are known to stimulate fibrogenesis. The process may be dependent on the genetic constitution of the host. Furthermore, regulatory cytokines that can suppress fibrogenesis, such as interferon γ (IFN-γ) or IL-12, may play a role in modulating the response.

While the above description focuses on granuloma formation and fibrosis of the liver, similar processes occur in urinary schistosomiasis. Granuloma formation at the lower end of the ureters obstructs urinary flow, with subsequent development of hydroureter and hydronephrosis. Similar lesions in the urinary bladder cause the protrusion of papillomatous structures into its cavity; these may ulcerate and/or bleed. The chronic stage of infection is associated with scarring and deposition of calcium in the bladder wall.

Immunomodulation is an essential mechanism in shaping the clinical and pathologic outcome of schistosomiasis. While most detailed immunologic analyses have been performed in experimental animals, enough evidence exists from studies in humans to delineate the suppression of T cell responses in association with active infections and a regulatory role for IL-10.

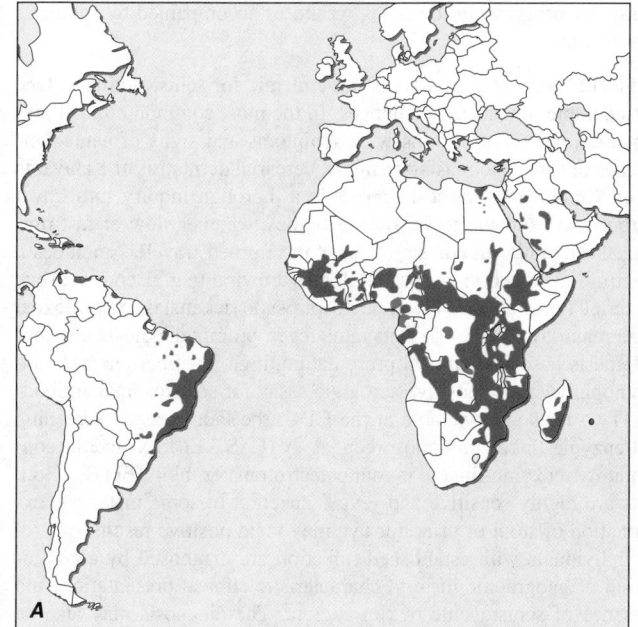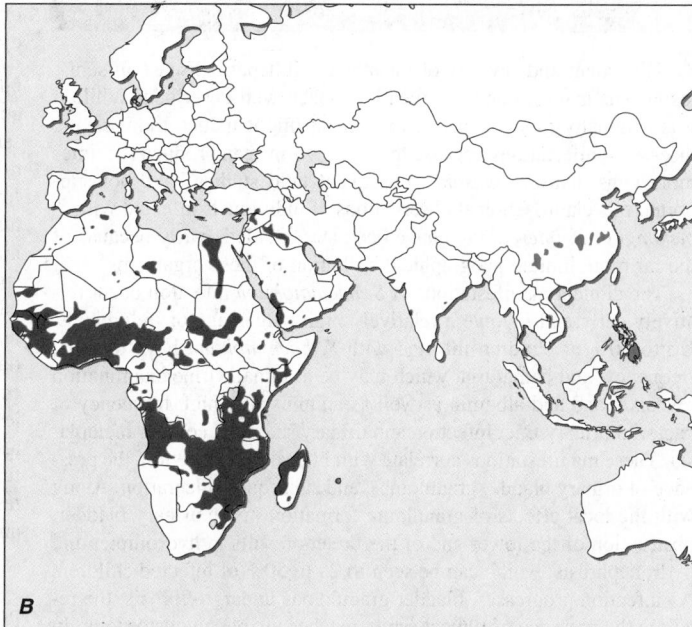

FIGURE 203-2 Global distribution of schistosomiasis. *A. S. mansoni* infection (*dark blue*) is endemic in Africa, the Middle East, South America, and a few Caribbean countries. *S. intercalatum* infection (*green*) is endemic in sporadic foci in West and Central Africa. *B. S. haematobium* infection (*purple*) is endemic in Africa and the Middle East. The major endemic countries for *S. japonicum* infection (*green*) are China, the Philippines, and Indonesia. *S. mekongi* infection (*red*) is endemic in sporadic foci in Southeast Asia.

Studies on immunity to schistosomiasis, whether innate or acquired, have expanded our knowledge of the components of these responses and the target antigens. The concept of innate immunity is illustrated by the inability of avian schistosomes, which cause swimmers' itch, to reach maturity in humans. The critical question, however, is whether humans acquire immunity to schistosomes. Epidemiologic evidence suggests the onset of acquired immunity during the course of infection in young adults. Curative treatment of infection divides populations in endemic areas into those who acquire reinfection rapidly (susceptible) and those who follow a protracted course (resistant). This difference may be explained by differences in transmission, immunologic response, or genetic susceptibility. The mechanism of acquired immunity involves antibodies, complement, and several effector cells, particularly eosinophils. Furthermore, the intensity of schistosome infection has been correlated with a region in chromosome 5. In several recent studies, a few protective schistosome antigens have been identified as vaccine candidates, but none has been evaluated in human populations to date.

CLINICAL FEATURES In general, disease manifestations of schistosomiasis occur in three stages, which vary not only by species but also by intensity of infection and other host factors, such as age and genetics. During the phase of cercarial invasion, a form of dermatitis may be observed. This so-called swimmers' itch occurs most often with *S. mansoni* and *S. japonicum* infections, manifesting 2 or 3 days after invasion as an itchy maculopapular rash on the affected areas of the skin. The condition is particularly severe when humans are exposed to avian schistosomes. This form of cercarial dermatitis is seen around the freshwater lakes in the northern United States, particularly in the spring. Cercarial dermatitis is a self-limiting clinical entity. During worm maturation and at the beginning of oviposition (i.e., 4 to 8 weeks after skin invasion), acute schistosomiasis or Katayama fever—a serum sickness–like syndrome with fever, generalized lymphadenopathy, and hepatosplenomegaly—may develop. Individuals suffering from acute schistosomiasis show a high degree of peripheral blood eosinophilia. Parasite-specific antibodies may be detected before schistosome eggs are identified in excreta. Acute schistosomiasis has become an important clinical entity worldwide because of increased travel to endemic areas. Travelers are exposed to parasites while swimming or wading in freshwater bodies and upon their return present with the acute manifestations. The course of acute schistosomiasis is generally benign, but deaths are occasionally reported in association with heavy exposure to schistosomes.

The main clinical manifestations of chronic schistosomiasis are species-dependent. Intestinal species (*S. mansoni*, *S. japonicum*, *S. mekongi*, and *S. intercalatum*) cause intestinal and hepatosplenic disease as well as several manifestations associated with portal hypertension. During the intestinal phase, which may begin a few months after infection and may last for years, symptomatic patients characteristically have colicky abdominal pain and bloody diarrhea. Patients may also report fatigue and an inability to perform daily routine functions and may show evidence of growth retardation. The severity of intestinal schistosomiasis is often related to the intensity of the worm burden. The disease runs a chronic course but rarely progresses to a functional level (e.g., malabsorption) or to anatomical lesions of the gut. The exception is colonic polyposis, which has been seen in some endemic areas, such as Egypt.

The hepatosplenic phase of disease manifests early (during the first year of infection, particularly in children) with enlargement of the liver due to parasite-induced granulomatous lesions. Hepatomegaly is seen in ~15 to 20% of infected individuals; it correlates roughly with intensity of infection, occurs more often in children, and may be related to specific HLA haplotypes. In subsequent phases of infection, presinusoidal blockage of blood flow leads to portal hypertension and splenomegaly. Moreover, portal hypertension may lead to varices at the lower end of the esophagus and at other sites. Patients with schistosomal liver disease may have right-upper-quadrant "dragging" pain during the hepatomegaly phase, and this pain may move to the left upper quadrant as splenomegaly progresses. Bleeding from esophageal varices may, however, be the first clinical manifestation of this phase. Patients may experience repeated bleeding but seem to tolerate its impact, since an adequate total hepatic blood flow permits normal liver function for a considerable period in schistosomal hepatomegaly. In late-stage disease, typical fibrotic changes occur along with liver function deterioration and the onset of ascites, hypoalbuminemia, and defects in coagulation. Intercurrent viral infections of the liver (especially hepatitis B and C) or nutritional deficiencies may well accelerate or exacerbate the deterioration of hepatic function.

The extent and severity of intestinal and hepatic disease in schistosomiasis mansoni and japonica have been well described. While it was originally thought that *S. japonicum* might induce more severe disease manifestations because the adult worms can produce ten times more eggs than *S. mansoni*, subsequent field studies have not supported this claim. Clinical observations of individuals infected with *S. mekongi* or *S. intercalatum* have been less detailed, partly because of the far more limited geographic distribution of these organisms.

The clinical manifestations of *S. haematobium* infection occur relatively early and involve a relatively high percentage of individuals. Up to 80% of children infected with *S. haematobium* have dysuria, frequency, and hematuria, which may be terminal. Urine examination reveals blood and albumin as well as an unusually high frequency of bacterial urinary tract infection and urinary sediment cellular metaplasia. These manifestations correlate with intensity of infection, the presence of urinary bladder granulomas, and subsequent ulceration. Along with the local effects of granuloma formation in the urinary bladder, obstruction of the lower end of the ureters results in hydroureter and hydronephrosis, which can be seen in 25 to 50% of infected children. As infection progresses, bladder granulomas undergo fibrosis; the result is the presence of typical sandy patches visible on cystoscopy. In many endemic areas, an association between squamous cell carcinoma of the bladder and *S. haematobium* infection has been observed. Such malignancy is detected in a younger age group than is transitional cell carcinoma. In fact, *S. haematobium* has now been classified as a human carcinogen.

Significant disease may occur in other organs during chronic schistosomiasis. Most important is disease in the lungs and central nervous system (CNS); other locations, such as the skin and the genital organs, are far less frequently affected. In pulmonary schistosomiasis, embolized eggs lodge in small arterioles, producing acute necrotizing arteriolitis and granuloma formation. During *S. mansoni* and *S. japonicum* infection, schistosome eggs reach the lungs after the development of portosystemic collateral circulation; in *S. haematobium* infection, ova may reach the lungs directly via connections between the vesical and systemic circulation. After the development of arteriolitis and granuloma formation, fibrous tissue deposition is detected and leads to endarteritis obliterans, pulmonary hypertension, and cor pulmonale. This clinical entity is an uncommon presentation during chronic schistosomiasis. The most frequent symptoms are cough, fever, and dyspnea; ascites and hemoptysis are less frequently encountered. Cor pulmonale may be diagnosed radiologically on the basis of prominent right side of the heart and dilation of the pulmonary artery. Frank evidence of right-sided heart failure may be seen in late cases.

CNS schistosomiasis is important but less common than pulmonary schistosomiasis. It characteristically occurs as cerebral disease due to *S. japonicum* infection. Migratory worms deposit eggs in the brain and induce a granulomatous response. The frequency of this manifestation among infected individuals in some endemic areas (e.g., the Philippines) is calculated at 2 to 4%. Jacksonian epilepsy due to *S. japonicum* infection is the second most common cause of epilepsy in these areas. *S. mansoni* and *S. haematobium* infections have been associated with transverse myelitis. This syndrome is thought to be due to eggs traveling to the venous plexus around the spinal cord. In schistosomiasis mansoni, transverse myelitis is usually seen in the chronic stage after the development of portal hypertension and portosystemic shunts, which allow ova to travel to the spinal cord veins. This proposed sequence of events has been challenged because of a few reports of transverse myelitis occurring early in the course of *S. mansoni* infection. More information is needed to confirm these observations. During schistosomiasis haematobia, ova may travel through communication between vesical and systemic veins, resulting in spinal cord disease that may be detected at any stage of infection. Pathologic study of lesions in schistosomal transverse myelitis may reveal eggs along with necrotic or granulomatous lesions. Patients usually present with acute or rapidly progressing lower-leg weakness accompanied by sphincter dysfunction.

DIAGNOSIS Physicians in areas not endemic for schistosomiasis face considerable diagnostic challenges. In the most common clinical presentation, a traveler returns with symptoms and signs of acute syndromes of schistosomiasis—namely, cercarial dermatitis or Katayama fever. Central to correct diagnosis is a thorough inquiry into travel history and exposure to freshwater bodies, whether slow or fast running. Differential diagnosis of fever in returned travelers includes a spectrum of infections whose etiologies are viral (e.g., Dengue fever), bacterial (e.g., enteric fever, leptospirosis), rickettsial, or protozoal (e.g., malaria). In cases of Katayama fever, prompt diagnosis is essential and is based on clinical presentation, high-level peripheral blood eosinophilia, and a positive serologic assay for schistosomal antibodies. Two tests are available at the CDC: the Falcon assay screening test/enzyme-linked immunosorbent assay (FAST-ELISA) and the confirmatory enzyme-linked immunoelectrotransfer blot (EITB). Both tests are highly sensitive and ~96% specific. In some instances, examination of stool or urine for ova may yield positive results.

Individuals with established infection are diagnosed by a combination of geographic history, characteristic clinical presentation, and presence of schistosome ova in excreta. The diagnosis may also be established with the serologic assays mentioned above or with those that detect circulating schistosome antigens. These assays can be applied either to blood or to other body fluids (e.g., cerebrospinal fluid). For stool examination, the Kato thick smear or any other concentration method generally identifies all but the most lightly infected individuals. Urine may be examined by microscopy of sediment or by filtration of a known volume through Nuclepore filters. Kato thick smear and Nuclepore filtration provide quantitative data on the intensity of infection, which is of value in assessing the degree of tissue damage and in monitoring the effect of chemotherapy. Finally, schistosome infection may be diagnosed by examination of tissue samples, typically rectal biopsies; other biopsy procedures (e.g., liver biopsy) are not needed, except in special circumstances.

Differential diagnosis of schistosomal hepatomegaly must include viral hepatitis of all etiologies, miliary tuberculosis, malaria, visceral leishmaniasis, ethanol abuse, and causes of hepatic and portal vein obstruction. Of patients with these conditions, only a few may present with organomegaly and relatively intact liver function. The differential diagnosis of hematuria in *S. haematobium* infection includes bacterial cystitis, tuberculosis, urinary stones, and malignancy.

℞ TREATMENT

Treatment of schistosomiasis depends on the stage of infection and the clinical presentation. Other than topical dermatologic applications for relief of itching, no specific treatment is indicated for cercarial dermatitis caused by avian schistosomes. Therapy for acute schistosomiasis or Katayama fever needs to be adjusted appropriately for each case. While antischistosomal chemotherapy is indicated, it does not address immediate pathologic changes. In severe acute schistosomiasis, management in an acute-care setting is necessary, with supportive measures and consideration of glucocorticoid treatment. Once the acute critical phase is over, specific chemotherapy is indicated. For all individuals with infection established by either the demonstration of schistosome eggs or positive serology, treatment to eradicate the parasite should be administered. The drug of choice is praziquantel, which—depending on the infecting species (Table 203-2)—is administered orally as 40 or 60 mg/kg in two or three doses over a single day. Praziquantel treatment results in parasitologic cure in ~85% of cases and reduces egg counts by >90%. Few side effects have been encountered, and those that do develop usually do not interfere with completion of treatment. The dependence on a single chemotherapeutic agent has raised the possibility of the development of resistance in the schistosomes; to date, such resistance does not seem to be clinically significant. Other antischistosomal chemotherapeutic agents are cur-

TABLE 203-2　*Drug Therapy for Human Trematode Infections*

Infection	Drug of Choice	Adult Dose and Duration
BLOOD FLUKES		
S. mansoni, *S. intercalatum,* *S. haematobium*	Praziquantel	20 mg/kg, 2 doses in 1 day
S. japonicum, S. mekongi	Praziquantel	20 mg/kg, 3 doses in 1 day
BILIARY (HEPATIC) FLUKES		
C. sinensis, O. viverrini, *O. felineus*	Praziquantel	25 mg/kg, 3 doses in 1 day
F. hepatica, F. gigantica	Triclabendazole	10 mg/kg once
INTESTINAL FLUKES		
F. buski, H. heterophyes	Praziquantel	25 mg/kg, 3 doses in 1 day
LUNG FLUKES		
P. westermani	Praziquantel	25 mg/kg, 3 doses per day for 2 days

rently considered only as alternatives when praziquantel is unavailable. The effect of antischistosomal treatment on disease manifestations varies by stage. Early hepatomegaly and bladder lesions are known to resolve following chemotherapy, but the late established manifestations, such as fibrosis, do not change. Additional management modalities are needed for individuals with other manifestations, such as hepatocellular failure or recurrent hematemesis. The use of these interventions is guided by general medical and surgical principles.

PREVENTION AND CONTROL　Since transmission of schistosomiasis is dependent on human behavior, it is theoretically possible to devise an effective preventive strategy. The geographic distribution of infections in endemic regions of the world is not clearly demarcated. It is therefore prudent for travelers to avoid contact with all freshwater bodies, irrespective of the speed of water flow or unsubstantiated claims of safety. Some topical agents, when applied to the skin, may conceivably inhibit cercarial penetration, but none of these agents is currently available. If exposure occurs, a follow-up visit with a health care provider is strongly recommended. Prevention of infection in inhabitants of endemic areas is a significant challenge. People of these regions use freshwater bodies for sanitary, domestic, recreational, and agricultural purposes. Several control measures have been used, including application of molluscicides, provision of sanitary water and means for sewage disposal, chemotherapy, and health education. Current recommendations to countries endemic for schistosomiasis emphasize the use of multiple approaches. Particularly with the advent of an oral, safe, and effective antischistosomal agent, chemotherapy has been most successful in reducing the intensity of infection and reversing disease. The duration of this positive impact depends on transmission dynamics of the parasite in any specific endemic region. The ultimate goal of research on prevention and control is the development of a vaccine. Although there are a few promising leads, this goal is probably not within reach during the next decade or so.

LIVER (BILIARY) FLUKES

Several species of biliary fluke infecting humans are particularly common in Southeast Asia and Russia. Other species are transmitted in Europe, Africa, and the Americas. On the basis of their migratory pathway in humans, these infections may be divided into the *Clonorchis* and *Fasciola* groups (Table 203-1).

CLONORCHIASIS AND OPISTHORCHIASIS　Infection with *Clonorchis sinensis*, the Chinese or oriental fluke, is endemic among fish-eating mammals in Southeast Asia. Humans are an incidental host; the prevalence of human infection is highest in China, Vietnam, and Korea. Infection with *Opisthorchis viverrini* and *O. felineus* is zoonotic in cats and dogs. Transmission to humans occurs occasionally, particularly in Thailand (*O. viverrini*) and in Southeast Asia and eastern Europe (*O. felineus*). Data on the exact geographic distribution of these infectious agents in human populations are rudimentary.

Infection with any of these three species is established by ingestion of raw or inadequately cooked freshwater fish harboring metacercariae. These organisms excyst in the duodenum, releasing larvae that travel through the ampulla of Vater and mature into adult worms in the bile canaliculi. Mature flukes are flat and elongated, measuring 1 to 2 cm in length. The hermaphroditic worms reproduce by releasing small operculated eggs, which pass with bile into the intestines and are voided with stools. The life cycle is completed in the environment in specific freshwater snails (the first intermediate host) and encystment of metacercariae in freshwater fish.

Except for late sequelae, the exact clinical syndromes caused by clonorchiasis and opisthorchiasis are not well defined. Since most infected individuals harbor a low worm burden, many are asymptomatic. Moderate to heavy infection may be associated with vague right-upper-quadrant pain. In contrast, chronic or repeated infection is associated with manifestations such as cholangitis, cholangiohepatitis, and biliary obstruction. Cholangiocarcinoma is epidemiologically related to *C. sinensis* infection in China and to *O. viverrini* infection in northeastern Thailand. This association has resulted in the classification of these infectious agents as human carcinogens.

FASCIOLIASIS　Infections with *Fasciola hepatica* and *F. gigantica* are worldwide zoonoses that are particularly endemic in sheep-raising countries. Human cases have been reported in South America, Europe, Africa, Australia, and the Far East. Recent estimates indicate a worldwide prevalence of 17 million cases. High endemicity has been reported in certain areas of Peru and Bolivia. In most endemic areas the predominant species is *F. hepatica*, but in Asia and Africa a varying degree of overlap with *F. gigantica* has been observed.

Humans acquire fascioliasis by ingestion of metacercariae attached to certain aquatic plants, such as watercress. Infection may also be acquired by consumption of contaminated water or ingestion of food items washed with such water. Acquisition of human infection through consumption of freshly prepared raw liver containing immature flukes has been reported. Infection is initiated when metacercariae excyst, penetrate the gut wall, and travel through the peritoneal cavity to invade the liver capsule. Adult worms finally reach the bile ducts, where they produce large operculated eggs, which are voided in the bile and through the gastrointestinal tract to the outside environment. The flukes' life cycle is completed in specific snails (the first intermediate host) and encystment on aquatic plants.

The clinical features of fascioliasis relate to the stage and intensity of infection. Acute disease develops during the parasites' migration (1 to 2 weeks after infection) and includes fever, right-upper-quadrant pain, hepatomegaly, and eosinophilia. Computed tomography of the liver may show migratory tracks. Symptoms and signs usually subside as the parasites reach their final habitat. In individuals with chronic infection, bile duct obstruction and biliary cirrhosis are infrequently demonstrated. No relation to hepatic malignancy has been ascribed to fascioliasis.

DIAGNOSIS　The diagnosis of infection with any of the biliary flukes depends on a high degree of suspicion, the elicitation of an appropriate geographic history, and stool examination for the characteristically shaped parasite ova. Additional evidence may be obtained by documenting peripheral blood eosinophilia or imaging the liver. Serologic testing is helpful, particularly in lightly infected individuals.

　TREATMENT

Drug therapy (praziquantel or triclabendazole) is summarized in Table 203-2. Patients with anatomical lesions in the biliary tract or malignancy are managed according to general medical guidelines.

INTESTINAL FLUKES

Two species of intestinal flukes cause human infection in defined geographic areas worldwide (Table 203-1). The large *Fasciolopis buski* (adults measure 2 by 7 cm) is endemic in Southeast Asia, while the smaller *Heterophyes heterophyes* is found in the Nile Delta of Egypt and in the Far East. Infection is initiated by ingestion of metacercariae attached to aquatic plants (*F. buski*) or encysted in freshwater or brackish-water fish (*H. heterophyes*). Flukes mature in human intestines, and eggs are passed with stools. Most individuals infected with intestinal flukes are asymptomatic. In heavy *F. buski* infection, diarrhea, abdominal pain, and malabsorption may be encountered. Heavy infection with *H. heterophyes* may be associated with abdominal pain and mucous diarrhea. The diagnosis is established by detection of the characteristically shaped ova in stool samples. The drug of choice for treatment is praziquantel (Table 203-2).

LUNG FLUKES

Infection with the lung fluke *Paragonimus westermani* (Table 203-1) and related species (e.g., *P. africanus*) is endemic in many parts of the world, excluding North America and Europe. Endemicity is particularly noticeable in West Africa, Central and South America, and Asia. In nature, the reservoir hosts of *P. westermani* are wild and domestic felines. In Africa, *P. africanus* has been found in other species, such as dogs. Adult lung flukes, which are 7 to 12 mm in length, are found encapsulated in the lungs of infected persons. In rare circumstances, flukes are found encysted in the CNS (cerebral paragonimiasis) or abdominal cavity. Humans acquire lung fluke infection by ingesting infective metacercariae encysted in the muscles and viscera of crayfish and freshwater crabs. In endemic areas, these crustaceans are consumed either raw or pickled. Once the organisms reach the duodenum, they excyst, penetrate the gut wall, and travel through the peritoneal cavity, diaphragm, and pleural space to reach the lungs. Mature flukes are found in the bronchioles surrounded by cystic lesions. Parasite eggs are either expectorated with sputum or swallowed and passed to the outside environment with feces. The life cycle is completed in snails and freshwater crustacea.

When maturing flukes lodge in lung tissues, they cause hemorrhage and necrosis, resulting in cyst formation. The adjacent lung parenchyma shows evidence of inflammatory infiltration, predominantly by eosinophils. Cysts usually measure 1 to 2 cm in diameter and may contain 1 or 2 worms each. With the onset of oviposition, cysts usually rupture in adjacent bronchioles—an event allowing ova to exit from the human host. Older cysts develop thickened walls, which may undergo calcification. During the active phase of paragonimiasis, lung tissues surrounding parasite cysts may contain evidence of pneumonia, bronchitis, bronchiectasis, and fibrosis.

Pulmonary paragonimiasis is particularly symptomatic in persons with moderate to heavy infection. Productive cough with brownish sputum or frank hemoptysis associated with peripheral blood eosinophilia is usually the presenting feature. Chest examination may reveal signs of pleurisy. In chronic cases, bronchitis or bronchiectasis may predominate, but these conditions rarely proceed to lung abscess. Imaging of the lungs demonstrates characteristic features, including patchy densities, cavities, pleural effusion, and ring shadows. Cerebral paragonimiasis presents as either space-occupying lesions or epilepsy.

DIAGNOSIS   Pulmonary paragonimiasis is diagnosed by the detection of parasite ova in sputum and/or stools. Serology is of considerable help in egg-negative cases and in cerebral paragonimiasis.

$\boxed{\text{R}}$ TREATMENT

The drug of choice for treatment is praziquantel (Table 203-2). Other medical or surgical management may be needed for pulmonary or cerebral lesions.

CONTROL AND PREVENTION OF TISSUE FLUKES

For residents of nonendemic areas who are visiting an endemic region, the only effective preventive measure is to avoid ingestion of local plants, fish, or crustaceans; if their ingestion is necessary, these items should be washed or cooked thoroughly. Instruction on water and food preparation and consumption should be included in physicians' advice to travelers (Chap. 108). Interruption of transmission among residents of endemic areas depends on avoiding ingestion of the infective stage of the helminths and appropriate disposal of feces and sputum to prevent the hatching of eggs in the environment. These two approaches rely greatly on socioeconomic development and health education. In countries where economic progress has resulted in financial and social improvements, transmission has decreased. The third approach to control in endemic communities entails selective use of chemotherapy for individuals posing the highest risk of transmission—i.e., those with heavy infections. The availability of praziquantel—a broad-spectrum, safe, and effective anthelmintic agent—provides a means for reducing the reservoirs of infection in human populations. However, the existence of most of these helminths as zoonoses in several animal species complicates control efforts.

FURTHER READING

CHAN HH et al: The clinical and cholangiographic picture of hepatic clonorchiasis. J Clin Gastroenterol 34:183, 2002

DOENHOFF MJ et al: Resistance of *Schistosoma mansoni* to praziquantel: Is there a problem? Trans R Soc Trop Med Hyg 96:465, 2002

DRUGS FOR PARASITIC INFECTIONS. Med Lett Drugs Ther 1:44, 2002

JUKES MC et al: Heavy schistosomiasis associated with poor school term memory and slower reaction times in Tanzanian school children. Top Med Int Health 2:104, 2002

LIU LX, HARINASUTA KT: Liver and intestinal flukes. Gastroenterol Clin North Am 25:627, 1996

MAHMOUD AAFM (ed): Schistosomiasis, in *Tropical Medicine: Science and Practice*, G Pasvol and S Hoffman (eds). London, Imperial College Press, 2001, pp 1–510

MAS-COMA MS et al: Epidemiology of human fascioliasis: A review and proposed new classification. Bull World Health Organ 77:340, 1999

ROSS AG et al: Schistosomiasis. N Engl J Med 346:1212, 2002

QUINNELL RJ: Genetics of susceptibility to human helminth infection. Int J Parasitol 33:1219, 2003

WORLD HEALTH ORGANIZATION: Prevention and control of schistosomiasis and soil-transmitted helminthiasis. Technical report series 912. Geneva, World Health Organization, 2002, pp 1–57

204 | CESTODES
A. Clinton White, Jr., Peter F. Weller

Cestodes, or tapeworms, are segmented worms. The adults reside in the gastrointestinal tract, but the larvae can be found in almost any organ. Human tapeworm infections can be divided into two major clinical groups. In one group, humans are the definitive hosts, with the adult tapeworms living in the gastrointestinal tract (*Taenia saginata*, *Diphyllobothrium*, *Hymenolepis*, and *Dipylidium caninum*). In the other, humans are intermediate hosts, with larval-stage parasites present in the tissues. Diseases in this category include echinococcosis, sparganosis, and coenurosis. For *Taenia solium*, the human may be either the definitive or the intermediate host.

The ribbon-shaped tapeworm attaches to the intestinal mucosa by means of sucking cups or hooks located on the scolex. Behind the scolex is a short, narrow neck from which proglottids (segments) form. As each proglottid matures, it is displaced further back from the neck by the formation of new, less mature segments. The progressively elongating chain of attached proglottids, called the *strobila*, constitutes the bulk of the tapeworm. The length varies among species. In some, the tapeworm may consist of more than 1000 proglottids and may be several meters long. The mature proglottids are hermaphroditic and produce eggs, which are intermittently released. Since eggs of the different *Taenia* species are morphologically identical, differences in the morphology of the scolex or proglottids provide the basis for diagnostic identification to the species level. Most human tapeworms require at least one intermediate host for complete larval development. After ingestion of the eggs or proglottids by an intermediate host, the larval oncospheres are activated, escape the egg, and penetrate the intestinal mucosa. The oncosphere migrates to tissues and develops into an encysted form known as a *cysticercus* (single scolex), a *coenurus* (multiple scolices), or a *hydatid* (cyst with daughter cysts, each containing several protoscolices). Ingestion by the definitive host of tissues containing a cyst enables a scolex to develop into a tapeworm.

TAENIASIS SAGINATA   The beef tapeworm *T. saginata* occurs in all countries where raw or undercooked beef is eaten. It is most prevalent in sub-Saharan African and Middle Eastern countries. *T. saginata asiatica* is a variant of *T. saginata* that is found in Asia and for which pigs are the intermediate host.

Etiology and Pathogenesis   Humans are the only definitive host for the adult stage of *T. saginata*. This tapeworm, which can reach 8 m in length, inhabits the upper jejunum and has a scolex with four prominent suckers and 1000 to 2000 proglottids. Each gravid segment has 15 to 30 uterine branches (in contrast to 8 to 12 for *T. solium*). The eggs are indistinguishable from those of *T. solium*; they measure 30 to 40 μm, contain the oncosphere, and have a thick brown striated shell. Eggs deposited on vegetation can live for months to years until they are ingested by cattle or other herbivores. The embryo released after ingestion invades the intestinal wall and is carried to striated muscle, where it transforms into a cysticercus. When ingested in raw or undercooked beef, this form can infect humans. After the cysticercus is ingested, it takes ~2 months for the mature adult worm to develop.

Clinical Manifestations   Patients become aware of the infection most commonly by noting passage of proglottids in their feces. The proglottids are often motile, and patients may experience perianal discomfort when proglottids are discharged. Mild abdominal pain or discomfort, nausea, change in appetite, weakness, and weight loss can occur with *T. saginata* infection.

Diagnosis   The diagnosis is made by the detection of eggs or proglottids in the stool. Eggs may also be present in the perianal area; thus, if proglottids or eggs are not found in the stool, the perianal region should be examined with use of a cellophane-tape swab (as in pinworm infection; Chap. 201). Distinguishing *T. saginata* from *T. solium* requires examination of mature proglottids or the scolex. Serologic tests are not helpful diagnostically. Eosinophilia and elevated levels of serum IgE may be detected.

℞ TREATMENT

A single dose of praziquantel (10 mg/kg) is highly effective.

Prevention   The major method of preventing infection is the adequate cooking of beef; exposure to temperatures as low as 56°C for 5 min will destroy cysticerci. Refrigeration or salting for long periods or freezing at −10°C for 9 days also kills cysticerci in beef. General preventive measures include inspection of beef and proper disposal of human feces.

TAENIASIS SOLIUM AND CYSTICERCOSIS   The pork tapeworm *T. solium* can cause two distinct forms of infection. The form that develops depends on whether humans are infected with adult tapeworms in the intestine or with larval forms in the tissues (cysticercosis). Humans are the only definitive hosts for *T. solium*; pigs are the usual intermediate hosts, although other animals may harbor the larval forms. *T. solium* exists worldwide but is most prevalent in Latin America, sub-Saharan Africa,

China, southern and Southeast Asia, and eastern Europe. Cysticercosis occurs in industrialized nations largely as a result of the immigration of infected persons from endemic areas.

Etiology and Pathogenesis   The adult tapeworm generally resides in the upper jejunum. The scolex attaches by both sucking disks and two rows of hooklets. Often only one adult worm is present, but that worm may live for years. The tapeworm, usually about 3 m in length, may have as many as 1000 proglottids, each of which produces up to 50,000 eggs. Groups of three to five proglottids are generally released and excreted into the feces, and the eggs in these proglottids are infective for both humans and animals. The eggs may survive in the environment for several months. After ingestion of eggs by the intermediate host, the larvae are activated, escape the egg, penetrate the intestinal wall, and are carried to many tissues, with a predilection for striated muscle of the neck, tongue, and trunk. Within 60 to 90 days, the encysted larval stage develops. These cysticerci can survive for months to years. Humans acquire infections that lead to intestinal tapeworms by ingesting undercooked pork containing cysticerci. Infections that cause human cysticercosis follow the ingestion of *T. solium* eggs, usually from close contact with a tapeworm carrier. Autoinfection may occur if an individual with an egg-producing tapeworm ingests eggs derived from his or her own feces.

Clinical Manifestations   Intestinal infections with *T. solium* may be asymptomatic. Epigastric discomfort, nausea, a sensation of hunger, weight loss, and diarrhea are infrequent. Fecal passage of proglottids may be noted by patients.

In cysticercosis, the clinical manifestations are variable. Cysticerci can be found anywhere in the body but are most commonly detected in the brain, skeletal muscle, subcutaneous tissue, or eye. The clinical presentation of cysticercosis depends on the number and location of cysticerci as well as the extent of associated inflammatory responses or scarring. Neurologic manifestations are the most common (Fig. 204-1). Seizures are associated with inflammation surrounding cysticerci in the brain parenchyma. These seizures may be generalized, focal, or Jacksonian. Hydrocephalus results from obstruction of cerebrospinal fluid (CSF) flow by cysticerci and accompanying inflammation or by CSF outflow obstruction from arachnoiditis. Signs of increased intracranial pressure, including headache, nausea, vomiting, changes in vision, dizziness, ataxia, or confusion, are often evident. Patients with hydrocephalus may develop papilledema or display altered mental status. When cysticerci develop at the base of the brain or in the subarachnoid space, they may cause chronic meningitis or arachnoiditis, communicating hydrocephalus, or strokes.

Diagnosis   The diagnosis of intestinal *T. solium* infection is made by the detection of eggs or proglottids, as described for *T. saginata*. In cysticercosis, diagnosis can be difficult. A consensus conference has proposed absolute, major, minor, and epidemiologic criteria for diagnosis (Table 204-1). Diagnostic certainty is possible only with definite demonstration of the parasite (absolute criteria). This task can be accomplished by histologic observation of the parasite in excised tissue, by funduscopic visualization of the parasite in the eye (in the anterior chamber, vitreous, or subretinal spaces), or by neuroimaging studies demonstrating cystic lesions containing a characteristic scolex. In most cases, diagnostic certainty is not possible. Instead, a clinical diagnosis is made on the basis of a combination of clinical presentation, radiographic studies, serologic tests, and exposure history.

Neuroimaging findings suggestive of neurocysticercosis constitute the primary major diagnostic criterion. These findings include cystic lesions with or without enhancement (e.g., ring enhancement), one or more nodular calcifications (which may also have associated enhancement), or focal enhancing lesions. Cysticerci in the brain parenchyma are usually 5 to 20 mm in diameter and rounded. Cystic lesions in the subarachnoid space or fissures may enlarge up to 6 cm in diameter and may be lobulated. For cysticerci within the subarachnoid space or ventricles, the walls may be very thin and the cyst fluid is often isodense

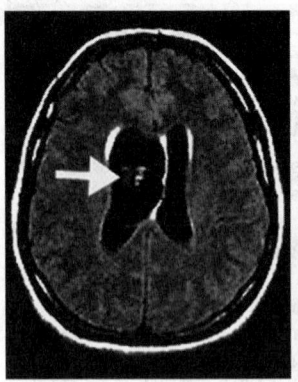 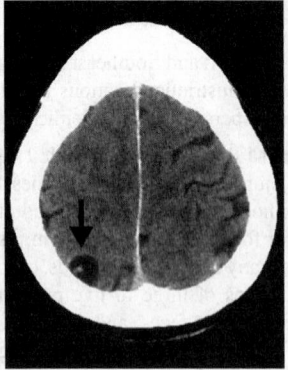 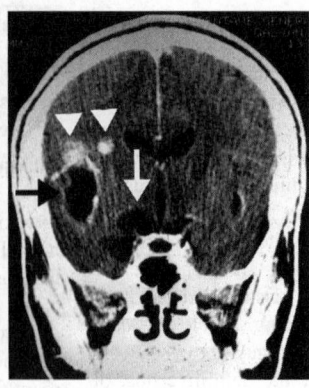

FIGURE 204-1 Neurocysticercosis is caused by *Taenia solium*. Neurologic infection can be classified on the basis of the location and viability of the parasites. When the parasites are in the ventricles, they often cause obstructive hydrocephalus. *Left:* MRI scan showing a cysticercus in the lateral ventricle, with resultant hydrocephalus. The arrow points to the scolex within the cystic parasite. *Center:* CT scan showing a parenchymal cysticercus, with enhancement of the cyst wall and an internal scolex (*arrow*). *Right:* Multiple cysticerci, including calcified lesions from prior infection (*arrowheads*), viable cysticerci in the basilar cisterns (*white arrow*), and a large degenerating cysticercus in the Sylvian fissure (*black arrow*). (*Modified with permission from JC Bandres et al: Clin Infect Dis 15:799, 1992. The University of Chicago Press.*)

with CSF. Thus, obstructive hydrocephalus or enhancement of the basilar meninges may be the only finding on computed tomography (CT) in extraparenchymal neurocysticercosis. Cysticerci in the ventricles or subarachnoid space are usually visible to an experienced neuroradiologist on magnetic resonance imaging (MRI) or on CT with intraventricular contrast injection. CT is more sensitive than MRI in identifying calcified lesions, whereas MRI is better for identifying cystic lesions and enhancement.

The second major diagnostic criterion is detection of specific antibodies to cysticerci. While most tests employing unfractionated antigen have high rates of false-positive and false-negative results, this problem can be overcome by using the more specific immunoblot assay. An immunoblot assay using lentil-lectin purified glycoproteins has >99% specificity and is highly sensitive. However, patients with single intracranial lesions or with calcifications may be seronegative. With this assay, serum samples provide greater diagnostic sensitivity than CSF. CSF may be useful when only unfractionated antigens are used. Antigen detection assays, especially those detecting antigen in the spinal fluid, may also improve diagnosis. However, these assays are not widely available, and the number of publications on their use is limited.

Studies have demonstrated that clinical criteria can aid in the diagnosis in selected cases. In patients from endemic areas who had single enhancing lesions presenting with seizures, a normal physical examination, and no evidence of systemic disease (e.g., no fever, adenopathy, or abnormal chest radiograph), the constellation of rounded CT lesions 5 to 20 mm in diameter with no midline shift was almost always caused by neurocysticercosis. Finally, spontaneous resolution or resolution after therapy with albendazole alone is consistent with neurocysticercosis.

Minor diagnostic criteria include neuroimaging findings consistent with but less characteristic of cysticercosis, clinical manifestations suggestive of neurocysticercosis (e.g., seizures, hydrocephalus, or altered mental status), evidence of cysticercosis outside the central nervous system (e.g., cigar-shaped soft tissue calcifications), or antibody in CSF detected by enzyme-linked immunosorbent assay (ELISA). Epidemiologic criteria include exposure to a tapeworm carrier or household member infected with *T. solium*, current or prior residence in an endemic area, and frequent travel to an endemic area.

Diagnosis is confirmed in patients with either one absolute criterion or a combination of two major criteria, one minor criterion, and one epidemiologic criterion (Table 204-1). A probable diagnosis is supported by the fulfillment of (1) one major criterion plus two minor criteria; (2) one major criterion plus one minor criterion and one epidemiologic criterion; or (3) three minor criteria plus one epidemiologic criterion. While the CSF is usually abnormal in neurocysticercosis, CSF abnormalities are not pathognomonic. Patients may have CSF

pleocytosis with a predominance of lymphocytes, neutrophils, or eosinophils. The protein level in CSF may be elevated; the glucose concentration is usually normal but may be depressed.

℞ TREATMENT

Intestinal *T. solium* infection is treated with a single dose of praziquantel (10 mg/kg). However, praziquantel can evoke an inflammatory response in the central nervous system if concomitant cryptic cysticercosis is present. Niclosamide (2 g) is also effective but is not widely available.

The management of neurocysticercosis focuses primarily on symptom-based treatment of seizures or hydrocephalus. Seizures can usually be controlled with antiepileptics. If parenchymal lesions resolve without development of calcifications and patients remain free of seizures, antiepileptic therapy can usually be discontinued after 2 years. Five placebo-controlled trials failed to identify any clinical advantage of antiparasitic drugs for parenchymal neurocysticercosis. However, trends toward faster resolution of neuroradiologic abnormalities were observed. Thus, some authorities favor use of antiparasitic drugs, including praziquantel (50 to 60 mg/kg daily in three divided doses for 15 days or 100 mg/kg in three doses given over a single day) or albendazole (15 mg/kg per day for 8 to 28 days). Both agents may exacerbate the inflammatory response around the dying parasite, exacerbating seizures or hydrocephalus. Thus, patients receiving these drugs should be carefully monitored. High-dose glucocorticoids can be used during treatment or if symptoms worsen. Since glucocorticoids induce first-pass metabolism of praziquantel and may decrease its antiparasitic effect, cimetidine should be coadministered to inhibit praziquantel metabolism.

For patients with hydrocephalus, the emergent reduction of intracranial pressure is the mainstay of therapy. In the case of obstructive hydrocephalus, the preferred approach is removal of the cysticercus via endoscopic surgery. However, this intervention is not always possible. An alternative approach is initially to perform a diverting procedure, such as ventriculoperitoneal shunting. Historically, shunts

---

TABLE 204-1 *Proposed Diagnostic Criteria for Human Cysticercosis, 2001*

1. Absolute criteria
   a. Demonstration of cysticerci by histologic or microscopic examination of biopsy material
   b. Visualization of the parasite in the eye by funduscopy
   c. Neuroradiologic demonstration of cystic lesions containing a characteristic scolex
2. Major criteria
   a. Neuroradiologic lesions suggestive of neurocysticercosis
   b. Demonstration of antibodies to cysticerci in serum by enzyme-linked immunoelectrotransfer blot
   c. Resolution of intracranial cystic lesions spontaneously or after therapy with albendazole or praziquantel alone
3. Minor criteria
   a. Lesions compatible with neurocysticercosis detected by neuroimaging studies
   b. Clinical manifestations suggestive of neurocysticercosis
   c. Demonstration of antibodies to cysticerci or cysticercal antigen in cerebrospinal fluid by ELISA
   d. Evidence of cysticercosis outside the central nervous system (e.g., cigar-shaped soft tissue calcifications)
4. Epidemiologic criteria
   a. Residence in a cysticercosis-endemic area
   b. Frequent travel to a cysticercosis-endemic area
   c. Household contact with an individual infected with *Taenia solium*

Note: ELISA, enzyme-linked immunosorbent assay.
Source: Modified from Del Brutto et al.

have usually failed, but low failure rates have recently been attained with treatment with antiparasitic drugs, chronic administration of glucocorticoids, or use of flow-sensitive shunts. Open craniotomy to remove the cysticerci is now required only infrequently. For patients with subarachnoid cysts or giant cysticerci, glucocorticoids are needed to reduce arachnoiditis and accompanying vasculitis. Most authorities recommend prolonged courses of antiparasitic drugs and shunting when hydrocephalus is present. In patients with cerebral edema and elevated intracranial pressure due to multiple inflamed lesions, glucocorticoids are the mainstay of therapy, and antiparasitic drugs should be avoided. For ocular and spinal medullary lesions, drug-induced inflammation may cause irreversible damage. Most patients should be managed surgically, although case reports have described cures with medical therapy.

Prevention Measures for the prevention of intestinal *T. solium* infection consist of the application to pork of precautions similar to those described above for beef with regard to *T. saginata* infection. The prevention of cysticercosis involves minimizing the opportunities for ingestion of fecally derived eggs by means of good personal hygiene, effective fecal disposal, and treatment and prevention of human intestinal infections.

ECHINOCOCCOSIS Echinococcosis is an infection caused in humans by the larval stage of *Echinococcus granulosus*, *E. multilocularis*, or *E. vogeli*. *E. granulosus*, which produces unilocular cystic lesions, is prevalent in areas where livestock is raised in association with dogs. This tapeworm species is found in Australia, Argentina, Chile, Africa, eastern Europe, the Middle East, New Zealand, and the Mediterranean region, particularly Lebanon and Greece. Molecular evidence suggests that *E. granulosus* strains may actually belong to more than one species; specifically, strains from sheep, cattle, pigs, horses, and camels probably represent separate species. *E. multilocularis*, which causes multilocular alveolar lesions that are locally invasive, is found in Alpine, sub-Arctic, or Arctic regions, including Canada, the United States, and central and northern Europe and Asia. *E. vogeli* causes polycystic hydatid disease and is found only in Central and South America. Like other cestodes, echinococcal species have both intermediate and definitive hosts. The definitive hosts are dogs that pass eggs in their feces. Cysts develop in the intermediate hosts—sheep, cattle, humans, goats, camels, and horses for *E. granulosus* and mice and other rodents for *E. multilocularis*—after the ingestion of eggs. When a dog ingests beef or lamb containing cysts, the life cycle is completed.

Etiology The small (5 mm long) adult *E. granulosus* worm, which lives for 5 to 20 months in the jejunum of dogs, has only three proglottids—one immature, one mature, and one gravid. The gravid segment splits to release eggs that are morphologically similar to *Taenia* eggs and are extremely hardy. After humans ingest the eggs, embryos escape from the eggs, penetrate the intestinal mucosa, enter the portal circulation, and are carried to various organs, most commonly the liver and lungs. Larvae develop into fluid-filled unilocular hydatid cysts that consist of an external membrane and an inner germinal layer. Daughter cysts develop from the inner aspect of the germinal layer, as do germinating cystic structures called *brood capsules*. New larvae, called *protoscolices*, develop in large numbers within the brood capsule. The cysts expand slowly over a period of years.

The life cycle of *E. multilocularis* is similar except that small rodents serve as the intermediate hosts. The larval form of *E. multilocularis*, however, is quite different in that it remains in the proliferative phase, the parasite is always multilocular, and vesicles without brood capsule or protoscolices progressively invade the host tissue by peripheral extension of processes from the germinal layer.

Clinical Manifestations Slowly enlarging echinococcal cysts generally remain asymptomatic until their expanding size or their space-occupying effect in an involved organ elicits symptoms. The liver and the lungs are the most common sites of these cysts. The liver is involved in about two-thirds of *E. granulosus* infections and in nearly all *E. multilocularis* infections. Since a period of years elapses before cysts enlarge sufficiently to cause symptoms, they may be discovered incidentally on a routine x-ray or ultrasound study.

Patients with hepatic echinococcosis who are symptomatic most often present with abdominal pain or a palpable mass in the right upper quadrant. Compression of a bile duct or leakage of cyst fluid into the biliary tree may mimic recurrent cholelithiasis, and biliary obstruction can result in jaundice. Rupture of or episodic leakage from a hydatid cyst may produce fever, pruritus, urticaria, eosinophilia, or anaphylaxis. Pulmonary hydatid cysts may rupture into the bronchial tree or peritoneal cavity and produce cough, chest pain, or hemoptysis. Rupture of hydatid cysts may lead to multifocal dissemination of protoscolices, which can form additional cysts. Rupture can occur spontaneously or at surgery. Other presentations are due to the involvement of bone (invasion of the medullary cavity with slow bone erosion producing pathologic fractures), the central nervous system (space-occupying lesions), the heart (conduction defects, pericarditis), and the pelvis (pelvic mass).

The larval forms of *E. multilocularis* characteristically present as a slowly growing hepatic tumor, with progressive destruction of the liver and extension into vital structures. Patients commonly complain of upper quadrant and epigastric pain, and obstructive jaundice may be apparent. The lesions may infiltrate adjoining organs (e.g., diaphragm, kidneys, or lungs) or may metastasize to the spleen, lungs, or brain.

Diagnosis Radiographic and related imaging studies are important in detecting and evaluating echinococcal cysts. Plain films will define pulmonary cysts of *E. granulosus*—usually as rounded masses of uniform density—but may miss cysts in other organs unless there is cyst wall calcification (as occurs in the liver). MRI, CT, and ultrasound reveal well-defined cysts with thick or thin walls. When older cysts contain a layer of hydatid sand that is rich in accumulated scolices, these imaging methods may detect this fluid layer of different density. However, the most pathognomonic finding, if demonstrable, is that of daughter cysts within the larger cyst. This finding, like eggshell or mural calcification on CT, is indicative of *E. granulosus* infection and helps to distinguish the cyst from carcinomas, bacterial or amebic liver abscesses, or hemangiomas. In contrast, ultrasound or CT of alveolar hydatid cysts reveals indistinct solid masses with central necrosis and plaquelike calcifications.

A specific diagnosis of *E. granulosus* infection can be made by the examination of aspirated fluids for protoscolices or hooklets, but diagnostic aspiration is not usually recommended because of the risk of fluid leakage resulting in either dissemination of infection or anaphylactic reactions. Serodiagnostic assays can be useful, although a negative test does not exclude the diagnosis of echinococcosis. Cysts in the liver elicit positive antibody responses in ~90% of cases, whereas up to 50% of individuals with cysts in the lungs are seronegative. Detection of antibody to specific echinococcal antigens by immunoblotting has the highest degree of specificity.

℞ TREATMENT

Therapy for cystic echinococcosis is based on considerations of the size, location, and manifestations of cysts and the overall health of the patient. Surgery has traditionally been the principal definitive method of treatment. Currently, ultrasound staging is recommended for *E. granulosus* infections (Fig. 204-2). For uncomplicated CE1 lesions and for some CE2 and CE3 lesions, PAIR (*p*ercutaneous *a*spiration, *i*nfusion of scolicidal agents, and *r*easpiration) is now recommended instead of surgery. PAIR is contraindicated for superficially located cysts (because of the risk of rupture), for cysts with multiple thick internal septal divisions (honeycombing pattern), and for cysts communicating with the biliary tree. For prophylaxis of secondary peritoneal echinococcosis due to inadvertent spillage of fluid during PAIR, the administration of albendazole (15 mg/kg daily in two divided

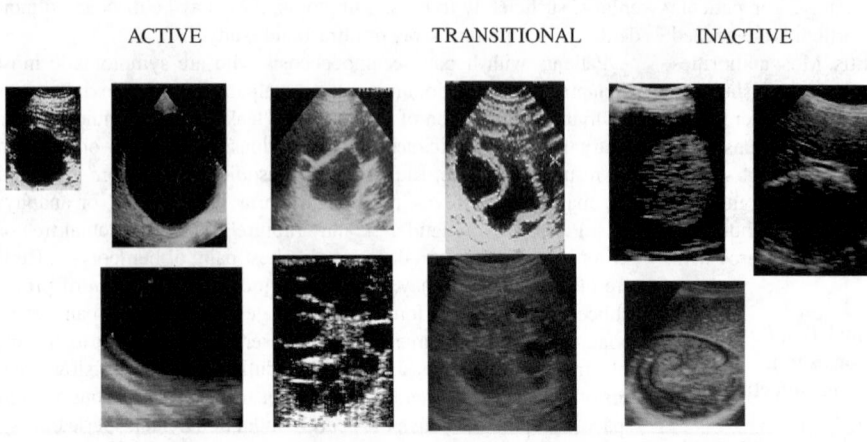

FIGURE 204-2 Management of cystic hydatid disease caused by *Echinococcus granulosus* should be based on viability of the parasite, which can be estimated from radiographic appearance. The ultrasound appearance includes lesions classified as active, transitional, and inactive. *Active* cysts include types CL (with a cystic lesion and no visible cyst wall), CE1 [with a visible cyst wall and internal echoes (snowflake sign)], and CE2 (with a visible cyst wall and internal septation). *Transitional cysts* (CE3) may have detached laminar membranes or may be partially collapsed. *Inactive cysts* include types CE4 (a nonhomogeneous mass) and CE5 (a cyst with a thick calcified wall).

doses) should be initiated at least 4 days before the procedure and continued for at least 4 weeks afterward. Ultrasound- or CT-guided aspiration allows confirmation of the diagnosis by demonstration of protoscolices in the aspirate. After aspiration, contrast material should be injected to detect occult communications with the biliary tract. Alternatively, the fluid should be checked for bile staining by dipstick. If no bile is found and no communication visualized, the contrast material is reaspirated, with subsequent infusion of scolicidal agents (usually either alcohol or hypertonic saline). Daughter cysts within the primary cyst may need to be punctured separately. In experienced hands, this approach yields rates of cure and relapse equivalent to those following surgery, with less perioperative morbidity and shorter hospitalization.

Surgery remains the treatment of choice for complicated *E. granulosus* cysts (e.g., those communicating with the biliary tract) or for areas where PAIR is not possible. For *E. granulosus*, the preferred surgical approach is pericystectomy, in which the entire cyst and the surrounding fibrous tissue are removed. The risks posed by leakage of fluid during surgery or PAIR include anaphylaxis and dissemination of infectious protoscolices. The latter complication has been minimized by careful attention to the prevention of spillage of the cyst and by soaking of the drapes with hypertonic saline. Infusion of scolicidal agents is no longer recommended because of problems with hypernatremia, intoxication, or sclerosing cholangitis. Albendazole, which is active against *Echinococcus*, should be administered adjunctively, beginning several days before resection and continuing for several weeks for *E. granulosus*. Praziquantel (50 mg/kg daily for 2 weeks), may hasten the death of the protoscolices. Medical therapy with albendazole alone for 12 weeks to 6 months results in cure in ~30% of cases and improvement in another 50%. In many instances of treatment failure, *E. granulosus* infections are subsequently treated successfully with PAIR or additional courses of medical therapy. Response to treatment is best assessed by serial imaging studies, with attention to cyst size and consistency.

Surgical resection remains the treatment of choice for *E. multilocularis* infection. Complete removal of the parasite continues to offer the best chance for cure. Ongoing therapy with albendazole for at least 2 years after presumptively curative surgery is recommended. Most cases are diagnosed at a stage at which complete resection is not possible; in these cases, albendazole treatment should be continued indefinitely, with careful monitoring. In some cases, liver transplantation has been used because of the size of the necessary liver resection.

However, continuous immunosuppression favors the proliferation of *E. multilocularis* larvae and reinfection of the transplant. Thus, indefinite treatment with albendazole is required.

Prevention In endemic areas, echinococcosis can be prevented by administering praziquantel to infected dogs, by denying dogs access to infected animals, or by vaccinating sheep. Limitation of the number of stray dogs is helpful in reducing the prevalence of infection among humans.

HYMENOLEPIASIS NANA Infection with *Hymenolepis nana*, the dwarf tapeworm, is the most common of all the cestode infections. *H. nana* is endemic in both temperate and tropical regions of the world. Infection is spread by fecal/oral contamination and is common among institutionalized children.

Etiology and Pathogenesis *H. nana* is the only cestode of humans that does not require an intermediate host. Both the larval and adult phases take place in the human. The adult—the smallest tapeworm parasitizing humans—is ~2 cm long and dwells in the proximal ileum. Proglottids, which are quite small and are rarely seen in the stool, release spherical eggs 30 to 44 μm in diameter, each of which contains an oncosphere with six hooklets. The eggs are immediately infective and are unable to survive for >10 days in the external environment. *H. nana* can also be acquired by the ingestion of infected insects (especially larval meal-worms and larval fleas). When the egg is ingested by a new host, the oncosphere is freed and penetrates the intestinal villi, becoming a cysticercoid larva. Larvae migrate back into the intestinal lumen, attach to the mucosa, and mature into adult worms over 10 to 12 days. Eggs may also hatch before passing into the stool, causing internal autoinfection with increasing numbers of intestinal worms. Although the life span of adult *H. nana* is only ~4 to 10 weeks, the autoinfection cycle perpetuates the infection.

Clinical Manifestations *H. nana* infection, even with many intestinal worms, is usually asymptomatic. When infection is intense, anorexia, abdominal pain, and diarrhea develop.

Diagnosis Infection is diagnosed by the finding of eggs in the stool.

℞ TREATMENT

Praziquantel (25 mg/kg once) is the treatment of choice, since it acts against both the adult worms and the cysticercoids in the intestinal villi.

Prevention Good personal hygiene and improved sanitation can eradicate the disease. Epidemics have been controlled by mass chemotherapy coupled with improved hygiene.

HYMENOLEPIASIS DIMINUTA *Hymenolepis diminuta*, a cestode of rodents, occasionally infects small children, who ingest the larvae in uncooked cereal foods contaminated by fleas and other insects in which larvae develop. Infection is usually asymptomatic and is diagnosed by the detection of eggs in the stool. Treatment with praziquantel results in cure in most cases.

DIPHYLLOBOTHRIASIS *Diphyllobothrium latum* and other *Diphyllobothrium* species are found in the lakes, rivers, and deltas of the northern hemisphere, Central Africa, and Chile.

Etiology and Pathogenesis The adult worm—the longest tapeworm (up to 25 m)—attaches to the ileal and occasionally to the jejunal mucosa by its suckers, which are located on its elongated scolex. The adult worm has 3000 to 4000 proglottids, which release ~1 million eggs daily into the feces. If an egg reaches water, it hatches and releases a free-swimming embryo that can be eaten by small freshwater crustaceans (*Cyclops* or *Diaptomus* species). After an infected crustacean containing a developed procercoid is swallowed by a fish, the larva migrates into the fish's flesh and grows into a plerocercoid, or sparganum larva. Humans acquire the infection by ingesting infected raw fish. Within 3 to 5 weeks, the tapeworm matures into an adult in the human intestine.

Clinical Manifestations Most *D. latum* infections are asymptomatic, although manifestations may include transient abdominal discomfort, diarrhea, vomiting, weakness, and weight loss. Occasionally, infection can cause acute abdominal pain and intestinal obstruction; in rare cases, cholangitis or cholecystitis may be produced by migrating proglottids. Because the tapeworm absorbs large quantities of vitamin B_{12} and interferes with ileal B_{12} absorption, vitamin B_{12} deficiency can develop. Up to 2% of infected patients, especially the elderly, have megaloblastic anemia resembling pernicious anemia and may exhibit neurologic sequelae of B_{12} deficiency.

Diagnosis The diagnosis is made readily by the detection of the characteristic eggs in the stool. The eggs possess a single shell with an operculum at one end and a knob at the other. Mild to moderate eosinophilia may be detected.

℞ TREATMENT

Praziquantel (5 to 10 mg/kg once) is highly effective. Parenteral vitamin B_{12} should be given if B_{12} deficiency is manifest.

Prevention Infection can be prevented by heating fish to 54°C for 5 min or by freezing it at −18°C for 24 h. Placing fish in brine with a high salt concentration for long periods kills the eggs.

DIPYLIDIASIS *Dipylidium caninum*, a common tapeworm of dogs and cats, may accidentally infect humans. Dogs, cats, and occasionally humans become infected by ingesting fleas harboring cysticercoids. Children are more likely to become infected than adults. Most infections are asymptomatic, but abdominal pain, diarrhea, anal pruritus, urticaria, eosinophilia, or passage of segments in the stool may occur. The diagnosis is made by the detection of proglottids in the stool. As in *D. latum* infection, therapy consists of praziquantel. Prevention requires anthelmintic treatment and flea control for pet dogs or cats.

SPARGANOSIS Humans can be infected by the sparganum, or plerocercoid larva, of a diphyllobothrid tapeworm of the genus *Spirometra*. Infection can be acquired by the consumption of water containing infected *Cyclops*; by the ingestion of infected snakes, birds, or mammals; or by the application of infected flesh as poultices. The worm migrates slowly in tissues, and infection commonly presents as a subcutaneous swelling. Periorbital tissues can be involved, and ocular sparganosis may destroy the eye. Surgical excision is used to treat localized sparganosis.

COENUROSIS This rare infection of humans by the larval stage (coenurus) of the dog tapeworm *Taenia multiceps* or *T. serialis* results in a space-occupying cystic lesion. As in cysticercosis, involvement of the central nervous system and subcutaneous tissue is most common. Both definitive diagnosis and treatment require surgical excision of the lesion. Chemotherapeutic agents generally are not effective.

FURTHER READING

DEL BRUTTO OH et al: Proposed diagnostic criteria for neurocysticercosis. Neurology 57:177, 2001

GARCIA HH et al: Current consensus guidelines for treatment of neurocysticercosis. Clin Microbiol Rev 15:747, 2002

KELLY R et al: Characteristics of ventricular shunt malfunctions among patients with neurocysticercosis. Neurosurgery 50:757, 2002

KERN P et al: European echinococcosis registry: Human alveolar echinococcosis, Europe, 1982–2000. Emerg Infect Dis 9:343, 2003

MENEZES DA SILVA A: Hydatid cyst of the liver—criteria for the selection of appropriate treatment. Acta Tropica 85:237, 2003

PAWLOWSKI ZS et al: Echinococcosis in humans: Clinical aspects, diagnosis, and treatment, in J Eckert et al (eds): *WHO/OIE Manual on Echinococcosis in Humans and Animals: A Public Health Problem of Global Concern.* World Organization for Animal Health, Paris, 2001

SINGH G, PRABHAKAR S: *Taenia solium Cysticercosis: From Basic Science to Clinical Science.* CABI Publishing, Wallingford, Oxon, UK, 2002

WORLD HEALTH ORGANIZATION INFORMAL WORKING GROUP ON ECHINOCOCCOSIS: Guidelines for treatment of cystic and alveolar echinococcosis in humans. Bull World Health Organ 74:231, 1996

——— PAIR puncture, aspiration, injection, re-aspiration: An option for the treatment of cystic echinococcosis. WHO/CDS/CSR/APH/2001.6. WHO, Geneva, 2001

205 MICROBIAL BIOTERRORISM
H. Clifford Lane, Anthony S. Fauci

Descriptions of the use of microbial pathogens as potential weapons of war or terrorism date from ancient times. Among the most frequently cited of such episodes are the poisoning of water supplies in the sixth century B.C. with the fungus *Calviceps purpurea* (rye ergot) by the Assyrians, the hurling of the dead bodies of plague victims over the walls of the city of Kaffa by the Tartar army in 1346, and the spreading of smallpox via contaminated blankets by the British to the native American population loyal to the French in 1767. Although the use of chemical weapons in wartime took place in the not-too-distant past (Chap. 206), the tragic events of September 11, 2001, followed closely by the anthrax attacks through the U.S. Postal System, dramatically changed the mindset of the American public regarding both our vulnerability to microbial bioterrorist attacks and the seriousness and intent of the Federal government to protect its citizens against future attacks.

Although the potential impact of a bioterrorist attack can be enormous, leading to thousands of deaths and extensive morbidity, acts of bioterrorism typically have their greatest impact through the fear and terror they generate. In contrast to biowarfare, where the primary goal is destruction of the enemy through mass casualties, an important goal of bioterrorism is to destroy the morale of a society through fear and uncertainty. While the actual biologic impact of a single act may be small, the degree of disruption created by the realization that such an attack is possible may be enormous. This was readily apparent with the impact on the U.S. Postal System and the functional interruption of the activities of the legislative branch of government following the anthrax attacks noted above. Thus, the key to the defense against these attacks is a highly functioning system of public health surveillance and education so that attacks can be quickly recognized and effectively contained. This is complemented by the availability of appropriate countermeasures in the form of diagnostics, therapeutics, and vaccines, both in response to and in anticipation of bioterrorist attacks.

The Working Group for Civilian Biodefense has put together a list of key features that characterize the elements of biologic agents that make them particularly effective as weapons (Table 205-1). Included among these are the ease of spread and transmission of the agent as well as the presence of an adequate database to allow newcomers to the field to quickly apply the good science of others to bad intentions of their own. Agents of bioterrorism may be used in their naturally occurring forms or they can be deliberately modified to provide maximal impact. Among the approaches to maximizing the deleterious effects of biologic agents are the genetic modification of microbes for the purposes of antimicrobial resistance or evasion by the immune system, creation of fine-particle aerosols, chemical treatment to stabilize and prolong infectivity, and alteration of host range through changes in surface proteins. Certain of these approaches fall under the category of *weaponization*, which is a term generally used to describe the processing of microbes or toxins in a manner that would ensure a devastating effect of a release. For example, weaponization of anthrax by the Soviets comprised the production of vast amounts of spores in a form that maintained aerosolization for prolonged periods of time; the spores were of sufficient size to enter the lower respiratory tract easily and could be delivered in a massive release, such as via a bomblet.

The U.S. Centers for Disease Control and Prevention (CDC) classifies potential biologic threats into three categories: A, B, and C (Table 205-2). Category A agents are the highest-priority pathogens. They pose the greatest risk to national security because they (1) can be easily disseminated or transmitted from person to person, (2) result in high mortality rates and have the potential for major public health impact, (3) might cause public panic and social disruption, and (4) require special action for public health preparedness. Category B agents are the second highest priority pathogens and include those that are moderately easy to disseminate, result in moderate morbidity rates and low mortality rates, and require specifically enhanced diagnostic capacity. Category C agents are the third highest priority. These include emerging pathogens, to which the general population lacks immunity, that could be engineered for mass dissemination in the future because of availability, ease of production, ease of dissemination, potential for high morbidity and mortality, and major public health impact. The recent emergence of a novel human coronavirus leading to outbreaks of severe acute respiratory syndrome (SARS) is one example of such an agent. It should be pointed out, however, that these designations are empirical, and, depending on evolving circumstances such as threat assessments, the priority rating of any given microbe or toxin could change.

TABLE 205-1   Key Features of Biologic Agents Used as Bioweapons

1. High morbidity and mortality
2. Potential for person-to-person spread
3. Low infective dose and highly infectious by aerosol
4. Lack of rapid diagnostic capability
5. Lack of universally available effective vaccine
6. Potential to cause anxiety
7. Availability of pathogen and feasibility of production
8. Environmental stability
9. Database of prior research and development
10. Potential to be "weaponized"

Source: From L Borio et al: JAMA 287:2391, 2002; with permission.

TABLE 205-2   CDC Category A, B, and C Agents

Category A
  Anthrax (*Bacillus anthracis*)
  Botulism (*Clostridium botulinum* toxin)
  Plague (*Yersinia pestis*)
  Smallpox (*Variola major*)
  Tularemia (*Francisella tularensis*)
  Viral hemorrhagic fevers
    Arenaviruses: Lassa, New World (Machupo, Junin, Guanarito, and Sabia)
    Bunyaviridae: Crimean Congo, Rift Valley
    Filoviridae: Ebola, Marburg
    Flaviviridae: Yellow fever; Omsk fever; Kyasanur Forest
Category B
  Brucellosis (*Brucella* spp.)
  Epsilon toxin of *Clostridium perfringens*
  Food safety threats (e.g., *Salmonella* spp., *Escherichia coli* 0157:H7, *Shigella*)
  Glanders (*Burkholderia mallei*)
  Melioidosis (*B. pseudomallei*)
  Psittacosis (*Chlamydia psittaci*)
  Q fever (*Coxiella burnetii*)
  Ricin toxin from *Ricinus communis* (castor beans)
  Staphylococcal enterotoxin B
  Typhus fever (*Rickettsia prowazekii*)
  Viral encephalitis [alphaviruses (e.g., Venezuelan, eastern, and western equine encephalitis)]
  Water safety threats (e.g., *Vibrio cholerae*, *Cryptosporidium parvum*)
Category C
  Emerging infectious diseases threats such as Nipah, hantavirus, and SARS coronavirus.

Source: Centers for Disease Control and Prevention and the National Institute of Allergy and Infectious Diseases.

CATEGORY A AGENTS

ANTHRAX (*BACILLUS ANTHRACIS*) (See also Chap. 122) ■ **Anthrax as a Bioweapon** Anthrax may be the prototypic disease of bioterrorism. Although rarely spread from person to person, it contains the other features of an ideal bioweapon outlined in Table 205-1. U.S. and British government scientists studied anthrax as a biologic weapon beginning approximately at the time of World War II (WWII). Offensive bioweapons activity including bioweapons research on microbes and toxins in the United States ceased in 1969 as a result of two executive orders by President Richard M. Nixon. The 1972 Biological and Toxin Weapons Convention Treaty outlawed research of this type worldwide. Clearly, the Soviet Union was in direct violation of this treaty until at least the dissolution of the Soviet Union in the late 1980s. It is well documented that during this post-treaty period, the Soviets produced and stored hundreds of tons of anthrax spores for potential use as a bioweapon. At present there is suspicion that research on anthrax as an agent of bioterrorism is ongoing by several nations and extremist groups. One example of this is the release of anthrax spores by the Aum Shrinrikyo cult in Tokyo in 1993. Fortunately, there were no casualties associated with this episode because of the inadvertent use of a nonpathogenic strain of anthrax by the terrorists.

The potential impact of anthrax spores as a bioweapon was clearly demonstrated in 1979 following the accidental release of spores into the atmosphere from a Soviet Union bioweapons facility in Sverdlosk, Russia. While actual figures are not known, at least 77 cases of anthrax were diagnosed with certainty, of which 66 were fatal. These victims appeared to have been exposed in an area within 4 km downwind of the facility. Deaths due to anthrax were also noted in livestock up to 50 km away from the facility. The interval between probable exposure and development of clinical illness ranged from 2 to 43 days. The majority of cases were within the first 2 weeks. Death typically occurred within 1 to 4 days following the onset of symptoms. It is likely that the widespread use of penicillin prophylaxis limited the total number of cases. The extended period of time between exposure and disease in some individuals supports the data from nonhuman primate studies suggesting the anthrax spores can lie dormant in the respiratory tract for at least 4 to 6 weeks. This extended period of microbiologic latency following exposure poses a significant challenge for management of victims in the postexposure period.

In September 2001, the American public was exposed to anthrax spores as a bioweapon delivered through the U.S. Postal System. The CDC identified 22 confirmed or suspected cases of anthrax as a consequence of this attack. These included 11 patients with inhalational anthrax, of whom 5 died, and 11 patients with cutaneous anthrax (7 confirmed), all of whom survived (Fig. 205-1). Cases occurred in individuals who opened contaminated letters as well as in postal workers involved in the processing of mail. A minimum of five letters mailed from Trenton, NJ, served as the vehicles for these attacks. One of these letters was reported to contain 2 g of material, equivalent to 100 billion to 1 trillion weapon-grade spores. This is an inoculum with a theoretical potential under optimal conditions of infecting up to 50 million individuals when one considers an LD_{50} of 10,000 spores. The strain used in this attack was the Ames strain. Although it was noted to have an inducible β-lactamase and to constitutively express a cephalosporinase, it was susceptible to all antibiotics standard for *B. anthracis*.

Microbiology and Clinical Features Anthrax is caused by *B. anthracis*, a gram-positive, nonmotile, spore-forming rod that is found in soil and predominantly causes disease in herbivores such as cattle, goats, and sheep. The long-lived spores of this organism can also be found in soil, and their stability makes them an ideal bioweapon. Anthrax spores can remain viable for decades, and their destruction in decontamination activities can be a challenge. Naturally occurring human infection is generally the result of contact with anthrax-infected animals or animal products such as goat hair. Studies performed in the 1950s using monkeys exposed to aerosolized anthrax suggested that ~10,000 spores were required to produce lethal disease in 50% of animals exposed to this dose (the LD_{50}). However, it has also been suggested that as few as one to three spores may be adequate to cause disease in some settings. Advanced technology is likely to be necessary to generate spores of the optimal size (1 to 5 μm) to travel to the alveolar spaces as a bioweapon.

The three major clinical forms of anthrax are gastrointestinal, cutaneous, and inhalational. *Gastrointestinal anthrax* is rarely seen and is unlikely to be the result of a bioterrorism event. The lesion of *cutaneous anthrax* typically begins as a papule following the introduction of spores through an opening in the skin. This papule then evolves to a painless vesicular stage followed by the development of a coal-black, necrotic eschar. It is the Greek word for coal (*anthrax*) that gives the organism and the disease its name. Cutaneous anthrax was ~20% fatal prior to the availability of antibiotics. *Inhalational anthrax* is the form most likely to be responsible for death in the setting of a bioterrorist attack. It occurs following the inhalation of spores that become de-

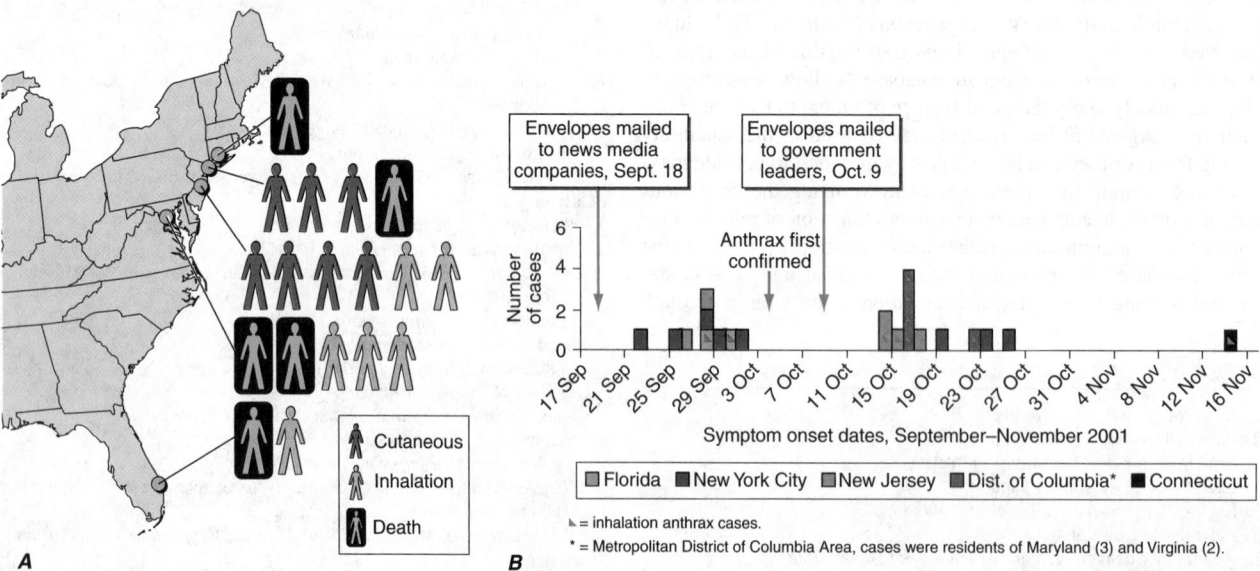

FIGURE 205-1 Confirmed anthrax cases associated with bioterrorism: United States, 2001. *A.* Geographic location, clinical manifestation, and outcome of the 11 cases of confirmed inhalational and 7 cases of confirmed cutaneous anthrax. *B.* Epidemic curve for the 18 confirmed cases of inhalational and cutaneous anthrax and additional 4 cases of suspected cutaneous anthrax. (*From DB Jernigan et al: Investigation of bioterrorism-related anthrax, US 2001: Epidemiologic findings. Emerg Infect Dis 8:1019, 2002; with permission.*)

posited in the alveolar spaces. These spores are phagocytosed by macrophages and transported to the mediastinal and peribronchial lymph nodes where they germinate, leading to active bacterial growth and elaboration of the bacterial products edema toxin and lethal toxin. Subsequent hematogenous spread of bacteria is accompanied by cardiovascular collapse and death. The earliest symptoms are typically a viral-like prodrome with fever, malaise, and abdominal and/or chest symptoms that rapidly progress to a moribund state. A characteristic finding is mediastinal widening and pleural effusions on chest x-ray (Fig. 205-2). While initially thought to be 100% fatal, the experiences at Sverdlosk in 1979 and in the United States in 2001 (see below) indicate that with prompt initiation of antibiotic therapy survival is possible. The characteristics of the 11 cases of inhalational anthrax diagnosed in the United States in 2001 following exposure to contaminated letters postmarked September 18 or October 9, 2001, are detailed in Table 205-3. These cases followed the classic pattern established for this illness, with patients presenting with a rapidly progressive course characterized by fever, fatigue or malaise, nausea or vomiting, cough, and shortness of breath. At presentation, the total white blood cell counts were ~10,000 cells/μL; transaminases tended to be elevated, and all 11 had abnormal findings on chest x-ray and computed tomography (CT). Pulmonary findings included infiltrates, mediastinal widening, and hemorrhagic pleural effusions. For cases in which the dates of exposure were known, symptoms appeared within 4 to 6 days. Death occurred within 7 days of diagnosis in the five fatal

cases (overall mortality rate 55%). Rapid diagnosis and prompt initiation of antibiotic therapy were key to survival.

℞ TREATMENT

Anthrax can be successfully treated if the disease is promptly recognized and appropriate therapy is initiated early. While penicillin, ciprofloxacin, and doxycycline are the currently licensed antibiotics for this indication, clindamycin and rifampin have in vitro activity against the organism and have been used as part of treatment regimens. Until sensitivity results are known, suspected cases are best managed with a combination of widely active agents (Table 205-4). Patients with inhalational anthrax are not contagious and do not require special isolation procedures.

Vaccination and Prevention The first successful vaccine for anthrax was developed for animals by Louis Pasteur in 1881. At present, the single vaccine licensed for human use is a product produced from the cell-free culture supernatant of an attenuated, nonencapsulated strain of *B. anthracis* (Stern strain), referred to as *anthrax vaccine adsorbed* (AVA). Clinical trials for safety in humans and efficacy in animals are currently under way to evaluate the role of recombinant protective antigen (one of the major components, along with lethal factor and edema factor, of *B. anthracis* toxins) as an alternative to AVA. Since

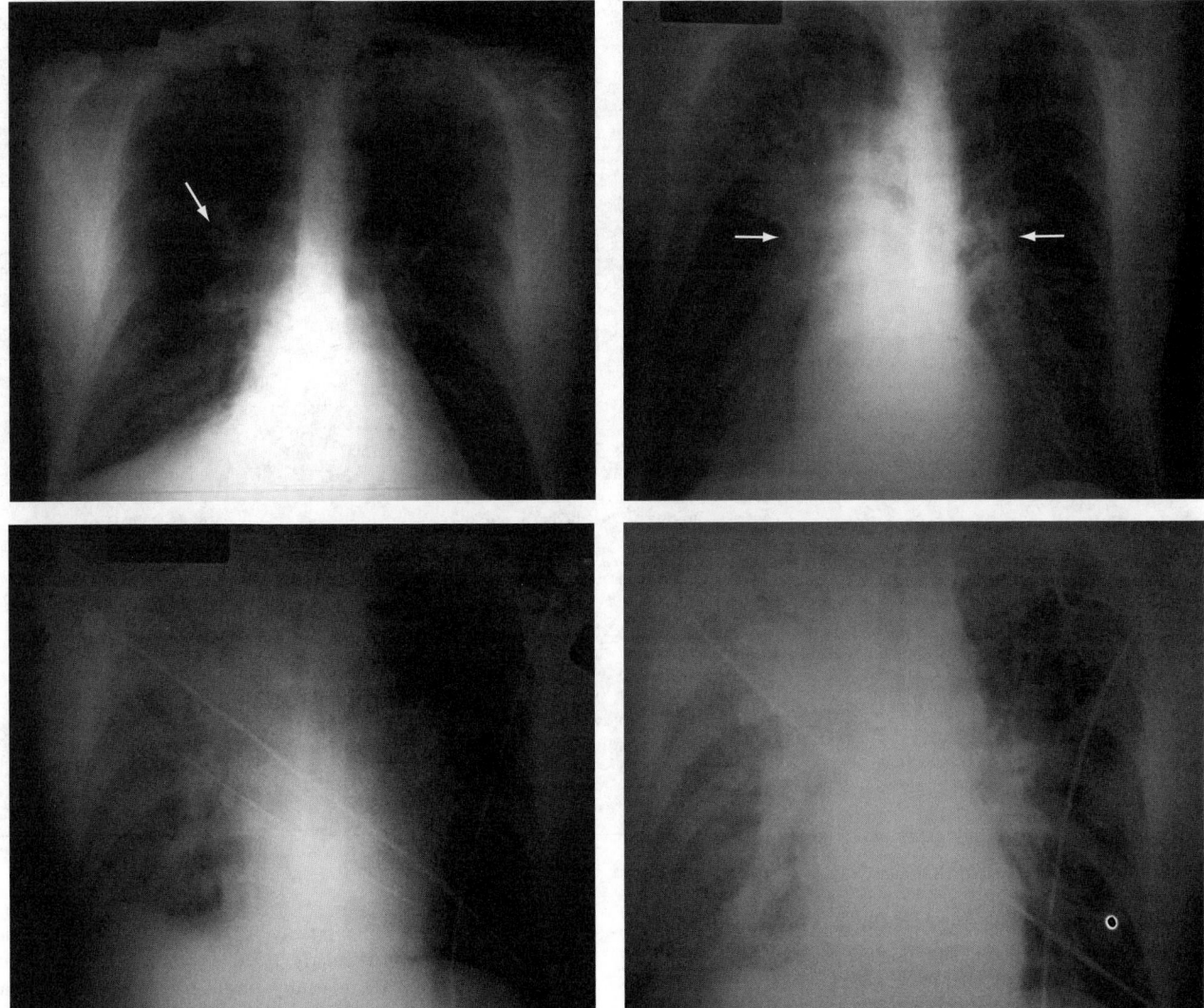

FIGURE 205-2 Progression of chest x-ray findings in a patient (Table 205-3, Patient 9) with inhalational anthrax. Findings evolved from subtle hilar prominence and right perihilar infiltrate to a progressively widened mediastinum, marked perihilar infiltrates, peribronchial cuffing, and air bronchograms. (*From L Borio et al: Death due to bioterrorism-related inhalational anthrax. JAMA 286:2554, 2001; with permission.*)

Case	Age/Sex	Location	Occupation	Initial Symptoms	Radiograph Findings CXR/CT	Initial WBC	Time Interval from 1st Symptom to Death, Days	Treatment[a]
FATAL CASES								
1	63 y/o man	FL	Photo editor, media company	Fever, malaise, fatigue, altered mental state	Widened upper mediastinum, pleural effusion	9400	8	Cefotaxime, ceftazidime, gentamicin, metronidazole, doxycycline, ampicillin, trimethoprim-sulfamethoxazole, penicillin G, levofloxacin, clindamycin
2	55 y/o man	DC	Postal worker	Fever, fatigue, myalgia, cough	Infiltrate, perihilar fullness, pleural effusion	10,300	5	Levofloxacin, diltiazem, insulin, mechanical ventilation
3	47 y/o man	DC	Postal worker	Nausea, vomiting, abdominal pain, syncope, cough	Perihilar infiltrate, mediastinal adenopathy, pleural effusion	13,300	6	Penicillin, ceftriaxone, rifampin, levofloxacin, mechanical ventilation
4	61 y/o woman	NY	Hospital worker	Malaise, myalgia, cough, chest pain, dyspnea, fatigue	Mediastinal adenopathy, pleural effusions	11,400	6	Levofloxacin, rifampin, gentamicin, nafcillin, ciprofloxacin, clindamycin, ceftazidime, mechanical ventilation, chest tubes
5	94 y/o woman	CT	Retired	Fever, fatigue, loss of appetite, cough, myalgia	Perihilar fullness, pleural effusion	8100	8	Vancomycin, ceftazidime, ampicillin, sulbactam, ciprofloxacin, clindamycin, thoracentesis, mechanical ventilation
NONFATAL CASES								
6	73 y/o man	FL	Mail handler, media company	Fever, fatigue, abdominal pain, vomiting, cough, dyspnea, conjunctivitis	Consolidation, pleural effusion	9900		Azithromycin, cefotaxime, ciprofloxacin
7	56 y/o woman	NJ	Postal worker	Fever, vomiting, diarrhea, cough, chest pain, dyspnea	Bibasilar infiltrates, mediastinal adenopathy, pleural effusion	8100		Levofloxacin, rifampin, ciprofloxacin, vancomycin, thoracentesis, chest tube
8	43 y/o woman	NJ	Postal worker	Fever, myalgia, vomiting, fatigue, cough, chest pain, dyspnea, headache	Perihilar consolidation, mediastinal adenopathy, pleural effusion	11,200		Levofloxacin, azithromycin, ciprofloxacin, clindamycin, ceftriaxone, doxycycline, thoracentesis X2
9	56 y/o man	DC	Postal worker	Fever, headache, malaise, sore throat, cough, dyspnea, nausea, vomiting	Bilateral hilar adenopathy, widened mediastinum, pleural effusion	7500		Ciprofloxacin, rifampin, clindamycin, diuretics, glucocorticoids, thoracentesis X3
10	56 y/o man	DC	Postal worker	Fever, headache, malaise, sore throat, nausea, photophobia, cough, dyspnea, chest pain	Widened mediastinum, bilateral hilar adenopathy, airspace disease, pleural effusion	9700		Ciprofloxacin, rifampin, clindamycin, glucocorticoids thoracentesis X2
11	59 y/o man	VA	Postal worker	Fever, sweats, myalgia, fatigue, headache, nausea, vomiting, abdominal pain, cough, chest pain	Mediastinal widening, mediastinal adenopathy, pleural effusion	9700		Ciprofloxacin, penicillin, rifampin, vancomycin, thoracentesis

[a] At anytime during the illness.
Note: CT, computed tomography; CXR, chest x-ray; WBC, white blood cell count.

the efficacy of AVA in a postexposure setting in humans has not been established, the current recommendation for postexposure prophylaxis is 60 days of antibiotics. Given the potential for *B. anthracis* to be engineered to express penicillin resistance, the empirical regimen of choice in this setting is either ciprofloxacin or doxycycline.

PLAGUE (*YERSINIA PESTIS*) (See also Chap. 143) ■ **Plague as a Bioweapon**
Although it lacks the environmental stability of anthrax, the highly

contagious nature and high mortality of plague make it a close to ideal agent of bioterrorism, particularly if delivered in a weaponized form. Occupying a unique place in history, plague has been alleged to have been used as a biologic weapon for centuries. The catapulting of plague-infected corpses into besieged fortresses is a practice that was first noted in 1346 during the assault of the city of Kaffa by the Tartars. There are some who believe this may have played a role in the start

TABLE 205-4 *Clinical Syndromes, Prevention, and Treatment Strategies for Diseases Caused by Category A Agents*

Agent	Clinical Syndrome	Incubation Period	Diagnosis	Treatment	Prophylaxis
Bacillus anthracis (anthrax)	Cutaneous lesion: Papule to eschar Inhalational disease: Fever, malaise, chest and abdominal discomfort Pleural effusion, widened mediastinum on chest x-ray	1–12 days 1–60 days	Culture, Gram stain, PCR, Wright stain of peripheral smear	Postexposure: Ciprofloxacin, 500 mg, PO bid × 60 d *or* Doxycycline, 100 mg PO bid ×60 d Amoxicillin, 500 mg PO q8h, likely to be effective if strain penicillin sensitive *Active disease:* Ciprofloxacin, 400 mg IV q12h *or* Doxycycline, 100 mg IV q12 *plus* Clindamycin, 900 mg IV q8h and/or rifampin, 300 mg IV q12h; switch to PO when stable ×60 d total *Antitoxin strategies:* Neutralizing monoclonal antibodies are under study	Anthrax vaccine adsorbed Recombinant protective antigen vaccines are under study
Yersinia pestis (pneumonic plague)	Fever, cough, dyspnea, hemoptysis Infiltrates and consolidation on chest x-ray	1–6 days	Culture, Gram stain, direct fluorescent antibody, PCR	Gentamicin, 2.0 mg/kg IV loading then 1.7 mg/kg q8h IV *or* Streptomycin, 1.0 g q12h IM or IV Alternatives include doxycycline, 100 mg bid PO or IV; chloramphenicol 500 mg bid PO or IV	Doxycycline, 100 mg PO bid (ciprofloxacin may also be active) Formalin-fixed vaccine (FDA licensed; not available)
Variola major (smallpox)	Fever, malaise, headache, backache, emesis Maculopapular to vesicular to pustular skin lesions	7–17 days	Culture, PCR, electron microscopy	Supportive measures; consideration for cidofovir, antivaccinia immunoglobulin	Vaccinia immunization
Francisella tularensis (tularemia)	Fever, chills, malaise, myalgia, chest discomfort, dyspnea, headache, skin rash, pharyngitis, conjunctivitis Hilar adenopathy on chest x-ray	1–14 days	Gram stain, culture, immunohistochemistry, PCR	Streptomycin, 1 g IM bid *or* Gentamicin, 5 mg/kg per day div q8h IV for 14 days *or* Doxycycline, 100 mg IV bid *or* Chlorphenid, 15 mg/kg IV qid *or* Ciprofloxacin, 400 mg IV bid	Doxycycline, 100 mg PO bid × 14 days *or* Ciprofloxacin, 500 mg PO bid × 14 days
Viral hemorrhagic fevers	Fever, myalgia, rash, encephalitis, prostration	2–21 days	RT-PCR, serologic testing for antigen or antibody Viral isolation by CDC or U.S. Army Medical Institute of Infectious Diseases (USAMRIID)	Supportive measures Ribavirin 30 mg/kg up to 2 g × 1, followed by 16 mg/kg IV up to 1 g q6h for 4 days, followed by 8 mg/kg IV up to 0.5 g q8h × 6 days	No known chemoprophylaxis Consideration for ribavirin in high-risk situations Vaccine exists for yellow fever
Botulinum toxin (*Clostridium botulinum*)	Dry mouth, blurred vision, ptosis, weakness, dysarthria, dysphagia, dizziness, respiratory failure, progressive paralysis, dilated pupils	12–72 h	Mouse bioassay, toxin immunoassay	Supportive measures including ventilation 5000–9000 IU equine antitoxin	Administration of antitoxin

Note: CDC, U.S. Centers for Disease Control and Prevention; FDA, U.S. Food and Drug Administration; PCR, polymerase chain reaction; RT-PCR, reverse transcriptase PCR.

of the Black Death pandemic of the fourteenth and fifteenth centuries in Europe. Given that plague was already moving across Asia toward Europe at this time, it is unclear whether such an allegation is accurate. During WWII, the infamous Unit 731 of the Japanese army was reported to have repeatedly dropped plague-infested fleas over parts of China, including Manchuria. These drops were associated with subsequent outbreaks of plague in the targeted areas. Following WWII, the United States and the Soviet Union conducted programs of research on how to create direct aerosols containing *Y. pestis* that could be used as a direct bioweapon leading to primary pneumonic plague. As mentioned above, plague was thought to be an excellent bioweapon due to the fact that in addition to causing infection in those inhaling the aerosol, significant numbers of secondary cases of primary pneumonic plague would likely occur due to the contagious nature of the disease and person-to-person transmission via respiratory aerosol. Secondary reports of research conducted during that time suggest that organisms remain viable for up to 1 h and can be dispersed for distances up to 10 km. While the offensive bioweapons program in the United States was terminated prior to production of sufficient quantities of plague organisms for use as a weapon, it is believed that Soviet scientists did manufacture quantities sufficient for such a purpose. It has also been reported that more than 10 Soviet Institutes and over 1000 scientists were working with plague as a biologic weapon. Of concern is the fact that in 1995 a microbiologist in Ohio was arrested for having obtained *Y. pestis* in the mail from the American Type Culture Collection, using a credit card and a false letterhead. In the wake of this incident, the U.S. Congress passed a law in 1997 requiring that anyone intending to send or receive any of 42 different agents that could potentially be used as bioweapons first register with the CDC.

Microbiology and Clinical Features   Plague is caused by *Y. pestis*, a non-motile, gram-negative bacillus that exhibits bipolar, or "safety pin," staining with Wright, Giemsa, or Wayson stains. It has had a major impact on the course of history, thus adding to the element of fear evoked by its mention. The earliest reported plague epidemic was in 224 B.C. in China. The most infamous pandemic began in Europe in the fourteenth century, during which time one-third to one-half of the entire population of Europe was killed. During a plague outbreak in India in 1994, it is estimated that 500,000 individuals fled their homes in fear of this disease.

The clinical syndromes of plague generally reflect the mode of infection. *Bubonic plague* is the consequence of an insect bite; primary *pneumonic plague* arises through the inhalation of bacteria. Most of the plague seen in the world today is bubonic plague and is the result of a bite by a plague-infected flea. Plague infection of rodents exists widely in nature, and each year thousands of cases of plague occur worldwide through contact with infected animals or fleas. Following inoculation of regurgitated bacteria into the skin by a flea bite, organisms travel through the lymphatics to regional lymph nodes, where they are phagocytized but not destroyed. Inside the cell, they multiply rapidly leading to inflammation, painful lymphadenopathy with necrosis, fever, bacteremia, septicemia, and death. The characteristic enlarged nodes, or *buboes*, give this form of plague its name. In some instances, patients may develop bacteremia without lymphadenopathy following infection, a condition referred to as *primary septicemic plague*. Extensive ecchymoses may develop due to disseminated intravascular coagulation, and gangrene of the digits and/or nose may develop in patients with advanced septicemic plague. It is thought that this appearance of some patients gave rise to the term *Black Death* in reference to the plague epidemic of the fourteenth and fifteenth centuries. Some patients may develop pneumonia (secondary pneumonic plague) as a complication of bubonic or septicemic plague. These patients may then transmit the agent to others via the respiratory route, causing cases of primary pneumonic plague. Primary pneumonic plague is the manifestation most likely to occur as the result of a bioterrorist attack, with an aerosol of bacteria spread over a wide area or a particular environment that is densely populated. In this setting patients would be expected to develop fever, cough with hemoptysis, dyspnea, and gastrointestinal symptoms 1 to 6 days following exposure. Clinical features of pneumonia would be accompanied by pulmonary infiltrates and consolidation on chest x-ray. In the absence of antibiotics, the mortality of this disease is on the order of 85%, and death usually occurs within 2 to 6 days.

℞ TREATMENT

Streptomycin, tetracycline, and doxycycline are licensed by the U.S. Food and Drug Administration (FDA) for the treatment of plague. Multiple additional antibiotics licensed for other infections are commonly used and are likely effective. Among these are aminoglycosides such as gentamicin, cephalosporins, trimethoprim/sulfamethoxazole, chloramphenicol, and ciprofloxacin (Table 205-4). A multidrug resistant strain of *Y. pestis* was identified in 1995 from a patient with bu-

bonic plague in Madagascar. While this organism was resistant to streptomycin, ampicillin, chloramphenicol, sulfonamides, and tetracycline, it retained its susceptibility to other aminoglycosides and cephalosporins. Given the subsequent identification of a similar organism in 1997 coupled with the fact that this resistance is plasmid-mediated, it seems likely that genetically modifying *Y. pestis* to a multidrug resistant form is possible. Unlike patients with inhalational anthrax (see above), patients with pulmonary plague should be cared for under conditions of strict respiratory isolation comparable to that used for multidrug resistant tuberculosis.

Vaccination and Prevention   A formalin-fixed, whole-organism vaccine was licensed by the FDA for the prevention of plague. That vaccine is no longer being manufactured, but its potential value as a current countermeasure against bioterrorism would likely have been modest at best as it was ineffective against primary pneumonic plague in animal studies. Efforts are under way to develop a second generation of vaccines that will protect against aerosol challenge. Among the candidates being tested are recombinant forms of the F1 and V antigens of *Y. pestis*. It is likely that doxycycline or ciprofloxacin would provide coverage in a chemoprophylaxis setting. Unlike the case with anthrax, in which one has to be concerned about the presence of spores, the duration of prophylaxis against plague need only extend to 7 days following exposure.

SMALLPOX (*VARIOLA MAJOR* AND *V. MINOR*) (See also Chap. 167) ■ **Smallpox as a Bioweapon**   Given that an effective vaccine exists for smallpox, it would not have been considered a good candidate as a bioweapon 30 years ago. However, with the cessation of immunization programs in the United States in 1972 and throughout the world in 1980 due to the successful global eradication of smallpox, close to 50% of the U.S. population is fully susceptible to smallpox today. Given its infectious nature and the 10 to 30% mortality in unimmunized individuals, the deliberate spread of this virus could have a devastating effect on our society and unleash a previously conquered deadly disease. It is estimated that an initial infection of 50 to 100 persons in a first-generation of cases could expand by a factor of 10 to 20 with each succeeding generation in the absence of any effective containment measures.

At the time that the World Health Organization (WHO) recommended that all immunization programs be terminated in 1980, it also recommended that remaining stocks of virus be destroyed and that samples be transferred to only two locations: one at the CDC in Atlanta, GA, in the United States and the other at the Institute of Virus Preparations in the Soviet Union. Several years later, it was recommended that these remaining two stocks be destroyed. However, these latter recommendations were reversed in the wake of increased concerns on the use of *Variola* as a biologic weapon and thus the need to maintain an active program of defensive research. Many of these concerns were based upon allegations made by former Soviet officials that extensive programs had been in place in that country for the production and weaponization of large quantities of smallpox virus. The dismantling of these programs with the fall of the Soviet Union led to fears that stocks of *V. major* may have made their way to other countries. In addition, accounts that efforts had been taken to produce recombinant strains of *Variola* that would be more virulent and more contagious than the wild-type virus have led to an increase in the need to be vigilant for the reemergence of this often fatal infectious disease.

Microbiology and Clinical Features   Smallpox is caused by one of two closely related viruses, *V. major* and *V. minor*. Both are double-strand DNA viruses and members of the Orthopoxvirus genus of the Poxviridae family. Infections with *V. minor* are generally less severe, with milder constitutional symptoms and lower mortality rates; thus *V. major* is the only one considered to be a viable bioweapon. Infection with *V. major* typically occurs following contact with an infected person from the time that a maculopapular rash occurs through the appearance of scabbing of the pustular lesions. Infection is thought to occur from inhalation of saliva droplets containing virus from the oropharyngeal exanthem. Contaminated clothing or linen can also spread infection.

Several days after exposure, a primary viremia is believed to occur that results in dissemination of virus to lymphoid tissues. A secondary viremia occurs ~4 days later that leads to localization of infection in the dermis. Approximately 12 to 14 days following the initial exposure the patient develops high fever, malaise, vomiting, headache, backache, and a maculopapular rash that begins on the face and extremities and spreads to the trunk (centripetal). The lesions are initially maculopapular and evolve to vesicles that eventually become pustules and then scabs. The oral mucosa also develops maculopapular lesions that evolve to ulcers. The lesions appear over a period of 1 to 2 days and evolve at the same rate. Although virus can be isolated from the scabs on the skin, the conventional thinking is that once the scabs have formed the patient is no longer contagious. Smallpox is associated with a 10 to 30% mortality, with patients typically dying of severe systemic illness during the second week of symptoms. Historically, ~5 to 10% of naturally occurring smallpox cases take either of two highly virulent atypical forms, classified as *hemorrhagic* and *malignant*. These are difficult to recognize because of their atypical presentations. The hemorrhagic form is uniformly fatal and begins with the relatively abrupt onset of a severely prostrating illness characterized by high fevers and severe headache and back and abdominal pain. Cutaneous erythema develops accompanied by petechiae and hemorrhages into the skin and mucous membranes. Death usually occurs within 5 to 6 days. The malignant form is frequently fatal and has an onset similar to the hemorrhagic form, but with confluent lesions developing more slowly and never progressing to the pustular stage.

R_x TREATMENT

Given the highly infectious nature of smallpox and the extreme vulnerability of contemporary society, patients who are suspected cases should be handled with strict isolation procedures. While laboratory confirmation of a suspected case by culture and electron microscopy is essential, it is equally important that appropriate precautions be employed when obtaining samples for culture and laboratory testing. All health care and laboratory workers caring for patients should have been recently immunized with vaccinia, and all samples should be transported in doubly sealed containers. Patients should be cared for in negative-pressure rooms with strict isolation precautions.

There is no licensed specific therapy for smallpox, and historic treatments have focused solely on supportive care. While several antiviral agents, including cidofovir, that are licensed for other diseases have in vitro activity against *V. major*, they have never been tested in the setting of human disease. For this reason it is difficult to predict whether or not they would be effective in cases of smallpox and, if effective, whether or not they would be of value in patients with advanced disease. Research programs studying the efficacy of new antiviral compounds against *V. major* are currently under way.

Vaccination and Prevention In 1796 Edward Jenner demonstrated that deliberate infection with cowpox could prevent subsequent infection with smallpox. Today, smallpox is a preventable disease following immunization with vaccinia. The current dilemma facing our society regarding assessment of the risk and/or benefit of smallpox vaccination is that the degree of risk that someone will deliberately and effectively release smallpox into our society is unknown. As a prudent first step in preparedness for a smallpox attack, virtually all members of the U.S. armed services have received primary or booster immunizations with vaccinia. In addition, tens of thousands of civilian health care workers who comprise smallpox-response teams at the state and local public health level have been vaccinated. The voluntary vaccination of other civilian first responders continues as part of a broader smallpox preparedness program.

Initial fears regarding the immunization of a segment of the American population with vaccinia when there are more individuals receiving immunosuppressive drugs and other immunocompromised patients than ever before have largely been dispelled as data are generated from the current military and civilian immunization campaigns. Adverse event rates for the first 450,000 immunizations are similar to

and, in certain categories of adverse events, even lower than those from historic data (Table 205-5). In addition, 11 patients with early stage HIV infection have been inadvertently immunized without problem. One significant concern during the recent immunization campaign, however, has been the description of a syndrome of myopericarditis, which was not appreciated during prior immunization campaigns with vaccinia.

TULAREMIA (*FRANCISELLA TULARENSIS*) (See also Chap. 142) ■ **Tularemia as a Bioweapon** Tularemia has been studied as an agent of bioterrorism since the mid-twentieth century, and it has been suggested that the outbreak of tularemia among German and Soviet soldiers during fighting on the Eastern Front during WWII might have been the consequence of a deliberate release. Unit 731 of the Japanese Army studied the use of tularemia as a bioweapon during WWII. Large quantities of *F. tularensis* were grown by the United States and were reportedly grown by the Soviet Union in the mid-1950s. It has also been suggested that the Soviet program extended into the era of molecular biology and that some strains were engineered to be resistant to common antibiotics. *F. tularensis* is an extremely infectious organism, and human infections have occurred from merely examining an uncovered petri dish streaked with colonies. Given these facts, it is reasonable to conclude that this organism might be utilized as a bioweapon through either an aerosol or contamination of food or drinking water.

Microbiology and Clinical Features While similar in many ways to anthrax and plague, tularemia, also referred to as rabbit fever or deer fly fever, is neither as lethal nor as fulminant as either of these other two category A bacterial infections. It is, however, extremely infectious, and as few as 10 organisms can lead to establishment of infection. Despite this fact, it is not spread from person to person. Tularemia is caused by *F. tularensis*, a small, nonmotile, gram-negative coccobacillus. Although it is not a spore-forming organism, it is a hardy bacterium that can survive for weeks in the environment. Infection typically comes from insect bites or contact with organisms in the environment. Large waterborne outbreaks have been recorded.

Humans can become infected through a variety of environmental sources. Infection is most common in rural areas where a variety of small mammals may serve as reservoirs. Human infections in the summer are often the result of insect bites from ticks, flies, or mosquitoes that have bitten infected animals. In colder months infections are most likely the result of direct contact with infected mammals and are most common in hunters. In these settings infection typically presents as a systemic illness with an area of inflammation and necrosis at the site

TABLE 205-5 *Complications from 438,134 Administrations of Vaccinia During the United States Department of Defense (DoD) Smallpox Immunization Campaign Initiated in December 2002*

Complication	Number of Cases	DoD Rate per Million Vaccinees (95% Confidence Interval)	Historic Rate Per Million Vaccinees
Mild or temporary:			
Generalized vaccinia, mild	35	67 (52, 85)	45 to 212[a]
Inadvertent inoculation, self	62	119 (98, 142)	606[a]
Vaccinia transfer to contact	28	53 (40, 69)	8 to 27[a]
Moderate or serious:			
Encephalitis	1	2.2 (0.6, 7.2)	2.6 to 8.7[a]
Acute myopericarditis	69	131 (110, 155)	100[b]
Eczema vaccinatum	0	0 (0, 3.7)	2 to 35[a]
Progressive vaccinia	0	0 (0, 3.7)	1 to 7[a]
Death[c]	1	1.9 (0.2, 5.6)	1 to 2[a]

[a] Based on adolescent and adult smallpox vaccinations from 1968 studies, both primary and revaccinations.
[b] Based on case series in Finnish military recruits given the Finnish strain of smallpox vaccine.
[c] Potentially attributable to vaccination; after lupus-like illness.
Source: From Grabenstein and Winkenwerder. *http://www.smallpox.mil/event/SPSafetySum.asp*

of tissue entry of the infection. Drinking of contaminated water may lead to an oropharyngeal form of tularemia characterized by pharyngitis with cervical and/or retropharyngeal lymphadenopathy (Chap. 142). The most likely mode of dissemination of tularemia as a biologic weapon would be as an aerosol. Approximately 1 to 14 days following exposure by this route one would expect to see inflammation of the airways with pharyngitis, pleuritis, and bronchopneumonia. Typical symptoms would include the abrupt onset of fever, fatigue, chills, headache, and malaise (Table 205-3). Some patients might experience conjunctivitis with ulceration, pharyngitis, and/or cutaneous exanthems. A pulse-temperature dissociation might be present. Approximately 50% of patients would show a pulmonary infiltrate on chest x-ray. Hilar adenopathy might also be present, and a small percent of patients could have adenopathy without infiltrates. Diagnosis is made by immunohistochemistry or culture of infected tissues or blood. Untreated, mortality rates range from 5 to 15% for cutaneous routes of infection and 30 to 60% for infection by inhalation. Since the advent of antibiotic therapy, these rates have dropped to <2%.

Rx TREATMENT

Both streptomycin and doxycycline are licensed for treatment of tularemia. Other agents likely to be effective include gentamicin, chloramphenicol, and ciprofloxacin (Table 205-4). Given the potential for genetic modification of this organism to yield antibiotic-resistant strains, broad-spectrum coverage should be the rule until sensitivities have been determined. As mentioned above, special isolation procedures are not required.

Vaccination and Prevention   There are no vaccines currently licensed for the prevention of infection with *F. tularensis*. While a live, attenuated strain of the organism has been used in the past with some reported success, there are inadequate data to support its widespread use at this time. Development of a vaccine for this agent is an important part of the current biodefense research agenda. In the absence of an effective vaccine, chemoprophylaxis with either doxycycline or ciprofloxacin appears to be a reasonable approach in individuals who have been exposed (Table 205-4).

VIRAL HEMORRHAGIC FEVERS (See also Chaps. 180 and 181) ■ **Hemorrhagic Fever Viruses as Bioweapons**   Several of the hemorrhagic fever viruses have been reported to have been weaponized by the Soviet Union and the United States. Nonhuman primate studies indicate that infection can be established with very few virions and that infectious aerosol preparations can be produced. Under the guise of wanting to aid victims of the latest Ebola outbreak, members of the Aum Shrinrikyo cult in Japan were reported to have traveled to central Africa in 1992 in an attempt to obtain Ebola virus for use in a bioterrorist attack. Thus, while there has been no evidence that these agents have ever been used in a biologic attack, there is clear interest in their potential for this purpose.

Microbiology and Clinical Features   The viral hemorrhagic fevers are a group of illnesses caused by any one of a number of similar viruses (Table 205-2). These viruses are all enveloped, single-strand RNA viruses that are thought to depend upon a rodent or insect host reservoir for long-term survival. They tend to be geographically restricted according to the migration patterns of their hosts. It is felt that Ebola has been responsible for the deaths of significant numbers of apes in sub-Saharan Africa. While humans are not a reservoir for these viruses, humans can become infected with them if they come into contact with an infected host or other infected animals. Person-to-person transmission has been documented for Ebola, Marburg, Lassa, and New World arenaviruses. While the modes of transmission for naturally occurring infections are largely unknown, these viruses have been shown in animal models to be highly infectious by the aerosol route. This, coupled with mortality rates as high as 90%, makes them excellent candidate agents of bioterrorism.

The clinical features of the viral hemorrhagic fevers may vary depending upon the particular agent (Table 205-4). Initial signs and symptoms typically include fever, myalgia, prostration, and diffuse intravascular coagulation with thrombocytopenia and capillary hemorrhage. A variety of different maculopapular or erythematous rashes may be seen. Leukopenia, temperature-pulse dissociation, renal failure, and seizures may also be part of the clinical presentation. Outbreaks of most of these diseases are sporadic and unpredictable. As a consequence it has been very difficult to study the pathogenesis and epidemiology in any detail. The diagnosis should be suspected in anyone with temperature >38.3°C for <3 weeks who also exhibits at least two of the following: hemorrhagic or purpuric rash, epistaxis, hematemesis, hemoptysis, or hematochezia in the absence of any other identifiable cause. In this setting, samples of blood should be sent to the CDC or the U.S. Army Medical Research Institute of Infectious Diseases (USAMRIID) for serologic testing for antigen and antibody as well as reverse transcriptase polymerase chain reaction (RT-PCR) testing for hemorrhagic fever viruses. All samples should be handled with double-bagging. Given how little is known regarding the human-to-human transmission of these viruses, appropriate isolation measures would include full barrier precautions with negative-pressure rooms and use of N95 masks or powered air-purifying respirators (PAPRs). Unprotected skin contact with cadavers has been implicated in the transmission of certain hemorrhagic fever viruses such as Ebola, so it is recommended that autopsies be performed using the strictest measures for protection and that burial or cremation be performed promptly without embalming.

Rx TREATMENT

There are no approved and effective antiviral therapies for this class of viruses (Table 205-4). While there are anecdotal reports of the efficacy of ribavirin, interferon α, or hyperimmune immunoglobulin, definitive data are lacking. The best data for ribavirin are in arenavirus (Lassa and New World) infections. In some animal models specific immunoglobulin has been reported to enhance disease progression, and thus these potential treatments must be approached with caution.

Vaccination and Prevention   A live attenuated virus vaccine is available in limited quantities for prevention of yellow fever. There are no other licensed and effective vaccines for these agents. Studies are currently under way examining the potential role of DNA, recombinant viruses, and attenuated viruses as vaccines for several of these infections. Among the most promising at present are vaccines for Argentine, Ebola, Rift Valley, and Kayasanur Forest viruses. Vaccines for Marburg and Lassa viruses are in preclinical testing.

BOTULISM TOXIN (*CLOSTRIDIUM BOTULINUM*) (See also Chap. 126) ■ **Botulism Toxin as a Bioweapon**   In a bioterrorist attack, botulinum toxin would likely be dispersed as an aerosol or as contamination of a food supply. While contamination of a water supply is possible, it is likely that any toxin would be rapidly inactivated by the chlorine used to purify drinking water. Similarly, toxin can be inactivated by heating any food to >85°C for >5 min. Without external facilitation, the environmental decay rate is estimated at 1% per minute, and thus the time interval between deposition and ingestion or inhalation needs to be rather short. The Japanese biologic warfare group, Unit 731, is reported to have conducted experiments on botulism poisoning in prisoners in the 1930s. The United States and the Soviet Union both acknowledged producing botulinum toxin, and there is some evidence that the Soviet Union attempted to create recombinant bacteria containing the gene for botulinum toxin. In records submitted to the United Nations, Iraq admitted to having produced 19,000 L of concentrated toxin—enough toxin to kill the entire population of the world three times over. By many accounts, botulinum toxin was the primary focus of the pre-1991 Iraqi bioweapons program. In addition to these examples of state-supported research into the use of botulinum toxin as a bioweapon, the Aum Shrinrikyo cult has unsuccessfully attempted on a least three occasions to disperse botulism toxin into the civilian population of Tokyo.

Microbiology and Clinical Features Unique among the category A agents for not being a live microorganism, botulinum toxin is one of the most potent toxins ever described and is thought by some to be the most poisonous substance in existence. It is estimated that 1 g of botulinum toxin would be sufficient to kill 1 million individuals if adequately dispersed. Botulinum toxin is produced by the gram-positive, spore-forming anaerobe *C. botulinum* (Chap. 126). Its natural habitat is soil. There are seven antigenically distinct forms of botulinum toxin, designated A to G. The majority of naturally occurring human cases are of types A, B, and E. Antitoxin directed toward one of these will have little to no activity against the others. The toxin is a 150-kDa zinc-containing protease that prevents the intracellular fusion of acetylcholine vesicles with the motor neuron membrane, thus preventing the release of acetylcholine. In the absence of acetylcholine-dependent triggering of muscle fibers, a flaccid paralysis develops. Although person-to-person spread does not occur, the ease of production of botulinum toxin coupled with its high morbidity and 60 to 100% mortality make it a close to ideal bioweapon.

Botulism can result from the presence of *C. botulinum* infection in a wound or the intestine, the ingestion of contaminated food, or the inhalation of aerosolized toxin. The latter two forms are the most likely modes of transmission for bioterrorism. Once toxin is absorbed into the bloodstream it binds to the neuronal cell membrane, enters the cell, and cleaves one of the proteins required for the intracellular binding of the synaptic vesicle to the cell membrane, thus preventing release of the neurotransmitter to the membrane of the adjacent muscle cell. Patients initially develop multiple cranial nerve palsies that are followed by a flaccid paralysis. The extent of the neuromuscular compromise is dependent upon the level of toxemia. The majority of patients experience diploplia, dysphagia, dysathria, dry mouth, ptosis, dilated pupils, fatigue, and extremity weakness. There are minimal true central nervous system effects, and patients rarely show significant alterations in mental status. Severe cases can involve complete muscular collapse, loss of the gag reflex, and respiratory failure. Recovery requires the regeneration of new motor neuron synapses with the muscle cell, a process that can take weeks to months. In the absence of secondary infections, which may be common during the protracted recovery phase of this illness, patients remain afebrile. The diagnosis is suspected on clinical grounds and confirmed by a mouse bioassay or toxin immunoassay.

Rx TREATMENT

Treatment for botulism is mainly supportive and may require intubation, mechanical ventilation, and parenteral nutrition (Table 205-4). If diagnosed early enough, administration of equine antitoxin may lead to a decrease in the level of nerve damage and severity of disease. At present antitoxins are available on a limited basis as a licensed bivalent product with activity against toxin types A and B and as an experimental product with activity against toxin type E. In the event of attack with another toxin type, an investigational antitoxin with activity against all seven toxin types is also available through the U.S. Army. A single dose of antitoxin is usually adequate to neutralize any circulating toxin. Given that these preparations are all derived from horse serum, one needs to be vigilant for hypersensitivity reactions, including serum sickness and anaphylaxis following their administration. Once the damage to the nerve axon has been done, however, there is little possible in the way of specific therapy, and vigilance for secondary complications during recovery is of the utmost importance. During the protracted recovery phase of botulism, patients may experience secondary infections. Due to their ability to worsen neuromuscular blockade, aminoglycosides and clindamycin should be avoided in the treatment of these infections.

Vaccination and Prevention A botulinum toxoid preparation has been used as a vaccine for laboratory workers at high risk of exposure and

in certain military situations; however, it is not currently available in quantities that could be used for the general population. At present, early recognition of the clinical syndrome and use of appropriate equine antitoxin is the mainstay of prevention of full-blown disease in exposed individuals. The development of human monoclonal antibodies as a replacement for equine antitoxin antibodies is an area of active research interest.

CATEGORY B AND C AGENTS

The category B agents include those that are moderately easy to disseminate and result in moderate morbidity and low mortality rates. A listing of the current category B agents is provided in Table 205-2. As can be seen, it includes a wide array of microorganisms and products of microorganisms. Several of these agents have been used in bioterrorist attacks, although never with the impact of the agents described above. Among the more notorious of these was the contamination of salad bars in Oregon in 1984 with *Salmonella typhimurium* by the Indian religious cult Rajneeshee. In this outbreak, which many consider to be the first bioterrorist attack against U.S. citizens, >750 individuals were poisoned and 40 were hospitalized in an effort to influence a local election.

Category C agents are the third highest priority agents in the biodefense agenda. These agents include emerging pathogens to which little or no immunity exists in the general population, such as the SARS coronavirus, that could potentially be engineered for mass dissemination in the future because of their availability in nature. These agents are characterized as being relatively easy to produce and disseminate and as having high morbidity and mortality rates as well as a major public health impact. There is no running list of category C agents at the present time.

PREVENTION AND PREPAREDNESS

As noted above, a numerous and diverse array of agents have the potential to be used in a bioterrorist attack. In contrast to the military situation with biowarfare, where the primary objective is to inflict mass casualties on a healthy and prepared militia, the objectives of bioterrorism are to harm civilians as well as to create fear and disruption among the civilian population. While the military needs only to prepare their troops to deal with the limited number of agents that pose a legitimate threat of biowarfare, the public health system needs to prepare the entire civilian population to deal with the multitude of agents and settings that could be utilized in a bioterrorism attack. This includes anticipating issues specific to the very young and the very old, the pregnant patient, and the immunocompromised individual. The challenges in this regard are enormous and immediate. While military preparedness emphasizes vaccines toward a limited number of agents, civilian preparedness needs to rely upon rapid diagnosis and treatment of a wide array of conditions.

The medical profession must maintain a high index of suspicion that unusual clinical presentations or clustering of rare disease may not be a chance occurrence but rather the first sign of a bioterrorist event. This is particularly true when such diseases occur in traditionally healthy populations, when surprisingly large numbers of rare conditions occur, and when diseases commonly seen in rural settings appear in urban populations. Given the importance of rapid diagnosis and early treatment for many of these conditions, it is important that the medical care team report any suspected cases of bioterrorism immediately to local and state health authorities and/or to the CDC (888-246-2675). Recent enhancements have been made to the public health surveillance network to facilitate the rapid sharing of information among public health agencies.

At present a series of efforts are taking place to ensure the biomedical security of the civilian population in the United States. The Public Health Service is moving toward a larger, more highly trained, fully deployable force. A National Pharmaceutical Stockpile (NPSP) has been created by the CDC to provide rapid access to quantities of pharmaceuticals, antidotes, vaccines, and other medical supplies that may be of value in the event of a biologic or biochemical terrorist event. The NPSP has two basic components. The first of these consists of eight 50-ton (45,360-kg) "push packages" that can be deployed anywhere in the United States within 12 h. These push packages are a preassembled set of supplies, pharmaceuticals, and medical equipment ready for immediate delivery to the field. They provide treatment for a variety of conditions given the fact that an actual threat may not have been precisely identified at the time of stockpile deployment. The contents of the push packs are constantly updated to ensure that they reflect current needs as determined by national security threat assessments; they include antibiotics for treatment of anthrax, plague, and tularemia as well as a cache of vaccine to deal with a smallpox threat. The second component of the NPSP comprises inventories managed by specific vendors and consists of the provision of additional pharmaceuticals, supplies, and/or products tailored to the specific attack.

The number of FDA-approved and -licensed drugs and vaccines for category A and B agents is currently limited and not reflective of the pharmacy of today. In an effort to speed the licensure of additional drugs and vaccines for these diseases, the FDA has proposed a new rule for the licensure of such countermeasures against agents of bioterror when adequate and well-controlled clinical efficacy studies cannot be ethically conducted in humans. Thus, for indications in which field trials of naturally occurring disease are not feasible, the FDA is proposing to rely on evidence solely from animal studies. For this rule to apply it must be shown that (1) there are reasonably well-understood pathophysiologic mechanisms for the condition and its treatment; (2) the effect of the intervention is independently substantiated in multiple animal species, including species expected to react with a response predictive for humans; (3) the animal study end point is clearly related

to the desired benefit in humans; and (4) the data in animals allow selection of an effective dose in humans.

Finally, an initiative referred to as Project BioShield has been established to facilitate biodefense research within the federal government, create a stable source of funding for the purchase of countermeasures against agents of bioterrorism, and create a category of "emergency use authorization" to allow the FDA to approve the use of unlicensed treatments during times of extraordinary unmet needs as might be present in the context of a bioterrorist attack.

While the prospect of a deliberate attack on civilians with disease-producing agents may seem to be an act of incomprehensible evil, history shows us that it is something that has been done in the past and will likely be done again in the future. It is the responsibility of health care providers to be aware of this possibility, to be able to recognize early signs of a potential bioterrorist attack and alert the public health system, and to respond quickly to provide care to the individual patient. Among the web sites with current information on microbial bioterrorism are *www.bt.cdc.gov*, *www.niaid.nih.gov*, *www.hopkinsbiodefense.org*, and *www.cns.miis.edu/research/cbw/index.htm*.

FURTHER READING

ALIBEK K, HANDELMAN S: *Biohazard: The Chilling True Story of the Largest Covert Biological Weapons in the World, Told from the Inside by the Man who Ran it.* New York, Random House, 1999

CRODDY E (with C Perey-Armendariz and J Hart): *Chemical and Biological Warfare: A Comprehensive Survey for the Concerned Citizen.* New York, Copernicus Books, 2001

GRABENSTEIN JD, WINKENWERDER W: United States military smallpox vaccination program experience. JAMA 289:3278, 2003

HENDERSON DA et al (eds): *Bioterrorism: Guidelines for Medical and Public Health Management.* JAMA and Archives Journals, AMA press, 2002

JERNIGAN JA et al: Bioterrorism-related inhalational anthrax: The first 10 cases reported in the United States. Emerg Infect Dis 7:933,2001

---

206 | CHEMICAL BIOTERRORISM
Charles G. Hurst, Jonathan Newmark, James A. Romano

The use of chemical warfare agents (CWAs) as weapons of terror against civilian populations is a potential reality that must be addressed by public health officials and by the medical profession. The use of sulfur mustard and nerve agents by Iraq against the Iranian military and Kurdish civilians, the sarin attacks in 1994–1995 in Japan, and the terrorist strikes of September 11, 2001, followed by the anthrax attacks in Florida, New York, and Washington, D.C., underscore this threat.

Many of the World War I (WWI) chemical agents, including chlorine, phosgene, and cyanide, are used in large amounts in industry. They are produced in chemical plants, stockpiled in large tanks, and travel up and down highways and railways in large tanker cars. The rupture of any of these by accident or purposefully could cause many injuries and deaths. Hazardous materials (HAZMATs), not used on the battlefield, can also be used as terrorist weapons. Some of these, including insecticides and ammonia, could wreak as much damage and injury as the weaponized chemical agents.

Military planners consider the WWI blistering agent, sulfur mustard, and the organophosphorus nerve agents as the most likely agents to be used on the battlefield. In a civilian or terrorist scenario, the choice widens considerably. Cyanide, a common chemical, causes symptoms within seconds and death in 5 to 10 min if not treated rapidly. Chlorine and phosgene have no specific antidotes but can require intensive care for weeks to months. Many believe these agents or one of the industrial HAZMATs will be the likely choice of terrorists.

Many mistakenly believe that chemical attacks will always be so

severe that little can be done except to bury the dead. History proves the opposite. Even in WWI, when intravenous fluids, endotracheal tubes, and antibiotics were unavailable, the mortality rate in U.S. forces on the battlefield from chemical warfare agents, chiefly sulfur mustard and the pulmonary intoxicants, was only 1.9%. This was far less than the mortality rate from conventional wounds (7%). In the 1995 Tokyo subway sarin incident, of the 5500 patients who sought medical attention at hospitals, 80% of whom were not actually symptomatic, only 12 died. Thus, it is prudent to attempt to understand the pathophysiology of the syndromes that these agents cause, with a view to treating all patients who present for care expeditiously and with an expectation of saving the vast majority. As we prepare to defend our civilian population from the effects of chemical terrorism, we must also consider that the concept of terrorism can itself produce sequelae in some individuals—physiologic and/or psychological effects that may resemble the effects of nonlethal exposures to CWAs. These effects are due to a general fear of chemicals, fear of decontamination, fear of protective ensemble, or other phobic reactions.

There may be difficulty in differentiating between stress reactions and nerve agent–induced organic brain syndromes. Knowledge of the behavioral effects of CWAs and their medical countermeasures is imperative in order to ensure that military and civilian medical and mental health organizations can deal with possible incidents involving weapons of mass destruction.

The agents of chemical terrorism together with their North Atlantic Treaty Organization (NATO) codes, their unique characteristics, and initial effects are summarized in Table 206-1. An outline of the approaches to decontamination and treatment of the agents of chemical terrorism is shown in Table 206-2. This chapter will restrict its discussion to vesicants and nerve agents, which are considered as a priority based on threat assessments and prior experiences in chemical warfare. For a more comprehensive listing and discussion of agents of

Agent	Agent Name	Unique Characteristics	Initial Effects
Nerve	Cyclohexyl sarin (GF) Sarin (GB) Soman (GD) Tabun (GA) VX	Miosis (pinpoint pupils) Copious secretions Muscle twitching/fasciculations	Miosis (pinpoint pupils) Blurred/dim vision Headache Nausea, vomiting, diarrhea Copious secretions/sweating Muscle twitching/fasciculations Breathing difficulty Seizures
Asphyxiant/blood	Arsine Cyanogen chloride Hydrogen cyanide	Possible cherry red skin Possible cyanosis Possible frostbite[a]	Confusion Nausea Patients may gasp for air, similar to asphyxiation but more abrupt onset Seizures prior to death
Choking/pulmonary-damaging	Chlorine Hydrogen chloride Nitrogen oxides Phosgene	Chlorine is a greenish-yellow gas with pungent odor Phosgene gas smells like newly mown hay or grass Possible frostbite[a]	Eye and skin irritation Airway irritation Dyspnea, cough Sore throat Chest tightness
Blistering/vesicant	Mustard/Sulfur mustard (HD, H) Mustard gas (H) Nitrogen mustard (HN-1, HN-2, HN-3) Lewisite (L) Phosgene oxime (CX)	Mustard (HD) has an odor like burning garlic or horseradish Lewisite (L) has an odor like penetrating geranium Phosgene oxime (CX) has a pepperish or pungent odor	Severe irritation Redness and blisters of the skin Tearing, conjunctivitis, corneal damage Mild respiratory distress to marked airway damage May cause death
Incapacitating/behavior-altering	Agent 15/BZ	May appear as mass drug intoxication with erratic behaviors, shared realistic and distinct hallucinations, disrobing and confusion Hyperthermia Mydriasis (dilated pupils)	Dry mouth and skin Initial tachycardia Altered consciousness, delusions, denial of illness, belligerence Hyperthermia Ataxia (lack of coordination) Hallucinations Mydriasis (dilated pupils)

[a] Frostbite may occur from skin contact with liquid arsine, cyanogen chloride, or phosgene.

Source: State of New York, Department of Health.

chemical terrorism, the reader is referred to Tables 206-1 and 206-2 as well as to the Centers for Disease Control and Prevention website at http://www.bt.cdc.gov/agent/agentlistchem.asp. Also, the antidote recommendations for exposure to cyanide are given in Table 206-3.

VESICANTS

SULFUR MUSTARD, NITROGEN MUSTARD, LEWISITE Sulfur mustard has been a military threat since it first appeared on the battlefield in Belgium during WWI. In modern times it remains a threat on the battlefield as well as a potential terrorist threat because of simplicity of manufacture and extreme effectiveness. Sulfur mustard accounted for 70% of the 1.3 million chemical casualties in WWI. Only sulfur mustard will be discussed here due to space constraints and because it is the prototypical vesicant or blistering agent (Table 206-1).

Mechanism Sulfur mustard constitutes both a vapor and a liquid threat to all exposed epithelial surfaces. Mustard's effects are delayed, appearing hours after exposure. Organs most commonly affected are the skin (with erythema and vesicles), eyes (ranging from mild conjunctivitis to severe eye damage), and airways (ranging from mild upper airway irritation, to severe bronchiolar damage). Following exposure to large quantities of mustard, precursor cells of the bone marrow are damaged, leading to pancytopenia and secondary infection. The gastrointestinal mucosa may be damaged, and there are sometimes central nervous system (CNS) signs of unknown mechanism. No specific antidotes exist; management is entirely supportive.

Mustard dissolves slowly in aqueous media, such as sweat, but once dissolved, it rapidly forms extremely reactive cyclic ethylene sulfonium ions, which reacts with cell proteins, cell membranes, and especially DNA in rapidly dividing cells. Mustard's ability to react with and alkylate DNA gives rise to the effects by which it has been characterized as "radiomimetic," similar to radiation injury. Mustard has many biological actions, but their actual mechanism of action is largely unknown. Much of the biological damage from mustard results from DNA alkylation and cross-linking in rapidly dividing cells: cor-

neal epithelium, basal keratinocytes, bronchial mucosal epithelium, gastrointestinal mucosal epithelium, and bone marrow precursor cells. This may lead to cellular death and inflammatory reactions. In the skin, proteolytic digestion of anchoring filaments at the epidermal-dermal junction may be the major mechanism of action resulting in blister formation. Mustard also possesses mild cholinergic activity, which may be responsible for effects such as early gastrointestinal and CNS symptoms.

Mustard reacts with tissue within minutes of entering the body. Its circulating half-life in unaltered form is extremely brief.

Clinical Features Topical effects of mustard occur in the skin, airways, and eyes, with the latter being most sensitive, followed by the airways. Absorbed mustard may produce effects in the bone marrow, gastrointestinal tract, and CNS. Direct injury to the gastrointestinal tract may also occur following ingestion of the compound through contamination of water or food.

Erythema is the mildest and earliest form of mustard skin injury (Table 206-1). It resembles sunburn and is associated with pruritus, burning, or stinging pain. Erythema begins to appear within 2 h to 2 days after vapor exposure. Time of onset depends on the severity of exposure, ambient temperature and humidity, and type of skin. The most sensitive sites are the warm moist locations and thin delicate skin, such as the perineum, external genitalia, axillae, antecubital fossae, and neck.

Within the erythematous areas, small vesicles can develop, which may later coalesce to form bullae. The typical bulla is large, dome-shaped, flaccid, thin-walled, translucent, and surrounded by erythema. The blister fluid, a transudate, is clear to straw-colored, which becomes yellow, tending to coagulate. The fluid does not contain mustard and is not itself a vesicant. Lesions from high-dose liquid exposure may develop a central zone of coagulation necrosis with blister formation at the periphery. These lesions take longer to heal and are more prone to secondary infection than the uncomplicated lesions seen at lower exposure levels. Severe lesions may require skin grafting.

TABLE 206-2 *Decontamination and Treatment of Chemical Terrorism*

Agent	Decontamination	First Aid	Other Patient Considerations
Nerve	Remove clothing immediately Gently wash skin with soap and water Do not abrade skin For eyes, flush with plenty of water or normal saline	Atropine before other measures Pralidoxime (2-PAM) chloride	Onset of symptoms from dermal contact with liquid forms may be delayed Repeated antidote administration may be necessary
Asphyxiant/blood	Remove clothing immediately if no frostbite* Gently wash skin with soap and water Do not abrade skin For eyes, flush with plenty of water or normal saline	Rapid treatment with oxygen For cyanide, use antidotes (sodium nitrate and then sodium thiosulfate)	Arsine and cyanogen chloride may cause delayed pulmonary edema
Choking/pulmonary-damaging	Remove clothing immediately if no frostbite* Gently wash skin with soap and water Do not abrade skin For eyes, flush with plenty of water or normal saline	Fresh air, forced rest Semi-upright position If signs of respiratory distress are present, oxygen with or without positive airway pressure may be needed Other supportive therapy, as needed	May cause delayed pulmonary edema, even following a symptom-free period that varies in duration with the amount inhaled
Blistering/vesicant	Immediate decontamination is essential to minimize damage Remove clothing immediately Gently wash skin with soap and water Do not abrade skin For eyes, flush with plenty of water or normal saline	Immediately decontaminate skin Flush eyes with water or normal saline for 10–15 minutes If breathing difficulty, give oxygen Supportive care	Mustard has an asymptomatic latent period There is no antidote or treatment for mustard Lewisite has immediate burning pain, blisters later Specific antidote British Anti-Lewisite (BAL) may decrease systemic effects of Lewisite Phosgene oxime causes immediate pain Possible pulmonary edema
Incapacitating/behavior-altering	Remove clothing immediately Gently wash skin with water or soap and water Do not abrade skin	Remove heavy clothing Evaluate mental status Use restraints as needed Monitor core temperature carefully Supportive care	Hyperthermia and self-injury are largest risks Hard to detect because it is an odorless and non-irritating substance Possible serious arrhythmias Specific antidote (physostigmine) may be available

a For frostbite areas, do NOT remove any adhering clothing. Wash area with plenty of warm water to release clothing.
Source: State of New York, Department of Health.

The primary airway lesion is necrosis of the mucosa with possible damage to underlying smooth muscle. The damage begins in the upper airways and descends to the lower airways in a dose-dependent manner. Usually, the terminal airways and alveoli are affected only as a terminal event. Pulmonary edema is not usually present unless the damage is very severe; in this case, it often becomes hemorrhagic.

The earliest effects from mustard, perhaps the only effects from a low concentration, involve the nose, sinuses, and pharynx. There may be irritation or burning of the nares, epistaxis, sinus pain, and pharyngeal pain. As the concentration increases, laryngitis, voice changes, and nonproductive cough develop. Damage to the trachea and upper bronchi leads to a productive cough. Lower airway involvement causes dyspnea, severe cough, and increasing quantities of sputum. Terminally, there may be necrosis of the smaller airways with hemorrhagic edema into the surrounding alveoli. Hemorrhagic pulmonary edema is rare.

Necrosis of airway mucosa causes "pseudomembrane" formation. These membranes may cause obstruction of the bronchi. During WWI, high-dose mustard exposure caused acute death via this mechanism in a small minority of cases.

The eyes are the organs most sensitive to mustard vapor injury. The latent period is shorter for eye injury than for skin injury and is also exposure concentration–dependent. After low-dose vapor exposure, irritation evidenced by reddening of the eyes may be the only effect. As the dose increases, the injury includes progressively more severe conjunctivitis, photophobia, blepharospasm, pain, and corneal damage (Fig. 206-1).

Ninety percent of eye casualties heal in 2 weeks to 2 months without sequelae. Scarring between the iris and lens may follow severe effects; this scarring may restrict pupillary movements and may predispose victims to glaucoma. The most severe damage is caused by liquid mustard. After extensive eye exposure, severe corneal damage with possible perforation of the cornea and loss of the eye can occur. In some individuals, chronic eye irritation, sometimes associated with corneal ulcerations, has been described 10 to 20 years after exposure.

The mucosa of the gastrointestinal tract is susceptible to mustard damage, either from systemic absorption or ingestion of the agent. Mustard exposure in small amounts will cause nausea and possible vomiting lasting up to 24 h. The mechanism of the nausea and vomiting is not understood, but mustard does have a cholinergic-like effect. The CNS effects of mustard, likewise, remain poorly defined. Large exposures can cause seizures in animals. Reports from WWI and Iran described the behavior of persons exposed to small amounts of mustard as sluggish, apathetic, and lethargic. These reports suggest that minor psychological problems could linger for a year or longer.

The causes of death in the majority of mustard poisoning cases are sepsis and respiratory failure. Mechanical obstruction via pseudomembrane formation and agent-induced laryngospasm is important in the first 24 h, but only in cases of severe exposure. From the third through the fifth day after exposure, a secondary bacterial pneumonia can be expected due to invasion of denuded necrotic mucosa. The third wave of death is caused by agent-induced bone marrow suppression, which peaks 7 to 21 days after exposure and causes death via sepsis.

℞ TREATMENT

A patient severely ill from mustard poisoning requires the general supportive care provided for any severely ill patient as well as the specific care given to a burn patient. Liberal use of systemic analgesics, maintenance of fluid and electrolyte balance and nutrition, use of appropriate antibiotics, and other supportive measures are necessary (Table 206-2).

The management of a patient exposed to mustard may range from simple, as in the provision of symptomatic care for a sunburn-like erythema, to complex, as in the provision of total management for a severely ill patient with burns, immunosuppression, and multisystem involvement. Before raw denuded areas of skin develop, especially with less severe exposures, topical cortisone creams or lotions may be of benefit. Some very basic research data point to the early use of anti-inflammatory preparations. Small blisters (<1 to 2 cm) should be left intact. Because larger bullae will eventually break, they should be carefully unroofed. Denuded areas should be irrigated three to four times daily with saline, other sterile solutions, or soapy water and then liberally covered with the topical antibiotic of choice, such as silver sulfadiazine or

TABLE 206-3 *Antidote Recommendations Following Exposure to Cyanide*

Patient	Mild (Conscious)	Severe (Unconscious)	Other Treatment
Child	If patient is conscious and has no other signs or symptoms, antidotes may not be necessary.	Sodium nitrate[a]: 0.12–0.33 mL/kg, not to exceed 10 mL of 3% solution[b] slow IV over no less than 5 min, or slower if hypotension develops *and* Sodium thiosulfate: 1.65 mL/kg of 25% solution IV over 10–20 min	For sodium nitrite–induced orthostatic hypotension, normal saline infusion and supine position are recommended. If still apneic after antidote administration, consider sodium bicarbonate for severe acidosis.
Adult	If patient is conscious and has no other signs or symptoms, antidotes may not be necessary.	Sodium nitrite[a]: 10–20 mL of 3% solution[b] slow IV over no less than 5 min, or slower if hypotension develops *and* Sodium thiosulfate: 50 mL of 25% solution IV over 10–20 min	

[a] If sodium nitrite is unavailable, administer amyl nitrite by inhalation from crushable ampules.
[b] Available in Pasadena Cyanide Antidote Kit, formerly Lilly Cyanide Kit.
Note: Victims whose clothing or skin is contaminated with hydrogen cyanide liquid or solution can secondarily contaminate response personnel by direct contact or through off-gassing vapors. Avoid dermal contact with cyanide-contaminated victims or with gastric contents of victims who may have ingested cyanide-containing materials. Victims exposed only to hydrogen cyanide gas do not pose contamination risks to rescuers. *If the patient is a victim of recent smoke inhalation (may have high carboxyhemoglobin levels), administer only sodium thiosulfate.*
Source: State of New York, Department of Health.

mafenide acetate, to a thickness of 1 to 2 mm. Some advocate sterile needle drainage of large blisters, collapsing the blister roof to form a sterile dressing. Mustard blister fluid does not contain sulfur mustard, only sterile tissue fluid. Health care staff should not fear possible contamination. If an antibiotic cream is not available, sterile petrolatum is useful. Modified Dakins solution (sodium hypochlorite 0.5%) was used both in WWI and in Iranian casualties (1984–1987) for field-expedient irrigation and antisepsis. Large areas of vesication require hospitalization, intravenous therapy, and whirlpool bath irrigation.

Systemic analgesics should be used liberally, particularly before manipulation of the patient. Monitoring of fluids and electrolytes is important in any sick patient, but it must be recognized that fluid loss is usually not of the magnitude seen with thermal burns. This may be because mustard burns, in general, are more superficial than thermal burns (no definitive data exist to support this supposition). Overly rigorous hydration seems to have precipitated pulmonary edema in a few Iranian casualties sent to European hospitals.

Conjunctival irritation from a low vapor exposure will respond to any of a number of available ophthalmic solutions after the eyes are thoroughly irrigated. A topical antibiotic applied several times a day will reduce the incidence and severity of infection. Animal laboratory data have shown remarkable results with commercially available topical antibiotic/glucocorticoid ophthalmologic ointments applied early. Topical glucocorticoids alone are not of proven value, but their use during the first few hours or days may significantly reduce inflammation and subsequent damage. Further use should be relegated to an ophthalmologist, who should be consulted in any case.

Vaseline or a similar substance should be applied regularly to the edges of the lids to prevent them from sticking together. Although topical analgesics may be useful initially if blepharospasm is too severe to permit an adequate examination, they have limited value.

A productive cough and dyspnea accompanied by fever and leukocytosis occurring within 12 to 24 h is indicative of a chemical pneumonitis. The clinician must resist the urge to use prophylactic antibiotics for this process. Infection often occurs on the third to fifth day and is signaled by an increased fever, pulmonary infiltrate, and an increase in sputum production with a change in color. Initial antibiotic therapy should await evidence of infection from Gram stain of sputum;

regimens can then be changed, if appropriate according to the results of sputum culture and sensitivity.

Intubation may be necessary if laryngeal spasm or edema makes it difficult or becomes life-threatening. Intubation permits better ventilation and facilitates suction of the necrotic and inflammatory debris. Early use of positive end-expiratory pressure (PEEP) or continuous positive airway pressure (CPAP) may be beneficial. Pseudomembrane formation may require fiberoptic bronchoscopy for suctioning of the necrotic debris.

Bronchodilators are of benefit for bronchospasm. If additional relief of bronchospasm is needed, glucocorticoids should be used. There is little evidence that the routine use of glucocorticoids is beneficial, except for additional relief of bronchospasm.

Leukopenia begins around day 3 with major systemic absorption. Marrow suppression peaks at 7 to 14 days. In the Iran-Iraq war, a white blood count of ≤200/μL usually resulted in death of the patient. Sterilization of the gut by nonabsorbable antibiotics should be considered to reduce the possibility of sepsis from enteric organisms. Cellular

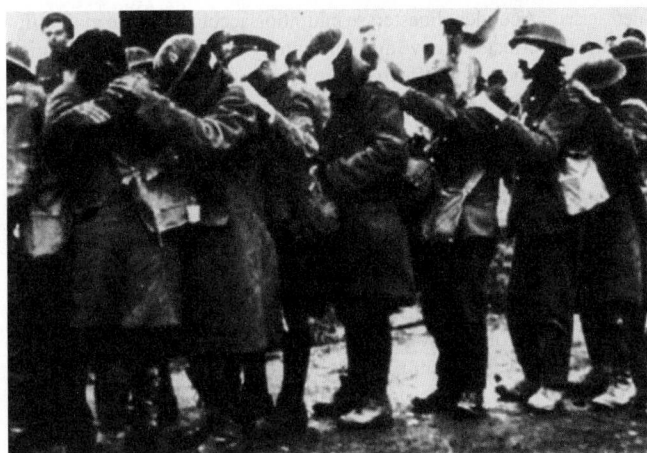

FIGURE 206-1 World War I photograph of troops exposed to sulfur mustard vapor. The vast majority of these troops survived with no long-term damage to the eyes; however, they were effectively rendered blind for days to weeks.

replacement (bone marrow transplants or transfusions) may be successful. In one study, granulocyte colony-stimulating factor produced a 50% reduction in the time for the bone marrow to recover in non-human primates exposed to sulfur mustard and should be considered in the case of human exposure. Medication for nausea and vomiting may be necessary for gastrointestinal side effects.

Excellent assessments of the contributions of DNA alkylation, inflammation, activation of proteolytic enzymes, or lipid peroxidation to the mustard injury have been developed in the past 15 years. Examples include (1) the demonstration up to 75% reduction of inflammation and tissue damage in the mouse ear swelling test by vanilloid compounds, and (2) the demonstration of 50 to 60% protection by *N*-acetylcysteine in the generation of free radicals within guinea pig lung exposed to mustard. In many cases, the demonstration of protection is dependent on the availability of sufficient amounts of drug with adequate half-lives. Strategies to enhance bioavailability include attachment of polyethylene glycol to the antioxidant drug/enzyme or delivery of the drug/enzyme in a liposome (or both).

NERVE AGENTS

The organophosphorus nerve agents are the deadliest of the chemical warfare agents. They work by inhibition of tissue synaptic acetylcholinesterase, creating an acute cholinergic crisis. Death ensues because of respiratory depression and can occur within seconds to minutes (Table 206-1).

The "classic" nerve agents include tabun (GA), sarin (GB), soman (GD), cyclosarin (GF), and VX. VR, similar to VX, was manufactured in the former Soviet Union (Table 206-1). The two-letter codes are a NATO international convention and convey no clinical implications. All of the nerve agents are organophosphorus compounds, which are liquid at standard temperature and pressure. The "G" agents evaporate at about the rate of water, except for GF, which is oily, and thus will probably have evaporated within 24 h after deposition on the ground. Their high volatility thus makes a spill of any amount a serious vapor hazard. In the Tokyo subway attack where sarin was used (see below), 100% of the symptomatic patients inhaled sarin vapor that spilled out on the floor of the subway cars. VX, an oily liquid, is the exception. Its low vapor pressure makes it much less of a vapor hazard but potentially a greater environmental hazard because it persists in the environment far longer.

The nerve agents tabun and sarin were first used on the battlefield by Iraq against Iran during the first Persian Gulf war, 1984–1987. Estimates of casualties from these agents range from 20,000 to 100,000. In 1994 and 1995, the Japanese cult Aum Shinrikyo used sarin in two terrorist attacks in Matsumoto and Tokyo.

Mechanism   Acetylcholinesterase inhibition accounts for the major life-threatening effects of nerve agent poisoning. Reversal of this inhibition by antidotal therapy is effective, proving that this is the primary toxic action of these poisons. At cholinergic synapses, acetylcholinesterase, bound to the postsynaptic membrane, functions as a turn-off switch to regulate cholinergic transmission. Inhibition of acetylcholinesterases causes the released neurotransmitter, acetylcholine, to accumulate abnormally. End-organ overstimulation, recognized by clinicians as cholinergic crisis, ensues (Fig. 206-2).

Clinical Features   Clinical effects of nerve agent exposure are identical for vapor and liquid exposure routes if the dose is sufficiently large. The speed and order of symptom onset will differ (Table 206-1).

Exposure of a patient to nerve agent vapor, overwhelmingly the more likely route of exposure in both battlefield and terrorist scenarios, will cause cholinergic symptoms in the order that the toxin encounters cholinergic synapses. The most exposed synapses on the integument of the human are in the pupillary muscles. Nerve agent vapor easily crosses the cornea, interacts with these synapses, and produces miosis, described by Tokyo subway victims as "the world going black." Rarely, this can also cause eye pain and nausea. Exocrine glands lo-

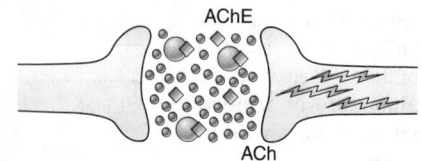

FIGURE 206-2   Schematic diagram of the pathophysiology of nerve agent exposure. Nerve agent (◇) binds to the active site of acetylcholinesterase (AChE), which is shown as floating free in space but is in reality a postsynaptic membrane-bound enzyme. As a result, acetylcholine (●), which is normally released from presynaptic membrane but not normally degraded, accumulates, and this leads (⚡) to organ overstimulation and cholinergic crisis.

cated in the nose, mouth, and pharynx next become exposed to the vapor, and cholinergic overload here causes increased secretions, rhinorrhea, excess salivation, and drooling. Next, toxin interacts with exocrine glands in the upper airway, causing bronchorrhea, and with bronchial smooth muscle, causing bronchospasm, the combination of which can cause hypoxia.

Once the victim has inhaled, vapor can passively cross the alveolar-capillary membrane, enter the bloodstream, and, incidentally and asymptomatically, inhibit circulating cholinesterases, particularly free butyrylcholinesterase and erythrocyte acetylcholinesterase, both of which can be assayed. Unfortunately, the assay may not be easily interpreted without a baseline, since cholinesterase levels vary enormously between persons and over time in an individual healthy patient.

Usually the first organ system to become symptomatic from blood-borne nerve agent exposure is the gastrointestinal tract, where cholinergic overload causes abdominal cramping and pain, nausea, vomiting, and diarrhea. After the gastrointestinal tract is involved, nerve agents affect the heart, distant exocrine glands, muscles, and brain. Because there are cholinergic synapses on both the vagal (parasympathetic) and sympathetic sides of the autonomic input to the heart, one cannot predict how heart rate and blood pressure will change. Remote exocrine activity will include oversecretion in the salivary, nasal, respiratory, and sweat glands—the patient will be "wet all over." Bloodborne nerve agents overstimulate neuromuscular junctions in skeletal muscles, causing fasciculations followed by frank twitching. If the process goes on long enough, ATP in muscle will eventually be depleted and flaccid paralysis will ensue, although this is never the first sign.

In the brain, since the cholinergic system is so widely distributed, bloodborne nerve agents, in sufficient doses, cause rapid loss of consciousness, seizures, and central apnea, leading to death within minutes. If respiration is supported, status epilepticus, which does not respond to usual anticonvulsants, may ensue (Chap. 349). If status persists, neuronal death and permanent brain dysfunction may occur. Even in mild nerve agent intoxication, patients may recover but experience weeks of irritability, sleep disturbance, and nonspecific neurobehavioral symptoms.

The time from exposure to development of the full-blown cholinergic crisis from nerve agent vapor inhalation can be minutes or even seconds; however, there is no depot effect. Since nerve agents have a short circulating half-life, improvement should be rapid with no subsequent deterioration if the patient is supported and, ideally, treated with antidotes.

Liquid exposure to nerve agents differs in speed and order of symptom onset. A nerve agent on intact skin will partially evaporate and partially begin to travel through the skin, causing localized sweating and then localized fasciculations when it encounters neuromuscular junctions. Once in muscle, it will cross into the circulation and cause gastrointestinal discomfort, respiratory distress, heart rate changes, generalized fasciculations and twitching, loss of consciousness, seizures, and central apnea. The time course will be much longer than with vapor inhalation; even a large, lethal droplet can take up to 30 min to have effect, and a small, sublethal dose could continue to take effect over 18 h. Clinical worsening that occurs hours after treatment has started is far more likely with liquid than with vapor exposure.

Additionally, miosis, practically unavoidable with vapor exposure, is not always present with liquid exposure and may be the last symptom to present in this situation. This is due to the relative insulation of the pupillary muscle from the systemic circulation.

Unless a nerve agent is removed by specific therapy (oximes), its binding to cholinesterase is essentially irreversible. Erythrocyte acetylcholinesterase activity recovers at about 1% per day. Plasma butyrylcholinesterase recovers more quickly and is a better guide to recovery of tissue enzyme activity.

℞ TREATMENT

Acute nerve agent poisoning is treated by decontamination, respiratory support, and three antidotes—an anticholinergic, an oxime, and an anticonvulsant (Tables 206-2 and 206-4). In acute cases, all of these forms of therapy may be given simultaneously.

Decontamination Decontamination of a vapor is theoretically not necessary, but in the Tokyo subway attack, sarin vapor trapped in the patients' clothing caused miosis in 10% of emergency personnel. Removal of clothing would have avoided most of this. Decontamination of liquid is accomplished in the military using the M291 skin decontamination kit, containing an active carbon impregnated with ion exchange resins (Ambergard) capable of absorbing liquid off the skin. Civilian agencies now stockpile this product, which is approved by the U.S. Food and Drug Administration (FDA). At hospitals, soap and copious amounts of water should suffice. Physical removal of the agent trumps all known decontamination solutions and lotions. In any even, decontamination must be accomplished before the patient enters the hospital facility to avoid contaminating the facility and its staff. In patients with contaminated wounds, extract from the wound potentially contaminated clothing and other foreign material that may serve as a depot for liquid agent.

Respiratory Support Death from nerve agent poisoning is almost always respiratory. Ventilation will be complicated by increased resistance and secretions. Atropine should be given before ventilation or as it begins as it will make ventilation far easier.

Antidotal Therapy ■ *ATROPINE* In theory, any anticholinergic could be used to treat nerve agent poisoning, but worldwide the choice is invariably atropine because of its wide temperature stability and rapid effectiveness, either intramuscularly or intravenously, and because inadvertent administration of this drug usually causes little CNS dysfunction (Table 206-4). Atropine rapidly reverses cholinergic overload at muscarinic synapses but has little effect at nicotinic synapses. Practically, this implies that atropine can quickly treat the life-threatening respiratory effects of nerve agents but will probably not help neuromuscular and possibly sympathetic effects. In the field, military personnel are given MARK I kits (Fig. 206-3A), which contain 2 mg atropine in autoinjector form for use intramuscularly. Civilian agencies are now stockpiling this FDA-approved product as well. One can only give full autoinjector doses and not divide them. The field-loading dose is 2, 4, or 6 mg, with retreatment every 5 to 10 min until the patient's breathing and secretions improve. The Iranians used larger doses initially during the Iran-Iraq war, in which oximes were in short supply. When the patient reaches a level of medical care where drugs can be given intravenously, this is the preferred route; in small children, this may be the preferred initial route of administration of atropine therapy. There is no upper bound to atropine therapy in a patient either intra-

muscularly or intravenously; however, a total average adult dose for a severely afflicted patient would usually be 20 to 30 mg.

In a mildly afflicted patient with miosis and no other systemic symptoms, atropine or homatropine eye drops may suffice for therapy. This will produce roughly 24 h of mydriasis. Frank miosis or imperfect accommodation may persist for weeks or even months after all other signs and symptoms have resolved.

TABLE 206-4 *Antidote Recommendations Following Exposure to Nerve Agents*

Patient Age	Antidotes Mild/Moderate Effects[a]	Antidotes Severe Effects[b]	Other Treatment
Infants (0–2 yrs)	Atropine: 0.05 mg/kg IM, or 0.02 mg/kg IV; and 2-PAM chloride: 15 mg/kg IM or IV slowly	Atropine: 0.1 mg/kg IM, or 0.02 mg/kg IV; and 2-PAM chloride: 25 mg/kg IM, or 15 mg/kg IV slowly	Assisted ventilation after antidotes for severe exposure. Repeat atropine (2 mg IM, or 1 mg IM for infants) at 5- to 10-min intervals until secretions have diminished and breathing is comfortable or airway resistance has returned to near normal. Phentolamine for 2-PAM-induced hypertension: (5 mg IV for adults; 1 mg IV for children). Diazepam for convulsions: (0.2 to 0.5 mg IV for infants <5 years: 1 mg IV for children >5 years; 5 mg IV for adults).
Child (2–10 yrs)	Atropine: 1 mg IM, or 0.02 mg/kg IV; and 2-PAM chloride[c]: 15 mg/kg IM or IV slowly	Atropine: 2 mg IM, or 0.02 mg/kg IV; and 2-PAM chloride[c]: 25 mg/kg IM, or 15 mg/kg IV slowly	
Adolescent (>10 yrs)	Atropine: 2 mg IM, or 0.02 mg/kg IV; and 2-PAM chloride[c]: 15 mg/kg IM or IV slowly	Atropine: 4 mg IM, or 0.02 mg/kg IV; and 2-PAM chloride[c]: 25 mg/kg IM, or 15 mg/kg IV slowly	
Adult	Atropine: 2 to 4 mg IM or IV; and 2-PAM chloride: 600 mg IM, or 15 mg/kg IV slowly	Atropine: 6 mg IM; and 2-PAM chloride: 1800 mg IM, or 15 mg/kg IV slowly	
Elderly, frail	Atropine: 1 mg IM; and 2-PAM chloride: 10 mg/kg IM, or 5 to 10 mg/kg IV slowly	Atropine: 2 to 4 mg IM; and 2-PAM chloride: 25 mg/kg IM, or 5 to 10 mg/kg IV slowly	

[a] Mild/moderate effects include localized sweating, muscle fasciculations, nausea, vomiting, weakness, dyspnea.
[b] Severe effects include unconsciousness, convulsions, apnea, flaccid paralysis.
[c] If calculated dose exceeds the adult IM dose, adjust accordingly.
Note: 2-PAM chloride is pralidoxime chloride or protopam chloride.
Source: State of New York, Department of Health.

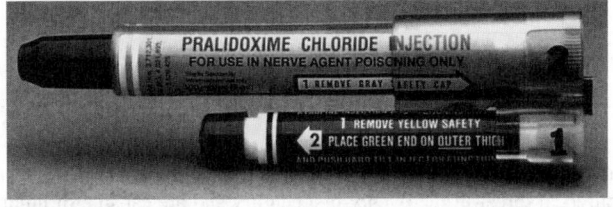

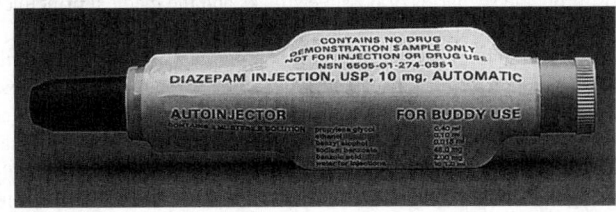

FIGURE 206-3 Antidotes to nerve agents. *A.* MARK I autoinjector set containing one 600-mg dose of 2-pralidoxime chloride and one 2-mg dose of atropine. Such sets are carried by all U.S. military forces in a potentially chemical battlefield and are now being stockpiled by civilian first responders. *B.* Diazepam 10-mg autoinjector. These are carried by all U.S. military forces in a potential chemical battlefield and are being stockpiled by civilian first responders.

OXIME THERAPY   Oximes are nucleophiles that reactivate the cholinesterase whose active site has been occupied and bound to nerve agent (Table 206-4). Therapy with oximes therefore restores normal enzyme function. Oxime therapy is limited by a second side reaction, called *aging*, in which a side chain on nerve agents falls off the complex at a characteristic rate. "Aged" complexes are negatively charged, and oximes cannot reactivate negatively charged complexes. The practical effect of this differs from one nerve agent to another since each ages at a characteristic rate. VX, for practical purposes, never ages, sarin ages in 3 to 5 h, and tabun ages over a longer period. All of these are so much longer than the patient's expected lifespan after untreated acute nerve agent toxicity that they may be ignored. Soman, on the other hand, ages in 2 min. Thus, after only a few minutes following exposure, oximes are useless in treating soman poisoning. The oxime used varies by country; the United States has approved and fielded 2-pralidoxime chloride (2-PAM Cl). MARK I kits (Fig. 206-3*A*) contain autoinjectors of 600 mg of 2-PAM Cl. Initial field loading doses are 600, 1200, or 1800 mg. Since blood pressure elevation may occur after administration of 45 mg/kg in adults, field use of 2-PAM Cl is restricted to 1800 mg, intramuscularly, per hour. During the time when more oxime cannot be given, atropine alone is recommended. In the hospital setting, 2.5 to 25 mg/kg of 2-PAM Cl intravenously has been found to reactive 50% of inhibited cholinesterase. The usual recommendation is 1000 mg through slow intravenous drip over 20 to 30 min, with no more than 2500 mg over a period of 1 to 1.5 h.

ANTICONVULSANT   Nerve agent–induced seizures do not respond to the usual anticonvulsants used for status epilepticus, including phenytoin, phenobarbital, carbamazepine, valproic acid, and lamotrigine (Chap. 349). The only class of anticonvulsants that has been shown to stop this form of status are the benzodiazepines. Diazepam is the only benzodiazepine approved for seizures in humans, although other FDA-approved benzodiazepines work well against nerve agent–induced seizures in animal models. Diazepam, therefore, is manufactured in 10-mg injectors for intramuscular use and given to U.S. forces for this purpose (Fig. 206-3*B*). Civilian agencies are stockpiling this field product (convulsive antidote for nerve agent, "CANA"), which is not generally used in hospital practice. Extrapolation from animal studies indicates that adults will probably require 30 to 40 mg diazepam, intramuscularly, to stop nerve agent–induced status epilepticus. In the hospital, or in a small child unable to receive the autoinjector, intra-

venous diazepam may be used at similar doses. The clinician may confuse seizures with the neuromuscular signs of nerve agent poisoning. In the hospital, early electroencephalography is recommended in order to distinguish between nonconvulsive status epilepticus, actual seizures, and postictal paralysis. Recent studies have shown that the most effective benzodiazepine in this situation is midazolam, which is not FDA-approved for seizures.

Peripheral neuropathy and the so-called intermediate syndrome, prominent long-term effects of insecticide poisoning, are not described in nerve agent survivors.

Recent research has explored approaches leading to a transient "immunity" or drugs that would provide protection against lethal nerve agents yet be devoid of side effects. A novel approach is to use enzymes to scavenge these highly toxic nerve agents before they attack their intended targets. The total body of studies has shown that if a scavenger is present at the time of nerve agent exposure, rapid reduction of toxicant levels is observed. This reduction is so rapid and profound that the need to administer a host of pharmacologically active drugs as antidotes is, in theory, eliminated.

FURTHER READING

AGENCY FOR TOXIC SUBSTANCES AND DISEASE REGISTRY (ATSDR): Managing Hazardous Materials Incidents, Vols I–III. Atlanta, GA, US Department of Health and Human Services, 2001

BROOMFIELD CA et al: Progress on the road to new nerve agent treatments. J Appl Toxicol 21:S43, 2001

KARALLIEDDE L et al: Possible immediate and long-term health effects following exposure to chemical warfare agents. Public Health 114:238, 2000

SIDELL FR: Clinical considerations in nerve agent intoxication, in *Chemical Warfare Agents*, SM Somani (ed). San Diego, California, Academic Press, 1992, pp 156–194

——— et al (eds): *Medical Aspects of Chemical and Biological Warfare, Vol I of Textbook of Military Medicine*. Washington, DC, Walter Reed Army Medical Center, Borden Institute, 1997. [Available on the website: *http://ccc.apgea.army.mil*]

SMITH WJ: Vesicant agents and antivesicant medical countermeasures: Clinical toxicology and psychological implications. Mil Psychol 14:145, 2002

STATE OF NEW YORK, DEPARTMENT OF HEALTH. *Chemical Terrorism Preparedness and Response Card*, #7002. August, 2002

US ARMY EDGEWOOD RESEARCH, DEVELOPMENT AND ENGINEERING CENTER: Technician EMS Course. Domestic Preparedness Training Program, Version 8.0. Aberdeen Proving Ground, Maryland, 1999

US ARMY MEDICAL RESEARCH INSTITUTE OF CHEMICAL DEFENSE, CHEMICAL CASUALTY CARE DIVISION: *Medical Management of Chemical Casualties Handbook*, 3d ed. Aberdeen Proving Ground, Maryland, 1999. [Available on the website: *http://ccc.apgea.army.mil*]

---

207   RADIATION BIOTERRORISM
Zelig A. Tochner, Ofer Lehavi, Eli Glatstein

Terror attacks using nuclear or radiation-related devices are an unequivocal threat in the twenty-first century and are capable of unique medical and psychological effects. In this chapter we will focus on the most probable scenarios of possible attacks and the medical principles of handling such threats.

There are two major categories of potential terrorist incidents with widespread radiologic consequences. The first is the use of radiologic dispersal devices. This could cause a purposeful dissemination of radioactive material without nuclear detonation by using conventional explosives with radionuclides, attacking fixed nuclear facilities, or attacking nuclear powered surface vessels or submarines. Malfunctioning nuclear weapons that are detonated with no nuclear yield (nuclear "duds") and/or installation of radionuclides in food or water are also a possible means of generating a terror attack. The second, and less probable, scenario is the actual use of nuclear weapons. Each scenario has its own medical aspects, including "conventional" blast or thermal injury, introduction to a radiation field, and exposure to either external or internal contamination from a radioactive explosion.

TYPES OF RADIOISOTOPIC RADIATION

Isotopes of atoms with uneven numbers of protons and/or neutrons are typically unstable; such isotopes discharge particles or energy to matter, a process that we define as *radiation*. The main radiation types are alpha, beta, gamma, and neutrons.

Alpha (α) radiation consists of heavy, positively charged particles containing two protons and two neutrons. Alpha particles are usually emitted from isotopes with an atomic number of ≥ 82, such as uranium or plutonium. Due to their large size, alpha particles have limited penetrating power. Fine obstacles such as cloth or human skin can usually stop them from penetrating into the body, and they represent a small risk to external exposure due to their limited penetration. If they somehow are internalized, then alpha particles can cause significant cellular damage within their immediate proximity.

Beta (β) radiation consists of electrons, which are small, light, negatively charged particles (about 1/2000 the mass of a neutron or proton). They can travel only a short finite distance in tissue, depending on their energy. Exposure to beta particles is common in many radiation accidents. Radioactive iodine, released in nuclear plant accidents, is the best known member of this group. Plastic layers and clothing can stop most beta particles, and their penetration is measured to be a few millimeters. A large quantum of energy to the basal stratum of the skin can cause a burn that is similar to a thermal burn and is treated as such.

Gamma (γ) rays and *x-rays* (both photons) are similar. Gamma rays are uncharged electromagnetic radiation discharged from a nucleus as a wave or photons of energy. X-rays are the result of abrupt mechanical deceleration of electrons striking a heavy target such as tungsten. Gamma and x-rays have similar properties, i.e., no charge and no mass, just energy. Both travel easily through matter, sometimes called *penetrating radiation*, and are the principal type of radiation to cause total-body exposure.

Neutrons (η) particles are heavy and uncharged, often emitted during nuclear detonation. They possess a wide energy range; their ability to penetrate tissues is variable, depending upon their energy. They are less likely to be present in most scenarios of radiation bioterrorism.

The ionization resulting from protons, electrons, and gamma rays is either a direct or indirect (i.e., mediated through water) effect of particles or photons on DNA. Ionization of DNA resulting from neutrons is secondary to the neutrons knocking electrons out of their atomic orbit and the formation of free radicals, which can also damage DNA directly.

The commonly used units of radiation are the rad and the gray (Gy). The rad (radiation absorbed dose) is energy deposited within living matter and is equal to 100 ergs/g of tissue. It is a simple concept but difficult to measure directly. The traditional rad has been replaced by the Système Internationale (SI) unit of the gray; 100 rad = 1 Gy.

TYPES OF EXPOSURE

Whole-body exposure represents deposition of radiation energy over the entire body. Alpha and beta particles have limited penetration and do not cause significant noncutaneous injury unless emission results from an internalized source. Whole-body exposure from gamma rays, x-rays, or neutrons, which can penetrate through the body (depending on their energy), can result in damage to multiple tissues and organs. The tissue damage is proportional to the radiation exposure of that organ or tissue.

External contamination is a result of fallout of radioactive particles that land on the body surface, clothing, skin, and hair. This is the dominant element to consider in the mass casualty situation resulting from a radioactive terrorist strike. The common contaminants will primarily emit alpha and beta radiation. Alpha particles do not penetrate beyond the skin and thus have minimal systemic effects. Beta emitters can cause significant cutaneous burns and scarring. Gamma emitters may not only cause local damage but can also cause whole-body radiation exposures and injury. The medical treatment is primarily decontamination of the body, including wounds and burns, to prevent the contamination from becoming internalized. Removing the contaminated clothing reduces the contamination significantly and is a first step in the decontamination process. Generally patients will not constitute a significant radiation hazard to health care providers, and life-saving treatment should not be delayed for fear of secondary contamination of the medical team. Any damage to health care personnel will depend directly on the duration of exposure and will be inversely proportional to the square of the distance from any radioactive source. Gowns that can be removed are essential to protect health-care personnel.

Internal contamination will occur when radioactive material is inhaled, ingested, or able to enter the body through open wounds or burns or via skin absorption. In principle, any externally contaminated casualty should be evaluated for internal contamination. Some isotopes may have toxic effects on specific target organs due to their chemical properties, in addition to radiologic injury. The respiratory system is the main portal of entrance for internal contamination, and the lung is the organ at greatest risk. Aerosol particles <5 μm can reach the alveoli, whereas larger particles will remain in proximal airways. The tiny particles can be absorbed by the lymphatic system or the bloodstream, continuing to irradiate (depending on their biologically active half-life) until being exhaled. Bronchial lavage is often helpful treat-

ment in this situation. Radioactive material entering the gastrointestinal (GI) tract will be absorbed according to its chemical structure and solubility. The insoluble radionuclides may affect the lower GI tract. Intact skin is normally a good barrier to most radionuclides. Penetration through the skin usually takes place when wounds or burns have altered the skin barriers. Therefore, any skin erosion should be cleaned and decontaminated promptly.

Absorbed radioactive materials will travel throughout the body. Liver, kidney, adipose tissue, and bone tend to bind and retain the radioactive material more than other tissues. The medical treatment includes preventing absorption, reducing incorporation, and enhancing elimination (see below).

Localized exposure means close contact between a highly radioactive source and a part of the body, causing discrete damage to the skin and deeper tissues, similar to a thermal burn. Later signs include epilation, erythema, moist desquamation, ulceration, blistering, or necrosis in proportion to exposure. Alopecia, transient or permanent, is dose-related and starts at cutaneous doses >3 Gy. Overt tissue damage can take weeks and even months to develop; the healing process can also be very slow and last for months. Long-term cutaneous changes, including keratosis, fibrosis, and telangiectasias, may appear years after the exposure. Treatment is based on analgesia and infection prophylaxis. Nevertheless, severe burns can often require grafting or even amputation. Long-term radiation effects are characterized by cell loss and cell death.

RADIOLOGIC DISPERSAL EVENTS

Radiologic dispersal incidents are generally of two types resulting from: (1) small, usually localized sources; or (2) wide dispersals over large areas. The radioactive materials can take the form of solid state, aerosol, gas, or liquid. They can be put into food or water, released from vehicles, or be spread by explosion. The principal route of exposure is usually by direct contact between the victim's skin and the radioactive particles, although internal contamination could occur if the material were inhaled or ingested. The radiation field is also a potential source of whole-body exposure. The psychosocial effects that accompany such an event are significant and are beyond the scope of this chapter. A list of radioactive materials, including information on their major properties and medical treatment, is shown in Table 207-1.

In a localized event, the amount and spread of the radioactive materials are usually limited and can be treated like a spill of hazardous material. Protective clothing prevents or minimizes the contamination of emergency responders.

The use of explosives coupled with a large amount of radioactive materials can result in wide dispersion of radiation, which is of far greater concern. Other potential sources of radiation are nuclear reactors, spent nuclear fuel, and transport vehicles. Less probable but still possible is the use of a large source of penetrating radiation without explosion. It is expected that most exposures would be low, and the principal health and psychosocial effects would be similar to the former scenario but on a larger scale.

Whenever an explosion is involved, conventional life-saving treatment should be given first priority. Only then should decontamination and specific treatment be given for the radiation exposure.

Silent exposure represents a scenario in which a powerful radiologic source could be hidden in a crowded place or radiologic materials spread without any awareness or announcement. It might take a long time to recognize the event and the source of exposure. One of the major clues to this situation is the appearance of unusual clinical manifestations in many individuals; such manifestations are often nonspecific and include symptoms of acute radiation sickness (see below) such as headache, fatigue, malaise, and opportunistic infections. GI phenomena such as diarrhea, nausea, vomiting, and anorexia may occur. Dermatologic symptoms (burns, ulceration, and epilation) and hematopoietic manifestations such as bleeding tendency, thrombocy-

Isotope Name	Symbol	Common Usage	Radiation Type $t_{1/2}$ Radiologic $t_{1/2}$ Biologic, days	Exposure Type	Mode of Contamination	Focal Accumulation in Body	Treatment
Manganese	Mn-56	Reactors, research laboratories	β, γ 2.6 h 5.7	External, internal	N/A	Liver	N/A
Cobalt	Co-60	Medical radiotherapy devices, commercial food irradiators	β, γ 5.26 y 9.5	External, internal	Lungs	Liver	Gastric lavage, purgatives; penicillamine in severe cases
Strontium	Sr-90	Fission product of uranium	β 28 y 18,000	Internal	Moderate GI tract	Bones—similar to calcium	Strontium, calcium, ammonium chloride
Molybdenum	Mo-99	Hospitals—scans	β, γ 66.7 h 3	External, internal	N/A	Kidneys	N/A
Technetium	Tc-99m	Hospitals—scans	β, γ 6.049 h 1	External, internal	IV administration	Kidneys, total body	Potassium perchlorate to reduce thyroid dose
Cesium	Cs-137	Medical radiotherapy devices	β, γ 30 y 70	External, internal	Lungs, GI tract, wounds, follows potassium	Renal excretion	Ion-exchange resins, Prussian blue
Gadolinium	Gd-153	Hospitals	β, γ 242 d 1000	External, internal	N/A	N/A	N/A
Iridium	Ir-192	Commercial radiography	β, γ 74 d 50	External, internal	N/A	Spleen	N/A
Radium	Ra-226	Instrument illumination, industrial applications, old medical equipment, former Soviet Union military equipment	α, β, γ 1602 y 16,400	External, internal	GI tract	Bones	$MgSO_4$ lavage, ammonium chloride, calcium alginates
Tritium	H-3	Luminescent gun sights, muzzle-velocity detectors, nuclear weapons	β 12.5 y 12	Internal	Inhalation, GI tract, wounds	Total body	Dilution with controlled water intake, diuretics
Iodine	I-131	Reactor accidents, thyroid ablators	β, γ 8.1 d 138	Internal	Inhalation, GI tract, wounds	Thyroid	Potassium/sodium iodide, propylthiouracil, methimazole
Uranium	U-235	Depleted uranium, natural uranium, fuel rods, weapons-grade material	α, (α, β, γ) 7.1×10^8 y 15	Internal	GI tract	Kidneys, bones	$NaHCO_3$, chelation with EDTA
Plutonium	Pu-239	Produced from uranium in reactors, nuclear weapons	α 2.2×10^4 y 73,000	Internal	Limited lung absorption, high retention	Lungs, bones, bone marrow, liver, gonads	Chelating with DTPA or EDTA
Americium	Am-241	Smoke detectors, nuclear weapon detonation fallout	α 458 y 73,000	Internal	Inhalation, skin wounds	Lungs, liver, bones, bone marrow	Chelating with DTPA or EDTA
Polonium	Po-210	Calibration source	α 138.4 d 60	Internal	Inhalation, wounds	Spleen, kidneys	Lavage, dimercaprol
Thallium	Th-232	Calibration source	α 1.41×10^{10} y 73,000	Internal	N/A	N/A	N/A
Phosphorus	P-32	Research laboratories, medical facilities	β 14.3 d 1155	Internal	Inhalation, GI tract, wounds	Bones, bone marrow, rapidly replicating cells	Lavage, aluminum hydroxide, phosphate

Note: N/A, not available; h, hours; y, years; GI, gastrointestinal

topenia, purpura, lymphopenia, or neutropenia are also possible and dose-related. Careful epidemiologic studies may be necessary to identify the source of such exposure.

NUCLEAR WEAPONS

The most likely scenario of nuclear terror would be the detonation of a single low-yield device. The estimated yield of such device is anywhere between 0.01 and 10 kiloton of TNT, although the probability would more likely be toward the lower yield. Coping with such an event is certainly possible. The effects of such an explosion are a combination of several components: ground shock, air blast, thermal radiation, initial nuclear radiation, residual nuclear radiation, crater formation, and radioactive fallout.

The nuclear detonation, like a conventional explosion, will produce a shock wave that can further damage structures and cause many casualties. In addition, the detonation can produce an extremely hot fireball that can ignite materials and cause severe burns. The detonation also releases an intense pulse of ionizing radiation, mainly gamma rays and neutrons. The radiation produced in the first minute is termed *initial radiation*, while the ongoing radiation due to fallout is termed *residual radiation*. Both types of radiation can cause acute radiation sickness (ARS; see below). The LD$_{50/30}$ (i.e., a dose that causes 50% mortality at 30 days) is ~4 Gy for whole-body exposure without medical support; with medical support, the LD$_{50/30}$ ranges between 8 and 10 Gy. Winds can carry fallout and contaminate large areas.

On top of its effects, a massive blast forms a crater in the soil and usually produces a ground shock compounding the damage and number of casualties. Inhalation of large amounts of radioactive dust causes pneumonitis that can lead to pulmonary fibrosis. Use of a mask covering the mouth and nose can be very helpful. The intense flash of infrared and visible light can cause either temporary or permanent blindness. Cataracts can develop months to years later among those who survive.

ACUTE RADIATION SICKNESS

Radiation interactions with atoms can result in ionization and the formation of free radicals that damage tissue by disrupting chemical bonds and molecular structures in the cell, including DNA. Radiation damage can lead to cell death; those cells that recover may be mutated and at higher risk for subsequent cancer. Cell sensitivity increases as the replication rate increases and the cell differentiation decreases. Bone marrow and mucosal surfaces of the GI tract, which have vast mitotic activity, are significantly more sensitive to radiation than slowly dividing tissues such as bones and muscles. Following exposure of either all or most of the human body to ionizing radiation, ARS can develop. The clinical manifestations of ARS reflect the dose and type of radiation as well as the part of the body exposed.

CLINICAL MANIFESTATIONS　ARS manifests as three major groups of signs and symptoms: gastrointestinal, hematopoietic, and neurovascular. There are four major stages in ARS: prodrome, latent phase, illness, and either recovery or death. The higher the radiation doses, the shorter and more severe each stage. The prodrome appears a few hours to 4 days postexposure; lasts between a few hours to a few days; and can include nausea, vomiting, anorexia, and diarrhea. At the end of the prodrome, ARS progresses to the latent phase. Minimal or no symptoms are present during the latent phase, which commonly lasts up to 2.5 weeks, but can last up to 6 weeks. The duration depends on the radiation dose, the health of the patient, and the coexisting illness or injury. Following the latent phase, the exposed person manifests illness that may eventuate in recovery or lead to death.

With exposure to doses <1 Gy, ARS is generally mild. At this dose symptoms can be minimal or nonexistent, even if the entire body is exposed to penetrating radiation. The clinical picture will mainly be transient depression of bone marrow that lasts up to 2 to 3 weeks and then recovers.

ARS is significantly more acute and severe with exposure to very high doses—>30 Gy. At this dose the prodrome appears in minutes and is followed by 5 to 6 h of latency before a cardiovascular collapse occurs secondary to irreversible damage to the microcirculation.

The type and dose of radiation and the part of the body exposed will determine not only the timing of the different stages of ARS but also the dominant clinical picture. At low radiation doses of 0.7 to 4 Gy, hematopoietic depression due to bone marrow suppression takes place and constitutes the main illness. The patient may develop infections and bleeding secondary to low leukocyte and platelet counts, respectively. The bone marrow will eventually recover in almost all patients if they are supported with transfusions and fluids; antibiotics are often needed in addition. With exposure to 6 to 8 Gy, the clinical picture is significantly more complicated. At these doses the bone marrow will not always recover and death may ensue. A GI syndrome may also accompany the hematopoietic manifestations and further worsen the patient's condition. Compromise of the absorptive layer of the gut alters absorption of fluids, electrolytes, and nutrients. GI injury can lead to diarrhea, hemorrhage, sepsis, and electrolyte and fluid imbalance in a patient whose blood counts are compromised for a period of weeks, often leading to death. Whole-body exposure to doses >9 to 10 Gy is almost always fatal. Crucial elements of the bone marrow simply will not recover. In addition to the GI syndrome associated with very large exposures, patients may develop a neurovascular syndrome; the latter dominates with whole-body doses >20 Gy. Vascular collapse, seizures, and death are usually seen. In this variant the prodrome and latent phase both shorten to a few hours.

℞ TREATMENT

The treatment of ARS is focused on maintaining homeostasis, giving damaged organs the chance to recover. Aggressive support is given to every damaged system. Treatment for the hematopoietic system includes mainly therapy for neutropenia and infection, transfusion and blood products as needed, and hematopoietic growth factors. The value of bone marrow transplantation in this situation is questionable. None of the transplants that were performed among the victims of the nuclear reactor accident in Chernobyl proved successful. Another major component of the treatment of ARS is partial or total parenteral nutrition, to bypass the damaged GI system. For blast and thermal injuries, standard therapy for trauma is given. Psychological support is essential in many cases.

MEDICAL MANAGEMENT OF RADIATION BIOTERRORISM

Victims of radiation bioterrorism can suffer from conventional thermal or blast injuries, exposure to radiation, and contamination by radioactive materials. Many will have combinations of the above, which can be synergistic and cause higher morbidity and mortality than when they occur alone. The number of casualties will be the major factor in determining the response of the medical system to an act of radiation bioterrorism. If only a few people are affected, then no significant changes and adaptation of the system are needed to treat the victims. However, if a terror attack results in a large number (hundreds or more) of casualties, then an organized disaster plan at the local and state levels must be invoked to deal with the crisis properly. Medical personnel should have a prior assignment and be prepared to function in a scenario with which they are familiar. Stockpiles of specific equipment and medications have to be preplanned (see the Centers for Disease Control and Prevention website—*http://www.bt.cdc.gov*). One needs to recognize that one of the goals of terrorists is to overwhelm medical facilities and to minimize the salvage of casualties.

Initial management consists of *primary triage and transportation* of the wounded to emergency rooms for treatment. The rationale behind the triage is to sort patients into classes according to the severity of injury, for the purpose of expediting clinical care and maximizing the use of the available clinical services and facilities. Triage requires determination of the level of emergency care needed. The higher the number and range of casualties, the more complex and difficult triage becomes. The mildly wounded and victims of contamination only can be sent to evacuation, registration with disaster response teams, and decontamination and treatment centers. In this way, the hospitals themselves can avoid being directly overwhelmed, and those who are severely wounded can receive better treatment. Emergency treatment will be administered initially according to the presence of conventional injuries such as wounds, trauma, and thermal or chemical burns. Individuals with such injuries should be stabilized, if possible, and immediately transported to a medical facility. Removing the victim's clothes and wrapping him or her in clean blankets or nylon sheets reduces both the exposure of the patient and the contamination risk to the staff. However, the possibility of contamination needs to be determined. Less severely injured victims should receive a preliminary decontamination before or during evacuation to a hospital.

One must remember that radionuclide contamination of the skin is commonly not an acute life-threatening situation to the patient or the personnel who care for the patient. Only powerful gamma emitters are likely to cause real damage from contamination. It is important to emphasize that exposure to a radiation field alone does not necessarily create any contamination. The exposed person, if not contaminated, is not radioactive and does not directly emit any radiation.

In order to protect the staff, protective gear (gowns, gloves, masks, and caps) should be used. NBC masks with filters and chemically pro-

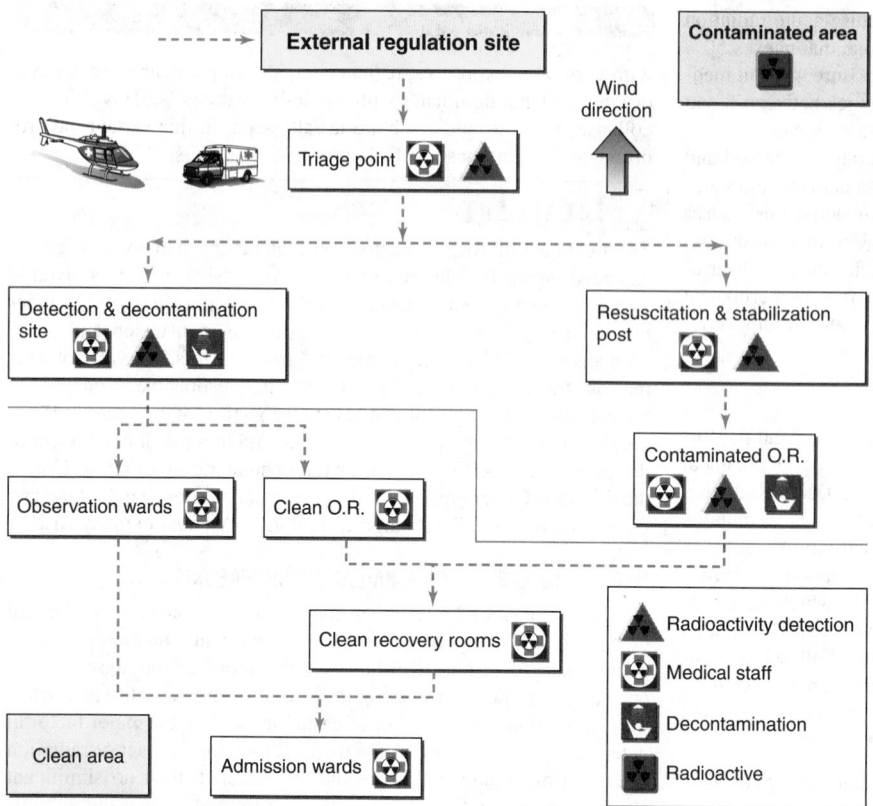

FIGURE 207-1 Flow chart of hospital triage. O.R., operating room.

Shielding with lead can be used as protection from small radioactive gamma sources. Geiger counters can detect gamma and beta radiation. Pocket chamber (pencil) dosimeters, film badges, and thermoluminescent dosimeters can measure accumulated exposure to gamma radiation. All of these detectors are in common use in medical facilities and should be used to help and define the level of contamination. Alpha radiation is harder to detect due to its poor penetration. An alpha scintillation counter, which is capable of detecting alpha radiation, is not commonly used in medical facilities.

GUIDELINES FOR HOSPITAL MANAGEMENT

Figure 207-1 illustrates a model for hospital arrangement for triage. Persons contaminated either externally or internally should be identified, externally decontaminated, and, if needed, treated immediately and specifically for internal contamination. In all other cases, the need for treatment of radiation injuries does not constitute a medical emergency. Early actions, such as blood sampling both for assessing the degree of severity of the exposure and for blood type and cross-matching for possible transfusion, need to be promptly taken if ARS is evident.

In the hospital entrance, a distinct decontamination area should be set up promptly. Separation between clean and contaminated areas is essential. Medical personnel in this area should wear protective gear as noted above. They also should be rotated in their assignments every 1 to 2 h to ensure minimal exposure to radiation. If patients are critically wounded and require either surgery or resuscitation, they need to pass directly to "contaminated" operating rooms or resuscitation sites for life-saving procedures. Once such patients are stable, they should then be decontaminated. It is important to obtain details concerning the exposure, to look for prodromal signs of radiation sickness, and to do a physical examination. One of the best ways to estimate exposure clinically is to measure the time of prodromal appearance. The earlier the prodromal signs and symptoms appear, the higher the dose of radiation exposure. A few laboratory tests need to be routinely taken, such as blood count and urinalysis. If internal contamination is suspected, specific treatment should be given, as outlined below.

tective overgarments provide excellent protection from contamination. Waterproof shoe covers are also important. Remaining in the contaminated area and dealing with life-saving procedures should take place according to the "ALARA" principle: as low as reasonably achievable. It is better to send many people for short exposure times than to send a few people for longer periods of time to do the same job.

Decontamination of victims should take place in the field prior to their arrival at medical facilities, but radiologic decontamination should never interfere with medical care. Removal of outer clothing and shoes will usually reduce the patient's contamination by 80 to 90%. Contaminated clothes should be carefully removed by rolling them over themselves, placing them in marked plastic bags, and removing them to a predefined area for contaminated clothes and equipment. A radiation detector should then be used to check for the presence of any residual radiologic contamination on the patient's body. In order to prevent internalization of the radioactive materials, one should cover open wounds prior to decontamination. Showering or washing of the entire skin and hair is very important. The skin is dried and reassessed for residual contamination until no radiation is found. Contamination-removing chemical agents are more than sufficient to remove radiologic contamination.

Wound decontamination should be as conservative as possible. The main goal is to prevent both extensive local damage and internal contamination through lacerated skin. The bandages should be removed and the wounds flushed. The wound should then be dried and assessed for radiation. This procedure can be repeated again and again until contamination is undetectable. Excision of contaminated wounds should be attempted only when surgically necessary.

In the hospital, staff can wear normal hospital barrier clothing, including two pairs of gloves, a gown, shoe covers, a head cover, and a face mask. Eye protection is recommended. Decontamination of medical personnel is obligatory following emergency treatment and decontamination of the patient. All protective clothing should be placed after use in a designated container for contaminated clothing.

Radiation intensity decays rapidly with the square of the distance from the source, and increasing the distance from the source and decreasing the time spent near it are basic principles of radiation safety.

TREATMENT

Treatment for internal radionuclide contamination should begin within hours of exposure. The goal is to leave the smallest amount of radionuclides as possible in the body. Treatment is given in order to reduce absorption and to enhance elimination and excretion. Many of the drugs for these indications are not approved by the U.S. Food and Drug Administration and are used as investigational drugs.

Clearance of the GI tract may be achieved by stomach lavage, emetics (such as apomorphine, 5 to 10 mg, or ipecac, 1- to 2-g capsules or 15 mL in syrup), or by using purgatives, laxatives, ion exchangers, and aluminum antacids. Prussian blue, 1 g tid for ≥3 weeks, is an ion exchanger used to treat cesium 137 internal contamination. Aluminum antacids (such as aluminum phosphate gel, 100 mL) may reduce strontium uptake in the gut if given immediately after exposure. Aluminum hydroxide, 60 to 100 mL, is less effective.

Prevention or reversal of radionuclide interaction with tissues can be done by blocking, diluting, mobilizing, and chelating agents. *Blocking agents* prevent entrance of radioactive materials. A good example is potassium iodide (KI), which blocks the uptake of radioactive iodine (^{131}I) by the thyroid. KI is most effective if taken within the first hour after exposure and is still effective 6 h after exposure. The effectiveness subsequently declines until 24 h after exposure; however, it is recommended that KI be taken up to 48 h postexposure. The KI dose is based on age, predicted thyroid exposure, and pregnancy and lactation status. Adults between the ages of 18 to 40 should receive 130 mg/d for 7 to 14 days if exposed to ≥10 cGy of radioactive iodine. Other thyroid-blocking agents include prophylthiouracil, 100 mg tid for 8 days, or methimazole, 10 mg tid for 2 days followed by 5 mg tid for 6 days, but they are somewhat less effective.

Diluting agents decrease the absorption of the radionuclide; for example, water may be used as a diluting agent in the treatment for tritium (^{3}H) contamination. The recommended amount is 3 to 4 L/d for at least 3 weeks.

Mobilizing agents are most effective when given immediately; however, they may be effective for up to 2 weeks after exposure. These include antithyroid drugs, parathyroid extract, glucocorticoids, ammonium chloride, diuretics, expectorants, and inhalants. All of them should induce the release of radionuclides from tissues.

Chelating agents can bind many radioactive materials, after which the complexes are excreted from the human body. In this regard, diethylenetriaminepentaacetic acid (DTPA) is superior to ethylenediamine tetraacetic acid (EDTA); it chelates plutonium, berkelium, californium, americium, curium, or any material with an atomic number >92. The dose is 1 g of Ca-DTPA or Zn-DTPA, dissolved in 250 mL of normal saline or 5% glucose, given intravenously over 1 hour daily for up to 5 days. DTPA can also be administrated by inhalation; 1 g is given in 1:1 dilution with water or saline over 15 to 20 min. Treating uranium contamination with DTPA is contraindicated, due to its synergistic damage to the kidneys.

Lung lavage can reduce radiation-induced pneumonitis and is indicated only when a large amount of radionuclide enters the lungs and has the potential for acute radiation injury. The procedure requires anesthesia. Table 207-2 summarizes the common treatment regimens for internal radionuclide contamination.

TABLE 207-2 *Common Drugs[a] for Treatment of Internal Contamination*

Medication	Administered for Radionuclides	Route of Administration	Dosage	Duration	Mechanism of Action
KI	Iodine-131	PO	130 mg/d for adults >40 with thyroid exposure >500 cGy 130 mg/d for adults 18–40 with thyroid exposure >10 cGy 130 mg/d for pregnant or lactating women with thyroid exposure >5 cGy 65 mg/d for children and adolescents 3–18 with thyroid exposure >5 cGy 32.5 mg/d for infants 1 month to 3 years with thyroid exposure >5 cGy 16 mg/d for neonates from birth to 1 month with thyroid exposure >5 cGy	7–14 days	Blocking agent
Zn-DTPA	Plutonium, trans-plutonium, yttrium, americium, curium	IV	1 g in 250 mL NS or 5% glucose, given in 1–2 h, *or* bolus over 3–4 min	Up to 5 days	Chelating agent
		Inhalation	1 g in 1:1 dilution with water or NS over 15–20 min		
		IM	1 g; not recommended because of pain		
Ca-DTPA	Plutonium, *trans*-plutonium, yttrium, americium, curium	IV	1 g in 250 mL NS or 5% glucose, given in 1–2 h, *or* bolus over 3–4 min	Up to 5 days	Chelating agent
		Inhalation	1 g in 1:1 dilution with water or NS over 15–20 min		
		IM	1 g; not recommended because of pain		
Bicarbonate	Uranium	IV	2 ampules sodium bicarbonate (44.3 meq each, 7.5%) in 1000 mL NS, 125 mL/L, *or* 1 ampule of sodium bicarbonate (44.3 meq, 7.5%) in 500 mL NS, 500 mL/h	Usually IV for the first 24 h, PO for additional 2 days; continuation of treatment for >3 days is rare and can be done according to titration of uranium amounts in the body	Increased excretion via the kidneys
		PO	2 tablets every 4 h until urine pH = 7–8, *or* 4 g (8 tablets) 3 tid		
Prussian blue	Cesium-137	PO	1 g tid with 100–200 mL water, up to 10 g/d	≥3 weeks titrated by urine and fecal bioassay and whole-body counting	Ion exchanger
Water	Tritium (H-3)	PO	>3–4 L per day	3 weeks	Excretion of water
Aluminum phosphate gel	Strontium	PO	100 mL immediately after exposure	Once	Decreased gut absorption
Aluminum hydroxide		PO	60–100 mL	Once	Decreased gut absorption

[a] Excluding KI, these drugs have not been approved for this purpose by the U.S. Food and Drug Administration at the time of publication.

Note: NS, normal saline

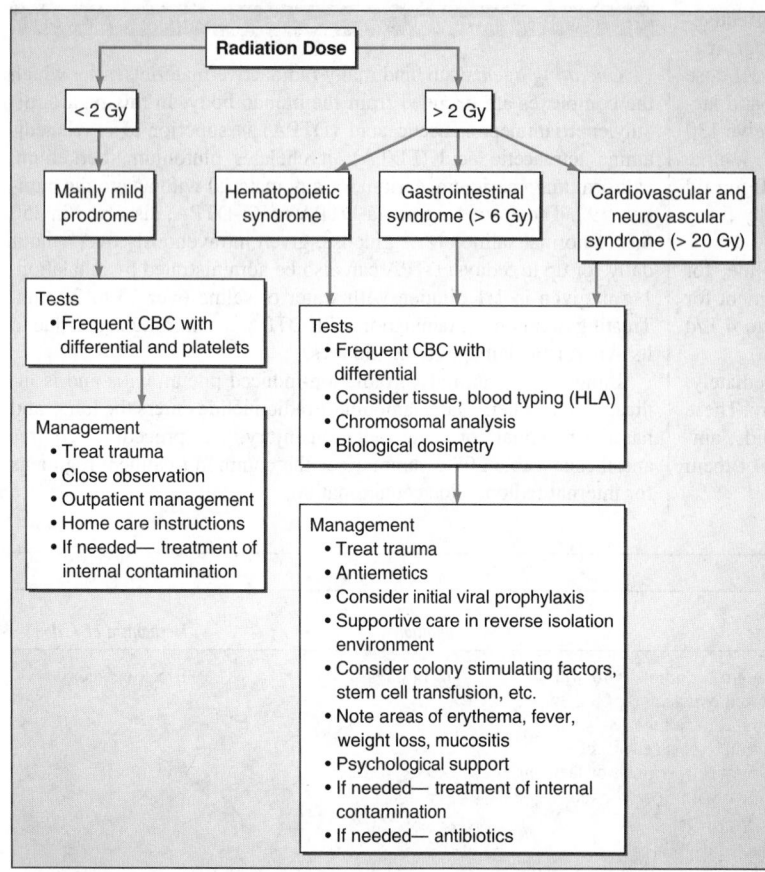

FIGURE 207-2 General guidelines for treatment of radiation casualties. CBC, complete blood count.

MEDICAL ASSAY OF THE RADIATION-EXPOSED PATIENT

One of the major difficulties in treating victims exposed to radiation is the determination of the amount of exposure. Clinical assessment of the patient is the best approach. Appearance of an early prodrome indicates high exposure to radiation. Victims who arrive at the hospital complaining of severe weakness, nausea, vomiting, diarrhea, or seizures probably will not survive despite support measures. Decontamination and the use of radiation-detection equipment are both very important. Few tests can be performed in order to estimate the radiation exposure and the contamination. Baseline laboratory tests should include a complete blood count with differential and platelet count, renal evaluation, and determination of electrolytes. Urine and stool samples should be obtained if internal contamination is suspected. Baseline samples should be taken and repeated every 24 h. Nasal swabs should be taken from each nostril for determination of inhalation of radionuclides. After exhalation, each swab is labeled and sealed in a plastic bag and sent for analysis to appropriate laboratories.

Follow-up complete blood counts including platelets are important on a daily basis as they reflect the bone marrow status. Patients exposed to 0.7 to 4 Gy will develop pancytopenia from as early as 10 days to as long 8 weeks postexposure. Lymphocytes show the most rapid decline, while other leukocytes and platelets decline less rapidly. Erythrocytes are the least vulnerable blood elements.

Absolute lymphocyte counts should be taken every 12 h for 3 days; they are the most valuable early indicator because they are recognized to be a sensitive marker for radiation damage and correlate with both the exposure and prognosis. A 50% drop in absolute lymphocyte count within the first 24 h indicates a significant injury. HLA typing is necessary whenever there is suspicion of irreversible bone marrow damage. Lymphocyte chromosomal analysis can detect radiation exposure as low as 0.03 to 0.06 Gy, and 15 mL of blood should be drawn early as possible in a heparinized collection tube and kept cool. Radiation-induced chromosomal aberrations in peripheral blood lymphocytes include dicentric chromosomes that last for a few weeks. By calibrating a dose-response curve, the radiation dose can be assessed.

Another method for estimating exposure is the micronucleus (MN/Mni) scoring, which is simple and fast but still empirical. An algorithm for the treatment of radiation casualties is provided in Figure 207-2.

FOLLOW-UP

It is desirable to continue follow-up in some circumstances, such as in cases of internal contamination, especially with exposure from uranium with its nephrotoxic properties; in cases of radiation exposure to distinct organs; and in cases where there is risk for carcinogenicity.

FURTHER READING

DAINIAK N: Hematologic consequences of exposure to ionizing radiation. Exp Hematol 30:513, 2002

Guidance for radiation accident management, Oak Ridge–associated universities. *http://www.orau.gov/reacts/guidance.htm*, updated 03/22/2002

JARRETT D et al (eds): *Medical Management of Radiation Casualties: Handbook.* AFRRI special publication 99-2. Bethesda, Md., Armed Forces Radiobiology Research Institute, 1999 (also available at *http://www.afrri.usuhs.mil.*)

Management of Terrorist Events Involving Radioactive Material. NCRP report no. 138. Bethesda, Md, National Council on Radiation Protection, 2001

METTLER FA JR, VOELZ GL: Major radiation exposure—what to expect and how to respond. N Engl J Med 346:1554, 2002

MOULDER JE: Report on an interagency workshop on the radiobiology of nuclear terrorism. Molecular and Cellular Biology of Moderate Dose (1–10 Sv) Radiation and Potential Mechanisms of Radiation Protection (Bethesda, Md, December 17–18, 2001). Radiat Res 158: 118, 2002

INTRODUCTORY COMMENTS

The following are tables of reference values for laboratory tests, special analytes, and special function tests. A variety of factors can influence reference values. Such variables include the population studied, laboratory methods and instrumentation, and even the type of container used for the collection of the specimen. Values supplied in this Appendix reflect typical reference ranges in adults. Pediatric reference ranges may vary significantly from adult values. The reference or "normal" ranges given in this appendix may therefore not be appropriate for all laboratories, and these values should only be used as general guidelines. Whenever possible, reference values provided by the laboratory performing the testing should be utilized in the interpretation of laboratory data.

In preparing the Appendix, the authors have taken into account the fact that the system of international units (SI, système international

d'unités) is used in most countries and in some medical journals. However, clinical laboratories may continue to report values in conventional units. Therefore, both systems are provided in the Appendix. The dual system is also used in the text except for (1) those instances in which the numbers remain the same but only the terminology is changed (mmol/L for meq/L or IU/L for mIU/mL), when only the SI units are given; and (2) most pressure measurements (e.g., blood and cerebrospinal fluid pressures), when the traditional units (mmHg, mmH_2O) are used. In all other instances in the text, the SI unit is followed by the conventional unit in parentheses.

Conversion from one system to another can be made as follows:

$$mmol/L = \frac{mg/dL \times 10}{atomic\ weight\ (or\ molecular\ weight)}$$

$$mg/dL = \frac{mmol/L \times atomic\ weight\ (or\ molecular\ weight)}{10}$$

A REFERENCE VALUES FOR LABORATORY TESTS

TABLE A-1 *Hematology and Coagulation*

Analyte	Specimen	SI Units	Conventional Units
Activated clotting time	WB	70–180 seconds	70–180 seconds
Activated protein C resistance (Factor V Leiden)	P	Not applicable	Ratio > 2.1
Alpha$_2$ antiplasmin	P	0.80–1.30	80–130%
Antiphospholipid antibody panel			
PTT-LA (lupus anticoagulant screen)	P	Negative	Negative
Platelet neutralization procedure	P	Negative	Negative
Dilute viper venom screen	P	Negative	Negative
Anticardiolipin antibody	S		
IgG		0–15 arbitrary units	0–15 GPL
IgM		0–15 arbitrary units	0–15 MPL
Antithrombin III	P		
Antigenic		220–390 mg/L	22–39 mg/dL
Functional		0.8–1.30 U/L	80–130%
Anti-Xa assay (Heparin assay)	P		
Unfractionated heparin		0.3–0.7 kIU/L	0.3–0.7 IU/mL
Low-molecular-weight heparin		0.5–1.0 kIU/L	0.5–1.0 IU/mL
Danaparoid (Orgaran)		0.5–0.8 kIU/L	0.5–0.8 IU/mL
Bleeding time (adult)		2–9.5 min	2–9.5 min
Bone Marrow: see Table B-3			
Carboxyhemoglobin	WB		
Nonsmoker		0–0.023	0–2.3%
Smoker		0.021–0.042	2.1–4.2%
Clot retraction	WB	0.50–1.00/2 h	50–100%/2 h
Cryofibrinogen	P	Negative	Negative
D-Dimer	P	<0.5 mg/L	<0.5 μg/mL
Differential blood count	WB		
Neutrophils		0.40–0.70	40–70%
Bands		0.0–0.10	0–10%
Lymphocytes		0.22–0.44	22–44%
Monocytes		0.04–0.11	4–11%
Eosinophils		0.0–0.8	0–8%
Basophils		0.0–0.03	0–3%
Erythrocyte count	WB		
Adult males		4.50–5.90 × 10^{12}/L	4.50–5.90 × 10^6/mm^3
Adult females		4.00–5.20 × 10^{12}/L	4.00–5.20 × 10^6/mm^3
Erythrocyte lifespan	WB		
Normal survival		120 days	120 days
Chromium labeled, half life (t$_{1/2}$)		25–35 days	25–35 days
Erythrocyte sedimentation rate	WB		
Females		1–25 mm/h	1–25 mm/h
Males		0–17 mm/h	0–17 mm/h

(continued)

Analyte	Specimen	SI Units	Conventional Units
Factor II, prothrombin	P	0.60–1.40	60–140%
Factor V	P	0.60–1.40	60–140%
Factor VII	P	0.60–1.40	60–140%
Factor VIII	P	0.50–2.00	50–200%
Factor IX	P	0.60–1.40	60–140%
Factor X	P	0.60–1.40	60–140%
Factor XI	P	0.60–1.40	60–140%
Factor XII	P	0.60–1.40	60–140%
Factor XIII screen	P	Not applicable	No deficiency detected
Factor inhibitor assay	P	<0.5 Bethesda Units	<0.5 Bethesda Units
Ferritin	S		
Male		30–300 μg/L	30–300 ng/mL
Female		10–200 μg/L	10–200 ng/mL
Fibrin(ogen) degradation products	P	<2.5 mg/L	<2.5 μg/mL
Fibrinogen	P	1.50–4.00 g/L	150–400 mg/dL
Folate (folic acid)	S, P		
Normal		7.0–39.7 nmol/L	3.1–17.5 ng/mL
Borderline deficient		5.0–6.8 nmol/L	2.2–3.0 ng/mL
Deficient		<5.0 nmol/L	<2.2 ng/mL
Excess		>39.7 nmol/L	>17.5 ng/mL
Glucose-6-phosphate dehydrogenase (erythrocyte)	WB	Not applicable	No gross deficiency
Ham's test (acid serum)	WB	Negative	Negative
Haptoglobin	S	0.16–1.99 g/L	16–199 mg/dL
Hematocrit	WB		
Adult males		0.41–0.53	41.0–53.0
Adult females		0.36–0.46	36.0–46.0
Hemoglobin			
Plasma	P	0.01–0.05 g/L	1–5 mg/dL
Whole blood:	WB		
Adult males		8.4–10.9 mmol/L	13.5–17.5 g/dL
Adult females		7.4–9.9 mmol/L	12.0–16.0 g/dL
Hemoglobin electrophoresis	WB		
Hemoglobin A		0.95–0.98	95–98%
Hemoglobin A_2		0.015–0.035	1.5–3.5%
Hemoglobin F		0–0.02	0–2.0%
Hemoglobins other than A, A_2, or F		Absent	Absent
Heparin-induced thrombocytopenia antibody	P	Negative	Negative
Homocysteine	P	0–12 μmol/L	0–12 μmol/L
Iron	S	5.4–28.7 μmol/L	30–160 μg/dL
Iron binding capacity	S	40.8–76.7 μmol/L	228–428 μg/dL
Leukocytes			
Alkaline phosphatase (LAP)	WB	Not applicable	13–133/100 neutrophils
Count (WBC)	WB	4.5–11 $\times$ 10^9/L	4.5–11.0 $\times$ 10^3/mm^3
Mean corpuscular hemoglobin (MCH)	WB	26.0–34.0 pg/cell	26.0–34.0 pg/cell
Mean corpuscular hemoglobin concentration (MCHC)	WB	310–370 g/L	31.0–37.0 g/dL
Mean corpuscular volume (MCV)	WB		
Male (adult)		78–100 fl	78–100 μm^3
Female (adult)		78–102 fl	78–102 μm^3
Methemoglobin	WB		Up to 1% of total hemoglobin
Osmotic fragility of erythrocytes	WB	Not applicable	Increased hemolysis as compared to normal control
Partial thromboplastin time, activated	P	22.1–35.1 s	22.1–35.1 s
Plasminogen	P		
Antigen		84–140 mg/L	8.4–14.0 mg/dL
Functional		0.80–1.30	80–130%
Plasminogen activator inhibitor 1	P	4–43 μg/L	4–43 ng/mL
Platelet aggregation	PRP		>65% aggregation in response to adenosine diphosphate, epinephrine, collagen, ristocetin, and arachidonic acid
Platelet count	WB	150–350 $\times$ 10^9/L	150–350 $\times$ 10^3/mm^3
Platelet, mean volume	WB	6.4–11 fl	6.4–11.0 μm^3
Prekallikrein assay	P	0.60–1.40	60–140%
Prekallikrein screen	P		No deficiency detected
Protein C	P		
Total antigen		0.70–1.40	70–140%
Functional		0.70–1.40	70–140%
Protein S	P		
Total antigen		0.70–1.40	70–140%
Functional		0.70–1.40	70–140%
Free antigen		0.70–1.40	70–140%
Prothrombin gene mutation G20210A	WB	Not applicable	Not present
Prothrombin time	P	11.1–13.1 s	11.1–13.1 s
Protoporphyrin, free erythrocyte	WB	0.28–0.64 μmol/L of red blood cells	16–36 μg/dL of red blood cells
Red cell distribution width	WB	0.115–0.145	11.5–14.5%

(continued)

Analyte	Specimen	SI Units	Conventional Units
Reptilase time	P	16–24 s	16–24 s
Reticulocyte count	WB	0.005–0.025 red cells	0.5–2.5% red cells
Reticulocyte hemoglobin content	WB	>26 pg/cell	>26 pg/cell
Ristocetin confactor (Functional von Willebrand factor)	P		
Blood group O		0.75 mean of normal	75% mean of normal
Blood group A		1.05 mean of normal	105% mean of normal
Blood group B		1.15 mean of normal	115% mean of normal
Blood group AB		1.25 mean of normal	125% mean of normal
Schilling test, orally administered vitamin B_{12} excreted in urine	U	Not applicable	7–40%
Sickle cell test	WB	Negative	Negative
Sucrose hemolysis	WB	<0.1	<10% hemolysis
Thrombin time	P	16–24 s	16–24 s
Total eosinophils	WB	70–140 × 10⁶/L	70–440/mm³
Transferrin receptor	S, P	9.6–29.6 nmol/L	9.6–29.6 nmol/L
Viscosity			
Plasma	P	1.7–2.1	1.7–2.1
Serum	S	1.4–1.8	1.4–1.8
Vitamin B_{12}	S, P		
Normal		185 pmol/L	>250 pg/mL
Borderline		92–185 pmol/L	125–250 pg/mL
Deficient		<92 pmol/L	<125 pg/mL
von Willebrand factor (vWF) antigen (factor VIII:R antigen)	P		
vWF multimers	P	Normal distribution	Normal distribution
White blood cells: see *Leukocytes*			

Note: P, plasma; PRP, platelet-rich plasma; S, serum; U, urine; WB, whole blood

TABLE A-2 *Immunology*

Analyte	Specimen	SI Units	Conventional Units
Autoantibodies			
Anti–adrenal antibody	S	Not applicable	Negative at 1:10 dilution
Anti–double stranded (native) DNA	S	Not applicable	Negative at 1:10 dilution
Anti–glomerular basement membrane antibodies	S		
Qualitative		Negative	Negative
Quantitative		<5 kU/L	<5 U/mL
Anti-granulocyte antibody	S	Not applicable	Negative
Anti-Jo-1 antibody	S	Not applicable	Negative
Anti-La antibody	S	Not applicable	Negative
Anti-mitochondrial antibody	S	Not applicable	Negative
Antineutrophil cytoplasmic autoantibodies, cytoplasmic (C-ANCA)	S		
Qualitative		Negative	Negative
Quantitative (Antibodies to proteinase 3)		<2.8 kU/L	<2.8 U/mL
Antineutrophil cytoplasmic autoantibodies, perinuclear (P-ANCA)	S		
Qualitative		Negative	Negative
Quantitative (Antibodies to myeloperoxidase)		<1.4 kU/L	<1.4 U/mL
Antinuclear antibody	S	Not applicable	Negative at 1:40
Anti-parietal cell antibody	S	Not applicable	Negative at 1:20
Anti-Ro antibody	S	Not applicable	Negative
Anti-platelet antibody	S	Not applicable	Negative
Anti-RNP antibody	S	Not applicable	Negative
Anti-Scl 70 antibody	S	Not applicable	Negative
Anti-Smith antibody	S	Not applicable	Negative
Anti–smooth muscle antibody	S	Not applicable	Negative at 1:20
Anti-thyroglobulin	S	Not applicable	Negative
Anti-thyroid antibody	S	<0.3 kIU/L	<0.3 IU/mL
Bence Jones protein, serum	S	Not applicable	None detected
Bence Jones protein, urine, qualitative	U	Not applicable	None detected in 50× concentrated urine
Bence Jones Protein, urine, quantitative	U		
κ		<0.03 g/L	<2.5 mg/dL
λ		<0.05 g/L	<5.0 mg/dL
β_2-Microglobulin			
	S	<2.7 mg/L	<0.27 mg/dL
	U	<120 μg/d	<120 μg/d

(continued)

Analyte	Specimen	SI Units	Conventional Units
C-reactive protein	S		
Routine		0.08–3.1 mg/L	0.08–3.1 mg/L
High sensitivity		0.02–8.0 mg/L	0.02–8.0 mg/L
C1-esterase-inhibitor protein	S		
Antigenic		0.12–0.25 g/L	12.4–24.5 mg/dL
Functional		Present	Present
Complement			
C3 (adults)	S	0.86–1.84 g/L	86–184 mg/dL
C4 (adults)	S	0.20–0.58 g/L	20–58 mg/dL
Total complement, EIA (adult)	S	63–145 kU/L	63–145 U/mL
Factor B	S	0.17–0.42 g/L	17–42 mg/dL
Cryoproteins	S	Not applicable	None detected
Immunofixation	S	Not applicable	None detected
Immunoglobulin, quantitation (adult)			
IgA	S	0.60–3.09 g/L	60–309 mg/dL
IgD	S	0–140 mg/L	0–14 mg/dL
IgE	S	24–430 μg/L	10–179 IU/mL
IgG	S	6.14–12.95 g/L	614–1295 mg/dL
IgG_1	S	2.7–17.4 g/L	270–1740 mg/dL
IgG_2	S	0.3–6.3 g/L	30–630 mg/dL
IgG_3	S	0.13–3.2 g/L	13–320 mg/dL
IgG_4	S	0.11–6.2 g/L	11–620 mg/dL
IgM	S	0.53–3.34 g/L	53–334 mg/dL
Joint fluid crystal	JF	Not applicable	No crystals seen
Joint fluid mucin	JF	Not applicable	Only type I mucin present
LE cell test	WB	Negative	Negative
Rheumatoid factor	S, JF	<30 kIU/L	<30.0 IU/mL
Serum protein electrophoresis	S	Not applicable	Normal pattern

Note: JF, joint fluid; P, plasma; S, serum; U, urine; WB, whole blood

TABLE A-3 *Clinical Chemistry*

Constituent	Specimen	SI Units	Conventional Units
Acetoacetate	P	<100 μmol/L	<1 mg/dL
Albumin	S	35–55 g/L	3.5–5.5 g/dL
Aldolase	S	0–100 nkat/L	0–6 U/L
α_1 antitrypsin	S	0.8–2.1 g/L	85–213 mg/dL
Alpha fetoprotein (adult)	S	<15 μg/L	<15 ng/mL
Aminotransferases	S		
Aspartate (AST, SGOT)		0–0.58 μkat/L	0–35 U/L
Alanine (ALT, SGPT)		0–0.58 μkat/L	0–35 U/L
Ammonia, as NH_3	P	6–47 μmol/L	10–80 μg/dL
Amylase	S	0.8–3.2 μkat/L	60–180 U/L
Angiotensin-converting enzyme (ACE)	S	<670 nkat/L	<40 U/L
Anion gap	S	7–16 mmol/L	7–16 mmol/L
Apolipoprotein A-1	S	1.2–2.4 g/L	119–240 mg/dL
Apolipoprotein B	S	0.52–1.63 g/L	52–163 mg/dL
Apo B/Apo A-1 ratio		0.35–0.98	0.35–0.98
Arterial blood gases			
$[HCO_3^-]$		21–28 mmol/L	21–30 meq/L
P_{CO_2}		4.7–5.9 kPa	35–45 mmHg
pH		7.38–7.44	
P_{O_2}		11–13 kPa	80–100 mmHg
β-Hydroxybutyrate	P	<300 μmol/L	<3 mg/dL
β-2-microglobulin	S	1.2–2.8 mg/L	1.2–2.8 mg/L
	U	≤200 μg/L	≤200 μg/L
Bilirubin	S		
Total		5.1–17 μmol/L	0.3–1.0 mg/dL
Direct		1.7–5.1 μmol/L	0.1–0.3 mg/dL
Indirect		3.4–12 μmol/L	0.2–0.7 mg/dL
Brain type natriuetic peptide (BNP)	P	Age and gender specific: <167 ng/L	Age and gender specific: <167 pg/mL
Calcium, ionized	WB	1.1–1.4 mmol/L	4.5–5.6 mg/dL
Calcium	S	2.2–2.6 mmol/L	9–10.5 mg/dL
CA-15-3	S	0–30 kU/L	0–30 U/mL
CA 19-9	S	0–37 kU/L	0–37 U/mL
CA 27-29	S	0–32 kU/L	0–32 U/mL
CA 125	S	0–35 kU/L	0–35 U/mL
Calcitonin	S		
Male		3–26 ng/L	3–26 pg/mL
Female		2–17 ng/L	2–17 pg/mL

(continued)

Constituent	Specimen	SI Units	Conventional Units
Carbon dioxide content (TCO$_2$)	P (sea level)	21–30 mmol/L	21–30 meq/L
Carbon dioxide tension (P$_{CO_2}$)	Arterial blood (sea level)	4.7–5.9 kPa	35–45 mmHg
Carbon monoxide content	WB	Symptoms with 20% saturation of hemoglobin	
Carcinoembryonic antigen (CEA)	S	0.0–3.4 ug/L	0.0–3.4 ng/mL
Ceruloplasmin	S	270–370 mg/L	27–37 mg/dL
Cholinesterase	S	5–12 kU/L	5–12 U/mL
Chloride	S	98–106 mmol/L	98–106 meq/L
Cholesterol: see Table A-7			
Coproporphyrins (types I and III)	U	150–460 μmol/d	100–300 μg/d
C-peptide	S	0.17–0.66 nmol/L	0.5–2.0 ng/mL
Creatine kinase (CK) (total)	S		
Females		0.67–2.50 μkat/L	40–150 U/L
Males		1.00–6.67 μkat/L	60–400 U/L
Creatine kinase-MB	S	0–7 μg/L	0–7 ng/mL
Creatine kinase relative index (ng/mL per total CK U/L) × 100	S	Method dependent	Method dependent
Creatinine	S	<133 μmol/L	<1.5 mg/dL
Erythropoietin	S	5–36 U/L	
Fatty acids, free (nonesterified)	P	0.28–0.89 mmol/L	<8–25 mg/dL
Ferritin	S		
Female		10–200 μg/L	10–200 ng/mL
Male		15–400 μg/L	15–400 ng/mL
Fibrinogen and fibrinogen split products: see Hematology and Coagulation			
Gamma glutamyltransferase	S	1–94 U/L	1–94 U/L
Glucose (fasting)	P		
Normal		4.2–6.4 mmol/L	75–115 mg/dL
Diabetes mellitus		>7.0 mmol/L	>125 mg/dL
Glucose, 2 h postprandial	P	<6.7 mmol/L	<120 mg/dL
Hemoglobin A$_{1c}$	WB	0.038–0.064 Hb fraction	3.8–6.4%
Homocysteine	P	4–12 μmol/L	4–12 μmol/L
Hydroxyproline	U, 24 hour	0–10 μmol/L	0–1.3 mg/d
Iron	S	9–27 μmol/L	50–150 μg/dL
Iron-binding capacity	S	45–66 μmol/L	250–370 μg/dL
Iron-binding capacity saturation	S	0.2–0.45	20–45%
Ketone (acetone)	S, U	Negative	Negative
Lactate dehydrogenase	S	1.7–3.2 μkat/L	100–190 U/L
Lactate	P, venous	0.6–1.7 mmol/L	5–15 mg/dL
Lactate dehydrogenase isoenzymes	S		
Fraction 1 (of total)		0.14–0.25	14–26%
Fraction 2		0.29–0.39	29–39%
Fraction 3		0.20–0.25	20–26%
Fraction 4		0.08–0.16	8–16%
Fraction 5		0.06–0.16	6–16%
Lipase	S	0–2.66 μkat/L	0–160 U/L
Lipids: see Table A-7			
Lipids, triglyceride: see Triglycerides			
Lipoprotein: see Table A-7			
Lipoprotein (a)	S	0–300 mg/L	0–30 mg/dL
Magnesium	S	0.8–1.2 mmol/L	1.8–3 mg/dL
Microalbumin urine			
24-h urine	U	<0.2 g/L or <0.031 g/24 h	<20 mg/L or <31 mg/24 h
Spot AM urine		<0.03 g albumin/g creatinine	<0.03 mg albumin/mg creatinine
Myoglobin	S		
Male		19–92 μg/L	
Female		12–76 μg/L	
5 Nucleotidase	S	0.02–0.18 ukat/L	0–11 U/L
N-telopeptide (cross linked), NTx	U	3–65 nmol/mmol creatinine	3–65 nmol/mmol creatinine
Osmolality			
	P	285–295 mmol/kg serum water	285–295 mosmol/kg serum water
	U	300–900 mmol/kg	300–900 mosmol/kg
Osteocalcin	S	3.1–14 μg/L	3.1–14 ng/mL
Oxygen content	WB, arterial (sea level)		17–21 vol%
	WB, venous arm (sea level)		10 to 16 vol%
Oxygen percent saturation (sea level)			
	WB, arterial	0.97 mol/mol	97%
	WB, venous, arm	0.60–0.85 mol/mol	60–85%
Oxygen tension (P$_{O_2}$)	WB	11–13 kPa	80–100 mmHg
pH	WB	7.38–7.44	
Parathyroid hormone–related peptide	S	<1.3 pmol/L	<1.3 pmol/L
Phosphatase, acid	S	0.90 nkat/L	0–5.5 U/L
Phosphatase, alkaline	S	0.5–2.0 nkat/L	30–120 U/L

(continued)

Constituent	Specimen	SI Units	Conventional Units
Phosphorus, inorganic	S	1.0–1.4 mmol/L	3–4.5 mg/dL
Porphobilinogen	U	None	None
Potassium	S	3.5–5.0 mmol/L	3.5–5.0 meq/L
Prealbumin	S	195–358 mg/L	19.5–35.8 mg/dL
Prostate-specific antigen (PSA)	S		
Female		<0.5 μg/L	<0.5 ng/mL
Male			
<40 years		0.0–2.0 μg/L	0.0–2.0 ng/mL
>40 years		0.0–4.0 μg/L	0.0–4.0 ng/mL
PSA, free, in males 45–75 years, with PSA values between 4 and 20 μg/L		>0.25 associated with benign prostatic hyperplasia (BPH)	>25% associated with BPH
Protein, total	S	55–80 g/L	5.5–8.0 g/dL
Protein fractions:	S		
Albumin		35–55 g/L	3.5–5.5 g/dL (50–60%)
Globulin		20–35 g/L	2.0–3.5 g/dL (40–50%)
Alpha$_1$		2–4 g/L	0.2–0.4 g/dL (4.2–7.2%)
Alpha$_2$		5–9 g/L	0.5–0.9 g/dL (6.8–12%)
Beta		6–11 g/L	0.6–1.1 g/dL (9.3–15%)
Gamma		7–17 g/L	0.7–1.7 g/dL (13–23%)
Pyruvate	P, venous	60–170 μmol/L	0.5–1.5 mg/dL
Sodium	S	136–145 mmol/L	136–145 meq/L
Transferrin	S	2.3–3.9 g/L	230–390 mg/dL
Triglycerides	S	<1.8 mmol/L	<160 mg/dL
Troponin I	S	0–0.4 μg/L	0–0.4 ng/mL
Troponin T	S	0–0.1 μg/L	0–0.1 ng/mL
Urea nitrogen	S	3.6–7.1 mmol/L	10–20 mg/dL
Uric acid	S		
Males		150–480 μmol/L	2.5–8.0 mg/dL
Females		90–360 μmol/L	1.5–6.0 mg/dL
Urobilinogen	U	1.7–5.9 μmol/d	1–3.5 mg/d
Vasoactive intestinal polypeptide	P	<75 ng/L	<75 pg/mL

Note: P, plasma; S, serum; U, urine; WB, blood

Analyte	Specimen	SI Units	Conventional Units
Adrenocorticotropin (ACTH)	P	1.3–16.7 pmol/L	6.0–76.0 pg/mL
Aldosterone (adult)			
Supine, normal sodium diet	S, P	55–250 pmol/L	2–9 ng/dL
Upright, normal sodium diet	S, P		2- to 5-fold increase over supine value
Supine, low-sodium diet	S, P		2- to 5-fold increase over normal sodium diet level
Random, low-sodium diet	U	6.38–58.25 nmol/d	2.3–21.0 μg/24 h
Androstenedione (adult)	S	1.75–8.73 nmol/L	50–250 ng/dL
C peptide (adult)	S, P	0.17–0.66 nmol/L	0.5–2.0 ng/mL
Cortisol			
Fasting, 8 AM–Noon	S	138–690 nmol/L	5–25 μg/dL
Noon–8 PM		138–414 nmol/L	5–15 μg/dL
8 PM–8 AM		0–276 nmol/L	0–10 μg/dL
Cortisol, free	U	55–193 nmol/24 h	20–70 μg/24 h
C-peptide (insulin)	S	0.26–0.62 nmol/L	0.78–1.89 ng/mL
Dehydroepiandrosterone (DHEA) (adult)			
Male	S	6.24–41.6 nmol/L	180–1250 ng/dL
Female		4.5–34.0 nmol/L	130–980 ng/dL
DHEA sulfate	S		
Male (adult)		100–6190 μg/L	10–619 μg/dL
Female (adult, premenopausal)		120–5350 μg/L	12–535 μg/dL
Female (adult, postmenopausal)		300–2600 μg/L	30–260 μg/dL
Deoxycorticosterone (DOC) (adult)	S	61–576 nmol/L	2–19 ng/dL
11-Deoxycortisol (adult) (compound S) (8:00 AM)	S	0.34–4.56 nmol/L	12–158 ng/dL
Dihydrotestosterone			
Male	S, P	1.03–2.92 nmol/L	30–85 ng/dL
Female		0.14–0.76 nmol/L	4–22 ng/dL
Dopamine	P	<475 pmol/L	<87 pg/mL
Dopamine	U	425–2610 nmol/d	65–400 μg/d
Epinepherine	P		
Supine (30 min)		<273 pmol/L	<50 pg/mL
Sitting		<328 pmol/L	<60 pg/mL
Standing (30 min)		<4914 pmol/L	<900 pg/mL

(continued)

Analyte	Specimen	SI Units	Conventional Units
Epinephrine	U	0–109 nmol/d	0–20 μg/d
Estradiol	S, P		
Female			
Menstruating			
Follicular phase		184–532 pmol/L	20–145 pg/mL
Mid-cycle peak		411–1626 pmol/L	112–443 pg/mL
Luteal phase		184–885 pmol/L	20–241 pg/mL
Postmenopausal		<217 pmol/L	<59 pg/mL
Male		<184 pmol/L	<20 pg/mL
Estrone	S, P		
Female			
Menstruating			
Follicular phase		55–555 pmol/L	1.5–15 pg/mL
Luteal phase		55–740 pmol/L	1.5–20 pg/mL
Postmenopausal		55–204 pmol/L	1.5–5.5 pg/mL
Male		55–240 pmol/L	1.5–6.5 pg/mL
Follicle-stimulating hormone (FSH)	S, P		
Female			
Menstruating			
Follicular phase		3.0–20.0 IU/L	3.0–20.0 U/L
Ovulatory phase		9.0–26.0 IU/L	9.0–26.0 U/L
Luteal phase		1.0–12.0 IU/L	1.0–12.0 U/L
Postmenopausal		18.0–153.0 IU/L	18.0–153.0 U/L
Male		1.0–12.0 IU/L	1.0–12.0 U/L
Fructosamine	S	1.61–2.68 mmol/L	1.61–2.68 mmol/L
Gastrin	S	<100 ng/L	<100 pg/mL
Glucagon	P	20–100 ng/L	20–100 pg/mL
Growth hormone (resting)	S	0.5–17.0 μg/L	0.5–17.0 ng/mL
Human chorionic gonadotropin (HCG) (nonpregnant)	S	<5 IU/L	<5 mIU/mL
17-Hydroxyprogesterone (adult)	S		
Male		0.15 nmol/L	5–250 ng/dL
Female			
Follicular phase		0.6–3.0 nmol/L	20–100 ng/dL
Midcycle peak		3–7.5 nmol/L	100–250 ng/dL
Luteal phase		3–15 nmol/L	100–500 ng/dL
Postmenopausal		≤2.1 nmol/L	≤70 ng/dL
5-Hydroindoleacetic Acid [5-HIAA]	U	10.5–36.6 μmol/d	2–7 mg/d
Insulin	S, P	14.35–143.5 pmol/L	2–20 μU/mL
17 Ketosteroids	U	10–42 μmol/d	3–12 mg/d
Luteinizing hormone (LH)	S, P		
Female			
Menstruating			
Follicular phase		2.0–15.0 U/L	2.0–15.0 U/L
Ovulatory phase		22.0–105.0 U/L	22.0–105.0 U/L
Luteal phase		0.6–19.0 U/L	0.6–19.0 U/L
Postmenopausal		16.0–64.0 U/L	16.0–64.0 U/L
Male		2.0–12.0 U/L	2.0–12.0 U/L
Metanephrine	P	Method dependent	Method dependent
Metanephrine	U	0.03–0.69 mmol/mol creatinine	0.05–1.20 μg/mg creatinine
Norepinephrine	U	89–473 nmol/d	15–80 μg/d
Norepinephrine	P		
Supine (30 min)		650–2423 pmol/L	110–410 pg/mL
Sitting		709–4019 pmol/L	120–680 pg/mL
Standing (30 min)		739–4137 pmol/L	125–700 pg/mL
Parathyroid hormone (PTH)	S	10–60 ng/L	10–60 pg/mL
Pregnanetriol	U	Age and sex dependent	Age and sex dependent
Progesterone	S, P		
Female			
Follicular		<3.18 nmol/L	<1.0 ng/mL
Midluteal		9.54–63.6 nmol/L	3–20 ng/mL
Male		<3.18 nmol/L	<1.0 ng/mL
Prolactin	S		
Female		0–20 μg/L	1.9–25.9 ng/mL
Male		0–15 μg/L	1.6–23.0 ng/mL
Renin (adult, normal sodium diet)	P		
Supine		0.08–0.83 ng/(L-s)	0.3–3.0 ng/(mL/h)
Upright		0.28–2.5 ng/(L-s)	1–9.0 ng/(mL/h)
Serotonin	WB	0.28–1.14 μmol/L	50–200 ng/mL
Serotonin	Platelet	0.7–2.8 amol/platelet	125–500 ng/10⁹ platelets
Sex hormone binding globulin (adult)	S		
Male			13–71 nmol/L
Female			18–114 nmol/L
Somatostatin	P	<25 ng/L	<25 pg/mL

(continued)

Analyte	Specimen	SI Units	Conventional Units
Somatomedin-C (IGF-1) (adult)	S		
16–24 years		182–780 μg/L	182–780 ng/mL
25–39 years		114–492 μg/L	114–492 ng/mL
40–54 years		90–360 μg/L	90–360 ng/mL
>54 years		71–290 μg/L	71–290 ng/mL
Testosterone, total, morning sample	S		
Female		0.21–2.98 nmol/L	6–86 ng/dL
Male		9.36–37.10 nmol/L	270–1070 ng/dL
Testosterone, unbound, morning sample			
Female, adult	S	6.9–107.5 pmol/L	0.2–3.1 pg/mL
Male, adult		416–1386 pmol/L	12.0–40.0 pg/mL
Thyroglobulin	S	0–60 μg/L	0–60 ng/mL
Thyroid binding globulin	S	206–309 μg/L	16–24 μg/dL
Thyroid hormone binding index (THBI or T₃RU)	S	0.83–1.17 mol ratio	0.83–1.17
(Free) thyroxine index	S	4.2–13	4.2–13
Thyroid stimulating hormone	S	0.5–4.7 mU/L	0.5–4.7 μU/mL
Thyroxine, total (T4)	S	58–140 nmol/L	4.5–10.9 μg/dL
Triiodothyronine, total (T3)	S	0.92–2.78 nmol/L	60–181 ng/dL
Thyroxine, free (fT4)	S	10.3–35 pmol/L	0.8–2.7 ng/dL
Triiodothyronine, free (fT3)	S	0.22–6.78 pmol/L	1.4–4.4 pg/mL
Vanillylmandelic Acid (VMA)	U, 24 h	7.6–37.9 μmol/d	0.15–1.2 mg/d
Vasoactive intestinal polypeptide (VIP)	P	<75 ng/L	<75 pg/mL

Note: P, plasma; S, serum; U, urine; WB, whole blood

Drug	Therapeutic Range Conventional Units	Therapeutic Range SI Units	Toxic Level Conventional Units	Toxic Level SI Units
Acetaminophen	10–30 μg/mL	66–199 μmol/L	>200 μg/mL	>1324 μmol/L
Amikacin				
Peak	25–35 μg/mL	43–60 μmol/L	>35 μg/mL	>60 μmol/L
Trough	4–8 μg/mL	6.8–13.7 μmol/L	>10 μg/mL	>17 μmol/L
Amitriptyline	120–250 ng/mL	433–903 nmol/L	>500 ng/mL	>1805 nmol/L
Amphetamine	20–30 ng/mL	148–222 nmol/L	>200 ng/mL	>1480 nmol/L
Antiepileptic drugs: see Table 348–8				
Barbiturates, most short-acting			>20 mg/L	>88 μmol/L
Bromide			>1250 μg/mL	>15.6 mmol/L
Carbamazepine	6–12 μg/mL	26–51 μmol/L	>15 μg/mL	>63 μmol/L
Chlordiazepoxide	700–1000 ng/mL	2.34–3.34 μmol/L	>5000 ng/mL	>16.7 μmol/L
Clonazepam	15–60 ng/mL	48–190 nmol/L	>80 ng/mL	>254 nmol/L
Clozapine	200–350 ng/mL	0.6–1 μmol/L		
Cocaine			>1000 ng/mL	>3300 nmol/L
Cyclosporine	Depends on timing after dose and transplant type with ranges of 100–400 ng/mL	Depends on timing after dose and transplant type with ranges of 83–333 nmol/L	Varies with time after dose and transplant type	Varies with time after dose and transplant type
Desipramine	75–300 ng/mL	281–1125 nmol/L	>400 ng/mL	>1500 nmol/L
Diazepam	100–1000 ng/mL	0.35–351 μmol/L	>5000 ng/mL	>17.55 μmol/L
Digoxin	0.8–2.0 ng/mL	1.0–2.6 nmol/L	>2.5 ng/mL	>3.2 nmol/L
Doxepin	30–150 ng/mL	107–537 nmol/L	>500 ng/mL	>1790 nmol/L
Ethanol			>300 mg/dL	>65 mmol/L
Behavioral changes	>20 mg/dL	>4.3 mmol/L		
Clinical intoxication	>100 mg/dL	>1 g/L		
Ethosuximide	40–100 μg/mL	283–708 μmol/L	>150 μg/mL	>1062 μmol/L
Flecainide	0.2–1.0 μg/mL	0.5–2.4 μmol/L	>1.0 μg/mL	>2.4 μmol/L
Gentamicin				
Peak	8–10 μg/mL	16.7–20.9 μmol/L	>10 μg/mL	>21 μmol/L
Trough	2–4 μg/mL	4.2–8.4 μmol/L	>4 μg/mL	>8.4 μmol/L
Ibuprofen	10–50 μg/mL	49–243 μmol/L	100–700 μg/mL	485–3395 μmol/L
Imipramine	125–250 ng/mL	446–893 nmol/L	>500 ng/mL	>1784 nmol/L
Lidocaine	1.5–6.0 μg/mL	6.4–26 μmol/L		26–34.2 μmol/L
CNS or			6–8 μg/mL	
Cardiovascular depression				>34.2 μmol/L
Seizures, obtundation, decreased cardiac output			>8 μg/mL	
Lithium	0.6–1.2 meq/L	0.6–1.2 nmol/L	>2 meq/L	>2 nmol/L
Methadone	100–400 ng/mL	0.32–1.29 μmol/L	>2000 ng/mL	>6.46 μmol/L
Methotrexate	Variable	Variable		
Low dose (1–2 weeks)			>9.1 ng/mL	>20 nmol/L
High dose (48 h)			>227 ng/mL	>0.5 μmol/L

(continued)

Drug	Therapeutic Range		Toxic Level	
	Conventional Units	SI Units	Conventional Units	SI Units
Morphine	10–80 ng/mL	35–280 nmol/L	>200 ng/mL	>700 nmol/L
Nitroprusside (as thiocyanate)	6–29 µg/mL	103–499 µmol/L		
Nortriptyline	50–170 ng/mL	190–646 nmol/L	>500 ng/mL	>1.9 µmol/L
Phenobarbital	10–40 µg/mL	43–170 µmol/L		
Slowness, ataxia, nystagmus			35–80 µg/mL	151–345 µmol/L
Coma with reflexes			65–117 µg/mL	280–504 µmol/L
Coma without reflexes			>100 µg/mL	>430 µmol/L
Phenytoin	10–20 µg/mL	40–79 µmol/L	>20 µg/mL	>79 µmol/L
Procainamide	4–10 µg/mL	17–42 µmol/L	>10–12 µg/mL	>42–51 µmol/L
Quinidine	2–5 µg/mL	6–15 µmol/L	>6 µg/mL	>18 µmol/L
Salicylates	150–300 µg/mL	1086–2172 µmol/L	>300 µg/mL	>2172 µmol/L
Theophylline	8–20 µg/mL	44–111 µmol/L	>20 µg/mL	>110 µmol/L
Thiocyanate				
After nitroprusside infusion	6–29 µg/mL	103–499 µmol/L		
Nonsmoker	1–4 µg/mL	17–69 µmol/L	>120 µg/mL	>2064 µmol/L
Smoker	3–12 µg/mL	52–206 µmol/L		
Tobramycin				
Peak	8–10 µg/mL	17–21 µmol/L	>10 µg/mL	>21 µmol/L
Trough	<4 µg/mL	<9 µmol/L	>4 µg/mL	>9 µmol/L
Valproic acid	50–150 µg/mL	347–1040 µmol/L	>150 µg/mL	>1040 µmol/L
Vancomycin				
Peak	18–26 µg/mL	12–18 µmol/L	>80–100 µg/mL	>55–69 µmol/L
Trough	5–10 µg/mL	3–7 µmol/L		

TABLE A-6 Vitamins and Selected Trace Minerals

Specimen	Analyte	SI Units	Conventional Units
Aluminum	S	<0.2 µmol/L	<5.41 µg/L
	U, random	5–30 µg/L	0.19–1.11 µmol/L
Arsenic			
	WB	0.03–0.31 µmol/L	2–23 µg/L
	U, 24 h	0.07–0.67 µmol/L	5–50 µg/d
Coenzyme Q10 (ubiquinone)	P	0.5–1.5 mg/L	0.5–1.5 µg/mL
Carotenoids	S	0.9–5.6 µmol/L	50–300 µg/dL
Copper			
	S	11–22 µmol/L	70–140 µg/dL
	U, 24 h	0.047–0.55 µmol/d	3–35 µg/d
Folic acid	RC	340–1020 nmol/L cells	150–450 ng/mL cells
Folic acid	S	7–36 nmol/L cells	3–16 ng/mL cells
Lead (adult)	S	<0.5–1 µmol/L	<10–20 µg/dL
Mercury			
	WB	3.0–294 nmol/L	0.6–59 µg/L
	U, 24 h	<99.8 nmol/L	<20 µg/L
Vitamin A	S	0.7–3.5 µmol/L	20–100 µg/dL
Vitamin B₁ (thiamine)	S	0–75 nmol/L	0–2 µg/dL
Vitamin B₂ (riboflavin)	S	106–638 nmol/L	4–24 µg/dL
Vitamin B₆	P	20–121 nmol/L	5–30 ng/mL
Vitamin B₁₂	S	148–590 pmol/L	200–800 pg/mL
Vitamin C (ascorbic acid)	S	23–57 µmol/L	0.4–1.0 mg/dL
Vitamin D₃, 1,25-dihydroxy	S	60–108 pmol/L	25–45 pg/mL
Vitamin D₃, 25-hydroxy (some labs report as a desirable level rather than a normal range)	P		
Summer		37.4–200 nmol/L	15–80 ng/mL
Winter		34.9–105 nmol/L	14–42 ng/mL
Vitamin E	S	12–42 µmol/L	5–18 µg/mL
Vitamin K	S	0.29–2.64 nmol/L	0.13–1.19 ng/mL
Zinc	S	11.5–18.5 µmol/L	75–120 µg/dL

Note: P, plasma; RC, red cells; S, serum; U, urine; WB, whole blood

TABLE A-7 Classification of LDL, Total, and HDL Cholesterol

LDL cholesterol	
<100	Optimal
100–129	Near or above normal
130–159	Borderline high
160–189	High
≥190	Very high
Total cholesterol	
<200	Desirable
200–239	Borderline high
≥240	High
HDL cholesterol	
<40	Low
≥60	High

Note: HDL, high-density lipoprotein; LDL, low-density lipoprotein
Source: Executive summary of the third report of the national cholesterol education program (NCEP) expert panel on detection, evaluation, and treatment of high blood cholesterol in adults (adult treatment panel III): JAMA 285:2486, 2001.

TABLE B-1 *Cerebrospinal Fluid[a]*

Constituent	SI Units	Conventional Units
Glucose	2.22–3.89 mmol/L	40–70 mg/dL
Lactate	1–2 mmol/L	10–20 mg/dL
Total protein		
Lumbar	0.15–0.5 g/L	15–50 mg/dL
Cisternal	0.15–0.25 g/L	15–25 mg/dL
Ventricular	0.06–0.15 g/L	6–15 mg/dL
Albumin	0.066–0.442 g/L	6.6–44.2 mg/dL
IgG	0.009–0.057 g/L	0.9–5.7 mg/dL
IgG index[b]	0.29–0.59	
Oligoclonal bands (OGB)	<2 bands not present in matched serum sample	
Ammonia	15–47 μmol/L	25–80 μg/dL
CSF pressure		50–180 mmH₂O
CSF volume (adult)	~150 mL	
Red blood cells	0	0
Leukocytes		
Total	0–5 mononuclear cells per mm³	
Differential		
Lymphocytes	60–70%	
Monocytes	30–50%	
Neutrophils	None	

[a] Since cerebrospinal fluid concentrations are equilibrium values, measurements of the same parameters in blood plasma obtained at the same time are recommended. However, there is a time lag in attainment of equilibrium, and cerebrospinal levels of plasma constituents that can fluctuate rapidly (such as plasma glucose) may not achieve stable values until after a significant lag phase.

[b] IgG index = CSF IgG(mg/dL) × serum albumin(g/dL)/Serum IgG(g/dL) × CSF albumin(mg/dL)

TABLE B-3 *Differential Nucleated Cell Counts of Bone Marrow Aspirates*

	Mean, %	Range, %	95% Confidence Intervals, %
Myeloid (total)	56.7		
Neutrophilic series (total)	53.6	49.2–65.0	33.6–73.6
Myeloblast	0.9	0.2–1.5	0.1–1.7
Promyelocyte	3.3	2.1–4.1	1.9–4.7
Myelocyte	12.7	8.2–15.7	8.5–16.9
Metamyelocyte	15.9	9.6–24.6	7.1–24.7
Band	12.4	9.5–15.3	9.4–15.4
Segmented	7.4	6.0–12.0	3.8–11.0
Eosinophilic series	3.1	1.2–5.3	1.1–5.2
Basophilic and mast cells	0.1	0–0.2	—
Erythroid (total)	25.6	18.4–33.8	15.0–36.2
Pronormoblasts	0.6	0.2–1.3	0.1–1.1
Basophilic normoblasts	1.4	0.5–2.4	0.4–2.4
Polychromatophilic normoblasts	21.6	17.9–29.2	13.1–30.1
Orthochromatic normoblasts	2.0	0.4–4.6	0.3–3.7
Lymphocytes	16.2	11.1–23.2	8.6–23.8
Plasma cells	1.3	0.4–3.9	0–3.5
Monocytes	0.3	0–0.8	0–0.6
Megakaryocytes	0.1	0–0.4	—
Reticulum cells	0.3	0–0.9	0–0.8
M:E ratio	2.3	1.5–3.3	1.1–3.5

Note: Data are from 12 healthy men.
Source: From SL Perkins: Normal blood and bone marrow values in humans, in GR Lee et al (eds): *Wintrobe's Clinical Hematology,* 10th ed, Philadelphia, Williams and Wilkins, 1999, pp 2738–2748, with permission.

TABLE B-2 *Urine Analysis*

	SI Units	Conventional Units
Acidity, titratable	20–40 mmol/d	20–40 meq/d
Ammonia	30–50 mmol/d	30–50 meq/d
Amylase		4–400 U/L
Amylase/creatinine clearance ratio [(Cl$_{am}$/Cl$_{cr}$) × 100]	1–5	1–5
Calcium (10 meq/d or 200 mg/d dietary calcium)	<7.5 mmol/d	<300 mg/d
Creatine, as creatinine		
Female	<760 μmol/d	<100 mg/d
Male	<380 μmol/d	<50 mg/d
Creatinine	8.8–14 mmol/d	1.0–1.6 g/d
Eosinophils	<100 eosinophils/mL	<100 eosinophils/mL
Glucose, true (oxidase method)	0.3–1.7 mmol/d	50–300 mg/d
5-Hydroxyindoleacetic acid (5-HIAA)	10–47 μmol/d	2–9 mg/d
"Microalbumin"	<0.02 g/L	<20 mg/L
Oxalate	228–684 μmol/d	20–60 mg/d
pH	5.0–9.0	5.0–9.0
Phosphate (phosphorus) (varies with intake)	12.9–42.0 mmol/d	400–1300 mg/d
Potassium (varies with intake)	25–100 mmol/d	25–100 meq/d
Protein	<0.15 g/d	<150 mg/d
Sediment		
Bacteria	Negative	
Bladder cells	Negative	
Broad casts	Negative	
Crystals	Negative	
Epithelial cell casts	Negative	
Granular casts	Negative	
Hyaline casts	0–5/low power field	
Red blood cell casts	Negative	
Red blood cells	0–2/high power field	
Squamous cells	Negative	
Tubular cells	Negative	
Waxy casts	Negative	
White blood cells	0–2/high power field	
White cell casts	Negative	
Sodium (varies with intake)	100–260 mmol/d	100–260 meq/d
Specific gravity	1.001–1.035	
Urea nitrogen	214–607 mmol/d	6–17 g/d
Uric acid (normal diet)	1.49–4.76 mmol/d	250–800 mg/d

TABLE B-4 *Stool Analysis*

	SI Units	Conventional Units
Bulk		
Wet weight	<197.5 (115 ± 41) g/d	<197.5 (115 ± 41) g/d
Dry weight	<66.4 (34 ± 15) g/d	<66.4 (34 ± 15) g/d
α₁ Antitrypsin	0.98 (±0.17) mg/g dry weight	0.98 (±0.17) mg/g dry weight
Coproporphyrin	600–1500 nmol/d	400–1000 μg/d
Fat		
Adult		<7 g/d
Adult on fat-free diet		<4 g/d
Fatty acid		
Free	0.01–0.10	1–10% of dry matter
Combined as soap	0.005–0.12	0.5–12% of dry matter
Nitrogen	<1.7 (1.4 ± 0.2) g/d	<1.7 (1.4 ± 0.2) g/d
Protein content	Minimal	Minimal
Urobilinogen	68–470 μmol/d	40–280 mg/d
Water	~0.65	~65%

TABLE C-1 *Renal Function Tests*

	SI Units	Conventional Units
Clearances (corrected to 1.72 m² body surface area)		
Measures of glomerular filtration rate (GFR)		
Inulin clearance (Cl)		
Males (mean ± 1 SD)	2.1 ± 0.4 mL/s	124 ± 25.8 mL/min
Females (mean ± 1 SD)	2.0 ± 0.2 mL/s	119 ± 12.8 mL/min
Endogenous creatinine clearance	1.5–2.2 mL/s	91–130 mL/min
Urea	1.0–1.7 mL/s	60–100 mL/min
Measures of effective renal plasma flow and tubular function		
p-Aminohippuric acid clearance (Cl$_{PAH}$)		
Males (mean ± 1 SD)	10.9 ± 2.7 mL/s	654 ± 163 mL/min
Females (mean ± 1 SD)	9.9 ± 1.7 mL/s	594 ± 102 mL/min
Concentration and dilution test		
Specific gravity of urine		
After 12-h fluid restriction	>1.025	>1.025
After 12-h deliberate water intake	≤1.003	≤1.003
Protein excretion, urine	<0.15 g/d	<150 mg/d
Specific gravity, maximal range	1.002–1.028	1.002–1.028
Tubular reabsorption, phosphorus	0.79–0.94 of filtered load	79–94% of filtered load

TABLE C-2 *Gastrointestinal Tests*

Test	SI Units	Conventional Units
Absorption tests		
D-Xylose: after overnight fast, 25 g xylose given in oral aqueous solution		
Urine, collected for following 5 h	33–53 mmol (or >20% of ingested dose)	5–8 g (or >20% of ingested dose)
Serum, 1 h after dose	1.7–2.7 mmol/L	25–40 mg/dL
Vitamin A: a fasting blood specimen is obtained and 200,000 units of vitamin A in oil is given orally	Serum level should rise to twice fasting level in 3–5 h	Serum level should rise to twice fasting level in 3–5 h
Bentiromide test (pancreatic function): 500 mg bentiromide (chymex) orally; p-aminobenzoic acid (PABA) measured		
Plasma		>3.6 (±1.1) μg/mL at 90 min
Urine	>50% recovered in 6 h	>50% recovered in 6 h
Gastric juice		
Volume		
24 h	2–3 L	2–3 L
Nocturnal	600–700 mL	600–700 mL
Basal, fasting	30–70 mL/h	30–70 mL/h
Reaction		
pH	1.6–1.8	1.6–1.8
Titratable acidity of fasting juice	4–9 μmol/s	15–35 meq/h
Acid output		
Basal		
Females (mean ± 1 SD)	0.6 ± 0.5 μmol/s	2.0 ± 1.8 meq/h
Males (mean ± 1 SD)	0.8 ± 0.6 μmol/s	3.0 ± 2.0 meq/h
Maximal (after SC histamine acid phosphate, 0.004 mg/kg body weight, and preceded by 50 mg promethazine, or after betazole, 1.7 mg/kg body weight, or pentagastrin, 6 μg/kg body weight)		
Females (mean ± 1 SD)	4.4 ± 1.4 μmol/s	16 ± 5 meq/h
Males (mean ± 1 SD)	6.4 ± 1.4 μmol/s	23 ± 5 meq/h
Basal acid output/maximal acid output ratio	≤0.6	≤0.6
Gastrin, serum	40–200 μg/L	40–200 pg/mL
Secretin test (pancreatic exocrine function): 1 unit/kg body weight, IV		
Volume (pancreatic juice) in 80 min	>2.0 mL/kg	>2.0 mL/kg
Bicarbonate concentration	>80 mmol/L	>80 meq/L
Bicarbonate output in 30 min	>10 mmol	>10 meq

TABLE C-3 *Circulatory Function Tests*

Test	SI Units (Range)	Conventional Units (Range)
Arteriovenous oxygen difference	30–50 mL/L	30–50 mL/L
Cardiac output (Fick)	2.5–3.6 L/m² of body surface area per minute	2.5–3.6 L/m² of body surface area per minute
Contractility indices		
Max. left ventricular *dp/dt (dp/dt)*/DP when DP = 5.3 kPa (40 mmHg)	220 kPa/s (176–250 kPa/s) (37.6 ± 12.2)/s	1650 mmHg/s (1320–1880 mmHg/s) (37.6 ± 12.2)/s
Mean normalized systolic ejection rate (angiography)	3.32 ± 0.84 end-diastolic volumes per second	3.32 ± 0.84 end-diastolic volumes per second
Mean velocity of circumferential fiber shortening (angiography)	1.83 ± 0.56 circumferences per second	1.83 ± 0.56 circumferences per second
Ejection fraction; stroke volume/end diastolic volume (SV/EDV)	0.67 ± 0.08 (0.55–0.78)	0.67 ± 0.08 (0.55–0.78)
End-diastolic volume	70 ± 20.0 mL/m² (60–88 mL/m²)	70 ± 20.0 mL/m² (60–88 mL/m²)
End-systolic volume	25 ± 5.0 mL/m² (20–33 mL/m²)	25 ± 5.0 mL/m² (20–33 mL/m²)
Left ventricular work		
Stroke work index	50 ± 20.0 (g·m)/m² (30–110)	50 ± 20.0 (g·m)/m² (30–110)
Left ventricular minute work index	1.8–6.6 [(kg·m)m²]/min	1.8–6.6 [(kg·m)/m²]/min
Oxygen consumption index	110–150 mL	110–150 mL
Maximum oxygen uptake	35 mL/min (20–60 mL/min)	35 mL/min (20–60 mL/min)
Pulmonary vascular resistance	2–12 (kPa·s)/L	20–130 (dyn·s)/cm⁵
Systemic vascular resistance	77–150 (kPa·s)/L	770–1600 (dyn·s)/cm⁵

Note: DP, diastolic pressure

Source: E Braunwald et al, *Heart Disease,* 6th ed. Philadelphia, Saunders, 2001, with permission

---

TABLE C-4 *Summary of Values Useful in Pulmonary Physiology*

	Symbol	Typical Values	
		Man Age 40, 75 kg, 175 cm Tall	Woman Age 40, 60 kg, 160 cm Tall
PULMONARY MECHANICS			
Spirometry—volume-time curves			
Forced vital capacity	FVC	4.8 L	3.3 L
Forced expiratory volume in 1 s	FEV_1	3.8 L	2.8 L
FEV_1/FVC	$FEV_1\%$	76%	77%
Maximal midexpiratory flow	MMF (FEF 25–27)	4.8 L/s	3.6 L/s
Maximal expiratory flow rate	MEFR (FEF 200–1200)	9.4 L/s	6.1 L/s
Spirometry—flow-volume curves			
Maximal expiratory flow at 50% of expired vital capacity	V_{max} 50 (FEF 50%)	6.1 L/s	4.6 L/s
Maximal expiratory flow at 75% of expired vital capacity	V_{max} 75 (FEF 75%)	3.1 L/s	2.5 L/s
Resistance to airflow			
Pulmonary resistance	RL/(R_L)	<3.0 (cmH₂O/s)/L	
Airway resistance	Raw	<2.5 (cmH₂O/s)/L	
Specific conductance	SGaw	>0.13 cmH₂O/s	
Pulmonary compliance			
Static recoil pressure at total lung capacity	Pst TLC	25 ± 5 cmH₂O	
Compliance of lungs (static)	CL	0.2 L cmH₂O	
Compliance of lungs and thorax	C(L + T)	0.1 L cmH₂O	
Dynamic compliance of 20 breaths per minute	C dyn 20	0.25 ± 0.05 L/cmH₂O	
Maximal static respiratory pressures:			
Maximal inspiratory pressure	MIP	>90 cmH₂O	>50 cmH₂O
Maximal expiratory pressure	MEP	>150 cmH₂O	>120 cmH₂O
LUNG VOLUMES			
Total lung capacity	TLC	6.4 L	4.9 L
Functional residual capacity	FRC	2.2 L	2.6 L
Residual volume	RV	1.5 L	1.2 L
Inspiratory capacity	IC	4.8 L	3.7 L
Expiratory reserve volume	ERV	3.2 L	2.3 L
Vital capacity	VC	1.7 L	1.4 L
GAS EXCHANGE (SEA LEVEL)			
Arterial O₂ tension	Pa_{O_2}	12.7 ± 0.7 kPa (95 ± 5 mmHg)	
Arterial CO₂ tension	Pa_{CO_2}	5.3 ± 0.3 kPa (40 ± 2 mmHg)	
Arterial O₂ saturation	Sa_{O_2}	0.97 ± 0.02 (97 ± 2%)	
Arterial blood pH	pH	7.40 ± 0.02	
Arterial bicarbonate	HCO_3^-	24 + 2 meq/L	
Base excess	BE	0 ± 2 meq/L	
Diffusing capacity for carbon monoxide (single breath)	DL_{CO}	0.42 mLCO/s per mmHg (25 mL CO/min per mmHg)	
Dead space volume	V_D	2 mL/kg body wt	
Physiologic dead space; dead space-tidal volume ratio	V_D/V_T		
Rest		≤35% V_T	
Exercise		≤20% V_T	
Alveolar-arterial difference for O₂	$P(A - a)_{O_2}$	≤2.7 kPa ≤20 kPa (≤20 mmHg)	

TABLE C-5 *Normal Values of Doppler Echocardiographic Measurements in Adults*

	Range	Mean
RVD (cm), measured at the base in apical 4-chamber view	2.6 to 4.3	3.5 ± 0.4
LVID (cm), measured in the parasternal long axis view	3.6 to 5.4	4.7 ± 0.4
Posterior LV wall thickness (cm)	0.6 to 1.1	0.9 ± 0.4
IVS wall thickness (cm)	0.6 to 1.1	0.9 ± 0.4
Left atrial dimension (cm), anteroposterior dimension	2.3 to 3.8	3.0 ± 0.3
Aortic root dimension (cm)	2.0 to 3.5	2.4 ± 0.4
Aortic cusps separation (cm)	1.5 to 2.6	1.9 ± 0.4
Percentage of fractional shortening	34 to 44%	36%
Mitral flow (m/s)	0.6 to 1.3	0.9
Tricuspid flow (m/s)	0.3 to 0.7	0.5
Pulmonary artery (m/s)	0.6 to 0.9	0.75
Aorta (m/s)	1.0 to 1.7	1.35

Note: IVS, interventricular septum; LV, left ventricle; LVID, left ventircular internal dimension; RVD, right ventricular dimension

Source: From A Weyman: *Principles and Practice of Echocardiography,* 2d ed, Philadelphia, Lea & Febiger, with permission.

D | MISCELLANEOUS

TABLE D-1 *Body Fluids and Other Mass Data*

	Reference Range	
	SI Units	Conventional Units
Ascitic fluid: see Chap . . .		
Body fluid		
Total volume (lean) of body weight	50% (in obese) to 70%	
Intracellular	0.3–0.4 of body weight	
Extracellular	0.2–0.3 of body weight	
Blood		
Total volume		
Males	69 mL per kg body weight	
Females	65 mL per kg body weight	
Plasma volume		
Males	39 mL per kg body weight	
Females	40 mL per kg body weight	
Red blood cell volume		
Males	30 mL per kg body weight	1.15–1.21 L/m² of body surface area
Females	25 mL per kg body weight	0.95–1.00 L/m² of body surface area
Body Mass Index	18.5–24.9 kg/m²	18.5–24.9 kg/m²

TABLE D-2 *Radiation-Derived Units*

Quantity	Old Unit	SI Unit	Name for SI Unit (and Abbreviation)	Conversion
Activity	curie (Ci)	Disintegrations per second (dps)	becquerel (Bq)	1 Ci = 3.7 × 10¹⁰ Bq 1 mCi = 37 mBq 1 μCi = 0.037 MBq or 37 GBq 1 Bq = 2.703 × 10⁻¹¹ Ci
Absorbed dose	rad	joule per kilogram (J/kg)	gray (Gy)	1 Gy = 100 rad 1 rad = 0.01 Gy 1 mrad = 10⁻³ cGy
Exposure	roentgen (R)	coulomb per kilogram (C/kg)	—	1 C/kg = 3876 R 1 R = 2.58 × 10⁻⁴ C/kg 1 mR = 258 pC/kg
Dose equivalent	rem	joule per kilogram (J/kg)	sievert (Sv)	1 Sv = 100 rem 1 rem = 0.01 Sv 1 mrem = 10 μSv

Bold number indicates the start of the main discussion of the topic; numbers with "f" and "t" refer to figure and table pages.

Cardiac transplantation (*Cont.*)
  posttransplant management
    allograft coronary artery disease, 1379
    infections, 1379
    malignancy, 1379
  results of, 1379, 1379f
  surgical techniques in, 1378
Cardiac tumors, **1420**
  clinical manifestations of, 1420
  fibroma, 1421
  lipoma, 1421
  metastases to heart, 1422
  myxoma, 1420–1421, 1421f
  papillary fibroelastoma, 1421
  primary, 1420, 1421t
  rhabdomyoma, 1421
  sarcoma, 1421
  treatment of, 1422
Cardiobacterium hominis, 867–868. *See also*
    HACEK organisms
  treatment of, 868, 868t
Cardiogenic shock, 1600t, 1603t, **1604, 1612**
  in acute fulminant myocarditis, 1616
  azotemia in, 247
  cardiac catheterization in, 1614
  clinical manifestations of, 1613
  compressive, 1604–1605
  coronary angiography in, 1614
  diagnosis of, 1613–1614
  echocardiography in, 1614
  electrocardiography in, 1614
  etiology of, 1613t
  hemodynamic values in, 1615t
  iatrogenic, 1617
  incidence of, 1612–1613
  intrinsic, 1604
  laboratory findings in, 1614
  in mitral regurgitation, 1616
  in myocardial infarction, 1456, 1604
  in myocardial rupture, 1616
  pathophysiology of, 1613, 1613f
  patient profile in, 1613
  prognosis in, 1616
  pulmonary artery catheterization in, 1614
  in right ventricular infarction, 1616
  timing of, 1613
  treatment of, 1604, 1614–1615, 1614f
    aortic counterpulsation, 1615
    reperfusion-revascularization, 1615, 1615f
    vasopressors, 1615
Cardiomyopathy, **1408.** *See also specific types*
  alcohol-induced, 2563
  classes of, 1408f
  diabetic, 2167
  etiology of, 1408t
  HIV-associated, 1108
  ischemic, 1408
  nausea and vomiting in, 220t
  peripartum, 34
  specific, 1408
  tachycardia-induced, 1345
Cardiopulmonary bypass
  platelet defects in, 678
  rewarming in hypothermia, 123–124, 124t
Cardiopulmonary resuscitation, 1621–1622
  in hypothermic cardiac arrest, 122
Cardiovascular collapse, **1618**
  clinical definition of forms of, 1618
  definition of, 1618, 1618t
Cardiovascular disease. *See also* Atherosclerosis;
    Heart disease
  in acromegaly, 1424
  alcohol-related, 2563
  aldosterone and, 2140–2141
  androgen therapy and, 2197
  approach to, **1301**
    pitfalls in, 1303
  in carcinoid, 1423–1424
  cardiac symptoms, 1301
  in chronic renal disease, 1657–1658, 1666
  death rates from, 1301
  in diabetes mellitus, 1422, 2166–2169
  diagnosis of, 1301–1302, 1302t
    electrocardiogram, 1302

embryonic and somatic stem cell therapy in,
    396
  epidemiology of, 1301
  family history and, 1302
  fear of, 1301
  functional impairment assessment in, 1302,
    1302t
  heart murmur and, 1302, 1303f
  in HIV infection, 1108
  hormone replacement therapy and, 30, 30t
  in hyperthyroidism, 1423
  in hypothyroidism, 1423
  malnutrition-related, 1422
  in Marfan syndrome, 2330
  natural history of, 1303
  New York Heart Association functional classifi-
    cation of, 1302t
  in obesity, 1423
  in pheochromocytoma, 1424
  physical examination for, **1304**
    abdominal examination, 1304
    extremities, 1304
    retinal examination, **1304**
  in rheumatoid arthritis, 1424
  in seronegative arthropathy, 1424
  smoking and, 2574
  in systemic lupus erythematosus, 1424, 1963–
    1964, 1963t
  in transplant patients, 1673
  treatment of, 1303
  in vitamin deficiencies, 1422–1423
  in women, 28, 29t, 30f
Cardiovascular system
  age-related changes in, 45t
  infections in cancer patients, 493
  late consequences of cancer, 584
  radiation-induced changes in, 487
  in sepsis, 1609
  in shock, 1601
Cardioversion
  for atrial fibrillation, 1346
  for atrial flutter, 1347
  for AV nodal reentrant tachycardia, 1347
  for tachyarrhythmias, 1356
  for ventricular tachycardia, 1352, 1457
  for Wolff-Parkinson-White syndrome, 1351
Carditis, rheumatic fever, 1978–1979
Caregivers, family. *See* Family caregivers
Caretaker genes, 448
Carey-Coombs murmur, 1310
Carmustine, 471t
  adverse effects of, 471t, 1558
  for astrocytoma, 2454
  for hematopoietic cell transplantation, 669
  for melanoma, 503
Carney syndrome, 1420, 2236
  pituitary tumor in, 2081
Carnitine deficiency, 2336t
Carnitine palmitoyltransferase deficiency, 2534
Caroli's disease, 1873
β-Carotene, 407–408
  adverse effects of, 70
  for cancer prevention, 443
  for erythropoietic protoporphyria, 328
  for protoporphyria, 2308
  supplementation with, 70
Carotenemia, 408
Carotenoderma, 238
Carotenoids, 407–408
Carotid artery
  common, ischemia in territory of, 2384
  internal
    dissection of, 2377
    ischemia in territory of, 2383–2384
  in migraine, 90
Carotid body, 210
Carotid cavernous fistula, 173
Carotid endarterectomy, 2377
Carotid pulse, 1304–1305
Carotid reflex, 126
Carotid sinus hypersensitivity
  syncope and, 126t, 127, 129
  treatment of, 130
Carotid sinus massage, 1344, 1347

Carotid sinus pressure, 1335, 1344
Carotid stenosis
  asymptomatic, 2377
  stroke and, 2377, 2381
  symptomatic, 2377
  syncope in, 128
  treatment of, 2377
Carotidynia syndrome, 86, 90
Carpal tunnel syndrome, 103, 2035, 2501, 2502t
  in pregnancy, 36
Carpenter syndrome, 426t
Carrier detection, hemophilia A, 682
Carteolol, 1473t
Cartilage, 2324
  in osteoarthritis, 2038–2039
Cartilage-hair hypoplasia syndrome, 352
Carvallo's sign, 1391
Carvedilol, 1473t
  adverse effects of, 1473t
  disposition of, 16t
  for heart failure, 1374–1375, 1374t
  for hypertension, 1473t
Casal's necklace, 405
Caseous necrosis, 956
Caspase, 1924
Caspofungin, 1178
  for aspergillosis, 1189t
  for candidiasis, 1187, 1187t
Cast(s)
  urinary, 250–251, 1649
    broad casts, 251
    major syndromes in nephrology, 247t
Castell's method, percussion for splenic dullness,
    346
Castleman's disease, 313, 643, 655
Cast nephropathy, 250
Cat(s)
  rabies, 1156
  toxoplasmosis, **1243**
Catagen, 275
Cataplexy, 154, 156t, 159, 159t
Cataracts, 171
  late consequences of cancer/cancer treatment,
    585
  surgical excision of, 171
Catatonia, 1625
Catecholamines
  myocardial contractility and, 1363
  in pheochromocytoma, **2148**
  as tumor marker, 439t
Caterpillar stings/dermatitis, 2607
Catfish, marine, 2597
Cat flea-associated rickettsiosis, 999t, 1003
Cathartic colon, 231
Catheter
  for hemodialysis access, 1665
  for peritoneal dialysis, 1667
Catheter ablation
  for arrhythmias, 1357
  for atrial fibrillation, 1346
  for atrial flutter, 1347
  for ventricular tachycardia, 1353
  for Wolff-Parkinson-White syndrome, 1351
Catheter-related infections
  in cancer patients, 491
  Candida, 1186–1187
  prostatitis, 1721
  Staphylococcus aureus, 11, 11f, 818
  in transplant recipient, 788
  urinary tract, 776–777, 1717, 1719
Catheter tip culture, 779
Cation-exchange resin, for hyperkalemia, 263
Cat-scratch disease, 308, 920, **930**
  clinical manifestations of, 929t, 930
  definition and etiology of, 930
  diagnosis of, 930
  epidemiology of, 930
  in HIV infection, 1119
  microbiology of, 930
  pathology of, 930
  risk factors for, 929t
  treatment of, 929t, 930
Cauda equina lesion, 2439

Topical Contents